CHILD AND ADOLESCENT PSYCHIATRY

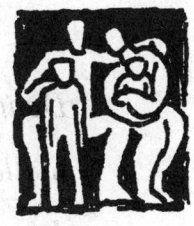

A Comprehensive Textbook

Second Edition

ADVISORY COMMITTEE

Dennis P. Cantwell, M.D.

Stella Chess, M.D.

James F. Leckman, M.D.

Dorothy Otnow Lewis, M.D.

David A. Tomb, M.D.

Elizabeth B. Weller, M.D.

Gabrielle Weiss, M.D.

CHILD AND ADOLESCENT PSYCHIATRY

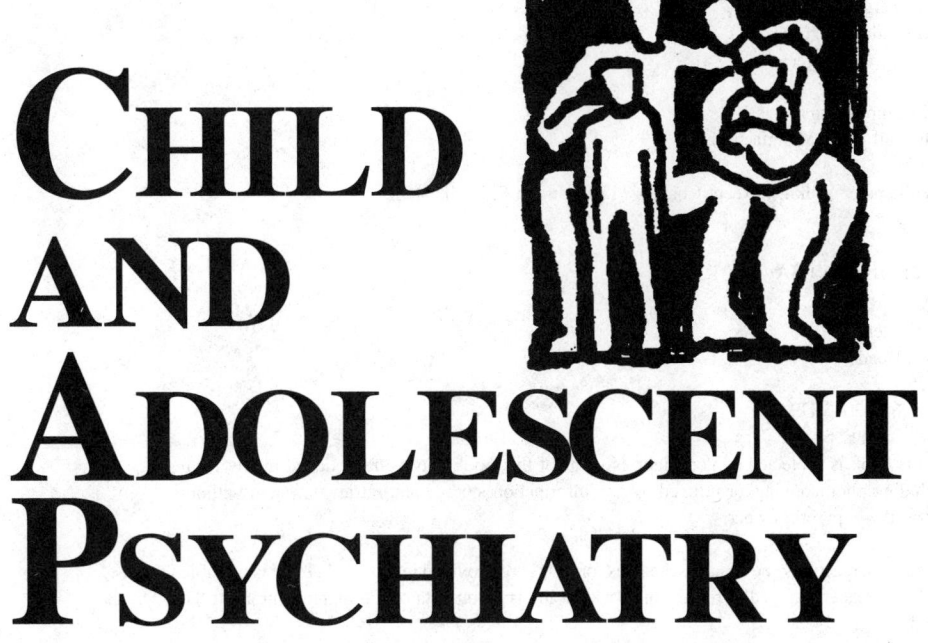

A Comprehensive Textbook

Second Edition

Edited by

Melvin Lewis M.B., B.S., F.R.C.Psych., D.C.H.

Professor of Child Psychiatry and Pediatrics
Yale Child Study Center
Yale University School of Medicine
New Haven, Connecticut

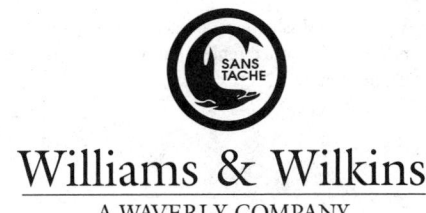

Williams & Wilkins
A WAVERLY COMPANY

BALTIMORE • PHILADELPHIA • LONDON • PARIS • BANGKOK
BUENOS AIRES • HONG KONG • MUNICH • SYDNEY • TOKYO • WROCLAW

Editor: David C. Retford
Project Manager: Barbara J. Felton
Copy Editors: Klemie Bryte, Bonnie Montgomery, Dominique van de Stadt
Designer: Wilma Rosenberger
Illustration Planner: Lorraine Wrzosek
Cover Designer: Wilma Rosenberger
Cover Artist: Eric Lewis
Typesetter: Maryland Composition
Printer/Binder: Maple Vail Book Manufacturing

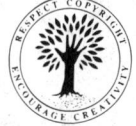

Printed in the United States of America

First Edition, 1991

Library of Congress Cataloging-in-Publication Data
Child and adolescent psychiatry : a comprehensive textbook / edited by
   Melvin Lewis.—2nd ed.
      p.   cm.
   Includes bibliographical references and index.
   ISBN 0-683-04955-0
   1. Child psychiatry.   2. Adolescent psychiatry.   I. Lewis,
Melvin, 1926–   .
   [DNLM: 1. Child Psychiatry.   2. Adolescent Psychiatry.   3. Mental
Disorders—in adolescence.   4. Mental Disorders—in infancy &
childhood.   WS 350 C53502 1996]
   RJ499.C4823   1996
   618.92′89—dc20
   DNLM/DLC
   for Library of Congress   95-23168
                                                               CIP

To purchase additional copies of this book, call our customer service department at **(800) 638-0672** or fax orders to **(800) 447-8438**. For other book services, including chapter reprints and large quantity sales, ask for the special sales department.

Canadian customers should call **(800) 268-4178** or fax **(905) 470-6780**. For all other calls originating outside of the United States, please call **(410) 528-4223** or fax us at **(410) 528-8550**.

Visit Williams & Wilkins on the Internet: **http://www.wwilkins.com** or contact our customer service department at **custserv@wwilkins.com**. Williams & Wilkins customer service representatives are available from 8:30 AM to 6:00 PM, EST, Monday through Friday, for telephone access.

ISBN 0-683-04955-0

90000

96 97 98 99 00
1 2 3 4 5 6 7 8 9 10

9 780683 049558

To
Dorothy, Eric, Gillian and Lu

Foreword to First Edition

On two previous occasions, including my Presidential Address to the American Psychiatric Association (1984), I delineated the requirements for a field of medical practice to be identified as an independent specialty. Among a number of requirements, I emphasized the need for a scientific base that is specific to the specialty, even though substantial reliance might be placed on the basic sciences of other specialties. I went on to point to the importance for clinicians in the specialty to have a unique set of knowledge and skills. I also stated that both the scientific base and the specific skills must have a degree of conceptual clarity to form the framework of a required educational curriculum. Child and adolescent psychiatry now has such an educational curriculum.

A specialty such as child and adolescent psychiatry also needs its own comprehensive textbook that conceptualizes the whole field for the reader. Such a textbook should combine information on the scientific bases and the techniques into an amalgam that enables the reader to acquire the up-to-date knowledge necessary for state-of-the-art practice. No easy task!

Approaching Lewis' volume precisely in the context of the above concepts, readers will acquire equal knowledge about what to do, when to do it, and, most importantly, why to do it. They will also become better practitioners whose actions will be based not on empiricism alone but on scientific evidence as well. Best of all, *Child and Adolescent Psychiatry* has the content and conceptual clarity needed for the education of new generations of students.

In addition to students of child and adolescent psychiatry, others concerned with the mental health of children and adolescents will find the text of great value. *Child and Adolescent Psychiatry* will be useful for experienced practitioners, pediatricians, psychologists, and neurologists, as well as allied professionals such as educators, nurses, social workers, lawyers, and policy planners. Some will find the scientific expositions of greater interest, others will focus on the practical clinical issues. All will gain a new opportunity for enlarging their knowledge and rounding out their clinical expertise through reading this intellectually satisfying and clinically informative book.

Child and Adolescent Psychiatry is more than a detailed primer for students of child and adolescent psychiatry. It is, in fact, a truly comprehensive reference manual for those who labor for the advancement of mental health for children and adolescents. Conceptually, scientifically, clinically, and pedagogically this book fills an important need in child and adolescent psychiatry. This was the goal for which Mel Lewis and the contributors strived with the hope of contributing to the greater achievements and happiness of new generations of our young. They have succeeded admirably in this goal.

George Tarjan, M.D.†
Professor Emeritus of Psychiatry
University of California, Los Angeles

PREFACE TO SECOND EDITION

Since the publication of the first edition of *Child and Adolescent Psychiatry: A Comprehensive Textbook* in 1991, research in child and adolescent psychiatry has been especially productive, and many advances in treatment have been made. These new research findings and clinical advances are the reason for this second edition. Every chapter in this second edition has been revised to ensure that new and up-to-date information is fully available to the reader. Many chapters consequently have been expanded and several completely new chapters have been added.

Among the enlarged and new chapters are chapters on developmental aspects of psychoneuroendocrinology (Anand and Nemeroff); neuroimaging of the brain (Peterson); the development of communication (Paul, Baker, and Cantwell); teratology and developmental effects of prenatal drug (alcohol, heroin, marijuana, and cocaine) exposure (Mayes and Granger); reactive attachment disorder (Richters, Volkmar, and Paul); eating disorders in infancy and childhood (Woolston); dissociative identity disorder/multiple personality disorder (Lewis and Yeager); a critical overview of the psychotherapies (Werry and Andrews); psychiatric issues in pediatric bone marrow and solid organ transplantation (Slater); the burned child (Stoddard); school consultation (Schwab-Stone); the role of the child expert in court-requested evaluation (Nordhaus and Solnit); ethics in the practice of child and adolescent psychiatry (Schetky); and a historical perspective on child and adolescent psychiatry (Bernstein).

During the past 5 years, a major change occurred also in the social and political environment of child and adolescent psychiatry in the United States—the change to "managed care" in health care delivery across the United States. By 1995 child and adolescent psychiatrists in ambulatory practice, hospitals, and academic settings were increasingly experiencing the stress of trying to offer the best care to their patients in the context of this corporate model of health care driven primarily by concerns for cost reduction. Some of the effects of this corporate model in the delivery of mental health care to children and their families are discussed in several of the chapters in this second edition, particularly in the chapters concerning hospital, day treatment, and residential care. The last word has yet to be written on this rapidly changing scene.

In 1994 the fourth edition of the *Diagnostic and Statistical Manual of Mental Disorders* (DSM-IV) was published. DSM-IV and ICD-10 are now more compatible with each other, although their differences are not trivial. Both systems are discussed and all DSM-IV modifications have been incorporated where appropriate into this second edition.

Again, we have continued to strive to provide a state-of-the-art, comprehensive, and useful account of contemporary child and adolescent psychiatry in a way that we hope is both intellectually satisfying and clinically useful to the reader.

I am enormously grateful to the 170 contributing authors for their unwavering commitment to excellence, their wonderful collegiality and enthusiasm, and the generous amounts of time and effort each has given to the work of revising, updating, enlarging, and, in some instances, creating the chapters in this second edition.

Once again I wish to express my thanks to the Advisory Committee (Drs. Cantwell, Chess, Leckman, Lewis, Tomb, Weller, and Weiss) for their wisdom and guidance, and to the staff at Williams & Wilkins for their unflagging efforts on behalf of the book. In particular, I owe a debt of gratitude to Barbara J. Felton for her management and production skills, to Wilma Rosenberger for her meticulous design, and to Klemie Bryte for her editing skills; each helped to keep the book on track and in trim at all times. Special thanks go to my secretary, Ann Chieppo, who assisted me in ways too many to mention. Lastly, I am, as ever, enormously grateful to my wife, Dorothy, for her continuing and loving support and her unsurpassed clarity of thought; to my daughter, Gillian, for her colorful insights; and to my son, Eric, for his artistic contributions to the cover and front matter.

Melvin Lewis, M.B., B.S., F.R.C.Psych., D.C.H.
Yale Child Study Center
New Haven, Connecticut
March 1996

PREFACE TO FIRST EDITION

Child and Adolescent Psychiatry presents an up-to-date, comprehensive, and useful account of child and adolescent psychiatry today. The book covers the field completely, from the migration of cells in the embryonic cortex to issues of world mental health. The book encompasses normal development, psychopathology, diagnosis, and treatment. International authorities have contributed scholarly chapters on virtually the complete syllabus for the modern child and adolescent psychiatrist.

The book contains nine sections: Normal Development; Development of Symptoms; Overview of Etiological Influences; Nosology and Classification; Diagnostic Assessment; Syndromes; Treatment; Child Psychiatry and Allied Professions (pediatrics, education, law, and public health); and Training and Research.

A unique feature is Section II, Development of Symptoms. Here, authorities were invited to describe their understanding of the actual development of cardinal symptoms encountered in child and adolescent psychiatry. Symptoms such as anxiety, depression, psychotic thinking, and violence, seen in a variety of different kinds of disorders, are explored in a manner similar to the way internal medicine would approach symptoms such as fever and pain. Another unusual feature of the book is its emphasis on the relevance of research findings to clinical experience. Clinical case illustrations highlight important aspects of the syndrome being described. The book also draws on many theories of development,

which are discussed in terms of their clinical relevance. The book will be useful to all specialists who try to help children and their families. There are subsections on child psychiatry and pediatrics, child psychiatry and education, child psychiatry and law, and child and adolescent psychiatry and public health. For the child psychiatry trainee and the young researcher, there are specific chapters on training and certification in child and adolescent psychiatry, new research techniques, and the ethics of research involving children.

The enthusiasm of the authors and their commitment to excellence is a source of great pleasure and pride to me. I am indebted to each of them. I wish to express special appreciation and gratitude to Doctors Dennis Cantwell, Stella Chess, James Leckman, Dorothy Otnow Lewis, David Tomb, Elizabeth Weller, and Gabrielle Weiss who comprised the Advisory Committee and whose advice was invaluable. I wish to thank the staff at Williams & Wilkins, including Nancy Collins, Carol Eckhart, Michael Fisher, John Gardner, Rebecca Marnhout, Anne Stewart Seitz, Steve Siegforth, Deborah Tourtlotte, and Chuck Zeller for their special combination of competence and enthusiasm. I also thank my secretary, Ann Chieppo, for her steadfast support and assistance in this immense task. Finally, I wish to thank my wife Dorothy for her clarity of thought and loving support.

Melvin Lewis

CONTRIBUTORS

Jean Adnopoz, M.P.H.
Associate Professor, Yale Child Study Center, Yale University School of Medicine, New Haven, Connecticut

John P. Alsobrook II, M.Phil.
Research Associate, Yale Child Study Center, Yale University School of Medicine, New Haven, Connecticut

K.J.S. Anand, M.B.B.S., Ph.D., F.A.A.P.
Assistant Professor of Pediatrics, Anesthesia, Psychiatry and Behavioral Sciences, Director of Research, Division of Critical Care Medicine, Director, Office for Research Promotion, Department of Pediatrics, Associate Investigator, Stress Neurobiology Laboratory, Emory University School of Medicine; Attending Pediatric Intensivist, Egleston Children's Hospital, Atlanta, Georgia

George M. Anderson, Ph.D.
Research Scientist, Director, Laboratory of Developmental Neurochemistry, Yale Child Study Center, Yale University School of Medicine, New Haven, Connecticut

Leah K. Andrews, M.B., Ch.B., F.R.A.N.Z.C.P.
Clinical Director, Child and Family Unit, Auckland Children's Hospital; Clinical Lecturer, Department of Psychiatry and Behavioural Science, University of Auckland School of Medicine, Auckland, New Zealand

Paula Armbruster, M.A., M.S.W.
Assistant Clinical Professor of Social Work, Director, Outpatient Services, Yale Child Study Center, Yale University School of Medicine, New Haven, Connecticut

Lorian Baker, Ph.D.
Research Psycholinguist, University of California, Los Angeles, Neuropsychiatric Institute, Los Angeles, California

Deborah C. Beidel, Ph.D.
Associate Professor of Psychiatry and Behavioral Sciences, Medical University of South Carolina, Charleston, South Carolina

Elissa P. Benedek, M.D.
Director, Research and Training, Center of Forensic Psychiatry, Clinical Professor of Psychiatry, University of Michigan Medical Center, Ann Arbor, Michigan

Ian Berg, M.D., F.R.C.P., F.R.C.Psych.
Senior Clinical Lecturer, Department of Psychological Medicine (Children), Leeds General Infirmary, Leeds, England

Dorothy M. Bernstein, M.D., M.S., M.A.
Clinical Professor of Psychiatry, University of Minnesota Medical School, Minneapolis, Minnesota

Boris Birmaher, M.D.
Associate Professor of Child Psychiatry, Western Psychiatric Institute and Clinic, University of Pittsburgh School of Medicine, Pittsburgh, Pennsylvania

Marc H. Bornstein, Ph.D.
Senior Research Scientist and Head, Child and Family Research, National Institute of Child Health and Human Development, Bethesda, Maryland

Andrew M. Boxer, Ph.D.
Assistant Professor of Psychiatry, University of Chicago, Chicago, Illinois

James R. Brasic, M.D., M.P.H.
Research Assistant Professor of Psychiatry, Coordinator of the Developmental Neurobiology Unit, New York University School of Medicine; Clinical Assistant, Department of Psychiatry, Bellevue Hospital Center, New York, New York

Monte Buchsbaum, M.D.
Professor of Psychiatry, Director, Neuroscience PET Laboratory, Mount Sinai School of Medicine, The Mount Sinai Hospital, New York, New York

Roger L. Cambor, M.D.
Clinical Assistant Professor of Psychiatry and Public Health, Cornell University Medical College, New York, New York

Dennis P. Cantwell, M.D.
Joseph Campbell Professor of Child Psychiatry, University of California, Los Angeles, Neuropsychiatric Institute, Los Angeles, California

Rochelle Caplan, M.D.
Associate Professor of Psychiatry, University of California, Los Angeles, School of Medicine, Los Angeles, California

Stella Chess, M.D.
Professor of Child Psychiatry, New York University Medical Center, New York, New York

Paul D. Clein, M.D.
Clinical Fellow, Division of Child and Adolescent Psychiatry, Johns Hopkins Medical Institutions, Baltimore, Maryland

Donald J. Cohen, M.D.
Director, Yale Child Study Center, Professor of Child Psychiatry, Pediatrics and Psychology, Yale University School of Medicine, New Haven, Connecticut

Lee Combrinck-Graham, M.D.
Stamford, Connecticut

James P. Comer, M.D.
Maurice Falk Professor of Child Psychiatry, Yale Child Study Center, Associate Dean, Yale University School of Medicine, New Haven, Connecticut

Henry P. Coppolillo, M.D.
Englewood, Colorado

Shauna B. Corbin, Ph.D.
Senior Psychologist, Emmanuel Convalescent Foundation, Aurora, Ontario, Canada

Anthony J. Costello, M.D.
Professor of Psychiatry, University of Massachusetts Medical Center, Worcester, Massachusetts

Roger D. Cox, Ph.D.
Clinical Associate Professor of Psychiatry, TEACCH Division, University of North Carolina at Chapel Hill, Chapel Hill, North Carolina

Fern J. Cramer-Azima, Ph.D.
Associate Professor, McGill University, Therapeutic Day Center for Emotionally Disturbed Children, Royal Victoria Hospital, Montreal, Quebec, Canada

Andre P. Derdeyn, M.D.

WOHDAN Professor of Psychiatry, Professor of Pediatrics, Chief, Division of Pediatric Psychiatry, University of Arkansas for Medical Sciences, Arkansas Children's Hospital, Little Rock, Arkansas

Susan Dobuler, M.S.W.

Clinical Instructor in Social Work, Yale Child Study Center, Yale University School of Medicine, New Haven, Connecticut

Felton Earls, M.D.

Professor of Human Behavior and Development, Department of Maternal and Child Health, Harvard School of Public Health; Professor of Child Psychiatry, Harvard Medical School, Boston, Massachusetts

Leon Eisenberg, M.D.

Maude and Lillian Presley Professor of Social Medicine, Professor Emeritus of Psychiatry, Harvard Medical School, Boston, Massachusetts

David Elkind, Ph.D.

Professor, Child Study, Department of Child Study, Tufts University, Medford, Massachusetts

Julian B. Ferholt, M.D.

Associate Clinical Professor of Psychiatry and Pediatrics, Yale Child Study Center, Yale University School of Medicine, New Haven, Connecticut

Matia Finn-Stevenson, Ph.D.

Research Scientist and Associate Director, Bush Center in Child Development and Social Policy, Yale University, New Haven, Connecticut

Victor J. Fischer, M.S.W., L.C.S.W.

Clinical Social Worker, Graduate School of Social Work and Social Research, Bryn Mawr College, Bryn Mawr, Pennsylvania; Director of Outpatient Services, Vera French Community Mental Health Center, Davenport, Iowa

Jan E. Fleming, M.D., F.R.C.P.C.

Associate Professor of Psychiatry, McMaster University; Director, Mood Disorders Program for Adolescents, Chedoke-McMaster Hospitals; Member, Centre for Studies of Children at Risk, Hamilton, Ontario, Canada

Brian W.C. Forsyth, M.B., Ch.B., F.R.C.P.(C.)

Associate Professor of Pediatrics, Yale Child Study Center, Yale University School of Medicine; Attending Pediatrician, Yale-New Haven Hospital, New Haven, Connecticut

Elliot M. Friedman, Ph.D.

Postdoctoral Fellow, Department of Psychiatry, University of California, San Diego, San Diego, California

H. Paul Gabriel, M.D.

Clinical Professor of Psychiatry, New York University Medical Center, New York, New York

Judy Garber, Ph.D.

Associate Professor, Department of Psychology and Human Development, Vanderbilt University, Nashville, Tennessee

Jessica Gaynor, Ph.D.

Assistant Clinical Professor, Department of Psychiatry, University of California at San Francisco, San Francisco, California

John P. Glazer, M.D.

Head, Section of Child and Adolescent Psychiatry, Director, Pediatric Consultation-Liaison Service, Departments of Psychiatry and Pediatrics, The Cleveland Clinic Foundation, Cleveland, Ohio

Ian S. Goldberg, M.D.

Clinical Assistant Professor of Psychiatry, New York University Medical Center, New York, New York

Paul N. Graffagnino, M.D.

Clinical Professor of Psychiatry, Associate Clinical Professor of Pediatrics, University of Connecticut School of Medicine, Farmington, Connecticut

Philip J. Graham, F.R.C.P., F.R.C.Psych.

Professor Emeritus, Developmental Psychiatry Section, Department of Psychiatry, University of Cambridge, Cambridge, England

Richard H. Granger, M.D.

Professor of Pediatrics, Yale Child Study Center, Yale University School of Medicine, New Haven, Connecticut

Arthur H. Green, M.D.

Clinical Professor of Psychiatry, Columbia University, College of Physicians and Surgeons; Medical Director, Therapeutic Nursery, and Senior Consultant, Family Center at Presbyterian Hospital New York, New York

Richard Green, M.D., J.D.

Professor Emeritus of Psychiatry, University of California, Los Angeles, School of Medicine, Los Angeles, California; Consulting Psychiatrist and Research Director, Gender Identity Clinic, Charing Cross Hospital, London, England; Senior Research Fellow, Institute of Criminology, University of Cambridge, Cambridge, England

Wayne Hugo Green, M.D.

Associate Professor of Clinical Psychiatry, Director of Training and Education, Division of Child and Adolescent Psychiatry, New York University School of Medicine; Director, Child and Adolescent Psychiatric Clinic, Bellevue Medical Center, New York, New York

Dorothy Grice, M.D.

Postdoctoral Fellow, Yale Child Study Center, Yale University School of Medicine, New Haven, Connecticut

R. Kevin Grigsby, D.S.W., L.C.S.W.

Associate Professor and Director of Research and Development, Telemedicine Center, Medical College of Georgia; Adjunct Associate Professor of Social Work, University of Georgia School of Social Work, Augusta, Georgia

H. Allen Handford, M.D.

Associate Professor and Chief, Division of Child Psychiatry, Pennsylvania State University College of Medicine, M.S. Hershey Medical Center, Hershey, Pennsylvania

Helen Hanesian, Ed.D.

Assistant Professor of Clinical Psychology, Columbia University College of Physicians and Surgeons; Psychologist, Pediatric Neuropsychiatry Service, Columbia-Presbyterian Medical Center, New York, New York

Elizabeth L. Hart, Ph.D.

Assistant Clinical Professor of Psychology in Psychiatry, Yale University School of Medicine, New Haven, Connecticut

Norris M. Haynes, Ph.D.

Associate Professor of Child Development, Psychology and Education, Yale Child Study Center and Department of Psychology, Yale Child Study Center, New Haven, Connecticut

Lily Hechtman, M.D., F.R.C.P.(C.)

Professor, Department of Psychiatry and Pediatrics, Director of Research, Division of Child Psychiatry, McGill University, Montreal Children's Hospital, Montreal, Quebec, Canada

Christopher Henrich, B.A.

Intern Teacher, North Shore Country Day School, Winnetka, Illinois

Jerry D. Heston, M.D.

Associate Professor of Psychiatry, Division of Child and Adolescent Psychiatry, Medical Director, Child and Adolescent Day Treatment Program, University of Tennessee College of Medicine, Memphis, Tennessee

Angela R. Holder, LL.M.

Clinical Professor of Pediatrics (Law), Yale University School of Medicine, New Haven, Connecticut

Michael Irwin, M.D.

Professor of Psychiatry, University of California, San Diego; Veterans Affairs Medical Center, San Diego, California

Todd M. Ivan, M.D.

Resident in Psychiatry, Cleveland Clinic Foundation, Cleveland, Ohio

Ian Ross Jenkins, M.D.

Clinical Assistant Professor, Department of Child and Adolescent Psychiatry, New York University-Bellevue, New York, New York

E. Roy John, Ph.D.

Professor of Psychiatry, Director, Brain Research Laboratories, Department of Psychiatry, New York University Medical Center, Nathan S. Kline Institute for Psychiatric Research, New York, New York

Anthony Kales, M.D.

Professor and Chairman, Department of Psychiatry, The Pennsylvania State University College of Medicine, Hershey, Pennsylvania

Diana Kaplan, Ph.D.

Clinical Instructor, Division of Child and Adolescent Psychiatry, New York University School of Medicine; Clinical Psychologist, Bellevue Hospital Center, New York, New York

Sandra J. Kaplan, M.D.

Associate Professor of Clinical Psychiatry, Cornell University Medical College; Associate Chairman, Department of Psychiatry for Child and Adolescent Psychiatry, North Shore University Hospital, Manhasset, New York

Javad H. Kashani, M.D.

Professor of Psychiatry, Psychology and Pediatrics, Director, Residency Training Section of Child Psychiatry, University of Missouri, Columbia, Columbia, Missouri

Alan E. Kazdin, Ph.D.

Professor of Psychology and Professor in the Child Study Center, Department of Psychology, Yale University School of Medicine, New Haven, Connecticut

Barbara K. Keogh, Ph.D.

Professor Emerita of Education, Graduate School of Education, Research Professor, Department of Psychiatry, University of California, Los Angeles, Los Angeles, California

Laurel J. Kiser, Ph.D.

Associate Professor of Psychiatry, Division of Child and Adolescent Psychiatry, University of Tennessee College of Medicine; Executive Director, Child and Adolescent Day Treatment Services, Memphis, Tennessee

Penelope Krener, M.D.

Professor of Psychiatry and Pediatrics, Chief, Division of Child, Adolescent and Family Psychiatry, University of California, Davis, Davis, California

Michael E. Lamb, Ph.D.

Head, Section on Social and Emotional Development, National Institute of Child Health and Human Development, Bethesda, Maryland

Cynthia G. Last, Ph.D.

Professor of Psychology, Director, Anxiety Treatment Center, Nova Southeastern University, Coral Springs, Florida

James F. Leckman, M.D.

Neison Harris Professor of Child Psychiatry and Pediatrics, Yale Child Study Center, Yale University School of Medicine, New Haven, Connecticut

Patricia K. Leebens, M.D.

Clinical Instructor, Yale Child Study Center, Yale University School of Medicine, New Haven, Connecticut; Attending Psychiatrist, River View Hospital for Children and Youth, Middletown, Connecticut

Robert J. Levine, M.D.

Professor of Medicine, Department of Internal Medicine, Yale University School of Medicine; Attending Physician, Yale-New Haven Hospital, New Haven, Connecticut

Melvin Lewis, M.B., B.S., F.R.C.Psych., D.C.H.

Professor of Child Psychiatry and Pediatrics, Yale Child Study Center, Yale University School of Medicine, New Haven, Connecticut

Dorothy Otnow Lewis, M.D.

Professor of Psychiatry, New York University School of Medicine, New York, New York

Richard Livingston, M.D.

Professor of Psychiatry, UMDNJ-New Jersey Medical School; Director of Child and Adolescent Psychiatry, UMDNJ Community Mental Health Center and United Children's Hospital, Newark, New Jersey

Paul J. Lombroso, M.D.

Associate Professor, Yale Child Study Center, Yale University School of Medicine, New Haven, Connecticut

Alexander R. Lucas, M.D.

Professor in Psychiatry, Mayo Medical School, Rochester, Minnesota

Steven Marans, M.S.W., Ph.D.

Harris Assistant Professor of Child Psychoanalysis, Yale Child Study Center, Yale University School of Medicine, New Haven, Connecticut

Judith Margolis, Ph.D.

Professor, California State University; Psychoeducational Consultant, Margolis Associates, Beverly Hills, California

Richard E. Mattison, M.D.

Associate Professor of Psychiatry, Division of Child Psychiatry, Washington University School of Medicine, St. Louis, Missouri

Linda C. Mayes, M.D.

Arnold Gessel Associate Professor of Child Development, Pediatrics and Psychology, Yale Child Study Center, Yale University School of Medicine, New Haven, Connecticut

John F. McDermott, Jr., M.D.

Professor Emeritus of Psychiatry, University of Hawaii School of Medicine, Honolulu, Hawaii

Edwin J. Mikkelsen, M.D.

Associate Professor of Psychiatry, Harvard Medical School; Medical Director, Mentor Clinical Care, Boston, Massachusetts; Consulting Child Psychiatrist, The Eunice Kennedy Shriver Center, Waltham, Massachusetts

Robert B. Millman, M.D.

Saul P. Steinberg Distinguished Professor of Psychiatry and Public Health, Cornell University Medical College, Director, Division of Substance Abuse Services, New York Hospital-Payne Whitney Psychiatry Clinic, New York, New York

Klaus Minde, M.D., F.R.C.P.(C.)

Chairman, Division of Child Psychiatry, Professor of Psychiatry and Pediatrics, McGill University; Director, Department of Psychiatry, Montreal Children's Hospital, Montreal, Quebec, Canada

Nancy E. Moss, Ph.D.

Assistant Clinical Professor, Yale Child Study Center, Yale University School of Medicine, New Haven, Connecticut

David A. Mrazek, M.D., F.R.C.Psych.

Chairman of Psychiatry and Behavioral Sciences, Children's National Medical Center, Professor of Psychiatry, Behavioral Sciences, and Pediatrics, The George Washington University School of Medicine, Washington, D.C.

Steven F. Nagler, M.S.W., A.C.S.W.

Assistant Clinical Professor, Yale Child Study Center, Yale University School of Medicine, New Haven, Connecticut

Alison Nash, Ph.D.

Associate Professor, Department of Psychology, State University of New York at New Paltz, New Paltz, New York

Charles B. Nemeroff, M.D., Ph.D.

Reunette W. Harris Professor and Chairman, Department of Psychiatry and Behavioral Sciences, Emory University School of Medicine, Atlanta, Georgia

Elaine Davidson Nemzer, M.D.

Clinical Assistant Professor of Psychiatry, Ohio State University College of Medicine, Columbus, Ohio

Barbara Nordhaus, M.S.W.

Assistant Clinical Professor of Social Work, Yale Child Study Center, New Haven, Connecticut

Barry Nurcombe, M.D., F.R.A.N.Z.C.P., F.R.A.C.P.

Professor and Director, Division of Child and Adolescent Psychiatry, Vanderbilt University School of Medicine, Nashville, Tennessee

Richard Oberfield, M.D.

Clinical Associate Professor of Psychiatry, New York University Medical Center, New York, New York

Daniel Offer, M.D.

Professor of Psychiatry and Behavioral Sciences, Director, Adolescent Research, Northwestern University Medical School, Chicago, Illinois

David R. Offord, M.D.

Professor of Psychiatry, Head, Division of Child Psychiatry, McMaster University; Research Director, Chedoke Division, Director, Centre for Studies of Children at Risk, Chedoke-McMaster Hospitals, Hamilton, Ontario, Canada

Edward M. Ornitz, M.D.

Professor of Child Psychiatry, University of California, Los Angeles, School of Medicine, Los Angeles, California

Harry Ostrer, M.D.

Professor of Pediatrics, Director, Human Genetics Program, New York University School of Medicine, Bellevue Hospital Center, New York, New York

Rhea Paul, Ph.D.

Professor, Department of Speech and Hearing Sciences, Portland State University, Portland, Oregon

David L. Pauls, Ph.D.

Associate Professor, Yale Child Study Center, Yale University School of Medicine, New Haven, Connecticut

Sean Perrin, Ph.D.

Postdoctoral Research Fellow, Anxiety Disorders Treatment Center, Nova Southeastern University, Coral Springs, Florida

Bradley S. Peterson, M.D.

Assistant Professor in Child Psychiatry, Yale Child Study Center, Yale University School of Medicine, New Haven, Connecticut

Theodore A. Petti, M.D., M.P.H.

Arthur B. Richter Professor of Child Psychiatry, Indiana University School of Medicine; Medical Director, Youth Services, Larue D. Carter Memorial Hospital, Indianapolis, Indiana

Cynthia R. Pfeffer, M.D.

Professor of Psychiatry, Cornell University Medical College, New York, New York; Chief, Child Psychiatry Inpatient Unit, The New York Hospital-Westchester Division, White Plains, New York

Jonathan H. Pincus, M.D.

Professor of Neurology, Chairman Emeritus, Georgetown University School of Medicine, Washington, D.C.

Richard R. Pleak, M.D.

Unit Chief, Child and Adolescent Day Hospital, Long Island Jewish Medical Center, Glen Oaks, New York; Assistant Professor of Psychiatry, Albert Einstein College of Medicine, Bronx, New York

Leslie Prichep, Ph.D.

Research Associate Professor of Psychiatry, Associate Director, Brain Research Laboratories, New York University Medical Center, Nathan S. Kline Institute for Psychiatric Research, New York, New York

Sally A. Provence, M.D.

Professor Emeritus of Pediatrics and Child Development, Yale Child Study Center, Yale University School of Medicine, New Haven, Connecticut
Deceased

Kyle D. Pruett, M.D.

Clinical Professor of Psychiatry, Yale Child Study Center, Yale University School of Medicine, New Haven, Connecticut

David B. Pruitt, M.D.

Professor of Psychiatry, Director, Division of Child and Adolescent Psychiatry, University of Tennessee, Memphis, College of Medicine, Memphis, Tennessee

Gary R. Racusin, Ph.D.

Associate Research Scientist, Department of Psychiatry, Yale Child Study Center, Yale University School of Medicine, New Haven, Connecticut

Naomi I. Rae Grant, M.B., B.S., F.R.C.P.(C.), F.R.C.Psych.

Professor Emerita, The University of Western Ontario, London, Ontario, Canada

Frank T. Rafferty, M.D.

Staff Psychiatrist, Gateway Center for Human Development, Brunswick, Georgia

Pasko Rakic, M.D., Sc.D.

Professor of Neuroscience, Section of Neurobiology, Yale University School of Medicine, New Haven, Connecticut

Kent Ravenscroft, M.D.

Associate Clinical Professor of Psychiatry, Georgetown and George Washington University Medical Schools; Faculty, International Institute of Object Relations Therapy, Washington, D.C.

Margot Moser Richters, Ph.D.

Clinical Child Psychologist, Reginald S. Lourie Center for Infants and Young Children, Rockville, Maryland

Mark A. Riddle, M.D.

Professor of Psychiatry and Pediatrics, Director, Division of Child and Adolescent Psychiatry, Johns Hopkins Medical Institutions, Baltimore, Maryland

Kenneth S. Robson, M.D.

Professor of Psychiatry, University of Connecticut School of Medicine, Farmington, Connecticut

David N. Rosen, LL.B.

Rosen & Dolan, P.C.; Lecturer, Yale Child Study Center, Yale University School of Medicine, New Haven, Connecticut

Andrew T. Russell, M.D.

Associate Professor of Psychiatry and Biobehavioral Sciences, University of California, Los Angeles, Neuropsychiatric Institute, Los Angeles, California

Diane H. Schetky, M.D.

Private Practice, Rockport, Maine; Associate Clinical Professor of Psychiatry, University of Vermini College of Medicine at Maine Medical Center, Portland, Maine

Kimberly A. Schonert-Reichl, Ph.D.

Assistant Professor, Department of Educational Psychology and Special Education, Faculty of Education, The University of British Columbia, Vancouver, British Columbia, Canada

David J. Schonfeld, M.D.

Associate Professor of Pediatrics, Yale Child Study Center, Yale University School of Medicine, New Haven, Connecticut

Eric Schopler, Ph.D.

Professor of Psychiatry and Psychology, University of North Carolina School of Medicine, Chapel Hill, North Carolina

John E. Schowalter, M.D.

Professor of Psychiatry, Albert J. Solnit Professor of Child Psychiatry and Pediatrics, Yale Child Study Center, Yale University School of Medicine, New Haven, Connecticut

Mary E. Schwab-Stone, M.D.

Harris Associate Professor of Child Psychiatry, Yale Child Study Center, Yale University School of Medicine, New Haven, Connecticut

Daniel J. Siegel, M.D.

Medical Director, Infant and Preschool Service, Division of Child and Adolescent Psychiatry, Department of Psychiatry and Biobehavioral Sciences, Clinical Faculty, University of California, Los Angeles, School of Medicine, Los Angeles, California

Larry B. Silver, M.D.

Clinical Professor of Psychiatry, Director of Training in Child and Adolescent Psychiatry, Georgetown University School of Medicine, Washington, D.C.

Jerome L. Singer, Ph.D.

Professor of Psychology and Child Study, Yale Child Study Center, Yale University School of Medicine, New Haven, Connecticut

Jonathan A. Slater, M.D.

Assistant Clinical Professor of Psychiatry, Columbia University; Director, Pediatric Consultation-Liaison Psychiatry, Babies and Children's Hospital, Columbia-Presbyterian Medical Center, New York, New York

Albert J. Solnit, M.D.

Sterling Professor Emeritus of Psychiatry and Pediatrics, Senior Research Scientist, Yale Child Study Center, New Haven, Connecticut

Frederick J. Stoddard, M.D.

Chief of Psychiatry, Shriners Burns Institute; Assistant Clinical Professor of Psychiatry, Harvard Medical School; Division of Child Psychiatry, Massachusetts General Hospital, Boston, Massachusetts

Elsa L. Stone, M.D.

Assistant Professor of Pediatrics, Yale University School of Medicine, New Haven, Connecticut

Jeffrey W. Summerville, M.Div., M.S.W., M.H.S.A.

Senior Partner, Mental Health Associates, Hamden, Connecticut

Hratch Svadjian, M.D.

Fellow in Child and Adolescent Psychiatry, Department of Psychiatry, The Ohio State University, Columbus, Ohio

Peter E. Tanguay, M.D.

Ackerly Professor of Child and Adolescent Psychiatry, Brigham Child Guidance Clinic, University of Louisville, Louisville, Kentucky

George Tarjan, M.D.

Professor Emeritus of Psychiatry, University of California, Los Angeles, Los Angeles, California
Deceased

Jacob Kraemer Tebes, Ph.D.

Associate Professor of Psychology in Psychiatry and Child Study, Yale Child Study Center, Yale University School of Medicine, The Consultation Center, New Haven, Connecticut

Lenore C. Terr, M.D.

Clinical Professor of Psychiatry, University of California, San Francisco, San Francisco, California

Douglas M. Teti, Ph.D.

Associate Professor, Department of Psychology, University of Maryland Baltimore County, Baltimore, Maryland

Alexander Thomas, M.D.

Professor of Psychiatry, New York University Medical Center; Director, Bellevue Psychiatric Hospital, New York, New York

Ross A. Thompson, Ph.D.

Professor, Department of Psychology, University of Nebraska, Lincoln, Nebraska

David A. Tomb, M.D.

Associate Professor of Psychiatry, University of Utah School of Medicine, Salt Lake City, Utah

Kenneth E. Towbin, M.D.

Director of Child and Adolescent Psychiatry Residency Training Program, Associate Professor of Psychiatry and Behavioral Science and Pediatrics, The George Washington University Medical Center, Washington, D.C.

Daniel M. Tucker, M.D.

National Institute of Mental Health Postdoctoral Research Fellow in Child Psychiatry, Yale Child Study Center, New Haven, Connecticut

Jeremy Turk, M.D.

Senior Lecturer, St. George's Hospital Medical School, London, England

Lawrence A. Vitulano, Ph.D.

Associate Clinical Professor of Psychology, Yale Child Study Center, Yale University School of Medicine, New Haven, Connecticut; Supervising Psychologist, Department of Children and Families, Middletown, Connecticut

Fred R. Volkmar, M.D.

Harris Associate Professor of Child Psychiatry, Pediatrics and Psychology, Yale Child Study Center, Yale University School of Medicine, New Haven, Connecticut

Judith S. Wallerstein, Ph.D.

Founder and Senior Consultant, Center for the Family in Transition, Corte Madera, California

Gabrielle Weiss, M.D., F.R.C.P.(C.)

Clinical Professor of Psychiatry, University of British Columbia; Staff Psychiatrist, British Columbia Children's Hospital, North Shore Hospital, West Vancouver, British Columbia, Canada

Elizabeth B. Weller, M.D.

Professor of Psychiatry, Pediatrics and Neuroscience, Department of Psychiatry, Ohio State University College of Medicine, Columbus, Ohio

Ronald A. Weller, M.D.

Professor of Psychiatry, Ohio State University College of Medicine, Columbus, Ohio

John Scott Werry, M.D.

Professor Emeritus of Psychiatry, University of Auckland, Auckland, New Zealand

Michael Will, M.D.

Faculty Research Fellow, Developmental Neurobiology Unit, Department of Psychiatry, New York University School of Medicine, Bellevue Hospital Center, New York, New York

Daniel T. Williams, M.D.

Associate Clinical Professor of Psychiatry, Columbia College of Physicians and Surgeons; Director, Pediatric Neuropsychiatry, Department of Child Psychiatry, Columbia-Presbyterian Medical Center, New York, New York

Julie J. Wiltsie Pugh, B.A.

Research Assistant, Department of Psychiatry, The Ohio State University, Columbus, Ohio

Stephen Wizner, J.D.

William O. Douglas Clinical Professor of Law, Yale University Law School, New Haven, Connecticut

Sula Wolff, F.R.C.P., F.R.C.Psych.

Honorary Fellow, Department of Psychiatry, University of Edinburgh, Edinburgh, Scotland

Joseph L. Woolston, M.D.

Associate Professor of Child Psychiatry, Yale Child Study Center, Yale University School of Medicine, New Haven, Connecticut

Alayne Yates, M.D.

Professor of Psychiatry, Director, Division of Child and Adolescent Psychiatry, University of Hawaii, Honolulu, Hawaii

Timothy Yates, M.D., F.R.C.P.(C.)

Associate Professor of Psychiatry and Pediatrics, Faculty of Medicine, University of Calgary; Staff Psychiatrist, Alberta Children's Hospital, Calgary, Alberta, Canada

Catherine A. Yeager, M.A.

Assistant Research Scientist, Assistant Director, Dissociative Disorders Clinic, Division of Child and Adolescent Psychiatry, New York University School of Medicine, New York, New York

J. Gerald Young, M.D.

Professor of Psychiatry, Division of Child and Adolescent Psychiatry, New York University School of Medicine, Bellevue Hospital Center, New York, New York

Edward F. Zigler, Ph.D.

Sterling Professor of Psychology, Yale University School of Medicine, New Haven, Connecticut

Kenneth J. Zucker, Ph.D.

Head, Child and Adolescent Gender Identity Clinic, Child and Family Studies Centre, Clarke Institute of Psychiatry, Toronto, Ontario, Canada

CONTENTS

SECTION VIII. CHILD PSYCHIATRY AND ALLIED PROFESSIONS

A/ Child Psychiatry and Pediatrics

SECTION IX. TRAINING, RESEARCH, ETHICS, AND HISTORY

SECTION I. NORMAL DEVELOPMENT
A/ Developmental Aspects of Biological Growth

1 GENES AND DEVELOPMENTAL NEUROBIOLOGY
James F. Leckman, M.D., and Paul J. Lombroso, M.D.

Human beings are complex living organisms that can be characterized by their appearance and behavior at each point in their life cycle. Many of these characteristics are uniquely human, such as the array of languages that facilitate interpersonal communication and that permit a meaningful interplay of ideas and emotions. Other characteristics, such as affection and aggression, are less distinctive and place our species as one among many that populate the earth. Scientific advances over the past 150 years clearly indicate that hereditary factors, which are transmitted from generation to generation, account for much of the observed variation among and within species. Although the complexities of human existence cannot be reduced simply to the effects of genes, it is inescapable that genetic factors provide the biological basis for many of our potentialities and vulnerabilities as human beings.

Our genetic endowment, as a species, is a unique collection of discrete units of heredity (genes) that for the most part are linearly arranged on 46 chromosomes (22 pairs of homologous chromosomes and two sex chromosomes) (Fig. 1.1). This collection of genes makes us both alike and different from other organisms. Although the precise genetic determinants of our interspecies similarities and differences are largely obscure, it is probable that many of the responsible genetic factors will be identified. For example, it may be possible to identify the genes that have contributed to the remarkable neuroanatomical and functional evolution of the cerebral neocortices across different mammalian species over the past 50 million years (Glezer et al., 1988; Puelles and Rubenstein, 1993).

Genetic factors also contribute to variations within species. A large number of physical and psychological traits, including gender, height, and intelligence, have been shown to be under at least partial genetic control. One need only examine the striking physical and psychological similarities between monozygotic (genetically identical) twins reared apart to recognize the powerful influence of genes in determining who we are (Juel-Nielsen, 1980; Shields, 1962). Some of these intraspecies differences, such as gender, are due to actual differences in the number and type of genes present in the individual (any gene on the Y chromosome is present only in males and is transmitted only from father to son). Other intraspecies differences are due to there being multiple forms (polymorphic alleles) of specific genes that are distributed within the population. Some of these variants are associated with disease states such as Huntington's disease, Marfan's syndrome, or sickle cell anemia, while others may contribute to traits such as blood type or eye color. Other intraspecies differences may depend on the sex of which parent passed on a particular piece of genetic material through the poorly understood process of genetic imprinting (Moore and Haig, 1991). The most dramatic example of imprinting concerns two distinctively different developmental disorders, Prader-Willi and Angelman's syndrome, that are due to alterations of DNA in the *same* general chromosomal region on chromosome 15 (Knoll et al., 1993).

Apart from interspecies and intraspecies variations, it is also important to recognize that differences within an individual member of a species can also be due to genetic factors. Simply put, this means that not all genes are active at the same time. For example, the hemoglobin genes that are active during fetal life are different from those that are active in adults. As we understand more of the biological determinants of the continuities and discontinuities of human development, it is likely that we will come to recognize an orderly unfolding of each individual's genetic potentialities.

The next two sections, "Genes" and "Regulation of Gene Function," present a condensed summary of some of the fundamental aspects of the structure and function of genes and gene products. Several excellent general references cover this material in greater depth (Freifelder, 1987; Watson et al., 1987).

GENES

The existence of discrete hereditary factors or genes was initially postulated by Mendel in 1865, but their importance was not appreciated until the early 1900s. As indicated above, genes are usually linearly arranged on chromosomes that are found in the nuclei of cells. Normally genes are extremely stable and are precisely copied during the chromosomal duplications that precede cell divisions (mitosis). Heritable changes in the structure of genes (mutations) can occur but are usually deleterious to the organism. This capacity for change can, in rare instances, lead to positive consequences, which serve as the basis for evolution.

Chemically, genes are composed of deoxyribonucleic acid (DNA). DNA is composed of a string of nucleotides (complex molecules that contain a sugar moiety, a phosphate group, and either a purine or a pyrimidine base) that are linked end to end. These linkages involve the phosphate group's connecting the $5'$ carbon atom of one sugar moiety to the $3''$ carbon atom of the next nucleotide. As a result, every nucleic acid chain has a direction determined by the orientation of its sugar-phosphate backbone. The two ends are designated $5''$ and $3''$ to indicate this orientation. Four separate nucleotides are found in DNA. Two contain purine bases (adenine and guanine), and two contain pyrimidine bases (thymine and cytosine) (Fig. 1.2).

Genetic information is conveyed by the specific nucleotide sequence of a particular DNA molecule. Most DNA molecules exist in a double helical structure composed of two polynucleotide chains held together by a series of hydrogen bonds between complementary base pairs (adenine is bonded to thymine and guanine to cytosine) (Fig. 1.3). This structure confers stability on the molecule and provides the basis for replication. Since each strand of DNA in the double helix is exactly complementary to the other, knowing the sequence of one strand immediately provides precise knowledge of the sequence of the other.

The sequence of complementary base pairs determines the order of the 20 different amino acids in proteins. As a consequence, the information contained in DNA provides the instructions that direct cells to grow and divide, set in motion developmental sequences that lead to orderly differentiation of cell types, and provide for the maintenance of a diversified population of cells that are necessary for the successful functioning of complex organisms.

The sequence of complementary base pairs, however, does not provide a direct template for protein synthesis. Instead, there is a complex

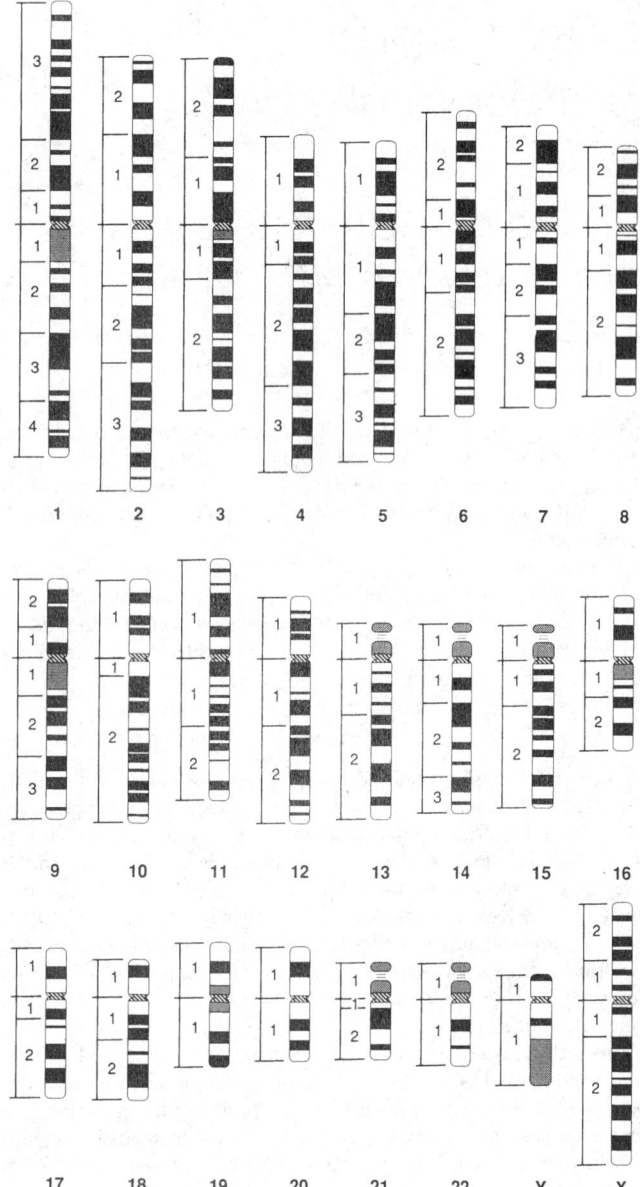

Figure 1.1.   Depiction of high-resolution banded human chromosomes. (Adapted from *Yale-HHMI Human Gene Mapping Library Chromosome Plots, Number 5.* New Haven, CT, Howard Hughes Medical Institute, 1989.)

series of events that depend on the transcription of the genetic code from DNA to messenger ribonucleic acid (mRNA). Messenger RNA is very similar in composition to DNA and can hybridize with complementary DNA sequences. All mRNA chains grow in a 5' to 3' direction and are single stranded. Mature mRNA conveys the information out of the nucleus and into the cytoplasm and serves as the template for protein synthesis.

The translation of a part of the genetic code into a specific amino acid sequence occurs at ribosomes (made of ribosomal RNA) located in either the cytoplasm or the endoplasmic reticulum. The genetic code is determined by the sequence of bases, with sets of three bases constituting one coding unit, or codon. At the ribosome, the codons of an mRNA molecule base pair with complementary anticodons of transfer RNA (tRNA), which contribute specific amino acids to the growing protein chain. This translation of the genetic code also occurs in a 5' to 3' direction. The basic elements of this "central dogma" of protein produc-

tion were first proposed by Crick in 1956 and remain fundamental to our understanding of these basic molecular events (Crick et al., 1961).

REGULATION OF GENE FUNCTION

According to some estimates, only about 1% of the genome is being expressed at a given time in higher eucaryotic cells (Watson et al., 1987). At any point in development and in any particular tissue, a different but overlapping set of genes is active. Some genes are constitutively expressed, while others are highly responsive to environmental changes. Regulation of gene function can occur at any one of the many steps required for gene expression (Fig. 1.4).

Transcriptional Factors

Transcription depends on a complex series of events that lead to the formation of mRNA. A central event is the binding of an RNA polymerase to specific promoter sites (highly conserved DNA sequences) that lie almost entirely outside (5' to) that portion of the gene that codes for the amino acid sequence. In addition to promoters, other DNA sequences have been identified that enhance transcription within certain tissues or cell types. These enhancers can function in either orientation and are often contained within the transcribed region of the gene.

Several classes of DNA-binding proteins, or transcription factors, that contribute to the regulation of certain genes have also been identified. The best characterized of these contain highly conserved polypeptide structures that are known to bind to specific DNA sequences. For example, homeobox genes contain a highly conserved DNA sequence of 180 nucleotides that code for a polypeptide with a helix-turn-helix structure that contains two α helices that bind in the major groove of the double helix of DNA (McGinnis et al., 1984). Other transcriptional factors have distinctive tertiary structures known as *zinc fingers* and *leucine zippers*, which bind to DNA (Landschultz et al., 1988; Miller, 1985).

Another set of factors that influence transcription involves steroid hormones acting in conjunction with cytosolic protein receptors (found only in certain cell types). After combining with the cytosolic receptors, the steroid-receptor complex enters the nucleus and binds to specific DNA regions, called responsive elements, to alter transcription (Evans, 1988).

Posttranscriptional Events

Transcribed RNA typically goes through a number of modifications before it is ready for export from the nucleus. These steps include the excision of specific regions of the message (introns) through the mechanism of splicing and the addition of long stretches of adenine nucleotides (the poly(A) tail). Differences in splice site selection and in the placement of the poly(A) tail have been demonstrated, indicating that alternate mRNAs can be derived from the same DNA sequence. This flexibility in mRNA formation may play an important role in the tissue-specific expression of some genes or may serve as the basis for differences in their expression over the course of development.

Translational Factors

The process of translating mature mRNA into proteins by ribosomes involves a complex series of events, some of which are under regulatory control. Although regulatory mechanisms at this level may seem unnecessary, they do provide a means of rapidly controlling how active cells are in the synthesis of gene products.

The stability of the mature mRNA once it has entered the cytosol is a critical determinant of how many copies of the protein will be synthesized by the ribosomal apparatus. Certain base sequences in the 3' untranslated region may influence the rate of degradation of some mRNAs.

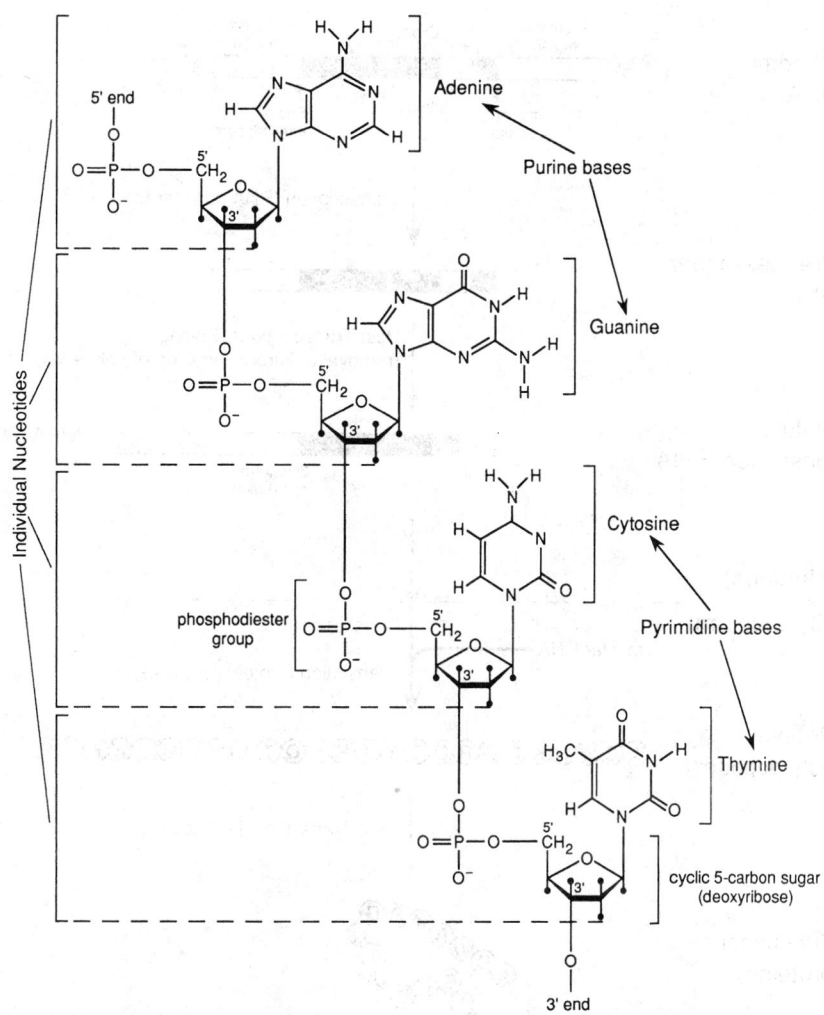

Figure 1.2. The chemical structure of DNA, showing the 3′-5′phosphodiester linkages that connect the nucleotides. (Adapted from Watson JD, Hopkins NH, Roberts JW, et al: *Molecular Biology of the Cell.* Menlo Park, CA, Benjamin/Cummings, 1987.)

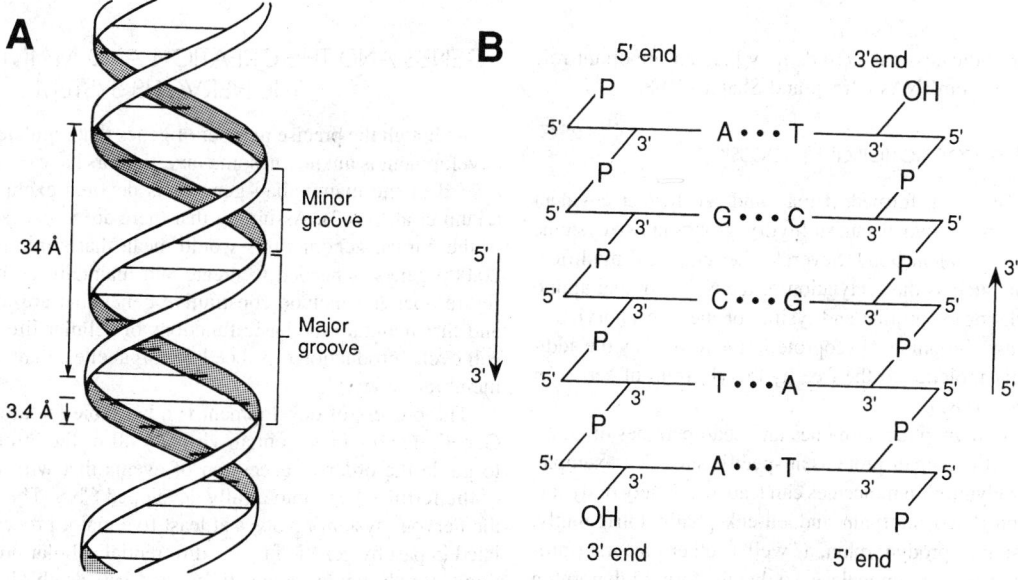

Figure 1.3. A, Diagram of the DNA double helix in its common form. **B,** A stylized drawing of a segment of DNA showing the antiparallel orientation of the complementary strands. (Adapted from Freifelder D. *Molecular Biology.* 2nd ed. Boston, Jones & Bartlett, 1987.)

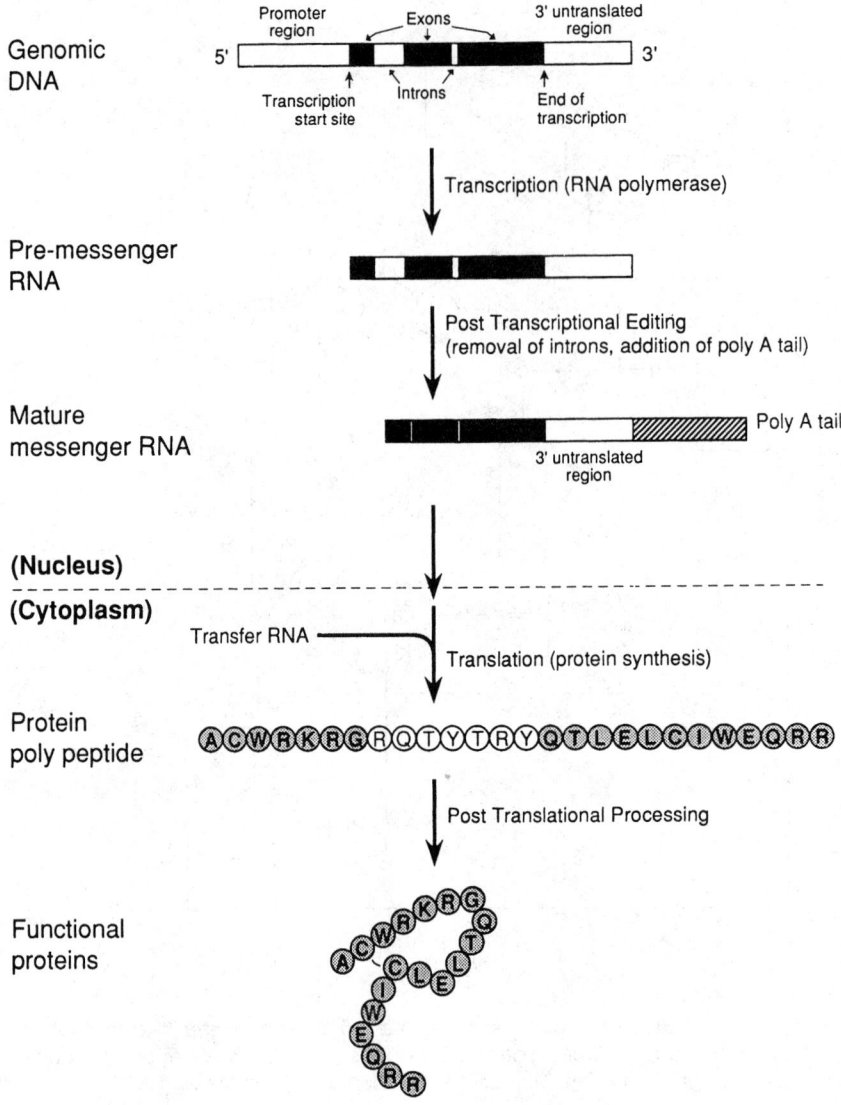

Figure 1.4. Sequence of events involved in gene expression.

Some evidence also indicates that steroids may play an important role in conferring stability to mRNAs (Brock and Shapiro, 1983).

Posttranslational Processing

Once a protein has been formed, it may undergo further covalent modification. For example, two distant sulfhydryl groups in two cysteine residues may form a covalent bond. Several other chemical modifications can also occur, such as the acetylation of the NH_2 terminal amino acids, the hydroxylation of proline and lysine, or the phosphorylation of serine, tyrosine, and threonine. Glycoproteins are formed by the addition of various sugar moieties to the free hydroxyl group of serine or threonine (Freifelder, 1987).

The formation of polypeptide hormones and neuropeptides often involves the cleavage of precursor proteins at specific sites. For example, the processing of prodynorphin molecules can lead to a variety of dynorphin moieties, α- and β-neoendorphin, and leu-enkephalin. Intriguingly, differential processing of prodynorphin, as well as other precursor proteins, in different tissues is commonplace, so that the form of dynorphin found in the anterior lobe of the pituitary is different from the form of dynorphin found in the neurointermediate lobe (Molineaux et al., 1986).

GENES AND THE CREATION AND MAINTENANCE OF THE NERVOUS SYSTEM

Although the precise number of genes that regulate CNS growth and development is unknown, some investigators have estimated that at least a third of the mammalian genome is devoted exclusively to this task (Hahn et al., 1982). Assuming that there are in excess of 50,000 genes in the human genome, this would mean that a minimum of 15,000 to 20,000 genes is needed to create and maintain the human CNS. This figure does not include constitutive genes that are universally present and that maintain the basic functions of cellular life (regulation of the cell cycle, production of subcellular organelles, maintenance of cellular membranes, etc.).

The process of development is a heritable feature of all organisms. Genetic factors must contain virtually all of the information necessary to guide the orderly succession of events that will transform portions of the fertilized egg into a fully developed CNS. The morphogenesis of the nervous system involves at least five major processes that are regulated in part by genetic factors: differential cellular proliferation, migration, growth, neural connectivity, and cell death (Jacobson, 1970). A fundamental understanding of these processes would require precise knowledge of (*a*) the developmental information relevant to the CNS that is encoded in the human genome, (*b*) how this information is regulated and utilized in ''morphogenetic'' time and space, and (*c*) how the products of these genes endow the differentiating and differentiated cells of the embryonic CNS with their functional characteristics (Davidson, 1986). We remain largely ignorant of the critical determinants of these processes.

Spatial Differentiation and Determination of Specific Cell Lineages

Interestingly, RNA synthesized by the mother during oogenesis provides the basis for most of the biosynthetic capacity of early embryos. This means that by the time of fertilization the egg has already been programmed to ensure the development of spatially distinct embryonic cell lineages. Literally thousands of mRNAs are formed during oogenesis, and in some species this set of maternal genes may constitute a majority of all genomic loci active in ontogeny (Davidson, 1986).

The maternal mRNAs persist until the blastula stage, when they are replaced by zygotic transcripts. Most of these transcripts are homologous with the maternal transcripts, but some are novel genes not included in the maternal set. An instructive example of this transition from maternal to zygotic transcripts concerns several evolutionarily conserved proteins that act as a trigger for cell divisions. In this case, studies have shown that the accumulation of the protein *cyclin* serves as the universal mitotic trigger for early cell divisions that are executed by maternally synthesized gene products, while later cell divisions after the transition to zygotic control depend on the production of a different trigger protein (O'Farrell et al., 1989).

Two other important classes of genes active at this point in development are segmentation and homeotic genes. These genes have been best characterized in *Drosophila*, where they determine the number and polarity of body segments and the identity and sequence of body segments (Gehring, 1987). Many of these genes are evolutionarily conserved and are present in the human genome.

Although the precise functions of these genes in mammalian development have not been fully established, they are known to be differentially expressed in the central and peripheral nervous systems, as well as in mesodermal derivatives (Graham et al., 1989). Intriguingly, some of these genes exist in multigene clusters related by duplication and divergence. In some instances the relative chromosomal position of the gene within a cluster corresponds to the domain of expression in the developing embryo (Fig. 1.5). Many of these genes code for DNA-binding proteins with a classical helix-turn-helix structure. As a consequence,

attention has focused on their potential role as transcription factors in organizing the differential expression of other effector genes that are ultimately responsible for establishing distinctive cellular phenotypes. Several closely related base sequences that bind these proteins have been identified. Interestingly, the majority of these sites have been found in the 5′ regulatory regions of other segmentation and homeotic genes, suggesting that there may be complex self-regulatory interactions between these genes (Levine and Hoey, 1988). There is also a strong likelihood that other effector genes will be identified that would confer the functional identity for a given class of cells. For example, these genes may be active in conferring the cellular identity of the polyclonal derivatives of the hematopoietic stem cells (Kongsuwan et al., 1988). Rakic has speculated that a similar mechanism may underlie the asymmetrical divisions of progenitor cells within the ventricular zone that lead to the polyclone of cells that exist within the radial units of the neocortex (Rakic, 1988b). Initial findings concerning the pattern of expression of some of these genes in the developing telencephalon offer limited support to this speculation (Boncinelli et al., 1993; Puelles and Rubenstein, 1993).

Another major issue concerns the mechanisms by which genes remain quiescent in some cell lineages or in a repressed configuration after a period of activity (Davidson, 1986). In this regard, it seems evident that at specific points in development specific genes are sequestered within heritable forms of chromatin complex that preclude transcription. Developmental repression of adult somatic cell genes is remarkably efficient. Ratios of 1:10,000,000 or more have been estimated for the level of globin and growth hormone transcripts in cells not expressing these genes, compared with those that are (Groudine and Weintraub, 1975; Ivarie et al., 1983). A related issue concerns early and random inactivation of one of the two X chromosomes in the cells of women. Although the mechanisms that underlie such events are poorly understood, they undoubtedly contribute to the range of phenotypic variation seen in women who have fragile X syndrome.

Migration of Neurons

The early embryonic development of the nervous system is characterized in part by the migration of populations of neurons. Examples of this phenomenon include the migration of neural crest cells to form elements of the peripheral nervous system (autonomic and sensory ganglia, glial cells, adrenomedullary cells) and the radial migration of neurons created in the ventricular zone to the cortical laminae. A range of

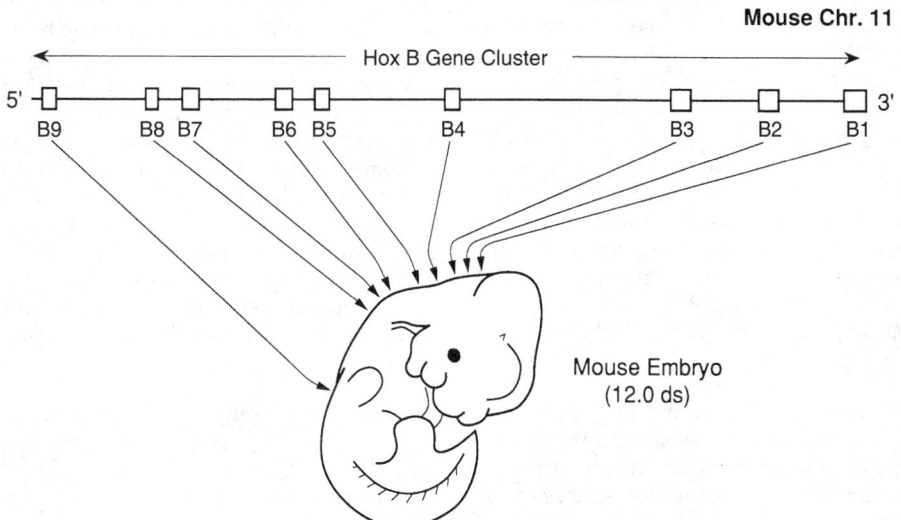

Figure 1.5. Correspondence between chromosomal position and gene expression (along the anterior-posterior axis of the mouse embryo) for the Hox B gene cluster. (Adapted from Graham A, Papalo-pulu N, Krumlauf R. The murine and drosophila homeobox gene complexes have common features of organization and expression. *Cell* 57:367–378, 1989.)

factors that mediate these events has been identified, including inherent directional preferences, chemotaxis, and differential adhesion (Purves and Lichtman, 1985). The role of genetic factors in controlling or influencing migration is unclear, although some inferences are possible based on the role of certain compounds involved in chemotaxis or adhesion. In the case of corticogenesis, it has been established that the newly formed neurons migrate along radial glial guides that stretch between the ventricular surface and the outer cortical surface (Rakic, 1988a). This suggests that certain recognition and adhesion molecules are necessary for this migratory process to occur (Hatten and Mason, 1986; Rakic, 1981, 1988b). The differential expression of these molecules is likely to be under genetic control, and genetically mediated defects in their structure and function are likely to be revealed in aberrant migratory patterns (as is seen in the ''weaver'' mouse mutant) (Rakic and Sidman, 1973a, 1973b).

Neural Connectivity and Survival

Developing nerve cells have the remarkable characteristic of being able to maintain contact with literally hundreds of other nerve cells by extending cellular processes over substantial distances. These contacts are undoubtedly of crucial importance in establishing and maintaining the functional integrity of the nervous system. These processes initially develop by way of local extension and retraction of specialized areas on the surface of the neurons, called growth cones. A variety of external signals may regulate the formation, maintenance, and/or degradation of these neuron-neuron connections, including mechanical guides, differential adhesiveness, the influence of electrical fields, and interaction with gradients of trophic substances (Kalil et al., 1986; Purves and Lichtman, 1985).

Once neuronal processes reach their target-field, the neurons acquire obligatory trophic dependencies. A given target-field, however, is able to support only a limited number of neurons, and the ''extra'' neurons are lost. For example, although nerve growth factor (NGF) does not attract sensory nerve fibers to their target-fields, it is intimately involved in the target-mediated survival of neurons. Indeed, from the first appearance of the neuronal processes in the target-field, there is a marked increase in the rate of transcription of the NGF gene and in the amount of NGF in the target-field. There is also a rapid appearance of cell-surface receptors for NGF on the sensory neurons (mediated by the transcription of the NGF receptor gene) (Davies et al., 1987).

Genetic factors are likely to play an important facilitatory role in neurite outgrowth and synaptogenesis throughout life. The dynamic equilibrium between neurite outgrowth and synaptogenesis versus neurite pruning and synapse withdrawal may well be crucial mechanisms that allow organisms to modify their behavior or ''learn'' as a result of experience. Although the precise genetic mechanisms that underlie these complex processes are not well understood, one mechanism may involve those genes that regulate the expression of molecules involved in neuron-neuron communication. For example, in vitro and in vivo studies have indicated that many neurotransmitters and neuromodulators, in addition to their communicative function in mature neural systems, play important roles in the development of these systems by promoting or inhibiting the growth of neural processes (Lipton and Kater, 1989).

THE ROLE OF EPIGENETIC AND ENVIRONMENTAL FACTORS

The development of the nervous system depends on epigenetic and environmental factors, as well as on genetic influences. At each level and stage of development, the microenvironments and macroenvironments of the organism play a crucial role. The unfolding of the genomic blueprint, with its complex sequences and patterns of gene expression, depends in large measure on the presence of transcriptional factors in the microenvironment of the nucleus. This means that our ability to separate out the relative contributions of genetic and epigenetic influ-

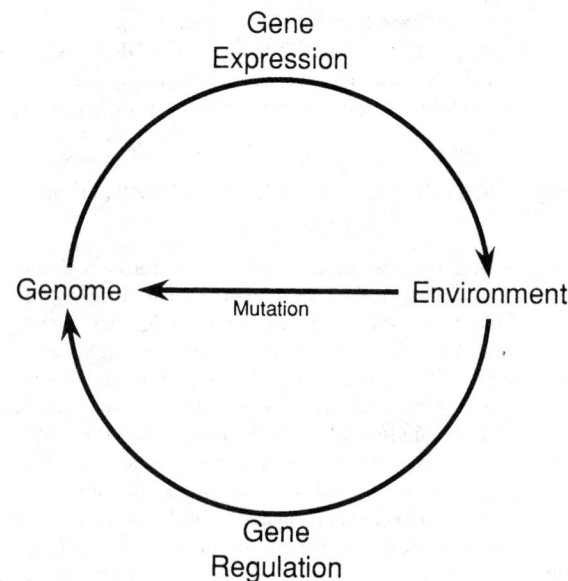

Figure 1.6. Gene-environment interactions. (Adapted from Purves D, Lichtman JW. *Principles of Neural Development.* Sunderland, MA, Sinauer, 1985.)

ences is difficult because the genes influence the developmental environment and the developmental environment influences the genes (Fig. 1.6).

At the macroenvironmental level, manipulation of sensory input can alter the structure and function of cytoarchitectonic areas of the cortex (Kalil et al., 1986; Rakic, 1988b). Although these external events are unquestionably translated into internal events that alter the microenvironment and disturb the balance of factors that permit neuronal outgrowth and survival, they underline the exquisite sensitivity of the developing nervous system to its external environment.

The sphere of influences acting on the nervous system continually enlarges during development (Purves and Lichtman, 1985). Assuming a ''good enough'' to support development, the cytoplasm of the egg, with its maternally derived biosynthetic apparatus, provides the initial milieu. Later local cellular interactions between neurons and glia and the functional activity of more distant neurons influence the multiple microenvironments of the discrete cell lineages. Finally, the nervous system is also shaped by wholly external events in the prenatal and postnatal world. The events in early family life, interactions with peers, and educational opportunities shape the course of development just as surely as the developing individual profoundly influences his or her environment. The developmental perspectives of psychoanalytic theory echo in the study of developmental neurobiology.

Some measure of persistent genetic and neural malleability must confer selective advantages. The generation of immunologically specific B and T cells, which allows us to respond to and remember novel antigens, provides a remarkable example of the conservation of genetic malleability (Weigert et al., 1978). The capacity of some individuals to survive and succeed in the face of persistent psychosocial adversity provides even more remarkable evidence of our persistent neural malleability.

PERSPECTIVES ON NEUROPSYCHIATRIC DISORDERS OF CHILDHOOD ONSET

The past decade has seen remarkable progress in the application of molecular genetic strategies to the study of neurological and neuropsychiatric disorders (Martin, 1989). Identification of the chromosomal locus for a number of autosomal-dominant, autosomal-recessive, and X-linked recessive disorders has been accomplished using restriction

Table 1.1.   Chromosomal Localization and Gene Abnormalities in Selected Psychiatric and Neurological Disorders

Genetic Disorder	Chromosomal Location	Genetic Defect (Gene Name)	Heterogeneity
Autosomal-dominant			
Charcot-Marie-Tooth disease			Nonallelic heterogenic
Type 1A	17p11.2–12	Gene duplication or point mutation (*PMP22*)	
Type 1B	1q22–23	Point mutation (myelin) P_0	
Type 1C	Unknown	Unknown	
Huntington's disease	4p16.3	Triplet repeat (*HD* or *IT15*)	None demonstrated
Spinocerebellar ataxia	6p24	Triplet repeat (*SCA1*)	None demonstrated
Myotonic dystrophy	19q13.3	Triplet repeat (*DM-1* or myotonin protein kinase)	None demonstrated
Familial Alzheimer's disease			Nonallelic heterogeneity
	14q24.3	Unknown	
	21q21	Unknown	
	19q	Unknown	
Neurofibromatosis			
Von Recklinghausen (*NFI*)	17q11.2	Deletions, insertions, translocations, and point mutations (neurofibromin)	None demonstrated
Acoustic neuroma (*NFI*)	22q	Translocations, point mutation (*NFI* gene)	None demonstrated
Familial amyloidotic polyneuropathy	18q11.2	Point mutation (transthyretin)	Allelic heterogeneity
Amyotrophic lateral sclerosis	21q21.1–22	Point mutation (SO dismutase)	Allelic heterogeneity
Hyperkalemic periodic paralysis	17q23–25	Point mutation (Na^+ channel)	Allelic heterogeneity
Benign familial neonatal convulsions	20q	Unknown	Nonallelic heterogeneity
Autosomal-recessive			
Gaucher's disease	1q21	Point mutation (glucocerebrosidase)	Allelic heterogeneity
Friedreich's ataxia	9p13–21.1	Unknown	None demonstrated
Ataxia-telangiectasia	14q32 and 11q23	Translocations (unknown)	Allelic heterogeneity
Wilson's disease	13q14.21	Unknown	None demonstrated
Prader-Willi syndrome	15q11–13	Deletions (candidate gene: *SNRPN*)	None demonstrated
Angelman syndrome	15q11–13	Deletions (unknown)	None demonstrated
Waardenburg syndrome	2q35	Point mutation, deletion (Pax-3)	None demonstrated
Williams syndrome	7q11.23	Deletions (elastin)	None demonstrated
Miller-Dieker syndrome	17p13.3	Deletions (lissencephaly-1)	None demonstrated
Retinoblastoma	13q14	Deletions, point mutations (*RB*)	Allelic heterogeneity
Von Hippel-Lindau	3p	Deletions (*VHL* gene)	None demonstrated
Attention deficit with hyperactivity disorder in patients with generalized resistance to thyroid hormone disorder	3p	Point mutations (thyroid receptor-beta gene)	Allelic heterogeneity
X-linked recessive			
Spinobulbar muscular atrophy (Kennedy syndrome)	Xp21.3	Triplet repeat (androgen receptor)	None demonstrated
Duchenne dystrophy	Xp21.21	Large deletion (dystrophin)	None demonstrated
Becker dystrophy	Xp21.21	Smaller deletion (dystrophin)	None demonstrated
Lesch-Nyhan syndrome	Xq27	Point mutations (HPRT deficiency)	Allelic heterogeneity
Fragile X syndrome	Xq27.3	Triplet repeat, deletions (*FMR-1*)	Allelic heterogeneity
Pelizaeus-Merzbacher disease	Xq21–22	Deletions, insertions, point mutations (proteolipid)	Allelic heterogeneity
Adrenoleukodystrophy	Xq28	Unknown	None demonstrated
Emery-Dreifuss dystrophy	Xq28	Unknown	None demonstrated
Kallmann syndrome	Xp22.3	Translocation (*KALIG-1*)	None demonstrated
Mitochondrial diseases with maternal transmission			
Mitochondrial myopathy	Mitochondria	Deletion in mitochondrial DNA	
Leber's hereditary optic atrophy	Mitochondria	Point mutation (NADH dehydrogenase)	
Kearns syndrome	Mitochondria	Deletion in mitochondrial DNA	

fragment length polymorphisms (Table 1.1). In some instances, such as Duchenne's muscular dystrophy, the abnormal gene has been cloned and the defective protein identified (Koenig et al., 1988).

Another remarkable example is that of fragile X syndrome, the second most common cause of mental retardation, which affects as many as 1 in 750 to 1,000 males and 1 in 500 to 750 females (Dykens et al., 1993; Chapters 46 and 96). Fragile X syndrome is transmitted from one generation to the next as an X-linked disorder. This X-linked transmission is highly unusual for two reasons. First, approximately 20% of the males who carry the abnormal gene are not mentally impaired. These men, called "normal transmitting males," can pass the abnormal gene to their daughters (who typically are not affected). However, their grandsons (the sons of these daughters) are at high risk for the full syndrome. This progression in severity is known as "anticipation" and relates to the usual molecular defect (a triplet repeat and associated methylation of CpG islands) found in the affected *FMR-1* genes (Fu et al., 1991). The "triplet repeat" refers to a repetitive sequence of three bases cytosine-guanine-guanine, or $(CGG)_n$, that can lengthen dramatically in affected individuals. Analyses of variations in length of the $(CGG)_n$ region in individuals *without* fragile X syndrome show remarkable variation in the number of repeats, from 6 to 54, with 29 repeats being the most frequent number in normal individuals (Fu et al., 1991). The extreme amplification of this CGG repeat sequence is the fragile X mutation site in the great majority of cases. Other family members may have numbers of CGG repeats that fall in between normal individuals and those who are fully affected with fragile X syndrome. These family members have CGG repeats that are in an intermediate zone, or between 54 and 200

repeats (Fu et al., 1991). Because this intermediate alteration has not been associated with the full fragile X phenotype, repeats in this range are called *pre-mutations* (Oberlé et al., 1991). This change from a pre-mutation to a full mutation accounts for the phenomenon of anticipation. In addition to the 200 to 1,000 CGG repeats in affected fragile X males, there are abnormalities in nearby regions called CpG "islands"; these structures are thought to play a role in gene regulation. These CpG islands are abnormally methylated in affected fragile X males (Oberlé et al., 1991). Methylation at the CpG islands correlates with the loss of expression of the *FMR-1* mRNA (Pieretti et al., 1991). The extreme variations in the CGG repeat sequence in affected fragile X individuals appear to induce methylation, which, in turn, down regulates the expression of the *FMR-1* mRNA, ultimately leading to the null mutation seen in fragile X males.

A second unusual feature of the inheritance of fragile X syndrome concerns the clinical status of the carrier females—more than a third of whom are themselves affected with some degree of mental impairment. These variations may be the result of the length of the CGG triplet repeat and the nature and extent of mosaicism (with regard to which X chromosome is inactivated) in brain-specific cell lineages early in development. These features focus attention on the poorly understood mechanisms involved in the germ line transmission of X chromosomes in females, and processes of X inactivation and reactivation.

In addition, the fine structure of the *FMR-1* genetic locus has been determined and "business end" of this gene has been partially characterized (Eichler et al., 1993). In one family a single base pair substitution in a highly conserved region of the *FMR-1* gene was associated with a full fragile X phenotype (De Boulle et al., 1993). This work has led to speculation that at some level aspects of intelligence are determined by protein RNA interactions (Siomi et al., 1994).

Studies of the pattern of expression of the *FMR-1* gene during development have clarified which areas of the brain are the most vulnerable in fragile X syndrome, including the basal forebrain (the same area that is affected in Alzheimer's disease) and the hippocampus (that is involved in short-term memory and sequential processing of information) (Abitbol et al., 1993). The results of these developmental neurobiological studies are consistent with both clinical/phenomenological studies (the profile of cognitive, speech, and language strengths and weaknesses seen in fragile X syndrome as well as associated psychopathology such as attention deficit hyperactivity disorder) and clinical neuroimaging studies (age-related volumetric changes have been detected in fragile X individuals in the hippocampus, for example) (Dykens et al., 1993; Riess et al., 1994). Finally, studies of homologous recombination have led to the successful development of animal models that resemble many of the clinical features seen in fragile X syndrome—setting the stage for even more detailed examination of the neurobiological consequences of the abnormal *FMR-1* gene (Dutch-Belgian Fragile X Consortium, 1994).

The fragile X story—unstable stretches of DNA composed of specific triplet repeats that can grow in number when transmitted from one generation to the next—has also led the way in understanding the molecular basis of more than five other inherited genetic disorders (Table 1.1) including Huntington's chorea, which involves a CAG repeat found in the coding region (Bates and Lehrach, 1994). As in fragile X syndrome, however, the reason for the genetic instability of these CG-rich areas remains unknown (Caskey et al., 1992).

Although the chromosomal locations of the genes responsible for manic-depressive illness and some familial forms of schizophrenia remain in doubt, there is reason for optimism that these disorders will yield some of their mysteries to determined molecular biologists. As reviewed in a later chapter (Chapter 29), these approaches are also likely to provide heuristically valuable insights into the pathobiology of other disorders of childhood onset, including Tourette's syndrome, some forms of obsessive compulsive disorder and attention deficit hyperactivity disorder, familial forms of dyslexia, and more pervasive developmental disorders such as autism.

Insights from genetics and developmental neurobiology are also likely to enhance our understanding of such diverse phenomena as idiosyncratic forms of autism, the adverse effects of prenatal drug exposures, the molecular impact of persistent psychosocial adversity, and why boys are at greater risk for a range of adverse psychopathological outcomes than are girls.

Autistic syndromes, particularly those associated with perinatal insults such as maternal rubella (especially when associated with deafness and/or blindness), phenylketonuria, and encephalitis, are likely to involve some alteration in the pattern of neural connectivity of the cortex. These disruptions in connectivity of neural circuits (as yet undefined) that are critical to the development of social cognition may be the neurobiological basis of some aspects of this disorder. Using embryonic ocular enucleation of primates as a model (Rakic and Williams, 1986), it may be reasonable to predict that certain architectonic areas of the cortex will be reorganized (with secondary changes in the surface features of that area) in some cases of autism.

In the case of prenatal drug exposure, such as to cocaine, it is likely that altered levels of dopamine or other neurotransmitters would affect the outgrowth and survival of specific neurites. This prediction is based on data that indicate that many of the neurotransmitters that are active in the mature brain also play important roles in the development, plasticity, and survival of individual neurons (Lipton and Kater, 1989). Given the elaborate homeostatic mechanisms active in neural systems, it is probable that some genetic factors may mediate the magnitude of these effects.

Finally, endocrine factors may be particularly important in determining gene expression. For example, the basic mechanisms by which expressions of parental hostility negatively affect developing organisms may be mediated in part by alterations of the microenvironment of cells and the action of stress-sensitive hormones such as the glucocorticoids, which can directly influence gene expression in a multiplicity of neural settings. Alternatively in males, the prenatal exposure of the developing brain to high levels of androgens undoubtedly has enduring structural and functional consequences that contribute to the increased vulnerability of boys to a range of maladaptive outcomes (Sikich and Todd, 1989).

References

Abitbol M, Menini C, Delezoide A-L, Rhyner T, Vekemans M, Mallet J: Nucleus basalis magnocellularis and hippocampus are the major sites of FMR-1 expression in human fetal brain. *Nature Gen* 4:147–152, 1994.

Bates G, Lehrach H: Trinucleotide repeat expansions and human genetic disease. *Bioessays* 16:277–284, 1994.

Boncinelli E, Gulisano M, Broccoli V: Emx and Otx in homeobox genes in the developing mouse brain. *J Neurobiol* 24:1356–1366, 1993.

Brock ML, Shapiro DJ: Estrogen stabilizes vitellogenin mRNA against cytoplasmic degradation. *Cell* 34:207, 1983.

Caskey CT, Pizzuti A, Fu Y-H, et al: Triplet repeat mutations in human disease. *Science* 256:784–789, 1992.

Crick FHC, Barnett L, Brenner S: General nature of the genetic code for proteins. *Nature* 192:1227, 1961.

Davidson EH: *Gene Activity in Early Development*. Orlando, FL, Academic Press, 1986.

Davies AM, Bandtlow C, Heumann R: Timing and site of nerve growth factor synthesis in developing skin in relation to innervation and expression of the receptor. *Nature* 326:353–357, 1987.

De Boulle K, Verkerk AJMH, Reyniers E, et al: A point mutation in the FMR-1 gene associated with fragile X mental retardation. *Nature Gen* 3:31–35, 1993.

Dutch-Belgian Fragile X Consortium: Fmr-1 knock out mice: A model to study fragile X mental retardation. *Cell* 78:23–33, 1994.

Dykens E, Hodapp RM, Leckman JF: *Development and Psychopathology in Fragile X Syndrome*. Newbury Park, CA, Sage Publications, 1993.

Eichler EE, Richards S, Gibbs RA, et al: Fine structure of the human FMR1 gene. *Hum Mol Genet* 2:1147–1153, 1993.

Evans RM: The steroid and thyroid hormone receptor superfamily. *Science* 240:889–895, 1988.

Freifelder D: *Molecular Biology*. Boston, Jones & Bartlett, 1987.

Gehring W: Homeoboxes in the study of development. *Science* 236:1245–1252, 1987.

Fu Y-H, Kuhl DP, Pizzuti A, et al: Variation of the CGG repeat at the fragile site results in genetic instability: Resolution of the Sherman paradox. *Cell* 67:1047–1058, 1991.

Fu Y-H, Ranjnarayan S, Dunne DW, et al: An unstable triplet repeat in a gene related to myotonic dystrophy. *Science* 225:1256–1258, 1992.

Glezer II, Jacobs MS, Morgane PJ: Implications of the "initial brain" concept for brain evolution in Cetacea. *Behav Brain Sci* 11:75–89, 1988.

Graham A, Papalopulu N, Krumlauf R: The murine and drosophila homeobox gene complexes have common features of organization and expression. *Cell* 57:367–378, 1989.

Groudine M, Weintraub H: Rous sarcoma virus activates embryonic globin genes in chicken fibroblasts. *Proc Natl Acad Sci USA* 72:4464, 1975.

Hahn WE, Van Ness J, Chaudhar N: Overview of the molecular genetics of mouse brain. In: Schmitt FO, Bird SJ, Bloom FE (eds): *Molecular Genetic Neuroscience*. New York, Raven Press, 1982, p. 332.

Hatten ME, Mason CA: Neuron-astroglia interactions in vitro and in vivo. *Trends Neurosci* 9:168–174, 1986.

Ivarie R, Schacter B, O'Farrell P: The level of expression of the rat growth hormone gene in liver tumor cells is at least eight orders of magnitude less than in anterior pituitary cells. *Mol Cell Biol* 3:1460, 1983.

Jacobson M: *Developmental Neurobiology*. New York, Holt, Rinehart & Winston, 1970.

Juel-Nielsen N: *Individual and Environment*. New York, International Universities Press, 1980.

Kalil RE, Dubin MW, Scott G, et al: Elimination of action potentials blocks the structural development of retinogeniculate synapses. *Nature* 323:156, 1986.

Knoll JH, Wagstaff J, Lalande M: Cytogenetic and molecular studies of Prader-Willi and Angelman syndromes: An overview. *Am J Hum Genet* 46:2–6, 1993.

Koenig M, Monaco AP, Kunkel LM: The complete sequence of dystrophin predicts a rod-shaped cytoskeletal protein. *Cell* 53:219–228, 1988.

Kongsuwan K, Webb E, Housiaux P, et al: Expression of multiple homeobox genes within diverse mammalian hemopoietic lineages. *EMBO J* 1988;7:2131.

Landschultz WH, Johnson PF, McKnight SL: The leucine zipper: A hypothetical structure common to a new class of DNA binding proteins. *Science* 140: 1759, 1988.

Levine M, Hoey T: Homeobox proteins as sequence-specific transcription factors. *Cell* 55: 537–540, 1988.

Lipton SA, Kater SB: Neurotransmitter regulation of neuronal outgrowth, plasticity and survival. *Trends Neurosci* 12:265–269, 1989.

Martin JB: Molecular genetic studies in the neuropsychiatric disorders. *Trends Neurosci* 12: 130–137, 1989.

McGinnis W, Levine MS, Hafen E, et al: A conserved DNA sequence in homeotic genes of the *Drosophila antennapedia* and bithorax complexes. *Nature* 308:428–433, 1984.

Mendel G: *Versuche uber Pflanzen-hybriden.* Brnn Moravia, Verh. D. Naturf Vereins, 1865.

Miller J: Repetitive zinc-binding domains in the protein transcription factor IIIA from *Xenopus oocytes. EMBO J* 4:1609, 1985.

Molineaux CJ, Hassen AH, Rosenberger JG, et al: Response of rat pituitary anterior lobe prodynorphin products to changes in gonadal steroid environment. *Endocrinology* 119:2297–2305, 1986.

Moore T, Haig D: Genomic imprinting in mammalian development: A parental tug-of-war. *Trends Genet* 7:45–49, 1991.

Oberlé I, Rousseau F, Heitz D, et al: Instability of a 550-base pair DNA segment and abnormal methylation in fragile X syndrome. *Science* 252: 1097–1110, 1991.

O'Farrell PH, Edgar BA, Lakich D, et al: Directing cell division during development. *Science* 246: 635–640, 1989.

Pieretti M, Zhang F, Fu Y-H, et al: Absence of expression of the FMR-1 gene in fragile X syndrome. *Cell* 66:817–822, 1991.

Puelles L, Rubenstein LR: Expression patterns of homeobox and other putative regulatory genes in the embryonic mouse forebrain suggest a neuromeric organization. *Trends Neurosci* 16:472–479, 1993.

Purves D, Lichtman JW: *Principles of Neural Development.* Sunderland, MA: Sinauer, 1985.

Rakic P: Neuronal-glial interactions during brain development. *Trends Neurosci* 4:184–187, 1981.

Rakic P: Defects of neuronal migration and the pathogenesis of cortical malformations. *Prog Brain Res* 73:15–37, 1988a.

Rakic P: Specification of cerebral cortical areas. *Science* 241:170–176, 1988b.

Rakic P, Sidman RL: Organization of cerebellar cortex secondary to deficit of granule cells in weaver mutant mice. *J Comp Neurol* 152:133–162, 1973a.

Rakic P, Sidman RL: Sequence of developmental abnormalities leading to granule cell deficit in cerebellar cortex of weaver mutant mice. *J Comp Neurol* 152:103–113, 1973b.

Rakic P, Williams RW: Thalamic regulation of cortical parcellation: An experimental perturbation of the striate cortex in rhesus monkeys. *Soc Neurosci Abstr* 12:1499, 1986.

Riess AL, Lee J, Freund L: Neuroanatomy of fragile X syndrome: The temporal lobe. *Neurology* 44:1317–1324, 1994.

Shields J: *Monozygotic Twins: Brought Up Apart and Brought Up Together.* London, England, Oxford University Press, 1962.

Sikich L, Todd RD: Are the neurodevelopmental effects of gonadal hormones related to sex differences in psychiatric illnesses. *Psychiatr Dev* 6: 277–310, 1988.

Siomi H, Choi M, Siomi M, et al: Essential role for KH domains in RNA binding: Impaired RNA binding mutation in the KH domain of FMR1 that causes fragile X syndrome. *Cell* 77:33–39, 1994.

Watson JD, Hopkins NH, Roberts JW, et al: *Molecular Biology of the Cell.* Menlo Park, CA, Benjamin/Cummings, 1987.

Weigert M, Gatmaitan L, Loh E, et al: Rearrangement of genetic information may produce immunoglobulin diversity. *Nature* 176:785–790, 1978.

2 DEVELOPMENT OF THE CEREBRAL CORTEX IN HUMAN AND NONHUMAN PRIMATES

Pasko Rakic, M.D., Sc.D.

The cerebral cortex in humans makes up about two-thirds of the neuronal mass and contains almost three-quarters of all our synapses. It is also the structure that most distinctively sets us apart from other species. Therefore, the principles governing the development of the cerebral cortex may hold the key to explaining the pathogenesis of many developmental neuropsychiatric disorders, as well as the evolution of human intelligence and creativity.

One of the most prominent features of the cerebral cortex in all mammalian species, but particularly in primates, is its distinct laminar pattern and parcellation into different cytoarchitectonic areas (Fig. 2.1). These areas are defined as regions of the cortex with distinct cellular, biochemical, connectional, and physiological characteristics. For example, individual cytoarchitectonic areas may process specific sensory information, control precise motor activity, or be involved primarily in complex cognitive functions, such as language, facial recognition, or spatial orientation. Comparison of the laminar pattern and cytoarchitectonic cortical maps in the three species illustrated in Figure 2.1 reveals several important points. First, the surface of the neocortex has expanded enormously during phylogeny. Obviously, the human brain did not evolve from any presently living species, but we need to account for the differences in size that have emerged from common ancestors (e.g., the surface of the human neocortex is 10 times larger than that of a macaque monkey and 1000 times larger than that of a rat). Second, during evolution, cytoarchitectonic areas do not expand uniformly (e.g., the primary visual cortex occupies $\frac{1}{5}$ of the neocortical surface in monkeys and only $\frac{1}{30}$ of that of humans). Third, new functional and anatomical areas are introduced during evolution (e.g., Broca's language areas in humans). Fourth, there are large variations in the sizes of cortical areas among individuals of the same species and between the two hemispheres in the same individual (e.g., the planum temporale is larger on the left side in most right-handed humans). However, despite these enormous differences in size of cortical surfaces and pattern of cytoarchitectonic maps, the thickness of the cortex has changed relatively little in phylogeny.

Understanding the development of the cerebral cortex and its expansion in size and complexity depends critically on answering some fundamental questions: When and where are cortical neurons generated? How is their number regulated in various species and in each individual? When and how are different cell phenotypes that constitute the cortex determined? How do postmitotic cells attain their proper laminar and areal position within the cortex? How are interspecies and intraspecies differences in cortical parcellation generated? Why does the surface of the cortex expand so enormously during evolution, while its thickness remains relatively constant? To what extent is the size of cytoarchitectonic areas determined innately, and could this size be changed by external stimulation? What are the mechanisms for the formation of complex connections between areas and with various subcortical structures? What is the role of various environmental factors, including functional activity and experience, in this process? How is the number and proportion of various classes of synapses in the cerebral cortex established? When does the susceptible period for structural and functional modifiability of cortical connections and cytoarchitectonic cortical maps end? Elucidation of these issues is an essential prerequisite for understanding the biological basis of neuropsychiatric disorders of genetic and developmental origin. Considerable progress has been made in defining and answering some of these questions.

The present chapter is based mostly on experimental studies of neocortical development in the macaque monkey, where the large size of the cerebrum and the presence of visible landmarks at its convoluted surface allow precise delineation of cortical areas, while its protracted

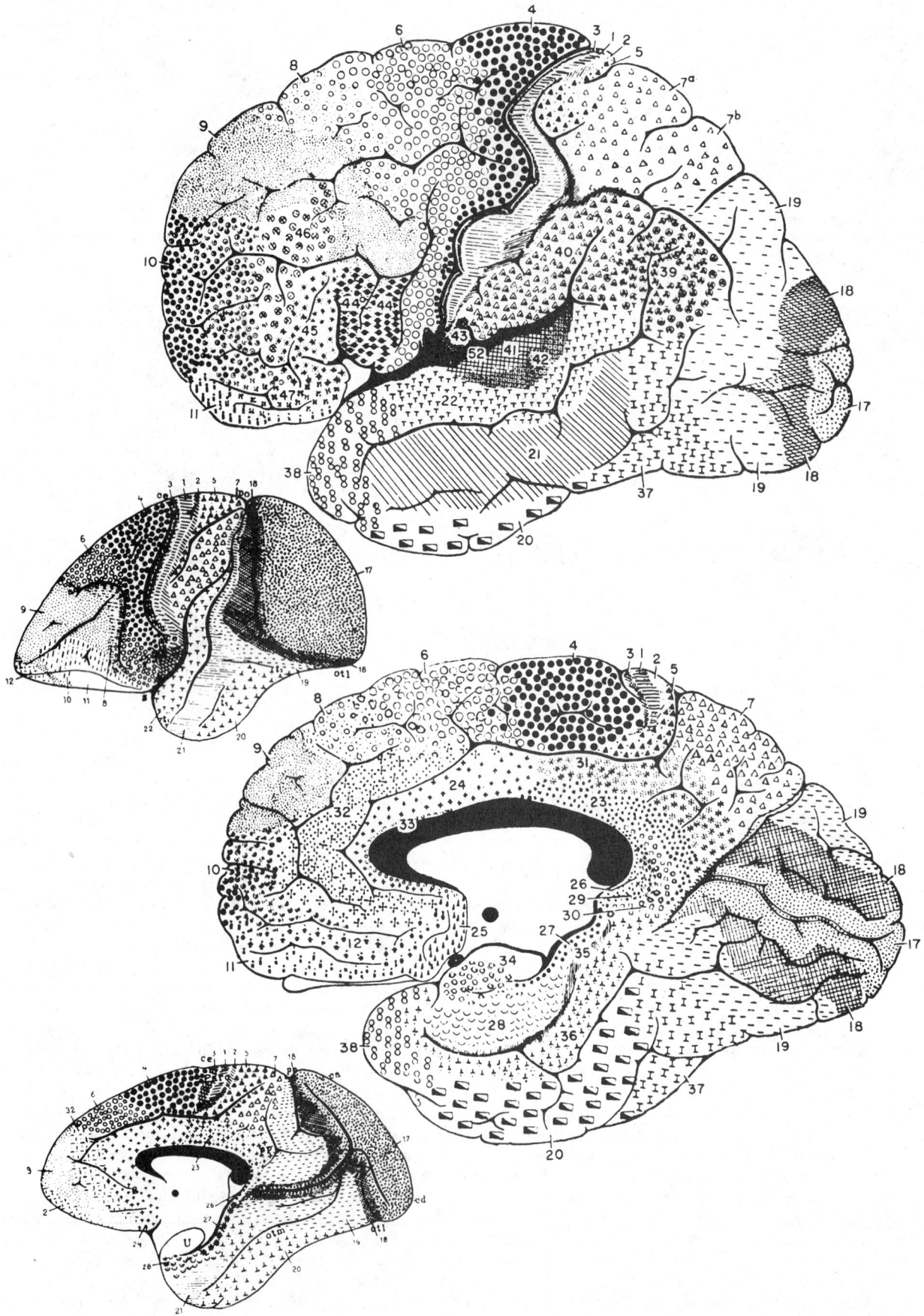

Figure 2.1.   Lateral (*upper figures*) and medial (*lower figures*) views of the cerebral hemisphere in human (*right*), macaque monkey (*left top*), and rat (*left bottom*), with schematic designation of individual cytoarchitectonic areas (Reproduced to approximate scale from Brodmann, 1909.)

development enables accurate timing of cellular events. We assume that the basic organization and principles of cortical development in primates are similar to that operating in nonprimate species. There are no known neurotransmitters, receptors, or ion channels in the human cortex that are not present in the rodent cortex. However, by virtue of its size, exceptionally prolonged postnatal development, and, in particular, the complex pattern of its cortico-cortical connections and elaborate parcellation of cytoarchitectonic areas, the cerebral cortex is the principal structure that makes us different from any other species. The organizational similarity of the cerebral cortex in the macaque monkey and human suggests that the same cellular and molecular mechanisms of development may apply to both species. Therefore, frequent comparisons of the developmental data available in these two primates are made in this chapter.

TIME OF NEURON ORIGIN

The cerebral cortex in the newborn child has well-delineated cortical layers, and it has been suspected that most cortical neurons in human cerebrum were generated before birth (Conel, 1939). However, only the method of marking permanently the time of DNA replication with ^{3}H-thymidine provided direct evidence and precise data on the onset and termination of corticogenesis in primates. The examination of adult macaque monkeys exposed to ^{3}H-thymidine during prenatal and postnatal ages revealed that the genesis of all cortical neurons is completed during the middle of gestation, which in this species lasts about 165 days (Rakic, 1974, 1988a). Cortical neurogenesis starts around the 40th embryonic day (E40) and lasts between 1 and 2 months, depending on the cytoarchitectonic area. For example, in the anterior cingulate cortex (Brodmann's area 24) neurogenesis stops at E70, while in the primary visual cortex (area 17) it stops at E100 (Fig. 2.2). Autoradiographic analysis of DNA labeling with ^{3}H-thymidine shows that neocortical neurons in macaque monkeys are not produced during the remainder of gestation (Rakic, 1974) or at any time after birth during the 30-year life span of this species (Rakic, 1985). Comparative cytological analysis indicates that in humans, with a gestational period of about 265 days, the first cortical neurons are also generated around E40, but their production lasts longer and continues until about E125 (Rakic, 1978, 1988a; Sidman and Rakic, 1973). Thus, unlike most mammalian species that have so far been examined, in which corticogenesis lasts until the time of birth or continues even shortly afterward, primates, including humans, acquire their full complement of cortical neurons mostly during the middle third of gestation (Fig. 2.3). It has been proposed that this stable population of neurons during adulthood may be a biological necessity, so that individual cognitive experience can be preserved in the synaptic assemblies through the decades of the primate life span (Rakic, 1985; Rakic and Kornack, 1992).

SITE OF NEURON ORIGIN

It has been suspected, on the basis of the high density of mitotic figures that can be observed near the ventricular surface in the human fetal cerebrum, that most cortical neurons might be produced there, rather than in the cortex itself (His, 1904). However, again the direct evidence for this hypothesis comes from ^{3}H-thymidine autoradiographic analysis. Examination of a series of macaque monkey embryos killed shortly after injection of the DNA precursor revealed that all neurons destined for the neocortex are produced in the proliferative zone near the cerebral ventricle (Rakic, 1975). This zone in the fetus is organized as a pseudostratified epithelium in which precursor cells divide asynchronously; their nuclei move away from the ventricular surface to synthesize DNA and move back to the surface to undergo another mitotic cycle (reviewed in Sidman and Rakic, 1973). Golgi, electron microscopic, and immunocytochemical analyses revealed that neuronal and glial cell lines coexist in the ventricular zone from the onset of corticogenesis (Levitt et al., 1981; Rakic, 1971, 1972). The early divergence

of these two basic cell types has been confirmed using retroviral gene transfer, which labels separate lineages of the precursor cells in the developing telencephalon (Cameron and Rakic, 1991; Luskin et al., 1988). Furthermore, as illustrated in Figure 2.4A, the ventricular zone in primates is divided by well-defined glial septa into columns of precursor or stem cells, termed "proliferative units" (Rakic, 1978). The number of stem cells in a proliferative unit is initially only 3–5, but increases up to more than 10 at later developmental stages (Rakic, 1988b). ^{3}H-Thymidine autoradiographic analysis indicates that around E40 proliferative units start producing postmitotic neurons, which migrate to their prespecified areal and laminar positions in the cortex (Rakic, 1974). The same method of analysis cannot be applied to human embryonic material, but the use of the various cytological criteria (Sidman and Rakic, 1982) and application of supravital DNA synthesis to slices of fetal brain tissue (Rakic and Sidman, 1968) indicate that the corresponding time point for the onset of corticogenesis in humans is 6 fetal weeks, or about E42.

NEURONAL CELL MIGRATION

Since all cortical neurons originate near the ventricular surface, they all must move to their final positions within the cortex, which develops in the outer territories of the cerebral wall, below the pia. A massive migration of neurons in primates, including humans, occurs during midgestation and coincides with the rapid growth of the cerebral wall in thickness and the initial buckling of its surface, which begins to form sulci and gyri. In fact, the phenomenon of neuronal cell migration was originally inferred from the analysis of the fixed brain of human embryos by Wilhelm His (1874). However, for the next hundred years little progress was made in terms of the underlying cellular and molecular mechanisms of this phenomenon. In the 1970s, a combination of Golgi, electron microscopic, and ^{3}H-thymidine autoradiographic analyses in nonhuman primates revealed that postmitotic neurons find their way through the intricate cellular lattice of the intermediate and subplate zones by following elongated shafts of nonneural elements called radial glial cells (Rakic, 1971, 1972). These elongated bipolar cells stretch their processes across the fetal cerebral wall from the beginning of corticogenesis, but appear most prominent during midgestation, when many of them temporarily stop dividing (Schmechel and Rakic, 1979). During the migratory period, cohorts of postmitotic cells originating in individual proliferative units follow a radial pathway consisting of single or, more often, multiple glial fibers, which form fascicles that span the developing cerebral wall (Fig. 2.5). While moving along the glial surface, migrating neurons may be in contact with many other axonal and dendritic processes, but nevertheless remain preferentially attached to glial fibers, which suggests a "gliophilic" mode of migration mediated by heterotypic adhesion molecules (Rakic, 1985; Rakic et al., 1994b). Several initial observations suggested that migrating neurons in all parts of the CNS may have the same binding affinity for the surface of radial glial cells (Rakic, 1981a). Although an occasional neuron may translocate from one to the other nearby radial glial fascicle (Rakic et al., 1974), a majority of migrating neurons do not follow any other classes of cellular processes that are present in the intermediate zone.

There is a class of postmitotic cells in the telencephalon, which do not obey glial constraints and usually move along tangentially oriented axonal fascicles. We suggested the term "neurophilic" to characterize the mode of migration of this class of cells (Rakic, 1985, 1990). Although lateral movement of postmitotic neurons has been observed in early studies (e.g., see bipolar cells situated in the intermediate zone in Figure 1 of Boulder Committee, 1970), it has attracted renewed attention after the use of retrovirus-mediated labeling of cell clones in the rodent telencephalon suggested widespread dispersion of some postmitotic cells (Walsh and Cepko, 1988), in addition to those whose movement is strictly radial (Luskin et al., 1988). However, the prevalence and significance of tangential migration in cortical ontogeny and phylogeny has not been settled. Recent studies in chimeric mice have provided

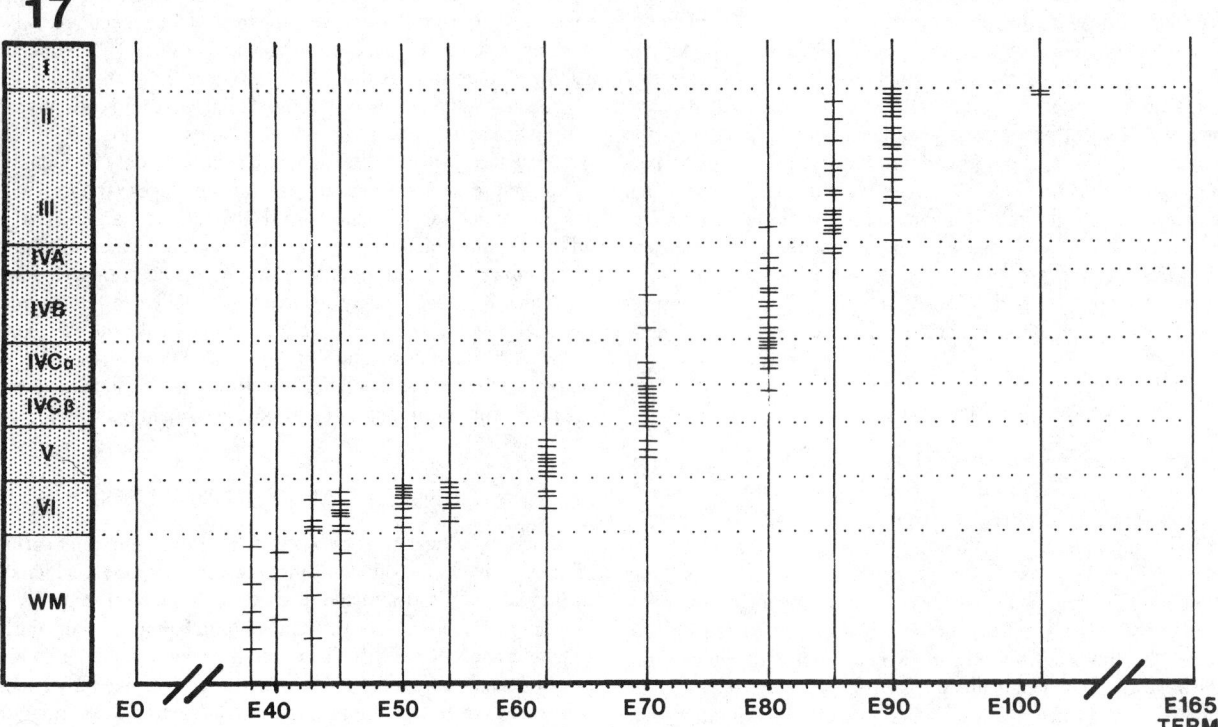

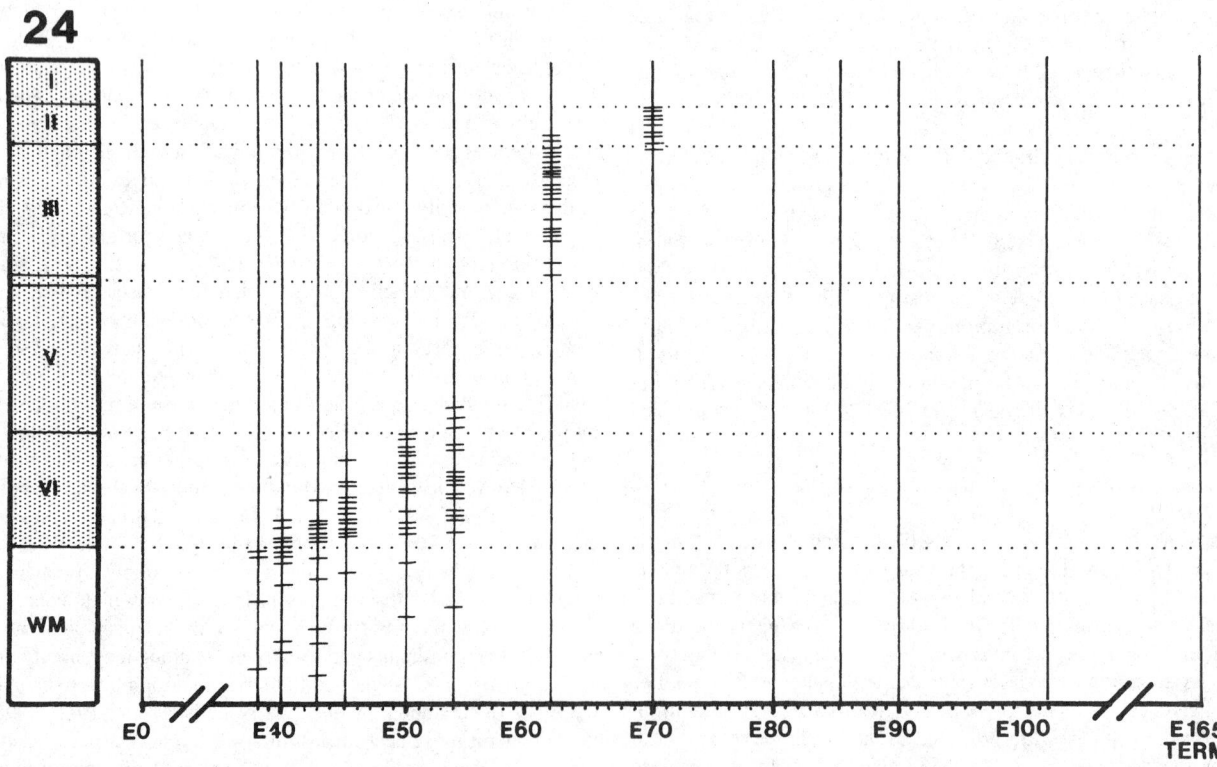

Figure 2.2.   Diagrammatic representation of the positions of heavily labeled neurons in the cortex of juvenile monkeys, each of which had been injected with ³H-thymidine at selected embryonic days: *top*, area 17; *bottom*, area 24 of Brodmann. On the *left side* of each diagram is a drawing of the cortex from cresyl violet-stained sections, in which subdivisions into cortical layers are indicated by *roman numerals*. Embryonic days (*E*) are represented on the *hori-* *zontal line*, starting on the *left* with the end of the first fetal month (*E27*) and ending on the *right* at term (*E165*). Positions of *vertical lines* (*left to right*) indicate the embryonic day on which one animal received a pulse of ³H-thymidine. On each *vertical line, short horizontal markers* indicate positions of all heavily labeled neurons encountered in one 2.5-mm-long strip of cortex. *WM,* white matter. (From Rakic, 1974 (top), 1976a (bottom).)

CORTICOGENESIS IN MACACA MULATTA AND HOMO SAPIENS

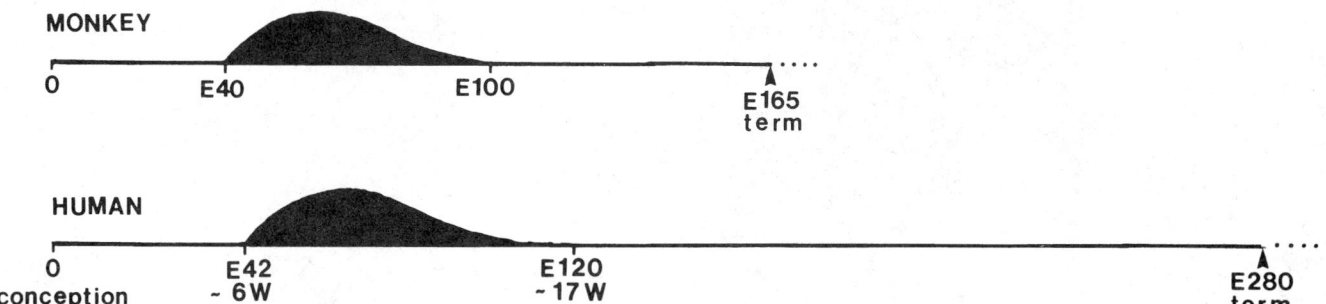

Figure 2.3. Diagrammatic representation of the time of neuron origin in rhesus monkey (*top*) and humans (*bottom*). The data for monkeys are obtained by ³H-thymidine autoradiography (Rakic, 1974), whereas the data for humans are based on the number of mitotic figures in the ventricular zone, supravital DNA synthesis, and the presence and density of migrating neurons in the intermediate zone of the fetal cerebrum. (Combined from Rakic, 1978; Rakic and Sidman, 1968; Sidman and Rakic, 1982.)

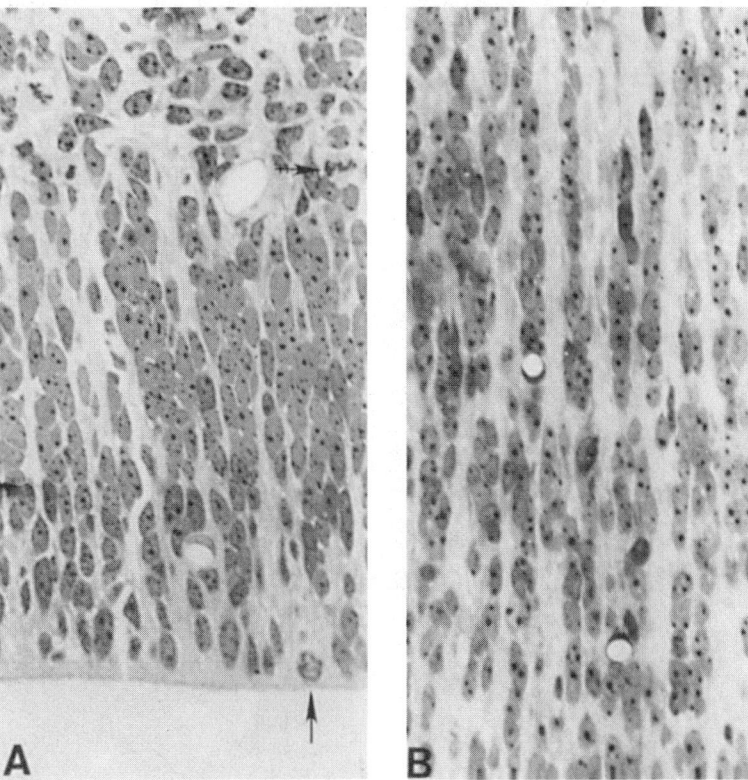

Figure 2.4. The radial organization of both ventricular zone and fetal cortical plate is best visible in cresyl violet-stained sections. **A.** Photomicrograph of an array of proliferative units within the ventricular zone of the occipital lobe in a 91-day-old monkey embryo. Most mitotic figures are located directly at the ventricular surface (*arrow*), although at this age some can be found in the subventricular zone (*crossed arrow*). **B.** Cortical plate in the occipital lobe of the same animal, showing ontogenetic columns composed of neurons that have originated from the set of proliferative units illustrated in **A.** Epon-embedded tissue, cut at 1 μm, stained with cresyl violet. (From Rakic, 1988a.)

direct evidence that in rodents an overwhelming majority of postmitotic neurons move radially to the cortex (Nakatsuji, et al., 1991; Tan and Breen, 1993). In ferret telencephalon, more than 83% of neurons appear to migrate radially (O'Rourke et al., 1992). In primates, it is likely that an even larger number of migrating neurons obey radial constraints imposed by an elaborate system of radial glial palisades (Rakic, 1988a; Kornack and Rakic, 1995). The spatiotemporal order of radially migrating neurons is usually preserved across the wide intermediate zone because postmitotic cells tend to remain in contiguity with a given radial

glial fascicle once they initiate their movement (Rakic, 1981a). The discovery of the glial-guided radial migration led to the proposal of the *radial unit hypothesis* (Rakic, 1988a) that has served as a useful working model in subsequent research on the cellular and molecular mechanisms involved in normal and abnormal cortical development (see later).

The universality of neuronal guidance by radial glial fibers in a variety of large brain structures has been supported by in vitro studies, which show that cross-matching between migrating neurons and radial glial cells obtained from different structures does not prevent differential

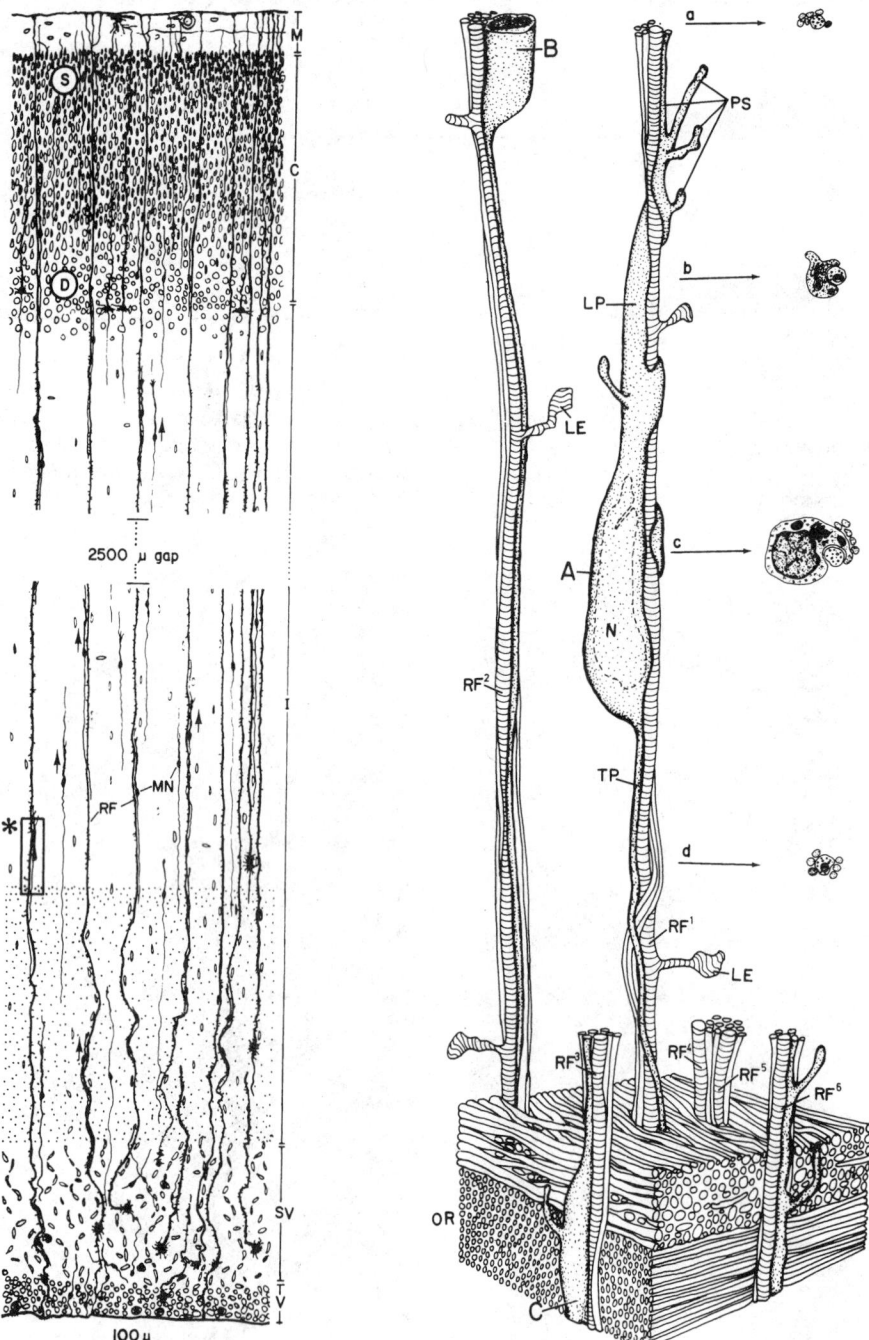

Figure 2.5. *Left,* Camera lucida drawing of the occipital cerebral wall of the monkey fetus at midgestation. The composite illustration is derived from a Golgi-impregnated section (*black profiles*) and from an adjacent section counterstained with toluidine blue (*outline of small nuclei*). The middle 2000 μm of the intermediate zone, similar in structure to the sectors drawn, is omitted. The *rectangle marked with an asterisk* shows the approximate position of the cell reconstruction seen in *B. C,* cortical plate; *I,* intermediate zone; *M,* molecular layer; *MN,* migrating neuron; *RF,* radial fiber; *SV,* subventricular zone; *V,* ventricular zone. *Right,* Three-dimensional reconstruction of migrating neurons, based on serial electron micrographs made at the level of the intermediate zone, indicated by the rectangle in *A.* The *lower portion* of the diagram contains parallel fibers of the optic radiation (*OR*), and the remainder is occupied by a more disposed fiber system. Except at the *lower portion* of the figure, most of these fibers are deleted from the diagram to expose the radial fibers (*striped vertical shafts RF*$^{1-6}$) and their relations to the migrating cells *A, B,* and *C.* The soma of migrating cell *A,* with its nucleus (*N*) and voluminous leading process (*LP*), is situated within the reconstructed space, except for the terminal part of the attenuated trailing process and the tip of the vertical ascending pseudopodium. Cross-sections of cell *A* in relation to the several vertical fibers in the fascicle are drawn at levels *a–d* at the *right side* of the figure. The perikaryon of cell *B* is cut off at the top of the reconstructed space, whereas the leading process of cell *C* is shown just penetrating between fibers of the optic radiation (*OR*) on its way across the intermediate zone. *LE,* lamellate expansions; *PS,* pseudopodia. (From Rakic, 1972.)

adhesion (Hatten and Mason, 1990). Initially, it was proposed, based on the observation in situ, that a single pair of binding, complementary molecules with gliophilic properties can account for the entire guidance phenomenon of radial migration (Rakic, 1981a). In the last decade, several candidates for recognition and adhesion molecules have been discovered and are being tested (e.g., Cameron and Rakic, 1994; Edelman, 1983; Hatten and Mason, 1986, 1990; Rakic et al., 1994b; Schachner et al., 1985). So far, accumulated evidence suggests it is likely that more than one class of surface molecules must be involved in neuronal cell migration to account for both recognition and adhesion (reviewed in Rakic et al., 1994b).

Considerable progress was also made in understanding the mechanism of the actual physical displacement of cell perikarya during translocation of the cells across the densely packed tissue. For example, it was shown that voltage- and ligand-gated ion channels on the leading process and cell soma of migrating neurons regulate the influx of calcium ions into migrating neurons, which, in turn, may trigger polymerization of cytoskeletal and contractile proteins essential for cell motility and translocation of the nucleus and surrounding cytoplasm (Komuro and Rakic, 1992, 1993). The composition of the receptor/channel complexes on the surface of migrating neurons is different from the composition they have after reaching their final destination (Farrant et al., 1994). These studies indicate that neuronal migration is a multifaceted developmental event, involving cell-cell recognition, differential adhesion, transmembrane signaling, and intracytoplasmic structural changes (Rakic et al., 1994b). Understanding the molecular mechanisms of neuronal migration may help to explain the pathogenesis of previously inexplicable genetic and acquired conditions, such as childhood epilepsy, mental retardation, schizophrenia or developmental dyslexia (Aicardi, 1991; Bloom, 1993; Galaburda et al., 1985; Palamini, 1991a; Volpe, 1987).

DEVELOPMENT OF THE TRANSIENT SUBPLATE ZONE

During embryonic and fetal development, the telencephalic wall consists of several cellular layers or zones that do not exist in the mature brain: ventricular zone, intermediate zone, subplate zone, cortical plate, and marginal zone (Fig. 2.6). Although most of these zones were well described and carefully characterized in the classical literature (e.g., His, 1904), the subplate zone has been recognized as a separate entity only recently (e.g., see review in Kostovic and Rakic, 1990). This zone consists of early-generated subplate neurons scattered among numerous axons, dendrites, glial fibers, and migrating neurons. Most of these subplate neurons eventually degenerate, but some persist in the adult cerebrum as a set of interstitial cells (Kostovic and Rakic, 1980; Luskin and Shatz, 1985). Migrating neurons traversing this zone remain attached to glial cell guides before entering the cortical plate to form radially oriented columns (Figs. 2.4B and 2.6). Although the existence of the subplate zone may provide an opportunity for interaction between migrating neurons, incoming afferent fibers, early-generated neurons, and the significance of these transient contacts is not fully understood.

One possibility, suggested soon after discovery of the subplate zone, was that it serves as a ''waiting'' compartment for afferents that are generated ahead of their neuronal targets and for cellular substrata for competition among cortical afferents (Rakic, 1977). Subsequent autoradiographic, electron microscopic, and histochemical studies in primates indicate that the axons observed in the subplate zone originate sequentially from the brainstem, basal forebrain, thalamus, and the ipsilateral and contralateral cerebral hemispheres (reviewed in Kostovic and Rakic, 1990). After a variable and partially overlapping period, these diverse fiber systems enter the cortical plate, while the subplate zone disappears, leaving only a vestige of cells scattered throughout the subcortical white matter that are known as interstitial neurons (Chun and Shatz, 1989; Kostovic and Rakic, 1980). A comparison between various species indicates that the size and relative duration of the transient subplate zone increases during mammalian evolution and culminates in human fetuses concomitantly with the enlargement of the cortico-cortical fiber systems (Kostovic and Rakic, 1990). The regional difference in the size, pattern, and resolution of the subplate zone correlates also with the pattern and size of cerebral convolutions (Goldman-Rakic and Rakic, 1984; Rakic, 1988b). Studies in developing macaque monkeys indicate that, contrary to prevailing notions, the subplate zone should not be considered a vestige of the phylogenetically old neural network (e.g., Marin-Padilla, 1978; Shatz et al., 1988). Rather, it is a new transient embryonic zone that expanded during the evolution of the cerebral cortex, most likely as a result of the increasing number of cortico-cortical connections and the elaboration of cerebral convolutions (Kostovic and Rakic, 1990). An abnormally large vestige of subplate neurons may form heterotopic masses in the form of a double cortex, and these are believed to be the source of intractable epileptic discharges in children (Palamini et al., 1991b). It was also suggested that migratory defects, which leave an abnormal cell population within the subplate zone, may be a source of abnormalities in some form of schizophrenia (Akbarian et al., 1993).

DETERMINATION OF NEURONAL PHENOTYPES

Immunocytochemical analyses in fetal monkeys provided the initial evidence that proliferative cells in the embryonic ventricular zone produce concomitantly both neurons and glial cell clones (Levitt et al., 1981). Furthermore, examination of the fate of the ^{3}H-thymidine-labeled cells suggests that multiple neural phenotypes are simultaneously produced and terminate either in the single or adjacent cortical layers (Rakic, 1988a). Therefore, after their last cell division, postmitotic neurons seem to become restricted in the repertoire of their possible fates. This is supported by several lines of evidence. For example, if neurons remain in ectopic positions near the cerebral ventricle (as a consequence of x-irradiation during embryonic stages) they nevertheless acquire the morphology and connections expected from the time of their origin (Jensen and Killackey, 1984). Likewise, ventricular cells transplanted from the embryos into the telencephalic wall of a newborn ferret migrate to the host cortex and assume laminar cortical positions, morphological characteristics, and a pattern of connections appropriate for the stage that they have achieved in the donor (McConnell, 1988). Callosal neurons send their axons to the contralateral hemisphere before its soma has entered layer II of the cortical plate (Schwartz et al., 1990). This early laminar commitment of cortical neurons is evident also in the reeler mutant mouse in which sequentially generated neurons assume a position in the cortical layers that is reversed compared to the normal mouse, but nevertheless differentiates into phenotypes expected from the time of their origin, rather than from their ectopic location (Caviness and Rakic, 1978). Recent analysis, in which RNA retrovirus-mediated gene transfer was used to mark the progeny of dividing cells, revealed that neurons of a different type originate from separate clones (Parnavelas et al., 1991). These findings collectively indicate that the range of morphologies and patterns of synaptic contacts of cortical neurons may be specified, in considerable measure, before they reach their final positions.

A survey of the emergence of the various transmitters and their receptors in the embryonic monkey telencephalon showed that, contrary to our expectations, most of them appear very early, prior to the formation of synapses. For example, α_1-adrenergic receptors are prominent in the ventricular and subventricular zones, up to midgestation, in conjunction with the intensive proliferation of cortical neurons, while, in contrast, β receptor subtype emerges in these zones only after the proliferation subsides and corticogenesis is completed (Lidow and Rakic, 1994). This sequence of developmental events suggests that α_1 sites may participate in promotion of cell proliferation while the β sites may participate in suppression of cell proliferation within the germinal zones of the fetal cerebrum. This suggestion is in harmony with the finding that cell division in vitro can be stimulated and inhibited by these two adrenergic subtypes, respectively. Since both ventricular and subventricular zones produce a variety of neuronal subtypes (McConnell, 1991; Parnavelas et al., 1991; Rakic, 1988a), it is possible that noradrenaline, or other

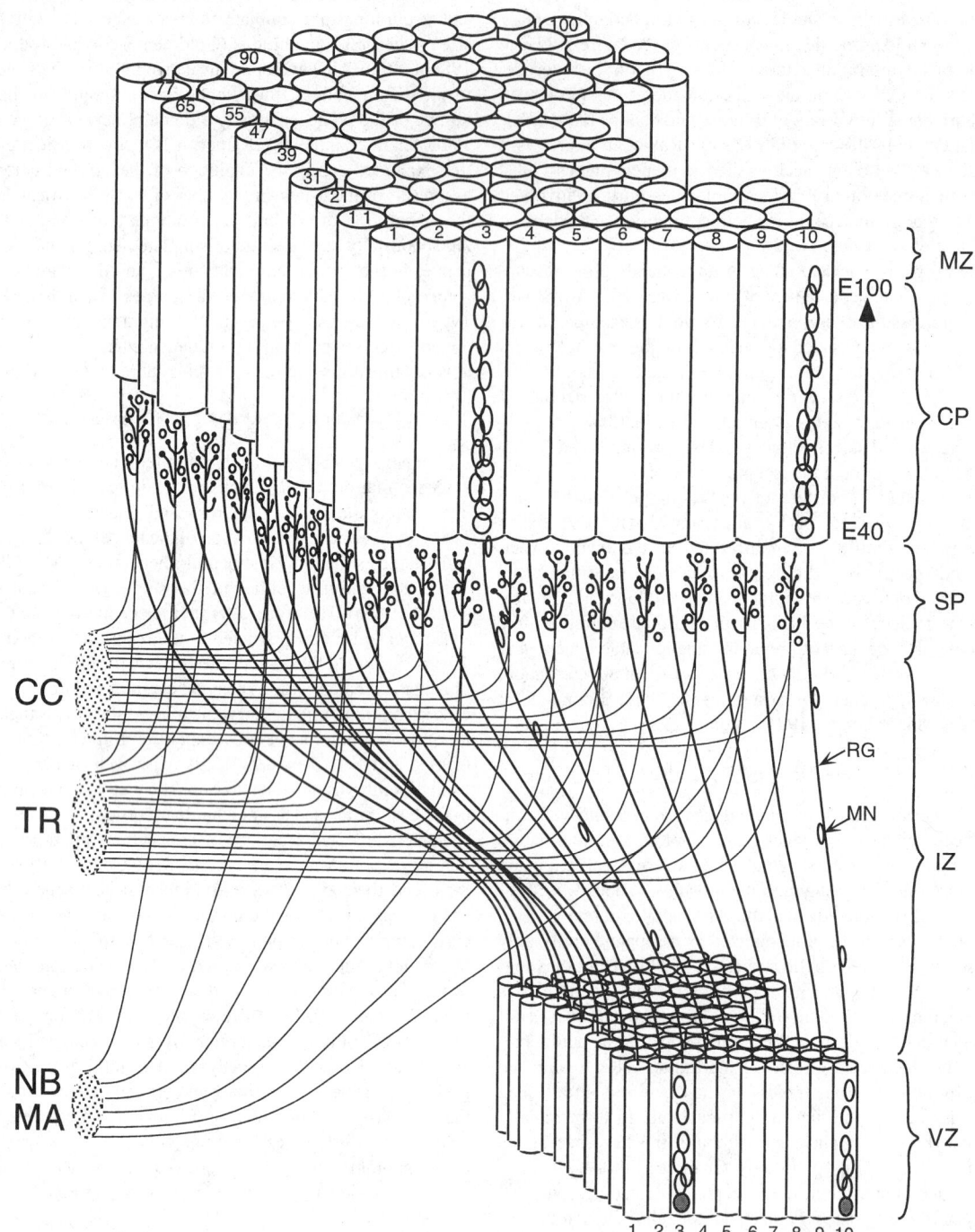

Figure 2.6. The relation between a small patch of the proliferative ventricular zone (*VZ*) and its corresponding area within the cortical plate (*CP*) in the developing cerebrum. Although the cerebral surface in primates expands and shifts during prenatal development, ontogenetic columns (*outlined by cylinders*) remain attached to the corresponding proliferative units by the grid of radial glial fibers. Neurons produced between E40 and E100 by a given proliferative unit migrate in succession along the same radial glial guides (*RG*) and stack up in reverse order of arrival within the same ontogenetic column. Each migrating neuron first traverses the intermediate zone (*IZ*) and then the subplate (*SP*) that contains interstitial cells and ''waiting'' afferents from the basal forebrain (*NB*), monoamine sub-cortical centers (*MN*), thalamic radiation (*TR*), and ipsilateral and contralateral cortico-cortical connections (*CC*). After entering the cortical plate, each neuron bypasses earlier-generated neurons and settles at the interface between the CP and marginal zone (*MZ*). As a result, proliferative units 1–100 produce ontogenetic columns 1–100 in the same position relative to one another without a lateral mismatch. Thus, the specification of cytoarchitectonic areas and topographic maps depends on the spatial distribution of their ancestors in the proliferative units, while the laminar position and phenotype of neurons within ontogenetic columns depends on the time of their origin. (Modified from Rakic, 1988a.)

neurotransmitters, can regulate the proliferation of various types of neurons already in the germinative epithelium. Both γ-aminobutyric acid (GABA) as well as GABA$_A$ receptor subtypes are expressed on migrating neurons before they reach their destination in the cortex (Schwartz and Meinecke, 1992). In vitro study indicates that these signaling molecules may play a role in differential cell death and, therefore, can influence the area- and layer-specific density of GABA-containing local circuit neurons (Vaccarino et al., 1995). These findings collectively demonstrate that the range of morphologies and patterns of connections of cortical neurons may be specified, in considerable degree, by various neuroactive molecules before postmitotic cells reach their final positions in the cerebral cortex.

ACQUISITION OF LAMINAR AND RADIAL POSITIONS

Since the genesis of cortical neurons in macaque monkeys does not start until E40 (Rakic, 1974) and in humans until a few days later (Sidman and Rakic, 1982) (Fig. 2.3), neuronal progenitors in the ventricular zone prior to that time produce only other progenitors. This so-called symmetric mode of cell division has been initially implied from the data on the kinetics of cell proliferation using ^{3}H-thymidine labeling of DNA in short-term experiments (Rakic, 1975). Thus, radioactivity uniformly became diluted in the ventricular zone 1 or 2 days following injection of the isotope. After E40, however, many progenitor cells begin to produce dissimilar daughters (by asymmetrical division), one of which becomes a postmitotic neuron, while the other may remain a stem cell or die (Fig. 2.7). The evidence that many stem cells in the proliferative units begin to divide asymmetrically came initially also from a ^{3}H-thymidine autoradiographic analysis, but this time using longer intervals following injections of isotope (Fig. 2.8). Examination of adult monkeys exposed to ^{3}H-thymidine between E40 and E100 revealed that the radioactivity of neurons, situated progressively more superficially in the cortex, diminished stepwise by halves (Rakic, 1988a). This finding indicated that, in a majority of mitotic divisions, one daughter cell remains in the proliferative unit and dilutes its radioactivity by subsequent divisions. Many divisions, however, must continue in a symmetrical mode, because a given proliferative unit, which might initially contain a single stem cell, contains several progenitor cells during later stages of corticogenesis. The concept of the gradual shift from a purely symmetrical mode of division to a mixture of symmetrical and asymmetrical modes in the telencephalic ventricular zone has received support from the use of double labeling methods, which enable the study of proliferation kinetics with two independent S phase markers (Takahashi et al., 1992, 1993). Therefore, proliferative units in the ventricular zone should be regarded as polyclones, and each ontogenetic column in the overlaying cortical plate should receive neurons from more than one clone. This model is supported by the distribution of ^{3}H-thymidine-labeled cells in the macaque monkey, which shows that, within the same column, intensely labeled and lightly labeled neurons (presumably from the same progenitor) can be interspersed among unlabeled neurons originating from a different progenitor within the same proliferative unit prior to or after an injection of ^{3}H-thymidine has been given (Fig. 2.8).

Eventually, all postmitotic cells generated in a given proliferative unit of the ventricular zone (Fig. 2.4A) form a morphologically identifia-

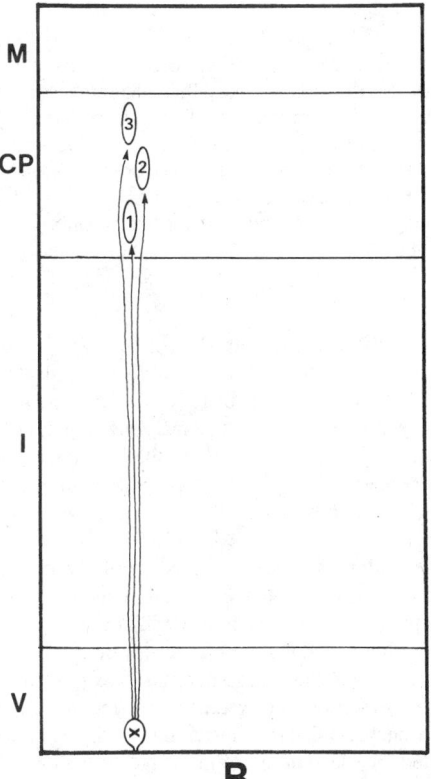

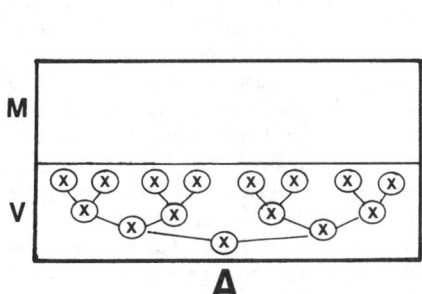

Figure 2.7. **A.** Schematic model of symmetrical cell divisions, which predominate before the 40th embryonic day (*E40*). At this early age, the cerebral wall consists of only the ventricular zone (*V*), where all cells proliferate, and the marginal zone (*M*), where they extend their radial processes. Symmetric division produces two progenitors during each cycle and causes lateral spread. **B.** Model of asymmetrical division, which becomes predominant, though not exclusive, in the monkey telencephalon after E40. During each asymmetrical division, progenation produces one postmitotic neuron that leaves the ventricular zone and another progenitor that remains within the proliferative zone. Postmitotic neurons migrate across the intermediate zone (*I*) and become arranged in the cortical plate (*CP*) in reverse order of their arrival (*1, 2, 3*). (From Rakic, 1991.)

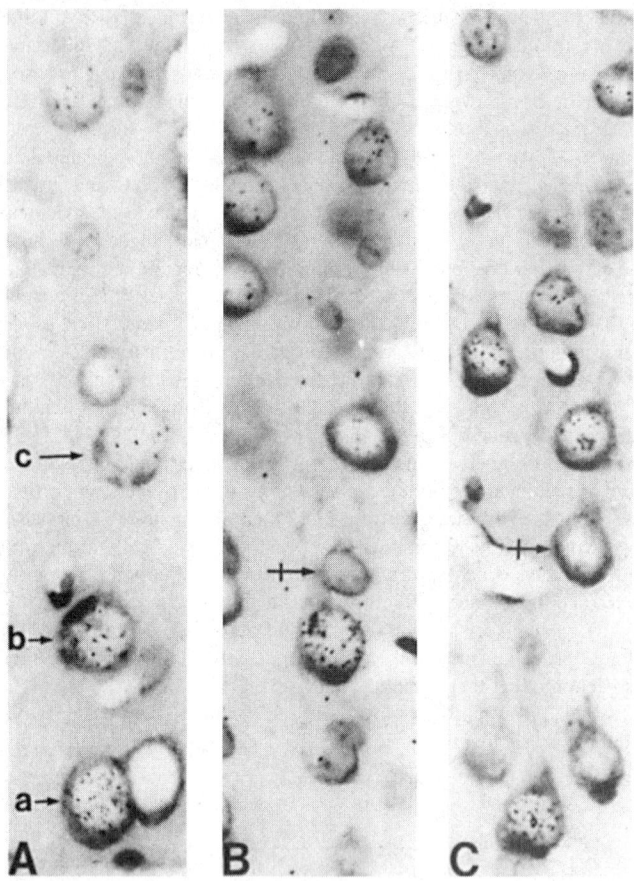

Figure 2.8. Microphotograph of three autoradiograms, showing neurons in the cortex of an adult monkey that was exposed to ³H-thymidine at E70. **A.** The most intensely radioactive neuron (*a*) lies deeper in the cortex than the two progressively less labeled, more superficially situated neurons (*b* and *c*). **B** and **C.** Unlabeled neurons (*crossed arrows* may be interspersed among radioactive neurons within the same ontogenetic column. Further explanation is in the text. (From Rakic, 1988a.)

ble stack of neurons in the cortical plate (Fig. 2.4*B*). These radially deployed neurons are easily distinguished and were variously termed ontogenetic or embryonic columns (Rakic, 1978, 1988b). The number of neurons in an ontogenetic column of the macaque monkey in the second half of gestation ranges between 70 in the anterior cingulate cortex (area 24), where neurogenesis lasts about 1 month, to more than 120 in the primary visual cortex (area 17), where neurogenesis lasts almost 2 months (see also Rakic, 1974, 1988b) (Fig. 2.2). However, the number of cells in the column is about 50% larger during midgestation and is eventually reduced by differential cell death, which in primates starts following completion of neurogenesis (Williams et al., 1987). Within each column, earlier generated neurons occupy deeper positions, and, therefore, those arriving to the cortex later must pass older neurons to become situated more superficially (Fig. 2.2). This relationship among cells with different birthdays, called the "inside-out" gradient of neurogenesis, was suspected by classical anatomists, but has been proven only after use of the ³H-thymidine autoradiographic method in a number of mammalian species (reviewed in Sidman and Rakic, 1973). The inside-out gradient of neurogenesis is particularly prominent in primates, in whom each daily injection of ³H-thymidine labels a more selective sample of cortical neurons than in rodents (Rakic, 1974). It is not clear why newly generated neurons must pass the older ones instead of piling up below each other, but one of several hypotheses is that this sequence enables feedback signals from older to arriving cells.

RADIAL UNIT HYPOTHESIS OF CORTICAL DEVELOPMENT

The finding that neurons in the cortex eventually form a morphologically identifiable stack of radially deployed neurons (Rakic, 1971,1972), subsequently termed also "ontogenetic" or "embryonic" columns, led to the postulate of the radial unit hypothesis of cortical development and evolution (Rakic 1978, 1988b, 1991). As described above and illustrated schematically in Fig. 2.6, the radial unit hypothesis predicts that the ventricular zone is a mosaic of proliferative units. These units produce cohorts of postmitotic neurons, most of which are gliophilic and, therefore, constrained in their migratory pathways, or otherwise prevented from randomly mixing while on their way to the cortex (Rakic, 1978, 1988a). If the two-dimensional, species-specific ventricular mosaic is translated over time via the radial glial scaffolding into a three-dimensional structure in the cortical plate, then the number of radial units in each species and individual may be, to some extent, specified already in the proliferative embryonic zones, before postmitotic cells come into contact with thalamic afferents (Fig. 2.6).

We suggested that an array of columns, or radially organized modules of synaptically interrelated neurons in the adult neocortex (Mountcastle, 1978; Szentagothai, 1987), may be a reflection of their developmental history (Rakic, 1978, 1988a). It was originally shown by Mountcastle that neurons situated within a single column in the somatosensory cortex are responsive to a specific modality and receptive field of stimulation. A similar anatomical and functional columnar organization was found in association cortices (Goldman and Nauta, 1976; Goldman-Rakic, 1987a; Mountcastle, 1978; Szentagothai, 1987). This striking columnar organization is also reflected in the pattern of thalamocortical and ipsilateral and contralateral cortico-cortical connections. The relatively constant size of such terminal fields among species with vastly different sizes of cerebral surface (Bagbee and Goldman-Rakic, 1982) supports the idea that during evolution the cortex expands by the addition of radial units rather than by enlargement of their size (Rakic, 1995).

The overall surface of the cerebral cortex, as well as the pattern of its cytoarchitectonic maps, displays a considerable degree of species-specific and individual differences (Filamonov, 1949). The radial unit hypothesis provides a model of how expansion of the cortex and its parcellation into various areas could occur during phylogenetic and ontogenetic development (Rakic, 1988a). Genetic control of the number of proliferative units at the ventricular surface is likely to set a limit on cortical size during both individual development and evolution of the species. However, a relatively small change in the timing of developmental cellular events may have large functional consequences by the process known as heterochrony in evolutionary biology (Gould, 1977). For example, a small change in the length or the number of cell cycles in the ventricular zone can result in large differences in the number of proliferative units (Rakic, 1988a). In the developing cerebrum, proliferation in the ventricular zone initially proceeds exponentially by the prevalence of symmetrical division, and, therefore, an additional round of mitotic divisions at that time can double the number of proliferative units and, consequently, double the number of radial ontogenetic columns (Rakic, 1991). According to this model, fewer than four extra rounds of cell divisions can account for the 10-fold difference in size of cortical surface between monkey and human (Fig. 2.7*A*). The thousandfold difference between mouse-size and human-size cerebral cortex can be achieved by the less than seven extra symmetrical divisions in the ventricular zone before the onset of corticogenesis. After the number of radial units is set and corticogenesis begins, many progenitors begin to divide asymmetrically, and, therefore, an extra round would have a negligible effect on the thickness of the cortex (Fig. 2.7*B*). According to this model, a 2–3 week longer period of corticogenesis (Rakic, 1995) in a human than in a macaque monkey enlarges the cortical thickness by only about 10–20%. In contrast, even a small delay of the onset of the second phase of corticogenesis has as an effect a large increase in the overall size of the cortical surface by increasing the number of proliferative units in the ventricular zone.

An attractive working hypothesis is that one set of regulatory genes that operates at early stages determines the proper mixture of symmetric-asymmetric types of cell divisions, as well as the total number of mitotic divisions at the ventricular surface. The dividing and/or generations of postmitotic cells then may interact with each other as they migrate with incoming afferents, and, thereby, generate variations in the composition of individual ontogenetic columns in different regions of the cerebral wall. It is likely that regulatory genes similar to those found in the fruit fly could operate in the mammalian telencephalon, and several candidates are currently being tested (e.g., Buffone et al., 1993; Lu et al., 1992; Proteus et al., 1991; Rubinstein et al., 1994).

If the protomap of the ventricular zone is translated via the radial glial scaffolding to the expanding cortical plate in the form of arrays of ontogenetic columns (Fig. 2.4*B*), then the number of units producing neurons for the cerebral cortex can be expected to vary among species and individuals. The rough estimation made by the author and his colleagues suggests that, in the macaque cerebrum, the total number of ontogenetic columns ranges between 15 and 20 million (Rakic, 1988a). In humans, this number must be at least 10 times larger and variation between individuals perhaps even greater.

PROTOMAP HYPOTHESIS OF CYTOARCHITECTONIC DIVERSITY

At present, it is not known how individual and species-specific cytoarchitectonic areas have emerged from the initially seemingly uniform cortical plate, but both intrinsic and extrinsic factors have been implicated. For example, one attractive hypothesis is that all cortical neurons are equipotential and that laminar and areal differences are induced by extrinsic influences exerted via thalamic afferents (Creutzfeldt, 1977). Indeed, the structural and functional homogeneity of the cortex emphasized by Lashley and his followers in the middle of this century (e.g., Lashley and Clark, 1946) has influenced also the thinking of many contemporary neuroembryologists (e.g., Killackey, 1990). The equipotentiality of the cortex appears to be supported by the ostensible similarity in the laminar pattern of cell distribution in various cortical areas and by the acknowledged resemblance of their synaptic circuitry (Eccles, 1984; Rakic and Singer, 1988; Szentagothai, 1987). This hypothesis also seems to be in harmony with reports that features of intraareal topographic maps can be altered by changing the input that comes from the receptors at the periphery (Van der Loos and Dorfl, 1978) and with findings that an essentially normal single-unit response with the visual receptive field properties can be elicited from the somatosensory cortex when input from the retina is experimentally rerouted to the somatosensory thalamus (Frost and Metin, 1985; Sur et al., 1988). Indeed, there is overwhelming evidence that many features of cortical organization are dependent on interaction with thalamic afferents. Perhaps the most dramatic examples in this category are formation of ocular dominance columns (Hubel et al., 1977; Rakic, 1976, 1977), barrel fields (Schlaggar and O'Leary, 1992; Van der Loos and Dorfl, 1978), or topographic maps of peripheral representation in the cerebral cortex (Mrzenich, 1988).

However, there is also considerable evidence that the cells generated within the cerebral vesicles contain some basic programs of their prospective species-specific cortical organization. To reconcile most of the existing experimental and descriptive data, we formulated a working model known as a *protomap hypothesis*, which suggests that the pattern of cytoarchitectonic areas emerge through synergistic, interdependent interactions between developmental programs intrinsic to cortical neurons and extrinsic signals supplied by specific input from the subcortical structures (Rakic, 1988a). According to this hypothesis, neurons of the embryonic cortical plate—indeed even the proliferative ventricular zone where they originate—set up a primordial species-specific cortical map of areas that preferentially attract appropriate afferents and have a capacity to respond to this input in a specific manner.

The initial indication that events in the ventricular zone foreshadow prospective regional differences in the overlaying cerebral mantle comes from ^{3}H-thymidine labeling of dividing cells, which shows that the ventricular region subjacent to area 17 produces more neurons per radial unit (Rakic, 1976b) and that area 17 substantially has a higher mitotic index (Kennedy and Dehay, 1993) than the adjacent area 18. Therefore, region-specific differences in production of the ventricular zone can be detected before neurons arrive at the cortex to be exposed to the input from periphery via thalamic afferents. In addition to the evidence for restriction of neuronal fates presented in the previous sections, it is worth mentioning that correct topological connections in anophthalmic mice and in early-enucleated animals can form in the absence of information from the periphery (Kaiserman-Abramoff et al., 1983; Olivaria and Van Sluyters, 1984; Rakic, 1988a). Finally, the primary visual cortex in monkey acquires a normal pattern of cytochrome oxidase (Kuljis and Rakic, 1990) and major neurotransmitter receptors (Rakic and Lidow, 1994) in the absence of any retinal input via the thalamus from the early embryonic stages.

The protomap hypothesis recently received support from several reports, which show the emergence of area-specific antigens in the cortex independent of thalamic input (e.g., Arimatsu et al., 1992; Barbe and Levitt, 1992; Ferri and Levitt, 1993; Levitt, 1994). Likewise, even specific functions can be restored only after transplantation of embryonic cells derived from the same, but not other, areas (Barth and Stainfield, 1994). Perhaps the most conclusive evidence in favor of the protomap hypothesis has been obtained by the use of transgenic mice combined with transareal transplantation. This approach has indicated that the expression of selective genes may occur exclusively in the region of the somatosensory cortex, irrespective of the type of afferents that arrived from the thalamus (Cohen-Tannudji et al., 1994). However, although the embryonic cerebral wall exhibits area-specific molecular differences, it should be underscored that the protomap in the embryonic cerebrum provides only a set of species-specific biological constraints. The precise position of interareal borders, the overall size of the cytoarchitectonic areas, and the details of cellular and synaptic characteristics of the adult cerebral cortex can be achieved through a cascade of reciprocal interactions between cortical neurons and cues from specific afferents arriving from a variety of extracortical sources (Rakic, 1988a). For example, the size of a given cytoarchitectonic area can be regulated by specific afferents originating from subcortical and other cortical areas (Rakic and Lidow, 1994; Rakic et al., 1991). This extracortical control can be exerted on the rate of cell elimination rather than on cell production in the ventricular zone. The concept of the protomap, therefore, involves both intrinsic and extrinsic regulation of cellular events that affect cortical parcellation; it assumes the presence of a larger number of participating neurons and synapses in the developing cortex from which the final pattern of the cytoarchitectonic map is carved.

OVERPRODUCTION OF NEURONS AND THEIR PROJECTIONS

With few exceptions, most brain structures in vertebrates have a larger number of neurons and axonal connections during development than in adulthood (for review, see Hamburger and Oppenheim, 1982; Williams and Herrup, 1988). In all parts of the brain so far studied, neurons, as well as their axons and dendrites, were found to be more numerous only during a well-defined phase of development (Easter et al., 1985; Purves, 1988; Rakic and Riley, 1983a; Rakic et al., 1994). The same basic phenomenon of initial exuberance has been observed during development of the cerebral cortex. Judging from the density of pyknotic (degenerating) cells, the visual cortex of fetal monkeys contains about 30% more neurons than that in adult monkeys (Williams et al., 1987). The elimination of cells occurs mostly during the second half of gestation, when the superficial cortical layers may lose 35–40% of the initial number of neurons that arrived at the cortical plate. In contrast, the deep cortical layers, which are formed earlier, lose less than 25% of the original number. The reason for the lamina-specific difference in the magnitude of neuronal death is not clear, but it may be significant

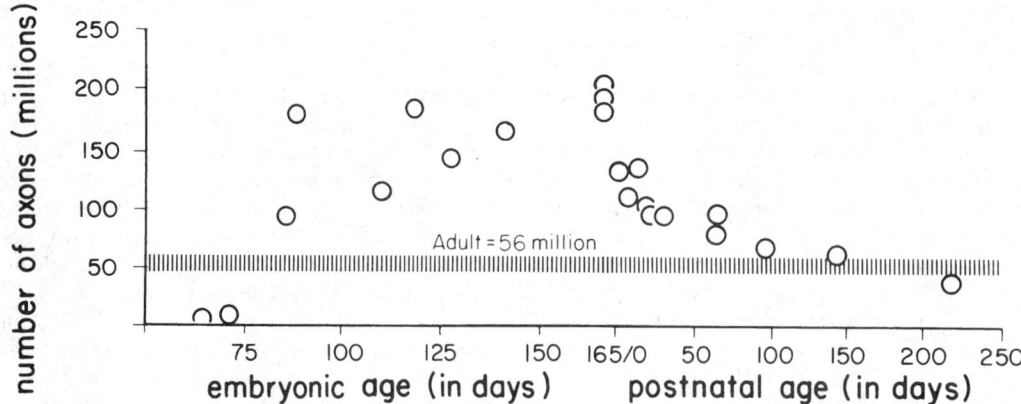

Figure 2.9. The estimated total number of axons in corpus callosum as a function of prenatal and postnatal ages in postconceptual days. *Each point* represents a single animal. Error values (<14%) are smaller than or equal to the *size of the dots* used to represent each data point. The *hatched line* indicates the average total number of callosal axons in eight adult monkeys. (From LaMantia and Rakic, 1990.)

that local circuit cortico-cortical systems that are predominantly situated in the superficial layers (that are generated later) lose more cells than cortico-subcortical efferent systems, which originate from the deep layers (that are generated early).

The phase of massive neuronal elimination from the primate cerebral cortex precedes the phase of axonal elimination in the large cortico-cortical fiber tracts. For example, the newborn monkey has about 190 million callosal axons, compared to less than 50 million in the adult (LaMantia and Rakic, 1990). A majority of these axons are eliminated during the first 3 postnatal weeks at the rate of 8 million per day or 50 per second. Therefore, callosal axons are lost at an estimated average rate of half a million per day or 5 per second, until the adult value is reached around puberty (Fig. 2.9). This enormous loss of callosal axons is not accompanied by a significant change in the number of cortical neurons during the same period. This apparent paradox can be explained, at least in part, by the fact that callosal neurons represent less than 1% of the total cortical cells. However, it should be noted that many collateral branches or secondary axons of callosal cells may be eliminated from neurons that survive to adulthood. Other classes of interhemispheric connections, such as the anterior and hippocampal commissures, are also lost at a similar rate during approximately the same time (LaMantia and Rakic, 1994, 1995). As discussed below, the number, pattern of distribution, or type of surviving neurons and axons can be modified at critical stages by the deletion of the neurons with which they have a direct synaptic relationship or more distant trophic dependence.

The biphasic development of cortical connections, which proceeds from initially diffuse to more sharply defined terminal fields, has been first and, perhaps, best documented in the primate visual area (Hubel et al., 1977; Rakic, 1976). Subsequently, a similar developmental scenario has also been shown in diverse structures in a variety of species (Easter et al., 1985; Innocenti, 1981; O'Leary, 1989; Purves, 1988). In primates, for example, terminals of the corticostriatal projections in the caudate nucleus are initially distributed in a diffuse manner, across wide territories, before synapses retract from the sites that eventually become occupied by later-arriving afferent systems (Goldman, 1978; Goldman-Rakic, 1981b). These two examples, one afferent (geniculocortical) and the other efferent (corticostriatal), reveal that the formation of both input and output to the cortex may be achieved through dynamic competitive cellular interactions that involve at least two well-defined steps. In the first step, several input systems project to the target structure in a diffuse and overlapping manner, without regard to its specific target area, the individual nerve cell, or its part. In the second phase, connections sort out and form more selective contacts with specific sets of neurons or their dendrites.

The functional significance of the large loss of axons in the cerebral

cortex is not fully understood. In primates it occurs after topographic and columnar organization has been achieved (LaMantia and Rakic, 1990; Schwartz and Goldman-Rakic, 1988) and, therefore, is not involved in establishing a basic pattern of connections. For example, in adult rhesus monkey, area 17 does not have callosal connections, and unlike the developing cat, this region is never interconnected (Kennedy and Dehay, 1993). Likewise, callosal axons in the prefrontal cortex precisely interconnect with appropriate areas in the middle of gestation, well in advance of the axonal loss phase that in this species occurs mostly postnatally (Schwartz and Goldman-Rakic, 1988). Therefore, axonal elimination in the cerebral cortex is probably involved in synaptic remodeling at the local rather than global level (LaMantia and Rakic, 1990). Indeed, as discussed below, loss of interhemispheric axons coincides with the period of rapid synaptic production rather than synaptic elimination.

OVERPRODUCTION OF CORTICAL SYNAPSES

In most structures of the vertebrate brain, where quantitative data have been obtained with reasonable accuracy, both the density of synapses and their total number are higher during one stage of development than in the adult state (e.g., Easter et al., 1985; Purves, 1988). The cerebral cortex is not an exception to that rule, and the magnitude of the overproduction in this structure is even more pronounced. A bewildering number of growing axons eventually must establish synaptic junctions with a specific neuron class in each cortical area or, even more precisely, with only a part of their body and dendritic tree. In the primate cerebral cortex this precise pattern of synaptic connectivity in the target structure is achieved through a marked overproduction and subsequent elimination. For example, the cerebral cortex in both human and macaque monkeys contains more synapses during infancy than in adulthood (Bourgeois and Rakic, 1993; Huttenlocher and de Courten, 1987; O'Kusky and Colonnier, 1984; Rakic et al., 1986; Zielinski and Hendrickson, 1992). In the newborn monkey, the density of synapses per unit volume of neuropil and their total number is approximately equal to the adult values. However, during the first 2–3 months of life, synaptic density continues to increase until it reaches about 40% more than in an adult (Fig. 2.10). The phase of high synaptic density lasts throughout adolescence and decreases significantly during sexual maturation, which in this species occurs during the 3rd year of life (Rakic et al., 1986, 1994a). The decline in number of synapses is due primarily to the elimination of asymmetrical junctions located on dendritic spines, while synapses on dendritic shafts and cell bodies remain relatively constant. The course of decline in density and absolute number of synapses is perhaps best documented for the macaque monkey primary visual cortex. The number

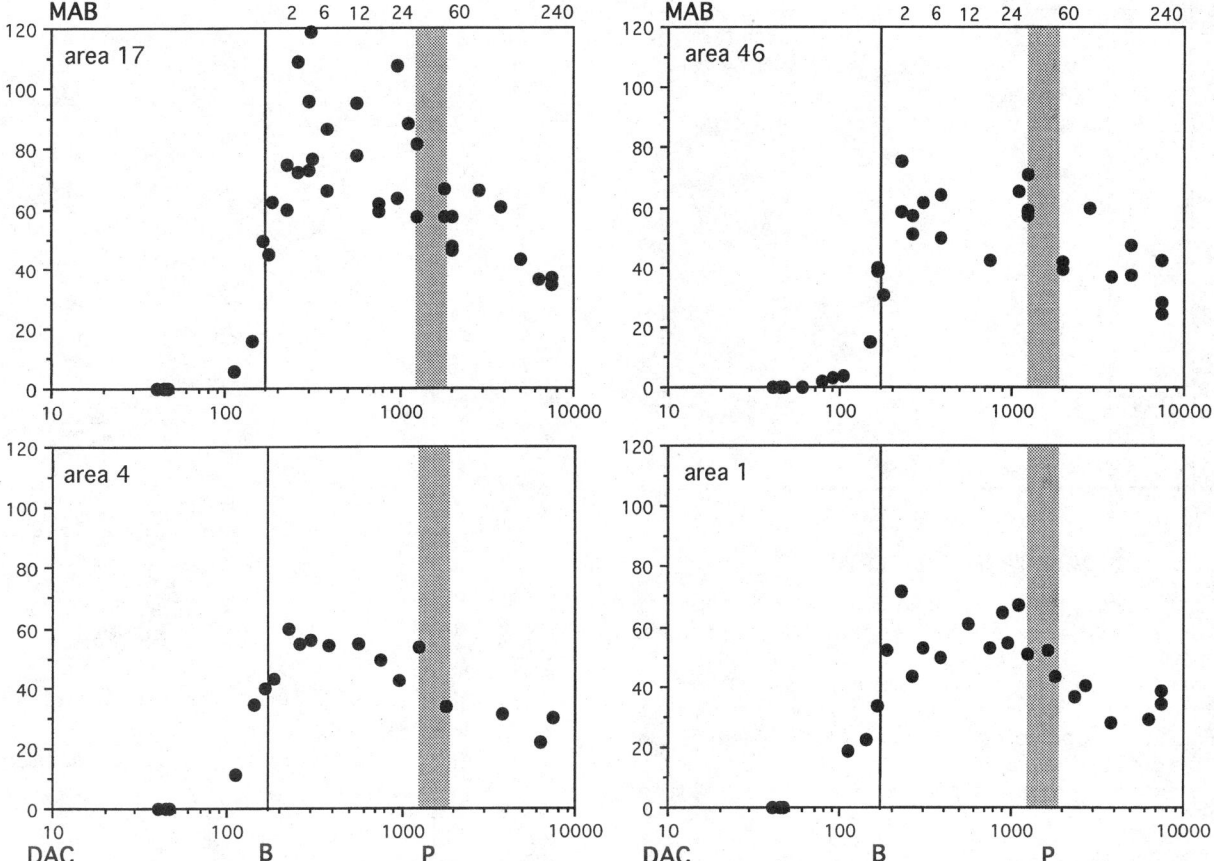

Figure 2.10. Histograms of the density of synapses per 100 μm^3 of neuropil in the primary visual (*area 17*), prefrontal association (*area 46*), primary motor (*area 4*), and primary somatosensory (*area 1*) at various ages. *Each black circle* represents the value obtained from a single electron microscopic probe (see Fig. 2.1), and data are corrected and transferred into N per volume according to the Anker and Cragg formula. The time is represented on a semilogarithmic scale. *MAB*, months after birth; *DAC*, days after conception; *B*, birth; *P*, days after puberty. (Data compiled from Bourgeois and Rakic, 1993; Bourgeois, Goldman-Rakic and Rakic, 1994; Zecevic and Rakic, 1991; Zecevic, Bourgeois and Rakic, 1984.)

of synapses lost in area 17 of a single cerebral hemisphere is about 1.8 × 10¹¹ (Bourgeois and Rakic, 1993). The magnitude of this loss is stunning when expressed as a loss of about 2500 synapses per second in the striate area of each hemisphere during a period of about 2–3 years.

Quantitative analysis of synaptogenesis in the motor (Zecevic et al., 1989), somatosensory (Zecevic and Rakic, 1991), visual (Bourgeois and Rakic, 1993), prefrontal (Bourgeois et al., 1994), and limbic (Grainger et al., 1995) cortex in macaque monkey indicates that a basic course of synaptogenesis, and, in particular, the ascending phase, occurs concomitantly (Fig. 2.10). Thus, contrary to the prevailing views, the entire population of synaptic junctions in the association Brodmann's area 46 matures concurrently with, rather than after, the primary sensory and motor areas. Although during this exponential phase there is a sequential accretion of some classes of synapses from diverse origins, overall the course of synaptogenesis is framed within a "window of time" centered on the exponential phase, which is common for all areas of the neocortex.

The cortical synapses in humans seem to form synchronously in diverse cortical areas also, although the available data initially suggested a delay in the rapid phase of synaptogenesis in the prefrontal, as compared to that in the visual striate, area (Huttenlocher, 1979; Huttenlocher and De Courten, 1987). However, if one eliminates the technical and procedural differences, the course of synaptogenesis in human and monkey is remarkably similar across the entire cortex. For example, when the data on synaptogenesis obtained from the human prefrontal (Huttenlocher, 1979) and human visual cortex (Huttenlocher and de Courten,

1987) were normalized and replotted to the maximum value of the curve on a semilogarithmic scale (Rakic et al., 1994a), both curves overlap, as they do in the monkey (Fig. 2.11). Moreover, by means of linear regression analysis, the two sets of values were fitted to a straight line, and statistical comparison between the two regression lines failed to reveal a significant difference in their slopes. It therefore appears that synaptogenesis both in humans and nonhuman primates proceeds synchronously in sensory and association cortex (Rakic et al., 1994a).

The time course of synaptogenesis in different cortical areas corresponds well with the changes occurring simultaneously in cerebral metabolism during development of both human and macaque cerebral cortex (Chugani et al., 1987; Jacob et al., 1994). In humans, the use of fluorodeoxyglucose, which indicates the level of metabolic activity in positron emission tomography, reveals that, after birth, metabolic activity also increases concurrently in prefrontal, motor, somatosensory, and visual cortex (Chugani et al., 1987). These studies lend support to the idea that maturation of diverse cortical areas in both monkey and human occurs simultaneously rather than in pronounced sequential order. Further, the synchrony in synaptogenesis observed in the nonhuman primate is in harmony with biochemical and functional data on cortical maturation in the same species. Biochemical studies (Goldman-Rakic and Brown, 1982) suggest that the concentrations of dopamine, noradrenaline, and serotonin increase rapidly in the cortex of the macaque monkey over the first 2 months and approach adult levels by the 5th month after birth. Recent studies of the accumulation of major neurotransmitter receptor sites in different cortical areas show that their maximum density

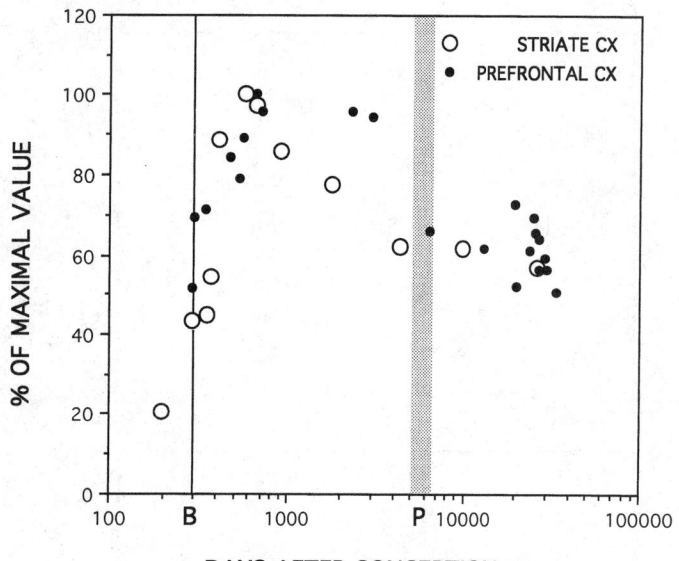

Figure 2.11. Synaptogenesis in human cerebral cortex. Synaptic density in the human striate area (*open, large circles*) and prefrontal cortex (*black, small circles*) based on the studies of Huttenlocker and Courten, 1987 and Huttenlocker, 1979, respectively. We replotted each point from their published data on a semilogarithmic scale as a function of conceptual age and normalized to the maximum value of the curve. Under these conditions, both curves overlap as they do in monkeys. For further explanation see text. (From Rakic et al., 1994a.)

is also reached between 2 and 4 months after birth in this species (Lidow et al., 1991; Lidow and Rakic, 1992). The curves of the increase in receptor density are very similar to those of synaptogenesis in all areas examined (Fig. 2.12). However, the phase of decline of receptor density appears to slightly precede the phase of synaptic decline. These observations from divergent cortical areas suggest that the initial formation and maintenance of synapses, as well as their biochemical maturation, may be determined by intrinsic signals, which are common to the entire cortical mantle.

The concurrent course of synaptogenesis and formation of neurotransmitter receptors in functionally different areas of the cerebrum is at variance with the tacit assumption, widespread in the literature, that development of cerebral cortex follows a hierarchical sequence of structural and functional development from the sensory to motor and, finally, to association cortex (originated by Flechsig, 1920; confirmed by Filimonov, 1949; Yakovlev and LeCourse, 1968; and reviewed in Greenfield, 1991). We argue that myelination of large axonal tracts is not a very useful criterion of functional maturation of a given cortical area and, furthermore, that hematoxylin staining of sections used to measure

Figure 2.12. Developmental changes in the overall changes (across all layers) in density of the synapses and specific binding of radioligands labeling a representative selection of neurotransmitter receptor subtypes in the prefrontal, primary, motor, somatosensory, and primary visual cortical regions of the developing rhesus monkey. For receptor densities, the *lines* were obtained by locally weighted least square fit with 50% smoothing (KALEIDA GRAPH, Synergy Software, Reading, PA) based on mean B$_{max}$ values obtained from the measurements of the entire cortical thickness in at least two animals at birth, 1, 2, 4, 8, 12, 36, and 60 months of age. Age is presented in postnatal days on a logarithmic scale. (The primary data are from Rakic et al., 1986; Lidow et al., 1991; and Lidow and Rakic, 1992.)

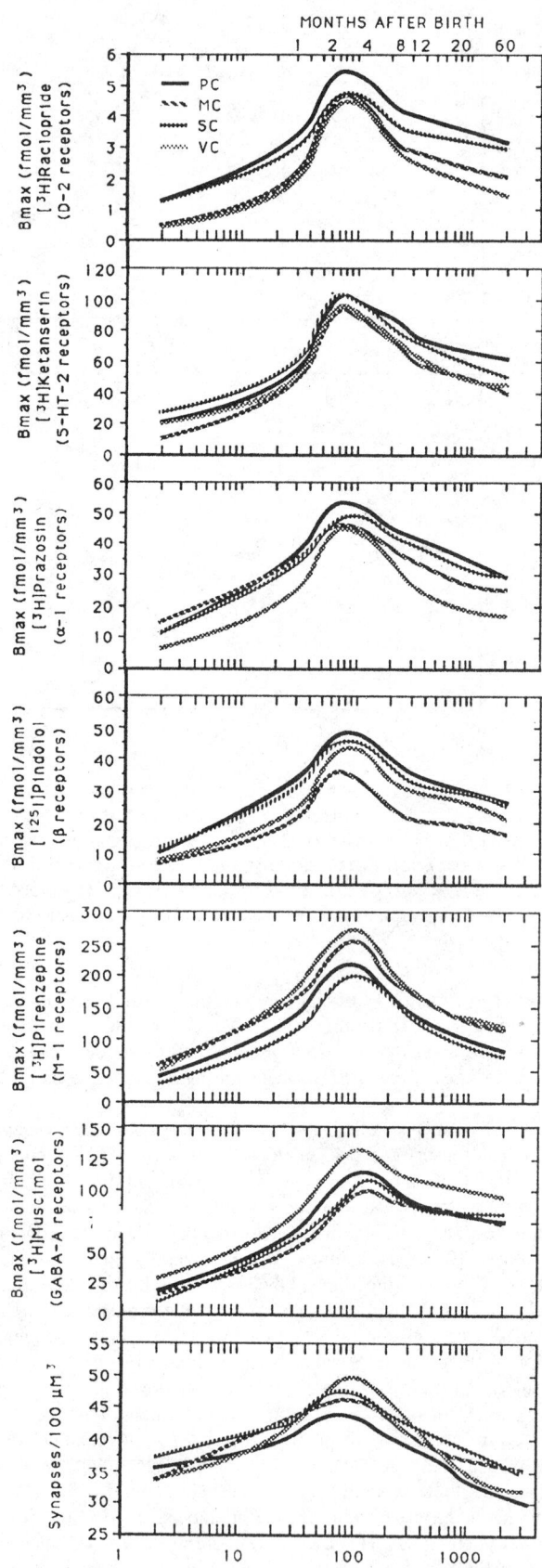

the amount of myelin is not a reliable quantitative method. There are clear exceptions to the hierarchical rule of cortical maturation even in these studies. For example, the corticospinal motor system is among the last to myelinate and becomes stained by hematoxylin only during the 2nd year of life, well after association pathways are myelinated (Yakovlev and LeCourse, 1978). On the other hand, concurrent structural (synaptic) and biochemical (neurotransmitters, receptors) maturation of the cortical mantle appears reasonable when one takes into account that integration of sensory, motor, limbic, and associative components are essential for even the simplest cortical functions (Goldman-Rakic, 1987a; 1988). This concept of concurrency becomes even more compelling when one considers the coupling between early maturation of the neuronal circuits of the cortex and the first expression of cognitive capacity that requires coordination of sensory and associational cortical areas (e.g., Spelke et al., 1994).

Isochronic development of anatomically and functionally diverse regions indicates that the establishment of cell-to-cell communication in this structure may be orchestrated by a single genetic or humoral signal. This phase of primate life may provide a long period of unparalleled opportunity for competitive, activity-driven stabilization among various initially overproduced intercortical and intracortical connections, which comprise the largest fraction of cortical synapses (Goldman-Rakic, 1987a). This period of supernumerary synapses in the cerebral cortex can be considered as a stage in life with maximal opportunity and minimal commitments, thus providing a window of enormous opportunity for the generation of cortical diversity beyond genes.

SYNAPTIC ELIMINATION AND FUNCTIONAL VALIDATION

Studies of the cerebral cortex in a variety of mammalian species support the hypothesis of competitive interactions as a mechanism of attaining point-to-point connectivity during segregation of initially more numerous and more diffuse projections (Easter et al., 1985; Edelman, 1988). The balance between overproduction and elimination of neurons and axons and competition between them determines the size and site of territories devoted to a given terminal field. The first, and perhaps the best documented, example of developmental processes, which proceeds from diffuse to sharply defined terminal fields is the primate binocular visual system (Hubel et al., 1977; Rakic, 1976a, 1977). This basic principle has since been shown in a variety of cortical areas (Easter et al., 1985; Innocenti, 1981; O'Leary, 1989; Shatz, 1983). Among the cellular mechanisms involved in the process of sorting out connections, selective, activity-dependent competition, which leads to selective elimination of inappropriate and less used synapses, is, perhaps, the most prominent. When it occurs during postnatal development and is associated with sensory stimulation, it is also known as the Hebbian mechanism or synaptic stabilization (Changeux, 1993; Hebb, 1949).

After the number and density of synapses in the cerebral cortex reach adult levels, they remain relatively stable throughout the life span in both humans and nonhuman primates (Huttenlocher and deCourten, 1987; Rakic et al., 1986, 1994a). Even though, obviously, we learn and acquire an enormous amount of information during adulthood, the number of synapses in the cerebral cortex during this period remains basically the same. From the crude quantitative analysis of the overall density and number of synapses, one cannot exclude the possibility that certain classes of synapses are constantly being produced while others are being eliminated in the same proportion (Rakic et al., 1986). However, the absence of profiles of immature synapses or their early forms, as well the lack of hard ultrastructural evidence for their degeneration under normal conditions, suggests that the turnover of synaptic population in primates must be either absent or negligible. Based on these findings, we argue that during infancy, childhood, and adolescence learning of the basic skills and formation of intellectual capabilities may be associated with considerable changes in population of synapses by both formation and elimination of selected synaptic junctions, as well

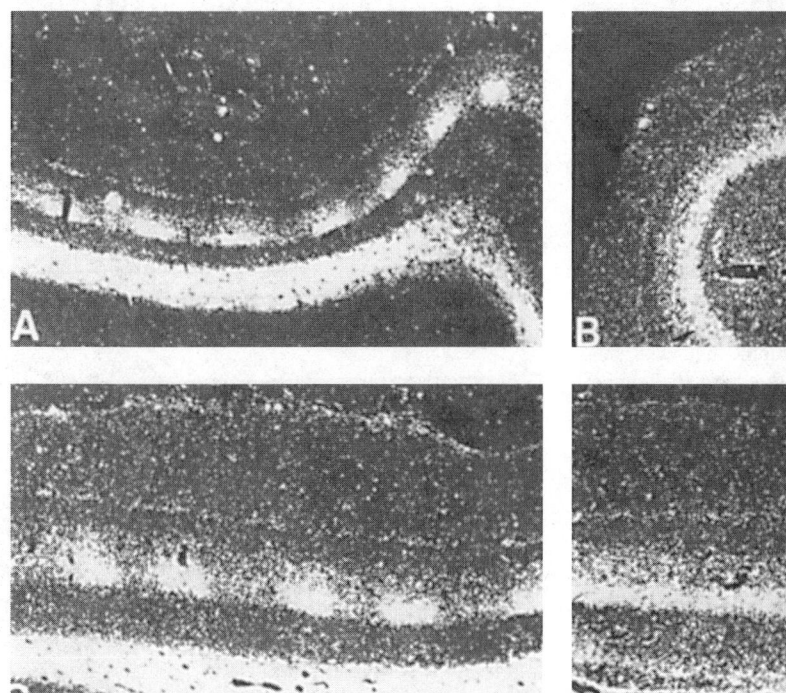

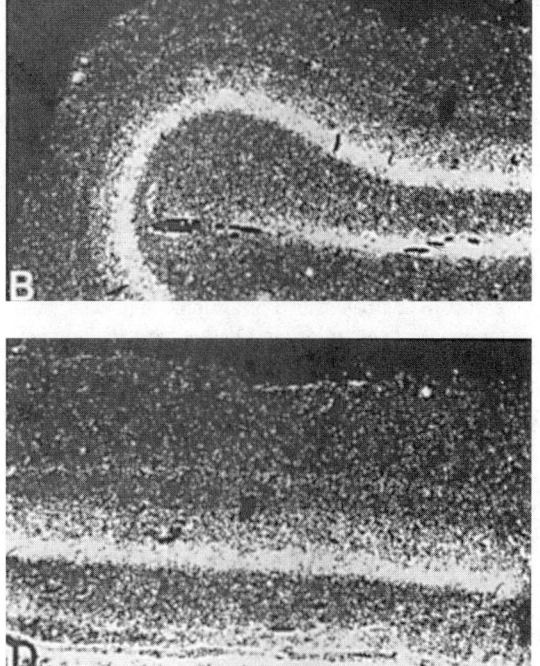

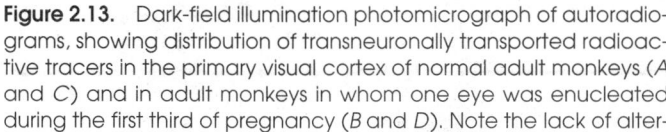

Figure 2.13. Dark-field illumination photomicrograph of autoradiograms, showing distribution of transneuronally transported radioactive tracers in the primary visual cortex of normal adult monkeys (*A* and *C*) and in adult monkeys in whom one eye was enucleated during the first third of pregnancy (*B* and *D*). Note the lack of alternating ocular dominance columns in the cortex of experimental animals. The distribution of silver grains over sublayers of layer IV remains similar to that in the control. See Figure 2.6 for the diagrammatic illustration of differential grain distribution in enucleated monkeys (From Rakic, 1983.)

as strengthening of their efficacy. In contrast, after puberty learning and memory probably depend primarily on changes in the strength of already existing synapses. It should be pointed out that this concept does not negate the capacity for functional plasticity that remains in the adult cerebral cortex (e.g., Merzenich, 1988) nor does it contradict the existence of competitive interactions based on strengthening of the selected connections in response to stimulation (Edelmen, 1987; Shatz, 1990). However, this hypothesis could explain substantial qualitative and quantitative differences in learning capability before and after sexual maturity. This mode of learning may be particularly important in primates, which depend on retention of acquired knowledge in the permanent set of neurons and their connections during a prolonged life span (Rakic, 1985).

The theory of competitive elimination of synapses during development of the cerebral cortex was initially obtained from studies of monocular eye deprivation, which resulted in a decrease in the size of ocular dominance columns subserving the occluded eye and enlargement of the functional eye (Hubel et al., 1977). This was the first clear anatomical evidence that the pattern of neuronal connectivity can be visibly changed by a short-time deprivation of function during the critical postnatal period of development. Even more dramatic changes are observed when the eye in a monkey fetus is enucleated before geniculocortical fibers have entered the cortical plate (Rakic, 1981a, 1983). In such cases, there is not a trace of ocular dominance columns in the visual cortex and, therefore, neurons that normally receive input from, and subserve, the left eye now receive input from the right eye (Fig. 2.13). Retinogeniculo-cortical connections fail to withdraw to appropriate territories even after blockade of electrical activity in one eye by tetrodotoxin (Dubin et al., 1986; Stryker and Harris, 1986). Some additional experiments done on the developing cerebral cortex are reviewed below to illustrate the extent of the changes in neuronal organization that can be induced by interference with the course of normal development.

EXPERIMENTAL MANIPULATION OF THE CORTICAL PROTOMAP

The cerebral cortex is basically an analyzer that makes association between diverse inputs originating from various sensory receptors communicated to its neurons via precisely and systematically organized thalamocortical connections. Although the information essential for developing a basic species-specific pattern of these connections must be imprinted in our genome, interference with normal interaction with the information derived from the periphery, where the stimulation arises, can have a devastating effect. The role of afferents in the development of cortical parcellation can be examined by altering the number of axons comprising specific thalamocortical systems at early embryonic stages and determining the size and cytoarchitectonic pattern in corresponding target areas of the cortex in adult animals. For example, binocular enucleation performed in monkey embryo around E60 reduces the number of geniculate neurons to less than one-half the number in age-matched controls without altering any other component in the thalamocortical system (Rakic, 1988a; Rakic et al., 1991). Furthermore, the occipital lobe in early enucleates displays dramatic and remarkably reproducible changes in the convolutions of the occipital operculum. These changes are milder in later-operated cases and cannot be induced by down-sizing geniculocortical input during the second half of gestation. Use of anterograde and retrograde transport of axonal tracers in early enucleates reveals the presence of topographically well-defined reciprocal connections of the occipital lobe with a vestige of the lateral geniculate nucleus (Rakic, 1988a).

In the specimens with an experimentally produced smaller lateral geniculate, area 17 is well differentiated from adjacent area 18, and its thickness and characteristic laminar pattern are surprisingly normal. However, the surface area and the total number of neurons in area 17 in the early-enucleated subjects are less than half those in age-matched controls (Rakic et al., 1991). Despite the drastically reduced number

of geniculocortical afferents, area 17 contained the normal number of neurons per unit volume of each layer and per each radial column. The distribution of major neurotransmitter receptors in early enucleates, in spite of some modification, retained the basic laminar pattern characteristic of area 17 (Rakic and Lidow, 1995). Furthermore, cytochrome oxidase blobs in layers II and III, which are thought to subserve color and form vision (Livingstone and Hubel, 1988), were segregated and maintained in the visual cortex of early binocular enucleates (Kuljis and Rakic, 1990). Finally, synaptic density per unit of neuropil, as revealed by quantitative electron microscopy, achieved normal range in all layers (Bourgeois and Rakic, unpublished). These results indicate that the basic cytological, synaptic, and biochemical characteristics of area 17 can develop in the absence of stimulation from the retina. However, the number of ontogenetic columns, and, therefore, the size of the surface of the visual cortex, is reduced to match the number of geniculocortical axons in the enucleated animals (Rakic, 1988a).

The reduction in size of area 17 in animals enucleated at early embryonic ages could result either from the creation of fewer radial columns or from an increase in their elimination (Fig. 2.14B). However, neither possibility seems likely since enucleation was performed after all proliferative units in the ventricular zone should have been formed, and cell death restricted to entire columns of cells has never been observed. It is possible, therefore, that the total number of ontogenetic columns in the cortices of animals that were operated on remained the same and that the adjacent cytoarchitectonic area, which normally receives input mainly from the adjacent thalamic nucleus (pulvinar), expanded (Fig.

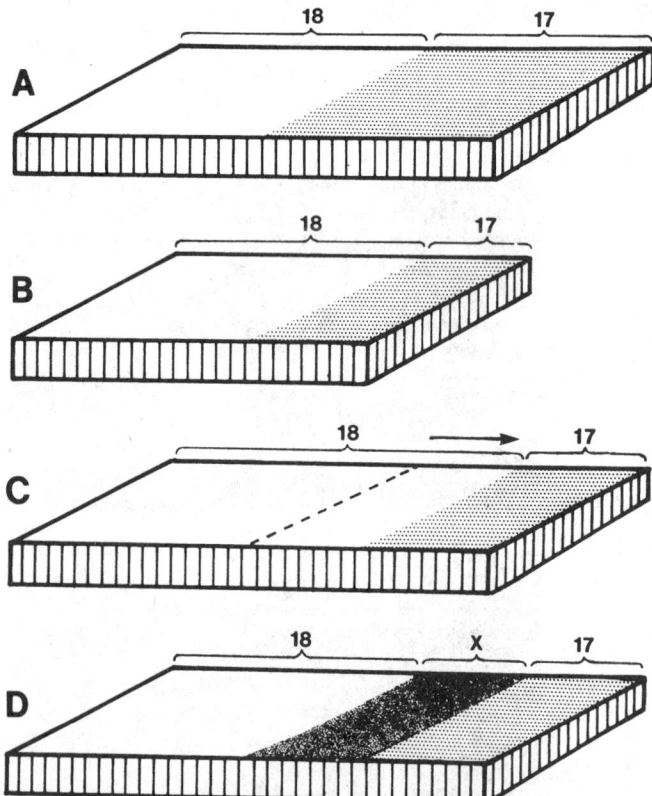

Figure 2.14. Schematic representation of the possible modes of decrease in the size of area 17 caused by experimental reduction of thalamic input. **A.** Relation between areas 17 and 18 in a normal animal. **B.** Differential cell death. **C.** Encroachment of adjacent area 18 into the territory of area 17. **D.** Formation of an abnormal cytoarchitectonic area (X) consisting of neurons genetically destined for area 17 that receive input characteristic for area 18. Further explanation is in the text. (From Rakic, 1988a.)

2.14*C*). Such changes would require respecification of neurons genetically programmed to become part of area 17 to accommodate input characteristic to area 18. This mismatch may create a "hybrid" cortex (*X* in Fig. 2.14*D*) that retains some characteristics of area 17, but takes on some features of area 18 as a result of receiving a different set of afferents (Rakic, 1988a). These findings may provide a hint about how a new type of cytoarchitectonic area can be introduced by input-target mismatching during evolution (Suner and Rakic, unpublished).

Regulation by thalamic input to the developing cortical plate is probably only one part of a complex interactive process that occurs during parcellation of the neocortex. For example, prenatal resection of the fetal cortex, which eliminates or decreases the amount of cortico-cortical input to the subplate zone at early stages, also affects the pattern of cortical convolutions in some unoperated areas on both sides (Goldman-Rakic, 1980; Goldman-Rakic and Rakic, 1984).

TIMING OF CORTICAL HISTOGENESIS IN HUMANS

Since our ultimate goal is to learn more about the development of the neocortex in humans, it is important to determine whether the development of the cortex in humans proceeds according to time schedules relative to birth and shares the same cellular and molecular mechanisms uncovered in nonhuman primates. A comparison of some of the morphological features of the cortex in human fetuses of different ages (e.g., Kostovic and Rakic, 1980, 1990; Poliakov, 1949, 1959, 1965; Rakic and Sidman, 1968; Sidman and Rakic, 1973) with those of the monkey may help to determine the corresponding time and sequence in these two species. Poliakov's comprehensive histological studies of cortical development in humans have been reviewed in more detail elsewhere (Sidman and Rakic, 1982) and are briefly summarized here and illustrated in Figure 2.15.

Stage I. Initial formation of the cortical plate (from approximately the 6th to 10th fetal week). During the 7th fetal week, postmitotic cells begin to migrate from the ventricular zone outward to form a new accumulation of cells at the junction of the intermediate and marginal zones. Already, by the middle of this period, synapses of unknown origin are present above and below the cortical plate (Molliver et al., 1973). This stage corresponds approximately to the level of cortical development found in the monkey fetus between E40 and E54, depending on the region.

Stage II. Primary condensation of the cortical plate (through approximately the 10th and 11th fetal weeks). At this stage the cortical plate increases in thickness, becomes more compact, and is clearly demarcated from the fiber-rich part of the intermediate zone, which seems to have fewer cells per unit volume, indicating that the first major wave of migration is almost spent (Fig. 2.15). The end of this stage corresponds approximately to the E55–E59 period in the monkey when the majority of efferent neurons of layers 6 and 5 are generated in most regions of the cortex.

Stage III. Bilaminate cortical plate (most pronounced during the 11th to the 13th fetal week). The uniform and compact cortical plate of the second stage becomes subdivided into an inner zone occupied mainly by cells with relatively large, somewhat widely spaced oval nuclei and an outer zone of cells with densely packed, darker, bipolar nuclei (Fig. 2.15). This heterogeneity results from the more advanced maturation of the deep-lying neurons that had arrived at the cortical plate during earlier developmental stages, plus the addition of a new wave of somas of immature neurons that take up more superficial positions. This period is also characterized by the appearance of the cell-sparse, fiber-rich subplate zone situated below the cortical plate. This transient embryonic zone in the human fetus is particularly wide in the regions subjacent to the association areas (Kostovic and Rakic, 1990). Stage III corresponds roughly to the level of development achieved in the monkey between E59 and E64.

Stage IV. Secondary condensation (from the 13th to the 15th fetal week). During this period of gestation, the ventricular zone becomes progressively thinner, while the subventricular zone remains relatively wide (Fig. 2.15). The cortical plate again becomes homogeneous in appearance and resembles, in a sense, a thickened version of Stage II. The reason for this change may be that, in Stage IV, most of the young neurons in the cortex become considerably larger as they differentiate, while relatively few new immature neurons enter the cortical plate. The result is a more uniform appearance. At the end of this stage, an accumulation of large cells appears below the cortical plate and the subplate zone enlarges further (Kostovic and Rakic, 1990). Depending on the cortical region, this stage appears in the monkey between E64 and E75.

Stage V. This prolonged stage of cortical maturation lasts from the 16th fetal week and continues well into the postnatal period. Morphological data are inadequate to determine for how long, and how many, neurons continue to migrate to the human neocortex after 16 weeks, and hence the line at the right side of the curve is dotted in Fig. 2.15. By the 5th lunar month, relatively few neuron precursors seem to be proliferating in the reduced ventricular zone of the human cerebral hemispheres, although many neurons that were generated prior to the 16th week have yet to reach the cortical plate. Comparison of the ^{3}H-thymidine autoradiographic results in the monkey (Rakic, 1974a, 1977) with comparable stages in humans (Kostovic and Rakic, 1990) indicates that probably all neurons of the human neocortex are generated before the middle of gestation. Toward term, the subplate zone dissolves, and, as the intermediate zone becomes myelinated and transforms into white matter, only a vestige of the subplate neurons remain as interstitial neurons (Kostovic and Rakic, 1980). After all cortical neurons have been generated and attained their final position, their differentiation, including formation of synapses, proceeds for a long time and reaches a peak only during the 2nd postnatal year. The subject of synaptogenesis in the cerebral cortex of both monkey and humans has been described in the preceding sections.

RELEVANCE TO MENTAL ILLNESS

It is generally agreed that many psychiatric and neurological disorders that become expressed in childhood and adolescence have a genetic and developmental background, but the exact time and place of the onset of a defective process has been difficult to place. Advances made in understanding normal cortical development provide insight into the pathogenesis of some inherited and acquired cortical malformations observed in animals and humans. However, the biological bases of many psychiatric disorders, such as schizophrenia, obsessive compulsive disorders, or various forms of congenital mental retardation have been more elusive. In such cases, methodological limitations allow even relatively large changes in the relative size of cortical areas or in the synaptic number to remain undetected. In other cases, the defect may be biochemical, but only quantitative analysis of the distribution of the involved molecules could reveal the effects. A few examples will be provided here of the visible and relatively well-defined disorders that are explicable in light of the present knowledge of corticogenesis that was reviewed on the preceding pages. These examples are selected because they also elucidate the main principles governing the development of the cerebral cortex.

One rare, but highly relevant, condition that affects the formation of the cortex is an absence of sensory input from the early stages of development. For example, it is surprising but well established that, when a child is born without retinas, area 17 has a normal thickness and lamination but a greatly reduced surface (Bolton, 1900; Brunquell et al., 1984). Although the cause of most cases of anophthalmia is unknown, the result is wholly explicable by findings from bilateral enucleation experiments (Rakic, 1988b; Suner and Rakic, unpublished), which indicate that this cortical abnormality is caused by a defect in eye formation during the first third of gestation. Experiments by the author and his colleagues, in which retinas are resected during the first third of gestation, provide a useful model to study the pathogenesis of secondary anophthalmia. So far, it has been learned that the visual cortex in these

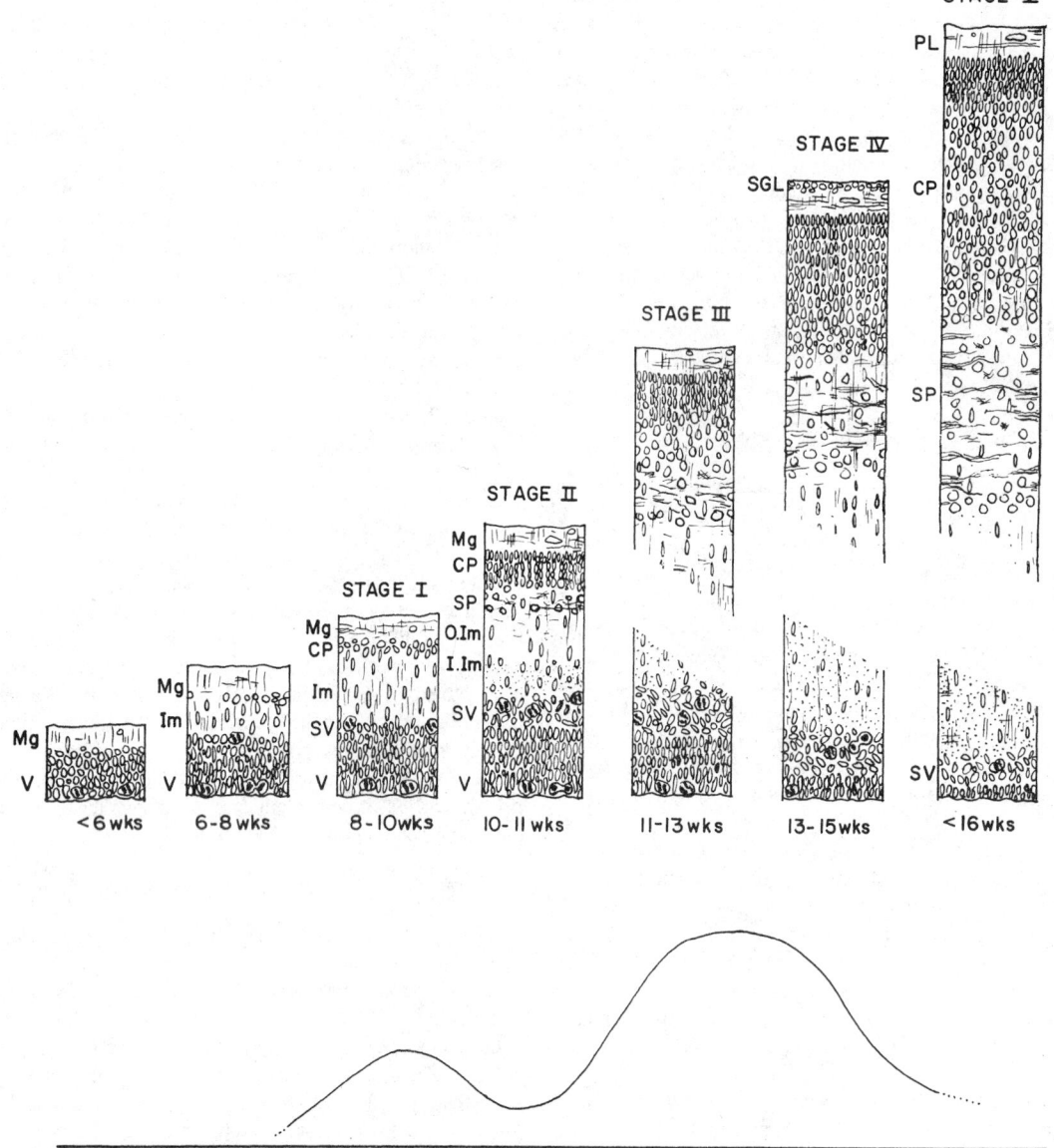

Figure 2.15. Semidiagrammatic drawings of the human cerebral wall at various gestational ages, listed in fetal *weeks below each column*. The stages refer specifically to an arbitrarily chosen area midway along the lateral surface of the hemisphere (detailed in Sidman and Rakic, 1982). In addition, the subplate zone, situated below the cortical plate, appears in the last three stages (Kostovic and Rakic, 1990). Because there is a gradient of maturation, as many as three of five stages of cortical development may be observed in different regions of the neocortex in the same fetal brain. In the *three columns on the right*, the intermediate zone is not drawn in full because the thickness of the cerebral wall has increased markedly compared with earlier stages and cannot fit into the drawing. The *curve below the drawing* schematically indicates waves of cell migration to the neocortex assessed by the density of migrating neurons in the intermediate zone. *CP*, cortical plate; *Im*, intermediate zone; *I.Im* and *O.Im*, inner and outer intermediate zones, respectively; *Mg*, marginal zone; *PL*, plexiform layer; *SGL*, subpial granular layer; *SP*, subplate zone; *SV*, subventricular zone; *V*, ventricular zone; *wks*, age in fetal weeks. (From Rakic, 1988b, with permission.)

animals develops a normal density of synapses and normal distribution and binding intensity of the major neurotransmitter receptors (Bourgeois and Rakic, unpublished; Rakic and Lidow, 1995). Other pertinent examples of cortical malformation are focal malformations found in both humans and mice, in which only a segment of the cortex confined to several radial units is highly disturbed and sharply delineated from adjacent areas (Nowakowski, 1984; Sherman et al., 1985), indicating that only cells originating from a small part of the ventricular zone have been affected. The classification of most cortical malformations in humans is traditionally based on the appearance of the cerebral cortex at autopsy. However, advances made in developmental neurobiology in the past decade allow some new interpretations. For example, according to the radial unit hypothesis, the pathogenesis of some cortical malformations can be classified into two major categories. The first category comprises malformations in which the number of radial units in the cortex is reduced, while the number of neurons within each ontogenetic column remains relatively normal. It can be expected that defects in this category result from an early-occurring event that alters the number of proliferative units at the time they are being formed in humans within the first 6 weeks of gestation. Once the number of proliferative units in the ventricular zone are established, albeit in fewer numbers, each unit can produce a normal or even greater number of neurons, which become crowded in the diminished cerebral vesicle. It could be expected that the cortex would have a smaller surface area in spite of a normal or enlarged thickness and the presence of massive neuronal ectopias in the white matter. These features are actually observed in some human malformations, such as lissencephaly and pachygyria (e.g., Volpe, 1987).

The second category consists of malformations in which the initial formation of radial units is not affected, while the number of neurons within ontogenetic columns is reduced. The defect in this category should begin after the 6th fetal week, when the normal complement of proliferative units has already been established. Such malformations can be caused by interference with cell proliferation via intrinsic (genetic) or extrinsic (irradiation or viral infections) factors. Diminished production of neurons in the proliferative units results in fewer neurons within ontogenetic columns, and the cortex is therefore thinner. The number of neurons in ontogenetic columns could also be affected by cell death or by a failure of their migration. In the latter case, some neurons may survive in ectopic positions within the white matter. All of this can be observed in the so-called polymicrogyric brain (e.g., Volpe, 1987). It should be recognized that cortical malformations may have features of only one or the other category, but in practice most show a mixture of both. The proposed classification suggests possible developmental mechanisms by separating defects of unit formation from defects of ontogenetic column formation. In support of the radial unit hypothesis and the concept of a cortical protomap, experimental and neuropathological data reveal that each step (formation of proliferative units, formation of ontogenetic columns, and formation of cytoarchitectonic areas) can be separately affected by genetic defects or by extrinsic factors. It can, therefore, be predicted that genetic alteration as well as mechanical, chemical, or viral lesions of distant but synaptically related structures that result in reduced input to the cortex would affect subsequent developmental events and provide the setting for new cell relationships, the net outcome of which could be the emergence of a unique cytoarchitectonic map.

Of particular relevance for the psychiatric disorders of adolescence may be abnormalities that are associated with the phases of synaptic overproduction and elimination. It is well established that many major psychoses, including schizophrenia, become manifest at the end of ado-lescence and in early adulthood. In addition, a growing number of studies of postmortem tissue samples from schizophrenics and of magnetic resonance images of the brains of living patients have provided a solid factual basis for morphological signs, such as enlarged ventricles, which predate the illness (Weinberger, 1987). The evidence for a genetic predisposition to schizophrenia (e.g., Kety et al., 1968) has naturally led investigators to consider the developmental antecedents of this major psychosis, and several hypotheses have invoked events related to synaptogenesis. For example, Feinberg (1982) proposed that schizophrenia may be caused by a ''fault in programs of synaptic elimination during adolescence.'' More recently, this concept has been elaborated in a computational model, which tests predictions relevant to particular symptoms in schizophrenia (Hoffman and McGlashan, 1993). However, in the absence of systematic data it has been speculated that the defect could be one of either excess pruning or the opposite, that is, failure of the normal pruning mechanisms such as described in this chapter.

More direct evidence for the possibility of excessive pruning comes from the recent studies of noninvasive methods in living patients (Pettegrew et al., 1993; Williamson et al., 1991). In these studies, the structural integrity of prefrontal cortex in drug naive schizophrenics shows excessive elimination of dendrites and axons. Complementing the in vivo studies, Selemon et al. (1994) found that there is a higher density of neurons per unit volume in prefrontal areas of schizophrenics compared with that in controls—a finding compatible with the loss of synaptic neuropil in schizophrenia. Glanz and Lewis (1993) have reported preliminary evidence of reduced synaptophysin labeling in the prefrontal cortex of schizophrenics. These studies indicate a pathological process at work in the various cortical regions of patients—findings that are compatible with a neurodevelopmental perspective. Although these changes occur at inflection points in the synaptogenesis curve, there is no direct evidence that they are causative in nature. It is likely, however, that knowledge of the normal course and mechanisms of synapse formation and the influence of various exogenous and endogenous events upon synapse stability and turnover are essential prerequisites to determining the locus and timing of etiological factors in diseases that affect the cortex and alter cognitive function. This is the ultimate justification for studies in nonhuman primates, where conditions are experimentally controlled and monitored.

References

Ackbarian S, Vinuela A, Kim JJ, et al: Distorted distribution of nicotinamide-adenine dinucleotide phosphate-diaphorase neurons in temporal lobe of schizophrenics implies anomalous cortical development. *Arch Gen Psychiatry* 50:178–187, 1993.

Arimatsu Y, Miyamoto M, Nihonmatsu I, et al: Early regional specification for a molecular neuronal phenotype in the rat neocortex. *Proc Natl Acad Sci USA* 89:8879–8883, 1992.

Barbe MF, Levitt P: Attraction of specific thalamic input by cerebral grafts depends on e molecular identity of the implant. *Proc Natl Acad Sci USA* 89: 3706–3710, 1992.

Barth TM, Stanfield BB: Homotopic, but not heterotopic, fetal cortical transplants can result in functional sparing following neonatal damage to the frontal cortex in rat. *Cereb Cortex* 4:271–278, 1994.

Bloom RE: Advancing a neurodevelopmental origin of schizophrenia. *Arch Gen Psychiatry* 50: 224–227, 1993.

Bolton JS: The exact histological localization of the visual area of the human cerebral cortex. *Philos Trans R Soc Lond Biol* 193:165–205, 1900.

Boulder Committee: Embryonic vertebrate central nervous system. Revised terminology. *Anat Rec* 166:257–261.

Bourgeois J-P, Rakic P: Changing of synaptic density in the primary visual cortex of the rhesus monkey from fetal to adult stage. *J Neurosci* 13: 2801–2820, 1993.

Bourgeois J-P, Jastreboff P, Rakic P: Synaptogenesis in the visual cortex of normal and preterm monkeys: Evidence for intrinsic regulation of synaptic overproduction. *Proc Natl Acad Sci USA* 86: 4297–4301, 1989.

Bourgeois J-P, Goldman-Rakic PS, Rakic P: Synaptogenesis in the prefrontal cortex of rhesus monkey. *Cereb Cortex* 4:78–79, 1994.

Brodmann K: *Vergleichende Localisationsationslehre der Grosshir-hinde.* Leipzig, Barth, 1909.

Brunquell PJ, Popole JH, Horton JC: Sex-linked hereditary bilateral anophthalmos. Pathologic and radiologic correlation. *Arch Ophthalmol* 102:108–113, 1984.

Buffone A, Kim HJ, Puelles L, et al: The mouse DLX-2 (Tes-1) Gbx-2 and Wnt-3 in the embryonic day 12.5 mouse forebrain defines potential transverse and longitudinal segmental boundaries. *Mech Dev* 40:129–140, 1993.

Bugbee NM, Goldman-Rakic PS: Columnar organization of cortico-cortical projections in squirrel and rhesus monkeys: Similarity of column width in species differing in cortical volume. *J Comp Neurol* 220:355–364, 1983.

Cameron RS, Rakic P: Glial cell lineage in the cerebral cortex: Review and synthesis. *Glia* 4: 124–137, 1991.

Cameron RS, Rakic P: Polypeptides that comprise the plasmalemmal microdomain between migrating neuronal and glial cells. *J Neurosci* 14: 3139–3155, 1994.

Caviness VS Jr, Rakic P: Mechanisms of cortical development: A view from mutations in mice. *Annu Rev Neurosci* 1:297–326, 1978.

Changeux J-P: A critical view of neuronal models of learning and memory. In: Anderson P (ed): *Memory Concepts.* Elsevier, Amsterdam. pp. 413–433, 1993.

Chugani HT, Phelps ME, Mazziotta JC: Positron emission tomography study of human brain functional development. *Ann Neurol* 22:487–497, 1987.

Chun JM, Shatz CJ: Interstitial cells of the adult neocortical white matter are the remnant of the early-generated subplate neuron population. *J Comp Neurol* 282:555–569, 1989.

Cohen-Tannoudji M, Babinet C, Wassef M: Early intrinsic regional specification of the mouse somatosensory cortex. *Nature* 368:460–463, 1994.

Conel JL: *The Postnatal Development of the Human Cerebral Cortex I. The Cortex of the Newborn.* Cambridge, MA, Harvard University Press, 1939.

Creutzfeldt OD: Generality of the functional structure of the neocortex. *Naturwissenschaften* 64: 507–517, 1977.

Dubin M, Start LA, Archer SM: A role for action-potential activity in the development of neuronal connections in the kitten retinogeniculate pathway. *J Neurosci* 6:1021–1036, 1986.

Easter S Jr, Purves D, Rakic P: The changing view of neural specificity. *Science* 230:507–511, 1985.

Eccles JC: The cerebral neocortex: A theory of its operation. In: Jones EG, Peters A (eds): *Cerebral Cortex* (Vol 2). New York, Plenum, 1984, pp. 1–36.

Edelman GM: Cell adhesion molecules. *Science* 219:450–457, 1983.

Edelman GM: *Neural Darwinism*. New York, Basic Books, 1987.

Farrant M, Feldmeyer D, Takahashi T, et al: NMDA-receptor channel diversity in the developing cerebellum. *Nature* 368:335–339, 1994.

Feinberg I: Schizophrenia: Caused by fault in programmed synaptic elimination during adolescence? *J Psychiatr Res* 17 (Suppl. 4):319–334, 1982.

Feinberg I, Korssko RL, Heller N: EEG sleep patterns as a function of normal. and pathological aging in man. *J Psychiatr Res* 5:107–144, 1967.

Ferri RT, Levitt P: Cerebral cortical progenitors are fated to produce region-specific neuronal populations. *Cereb Cortex* 3(3):187–198, 1993.

Filimonov IN: Cortical cytoarchitecture general concepts. Classification of the architectonic formations. In: Sarkisov SA, Filimonov IN, Preobrazenskaya NS (eds): *Cytoarchitecture of the Cerebral Cortex in Man*. Moscow, Medgiz, 1949, pp. 11–32.

Flechsig P: *Anatomie des Menschlichen Gehirns und Ruckenmarks auf Myelogenetischer Grundlage*. Thieme, Leipzig, 1920.

Frost DO, Metin C: Introduction of functional retinal projections to the somatosensory system. *Nature* 317:162–164, 1985.

Galaburda AM, Sherman GF, Rosen GD, et al: Developmental dyslexia: Four consecutive patients with cortical abnormalities. *Ann Neurol* 18:222–223, 1985.

Glantz LA: Synaptophysin immunoreactivity is selectively decrease in the prefrontal cortex of schizophrenic subjects. *Soc Neurosci Abstr* 19:201, 1993.

Goldman PS: Neuronal plasticity in primate telencephalon: Anomalous crossed cortico-caudate projections induced by prenatal removal of frontal association. *Science* 202:768–776, 1978.

Goldman PS, Nauta WJH: Columnar organization of association and motor cortex: Autoradiographic evidence for cortico-cortical and commissural columns in the frontal lobe of the newborn rhesus monkey. *Brain Res* 122:369–385, 1977.

Goldman-Rakic PS: Morphological consequences of prenatal injury to the primate brain. *Prog Brain Res* 53:3–19, 1980.

Goldman-Rakic PS: Development and plasticity of primate frontal association cortex. In: Schmitt FO, Worden FG, Dennis SG, et al (eds): *The Organization of the Cerebral Cortex*. Cambridge, MA, MIT Press, 1981a, pp. 69–97.

Goldman-Rakic PS: Prenatal formation of cortical input and development of cytoarchitectonic compartments in the neostriatum of rhesus monkey. *J Neurosci* 1:721–735, 1981b.

Goldman-Rakic PS: Circuitry of primate prefrontal cortex and regulation of behavior by representational memory. In: Mountcastle VB, Plum F, Geiger SR (eds): *Handbook of Physiology* 5, Part 1, Ch 9. 1987a, pp. 373–417.

Goldman-Rakic PS: Development of cortical circuitry and cognitive functions. *Child Dev* 58:642–691, 1987b.

Goldman-Rakic PS: Topography of cognition: Parallel distributed networks in primate association cortex. *Annu Rev Neurosci* 11:137–156, 1988.

Goldman-Rakic PS, Brown RM: Postnatal development of monoamine content and synthesis in the cerebral cortex of rhesus monkeys. *Dev Brain Res* 4:339–349, 1982.

Goldman-Rakic PS, Rakic P: Experimental modification of gyral patterns. In: Geschwind N, Galaburda AM (eds): *Cerebral Dominance: The Biological Foundation*. Cambridge, MA, Harvard University Press, 1984, pp. 179–192.

Gould SJ: *Ontogeny and Phylogeny*. Cambridge, MA, Belknap Press, 1977.

Granger B, LeSurd AM, Rakic P, et al: Tempo of neurogenesis and synaptogenesis in the primate cingulate mesocortex: Comparison with neocortex. *J Comp Neurol*, submitted.

Greenfield PM: Language, tools and brain: the ontogeny and phylogeny of hierarchically organized sequential behavior. *Behav Brain Sci* 14:531–595, 1991.

Hamburger V, Oppenheim RW: Naturally occurring neuronal death in vertebrates. *Neuroscience* 1:39–55, 1982.

Hatten ME, Mason CA: Neuron-astroglia interactions in vitro and in vivo. *Trends Neurosci* 9:168–174, 1986.

Hatten ME, Mason CA: Mechanism of glial-guided neuronal migration in vitro and in vivo. *Experientia* 46:907–916, 1990.

Hebb DO: *The Organization of Behavior*. Wiley, New York, 1949.

His W: *Unserer Koperform und das Physiologishe Problem inrer Enstehung*. Leipzig, Engelman, 1874.

His W: *Die Entwicklung des Monschlichen Gehirns Wahrend der Ersten Monate*. Leipzig, Hirzel, 1904.

Hoffman RE, McGlashan TH: Parallel distributed processing and the emergence of schizophrenic symptoms. *Schizophr Bull* 19:119–140, 1993.

Hubel DH, Wiesel TN, LeVay S: Plasticity of ocular dominance columns in monkey striate cortex. *Philos Trans R Soc Lond Biol* 278:377–409, 1977.

Huttenlocher PR: Synaptic density in human frontal cortex-developmental changes and effects of aging. *Brain Res* 163:195–205, 1979.

Huttenlocher PR, deCourten C: The development of synapses in striate cortex of man. *Hum Neurobiol* 6:1–9, 1987.

Innocenti GM: Growth and reshaping of axons in the establishment of visual connections. *Science* 212:824–827, 1981.

Jacob B, Chugani HT, Vivekanand A, et al: Developmental changes in brain metabolism in sedated rhesus macaques and vervet monkeys revealed by positron emission tomography. *Cereb Cortex*, in press.

Jensen KF, Killackey HP: Subcortical projections from ectopic neocortical neurons. *Proc Natl Acad Sci USA* 81:964–968, 1984.

Johnson J, Van der Kooy D: Protooncogene expression identifies a columnar organization of the ventricular zone. *Proc Natl Acad Sci USA* 86:1066–1070, 1989.

Kaiserman-Abramoff IR, Graybiel AM, Nauta WJH: The thalamic projection to cortical area 17 in a congenitally anophthalmic mouse strain. *Neuroscience* 5:41–52, 1980.

Kennedy H, DeHay C: Cortical specification of mice and men. *Cereb Cortex* 3:171–186, 1993.

Kety SS, Rosenthal D, Wender PH, et al: The types and prevalence of mental illness in biological families of adopted schizophrenics. In: Rosenthal D, Kety SS (eds): *Transmission of Schizophrenia*. Oxford, Pergamon, 1968, pp. 345–362.

Killackey HP: Neocortical expansion: An attempt toward relating phylogeny and ontogeny. *J Cog Neurosci* 2:1–17, 1990.

Komuro H, Rakic P: Specific role of N-type calcium channels in neuronal migration. *Science* 257:806–809, 1992.

Komuro H, Rakic P: Modulation of neuronal migration by NMDA receptors. *Science* 260:95–97, 1993.

Kornack DR, Rakic P: Radial and horizontal deployment of clonally related cells in the primate neocortex: Relationship to distinct mitotic lineages. *Neuron* 15:311–321, 1995.

Kostovic I, Rakic P: Cytology and time of origin

of interstitial neurons in the white matter in infant and adult human and monkey telencephalon. *J Neuron* 9:219–242, 1980.

Kostovic I, Rakic P: Developmental history of transient subplate zone in the visual and somatosensory cortex of the macaque monkey and human brain. *J Comp Neurol* 297:441–470, 1990.

Kuljis RO, Rakic P: Hypercolumns in the monkey visual cortex can develop in the absence of cues from photoreceptors. *Proc Natl Acad Sci USA* 87:5303–5306, 1990.

LaMantia AS, Rakic P: Axon overproduction and elimination in the corpus callosum of the developing rhesus monkey. *J Neurosci* 10:2156–2175, 1990.

LaMantia AS, Rakic P: Axon overproduction and elimination in the anterior commissure of the developing rhesus monkey. *J Comp Neurol* 340:328–336, 1994.

LaMantia MS, Rakic P: Organization and development of the hippocampal commissure in primates: Overproduction and elimination of commissural axons in infant rhesus monkeys. *Dev Brain Res*, submitted, 1995.

Lashley KS, Clark G: The cytoarchitecture of the cerebral cortex of Ateles: A critical examination of cytoarchitectonic studies. *J Comp Neurol* 85:223–305, 1946.

Levitt P: Experimental approaches that reveal principles of cerebral cortical development. In: *The Cognitive Neurosciences*. Cambridge, MA, MIT Press, 1994, pp. 147–163.

Levitt P, Cooper ML, Rakic P: Coexistence of neuronal and glial precursor cells in the cerebral ventricular zone of the fetal monkey: An ultrastructural immunoperoxidase analysis. *J Neurosci* 1:27–39, 1981.

Lidow MS, Rakic P: Postnatal development of monoaminergic neurotransmitter receptors with primate neocortex. *Cereb Cortex* 2:401–415, 1992.

Lidow MS, Rakic P: Unique profiles of α-1, α-2, and β-adrenergic receptors in the developing cortical plate and transient embryonic zones of the rhesus monkey. *J Neurosci* 14:4064–4078, 1994.

Lidow MS, Goldman-Rakic PS, Rakic P: Synchronized overproduction of neurotransmitter receptors in diverse regions of the primate cerebral cortex. *Proc Natl Acad Sci USA* 88:10218–10221, 1991.

Livingstone MS, Hubel DH: Segregation of form, color, movement and depth: Anatomy, physiology and perception. *Science* 240:740–749, 1988.

Lu S, Bogorad LD, Murtha MT, et al: Expression pattern of a mourine homeobox gene, Dbx, displays extreme spatial restriction in embryonic forebrain and spinal cord. *Proc Natl Acad Sci USA* 89:8053–8057, 1992.

Luskin MB, Shatz DJ: Studies of the earliest generated cells of the cat's visual cortex: Cogeneration of subplate and marginal zones. *J Neurosci* 5:1062–1075, 1985.

Luskin MB, Pearlman AL, Sanes JR: Cell lineage in the cerebral cortex of the mouse studied in vivo and in vitro with a recombinant retrovirus. *Neuron* 1:635–647, 1988.

Marin-Padilla M: Dual origin of the mammalian neocortex and evolution of the cortical plate. *Anat Embryol* 152:109–126, 1978.

McConnell SK: Development and decision-making in the mammalian cerebral cortex. *Brain Res Rev* 13:1–23, 1988.

Menezes JRL, Luskin MB: Expression of neuron-specific tubulin defines a novel population in the proliferative layers of the developing telencephalon. *J Neurosci* 14:5399–5416, 1994.

Merzenich MM, Recanzone G, Jenkins WM, et al: Cortical representation plasticity. In: *Neurobiology of Neocortex*. New York, Wiley, 1988, pp. 41–67.

Molliver ME, Kostovic I, Van der Loos H: The

development of synapses in cerebral cortex of the human fetus. *Brain Res* 50:403–407, 1973.

Mountcastle VB: An organizing principle for cerebral function: The unit module and the distributed system. In: Schmitt FO, Worden FG (eds): *The Neurosciences: Fourth Study Program.* Cambridge, MA, MIT Press, 1979, pp. 21–42.

Nakatsuji M, Kadokawa Y, Suemori H: Radial columnar patches in the chimeric cerebral cortex visualized by use of mouse embryonic stem cells expressing b-galactosidase. *Dev Growth Differ* 33: 571–578, 1991.

Nowakowski RS: The mode of inheritance of a defect in lamination in the hippocampus of BALB/c mice. *J Neurogenet* 1:249–258, 1984.

O'Kusky J, Colonnier MA: Laminar analysis of the number of neurons, glia and synapses in the visual cortex (area 17) of the adult macaque monkey. *J Comp Neurol* 210:278–290, 1982.

O'Leary DDM: Do cortical areas emerge from a protocortex? *Trends Neurosci* 12:400–406, 1989.

Olivaria J, Van Sluyters RC: Callosal connections of the posterior neocortex in normal-eyed, congenitally anophthalmic and neonatally enucleated mice. *J Comp Neurol* 230:249–268, 1984.

O'Rourke NA, Dailey ME, Smith SJ, et al: Diverse migratory pathways in the developing cerebral cortex. *Science* 258:299–302, 1992.

Palamini A, Anderman F, Aicardi J, et al: Diffuse cortical dysplasia, or the "double cortex" syndrome. *Neurology* 41:1656–1662, 1991a.

Palamini A, Anderman F, Olier A, et al: Focal neuronal migration disorders and intractable partial epilepsy: Results of surgical treatment. *Ann Neurol* 30:750–757, 1991b.

Parnavelas JG, Barfield JA, Franke E, et al: Separate progenitor cells give rise to pyramidal and nonpyramidal neurons in the rat telencephalon. *Cereb Cortex* 1:463–491, 1991.

Pettegrew JW, Keshavan MJ, Minshew NJ: [31]P nuclear magnetic resonance spectroscopy: Neurodevelopment and schizophrenia. *Schizophr Bull* 19: 35–53, 1993.

Poliakov GI: Structural organisation of the human cerebral cortex during ontogenetic development. In: Sarkisov SA, Filimonov IN, Preobrazenskaya NS (eds): *Cytoarchitectonic of the Cerebral Cortex in Man.* Moscow, Medgiz, 1949, pp. 33–92.

Poliakov GI: Progressive neuron differentiation of the human cerebral cortex in ontogenesis. In: Sarkisov SA, Preobrazenskaya SN (eds): *Development of the Central Nervous System.* Moscow, Medgiz, 1959, pp. 11–26 (in Russian).

Poliakov GI: Development of the cerebral neocortex during the first half of intrauterine life. In: Sarkisov SA (ed): *Development of the Child's Brain.* Leningrad, Medicina, 1965, pp. 22–52 (in Russian).

Proteus MH, Brice EJ, Buffone A, et al: Isolation and characterization of a library of cDNA clones that are preferentially expressed in the embryonic telencephalon. *Neuron* 7:221, 1991.

Purves D: *Body and Brain. A Trophic Theory of Neural Connections.* Cambridge, MA, MIT Press, 1988.

Rakic P: Guidance of neurons migrating to the fetal monkey neocortex. *Brain Res* 33:471–476, 1971.

Rakic P: Mode of cell migration to the superficial layers of fetal monkey neocortex. *J Comp Neurol* 145:61–84, 1972.

Rakic P: Neurons in the monkey visual cortex: Systematic relation between time of origin and eventual disposition. *Science* 183:425–427, 1974.

Rakic P: Timing of major ontogenetic events in the visual cortex of the rhesus monkey. In: Buchwald NA, Brazier N (eds): *Brain Mechanisms in Mental Retardation.* New York, Academic Press, 1975, pp. 3–40.

Rakic P: Prenatal genesis of connections subserving ocular dominance in the rhesus monkey. *Nature* 261:467–471, 1976a.

Rakic P: Differences in the time of origin and in eventual distribution of neurons in areas 17 and 18 of the visual cortex in the rhesus monkey. *Exp Brain Res Suppl* 1:244–248, 1976b.

Rakic P: Prenatal development of the visual system in the rhesus monkey. *Philos Trans R Soc Lond Biol* 278:245–260, 1977.

Rakic P: Neuronal migration and contact interaction in primate telencephalon. *Postgrad Med J* 54: 25–40, 1978.

Rakic P: Genetic and epigenetic determinants of local neuronal circuits in the mammalial central nervous system. In: Schmitt FO, Worden FG (eds): *Neurosciences: Fourth Study Program.* Cambridge, MA, MIT Press, 1980, pp. 109–127.

Rakic P: Neuronal-glial interaction during brain development. *Trends Neurosci* 4:184–187, 1981a.

Rakic P: Development of visual centers in the primate brain depends on binocular competition before birth. *Science* 214:928–931, 1981b.

Rakic P: Geniculo-cortical connections in primates: Normal and experimentally altered development. *Prog Brain Res* 58:393–404, 1983.

Rakic P: Limits of neurogenesis in primates. *Science* 227:154–156, 1985.

Rakic P: Specification of cerebral cortical areas. *Science* 241:170–176, 1988a.

Rakic P: Defects of neuronal migration and pathogenesis of cortical malformations. *Prog Brain Res* 73:15–37, 1988b.

Rakic P: Radial unit hypothesis of cerebral cortical evolution. *Exp Brain Res Suppl* 21:25–43, 1991.

Rakic P: A small step for the cell—A giant leap for mankind: A hypothesis of neocortical expansion during evolution. *Trends Neurosci* 18:383–388,1995.

Rakic P, Kornack DR: Constraints on neurogenesis in adult primate brain: An evolutionary advantage? In: Cuello AC (ed): *Neuronal Cell Death and Repair. Restorative Neurology 6.* Amsterdam, Elsevier, 1993, pp. 257–266.

Rakic P, Lidow M: Distribution and density of neurotransmitter receptors in the absence of retinal input from early embryonic stages. *J Neurosci* 15:2561–2574, 1995.

Rakic P, Riley KP: Overproduction and elimination of retinal axons in the fetal rhesus monkey. *Science* 209:1441–1444,1983a.

Rakic P, Riley KP: Regulation of axori numbers in the primate optic nerve by prenatal binocular competition. *Nature* 305:135–137, 1983b.

Rakic P, Sidman RL: Supravital DNA synthesis in the developing human and mouse brain. *J Neuropathol Exp Neurol* 27:246–276, 1968.

Rakic P, Singer W: *Neurobiology of the Neocortex.* New York, Wiley, 1988.

Rakic P, Stensaas LJ, Sayre EP: Computer-aided three-dimensional reconstruction and quantitative analysis of cells from serial electronmicroscopic images of fetal monkey brain. *Nature* 250:31–34, 1974.

Rakic P, Bourgeois J-P, Eckenhoff ME: Concurrent overproduction of synapses in diverse regions of the primate cerebral cortex. *Science* 232:232–235, 1986.

Rakic P, Suner I, Williams RW: Novel cytoarchitectonic areas induced experimentally within primate striate cortex. *Proc Natl Acad Sci USA* 88: 2083–2087, 1991.

Rakic P, Bourgeois J-P, Goldman-Rakic PS: Synaptic development of the cerebral cortex: Implication for learning, memory, and mental illness. *Prog Brain Res* 102:219–235, 1994a.

Rakic P, Cameron RS, Komuro H: Recognition, adhesion, transmembrane signaling, and cell motility in guided neuronal migration. *Curr Opin Neurobiol* 4:63–69, 1994b.

Rubinstein JLR, Martinez S, Shimamura K, et al: The embryonic vertebrate forebrain: The prosomeric model. *Science* 266:578–580, 1994.

Sanes JR: Analyzing cell lineages with a recombinant retrovirus. *Trends Neurosci* 12:21–28, 1989.

Schachner M, Faissner A, Fischer G: Functional and structural aspects of the cell surface in mammalian nervous system development. In: Edelman GM, Gall WE, Thiery JP (eds): *The Cell in Contact: Adhesions and Junctions as Morphogenetic Determinants.* New York, Wiley, 1985.

Schlagger BL, O'Leary DDM: Potential of visual cortex to develop an array of functional units unique to somatosensory cortex. *Science* 252:1556–1560, 1992.

Schmechel DE, Rakic P: Arrested proliferation of radial glial cells during midgestation in rhesus monkey. *Nature* 227:303–305, 1979.

Schwartz ML, Goldman-Rakic PS: Prenatal specification of callosal connections in fetal monkey. *J Comp Neurol* 307:144–162, 1991.

Schwartz ML, Meinecke DL: Early expression of GABA-containing neurons in the prefrontal visual cortices of rhesus monkeys. *Cereb Cortex* 2:16–37, 1992.

Schwartz ML, Rakic P, Goldman-Rakic PS: Early phenotype of cortical neurons: Evidence that a subclass of migrating neurons have callosal axons. *Proc Natl Acad Sci USA* 88:1354–1358, 1991.

Selemon LD, Rajkowska G, Goldman-Rakic PS: Cytologic abnormalities in area 9 of the schizophrenic cortex. *Soc Neurosci Abstr* 19:367, 1993.

Shatz CJ: Prenatal development of cat's retinogeniculate pathway. *J Neurosci* 3:482–499, 1983.

Shatz CJ: Impulse activity and patterning of connections during CNS development. *Neuron* 5:1–10, 1990.

Shatz CJ, Chun JJM, Luskin MB: The role of the subplate in the development of mammalian telencephalon. In: Peters A, Jones EG (eds): *Cerebral Cortex.* New York, Plenum, 1988, pp. 35–38.

Sherman GF, Galaburda AM, Geschwind N: Cortical anomalies in brains of New Zealand mice: A neuropathologic model of dyslexia. *Proc Natl Acad Sci USA* 82:8072–8074, 1985.

Sidman RL, Rakic P: Neuronal migration with special reference to developing human brain: A review. *Brain Res* 62:1–35, 1973.

Sidman RL, Rakic P: Development of the human central nervous system. In: *Histology and Histopathology of the Nervous System.* Haymaker W, Adams RD (eds): Springfield, IL, Charles C Thomas, 1982, pp. 3–145.

Spelke ES, Vishton P, VonHofsten C: Object perception, object-directed action, and physical knowledge in infancy. In: Gazzaniga M (editor-in-chief): *Cognitive Neurosciences.* Cambridge, MA, MIT Press, 1994, pp. 165–179.

Staindler DA, Cooper NGF, Faissner A: Boundaries defined by adhesion molecules during development of the cerebral cortex. *Dev Biol* 131:407–418, 1989.

Stryker MP, Harris WA: Binocular impulse blockade prevents the formation of ocular dominance columns in cat visual cortex. *J Neurosci* 6: 2117–2133, 1986.

Sur M, Garraghty PE, Roe AW: Experimentally induced visual projections in auditory thalamus and cortex. *Science* 242:1434–1441, 1988.

Szentagothai J: The neuronal network of the cerebral cortex: A functional interpretation. *Prog Brain Res* 201:219–248, 1987.

Takahashi T, Nowakowski RS, Caviness VS: BUdR as an S-phase marker for quantitative studies of cytokinetic behavior in the murine cerebral ventricular zone. *J Neurocytol* 21:183–197, 1992.

Takahashi T, Nowakowski RS, Caviness VS:

Cell cycle parameters and patterns of nuclear movement in the neocortical proliferative zone of the fetal mouse. *J Neurosci* 13:820–833, 1993.

Tan S-S, Breen S: Radial mosaicism of the mouse neocortex revealed by X-irradiation of a A-lacZ transgene. *Nature*, submitted.

Vaccarino FM, Schwartz ML, Hartigan D, et al: Effect of basic fibroblast growth factor on the genesis of excitatory and inhibitory neurons in primary cultures of cells from mammalian telencephalon. *Cereb Cortex*, in press.

Van der Loos H, Dorfl J: Does the skin tell the somatosensory cortex how to construct a map of the periphery. *Neurosci Lett* 7:23–30, 1978.

Volpe JJ: *Neurology of the Newborn* (2nd ed). Philadelphia, Saunders, 1987.

Walsh C, Cepko CL: Clonally related cortical cells show several migration patterns. *Science* 241: 1342–1345, 1988.

Weinberger DR: Implications of normal brain development for the pathogenesis of schizophrenia. *Arch Gen Psychiatry* 44:464–669, 1987.

Williams RW, Herrup K: Control of neuron number. *Annu Rev Neurosci* 278:344–352, 1988.

Williams RW, Ryder K, Rakic P: Emergence of cytoarchitectonic differences between areas 17 and 18 in the developing rhesus monkey. *Abstr Soc Neurosci* 13:1044, 1987.

Williamson P, Drost D, Stainly J, et al: Localized phosphorus 31 magnetic resonance spectroscopy in chronic schizophrenic patients and normal controls. *Arch Gen Psychiatry* 48:578, 1991.

Yakovlev PI, Lecours AR: The myeloarchitectonic cycles of regional maturation of the brain. In: Minkowsky A (ed): *Regional Development of the Brain in Early Life*. Oxford, UK, Blackwell, 1967, pp. 3–70.

Zecevic N, Rakic P: Synaptic density in motor cortex of rhesus monkey during fetal and postnatal life. *Dev Brain Res* 50:11–32, 1989.

Zecevic N, Bourgeois J-P, Rakic P: Changes in synaptic density in motor cortex of rhesus monkey during fetal and postnatal life. *Dev Brain Res* 50: 11–32, 1989.

Zielinski BS, Hendrickson A: Development of synapses in macaque monkey striate cortex. *Vis Neurosci* 8:491–504, 1992.

3 NEUROBIOLOGY OF NEUROPSYCHIATRIC DISORDERS

George M. Anderson, Ph.D., and Donald J. Cohen, M.D.

As advances in basic neuroscience have led to a better understanding of brain functioning, the potential for understanding the alterations that may exist in neuropsychiatric disorders has become increasingly real. Elucidation of causative factors in parkinsonism, Alzheimer's, and other neuropsychiatric disorders as well as the gains in efficacy and specificity of neuropharmacological agents further encourage the notion that the biological bases of childhood neuropsychiatric disorders can be ascertained. Although biological psychiatry is not without its difficulties, and some inherent limitations, the approach holds great promise.

Biological psychiatry has two main purposes: the identification of useful markers of disorders and the determination of etiology. These goals are not mutually exclusive: In most cases, hypotheses concerning etiology serve to direct the search for markers. Markers can be sought that reflect either the state of an illness or the trait of being predisposed toward an illness. State markers are not necessarily genetically influenced and should revert to normal on recovery or remission. They are presumably not related to the most basic etiological alteration but to some aspect of symptom mediation. Trait markers can be considered to be associated in some way with the genetic alteration; they are present before, during, and after illness; and they are present in family members of probands with heritable illness. The association of a trait marker with illness could be coincidental, due to genetic linkage. Although such a marker might be extremely useful for pedigree analysis and gene localization, it would in itself give little or no information as to etiology.

Trait markers may be dichotomous, discrete, or continuous. Much of the work of biological psychiatry has been directed, implicitly or explicitly, toward finding trait markers in continuous variables that have been hypothesized to be related to etiological alterations. Preferably, a marker is easily and reliably measured, with little overlap existing between normal and affected groups. A trait marker would be expected to be useful in diagnosis, subtyping, family and genetic studies, establishing prognosis, and selecting therapy.

The second goal—the elucidation of etiology—holds the promise of cure. Studies of etiology have typically examined several variables related to a neurotransmitter system that has been postulated to be altered or dysfunctional. The goals of this endeavor include the development of more sensitive and specific markers, the use of new, rational interventions, and the determination of protein and genetic alterations.

METHODOLOGY

The strategies employed in biological psychiatry can be grouped into four types: (*a*) measurement of neurotransmitters, metabolites, and neurotransmitter-related enzymes; (*b*) measurement of neurotransmitter receptors (number, affinity, and functioning); (*c*) neuroendocrine studies; and (*d*) brain imaging studies.

The neurotransmitters and their metabolites have been measured in postmortem brain tissue, cerebrospinal fluid (CSF), plasma and blood elements, and urine. Enzymes have been determined in the brain, CSF, and blood, while receptor measurements have been carried out with brain and blood specimens. Neuroendocrine studies typically measure blood hormone concentrations after administration of releasing or inhibitory agents. Brain-imaging studies have employed computed tomography (CT), magnetic resonance imaging (MRI), positron emission tomography (PET), and single-photon emission computed tomography (SPECT) to examine neuroanatomical structure, blood flow, and receptor binding. With all approaches, a critical issue is to what extent the measure provides information about the central neurotransmitter system of interest. This is true for measurements made in the brain and becomes even more problematic when measurements are made in peripheral fluids and tissue. The degree of correlation between a particular measure and central neurotransmitter functioning is difficult to assess and depends upon the specific measure and system under study.

Neurotransmitter Systems

Several neurotransmitters have been hypothesized to be involved in childhood neuropsychiatric disorders (Cohen and Young, 1977; Rasmusson et al., 1990; Rogeness et al., 1992; Young et al., 1983, 1984). Most extensively studied have been the three monoamine transmitters, serotonin (5-hydroxytryptamine, or 5-HT), dopamine (DA), and norepinephrine (NE). Other systems studied include opioid peptides, γ-aminobutyric acid (GABA), and acetylcholine (ACh). The emphasis on monoamines has been a result of both the importance of these systems in mediating behavioral phenomena and the marked effects of pharmacological agents known to affect monoamine functioning.

The metabolism of serotonin (5-HT) is depicted in Figure 3.1. Interest in central 5-HT functioning derives from 5-HT's important role in processes as diverse and important as sleep, mood, appetite, perception, and hormone secretion. Serotonin is produced after hydroxylation and decarboxylation of the essential amino acid tryptophan. Cell bodies of 5-HT-containing neurons are located in the raphe nuclei of the hindbrain and project to nearly all areas of the central nervous system (Green, 1988; Iverson and Iverson, 1981).

The metabolism of the catecholamines, NE and DA, is shown in Figure 3.2. DA is synthesized from tyrosine, also after hydroxylation and

TRYPTOPHAN

Tryptophan Hydroxylase

5-HYDROXYTRYPTOPHAN
(5-HTP)

L-Aromatic Amino Acid
Decarboxylase (AADC)

5-HYDROXYTRYPTAMINE
(5-HT) (SEROTONIN)

Monoamine Oxidase (MAO)

5-HYDROXYINDOLEACETIC
ACID
(5-HIAA)

Figure 3.1. Synthesis and catabolism of the indolamine neurotransmitter serotonin.

decarboxylation, and is found in highest concentration in the midbrain, although extensive cortical projections also occur. DA has been shown to be critical in reward, modulating movement, and in cognition (Iverson and Alpert, 1982; Moore and Bloom, 1978; Randrup and Munkvad, 1974). NE is produced from DA by the action of the enzyme dopamine β-hydroxylase (DBH). Nearly all NE-containing neurons project from the locus ceruleus and innervate midbrain and cortical areas. Stress responses, central and peripheral arousal, and learning and memory are all critically modulated by noradrenergic neurons (Amaral and Sinnamon, 1977; Iverson and Iverson, 1981). The three monoamine systems are highly functionally interrelated, making direct connections as well as often simultaneously modulating other transmitter systems.

Assessment of Neurotransmitter Functioning

Some general considerations regarding the various sample types, as well as specific advantages and limitations of specific measures, need to be kept in mind when designing and evaluating neurobiological studies of neuropsychiatric disorders.

POSTMORTEM BRAIN

Analysis of postmortem brain tissue allow the most direct access to the systems of interest. One can measure levels of neurotransmitters, their precursors and metabolites, associated enzymes (both synthetic and catabolic), reuptake sites, and presynaptic and postsynaptic receptor

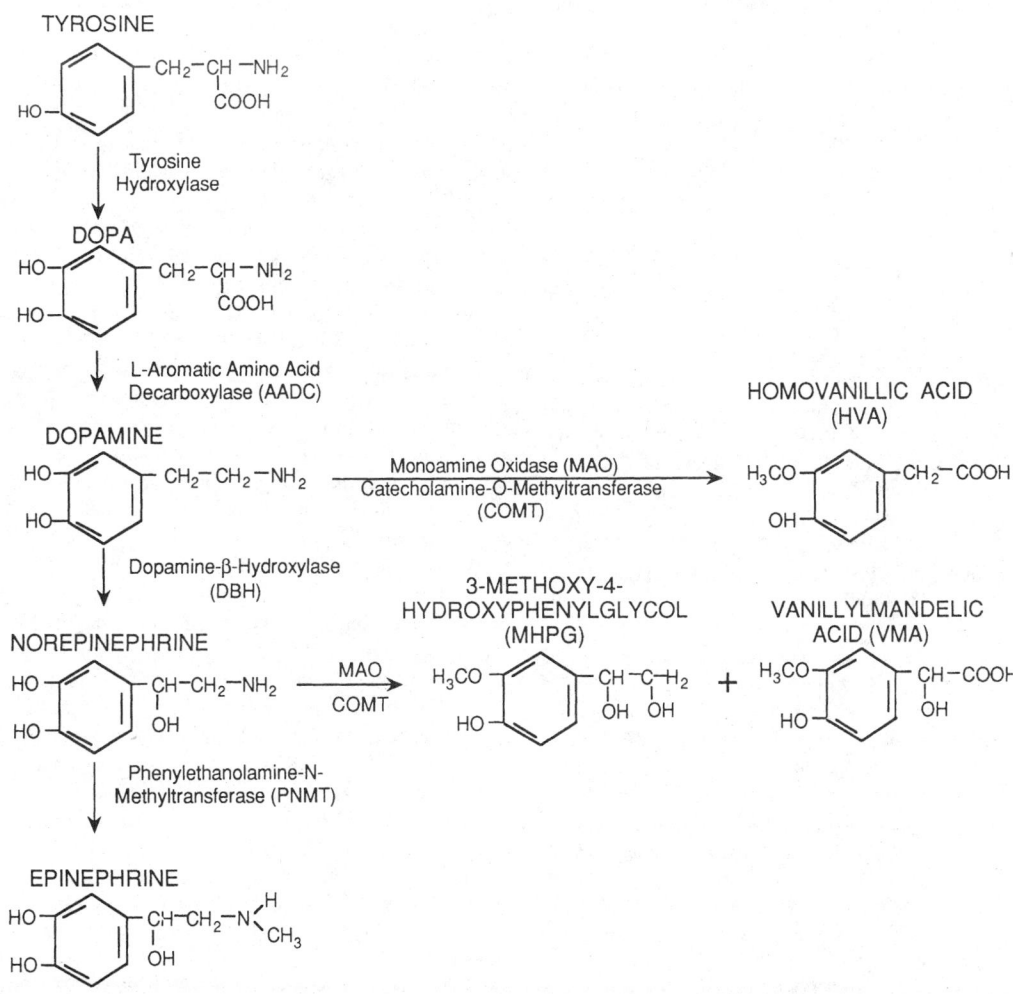

Figure 3.2. Synthesis and catabolism of the catecholamine neurotransmitters norepinephrine and dopamine.

sites. This approach has been extensively employed in the study of such neuropsychiatric disorders as Alzheimer's disease, Parkinson's disease, and Huntington's disease, as well as schizophrenia and depression (Arai et al., 1984; Korpi et al., 1986; Lee et al., 1978). The anatomical resolution and the wide range of neurotransmitter-related analytes have made postmortem studies of paramount importance. Yet there are some disadvantages inherent in this approach, including postmortem degradation, subject recruitment, control matching, and the fundamental limitation arising from an inability to measure functionality (Perry and Perry, 1983).

CEREBROSPINAL FLUID

Measurements of transmitters, metabolites, and enzymes in CSF have been considered to be the next best thing to postmortem analyses. Although a number of the compounds measured in CSF have been shown to be derived predominantly from the brain, other analytes are thought to originate from spinal cord metabolism or to diffuse into the CSF from the blood (Garelis et al., 1974). Even when compounds are solely of brain origin, lumbar CSF concentrations are affected by clearance rates. The greatest limitation of CSF measures is their failure to provide information regarding anatomical localization. A resultant practical shortcoming is that only global or marked changes in brain neurochemistry can be expected to be detected.

The DA metabolite homovanillic acid (HVA) has been extensively assayed in CSF and is thought to be substantially derived from brain metabolism of DA (Elchisak et al., 1978; Elsworth et al., 1987; Garelis and Sourkes, 1973; Sourkes, 1973). However, CSF levels of NE and the NE metabolite 3-methoxy-4-hydroxyphenylglycol (MHPG) appear to primarily reflect NE metabolism in the spinal cord (Kopin et al., 1983; Ziegler et al., 1977). Similarly, the 5-HT metabolite 5-hydroxyindoleacetic acid (5-HIAA) is apparently predominantly of spinal cord origin (Bulat, 1977; Moir et al., 1970; Wier et al., 1973). It is often unclear to what extent peptides and amino acids measured in lumbar CSF reflect brain, spinal cord, and peripheral metabolism.

BLOOD AND URINE

Measurements of monoamine metabolites in blood and urine have been performed widely; however, the issue of peripheral versus central contribution is problematic. It is clear that the vast majority of plasma and urine 5-HIAA is of peripheral origin, arising from the catabolism of 5-HT produced in the enterochromaffin cells of the intestine (Udenfriend et al., 1956). This has limited the utility of measurements of blood and urine 5-HIAA levels to those situations where the rate of gut 5-HT synthesis is of interest. Urine 5-HT has been rarely measured, as it too probably reflects only gut synthesis of 5-HT. Blood levels of 5-HT have been more frequently studied due to 5-HT's localization in platelets. Similarities between platelet and neuronal uptake, storage, and release of 5-HT have made the platelet of special interest (DePrada et al., 1988; Pletscher, 1988; Sneddon, 1973). Findings in autism have further stimulated research in the area.

Plasma and urine HVA concentrations have been widely determined in an attempt to assess central DA functioning (Bowers, 1991). Recent studies have attempted to ascertain the central contribution to plasma (and urine) levels. Known sources of peripheral DA and HVA include the sympathetic nervous system, the adrenal glands, and the kidney. When peripheral DA synthesis and metabolism are inhibited with debrisoquin, a peripherally acting monoamine oxidase inhibitor and neuronal blocker, plasma and urine HVA levels decrease to about 50% of baseline, indicating that at least half of the measured HVA originates in the periphery (Maas et al., 1985; Riddle et al., 1986). Changes in the norepinephrine metabolite MHPG after debrisoquin administration are even more marked, indicating that less than 25% of plasma or urine MHPG is of central origin (Kopin et al., 1988). Investigators have also measured plasma and urine levels of the catecholamines themselves. It is clear that all plasma and urine NE arises from the adrenal glands and

sympathetic nervous system. However, the tight coupling between the central norepinephrine neurons and the sympathetic nervous systems suggests that plasma and urine NE might still be useful indices of central noradrenergic functioning. Unfortunately, clearance and catabolism affect the measured levels of the monoamines and their metabolites. Urine measurements can actually offer advantages in that differences in clearance are less a problem than with plasma. Urine samples can be more easily obtained, although it is difficult to observe acute (less than 1–2-hour) changes.

Neurochemical analyses of blood and urine have been made both in unperturbed (baseline) situations and after administration of centrally acting agents; the latter approach bears strong resemblance to neuroendocrine challenge studies. These neuroendocrine studies have attempted to assess central 5-HT, DA, NE, and opioid functioning by determining plasma levels of growth hormone, prolactin, cortisol, and other hormones after administration of challenge agents. A number of factors tend to confound the neuroendocrine approach, including pulsatile and fluctuating release, poor specificity of the challenge agents, and the difficulty in relating findings in the hypothalamus, pituitary, or adrenal gland (or thyroid gland) to etiology.

The numbers and affinities of a range of neurotransmitter receptors have been measured on blood elements. Platelet serotonergic ($5-HT_2$) and adrenergic (α_2) receptors, platelet 5-HT uptake sites (imipramine-binding sites), and white blood cell adrenergic (β) receptor sites have been measured using radioactively labeled ligands. The measurement of receptor function has been less prevalent, although a host of studies have examined the platelet uptake of tritiated 5-HT and binding of reuptake inhibitors.

CLINICAL STUDIES

Neurobiology of Normal Development

Many recent exciting advances have led to a better picture of neuronal development, both at the cellular level and in relation to cell-cell interactions and complex circuit assembly. Animal studies have examined the ontogeny of neurotransmitter synthesis, storage, release, and uptake, as well as receptor number, affinity, and coupling. Work on the developing primate brain has been most informative as to what changes may be occurring during different periods of childhood (Kandel and Schwartz, 1981; Purves and Litchman, 1986; Rakic, 1988; Shepherd, 1983).

Studies of neurotransmitter ontogeny in psychiatrically normal children have predominantly dealt with the measurement of neurotransmitters, metabolites, and associated enzymes in CSF, blood, and urine. These studies have helped to establish normative ranges for contrasting with values seen in neuropsychiatric disorders and have also served to point out periods of change and to allow the validity of animal models to be assessed.

A large study of CSF monoamine precursors and metabolites in children treated for leukemia found large decreases in HVA and 5-HIAA over childhood and adolescence. Mean values for HVA in subjects ages 2–5, 6–11, and 12–17 years decreased from 92 to 62 to 44 ng/ml, respectively, while 5-HIAA declined from 30 to 21 to 17 ng/ml, respectively. Changes in the precursors were substantially less. The multiple lumbar punctures performed allowed an estimation of mean intraindividual variation of 20–25% to be made (Riddle et al., 1986). The ontogenetic declines in HVA and 5-HIAA levels have also been observed in developing (12–42-day-old) rat pups. Changes in CSF metabolite levels tended to parallel declining brain metabolite levels, while levels of total brain monoamine levels (DA and 5-HT) increased (Shaywitz et al., 1985). Studies of CSF metabolite ontogeny in humans have been extended to the neonatal period, where even higher levels of 5-HIAA, HVA, tryptophan, and tyrosine are seen (Anderson et al., 1985). Mean levels of 5-HIAA and HVA in newborns were 143 and 184 ng/ml, respectively, substantially higher than in the 2–5-year-old period. Neonatal levels of MHPG were also significantly higher (27 ng/ml) than those seen in 2–5-year-olds, although unlike 5-HIAA and HVA, MHPG levels did not decline further after the period of 2–5 years of age. Another compound with an early, rapid maturational decline is the other DA metabolite, 3,4-dihydrophenylacetic acid (DOPAC) (Anderson et al., 1988). Although the causes of the maturational declines are not clear, the dissociation between the ontogenies of DOPAC (with its early, rapid decline) and HVA (with its more gradual decline) would indicate that transport and clearance changes are not major determinants.

These studies of normal neurochemical ontogeny provide a context when examining levels seen in childhood disorders and after neonatal drug exposure. In studies of CSF levels of monoamine and metabolites in neonates exposed prenatally to cocaine, signficantly lower levels of the dopamine metabolite HVA were seen in the exposed infants (Needlman et al., 1993). Further studies are needed to see whether this decrease persists over the first months and years of life. A short lasting decrease may be due simply to an acute pharmacological effect; longer lasting reductions in HVA would probably be a result of reductions in dopamine innervation.

Blood concentrations and urinary excretion rates of the catecholamines and their metabolites are generally observed to decline over childhood (Dalmaz and Peyrin, 1982; Gitlow et al., 1968). This is apparently due both to decreasing synthesis and to increasing activity of the catabolic enzymes monoamine oxidase (MAO) and catechol-*O*-methyltransferase (COMT) (Young et al., 1984). It is not clear whether the decreasing synthesis corresponds to decreasing functional release. Definite statements about relative central and peripheral contributions to plasma or urine catecholamine metabolite levels cannot be made, although the situation in childhood does not appear to be more favorable than in adulthood. Blood levels of 5-HT have been observed to decrease with age; however, when concentrations are expressed as $ng/10^9$ platelets, levels are constant down to the youngest subjects examined (neonates) (Anderson et al., 1987). This suggests that platelet uptake and storage of 5-HT are fully developed in early childhood.

Attention Deficit Hyperactivity Disorder

The symptomatology of attention deficit hyperactivity disorder (ADHD) includes inattention, distractibility, and impulsivity, with or without hyperactivity (Carey, 1988; Shaywitz and Shaywitz, 1982, 1992). Early work focused on the presence of this behavioral pattern in children who had suffered from encephalitis or brain damage. Although the idea that there existed some sort of minimal brain damage (MBD) led to the use of MBD as a diagnostic category, no consistent or specific abnormality was demonstrated. The behavioral sequelae of encephalitis along with the remarkable effects of stimulants on ADHD children have led to a long-standing and continuing interest in the role of DA. Family and twin studies have supported the idea that there exists an inherited biological component to some forms of the disorder (Pauls et al., 1983).

A large number of neurobiological studies have been carried out; the majority involve the measurement of neurotransmitter metabolites in blood and urine, either at baseline or after pharmacological perturbation. Several neuroendocrine challenges have been performed, while there are only a limited number of studies involving receptor assessment (Hunt et al., 1982; Shekim et al., 1994) or brain-imaging (Geidd et al., 1994; Hynd et al., 1991, 1993; Lou et al., 1989, 1990).

SEROTONIN

Interest in a role for 5-HT in ADHD was stimulated by early reports of decreased platelet 5-HT in affected children. Subsequent studies have not replicated this finding and have found normal levels of platelet and urine 5-HIAA (Zametkin and Rapoport, 1987a), as well as normal numbers and affinities of platelet imipramine-binding sites in ADHD subjects (Weizman et al., 1988). In addition, studies of CSF 5-HIAA have not found differences between ADHD and control subjects. On the whole, the neurochemical research and the minimal treatment response to serotonergic agents have tended to make it seem less likely that a 5-HT alteration is etiologic. However, as a recent review makes clear, the role of 5-HT in disruptive behaviors deserves further consideration (Anderson, 1993; Zubieta and Alessi, 1993).

DOPAMINE/NOREPINEPHRINE

The two catecholamines have been extensively studied in ADHD; most of the work has been prompted by neuropharmacological observations. The ameliorative effects of the stimulants methylphenidate, amphetamine, and pemoline have strongly implicated DA. However, agents thought to be specific for NE, such as clonidine and desipramine, can also be of benefit (Biederman et al., 1986; Donnelly et al., 1986; Zametkin and Rapoport, 1987b), and the stimulants also tend to enhance NE functioning. The hypodopaminergic hypothesis also has been questioned due to the relatively benign or slightly beneficial effects of DA blockers; a complex role for noradrenergic involvement is suggested by the beneficial effects of desmethylimipramine and clonidine, drugs that might be expected to produce opposite effects on NE functioning. Clinical studies of more specific adrenergic agents such as guanfacine (Arnsten and Contant, 1992) should provide a better understanding of the role of NE in ADHD-related behaviors.

Although the neurochemical evidence is extensive, it fails to conclusively support either NE or DA involvement (Zametkin and Rapoport, 1987a). The limited CSF data suggest a possible lowering of HVA in ADHD. Baseline measurements of NE in serum, MHPG in plasma, HVA in plasma and urine, and DA in urine have not revealed differences between ADHD and control subjects. The data with respect to MHPG and NE in urine are less consistent, with MHPG excretion, for instance, being reported to be decreased, unchanged, or increased in ADHD (Baker et al., 1993; Zametkin and Rapoport, 1987a). Platelet levels of MAO activity have been reported to be unchanged or decreased in ADHD, and platelet α_2-adrenergic receptors are reported to be lower in ADHD (Shekim et al., 1994), while serum DBH was similar in ADHD and control subjects. Urine or plasma levels of NE, MHPG, DA, and HVA have also been measured after administration of stimulants or tricyclic antidepressants. Although neurochemical changes are observed after the drug treatment (e.g., lowered MHPG with desipramine, increased NE with yohimbine), no conclusive differences in neurochemical response to the agents have been shown between ADHD and control subjects. Neuroendocrine studies in ADHD are limited and provide no definite information regarding possible group differences.

In summary, the neurochemical and neuroendocrine data are inconclusive, although neuropharmacological evidence is fairly suggestive of alterations in either (or both) dopaminergic or noradrenergic functioning. The general difficulty regarding nosology and syndrome definition has probably contributed to the lack of clarity, as has the fact that central DA and NE systems are highly interrelated. One line of evidence that strongly supports a focus on dopaminergic functioning is recent work on cerebral blood flow. In SPECT imaging studies using ^{133}Xe to measure regional cerebral blood flow, hypoperfusion was observed in striatal regions in ADHD children (Lou et al., 1989, 1990). The hypoperfusion is presumed to reflect reduced metabolism and neuronal activity in the striatum. The low perfusion was partially reversed after administration of methylphenidate; both the neuroanatomical and neuropharmacological data suggest decreased dopamine functioning. This is consistent with an animal model for ADHD produced by 6-hydroxydopamine treatment of neonatal rat pups (Lipton et al., 1980; Shaywitz et al., 1976). Recent imaging studies have also observed decreased corpus callosum volumes (Geidd et al., 1994; Hynd et al., 1991) and decreased caudate asymmetry (Hynd et al., 1993) in ADHD subjects. Further imaging research employing other measures of cerebral metabolism and dopaminergic-specific agents should be informative. Finally, the lack of postmortem data in ADHD, somewhat surprising given the high incidence of the disorder, should be remedied so that a wide range of DA-related (and NE-related) aspects of brain functioning can be addressed.

Autism

Autism is a pervasive developmental disorder with disturbances in social relations, language, and communication (Cohen and Donnellan, 1987). The three monoamine transmitters have been well studied in autistic children, and some work has also been carried out in relation to the opioid transmitters.

NOREPINEPHRINE

Apparent disturbances in arousal and attention have suggested possible involvement of altered noradrenergic functioning. Studies of NE, NE metabolite levels, and NE-related enzymes have in general found similar levels and activities in autistic and control groups (Anderson, 1987). Two reports of CSF concentrations of MHPG in autistic and control subjects were unremarkable. Levels of MHPG in plasma and urine also do not appear to be altered in autism. Although increased plasma NE and decreased urine NE have been reported in autism, more recent research has found normal urinary NE, as well as normal levels of MHPG and the peripheral metabolite vanillylmandelic acid (VMA) in autism (Minderaa et al., 1994). Study of the catechol-related enzymes DBH, COMT, and MAO has not been conclusive, as variable findings have been reported (Anderson, 1987). One can tentatively conclude, based on CSF MHPG measurements and the more recent studies of plasma or urine NE, MHPG, and VMA, that basal functioning of both central and peripheral noradrenergic systems are not greatly altered in autism. Specific or local alterations in noradrenaline neural transmission cannot, however, be ruled out.

DOPAMINE

A case for altered DA functioning in autism can be made, based on its clear role in mediating motoric disturbances (e.g., stereotypies) and the observation that DA blockers are effective in treating some aspects of autism. The majority of relevant neurochemical studies have examined levels of HVA (Anderson, 1987). The concentration of HVA in CSF has been reported to be slightly decreased, apparently normal, or significantly (approximately 50%) increased in autism. The most recent study, controls selected from patients undergoing myelography, did not find any difference between autistic and control subjects (Narayan et al., 1993). Measurements of HVA in urine have been in disagreement, with some groups reporting increased excretion and others reporting normal excretion in autism. The only study of plasma HVA reported similar levels in autistic and control subjects (Minderaa et al., 1989). Other relevant measures include urinary DA, reportedly normal in autism, and plasma prolactin, which also has been reported to be normal in autistic subjects (McBride et al., 1989; Minderaa et al., 1989). To summarize, the majority of studies report normal DA metabolism and normal baseline levels of prolactin, a hormone under strong inhibitory control by the tuberoinfundibular DA system. The bulk of the studies suggest that central dopaminergic functioning, to the extent it can be assessed by the measures employed, is normal in autism.

SEROTONIN

Initial interest in a role for 5-HT in autism stemmed in part from the powerful effects of serotonergic agents, such as lysergic acid diethylamide, on perception. Research in the area was further stimulated by, and has continued to evolve around, the early studies of Freedman of elevated 5-HT in blood of autistic children (Hanley et al., 1977; Schain and Freedman, 1961). Relatively recent reports of the presence of 5-HT receptor antibodies in the CSF of autistic patients (Todd and Ciaranello, 1985) and of beneficial effects after treatments with the serotonergic agent fenfluramine (Campbell, 1988; Ritvo et al., 1986) also heightened interest in the role of 5-HT in autism. At this time, it should be pointed out that careful follow-up studies have not replicated either the autoantibody finding (Yuwiler et al., 1992) or the early reports of

fenfluramine's benefits (Leventhal et al., 1993; Stern et al., 1990; Varley and Holm, 1990).

Although most of the 5-HT-related research has focused on the hyperserotonemia of autism, a number of studies of CSF 5-HIAA and several neuroendocrinological studies of central 5-HT functioning have been reported (Anderson, 1987; Anderson and Hoshino, 1987). CSF studies are in general agreement that few or no differences exist between autistic and control groups' mean levels of 5-HIAA (see Anderson, 1994, for overview). Two neuroendocrine studies have involved the measurement of growth hormone, prolactin, or cortisol after challenge with either fenfluramine (McBride et al., 1989) or the 5-HT precursor 5-hydroxytryptophan (5-HTP) (Hoshino et al., 1984). Both studies report a lowering or blunting of the prolactin response to the serotonergic challenge, suggesting a possible alteration in central 5-HT functioning either presynaptically or postsynaptically.

The bulk of the 5-HT-related studies directly deal with, or can be related to, the characterization or elucidation of the hyperserotonemia of autism (Anderson et al., 1990). The basic finding of elevated platelet 5-HT is robust and well replicated. Increased levels are observed regardless of whether concentrations are expressed as amount per volume of blood (e.g., nanograms per milliliter) or as amount per number of platelets (nanograms per 10^9 platelets); in addition, platelet counts and size distribution have been reported to be normal in autism. Although most studies have measured total whole blood 5-HT, the several studies that assayed 5-HT in isolated platelets also observed increased group means in autistic subjects. This is certainly expected, given that nearly all (>99%) of blood 5-HT is found sequestered in the platelets.

Although the basic finding of a group mean increase of typically 50% in autistic subjects is well established, the relationship of blood 5-HT to the behavioral aspects of autism and the distribution of the measure in the autistic group are not clear. Serotonin levels have not been consistently correlated with degree of mental retardation or other symptomatology. In a group of 21 well-studied, unmedicated autistic individuals, the distribution of blood 5-HT levels was apparently normal, suggesting that the group mean increase was not due to a subgroup of hyperserotonemic individuals (Anderson et al., 1987). The possibility of a multimodal distribution cannot be ruled out, however, given the size of the group examined.

Unfortunately, although the typical group mean increase observed is relatively robust, the large degree of overlap with the normal population has prevented the use of blood 5-HT levels in screening or diagnosis of autism. Numerous investigators have been intrigued, however, by the possibility of discovering the cause(s) of the elevation (Anderson et al., 1990; Hanley et al., 1977; Young et al., 1982; Yuwiler et al., 1985). It has been hoped that understanding of the mechanism of hyperserotonemia would lead to the development of more specific and useful markers, elucidation of the central nervous system abnormality, and useful approaches to the treatment of the condition.

Two main possibilities have been considered as potential causes of the hyperserotonemia: (a) increased exposure of the platelets to free 5-HT as a result of either decreased catabolism or increased synthesis of 5-HT and (b) altered platelet handling of 5-HT. The issue of decreased catabolism of 5-HT has been examined by measurements of platelet MAO activity and by measuring monoamine substrates and metabolites. These studies have strongly suggested that MAO activity, and hence 5-HT catabolism, is not altered in autism (Anderson, 1990). The normal excretion rates observed for 5-HIAA in autistic subjects in most, but not all, studies also strongly indicate that 5-HT synthesis is not increased in autism.

While these data strongly suggest that 5-HT metabolism is unaltered in autism, they do not definitely indicate whether or not the circulating platelet is exposed to increased levels of 5-HT. This issue can be addressed most directly by determining plasma free levels of 5-HT. When high performance liquid chromatography (HPLC) was used to determine platelet-poor plasma 5-HT levels in autistic subjects, the levels were similar to those seen in normal controls (Cooke et al., 1988). Urinary excretion rates for 5-HT in autistic subjects have also been measured, and the group mean was found to be similar to or slightly lower than that seen for normal subjects (Anderson et al., 1989). These more direct measures of plasma 5-HT levels, as well as the evidence regarding 5-HT metabolism, indicate that the platelet is not exposed to increased concentrations of 5-HT. This, in turn, strongly implies that the platelet's handling of 5-HT is altered in autism. Accumulated evidence warrants focusing research on platelet uptake, storage, and release of 5-HT.

Despite work in a number of laboratories, no consensus has been reached concerning relative rates of 5-HT uptake by platelets from autistic and normal subjects. Rates in autistic individuals have been reported to be higher than, similar to, and lower than those in normal subjects (Anderson et al., 1990). The studies have been more consistent in not finding differences in the affinities for uptake in the two groups. Researchers have also examined the number (B_{max}) and affinity (K_d) of the platelet imipramine-binding sites in autistic and normal individuals (Anderson et al., 1984; Weizman et al., 1987). In neither study were significant group differences seen in either measure of imipramine binding, which is now thought to occur directly at the plasma membrane 5-HT uptake site (Humphreys et al., 1988). The question of altered efflux has been studied in some detail after an initial report indicated that platelets from autistic subjects have a greater efflux of preloaded tritiated 5-HT during in vitro incubation. In a multicenter study, the consensus was that autistic and normal groups had similar mean efflux rates (Boullin et al., 1982).

A study by Safai-Kutti et al. (1985) addressed the question of in vivo platelet secretion by measuring plasma levels of β-thromboglobulin (BTG) and platelet factor 4 (PF4), two platelet-specific secretory proteins found in platelet α-granules. Plasma levels of these two proteins are considered to be indicative of the amount of in vivo platelet activation and secretion. They also determined bleeding times, a measure of in vivo platelet function. The autistic group was observed to have substantially lower mean plasma levels of BTG and PF4, as well as increased bleeding times, suggesting that the platelets of the autistic subjects were less responsive to physiological stimulation. McBride et al. (1989) have examined the 5-HT$_2$ receptor-mediated augmentation of adenosine diphosphate (ADP)-induced platelet aggregation and found lower 5-HT augmentation in the autistic group than in the normal subjects. In addition to the blunted augmentation response, the autistic group had lower numbers (B_{max}) of 5-HT$_2$ receptors detected by iodinated lysergic acid diethylamide binding. Interestingly, there was an inverse correlation between 5-HT augmentation and platelet 5-HT levels, with the less-responsive platelets having a higher-5-HT content.

The identification of the platelet alteration responsible for the hyperserotonemia of autism should prove useful in several ways. It would be expected that assessment of the altered function would provide a marker with less overlap with the normal population than the multidetermined measure of blood 5-HT. Determination of the specific protein(s) involved should lead directly to gene probes and chromosomal location. This, in turn, should prove useful in neonatal screening, subtyping, and more powerful genetic and family studies. Work of this sort might also allow early intervention and improved treatment. Finally, characterization of the physiological alteration would provide a basis for focusing studies of brain neurochemistry and should, as well, suggest modes of neuropharmacological intervention. The confidence that one can have in the basic finding of hyperserotonemia in autism and the potential benefits to be derived from its explication make further research in this area of interest.

OTHER STUDIES

Although there has been considerable speculation regarding a role for opioid peptides in autism and related behaviors (Chamberlain and Herman, 1990; Panksepp et al., 1980), studies of plasma levels of opioid peptides have not revealed consistent or replicated differences (Anderson and Hoshino, 1987; Sandman, 1992), and studies with opioid antago-

nists are not conclusive. Two studies of CSF endorphins have found increased levels in the CSF of autistic individuals (Gillberg et al., 1985; Ross et al., 1987), and it should be mentioned that plasma endorphins are not centrally derived but rather can be considered peripheral stress hormones.

Imaging studies have reported a number of intriguing findings in at least a portion of autistic subjects. CT scan studies suggest ventricular enlargement is present in some autistic subjects (Campbell et al., 1982; Gillberg and Svendsen, 1983); MRI studies have reported ventricular enlargement and basal ganglia abnormalities (Gaffney and Tsai, 1987), as well as hypoplasia of the vermis of the cerebellum (Courchesne et al., 1988). Neuropathological studies have found changes in the limbic system and cerebellum (Bauman and Kemper, 1984; Ritvo et al., 1986), while PET scans using [^{19}F]fluorodeoxyglucose to assess local brain metabolism have indicated increased temporal lobe metabolism (Rumsey et al., 1985). Recent imaging studies have not lent much support to the idea that ventricular enlargement is often present or that consistent morphological changes are present in specific brain areas (see Minshew and Dombrowski, 1994).

Tourette's Disorder

Tourette's disorder is a persistent familial neuropsychiatric disorder characterized by multiple motor and phonic tics that tend to wax and wane in severity (Chappell et al., 1990; Leckman et al., 1987; Shapiro et al., 1988). Knowledge of the disorder has grown dramatically in the past 10–20 years; a clearer picture of the clinical phenomena and an increased awareness of the disorder have allowed better diagnosis and more systematic neurobiological research. Neuroanatomical and neuropharmacological considerations have prompted a number of neurochemical studies with a focus on the monoamines DA, 5-HT, and NE (Kurlan, 1992; Leckman et al., 1994).

DOPAMINE

A role for DA is suggested by the amelioration of tics by neuroleptics, the exacerbation of symptomatology after administration of stimulants, and the importance of DA pathways in mediating motoric behavior. The measurement of HVA in CSF has not revealed consistent differences between mean levels in Tourette's and control groups. Only limited data are available comparing plasma or urine levels of HVA; however, group differences have not been apparent. Studies of postmortem brain from a small number of Tourette's patients have given conflicting results. Singer and colleagues (1991) have found increased densities of the dopamine transporter in basal ganglia regions and have suggested that the increased densities are a reflection of increased dopamine innervation within the striatum. However, observations of the normal striatal levels of dopamine, homovanillic acid, and tyrosine hydroxylase do not support this idea (Anderson et al., 1992).

The notion that hypersensitive central DA receptors may be etiological in Tourette's has prompted attempts at receptor modulation by administration of dopaminergic agents (Friedhoff, 1982). Other than the observation of normal baseline plasma prolactin levels, little neuroendocrinological assessment of central DA receptors has been performed. In a PET study of [^{11}C]-3-N-methylspiperone binding in seven individuals with Tourette's disorder, the DA receptor (D$_2$) number appeared to be normal (Singer et al., 1985). Similarly, in a recent PE study of DA turnover and ^{11}C-raclopride binding, no striatal alterations were seen in Tourette's subjects (Turjanski et al., 1994).

NOREPINEPHRINE

The importance of noradrenergic projections from the locus ceruleus in controlling states of arousal, as well as reports of symptom amelioration after treatment with the α_2-agonist clonidine (Leckman et al., 1985, 1991), are suggestive evidence for altered noradrenergic functioning in Tourette's disorder. Measurements of NE and MHPG in CSF have generally found similar mean levels in affected and control groups. There are several reports of lowered urinary excretion of MHPG in Tourette's disorder; however, this finding has not been consistently replicated. Although measurements of plasma MHPG (Leckman et al., 1986) and platelet α_2-adrenergic receptors and plasma NE (Silverstein et al., 1984) after clonidine administration or withdrawal have been relevant to the phenomena of rebound and modulation of receptor sensitivity, they provide no definitive information concerning possible etiologic alterations in Tourette's disorder. Assessment of the sympathetic nervous system by measurement of autonomic cardiovascular measures has not revealed any substantial differences in the Tourette's group (van Dijk et al., 1992). However, studies of plasma, urinary, and CSF stress hormones before and after a lumbar puncture clearly suggest that at least some Tourette's patients have an increased stress response (Chappell et al., 1994).

SEROTONIN

Interest in a role for 5-HT has increased due to the strengthened connection between Tourette's disorder and obsessive compulsive disorder (Grad et al., 1987; Montgomery et al., 1982; Nee et al., 1982; Pauls et al., 1986). Effective treatment of obsessive compulsive symptoms in Tourette's patients with the serotonergic uptake inhibitors fluvoxamine and fluoxetine has further stimulated research on the connection between the disorders and symptoms (Riddle et al., 1992). Earlier studies of CSF 5-HIAA reported normal or slightly lowered levels in Tourette's disorder; a more recent study found significantly lowered CSF 5-HIAA in the group of Tourette's patients with prevalent obsessive compulsive symptoms (Leckman et al., 1988). No studies of 5-HT receptor functioning have been carried out in Tourette's patients, and early reports of benefit from 5-HTP have not been replicated (Van Woert et al., 1982).

Recent research on postmortem brain tissue has found decreases in 5-HT, 5-HIAA, and tryptophan across nearly all cortical and subcortical areas in the Tourette's patients (Akbari et al., 1993; Anderson et al., 1992). In addition, increased levels of the 5-HT$_{1A}$ receptor were found in most cortical areas examined. Further postmortem research is necessary in order to replicate the findings; however, the results do tend to increase the possibility that 5-HT may be a factor in the symptomatology of Tourette's disorder. In other indolamine-related research, Durson et al. (1994) have reported increased levels of plasma kynurenine in Tourette's patients and have suggested that this may reflect a shunting of tryptophan metabolism away from the production of 5-HT.

OTHER STUDIES

The importance of ACh and GABA in basal ganglia neural transmission has led to treatment studies using choline and other cholinergic agents (Stahl and Berger, 1981), as well as GABA-ergic agents (Mondrup et al., 1985). However, studies of CSF acetylcholinesterase (Singer et al., 1984) and CSF GABA have not found group differences. Reports of increased red blood cell choline have continued to appear (Sallee et al., 1992) and muscarinic receptor binding in white blood cells has been reported to be drastically lowered in Tourette's disorder (Rabey et al., 1992).

Immunohistochemical study of met-enkephalin, substance P, and dynorphin in basal ganglia areas of postmortem brain has suggested that dynorphin is reduced in the lateral globus pallidus in Tourette's disorder, while the other peptides appear normal (Haber et al., 1986; Haber and Wolfer, 1992). In contrast, levels of dynorphin measured in CSF have been reported to be elevated in Tourette's subjects (Leckman et al., 1988). In other studies of opioid systems in Tourette's disorder, small treatment effects were seen with naloxone (Chappell et al., 1992) while little effect was seen after the administration of the κ agonist, spiradoline (Chappell et al., 1994).

The amino acid neurotransmitters have been little studied. In the one study of central excitatory amino acids, postmortem brain levels of glutamate were reported to be lowered in the three projection areas of the subthalamic nucleus (Anderson et al., 1992). It was hypothesized that this might lead to disinhibition of the thalamocortical circuit. This would tend to place Tourette's in the group of hyperkinetic movement disorders including Huntington's disorder and hemiballismus. Further research is needed to clarify basal ganglia functioning in Tourette's disorder; recent imaging studies (George et al., 1992; Peterson et al., 1993; Riddle et al., 1992) and the postmortem research have provided interesting leads to consider with respect to the functioning of cortico-striato-pallido-thalamocortical pathways.

SUMMARY AND FUTURE RESEARCH DIRECTIONS

The underlying mechanisms that regulate the unfolding maturation of the central nervous system are presumably regulated by genetic factors concerned with the timing of expression of particular genes; findings concerning homeobox genes and other regulators now are providing ways of approaching this biology of maturation that are also relevant to the investigation of the onset of specific disorders at certain phases of brain maturation (e.g., Tourette's syndrome around the early school-age years and obsessive compulsive disorder several years later). Many steps from genetic to neuronal functioning have been characterized for model systems, including the localization, cloning, and sequencing of the genes for important enzymes and receptor systems; assessment of gene activity through measurement of messenger RNA; elucidation of the steps involved in synthesis, storage, release, and reuptake of transmitter compounds; mechanisms of coupling between transmitter and receptors; and the cascade of events that follows upon receptor stimulation (alterations in membrane channels and other membrane changes, reconfiguration of receptors, and activation of second-messenger systems). The neurochemical point of view on brain functioning is increasingly being integrated with other perspectives, including the neuroanatomical, neurophysiological, and developmental.

Molecular biology has provided powerful new methods for clarifying the various stages in neural function and transmission. It is thus natural to appraise the role of more traditional approaches to neurochemical study, including measurements of neurotransmitters, enzyme systems, specific proteins, and metabolites. There are sound reasons for the continued prominence of the neurochemical approach: the role of neurochemical research in understanding drug action, the search for mechanisms underlying the range of expression of specific genes, and the recognition that for many disorders there are likely to be polygenic contributions as well as gene-environment interactions that are expressed in neurochemical systems. Also, the detection of chemical abnormalities may provide information critical to detecting the relevant gene(s) in a disorder whose genetics are obscure and for which there are no known biological markers. For example, the finding of an altered neuron-related protein using methods such as two-dimensional giant gel electrophoresis can swiftly be exploited through available techniques to identify the genetic locus and thus the underlying gene(s). The study of neurochemical factors in the course of normal and deviant development will probably play increasingly important roles as genetic factors are elucidated and we begin to understand the ways in which genes are expressed or modified.

Neurochemical concepts underlie and are being enriched by the availability of methods of brain imaging such as PET, magnetic resonance spectroscopy (MRS) and SPECT that provide information about brain functioning. With the discovery of more specific ligands for different types of receptors (e.g., the D$_2$ dopamine receptor), it is becoming possible to perform neuropharmacological studies (e.g., localization of receptors and determination of receptor numbers, affinities, and occupancy) in humans using SPECT that previously were feasible only with isolated brain slices. The detection of specific sites of neurochemical abnormality in postmortem brain specimens, in turn, may provide suggestions for where to look in human brain using brain-imaging techniques.

There is, however, a tremendous gap between the basic research understanding of brain maturation and function and the clinical investigation of specific disorders in children and adolescents. This gap is the result of various factors, including the the paucity of research programs capable of mounting sophisticated neurobiological research with well-assessed and well-treated children and ethical and practical concerns in performing research with children and adolescents. Also critical is the limitation of valid and reliable methodology for the study of neurochemical factors that reflect CNS functioning. The search for profound alterations in a specific neurochemical system (such as the DA system) reflected in static measurements of metabolites (such as HVA) in CSF or other bodily fluids has, so far, been unavailing. This does not preclude better fortune over the next years as other compounds are assessed in CSF, blood, and urine. However, a trend to greater emphasis on receptor assessment, postmortem studies, and brain-imaging studies is evident. It is far too early for research to fixate on one approach, level, or system; to the contrary, it is through the integration of various approaches that we are most likely to understand the biological basis of childhood neuropsychiatric disorders.

References

Akbari HM, Anderson GM, Pollak ES, et al: Serotonin receptor binding and tissue indoles in postmortem cortex of Tourette's syndrome individuals. *Soc Neurosci Abstr* 19:838, 1993.

Amaral DG, Sinnamon HM: The locus coeruleus: Neurobiology of a central noradrenergic nucleus. *Prog Neurobiol* 9:147, 1977.

Anderson GM: Monoamines in autism: An update of neurochemical research on a pervasive developmental disorder. *Med Biol* 65:67, 1987.

Anderson GM: Review of the role of serotonin in disruptive behavior [Editorial]. *J Child Adolesc Psychopharmacol* 3:vii–ix, 1993.

Anderson GM: Studies on the neurochemistry of autism. In: Bauman ML, Kemper TL (eds): *The Neurobiology of Autism*. Baltimore, Johns Hopkins University Press, pp. 227–242, 1994.

Anderson GM, Hoshino Y: Neurochemical studies of autism. In: Cohen DJ, Donnellan A (eds): *Handbook of Autism and Pervasive Developmental Disorders*. New York, VH Winston, 1987, p. 166.

Anderson GM, Freedman DX, Cohen DJ, et al: Whole blood serotonin in autistic and normal subjects. *J Child Psychol Psychiatry* 28:885, 1987.

Anderson GM, Hoder EL, Shaywitz BA, et al: Neurotransmitter precursors and metabolites in cerebrospinal fluid of human neonates. *Dev Med Child Neurol* 27:207, 1985.

Anderson GM, Horne WC, Chatterjee D, et al: The hyperserotonemia of autism. *Ann NY Acad Sci* 600:331, 1990.

Anderson GM, Minderaa RB, Cho SC, et al: The issue of hyperserotonemia and platelet serotonin exposure: A preliminary study. *J Autism Dev Disord* 19:349, 1989.

Anderson GM, Minderaa RB, van Bentem PPG, et al: Platelet imipramine binding in autistic subjects. *Psychiatry Res* 11:133, 1984.

Anderson GM, Riddle MA, Hoder EL, et al: The ontogeny of 3,4-dihydroxyphenylacetic acid (DOPAC) in human cerebrospinal fluid. *J Neurol Neurosurg Psychiatry* 51:1100, 1988.

Arai H, Kosaka K, Iizuka R: Changes of biogenic amines and their metabolites in postmortem brains from patients with Alzheimer-type dementia. *J Neurochem* 43:388, 1984.

Arnsten AF, Contant TA: Alpha-2 adrenergic agonists and their metabolites in postmortem brains from patients with Alzheimer-type dementia. *J Neurochem* 43:388, 1992.

Baker GB, Bornstein RA, Douglass AB, et al: Urinary excretion of MHPG and normetanephrine in attention deficit hyperactivity disorder. *Mol Chem Neuropathol* 18:173–178, 1993.

Bauman M, Kemper TL: Histoanatomic observations of the brain in early infantile autism. *Neurology* 35:866–874, 1984.

Biederman J, Gastfriend DR, Jellinek MS: Desipramine in the treatment of children with attention deficit disorder. *J Clin Psychopharmacol* 6:359, 1986.

Bouillin DJ, Freeman BJ, Geller E, et al: Efflux of platelet ^{3}H-serotonin in autistic and normal subjects: Toward the resolution of conflicting findings. *J Autism Dev Disord* 12:97, 1982.

Bowers MB Jr: Characteristics of psychotic inpatients with high or low HVA levels at admission. *Am J Psychiatry* 148:240–243, 1991.

Bulat M: On the cerebral origin of 5-hydroxyindoleacetic acid in the lumbar cerebrospinal fluid. *Brain Res* 122:388, 1977.

Campbell M: Annotation: Fenfluramine treatment of autism. *J Child Psychol Psychiatry* 29:1, 1988.

Campbell M, Rosenbloom S, Perry R, et al: Computerized axial tomography in young autistic children. *Am J Psychiatry* 139:510, 1982.

Carey WB: A suggested solution to the confusion in attention deficit diagnosis. *Clin Pediatr* 27:348, 1988.

Chamberlain RS, Herman BH: A novel biochemical model linking dysfunctions in brain melatonin, proopiomelanocortin peptides, and serotonin in autism. *Biol Psychiatry* 290:773–793, 1990.

Chappell PB, Leckman JF, Pauls D, et al: Biochemical and genetic studies of Tourette's syndrome. In: Deutsch S (ed): *Basic Neuroscience in Child Psychiatry*. New York, Plenum, 1990.

Chappell PB, Leckman JF, Riddle MA, et al: Neuroendocrine and behavioral effects of naloxone in Tourette syndrome. In: Chase TN, Friedhoff AJ, Cohen DJ (eds): *Advances in Neurology—Tourette's Syndrome: Genetics, Neurobiology, and Treatment* (Vol 58). New York, Raven Press, pp. 253–262, 1992.

Chappell PB, Leckman JF, Scahill LS, et al: Neuroendocrine and behavioral effects of the selective kappa agonist spiradoline in Tourette's syndrome: A pilot study. *Psychiatry Res* 47:267–280, 1993.

Chappell PB, Riddle MA, Anderson GM, et al: Enhanced stress responsivity of Tourette syndrome patients undergoing lumbar puncture. *Biol Psychiatry* 36:35–43, 1994.

Cohen DJ, Donnellan A (eds): *Handbook of Autism and Developmental Disorders*. Silver Spring, MD, VH Winston, 1987.

Cohen DJ, Leckman JF: Developmental psychopathology and neurobiology of Tourette's syndrome. *J Am Acad Child Adolesc Psychiatry* 33:2–15, 1994.

Cohen DJ, Young JG: Neurochemistry and child psychiatry. *J Am Acad Child Psychiatry* 16:353, 1977.

Cooke EH, Leventhal BL, Freedman DX: Free serotonin in plasma: Autistic children and their first degree relatives. *Biol Psychiatry* 24:488, 1988.

Courchesne E, Yeung-Courchesne R, Press GA, et al: Hypoplasia of cerebellar vermal lobules VI and VII in autism. *N Engl J Med* 318:1349, 1988.

Dalmaz Y, Peyrin Z: Sex-differences in catecholamine metabolites in human urine during development and at adulthood. *J Neural Transm* 54:193, 1982.

DePrada M, Cesura AM, Laundy JM, et al: Platelets as a model for neurons. *Experientia* 44:115, 1988.

Donnelly M, Zametkin AM, Rapoport IL, et al: Treatment of childhood hyperactivity with desipramine: Plasma drug concentration, cardiovascular effects, plasma and urinary catecholamine levels, and clinical response. *Clin Pharmacol Ther* 39:72, 1986.

Dursun SM, Farrar G, Handley SL, et al: Elevated plasma kynurenine in Tourette syndrome. *Mol Chem Neuropathol* 21:55–60, 1994.

Elchisak MA, Polinsky RI, Ebert MH, et al: Contribution of plasma homovanillic acid (HVA) to urine and cerebrospinal fluid HVA in the monkey and its pharmacokinetic disposition. *Life Sci* 23:2339, 1978.

Elsworth ID, Leahy DI, Roth RH, et al: Homovanillic acid concentrations in brain, CSF and plasma as indicators of central dopamine function in primates. *J Neural Transm* 68:51, 1987.

Friedhoff AJ: Receptor maturation in pathogenesis and treatment of Tourette syndrome. In: Friedhoff AI, Chase TN (eds): *Advances in Neurology: Gilles de la Tourette Syndrome* (Vol 35). New York, Raven Press, 1982, p. 130.

Gaffney GR, Tsai LY: Magnetic resonance imaging of high level autism. *J Autism Dev Disord* 17:433, 1987.

Garelis E, Sourkes TL: Sites of origin in the central nervous system of monoamine metabolites measured in human cerebrospinal fluid. *J Neurol Neurosurg Psychiatry* 36:625, 1973.

Garelis E, Young SN, Lal S, et al: Monoamine metabolites in lumbar CSF: The question of their origin in relation to clinical studies. *Brain Res* 79:1, 1974.

George E, Young SN, Lal S, et al: Monoamine metabolites in lumbar CSF: The question of their origin in relation to clinical studies. *Brain Res* 79:1, 1974.

Gillberg C, Svendsen P: Childhood psychosis and computed tomographic brain scan findings. *J Autism Dev Disord* 13:19, 1983.

Gillberg C, Terenius L, Lonnerholm G: Endorphin activity in childhood psychosis. *Arch Gen Psychiatry* 42:780–783, 1985.

Gitlow SE, Mendlowitz M, Wilk K, et al: Excretion of catecholamine catabolites by normal children. *J Lab Clin Med* 72:612, 1968.

Grad LR, Pelcovitz D, Olson M, et al: Obsessive-compulsive symptomatology in children with Tourette's syndrome. *J Am Acad Child Adolesc Psychiatry* 26:69, 1987.

Green AR (ed): *Neuropharmacology of Serotonin*. New York, Oxford University Press, 1988.

Haber SN, Wolfer D: Basal ganglia peptidergic staining in Tourette syndrome: A follow-up study. In: Chase TN, Friedhoff AJ, Cohen DJ (eds): *Advances in Neurology—Tourette's Syndrome: Genetics, Neurobiology, and Treatment* (Vol 58). New York, Raven Press, pp. 145–150, 1992.

Haber SN, Kowall NW, Vonsattel JP, et al: Gilles de la Tourette's syndrome: A postmortem neuropathological and immunohistochemical study. *J Neurol Sci* 75:225, 1986.

Hanley HG, Stahl SM, Freedman DX: Hyperserotonemia and amine metabolism in autistic and retarded children. *Arch Gen Psychiatry* 34:521, 1977.

Hoshino Y, Tachibana R, Watanabe M, et al: Serotonin metabolism and hypothalamic-pituitary function in children with infantile autism and minimal brain dysfunction. *Jpn J Psychiatry* 26:937–945, 1984.

Humphreys GI, Levin I, Rudnick G: Antidepressant binding to the porcine and human platelet serotonin in transporter. *Mol Pharmacol* 33:657, 1988.

Hunt RD, Cohen DI, Shaywitz SE, et al: Strategies for study of the neurochemistry of attention deficit disorder in children. *Schizophr Bull* 8:236, 1982.

Hynd GW, Hern KL, Novey ES, et al: Attention deficit hyperactivity disorder and asymmetry of the caudate nucleus. *J Child Neurol* 8:339–347, 1993.

Hynd GW, Semrud-Clikeman M, Lorys AR, et al: Corpus callosum morphology in attention deficit hyperactivity disorder: Morphometric analysis of MRI. *J Learn Disabil* 24:141–146, 1991.

Iverson SD, Alpert JE: Functional organization of the dopamine system in normal and abnormal behavior. In: Friedhoff AJ, Chase TN (eds): *Advances in Neurology: Gilles de la Tourette Syndrome* (Vol 35). New York, Raven Press, p. 69, 1982.

Iverson SD, Iverson LL: *Behavioral Pharmacology* (2nd ed). New York, Oxford University Press, 1981.

Kandel ER, Schwartz JH: *Principles of Neural Science*. New York, Elsevier/North Holland, 1981.

Kopin IJ, Bankiewicz K, Harvey-White J: Effect of MPTP-induced Parkinsonism in monkeys on the urinary excretion of HVA and MHPG during debrisoquin administration. *Life Sci* 43:133, 1988.

Kopin IJ, Gordon EK, Jimerson DC, et al: Relation between plasma and cerebrospinal fluid levels of 3-methoxy-4-hydroxyphenethyleneglycol. *Science* 219:73, 1983.

Korpi ER, Kleinman JE, Goddman SI, et al: Serotonin and 5-hydroxy-indoleacetic acid in brains of suicide victims. *Arch Gen Psychiatry* 43:594, 1986.

Kurlan R: The pathogenesis of Tourette's syndrome. *Arch Neurol* 49:874, 1992.

Leckman IF, Detlor I, Harcherik DF, et al: Short and long term treatment of Tourette's syndrome with clonidine: A clinical perspective. *Neurology* 35:343, 1985.

Leckman JF, Hardin MT, Riddle MA, et al: Clonidine treatment of Gilles de la Tourette's syndrome. *Arch Gen Psychiatry* 48:324–328, 1991.

Leckman JF, Ort S, Caruso HA, et al: Rebound phenomena in Tourette's syndrome after abrupt withdrawal of clonidine: Behavioral, cardiovascular, and neurochemical effects. *Arch Gen Psychiatry* 43: 1168. 1986.

Leckman JF, Riddle MA, Berrettini WH, et al: Elevated CSF levels of dynorphin A (1-8) in Tourette's syndrome. *Life Sci* 43:2015, 1986.

Leckman JF, Walkup IT, Riddle MA, et al: Tic disorders. In: Meltzer HY (ed): *Psychopharmacology: The Third Generation of Progress*. New York, Raven Press, 1987, p. 1239.

Lee T, Seeman P, Rajput A: Receptor basis for dopaminergic supersensitivity in Parkinson's syndrome. *Nature* 273:59, 1978.

Leventhal BL, Cook EH Jr, Morford M, et al: Clinical and neurochemical effects of fenfluramine in children with autism. *J Neuropsychiatr Clin Neurosci* 5:307–315, 1993.

Lipton SV, McGough TP, Shaywitz BA: Effects of apomorphine on escape performance and activity in developing rat pups treated with 6-hydroxydopamine. *Pharmacol Biochem Behav* 13:371, 1980.

Lou HC, Henriksen L, Bruhn P, et al: Striatal dysfunction in attention deficit and hyperkinetic disorder. *Arch Neurol* 46:48, 1989.

Lou HC, Henriksen L, Bruhn P: Focal cerebral dysfunction in developmental learning disabilities. *Lancet* 335:8, 1990.

Maas IW, Contreras SA, Bowden CL, et al: Effects of debrisoquin on CSF and plasma HVA concentrations in man. *Life Sci* 36:2163, 1985.

Martineau J, Barthelemy C, Jouve J, et al: Monoamines (serotonin and catecholamines) and their derivatives in infantile autism: Age-related changes and drug effects. *Dev Med Child Neurol* 34:593–603, 1992.

McBride PA, Anderson GM, Hertzig ME, et al: Serotonergic responsivity in male young adults with autistic disorder: Results of a pilot study. *Arch Gen Psychiatry* 46:213, 1989.

Minderaa RB, Anderson GM, Volkmar FR, et al: Neurochemical study of dopamine functioning in autistic and normal subjects. *J Am Acad Child Adolesc Psychiatry* 23:190, 1989.

Minderaa RB, Anderson GM, Volkmar FR, et al: Noradrenergic and adrenergic functioning in autism. *Biol Psychiatry* 36:237, 1994.

Minshew NJ, Dombrowski SM: In vivo neuroanatomy of autism: Neuroimaging studies. In: Bauman ML, Kemper TL (eds): *The Neurobiology of Autism*. Baltimore, Johns Hopkins University Press, pp. 66–85, 1994.

Moir ATB, Ashcroft GW, Crawford TBB, et al: Cerebral metabolites in cerebrospinal fluid as a biochemical approach to the brain. *Brain* 93:357, 1970.

Mondrup K, Dupont E, Braendgaard H: Progabide in the treatment of hyperkinetic extrapyramidal movement disorders. *Acta Neurol Scand* 72:341, 1985.

Montgomery MA, Clayton PJ, Friedhoff AJ: Psychiatric illness in Tourette syndrome patients and first degree relatives. In: Friedhoff AJ, Chase TN (eds): *Advances in Neurology: Gilles de la Tourette Syndrome* (Vol 35). New York, Raven Press, 1982, p. 335.

Moore RY, Bloom FE: Central catecholamine neuron systems: Anatomy and physiology of the dopamine systems. *Annu Rev Neurosci* 1:129, 1978.

Narayan M, Srinath S, Anderson GM, et al: Cerebrospinal fluid levels of homovanillic acid and 5-hydroxyindoleacetic acid in autism. *Biol Psychiatry* 33:630–635, 1993.

Nee LE, Polinsky RJ, Ebert MH: Tourette syndrome: Clinical and family studies. In: Friedhoff AJ, Chase TN (eds): *Advances in Neurology: Gilles de la Tourette Syndrome* (Vol 35). New York, Raven Press, 1982, p. 291.

Needlman R, Zuckerman B, Anderson GM, et al: CSF monoamine precursors and metabolites in human neonates following in utero cocaine exposure: A preliminary study. *Pediatrics* 92:55–60, 1993.

Panksepp J, Herman B, Vilberg T, et al: Endogenous opioids and social behavior. *Neurosci Biobehav Rev* 4:473–487, 1980.

Pauls DL, Shaywitz SE, Kramer PL, et al: Demonstration of vertical transmission of attention deficit disorder. *Ann Neurol* 14:563, 1983.

Pauls DL, Towbin KE, Leckman JF, et al: Evidence supporting a genetic relationship between Gilles de la Tourette's syndrome and obsessive compulsive disorder. *Arch Gen Psychiatry* 43:1180, 1986.

Perry EK, Perry RH: Minireview: Human brain neurochemistry—Some postmortem problems. *Life Sci* 33:1733, 1983.

Peterson BS, Riddle MA, Cohen DJ, et al: Reduced basal ganglia volumes in Tourette's syndrome using three-dimensional reconstruction techniques from magnetic resonance images. *Neurology* 43: 941–949, 1993.

Pletscher A: Platelets as models: Use and limitations. *Experientia* 44:152, 1988.

Purves D, Litchman JW: *Principles of Neural Development*. New York, Sinaver, 1986.

Rabey JM, Lewis A, Graff E, et al: Decreased (3H) quinuclidinyl benzilate binding to lymphocytes in Gilles de la Tourette syndrome. *Biol Psychiatry* 31:889–895, 1992.

Rakic P: Specification of cerebral cortical areas. *Science* 241:170, 1988.

Randrup A, Munkvad I: Pharmacology and physiology of stereotyped behavior. *J Psychiatr Res* 11: 1, 1974.

Rasmusson AM, Riddle MA, Leckman JF, et al: Neurotransmitter assessment in neuropsychiatric disorders of childhood. In: Deutsch S, Weizman A, Weizman R (eds): *Application of Basic Neuroscience to Child Psychiatry*. New York, Plenum, 1990, pp. 33–59.

Riddle MA, Anderson GM, McIntosh S, et al: Cerebrospinal fluid monoamine precursor and metabolite levels in children treated for leukemia: Age and sex effects and individual variability. *Biol Psychiatry* 21:69, 1986.

Riddle MA, Leckman JF, Cohen DJ, et al: Assessment of central dopaminergic function using plasma-free homovanillic acid after debrisoquin administration. *J Neural Transm* 67:31, 1986.

Riddle MA, Rasmusson AM, Woods SW, et al: SPECT imaging of cerebral blood flow in Tourette's syndrome. In: Chase TN, Friedhoff AJ, Cohen DJ (eds): *Advances in Neurology—Tourette's Syndrome: Genetics, Neurobiology, and Treatment* (Vol 58). New York, Raven Press, pp. 207–211, 1992.

Ritvo ER, Freeman BJ, Scheibel AB: Lower Purkinje cell counts in the cerebella of four autistic subjects: Initial findings of the UCLA-NSAC autopsy research report. *Am J Psychiatry* 143:862, 1986.

Ritvo ER, Freeman BJ, Yuwiler A, et al: Fenfluramine treatment of autism: UCLA collaborative study of 81 patients at nine medical centers. *Psychopharmacol Bull* 22:133, 1986.

Rogeness GA, Javors MA, Pliszka SR: Neurochemistry and child and adolescent psychiatry. *J Am Acad Child Adolesc Psychiatry* 31:765, 1992.

Ross DL, Klykylo WM, Anderson GM: Cerebrospinal fluid indoleamine and monoamine effects of fenfluramine treatment of infantile autism. *Ann Neurol* 18:394, 1985.

Rumsey JM, Duora R, Grady C, et al: Brain metabolism in autism: Resting cerebral glucose utilization rates as measured with positron emission tomography. *Arch Gen Psychiatry* 42:448, 1985.

Safai-Kutti S, Kutti J, Gillberg C: Short communication: Impaired in vivo platelet reactivity in infantile autism. *Acta Pediatr Scand* 74:799, 1985.

Sallee FR, Kopp U, Hanin I: Controlled study of erythrocyte choline in Tourette syndrome. *Biol Psychiatry* 31:1204–1212, 1992.

Sandman CS: Various endogenous opioids and autistic behavior: A reponse to Gillberg [Letter to the Editor]. *J Autism Dev Disord* 22:132–133, 1992.

Schain RJ, Freedman DX: Studies on 5-hydroxyindole metabolism in autistic and other mentally retarded children. *J Pediatr* 58:315, 1961.

Shapiro AK, Shapiro E, Young JG, et al: *Gilles de la Tourette Syndrome* (2nd ed). New York, Raven Press, 1988.

Shaywitz BA, Anderson GA, Cohen DJ: Cerebrospinal fluid (CSF) and brain monoamine metabolites in the developing rat pup. *Dev Brain Res* 17: 225, 1985.

Shaywitz BA, Klopper JH, Yager RD, et al: Paradoxical response to amphetamine in developing rat pups treated with 6-hydroxydopamine. *Nature* 261: 153, 1976.

Shaywitz SE, Shaywitz BA: Biological influence in attentional disorders. In: Levine MD, Carey WB, Crocker AC, et al (eds): *Developmental Behavioral Pediatrics*. Philadelphia, Saunders, 1982, p. 746.

Shaywitz SE, Shaywitz BA: *Attention Deficit Disorder Comes of Age*. Austin, Pro-Ed, 1992.

Shekim WO, Bylund DB, Hodges K, et al: Platelet alpha 2-adrenergic receptor binding and the effects of *d*-amphetamine in boys with attention deficit hyperactivity disorder. *Neuropsychobiology* 29: 120–124, 1994.

Shepherd G: *Neurobiology*. New York, Oxford University Press, 1983.

Silverstein F, Smith CB, Johnston MV: Effect of clonidine on platelet alpha adrenoreceptors and plasma norepinephrine of children with Tourette syndrome. *Dev Med Child Neurol* 27:793, 1984.

Singer HS, Hahn IH, Moran TH: Abnormal dopamine uptake sites in postmortem striatum from patients with Tourette's syndrome. *Ann Neurol* 30: 558–562, 1991.

Singer HS, Oshida L, Coyle JT: CSF cholinesterase activity in Gilles de la Tourette's syndrome. *Arch Neurol* 41:756, 1984.

Singer HS, Wong DF, Tiemeyer M, et al: Pathophysiology of Tourette syndrome: A positron emission tomographic and postmortem analysis. *Ann Neurol* 18:416, 1985.

Sneddon JM: Blood platelets as a model for monoamine-containing neurons. *Prog Neurobiol* 1: 151, 1973.

Sourkes TL: On the origin of homovanillic acid (HVA) in the cerebrospinal fluid. *J Neural Transm* 34:153, 1973.

Stahl SM, Berger PA: Physostigmine in Tourette syndrome: Evidence for cholinergic underactivity. *Am J Psychiatry* 138:240, 1981.

Stern LM, Walker MK, Sawyer MG, et al: A controlled, crossover trial of fenfluramine in autism. *J Child Psychol Psychiatry* 31:569–585, 1990.

Todd RD, Ciaranello RD: Demonstration of inter- and intraspecies differences in serotonin binding sites by antibodies from an autistic child. *Proc Natl Acad Sci USA* 82:612, 1985.

Turjanski N, Sawle GV, Playford ED, et al: PET studies of the presynaptic and postsynaptic dopaminergic system in Tourette's syndrome. *J Neurol Neurosurg Psychiatry* 57:688–692, 1994.

Udenfriend S, Titus E, Weissbach H, et al: Biogenesis and metabolism of 5-hydroxyindole compounds. *J Biol Chem* 219:335, 1956.

van Dijk JG, Koenderink M, Kramer CG, et al: Non-invasive assessment of autonomic nervous function in Gilles de la Tourette's syndrome. *Clin Neurol Neurosurg* 94:157–190, 1992.

Van Woert MH, Rosenbaum D, Enna SJ: Overview of pharmacological approaches to therapy for Tourette syndrome. In: Friedhoff AJ, Chase TN (eds): *Advances in Neurology: Gilles de la Tourette Syndrome* (Vol 35). New York, Raven Press, 1982, p. 369.

Varley CK, Holm VA: A two-year follow-up of autistic children treated with fenfluramine. *J Am Acad Child Adolesc Psychiatry* 29:137–140, 1990.

Weir RL, Chase TN, Ng LKY, et al: 5-Hydroxyindoleacetic acid in spinal fluid: Relative contribution from brain and spinal cord. *Brain Res* 52:409, 1973.

Weizman A, Bernhout E, Weitz R, et al: Imipramine binding to platelets of children with attention deficit disorder with hyperactivity. *Biol Psychiatry* 23:491, 1988.

Weizman A, Goren N, Tyans S, et al: Platelet [3H]imipramine building in autism and schizophrenia. *Psychopharmacology* 91:101, 1987.

Young JG, Cohen DJ, Anderson GM, et al: Neurotransmitter ontogeny as a perspective for studies of child development and pathology. In: Shopsin B, Greenhill L (eds): *The Psychobiology of Childhood: A Profile of Current Issues*. New York, Spectrum, 1984, p. 51.

Young JG, Cohen DJ, Shaywitz BA: Molecular pathology in the childhood psychoses. In: Wing JK (ed): *Handbook of Psychiatry* (Vol 3). London, Cambridge University Press, 1983, p. 229.

Young JG, Kavanaugh ME, Anderson GM, et al: Clinical neurochemistry of autism and associated disorders. *J Autism Dev Disord* 12:147, 1982.

Yuwiler A, Geller E, Ritvo E: Biochemical studies of autism. In: Lajtha E (ed): *Handbook of Neurochemistry*. New York, Plenum, 1985, p. 671.

Yuwiler A, Shih JC, Chen CH, et al: Hyperserotonemia and antiserotonin antibodies in autism and other disorders. *J Autism Dev Disord* 22:33–45, 1992.

Zametkin AJ, Rapoport JL: Neurobiology of attention deficit disorder with hyperactivity: Where have we come in 50 years? *J Am Acad Child Adolesc Psychiatry* 26:676, 1987a.

Zametkin AJ, Rapoport JL: Noradrenergic hypothesis of attention deficit disorder with hyperactivity: A critical review. In: Meltzer HY (ed): *Psychopharmacology: The Third Generation of Progress*. New York, Raven Press, 1987b, p. 837.

Ziegler MG, Wood JH, Lake CR, et al: Norepinephrine and 3-methoxy-4-hydroxyphenylglycol gradients in human cerebrospinal fluid. *Am J Psychiatry* 134:565, 1977.

Zubieta JK, Alessi NE: Is there a role of serotonin in the disruptive behavior disorders? A literature review. *J Child Adolesc Psychopharmacol* 3:11–35, 1993.

4 DEVELOPMENTAL ASPECTS OF NEUROPHYSIOLOGY

Edward M. Ornitz, M.D.

During the developmental progression from infancy through early and later childhood to adolescence, the striking behavioral, emotional, and cognitive changes with which child psychiatrists are familiar accompany neuroanatomical indices of complex brain growth patterns. These include gross measures of brain growth, such as linked brain weight and head circumference measurements (human brain weight is proportional to the cube of head circumference) (Epstein, 1979, 1986), thickness of cerebral cortex and size of pyramidal cells (Rabinowicz et al., 1977), progression of regional myelination of specific brain areas (Yakovlev and Lecours, 1967), neuronal density in frontal cortex (Huttenlocher, 1979; Rabinowicz, 1986), synaptic density in frontal (Huttenlocher, 1979) and visual (Huttenlocher et al., 1982) cortex, and dendritic and axonal differentiation of prefrontal cortex neurons (Mrzljak et al., 1990).

Two types of maturational brain changes occur. There are progressive changes across the childhood and adolescent years, and there are maturational growth spurts at particular ages. From infancy to adulthood, there are progressive increases in brain weight (e.g., Huttenlocher, 1979), head circumference (Epstein, 1979, 1986), and cerebral cortical thickness (Rabinowicz, 1986; Rabinowicz et al., 1977), and a progressive decrease in neuronal density in cerebral cortex (Huttenlocher, 1979; Rabinowicz, 1986) and other cortical and subcortical regions (Rabinowicz, 1986). The decrease in neuronal density is precipitous before birth, with a slower decrease to about 6–15 months, after which time adult values are reached (Rabinowicz, 1986). Synaptic density increases from birth to 8 months of age in visual cortex (Huttenlocher et al., 1982) and to about 12 months of age in frontal cortex (Huttenlocher, 1979) and then progressively declines to adult values, which are obtained around 11 years of age. The dendritic and axonal architecture in prefrontal cortex appears to mature about the same time (Mrzljak et al., 1990).

These progressive changes in postnatal brain structure seem to involve two overlapping phases, a more rapid one occurring between birth and 1–3 years and a slower one occurring between 1 and 11 years of age with continuing changes during adolescence and young adulthood. The manifestation of these changes in prefrontal cortex are of particular importance because of their association with stages of cognitive development during childhood (Goldman-Rakic, 1987). The earlier prefrontal cortical phase involves the persistence of granular layer IV (which becomes dysgranular in the adult brain), the gradual disappearance of the subplate zone (a transient fetal-neonatal zone associated, in frontal cortex, with prolonged postnatal growth of cortico-cortical pathways) during the first 6 months of postnatal life, and overproduction of cortico-cortical axons associated with excessive synaptogenesis (Goldman-Rakic, 1987; Kostovic, 1990). In general, during this early childhood phase of progressive frontal cortical maturation, the transient preterm pattern is transformed into the "structurally adult-like pattern of cortical organization" (Kostovic, 1990). The early phase is also associated with complex changes in frontal cortical cholinergic receptor function, marked by changing acetylcholine esterase (AChE) activity (see Kostovic, 1990). During the later childhood to adolescent progressive phase, the gradual increase in AChE reactivity in layer III pyramidal neurons has been associated with the innervation of cortical association neurons, synaptic reorganization, and cognitive development (Kostovic, 1990).

Some of these progressive increments or decrements in brain growth measures are not smooth; rather, they are characterized by spurts and lags in development, resulting in peaks and troughs of brain growth at particular age periods. Detailed analyses of the rate of brain weight and head circumference change have suggested peaks in brain growth rates around ages 3, 7, 11–12, and 15 years, with troughs in the intervening years (Epstein, 1974a, 1979; Thatcher, 1980). In the most recent reconsideration of the brain weight and head circumference data, Epstein (1986) concluded that the peaks in brain growth rates were statistically significant at 7, 11–12, and 15 years for male brains. Using a different statistical approach, McCall et al. (1983) were able to confirm the significance of only the 15-year-old peak. However, detailed neuroanatomical studies of cortical thickness, pyramidal cell development, neuronal density, and myelination document the validity of the earlier stages. Progressive increases in cortical thickness are interrupted by maturational troughs at 2 years and 6 years, which are followed by accelerated growth between 2 and 4 years and 6 and 10 years (Rabinowicz, 1986; Rabinowicz et al., 1977). (This is a general statement. Particular cortical regions vary somewhat in the timing of these troughs and/peaks in rates of cortical thickening.) Pyramidal cell size and shape also show two periods of accelerated change, between 15 months and 2 years and between 8 and 10 years (Rabinowicz et al., 1977), and neuronal density, which reaches adult values by 15 months of age, shows a consistent small peak of cell density around 6 years of age in frontal, parietal, temporal, and limbic cortex (Rabinowicz, 1986). From the cortical thickness, pyramidal cell size and shape, and neuronal density data, Rabinowicz (1986) concluded that (a) an important period in cortical maturation occurs between 15 and 24 months and (b) a period of cortical ''remodeling'' takes place between 6 and 8 years. He also referred to unpublished data that suggested additional periods of ''cortical remodeling'' between 10 and 12 years and around 18 years.

Myelination proceeds at different rates for different brain regions, but, in general, myelination of most tracts is completed at or before 2–3 years of age. The reticular formation, the nonspecific thalamic radiations, and the great cerebral commissures are not completely myelinated until between 8 and 10 years of age. Myelination of the intracortical association areas continues into the second and third decades (Lecours, 1982; Yakovlev and Lecours, 1967). (A more recent study suggests earlier maturation of myelination (Brody et al., 1987), but data are available to only 2 years of age.) Myelination of the superior medullary lamina of the parahippocampal gyrus shows a progressive increase throughout childhood. Axons in the superior medullary lamina connect limbic and cortical structures and, hence, ''could play some role in the corticolimbic integration of emotional behaviors with cognitive processes'' (Benes et al., 1994).

In general, there appear to be four periods of major structural change in brain development, which punctuate the progressive increases and decreases in the size of the brain and its substructures at both the macroscopic and microscopic levels. The first takes place during early childhood, between about 15 months and 4 years of age. The second occurs during or toward the end of late childhood, sometime between 6 and 10 years of age. The third is associated with prepuberty, and the fourth, at least in males, occurs in mid-adolescence. Epstein (1974b) has suggested correlations between these accelerated periods of brain growth and spurts in mental age occurring during the same time periods. Although some critics have found these correlations to be unconvincing because of a paucity of behavioral data (Fischer and Silvern, 1985) and an inability to confirm concordance between spurts in brain and mental growth statistically (McCall et al., 1983), it is noteworthy that the first of these periods of brain growth overlaps the Piagetian mental stages of sensorimotor and preoperational behavior, while the second coincides with the Piagetian stage of concrete operations, and the third and fourth overlap the Piagetian stage of formal operations (Inhelder and Piaget, 1958). Thus the stages of brain growth seem to occur in association with signifi-

cant mental developments that involve important advances in both cognitive and emotional functions.

Developmental neurophysiology, the subject of this chapter, focuses on the functional correlates of the structural brain changes that occur during development. These changes in brain function should relate to the behavioral changes occurring during the developmental progression from infancy, through childhood, to adolescence and adulthood. Neurophysiologic studies of development fall into two broad categories: the study of the brain in its resting state and the study of the brain perturbed by external stimuli. The former involves primarily studies of changes in EEG frequencies in the waking state and changes in sleep parameters, notably the tonic and phasic components of rapid eye movement (REM) sleep. The latter includes the startle response and its modulation, nystagmus evoked by vestibular stimulation, and exogenous and endogenous event-related potentials. This review is limited for the most part to studies that encompass all or the greater part of childhood, from the preschool period to adolescence, and provide quantitative data permitting the evaluation of maturational changes. Studies from early infancy are included only when comparable data are available later during childhood. The many important studies confined to the newborn and very young infant are not included; an excellent review of these can be found in Graham et al. (1983) in the context of orienting responses.

DEVELOPMENTAL CHANGES IN THE EEG

Niedermeyer (1993) provides an excellent comprehensive review of *qualitative* descriptions of the maturation of the EEG, including EEG patterns in the premature and full-term newborn. This chapter focuses on *quantitative* studies of changes in EEG frequencies with maturation. Developmental EEG studies have utilized hand measurement of EEG frequencies (Eeg-Olofsson, 1980; Lindsley, 1936, 1939; Petersen and Eeg-Olofsson, 1971), analogue frequency analysis (Matousek and Petersen, 1973), and spectral analysis (Matthis et al., 1980; Thatcher et al., 1987).

In general, regardless of the method used, EEG maturation between about 5 and 11 years of age has been characterized by a reduction in slower frequencies (those in the delta and theta bands) and an increase in higher frequencies (primarily the alpha band) (Eeg-Olofsson, 1980; Matousek and Petersen, 1973; Mattis et al., 1980). Some of the slower frequencies tend to increase from 1 to between 5 and 8 years of age and then decrease to 15 years of age (Petersen and Eeg-Olofsson, 1971). Theta activity shows a developmental peak at 4 years of age (Matousek and Petersen, 1973). The frequency of the more extensively studied occipital alpha rhythm increases progressively from 3 months of age to adulthood (Lindsley, 1936, 1939; Petersen and Eeg-Olofsson, 1971). The relative spectral power of alpha in the 9.5- to 12.5-Hz band increases between 4 and 11 years of age (Matthis et al., 1980), the amplitude of 9.5- to 12.5-Hz alpha increases from 1 to 21 years of age (Matousek and Petersen, 1973), and the mean absolute phase of 7- to 13-Hz alpha increases from birth to adulthood (Thatcher et al., 1987). Most of these progressive increases in alpha activity are exponential, with rapid increases from birth to about 5 or 6 years of age, followed by slower rates of change to adulthood; these changes closely parallel a similar exponential growth curve for brain weight (Huttenlocher, 1979).

The progressive developmental changes in alpha activity are punctuated by spurts and lags. Epstein (1979, 1980, 1986) has analyzed the developmental EEG data of Matousek and Petersen (1973) in terms of biennial increments of change and demonstrated EEG developmental stages with peaks of alpha activity around 4, 7–8, 11–12, and 15 years, and intervening troughs at 6, 9–10, and 13 years. These EEG developmental stages coincide quite well with the brain growth stages based on analyses of brain weight-head circumference data, cortical thickness data, pyramidal cell dimensions, and neuronal density changes, as described earlier. The well-defined trough in the development of alpha activity at 6 years, followed by the peak at 7–8 years (Epstein, 1980, 1986), coincides with the beginning of a brain development stage that

Rabinowicz (1986) describes as "a remodeling of the cortex." This restructuring of cortical substance involves a relative decrease in cortical thickness, a corresponding decrease in length and increase in width of the Betz cells, and an increased cell density. Thus, functional and structural brain changes coincide at a critical age in child development, the age that for most children is associated with the readiness to learn in a school setting, or, in Piagetian terms, to engage in operational thinking.

Using measures of EEG coherence and phase, Thatcher et al. (1987) confirmed EEG periods of growth and change around 4–6, 8–10, 11–14, and 15 years and demonstrated hemispheric differences in participation in these developmental stages. The 4- to 6-years period involves spurts in left hemispheric (frontal-occipital and frontal-temporal) coupling and right frontal pole pairing, while the 8- to 10-years period is notable for accelerated development of right hemispheric (frontal-temporal) connections. The preadolescent and adolescent periods are bilateral, involving primarily frontal lobe connections. Comparison of the Thatcher et al. (1987) findings and further mathematical analysis of the Matousek and Petersen (1973) data by Hudspeth and Pribram (1990) showed "a striking similarity to the timing and sequencing" of the EEG growth spurts (Thatcher, 1991).

Although relatively little is known about the development of hemispheric differences, it is most interesting to note recent evidence of a developmental shift in dendritic prominence (total dendritic length) from the right to left motor speech areas (Simonds and Scheibel, 1989). This shift to left-sided primacy of language-related areas occurs during the same 4- to 6-years period during which the spurt in left frontal-temporal EEG coupling occurs (Thatcher et al., 1987). This ontogenetic shift in hemispheric structure and function parallels an evolutionary trend toward lateralization of auditory cortex (Thatcher, 1980).

DEVELOPMENT OF SLEEP PATTERNS

Between birth and late adolescence the total time spent asleep is reduced from about 16 to about 8 hours (Roffwarg et al., 1966). Of greater interest for the neurophysiology of development is the fact that REM sleep accounts for 50% of total sleep time at birth but only 20% by 3 years, at which time adult values are approached.

The anlage of the REM state makes its appearance in the fetus before birth. By 28–30 weeks it is possible to begin to identify REM and non-REM sleep states (Parmelee and Stern, 1972). At birth REM sleep is relatively "undifferentiated" in comparison with REM sleep in older children (Emde and Metcalf, 1970). Two major changes mark the differentiation of REM sleep within the first 3 months of life: Starting at approximately 2½ months of age, sleep begins with a non-REM instead of a REM period (Emde and Metcalf, 1970), and the initial high variability in physiological patterning of neonatal REM sleep becomes organized, so that behavioral and electrophysiological events uncharacteristic of REM sleep become segregated out of REM sleep and into drowsy and non-REM states. For example, EEG activity during REM sleep in the frequency range of stage 2 sleep spindles in 6- to 8-month-old babies is significantly reduced by 19–45 months (Ornitz et al., 1971). Concomitant with this increasing organization, there is a decrease in REM period length and in the percent of total sleep time occupied by REM sleep (Parmelee and Stern, 1972; Roffwarg et al., 1966) to approximately 40% by 3–5 months of age and to 30% by 6–23 months (Roffwarg et al., 1966). By 3 years, while total sleep time has decreased from 16 to 11 hours per day, REM sleep time has decreased from 8 to about 2 hours per day (Roffwarg et al., 1966). REM sleep is an activated state of consciousness, with a low-amplitude, high-frequency EEG similar to the waking EEG record and a tonic muscular atonia, punctuated by phasic motor and autonomic behavior such as the bursts of rapid eye movements, twitching movements of the extremities, and increased fluctuations of cardiovascular and respiratory activity, and phasic inhibition of responses to sensory input. Roffwarg et al. (1966) suggested that the REM state serves the newborn and young infant as an endogenous source

of stimulation when less exogenous stimulation is available. It is notable that the sum of waking time (8 hours) and REM sleep time (8 hours) in the newborn is almost the same as the sum of waking time (13.5 hours) and REM sleep time (2 hours) in the 5- to 9-year-old child, supporting the idea that one function of REM sleep during early development is to compensate for reduced time awake. It is most noteworthy, however, that the percent of total sleep time required for REM sleep has decreased to the adult level around 3 years of age, the time of completion of myelination of many subcortical pathways and of the first major spurt in brain growth.

The ontogenetic changes in the percent of REM sleep time are accompanied by developmental changes in the phasic motor activity of REM sleep. After adjustment for the differences in the time of night during which REM sleep episodes occur in the course of early childhood development, Tanguay et al. (1976) showed that the rapid eye movements of REM sleep clustered significantly more tightly into bursts with increasing age from 3 months to about 6½ years. This increasing organization of eye movement activity is accompanied by increasing inhibition of the relative amplitude of evoked responses to auditory stimuli during the eye movement bursts, with increasing age from 6 months to about 6½ to 9 years, during which time adult levels of phasic inhibition are reached (Ornitz, 1972; Ornitz et al., 1969). Hence neither the phasic motor excitation nor the phasic sensory inhibition of REM sleep are well defined in early infancy; however, these concurrent neurophysiologic processes develop rapidly during early childhood and mature after the preschool period. The phasic activity of REM sleep is generated in the parapontine reticular formation and mediated by the medial vestibular nucleus (MVN) (Pompeiano, 1967a, 1967b, 1980). The contribution of the MVN, a central vestibular structure, to the development of phasic motor activity during REM sleep is particularly interesting, as will be seen in the next section where we consider the developmental changes in vestibular function in the waking child.

The functions of the phasic events of REM sleep have rarely been discussed. However, these short, intermittent, recurrent periods of very intense motor activation (e.g., bursts of rapid eye movements, twitching of the muscles of the middle ears, vibrissae, and extremities) are embedded in the longer REM sleep periods, whose function is thought to be the activation of the brain during sleep without arousal of the organism (Vertes, 1984, 1986). This view is consistent with that of Roffwarg et al. (1966), who, as noted above, postulated that REM sleep "serves as an endogenous source of stimulation" in early infancy. Presumably, the need for such endogenous stimulation becomes less with maturation during childhood, as waking time increases and the quality of waking life becomes increasingly active. Hence as the percent of REM sleep time declines precipitously during the first 3 years of early childhood (Roffwarg et al., 1966), the phasic motor activity of REM sleep becomes more concentrated in discrete periods of time (Tanguay et al., 1976), and the phasic sensory inhibition becomes more pronounced (Ornitz, 1972; Ornitz et al., 1969). The increase in phasic sensory inhibition with maturation may serve to protect the developing child from the waking effect of exogenous stimulation at the time of the most intense motor excitation.

A change in the sleep EEG pattern of non-REM sleep also occurs around 3 years of age. The percent time and number of the 12- to 14-Hz sleep spindles and the duration of the spindles during stage 2 sleep all decrease from 4 months of age, reaching minimal values at 3½ years, and then increase between 4 and 5 years of age (Tanguay et al., 1975). Spindle rhythms are thought to be generated in reticular thalamic neurons that project to thalamocortical neurons, and brainstem reticular activity blocks the generation of EEG spindling by inhibitory projections to the reticular thalamic neurons (Steriade, 1988). Perhaps the decrease in EEG spindles around 3½ years of age reflects a peak period of brainstem reticular or reticular thalamic activity associated with the first major spurt in brain maturation.

DEVELOPMENTAL CHANGES IN VESTIBULAR NEUROPHYSIOLOGY

Vestibular reflexes serve primarily to stabilize gaze during head movements and maintain equilibrium during body movements and are influenced by, and interact with, visual and proprioceptive inputs. The development of these aspects of vestibular reflexes are addressed in this section. Other functional roles for vestibular reflexes, such as compensation for changes in the direction of the force of gravity and maintenance of tonic muscular tone (Baloh and Honrubia, 1979), have not been systematically studied in the human child and are not considered here.

Vestibular function is most readily studied by quantifying changes in the vestibulo-ocular reflex (VOR). Quantification of the VOR is facilitated by measurement of certain parameters of the ocular nystagmus induced by angular acceleration, and understanding of human vestibular function and its development has depended primarily upon this approach. The nystagmus consists of alternating slow and fast conjugate deviations of the eyes. The velocity of the slow deviation in the opposite direction to that of the acceleration reflects vestibular activity. The VOR is the output of a first-order open-loop control system, best characterized by its gain and time constant. In response to constant or impulsive accelerations, the gain is the nystagmus slow-component velocity (SCV) relative to the head acceleration or to the sudden change in velocity. The time constant (the exponential rate of change of the SCV in response to the acceleration) reflects the viscoelastic properties of the cupula (peripheral time constant) and the effect of a central integrator that prolongs the peripheral time constant to that of the nystagmus. In response to sinusoidal accelerations, the gain is the nystagmus SCV relative to the head velocity, and the time constant can be computed from the phase shift between nystagmus and head velocities (Honrubia et al., 1982).

The vestibular system is both anatomically complete and functionally responsive at or before birth. Histologically, the vestibular apparatus appears complete in the human fetus at $9\frac{1}{2}$ weeks of gestation (Hooker, 1952). The large neurons of the vestibular nuclei are "unquestionably functional" at 21 weeks of gestation (Humphrey, 1965). The myelination of the vestibular system is well advanced at 6 months of gestation (Langworthy, 1933). The endolymphatic and bony labyrinths (Dayal et al., 1973) and the number of myelinated vestibular nerve fibers (Bergstrom, 1973) and vestibular hair cells (Rosenhall, 1972) are mature at birth. Newborn infants respond to acceleration, the slow component of nystagmus deviating in the expected direction (i.e., opposite to that of the acceleration) (Tibbling, 1969), although the fast component, which is of pontine origin (Cohen, 1972), may not occur.

There are functional changes in the vestibular system during development from early infancy to adolescence that suggest considerable plasticity of the nervous system during childhood. Vestibular responses to an equivalent stimulus, be it caloric or rotational, differ markedly in preadolescent children from that found in adults (Conraux and Collard, 1970; Jongkees and Gasthuis, 1973). The responses of children to vestibular stimulation are not only different from the responses of adults but also differ within the childhood age span, with the most marked maturational changes taking place in preschool children (Ornitz, 1985; Ornitz et al., 1979). During the 1st year of life, the vestibular system is functioning at its highest level of reactivity, a level that decreases with subsequent development. At the same time, suppression of the VOR by visual fixation is minimal or absent (Ornitz and Honrubia, 1988). The peaking of vestibular activity during the 1st year of life is associated with overflow phenomena in the form of behaviors such as rocking and is followed by a subsequent rapid decrement in vestibular reactivity. These features of the maturation of vestibular function suggest that important modifications of vestibular mechanisms take place rapidly during the first few years of life and continue to do so, albeit at a slower pace, throughout childhood (Ornitz, 1983, 1988).

Those studies that have measured appropriate nystagmus parameters (i.e., the SCV or its expression as VOR gain) have demonstrated the following developmental sequence. Nystagmus is present in the full-term newborn, subject to sufficient arousal, and also in the premature and small-for-dates neonate. Nystagmus is weaker in the latter groups, but after several months of postnatal life the differences are no longer apparent. The maximum intensity of the vestibular response probably occurs by 6 months, and it is about this time that spontaneous vestibular self-stimulation first occurs, indicating a period of heightened vestibular reactivity. After the 1st year, the intensity of vestibular nystagmus and spontaneous vestibular behavior decrease rapidly until about 30 months of age, following which there is a gradual decrease toward adult values between 7 and 10 years. This decrease in the intensity of the vestibular response (reduced velocity of nystagmus and reduced VOR gain) is associated with increasing time constants (Ornitz, 1985; Ornitz et al., 1985). The association of decreasing gain with increasing time constants during development suggests that the immature human vestibular system is characterized by relatively deficient modulation of vestibular reflexes. It can be postulated that the decreasing gain reflects increasing modulation of vestibular function with development and that increasing time constants reflect the development of the modulating mechanisms. Both pharmacologic (Blair and Gavin, 1979) and neurophysiologic (Buettner et al., 1978) investigation suggest that the modulating mechanisms reside in reverberating brainstem reticular formation neuronal networks.

Studies of the development of vestibular adaptation to constant acceleration also suggest that the postnatal development of the vestibular system involves central mechanisms. The adaptive process that shapes the time course of the total nystagmus response to constant angular acceleration begins during the decline of the postacceleration primary nystagmus and is amplified during the subsequent secondary nystagmus (nystagmus with slow components in the opposite direction to that of the primary nystagmus) (Malcolm et al., 1970). The maximum SCV in all adults occurs at the same time during secondary nystagmus, regardless of stimulus magnitude (Sills et al., 1978). Sills et al. (1978) attribute this consistency to a central, stimulus-independent process. In children, the maximum SCV during secondary nystagmus varies according to age and by 10 years of age is close to the values of Sills et al. for adults (Ornitz, 1983). These data, together with developmental changes in secondary nystagmus/primary nystagmus peak SCV ratios (Ornitz et al., 1979), show strong age-dependent effects on adaptation during the childhood years. The maturational changes in VOR gain and time constant (Ornitz et al., 1985), vestibular adaptation (Ornitz, 1983; Ornitz et al., 1979), and visual-vestibular interaction (Ornitz and Honrubia, 1988) all support the notion that the postnatal development of the human vestibular system involves central modulating mechanisms.

The above considerations apply to the development of the mechanisms underlying the slow components of nystagmus, which originate in the vestibular nuclei and are modulated by brainstem reticular formation (BSRF) activity. The fast components, on the other hand, are generated in the BSRF, more specifically in the parapontine reticular formation (PPRF) (Cohen, 1972). The likelihood of generating fast components in response to near-threshold vestibular stimulation increases progressively from early childhood to young adulthood (Fuster et al., 1994). Since the same PPRF neurons generate both vestibular fast components and saccades, the maturation of fast component activity may parallel the fine tuning of saccade-mediated vestibulo-ocular mechanisms, which mature throughout childhood. Since the gain of the slow component decreases with development while the fast component and saccadic activity increase, it can be postulated that, with maturation, vestibular responsivity is modified by visuovestibular interaction (Ornitz and Honrubia, 1988). This developing interaction is, in turn, mediated by the development of the same BSRF circuits in the PPRF, which lengthen the nystagmus time constant and modulate vestibular output (see discussion in Fuster et al., 1994).

For more complete reviews of the development of vestibular function during childhood, see Ornitz (1983, 1988).

DEVELOPMENTAL CHANGES IN STARTLE MODULATION

The magnitude of the startle blink reflex in the human adult can be modulated by nonstartling prestimulation in three ways (Anthony, 1985; Graham, 1975). Inhibitory modulation of the startle response to an intense sudden stimulus follows brief (20-msec), low intensity, nonstartling stimuli presented at short intervals (30–240 msec) prior to the startling stimulus (Graham, 1975; Graham and Murray, 1977). At these short prestimulation intervals, the same amplitude inhibition may (Graham and Murray, 1977) or may not (Blumenthal and Levey, 1989) occur when the prestimulation is sustained continuously throughout the warning interval, depending on the prestimulation intensity and other experimental parameters. Facilitation of startle magnitude follows longer (>1400 msec) prestimuli that are sustained continuously throughout the prestimulation interval preceding the startling stimulus (Graham, 1975; Graham et al., 1975). Facilitation following these long, sustained prestimuli can occur in experimental designs in which the prestimulation interval is constant or is variable in duration (Anthony, 1985; Graham, 1975; Graham et al., 1975). In contrast, a brief (20-msec) stimulus presented 2000 msec prior to the startling stimulus induces startle facilitation only in the context of variable prestimulation intervals and not when the prestimulation interval is constant (Graham, 1975; Graham et al., 1975). Because of the uncertainty associated with the variable prestimulation intervals, the facilitating effect was attributed to an orienting-attentional mechanism. Subsequent research has shown that in the adult human a third type of startle modulation involving nonstartling prestimulation is due to orienting-attentional influences, and the effect can be facilitatory or inhibitory, depending on whether attention is directed toward or away from either the prestimulus or the startling stimulus (Anthony, 1985).

Inhibitory startle modulation is a brainstem function involving the processing of sensory input. Startle inhibition by prestimulation is mediated by an inhibitory pathway in the brainstem tegmentum as demonstrated by lesion (Leitner and Cohen, 1985; Leitner et al., 1981) and stimulation (Saitoh et al., 1987) studies in the rat. This pathway impinges on the primary startle pathway (Davis et al., 1982) at, or prior to, the medial pontomedullary reticular formation (Wu et al., 1988). As with the modulation of vestibular responses by polysynaptic brainstem reticular formation neuronal networks (Buettner et al., 1978) as described above, startle modulation also matures between 6 and 10 years of age (Ornitz et al., 1986, 1990, 1991). Thus, a synchronous maturational effect involves two related functions, startle and vestibular modulation, since the motor component of the startle blink reflex, the facial motoneuron, receives vestibular projections (to the facial nucleus) (Shaw and Baker, 1983). Their suggested role is the coordination of facial movements, including blinking, with eye and head movements, all of this being motor activity, modulated in the brainstem, that is involved in the response to sudden sensory input.

Systematically collected data on startle modulation by prestimulation from infancy throughout childhood are available for only experimental paradigms that have not attempted to manipulate the direction of attention (Ornitz et al., 1986, 1990, 1991). (Graham and her colleagues have carried out such experiments during the 1st year of life and have reported on differences from adult responses (Anthony and Graham, 1983, 1985; Balaban et al., 1985, 1989; Graham et al., 1981). Anthony and Putnam (1985) compared startle modulation effects in 5-year-olds and adults.) Prior to about 4 years of age, inhibitory startle modulation is characterized by fluctuating weak inhibition (25% response inhibition in 2- to 6-month-olds (Graham et al., 1981)), nonsignificant facilitation (17% response increase in 15-month-olds (Balaban et al., 1989)), and, again, weak inhibition (23% response inhibition) in 3-year-old boys (Ornitz et al., 1986). In 4-year-old girls and boys there is nonsignificant startle amplitude facilitation (about 10 and 22%, respectively) 120 msec following prestimulation. In 5-year-old boys, 30% response inhibition has developed. By 8 years, both girls and boys show strong significant response inhibition, 50 and 75%, respectively, approximating adult values. Simi-

lar developmental response patterns occur following prestimulation at 250 msec (Ornitz et al., 1986, 1991). Facilitatory startle modulation in response to prolonged sustained prestimulation follows a similar developmental course (Ornitz et al., 1986, 1991).

Both inhibitory and facilitatory startle modulation show, respectively, significant peak losses in startle inhibition and peak gains in startle facilitation at about $4\frac{1}{2}$ years of age, followed by a progressive increase in inhibition and decrease in facilitation until 8 years of age, when mature values are obtained (Ornitz et al., 1986, 1990).

Startle can also be modulated by habituation. There is only one developmental study of startle modulation by habituation (Zametkin et al., 1979). In response to glabellar taps, the number of reflex blinks to habituation increased from the 1st year of life until 3–5 years of age. Habituation recurred at 6 years of age and became progressively stronger until adulthood. Hence startle modulation by habituation shows the same loss of inhibitory modulation around $4\frac{1}{2}$ years of age as does startle modulation by prestimulation.

Inhibitory startle modulation matures during a critical period of human neurologic growth and development that is characterized by many important structural brain and functional neurophysiological changes, as described above. Myelination of the brainstem reticular formation and the great cerebral commissures is not completed until sometime between 8 and 10 years (Yakovlev and Lecours, 1967). Rabinowicz (1986) describes a period of cortical "remodeling" characterized by changes in cortical thickness, pyramidal cell size and shape and neuronal density that occurs between 6 and 8 years. Epstein (1986) describes a peak of brain growth (inferred from head circumference data) at 7 years, which he attributes to increased neuronal arborization. Epstein (1979, 1980, 1986) has demonstrated several peaks of alpha activity in the developmental EEG data of Matousek and Petersen (1973), one of which is a well-defined trough of alpha activity at 6 years, followed by a peak at 7–8 years. Between 8 and 10 years, EEG coherence and phase studies suggest accelerated development of right hemispheric frontotemporal connections (Thatcher et al., 1987).

All of these structural and functional changes in the human nervous system occur during that period of childhood when children are able to engage meaningfully in learning and, in most cultures, are enrolled in school. This is approximately the Piagetian period of concrete operations (Inhelder and Piaget, 1958), during which time the child's concept of reality becomes less egocentric and less anthropomorphic, permitting the initial development of logical thinking. Hence the maturation of inhibitory mechanisms in the brainstem that damp the response to strong external stimuli and the reduction of excitation following sustained stimulation (sensory modulation) parallel the development of cortical (cognitive) processes that require the capacity of the child to separate affectively and conceptually from external objects and events, a capacity that would seem to require inhibitory functions. In fact, tests of frontal lobe functions indicate an accelerated development of the capacity to inhibit the retroactive interference of a stimulus set upon the recall of a prior stimulus set during this period of childhood (Passler et al., 1985).

DEVELOPMENT OF EVENT-RELATED POTENTIALS

Event-related potentials (ERPs) are responses to stimuli in the EEG that may be exogenous or endogenous. The exogenous ERPs are always elicited by external events, and their response characteristics (e.g., latency and amplitude) vary with the physical parameters of the stimuli. The endogenous ERPs are nonobligatory responses to stimuli, may occur in the absence of an expected stimulus, and are relatively unaffected by the physical parameters of the stimulus (Donchin et al., 1978). Hence the exogenous ERPs represent relatively lower levels of sensory processing (stimulus registration), while the endogenous ERPs represent relatively higher levels of processing of the information conveyed by sensory stimuli (e.g., expectation, importance or relevance of the stimulus, recognition of novelty).

Exogenous Event-related Potentials

The extensive literature prior to 1978 on the maturation of exogenous ERPs during childhood has been thoroughly reviewed by Klorman et al. (1978). They found that, in general, the latencies of these responses to auditory, visual, and somatosensory stimuli decreased rapidly during the 1st year of life and changed more slowly or not at all from early childhood to adolescence. Since the exogenous ERP components are characterized by latencies less than 100 msec, the more marked decreases in latency during the 1st year were attributed to the early completion of myelination of specific thalamocortical sensory pathways. In contrast, the endogenous ERP components, which have longer latencies, show maturational changes throughout childhood, and these changes were attributed to the much later myelination of nonspecific brainstem and reticular thalamic pathways (Klorman et al., 1978). However, in the auditory system Eggermont (1992) has shown that the *rate* of maturation (during the first 2 years) of P2 and N2, ERP components occurring around 200 msec that have endogenous ERP characteristics, is the same as the rate of maturation of wave 5 of the exogenous brainstem auditory evoked response, suggesting similar developmental rates of myelination and synaptic activity of brainstem and more rostral auditory pathways.

The exogenous ERPs occur in all sensory modalities and include the brainstem auditory-evoked response, the somatosensory-evoked potentials, and the pattern reversal visual-evoked potentials.

The *brainstem auditory-evoked response* (*BSAER*) is composed of a series of five waves with peak latencies from about 1 to 6 msec (in adults). Based on experimental animal and clinical patient studies (see review by Fabiani et al., 1979), these peaks represent auditory transmission from the auditory nerve (wave 1), through the cochlear nucleus (wave 2), the superior olivary complex (wave 3), to more rostral regions of the brainstem (waves 4 and 5). Thus, wave 1 represents peripheral auditory transmission, and the remaining components represent progressive central auditory transmission through the brainstem. With maturation during infancy and early childhood, the latencies of the several BSAER components shorten but at different rates. The peripheral transmission (wave 1) matures early, reaching the adult latency between the 6th week (Salamy and Mckean, 1976) and the 2nd month (Mochizuki et al., 1983) of postnatal life. The central transmission time, measured as the brainstem transmission time between waves 1 and 5, matures more slowly. Adult values are approached between ages 3 and 5 years (Fabiani et al., 1979; Mochizuki et al., 1983) and finally reached at 8 years (Fabiani et al., 1984), the same time that another measure of brainstem development, startle modulation, matures (Ornitz et al., 1986, 1990, 1991).

Developmental amplitude changes in BSAER components have received less attention than latency changes (Jiang et al., 1993). Jiang et al. (1993) have observed an increase in wave 5 amplitude from birth to 5 years of age, followed by a gradual decrease in amplitude toward adult values. This peak of BSAER activity coincides developmentally both with the peak loss of inhibitory prestimulation modulation of startle (PMS) and the peak increment of facilitatory PMS (see above) and the peak increment of the P300 component of the auditory event-related potential (see below). The implications of these several manifestations of heightened responsivity to sensory stimuli are discussed later in this chapter.

The *somatosensory-evoked potentials* (*SEP*) comprise a series of scalp-recorded negative and positive peaks that vary in peak latency from about 20 to 200 msec following electrical stimulation of the fingers or the median nerve at the wrist (Klorman et al., 1978). Desmedt and his colleagues (Desmedt et al., 1980) have carried out the most extensive studies of the maturation of the SEP, focusing on the negative neonatal component with a peak latency of about 30 msec and a duration of over 15 msec. By adulthood, this broad, prominent peak has evolved into a narrow, smaller negative component with a peak latency of 22 msec and a duration of less than 5 msec (Desmedt et al., 1980). To assess the significance of these changes in terms of the known increase in

conduction velocity with maturation, it is necessary to consider the *onset* latency of this SEP component in relation to body growth. When the onset latency is divided by body length, the resulting negative exponential function shows a rapid decrease in conduction time relative to somatosensory pathway length, from 46 msec/m in the newborn to less than 20 msec/m by 1 year of age to a mature (adult) value of 11 msec/m by 8 years of age (Desmedt et al., 1980). These maturation changes in overall conduction times along the entire somatosensory pathway reflect maturational changes in both peripheral and central conduction velocities. Desmedt et al. (1980) have estimated the peripheral conduction velocity at birth to be about 27 m/sec; adult values around 65 m/sec are obtained by 1 or 2 years of age. In contrast, the central conduction velocity of the SEP is about 10 m/sec at birth and reaches an adult value of 50 m/sec by 8 years of age. Hence the SEP shows a similar maturational progression to that of the BSAER: rapid maturation of the peripheral system and slower maturation of the central brainstem pathway. For both systems, about the 8th year appears to be a critical period for brainstem maturation.

The *visual-evoked potentials* (*VEP*) can be evoked in the EEG by simple flashes or by more complex visual stimuli. Because of the variability of the evoked response to flashes, most modern investigations of the VEP utilize the method of pattern reversal. The pattern reversal VEP is evoked by, for example, the alternating dark and light squares of a checkerboard pattern. Developmental studies carried out prior to 1978 utilized the flash-evoked VEP method, and reviews of these early studies suggested both latency increases (Klorman et al., 1978) and decreases (Moskowitz and Sokol, 1983) with increasing age during childhood. Using the pattern reversal VEP and measuring the consistent prominent positive component at 100–120 msec in adults, Moskowitz and Sokol (1983) found that the latency in response to a pattern of large checks decreased rapidly during the 1st year of life, reaching adult values at about 1 year of age. In response to a pattern of small checks, developmental changes were slower, so that by 5 years of age adult values were still not obtained. Similar developmental differences in response to the two sizes of checks were also observed in earlier studies (Sokol and Jones, 1979) and Spekreijse (1978) found that the latency for VEP responses to small checks matured at about 10 years of age.

The source of the differential developmental response to large and small pattern elements is not well understood. Moskowitz and Sokol (1983) have drawn attention to reviews of the neurophysiologic and neuroanatomical evidence for the presence of two parallel pathways from the retina to the lateral geniculate nucleus to the visual cortex that process different aspects of visual input. One system consists of cells (Y cells) that respond with short latencies to *transient* events and functions, to detect movement and gross patterns; the second system is comprised of cells (X cells) that respond with long latencies to *sustained* input and functions, to discriminate fine patterns (Breitmeyer and Ganz, 1976; Lennie, 1980). Moskowitz and Sokol (1983) suggest that it is the short latency, transient system, which responds to large patterns, that matures rapidly, and the long latency, sustained system, which responds to small patterns, that matures more slowly. However, neuroanatomical studies of the human lateral geniculate nucleus (LGN) (Hickey, 1977) and neurophysiologic studies of the kitten LGN (Daniels et al., 1978) suggest that it is the sustained (X cell) system that matures earlier and the transient (Y cell) system that matures later. These results are not completely comparable to those of Moskowitz and Sokol (1983) because the time course for the increase in size of human LGN cells in both systems (adult size is attained by cells associated with the sustained system by 12 months of age and by cells associated with the transient system by 24 months) is much shorter than the time course for development of VEPs in response to large and small checks (mature responses by 1 year and by 5–10 years of age, respectively).

The issue of differential development of transient and sustained response systems is important because the dual functioning of these two systems seems to be a characteristic of a more general principle of the processing of sensory information in the nervous system (Graham et al., 1981). In the auditory modality Graham and Murray (1977) have proposed that inhibitory and facilitatory startle modulation (see description in the previous section) are associated with two neuronal systems, described by Gersuni (1971), that transmit auditory information about transient and sustained events. Neurons in the auditory system capable of detecting the onset of a signal (transient event) with great precision (short-time constant neurons) and other neurons capable of temporal accumulation of information (sustained event) about the signal (long-time constant neurons) are found in both the cochlear nucleus (Radionova, 1971) and the inferior colliculus (Gersuni et al., 1971). In contrast to the early development during infancy of VEP responses to large checks, which Moskowitz and Sokol (1983) associate with the transient system, inhibitory startle modulation, which Graham and her colleagues (Graham and Murray, 1977; Graham et al., 1981) also associate with the transient system, develops late during childhood (Graham et al., 1981; Ornitz et al., 1986, 1991). For both the visual system (Breitmeyer and Ganz, 1976) and the auditory system (Gersuni, 1971), the transient system is responsive to novel patterns, stimulus onsets, or other aspects of environmental change, while the sustained system is involved with more elaborate processing and analysis of the information in the stimulus. For visual responses to nonstartling stimuli, there is agreement that the transient system (Y cells) also functions to inhibit (or regulate the tonic inhibition of) the activity of the sustained system (X cells) (Breitmeyer and Ganz, 1976; Lennie, 1980) in order to adjust information processing to the requirements of response to new input. For responses to startling stimuli, it has been suggested that the transient system inhibits responses to new input in order to protect information processing (i.e., processing of sustained stimuli) from distraction by responses to new sensory input (Graham and Murray, 1977). These somewhat contradictory hypotheses and the differing developmental sequences should generate fruitful research concerning the neurophysiology underlying the development of attentional mechanisms and cognitive processes in different sensory systems during childhood.

Studies of the pattern onset visual-evoked potential have identified a striate cortex component, which changes as a function of age. A single positive peak at about 130 msec in children under 8 years of age evolves into a negative-positive complex with peak latencies of about 100 and 150 msec between 9 and 16 years of age (Ossenblok et al., 1992). This change is attributed by Ossenblok et al. to the changes in synaptic connectivity in striate cortex that occur in comparable age periods (Huttenlocher et al., 1982).

A general characteristic of the maturation of the auditory, somatosensory, and visual exogenous event-related potentials is the presence of at least two developmental sequences, a rapid maturational progression that is completed during the 1st or 2nd year of life and a slower progression that is not completed until after 5 years of age and that may extend more slowly until 8–10 years of age. Eggermont (1988) has provided a mathematical model that represents the developmental latency changes as the sum of a series of decaying exponential functions that apply equally to the three stimulus modalities. The time constants derived from these functions describe these two different rates of development of the exogenous ERPs as well as a third very rapid developmental process during the first few weeks of life.

Endogenous Event-related Potentials

Many endogenous ERPs have been described in experiments designed to require meaningful responses to stimuli. These include negative and positive ERP components of different latencies and durations. The earlier (<300 msec) negative and positive components tend to reflect various aspects of orienting to stimuli, while later (>300 msec) components tend to reflect utilization of the information contained in stimuli (Hillyard and Picton, 1987).

Several prominent negative endogenous ERP components have been identified. Wave N1 (peak latency around 100 msec) is sensitive to transient aspects of stimuli (Naatanen and Picton, 1987) and reflects feature detection (Naatanen et al., 1988), increasing in amplitude with increasing confidence in correct detection (Hillyard and Kutas, 1983). Developmentally, in 175 normal subjects of both sexes, the latency (but not the amplitude) of wave N1 in response to auditory stimuli decreased linearly from 4 to 16 years of age (Fuchigami et al., 1993). In a smaller study (40 subjects between 7 and 20 years of age) limited to girls, Johnson (1989) found neither amplitude nor latency changes in wave N1 with maturation in response to *auditory* stimuli, while demonstrating a linear latency decrement (but no amplitude changes) in response to *visual* stimuli, in wave N1 across the same age range.

Component Nd, the difference negativity, also referred to as the processing negativity, overlaps wave N1 when an attended auditory stimulus is differentiated from an ignored stimulus (Naatanen and Picton, 1987). This increased and more prolonged negativity reflects an early stage of stimulus processing that preferentially extracts information from the attended auditory stimulus (Hillyard and Hansen, 1986; Hillyard and Kutas, 1983; Hillyard and Picton, 1987). In response to visual stimuli, an analogous ERP component NA has been associated with stimulus recognition and compared to the auditory processing negativity (Ritter et al., 1983, 1988). The processing (also known as mismatch) negativity (peak latency about 150–200 msec) reflects a response to relationships between two stimuli (Naatanen and Picton, 1987), evaluating novel or deviant stimuli against the background of standard or expected stimuli (Naatanen et al., 1989). In preadolescent children, compared with adolescents and young adults, this mismatch or processing negativity in response to targeted longer-duration syllables interspersed among "irrelevant" shorter-duration syllables is significantly smaller, suggesting a neurophysiological correlate of the child's reduced efficiency in directing attention among competing inputs (Berman et al., 1990; Friedman, 1991).

Wave N2 (peak latency about 200 msec) also reflects registration of stimulus deviance from a steady-state background (Hillyard and Kutas, 1983). It seems to reflect a stage of discriminative stimulus processing, associated with stimulus classification (Ritter et al., 1983), that precedes the further processing associated with later ERP components (Hillyard and Picton, 1987). A late slow wave with negative polarity that develops around 1200 msec and persists beyond 2700 msec has been associated with increasing conceptual difficulty (Ruchkin et al., 1988).

Wave N2 has been studied developmentally. It was first described in 5- to 11-year-old children by Symmes and Eisengart (1971) as a large negative wave in response to attention-getting stimuli and later referred to as Nc by Courchesne (1977, 1978), who described it both in response to surprising or novel stimuli and also to target stimuli that must be discriminated from background stimuli (Courchesne et al., 1987). This negative ERP component is large and long in latency, between 4 and 7 months of age, after which time there is a progressive reduction in amplitude and latency throughout childhood and adolescence (Courchesne, 1978; Courchesne et al., 1987; Friedman et al., 1984; Fuchigami et al., 1993; Enoki et al., 1993). (Fuchigami et al. (1993) did not find developmental amplitude changes in N2, which, however, was measured peak-to-peak from the preceding wave P2.) By late adolescence, this wave has assumed the adult form of wave N2 (Friedman et al., 1984). Its latency is about 700 msec in infancy, 400 msec during childhood (Courchesne et al., 1987), and 200–250 msec in adolescence (Friedman et al., 1984; Enoki et al. 1993). Its changing stimulus parameters seem to parallel the changing perceptual styles and interests that occur with maturation. In this regard, it is noteworthy that children under 13 years of age show a similar wave N2 to that of adolescents and adults in response to the requirement to identify a target stimulus, but show a large delayed negative wave in response to surprising novel stimuli (see Figure 7 in Courchesne, 1978, where the large N2 in preadolescent children in response to novel stimuli was labeled Nc). Although described as a special ERP component found in childhood and given a special label (Courchesne, 1977; Courchesne et al., 1987), there seems to be little reason not to consider this component as a developmental precursor of wave N2, with a changing configuration throughout its developmental course (see also discussion in Friedman et al., 1984). In both children (Courchesne, 1978) and adults (Knight, 1984), it has a predominantly frontocentral scalp topography and increases in amplitude when elicited in response to novel as compared to target stimuli. Hence wave N2, which reflects stimulus classification, undergoes striking developmental changes in both latency and amplitude. Its developmental precursor, Nc, seems to reflect the earliest ERP evidence of cognitive processing since as early as 4–7 months of age it shows increased amplitude and longer latency in response to infrequent compared to frequent events (Courchesne et al., 1981; Karrer and Ackles, 1987). It is during this period, the first 6 months of postnatal life, that major changes in frontal cortical laminar structure and cortico-cortical connectivity occur (Kostovic, 1990).

A plethora of positive endogenous ERP components have also been described. These include the P3a, the slow wave, frontocentral positivities, and the P300 (Donchin and Coles, 1988; Fabiani et al., 1987; Ruchkin et al., 1988). Of these, the P300, also labeled P3 and P3b, has received the greatest experimental attention and theoretical analysis (see reviews by Donchin and Coles, 1988; Donchin et al., 1986a, 1986b; Fabiani et al., 1987; Johnson, 1988) and is the only positive ERP component to have received serious developmental investigation in children and adolescents (Courchesne, 1978, 1983; Courchesne et al., 1987; Finley et al., 1985; Friedman et al., 1984; Goodin et al., 1978; Martin et al., 1988a, 1988b).

The P300 is a positive peak in the ERP, occurring from somewhat less than 300 msec to nearly 1000 msec after a stimulus (Hillyard and Kutas, 1983) with maximum amplitude over the parietal scalp. Human neurosurgical/neurophysiologic studies have suggested multiple generators of the P300, particularly the medial temporal lobe (Halgren, 1988), the temporal-parietal junction (Knight et al., 1989), the frontal lobe (Wood and McCarthy, 1985), and the thalamus (Velasco et al., 1986; Yingling and Hosobuchi, 1984). Lesion studies in the monkey suggest that noradrenergic projections to these structures from the locus coeruleus are important in the generation and modulation of the scalp-recorded P300 (Pineda et al., 1989).

The amplitude of P300 increases with increasing relevance of a task associated with a stimulus and with decreasing probability that the stimulus will occur (Donchin et al., 1986a, 1986b). Hence P300s are usually elicited in experiments in which the subject is asked to identify certain stimuli (e.g., higher pitched tones) that occur infrequently during a series of frequently occurring and ignored stimuli (e.g., lower pitched tones). More generally, the peak amplitude of the P300 appears to be responsive to the distinctiveness of stimuli, reflecting the mental evaluation of surprising events, and hence to reflect mental activity associated with revisions of the subject's current model of the environment (Donchin and Coles, 1988; Donchin et al., 1986b). The peak latency of P300 is thought to reflect the time required to categorize stimuli (Hillyard and Kutas, 1983) and thus to update the subject's model of the environment (Donchin and Coles, 1988; Donchin et al., 1986b). More difficult discriminations result in longer latencies (Donchin et al., 1986b), suggesting that the level of mental abstraction utilized in performing a task may be reflected in the peak latency of P300 (Donchin et al., 1986a). Johnson (1988) has discussed the control of P300 amplitude and latency in the context of information theory: The degree to which P300 amplitude and latency are affected by stimulus probability and task relevance (which is affected by task and stimulus complexity as well as stimulus value) is modified by the degree to which the subject is uncertain about having correctly identified the stimulus. Greater uncertainty means that a smaller proportion of information is transmitted; this is reflected in decreased amplitude and increased latency.

Hence in the human adult, the P300 wave reflects a considerable degree of information processing, becoming larger and occurring earlier as a greater proportion of information is transmitted, that is, as prior uncertainty is resolved by a stimulus or, in information theory terms (Shannon and Weaver, 1963), as equivocation is reduced (Hillyard and Kutas, 1983; Johnson, 1988).

Developmentally, the P300, which is not present in infancy (Courchesne et al., 1981), has been demonstrated in response to infrequently presented target stimuli in 3-year-old children (Courchesne, 1983; Courchesne et al., 1987). Its small amplitude increases to maximum values between 3.7 and 6 years of age, after which amplitude may decrease to adult values between 10 and 13 years of age (Courchesne, 1983, 1978; Courchesne et al., 1987; Wijker et al., 1989), show no further change until adulthood (Fuchigami et al., 1993; Mullis et al., 1985; Martin et al., 1988b), or actually increase (Polich et al., 1990). Although differential effects of target stimulus probabilities, stimulus modality, or the nature of the required response to the target stimulus have been proposed to explain these differences, perusal of the above literature revealed no consistent relationship between these experimental variables and the discrepant developmental results. In one study (Johnson, 1989), both visual and auditory stimuli and two types of responses to target stimuli were used. Stimulus modality had no effect on P300 amplitude between 7 and 20 years of age, but P300 amplitude decreased with age when the subjects were asked to press a button to the target stimuli and showed no developmental effect when subjects were asked to count the targets. In response to orthographic and phonological targets, a developmentally maximum amplitude occurred around 11 years of age (Taylor, 1993), followed by a decrease in P300 amplitude until young adulthood.

Regardless of the developmental course of P300 amplitude changes following the preschool period, the earliest manifestation of increased P300 amplitude in response to target stimuli relative to background stimuli, i.e., information processing, occurs sometime between 3 and 5 years of age (Courchesne et al., 1987). This developmental neurophysiological landmark coincides with the developmental peak loss of inhibitory startle modulation and the associated peak increment of facilitatory startle modulation (Ornitz et al., 1986; Ornitz et al., 1990, 1991), the developmental peak dishabituation of the startle blink (Zametkin et al., 1979), and an early maturational period of EEG changes characterized by developmental peaks of theta (Matousek and Petersen, 1973) and alpha (Epstein, 1979, 1980, 1986) activity and coherence and phase changes suggesting increased left fronto-occipital and frontotemporal coupling and right frontal pole pairing (Thatcher et al., 1987). Hence the P300, reflecting responsiveness to the distinctiveness of stimuli and the transmission of information, becomes functional during a major developmental period of functional cortical reorganization (reflected in EEG changes) and reduced brainstem control over response to sensory input (reduced inhibitory and increased facilitatory startle modulation). This constellation of endogenous ERP, EEG, and startle modulation changes, peaking around 4–5 years of age, coincides with the Piagetian mental stage of preoperational behavior and may reflect or be part of a neurophysiologic developmental stage that underlies the heightened awareness and capacity to absorb new information from the environment and the relative inability to modulate reactions to the environment that is so characteristic of the preschool child. This preschool stage of neurophysiologic development follows the end of the first major period of structural brain maturation, which occurs between 15 months and 4 years and includes accelerated increases or changes in brain weight (Epstein, 1979), cortical thickness (Rabinowicz et al., 1977), pyramidal cell size and shape (Rabinowicz, 1977), neuronal density (Rabinowicz, 1986), and completion of myelination of the sensory-specific thalamic radiations (Lecours, 1982; Yakovlev and Lecours, 1967). It precedes the second period of brain growth and restructuring, which begins around 6 years of age (Epstein, 1986; Rabinowicz, 1986).

The latency of P300 follows a different developmental pattern than that of amplitude. It decreases exponentially with maturation in response to both target and background stimuli, from over 800 msec in 3-year-olds to 300–400 msec in adolescents and young adults (Courchesne, 1978; Courchesne et al., 1987; Finley et al., 1985; Fuchigami et al., 1993; Goodin et al., 1978; Howard and Polich, 1985; Johnson, 1989; Martin et al., 1988a, 1988b; Taylor, 1993). Unlike P300 amplitude, the maturational changes in latency are continuous from the earliest demonstration of the P300 response and seem to be independent of the response to the target (Johnson, 1989). According to the interpretation of P300 latency as reflecting the time required to categorize stimuli (Hillyard and Kutas, 1983), the decrease in P300 latency with maturation may index the development of this aspect of information processing. The decrease in P300 latency between 5 and 14 years of age also correlates strongly with increasing scores on tests measuring memory span (Howard and Polich, 1985; Polich et al., 1990), and in 4- to 7-year-olds, P300 latencies are significantly shorter in children with IQs greater than 140 (Martin et al., 1993).

Recent attempts to apply topographical analyses (variations in ERP waveforms across scalp locations) to developmental changes in ERPs during complex cognitive tasks (picture matching and continuous recognition memory) have led to the conclusion that by 7 years of age the longer latency ERPs, P300, and a negative deflection at 400 msec (probably a variant of wave N2) are similar in children and young adults, except for the longer latencies in children, reflecting the reduced efficiency in speed of stimulus evaluation and information processing (Friedman, 1991; Friedman et al., 1988). A recent innovation in developmental ERP studies has utilized topographical analysis of long-latency ERP changes in response to tasks which measure the cognitive transitions from the Piagetian preoperational stage (2–7 years) to the stage of concrete operations (7–11 years) and from the latter to the stage of formal operations (11–15 years). In this complex study, Stauder (1992) recorded ERPs to pictorial analogues of the Piagetian liquid conservation task in 5- to 7-year-olds and to pictorial analogues of the Raven Standard Progressive Matrices in 9- to 11-year-olds. In the younger children, the transition from nonconservation (preoperational level) to conservation (stage of concrete operations) was associated with a reduction in a broad late (up to 1000 msec) ERP positivity over frontal electrode sites. In the older children, the transition to improved performance on the Standard Progressive Matrices (at the onset of the stage of formal operations) was associated with the reduction of a broad late (700–2000 msec) negativity in the ERP in the more anterior scalp locations. This demonstration of ERP changes in response to actual performance on tasks indexing developmental transitions is currently the most direct approach to the neurophysiology of cognitive development. These findings of neurophysiological transitions between developmental stages are congruent with the delineation of the three neurophysiological stages described in this chapter and with their relationship to the three Piagetian stages of preoperational behavior, concrete operations, and formal operations. The ERP topographical findings also point to the predominance of frontal cortical structural and functional change during childhood, a progressive development that is accompanied by the changing response to tests of frontal lobe functioning throughout childhood (Welsh and Pennington, 1988; Levin et al., 1991).

SUMMARY AND OVERVIEW OF DEVELOPMENTAL NEUROPHYSIOLOGY

Neurophysiologic development during childhood must be considered against the background of what is known about the maturation of the structure of the human brain. Both brain maturation and neurophysiologic development are characterized by progressive changes throughout long periods of childhood and by accelerations, usually followed or preceded by decelerations, in the rate of change, resulting in peaks and troughs of both structural and functional change. While there is a tendency for the neurophysiologic spurts in development to coincide with structural spurts in maturation, there may be lags, such that important periods of functional change occur during slowdowns in structural growth or between periods of structural reorganization.

Following very rapid developmental and structural changes occurring from the end of gestation through the early weeks of postnatal life (not considered in this chapter), there are two major progressive structural sequences.

The first and more rapid takes place between birth and 1–3 years and includes general reductions in neuronal densities, increases in synaptic densities, and completion of myelination of the sensory-specific thalamic radiations. Many important early progressive neurophysiologic changes are associated with these structural developments. These include the marked reduction in REM sleep time and the rapid early reductions in BSAER transmission time, peripheral conduction velocity, and latency of VEPs in response to large pattern changes.

The second progressive sequence of neuroanatomical change is slower and includes a gradual increase in brain weight and cerebral cortical thickness from infancy to adulthood, a decrease in synaptic density between 1 and 11 years of age, and continuing myelination of the reticular formation, nonspecific thalamic radiations, and cerebral commissures until 8–10 years, and of the intracortical association areas until the second and third decades of life. Associated neurophysiologic events include progressive increases in EEG alpha activity between infancy and adulthood and decreases in activity of slower EEG frequencies between 5 years and adulthood; increased organization of the phasic motor activity and phasic sensory inhibition during REM sleep between infancy and 9 years of age; progressive changes in vestibular function (increased gain, prolongation of time constants, and changes in adaptation) between infancy and 10 years of age; further reduction in BSAER transmission time, SEP central conduction velocity, and VEP latency in response to fine pattern changes between early childhood and 8 to 10 years of age; and reduction of amplitude and latency of the N2 component and latency of the P300 component of the event-related potential between infancy and adolescence.

The progressive changes in brain growth are punctuated by four maturational spurts. The first takes place between about 15 months and 4 years of age. It includes an acceleration in cerebral cortical thickening and changes in pyramidal cell size and shape. Associated neurophysiologic changes include a spurt in EEG alpha activity and a developmental peak of theta activity at the end of this period.

The second spurt in brain maturation takes place between 6 and 10 years of age. Brain changes include a second acceleration in the rate of cerebral cortical thickening, a small increment in cortical and subcortical neuronal density, and further changes in pyramidal cell size and shape. Myelination of reticular tissue is also completed during this period. Associated neurophysiologic activity includes a spurt in EEG alpha activity and a peak in EEG coherence and phase, suggesting accelerated development of right hemispheric frontal-temporal connections. During this second major spurt in brain growth and change, the developmental progressions of several important neurophysiologic functions are completed. The organization of rapid eye movements into bursts and phasic sensory inhibition during REM sleep, the gain and time constant of vestibular nystagmus, the modulation of startle by inhibitory and facilitatory prestimulation, the central transmission time of the BSAER, the central conduction velocity of the SEP, and the latency of the VEP in response to fine patterns all reach adult values. Hence by the end of this second spurt in structural and functional brain development, at around 10 years of age, many significant subcortical functions have matured, and accelerated development of some measures of cortical activity have taken place. This period coincides with the Piagetian period of concrete operations, that is, the beginnings of logical thinking (see Chapter 11). Many of the mature subcortical mechanisms are of an inhibitory nature, suggesting a relationship between the capacity to inhibit and the readiness for higher cognitive processes. During this period, there is an accelerated development of the ability to inhibit the retroactive interference of a second set of stimuli upon the recall of a prior set. This is a frontal lobe function. It is suggested that the developing capacity to inhibit, which is requisite for frontal lobe mediated cognition, may be linked to the development of subcortical inhibitory mechanisms.

Prior to the second maturational spurt in brain growth and change, and following the first such spurt (i.e., between 4 and 6 years), there is an important period of neurophysiologic development characterized by a particular constellation of EEG, ERP, and startle physiology changes. Initiated around 4 years of age by developmental peaks in EEG alpha and theta activity and changes in EEG coherence and phase suggesting advances in frontal cortex connectivity, this period is notable for a peak increment in event-related potential activity ranging from the exogenous wave 5 of the BSAER to the endogenous P300 and a concurrent peak deficit in inhibitory startle modulation. This stage of neurophysiologic development involving increased reactivity to stimuli at both cortical and subcortical levels, occurring between an earlier period of cortical maturation and a later period of cortical "remodeling" (per Rabino-wicz), coincides with the Piagetian stage of preoperational behavior. The neurophysiologic characteristics suggest the heightened awareness coupled with the inability to inhibit that characterize the preschool child.

Brain weight changes and histological evidence for cortical remodeling suggest two additional spurts in brain maturation and change around puberty and during mid-adolescence. These late brain growth periods are also accompanied by neurophysiologic changes manifested by peaks of EEG alpha activity and changes in coherence and phase measures involving frontal cortex connectivity. During adolescence, the progressive changes in the ERP components N2 and P300 terminate in adult values.

An overview of the relationships between neurophysiologic development and brain growth suggests a general but not absolute concordance. There is evidence for considerable plasticity in neurophysiologic development, such that important developmental neurophysiologic changes occur long after structural change seems to be complete (as exemplified by the course of vestibular development) or during lulls in structural change. A major component of plasticity in neurophysiological development may also be attributed to neuronal plasticity in the case of cerebral cortex. Here there is overproduction and redundancy of synaptic connections early in childhood, with synapse elimination with maturity. Huttenlocher (1990) has suggested that neural plasticity can be understood as the incorporation of some of the excessive synaptic contacts into functioning systems. These synaptic contacts become stabilized, while "labile contacts that fail to be incorporated" are eliminated. Developmental neurohistological studies in primates indicate a similar early synaptic excess followed by elimination of excessive synapses with maturity (Goldman-Rakic, 1987). Similar cognitive functions of delayed response in the monkey and object permanence in the infant emerge during the period of synaptic excess; Goldman-Rakic (1987) has suggested that while a critical mass of synapses is associated with the emergence of this type of cognition, "mature capacity may depend upon the [later] elimination of excess synapses."

An overview of the relationships between neurophysiologic development and behavior suggests three significant stages that, not surprisingly, coincide with the preschool- and school-age periods of childhood and early adolescence. Between 3 and 5 years, there is a neurophysiologic stage of increased receptivity coupled with disinhibition in response to environmental stimuli. Between 6 and 10 years, there is a neurophysiologic stage of increased inhibition in response to stimuli, coupled with increasing development of neurophysiologic indices of information processing. In early adolescence, there is a third stage of development during which there is neurophysiologic evidence for further development of intracortical, particularly frontal, connectivity and final maturation of event-related potential indices of information processing. These three neurophysiologic stages coincide with the Piagetian stages of preoperational behavior, concrete operations, and formal operations. Hence the developing neurophysiologic capacity to register, process, and extract information from stimuli, coupled with the increasing ability to inhibit responses to stimuli, appears to underlie the changing style of learning that progresses from the egocentric (preschool child) to the more objective but concrete (school child) and finally to abstract thinking (adolescence).

Acknowledgments. *The author's work cited in this chapter was funded by National Institutes of Health Grants HD-14193 and EY02612, National Institute of Mental Health Grants MH-26798 and MH-39065, and the Alice and Julius Kantor Charitable Trust. Marie Chia prepared the manuscript.*

References

Anthony BJ: In the blink of an eye: Implications of reflex modification for information processing. In: Ackles PK, Jennings JR, Coles MGH (eds): *Advances in Psychophysiology* (Vol 1). Greenwich, London, JAI Press, 1985, pp. 167–218.

Anthony BJ, Graham FK: Evidence for sensory-selective set in young infants. *Science* 220:742–744, 1983.

Anthony BJ, Graham FK: Blink reflex modification by selective attention: Evidence for the modulation of "automatic" processing. *Biol Psychol* 21:43–59, 1985.

Anthony BJ, Putnam LE: Cardiac and blink reflex concomitants of attentional selectivity: A comparison of adults and young children. *Psychophysiology* 22:508–516, 1985.

Balaban MT, Anthony BJ, Graham FK: Modality-repetition and attentional effects on reflex blinking in infants and adults. *Infant Behav Dev* 8:443–457, 1985.

Balaban MT, Anthony BJ, Graham FK: Prestimulation effects on blink and cardiac reflexes of 15-month human infants. *Dev Psychobiol* 22:115–127, 1989.

Baloh RW, Honrubia V: *Clinical Neurophysiology of the Vestibular System.* Philadelphia, FA Davis, 1979.

Benes FM, Turtle M, Khan Y, et al: Myelination of a key relay zone in the hippocampal formation occurs in the human brain during childhood, adolescence, and adulthood. *Arch Gen Psychiatry* 51:477–484, 1994.

Bergstrom B: Morphology of the vestibular nerve. II: The number of myelinated vestibular nerve fibers in man at various ages. *Acta Otolaryngol (Stockh)* 76:173–179, 1973.

Berman S, Friedman D, Cramer M: Age-related changes in processing negativity during selective attention to speech sounds and pure tones. In: Brunia CHM, Gaillard AWK, Kok A (eds): *Psychophysiological Brain Research* (Vol 2). The Netherlands, Tilburg University Press, 1990, pp. 147–151.

Blair SM, Gavin M: Modifications of vestibulo-ocular reflex induced by diazepam. *Arch Otolaryngol* 105:698–701, 1979.

Blumenthal TD, Levey BJ: Prepulse rise time and startle reflex modification: Different effects for discrete and continuous prepulses. *Psychophysiology* 26:158–165, 1989.

Breitmeyer BG, Ganz L: Implications of sustained and transient channels for theories of visual pattern making, saccadic suppression, and information processing. *Psychol Rev* 83:1–36, 1976.

Brody BA, Kinney HC, Kloman AS, et al: Sequence of central nervous system myelination in human infancy. I: An autopsy study of myelination. *J Neuropathol Exp Neurol* 46:283–301, 1987.

Buettner UW, Buttner U, Henn V: Transfer characteristics of neurons in vestibular nuclei of the alert monkey. *J Neurophysiol* 41:1614–1628, 1978.

Cohen B: Origin of quick phases of nystagmus. In: Brodal A, Pompeiano O (eds): *Basic Aspects of Central Vestibular Mechanisms.* Amsterdam, Elsevier, 1972.

Conraux C, Collard M: L'electronystagmographie chez l'enfant. *Acta Otorhinolaryngol Belg* 24:363–369, 1970.

Courchesne E: Event-related brain potentials: Comparison between children and adults. *Science* 197:589–592, 1977.

Courchesne E: Neurophysiological correlates of cognitive development: Changes in long-latency event-related potentials from childhood to adulthood. *Electroencephalogr Clin Neurophysiol* 45:468–482, 1978.

Courchesne E: Cognitive components of the event-related brain potential: Changes associated with development. In: Gaillard AWK, Ritter W (eds): *Tutorials in ERP Research: Endogenous Components.* Amsterdam, North-Holland, 1983, pp. 329–344.

Courchesne E, Elmasian R, Yeung-Courchesne R: Electrophysiological correlates of cognitive processing: P3b and Nc, basic, clinical, and developmental research. In: Halliday AM, Butler SR, Paul R (eds): *A Textbook of Clinical Neurophysiology.* New York, Wiley, 1987, pp. 645–676.

Courchesne E, Ganz L, Norcia AM: Event-related brain potentials to human faces in infants. *Child Dev* 52:804–811, 1981.

Daniels JD, Pettigrew JD, Norman IL: Development of single-neuron responses in kitten's lateral geniculate nucleus. *J Neurophysiol* 41:1373–1393, 1978.

Davis M, Gendelman DS, Tischler MD, et al: A primary acoustic startle circuit: Lesion and stimulation studies. *J Neurosci* 2:791–805, 1982.

Dayal VS, Farkashidy J, Kokshanian A: Embryology of the ear. *Can J Otolaryngol* 12:136, 1973.

Desmedt JE, Brunko E, Debecker J: Maturation and sleep correlates of the somatosensory evoked potential. *Prog Clin Neurophysiol* 7:146–161, 1980.

Donchin E, Coles MGH: Precommentary: Is the P300 component a manifestation of context updating? *Behav Brain Sci* 11:357–374, 1988.

Donchin E, Karis D, Bashore TR, et al: Cognitive psychophysiology and human information processing. In: Coles MGH, Donchin E, Porges SW (eds): *Psychophysiology: Systems, Processes, and Applications.* New York, Guilford, 1986a, pp. 244–267.

Donchin E, Kramer AF, Wickens C: Applications of brain event-related potentials to problems in engineering psychology. In: Coles MGH, Donchin E, Porges SW (eds): *Psychophysiology: Systems, Processes, and Applications*. New York, Guilford, 1986b, pp. 702–718.

Donchin E, Ritter W, McCallum WC: Cognitive psychophysiology: The endogenous components of the ERP. In: Callaway E, Tueting P, Koslow SH (eds): *Event-Related Brain Potentials in Man*. New York, Academic Press, 1978, pp. 349–412.

Eeg-Olofsson O: Longitudinal development course of electrical activity of brain. *Brain Dev* 2:33–44, 1980.

Eggermont JJ: On the rate of maturation of sensory evoked potentials. *Electroencephalogr Clin Neurophysiol* 70:293–305, 1988.

Eggermont JJ: Development of auditory evoked potentials. *Acta Otolaryngol (Stockh)* 112:197–200, 1992.

Emde RN, Metcalf DR: An electroencephalographic study of behavioral rapid eye movement states in the human newborn. *J Nerv Ment Dis* 150:376–386, 1970.

Enoki H, Sanada S, Yoshinaga H, et al: The effects of age on the N200 component of the auditory event-related potentials. *Cogn Brain Res* 1:161–167, 1993.

Epstein HT: Phrenoblysis: Special brain and mind growth periods. I: Human brain and skull development. *Dev Psychobiol* 7:207–216, 1974a.

Epstein HT: Phrenoblysis: Special brain and mind growth periods. II: Human mental development. *Dev Psychobiol* 7:217–224, 1974b.

Epstein HT: Correlated brain and intelligence development in humans. In: Hahn ME, Jensen C, Dudek BC (eds): *Development and Evolution of Brain Size*. New York, Academic Press, 1979, pp. 111–131.

Epstein HT: EEG developmental stages. *Dev Psychobiol* 13:629–631, 1980.

Epstein HT: Stages in human brain development. *Dev Brain Res* 30:114–119, 1986.

Fabiani M, Gratton G, Karis D, et al: Definition, identification, and reliability of measurement of the P300 component of the event-related brain potential. In: Ackles PK, Jennings JR, Coles MGH (eds): *Advances in Psychophysiology: A Research Annual* (Vol 2). Greenwich, London, JAI Press, 1987, pp. 1–78.

Fabiani M, Sohmer H, Tait C, et al: A functional measure of brain activity: Brain stem transmission time. *Electroencephalogr Clin Neurophysiol* 47:483–491, 1979.

Fabiani M, Sohmer H, Tait C, et al: Mathematical expression of relationship between auditory brainstem transmission time and age. *Dev Med Child Neurol* 26:461–465, 1984.

Finley WW, Faux SF, Hutcheson J, et al: Long-latency event-related potentials in the evaluation of cognitive function in children. *Neurology* 35:323–327, 1985.

Fischer KW, Silvern L: Stages and individual differences in cognitive development. *Annu Rev Psychol* 36:613–648, 1985.

Friedman D: The endogenous scalp-recorded brain potentials and their relationship to cognitive development. In: Jennings JR, Coles MGH (eds): *Handbook of Cognitive Psychophysiology*. New York, Wiley, 1991, pp. 621–656.

Friedman D, Brown C, Vaughan HG, et al: Cognitive brain potential components in adolescents. *Psychophysiology* 21:83–96, 1984.

Friedman D, Sutton S, Putnam L, et al: ERP components in picture matching in children and adults. *Psychophysiology* 25:570–590, 1988.

Fuchigami T, Okubo O, Fujita Y, et al: Auditory event-related potentials and reaction time in children: Evaluation of cognitive development. *Dev Med* 35:230–237, 1993.

Fuster MM, De Traversay J, Ornitz EM: Maturation of the fast component of vestibular nystagmus during childhood and young adulthood. *Acta Otolaryngol (Stockh)* 114:239–244, 1994.

Gersuni GV: Temporal organization of the auditory function. In: Gersuni GV (ed): *Sensory Processes at the Neuronal and Behavioral Levels* (Rose J, trans). New York, Academic Press, 1971, pp. 85–114.

Gersuni GV, Altman JA, Maruseva AM, et al: Functional classification of neurons in the inferior colliculus of the cat according to their temporal characteristics. In: Gersuni GV (ed): *Sensory Processes at the Neuronal and Behavioral Levels* (Rose J, trans). New York, Academic Press, 1971, pp. 157–179.

Goldman-Rakic PS: Development of cortical circuitry and cognitive function. *Child Dev* 58:601–622, 1987.

Goodin DS, Squires KC, Henderson BH, et al: Age-related variations in evoked potentials to auditory stimuli in normal human subjects. *Electroencephalogr Clin Neurophysiol* 44:447–458, 1978.

Graham FK: The more or less startling effects of weak prestimulation. *Psychophysiology* 12:238–248, 1975.

Graham FK, Murray GM: Discordant effects of weak prestimulation on magnitude and latency of the reflex blink. *Physiol Psychol* 5:108–114, 1977.

Graham FK, Anthony BJ, Zeigler BL: The orienting response and developmental processes. In: Siddle D (ed): *Orienting and Habituation: Perspectives in Human Research*. New York, Wiley, 1983, pp. 371–430.

Graham FK, Putnam LE, Leavitt LA: Lead-stimulation effects on human cardiac orienting and blink reflexes. *J Exp Psychol* 104:161–169, 1975.

Graham FK, Strock BD, Zeigler BL: Excitatory and inhibitory influences on reflex responsiveness. In: Collins WA (ed): *Aspects of the Development of Competence* (Vol 14, The Minnesota Symposium on Child Psychology). Hillsdale, NJ, Erlbaum, 1981, pp. 1–38.

Halgren E: The P3: A view from the brain. *Behav Brain Sci* 11:383–385, 1988.

Hickey TL: Postnatal development of the human lateral geniculate nucleus: Relationship to a critical period for the visual system. *Science* 198:836–838, 1977.

Hillyard SA, Hansen JC: Attention: Electrophysiological approaches. In: Coles MGH, Donchin E, Porges SW (eds): *Psychophysiology: Systems, Processes and Applications*. New York, Guilford, 1986, pp. 227–243.

Hillyard SA, Kutas M: Electrophysiology of cognitive processing. *Annu Rev Psychol* 34:33–61, 1983.

Hillyard SA, Picton TW: Electrophysiology of cognition. In: Mountcastle VB, Plum F, Geiger SR (eds): *Handbook of Physiology: A Critical, Comprehensive Presentation of Physiological Knowledge and Concepts. Sect 1: The Nervous System. Volume 5: Higher Functions of the Brain (Part 2)*. Bethesda, MD, American Physiological Society, 1987, pp. 519–584.

Honrubia V, Jenkins HA, Baloh RW, et al: Evaluation of rotary vestibular tests in peripheral labyrinthine lesions. In: Honrubia V, Brazier MAVB (eds): *Nystagmus and Vertigo: Clinical Approaches to the Patient with Dizziness*. New York, Academic Press, 1982, pp. 57–77.

Hooker D: *The Prenatal Origin of Behavior*. Lawrence, KA, University of Kansas Press, 1952.

Howard L, Polich J: P300 latency and memory span development. *Dev Psychol* 21:283–289, 1985.

Hudspeth WJ, Pribram KH: Stages of brain and cognitive maturation. *J Educ Psychol* 82:881–884, 1990.

Humphrey T: The embryologic differentiation of the vestibular nuclei in man correlated with functional development. In: *International Symposium on Vestibular and Oculomotor Problems*. Tokyo, Japan, 1965, p. 51.

Huttenlocher PR: Synaptic density in human frontal cortex. Developmental changes and effects of aging. *Brain Res* 163:195–205, 1979.

Huttenlocher PR: Morphometric study of human cerebral cortex development. *Neuropsychologia* 28:517–527, 1990.

Huttenlocher PR, de Courten C, Garey LJ, et al: Synaptogenesis in human visual cortex—Evidence for synapse elimination during normal development. *Neurosci Lett* 33:247–252, 1982.

Inhelder B, Piaget J: *The Growth of Logical Thinking from Childhood to Adolescence* (Parsons A, Milgram S, trans). New York, Basic Books, 1958.

Jiang ZD, Zhang L, Wu YY, et al: Brainstem auditory evoked responses from birth to adulthood: Development of wave amplitude. *Hearing Res* 68:35–41, 1993.

Johnson R Jr: The amplitude of the P300 component of the event-related potential: Review and synthesis. In: Ackles PK, Jennings JR, Coles MGH (eds): *Advances in Psychophysiology* (Vol 3). Greenwich, London, JAI Press, 1988, pp. 69–138.

Johnson R Jr: Developmental evidence for modality-dependent P300 generators: A normative study. *Psychophysiology* 26:651–667, 1989.

Jongkees LBW, Gasthuis W: La fonction de l'organe vestibulaire du nouveau-ne et de l'enfant. *J Fr Otorhinolaryngol* 22:97–101, 1973.

Karrer R, Ackles PK: Visual event-related potentials of infants during a modified oddball procedure. In: Johnson R, Rohrbaugh JW, Parasuraman R (eds): *Current Trends in Event-Related Potential Research* (EEG Suppl. 40). New York, Elsevier Science, 1987, pp. 603–608.

Klorman R, Thompson LW, Ellingson RJ: Event-related brain potentials across the life span. In: Callaway E, Tueting P, Koslow SH (eds): *Event-Related Brain Potentials in Man*. New York, Academic Press, 1978, pp. 511–570.

Knight RT: Decreased response to novel stimuli after prefrontal lesions in man. *Electroencephalogr Clin Neurophysiol* 59:9–20, 1984.

Knight RT, Scabini D, Woods DL, et al: Contributions of temporal-parietal junction to the human auditory P3. *Brain Res* 502:109–116, 1989.

Kostovic I: Structural and histochemical reorganization of the human prefrontal cortex during perinatal and postnatal life. *Prog Brain Res* 85:223–240, 1990.

Langworthy OR: Development of behavior patterns and myelinization of nervous system in human fetus and infant. *Contrib Embryol* 24:1, 1933.

Lecours A-R: Correlates of developmental behavior in brain maturation. In: Bever TG (ed): *Regressions in Mental Development: Basic Phenomena and Theories*. Hillsdale, NJ, Erlbaum, 1982, pp. 267–298.

Leitner DS, Cohen ME: Role of the inferior colliculus in the inhibition of acoustic startle in the rat. *Physiol Behav* 34:65–70, 1985.

Leitner DS, Powers AS, Stitt CL, et al: Midbrain reticular formation involvement in the inhibition of acoustic startle. *Physiol Behav* 26:259–268, 1981.

Lennie P: Parallel visual pathways: A review. *Vision Res* 20:561–594, 1980.

Levin HS, Culhane KA, Hartmann J, et al: Developmental changes in performance on tests of purported frontal lobe functioning. *Dev Neuropsychol* 7:377–395, 1991.

Lindsley DB: Brain potentials in children and adults. *Science* 84:354, 1936.

Lindsley DB: A longitudinal study of the occipital alpha rhythm in normal children: Frequency and amplitude standards. *J Genet Psychol* 55:197–213, 1939.

Malcolm R, Melvill-Jones G: A quantitative study of vestibular adaptation in humans. *Acta Otolaryngol (Stockh)* 70:126, 1970.

Martin F, Delpont E, Suisse G, et al: Long latency event-related potentials (P300) in gifted children. *Brain Dev* 15:173–177, 1993.

Martin LJ, Barajas JJ, Fernandez R: Auditory P3 development in childhood. *Scand Audiol Suppl* 30: 105–109, 1988a.

Martin L, Barajas JJ, Fernandez R, et al: Auditory event-related potentials in well-characterized groups of children. *Electroencephalogr Clin Neurophysiol* 71:375–381, 1988b.

Matousek M, Petersen I: Frequency analysis of the EEG in normal children and adolescents. In: Kellaway P, Petersen I (eds): *Automation of Clinical Electroencephalography*. New York, Raven Press, 1973, pp. 75–102.

Matthis P, Scheffner D, Denninger CHR, et al: Changes in the background activity of the electroencephalogram according to age. *Electroencephalogr Clin Neurophysiol* 49:626–635, 1980.

McCall RB, Meyers ED, Hartman J, et al: Developmental changes in head-circumference and mental-performance growth rates: A test of Epstein's phrenoblysis hypothesis. *Dev Psychobiol* 16: 457–468, 1983.

Mochizuki Y, Ohkubo GH, Motomura T: Development of human brainstem auditory evoked potentials and gender differences from infants to young adults. *Prog Neurobiol* 20:273–285, 1983.

Moskowitz A, Sokol S: Developmental changes in the human visual system as reflected by the latency of the pattern reversal VEP. *Electroencephalogr Clin Neurophysiol* 56:1–15, 1983.

Mrzljak L, Uylings HBM, Van Eden CG, et al: Neuronal development in human prefrontal cortex in prenatal and postnatal stages. *Prog Brain Res* 85: 185–222, 1990.

Mullis RJ, Holcomb PJ, Diner BC, et al: The effects of aging on the P3 component of the visual event-related potential. *Electroencephalogr Clin Neurophysiol* 62:141–149, 1985.

Naatanen R, Picton T: The N1 wave of the human electric and magnetic response to sound: A review and an analysis of the component structure. *Psychophysiology* 24:375–425, 1987.

Naatanen R, Paavilainen P, Alho K, et al: Do event-related potentials reveal the mechanism of the auditory sensory memory in the human brain? *Neurosci Lett* 98:217–221, 1989.

Naatanen R, Sams M, Alho K, et al: Frequency and location specificity of the human vertex N1 wave. *Electroencephalogr Clin Neurophysiol* 69: 523–531, 1988.

Niedermeyer E: Maturation of the EEG: Development of waking and sleep patterns. In: Niedermeyer E, Lopes da Silva F (eds): *Electroencephalography: Basic Principles, Clinical Applications and Related Fields*. Baltimore, Williams & Wilkins, 1993.

Ornitz EM: Development of sleep patterns in autistic children. In: Clemente CD, Purpura D, Mayer F (eds): *Sleep and the Maturing Nervous System*. New York, Academic Press, 1972, pp. 363–381.

Ornitz EM: Normal and pathological maturation of vestibular function in the human child. In: Romand R (ed): *Development of Auditory and Vestibular Systems*. New York, Academic Press, 1983, pp. 479–536.

Ornitz EM: Maturation of the vestibulo-ocular reflex during infancy and childhood. In: Igarashi M, Black FO (eds): *Vestibular and Visual Control on Posture and Locomotor Equilibrium*. Basel, Karger, 1985, pp. 241–245.

Ornitz EM: Development of the vestibular system. In: Meisami E, Timiras PS (eds): *Handbook of Human Growth and Developmental Biology. Vol 1: Neural, Sensory, Motor, and Integrative Development. Part B: Sensory, Motor and Integrative Development*. Boca Raton, FL, CRC Press, 1988, pp. 11–32.

Ornitz EM, Honrubia V: Developmental modulation of vestibular-ocular function. *Adv Otorhinolaryngol* 41:36–39, 1988.

Ornitz EM, Atwell CW, Walter DO, et al: The maturation of vestibular nystagmus in infancy and childhood. *Acta Otolaryngol (Stockh)* 88:244–256, 1979.

Ornitz EM, Guthrie D, Kaplan AR, et al: Maturation of startle modulation. *Psychophysiology* 23: 624–634, 1986.

Ornitz EM, Guthrie D, Lane SJ, et al: Maturation of startle facilitation by sustained prestimulation. *Psychophysiology* 27:298–308, 1990.

Ornitz EM, Guthrie D, Sadeghpour M, et al: Maturation of prestimulation-induced startle modulation in girls. *Psychophysiology* 28:11–20, 1991.

Ornitz EM, Kaplan AR, Westlake JR: Development of the vestibulo-ocular reflex from infancy to adulthood. *Acta Otolaryngol (Stockh)* 100:180–193, 1985.

Ornitz EM, Ritvo ER, Lee YH, et al: The auditory evoked response in babies during REM sleep. *Electroencephalogr Clin Neurophysiol* 27:195–198, 1969.

Ornitz EM, Wechter V, Hartman D, et al: The EEG and rapid eye movements during REM sleep in babies. *Electroencephalogr Clin Neurophysiol* 30: 350–353, 1971.

Ossenblok P, Reits D, Spekreijse H: Analysis of striate activity underlying the pattern onset EP of children. *Vision Res* 32:1829–1835, 1992.

Parmelee AH Jr: Development of states in infants. In: Clemente CD, Mayer FE, Purpura DP (eds): *Sleep and the Maturing Nervous System*. New York, Academic Press, 1972, pp. 199–228.

Passler MA, Isaac W, Hynd GW: Neuropsychological development of behavior attributed to frontal lobe functioning in children. *Dev Neuropsychol* 1: 349–370, 1985.

Petersen I, Eeg-Olofsson O: The development of the electroencephalogram in normal children from the age of 1 through 15 years. *Neuropaediatrie* 2: 247–304, 1971.

Pineda JA, Foote SL, Neville HJ: Effects of locus coeruleus lesions on long-latency, event-related potentials in monkey. *J Neurosci* 9:81–93, 1989.

Polich J, Ladish C, Burns T: Normal variation of P300 in children: Age, memory span, and head size. *Int J Psychophysiol* 9:237–248, 1990.

Pompeiano O: The neurophysiologic mechanisms of the postural and motor events during desynchronized sleep. *Res Nerv Ment Dis* 45:351–423, 1967a.

Pompeiano O: Sensory inhibition during motor activity in sleep. In: Yahr MD, Pupura DP (eds): *Neurophysiological Basis of Normal and Abnormal Motor Activities*. New York, Raven Press, pp. 323–372, 1967b.

Pompeiano O: Cholinergic activation of reticular and vestibular mechanisms controlling posture and eye movements. In: Hobson JA, Brazier MA (eds): *The Reticular Formation Revisited: Specifying Function for a Nonspecific System*. (Vol 6, International Brain Research Organization Monograph Series). New York, Raven Press, 1980, pp. 473–512.

Rabinowicz T: The differentiated maturation of

the cerebral cortex. In: Falkner F, Tanner JM (eds): *Human Growth, A Comprehensive Treatise*. New York, Plenum, 1986, pp. 385–410.

Rabinowicz T, Leuba G, Heumann D: Morphologic maturation of the brain: A quantitative study. In: Berenberg SR (ed): *Brain Fetal and Infant: Current Research on Normal and Abnormal Development*. The Hague, Martinus Nijhoff, 1977, pp. 29–51.

Radionova EA: Two types of neurons in the cat's cochlear nuclei and their role in audition. In: Gersuni GV (ed): *Sensory Processes at the Neuronal and Behavioral Levels* (Rose J, trans). New York, Academic Press, 1971, pp. 135–155.

Ritter W, Simson R, Vaughan HG Jr: Event-related potential correlates of two stages of information processing in physical and semantic discrimination tasks. *Psychophysiology* 20:168–179, 1983.

Ritter W, Simson R, Vaughan HG Jr: Effects of the amount of stimulus information processed on negative event-related potentials. *Electroencephalogr Clin Neurophysiol* 69:244–258, 1988.

Roffwarg HP, Muzio JN, Dement WC: Ontogenetic development of the human sleep-dream cycle. *Science* 152:604–619, 1966.

Rosenhall U: Vestibular macular mapping in man. *Ann Otol Rhinol Laryngol* 81:339–351, 1972.

Ruchkin DS, Johnson R, Mahaffey D, et al: Toward a functional categorization of slow waves. *Psychophysiology* 25:339–353, 1988.

Saitoh K, Tilson HA, Shaw S, et al: Possible role of the brainstem in the mediation of prepulse inhibition in the rat. *Neurosci Lett* 75: 216–222, 1987.

Salamy A, Mckean CM: Postnatal development of human brain stem potentials during the first year of life. *Electroencephalogr Clin Neurophysiol* 40: 418–426, 1976.

Shannon CE, Weaver W: *The Mathematical Theory of Communication*. Urbana, IL, University of Illinois Press, 1963.

Shaw MD, Baker R: Direct projections from vestibular nuclei to facial nucleus in cats. *J Neurophysiol* 50:1265–1280, 1983.

Sills AW, Honrubia V, Baloh RW: Is the adaptation model a valid description of the vestibulo-ocular reflex? *Biol Cybern* 30:209–220, 1978.

Simonds RJ, Scheibel AB: The postnatal development of the motor speech area: A preliminary study. *Brain Lang* 37:42–58, 1989.

Sokol S, Jones K: Implicit time of pattern evoked potentials in infants: An index of maturation of spatial vision. *Vision Res* 19:747–755, 1979.

Spekreijse H: Maturation of contrast EPs and development of visual resolution. *Arch Ital Biol* 116: 358–369, 1978.

Stauder JEA: Event related brain potentials and cognitive development during childhood. Doctoral dissertation, University of Amsterdam, 1992, pp. 1–135.

Steriade M: New vistas on the morphology, chemical transmitters and physiological actions of the ascending brainstem reticular system. *Arch Ital Biol* 126:225–238, 1988.

Symmes D, Eisengart MA: Evoked response correlates of meaningful visual stimuli in children. *Psychophysiology* 8:769–778, 1971.

Tanguay PE, Ornitz EM, Forsythe AB, et al: Rapid eye movement (REM) activity in normal and autistic children during REM sleep. *J Autism Child Schizophr* 6:275–288, 1976.

Tanguay PE, Ornitz EM, Kaplan A, et al: Evolution of sleep spindles in childhood. *Electroencephalogr Clin Neurophysiol* 38:175–181, 1975.

Taylor MJ: Maturational changes in ERPs to orthographic and phonological tasks. *Electroencephalogr Clin Neurophysiol* 88:494–507, 1993.

Thatcher RW: Neurolinguistics: Theoretical and

evolutionary perspectives. *Brain Lang* 11:235–260, 1980.

Thatcher RW: Maturation of the human frontal lobes: Physiological evidence for staging. *Dev Neuropsychol* 7:397–419, 1991.

Thatcher RW, Walker RA, Giudice S: Human cerebral hemispheres develop at different rates and ages. *Science* 236:1110–1113, 1987.

Tibbling L: The rotatory nystagmus response in children. *Acta Otolaryngol (Stockh)* 68:459, 1969.

Velasco M, Velasco F, Velasco AL, et al: Subcortical correlates of the P300 potential complex in man to auditory stimuli. *Electroencephalogr Clin Neurophysiol* 64:199–210, 1986.

Vertes RP: Brainstem control of the events of

REM sleep. *Prog Neurobiol* 22:241–288, 1984.

Vertes RP: A life-sustaining function for REM sleep: A theory. *Neurosci Biobehav Rev* 10:371–376, 1986.

Welsh MC, Pennington BF: Assessing frontal lobe functioning in children: Views from developmental psychology. *Dev Neuropsychol* 4:199–230, 1988.

Wijker W, Molenaar PCM, van der Molen MW: Age-changes in scalp distribution of cognitive event-related potentials elicited in an oddball task. *J Psychophysiol* 3:179–189, 1989.

Wood CC, McCarthy G: A possible frontal lobe contribution to scalp P300. *Soc Neurosci Abstr* 11:879, 1985.

Wu M-F, Suzuki SS, Siegel JM: Anatomical distribution and response patterns of reticular neurons active in relation to acoustic startle. *Brain Res* 457:399–406, 1988.

Yakovlev PI, Lecours A-R: The myelogenetic cycles of regional maturation of the brain. In: Minkowski A (ed): *Regional Development of the Brain in Early Life*. Oxford, United Kingdom, Blackwell, 1967, pp. 3–70.

Yingling CD, Hosobuchi Y: A subcortical correlate of P300 in man. *Electroencephalogr Clin Neurophysiol* 59:72–76, 1984.

Zametkin AJ, Stevens JR, Pittman R: Ontogeny of spontaneous blinking and of habituation of the blink reflex. *Ann Neurol* 5:453–457, 1979.

5 DEVELOPMENTAL ASPECTS OF PSYCHONEUROIMMUNOLOGY

Michael Irwin, M.D., and Elliot M. Friedman, Ph.D.

Psychoneuroimmunology describes the study of interactions among behavior, the psyche, the central and peripheral nervous systems, and the immune system. One hypothesis guiding research in this relatively new field is that these interactions underlie the effects that psychological experiences such as stress can exert on health. During the course of the past two decades, it has become clear that both acute and chronic psychological stress can influence the numbers and functional capacities of multiple immune cells. It is also evident that the immune system of the developing organism is particularly sensitive to stress. Psychological perturbation occurring in infancy or before birth can alter the developmental course of the immune system and result in altered immune responses in later life. This chapter reviews experimental evidence concerning the neural and endocrine pathways by which the central nervous system may regulate immune function as well as the short- and long-term immunological effects of early psychological experiences. Preclinical and clinical investigations are also presented to document the influence of both stressors and psychosocial processes on immunity. Before beginning the discussion of interactions among the brain, behavior, and immunity, we provide a brief overview of the immune system.

OVERVIEW OF THE IMMUNE SYSTEM

The immune system functions to discriminate "self" from "nonself" cells, protecting the organism from invasion by pathogens such as viruses and bacteria or from abnormal internal cells such as cancer cells (Cohn, 1985; Hood et al., 1985). These functions are closely regulated and performed without damage to the host, although an overresponsive immune system is purported to lead to autoimmune disease in which the organism's own tissues are attacked (Cohen, 1988; Morimoto et al., 1987; Paul, 1984; Strakosch et al., 1982; Talal, 1980).

The organs of the mammalian immune system include the thymus, spleen, and lymph nodes (Hood et al., 1985; Paul, 1984). The working cells of the immune system are represented by three distinct populations: T cells, B cells, and natural killer (NK) cells (Hood et al., 1985; Paul, 1984; Ritz, 1989).

Immune responses are typically divided into two important components: cellular immunity and humoral responses (Gilliland, 1983; Nossal, 1987; Paul, 1984). There is evidence that T cells and B cells interact and cooperate in many cellular immune responses and in most humoral immune responses, although cellular immunity is thought to be mediated primarily by T lymphocytes and humoral responses by B lymphocytes and their soluble products (Hood et al., 1985).

The T lymphocytes develop from stem cells in the bone marrow and migrate to the thymus where they mature into several subsets including the cytotoxic T cell, T-helper cell, and T-suppressor cell (Hood et al., 1985). These T cells circulate into the periphery and are found in the lymph nodes, blood vessels, and spleen. Briefly, the cytotoxic T cell is characterized by its ability to seek out and destroy either cells infected with viruses or tumor cells that have acquired foreign nonself antigens (Henney and Gillis, 1984; Zinkernagal and Doherty, 1979). In the development of the cytotoxic T-cell response, a foreign antigen is first encountered and incorporated onto the surface of an antigen-presenting cell such as a macrophage. After the antigen is presented to the T cell, recognized, and bound by a specific receptor on the T cell, then the T cell multiplies and becomes capable of attacking any cell that presents that specific foreign surface-antigen (Henney and Gillis, 1984). Other types of T lymphocytes such as the T-helper cells secrete interleukin-2 (IL-2) and regulate the proliferative response of the T cell to antigenic stimulation (Henney and Gillis, 1984). Reexposure of the cytotoxic T cell to an antigen produces a more rapid and extensive reaction than that found upon initial presentation.

The B cell is primarily involved in the humoral response. Like the T cell, the B cell arises from a precursor stem cell in the bone marrow, although in humans its site of maturation remains unknown (Hood, et al., 1985). Following initial antigen processing by the macrophage, the antigen-major histocompatibility complex (MHC) on the accessory cell surface engages the receptors of an appropriate T-helper cell antigen and the macrophage releases interleukin-1 (IL-1). Thus stimulated, the T-helper cell proliferates, forming a clone, and secretes factors such as IL-2, which stimulate T-cell and B-cell growth. The activated B cell in turn proliferates and differentiates into plasma cells that synthesize and secrete antigen-specific antibodies, of which the five major classes of immunoglobulins (Ig) are IgM, IgG, IgA, IgE, and IgD (Goodman, 1991). IgM is produced soon after antigenic stimulation. Cytokines liberated by activated T-helper cells, such as IL-4 and IL-5, subsequently promote the switch from IgM production by plasma cells to the production of other isotypes such as IgG (Nossal, 1987; Oppenheim et al., 1991). IgA is found primarily in the secretions of the body (i.e., nasal mucus, saliva, etc.). IgE in combination with a specific antigen binds to mast cells and mediates the immediate hypersensitivity response.

IgE may also be important in the development of allergic reactions (Oppenheim et al., 1991). The function of IgD is not known, although its prominence on B-cell surfaces during certain stages of development suggests that it may be involved in cell differentiation (Goodman, 1991).

In addition to the T and B cells, a distinct subpopulation of lymphocytes comprised of NK cells has been described. The NK cell is immunologically nonspecific and does not require sensitization to specific antigens to perform its cytotoxic activity (Herberman, 1980; Lotzova and Herberman, 1986; Trinchieri, 1989). Thus, the NK cell responds to a variety of cell surface markers, as long as the markers differ from self markers, and lyses a wide variety of cell types. While the role of the NK cell in tumor surveillance remains controversial (Lotzova and Herberman, 1986; Ritz, 1989), substantial evidence has demonstrated the importance of the NK cell in the control of herpes and cytomegalovirus infections in humans (Biron et al., 1989; Padgett et al., 1968; Ritz, 1989; Sullivan et al., 1980) and animals (Bancroft et al., 1981; Bukowski et al., 1985; Habu et al., 1984).

Regulation of immune responses involves the secretion of cellular factors or lymphokines (Oppenheim et al., 1991). These lymphokines together form a network of regulatory signals that show considerable overlap in activity and patterns of synergism as well as antagonism. For example, the lymphokine IL-1 is produced by nearly all immunologic cell types including NK cells, T and B lymphocytes, brain astrocytes, microglia, and macrophages (Dinarello and Mier, 1987). IL-1 acts mainly as an endogenous adjuvant serving as a cofactor during lymphocyte activation, inducing the synthesis of other lymphokines and the activation of resting T cells (Dinarello and Mier, 1987). For example, IL-1 stimulates T lymphocytes to synthesize and release IL-2, and IL-1 further acts on NK cells to induce the expression of the IL-2 receptor. Binding of IL-2 by its receptor on the NK cell is a crucial step in the activation of such cytotoxic cells (predominantly large granular lymphocytes) to form lymphokine-activated killer cells that are able to lyse a wide range of target cells in a non-MHC-restricted manner (Henney and Gillis, 1984).

MEASURES OF IMMUNE FUNCTION

The immune system can be evaluated by measures that assess the *number* of different cell types as well as the *function* of various components of cellular and humoral immunity. To quantitate the number of cells in various subpopulations, specific monoclonal antibodies are available that bind to unique surface markers on cell types such as T-helper, T-suppressor, and NK cells (Bernard and Boumsell, 1984). While enumeration of cell types reveals the balance of different cell types needed for the optimal immune response, numbers of different cell types do not necessarily correlate with functional capacity, and changes of cell numbers in the peripheral circulation may merely reflect a redistribution of cell types from various immune compartments (Murray et al., 1992).

Measurement of the function of the immune system can involve in vivo and in vitro techniques. Two examples of in vivo assays of immunity are measurement of the delayed-type hypersensitivity (DTH) response following administration of skin tests and measurement of antibody responses to a specific antigen. Both techniques provide valuable data about the physiological response of the organism to an antigenic challenge, and they have been proposed to be more relevant in the clinical assessment of immunocompetence than in vitro measures of immune function. However, these assays are expensive to perform, and because subsequent immunologic evaluations are altered by primary immunization, they cannot be utilized in longitudinal studies.

An indirect assessment of cellular immune function includes the measurement of antibody titers to latent viruses (Glaser et al., 1985). The cellular immune response is thought to be important in controlling latent viral infections, and reactivation of such viruses as herpes viruses can occur during conditions in which cellular immunity is compromised.

In turn, synthesis of virus or viral proteins is increased and elevations in antibody titers are detected in serum.

Two in vitro correlates of cellular immune function, mitogen-induced lymphocyte proliferation and NK cell activity, have been widely used to assess cell-mediated immune function. Both of these assays evaluate the function of cells outside the body. Mitogen-induced lymphocyte stimulation determines the proliferative capacity of lymphocytes following activation in vitro either with plant lectins such as concanavalin A (ConA) or phytohemagglutinin (PHA), which predominantly activate the T lymphocyte to divide, or with pokeweed mitogen that induces proliferation of B cells (Keller et al., 1981). The proliferative response is quantitated by the cellular incorporation of radioactively labeled thymidine or idoxuridine into newly synthesized DNA.

The other frequently used in vitro assessment of cellular immunity involves measurement of NK activity. Assay of NK lytic activity is carried out by the coincubation of isolated ''effector'' lymphocytes with radioactively labeled ''target'' tumor cells. The release of radioactivity by the lysed target cells is proportionate to the activity of the effector NK cells (Herberman and Ortaldo, 1981; Irwin et al., 1987).

Humoral immune function is generally assessed by the measurement of plasma concentrations of specific immunoglobulins, particularly IgM and IgG. Typically, enzyme-linked immunosorbent assays (ELISAs) are utilized. Immunoglobulin levels in serum provide an index of B-cell responses, but do not assess the mechanisms by which these responses are regulated (Schleifer et al., 1986).

Assay of levels of lymphokines (IL-1, IL-2, and interferon) in the plasma or following lymphocyte stimulation has been recently employed to quantitate possible alterations in the regulation of these cellular factors important in humoral and cellular immune responses (Glaser et al., 1990). IL-1 promotes lymphocyte differentiation via increased expression of IL-2 receptors, whereas IL-2 provides a signal for the proliferation and differentiation of immune cells (Oppenheim et al., 1991). Assay of these lymphokines is proposed to provide information about the immunologic mechanisms that may be related to changes in ex vivo measures such as lymphocyte proliferation or NK activity (Glaser et al., 1990; Maes et al., 1991).

MECHANISMS OF IMMUNOMODULATION

Autonomic Nervous System

The autonomic nervous system is one pathway for communication from the brain to cells of the immune system. Anatomical studies have revealed an extensive presence of autonomic fibers in both primary and secondary lymphoid organs (Bulloch and Pomerantz, 1984; Felten and Olschowka, 1987; Felten et al., 1981, 1984, 1985; Kendall and al-Shawaf, 1991; Leposavic et al., 1992), innervating both the vasculature and the parenchyma of the tissues. In a pattern of classic anatomical connection, preganglionic cell bodies located in the intermediolateral cell column of the spinal cord synapse with the ganglionic cells that are found either in the sympathetic chain or in collateral ganglia (Felten et al., 1987). Immunohistochemical studies have demonstrated that nerve fibers enter the lymphoid organs, such as the spleen, along with the vasculature and branch into the parenchyma (Felten et al., 1985) and areas in which lymphocytes (primarily T cells) reside (Ackerman et al., 1987; Felten et al., 1985). These noradrenergic fibers are not only adjacent to sites where T cells congregate but, at the electron microscopic level, end in synapse-like contacts with lymphocytes in the spleen (Felten and Olschowka, 1987). Together these observations establish an anatomical link between the brain and the immune system.

It has been hypothesized that the development and differentiation of lymphoid tissue are guided by the autonomic nervous system (Ackerman et al., 1987; Bullock, 1985; Bulloch et al., 1987). For example, the thymus was reported to be penetrated by vagal fibers before its immune and endocrine functions develop (Hammar, 1935). Furthermore, in the spleen, development of catecholaminergic nerves in the periarteriolar lymphatic sheaths parallels changes in T-cell compartmentalization (Ackerman et al., 1987), suggesting that norepinephrine influences lymphocyte movement into the spleen and the development of T- and B-cell compartments shortly after birth. Sympathetic innervation of the spleen may also be essential for the development of splenic immune cell function. Fischer 344 rats that were chemically sympathectomized with the neurotoxin 6-hydroxydopamine (6-OHDA) in the 1st week of life showed impaired NK cytotoxicity, mitogen-stimulated lymphocyte proliferation, and antibody responses lasting up to 3 months, in some cases, compared with saline-treated controls (Ackerman et al., 1991; Madden et al., 1993).

In the adult animal, norepinephrine appears to act as a neurotransmitter in the spleen. Norepinephrine is released within the spleen; early studies by von Euler (1946) found that splenic nerve stimulation yields a release of norepinephrine. Furthermore, in vivo dialysis techniques documented a 1 μM concentration of norepinephrine in the rat spleen (Felten et al., 1986), a concentration that is more than 100-fold higher than that in blood, suggesting local release of norepinephrine within the spleen.

Lymphocytes have been found to receive signals from sympathetic neurons by adrenoreceptor binding of norepinephrine, epinephrine, and dopamine (Aarons and Molinoff, 1982; Bidart al., 1983; Brodde et al., 1981; Miles et al., 1984; Motulsky and Insel, 1982; Williams et al., 1976). These β-receptors are linked to adenylate cyclase (Katz et al., 1982; Strom et al., 1977; Watson, 1975) and appear to have a functional role in the modulation of cellular immunity. In vitro incubation of lymphocytes with varying concentrations of either norepinephrine or epinephrine decreases NK activity (Hellstrand et al., 1985) and mitogenic responses (Hadden et al., 1970). As preincubation with a β-antagonist reverses the inhibitory effects of norepinephrine in vitro (Hellstrand et al., 1985), β-adrenoreceptor binding is believed to mediate an inhibition of cellular immunity (Livnat et al., 1985).

In vivo studies have shown that either surgical denervation of the spleen or chemical sympathectomy with 6-OHDA produces an augmented antibody response to thymus-dependent antigens such as sheep red blood cells (Besedovsky et al., 1979), an enhanced plaque-forming cell response to thymus-independent antigens (Miles et al., 1981), and altered T- and B-cell responsiveness to mitogen stimulation (Hall and Goldstein, 1981; Livnat et al., 1985). Others have found in animals and humans that infusion of adrenergic agonists results in a down-regulation of β-adrenergic receptors in circulating mononuclear cells (Aarons and Molinoff, 1982; Krall et al., 1980) and acute changes in NK cell function and lymphocyte responses to mitogens and a specific antigen (Heilig et al., 1993; Livnat et al., 1985; Pezzone et al., 1992; Schledowski et al., 1993; Tonnesen et al., 1984). Endogenous release of sympathetic catecholamines appears to mediate the immunomodulatory effects of acute stress. Animals exposed to aversive stress or central doses of neuropeptides such as corticotropin-releasing hormone (CRH) that activate sympathetic outflow show suppression of cellular immunity or in vivo specific antibody responses that can be reversed by autonomic blockade (Irwin et al., 1988) or chemical sympathectomy (Irwin et al., 1990). Pharmacologic blockade of β-adrenergic receptors restores suppressed splenic lymphocyte responses to ConA produced by foot shock stress and conditioned immunosuppression (Cunnick et al., 1990; Luecken and Lysle, 1992).

Chronic elevation of sympathetic tone has also been found to mediate a reduction of immunity (Irwin et al., 1991). In animals, for example, induction of a chronic hyperadrenergic state (experimental congestive heart failure or 2-week infusion of the β-agonist isoproterenol) reduces NK activity, in vivo antibody responses, and lymphocyte proliferation (Waltman et al., 1992). Similar to findings following acute stress, the immunosuppressive effect of chronic elevated sympathetic tone is completely antagonized by β-receptor blockade. In humans, chronic elevated sympathetic tone as reflected by circulating concentrations of neuropeptide Y may also contribute to the modulation of immune function during severe life stress and depression (Irwin et al., 1991). Neuropeptide Y

is present in peripheral sympathetic nerves and is released following emotional stress, potentiating the effects of vasoactive catecholamines and other pressor substances (Romano et al., 1991). Irwin et al. (1991) have shown that plasma concentrations of neuropeptide Y are elevated in depressed patients as well as in aged individuals and persons undergoing severe Alzheimer caregiver stress. Furthermore, activation of the sympathetic nervous system and release of neuropeptide Y is associated with a reduction of natural cytotoxicity in depression and life stress. Additional findings also support the hypothesis that elevated sympathetic activity in depression is associated with immune alterations. In depressed patients, excretion of 3-methoxy-4-hydroxyphenylglycol (MHPG) has been used as an index of total body noradrenergic turnover or sympathetic activity, and MHPG excretion was inversely related with lymphocyte proliferative responses in depressed patients (Maes et al., 1989). Together, these data suggest that elevated sympathetic tone in patients with major depressive disorder and/or in persons undergoing life stress is inversely correlated with cellular immune function.

Neuroendocrine Influences on Immunity

ADRENAL AXIS

The neuroendocrine system might also exert influence on immune responses. The secretion of corticosteroids has long been considered as the mechanism of stress-induced and/or depression-related suppression of immune function (Cupps and Fauci, 1982; Munck et al., 1984; Parrillo and Fauci, 1978; Riley, 1981; Selye, 1976). Specific intracytoplasmic corticosteroid receptors have been identified in normal human lymphocytes (Lippman and Barr, 1977), and these receptors bind corticosteroids and appear to play a role in the regulation of cellular function through modulation of cyclic AMP levels (Parker et al., 1973). In vitro studies have further demonstrated that glucocorticoids act to inhibit interleukin-2 production in vitro with resulting suppression of lymphocyte responses to mitogenic stimulation (Gillis et al., 1979), natural killer cell activity (antibody-dependent cytotoxicity is relatively refractory to glucocorticoids) (Parrillo and Fauci, 1978), and the differentiation and function of macrophages (Baybutt and Holsboer, 1990).

Even though pharmacologic data from in vitro and in vivo studies demonstrated that corticosteroids suppress a number of parameters of immunity (Cupps and Fauci, 1982), increased adrenocortical activity is not always correlated with changes in immune function in an organism responding to aversive stressors. For example, acute administration of either forced immobilization (Irwin and Hauger, 1988) or audiogenic stress (Irwin et al., 1989) produces an activation of adrenal steroid secretion but does not alter immune function as measured by natural killer cell activity. Likewise with repeated exposure to the stressor, pituitary adrenal activation is dissociated from a reduction in cytotoxicity (Irwin and Hauger, 1988; Irwin et al., 1989). Finally, stress-induced suppression of lymphocyte function following unpredictable, unavoidable tail shock occurs both in adrenalectomized (Keller et al., 1983) and in hypophysectomized animals (Keller et al., 1988). Nevertheless, stress-related reductions of lymphocyte and antibody responses in which adrenal activation clearly participates have been reported (Cunnick et al., 1990; Dobbs et al., 1993). A possible resolution of these discrepancies may lie in the site of action for adrenal corticoids. Stress-induced decreases in splenocyte mitogen responses can be abolished by pharmacologic blockade of β-adrenergic receptors, but the responses of peripheral blood lymphocytes are only partially restored (Cunnick et al., 1990; Pezzone et al., 1992). In contrast, adrenalectomy prevents stress-induced inhibition of mitogenic responses in peripheral blood, but not splenic lymphocytes in rats, and use of the glucocorticoid receptor antagonist RU486 attenuates stress-induced reductions in antibody responses to herpes simplex virus in mice (Pezzone et al., 1992).

Clinical research has found no relationship between adrenocortical activity and immunity in depressed patients and in stressed persons. In depressed patients, decreased lymphocyte responses to mitogens are not associated with dexamethasone nonsuppression (Kronfol and House, 1985) or with increased excretion rates of urinary free cortisol (Kronfol et al., 1986). Furthermore, in bereavement in which a reduction of natural killer activity has been demonstrated, this immunologic change occurs even in subjects who had plasma cortisol levels comparable to those of control subjects (Irwin et al., 1988).

OPIOID PEPTIDES

Pharmacologic evidence has shown that some cells of the immune system have opioid receptors, although the data remain tentative and fragmentary and few studies have reported on the saturability or stereospecificity of these binding sites (Sibinga and Goldstein, 1988). Opioid binding on immune cells was first suggested by the finding that nanomolar concentrations of opioids affect active rosetting of human T lymphocytes (Wybran et al., 1979). Morphine inhibits rosetting, whereas met-enkephalin stimulates it and both effects are blocked by naloxone. Using radiolabeling techniques, specific opioid binding on human phagocytic leukocytes (Falke et al., 1985; Farrar, 1984; Lopker et al., 1980), platelets (Mehrishi and Mills, 1983), and lymphocytes (Ausiello and Roda, 1987; Mehrishi and Mills, 1983) has been demonstrated.

Endogenous opioid peptides are able to influence in vitro the function of most cell types of the immune system; both inhibitory and immunoenhancing effects of opioid peptides have been described. Johnson et al. (1982) found that α-endorphin, met-enkephalin, and leu-enkephalin (all with approximately equal potency) decrease the proliferation and antibody production of splenocytes in the plaque-forming assay, an effect that is blocked by naloxone. Confirming these results, Heijnen et al. (1986) demonstrated that (des-Tyr) β-endorphin is also active in suppressing the plaque-forming cell response. PHA-induced proliferation is affected by opioid peptides, although both stimulatory (Bocchini et al., 1983; Farrar, 1984; Gilman et al., 1982) and inhibitory effects (McCain et al., 1986; Puppo et al., 1985) have been reported, and these opioid effects on mitogen-induced lymphocyte proliferation and interleukin-2 production are not blocked by the specific opiate antagonist naloxone (Gilmore and Weiner, 1988).

A naloxone reversible enhancement of human natural cytotoxicity by very low concentrations of β-endorphin (10 fM) and of met-enkephalin (10 pM) has also been reported. However, some studies have described an inverted U-shaped dose response for β-endorphin and a bidirectional effect of the enkephalins and selective opiate agonists on human NK activity; subjects with ''low'' (below the median) NK activity show stimulation with enkephalin, whereas the cytolytic activity of cells from the ''high'' group is inhibited by similar doses of enkephalin (Oleson and Johnson, 1988). Recent evidence suggested that endorphins modulate NK activity through the (6–9) amino acid region (i.e., the α-helix portion of β-endorphin) (Kay et al., 1987).

Systemic administration of opioids as well as the release of opiate peptides following stress appear to modulate changes of NK cytotoxicity in animals, although the physiological importance of opioid modulation of other in vitro correlates of immune function cannot yet be adduced with confidence. In rats repeatedly administered intermittent inescapable foot shock over 4 consecutive days (Shavit et al., 1984), a significant suppression of NK activity occurs that can be completely antagonized by the preadministration of naltrexone. Unconditioned (foot shock) and conditioned suppression of lymphocyte proliferation responses can be attenuated by naltrexone (Lysle et al., 1992). Daily injection of morphine for 4 days at doses of 10, 30, or 50 mg/kg produces a similar suppression of cytotoxicity (Shavit et al., 1984, 1986). In contrast, inhibition of NK cytotoxicity in a forced-swimming paradigm was unaffected by pretreatment with naltrexone (Ben-Eliyahu et al., 1990), and naltrexone dose dependently aggravated reductions in primary and secondary antibody responses to sheep red blood cells induced by restraint stress (Ray et al., 1992).

Nevertheless, direct peripheral effects of opioid agonists on the immune system are also possible, because opioid agonists bind on specific receptors on cells of the immune system (Carr et al., 1988). Indeed, experimental and correlative evidence suggest that peripheral increases of endogenous circulating concentrations of β-endorphin stimulate NK activity, similar to the findings generated in vitro. In the rat, release of β-endorphin into the plasma following acute exposure to forced immobilization are correlated with immediate, poststress increases of splenic NK activity (Irwin and Hauger, 1988). Likewise, clinical research has found that exercise-induced enhancement of NK cytotoxicity is completely antagonized by the preadministration of the opiate antagonist naloxone (Fiatarone et al., 1988). Finally, plasma levels of β-endorphin are positively correlated with NK activity in depressed patients (Darko et al., 1992).

ADRENOCORTICOTROPIC HORMONE

A receptor for adrenocorticotropic hormone (ACTH) has been identified on lymphocytes, also raising the possibility that some aspects of altered lymphocyte function in depression are regulated by this peptide. In vitro studies have shown that ACTH inhibits the antibody response at an early state in the antibody response (Johnson et al., 1992). In regard to cellular immunity, McGlone et al. (1991) have recently evaluated the effects of ACTH administered in vitro and in vivo on NK cell function. Exogenous, peripheral administration of ACTH at physiological concentrations increases both NK activity and IL-2-stimulated NK cytotoxicity compared with levels in saline control subjects. Because in vitro doses of ACTH have no effect on NK activity (McGlone et al., 1991), the action of this peptide in vivo is likely caused by an indirect mechanism, i.e., alteration of leukocyte traffic or suppression of central CRH. Finally, one clinical study of 26 depressed patients failed to demonstrate an association between plasma concentrations of ACTH and lymphocyte proliferation (Darko et al., 1989), although the effects of ACTH on NK activity have not yet been evaluated.

PROLACTIN

A direct involvement of prolactin in the regulation of the immune system has been proposed. Prolactin receptors have been found on T and B lymphocytes (Russell et al., 1985), and prolactin induces a marked enhancement of NK activity (Nagy et al., 1983). In hypophysectomized rats as well as in animals treated with bromocriptine, a dopamine agonist that inhibits prolactin secretion, impairment of both humoral and cell-mediated immune response has been demonstrated. This impairment can be reversed by treatment with exogenous, physiologic doses of prolactin (Bernton et al., 1988). In addition, antibodies to prolactin have been reported to inhibit lymphocyte proliferation (Hartmann et al., 1989). Preliminary observations by Darko et al. (1989) have found that plasma levels of prolactin positively correlated with T-cell mitogen proliferation, although Clodi et al. (1992) failed to show any immune alteration as reflected by serum concentrations of immunoglobulin, IL-1, soluble IL-2 receptor, lymphocyte subsets, or NK activity in patients with prolactinomas. Chronic prolactin elevation may lead to adaptive changes that effectively abolish the immunomodulatory effects of prolactin.

GROWTH HORMONE

Growth hormone is a polypeptide that plays a pivotal role in growth and development. In addition to its endocrine and metabolic effects, growth hormone is likely to have significant effects on the immune system, particularly T-cell development (Weigent and Blalock, 1990). In growth hormone-deficient mouse strains, hematopoietic and B-cell progenitor deficiencies, marked atrophy of the cortical region of the thymus, and an impairment of cell-mediated immunity have been found and can be reversed by treatment with growth hormone (Dumont et al., 1979; Murphy et al., 1992). Likewise, thymic size in the aged rat can be increased by growth hormone (Kelley et al., 1986). In adult rats, growth hormone is reported to stimulate macrophage superoxide release (Edwards et al., 1992) and to confer resistance to bacterial infection

(Edwards et al., 1992). In contrast with these observations, Cross et al., (1992) have indicated that hypopituitary mice lag behind heterozygous littermates with respect to development of immunocompetence but that normal immune responsiveness does fully develop. Exploratory clinical studies in depression have failed to identify any relationship between growth hormone and immune function (Darko et al., 1989), although the number of depressed subjects studied is small.

SEROTONIN

Substantial evidence has demonstrated that serotonergic systems are altered in depression, and recent in vitro data have shown that serotonin modulates lymphocyte proliferation and NK activity. For example, serotonin suppresses lymphocyte response to PHA in vitro (Bonnet et al., 1984), whereas the addition of serotonin to enriched mononuclear cells induces a 2-fold, dose-dependent enhancement of NK activity, similar to the stimulation induced by IL-2 (Hellstrand and Hermodsson, 1987). The induction of NK activity is monocyte dependent and likely mediated by specific binding of serotonin at the $5\text{-}HT_1$ receptor on the monocyte; the enhancing properties of serotonin are mimicked by the $5\text{-}HT_1$-specific receptor agonist 8- hydroxypropylamino tetralin (8-OH DPAT) and completely antagonized by the serotonin receptor antagonist cyproheptadine. Clinical studies have not yet characterized whether expression and regulation of the $5\text{-}HT_{1A}$ receptor on monocytes is altered in depressed patients, and it is not known whether monocyte $5\text{-}HT_{1A}$ activity has a role in the reduction of NK activity in depression.

Role of Central Nervous System

In 1982, Geschwind and Behan advanced intriguing correlational data suggesting an increased incidence of immune-related disorders such as rheumatoid arthritis and diabetes in individuals who are strongly left-handed and/or whose immediate relatives are strongly left-handed. These relationships were observed in both clinical and general populations (Geschwind and Behan, 1982). While no causal relationships can be established from these data, they do suggest an association between brain structure and immune function.

Experimental evidence now exists indicating that the brain can influence immune function, probably by coordinating the autonomic nervous system and neuroendocrine pathways. Early experiments placed electrolytic or other destructive lesions in the hypothalamus and demonstrated alterations in lymphoid tissue architecture (Cross et al., 1980; Isakovic and Jankovic, 1973), either impairment or enhancement of lymphoid cell activation (Brooks et al., 1980; Keller et al., 1980; Roszman et al., 1982), impairment of delayed-type hypersensitivity (Macris et al., 1970; Stein et al., 1976), and suppression of natural killer cell activity (Cross et al., 1984). Fewer focal lesions in cortical tissue have revealed not only that cellular and humoral immune responses are modulated by ablation of parieto-occipital neocortex, but also that these effects are observed only following right hemisphere lesions (Barneoud et al., 1987).

Consistent with the cortical lesions studies, Kang et al. (1991) reported that women with extreme right frontal activation (measured by electroencephalography) had lower levels of NK activity than did left frontally activated individuals. These observations are intriguing in light of psychophysiological evidence that emotions are asymmetrically processed in frontal cortex, with negative emotions (e.g., disgust) producing greater relative right frontal activation and positive emotions (e.g., amusement) producing greater relative left frontal activation (Wheeler et al., 1993). Furthermore, clinical depression or a history of clinical depression are both associated with decreased relative left frontal activation (Henriques and Davidson, 1991; Henriques and Davidson, 1990).

Additional studies have examined cellular immune responses following the administration of either pharmacological agents or neuropeptides, which are capable of changing central nervous system activity. For example, depletion of CNS catecholamines by central injection of the neurotoxin 6-hydroxydopamine into the cisterna magna impairs the primary antibody immune response (Cross and Roszman, 1988; Cross et al., 1986) by inducing T-suppressor cell activity (Cross et al., 1988).

Opiate-induced modulation of NK cytotoxicity is also mediated in part by the central nervous system. A reduction of splenic NK activity is achieved by the administration of a dose of morphine that is a thousand times smaller given into the cerebral ventricle than that required when given systemically (Shavit et al., 1986). Peripheral administration of a morphine analogue (one that does not cross the blood-brain barrier to enter the central nervous system) is not effective in altering NK activity (Shavit et al., 1986). Moreover, intracerebral infusion of morphine into the periaqueductal gray matter, but not into other brain regions, produces a suppression of splenic NK activity (Weber and Pert, 1989). Finally, peripheral administration of naltrexone has been shown to block conditioned suppression of lymphocyte proliferation responses, but *N*-methyl-naltrexone, which does not cross the blood-brain barrier, is unable to reverse the suppression (Lysle et al., 1992).

Corticotropin-releasing factor (CRF) has been postulated to be a physiological central nervous system regulator that integrates biological responses to stress (Axelrod and Resine, 1984; Taylor and Fishman, 1988). Its role in modulating immune function through a central site of action has been recently examined (Irwin et al., 1987). In addition to its well-established role as a hypothalamic regulator of the pituitary secretion of ACTH and β-endorphin (Vale et al., 1981), CRF is also found to act in the central nervous system at extrahypothalamic sites, inducing an increase in the firing rate of the locus ceruleus (Valentino et al., 1983), activating the autonomic nervous system as reflected by increased plasma concentrations of norepinephrine and epinephrine (Fisher et al., 1982), and producing a pattern of behavioral responses such as decreased feeding and increased locomotor activity (Britton et al., 1982; Sherman and Kalin, 1985; Sutton et al., 1982). Moreover, central administration of CRF induces a dose-dependent suppression of splenic NK activity (Irwin et al., 1987), which is mediated by central activation of the sympathetic nervous system (Irwin et al., 1988). Finally, recent data suggested a physiological role for the release of central endogenous CRF in stress-induced suppression of cellular immunity; central administration of an antiserum to CRF completely antagonizes the effects of inescapable shock on splenic NK activity and lymphocyte proliferation (Irwin et al., 1990; Saperstein et al., 1992). Consistent with the previous findings that show that activation of the pituitary adrenal axis is dissociated from acute stress-induced changes in cellular immunity (Keller et al., 1983, 1988), peripheral administration of antiserum to CRF antagonizes stress-induced release of ACTH and corticosterone but has no effect on the suppression of NK activity (Irwin et al., 1990).

There is a growing literature devoted to the impact of the immune response and soluble immune response modifiers on brain function and behavior. Interleukin-1 is an immune response modifier that has received a large amount of attention because of its pleiotropic physiological and behavioral effects. This cytokine, when introduced into the brain, induces slow wave sleep (Krueger and Obal, 1993), increased release of hypothalamic CRH (Sapolsky et al., 1987), and increased circulating concentrations of ACTH (Vale et al., 1981). Since IL-1 plays a crucial role in regulating a number of immunological responses (Dinarello and Mier, 1987), Sundar et al. (1990) and Brown et al. (1991) have investigated whether central administration of IL-1 would affect immunity, and both groups demonstrated that central doses of IL-1 (3.1–12.4 fmol) rapidly reduce ex vivo cellular immune responses such as NK cell activity, lymphocyte proliferative response to PHA, IL-2 production, and macrophage IL-1 secretion. Importantly, the effects of central IL-1 on immune function are blocked by the administration of an antibody to CRH, indicating that IL-1β likely mediates immunosuppression via central release of CRH (Saperstein et al., 1992; Sundar et al., 1989). Consequently, the pathways by which IL-1 regulates peripheral immune function are similar to mechanisms involved in central CRH suppression of immunity. Administration of a ganglionic blocker abrogates the effects of IL-1 (Sundar et al., 1990), similar to observations that autonomic and sympathetic nervous mechanisms mediate CRH-induced suppression of NK activity (Irwin et al., 1988, 1990).

STRESS AND IMMUNITY: PRECLINICAL STUDIES

Aversive Stressors and Disease Susceptibility

Many workers have identified links between the stress associated with physical and psychological stimuli and the increased susceptibility of animals to a number of immune-related disorders such as infectious and neoplastic disease (Griffin, 1989). To evaluate altered resistance to infections, a number of different aversive stressors have been used in rodents. Psychosocial stimulation of animals involving either avoidance conditioning, physical restraint, or auditory stimulation is associated with decreased resistance to herpes simplex, coxsackie B, poliomyelitis, or vesicular stomatitis virus, and tuberculosis (Friedman and Glasgow, 1966). High population density affects the susceptibility of mice to the malarial parasite *Plasmodium berghei* (Plaut et al., 1969), and isolation housing is associated with increased risk of encephalomyocarditis virus infections (Friedman et al., 1969). Restraint stress was recently reported to diminish cellular immune and inflammatory responses to viral infection in mice (Hermann et al., 1994), an effect that is mediated by corticosterone and catecholamines (Dobbs et al., 1993). It appears that both the virulence of the organism as well as the psychophysiological state of the animal affects disease risk. If the infectious agent produces a chronic or insidious infection and the animals are stressed at the time of exposure, then symptoms of disease are more likely (Ader, 1983; Friedman et al., 1965; Griffin, 1989). Preliminary research with macaque monkeys infected with simian immunodeficiency virus (SIV) found that early psychosocial factors, such as rearing condition (i.e., with mother or with peers) and the number of changes in housing (i.e., from a familiar social group to an unfamiliar group or to isolation) were significantly correlated with disease-related variables such as latency to leukopenia, weight loss, and survival (Capitanio and Lerche, 1991).

Findings from studies of the role of stress in susceptibility to neoplastic disease are heterogeneous, depending upon the age and species of the animal, the type of tumor (viral or chemically induced), the timing of the stressor in relation to tumor inoculation, and the quality of the stressor (inescapable or escapable) (Griffin, 1989; Justice, 1985; Riley, 1981; Sklar and Anisman, 1981). In general, it appears that simultaneous exposure of rats or mice to inescapable shock and tumor cells facilitates tumor growth, while administration of the stressor before implantation inhibits its growth (Shavit et al., 1985). Exposure to escapable shock has no impact on tumor development (Shavit et al., 1985).

Effects of Stressors on Immune Responses

Behavioral responsiveness to inescapable aversive stimulation has provided an animal model to investigate clinical depression (Irwin et al., 1989). Aversive stressors such as sound exposure (Irwin et al., 1989; Monjan and Collector, 1977), rotation (Kandil and Borysenko, 1987; Riley, 1981), intermittent shock (Keller et al., 1981, 1983; Shavit et al., 1984), and forced immobilization (Irwin and Hauger, 1988) have been shown to affect lymphocyte responses to mitogen stimulation and/or NK activity in a manner that depends on their dose- and time-response profiles. For example, using an audiogenic stressor repeated at daily intervals, Irwin et al. (1989b) have replicated the findings of Monjan and Collector (1977) who found that the initial stress-induced immune suppression is followed by an increase or enhancement of natural cytotoxicity. Keller et al. (1981) have demonstrated a relationship between the intensity of an acute stressor and the degree of suppression of T-cell function. A progressive decrease of PHA-induced stimulation is found in animals who receive apparatus, low-level tail shock, or high-level electric tail shock, respectively, as compared to home cage controls (Keller et al., 1981).

Cellular in vivo immune responses and antibody responses are also altered by aversive stressors. Delayed-type hypersensitivity reaction is

decreased in mice exposed to heat stress (Pitkin, 1965) and the graft-versus-host response is suppressed in animals subjected to limited feeding (Amkraut et al., 1973), an effect that is independent of adrenocortical levels (Amkraut et al., 1973). Reduced antibody responses are found in monkeys exposed to a number of aversive stimuli (Felsenfeld et al., 1966; Hill et al., 1967), in mice housed in high- versus low-density grouping (Solomon, 1969), and in mice subjected to changes in housing condition (either from individual to group housing or from a group to the return to an individual cage) (Edwards et al., 1980). Similar to the effects of stressor timing on susceptibility to infectious or neoplastic disease, restraint produces a significant reduction in antibody response to sheep red blood cells only if the stress is applied before the time of immunization; there is no change in antibody production when the stress is applied after antigen injection (Okimura et al., 1986).

Modulation by Psychological Factors

In addition to the effects of stressor characteristics, the psychological response of the animal to the stressor has been related to the immunologic consequences of the stress. Laudenslager et al. (1983) found that rats exposed to inescapable uncontrollable electric tail shock have reduced lymphocyte activity, whereas animals that receive the same total amount of shock but are able to terminate it did not show altered immunity. Furthermore, Mormede et al. (1989) reported that even stressor predictability, in the form of a warning stimulus preceding inescapable foot shock, completely reverses the shock-induced suppression of lymphocytes. Consistent with the hypothesis that fear ultimately determines the amount of immunosuppression induced by aversive stimuli, a non-aversive stimulus that is associated with electric shock can be conditioned to impair lymphocyte proliferation independent of the direct effect of the physically aversive stimulation (Lysle et al., 1988, 1992).

Immunological Consequences of Early Life Experiences

Infancy has been suggested to be a period of life during which the organism is particularly sensitive to psychological perturbation, and stressful experiences during this period may have long-term physiological impact. Early life experiences such as premature maternal separation produce alterations in many processes regulated by the hypothalamus, including body temperature, sleep, metabolic rate, and maturation of autonomic processes (Ackerman et al., 1979; Hofer, 1984). There is now evidence that the physiological effects of these experiences also include changes in immune function.

Because of their social nature, nonhuman primates have been the subjects of many studies involving the effects of psychological stress on immune responses in young animals (see Coe, 1993, for review). One of the earliest studies reported that lymphocyte proliferation responses to stimulation with ConA and PHA were reduced in two pairs of infant pigtail macaques undergoing separation from their peers (Reite et al., 1981). This effect was later reproduced in infant bonnet macaques briefly separated from their mothers (Laudenslager et al., 1982). In both of these studies, lymphocyte responses were reduced for the 2-week period of separation and returned to their original levels following reunion.

Since that time, numerous experiments involving multiple species of New and Old World nonhuman primates have replicated these early findings and have extended them to other measures of immunity including lymphocyte subset numbers, levels of complement proteins and immunoglobulins, macrophage chemiluminescence, and DTH responses (Boccia et al., 1989; Coe et al., 1988a, 1988b; Friedman et al., 1991; Gordon et al., 1992; Gust et al., 1992; Laudenslager et al., 1990). Immune responses and cell numbers have proven to be sensitive to psychosocial stressors ranging from mother-infant separation to the formation of novel social groups.

Some of these studies have also shown, however, that animals' physiological responses to these stressors are influenced by a number of psychological factors. The largest stress-related differences in immune function are typically found in the monkeys that are observed to have the most severe behavioral responses to both experimental (Laudenslager et al., 1990) and natural stressors (Laudenslager et al., 1993). The magnitude of change in immune function following psychosocial stress also depends on several factors, including the time at which immunity is measured, the environment in which the animal experiences the stressor, and the age of the animal at the time of the stressor (Coe, 1993). Stress-related reductions in antibody responses to a bacteriophage, for example, are attenuated in monkeys housed with familiar, but not unfamiliar, companions or in a familiar location for the duration of the separation (Coe, 1993).

Longitudinal assessments of immunity have revealed that early life experiences like those described above may have long-term immunological consequences. Pigtail monkeys briefly separated from their mothers during the 1st year of life showed greater reductions in lymphocyte proliferation responses as adults than did control monkeys (Laudenslager et al., 1985). In 40-day-old rats separated from their mothers on postnatal day 15, lymphocyte responses are lower than responses in rats that remained with their mothers until day 22 (Ackerman et al., 1988). Mice that were maternally deprived and weaned at 15 days postpartum show a depressed antibody response to sheep erythrocyte immunization at 7 and 8 weeks of age, but no differences in body weight or adrenal weight. Finally, preliminary evidence suggests that rats prematurely separated 100 days after weaning may show greater susceptibility to severe respiratory infection (Schleifer et al., 1986).

Several reports have provided additional data that tumor growth in the adult animal is effected by early life experience. Daily handling of mice prior to weaning leads to increased rates of mortality following implantation of a lymphoid leukemia (Levine and Cohen, 1959), and handling of rats during the first 3 weeks of life affects the growth of a carcinosarcoma (Ader and Friedman, 1965).

More chronic early life experiences such as rearing environment have been shown to exert long-term influence on the immune system. Infant rhesus monkeys reared in a nursery by human hands for the first 6 months of life showed greater lymphocyte responses to stimulation with ConA than did monkeys reared with their mothers (Coe et al., 1989). These differences persisted through 2.5 years of age, despite the fact that both groups of monkeys were housed with peers after their 1st year (Coe et al., 1989). The augmented lymphocyte responses, which contrast with the reduced responses typically reported following acute stress, may be the product of an abnormally high T-helper to T-suppressor cell ratio in nursery-reared monkeys (Lubach et al., 1994).

New evidence suggests that early vulnerability to environmental stressors may begin before birth. Rhesus monkey neonates whose mothers experienced psychosocial stress or ACTH treatment during pregnancy exhibited abnormal postnatal development of neuromotor reflexes (Schneider and Coe, 1993; Schneider et al., 1992). Ongoing studies indicate that these monkeys also exhibit reduced lymphocyte proliferation responses in mixed lymphocyte reactions, reduced cytotoxic responses, and altered lymphocyte β-adrenergic receptor expression (Coe, 1993).

STRESS AND IMMUNITY: CLINICAL STUDIES

Limitations of Current Studies

No study has yet delineated a causal chain showing that severe life stress or a particular psychological state produced an immunologic response that then resulted in an altered clinical outcome. In one of the few prospective studies in this area, Cohen et al. (1991) recently showed that psychological stress was associated in a dose-response manner with an increased risk of acute infectious respiratory illness. Importantly, this association was due to increased rates of infection rather than to an increased frequency of symptoms after infection. However, measures of cellular immune function were not obtained.

To understand the relationship between stress and disease, all the processes involved in an "X" to "Y" to "Z" model must be studied (Elliot and Eisdorfer, 1982). Some studies, like that of Cohen et al., have shown that life events and psychological processes influence the development of disease, whereas other studies have demonstrated that psychological processes result in immune changes. Neither approach alone is sufficient, since these psychosocial factors could produce independent and unrelated effects both on immune function and on disease states (Ader, 1987). Prospective studies are needed that examine all these links simultaneously (Braveman, 1987). Furthermore, in vitro immune measures may not accurately reflect immunologic competence in vivo and, thus, may not be useful predictors of increased illness susceptibility (Calabrese et al., 1987; Hood et al., 1985). For example, a decrease in one immune parameter such as NK activity might be compensated by increased numbers or function of other cell types with no resultant increased risk for acute viral infections. Despite these caveats regarding biological relevance, changes in the immune system in persons undergoing stress may have clinical implications, and the hypothesis is presented that immunologic alterations mediate the relationship between stressful life events and poor health outcome.

Life Stress and Immunologically Mediated Disease

MORBIDITY AND MORTALITY IN BEREAVEMENT

In the past 20 years, studies of conjugal bereavement have demonstrated an elevated mortality rate among bereaved spouses that varies with age, sex, and time elapsed after the loss (Bowling and Benjamin, 1985; Clayton, 1974; Cox and Ford, 1964; Ekblom, 1963; Kaprio et al., 1987; Kraus and Lilienfeld, 1959; Mellstrom et al., 1982; Parkes et al., 1969; Rees and Lutkins, 1967; Ward, 1976; Young et al., 1963). The results are heterogeneous, although there appears to be an increased mortality during the early periods succeeding the loss, particularly among the middle-aged to older widowers (Helsing et al., 1981). Besides an increase in mortality, widowhood is associated with the onset of specific immune-related medical disorders such as influenza and pneumonia as well as other diseases, including cardiovascular problems (Jacobs and Ostfeld, 1977; Klerman and Izen, 1977; Parkes, 1970), possible increases in physician consultations and hospitalizations (Maddison and Viola, 1968; Mor et al., 1986; Parkes, 1964), and decreases in general well-being (Maddison and Viola, 1968; Parkes, 1970).

DEPRESSION AND ILLNESS

Disease might be more likely to occur in settings in which object loss and depression occur. Among 42 patients admitted to a general medical service, 31 of these patients had experienced the onset of their illness within 1 week of a significant loss (Schmale and Iker, 1966a, 1966b). In addition, a composite of available data suggests an association between depressive profiles and the development of cancer. In 40 women hospitalized for cone biopsies having class III Pap smears, feelings of hopelessness identified at patient interview correctly classified 8 of the 14 women with cancer and 23 of the 26 women without cancer (Schmale and Iker, 1966). In a 10-year longitudinal study, feelings of hopelessness and depression at baseline are associated with an increased incidence of cancer among 1353 persons examined in a Yugoslav village (Grossarth-Maticek et al., 1985). Finally, the Western Electric Health Study has demonstrated, with 20 years of follow-up, an association between depression as measured by the Minnesota Multiphasic Personality Inventory and an increased incidence in mortality for cancer (Persky et al., 1987). Even after adjustment for age, number of cigarettes smoked, alcohol intake, occupational status, and family history of cancer, the relationship between depressive personality and cancer persisted. One recent study found, however, that depressive symptoms are not significant predictors of cancer morbidity with or without adjustment for age, sex, marital status, smoking, family history of cancer, and hypertension (Zonderman et al., 1989). In general, the findings of increased cancer incidence in clinically depressed patients are consistent with a "null or weak relationship" (Fox, 1989). Nevertheless, several follow-up studies have demonstrated a relationship between affective disorders and clinical depression and increased cancer morbidity and mortality, particularly in male patients over age 40 who had primary diagnoses of affective disorders (Kerr et al., 1969; Varsamis et al., 1972; Whitlock and Sisking, 1979).

The promise of recent investigations has suggested that psychiatric interventions that reduce psychological distress may have beneficial effects on cancer survival. Spiegel (1989) found that group psychotherapy of breast cancer patients improved quality of life and extended life expectancy for patients with metastatic breast cancer, and Fawzy et al. (1990) showed that other types of cancer patients improve both psychologically as well as immunologically with psychosocial group therapy.

CHILD STUDIES

The relationship between life events and occurrence of medical disease in children has been less extensively studied than that in adults. However, the onset and course of several immune-related diseases have been linked to stressful life experiences. Bronchial asthma and allergic rhinitis, two disorders thought to be mediated by humoral immune responses, occur more frequently in children undergoing life events who have limited abilities to cope psychologically with these changes (Czubalski and Zawisza, 1976; DeAraujo et al., 1973; Holmes et al., 1951; Knapp, 1969). Streptococcal infections and increased antibodies to streptolysin O are more likely in members of families in which high levels of stress are noted (Meyer and Haggerty, 1962). Serious, and often fatal, viral infections have been found in emotionally deprived children (Spitz, 1965).

The role that psychological and emotional factors play in increasing the susceptibility of youngsters to cancers is not yet known, although Greene and Miller (1958) and Jacobs and Charles (1980) have conducted investigations of the relationship of such factors to the onset of leukemia and lymphoma in children and adolescents and found that experiencing separation and loss appears to be one of multiple factors associated with the development of leukemia in children. For example, of 33 patients with lymphocytic and myelogenous leukemia, 31 are found to have experienced one or more losses or separations in the 2-year period prior to the onset of their illness, with half of these experiences occurring in the 6 months prior to that time (Greene and Miller, 1958).

Life Events and Immune Changes

While there has often been disagreement about the existence of changes in immunity related to life stressors, a recent meta-analysis of the relationship between stress and immunity concluded that there is substantial evidence for stress-induced modulation of the numbers and functional capacities of multiple immune cell types (Herbert and Cohen, 1993). Important variables influencing immunity included stressor duration and the extent to which the stressor involved social (e.g., loss of spouse) rather than nonsocial (e.g., loss of job) events (Herbert and Cohen, 1993). A more detailed consideration of the types of stressors that have been linked to altered immunity follows.

CLINICAL STUDIES OF BEREAVEMENT

Clinical studies of immune function in bereaved subjects have demonstrated altered immunity, including suppression of lymphocyte responses to mitogenic stimulation, reduced natural killer cell activity, and alterations of T-cell subpopulations. The relationship between bereavement and immunological functioning was first reported by Bartrop et al. (1977) who compared measures of lymphocyte responses to mitogen stimulation between 26 men and women whose spouses had died and 26 age- and sex-matched control subjects. At both 3 and 6 weeks after the death of the spouses, during which time active bereavement occurs, T-cell responses to low doses of PHA and ConA were reduced

in the bereaved group. T- and B-cell numbers did not differ between groups. Using several specific antigens (streptokinase, mumps antigen, and purified protein derivative of tuberculin), delayed hypersensitivity reactions on routine skin testing were also not different. In a prospective study, Schleifer et al. (1983) replicated the earlier findings, demonstrating a significant suppression of lymphocyte responses during the first 2 months following the death of a spouse and an intermediate level of mitogen responsiveness during the 4- to 14-month period after bereavement.

Other in vitro parameters of cell-mediated immune function are also found to be altered during bereavement. Measures of natural killer cell cytotoxicity, total lymphocyte counts, and T-helper and T-suppressor cell numbers were compared among three groups of women: those whose husbands were dying of lung cancer, those whose husbands had recently died, and women whose husbands were in good health (Irwin et al., 1987a, 1987b). In the groups who were undergoing moderate or severe life stress (comprised significantly by women anticipating or breaving the death of their spouse), a reduction of natural killer cell activity was found compared with the values in the low stress, nonbereaved comparison subjects. Neither the absolute number of lymphocytes nor the number of T-cell subpopulations, including number of T-helper, T-suppressor/cytotoxic cells and ratio of T-helper to T-suppressor/cytotoxic cell, is different between the groups.

Psychological responses, not merely the event, might contribute to the immune changes in bereavement. Consistent with this hypothesis, severity of depressive symptoms is correlated with reduced natural killer cell activity, a loss of T-suppressor/cytotoxic cells, and an increase in the ratio of T-helper to T-suppressor/cytotoxic cells (Irwin et al., 1987a). Using various measures of humoral and cell-mediated immunity, Linn et al. (1984) found reduced lymphocyte responses to the mitogen PHA only in bereaved subjects who had high depression scores but not in those bereaved subjects who had few signs of depression. Other immunologic measures, including lymphocyte responses to ConA and pokeweed mitogen, serum levels of IgG, IgA, and IgM, in vivo responses to skin tests, and neutrophilic chemotaxis, are comparable to those found in the controls.

EFFECTS OF EXAMINATION STRESS

Relatively minor aversive events such as the stress of academic examinations are also associated with altered immunity. Dorian et al. (1982) reported higher white blood cell counts, an increased absolute lymphocyte count, a reduction in PHA reactivity, and a reduction in plaque-forming cell response (an index of B-cell function) in 8 psychiatry trainees taking their oral examinations compared with the values in 16 psychiatrists not taking examinations. In a series of other studies conducted by Kiecolt-Glaser et al. (1984), the initial observations of examination-related alterations of cellular immunity have been confirmed and extended. Medical students demonstrated significantly lower levels of natural killer cell activity and of blastogenesis (in response to both ConA and PHA) during final examinations compared with levels of baseline samples taken 1 month earlier (Kiecolt-Glaser et al., 1984). Additionally, the students exhibited stress-related decreases in the percentages of total T lymphocytes, helper T lymphocytes, and suppressor T cells (Glaser et al., 1985) and significant increases in plasma levels of IgG, IgM, and IgA (Glaser et al., 1986). Moreover, these researchers have speculated that these immunologic changes may be important for the control of recurrent latent herpes virus infections and found that antibody titers to Epstein-Barr virus (EBV), cytomegalovirus (CMV), and herpes simplex virus (HSV) are significantly increased during the 1st day of examination compared with either the month before examination or upon return from summer vacation (Kiecolt-Glaser et al., 1984). The same stressor was also associated with significant decreases in the number and synthesis of IL-2 receptors on peripheral blood leukocytes and with increased release of IL-2 by these cells (Glaser et al., 1990).

CHRONIC STRESS AND IMMUNE DYSFUNCTION

In addition to the effects of acutely occurring severe, as well as relatively minor, aversive events, chronic stressors that last 1 or more years have also been found to result in alterations in immune function. The stresses of Alzheimer's disease caregiving often place family members at risk for depression (Eisdorfer et al., 1983) and are associated with decreased life satisfaction (George and Gwyther, 1986) and increased levels of psychiatric symptoms (George and Gwyther, 1986). Furthermore, immunologic analyses have revealed significantly higher antibody titers to EBV and reduced percentages of total T lymphocytes and helper T cells in 34 Alzheimer caregivers versus those values in 34 matched control subjects (Kiecolt-Glaser et al., 1987). Neither T-suppressor cells nor numbers of natural killer cells differed between the two groups. These changes in immunity may have health consequences, as Alzheimer caregiving has also been associated with significant increases in episodes of infectious illness and illness-associated physician visits (Kiecolt-Glaser et al., 1991).

The stress of job loss and long-term unemployment has also been found to be associated with psychologic distress and reduced cellular immune responses as measured by a decrease in lymphocyte reactivity to PHA and purified protein derivative (PPD) in vitro (Arnetz et al., 1987).

COPING AND SOCIAL SUPPORT

Style of coping and quality of social support are postulated as determinants of whether severe adversities such as bereavement or caregiving become translated into psychological and physical morbidity. In this regard, discord or dissatisfaction within the marital relationship are found to have effects on immune function (Kiecolt-Glaser et al., 1987); poor marital quality is associated with reduced immunologic functioning (lower percentages of natural killer and helper cells, poor mitogen responsiveness, and higher percentages of antibody titers to some herpes viruses) among married women (Kiecolt-Glaser et al., 1987) and married men (Kiecolt-Glaser et al., 1988).

Despite a demonstrated link between coping and psychological adjustment during stress, few studies have evaluated the role of coping responses as defined by Lazarus et al. (1984) in mediating stress-induced alterations in immune function. Instead, most studies have evaluated coping responses indirectly, postulating that a diminished capacity to adapt, as indicated by psychiatric symptoms, is a measure of coping. For example, Locke et al. (1985) rated the severity of life events in 114 students and on the basis of these reports and measures of psychiatric symptoms divided the sample into four groups: low stress/low symptoms, high stress/high symptoms, high stress/low symptoms, and low stress/high symptoms. Those subjects with few psychological symptoms in the face of large amounts of stress ("good copers") have significantly higher natural killer cell activity than those experiencing high levels of both symptoms and stress. Temoshok (1986) has also found that one factor influencing survival among AIDS patients is the degree of control they experienced over their lives; those who felt they could exert little control died more quickly. Finally, consistent with the findings generated in preclinical studies, administration of an uncontrollable (but not controllable) stress produces greater elevations in the plasma concentration of ACTH and epinephrine in humans (Breier et al., 1987).

DEPRESSION AND IMMUNE CHANGES

Psychological response to distressing life events is an important correlate of immune dysfunction in persons undergoing severe life stress, and it has been hypothesized that psychological depression or anxiety may itself be associated with immune change (see Chapters 33 and 60). Herbert and Cohen (1993) recently conducted a meta-analysis of studies of depression and immunity and concluded that depression is significantly related to impaired cellular immunity with severity of depressive symptoms associated with greater decreases in immune cell numbers and activity (Herbert and Cohen, 1993).

To clarify the role of depression in impairing cell-mediated immunity, several studies have compared immune responses between depressed patients and control subjects. Cappel et al. (1978) reported that PHA responses are lower in psychotically depressed patients during the 1st days of illness than following clinical remission. Kronfol et al. (1983) replicated these observations in 26 drug-free depressed patients and found blunted lymphocyte responses to mitogenic stimulation with ConA, PHA, and pokeweed during depression. Schleifer et al. (1984) also found suppressed lymphocyte reactivity in severely depressed patients and further described abnormalities of lymphocyte subpopulations in depression: absolute and T- and B-lymphocyte cell counts are reduced, although relative percentages are unchanged. Since no differences in immune measures have been found between mildly depressed outpatients and control subjects (Schleifer et al., 1985), Schleifer et al. have concluded that the severity of depressive symptoms is an important factor associated with altered lymphocyte responses in depression.

Extending these observations of altered lymphocyte proliferation responses in depression, Irwin et al. (1987b) measured the cytolytic activity of peripheral lymphocytes in two groups of subjects: medication-free, hospitalized, acutely depressed patients and age- and sex-matched control subjects studied on the same day as the patients. Natural killer cell activity was significantly lower in the depressed patients compared with that in the control subjects, a finding that has been replicated by Urch et al. (1988) and by Mohl et al. (1987). In addition, severity of depressive symptoms was correlated with a reduction in natural killer cell activity.

In an attempt to understand why some (but apparently not all) patients with major depression show immune changes, the contribution of other factors that might affect immunity in depressed patients has been studied. Schleifer et al. (1989) have examined the role of age in the relationship between depression and altered immunity. Employing an extensive assessment of the immune system, including enumeration of T-lymphocyte subsets, assay of natural killer cell activity, and measurement of mitogen-induced lymphocyte stimulation, significant age-related differences between depressed patients and control subjects were found for numbers of T-helper lymphocytes and for mitogen responses. Age-related increases in T-helper cells and in mitogen responses were found in the control subjects, whereas advancing age was associated with no changes in the number of T-helper cells and decreased lymphocyte responses in depressed patients. These findings suggest that age as well as severity of depression are important correlates of immune changes in depression; immune changes in major depressive disorder are present mainly in elderly, severely depressed patients.

In addition to the independent contribution of age to depression-related changes in immunity, alcohol consumption is also reported to play a role in further reducing cellular immunity in depressed patients. Alcohol use, even in moderate doses, is associated with alterations in cell-mediated immune function such as natural killer cell activity. The contribution of alcohol use to produce a greater decrement in immunity in depressed patients with histories of alcohol abuse compared with that in depressed patients without such alcoholism has been compared (Irwin et al., 1990). Consistent with earlier reports, natural killer cell activity was significantly lower both in depressed and in alcoholic patients (compared with that in controls). Perhaps of more interest, patients with dual diagnoses of either alcohol abuse and secondary depression or depression with a history of alcohol abuse demonstrate a further decrease in natural killer cell activity compared with that found in patients with either depression or alcoholism alone.

Alterations in T-cell subpopulations have also been characterized in depressed patients compared with that in control subjects. Consistent with the findings of Irwin et al. (1987b), who found a relationship between severity of depressive symptoms and an increase in the ratio of T-helper to T-suppressor/cytotoxic cells in bereaved women, Syvalahti et al. (1985) found that depressed patients have a lower percentage of T-suppressor/cytotoxic cells and a higher ratio of T-helper to T-suppressor/cytotoxic cells than that of the control subjects. However, other studies have found no depression-related differences in quantitative measures of lymphocytes including number of T cells, B cells, T-helper, T-suppressor, and natural killer cells (Darko et al., 1989; Wahlin et al., 1984).

Beyond the use of more sophisticated measures of immune cell function, future investigations need to test the clinical relevance and biologi-cal significance of depression-related changes in the immune system. Furthermore, preclinical and clinical studies of the mechanisms that underlie changes in depression in such biological parameters as measures of immunity will help identify the pathways of communication among the nervous, endocrine, and immune systems.

Acknowledgments. *This work was supported by National Institutes of Mental Health Grants MH18399, MH46867, and MH44275, and by VA Merit Review (M.I.).*

References

Aarons RD, Molinoff PB: Changes in the density of beta adrenergic receptors in rat lymphocytes, heart, and lung after chronic treatment with propranolol. *J Pharmacol Exp Ther* 221:439–443, 1982.

Ackerman KD, Bellinger DL, Felten SY, et al: Ontogeny and senescence of noradrenergic innervation of the rodent thymus and spleen. In: Ader R, Felten DL, Cohen N (eds): *Psychoneuroimmunology* (2nd ed). San Diego, Academic, 1991, pp. 72–115.

Ackerman KD, Felten SY, Bellinger DL, et al: Noradrenergic sympathetic innervation of spleen and lymph nodes in relation to specific cellular compartments. *Prog Immunol* 6:588–600, 1987.

Ackerman KD, Felten SY, Bellinger DL, et al: Noradrenergic sympathetic innervation of the spleen: III. Development of innervation in the rat spleen. *J Neurosci Res* 18:49–54, 1987.

Ackerman SH, Hofer MA, Weiner H: Sleep and temperature regulation during restraint stress in rats is affected by prior maternal separation. *Psychosom Med* 41:311–319, 1979.

Ackerman SH, Keller SE, Schleifer SJ, et al: Brief communication: Premature maternal separation and lymphocyte function. *Brain Behav Immun* 2:161–165, 1988.

Ader R: Developmental psychoneuroimmunology. *Dev Psychobiol* 16(4):251–267, 1983.

Ader R: Clinical implications of psychoneuroimmunology. *Dev Behav Pediatr* 8:357–358, 1987.

Ader R, Friedman SB: Differential early experiences and susceptibility to transplanted tumor in the rat. *J Comp Physiol Psychol* 59(3):361–364, 1965.

Amkraut AA, Solomon GF, Kasper P, et al: Stress and hormonal intervention in the graft-versus-host response. In: Jankovic BD, Isakovic K (eds): *Microenvironmental Aspects of Immunity*. New York: Plenum, 1973, pp. 667–674.

Arnetz BB, Wasserman J, Petrini B, et al: Immune function in unemployed women. *Psychosom Med* 49:3–12, 1987.

Ausiello CM, Roda LG: Leuenkephalin binding to cultured human T lymphocytes. *Cell Biol Int Rep* 8:97, 1987.

Axelrod J, Resine TD: Stress hormones: Their interaction and regulation. *Science* 224:452–459, 1984.

Bancroft GJ, Shellam GR, Chalmer JE: Genetic influences on the augmentation of natural killer cells (NK) during murine cytomegalovirus infection: Correlation with patterns of resistance. *J Immunol* 124:988–994, 1981.

Barneoud P, Neveu PJ, Vitiello S, et al: Functional heterogeneity of the right and left cerebral neocortex in the modulation of the immune system. *Physiol Behav* 41:525–530, 1987.

Baybutt HN, Holsboer F: Inhibition of macrophage differentiation and function by cortisol. *Endocrinology* 127:476–480, 1990.

Ben-Eliyahu S, Yirmiya R, Shavit Y, et al: Stress-induced suppression of natural killer cell cytotoxicity in the rat: A naltrexone-insensitive paradigm. *Behav Neurosci* 104:235–238, 1990.

Bernard A, Boumsell L: The clusters of differentiation (CD) defined by the First International Workshop on Human Leukocyte Differentiation Antigens. *Hum Immunol* 11:1–10, 1984.

Bernton EW, Meltzer MS, Holaday JW: Suppression of macrophage activation and T-lymphocyte function in hypoprolactinemic mice. *Science* 239:401–404, 1988.

Besedovsky HO, del Rey A, Sorkin E, et al: Immunoregulation mediated by the sympathetic nervous system. *Cell Immunol* 48:346–355, 1979.

Bidart JM, Motte PH, Assicot M, et al: Catechol-o-methyltransferase activity and aminergic binding site distribution in human peripheral blood lymphocyte subpopulations. *Clin Immunol Immunopathol* 26:1, 1983.

Biron CA, Byron KS, Sullivan JL: Severe herpes virus infections in an adolescent without natural killer cells. *N Engl J Med* 320:1731–1735, 1989.

Bocchini G, Bonanno G, Canivari A: Influence of morphine and naloxone on human peripheral blood. *Drug Alcohol Depend* 11:233, 1983.

Boccia ML, Reite M, Kaemingk K, et al: Behavioral and autonomic responses to peer separation in pigtail macaque monkey infants. *Dev Psychobiol* 22:447–461, 1989.

Bonnet M, Lespinats G, Burtin C: Histamine and serotonin suppression of lymphocyte response to phytohemagglutinin and antigen. *Cell Immunol* 83:280, 1984.

Bowling A, Benjamin B: Mortality after bereavement: A follow-up study of a sample of elderly widowed people. *Biol Soc* 2:197–203, 1984.

Braveman N: Immunity and aging: Immunological and behavioral perspectives. In: Riley MW, Matarazzo JM, Baum A (eds): *The Aging Dimension*. Hillsdale, NJ, Erlbaum, 1987.

Breier A, Albus M, Pickar D, et al: Controllable and uncontrollable stress in humans: Alterations in mood and neuroendocrine and psychophysiological function. *Am J Psychiatry* 144:1419–1425, 1987.

Britton KT, Koob GF, Rivier J, et al: Intracerebroventricular corticotropin-releasing factor enhances the behavioral effects of novelty. *Life Sci* 31:363–367, 1982.

Brodde OE, Engel G, Hover D, et al: The beta-adrenergic receptor in human lymphocytes. *Life Sci* 29:2189–2198, 1981.

Brooks WH, Cross RJ, Roszman TL, et al: Neuroimmunomodulation: Neural anatomical basis for impairment and facilitation. *Ann Neurol* 12:56–61, 1980.

Brown R, Li Z, Vriend CY, et al: Suppression of splenic macrophage interleukin-1 secretion following intracerebroventricular injection of interleukin-1β: Evidence for pituitary-adrenal and sympathetic control. *Cell Immunol* 132:84–93, 1991.

Bukowski JF, Warner JF, Dennert G, et al: Adoptive transfer studies demonstrating the antiviral affect of natural killer cells in vivo. *J Exp Med* 131:1531–1538, 1985.

Bulloch K: Neuroanatomy of lymphoid tissue: A review. In Guillemin R, Cohn M, Melnechuk T (eds): *Neural Modulation of Immunity*. New York: Raven, 1985, pp. 111–141.

Bulloch K, Pomerantz W: Autonomic nervous system innervation of thymic-related lymphoid tissue in wild-type and nude mice. *J Comp Neurol* 228:57–68, 1984.

Bulloch K, Cullen MR, Schwartz RH, et al: Development of innervation within syngeneic thymus tissue transplanted under the kidney capsule of the nude mouse: A light and ultrastructural microscope study. *J Neurosci Res* 18:16–27, 1987.

Calabrese JR, Kling MA, Gold PW: Alterations in immunocompetence during stress, bereavement and depression. *Am J Psychiatry* 144:1123–1134, 1987.

Capitanio JP, Lerche NW: Psychosocial factors and disease progression in simian AIDS: A preliminary report. *AIDS* 5:1103–1106, 1991.

Cappel R, Gregoire F, Thiry L, et al: Antibody and cell-mediated immunity to herpes simplex virus in psychiatric depression. *J Clin Psychiatry* 39:266–268, 1978.

Carr DJ, Bost KL, Blalock JE: The production of antibodies which recognize opiate receptors on murine lymphocytes. *Life Sci* 42:2615–2624, 1988.

Clayton PJ: Mortality and morbidity in the first year of widowhood. *Arch Gen Psychiatry* 30:747–750, 1974.

Clodi M, Svoboda T, Kotzmann H, et al: Effect of elevated serum prolactin concentrations on cytokine production and natural killer cell activity. *Neuroendocrinology* 56:775–779, 1992.

Coe CL: Psychosocial factors and immunity in nonhuman primates: A review. *Psychosom Med* 55:298–308, 1993.

Coe CL, Lubach GR, Ershler WB, et al: Effect of early rearing on lymphocyte proliferation responses in rhesus monkeys. *Brain Behav Immun* 3:47–60, 1989.

Coe CL, Rosenberg LT, Levine S: Prolonged effect of psychological disturbance on macrophage chemiluminescence in the squirrel monkey. *Brain Behav Immun* 2:151–160, 1988a.

Coe CL, Rosenberg LT, Levine S: Effect of maternal separation on the complement system and antibody responses in infant primates. *Int J Neurosci* 40:289–302, 1988b.

Cohen IR: The self, the world and autoimmunity. *Sci Am* 258:52–60, 1988.

Cohen S, Tyrell DA, Smith AP: Psychological stress and susceptibility to the common cold. *N Engl J Med* 325:606–656, 1991.

Cohn M: What are the ''must'' elements of immune responsiveness? In: Guillemin R, Cohn M, Melnechuk T (eds): *Neural Modulation of Immunity*. New York: Raven, 1985, pp. 3–25.

Cox PR, Ford JR: The mortality of widows shortly after widowhood. *Lancet* 1:163–164.

Cross RJ, Roszman TL: Central catecholamine depletion impairs in vivo immunity but not in vitro lymphocyte activation. *J Neuroimmunol* 19:33–45, 1988.

Cross RJ, Brooks WH, Roszman TL: Hypothalamic-immune interactions. I. The acute effect of anterior hypothalamic lesions on the immune response. *Brain Res* 196(1):79–87.

Cross RJ, Brooks WH, Roszman TL: Modulation of T-suppressor cell activity by central nervous system catecholamine depletion. *J Neurosci Res* 18:75–81.

Cross RJ, Bryson JS, Roszman TL: Immunologic disparity in the hypopituitary dwarf mouse. *J Immunol* 148:1347–1352, 1992.

Cross RJ, Jackson JC, Brooks WH, et al: Neuroimmunomodulation: Impairment of humoral immune responsiveness by 6-hydroxydopamine treatment. *Immunology* 57:145–152, 1986.

Cross RJ, Markesbery WR, Brooks WH, et al: Hypothalamic immune interactions: Neuromodulation of natural killer activity by lesioning of the anterior hypothalamus. *Immunology* 51:399–405, 1984.

Cunnick JE, Lysle DT, Kucinski BJ, et al: Evidence that shock-induced immune suppression is mediated by adrenal hormones and peripheral β-adrenergic receptors. *Pharmacol Biochem Behav* 36:645–651, 1990.

Cupps TR, Fauci AS: Corticosteroid-mediated immunoregulation in man. *Immunol Rev* 65:133–155, 1982.

Czubalski K, Zawisza E: The role of psychic factors in patients with allergic rhinitis. *Acta Otolaryngol* 81:484, 1976.

Darko DF, Gillin JC, Risch SC, et al: Mitogen-stimulated lymphocyte proliferation and pituitary hormones in major depression. *Biol Psychiatry* 26:145–155, 1989.

Darko DF, Irwin MR, Risch SC, et al: Plasma beta-endorphin and natural killer cell activity in patients with major depression. *Psychiatry Res* 4:111–119, 1992.

DeAraujo G, Van Arsdel PP, Holmes TH, et al: Life change, coping ability and chronic intrinsic asthma. *J Psychosom Res* 17:359, 1973.

Dinarello CA, Mier JW: Medical Intelligence: Current concepts: Lymphokines. *N Engl J Med* 317:940–945, 1987.

Dobbs CM, Vasquez M, Glaser R, et al: Mechanisms of stress-induced modulation of viral pathogenesis and immunity. *J Neuroimmunol* 48:151–160, 1993.

Dorian B, Garfinkel P, Brown G, et al: Aberrations in lymphocyte subpopulations and function during psychological stress. *Clin Exp Immunol* 50:132–138, 1982.

Dumont F, Robert F, Bischoff P: T and B lymphocytes in pituitary dwarf Snell-Bagg mice. *J Immunol* 38:23, 1979.

Edwards CK, Arkins S, Yunger LM, et al: The macrophage-activating properties of growth hormone. *Cell Mol Neurobiol* 12:499–510, 1992.

Edwards CK, Ghiasuddin SM, Yunger LM, et al: In vivo administration of recombinant growth hormone or gamma interferon activates macrophages: Enhanced resistance to experimental *Salmonella typhimurium* infection is correlated with generation of reactive oxygen intermediates. *Infect Immun* 60:2514–2521, 1992.

Edwards EA, Rahe RH, Stephens PM, et al: Antibody response to bovine serum albumin in mice: The effects of psychosocial environmental change. *Proc Soc Exp Biol Med* 164:478–481, 1980.

Eisdorfer C, Kennedy G, Wisnieski W, et al: Depression and attributional style in families coping with the stress of caring for a relative with Alzheimer's disease. *Gerontologist* 23:115–116, 1983.

Ekblom B: Significance of sociopsychological factors with regard to risk of death among elderly persons. *Acta Psychiatr Scand* 29:627–633, 1963.

Falke NE, Fischer EG, Martin R: Stereospecific opiate binding in living human polymorphonuclear leucocytes. *Cell Biol Int Rep* 9:1041, 1985.

Farrar WL: Endorphin modulation of lymphokine activity. In Fraioli F, Isidori I, Mazzetti M (eds): *Opioid Peptides in the Periphery*. Amsterdam: Elsevier, 1984, p. 159.

Fawzy FI, Kemeny ME, Fawzy NW, et al: A structured psychiatric intervention for cancer patients. *Arch Gen Psychiatry* 47:729–935, 1990.

Felsenfeld O, Hill CW, Greer WE: Response of *Cercopithecus aethiops* to cholera vibrio lipopolysaccharide and psychological stress. *Trans R Soc Trop Med Hyg* 60:514–518, 1966.

Felten DL, Felten SY, Bellinger DL, et al: Noradrenergic sympathetic neural interactions with the immune system: Structure and function. *Immunol Rev* 100:225–260, 1987c.

Felten DL, Felten SY, Carlson SL, et al: Noradrenergic and peptidergic innervation of lymphoid tissue. *J Immunol* 135:755s–765s, 1985.

Felten DL, Livnat S, Felten SY, et al: Sympathetic innervation of lymph nodes in mice. *Brain Res Bull* 13:693–699, 1984.

Felten DL, Overhage JM, Felten SY, et al: Noradrenergic sympathetic innervation of lymphoid tissue systems. *Brain Res Bull* 7:595–612, 1981.

Felten SY, Olschowka J: Noradrenergic sympathetic innervation of the spleen. II. Tyrosine hydroxylase (TH)-positive nerve terminals form synaptic-like contacts on lymphocytes in the splenic white pulp. *J Neurosci Res* 18:37–48, 1987.

Felten SY, Housel J, Felten DL: Use of in vivo dialysis for evaluation of splenic norepinephrine and serotin. *Soc Neurosci Abstr* 12:1065, 1986.

Fiatarone MA, Morley JE, Bloom ET, et al: Endogenous opioids and the exercise-induced augmentation of natural killer cell activity. *J Lab Clin Med* 112:544–552, 1988.

Fisher LA, Rivier J, Rivier C, et al: CRF: Central effects on mean arterial pressure and heart rate in rats. *Endocrinology* 110:2222–2224, 1982.

Fox BH: Depressive symptoms and risk of cancer. *JAMA* 262:1231, 1989.

Friedman EM, Coe CL, Ershler WB: Time-dependent effects of peer separation on lymphocyte proliferation responses in juvenile squirrel monkeys. *Dev Psychobiol* 24:159–173, 1991.

Friedman SB, Glasgow LA: Psychologic factors and resistance to infectious disease. *Pediatr Clin North Am* 13:315–355, 1966.

Friedman SB, Ader R, Glasgow LA: Effects of psychological stress in adult mice inoculated with Coxsackie B viruses. *Psychosom Med* 27:361–368, 1965.

Friedman SB, Glasgow LA, Ader R: Psychosocial factors modifying host resistance to experimental infections. *Ann NY Acad Sci* 164:381–392, 1969.

George LK, Gwyther LP: Caregiver well-being: A multidimensional examination of family caregivers of demented adults. *Gerontologist* 26:253–259, 1986.

Geschwind N, Behan P: Left-handedness: Association with immune disease, migraine, and developmental learning disorder. *Proc Natl Acad Sci USA* 79:5097–5100, 1982.

Gilliland BC: Introduction to clinical immunology. In: Petersdorf RG, Adams RD, Brunwald E (eds): *Principles of Internal Medicine*. New York: McGraw-Hill, 1983, pp. 344–354.

Gillis S, Crabtree GR, Smith KA: Glucocorticoid-induced inhibition of T cell growth factor production. I. The effect on mitogen-induced lymphocyte proliferation. *J Immunol* 123:1624–1631, 1979.

Gilman SC, Schwartz JM, Milner RJ, et al: β-Endorphin enhances lymphocyte proliferative responses. *Proc Natl Acad Sci USA* 79:4226–4230, 1982.

Gilmore W, Weiner LP: β-Endorphin enhances interleukin-2 (IL-2) production in murine lymphocytes. *J Neuroimmunol* 18:125, 1988.

Glaser R, Kennedy S, Lafuse WP, et al: Psychological stress-induced modulation of interleukin-2 receptor gene expression and interleukin-2 production in peripheral blood leukocytes. *Arch Gen Psychiatry* 47:707–712, 1990.

Glaser R, Kiecolt-Glaser JK, Speicher CE, et al: Stress, loneliness and changes in herpes virus latency. *J Behav Med* 8:249–260, 1985.

Glaser R, Kiecolt-Glaser JK, Stout JC, et al: Stress-related impairments in cellular immunity. *Psychiatry Res* 16:233–239, 1985.

Glaser R, Mehl VS, Penn G, et al: Stress-associated changes in plasma immunoglobulin levels. *Int J Psychosom* 33:41–42, 1986.

Goodman JW: Immunoglobulin structure and function. In: Stites DP, Terr AI (eds): *Basic and Clinical Immunology* (7th ed). East Norwalk, CT: Appleton & Lange, 1991, pp. 109–121.

Gordon TP, Gust DA, Wilson ME, et al: Social separation and reunion affects immune system in juvenile rhesus monkeys. *Physiol Behav* 51:467–472, 1992.

Greene WA, Miller G: Psychological factors and reticuloendothelial disease. IV: Observations on a group of children and adolescents with leukemias: An interpretation of disease development in terms of mother-child unit. *Psychosom Med* 10:124–144, 1958.

Griffin JFT: Stress and immunity: A unifying concept. *Vet Immunol Immunopathol* 20:263–312, 1989.

Grossarth-Maticek R, Bastinans J, Kanazir DT: Psychosocial factors as strong predictors of mortality from cancer, ischemic heart disease, and stroke. *J Psychosom Rev* 33:129–138, 1985.

Gust DA, Gordon TP, Wilson ME, et al: Removal from natal social group to peer housing affects cortisol levels and absolute numbers of T cell subsets in juvenile rhesus monkeys. *Brain Behav Immun* 6:189–199, 1992.

Habu S, Akamatsu K, Tamaoki N, et al: In vivo significance of NK cells on resistance against virus (HSV-1) infections in mice. *J Immunol* 133:2743–2747, 1984.

Hadden JW, Hadden EM, Middleton E: Lymphocyte blast transformation. I. Demonstration of adrenergic receptors in human peripheral lymphocytes. *J Cell Immunol* 1:583–595, 1970.

Hall NR, Goldstein AL: Neurotransmitters and the immune system. In: Ader R (ed): *Psychoneuroimmunology*. New York: Academic, 1981, pp. 521–544.

Hammar JA: Konstitutionsanatomische Studien uber die Neurotisierung des Menschenembryos. IV: Uber die Innervationsverhaltnisse der Inkretorgane und der Thymus bis in den 4 Fotalmonat. *Z Mikrosk Anat* 38:253–293, 1935.

Hartmann DP, Holaday JW, Bernton EW: Inhibition of lymphocyte proliferation by antibodies to prolactin. *FASEB J* 3:2194–2202, 1989.

Heijnen CJ, Bevers C, Kavelaars A, et al: Effect of α-endorphin on the antigen-induced primary antibody response of human B cells in vitro. *J Immunol* 136:213, 1986.

Heilig M, Irwin M, Grewal I, et al: Sympathetic regulation of T-helper cell function. *Brain Behav Immun* 7:154–163, 1993.

Hellstrand K, Hermodsson S: Role of serotonin in the regulation of human natural killer cell cytotoxicity. *J Immunol* 139:869–875, 1987 (Abstract).

Hellstrand K, Hermodsson S, Strannegrård Ö: Evidence for a β-adrenoceptor-mediated regulation of human natural killer cells. *J Immunol* 134:4095–4099, 1985.

Helsing KJ, Szklo M, Comstock EW: Mortality after bereavement. *Am J Public Health* 71:802–809, 1981.

Henney CS, Gillis S: Cell-mediated cytotoxicity. In: Paul WE (ed): *Fundamental Immunology*. New York: Raven, 1984, pp. 669–684.

Henriques JB, Davidson RJ: Regional brain electrical asymmetries discriminate between previously depressed and healthy control subjects. *J Abnorm Psychol* 99:22–31, 1990.

Henriques JB, Davidson RJ: Left frontal hypoactivation in depression. *J Abnorm Psychol* 100: 535–545, 1991.

Herberman RB: *Natural Cell Mediated Immunity against Tumors.* New York, Academic, 1980.

Herberman RB, Ortaldo JR: Natural killer cells: Their role in defenses against disease. *Science* 214: 24–30, 1981.

Herbert TB, Cohen S: Depression and immunity: A meta-analytic review. *Psychol Bull* 113:472–486, 1993.

Herbert TB, Cohen S: Stress and immunity in humans: A meta-analytic review. *Psychosom Med* 55:364–379, 1993.

Hermann G, Tovar CA, Beck FM, et al: Restraint stress differentially affects the pathogenesis of an experimental influenza viral infection in three inbred strains of mice. *J Neuroimmunol* 47:83–94, 1994.

Hill CW, Greer WE, Felsenfeld O: Psychological stress, early response to foreign protein, and blood cortisol in vervets. *Psychosom Med* 29:279–283, 1967.

Hofer MA: Relationships as regulators: A psychobiologic perspective on bereavement. *Psychosom Med* 46:183–197, 1984.

Holmes TH, Treuting T, Wolff HG: Life situations, emotions and nasal disease. *Psychosom Med* 13:71, 1951.

Hood LE, Weisman IL, Wood WB, et al: *Immunology.* Menlo Park, CA, Benjamin Cummings, 1985.

Irwin MR, Gillin JC: Impaired natural killer cell activity among depressed patients. *Psychiatry Res* 20:181–182, 1987.

Irwin MR, Hauger RL: Adaptation to chronic stress: Temporal pattern of immune and neuroendocrine correlates. *Neuropsychopharmacology* 1: 239–242, 1988.

Irwin MR, Britton KT, Vale W: Central corticotropin-releasing factor suppresses natural killer cytotoxicity. *Brain Behav Immun* 1:81–87, 1987.

Irwin MR, Brown M, Patterson T, et al: Neuropeptide Y and natural killer cell activity: Findings in depression and Alzheimer caregiver stress. *FASEB J* 5:3100–3107, 1991.

Irwin MR, Caldwell C, Smit TL, et al: Major depressive disorder, alcoholism, and reduced natural killer cell cytotoxicity: Role of severity of depressive symptoms and alcohol consumption. *Arch Gen Psychiatry* 47:713–719, 1990.

Irwin MR, Daniels M, Risch SC, et al: Plasma cortisol and natural killer cell activity during bereavement. *Biol Psychiatry* 24:173–178, 1988.

Irwin MR, Daniels M, Smith TL, et al: Life events, depressive symptoms, and immune function. *Am J Psychiatry* 144:437–441, 1987a.

Irwin MR, Daniels M, Smith TL, et al: Impaired natural killer cell activity during bereavement. *Brain Behav Immun* 1:98–104, 1987b.

Irwin MR, Hauger RL, Brown M, et al: Corticotropin-releasing factor activates autonomic nervous system and reduces natural killer cytotoxicity. *Am J Physiol* 255:R744–R747, 1988.

Irwin MR, Hauger RL, Jones L, et al: Sympathetic nervous system mediates central corticotropin-releasing factor induced suppression of natural killer cytotoxicity. *J Pharmacol Exp Ther* 255:101–107, 1990.

Irwin MR, Segal DS, Hauger RL, et al: Individual behavioral and neuroendocrine differences in responsiveness to audiogenic stress. *Pharmacol Biochem Behav* 32:913–917, 1989.

Irwin MR, Vale W, Rivier C: Central corticotropin-releasing factor mediates the suppressive effect of stress on natural killer cytotoxicity. *Endocrinology* 126:2837–2844, 1990.

Isakovic K, Jankovic BD: Neuroendocrine correlates of immune response. II: Changes in the lymphatic organs of brain lesioned rats. *Int Arch Allergy Immunol* 45:373–384, 1973.

Jacobs S, Ostfeld A: An epidemiological review of the mortality of bereavement. *Psychosom Med* 39: 344–357, 1977.

Jacobs TJ, Charles E: Life events and the occurrence of cancer in children. *Psychosom Med* 42: 11–24, 1980.

Johnson HM, Downs MO, Pontzer CH: Neuroendocrine peptide hormone regulation of immunity. In: Blalock JE (ed): *Neuroimmunoendocrinology* (2nd ed). Basel: Chem Immunol, 1992, pp. 49–53.

Johnson HM, Smith EM, Torres BA, et al: Regulation of the in vitro antibody response by neuroendocrine hormones. *Immunology* 79:4171–4174, 1982.

Justice A: Review of the effects of stress on cancer in laboratory animals: Importance of time of stress application and type of tumour. *Psychol Bull* 98:108–138, 1985.

Kandil O, Borysenko M: Decline of natural killer cell target binding and lytic activity in mice exposed to rotation stress. *Health Psychol* 6(2):89–99, 1987.

Kang D, Davidson RJ, Coe CL, et al: Frontal brain asymmetry and immune function. *Behav Neurosci* 105:860–869, 1991.

Kaprio J, Koskenvuo M, Rita H: Mortality after bereavement: A prospective study of 95,647 widowed persons. *Am J Public Health* 77:283–287, 1987.

Katz P, Zaytoun AM, Fauci AS: Mechanisms of human cell-mediated cytotoxicity. I: Modulation of natural killer cell activity by cyclic nucleotides. *J Immunol* 129:287–296, 1982.

Kay N, Morley JE, van Ree JM: Enhancement of human lymphocyte natural killing function by non-opioid fragments of β-endorphin. *Life Sci* 40: 1083–1087, 1987.

Keller SE, Schleifer SJ, Liotta AS, et al: Stress-induced alterations of immunity in hypophysectomized rats. *Proc Natl Acad Sci USA* 85:9297–9301, 1988.

Keller SE, Stein M, Camerino MS, et al: Suppression of lymphocyte stimulation by anterior hypothalamic lesions in the guinea pig. *Cell Immunol* 52: 334–340, 1980.

Keller SE, Weiss JM, Schleifer SJ, et al: Suppression of immunity by stress: Effect of a graded series of stressors on lymphocyte stimulation in the rat. *Science* 213:1397–1400, 1981.

Keller SE, Weiss JM, Schliefer SJ, et al: Stress-induced suppression of immunity in adrenalectomized rats. *Science* 221:1301–1304, 1983.

Kelley KW, Brief S, Westly HJ, et al: GH3, pituitary adenoma cells can reverse thymic aging in rats. *Proc Natl Acad Sci USA* 83:5663–5667, 1986.

Kendall MD, al-Shawaf AA: Innervation of the rat thymus gland. *Brain Behav Immun* 5:9–28, 1991.

Kerr TA, Schapiro K, Roth M: Relationship between premature death and affective disorders. *Br J Psychiatry* 115:1277–1282, 1969.

Kiecolt-Glaser JK, Dura JR, Speicher CE, et al: Spousal caregivers of dementia victims: Longitudinal changes in immunity and health. *Psychosom Med* 53:345–362, 1991.

Kiecolt-Glaser JK, Fisher LD, Ogrock P, et al: Marital quality, marital disruption, and immune function. *Psychosom Med* 49:13–34, 1987.

Kiecolt-Glaser JK, Garner W, Speicher C, et al: Psychosocial modifiers of immunocompetence in medical students. *Psychosom Med* 46:7–14, 1984.

Kiecolt-Glaser JK, Glaser R, Dyer C, et al: Chronic stress and immunity in family caregivers of Alzheimer's disease victims. *Psychosom Med* 49: 523–535, 1987.

Kiecolt-Glaser JK, Kennedy S, Malkoff S, et al: Marital discord and immunity in males. *Psychosom Med* 50:213–219, 1988.

Klerman GL, Izen J: The effects of bereavement and grief on physical health and general well-being. *Adv Psychosom Med* 9:63–104, 1977.

Knapp PH: The asthmatic and his environment. *J Nerv Ment Dis* 149:133, 1969.

Krall JF, Connelly M, Tuck ML: Acute regulation of β adrenergic catecholamine sensitivity in human lymphocytes. *J Pharmacol Exp Ther* 214: 554–560, 1980.

Kraus AS, Lilienfeld AM: Some epidemiologic aspects of the high mortality rate in the young widowed group. *J Chronic Dis* 9:207–217, 1959.

Kronfol Z, House JD: Depression, hypothalamic-pituitary adrenocortical activity and lymphocyte function. *Psychopharmacol Bull* 21:476–478, 1985.

Kronfol Z, Hover JD, Silva J, et al: Depression, urinary free cortisol excretion, and lymphocyte function. *Br J Psychiatry* 148:70–73, 1986.

Kronfol Z, Silva J, Greden J, et al: Impaired lymphocyte function in depressive illness. *Life Sci* 33: 241–247, 1983.

Krueger JM, Obal F: Growth hormone-releasing hormone and interleukin-1 in sleep regulation. *FASEB J* 7:645–652, 1993.

Laudenslager ML, Capitanio JP, Reite M: Possible effects of early separation experiences on subsequent immune function in adult macaque monkeys. *Am J Psychiatry* 142:862–864, 1985.

Laudenslager ML, Held PE, Boccia ML, et al: Behavioral and immunological consequences of brief mother-infant separation: A species comparison. *Dev Psychobiol* 23:247–264, 1990.

Laudenslager ML, Rasmussen KL, Berman CM, et al: Specific antibody levels in free-ranging rhesus monkeys: Relationships to plasma hormones, cardiac parameters, and early behavior. *Dev Psychobiol* 26: 407–420, 1993.

Laudenslager ML, Reite ML, Harbeck RJ: Suppressed immune response in infant monkeys associated with maternal separation. *Behav Neural Biol* 6: 40–48, 1982.

Laudenslager ML, Ryan SM, Drugan RC, et al: Coping and immunosuppression: Inescapable but not escapable shock suppresses lymphocyte proliferation. *Science* 221:568, 1983.

Lazarus RS, Folkman S: *Stress, Appraisal and Coping.* New York: Springer, 1984.

Leposavic G, Micic M, Ugresic N, et al: Components of sympathetic innervation of the rat thymus during late fetal and postnatal development: Histofluorescence and biochemical study. Sympathetic innervation of the rat thymus. *Thymus* 19:77–87, 1992.

Levine S, Cohen C: Differential survival to leukemia as a function of infantile stimulation in DBA/Z mice. *Proc Soc Exp Biol Med* 102:53–54, 1959.

Linn MN, Linn BS, Jensen J: Stressful events, dysphoric mood and immune responsiveness. *Psychol Rep* 54:128–129, 1984.

Lippman M, Barr R: Glucocorticoid receptors in purified subpopulations of human peripheral blood lymphocytes. *J Immunol* 118:1977–1981, 1977.

Livnat S, Felten SY, Carlson SL, et al: Involvement of peripheral and central catecholamine systems in neural-immune interactions. *J Neuroimmunol* 10:5–30, 1985.

Locke SE, Krause L, Leserman L, et al: Life change stress, psychiatric symptoms, and NK activity. *Psychosom Med* 46:441–453, 1984.

Lopker A, Abood LG, Hoss W, et al: Stereoselective muscarinic acetylcholine and opiate receptors in human phagocytic leukocytes. *Biochem Pharmacol* 29:1361, 1980.

Lotzova E, Herberman RB: *Immunobiology of NK Cells II.* Boca Raton, FL, CRC Press, 1986.

Lubach GR, Coe CL, Ershler WB: Effects of early rearing environment on immune responses of infant rhesus monkeys. *Brain Behav Immun* 1994, in press.

Luecken LJ, Lysle DT: Evidence for the involvement of β-adrenergic receptors in conditioned immunomodulation. *J Neuroimmunol* 38:209–220, 1992.

Lysle DT, Cunnick JE, Fowler H, et al: Pavlovian conditioning of shock-induced suppression of lymphocyte reactivity: Acquisition, extinction, and preexposure effects. *Life Sci* 42:2185–2194, 1988.

Lysle DT, Luecken LJ, Maslonek KA: Modulation of immune status by a conditioned aversive stimulus: Evidence for the involvement of endogenous opioids. *Brain Behav Immun* 6:179–188, 1992.

Macris NT, Schiavi RC, Camerino M: Effect of hypothalamic lesions on immune processes in the guinea pig. *Am J Physiol* 219:1205–1209, 1970.

Madden KS, Ackerman KD, Livnat S, et al: Neonatal sympathetic denervation alter the development of natural killer (NK) cell activity in F344 rats. *Brain Behav Immun* 7:344–351, 1993.

Maddison DC, Viola A: The health of widows in the year following bereavement. *J Psychosom Res* 12:297–306, 1968.

Maes M, Bosmans E, Suy E, et al: Impaired lymphocyte stimulation by mitogens in severely depressed patients. A complex interface with HPA axis hyperfunction, noradrenergic activity and the ageing process. *Br J Psychiatry* 155:793–798, 1989.

Maes M, Bosmans E, Suy E, et al: Depression-related disturbances in mitogen-induced lymphocyte responses and interleukin-1β and soluble interleukin-2 receptor production. *Acta Psychiatr Scand* 84:379–386, 1991.

McCain HW, Lamster IB, Bilotta J: Modulation of human T-cell suppressor activity by beta endorphin and glycyl-L-glutamine. *Int J Immunopharmacol* 8:443, 1986.

McGlone JJ, Lumpkin EA, Norman RL: Adrenocorticotropin stimulates natural killer cell activity. *Endocrinology* 129:1653–1658, 1991.

Mehrishi JN, Mills IH: Opiate receptors on lymphocytes and platelets in man. *Clin Immunol Immunopathol* 27:240–249, 1983 (Abstract).

Mellstrom D, Nilssom A, Olden A, et al: Mortality among the widowed in Sweden. *Scand J Soc Med* 10:33–41, 1982.

Meyer RJ, Haggerty RJ: Streptococcal infections in families: factors altering individual susceptibility. *Pediatrics* 29:539–549, 1962.

Miles K, Atweh S, Otten G, et al: Beta-adrenergic receptors on splenic lymphocytes from axotomized mice. *Int J Immunopharmacol* 6:171, 1984.

Miles K, Quintans J, Chelmicks-Schoor E, et al: The sympathetic nervous system modulates antibody response to thymus independent antigens. *J Neuroimmunol* 1:101–105, 1981.

Mohl PC, Huang L, Bowden C, et al: Natural killer cell activity in major depression (letter). *Am J Psychiatry* 144:1619, 1987.

Monjan AA, Collector MI: Stress-induced modulation of the immune response. *Science* 196:307–308, 1977.

Mor V, McHornney C, Sherwood S: Secondary morbidity among the recently bereaved. *Am J Psychiatry* 143:158–163, 1986.

Morimoto C, Hafler DA, Weiner HL, et al: Selective loss of the suppressor-inducer T-cell subset in progressive multiple sclerosis: Analysis with anti-2H4 monoclonal antibody. *N Engl J Med* 316:67–72, 1987.

Motulsky HJ, Insel PA: Adrenergic receptors in man: Direct identification, physiologic regulation, and clinical alterations. *N Engl J Med* 307:18–29, 1982.

Munck A, Guyre PM, Holbrook NJ: Physiological functions of glucocorticoids in stress and their relation to pharmacologic actions. *Endocr Rev* 5:25–44, 1984.

Murphy WJ, Durum SK, Anver MR, et al: Immunologic and hematologic effects of neuroendocrine hormones: Studies on DW/J dwarf mice. *J Immunol* 148:3799–3805, 1992.

Murray DR, Irwin M, Rearden CA, et al: Sympathetic and immune interactions during dynamic exercise: Mediation via beta2-adrenergic dependent mechanism. *Circulation* 83:203–213, 1992.

Nagy E, Berczi I, Friesen HG: Regulation of immunity in rats by lactogenic and growth hormones. *Acta Endocrinol* 102:351–357, 1983.

Nossal GJ: Current concepts: Immunology: The basic components of the immune system. *N Engl J Med* 316:1320–1326, 1987.

Okimura T, Satomi-Sasaki Y, Ohkuma S: Stress and immune responses. II: Identification of stress-sensitive cells in murine spleen cells. *Jpn J Pharmacol* 40:513–525, 1986.

Oleson DR, Johnson DR: Regulation of human natural cytotoxicity by enkephalins and selective opiate agonists. *Brain Behav Immun* 2:171–186, 1988.

Oppenheim JJ, Ruscetti FW, Faltynek C: Cytokines. In: Stites DP, Terr AI (eds): *Basic and Clinical Immunology* (7th ed). Norwalk, CT, Appleton & Lange, 1991, pp. 78–100.

Padgett GA, Reiquam CW, Henson JB, et al: Comparative studies of susceptibility to infection in the Chediak-Higashi syndrome. *J Pathol Bacteriol* 95:509–522, 1968.

Parker CW, Huber MG, Baumann ML: Alterations of the cyclic AMP metabolism in human bronchial asthma. III. Leukocyte and lymphocyte responses to steroids. *J Clin Invest* 52:1342, 1973.

Parkes CM: Effects of bereavement on physical and mental health: A study of the medical records of widows. *Br Med J* 2:274–279, 1964.

Parkes CM: The first year of bereavement: A longitudinal study of the reaction of London widows to the death of their husbands. *Psychiatry* 33:444–467, 1970.

Parkes CM, Benjamin B, Fitzgerald R: Broken heart: Statistical study of increased mortality among widowers. *Br Med J* 1:740, 1969.

Parrillo JE, Fauci AS: Comparison of the effector cells in human spontaneous cellular cytotoxicity and antibody-dependent cellular cytotoxicity: Differential sensitivity of effector cells to in vivo and in vitro corticosteroids. *Scand J Immunol* 8:99–107, 1978.

Paul WE: The immune system: An introduction. In: Paul WE (ed): *Fundamental Immunology*. New York: Raven, 1984, pp. 3–22.

Persky VS, Kempthorne-Rawson J, Shekelle RB: Personality and risk of cancer: 20-year follow-up of the Western Electric Study. *Psychosom Med* 49:435–449, 1987.

Pezzone MA, Rush KA, Kusnecov AW, et al: Corticosterone-independent alteration of lymphocyte mitogenic function by amphetamine. *Brain Behav Immun* 6:293–299, 1992.

Pitkin DH: Effect of psychological stress on the delayed hypersensitivity reaction. *Proc Soc Exp Biol Med* 120:350–351, 1965.

Plaut SM, Ader R, Friedman SB, et al: Social factors and resistance to malaria in the mouse: Effects of group vs. individual housing on resistance to *Plasmodium berghei* infection. *Psychosom Med* 31:536–552, 1969.

Puppo F, Corsini G, Mangini P, et al: Influences of β-endorphin on phytohemagglutinin-induced lymphocyte proliferation and on the expression of mononuclear cell surface antigens. *Immunopharmacology* 10:119, 1985.

Ray A, Mediratta PK, Sen P: Modulation by naltrexone of stress-induced changes in humoral immune responsiveness and gastric mucosal integrity in rats. *Physiol Behav* 51:293–296, 1992.

Rees WD, Lutkins SG: Mortality of bereavement. *Br Med J* 4:13, 1967.

Reite M, Harbeck R, Hoffman A: Altered cellular immune response following peer separation. *Life Sci* 29:1133–1136, 1981.

Riley V: Psychoneuroendocrine influences on immunocompetence and neoplasia. *Science* 212:1100–1109, 1981.

Ritz J: The role of natural killer cells in immune surveillance. *N Engl J Med* 320:1748–1749, 1989.

Romano TA, Felten SY, Felten DL, et al: Neuropeptide-Y innervation of the rat spleen: Another potential immunomodulatory neuropeptide. *Brain Behav Immun* 5:116–131, 1991.

Roszman TL, Cross RJ, Brooks WH, et al: Hypothalamic immune interactions. II: The effect of hypothalamic lesions on the ability of adherent spleen cells to limit lymphocyte blastogenesis. *Immunology* 45:737–742, 1982.

Russell DH, Kibler R, Matrisian L, et al: Prolactin receptors on human T and B lymphocytes. Antagonism of prolactin binding by cyclosporin. *J Immunol* 134:3027–3031, 1985.

Saperstein A, Brand H, Audhya T, et al: Interleukin 1β mediates stress-induced immunosuppression via corticotropin-releasing factor. *Endocrinology* 130:152–158, 1992.

Sapolsky R, Rivier C, Yamamoto G, et al: Interleukin-1 stimulates the secretion of hypothalamic corticotropin-releasing factor. *Science* 238:522–524, 1987.

Schledowski M, Falk A, Rohne A, et al: Catecholamines induce alterations of distribution and activity of human natural killer (NK) cells. *J Clin Immunol* 13:344–351, 1993.

Schleifer SJ, Keller SE, Bond RN, et al: Major depressive disorder and immunity: role of age, sex, severity, and hospitalization. *Arch Gen Psychiatry* 46:81–87, 1989.

Schleifer SJ, Keller SE, Meyerson AT, et al: Lymphocyte function in major depressive disorder. *Arch Gen Psychiatry* 41:484–486, 1984.

Schleifer SJ, Keller SE, Meyerson AT, et al: Depression and immunity: Lymphocyte function in ambulatory depressed patients, hospitalized schizophrenic patients, and patients hospitalized for herniorrhaphy. *Arch Gen Psychiatry* 42:129–133, 1985.

Schleifer SJ, Scott B, Stein M, et al: Behavioral and developmental aspects of immunity. *J Am Acad Child Adolesc Psychiatry* 26:751–763, 1986.

Schmale AH, Iker H: Hopelessness as a predictor of cervical cancer. *Soc Sci Med* 5:95–100, 1966a.

Schmale AH, Iker H: The affect of hopelessness and the development of cancer. I: Identification of uterine cervical cancer in women with atypical cytology. *Psychosom Med* 28:714–721, 1966b.

Schneider ML, Coe CL: Repeated social stress during pregnancy impairs neuromotor development of the infant primate. *J Dev Behav Pediatr* 14:81–87, 1993.

Schneider ML, Coe CL, Lubach GR: Endocrine activation mimics the adverse effects of prenatal stress on the neuromotor development of the infant primate. *Dev Psychobiol* 25:427–439, 1992.

Selye H: *Stress in Health and Disease*. Boston: Butterworth, 1976.

Shavit Y, Depaulis A, Martin FC, et al: Involvement of brain opiate receptors in the immune suppressive affect of morphine. *Proc Natl Acad Sci USA* 83:7114–7117, 1986.

Shavit Y, Lewis JW, Terman GW, et al: Opioid peptides mediate the suppressive effect of stress on natural killer cell cytotoxicity. *Science* 223:188–190, 1984.

Shavit Y, Terman GW, Lewis JW, et al: Effects of footshock stress and morphine on natural killer lymphocytes in rats: Studies of tolerance and cross-tolerance. *Brain Res* 372:382, 1986.

Shavit Y, Terman GW, Martin FC, et al: Stress,

opioid peptides, the immune system, and cancer. *J Immunol* 135:834s–837s, 1985.

Sherman JE, Kalin NH: ICV-CRH potently affects behavior without altering antinociceptive responding. *Life Sci* 39:433–441, 1985.

Sibinga NES, Goldstein A: Opioid peptides and opioid receptors in cells of the immune system. *Annu Rev Immunol* 6:219–249, 1988.

Sklar LS, Anisman H: Stress and cancer. *Psychol Bull* 89:369–406, 1981.

Solomon GF: Stress and antibody response in rats. *Int Arch Allergy* 35:97–104, 1969.

Spiegel D, Bloom J, Kraemer HC, et al: The beneficial effect of psychosocial treatment on survival of metastatic breast cancer patients: A randomized prospective study. *Lancet* 10:888–891, 1989.

Spitz RA: *The First Year of Life.* New York: International University Press, 1965.

Stein M, Schiavi RC, Camerino M: Influence of brain and behavior on the immune system. *Science* 191:435–440, 1976.

Strakosch CR, Wenzel BE, Row VV, et al: Immunity of autoimmune thyroid disease. *N Engl J Med* 307:1499–1506, 1982.

Strom TD, Lundin AP, Carpenter CB: Role of cyclic nucleotides in lymphocytes activation and function. *Prog Clin Immunol* 3:115–153, 1977.

Sullivan JL, Byron KS, Brewster FE, et al: Deficient natural killer activity in X-linked lymphoproliferative syndrome. *Science* 210:535, 1980.

Sundar SK, Becker KJ, Cierpial MA, et al: Intracerebroventricular infusion of interleukin-1 rapidly decreases peripheral cellular immune responses. *Proc Natl Acad Sci USA* 86:6398–6402, 1989.

Sundar SK, Cierpial MA, Kilts C, et al: Brain IL-1-induced immunosuppression occurs through activation of both pituitary-adrenal axis and sympathetic nervous system by corticotropin-releasing factor. *J Neurosci* J:3701–3706, 1990.

Sutton RE, Koob GF, LeMoal M, et al: Cortico-

tropin releasing factor produces behavioral activation in rats. *Nature* 297:331–333, 1982.

Syvalahti E, Eskola J, Ruuskanen O, et al: Non-suppression of cortisol and immune function in depression. *Prog Neuropsychopharmacol Biol Psychiatry* 9:413–422, 1985.

Talal N: Autoimmunity. In: Fudenberg HH, Stites DP, Caldwell JL (eds): *Basic and Clinical Immunology.* Los Altos: Lane, 1980, p. 220.

Taylor AI, Fishman LM: Corticotropin releasing hormone. *N Engl J Med* 319:213–222, 1988.

Temoshok L, Fox BH: Temoshok L, Fox BH (eds): *International Issue Advances,* 1986.

Tonnesen E, Tonnesen J, Christensen NJ: Augmentation of cytotoxicity by natural killer cells after adrenaline administration in man. *Acta Pathol Microbiol Immunol Scand Sect C* 92:81–83, 1984.

Trinchieri G: Biology of natural killer cells. *Adv Immunol* 47:187–376, 1989.

Urich A, Muller CH, Aschauer H, et al: Lytic effector cell function in schizophrenia and depression. *J Neuroimmunol* 18:291–301, 1988.

Vale W, Spiess J, Rivier C, et al: Characterization of a 41-residue ovine hypothalamic peptide that stimulates secretion of corticotropin and beta-endorphin. *Science* 213:1394–1397, 1981.

Valentino RJ, Foote SL, Aston-Jones G: Corticotropin-releasing factor activates noradrenergic neurons of the locus coeruleus. *Brain Res* 270:363–367, 1983.

Varsamis J, Zuchowski T, Main KK: Survival rate and causes of death of geriatric psychotic patients. *Can Psychiatry Assoc J* 17:17–21, 1972.

von Euler US: The presence of a substance with sympathin E properties in spleen extracts. *Acta Physiol Scand* 11:168, 1946.

Wahlin A, von Knorring L, Roos G: Altered distribution of T lymphocyte subsets in lithium-treated patients. *Neuropsychobiology* 11:243, 1984.

Waltman TJ, Irwin MR, Harris TJ, et al: Cell

mediated immunity in rats with congestive heart failure. *Proc Am Heart Assoc* 65:19203, 1992.

Ward AWM: Mortality of bereavement. *Br Med J* 1:700–702, 1976.

Watson JJ: The influence of intracellular levels of cyclic nucleotides on cell proliferation and the induction of antibody synthesis. *J Exp Med* 141:97–111, 1975.

Weber RJ, Pert A: The periaqueductal gray matter mediates opiate-induced immunosuppression. *Science* 245:188–190, 1989.

Weigent DA, Blalock JE: Growth hormone and the immune system. *Prog Neuroendocrinimmunol* 3:231, 1990.

Wheeler RE, Davidson RJ, Tomarken AJ: Frontal brain asymmetry and emotional reactivity: A biological substrate of affective style. *Psychophysiology* 30:82–89, 1993.

Whitlock FA, Sisking M: Depression and cancer: A follow-up study. *Psychol Med* 9:747–752, 1979.

Williams LT, Snyderman R, Lefkowitz RJ: Identification of β-adrenergic receptors in human lymphocytes by $(-)[^3H]$alprenolol binding. *J Clin Invest* 57:149–155, 1976.

Wybran J, Appelboom T, Famaey J, et al: Suggestive evidence for receptors for morphine and methionine-enkephalin on normal human blood T lymphocytes. *J Immunol* 123:1068–1070, 1979.

Young M, Benjamin B, Wallis C: The mortality of widowers. *Lancet* 2:454, 1963.

Zinkernagal RM, Doherty PC: MHC-restricted cytotoxic T cells: Studies on the biological role of polymorphic transplantation antigens determining T-cell restriction-specificity, function, and responsiveness. *Adv Immunol* 27:51–177, 1979.

Zonderman AB, Costa PT Jr, McCrae RR: Depression as a risk for cancer morbidity and mortality in a nationally representative sample. *JAMA* 262:1191–1195, 1989.

6 DEVELOPMENTAL PSYCHONEUROENDOCRINOLOGY

K.J.S. Anand, M.B.B.S., D.Phil., and Charles B. Nemeroff, M.D., Ph.D.

BACKGROUND

The unique biologic and behavioral characteristics of newborns, infants, and children in different stages of development imply important differences between adult neuroendocrine processes and those occurring during development. Not only is the neuroendocrine system functioning and capable of dynamic responses to the changing environment, but in the early stages of development it can undergo long-lasting and permanent changes as a result of these early influences. Clear understanding of the developmental aspects of psychoneuroendocrinology would require investigations at the embryological, fetal, neonatal, and later developmental stages and at the molecular, cellular, and architectural levels of organization in the anatomical, neurochemical, neurophysiologic, behavioral, and clinical aspects of the brain and the endocrine system. This may seem a mammoth undertaking, but is very likely to be remarkably productive.

In this chapter, we review the current literature on neuroendocrinology and childhood behavior and ask the question: How do these neuronal cell populations, pathways, neurotransmitters, and regulatory and other physiologic mechanisms develop and interact with the developing endocrine system. This approach carries the basic assumption that the same anatomical and physiological processes, albeit immature, are used in the developing brain and endocrine system as those in the adult organism. Therefore, our purpose may be reduced to investigating how they function in the immature state and during different stages of development. However, this approach may be fraught with several difficulties.

First, the presently accepted view of neuroendocrine functions may be incorrect and incomplete, and searching for their ontogeny may lead to a compounding of these errors. Second, it is entirely possible, and perhaps likely, that the fetus and neonate use neuroendocrine mechanisms that are vastly different from those in the adult. Their repertoire of behavior and responses to stress is certainly different. Neuronal cell populations, connecting pathways, neurotransmitters, and other physiologic mechanisms may exist transiently during development and be lost in the adult brain and endocrine system. In addition, neuroendocrine mechanisms that have limited roles in the adult may indeed have sweeping and pluripotent roles in altering the development of the neuroendocrine system and, secondarily, altering cognitive processes and behavior during childhood. This highly complex and vulnerable system generates enormous possibilities for altered and abnormal development or altered regulation, with important implications for the practice of child and adolescent psychiatry.

Neuroendocrine Regulation of Brain Development

Developmental events in the CNS are regulated by a variety of genetic mechanisms, ionic gradients, neuroendocrine factors, and paracrine influences. Neuroendocrine factors that control the migration, differentiation, and maturation of neuronal cell populations include thyroid hormones, glucocorticoids, androgens and estrogens, and several neuropeptides. Much of the research on neurobiological development and the basic mechanisms of psychoneuroendocrinology has been performed in rodent species (rats, mice). Apart from logistic reasons such as laboratory cost and convenience, short gestation, and simple breeding and rearing conditions, two other reasons contribute to this choice. First, the cellular, molecular, and architectural events in the development of the central nervous system follow remarkably similar patterns in the human and rodent species. Some of the relevant data illustrating this interspecies correlation is summarized in Table 6.1. The rat brain at birth (P0) is at the same developmental stage as the brain of a 24-week-gestation human premature infant, and at 10 days of age (P10) the rat brain corresponds to the brain of a full-term newborn infant (Bass et al., 1977; Eayrs, 1968). Second, the behavior of infant and adult rats has been investigated in much greater detail than that in any other species. The rich repertoire of cognitive and behavioral tests that have been validated and published allow meaningful correlations between neurobiological events and mechanisms, experimental paradigms, drug therapies, and the resulting (often quantifiable) behavioral changes. A powerful combination of these investigative advantages makes rodents the primary choice for developing animals models of human psychiatric and behavioral disorders. This chapter therefore focuses much of the discussion on developmental aspects of psychoneuroendocrinology in rodent and human species.

THYROID HORMONES

Thyroid hormones influence brain development in three phases during fetal and neonatal life. Phase I includes the influence of maternal thyroid hormones, which extends up to 17 days of gestation in the rat and 10–12 weeks gestation in the human. A significant proportion of brainstem and cerebral neurogenesis occurs during this period, and the role of thyroid hormones is presently undefined. Placental transport of thyroid hormones occurs in humans (Vulsma et al., 1989) and rats (Morreale de Escobar et al., 1990), with localization in the fetal brain as early as E12 in the rat (Porterfield and Hendrich, 1992) and 10 weeks gestation in the human fetus (Ferreiro et al., 1988). The fetal brain selectively accumulates thyroid hormones (triiodothyronine (T_3) > thyroxine (T_4)), and thyroid hormone receptors are present from E14 in the rat (Perez-Castillo et al., 1985) and the first trimester of human

gestation (Bernal and Pekonen, 1984). The synthesis of transthyretin in the choroid plexus may regulate the transport of thyroxine across the blood-brain barrier (Schreiber et al., 1990), where it is selectively deiodinated to form T_3. Destruction of the fetal and maternal thyroid gland in midgestation results in decreased mRNA and protein synthesis in the brain (Holt et al., 1973) with specific reductions in mRNAs for Mb5 and Ma1 tubulin isotypes (Stein et al., 1989). Treatment of pregnant rats from E7 with propylthiouracil was associated with delayed cell accumulation in mesencephalic and motor nuclei (Narayanan and Narayanan, 1985). These experimental observations were correlated with cognitive deficits and delayed motor skills in children exposed to maternal hypothyroidism in early gestation (Letarte and Garagorri, 1989; Rovet, 1986).

During phase II (E17–E21 in rats, 12–40 weeks gestation in humans), the fetal and maternal thyroid glands are active sources of thyroid hormones. The partial neurogenesis, neuronal migration, neurite formation, and synaptogenesis occurring in this period are exquisitely sensitive to the presence of thyroid hormones. Potter et al. (1986) found that reduced brain growth due to maternal hypothyroidism was restored to normal in sheep fetuses after the onset of fetal thyroid function. Although maternal hypothyroidism could alter fetal brain development by nonspecific mechanisms such as altered maternal metabolism and compromised nutrient availability, decreased placental growth, circulation, or function, or indirectly, by altering the regulation of trophic hormones (growth hormone, IGF-1, IGF-II), it is now well-accepted that these effects are specific and mediated directly by effects of thyroid hormones on the growth and maturation of neuronal cell populations (Porterfield and Hendrich, 1993).

In phase III, which follows birth, brain development is entirely dependent on the activity of the neonatal thyroid gland. The small amounts of thyroid hormones present in milk are insufficient to support normal brain development (Mallol et al., 1982). Hypothyroid states in this phase mostly affect neuronal maturation and development in the forebrain cerebellum, together with myelination and glial cell proliferation and maturation throughout the nervous system. This critical period extends from birth to P21 in the rat and up to 2 years in the human, and serious and permanent brain damage will result from thyroid deficiencies in this period. Several lines of evidence emphasize the importance of thyroid hormones in the regulation of protein synthesis in neuronal and glial cells (Dussault and Ruel, 1987). Thyroid hormones function as a time clock in phase III, terminating neuronal proliferation and stimulating differentiation, particularly in the rat cerebellum. Triiodothyronine regulates the expression of the neurotrophic factor, neurotrophin-3 (NT-3), in cerebellar granule cells in vivo and in cell culture (Lindholm et al., 1993). Purkinje cells do not express NT-3 but do express trkC, the

Table 6.1. Correlation of Rat and Human Brain Development

Developmental Feature	Rat[a]	Human	References
Morphology of the spinal cord (Nissl stain, etc.)	E15	6 weeks	Marti et al., 1987
	E17	8 weeks	Marti et al., 1987
In-growth of afferent fibers	E14–E15	7–10 weeks	Okado et al., 1982
Substantia gelatinosa cells born	E16	14 weeks	Marti et al., 1987
			Nornes and Das, 1974
Lamination in the spinal cord	E17	13 weeks	Rizvi et al., 1987
			Marti et al., 1987
First movements	E16	7–8 weeks	Narayanan et al., 1971
			De Vries et al., 1982
Motoneurone death	E15–P1	11–25 weeks	Nornes and Das, 1974
			Oppenheim, 1987
Nociceptive neurotransmitters	E16–E18	8–10 weeks	Marti et al., 1987
Increased neurotransmitter and receptor expression	E20–E21	26–30 weeks	Charnay et al., 1984
		36–40 weeks	Loizou, 1972
			Okado et al., 1984
Exaggerated cutaneous reflexes	Up to P10	Up to 1 year	Fitzgerald and Gibson, 1984
			Prendergast and Shusterman, 1982
Corticospinal tract maturation	P7–P10	1–2 years	Schreyer and Jones, 1982
			Prendergast and Shusterman, 1982

[a] Age of the rat fetus: E, embryological day; E0/E21, day of fertilization/birth; P, postnatal day.

Table 6.2. Effects of Thyroxine and Corticosterone on Postnatal Brain Development in Rats

Developmental Features	Thyroid Deficiency	Treatment with Thyroxine	Treatment with Corticosterone
Postnatal cell formation			
Final cell number	Normal	Deficit	Deficit
Rate of cell acquisition	Retarded	No effect P0–P7	Retarded P0–P7
Period of rapid cell division	Prolonged (cerebellum)	Premature termination	Normal
Biochemical maturation			
Conversion of glucose to amino acids	Retarded	Advanced	Normal
Metabolic compartmentation present	Retarded	Advanced	—
Neuronal differentiation			
Dendritic arborization	Retarded	Accelerated	Transiently decreased
Dendritic spine formation	Retarded	Accelerated	Transiently decreased
Synaptogenesis	Retarded	Accelerated, but final number decreased	—
Behavioral changes			
Development of innate behavioral patterns	Retarded	Advanced	Retarded
Performance tests of adaptive behavior	Impaired	Impaired	Normal

Adapted and modified from Balazs R: Hormonal influences on brain development. *Biochem Soc Spec Publ* 1:39–57, 1973.

putative neuronal receptor for NT-3. Exposure of cerebellar Purkinje cells to NT-3 produced by T_3-stimulated granule cells induces hypertrophy and neurite sprouting of the Purkinje cells and upregulates the mRNA for 28-kDa calbindin, the calcium-binding protein (Lindholm et al., 1993). Myelination of central tracts by oligodendrocytes is preceded by the transient expression of nuclear T_3-receptors, which are absent before the critical period of active myelination (Besnard et al., 1994). Discovery of these cellular mechanisms in neuronal and glial cells have begun to define the important role of thyroid hormones in normal and abnormal brain development (Table 6.2).

GLUCOCORTICOIDS

Glucocorticoids appear to have a dual role in the developing brain, with inhibitory effects on the proliferation and growth of neuronal and glial cell populations, together with stimulatory effects on the synthesis of certain neurotransmitters and maturation of neuronal function (see Table 6.2). Although direct effects of glucocorticoids on early brain development have not been demonstrated, low doses may potentiate the production of nerve growth factor (NGF), as well as the genomic and nongenomic effects of NGF and other trophic factors (Greene et al., 1983; Perez-Polo et al., 1977). Glucocorticoids accelerate the mechanisms of transmitter synthesis and release, synaptic maturation, and the electrolyte distribution across neuronal membranes (Baethmann, 1985; Puro, 1983). Direct effects on neuronal maturation in the cerebral cortex (Chubakov et al., 1986), reticular formation (Avanzino et al., 1983), limbic system (Telegdy and Vermes, 1975), and spinal cord occur (Hall et al., 1978). These widespread changes may be related to glucocorticoid effects on the maturation of intracellular signaling, enzyme activity (e.g., Na^+/K^+-ATPase, glutamine synthetase, tryptophan synthetase), and neurotransmitter synthesis (Baethmann, 1985; Leret et al., 1993; Slotkin et al., 1993; Telegdy and Vermes, 1975).

Large doses of glucocorticoids given postnatally will suppress growth and cell division, particularly in glial cells and in cerebellar neurons. These effects are mediated by inhibition of DNA synthesis, and the production of myelin and gangliosides, leading to the developmental delay of several behavioral milestones (Dussault and Ruel, 1987). Further studies on the development and distribution of glucocorticoid receptor subtypes and their genomic effects in neuronal and glial cells (O'Banion et al., 1994) will help to further define the developmental roles of glucocorticoids.

GONADAL STEROIDS

Gonadal steroid hormones including the androgens, progestins, and estrogens regulate the developmental mechanisms leading to sexual dimorphism in the mammalian central nervous system. These observations were first suggested by Pffaf (1966) from morphological changes in the adult male rat following neonatal castration and were supported by the pioneering studies of Raisman and Field (1971). There are well-defined sensitive periods for the development of sexually dimorphic behavior in many animal species, and these changes are sex hormone (mostly androgen) dependent. For example, for a permanent feminizing effect, the castration of male rat pups must occur within the first few days after birth and not later than P7, whereas androgen therapy in female rat pups has long-term masculinizing effects if given during the same period (Bermant and Davidson, 1974). The changes produced in the CNS relate not only to sexual behavior, but also to other forms of behavior that differ between the sexes. The critical periods for sexually dimorphic brain development vary between species and do not bear a constant relationship to birth (being prenatal in guinea pig and rhesus monkey, perinatal in the dog, and postnatal in the rat, mouse, hamster, and ferret) (Goy and McEwen, 1980). Raisman and Field's studies (1973) described the differential neuronal development in the preoptic area and hypothalamus, with differences in synaptogenesis, dendritic arborization, and cellular features such as the size of the nucleus.

The actions of gonadal steroids on the developing brain are mediated by specific classes of receptors, presumed to modulate protein synthesis by altering genomic transcription (Beyer and Feder, 1987). It is likely that the distribution of these receptor classes would correspond with sexually dimorphic areas in the brain, including those implicated in the regulation of sexual behavior, gonadotropin secretion, and other gender-specific social behavior (Baum, 1986; MacLusky et al., 1987). Testosterone implants in the female rat CNS were associated with the marked growth and differentiation of neurons in the sexual dimorphic nucleus of the preoptic area and the spinal nucleus supplying the bulbocavernosus muscle, whereas castration of male rats at birth resulted in significant decreases in the size of these areas. Transplantation of the sexual dimorphic nucleus to the brains of castrated male rats restored mating behavior and gonadotropin regulation (Arushanyan and Borovkova, 1989). In addition to gender differences in gross volume of the brain, sexual dimorphism has been reported in the planum temporale, corpus callosum, amygdala, and cerebellum (Baum, 1986; Beyer and Feder, 1987; MacLusky et al., 1987). The sexually dimorphic features of the human brain are summarized in Table 6.3.

Androgenic and estrogenic effects on brain growth (globally) and neuronal differentiation in sexually dimorphic areas may be mediated either directly or secondary to their effects on glial cells. For example, exposure to estrogens stimulates astrocytes to participate in the remodelling of hypothalamic neurons that control pituitary function. Glial cells may modulate neuroendocrine actions by synthesizing and releasing trophic factors such as insulin-like growth factor-1 (IGF-1) or transforming growth factor-α (TGF-α), which may regulate the release of hypothalamic factors (e.g., luteinizing hormone-releasing hormone (LHRH))

Table 6.3. Sexual Dimorphism of the Human Brain

Dimorphic Features	Sex Differences
Global characteristics	
Brain weight	M > F, by 10–15%
Brain volume	M > F, by 10–15%
Dendritic arborization	M > F, at birth
Hypothalamus	
Sexually dimorphic nucleus	M > F
Suprachiasmatic nucleus	M ≥ F
Thalamus	
Massa intermedia	Present in F > M
Cerebral cortex	
Heschl's gyrus	Different morphology in M/F
Anterior end of sylvian fissure	Located more anterior in M
Planum temporale	L > R in M, L = R in F
Posterior frontal opercular sulcus	Different morphology in M/F
Corpus callosum	
Genu, splenium	M > F
Isthmus	F > M

directly, or by actions on other neurons or glial cells (Duenas et al., 1994). In the rat arcuate nucleus, gonadal steroids caused a marked upregulation of IGF-1-like immunoreactivity in astrocytes and tanycytes, associated with permanent changes in the morphology of the arcuate nucleus (Duenas et al., 1994). Further studies to define the precise cellular changes produced by gonadal steroids in the developing brain, together with the genomic and nongenomic mechanisms of these effects, should be related to the gender-specific differences in male and female behavior. Only then will we understand the biological basis for developmental abnormalities in gender-derived social behavior.

Development of the Pituitary Gland

The anatomical origin of the pituitary occurs from the hypophyseal placode, a thickening of the midline somatic ectoderm which is rostrally continuous with the neural crest (Schwind, 1928). With the closure of the neural tube and formation of the mouth, this hypophyseal placode comes to lie ventral to the floor of the forebrain vesicle in the region of the infundibulum and medial eminence, just rostral to the anterior end of the notochord (Schwind, 1928). The earliest molecular markers for the hypophyseal placode include the mRNAs for the α-glycoprotein subunit of the gonadotropins and the β-thyroid-stimulating hormone subunit (β-TSH), expressed on E11 when the anterior neuropore is just closing (Simmons et al., 1990). This is followed by evagination of the infundibulum from the floor of the developing hypothalamus and the formation of Rathke's pouch by E13. A day later, β-TSH mRNA are localized to the most anterior part of anterior lobe, with proopiomelanocortin (POMC) mRNA expressed in cells just caudally. By E17, ventrally located cells in the anterior lobe first express the mRNAs for luteinizing hormone (LH) and follicle-stimulating hormone (FSH), followed by the expression of growth hormone (GH) and prolactin (PRL) transcripts by E18 (Swanson, 1992).

During the next 2 weeks of development, cells expressing GH mRNA proliferate much faster than those containing PRL, indicating a differential genetic regulation of these cell types. The expression of these hormones is preceded by the synthesis of Pit-1 mRNA and protein on E15, a specific transcription factor that upregulates the transcription rates of both GH and PRL genes (Ingraham et al., 1988). Pit-1 is expressed in somatotropes, lactotropes, and thyrotopes and also serves as a growth factor for each of these cell types (Simmons et al., 1990). Another nuclear transcription factor belonging to the leucine zipper family, called thyrotroph embryonic factor (TEF) and expressed on E13, increased the transcription rate of the β-TSH gene (Drolet et al., 1991). Thus, these transcription factors play an important role in the cell- and tissue-specific expression of the anterior pituitary hormones, and their spaciotemporal patterns correspond with the expression of the hormonal genes that they regulate.

HYPOTHALAMIC-PITUITARY-ADRENOCORTICAL AXIS

Ontogeny of the Hypothalamic-Pituitary-Adrenal Axis

In the rat fetus, CRF-immunoreactive nerve terminals can be detected in the anterior regions of the median eminence from E18 (Bugnon et al., 1982), followed by proliferation and growth of CRF-immunoreactive fibers and nerve terminals into the developing pituitary. This period is also associated with the proliferation of pituitary cells expressing the POMC gene, although it is unknown whether the maturing CRF-containing median eminence nerve terminals have any effect on the differentiation of these cells. CRF mRNA was detected in the ventral neuroepithelial lobe of the fetal hypothalamus on day 17 of gestation, prior to the formation of a morphologically distinct PVN (Grino et al., 1989). Hypothalamic CRF mRNA levels increased markedly on E19 and E20, with simultaneous increases in POMC gene transcription and fetal circulating ACTH levels (Grino et al., 1989a, 1989b). Following birth on E21, CRF immunostaining is temporarily absent from the hypothalamic median eminence, probably related to the stress of parturition, because CRF perikarya in the PVN and CRF-containing fibers in the median eminence can be detected by 12 hours after birth (Bugnon et al., 1982). In newborn rats from P0 to P7, the hypothalamic CRF and pituitary ACTH concentrations are approximately 10% of those in adult rats and increase progressively to adult concentrations by 45 days after birth (Walker et al., 1986). A targeted mutation in the CRF gene produced CRF-deficient mice, which manifested lung hypoplasia during fetal life. Despite severe glucocorticoid deficiency, these mice exhibited normal growth, fertility, and longevity in postnatal life (Muglia et al., 1995).

Corticotropin-Releasing Factor Regulation of the Hypothalamic-Pituitary-Adrenocortical Axis

Within minutes after exposure of pituitary cells to corticotropin-releasing factor (CRF) in vivo or in vitro, a dose-dependent increase in the secretion of POMC-related pituitary hormones occurs, including adrenocorticotropic hormone (ACTH) and β-endorphin (Aguilera et al., 1986; Rivier and Plotsky, 1986). ACTH secretion following adrenalectomy or acute stress can be greatly decreased by intravenous injection of α-helical CRF$_{9-41}$, a CRF receptor antagonist, or neutralization with CRF-antiserum, or destruction of the paraventricular nucleus (PVN) of the hypothalamus (Rivier and Plotsky, 1986; Rivier et al., 1982). These data, taken together with the CRF responses to stress, adrenalectomy, and corticosteroid replacement support the hypothesis that release of endogenous CRF from the paraventricular nucleus regulates the secretory activity of pituitary corticotropes (Rivier and Plotsky, 1986). CRF may mediate the ACTH response to stressors with a more "psychological" component, whereas both CRF and vasopressin may be involved in the increased ACTH responses to physical stressors (Mason, 1971; Pich et al., 1993). Both norepinephrine and epinephrine augment cyclic AMP production and the ACTH responses to CRF in pituitary cells (Abou-Samra et al., 1986; Aguilera et al., 1986). A similar synergism occurs between CRF and vasopressin on ACTH release (Aguilera et al., 1986). Thus, a variety of neuroendocrine factors have important roles in the regulation of ACTH secretion.

Control of ACTH secretion is mediated by the feedback inhibition of cortisol in primates (corticosterone in rodents); removal of this feedback by adrenalectomy causes 3-fold increases in CRF mRNA expression and 4- to 7-fold increases in arginine vasopressin (AVP) mRNA expression in PVN neurons (Bradbury et al., 1994; Byer et al., 1988), together with large increases in the synthesis of ACTH (Fig. 6.1). Feedback inhibition of ACTH release by corticosterone can be divided into rapid and delayed effects, that are partially reversed by exposing pituitary corticotropes to CRF, vasopressin, angiotensin II, and norepinephrine (Abou-Samra et al., 1986; Levin et al., 1988). The rapid effects on ACTH secretion occur within minutes due to direct steroid effects on ACTH release mechanisms, and the delayed effects occur over hours and days mediated by the inhibition of CRF mRNA expression in the PVN, decreased CRF release from the median eminence, altered CRF receptor-mediated signal transduction, decreased POMC gene transcription and ACTH synthesis in the pituitary (Dallman et al., 1994). Chronic in vivo or in vitro exposure to high CRF concentrations desensitize corticotroph secretory responses by down-regulation of CRF receptor number (Aguilera et al., 1987; Axelrod and Reisine, 1984). In addition to potentiating CRF-stimulated ACTH secretion, vasopressin may also modulate CRF-induced desensitization and down-regulation of CRF receptors in the anterior pituitary (Aguilera et al., 1987). Occupancy of the high affinity (type I or mineralocorticoid (MR)) receptors by low plasma concentrations of corticosterone decreases CRF and AVP expression in PVN cells and normalizes the basal ACTH secretion in the morning, but occupancy of both MR and low affinity glucocorticoid receptors (GR) is required to reduce the peak ACTH secretion in the evening (Bradbury et al., 1994; Byer et al., 1988; Kwak et al., 1993). Specific MR antagonists increase the basal ACTH secretion, whereas both MR and GR antagonists will increase ACTH secretion during the circadian peak or following stress (Dodt et al., 1993; Ratka et al., 1989).

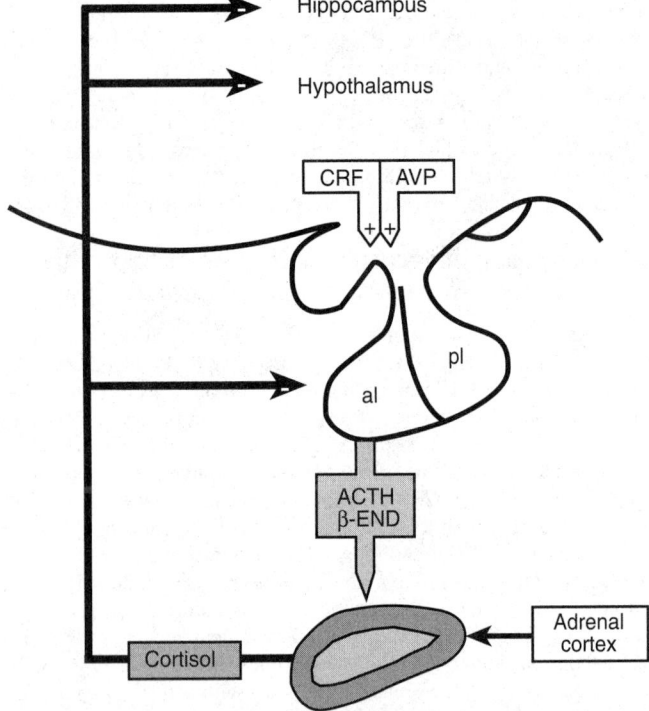

Figure 6.1. The hypothalamic-pituitary-adrenocortical axis. *CRF*, corticotropin-releasing factor; *AVP*, arginine vasopressin; *al*, anterior lobe of pituitary; *pl*, posterior lobe of pituitary; *ACTH*, adrenocorticotropic hormone; *β-END*, β-endorphin (negative feedback inhibition is mediated by corticosterone in the rodent species and cortisol in the human species).

Distribution of Corticotropin-Releasing Factor in the Brain

Although the main physiologic function of CRF is to act as the cephalic representative of the hypothalamic-pituitary-adrenal (HPA) axis, the biological role of the peptide involves widespread CNS effects on autonomic, immune, and behavioral functions. CRF immunoreactivity has been localized in hypothalamic and extrahypothalamic structures of the CNS (Bloom et al., 1982; Swanson et al., 1983, 1986). In addition to CRF-containing cell bodies in the hypothalamic PVN, CRF-containing neurons and nerve terminals occur in the central nucleus of the amygdala, parabrachial area and substantia innominata, bed nucleus of the stria terminalis, and the locus coeruleus and olfactory bulb. Bipolar cerebrocortical cells containing CRF (presumably interneurons) also occur, mainly in layers III and IV of the neocortex (Swanson et al., 1986). The pattern for CRF receptor distribution in the primate and rodent brain can be differentiated by the very high CRF density of binding sites in the primate prefrontal, orbital, and insular cortices (DeSouza et al., 1985; Millan et al., 1986: Wynn et al., 1984). These are phylogenetically mature brain regions and control higher cortical functions of primates. Hypothalamic CRF neurons are present throughout the parvocellular division of the PVN, particularly in a dorsomedial cell condensation just ventral to the anterior commissure, and project to the median eminence. The magnocellular division contains only a few CRF cell bodies, and these are functionally associated with vasopressinergic and oxytocinergic neurons (Swanson et al., 1986). Good correspondence was noted between the distribution of CRF neurons, CRF binding sites, and in situ hybridization of CRF receptor mRNA (De Souza, 1987; Perrin et al., 1993). The abundance of CRF neurons in extrahypothalamic brain regions, together with its electrophysiological effects, suggests a neurotransmitter role for CRF, which modulates affective behavior and visceral responses (Menzaghi et al., 1994), these relevant data are summarized in Table 6.4.

In summary, the direct CNS effects of CRF not only trigger a cascade of hormonal events with ACTH release and increased adrenomedullary release of catecholamines via stimulation of hypothalamic sympathetic outflow, leading to significant changes in cardiovascular, gastrointestinal, metabolic, and immune function, but also mediate the appropriate behavioral responses to physical and psychological stressors.

Regulation of Corticotropin-Releasing Factor Receptors

Localization of the CRF receptor using homogenate-binding assays and autoradiography techniques (DeSouza et al., 1985; Hauger et al., 1987, 1988a; Wynn et al., 1984) together with its molecular characterization (Perrin et al., 1993) has allowed systematic investigation of its regulation. Activation of CRF receptors is associated with stimulation of adenylate cyclase activity and consequent increases in cyclic AMP levels (Aguilera et al., 1986) in pituitary cells, in orbital and frontal

Table 6.4. Behavioral Effects of Corticotropin-Releasing Factor

Behavior following CRF Administration	Behavior following CRF Receptor Antagonism or CRF Passive Immunization
Increased locomotor activity in familiar environments	Reversed stress- and drug-induced anorexia
Decreased exploration of unfamiliar environments	Decreased stress-induced fighting
Decreased response to operant conflict	Reversed defensive withdrawal (induced by stress, drugs, or genotype) and restored exploratory behavior
Enhanced stress-induced freezing	Attenuated stress-induced freezing
Decreased food intake	Blocked fear-potentiated startle
Disrupted sexual behavior	Decreased acquisition of conditioned emotional response
Enhanced acoustic startle response	Reduced defensive burrowing
Conditioned fear and aversion	Prevented stress-induced sensitization
Disrupted sleep rhythms	
Increased frequency of grooming and defensive burrowing	
Induced seizures at high doses	

Adapted from Koob GF, Heinrichs SC, Menzaghi F, et al: Corticotropin releasing factor, stress and behavior. *Semin Neurosci* 6:221–229, 1994.

cortical neurons, and in the amygdala, but not in the pons where CRF binding sites are absent (Millan et al., 1986; Wynn et al., 1984).

The expression of pituitary CRF receptors is altered by physiological variations in circulating glucocorticoid levels and is associated with the delayed corticosteroid inhibition of ACTH transcription and release. Exogenous corticosterone administration produces a dose-dependent reduction in CRF receptor binding density in the anterior pituitary, thus contributing to the feedback inhibition of ACTH secretion (Hauger et al., 1987). Adrenalectomy causes a decrease in CRF-stimulated adenylate cyclase activity and a down-regulation of pituitary CRF receptors, prevented by corticosteroid replacement in adrenalectomized rats (Aguilera et al., 1986; Wynn et al., 1984). The hypersecretion of CRF from hypothalamic neurons results in a homologous, ligand-induced down-regulation of CRF receptor numbers and desensitization of the adenylate cyclase-linked signal transduction. Nevertheless, CRF receptor regulation is dissociated from ACTH responsiveness in the postadrenalectomy period based on the observation that in vivo and in vitro ACTH responses to CRF are greater following adrenalectomy, despite the loss of pituitary CRF receptors (Aguilera et al., 1986). In contrast to these changes in the pituitary, CRF receptors in other parts of the brain are unchanged following very high doses of corticosterone or removal of the adrenal glands (Hauger et al., 1987). Release of ACTH and corticosteroids following acute stress does not alter CRF receptor density in the pituitary, although chronic stress causes down-regulation of pituitary CRF receptors, temporally related to the progressive normalization of ACTH secretion during chronic stress (Hauger et al., 1988). Pituitary ACTH responses to novel stressors or intravenous CRF injection were markedly accentuated in chronically stressed animals, compared with the ACTH responses of nonstressed control animals (Hauger et al., 1988). In vitro CRF-stimulated cyclic AMP and ACTH release from pituitary cells is reduced following chronic stress, a discrepancy explained by the concomitant effects of vasopressin release in vivo, which reverses the desensitization of pituitary cells to resemble those of nonstressed controls (Hauger et al., 1988). Thus, vasopressin, norepinephrine, and other neurotransmitters may contribute to the in vivo sensitization of ACTH responses to novel stressors in chronically stressed animals.

Hypothalamic-Pituitary-Adrenal Axis Responses to Stress

STRESS HYPORESPONSIVE PERIOD

ACTH release from fetal or neonatal pituitary glands can be demonstrated in vitro following CRF stimulation (Dupouy and Chatelain, 1983; Hary et al., 1984), though the HPA axis in vivo remains relatively hyporesponsive to stress for 2 weeks after birth in rats (Levine, 1970; Sapolsky and Meaney, 1986; Walker et al., 1986a, 1986b). The threshold for pituitary-adrenal responsiveness is particularly high in the 24–72 hours after birth, with progressive decreases in the subsequent weeks. Following the increased transcription of hypothalamic CRF mRNA and pituitary POMC mRNA levels in rat fetuses from E17 to E20, CRF and POMC gene transcription decreases markedly during the perinatal period (Grino et al., 1989a, 1989b). A progressive increase in POMC mRNA expression occurs in the rat neurointermediate lobe of the pituitary from P1 to P21, which is corticosteroid insensitive due to an absence of glucocorticoid receptors. This implies a greater glucocorticoid negative feedback in the perinatal period, leading to secondary inhibition of the expression of CRF mRNA expression in PVN neurons (Grino et al., 1989a, 1989b).

The hypothesis that the stress-hyporesponsive period results from increased corticosteroid inhibition of the HPA axis was supported by the demonstration of enhanced sensitivity to negative feedback, in vivo and in vitro, to CRF-induced pituitary ACTH release in neonatal rats (Walker et al., 1986). Adrenalectomy of perinatal rat pups was associated with normal ACTH responses to ether stress, though the levels of POMC mRNA in the anterior pituitary after adrenalectomy were lower

at P7 than at P14 (Grino et al., 1989a, 1989b). Thus, the relative hyporesponsiveness of the anterior pituitary during the perinatal period may be explained by both decreased sensitivity to CRF stimulation and increased sensitivity to corticosteroid negative feedback.

Previous data suggested that β-endorphin responses to CRF stimulation in pituitary cells were similar in 7- and 14-day-old rats (Grino et al., 1989a), though CRF mRNA expression in the PVN increases significantly in 14-day-old rats and remains unchanged in 7-day-old rats following adrenalectomy, an effect reversed by daily CRF injections (Grino et al., 1989a, 1989b). Consequently, the stress hyporesponsive period may result from immature corticosteroid regulation of CRF gene expression in the hypothalamus, perhaps due to the immaturity of afferent inputs to CRF neurons in the neonatal PVN. The ontogeny of CRF receptors in the CNS does not explain the stress hyporesponsive period. Detectable numbers of CRF receptors (40% of receptor density in the adult rat) were measured in the E17 rat CNS (Insel et al., 1988). CRF receptor concentrations increased progressively in the brain until P8, when the receptor density was 312% of adult levels, and then declined to typical adult levels by P21 (Insel et al., 1988). The highest densities of fetal CRF receptors were found in the striatum, whereas after birth CRF binding increased progressively to reach its maximum in the cerebral cortex (Insel et al., 1988). Fetal CRF receptors are coupled to adenylate cyclase-linked signal transduction from E17, and postnatal development is characterized by progressive increases in the percentage of CRF receptors coupled via the stimulatory G-protein to the adenylate cyclase catalytic subunit, with maximum coupling noted in the CNS of adult rats (Insel et al., 1988). The relative hyporesponsiveness of the HPA axis during the perinatal period has not been documented in the human neonate, though the CNS maturity of the newborn rat (at P0) corresponds to that of the premature infant at 24 weeks gestation (data summarized in Table 6.1).

STRESS RESPONSES IN HUMAN NEONATES

The hormonal responses of human neonates to surgical operations performed under minimal or no anesthesia were characterized by substantial increases in plasma catecholamines, which had returned to preoperative values by 6 hours after surgery (Anand et al., 1985a, 1985b). Responses of the HPA axis to surgical stress were related to significant perioperative increases in plasma cortisol concentrations in term neonates and increases in the precursor steroid hormones (11-deoxycortisol, 11-deoxycorticosterone, 17-hydroxyprogesterone, and progesterone) in premature neonates (Anand et al., 1987, 1988). In term neonates undergoing circumcision without anesthesia, plasma cortisol values increased markedly during and after the procedure (Gunnar et al., 1981; Masciello, 1990; Stang et al., 1988; Talbert et al., 1976).

Fentanyl anesthesia in preterm babies undergoing major surgery produced substantial reductions in hormonal responses to surgery, as indicated by significant decreases in plasma epinephrine, norepinephrine, glucagon, aldosterone, corticosterone, and other steroid hormone responses. The hormonal responses of neonates receiving minimal anesthesia were associated with significant increases in blood glucose, lactate, and pyruvate; these metabolic changes were prevented in neonates receiving opioid analgesia, together with endogenous protein breakdown and the postoperative complications after surgery (Anand et al., 1987). Similar responses were observed in full-term neonates receiving halothane anesthesia for moderate surgical stress (Anand and Aynsley-Green, 1988; Anand et al., 1988).

In neonates undergoing cardiac surgery, anesthetic management with halothane and low-dose morphine was associated with substantial catecholamine, corticosteroid, β-endorphin, and glucagon responses during and after cardiac surgery; these responses were blunted in neonates given high dose sufentanil anesthesia (Anand and Hickey, 1992). Metabolic stress responses between the two groups were strikingly different, with decreased hyperglycemia and lactic acidosis in neonates given opioid anesthesia. The incidence of metabolic, infectious, and cardiovascular complications postoperatively was decreased, together with a significant reduction in postoperative mortality in neonates given sufentanil (Anand and Hickey, 1992).

EFFECTS OF EARLY HANDLING AND MATERNAL DEPRIVATION

The handling of rat pups in the 1st week after birth (or for 21 days, in some studies) results in adult rats with decreased behavioral inhibition in novel environments and decreased HPA responses to a variety of stressors (Ader and Grota, 1969; Levine, 1957, 1962; Levine et al., 1967; Meaney et al., 1989). Handled rats (H) had decreased ACTH and corticosterone responses as compared with nonhandled rats (NH) in response to a variety of stressors (Hess et al., 1969; Meaney et al., 1989, 1991; Viau et al., 1993). Lower peak plasma levels and a faster return to baseline in H rats lead to substantial differences between the integrated plasma hormone responses of H and NH rats, and these differences persisted over the entire life of these animals (Meaney et al., 1988, 1991). These studies showed no differences between the H and NH groups in the adrenal sensitivity to ACTH, the pituitary sensitivity to CRF, the metabolic clearance of ACTH or corticosterone, the plasma levels of corticosterone-binding globulin, or in the basal ACTH or corticosterone levels at any point in the diurnal cycle. These data suggested that long-term effects of neonatal handling were related to neuroendocrine changes above the level of the pituitary. Subsequent studies demonstrated that differences in the HPA axis responses of H and NH rats resulted from increased negative-feedback inhibition in H rats, secondary to an increased expression of glucocorticoid receptors in the hippocampus and median prefrontal cortex of H compared with NH animals (Meaney et al., 1985, 1987, 1989; O'Donnell et al., 1994; Sarrieau et al., 1988). Chronic corticosteroid treatment (for 5 days) in H and NH rats reversed their differences in both the hippocampal glucocorticoid receptor density and the HPA axis responses to stress (Meaney et al., 1985). Thus, it appears that up-regulation of glucocorticoid receptors in the hippocampus is a critical determinant of the decreased HPA stress responses in the adult rat subjected to neonatal handling. Hippocampal lesions result in increased CRF and AVP mRNA expression in the hypothalamus and increased corticosterone responses to stress (Herman et al., 1989; Jacobson and Sapolsky, 1991; Sapolsky et al., 1984).

Prolonged separation from the mother during the neonatal period results in a loss of maternal care, including the nutritional and thermal needs of the rat pup. Rat pups separated from their mothers in the first 3 weeks after birth exhibited higher basal corticosterone levels and greater corticosterone responses to acute stress than nonseparated controls (Thomas et al., 1968). Rat pups separated from their mothers for 0, 15, 30, 60, 180, and 360 minutes each day from P2 to P14 showed markedly different HPA responses to stress during adulthood (Plotsky and Meaney, 1993). Rats separated for 0 and 15 minutes each day behaved like the NH and H rats, respectively, as described above; rats separated for 180–360 minutes each day showed significantly increased ACTH and corticosterone responses compared with the H and NH groups. These adult rats (following 180 min/day neonatal separation) showed a marked increases in CRF mRNA in paraventricular neurons in the hypothalamus, increased CRF peptide content in the median stalk, and early escape from a dexamethasone suppression test, thus suggesting a hypothalamic mechanism for the increased ACTH and corticosterone responses to stress (Plotsky and Meaney, 1993). Glucocorticoid receptor density was significantly reduced in the hypothalamus, hippocampus, and frontal cortex of adult animals exposed to neonatal stress, which may be related to the decreased negative feedback sensitivity in the HPA axis of these rats (Meaney et al., 1994).

The excessive and prolonged duration of HPA axis responses to stress in these animals may damage hippocampal neurons from prolonged exposure to stress-induced elevations of plasma corticosterone concentrations. In addition to their immunosuppressive and metabolic effects, high circulating levels of glucocorticoids accelerate the loss of hippo-

campal neurons, leading to cognitive and memory impairments, stress, and perhaps anxiety and mood disorders during adult life (McEwen, 1994; Sapolsky et al., 1986). Glucocorticoid hypersecretion was associated with the loss of type II glucocorticoid receptors in chronically stressed rats, aged rats, and AVP-deficient Brattleboro rats (Sapolsky et al., 1986). These long-term effects may result from the impaired feedback inhibition mechanisms mediated by hippocampal neurons, leading to increased expression of CRF and AVP in hypothalamic neurons and increased release of CRF/AVP in response to acute stress, with consequently increased ACTH and corticosterone responses (Dallman et al., 1993; Meaney et al., 1993; Plotsky and Sawchenko, 1987; Plotsky et al., 1986; Sapolsky et al., 1986). The transition from low to high serum corticosterone concentrations within the range of physiologic circadian changes or from high basal to stressed values, increased the susceptibility of hippocampal neurons to excitotoxic damage (quantitated by increased neuron loss, τ immunoreactivity and spectrin proteolysis, as well as qualitative changes in neuronal and dendritic morphology) in the CA3 region of the hippocampus (Stein-Behrens et al., 1994).

As summarized in Table 6.4, central administration of CRF in nonhuman primates causes behavioral changes almost identical to those observed in primate models of depression involving the separation of neonatal monkeys from their mothers (Kalin and Takahashi, 1988). Several lines of evidence suggest that the hypothalamic hypersecretion of CRF may result from maternal deprivation and predispose to the development of depression in adulthood (Gold et al., 1988). Our group has obtained evidence for this phenomenon in both rodents (Owens et al., 1994) and nonhuman primate (Coplan et al., 1995) studies. Prolonged alterations were observed in the cerebrospinal fluid (CSF) CRF concentrations in infant and young monkeys following maternal stress due to variable foraging conditions (Coplan et al., 1995). Clinical correlates of these experiments may be obtained from victims of sexual or physical abuse, poor parenting, and exposure to other stressful life events (Goodyear, 1994; Mullen et al., 1993).

Alterations in Childhood Psychiatric/Behavioral Disorders

CHILDHOOD SHYNESS

Shyness was defined by Kagan et al. (1988) as an initial avoidance of and/or prolonged behavioral restraint to an unfamiliar event. Excessive shyness in young children often persists into adulthood in the form of excessive anxiety, social avoidance/isolation, and panic and mood disorders, which may lead to severe psychological impairment. In pathologically shy children, hypothalamic and amygdala-mediated responses to novel situations are hyperreactive. Increased sympathetic nervous system activity was documented in shy and inhibited children exposed to unfamiliar events, by their increased heart rate, pupillary dilation, and peripheral norepinephrine responses, also correlated with high morning levels of salivary cortisol (Kagan, 1982; Kagan et al., 1988).

It is likely that shyness may result from the diathesis of an abnormally low threshold for limbic-hypothalamic responsivity to novel stimuli or stress. Because CRF is a primary regulator of limbic sites stimulating the sympathoadrenomedullary axis and the HPA axis, CRF may be involved in the pathogenesis of severe childhood shyness. CRF hypersecretion may cause behavioral inhibition and pathological pituitary-adrenal, catecholamine, and cardiovascular responses in shy children. CRF overdrive in the CNS may be a common pathogenetic mechanism for childhood shyness and major depression in adults (Gold et al., 1988).

MAJOR DEPRESSIVE DISORDER

Chronic hyperactivity of the HPA axis occurs in adults with a major depressive disorder (MDD), which is due at least in part to CRF hypersecretion. Pathophysiological alterations of the HPA axis in depression during the acute phase of illness include hypersecretion of cortisol, increased amplitude of each cortisol secretory episode, and an early onset (i.e., phase-advance) of the nocturnal quiescent period and of the subsequent increase toward the morning peak for ACTH/cortisol circadian rhythms. In addition, alterations in corticosteroid feedback, as evidenced by nonsuppression of plasma cortisol levels in response to the synthetic glucocorticoid dexamethasone, decreased ACTH responses to intravenously administered CRF, and increased CSF concentrations of CRF occur, together with down-regulation of the number of CRF receptor sites in the frontal cortex of depressed suicidal patients (Gold et al., 1988; Hauger et al., 1989; Nemeroff et al., 1988; Owens et al., 1995). Although some of these HPA axis abnormalities are not unique to depression, their presence in acutely depressed patients suggests that the effects of CRF hypersecretion at hypothalamic and extrahypothalamic levels may contribute to the pathogenesis of depression. This overactivity of the HPA axis is a reversible, state-dependent secretory disturbance, which normalizes following a recovery from depression. Therefore, these neuroendocrine changes are indicative of a state of stress maladaptation, supporting the hypothesis that pathological stress responses contribute to the pathogenesis of depression (Anisman, 1984).

There is currently considerable debate over the issue of whether the HPA axis of prepubertal children and adolescents with MDD resembles the overactive HPA axis of adult patients with depression. A preliminary study suggested that cortisol hypersecretion can occur in prepubertal children with endogenous depression (Puig-Antich et al., 1979), though this was not confirmed in a subsequently large published longitudinal study of 45 prepubertal children with MDD (Puig-Antich et al., 1989). The 24-hour mean cortisol secretion, the circadian peak and nadir for cortisol, and the timing of the early morning increase in cortisol secretion in adolescents with MDD were not significantly different from psychiatrically well adolescents (Dahl et al., 1989). Our group found that adolescents hospitalized for major depression exhibited high rates of dexamethasone nonsuppression; these responses normalized after recovery from MDD (Evans et al., 1987). These data indicate that state-dependent changes in the HPA axis occur in hospitalized prepubertal children and adolescents with MDD, though the clinical significance of these changes and their role in the pathogenesis of MDD remain obscure.

CHILDHOOD AUTISM

Autism is a developmental neuropsychiatric syndrome characterized by the early childhood onset of severe disturbances in language, cognitive development, absence of object relatedness, social withdrawal, idiosyncratic affective states, motoric stereotypes, and increased locomotor behavior. In a landmark neurochemical study, Schain and Freedman (1961) demonstrated that circulating levels of serotonin (5-HT) were markedly elevated in autistic children. Further investigations revealed that blood 5-HT concentrations were elevated in 30% of children with clinically defined (DSM-III criteria) autism. Several mechanisms may account for this finding, ranging from abnormal metabolism of serotonin in the gut, to the properties of platelets that transport serotonin, to CNS mechanisms that control these processes. Systematic studies of peripheral serotonin production, gut motility, and blood flow; platelet numbers, size, storage capacity, and half-life; hormones or other endogenous mediators that may alter the serotonin transporter on platelet membranes; or the central dysregulation of serotonergic pathways; all could contribute to defining the etiopathogenesis of autism. However, in most studies published subsequently, the patient populations were not defined by hyperserotoninemia but by the clinical features of autism. A great deal of research that focused on defining the abnormal serotonergic mechanisms in autism did not even measure blood serotonin concentrations. This is important because only 30% of clinically defined autistic children have hyperserotoninemia, and the percentage in any subpopulation may range from 0 to 100. Therefore, separate studies measuring a variable relevant to the mechanism of hyperserotoninemia will differ quantitatively in accordance with the unknown proportion of hyperserotoninemics in the study population, leading to different, or even opposing, con-

clusions. Much of the confusion in this area can be avoided if study populations are defined by their etiological diagnosis rather than by their clinical diagnosis (Yuwiler, 1995).

Fenfluramine given in low doses acutely increased central 5-HT neurotransmission via stimulation of 5-HT release, inhibition of presynaptic 5-HT reuptake, and interaction at postsynaptic 5-HT receptors as a weak agonist (Costa et al., 1971). High-dose or chronic fenfluramine administration exerts neurotoxic effects on presynaptic 5-HT nerve terminals, with a sustained depletion of neuronal 5-HT stores (Costa et al., 1971; Garrattini et al., 1975). Fenfluramine therapy in autistic children resulted in significant clinical improvement and was correlated with 50% reduction in blood serotonin levels (Ritvo et al., 1984), though these findings were not replicated in subsequent studies. Fenfluramine-induced changes in pituitary prolactin secretion were used to measure serotonergic responsivity in male autistic children (McBride et al., 1989). Prolactin responses to fenfluramine were blunted in autistic patients, together with a marked reduction in the magnitude of 5-HT-amplified platelet aggregation and decreased numbers of $5-HT_2$ receptors in the platelets of autistic children (McBride et al., 1989). It is plausible that autism may be characterized by hyperserotoninemia and the desensitization of brain serotonergic systems to 5-HT agonists. Decreased activity in serotonergic pathways in autistic patients may explain a number of their clinical findings and suggests that drugs augmenting central serotonergic neurotransmission may be therapeutic. A concordance between serotonergic mechanisms in peripheral blood platelets and in the CNS has never been proven conclusively, although it is frequently assumed in mechanistic and therapeutic studies.

Stress responses of the HPA axis may be abnormal in autistic children. Cortisol secretion in response to insulin-induced hypoglycemia in autistic children is elevated and prolonged compared with that in control children (Maher et al., 1975). Because the regulation of hypothalamic CRF release involves stimulatory input from serotonergic neurons (via $5-HT_2$ receptors), the abnormal cortisol responses to hypoglycemia may reflect abnormalities in central serotonergic neurotransmission (Calogero et al., 1989). Fenfluramine administration reduces hypothalamic CRF concentrations, presumably by stimulating CRF release, and increases CRF concentrations in the hippocampus, midbrain, and spinal cord (DeSouza et al., 1989). The clinical improvement noted with fenfluramine therapy in autistic children may be partially related to the normalization of CRF-mediated mechanisms essential for stress adaptation.

Some of the behavioral and motoric symptoms in autism suggest abnormalities in dopamine (DA) neurotransmission. Increased CSF concentrations of the principal DA metabolite homovanillic acid (Cohen et al., 1977) and decreased GH responses to L-dopa were documented in some autistic children (Deutsch et al., 1985), suggesting that dopaminergic mechanisms influencing GH release may be desensitized in autism. Conversely, the GH responses to insulin-induced hypoglycemia, mediated via the catecholaminergic, serotonergic, and glucoreceptor stimulation of PVN neurons, were prolonged in autism (Deutsch et al., 1986). These disparate neuroendocrine manifestations of childhood autism indicate the need for much greater precision in neurobiologic studies investigating the mechanisms of this neuropsychiatric disorder, with particular focus on regulation of the HPA axis and the somatotrophic axis. Certainly brain imaging studies, both structural and functional, could play a pivotal role in elucidating the pathophysiology of this devastating disorder.

THE SOMATOTROPHIC AXIS

Ontogeny of the Somatotrophic Axis

GHRF immunoreactivity can be measured in the infundibular nucleus of the hypothalamus from 18-week-old human fetuses (Bresson et al., 1984). However, GHRF neurons in the arcuate nucleus cannot be detected until 29 weeks of gestation (Bloch et al., 1984). Consequently, fetal GH regulation may not involve GHRF until mid- to late gestation. In the feline CNS, GHRF terminals are sparse in the median eminence at 15 days postpartum, followed by their rapid proliferation in the 1st month after birth (Bugnon et al., 1983). Fetal sheep have higher circulating concentrations of GH as compared with that in neonatal sheep, associated with the maximum GH responses to GHRF in fetal sheep from 71 to 135 days of gestation (Gluckman, 1984; Ohmura et al., 1984). In the human species, GH responses to GHRF are fairly constant throughout puberty and adulthood. The sensitivity of the pituitary somatotroph to GHRF does not change after early childhood; therefore, it is likely that gradual reduction of GH secretion with age is secondary to decreases in hypothalamic GHRF release (Gelato and Merriam, 1986).

Distribution of Growth Hormone-Releasing Factor in the Brain

After Vale et al. (1981) reported the isolation, sequencing, and synthesis of a 41-amino acid ovine hypothalamic peptide CRF that stimulated pituitary ACTH and β-endorphin secretion (Vale et al., 1981), the same group (Rivier et al., 1982) and another group (Guillemin et al., 1982) independently identified and sequenced growth hormone-releasing factor (GHRF) from tissue extracts of pancreatic islet cell tumors from two patients with acromegaly (Guillemin et al., 1982; Rivier et al., 1982). Further research has characterized the distribution of hypothalamic neurons containing these peptides, together with the localization of receptor sites for these regulatory factors in the pituitary gland and other parts of the CNS.

Although CRF, somatostatin, and thyrotropin-releasing hormone (TRH) are widely distributed in the mammalian CNS, GHRF has a much more limited CNS localization in human and nonhuman primates and in rodents (Bloch et al., 1983: Merchethaler et al., 1984). GHRF-immunoreactive cell bodies are primarily located in the arcuate and ventromedial nuclei of the hypothalamus and project GHRF-containing nerve terminals in the median eminence. Other tissues that express GHRF include the placenta and parts of the gastrointestinal tract (e.g., in the gastric antrum colocalized with the peptide gastrin and upper intestinal tract).

The only nonhypophysial behavioral effect thus far identified for GHRF is its ability to stimulate food intake when injected intracerebroventricularly (ICV) (Vaccarino et al., 1985). ICV GHRF does not alter other behaviors such as locomotor activity or arousal, while the intravenous administration of GHRF releases GH without stimulating feeding behavior (Vaccarino et al., 1985). The regulation of appetite is a central action of GHRF that may facilitate GH-induced somatic growth in children and adolescents.

Regulation of GHRF Receptors

Specific high-affinity ($K_d = -0.1$ μM) receptor sites for GHRF were demonstrated in the anterior pituitary and in other organs including the exocrine pancreas, where GHRF stimulates pancreatic enzyme secretion (Seifert et al., 1985). Although GHRF receptors in the pituitary are specific for GHRF, other endogenous mediators such as vasoactive intestinal peptide (VIP) also demonstrate high affinity binding to pancreatic GHRF receptors (Pandol et al., 1984; Seifert et al., 1985). Similar to other hypothalamic releasing hormones, the binding of GHRF to its receptor stimulates adenylate cyclase activity, leading to increases in intracellular cyclic AMP concentrations, which mediate GHRF-stimulated GH release (Harwood et al., 1984). In addition, GHRF promotes the phosphorylation of phosphatidylinositol, suggesting that post-GHRF receptor mechanisms may involve intracellular calcium influx as a second messenger (Canonico et al., 1983). It is likely that GHRF-stimulated GH release may involve multiple signal transduction systems. At the present time, there is no known synergy between GHRF and other hypothalamic factors in the regulation of GH release, with the exception of somatostatin, which inhibits GH release (see below).

Despite the absence of CRF-mediated GH release, the HPA axis modulates the somatotrophic axis by multiple mechanisms, via the central effects of adrenocortical hormones. In vitro experiments have shown that glucocorticoids increase GH gene transcription, increase GH content and release, and enhance GH responses to GHRF from pituitary somatotrophs. In vivo, corticosteroids suppress somatic growth and GH responses to various stimuli (Evans et al., 1982; Gelato and Merriam, 1986; Wehrenberg et al., 1983). The GHRF-binding capacity of the anterior pituitary is decreased by adrenalectomy, and dexamethasone administration results in a large increase in the number of pituitary GHRF receptors in adrenalectomized rats (Seifert et al., 1985). The physiologic role of this interaction was substantiated by a similar increase in GHRF-binding capacity in animals with intact adrenal glands, suggesting that the HPA axis is part of a larger hypothalamic neural network that mediates feeding, growth, and energy balance (Dallman et al., 1994; Seifert et al., 1985). Within this network, corticosteroids may enhance the responsivity of pituitary somatotrophs by upregulating GHRF receptors. Stress-mediated glucocorticoid release may exert a negative effect on GH secretion, in order to inhibit feeding and other restorative behaviors. The central actions of GHRF, such as the stimulation of food intake, may also be modulated by the stress-related or baseline secretion of glucocorticoids.

Similar to other transmitter systems, prolonged exposure to hypothalamic releasing factors results in homologous desensitization of their secretory responses and is associated with a concurrent down-regulation of their specific receptors (Catt et al., 1979). Thus, prolonged exposure to GHRF stimulation in vivo or in vitro leads to a significant blunting of the resulting GH responses, associated with GHRF receptor downregulation (Bilezikjian et al., 1986; Ceda and Hoffman, 1985; Wehrenberg et al., 1986). The in vitro desensitization of GH secretory responses during prolonged exposure to increased GHRF levels does not correspond with the loss of pituitary GHRF receptors (Bilezikjian et al., 1986). Pituitary somatotrophs become less sensitive to GHRF due to the depletion of GHRF-sensitive intracellular GH pools. Such desensitized pituitary somatotrophs can respond to very high levels of GHRF, indicating that chronic GHRF infusions may have a therapeutic role in disorders of growth (Bilezikjian et al., 1986).

Regulation of Growth Hormone Secretion

SOMATOSTATIN

The oscillatory interactions between GHRF and somatostatin are responsible for the regulation of GH release (Fig. 6.2). The pulsatile secretion of GH results from GHRF pulses released by hypothalamic GHRF neurons, whereas the intermittent secretion of hypothalamic somatostatin causes the variability in the magnitude of GH pulses secreted in response to GHRH. The peaks of GH secretion result from the coincidence of a GHRH peak and a somatostatin nadir from the hypothalamus, and the troughs of serum GH concentrations correlate with the peaks of somatostatin release from the hypothalamus (Gelato and Merriam, 1986; Hartmann et al., 1993). This regulation is illustrated by a sustained increase in GH secretion for several hours in response to a continuous infusion of GHRF during immunoneutralization of somatostatin. In the absence of pretreatment with the somatostatin antiserum, the same GHRF infusion resulted in pulsatile GH release (Wehrenberg et al., 1986).

The in vitro exposure of pituitary cells to somatostatin resulted in a dose-dependent inhibition of GHRF-stimulated cyclic AMP accumulation and adenylate cyclase activity (Harwood et al., 1984). Although this may be the primary mechanism for somatostatin effects, the ID_{50} for somatostatin inhibition of GH responses to GHRF is 1000-fold less than ID_{50} values for the inhibitory effects of somatostatin on GHRF-stimulated cyclic AMP production. Endogenous somatostatin does not influence the down-regulation of pituitary GHRF receptors induced in vivo by a GHRF infusion, suggesting that somatostatin does not regulate

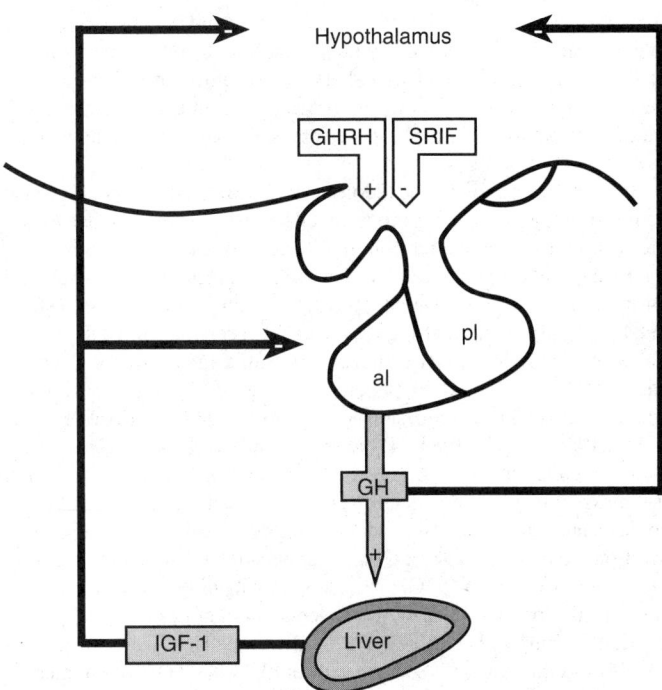

Figure 6.2. The somatotrophic axis. *GHRH,* growth hormone releasing hormone; *SRIF,* somatostatin; *al,* anterior lobe of pituitary; *pl,* posterior lobe of pituitary; *GH,* growth hormone; *IGF-1,* insulin-like growth factor-1.

GHRF receptor sites (Wehrenberg et al., 1986). The partial decreases in GHRF-induced cyclic AMP production cannot fully explain the somatostatin-induced suppression of GH secretion; somatostatin most likely blocks somatotrophic responsivity to GHRF by acting at postreceptor sites distal to the second messenger (e.g., protein kinase phosphorylation), in addition to inhibiting adenylate cyclase. Further studies may define the precise cellular mechanisms for somatostatin-mediated decreases in GH secretion.

EFFECTS OF CRF

Somatostatin can centrally inhibit CRF release and prevent stress-induced ACTH and epinephrine secretion (Brown et al., 1984). Activation of somatostatin receptors on pituitary cells may decrease ACTH responses to CRF (Axelrod and Reisine, 1984). Alternatively, high circulating levels of glucocorticoids in depressed patients may decrease CNS somatostatin release, leading to disinhibition of the HPA axis. The nonsuppression of plasma cortisol levels after dexamethasone in depressed patients was correlated with low CSF somatostatin concentrations (Rubinow, 1986). These data substantiate a pathophysiological relationship between somatostatin and the HPA axis in depressed patients.

CRF directly stimulates somatostatin secretion from cultured fetal brain cells (Peterfreund and Vale, 1983). Although CRF has no direct inhibitory effects on pituitary GH secretion, the ICV injection of CRF suppresses basal GH secretion, morphine-stimulated GHRF release, and GH responses to intravenous GHRF (Rivier and Vale, 1985). Immuno-neutralization of endogenous somatostatin abolishes CRF-induced suppression of basal and dynamic GH secretion, whereas the ICV administration of a CRF-receptor antagonist (α-helical CRF$_{9-41}$) abolishes the inhibition of GH secretion after acute stress (Rivier and Vale, 1985). Therefore, central CRF hypersecretion in pathophysiological states may alter the regulation of GH secretion by GHRF by stimulating the release of somatostatin. Hyperglycemia in normal human subjects can result in GH hyposecretion and can also inhibit pituitary GH responses to GHRF (Gelato and Merriam, 1986). Hypothalamic somatostatin release in re-

sponse to hyperglycemia may be involved in these effects on the responsiveness of pituitary somatotrophs. These interactions further substantiate the view that the HPA axis and the somatotrophic axis are embedded within a hypothalamic neural network controlling growth, metabolism, and energy balance.

Disorders of the Somatotrophic Axis during Childhood

GROWTH HORMONE DEFICIENCY

Monosodium glutamate treatment of neonatal rats results in destruction of the arcuate nucleus and its GHRF neurons leading to GH hyposecretion and growth failure, which is reversible by exogenous GHRF administration (Millard et al., 1982; Nemeroff et al., 1977; Wehrenberg et al., 1984). Exogenous GHRF does not stimulate cyclic AMP production or GH secretion from pituitary cells of the "lit/lit" dwarf mouse, an animal model of pituitary GH deficiency (Jansson et al., 1986). The somatotrophs of lit/lit mice were unresponsive to GHRF, though in vitro pituitary GH release was stimulated by dibutyryl cyclic AMP, forskolin, and cholera toxin. These data suggest that the catalytic and regulatory subunits (G_s) of adenylate cyclase and the GH release pathway distal to adenylate cyclase can be activated in pituitary somatotrophs from the lit/lit mouse (Jansson et al., 1986). The GHRF challenge test is being utilized to distinguish GH deficiency states due to hypothalamic versus pituitary defects. For example, a functional GH response to an injection of GHRF in patients with growth impairment would indicate the presence of hypothalamic GH deficiency (Gelato and Merriam, 1986). If an intrinsic pituitary defect is excluded, treatment with exogenous GHRF potentially could be used to restore normal growth.

PSYCHOSOCIAL DWARFISM

Psychosocial dwarfism is defined as a syndrome of reversible growth failure and developmental delay characterized by reduced statural growth and hyposecretion of GH (Powell et al., 1967). The diagnostic criteria proposed for psychosocial dwarfism include: (*a*) onset between 2 to 3 years of age; (*b*) delayed bone age and linear growth retardation (<3rd percentile) without signs of malnutrition; (*c*) decreased basal secretion of GH and somatomedin; (*d*) blunted GH responses to secretory stimuli; (*e*) behavioral changes such as bizarre patterns of food intake, sleep disorders, temper tantrums, withdrawal, delayed cognitive development, etc.; and (*f*) parental deprivation secondary to psychiatrically disturbed and abusive parents (Green et al., 1987).

Endocrinologic studies of these patients demonstrated pathologically low fasting GH levels, and reduced GH responses to insulin-induced hypoglycemia, arginine infusion, or exercise, when the patients were in the deprived environment (Green et al., 1987; Money et al., 1976; Powell et al., 1967a, 1967b). Sleep studies in children suffering from psychosocial dwarfism showed increased stage I sleep, a large reduction in slow-wave sleep (SWS) due to the absence of stage IV sleep, and a decrease in the total sleep period (Guilhaume et al., 1982). The SWS phase of sleep is primarily associated with nocturnal GH secretion; therefore, growth failure occurs from the lack of this physiologic stimulus for GH secretion. The regulation of GH secretion in psychosocial dwarfism is very sensitive to the child's environment. For example, during a hospital admission or when the child is placed in a beneficial nurturing environment, basal GH secretion and dynamic GH responses normalize rapidly, with initiation of bone growth. If the child returns to the socially deprived environment, GH hyposecretion recurs (Powell et al., 1967a, 1967b). Normalization of the diminished circulating levels of serum somatomedins occurs in children with psychosocial dwarfism after hospitalization (D'Ercole et al., 1977).

Maternal deprivation by physical separation or by maternal anesthesia were used to develop an animal model of psychosocial dwarfism in preweaning rat pups. The relative lack of active tactile interaction between the rat pups and their mothers decreased the circulating serum GH concentrations, metabolic activity of brain and peripheral tissue, and ornithine decarboxylase (ODC) activity, an index of organ growth and differentiation. These changes were rapidly reversed when the pups were returned to their mother (Kuhn et al., 1978). Because maternal deprivation did not alter serum concentrations of corticosterone or prolactin, it is unlikely that hyposecretion of GH resulted largely from the effects of stress. Exogenous GH or placental lactogen, combined with normal feeding of these pups, did not reverse the reduced brain and peripheral ODC levels in the absence of the mother. Conversely, vigorous stroking of the separated rat pups or the presence of an awake mother who cannot nourish due to ligated nipples were found to restore growth and maturation (Kuhn et al., 1979). Kuhn et al. (1990) have further reported that prolonged periods of maternal separation (>2 hours) results in a suppression of plasma growth hormone, whereas brief periods of separation (i.e., 15 minutes) or handling lead to increases in plasma GH concentrations. Thus, differential environmental conditions during early life may have widely different neuroendocrine effects; there is some evidence that these neuroendocrine changes persist for the entire life of the individual (Meaney et al., 1994).

GH hyposecretion and subsequent tissue insensitivity to GH in human psychosocial dwarfism may result from the psychogenic suppression of GHRF secretion in the CNS and/or the excessive release of brain somatostatin in the absence of active mothering behavior. This hypothesis was originally proposed by Powell et al. (1967), when they stated that "the emotional disturbance in these children may have had an adverse effect upon release of pituitary trophic hormone via the central nervous system." A state-dependent decrease in the basal secretion of corticosteroids is present in children with psychosocial dwarfism, which can be reversed by exogenous ACTH administration (Powell et al., 1967a, 1967b). Although ACTH secretion may be deficient, adrenocortical sensitivity to ACTH is intact in psychosocial dwarfism. Early maternal separation leads to marked and long-term increases in the sensitivity of the HPA axis to mild or moderate stressors, secondary to decreased feedback inhibition of PVN neurons expressing CRF and AVP (Meaney et al., 1994) and to CNS CRF neurons as well (Coplan et al., 1995), as described above.

MAJOR DEPRESSIVE DISORDER

Diurnal hypersecretion of GH occurs in adult patients with endogenous depression, with a phase-advanced circadian timing of GH secretion (Linkowski et al., 1987; Mendelwicz et al., 1985). This abnormality persists despite a therapeutic response to antidepressants or following complete recovery in remitted patients who are off antidepressants (Jarrett et al., 1990). The GH responses to insulin-induced hypoglycemia, clonidine, desmethylimipramine (DMI), and zimelidine (but not to the dopamine agonists amphetamine, L-dopa, or apomorphine) have been consistently shown to be reduced during depression. In adult patients with MDD, the blunting of GH responsiveness to these stimuli persists despite clinical remission and response to therapy (Amsterdam et al., 1987; Charney et al., 1982; Siever and Uhde, 1984).

Further, some, but not all, investigators have reported that GH responses to GHRF are significantly reduced in adult patients with MDD as compared with those in healthy controls (Krishnan et al., 1987; Lesh et al., 1987; Risch et al., 1988); the blunting of GH responses to GHRF may persist for years after recovery from depression (Risch and Hauger, 1988). Decreased GH secretion in major depression may either result from desensitization of pituitary somatotrophs by excessive release of GHRF, or from somatostatin hypersecretion in the depressive state. Based on preclinical studies, CRF hypersecretion in depression could suppress basal GH secretion and dynamic GH responses by stimulating the excessive release of somatostatin from extrahypothalamic and hypothalamic sites. However, our studies indicated that GH responses to GHRF are not decreased and may actually be increased in depression

(Krishnan et al., 1987). This conflicting finding and the observation that major depression is associated with an episodic daytime hypersecretion of GH would suggest that hypothalamic somatostatin secretion is reduced, a hypothesis consistent with the measurement of low somatostatin concentrations in the CSF of depressed patients (Rubinow et al., 1983).

Prepubertal children and adolescents with major depression also demonstrate some abnormalities in GH secretion. In contrast to depressed adults, prepubertal children secrete excessive GH during the total sleep period in the acute episode of endogenous depression and during remission (Puig-Antich, 1987; Puig-Antich et al., 1984a, 1984b, 1984c, 1984d). Abnormal regulation of GH secretion in MDD is supported by the reduced GH responses to insulin-induced hypoglycemia and DMI in depressed prepubertal children and adolescents; these changes persist during remission (Puig-Antich, 1987; Puig-Antich et al., 1984a, 1984b, 1984c, 1984d; Ryan et al., 1988). Deficient GH responses were not correlated with the severity or other features of MDD, though the maximum reduction of GH responses to DMI were measured in adolescents who had made a suicide attempt or had prominent suicidal ideation (Ryan et al., 1988). Clinical application of these data suggests that trait dysregulation of GH secretion may identify depressed adolescents at risk for suicide. State-dependent abnormalities in the HPA axis of adult patients with depression were also associated with suicidal tendencies (Arato et al., 1988; Nemeroff et al., 1988). Despite numerous studies in this area, it remains unclear whether these alterations in the somatotrophic axis play any precise role in the etiology or pathophysiology of MDD.

HYPOTHALAMIC-PITUITARY-THYROID AXIS

The effects of thyroid hormones on the development of the brain are described in the first part of this chapter and are summarized in Table 6.2. This section will examine the ontogeny of the hypothalamic-pituitary-thyroid (HPT) axis and describe the neuroendocrine regulation of thyroid function under basal conditions and during acute stress, as well as discuss some of the psychiatric correlates of abnormal thyroid function (Fig. 6.3).

Regulation of the HPT Axis

The major thyroid gland hormones are T_3 and T_4, both of which are released from the thyroid gland. However, about 90% of plasma T_3 is derived from the deiodination of T_4 in the CNS and peripheral tissues. The biological activity of T_3 is much greater than T_4, and >99% of both hormones are bound in serum to proteins such as thyroxine-binding globulin (TBG), albumin, and prealbumin; thus, <1% of the circulating concentrations of these hormones are unbound and biologically active. The biological activity of these hormones in the brain is closely regulated by uptake across the blood-brain barrier (Schreiber et al., 1990) and the activity of the enzyme 5′-deiodinase-II, which converts T_4 to T_3 in neuronal and glial cells (Leonard, 1990).

Biosynthesis and release of T_3 and T_4 are controlled by TSH secreted from the anterior pituitary, and the biosynthesis and release of TSH is regulated by TRH secreted from nerve terminals in the median eminence into the hypothalamohypophysial portal venous system. Dopamine is a potent inhibitor of TSH synthesis and release and blunts the pituitary responses to TRH with consequent decreases in serum T_3 and T_4 (Kaptein et al., 1980). Homeostatic control within the HPT axis is maintained by the feedback inhibition of TSH biosynthesis and release, mediated mostly by the biologically active circulating concentrations of T_3 and to a lesser extent T_4. T_3 also selectively reduces TRH biosynthesis in the PVN (Segerson et al., 1987a, 1987b), which may provide another means for homeostatic control of the HPT axis. The secretion of TSH and TRH is under complex control and can be modified by alterations in the activity of several neurotransmitter systems (Jacobowitz, 1988; Morley, 1981).

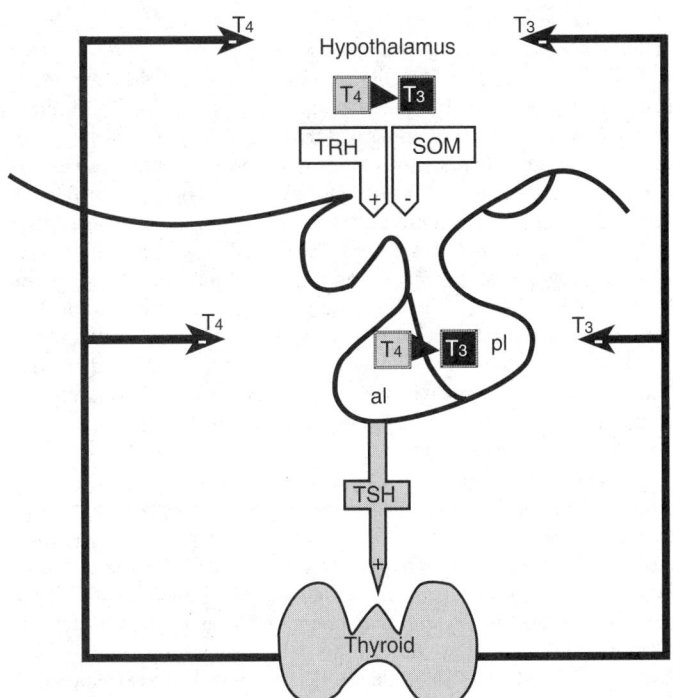

Figure 6.3. The hypothalamic-pituitary-thyroid axis. *TRH,* thyrotropin-releasing hormone; *SOM,* somatostatin; *al,* anterior lobe of pituitary; *pl,* posterior lobe of pituitary; *TSH,* thyroid-stimulating hormone; T_3, triiodothyronine; T_4, thyroxine.

Effects of T_3 and T_4 in the brain are controlled by 5′-deiodinase-II activity, which has been localized only in the brain, pituitary, brown adipose tissue, and placenta. 5′-Deiodinase-II activity in the brain increases 3- to 5-fold within 24 hours of thyroidectomy and decreases by 80–90% within a few hours after injection of a saturating dose of T_3, suggesting that the enzyme is responsible for a homeostatic mechanism by which intracellular T_3 levels are maintained within narrow limits (Leonard, 1990). Thyroid hormone-related changes in enzyme activity are due to changes in the half-life of the enzyme and do not depend on changes in the rates of transcription or translation (Leonard, 1990). Thus, it is likely to expect that thyroid hormones play important roles in the normal development and functioning of the intact brain. The impact of thyroid function on brain development has been described above, and support for the effects of T_3 and T_4 on brain function is obtained from significant changes in the EEG and evoked potentials (Pohunkova et al., 1989; Sulc et al., 1990), from the observation of specific behavioral changes during thyroid disease, and from reports of alterations in the HPT axis in certain psychiatric disorders.

Ontogeny of the Pituitary-Thyroid Axis

With its expression on E11, the mRNA for β-TSH forms one of the earliest molecular markers for the developing hypophyseal placode (Simmons et al., 1990). By E14, the mRNA for β-TSH is localized in the anterior-most cells of the developing anterior pituitary. The TEF, expressed on E13, specifically increases the transcription rate of the β-TSH gene in these cells (Drolet et al., 1991). The mRNA for TRH is first detected in the hypothalamus on E14 and is localized in parvocellular neurons of the PVN and other hypothalamic neurons by E16 (Burgunder and Taylor, 1989; Segerson et al., 1987a). The expression of TRH mRNA reaches an adult pattern of distribution in hypothalamic and extrahypothalamic sites by P21 in the rat (Burgunder and Taylor, 1989). Exposure of immature and adult rats to hypothermia upregulates TRH mRNA expression in the PVN; however, this effect is not seen at the circadian peak of TRH mRNA levels at the onset of darkness (Zoeller et al., 1990).

Effects and Regulation of TRH Secretion

Regulation of TRH secretion by parvocellular neurons in the PVN occurs by negative feedback inhibition. The mechanisms for feedback inhibition mediated by T_3 and T_4 develop and mature between E20 and P7 in the neonatal rat (Taylor et al., 1990). High levels of TRH mRNA in the PVN were noted in animals that were chemically thyroidectomized and reverted to baseline after treatment with T_3 (Koller et al., 1987; Segerson et al., 1987b). Regulation of TRH expression is primarily controlled by the direct action of T_3 in PVN neurons and is independent of TSH, other pituitary hormones, and catecholamine input to the hypothalamus (Dyess et al., 1988; Zoeller et al., 1988). Support for the primary role of T_3 in feedback inhibition of TRH is provided by transcripts encoding for the α_1- and β_1-thyroid receptor genes in parvocellular neurons of the PVN (Bradley et al., 1990).

TRH is the primary regulator of TSH secretion from the anterior pituitary, and it also stimulates prolactin release. The concentrations of TRH are highest in the median eminence, though substantial concentrations of TRH are localized in extrahypothalamic brain areas including the brainstem, midbrain, preoptic area, septum, basal ganglia and the cerebral cortex, where TRH apparently functions as a neurotransmitter and neuromodulator (Timiras and Nzekwe, 1989). TRH effects on anterior pituitary cells are mediated via the phosphoinositol second messenger system; other forms of signal transduction may be involved in the nonpituitary effects of TRH. The neurotransmitter role for TRH is thought to explain widespread changes in behavior and brain functions, such as the antagonism of hibernation and the sedation and hypothermia induced by centrally acting depressants, e.g., barbiturates, ethanol and anesthetics. In addition, TRH increases body temperature, reduces food intake, stimulates locomotor activity, increases blood pressure and respiratory rate, causes arousal and EEG activation, increases gastric motility and has antinociceptive effects. These effects may be produced directly or by interaction with a variety of monoamine and peptide neurotransmitters (Griffith, 1985; Nemeroff et al., 1984; Timiras and Nzekwe, 1989; Vaccari, 1988). In human subjects, TRH appears to increase the sense of well-being, motivation, relaxation, and coping capacity. These effects were noted in normal subjects and patients with neurological (Parkinson's disease) or psychiatric disorders (depression, schizophrenia, autism) (Loosen, 1988a, 1988b; Loosen and Prange, 1984; Prange et al., 1979), although it is often difficult to separate the direct behavioral effects of TRH from its endocrine effects leading to secondary changes in behavior, as well as its interactions with various other neurotransmitter systems (Griffith, 1985; Nemeroff et al., 1984).

Thyroid Hormone Receptors

The effects of thyroid hormones (T_3 and T_4) on the developing and adult brain are mediated by a specific class of intracellular nuclear receptors, found on both neuronal and glial cells (Evans, 1988). Although both T_3 and T_4 bind to the nuclear thyroid receptor, most of the biological activity results from T_3 and $\geq 80\%$ of the T_3 is derived from the β-deiodination of T_4 in the neuronal cell (Dussault and Ruel, 1987). The homology between steroid and thyroid receptors suggests that these belong to a superfamily of nuclear receptors containing three functional domains that mediate hormone binding, DNA binding, and transcription (Evans, 1988; Evans and Arriza, 1989; Samuels et al., 1989). The binding affinity of these receptors for T_3 is about 10 times their affinity for T_4, a factor that roughly parallels the in vivo potency ratio for these two hormones (Komisaruk et al., 1986).

The expression of thyroid hormone receptors in the human brain precedes the prenatal increase in serum T_3 levels and the peak growth spurt in neuronal differentiation and glial replication (Komisaruk et al., 1986; Kuhn and Schanberg, 1984). High densities of thyroid receptors are expressed in the developing brain from early gestation, with preferential localization on neurons rather than glial cells. Specific T_3-binding sites were barely detectable at 10 weeks gestation and increased 10-fold by 16 weeks gestation in the human fetus. Similar increases occurred around birth in rat pups and reach peak levels at P9 (Dussault and Ruel, 1987; Komisaruk et al., 1986; Kuhn and Schanberg, 1984). The abundant expression of thyroid hormone receptors in early gestation underlines the important role of T_3 and T_4 in controlling the normal development of the immature mammalian brain.

HPT Axis Responses to Stress

Acute stress in the form of critical illness, surgical operation, starvation, burns, or severe systemic diseases produces the ''sick euthyroid syndrome'' in all age groups. This includes decreased plasma concentrations of T_3, low or normal total and free T_4, normal TSH, and significantly increased plasma reverse T_3 concentrations (Brandt et al., 1976; Fisher, 1990; Weissman, 1990). Serum TSH responses to exogenous TRH appeared normal after surgical stress, but the maximal TRH-induced increase in TSH and the integrated TSH responses were reduced in critically ill postoperative patients (Zaloga et al., 1985). Pituitary hyporesponsiveness to TRH stimulation was directly correlated with serum dopamine concentrations, and with clinical outcome following critical illness (McLarty et al., 1975; Philips et al., 1984; Silberman et al., 1988). These findings were confirmed in a recent study, in which the plasma concentrations of cortisol, T_3 and TSH were found to be the most accurate predictors of mortality following critical illness (Rothwell and Lawler, 1995). These findings indicate that pathological alterations in the HPT axis and thyroid function in response to acute stress are associated with marked increases in illness severity and poor outcome.

Behavioral Manifestations of Thyroid Dysfunction

HYPOTHYROIDISM

Infants with untreated congenital hypothyroidism show profound mental retardation with specific motor and sensory abnormalities, in addition to the physical stigmata and metabolic characteristics of cretinism (Fisher, 1986). Severe deficits in IQ occur in >80% of hypothyroid infants who received delayed treatment, and only 15% of infants who received early treatment with thyroxine (Klein et al., 1972). The degree of thyroid deficiency and the age of the patient at the time treatment is begun determine the intellectual prognosis and the effectiveness of therapy (Dussault, 1986; New England Collaborative Study, 1981). Even in patients with normal or near normal intellectual development, impaired brain development may be manifested in the form of clumsiness (33%), behavior disorders (23%), speech disorders (20%), learning deficits (26%), and poor motor coordination in the majority of children (MacFaul et al., 1978). Older children and adolescents may show a variable deterioration in school performance, although some adult symptoms may also be present (Fisher, 1986).

Acquired hypothyroidism in adults is manifested primarily by impaired cognition, often associated with depression, fatigue, and anxiety, and occasionally the development of psychosis (Reitan, 1963; Schon et al., 1961; Whybrow et al., 1969). In some patients, the overt psychiatric disorders may precede the onset of hypothyroid signs and symptoms and may go unrecognized until the failure of therapy with psychotropic drugs (Reed and Bland, 1977).

HYPERTHYROIDISM

The behavioral manifestations of hyperthyroidism are limited to the patients being tense, agitated, confused, and remarkably restless. These signs may often be mistaken for attention deficit hyperactivity disorder (ADHD) and other behavioral disorders in school-age and some preschool children and as mania, panic disorder, or generalized anxiety disorders in adults.

Thyroid Function in Major Depressive Disorder

The HPT axis is as important for the maintenance of normal affective state and behavior as it is for cognition. As noted above, depression

occurs commonly in patients with hypothyroidism. Conversely, approximately 30% of euthyroid depressed patients show a decreased TSH secretory response to TRH administration, and some of these may have subclinical hypothyroidism (Gold et al., 1981; Loosen, 1992). Antithyroid antibodies were found in 20% of psychiatric inpatients with prominent depressive symptoms (Nemeroff et al., 1985) and 9% of patients with unipolar depression (Joffe et al., 1987). Although the endocrine effects of treatment with antidepressants cannot be separated, most studies have shown a significant improvement in thyroid function with remission in depressed patients (Loosen, 1992). This was first suggested by Whybrow et al. (1972), who found that improved thyroid function before treatment in depressed patients was positively correlated with a rapid response to treatment with imipramine. Decreased thyroid function noted in patients with rapid cycling bipolar disorder has shown a clinical response to treatment with high-dose T_4 in preliminary studies (Bauer and Whybrow, 1990).

Decreased TSH responses to TRH in depressed patients were not correlated with their age or somatic measures, the severity of depression or treatment history, or the increased activity of thyroid hormones, corticosteroids, somatostatin, or dopamine. Decreased TSH responses could not be correlated with clinical factors such as primary or secondary depression, unipolar or bipolar subgroups, and patients who were acutely ill or in remission. However, the primary clinical importance of decreased TRH-induced TSH responses derives from their association with a history of violent suicidal behavior and an increased risk of suicide (Loosen, 1988a, 1988b). Repeated TRH tests may be useful for prognostic purposes, although these data have not been validated and require cautious interpretation (Loosen, 1992). The data begin to suggest some similarities between the endocrine correlates of critical physical illness (see above) and severe psychiatric disorders, a concept that may generate a host of interesting hypotheses for future research.

HYPOTHALAMIC-PITUITARY-GONADAL AXIS

Ontogeny of the Pituitary-Gonadal Axis

Neurons expressing gonadotropin-releasing hormone (GnRH) first develop anteriorly in the olfactory placode and migrate posteriorly to reach the median basal hypothalamus by 9–11 weeks of gestation in the human fetus. The development and migration of these neurons are altered in patients with Kallman's syndrome (hypogonadotropic hypogonadism and hyposmia) associated with a Xp22.3 deletion of the X chromosome (Handelin et al., 1993; Schwanzel-Fukuda et al., 1989). In the normal human fetus, GnRH mRNA is expressed in the fetal hypothalamus from about 10 weeks gestation, and the developing pituitary gland contains β-FSH from 10 to 15 weeks of gestation. The mRNA for the α-glycoprotein subunit of gonadotropins forms one of the earliest molecular markers for the hypophyseal placode, expressed on E11 in the rat fetus, when the anterior neuropore is just closing (Simmons et al., 1990). By E17 in rats, ventrally located cells in the anterior lobe first express the mRNAs for LH and FSH (Swanson, 1992). The hypothalamic-hypophyseal portal circulation develops at about midgestation in most species, leading to a marked increase in gonadotropin secretion (Gluckman et al., 1981). The increased concentration of gonadotropins in peripheral plasma is responsible for the testicular and ovarian maturation that occurs after midgestation. Sheep fetuses exposed to a long-acting GnRH agonist in the latter half of gestation showed the absence of pituitary gonadotrophs and reduced testicular growth at birth (Thomas et al., 1994). Steroidogenic factor 1 (SF-1), an orphan nuclear receptor, regulates the development of gonadotroph in the pituitary as well as the enzymes that produce sex steroids in the adrenal gland and gonads. In SF-1 knockout mice, pituitary cells lacked the expression of gonadotroph-specific factors including LHβ, FSHβ, and the GnRH receptor (Ingraham et al., 1994).

During the third trimester, the expression of steroid receptors in the hypothalamus is associated with the onset of feedback inhibition and a resulting decrease in the secretion of gonadotropins. At birth, the fetal hypothalamus is released from the control of high maternal plasma estrogen concentrations, and gonadotropin secretion increases substantially within 2–4 days after birth. Episodic peaks of gonadotropin secretion can be detected for 2–4 years after birth, often associated with the secretion of gonadal steroid hormones in the pubertal range (Stein, 1992).

Neuroendocrine Regulation of Puberty

Puberty is a sequence of events characterized by the secretion of pituitary and gonadal hormones leading to the development of secondary sexual characteristics, gametogenesis, reproductive function, and transformation of the child's appearance to the dimorphic adult state. Regulation of the onset of this epochal life event involves the complex interaction of several neuroendocrine mechanisms, many of which are susceptible to modulation by genetic, psychological, behavioral, dietary, and environmental factors. Some of these regulatory neuroendocrine mechanisms include: (*a*) changes in the sensitivity of the hypothalamus to inhibitory steroid feedback, (*b*) synchronization of the GnRH secreting hypothalamic neurons leading to a summation of the stimuli producing the secretion of gonadotropins (FSH, LH) from the pituitary, (*c*) development of the secretory capacity of pituitary gonadotrophs, (*d*) removal of inhibitory influences of nongonadal origin (e.g., melatonin), and (*e*) proposed decreases of the inhibitory influences from higher brain centers. Other somatic and endocrine factors include the amount and distribution of body fat mass (de Ridder et al., 1992), the levels of sex-hormone binding globulin (SHBG) (Mendel, 1989; Siiteri et al., 1972), ovarian estrogen secretion in response to LH (Garibaldi et al., 1993), and the effects of other pituitary hormones and cytokines (Chrandrashekar et al., 1988; Hall et al., 1992).

CONTROL OF GONADOTROPIN SECRETION

Stimulation of the pituitary gonadotrophs by the hypothalamic decapeptide GnRH released into the hypophyseal portal system leads to the characteristic secretion of FSH and LH pulses as measured in peripheral plasma (Apter et al., 1993) (Fig. 6.4). The pulsatile secretion of GnRH most likely results from intrinsic mechanisms within the network of GnRH-secretory neurons (Mellon et al., 1990), though the frequency of GnRH pulses and synchronization of individual GnRH neurons may depend on other hypothalamic and extrahypothalamic factors (Styne, 1994). In normal children, increased gonadotropin secretion occurs for a period of 2–4 years after birth followed by a period of quiescence, which is known as the juvenile phase. At the onset of puberty, the GnRH secretion increases again with marked accentuation of the magnitude and duration of gonadotropic hormone pulses (Grumbach and Styne, 1992). Other pituitary hormones may also alter the secretion of gonadotropins. Studies in transgenic mice overexpressing the human GH gene suggested that GH altered the pituitary sensitivity to GnRH and/or increased pituitary gonadotropin synthesis and secretion (Chrandrashekar et al., 1988, 1989). Decreased body weight, testicular weight, and development following thymectomy in animals was related to the stimulation of hypothalamic LHRH secretion and pituitary LH release by thymosin-β4 (Comsa, 1973; Hall et al., 1992). Conversely, the blockade of LHRH receptors in neonatal rats (P1–P5) permanently impaired the development of the thymus and maturation of T lymphocytes and inhibited normal sexual maturation (Morale et al., 1991).

Inhibition of gonadotropin secretion results from feedback inhibition of sex steroid hormones and inhibin (which suppresses FSH secretion only) and control from higher brain centers. In patients without gonads (e.g., patients with Turner's syndrome, agenesis of the ovary) or in castrated animals, the pattern of gonadotropin secretion during infancy and childhood is qualitatively similar to that of normal children, but the baseline and peak serum levels of gonadotropin pulses are increased significantly (Conte et al., 1975). The absence of gonads does not alter

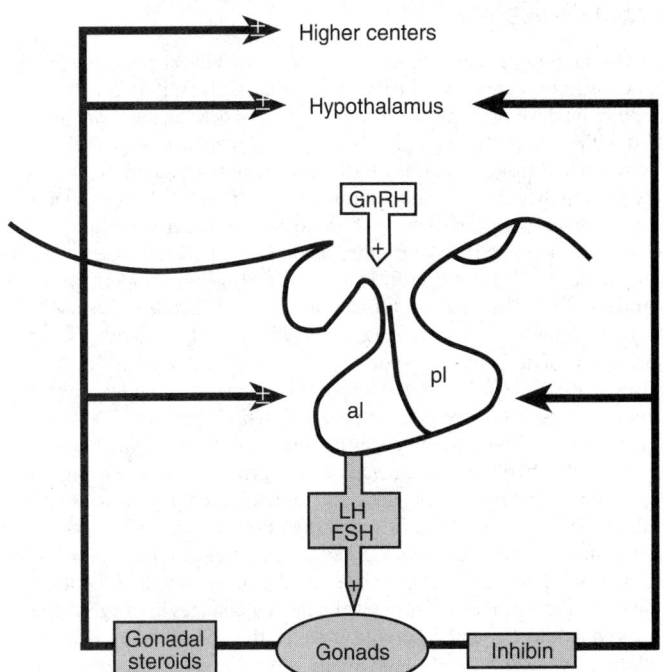

Figure 6.4. The hypothalamic-pituitary-gonadal axis. *GnRH*, gonadotropin-releasing hormone; *al*, anterior lobe of pituitary; *pl*, posterior lobe of pituitary; *LH*, luteinizing hormone; *FSH*, follicle-stimulating hormone.

the qualitative pattern of increased gonadotropin secretion during infancy or puberty and the quiescent phase during childhood, but the quantitative increases in the magnitude of gonadotropin secretion implicate the inhibitory feedback of gonadal steroid hormones (Grumbach and Styne, 1992). Increased plasma cortisol also decreases the pulsatile secretion of LH and GnRH, implying its role in stress-associated menstrual disturbances (Saketos et al., 1993).

Inhibitory control from higher brain centers is thought to be responsible for mediating the juvenile phase, which occurs in a steroid-independent manner, although the mechanisms and precise loci mediating this control of gonadotropin secretion are presently unknown. Loss of this control is demonstrated in patients who develop chronic increases in intracranial pressure (e.g., secondary to hydrocephalus or subarachnoid cysts) with the onset of central precocious puberty (CPP), which is reversed by surgical procedures (e.g., ventriculoperitoneal shunt placement) that normalize the intracranial pressure. Rare patients with hamartomas of the tuber cinereum, which often contain ectopic GnRH-secreting neurons, also present with central precocious puberty because these ectopic neurons do not receive the descending inhibitory control from higher brain centers (Grumbach and Styne, 1992). Thus, the onset of CPP may be related to the disinhibition of hypothalamic GnRH neurons resulting from the absence of control from higher brain centers.

Both of the gonadotropins, LH and FSH, can be measured by specific radioimmunoassays, although recent interest in measuring the biologically active component of LH (by testosterone production in rat Leydig cells) and FSH (by aromatase activity in rat Sertoli cells) has demonstrated different patterns of changes from those of the immunoreactive hormones (Beitins and Padmanabhan, 1991; Kletter et al., 1993). These data revealed that plasma concentrations of biologically active LH may increase manyfold and were not associated with corresponding changes in immunoreactive LH concentrations. Comparison of biologically active and immunoreactive FSH concentrations in serum did not show such striking differences (Kletter et al., 1993). The role of bioactive gonadotropins in the regulation of the normal and abnormal HPG axis remains speculative.

ONSET OF PUBERTY

The amplitude and frequency of nocturnal GnRH pulses from the hypothalamus increase gradually and progressively well before the onset of pubertal development (Apter et al., 1993). These changes are associated with increased production of pituitary gonadotropins and episodic increases in estrogen and testosterone secretion from the immature gonads. In prepubertal boys, early morning testosterone levels of ≥ 0.7 nmol/liter were accurate predictors of the onset of puberty within 12–15 months (Wu et al., 1993). Another predictor of pubertal onset was the magnitude of LH secretion in response to exogenous GnRH (100 mg intravenously). Although significant increases in serum LH concentrations were predictive of pubertal onset within 6–12 months, the wide variability of individual responses was associated with a number of false-positive and false-negative results (Crowley and Jameson, 1992). Longer-acting and more potent analogs of GnRH activity may be more accurate in determining the onset of puberty (Cuttler et al., 1993).

Normal pubertal development is characterized by a complex interaction of gonadal steroids, gonadotropins, SHBG, and body mass composition (de Ridder et al., 1990; Frisancho and Flegel, 1982). The amplitude of nocturnal GnRH pulses is markedly accentuated at the onset of puberty, leading to significant increases in the magnitude and duration of gonadotropic hormone pulses, developmental changes in the gonads and the production of gonadal steroids. Initially, the GnRH and gonadotropic pulses occur at the onset of sleep and progressively increase to cover the entire night (Grumbach and Styne, 1992; Morales et al., 1992). Developmental changes in monopolar and bipolar LHRH-immunoreactive neurons located in the medial septal-preoptic area and the diagonal band of Broca in male syrian hamsters were related to the onset of puberty (Urbanski et al., 1992), although the mechanisms mediating these morphological changes remain unknown. In normal girls, control of the onset of puberty and the maturation of negative feedback control of the HPG axis are partially independent, thus allowing ''catch up'' pubertal maturation in girls with a late onset of puberty (de Ridder et al., 1992).

The change in GH secretion during the pubertal growth spurt is closely associated with the stages of puberty. Plasma concentrations of both LH and GH measured in normal boys and girls (7.2–14.6 years age) showed increases in the amplitude and frequency of nocturnal pulses with the progression of puberty (Van de Waal et al., 1991; Bourouignon, 1991). The coordination of the pubertal growth spurt and pubertal development may occur via neuroendocrine mechanisms at the hypothalamus and/or pituitary. Little is known of these mechanisms apart from GH effects on the pituitary sensitivity to GnRH and/or increased pituitary gonadotropin secretion (Chrandrashekar et al., 1988, 1989) The role of endocrine and paracrine factors *other than gonadotropins* in regulating the production of gonadal estrogens was suggested in a recent study of early central precocious puberty in girls (Garibaldi et al., 1993). For example, interleukin-1 (IL-1) altered the expression of LH receptors in the rat ovary, and interferon-α was capable of suppressing estrogen and progesterone release (Hall et al., 1992). These data indicate that a complete understanding of the mechanisms controlling the onset of puberty is not presently available.

After the onset of puberty, gonadotropin secretion during the daytime increases, associated with progressive decreases in the nocturnal gonadotropin secretion that is characteristic of early puberty. The later stages of puberty are identified by the lack of diurnal variation in gonadotropin secretion and the development of positive feedback between ovarian estrogen secretion and pituitary LH release to stimulate normal ovulation at the peak of the LH surge (Morales et al., 1992).

Disorders of Hypothalamic-Pituitary-Gonadal Function

ANOREXIA NERVOSA AND BULIMIA

Anorexia nervosa is behaviorally defined as weight loss of $\geq 15\%$ below expected body weight, associated with an intense fear of weight gain, an abnormal body image, and amenorrhea. Bulimia is characterized by recurrent episodes of binge-eating followed by purging behavior such as self-induced vomiting, use of laxatives, diuretics, strict dieting, or vigorous exercise (Kennedy and Garfinkel, 1987). These two disorders have considerable overlap: They first appear during adolescence and young adulthood, are often accompanied by major depression, and have characteristic abnormalities in neuroendocrine function (Bruch, 1973; Kennedy and Garfinkel, 1987). The etiology of anorexia nervosa and bulimia most likely involves complex interactions between the endocrine system, CNS, and psychological and social factors. A great deal of recent research has examined the hypothesis that primary hypothalamic abnormalities may lead or predispose to the combination of behavioral disorders and neuroendocrine pathophysiology that characterize anorexia nervosa and bulimia. Their neuroendocrinology may be comparable because both cause similar behavioral and psychological disturbances (such as a morbid fear of obesity, distorted body image, poor impulse control, anxiety, and depression).

The weight loss in anorexia nervosa is preceded by amenorrhea, a clinical finding also noted in underweight bulimic patients, but not in those of normal weight (Boyar et al., 1974; Halmi and Sherman, 1975; Marshall and Kelch, 1979). The amenorrhea in both disorders is attributed to hypothalamic hypogonadism and it may or may not be reversed by the restoration of weight gain. Basal circadian levels of LH and FSH are decreased in pubertal women with anorexia nervosa to plasma levels typical of the prepubertal period (Boyar et al., 1974; Halmi and Sherman, 1975; Marshall and Kelch, 1979). Exogenous administration of GnRH results in the normal release of LH and FSH, suggesting that the pituitary is intact and that the abnormality exists at the level of the hypothalamus. The hypothesis that the site of the neuroendocrine dysfunction is at or above the hypothalamus, however, does not confirm whether weight loss, protein-calorie malnutrition, or a primary CNS defect results in amenorrhea. CRF hypersecretion may contribute to the hyposecretion of gonadotropins (Olster and Ferin, 1987; Rivier and Vale, 1984). For example, ICV administration of CRF produces a dose-dependent decrease in pituitary LH secretion (without any effects on FSH secretion) (Rivier and Vale, 1984). The stress-induced suppression of LH secretion can be abolished by the central administration of CRF antagonists (Rivier et al., 1986). Therefore, intrahypothalamic CRF hypersecretion may inhibit GnRH neurons in the arcuate nucleus, via mechanisms that have not been identified yet.

The HPA axis is hyperactive in anorexia nervosa, based on the observations of elevated basal cortisol secretion, increased cortisol responses to stress, an increased number of cortisol secretory episodes per day, and decreased feedback inhibition (based on abnormal dexamethasone suppression test). As patients gain weight, the rate of cortisol secretion normalizes and feedback inhibition is restored, suggesting this defect is state-dependent (Kennedy and Garfinkel, 1987). Abnormal dexamethasone suppression tests are also characteristic of depression, bulimia without weight loss, late-stage Alzheimer's disease, and protein-calorie malnutrition. Increased plasma cortisol concentrations may reflect both a decreased metabolism and increased HPA axis activity, the latter further suggested by increased CSF levels of CRF in underweight patients (Kaye et al., 1987). Increased plasma cortisol levels also occur in starved human subjects who do not have anorexia nervosa or depression (Fichter and Pirke, 1986; Pahl et al., 1985). A generalized reduction in metabolic rate occurs as a physiological adaptation to protein-calorie malnutrition and cachexia. Anorexia nervosa, bulimia, and MDD share not only neuroendocrine abnormalities but also anorexia, amenorrhea, decreased libido, hyperactivity, agitation, and depression. Thus, it is likely that hypercortisolism, an abnormal dexamethasone suppression test, and hypersecretion of CRF in various neuropsychiatric syndromes reflect a common CRF-mediated stress pathophysiology rather than being etiological factors unique to any particular disorder.

Patients with anorexia nervosa have increased GH levels; these are restored to normal with increased caloric intake (Kennedy and Garfinkel, 1987). Increased secretion of GH occurs in protein-calorie malnutrition with chronic hypoglycemia, thereby further supporting the hypothesis that neuroendocrine abnormalities in these two conditions are related to reduced caloric intake. Diminished GH responses to insulin-induced hypoglycemia and L-dopa, and increased GH responses to GHRF (but not clonidine), occur in anorexic patients (Brambilla et al., 1989).

Other neuroendocrine disturbances in eating disorders do not suggest that their etiology is related to central neuroendocrine dysfunction (Kennedy and Garfinkel, 1987). Thyroid function is characterized by a reduction in peripheral T_3 concentrations and increased concentrations of the inactive reverse T_3 in the face of normal circulating levels of TSH and T_4. These changes in thyroid hormones result from the decreased hepatic deiodination of T_4 to T_3, typical of catabolic states. The low T_3 decreases the metabolic degradation of cortisol because T_3 replacement in anorexic patients results in a shorter half-life for cortisol. The TSH response to TRH is also blunted in bulimia, similar to the responses seen in MDD, while anorexic patients exhibit a delayed but not blunted TSH response.

Patients with anorexia nervosa exhibit defects in urinary dilution and concentration that result from abnormal secretion of AVP (Gold et al., 1983; Nishita et al., 1989). Cold intolerance is characteristic of anorexia nervosa and may be related to a central defect in temperature regulation in the hypothalamus. Anorexic patients also manifest various abnormalities of monoamine secretion (Kennedy and Garfinkel, 1987). Decreased CNS noradrenergic activity and turnover may be a trait marker for anorexia nervosa, as suggested by decreased urinary, plasma, and CSF concentrations of 3-methoxy-4-hydroxy-phenylglycol (MHPG, a metabolite of noradrenaline); low CSF levels of noradrenaline; decreased CSF and urinary homovanillic acid (HVA)—which remain unchanged with long-term recovery. Decreased CSF and urinary concentrations of 5-hydroxyindoleacetic acid (5-HIAA, a metabolite of serotonin), which normalize with weight gain, suggest state-associated disturbances of serotonin metabolism, in contrast to the state-independent changes in noradrenaline metabolism. Bulimic patients also have decreased central noradrenaline and serotonin function, which can precede, accompany, or follow behavioral changes. Their role in the etiology of eating disorders remains uncertain because similar changes in neurotransmitter metabolism may result from caloric deprivation or weight loss per se. However, it is of interest that several of the selective serotonin reuptake inhibitors such as fluoxetine have been demonstrated, in double blind placebo controlled clinical trials, to be efficacious in the treatment of bulimia.

HYPOTHALAMIC OBESITY

A number of endocrine and genetic causes can lead to hypothalamic obesity, including Cushing's disease, polycystic ovary syndrome, castration, and Prader-Willi syndrome, to name a few. Although hypothalamic obesity was described over 100 years ago (Bray and Gallagher, 1975), recent studies using stereotaxic lesions have shown that small lesions in the paraventricular nucleus (Fukushima et al., 1987) or the ventromedial nucleus (VMN) of the hypothalamus (Parkinson and Weingarten, 1990) can produce hypothalamic obesity. Lesions in the PVN produce hyperphagia leading to obesity (prevented by limiting caloric intake) whereas VMN lesions cause obesity by complex alterations in autonomic function (increased parasympathetic activity and decreased sympathetic activity) (Bray, 1992). Following a VMN lesion, vagal efferent activity increases acutely (with increased insulin secretion), the thermogenic component of sympathetic activity decreases (Bray et al., 1990; Sakaguchi et al., 1988), and GH secretion decreases because of injury to GHRH-producing cells (Bernardis and Frohman, 1970). These neuroendocrine changes lead to decreased energy expenditure for growth or temperature regulation and increased retention of ingested calories as fat. In humans, hypothalamic obesity is often associated with impaired diurnal rhythms, somnolence, and abnormalities in temperature control (Bray, 1992). Prader-Willi syndrome, characterized by hypogonadism, central obesity, delayed puberty, hypotonia, and mild mental retardation, is associated with deletions or translocations on chromosome 15 or with a normal karyotype. Obesity in these patients is related to a remarkable hyperphagia and hypoactivity. Behavioral difficulties also include cognitive and language problems, temper tantrums in infancy, and poor

relationships with peers (Butler, 1990; Cassidy and Ledbetter, 1989). Thus, central or peripheral abnormalities in the HPG axis may lead to altered caloric intake and metabolism and should be considered in obese patients with behavioral and psychiatric illnesses.

PRECOCIOUS PUBERTY

Pubertal development before the age of 8 years is defined as precocious puberty. The etiology of precocious puberty can be classified into peripheral, central and combined causes. Central precocious puberty results from the premature activation of the HPG axis by GnRH or gonadotropins. Peripheral precocious puberty is a gonadotropin-independent process that results from the excessive production of adrenal or gonadal steroids or from ingestion of exogenous sex steroids. Combined precocious puberty involves activation of the HPG axis following abnormal production of sex steroids in the adrenal glands or gonads. The diagnosis and treatment of precocious puberty is not discussed any further in this chapter; the interested reader may refer to several recent reviews (e.g., Breyer et al., 1993; Pescovitz, 1990; Stein, 1992).

Behavioral disturbances, development of breasts and pubic hair, accelerated growth with premature epiphyseal closure are common early manifestations of precocious puberty. Children with precocious puberty often have poor self-esteem and difficulty with peer and parental relationships (Jackson and Ott, 1990) and may be at high risk for sexual abuse because of their cognitive and emotional immaturity.

TRANSSEXUALITY AND HOMOSEXUALITY

The neurobiologic basis for sexual and behavioral orientations has been investigated for several decades. Sex hormones are thought to be the major biological determinants of sexual orientation because of their well-known effects on somatic sexual differences and the development of sexual dimorphism in the brain (Witelson, 1991). Despite recent advances in neurobiology and behavior, the relative importance of biological and psychosocial factors and their complex interactions in the development of sexual orientation are poorly understood. Studies associating sexual orientation with systemic sex hormone levels during adolescence and adulthood yielded largely negative results, especially in men (Meyer-Bahlberg, 1984, 1991). Psychoneuroendocrine research on transsexuality and homosexuality is therefore focused on the role of prenatal or perinatal sex hormones on the development of structural sex differences in the brain and on the gender-specific repertoires of reproductive and nonreproductive behaviors (Gerall et al., 1992; MacLusky and Naftolin, 1981; Tallal and McEwen, 1991).

In many species, the hypothalamus and adjacent areas of the brain undergo sexual differentiation following exposure to sex steroids at a species-specific sensitive interval during the perinatal period (MacLusky and Naftolin, 1981). Sex differences noted in the human brain are listed in Table 6.3 above. The sexually dimorphic nucleus (SDN), located in the preoptic area of the hypothalamus, is thought to be involved in sexual orientation and gender identity; its size is 2.5 times greater in men and contains twice as many neurons as compared to the number in women (Gladue et al., 1984). The size, number, and morphology of neurons in the SDN are determined by exposure to sex hormones in the perinatal period (Gorski et al., 1978). Small-sized SDNs were found in the brains of transsexuals as compared to heterosexual men (Swaab and Hofman, 1988), suggesting a role for this nucleus in male homosexuality.

Some of these structural sexual differences in the brain can be produced by exposure of the female fetus or newborn to androgenic hormones. Postnatal treatment of female gerbils with testosterone (or diethylstilbestrol (DES)) increased the relative sizes of the SDN and suprachiasmatic nucleus (SCN), whereas similar treatment during adulthood had no effect. Increase in the size of the left SDN was associated with male-type courtship vocalizations (Holman and Hutchison, 1991). The effects of testosterone are located in sexually dimorphic areas of the hypothalamus and the limbic areas associated with reproductive functions (Wozniak et al., 1992). Administration of testosterone with an aromatase cytochrome P-450 inhibitor or an estrogen antagonist abolishes the effects of testosterone on sexual behavior. The mechanism of action of testosterone and other androgens therefore appears to depend on their in situ aromatization in these areas (Hutchison and Beyer, 1994). Further, the expression of aromatase mRNA in the mouse diencephalon was significantly increased by testosterone via transcriptional control (Yamada et al., 1993). This mechanism may also explain why the prenatal exposure to DES, an estrogen, has behavioral and morphological consequences similar to those of androgen exposure (Hines et al., 1982). The control of reproductive behaviors by neuroendocrine mechanisms remains under active investigation.

The importance of these findings results from the exposure of human fetuses to DES, which is thought to be related to altered sexual behavior and the development of homosexual orientation (Meyer-Bahlburg et al., 1995). Human females exposed to prenatal androgens because of congenital adrenal hyperplasia or DES were more masculine in their childhood behavior than their own sisters or unrelated control subjects, with increased physical activity; increased preference for rough-and-tumble and pursuit play and male-typical toys and activities; and a decreased preference for parental doll play, and female-typical toys and activities. These girls were also more likely to emphasize careers over childbearing in their fantasies about adult life (Berenbaum and Snyder, 1995; Dittmann, 1989; Ehrhart and Baker, 1974; Money and Ehrhardt, 1972). Similarly, atypical gender role behavior during childhood was documented by history in about two-thirds of homosexual men and women, interpreted as having crossed the line into the other gender's role-play and identity during childhood (Bell et al., 1981; Whitam and Mathy, 1986). To some extent, the neuropsychological differences between homosexual and heterosexual men resemble those found between heterosexual men and women (Gladue et al., 1990; McCormick and Witelson, 1991).

We must emphasize that, even if a neuroendocrine basis for sexual orientation is confirmed, this may apply to only two-thirds or some such proportion of homosexual men and women and that the importance of learning, psychosocial role models, and other cultural factors is not diminished by these hypotheses or supporting data.

FUTURE DIRECTIONS FOR DEVELOPMENTAL PSYCHONEUROENDOCRINOLOGY

The past decade has witnessed remarkable advances in neuroscience in general, and in molecular neurobiology and structural and functional brain imaging in particular. Both of these approaches can be applied to developmental psychoneuroendocrinology, both basic and clinical, with the result being an incremental advance in our knowledge of developmental neuroscience, a discipline that has always lagged behind the rest of neuroscience because essentially in development the CNS, particularly the brain, is different virtually on a daily basis. As such, neuroanatomists, neurochemists, and behaviorists have to some extent steered clear from this complicated and difficult to untangle area because the CNS substrate changes so rapidly. Indeed, we still do not have at our disposal a high resolution developmental brain atlas for most mammals, including humans.

Measurement of the expression of various genes encoding for neurotransmitters, neurotransmitter-linked enzymes, and neurotransmitter receptors and their regulation in development is sorely needed. This will undoubtedly help understanding of complex phenomena such as the timing of puberty, maturation of the stress response, and the pathophysiology of a variety of important clinical disorders such as anorexia nervosa, precocious puberty, and even complex behavioral alterations such as sexual preference.

Perhaps the greatest promise for clinical studies to help us elucidate the pathophysiology of childhood disorders, such as autism, affective disorders, anxiety disorders, eating disorders, and ADHD, lies with functional brain imaging. Techniques such as single proton emission computed tomography (SPECT) and positron emission tomography (PET), if determined to be safe for use in children and adolescents, will provide the ability to measure not only functional brain activity at basal levels but after response to various stimuli. Such techniques as glucose utilization or cerebral blood flow measurements will provide novel information on regional brain activity in these disease states, and we will also be able to study the dynamics of neurotransmitter and hormonal receptor regulation. These methods, combined with structural brain imaging, will undoubtedly point to particular brain regions that need to be further scrutinized in these devastating disorders. In addition, reproducible abnormalities established using functional brain imaging in symptomatic patients can then be followed after treatments for these disorders to determine whether markers for such disorders can be identified. There is little doubt that the next decade will bring remarkable achievements in this area, far beyond what we might have even imagined two decades ago.

Acknowledgments. *The authors are supported by National Institute of Mental Health Grants MH-42088, MH-39415, MH-40524, and MH-51761 and a CRC Scholar Grant from Emory-Egleston Children's Research Center.*

References

Abou-Samra A-B, Catt KL, Aguilera G: Biphasic inhibition of adreno-corticotropin release by corticosterone in cultured anterior pituitary cells. *Endocrinology* 119:972, 1986.

Ader R, Grota LJ: Effects of early experience on adrenocortical reactivity. *Physiol Behav* 4:303–305, 1969.

Aguilera G, Millan MA, Hauger RL, et al: Corticotropin-releasing factor receptors: Distribution and regulation in brain, pituitary, and peripheral tissues. *Ann NY Acad Sci* 512:48–66, 1987.

Aguilera G, Wynn PC, Harwood JP, et al: Receptor-mediated actions of corticotropin-releasing factor in pituitary gland and nervous system. *Neuroendocrinology* 43:79–88, 1986.

Amsterdam JD, Schweizer E, Winokur A: Multiple hormonal responses to insulin induced hypoglycemia in depressed patients and normal volunteers. *Am J Psychiatry* 144:170–175, 1987.

Anand KJS, Aynsley-Green A: Measuring the severity of surgical stress in newborn infants. *J Pediatr Surg* 23:297–305, 1988.

Anand KJS, Brown MJ, Bloom SR, et al: Studies on the hormonal regulation of fuel metabolism in the human newborn infant undergoing anaesthesia and surgery. *Horm Res* 22:115–128, 1985.

Anand KJS, Causon RC, Christofides ND, et al: Can the human neonate mount an endocrine and metabolic response to surgery? *J Pediatr Surg* 20:41–48, 1985.

Anand KJS, Sippell WG, Aynsley-Green A: Randomized trial of fentanyl anaesthesia in preterm babies undergoing surgery: Effects on the stress response. *Lancet* i:243–248, 1987.

Anand KJS, Sippell WG, Schofield NM, et al: Does halothane anaesthesia decrease the metabolic and endocrine stress responses of newborn infants undergoing operations? *Br Med J* 296:668–672, 1988.

Anisman H: Vulnerability to depression: Contribution of stress. In: Post RM, Ballenger JC (eds): *Neurobiology of Mood Disorders.* Baltimore, Williams & Wilkins, 1984, pp. 407–431.

Apter D, Butzow TL, Laughlin GA, et al: Gonadotropin-releasing hormone pulse generator activity during pubertal transition in girls: Pulsatile and diurnal patterns of circulating gonadotropins. *J Clin Endocrinol Metab* 76:940–949, 1993.

Arato A, Banki CM, Nemeroff CB, et al: Hypothalamic-pituitary-adrenal axis and suicide. *Ann NY Acad Sci* 515:263–271, 1988.

Arushanyan EB, Borovkova GK: Psychotropic properties of ovarian estrogens (review). *Neurosci Behav Physiol* 19:57–66, 1989.

Avanzion GL, Celasco G, Cogo CE, et al: Actions of microelectrophoretically applied glucocorticoid hormones on reticular formation neurones in the rat. *Neurosci Lett* 38:45–49, 1983.

Axelrod J, Reisine TD: Stress hormones: Their interaction and regulation. *Science* 224:452, 1984.

Baethmann A: Steroids and brain function. In: James HE, Anas NG, Perkins RM (eds): *Brain Insults in Infants and Children.* Orlando, FL, Grune & Stratton, 1985, pp. 3–17.

Balazs R: Hormonal influences on brain development. *Biochem Soc Spec Publ* 1:39–57, 1973.

Bass NH, Pelton EW, Young E: Defective maturation of cerebral cortex: An inevitable consequence of dysthyroid states during early postnatal life. In: Grave GD (ed): *Thyroid Hormones and Brain Development.* New York, Raven Press, 1977, pp. 199–214.

Bauer MS, Whybrow PC: Rapid cycling bipolar affective disorder. II: Treatment of refractory rapid cycling with high-dose levothyroxine: A preliminary study. *Arch Gen Psychiatry* 47:435–440, 1990.

Baum M: Gender dimorphism in the brain. *Natl Inst Drug Abuse Res Monogr* 65:49–57, 1986.

Beitins IZ, Padmanabhan V: Bioactivity of gonadotropins. *Endocrinol Metab Clin North Am* 20:85–120, 1991.

Bell AP, Weinberg MS, Hammersmith SK: *Sex-

ual Preference: Its Development in Men and Women. Bloomington, Indiana University Press, 1981.

Berenbaum SA, Snyder E: Early hormonal influences on childhood sex-typed activity and playmate preferences: Implications for the development of sexual orientation. *Dev Psychol* 31(1):31–42, 1995.

Bermant G, Davidson JM: *Biological Bases of Sexual Behavior.* New York, Harper & Row, 1974.

Bernal J, Pekonen F: Ontogenesis of the nuclear 3,5,3′-triiodothyronine receptor in the human fetal brain. *Endocrinology* 114:677–679, 1984.

Bernardis LL, Frohman LA: Effect of lesion size in the ventromedial hypothalamus on growth hormone and insulin levels in weanling rats. *Neuroendocrinology* 6:319–328, 1970.

Besnard F, Luo M, Miehe M, et al: Transient expression of 3,5,3′-triiodothyronine nuclear receptors in rat oligodendrocytes: In vivo and in vitro immunocytochemical studies. *J Neurosci Res* 37: 313–323, 1994.

Beyer C, Feder HH: Sex steroids and afferent input: Their roles in brain sexual differentiation. *Ann Rev Physiol* 49:349–364, 1987.

Bilezikjian LM, Seifert H, Vale W: Desensitization to growth hormone-releasing factor (GRF) is associated with down-regulation of GRF-binding sites. *Endocrinology* 118:2045–2052, 1986.

Bloch B, Brazeau P, Ling N, et al: Immunohistochemical detection of growth hormone-releasing factor in brain. *Nature* 301:607–608, 1983.

Bloch B, Gaillard RC, Brazeau P, et al: Topographical and ontogenetic study of the neurons producing growth hormone-releasing factor in human hypothalamus. *Regul Pept* 8:21–31, 1984.

Boom FE, Battenberg EL, Rivier J, et al: Corticotropin releasing factor (CRF): Immunoreactive neurons and fibers in rat hypothalamus. *Regul Pept* 4: 43–48, 1982.

Bourouignon J: Growth and timing of puberty: Reciprocal effects. *Horm Res* 36:131–135, 1991.

Boyar RM, Katz J, Finkelstein JW, et al: Anorexia nervosa: Immaturity of the 24-hour luteinizing hormone secretory pattern. *N Engl J Med* 291: 861–865, 1974.

Bradbury MJ, Akana SF, Dallman MF: Roles of type I and II corticosteroid receptors in regulation of basal activity in the HPA axis during the diurnal trough and peak: Evidence for a non-additive effect of combined receptor occupation. *Endocrinology* 134:1286–1296, 1994.

Bradley DJ, Young WS III, Weinberger C: Differential expression of α and β thyroid hormone receptor genes in rat brain and pituitary. *Proc Natl Acad Sci USA* 86:7250–7254, 1989.

Brambilla F, Ferrari E, Cavagnini F, et al: Adrenoceptor sensitivity in anorexia nervosa: GH response to clonidine or GHRH stimulation. *Biol Psychiatry* 25:256–264, 1989.

Brandt MR, Kehlet H, Skovsted L, et al: Rapid decrease in plasma-triiodothyronine during surgery and epidural analgesia independent of afferent neurogenic stimuli and of cortisol. *Lancet* December 18, 1333–1336, 1976.

Bray GA: Genetic, hypothalamic and endocrine features of clinical and experimental obesity. *Prog Brain Res* 93:333–341, 1992.

Bray GA, Gallagher TF: Manifestations of hypothalamic obesity in man: A comprehensive investigation of eight patients and a review of the literature. *Medicine* 54:301–330, 1975.

Bray GA, Fisler JS, York DA: Neuroendocrine control of the development of obesity: Understanding gained from studies of experimental animal models. *Front Neuroendocrinol* 11(2):128–181, 1990.

Bresson IL, Clavequin MC, Fellman D, et al: Ontogeny of the neuroglandular system revealed with hp GRF-44 antibodies in human hypothalamus. *Neuroendocrinology* 39:68–73, 1984.

Breyer P, Haider A, Pescovitz OH: Gonadotropin-releasing hormone agonists in the treatment of girls with central precocious puberty. *Clin Obstet Gynecol* 36:764–772, 1993.

Brown MR, Rivier C, Vale W: Central nervous system regulation of adrenocorticotropin secretion: Role of somatostatins. *Endocrinology* 114: 1546–1549, 1984.

Bruch H: *Eating Disorders: Obesity, Anorexia Nervosa, and the Person Within.* New York, Basic Books, 1973.

Bugnon C, Fellmann D, Gouget A, et al: Ontogeny of the corticoliberin neuroglandular system in rat brain. *Nature* 298:159–161, 1982.

Bugnon C, Gouget A, Fellman D, et al: Immunocytochemical demonstration of a novel peptidergic neurone system in the cat brain with an anti-growth hormone-releasing factor serum. *Neurosci Lett* 38: 131–137, 1983.

Burgunder J-M, Taylor T: Ontogeny of thyrotropin-releasing hormone gene expression in the rat diencephalon. *Neuroendocrinology* 49:631–640, 1989.

Butler MG: Prader-Willi syndrome: Current understanding of cause and diagnosis. *Am J Med Genet* 35:319–332, 1990.

Byer HS, Matta SG, Sharp BM: Regulation of the messenger ribonucleic acid for corticotropin-releasing factor in the paraventricular nuclei and other brain sites in the rat. *Endocrinology* 123:2117–2123, 1988.

Cabrera TM, Levy AD, Li Q, et al: Prenatal methamphetamine attenuates serotonin mediated renin secretion in male and female rat progeny: Evidence for selective long-term dysfunction of serotonin pathways in brain. *Synapse* 15:198–208, 1993.

Cabrera TM, Yracheta JM, Li Q, et al: Prenatal cocaine produces deficits in serotonin mediated neuroendocrine responses in adult rat progeny: Evidence for long-term functional alterations in brain serotonin pathways. *Synapse* 15:158–168, 1993.

Calogero AE, Bemardini R, Margioris AN, et al: Effects of serotonergic agonists and antagonists on corticotropin-releasing hormone secretion by explanted rat hypothalami. *Peptides* 10:189–200, 1989.

Canonico PL, Cronin MJ, Thorner MO, et al: Human pancreatic GRF stimulates phosphatidylinositol labeling in cultured anterior pituitary cells. *Am J Physiology* 245:E587–590, 1983.

Cassidy SB, Ledbetter DH: Prader-Willi syndrome. *Neurol Clin* 7(1):37–56, 1989.

Catt KJ, Harwood JP, Aguilera G, et al: Hormonal regulation of peptide receptors and target cell responses. *Nature* 280:109–114, 1979.

Ceda GP, Hoffman AR: Growth hormone-releasing factor desensitization in rat anterior pituitary cells in vitro. *Endocrinology* 116:1334–1340, 1985.

Chandrashekar V, Bartke A, Wagner TE: Endogenous human growth hormone (GH) modulates the effect of gonadotropin-releasing hormone on pituitary function and the gonadotropin response to the negative feedback effect of testosterone in adult male transgenic mice bearing the human GH gene. *Endocrinology* 123:2712–2722, 1988.

Chandrashekar V, Bartke A, Wagner TE: Interactions of human growth hormone and prolactin on pituitary and Leydig cell function in adult transgenic mice expressing the human growth hormone gene. *Biol Reprod* 44:135–140, 1989.

Charney DS, Heninger GR, Ternberg DE: Adrenergic receptor sensitivity in depression: Effects of clonidine in depressed patients and healthy subjects. *Arch Gen Psychiatry* 39:290–294, 1982.

Checkley SA, Slade AP, Shur E: Growth hormone and other responses to clonidine in patients with endogenous depression. *Br J Psychiatry* 138: 51–55, 1981.

Chubakov AR, Gromova EA, Konovalov GV, et al: The effects of serotonin on the morphofunctional development of rat cerebral neocortex in tissue culture. *Brain Res* 294:211–223, 1986.

Cohen DJ, Caparulo BK, Shaywitz BA, et al: Dopamine and serotonin metabolism in neuropsychiatrically disturbed children: CSF homovanillic acid and 5-hydroxy indoleacetic acid. *Arch Gen Psychiatry* 34:545–550, 1977.

Comsa J: Thymus replacement and HTH, the homeostatic thymic hormone. In: Luckey TD (ed): *Thymic Hormones.* Baltimore, University Park Press, 1973.

Conte FA, Grumbach MM, Kaplan SL: A diphasic pattern of gonadotropin secretion in patients with the syndrome of gonadal dysgenesis. *J Clin Endocrinol Metab* 40:670–675, 1975.

Coplan JD, Andrews MW, Rosenblum LA, et al: Persistent elevations of cerebrospinal fluid concentrations of corticotropin-releasing factor in adult non-human primates exposed to early life stressors: Implications for the pathophysiology of mood and anxiety disorders. *Proc Natl Acad Sci USA,* in press.

Costa E, Groppetti A, Revuelta A: Action of fenfluramine on monoamine stores of rat tissue. *Br J Pharmacol* 41:57–64, 1971.

Crowley WF Jr, Jameson JL: Clinical counterpoint: Gonadotropin-releasing hormone deficiency: Perspectives from clinical investigation. *Endocr Rev* 13:635–640, 1992.

Cuttler L, Rosenfield RL, Ehrmann DA, et al: Maturation of gonadotropin and sex steroid responses to gonadotropin-releasing hormone agonist in males. *J Clin Endocrinol Metab* 76:362–366, 1993.

Dahl R, Puig-Antich J, Ryan N, et al: Cortisol secretion in adolescents with major depressive disorder. *Acta Psychiatr Scand* 80:18–26, 1989.

Dallman MF, Akana SF, Bradbury MJ, et al: Regulation of the hypothalamo-pituitary-adrenal axis during stress: Feedback, facilitation and feedback. *Semin Neurosci* 6:205–213, 1994.

Dallman MF, Akana SF, Scribner KA, et al: Stress, feedback and facilitation in the hypothalamo-pituitary-adrenal axis. *J Neuroendocrinol* 4: 517–526, 1993.

Delemarre-van de Wall L, Wennick J, Odink R: Gonadotropin and growth hormone secretion throughout puberty. *Acta Paediatr Scand Suppl* 372: 26–31, 1991.

D'Ercole AJ, Underwood LE, Van Wyk JJ: Serum somatomedin-C in hypopituitarism and in other disorders of growth. *J Pediatrics* 90:375–381, 1977.

de Ridder CM, Bruning PF, Zonderland ML: Body fat mass, body fat distribution and plasma hormones in early puberty in females. *J Clin Endocrinol Metab* 70:888–893, 1990.

de Ridder CM, Thijssen JHH, Bruning PF, et al: Body fat mass, body fat distribution, and pubertal development: A longitudinal study of physical and hormonal sexual maturation of girls. *J Clin Endocrinol Metab* 76:442–446, 1992.

DeSouza EB: Corticotropin releasing factor receptors in the rat central nervous system: Characterization and regional distribution. *J Neurosci* 7: 88–100, 1987.

DeSouza EB, Insel TR, Perrin MH, et al: Corticotropin-releasing factor receptors are widely distributed within the rat central nervous system: An autoradiographic study. *J Neurosci* 5:3189–3203, 1985.

DeSouza EB, Zaczek R, Owens M, et al: Effects of fenfluramine treatment on CRF activity in rat brain. *Soc Neurosci Abstr* 15:800, 1989.

Deutsch SI, Campbell M, Perry R, et al: Plasma growth hormone response to insulin-induced hypoglycemia in infantile autism: A pilot study. *J Autism Dev Disord* 16:59–68, 1986.

Deutsch SI, Campbell M, Sahar EJ, et al: Plasma growth hormone response to oral L-dopa in infantile autism. *J Autism Dev Disord* 15:205–212, 1985.

Dodt C, Kern W, Fehm HL, et al: Antimineralocorticoid canrenoate enhances secretory activity of the hypothalamus-pituitary-adrenocortical (HPA) axis in humans. *Neuroendocrinology* 58:570–574, 1993.

Dorner G: Neuroendocrine response to estrogen and brain differentiation in heterosexuals, homosexuals, and transsexuals. *Arch Sex Behav* 17:57–75, 1988.

Duenas M, Luquin S, Chowen JA, et al: Gonadal hormone regulation of insulin-like growth factor-I-like immunoreactivity in hypothalamic astroglia of developing and adult rats. *Neuroendocrinology* 59:528–538, 1994.

Dupouy JP, Chatelain A: In vitro effects of corticosterone, synthetic ovine corticotropin releasing factor and arginine vasopressin on the release of adrenocorticotrophin by fetal rat pituitary glands. *J Endocrinol* 101:339–344, 1983.

Dussault JH: The thyroid in infancy and childhood. Congenital hypothyroidism. In: Ingbar SH, Braverman LE (eds): *The Thyroid*. Philadelphia, Lippincott, 1986, pp. 1393–1404.

Dussault JH, Ruel J: Thyroid hormones and brain development. *Annu Rev Physiol* 49:321–324, 1987.

Dyess EM, Segerson TP, Liposits Z, et al: Triiodothyronine exerts direct cell-specific regulation of thyrotropin-releasing hormone gene expression in the hypothalamic paraventricular nucleus. *Endocrinology* 123:2291–2297, 1988.

Eayrs JT: Developmental relationship between brain and thyroid. In: Michael RP (ed): *Endocrinology and Human Behavior*. London, Oxford University Press, 1968, pp. 239–255.

Essence of stress [Editorial]. *Lancet* 344:1713–1714, 1994.

Evans DL, Nemeroff CB, Haggerty JJ Jr, et al: Use of the dexamethasone suppression test with DSM-III criteria in psychiatrically hospitalized adolescents. *Psychoneuroendocrinology* 12:203–209, 1987.

Evans RM: The steroid and thyroid hormone receptor superfamily. *Science* 240:889–895, 1988.

Evans RM, Arriza JL: A molecular framework for the actions of glucocorticoid hormones in the nervous system. *Neuron* 2:1105–1112, 1989.

Evans RM, Bimberg NC, Rosenfeld MG: Glucocorticoid and thyroid hormone transcriptionally regulate growth hormone gene expression. *Proc Natl Acad Sci USA* 79:7659–7662, 1982.

Ferreiro B, Bernal J, Goodyer CG, et al: Estimation of nuclear thyroid hormone receptor saturation in human fetal brain and lung during early gestation. *J Clin Endocrinol Metab* 67:853–856, 1988.

Fichter MM, Pirke KM: Effect of experimental and pathological weight loss upon the hypothalamo-pituitary-adrenal axis. *Psychoneuroendocrinology* 11:295–305, 1986.

Fisher DA: Acquired juvenile hypothyroidism. In: Ingbar SH, Braverman LE (eds): *The Thyroid*. Philadelphia, Lippincott, 1986, pp. 1230–1238.

Fisher DA: Euthyroid low thyroxine (T_4) and triiodothyronine (T_3) states in prematures and sick neonates. *Pediatr Clin North Am* 37:1297–1312.

Frisancho AR, Flegel PN: Advanced maturation with centripetal fat pattern. *Hum Biol* 54:717–727, 1982.

Garibaldi LR, Aceto T Jr, Weber C, et al: The relationship between luteinizing hormone and estradiol secretion in female precocious puberty: Evaluation by sensitive gonadotropin assays and the leuprolide stimulation test. *J Clin Endocrinol Metab* 76:851–860, 1993.

Garrattini S, Buczko W, Jori A, et al: The mechanism of action of fenfluramine. *Postgrad Med J* 51(suppl I):27–34, 1975.

Gelato MC, Merriam GR: Growth hormone releasing hormone. *Ann Rev Physiol* 48:569–591, 1986.

Gerall AA, Moltz H, Ward IL: *Handbook of Behavioral Neurobiology*. Vol II: *Sexual Differentiation*. New York, Plenum, 1992.

Glotzbach SF, Edgar DM, Boeddiker M, et al: Biological rhythmicity in normal infants during the first 3 months of life. *Pediatrics* 94:482–490, 1994.

Glotzbach SF, Edgar DM, Boeddiker M, et al: Biological rhythmicity in preterm infants prior to discharge from neonatal intensive care. *Pediatrics* 95:231–240, 1995.

Gluckman PD: Functional maturation of the neuroendocrine system in the perinatal period: Studies of the somatotropic axis in the ovine fetus. *J Dev Physiol* 6:301–312, 1984.

Gluckman PD, Grumbach MM, Kaplan SL: The neuroendocrine regulation and function of growth hormone and prolactin in the mammalian fetus. *Endocr Rev* 2:363–395, 1981.

Gold MS, Pottash ALC, Extein I: Hypothyroidism and depression. *JAMA* 245:1919–1922, 1981.

Gold PW, Goodwin FK, Chrousos GP: Clinical and biochemical manifestations of depression. *N Engl J Med* 319:348–420, 1988.

Gold PW, Gwirtsman H, Avgerinos PC, et al: Abnormal hypothalamic-pituitary-adrenal function in anorexia nervosa: Pathophysiologic mechanisms in underweight and weight-corrected patients. *N Engl J Med* 315:1335–1342, 1986.

Gold PW, Kaye W, Robertson GL, et al: Abnormal regulation of arginine vasopressin in plasma and cerebrospinal fluid of patients with anorexia nervosa. *N Engl J Med* 308:1117–1123, 1983.

Goodyear IM: Developmental psychopathology: The impact of recent life events in anxious and depressed school-age children. *J R Soc Med* 87:327–329, 1994.

Goy RW, McEwen BS: *Sexual Differentiation of the Brain*. Cambridge, MA, MIT Press, 1980.

Green WH, Deutsch SI, Campbell M: Psychosocial dwarfism, infantile autism, and attention deficit disorder. In: Nemeroff CB, Loosen PT (eds): *Handbook of Clinical Psychoneuroendocrinology*. New York, Guilford Press, 1987, pp. 109–142.

Greene LA, Bernd P, Black MM, et al: Genomic and non-genomic actions of nerve growth factor in development. In: Changeux JPO, Glowinski J, Imbert M, et al. (eds): *Molecular and Cellular Interactions Underlying Higher Brain Functions*. London, Academic Press. *Progress in Brain Research* 58:347–357, 1983.

Griffith EC: TRH: Endocrine and central effects. *Psychoneuroendocrinology* 10:225–235, 1985.

Grino M, Burgunder JM, Eskay RL, et al: Onset of glucocorticoid responsiveness of anterior pituitary corticotrophs during development is scheduled by corticotropin-releasing factor. *Endocrinology* 124:2686–2692, 1989a.

Grino M, Young WS III, Burgunder JM: Ontogeny of expression of the corticotropin-releasing factor gene in the hypothalamic paraventricular nucleus and of the proopiomelanocortin gene in rat pituitary. *Endocrinology* 124:60–68, 1989b.

Gruen PG, Sachar EJ, Altman N, et al: Growth hormone responses to hypoglycemia in post-menopausal depressed women. *Arch Gen Psychiatry* 32:31–33, 1975.

Grumbach MM, Styne DM: Puberty: Ontogeny, neuroendocrinology, physiology and disorders. In: Wilson JD, Foster DW (eds): *Williams Textbook of Endocrinology*. Philadelphia, WB Saunders, 1992, pp. 1139–1221.

Guilhaume A, Benoit O, Gourmelen M, et al: Relationship between sleep stage IV deficit and reversible HGH deficiency in psychosocial dwarfism. *Pediatr Res* 16:299–303, 1982.

Guillemin R, Brazeau P, Bohlen P, et al: Growth hormone-releasing factor from a human pancreatic tumor that caused acromegaly. *Science* 218:585–587, 1982.

Hall ED, Baker T, Riker WF: Glucocorticoid effects on spinal cord function. *J Pharmacol Exp Ther* 206:361–370, 1978.

Hall NRS, O'Grady MP, Menzies RA: Thymic regulation of the hypothalamic-pituitary-gonadal axis. *Int J Immunopharmacol* 14:353–359, 1992.

Halmi KA, Sherman BM: Gonadotropin response to LH-RH in anorexia nervosa. *Arch Gen Psychiatry* 32:875–878, 1975.

Handelin JP, Levilliers J, Young J, et al: Xp22.3 deletions in isolated familial Kallmann's syndrome. *J Clin Endocrinol Metab* 76:827–831, 1993.

Harris GW: Neural control of the pituitary gland. *Physiol Rev* 28:139, 1948.

Hartman ML, Velduis JD, Thorner MO: Normal control of growth hormone secretion. *Horm Res* 40:37–47, 1993.

Harwood JP, Grewe C, Aguilera G: Actions of growth hormone-releasing factor and somatostatin in adenylate cyclase and growth hormone release in rat anterior pituitary. *Mol Cell Endocrinol* 37:277–284, 1984.

Hary L, Dupouy JP, Chatelain A: Effect of norepinephrine on the pituitary adrenocorticotrophic activation by ether stress and on the in vitro release of ACTH by the adenohypophysis of male and female newborn rats. *Neuroendocrinology* 39:105–113, 1984.

Hauger RL, Millan MA, Catt KJ, et al: Differential regulation of brain and pituitary corticotropin-releasing factor receptors by corticosterone. *Endocrinology* 120:1527–1533, 1987.

Hauger RL, Millan MA, Lorang M, et al: Corticotropin-releasing factor receptors and pituitary adrenal responses during immobilization stress. *Endocrinology* 123:396–405, 1988a.

Hauger RL, Risch SC, Millan M, et al: Corticotropin-releasing factor regulation of the pituitary-adrenal axis and the central nervous system. In: Michels R (ed): *Psychiatry: Psychobiological Foundations of Clinical Psychiatry* (Vol 3). New York, Lippincott, 1989, pp. 1–22.

Hauger RL, Scheinin M, Siever LJ, et al: Dissociation of norepinephrine turnover from alpha-2 responses after clorgiline. *Clin Pharmacol Ther* 43:32–38, 1988b.

Henkin RI: The role of adrenal corticosteroids in sensory processes. In: Blaschko, Sayers, Smith (eds): *Handbook of Physiology-Endocrinology* (Vol 6). Baltimore, Williams & Wilkins, 1975, pp. 209–230.

Herman JP, Schafer MK-H, Young EA, et al: Evidence for hippocampal regulation of neuroendocrine neurons of the hypothalamo-pituitary-adrenocortical axis. *J Neurosci* 9:3072–3082, 1989.

Hess JL, Denenberg VH, Zarrow MX, et al: Modification of the corticosterone response curve as a function of handling in infancy. *Physiol Behav* 4:109–112, 1969.

Holman SD, Hutchison JB: Lateralized action of androgen on development of behavior and brain sex differences. *Brain Res Bull* 27:261–265, 1991.

Holt AB, Cheek DB, Kerr GR: Prenatal hypothyroidism and brain composition in primates. *Nature* 243:413–414, 1973.

Hutchison JB, Beyer C: Gender-specific brain formation of oestrogen in behavioural development. *Psychoneuroendocrinology* 19:529–541, 1994.

Ingraham HA, Chen R, Mangalam HJ, et al: A tissue-specific transcription factor containing a homeodomain specifies a pituitary phenotype. *Cell* 55:519–529, 1988.

Ingraham HA, Lala DS, Ikeda Y, et al: The nuclear receptor steroidogenic factor 1 acts at multiple levels of the reproductive axis. *Genes Dev* 8: 2302–2312, 1994.

Insel TR, Battaglia G, Fairbanks DW, et al: The ontogeny of brain receptors for corticotropin-releasing factor and the development of their functional association with adenylate cyclase. *J Neurosci* 8: 4151–4158, 1988.

Jackson PL, Ott MJ: Perceived self-esteem among children diagnosed with precocious puberty. *J Pediatr Nurs* 5:190–203, 1990.

Jacobson L, Sapolsky RM: The role of the hippocampus in feedback regulation of the hypothalamic-pituitary-adrenal axis. *Endocr Rev* 12:118–134, 1991.

Jakobowitz DM: Multifactorial control of pituitary hormone secretion: The "wheels" of the brain. *Synapse* 2:186–192, 1988.

Jansson J-O, Down TR, Beamer WG, et al: Receptor-associated resistance to growth hormone-releasing factor in dwarf "little" mice. *Science* 232: 511–512, 1986.

Jarrett DB, Miewald JM, Kupfer DJ: Recurrent depression is associated with a persistent reduction in sleep-related growth hormone secretion. *Arch Gen Psychiatry* 47:113–118, 1990.

Kagan J: Heart rate and heart rate variability as signs of a temperamental dimension in infants. In: Izard C (ed): *Measuring Emotions in Infants and Children*. Cambridge, Cambridge University Press, 1982, pp. 38–66.

Kagan J, Reznick JS, Snidman N: Biological bases of childhood shyness. *Science* 240:167–171, 1988.

Kalin NH, Takahashi LK: Altered hypothalamic-pituitary-adrenal regulation in animal models of depression. In: Gild PW, Chrousos G (eds): *The Hypothalamic-Pituitary-Adrenal Axis*. New York, Raven Press, 1988, pp. 67–70.

Kaptein EM, Spencer CA, Kamiel MB, et al: Prolonged dopamine administration and thyroid hormone economy in normal and critically ill subjects. *J Clin Endocrinol Metab* 51:387–393, 1980.

Kaye WH, Gwirtsman HE, George DT, et al: Elevated cerebrospinal fluid levels of immunoreactive corticotropin-releasing hormone in anorexia nervosa: Relation to state of nutrition, adrenal function, and intensity of depression. *J Clin Endocrinol Metab* 64: 203–208, 1987.

Keller-Wood ME, Dallman MF: Corticosteroid inhibition of ACTH secretion. *Endocr Rev* 5:1–24, 1984.

Kennedy SH, Garfinkel PE: Disorders of eating. In: Nemeroff CB, Loosen PT (eds): *Handbook of Clinical Psychoneuroendocrinology*. New York, Guilford Press, 1987.

Klein AH, Meltzer S, Kenny FN: Improved diagnosis of congenital hypothyroidism treated before age 3 months. *J Pediatr* 81:912–915, 1972.

Kletter GB, Padmanabhan V, Brown MB, et al: Serum bioactive gonadotropins during male puberty: A longitudinal study. *J Clin Endocrinol Metab* 76: 432–438, 1993.

Koller KJ, Wolff RS, Warden MK, et al: Thyroid hormones regulate levels of thyrotropin-releasing mRNA in the paraventricular nucleus. *Proc Natl Acad Sci USA* 84:7329–7333, 1987.

Komisaruk BR, Siegel HI, Cheng MF, et al (eds): Reproduction: A behavioral and neuroendocrine perspective. *Ann NY Acad Sci* 474, 1986.

Koob GF, Heinrichs SC, Menzaghi F, et al: Corticotropin releasing factor, stress and behavior. *Semin Neurosci* 6:221–229, 1994.

Krishman KRR, Manepalli AN, Ritchie JC, et al: Growth hormone releasing factor stimulation test in depression. *Am J Psychiatry* 145:90–92, 1987.

Kuhn C, Schanberg S: Hormones and brain development. In: Nemeroff CB, Dunn AJ (eds): *Peptides, Hormones, and Behavior*. New York, Spectrum, 1984, pp. 775–822.

Kuhn CM, Butler ST, Schanberg SM: Selective depression of serum growth hormone during maternal deprivation in rat pups. *Science* 201:1034–1036, 1978.

Kuhn CM, Evoniuk G, Schanberg SM: Loss of tissue sensitivity to growth hormone during maternal deprivation in rats. *Life Sci* 25:2089–2097, 1979.

Kuhn CM, Pauk J, Schanberg SM: Endocrine responses to mother-infant separation in developing rats. *Dev Psychobiol* 23:395–410, 1990.

Kwak S, Morano MI, Young EA, et al: The diurnal CRF mRNA rhythm in the hypothalamus: Decreased expression in the evening is not dependent on endogenous glucocorticoids. *Neuroendocrinology* 57:96–105, 1993.

Leonard JL: Identification and structure analysis of iodothyronine deiodinases. In: Greer MA (ed) *The Thyroid Gland*. New York, Raven Press, 1990, pp. 285–305.

Leret ML, Gonzalez MI, Arahuetes RM: Effect of maternal adrenal deprivation on the content of catecholamines in fetal brain. *Life Sci* 52:1609–1615, 1993.

Lesh KP, Erb A, Pfuller H, et al: Attenuated growth hormone response to growth hormone-releasing hormone in major depressive disorder. *Biol Psychiatry* 22:1495–1499, 1987.

Letarte J, Garagorri JM: Congenital hypothyroidism: Laboratory and clinical investigation of early detected infants. In: Collu R, Ducharme JR, Guyda HJ (eds): *Pediatric Endocrinology*. New York, Raven Press, 1989, pp. 449–471.

Levin N, Shinsako J, Dallman MF: Corticosterone acts on the brain to inhibit adrenalectomy-induced adrenocorticotropin secretion. *Endocrinology* 122:694–701, 1988.

Levine S: Infantile experience and resistance to physiological stress. *Science* 126:405, 1957.

Levine S: Plasma-free corticosteroid response to electric shock in rats stimulated in infancy. *Science* 135:795–796, 1962.

Levine S: The pituitary-adrenal system and the developing brain. *Prog Brain Res* 32:79–100, 1970.

Levine S, Haltmeyer GC, Karas GC, et al: Physiological and behavioral effects of infantile stimulation. *Physiol Behav* 2:55–63, 1967.

Lindholm D, Castren E, Tsoulfas P, et al: Neurotrophin-3 induced by tri-iodothyronine in cerebellar granule cells promotes Purkinje cell differentiation. *J Cell Biol* 122:443–450, 1993.

Linkowski P, Mendlewicz J, Kerkhofs M, et al: 24-hour profile of adrenocorticotropin, cortisol and growth hormone in major depressive illness: Effect of antidepressant treatment. *J Clin Endocrinol Metab* 65:141–151, 1987.

Loosen PT: Thyroid function in affective disorders and alcoholism. *Endocrinol Metab Clin North Am* 17:55–82, 1988a.

Loosen PT: TRH: Behavioral and endocrine effects in man. *Prog Neuropsychopharmacol Biol Psychiatry* 12(suppl):S87–S117, 1988b.

Loosen PT: Effects of thyroid hormones on central nervous system in aging. *Psychoneuroendocrinology* 17:355–374, 1992.

Loosen PT, Prange AJ Jr: Hormones of the thyroid axis and behavior. In: Nemeroff CB, Dunn AJ (eds): *Peptides, Hormones and Behavior*. New York, Spectrum, 1984, pp. 533–577.

MacFaul R, Dorner S, Brett EM, et al: Neurological abnormalities in patients treated for hypothyroidism from early life. *Arch Dis Child* 53:611–619, 1978.

MacLusky NJ, Clark AS, Naftolin F, et al: Estrogen formation in the mammalian brain: Possible role of aromatase in sexual differentiation of the hippocampus and neocortex. *Steroids* 459–474, 1987.

Maher KR, Hauper JF, Mackay A, et al: Peculiarities in the endocrine response to insulin stress in early infantile autism. *J Nerv Ment Dis* 161:180–189, 1975.

Mallol J, Obregon MJ, Morreale de Escobar G: Analytical artifacts in radioimmunoassay of L-thyroxin in human milk. *Clin Chem* 28:1277–1282, 1971.

Marshall JC, Kelch RP: Low dose pulsatile gonadotropin-releasing hormone in anorexia nervosa: A model of human pubertal development. *J Clin Endocrinol Metab* 49:712–718, 1979.

Mason JW: A re-evaluation of the concept of "non-specificity" in stress specificity in stress theory. *J Psychiatr Res* 8:323–333, 1971.

McBride PA, Anderson GM, Hertzig ME, et al: Serotonergic responsivity in male young adults with autistic disorder. *Arch Gen Psychiatry* 46:213–221, 1989.

McEwen BS: The plasticity of the hippocampus is the reason for its vulnerability. *Semin Neurosci* 6: 239–246, 1994.

McLarty DG, Ratcliffe WA, McColl K, et al: Thyroid hormone levels and prognosis in patients with serious non-thyroidal illness. *Lancet* 2: 275–276, 1975.

Meaney MJ, Aitken DH, Bhatnagor S, et al: Postnatal handling attenuates neuroendocrine, anatomical, and cognitive impairments related to the aged hippocampus. *Science* 239:766–768, 1988.

Meaney MJ, Aitken DH, Bodnoff SR, et al: Early, postnatal handling alters glucocorticoid receptor concentrations in selected brain regions. *Behav Neurosci* 99:760–765, 1985.

Meaney MJ, Aitken DH, Sapolsky MR: Thyroid hormones influence the development of hippocampal glucocorticoid receptors in the rat: A mechanism for the effects of postnatal handling on the development of the adrenocortical stress response. *Neuroendocrinology* 45:278–283, 1987.

Meaney MJ, Aitken DH, Sapolsky MR: Environmental regulation of the adrenocortical stress response in female rats and its implications for individual differences in aging. *Neurobiol Aging* 12:31–38, 1991.

Meaney MJ, Aitken DH, Sharma S, et al: Postnatal handling increases hippocampal type II, glucocorticoid receptors and enhances adrenocortical negative-feedback efficacy in the rat. *Neuroendocrinology* 51:597–604, 1989.

Meaney MJ, Aitken DH, Viau V, et al: Neonatal handling alters adrenocortical negative feedback sensitivity and hippocampal type II glucocorticoid receptor binding in the rat. *Neuroendocrinology* 50: 597–604, 1989.

Meaney MJ, Bhatnagar S, Diorio J, et al: Molecular basis for the development of individual differences in the hypothalamic-pituitary-adrenal stress response. *Cell Mol Neurobiol* 13:321–347, 1993.

Meaney MJ, Tannenbaum B, Francis D, et al: Early environmental programming hypothalamic-pituitary-adrenal responses to stress. *Semin Neurosci* 6:247–259, 1994.

Mellon PL, Windle JJ, Goldsmith PC, et al: Immortalization of hypothalamic GnRH neurons by genetically targeted tumorigenesis. *Neuron* 5:1–10, 1990.

Mendel CM: The free hormone hypothesis: A physiologically based mathematical model. *Endocr Rev* 10:232–274, 1989.

Mendlewicz J, Linkowski P, Kerkhofs M, et al: Diurnal hypersecretion of growth hormone in depression. *J Clin Endocrinol Metab* 60:505–512, 1985.

Menzaghi F, Heinrichs SC, Pich EM, et al: Involvement of hypothalamic corticotropin-releasing factor neurons in behavioral responses to novelty in rats. *Neurosci Lett* 168:139–142, 1994.

Merchethaler I, Vigh S, Schally AV, et al: Immunocytochemical localization of growth hormone-releasing factor in the rat hypothalamus. *Endocrinology* 114:1082–1085, 1984.

Metcalf G, Jackson IMD (eds): Thyrotropin-releasing hormone. Biomedical significance. *Ann NY Acad Sci* 553:1–532, 1989.

Meyer-Bahlburg HFL: Psychoendocrine research on sexual orientation. Current status and future options. *Prog Brain Res* 61:375–398, 1984.

Meyer-Bahlburg HFL: Can homosexuality in adolescents be treated by sex hormones. *J Child Adolesc Psychopharmacol* 1:231–235, 1991.

Meyer-Bahlburg HFL, Ehrhardt AA, Rosen LR, et al: Prenatal estrogens and the development of homosexual orientation. *Dev Psychology* 31(1):12–21, 1995.

Millan MA, Jacobowitz DM, Hauger RL, et al: Distribution of corticotropin-releasing factor receptors in primate brain. *Proc Natl Acad Sci USA* 83: 1921–1925, 1986.

Millard WJ, Martin JB Jr, Audet J, et al: Evidence that reduced growth hormone secretion observed in monosodium glutamate-treated rats is the result of a deficiency in growth hormone-releasing factor. *Endocrinology* 110:540–550, 1982.

Money J, Annecillo C, Werlwas J: Hormonal and behavioral reversals in hyposomatotropic dwarfism. In: Sachar EJ (ed): *Hormones, Behavior, and Psychopathology.* New York, Raven Press, 1976, pp. 243–261, 1976.

Morale MC, Batticane N, Bartoloni G, et al: Blockade of central and peripheral luteinizing hormone-releasing hormone (LHRH) receptors in neonatal rats with a potent LHRH-antagonist inhibits the morphofunctional development of the thymus and maturation of the cell-mediated and humoral immune responses. *Endocrinology* 128:1073–1080, 1991.

Morales AJ, Hjolden JP, Murphy AA: Pediatric and adolescent gynecologic endocrinology. *Curr Sci* 860–866, 1992.

Morley JE: Neuroendocrine control of thyrotropin secretion. *Endocr Rev* 2:396–436, 1981.

Morreale de Escobar G, Calvo R, Obregon MJ, et al: Contribution of maternal thyroxine pools in normal rats near term. *Endocrinology* 126: 2765–2767, 1990.

Muglia L, Jacobson L, Dikkes P, et al: Corticotropin-releasing hormone deficiency reveals major fetal but not adult glucocorticoid need. *Nature* 373: 427–432, 1995.

Mullen PE, Martin JL, Anderson JC, et al: Childhood sexual abuse and mental health in adult life. *Br J Psychiatry* 163:721–732, 1993.

Narayanan CH, Narayana Y: Cell formation in the motor nucleus and mesencephalic nucleus of the trigeminal nerve of rats made hypothyroid by propylthiouracil. *Exp Brain Res* 59:257–266, 1985.

Nemeroff CB, Kalivas PW, Golden RN, et al: Behavioral effects of hypothalamic hypophysiotropic hormones, neurotensin, substance P and other neuropeptides. *Pharmacology* 24:1–56, 1984.

Nemeroff CB, Konkol RJ, Bissette G, et al: Analysis of the disruption in hypothalamic-pituitary regulation in rats treated neonatally with monosodium L-glutamate (MSG): Evidence for the involvement of tuberoinfundibular cholinergic and dopaminergic systems in neuroendocrine regulation. *Endocrinology* 101:613–622, 1977.

Nemeroff CB, Owens MJ, Bissette G, et al: Reduced corticotropin releasing factor binding sites in the frontal cortex of suicide victims. *Arch Gen Psychiatry* 45:557–562, 1988.

New England Congenital Hypothyroidism Collaborative: Effects of neonatal screening for hypothyroidism: Prevention of mental retardation by treatment before clinical manifestation. *Lancet* ii: 1095–1098, 1981.

Nishita JK, Ellinwood EH Jr, Rockwell WJK, et al: Abnormalities in the response of plasma arginine vasopressin during hypertonic saline infusion in patients with eating disorders. *Biol Psychiatry* 26: 73–86, 1989.

O'Banion MK, Young DA, Bohn MC: Corticosterone-responsive mRNAs in primary rat astrocytes. *Mol Brain Res* 22:57–68, 1994.

O'Donnell D, Larocque S, Seckl JR, et al: Postnatal handling alters glucocorticoid, but not mineralocorticoid mRNA expression in the hippocampus of adult rats. *Mol Brain Res*, 26:242–248, 1994.

Ohmura E, Janssen A, Cherncick V, et al: Human pancreatic growth hormone releasing factor (hpGRF-1-40) stimulates GH release in the ovine fetus. *Endocrinology* 114:299–301, 1984.

Olster DH, Ferin M: Corticotropin-releasing hormone inhibits gonadotropin secretion in the ovariectomized rhesus monkey. *J Clin Endocrinol Metab* 65:262–267, 1987.

Otten U, Thoenen H: Effect of glucocorticoids on nerve growth factor-mediated enzyme induction in organ cultures of rat sympathetic ganglia: Enhanced response and reduced time requirement to initiate enzyme induction. *J Neurochem* 29:69–75, 1977.

Pahl J, Pirke KM, Schweiger U, et al: Anorectic behavior, mood, and metabolic and endocrine adaptation to starvation in anorexia nervosa during inpatient treatment. *Biol Psychiatry* 20:874–887, 1985.

Pandol SJ, Seifert H, Thomas MW, et al: Growth hormone releasing factor stimulates pancreatic enzyme secretion. *Science* 225:326–329, 1984.

Parkinson WL, Weingarten HP: Dissociative analysis of ventromedial hypothalamic obesity syndrome. *Am J Physiol* 259:R829–R835, 1990.

Perez-Castillo A, Bernal J, Ferreiro B, et al: The early ontogenesis of thyroid hormone receptor in the rat fetus. *Endocrinology* 177:2457–2461, 1985.

Perez-Polo JR, Hall K, Livingston K, et al: Steroid induction of nerve growth factor synthesis in cell culture. *Life Sci* 21:1535–1544, 1977.

Perrin MH, Donaldson CJ, Chen R, et al: Cloning and functional expression of a rat brain corticotropin-releasing factor (CRF) receptor. *Endocrinology* 133: 3058–3061, 1993.

Pescovitz OH: Precocious puberty. *Pediatr Rev* 11:227–237, 1990.

Peterfreund RA, Vale WW: Ovine corticotropin-releasing factor stimulates somatostatin secretion from cultured brain cells. *Endocrinology* 112:1275, 1983.

Pfaff D: Morphological changes in the brains of adult male rats after neonatal castration. *J Endocrinol* 36:415–416, 1966.

Phillips RH, Valente WA, Caplan ES, et al: Circulating thyroid hormone changes in acute trauma: Prognostic implications for clinical outcome. *J Trauma* 24:116–119, 1984.

Pich EM, Heinrichs SC, Rivier C, et al: Blockade of pituitary-adrenal axis activation induced by peripheralimmunocentralization of corticotropin-releasing factor does not affect the behavioral response to social defeat stress in rats. *Psychoneuroendocrinology* 18:495–507, 1993.

Plotsky OM, Otto S, Sapolsky MR: Inhibition of immunoreactive corticotropin-releasing factor secretion into the hypophysial-portal circulation by delayed glucocorticoid feedback. *Endocrinology* 119: 1126–1130, 1986.

Plotsky PM, Meaney MJ: Early, postnatal experience alters hypothalamic corticotropin-releasing factor (CRF) release in adult rats. *Mol Brain Res* 18: 195–200, 1993.

Plotsky PM, Sawchenko PE: Hypophysial-portal plasma levels, median eminence content and immunohistochemical staining of corticotropin releasing factor, arginine vasopressin and oxytocin following pharmacological adrenalectomy. *Endocrinology* 120:1361–1369, 1987.

Pohunkova D, Sulc J, Vana S: Influence of thyroid hormone supply on EEG frequency spectrum. *Endocrinol Exp* 23:251–258, 1989.

Porterfield SP, Hendrich CE: Tissue iodothyronine levels in fetuses of control and hypothyroid rats at 13 and 16 days gestation. *Endocrinology* 131: 195–200, 1992.

Porterfield SP, Hendrich CE: The role of thyroid hormones in prenatal and neonatal neurological development—Current perspectives. *Endocrinol Rev* 14(1):94–106, 1993.

Potter BJ, McIntosh GH, Mano MT, et al: The effect of maternal thyroidectomy prior to conception on foetal brain development in sheep. *Acta Endocrinol* 112:93–99, 1986.

Powell GF, Brasel JA, Blizzard MR: Emotional deprivation and growth retardation simulating idiopathic hypopituitarism. I: Clinical evaluation of the syndrome. *N Engl J Med* 276:1271–1278, 1967.

Powell GF, Brasel JA, Raiti S, et al: Emotional deprivation and growth retardation simulating idiopathic hypopituitarism. II: Endocrinologic evaluation of the syndrome. *N Engl J Med* 276:1279–1283, 1967.

Puig-Antich J: Affective disorders in children and adolescents: Diagnostic validity and psychobiology. In: Meltzer HY (ed): *Psychopharmacology: The Third Generation of Progress.* New York, Raven Press, 1987.

Puig-Antich J, Chambers W, Halpern F, et al: Cortisol hypersecretion in prepubertal depressive illness: A preliminary report. *Psychoneuroendocrinology* 4:191–197, 1979.

Puig-Antich J, Dahl R, Ryan N, et al: Cortisol secretion in prepubertal children with major depressive disorder. *Arch Gen Psychiatry* 46:801–809, 1989.

Puig-Antich J, Novancenko H, Davies M, et al: Growth hormone secretion in prepubertal major depressive children: I. *Arch Gen Psychiatry* 41: 455–460, 1984a.

Puig-Antich J, Novancenko H, Davies M, et al: Growth hormone secretion in prepubertal major depressive children: II. *Arch Gen Psychiatry* 41: 463–466, 1984b.

Puig-Antich J, Novancenko H, Davies M, et al: Growth hormone secretion in prepubertal major depressive children: III. *Arch Gen Psychiatry* 41: 471–475, 1984c.

Puig-Antich J, Novancenko H, Davies M, et al: Growth hormone secretion in prepubertal major depressive children: IV. *Arch Gen Psychiatry* 41: 479–483, 1984d.

Raisman G, Field P: Sexual dimorphism in the neutrophil of the preoptic area of the rat and its dependence on neonatal androgen. *Brain Res* 54:1–29, 1971.

Raisman G, Field P: Sexual dimorphism in the preoptic area of the rat. *Science* 173:731–733, 1971.

Ratka A, Sutrano W, Bloemers M, et al: On the role of mineralocorticoid (type I) and glucocorticoid (type II) receptors in neuroendocrine regulation. *Neuroendocrinology* 50:117–123, 1989.

Reed K, Bland RD: Masked ''myxedema madness.'' *Acta Psychiatr Scand* 56:421–526, 1977.

Reitan MR: Intellectual functions in myxedema. *Arch Neurol Psychiatry* 69:436–449, 1963.

Restrepo C, Armario A: Chronic stress alters pituitary-adrenal function in prepubertal male rats. *Psychoneuroendocrinology* 12:393–398, 1987.

Risch SC, Hauger RL: Persistent growth hormone dysfunction in depression. Abstract at World Psychiatric Association Regional Symposium, Washington, DC, October 13–16, 1988, (Abstract 57).

Risch SC, Ehlers C, Janowsky DS: Human growth hormone releasing factor infusion effects on plasma growth hormone in affective disorder patients and normal controls. *Peptides* 9:45–48, 1988.

Ritvo ER, Freeman BJ, Yuwiler A, et al: Study of fenfluramine in outpatients with the syndrome of autism. *J Pediatr* 105:823–828, 1984.

Rivier C, Plotsky PM: Mediation by corticotropin releasing factor (CRF) or adenohypophysial hormone secretion. *Annu Rev Physiol* 48:475, 1986.

Rivier C, Vale W: Influence of corticotropin-releasing factor on reproductive functions in the rat. *Endocrinology* 114:914–921, 1984.

Rivier C, Vale W: Involvement of corticotropin-releasing factor and somatostatin in stress-induced inhibition of growth hormone secretion in the rat. *Endocrinology* 117:2478–2482, 1985.

Rivier C, Rivier J, Vale W: Stress-induced inhibition of reproductive functions: Role of endogenous corticotropin-releasing factor. *Science* 231:607–608, 1986.

Rivier J, Spiess J, Thorner M, et al: Characterization of a growth hormone-releasing factor from a human pancreatic islet tumor. *Nature* 300:276–278, 1982.

Rothwell PM, Lawler PG: Prediction of outcome in intensive care patients using endocrine parameters. *Crit Care Med* 23:78–83, 1995.

Rovet JF: A prospective investigation of children with congenital hypothyroidism identified by neonatal thyroid screening in Ontario. *Can J Public Health* 77:164–173, 1986.

Rubinow DR: Cerebrospinal fluid somatostatin and psychiatric illness. *Biol Psychiatry* 21:341–351, 1986.

Rubinow DR, Gold PW, Post MR: CSF somatostatin in affective illness. *Arch Gen Psychiatry* 40:403–412, 1983.

Ryan ND, Puig-Antich J, Rabinovich H, et al: Growth hormone response to desmethylimipramine in depressed and suicidal adolescents. *J Affect Disord* 15:323–337, 1988.

Sachar EJ, Frantz AG, Ahman N, et al: Growth hormone and production in unipolar and bipolar depressed patients: Responses to hypoglycemia and L-dopa. *Am J Psychiatry* 130:1362–1367, 1973.

Sakaguchi T, Bray GA, Eddlestone G: Sympathetic activity following paraventricular or ventromedial hypothalamic lesions in rats. *Brain Res Bull* 20(2):461–465, 1988.

Saketos M, Sharma N, Santoro NE: Suppression of the hypothalamic-pituitary-ovarian axis in normal women by glucocorticoids. *Biol Reprod* 49:1270–1276, 1993.

Samuels HH, Forman BB, Horowitz ZC, et al: Regulation of gene expression by thyroid hormone. *Annu Rev Physiol* 51:623–639, 1989.

Sapolsky MR, Meaney MJ: Maturation of the adrenocortical stress response: Neuroendocrine control mechanisms and the stress hyporesponsive period. *Brain Res Rev* 11:65–76, 1986.

Sapolsky MR, Krey LC, McEwen BS: Glucocorticoid-sensitive hippocampal neurons are involved in terminating the adrenocortical stress response. *Proc Natl Acad Sci USA* 81:6174–6177, 1984.

Sapolsky MR, Krey LC, McEwen BS: The neuroendocrinology of stress and aging: The glucocorticoid cascade hypothesis. *Endocr Rev* 7:284–306, 1986.

Sarrieau A, Sharma S, Meaney MJ: Postnatal development and environmental regulation of hippocampal glucocorticoid and mineralocorticoid receptors in the rat. *Dev Brain Res* 43:158–162, 1988.

Schain RJ, Freedman DX: Studies on 5-hydroxyindole metabolism in autistic and other mentally retarded children. *J Pediatr* 58:315–320, 1961.

Schon M, Sutherland AM, Rawson RW: Hormones and neuroses: The psychological effects of thyroid deficiency. In: *Proceedings of the Second World Congress on Psychiatry*. Montreal, McGill University Press, 1961.

Schreiber G, Aldred AR, Jaworowski A, et al: Thyroxine transport from the blood to brain via transthyretin synthesis in chorioid plexus. *Am J Physiol* 258:R338–R345, 1990.

Schwanzel-Fukuda M, Bick MD, Pfaff DW: Luteinizing hormone-releasing hormone (KHRH)-expressing cells do not migrate normally in an inherited hypogonadal (Kallmann) syndrome. *Mol Brain Res* 6:311–326, 1989.

Schwind J: The development of the hypophysis cerebri of the albino rat. *Am J Anat* 41:295–319, 1928.

Segerson TP, Hoefler H, Childers H, et al: Localization of thyrotropin-releasing hormone prohormone messenger ribonucleic acid in rat brain by in situ hybridization. *Endocrinology* 121:98–107, 1987a.

Segerson TP, Kaur J, Wolfe HC, et al: Thyroid hormone regulates TRH biosynthesis in the paraventricular nucleus of the rat hypothalamus. *Science* 238:78–82, 1987b.

Seifert H, Perrin M, Rivier J, et al: Growth hormone-releasing factor binding sites in rat anterior pituitary membrane homogenates: Modulation by glucocorticoids. *Endocrinology* 117:424, 1985.

Siever LJ, Uhde TW: New studies and perspectives on the noradrenergic receptor system in depression: Effects of the alpha-adrenergic agonist clonidine. *Biol Psychiatry* 19:131–156, 1984.

Siiteri PK, Ashby B, Schwartz B, et al: Mechanism of estrogen action studies in the human. *J Steroid Biochem* 3:456, 1972.

Silberman H, Eisenberg D, Ryan J, et al: The relations of thyroid indices in the critically ill patient to prognosis and nutritional factors. *Surg Gynecol Obstet* 166:223–238, 1988.

Simmons DM, Voss JW, Ingraham HA, et al: Pituitary cell phenotypes involve cell-specific Pit-1 mRNA translation and synergistic interactions with other classes of transcription factors. *Genes Dev* 4:695–711, 1990.

Slotkin TA, McCook EC, Seidler FJ: Glucocorticoids regulate the development of intracellular signaling: Enhanced forebrain adenylate cyclase catalytic subunit activity after fetal dexamethasone exposure. *Clin Res Bull* 32:359–364, 1993.

Soya H, Suzuki M: Somatostatin rapidly restores rat growth hormone (GH) release response attenuated by prior exposure to human GH-releasing factor in vitro. *Endocrinology* 122:2492–2498, 1988.

Stein DA: Southwestern internal medicine conference: New developments in the diagnosis and treatment of sexual precocity. *Am J Med Sci* 303:53–71, 1992.

Stein SA, Shanklin DR, Adams PM, et al: Thyroid hormone regulation of specific mRNAs in the developing brain. In: Delong GR, Robbins J, Condliffe PG (eds): *Iodine*. New York, Plenum, 1989, pp. 59–78.

Styne DM: Physiology of puberty. *Horm Res* 41(suppl):3–6, 1994.

Sulc J, Pohunkova D, Vana S: EEG frequency spectrum and the saturation with thyroid hormones. *Acta Nerv Superior* 32:74XXIS, 1990.

Swanson LW: Spatiotemporal patterns of transcription factor gene expression accompanying the development and plasticity of cell phenotypes in the neuroendocrine system. In: Joosse J, Buijs MR, Tilders FJH (eds): *Progress in Brain Research* (Vol 92). New York, Elsevier, 1992, pp. 87–113.

Swanson LW, Sowchenko PE, Lind RW: Regulation of multiple peptides in CRF parvocellular neurosecretory neuron: Implications for the stress response. In: Hokfelt T, Fuke K, Perow B (eds): *Progress in Brain Research* (Vol 68). New York, Elsevier, 1986, pp. 169–190.

Swanson LW, Sowchenko PE, Rivier J, et al: The organization of ovine corticotropin-releasing factor (CRF) immunoreactive cells and fibres in the rat brain: An immunohistochemical study. *Neuroendocrinology* 36:165–186, 1983.

Tallal P, McEwen BS: Neuroendocrine effects on brain development and cognition. *Psychoneuroendocrinology* 16:1–3, 1991.

Taylor T, Gyves P, Burgunder J-M: Thyroid hormone regulation of TRH mRNA levels in rat paraventricular nucleus of the hypothalamus changes during ontogeny. *Neuroendocrinology* 52:262–267, 1990.

Telegdy G, Vermes I: Effect of adrenocortical hormones on activity of the serotonergic system in limbic structures in rats. *Neuroendocrinology* 18:16–26, 1975.

Thomas EB, Levine S, Arnold WJ: Effects of maternal deprivation and incubator rearing on adrenocortical activity in the adult rat. *Dev Psychobiol* 1:21–23, 1968.

Thomas GB, McNeilly AS, Gibson F, et al: Effects of pituitary-gonadal suppression with a gonadotrophin-releasing hormone agonist on fetal gonadotrophin secretion, fetal gonadal development and maternal steroid secretion in the sheep. *J Endocrinol* 141:317–324, 1994.

Timiras PS, Nzekwe EU: Thyroid hormones and nervous system development. *Biol Neonate* 55:376–385, 1989.

Urbanski HF, Doan A, Perice M, et al: Maturation of the hypothalamo-pituitary-gonadal axis of male syrian hamsters. *Biol Reprod* 46:991–996, 1992.

Vaccari A: Teratogenic mechanism of dysthyroidism in the central nervous system. *Prog Brain Res* 73:71–86, 1988.

Vaccarino FJ, Bloom FE, Rivier J, et al: Stimulation of food intake in rats by centrally administered hypothalamic growth hormone-releasing factor. *Nature* 314:167–168, 1985.

Vale W, Spiess J, Rivier C, et al: Characterization of a 41-residue ovine hypothalamic peptide that stimulates secretion of corticotropin and beta-endorphin. *Science* 213:1394–1397, 1981.

Viau V, Sharma S, Plotsky PM, et al: The hypothalamic-pituitary-adrenal response to stress in handled and nonhandled rats: Differences in stress-induced plasma ACTH secretion are not dependent upon increased corticosterone levels. *J Neurosci* 13:1097–1105, 1993.

Vulsma T, Gons MH, de Vijlder J: Maternal-fetal transfer of thyroxine in congenital hypothyroidism due to a total organification defect of thyroid agenesis. *N Engl J Med* 321:13–16, 1989.

Walker C-D, Perrin M, Vale W, et al: Ontogeny of the stress response in the rat: Role of the pituitary and the hypothalamus. *Endocrinology* 118:1445–1451, 1986.

Walker C-D, Sapolsky MR, Meaney MJ, et al: Increased pituitary sensitivity to glucocorticoid feedback during the stress nonresponsive period in the neonatal rat. *Endocrinology* 119:1816–1821, 1986.

Walsh BT, Lo ES, Cooper T, et al: Dexamethasone suppression test and plasma dexamethasone levels in bulimia. *Arch Gen Psychiatry* 44:797–800, 1987.

Wehrenberg WB, Baird A, Ling N: Potent interaction between glucocorticoids and growth hormone-releasing factor in vivo. *Science* 221:556–558, 1983.

Wehrenberg WB, Bloch B, Chong-Li Z, et al:

Pituitary response to growth hormone-releasing factor in rats with functional or anatomical lesions of central neuron system that inhibit endogenous growth hormone secretion. *Regul Pept* 8:1–8, 1984.

Wehrenberg WB, Seifert H, Bilezikjian LM, et al: Down-regulation of growth hormone releasing factor receptors following continuous infusion of growth hormone releasing factor in vivo. *Neuroendocrinology* 43:266–268, 1986.

Weissman C: The metabolic response to stress: An overview and update. *Anesthesiology* 73:308–327, 1990.

Whitman FL, Mathy RM: *Male Homosexuality in Four Societies: Brazil, Guatemala, the Philippines, and the United States.* New York, Praeger, 1986.

Whybrow PC, Copen A, Prange AJ, et al: Thyroid function and the response to liothyronine in depression. *Arch Gen Psychiatry* 26(3):242–245, 1972.

Whybrow PC, Prange AJ, Treadway CR: The mental changes accompanying thyroid gland dysfunction. *Arch Gen Psychiatry* 20:48–63, 1969.

Witelson SF: Neural sexual mosaicism: Sexual differentiation of the human temporo-parietal region for functional asymmetry. *Psychoneuroendocrinology* 16:131–153, 1991.

Wozniak A, Hutchison RE, Hutchison JB: *Neurosci Lett* 146:191–194, 1992.

Wu FCW, Brown DC, Butler GE, et al: Early morning plasma testosterone is an accurate predictor of imminent pubertal development in prepubertal boys. *J Clin Endocrinol Metab* 76:26–31, 1993.

Wynn PC, Hauger RL, Holmes MC, et al: Brain and pituitary receptors for corticotropin releasing factor: Localization and differential regulation after adrenalectomy. *Peptides* 5:1077–1084, 1984.

Yamada K, Harada N, Tamaru M, et al: Effects of changes in gonadal hormones on the amount of aromatase messenger RNA in mouse brain diencephalon. *Biochem Biophys Res Commun* 195:462–468, 1993.

Yuwiler A: Diagnosis and the hunt for etiology [Editorial]. *Soc Biol Psy* 37:1–3, 1995.

Zaloga GP, Chernow B, Smallridge RC, et al: A longitudinal evaluation of thyroid function in critically ill surgical patients. *Ann Surg* 201:456–464, 1985.

Zoeller RT, Kabeer N, Albers HE: Cold exposure elevates cellular levels of messenger ribonucleic acid encoding thyrotropin-releasing hormone in paraventricular nucleus despite elevated levels of thyroid hormones. *Endocrinology* 127:2955–2962, 1990.

Zoeller RT, Wolff RS, Koller KJ: Thyroid hormone regulation of messenger ribonucleic acid encoding thyrotropin (TSH)-releasing hormone is independent of the pituitary gland and TSH. *Mol Endocrinol* 2:248–252, 1988.

7 BRAIN AND BEHAVIOR
John Scott Werry, M.D.

"The boundary between biology and behavior is arbitrary and changing. It has been imposed not by the natural contours of the disciplines but by lack of knowledge" (Kandel, 1991b).

It is not the purpose of this chapter to review in detail the nature of brain structure and function, nor behavior minutely dissected, both of which are covered in other sections of this volume and in specialized reviews and texts such as Kandel et al. (1991), Jacobson (1991), Lezak (1995), Lishman (1987), Orbach (1982), and Rothenberger (1990). Rather, discussion is restricted to a broad-brushed canvas of the relationship between brain and behavior (used in its widest meaning), concentrating on the principles that are germane to child and adolescent psychiatry. In so doing, certain points must be borne in mind.

First, child and adolescent psychiatry is, above all, concerned with developing behavior and biology, which though continuing throughout the life span will not again do so at such a fast pace until the last of the Seven Ages of Man (this time negatively). Put another way, it is not that development is irrelevant to mature life; it is just that the pace is slow enough for it to be conveniently ignored, while with children and youth the fact is obtrusive and inescapable.

Second, scientific knowledge applicable to brain and behavior is now so vast and developing so rapidly that no one person can hope to grasp more than an inkling of their interrelationship. Nevertheless, though knowledge (especially in molecular biology) is expanding rapidly, there is still a remarkable continuity of knowledge in neuroscience, as revealed by scholarly texts that have a sense of history such as Kandel et al. (1991). Thus, what was learned in medical school or in residency training is far from totally obsolete or useless in understanding brain and behavior today and puts the fundamental principles within the grasp of any child psychiatrist or mental health professional with a training in human biology.

Third, despite all the advances, there is still a yawning gap between the laboratory and clinical practice. Most clinical decisions must be made with an imperfectly garnered, largely pragmatic data set that at best touches only lightly on brain-behavior functions. This knowledge gap often produces two extreme positions—those who crudely crash it and see a disordered brain behind everything clinical, and those who, apart from an occasional perfunctory genuflection to the brain, act as if all behavior is determined solely by intrapsychic, interpersonal, or (nowadays) intrafamilial processes. In fact, a good grasp of brain-behav-

ior relationships is one of the unique things that psychiatrists bring to the multidisciplinary team and is a way to command respect for this complex area of science without overvaluing its role in clinical decisions.

Finally, looking at the development of biological psychiatry since 1950, it is not hard to see that in some areas etiological breakthroughs that will radically affect clinical practice are imminent. Most of these will affect the major psychiatric disorders (such as obsessive compulsive disorder, schizophrenia, and Tourette's disorder), which form only a small (but important) part of child and adolescent psychiatry. Perhaps more important in terms of its larger clinical applicability, better understanding will come too of the genetic and molecular biological basis of *human variability* (see Chapters 1–6) and how its derived macrofunctions like temperament, cognition, and other developmental abilities interact with experience to create psychopathology (e.g., Lewis, 1992; Shaw and Bell, 1993; Taylor, 1991). From this knowledge, it is but one step to biologically based modifications, some therapeutic, but most excitingly, some preventive, in a true pediatric psychopharmacology. For this, if no other reason, the child and adolescent psychiatrist must try to stay abreast of developments in brain-behavior relationships.

GENERAL PRINCIPLES
Concepts of Brain-behavior Relationships

The best way to introduce fundamental concepts is by way of a historical review. The notion that the brain influences behavior is fairly recent, appearing significantly only with 19th century phrenology (Kandel, 1991a). Before that, humoral (i.e., endocrinological) theories, derived from Greek medicine, seem to have predominated and gave such words as sanguine, melancholy, and choleric. Some of the basic ideas about how the brain influences behavior (and vice versa) arose over 150 years ago.

LOCALIZATION VERSUS EQUIVALENCE

The phrenologists who mapped 35 higher brain functions, such as benevolence, hope, conjugality, and secretiveness, to specific bumps on the skull were the first exponents of one of the two recurring themes in neurobehavior theory: *localization of function.* According to Kandel

(1991a), the phrenologists were debunked by Flourens, who removed parts of the brains of animals and, finding no site-specific change in behavior, simultaneously created the other evergreen theme, *equivalence*, which holds all parts of the brain to be capable of performing any function. The reader should note these two themes of localization and equivalence well, since they still continue to leapfrog each other in popularity, especially in the area of higher functions like cognition and emotion. It appears that we are well into another localization era, derived from developments in pharmacology, neurotransmitter physiology, and organ imaging, but it was not always so. The prime example of a persistent equivalence view in child psychopathology is that of minimal brain damage/dysfunction, in which it is the *amount* of brain damage, not its site, that is believed to determine the syndrome. As positron-emission tomography (PET) scans have shown, both views are correct and complementary—many functions are localized but their learning, execution, or integration with others requires most of the brain to be involved.

HARD AND SOFT EFFECTS

Many years ago Teuber (1960) drew attention to another important concept associated particularly with abnormal brain function, that of the *hard*, or *deterministic*, view in which the brain is seen as totally determining observed behavior. This view was popular in the eugenics era around the turn of the 19th century and, in child psychiatry, after the encephalitis pandemic of the 1920s in what we now call conduct disorder. A more modern example is seen among those who explain behavior in children, especially younger ones, entirely on the basis of temperament via such concepts as "the difficult child syndrome" without reference to the flow-on effects of interactions between parent and difficult infant, infant and difficult parent, or both (Shaw and Bell, 1993; see Chapter 13).

The opposite of the hard is the *soft* view, in which the brain is seen as irrelevant before the much more powerful influence of experience, a view that seems to have dominated much of child psychopathology research between 1940 and 1970 and is today seen in the thinking of far too many child mental health professionals in (unwitting) parent-blaming.

In fact hard and soft views are less categorical than extreme poles of a single axis, so that intermediate views (e.g., Eisenberg, 1957; Lewis, 1992; Lewis et al., 1989; Shaw and Bell, 1993) emphasize that behavior is a downstream endpoint in the interaction between brain function and experience. This view is the most sensible and valid one. It might suggest though, as indeed it seems at times to do, that in view of the enormous variation in human experience and the transactional effect of development, detection of any meaningful relationships between brain function and behavior in children will be impossible—that is, each child is unique. Science does not accept this view and seeks to reduce experience to a manageable number of types, as indeed do most developmental theories, whatever their theoretical orientation, for example, attachment or social learning (Shaw and Bell, 1993).

The Brain

HOW THE BRAIN WORKS

As detailed in the previous chapters of this section, the brain consists of billions of cells and their processes—neuronal, which do the work of the brain, and glial, which support, nourish, and clean up the neurons. The principles of neuronal function and synaptic transmission have already been described in previous chapters in this section and/or are too well known to need detailing. More important for the purposes of this chapter is how these individual cells are organized to do the work of the brain. There are two main ways of operating: point-to-point or one-way traffic, rather like telegraph or fax systems. The other is more like the telephone, in which communication goes back and forth between sender and receiver, though in the brain, two electrically separate cables are used. The back-and-forth telephone model is much more characteristic of most brain function than the telegraph model. What were formerly

thought of as unidirectional way stations like the thalamus or basal ganglia are now known to transmit, receive, and *modulate* in a perpetual dialogue. Since axonal and synaptic transmission is so ultrarapid, it is clear that some kind of way of keeping things alive and active is needed for slower processes like memory, thinking, worrying, and the like. This is achieved by reverberating circuits, some of which, like the Papez or emotional/memory circuit, are very extended. Individual neurons and their processes become organized partly by genetic programming and partly by experience, into units called cell assemblies (Hebb, 1949), which are very like integrated circuits or chips. These become the functional units in much of the brain's actions, though they do have connections in parallel and series outside these assemblies, very importantly, allowing for cross-talk.

DEVELOPMENT OF THE BRAIN

This is discussed in detail in this book (Chapter 2) and elsewhere (Casaer, 1993; Ebels, 1980; Jacobson, 1991; Kandel et al., 1991). Life begins as a single cell, yet the billions of neurons are created, basically differentiated, and crudely in place by birth and are nonreplaceable. However, from later fetal life on, the process shifts from skeletal construction to one of embellishment or differentiation and fine-tuning. Modern developmental neurobiology holds that most of the fundamental organization and architecture of the brain, differentiation of neurons, and axonal development is preprogrammed and uninfluenced by anything but adverse and physical environmental experiences, yet it is also estimated that there are sufficient genes to program only a fifth of the brain's neurons, leaving huge areas of flexibility upon which experience can work and that form the basis of learning.

Postnatally, the most significant developments in the brain are: (*a*) the development of *interconnections* shown microscopically by an enormous proliferation of dendritic and axonal processes and (*b*) *myelination* of axons, which greatly enhances the speed and efficiency of nerve conduction (Ebels, 1980). Though approximately 75% of brain growth (as shown by weight) occurs by the age of 2 years (Carmichael, 1990), these two processes of differentiation continue (Casaer, 1993), though at a decelerating rate, until adulthood. Even thereafter, increase in myelin density (Kolb and Whishaw, 1980) and axonal and dendritic growth continue throughout life until final senescence. This means that at the level of cell assembly organization or complex circuitry the brain is actually in a constant state of change, and this is probably one mechanism by which learning occurs (see below).

DISRUPTIONS IN BRAIN DEVELOPMENT

As can be seen from earlier chapters, the initial process of neurogenesis and development of brain architecture is a highly complex and surprisingly rapid process. It is obvious that brain development should be most susceptible to disruption during the most rapid phase of neurogenesis and organization, when any disruptions may have gross and catastrophic results, such as congenital malformations and severe mental retardation. As pointed out in Chapter 2, there are two major types of disruptions of normal development—pathogenic "software" due to abnormal genes/chromosomes and errors in execution of the genetic programming induced by subtle changes in the intrauterine environment, such as those induced by viral infections or biochemical abnormalities, for example, from alcohol, tobacco and drug abuse, maternal malnutrition, placental dysfunction, maternal vomiting, and even stress (Leckman et al., 1990; Taylor, 1991; see Chapter 6). Being highly specialized in function, neurons are exquisitely sensitive to such changes in the biochemical environment—its acidity, ionic composition, and supply of essential nutrients, particularly oxygen and glucose. Both of the latter are vulnerable to marked change in blood levels (e.g., during abnormalities of pregnancy and delivery) and in demand according to the brain activity, which is never zero, since a mature neuron maintains a basal tonic level of readiness for action that is essential to normal function. As knowledge grows about the surprisingly early and critical role in initial brain organization of neurotropic messengers, most of which are normal biochemical substances that will later fulfill endocrine, e.g., androgens (Peterson et al., 1992; see Chapters 6 and 18), and neurotransmitter (Casaer, 1993) function, concern must mount about the possibilities of subtle brain disruptions. For example, Casaer (1993) points out that receptors in the cerebellum become sensitive to γ-aminobutyric acid (GABA) before its actual productive and, more importantly, inactivation mechanisms develop. He argues that benzodiazepines given to the mother might therefore have powerful effects in fetal life.

Injury and local brain disease can also result in direct loss of nervous tissue so that, after these prenatal pathogens, the most dangerous point is often assumed to be birth. However, the most destructive force at this time is not direct injury to the brain, but that induced by anoxia and hypoglycemia, especially when combined with prematurity (Werry, 1986). Modern advances in obstetrical and neonatal care have greatly reduced the frequency of this kind of brain disruption, and it is possible that postnatal head injury is now more of a threat to brain development in children.

Much of the controversy about brain and behavior (reviewed by Kreusi, 1990; Rutter, 1982; Taylor, 1991; Werry, 1986) does not involve gross and obvious abnormalities of development usually resulting in one or more of the neurological "big three" (mental retardation, cerebral palsy, and epilepsy), but rather focuses on the role, compared with that of the social environment, of minor congenital abnormalities or prenatal, perinatal, and postnatal insults to the brain (Taylor, 1991) in the production of extreme temperamental types like the "difficult child" or psychiatric disorders like attention deficit hyperactive disorder (ADHD), developmental learning, tic and obsessive compulsive disorders (Leckman et al., 1990), and schizophrenia (Werry and Taylor, 1993). For example, there is a close association between social advantage and school performance, but how much actual physical brain development directly contributes to this is unclear (Madge and Tizard, 1980). One study of children who had marasmus showed that malnutrition and, presumptively, the resultant brain maldevelopment have some effect independent of social environment. The effect on IQ was small, but there were much larger effects on more subtle cognitive functions such as attention and also on emotional stability (Galler et al., 1983a, 1983b, 1985). This along with other evidence suggests that effects may be there but less obvious (Taylor, 1991).

RECOVERY FROM BRAIN DISRUPTIONS

General Principles

Despite the above litany of risk factors, one thing is clear about most brain disruptions—there is no simple relationship between brain insult and brain development (Taylor, 1991). For one thing, there is both a high threshold to injury (Taylor, 1991) and a strong tendency to recovery or increasing attenuation (Kreusi, 1990). The basis of this is disputed and probably multifactorial. One factor could be surplus neurons since, as noted above, there is a large redundancy of neurons (as high as 50%) gradually lost by adulthood through neuronal death due to disuse (Casaer, 1993). Some is due to cleanup of the products of inflammation, necrosis, trauma, bleeding, and so on. Loss of neurons may be compensated to some degree by development of more dendritic processes, thus getting a bigger bang for the neuronal buck, as it were. Such development, however, is an active process that requires stimulation and so lends plausibility to the hypothesis that active rehabilitation/learning programs should have a role to play in repairing brain insults. But probably the most important factor is that of parallel functions; when one way is obstructed, there is always another. In the brain, this parallelism is derived in part from the fact that chains of neurons are probably connected in series *and* in parallel. But it is not only neurons that exhibit parallelism; so too do the elementary subfunctions of higher information processing, so that "neural processing for a given function is distributed within the brain and handled at several sites" (Kandel, 1991a). However, this principle is limited and least true of, for instance, motor or sensory

ones, functions that are simple or highly specific and sharply topographically localized with point-to-point representation.

Age and Recovery

It is often held that brain injury occurring early in life has a better prospect of recovery. Certainly, all the prospective studies of putatively brain-damaging prenatal and perinatal situations have shown that many initial effects are often largely undetectable by the start of school (Kreusi, 1990; Rutter, 1981; Werry, 1986). The counterview is that of critical periods, well-demonstrated in the area of the development of vision, where early disruption (e.g., strabismus) can lead to functional blindness (see Chapter 2). In a review of the empirical evidence, Fletcher and Satz (1983) concluded that the only thing that makes early damage look less disabling is the increased length of time between assessment of function and damage, or, in short, that *time after injury, not age*, may be the critical determinant of recovery. In fact, they concluded that there is some evidence that early damage may be more serious than later damage. Taylor (1991) also points out that regrowth and reconnection may not always be beneficial, but may produce new anomalies and that the early consequences (notably motor problems) may be different from the late one (cognitive) and require more subtle detection methods.

Nevertheless, some degree of recovery continuing for a long time is almost inevitable and may give intensive rehabilitative treatments a credibility that they do not deserve.

EXPERIENCE AND THE BRAIN

So far the emphasis has been on disruptions in the brain, but what evidence is there that experience may influence brain development? Animal experiments have shown that the weight of the brain, complexity of dendrites, and synaptic size are all significantly greater in animals exposed to an enriched environment and that these morphological changes are matched by improved performance. The increases are greatest if stimulation is given early in life but are still apparent even if applied later (Kolb and Whishaw, 1980).

Kandel (1991b) summarizes the process of brain development thus: Synapse formation is largely under genetic control, but when in place, synapses require appropriate environmental stimulation for their activation and fine-tuning. Some of this activation may have a critical time frame (such as the development of binocular vision, affection bonds, or fluency in a language). After the laying down of synapses, experience works throughout the life span primarily by influencing the effectiveness of these synapses—downgrading some (unlearning) and upgrading others (learning). This view of *synaptic strength*, which is attributable to Hebb (1949), has much experimental support but does not take account of the fact that the neuronal processes are actually in a constant state of growth, with synapses disappearing and reorganizing. It seems likely that the concept of synaptic strength is conceptually correct but anatomically incorrect. However, it matters little for our purposes; the important and obvious thing is that experience alters the brain.

METHODS OF STUDYING BRAIN FUNCTION

No attempt will be made to cover these in detail. For more detail see other sections and chapters of this book (e.g., Chapter 8) and Rutter (1981, 1982), Taylor (1991), and Werry (1986). In humans, because of obvious ethical constraints, natural clinical states such as disease, injury, malformation, and so on must be utilized. Unless the patient dies, the full extent of the abnormality is rarely known, and the child psychiatry literature is full of methodologically pitiful studies that have aggregated "brain-injured" children when there is good reason to suspect that the site, extent, and nature of the brain damage differed widely. Even in disorders of similar etiology like head injury (Chapter 59), the variation in brain damage can be enormous, not only because of differences in the site and force of the impact but also because of variable disseminated or far-distant effects like deceleration, contrecoup, shearing, and torsion effects. Add to all this the variation in postinjury experience, and the situation can be seen to be most complex. Only large single effects are likely to be detectable in the usual-size sample of considerably less than 100 subjects.

Clinical Methods (History and Examination)

These are the most popular, yet among the poorest since they are often unreliable, of unknown validity, only lightly correlated with brain damage, and subject to errors of detection, especially for areas of the brain that are of most interest in psychopathology. Much of the study of brain function in child psychiatry before 1980 falls in this category and is quite error-prone (Rutter, 1981; Werry, 1986).

Psychophysiology

In more recent years, the crude and largely noncontributory technique of electroencephalography has been replaced by more functionally oriented methods like evoked potentials and other techniques (see Chapters 8 and 124), many of which have attained great sophistication through computer averaging, mathematical analysis like power spectral analysis, and a general growth in knowledge about each of the components of the characteristic waveform. In general, evoked potentials (Chapters 8 and 124) are most suited to studies of general brain states such as arousal and vigilance or gross intactness of the sensory apparatus and brain as a whole. However, they have also offered some useful if very technical information on the development of certain brain processes like attention (Lincoln et al., 1990) and for the functional analysis of pharmacological effects such as that of the stimulants (Coons et al., 1987).

Anatomical Pathology

These methods are largely limited to postmortem studies, and death is a rare event in most children with psychiatric disorders. It is of interest that good autopsy reports of disorders like autism are only just emerging.

Organ Imaging

Traditional methods, such as ventriculography, of very limited (gross anatomical pathology) and somewhat dangerous nature, are now giving way to exciting developments beyond computed tomography (CT), like magnetic resonance imaging (MRI) and the much more cumbersome PET (Kuperman et al., 1990; Martin and Brust, 1991) (see also Chapters 8 and 124). The latter (PET) is particularly exciting as a research tool for child psychiatry where gross neuropathology seems largely irrelevant, because it is a functional rather than an anatomical test. Despite all these new methods of studying the human brain, so far the clinical yield in child psychiatry has not been too impressive except for what it has ruled out as causes and for clear indications that the role of brain factors in etiology of psychopathology is probably much more extensive than formerly believed (Bertier et al., 1993; Hendren et al., 1991; Kuperman et al., 1990; Leckman et al., 1992).

Neuropsychology

Child psychiatry has had a long association with neuropsychology, since at least the days of Strauss and Lehtinen (1947). There is good reason for this, namely, the close relationship between school and clinic and the common association of behavioral and learning problems. Neuropsychology is now an advanced science typified in texts such as Lezak (1995), Kolb and Whishaw (1980), and Hynd and Obrzut (1981), to name but a few. While such tests are extremely helpful in the assessment of major brain disorder, their role in most of the problems seen in child and adolescent psychopathology remains, at best, controversial (Feagans, 1983; Taylor, 1991; Werry, 1986). Much of the problem lies in the unknown reliability and validity of the tests in the detection and localization of brain disorders. Often they seem to have acquired a quasi-neurological status that they do not deserve, especially in the area of learning disabilities (Feagans, 1983; Werry, 1986).

Biochemical/Pharmacological Studies

This is a rapidly developing area. The past tendency to rely primarily on the analysis of blood, cerebrospinal fluid, and other body fluids has increasingly been replaced by the active chemical probe of function in a manner analogous to the increasing use of evoked potentials in the electrophysiology field. The most useful instruments for this probe are pharmacological substances, ever increasing in number and specificity. This is well illustrated in modern theories of schizophrenia and major depression and in child psychiatry of autism, Tourette's disorder, and ADHD (Zametkin and Rapoport, 1987; Chapter 3). However, there are limitations to this approach; few drugs or their target receptors are specific to one functional area or system. The complex interactive nature of brain function, with the convergence of many different pathways at the effector level, may result in confusion of downstream or compensatory effects for the primary disturbance. Some of these may be responsible for the fact that the biochemical theories of schizophrenia and depression do not seem to this reviewer to have advanced much since the cellular actions of the drugs used in their management became known more than 25 years ago.

Genetic Studies

Good summaries of this area can be found in Propping and Hebebrand (1990), Kreusi (1990), Shields (1980), and Chapters 1 and 29. The most important methods are family pedigree studies, twin studies, and naturally occurring experiments such as chromosomal abnormalities. The finding of some genetic role in the etiology of behavior or cognitive disorders like autism (Propping and Hebebrand, 1990), ADHD (Goodman and Stevenson, 1989b), or Tourette's disorder (Leckman et al., 1992) permits an *inference* that the brain is affected. However, in the last few years the tremendous strides in molecular biology have opened up the imminent possibility of deriving direct *causative* relationships. The best example of this is Huntington's disease, where the genetic location has been established, though not the precise biochemical mechanism.

Summary

Methods of studying brain function, though individually often alluring and sophisticated, still have a long way to go before they can help in pinpointing any role brain function might have in understanding and treating the complex dysfunctions seen in child and adolescent psychiatry. There is an additional problem with children. Many of the indicators of brain dysfunction so useful in adults represent loss of function, whereas in children the problem is one of failure to develop a function (e.g., enuresis) or, more commonly, slower or imperfect development (e.g., motor incoordination, dysphasia). Put another way, abnormality is often developmental or chronological and quantitative rather than qualitative. In this context it is hard to know whether the "abnormality" is merely a lag in development, a developmental variation (that can have experiential as well as physical causes), or a true abnormality. For example, it is said that both Einstein and Churchill began to talk very late, yet clearly they had very good brain function. Or again, many of the so-called soft neurological signs, such as sensorimotor incoordination, are in fact merely the kinds of function seen in somewhat younger children, and their status as true neurological indicators is unclear (Tupper, 1987; Chapter 42).

Behavior

CLASSIFICATION OF BEHAVIOR

So far the talk has been largely of the *brain*. Now discussion moves to *behavior*, defined in the broad way of child psychiatry to encompass all activity of the organism beyond simple physiological functions necessary to sustain life. There are certain conventions in classifying brain functions that offer a point of convergence with the behavior side of the brain-behavior equation. The neurological view, derived largely from the study of disease and the ability to detect these diseases with simple clinical examinations, has typically been input (sensation/perception), output (motor), and in between (association). The latter, being much more complex and less reachable, has remained more elusive to study, yet this is the area of greatest interest to psychiatry. Neuropsychiatry has therefore developed somewhat different classifications, which are more dissected, more functional, less topographical, and more oriented to psychological theory, though compatible with the neurological view. One of these taxonomies of behavior is as follows (Lezak, 1995):

1. *Information processing or intellectual function*, further subdivided into *receptive function* (acquisition, processing, classification, and integration of information), *memory and learning* (storing and recall of information), *thinking* (organization and reorganization of information), and *expressive functions* (communication and enacting of information). *Mental activity*, though closely allied to intellectual function, is not considered a basic function since it has no clear behavioral end product but is concerned with the efficiency of intellectual function, including attention, level of consciousness, and activity rate or speed.
2. *Emotionality* (feelings, motivation). This is one of the traditional domains of psychiatry, though some of the previously popular theories, like Freud's, still require scientific validation.
3. *Executive/control function.* These are capacities which enable a person to engage in independent, purposive, self-serving behavior successfully (Lezak 1995).

A survey of these three areas shows how germane they all are to child and adolescent psychiatry and how artificial are divisions among child psychiatry, pediatric neurology, and neuropsychology. If psychiatry can claim any particular specialization within this area, it must be to whole organism function, but even that is an artifact of poor medical practice, which has aimed to separate patient from illness, mind from body. However, it would be idle to claim that this classification of behavior is complete or satisfactory for much that concerns child psychiatry, since it is essentially intraorganismic and pays little credence to the context in which behavior occurs, the stimuli that elicit it, or its social interactive, systemic, or developmental properties (Shaw and Bell, 1993).

DEVELOPMENT OF BEHAVIOR

In view of extensive coverage in Section ID of this volume, it is unnecessary to do other than summarize the main principles of child development here. If one tried to isolate the main themes in development, they would include the following.

Loss of Much Stereotyped Reflexive Behavior

The neonate and young infant have a series of preprogrammed behaviors, many necessary for survival, like the rooting and sucking reflexes, which are lost in a few months. Other studies, particularly by ethologists (e.g., Bowlby), have identified other reflexes, like stranger and separation anxiety, that prevent the newly mobile immature organism from straying from protecting caretakers, or the smiling reflex, and have shown how these initially automatic reflexes become the basis of socialization as they lose their automaticity. Compared with most other species, the human baby has relatively few of these automatic behaviors, and it is thought that this is because this places fewer obstacles in the way of the rapid development of complex and flexible behaviors, such as most intellectual and social function. However, there is still considerable debate as to precisely how much of behavior, especially in infants and younger children, is deterministic, for example, the exact role of temperament and gender differences (Chapters 13 and 18).

Differentiation of Behavior

Throughout development there is a movement away from gross, poorly targeted behavior involving most of the organism toward highly specialized, focused activities. Examples of this progression can be seen in motor behavior, from the whole body, flailing behavior of the infant to the finely coordinated activities of the watchmaker or musician. But this is equally true of every subcategory of intellectual, executive, and emotional behavior, though perhaps least striking in the latter.

Internalization of Behavior

Impulsive gross motor or emotional reactions to stimuli decrease in frequency because more and more behavior occurs unseen, as incoming and self-generated information is processed internally by thinking, as developmental epistemologists like Piaget have described. But this is also seen in the gradual reduction in motor activity level (and hence of hyperactivity) throughout childhood.

Higher-Order Contingencies

More and more, behavior becomes governed by a set of complex rewards and punishments—problem solving, intellectual/aesthetic satisfaction, and, above all, social responses—and less and less by primary self-survival needs. Both behaviorists and psychoanalysts, among others, have described this process in their developmental theories.

The pace of this development varies with the function. For example, the acquisition of language and vocabulary between the ages of 1 and 3 years is truly astounding (Howlin, 1980), as is the acquisition of reading skills at the start of school, whereas the process of intellectual development outlined by Piaget occurs more gradually. As a general rule, the more complex the function (e.g., social behavior; very finely coordinated motor skills, as in violin playing), the longer the process is likely to be. Of course, too, the pace begins to decelerate and ultimately even reverse as adult life proceeds to its inevitable conclusion.

It is also apparent that many primitive or immature levels of behavior do not disappear completely. It is not only the infant who has temper tantrums or who will ignore any rights of others in egocentric pursuit, but in most adults these would be expected to emerge only in disaster situations or when the power of the brain is diminished due to alcohol intoxication or dementia.

BRAIN AND BEHAVIOR

Having described both brain and behavior, now it is time to try to relate the two to each other and to look at their interaction.

Brain Anatomy and Behavior

One approach to the question, ''How do we know the brain affects behavior and in what way?'' is to look at the relationship between brain anatomy and behavior. Much of the knowledge applicable to humans in this area is understandably derived from disease or other abnormal states, for the very good reasons that animal work has limited extrapolation, and studies of normal function are more difficult to relate precisely to brain function. The problem is even more difficult with children and adolescents whose brains are still immature, and the ways of relating any deviations in development to brain states are handicapped by the lack of good information about exactly what is truly abnormal and what is simply within normal variation.

GENERAL PRINCIPLES

Comparative anatomical studies show that the amount and complexity of brain development, especially in the cerebral cortex, is closely related to the complexity of behavior, both reaching their highest development in the human species. There are strong parallels between the developmental state of the brain and the development of behavior in humans, especially in early childhood. At birth, the cerebral cortex consists of small, underdeveloped neurons, with few dendrites especially in the newer parts of the brain (Casaer, 1992). The process of dendrite differentiation and axonal myelination occurs rapidly during the first few years, though it continues to some degree into adult life.

The brain and certain specific behaviors can be seen to be topographically linked in animal experiments, and in humans, not only in disease states but also in normal development. For example, the smiling response in infants coincides with the myelination of the visual cortex (Casaer, 1991). The linkage is closest for simple input and output functions. Complex functions like thinking involve many parts of the brain and, further, are subject to the principle of parallelism of functions discussed above. This means that topography is less well defined in these behaviors in development and in disease states, though still discernible at times.

Much function is asymmetrical, and this asymmetry is reflected in anatomical asymmetry. For example, the left hemisphere, which subserves much language function, is heavier than the right in most individuals, especially males, with those areas concerned specifically with language being larger in the dominant hemisphere than in the nondominant hemisphere. On the other hand, areas concerned with visuospatial function, subserved largely in the nondominant hemisphere, are larger there than in the dominant hemisphere (Lezak, 1995).

Brain Topography and Behavioral Function

The precise relationship between specific brain areas and behavior will now be reviewed. Much of what follows is set out in Lezak (1995), Lishman (1987), and Kandel et al. (1991). In child psychopathology, the reviews by Lewis (1992) and Taylor (1991) are among the most germane in trying to relate topography to behavior. Only those areas concerned with higher functions will be discussed. A word of warning is needed though. Most of the data come either from animal studies or, in humans, from brain disorders in adults when differentiation of function is long established. It is not clear how true the findings are of children, especially when the damage occurs very early in life when there is greater opportunity for utilization of alternative pathways and also development of alternative adaptational behaviors (Taylor, 1991).

DIENCEPHALON

This is the only midline structure to be discussed and includes the thalamus and hypothalamus. The thalamus is the Grand Central Station of sensation, through which sensory information passes on its way to the cortex and allied nuclei, but there are also important return circuits. It is involved in sensory processing (crossed), local sensorimotor integration, memory, emotion, attention, and alerting. Deficits associated with thalamic lesions are less absolute than are subtle but important impairments, like a decrease in verbal fluency (with left-sided deficits) and difficulty with pattern recognition (with right-sided deficits).

As is well known, the hypothalamus is concerned with autonomic and endocrine functions and thus is intimately involved in the expression of emotion (including stereotyped responses like rage) and motivational states like sexual drive and aggression (Lewis, 1992).

BASAL GANGLIA

These modulate motor and some autonomic functions by varying tone and producing synchrony of movement, but are also involved in intellectual functions too, especially the maintenance of attention. Their function is probably better described as one of generally maintaining and regulating motor and information flow and cerebral activity through reverberating circuits between cortex (especially the frontal region) and basal ganglia. Impairments here are most easily demonstrated in the classical movement disorders of parkinsonism, athetosis, chorea, and dystonias, but disorders of intellectual function are also seen in basal ganglion disorders. In parkinsonism there is rigidity of attention and inflexibility of cognition, qualitatively rather similar to the motor disorder (Lezak, 1995). Perhaps of more interest to child and adolescent psychiatrists (apart from drug-induced parkinsonism) is obsessive compulsive disorder (OCD). Though ordinarily thought of as an anxiety disorder, OCD has strong cognitive components that exhibit some of the same kind of rigidity seen in parkinsonism, except that in this case the rigidity is not one of tone but of a circularity or positive feedback loop of thinking. But just as parkinsonism has both motor and cognitive components, so has OCD at times, in the well-known concurrence of obsessive thinking in Tourette's disorder and postencephalitic parkinsonism (Leckman et al., 1993; Rapoport, 1988). It is therefore not surprising that recent research suggests that in OCD there may be an abnormality of the circuit between the frontal lobes, the basal ganglia, and the thalamus (Cohen and Leckman, 1994; Rapoport, 1988).

THE AMYGDALA

These are bilaterally paired nuclei deep within the cerebral hemispheres and in close relationship with the older olfactory brain. Not surprisingly, their strongest topographical link is to fear-provoked aggression (Lewis, 1992). But, as with the basal ganglia, lesions of the amygdala have more widespread effects—disturbances of control, spontaneity, and flexibility of affect and cognition.

WHITE CEREBRAL MATTER (LARGELY FIBERS)

This consists primarily of three types of fibers: association fibers, linking parts of the cortex together; commissure fibers, connecting the hemispheres; and projection fibers, linking cortex to distant parts. The effects of disorders of association fibers depend on the tightness of the fiber organization, the specificity of the function, and the extent of the lesion. For example, lesions of the tightly bound left arcuate fasciculus linking Broca's area (frontal) and Wernicke's area (parietal) produce construction aphasia in which the patient understands and expresses language well, but cannot repeat phrases accurately and tends to use inappropriate words (Kandel, 1991a). In most instances, however, damage to the association areas results in subtle defects of integration of higher function between the areas affected and, as a consequence, a more general, less specific type of impairment (Lezak, 1995). Abnormalities and lesions of the corpus callosum are often surprisingly silent (Taylor, 1991), perhaps because of alternative and possibly more usual vertical interconnections through the thalamus. However, neuropsychological tests show that slowing and some impairment of tasks that rely on integration of functions between hemispheres is often present.

On the other hand, projection fiber lesions such as those of the internal capsule are likely to have predictable and obvious results, like hemiplegia, since most are involved in highly specific point-to-point representation.

CEREBRAL CORTEX

Lezak (1995) points out that cortical functions can be thought of as roughly organized along two dimensions: lateral (left/right) and frontal/posterior. It is important to state early on that this topography becomes considerably inaccurate when the function concerned involves much of the brain that PET scans have shown is often the case, especially in any complex or novel task (Martin and Brust, 1991).

Asymmetrical Functions

In addition to similar but crossed primary sensory and motor functions, both hemispheres have specialization of function. In general, the left or dominant hemisphere is concerned with verbal and language functions, and this includes the storage of such information in the memory systems of the temporal lobes. The right hemisphere is concerned with nonverbal, including spatial, information. But these distinctions are not absolute, and the idea of dominance itself is misleading since specialization of function in each hemisphere is more accurate (Taylor, 1991). For example, the "poor relation" right hemisphere may actually be the one that enriches brain function and experience in general. For example, much of the melody of speech, humor, lateral or intuitive thinking, imagination, artistry and music, and the visuospatial aspects of mathematics may be quite dependent on the nondominant or right hemisphere, as may attention itself. There are gender differences in right and left hemispheric organization, primarily, in females, later developing and less marked laterality (e.g., of language functions) that is accompanied by less marked morphological differences in the two hemispheres (D.D. Kelly, 1991; Lezak, 1995). At a functional level these differences are also matched by differences in the cognitive styles of men and women—men are better at advanced mathematics, less verbally fluent, and better visuospatially, though these anatomical, organizational, and functional differences are relative, and there are large areas of overlap between the two sexes (Lezak, 1995). How these gender differences arise is still a mystery. The politically fashionable view is that these are the result of socialization; but there is now clear evidence that there are gender differences in endocrine secretion beginning early in fetal life (Peterson et al., 1992) when the brain is first developing and that these are related to sexual dimorphism in the brain (Lewis, 1992) though what relationship these have to nonsexual behavior is unclear (see Chapter 18). In child psychiatry, one of the more durable areas involving asymmetry of function is that of learning disorders, where failure to develop asymmetry is posited to lie behind some cases of dyslexia (Duane, 1989), though considerable skepticism about this rather durable theory is needed since reading is a most complex process (Snowling, 1991).

Frontal/Posterior Dimension

The frontal lobes are most concerned with motor and executive functions like speaking, organizing, and planning complex activities. Defects lead to aphasias, certain kinds of apraxias (inability to plan and execute sequences of movements such as dressing), deficits of attention and the planning and execution of complex behavior (Lezak, 1995; Rothenberger, 1990). The parietal, occipital, and parts of the temporal lobes have largely sensory functions, including complex interpretations of sensory data in light of experience and integration of these data across modalities. Deficits here lead to agnosias and receptive aphasias.

TEMPORAL LOBES AND THE LIMBIC SYSTEM

These are of special interest in psychiatry because of their well-demonstrated emotional and memory function, but they also have sensory functions associated with visceral sensations, olfaction, hearing, and speech. Organizationally, they have close links to midline structures concerned with emotional expression (e.g., the hypothalamus) and memory (e.g., the nucleus basalis of Meynert (Cote, 1991)), as well as to the cortex as a whole. Stimulation of this region during surgery or by an irritable focus can produce schizophrenic-like positive symptoms such as déjà vu and visceral or other hallucinations, giving strength to the postulate that dysfunction of the left temporal lobe is involved in schizophrenia (Crowe, 1992). Destructive lesions can result in negative symptoms or deficits, such as amnesias, and agnosias, such as impaired sound discrimination, amusia, and receptive dysphasias. Emotional disturbances of blandness similar to the negative states of schizophrenia or of poor regulation (e.g., irritability, panics, anxiety, obsessions) are also characteristic.

LONGITUDINAL SYSTEMS

The most important one for psychiatry is the reticular system of the more rostral brainstem, which has projections throughout the cortex. This system is much more complicated than originally thought, containing homeostatic, postural, activating (noradrenergic), and incoming information-modulating (serotonergic and dopaminergic) sections (J.P. Kelly, 1991).

Factors Affecting Brain and Behavior

More detailed discussions appropriate to each disorder and to brain damage syndromes in general can be found elsewhere in this book and in other reviews (Gudex and Werry, 1990; Kreusi, 1990; Rutter 1981, 1982; Taylor, 1991; Werry, 1986). Here, discussion is restricted to factors that have general effects on brain-behavior relationships or that illustrate particular points. Much of what follows relates to major brain abnormalities and hence should be applied with caution to lesser or more uncertain lesions or to normal states. The caveat about the validity of these largely adult-derived data in children also applies.

LOCALIZED VERSUS GENERALIZED DAMAGE

Lipowski (see Gudex and Werry, 1990) has classified brain-behavior syndromes as partial (or localized) and generalized, and this typology has been applied to organic brain disorders in children (Gudex and Werry, 1990). The amnestic disorders and some types of personality change due to a general medical condition (e.g., frontal or temporal lobe syndromes) are examples of partial disorders, while dementia and delirium are examples of generalized syndromes.

Partial Syndromes

In child psychiatry those of particular interest are the so-called "temporal lobe" syndromes of explosive, aggressive behavior said to be associated with temporal lobe epilepsy or inferred to represent temporal lobe dysfunction from the behavior itself or its putative response to anticonvulsants (Kandel, 1991a; see also Chapter 59). The validity of this syndrome is still disputed, especially in children (Hermann and Whitman, 1984; Kreusi, 1990; Lewis et al., 1989; Rutter, 1981), and though there were allusions to it in DSM-III in the text, it does not appear in DSM-IV, where classifications of personality change due to medical conditions are defined strictly behaviorally rather than etiologically. However, the idea is not likely to die so easily (see Taylor, 1991, and Chapter 59 for a fuller discussion). Other possible examples of localized or partial syndromes (equally disputed as to whether and where) are developmental language (right temporal lobe), learning and motor skills disorders (Duane, 1989; Feagans, 1983; Silver, 1989; Taylor, 1991; Werry et al., 1990), and ADHD (Rothenberger, 1990; Taylor, 1991; Zametkin and Rapoport, 1987). In adult disorders that also occur in children, organ-imaging techniques suggest a dysfunction of frontobasal ganglia circuits in OCD and Tourette's disorder (Cohen and Leckman, 1994; Rapoport, 1988) and of the temporal lobe in panic disorder (Kandel, 1991a), whereas schizophrenia seems to have both temporal lobe and frontal lobe possibilities (Werry and Taylor, 1994). So far, however, though encouraging, these are only isolated findings, and conclusive evidence of localized or partial syndromes in child psychiatry remains elusive.

Generalized Syndromes

In contrast to syndromes in adults, generalized syndromes like dementia and delirium, so topical in adult psychiatry, are little studied in children (Gudex and Werry, 1990; Volkmar, 1992). In adults, generalized brain disorders are marked by decline in all higher functions, though the precise pattern depends on how much and which parts of the brain and which localized functions are affected as well (Albert, 1981). In child and adolescent psychiatry, degenerative disorders are rare, and greater interest centers on mental retardation, the effects of anoxia at birth, and postnatal head injury. It seems logical to expect that, as in dementia, there should be a general reduction in the overall number of neurons. In Down syndrome, brain size is reduced by about 25% (though interestingly this is not true until ages 3–5, suggesting a failure of the brain to develop), and there is also a reduction in the complexity of convolutions so essential to accommodate the increased number of neurons and processes in the human cerebral cortex. At a microscopic level, there appears to be little localization of pathology (Propping and Hebebrand, 1990), so that all this suggests that severe mental retardation can be viewed as a generalized syndrome.

While gross brain damage/disorder occurring prenatally or perinatally can result in mental retardation, long-term follow-up studies suggest that the effects of the much commoner milder degrees of anoxia are difficult to detect after the first few years of life, when the compensatory effect of a felicitous environment seems to override the more obvious effects of generalized brain damage (Rutter, 1981; Werry, 1986). More subtle, difficult to detect effects like attentional and learning disorders remain a strong possibility (Feagans, 1983; Taylor, 1991); most such learning disorders would be localized, not generalized, syndromes (Duane, 1989).

Head injuries (see Chapter 59) in children and adolescents are frequent—40,000 in the United Kingdom in 1985 (Middleton, 1989)—and provide opportunities to study brain-behavior relationships in a generalized context because, in addition to local and contrecoup lesions, head injury often produces widespread permanent microscopic effects (Lezak, 1995; Taylor, 1991) as a result of acceleration and torsion effects. Such generalized effects in adults are well described and can be summarized as a decline in mental efficiency affecting attention, speed of mental processes, cognitive efficiency, and, when severe, high-level intellectual functions like abstract reasoning. In turn, this often is accompanied by irritability, fatiguability, and loss of initiative (Lezak, 1995). In children, in addition, there is evidence that the risk of development of any psychiatric disorder is increased, suggestive of some general effect (Taylor, 1991; Chapter 59). Fortunately, severe injury is infrequent in children and adolescents, and most of the injuries are mild. Middleton (1989) criticizes the belief that mild injuries are without long-term sequelae, pointing to problems of methodology in some studies and to the existence of contrary evidence. Development of the brain continues into adolescence, and there is a change in the relative importance of areas of the brain toward those concerned with higher levels of cognitive function. It has therefore been posited that there may well be ''sleeper,'' or delayed, effects that will become apparent only later. In any case, much of the more recent work in adults has shown that the changes listed above are detectable for several months after even a mild concussion (Middleton, 1989), suggesting it would be unwise at this stage to take too sanguine a view of head injury in children and adolescents.

In summary, then, generalized brain disorder probably results in generalized cognitive and behavioral changes, of a degree and permanence depending on the amount involved.

Much more controversial are other possible generalized (or localized) brain-behavior syndromes that are not due to frank brain pathology but to normal variations such as temperament and certain behavioral traits like high activity or asociability. Much of the research in this area depends for its biological underpinnings on genetic studies, especially of twins (Garrison and Earls, 1987). For example, the studies by Goodman and Stevenson (1989b) suggest that activity level has a strong genetic base (50% of the variance) and that even anxiety/withdrawal and somatizing traits may also have some hereditary base (Goodman and Stevenson, 1989b). In the end, genes operate through specific cellular effects, and if temperamental and personality trait variations are biologically influenced, the brain seems the most logical vehicle.

AGE

Age is of critical interest in child and adolescent psychiatry. One of the more durable beliefs about brain-behavior relationships is that of plasticity; the effects of any abnormalities of brain structure or function are said to be less serious the younger they occur. But there is an equally durable but opposite view that there are critical periods for the development of normal function, which, if missed or impaired, result in permanent disabilities. This is best illustrated by strabismus, which, if not corrected in the first few years of life, results in amblyopia. There is evidence to suggest that the popular idea that younger age reduces the risk of severity or durability of disability may well be false (Fletcher and Satz, 1983; Middleton, 1989). Further, the notion of sleeper, or delayed, effects emerging only later as a function of development of more complex cognitive and other brain functions must be borne in mind. In his review, Taylor (1991) expresses concern about the failure

of neurologists, child psychiatrists, developmental psychologists, and others to get together on this issue, pointing out, for example, that the best studies of head injury were done more than 20 years ago and before modern organ-imaging techniques could pinpoint the amount and location of damage so critical to meaningful study.

GENDER

Nearly all the putative brain-behavior syndromes in children, such as ADHD, learning and developmental language disorders, autism, schizophrenia, and Tourette's disorder, have appeared markedly in excess in boys. This may well reflect the sexual dimorphism of brain anatomy and development (Peterson et al., 1992) discussed above under Asymmetrical Functions, such as, in females, later and less complete development of dominance, lesser differences in size between right and left hemispheres, and/or in males, greater vulnerability to damage (D.D. Kelly, 1991). Also interesting is animal and clinical research on disorders like Turner's syndrome and on androgen sensitivity in the development of sexual preference and gender identity (see Chapters 18 and 56), and developmental research on other kinds of behavior, such as aggressiveness or activity level, that are observed to be different in the two sexes (e.g., Goodman and Stevenson, 1989a; Lewis, 1992), even early in life (Garrison and Earls, 1987). Research into gender identity, sex-typed behavior, and sexual preference in animals and humans with chromosomal or endocrine anomalies like Turner's syndrome or androgen insensitivity suggests that brain factors are influential, especially in the prenatal period (Garrison and Earls, 1987; D.D. Kelly, 1991; Rutter, 1980), but so are environmental factors, as shown by reassigning the gender of babies after events not involving prenatal factors (e.g., accidental amputation of the penis) (D.D. Kelly, 1991; Rutter, 1980). Nevertheless, the very early demonstration of sexual dimorphism (e.g., in androgen levels) in the fetus when the brain is first developing (Peterson et al., 1992) and clear differences in behavior (e.g., in activity level) in male and female infants suggest that brain-behavior relationships get off to a somewhat different start in the two sexes. How much they then diverge further or converge on the basis of experience is a most important question.

ETIOLOGY

While different etiologies produce different brain-behavior effects—for example, those of trisomy 21, head injury, and disorders of the temporal lobe all differ—there is good reason to posit that these differences will in the end be better explained by precise knowledge of the regions and functions of the brain affected and the pace and durability of any pathological changes (Rutter, 1980, 1981; Werry, 1986). Quite apart from the needs of treatment, it thus makes good sense to identify etiology as an important defining variable in brain-behavior relationships and to utilize what is known about the general and anatomic pathology (e.g., amount of extravasation, toxicity, and regional vulnerability of the brain) to generate hypotheses about brain-behavior relationships, and then to relate these to clinical facts. This is one of the main approaches in current neuropsychology, which increasingly eschews such global concepts as ''brain damage,'' dementia, intelligence, and so on (Albert, 1981; Lezak, 1995); instead, etiology is seen as often having strong functional implications. However, Taylor's (1991) extensive critical review of etiology shows that in children this is full of methodological complexities, few of which have characterized past studies, such as accurate delineation of areas of dysfunction (many of which are biochemical, not anatomical), precise and comprehensive measures of psychological function, and controlling for environmental and developmental effects.

EXPERIENCE

It is probably unnecessary in child psychiatry to highlight the role of experience in shaping and modifying brain-behavior relationships.

This review and others have given instances in which the outcome of any brain state or dysfunction has been demonstrated to be influenced by experience, for example, limbic dysfunction and violent behavior (Lewis, 1992; Lewis et al., 1989), sexual preference and the reassigning of gender (Chapter 18 and D.D. Kelly, 1991), and the attenuation of long-term effects of perinatal anoxia (Rutter, 1980, 1981; Werry, 1986). There is also no doubt that experience can produce permanent change in normal brain structure and function; that is what learning and long-term memory must be. For example, though the postcentral gyrus sensory map of the brain is basically similar in all humans, animal experiments have shown that this map can be changed quite significantly by immobilizing some fingers and exercising the others, or by sectioning a nerve (Kandel, 1991b). This process of ''reassigning'' brain areas seems to be a general property of the nervous system.

At a cellular level, reassignment, learning, and memory are thought to be achieved to a significant degree by alteration of synaptic transmission—increasing or decreasing the sensitivity or effective number of active presynaptic release sites or postsynaptic receptors (Kandel, 1991b). The way that this is brought about is probably complex and not necessarily homogeneous. For example, the elaboration of dendritic processes would increase the number of receptors, while biochemical changes at any one synapse could result in changes in the ratio of active to inactive receptors. However, it would be naive to go as far as Flourens or Lashley (see ''Concepts of Brain-Behavior Relationships'' above and Kandel, 1991a), or far too many professionals working with children, to think that experience or retraining programs can overcome any or all brain dysfunctions (Taylor, 1991). It seems likely that certain regions of the brain where localization is well developed and not replicated and/or the amount of residual brain left after damage will limit the extent and scope of experience (Taylor, 1991).

A Clinical Example

The clinical cogency of brain-behavior relationships and the principles outlined above will be illustrated now with one brief example, Tourette's disorder, largely because it has some of the most elegant hypotheses of brain-behavior interactions among child and adolescent disorders. What follows is described in more detail later in this monograph (Chapter 57) and elsewhere (Cohen and Leckman, 1994; Leckman et al., 1990, 1992, 1993; Peterson et al., 1992). Here the emphasis is on illustrating clinical relevance of principles, rather than on the disorder itself.

The behavior that brings the patient with Tourette's disorder to the clinician is unwanted, involuntary, repetitive, purposeless, stereotyped motor and vocal acts (tics), which may take quite complex forms in severe cases and can be socially disabling. These acts are often preceded by premonitory urges (Leckman et al., 1993). The disorder is often accompanied by other behavioral difficulties of a disinhibited, impulsive, or obsessive compulsive kind (see Chapter 57).

Pedigree and twin studies have suggested that Tourette's disorder is the product of a single major autosomal gene, but that the frequency in identical twins is only 50% (Hyde et al., 1992; Leckman et al., 1990). Also, that the disorder is commoner in boys, its severity varies across and within individuals, and there is an increased frequency of other disorders, notably OCD and ADHD in relatives.

These mostly clinical observations raise a number of questions that epitomize the nature of brain-behavior relationships in child psychopathology: What is the action of Tourette's disorder genes on the developing brain? Where do they act? What makes males more susceptible? What are the risk and protective factors determining whether or not, how severely, and which of the interrelated disorders appear clinically? How do these protective/risk factors operate on the brain? What is it that influences the day-to-day and minute-to-minute frequency of the symptoms in any one individual? Why does it take several years before the disorder emerges? While no definitive answers are yet available to any of these questions, there are some promising hypotheses and leads.

Simplistically, tic disorders (and OCD) seem to reflect neuronal circuits that reverberate instead of switching off—a failure to self-inhibit (Leckman et al., 1993). Genes lay down the fundamental anatomical organization of the brain, and minor variations in this could lead to the propensity of some microcircuits to be driven by some ectopic or rogue pacemaker and/or to be over-readily excited by incidental brain activity. Research suggests that the anatomical substrate may lie in the cortico-striato-cortico-thalamic system that regulates the planning and performance of motor behavior (Leckman et al., 1993). This could explain why the disorder manifests both cognitive (premonitory urges) and complex motor (tics) symptoms and also why there may be a particular somatic distribution to both (Leckman et al., 1993).

The increased frequency in males is of interest because it is characteristic of a number of psychiatric (and physical) disorders and is intimately related to the controversial question of sexual dimorphism of the brain discussed above. There is now evidence that testicular hormones begin to be secreted as early as the 8th week of fetal life, at a time when the brain is undergoing its major initial development, and are thought to play a major part in sensitizing certain regions to sex hormones (Peterson et al., 1992). The way in which this could predispose males to Tourette's disorder and induce it in childhood and adolescence as androgen secretion increases is outlined with supporting evidence in Peterson et al. (1992). The delays in onset of the disorder can be explained, in part, by this rise in secretion, but also by maturation and/or experiential realigning of brain architecture, which as already noted is most active during early life but continues at a negatively decelerating rate until death. The development of the brain is also dependent on a continued optimum biochemical environment and this is vulnerable to disruption. Two such disruptive factors, maternal vomiting during the first trimester and maternal stress, were shown in one study to influence the severity of tics in those with established Tourette's disorder (Leckman et al., 1990). Another risk factor, observed in identical twins, is lower birth weight (Hyde et al., 1992), suggesting that the power of one twin to get a better share of placental nutriments is a factor in the impact of genes on brain development. Maternal drug, tobacco, and alcohol use are universal ambients also known to alter the fetal environment and fetal development, though their role in Tourette's disorder awaits clarification (Leckman et al., 1992).

The influence of psychosocial variables in Tourette's disorder in postnatal life is widely assumed; but as in many other disorders, study of these variables would benefit from the same degree of rigor that now typifies biological studies—anxiety and/or stress may precipitate or make tics worse and they may be suppressed for variable periods with effort and are more prominent in relaxed or drowsy states (see Chapter 57). How these might work at a psychophysiological level needs clarification, though one obvious mechanism is through concomitant variations in neurotransmitters like noradrenalin, dopamine, and serotonin (5-hydroxytryptamine (5-HT)) and neuropeptides, all of which have modulating actions on brain activity additional to any specific transmitter actions (see Chapter 3).

In summary, Tourette's disorder illustrates how genes, gender, maternal stress, and uterine environment might alter brain microstructure and microorganization, making some individuals vulnerable to develop the disorder. The trigger for the emergence of the disorder might be the maturation of ''capable'' pathways, the rise of sex hormones, and as posited by Weinberger (1987) for schizophrenia, development-specific stresses that activate at risk pathways. Temperamental variables that increase anxiety-proneness may also make individuals more vulnerable. Once the disorder is established, its severity will be influenced by variations in levels in arousal, which in turn will be influenced by what is happening to the child or adolescent on a moment-to-moment basis. The content of vocal tics will reflect the child's learned vocabulary, and educational, supportive, and behavioral programs suggest that even presumptively biogenic mechanisms can be influenced to some degree by purely psychosocial variables. In the end, all factors—biogenic or psychogenic—operate through a final common brain pathway to express the disorder as clinicians recognize it.

Tourette's disorder illustrates the power of the biological substrate in this equation, but other disorders could have been chosen equally to illustrate the power of the environment. It is, however, not either/or, but a question of variation in the mix of these two factors and where current knowledge indicates therapeutic intervention may best be made. There is, however, a need in research on psychosocial variables to move beyond correlational studies, to be cast more precisely, and to be tied functionally to variations in brain function, otherwise their credibility in this equation may be diminished, which would be most unfortunate.

CONCLUSIONS

In this chapter, it is shown that the brain is an inordinately complex and wondrous mechanism. Its functions are both sharply localized and generalized, depending on the complexity of the function and the number of different regions of the brain necessary to that function. In a way, however, even the generalized functions seem composed of parallel or interacting localized functions so complex that they only *seem* generalized. Sharply localized functions like speech or fine motor movements are vulnerable to disruption in disease states, but parallel function protects a lot of higher functions from greater devastation from disease or injury.

Development is a major variable, of relevance in terms of both brain morphology and the unveiling of complex functions. It also protects the brain before and during birth in that the undeveloped state of the cortex particularly makes it more resistant to pressure and anoxia (Werry, 1986). While much of the process of brain development is preprogrammed, inexorable, and with clear limits, experience plays a vital role, especially in more subtle aspects of morphological and biochemical differentiation, shaping, and reshaping. The behavioral analogue of this we call learning, which is a lifelong process, not confined to childhood or adolescence. While there is now a large body of knowledge linking brain function and topography to behavior, much of this is derived from adults, animals, and disease states of little relevance to child and adolescent psychiatry. It does, however, enable hypotheses to be made about possible relationships and indicate meaningful lines of research.

As Kandel (1991b) points out, the separation of brain and behavior reflected in the divorce of neurology and psychiatry in the mid-20th century was due largely to the limitations of our knowledge and becomes increasingly obsolete. Rapid developments in molecular biology, neuropsychology, and other neuro- and behavioral sciences are closing this gap, though this may be more apparent at a research and theoretical than at a clinical level. However, such is the pace of development of new knowledge that it is not too fanciful to predict that presumptively *major brain disorders* like autism, obsessive compulsive and Tourette's disorders, and schizophrenia will yield their secrets and cause a major shift in the focus and thinking in much of child and adolescent psychiatry since many of these disorders are neurodevelopmental with origins in childhood or even in fetal life. But this will be but part of the shift. Soon to be revealed too will be the biological (especially the polygenetic) basis of a major preoccupation of child psychiatry, *variations of normal* behavior/personality like temperament, hyperactivity, anxiety threshold, and so on. Then doctors will surely be asked to change this or that characteristic in children, probably through pharmacological or molecular biological means. Trained as they are in human biology in health and disease and steeped in the ethical traditions of medicine, child psychiatrists must accept the responsibility to serve as a bridge to knowledge about brain and behavior so that the clinical picture of the child may be fuller and richer, yet keeping the treatment always in the child's best interests as a unique human being.

References

Albert MS: Geriatric neuropsychology. *J Consult Clin Psychol* 48:835, 1981.

Berthier ML, Bayes A, Tolosa ES: Magnetic resonance imaging in patients with concurrent Tourette's disorder and Asperger's syndrome. *J Am Acad Child Adolesc Psychiatry* 32:633–639, 1993.

Carmichael A: Physical development and biological influences. In: Tonge B, Burrows GD, Werry JS (eds): *Handbook of Studies in Child Psychiatry.* Amsterdam, Elsevier, 1990.

Casaer P: Old and new facts about perinatal brain development. *J Child Psychol Psychiatry* 34:101–109, 1993.

Coons H, Klorman R, Borgstedt AD: Effects of methylphenidate on adolescents with a childhood history of attention deficit disorder. II: Information processing. *J Am Acad Child Adolesc Psychiatry* 26:368, 1987.

Cohen DJ, Leckman JF: Developmental psychopathology and neurobiology of Tourette's syndrome. *J Am Acad Child Adolesc Psychiatry* 33:2–15, 1994.

Cote L: Aging of the brain and dementia. In: Kandel ER, Schwartz JH, and Jessell TM (eds): *Principles of Neural Science* (3rd ed). New York, Elsevier, 1991.

Crowe TJ: Temporal lobe asymmetries as the key to the etiology of schizophrenia. *Schizophr Bull* 16:433–442, 1990.

Duane DD: Neurobiological correlates of learning disorders. *J Am Acad Child Adolesc Psychiatry* 28:314, 1989.

Ebels EJ: Maturation of the central nervous system. In: M Rutter (ed): *Developmental Psychiatry.* London, Heinemann, 1980.

Eisenberg L: Psychiatric implications of brain damage in children. *Psychiatr Q* 31:72, 1957.

Feagans L: A current view of learning disabilities. *J Pediatr* 102:487, 1983.

Fletcher JM, Satz P: Age plasticity and equipotentiality: A reply to Smith. *J Consult Clin Psychol* 51:763, 1983.

Galler JR, Ramsey F, Solimano G, et al: The influence of early malnutrition on subsequent behavioral development. I: Degree of impairment in intellectual performance. *J Am Acad Child Psychiatry* 22:8, 1983a.

Galler JR, Ramsey F, Solimano G, et al: The influence of early malnutrition on subsequent behavioral development. II: Classroom behavior. *J Am Acad Child Psychiatry* 22:16, 1983b.

Galler JR, Ramsey F, Solimano G: The influence of early malnutrition on subsequent behavioral development. V: Child's behavior at home. *J Am Acad Child Psychiatry* 24:58, 1985.

Garrison WT, Earls FJ: *Temperament and Child Psychopathology.* New York, Sage, 1987.

Goodman R, Stevenson J: A twin study of hyperactivity. I: An examination of hyperactivity scores and categories derived from the Rutter teacher and parent questionnaires. *J Child Psychol Psychiatry* 30:671, 1989a.

Goodman R, Stevenson J: A twin study of hyperactivity. II: The aetiological role of genes, family relationships and perinatal adversity. *J Child Psychol Psychiatry* 30:671, 1989b.

Gudex M, Werry JS: Organic and substance use disorders. In: Tonge B, Burrows GD, Werry JS (eds): *Handbook of Studies in Child Psychiatry.* Amsterdam, Elsevier, 1990.

Hebb DO: *The Organization of Behavior.* New York, Wiley, 1949.

Hendren RL, Hodde-Vargas JE, Vargas LA, et al: Magnetic resonance imaging of severely disturbed children—A preliminary study. *J Am Acad Child Adolesc Psychiatry* 30:466–470, 1991.

Hermann BP, Whitman S: Behavioral and personality correlates of epilepsy: A review, methodological critique, and conceptual model. *Psychol Bull* 95:452, 1984.

Howlin P: Language. In: Rutter M (ed): *Developmental Psychiatry.* London, Heinemann, 1980.

Hyde TM, Aaronson BA, Randolph C, et al: Relationship of birth weight to the phenotypic expression of Gilles de la Tourette's syndrome in monozygotic twins. *Neurology* 42:652–658, 1992.

Hynd GW, Obrzut JE: *Neuropsychological Assessment and the School Age Child: Issues and Procedures.* New York, Grune & Stratton, 1981.

Jacobson M: *Developmental Neurobiology* (3rd ed). New York, Plenum, 1991.

Kandel ER: Brain and behavior. In: Kandel ER, Schwartz JH, Jessell TM (eds): *Principles of Neural Science* (3rd ed). New York, Elsevier, 1991a.

Kandel ER: Cellular mechanisms of learning and the biological basis of individuality. In: Kandel ER, Schwartz JH, Jessell TM (eds): *Principles of Neural Science* (3rd ed). New York, Elsevier, 1991b.

Kandel ER, Schwartz JH, Jessell TM: *Principles of Neural Science* (3rd ed). New York, Elsevier, 1991.

Kelly DD: Sexual differentiation of the nervous system. In: Kandel ER, Schwartz JH Jessell TM (eds): *Principles of Neural Science* (3rd ed). New York, Elsevier, 1991.

Kelly JP: The brain stem and reticular core: Integration of sensory and motor systems. In: Kandel ER, Schwartz JH, and Jessell TM (eds): *Principles of Neural Science* (3rd ed). New York, Elsevier, 1991.

Kolb B, Whishaw IQ: *Fundamentals of Human Neuropsychology.* San Francisco, Freeman, 1980.

Kreusi MJP: Biological risk factor in the aetiology of childhood psychiatric disorders. In: Tonge B, Burrows GD, Werry JS (eds): *Handbook of Studies in Child Psychiatry.* Amsterdam, Elsevier, 1990.

Kuperman S, Gaffney GR, Hamdan-Allen G, et al: Neuroimaging in child and adolescent psychiatry. *J Am Acad Child Adolesc Psychiatry* 29:159–172, 1990.

Leckman JF, Dolnansky ES, Hardin, MT, et al: Perinatal factors in the expression of Tourette's syndrome: An exploratory study. *J Am Acad Child Adolesc Psychiatry* 29:220–226, 1990.

Leckman JF, Pauls DL, Peterson BS, et al: Pathogenesis of Tourette syndrome: Clues from the clinical phenotype and natural history. In: Chase TN, Friedhoff AJ, Cohen DJ (eds): *Advances in Neurology* (Vol 58). New York, Raven Press, 1992.

Leckman JF, Walker DE, Cohen DJ: Premonitory urges in Tourette's syndrome. *Am J Psychiatry* 150:98–102, 1993.

Lewis DO: From abuse to violence. Psychophysiological consequences of maltreatment. *J Am Acad Child Adolesc Psychiatry* 31:383–391, 1992.

Lewis DO, Lovely R, Yeager C, et al: Towards a theory of genesis of violence: A follow-up study of delinquents. *J Am Acad Child Adolesc Psychiatry* 28:431–436, 1989.

Lezak MD: *Neuropsychological Assessment* (3rd ed). New York, Oxford University Press, 1995.

Lincoln AJ, Courchense E, Elmasian R: Considerations of the study of neurophysiological correlates of developmental psychopathology. In: Rothenberger A (ed): *Brain and Behavior in Child Psychiatry*. Heidelberg, Springer Verlag, 1990.

Lishman WA: *Organic Psychiatry: The Psychological Consequences of Cerebral Disorder* (2nd ed). Oxford, Blackwell Scientific Publications, 1987.

Madge N, Tizard J: Intelligence. In: Rutter M (ed): *Developmental Psychiatry*. London, Heinemann, 1980.

Martin JH, Brust JCM: Imaging the living brain. In: Kandel ER, Schwartz JH, Jessell TM (eds): *Principles of Neural Science* (3rd ed). New York, Elsevier, 1991.

Middleton J: Thinking about head injuries in children. *J Child Psychol Psychiatry* 30:663, 1989.

Orbach J: *Neuropsychology after Lashley*. Hillsdale, NJ, Erlbaum, 1982.

Peterson BS, Leckman JF, Scahill L, et al: Steroid hormones and CNS sexual dimorphisms modulate symptom expression in Tourette's syndrome. *Psychoendocrinology* 17:553–563, 1992.

Propping P, Hebebrand J: Genetic aspects of brain maturation and behavior. In: Rothenberger A (ed): *Brain and Behavior in Child Psychiatry*. Heidelberg, Springer Verlag, 1990.

Rapoport JL: The neurobiology of obsessive-compulsive disorder. *JAMA* 260:2888, 1988.

Rothenberger A: The role of the frontal lobes in child psychiatric disorders. In: Rothenberger A (ed): *Brain and Behavior in Child Psychiatry*. Heidelberg, Springer Verlag, 1990.

Rutter M: Psychosexual development. In: Rutter M (ed): *Developmental Psychiatry*. London, Heinemann, 1980.

Rutter M: Psychological sequelae of brain damage in children. *Am J Psychiatry* 138:1533, 1981.

Rutter M: Syndromes attributed to "minimal brain dysfunction." *Am J Psychiatry* 139:1, 1982.

Shaw DS, Bell RQ: Developmental theories of parental contributions to antisocial behavior. *J Abnorm Child Psychol* 21:493–518, 1993.

Shields J: Genetics and mental development. In: Rutter M (ed): *Developmental Psychiatry*. London, Heinemann, 1980.

Silver LB: Learning disabilities: Introduction. *J Am Acad Child Adolesc Psychiatry* 28:309, 1989.

Snowling MJ: Developmental reading disorders. *J Child Psychol Psychiatry* 32:49–77, 1991.

Strauss A, Lehtinen L: *Psychopathology and Education of the Brain Injured Child*. New York, Grune & Stratton, 1947.

Taylor E: Developmental neuropsychiatry. *J Child Psychol Psychiatry* 32:3–48, 1991.

Teuber HL: The premorbid personality and reaction to brain damage. *Am J Orthopsychiatry* 30:322, 1960.

Tupper DE: *Soft Neurological Signs*. New York, Grune & Stratton, 1987.

Volkmar FR: Childhood disintegrative disorder: Issues for DSM-IV. *J Autism Dev Dis* 22:625–642, 1992.

Weinberger DR: Implications of normal brain development for the pathogenesis of schizophrenia. *Arch Gen Psychiatry* 44:660–669, 1987.

Werry JS: Biological factors. In: Quay HC, Werry JS (eds): *Psychopathological Disorders of Childhood* (3rd ed). New York, Wiley, 1986.

Werry JS, Taylor E: Schizophrenia and allied disorder. In: Rutter M, Hersov L, Taylor E (eds): *Child and Adolescent Psychiatry: Modern Approaches* (3rd ed). Oxford, Blackwell Scientific Publications, 1994.

Werry JS, Scaletti R, Mills F: Sensory integration and teacher-perceived learning disorders: A controlled intervention trial. *Aust J Pediatr Child Health* 26:31–35, 1990.

Zametkin AJ, Rapoport JL: The neurobiology of attention deficit disorder with hyperactivity: Where have we come in 50 years? *J Am Acad Child Adolesc Psychiatry* 26:676, 1987.

8   Neuroimaging in Developmental Neuropsychiatric Disorders

Bradley S. Peterson, M.D., and Daniel M. Tucker, M.D.

The use of novel imaging modalities in the study of normal and pathological central nervous system structure and function in childhood developmental disorders is, like the subject of its study, still in its infancy. Concern for subject safety has appropriately delayed neuroimaging studies of children relative to those of adult disorders. With the ensuing reassurance of the safety of some imaging modalities, like magnetic resonance imaging (MRI), however, studies of brain structure in children are now being conducted on a larger scale. Functional imaging studies such as positron emission tomography (PET) and single photon emission computed tomography (SPECT) still typically require some degree of radiation exposure, although newer imaging modalities like functional MRI may make much more feasible the safe study of brain function in children throughout normal and pathological development. Despite the existing limitations of neuroimaging studies in children, advances nevertheless have been made in the understanding of brain structure and function in normal growth and in illness, and some indication of the potential for what questions imaging studies can pose, and the kinds of answers that can be anticipated in the study of children, are now evident. Broad features of the advances made thus far in understanding normal central nervous system development and the biological substrate of several common neuropsychiatric disorders of childhood are reviewed. Major pathophysiologic implications of the imaging findings are presented, insofar as they indicate how neuroimaging can inform our understanding of normal and pathological brain development. The physical bases of the most common imaging modalities are only briefly reviewed. More complete accounts can be found elsewhere (Keshevan et al., 1991; Oldendorf and Oldendorf, 1991; Volkow et al., 1991).

IMAGING MODALITIES

CT Scanning

The development and widespread application in the mid-1970s of axial computed tomography (CT) first heralded the advent of neuroimaging in neuropsychiatric disorders. CT scanning utilizes x-radiation, however, which has limited the use of CT in the research of childhood disorders. In the acquisition of a CT image, an x-radiation source is physically rotated many times around the subject's head. The varying strength of the x-radiation that passes through the head, which is determined by characteristics of the tissue through which it passes, is then measured multiple times and at multiple angles through the cranium. Computer processing methods then reconstruct the image through calculation of attenuation coefficients for each portion of the brain, and those coefficients are then assigned intensity values, which produces light and dark areas (contrast) in the brain image. CT scan resolution is approximately 1 mm, although the imaging plane is limited to axial sections. Tissue contrast does not even begin to approach that of MRI, which accounts for the favored use of MRI in neuroimaging studies.

MRI

MRI scanning capability has been widely available clinically since the early 1980s, although the "resonance" properties of certain nuclei placed in magnetic fields had been known for decades prior to the first acquisition of MR images as we know them. Among the nuclei sharing the property of resonance is the most common nucleus in biological tissues, hydrogen, which makes the imaging of brain tissue possible. When placed in a strong magnetic field, the hydrogen nucleus, which otherwise is randomly oriented with its axis of spin pointed in any direction, instead orients its axis parallel to the external magnetic field. In addition to the usual nuclear spin, this nucleus now also has another motion, that of *precession* around an axis parallel to the magnetic field, similar to a spinning top or a gyroscope (Fig. 8.1). While the magnetic field is maintained, a very brief radiofrequency pulse is then emitted from a coil apparatus around the subject's head. The frequency of the applied pulse is carefully chosen to be precisely the frequency that is most efficiently absorbed by the nucleus, its "resonance" frequency. This happens to match precisely the frequency of precession of the nucleus.

Absorption of the resonant frequency signal tips the spin axis toward a plane perpendicular to the precessional axis, in effect increasing the magnitude of the precessing motion. This "excited" nucleus then begins to tip its spin axis back toward the precessional axis, while continuing to precess because of the continued presence of the external magnetic field. The rate at which the nucleus returns to align itself back toward its precessional axis is determined in part by its immediate physical environment, the nuclei surrounding it. The nuclear spin creates in the nucleus a small magnetic field that, as the nucleus precesses, in turn constitutes a moving electrical charge and therefore a new radiofrequency signal. Thus, the scanner's radiofrequency pulse excites and tips a precessing nucleus, which then dissipates the absorbed energy as a second radiofrequency signal distinct from the first, and which carries in its rate of return toward its precessional axis information about its unique physical environment. In effect, each precessing nucleus becomes a radiotransmitter whose broadcasted signal specifies the location of the nucleus and the nature of its immediate physical environment.

Highly specialized signal processing techniques are needed to discern this newly emitted signal and to decode the information that it contains about the excited, resonating nuclei. It is the development and application of these signal analytic and image processing techniques that made MR imaging possible. These signal analytic techniques rely on Fourier analysis of the signal to transform into spatial coordinates the many complex radiofrequency waveforms emitted by the excited nuclei. In addition to providing spatial coordinates of nuclei, these image processing methods must also provide qualitative information that differentiates one nucleus from another. Without this qualitative information, spatial localization would provide simply a visually uniform map of hydrogen nucleus localization. Image processing techniques provide qualitative information about hydrogen nuclei, which appears as contrast between different portions of the image, by extracting from the signal emitted by excited nuclei information about their differing tissue environments.

The image processing techniques provide this qualitative information of tissue environment by breaking down each signal into one component that is parallel to the precessional axis of the nucleus and the magnetic field, and another component that lies in the transverse plane perpendicular to that axis. These signal components vary in time as the excited, precessing nucleus returns toward its precessional axis. Because these time-varying components of the radiofrequency signal are the electromagnetic consequence of the nucleus moving from a higher to a lower energy state as it precesses, they are referred to as "relaxation" times. The rate of relaxation along the axis parallel to the magnetic field is called "T_1," and that within the transverse plane perpendicular to this axis is called "T_2." These relaxation times vary according to the tissue characteristics in which the nucleus resides. Intensity values are assigned to specific combinations of T_1 and T_2 values, and images are constructed based on these intensity value assignments for each picture element (pixel) on the screen. Thus, T_1 and T_2 are the determinants of tissue contrast in MR images.

Because the tissue characteristics determine T_1 and T_2 relaxation times, different tissue characteristics can be emphasized on an MR image simply by varying the intensity values assigned to each combination of T_1 and T_2 times. Thus, the water content of cerebrospinal fluid (CSF)

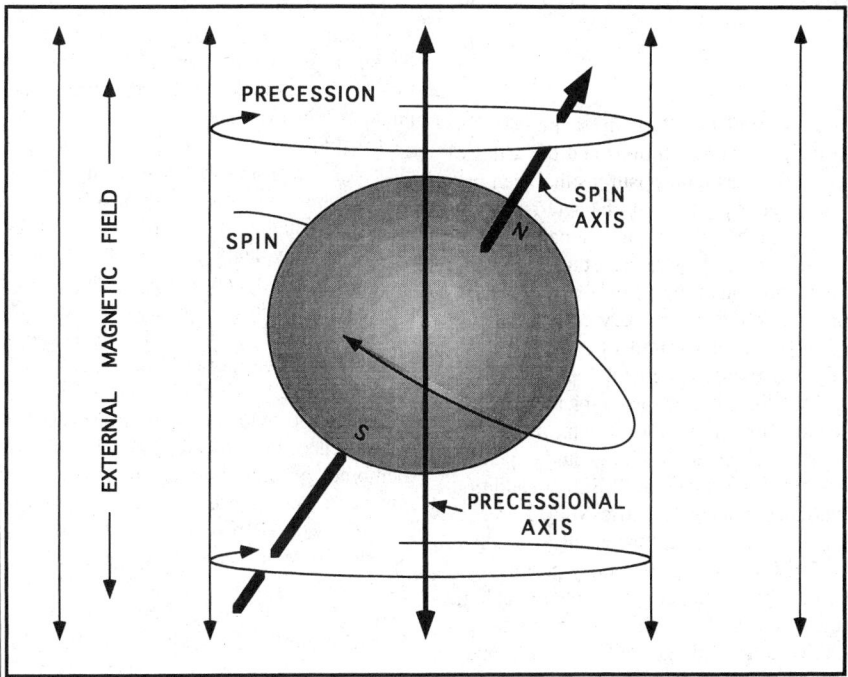

Figure 8.1. Precession of nuclei occurs when certain spinning nuclei are placed in an external magnetic field. The precession occurs around an axis parallel to the lines of force of the magnetic field. When an appropriate external radiofrequency pulse is applied to the precessing nuclei, the magnitude of the precession increases, effectively tipping the nuclear spin axis toward the transverse plane perpendicular to the precessional axis and the lines of force of the external magnetic field.

or the fat content of white matter myelin can be varyingly emphasized or deemphasized, depending upon the clinical or investigative need. The excellent tissue contrast that MR imaging produces, its excellent in-plane and between-plane resolution (which is now on the order of 1 mm), and its safety make MRI a useful clinical and research tool.

PET

PET involves the imaging of radiolabeled tracers that emit positrons. When the tracers are injected or inhaled, the positrons emitted from the tracers soon (within a 3-mm distance from the tracer molecule) collide with electrons. The colliding positrons and electrons annihilate one another, producing two gamma rays that are emitted at 180° trajectories from one another. These two gamma rays then pass out of the tissue and are recorded by detectors in the axial plane surrounding the subject. The precise localization of the origination of the gamma rays can be determined by noting which detections occur simultaneously at 180° orientations (Reba, 1993).

This site of gamma ray origination will vary depending upon the pharmacological properties of the particular radiotracer used. Some tracers, for instance, are primarily confined to intravascular space, and the localization of gamma ray origination can be assumed to reflect the distribution of blood vessels. Other tracers, like 2-deoxyglucose, are taken up by neurons and phosphorylated. Because the phosphorylated deoxyglucose cannot be metabolized further, the accumulating tracer reflects the degree of activity of the neurons containing them, which is then measured in the amount of radioactivity detected in that particular brain region. Additional tracer types include ligands for specific neurotransmitter receptors. Raclopride, for instance, is a D_2 receptor ligand. The isotopes that are incorporated into the various tracers have short half-lives, that for ^{15}O (incorporated in water for blood flow studies) being 2 minutes, that for ^{11}C (incorporated, for instance, into raclopride for dopamine D_2 receptor studies) being 20 minutes, and that for ^{18}F (incorporated into deoxyglucose for metabolic studies) being 110 minutes. In-plane resolution of the newer PET scanners is approximately 3 mm for ^{18}F-labeled tracers, and 8 mm for ^{15}O-labeled ones, the difference being due to differences in the distance between origination and annihilation of the positrons from each of the isotopes in their differing tissue compartments.

SPECT

SPECT imaging is functionally similar to PET, the primary differences between the two being their spatial resolutions and the kinds of tracers they employ. Whereas PET tracers emit positrons that then produce gamma rays, SPECT tracers emit photons of characteristic energies. Each photon is emitted in a manner that is directionally random and temporally independent of any other photon release, thus accounting for the "single photon emission" portion of the SPECT acronym. Specifics of the photon detection system are the primary determinants of resolution of any particular SPECT scanner. Currently the spatial resolution of SPECT, though rapidly improving, is still (at approximately 8 mm) inferior to that of PET. SPECT ligands, however, typically incorporate long-lived isotopes of technetium and iodine, which, unlike PET ligands, do not need to be synthesized on-site in a large and expensive cyclotron. This is a major cost-saving advantage of SPECT. In addition, the development of new, pharmacologically specific SPECT tracers, such as highly specific dopamine reuptake receptor ligands (Laruelle et al., 1993), make the future of SPECT imaging extremely promising.

Although new radiotracers may be developed whose pharmacologic properties and half-life offer the potential of reducing the radiation exposure for children who might in the future undergo PET or SPECT imaging, the need for radiation exposure in these imaging modalities will never be eliminated entirely. Reducing total radiation exposure will likely make PET and SPECT imaging safe for the clinical investigation of children who have severe neuropsychiatric illnesses, but the persistence of radiation exposure, no matter how minimal, is also likely to

make the recruitment of normal control children for research protocols prohibitively difficult. The development of novel experimental designs that would contrast various disease groups could in the future, however, make the combination of clinical and research protocols possible.

Functional MRI

The first reports characterizing changes on MR images during specific cognitive tasks appeared in 1991 (Belleveau et al., 1991). The changes on the MRI scans, which consist of subtle regional intensity changes during task activation, are now believed to track blood flow-related phenomena. It also appears that the spatial and temporal resolutions of this technique surpass conventional PET and SPECT imaging capabilities. The regional image intensity changes appear to derive from changes in the contents of oxyhemoglobin and deoxyhemoglobin present during the task, compared with their contents during the control state. Decreases in deoxyhemoglobin concentration during task performance increases the strength of the radiofrequency signal emitted by the underlying tissue, producing an increased regional image intensity. Images acquired during task activation can be compared with appropriate control images to determine which pixel intensities (and, presumably, which regional cerebral blood flow (rCBF) values) have changed during the task (for an excellent review of functional MRI (fMRI), see Cohen and Bookheimer, 1994).

Magnetic Resonance Spectroscopy (MRS)

The principles of MRS are predicated and build upon those of MRI. Instead of imaging primarily hydrogen nuclei, however, MRS can also image other nuclei that exhibit magnetic resonance. Magnetic resonance depends upon having a net nuclear spin, which entails that only nuclei having odd-numbered protons will demonstrate magnetic resonance. These nuclei include ^1H, ^{13}C, ^{19}F, ^{23}Na, and ^{31}P. Each of these nuclei, because they vary in atomic weight, have unique resonant frequencies in any given magnetic field, and thus the MR scanner's excitatory radiofrequency pulse can selectively excite any one of these nuclei simply by applying the radiofrequency pulse of the appropriate frequency. As the excited nuclei relax, the radiofrequency signal that they in turn emit is, like that emitted in MR imaging, in part determined by the physical environments immediately surrounding those nuclei. The frequency of the signal is altered slightly, producing a "chemical shift" fingerprint that is characteristic for the specific molecules in which the resonant nuclei are incorporated.

In addition to the nuclei that are selectively excited, another difference of MRS from MRI includes the requirement of stronger and more homogenous magnetic fields in MRS, which allows the preservation and discrimination of the subtle radiofrequency chemical shifts. Imaging in MRS also typically requires the use of surface coils, which localizes the region of interest to a volume of tissue near the cortical surface, although newer image processing methods make possible the imaging of larger regions of interest. The areas under specific spectral peaks then reflect the concentrations of the specific molecules generating the peaks.

Although all potential uses of MRS are still unknown, the technique promises to provide detailed information on regional brain metabolism of high energy phosphates like adenosine triphosphate (ATP), regional membrane phospholipid metabolism, electrolyte balance, and the metabolism of carbohydrates, amino acids, and lipids. The numerous current limitations of MRS include poor spatial and temporal resolution, poor chemical detection sensitivity, and the limited number of biologically relevant nuclei that can be imaged (Keshavan et al., 1991).

IMAGING OF THE NORMAL CENTRAL NERVOUS SYSTEM

Normal Development

Studies of changes in cerebral morphology and function associated with normal development are of vital importance for the proper design and interpretation of studies that are intended to elucidate the pathophys-iological mechanisms leading to disease in children and adolescents. Knowing the strongest correlates of regional brain volume allows, for instance, the recruitment of the appropriate contrast groups to control for the presence of potentially confounding variables that could obscure the true relationships between variables of hypothesized etiological sig-nificance and measures of the disease process in question. More broadly stated, no advances in our understanding of disease processes can be possible without first understanding normal development.

STRUCTURAL IMAGING

The changes in normal brain structure associated with development are only beginning to be defined (Fig. 8.2). The first reports of develop-mental changes detected radiographically came from Jernigan and asso-ciates (1990), who used semiautomated techniques that separated gray and white matter from each other and from CSF on MRI scans. Methods of defining anterior, posterior, superior, and inferior brain regions were referenced to standard brain landmarks (the anterior and posterior com-missures). In 58 subjects between the ages of 8 and 80, a linear decrease in supratentorial volumes was noted, with a concomitant increase in both cortical and ventricular CSF volumes (Jernigan et al., 1991a). A curvilinear decrease in cortical gray matter with age was also noted. In 39 children and young adults between the ages of 8 and 35 years, using identical image analytic techniques, significant linear *increases* were detected in both anterior and posterior regions of the superior cerebral divisions (r = 0.28–0.40), but not in inferior brain regions. The superior regions were smaller in females. When considering developmental changes in cortical (as opposed to entire cerebral) volume, however, decreases in both of the superior regions, and larger CSF spaces, were seen with increasing age. Subcortical gray matter structures like the basal ganglia appeared to *decrease* in size with age as well (Jernigan et al., 1990, 1991b); age-related basal ganglia volume reductions may be proportionally greater than those of overall brain volume (Murphy et al., 1992). Age-related increases in the volume of the temporal horns of the lateral ventricles, and decreases in hippocampal volume, have also been reported (Lim et al., 1990).

Whole brain volumes have been shown to correlate modestly, though

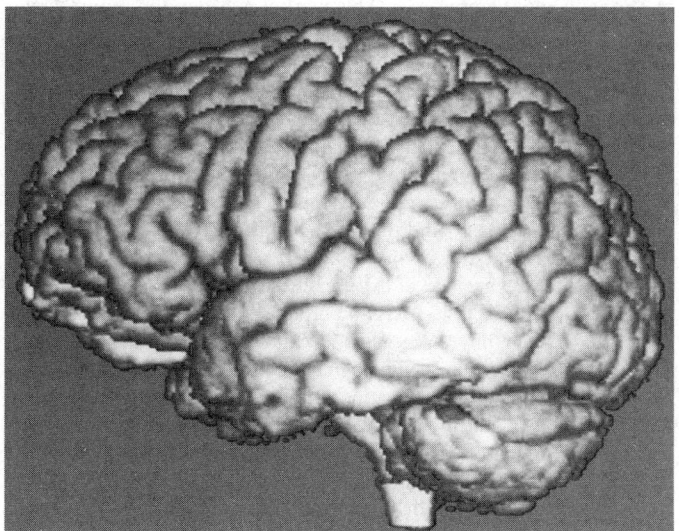

Figure 8.2. Three-dimensional cortical surface rendering for ana-tomical studies. Cortical surface can now be visualized with enough detail to permit preliminary analyses of regional cortical volumes based upon cortical division according to gyral and sulcal anat-omy. (Courtesy of the author and publisher (Schultz R and Chakra-borty A, in press).) See color plate.

significantly, with brain size in normal adult subjects. Willerman et al. (1991) demonstrated correlations (r = 0.35–0.51) between MRI measures of brain volume and IQ in 40 young adults, correlations that persisted even after controlling for body size. These findings were con-firmed and extended in another MRI study of 67 normal adults (mean age 38 ± 16 years) (Andreasen et al., 1993). Full-scale IQ correlated with overall brain volume (r = 0.36–0.38), and specifically with cere-bral gray (r = 0.31) but not white matter. These correlations controlled for the effect of subject height on brain volume, but did not assess cortical subregions to address whether specific brain region volumes in particular contribute most to overall intelligence. The authors duly note that, despite the significant correlations, the volumes measured account for only 12–30% of the overall variance in IQ scores, suggesting the importance of other, as yet unknown, neurobiological determinants of general intelligence.

FUNCTIONAL IMAGING

Concerns about radiation exposure in children understandably have limited radionuclide studies of age-related changes in cerebral blood flow and metabolism in early development. Blood flow was studied with SPECT in 30 neonates who either had been deemed at risk for developing cerebral palsy (because of low birth weight, asphyxia, or hypoglycemia) or who had suffered neonatal seizures (Rubinstein et al., 1989). All infants, however, had normal neurological and EEG examina-tions. A distinct pattern of development of cerebral perfusion was ob-served, in which prominent thalamic but low cortical perfusion was seen prior to a gestational age (GA) of 40 weeks. At a GA of 40 weeks, the continued thalamic perfusion was accompanied by an increasing flow to the parietal cortex, followed by prominent occipital perfusion at a GA of 44 weeks. Parietal and occipital flow then predominated by age 2 months and persisted until 6 months postpartum, when frontal activity was first seen. Flow to all cortical regions appeared relatively uniform by the age of 1 year. Thus, initial (preterm) thalamic perfusion, and presumably the associated thalamic synaptic activity producing it, ap-pears to be followed by an orderly and progressive recruitment of telen-cephalic neocortical regions in the 1st year of life.

In a cross-sectional study of blood flow in 42 children, ages 2 days to 19 years, rCBF was measured using either ^{133}Xe injection or inhala-tion during SPECT imaging (Chiron et al., 1992). All absolute rCBF values at birth were lower than adult values and increased thereafter to maximum levels at an age of 5–6 years, peaking at an average of 70% above adult values. All regional blood flow values gradually decreased thereafter, reaching adult levels by the age of 15 years. When regional values were normalized by the average global CBF, values were low at birth when compared with normalized adult values, increased until the age of 2 years, and then remained essentially at adult levels thereafter.

[18]F-Labeled deoxyglucose (FDG) PET studies of developmental changes in cerebral metabolism are consistent with these blood flow studies, demonstrating low metabolic rates at birth that rise quickly to adult values around the age of 2 years and that continue to rise until the age of 9 years. Rates decline gradually thereafter, reaching adult levels again in early adulthood (Chugani et al., 1987). Presumably the developmental changes in rCBF and regional metabolism in children reflect in part maturational changes that include axonal and dendritic growth, synaptogenesis, myelination, and angiogenesis. This presump-tion is substantiated by the global nature of the absolute changes in flow and metabolism and the attainment of normalized values early in life.

A preliminary MRS study of phosphorous compounds and metabolite concentrations was performed in 16 normal living neonates, 17 infants, and 28 adults (Buchli et al., 1994). Analyses of metabolite concentra-tions clearly indicated that ATP levels nearly double between neonatal and adult life. Although of uncertain physiological significance alone, these studies indicate the potential for safe imaging procedures to eluci-date brain structural, functional, and biochemical changes throughout normal and pathological development.

Studies of Normal Cerebral Asymmetries

In addition to beginning the documentation of general changes in cerebral structure and function through childhood development, neuroimaging studies have also begun the in vivo investigation of other more subtle brain characteristics, such as normal cerebral asymmetries, that have become increasingly important in theories of pathogenesis of numerous developmental disorders, including schizophrenia, Tourette's syndrome, and dyslexia.

TEMPORAL LOBE STRUCTURES

Numerous studies have documented normal asymmetries in the temporal lobe and in its substructural components. In 52 normal subjects, ages 20–40, volumetric measurements of the anterior temporal lobe and hippocampus demonstrated, in right-handed subjects only, larger right-sided structures compared with the left. The laterality differences were small in magnitude (4–10%) but statistically significant. Asymmetries were not detected in the left-handed subjects, and no age or sex differences in asymmetry were seen (Jack et al., 1989). Using MRI pulse sequences that provided higher resolution, and employing anatomic region-defining methods of probably greater rigor, normal hippocampal asymmetry was confirmed, and an additional normal right-larger-than-left asymmetry of the amygdaloid complex was described in 11 predominantly right-handed adults, aged 20–59 (Watson et al., 1992). These neuroimaging studies corroborate histopathological reports of asymmetry in the human amygdaloid complex (Murphy et al., 1987).

Another portion of the temporal lobe that has been shown to be structurally lateralized is the planum temporale. The planum, in fact, is the structure in which asymmetries were first described in postmortem reports (Geschwind, 1972; Geschwind and Levitsky, 1968). Because the planum is thought to subserve important aspects of language, and because of the lateralization of language functions in the human central nervous system, asymmetry of the planum has been the object of increasingly intense study (Galaburda, 1993). A larger left-sided planum has been described in normal children and adults in numerous MRI studies (Hynd et al., 1990; Kushch et al., 1993; Larsen et al., 1990; Leonard et al., 1993; Schultz et al., 1994). Semiautomated methods of cortical and sulcal definition have also demonstrated normal asymmetries in portions of the temporal and parietal lobes, particularly in the lengths of certain portions of the Sylvian fissure and central sulcus (Falk et al., 1991). Asymmetries of other cortical regions, especially along the cerebral convexities, have not been studied extensively, primarily due to the high individual variability in the presence and location of sulcal landmarks that makes the valid and reliable parcellation of cortex into smaller subregions extremely difficult (Ono et al., 1990).

BASAL GANGLIA

In a study of 14 normal right-handed adults, the putamen and globus pallidus volumes on MRI scans were shown to be approximately 10% larger on the left than on the right, while caudate nucleus volumes were approximately 4% larger on the right (Fig. 8.3). When an additional four left-handed subjects were included in the analyses, correlations were noted between the degree of basal ganglia asymmetry and the degree of functional cerebral dominance (as measured by a standard handedness survey) (Peterson et al., 1993b). These findings corroborate a previous postmortem report of humans between the ages of 26 weeks gestation to 86 years, in which globus pallidus volumes were found to be approximately 5% larger on the left than on the right. The asymmetries seemed to be present even in fetal brains (Kooistra and Heilman, 1988). In this study, too, the degree and direction of structural CNS asymmetry correlated with antemortem handedness. The normal putamen asymmetries described by Peterson and colleagues (1993b) were confirmed in an MRI study of children (Singer et al., 1993), as were the normal caudate nucleus asymmetries (Castellanos et al., 1994). Other asymmetries of subcortical brain regions reported in postmortem studies, such

as those of the posterior thalamus (Geschwind and Levitsky, 1968), have not yet been confirmed in imaging studies.

RELAXATION TIME ASYMMETRIES

As already discussed, T_1 and T_2 relaxation times are tissue characteristics reflecting the recovery of the bulk nuclear magnetization from hydrogen nuclei that have been excited by an appropriate radiofrequency pulse during MR imaging. The relaxation times determine how much nuclear magnetic resonance (NMR) signal is recorded for each tissue. Relaxation time differences between different tissues thus are the basis of tissue contrast in MR images. T_2 relaxation times measured in 14 right-handed adults were determined bilaterally in basal ganglia nuclei, the anterior and posterior thalamus, insular cortex, amygdala, the cingulum gray and white matter, frontal and occipital white matter, the red nucleus, and the substantia nigra pars reticularis (Peterson, Gore, et al., 1994). Right-left differences were seen in every region, with all right-sided regions except the red nucleus having the longer T_2 times. Effects were small in magnitude (2–5%) but statistically highly significant. These normal T_2 time asymmetries suggest that the determinants of basic tissue characteristics differ between the two sides of the brain from cortex to brainstem, and that those tissue differences are evident over very short distances across the midline. These findings should be regarded as preliminary until confirmed in a larger number of subjects.

BLOOD FLOW

Despite the considerable data potentially available on normal rCBF and cerebral metabolism from prior PET research, very few studies have thus far actually assessed whether blood flow is asymmetrically distributed between the two hemispheres, either globally or regionally. One early study has reported a 5–10% greater blood flow to the left hemicerebrum in right-handed subjects at rest, while oxygen extraction and cerebral blood volume did not seem to differ between hemispheres (Perlmutter et al., 1987). Whether this apparent asymmetry in CBF changes through development is unknown.

Imaging of Normal Mental Processes

One of the exciting developments in functional neuroimaging is the emerging elucidation of brain regions that subserve any of a wide array of normal cognitive processes. This work was begun in the PET arena and was made possible by the advent of radiotracers like ^{15}O-labeled water, whose very short half-lives and consequently favorable safety profiles made possible repeated tracer administration and repeated scannings within the same subjects. Regional blood flow and metabolic rates determined from images that were acquired during well-defined mental tasks could then be compared to flows and rates measured on images acquired during control conditions. Significant changes in metabolism during task activation could then be presumed to be due to activation of brain regions uniquely involved in the neuronal processes subserving the task. Primarily because of the ever-present concerns about radiation exposure, these PET task activation protocols have never been applied to the study of cognitive processes in children.

An even more recent technological advance in functional imaging has been adapting the task activation paradigms developed in PET during the acquisition of functional MR images. MR scans are first acquired during states of cognitive task activation and during rest. Regional signal intensities are then compared between the two sets of images by color-coding pixels according to their degree of statistically significant change during the two states. Those color-coded statistical maps can then be overlaid on an anatomical image acquired in exactly the same locations, to determine which regions are activated during the task. Although the physiological basis of the change in MR signal intensities during task activation are still not entirely known, the changes appear to track blood flow-related phenomena. Currently those phenomena are thought to involve changes in the oxygenation status of hemoglobin that are associ-

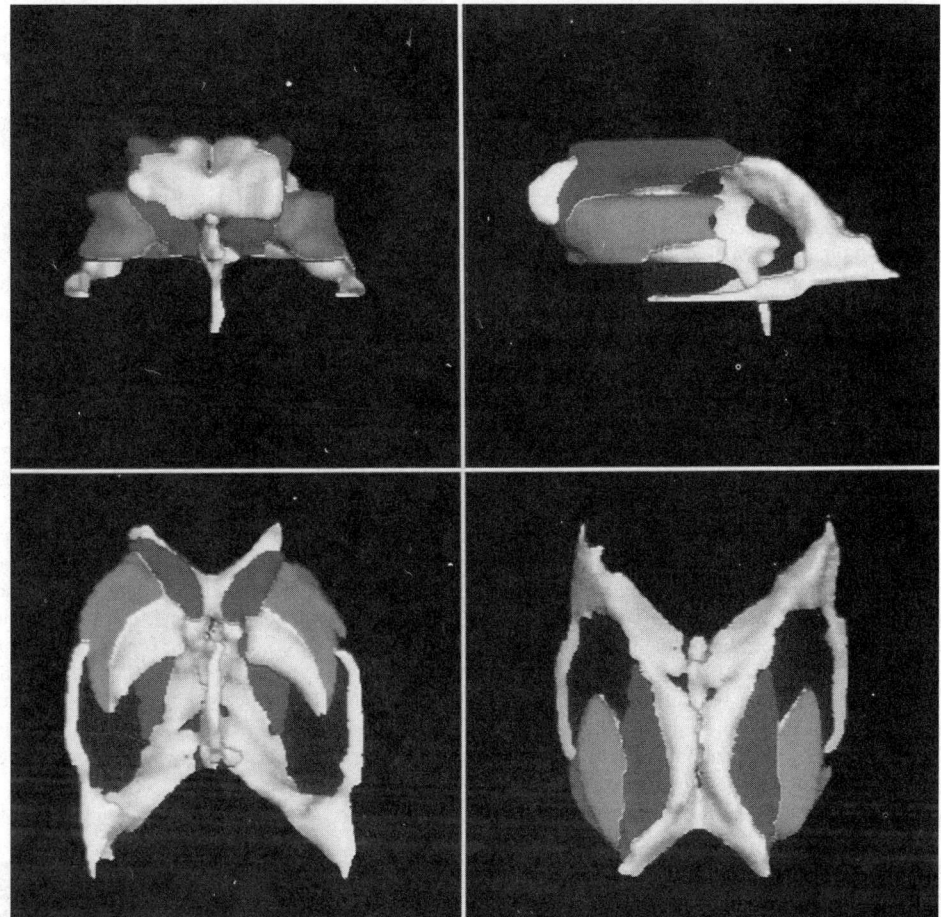

Figure 8.3. Three-dimensional views of basal ganglia and lateral ventricles. Basal ganglia circumscribed in two-dimensional format have been viewed in computer three-dimensional reconstructions (ISG Technologies, Toronto, Canada). Portrayed here are anterior (*upper left*), lateral (*upper right*), inferior (*lower left*), and superior (*lower right*) views. The three-dimensional relationships of the lateral ventricles (*white*), caudate (*red*), putamen (*green*), and globus pallidus (*white*) can be seen in each of the representations. See color plate.

ated with changes in metabolic demand during task activation (Kwong et al., 1992). This technique is still in its relative infancy, and many technical difficulties need to be overcome before fMRI can realize its full potential in the study of normal and pathological neural processes. Its apparent total safety, however, offers the future promise of being able to study cognitive processes throughout child development.

PET AND SPECT

Arguably, the most elegant PET studies of normal cognitive processes have come from the former Washington University-St. Louis group of Petersen, Fox, and their colleagues. Using task activation paradigms, they have begun to unravel the neurobiologic underpinnings of human language in general, and of lexical processing in particular. Their initial task activation paradigms involved the kinds of activation and control states described in Table 8.1.

Notice that the active state of one level of analysis serves as the control state for the next level of analysis. This experimental design allowed the dissection of the brain-based regional substrates for each of the cognitive components of the sensory perception, motoric production, and semantic understanding of words. These task activations were moreover conducted for both visual and auditory input, allowing the comparison of the neural bases of reading and audition. Words presented *passively* activated primary and secondary sensory-processing areas. Written words activated visual cortex, and aurally presented words activated auditory cortex.

Table 8.1. Language Task Activation Paradigms

Control State	Active State	Added Cognitive Compound
Gaze fixation only	Passive words	Passive sensory processing, automatic word-level coding
Passive words	Repeat words	Articulatory coding, motor programming, and output
Repeat words	Generate verbs	Semantic/syntactic association, selection for action

The lexical processing tasks used in PET studies of the neural bases of language are likely to be adapted with increasing frequency to the study of other cognitive systems. Each active state has an appropriate control state, which together help isolate the various components of a conceptual and neural processing heirarchy. Reproduced with permission, from Petersen SE, Fiez JA: The processing of single words studied with positron emission tomography. *Ann Rev Neurosci* 16:509–530, 1993. © by Annual Reviews, Inc.

Word *repetition*, in turn, activated brain regions believed to be involved in motor coding and programming, such as the primary sensorimotor cortex, the supplementary motor area, the lateral premotor region, and portions of the cerebellum, regardless of the sensory modality in which the words were presented. Actively *generating* verbs appeared to activate portions of the anterior cingulate cortex, the left anterior inferior prefrontal cortex, and the right inferior cerebellum.

Similar experimental designs have been useful in dissecting the brain regions involved in processing the lexical and semantic (meaning) aspects of language. Many other similar studies have been performed with PET and, to a lesser extent, SPECT. These include (to name a few) studies of motor control (Colebatch et al., 1991; Roland et al., 1982; Shibasaki et al., 1993), attention (Corbetta et al., 1993; Pardo et al., 1991), mood (Schneider et al., 1993), and sensory perception (Burton et al., 1993; Jones et al., 1991; Lueck et al., 1989) (Fig. 8.4).

FUNCTIONAL MRI

Many of the fMRI studies of cerebral activation thus far have adapted experimental designs from previous PET research. These ''replication'' studies help to validate the techniques of fMRI and provide a starting point from which can evolve other applications that may potentially even surpass the capabilities of PET imaging. Cerebral activation using fMRI, for example, can often be visualized in a single individual's scan, in contrast to the current need for averaging over multiple subjects in PET imaging. In addition to replicating previous PET study findings, other validation studies of fMRI that are underway include imaging the same subjects during the same task activation protocols using both PET and fMRI (Fried et al., 1994) and confirming the cortical activation seen on fMRI during intraoperative electrophysiological recording (Puce et al., in press).

The earliest studies of fMRI simply demonstrated activation of sensory cortex in response to photic and somatosensory stimulation (Belliveau et al., 1991; Blamire et al., 1992; Kwong et al., 1992; Ogawa et al., 1992) and then motor cortex activation during the performance of motor tasks (Constable et al., 1993; Rao et al., 1993; Schad et al., 1993). Adaptations of the PET language experiments have also confirmed frontal cortex activation during verb generation in humans (McCarthy et al., 1993) (Fig. 8.5). More recent fMRI applications include studies of cerebellar activation during a complex pegboard problem-solving task (Kim et al., 1994), visual cortex activation during mental imagery (Le

Bihan et al., 1993), and visual cortex activation during photic stimulation in schizophrenics compared with controls (Renshaw et al., 1994).

DEVELOPMENTAL NEUROPSYCHIATRIC DISORDERS

When compared with the imaging of adult disorders, the use of neuroimaging technologies to study childhood disorders has been relatively neglected. The reasons for this relative neglect are, not surprisingly, multiple. Successful neuroimaging enterprises are inevitably expensive, and they require a large interdisciplinary team of radiologists, physicists, clinicians, and other support staff. In addition, the initial safety uncertainties of some of the techniques made clinicians and parents understandably cautious of imaging children, although the safety of MRI is now well established, making large-scale structural studies more feasible. Safety concerns, however, still generally apply to PET and SPECT imaging in children. Finally, the appreciation of the importance of understanding developmental processes for improving the understanding of adult disease is probably still esoteric; many neuroscientists and neuroimagers seem tacitly to regard adulthood and adult illnesses as static entities, and children and their illnesses as the same as adults and their illnesses, though in miniature. Consequently, the major contributions from neuroimaging in understanding disease have been made in the fields of adult schizophrenia and, possibly, in adult obsessive compulsive disorder (OCD). Efforts in functional imaging have been particularly productive. Ironically, these disorders are nearly paradigmatic in terms of being developmental in nature, meaning that both are characteristically of adolescent or early adult onset, childhood variants appear to be common, and their pathophysiologies are thought to include determinants that either occur early in development or that are significantly influenced by normal CNS maturational events. Consequently, the fol-

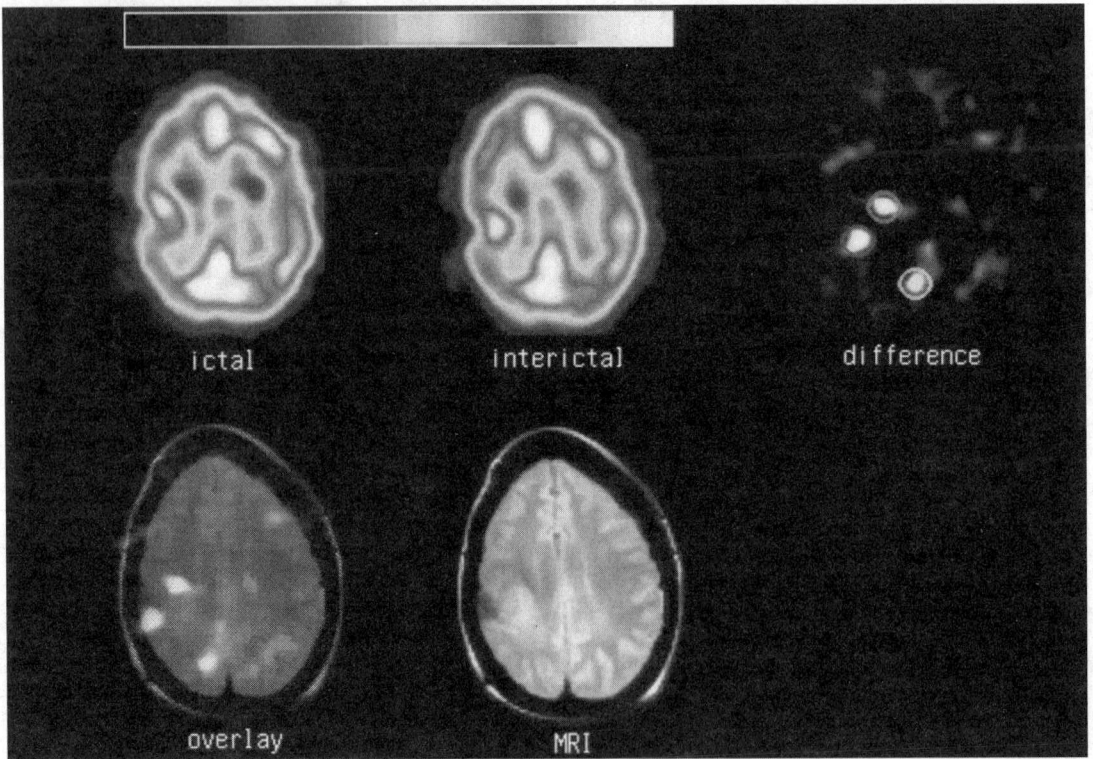

Figure 8.4.   Functional image subtraction techniques employed in HMPAO SPECT imaging. Image subtraction techniques now have been applied in nearly all functional imaging modalities, including SPECT. This figure demonstrates the utility of subtraction techniques in identifying seizure foci in a female patient having a childhood onset of complex partial seizures. The seizures were resistant even to surgical resection of the anterior portion of her right temporal lobe. Both the *ictal* and *interictal* scans demonstrate only the surgical defect. Subtraction (*difference*) of these scans, however, identifies three foci of increased metabolic activity possibly representing seizure activity, the locations of which are evident when the subtraction images are overlaid (*overlay*) on a coregistered MRI scan. See color plate. (Courtesy of Paul Hoffer, Professor, Yale University School of Medicine, Division of Diagnostic Radiology.)

lowing review will include adult studies of these particular disorders, as well as studies of disorders that are regarded as more quintessentially of childhood onset (Table 8.2).

Autism

Ventricular Size. Early CT studies first reported enlarged ventricular systems in autistic adults and children (Campbell et al., 1982; Da-

masio et al., 1980; Rosenbloom et al., 1984). MRI scans of 13 autistic children were compared with those of 33 controls who had been imaged as part of a neurological evaluation (Gaffney et al., 1989). Image acquisitions were therefore nonuniform, head position was not standardized, important clinical data such as IQ and handedness were not available, and regional measures were obtained from only a single axial section. Ventricular size was found to be 60% larger in the autistic subjects. Given the methodologic limitations, these findings should be regarded

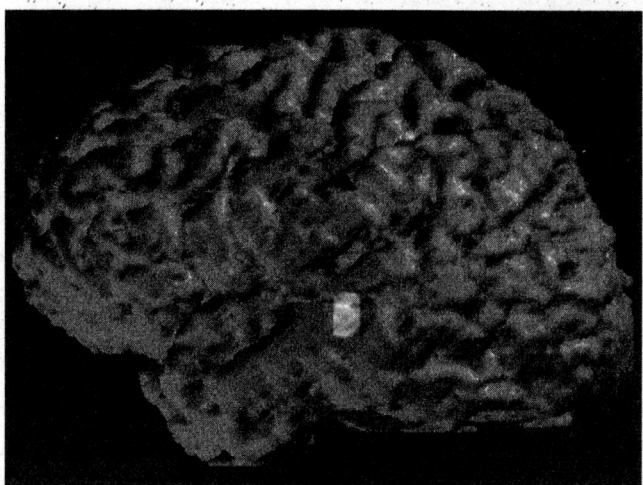

Figure 8.5. Functional MRI of language systems. An fMRI activation map has been superimposed on a three-dimensional brain rendering to demonstrate regional cortical activation during a language task relative to a control state. The language task involves judging whether a visually presented name correctly identifies a simultaneously displayed picture. Images acquired during times when the name correctly identifies the picture are compared with images acquired during times when the "name" presented is a nonsense word and the picture presented is a nonsense figure. The region of activation that this protocol yields (*represented by green shading*) is in the left posterior temporal lobe posterior to the sylvian fissure, in regions of the brain thought to subserve language functions. See color plate. (Courtesy of John Gore, Professor, Yale University School of Medicine, Division of Diagnostic Radiology.)

Table 8.2. Summary of Major Neuroimaging Findings in Developmental Disorders

Condition	CSF	Cortex	Subcortex	Other
Normal	Cortical and ventricular CSF increase with age	Whole brain volume may increase with age in children Supratentorial volume and gray matter decrease with age in children and adults R > L hemispheric blood flow in adults Temporal lobe volumes may decrease with age R > L temporal lobe asymmetries (amygdala and hippocampus) L > R planum temporale R > L T_2 time asymmetries throughout cerebrum	Basal ganglia volumes decrease with age Normal L > R basal ganglia asymmetries R > L T_2 time asymmetries in basal ganglia and thalamus	Thalamic perfusion prenatally progresses to partietal, then occipital, then frontal regions over the 1st year of life All absolute rCBF's and metabolism low at birth, increase to max between ages 5 and 9, and decrease thereafter to adult levels by late adolescence ATP levels double between birth and adulthood
Autism	Possibly increased cortical and ventricular CSF	High frequency of regional structural abnormalities that include localized parietal and frontal volumes loss, localized pachygyria, and mucrogyria and macrogyria, suggestive of neuronal migration abnormalities Diffuse regional abnormalities in rCBF and metabolism many correspond to the presence of regional structural abnormalities MRS studies suggest hypermetabolism and abnormal cell membrane metabolism in prefrontal cortex Possibly altered size of vermian lobules VI and VII. Hypoplastic and hyperplastic subtypes may exist No alterations in cerebellar blood flow have been seen	None described	Possibly reduced size of midbrain and medulla

(continued)

Table 8.2. *continued*

Condition	CSF	Cortex	Subcortex	Other
Fragile X	Increased 4th ventricle size	Bilaterally increased hippocampal volumes Bilaterally decreased size of the superior temporal gyrus Hippocampal and superior temporal gyrus volume changes may correlate with increasing age Size reductions of vermian lobules VI and VII that may correlate with sex-specific differences in the degree of genetic loading	None described	None
Down's syndrome	None described	Decreased whole brain and gray matter volumes, with a disproportionately large reduction in frontal gray matter volume Abnormal regional intercorrelations of frontal and parietal cortices Reduced cerebellar volumes, and reduced size of all vermian lobules	Relative sparing of lenticular nucleus and diencephalon	Reduced size of the anterior regions of the corpus callosum
Schizophrenia	Increased cortical CSF and increased ventricle-brain ratio (VBR) Increased size of temporal horn of left lateral ventricle Ventricular size in at-risk individuals appears to be determined by the interaction of genetic and environmental risk factor exposure	Decreased metabolism and rCBF in frontal cortex Possibly reduced frontal volumes Reduced volumes of anterior superior temporal gyrus (auditory association cortex), and possibly increased rCBF during auditory hallucinations Possibly reduced amygdala and hippocampus (especially gray matter) volumes Possibly reduced asymmetries of temporal lobe and cortical surface Inconsistent reports of increased size of all cerebellar vermian lobules	Variable volumetric changes in basal ganglia, possibly increased Decreased metabolism and rCBF in basal ganglia that may normalize with treatment Reduced basal ganglia volumetric and metabolic asymmetries Increased right-sided basal ganglia metabolism with neuroleptics Inconsistent findings of increased striatal dopamine receptor density Thalamic "lesions", especially on the right	None
Obsessive-compulsive disorder	Inconsistent CSF findings	Increased metabolism and rCBF to orbitofrontal cortex that correlates with symptom severity, increases during symptom provocation, and normalizes with treatment Possible abnormalities in T_1 asymmetries in orbitofrontal cortex and anterior cingulum	Probable caudate nucleus reduction and metabolic abnormalities Increased rCBF to right caudate during symptom provocation Possibly abnormal caudate nucleus volume asymmetries, and T_1 time asymmetry abnormalities in caudate and lenticular nuclei	None
Tourette's syndrome	Possibly enlarged ventricles with abnormal asymmetires	Possibly reduced metabolism in frontal, cingulate, and insular cortices Abnormal T_2 asymmetries in frontal white matter	Left-sided lenticular nucleus volume reductions and absence of asymmetry in children and adults Reduced basal ganglia metabolism, more pronounced in ventral portions Abnormal T_2 asymmetries in basal ganglia Increased presynaptic dopamine uptake sites	Reduced midsagittal cross-sectional area of the corpus callosum in adults Possibly abnormal T_2 times in red nucleus and amygdala
Attention deficit hyperactivity disorder	No obvious ventricular size abnormalities	Possibly sulcal widening Variable functional findings, including: reduced metabolic rates in sensorimotor, auditory, and occipital regions in adolescents; reductions in global rates and regional normalized rates in premotor and sensorimotor regions in adults	Possibly reduced left lenticular nucleus volumes in ADHD subjects when present comorbidly with TS Possibly reduced striatal metabolism in adolescents Possibly reduced right caudate nucleus volumes	Reduced cross-sectional area of corpus collosum subregions, variably seen in anterior (genu, rostrum) and posterior (rostral body, isthmus, spenium) portions
Dyslexia	None described	Varying reports of abnormal asymmetries in the planum temporale Tissue may be distributed differently between the temporal and parietal banks of the planum in dyslexic subjects Multiple Heschl's gyri often seen on either side in the planum temporale Metabolic activation of the left posterior planum may be reduced, and activation of medial portions may be increased bilaterally during phonological processing tasks	None described	None

See the corresponding portions of the text for a more complete discussion of these summary findings and citations of the studies reporting them.

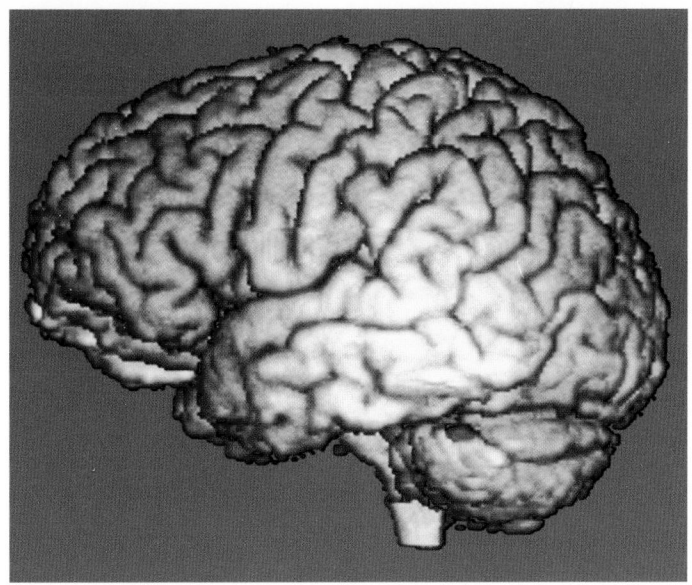

Figure 8.2.

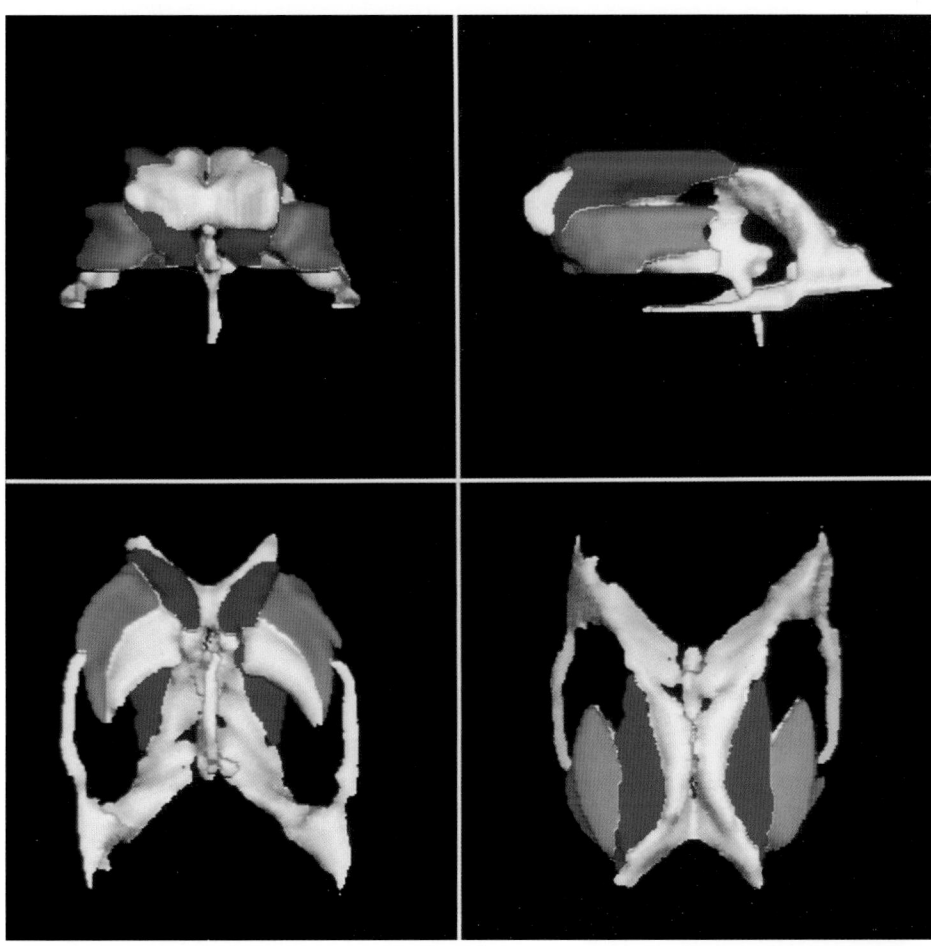

Figure 8.3.

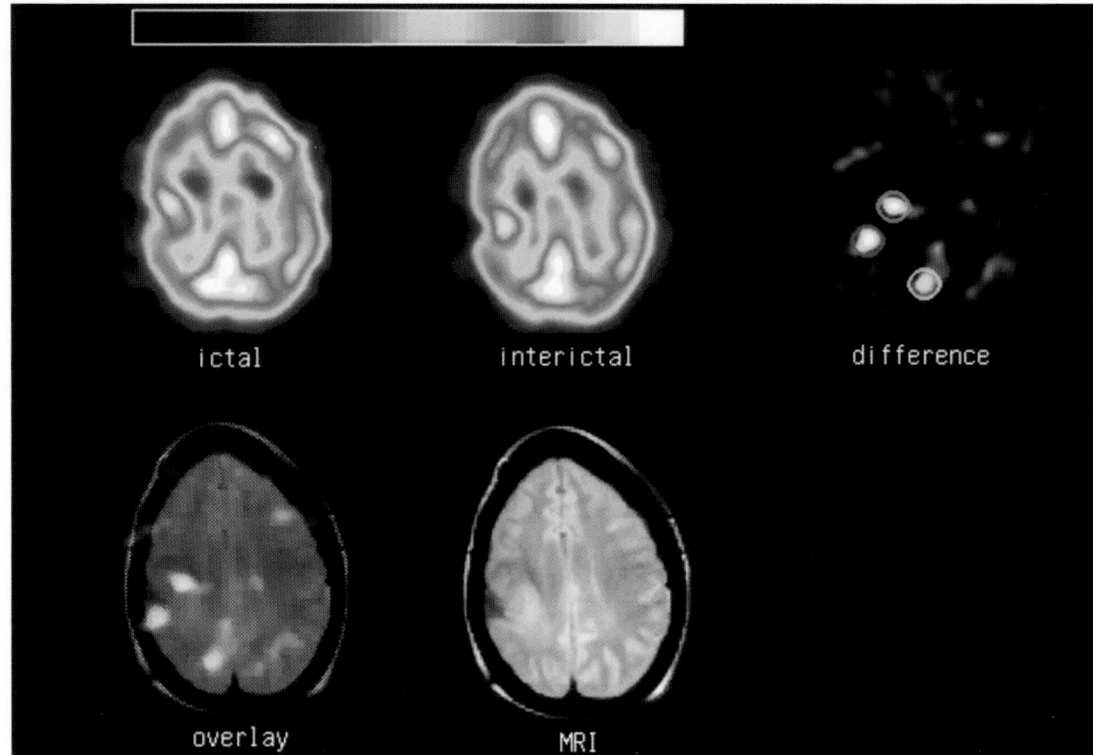

Figure 8.4.

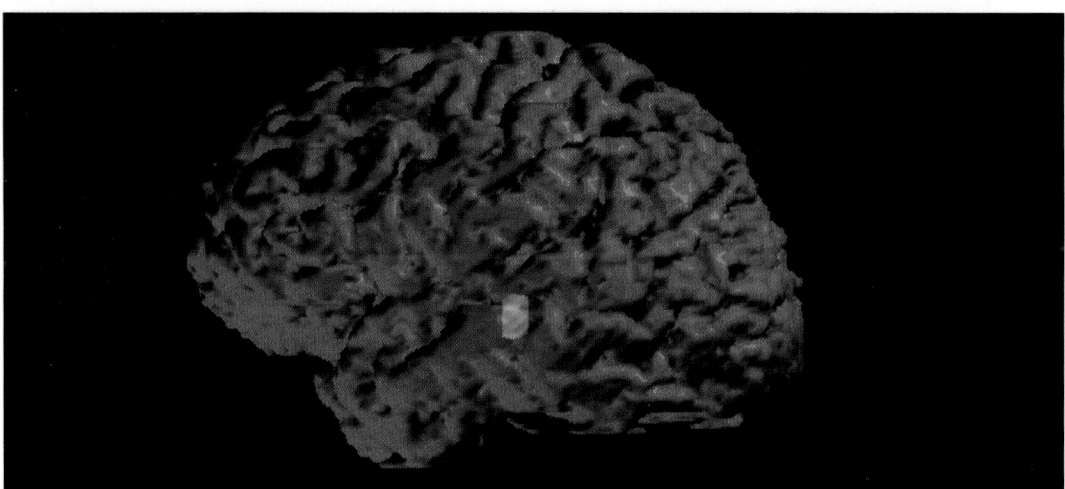

Figure 8.5.

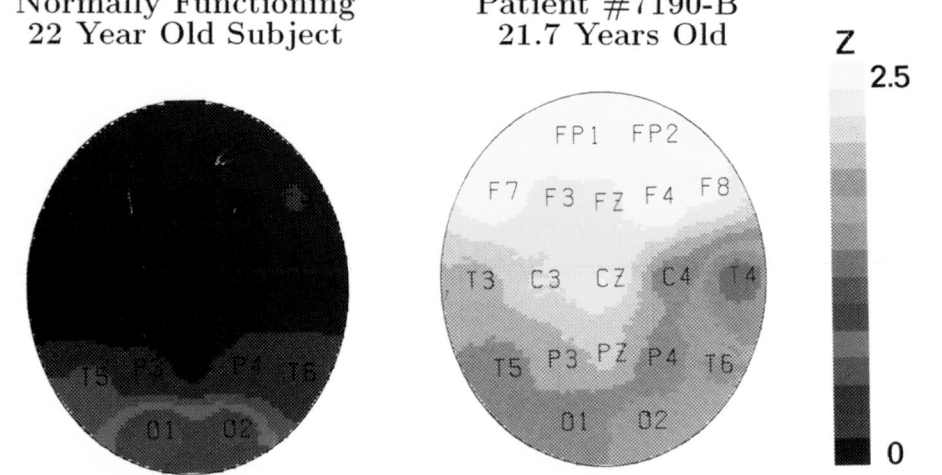

Figure 124.8C

as preliminary. A technically superior MRI study of 22 male adolescent and adult autistic patients and 20 male community control subjects reported significantly larger lateral ventricles in the autistic group, although total cerebral and parenchymal volumes were significantly greater and performance IQ was significantly lower in the autistic subjects, thereby confounding interpretaton of the ventricular findings (Piven et al., 1995).

Regional Cortical Abnormalities. Although no consistent cortical abnormalities have been found, a high incidence of regional abnormalities have been described in varying regions of the cerebral cortex in autistic subjects. Courchesne and colleagues, for instance, provided non-quantitative assessments of the parietal lobe in autistic subjects, reporting various subtle abnormalities in 9 (43%) of 21 subjects, while none were found in 12 control subjects. Abnormalities included apparent volume loss in the gray and white matter of the parietal lobe that occasionally extended into the frontal and occipital lobes (Courchesne et al., 1993). It is unclear from this report whether these cortical findings were based on a review of the scans that was entirely blind to subject diagnosis. In addition, the findings have not yet been replicated. Another investigation of 13 high-functioning male autistic and 13 matched control subjects detected cortical malformations in 7 of the autistic and in none of the control subjects (Piven et al., 1990). Malformations included polymicrogyria in 5, schizencephaly and macrogyria in 1, and macrogyria in another subject. Because neuronal migration abnormalities are thought to produce the kinds of cortical abnormalities described, the findings suggest that disturbances in neuronal migration during early CNS development could play some pathophysiological role in at least some autistic individuals. Moreover, if findings of neuronal migration abnormalities are replicated, they would suggest that the pathophysiological insult in autism occurs sometime in the first 6 months of gestation.

PET studies have not demonstrated consistent regional abnormalities in blood flow or metabolism, although inconsistent regional abnormalities in metabolism have been seen throughout the cortex (Horwitz et al., 1988; Rumsey et al., 1985). One SPECT study of 21 autistic children did not detect any blood flow abnormalities when compared with 14 children with language disorder, although the limitations of SPECT resolution does not preclude the possibility that real group differences could have gone undetected (Zilbovicius et al., 1992).

Functional and structural imaging modalities have been combined in a small number of autistic subjects to help localize regions of cortical abnormality. Of 13 mentally retarded, autistic children, 4 had regional abnormalities on both PET and either CT or MRI, and two additional patients had abnormal PET or MRI scans, but not both (Schifter et al., 1994). PET abnormalities included primarily localized regions of hypometabolism in cortical association areas, especially in the parietal, occipital, and temporal areas. In three of the five scans showing structural abnormalities, those abnormalities consisted of focal pachygyria, which again is suggestive of a neuronal migration abnormality. Two of the three structural abnormalities were detected only as a consequence of metabolic abnormalities having first been detected in those regions on the PET scans. Although this study highlights the potential usefulness of combined structural and functional imaging applications within single subjects, as well as the possible etiologic importance of neuronal migration abnormalities in autism, these conclusions must be still be regarded as preliminary, since the findings are based on a small number of subjects in the absence of a control group.

A preliminary MRS study compared the high energy phosphate and membrane phospholipid metabolism in the prefrontal cortex of 11 high-functioning autistic adolescents and adults with that of 11 normal control subjects matched by age, gender, IQ, race, and socioeconomic status (Minshew et al., 1993). Although the understanding of the physiological significance MRS data is still rapidly evolving, this early study seems to indicate hypermetabolism in the dorsal prefrontal cortex of high-functioning autistic subjects. Furthermore, within the autistic group, performance on neuropsychological tasks correlated with metabolite levels

in this prefrontal region, a portion of the cortex that is believed to subserve the performance of these particular tasks. In addition, the data provided evidence for undersynthesis and enhanced degradation of cell membranes, the significance of which is still unknown.

Posterior Fossa Abnormalities. Considerable excitement in the study of autism followed initial reports of hypoplasia of certain cerebellar subregions, vermian lobules VI and VII, as visualized on MRI scans. In an initial report of the midsagittal cross-sectional area of cerebellar vermian lobules VI and VII in 18 autistic and 12 normal control subjects, vermian lobule size averaged 19% smaller in the autistic subjects (Courchesne et al., 1988). In a subsequent report, cerebellar volume estimates and vermian lobule cross-sectional areas were measured in 10 autistic and 8 control subjects, a sample that overlapped somewhat that of Courchesne (1988). Cerebellar volume was reduced by 12% and the superior-posterior vermis size was reduced by 20% in the autistic subjects compared with the controls (Murakami et al., 1989). These initial neuroradiologic findings were exciting primarily because they were the first reports of structural pathology imaged in the actual brain substance of living autistic subjects (as opposed to reported abnormalities of the ventricular system) and because the findings were consistent with histopathological reports of reduced numbers of cerebellar Purkinje and granule cells in autistic subjects (Bauman and Kemper, 1985; Ritvo et al., 1986).

Despite the initial excitement generated by these findings, subsequent studies have had difficulty confirming cerebellar hypoplasia (Hashimoto et al., 1992; Ritvo and Garber, 1988). One MRI study of 13 autistic and 28 control children failed to find group differences in the size of the vermal lobules, the fourth ventricle, or pons (Kleiman et al., 1992), and another MRI study of 15 high functioning autistic and 15 matched control subjects failed to find group differences when lobule size was adjusted for age, IQ, and brain cross-sectional area in the midsagittal plane (Piven et al., 1992). Alterations in cerebellar blood flow or metabolism have not yet been detected (Chris-Heh et al., 1989).

Subsequently, the investigators who initially reported the cerebellar findings in autism reviewed their data, studied additional subjects (bringing total sample size to 50), and performed a meta-analysis of prior MRI studies of cerebellar size in autism (bringing the meta-analysis sample size to 88) (Courchesne et al., 1994a, 1994b). They concluded that the failure to replicate the findings of hypoplasia was in part due to subject sample sizes that were too small to detect the magnitude of the group differences that they previously had found. They also suggested that the distribution of sizes of cerebellar lobule VI-VII is bimodal, with a large subgroup of autistic subjects having small lobules, and a smaller subgroup having larger lobules, when compared with normal subjects. Although the graphical representation of their data may indeed suggest that the size of lobule VI-VII is bimodally distributed in autistic subjects, it must be cautioned that the frequency distribution of cerebellar volumes could be changed into a merely skewed distribution having a greater than average variance, simply by including two or more subjects who have lobule sizes falling in the region of the distribution that interfaces the hypoplastic and hyperplastic subtypes (i.e., the feature making the distribution appear bimodal appears statistically very unstable). Therefore, the ''findings'' based on this assumption of bimodality must be considered post hoc, exploratory, and preliminary. The cerebellar abnormalities, whether they are hypoplastic or hyperplastic in nature, require confirmation. If confirmed, their pathophysiological significance is still unclear. They could, for example, represent some central pathological abnormality in autism. The findings could also be regarded, however, as reflecting a more distal marker for some other more central pathophysiologic insult occurring early during central nervous system development, when the cerebellar lobules and many other important brain regions are actively being formed.

Other posterior fossa abnormalities that have been reported include reduced size of the midbrain and medulla in 12 mentally retarded autistic and 15 retarded nonautistic children compared with 14 control subjects (cerebellar vermis lobule sizes did not differ between groups in this study) (Hashimoto et al., 1992). Although the significance of these yet unreplicated findings is unknown, they may, like cerebellar vermian size, be a marker for earlier developmental brain injury. They may also represent correlates of previously reported abnormalities in neurotransmitter regulation in autistic subjects, since the majority of neurotransmitter systems arise from the brainstem.

SPECIFIC MENTAL RETARDATION SYNDROMES

Mental retardation syndromes have been grossly understudied, largely because of ethical and legal concerns regarding any potential adverse effects from imaging procedures in children whose ability to provide informed consent may be compromised. Heterogeneity of mental retardation syndromes has also complicated the interpretability of findings and slowed research in this important area. With the beginning elucidation of homogeneous genetic subtypes of retardation syndromes, as has happened with fragile X and Down's syndromes, specifying the precise neurobiologic effects of very specific genetic defects may now be possible. Despite the relative etiologic homogeneity of these syndromes, finding appropriate contrast groups still proves to be a methodologic conundrum, since important potential confounding variables such as IQ are likely to correlate with structural and functional measures throughout the cerebrum. In addition, studying other subnormal IQ subjects as a contrast group is likely to include other genetic and nongenetic syndromes that may spuriously affect the comparison of patient and control groups. The first structure studied in both fragile X and Down's syndromes was the cerebellum, which was largely prompted by the prior findings of cerebellar abnormalities in autism, a heterogeneous developmental disorder that shares several clinical features with these more homogeneous disorders.

Fragile X Syndrome

The Posterior Fossa. Few neuroimaging studies have been conducted in fragile X research. The largest and most rigorous study has been that of Reiss et al. (1991a, 1991b, 1994). When compared with age, sex, and IQ-matched normal control subjects and with others having a variety of "neurobehavioral or developmental" disorders, 14 male fragile X subjects were noted to have reduced midsagittal cross-sectional areas of the posterior cerebellar vermis, lobules VI and VII in particular. The fourth ventricle was increased in size, which is consistent with a reduced size of the adjacent cerebellar vermis. Vermian size in 12 females heterozygous for the fragile X mutation was intermediate between the sizes seen in fragile X males and those seen in control subjects. This would suggest some degree of dose-response relationship between the degree of genetic loading and the manifestation of both clinical phenotype and brain-based morphology, since fragile X males, who are by definition homozygotes, are more clinically and neuropsychologically impaired than are female heterozygotes. That the findings of vermian size reductions persist even when compared with developmentally delayed children suggests that the cerebellar findings are not simply associated with just any behavioral or developmental disturbance and that the findings have some degree of specificity in fragile X. The similarities of the findings to those in autism, however, of course indicate some degree of nonspecificity, and also raise the question of whether the findings in autism could be attributable in part to the inclusion of misdiagnosed fragile X subjects.

Temporal Lobe. Fragile X subjects also appear to have proportionately larger hippocampal volumes bilaterally when compared with a heterogeneous group of other age- and IQ-matched, developmentally delayed children (Reiss et al., 1994). The hippocampus was studied for two reasons: (*a*) the hippocampus is thought to subserve in part certain cognitive functions in which fragile X subjects are typically deficient, such as memory, attention, affect, sensory response, and socialization; (*b*) expression of the mouse homologue of the fragile X mental retardation 1 gene was reported to be most concentrated in the granular layers

of both the cerebellum and hippocampus (Hinds et al., 1993), and messenger RNA expression in human fetal brains was greatest in the pyramidal neurons of the hippocampus and the cholinergic neurons of the nucleus basalis (Abitbol et al., 1993). In addition to the hippocampal volume increases, volume decrements were seen in the superior temporal gyrus, a region involved in auditory and language processing. Decreasing size of the superior temporal gyrus and increasing size of the hippocampus bilaterally correlated strongly with increasing age in fragile X but not in control subjects, suggesting the possibility of ongoing neurobiologic degeneration in the disorder, although the authors correctly note that only longitudinal prospective studies can address this hypothesis directly.

Down's Syndrome

Cerebral Cortex. The first MRI study of Down's syndrome (DS) involved only three adolescent subjects (Jernigan and Bellugi, 1990). Comparison groups included 14 normal control subjects (ages 8–32) and 6 adolescents with Williams syndrome (WS). WS is a rare genetic disorder producing characteristic facies and neuropsychological deficits that include mental retardation with a relative sparing of linguistic ability. Sample size was increased in a later report to include 6 DS, 9 WS, and 21 normal subjects (Jernigan et al., 1993). In both studies, overall brain volume was significantly reduced in DS and WS patients compared with normals, consistent with postmortem and CT studies of DS adults (Schapiro et al., 1992; Solitaire and Lamarche, 1967). An important caveat is that brain volume comparisons did not control for subject height, which is known to correlate with brain volume in normal subjects and which could be an important confound, given the generally smaller stature of DS and WS subjects compared to same-age norms. Total cerebral gray matter was also reduced equally in both DS and WS subjects. Subregion analyses, however, revealed that the DS subjects had less gray matter in the frontal cortex than did either the WS or normal control subjects, suggesting a greater hypofrontality in DS. In addition, DS gray matter of the limbic region relative to whole brain gray matter volume also was reduced in DS compared with WS and normal subjects, and it exhibited some degree of specificity, as the limbic gray matter of WS patients did not differ from that of normal subjects. The temporolimbic gray matter reductions in DS appeared larger on the left than on the right side.

Consistent with these findings of DS frontal cortex volume reduction were findings of reduced midline cross-sectional area of the anterior corpus callosum in these same DS, WS, and normal control subjects (Wang et al., 1992). The anterior region of the corpus callosum is the portion through which the interhemispheric fibers of the prefrontal cortex pass (Lamantia and Rakic, 1990). Whether the cortical and callosal findings represent a hypoplastic (failure to develop) or an atrophic (degenerative) process is unknown. Histopathological studies demonstrating smaller structures in midterm fetuses (Schmidt-Sidor et al., 1990), and the presenile cortical degeneration in DS that is associated with the accumulation of amyloid plaques and neurofibrillary tangles, suggest that the cortical imaging findings could be both hypoplastic and degenerative in nature. Cortical and ventricular CSF appears to increase in older DS subjects compared with normal and younger DS subjects, again suggesting degenerative processes in aging DS subjects (Schapiro et al., 1992).

Preliminary PET studies may be consistent with these morphological findings. Although global and regional CBF and metabolism studies surprisingly have not in general demonstrated differences between DS and normal control subjects, the patterning of regional intercorrelations of cerebral metabolism may be altered in DS. Metabolic patterns involving frontal and parietal regions, and language systems in particular, appear to be abnormal (Horwitz et al., 1990). These structural and functional findings are thought to reflect the language disability commonly seen in DS.

Posterior Fossa. Again, largely because of the previous findings of reduced vermian size in autism, the first brain region studied in Down's syndrome was the cerebellar vermis. Overall cerebellar volume and the sizes of all vermian lobules were reduced in DS compared with normal control subjects (Jernigan et al., 1990, 1993). WS individuals, in contrast, appeared to have specifically enlarged vermian lobules VI and VII, both in absolute value and in relation to the size of the remaining vermis. The whole brain and cerebellar volume reductions in DS were consistent with previous histopathological findings (Crome et al., 1966). The apparently hypoplastic and hyperplastic vermian lobules seen in these two severe developmental disorders lend some credence to the possibility of hypoplastic and hyperplastic vermian lobule subtypes in autism, which is undoubtedly a heterogeneous group of severe developmental disorders.

Subcortex. Absolute volumes of the lenticular nucleus and diencephalon (thalamus and hypothalamus) in the Jernigan studies (1990, 1993) did not differ between DS and normal control subjects, while volumes in WS were decreased in proportion to their overall brain gray matter volume reductions. These findings suggest a relative sparing of subcortical motor and sensory systems in DS, relative to DS cortical deficits.

Schizophrenia

Neuroimaging studies have made important contributions to understanding the neurobiology of schizophrenia. The early CT studies of schizophrenia in the late 1970s and early 1980s that demonstrated enlarged ventricular volumes were, along with the proven efficacy of chlorpromazine in schizophrenia treatment, of central importance in establishing the biological basis of the disorder and marked an important turning point in the history of psychiatry.

Frontal Cortex. From the early CT studies of ventricular size, progress in the neuroimaging of schizophrenia included demonstration of increased CSF volumes in the cerebral sulci (Gur et al., 1991). Reduced volumes of the frontal cortex (e.g., Andreasen et al., 1986) have not been consistently replicated (e.g., Andreasen et al., 1990), likely due to methodological difficulties in consistently defining the region of interest and to structural and functional heterogeneity within that portion of the cortex. The study that has employed the most methodologically rigorous morphometrics of the frontal cortex in 52 schizophrenic adults and 90 normal control subjects demonstrated a specific decrease in frontal lobe volume of the schizophrenics that persisted even after controlling for smaller brain volumes in that group (Andreasen et al., 1994).

Functional studies have been reasonably consistent in demonstrating reduced blood flow and metabolism to the frontal cortex in schizophrenia (e.g., Buchsbaum et al., 1992); they have in addition suggested that the hypofrontality is related to the presence of negative symptoms and not to previous neuroleptic treatment (Andreasen et al., 1992; Berman et al., 1992; Wolkin et al., 1992). Preliminary studies of monozygotic twins discordant for the presence of schizophrenia furthermore suggest that the hypofrontality of schizophrenia is of nongenetic origin (Berman et al., 1992).

Temporal Lobe Structures. Structural studies of temporolimbic cortex have been more successful than structural studies of frontal cortex in consistently demonstrating regional abnormality. Reduced volumes of the anterior superior temporal gyrus on the left, presumably the neural substrate of auditory association cortex, correlated with ratings of hallucination severity (Barta et al., 1990). Others subsequently confirmed abnormalities in the left-sided superior temporal gyrus (e.g., Shenton et al., 1992). Volume reductions in more mesial structures, like the amygdala and hippocampus, have also been reported in schizophrenia (e.g., Bogerts et al., 1990; Breier et al., 1992; Suddath et al., 1990), and some degree of disease specificity for the gray matter volume reductions in these areas has been demonstrated (Schlaepfer et al., 1994). Reduced volumes of temporal lobe structures generally corroborate similar findings from postmortem studies of schizophrenia (Bogerts et al., 1985; Brown et al., 1986; Colter et al., 1987).

Findings from functional imaging studies of the temporal lobe and limbic regions have been less consistent than functional studies of frontal cortex. Both increased and decreased metabolism have been reported in the temporal lobe (DeLisi et al., 1989; Jernigan et al., 1985; Tamminga et al., 1992) and in the anterior cingulate cortex (Tamminga et al., 1992). Positive correlations with symptom severity have been noted in the parahippocampal gyrus (Liddle et al., 1992; Musalek et al., 1989), hippocampus and amygdala (DeLisi et al., 1989; Musalek et al., 1989), and in Broca's area during auditory hallucinations (McGuire et al., 1993).

Posterior Fossa. The cerebellar vermis has been measured on the MR images of 30 adult male schizophrenic and 11 normal control subjects (Nasrallah et al., 1991). Contrary to the hypothesis that vermian lobules would be reduced in schizophrenia, as they were initially reported to be in autism, the sizes of all vermian lobules were actually found to be larger in the schizophrenic group. The group comparisons did not control for the possible confounding effects of differences in overall brain volume. These findings of increased vermian lobule sizes were not confirmed in a larger MRI study of 36 schizophrenic and 51 normal control subjects (Aylward et al., 1994). Brainstem volumes also did not differ between groups. These conflicting results may be due to diagnostic heterogeneity or to differences in imaging and morphometric procedures.

Basal Ganglia. Alterations in basal ganglia morphology have been reported in schizophrenia, although findings have been somewhat inconsistent. Several investigators have found either no differences between the basal ganglia of schizophrenic compared to control subjects or else trends toward volume reduction (e.g., DeLisi et al., 1991). Reports of increased basal ganglia volumes have been more common, however (Elkashef et al., 1994; Jernigan et al., 1991c; Swayze et al., 1992). The finding of structural enlargement runs counter to the usual pattern in neurobiology, in which disease is generally associated with smaller structures; the replication of this rather unusual finding several times within the same disorder tends to speak to its validity. Increased striatal volumes, more pronounced on the left, and increased globus pallidus volumes, especially on the right, have also been reported in a postmortem study (Heckers et al., 1991).

Functional studies have generally documented decreased metabolism and blood flow in the basal ganglia of schizophrenic subjects (Buchsbaum et al., 1987, 1992a; Early et al., 1989; Siegel et al., 1993). Low metabolic rates in the striatum may predict positive clinical response to neuroleptics (Buchsbaum et al., 1992b), and indeed neuroleptic treatment appears to increase basal ganglia metabolism (Buchsbaum et al., 1987; Szechtman et al., 1988) and possibly basal ganglia volumes as well (Chakos et al., 1994).

Although postmortem studies have suggested an increased density of D_2 receptors in the caudate and putamen of schizophrenic subjects, including those never treated with neuroleptic medication (Seeman and Niznik, 1990), the findings from receptor imaging studies of the dopamine D_2 receptor system in schizophrenia have thus far been inconclusive. A $[^{11}C]N$-methyl-spiperone (NMSP) PET study has demonstrated a 2- to 3-fold increase in D_2 receptor density in the caudate nuclei of 15 schizophrenic compared with 11 normal control subjects (Wong et al., 1986). Mean striatal D_2 receptor densities were not found to differ, however, between neuroleptic-naive schizophrenic and control subjects in two studies using $[^{11}C]$raclopride as the radioligand tracer (Farde et al., 1990; Hietala et al., 1994). Despite these negative findings, there was some evidence for D_2 receptor density abnormalities in the striata of a subset of these schizophrenic subjects (Hietala et al., 1994). Differing pharmacokinetics of the two ligands used in these PET studies may account for the differences in their findings. Seeman and colleagues (1993) have presented data suggesting, for instance, that the study differences may be attributable to the differing binding affinities of the two radioligands to the numerous subtypes of dopamine receptor. Using postmortem tissue from elderly schizophrenic subjects, they demonstrated a 6-fold increase in striatal D_4 receptors of schizophrenic subjects compared with tissue from normal controls. Because NMSP has a greater binding affinity for D_4 receptors than does raclopride, the PET findings of increased dopamine receptors in schizophrenia using NMSP but not raclopride may be due to binding of NMSP to both D_2 and D_4 receptors. In addition to these pathophysiological studies, receptor ligand-based imaging has been initiated in neuropharmacological studies of antipsychotic medications, which may lead to important treatment refinements in psychotic disorders (Sedvall, 1990).

Thalamus. Neuroimaging evidence for thalamic involvement in the pathophysiology of schizophrenia is recent. Using novel image processing techniques adapted from PET studies, Andreasen and her colleagues (1994) have warped individual brain scans to uniform coordinates defined by a ''bounding box'' in three dimensions and then added together in their respective groups the images of 39 male patients and 47 normal male control subjects, to derive an ''average brain'' for each group. The brightness of each corresponding pixel of the two group-averaged brain images were compared. The major differences between the two averaged brains was primarily in the right hemithalamus and in the white matter tracts (the internal capsule) adjacent to it. Although the data are compelling and the image processing techniques are ingenious, the findings, of course, require replication. Nevertheless, the findings suggest an important role for the thalamus in the pathophysiology of schizophrenia. The authors suggest that thalamic lesions could produce a loss of sensory gating in the illness, with a consequent flooding of cortical centers with sensory stimuli and an attendant fragmentation of thought processes experienced as delusions and hallucinations.

Abnormal Cerebral Asymmetries. One of the most robust and recent constellations of findings in the neuroimaging of schizophrenia concerns the absence or loss of normal structural and functional brain asymmetries. Perhaps the strongest structural asymmetry findings in schizophrenia are volumetric studies of the temporal lobe, which include postmortem reports of increased size of the temporal horn of the left lateral ventricle (Crow et al., 1989) and varying reports of lateralized abnormalities in temporal lobe substructures like the superior temporal gyrus, hippocampus, and amygdala (Barta et al., 1990; Bogerts et al., 1990). Schizophrenic subjects, in addition, have been reported to have, in comparison to normal control subjects, less structural lateralization of their basal ganglia (Breier et al., 1992; Elkashef et al., 1994) and of numerous cortical subregions (Bilder et al., 1994). These abnormalities in structural asymmetries may have functional correlates in the disorder, as abnormal asymmetries in cortical and subcortical blood flow and metabolic rates have been reported quite consistently in those functional studies that have examined it (Buchsbaum et al., 1992a; Early et al., 1989; Siegel et al., 1993; Szechtman et al., 1988). Neuroleptics may affect striatal metabolism asymmetrically, preferentially increasing right-sided activity (Buchsbaun et al., 1992b; Szechtman et al., 1988). Although dopamine D_2 receptor density asymmetries in the putamen have been reported (Farde et al., 1990), this finding has not yet been confirmed (Hietala et al., 1994).

The pathophysiologic implication of these apparent asymmetry aberrancies is still unknown. Normal lateralization of the CNS appears to be under both genetic and nongenetic control, and abnormal lateralization in schizophrenia conceivably could be due to disturbances in either. Nongenetic determinants of normal lateralization appear to include prenatal neurohormones, sex steroids in particular (Geschwind and Galaburda, 1987). Animal models of cerebral lateralization have suggested that maternal stress during pregnancy can dramatically alter cerebral structural lateralization (Fleming et al., 1986), as well as the lateralization of important neurotransmitter systems such as dopamine (Fride and Weinstock, 1989). Maternal stress may induce these changes in lateralization by altering the magnitude and timing of sex hormone surges during critical periods of lateralizing prenatal central nervous system development (Ward, 1984).

One particularly elegant imaging study of schizophrenia deserves special mention with regard to these issues of perinatal stress; the study potentially may have importance in better understanding the pathophysiology of the disorder, even though it does not directly examine cerebral lateralization. Cannon et al. (1993) studied the importance that gene-environment interactions may have in determining features of brain structure in schizophrenia by assessing varying degrees of genetic loading for schizophrenia in the context of varying degrees of perinatal risk and obstetrical complication. A cohort of adolescents evaluated initially at age 15 were classified as having one (N = 72), two (N = 25), or no (N = 60) parents with schizophrenia. Their obstetrical records were reviewed for perinatal and obstetrical complications. All subjects then underwent CT scanning in midadulthood, and the volumes of their lateral ventricles were assessed. Significant interactions were detected between the degree of genetic risk for each subject and the severity of obstetrical complications in predicting the size of the ventricular system. These findings suggest that *both* genes *and* environment are important in the determination of cerebral structures in high-risk individuals and, furthermore, that genes and environment are *interactive* in their effects on cerebral development. Although these findings apply to individuals at high genetic risk for schizophreniform illness, and thus may not necessarily be directly applicable to individuals who actually develop the illness, and although the CT scans do not provide anatomic information anywhere near the quality of modern MRI scans, the general approach to assessing gene-environment interactions in the determination of neurobiological substrate will likely be an increasingly important program of research in the neuroimaging of developmental psychopathologies.

Obsessive Compulsive Disorder

Ventricular System. Reports of ventricular size in OCD have been inconsistent in their findings. The first CT study of 10 OCD adults reported no ventricular enlargement, cortical atrophy, or other consistent gross morphologic abnormality (Insel et al., 1983). The next CT study of 16 adolescents with OCD, however, found significantly higher mean ventricle:brain ratios than in matched control subjects (Behar et al., 1984), although this was not later confirmed in 12 adults (Kellner et al., 1991).

Cortical Regions. Numerous PET and SPECT studies have consistently shown increased metabolism and blood flow in the orbitofrontal cortex of OCD subjects (Baxter et al., 1987, 1988; Machlin et al., 1991; Nordahl et al., 1989; Rubin et al., 1992; Swedo et al., 1989, 1992). Hypermetabolism has been reported in several additional brain regions, including the anterior cingulum (Rauch et al., 1994; Swedo et al., 1989), right sensorimotor cortex (Swedo et al., 1989), and dorsal parietal cortices (Rubin et al., 1992). Only one of these studies imaged adult OCD subjects who specifically were determined to have had a childhood onset of illness, and in that study symptom severity was seen to correlate with prefrontal and orbitofrontal metabolism (Swedo et al., 1989, 1992). Depression comorbidity did not appear to be responsible for the elevated metabolic rates in frontal cortex (Baxter et al., 1990).

Several investigators have found not only that regional frontal hypermetabolism normalizes in response to successful antiobsessional therapies (Baxter et al., 1987, 1990, 1992; Hoehn-Saric et al., 1991; Swedo et al., 1992), but that the degree of OC symptom improvement also correlates with the decrement in orbitofrontal metabolic activity (Baxter et al., 1992; Swedo et al., 1992). In addition, a ^{33}Xe study in 10 OCD patients demonstrated a symptom exacerbation that correlated with an increase in frontal cortex rCBF after administration of meta-chlorophenylpiperazine (m-CPP), a serotonin agonist (Hollander et al., 1991). Similarly, symptom provocation during ^{15}O-labeled CO_2 gas inhalation by 8 OCD patients demonstrated increases in rCBF compared with the resting state in the left anterior cingulate and bilateral orbitofrontal cortices (Rauch et al., 1994).

Basal Ganglia. Reduced caudate nucleus volumes were initially reported in CT images of 10 young adult OCD males, compared with age- and sex-matched control subjects (Luxenberg et al., 1988). An MRI study of 12 OCD patients, however, then failed to confirm caudate nucleus volume reduction and in addition found no morphologic abnormalities in the cingulum, corpus callosum, or ventricular size (Kellner et al., 1991). An MRI study of 20 OCD adults found an *increased* volume of the head of the right caudate nucleus compared with that of normal control subjects, but these volumes were not corrected for the overall brain sizes of the subjects (Scarone et al., 1992). The most methodologically rigorous MRI study to date of caudate nucleus volumes in 26 adult OCD and 26 normal controls recently reported a significant 11% bilateral volume reduction in the OCD group (Robinson et al., 1995). Higher signal intensity values in the left compared to the right caudate have been reported in adult OCD subjects, but not in normal controls (Calabrese et al., 1993).

Two PET studies reported hypermetabolism of the caudate (Baxter et al., 1987, 1988). Three others, however, reported no group differences (Nordahl et al., 1989; Swedo et al., 1989, 1992), and one SPECT study reported bilaterally decreased caudate rCBF (Rubin et al., 1992). Symptom provocation may increase rCBF to the right caudate nucleus (Rauch et al., 1994). Effective treatment of OCD, whether from medication or behavioral therapy, has been associated with a decrease in normalized metabolic rates of the right caudate nucleus, compared with no changes in metabolism seen in nonresponders and normal control subjects (Baxter et al., 1992). Changes in right caudate metabolic rates during treatment, moreover, correlated with changes in OC symptom severity ratings.

Although demonstrations of flow and metabolism changes in the caudate and orbitofrontal cortex during treatment and symptom provocation are important findings, it must be cautioned that, as with all statistical associations, group differences and change measures do not demonstrate causality. It is possible, for instance, that subcortical and cortical group differences represent a *response* to the presence of obsessions and compulsions. The findings could, for example, represent inhibitory or compensatory mechanisms of the orbitofrontal cortex and caudate nucleus that manifest in functional images during an attempt to suppress obsessions or resist compulsions. Symptom provocation would then increase and effective treatment would decrease the need for these inhibitory processes. Thus, imaging findings should not be regarded as providing proof that the metabolically more active regions of interest are the brain centers generating OC symptoms.

Abnormal Asymmetries. Cerebral asymmetries in OCD have not been studied extensively. T_1 asymmetry differences in 13 OCD subjects, however, were reported in the frontal white matter, and T_1 asymmetry indices in the orbital frontal cortex, anterior cingulum, and lenticular nucleus correlated strongly with symptom severity (Garber et al., 1989). As already noted, abnormal asymmetries have been reported for caudate nucleus volumes (Scarone et al., 1992) and T_1-weighted image signal intensities (Calabrese et al., 1993).

Tourette's Syndrome

Ventricular Size. An initial CT study of children with Tourette's syndrome (TS) reported ventricular enlargement and asymmetry in 4 of 20 patients, although volumes of the ventricles and other brain regions were not reported (Harcherik et al., 1985). A later MRI study found trends toward ventricular enlargement and a statistically significant increase in the variance of ventricular volumes bilaterally (Peterson et al., 1993b).

Basal Ganglia. Lenticular nucleus volume reductions were first reported in an MRI study of 14 medication-free, neuroleptic-naive, adult TS patients and 14 individually matched normal control subjects (Peterson et al., 1993b). The volume reductions, nearly 11% on the left and 4% on the right side, attained statistical significance only on the left, and volume reductions in both the globus pallidus and putamen nuclei (which together comprise the lenticular nucleus) seemed to contribute equally to the group differences.

From this first report alone, it is impossible to exclude the possibility that the basal ganglia volume differences are the consequence of plastic changes in the adult TS CNS due to having had a chronic neuropsychiatric disorder since early childhood. The predominantly left-sided reduction, however, has been confirmed in a cohort of 37 children with TS,

which speaks against the likelihood that the differences are a plastic response to the presence of chronic illness (Singer et al., 1993). The confirmation also places the determination of the morphological changes at an earlier period of development, into early childhood at least, and perhaps even before, into fetal or perinatal life.

TS functional imaging studies generally corroborate basal ganglia pathology. An FDG PET study reported a 15% decrement in nonnormalized glucose utilization in the frontal, cingulate, and insular cortices, as well as in the "inferior corpus striatum" (Chase et al., 1986). A technically superior study also found hypometabolism in the ventral striatum, specifically in the nucleus accumbens, ventromedial caudate, and left anterior putamen (Braun et al., 1993; Stoetter et al., 1992). An increased number of presynaptic dopamine uptake sites in the basal ganglia has been reported in a preliminary study of 5 unmedicated TS subjects (Malison et al., in press); D_2/D_3 receptor availability, however, has not been found to differ from control levels (George et al., 1994).

Cortical Regions. An FDG PET study of 12 TS adults reported decreases in metabolic rates in the frontal and cingulate cortices (Chase et al., 1986). A significant inverse correlation between the severity of both motor and vocal tics and glucose utilization in these same regions was also seen. A more recent FDG PET study using a higher resolution scanner in 16 medication-free TS adults reported decreased glucose utilization in the orbitofrontal, parahippocampal (entorhinal), and inferior insular cortices, as well as in the midbrain (Braun et al., 1993; Stoetter et al., 1992). A SPECT blood flow study found differences in frontal lobe/basal ganglia ratios in "pure TS" compared with TS subjects who had comorbid OCD, although the differences were not statistically significant (George et al., 1992).

Abnormal Asymmetries. Adult TS subjects appear to lack the volumetric asymmetries seen in normal basal ganglia (Peterson et al., 1993b). TS subjects appear to have either reduced or reversed asymmetries in their globus pallidi, lenticular nuclei, and total basal ganglia volumes. Basal ganglia asymmetry abnormalities have been confirmed in TS children (Singer et al., 1993), who have been noted to lack normal asymmetry in the putamen and in the lenticular nuclei. Subgroup analyses seem to indicate that TS males in particular have smaller left putamen, lenticular, and globus pallidus nuclei compared with normal subjects, which may account for the loss of normal left-larger-than-right asymmetries. TS subjects with comorbid attention deficit hyperactivity disorder (ADHD) have also been reported to have a smaller left globus pallidus than either the TS subjects without ADHD or the control subjects.

An MRI study of 10 TS monozygotic twin pairs who were concordant for the presence of tic disorders but discordant for tic symptom severity demonstrated reduced right caudate nucleus volume in the cotwin with the more severe tic syndrome. Given the previous findings of reduced right caudate nucleus volumes in ADHD (Castellanos et al., 1994) and bilateral reduction in OCD (Robinson et al., 1995), it is unfortunate that ADHD and OCD comorbidity in these MZ twins was not characterized. Nevertheless, the findings suggest that right caudate nucleus volume reductions, if real, are attributable to nonshared environmental determinants, and not to the effects of the TS gene (Hyde et al., 1995). This same group also replicated in the MZ twin group previous findings that the co-twin with the greater symptom severity had the lower birthweight (Leckman et al., 1987; Hyde et al., 1992), providing indirect evidence for the importance of perinatal events in the pathophysiology of TS brain structure and symptom severity.

Altered T_2 relaxation time asymmetries have been noted in the TS insular cortex and frontal white matter and in the putamen and caudate nuclei. T_2 times appear to be shorter in the TS right amygdala and right red nucleus, with similar trends seen in the corresponding left-sided structures (Peterson, Gore et al., 1994). Because the determinants of relaxation times are many and complex, it is at this time impossible to say precisely what is responsible for the abnormal asymmetries. Nonetheless, the group differences in TS T_2 relaxation time asymmetries are consistent with the hypothesis of altered CNS lateralization in the disorder.

Lastly, TS subjects appear to have an exaggerated lateral ventricular asymmetry compared with normal control subjects (Peterson et al., 1993b). TS right ventricle volumes may be as much as 26% larger on the right than on the left. The significance of these findings is still unknown, although it could indicate the presence either of a right hemisphere cortical abnormality producing a "hydrocephalus ex vacuo" or else a left-sided parenchymal hypertrophy causing relatively smaller left lateral ventricles. The bilateral trend toward larger ventricles favors the former interpretation.

Corpus Callosum. It has been hypothesized that the alteration of structural lateralization found in TS basal ganglia might also be seen in other lateralized cerebral structures (Peterson, Leckman et al., 1994). Given the massive funneling of interhemispheric axons through the corpus callosum (CC) and the subsequent potential sensitivity of CC size as an index of change in cortical anatomy, it was hypothesized that those changes in cerebral asymmetries, if present, might be reflected as changes in TS CC morphology. In the same 14 adult TS subjects in whom the basal ganglia structural asymmetries and T_2 time asymmetry abnormalities were first described, overall CC size was decreased by nearly 20% in the TS group (Peterson, Leckman et al., 1994). Subregional areas appeared all to be reduced to a similar degree, and decreases in both curvilinear length and width of the CC appeared to be responsible for overall size reductions. Preliminary shape analyses also suggested that TS CCs are generally less curved than those of normal subjects. The CC size reductions suggest that structural interhemispheric connectivity may be aberrant in the TS CNS, and they provide further indirect supportive evidence that TS cerebral lateralization may be aberrant.

The basal ganglia volume reductions and hypometabolism seen in TS are suggestive of some kind of CNS developmental abnormality. The apparent morphological abnormalities in more than one set of brain regions (in the basal ganglia and CC at least) would suggest that the underlying pathoetiologic processes impact on the developing TS CNS diffusely. The CC findings certainly suggest that disturbances in cortical connectivity may be widespread in TS, and that other cortical and subcortical abnormalities in both structure and function should be sought. The differences on performance of lateralized behavioral tasks (Yazgan et al., in press), the apparently common occurrence of lateralized neurological soft signs in TS subjects (Sweet et al., 1973), and the preliminary findings of altered asymmetries of tissue magnetic resonance characteristics in numerous regions of the cerebrum support the contention that the pathoetiologic determinants of TS affect the cerebrum diffusely.

The similarity of the TS neuroimaging findings to those seen in schizophrenia raises the issue of the specificity of aberrant CNS lateralization in those illnesses. It is possible that abnormal asymmetries may be specific to certain brain structures in certain disorders, and if enough brain regions are sampled, the unique constellation of abnormally lateralized structures that distinguishes any given disorder can be ascertained. It is also possible, on the other hand, that abnormal CNS lateralization is not unique to TS or schizophrenia, and that it instead may contribute to the expression of a constitutional vulnerability for developing a given illness. It may be, for instance, that prenatal stressors contribute both to abnormal CNS lateralization and to more severe symptom expression in both TS *and* schizophrenia, and that in the absence of prenatal stressors, the illnesses would be expressed as symptomatically mild variants, or as no disease at all. Studies of monozygotic twins with TS and schizophrenia, for example, demonstrate the importance of prenatal stressors in the determination of symptom severity discordances between the co-twins (Berman et al., 1992; Hyde et al., 1992; Leckman et al., 1987).

Attention Deficit Hyperactivity Disorder

Ventricular Size. An initial CT study of 35 ADHD children failed to find differences from normal subjects in ventricular size or asymmetry or in hemispheric width (Shaywitz et al., 1983). Another CT study of 24 young ADHD adults also found no ventricular enlargement, but did

report significantly increased sulcal widening, suggesting the presence of cortical atrophy. Seven of the 24 ADHD subjects had a history of alcohol abuse, but the incidence of sulcal widening was not disproportionately greater in this group compared with those without an alcohol history.

Cortical Regions. The first ^{18}Xe PET study from Denmark assessed 13 children with ADHD, the majority of whom had significant comorbid neurological deficits or a history of CNS insult. Significantly reduced metabolic rates were seen in the left sensorimotor, primary auditory, and occipital regions (Lou et al., 1989). Because of ethical concerns in the United States about exposing children to radioactivity, the first FDG PET study of ADHD here imaged 25 adults who had persistent ADHD since childhood and who also had offspring with ADHD (Zametkin et al., 1990). Compared with 50 unmatched normal control subjects, the ADHD group had reduced cerebral metabolism globally, as well as hypometabolism in the premotor and somatosensory cortices when regional metabolism was normalized by the global glucose metabolic values. It is possible that the findings of sulcal widening, if confirmed, could represent a structural defect underlying these early PET findings of global hypometabolism in ADHD adults. Another FDG-PET study then imaged 10 adolescents with ADHD, 4 of whom had learning disabilities, and compared them with 10 control subjects, 7 of whom were nonaffected siblings of ADHD children (Zametkin et al., 1993). Global reduction in metabolism was not confirmed in this group, possibly due to statistical power that was low compared with the prior adult study or possibly because of developmental changes in the ADHD central nervous system. In the adolescent sample, normalized regional metabolic rates were lower in the left anterior frontal, right temporal, left thalamic, and right hippocampal regions. Metabolism in the left frontal region correlated negatively with numerous symptom severity measures.

Corpus Callosum. MRI studies of the corpus callosum in ADHD have reported either smaller genu and isthmus regions (Hynd et al., 1991), smaller rostrum and rostral body (Giedd et al., 1994), or smaller splenia (Semrud-Clikeman et al., 1994) than the corresponding structures in normal control subjects. The differences between studies in regional findings may be due to different pulse sequences, the presence or exclusion of comorbid illnesses, the matching (or not) of control subjects, and methods of corpus callosum subdivision. Nevertheless, the callosum subregions in which group differences have been reported contain interhemispheric axons connecting frontal, supplementary motor, and parietal cortices, regions thought to subserve motor and attentional systems, suggesting that disturbances in these systems could mediate the symptoms of motoric hyperactivity and inattention.

Basal Ganglia. An MRI basal ganglia volumetric study of 37 Tourette syndrome children looked at the subgroup of 18 TS children who had comorbid ADHD, and found significantly smaller left globus pallidus and left lenticular nucleus volumes than was seen in either the normal or the non-ADHD TS group (Singer et al., 1993). The TS + ADHD group also evidenced a loss of lenticular asymmetry compared with that of the control subjects. Children with ADHD alone have been reported to lack the right-larger-than-left caudate nucleus asymmetry seen in normal control subjects (Castellanos et al., 1994), again raising the question concerning the specificity of aberrant structural asymmetries seen in various developmental neuropsychiatric disorders. Lastly, the Danish ADHD PET study reported reduced metabolic rates in the striata of ADHD children, further implicating caudate nucleus in ADHD pathophysiology (Lou et al., 1989).

Dyslexia

Planum Temporale. The planum temporale is a triangular-shaped region located within the depths of the sylvian fissure on the upper surface of the temporal lobe, extending onto the inferior surface of the parietal lobe. The planum temporale has been of long-standing interest in the study of dyslexia because of the considerable experimental evidence that dyslexia results from disordered language (in particular, phonetic) processing and because phonetic processing is thought to be subserved by regions in or around the planum (Kinsbourne et al., 1991; Shaywitz et al., 1992). The lateralization of language systems to the left hemisphere, moreover, has generally been associated with the structural lateralization of the planum reported in postmortem and neuroradiologic studies. It thus follows that, if the planum were involved in phonological processing, then the impaired phonological processing of dyslexic subjects might be associated with structural alterations in the planum and possibly with abnormal structural lateralization in the region as well.

Numerous imaging studies have assessed planum structure in dyslexic subjects, although they have differed in the degree to which they controlled for important subject characteristics thought to influence planum morphology, such as age, body and brain size, IQ, and handedness (an index of cerebral dominance and functional lateralization). These studies have also varied considerably in their methods of planum definition, with the earliest studies measuring thick axial or coronal sections that provide poor resolution relative to contemporary standards, and poor visualization of perisylvian anatomy that is probably instead best measured in the sagittal plane. No studies have yet employed revisualization of the planum in multiple planes, which would likely provide the best definition of this anatomically diffuse structure. These important methodologic differences may account for some of the differences in the findings reported for planum structure in dyslexia (Hynd and Semrud-Clikeman, 1989; Leonard et al., 1993; Schultz et al., 1994).

Several MRI studies have confirmed the absence or reversal in dyslexia of the leftward asymmetry of the planum seen in normal subjects. The abnormal asymmetries in some studies appear to be due to smaller left-sided structures (Hynd et al., 1990; Jernigan et al., 1991; Kushch et al., 1993), and in other studies appear to be due to larger right-sided plana (Larsen et al., 1990). In one study, the magnitude of planum asymmetry correlated with reading comprehension scores in the dyslexic but not in the control subjects (Kushch et al., 1993), suggesting that the structural abnormalities might have functional correlates that are pertinent to phonological processing deficits in the dyslexic group. Other studies have failed to replicate findings of group differences in hemispheric asymmetry (Leonard et al., 1993; Schultz et al., 1994).

A more recent study has transformed the discussion of the comparison of planum size between cerebral hemispheres to a discussion of a comparison of the sizes of subregions of the planum within the same cerebral hemisphere. Leonard and colleagues (1993), for instance, have reported that the distribution of planum tissue appears to be shifted from the parietal to the temporal banks in dyslexic compared to normal control subjects. These investigators have also presented evidence that dyslexia is associated with the presence in the planum of minor structural anomalies and ectopias, such as multiple Heschl's gyri on both the left and the right. Heschl's gyrus is an important relay center in auditory processing pathways.

Rumsey and colleagues (1992, 1994) used ^{15}O-labeled water as a PET tracer to study cerebral blood flow during linguistic task activation paradigms. During syntactical tasks, normal readers and dyslexics both activated left middle and anterior portions of the temporal and inferior frontal regions, and the change in blood flow correlated with task performance in the control subjects (Rumsey et al., 1994). During phonological processing tasks, in contrast, only normal control and not dyslexic subjects activated posterior portions of the planum that included the left temporoparietal cortex near the angular gyrus, the region believed to be most specifically involved in phonological processing (Rumsey et al., 1992). In another PET study, FDG metabolism was shown to be higher bilaterally in the medial temporal lobe during specific phonological processing tasks in adult dyslexic subjects (Hagman et al., 1992). Despite the inconsistencies in the directionality of the group differences in functional studies and the inconsistencies of the structural studies, these findings taken together suggest that the planum temporale subserves phonological processing tasks in normal subjects and that both the structural and functional abnormalities in this region may produce the clinical deficits seen in dyslexia.

FUTURE DIRECTIONS OF NEUROIMAGING IN DEVELOPMENTAL NEUROPSYCHIATRIC DISORDERS

Imaging Technologies

The next major advances in the neuroimaging of childhood neuropsychiatric disorders will likely include significant progress in functional imaging, possibly in conventional PET and SPECT studies using patient contrast groups imaged with novel radioligands having short half-lives and a high degree of neurochemical specificity. Progress in the functional imaging of children will also be made using newer imaging modalities like fMRI, and these preliminary studies already are underway. Other advances will continue to be made in structural imaging. The application in structural MRI of new pulse sequences and high magnetic field strengths will provide, in briefer imaging times, an improved resolution of increasingly smaller regions of interest. Recent applications of new imaging protocols, for instance, have been able to achieve in-plane resolution of several hundred μm, permitting the identification of specific myeloarchitectonic regions of the human brain (Clark et al., 1992). The application of high field strengths will provide imaging resolutions on the order of 100 μm, which will permit in the foreseeable future the visualization of individual nerve fiber bundles and possibly of individual cortical columns. Although the precise role of MR spectroscopy in the future imaging of children is unclear, it is a technology that will undoubtedly be applied with increasing frequency to the study of childhood disorders. Another arena of exciting technological advance has been in high-resolution electroencephalography that is used in conjunction with MRI, which offers the promise of imaging brain electrical change with a temporal resolution of milliseconds and a spatial resolution comparable to current MRI standards (see, for example, Givens et al., 1991). Important progress will also be made in the study of brain structure/function relationships within and across developmental stages by acquiring structural and functional images in the same subjects.

Broadening the Scope of the Disorders Studied

Despite the high prevalence and morbidity of many childhood developmental neuropsychiatric disorders, such as depression, conduct disorder, anxiety disorders, and pervasive developmental disorders, and despite the known importance of biological, environmental, and developmental determinants in each, no imaging studies of these disorders in children have yet been reported. Neuroimaging will undoubtedly be an increasingly important tool in the future study of the brain-based mediators of the family-genetic and environmental determinants of the clinical phenotype for each of these illnesses.

Studying the Determinants of Neurobiological Substrate

Aside from technical advances in neuroimaging, new directions in the imaging of childhood disorders will involve the novel application of more standard clinical investigative tools to help delineate through imaging the genetic and nongenetic determinants of the neurobiological substrate of childhood disorders. Stratifying subjects with respect to the degree of genetic risk (using family-genetic data or genetic markers) and with respect to the degree of exposure to known nongenetic risks (such as prenatal and obstetrical complications) will permit the ascertainment of the effects of genetic and nongenetic factors on the neurobiological substrate of these disorders.

For the vast majority of complex neuropsychiatric disorders, the effects of these factors will likely be most evident in their interactions. A given nongenetic risk factor may exert its effect on neurobiologic substrate, for instance, only in the context of some threshold of genetic risk or vulnerability to developing the disorder. Conversely, nongenetic determinants appear to have varying degrees of importance in the pathophysiology of childhood neuropsychiatric disorders. Exposure to a nongenetic risk factor during a period of developmental vulnerability may alone be sufficient to produce a specific disorder and its corresponding substrate; alternatively, an environmental exposure may predispose to any number of disorders, in which case the child's specific genetic and other constitutional endowments will determine which particular disorder is manifested. Only careful clinical and biological characterization will permit the kind of dissection of pathophysiology that will discern the effects of these numerous determinants on neurobiological substrate and disease phenotype.

Longitudinal Studies

Finally, perhaps the most important scientific information to be obtained in imaging childhood neuropsychiatric disorders will derive from longitudinal studies of brain structure and function through normal and pathological development. The importance of studying developmental changes in brain structure and function in normal children for the improved understanding of pathological brain development cannot be overemphasized. Longitudinal imaging studies are understandably less feasible than simple cross-sectional studies, given the potential difficulties inherent in longitudinal research with patient compliance and current concerns about radiation exposure with PET and SPECT. Nonetheless, longitudinal imaging studies are necessary to determine whether individual and group differences seen in disease states are a cause or a consequence of the disease. Longitudinal studies are also necessary to begin discerning the effects that normal CNS maturation has on the unfolding of the clinical expression of a disease at characteristic times and in characteristic manners at varying stages of development. Sizeable longitudinal studies, combined with careful clinical and biological subject characterization, will thus permit the beginning elucidation of the mechanisms whereby genetic and environmental risk, in the context of normal and pathological CNS maturation, interact to produce a particular neurobiological substrate and a subsequently unique clinical phenotype.

Acknowledgments. *Portions of this work appear in Peterson B: Neuroimaging in child and adolescent psychiatric disorders. J Am Acad Child Adolesc Psychiatry, in press. This work was supported in part by grants MH49351, MH18268, MH30929, MH01232-01, NIH RR06022, and HD03008. The authors are grateful to Drs. John Gore, Paul Hoffer, and Robert Schultz for their contributions of the glossy prints that appear in this chapter.*

References

Abitbol M, Menini C, Delezoide A-L, et al: Nucleus basalis magnocellularis and hippocampus are the major sites of FMR-1 expression in the human fetal brain. *Nat Genet* 4:147–153, 1993.

Andreasen NC, Arndt S, Swayze V II, et al: Thalamic abnormalities in schizophrenia visualized through magnetic resonance image averaging. *Science* 266:294–298, 1994.

Andreasen NC, Ehrhardt JC, Swayze VW II, et al: Magnetic resonance imaging of the brain in schizophrenia: The pathophysiologic significance of structural abnormalities. *Arch Gen Psychiatry* 47:35–44, 1990.

Andreasen NC, Flaum M, Swayze V, et al: Intelligence and brain structure in normal individuals. *Am J Psychiatry* 150:130–134, 1993.

Andreasen NC, Flashman L, Flaum M, et al: Regional brain abnormalities in schizophrenia measured with magnetic resonance imaging. *JAMA* 272:1763–1769, 1994.

Andreasen NC, Nasrallah HA, Dunn V, et al: Structural abnormalities in the frontal system in schizophrenia. *Arch Gen Psychiatry* 43:136–144, 1986.

Andreasen NC, Rezai K, Alliger R, et al: Hypofrontality in neuroleptic-naive patients and in patients with chronic schizophrenia. *Arch Gen Psychiatry* 49:943–958, 1992.

Aylward EH, Reiss A, Barta PE, et al: Magnetic resonance imaging measurement of posterior fossa structures in schizophrenia. *Am J Psychiatry* 151:1448–1452, 1994.

Barta P, Pearlson G, Richards S, et al: Reduced superior temporal gyrus volume in schizophrenia: Relationship to hallucinations. *Am J Psychiatry* 147:1457–1462, 1990.

Bauman M, Kemper T: Histoanatomic observations of the brain in early infantile autism. *Neurology* 35:866–874, 1985.

Baxter L, Phelps M, Mazziotta J, et al: Local cerebral glucose metabolic rates in obsessive-compulsive disorder: A comparison with rates in unipolar depression and in normal controls. *Arch Gen Psychiatry* 44:211–218, 1987.

Baxter LR, Schwartz JM, Bergman KS, et al: Caudate glucose metabolic rate changes with both drug and behavior therapy for obsessive-compulsive disorder. *Arch Gen Psychiatry* 49:681–689, 1992.

Baxter L, Schwartz J, Guze B, et al: PET imaging in obsessive compulsive disorder with and without depression. *J Clin Psychiatry* 51:61–69, 1990.

Baxter L, Schwartz J, Mazziotta J, et al: Cerebral glucose metabolic rates in nondepressed patients with obsessive-compulsive disorder. *Am J Psychiatry* 145:1560–1563, 1988.

Behar D, Rapoport J, Berg C, et al: Computerized tomography and neuropsychological test measures in adolescents with obsessive-compulsive disorder. *Am J Psychiatry* 141:363–369, 1984.

Belleveau JW, Kennedy DN, McKinstry RC, et al: Functional mapping of the human visual cortex by magnetic resonance imaging. *Science* 254:716–718, 1991.

Benkelfat C, Nordahl T, Semple W, et al: Local cerebral glucose metabolic rates in obsessive-compulsive disorder. *Arch Gen Psychiatry* 47:840–848, 1990.

Berman KF, Torrey F, Daniel DG, et al: Regional cerebral blood flow in monozygotic twins discordant and concordant for schizophrenia. *Arch Gen Psychiatry* 49:927–934, 1992.

Bilder RM, Wu H, Bogerts B, et al: Absence of regional hemispheric volume asymmetries in first-episode schizophrenia. *Am J Psychiatry* 151:1437–1447, 1994.

Blamire AM, Ogawa S, Ugurbil K, et al: Dynamic mapping of the human visual cortex by high-speed magnetic resonance imaging. *Proc Natl Acad Sci USA* 89:11069–11073, 1992.

Bogerts B, Ashtari M, Degreef G, et al: Reduced temporal limbic structure volumes on magnetic resonance images in first episode schizophrenia. *Psychiatry Res Neuroimaging* 35:1–13, 1990.

Bogerts B, Meertz E, Schonfeldt-Bausch R: Basal ganglia and limbic system pathology in schizophrenia: A morphometric study of brain volume and shrinkage. *Arch Gen Psychiatry* 42:784–791, 1985.

Braun A, Stoetter B, Randolph C, et al: The functional neuroanatomy of Tourette's syndrome: An FDG-PET study. I: Regional changes in cerebral glucose metabolism differentiating patients and controls. *Neuropsychopharmacology* 9:277–291, 1993.

Breier A, Buchanan RW, Elkashef A, et al: Brain morphology and schizophrenia. A magnetic resonance imaging study of limbic, prefrontal cortex, and caudate structures. *Arch Gen Psychiatry* 49:921–926, 1992.

Brooks D, Turjanski N, Sawle G, et al: PET studies on the integrity of the pre and postsynaptic dopaminergic system in Tourette syndrome. In: Chase TN, Friedhoff AJ, Cohen DJ (eds): *Advances in Neurology-Tourette's Syndrome: Genetics, Neurobiology, and Treatment* (Vol 58). New York, Raven Press, 1992, pp. 227–231.

Brown R, Colter N, Corsellis JAN, et al: Postmortem evidence of structural brain changes in schizophrenia. *Arch Gen Psychiatry* 43:36–42, 1986.

Buchli R, Martin E, Boesiger P, et al: Developmental changes of phosphorus metabolite concentrations in the human brain: A ^{31}P magnetic resonance spectroscopy study in vivo. *Pediatr Res* 35:431–435, 1994.

Buchsbaum MS, Haier RJ, Potkin SG, et al: Frontostriatal disorder of cerebral metabolism in never-medicated schizophrenics. *Arch Gen Psychiatry* 49:935–942, 1992a.

Buchsbaum MS, Ingvar DH, Kessler R, et al: Cerebral glucography with positron tomography. *Arch Gen Psychiatry* 39:251–259, 1987.

Buchsbaum MS, Potkin SG, Siegel BV, et al: Striatal metabolic rate and clinical response to neuroleptics in schizophrenia. *Arch Gen Psychiatry* 49:966–974, 1992b.

Burton H, Videen TO, Raichle ME: Tactile-vibration-activated foci in insular and parietal-opercular cortex studied with positron emission tomography: Mapping the second somatosensory area in humans. *Somatosens Mot Res* 10:297–308, 1993.

Calabrese G, Colombo C, Bonfanti A, et al: Caudate nucleus abnormalities in obsessive-compulsive disorder: Measurements of MRI signal intensity. *Psychiatry Res Neuroimaging* 50:89–92, 1993.

Campbell M, Rosenbloom S, Perry R, et al: Computerized axial tomography in young autistic children. *Am J Psychiatry* 139:510–512, 1982.

Cannon TD, Mednick SA, Parnas J, et al: Developmental brain abnormalities in the offspring of schizophrenic mothers. I: Contributions of genetic and perinatal factors. *Arch Gen Psychiatry* 50:551–564, 1993.

Castellanos FX, Giedd JN, Eckburg P, et al: Quantitative morphology of the caudate nucleus in attention deficit hyperactivity disorder. *Am J Psychiatry* 151:1791–1796, 1994.

Chakos MH, Lieberman JA, Bilder RM, et al: Increase in caudate nuclei volumes of first-episode schizophrenic patients taking antipsychotic drugs. *Am J Psychiatry* 151:1430–1436, 1994.

Chase T, Geoffrey V, Gillespie M, et al: Structural and functional studies of Gilles de la Tourette syndrome. *Rev Neurol* 142:851–855, 1986.

Chiron C, Raynaud C, Mazière B, et al: Changes in regional cerebral blood flow during brain maturation in children and adolescents. *J Nucl Med* 33:696–703, 1992.

Chris-Heh CW, Smith R, Wu J, et al: Positron emission tomography of the cerebellum in autism. *Am J Psychiatry* 146:242–245, 1989.

Chugani HT, Phelps ME, Mazziotta JC: Positron emission tomography study of human brain functional development. *Ann Neurol* 22:487–497, 1987.

Cohen MS, Bookheimer SY: Localization of brain function using magnetic resonance imaging. *Trends Neurosci* 17:268–277, 1994.

Colebatch JG, Deiber M-P, Passingham RE, et al: Regional cerebral blood flow during voluntary arm and hand movements in human subjects. *J Neurophysiol* 65:1392–1401, 1991.

Colter N, Battal S, Crow TJ, et al: White matter reduction in the parahippocampal gyrus of patients with schizophrenia. *Arch Gen Psychiatry* 44:1023, 1987.

Constable RT, McCarthy G, Allison T, et al: Functional brain imaging at 1.5 T using conventional gradient echo MR imaging techniques. *Magn Reson Imaging* 11:451–459, 1993.

Corbetta M, Miezin FM, Shulman GL, et al: A PET study of visuospatial attention. *J Neurosci* 13:1202–1226, 1993.

Courchesne E, Press GA, Corchesne RY: Parietal lobe abnormalities detected with MR in patients with infantile autism. *Am J Roentgenol* 160:387–393, 1993.

Courchesne E, Saitoh O, Yeung-Courchesne R, et al: Abnormality of cerebellar vermian lobules VI and VII in patients with infantile autism: Identification of hypoplastic and hyperplastic subgroups with MR imaging. *Am J Roentgenol* 162:123–130, 1994a.

Courchesne E, Townsend J, Saitoh O: The brain in infantile autism: Posterior fossa structures are abnormal. *Neurology* 44:214–223, 1994b.

Courchesne E, Yeung-Courchesne R, Press GA, et al: Hypoplasia of cerebellar vermal lobules VI and VII in autism. *N Engl J Med* 318:1349–1354, 1988.

Crome L, Cowie V, Slater E: A statistical note on cerebellar and brain-stem weight in mongolism. *J Ment Defic Res* 10:69–72, 1966.

Crow T, Ball J, Bloom S, et al: Schizophrenia as an anomaly of development of cerebral asymmetry. *Arch Gen Psychiatry* 46:1145–1150, 1989.

Damasio H, Maurer RG, Damasio AR, et al: Computerized tomographic scan findings in patients with autistic behavior. *Arch Neurol* 37:504–510, 1980.

de Lacoste M-C, Horvath D, Woodward D: Possible sex differences in the developing human fetal brain. *J Clin Exp Neuropsychol* 13:831–846, 1991.

DeLisi LE, Buchsbaum MS, Holcomb JJ, et al: Increased temporal lobe glucose use in chronic schizophrenic patients. *Biol Psychiatry* 25:835–851, 1989.

DeLisi LE, Hoff AL, Schwartz JE, et al: Brain morphology in first-episode schizophrenic-like psychotic patients: A quantitative magnetic resonance imaging study. *Biol Psychiatry* 29:159–175, 1991.

Early TS, Reiman EM, Raichle ME, et al: Left globus pallidus abnormality in never-medicated patients with schizophrenia. *Proc Natl Acad Sci USA* 84:561–563, 1989.

Elkashef AM, Buchanan RW, Gellad F, et al: Basal ganglia pathology in schizophrenia and tardive dyskinesia: An MRI quantitative study. *Am J Psychiatry* 151:752–755, 1994.

Falk D, Hildebolt C, Cheverud J, et al: Human cortical asymmetries determined with 3D MR technology. *J Neurosci Methods* 39:185–191, 1991.

Farde L, Wiesel FA, Stone-Elander S, et al: D$_2$ dopamine receptors in neuroleptic-naive schizophrenic patients: A positron emission tomography study with ^{11}C raclopride. *Arch Gen Psychiatry* 47:213–219, 1990.

Fleming B, Anderson R, Rhees R, et al: Effects of prenatal stress on sexually dimorphic 21 asymmetries in the cerebral cortex of the rat. *Brain Res Bull* 16:395–398, 1986.

Fride E, Weinstock M: Prenatal stress increases anxiety related behavior and alters cerebral lateralization of dopamine activity. *Life Sci* 42:1059–1065, 1988.

Fried I, Nenov VI, Ojemann S, et al: Functional MRI and PET imaging of motor and visual cortices for neurosurgical planning in epilepsy patients [Abstract]. *Epilepsia* 35(suppl):24, 1994.

Gaffney GR, Kuperman S, Tsai LY, et al: Forebrain structure in infantile autism. *J Am Acad Child Adolesc Psychiatry* 28:534–537, 1989.

Galaburda AM: The planum temporale [Editorial]. *Arch Neurol* 50:457, 1993.

Garber J, Ananth J, Chiu L, et al: Nuclear magnetic resonance study of obsessive-compulsive disorder. *Am J Psychiatry* 146:1001–1005, 1989.

George M, Robertson MM, Costa DC, et al: Dopamine receptor availability in Tourette's syndrome. *Psychiatry Res Neuroimaging* 55:193–203, 1994.

George M, Trimble M, Costa D, et al: Elevated frontal cerebral blood flow in Gilles de la Tourette syndrome: A ^{99}Tc^m-HMPAO SPECT study. *Psychiatry Res Neuroimaging* 45:143–151, 1992.

Geschwind N: Language and the brain. *Sci Am* 226:340–348, 1972.

Geschwind N, Galaburda AM: *Cerebral Lateralization: Biological Mechanisms, Associations, and Pathology*. Cambridge, MA, MIT, 1987.

Geschwind N, Levitsky W: Left-right asymmetries in temporal speech region. *Science* 161:186–187, 1968.

Giedd J, Castellanos F, Casey B, et al: Quantitative morphology of the corpus callosum in attention deficit hyperactivity disorder. *Am J Psychiatry* 151:665–669, 1994.

Givens A, Le J, Brickett P, et al: Seeing through the skull: Advanced EEGs use MRIs to accurately measure cortical activity from the scalp. *Brain Topogr* 4:125–131, 1991.

Gur RE, Mozley PD, Resnick SM, et al: Magnetic resonance imaging in schizophrenia: Volumetric analysis of brain and cerebrospinal fluid. *Arch Gen Psychiatry* 48:407–412, 1991.

Hagman JO, Wood F, Buchsbaum MS, et al: Cerebral brain metabolism in adult dyslexic subjects assessed with positron emission tomography during performance of an auditory task. *Arch Neurol* 49:734–739, 1992.

Harcherik D, Cohen D, Ort S, et al: Computed tomographic brain scanning in four neuropsychiatric disorders of childhood. *Am J Psychiatry* 142:731–734, 1985.

Hashimoto T, Murakawa K, Mizaki M, et al: Magnetic resonance imaging of the brain structures in the posterior fossa in retarded autistic children. *Acta Paediatr* 81:1030–1034, 1992.

Hashimoto T, Tayama M, Miyazaki M, et al: Reduced brainstem size in children with autism. *Brain Dev* 14:94–97, 1992.

Heckers S, Heinsen H, Heinsen YC, et al: Cortex, white matter and basal ganglia in schizophrenia: A volumetric postmortem study. *Biol Psychiatry* 29:556–566, 1991.

Hietala J, Syvälahti E, Vuoriio K, et al: Striatal D$_2$ dopamine receptor characteristics in neuroleptic-naive schizophrenic patients studied with positron emission tomography. *Arch Gen Psychiatry* 51:116–123, 1994.

Hinds HL, Ashley CT, Sutcliffe JS, et al: Tissue specific expression of FMR-1 provides evidence for a functional role in fragile X syndrome. *Nat Genet* 3:36–43, 1993.

Hoehn-Saric R, Pearlson G, Harris G, et al: Effects of fluoxetine on regional cerebral blood flow in obsessive-compulsive patients. *Am J Psychiatry* 148:1243–1245, 1991.

Hollander E, DeCaria C, Saoud J, et al: M-CPP-activated regional cerebral blood flow in obsessive-compulsive disorder. *Biol Psychiatry* 29:170A, 1991.

Horwitz B, Rumsey JM, Grady CL, et al: Metabolic landscape in autism: Intercorrelations of regional glucose utilization. *Arch Neurol* 45:749–755, 1988.

Horwitz B, Schapiro MB, Grady CL, et al: Cerebral metabolic pattern in young adult Down's syndrome subjects: Altered intercorrelations between regional rates of glucose utilization. *J Ment Defic Res* 34:237–252, 1990.

Hyde T, Aaronson B, Randolph C, et al: Relationship of birth weight to the phenotypic expression of Gilles de la Tourette's syndrome in monozygotic twins. *Neurology* 42:652–658, 1992.

Hyde T, Stacey M, Coppola R, et al: Cerebral morphometric abnormalities in Tourette's syndrome: A quantitative MRI study of monozygotic twins. *Neurology* 45:1176–1182, 1995.

Hynd GW, Semrud-Clikeman M: Dyslexia and brain morphology. *Psychol Bull* 106:447–482, 1989.

Hynd GW, Semrud-Clikeman M, Lorys AR, et al: Brain morphology in developmental dyslexia and attention deficit disorder/hyperactivity. *Arch Neurology* 47:919–926, 1990.

Hynd G, Semrud-Clikeman M, Lorys A, et al: Corpus callosum morphology in attention deficit-hyperactivity disorder: Morphometric analysis of MRI. *J Learn Disabil* 24:141–146, 1991.

Insel T, Donnelly E, Lalakea M, et al: Neurological and neuropsychological studies of patients with obsessive-compulsive disorder. *Biol Psychiatry* 18:741–751, 1983.

Jack CR, Twomey CK, Zinsmeister AR, et al: Anterior temporal lobes and hippocampal formations: Normative volumetric measurements from MR images in young adults. *Radiology* 172:549–554, 1989.

Jernigan TL, Bellugi U: Anomalous brain morphology on magnetic resonance images in Williams syndrome and Down syndrome. *Arch Neurol* 47:529–533, 1990.

Jernigan TL, Archibald SL, Berhow MT, et al: Cerebral structure on MRI. Part I: Localization of age-related changes. *Biol Psychiatry* 29:55–67, 1991b.

Jernigan TL, Bellugi U, Sowell E, et al: Cerebral morphologic distinctions between Williams and Down syndromes. *Arch Neurol* 50:186–191, 1993.

Jernigan TL, Press GA, Hesselink JR: Methods for measuring brain morphologic features on magnetic resonance images. Validation and normal aging. *Arch Neurol* 47:27–32, 1990.

Jernigan TL, Sargent T III, Pfefferbaum A, et al: 18-Fluorodeoxyglucose PET in schizophrenia. *Psychiatry Res* 16:317–329, 1985.

Jernigan TL, Trauner DA, Hesselink JR, et al: Maturation of human cerebrum observed in vivo during adolescence. *Brain* 114:2037–2049, 1991a.

Jernigan TL, Zisook S, Heaton RK, et al: Magnetic resonance imaging abnormalities in lenticular nuclei and cerebral cortex in schizophrenia. *Arch Gen Psychiatry* 48:881–890, 1991c.

Jones AKP, Brown WD, Friston KJ, et al: Cortical and subcortical localization of response to pain in man using positron emission tomography. *Proc R Soc Lond B Biol Sci* 244:39–44, 1991.

Kellner C, Jolley R, Holgate R, et al: Brain MRI in obsessive-compulsive disorder. *Psychiatry Res* 36:45–49, 1991.

Keshavan MA, Kapur S, Pettegrew JW: Magnetic resonance spectroscopy in psychiatry: Potential, pitfalls, and promise. *Am J Psychiatry* 148:976–985, 1991.

Kim S-G, Uǧurbil K, Strick PL: Activation of a cerebellar output nucleus during cognitive processing. *Science* 265:949–951, 1994.

Kinsbourne M, Rufo DT, Gamzu E, et al: Neuropsychological deficits in adults with dyslexia. *Dev Med Child Neurol* 33:763–775, 1991.

Kleiman MD, Neff S, Rosman NP: The brain in

infantile autism: Are posterior fossa structures abnormal? *Neurology* 42:753–760, 1992.

Kooistra C, Heilman K: Motor dominance and lateral asymmetry of the globus pallidus. *Neurology* 38:388–390, 1988.

Kushch A, Gross-Glenn K, Jallad B, et al: Temporal lobe surface area measurements on MRI in normal and dyslexic readers. *Neuropsychologia* 31: 811–821, 1993.

Kwong KK, Belliveau JW, Chesler DA, et al: Dynamic magnetic resonance imaging of human brain activity during primary sensory stimulation. *Proc Natl Acad Sci USA* 89:5675–5679, 1992.

Lamantia A-S, Rakic P: Cytological and quantitative characteristics of four cerebral commissures in the rhesus monkey. *J Comp Neurol* 291:520–537, 1990.

Larsen JP, Høien T, Lundberg I, et al: MRI evaluation of the size and symmetry of the planum temporale in adolescents with developmental dyslexia. *Brain Lang* 39:289–301, 1990.

Laruelle M, Baldwin R, Malison R, et al: SPECT imaging of dopamine and serotonin transporters with [¹²³I]β-CIT: Pharmacological characterization of brain uptake in nonhuman primates. *Synapse* 13: 295–309, 1993.

Le Bihan D, Turner R, Zeffiro TA, et al: Activation of human primary visual cortex during mental imagery. In: *Functional MRI of the Brain*. Arlington, VT, Society of Magnetic Resonance in Medicine, 1993, pp. 191–195.

Leckman J, Dolnansky E, Hardin M, et al: Perinatal factors in the expression of Gilles de la Tourette's syndrome: An exploratory study. *J Am Acad Child Adolesc Psychiatry* 29:220–226, 1990.

Leckman J, Price R, Walkup J, et al: Nongenetic factors in Gilles de la Tourette's syndrome [Letter]. *Arch Gen Psychiatry* 44:100, 1987.

Leonard CM, Voeller KKS, Lombardino LJ, et al: Anomalous cerebral structure in dyslexia revealed with magnetic resonance imaging. *Arch Neurol* 50: 461–469, 1993.

Liddle PF, Friston KJ, Frith CD, et al: Patterns of cerebral blood flow in schizophrenia. *Br J Psychiatry* 160:179–186, 1992.

Lim KO, Zipursky RB, Murphy GM, et al: In vivo quantification of the limbic system using MRI: Effects of normal aging. *Psychiatry Res Neuroimaging* 35:15–26, 1990.

Lou H, Henriksen L, Bruhn P, et al: Striatal dysfunction in attention deficit and hyperkinetic disorder. *Arch Neurol* 46:48–52, 1989.

Lueck CJ, Zeki S, Friston KJ, et al: The colour centre in the cerebral cortex of man. *Nature* 340: 386–389, 1989.

Luxenberg J, Swedo S, Flament M, et al: Neuroanatomical abnormalities in obsessive-compulsive disorder detected with quantitative x-ray computed tomography. *Am J Psychiatry* 145:1089–1093, 1989.

Machlin S, Harris G, Pearlson G, et al: Elevated medial-frontal cerebral blood flow in obsessive-compulsive patients: A SPECT study. *Am J Psychiatry* 148:1240–1242, 1991.

Malison RT, McDougle CJ, van Dyck CH, et al: [¹²³I]β-CIT SPECT imaging demonstrates increased striatal dopamine transporter binding in Tourette's syndrome. *Am J Psychiatry*, in press.

McCarthy G, Blamire AM, Rothman DL, et al: Echo-planar magnetic resonance imaging studies of frontal cortex activation during word generation in humans. *Proc Natl Acad Sci USA* 90:4952–4956, 1993.

McGuire PK, Shah GMS, Murray RM: Increased blood flow in Broca's area during auditory hallucinations in schizophrenia. *Lancet* 342:703–706, 1993.

Minshew NJ, Goldstein G, Dombrowski SM, et al: A preliminary ³¹P MRS study of autism: Evidence for undersynthesis and increased degradation of brain membranes. *Biol Psychiatry* 33:762–773, 1993.

Murakami JW, Courchesne E, Press GA, et al: Reduced cerebellar hemisphere size and its relationship to vermal hypoplasia in autism. *Arch Neurol* 46: 689–694, 1989.

Murphy DGM, DeCarli C, Schapiro MB, et al: Age-related differences in volumes of subcortical nuclei, brain matter, and cerebrospinal fluid in healthy men as measured with magnetic resonance imaging. *Arch Neurol* 49:839–845, 1992.

Murphy GM, Inger P, Mark K, et al: Volumetric asymmetry in the human amygdaloid complex. *J für Hirnforschung* 28:281–289, 1987.

Musalek M, Podreka I, Walter H, et al: Regional brain function in hallucinations: A study of regional cerebral blood flow with 99m-Tc-HMPAO-SPECT in patients with auditory hallucinations, tactile hallucinations, and normal controls. *Compr Psychiatry* 30: 99–108, 1989.

Nasrallah H, Loney J, Olson S, et al: Cortical atrophy in young adults with a history of hyperactivity in childhood. *Psychiatry Res* 17:241–246, 1986.

Nasrallah HA, Schwarzkopf SB, Olson SC, et al: Perinatal brain injury and cerebellar vermal lobules I–X in schizophrenia. *Biol Psychiatry* 29:567–574, 1991.

Nordahl T, Benkelfat C, Semple W, et al: Cerebral glucose metabolic rates in obsessive-compulsive disorder. *Neuropsychopharmacology* 2:23–28, 1989.

Ogawa S, Tank DW, Monon R, et al: Intrinsic signal changes accompanying sensory stimulation: Functional brain mapping with magnetic resonance imaging. *Proc Natl Acad Sci USA* 89:5951–5955, 1992.

Oldendorf W, Oldendorf W Jr (eds): *MRI Primer*. New York, Raven Press, 1991.

Ono M, Kubik S, Abernathey CD: *Atlas of the Cerebral Sulci*. New York, Thieme, 1990.

Pardo JV, Fox PT, Raichle ME: Localization of a human system for sustained attention by positron emission tomography. *Nature* 349:61–64, 1991.

Perlmutter JS, Powers WJ, Herscovitch P, et al: Regional asymmetries of cerebral blood flow, blood volume, and oxygen utilization and extraction in normal subjects. *J Cereb Blood Flow Metab* 7:64–67, 1987.

Petersen SE, Fiez JA: The processing of single words studied with positron emission tomography. *Annu Rev Neurosci* 16:509–530, 1993.

Petersen SE, Fox PT, Posner MI, et al; Positron emission tomographic studies of the cortical anatomy of single-word processing. *Nature* 331:585–589, 1988.

Peterson B, Gore J, Riddle M, et al: Abnormal T₂ relaxation time asymmetries in Tourette's syndrome. *Psychiatry Res Neuroimaging* 55:205–221, 1994.

Peterson B, Leckman J, Duncan J, et al: Corpus callosum morphology from magnetic resonance images in Tourette's syndrome. *Psychiatry Res Neuroimaging* 55:85–99, 1994.

Peterson B, Riddle M, Cohen D, et al: Reduced basal ganglia volumes in Tourette's syndrome using three-dimensional reconstruction techniques from magnetic resonance images. *Neurology* 43:941–949, 1993a.

Peterson B, Riddle M, Cohen D, et al: Human basal ganglia volume asymmetries on magnetic resonance images. *Magn Reson Imaging* 11:493–498, 1993b.

Piven J, Arndt S, Bailey J, et al: An MRI study of brain size in autism. *Am J Psychiatry* 152: 1145–1149, 1995.

Piven J, Berthier ML, Starkstein SE, et al: Magnetic resonance imaging evidence for a defect of cerebral cortical development in autism. *Am J Psychiatry* 147:734–739, 1990.

Piven J, Nehme E, Simon J, et al: Magnetic resonance imaging in autism: Measurement of the cerebellum, pons, and fourth ventricle. *Biol Psychiatry* 31:491–504, 1992.

Puce A, Constable T, Luby ML, et al: Functional magnetic resonance imaging of sensory and motor cortex: Comparison with intraoperative localization. *J Neurosurg*, in press.

Rao SM, Binder JR, Bandettini PA, et al: Functional magnetic resonance imaging of complex human movements. *Neurology* 43:2311–2318, 1993.

Rauch S, Jenike M, Alpert N, et al: Regional cerebral blood flow measured during symptom provocation in obsessive-compulsive disorder using oxygen 15-labeled carbon dioxide and positron emission tomography. *Arch Gen Psychiatry* 51:62–70, 1994.

Rebe RC: PET and SPECT: Opportunities and challenges for psychiatry. *J Clin Psychiatry* 54(suppl):26–32, 1993.

Reiss AL, Aylward E, Freund LS, et al: Neuroanatomy of fragile X syndrome: The posterior fossa. *Ann Neurol* 29:26–32, 1991a.

Reiss AL, Freund L, Tseng JE, et al: Neuroanatomy in fragile X females: The posterior fossa. *Am J Hum Genet* 49:279–288, 1991b.

Reiss AL, Lee J, Freund L: Neuroanatomy of fragile X syndrome: The temporal lobe. *Neurology* 44:1317–1324, 1994.

Renshaw PF, Yurgelun-Todd DA, Cohen B: Greater hemodynamic response to photic stimulation in schizophrenic patients: An echo planar MRI study. *Am J Psychiatry* 151:1493–1495, 1992.

Riddle M, Rasmusson A, Woods S, et al: SPECT imaging of cerebral blood flow in Tourette syndrome. In: Chase TN, Friedhoff AJ, Cohen DJ (eds): *Advances in Neurology-Tourette's Syndrome: Genetics, Neurobiology, and Treatment* (Vol 58). New York, Raven Press, 1992, pp. 207–211.

Ritvo ER, Garber HJ: Cerebellar hypoplasia and autism. *N Engl J Med* 319:1152, 1988.

Ritvo ER, Freeman BJ, Scheibel AB, et al: Lower Purkinje cell counts in the cerebella of four autistic subjects: Initial findings of the UCLA-NSAC autopsy research report. *Am J Psychiatry* 143:862–866, 1986.

Robinson D, Wu H, Munne RA, et al: Reduced caudate nucleus volume in obsessive-compulsive disorder. *Arch Gen Psychiatry* 52:393–398, 1995.

Roland PE, Meyer E, Shibasaki T, et al: Regional cerebral blood flow changes in cortex and basal ganglia during voluntary movements in normal human volunteers. *J Neurophysiol* 48:467–480, 1982.

Rosenbloom S, Campbell M, George AE, et al: High resolution CT scanning in infantile autism: A quantitative approach. *J Am Acad Child Psychiatry* 23:72–77, 1984.

Rubin R, Villanueva-Meyer J, Ananth J, et al: Regional xenon 133 cerebral blood flow and cerebral technetium 99m HMPAO uptake in unmedicated patients with obsessive-compulsive disorder and matched normal control subjects. Determination by high-resolution single-photon emission computed tomography. *Arch Gen Psychiatry* 49:695–702, 1992.

Rubinstein M, Denays R, Ham HR, et al: Functional imaging of brain maturation in humans using iodine-123 iodoamphetamine and SPECT. *J Nucl Med* 30:1982–1985, 1989.

Rumsey JM, Andreason P, Zametkin AJ, et al: Failure to activate the left temporoparietal cortex in dyslexia: An oxygen 15 positron emission tomographic study. *Arch Neurol* 49:527–534, 1992.

Rumsey JM, Duara R, Grady C, et al: Brain metabolism in autism: Resting cerebral glucose utilization rates as measured with positron emission tomography. *Arch Gen Psychiatry* 42:448–455, 1985.

Rumsey JM, Zametkin AJ, Andreason P, et al: Normal activation of frontotemporal language cortex in dyslexia, as measured with oxygen 15 positron emission tomography. *Arch Neurol* 51:27–38, 1994.

Scarone S, Colombo C, Livian S, et al: Increased right caudate nucleus size in obsessive-compulsive disorder: Detection with magnetic resonance imaging. *Psychiatry Res Neuroimaging* 45:115–121, 1992.

Schad LR, Trost U, Knopp MV, et al: Motor cortex stimulation measured by magnetic resonance imaging on a standard 1.5 T clinical scanner. *Magn Reson Imaging* 11:461–464, 1993.

Schapiro MB, Haxby JV, Grady CL: Nature of mental retardation and dementia in Down syndrome: Study with PET, CT, and neuropsychology. *Neurobiol Aging* 13:723–734, 1992.

Schifter T, Hoffman JM, Hatten HP, et al: Neuroimaging in infantile autism. *J Child Neurol* 9:155–161, 1994.

Schlaepfer TE, Harris GJ, Tien AY, et al: Decreased regional cortical gray matter volume in schizophrenia. *Am J Psychiatry* 151:842–848, 1994.

Schmidt-Sidor B, Wisniewski K, Shepard T, et al: Brain growth in Down syndrome subjects 15 to 22 weeks of age and birth to 60 months. *Clin Neuropathol* 9:181–190, 1990.

Schneider F, Gur RC, Jaggi JL, et al: Differential effects of mood on cortical cerebral blood flow: A ^{133}xenon clearance study. *Psychiatry Res* 52:215–236, 1994.

Schultz RT, Cho NK, Staib LH, et al: Brain morphology in normal and dyslexic children: The influence of sex and age. *Ann Neurol* 35:732–742, 1994.

Sedvall GC: PET imaging of dopamine receptors in human basal ganglia: Relevance to mental illness. *Trends Neurosci* 13:302–308, 1990.

Seeman P, Niznik HB: Dopamine receptors in Parkinson's disease and schizophrenia. *FASEB* 4:2737–2744, 1990.

Seeman P, Guan H-C, Van Tol HHM: Dopamine D$_4$ receptors elevated in schizophrenia. *Nature* 365:441–445, 1993.

Semrud-Clikeman M, Filipek PA, Biederman J, et al: Attention-deficit hyperactivity disorder: Magnetic resonance imaging morphometric analysis of the corpus callosum. *J Am Acad Child Adolesc Psychiatry* 33:875–881, 1994.

Shaywitz B, Shaywitz S, Byrne T, et al: Attention deficit disorder: Quantitative analysis of CT. *Neurology* 33:1500–1503, 1983.

Shaywitz SE, Escobar MD, Shaywitz BA, et al: Evidence that dyslexia may represent the lower tail of a normal distribution of reading ability. *N Engl J Med* 326:145–150, 1992.

Shenton ME, Kikinis R, Jolesz FA, et al: Left-lateralized temporal lobe abnormalities in schizophrenia and their relationship to thought disorder: A computerized, quantitative MRI study. *N Engl J Med* 327:604–612, 1992.

Shibasaki H, Sadato N, Lyshkow H, et al: Both primary motor cortex and supplementary motor area play an important role in complex finger movement. *Brain* 116:1387–1398, 1993.

Shifter T, Hoffman JM, Hatten HP, et al: Neuroimaging in infantile autism. *J Child Neurol* 9:155–161, 1994.

Siegel BV, Buchsbaum MS, Bunney WE, et al: Cortical-striatal-thalamic circuits and brain glucose metabolic activity in 70 unmedicated male schizophrenic patients. *Am J Psychiatry* 150:1325–1336, 1993.

Singer H, Reiss A, Brown J, et al: Volumetric MRI changes in basal ganglia of children with Tourette's syndrome. *Neurology* 43:950–956, 1993.

Solitare GB, Lamarche JB: Brain weight in the adult mongol. *J Ment Defic Res* 11:79–84, 1967.

Stoetter B, Braun A, Randolph C, et al: Functional neuroanatomy of Tourette syndrome: Limbic-motor interactions studied with FDG PET. In: Chase TN, Friedhoff AJ, Cohen DJ (eds): *Advances in Neurology-Tourette's Syndrome: Genetics, Neurobiology, and Treatment* (Vol 58). New York, Raven Press, 1992, pp. 213–226.

Suddath RL, Christison GW, Torrey EF, et al: Anatomical abnormalities in the brains of monozygotic twins discordant for schizophrenia. *New Engl J Med* 322:789–794, 1990.

Swayze VW, Andreasen NC, Alliger RJ, et al: Subcortical and temporal structures in affective disorder and schizophrenia: A magnetic resonance imaging study. *Biol Psychiatry* 31:221–240, 1992.

Swedo S, Pietrini P, Leonard H, et al: Cerebral glucose metabolism in childhood-onset obsessive-compulsive disorder. Revisualization during pharmacotherapy. *Arch Gen Psychiatry* 49:690–694, 1992.

Swedo S, Schapiro M, Grady C, et al: Cerebral glucose metabolism in childhood-onset obsessive-compulsive disorder. *Arch Gen Psychiatry* 46:518–523, 1989.

Sweet RD, Solomon GE, Wayne H, et al: Neurological features of Gilles de la Tourette's syndrome. *J Neurol Neurosurg Psychiatry* 36:1–9, 1993.

Szechtman H, Nahmias C, Garnett S, et al: Effect of neuroleptics on altered cerebral glucose metabolism in schizophrenia. *Arch Gen Psychiatry* 45:523–532, 1988.

Tamminga CA, Thaker GK, Buchanan R, et al: Limbic system abnormalities identified in schizophrenia using positron emission tomography with fluorodeoxyglucose and neocortical alterations with deficit syndrome. *Arch Gen Psychiatry* 49:522–530, 1992.

Volkow ND, Brodie J, Bendriem B: Positron emission tomography: Basic principles and applications in psychiatric research. *Ann NY Acad Sci* 620:128–144, 1991.

Wang PP, Doherty S, Hesselink JR, et al: Callosal morphology concurs with neurobehavioral and neuropathological findings in two neurodevelopmental disorders. *Arch Neurol* 49:407–411, 1992.

Ward IL: The prenatal stress syndrome: Current status. *Psychoneuroendocrinology* 9:3–11, 1984.

Watson C, Andermann F, Gloor P, et al: Anatomic basis of amygdaloid and hippocampal volume measurement by magnetic resonance imaging. *Neurology* 42:1743–1750, 1992.

Willerman L, Schultz R, Rutledge JN, et al: In vivo brain size and intelligence. *Intelligence* 15:223–228, 1991.

Wolkin A, Sanfilipo M, Wolf AP, et al: Negative symptoms and hypofrontality in chronic schizophrenia. *Arch Gen Psychiatry* 49:959–965, 1992.

Wong DF, Wagner HN, Tune LE, et al: Positron emission tomography reveals elevated D$_2$ receptors in drug-naive schizophrenics. *Science* 234:1558–1563, 1986.

Yazgan MY, Peterson B, Wexler BE, et al: Behavioral laterality in individuals with Gilles de la Tourette's syndrome and basal ganglia alterations: A preliminary report. *Biol Psychiatry*, in press.

Zametkin A, Liebenauer L, Fitzgerald G, et al: Brain metabolism in teenagers with attention-deficit hyperactivity disorder. *Arch Gen Psychiatry* 50:333–340, 1993.

Zametkin A, Nordahl T, Gross M, et al: Cerebral glucose metabolism in adults with hyperactivity of childhood onset. *N Engl J Med* 323:1361–1366, 1990.

Zilbovicius M, Garreau B, Tzourio N, et al: Regional cerebral blood flow in childhood autism: A SPECT study. *Am J Psychiatry* 149:924–930, 1992.

B/ Major General Theories of Child and Adolescent Development

9 COGNITIVE-BEHAVIORAL APPROACHES

Alan E. Kazdin, Ph.D.

Behavior modification, or behavior therapy, refers to an approach toward the assessment, evaluation, and alteration of behavior.[1] The approach focuses on the treatment of clinical problems and development of adaptive functioning in everyday life. Although many people may associate behavior modification with a specific form of treatment, in fact several different *treatment techniques* are embraced by the approach. The different techniques can be applied to many *different clinical disorders and maladaptive behaviors*. Applications often focus on anxiety, affective, conduct and oppositional-defiant, eating, stereotyped movement, speech and language, developmental, and many other disorders. In addition, behavioral techniques often are used to improve a

[1] The terms *behavior modification* and *behavior therapy* are used synonymously in the present chapter. Historically, these terms have been delineated on the basis of theoretical approaches, constituent treatment techniques, the manner in which the techniques are applied, and the countries in which the techniques have emerged (Franzini and Tilker, 1972; Keehn and Webster, 1969; Krasner, 1971; Yates, 1970). Yet, the distinction and its basis have not been adopted in a consistent fashion.

variety of behaviors in everyday life outside the context of psychiatric disorder such as promoting healthy lifestyles (eating nutritious foods, exercising), adhering to medical regimens, interacting prosocially with peers, managing and controlling pain and headache, and others.

The range of *persons and populations* to which different techniques have been applied is also broad and includes children, adolescents, and adults in everyday settings, such as at home, school, and work, and special populations, such as psychiatric patients, prisoners, nursing home residents, and others. Behavior modification also includes many *different theories about clinical problems* and how they emerge and are maintained. The theories vary in their explanation of behavior and the role they accord the influence of processes within the individual (e.g., thoughts, beliefs, perceptions) or processes resulting from events in the environment (e.g., cues, feedback, and consequences for behavior). In short, behavior modification encompasses many treatments, clinical problems, populations, and conceptual views.

The present chapter discusses behavior modification as an approach toward clinical dysfunction and traces its development over the 40 years since its inception. The chapter examines characteristics of the approach, the conceptual and laboratory foundations, and the current status of the behavioral approaches in contemporary clinical work with children and adolescents.

FOUNDATIONS OF BEHAVIOR MODIFICATION

There are many paths leading to the emergence of contemporary behavior modification (Kazdin, 1978). Although these cannot be elaborated here, a few lines of influence are especially noteworthy.

Experimental Animal Research

CLASSICAL CONDITIONING

The roots of behavior modification can be traced to laboratory research in physiology in the 1800s and 1900s. Among the many influences, the work of the Russian physiologist, Ivan P. Pavlov (1849–1936) is particularly significant. Pavlov studied digestion, especially reflex responses and how they were influenced by substances placed in the digestive system. Pavlov stimulated various portions of an animal's digestive system with food or food powder and observed the physiological reactions. As part of his studies, he found that gastric secretions were stimulated when animals—in this case dogs—merely saw the food or heard the preparation of the food. This was significant because it suggested that digestive processes could be stimulated even without direct physical stimulation. Pavlov viewed this process to be the result of the animal's experience in the laboratory, i.e., learning. He shifted his research to study how connections were made between various environmental stimuli (sights and sounds) and reflex reactions such as salivation in response to food (Pavlov, 1906, 1927).

The type of learning that Pavlov studied has been referred to as *classical or respondent conditioning*. Classical conditioning is concerned with stimuli that evoke responses. Certain stimuli in one's environment (such as noise, shock, light, and the taste of food) *elicit* reflex responses. These reflex reactions are referred to as *respondents*, or unconditioned responses. Respondents frequently are considered involuntary or automatic responses that are not under control of the individual. The connection between the unconditioned stimulus and the response is automatic, i.e., not learned. However, reflex behavior sometimes occurs in response to a stimulus that does not automatically elicit the response.

Through classical conditioning, a stimulus that is neutral (that is, does not elicit a particular reflex) can be made to elicit a reflex response. In a simple arrangement to achieve this, the neutral stimulus (referred to as a conditioned stimulus) is paired with a stimulus that elicits a reflex response (an unconditioned stimulus). If the conditioned stimulus is consistently paired with an unconditioned stimulus, the conditioned stimulus alone can elicit the response (referred to as a conditioned response). The process whereby new stimuli gain the power to elicit respondent behavior is called classical or respondent conditioning.

Pavlov's work was significant because of both his specific findings and methods of investigation. His findings suggested one way in which behaviors can be learned. The concepts of conditioning from his laboratory work were extended to explain virtually all learning, including such broad areas as the learning of language, acquisition of knowledge, and the development of deviant and maladaptive behavior (e.g., alcoholism). It is clear today that the concepts were overextended because they do not give accurate or complete accounts of these areas. Also, more recent research has shown that conditioning itself is more complex than originally thought (e.g., certain kinds of connections are more easily learned than others, and pairing stimuli does not automatically lead to learning) (Rescorla, 1988). However, the significant contribution was the scientifically and learning-based explanation of behavior. The clear demonstration of the process of learning under well-controlled conditions helped foster more elaborate studies of different kinds of learning.

Another significant feature of Pavlov's work was the method of his experiments. Pavlov used precise methods that permitted careful observation and quantification of what he was studying. For example, in some of his studies, drops of saliva were counted to measure the conditioned reflex. His meticulous laboratory notes and rigorous methods helped greatly to advance a scientific approach toward the study of behavior. Because his methods were described so clearly, they could be used by others. Also, the *zeitgeist* was to apply the scientific approach to diverse areas of inquiry beyond physiology. Pavlov seemed to exemplify scientific values and hence served as a model to others. His receipt of the Nobel Prize (1904) in physiology for his research on digestion increased the visibility of his work and adoption of his methods.

OPERANT CONDITIONING

Another type of learning that did not involve reflex responses was also under investigation. Investigators were evaluating the impact of different consequences on developing new behavior (Kazdin, 1978). Along these lines, the work of Edward L. Thorndike (1874–1949) is noteworthy. Thorndike was concerned with the learning of new behaviors, rather than establishing new connections of reflex behavior. Among his many animal experiments, the most well known are the puzzle-box experiments with cats.

Thorndike placed a hungry cat into a box and recorded the amount of time it took the animal to escape by moving a barrier. A small piece of food was placed outside the box and provided an incentive to learn to escape. With repeated trials, Thorndike found that it took less and less time for the animal to escape. Eventually, as soon as the cat was placed in the box, it removed the barrier, escaped, and ate the food reward. From many similar experiments and observations, Thorndike (1932) formulated laws or principles of behavior. The most significant of these was the *Law of Effect*, which noted that consequences that follow behavior helped learning. The rewards (e.g., food for the cat after escape) provided consequences that increased learning of the behavior. Thorndike's emphasis on the consequences of behavior was significant and previewed subsequent developments in laboratory and applied research.

B.F. Skinner (1904–1990) was influenced by Pavlov and Thorndike and also conducted a number of animal laboratory studies. Skinner's paradigm followed the type of learning of Thorndike and explored the impact of various consequences on behavior. Skinner helped clarify this type of learning and the differences from respondent conditioning studied by Pavlov. Skinner noted that many behaviors are *emitted* spontaneously and are controlled primarily by their consequences. He referred to such behaviors as *operants* because they are responses that operate (have some influence) on the environment. Operant behaviors are strengthened (increased) or weakened (decreased) as a function of the events that follow them. Most behaviors performed in everyday life are operants. They are not reflex responses (respondents) controlled by eliciting stimuli. Examples of operant behaviors include reading, walk-

Table 9.1. Summary of Basic Principles of Operant Conditioning

Principle	Characteristic Procedure and Its Effect on Behavior
Reinforcement	Presentation or removal of an event after a response that increases the frequency of the response.
Punishment	Presenation or removal of an event after a response that decreases the frequency of the response.
Extinction	No longer presenting a reinforcing event after a response which decreases the frequency of the previously reinforced response.
Stimulus control	Reinforcing the response in the presence of one discrimination stimulus but not in the presence of another. This training procedure increases the frequency of the response in the presence of the former stimulus and decreases the frequency of the response in the presence of the latter stimulus.

ing, working, talking, nodding one's head, smiling, or any response freely emitted (Skinner, 1953). Operants are distinguished by virtue of being controlled (influenced) by their consequences. The process of learning operant behaviors is referred to as *operant conditioning.*

Several types of consequences and principles were developed to explain how operant behaviors can be developed and altered (Skinner, 1938). The major relations that were investigated can be seen in the principles of operant conditioning highlighted in Table 9.1. These principles provide general statements about the relations between behaviors and environmental events. Investigations of these principles began with laboratory animals (e.g., rats, pigeons) engaging in simple responses (e.g., pressing a lever) under highly controlled conditions. Current applications of the general principles bear very little resemblance to these experimental beginnings.

As with Pavlov, the significance of Skinner's work also stemmed from the approach toward the study of behavior. His method included the focus on overt behavior, the assessment of frequency of behavior over extended periods, and the study of one or a few organisms at one time. The goal was to identify the variables that influenced behavior by the careful and intensive study of one or two subjects. The specific methodological approaches of Pavlov and Skinner and their contemporaries were quickly seized in the context of clinical work, as we shall see later.

Behaviorism in America

The late 1800s and early 1900s reflect a broader orientation, of which significant contributors such as Pavlov and Thorndike, and later Skinner, were a part. Increased interest in the scientific method was evident in diverse areas of work. Research on infrahuman species was particularly important at the time as well. The context for this in part was the influence of Charles Darwin, whose works on evolution such as the *On the Origin of Species by Means of Natural Selection* (1859) and *The Descent of Man* (1871) had suggested the continuity of species and the relevance of animal behavior.

Psychological research in America was greatly influenced by the larger movement toward more objective methods of studying behavior, as well as the specific contributions of Pavlov and his contemporaries. In America, a movement in psychology, referred to as behaviorism, was crystallized by John B. Watson (1878–1958) who was interested in animal psychology and in applying methods from animal research to study human behavior. He criticized psychology because of the use of subjective methods such as introspection, in which mental phenomena (e.g., thoughts and feelings) were studied by asking people to report on their private experience. This method of study, Watson noted, was not objective or scientific.

Watson was greatly influenced by the work of Pavlov and his contemporaries and transplanted concepts and methods of conditioning to American psychology. He argued a new "behaviorist" approach for psychology (1913, 1919), which influenced greatly the shape of psychology. His writings explained many different topics and accorded learning

a critical role. Some of his claims suggested that learning could entirely shape human behavior. In addition, conditioning was used as the basis for explaining virtually all behavior that was acquired as part of development. Watson's purpose was to convey that the concepts of conditioning and scientific methods could be applied to the study of behavior. Many of his specific statements about human behavior and its development were extreme and went well beyond what was known at the time. Yet, his major contribution was in moving psychology toward the scientific study of behavior.

EMERGENCE OF BEHAVIOR MODIFICATION

The emergence of behavior modification as an approach toward treatment and clinical work can be considered from at least two interrelated perspectives. The initial perspective is the extension of the concepts of conditioning and scientific methods to clinical work. A second perspective pertains to the dissatisfaction with prevailing approaches toward diagnosis, assessment, and treatment at the time behavior modification emerged.

Clinical Extensions

Respondent and operant conditioning were used as a basis to conceptualize personality, psychotherapy, and behavior change. Also, concepts were used to develop new techniques for treating adults and children for a host of psychological and behavioral problems. Only a few of the many steps leading to contemporary work can be illustrated here.

RESPONDENT CONDITIONING

A historically significant example that attempted to show the importance of respondent conditioning was provided by Watson and Rayner (1920), who conditioned a fear reaction in an 11-month-old boy named Albert. Albert freely played with a white rat without any adverse reaction. Prior to the study, the investigators noted that a loud noise (unconditioned stimulus) produced a startle and fear reaction (unconditioned response) in Albert. In contrast, a white rat given to Albert to play with did not elicit any adverse reaction. The investigators wished to determine if the startle reaction could be conditioned to the presence of the white rat. To condition the startle reaction, the presence of the white rat (neutral or conditioned stimulus) was immediately followed by the noise. Whenever Albert reached out and touched the rat, the noise sounded, and Albert was startled. Over a period of 1 week, the presence of the rat and the noise were paired only seven times. Finally, the rat was presented without the noise, and Albert fell over and cried. The conditioned stimulus elicited the fear response (conditioned response). Moreover, the fear generalized to other objects he was not afraid of previously (e.g., a rabbit, dog, Santa Claus mask, sealskin coat, and cotton wool). This suggested that fears can be acquired through respondent conditioning.[2]

The original report about Albert was only a first step, and the full significance of the demonstration was accentuated 3 years later by M.C. Jones, a student working under the advice of Watson. Jones (1924a) reported the case of Peter, a 34-month-old-boy whose case was a natural sequel to that of Albert. Essentially, Peter was afraid of the diverse stimuli that Albert had been conditioned to fear. The task was to develop

---

[2] The case was extremely significant because it was regarded as providing clear evidence that fears can be conditioned. The implications of such an interpretation were great, suggesting at once that learning might account for fears and avoidance behavior and, by implication, that such behaviors might be overcome by alternative learning experiences. The significance of the case is especially noteworthy because the phenomena that were demonstrated proved difficult to replicate (Bregman, 1934; English, 1929). Moreover, the original study itself is usually inaccurately cited, so that the actual findings are misrepresented (Harris, 1979). Finally, whether the study demonstrated respondent conditioning as usually conceived can be easily challenged by examining the actual procedures that were used (Kazdin, 1978). Notwithstanding these critical issues, the case exerted major impact.

ways to overcome Peter's fears. Because a rabbit elicited greater fear than other stimuli in the testing situation, it was used as the feared object during treatment. Several procedures were used to overcome fear, primarily the gradual presentation of the rabbit to Peter under nonthreatening conditions. While Peter ate, the caged rabbit was gradually brought closer to him without eliciting fear. The purpose was to associate pleasant stimuli (food) and responses (eating) with the feared object. Eventually, Peter did not react adversely when the rabbit was free to move outside of the cage, and he actually played with it.

In addition to the successful treatment of Peter, Jones (1924b) published a more extensive report that included several different methods of treating institutionalized children who had a variety of fears (e.g., being left alone, being in a dark room, and being near small animals). Two methods appeared to be particularly successful, namely, direct conditioning, in which a feared object was systematically and gradually associated with positive reactions (e.g., as had been done with Peter), and social imitation, in which nonfearful children modeled fearless interaction with the stimulus.

The demonstrations by Watson, Rayner, and Jones that fears could be conditioned and deconditioned were of obvious significance by themselves. In addition, the investigators were explicit in pointing out the implications of the findings for existing conceptions of psychopathology. For example, Watson and Rayner (1920) scoffed at the psychoanalytic interpretations that might be applied to Albert's newly acquired fear, despite the fact that the fear had been conditioned in the laboratory. Thus, the demonstrations of the conditioning and deconditioning of fear were placed in the larger arena of psychopathology and its treatment and were posed as a challenge to existing approaches.

Another early extension of respondent conditioning was in the treatment of enuresis (bed wetting). Enuresis can be conceptualized as a failure of certain stimuli (bladder cues) to elicit a response (waking) so the individual can get up and urinate appropriately. To condition waking to the bladder cues (distension), a stimulus which elicits waking is required. O.H. Mowrer and W.A. Mowrer (1938) devised an apparatus to classically condition waking to the cues that precede urination while the child is asleep. The apparatus included a liquid-sensitive pad, which is placed in the child's bed. As soon as the child urinates, a circuit is closed and an alarm is activated. The alarm serves as an unconditioned stimulus that eventually elicits waking prior to urination and sounding of the alarm. The procedure results in control of urination and permits the individual to sleep through the night without urination. This procedure, an effective technique for enuresis, was actually available prior to the 1930s. Historically, its reemergence was significant because the procedure was couched in terms of classical conditioning and hence viewed as a learning-based approach to treatment.

Another, more contemporary, extension of classical conditioning to clinical work was completed by Joseph Wolpe (1958), who developed a procedure for the treatment of anxiety. Wolpe, a physician working in South Africa, conducted experiments with laboratory animals (cats) in which he was investigating anxiety and avoidance reactions. Wolpe investigated a phenomenon referred to as *experimental neuroses*, which consists of an experimentally induced state in which animals show agitation, disruption of behavior, and other signs that resemble anxiety in humans. Experimental neuroses had been studied for some time, beginning in Pavlov's laboratory. Wolpe's special contribution was to develop a procedure to overcome anxiety in the cats he studied and then to extend the method to treat humans with anxiety disorders.

After anxiety had been developed, Wolpe exposed animals gradually to situations that elicited anxiety. When the animals were exposed to the situation (room) in which anxiety had been developed, the animals showed severe signs of anxiety and would not engage in any other behaviors. Wolpe exposed the animals to cues (other rooms) that only resembled the original situation. With less avoidance and agitation due to a reduced dose of anxiety-provoking stimuli, Wolpe encouraged the animals to engage in other responses such as eating. He reasoned that exposure to a series of anxiety-provoking situations while engaging

in other competing responses gradually would overcome the anxiety. Anxiety was reduced, and continuation of this procedure led to its elimination.

An especially significant step was to use the information derived from experiments with cats to develop a technique for human anxiety. Wolpe developed a treatment, referred to as *systematic desensitization*, in which humans were exposed in real life or in imagination to situations that provoked anxiety. They were exposed to a graduated series of stimuli. To overcome anxiety, Wolpe trained clients to become deeply relaxed so that exposure to mild representations of the anxiety-provoking situation might cause only very little anxiety. Relaxation would overcome small amounts of anxiety as each situation or imagined scene was paired with relaxation. Over time, the individual could be exposed to or imagine situations that provoked greater anxiety. Relaxation would overcome these anxious responses as well. Eventually, the individual would no longer be anxious in response to the situation that originally provoked anxiety.

The procedure was conceptualized from the standpoint of classical conditioning. Certain cues or stimuli in the environment elicit anxiety or fear. The fear could be altered by conditioning an alternative response (relaxation) that is incompatible with fear. As relaxation becomes associated with the imagined scenes, the capacity of the stimuli to elicit anxiety is eliminated. Altering the valence of the capacity of stimuli to elicit reactions adheres closely to the respondent conditioning paradigm.

Wolpe (1958) reported use of this technique in various forms with over 200 patients. He claimed that the treatment had been effective. Uncontrolled case studies are not acceptable scientifically because the basis for the change cannot be determined. Yet, Wolpe's technique and claims eventually stimulated a great deal of research on the effects of systematic desensitization. From a broader perspective, Wolpe's work was quickly assimilated because of other influences such as his reliance on animal laboratory methods, his use of learning concepts, and his concerns over objective bases of developing treatments.

The above illustrations sample a few of the more visible extensions of respondent conditioning to clinical problems. Diverse clinical and educational extensions emerged soon after classical conditioning research developed (Kazdin, 1978). Thus, there was a rapid diffusion of the concepts into multiple areas of applied work.

OPERANT CONDITIONING

The control that rewarding consequences exerted over behavior was not a new insight identified by laboratory research on operant conditioning. However, the lawful effects on behavior that were demonstrated in the laboratory were eventually extended from infrahuman species to humans (Lindsley, 1955, 1960). Some of the early laboratory work seemed to have clinical relevance. For example, laboratory studies were conducted with hospitalized psychotic patients who performed on various apparatus daily to earn small rewards (e.g., money, pictures). The purpose was to examine response patterns under various arrangements of rewarding consequences. The results showed that response patterns of psychiatric patients differed from patterns that had been evident in "normal" adults. Also, performance on the laboratory apparatus was often interrupted by pauses in which psychotic symptoms (e.g., vocal hallucinatory behaviors) could be observed. These observations suggested that the operant conditioning paradigm might be an objective way to study psychotic behavior. Perhaps of even greater significance was the finding that responding to laboratory tasks occasionally resulted in a reduction of symptoms (e.g., staring into space) both in the laboratory and on the hospital ward (King et al., 1960; Lindsley, 1955). This suggested clearly that symptoms might be altered in important ways by increases in operant responding.

Laboratory extensions of operant conditioning were made to study the behavior of many populations such as mentally retarded and autistic children. In most of the studies, the goals were merely to use operant conditioning laboratory methods to investigate how special populations responded. Operant conditioning methods were soon extended to human behavior outside of the laboratory. Quite simple demonstrations suggested that important behaviors might be influenced greatly by environmental consequences.

Several demonstrations were completed in the 1960s to examine direct extensions in applied settings. For example, demonstrations with hospitalized adult patients showed in controlled evaluations that symptoms as well as self-care and social behaviors could be readily altered (Ayllon and Azrin, 1965; Ayllon and Haughton, 1964; Ayllon and Michael, 1959). These demonstrations and many others like this indicated that human behavior in applied settings and various clinical problems could be altered by changing the consequences (e.g., attention and praise of other persons such as staff) (Eysenck, 1959; Ullmann and Krasner, 1965). The idea of using consequences to change behavior was not new, given the many applications of rewarding and punishing consequences for behavior throughout civilization. What was new was the application under a variety of special conditions and with careful assessment of behavior. The early extensions of operant conditioning principles to human behavior merely began an area of research.

Traditional Approaches toward Deviant Behavior

The development of laboratory research and the scientific study of behavior were significant ingredients underlying the development of behavior modification. No less significant was the emerging dissatisfaction with conceptualizations of clinical dysfunction, personality, and behavior that dominated mental health-related fields such as clinical psychology, psychiatry, and social work.

INTRAPSYCHIC APPROACHES

Traditionally, personality had been viewed by many theorists as an assortment of psychological forces inside the individual (Hall and Lindzey, 1978). Although these forces vary, depending upon specific theories of personality, they generally consist of such psychological factors as drives, impulses, needs, motives, conflicts, and traits. The traditional approach toward understanding behavior, both abnormal and normal, can be referred to as *intrapsychic* because psychological forces within the individual are accorded the crucial role. "Normal" behavior generally represents a socially acceptable expression of intrapsychic forces. On the other hand, "abnormal" behavior reflects disordered personality development or psychological processes.

Many different intrapsychic theories have been proposed to account for personality. Certainly, the most influential intrapsychic theory of personality is *psychoanalysis*, proposed by Sigmund Freud (1856–1939). Freud explained behavior by referring to manifestations of unconscious personality processes. Understanding behavior required a careful scrutiny of personality to determine the meaning of behavior, that is, what motives behavior represents. The psychological processes and motives behind behavior were regarded as existing in the individual. Freud's view of personality describes behavior in terms of psychological energies or motivating forces, drives, and impulses, and their interrelation. Growth and psychological development were traced to psychological impulses and their expression at various stages early in the child's development. Diverse behavior can be traced to the expression of a few psychological forces.

The development of psychoanalytic theory provided several important contributions to understanding behavior. First, the view advanced the notion that behavior is *determined*. This means that behavior, whether deviant or normal, is not random but can be traced to specific causes. For example, Freud suggested that abnormal behavior, habits, dreams, slips of the tongue, and indeed all facets of behavior often could be traced to intrapsychic processes formed early in child development. Second, psychoanalytic theory stimulated other theories on the psychological bases of behavior. Many of Freud's disciples began to develop their own intrapsychic theories; others developed theories that com-

pletely challenged the basic tenets of psychoanalysis. Third, psychoanalytic theory stimulated the development of psychological forms of treatment. If psychological forces caused emotional disturbance, psychologically based treatments might be required to alter these forces. Psychoanalytic treatment began as a method of uncovering and resolving intrapsychic processes that were assumed to underlie behavior. The primary method of treatment was talking with a therapist and working through various impulses, conflicts, defenses, and unresolved childhood experiences.

Intrapsychic approaches toward clinical problems generated a number of psychotherapy techniques. Various forms of psychotherapy have been applied to help people resolve the underlying causes presumed to account for their distress and abnormal behavior. Treatments based on intrapsychic views tend to focus on bringing to light underlying feelings, motives, and thoughts that are considered to be responsible for behavior. The primary agent for change is talk, expression of feelings, and the development of a close relationship with the therapist. Clients are encouraged to understand their own motives and to express thwarted feelings.

DISSATISFACTION

Criticisms toward intrapsychic approaches, especially psychoanalysis, grew in the 1950s and 1960s. The objections focused on the difficulty in verifying many of the claims of psychoanalysis empirically, inconsistencies within the theory itself and the therapeutic procedures derived from the theory, the neglect of social and cultural influences on behavior, and the lack of empirical support (Kazdin, 1978; Salter, 1952; Stuart, 1970). Perhaps most significant was the fact that psychoanalytic views did not seem to be based on research or easily subjected to scientific inquiry. With behaviorism on the increase, there was a need for and strong interest in approaches that were more amenable to scientific research.

It was not merely the intrapsychic view or general approach that was subject to criticism. Considerable dissatisfaction was voiced over traditional forms of psychotherapy and their focus on intrapsychic processes. In the early 1900s psychoanalysis and psychoanalytically oriented psychotherapy dominated clinical practice. In the 1940s and 1950s, many researchers began to question and criticize the effects of these techniques. In 1952, Hans Eysenck published a paper that expressed dissatisfaction with traditional treatments. Eysenck reviewed contemporary research and claimed that the evidence did not support the efficacy of psychotherapy. He noted that providing psychotherapy seemed to be no more effective than simply leaving people alone (no treatment). Eysenck's paper and subsequent revisions in the 1960s yielded a simple conclusion, namely, that traditional forms of treatment did not seem to work. His evaluation of the available research and the overall conclusion were very actively debated.

Eysenck had also suggested that learning-based treatments were more effective than traditional forms of treatment. There was no firm evidence at this time to provide a clear basis for this claim. Yet, the claim helped polarize the field in different ways. To those interested in traditional psychotherapy, these papers served as a challenge to conduct the needed research to see if, or to show that, the treatments really were effective. To those dissatisfied with traditional approaches, Eysenck's work helped point the way to learning-based approaches.

Over the last 35 years, a tremendous amount of research has emerged on the effects of psychotherapy (Bergin and Garfield, 1994). The findings vary among the different types of treatment and clinical problems to which they are applied and hence cannot be easily summarized. Generally, large-scale evaluations have suggested that psychotherapy often leads to positive changes in behavior (Brown, 1987). In contrast to Eysenck's earlier claim, treatment is usually significantly better than no treatment. Yet, currently over 400 different forms of psychotherapy have been identified for adults (TB Karasu, personal communication) and well over 230 for children and adolescents (Kazdin, 1988). The fact remains that very few of these have been studied at all. Consequently, the effectiveness of most treatments has not been established empirically.

General Comments

The dissatisfaction extends beyond the psychoanalytic approach as a model of clinical dysfunction and the effectiveness of alternative forms of psychotherapy. Other areas of dissatisfaction include the conceptual bases, utility, and validity of alternative assessment (e.g., projective techniques) and diagnostic approaches. These sources of dissatisfaction are rich topics in their own right and cannot be elaborated here. From the standpoint of the history of behavior modification, the critical point to note is that the dissatisfaction served as a critical backdrop for a new approach toward clinical dysfunction.

It is important to acknowledge that much of the behavioral portrayal of intrapsychic approaches to clinical dysfunction were simplified views that painted the disease model and its implications as relatively extreme. For example, in criticizing the disease model early in the formation of behavior therapy, there was little acknowledgement or appreciation of the complex and diverse disease models that medicine embraces (Buss, 1966). A bacterial disease model was adopted for criticism by proponents of behavior therapy who criticized psychodynamic approaches; this disease model oversimplifies psychodynamic views. Similarly, specific phenomena within the intrapsychic approach were oversimplified for purposes of argument. For example, proponents of behavior modification were apt to note that an intrapsychic approach predicted symptom substitution (Ullmann and Krasner, 1965). The absence of symptom substitution or improvements in nontreated areas following treatment were taken to provide strong evidence against an intrapsychic view. Absent from the bulk of behavioral discussions at the time was recognition that symptom substitution was not invariably predicted by intrapsychic views, a point noted by Freud (1936).

In the development of behavior therapy as a movement, it was critical to establish differences between old and new. In the process, both the old (traditional intrapsychic approaches) and new (behavior modification) tended to be polarized. With the benefit of a historical perspective, it is now clear that the "new" was not all that new and much of the "old" was cast aside too quickly. Nevertheless, the polarities served a critical dialectic function. As psychology had grown as a science, experimental findings about behavior and its development had little impact on the dominant positions within clinical work. Specific psychological constructs, as well as the approach of scientific research, provided viable alternatives that address many of the criticisms of prevailing approaches. The strengths of behavior modification as an alternative paradigm or approach were expressly in those areas where the intrapsychic approach appeared weak, namely, specificity of treatment and empirical outcome research.

CONTEMPORARY BEHAVIOR MODIFICATION

By the early 1960s, behavior therapy had become a formal movement as ideas spread across different conceptual and geographical boundaries. Behavior therapy consisted of several different developments, including varied theoretical approaches and treatment techniques. However, common denominators of the approach can be identified.

Characteristics of Behavior Modification

PRIMACY OF BEHAVIOR

Within behavior modification, overt behavior plays a major part in the assessment, treatment of clinical dysfunction, and evaluation of treatment. Whenever possible, clinical problems are operationalized in terms of overt behavioral referents. Thus, symptoms or groups of several symptoms that go together (syndromes or disorders) are conceptualized in terms of behavior. Although emphasis is placed on behavior or what a person does, this does not mean that problems are viewed solely in terms of overt actions. How people feel (affect) and think (cognition) also are important and often central to the specific problems brought to treatment. For example, depressed persons often feel sad (affect), believe they cannot do anything right (cognition), and engage in few activities (behaviors) in their everyday lives. Although affect, cognition, and behavior are important, behavioral treatments give primary attention to behavior as a means of altering the clinical problem. In the treatment process, a depressed patient may be encouraged to engage in specific activities involving interactions with others and in setting goals for accomplishing tasks. Increases in activity and completion of tasks are some of the behaviors found to alter depressive symptoms, including the many feelings and thoughts that comprise depression. Consequently, the approach often focuses on behavior both as an end in itself and as a means of changing affect and cognition.

IMPORTANCE OF LEARNING

An assumption of behavior modification is that behaviors of interest in the context of therapeutic, educational, social, and other settings can be altered by providing new learning experiences. Understandably, the approach has drawn heavily on learning theories and research in psychology. Behavioral treatments essentially provide special learning experiences to alter deviant or clinically maladaptive behavior and to increase adaptive behavior.

In noting that new learning experiences can change behavior, it is important not to overstate the claim. Proponents of behavior modification do *not* adhere to the views that all behaviors are learned and all behaviors can be changed through learning. Diverse biological, behavioral, social, cultural, and other factors converge to influence behavior. The influences that control behavior for most disorders are not fully understood. The key feature of the behavioral approach is recognition of the plasticity of behavior or the amenability of behavior to change when systematic learning experiences are provided. Whether providing new learning experiences will effectively alter behavior can be determined only empirically. The assumption that learning experiences can alter behavior has proven to be extremely helpful in developing effective treatments. Learning research often suggests what to do in treatment to achieve behavior change.

DIRECTIVE AND ACTIVE TREATMENTS

Behavior modification techniques usually rely on directive and active treatments. This means that persons who come for treatment are given specific directions for procedures they are to perform. This does not mean that clients are simply told what to do. Indeed, the client often plays an important role in negotiating and implementing the plan of action to change behavior. Behavioral techniques do not rely on therapeutic processes such as talking about one's problem to relieve emotional distress or insight or the therapeutic relationship as the mechanism through which change occurs. During the course of treatment these elements may be important and have beneficial effects. Yet, talking about one's problems is not viewed as the most effective way of producing behavior change. Rather, explicit training experiences are prescribed in treatment.

Treatment sessions are frequently used as the context in which actions for change are planned and often carried out. Often the actions or activities are assigned to persons as "homework" in which specific activities are carried out to help achieve the desired changes. Therapeutic change in behavior modification is conceptualized as *learning new behaviors* that are to be performed in everyday life. Specific and direct activities serve as the basis for developing these new behaviors.

IMPORTANCE OF ASSESSMENT AND EVALUATION

A central characteristic of behavior modification is a commitment to assessment and evaluation of alternative treatments. In research, behavior modification places major emphasis on measuring outcome and evaluating treatment in controlled studies to decide if alternative treatments are effective and which variations of treatment are more effective than others. The emphasis on outcome research to investigate treatment has been a hallmark of the approach. In clinical work with individual clients, evaluation is also very important. In this context, evaluation refers to measuring the affect, cognition, and behavior of interest to monitor the progress the client makes during the course of treatment. The evaluation of treatment involves different components.

First, the behaviors that are to be altered are carefully assessed. The assessment may consist of several different ways of measuring the problem or desired behavior including direct observation of how the child performs at home and at school, evaluations by significant others (parents, peers), and evaluations by the clients themselves. The assessment is central for identifying the extent and nature of the problem.

Second, the goals and the means to obtain them are usually well specified. Before treatment the therapist conducts an evaluation to identify what the problem is, how the client and others are affected by it, and the circumstances under which the problem emerges. The evaluation tends to focus on details of the symptoms or behaviors, the conditions associated with their performance (e.g., setting, antecedents, consequences), and resources in the child's repertoire and environment that might be mobilized in specific treatment strategies. Once the problem is identified and assessed, the procedures and the goals toward which they will be directed can be specified. The explicit nature of the procedures and goals is an important characteristic of behavior modification.

Third, the effects of treatment are assessed to determine if the desired outcomes have been obtained. Specific techniques of evaluating change in the individual case are often used to permit identification of the effects of treatment and the extent to which clinically important changes have been achieved (Barlow et al., 1984; Kazdin, 1982). Evaluation of progress in treatment is also facilitated by having clearly specified goals and procedures.

USE OF PERSONS IN EVERYDAY LIFE

Behavioral techniques often are carried out at home, at school, in various institutional settings (psychiatric hospitals), and in the community, rather than in a therapist's office. Persons who are responsible for the care, management, and education of children, such as parents, teachers, relatives, or persons who can exert influence in their daily contact such as peers and siblings, are often involved to help with the behavior change program. These individuals are occasionally referred to as *paraprofessionals* because they work along with professionals in achieving therapeutic change.

Paraprofessionals who are in frequent contact with the client can observe the behaviors in the actual situations in which they are performed so they are in the best position to focus on behavior as it is actually occurring. For example, in applications with children, parents, teachers, and peers frequently are trained in behavior change techniques (Kazdin, 1994). Because these persons are in direct contact with the client at home and at school, they are likely to be in a better position to change behaviors of interest (e.g., tantrums, oppositional behavior, completion of homework).

CASE ILLUSTRATION

The above features of the behavioral approach are quite general. An illustration may convey more concretely how some of the characteristics are reflected in actual practice. Consider as an example the case of a 12½-year-old girl named Tammy who was admitted to an 18-bed psychiatric inpatient unit for children, ages 6–12 (Esveldt-Dawson et al., 1982). She was referred for evaluation because of the presence of several symptoms including "nervousness," chronic constipation, abdominal pains, and school failure. The onset of the symptoms occurred approximately 4 years earlier and was coincident with the beginning of her alleged sexual abuse by her blind, 75-year-old grandfather. The molestation by the grand-

father apparently had continued over a period of approximately 4 years and was terminated before hospitalization. Prior to this experience, Tammy's academic performance was above average (B grade average) and her school attendance was excellent. Since the experiences with her grandfather, her school performance deteriorated and her symptoms emerged.

Tammy lived with her parents and four older sisters. She grew up without any significant illness or developmental delays. Her Weschler Intelligence Scale for Children-Revised (WISC-R) IQ was within the normal range (full scale = 95). There had been chronic sources of stress in the home. Her mother had a history of alcohol abuse and attempted suicide. Early in Tammy's development, the father was in the military and frequently away from home for extended periods. Her mother and father suffered marital disharmony for protracted periods, including divorce and remarriage to each other.

Prior to and immediately after admission, information was obtained from direct interviews with Tammy and her parents. The primary symptoms evident in the interviews were anxiety, marked self-consciousness, avoidance of men, and preoccupation with her past behaviors. Additional symptoms that were evident but less marked included loss of interest and pleasure in the usual activities, feelings of guilt, impairment of functioning at school, and somatic complaints. The principal diagnosis (Axis I) was anxiety disorder, specifically, overanxious disorder (DSM-III). The diagnosis was supported by multivariate diagnosis based on parent completed ratings on the Child Behavior Checklist (CBCL) (Achenbach and Edelbrock, 1983). In general, her CBCL reflected high internalizing dysfunction. Tammy's profile was closest to the empirically derived cluster referred to as anxious-obsessive-aggressive.

A behavioral approach was used in the hospital to treat problem areas revealed through the diagnosis. Salient symptom areas were anxiety and avoidance, particularly associated with school and unfamiliar men. In the presence of men she exhibited withdrawal and severe anxiety that was visibly evident and was attributed to her sexual contact with her grandfather. The selection of anxiety associated with school and unfamiliar men was based on information obtained daily in interactions in the hospital, her impaired functioning, and the relation of these problems to the clinical picture when she was initially referred for treatment.

To assess anxiety toward school and men, several role-play situations were devised. The situations pertaining to men included: asking a man for a donation to a hospital, asking a salesman for help in trying on shoes, meeting a new male therapist, welcoming a peer's father on the inpatient unit, and sitting next to a male usher at a dinner. Anxiety pertaining to school situations included: receiving a poor mark on an assignment, being excluded by peers during an art project, speaking in front of class, being unjustly accused of cheating by the teacher, and being sent to the principal for tardiness.

The situations required 15 minutes to complete through a role-play test each day and were administered by a therapist (female psychiatric resident) taking the role of the person(s) in the situation. Tammy was encouraged to respond as she normally would. The behaviors Tammy performed while enacting these role-play situations were observed daily from behind a one-way mirror. Several behaviors related to anxiety and social functioning were assessed (e.g., nervous mannerisms, stiffness). Tammy was also asked to rate her own level of anxiety. Appropriate eye contact, expression of affect, body movements, and overall social skills were also rated.

After several days of assessment, training was initiated by the therapist. Training consisted of providing instructions, therapist modeling, coaching, feedback, and social reinforcement to develop specific behaviors within each role-play situation. Training was introduced in a multiple-baseline design across different behaviors. This design consists of introducing the intervention to one behavior while continuing to collect data on all behaviors of interest. In turn, the intervention was applied to each behavior. The relation between the intervention and change can be inferred in this fashion; in addition, weak or ineffective interventions can be detected and altered quickly as needed (Kazdin, 1982).

The effects of training can be seen in Figure 9.1, which shows

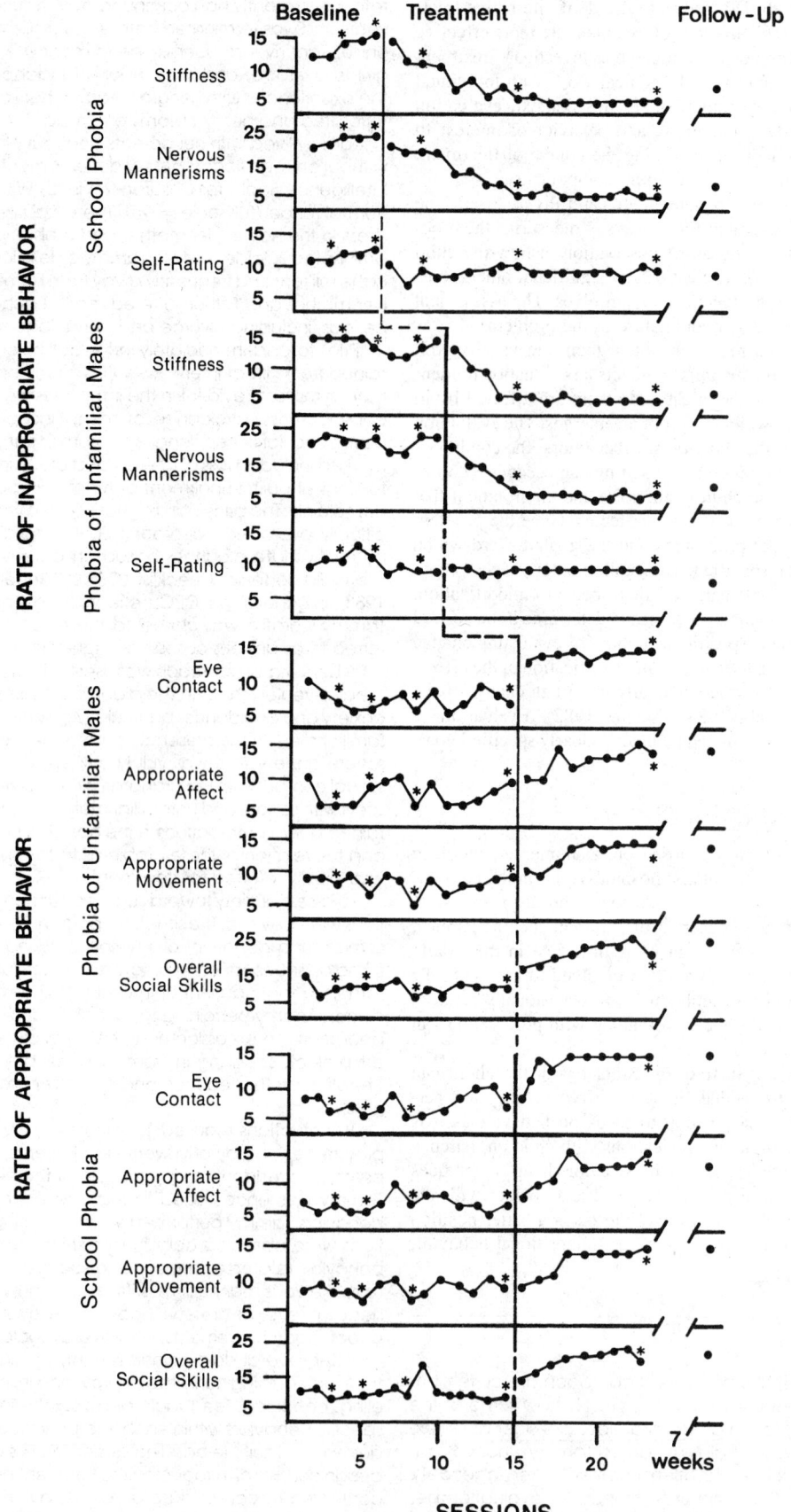

Figure 9.1. Rates of appropriate and inappropriate behaviors across experimental conditions in daily assessments and probes (evaluations by a second rater indicated by *asterisks*). (From Esveldt-

Dawson K, Wisner KL, Unis AS, Matson JL, Kazdin AE: Treatment of phobias in a hospitalized child. *J Behav Ther Exp Psychiatry* 13:77–83, 1982.)

that inappropriate behaviors decreased and appropriate behaviors increased as training was introduced. Additional measures not represented in the figure were included. At five different points over the course of assessment and treatment, an interview was scheduled with an unfamiliar male (one of three males introduced as doctors of the hospital who rotated among the interviews). Each asked mundane questions as part of the brief interview. The interview was rated from behind a one-way mirror to assess nervous mannerisms, stiffness, and other behaviors beyond the confines of the role-play test. Over the course of treatment, these behaviors also reflected reductions in anxiety. Finally, ratings of videotapes of baseline and treatment sessions were made by direct-care staff who were naive to the conditions sampled in the tapes. Staff rated Tammy's discomfort as lower and her sociability as higher for the treatment tape. In general, the data indicated changes were achieved. The qualitative changes in affect, approach behavior in social situations, conversations with adults, and overall functioning were dramatic but not easily documented. Follow-up contact 7 and 21 weeks after discharge and treatment termination indicated that school attendance, academic performance, and interactions with adults and peers had improved.

Several features of the behavioral approach can be seen in the case of Tammy and her treatment. The focus on her behavior, the use of active treatments to reduce anxiety, and an effort to affect behavior in and draw from everyday situations are primary examples. Perhaps less dramatically illustrated but even more important was the effort to evaluate Tammy's progress. The central question is whether the treatment is achieving the desired ends. The data gathered about Tammy's progress were obtained to address this question.

Current Status

Although the case conveys several characteristics outlined previously, it samples a small segment of behavioral approaches. The reason has to do with the diverse views and techniques the field embraces. Behavior modification is not a uniform or monolithic position. At the inception of the field, many independent attempts to provide a scientific and learning-based foundation for psychotherapy were unified under the rubrics *behavior modification* and *behavior therapy*. The justification for unifying different developments was the common reaction against the prevailing views in psychiatry and clinical psychology and the adherence to learning theory, broadly conceived. Differences within the areas of behavior modification were minimized or ignored for the purpose of developing a relatively unified movement to oppose the traditional intrapsychic model of abnormal behavior and its treatment.

After behavior therapy emerged, individual approaches within the field developed and differences among the approaches became more marked. The diversity can be illustrated by examining the manifold conceptual approaches upon which behavioral techniques rely. Major approaches include a stimulus-response (S-R) mediational view, applied behavior analysis, and cognitive behavior modification. The S-R mediational view consists primarily of the application of learning concepts and emphasizes stimulus-response pairing, as derived from the contiguity learning views of Pavlov, Guthrie, Mowrer, and others. Intervening variables and hypothetical constructs are relied on to account for behavior. Illustrative of this general theoretical approach are techniques such as systematic desensitization and flooding, which focus on extinguishing the underlying anxiety that accounts for and sustains avoidant behavior. Characteristic of this approach is an attempt to link mediational constructs to antecedent stimuli and responses that can be readily operationalized.

Applied behavior analysis is quite different as an approach within behavior therapy because it draws primarily on the substantive and methodological heritage of operant conditioning and the experimental analysis of behavior. Emphasis is placed on antecedent and consequent events; mediational states, private events, and cognitions are avoided. Treatment focuses on altering antecedents and consequences in order to alter the target behavior. A unique methodological approach also characterizes applied behavior analysis and includes the experimental evaluation of the performance of individuals using intrasubject-replication designs, usually in place of between-group designs. Applied behavior analysis includes a variety of techniques based on reinforcement, punishment, extinction, stimulus, control, and other principles derived from laboratory research (Kazdin, 1994).

COGNITIVE BEHAVIOR THERAPY

Cognitive behavior therapy is an approach that stresses thoughts, beliefs, and the assumption that people actively shape their own environment. Maladaptive behavior is viewed as resulting from faulty cognitions; therapy focuses on eliminating these cognitions and replacing them with thoughts and self-statements that will promote more adaptive behavior. Although behavior is viewed as a result of cognitive symbolic processes, often behavioral methods are used to alter these cognitive processes, such as practicing and receiving reinforcing consequences for making self-statements that promote the desired behaviors. Among the alternative positions, cognitively based paradigms have received the greatest attention within the past 15 years.

Cognitive and behavioral views of human functioning, clinical problems, and intervention have merged. In fact, the field is more aptly characterized by reference to *cognitive behavior therapy* rather than to behavior therapy (see Craighead et al., 1994; Kendall, 1991). Cognitive behavior therapy includes many conceptual views and interventions. Given the diversity of views, techniques, it is not really possible to characterize the field in ways that address the substantive content or focus of the field. For example, *behavior therapy* with or without cognitive as a modifier is not defined by any circumscribed conceptual views, intervention techniques, or singular roots (e.g., the laws and principles of learning). Although learning theory and findings have been especially useful, the domain has expanded, so that behavior modification has been defined more generally as treatment based on experimental findings from the psychology and social sciences.

CONTEMPORARY CHARACTERISTICS

Because of the expanded definition of the field and the development of alternative and often diametrically opposed conceptual interpretations of behavior and therapeutic change, few characteristics of the field can be set forth that encompass all factions. Currently, the distinguishing characteristics of behavior therapy appear to lie in its approach to treatment and its conceptualization rather than in a specific theoretical basis or set of techniques. In general, behavior therapy tends to

1. Focus on current rather than historical determinants of behavior;
2. Emphasize overt behavior change as a major criterion in evaluating treatment;
3. Rely on basic research from psychology to generate hypotheses about treatment and specific techniques;
4. Specify treatment in objective and operational terms so that the procedures can be repeated;
5. Specify the target behavior and the techniques for measuring outcome.

In addition to these characteristics, current behavior therapy still rejects the major tenets of intrapsychic approaches. However, the major *positive* characteristics that distinguish behavior therapy reflect more of a general scientific approach toward treatment and clinical practice rather than a particular conceptual stance or set of theoretical propositions. An empirical approach toward treatment has extended to many treatments and reflects a broader movement within therapy research (Bergin and Garfield, 1994).

PROLIFERATION OF INTERVENTION FOCI

Behavioral techniques have been applied to the many dysfunctions, disorders, and problems of living that bring youth and adults to psychotherapy. Within the broad area of clinical dysfunction, behavior therapy has been able to expand well beyond traditional domains. For example, behavioral treatments provide specific interventions to improve the functioning of such populations as autistic children and youth with various levels of mental retardation, areas where traditional therapy have had limited applicability (see Kazdin, 1994).

Perhaps more noteworthy is that behavioral techniques have extended well beyond the usual domains of clinical dysfunction. Three factors have contributed to these extensions. First, the principles and procedures (e.g., reinforcement, extinction) on which many behavioral techniques have wide applicability across populations (e.g., preschoolers in day care, geriatric patients). Second, the strong commitment to assessment and outcome evaluation interfaces well with concerns of accountability. Third, many of the techniques are conceptually simple and as a result have an appeal in many applied settings. The conceptual simplicity is often deceptive because many of the procedures work only when well-specified parameters of administration are carefully adhered to.

Behavior therapy with children and adolescents illustrates the scope of applications. As examples, behavioral interventions have been applied to treat a wide range of youth with acute or chronic medical illness and injury, to reduce anxiety and pain associated with invasive medical procedures, to improve adherence and compliance with medical regimens (e.g., among dialysis and diabetic patients), and to improve a variety of habits in everyday life (e.g., use of seat belts, eating nutritious meals, maintaining dental hygiene) (see Peterson et al., 1994). Major and large-scale applications of behavioral techniques have emerged in relation to education and academic performance, athletic performance, traffic safety (e.g., reducing accidents), and in business and industry (e.g., to manage employee performance to reduce accidents). In addition, a variety of prevention techniques have been applied to youth (e.g., to avert academic dysfunction, substance use and abuse). In general, altering behavior is a goal of many facets of society (government, law, child rearing, education). Given the extension of behavioral techniques deeply into many of these areas, the use of the term behavior ''therapy'' to characterize the field has become a misnomer.

Developmental Considerations

Description of the development of behavior therapy, alternative approaches, and characteristics of behavioral interventions has neglected to consider the role of child development. Behavioral approaches do not neglect developmental issues and considerations. At the same time, there is no overarching single developmental perspective or theoretical base that permeates treatment.

As already noted, behavioral approaches encompass many different views about dysfunction and intervention. Thus, one would not expect that these views consider developmental issues in the same way. The common theme of behavioral approaches is that principles of behavior can be identified and utilized as the basis of therapeutic change. Although the translation of these to practice might well take into account exigencies of development, the principles are not fundamentally different. At the other side of the spectrum are behavioral views that accord development a central role in terms of what techniques might be appropriate. For example, cognitively based procedures attempt to draw upon developmental psychology in substance and application.

There are manifold ways in which development is considered. These include the focus of interventions, the translation of alternative techniques to suit children and adolescents, cognitive developmental issues, and conceptualization of dysfunction.

FOCUS OF DYSFUNCTIONS ARISING IN CHILDHOOD

Behavioral techniques have been applied to the full range of dysfunctions that emerge in infancy, childhood, and adolescence. The intervention research is rather extensive in terms of the breadth of focus among disorders including mental retardation, attention deficit-hyperactivity, conduct and oppositional, anxiety, eating, speech and language, stereo-

typed movement, and other disorders (Mash and Barkley, 1989). The applications to children and problems that emerge in childhood have been sufficiently active to delineate an area of research as *child behavior therapy* (Marholin, 1978; Ross, 1981) with its own journal (*Child and Family Behavior Therapy*). The focus on children as part of treatment and delineation of a special area has naturally led the field to greater specialization in considering the problems, needs, and issues that emerge in development.

ADAPTATION OF TREATMENTS

General principles that describe influences on behavior may be applicable across the developmental spectrum. Nevertheless, how these are implemented and the points of intervention to maximize efficacy might well vary as a function of development. Behavioral treatments often consider development in the context of implementation of many procedures. For example, among children, two obviously critical sources of influence are the family and peers. The use of behavioral techniques based on alternative social learning procedures are often conducted in ways to capitalize on the sensitivity of children to the influence of family and peers. Thus, major treatment modalities are based on using family members to alter behavior of the child. Parent management training, as one illustration, has been used with a very wide range of young children whose dysfunctions include mental retardation, conduct and oppositional disorders, anxiety disorders, eating disorders, enuresis, and encopresis, to mention a few. The principles and practices (e.g., reinforcement, extinction, shaping) are applied by parents because of their special position in relation to the child. Parent management training is probably the most well-investigated of all therapy techniques for children in light of an extraordinary number of controlled outcome trials (e.g., Kazdin, 1985; Miller and Prinz, 1990).

Peers also play a pivotal role in behavioral interventions for children and adolescents. These applications take advantage of findings that children are interested in serving in the capacity of behavior change agents for their peers, profit greatly from the experience in terms of their own learning and therapeutic change, and respond as well or better to peer-based programs as to programs administered by adults (Kazdin, 1994). Developing programs for groups of children are often used as well, particularly in classroom settings where peer influences are mobilized to augment behavior change (Strain, 1981).

COGNITIVE DEVELOPMENT

An area of behavioral research that makes relatively strong contact with developmental research is cognitive treatment of childhood dysfunction (Shirk, 1988). The development and emergence of cognitive processes is a central area of basic research in developmental psychology. At the same time, clinical researchers have been interested in using cognitively based interventions to effect behavior change. The importance of considering cognitive development and the integration of this information have been evident in several applications.

For example, Spivack and Shure (1982) have identified several cognitive problem-solving skills (e.g., generating alternative solutions, means-ends thinking) that underlie interpersonal behavior. They have developed intervention techniques to develop these cognitive skills in children both for the purpose of treatment and prevention of childhood dysfunction. Interestingly, the specific cognitive processes vary in their significance in relation to child adjustment at different ages and consequently can receive different emphases. The findings come from studying cognitive development and integrating development differences into treatment programs for youth of different ages.

CONNECTING DEVELOPMENTAL PROCESSES, OUTCOMES, AND INTERVENTIONS

Early in behavior therapy, there was relatively little interest in understanding many of the processes leading to clinical dysfunction. One of the reasons was a broader reaction against speculative processes discussed in intrapsychic approaches which rarely led to empirical tests and could not be well verified in relation to dysfunction (e.g., depression is the result of aggression directed inwardly; regression and fixation or unresolved conflicts lead to dysfunction). The types of processes posed in broader fields of psychology and psychiatry and methods to assess process-outcome connections have evolved considerably. Along with that, behavior therapy researchers have taken greater interest in examining the factors leading to dysfunction. The goal, of course, is to identify critical processes and to predict how they lead to dysfunction. From that, interventions can be developed to target key processes.

For example, Patterson and his colleagues (1989, 1992) have proposed and validated a developmental model of antisocial behavior. The model focuses on the progression of antisocial behavior, beginning with early family influences in the home and including interactions with peers and involvement in delinquent behavior. Research has shown how specific child-rearing practices contribute to escalation of aggression and antisocial behavior in the home, how these are part of a larger sequence of events involving the family (e.g., stress) and the adverse outcomes to which these lead (e.g., in relation to the child's self-esteem, dysfunctional peer relations, and poor school performance). The work has underscored the importance of child-rearing practices as one point of intervening to disrupt the processes.

As another example, cognitive processes have been shown to underlie aggressive behavior among children and adolescents. As an illustration, Dodge et al. have identified a significant *attributional bias* among aggressive children and adolescents (e.g., Dodge et al., 1990; Dodge and Somberg, 1987). Aggressive youth tend to view ambiguous situations (where the intention of others is unclear) as hostile. The attribution of hostility to others helps to precipitate aggressive acts that are merely retaliatory from the standpoint of the aggressive child. These acts, however, do not seem justified in the views of the child's peers. Peer rejection appears to follow aggressive behavior. The reactions of the peers and their dislike of and isolation from the aggressive child provide additional cues to the aggressive child that the environment is hostile. Thus, a vicious circle of aggressive behavior and untoward peer reactions can be sustained. Research such as the work on attributional bias serves to identify potential points of intervention to interrupt aggressive behavior. A number of cognitive behavioral techniques based on this type of research have been effective (Durlak et al., 1991). The goal of the research is to develop techniques that draw on theory and supporting research on factors leading to dysfunction. In principle, this has always been the goal of intervention research. The insistence on data at each stage is the primary contribution of contemporary research.

GENERAL COMMENTS

The areas discussed merely illustrate developmental considerations in behavioral research. Developmental psychology is an area that provides a research base from which behavioral research can draw. Developmental psychology charts the affective, cognitive, and behavioral processes that may be critical for treatment. Although behavioral approaches consider development in many different ways, the integration of development and treatment is rather weak.

The hiatus between developmental theory and research and treatment is difficult to bridge for behavioral and nonbehavioral views. Usually general abstractions are discussed such as considering sensitive (critical periods), emergent processes, and other global developmental concepts. Thus, a developmental perspective for many approaches, including behavioral approaches, has more to do with a general view than with a rigorous integration of theory and findings from developmental research. This does not mean that the influence of developmental theory and

research is minor or that interventions as currently practiced are not informed by research. However, upon scrutiny, the specific use of developmental findings in the treatment process is difficult to discern among alternative approaches.

CONCLUSIONS

When behavior therapy first emerged as a formal movement, it encompassed different conceptual positions and treatment techniques. However, the differences at the inception of the movement were deemphasized to promote the important common characteristics, namely, treatment procedures based on learning and a conceptual alternative to the intrapsychic approaches. Early definitions stressed the ties of behavior therapy to learning theory and conditioning principles as a common ingredient. When behavior therapy first developed, it enjoyed the illusive clarity often associated with youth. The polarity of intrapsychic and behavioral approaches seemed clear, whether discussed at the broad conceptual level (e.g., psychoanalytic versus behavioral theories) or in relation to specific clinical phenomena (e.g., symptom substitution). Also, the foundation of "learning theory," although often debated, was considered by proponents of behavior modification to provide much firmer ground than the conceptual quicksand psychoanalysis offered. Over the years, theory, research, and clinical experience has altered in many ways critical features of the approach. Although learning has represented a critical emphasis, ambiguities at the theoretical level in the most basic paradigms such as classical conditioning have made the foundations less clear. Also, the relation of specific behavioral techniques to learning theories or laboratory paradigms are more readily acknowledged as strained. The intolerance of psychodynamic approaches has tempered. The move toward cognitive views within behavior modification has been coupled with a broader orientation toward integration of many theoretical approaches. Rapprochement and integration of previously adversarial approaches are actively discussed and advocated (Norcross and Goldfried, 1992). The goal of developing a clear and distinct behavioral approach has become subservient to the task of understanding clinical phenomena and drawing upon and testing diverse theoretical views.

Contemporary developments within behavior modification, beyond the scope of the present chapter, convey that the field has developed remarkably in the four decades since its formal inception. The field cannot be characterized accurately by pointing to a particular set of theories or domain of psychology as the basis of treatment. A major characteristic of contemporary behavior modification is an empirical approach to intervention and its evaluation. Interestingly, this common feature of the approaches within behavior modification reflects the general methodological tenets of behaviorism to which the overall movement can be traced. Within the general methodological approach, diversity within the field is encouraged at both the conceptual and the technical levels. Approaches are welcome as long as they are amenable to empirical evaluation. On the other hand, behavior modification is not a blind empiricism as applied to psychotherapy because many techniques and procedures draw heavily from scientific psychology, and learning theories in particular. Further, advancing research techniques often generate their own theoretical approaches, which are subjected to further validation. The present chapter has traced the major developments that led to the emergence of behavior modification as an overall movement and approach toward therapy.

Acknowledgment. *Completion of this chapter was facilitated by Research Scientist Award MH00353 and Grant MH35408 from the National Institute of Mental Health.*

References

Achenbach TM, Edelbrock CS: *Manual for the Child Behavior Checklist and Revised Child Behavior Profile*. Burlington, VT, University Associates in Psychiatry, 1983.

Ayllon T, Azrin NH: The measurement and reinforcement of behavior of psychotics. *J Exp Anal Behav* 8:356–383, 1965.

Ayllon T, Haughton E: Modification of symptomatic verbal behavior of mental patients. *Behav Res Ther* 2:87–97, 1964.

Ayllon T, Michael J: The psychiatric nurse as a behavioral engineer. *J Exp Anal Behav* 2:323–334, 1959.

Barlow DH, Hayes SC, Nelson RO: *The Scientist-Professional: Research and Accountability in Clinical and Research Settings*. New York, Pergamon, 1984.

Bergin AE, Garfield SL (eds): *Handbook of Psychotherapy and Behavior Change* (4th ed). New York, Wiley, 1994.

Bregman EP: An attempt to modify the emotional attitudes of infants by the conditioned response technique. *J Gen Psychol* 45:169–198, 1934.

Brown J: A review of meta-analyses on psychotherapy outcome research. *Clin Psychol Rev* 7:1–23, 1987.

Buss AH: *Psychopathology*. New York, Wiley, 1966.

Craighead L, Craighead WE, Kazdin AE, et al: *Cognitive and Behavioral Interventions: An Empirical Approach to Mental Health Problems*. Needham Heights, MA, Allyn & Bacon, 1994.

Darwin C: *On the Origin of Species by Means of Natural Selection*. London, Murray, 1859.

Darwin C: *The Descent of Man*. New York, Appleton, 1871.

Dodge KA, Somberg DR: Hostile attributional biases among aggressive boys are exacerbated under conditions of threats to the self. *Child Dev* 58:213–224, 1987.

Dodge KA, Price JM, Bachorowski J, et al: Hostile attributional biases in severely aggressive adolescents. *J Abnorm Psychol* 99:385–392, 1990.

Durlak JA, Fuhrman T, Lampman C: Effectiveness of cognitive-behavioral therapy for maladapting children: A meta-analysis. *Psychol Bull* 110:204–214, 1991.

English HB: Three cases of the conditioned fear response. *J Abnorm Soc Psychol* 24:221–225, 1929.

Esveldt-Dawson K, Wisner KL, Unis AS, et al: Treatment of phobias in a hospitalized child. *J Behav Ther Exp Psychiatry* 13:77–83, 1982.

Eysenck HJ: The effects of psychotherapy: An evaluation. *J Consult Psychol* 16:319–324, 1952.

Eysenck HJ: Learning theory and behaviour therapy. *J Ment Sci* 105:61–75, 1959.

Eysenck HJ (ed): *Experiments in Behaviour Therapy*. New York, Macmillan, 1964.

Franzini LR, Tilker HA: On the terminological confusion between behavior therapy and behavior modification. *Behav Ther* 3:279–282, 1972.

Freud S: *The Problem of Anxiety* (Bunker HA, trans). New York, Norton, 1936.

Hall CS, Lindzey G: *Theories of Personality* (3rd ed). New York, Wiley, 1978.

Harris B: Whatever happened to Little Albert? *Am Psychol* 34:151–160, 1979.

Jones MC: A laboratory study of fear: The case of Peter. *Pediatr Semin* 31:308–315, 1924.

Jones MC: The elimination of children's fears. *J Exp Psychol* 7:382–390, 1924.

Kazdin AE: *History of Behavior Modification: Experimental Foundations of Contemporary Research*. Baltimore, University Park Press, 1978.

Kazdin AE: *Single-Case Research Designs: Methods for Clinical and Applied Settings*. New York, Oxford University Press, 1982.

Kazdin AE: *Treatment of Antisocial Behavior in Children and Adolescents*. Homewood, IL, Dorsey Press, 1985.

Kazdin AE: Child psychotherapy: *Developing and identifying effective treatments*. Elmsford, NY, Pergamon, 1988.

Kazdin AE: *Behavior Modification in Applied Settings* (5th ed). Pacific Grove, CA, Brooks/Cole, 1994.

Keehn JD, Webster CD: Behavior therapy and behavior modification. *Can Psychol* 10:68–73, 1969.

Kendall PC (ed): *Child and Adolescent Therapy: Cognitive-Behavioral Procedures*. New York, Guilford, 1991.

King GF, Armitage SG, Tilton JR: A therapeutic approach to schizophrenics of extreme pathology: An operant-interpersonal method. *J Abnorm Soc Psychol* 61:276–286, 1960.

Krasner L: Behavior therapy. In: Mussen PH (ed): *Annu Rev Psychol* (Vol 22). Palo Alto, CA, Annual Reviews, 1971.

Lazarus AA: Has behavior therapy outlived its usefulness? *Am Psychol* 32:550–554, 1977.

Lindsley OR: Operant conditioning methods applied to research in chronic schizophrenia. *Psychiatr Res Rep* 5:118–139, 1955.

Lindsley OR: Characteristics of the behavior of chronic psychotics as revealed by free-operant conditioning methods. *Dis Nerv Syst (Monograph Supplement)* 21:66–78, 1960.

Marholin D III (ed): *Child Behavior Therapy*. New York, Gardner Press, 1978.

Mash EJ, Barkley RA (eds): *Treatment of Childhood Disorders*. New York, Guilford, 1989.

Miller GE, Prinz RJ: Enhancement of social learning family interventions for child conduct disorder. *Psychol Bull* 108:291–307, 1990.

Mowrer OH, Mowrer WM: Enuresis: a method for its study and treatment. *Am J Orthopsychiatry* 8:436–459, 1938.

Norcross JC, Goldfried MR (eds): *Handbook of Psychotherapy Integration*. New York, Basic Books, 1992.

Patterson GR, DeBaryshe BD, Ramsey E: A developmental perspective on antisocial behavior. *Am Psychol* 44:329–335, 1989.

Patterson GR, Reid JB, Dishion TJ: *Antisocial Boys*. Eugene, OR, Castalia, 1992.

Pavlov IP: The scientific investigation of the psychical faculties or processes in the higher animals. *Science* 24:613–619, 1906.

Pavlov IP: *Conditioned Reflexes: An Investigation of the Physiological Activities of the Cerebral Cortex*. London, Oxford University Press, 1927.

Peterson L, Sherman DD, Zink M: Applications to pediatric psychology. In: Craighead L, Craighead WE, Kazdin AE, Mahoney MJ (eds): *Cognitive and Behavioral Interventions: An Empirical Approach to Mental Health Problems*. Needham Heights, MA, Allyn & Bacon, 1994, pp. 359–375.

Rescorla RA: Pavlovian conditioning: It's not what you think it is. *Am Psychol* 43:151–160, 1988.

Ross AO: *Child Behavior Therapy: Principles, Procedures, and Empirical Basis*. New York, Wiley, 1981.

Salter A: *The Case against Psychoanalysis*. New York, Holt, 1952.

Shirk SR (ed): *Cognitive Development and Child Psychotherapy*. New York, Plenum, 1988.

Skinner BF: *The Behavior of Organisms*. New York, Appleton-Century-Crofts, 1938.

Skinner BF: *Science and Human Behavior*. New York, Free Press, 1953.

Spivack G, Shure MB: The cognition of social adjustment: Interpersonal cognitive problem-solving thinking. In: Lahey BB, Kazdin AE (eds). *Advances in Clinical Child Psychology* (Vol 5). New York, Plenum, 1982, pp. 323–372.

Strain PS (ed): *The Utilization of Classroom Peers as Behavior Change Agents*. New York, Plenum, 1981.

Stuart RB: *Trick or Treatment: How and When Psychotherapy Fails*. Champaign, IL, Research Press, 1970.

Thorndike EL: *The Fundamentals of Learning*. New York, Teachers College, 1932.

Ullmann LP, Krasner L (eds): *Case Studies in Behavior Modification*. New York, Holt, Rinehart & Winston, 1965.

Watson JB: Psychology as the behaviorist views it. *Psychol Rev* 20:158–177, 1913.

Watson JB: *Psychology from the Standpoint of a Behaviorist*. Philadelphia, PA, Lippincott, 1919.

Watson JB, Rayner R: Conditioned emotional reactions. *J Exp Psychol* 3:1–14, 1920.

Wolpe J: *Psychotherapy by Reciprocal Inhibition*. Stanford, CA, Stanford University Press, 1958.

Wolpe J, Lazarus AA: *Behavior Therapy Techniques: A Guide to the Treatment of Neurosis*. New York, Pergamon, 1966.

Yates AJ: *Behavior Therapy*. New York, Wiley, 1970.

10 ATTACHMENT THEORY AND RESEARCH

Ross A. Thompson, Ph.D.

Although Freud in 1940 described the mother-infant relationship as "unique, without parallel, established unalterably for a whole lifetime as . . .the prototype of all later love relations" (p. 45), he was not the first to speculate about the importance of mother-infant attachment. For centuries parents have recognized their special place in the lives of young offspring, and because infants are so vulnerable and dependent, philosophers, practitioners, and (later) psychologists have been concerned with the quality of parental care that provides a secure foundation for healthy psychological development. It is only in the past two to three decades, however, that their ideas have been systematically tested by developmental researchers, and the interesting and provocative findings from their studies have contributed to making attachment theory one of the most exciting fields of contemporary developmental study, addressing enduring questions concerning infant-parent relationships. Moreover, the applications of attachment research to the understanding of developmental psychopathology (Crittenden, 1992; Erickson et al., 1992), social policies concerning early child care (Belsky, 1986, 1988), and judicial efforts to address a child's "best interests" in custody disputes (Waters and Noyes, 1983–1984) underscore the practical as well as theoretical value of this literature. In a sense, attachment theory and research have provided developmental scholars with an unprecedented opportunity to empirically evaluate theoretical views of the importance of parental care for early psychological development, and to explore diverse important applications of this research.

Attachment can be defined as an enduring emotional bond uniting one person (or animal) with another, and attachments are commonly manifested in efforts to seek proximity and contact to the attachment figure, especially when the individual is under stress. Current theories of attachment underscore its evolutionary origins to promote the protection and nurturance of the young and thus contribute to species survival. Applied to human behavior, attachment is also regarded as an important psychological catalyst for the early emergence of trust in others and understanding of self. As a consequence, attachment theory unites interests in evolutionary biology and developmental psychology in understanding early parent-offspring bonding.

In succinctly summarizing this exciting field, my purpose is to provide an orienting introduction to the theoretical views, research methodologies and findings, ongoing controversies, applications, and emergent trends that characterize contemporary attachment theory and research (the reader will also be directed to major papers and current review sources for further information). In so doing, my goal is to highlight both what we do and do not know about the origins, correlates, and sequelae of early attachment relationships, and their relevance to applied problems of early psychological development. A dual focus on the substance and limitations of our knowledge is important because theoretical views of the importance of the infant-mother relationship have a long heritage in psychology and may lead us to believe that we know more about this phenomenon than we really do. If nothing else, recent research has provided convincing evidence that when we consider seriously the mutual influences of the quality of parental care, the child's characteristics, the ecology of early development, and the consistency of caregiving influences on early attachment relationships, this phenomenon appears to be far more complex than traditional theoretical views might portray. It is this complexity, and the research agenda it provides, that makes this field of research both exciting and compelling.

THE THEORETICAL LEGACY: DEVELOPMENTAL PSYCHOLOGY, EVOLUTIONARY BIOLOGY, AND OBJECT RELATIONS THEORY

In Freud's view (as well as that of his followers), the mother is important to the baby as the provider of basic satisfactions, most notably related to the relief of hunger, cold, and other discomfort. This secondary drive formulation was later adopted (in modified form) by early learning theorists, who argued that the mother assumed the status of secondary reinforcer due to her frequent association with primary reinforcers (e.g., food, warmth, etc.). The problem with both formulations is that they could not adequately explain research findings that revealed the baby's need for human contact and nurturance, independent of the relief of basic physical needs. Why, for example, did Harlow's (1958) mother-deprived rhesus infants prefer contact with a terry cloth-covered wire surrogate that provided "contact comfort" over a bare wire surrogate that provided food? Why did institutionalized infants fail to thrive in orphanages where their physical needs were satisfied by a large, varying staff of caregivers (Spitz, 1945)?

Into this theoretical dilemma arrived John Bowlby, a psychoanalytic psychiatrist who sought to update psychoanalytic formulations in light of current advances in developmental psychology and evolutionary biology (Karen, 1994). Bowlby (1969/1983, 1973) borrowed from contemporary evolutionary thinking to argue that infant-mother attachment develops not just because of the mother's association with gratifications but due to species-typical behavioral patterns that evolved to promote infant survival. In the savannah grasslands of human evolution, Bowlby reasoned, there would have been survival advantages for vulnerable and

defenseless human young to seek the protective proximity of responsive conspecific adults, especially when they were distressed, alarmed, or in danger, and processes of evolutionary adaptation may account for why infants develop emotional attachments to responsive adults that motivate such proximity and contact-seeking efforts. Young who are motivated to stay close to such adults in these circumstances are less likely to fall victim to predators, become lost, or suffer other calamities that, in the end, may undermine reproductive success, and thus it is normative for infants to develop attachments to their caregivers in species-typical rearing conditions. In a sense, Bowlby proposed that infants are predisposed virtually from birth to respond socially to social partners as part of this survival-enhancing motivational system, and he borrowed ideas from engineering control systems theory (updating the hydraulic energy model of psychoanalysis) to explain the dynamic functioning of this system. Finally, Bowlby provided a developmental perspective to his analysis by using insights from developmental psychology (especially Piaget's cognitive theory) to explain the growth of the baby's discrimination of and emotional investment in the parent, the increasing sophistication of the infant's attachment behavioral repertoire, and the child's developing understanding of the relationship with the parent.

Attachment theorists have been as interested in the significance of individual differences as in the normative unfolding of attachment processes, and as a clinician, Bowlby was concerned with the long-term consequences of variations in the quality of infant-parent attachment. He and another early attachment theorist, Mary Ainsworth (1973), argued that the quality of these attachment relationships varies on a dimension of security, and that infants develop security in their caregivers based on their prior experiences of sensitive, helpful, responsive care (cf. Erikson's (1963) concept of "basic trust"). The secure attachment that results is adaptive—in both an evolutionary and a psychological sense—because it derives from the infant's confidence that his or her help-seeking signals will receive a prompt and appropriate adult response. If infants experience sensitive care only inconsistently or sporadically, or if their care is regularly insensitive or unresponsive, they develop insecure attachments, and Bowlby (1973) believed that many adult personality disorders could be traced to the early development of insecure attachment. Indeed, in his view, an important part of the therapeutic process is to assist the client in developing secure attachments (such as to the therapist) while simultaneously examining the contemporary ramifications of earlier, insecure attachment relationships. Such a view has recently been revived in current studies of adults' representations of their early experiences of childhood care (Main, 1991; Main and Hesse, 1990).

The formulations of object relations theory can thus be found in Bowlby's portrayal of the sequelae of early attachments, and object relations formulations have become more influential in attachment theory recently with researchers' interests in studying the later outcomes of secure or insecure infant attachments. According to several current theorists (Bretherton, 1990; Main et al., 1985; Sroufe and Fleeson, 1986), attachment relations exist not only as a behavioral system characterizing infant-parent relationships but also as a conceptual system governing significant social ties throughout the life span, with the emotions and expectations (secure or insecure) arising out of infant-parent relationships forming the basis for rudimentary conceptual representations of self and others in the years that follow. These "working models" or "states of mind" (Bowlby, 1973; Bretherton, 1990; Main, 1992; Main et al., 1985) of self and significant caregivers are portrayed by theorists as interpretive filters through which self-understanding and understanding of important relationships are processed, while operating generally out of conscious awareness. Because of this, they are thought to be relatively stable over developmental time, and individual differences in such working models may thus not only foster consistent, long-term characteristics in parent-child relationships but, as they are maintained, also intergenerational continuities in caregiving tendencies as offspring internalize roles of caregiver and of care-recipient (Sroufe and Fleeson, 1986). Such a view is also consistent with the notion that psychosocial development is characterized by a "continuity of adaptation" (Sroufe, 1979) in which a child's success in meeting early developmental challenges (such as forming a secure attachment) provides a strong or weak foundation for subsequent developmental challenges. In each case, a secure attachment in infancy provides the basis for more successful psychosocial functioning in later years and conceptions of self as lovable and others as trustworthy, while an insecure attachment affords a much weaker psychosocial beginning and different forms of self and other-understanding. In these ways, concepts from object relations theory significantly inform attachment theorists' views of the sequelae of early secure or insecure attachments.

Taken together, Bowlby's theoretical insight was to wed contemporary thinking in developmental psychology with evolutionary biology to provide fresh explanations for important psychoanalytic insights concerning the importance of the mother-infant relationship. By also departing from analytic notions that were either untestable or inconsistent with research findings (e.g., secondary drive, psychic energy), Bowlby's formulation stimulated research on issues of long-standing interest in a theoretical context that was more consistent with current thinking in the behavioral and developmental sciences.

By and large, Bowlby's attachment theory has well-served the field during the past 2 decades, although important shortcomings have more recently become apparent. For example, the evolutionary model used by Bowlby is now more than 20 years old, and current thinking emphasizes that organisms are equipped with a variety of adaptive behavioral patterns that are employed contingently on ecological demands and other life circumstances (Hinde, 1982; Lamb et al., 1985; Trivers, 1985). Thus, contrary to the view that evolutionary processes have equipped infants with a single adaptive attachment pattern (i.e.. a "secure" attachment) that is based on a species-typical style of sensitive parental care, different patterns of infant attachment behavior can be considered adaptive in different caregiving contexts and in relation to different styles of parental care (Hinde, 1982). This has important practical as well as theoretical implications because it means that "insecure" attachment behavior may not always mean the same thing in different caregiving conditions (Levine and Miller, 1990). On another note, recent research findings concerning the development of self-referent beliefs of infants and young children could be fruitfully incorporated into theoretical portrayals of the developing "working models" of young children and their consequences emerging from attachment relationships (Thompson, 1991a, in press). This is an important task because developmental researchers have found that young children have a rather impoverished conceptual understanding of self and other in the early years, and it remains to be shown how these beliefs can form the basis for the characterological forms of self-understanding of later years hypothesized by attachment theorists. On the whole, however, Bowlby's attachment theory remains a provocative and insightful catalyst for further research on attachment processes in infancy and later life.

RESEARCH METHODS

The value of these theoretical formulations would have remained limited, however, without the concurrent emergence of empirical tools for assessing individual differences in the security of infant-parent attachment. Along with her contributions to the conceptualization of these differences, Ainsworth's major contribution to attachment research was the creation of the Strange Situation procedure (Ainsworth et al., 1978), a 21-minute laboratory assessment that has become the predominant procedure for assessing the security of attachment in infancy. It is difficult to overemphasize the contribution of this assessment procedure to attachment research. Because it provided developmentalists with a semistandardized, easy to use, and readily scorable means of studying a phenomenon that was long assumed to be fundamentally important to early sociopersonality development, the availability of the Strange Situation (together with Bowlby's provocative theorizing) virtually unleashed an unprecedented amount of research on attachment. This reli-

ance on a single methodology also permits the comparability of diverse studies on attachment using different samples observed in the Strange Situation, and this is a benefit rarely enjoyed by students of early social development. But this reliance also has its risks. "Security of attachment" in infancy has been, until recently, synonymous with Strange Situation behavior, even though the latter may be influenced by factors (e.g., experiential history, etc.) that are independent of the quality or security of the parent-infant relationship (Lamb et al., 1985; LeVine and Miller, 1990).

The Strange Situation is designed to create a condition in which critical features of an infant's rudimentary "working model" of the caregiver's helpfulness and accessibility will be revealed behaviorally. Because attachment behavior is instigated when babies are distressed or alarmed, the Strange Situation creates gradually escalating stress for the baby to heighten the child's need for the parent's assistance over the course of seven 3-minute laboratory episodes. After a brief introduction to the setting followed by an initial episode in which the infant plays with toys in the mother's presence (episode 2), a stranger enters the room and plays with the baby (episode 3), after which the mother leaves the baby in the company of the stranger (episode 4). Mother and child are reunited (and the stranger departs) in episode 5, but stress is further incremented by a second separation period with the baby alone (episode 6), and the stranger's subsequent return to the room while mother remains absent (episode 7). Mother and infant are reunited a second time in episode 8, at which time the stranger again departs. Thus, by altering the social setting of the laboratory playroom, the Strange Situation heightens the child's need for the parent's support and assistance and, consistent with the evolutionary model, variations in the security of the infant's attachment to the parent are thought to be revealed most clearly (see Ainsworth et al., 1978, for further details).

Attachment researchers focus particular attention on the two reunions (episodes 5 and 8) during which these variations are most apparent. Infants who are deemed securely attached (group B) greet the parent's return with relatively unequivocal pleasure, conveyed either through proximity and contact-seeking efforts or through distal interactive behavior (e.g., smiling, proffering a toy, etc.). These behavioral reactions are thought to reflect underlying confidence that the parent will be accessible and helpfully responsive to their needs for comfort or assistance. Alternatively, infants may be deemed insecurely attached and assigned instead to one of three other groups. Insecure-avoidant (group A) infants either conspicuously avoid the parent during reunions or, more commonly, mingle avoiding or ignoring the parent with more positive reunion greetings (e.g., a markedly delayed look and proffer of toy). Insecure-resistant (group C) babies combine proximity- and contact-seeking activities with angry, rejecting reunion behavior, or alternatively show extreme passivity during reunions. Finally, a new classification—insecure-disorganized/disoriented (group D)—is characterized during reunions not by any distinct behavioral style but by incoherent, confused, or inconsistent behavioral patterns (e.g., approaching parent with head averted) (Main and Solomon, 1986, 1990). In each case, the behavioral reactions indexing insecure attachment are thought to be reflections of uncertainty or ambivalence concerning the parent's helpfulness following stressful separations, or an expectation that the parent will be unhelpful during reunion.

These classifications can be assigned accurately and reliably by well-trained researchers who have worked with an experienced rater and are acquainted with the range of infant behavior that can be observed in this procedure. In most middle-class samples, the large majority (approximately 65%) of infants are deemed securely attached; this proportion tends to be lower in lower-income samples and is markedly depressed in many clinical samples. This is true whether infant-mother or infant-father attachments are studied or, for that matter, attachment relationships with any regular caregiver in the baby's life. As attachment theory predicts, infants develop emotionally meaningful attachments to each of the variety of adults who assume a regular caregiving role, including mothers, fathers, and regular baby sitters and day-care workers (Howes and Hamilton, 1992). Although these attachments usually vary independently in their security (e.g., an infant may be secure with mother and insecure with father, or the reverse), there is sometimes convergence between these different attachment relationships (Fox et al., 1991).

Alternative Approaches

Research using the Strange Situation accounts for most of the literature concerning the security of attachment in infancy, but this procedure is limited to samples of infants between 11 and 24 months of age. After 2 years, brief separations from the mother do not have the same impact on the child's attachment behavior because separations are usually much less stressful. As a consequence, attachment researchers have recently explored several alternative methodologies that are appropriate for older children or can be used with a broader range of ages.

One alternative is a parent- or observer-report instrument called the Attachment Q-sort, in which individuals who are familiar with the child can systematically describe the child's attachment-related characteristics (Waters and Deane, 1985). The Attachment Q-sort consists of 90 brief behavioral descriptors written on cards (e.g., "easily comforted by adult") that are sorted by the rater into one of nine piles, depending on how accurately they describe the child. Thus, cards sorted into pile 1 are "very much unlike the child," while those put into pile 9 are "very much like the child," and so forth. After the sorting is completed, cards are scored (i.e., cards in pile 9 are each assigned a score of 9, cards in pile 8 receive scores of 8, etc.), and the entire card set can then be correlated with a criterion Q-sort that describes the characteristics of a securely attached child. The higher the correlation, presumably, the more securely attached a child is. Alternative criterion Q-sorts also exist for dependency and sociability. Although the Q-sort approach is necessarily susceptible to the biasing influences of any observer-report procedure—that is, it indexes an observer's perceptions of the child's behavior, not necessarily the behavior itself—it benefits from the observer's detailed and long-term knowledge of the child and provides the most versatile means of indexing attachment security in children of various ages. Indeed, the Q-sort developed by Waters and Deane (1985) is suitable for children from infancy through early childhood and can be used in longitudinal as well as cross-sectional studies; in infancy, Q-sort scores often concord well with Strange Situation classifications (Vaughn and Waters, 1990). However, defining a suitable threshold correlation with the criterion Q-sort for a securely attached child has proven to be difficult. Some researchers use an empirical threshold from previous attachment research (e.g., children with the highest 65% of the correlations in the sample are regarded as securely attached), while others establish an a priori threshold (e.g., a correlation of 0.36 or larger); some procedural consistency will be necessary before studies using this method can be compared and evaluated.

Other researchers have sought to develop direct behavioral measures of attachment suitable for older children (Greenberg et al., 1990). Among the more notable efforts is a procedure for 6-year-olds devised by Main, Cassidy, and their colleagues (Cassidy, 1988; Cohn, 1990; Main and Cassidy, 1988). The procedure begins with the family together watching a short film of a child during a 10-day separation from his parents and is followed by an hour-long separation of parents and child during which the child plays with a female stranger and responds to a "separation anxiety interview." Observations of the subsequent parent-child reunion provide the primary basis for classifying 6-year-olds' attachment security, borrowing the strategy of the Strange Situation. Attachment classifications for 6-year-olds include a secure category as well as insecure-avoidant and insecure-ambivalent (or resistant) classifications. New for this age are additional classifications for insecure-controlling and insecure-unclassified attachments (Main and Cassidy, 1988).

Finally, attachment theorists with a special interest in adolescents' and adults' representations of attachment processes have developed an interview procedure called the Adult Attachment Interview that systematically assesses the adult's recollections of the earlier parent-child rela-

tionship they experienced, including memories of security and comfort, acceptance by their own parents, feelings of rejection, fears of abandonment, and similar phenomena (Kobak et al., 1993; Main, 1991; Main and Goldwyn, 1984; Main et al., 1985). Based on their responses to interview questions, adults are classified either "autonomous," "dismissing of attachment," "preoccupied with attachment," or "unresolved," and interviews are analyzed in other ways pertaining to the quality, emotional tone, and coherence of the adult's representations of relationships with each parent.

Research using the Adult Attachment Interview has yielded provocative findings indicating that differences in adults' representations of attachment are associated with variations in parental sensitivity and in the security of attachment in offspring: adults with autonomous (i.e., secure) representations tend to be more sensitive and to have infants with more secure attachments, compared with adults with dismissing, preoccupied, or unresolved classifications (Fonagy et al., 1991; van IJzendoorn, in press). It is yet unclear whether this arises because early patterns of care as a child have long-term effects on parenting capacity—consistent with current interest in the intergenerational transmission of parenting (van IJzendoorn, 1992)—or whether contemporary attachment representations are part of the self-referential beliefs and attitudes that are shaped throughout life and which guide parenting in complex ways (Goodnow and Collins, 1990). Probably both processes are involved and, it is hoped, will be elucidated in future research employing the Adult Attachment Interview and other measures of parenting beliefs (Thompson, in press).

These exciting methodological advances attest to the fact that attachment researchers have clearly moved beyond their initial concern with infancy to consider attachment processes throughout the life span. Moreover, studies using the Adult Attachment Interview and the Attachment Q-set indicate that these measures have promising validity and reliability and suggest important conceptual and developmental links to processes of attachment in infancy. This early literature is promising, but the focus of the research review that follows is with the more substantive literature on infant attachment as it is appraised in the Strange Situation procedure. This research raises significant issues about attachment processes, however, that have lifelong importance.

SECURITY OF ATTACHMENT: ANTECEDENTS, STABILITY, AND SEQUELAE

Consistent with traditional formulations of infant-parent attachment and the theoretical model developed by Bowlby and his followers, most of the research on the security of attachment has focused on several basic questions (for comprehensive reviews of this research, see Lamb et al., 1984, 1985; Thompson, in press; Thompson and Lamb, 1986). First, what are the antecedents of individual differences in attachment security, and in particular, are they associated with variations in the caregiver's sensitivity, helpfulness, and accessibility (as predicted by attachment theory)? Second, once consolidated, how stable are differences in the security of attachment over time? These differences are likely to have a more profound effect on early sociopersonality development if they exert a consistent influence throughout the early years rather than changing over time. Third, what are the predictable sequelae of a secure or insecure attachment in infancy and, equally (or more) important, by what processes do these consequents occur? The reader will recognize that although these issues are central to the formulations of attachment theory, they also encompass long-standing theoretical questions concerning developmental continuity and the importance of early experiences. This helps to account for the widespread interest of developmental scholars in attachment research.

Antecedents

Consistent with theoretical expectations, attachment researchers have found that infants who become securely attached experience more optimal maternal care in the 1st year than do those who become insecurely attached. In general, the mothers of securely attached infants tend to act more positively, harmoniously, responsively, and sensitively toward their babies compared with the mothers of insecurely attached infants (Isabella, 1993, 1995). Using more extreme comparison groups, a number of researchers have found that the large majority of infants experiencing parental maltreatment are insecurely attached, when compared with matched nonmaltreated control groups. These findings substantiate the validity of the Strange Situation as an index of infant-mother attachment as well as confirming several important predictions of attachment theory. Finally, as noted earlier, there is also evidence that the parents of securely and insecurely attached infants themselves differ in their security and in their recollections and representations of the care they received as children (Fonagy et al., 1991; van IJzendoorn, in press), although the reason for this association remains to be elucidated.

Although the quality of early care is an important influence on the security of attachment, it is obviously not the only important influence. Others include the caregiving involvement of the father and the extent of parental satisfaction with the marital relationship, the impact of socioeconomic stress on the family, social support to the mother, and the infant's own temperamental characteristics (see Jacobson and Frye, 1991; Thompson, in press; Vaughn et al., 1992). These findings indicate that the security of attachment is shaped not only by the quality of maternal care, but also by the reciprocal influences of each parent, the baby, the family network, and the broader ecological circumstances in which they live. The importance of adopting a broad, rather than narrow, view of the antecedents of attachment security is underscored by a meta-analysis of attachment research by Goldsmith and Alansky (1987), who found that maternal caregiving quality and infant temperament alone each accounted for a meaningful but small proportion of the variance in the security of attachment. While the emotional climate of maternal care is important, that climate is influenced by many other aspects of the child's life circumstances.

This view is affirmed by cross-cultural studies of attachment, which have found considerable variation between cultures and subcultural groups in the relative proportions of secure and insecure attachments (Thompson, in press; Sagi and Lewkowicz, 1987; van IJzendoorn and Kroonenberg, 1988). For example, insecure-avoidant attachments are uncommon but insecure-resistant attachments occur more frequently than in America among samples of infants raised in Japan and on traditional Israeli kibbutzim. By contrast, avoidant attachments are more common among West German than American infants. However, there is also considerable variation within, as well as between, these cultural groups (van IJzendoorn, 1990). Why do these differences exist? Although researchers disagree, most believe that cultural differences in the normative conditions of early infant care (e.g., frequency of contact with strangers, regularity of separations from mother) and/or in child-rearing prescriptions (e.g., parental independence-training) may help account for these differences. Because the Strange Situation, which was originally designed for middle-class American infants, includes experiences with strangers and separations, it may provide an unusually stressful experience for some infants from other cultures, such as for Japanese infants who have had little prior experience with maternal separations. As a consequence, the Strange Situation may not appropriately or validly assess the security of attachment for infants from these settings. Some babies may act insecurely when they are overwhelmingly distressed, for example, but the infant-parent relationship may generally be secure. These studies not only suggest, therefore, that cultural and subcultural child-rearing norms may foster meaningful variations in normative patterns of attachment, but also that an infant's experiential background must be considered very carefully in evaluating the validity of the Strange Situation as an assessment of the security of attachment.

Stability

Despite a theoretical legacy positing that infantile attachments, once consolidated, should remain relatively stable over time because they take

shape during a period of heightened sensitivity to caregiving influences during the 1st year, the empirical evidence is actually quite mixed. In studies of infants from low-income as well as middle-class homes, the proportion of infants with stable attachments over a 6- to 8-month period in the 2nd year ranged from 48 to 96% in test-retest assessments (Thompson, in press). Although some stability estimates are rather high, they characterize stability in infant behavior over only a few months. It appears that the security of attachment can, and does, change normatively during the 2nd year.

Equally important, however, is additional research evidence that changes in attachment are theoretically predictable: They are linked to circumstances that might precipitate changes in the infant-mother relationship. In a study of low-income families (Vaughn et al., 1979), for example, attachment security changed in response to financial, legal, and social stresses on the family; in another study of middle-class families (Thompson et al., 1982), changes occurred in response to significant transitions in caregiving arrangements for the baby. In short, although changes in the security of attachment are normative, they are neither haphazard nor random but are predictably linked to family events that might force a renegotiation of familiar patterns of mother-infant interaction. This is, in fact, exactly what we would expect to find if the Strange Situation sensitively appraises normative fluctuations in attachment relationships in infancy, although considerably more research is necessary to specify the conditions underlying change, and continuity, in attachment.

Such a conclusion is unsurprising, given the variety of antecedent influences shaping the security of attachment outlined earlier. Because infants are embedded in a complex social ecology, changes in that ecology are likely to influence their attachment relationships. But these findings also indicate that the security of attachment reflects the current—but not necessarily enduring—status of the infant-parent relationship, and efforts to predict whether the current status of this relationship will endure or change must take into account the consistency of the conditions of care experienced by the child. When caregiving conditions remain consistent, attachment relationships are more likely to remain the same (for an example, see Main and Cassidy, 1988); when conditions of care change appreciably, the security of attachment is more likely to change also. This makes it very difficult to define a level of normative stability in attachment relationships in the early years. As a general rule, however, flexibility rather than resiliency of early attachments seems to be true, and although this view is contrary to some theoretical expectations, it is optimistic with respect to the possibility of intervening into dysfunctional infant-parent dyads by changing familiar patterns of interaction or the broader ecological conditions in which they live (see, for example, Lieberman et al., 1991).

Sequelae

Perhaps the most important and controversial propositions of attachment theory pertain to the predicted associations between attachment security in infancy and later psychosocial functioning, partly because developmental researchers have rarely found early socioemotional measures with long-term predictive utility. Perhaps for this reason, a large number of researchers have explored the links between the security of infant-parent attachment and measures of cognitive, social, and personality functioning in the preschool and grade school years, with provocative results. There is considerable evidence that securely attached infants are more sociable with unfamiliar adults, more cooperative with parents, show greater exploratory competence, and may also get along better with peers compared to insecurely attached infants, in both contemporaneous and follow-up assessments (Thompson, in press). Although these research findings are undisputed, attachment researchers disagree concerning their interpretation. On one hand, these results may confirm long-standing theoretical views of infancy as a formative period of developing psychosocial competencies and emergent personality organization. From this perspective, a secure attachment in infancy provides a firmer psychological foundation for the subsequent developmental challenges of the preschool and grade school years, rendering securely attached infants better prepared to establish positive social relations with peers, cooperate prosocially with adults, and develop successful cognitive and academic skills because of the emergent personality processes that have begun to take shape.

On the other hand, some researchers have noted that the predictive association between attachment security and later psychosocial functioning is most apparent when there is considerable stability over time in the child's conditions of care, sometimes through sample selection procedures. By contrast, when there is evidence for significant change in caregiving influences over time (such as when parents separate or substitute care changes markedly), security of attachment in infancy does not strongly predict the child's later behavior (see, for example, Erickson et al., 1985). They have concluded that consistency in ongoing caregiving supports for healthy psychological functioning, rather than an early secure attachment per se, accounts for later positive adjustment (Lamb et al., 1984, 1985; Thompson, 1991a; Thompson and Lamb, 1986). In this view, the kind of sensitive, harmonious parental care that fostered a secure attachment in infancy will, if maintained over time, also promote sociability, prosocial behavior, and competence in the preschool and grade school years. Conversely, insensitive parental care that initially heightens attachment insecurity may, if maintained, also undermine other aspects of psychosocial competence in later years. From this perspective, therefore, the locus of psychosocial continuity in attachment studies may not be in the formative effect of an early secure or insecure attachment, because that relationship may change over time. Instead, it may derive from an ongoing interaction between the child and the caregivers, each of whom contributes to maintaining and supporting—and sometimes changing—behavioral tendencies established in infancy. An earlier insecure attachment may not necessarily predispose a child to later difficulty, for example, if caregiving conditions become more supportive (Lieberman et al., 1991).

Although there are significant differences in these explanations for developmental continuity (with different implications for intervention), each confirms that the maintenance of stable individual differences in psychosocial functioning from infancy to childhood is a joint function of the child and the caregiving context. In the end, considerably more research is required to determine precisely how influences from infancy affect later behavior as well as the relative plasticity of these influences, and this is a research task that is both challenging and enticing.

Taken together, research findings concerning the antecedents, stability, and sequelae of individual differences in the security of attachment confirm certain theoretical expectations while questioning others. While affirming the origins of attachment security in the emotional climate of maternal care, current research underscores the multifaceted, interactive influences on infant attachments and the flexibility of this behavioral system over time and as a predictor of later behavior. To be sure, developmental consolidations in attachment relations in childhood and adolescence may contribute to greater stability in individual differences with increasing age (due, in part, to the growth and consolidation of self-referent beliefs) and their stronger links to other aspects of psychological functioning (Thompson, 1991a, in press). This accounts, in part, for growing scholarly interest in attachment processes in later years. But attachment relationships in infancy seem to provide a provisional, rather than necessarily enduring, basis for later psychological growth. This view has, we shall see, significant practical implications.

APPLICATIONS OF ATTACHMENT THEORY AND RESEARCH

Given the amount of interest they have generated among developmental scholars, it is perhaps unsurprising that formulations of attachment theory have found important applications in child clinical therapy, law, and child and family policy. In this final substantive section, three domains of research applications are outlined to illustrate some of the practical implications of this field of study.

Attachment and Infant Day Care

Because of increasing numbers of dual-career families, single parents, and teenage mothers, the demand for infant care services has grown dramatically, along with the concerns of child advocates. High-quality infant day care is extremely expensive to provide, and concern has focused primarily on the consequences of the day care experience for infant-parent attachment. Owing to the repeated experience of daily separation from the mother, some developmentalists have been concerned that day care experience in the 1st year will prove deleterious to the security of attachment and perhaps also impair psychosocial development in the preschool years.

These concerns were articulated (and widely publicized) by Jay Belsky (1986, 1988), a developmental psychologist who concluded from his own review of the research on infant day care that early (i.e., occurring in the 1st year) and extended (i.e., more than 20 hours weekly) day care experience is a "risk factor" for the development of insecure infant-parent attachments, especially insecure-avoidant attachments. Furthermore, Belsky noted that preschool children who experienced extended amounts of day care in infancy tended to behave more aggressively and noncompliantly than preschoolers without this experience. This conclusion is, according to Belsky, "strikingly consistent" with the formulations of attachment theory concerning the association between insecure attachment and later psychosocial difficulties. Thus in his view, early and extended day care experience heightens the possibility not only of insecure infant-parent attachment but also of its sequela, antisocial behavior in the preschool years.

Belsky's conclusions have been criticized for a number of reasons (Clarke-Stewart, 1989; Thompson, 1991b). First, critics have argued that avoidant behavior in the Strange Situation may not always indicate an insecure attachment for day care infants, but instead that certain infants are unperturbed by the separation episodes and do not need their mothers' assistance. Indeed, to some reviewers (Clarke-Stewart, 1989), their avoidant behavior may reflect maturity in coping with the demands of the Strange Situation in light of their greater experience with maternal separations. At the least, critics argue, the experiential background of infants in day care must be considered very carefully in interpreting their Strange Situation behavior, especially because this procedure was originally designed for home-reared infants. A similar argument has been made, as earlier noted, in interpreting cross-cultural findings. Second, critics have also noted that the difference between day care infants and those who are exclusively home-reared in their relative proportions of insecure attachments is small (roughly 8–16% higher in day care samples). In view of the fact that the majority of day care infants are securely attached, they argue, it does not seem justified to deem early day care experience a "risk factor" for attachment insecurity. Third, many critics have pointed out that day care effects may have more to do with the quality of care than age of onset; in one Swedish study, for example, infants who experienced early day care that was of uniformly high quality showed significantly better later cognitive and psychosocial outcomes (Andersson, 1989, 1991). Fourth, and finally, critics have noted that preschoolers with early, extended day care experience show heightened prosocial as well as antisocial behavior: Day care experience broadens their repertoire of social skills, both positive and negative. This conclusion diminishes somewhat the concerns about the long-term negative sequelae of early day care experience.

In general, although there are many reasons to be concerned about infant day care and its quality, the likelihood of an increased risk of insecure attachment and later psychosocial difficulty does not appear warranted by the research evidence (Thompson, 1991b). However, attachment theory has contributed to a clearer articulation of the concerns of child advocates about the developmental consequences of early day care experience, and this has fostered advocacy efforts to improve the availability (and affordability) of high-quality, development-enhancing infant day care centers. In a sense, while early, extended day care experience per se does not seem to have the negative consequences that have concerned some scholars, attachment theory informs efforts to define the ingredients of high-quality infant day care and its effects on early development.

Attachment and Child Custody Decisions

Insights from attachment theory have also contributed to judicial efforts to articulate concepts like the "best interests of the child" and "psychological parenting" as they influence child custody decision-making (Waters and Noyes, 1983–1984). This is a significant contribution because lawyers, judges, and other legal experts are often ill-equipped to make the kinds of relational, person-centered judgments required when parents divorce and are in conflict over the custody of offspring, or when parents, grandparents, or other parties vie for the custody of children. Because judicial precedent provides little guidance in such situations, judges often make their decisions based on their personal values about the family, raising questions about whether their judgments are truly objective, impartial, and reliable (Mnookin, 1975).

Although the formulations of attachment theory obviously cannot lead directly to valid judgments for specific custody disputes, they can offer broad guidelines concerning parent-child relationships to inform judicial considerations (Thompson, 1986). These include (*a*) a focus on parenting roles that are based on their psychological, rather than exclusively biological, significance to the child, and thus including consideration of the importance of nonparental caregivers and consideration of different parental roles in child care; (*b*) a recognition that children of all ages develop attachments to multiple regular caregivers, even though these attachments may vary in their relative security and salience to the child; (*c*) an appreciation that the distinction between primary and secondary caregiving roles (regardless of the caregiver's gender) may be important to very young children because of their dependency on basic caregiving ministrations, even though this distinction may not satisfactorily inform custody decision-making at later ages (Thompson, 1986); and (*d*) underscoring the child's need to maintain ties to noncustodial caregivers through an ongoing visiting relationship, even though this may be difficult for the custodial parent. In some respects, these guidelines are contrary to earlier legal traditions governing child custody disputes (such as presumptions in favor of biological mothers when children were in their "tender years"), as well as some contemporary theoretical proposals (such as Goldstein et al.'s (1973) recommendation that noncustodial parental visiting be entirely under the control of the custodial parent). But insofar as they are based on the results of well-designed empirical research and theory, they offer a somewhat more valid framework for custody decision-making than the subjective valuations of individual judges. In this respect, the contributions of attachment theory to judicial thinking are heuristic rather than dispositive.

Attachment and Child Clinical Intervention

Among the most exciting applications of attachment theory are current efforts to apply theory and research from this field to the understanding and treatment of child clinical disorders. This is especially true because the study of early mental health is still in its infancy, and thus the growth of attachment theory has coincided with the emergence of theoretical and clinical models of socioemotional disorders in the infancy and preschool years. And with attachment theorists' concerns about early patterns of social interaction, psychosocial functioning, and the prediction of later behavioral problems from early social relationships, there is a natural affinity with the etiologic, diagnostic, and therapeutic concerns of child clinicians.

The applications of attachment theory to clinical intervention raise concerns, however, about the foundation of empirical research required to support well-conceived therapeutic endeavors. On one hand, the heuristic value of attachment theory to child clinical concerns is substantial: Ideas from attachment research can provide a valuable interpretive structure for thinking about children's problems, along with other etiological

models. The importance of parental warmth and sensitivity, the significance of the child's feelings of security in the parent's helpfulness and accessibility when under stress, the multidimensional influences (via baby, mother, and family ecology) on the security of attachment, and the possibility of relatively enduring "working models" of attachment emerging from early relationships with caregivers can significantly inform how child clinicians perceive the difficulties of their clients and strive to assist them. In addition, an emerging literature in developmental psychopathology is identifying the attachment-related correlates of child clinical conditions, ranging from child maltreatment to Down's syndrome to conduct disorders. With respect to treatment, moreover, attachment theory offers powerful heuristics related to the impact of attachment representations in the parenting behavior of adults, the emergence of social expectations related to attachment security in young children that may bias their encounters with others, and the "working models" of self and other that may be a consequence of differences in the security of attachment. Because of these heuristic contributions (some of which are not exclusive to attachment theory), several intervention strategies for infants and parents that have considerable potential value have been designed (see Fraiberg, 1980: Greenspan and Lieberman, 1988; Lieberman and Pawl, 1988, 1994; Marvin, 1992).

Some applications of attachment theory must be framed considerably more cautiously, however. Does existing research support the conclusion, for example, that an insecure attachment itself requires "remediation of the early competencies that were not obtained" (Peterson, 1987, p. 803)? How broadly should the diagnostic concept "disorders of attachment" (Greenspan and Lieberman, 1988; Lieberman and Pawl, 1988; Zeanah et al., 1994) be defined? Should researchers assume an ethical responsibility of informing parents of the risk status of their offspring merely because they have been found to be insecurely attached in the Strange Situation, as one research group has done (Nezworski et al., 1988)? In what ways does an insecure attachment define "risk status" for a baby? In addressing such questions, there are several reasons why thoughtful applications of attachment theory and research to problems of early mental health require careful reflection and the integration of attachment-based formulations with other etiologic models of developmental psychopathology.

First, the results of research with nonclinical samples, reviewed above, indicate that there is considerable flexibility, rather than resiliency, to attachment system functioning in the early years of life. Rather than foreshadowing inevitable subsequent difficulties, an insecure attachment is related only conditionally and provisionally to later psychosocial problems (compare Bates and Bayles, 1988; Erickson et al., 1985; Fagot and Kavanagh, 1990; Lewis et al., 1984). As noted earlier, infant attachments have predictive value largely when there is consistency in caregiving influences over time that help to maintain early characteristics in offspring. This mandates a focus on family functioning, rather than on infant status alone, in infant mental health efforts. Second, because Strange Situation assessments index the security of attachment but also other influences (as noted in the cross-cultural and day care studies), clinicians should be cautious in making individualized assessments of either infant functioning or the infant-parent relationship based on the Strange Situation alone. Convergent assessments in which attachment procedures may be one component are warranted. Finally, although concepts like "working models" of attachment representations are heuristically powerful, very little is known about the developmental origins of individual differences in these representations in children and adults. Even though there are influential theoretical models positing that adult representations of attachment are directly linked to early experiences of care—and help to account for controversy concerning the "intergenerational transmission" of parenting—these theoretical models have not yet been adequately tested. This warrants caution in making assumptions about the bases of these attachment representations, which are likely to be quite complex.

It should be clear that there are valuable applications of attachment theory and research to the concerns of child clinicians, and these applications are already apparent in the design of early intervention programs and the portrayal of problems of infant mental health. Although the formulations of attachment theory are of considerable heuristic value, however, substantially more research (with clinical as well as nonclinical samples) is required to specify more clearly the meaning of security or insecurity of early attachment and its contemporary and subsequent significance.

CONCLUSIONS

Summarizing theory and research in parent-child attachment several years ago would have meant a more exclusive focus on basic developmental studies of infancy, and part of what has contributed to a renaissance in attachment work during the past few years has been an extension of thinking to attachment processes in preschool and in later years, the relevance of this work to social policies concerning children and families, and the applications of attachment research to clinical issues. As a consequence, developmental researchers, clinicians, and other practitioners have a considerable research agenda for building upon the provocative findings of studies reviewed in this chapter. Given the continuing contributions of Bowlby's insightful theory, there is good reason for optimism concerning the future contributions of attachment theory and research.

References

Ainsworth MDS: The development of infant-mother attachment. In: Caldwell BM, Ricciuti H (eds): *Review of Child Development Research* (Vol 3). Chicago, University of Chicago Press, 1973, pp. 1–94.

Ainsworth MDS, Blehar MC, Waters E, et al: *Patterns of Attachment.* Hillsdale, NJ, Erlbaum, 1978.

Andersson BE: Effects of day-care on cognitive and socioemotional competence of thirteen-year-old Swedish schoolchildren. *Child Dev* 63:20–36, 1992.

Andersson BE: Effects of public day-care—A longitudinal study. *Child Dev* 60:857–866, 1989.

Bates JE, Bayles K: Attachment and the development of behavior problems. In: Belsky J, Nezworski T (eds): *Clinical Implications of Attachment.* Hillsdale, NJ, Erlbaum, 1988, pp. 253–299.

Belsky J: Infant day care: A cause for concern? *Zero to Three* 6:17, 1986.

Belsky J: The "effects" of infant day care reconsidered. *Early Child Res* 3:235–272, 1988.

Belsky J, Nezworski T (eds): *Clinical Implications of Attachment.* Hillsdale, NJ, Erlbaum, 1988.

Bowlby J: *Attachment and Loss. Vol 1: Attachment.* New York, Basic Books, 1969 (second edition published 1983).

Bowlby J: *Attachment and Loss. Vol 2: Separation.* New York, Basic Books, 1973.

Bretherton I: Open communication and internal working models: Their role in the development of attachment relationships. In: Thompson RA (ed): *Socioemotional Development* (Nebraska Symposium on Motivation, Vol 36). Lincoln, NE, University of Nebraska Press, 1990.

Cassidy J: Child-mother attachment and the self in six-year-olds. *Child Dev* 59:121–134, 1988.

Clarke-Stewart KA: Infant day care: Maligned or malignant? *Am Psychol* 44:266–273, 1989.

Cohn DA: Child-mother attachment of six-year-olds and social competence at school. *Child Dev* 61: 152–162, 1990.

Crittenden PM: Treatment of anxious attachment in infancy and early childhood. Dev Psychopathol 4: 575–602, 1992.

Erickson MF, Korfmacher J, Egeland BR: Attachments past and present: Implications for therapeutic intervention with mother-infant dyads *Dev Psychopathol* 4:495–507, 1992.

Erickson MF, Sroufe LA, Egeland B: The relationship between quality of attachment and behavior problems in preschool in a high-risk sample. In: Bretherton I, Waters E (eds): *Growing Points in Attachment Theory and Research* (Monographs of the Society for Research in Child Development). Chicago, University of Chicago Press, 1985, pp. 147–166.

Erikson EN: *Childhood and Society* (2nd ed). New York, Norton, 1963.

Fagot B, Kavanagh K: The prediction of antisocial behavior from avoidant attachment classifications. *Child Dev* 61:864–873, 1990.

Fonagy P, Steele H, Steele M: Maternal representations of attachment during pregnancy predict the organization of infant-mother attachment at one year of age. *Child Dev* 62:891–905, 1991.

Fox NA, Kimmerly NL, Schafer WD: Attachment to mother/attachment to father: A meta-analysis. *Child Dev* 62:210–225, 1991.

Fraiberg S (ed): *Clinical Studies in Infant Mental Health: The First Year of Life.* New York, Basic Books, 1980.

Freud S: *An Outline of Psychoanalysis.* New York, Norton, 1940.

Goodnow JJ, Collins WA: *Development According to Parents: The Nature, Sources, and Consequences of Parents' Ideas.* Hillsdale, NJ, Erlbaum, 1990.

Greenberg MT, Cicchetti D, Cummings M (eds): *Attachment in the Preschool Years.* Chicago, University of Chicago Press, 1990.

Greenspan SI, Lieberman AF: A clinical approach to attachment. In: Belsky J, Nezworski T (eds): *Clinical Implications of Attachment.* Hillsdale, NJ, Erlbaum, 1988, pp. 387–424.

Goldsmith NH, Alansky JA: Maternal and infant temperamental predictors of attachment: A meta-analytic review. *J Consult Clin Psychol* 55:805–816, 1987.

Goldstein J, Freud A, Solnit AJ: *Beyond the Best Interests of the Child.* New York, Free Press, 1973.

Harlow NF: The nature of love. *Am Psychol* 13: 673–685, 1958.

Hinde RA: Attachment: Some conceptual and biological issues. In: Stevenson-Hinde J, Murray Parkes C (eds): *The Place of Attachment in Human Behavior.* New York, Basic Books, 1982, pp. 60–76.

Howes C, Hamilton CE: Children's relationships with child care teachers: Stability and concordance with parental attachments. *Child Dev* 63:867–878, 1992.

Isabella RA: Origins of attachment: Maternal interactive behavior across the first year. *Child Dev* 64:605–621, 1993.

Isabella RA: The origins of infant-mother attachment: Maternal behavior and infant development. In: Vasta R (ed): *Annals of Child Development.* London, Jessica Kingsley Publishers, Ltd., 1995, pp. 57–82.

Jacobson SW, Frye KF: Effect of maternal social support on attachment: Experimental evidence. *Child Dev* 62:572–582, 1991.

Karen R: *Becoming Attached.* New York, Warner Books, 1994.

Kobak RR, Cole HE, Ferenz-Gillies R, et al: Attachment and emotion regulation during mother-teen problem solving: A control theory analysis. *Child Dev* 64:231–245, 1993.

Lamb ME, Thompson RA, Gardner W, et al: *Infant-Mother Attachment.* Hillsdale, NJ, Erlbaum, 1985.

LeVine RA, Miller PM: Commentary. *Hum Dev* 33:73–80, 1990.

Lewis M, Feiring C, McGuffog C, et al: Predicting psychopathology in six-year-olds from early social relations. *Child Dev* 55:123–136, 1984.

Lieberman AF, Pawl JH: Clinical applications of attachment theory. In: Belsky J, Nezworski T (eds): *Clinical Implications of Attachment.* Hillsdale, NJ, Erlbaum, 1988, pp. 327–351.

Lieberman AF, Pawl JH: Infant-parent psychotherapy. In: Zeanah CH (ed): *Handbook of Infant Mental Health.* New York, Guilford, 1994, pp. 427–442.

Lieberman AF, Weston DR, Pawl JH: Preventive intervention and outcome with anxiously attached dyads. *Child Dev* 6:199–209.

Main M: Metacognitive knowledge, metacognitive monitoring, and singular (coherent) vs. multiple (incoherent) model of attachment: Findings and directions for further research. In: Murray Parkes C, Stevenson-Hinde J, Marris P (eds): *Attachment Across the Life Cycle.* London, Routledge, 1991, pp. 127–159.

Main M, Cassidy J: Categories of response to reunion with the parent at age 6: Predictable from infant attachment classifications and stable over a 1-month period. *Dev Psychol* 24:415–426, 1988.

Main M, Goldwyn R: Predicting rejection of her infant from mother's representation of her own experience: Implications for the abused-abusing intergenerational cycle. *Child Abuse Neglect* 8:203–217, 1984.

Main M, Hesse E: Parents' unresolved traumatic experiences are related to infant disorganized attachment status: Is frightened and/or frightening parental behavior the linking mechanism? In: Greenberg MT, Cicchetti D, Cummings EM (eds): *Attachment in the Preschool Years.* Chicago, University of Chicago Press, 1990, pp. 161–182.

Main M, Solomon J: Discovery of an insecure disorganized/disoriented attachment pattern. In: Brazelton TB, Yogman MW (eds): *Affective Development in Infancy.* Norwood, NJ, Ablex, 1986, pp. 95–124.

Main M, Solomon J: Procedures for identifying infants as disorganized/disoriented during the Ainsworth Strange Situation. In: Greenberg MT, Cicchetti D, Cummings EM (eds): *Attachment in the Preschool Years.* Chicago, University of Chicago Press, 1990, pp. 121–160.

Main M, Kaplan K, Cassidy J: Security in infancy, childhood, and adulthood: A move to the level of representation. In: Bretherton I, Waters E (eds): *Growing Points in Attachment Theory and Research (Monographs of the Society for Research in Child Development).* Chicago, University of Chicago Press, 1985, pp. 66–104.

Marvin RS: Attachment and family systems-based intervention in developmental psychopathology. *Dev Psychopathol* 4:697–711, 1992.

Mnookin RH: Child-custody adjudication: Judicial functions in the face of indeterminacy. *Law Contemp Prob* 39:226–293, 1975.

Nezworski T, Tolan WJ, Belsky J: Intervention in insecure infant attachment. In: Belsky J, Nezworski T (eds): *Clinical Implications of Attachment.* Hillsdale, NJ, Erlbaum, 1988, pp. 352–386.

Peterson L: Introduction to the special series. *J Consult Clin Psychol* 55:803–804, 1987.

Sagi S, Lewkowicz KS: A cross-cultural evaluation of attachment research. In: Tavecchio LWC, van IJzendoorn MH (eds): *Attachment in Social Networks*. Amsterdam, Elsevier Science, 1987, pp. 427–459.

Spitz RA: Hospitalism: An inquiry into the genesis of psychiatric conditions in early childhood. *Psychoanal Study Child* 1:53–74, 1945.

Sroufe LA: The coherence of individual development. *Am Psychol* 34:834–841, 1979.

Sroufe LA, Fleeson J: Attachment and the construction of relationships. In: Hartup WW, Rubin Z (eds): *Relationships and Development*. Hillsdale, NJ, Erlbaum, 1986, pp. 51–71.

Thompson RA: Fathers and the child's "best interests": Judicial decision-making in custody disputes. In: Lamb ME (ed): *The Father's Role: Applied Perspectives*. New York, Wiley, 1986, pp. 61–102.

Thompson RA: Construction and reconstruction of early attachments: Taking perspective on attachment theory and research. In: Keating DP, Rosen N (eds): *Constructivist Perspectives on Atypical Development and Developmental Psychopathology*. Hillsdale, NJ, Erlbaum, 1991a, pp. 41–67.

Thompson RA: Infant day care: Concerns, controversies, choices. In: Lerner JV, Galambos N (eds): *Employed Mothers and their Children*. New York, Garland Press, 1991b, pp. 9–36.

Thompson RA: Early sociopersonality develop-ment. In: Damon W (ed): *Handbook of Child Psychology* (5th ed.) Vol 4. Social, emotional, and personality development (Eisenberg N, vol ed). New York, Wiley.

Thompson RA, Lamb ME: Infant-parent attachment: New directions for theory and research. In: Baltes PB, Featherman DL, Lerner RM (eds): *Lifespan Development and Behavior* (Vol 7). Hillsdale, NJ, Erlbaum, 1986, pp. 1–41.

Thompson RA, Lamb ME, Estes D: Stability of infant-mother attachment and its relationship to changing life circumstances in an unselected middle-class sample. *Child Dev* 53:144–148, 1982.

Trivers R: *Social Evolution*. Menlo Park, CA, Benjamin/Cummings, 1985.

van IJzendoorn MH: Developments in cross-cultural research on attachment: Some methodological notes. *Hum Dev* 33:39, 1990.

van IJzendoorn MH: Intergenerational transmission of parenting: A review of studies in nonclinical populations. *Dev Rev* 12:76–99, 1992.

van IJzendoorn MH: The association between adult attachment representations and infant attachment, parental responsiveness, and clinical status: A meta-analysis on the predictive validity of the adult attachment interview. *Psychol Bull*, in press.

van IJzendoorn MH, Kroonenberg PM: Cross-cultural patterns of attachment: A meta-analysis of the Strange Situation. *Child Dev* 59:147–156, 1988.

Vaughn B, Waters E: Attachment behavior at home and in the laboratory: Q-sort observations and Strange Situation classifications of one-year-olds. *Child Dev* 61:1965–1973, 1990.

Vaughn B, Egeland B, Sroufe LA, et al: Individual differences in infant-mother attachment at twelve and eighteen months: Stability and change in families under stress. *Child Dev* 50:971–975, 1979.

Vaughn BE, Stevenson-Hinde J, Waters E, et al: Attachment security and temperament in infancy and early childhood: Some conceptual clarifications. *Dev Psychol* 28:463–473, 1992.

Waters E, Deane KE: Defining and assessing individual differences in attachment relationships: Q-methodology and the organization of behavior in infancy and early childhood. In: Bretherton I, Waters E (eds): *Growing Points in Attachment Theory and Research* (Monographs of the Society for Research in Child Development). Chicago, University of Chicago Press, 1985, pp. 41–65.

Waters E, Noyes DM: Psychological parenting vs. attachment theory: The child's best interests and the risks in doing the right things for the wrong reasons. *NYU Rev Law Soc Change* 12:505–515, 1983–1984.

Zeanah CH Jr, Mammen OK, Lieberman AF: Disorders of attachment. In: Zeanah CH (ed): *Handbook of Infant Mental Health*. New York, Guilford, 1994, pp. 332–349.

11 THEORIES OF COGNITIVE DEVELOPMENT

Timothy Yates, M.D.C.M., F.R.C.P.(C.)

Part 1: Developmental Theories

Theories of cognitive development help clinicians to see the world through the eyes of children and show clinicians how children invest their experiences with meaning in age-specific ways. Critical events—abuse, divorce, or death of parents—have different implications for the developing self from phase to phase, and emotional conflicts manifested in later life often remain structured according to their point of origin in earlier development. Since interpersonal and emotional developmental deviations are part of virtually all clinical problems, knowledge of cognitive development points the psychiatrist toward the fundamental dynamics of the disturbance and informs his or her attempts at remediation.

The field of cognitive psychology explores how the mind makes knowledge from experience and how it organizes knowledge as "representational structures." As a subset of cognitive psychology, cognitive development looks at how these structures are transformed over the life span. This chapter outlines the principal streams of cognitive developmental theory and demonstrates their relevance to affective and interpersonal development and to the puzzling clinical problem of autism.

INTRODUCTION OF TERMS

Cognition

Since there is no generally agreed-upon definition of cognition, let us begin by looking at some current views and the questions each provokes and addresses. Gregory (1987, p. 149) called cognition "the use and handling of knowledge." This metaphor of knowledge as a substance invites the questions: Of what is it made? Handled by what? Others (Flavell et al., 1993; Vygotsky, 1986) consider cognition to be "higher mental processes." This view shifts the focus from knowledge as substance to thought as activity and raises different questions: How does a mental process act? Is knowledge "handled" by higher mental processes? Finally, Kegan (1982) and Bruner (1990) see cognition as "meaning-making" which has affective and personal connotations. New questions arise: How are feeling and thinking related? How is personal meaning related to knowledge?

Some (Sternberg, 1984) see cognitive development as the increasing speed and sophistication of mental processes, independent of one's store of knowledge; others (Chi, 1988) believe that the contents of knowledge play an essential role in development. Some include affect to explain cognitive development (Case, 1985), others do not (JR Anderson, 1983). Indeed, Flavell (1993) contends that *all* psychological activity may, in some sense, be seen as cognitive. Clearly, there are significant differences of opinion about what cognition is and how it develops.

To start, let us make some distinctions among the psychological activities of cognition, affect, sensation, and perception. To distinguish the first two, Piaget argued that affect is an energizing force that is organized and channelled by cognition the way a car engine structures and directs the energy provided by gasoline (Cowan, 1981). Piaget's distinction is a qualitative one: Cognition is structure; affect is energy. Those who view cognition as the processing of information distinguish it from sensation and perception quantitatively by the time it takes to process a stimulus from input to output: the more time taken, the more complex the mediating events, and therefore, the more "cognitive" the process. Taking both views together then, cognition may be characterized on the one hand by *structure* and on the other by *complexity*.

Development

The term "development" denotes a sequential increase in the structural and/or functional complexity of a system. *Structures* are inferred organizational properties, underlying a given behavior, that change systematically with age. Development of structure means that a system becomes organized in a more complex way while development of function implies that it manages more complex arrays of information. It is likely that a change in functional (or processing) complexity entails an increase in structural (or architectural) complexity and vice versa.

Development also implies an alternation of *differentiation* and *integration* (or *coordination*) (Werner, 1948). For example, in biology, unspecialized precursor cells differentiate during development into several types of specialized offspring. These, in turn, integrate their specialized functions to form organs, which, at a higher level, organize themselves into organ systems. In psychological development, sensory and symbolic stimuli are taken in by the child and become *mental representational structures*. Representations combine to form complex arrangements that, in turn, differentiate and recombine into ever more integrated and complex structures that then influence the selection and handling of further input. We shall meet examples of these as "structures-of-the-whole," "cognitive architectures," and so on. The concept of a mental representation is fundamental, but it is ambiguous. Here we define representations as "the internalized schemas or frames of reference which the child uses in his interaction with the external world" (Deregowski, 1977, p. 219). Further nuances of the term are encountered below, in the discussion of autism.

Stages

Often a developmental theory is presented as a series of *stages*. Stage theories imply discontinuous development: Periods of stability and consolidation alternate with periods of instability and transition. They also imply qualitative changes in cognition from stage to stage. This is controversial. Some believe stages reflect a natural rhythm in the developing organism; others see them as artifacts of the method or the bias of the investigator. Theories based on a biological metaphor, Piaget's, for example, tend to be set in stages, while nonstage theories have a more social-learning pedigree.

In a Piagetian-type stage theory, each stage organizes all cognitions in a characteristic way at any point in the life span. Each stage entails the hierarchical integration and transformation of the preceding ones; each earlier one becomes a subset of the next later one. Stages succeed one another in an invariant sequence of transformations; a step cannot be skipped, nor does the culture change the sequence. Stages are universal; the culture may vary the content, but not the structure. Finally, each stage achieves its full range only upon completion; most activities in a stage are incomplete and contribute to the final version. The theories of Piaget, the neo-Piagetians (Case, 1985, 1991) and some Piaget-based social-cognitive (Selman, 1980), moral (Kohlberg, 1969) and self-developmental (Kegan, 1982; Noam, 1988) theories are stage theories.

Nonstage theories are represented in this chapter by some information-processing (Anderson, 1983) and learning-based theories (Chi, 1988). In these, development is continuous; they do not distinguish points of qualitative change in cognition nor alternating periods of relative stability and instability. They explain the apparently discontinuous changes of cognitive development as the cumulative effect of small increments of learning. They do not require invariant sequencing or central processing structures that organize disparate domains of knowledge according to a single blueprint.

Sternberg and Berg (1992) identify six distinguishable theories of cognitive development—Piagetian, sociocultural (contextual), information-processing, neo-Piagetian, learning, and psychometric. In this chapter the first four are presented under their own headings while one learning-based theory (Chi et al., 1988) is mentioned in passing. The reader is referred to Sternberg and Berg for discussion of psychometric theory.

JEAN PIAGET: THE GENEVA SCHOOL

Piaget's Goals and Methods

Piaget was the first to systematically study the "qualitative development of intellectual structures" (Flavell, 1963, p. 15). As a child, he had been a somewhat solitary prodigy with an interest in natural history and published his first article, on a species of sparrow, at age 10. He discovered philosophy and psychology in adolescence and, after graduating in biology, worked with Simon in Paris doing standardized intelligence tests on children. He became interested in the reasoning children of different ages used to explain their answers, both correct and incorrect, and saw a connection between the development of logical thinking in children and the philosophical problem of knowledge—epistemology.

Curious about the evolution of the capacity for reasoning, Piaget interviewed children in detail about their ways of knowing, applying techniques from psychoanalysis and clinical psychology. His "clinical method" allowed more flexible interaction than did formal laboratory procedures. Piaget augmented his early experimental work by systematically observing his own children in their home and posing naturalistic tasks at intervals throughout their childhood. On the basis of these observations, and other, more formal ones, he made inferences about the development of children's capacity to think in terms of formal logic, which he believed to be the basis of cognitive structure. He called this approach "genetic epistemology."

Heredity and the "Functional Invariants"

Piaget believed psychological organization to be the end toward which biological development is directed (Langer, 1969). The biological bases of the theory were the notions of specific and general heredity. Specific heredity allotted to each member of a species a common physical apparatus that would function in a consistent, species-specific manner in an adequate environment (Ginsberg, 1985). General heredity ensured what Piaget called the *functional invariants—organization* and *adaptation*.

ORGANIZATION: SCHEMES AND STRUCTURES

Piaget proposed that humans are innately predisposed to organize whatever is taken in by the nervous system. In doing so, the individual constructs *schemes*, which are "the internal representation . . .of some generalized class of situations, enabling the organism to act in a coordinated fashion over a whole range of analogous situations" (Gregory, 1987, p. 696). Schemes combine to form comprehensive *structures-of-the-whole* organized, as we shall see, in a stage-specific logical form.

ADAPTATION: ASSIMILATION, ACCOMMODATION, AND EQUILIBRATION

Adaptation is subdivided into the complementary processes of *assimilation* and *accommodation*, by means of which the organism creates and adapts to new knowledge. During assimilation, the organism adapts by organizing novel stimuli according to schemes already in its repertoire. Accommodation occurs when the cognitive apprehension of a novel stimulus causes the scheme to expand or alter its organizational structure. An infant with a scheme for grasping will attempt to grasp everything in sight, that is, to assimilate newly encountered objects as "things-to-be-grasped." At the same time, different shapes and sizes of objects oblige the grasping scheme to enlarge and diversify so as to accommodate the variety of things-to-be-grasped. With each new encounter, these processes work together until the novelty, which has temporarily unbalanced the cognitive organization, has been adapted to, a new equilibrium is established and new knowledge has been created. The rebalancing tendency is *equilibration*, which is the fundamental developmental transition process. In this way, the child could be said to construct his or her own knowledge.

Piaget's Stage Sequence of Development

Piaget proposed cognitive development to be a structural evolution. The child continuously adapts to and organizes events by assimilating and accommodating. Schemes are constructed, enlarged, combined, and coordinated to form ever more comprehensive and complex structures. These structures ultimately form a structure-of-the-whole that, in each stage, organizes experience across all domains of knowledge. This sets the stage for a qualitative leap to a new structure of thinking, and the process is repeated as the old structure is folded into the newly forming one. This occurs in four stages.

THE SENSORIMOTOR STAGE (BIRTH THROUGH 18–24 MONTHS)

The infant's first strategies for organizing experience are innate reflexes such as grasping or rooting. During this stage, the infant will transform his or her reflexes into self-generated schemes of action. However, sensorimotor cognition is still nonsymbolic; it can only operate upon an environment that is immediately apprehended by the senses and the motor system. By the end of this stage, the scene will be set for the transition from a biological to a psychological basis for thought with the acquisition of conceptual representations.

The transformation of reflex to scheme begins as the neonate, enacting its reflexive organization, interacts with the environment. As something touches its palm, it grasps; as something touches its lips, it sucks, and so on. The more experience the child has of grasping, the stronger the grasping tendency. The stronger this tendency is, the more things the child will grasp and the greater the variety of things assimilated as "graspable." The child accommodates by using different grasps for different things. As the grasping begins to differentiate, a scheme of grasping is constructed.

Early in the 2nd month, elementary schemes emerge as the infant experiences feedback from its own body. For example, although thumb-sucking behavior was innate, it is now repeated in an intentional way. Piaget called these first schemes *primary circular reactions*—"primary" because they involve the infant's own body, circular because an action-reaction loop is set up. During the middle third of the 1st year, the infant begins to interact with the external world in the same way, constructing *secondary circular reactions*. For example, coordination of two schemes, such as gazing and reaching, begins to occur. A random arm movement causes a mobile over the crib to move, creating an interesting visual effect. Soon the movements become less random. The infant's arm causes the mobile to move, and the pleasure generated causes the infant to do it again, establishing a circularity. Toward the close of the 1st year, the infant begins to explore, rather than merely respond. In one celebrated sequence, Piaget interposed his hand between that of his son, Laurent, and a matchbox that fascinated him. At 7½ months, after earlier unsuccessful trials, Laurent actively attempted to push aside the obstructing hand to reach for the matchbox (Piaget, 1952). Using the "means" of removing the obstacle, the hand, to attain an "end," the matchbox, marks the beginning of complex intentional behavior and of an appreciation of causality.

During the first half of the 2nd year, infants become more intentional in their explorations. Instead of seeking to reproduce exactly the previous effect, they deliberately vary the procedure so as to cause slight differences each time. Laurent, dropping different objects, varied the position of his arm upon release each time. He would repeat the procedure exactly for a few trials, as if to confirm an observation, and then resume his variations. "This interest in novelty for its own sake is called a *tertiary circular reaction*" (Ginsburg and Opper, 1969, p. 58, emphasis added).

The acquisition of the *symbolic* (or *semiotic*) *function* in the last half of the 2nd year marks a major developmental advance. The child begins to use symbolic play and language to represent its experience. The transition to symbolic mental representation begins with symbolic physical representation. Piaget's daughter Lucienne, at the age of 16 months, was presented with a matchbox containing a watch chain. She had learned from previous experience either to reach in and remove it or to invert the box to make it fall out. This time Piaget narrowed the opening so that she could not reach in, nor would it fall out. Lucienne stared at the narrow opening and opened her mouth successively wider and wider. Piaget saw this as a sensorimotor representation of her awareness of the opening and the space beneath it. "Soon after this phase of plastic reflection, Lucienne pulls so as to enlarge the opening. She succeeds and grasps the chain" (Piaget, 1952, pp. 337–338). Very soon, symbols—words—become available to express this knowledge. Piaget wrote of T. at nearly 18 months, "'No more' meant going away, then throwing something on the ground and was then used of something that was overturned (without disappearing). He thus said 'no more' to his blocks" (Piaget, 1951, p. 218).

THE PREOPERATIONAL STAGE (2 THROUGH 5–7 YEARS)

Achievement of the symbolic function ushers in the preoperational period. This stage has also been called the intuitive or prelogical period and is contrasted with subsequent stages wherein thought is organized logically. Since Piaget was particularly interested in the development of logical thought, he seems to dwell more upon children's cognitive limitations during this period than on their accomplishments.

Object Permanence and Centration

At 10 months Jacqueline could retrieve a toy Piaget had twice put under a cover as she watched. However, if he subsequently put it under an adjacent cover, also as she watched, she looked under the first cover the moment the toy disappeared from view. At 18 months, playing the same game with a coin, Jacqueline watched as her father concealed the coin in his hand, moved his hand from A to B to C, and showed it to her, empty. She pushed aside his hand and searched sequentially in A, B, and, triumphantly, in C. For her, the object now has a permanence beyond sensorimotor apprehension.

This achievement of *object permanence* is a Copernican event for the toddler in that he or she can now manipulate images and words internally. However, the relationship of one representation to another is not yet fixed, and magical thinking—what Piaget called *transductive logic*—is the norm. "This kind of reasoning proceeds from particular to particular. *Centering* on one salient element of an event, the child proceeds irreversibly to draw as conclusion from it some other, perceptually compelling happening" (Flavell, 1963, p. 160, emphasis added).

The child's understanding of things, once subject to its sensations and motor activity, is now dominated by its perceptions. Piaget argued that children tend to center their thinking on one dimension of a problem and have difficulty systematically coordinating it with another. At 2 years, 7½ months, Jacqueline saw her younger sister in a bathing suit and cap and asked, "'What's the baby's name?'" Her mother explained that it was a bathing costume, but J. pointed to L. herself and repeated the question several times. But as soon as L. had her dress on again, J. exclaimed very seriously, 'It's Lucienne again,'" as if Lucienne had become a different person upon changing her clothes (Piaget, 1951). Jacqueline had "centered" on the novel clothing and could not "decenter" so as to recognize her sister.

Egocentrism

An important extension of centration is the controversial notion of *egocentrism*—the apparent inability to see things, at first perceptually and later cognitively, from another's point of view. In a famous experiment, Piaget stood children on the opposite side of a tabletop model of three quite different mountains. He asked each child to indicate how the child thought he, the experimenter, saw the mountains in relation to one another. Young preoperational children maintained that the experimenter saw the model as they did in spite of their 180° difference in perspective. It seemed as if the child believed her or his own point of view to be the only possible one.

Piaget extrapolated perceptual egocentrism into the social-cognitive arena and suggested a concomitant conceptual and affective egocentrism that limits the preschool child's capacity for what has become known as *social perspective-taking*, that is, understanding another's psychological point of view (Selman, 1980). Elkind (1970, 1978) proposed that interpersonal egocentrism accounted for limits in social cognition at different stages of development. He saw egocentrism as a way of measuring how a child is moving toward adult thinking along three parameters—distinguishing transient from permanent phenomena, objective from subjective phenomena, and universal from particular phenomena. For example, an instance of subjective-objective egocentrism in the sensorimotor stage would be the child's incapacity to distinguish an object from her or his own sensory impressions of it. When something is no longer seen, it would no longer exist. Upon acquiring object permanence, people and things, like Jacqueline's coin, endure in the child's memory and so become "real." The capacity to make symbolic mental representations frees the child from sensorimotor egocentrism but creates preoperational egocentrism. For example, problems young children have with sharing can be traced to transient-permanent egocentrism. The use by another child of one child's toy may cause great distress because the owner does not distinguish the temporary possession by the second child from his own more permanent one and experiences the toy as having been taken away permanently.

Critique of Egocentrism

Donaldson (1978) challenged Piaget's assertions about early egocentrism because she believed the tasks posed were too abstract. She cited a study in which preschool children were given a modified version of Piaget's "mountains" task without changing its logical structure. The task was presented in the form of a story/game of hiding a boy doll from policemen dolls standing at various vantage points. Under these conditions, decentration is found in children as young as 2 years, pointing, among other things, to the power of a familiar framework such as a game or story as an aid to reasoning. Other studies show the capacity for both perceptual and conceptual perspective-taking at 3 years (Borke, 1975; Zahn-Waxler et al., 1977).

The degree of egocentrism attributed to a preschooler thus depends upon how the task is presented. If small variations in experimental procedure yield larger variations in the age at which a task is mastered, a Piagetian age-specific logical structure is harder to defend. As we shall see, information processing methodology determines how many steps are needed to solve a problem. Looked at this way, many logically similar tasks have very different cognitive demands. Sociocultural theorists would interpret the discrepancy between the "mountains" task and the "boy-hiding-from-policeman" version as supporting their developmental premise that children learn by having their problem-solving efforts "scaffolded" by helpful adults, often as narrative (Bruner, 1992).

CONCRETE OPERATIONAL STAGE (6–11 YEARS)

What are the "operations" to which toddlers are "pre-operational," and which for schoolchildren are "concrete"?

A preoperational child, shown a collection of colored wooden blocks and asked if there are more wooden blocks than red ones, may reply that there are more red ones. A concrete operational child who can classify understands that "red blocks" is a subclass of "wooden blocks" and is not fooled. A preoperational child, told that Billy is taller than David and that Susan is taller than Billy, may not be sure that Susan is taller than David. A concrete operational child can arrange a series of things according to any one of their several properties, or, in Piaget's terms, can seriate. He or she can form one series of Susan, David, and Billy according to height and a different one according to weight, given the information. A preoperational child who sees a liquid being poured from a short, broad container into a tall, slender one is liable to center on the dimension of height and proclaim the latter to contain more liquid, even though he can see that the same amount of liquid went into both containers. A concrete operational child can mentally reverse the act of pouring and understands that the volume was conserved. For Piaget, a *mental operation* is "any representational act

which is part of an organized network of related acts" (Flavell, 1963, p. 166). The three discussed above—classification, seriation, and conservation—are among the most important mental operations. With classification, recursive relations can be constructed, and concepts can be nested vertically in a branching hierarchy. Seriation permits things to be ordered horizontally in lists and rows according to their properties. Conservation stabilizes transformations because the child can "reverse the film" and mentally restore the transformed situation to its original form, conserving continuity.

Once stability of operations has been achieved, the child's representations are connected logically in orderly ways, rather than in the apparently inconstant, intuitive way of the preschooler. As concepts begin to override percepts, the world ceases to be magical and takes on order and predictability. The limit is that children can operate only upon concrete objects, present or experienced.

School-Age Egocentrism

Preoperational egocentrism embedded the child in symbols—language had become reified; words were not distinguished from things. The stage of concrete operations allows the child to construct the world as rule-bound and predictable and so to make assumptions and form hypotheses. This capacity to reason from assumptions to hypotheses puts words back at the service of their referents but, according to Elkind, ensnares the child in the concrete operational version of egocentrism. Hypotheses are reified, seen as if they were facts, and "as a consequence such youngsters often operate according to what might be called *assumptive realities*, assumptions about reality that children make on the basis of limited information and which they will not alter in the face of . . .contradictory evidence" (Elkind, 1970, p. 55). Elkind (1978) tells the story of an 8-year-old accustomed to leaving his toothbrush on the bathroom counter. His mother, while tidying, replaced it in the holder where it belonged. The child did not find it where he expected and complained it had been stolen. Because he took his hypothesis for fact, he did not look further for it. When shown its new location, he concluded that the thief returned it rather than considering that perhaps his hypothesis was incorrect.

FORMAL OPERATIONAL STAGE (11 TO ADULTHOOD)

An observer may ask a young subject to indicate whether what she (the observer) says about a solid-colored poker chip she holds is true, false, or uncertain. She may say, "Either the chip in my hand is green, or it is not green," or, "The chip in my hand is green, and it is not green." During some trials the chip is concealed, and during others it is not. School-age children tend to depend upon the physical, visible evidence of the actual chip to judge the truth of the statements—the "greenness" standard. Adolescents can focus on the formal propositional nature of the statements themselves and recognize that the first statement is true, and the second false, irrespective of the color of the chip (Osherson and Markman, 1975).

This experiment captures an essential difference between the thought processes of a concrete operational school-age child and a formal operational adolescent. The adolescent's thought is not structured by the percept or the concept of the actual object in question. The younger child can form hypotheses about what *is*—empirico-deductive reasoning; the older can hypothesize about what *could be*—hypothetico-deductive reasoning. Formal operations are the culmination of cognitive development for Piaget since they form the backbone of logical, and hence scientific, thought. Others believe that cognitive development extends beyond formal operations (see Summary).

Adolescent Egocentrism

The capacity of the adolescent to conceptualize his or her own thought allows the adolescent to distinguish hypotheses from facts but embeds the adolescent in new and more complex egocentrisms. The adolescent can, recursively, think about thinking, taking his or her own and others' thoughts as object. However, Elkind (1970) maintains that since the teen "fails to differentiate between what others are thinking about and his own mental pre-occupations, he assumes that other people are [for example] as obsessed with his behavior and appearance as he is himself" (p. 67). This objective-subjective egocentrism leaves the teen feeling as if he or she is continually performing before an imaginary audience. Deriving from this feeling is the universal-particular egocentrism that he or she is unique; never before has anyone felt the burden of youth as acutely. However adequate an explanation egocentrism may be for adolescent self-consciousness, it represents one of the first attempts to provide a cognitive basis for what had hitherto been explained only psychodynamically. Finally, unlike earlier forms of egocentrism, that of adolescence is dispelled by experience rather than by an increase in the complexity of the cognitive apparatus.

Critique and Comment

Piaget's theory still generates debate about its ongoing relevance. David Cohen (1983, p. 152) believes "it is time psychologists ceased being so obsessed with him. It is not that he should be burned but that he should be buried." By contrast, Mike Anderson (1992, p. 115) contends, "it is safe to say, as yet, nothing has replaced Piagetian theory as a general theory of cognitive development."

Piagetian theory draws attention to the commonalities of cognition across domains at a given age, and to the child as active constructor of his or her own experience. It also explains why children can solve some logical problems spontaneously at a certain age, but not earlier, even with instruction. It does not explain discrepancies in performance on different but logically similar tasks nor does it account for improvements, with instruction, in performance on tasks that were theoretically beyond the logical competence of the child. These facts argue against structures-of-the-whole. Finally, since Piaget based all cognition on logico-mathematical structures, he did not account well for development of other forms of cognition. Because children's thinking could be parsed in terms of logical structures, that does not necessarily mean that is how children represent things to themselves. It seemed to some that "Piaget's theory was better equipped for representing the structure in the mind of logicians than the structure in the minds of young children" (Case, 1992, p. 6).

To sum up, Piaget's work evokes a metaphor of the child as scientist, exploring his or her environment and constructing representations, based on logical principles, that organize their experience. Representations are tested by their ability to assimilate novel experiences. If they cannot, accommodation helps form more adequate ones and cognitive equilibrium is restored. More complex representations (and combinations of representations) extend a child's range of interactions and increase encounters with novelty, and so on. Interestingly, this image of a somewhat solitary investigator with the world for a laboratory, resembles Piaget himself as a child.

VYGOTSKY: THE SOCIOCULTURAL APPROACH

The Russian psychologist Lev Vygotsky was broadly educated in literature and philosophy and a committed Marxist. He worked during the early years of Soviet communism when the capacity for transformation of the individual by the social order was a central philosophical and political issue. Where Piaget saw young scientists exploring the world of things, Vygotsky saw children immersed in a complex sociocultural system based on a shared set of symbols for organizing and interpreting experience. The child develops by imitating and "internalizing" culturally based forms of behavior used by others in interaction with him. Therefore, all cognitive processes appear first on the interpsychological (social-cultural) level and then on the intrapsychological (individual) level. "Piaget believed that intelligence matured from the inside and directed itself outward. Vygotsky, in contrast, believed that intelligence begins in the social environment and directs itself inward" (Sternberg, 1990, p. 242).

Vygotsky's Genetic Method

The foundation of Vygotsky's thought is his "genetic method." As in Piaget's "genetic epistemology," the term "genetic" here means to understand a phenomenon in terms of how it developed. Therefore, before one can understand individual development, one must appreciate human biological organization in terms of its evolutionary origins and the requirements and values of one's culture in terms of its history. On this basis, Vygotsky rooted cognitive development in three "genetic domains"—phylogenesis (evolution), cultural history, and ontogenesis (individual development)—each with its own line of development. Developmental change in each line is due to the emergence of new forms of *mediation*, that is, *tools* and *signs*. For example, the emergence of tool use in primates marked a phylogenetic discontinuity whence, from that point on, anthropology explained human development better than biology.

Internalization, Semiotic Mediation, and Decontextualization

In Vygotsky's terms, both culture and cognition are *semiotically mediated*, that is, expressed through, and shaped by, signs and symbols. Tools are used in the physical world to shape materials, and, by analogy, signs are "psychological tools," inwardly directed, to shape the form of thought, whether one's own or others'. Individual cognitive development takes place when the culture's psychological tools—mainly language—are transmitted to, and internalized by, the child. *Internalization* is, for the individual, "the process of gaining control over external sign forms" (Wertsch, 1989, p. 65). Since developmental transitions occur with a change in the form of semiotic mediation, Vygotsky examined "the representational systems . . .needed to participate in . . .[social] processes—hence his emphasis on the internalization of *speech*. In contrast, Piaget's focus on the young child's interaction with physical reality led him to examine the representational systems required to manipulate objects" (Wertsch, 1989, p. 62).

At birth, each person has a set of biologically given *elementary mental processes*—memory, attention, and so on—analogous to the same capacities in other species. Cognitive development is the supersession of elementary mental processes by "higher," culturally based, ones that are uniquely human. "Elementary attention," for example, is stimulus-bound and reacts automatically to signals from the environment. The higher level "voluntary attention" is semiotically mediated—regulated by *inner speech*—selective and self-activated. In the same way, elementary, holistic, "integral perception" becomes the higher, sequential, "analytic perception." Similarly, "early memory" becomes "logical memory" with "the internalization of a language with which to represent logical problems" (Case, 1985, p. 72).

Higher mental functions, in turn, are subdivided into *rudimentary* and *advanced* ones by the degree of "*decontextualization* of mediational means" (Wertsch, 1989, pp. 56–57, emphasis added). Decontextualization simply means the capacity someone acquires to use cultural signs independent of any particular referent or setting. For example, when a child first learns to count, he or she can do so only with particular things; numbers (the "mediational means") cannot be manipulated in the absence of a concrete referent. This is a rudimentary higher process. Numbers must be decontextualized before the child can understand 2 + 2 = 4, irrespective of what is counted. Decontextualization allows the individual to attain advanced forms of higher mental functioning, which, in the history of populations, provides the possibility of sociocultural change.

Speech and Activity: Social, Egocentric, and Inner Speech

Prior to their coming together in cognition, Vygotsky believed thought and speech had independent origins. In the first 2 years of life, children use vocal activity for social contact and emotional expression—"pre-intellectual speech." Nevertheless, during this period they can problem solve and act in goal-directed ways unmediated by language—"pre-verbal thought." However, the child's language soon begins to include "syntactic and logical forms which have parallels in the child's problem-solving activity but are not linked to them in any systematic or useful way" (Meadows, 1993, p. 245). This is so-called *egocentric speech*, which develops further as children start to use language to help with problem-solving and "can be heard to talk themselves through problems or to count by using their fingers as aids. Finally, such aids are internalized and problem-solving thought uses internal dialogue, while language can be used more to reflect on and develop thought than as a prop to support problem-solving" (p. 245).

Egocentric speech has characteristics of both inner and social speech. For example, a child assembling a puzzle might say to himself "Now where does that piece go?" For Piaget, this bit of egocentric speech is a by-product of the principal cognitive process that is taking place internally. It will become social speech as a result of the child's interactions with others. Vygotsky, however, believed that egocentric speech is not only social in origin but also essential for mature thought. Young children "must essentially talk to themselves using their speech to guide thought and behavior. With development, the self-regulatory function of language changes so that children can direct their behavior using inner speech" (Bjorklund, 1989, p. 141). Egocentric speech is a form of "self-scaffolding" and a vital intermediate step between social speech and inner speech. Ultimately, self-talk is no longer articulated and becomes inner speech, the internal conversation used in problem-solving. Inner speech as a means of problem-solving is central in cognitive behavior modification (Meichenbaum, 1977).

Social speech has an earlier, *indicative* and a later, *symbolic* function. Indicative speech is highly contextualized; adult, child, and object must all be physically present, as when an adult uses words to draw the child's attention to a particular object in their shared environment. By contrast, symbolic speech abstracts (decontextualizes) properties of an object so that it may be categorized with others of its type. Further abstraction allows connections among categories and so on. To understand how this faculty develops, Vygotsky posed a block-sorting task to children of different ages. On the bottoms of a particular category in an assortment of blocks of different colors, shapes, and sizes, he wrote a nonsense word. He upturned one and asked children to sort those that they believed would have the same word on the bottom. When each child was done, he showed each child the bottom of an unselected piece, either with the same word on it but differing in some way or one that seemed to resemble those selected but had a different word on it, and asked the child to try again. He determined that young children tend to sort into idiosyncratic, unorganized heaps; older ones into complexes where there is an obvious relation among the blocks but not a "logical" one; and finally, in the oldest, sufficient capacity for generalization and decontextualization that allows sorting on the basis of true concepts. "Higher, uniquely human forms of psychological social interactions are possible only because thinking reflects reality in a generalized way (Vygotsky, 1934, pp. 11–12). "The stages in the development of *generalization* are directly linked to stages in the development of social interaction" (Wertsch, 1989, p. 96).

The internalization of speech and its decontextualization forms and transforms cognition. As the child internalizes, decontextualizes, and generalizes, the child gains control over his or her cognition. The child becomes more aware that he or she is thinking and problem-solving and that others are too. This awareness increases cognitive control, efficiency, and effectiveness. He or she can interact with the culture in ever more sophisticated ways as a storehouse for vast amounts of symbolically mediated knowledge. In doing so the child is not only acquiring knowledge but developing cognitively.

Zone of Proximal Development

Vygotsky's model of development brings the connection between knower and learner onto center stage. Such a connection may begin when a child brings his or her *intra*psychological resources (knowledge) to bear upon a problem that he or she cannot solve. The adult has to set up an *inter*psychological space such that the child can, with help, learn to solve the problem. Internalization will allow the child to solve the same problem the next time, unaided, and generalization will allow the child to approach other problems similar to it (see Sternberg's "selective encoding" below). Early on, the intersubjective space through which learning passes is context-bound and informal; later, with a shared set of linguistic meanings established, learning can be more formal and decontextualized, as in school. However it is structured, "the distance between the actual developmental level as determined by independent problem-solving and the level of potential development as determined through problem-solving under adult guidance or in collaboration with more capable peers" is termed the *zone of proximal development* (Vygotsky, 1978, p. 86).

"In order to understand the role of verbal mediation in volitional, intrapsychological functioning, [Vygotsky] argued that one must examine speech on the interpsychological plane. In particular, one must view such phenomena as the use of directives or commands by adults to regulate children" (Wertsch, 1989, p. 92). Experimenters who looked at the techniques of effective mother-child instructional interaction noted that the most successful mothers titrated their level of involvement to the child's apparent need. When the child began to fail, a little more instruction was added; as the child succeeded, the parent stood back. "One sets the game, provides a *scaffold* to assure that the child's ineptitudes can be rescued by appropriate intervention, and then removes the scaffold part by part as the reciprocal structure can stand on its own" (Bruner, 1983, p. 60). Scaffolding is useful for instruction and also provides a narrative structure so that, in a clinical setting, a child can be helped to become aware of what she knows but could not say (Meadows, 1993). For example, suppose a 6-year-old girl tells her father she has misplaced her boots. Father helps her to reconstruct her activities throughout the day until the moment when she becomes aware, in retrospect, where she left them (Wertsch, 1988). Even though the father did not have the necessary information, he had a systematic strategy for accessing it. The child had the information but, as yet, no strategy. Next time she misplaces something, she may say aloud to herself "Now, let's see, where did I have it last?"

Jaan Valsiner extends the zone of proximal development (ZPD) concept to a tripartite arrangement including a "zone of free movement" (ZFM) and a "zone of promoted action" (ZPA) (Valsiner, 1989). The ZFM "specifies the structure of the environment that is functionally available to the developing child at a given time" (p. 165). Initially it limits the child's actions but, as it is internalized, it is susceptible to internal modification as reason and affects are brought to bear on it. The ZPA "is the set of activities, objects or areas . . .within which actions are facilitated by 'social others'" (p. 165). With internalization, these become the person's norms and expectations and shape future goal-oriented acting and planning. They too, are subject to internal modification. The ZPD, in this context, "captures those psychological functions that . . .are in the process of turning from the realm of the possible to that of the actual, with the help of other people" (p. 165). "In general, it is the ZFM-ZPA-ZPD complex that constitutes the description of the process by which child development takes place" (p. 165).

"Because an adult and a child operating in the zone of proximal development often bring divergent situation definitions to a task setting, they may be confronted with severe problems of establishing and maintaining intersubjectivity. The challenge to the adult is to find a way to communicate with the child such that the latter can participate . . .in interpsychological functioning and can eventually come to define the task setting in a new, culturally appropriate way" (Wertsch, 1989, p. 161). This is a succinct characterization of the central task of child psychiatry and psychotherapy.

Thought as Narrative

Jerome Bruner (1990), for decades the major American exponent of the sociocultural view, views the child as a natural maker of meaning and an apprentice storyteller. He was dismayed that the "cognitive revolution" (below) had reduced cognition to computation and that the computer metaphor had centered development on the private "processing of information" rather than the public and interactional "construction of meaning." He proposed a "cultural psychology" "organized around those meaning-making and meaning-using processes that connect man to culture. . . .by virtue of participation in culture, meaning is rendered *public* and *shared*" (pp. 12–13).

In Bruner's view, the computational model left no room for *intentionality*—the mind's predisposition to think *about* x, to wish *for* y or to believe *that* z. For many, intentionality is constitutive of mind; without intentionality the individual cannot be seen as an agent, and without *agency* there can be no meaning. Bruner, therefore, concerned himself not with objectivized "behavior" but with intentional "action," specifically, with "action situated in a cultural setting, and in the mutually interacting intentional states of the participants" (p. 19). These interacting intentional states form the culture and provide an interpretive system for the making of meaning. The form of this interpretive system is *narrative*.

Narrative implies a sequence of happenings, told from someone's point of view, that explains events in terms of the intentional states of the actors. It is a culture's way of interpreting events, especially "noncanonical"—extraordinary—events: It is both everyday conversation and the nightly news. Narrative "mediates between the canonical [expected] world of culture and the more idiosyncratic world of [one's] beliefs, desires and hopes" (p. 52). People make meaning as narrative both by innate predisposition and cultural facilitation. There are "certain classes of meaning to which human beings are innately tuned and for which they actively search" (p. 72). "Narrative structure is even inherent in the *praxis* of social interaction before it achieves linguistic expression" (p. 77). That is, "social understanding, however abstract it may become, always begins as praxis in particular contexts. . . .the child learns to play a part in everyday family 'drama' *before* there is any telling or justifying or excusing required" (p. 85) (see also Dunn, 1988). Margaret Donaldson (above, 1978) and others showed how logically competent very young children can be when propositions are embedded in a story. Similarly, some have proposed that children younger that 4 years do not have a "theory of mind"—a representation of what another person may be thinking—because they do not seem to understand deception in stories told them by an experimenter (Leslie, 1987; Perner, 1991). However, Chandler found that, if children were *participants* in the deception, between 2 and 3 years they showed an awareness of others' false beliefs (Chandler et al., 1989). Others dispute this (Perner, 1991, p. 311). We will revisit "theory of mind" and Bruner's idea of innate narrativity in our discussion of a cognitive theory of autism.

So then, both the culture as a whole, and children as individuals, organize experience as narrative, and the two levels of meaning-making interact recursively. The culture teaches a child to tell a good story as part of growing up. Most responses to questions in the to-and-fro of the family are, and are expected to be, in the form of a story, often to justify one's actions (and to displace blame onto the nearest sibling). Katherine Nelson described Emily's evolving narrative competence between 18 months and 3 years of age (Nelson, 1989). Time and again her evolving speech seemed "impelled by a need to get things organized in an appropriate serial order, to get them marked for their specialness to take some sort of stance on them" (Bruner, 1990, p. 89). "In time she imports another genre into her narratives—problem-solving" (p. 94). This last is a direct challenge to the Piagetians and information processing theorists for whom problem-solving is the foundation of cognitive development.

What becomes of the self if we "story" ourselves rather than conceptualize ourselves? In Bruner's cultural psychology, the self is not so much a "pure and enduring nucleus" of identity but a "distributed self" that is "the sum and swarm of participations" (p. 107). The idea of psychotherapy as a form of renarratizing one's life has influenced both psychoanalysis (Schafer, 1983; Spence, 1982) and family systems therapy (White and Epston, 1990).

INFORMATION-PROCESSING APPROACH

The Child's Mind as a Computational Device

The third contemporary explanation of cognitive development is that of information-processing (IP) theory. IP theory is not tied to the work of a single pioneer investigator, so it is not as unitary as Piaget's or Vygotsky's. It proposed originally to explain how an adult starts from knowing nothing about a subject and ends up knowing a great deal—the "novice-to-expert transition." It has only recently offered explanations of children's thinking and so is a newcomer to the family of developmental theories.

Information-processing theories of development "focus on the information that children represent, the processes that they use to transform the information, and the memory limits that constrain the amount of information they can represent and process" (Siegler, 1991). The goal is to construct a comprehensive model of the mind—a *cognitive architecture*—that accounts for the "sort of general information-processing capacities a mind must have in order to do the many things it does" (Stillings et al., 1991, p. 17). The mind is seen to be, essentially, a problem-solving device, and cognitive scientists have constructed computer-based cognitive architectures to synthesize and extrapolate the findings of experimental psychologists (McClelland and Rumelhart, 1986; Newell, 1990). The developmental task of IP theory is to account for the enormous increase, from birth to maturity, in the complexity of a person's knowledge organization and processing capacity.

Data, Information, and Knowledge

It is important, first, to distinguish among data, information, and knowledge. In the world of artificial intelligence, *data* are simply "facts without context in a form . . .that can be entered into a computer" (Thro, 1991, p. 76). Once entered, "Human organization and interpretation give data context and meaning, producing *information*" (p. 76). If information may be distinguished from data by meaning, knowledge may be distinguished from information by longevity and purpose: *Knowledge* is the "representation of facts (including generalizations) and concepts organized for future use, including problem-solving" (Gregory, 1989, p. 410).

A data-processing system must be able to transform input into an internal representation it can operate upon, that is, to *encode*. It must be able to hold new information "onscreen" for appraisal, to transform it into knowledge by connecting it with prior knowledge, and have the storage capacity to keep the new knowledge for future use. By analogy, in order to learn, children must first be able to transform a stimulus into information by encoding it as a mental representation. They then must hold the representation in a sort of active memory while retrieving relevant knowledge from their accumulated store. The new information is brought together with the "old" knowledge and, if it is deemed important to the ongoing life of the child, the information will be stored, in the context of related knowledge, for future use. The input system will be freed up for new data. This outline constitutes a simplified cognitive architecture.

Information processors and Piagetians agree that children actively modify their own cognition, but disagree about how. The former analyzed standard Piagetian tasks, for example, the balance-beam task, in terms of the problem-solving steps required instead of analyzing their logical form as Piaget did. In this task, children of different ages are asked to predict which side of a balance beam will go down as weights and their distances from the fulcrum are varied. The child's performance is measured in terms of his or her processing capacity relative to the *processing demands*—the number of discrete cognitive operations—of the task. The older the child, the better the ability to predict correctly as variations of weights and distance become more complex. These age differences suggest that many tasks that shared a similar logical form imposed quantitatively different processing demands. Many cognitive architectures have been constructed to explain how children go about solving such problems; five are presented below.

CLASSICAL PROCESSING MODEL

In 1956 George Miller wrote the landmark paper ''The Magical Number Seven Plus or Minus Two: Some Limits on Our Capacity to Process Information.'' He argued that ''humans are limited to remembering approximately seven items (plus or minus two) in their immediate memory. However, by *chunking* items into composite units, a large amount of information could be contained in seven units'' (Miller, 1989, p. 276). For example, it would be too difficult for most people to repeat back the 13 digit series 7472462121945 without a strategy. However, if one associated 747 with the aircraft, 246 with the first three even numbers, 212 as the boiling point of water in°F, and 1945 as the end of World War II, the original 13 units become 4 and the task is manageable.

Miller's paper gave the newborn movement a name and delineated its central metaphor—*processing capacity.* He identified ''immediate memory'' as the locus of information processing and proposed chunking to be the principal strategy for increasing available processing space. Chunks are aggregates of related facts, concepts, or percepts. Chunks become larger and more complex with experience and are often hierarchically integrated, one inside another, like Russian dolls, so as to take up less processing space. Development may be seen as the increasing capacity of this ''immediate'' or *short-term memory*—now called ''working memory.'' If so, is this due to biological maturation or increasingly effective and sophisticated strategies to chunk information? Clearly one's general knowledge base and specific knowledge of memory strategies influence this capacity (Chi et al., 1982).

Let us follow an item of information through the system according to a version of this classic model (Atkinson and Shiffrin, 1968). The stimulus, for example, an auditory or visual sensation, passes first into a modality-specific *sensory register* — ''echoic store'' for sound, ''iconic store'' for sight—where, in milliseconds, it is scanned for pattern recognition, tagged as relevant, and transferred into *short-term memory.* In an adult, it may stay there up to 15–30 seconds in the form of five to nine (''seven plus or minus two'') units. It may be lost, or it may stay longer if some deliberate strategy—*control process*—is used to keep it active. One such process is ''rehearsal,'' wherein a person might repeat the input (e.g., a telephone number) to himself. This new information may be interpreted as insignificant and forgotten, cause a behavioral response, be stored in *long-term memory,* or remain in short-term memory and undergo further processing. These possibilities may be represented as a flow diagram (Fig. 11.1).

In the classic model, the place where new information is held, awaiting further processing, is simply ''short-term memory.'' This concept has recently become the more comprehensive *working memory* (Baddely, 1986). Briefly, it consists of an attentionlike, central executive that manages both an ''articulatory loop'' system, associated with the reception of phonological information and the production of speech, and a visuospatial ''scratch-pad'' for encoding images (Eysenck, 1990). Working memory is the principal arena of cognition, and its processing capacity determines the sophistication of problem-solving. In many IP theories, changes in this capacity account for development.

SEMANTIC ORGANIZATION: NETWORKS AND PRODUCTION SYSTEMS

Information processing may also be rendered as a series of *production systems,* as in a computer program (Anderson, 1983; Newell, 1990; Newell and Simon, 1972). Production systems are rule-based mental representations in the form of condition-action (''if . . .then'') statements stored in long-term memory. If condition ''A'' is held in working memory and matches a rule for action in long-term memory, then the unit acts to produce an output that in turn may trigger another production system, and so on. For example, a student reading a text may bring into operation the production system ''If the sentence is important, then underline it'' followed by ''If the book isn't yours, don't mark it up.'' There can be a great many of these nested within one another to make up a ''program'' of great recursive complexity. A more current version of the flow-diagram representation described above is a network type of architecture also based on production systems. One such is the propositional network of J.R. Anderson (1983), which he called ACT*, an acronym for ''adaptive control of thought.''

Anderson proposed an architecture based upon two fundamental types of knowledge—*declarative knowledge* and *procedural knowledge.* Declarative knowledge is ''knowing that''; it is knowledge of facts and concepts, such as the date and significance of a historical event. It may be stored as languagelike representations (propositions) or perceptionlike representations (images) (Stillings et al., p. 18). Procedural knowledge is ''knowing how'' to do things, such as read a book or ride a bicycle. It contains elements of declarative knowledge that have been *proceduralized.* That is, copies of elements of declarative knowledge have been integrated into production systems so that one can access this information from production memory automatically and instantaneously rather than consciously searching declarative memory each time the information is needed. Once proceduralized, however, retrieval of these declarative elements requires conscious, focused attention, that is, *controlled* processes. Procedural knowledge operates by *automatic* processes that are unconscious and make no demands on working memory (Schneider and Schiffrin, 1977). Developmentally, the more we proceduralize our knowledge, the more we can do simultaneously and the more complex the tasks we can manage.

As above, let us follow an item of information through this system. To begin with, an external stimulus or an internal computation is encoded in working memory which, in ACT*, is not separate but designates the currently active part of declarative memory. Information may enter declarative memory as a proposition, image, or representation of a sequence of events. The declarative system is made up of propositions: ''I need to study tonight to pass tomorrow's exam.'' Production systems form the procedural component: ''If invited out tonight, then decline.''

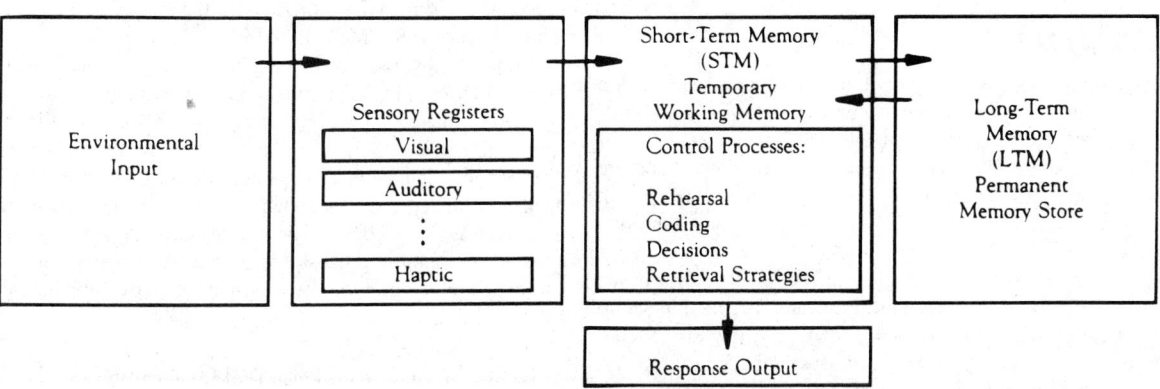

Figure 11.1. Flow of information through the memory system. (From Atkinson RC, Shiffrin RM: *The Control of Short Term Memory.* Copyright © 1971 by Scientific American, Inc. All rights reserved.)

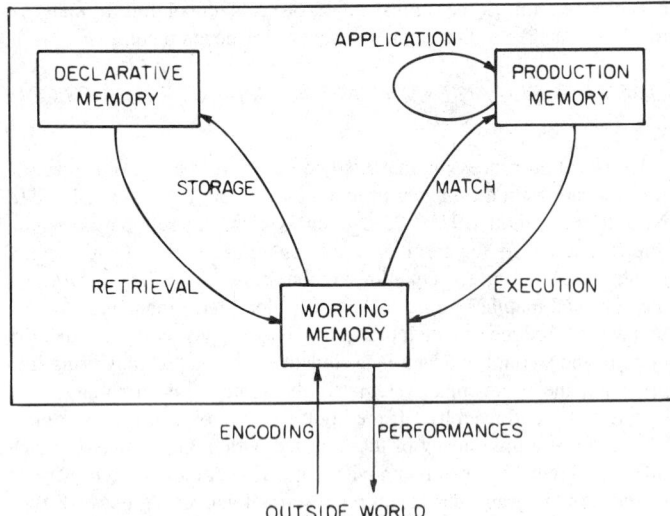

Figure 11.2. A general framework for the ACT production system. (From Anderson JR: *The Architecture of Cognition.* Cambridge, MA, Harvard University Press, 1983, p. 19.)

"For a production to apply, the clauses specified in its condition must be matched against the information active in working memory. This information is part of the system's *declarative* component . . .[and] must be retrieved from long-term memory" (Anderson, 1983, pp. 10–11) (Fig. 11.2). If more than one rule may apply, as above with the "underlining" dilemma, preference may be given to the one that most closely matches the goals currently in working memory (therefore, underline) or, since whenever a rule is applied successfully it is strengthened and more likely to be called up again, the prohibition against defacing library books might override the immediate goal (therefore don't).

Knowledge is represented in declarative memory as a network of *nodes*, and relations among them, or *links*. In Anderson's scheme, "The nodes of the propositional network stand for ideas, and the linkages among the nodes represent associations among those ideas" (Best, 1989, p. 249). Retrieval of ideas or images from long-term memory involves *spreading activation* (Collins and Loftus, 1975; Quillian, 1968). "Activation controls the rate of information processing. . . .Activation spreads through the declarative network along paths from original sources to associated concepts. A piece of information will become active to the degree that it is related to current sources of activation" (Anderson, 1983, p. 86). The "firing" (or not) of a node influences the ongoing direction of the activation. Particular nodes may be more or less easily involved in this chain reaction, depending on the relevance of their content to the current situation and the closeness of their association to already activated nodes.

NEURAL NETWORKS AND "CONNECTIONISM"

Anderson's production system model has been criticized as too "computerized" and remote from the way people actually think (Gardner, 1985). In Anderson's ACT*, as in the classical model, "sets of symbols are moved about from one memory store to another, and are processed by explicit rules applied in sequence" (Eysenck, 1991, p. 66). While this is how digital computers work, it may not be how the brain (usually) works.

Initially, it seemed promising to build a model of cognition based on rules and symbols. However, when programmers first tried to set up software to do things that brains seemed to do easily, they discovered that the simpler the task for a human, the harder it seemed for a computer. A program for college-level calculus was easier to write than for grade-school math and it was virtually impossible to write one to manipulate an infant's blocks. So too, when programmers tried to write rule-based

programs based on human experts' experience-derived knowledge in their field, they found that the experts could not articulate their rules to solve any but the simplest problems; they seemed to operate more by a combination of intuition and rules with multiple exceptions than by formal logic. These setbacks moved some cognitive scientists to look to the structure of the brain to inform the design of their cognitive architectural software. These revolutionary cognitive architectures are called *neural networks*.

The basic design of a neural network is simply a layer of input processing units, or "neurons," a layer of "connecting" neurons, and a layer of output neurons. Data are taken in and passed to the connecting layer, which has a myriad of interconnections among its elements. "Each neuron takes in signals from other neuronlike components, adds them up, and decides on the basis of the answer whether to send out a signal of its own. In a way the neural units . . .are analogous to people in a jury talking amongst themselves, trying to influence each other to decide one way or another . . ." (Allman, 1989, p. 12). At some point, output ensues. The relative success or failure of the output in solving the problem at hand constitutes new input, and particular connecting pathways are strengthened—*weighted*—or weakened as a consequence—hence "connectionism" to characterize this approach to cognitive architecture. Like humans, the system learns from examples, by trial and error.

Knowledge is represented as the sum of all these connections at any given moment. It is therefore "distributed," that is, spread throughout the network; there is no "central processor" nor distinct memory bank. So too, most or all elements of the system are necessarily active at the same moment as activation spreads among millions of neurons simultaneously, that is, the system works in parallel rather than in sequence. Given these characteristics, one of the most developed connectionist architectures is called "parallel distributed processing" (McClelland and Rumelhart, 1986). By entering lists of verbs and their past tenses, Rumelhart and McClelland (1986) "taught" a neural network system to change the present-tense form of a verb to its past-tense form and found that, "though it wasn't designed to do so, this neural network made the same kinds of mistakes that children make when they are learning verbs" (Allman, 1989, pp. 36–37).

Neural networks explain better than conventional, rule-based architectures how we make inductive inferences and generalize. As the number of input neurons is virtually limitless all sorts of subtle contextual variations can be encoded so as to enormously increase the capacity to adapt to shifting circumstances and act on incomplete information. Connections resemble rules in that antecedent circumstances influence subsequent ones, but the influence is virtually indeterminate since one can never be sure, from instance to instance, how all the inputs will add up. Connections are probabilistic rather than deterministic; rules impose hard constraints, connections soft ones. Parenthetically, neural networks also undergird applications of "fuzzy logic," a new form of artificial intelligence that allows nonhuman systems essentially to program themselves, taking as input partial truths and incomplete information the processing of which has hitherto been the unique property of the human mind (Kosko, 1993; McNeil and Freiberger, 1993).

Connectionist models may explain more precisely Piaget's concepts of assimilation and accommodation. "Assimilation can be interpreted in terms of the tendency of an interactive network to settle into the most appropriate of its stable (attractor) states . . .when input is presented to it; in Piaget's language, this is the schema to which the experience has been assimilated. Accommodation can be interpreted as the changes in activations as well as weights that occur in order to assimilate the experience. . . .these processes can actually be designed into networks and observed under a variety of scenarios" (Bechtel and Abrahamsen, 1991, p. 271).

Mike Anderson's Minimal Cognitive Architecture

Australian Mike Anderson (1992)—no relation to J.R. Anderson—has proposed a "minimal cognitive architecture" that accounts both for individual differences in intelligence and for cognitive development on the basis of an interaction of *generality* and *modularity* in mental functioning. We will come back to this in the neo-Piagetian model of Robbie Case.

Anderson begins by noting that individuals differ in data processing speed, measured neurophysiologically as "inspection time" (IT), "reaction time" (RT) and "average evoked potential" (AEP). AEP is derived mathematically from EEG tracings while IT and RT are simply measures of how much time it takes subjects to make choices on the basis of rapidly presented sensory stimuli. Although controversial, these measures may represent a sort of general neuronal efficiency, and all correlate well with IQ and other measures of cognitive ability. A person's relative performance on cognitive tests remains more or less constant throughout life so that differences in processing speed are likely biologically based. Anderson postulates a "wired-in" *basic processing mechanism (BPM)* that carries out general computation and varies in speed from person to person. This would account for some individual differences in intelligence (Fig. 11.3).

On the other hand, there are some things that everyone can do about the same, irrespective of IQ, and that computers find very difficult. For example, virtually from birth, all can extract the features of three-dimensional space, encode phonological information, and organize their own and others' utterances as language. These abilities do not correlate with processing speed, and Anderson suggests these are, like the BPM, part of our genetic inheritance. However, unlike the BPM, they do not vary in efficiency, but operate in an all-or-none fashion. He calls them *modules*. They come "on-line" at different points as we mature.

People differ in their talents and, often, a particular talent is associated with other talents: some people are better at art, others at math; and, if they are good at math, they are likely to be musical. Indeed, during World War II, musicians were put to work as cryptographers simply because they were handy, but they turned out to have unusual gifts for unraveling codes. Standard IQ tests recognize such differences by sorting cognitive abilities into two piles—verbal and performance. Correspondingly, Anderson proposes two *specific processors*, which are, "function-specific knowledge-acquisition mechanisms" (p. 118). One generates "problem-solving algorithms" for verbal/propositional input (SP1) and the other for visuospatial input (SP2) the way computer languages such as LISP and FORTRAN are each designed to process

a different sort of data. SPs are "experience-dependent" in that they need experience to develop as processing mechanisms. They must "borrow" from the general computational capacity of the BPM to process information so their development is also dependent upon the BPM's processing speed. By contrast, modules are "experience expectant," that is, they need only exposure to an experience (perhaps during a "sensitive period") to unfold. Knowledge is acquired either by thought-mediated learning (Fig. 11.3, *Route 1*) or by the age-related activation of phylogenetically given modules (Fig. 11.3, *Route 2*).

Finally, there are things that some cannot do irrespective of intelligence. For example, dyslexics, even with a high IQ, cannot decode certain types of language-based information. In some cases there may be a fault in SP1, in others a defect in the module for phonological encoding. These possibilities are not mutually exclusive, as there are types of dyslexia that are better explained as processing problems and others better explained as pure or modular defects.

For Mike Anderson, development happens in two distinct ways: (*a*) the acquisition of new competencies and (*b*) the elaboration of knowledge (Fig. 11.3). "The maturation of modules is the primary cause of cognitive development" (p. 207). For example, the maturation of language-related modules brings a new set of processing competencies to all. "Suddenly having access to linguistic representations will result in a discontinuity of development that is unrelated to individual differences in intelligence. However, elaborating one's knowledge of the world by using this new competence—for example, by building vocabularies—will be constrained by the basic processing mechanism and the specific processors. Thus, individual differences in intelligence will have an effect on the elaboration of knowledge but not on the acquisition of new competencies" (p. 121).

Components of Cognition

Robert Sternberg's (1984) Triarchic Theory provides conceptual tools for an analysis of what constitutes intelligent behavior. One subtheory of the triarchy describes what goes on "inside one's head" to produce intelligent behavior, another describes what makes one's behavior intelligent in a given setting, and the third describes one's experience at the interface between the "head" and the "setting," as performance is being automatized. The "setting-specific" element acknowledges that

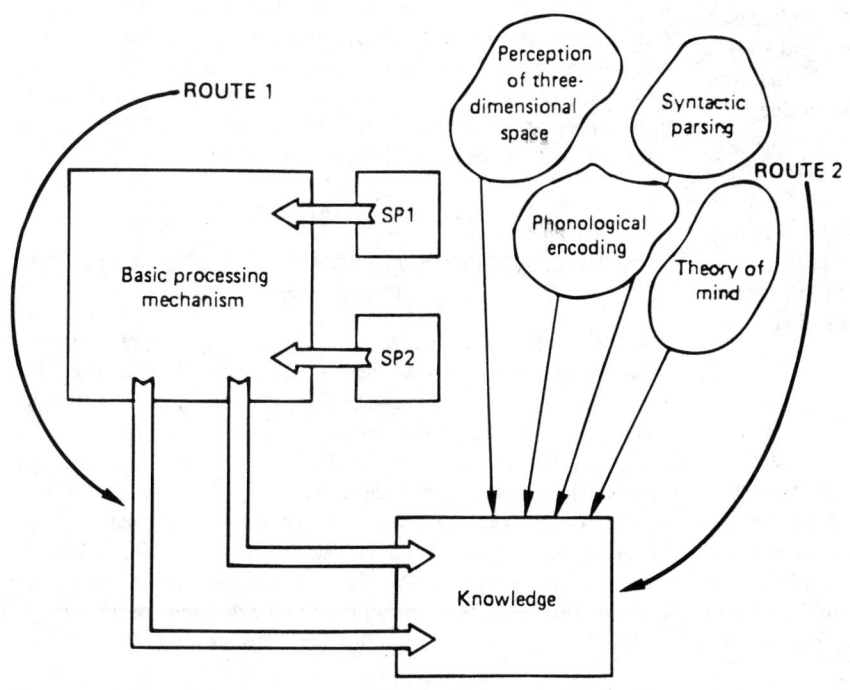

Figure 11.3. A diagram of Mike Anderson's model of cognitive structures. *SP*, specific processor. (From Anderson JR: *The Architecture of Cognition*. Cambridge, MA, Harvard University Press, 1983, p. 107.)

IQ tests, for example, do not necessarily predict successful performance in the individual's real life. The "interface" element draws attention to the degree of novelty of an experience: It must be interesting or compelling enough to engage the intelligence but also within the cognitive reach of the individual. The "head" element is the only one to develop and is the one to be discussed further here.

The "head" part is the so-called componential subtheory and describes the interaction among three information-processing *components*: A component is "an elementary information process that operates on internal representations of objects or symbols" (p. 164). Sternberg's three groups of components are (*a*) *performance components*, (*b*) *knowledge acquisition components*, and (*c*) *metacomponents*. The last sits "above" the other two and deploys them to solve a given problem. For example, "problem recognition" is a metacomponent that determines whether a given problem is familiar, and if so, of what generic type it is. Once this is determined, performance components, such as "encoding"—organizing the input to fit existing procedures—are selected to implement the decision to solve the problem according to its type. Knowledge acquisition components, such as "selective encoding," must distinguish information relevant to solving the type of problem from all the data available. If relevant knowledge is missing, this component mobilizes strategies to acquire it. "Selective combination" puts together the bits of relevant data encoded and "selective comparison" brings "old" knowledge to bear on the newly encoded and combined information. When faced with a novel problem, competent adults spend proportionately more time than 7-year-olds encoding the terms of the problem. The child's strategy of jumping right in lowers the working memory load but is ultimately less efficient because important factors are not encoded (Sternberg and Rifkin, 1979). Gifted children, like adults, spend more time encoding and are generally more efficient at using other knowledge acquisition components (Sternberg and Davidson, 1983).

Sternberg accounts for development in terms of changes in function of these information-processing components, particularly the metacomponents. The better the metacomponents become at strategically deploying the resources of the other two, the more sophisticated the cognition. Cognitive development also occurs as "the functioning of a given componential subsystem for a particular task domain proceeds from "controlled" to "automatic" (Sternberg, 1984, p. 173). Controlled processing implies a hierarchical directing of the performance and knowledge acquisition components by the metacomponents. Controlled processing is of limited capacity, but can access the entire knowledge base. It operates serially, and because it is a conscious process, it is costly in terms of space in working memory. Automatic processing is less costly and nonhierarchical: All three types of components now operate at the same level, which means that the strategies originally used consciously by the metacomponents are now automatic. This allows parallel processing, but there is limited access to stored information. New information is processed in a controlled manner, while familiar information is processed automatically.

Development of Processing Capacity

In information-processing models, development is toward faster processing and greater organizational complexity of cognitive architecture. A cognitively mature person can manage more information per unit of time and deal better with complex and ambiguous information than an immature one. Infants cannot handle complex information as well as older children, because they would have to "attend to and interrelate more pieces of information than their working memory

capacities can handle" (Flavell, 1985, p. 85). With experience, elements of a task are chunked into aggregates and processes automatized, which allows more attention for conscious, reflective thinking and problem-solving.

Information Processing and Piagetian Models Compared

In both Piagetian and information processing models, cognition entails mental representation, but representations are organized differently in each. Piagetian structures are age-specific and explain consistent performance across cognitive domains. However, Piagetians were obliged to recognize that the theory did not account well for uneven performance across tasks with the same apparent logical structure—*horizontal décalage*. For example, a child may be able to pass a conservation of number problem at age 5 but not pass a conservation of volume task until age 9 or 10. Information processors emphasize task and domain specificity, that is, the encoding of the task as of one type or another draws together and organizes knowledge to solve it. Cognitive representations have their origins and applications in particular domains. For example, the capacity to perform certain mental operations in the domain of mathematics does not mean that the child can transfer this capacity to the spatial domain: décalages are discrepancies in domain-specific knowledge and likely also reveal discrepant processing demands, concealed by apparent similarities in logical structure. However, with the exception of Mike Anderson and, as we shall see, Robbie Case, both Piagetian and IP theorists constructed general models of the mind, that is, some sort of central processor or logical "structure-of-the-whole" upon which learning and development are based.

Critique of Information Processing as a Developmental Theory

Patricia Miller (1989) noted that, while changes in processing capacity have been clearly described in adults as they go from novice to expert, development from child to adult may not proceed in the same way. Siegler does not see this to be a problem. Investigators, he believes, "can better understand the development of children's thinking when [they] know where that thinking is headed" (Siegler, 1986, p. 63). Miller also felt that there has been relatively little application of IP theory to the understanding of emotions, motivation, and social development. Recently, however IP theory has been brought to bear on explaining autism (see below). So too, Case's neo-Piagetian theory may also be characterized as an IP theory, and it has been applied to social and emotional development (see below) (Case, 1988).

NEO-PIAGETIAN THEORY

The Response to Piaget and the Responses to the Response

Case (1992) has summarized the recent history of, and intellectual influences on, the most current theories of cognitive development. First, in reaction to the inadequacies of Piaget's "monolithic, universal and endogenous" system (p. 10), other investigators—"empiricists"—began to study task-specific learning and avoided hypothesizing about how the development of different competencies might resemble one another. As one would expect, these projects explained some of what the Piagetian enterprise could not, but did not account for the similarities among children of divergent cultures and common, age-specific constraints on learning. This impasse prompted three, quite different, responses.

The "neonativist" groups, influenced by Chomsky's notion of innate structures for language acquisition, proposed that cognitive development was based upon the maturing of "wired-in" modules (Herschfeld and Gelman, 1994). These predisposed children to attend to, and take in, certain types of stimuli (as described in the sections on Mike Anderson and Jerome Bruner). Howard Gardner (1983), for example, suggested there were, in fact, seven different intelligences—musical, logical, verbal, spatial, kinesthetic, intrapersonal, and interpersonal—each essentially modular. This architecture likely has a central processor of some sort but individual differences and developmental change are inherent in the modules.

The "new learning (neoassociationist)" theory put forth a model of development similar to the novice-to-expert transition in adult learning. Development is learning-based and is cumulative. As children acquire more experience in a domain, "they begin to form new connections (whether conceptual, procedural or purely associationistic) among the basic elements of which the domain is comprised. These . . .lead to the integration of knowledge structures that were previously discrete. Once integrated, new knowledge structures or networks lead to new [problem-solving] strategies . . .and to new memorial capacities" (Case, 1992, p. 14). Micheline Chi (1988), a pioneer in this approach, did a fascinating study on a 5-year-old dinosaur expert, demonstrating a reciprocity between knowledge structures and learning strategies (Chi and Koeske, 1983).

Finally, the "neo-Piagetian" groups proposed that there are domain-specific cognitive structures that develop more or less independently. Like task-specific structures, they are dependent on the context of learning and the child's previous experience: Like Piagetian ones, their application is broad within their domain. Their pattern of development is hierarchical and recursive (Fig. 11.5), and they are constrained, at any given age, by maturational limitations on the size of working memory and/or the speed of processing.

Robbie Case

A well-regarded example of the neo-Piagetian synthesis is the work of Robbie Case (1985). Case supported the Piagetian notion of age-related, general cognitive structures evolving in an invariant sequence, but also believed that problem-solving strategies and working memory limitations had to be taken into account. Significantly, he incorporated affect as an important element in his approach. More recently, his work (Case, 1992) has addressed the question of modularity. That is, is the mind best understood as a general information processing device that stretches across domains to approach problems with the same tools or is it a system of phylogenetically shaped modules whose components are each dedicated to processing only particular kinds of data or information?

EXECUTIVE CONTROL STRUCTURES

Case (1985) proposed that a child's cognitions are composed of schemes representing "patterns of stimulation," called *state representations*, and schemes representing mechanisms of transforming these states, called *operations*. The activation of a scheme is attended by an affect: positive, negative, or neutral. From the 2nd month of life, children have some control over and attempt to optimize their affective experience. They do this by organizing schemes to represent (*a*) a particular, recurrent state, the *problem representation*; (*b*) an anticipated state of greater pleasure, the *objective*; and (*c*) the operation that will produce this transition, the *strategy*. These three elements are combined to form *executive control structures*, which are basic problem-solving structures analogous to production systems.

Case applied the concept of executive control structures to the well-known "juice problem" (Noelting, 1975). In this problem, children are asked to compare two lines of small cups, each line containing some

PROBLEM SITUATION
- Two sets of cups, each set with some juice cups and some water cups.

OBJECTIVE
- Determine the set with a lot of juice.

STRATEGY
- Scan each line of juice cups. Pick the set where the line of juice cups is long.

A

PROBLEM SITUATION
- Two sets of cups, each set with some juice cups and some water cups.
- Each line of juice cups is approximately the same length.

OBJECTIVES
- Determine the set with the greater juiciness.
- Determine the set with the greater number of juice cups.

STRATEGY
1. Count each line of juice cups. Note the line with the bigger number.
2. Assume that the line with the bigger number will taste juicier. Pick it.

B

Figure 11.4. The executive control structure for solving the second problem. **A,** Four-year-old control structure. **B,** Six-year-old control structure. (From Sternberg RJ (ed): *Mechanisms of Cognitive Development.* Copyright © 1984 by WH Freeman and Company. Reprinted by permission.)

cups filled with juice and some filled with water. One line has a large number of juice cups and a few water cups. The other has a small number of juice cups and the same number of water cups as the first, so that it is shorter in length than the other line. The children are asked which line, when mixed together, will taste "juicier." Four-year-olds guess (correctly) the first, because "there's a lot there." This is the earliest that children can solve this problem. At 6, children can go one better. In this situation the lines of cups are made of equal length, and the same question is posed. By counting juice cups on each side, the children confidently pick the side with the greater number. The executive control structures assembled for the juice problem, for each age group, appear in Figure 11.4.

The 6-year-old's structure is actually two hierarchically integrated structures. It is more quantitatively fine-tuned than the earlier one, more "dimensional." Case (1984) used this analysis to contrast the cognitive organization of 4-year-olds with that of 6-year-olds. For Case, the "4 to 6" transition is a stage transition, one of three linking his four stages. At 6, two different, earlier executive control structures have been coordinated and hierarchically integrated. As a result, a qualitative differentiation occurs, wherein a new way of thinking emerges—a *quantitative dimension* of thought. This capacity to, as it were, dimensionalize applies not only to the task at hand; once this dimensional structure is established, the child applies it to a wide variety of tasks. Case calls this higher-level knowledge organization a *central conceptual structure*. It is central in that it can be applied to a broad range of tasks, analogous to, although perhaps less comprehensive than, Piaget's structures-of-the-whole.

CENTRAL CONCEPTUAL STRUCTURES

As in the information-processing and sociocultural models, respectively, executive control structures are task and culture specific. As in the Piagetian model, they are transformed according to a "general and universal" sequence of stages throughout development. This takes place stepwise in four age-specific stages—*sensorimotor, relational, dimen-*

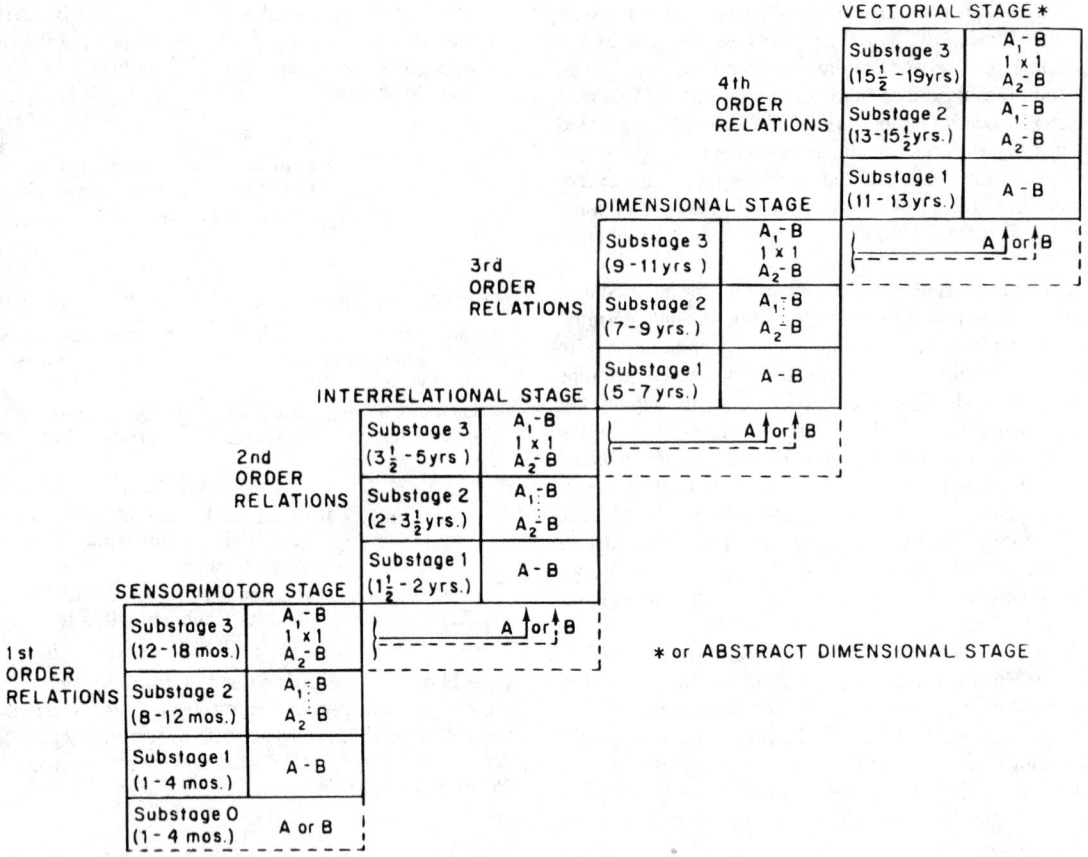

Figure 11.5. The neo-Piagetian system of Robbie Case. (From Case R: The whole child: Toward an integrated view of young children's cognitive, social, and emotional development. In: Pellegrini AD (ed): *Psychological Bases for Early Childhood Education.* New York, Wiley, 1988, p. 159.)

sional, and *vectorial*—as depicted in Figure 11.5. Case's sensorimotor stage, like Piaget's, describes a physical, sensory representational system. The relational stage is characterized by a global, nonquantified world view of "up-down," "big-little," "high-low," and the like. It is "either-or," "pass-fail." The dimensional stage is full of measurement and shadings of "this much" more or "that much" taller. The vectorial stage allows the representation of real or hypothetical quantity, which has, as it were, both magnitude and direction. It permits the representation of a multiplicative relationship between two forces.

The Mechanism of Development: Stage and Substage Transition

Stage transition occurs as executive control structures assembled during the previous stage, different in form and function, are hierarchically integrated. Stages are distinguished from one another by the kind of elements of which the executive control structures are made up. For example, when the "counting" element is integrated with the "relative amount" element, a whole new type of element, a dimensional one, has been constructed. This is the difference between a 4-year-old's approach to the juice problem and a 6-year-old's.

Substage transition also occurs by integration of executive structures, but the integration need not be hierarchical, nor need the elements be different. Within each stage there is a universal, age-specific sequence of three substages—*unifocal, bifocal,* and *elaborated coordination*—differentiated by the number of bits of information they represent and how these bits are organized. Within the dimensional stage, substages unfold, coordinating two, then three, then four elements. This allows more complex dimensionality in that different sets of counting

and relative amount units can be coordinated but does not produce a qualitative transformation as at the stage shift from relational to dimensional thought (Fig. 11.6). Stage transition (Fig. 11.5) is the natural outcome of substage transition (Fig. 11.6). Substage transition is the natural outcome of a growth in the capacity of working memory. Working memory is made up of space for executing cognitive operations and space for short-term storage and retrieval of relevant, but temporarily inactive, elements of the problem.

Logically, working memory can grow either by some sort of maturational increase in short-term storage space or by becoming able to process more efficiently so that less space is taken up by executing cognitive operations. Although practice does increase precision of representation and operational efficiency, it cannot entirely account for the process of development. Physical maturation, perhaps in the form of increasing myelinization, may be ultimately rate limiting. Case (1992b) describes some promising correlations between his developmental timetable and frontal lobe EEG changes.

Case's recent work (1992) stays true to its neo-Piagetian roots, as above, but incorporates elements from neonativist theory (modules), neoassociationist theory (domain-specific learning), and sociocultural theory (Vygotsky). He begins with the premise that children's cognition is innately modular and domain-specific including social, verbal, numerical, and spatial domains, at least. Each module is unique in the organization of its contents and its processing style. At the heart of children's conceptual systems is the central conceptual structure, which undergoes qualitative shifts at certain ages throughout development. Central conceptual structures are semantic networks that need domain-specific experience to develop both the nodes and the links between them. Culturally specific experience, especially academic learning, becomes more

Begin reading from bottom panel

DIMENSIONAL STAGE

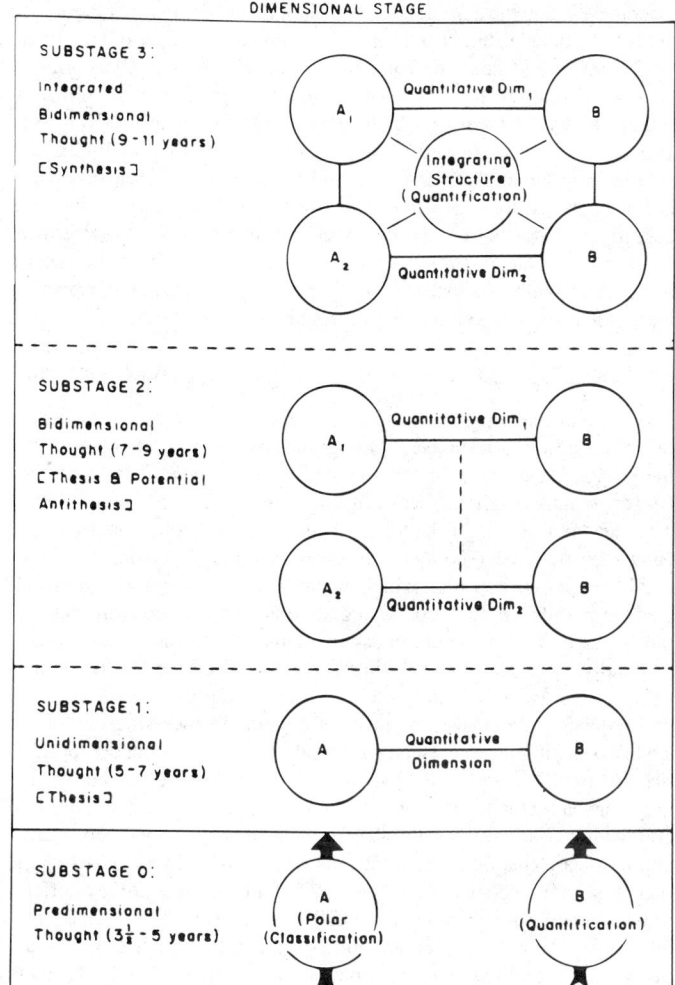

Figure 11.6. Substages within Case's dimensional stage. (From Case R: The whole child: Toward an integrated view of young children's cognitive, social, and emotional development. *Dim*, dimension. In: Pellegrini AD (ed): *Psychological Bases for Early Childhood Education*. New York, Wiley, 1988, p. 157.)

important in filling these structures as the child becomes more cognitively advanced. Although there is no intrinsic limit to the growth of these structures in adulthood, there are maturational constraints on the rate of development of children's central conceptual structures. These constraints limit the capacity of executive structures and/or working memory. Finally, consonant with classical Piagetian theory, these structures are actively constructed by the child, grow by differentiation and coordination (integration) of existing structures, undergo qualitative changes by structural reworking, and become more powerful, abstract, and complex with development.

"Case proposes a multilevel cognitive system, with levels ranging from the very general to the specific. . . .An increase in capacity (*general* systemwide change), along with . . .particular experiences . . .leads to a change in the central conceptual structures. These . . .are at an *intermediate* level of generality; each is a representational system of a domain of knowledge such as number or space. These structures interpret specific tasks and affect the problem-solving procedures for these tasks (*specific*-level change). By including systems that vary in generality, Case accounts for both the evenness and unevenness of cognitive development" (Flavell et al., 1993, p. 14).

Part 2: Applications of Cognitive-Developmental Theory to Affective Development and Clinical Practice

A NEO-PIAGETIAN VIEW OF SOCIAL-EMOTIONAL DEVELOPMENT

Cognitive Dimensions of Early Affective Relationships

A neo-Piagetian viewpoint has been brought to bear on early object relationships and "the vital issues that must be negotiated at different stages of development, if these early relationships are to form a basis of healthy functioning in later life" (Case, 1988, p. 155). Two of the most important questions upon which the thinking of psychodynamic psychiatrists and cognitive developmentalists is converging are (*a*) How do children represent the affectively powerful transactions that take place with their earliest caretakers? and (*b*) How do these representations evolve in the course of children's development? For a start, it is assumed that the cognitive construction of both the social and inanimate world is subject to equivalent constraints based on the child's general level of cognitive development. "In particular, it is assumed the *level of relationship* children can encode, and the *complexity of event* they can understand which entails such a relationship, increases with age at approximately the same rate, and according to the same epigenetic schedule" (Case, 1988, p. 162).

THE SOCIAL-COGNITIVE DIMENSIONS OF JEALOUSY

Hayward (1986) examined the development of jealousy in children using Case's framework. She studied children between 1 and 5 years of age—Case's relational stage—during which the child enters the world of physical and social *systems*, whereas in the previous stage they had occupied the world of physical and social *objects*.

By 18 months, children can regulate their proximity to mother and generate feelings of security. They can also monitor mother's relationship with others and the affective consequences. These two capacities exist independently of each other. During the first relational substage, 18–24 months, children coordinate these two previously unconnected relationships and recognize the higher-order relationship between them. They become aware that mother's involvement with another limits her availability to them. The affective consequence is jealousy.

In the next substage, between 2 and 3½ years, the child correlates two schemes in the same domain, in this case, the social-emotional domain. This means that a 3-year-old, threatened with feelings of displacement by a newborn sibling, can bring new strategies to bear on the problem if assisted to by a sensitive environment. Suppose, for example, the mother sets up a new type of relationship with the toddler that excludes the baby, in a complementary way, on occasions when the 3-year-old may feel left out. One way might be to ask the child to draw a picture, perhaps at the baby's feeding time. At this age, the child can coordinate (*a*) the new relationship as "mother's big girl" who can do something the infant cannot (i.e., draw) with (*b*) the relationship between mother and infant, from which she feels excluded. She can now comprehend that the new relationship compensates for the relative loss of the old one as "mother's baby." Indeed, the new-found status still allows for cuddling with mother when the infant's feeding time is over.

By the end of the relational stage, the child is capable of an elaborated coordination of relationships. The child, now 5, not only can compensate for a displacement by forming a new quality of relationship with mother but also can enter into a complementary relationship with the rival by emulating mother's caregiving. This, in turn, is likely to elicit praise from mother and perhaps even an independently gratifying response from the infant. This developmental sequence is diagrammed in Figure 11.7.

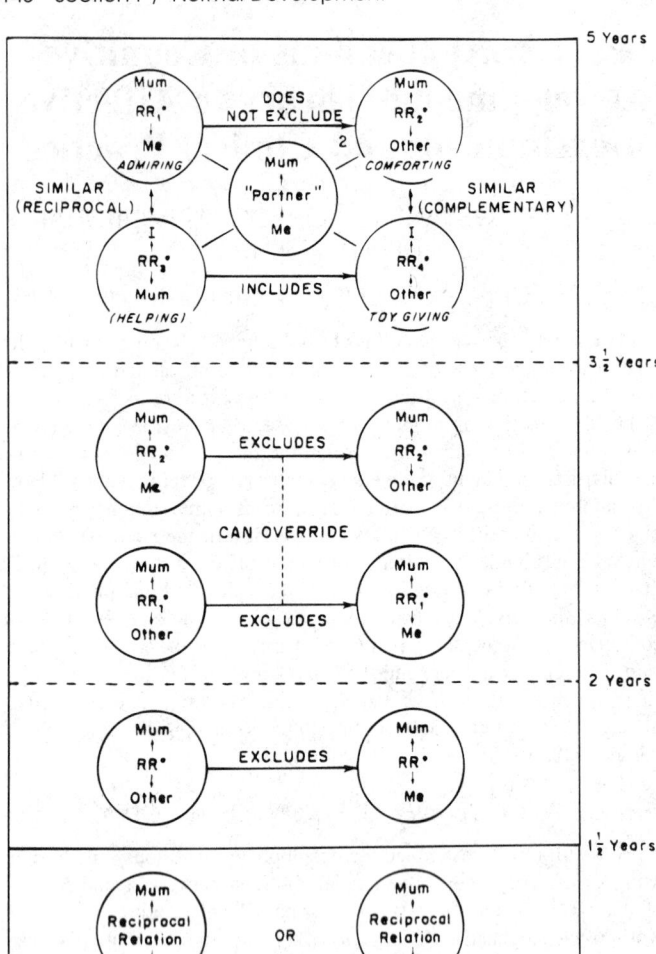

Figure 11.7. Substages in the development of jealousy and sharing during Case's relational stage. (From Case R: The whole child: Toward an integrated view of young children's cognitive, social, and emotional development. In: Pellegrini AD (ed): *Psychological Bases for Early Childhood Education.* New York, Wiley, 1988, p. 157.)

Hayward notes that the sequence proposed in Figure 11.7 depends upon (*a*) the "rival" being different from the self in some way that is an analogue of the self's difference from mother and (*b*) the mother's willingness to allow the older child a partnership relationship with her. If these conditions are not met, jealousy may well intensify by the end of the period. Strategic and systemic therapists will recognize this process as one of reframing. Ongoing redefinitions of the relationship between children and parents should occur naturally in growing up and are essential for a mature sense of self.

COGNITIVE ASPECTS OF EMPATHY: IMPLICATIONS FOR DEVELOPMENT

Kohut (1971) described empathy as "a mode of cognition which is specifically attuned to the perception of complex psychological configurations" (p. 300). He indicted parental "empathic failure" during early childhood as the cause of adult narcissistic disturbances and believed the therapist's empathic attunement to the patient is essential for the successful treatment. What Staub (1987, p. 106) calls *participatory empathy*—"a joining of the other"—is seen as an essential meliorating factor in psychotherapy generally (Havens, 1986; Marcia, 1987).

Virtually all developmentalists agree that parental empathy is absolutely necessary for the social, personal, and moral development of the child (Feshbach, 1987; Staub, 1987). Hobson (1993) cites an innate

incapacity for affect perception and responsivity as the fundamental reason why autistic children cannot fathom the minds of others (see below). Gender differences in the development of empathy (Hoffman, 1977) are also central to women-centered developmental theories in general (Jordan et al., 1991) and moral ones in particular (Gilligan, 1982). Other such theories, which emphasize self-sufficiency (Kohlberg, 1969), have been criticized for a masculine bias (Gilligan, 1982).

Empathy has both an affective and cognitive component. Empathy is both a "vicarious affective response to another person" and "the cognitive awareness of another person's internal states" (Hoffman, 1984, p. 103). The cognitive aspect of empathy is somewhat like social perspective-taking so that "empathy development must correspond at least partly to the development of a cognitive sense of others" (p. 108).

A Social-Cognitive View of Empathy Development

Hoffman suggests that empathy originates in infancy as a quasi-reflexive affective response, but cognition is required for its development (Hoffman, 1984). In social-cognitive development, children need first to acquire a reliable sense of others as separate physical entities. Then they must distinguish their own internal states from those of others. Next they must become aware of others as having personal identities and life experiences within which the immediate situation is contextualized. In parallel to these social-cognitive developments, Hoffman proposes stages in the development of empathy. Hoffman calls infants "globally empathic"; they cry in response to the crying of other infants in a passive and involuntary way, "based on the pull of surface cues and requiring the shallowest level of cognitive processing" (p. 112). Toddlers distinguish themselves from others physically but do not reliably distinguish their own internal states from those of others so that they may attempt to comfort others with what they themselves find comforting, as in a 13-month-old offering a distressed adult a doll. Older children learn that others' feelings may differ from theirs, based on the others' separate needs and situation. With language, the range of affects to which they can respond empathically increases, and they can eventually empathize with several emotions, even conflicting ones, simultaneously. Later, children can empathize on the basis of being told about someone's plight, even in the person's absence. For prepubertal children, others clearly have separate identities and histories; others have feelings not only in the immediate situation but also in their larger life experience. With the ability to group people into categories, children may then empathize with entire groups or classes of people, which, Hoffman feels, may be the most advanced form of empathic distress.

Hoffman, like Piaget, took a risk matching ages to stages. Others have shown evidence of adultlike empathy in very young children. Trevarthen (1982) suggests that "A rudimentary awareness of the subjective states of others may appear as early as 1 year of age . . . when infants and toddlers make efforts to achieve joint intentionality with another by trying to direct another's attention (e.g., pointing to an object and vocalizing) . . . they are demonstrating that the subjective states of others are different and can potentially be shared" (p. 136). This is "primary intersubjectivity." According to Thompson (1987), "once children have imbued emotional signals with emotional meaning, the development of "secondary intersubjectivity" fosters the mutual sharing of emotional conditions" (p. 136).

A NEO-PIAGETIAN STUDY OF EMPATHY

Bruchkowsky (1989) offers a developmental analysis of empathy based on Case's theory. In her study, children of 4, 6, and 10 years were presented with videotapes of peers enacting emotionally distressing situations. One situation depicted a little girl, Mary, and her dog playing together; shortly afterward, the dog was killed offscreen by a car. The subjects were asked, "How do you feel?" "How do you think Mary is feeling?" and "Why is she feeling that way?" Analysis of facial expression during the showing was performed to cross-validate the verbal responses.

Bruchkowsky found no significant age differences in the accuracy of emotional attributions: The children did not differ in terms of what they appeared to feel, what they said they felt, and what they said the other felt. As predicted, 4- and 6-year-olds could attribute only one affect, while 10-year-olds could attribute two or more. Bruchkowsky found a "stable developmental progression" in children's reports of why Mary felt as she did (empathic cognitions). Some 4-year-olds couldn't construct any explanation for their affective labeling of the other's reaction. They would say things like, "Mary was sad because it was raining." These children were considered "pre-empathic." Most 4-year-olds, however, were able to offer an explanation for Mary's feelings. They focused on external and salient features of the situation: "Mary was sad because her dog died." These children could coordinate (*a*) Mary's perceived affective reaction with "sad" and (*b*) "sad" with "her dog died."

Most 6-year-olds referred to an internal dimension of the other's affective experience in addition to the external event: "Mary was sad because her dog died, and she will miss it." Ten-year-olds focused on and coordinated two intrinsic dimensions of the other's affective experience: "Mary was sad because her dog died and she loved him and she will miss him." Some offered as well a coordination of two opposing affects over time: "Mary was sad because at first she was playing with her dog and she was happy, then her dog was run over by a car and she was sad." In sum, only external cues elicited a response at first, then one internal state was inferred, then two were inferred and coordinated in an elaborated manner. Age differences in children's empathic cognitions depended on a progressive increase in the capacity to coordinate from one to two to four elements. Case's theory, as an example of a cognitive developmental theory designed on the basis of problem-solving with physical tasks can also provide an account for the development of social relationships as well as their maldevelopment (McKeough et al., 1994).

DEVELOPMENT OF SOCIAL COGNITION

Social Versus Nonsocial Cognition

Social cognition is distinguished from nonsocial cognition by the inherent intentionality of humans; people (including oneself) think, feel, and cause things to happen. Both oneself and others may conceal intentions and harbor ambivalences. Thoughts about others are virtually always informed by affects, by the social context of interactions, and by the need to separate one's own thoughts from those of others. This similarity between the knower and the known poses new cognitive challenges. Working out issues of cause and effect where one's way of thinking influences the way one's object of thought thinks and behaves is quite different from sorting out causality with a crib mobile or hidden coins. Other human beings can establish "mutually intentional relations" with the child. "It is this mutuality of conduct and communication that distinguishes social from merely physical events and that engenders (and requires) a special sort of understanding. The developmental study of social cognition is, in part, a study of this understanding as it grows and changes in the child" (Damon, 1981, p. 159). There is a reciprocity between social and cognitive development: Cognitive skills mediate social interaction, which in turn provides the context for further cognitive development.

On the other hand, social cognition holds to many of the same developmental sequences as nonsocial cognition. For example, it proceeds from centration on particular external, perceptually salient events and objects of thought to decentration and the capacity to comprehend multiple interacting factors and internal, conceptual events. The child becomes able to conserve the identities of things and people—the self no less than others—over time and through transformations. Abstract and hypothetical thinking about self and others allows inferences about present relationships and internal activities, as well as hypotheses about future states of the self, those of others and relationships.

The Structure of Social Perspective-Taking

One form of social cognition is Selman's social perspective-taking, which entails the capacity to conceptualize self and other and the relationship between them. Selman's (1980) structural model is essentially Piagetian and depicts such a stage-developmental sequence in *concepts of persons* (e.g., "undifferentiated") and *concepts of relationships* (e.g., "egocentric"). The capacity for social perspective-taking has implications for the development of all social relationships, particularly empathy and moral judgment.

LEVEL 0: UNDIFFERENTIATED AND EGOCENTRIC PERSPECTIVES (3–6 YEARS)

A preschool child's concept of persons does not differentiate objective-physical from subjective-psychological states of self and other. There is confusion between acts and feelings and between intended and unintended behavior. Concepts of relations are egocentric in that the preschooler attributes his or her own perspective to the other person. The other is distinguished from oneself, but no commonality is established.

LEVEL 1: DIFFERENTIATED AND SUBJECTIVE PERSPECTIVES (5–9 YEARS)

The child's concept of persons now differentiates the physical from the psychological. The other is seen as having a "unique, subjective, covert psychological life" (Selman, 1980, p. 38), although it is seen as unitary, in that multiple feelings and internal conflicts cannot be recognized. The child's concepts of relations are one-way rather than mutual. It is the physical entity of a gift that makes someone happy, not the thought behind it; the intentionality of giving is not yet appreciated. Subjective attributions are made about another if the other is in a situation familiar to the child, by the reasoning "same situation equals same viewpoint."

LEVEL 2: SELF-REFLECTIVE/SECOND-PERSON AND RECIPROCAL PERSPECTIVES (6–12 Years)

The later school-age child can see his or her own thoughts, feelings, and actions from another's perspective. This second-person perspective allows for reciprocity. However, although each can see self and other, he or she cannot yet see the relationship system between them as an entity distinguishable from the individuals that constitute it. Actions can be seen as different from intentions, and feelings can be seen as multiple and contradictory. Concepts of relations are reciprocal in that the child can differentiate self from other at a psychological level and not merely at the level of overt behavior. Attributions are made with uncertainty, since the other is now seen as having an inner life distinct from one's own and may dissemble.

LEVEL 3: THIRD-PERSON AND MUTUAL PERSPECTIVES (10–15 YEARS)

Adolescence awakens the possibility of taking an observer position to the two-party reciprocity of the previous stage. This third-party perspective allows a clearer vision of the mutuality of individual perspectives. Adolescents "see themselves as both actors and objects, simultaneously acting and reflecting on the effects of action on themselves, reflecting upon the self in interaction with the self" (Selman, 1980, p. 39). Thus, the observing ego is born. The concept of relations is a third-person or "generalized other" perspective from which one can coordinate, simultaneously, the perspectives of all parties in interaction, including the self and the social system in which all are embedded.

LEVEL 4: IN-DEPTH AND SOCIETAL-SYMBOLIC PERSPECTIVES (12 YEARS TO ADULTHOOD)

One gradually learns that the observing ego cannot always comprehend the complexity of internal relations, that something is always hidden. At this stage the idea of a personal unconscious emerges. When younger, a child may have been able to understand that someone may do something he doesn't want to; now the child can see that the other may not understand why. Relations are understood to go beyond the third-party stance of the previous stage and can be seen as systems of perspectives in relation to one another. This allows for a "generalized other" perspective of the interplay of multiple social forces and of the participation of self and other in the formation of this "generalized other" point of view. Coming full circle from infancy, one can recognize the possibility of an inner, unspoken mutuality among people.

Selman and Schultz (1990) applied the stages of social perspective-taking to observations of children forming peer relationships and negotiating (or not) conflicts that arise in working together. If one child has something the other wants, the child at level 0 will act impulsively and, for example, try to take it away. At level 1 a child will likely try to influence the other, perhaps by a demand, to get what he wants. The effect of the loss on the other is not a consideration. At level 2, the child is aware he will have to influence the other's mental state and attempt to persuade or bargain. At level 3 the child can reflect on both their mental states and suggest compromises that may satisfy both. This work provides a useful guide to social-skills training and education.

Development of Emotional Understanding

Nannis (1988) has analyzed the sequential development of the ways that children reason about their feelings. She examines children's explanations of their feelings and the focus of control of those feelings.

Initially, feelings are seen as inherent in the situation eliciting them. Getting a gift creates happiness in itself; the inner response of the child is not invoked as an explanation. The control of the feeling is equally external; the gift causes a smile in the recipient, virtually without his or her participation. Next, feelings are seen as internal, although located somewhat concretely within the child, almost like a body organ. The child experiences little control since the body is represented as a receptacle into which feelings are put. At the next point in development, feelings are understood as being diffuse within the person rather than concrete things in a concrete body. Feelings are now experienced as being influenced by the self, they have become conceptualized. Finally, the most complex conception of affects moves the self to center stage. "Feelings involve the regulation and integration of internal processes and external events. Feelings are part of a system with universal laws or principles. The self has gone from receptacle, to regulator, to mediator" (Nannis, 1988, pp. 102–103). There are close parallels between this sequence and that of Selman's stages of social perspective-taking.

Multiple Feelings

Harter (1983) questioned preoperational and concrete operational children about their understanding of multiple feelings. She discovered that younger children simply could not conceive of experiencing two emotions, perhaps because they locate them physically, in the facial expression. Slightly older children could manage them sequentially, usually opposite feelings (e.g., first happy, then sad). The oldest ones could conceive of experiencing two feelings simultaneously, usually of the same valence. She accounted for this development by the acquisition of Piaget's operations of conservation and classification. Conservation allows the child to decenter from perceptions so that he can conceive of two affects experienced simultaneously, even if both facial expressions cannot be present at the same time. Classification permits the same object to be classified differently according to its different properties. Thus, different aspects of oneself might have different feelings simultaneously. Nannis maintains that these differing parts of the self must also become integrated into a whole without loss of the contradictory parts. Her impression is that a clinical population has more problem with such ambivalence than a nonclinical one.

Development of Moral Reasoning

In general terms, moral development involves increasing the complexity of one's perspective-taking, sense of intentionality, and capacity for coordinating complex and often contradictory arrangements of factors. It also entails a diminishing of one's egocentrism and a better capacity to interiorize one's own and others' motives. Piaget applied his ideas on the development of logical thought to the evolving capacity of the child to make moral judgments. He proposed stages of moral reasoning to parallel his stages of cognitive development. These were elaborated extensively by Kohlberg and critiqued trenchantly from a feminist point of view by Carol Gilligan. This is discussed elsewhere (Chapter 17).

CLINICAL-DEVELOPMENTAL INTEGRATION

Some clinician theorists have organized the processes and stages of self-development on a Piagetian framework. Among the best articulated of these "clinical-developmental" approaches are those of Robert Kegan and Gil Noam. Their work is informed by Kohlberg's and by Selman's social perspective-taking and the views of psychodynamic ego psychologists, Erikson and Loevinger.

Robert Kegan: The Evolving Self

THE SUBJECT-OBJECT BALANCE

Robert Kegan (1982) proposed development to be an evolution in the ways persons make meaning from experience and the self to be the structure within which one's meaning is made. The self is *embedded*, from infancy, in limited cognitive frames of reference to which it is *subject*: It cannot make them an *object* of cognitive operations. Development entails sequential differentiation or *disembedding* of the self from these cognitive frames by a process similar to Piaget's idea of decentration. As the self disembeds from early paradigms, it necessarily becomes embedded in new ones, albeit more differentiated structures that can operate cognitively on earlier ones.

Early in development, for example, a child's self is subject to his or her perceptual processes. When a preschooler looks at something from one position and then another, he or she is likely to say that the object has changed size or shape. For the preschooler, it is not his or her perception that changed, it is the thing itself: The child *is*, in a sense, his or her perceptions. Soon the preschooler will be able to perceptually conserve (in Piaget's sense) the physical object in the face of a change of position and will know that the object remains constant as he or she moves around it. The child will then become a self that can *have* perceptions, that is, take them as object of a perceptually disembedded self. Each of Kegan's stages of self development is in the form of a particular balance between what the self is subject to and what it can take as object. This balance is analogous to the equilibration that produces Piaget's structures-of-the-whole.

Personal meaning-making takes place within a psychosocial matrix analogous to the "holding environment" that Winnicott (1972) described as being characteristic of infancy. Kegan extends the concept of holding environments throughout the life span, calling them *cultures of embeddedness*. To understand a person fully, one must be aware of his or her undifferentiated (embedded) self as well as the individuated one. The "person" is the sum of the individuated and the embedded selves; one can understand a person, only if one also understands the culture of embeddedness in which he or she is held.

CONFIRMATION, CONTRADICTION, AND CONTINUITY

Adaptation is a lifelong balancing act between the need to be a distinct and unique self—*independence*—and the equal and often contradictory need to be connected to others, to belong—*inclusion*. Each developmental stage requires the culture to *confirm* the self's organization, and yet experience continually poses discrepancies that challenge the child's cognitive paradigm, moving the child to ask himself questions. The culture allows *contradictions*, as well as confirmations. If the balance favors independence, the culture poses the issue of inclusion, and vice versa. Finally, the culture must provide cognitive and emotional *continuity* to anchor the developing individual during necessary periods of imbalance.

TRANSFORMATIONS IN THE SUBJECT-OBJECT BALANCE

The mechanism of stage transition lies in the interaction of the child with both the confirming and contradicting elements of the culture of embeddedness. Intrinsically, "every developmental balance involves—a built-in falsehood or subjectivity which forms the seed of its own undoing. Given enough experience with the world, assimilative defenses which have not had to become all-powerful, holding environments which can let go of one balance and recognize another" (Kegan, 1982, p. 223), then each subject-object balance will eventually disintegrate, and a new one replace it. The experience of disembedding may be frightening and painful, as is any form of differentiation or individuation, in that in a very real sense, one leaves a part of one's "self" behind. Both anxiety over the lost equilibrium and grieving for the lost "self" require a nurturing and consistent culture of embeddedness for their resolution.

Kegan believes that the therapeutic situation provides a culture of embeddedness and that it must first confirm the self-structure presented and then pose contradictions, not as opposition or confrontation, but as alternatives. All this must be done in a firm continuity of relationship. In this way, therapy provides a natural setting that allows the patient to attain a more differentiated stage of development. Kegan's system is an elegant application of Piaget to personal development but does not address in depth the origins of psychopathology. This is explored more fully in the work of Gil Noam.

Gil Noam: The Theory of Biography and Transformation

THE LIMITATIONS OF PIAGETIAN THEORY

Gil Noam (1988) believes that one must go beyond classical Piagetian thinking to understand aberrations of personality development. In the Piagetian system, "each structural transformation leads to a synthesis of all earlier structures into a new whole. However when applied to the development of self and personality, this view systematically screens out such phenomena as disintegration and structural discrepancies" (p. 277). There seems to be no place for incomplete integration such as Laing's (1965) "divided self" or Winnicott's (1972) "false self." Noam frames the question for developmental psychopathology in terms of which structures go forth with development, which do not, and why.

BIOGRAPHY AND TRANSFORMATION

If psychodynamics emphasizes the biographical event at the expense of structural transformation, then cognitive development emphasizes structural transformation at the expense of personal history. By way of balance, Noam calls his approach the theory of "biography and transformation." *Biography* refers both to the contents of one's life history and the continuing influence of unintegrated earlier structures. *Transformation* resides in the continuing developmental momentum of the self-structures, even when some aspects remain under the influence of earlier constructions. The intrapsychic self is made up of internalizations of the interpersonal. However, the original interpersonal perspective alters as it becomes an internal perspective. A "strong" self is characterized by the ongoing integration of earlier self-constructions with the most mature structure at each developmental transition. A "fragile" self is beset by "simultaneous multiple interpretations of reality ('divided self' [or encapsulation]), or with an 'as if' integration, which represents an

internally consistent, yet alienated self (a 'false self' [or problem pathway])" (Noam, 1988, p. 296).

Each stage transition, in the Piagetian tradition, is a point of disequilibration, when accommodation dominates assimilation. At these times, Noam postulates, an innate human drive for self-integration generalizes the accommodative capacity to include previously unintegrated material in the most mature self-organization. If this happens, the old material becomes content in the new structure. If not, encapsulations form or persist. Development does not always improve mental health. "Because each stage transition is a form of internalization, there exists the possibility of a paradoxical outcome: from the perspective of self-development the person can have achieved greater complexity and broader self-awareness, while from the perspective of self-cohesion the person can . . .have a more complex 'false self'" (Noam, 1988, p. 294).

ENCAPSULATIONS AND PROBLEM PATHWAYS: THE ORIGINS OF PSYCHOPATHOLOGY

Experiences that cannot be integrated into the current self-representation remain in structures that do not develop beyond their developmental point of origin. These pockets of early affective-cognitive meaning do not become enfolded into the subsequent stage and so are called *encapsulations*. They persist in the form of themes and attributions about the self and important relationships. Some encapsulations remain utterly untransformed by subsequent development and persist in their original, primitive structure. Others become partially integrated and structurally transformed with ongoing cognitive development but as deviant *problem pathways*. They are concealed within the most advanced developmental positions and experienced as current and often ego-syntonic issues.

Why do some early self-constructions resist integration? Noam's response, like Kegan's, is that the fear, engendered by the loss involved in letting go of old self-constructions, outweighs the anticipated benefits of further development. Stage transition entails giving up the affectively charged internalizations that are the existing self-structures. This may be experienced as loss or feared as personal disintegration and attended by anxiety and grief. A noxious interpersonal environment, for example, may promote "destructive loyalties to important others and to an old self" so that encapsulations are formed (1988, p. 293).

THERAPY

Therapy, which is a process of induced disequilibrium, allows some self-reorganization and "weaving in" of unintegrated material. In therapy, as in life, content is organized around core themes—interpersonal and intrapsychic material perceived as recurring patterns in one's biography. They form a bridge between the most mature self and encapsulations. The therapist must be able to identify the central themes in therapy, assess the most mature stage of self-organization, and facilitate integration of unintegrated elements from earlier periods, thus promoting the development of a strong self.

Cognitive Developmental Explanations of Autism

Ever since Kanner (1943) described autism, as a "primary disturbance of affective contact," the nature of the developmental deviation has been an enduring clinical puzzle in child psychiatry. Although autism undoubtedly has a genetic-neurological basis, the question remains: By which psychological pathway it is expressed? There is much evidence to support Kanner's intuition of a primary disturbance of affective development (Hobson, 1989, 1993). However, recent work makes an equally strong case for a primary disturbance of cognitive development (Baron-Cohen et al., 1985; Bruner, 1993; Frith, 1989, 1991; Happé, 1991; Perner, 1991; Sternberg, 1987).

THE NATURE OF SOCIAL RELATEDNESS IN AUTISM

Autism entails characteristic impairments in the capacity for social relations. Interpersonal communication, if present, is repetitive and self-absorbed or instrumental and literal, without regard for social context; that is, the *pragmatics* of communication are impaired. For example, Langdell found autistic children unable to modify their account of an event regardless of whether or not they knew if the listener had witnessed it (Langdell, 1980). A particular autistic child may, with age, learn to communicate with others but "an inability to participate in two-way reciprocal social interaction persists throughout the lives of autistic people" (Baron-Cohen, 1988, p. 384).

A PRIMARY DISTURBANCE OF THEORY OF MIND

Baron-Cohen (1988, 1989) argues that a disturbance of affective development is not primary in autism. Autistic children have emotional responsivity and they do not avoid eye contact nor physical closeness with others; they simply do not seek it out as normal children do (Hermelin and O'Connor, 1970). Autistic children can also show preferential attachment: There is little to distinguish them from developmentally delayed controls in the "strange situation," the standard experimental setup for attachment studies (Sigman et al., 1986). On the other hand, one of the landmarks of infant development is "protodeclarative pointing" where the infant, who "knows" from early on how to track mother's gaze, coordinates this with pointing to something of interest that he wishes to direct the attention of the mother toward. The capacity for "shared attention" suggests the infant intuits that its mother has a mind too. Shared attention is a staple of normal mother-infant interaction and is conspicuously absent in autistic infants.

Baron-Cohen et al. (1985) argue that the primary deficit in autism is an innately impaired capacity to develop a "theory of mind." A child who has a theory of mind understands that "people have minds and mental states, and that mental states relate to behaviour" (Baron-Cohen, 1993, p. 59). Without this, children cannot represent to themselves the mental states (representations) of others and use that to predict their behavior. Since they cannot represent to themselves others' mental representations, they cannot form *metarepresentations* and therefore do not have a theory of mind. Mike Anderson has suggested that there may be a "theory of mind" module that is dysfunctional or absent in autistic people (Anderson, 1992).

Normally children come to understand that they share with others the capacity to be intentional. Intentionality is the mind's inherent tendency to form mental representations. As we have seen, it is manifested as "aboutness"—our thoughts, wishes, beliefs and so on are directed *at* some object. In the language of cognitive science, "Insofar as the information contained in and processed by an information-processing system is about anything—that is, insofar as it functions representationally—the states and processes of that system are intentional" (Stillings et al., 1987, p. 317). The shared attention of mother and child as they point together is based on their mutual representation of each other's intentions. Insofar as children can imagine what another thinks and apply this knowledge socially, they can be said to have a theory of mind.

Baron-Cohen and others devised an ingenious experiment to look at children's theory of mind (Baron-Cohen et al., 1985). Normal children, children with Down's syndrome, and autistic children, matched for mental age, watched a scenario in which two dolls, Sally (beside a basket holding a marble) and Anne (beside a box) are depicted together. Sally puts the marble in her basket and leaves the scene. While Sally is "offstage" Anne removes the marble from Sally's basket and puts it in her box. Sally returns and the child is asked "Where will Sally look for her marble?" Most of the nonautistic children answered correctly "In the basket." By contrast, 80% of the autistic children indicated the box (as would children under 4 years). The authors believed the results demonstrated that autistic children, irrespective of their intellectual capacities, have a specific problem inferring the mental states of others.

What of the 20% of autistic children who "passed" the Sally-Anne marble experiment? Baron-Cohen (1989) called the capacity to attribute belief to another "first-order belief attribution" and recognized that some (the oldest) autistic children could do this. He devised a more

complex study to explore "second-order belief attribution," that is, the ability to represent to oneself what a second person believes a third person believes. The scenario was a toy village with a park, two houses, a church, and four people. John and Mary are in the park when the ice cream man comes along in his van. John wants an ice cream but has no money and has to go home to fetch some. The ice cream man assures John that he will still be at the park when John returns. Mary stays in the park. However, the ice cream man then decides to drive to the church to try and sell ice cream there. On the way he passes John and tells him where he is going. Mary, who sees nothing of this, goes later to John's house and his mother tells her that he has gone to buy ice cream. The question is then posed to the child "Where does Mary think John has gone to buy ice cream?" To answer correctly the child has to understand what Mary believes about where John believes the ice cream man is. None of the autistic children (mean age 15 years, mean nonverbal mental age (M.A.) 10.7 years) answered correctly while 90% of normal (age 7) and 60% of Down's syndrome children (age 14, M.A. 6.8 years) got it. Since Baron-Cohen controlled for memory capacity, intellectual ability, and motivational factors, he believes the best explanation for the results is to postulate a specific delay in the development of a (second-order) theory of mind.

To investigate the specificity of this cognitive limitation, they showed three different four-panel comic strips to the same groups of children (Baron-Cohen et al., 1986). Each strip tested a specific kind of causal reasoning. The first (a "mechanical" story) depicted a balloon carried away from someone's hand, landing in a tree, and bursting when punctured by a sharp branch. The second (a "behavioristic" story) involved a child going into a candy store, buying candy, and leaving. The third (a "mentalistic" story) showed a child putting a candy in a box, then going out to play. Unseen by him, his mother removes the candy and eats it. The child returns, opens the box, and looks surprised. Despite a lower mental age, Down's syndrome children understood the mentalistic story better than autistic children. The two groups performed the same on the behavioral one, and the Down's group worst on the mechanical one. Frith concluded that *mentalizing* is a different sort of reasoning from causal or behavioral reasoning. By "mentalizing" Frith means both the ability and the drive to "predict relationships between external states of affairs and internal states of mind"—not unlike intentional reasoning (Frith, 1989, pp. 156–157).

THEORY OF MIND AND METAREPRESENTATION

Josef Perner (1991) distinguishes theory of mind from the capacity for metarepresentation. He argues that, while autistic children may have difficulties knowing other minds, there is evidence that they can form representations of representations. In one experiment, children took a picture of a doll in a blue dress. While the picture was developing, the doll was changed into a yellow dress. Before being shown the developed photo, the child was asked what color the dress was in the photo; 15 of 16 autistic children replied, correctly, blue. Yet they failed a matching false belief task that had the doll's friend seeing her in blue, and, while the friend was away, changing into yellow. Only 4 of the 16 autistic children answered that the friend would still think the doll was in blue. Since they can represent to themselves a photographic image, which is itself a representation, they can be said to be able to metarepresent. Perner holds that such results militate against a general metarepresentational deficit. Much in this debate depends upon what one means by "representation." Sometimes representation refers to the *relationship* between a thing and the copy or symbol that stands for it, but at other times it refers to the *content* of the copy itself. For example, any 2-year-old could tell you a photograph of, say, a horse, is a representation of the horse in the second sense, but not until age 4 could the child explain that the likeness of the horse in the photograph stood *in a representational relationship* to a horse (Perner, 1991, p. 17). Perner (1993) proposes that autistic children can metarepresent in the sense of content but not in the sense of representational relationship.

Since then, Baron-Cohen (1993) has collated research on the comparative abilities of normal, retarded, and autistic children to understand others' mental representations by knowledge category. For example, there is almost no difference from the other groups in the capacity of autistic children to represent to themselves what others are perceiving; in other words, they know a picture on a table upside down to them would be right side up to someone standing opposite them. On the other hand, it is progressively more difficult for them to understand what others desire or imagine, pretend, and finally, believe. These findings also address Perner's contention that autism does not entail a total absence of metarepresentational capacity.

MENTALIZING AND COGNITIVE COHERENCE

Frith proposed a more general problem of cognitive integration as the basis for autism. She saw the autistic person as unable to "pull together disparate information into a coherent pattern" (Frith, 1989, p. 157). She proposed that autism is a disconnection between central information processing and peripheral processing, causing a "lack of central coherence." Since meaning derives from a sense of what is relevant based on a consistent and coherent basis for interpretation of physical and mental events, autistic people cannot process new information consistently or "canonically." Frith suggests this also explains the peculiar pattern of intellectual abilities in some autistic people, such as the idiot savant phenomenon, and repetitive behaviors and stereotypies such as echolalia and pronominal reversal. For example, to explain pronominal reversal, Frith argues "autistic children are subject only to a drive for local not global coherence. They only pull together a very limited amount of information at one time. Normal children, in contrast, take into account a much larger amount of information. They understand how pronouns relate to previously used, or mutually understood, nouns. Therefore they use the name or pronoun, whichever serves best in the cohesion of discourse" (Frith, 1989, p. 127). The "iceberg," of which these symptoms are the tip, is a "lack of appreciation of wider meaning including the speaker's intentions" (Frith, 1989, p. 127).

STERNBERG'S COMPONENTIAL SUBTHEORY AND AUTISM

Sternberg casts the basis of autism in terms of deviance in the knowledge acquisition components of cognition. These components have two principal functions—to organize and acquire information to deal with novelty and to automatize information processing to deal with a familiar task. Sternberg posits that autistic children do not selectively encode and compare information in a way susceptible to consensual validation and do not selectively combine information to create inner coherence of experience. "In autism, the three selective processes are applied in a way that is, to the rest of the world, "misselective. The child parses certain domains, and especially the verbal domain in a way that is different from everyone else" (Sternberg, 1987, p. 693). Sternberg does not explain what causes the autistic child's knowledge acquisition components to malfunction.

AUTISM AS A FAILURE OF NARRATIVITY

Jerome Bruner and Carol Feldman (1993) agree that there is a failure in the autistic child's theory of mind, but they identify a more fundamental deficit. They point to experimental evidence that the autistic child "is incapable of (or highly resistant to) organizing interpersonal encounters into a canonical form that captures . . . regularities in the way in which people's intentional states are situated in typical situations, are expressed in typical action sequences, and require reciprocal response from those who are interacting with them" (p. 286). If so, autistic children cannot create, with others, zones of proximal development and are deprived of the interpersonal "scaffolding" that promotes the development of internalized cognitive structures—in this case, the structures that enable one to construct a coherent self-narrative.

Structures of canonical sequences, or *formats*, depend upon the ca-

pacity to consistently represent the other's mental state. Bruner and Feldman do not believe, however, that the innate capacity to intuit another's mental state, which they believe to be impaired in autism, entails a theory of mind. They suggest that a theory of mind might follow from the application of the child's innate predisposition to interact and develop representations of cultural formats. "Some autistic children could follow narrative sequences, even those involving intentional states, when such narratives were well scaffolded by pictures and stories told by others" (p. 287). They invoke the Sigman-Feldman "computational surmise" to explain the more adequate functioning of higher-level autistic people such as those with Asperger's syndrome. This is that these intelligent children and adults reason their way through interpersonal situations as others would reason through a math problem; they "convert the personal world of intention-regulated social experience into an impersonal world of causally-driven events" (p. 288). In other words, going back to the reasoning task using comic strips (above), these people could often successfully apply mechanical or behavioral thinking to an intentional situation and obscure the fact that they were not truly thinking in an intentional way. Since it takes more time to reason through interpersonal situations than to intuit a response, these children always seem "out of synch" in social exchanges.

RELEVANCE THEORY AND AUTISM

Francesca Happé (1991) applied Sperber and Wilson's (1986) Relevance Theory of communication to the failure of pragmatics in autism. Briefly, this theory maintains, first, that "our attention automatically turns to what seems relevant in the environment" (p. 226). Relevance, here, is maximal cognitive gain for minimal cognitive effort. Because it is costly to process new input piecemeal, when a communication is directed toward him or her, a person they tends to supply the context that makes the least demand on his or her information-processing system, rather like the infant's tendency to attempt to assimilate new data into existing schemes. Secondly, all acts of *ostensive-inferential* communication—communication that points back toward its intent to communicate—imply their own optimal relevance to the listener. For example, if someone speaks to you, this act implies that they think that what they say will have some bearing on your life so that you will put what they said in an appropriate context. They may be mistaken, of course (Tannen, 1990), but that does not invalidate the principle. The need for a "theory of mind" is evident.

The selection of an appropriate context requires the sharing between audience and speaker of a mutual, usually canonical, set of assumptions about their world and their relation to each other including the speaker's purpose in initiating an act of communication. Happé adduces evidence that autistic children not only do not attend to what is canonically relevant but often attend to irrelevancies instead. For example, they may organize their responses to the teacher's dress instead of what is being taught. Frith's hypothesis of a lack of central processing coherence could explain this but Happé allows two other possibilities. First, the autistic person's cost of processing irrelevancies could be so low that there is no quantitative basis for choice of relevance. Normally, "new, unconnected information that could only be processed piecemeal would not be worth processing. . . . But what if such piecemeal processing were not too costly? . . . in some autistic people the same cognitive architecture that allows extraordinarily good rote memory, and even outstanding 'savant' abilities, could lead to . . . abnormally low . . . processing costs." (Happé, 1991, p. 228). The third possibility is that autistic people have a different memory organization and the processing paths of least effort are so idiosyncratic that communication with a nonautistic person, who assumes canonicality, breaks down.

SUMMARY: CHILDHOOD'S END

As a child develops cognitively, she or he can move beyond the observed to the inferred, beyond percept to concept, beyond concrete to abstract, and beyond intuitive knowing to conscious reflection. The child becomes aware that events can have internal and symbolic meaning beyond their external and literal significance. As she or he invests events with meaning, the child can go beyond content to appreciate formal resemblances, patterns, and processes. As the child reflects on patterns and processes, she or he can reflect on systems, including social systems. Older children can reflect on their own patterns and processes and how they relate to those of others and to those of the larger social world.

As a child becomes aware of himself or herself as part of a larger world—call it decentration, disembedding, or social perspective-taking—the universal enters the personal: The "I" becomes at once smaller and larger. With differentiation, the subjective "I" encompasses less of an ever more complex array of possibilities, yet, as a child internalizes experience, his or her sense of self grows in ways hitherto unimaginable. However, in each moment of transition, he or she may become aware that, to gain a new sense of self, an old one, usually quite comfortable, must be given up. This may be frightening, the more so because the child does not know why he or she feels anxious, and the caregivers are often equally puzzled. Yet the adults that form the child's "holding environment" must be intuitively, if not consciously, aware of these developmental anxieties and support the child in his or her journey from the global undifferentiated "I" of infancy to the smaller but more integrated "I" of true adulthood.

Development also entails an ever-increasing capacity to draw distinctions. Drawing distinctions sets up tensions, which, when resolved, are replaced by new distinctions and new tensions. Integrating the new into the familiar and transforming the familiar into the new, creating a more complex familiarity, is the task of a lifetime. The dialectics of development—differentiation and integration, assimilation and accommodation, being "a part of" or "apart from"—operate throughout the life cycle.

Later adulthood often brings an awareness that life is more process than achievement. For this awareness to happen, Michael Basseches (1984) believes that formal operations, Piaget's last word, must be superseded by "dialectical" thinking. Formal thinking ultimately requires static entities and fixed relationships: It is designed to avoid contradiction. Dialectical thinking does not push for closure; it needs contradiction and creates a lifelong interplay of contrasting ideas (Carse, 1986). By old age, the self may become less dependent upon externals, and integrity comes to rest in a sense that one's life is "the accidental coincidence of but one life cycle with but one segment of history; and that for [one] all human integrity stands and falls with the one style of integrity of which [one] partakes" (Erikson, 1959, p. 98).

Acknowledgments. *I am deeply indebted to Professor Anne McKeough of the Department of Educational Psychology, University of Calgary, for her invaluable contribution to my cognitive development.*

References

Allman WF: *Apprentices of Wonder: Inside the Neural Network Revolution.* New York, Bantam, 1989.

Anderson JR: *The Architecture of Cognition.* Cambridge, MA, Harvard University Press, 1983.

Anderson M: *Intelligence and Development: A Cognitive Theory.* Oxford, Blackwell, 1992.

Atkinson R, Shiffrin RM: Human memory: A proposed system and its control processes. In: Spence K, Spence J (eds): *The Psychology of Learning and Motivation: Advances in Research and Theory* (Vol 2). New York, Academic Press, 1968.

Baddely AD: *Working Memory.* Oxford, Oxford University Press, 1986.

Baron-Cohen S: Social and pragmatic deficits in autism. *J Autism Dev Disord* 18(3):379, 1988.

Baron-Cohen S: The autistic child's theory of mind: A case of specific developmental delay. *J Child Psychol Psychiatry* 30(5):285, 1989.

Baron-Cohen S: From attention-goal psychology to belief-desire psychology: The development of a theory of mind and its dysfunction. In: Baron-Cohen S, Tager-Flusberg H, Cohen DJ (eds): *Understanding Other Minds: Perspectives from Autism.* Oxford, Oxford University Press, 1993, p. 59.

Baron-Cohen S, Leslie AM, Frith U: Does the autistic child have a "theory of mind"? *Cognition* 21:37, 1985.

Baron-Cohen S, Leslie AM, Frith U: Mechanical, behavioural and intentional understanding of picture stories in autistic children. *Br J Dev Psychol* 4:113, 1986.

Basseches M: *Dialectical Thinking and Adult Development.* Norwood, NJ, Ablex, 1984.

Bechtel W, Abrahamsen A: *Connectionism and the Mind: An Introduction to Parallel Processing in Networks.* Oxford, Blackwell, 1991.

Best J: *Cognitive Psychology* (2nd ed). St. Paul, MN, West Publishing, 1989.

Bjorklund DF: *Children's Thinking: Developmental Function and Individual Differences.* Pacific Grove, CA, Brooks/Cole, 1989.

Borke H: Piaget's mountains revisited: Changes in the egocentric landscape. *Dev Psychol* 11:240, 1975.

Bruchkowsky M: *Affect and Cognition in the Development of Empathy in Middle Childhood.* Unpublished doctoral dissertation, Toronto, Ontario, University of Toronto, 1989.

Bruner JS: *Child's Talk.* New York, Norton, 1983.

Bruner JS: *Acts of Meaning.* Cambridge, MA, Harvard University Press, 1990.

Bruner JS, Feldman C: Theories of mind and the problem of representation in autism. In: Baron-Cohen S, et al (eds): *Understanding Other Minds: Perspectives from Autism.* Oxford, Oxford University Press, 1993, p. 267.

Carse JP: *Finite and Infinite Games.* New York, Ballantine Books, 1986.

Case R: The process of stage transition: A neo-Piagetian view. In: Sternberg RJ (ed): *Mechanisms of Cognitive Development.* New York, Freeman, 1984, pp. 20–44.

Case R: *Intellectual Development: Birth to Adulthood.* Orlando, FL, Academic Press, 1985.

Case R: The whole child: Toward an integrated view of young children's cognitive, social, and emotional development. In: Pellegrini AD (ed): *Psychological Bases for Early Education.* New York, Wiley, 1988.

Case R: *The Mind's Staircase: Exploring the Conceptual Underpinnings of Children's Thought and Knowledge.* Hillsdale, NJ, Erlbaum, 1992a.

Case R: The role of the frontal lobes in the regulation of cognitive development. *Brain Cogn* 20:51, 1992b.

Chandler M, Fritz AS, Hala S: Small-scale deceit: Deception as a marker of two-, three-, and four-year-olds' theories of mind. *Child Dev* 60:1263, 1989.

Chi MTH, Koeske RD: Network representation of a child's dinosaur knowledge. *Dev Psychol* 19:29, 1983.

Chi MTH, Glaser R, Farr MJ: *The Nature of Human Problem Solving.* Hillsdale, NJ, Erlbaum, 1988.

Cohen D: *Piaget: Critique and Reassessment.* London, Croom Helm, 1983.

Collins AM, Loftus EF: A spreading activation theory of semantic processing. *Psychol Rev* 82: 407–428, 1975.

Cowan PA: Preface. In: Piaget J: *Intelligence and Affectivity: Their Relationship During Child Development* (Brown TA, Kiegi CE, trans and eds). Palo Alto, Annual Reviews Inc., 1981, p. xi.

Damon W: Exploring children's social cognition on two fronts. In: Flavell J, Ross L (eds): *Social Cognitive Development: Frontiers and Possible Futures.* New York, Cambridge University Press, 1981.

Deregowski JB: Pictures, symbols and frames of reference. In: Butterworth G (ed): *The Child's Representation of the World.* New York, Plenum, 1977.

Donaldson M: *Children's Minds.* Glasgow, Fontana/Collins, 1978.

Dunn J: *The Beginnings of Social Understanding.* Cambridge, MA, Harvard University Press, 1988.

Elkind D: *Children and Adolescents: Interpretive Essays on Jean Piaget.* New York, Oxford University Press, 1970.

Elkind D: *The Child's Reality: Three Developmental Themes.* Hillsdale, NJ, Erlbaum, 1978.

Erikson E: *Identity and the Life Cycle.* New York, International Universities Press, 1959.

Eysenck MW (ed): *The Blackwell Dictionary of Cognitive Psychology.* Oxford, Basil Blackwell, 1990.

Feshbach ND: Parental empathy and child adjustment/maladjustment. In: Eisenberg N, Strayer J (eds): *Empathy and Its Development.* Cambridge, Cambridge University Press, 1987, p. 271.

Flavell JH: *The Developmental Psychology of Jean Piaget.* New York, Van Nostrand, 1963.

Flavell JH, Miller PH, Miller SA: *Cognitive Development* (3rd ed). Engelwood Cliffs, NJ, Prentice-Hall, 1993.

Frith U: *Autism: Explaining the Enigma.* Oxford, Blackwell, 1989.

Frith U (ed): *Autism and Asperger Syndrome.* Cambridge, Cambridge University Press, 1991.

Gardner H: *The Mind's New Science.* New York, Basic Books, 1985.

Gilligan C: *In a Different Voice.* Cambridge, Harvard University Press, 1982.

Ginsberg H: Jean Piaget. In: Kaplan H, Sadock B (eds): *Comprehensive Textbook of Psychiatry* (Vol 1, 4th ed). Baltimore, Williams & Wilkins, 1985.

Ginsburg H, Opper S: *Piaget's Theory of Intellectual Development: An Introduction.* Engelwood Cliffs, NJ, Prentice-Hall, 1969.

Gregory RL: *The Oxford Companion to the Mind.* Oxford, Oxford University Press, 1987.

Happé FGE: The autobiographical writings of three Asperger syndrome adults: Problems of interpretation and implications for theory. In: Frith U (ed): *Autism and Asperger Syndrome.* Cambridge, Cambridge University Press, 1991, p. 207.

Harter S: Children's understanding of multiple emotions: A cognitive developmental approach. In: Overton W (ed): *The Relationship between Social* and Cognitive Development. Hillsdale, NJ, Erlbaum, 1983.

Havens L: Making Contact. Cambridge, MA, Harvard University Press, 1986.

Hayward S: A Developmental Study of Jealousy: The Social Triangle and Its Effects on the Developing Child. Unpublished doctoral dissertation, Toronto, Ontario, University of Toronto, 1986.

Herschfeld L, Gelman A: Mapping the Mind. Cambridge, Cambridge University Press, 1994.

Hermelin B, O'Conner N: Psychological Experiments with Autistic Children. Oxford, Pergamon, 1970.

Hobson JP: Beyond cognition: A theory of autism. In: Dawson G (ed): Autism: New Perspectives on Diagnosis, Nature and Treatment. New York, Guilford, 1989, p. 22.

Hobson JP: Understanding persons: The role of affect. In: Baron-Cohen S, Tager-Flussberg H, Cohen DJ (eds): Understanding Other Minds: Perspectives from Autism. Oxford, Oxford University Press, 1993.

Hoffman ME: Sex differences in empathy and related behaviors. Psychol Bull 84(4):712–722, 1977.

Hoffman ME: Interaction of affect and cognition in empathy. In: Izard C, Kagan J, Zajonc R (eds): Emotions, Cognition and Behavior. Cambridge, Cambridge University Press, 1984.

Jordan JV, Kaplan AG, Baker Miller J, et al: Women's Growth in Connection: Writings from the Stone Center. New York, Guilford, 1991.

Kanner L: Autistic disturbances of affective contact. Nerv Child 2:217, 1943.

Kegan R: The Evolving Self. Cambridge, MA, Harvard University Press, 1982.

Kohut H: The Analysis of the Self. New York, International University Press, 1971.

Kohlberg L: Stage and sequence: The cognitive-developmental approach to socialization. In: Goslin DA (ed): Handbook of Socialization Theory and Research. Chicago, Rand McNally, 1969.

Kosko B: Fuzzy Thinking: The New Science of Fuzzy Logic. New York, Hyperion, 1993.

Laing RD: The Divided Self. Harmondsworth, UK, Penguin Books, 1965.

Langdell T: Pragmatic aspects of autism: Or why is 'I' a normal word. Unpublished paper presented at the BPS Developmental Psychology Conference, Edinburgh, 1980. (In: Baron-Cohen S: Social and pragmatic deficits in autism. J Autism Dev Disord 18(3):386, 1988.)

Langer J: Theories of Development. New York, Holt, Rinehart & Winston, 1969.

Leslie AM: Pretense and representation: The origins of "theory of mind." Psychol Rev 94: 412–426, 1987.

Marcia J: Empathy and psychotherapy. In: Eisenberg N, Strayer J (eds): Empathy and Its Development. Cambridge, Cambridge University Press, 1987, p. 81.

McClelland JL, Rumelhart DE, the PDP Research Group: Parallel Distributed Processing: Explorations in the Microstructure of Cognition. Vol 2: Psychological and Biological Models. Cambridge, MA, MIT Press/Bradford Books, 1986.

McKeough A, Yates T, Marini A: Intentional reasoning: A developmental study of behaviorally aggressive and normal boys. Dev Psychopathol 6: 285–304, 1994.

McNeil D, Freiberger P: Fuzzy Logic. New York, Simon & Schuster, 1993.

Meadows S: The Child as Thinker: The Development and Acquisition of Cognition in Childhood. London, Routledge, 1993.

Meichenbaum D: Cognitive Behavior Modification: An Integrative Approach. New York, Plenum, 1977.

Miller G: The magical number seven, plus or minus two: Some limits on our capacity to process information. Psychol Rev 63:81–97, 1956.

Miller PH: Theories of Developmental Psychology (2nd ed). New York, Freeman, 1989.

Nannis E: Emotional understanding and child psychotherapy. In: Shirk S (ed): Cognitive Development and Child Psychotherapy. New York, Plenum, 1988.

Nelson K (ed): Narratives from the Crib. Cambridge, MA, Harvard University Press, 1989.

Newell A: Unified Theories of Cognition. Cambridge, MA, Harvard University Press, 1990.

Newell A, Simon HA: Human Problem Solving. Englewood Cliffs, NJ, Prentice-Hall, 1972.

Noam G: The theory of biography and transformation: Foundation for clinical-developmental therapy. In: Shirk S (ed): Cognitive Development and Child Psychotherapy. New York, Plenum, 1988, pp. 273–317.

Noelting G: Stages and mechanisms in the development of the concept of proportionality in the child and adolescent. In: International Interdisciplinary Conference on Piagetian Theory and Its Implications for the Helping Professions: Piagetian Theory and Its Implications for the Helping Professions. Los Angeles, University of Southern California, 1975.

Osherson D, Markman E: Language and the ability to evaluate contradictions and tautologies. Cognition 2:213–226, 1975.

Perner J: The theory of mind deficit in autism: Rethinking the metarepresentational theory. In: Baron-Cohen S, Tager-Flusberg H, Cohen DJ (eds): Understanding Other Minds: Perspectives from Autism. Oxford, Oxford University Press, 1993, p. 112.

Perner J: Understanding the Representational Mind. Cambridge, MA, MIT Press, 1991.

Piaget J: Play, Dreams and Imitation in Childhood. London, Routledge & Kegan Paul, 1951.

Piaget J: The Origins of Intelligence in Children. New York, International Universities Press, 1952.

Quillian MR: Semantic memory. In: Minsky M (ed): Semantic Information Processing. Cambridge, MA, MIT Press, 1968.

Rumelhart DE, McClelland JL, the PDP Research Group: Parallel Distributed Processing: Explorations in the Microstructure of Cognition. Vol 1: Foundations. Cambridge, MA, MIT Press/Bradford Books, 1986.

Schafer R: The Analytic Attitude. New York, Basic Books, 1983.

Schneider W, Schiffrin RM: Controlled and automatic information processing. I: Detection, search and attention. Psychol Rev 84:1–66, 1977.

Selman R: The Growth of Interpersonal Understanding. New York, Academic Press, 1980.

Selman RL, Schultz LH: Making a Friend in Youth. Chicago, University of Chicago Press, 1990.

Siegler RS: Children's Thinking. Englewood Cliffs, NJ, Prentice-Hall, 1986.

Sigman M, Mundy P, Sherman T, et al: Social interactions of autistic, mentally retarded, and normal children and their caregivers. J Child Psychol Psychiatry 27:647, 1986.

Spence DP: Narrative Truth and Historical Truth: Meaning and Interpretation in Psychoanalysis. New York, Norton, 1982.

Sperber D, Wilson D: Relevance: Communication and Cognition. Oxford, Blackwell, 1986.

Staub E: Commentary on Part 1. In: Eisenberg N, Strayer J (eds): Empathy and Its Development. Cambridge, Cambridge University Press, 1987, p. 105.

Sternberg RJ: Mechanisms of cognitive development: A componential approach. In: Sternberg RJ (ed): Mechanisms of Cognitive Development. New York, Freeman, 1984.

Sternberg RJ: A unified theoretical perspective on autism. In: Cohen DJ, Donnellan A, Paul R (eds): Handbook of Autism and Pervasive Developmental Disorders. New York, Wiley, 1987.

Sternberg RJ: Metaphors of Mind: Conceptions of the Nature of Intelligence. Cambridge, Cambridge University Press, 1990.

Sternberg RJ, Berg CA (eds): Intellectual Development. Cambridge, Cambridge University Press, 1992.

Sternberg RJ, Davidson JE: Insight in the gifted. Educ Psychol 18:52–58, 1983.

Sternberg RJ, Rifkin B: The development of analogical reasoning processes. J Exp Child Psychol 27: 195–232, 1979.

Stillings NA, Feinstein MH, Garfield JL, et al: Cognitive Science: An Introduction. Cambridge, MA, MIT Press, 1987.

Tannen D: You Just Don't Understand: Women and Men in Conversation. New York, William Morrow, 1990.

Thompson RA: In: Eisenberg N, Strayer J (eds): Empathy and Its Development. Cambridge, Cambridge University Press, 1987, p. 141.

Thro E: The Artificial Intelligence Dictionary. San Marcos, CA, Microtrend Books, 1991.

Trevarthen C: The Primary motives for cooperation and understanding. In: Butterworth G, Light P (eds): Social Cognition: Studies of the Development of Understanding. Brighton, Harvester, 1982, p. 136.

Valsiner J (ed): Child Development in Cultural Context. Gottingen, Hogrefe and Huber, 1989.

Vygotsky L: Mind in Society: The Development of Higher Psychological Processes. Cambridge, MA, Harvard University Press, 1978.

Vygotsky LS: Thought and Language (Kozulin A, trans and ed). Cambridge, MA, MIT Press, 1986.

Werner H: The Comparative Psychology of Mental Development. New York, International Universities Press, 1948.

Wertsch JV: A sociocultural approach to cognition. Paper presented at "Colloquium on Cognition and Learning," Department of Educational Psychology, University of Calgary, September 1988.

Wertsch JV: Vygotsky and the Social Formation of Mind. Cambridge, MA, Harvard University Press, 1989.

White M, Epston D: Narrative Means to Therapeutic Ends. New York, Norton, 1990.

Winnicott DW: The Maturational Processes and the Facilitating Environment. London, Hogarth, 1972.

Zahn-Waxler C, Radke-Yarrow M, Brady-Smith J: Perspective-taking and prosocial behaviour. Dev Psychol 13:87–88, 1977.

12 CHILD PSYCHOANALYTIC THEORIES OF DEVELOPMENT

Steven Marans, M.S.W., Ph.D., and Donald J. Cohen, M.D.

The central concern of the theory of child psychoanalysis is the understanding of emotional life—the experiences of loving, hating, pain, pleasure, longing, guilt, and concern—and its representation in the child's mind. Psychoanalytic investigation focuses on how children develop into individuals with their own minds, feelings, and desires and how they become engaged with their parents and others who become important to them. The emphases of child analysis are the internal and private experiences of children, from the first months of life through adolescence; the ways in which bodily and environmental processes influence inner life and the child's perceptions of the outer world; the ways in which children represent their experiences and their selves; and the mutual interactions between reality and fantasy, inner and outer, adaptation to the shared world of reality and appreciation of personal desires and needs. The theory of child analysis involves cultural and personal history—familial and social influences that have their origin before the birth of the child and that are conveyed to the child through the particular social expectations and caregiving of parents and society as well as the enduring effects of experience and the continuities and discontinuities in the child's outer and inner life.

Psychoanalytic theories of development begin with somatic experiences and processes, the infant's bodily sensations and ability to attend to and regulate the impact of internal and external stimulation. With maturation, these inherent functions become elaborated into increasingly sophisticated forms of organization of the child's perceptions of himself or herself and others. The physical requirements of the young infant and the parents' emotional investment in the infant's well-being are paradigmatic for the unfolding relationships that serve as the context in which neurologically based systems unfold. At each phase of development, *maturing* biological demands and capacities assume meaning and find expression in the constructs, including the conscious and unconscious fantasies, that the child *develops* to make sense of himself or herself and the world around. The child's functioning at any one point reflects the mutual interactions between many forces; in turn, the child's history and current functioning set the stage for the emergence of capacities and vulnerabilities in subsequent phases of personal development (Erikson, 1959; Freud, 1966; Klein, 1958).

Throughout childhood, the processes of maturation and development reflect the interaction between biology and endowment—genetically transmitted characteristics, constitution, and the programming for physical change—as well as experience (in the family and broader social world) and the workings of the child's mental apparatus, as such. The charting of the mutual influences between psyche and soma and their representation in mental life provides a framework for understanding both normal development and illness (A. Freud, 1965).

DATA OF CHILD PSYCHOANALYTIC THEORY

Child psychoanalytic theories of development have grown out of clinical experiences and research with children in varied settings, including (a) the home, well-baby clinics, school, and group living arrangements (Bowlby, 1969, 1973; A. Freud and Burlingham, 1973; Hellman, 1962, 1983; Mahler et al., 1975; Stern, 1985); (b) institutional settings (Provence and Lipton, 1962; Robertson and Robertson, 1958, 1971; Spitz, 1945); (c) medical or rehabilitative settings (Burlingham, 1961,

1979; Earle, 1979; Fraiberg, 1968; Freud, 1952; Furman et al., 1968; Moran, 1984; Schowalter and Lord, 1972); (d) the course of determining custody and placement disposition (Goldstein et al., 1973, 1979, 1986; Solnit, Nordhaus and Lord, 1992); and (e) child psychoanalytic treatment (Anthony, 1980; Bornstein, 1953; Freud, 1945; Frijling-Schreuder, 1969; Marans, 1993b; Meers, 1970; Neubauer, 1987; Sandler et al., 1975; Target and Fonagy, 1994).

Similar to Freud's earliest work, child psychoanalytic theories of development have evolved primarily out of a clinical perspective on infants and children with difficulties. Within the context of clinical care, psychoanalytic observations of children focus on the interplay of features of emotional presentation, cognition, modes of communication, physical activity, themes of play, and discussion and patterns of interaction. However, whether in the "unstructured" hours of ongoing psychotherapy or in observations of children in other settings, child psychoanalytic investigators generally proceed by careful observation of the ways in which the child's interests, concerns, and patterns of functioning unfold. They integrate the data with information from caregivers about current and past life experiences. The data are used to develop multiple hypotheses regarding (a) implications of the child's biological "equipment" and its impairment on the tasks of development, (b) areas of strength and preferred modalities for adaptation, (c) specific developmental tasks and various ways in which they are negotiated, (d) areas of vulnerability in the path of development, (e) implications of various life events on the course of development, (f) the nature of unconscious conflict, and (g) defense activity and conflict resolution.

Psychoanalytic theories of development have evolved over the past decades in response to new observations and concepts. Using available observational and historical information, the psychoanalyst attempts to reconstruct a narrative history of the child's life, a portrait of the child's inner experiences, relationships and modes of representing himself or herself and others. There is no one uniform, systematized theory in which all major concepts are formally defined; rather, child psychoanalysis as theory consists of a range of related theoretical perspectives. While these share an orientation on inner emotional experience and developments, they differ, to a greater or lesser degree, in particular conceptual emphases. Relating these perspectives to a specific child or phenomenon may highlight theoretical divergences or, alternatively, may be seen to provide a sense of the complexity of development and emotional life.

CATEGORIES OF EXPERIENCE

Psychoanalytic concepts of early development have long been organized according to a hierarchy of dominant bodily zones. The delineation of oral, anal, phallic, narcissistic, and oedipal phases was meant to map out processes of development from the infant's earliest dependence on the mother to the adult's relative independence and autonomy. The goal of these theoretical constructs was to provide a framework for organizing observations. However, the broadening scope of observations of the development of relationships, concepts about the self, cognition, and the like, highlighted a tension within the theory between the notion of continuity and discontinuity of experience. While there are nodal points that mark out different experiences in different periods of life—reflecting a degree of discontinuity—the concept of "stages" as defined by bodily zones is limited when we observe the overlapping of psychological experiences from one period of life to another, or, rather, the underlying continuities. The goal of contemporary "phase theory" is to explicate major modes of psychological organization and changes from one epoch to another. In addition, the theory tries to describe and understand the personal and shared meanings of experiences and tasks that are salient in a given period of life as well as those that continue to exert influence from earlier periods.

0–18 Months ("Oral" Phase)

Contemporary psychoanalytic theories focus on the ways in which biological processes in this earliest period of development come to have psychological meaning in the infant's rudimentary sense of the self as distinct from others. That is, how do the infant's bodily sensations contribute to the emergence of an internal, psychological "self" that experiences the body and increasingly guides its actions?

During the 1st months of life, the mouth plays a central role in shaping the infant's earliest images of himself or herself in the context of the world. In addition to its role in eating and sustaining life, the baby uses his or her mouth—in activities of sucking, licking, and biting—as a central organ of perceiving, regulating, and altering sensations. In the absence of hunger, the infant mouths fingers, toes, toys, pacifiers, and mother's breast to self-soothe at once, experiencing the various physical properties and decreasing his or her distress. Similarly, his or her crying when uncomfortable or making high-pitched squeals to attract mother's attention leads him or her to represent the communicative power of the mouth.

The experiences associated with orality—pleasure in the satisfaction of urges and discomfort when satisfaction is not immediately available—continue to be central to psychoanalytic conceptualizations about early development. In addition, the contributions of early infant research (Emde, 1982; Klaus and Kennel, 1976; Spitz, 1965; Stern, 1985) have focused on a broader range of inborn processes and their influence on the infant's earliest experience of the body and emergence of a "self." The study of variations in the sensorimotor system (sight, audition, reflexes, muscle tone) and state regulation (sleep/wake cycles, quiet/alert periods, withdrawal, gaze, responsivity to comforting) have emphasized the contribution of these "non-oral" intrinsic factors to early patterns of mediating endogenous/instinctual or external/environmental stimulation (Mayes and Cohen, 1994).

From the beginning of life, the infant's relationship with his or her caregivers organizes the ways in which bodily requirements, inborn processes, and constitutional and instinctual urges find expression. The mother's investment in the infant's bodily needs sensitizes her to the ways she can help diminish the potential for discomfort. Maternal involvement and intimate contact with the infant's body—feeding, cleaning, holding, cooing, and so forth—reflect the mother's earliest attachment (Bowlby, 1969; Freud, 1974; Greenacre, 1957; Klein, 1958; Mahler et al., 1975); she "reads" the infant's cues according to the recognition of specific sources of pleasure and discomfort. In addition, the mother attributes emotional meaning to gross and subtle changes in the infant's presentation. This guides her response and progressively conveys to the child a sense of meaningfulness of her actions and affection. Inborn hypersensitivities to various stimuli—touch, sound, gastrointestinal, and the like—complicate the mother's task of learning how to understand and establish reliable means of responding to her infant's needs. The infant's neurological maturation—for example, decreasing the prominence of colic or ease of startling and becoming distressed by noise—and the mother's increased experience often offset difficulties in the early mother-child relationship. It is important to note that the tremendous variation of inborn characteristics in state regulation may play as crucial a role in the infant's early adaptation as the contributions of possible conflicts the mother or father may have about various aspects of parenthood (Furman, 1993; Kestenberg, 1956, 1980; Winnincott, 1962).

The mother's efforts to maximize her infant's comfort and relieve his or her distress take over where the infant is not yet able to soothe himself or herself. By ensuring that the baby is not overwhelmed by discomfort, the mother contributes to the child's experience of effectance; *his* or *her* activities can make things happen that alter the child's own bodily sensations. Repetition of patterns of maternal care, in turn, influences and reinforces those behaviors of the infant that promote pleasure and satisfaction of needs. While diminishing physical tension (between need and gratification) and maximizing pleasure appear to be essential tasks during this period of development, experiences of frustration and discomfort are equally significant in the baby's maturation and development. In fact, the sequence of discomfort followed by relief is mediated, in part, by the absence and appearance of the caregiver and contributes to the infant's growing capacity to more clearly delineate between "me/not me." The discrepancy between the experience of need and satisfaction may include nuances of interaction-failure to elicit a smile, a cuddle, soothing or playful tone of voice, or physical proximity, as well as hunger or physical discomfort from a soiled diaper. Beginning with the buccal mucosa as a junction between inner and outer, sensations associated with repeated sequences of coordinated activity—sucking, biting, licking, swallowing, looking, listening, touching—foster the infant's capacity to locate and identify the origins of percepts and contribute to the delineation of body boundaries. While the infant's recognition of the mother's face is observable from the earliest weeks of life (Mayes, 1989; 1993), by the middle of the 1st year his or her response to her is no longer dominated by the satisfaction of bodily needs. With the appreciation of physical separateness, the infant links the pleasure associated with her ministrations to the person of the mother in her own right. Her presence itself is a source of pleasure and satisfaction: her absence is a source of anxiety. He or she will look at mother to see if a situation is safe or dangerous and, by this process of *social referencing* of the meaning of situations, the baby will be socialized into the family. He or she will learn about the parents' specific ways of responding (muting or exaggerated, calm or fearful), including how they deal with closeness and separation. The child's protests at being handled by others, his or her distress on seeing people other than mother (stranger anxiety), and his or her upset on separations from her stem from the infant's feeling that "not here" is "gone forever." With the delineation of boundaries, the infant views mother as a bridge between himself or herself and the world. In her absence, he or she may appear panic-stricken and "disoriented as if he/she had lost his connection with his/her newfound world and with emerging feelings of 'self'" (Fraiberg, 1959). From within the dyadic relationship, how the mother acts on leaving and how she feels on return will exacerbate or diminish the child's worries.

Games of peek-a-boo, experimenting with hiding and finding objects, and repeated experiences of parents coming and going help the infant on his or her way to establishing object permanence (Piaget, 1952, 1954), the ability to conceive that things continue to exist even when hidden, that "not here" is "maybe there." The ability to mentally "hold on to," or internally represent images of the parents in their absence contribute to the infant's exploration of the world beyond the lap as the child begins to stand, cruise, and then take his or her first steps. The toddler's ability to move away from the parents under his or her own steam provides a vivid experience of physical separateness from them well beyond the earlier activities of averting gaze or arching away from mother's body when held. While needing periodically to check back with the parents, or "refuel" (Mahler et al., 1975), the toddling infant's explorations contribute to his or her inner definition of "self," that is, what the toddler can do in relation to his or her body and in relation to the central figures in his or her life (Freud, 1965). Increased dexterity, language acquisition, and rudimentary cause-effect thinking provide the tools for this research. Optimally, the young child's investment in these burgeoning capacities leads to the child's "love affair with the world" (Greenacre, 1957), in which the pleasure of mastery facilitates the elaboration of these capacities. Alternatively, gross disruptions in the dyadic relationship, including prolonged separations between mother and child, mother's emotional unavailability due to severe depression, and physical abuse, may lead to the earliest expressions of psychopathology, such as failure to thrive, anaclitic depression, hypersensitivity to stimulation, and extreme wariness in interactions with others.

The child's psychological differentiation and separation from the parents is accompanied by tension, sadness, and anxiety as well; he or she may sometimes find "walking away," or being walked away from, a painful experience. The young child often turns to a specific soft blanket or cuddly toy, especially invested with attributes of the mother, to hold and fondle in her absence. Unlike the real mother of separation, these transitional objects (Winnicott, 1953, 1965, 1971) can be controlled and literally held on to by the toddler when the mother is too far away. The capacity to evoke mental images of the self and parents and memories of satisfaction of needs and possible sequences of events are crucial achievements in this phase and have broad implications for the young child's capacity to remember and to anticipate interactions with the world. From suckling at the breast to first steps and from random smiling and cooing to words and conversation, the infant's developing organization of "self" as distinct from the body is matched by an accompanying elaboration of mental schemas—conscious and unconscious fantasies—of his or her relationship to the central figures in his or her life. The increased specificity of feelings, both pleasurable and frustrating, associated with the parents during infancy form a foundation on which internal mental structures and attachments to others will gain complexity in subsequent phases of development.

18–36 Months ("Anal" Phase)

This phase of development obviously owes its designation to the role of elimination and toilet training in early childhood. The capacity to control defecation and urination and the demands of the parents to do so have been seen as *paradigmatic* for a range of tasks and struggles the child encounters with regard to his or her body, relationships, impulses, and fantasies.

In addition to the toddler's continued exploration of the world around him or her, heightened anal sensations in the period of development also promote the toddler's appreciation for the separateness between himself or herself and caregivers. Central nervous system maturation underlies the increased awareness of rectal pressure and anal sensitivity; psychologically, the child's attention becomes focused on yet another area of the body where there is an interface between inner and outer. In defecation and urination, the child experiences a complex process involving bodily feelings, self-control, action, and perception. He or she feels and sees how what is originally *inside* can become *outside*, along with a sense of what was previously *hidden* being *public* and *shared*. Defecating and urinating are no longer simple processes that occur in response to physical pressure; they assume meaning as sources of pleasure that the toddler can control.

The ability to label and identify parts of the body is concurrent with the ability to regulate pleasurable sensations through holding and releasing feces and urine; these capacities permit the elaboration of an internal set of representations of the self. A distance is established between the body and the self that experiences the body. As the child represents himself or herself as an object that can be perceived, the child naturally begins to compare his or her body with that of others. This capacity to compare leads to the child's appreciation of anatomical differences between the sexes and between child and adult.

Recognition of separateness and specific differences in the body and abilities between the child and adult caregivers (and other children) is crucial in the child's development of "reality testing" and sense of self. In addition, this recognition is also a source of considerable conflict and anxiety. Under the sway of powerful sexual and aggressive desires, the toddler seeks immediate satisfaction of urges that his or her developing capabilities alone cannot always deliver. In addition to the motivation provided by need satisfaction—seen throughout development—the

child now experiences the satisfaction of his or her needs as related to his or her own degree of control and effectiveness. The child's awareness that he or she does not share the powers of the parents increases the intensity of the wish for effectiveness; awareness of dependency is often at odds with the wish for autonomy and omnipotent control. Parents are then frequently confronted with a toddler who is inconsolable about his or her inability to accomplish a given task or satisfy a need. The child may loudly protest what he or she can't accomplish alone and angrily refuse all parental attempts of assistance. The young child crumpling to the floor in tears is a poignant illustration of the struggle between the competing aims of independence and dependence. In this phase, anxiety experienced on occasions of separation from parents is an additional marker of the child's comparison of his or her competence with the parents' and his or her continued need to rely on them for care, safety, and affection. In earlier separations the infant was frightened and disoriented due to an inability to conceptualize the existence of the mother or father in their absence. In this later period of development, however, the child may believe that by his or her voracious demands, anger, and frustration and moves toward independent power the child has become the agent of their destruction. Until reunited with mother, the child imagines that she has gone away forever and feels completely alone, bereft, and guilty.

In this period, words can now substitute for actions; remembering simple sequences of events can help the child anticipate the immediate future, and increased coordination can broaden the range of pleasurable physical activities. These capacities promote the young child's sense of effectiveness and offer potential diversion from the intensity of needs and impulses that were previously satisfied only by the parents' immediate response. The child can now tell the mother that he or she is hungry instead of simply crying. And when told by the mother to "wait for a few minutes" the child may be able to mobilize defenses against feeling hurt and sustain the wait by rolling cars on the floor, knowing that "a few minutes" means not *too* long. Alternatively, the child may again use language to implore mother to hurry or crash the cars or other toys as a way of displacing/deflecting the anger felt toward her for not responding to his or her needs quickly enough.

While the child is able to tolerate greater amounts of frustration, relative to earlier phases, parental demands to do more or wait just a bit longer introduce conflicts that further the cause of mediating between impulses and action. The child's fear of losing the parent as the result of destructive urges and the wish to please the parent and receive praise are powerful contingencies that often fly in the face of aims of immediate gratification and absolute autonomy. The toddler's alternation between compliance with and obstinate defiance of parental rules, and the attendant tantrums, expresses struggles between passivity and activity, love and hate. As parents expect more from a child in the areas of toileting, self-feeding habits, waiting for help, and attention, for example, they are setting goals for which the child will reach. When they are achieved, the child is proud of himself or herself and enjoys the admiration of the parents; when the demands are too difficult, the child may feel frustrated, humiliated, or in danger of losing the parents' love.

Development in language and symbolization, object permanence, and cause-effect thinking sets the stage for the child to elaborate the "representational world" (Sandler and Joffe, 1962). Within psychoanalytic theory, "self" and "object" representations refer to the organization of the variety of composite images of himself or herself and others that the child has internally constructed on the basis of experiences, urges, and feelings. These concepts are never articulated in consciousness as a sum total but, rather, are expressed as parts in the child's ever-changing fantasies, attitudes, and behavior. At times the child may comply with the parents' requests in response to his or her inner view of them as wonderful and all-giving. Alternatively, the child's tirades against them may reflect a feeling that they are frustrating figures who are set on depriving him or her of pleasure. They may be seen as sources of safety and comfort or as obstacles in the path toward independence. Simultaneously, the child has rapid shifts in feelings about himself or herself—at one moment victorious and able, at another frightened and helpless. Moreover, the child may oscillate between views of himself or herself and parents as all good or all bad, determined by experiences of the child's own and by his parents loving and destructively hostile urges.

While the child struggles—internally and externally—with these varying attitudes, the flexibility of the representational world produces greater self-reliance. Now the child's ability to recall loving images of the parents in their absence allows for longer periods of independent activity, sustained by the confident expectation that needs will ultimately be satisfied (Mahler et al., 1975). Second, internalized standards, both prohibitive and encouraging, serve as referents in determining consequences of action (i.e., trial action in thought). Finally, in the absence of real gratification of wishes, impulses and feelings can find expression/discharge in the manipulation of self-object interactions in fantasy. Here, *conscious fantasying* involves daydreams in which real experiences can be altered or replaced entirely by more gratifying, wish-fulfilling imaginative scenarios. These mental operations involved in fantasying support the child's capacity to tolerate increasing frustration, whether from his or her own limitations or those imposed by the environment. The young child can now "hold on to" a variety of representations and "play" with them, or pretend. He or she can use imagination for escaping from unbearable disappointment in reality, altering current feeling states and planning courses of future action. In a broader context *unconscious fantasies* and their conscious derivatives give expression to the child's deeply felt longings, conflicts aroused by forbidden urges, attempts at resolving conflicts, and preparation for or postponement of action. As such, fantasies may be a source of pleasure and anxiety. When unconscious fantasies give form to unacceptable impulses and wishes, defensive operations will be employed to disguise them before they find expression in conscious thought.

In this phase, fantasies and activities that serve to diminish anxiety, when these aims and wishes are at odds with reality or internalized standards, expand and become more identifiable to the observer. The child's growing disaffection with messiness and disorder, for example, is a signal accomplishment in the anal phase and reflects an active repudiation of pleasurable activities that are in opposition to parental attitudes (reaction formation). By complying with these external demands, the child avoids disapproval and reaps the satisfaction of adult approval. Initially having to yield control of his or her body to the expectations of others, the child's growing identification with parental demands and responses make them his or her own. While vulnerable to reexternalization, the conflict between competing aims is now internal, belonging to the child alone. Anxiety associated with the dangers of aggressivity and from the conflict between loving and hating may be dealt with via various imaginative mental processes for mobilizing fantasies, which counteract other more frightening fantasies or which modulate anxieties in other ways. These "defensive processes" or *mechanisms of defense* (Freud, 1966) include the child's disavowal of a particular feeling or aspect of reality (denial), a sense that the feeling belongs to someone else (projection), or shifting the target of feelings from parents to himself or herself, to others, or to a toy (displacement). Hostile impulses that run counter to the love the child feels toward parents, for example, are disowned. Being fearful of others' hatred or frightened of monsters and noises in the night is a preferable alternative to the imagined destruction of loved figures on whom the child depends. These mental activities allow the child to express competing feelings of love and hate without needing to relegate them to completely separate images of himself or herself or the parent (Marans et al., 1993c; Mayes and Cohen, 1993). Real competence in communicating and acting on needs independently and the continued experience of the parent's availability promote a psychological "rapprochement" (Mahler et al., 1975). The child can begin to tolerate an ambivalent attitude toward himself or herself and the parents, between love and hatred, and between total dependence and self-reliance. In this phase, the child's recognition of others as separate entities and ability to appreciate the specificity of his

or her own feelings toward them extends to a capacity to empathize with their feelings as well. These achievements are seen in expressed concern for and questions about parental moods and in the designation of feelings to figures used in play.

In the 1st year of life, physical objects were mouthed and handled as the infant explored their properties as well as the bodily sensations aroused in the process. These activities, as described earlier, aided the infant's delineation of body boundaries (Hoffer, 1949). In the latter part of the 2nd and in the 3rd year, the child uses toys and other play items for the extensive representation and elaboration of daily experiences and fantasies, as well as for the purpose of engaging the caregivers in pleasurable interaction. Moving cars across the floor, carrying and feeding baby dolls, manipulating puppets, and imitating parental activities constitute rehearsals, reworking of experiences, and trying on new roles. They also are precursors to the development of imaginative/pretend play in which the child will employ complex narrative structures or story lines to elaborate these roles and fantasy scenarios. At age 3 there is a gradual move in the child's view of other children as playthings or things that get in the way of personal pursuits. Increasingly, children not only play side by side but turn to one another as companions and partners in shared activities that are more fun because they are social. Here, the capacity to generalize symbolic representation and empathize with the feelings of others serves as a common basis on which the fantasy configurations of each partner can be mutually enriched and enacted in play.

The achievements in this phase of development expand the young child's range of possible pleasures and the complexity of conflicts. Increased capacity for independent functioning is a source of pride in mastery, while the appreciation of separateness/reality highlights limitations and the vulnerability of being little and dependent. Ownership of the body and insistence of bodily urges (drive pressures) are in conflict with the child's sense of the contingent nature of the relationship with his or her parents. That is, the push to give expression to his or her own will is at odds with the desire to please the objects of his or her love by submitting to their requirements. As external controls and rewards become internalized, so too do the capacities to retain and elaborate various representations of self and significant others. Whether serving configurations of fantasy or memories of reality, the capacity for representation offers the young child an inner frame of reference that can be a resource for increased frustration tolerance, substitute forms of gratification, trial action in thought, self-esteem, and the companionship of important people regardless of their presence or absence. As the central tasks of the anal phase of development merge into those of subsequent stages, the groundwork is laid for further elaboration of relationships and capacities both within and outside of the context of the child's family.

36–48 Months ("Genital-Narcissistic" Phase)

A transitional phase of development has been posited between the anal and oedipal periods. This phase is characterized by an increasing crystallization of gender and concurrent preoccupation with appearance, anatomical differences, and sensations arising from the phallus and testicles, in boys, and the vagina and clitoris, in girls.

The child's assumption of a specific gender identity—the core sense of being a boy or a girl—obviously has its roots in the 1st year or two of life. Early genderization during infancy is the result of multiple, interacting forces, including differential treatment of girls and boys by parents and others; the anatomically distinctive sensations arising from the genitals in the course of parental handling, elimination, and self-stimulation (including penile erection, clitoral stimulation, and the sensations accompanying defecation and urination); and other biological factors, including genetic and endocrine influences on brain and behavior. By age 3, children generally are quite clear that they are either a girl or boy and are aware of the types of play activities, dress, and the like expected of children of their sex. Attempts to alter assigned sexuality after this time, for example, for children with anomalous genitalia, usually are not successful. As a psychologically organizing internal construct, however, gender may not be sharply dichotomous, for either boy or girl, during the 1st years of life or even much later. Indeed, psychoanalysts have long appreciated that there is a spectrum of gender-related experiences throughout the course of development that may be considered normative bisexuality—the desire for some of the attributes and opportunities of the opposite sex.

Consistent with the psychoanalytic theory of psychosexual stages as developed in relation to the oral and anal phases, "phallic narcissism" (Burgner and Edgcumbe, 1975) has been used to designate the central zone of sexual sensations during this phase of development. However, the emphasis on the phallus does not recognize the girl's prideful and pleasurable experiences of her genitals or the anatomical distinctions that are felt by both girls and boys. A more suitable designation for this psychosexual phase, which arises around age 3, might thus be "genderized, genital narcissism," a period in which children become progressively more aware of the pleasurable sensations in their genitals as well as tensions arising from the genital zone, take pleasure in displaying and being appreciated for their genitality, and experience themselves as having a core gender identity, that is, when all goes well, consistent with their anatomical identity. During this phase, both boys and girls may show off their genitals (enjoying how far they can urinate or lifting their skirts) and engage in more focused and sometimes more persistent masturbation (occasionally leading to genital irritation and a cycle of concern by both the parents and the child). While the genitals may be a leading edge of narcissistic investment, during this phase children feel a generalized pride in their bodies and what they can do in rough and tumble play, learning new skills on the jungle gym, displaying their fine and gross motor skills and coordination, and gaining parental attention through exhibitionism (such as dressing up in mother's clothes, clowning, or performing new feats of skill).

As with each phase, there are dilemmas faced by children during this period that are directly related to the developmental achievements. A child whose self-esteem is closely related to the beauty, power, and pleasures of the body may feel hurt, rejected, and enraged by not being noticed or mirrored by his or her parents or from failure in learning or performing some tasks for which the child may still be too immature or small. While the anal phase was characterized by struggles concerning control, the phase of genital (bodily) narcissism may be burdened by struggles with siblings with whom the child may be rivalrous and with parents concerning issues of competence. The child may be unmindful of or angered by the recognition of his or her personal limitations. The parents' imposition of rules or even their offers of help may be felt by a child as demeaning, and sensitive parents may try to disguise their assistance or attribute the achievements to the child to foster the narcissistic delight in mastery.

There is a gradual transition rather than a sharp boundary between the psychological issues of genderized, genital narcissism—prideful exhibitionism delight, pleasure, and sense of achievement as a girl or as a boy—and the issues of the oedipal phase. In some ways, this boundary is crossed as boys become more worried about the loss of their prized genitalia and girls express more concern about the adequacy of theirs, along with a range of increasingly complex feelings about the roles of the male and female parents.

4–6 Years ("Oedipal" Phase)

Within contemporary psychoanalytic theory, *oedipal phase* refers to a range of concerns about loving, sexual/rivalrous, and aggressive attitudes toward the same and different-sex parent, which are correlated intrapsychically to the consolidation of mental structures. The achievements of this phase are a consequence of the advance of multiple forces—cognitive, affective, social, bodily—and provide a template for perceptions about the self and intimate relations with others for future development. If the child was an "explorer" in earlier periods of devel-

opment, the oedipal child is best described as a "scientist," curious, developing hypotheses, and experimenting in thought and play about (*a*) his or her relations with parents, (*b*) their relationship with each other, and (*c*) how his or her mind works.

PRECONDITIONS

During the 1st years of life, the child moves though several phases of development, which have been characterized in relation to the "leading" bodily zone (oral, anal, genital). Within psychoanalytic theory of development, the various tasks, concerns, and processes of these phases lead to a phase of mental integration involving economic factors (biologically driven urges), the direction of love and hate, and the relationship between unconscious and conscious thoughts and feelings in the context of the realities of daily life. The preconditions for the child's successful move into the oedipal phase and its optimal negotiation include overlapping, mutually influencing "preoedipal" achievements in areas such as the following ones:

1. Social relations: Good primary attachments to parents, representations of mother and father as separate and good, sense of self as the locus of initiatives that are successful, and capacity for empathizing with the feelings of others.
2. Cognition: The ability to represent abstractions and to call on these in assuming various social roles, taking the perspective of others, tolerating mixed feeling about self and others, appreciating the rights and responsibilities of oneself and others, and sensing that oneself and others can act and feel differently at different times.
3. Moral: A developing sense of right and wrong, good and bad, recognizing the link between actions and their consequences in relation to parents (approval and pleasure versus disapproval and anger) and to the self (well-being and pride versus shame and guilt).
4. Physical: The capacity for fine and gross motor coordination for pleasurable and playful activities such as running, jumping, and climbing, as well as self-care (toileting oneself, brushing teeth, handwashing) and imitating adult behavior in play (cooking, driving a car, caring for a baby, building).
5. Emotional: The development of a wide range of feelings (including excitement, happiness, sadness, remorse, fear, disappointment, pride, anger, envy, love, and hate) that can be distinguished, expressed, and communicated to others.
6. Mental: The capacity for remembering personal history, realizing that dreams and imagination come from within oneself, perceiving complex social situations involving causality and time sequences, and developing narrative structures that organize inner and external experiences.
7. Biological: A hypothesized biological state that is analogous to the maturation of psychosexual zones (oral, anal, and genital) and to biological changes seen in puberty, which is now represented primarily in relation to emotions—intensified affective and sexualized longings (love) and raw expression of rivalry and aggression (hate). These are directed to the same/opposite sex parents during the oedipal phase and later are expressed in adolescence toward peers.

When the preconditions are in place, the 4- to 6-year-old child moves naturally into the oedipal phase, as evidenced by new integrations of self and others. During this period the child recognizes that he or she is the child of his or her parents and that the parents have a relationship to each other that is not solely related to their roles as parents. Appreciating their strong feelings for each other, the child wishes to remain with them as in his or her previous fantasies—the center of their lives. The child knows that this position can be recaptured, if only for a while, through being very good, attractive, and clever or through being very naughty, destructive, and demanding. In addition, the child understands that he or she cannot be the only person for mother or father. Ultimately, the oedipal phase child recognizes the complexity of mother and father as full people. Whereas previously they were seen as either all good or all bad, depending on the child's state of frustration/satisfaction, increasingly, as a result of improved cognitive abilities, he or she feels the need to understand them as autonomous individuals, separate and in relation to himself or herself, to each other, and to others both in and outside of the family.

TRIADIC RELATIONS AND THE PRIMAL SCENE

The classical oedipal phase within psychoanalysis in its boldest expression related to one aspect of the Greek myth: the murder of the father by the son and sexual union between son and mother. This mythic beginning for the theory of the oedipal phase had the virtue of drama and suggestiveness but the vice of oversimplifying the phenomenology. The child in the oedipal myth didn't know who was being murdered, and the remorse came later. The struggles of the oedipal phase are painful just because of the child's knowledge and continued love for both parents. He or she is confronted with amorous longings and rivalrous wishes *and* the desire to work out possible compromises—how to be powerful and central, to feel proud of achievements, and at the same time to have the continuing secure presence of both parents (Marans et al., 1993c).

Crucial to the challenges of this phase is the fact that the girl's wish to exclusively possess her father, and the boy, his mother, cannot and will not find immediate gratification in reality. In order to sustain his or her quest, the oedipal child must be capable of suspending disbelief of denying that he or she is small and cannot enjoy the privileges and pleasures of the grownups (Freud, 1974a). However, the child is burdened in this quest by anxieties and real deficiencies that must be denied, lessened, or worked through if the child's invincibility is to be maintained (Peller, 1954). Boys and girls must find ways to explain why they do not win the ''exclusive'' position in the opposite-sex parent's life in spite of attempts to woo the parent (by impressing the parent with physical and intellectual competence as well as charm).

Oedipal children are confronted by their exclusion from the parents' special relationship even though each parent may acknowledge how big, strong, attractive, or smart the young suitor might be. A hallmark of this phase is the child's capacity for *triadic relations*: the representation of the parents' relationship with each other and with him or her as *their* child. The child's theories about the parents' relationships with each other in his absence (*primal scene fantasies*) are based on observations of their affective ties as well as on projection of the child's own intense sexual and aggressive urges. Primal scene fantasies are a source of excitement and danger—in the child's view of sexual intercourse as violent—and of narcissistic hurt as well, representing the ultimate adult activity from which the child is excluded. Oedipal children must turn from a passive role in which they might fall prey to dangers and disappointments to an active one in which they can feel as though they are the masters of their own fate (Freud, 1917). In this task they increasingly turn to fantasy and its expression in play.

REPRESENTATIONS IN PLAY

The child of this age has an increased capacity for reality testing; in addition, he or she continues to have the facility for magical thinking as well as more advanced capacities for guiding integration of competing wishes and aims. His or her ability for daydreaming, fantasy, and pretend play allows greater access to wishes that do not need to be compromised too quickly by reality. The child is thus protected in fantasy from the recognition of ultimate frustration. An increased capacity for symbolic representation opens the door to more elaborate forms of binding anxiety and expressing bodily urges in thought and imaginative activities (Marans et al., 1993a). Advances in cognitive and motor skills yield functional pleasure, minimize anxieties, and compensate for felt inadequacies in comparison with the adults with whom he or she competes (Peller, 1954).

Oedipal children can move fluidly through a range of themes determined by the urgency of what is uppermost in their minds, whether exciting, pleasurable, or fearful. The child's push toward mastery combines with curiosity to arrive at solutions in play in which theories may be tested and explored. Do babies come from eating special, magical foods? Do mommy and daddy hurt each other when they are in their bed together without me? (Cohen et al., 1987; Marans, 1993b).

The oedipal child's play, in particular, reflects a plasticity of representations employed in the service of creating and maintaining the illusion of wish fulfillment and invincible mastery. The guiding motif of the child's creativity is contained in the oedipal wish and in attempts to ward off its attending dangers and disappointing confrontation with reality. The child in this phase of development is able to juggle the inconsistencies he or she perceived both *within* fantasies and *between* fantasies and reality. There is equal flexibility as the constituent themes of the oedipal phase seek expression in fantasy and play. At one moment aggressive competition with the rival may be uppermost as the child assumes the role of the strongest, most attractive and competent member of the family. The same role may simultaneously give expression to the child's exhibitionistic impulses or wish to protect and care for the object of his or her longings. The play may easily shift from themes of power and strength to scenarios involving the production and feeding of babies. Repeated crashing of toy cars may at one moment express the child's concerns about aggression and bodily intactness. With additional features and elaboration, the same play may articulate the child's fantasies about sexual intercourse. In this latter context, the child's curiosity about the contents and activities behind closed dollhouse doors or in closets and bedrooms may at once give vent both to sexual excitement and to disappointment at being excluded from parental activities. Equally, increased interest in theories regarding the origin of babies, sexually exciting sensations focused on genitals, and anatomical differences and comparisons of physical attributes between sexes and between adult and child versions (same sex) will be expressed in the oedipal child's fantasies and imaginative play (Marans et al., 1993a). Reality events in the child's life—accidents and injuries, as well as surprises and pleasures—are dexterously integrated into fantasies as they stimulate, organize, and accentuate the specific themes with which the child struggles (Cohen et al., 1987; Neubauer, 1987; Solnit, 1987).

Infantile Neurosis

The powerful wish to get rid of the same-sex parent and assume his or her role in an exclusive, intimate relationship with the opposite-sex ''partner'' is also fraught with tension as the child struggles with love and hate felt toward the rival. The experience of hurt, tension, and uncertainty during this phase leads to the achievement of internalized conflict. The child now has the capacity for neurosis, that is, an internal struggle between opposing forces (wishes versus personal values, desires versus parental attitudes and opposing desires). The *infantile neurosis* is theoretically the paradigmatic form for age-appropriate mental disorders engaged by oedipal phase structures. It is expressed by the appearance of regressive behaviors and fears—obsessive-compulsive symptoms, enuresis, encopresis, thumb-sucking, phobias, separation difficulties, nightmares, frequent battling with parents—that are common in this period of development and serve the child's attempts to withdraw from or displace the conflicts aroused by the intensity of his or her oedipal longings. Similarly, in imaginative play, the child will change the narrative script when it is unable to maintain an adequate distance from painful reality or anxiety stemming from conflicts. For example, the role of a given protagonist may be elaborated in order to add dimensions that would compensate for the child's intruding sense of vulnerability (e.g., the policeman who is battling robbers is transformed into Superman). Alternatively, the specific role and theme in the play may be abandoned altogether as the child shifts to ones more congenial to the maintenance of pleasure and the prospect of mastery. This shift might be seen in the child's assuming the voice and behavior of a baby, in provocative messing, or in destruction of play materials. However, the child might equally turn to an intensification and insistent involvement in the fantasy, becoming narrower in his or her range of play while trying to overcome anxiety in the repetition of a singular theme.

In these varied ways, the child's internal conflicts and their representation in fantasy, symptoms, and imaginative play constitute the child's research about the self and others. Expanding experience in a broader social context (chiefly through the introduction of nursery and school programs) fosters increased psychological independence. Organized and regular group experiences offer a broader context in which the conflicts and tasks of the oedipal phase of development may be worked through. The capacity and opportunity to engage with peers increases the range of play activities in which fantasies and skills may be "tried on." Co-operative play (in which role assignment, turn taking, and mutual elaboration of narrative/story line are component parts) often revolves around themes regarding

1. Exploration of and acquisition of knowledge about physical properties of things and various characteristics of the environment
2. The child's sense of place within the family
3. Size, strength, capacities/competence
4. Theories and feelings about babies and their origins
5. Anatomical differences and attributes of both sexes
6. Curiosity and excitement associated with genital sensations
7. Competition and rivalry
8. Destructive aggressivity
9. Consequences of wishes and actions

Relationships with children and adults outside of the family capitalize on and promote the youngster's greater frustration tolerance, reliance on increased intellectual and physical capacities, and confidence in the ability to function—with pleasure—in the absence of parents. In addition, the world beyond the family affords the child with a broader range of stimulation and opportunities for using new skills such as reading, writing, and problem solving in the classroom setting.

While giving rise to considerable anxiety, the oedipal child's experiments in thought and pretend play serve to integrate representations of the self and others. The conflict between loving and hating leads the child to further consolidate and integrate the images of the "good" and "bad" parents into representations of them as whole, autonomous people who have relationships beyond the dyadic parent-child configuration. In muting the intensity of oedipal longings, the child strives to live up to the ideal of being like the rival parent (*ego ideal*) and to identify with their rules and values (*superego*). These achievements of internalization allow the child to desist in overt rivalry with the same-sex parent, to feel that he or she hasn't lost out in the struggles but has in fact taken on the role of the parent internally, and serve as reparative structures for anxiety, frustration, and the hurt narcissism that accompanied the more raw competition. The child's feelings of wounded pride and anxiety serve as "signal affects" and alert the child to how he or she is feeling in response to specific thoughts and actions (in the past, present, and future) and lead to the child's capacity to observe himself or herself and establish theories of how his or her mind works.

THEORIES OF MIND

The "theories" the child develops organize internal experience of affects, bodily urges, memories, parental rules, and praise and personal ideals and provide structure and cohesion for the child's perceptions of self and others. They are tested and elaborated in fantasy, play, and daily life and draw on the many new roles the child assumes in relationship to the parents, as a friend to peers, as a sibling, as a student in the classroom, and the like (Mayes and Cohen, 1994). The child's theories of how his or her mind works—what makes the child worry, and how does the child enhance good feelings about himself or herself through fantasy, imaginative play, and direct action—lead to decreased egocentricity and increased self-observation (Marans et al., 1993c). The ability to manipulate ideas and feelings in preparation for action and the capacity to take the perspective of parental representations allow the child to

postpone gratification, to balance urges with ideals that are now the child's own. Achievements in delaying immediate satisfaction and identifying the principles of justice/morality are expressed in the child's social play with companions, where he or she is able to see the world from the view of the other—not grabbing toys, taking turns, playing by implicit rules, developing narratives from shared fantasies—and accepting the fact that he or she is not alone in having important needs. The child's new capacities are also apparent in the child's recognition of the difference between play and work and in his or her sense that industriousness/perseverance brings its own rewards and personal satisfaction. While parents' approval and praise (and the admiration of other adults and peers) remain important to the oedipal child, the child's ability to refer internal theories about himself or herself—sources of pleasure, memories, ideals, positive and negative consequences of thoughts and actions—allows the child to give up a singular reliance on external sources of reward/response for the regulation of self-esteem (Marans et al., 1993b, 1993c; Mayes and Cohen, 1994).

7–10 Years ("Latency" Phase)

The term *latency* refers to a decrease in the prominence of preoedipal and oedipal striving in terms of both intensity and direction. While they do not go completely underground, the degree of preoccupation with sexual impulses and interests that are explicitly connected with the assumption of parental roles is significantly diminished. In fact, it would seem that in the sexual curiosity, excitement, and joking that can be observed among latency-age children, notions about parents as sexual objects/beings must be denied or avoided. Activities and attitudes seen as infantile—dependency on parents, fearfulness, and the like—also need to be avoided at all costs. In the face of conflicts established in the preoedipal and oedipal phases, infantile and incestuous longings are repressed, and a widening array of adaptive defenses, including intellectualization, humor, identification, obsessional interests, and sublimation, are utilized to support the diversion and alteration of the original impulses (Bornstein, 1951; Freud, 1968).

The continued consolidation of intellectual, sensorimotor, and social skills and opportunities affords the latency child with a variety of pathways for the sublimated expression of urges that dominated earlier phases of development. For example, friendships and group affiliation can serve as an alternative to the exclusive, close tie to the parents while further facilitating the child's exploration of the world outside of the family. The intense interest and curiosity about the origins of babies, the intimate life of parents, and the mysteries of sexual differences can now be employed for and shaped by the challenges of learning that occur in both school and extracurricular activities. Competitive strivings central in the oedipal phase of development can find expression in games and in relationships with peers. Exhibitionistic impulses find a broader range of vehicles and audiences in the performance of intellectual tasks and mastery of athletic and creative pursuits. In addition, the demands and rewards associated with a relatively stable conscience (or superego) are increasingly exercised in the latency-age child's interests and activities. While not without breaches, as seen in cheating and insensitivity to peers and family members, insistence on following the "rules of the game," empathy with the feelings of others, and a clear sense of right and wrong are hallmarks of the child's establishment in latency. Similarly, descriptively obsessional interests in orderliness, collecting (as in hobbies), and details of functional relationships and properties of physical phenomena serve reaction formations that derive from both benign and prohibitive aims of the superego. These elaborations of defensive and adaptive functions are only possible with and equally reflective of the development of more sophisticated cognitive processes involving the introduction of operational thought.

Optimally, the latency-age child achieves greater autonomy with respect to aspects of daily living such as hygiene, dressing, looking after possessions, and the like. The ability to engage in operational thinking and problem solving, in conjunction with the capacity for increased frustration tolerance, broaden the range of potential achievements and attendant satisfaction. These accomplishments enrich the child's interaction with peers, who are viewed as partners and ''best friends'' as well as new objects of identification, admiration, and competition.

The central threat to the latency-age child is the reemergence or breakthrough of the original sexual and aggressive fantasies of the oedipal phase, particularly when associated with the impulse to masturbate. Sleeping difficulties; nightmares; worries about burglars, bodily injury, and death; and the ease of regression to earlier modes of relating to parents (struggles over food, self-care, household responsibilities, and the like) may be some of the behavioral phenomena that accompany the child's attempts to defend against and give expression to the residual or persistent intensity of oedipal conflicts in the early period of latency. The elaboration of cognitive capacities, peer group involvement, and academic and extracurricular interests facilitates the late-latency child's sublimation of previous trends in action and fantasy and promotes greater distance from the original objects of oedipal longings. Alternately, these achievements are subject to neurotic interference; school failure is not necessarily an outcome of learning disabilities, and isolation from the peer group is not alone determined by athletic skills, looks, or abundance of toys.

Adolescence (12–20+ Years)

Adolescence is one of the most dramatic phases in the course of development, marked by profound changes in biological, psychological, and social functioning. Preceded by a period between ages 10 to 12 in which there is renewed interest in anatomical differences, sexual curiosity, and masturbation (preadolescence), the transition into *early adolescence* (12–14 years) is introduced by the endocrinological and biological processes of puberty. With much greater intensity, these processes focus the young adolescent's attention on concerns about bodily changes and sexual sensations. The primary and secondary sexual characteristics—growth spurt, voice changes, menarche, nocturnal emissions, breast development, and pubic, axillary, and facial hair—associated with pubertal maturation are often greeted with a mixture of pleasure and trepidation. Preoccupations with comparisons of the rate of changes in others; the intensification of exciting genital sensations and the compelling need for masturbation as a source of relief; and the increased conscious awareness of sexually arousing yet conflictual fantasies, precipitating the urge for and accompanying masturbation, may all arouse a tremendous amount of anxiety for the young adolescent (Blos, 1970; Dahl, 1993; Kestenberg, 1980).

While physical maturation heralds the entry into manhood and womanhood, the changes can be experienced as happening too quickly or not quickly enough. These feelings may be manifested in the exhibitionism, embarrassment, and secretive behaviors seen in the young adolescent's attitudes toward his or her body. In either event, pubescent children may be impressed and made anxious by the lack of control of their own bodies. Menarche and the first nocturnal emission are dramatic, paradigmatic events for the real absence of control that characterizes this phase of development. The young adolescent's relationships with his or her parents may be equally tumultuous as rapid shifts between longings to remain close and dependent and requirements for privacy and strivings for autonomy are experienced. These struggles are often played out around old issues having to do with bodily care and hygiene, cleanliness and orderliness of personal property, insensitivity to the feelings and needs of others, and intense preoccupation with immediate satisfaction of one's own needs (Blos, 1962; Freud, 1958; Laufer, 1985; Ritvo, 1984).

By *mid-adolescence* (14–16 years) maturation levels off; all girls are now in menarche, boys are able to ejaculate, and both have attained secondary sexual characteristics. Physical maturation potentiates the conflictual nature of incestuous fantasies that reemerge during adolescence. Unlike the 4- to 6-year-olds, the young person by midadolescence is confronted with the reality that he or she now possesses the equipment

necessary for carrying out both sexual and aggressive wishes. The adolescent's provocative and battling stance toward the same-sex and both parents reflects renewed oedipal competition and repudiation of both oedipal and preoedipal longings. Disregard for family rules at this point may reflect desperate attempts to achieve emotional distance from parents. However, behaviors that ''test limits'' are now often implicit invitations for parents to remain involved and take charge; the adolescent's subsequent outrage maintains his or her explicit objection to any parental interference with his or her freedom.

The complexity and difficulties of family relations further stimulate and support the adolescent's activities outside of the home. He or she finds refuge from the claustrophobic pull of family ties in intellectual, athletic, musical, and political interests and potentially in illicit drug use, drinking, and crime as well. Similarly, as the adolescent withdraws from his or her parents, the intensity of the attachment to them is shifted to peer group relations, including same-sex and opposite-sex relationships. Opposite-sex pairing and dating serve as (*a*) sexual and emotional experiments in intimacy, (*b*) a gauge of masculinity and femininity, (*c*) an opportunity to try on (in reality as opposed to imaginative play) adult relationships, (*d*) an escape from fantasied or real incestuous and homosexual activity, or (*e*) a marker of conquest and competence, to be appreciated by an audience of peers. In addition to tighter affiliations with peers, social expectations and the push for mastering anxiety associated with dependency on parents spur the adolescent toward real independent functioning. In this the adolescent must recognize that the craving for independence implies truly relying on his or her own abilities rather than on parents.

By *late adolescence* (17–20+), involvement in relatively stable peer groups, academic and extracurricular activities and interests, some degree of financial reward for responsibilities associated with jobs, and the like reflect the adolescent's emancipation from the roles and requirements of earlier phases of development. The degree of successful engagement in life beyond the relationship with the parents may be a gauge of the extent to which the adolescent is able to emotionally disengage from and mourn the passing of his or her reliance on these powerful figures.

There is perhaps no more powerful example and test of the adolescent struggle for autonomy from parents—the breaking of preoedipal and oedipal ties—than the fantasied and real search for a new, typically heterosexual partnership. In late adolescence the young person is very aware of the difference between the love felt toward a new heterosexual partner and the earlier experiences of experimentation. The girl is no longer primarily interested in conquests or in simply owning and overpowering the man; the boy is no longer singularly guided by his need to prove his powers of seduction, his masculinity, and his repudiation of homosexual aims. Both are caught up in the desires that had been previously in the domain of oedipal fantasies. Longings for physical intimacy, for exclusive attachment, and to protect and be protected, to admire and be admired, can find full expression in the courtships of adolescence. This new experience of closeness and trust is the essential climate for surrender to the heterosexual partner in which earlier components of the attachment to parents—dependency, passivity, exclusivity, jealousy, physical intimacy, and so on—may be subsumed. Again, the extent to which these and other longings (such as unresolved childhood wishes to possess the anatomy and prerogatives or the opposite sex) remain predominantly and conflictally tied to their original objects, the parents, will determine option for and depth of new, heterosexual partnerships.

While many, and perhaps most, adolescents experience some degree of sexual interest in individuals of the same sex and may engage in some degree of arousing physical contact (such as mutual masturbation or sexual display), their fantasy lives and primary objects of sexual arousal are heterosexual. Typical homosexual experimentation occurs in the context of primarily heterosexual interests. During the usual course of development, heterosexual orientation appears to be based on biological factors that are shaped during gestation and the 1st months of life and that are reinforced by social experiences in the family and peer group, as well as the developmental sequences of the psychosexual phases. A sizeable number of adolescents, however, are primarily involved in thinking about and being aroused by individuals of the same sex; they are not turned on by individuals of the opposite sex. For some, the recognition of the direction of their attraction is clear during the earlier school-age years (latency); for others, the intensity and singularity of homosexual object choices become clear only during early adolescence or somewhat later. There are probably a variety of determinants of homosexual orientation in both males and females; biological factors have been suggested, as well as interactions between constitutional and familial patterns of interaction. There is also a range of variants of homosexuality in adolescence, which for clinical purposes need to be differentiated: Homosexuality may represent a defense against aggression or a negative resolution of oedipal conflicts (i.e., focusing longings for intimacy with the same-sex parent as a way of warding off anxiety associated with incestuous wishes involving the opposite-sex parent), it may be an exaggeration of bisexuality or emerge in specific environmental contexts (e.g., in seminaries or boarding schools), or it may represent the adolescent's immutable and well-integrated sexual orientation, as authentically a part of the adolescent's self as is heterosexuality.

The developmental tasks for homosexual adolescents are complicated by both internal and external factors. The youth's discovery that he or she is excited by and attracted to individuals of the same sex runs counter to what the adolescent may have expected and the experiences of his or her peer group. This feeling of being different compounds the usual feelings of estrangement and secrecy of adolescent sexual development. The homosexual adolescent also usually has no peer with whom to share, in locker room or girl-to-girl intimate chats, the emerging sense of being a sexual person. The homosexual adolescent also lacks socially sanctioned opportunities for sexual experimentation, for finding suitable intimacy, for using the pairing of adolescence to move away from the parental ties. In his or her loneliness, the homosexual adolescent may try to deny sexuality altogether and attempt to be celibate; may attempt to engage heterosexual friends in sexual relations that the other youngster feels initially are experimentation but that for the homosexual takes on more intense, crushlike importance; or may feel the need to engage in brief encounters that may be dangerous psychologically and with the increased risk of HIV infection (Isay, 1989).

The capacity for more mature, intimate relationships in the latter part of adolescence by no means guarantees their permanence. The task of consolidating the sense of self continues to find expression in shifting interests and ideals; the extent to which they mesh with those of the chosen partner will, in part, determine the success or failure of the relationship at any given time. In addition, the amount of emotional energy available for intimate ties with others may fluctuate as the adolescent becomes increasingly involved in making plans for the future. That these may involve the young person's physical departure from home and community often contributes to the ending of significant intimate relationships. Even more important is the adolescent's psychological departure from and break with the familiar, as he or she moves further into the realization of independent strivings and autonomous functioning. These are not without considerable practicing, uncertainty, and anxiety, as the adolescent anticipates the breadth or limitations—determined by individual strengths as well as multiple social factors—of opportunities available in the world beyond the family.

Adolescence has long been described as a period of inner turmoil in which the onslaught of biological changes, intensified sexual and aggressive urges, and shifting social relations and responsibilities make the search for a cohesive self a ubiquitous, crisis-laden struggle. Given the reality of the multiple variations in the appearance and behavior of teenagers observed on the streets and in the malls and schools of inner cities, working class neighborhoods, and upper-middle-class communities, can there be a central theory of adolescent development? While there are "typical" preschool- and school-age children, what can be said about adolescent development that is true to the tremendous varia-

tions seen in this period? The task of a psychoanalytic theory of adolescent development is to delineate those processes that (*a*) are generally found in adolescents, regardless of surface differences in behavior, and (*b*) allow for the broad variations in personal and social situations, explaining why adolescents operate in the context of their families and neighborhoods on the one hand, and in relation to their personal, inner lives on the other. While there are other approaches to understanding the problems and achievements of this phase of development, the psychoanalytic task is primarily to understand the meaning of the inner experiences of adolescents and their links to behavioral and life choices.

PSYCHOANALYTIC PHENOMENOLOGY OF ADOLESCENCE

From the psychoanalytic perspective, the phenomenology of adolescence centers around an array of reorganizations of inner life. The primary reorganization concerns the representation of the bodily and sexual experiences: Early in puberty the child initially feels that these new experiences are external to the self, but when all goes well, he or she gradually integrates the mature sexual body as a source of pride and pleasure. Concurrent with the reorganization of the representation of the body in its mature sexuality and size, there are psychological reorganizations in relation to drives (especially the modulation of aggression and the fusion between aggression and tenderness), values (especially the assumption of personal values that differ from those of parents), concepts of time (especially the adolescent's sense of having a personal history and a future that he or she can more or less envision), and the self and relations to others (especially the possibility for sharing intimate experiences outside the family and the giving and receiving of sexual pleasure). Each of these reorganizations rests upon the achievement of various preconditions during earlier phases of development, good enough physical and cognitive functioning, ongoing support from the family and other adults, particularly teachers, and good fortune in finding friends and avoiding irreparable injury.

While most adolescents do not experience psychiatric disorders (Rutter et al., 1976), this phase represents a period of increased prevalence of a broad range of psychiatric and behavioral disturbances, including affective disorders, anorexia, suicide, and accidents. For children who are vulnerable because of preexisting difficulties, such as chronic medical illness, emotional difficulties, cognitive delays, or the burdens of poorly resolved earlier neurotic conflicts, the entry into adolescence, with the push toward autonomy and new social expectations, may herald major upheavals in previously stable patterns of medical care or parent-child relations.

The Experience and Representation of the Body

Preoccupation with the body is a prominent characteristic of adolescence. Normal young adolescents devote considerable attention to ensuring its attractiveness to others. Yet the body may also be punished, mutilated, and destroyed by the adolescent who is experiencing turmoil. The balance between the adolescent's love and hatred for his or her body, between self-care and self-destruction, may shift rapidly, repeatedly, and precipitously. The adolescent will use his or her body as the stage for enacting pride or shame, joy or despair, a sense of being beautiful or of being horrid. The body may be seen as another, to be treated respectfully or thoughtlessly; as a persecutor, to be ignored or attacked; as a lover, to be caressed and narcissistically exhibited.

Psychologically, the adolescent may experience the rapid changes in his or her body in a passive mode that may reverberate with earlier experiences of humiliation or dependence. Here again, the adolescent may feel that he or she is forced to "learn to accept" what is not under his or her control. The adolescent may try to deny what is happening to his or her body and hold on to the interests and social forms of latency. Or he or she may feel comfortable with its increasing potentialities, secure that what nature has in store is consistent with previous good experiences. Or, most commonly, the adolescent may react to the changes in body and drives with a mixture of anxiety and exhilaration, of acceptance of what is in store along with a push toward mastery in which passive is turned into active. In trying to take active control over the passive experiences of puberty, the adolescent may try to improve upon nature—to decorate his or her body with hairdos, special clothing, makeup, and tattoos; to improve the appearance of the body's shapes by weight lifting, dieting, or gaining weight to increase muscle bulk; or to distort the body's appearance, to make what the child feels is passively weird (in his or her own eyes) into actually weird, through second-hand clothing, wild hair, multiple earrings, long hair, or whatever else the peer group, at a particular moment, has defined as hip, in, or cool. Through such stage design, the adolescent reorganizes his or her representation of the body and the meanings of its various parts in relation to others, including same- and opposite-sex peers and parents. When not carried too far, the experimentation allows the child to take responsibility, to own his or her body in its new form, smells, and modes of arousal.

For the vulnerable adolescent, the manipulation of the body as a thing may become a preoccupation. The adolescent may feel that life is unbearable because her nose is too long, his penis is too small, or she or he is too tall or too short. The reorganization of the body representation may also become enmeshed in the reorganization of family relations or other changes in self, leading, along with other determinants, to anorexia, bulimia, self-mutilation, or obesity. When the body becomes the expression of neurotic and intrafamilial conflicts, the reorganization of the self revolves around representations of the body: who owns the body, who is responsible for it, and who enjoys its pleasures and feels its attacks.

Sexuality: from Autoeroticism to Shared Intimacy

Psychoanalytic theory emphasizes the role of sexuality—of pleasurable experiences through the body—from the 1st months of life. Autoeroticism and sexuality continue throughout each of the psychosexual phases, with pleasures felt in specific zones (oral, anal, genital), and in the activity of the body and its musculature as a whole. Puberty heightens the role of sexuality in conscious and unconscious life and focuses sexual feelings on the genitals. As with sexuality in general, psychoanalytic theory recognizes the child's ability to provide himself or herself with sexual pleasures through his or her own activity and fantasy, from the 1st years of life. With puberty, sexual self-gratification through masturbation and self-regulated fantasy becomes central to the definition of selfhood and the relations between self and others. Adolescent masturbation is an achievement: It includes physical maturation and the capacity for erection/ejaculation or vaginal/clitoral orgasm, the capacity to imagine and sustain fantasies that are pleasurable enough to lead to climax, and the maturity to delay satisfaction, to plan for and carry out masturbatory activities at suitable, private times.

Adolescent masturbation, as a physical act, is accompanied by rich internal processes that have been conceptualized as "masturbatory fantasies." The adolescent is aware of the conscious story, major themes and images, and cast of characters. Often, these conscious elements are based on current experiences with peers, popular movie star images, and materials such as magazines and the like, as well as on powerful experiences that the adolescent may actually have had earlier (including beatings, active or passive sexual encounters, and primal scene fantasies and observations).

Psychoanalysts such as the Laufers (1987) have postulated that adolescents generally have a fixed and limited number of *central masturbatory fantasies*—fantasies that are not fully conscious or conscious at all and that underlie the structure or affects of the conscious fantasies. These central masturbatory fantasies may provide a paradigmatic form or emotional tone to the experienced or conscious fantasy—for example, sadomasochistic features, incestuous impulses, teasing, perversity, or passive longings—that may be uncomfortable or the source of anxiety within the conscious masturbatory experience. The central masturbatory fanta-

sies are integrative; they bring current sexual urges together with the child's earlier experiences with being cared for by the mother (tactile, oral, anal), his or her fantasies during the oedipal phase and in relation to primal scene, and the pleasures of genderized genitality and latency-age masturbation and excitements.

When development along the line from autoeroticism to adolescent sexuality has gone well, masturbation provides opportunities for rehearsing sexual behavior, expressing and receiving affection, and trying on the different active and passive roles needed for mutuality in love-making (including how to hold back on orgasm until just the right moment). Probably few adolescents are completely without guilt concerning masturbation; understanding the sources of this guilt reveals the ways in which adolescents may feel that sexuality is the appropriation of parental rights, that their fantasies run counter to their values, especially in relation to aggressively being out of control or oedipally prohibited. Adolescents who are too anxious about sexuality or too frightened by aspects of their masturbatory fantasies may try to abstain completely; other adolescents may compulsively and guiltily engage in masturbation, increasing their guilt and thus the tension that leads to masturbation. Through trying to titrate their involvement in masturbation, adolescents reorganize their representations of control over their sexual desires. They learn they can turn on, delay, and discharge their sexual feelings, more or less at will.

Reorganization of the Self

The "self" has many meanings: It can be understood theoretically as the locus for the integration of intention, abilities, desires, and values; as a mental structure that coordinates the other agencies of the mind; as an internal, conscious and unconscious "representation" of the individual's feelings, ambitions, and goals; or as a component of an individual's experience, quality of experience, and personal identity, which has continuity over time, space, and feeling states. The concept of self has a sense of individuality, distinctiveness, and boundaries—of the separateness of the person from others. Being true to oneself is a value, but self-valuation carried to self-preoccupation is self-absorption and selfishness at the expense of others. On the other hand, giving oneself to others and feeling other's needs as though they were one's own may be enriching of the self as long as one doesn't lose track of one's own self-interests. The concept of self is recursive, as captured by phenomena such as self-consciousness and self-awareness, as well as by processes such as taking, or not taking, care of oneself.

Adolescents take their selves seriously: They wonder who they really are, how they are different from their parents, how they became who they find themselves to be, what they are becoming. They enjoy losing themselves in crowds and finding themselves in "deep and meaningful" relationships. They search for their true values and refuse to compromise, fearful that any loss of the high ground will lead to the slippery slope of loss of their hard-earned individuality. They become abstractly conceptual, wondering about how their minds work, about their values, authenticity, and politics. They may feel that they are obligated and may even have the ability to make a difference, to reduce the suffering or wrongs of the world; or, just the opposite, they may explain to themselves that, "the world being the way it is," there is nothing they can do but simply get by, get even, go along, drop out, or have a good time. Whatever side of the polarity of involvement in the broader social world that they select, they are likely to think about their choices "philosophically," in categories of value and history rather than solely or consciously in relation to what their parents believe and they have been taught.

This reorganization of the self involves a heightened cathexis or direction of attention to the internal world (e.g., feeling states and impulses); alternations in the regulation of narcissism; and, concurrently, revaluation of relationships with friends and partners in intimacy (object relations). These closely intertwined processes are closely associated with sexuality. For example, the adolescent's experience of a crush—of the enchantment of another—at the same time expresses and affects several domains: The adolescent recognizes the power of the other; he or she feels a loss of self-sufficiency and self-control; he or she experiences an enhancement of self through fantasied union with the desired other. Through idealizations and crushes, the adolescent finds ways of dealing with the depressive feelings associated with loss of earlier relations with the parents. When these intertwined processes of reorganization are successful, and the adolescent is fortunate, the adolescent increasingly feels a consolidation of his or her personal identity as a sexual, competent, and reliable individual.

Relations with parents provide a testing ground and launching pad for the reorganization of the adolescent's self. By approaching his or her parents with worries and then striking out at them for intruding or not understanding, the adolescent, who may seem at such times to be paranoid, learns how far he or she has moved toward feeling secure in his or her own abilities to deal with impulses and frustration. Adolescents need to learn how far they can go on their own and also how they can return, when need be, to the security of the preadolescent relations with the father and mother. As they move away and back toward the dependency, adolescents may provoke battles about issues that are of relatively little obvious consequence. In the process of negotiating rules about when to be home at night, whether he or she has carried out the garbage as promised, and the appropriate length of hair or density of makeup, the adolescent boy and girl learn about the modulation of their rage at their parents (in their role as symbols of their own dependency longings) and whether the parents can survive their aggression (in their role as representatives of the adolescent's own abilities to hold together when overwhelmed). When parents break down under the pressure of unremitting aggression, adolescents do not feel victorious. They may feel panicked. And in their distress, they may feel compelled to attack, insisting that the parents be strong, or withdraw in an angry and depressive huff.

Within the family, the adolescent's struggle for self-definition may set off varied reverberations with parents. Parents may feel envious of the youngster's freedom and experimentation, particularly sexual freedoms, or may anxiously overreact to their fantasies of what their child is engaged in. The mother who pounds at the bathroom door when her son stays inside too long knows, and yet does not know, what has happened to her little boy. The sexually mature adolescent daughter may arouse incestuous fantasies in her father, who then, through projection and displacement, engages her defensively in battles about boyfriends and morality. Parents may establish rules that are harshly enforced as externalizations and barriers to the enactment of forbidden (and not fully unconscious) fantasies. Alternatively, parents may vicariously enjoy the exploits of adolescence and too easily relinquish the parental role; they may be too understanding or may implicitly encourage their child's promiscuity, drinking, and fast driving while explicitly condemning him or her for getting into trouble.

Adolescent Disturbances

The phenomenological processes of adolescence that move toward consolidation of the self in its many facets also are vulnerable to multiple different types of disorder, from within the adolescent's own bodily changes and mental processes and from the outside world.

There are special burdens to adolescent development that arise from the timing of puberty or its results: precocious puberty, which marks out a child as sexually mature or too tall before he or she is ready, or delayed puberty, which prevents a child from entering fully into the experiences of his or her peers in the discovery of sexuality. There are other burdens that represent the carrying over into adolescence of the sensitivities, conflicts, and poor resolutions of earlier phases: inability to tolerate frustration, predisposition to anxiety, tendency to deal with tension by impulsive activity, and lack of an internal sense of security in relations with parents and within the self. And there are burdens that arise specifically in response to the emergent issues of adolescence: the strength of sexual drives, the preoccupation with fantasies, guilt over sexuality and aggression, and troubles coping with the maturing body.

Given the complexity of the developmental tasks involved in reorga-

nization of the self and its representations of the body and others and the modulation of aggression, sexuality, and narcissism, it is no surprise that there is a marked increase in many psychiatric disorders concurrent with puberty. These include affective disorders, particularly depression; personality disorders, which reflect difficulties in self and object representations; disorders of appetite (such as anorexia and bulimia); and frank schizophrenia. Adolescents also demonstrate breakdowns that elude categorical diagnosis and include dramatic and life-threatening symptoms, in various combinations: self-destructiveness, brooding despair, complete social withdrawal, sexual promiscuity and perversity, addictions, immobilizing preoccupations, seeking out and experimenting with danger, and the like. Psychoanalytic investigation of these disorders involves placing the child's inner experiences in the context of his or her personal development and understanding the developmental meaning of the symptoms and activities. Since adolescents are often deeply interested in understanding the lives they are living, they can be engaged, as younger children may not, in reconstructing their histories and reflecting on their experiences; thus, therapeutic work may be in keeping with the developmental tasks faced by all adolescents of finding new representations through reorganization of the self.

Just as adolescence presents difficult tasks of development for each agency of the mind, the achievement of adolescence, as defined by the success of reorganizations, leaves the adolescent with a sense of pride and vigor. Competent, attractive adolescents evoke adult fantasies concerning youth and potentiality, as well as envy and yearning. The image of adolescence in literature—adventurous, seeking, seductive, vulnerable, and emotionally alive and open to new experience—captures the achievements of adolescence and also how the development of adolescents, as the next generation, is intertwined with that of their parents, as reminders of fulfilled longing as well as bearers of hope.

PSYCHOANALYTIC THEORY: DOMAIN, CONCEPTS, AND THEORETICAL INTENTIONS

The primary domain of psychoanalytic theory is the child's inner world, mental functioning, and internal experiences, as they elaborate over the course of development. Psychoanalysts are mostly interested in the personal, private, and intimate experiences of life—in emotions, feelings, thoughts, wishes, dreamlike states, daydreams, worries, yearnings, pleasures—and how the person becomes aware of these experiences, allows for their unfolding, pushes them outside of consciousness, shares and hides them. Secondarily, psychoanalysis is interested in behavior—in what children do—and the relations between the inner world and action, particularly how the child experiences his or her own action and the actions of others. Psychoanalysis focuses on the child's understanding of his or her own life, of the ways in which the child comes to represent and make sense of his or her inner world and the minds and actions of others. In these ways, psychoanalysis is particularly concerned with highly individualized, detailed, and rich descriptions of mental processes. The major concepts of psychoanalysis are aimed at providing categories and approaches for such descriptions, charting the major domains of experience over the course of development.

Closely related to this descriptive and in many ways historical undertaking, psychoanalytic theory also concerns origins and determinants. The "explanatory" theories of psychoanalysis consist of a range of perspectives, some of which are already outlined by Freud in his classical writings and others that have been described by theorists over the past decades. Freud's primary perspectives were the cathartic (the purging of the mental apparatus of negative experiences by abreaction, closely related to hypnosis and the so-called talking cures), economic (the distribution of psychic forces and the effects of their being pent up or discharged), dynamic (the conflict between wishes and prohibitions and their expression in symptoms), topographic (the distinction between conscious, preconscious, and unconscious mental processes), and structural (the functions of the ego, id, and superego) theories. These theories have been applied and remain useful within child psychoanalysis as well. They have been augmented by perspectives that emphasize development (the emergence of new structures and the changes in each of the classical perspectives over the course of maturation), developmental lines, the organizing role of the self, the importance of social relations (object relations), and the complexities of proverbial experience and mother-child relations.

Alongside the psychological perspectives to explanation or understanding of mental life, psychoanalytic theory has recognized the importance of general theories of psychology (Fonagy, 1991;Fonagy et al., 1993; Mayes and Cohen, 1994), originally conceptualized as autonomous ego functions and adaptation (Hartmann, 1939), and the role of biological processes—genetic (Peterson et al., 1995), endocrine (Moran, 1984; Moran and Fonagy, 1987), and constitutional (Mayes and Cohen, 1993)—and the general health and experiences of illness (Lewis, 1994; Moran, 1984) of the individual throughout the course of maturation.

The range of concepts within psychoanalysis is thus enormously broad, encompassing descriptive, historical, and narrative conceptions; multiple perspectives on causation and explanation; and associated conceptions of the roles of learning, adaptation, the environment, and the physical body in mental life. Core psychoanalytic concepts can be illustrated by the central role of conscious and unconscious fantasy as a common pathway for the representation and integration of experiences.

Within child psychoanalysis, conceptual disagreements have revolved around emphasis, timing, and the terminology used to describe normal development and its relationship to clinical phenomena. In this area, the contrasting views of Anna Freud and Melanie Klein and their adherents have been central in the development of child psychoanalytic theory.

With her monograph *The Ego and Mechanisms of Defense* (1966), Anna Freud (1895–1982) became a major contributor to the emerging field of ego psychology and established a new, developmental viewpoint on the broad range of mental functions (intellectualization, sublimation, displacement, reaction formation, identification, turning passive into active, humor, etc.) that individuals can mobilize to reduce anxiety, cope with psychic conflict, or modulate the pain associated with failures in the environment or in one's own achievements. Her work was closely related to the work of Heinz Hartmann, whose *Ego Psychology and the Problem of Adaptation* (1939) was the first systematic exposition of psychoanalytic ego psychology and the concept of the nonconflictual sphere of functioning (memory, reality testing, perception, etc.).

Over the course of decades, Anna Freud articulated a broad, descriptive approach to the charting of the course of children's development and the contributions of biological and experimental determinants. In particular, she emphasized the importance of direct observation and the need to relate theory to observable phenomena; she eschewed speculation about inner life and fantasies that could not be confirmed by the child's own constructions in play or speech. For Anna Freud, conflict among the agencies of mental functioning is not expressed only in symptoms but also in the course of adaptation. She conceptualized the mutually enriching roles of sexual and aggressive instinctual urges in many areas of life; these unfold in relation to the child's parents and the realities of the child's satisfactions and the quality and continuity of responsive caregiving. Anna Freud gave a role to anxiety and tensions as expectable during the course of development, with each developmental phase having modal developmental tasks and specific, normative types of anxiety. She strove to create a developmental point of view, analogous to Sigmund Freud's structural, dynamic, topographic, genetic, and adaptive viewpoints, that recognized that along with maturation there are changes in the functioning of the basic mechanisms of the mind (the functions of the ego, the available mechanisms of defense, the complexity and symbolization of fantasy, the experience of the superego and guilt, etc.). This developmental perspective distinguished disturbances of development (in the emergence of basic capacities for reality testing, memory, social relating, synchronization of functions, unfolding of cognitive abilities, and the physical apparatus) from disturbances that reflected internalized conflict and neurosis.

Psychoanalysts influenced by Klein have felt that Anna Freud was excessively interested in the "surface" markers of children's fantasy life, that she paid too much attention to the influence of the external world of the child, and that she overemphasized the role of adaptation in the course of development. In addition, Kleinian critics feel that Anna Freud undervalued the implications of primitive unconscious fantasies occurring in the 1st year of life and question the usefulness of her formulation in conducting "deeper" clinical work, particularly with the most severely disturbed patients. Indeed, throughout her career Anna Freud emphasized that the child patient continued to live within the family and that the realities of this life were critical to his or her psychological development, as were the realities of his or her physical and intellectual endowment. As such, the fantasy life of the child was described by Anna Freud as reflecting the mutual influences of factors from these domains and organized according to the unfolding hierarchy of mental functions.

Beginning her work in child analysis at roughly the same time as Anna Freud, Melanie Klein (1882–1960) emphasized that instinctual life was shaped from its initiation by the mother-child relationship, not only by the contributions of particular erotogenic zones, and that aggressive as well as sexual forces were operative from within the 1st months of life. Klein portrayed the inner life of infants as actively organizing their experiences of sexual and aggressive urges in specific and rich fantasies (Klein, 1984a, 1984b). She described the earliest phase of life in relation to "paranoid" feelings and being persecuted and the next phase centering around the child's "depressive" guilt for aggression directed at the mother (Klein, 1984b). The working through of this normal depressive phase was, in Klein's theory, an essential step in early development and was a continuing process at various points in life. An important aspect of working through the depressive position was not only acknowledgment of responsibility but also the psychological process of "reparation," of making amends to the fantasied mother who was the object of the infant's attacks. Unlike for Anna Freud, for Melanie Klein envy and jealousy as well as the components of the oedipal phase were present during the 1st year of life. In her broadest metapsychology, Klein adhered to and elaborated Freud's "dual instinct theory" of primary life (eros) and death (thanatos) drives and their instantiation in primitive emotional development, while other psychoanalysts have jettisoned Freud's conceptualization of the death instinct.

In large part, controversies stirred by Klein's work related to the precocious timetable she envisioned for the emergence of capacities for fantasy and complex conflict and to her use of pathological terms to describe normative developmental phenomena. Her ideas, however, provide psychoanalysis with an array of clinically useful constructs concerning fragmentation, splitting, projective identification, and the central role of aggression in fantasy as substrate for experiencing the world and organizing the self. Clinicians working with severely disturbed patients (such as schizophrenics) and in situations where individuals are regressed in their functioning (such as borderline patients in analysis and psychotherapy) have found her ideas especially useful.

At present, there is no fully integrated metapsychology that systematically relates the different levels and approaches to psychoanalytic explanation. Instead, the varying theories and concepts resemble a complex historical geography, rather like an atlas in which topographic, hydrological, agricultural, military, population, transportation, and other multicolored maps are presented, page after page. There is no single, correct map of the earth; rather, there are different maps for different purposes. Nor is there a unifying geography of the economic, dynamic, topographic, structural, and developmental contours of the mind over the course of individual development. Instead, psychoanalysis provides the explorer with varied sets of signposts and pathways, with assistance in finding one's way into and out of the otherwise overwhelmingly complex and confusing spaces of the child's inner life.

Psychoanalytic theory has perhaps made its major contributions in relation to understanding the difficulties of children suffering from emotional disorders. The validation of psychoanalytic understanding occurs most convincingly in the context of psychoanalytic therapy. In fact, much of psychoanalytic research has involved reporting clinical material from single cases or from groups of children with related problems. Critics argue, however, that psychoanalytic propositions employed in treatment have been developed with a lack of scientific rigor (Grunbaum,

1984; Kazdin, 1988; Popper, 1963). The broad justification for the use of single case narratives as a database for theory is that they provide a detailed account of the treatment process that is especially suitable for capturing the complexity, variation, and individuality of a particular child's inner life. The single case report generally attempts to highlight and explicate variables that are likely to be seen in other cases. Problems involved in demonstrating the generalizability of findings from single cases include (a) the reliability of the observations, (b) inability to replicate the findings by going back and looking again, and (c) how clinical material should be presented (e.g., verbatim accounts of single hours versus broad descriptive phenomenology versus an emphasis on metapsychological terminology) (Marans, 1989). Finding ways of reliably documenting observations for critical study is an important task for psychoanalytic investigators.

For the last several decades, academically oriented child analysts have recognized the limitations of the narrative, single case report and have attempted to develop (a) schemes for classifying and organizing data (e.g., the Hampstead index (Sandler, 1962) and the Hampstead Diagnostic Profile (A. Freud, 1965)), (b) controlled studies of psychoanalytic treatment and outcome (e.g., Heinecke and Ramsey-Klee, 1986; Moran and Fonagy, 1987), and (c) reliable ratings of children's presentations of clinical and experimental settings using direct observation and recording of children's sessions with analysts (e.g., Cohen et al., 1987; Marans et. al., 1993b). In a major study of over 700 hundred cases of child psychoanalysis and psychotherapy conducted at the Anna Freud Centre, charts were reviewed and assessed across multiple domains. Examining changes in DSM-III-R diagnoses and levels of adaptation as measured by the Children's Global Assessment Scale (CGAS), the study identified predictors of improvement and showed that severe or pervasive pathology requires intensive analytic treatment (Target and Fonagy, 1994). In addition to this retrospective chart review approach, researchers at the Anna Freud Centre have developed a manual of child psychoanalytic treatment and have devised a prospective, controlled study that will examine both process and outcome in three groups of treatment subjects.

Common to each of these research efforts is the development of measures that are based on operational definitions of theoretical constructs that are derived from clinical observations. Continued development of strategies that combine the use of narrative process notes, videotaped clinical encounters, manualized treatments, and the application of nonanalytic, standardized measures of diagnosis and adaptive functioning (e.g., the Vineland Adaptive Behavior Scales (Sparrow et al., 1984)) will further psychoanalytic efforts at investigating the developing mind of the child. As psychoanalytic knowledge continues to be enriched by detailed case reports, child psychoanalytic research has developed increasingly sophisticated approaches to systematic research methodology. However, enormous challenges remain as psychoanalytic researchers attempt to retain the breadth and complexity of the psychoanalytic conceptual system while trying to achieve greater clarity and precision in describing the phenomena associated with the inner life of the child as well as the child's experience of the external world.

In addition to its value within the field of psychotherapy, psychoanalytic theory has provided developmental psychology with many major concepts and hypotheses, including the central importance of early mother-child experiences, attachment and separation, the role of anxiety and mechanisms of defense in normal development, and the developmental point of view on emotions and internal representations of the self and others (Mayes et al., 1993). Systematic research outside of the therapeutic situation has supported the heuristic value of many of the concepts of psychoanalytic clinical theory. There is thus a mutual enrichment between the clinical and empathic study of individual children and rigorous research paradigms. In the future, psychoanalytic theory will continue to be elaborated by intensive, well-reported clinical investigation with individual children, as well as by advances within developmental biology and child development.

Similarly, the application of child psychoanalytic principles of development outside of the consulting room continues to lead to the creation of innovative programs and interventions that address a broad range of problems confronting children and their families. The legacy of applied psychoanalysis in the war nurseries operated by Anna Freud and her colleagues during World War II (Freud and Burlingham, 1954) is continued in the pioneering work of the School Development Project initiated by Dr. James Comer who has employed psychoanalytic principles of child development in a hugely successful program that engages parents, teachers, and mental health professionals in transforming schools into forums for enhancing self-esteem and family empowerment (Comer, 1990; Comer and Haynes, 1992). As a national model for collaboration between mental health and law enforcement professionals, the Child Development-Community Policing Program, trains police officers in psychoanalytic principles of development and human functioning and establishes a 24-hour/day consultation service for children exposed to community violence. The program extends the effectiveness of police professionals in their interactions with children and families while increasing the knowledge of their psychoanalytic colleagues about the psychological phenomena associated with violent trauma and about new ways of delivering psychological services for inner-city children and families (Marans and Cohen, 1993; Marans, 1994). Similarly, psychoanalytic attention paid to victims of violence and abuse (Pynoos, 1988, 1989; Terr, 1991) and international work with children caught up in the terror of war (Garberino, 1992; Simon and Apfel, in press) have made enormous contributions to our understanding of the developmentally specific and complex phenomena associated with trauma and posttraumatic stress disorder. Where the work of the Robertsons and Edith B. Jackson was responsible for the ways in which we view and deal with the hospitalizations of pediatric patients (Robertson and Robertson, 1958), the development of consultation liaison services as part of standard pediatric practice (Lewis, 1991, 1994) continues to draw on and develop our understanding of the synergistic relationship between physical and psychological health.

The field of child psychoanalysis encompasses a broad range of clinical inquiry, theoretical conceptualizations, and their applications drawing on detailed observations of the interaction of endowment, maturational and developmental forces, affect regulation, cognitive capacities, and social relationships. Whether the psychoanalyst meets with the child in the consulting room, on pediatric wards, in institutional settings, in custody/placement evaluations, or on the streets of our inner cities, the work is defined by an appreciation of the complex relationship between the inner life of urges, conflicts, defenses, and sense of self that are represented in fantasy, modes of relating, behavior, and adaptive capacities. By attending to the details of the children's experience of themselves and their perspectives of the world and others, psychoanalysts will continue to contribute to our knowledge about the developing mind of the child and enhance the ways in which clinical practice, program development, and social policy optimize children's developmental potential.

Acknowledgments. *The authors wish to express their gratitude to Drs. Robert Evans, Allen Marans, and Albert Solnit for their contributions.*

References

Anthony EJ: The family and the psychoanalytic process in children. *Psychoanal Study Child* 35:3, 1980.

Blos P: *On Adolescence.* New York, Free Press, 1962.

Blos P: *The Young Adolescent.* New York, Free Press, 1970.

Bornstein B: On latency. *Psychoanal Study Child* 6:279, 1951.

Bornstein B: Fragments of an analysis of an obsessional child. *Psychoanal Study Child* 8:313, 1953.

Bowlby J: *Attachment and Loss.* Vol 1: *Attachment.* New York, Basic Books, 1969.

Bowlby J: *Attachment and Loss.* Vol 2: *Separation.* New York, Basic Books, 1973.

Burgner M, Edgcumbe R: Phallic-narcissistic phase: A differentiation. *Psychoanal Study Child* 30: 161, 1975.

Burlingham D: To be blind in a sighted world. *Psychoanal Study Child* 34:5, 1979.

Cohen D, Marans S, Dahl K, et al: Analytic discussions with oedipal children. *Psychoanal Study Child* 45:89, 1987.

Comer JP: African-American children and the school. In: Lewis M (ed): *Child and Adolescent Psychiatry: A Comprehensive Textbook*. Baltimore: Williams & Wilkins, 1991, pp. 1084–1091.

Comer JP, Haynes NM: Helping black children succeed: The significance of some social factors. In: Lomotey K (ed): *Going to School: The African American Experience*. Albany, NY, State University of New York Press, 1990, pp. 103–112.

Earle E: The psychological effects of mutilating surgery. *Psychoanal Study Child* 34:527, 1979.

Emde R: Toward a psychoanalytic theory of affect. In: Greenspan S, Pollock G (eds): *Infancy and Early Childhood*. Washington, DC, National Institute of Mental Health, 1982.

Erikson E: *Identity and the Life Cycle*. New York, International Universities Press, 1959.

Fonagy P, Steele M, Moran G, et al: Measuring the ghost in the nursery: An empirical study of the relation between parents' mental representations of childhood experiences and their infants' security of attachment. *J Am Psychoanal Assoc* 41(4):957–989, 1993.

Fonagy P, Steele M, Steele H, et al: The capacity for understanding mental states: The reflective self in parent and child and its significance for security of attachment. Special Issue: The effects of relationships on relationships. *Infant Ment Health J* 12(3):201–218, 1991.

Fraiberg S: *The Origins of Intelligence in Children*. New York, International Universities Press, 1952.

Fraiberg S: *The Magic Years*. New York, Scribner, 1959.

Fraiberg S: *Insights from the Blind*. New York, Basic Books, 1968.

Freud A: Indications for child analysis. *Psychoanal Study Child* 1:127, 1945.

Freud A: The role of bodily illness in the mental life of children. *Psychoanal Study Child* 7:42, 1952.

Freud A: Adolescence. *Psychoanal Study Child* 13:255, 1958.

Freud A: *The Writings of Anna Freud*. Vol 6: *Normality and Pathology*. New York, International Universities Press, 1965.

Freud A: *The Writings of Anna Freud*. Vol 2: *The Ego and Mechanisms of Defense*. New York, International Universities Press, 1966. (Originally published 1936.)

Freud A: On certain difficulties in the pre-adolescent relation to his parents. In: *The Writings of Anna Freud* (Vol 4). New York, International Universities Press, 1968. (Originally published 1949.)

Freud A, Burlingham D: Infants without families. In: *The Writings of Anna Freud* (Vol 3). New York, International Press, 1973.

Freud S: A childhood recollection from Dichtung and Wahrheit. In: Strachey J (ed): *The Standard Edition of the Complete Psychological Works of Sigmund Freud* (Vol 17). London, Hogarth Press. (Originally published 1917.)

Freud S: Beyond the pleasure principle. In: Strachey J (ed): *The Standard Edition of the Complete Psychological Works of Sigmund Freud* (Vol 18). London, Hogarth Press, 1974a. (Originally published 1920.)

Freud S: On narcissism. In: Strachey J (ed): *The Standard Edition of the Complete Psychological Works of Sigmund Freud* (Vol 14). London, Hogarth Press, 1974b. (Originally published 1914.)

Furman E, Solnit AJ, Lang JL, et al: Symposium:

Child analysis and pediatrics. *Int J Psychoanal* 49:276, 1968.

Garbarino J, Dunbrow N, Kostelny K, et al: *Children in Danger: Coping with the Consequences*. San Francisco, Jossey-Bass, 1992.

Goldstein J, Freud A, Solnit AJ: *Beyond the Best Interests of the Child*. New York, Free Press, 1973.

Goldstein J, Freud A, Solnit AJ, et al: *Before the Best Interests of the Child*. New York, Free Press, 1979.

Goldstein J, Freud A, Solnit AJ, et al: *In the Best Interests of the Child*. New York, Free Press, 1986.

Greenacre P: The childhood of the artist: Libidinal phase development and giftedness. *Psychoanal Study Child* 12:27, 1957.

Grunbaum A: *The Foundations of Psychoanalysis*. Berkeley, CA, California University Press, 1984.

Hartmann H: *Ego Psychology and the Problem of Adaptation*. New York, International University Press, 1939.

Heinicke C, Ramsey-Klee DM: Outcome of child psychotherapy as a function of frequency of session. *J Am Acad Child Adolesc Psychiatry* 25:247–253, 1986.

Hoffer W: Mouth, hand and ego integration. *Psychoanal Study Child* 3/4:49, 1949.

Isay R: *Being Homosexual: Gay Men and Their Development*. New York, Farrar, Straus, Giroux, 1989.

Kasdin A: *Child Psychotherapy*. New York, Pergamon, 1988.

Kestenberg J: On the development of maternal feelings in early childhood. *Psychoanal Study Child* 11:257, 1956.

Kestenberg J: Eleven, twelve, thirteen: Years of transition. In: Pollock G, Greenspan S (eds): *The Course of Life* (Vol 2). Washington, DC, National Institute of Mental Health, 1980.

Klaus M, Kennel J: *Maternal-Infant Bonding*. St. Louis, Mosby, 1976.

Klein M: On the development of mental functioning. *Int J Psychoanal* 39:84, 1958.

Klein M: *Envy and Gratitude and Other Works 1946–1969*. London, Hogarth Press, 1984a.

Klein M: *Love, Guilt and Reparation and Other Works 1921–1945*. London, Hogarth Press, 1984b.

Laufer M: Adolescence and psychosis. *Int J Psychoanal* 67:267, 1985.

Laufer M, Laufer E: *Adolescence and Developmental Breakdown*. New Haven, CT, Yale University Press, 1987.

Lewis M: Introduction to hospital consultation-liaison in pediatrics. In: Lewis M (ed): *Child and Adolescent Psychiatry: A Comprehensive Textbook*. Baltimore: Williams & Wilkins, 1991, pp. 941–944.

Lewis M: Consultation process in child and adolescent psychiatric consultation-liaison in pediatrics. In: Lewis M, King R (eds): *Consultation-Liaison in Pediatrics, Child and Adolescent Psychiatric Clinics of North America*. Philadelphia, Saunders, 1994, pp. 439–448.

Mahler M, Pine F, Bergmann A: *The Psychological Birth of the Human Infant*. New York, Basic Books, 1975.

Marans S: Psychoanalytic psychotherapy with children: Current research trends and challenges. *J Am Acad Child Adolesc Psychiatry* 28:669–674, 1989.

Marans S: From enactment to play to discussion: The analysis of a young girl. In: Solnit AJ, Neubauer PB, Cohen DJ (eds): *The Many Meanings of Play in Child Psychoanalysis*. New Haven, CT, Yale University Press, 1993b, pp. 183–200.

Marans S: Community violence and children's development: Collaborative interventions. In: Chi-

land C, Young JG (eds): Northvale, NJ, Aaronson, 1994, pp. 109–124.

Marans S, Cohen DJ: Children and inner-city violence: Strategies for intervention. In: Leavitt L, Fox N (eds): *Psychological Effects of War and Violence on Children*. Hillsdale, NJ, Erlbaum, 1993, pp. 218–301.

Marans S, Dahl K, Marans W, et al: Discussion with oedipal children: Aggressivity in play. In: Solnit AJ, Neubauer PB, Cohen DJ (eds): *The Many Meanings of Play in Child Psychoanalysis*. New Haven, CT, Yale University Press, 1993c, pp. 275–296.

Marans S, Mayes LC, Colonna A: Psychoanalytic views of children's play. In: Solnit AJ, Neubauer PB, Cohen DJ (eds): *The Many Meanings of Play in Child Psychoanalysis*. New Haven, CT, Yale University Press, 1993a, pp. 9–28.

Mayes LC: Investigations of learning processes in infants. *Semin Perinatol* 13:437, 1989.

Mayes LC, Cohen DJ: The role of constitution in psychoanalysis. In: Moore B (ed): *Concepts in Psychoanalysis*, New Haven, CT, Yale University Press, 1995, pp. 271–272.

Mayes LC, Cohen DJ: The social matrix of aggression: Enactments and representation of loving and hating in the first years of life. *Psychoanal Study Child* 48:150, 1993.

Mayes LC, Cohen DJ, Klin A: Desire and fantasy: A psychoanalytic perspective on theory of mind and autism. In: Baron-Cohen S, Tager-Flusberger H, Cohen DJ (eds): *Understanding Other Minds: Perspectives from Autism*. Oxford University Press, London, 1993.

Meers D: Ghetto culture, symptom formation and ego anomalies in childhood. *Psychoanal Study Child* 25:209, 1970.

Moran G: Psychoanalytic treatment of diabetic children. *Psychoanal Study Child* 39:407, 1984.

Moran G: Psychoanalytic treatment of diabetic children. *Psychoanal Study Child* 39:407–447, 1984.

Moran G, Fonagy P: Psychoanalysis and diabetic control. *Br J Med Psychol* 60:357–372, 1987.

Neubauer P: The many meanings of play: Introduction. *Psychoanal Study Child* 42:3, 1987.

Peller L: Libidinal phases, ego development and play. *Psychoanal Study Child* 9:148, 1954.

Peterson B, Leckman J, Cohen D: Tourette's syndrome: A genetically predisposed and an environmentally specified developmental psychopathology. In: Cicchetti D, Cohen D (eds): *Developmental Psychopathology Theory: Methods* (Vol 1). 1995.

Piaget J: *The Origins of Intelligence in Children*. New York, International Universities Press, 1952.

Piaget J: *The Construction of Reality in Children*. New York, Basic Books, 1954.

Popper K: *Conjectures and Refutations*. New York, Basic Books, 1963.

Provence S, Lipton R: *Infants in Institutions*. New York, International Universities Press, 1962.

Pynoos RS, Nader K: Psychological first aid and treatment approaches to children exposed to community violence: Research implications. *J Traumatic Stress* 1(4):455–473, 1988.

Pynoos RS, Nader K: Children's memory and proximity to violence. *J Am Acad Child Adolesc Psychiatry* 28(2):236–241, 1989.

Ritvo S: Images and uses of the body in psychic conflict: Adolescent eating disorders. *Psychoanal Study Child* 39:449, 1984.

Robertson J, Robertson J: *Young Children in Hospital*. New York, Basic Books, 1958.

Rutter M, Graham P, Chadwick O, et al: Adolescent turmoil: Fact or fiction? *J Child Psychol Psychiatry* 17:35, 1976.

Sandler J: Hampstead Index as an instrument of psychoanalytic research. *Int J Psychol* 43:287, 1962.

Sandler J, Joffe W: The concept of the representational world. *Psychoanal Study Child* 17:128, 1962.

Sandler J, Kennedy H, Tyson R, et al: Discussions on transference: The treatment situation and technique in child psychoanalysis. *Psychoanal Study Child* 30:409, 1975.

Schowalter J, Lord R: On the writings of adolescents in a general hospital ward. *Psychoanal Study Child* 27:181, 1972.

Simon B, Apfel R (eds): *Minefields in Their Hearts: The Mental Health of Children in War and Communal Violence*. New Haven, CT, Yale University Press, in press.

Solnit AJ: A psychoanalytic view of play. *Psychoanal Study Child* 42:205, 1987.

Solnit AJ, Nordhaus B, Lord R: *When Home is No Haven*. New Haven, CT, Yale University Press, 1992.

Sparrow S, Balla DA, Cicchetti D: *Vineland Adaptive Behavior Scales*. Circle Pines, MN, American Guidance Service, 1984.

Spits R: Hospitalism: An inquiry into the genesis of psychiatric conditions in childhood. *Psychoanal Study Child* 1:53, 1945.

Spitz R: *The First Year of Life*. New York, International Universities Press, 1965.

Stern D: *The Interpersonal World of the Infant*. New York, Basic Books, 1985.

Target M, Fonagy P: Efficacy of psychoanalysis for children with emotional disorder. *J Am Acad Child Adolesc Psychiatry* 33(3):361–371, 1994.

Terr LC: Childhood traumas: An outline and overview. *Am J Psychiatry* 148(1):10–20, 1991.

Winnicott DW: *The Maturational Process and the Facilitating Environment*. New York, International Universities Press, 1965.

Winnicott DW: *Playing and Reality*. New York, Basic Books, 1971.

13 TEMPERAMENT

Stella Chess, M.D., and Alexander Thomas, M.D.

Recent decades' major studies of normal and pathological development have clearly identified the importance of empirical and theoretical formulations of temperament. Every professional worker who needs to understand the behavioral patterns of any person—infant, toddler, school-age child, adolescent, young adult, or adult of later years—must have knowledge of the role of an individual's temperament characteristics. Clinical professionals who specialize in working with children, in line with the findings of contemporary research, must identify and attend to temperament for many reasons: child psychiatrists, to aid in the conceptualization, prevention, and treatment of behavior disorders; educators, to devise strategies to facilitate children's and adolescents' school functioning and the education of handicapped children; pediatricians and nurses, to promote successful medical management (Chess and Thomas, 1986).

A committee of the Institute of Medicine has emphasized an additional reason for the importance of temperament research: "Recent attention to biologically endowed characteristics of children and an emphasis on children's contribution to their own development have led to tremendous research emphasis on early temperament . . . . Temperamental qualities are important because they promise to link genetic and neurophysiologic characteristics with socially relevant behavioral patterns" (Institute of Medicine, 1989, p. 77).

This chapter's discussion of the importance of temperament has three major foci. First is the summary of our methods of data collection and the identification, definition, and ratings of distinct categories of temperament. We then report the empirical findings on the significance of temperament categories for normal and deviant psychological development. Some theoretical and practical implications of these findings are indicated. In addition, the studies of developmental psychiatrists, psychologists, pediatricians, educators, and nurses in recent years confirming our findings are presented (Carey and McDevitt, 1989; Chess and Thomas, 1986; Porter and Collins, 1982).

The second section deals with the wealth of new data produced by a growing number of research units and workers who have raised controversial methodologic and conceptual questions related to our own findings and basic formulations. A number of these controversies and challenges to our initial methods and concepts of temperament are summarized. The final section concludes the chapter with ideas on new research directions.

OUR BASIC FINDINGS, THEIR UNDERLYING CONCEPTS, AND THE IMPLICATIONS OF TEMPERAMENT

Our interest in the study of temperament arose primarily from our practice in the 1940s and early 1950s. At that time, the dominant theo-

retical formulations attributed exclusive etiologic importance for both healthy and pathologic psychological development to environmental forces—first and foremost the influence of the mother or other primary caretaker. Depending on one's particular conceptual viewpoint, also included were other intrafamilial and extrafamilial environmental factors. Individual differences in behavioral style, a phenomenon evident even in the neonate and young infant, were, with few exceptions, either ignored, minimized, or categorized as secondary reactive effects on the caretakers' attitudes and practices.

However, as clinicians, we saw many cases in which this one-sided environmentalist approach could not, at least to our satisfaction, explain adequately the child's, adolescent's, or adult's personality structure or developmental course. Beyond the influence of family and the larger environment, something was missing. It was our hypothesis that at least one significant gap in our clinical evaluations resulted from failure to assign the child an active as well as a reactive role. Development then would reflect the continuous dynamic interaction between the individual and the environment at all age periods.

These clinical experiences made it imperative to initiate a systematic study of individual behavioral styles. The literature revealed many pertinent reports of specific aspects of behavioral individuality, but none that had attempted a systematic comprehensive study of this phenomenon or provided a methodology adequate for such an endeavor (Thomas et al., 1968, pp. 5–8). It was clear to us that a prospective longitudinal study was required, from which we could gather data of sufficient scope and pertinence to test our hypothesis. With this commitment, we launched the New York Longitudinal Study (NYLS) in 1956.

We conceptualized temperament as representing the *how*, or style of behavior, as contrasted to the *why*, or motivations and goals of behavior, and the *what*, or perceptions, abilities, and talents of the individual. Two children may dress themselves or ride a bicycle with the same dexterity and have the same motives for engaging in this behavior. Two adolescents may display similar learning ability and intellectual interests, and their academic roles may coincide. Two adults may show the same reason for devoting themselves to their jobs. These behaviors reflect their motivations and abilities. Yet these two children, adolescents, or adults may differ significantly with regard to the quickness with which they move; the ease with which they approach a new physical environment, social situation, or task; and the effort required by others to distract them when they are absorbed in an activity. These variations reflect differences in their temperament characteristics. Or, in other instances, temperaments may be similar, and abilities or motivations may differ. This analysis of behavior into the *how, why,* and *what* had also been suggested by several developmental psychologists, especially by Cattell (1950), and Guilford (1959), and a number of important studies of motivations and abilities had been undertaken by them and other workers. But investigations of the nature and significance of temperament and of the relationship of temperament to motivations were still lacking.

Methodology

Our research into temperament required an anterospective longitudinal study, that is, the gathering and analysis of behavioral data on the same group of children at sequential age periods. By contrast, cross-sectional studies evaluate matched samples of same-age subjects. They then study other age periods through examination of other samples of different ages. Such studies can identify group trends on one or more variables over time, but they cannot trace the developmental course of individual subjects over time. For example, a series of cross-sectional studies may show a certain average change in a specific variable from one age period to another. But with this method, one subject may change from high to low over time, another from low to high, and still another show no change. The cross-sectional study cannot identify such differences in individuals over time and cannot, therefore, identify and analyze patterns of continuity and change in a behavioral attribute, such as temperament, in any given person. Only a longitudinal study, which follows the developmental course of the same group of subjects over time, can hope to explore individual patterns of change and continuity and their meaning.

A prospective study, in which data are collected at the time or very close to the time of their occurrence, is also essential. A number of studies have revealed significant distortions in the accuracy of parents' retrospective reports on the early behavioral history of their children, even when the child's development has been normal (Haggard et al., 1963; Robbins, 1963; Wenar, 1963). The problem is the same with adults' recall of their earlier life. Vaillant (1977) reports this vividly from his findings of the Harvard Grant Study: "How then may we obtain truth about the adult life cycle? Clearly, it must be studied prospectively. It is all too common for caterpillars to become butterflies and then to maintain that in their youth they had been little butterflies. Maturation makes liars of us all" (p. 197).

The Parent as a Source of Research Data

In starting the NYLS, we had to determine the nature and source of our raw data. We consulted the literature, several sophisticated research neuropsychologists, and developmental psychologists, without success. The answer came, as so often happens, when our first approach failed. We instructed a group of parents to apply a simple procedure that would, we thought, form individual reflex patterns for their newborns. This did not succeed. Each parent followed this method and reported to us the details of each infant's reactions. As the parents talked about their babies' behaviors during sleep, feeding, and other daily routines, a clear picture of individuality in these newborns did emerge. This gave us the opportunity to devise questions and listening skills needed to turn generalities and subjective statements into specifics and objective data.

It became clear to us that the primary child caregivers, usually the parents, were indeed a unique and comprehensive source of information on their infants' behavioral styles. The parents, with their continuous involvement with their infants, could observe and report to us on all the details of their babies' behavior within all the routines of daily life. They could also describe the child's sequence of reactions to anything new and different—the first bath, a new food, a stranger, an illness, a move to a new home, and so on. By contrast, an outside observer coming into the home for a few hours could catch only a slice of the overall behavioral repertoire of the child, and that slice might not even be typical if some unusual situation and stimulus had just occurred.

But parents can be biased in their perception and interpretation of their child's behavior and in how they report it. Our interview protocol therefore focused on obtaining detailed, factual, and descriptive items of behavior. For example, if a mother reported, "He doesn't like cereal," we would press her gently and firmly for a detailed description of exactly how the baby behaved to make the mother conclude that he "didn't

like cereal." We also paid special attention in our interview protocol to any new events in the child's life. Here, we did not stop with the description of the child's initial reaction to the new but also asked, "What did you (the parent) do when the baby responded so-and-so?" and then, "How did the baby respond to what you did?" and then, "What did you do next?" and so on until the whole sequence of the child's reaction to the new and the parent's handling of this reaction had been reported. In this way we obtained richly detailed data not only on the child's behavior but also on the parents' patterns of child care.

Originally, we explored the possibility of obtaining data from the neonatal period onward. However, a pilot study, confirmed by a search of the literature, showed that the newborn infant's behavior varied significantly from day to day, even from hour to hour. Data collection and analysis at that age would be an exceedingly demanding and complex process. We further determined that the infant's behavioral characteristics usually began to show definiteness and consistency of patterning between the 4th and 8th week of life. Therefore, our initial interview with the parents was scheduled when the child was 2–3 months of age.

We gathered the NYLS sample over a period of 5 years, starting in 1956. The families were obtained through personal contact and included only if they were willing to participate in the study for at least a 10-year period. (But, in fact, all the parents have cooperated with our project for many years.) We included younger children born to families in the study, if this occurred during the period of our sample collection. The inclusion of siblings made possible a number of comparisons of the development of brothers and sisters growing up in the same household.

The sample comprised middle- and upper-middle-class families living in the New York areas, and with a few exceptions, all the parents were born in the United States. Such a homogeneous sociocultural group was desirable for the study of innate behavioral differences in the children because it minimized the influences that could be introduced by substantial sociocultural variability. The use of such a homogeneous group does not, of course, eliminate differences in environmental influences. Our study protocols did give appropriate attention to such phenomena as trauma, unusual events, and idiosyncratic parental attitudes. In a heterogeneous group it would have been more difficult to decide whether observed individual differences in behavior resulted from differences in temperament or differences in sociocultural background.

On the other hand, the use of a relatively homogeneous sample limits the possibility of generalizing the findings to other populations of different economic, cultural, and racial status. To deal with this issue, we initiated a second longitudinal study of 95 children born in New York of unskilled and semiskilled working-class Puerto Rican families. This group was also followed longitudinally from early infancy through childhood, using the same approach to data collection and analysis as in the NYLS. In addition, a number of projects based upon our findings have been undertaken in research centers in this country and abroad, utilizing a variety of populations with significant sociocultural differences from our NYLS subjects. These studies, as well as our own Puerto Rican population project, have made possible a number of significant comparisons with the NYLS study, as will be indicated below. In the discussion of our findings that follows, the reports will be from our major study, the NYLS, unless otherwise indicated.

Data Collection

Our original NYLS sample comprised 138 children from 85 families. Five subjects were lost to the study after one or two interviews in the infancy period, when the families moved to areas distant from New York, and our resources did not allow us to travel to their new homes. None of the data from these five infants was used in any of our analyses. No further attrition of the sample occurred until the present follow-up of the sample in their mid- and late twenties, when four subjects dropped out for personal reasons. This gives us a retention rate of 97% over this 25–30-year period. All the other 129 subjects and their parents have continued to be fully cooperative with our interviews and other procedures.

Our semistructured parent interviews were conducted at 3-month intervals during the first 18 months of life, then at 6-month intervals until 5 years of age, and then yearly until 8 or 9 years of age. In adolescence the subjects were interviewed directly and their parents separately, and the same procedures were followed in the 18- and 22-year age period. In the most recent follow-up the subjects were interviewed again, but not their parents, because at this age period the subjects now live mostly away from their parents. We judged that by this time most parents would not have the wealth of data to supply that they had in the childhood and adolescent years.

Data were also collected from nursery schools, kindergarten, and the 1st grade, through yearly interviews with teachers and yearly school observations lasting 1–2 hours, conducted by one of our staff members sitting in a corner of the classroom.

Standard psychometric testing was carried out when each child was 3 years old and again at 6 years. A running account of the child's behavior and verbal responses to the testing was made by a staff observer seated in the rear of the testing room. This procedure permitted us to gain standard IQ scores and also to record the style of the child's responses to the demands for task performance made by the sequential items of the psychometric test.

When each child was 3 years old, a special structured interview to elicit information regarding parental practices and attitudes was held in the child's home with the mother and father, separately but simultaneously. These interviews were collected and taped by two staff members who had no previous contact with the parents. Immediately following the interviews, the interviewers rated each parent on a number of categories related to parental attitudes and practices.

THE CLINICAL SAMPLE

A major goal of the NYLS was the determination of the functional significance of temperament for the origins and evolution of behavior disorders. At the time, each parent was told that the research staff included an experienced child psychiatrist (S.C.) who would be ready to provide psychiatric consultation and advice if behavioral difficulties of any kind occurred at any point in the child's development. Thus, whenever a parent or teacher expressed concern about some aspect of the child's behavior, the interviewer immediately transmitted this information to the child psychiatrist. Not every child whose behavior was brought to notice in this way was clinically studied. In many instances the reported problems represented age-specific behaviors that, though troublesome, were not deviant. In some of these cases, it appeared clear that the problem was a simple one that involved the parents' unintentional inappropriate routines in managing the child. In such instances, parents accepted simple suggestions from the psychiatrist, transmitted through the interviewer, and modified their undesirable child care practices. As a result, both the "problem" and the parental concerns disappeared.

In other cases, however, the parents would or could not carry out such simple recommendations, and the child's undesirable patterns of functioning persisted or became worse. When this happened, a standard clinical evaluation was conducted in a manner identical with a standard consultation, as it would be carried out either with a private patient or with a case presenting at a child guidance clinic. In 75% of the cases, both parents participated in the clinical workup, but in the remainder only the mother was seen, because of either the father's unavailability or refusal to attend.

Special neurological or psychological studies were undertaken when a child's history and the psychiatric findings made this advisable. If the presenting complaint involved aspects of school or nursery school functioning, the teachers were reinterviewed, and additional observations of the child were carried out in the school setting.

When such a clinical evaluation indicated the presence of a significant behavior problem, a diagnosis was made, including severity. When the American Psychiatric Association DSM-III-R categories became available, all diagnoses were formulated to correspond to that manual.

Following the diagnostic evaluation, the child's anterospective information was reviewed, available by virtue of the child's having been a par-

ticipant in the longitudinal study. No diagnosis was changed because of this review, but in each case, the formulation of the dynamics, of the pathogenic child-environment interaction, and the ontogenesis of the behavior problem was derived from a composite of clinical and research information. A decision was then made as to the advisability of direct treatment of the child, parent guidance, or other patterns of therapeutic intervention, and the choice was then suggested to the parents and arranged.

Though our routine data collection protocols did not involve the gathering of new data between the middle childhood period and adolescence, we did pursue a continuing evaluation of each clinical case at regular intervals. This special follow-up was discontinued only if the child showed a complete and sustained recovery from his or her difficulties.

Data Analysis

There are two basic methods of research data analysis: the qualitative (clinical) and the quantitative. The qualitative approach has been traditionally utilized in psychiatry and other fields of medicine, as well as in psychology, biology, and epistemology; to name only a few, there are Darwin, Pasteur, Bernard, Virchow, Kraepelin, Freud, Bleuler, and Piaget. Since by virtue of our training and practice as clinicians we shared this research tradition, our data collection was primarily qualitative: parent and teacher interviews, narrative description of the child's behavior at school and during an IQ test, and special interviews with the parent when the child was 3 years old. In other words, our primary data were not obtained through scores or other methods of quantitative ratings. The rigors and restrictions of such primarily quantitative methods of data collection would have precluded the identification of meaningful subtleties in the developmental course of individual children.

However, we realized that our qualitative studies of the NYLS information also required the analytic power of statistical methods to provide reliable comparisons of quantitative ratings from different sources of data and at different periods. We were clear that both objective qualitative and quantitative ratings were necessary to identify consistencies and changes in any child's characteristics over time and to trace the vicissitudes of and influences on the child's developmental course. We ourselves could not accomplish the task of converting our qualitative data into quantitative scores. We turned to Dr. Herbert Birch, who had already achieved a brilliant career through behavioral studies that involved both qualitative and quantitative analysis. Dr. Birch conducted an inductive content analysis (essentially a qualitative procedure) of the four parent interview protocols of each of our first 22 NYLS subjects for the 1st year of life. He defined nine categories of temperament, established scoring criteria for each category, and determined a method of rating each item of behavior in each interview. He formulated the criteria for a three-point rating scale for each item (high, medium, low). The item scores for each category for each subject in any one interview were combined and then divided by the total number of items to give a weighted score.

It is of interest that almost all the nine categories defined independently by Dr. Birch corresponded closely to our formulations by our qualitative study of parent interviews. Dr. Birch added several categories of interest that we had not identified, such as rhythmicity and sensory threshold. His unique contribution served to transform our narrative data into categories with precise definitions and criteria for the scoring of behavioral items that could then be rated quantitatively for each temperament category. This then made our many quantitative and qualitative data analyses possible as our longitudinal study progressed and gathered meaningful data at sequential age periods of our NYLS and related studies. Dr. Birch himself continued as a senior member of our research team until his untimely death in 1973 and contributed a number of important theoretical and practical contributions to our study.

TEMPERAMENT CATEGORIES

The nine categories and their definitions are as follows:

1. *Activity level:* The motor component present in a given child's functioning and the diurnal proportion of active and inactive periods.

2. *Rhythmicity (regularity):* The predictability and/or unpredictability in time of any function. It can be analyzed in relation to the sleep-wake cycle, hunger, feeding pattern, or elimination schedule.
3. *Approach or withdrawal:* The nature of the initial response to a new stimulus, be it a new food, a new toy, or a new person. Approach responses are positive, whether displayed by mood expression (smiling, verbalizations, and the like) or motor activity (swallowing a new food, reaching for a new toy, active play, and so on). Withdrawal reactions are negative, whether displayed by mood expression (crying, fussing, grimacing, verbalizations, or the like) or motor activity (moving away, spitting new food out, pushing new toy away, and so forth).
4. *Adaptability:* Responses to new or altered situations. One is not concerned with the nature of the initial responses, but with the ease with which they are modified in a desired direction.
5. *Threshold of responsiveness:* The intensity level of stimulation that is necessary to evoke a discernible response, irrespective of the specific form that the response may take or the sensory modality affected. The behaviors utilized are those concerning reactions to sensory stimuli, environmental objects, and social contacts.
6. *Intensity of reaction:* The energy level of response, irrespective of its quality or direction.
7. *Quality of mood:* The amount of pleasant, joyful, and friendly behavior, as contrasted with unpleasant, crying, and unfriendly behavior.
8. *Distractibility:* The effectiveness of extraneous environmental stimuli in interfering with or altering the direction of the ongoing behavior.
9. *Attention span and persistence:* These two categories are related. Attention span concerns the length of time a particular activity is pursued by the child. Persistence refers to the continuation of an activity in the face of obstacles to the maintenance of the activity direction.

Qualitative analysis, supplemented by factor analyses, led us to formulate in addition three constellations of temperament made up of various combinations of the individual categories, which appeared to have functional significance. These are

1. *Easy temperament:* Typically this comprises the combination of biological regularity, approach tendencies to the new, quick adaptability to change, and a predominantly positive mood of mild or moderate intensity. This group comprised approximately 40% of the study population.
2. *Difficult temperament:* This is the opposite of easy temperament, namely, biological irregularity, withdrawal tendencies to the new, slow adaptability to change, and frequent negative emotional expressions of high intensity. This group comprised approximately 10% of the study population.
3. *Slow-to-warm-up temperament:* This category comprises withdrawal tendencies to the new, slow adaptability to change, and frequent negative emotional reactions of low intensity. Such individuals are often labeled ''shy.'' This group comprised approximately 15% of the study population.

It is apparent that the group of temperamentally easy children are indeed easy for the caregiver to manage. They are also children who typically adapt quickly and positively to new situations and demands. The temperamentally difficult child, by contrast, though normal, is difficult to manage and often finds adaptation to the new distressing and stressful. The slow-to-warm-up child may also present difficulties in management, but since his or her negative reactions to new foods, places or people are expressed mildly, rather than with the violent intensity of the difficult child, caregivers and teachers can usually tolerate this slow-to-warm-up behavior and give the child time to make a gradual adaptation to the new.

As can be seen from the percentages given above, not all children fit into these three temperament groups. This results from the varying and different combinations of temperament traits manifested by individual children. Also, among those children who do fit one of these three

patterns, there is a wide range in degree of manifestation. Some are extremely easy children in practically all situations; others are relatively easy in some situations but vary in their reactions to others. A few children are extremely difficult with all new situations and demands; others show only some of these characteristics, and only relatively mildly. For some children it is highly predictable that they will warm up slowly in any new situation; others warm up slowly with certain types of new stimuli or demands but warm up quickly in others.

It should be emphasized that the various temperament categories and constellations all represent variations within normal limits. Any child may be easy, difficult, or slow-to-warm-up temperamentally, have a high or low activity level, be distractible with low persistence or the opposite, or show any other relatively extreme rating score for a specific temperament attribute. However, such amodal ratings are not criteria of psychopathology but rather an indication of the wide range of behavioral styles exhibited by normal children, adolescents, or adults.

We have been able to rate our NYLS subjects on the nine categories and three constellations at all age periods in childhood, adolescence, and now into early adult life. Of course, the patterns of behavior change and become increasingly complex at sequential age periods. Therefore, the criteria for rating temperament must reflect these behavioral changes. Thus, behavioral items for scoring temperament in infancy will focus on sleep and feeding schedules, the first reactions to the bath, adaptation to new foods and new people, loudness and frequency of crying and laughter, distractibility during feeding, and so on. During the toddler stage, data collection will concentrate on peer reactions, play patterns, distractibility, and persistence when playing with a new game or toy. In the older child, the adaptation to school, parties, family, peers, play, and task-oriented activities are of interest. In the adolescent and adult, the identification of temperament is more complex because of the increasing individual variation in activities, such as athletics, hobbies and special interests, social life, school curriculum, and job experiences.

However, by now, we and other research centers have developed temperament interviews and questionnaires appropriate to the different age groups through early adult life (Chess and Thomas, 1986, pp. 115–147). We have found it possible to rate temperament in a number of other populations that we have studied: children born in New York of unskilled and semi-skilled working-class parents born in Puerto Rico; premature children with birth weights ranging from 1000 to 1750 g; children with mildly retarded intellectual levels but without gross evidence of motor dysfunction; and a large group of children with various handicaps due to congenital rubella.

Our findings have also been confirmed in a large number of research centers in this country and abroad (Maziade et al., 1984, 1990; Porter and Collins, 1982). Many investigators and clinicians use our categories as we have defined them; some others have introduced modifications or additional patterns of temperament (Cameron et al., 1989; Kagan, 1989). Because the interview and item-scoring method we evolved is time consuming, a number of relatively brief questionnaires have been developed to cover the sequential age periods of childhood, adolescence, and early adult life. These questionnaires are now widely used in temperament research and have the advantage of economy of time in administration and scoring. They do have the disadvantages of demanding forced choice responses and of not permitting the exploration of specific areas that the parent or other respondent might be able to emphasize in an interview.

The Validity of the Parents' Reports

Controversy exists in the temperament research field as to the accuracy of parents' reports of their child's behavior, whether by interview or questionnaire. There is no doubt that some or many parents will have subjective biases or a defensiveness may distort their perceptions and reports. On the other hand, the mother and father are in the special position of being familiar with the child's behavior over long periods of time, an asset that is very valuable in rating a number of temperament categories. This special knowledge is shared with teachers and pediatricians, who get to know the children under their care with the passage of time.

We ourselves tested the accuracy of the parents' interview reports in the infancy period by obtaining, in 18 cases, detailed reports of the child's behavior in the home by two independent trained observers. The observations were made on separate days, lasted 2–3 hours each, and were done within 2 weeks of a parent interview. In five other infants, only one observation was possible. These observations were scored for temperament, using the same method as for the parent interviews. A significant positive correlation, though not a perfect agreement, was found between observer and parent reports (Thomas et al., 1963, pp. 53–55).

In addition, many spot checks of the study children's behavior were possible, inasmuch as most of the interviews were done in the home. Close agreement between these spot observations and the parental report was uniformly found.

Additionally, a number of reports from other centers (Bates and Bayles, 1984, pp. 111–130: Matheny et al., 1987, pp. 323–331; Rutter, 1987, pp. 443–458) have indicated a strong objective component in the mother's report and the findings of an objective observer (Crockenberg and Acredolo, 1983, p. 61–72: Vaughn et al., 1981, pp. 1–17). In almost all these comparative studies, however, it is assumed that the independent observer's report should be used as the standard, accurate description of the child's typical behavior, against which the mother's report is to be judged. However, even professionally trained observers can have unconscious, theoretical, idiosyncratic, or cultural biases. Their observations also are typically of short duration. Further, the presence of a strange observer may make some mothers self-conscious and alter their behavior with the children, which in turn alters the child's behavior that the observer records.

In our judgment, the parents' report still represents the best single source of information on the child's temperament, when the data supplied are concrete, descriptive terms of behavior. It would be useful to develop a systematic protocol for independent observations, which would minimize the problems indicated in the preceding paragraph and thus could correct the biases found in some parental reports. Most useful would be the identification of specific biological markers for the different temperament traits. Encouraging work in this direction is already under way and is noted below. Reports from teachers and pediatricians who have experienced repeated contact with children are another valuable source for temperament data. Bates emphasizes this issue: ''We have known for some time that parental diaries are the best way to measure emerging language abilities. . . . after all, parents are with the child in many different situations, including those of highly predictable routine settings that are the birthplace of early words (e.g. feeding, bathing, going to bed). . . .'' (Bates E et al., 1994).

Goodness or Poorness of Fit

For each subject who required evaluation of a possible clinical behavior disorder, we compiled the already existing data regarding the subject's temperament characteristics and also from the parents and teacher. We identified expectations and demands on the child. From the evaluations that traced each child's healthy or pathological psychologic development, we formulated our conceptualization of ''goodness of fit'' or ''poorness of fit.'' We found that goodness of fit results when the functioning of the parents or others in the environment with respect to their expectations or demands of the child are in *consonance* with the child's temperament characteristics and capabilities. With such a goodness of fit, a child's optimal development in a progressive direction was possible. Conversely, poorness of fit involved discrepancies and *dissonances* between environmental opportunities and demands on the one hand and the child's capacities and temperament characteristics on the other. Under such circumstances, distorted and maladaptive functioning occurred. Goodness or poorness of fit was never an abstraction but was always determined in terms of the values and demands of a given culture or socioeconomic group.

It should be emphasized that this does not imply an advocacy of eliminating all stress and conflict. Quite the contrary. They are inevitable concomitants of the developmental process, in which new expectations and demands for change and progressively higher levels of functioning occur continuously as the child grows older. Demands, stresses, and conflicts, when consonant with the child's developmental potentials and capacities for mastery, may be constructive in their consequences and should not be considered inevitable causes of a behavior disorder. The issue involved in disturbed behavioral functioning is rather one of *excessive* stress resulting from poorness of fit.

This concept of a dynamic integration between temperament and environment as conceptualized by goodness or poorness of fit can be easily seen by researchers and clinicians in a wealth of illustrations (Chess and Thomas, 1986). To give one example, we can spell out the type of fit through the temperament category of motor activity level. The high-activity child whose outlets for exercising muscles are insufficient will become restless, impulsive, and difficult to manage. At home such a child may become a nuisance, and at school a disciplinary problem, if there is a demand to sit still for long periods of time. All too often, when this happens the child will be criticized and punished by an unsympathetic teacher, which will only intensify the disturbance. What emerges is a designated ''bad boy'' or ''bad girl'' with a derogatory self-image. This sequence is an outcome of significant poorness of fit. If, on the other hand, thoughtful parents and teachers recognize the child's need for adequate motor activity, the story will be different. The parents can seek out playground programs that emphasize active play and will not expect the child to sit quietly through a long religious attendance or a prolonged automobile ride. The teacher can also give the child a class responsibility that involves a good deal of motor activity, such as inventing brief errands when he or she notices that the youngster is particularly restless.

The importance of cultural expectations in the consequences for high-activity level children can be dramatized in the contrasting findings in the middle-class NYLS children and the Puerto Rican working-class (PRWC) children living in the congested and underprivileged East Harlem section of New York City. Of the PRWC children who had developed behavior disorders before the age of 9, half had high activity levels. They presented symptoms of excessive and uncontrolled motor activity. By contrast, only one NYLS youngster displayed these symptoms, and this was a brain-damaged child. The PRWC families usually had relatively large numbers of children and lived in small apartments with little space for the constructive motor activity the highly active children required. Furthermore, these very children were more likely to be cooped up at home, for their mothers feared that running around in the unsafe streets could bring a special danger of accidents. Safe playgrounds and recreational resources were meagerly available for these families, and the many household responsibilities did not permit mothers to sit for long periods safeguarding their children's outdoor play. These high-activity children were exposed to poorness of fit, excessive stress, and a high risk for behavior disorder development. By contrast, the NYLS families lived in spacious apartments or private homes with backyards, with safe streets and playgrounds also available. The high-activity children in these middle-class families therefore had ample opportunities to exercise their need for motor activity safely. Consequently, clashes with caregivers on this score were few, and a goodness of fit with low risk for pathogenic excessive stress existed. A further variation in the goodness of fit was found in Kokwet, a rural African farming community. Functioning features of the infants' niche, particularly with regard to the structuring of sleep, were delineated by ethnographic methods, and it was found that individual differences in rhythmicity were not of great significance in that context—willingness to be soothed by back-carrying and other techniques available to sibling caretakers are critical components in being an ''easy baby'' in Kokwet (Super and Harkness, 1986).

Any amodal child's temperament trait or constellation, such as the difficult or slow-to-warm-up patterns, may endow daily behavior episodes with much potential for confrontation. Some parents may label the youngster as a psychopathological or "bad" child. If such a parent or other authority insists that the child conform fully to the culturally expected norm, there is the formation of excessive stress and a poorness of fit. Should, by contrast, the parents understand the temperament characteristic, the parents or others will accept the fact that the behavior is basically normal and healthy. Through patience and the type of helpfulness to the child that conforms both to the temperament necessities and minimum cultural expectations, then excessive demands will not be imposed, and a goodness of fit will result.

Goodness or poorness of fit can at times also involve issues other than temperament. For example, Hunt has emphasized what he calls "the problem of match" between the child's cognitive capacity and the demands made on him or her. If the demand is dissonant with the cognitive level, the child shows "withdrawal and distress, and often tears"; if consonant, the task is performed with "interest and joyful excitement" (p. 34). In an attempt to understand both typical human development and individual differences within the same theoretical framework, Sandra Scarr has concluded that, despite a wide range of environmental opportunities, emotional supports, and genetic variation, most children grow up to be individually different based on their genotypes (Scarr, 1992, 1994). Melvin Lewis, in his discussion of chronic illness as a psychological risk factor, has noted that the temperament model of "goodness of fit" can be applied also to chronically ill children and their families (Lewis, 1994).

Continuity or Change in Temperament

Our search for categories and ratings of individual differences in temperament initially started with infants and young children. In those first years of inquiry, we assumed that specific individual temperament characteristics would remain constant throughout life. The boisterous baby would become the vigorous adult; the shy child would be, in adulthood, the quiet grown-up; the youngster who moved toward most new activities would in middle childhood, in adolescence, and as a mature person be rather the "joiner" than otherwise.

But as our young children became older, we have found that such continuities have not always been the case. And, in reflection, how could it be so? All other psychologic phenomena, such as intellectual competence, coping mechanisms, adaptive patterns, and value systems, can and do change over time. How could it be otherwise for temperament? The possibility of change of temperament over time, as well as other psychological factors, would be inevitable from our fundamental commitment to an interactionist viewpoint, in which individual behavioral development is conceived as a constantly evolving and changing process of organism-environment interaction over time. As one example, a child's earlier characteristic expression of temperament may be blurred at later specific age periods by routinization of functioning. This infant who showed marked withdrawal from the bath, new foods, and new people may, a year or two later, show positive responses to these same situations because of repeated exposure and final adaptation. Then, at some subsequent age periods, if the youngster experiences few new situations, the infant withdrawal reactions will not be evident. If, however, at some later age period the child or adolescent is exposed again to a number of new unfamiliar situations, the withdrawal behavior reactions may be evident again.

We have now made some headway in our examination of this issue of consistency and change of temperament over time (Chess and Thomas, 1984, pp. 261–272; Thomas and Chess, 1977, pp. 155–174). The quantitative ratings of the temperament categories of this NYLS sample have been calculated statistically for the interyear correlations for the first 5 years. We have found significant correlations from one year to another for almost all temperament categories, but as the time span for the comparisons is increased from 1 year to 2, 3, or 4 years, the number of significant correlations decreased. Our interpretation is that this substantial change of temperament over time reflects the increasing environmental influence upon the child's functioning. Also, changing biological patterns of maturation of development over time

may also modify various temperament characteristics.

A recent analysis compared the temperament ratings of the NYLS sample in early childhood with the ratings of the early adult life follow-up period (Chess and Thomas, 1984, pp. 96–97). The difficult-easy temperament score of the sample at age 3 found a relationship to the early adult life period. (A difficult-easy temperament rating is calculated by adding the five scores of rhythmicity, approach-withdrawal, adaptability, intensity, and quality of mood and dividing by five.) Quantitative comparisons of individual temperament categories of early childhood with early adult life did not show any significant correlations. However, individual subjects in some cases did by qualitative studies suggest significant and sometimes even dramatic consistency in one or another temperament category from early childhood to early adult life (Chess and Thomas, 1984, pp. 261–272).

McDevitt (1986) has recently reviewed and summarized reports of continuity and discontinuity of temperament, including his own work, that of others, and ours. He concluded that, within the period of early childhood, temperament has moderate to high stability. However, individual characteristics continue to be stable into childhood, and global measures of difficulty demonstrate significant links to teen and young adult periods (p. 35). He also comments that continuities in temperament are more easily detected as the level of analysis becomes less specific and more global. Conversely, with increase in the generality of a measure, its ability to provide useful theoretical or clinical information decreases (p. 36). We certainly agree with McDevitt's observations. In the collection of temperament data we have always formulated our protocols and questionnaires in terms of basic concerns for the details of specific and contextual situations in which a subject's behavioral characteristics have been expanded.

We can also add that McDevitt's desirable criteria for enhancing the detection of continuities in temperament also provide more useful clinical and theoretical information for detecting discontinuities of temperament.

Biological Issues in Temperament Research

A number of findings lead most of us to the opinion that the evidence supports the concept of a biological origin for temperament. A review of these findings is summarized here.

Individual characteristics in temperament are apparent within the first few months of life, and these differences become dramatic by the latter half of the 1st year of life. No consistent qualities in parental practices and attitudes have been found in various research samples that could account for this variability in temperament (Thomas and Chess, 1977, pp. 137–138). We also compared the temperament scores of our NYLS infants with those in our working-class Puerto Rican families—two groups with marked culturally divergent approaches to child care—and found no dramatic differences in temperament distribution (Thomas and Chess, 1977, pp. 146–148). Along the same lines, Korner (1973) has reviewed the research literature that indicates that even in infancy, parents, especially mothers, treat girls dissimilarly from boys. Yet our study and others found only very modest sex differences in temperament scores in boys versus girls, indicating that temperament individuality in young children is not shaped by any variability in parental attitudes and practices based on the sex of the child (Chess and Thomas, 1984, pp. 89–95). A final bit of evidence comes from the study of infants born prematurely, in which temperament data were collected and analyzed as in the NYLS. In these premature infants, the parents were realistically concerned and even anxious as to whether their children would develop normally or suffer some permanent brain injury, as some of the children actually did. Yet in spite of these parental anxieties, the temperament scores for these premature infants were not significantly disparate from those of the full-term infants in the NYLS (M. Hertzig, personal communication, 1984).

These studies provide circumstantial evidence challenging any concept that infant temperament is primarily determined by the parents' attitudes and practices. Positive evidence in the same direction is provided by two major studies, which have demonstrated a definite genetic factor in shaping individual likeness or unlikeness in temperament. Both studies used the classic method whereby the intrapair differences in a group of monozygotic twins, who are 100% genetically similar, are compared with the intrapair differences in a group of same-sex but heterozygotic twins, who are, on the average, 50% genetically similar.

In one study conducted in Bergen, Norway, a sample of 50 same-sex twin pairs was collected (Torgersen and Kringlen, 1978). On the basis of blood typing, 34 pairs were identified as monozygotic and 16 as dizygotic. Behavioral interviews were obtained with the mother when the infants were 2 months old and again when they were 9 months. The translated NYLS interview protocol was used, and the data item scored for our nine temperament categories. At 2 months of age there were statistically significant intrapair differences between the two groups of twins only in rhythmicity, sensory threshold, and intensity. At 9 months, however, the differences between the two groups was statistically significant for all nine categories, in seven reaching the .001 level. In all categories, the monozygotic twin pairs were more similar to each other than were the dizygotic twins. The investigators also examined the possibility that the mothers of monozygotic twins might treat the infants more similarly and report their behavior as more alike than it really was. However, neither at 2 months nor at 9 months did the majority of mothers have any definite opinion regarding the zygosity of their twins. The investigators judged that the marked increase in positive findings from 2 to 9 months possibly reflected the residual effect of the pregnancy and the birth process on the infant's behavior at 2 months. Their reasonable hypothesis was that these residual effects had disappeared by 9 months, at which time the definitive expression of temperament was clearer.

Another genetic study has been reported by Buss and Plomin (1975) from the University of Colorado. They used a different categorization of temperament, namely, activity, emotionality, sociability, and impulsivity. They employed a short questionnaire, and most of the items were general in nature. A sample of 139 pairs of same-sex twins was used, with an age range of 1–9 years. The intrapair correlations were significantly higher for the monozygotic versus the dizygotic twins for their temperament categories, except impulsivity, again indicating a genetic factor for the other three categories.

In addition, a long-term longitudinal study of twins, initiated in 1971 at the University of Louisville, has found that initial analysis, performed at age 12 months, showed monozygotic twins more concordant than dizygotic twins for individual temperaments. This was also true for the profile of factor scores at one point in time as well as age-to-age change in factor scores. The authors conclude that this suggested a genetic influence on developmental change itself (Wilson and Matheny, 1986).

Recently, Ebstein et al. (1996) demonstrated that higher than average Novelty Seeking scores (as measured by the tridimensional personality questionnaire (Cloninger et al., 1993) for the domain of Novelty Seeking in human temperament appear to be associated with the 7 repeat allele in the locus for the D4 dopamine receptor gene (D4DR). Similarly, Benjamin et al., (1996) demonstrated in ethnically disparate populations an association of the longer repeat D4DR alleles with the personality characteristics related to Novelty Seeking (being impulsive, exploratory, fickle, excitable quick-tempered, and extravagant), and that D4DR accounted for about 10% of the genetic variance, i.e., that Novelty Seeking is partially mediated by genes and that D4DR polymorphism accounts for some (but not all) of the genetic effects. Ebstein et al. noted that the combined findings of both studies provide "the first replicated association between a specific genetic locus involved in neurotransmission and a normal personality trait" (p. 78).

As significant as these genetic studies are, they explain only part of the variance with determination of temperament individuality. Other biological nongenetic factors, such as hormonal or other aspects of the prenatal environment or the birth process, may also be important. Also, a genetic influence in no way implies fixed predetermination and immutability of temperament, any more than it does any other psychological or physical characteristic of an organism. Phenotypic characteristics, as emphasized by modern geneticists, are always the final product of the continuously evolving interaction between genetic and environmental factors (Dobzhansky, 1962).

A promising pioneering study of the relationship of temperament to various physiological and hormonal factors has been developed by Jerome Kagan and his associates (1988) at Harvard University. This group used a sample of 60 children classified at 21 months as behaviorally inhibited, and 60 who were uninhibited. (Their criteria for uninhibited-inhibited correspond closely to those for our temperament category of approach/withdrawal.) At age $5\frac{1}{2}$ years, the children originally evaluated as inhibited when compared with the uninhibited group were more inhibited with peers in both laboratory and school, as well as with an adult examiner, and more cautious in a situation of mild risk. The earlier finding of a relatively high and stable heart rate in the inhibited children was present at 21 months and again at $5\frac{1}{2}$ years. Salivary cortisol levels were also higher in these same children at 21 months and $5\frac{1}{2}$ years. The inhibited children also had tonically larger pupils when exposed to cognitive stress than did the uninhibited children at the same age periods. However, in reassessment at age $7\frac{1}{2}$, developmental influences toward change may have appeared. While continuing to be behaviorally either socially withdrawing or socially interactive, as before, the absolute heart rate and cortisol level in the saliva were not as discriminating as they had been 2 years earlier (Kagan et al., 1988).

Kagan, in an extensive publication (1989), speculates that most inhibited children were born with a lower threshold for limbic-hypothalamic arousal to unexpected changes in the environment. He strengthens his speculation or hypothesis by citing a number of animal studies with comparable data (p. 161). Kagan's biological findings and speculations further indicate that the interaction of temperament and environment has biological roots, and he mentions a number of situations that can enhance or modify such interactional processes. We agree with his formulation that psychologists who begin to assess the interaction between experience and temperament will begin to synthesize inherent biological states with environmental events (p. 173).

Kagan's formulation has been confirmed by Gunnar and her coworkers, who demonstrated that infants who showed more of the normative response to heel stick blood drawn in the newborn period cried more, showed larger increases of cortisol and greater decreases in vagal tone, were reported by parents to be less negative in temperament at 6 months of age (Gunnar, 1994).

Temperament and Personality

We do not advocate a temperament theory of personality (Thomas et al., 1968, pp. 182–184). Temperament is one of the significant factors in development, but is not identical with personality.

It is true that, in the very young infant, temperament characteristics do seem to be the whole personality, but as the child grows older, a host of other factors enter, which all contribute to personality development. Judd Marmor (1983), a leading student of personality theory, has enumerated the types of variables that must be considered: faulty parenting; temperament; the diversity of personality patterns and culturally acquired value systems and expectations of the parents; economic, racial, and ethnic realities; dietary adequacy or inadequacy; and the nature of relationships with siblings, extended family members, peers, teachers, and other individuals. He concludes, "We begin to get a glimpse of how difficult it is to accurately trace the origins of specific personality patterns at all, let alone to try to derive them from just one or two variables" (p. 856).

PRACTICAL IMPLICATIONS

The functional significance of temperament holds the promise for the prevention, management, and treatment of many behavior disorders of children. Parents, mental health professionals, teachers, pediatricians, and nurses can identify and recognize the behavioral individuality of children's temperament characteristics (Chess and Thomas, 1986). Then the formulation "Know, help, and treat each child as an individual" can become a meaningful concept instead of a mechanical cliche. For the parents who believed that they were responsible for a deviation in their child from a conventional norm, the knowledge of the part played by the child's temperament may relieve them of a needless oppressive burden of guilt and anxiety. At the same time, parents may figure out for themselves or be helped by other professionals as to how to reach the optimal approach for each pattern of temperament, instead of relying on global characterizations and blanket judgments applied to all children indiscriminately. Clear-cut objective insight into the child's temperament and its implications is now substituted for speculative assumptions of complex psychodynamic mechanisms. The parent or teacher of a child who sometimes cannot attain the expected norm of behavior should not brand this youngster as "bad," "sick," "willful," or "disobedient." Such negative judgments distort the child's self-image, create inappropriate defenses, and can lead only to a self-fulfilling prophecy. On the contrary, if the parent or teacher does respect the child's behavioral style, the youngster can then learn self-confidence and insight into the positive significance of that particular behavioral individuality.

The paradigm of goodness or poorness of fit provides a framework for the prevention or treatment of childhood behavior disorders through the valuable tool of parent guidance. The rationale of such a guidance procedure is first to collect the data and analyze the dynamics of goodness or poorness of fit. The specific area or areas are identified as the centers of unhealthy parent-child interaction, and these are then described to the parents, and alternative handling is outlined.

In the NYLS a number of parents, perhaps at least 50%, were eager and able to carry through the program of behavioral change recommended to them. In such cases, only several discussions were necessary for its full implementation. In others, the parents rejected a temperament interpretation, insisting on a malevolent motivation, and pursued an unchanged approach. In these cases the child continued to respond to the excessive stress and developed or retained a behavior disorder (Chess and Thomas, 1986, pp. 159–181).

Inevitably, the guidance sessions did reveal misconceptions, confusions, defensiveness, anxiety, or guilt in a number of cases. Additional discussions were then required for clarification of those parental attitudes and practices that interfered with the child's desirable development. In some cases, parents did respond positively to this new knowledge with amelioration of their disturbed previous reactions. In other instances, however, psychopathology in the parents appeared to be so rigidly fixed as to prevent their making changes in their daily handling of their child.

The failure of parent guidance then leaves only the recommendation for direct psychotherapy for the child. At times it was clear from the start that we were dealing with parental pathology that made parent guidance unsuitable as an intervention of choice, and direct psychotherapy was immediately recommended.

A number of studies explored by Barbara Keogh (1982) and Roy Martin (1989) have reported the usefulness for many teachers of examining their pupils' classroom activities in the light of the functional significance of the children's temperament characteristics. Similarly, a number of pediatricians and nurses have found that the recognition of their patients' temperament characteristics was frequently helpful both in treatment and in well-child care (Chess and Thomas, 1986).

CONTROVERSIAL TEMPERAMENT ISSUES

The introductory section of this chapter comments that a growing number of research units and workers, especially in this country, whose concerns are with temperament studies have raised many controversial methodological and conceptual issues. Also, many workers are posing exciting and fruitful new theoretical and practical questions to be answered by future research.

These voluminous contributions to the literature are too numerous for us to present in detail. Several extensive, detailed reviews of this literature can be recommended to the interested reader (Bates, 1987; Kohnstamm et al., 1989; Plomin and Dunn, 1986).

Definitions and Conceptualization of Temperament

A scholarly historical review of the meaning of the term *temperament*, starting from Hippocrates and Galen, has been presented by Kagan

(1989, pp. 107–127). He dates contemporary theorists from the 1950s. Our own formulation, starting in the late 1950s, is detailed above.

The British psychologist Eysenck (1953) has posited four temperament types formed from the conjunction of two orthogonal dimensions: extraversion-introversion and emotional lability-stability. Eysenck's conceptions have been influential, especially in European centers, in contrast to their influence in the United States. They can be criticized on several grounds: (a) His categories are abstract, comprise global judgments, and are unsupported by empirical evidence; and (b) he also combines several of his temperament categories, which then become broad pathological or normal personality types. For example, the combination of extroversion and lability is designated hysteria and criminality, and the combination introversion and lability becomes dysthymia. The combinations of introversion and stability and of extroversion and stability are classified as normal personality.

The studies of temperament in East European centers have been traditionally shaped by the Pavlovian biological concept of strength versus weakness of the central nervous system. Temperament was then determined by the intensity of excitation and stimulation required to evoke behavioral reaction. The strong nervous system required only a mild degree of stimulation to produce a response, while the weak nervous system responded only to a high degree of stimulation (Strelau, 1983). A most significant modification of the previously dominant Russian Pavlovian schools has been formulated by the leading Polish psychologist Jan Strelau. Strelau and his coworkers, such as Eliasz, now present a neo-Pavlovian model that focuses on the interaction of biological and environmental factors. Strelau and Eliasz now formulate a biological-temperamental personality-interactional process, which breaks with the traditional Pavlovian typologies and turns instead to a dynamic psychological developmental model. There are a number of similarities between their formulations and the concepts of various Western temperament workers, especially with our own work.

Strelau and coworkers, however, are committed to concepts that differ from the basic approaches of most American sources. While their theory of temperament has several sources, they aver that it could not have developed without the basis of Pavlovian typology. With his neo-Pavlovian view, Strelau emphasizes "reactivity as a primary feature of temperament" (1983, p. 176), and the classification of reactivity is based on the concept of individual differences in both degree and intensity (magnitude or amplitude) of expression.

This then provides Strelau's Reactivity Rating Scales, for example, for the nursery school child, in which specific behavioral items are rated by lowest to highest degrees of intensity. Our assessment of this scale immediately brings to mind specific Chess-Thomas temperament categories. For example, the items "cannot concentrate on current activity, engages in conversation with others, looks at their work" we would rate as high distractibility; "is timid in the presence of an unknown adult (reddens, averts gaze, answers with monosyllables" we would rate as high withdrawal, and so on (Strelau, 1983, pp. 342–343). We and others agree with Strelau's interactional concept and his emphasis on specific items of behavior. However, his stated categories of temperament are basically different from ours or those of other American research units. We have met with Strelau and Eliasz to explore the question of reconciling these two systems of temperament categorization. This goal appears quite possible and, if successful, would be most valuable.

We have discussed Strelau's views at some length because his specific structures of conceptualizations and methodology of temperament are promising for research and empirical work and influential in many European centers.

American Definitions and Conceptualizations

A number of these issues have been summarized by a group of influential workers in a roundtable in *Child Development* (Goldsmith et al., 1987). Buss and Plomin, the behavioral geneticists, consider temperament to be a set of inherited personality traits. They also formulate the basic interactionist concept of goodness of fit but use the terms "matches" and "mismatches" between person and environment. In the roundtable, Robert Hinde, the prominent ethologist, sharply criticizes Buss and Plomin's concept of genetic basis, which he calls a "discredited dichotomy distinguishing between innate and learned behavior." Hinde points out that heritability may change with age, sample, or environment (p. 522).

In the roundtable, the developmental psychologist Mary Rothbart formulated an intriguing concept of temperament "as relatively stable, primarily biologically based individual differences in reactivity and self regulation." She enumerates specific-reactivity biological responses and describes modulation of several processes by self-regulation. She then lists various behavioral phenomena inferred from biological individual differences and states that these variables show clear similarities to those studied by Thomas and Chess and others. Her hypotheses have heuristic value for biological correlations of temperament (Rothbart, 1987, p. 510). Her temperament categories, however, have as yet ignored the important traits of distractibility, persistence, and adaptability.

The psychologist Hill Goldsmith, in collaboration with Joseph Campos, has proposed a definition that identifies temperament as "individual differences in the probability of experiencing and expressing primary emotions and arousal." The two confine their definition to the behavioral level to facilitate empirical investigation (Goldsmith et al., 1987, pp. 510–511). The primary emotions are certainly major important aspects of temperament, and Goldsmith and Campos's emphasis on the meaningfulness of social contexts and the facilitation of empirical investigation is noteworthy. However, we would consider that emotion-based temperament categories ignore other important traits, such as activity level, adaptability, distractibility, and persistence.

Hinde has pointed up correctly some confusion in our own definition, which requires clarification. We distinguish temperament from motivation. Hinde points out that the example we provide of the neophobic child clinging to its mother seems motivational in essence (Goldsmith et al., 1987, p. 523). Certainly the slow-to-warm-up child (shy) is motivated to relieve distress by seeking support from the mother. The child's wariness, however, is a primary response of distress due to an unfamiliar circumstance, which evokes a negative temperament response that is nonmotivational. Once this distress has been experienced, then the child is motivated to alleviate his or her distress. This motivation we would then interpret as a secondary rather than primary phenomenon.

Finally, in the roundtable, Robert McCall, the developmental psychologist, has commented that temperament researchers should not be troubled by their inability to agree to a common definition of temperament (Goldsmith et al., 1987). He points out that we do not have a very good definition of intelligence, but this has stopped no investigator from studying it. His point is cogent: He believes definitions to be not valid or invalid, confirmable or refutable, but rather, either more or less useful (Goldsmith et al., 1987). We ourselves, and many others, have affirmed our definition because of its valuable theoretical and clinical usefulness, as detailed above.

Validity of Temperament Data

In the first section of this chapter, there is a discussion of the validity of parental interviews of child behavior as a source of temperament data, which summarized the controversy over the accuracy of parents' reports in the temperament research field. After this review, we concluded that the parents' report still represented the best single source of information on the child's temperament, when the data supplied are concrete descriptive items of behavior (McDevitt, 1989, p. 196). Many relatively sophisticated questionnaires for the infant and toddler period are now available. In addition, questionnaires have been developed for the adolescent period (Lerner et al., 1982) and early adult life (Thomas et al., 1982), and these questionnaires have served to gather useful temperament data. However, the "standardization and analysis of the reliability and validity of the newer questionnaires are necessary to advance in the field" (Institute of Medicine, 1989, p. 78). This latter comment is indeed an important goal for temperament research. Going beyond the value of questionnaires, the Institute of Medicine report cites a number of laboratory-based methods to assess temperament measures and states

that although these approaches are "time-consuming and relatively expensive," they "offer an objectivity and precision unmatched by the questionnaire and interview approaches" (p. 78). However, the question still remains whether parental interviews, properly conducted, can offer a range of data and behavioral time sequences that matches or supports laboratory-based approaches. Kagan (1989) has also emphasized that "The most serious problem in contemporary research on temperament is the habit of gathering only one source of evidence" (p. 175). He has conducted his own temperament study with a combination of methods. We agree emphatically with his caveat regarding the limiting of data gathering to a single source. Our own NYLS study has gathered data during the childhood period from parental interviews, teacher interviews and classroom observations, behavioral observations of psychometric tests, and a standardized clinical workup for any subjects exhibiting deviant behavior. In early adult life, we have also included parent interviews, subject interviews, and self-report questionnaires. Objective and precise laboratory approaches offer objectivity and precision, but a full picture of the individual is lacking if one gathers only one source of evidence.

Consistency and Inconsistency over Time

Again, we have commented on this controversy above, and McDevitt's (1986, pp. 35–36) summary, mentioned above, is useful.

McCall (1986) is concerned that the study of individual differences holds the danger of a one-sided search for continuity. He asserts that the essence of development of any function is both continuity and change. McCall's challenge is that "we should be just as vigorous in describing change, whether in individual differences or developmental functions and whether in mental development or temperament, as we are in the search for stability and continuity" (p. 16). We have previously reported a clinical impression of several patterns of temperament in our NYLS sample over the years: (a) consistency over time, (b) consistency in some aspects of temperament at one period and other aspects at another time, (c) distortion of the expression of temperament over time, (d) consistency in temperament but qualitative change in temperament-environment interaction, and (e) change in a conspicuous temperament characteristic over time. These impressionistic findings are suggestive enough to require detailed organized examination of the data. This is now under way.

Difficult Temperament (or the Difficult Child)

We have called attention over the years to the special functional significance of the temperament cluster we have termed "the difficult child," starting with our first detailed report (Thomas et al., 1968, pp. 75–84). We summarize here the concept of the difficult child and the data from which it emerged so that the criticisms of it may be clear. We have found that the constellation of irregularity, withdrawal tendency, predominantly negative mood, slow adaptability, and high intensity appeared in about 10% of the NYLS population, but represented about 24% of the behavior disorders that had emerged up to age 9. We coined the term "the difficult child" and found further that by age 9, of all the difficult children, 70% had developed a behavior disorder and 30% had not (Thomas et al., 1968, pp. 35–47). This indicated to us that, at least in middle-class Western society, the temperament features of this group resulted in poorness of fit in meeting cultural demands for socialization and task mastery at home, in school, and/or with the peer group. Examining the 30% who functioned well, we found that, either spontaneously or with guidance, these children had been provided with opportunities to familiarize and adapt at their own slow pace and had not been denigrated for their negative mood even when it had been expressed with high intensity. With familiarization, negative mood changed to positive acceptance and paired with high intensity, earned the positive titles "zest" and "ebullience." Further, these youngsters did achieve developmentally expected social habits, made friends, and demonstrated developmentally expected accomplishments.

Several child psychiatrists have questioned whether such a child's behavioral cluster was in fact due to temperament. They suggested that this really constituted a behavior problem and not a temperament risk factor (Graham and Stevenson, 1987). If such an interpretation were correct, this would assume that it was the child's difficult behavior that was primarily responsible for the parents' distressed and often confused behavior. In addition, some of the participants in the roundtable referred to above, such as Rothbart and Goldsmith, have expressed their skepticism of the usefulness of the concept of difficult temperament (Goldsmith et al., 1987, p. 521). John Bates, the temperament researcher and clinician, has also expressed similar doubts regarding difficult temperament (1980, 1989). But it is of interest that Bates, in the same chapter, describes a child with difficult temperament with special expression of marked negative intensity, who was managed badly by her mother, resulting in poorness of fit and the child's development of severely disturbed behavior. Bates, acting as a clinician, handled the case with parent guidance. The mother responded positively to the specific recommendations for changing her behavior, and the child improved significantly (Bates, 1989, pp. 345–346). Plomin points to the possibility of other temperament qualities such as frequent temper tantrums and high activity as being causes of parental concern and sees little value in the particular cluster of the difficult child.

In contrast, William Carey (1989), a pediatrician who has both applied the concept of temperament clinically with his patients and carried out research into the clinical relevance of several temperament qualities, has found important links with colic, night awakening, and other common pediatric complaints (Carey, 1989, pp. 58–59). Having obtained data on the children's temperament traits by questionnaires, he kept watch on those with the difficult child cluster so as to prevent poorness of fit and behavior disorder. Yet he cautions against labeling a child as such to parents lest the pediatrician cause difficulties that might not otherwise arise, or even create a self-fulfilling prophecy (Carey, 1986, pp. 228–229).

With a sharply divergent approach, Turecki (1989), a psychiatrist, runs a clinic called "The Difficult Child" and has written a book with the same title. Turecki's interest in the difficult child was sparked by his own daughter, who fulfilled this description both in her behavior and in the anguish her parents experienced in her early years. Once he had become familiar with the concept of temperament individuality, he applied the term "the difficult child" to mean any child-parent combination in which one or more of the child's temperament traits were dissonant with parental handling, thus forming a poorness of fit, which he altered through parent guidance, including the use of parent groups. In his terms, low threshold may be the hallmark of a difficult child if the parents feel victimized by the daily battle about getting dressed for school instead of recognizing that the child is truly in discomfort and needs softer clothing rather than rough orders. From the positive response of parents to Turecki's clinic and book, they appear to have no objection to having the term "difficult child" applied to their own child.

Finally, a number of studies have shown that a high- or low-risk factor for difficult temperament is determined by specific cultural value systems. Middle-class and also many working-class parents in the United States expect specific adaptations for the child's socialization that may be stressful for children with a difficult temperament. By contrast, similar children from different cultures may have fewer or different value systems and expectations and thereby socialize with less difficulty and stress (deVries, 1984; Korn and Gannon, 1983; Super and Harkness, 1981).

Qualitative (Clinical) and Quantitative Analysis

Sometimes the statistician looks down upon the clinician's concepts, which appear to be based upon "unscientific," crude, untidy, and even subjective observations and tabulations. By contrast, some clinicians may be convinced that their personal clinical experience is a sufficient proof and ignore statistical methods, with their neatness, tidiness, and tests of statistical significance.

Quantitative and qualitative methods each have their own different strengths and weaknesses. In combination they make for the most powerful approach to the analysis of a body of data. We have applied this qualitative-quantitative combination to the analysis of the data on tem-

perament and behavior disorder development in the NYLS anterospective longitudinal study (Chess and Thomas, 1984).

Over the years, we have tried to keep abreast of the increasing projects of temperament researchers. Recently, we have gained a distinct impression of a trend of emphasis in temperament studies: The majority of researchers seem to be concentrating on statistical analyses, and only a relatively few respect and appreciate the utilization of qualitative data analyses (Malhotra, 1989, pp. 91–96; Weisbluth, 1989, pp. 113–116).

The mathematical precision of statistical methods in behavioral studies, especially when these rely on the speed and accuracy of computer programs, all too often give an aura of authority and certainty to the results of the analyses that may be misleading (Kraemer, 1981, p. 310). For example, Plomin and Daniels (1984) suggested the use of hierarchical multiple regression to statistically assess temperament-environment interaction. They employed systematic statistical searches for interaction effects. Plomin and Daniels (1984) concluded that "so far, it is considerably easier to talk about temperament interactions than it is to find them" (p. 161). But the complexities and variables for such interactions are such that a multiple regression or even more complex statistical method is bound to be a dead end. Rutter (1980) reminds us that "attention must be paid to the specificities of person-situation interactions . . . . It may be suggested that it is preferable to take an idiographic approach which explicitly focuses on the individuality of human beings" (p. 5). Lerner et al. (1986) also remind us that it is not possible to specify in advance the particular features of the context that will exist in a given child's life at any specific time. It follows that we may speak only probabilistically of the effects of a given child on his or her context or of the feedback the child is likely to receive (pp. 99–100).

But if we use an idiographic approach toward temperament-environment interactions, we may be able to find them despite the inability of the statisticians to do so. A few examples can be given of experienced and sophisticated researchers who include a qualitative idiographic approach in their analyses and have been able to find meaningful and heuristically important temperament-environment interactions in the goodness of fit or match-mismatch concept. Examples include Caspi et al. (1988), Chess and Thomas (1984), Lerner et al. (1986), Greenspan (1981, p. 204), Murphy (1981, p. 168), and Super and Harkness (1981).

With regard to Plomin and Daniels's paper, we do respect a number of their significant quantitative studies. The point is, however, that they limit their search for temperament-environment interaction to statistical strategies and report failure of the concept since they cannot recommend a promising qualitative approach. Our concern is that all too many developmental researchers are committed at this time to the single track of statistical analysis.

NEW DIRECTIONS AND OVERVIEW

A number of the controversial issues discussed in the previous section have indicated new directions for temperament work. Beyond these, the expanding temperament literature has raised many new exciting ideas and challenges for current and future theoretical and practical activity. So many new directions come to mind that this section can only enumerate them briefly. There are discussions in this chapter of stability and change in temperament and of some of the steps being taken to explore the facts and their meanings. Dunn (1986) attempts to refine the questions to be asked. She distinguishes factors affecting different children, such as dimensions of temperament, developmental stages, and endogenous or exogenous sources of variation. She posits that causes of stability may differ for dimensions of temperament and for individual children. Some children may be "stable" in particular dimensions of temperament because they actively seek out specific types of social environment. Others may remain stable because their parents encourage certain styles of behavior. She highlights the question of the processes that are involved in the patterns of stability and change (p. 166).

Such questions, and others, emphasize the need for greater accuracy and comprehensiveness in the collection of temperament data. A dozen questionnaires have been devised for sequential age periods, from infancy to early adult life. A number of direct observational and laboratory techniques have been elaborated. Parental interviews and interview protocols for adolescents and young adults are available. Clinical observations by psychiatrists, pediatricians, and nurses and classroom observations by teachers are all sources of useful temperament data. All these methods require further refinement, standardization, and analysis of their reliability and validity. A further important task is the challenge to integrate and combine these separate sources of information, giving full value to the differences in behavior in different situations.

"Longitudinal studies are the lifeblood of temperament research" (Institute of Medicine, 1989, p. 79). Such projects, together with cross-cultural studies, promise to expand our insights into normal and pathological development, as well as to provide opportunities for refinement and application of the concept of goodness of fit. The genetic temperament studies of Buss and Plomin (1975) and Torgersen and Kringlen (1978) and the psychobiological studies of Kagan and his associates (1988) have opened the exploration of the biological basis of temperament. Important practical applications of temperament research for both prevention and treatment will be of value to clinicians and educators (Chess and Thomas, 1986), and these are being expanded.

Recent additions to temperament research are the pioneering community parenting projects, emphasizing temperament, that are ongoing in California, Oregon, and Vancouver, Canada (Andersen, 1994). These programs point to exciting horizons for the enhancement of healthy child development and the prevention of behavior disorder in high-risk children with difficult temperament (Cameron and Rice, 1986; J Rahe, personal communication, 1990; Smith, 1994).

We, the clinical arm of the NYLS study, have already embarked on several projects to ask retrospective questions for which the early data were anterospectively gathered. For example, we are exploring such issues as the clinical role of intrusiveness and/or detachment of parents as regards their children, environmental factors that have occurred concurrently with marked changes in temperament, and factors that may have contributed to temperament stability.

We present our basic conceptual theme as a final overview: As we have considered the developmental course of our NYLS subjects, what has come to the fore has been the diversity of interactional processes and personality outcome, so clearly unique as these youngsters matured from infancy to childhood, through adolescence, and into early adult life. The capacity for flexibility, adaptability, and mastery in the face of all kinds of adverse and stressful life experiences has been equally striking. We have also been impressed that our preventative and therapeutic interventions have made differences at all age periods.

References

Anderson CJ: Parent support groups. In: Carey WB, McDevitt S (eds): *Prevention and Early Intervention. A Festschrift for Stella Chess and Alexander Thomas.* New York, Brunner/Mazel, 1994, pp. 267–275.

Bates JE: The concept of difficult temperament. *Merrill-Palmer Q* 26:299–319, 1980.

Bates JE: Temperament in infancy. In: Osofsky JD (ed): *Handbook of Infant Development* (2nd ed). New York, Wiley, 1987, pp. 1101–1149.

Bates JE: Application of temperamental concepts. In: Kohnstamm GA Bates JE, Rothbart MK (eds): *Temperament in Childhood.* New York, Wiley, 1989.

Bates JE, Bayles K: Objective and subjective components in mothers' perceptions of their children from age 6 months to 3 years. *Merrill-Palmer Q* 30: 111, 1984.

Bates JE, Wachs TD, Emde RN: Toward practical uses for biological concepts of temperament. In: Bates JE, Wachs T (eds): *Temperament. Individual Differences at the Interface of Biology and Behavior.* Washington, DC, American Psychological Association, 1994, pp. 275–305.

Benjamin J, Greenberg B, Murphy DL, et al: Population and familial association between the D4 dopamine receptor gene and measures of Novelty Seeking. *Nature Genet* 12:81–84, 1996.

Bruch H: Parent education on the illusion of omnipotence. *Am J Orthopsychiatry* 24:723, 1954.

Buss AN, Plomin R: *A Temperament Theory of Personality.* New York, Wiley, 1975.

Cameron JR, Rice DC: Developing anticipatory guidance programs based on early assessment of infant temperament. Two tests of a prevention model. *J Pediatr Psychol* 11:221–234, 1986.

Cameron JR, Hansen R, Rosen D: Preventing behavior problems in infancy through temperament assessment and parental support programs. In: Carey WB, McDevitt SC (eds): *Clinical and Educational Applications of Temperament Research.* Berwyn, PA, Swets North America, 1989.

Carey WB: Temperament in pediatric practice. In: Chess S, Thomas A (eds): *Temperament in Clinical Practice.* New York, Guilford Press, 1986, pp. 218–239.

Carey WB: Temperament risk factors in general pediatric practice. In: Carey WB, McDevitt SC (eds): *Clinical and Educational Applications of Temperament Research.* Berwyn, PA, Swets North America, 1989.

Carey WB, McDevitt SC (eds): *Clinical and Educational Applications of Temperament Research.* Berwyn, PA, Swets North America, 1989.

Caspi A, et al: Moving away from the world: Life course patters of shy children. *Dev Psychol* 24: 824–831, 1986.

Cattell RB: *Personality: A Systematic and Factual Study.* New York, McGraw-Hill, 1950.

Chess S, Thomas A: *Origins and Evolution of Behavior Disorders.* New York, Brunner/Mazel, 1984.

Chess S, Thomas A: *Temperament in Clinical Practice.* New York, Guilford Press, 1986.

Cloninger CR, Svrakic DM, Przybeck TB: A psychobiological model of temperament and character. *Arch Gen Psychiatry* 50:975–990, 1993.

Crockenberg S, Acredolo C: Infant temperament ratings: A function of infants, or mother, or both? *Infant Behav Dev* 6:61, 1983.

deVries MW: Temperament and infant mortality among the Massai of East Africa. *Am J Psychiatry* 141:1189–1194, 1984.

Dobzhansky T: *Mankind Evolving.* New Haven, CT, Yale University Press, 1962.

Dunn J: Issues for future research. In: Plomin R, Dunn J (eds): *The Study of Temperament: Changes, Continuities and Challenges.* Hillsdale, NJ, Erlbaum, 1986, pp. 163–171.

Ebstein RP, Novick O, Umansky R, et al: Dopamine D4 receptor (D4DR) exon III polymorphism associated with the human personality trait of novelty seeking. *Nature Genet* 12:78–80, 1996.

Eysenck HJ: *The Structure of Human Personality.* London, Methuen, 1953.

Goldsmith HH, et al (Covenar) Roundtable: What is temperament? Four approaches. *Child Dev* 58:510, 1987.

Graham P, Stevenson J: Temperament and psychiatric disorders: The genetic contribution to behavior in childhood. *Aust NZ J Psychiatry* 21:267–274, 1987.

Greenspan SI: *Psychopathology and Adaptation in Infancy and Early Childhood.* New York, International Universities Press, 1981.

Guilford JP: *Personality.* New York, McGraw-Hill, 1959.

Gunnar MR: Psychoendocrine studies of temperament and stress in early childhood: Expanding current models. In: Bates JE, Wachs TD (eds): *Temperament. Individual Differences at the Interface of Biology and Behavior.* Washington, DC, American Psychological Association, 1994, pp. 175–198.

Haggard EA, Brekstad A, Skard AG: On the reliability of the amnestic history. *J Abnorm Soc Psychol* 66:221, 1963.

Hinds R: Comment. In: Goldsmith H, Buss AH, Plomin R, et al (eds): What is temperament? Four approaches. *Child Dev* 58:505–529, 1987.

Hunt JV: Implications of plasticity and hierarchical achievements for the assessment of development and risks of mental retardation. In: Sawin DB, Hawkins RC, Walker LO, et al (eds): *Exceptional Child.* New York, Brunner/Mazel, 1980, p. 34.

Institute of Medicine: *Research on Children and Adolescents' Mental, Behavioral and Developmental Disorders: Mobilizing a National Initiative.* Washington, DC, National Academy Press, 1989.

Kagan J: *Unstable Ideas, Temperament, Ideas and Self.* Cambridge, MA, Harvard University Press, 1989.

Kagan J, Resnick JS, Snidman N, et al: Childhood derivatives of inhibition and lack of inhibition to the unfamiliar. *Child Dev* 59:1580–1589, 1988.

Keogh BK: Children's temperament and teachers' decisions. In: Pater R, Collins G (eds): *Temperamental differences in infants and young children.* Ciba Foundation Symposium 89, pp. 269–279, 1982.

Kohnstamm GA, Bates JE, Rothbart MK (eds): *Handbook of Temperament in Childhood.* London, Wiley, 1989.

Korn SJ, Gannon S: Temperament, cultural variation and behavior disorder in preschool children. *Child Psychiatry Hum Dev* 13:203–212, 1983.

Korner AF: Sex differences in newborns, with special references to differences in the organization of oral behavior. *J Child Psychol Psychiatry* 14:1929, 1973.

Kraemer HC: Coping strategies in psychiatric clinical research. *J Consult Clin Psychol* 49: 309–319, 1981.

Lerner RM, Lerner JV, Windle M, et al: Children and adolescents in their contexts: Tests of a goodness of fit model. In: Plomin R, Dunn (eds): *The Study of Temperament: Changes, Continuities and Challenges.* Hillsdale, NJ, Erlbaum, 1986, pp. 99–144.

Lerner RM, Palermo M, Spiro A, et al: Assessing the dimensions of temperamental individuality across the life-span. The dimension of temperament survey (DOTS). *Child Dev* 53:149–159, 1982.

Lewis M: Chronic illness as a psychological risk factor in children. In: Carey WB, McDevitt S (eds): *Prevention and Early Intervention.* New York, Brunner/Mazel, 1994, pp. 103–112.

Marmor J: Systems thinking in psychiatry: Some theoretical and clinical applications. *Am J Psychiatry* 140:833–838, 1983.

Martin R: Temperament and education: implications for underachievement and learning disabilities. Chapter 2. In: Carey WB, McDevitt SC (eds): *Clinical and Educational Applications of Temperament Research*. Berwyn, PA, Swets North America, 1989.

Matheny AP, Wilson RW, Thoben AS: Home and mother: Relations with infant temperament. *Dev Psychol* 23:323, 1987.

Maziade M, Boudreault M, Thivierge J, et al: Infant temperament: SES and gender differences and reliability of measurement in a large Quebec sample. *Merrill-Palmer Q* 30:111, 1984.

Maziade M, Caron C, Côté R, et al: Extreme Temperament and Diagnosis: A Study in a Psychiatric Sample of Consecutive Children. *Arch Gen Psychiatry* 47:477–484, 1990.

McCall RB: Issues of stability and continuity in temperament research. In: Plomin R, Dunn J (eds): *The Study of Temperament: Changes, Continuities and Challenges*. Hillsdale, NJ, Erlbaum, 1986.

McDevitt S: Continuity and discontinuity of temperament. In: Plomin R, Dunn J (eds): *The Study of Temperament Changes, Continuities and Challenges*. Hillsdale, NJ, Erlbaum, 1986.

McDevitt S: Clinical applications of temperament research in children: Implications and directions for the future. Chapter 20. In: Carey WB, McDevitt SC (eds): *Clinical and Educational Applications of Temperament Research*. Berwyn, PA, Swets North America, 1989.

Malhotra S: Varying risk factors and outcomes: An Indian perspective. Chapter 9. In: Carey WB, McDevitt SC (eds): *Clinical and Educational Applications of Temperament Research*. Berwyn, PA, Swets North America, 1989.

Murphy LB: Explorations in child personality. In: Robins A, Aronoff J, Barclay AM, et al (eds): *Further Explorations in Personality*. New York, International Universities Press, 1981.

Plomin R, Daniels D: The interaction between temperament and environment: Methodological considerations. *Merrill-Palmer Q* 30:149–162, 1984.

Plomin R, Dunn J (eds): *The Study of Temperament: Changes, Continuities and Challenges*. Hillsdale, NJ, Erlbaum, 1986.

Porter R, Collins GM: Temperamental differences in infants and young children. CIBA Symposium 89. London, Pitman, 1982.

Robbins L: The accuracy of parental recall of aspects of child development and child rearing practices. *J Abnorm Soc Psychol* 66:261, 1963.

Rothbart MK: In: Goldsmith HH (Covenar) Roundtable: What is temperament? Four approaches. *Child Dev* 58:510, 1987.

Rutter M: Introduction. In: Rutter M (ed): *Scientific Foundations of Developmental Psychiatry*. London, Heinemann, 1980, pp. 1–7.

Rutter M: Temperament, personality and personality disorder. *Br J Psychiatry* 150:443–458, 1987.

Scarr S: Presidential address. Developmental theories for the 1990's: Development and individual differences. *Child Dev* 63:1–19, 1992.

Scarr S: Genetics and individual differences. In: Carey WB, McDevitt S (eds): *Prevention and Early Intervention*. New York, Brunner/Mazel, 1994, pp. 170–178.

Smith B: The temperament program: Community based prevention of behavior disorders in children. In: Carey WB, McDevitt S (eds): *Prevention and Early Intervention*. New York, Brunner/Mazel, 1994, pp. 257–266.

Strelau J: *Temperament Personality Activity*. New York, Academic Press, 1983.

Super CM, Harkness S: Figure, ground and gestalt: The cultural context of the active individual. In: Lerner RM, Busch-Rossnagel NA (eds): *Individuals as Producers of Their Development*. New York, Academic Press, 1981, pp. 69–86.

Super CM, Harkness S: Temperament and development and culture. Chapter 10. In: Plomin R, Dunn J (eds): *The Study of Temperament: Changes, Continuities, and Challenges*. Hillsdale, NJ, Erlbaum, 1986.

Thomas A, Chess S: *Temperament and Development*. New York, Brunner/Mazel, 1977.

Thomas A, Chess S: Genesis of behavior disorders: From infancy to early adult life. *Am J Psychiatry* 141:1–9, 1984.

Thomas A, Chess S, Birch HG, et al: *Behavioral Individuality in Early Childhood*. New York, New York University Press, 1963.

Thomas A, Chess S, Birch HG: *Temperament and Behavior Disorders in Children*. New York, New York University Press, 1968.

Thomas A, Mittleman M, Chess S, et al: A temperament questionnaire for early adult life. *Educ Psychol Meas* 42:591–600, 1982.

Torgersen AM, Kringlen E: Genetic aspects of temperamental differences in infants. *J Am Acad Child Psychiatry* 17:433–434, 1978.

Turecki S: *The Difficult Child* (rev ed). New York, Bantam, 1989.

Vaillant GE: *Adaptation to Life*. Boston, Little, Brown, 1977.

Vaughn BE, Taraldson BJ, Chrichton L, et al: The assessment of infant temperament: A critique of the Carey Infant Temperament Questionnaire. *Infant Behav Dev* 4:1, 1981.

Weisbluth M: Sleep temperament interactions. Chapter 11. In: Carey WB, McDevitt SC (eds): *Clinical and Educational Applications of Temperament Research*. Berwyn, PA, Swets North America, 1989, pp. 113–116.

Wenar C: The reliability of developmental histories. *Psychosom Med* 25:505–509, 1963.

Wilson RS, Matheny AP Jr: Behavior genetics research in input temperament: The Louisville Temperament Study. Chapter 7. In: Plomin R, Dunn J (eds): *The Study of Temperament: Changes, Continuities and Challenges*. Hillsdale, NJ, Erlbaum, 1986.

14 DEVELOPMENT OF ATTENTION, PERCEPTION, AND MEMORY

Daniel J. Siegel, M.D., and Barry Nurcombe, M.D., F.R.A.C.P.

Attention, perception, and memory are often affected by childhood psychopathology, yet we have only a patchy understanding of the normal development of these cognitive functions. Research is complicated by the interaction, coincidence, and multidimensional nature of the three functions and by the instability of contemporary developmental theory. Interaction, coincidence, and multidimensionality hamper the testing of unconfounded processes, whereas developmental theory provides no clear guide to the particular assessments that should be combined to yield a comprehensive evaluation of the three functions. Such disclaimers notwithstanding, this chapter attempts to define the three processes, summarize what is known about their normal development, and review their neurobiology and psychopathology.

DEFINITIONS

Attention is the act or faculty of mental selection by which a significant object or idea is located, examined, and responded to. Following arousal and orientation, attention involves the serial but overlapping processes of selective scanning, orientation, sustained concentration, and reflective responding.

Perception refers to the immediate awareness or recognition of a sensory impression. Although the interpretation of a sensory impression is properly referred to as *apperception*, the term ''perception'' is commonly applied to both the awareness of and the interpretation of sensory stimuli.

Memory is the act or faculty of registering, retaining, or recalling the mental representation of an object, event, or concept.

The three processes operate in concert. Without memory and selective attention, apperception would not be possible. The search for and location of objects requires durable mnemonic representations, for it is through them that objects are recognized; whereas without attention and perception, memories could not be registered. Attention, perception, and memory are inextricably entwined. The next section of this chapter discusses the development of infant cognition in terms of a composite of the three faculties.

INFANT COGNITION

Since Fantz's (1958) groundbreaking studies of visual perception, research into infant cognition has exploded. Aside from its practical significance, the study of infancy illuminates issues of profound philosophical import (Bornstein, 1992). Is the baby a *tabula rasa*, shaped primarily by experience? Empiricists from Berkeley and Locke to von Helmholtz, James and Skinner have propounded this view. Conversely, does the infant bring into the world an innate categorical knowledge that organizes experience, as the nativist tradition of Descartes, Kant, Gibson, and Chomsky would have it? How do nature, nurture, and maturation interact? Developmental psychologists have begun to address these fundamental questions (see reviews by Acredolo and Hake, 1982; Aslin et al., 1983; Banks and Salapatek, 1983; Bornstein, 1992; Harris, 1983; Hirschman et al., 1982; and Olson and Sherman, 1983).

Methodology

An infant cannot respond verbally or reflect upon experience; consequently, researchers have relied upon the following indirect techniques to explore early cognition: electrophysiological measures; habituation responses; preferential looking, reaching, tasting, and smelling; and classical and operant conditioning.

A visual cortical evoked potential can be detected as early as 25 weeks gestation; by 40 weeks, it resembles in pattern that of the adult. The amplitude of the visual evoked potential increases up to 3 years, then gradually decreases until adulthood (Berg and Berg, 1979). Auditory evoked potentials can also be detected during the third trimester (Scibetta et al., 1971). Do these electrocortical phenomena mean that the fetus perceives sensation? Not necessarily.

A number of infant autonomic responses have been examined in the search for indices of infant attention. For example, from the first weeks of life, alert infants respond to novel auditory and visual stimulation with sustained cardiac deceleration (Sameroff et al., 1973; Schachter et al., 1971). Cardiac deceleration has been related by Graham and Clifton (1966) to the orienting response that accompanies intake of information (Sokolov, 1963). After the infant becomes habituated to a stimulus, that is, recognizes the stimulus to be familiar, the heart no longer slows.

Infant attention has been associated with (*a*) orientation to salient novel stimulus cues (Fagan, 1977) and (*b*) intensity of regard (Kagan and Lewis, 1965). McCall and Kagan (1967) have related cardiac deceleration to a recognition of the discrepancy between unfamiliar and familiar stimuli. Habituation, in contrast, implies that the infant has a prior mental representation of a stimulus or class of stimuli and that new presentations are matched against it.

Imaginative research techniques have been designed to study infant perception. For example, orientation to novel stimuli has been investigated by observing eye movement and facial expression (e.g., Salapatek and Kessen, 1966), preferential head turning, visual fixation, smiling, and reaching (e.g., Fantz, 1958). Visual fixation, cardiac orientation response, and sucking rate decrease as the infant habituates to a stimulus. By exploiting these phenomena, researchers can test the infant's capacity to perceive discrepancies between familiar and novel stimuli (e.g., Caron et al., 1979). Operant conditioning has been used for the same purpose (e.g., Bower, 1966a, 1966b). High amplitude sucking, for example, has been used by Eimas (1975) as an index of familiarity to a conditioned stimulus. Classical conditioning has also been used, for example, to investigate an infant's capacity to locate objects in space (e.g., Acredolo, 1978). By these ingenious means, researchers have investigated infant hearing, vision, taste, olfaction, cutaneous sensation, and cross-modal transfer.

Auditory Perception

In the third trimester fetus, external sounds evoke movement, cardiac acceleration, and electrocortical responses (Bench, 1978), while the neonate reacts to loud or sudden sounds with a generalized startle response; however, an infant's intensity threshold is higher than that of an adult, especially for the lower and higher frequencies. Hearing at low and high frequencies continues to improve during the first 20 years of life (Trehub et al., 1989).

The rudiments of hemispheric specialization are apparent soon after birth: lateral asymmetries in the auditory evoked potential can be produced by speech stimuli (Molfese and Molfese, 1978). The infant is specially receptive to sounds in the human frequency range (Hutt et al., 1968) and to sounds with intonational patterns similar to those of speech (Eisenberg, 1979). Condon and Sander (1974) report that infants move in rhythm to the stress patterns of speech. Infants under 6 months of age have been found to discriminate between a number of speech consonants (Eimas, 1975). These important findings suggest that the infant has an inherent tendency to perceive those categorical discriminations that are fundamental to phonological development and that speech processing differs from that for other sounds. By the 6th month, infants can differentiate most of the acoustic contrasts required for phonological development (Lynch et al., 1992).

Visual Perception

Although the neonate has some visual acuity, adult levels are not attained until 6 months (Lewis et al., 1978). Fantz (1958) was the first to show that neonates see patterns; it has subsequently been established that they tend to fixate upon high contrast features within geometric forms (Salapatek, 1975). As the infant develops, increasingly more complex patterns are preferred (De Loache et al., 1978). By 1 month, the infant has begun to recognize the mother's face, and by 2 months, moving eyes are of special interest (Girton, 1979; Mauer and Salapatek, 1976). In the 2-month-old infant, complex patterns evoke electrocortical responses that may represent a shift from subcortical to cortical processing (Hoffmann, 1978). Field (1979) has shown that infants attempt to modulate the effect of highly arousing stimuli (e.g., animated faces) by averting their eyes. The perception of faces and emotional expressions appears to play a central role in the development of affect regulation during the 1st year of life (Schore, 1994).

As language reflects, adults perceive the continuous spectrum as though it were divided into different colors. Is color categorization an inherent propensity, or is it molded developmentally by the arbitrary discriminations imposed by such words as "red," "blue," and "green"? In short, does the infant perceive categorically? Bornstein et al. (1976a, 1976b) found that 4-month-old babies discriminated green from blue, but treated a second blue as similar to the first, even though the contrasted green and blue were at a distance equal in wavelength from the central blue. Like adults, babies tend to perceive the color spectrum in shades of red, yellow, green, and blue (Bornstein, 1981). However, form and color are not integrated as wholes until 6 months (Cohen, 1979).

The 3-month-old infant already has the rudiments of shape constancy, size constancy, and preferential orientation to the vertical (Bornstein, 1984; Bower, 1966a, 1966b; Caron et al., 1978; Hayes and Watson, 1981). Infants of 4 months are sensitive to symmetry (Bornstein, 1992). However, it is not until the 2nd year of life that babies use landmarks to locate themselves in space, an ability probably facilitated by crawling (Benson and Uzgiris, 1985). Coldren and Colombo (1994) have recently found that 9-month-old infants can process compound stimuli in a dimensional manner and that they can solve discrimination-learning problems by the categorical selection and testing of perceptual features.

Visual accommodation, ocular convergence, and motion parallax are used as depth perception cues within the first 6 months. Field (1977) has demonstrated preferential reaching for near objects as early as 3 months. Head retraction to looming objects (which appear to move toward the infant on a collision course) has been noted in early infancy (e.g., Ball and Tronick, 1971); However, there has been controversy whether the head movement represents innate fear or innate interest. According to the index of heart rate change, infants as young as 2 months of age can perceive a visual cliff illusion (Campos et al., 1970; Gibson and Walk, 1960).

Taste and Smell

Neonates show their preference for sweetened water by smiling and sucking in longer bursts, with shorter pauses (Crook, 1978; Lipsitt et al., 1976). Sour or bitter fluids, in contrast, evoke lip pursing or grimacing. Similar responses have been noted in anencephalic infants, suggesting that the movements are of subcortical origin (Steiner, 1979). Newborns are able to detect strong smells (Engen and Lipsitt, 1965), to discriminate their mother's breast pads (McFarlane, 1975), and to grimace at unpleasant odors (Steiner and Finnegan, 1975). The grimacing response, which is found in anencephalic infants, is probably a subcortical reflex. Ruff (1990) found that mouthing predominated as a perceptual tool during the first 6 months, but that it was displaced by fingering during the second 6 months.

Cutaneous Sensation

The mouth and genitals of the fetus become sensitive to touch during the first trimester and are followed by the palms, the soles, and the rest of the body. Thus, before birth, the structural and functional basis of skin sensation has already been established. The motor responses of the neonate to different cutaneous stimuli can be assessed by a number of neurological tests (e.g., the rooting, sucking, and plantar reflexes). Emde et al. (1971) and Anders and Chalemian (1974) noted that neonates fuss and cry during and after circumcision, suggesting that they are capable of experiencing pain.

Intermodal Perception

Piaget (1971) theorized that the coordination of the senses to form integrated perceptions could be achieved only after multiple parallel sensory experiences. In contrast, Gibson (1969), Bruner and Koslowski (1972), and Bower (1977) have hypothesized that early perception is diffuse and that perceptual specificity evolves from global sensory impressions.

Mendelson and Haith (1976) and Muir and Field (1979) have found that neonates will turn their heads and eyes in search of sustained sounds. Spelke (1979a, 1979b) has demonstrated that 4-month-old infants prefer to look at films in which sound is synchronized with action (compared with films that are out of synchrony). Spelke and Owsley (1979) have shown that 4-month-olds associate a parental voice with the visual image of that parent. Meltzoff and Borton (1979) have demonstrated mouth-eye cross-modal transfer as early as 1 month; and Lewkowicz and Turkewitz (1980) have found evidence that 3-week-old babies associate loudness and brightness. The global sensation theory appears to have been strongly supported; however, there is also evidence that premature babies are delayed in the capacity for cross-modal transfer (Rose et al., 1978).

Summary

Neonates can hear, see, smell, taste, and feel. The rudiments of hemispheric lateralization appear quite early, along with a particular sensitivity to speech and to the categorical distinctions associated with human phonological development. As they grow, infants prefer increasingly complex visual patterns, show a special liking for animated faces, exhibit shape and size constancy, and perceive color categorically. Early sensation appears to be global, but perceptual specificity evolves rapidly during the 1st year. In brief, nativist theory has been strongly supported by recent research; however, the complex interaction between learning and postnatal neural maturation requires elaboration.

PERCEPTUAL DEVELOPMENT

Of all developmental theorists, Gibson (1969) puts the greatest emphasis upon perception. To her, the child is an active perceiver, primed by species-specific genetic evolution to explore the environment and select what is required for adaptation. In contrast to Piaget who postulates that children construct their own representational worlds, Gibson describes the child as extracting available information from the stimulus field. The information elicited can vary from concrete (perceiving an object, for example) to abstract (as in the apperception of a melodic pattern). Perception grades imperceptibly into conceptualization as the child learns the distinctive features of particular objects (such as the mother's face), the common features of similar objects (such as the genus of dogs), and the deep structure of stimulus arrays (such as the syntax of a sentence). Perceptual processes would not be possible without search strategies, selective attention, and the exclusion of irrelevant input. According to Gibson, perceptual differentiation proceeds in linear fashion, not in stages.

Gibson et al. (1962) found that perceptual acuity for letterlike shapes increases from 4 to 8 years of age, but that, at all ages, children are able to discriminate, in order of difficulty: (1) figural breaks (e.g., *C* vs. *O*); (2) rotations and reversals (e.g., *b* vs. *P* vs. *d*); and (3) transformations (e.g., *H* vs. *N*). Bornstein and Stiles-Davis (1984) found that, between 4 to 6 years, vertical symmetry begins to assume precedence over horizontal and oblique symmetries, as is the case with adults. Gibson's theory of perceptual development has implications for the acquisition of reading skills. For example, poor readers exhibit the following phenomena:

1. *Literal decoding.* Poor readers tend to read word for word, without extracting meaning (Ryan, 1979).
2. *Poor comprehension.* In that they tend to be oblivious to contradictions or ambiguities in written material, poor readers seem not to monitor what they read for meaning (e.g., Paris and Myers, 1981).
3. *Poor strategies for the abstraction of meaning.* Poor readers have difficulty abstracting the gist of a story (Owings et al., 1980). Young children and older poor readers may be unaware of the purpose of reading, and unable to apply such *metacognitive strategies* as scanning rapidly for meaning, and looking for syntactic and semantic cues. Metacognition transcends concrete perception and will be considered further in the development of attention and memory. It has important implications for remedial reading (Ryan, 1979).

DEVELOPMENT OF ATTENTION

Clinicians often speak of attention as if it were unitary and distinct. On the contrary, attention is a multidimensional construct composed of such phenomena as strategic scanning, the exclusion of irrelevant stimuli, sustained attention, divided attention, the inhibition of impulsive action, and the selection and monitoring of response. It is not possible to design a test that taps a "pure" attentional faculty. Furthermore, children are unlikely to attend unless they know why they should, unless they find the task interesting or rewarding and unless they are able to distinguish figure from ground and signal from noise.

Under the age of 5 years, children's attention is captured by the salient features of a novel stimulus; attention is thus said to be *stimulus bound*. Between 5 and 7 years, a shift occurs: attention comes under the control of inner processes, such as selective search strategies. As children mature, they become more systematic, more flexible, and less egocentric (i.e., more *decentered*). In essence, older children know when and how to attend. Poor learners, conversely, spend inadequate time "on task," lack cognitive strategies for analyzing task demands, and mobilize insufficient effort to succeed (Zelniker and Jeffrey, 1979). The metacognitive processes that facilitate attention overlap those relevant to perception and memory.

Given the frequent reference to defective attention in child and adolescent psychiatry, surprisingly little is known about its normal development. Reaction time, the capacity for vigilance and sustained attention, and the control of impulsive responses, improve up to 12 years. Thereafter, although reaction time stabilizes, accuracy continues to advance as more efficient search strategies are acquired (Salkind and Nelson, 1980). In one of the few studies that have provided age-normalized data, Levy (1979) found that, from 3 to 8 years, measures of sustained attention, reaction time, and motor inhibition showed strong age and social class effects and that the three measures improved exponentially between 4 and 6 years of age. Multivariate analysis subsequently isolated a generalized "attention" factor upon which reaction time and continuous performance loaded heavily and which was separable from motor inhibition. A measure of motor activity was later found to be correlated with the attention factor. Subsequently, a study of clinic-referred children demonstrated that the clinical sample performed significantly more poorly than normal children of the same age on measures of attention, motor inhibition, and activity. However, when performance was related to age, the performance curves of the clinic sample paralleled those of the normal children. This study suggests that the diagnosis of attention deficit may be problematic in children younger than 5 years, since, between 4 and 5 years, normal children show marked variation in activity level, in the capacity for sustained attention, and in motor inhibition; furthermore, in the transitional period between 4 and 6 years of age, social class has a powerful effect on the capacity for sustained and selective attention.

In an extensive review of research into the development of attention, Taylor (1980) concludes that little is known of the development of the capacity for divided attention, other than that it improves with age. It appears that older children are better able to resist distraction by stimuli irrelevant to the task at hand. Younger children find distractions harder to ignore, to the extent that the stimuli are salient, novel, or similar to the stimulus that is relevant to the task.

Barkley (1988) has discussed the importance of motivation in regard to attention. The capacity for sustained, selective attention and for reflective, nonimpulsive responding is affected by both maturation and learning. A child who has neither been expected to concentrate, nor praised for doing so, is likely to be slow in acquiring the capacity for sustained, reflective attention. However, if a generally inattentive child has previously had the benefit of adequate models and consistent reinforcement, it is more likely that the origin of the problem lies in the neural substrate. Two causative hypotheses have been advanced: (a) the sensory analyzers mediating selective attention might be abnormal or (b) the neural links between memory, punishment, and reinforcement might be defective. (For further discussion of the development of inattention, see Chapter 26.)

Mirsky et al. (1991) propose that attention has the following components: *focus*, *sustain*, and *shift*. Focussing is the selection of target information for enhanced processing. Sustaining refers to the maintenance of focus and alertness over time. Shifting is the changing of focus in a flexible, adaptive manner. The validity of the three components of attention has been supported by multivariate studies of the attention performance scores of both adults and children. Sohlberg and Mateer (1989) hypothesize that attention is a multidimensional cognitive capacity with five levels: focussed attention, sustained attention, selective attention, alternating attention, and divided attention. The upper levels require controlled processing, whereas the lower levels are automatic.

DEVELOPMENT OF MEMORY

The term "memory" has connotations ranging from the act of recalling a personally experienced event (*autobiographical memory*) to the automatized repetition of a learned behavior (*procedural memory*). Memory is inextricably linked to other cognitive processes such as attention, perception, categorization, schematization, consciousness, and metamemory (which assesses the origin and accuracy of memory). The development of memory is not separable from that of cognition in general. Interpersonal experience as well as neuronal maturation directly influence different forms of memory.

Forms of Memory

INFORMATION PROCESSING

Memory has been studied from the perspective of information processing. In this view, sensory input impacts sensory registers, producing a short-lived *sensory memory* (less than 250 msec). At this stage, information is scanned by attentional processes and a small proportion placed in short-term ("working") memory. Without active processing, short-term memory decays after about 30 seconds. After attention and processing (e.g., by classification or rehearsal), information in short-term memory can be deposited in long-term memory for an indefinite period.

Encoding refers to the transfer of information from sensory registers to short-term memory and then to long-term memory. *Storage* refers to the capacity of the mind to represent information and have it potentially available for later access. *Retrieval* is the accessing of information from storage. Retrieval processes activate behavior, emotion, and verbal output, which leads to *recounting*.

The recounting of autobiographical events often takes the form of a narrative and is related to the capacity to retrieve items from memory storage, to sequence them in story form, and to communicate them to a listener. Recounting, thus, involves both cognition and discourse.

EARLY AND LATE MEMORY

Cognitive psychologists have described two forms of retrieval: *direct* and *indirect*. Direct retrieval includes free recall (at which young children are poor) and recognition (at which they are much better). Indirect retrieval acts on processes and representations that convey a general pattern of action (e.g., long-term memory, sensory imaging) (Siegel, 1995a).

Retrieval can be conceptualized as the reactivation of a neural net configuration similar to that activated at the time of encoding. Memory is reconstructive, not reproductive. Encoding, storage, and retrieval are influenced by organizing processes such as attention, perception, and schematization. From a developmental viewpoint, the brain's ability to store experience as neural representations with the potential for reactivation is dependent on the sophistication of encoding, storage, and retrieval. Access to stored representations (i.e., the activation of latent neural net configurations) will also be dependent on retrieval. Thus, the inability of young children to recall aspects of an experience directly may mean that it was never encoded or that it was encoded and stored but that reactivation is impaired by immature retrieval strategies.

Given the distinction between early, nondeclarative memory and late, declarative memory, one must be clear about what kind of memory is being discussed. Emotional learning and behavioral learning occur early. Childhood amnesia, for example, affects memory up to about 3 years of age. Childhood amnesia refers to an impairment of the access to declarative autobiographical memory, whereas nondeclarative (emotional and behavioral) memory may be intact.

Clinicians and researchers have focused on the development of declarative memory. However, early emotional and behavioral learning also influence child development. Attachment theory (Bowlby, 1969; Main, 1991) derives its constructs from the idea that, after repeated patterns of relating, an infant constructs mental models of attachment. These mental models organize the infant's behavioral and emotional responses, and, later, influence declarative memory, self-reflection, and autobiographical memory.

Past maltreatment can affect nondeclarative memory. The retrieval of early learned emotional-behavioral responses may be triggered in adulthood by emotional states similar to those that applied in early childhood. This could explain the transgenerational transfer of child abuse, and the perpetrator's unawareness of its origin. Some of the symptoms of posttraumatic stress disorder (e.g., intrusive memories, avoidance, startle response, traumatic amnesia) could be explained on the basis of the impaired explicit memory and intact implicit memory of traumatic experiences (Siegel, 1995b).

Domains of Memory Development

STRATEGIES

Immature memory strategies limit the young child's ability to encode and store memory and to retrieve it in declarative form. As memory strategies develop, the mind becomes better able to encode, store, and retrieve memories. Young children often require help with retrieval cues, whereas older children may be capable of both free recall and effective access to relevant memories.

Encoding and storage strategies are potentially conscious activities that facilitate encoding and storage. They include looking, pointing (to direct attention), naming, and talking about things. Strategies become more complex, flexible, and specific with maturation. *Rehearsal strategies* help to move items from short-term memory to long-term memory. *Organizational strategies*, such as clustering, establish associational links that facilitate storage. *Elaborational strategies* add meaning to presented items to enhance storage. Finally, the development of efficient strategies to allocate cognitive resources facilitates encoding. The evolution of these complex processes allows the child to search memory more intelligently, efficiently, flexibly, systematically, and exhaustively. As children develop, they tailor the strategy of retrieval to the task at hand.

Research suggests that some memory strategies can be taught. However, many children continue to rely on techniques they have acquired spontaneously in the course of development.

KNOWLEDGE

Memory is not a photocopy machine. What people already know influences what they can learn and remember. Encoding and storage are constructive; retrieval is reconstructive. Memory is organized in part by schemata or concepts that are in flux between organization and reorganization. Neural net representations carry meaning that is fundamental to schematization. Thus, retrieval may involve memory reactivation and cognitive inference, both of which bridge the gaps that block retrieval.

As the child develops, new knowledge schemata and structures shape memory. The constructive aspect of memory is exemplified by memory for events. Event memory is influenced by general schemata. For example, the memory of something occurring at school is influenced by the generic memory of a typical day at school. The predominance of general schemata in early childhood retrieval may be explained by the late maturation of the hippocampus and related brain regions.

Indirect forms of retrieval include *priming*, that is, behavioral learning independent of conscious awareness of prior experience. The speed at which a task is learned is affected by priming. The indirect recall characteristic of infancy and early childhood is known as *early memory*, *procedural memory*, *nondeclarative memory*, or *implicit memory*, terms that are regarded as synonymous in this chapter. Implicit memory is multifaceted; it embraces behavioral learning, emotional learning, and priming.

In contrast, direct recall is known as *late memory*, *episodic memory*, *semantic memory*, *declarative memory*, or *explicit memory*. These terms overlap in meaning and refer to a general kind of recall known as "remembering." Remembering involves the recall of facts or concepts (semantic memory) and the recall of personally experienced events (episodic memory). Semantic and episodic memory are usually explicit or declarative, that is, recountable in words or other symbols. (For further discussion of information processing, see Chapter 11.)

Maturation of Memory

The mature brain contains over 20 billion neurons. At birth the number is greater. The neuronal pruning occurring during infancy and early childhood is genetically and experientially determined. On the other hand, the number of synapses increases markedly during the early years until each neuron is connected to thousands of other neurons. Neurons interconnect in parallel distributions known as neural networks. Cognitive processes derive from parallel processing in neural nets. A mental "representation" is thought to be based in a neural-net activation pattern. A "process" is a neural activity that acts on representations and transforms them, creates new connections, or extracts common features from different representations (i.e., generalizations, similarities, or dif-

ferences). Cognitive "structures" are complex functions that have repeated patterns of action, such as focal attention or long-term memory.

Cognitive processes can represent cognitive processes. This process, metacognition, develops during the preschool and elementary school years. One form of metacognition—metamemory—allows the child to understand memory itself. Metamemory conveys knowledge about how memory works as well as how to monitor and regulate it. Metamemory embraces the assessment of current memory state, the selection of strategies, and the evaluation of progress toward cognitive goals. An example of metamemory would be the subjective sensation of hunting for a memory and then recalling it.

The capacity to locate the origin of a memory is called *source monitoring*. One form of source metamemory, *reality monitoring*, is the process by which the mind determines if a memory is external or imaginary in origin. Reality monitoring becomes more efficient in later childhood (Johnson, 1991).

Memory Capacity

If the energy resources allocated to information processing are limited, then the operation of intentional, nonautomatic processes will limit the resources available for other cognitive processes. Thus, in a young child, immature storage and retrieval drains resources from and restricts other memory processes (Fivush and Hudson, 1990).

Cognitive development enhances memory capacity by freeing resources for use in other mnemonic activities. For example, as strategies become automatized, storage capacity and retrieval efficiency increase. The automatization of metamemory together with the way that knowledge structures provide individualized scaffolds for storage and retrieval contribute to the uniqueness of each child's memory development. The full development of memory, thus, depends upon an interaction among strategies, knowledge, metamemory, and capacity (Flavell et al., 1993). The next section illustrates this complex interplay.

Development of Autobiographical Memory

MEMORY, SELF, AND TIME

Autobiographical memory refers to memory of the self at a particular time in the past. The terms *explicit memory*, *declarative memory*, and *late memory* embrace episodic or autobiographical memory. However, it is unclear whether autobiographical memory is different from semantic memory for facts and ideas. The retrieval of a particular autobiographical memory conveys a profile of representations of sensations, emotions, facts, and self-in-the-past.

INFANTILE AMNESIA

The maturation of autobiographical memory involves an interaction among language, social interaction, self-concept, and sense of time. The earliest form of declarative memory is *generic event memory*. Children construct generalized patterns that represent familiar, oft-repeated events. As a result, new experiences are processed in accordance with generic memory. Encoding, thus, is biased by expectations based on preexisting structures, while accurate retrieval is biased insofar as retrieval scanning is influenced by generic memory. Generic event scripts may be associated with preevent and postevent suggestibility (Ceci and Bruch, 1993).

The immaturity of autobiographical memory in infancy and early childhood is associated with infantile and childhood amnesia. Freud (1963) proposed that infantile amnesia was due to an active repression of early experience. The encoding deficit theory (Wetzler and Sweeney, 1986) proposes a lack of attention to experiential detail, with impaired encoding and blocked retrieval. A third view (Pillemer and White, 1989) hypothesizes a discrepancy between encoding state and retrieval state, in that prelinguistic encoding is incompatible with more mature cognitive and language-based retrieval. Freud suggested that the repression barrier lifts at 8 years of age. The encoding deficit and the encoding-retrieval discrepancy theories propose 5 years of age for the termination of childhood amnesia. Fitzgerald (1991) contends that autobiographical memory emerges at 3 years of age. This early, implicit memory, which is intact during "childhood amnesia" may influence play therapy and transference experiences within psychotherapy (Lewis, 1995).

Children begin to tell stories of their experiences at about 3 years of age. In fact, in childhood, autobiographical memory is expressed primarily in narrative form.

NARRATIVE AND AUTOBIOGRAPHICAL MEMORY

Autobiographical memory and narrative capacity intertwine. Narrative is a social interaction in the form of a discourse between people in which the teller takes account of the listener's interests and expectations while recounting a temporal sequence of events together with the intentions of the characters in the story. The basis of narrative capacity, like Vygotsky's (1978) notion of thought as internalized dialogue, is the facilitation of personal relationships. Parents help their children to construct narratives; thus, a lack of exposure to coconstruction and memory talk could lead to an impairment of narrative memory. Children classified in infancy as avoidantly attached subsequently tend to exhibit a deficit in autobiographical memory that is correlated with similar deficiencies in their parents (Main, 1991). Further research is required to determine whether the correlation is causal in nature.

Autobiographical recounting necessitates an interplay between language, social skills, self-concept, and temporality. Language development allows memory to be expressed in communicable form, as does the capacity to draw pictures.

As language and social competence mature, the child's sense of self and capacity to reflect on selfness enhance autobiographical memory. Theoretically, self-reflection enables the elaboration of memory as "self" experience. Both encoding and retrieval may be organized by the self-concept. In other words, self-reflection interacts with social interaction and language in the reciprocal facilitation of autobiographical memory. The capacity for sequencing or temporality is also involved. A child's sense of time and order develop throughout the preschool- and early school-age years. As temporality develops, the sense of self-in-time begins to shape autobiographical memory. A sense of personal continuity thus emerges, permitting new experiences to be processed from a temporal perspective.

NEUROBIOLOGY OF ATTENTION AND MEMORY

Attention

Margulies (1985) proposes that the hippocampus mediates selective attention. Features or patterns abstracted from sensory data are conveyed to the hippocampus and matched against a cognitive "map" in order to determine whether a particular stimulus is noteworthy. Noteworthiness is determined in accordance with such criteria as novelty, salience, and emotional valence. The threshold and propensity of hippocampal selectivity may be modulated on a phasic basis (by norepinephrine), on a diurnal basis (by serotonin), or on a long-term basis (by corticosteroids). Once a stimulus is selected as noteworthy, efferents flow from the hippocampus to the medial septum (where spatial localization is determined) and the nucleus accumbens (which interrupts thought and allows the integration of the noteworthy stimulus into behavior). The organism, thus, can change the direction of attention toward the new stimulus.

Hunt et al. (1987) and Zametkin and Rapoport (1987) regard the noradrenergic theory of attention deficit disorder as the strongest current contender. According to this theory, attention deficit and hyperactivity are due to an increase in noradrenergic transmission, possibly emanating from the locus coeruleus. Such an increase could be due to a variety of processes (e.g., heightened postsynaptic receptor sensitivity, or increased presynaptic production or release). It is unclear how the noradrenergic hypothesis of attention deficit fits the hippocampal theory of selective attention; perhaps a tonically high noradrenergic state causes a reduction of the hippocampal threshold to stimuli, leading to increased distractibility.

Mirsky et al. (1991) refer their three proposed components of attention—focus, sustain, and shift—to different brain systems. Focussing and execution are related to the superior temporal and inferior parietal cortices and to the corpus striatum. Sustained vigilance is related to the mesopontine reticular formation and to the midline and reticular thalamic nuclei. The capacity to shift from one salient aspect of the environment to another is associated with the prefrontal cortex.

Memory

Implicit memory is thought to be associated with the function of the basal ganglia, amygdala, and, possibly, the motor and somatosensory cortices. Recent research suggests that the medial temporal lobe is the key to declarative, autobiographical memory. Within the medial temporal lobe is the hippocampus, one of the few brain regions that undergo postnatal neurogenesis. In humans, hippocampal neurogenesis may occur up to 2 years of age, while synaptogenesis continues even longer. Hippocampal neurogenesis coincides with the period of childhood amnesia.

In nonhuman primates and other mammals, the hippocampus has a central role in environmental memory, such as the ability to learn a maze. Environmental memory requires spatial and temporal competence. Learning involving the hippocampus permits context-dependent encoding and retrieval. The hippocampus is thought to be associated with cognitive "maps" that structure time, space, and sense of self in such a way as to facilitate autobiographical memory.

In humans, clinical disorders caused by lesions to the hippocampus impair declarative memory, whereas implicit memory remains intact (Squire, 1992). In the absence of hippocampal processing, a form of learning is possible, but it lacks an explicit sense of time, self, or context. Infants exhibit implicit memory postnatally, develop generic event memory, and then, by 3 years of age, autobiographical memory emerges. Context-free, generic memories may be a function of an immature hippocampus. As postnatal neurogenesis and synaptogenesis establish full hippocampal function, memories incorporating time, place, and self become possible.

Social interactions that stimulate the communication of a sense of self and time may both depend on hippocampal maturation and also stimulate its further development. Individual differences in autobiographical memory capacity may thus reflect the interdependency of social interaction, cognition, and neural substrate. Autobiographical memory and narrative reflect a transaction between experience and brain function.

Recent research has illuminated the cellular substrate of episodic memory. Neurochemical explanations must account for the extraordinary associativity, durability, efficiency, capacity, and rapidity of memory. Some, at least, of those qualities are consistent with long-term potentiation of the hippocampus by brief bursts of high-frequency stimulation.

Long-term potentiation is associated with the opening of calcium ion channels by glutamate, an excitatory neurotransmitter. Calcium ions enter the neuron and function as a second messenger system, activating intracellular kinases, proteases, and lipases. The consequent degradation of cytostructural proteins and membrane phospholipids is thought to promote an increase in the number of excitatory receptors, changes in the shape of dendritic spines, and a proliferation of dendritic synapses. These structural and functional alterations would be consistent with long-term potentiation. Furthermore, the coincident activation of multiple sensory synapses on the one association neuron (or set of neurons) could provide a neural basis for cross-modal perception.

It has recently been discovered that the serotonergic stimulation of neurons elevates intracellular levels of cyclic AMP (cAMP). When a critical level of cAMP is exceeded, the nuclear cyclic response element binding (CREB) gene is activated (by phosphorylation). CREB transcription proteins then activate other genes, which in turn activate memory storage (by an as yet unknown mechanism).

DEVELOPMENTAL PSYCHOPATHOLOGY OF ATTENTION, PERCEPTION, AND MEMORY

Although neither attention, nor perception, nor memory is ever exhibited in isolation, in different forms of developmental psychopathology, it is possible to discern defect, hypertrophy, and deviance of each of these functions.

Disorders of Attention

DEFICIENT ATTENTION

Attention deficit is thought to be the cardinal sign of attention deficit disorder, a condition characterized in part by distractibility, difficulty following instructions, difficulty sustaining attention on an imposed task, heedlessness, impulsiveness, and recklessness. Douglas (1983) has described how poor attention and impulsivity can impede the acquisition of concepts, learning strategies, and effectance motivation. However, despite the confidence with which attention deficit disorder is customarily diagnosed, there are many questions concerning the homogeneity and categorical distinctness of this disorder (Taylor, 1988). As described previously, since the capacity for sustained and selective attention increases markedly between 48 and 54 months (Levy, 1979), the diagnosis should be cautiously made in children younger than 4 years of age. It is unclear how inclusive or exclusive the diagnostic criteria for this condition should be; as a result, the estimated prevalence of the condition varies between Europe (where it is relatively low) and North America (where it is much higher). As Rutter (1983) points out, inattention and overactivity are encountered in many situations, from pain, fatigue, illness, and transient emotional upset, to psychopathological conditions such as mania, major depression, panic disorder, schizophrenia, intoxication, and confusional states. Furthermore, as previously discussed, attention is not a unitary phenomenon. Not surprisingly, it is unclear whether oppositional defiant disorder, conduct disorder, and attention deficit disorder are distinct, coterminous, or coincidental. Douglas (1983) notes that, although attentional problems are often associated with impulsivity, poor arousal modulation, and an inclination to seek immediate reinforcement, it has not been clearly established that defective attention is the basic dysfunction of attention deficit disorder.

Defective attention has also been found in children at high risk for developing schizophrenia (Mednick et al., 1978); however, the relationship between this phenomenon and later schizophrenia is unclear. (For further discussion of inattention, see Chapter 26.)

HEIGHTENED ATTENTION

Hypervigilance and narrowing of attention occur in situations involving focussed fear (e.g., watching a horror movie), night terrors, paranoid conditions (rare in childhood), and in some acute schizophrenic states. Attention fluctuates in delirium and is diminished particularly at night and in situations associated with reduced sensory stimulation. Heightened attention may be associated with perceptual illusions; for example, the anxious or phobic child who mistakes nocturnal rustlings for the approach of an intruder. Cocaine and stimulant abuse are associated with exaggerated, fixed concentration.

Disorders of Perception

Ludwig (1980) classifies perceptual abnormalities as follows:

1. False perceptions independent of reality
2. False perceptions dependent upon reality
3. False perceptions that stem from sensory deficit or dysfunction

INDEPENDENT FALSE PERCEPTIONS

Independent false perceptions take the form of *hallucinations* or *pseudohallucinations*.

A *hallucination* is a perception that has no basis in objective reality. Hallucinations vary in sensory modality, in form (from amorphous to organized), in intensity (e.g., loud or soft), in clarity (vague or clear), in spatial location (internal or external, near or far), and in the degree of conviction or urgency they convey.

Epileptic auras and temporal lobe seizures may be associated with poorly formed auditory, olfactory, or visceral hallucinations. Panoramic visions may be described. Delirium is typically associated with poorly formed, unpleasant, visual, auditory, or cutaneous hallucinations. Cerebral space-occupying lesions may be associated with intense, compelling hallucinations, and with bizarre phenomena such as negative hallucinations, autoscopy, the perception of a *doppelgänger*, distortions of the body image, depersonalization, and déjà vu experiences. The hallucinations that result from the ingestion of hallucinogens tend to be associated with profound distortions of sensory perception and affective experience and subsequently with traumatic "flashbacks" (intrusive memories of the hallucinatory state).

Schizophrenia is typically associated with unpleasant auditory hallucinations that emerge from amorphous perceptual distortions and take the form of conversations, commands, commentaries on the subject's actions, or echoing of the subject's thoughts. In paranoid states, auditory hallucinations tend to be accusatory, degrading, controlling, or laudatory in nature and consistent with the patient's delusional beliefs.

Disorganized auditory or visual hallucinations are sometimes encountered in mania; whereas in melancholia, depressive hallucinations (relatively rare in adolescence) are consistent with the prevailing delusions of guilt and self-abasement.

Cantor et al. (1982) contend that preschool children can manifest schizophrenia, but this condition is exceptionally rare before 7 years of age and quite uncommon before adolescence. There has been some uncertainty whether autistic children are prone to develop hallucinatory psychotic disintegration in late childhood or adolescence (Petty et al., 1984). The hallucinations in such conditions are relatively unsystematized and perceived as alien, commanding, or threatening in nature.

Pseudohallucinations are experienced in the form of heightened internal thought or images. Pseudohallucinations convey less conviction than true hallucinations, and have a content directly related to the individual's psychic predicament. For example, a sexually traumatized adolescent may have recurrent vivid memories ("flashbacks") of being attacked, with accompanying conversations and visual imagery; or a miserable, lonely child may have an image of a deceased relative speaking words of consolation. Pseudohallucinations are common in the overlapping conditions of hysterical psychosis, dissociative disorder, and posttraumatic stress disorder. Care should be taken to distinguish these common conditions from schizophrenia and temporal lobe epilepsy, with which they are frequently confused. (For further discussion of the development of psychotic thinking, see Chapter 25.)

DEPENDENT FALSE PERCEPTIONS

An illusion is sensation given a false interpretation, that is, the erroneous perception of a real experience. Auditory and visual illusions are characteristic of intense emotional states (e.g., religious conversion) and physical deprivation (e.g., hunger, thirst, or fatigue). They are also encountered in delirium, intoxication (especially with hallucinogens), epilepsy, hysteria, and acute psychotic conditions. The phenomena of depersonalization, derealization, déjà vu, body image distortion, and alteration of the sense of time are commonly associated with anxiety in adolescence, but are also found in intoxication with hallucinogens, and in epilepsy, hysteria, and psychosis.

FALSE PERCEPTIONS ASSOCIATED WITH SENSORY DEFICIT OR DEPRIVATION

Deafness and blindness may be associated with misperception, especially when the individual is delirious, deprived of sensory input, or affected by certain medications (e.g., salicylates).

HEIGHTENED PERCEPTION

Eidetic imagery has the clarity of real perception and is perceived as though external to the viewer. The propensity to generate accurate, vivid, perceptual memories of events may be a normal variant. It could conceivably interact with stress or metabolic instability to generate visual hallucinations.

PERCEPTUAL IMPAIRMENT

The association between perceptual impairment and reading retardation has been a topic of investigation and debate for many years. Is dyslexia fundamentally a perceptual disorder? Or is the perceptual immaturity associated with dyslexia secondary to higher-order language dysfunction? Or do children with perceptual disorder represent a subgroup of dyslexics? These issues are discussed in Chapter 48, "Developmental Learning Disorder."

Disorders of Memory

Disturbances of memory in children can range from an inhibition of semantic recall and impairment of encoding occurring after head trauma, to an impairment of the retrieval of autobiographical memory in posttraumatic stress disorder. The intricate relationships among attention, perception, schematization, and memory suggest that impairment in a variety of cognitive processes could affect memory. Thus, the clinical assessment of memory in a child requires a broad developmental profile including cognitive development, experiential history, family functioning, and school environment.

Memory dysfunction can be present in any of the domains of memory described earlier in this chapter. Thus, clinicians encounter deficits in encoding, short-term memory, access to long-term memory, or retrieval of autobiographical or semantic memory. Cases have been described in which implicit memory is intact but explicit memory impaired. Hippocampal lesions, Korsakoff's syndrome, hypnotic amnesia, the aftermath of surgical anesthesia, the side effect of benzodiazepines, and childhood amnesia are associated with this kind of mnemonic disassociation. Memory disturbances can involve a loss of previously attained memory, temporary abnormalities in established functions, or maturational delay. Because memory is embedded in cognition as a whole, specific learning disorder, mental retardation, language disorder, attention deficit disorder, and organic brain disorder are all associated with memory dysfunction.

Depending on the location and extent of brain pathology, neurological disorders can present with a variety of memory abnormalities. Disorders leading to dementia may produce impairment of the encoding and retrieval of both short-term and long-term memory. Examples of such disorders are infections (e.g., subacute sclerosing panencephalitis, Jakob-Creutzfeldt disease, AIDS), metabolic disorder (e.g., Tay-Sachs disease, Wilson's disease), neurocutaneous degenerative disorders (e.g., Sturge-Weber syndrome, neurofibromatosis, tuberous sclerosis), and toxic syndromes (e.g., lead encephalopathy).

Head injury can produce anterograde and retrograde amnesia. Retrograde amnesia is thought to be due to disruption of the cortical consolidation required to establish long-term memory.

Seizure disorders can be associated with defects in memory. Generalized seizures impair the retrieval of recently experienced events. Partial complex seizure disorder (temporal lobe epilepsy) causes a disturbance in verbal recall and encoding. Preictal (aura) states are associated with dissociative symptoms (derealization, distortions in the sense of time, perceptual distortion). Ictal and postictal states can impair attention, language processing, and memory retrieval.

Other neurological disorders affecting memory include viral infection (e.g., herpes encephalitis), multiple sclerosis, and brain tumor. The location of the lesion determines the nature of the memory pathology.

Experiential factors affecting memory include attachment disruption and psychological trauma. Culture, family environment, and school all shape memory development. The family's encouragement of intellectual achievement, memory talk, and the shared construction of stories stimulate the domains of memory development: strategies, knowledge, metamemory, and memory capacity.

As described earlier, attachment research suggests that two groups (avoidantly attached children, dismissing adults) exhibit a paucity of autobiographical narrative and diminished access to episodic memory (Main, 1991). These nonclinical studies suggest that, in the United States, at least 10% of the population has impaired access to autobiographical memory. The factors that mediate this impairment are unclear. It is possible that the remote or rejecting parents who have avoidantly attached offspring fail to stimulate their children by telling, sharing, and listening to stories. Another possibility is that the association is genetic.

A failure to tell stories may aggravate psychological trauma. If parent and child cannot talk about the child's frightening experience—for example, if the parent is too misguided, preoccupied, oblivious, or compromised to do so—the child may be at risk of posttraumatic stress disorder. Posttraumatic amnesia is a controversial matter. The mental mechanisms known by clinicians as repression, dissociation, and distortion require empirical validation and clarification. Repression has been ascribed to the automatization of conscious suppression: Encoding has occurred but retrieval is blocked. Dissociation is akin to the divided attention and altered consciousness observed in hypnotic states. The subject's mental state at the time of encoding can influence later accessibility to retrieval. Divided attention research using dichotic listening methodology has shown that implicit memory may be intact in the nonattending ear. If a child learns to adapt to trauma by means of autohypnotic division of attention and dissociation, implicit memory may be intact, whereas explicit, narrative memory is impaired (Siegel, 1995b).

Since memory is reconstructive, not reproductive, error and distortion are possible. Both adults and children are subject to preevent biasing and postevent suggestion, for example, by the use of leading questions, persuasion, coercion, or group pressure. After repeated suggestive questioning, a child may begin to construct memories that are consistent but false. This is a serious problem in the investigation of allegations of abuse, particularly with regard to preschool children who have difficulty providing sequential narratives and who often require a certain amount of leading (Ceci and Bruck, 1993; Goodman and Bottoms, 1993).

CONCLUSION

At the beginning of the chapter, it was suggested that the unstable nature of contemporary developmental theory has impeded research into attention, perception, and memory. Kuhn (1988) and Horowitz (1987) have discussed why and how this is so.

Prior to 1960, the dominant model in developmental psychology was behaviorist. In the study of memory, for example, behaviorists might examine the learning of paired nonsense syllables, stripping the mnemonic task of meaning and context, and hoping, thus, to tap the fundamental processes involved. Behaviorists viewed development as the cumulative acquisition of units of behavior under the control of the environment, and they eschewed theorizing about internal ("black box") processes.

During the 1960s, the constructivist model of Jean Piaget became increasingly influential. In Piagetian theory, development was regarded as the outcome of an interaction between the individual and the physical environment. Through this interaction, the child acquired mental structures that direct the search for meaning and undergo sweeping qualitative reorganizations at different points of development.

The conflict between behaviorists and constructivists held center stage during the 1960s, but, eventually, disillusion set in with both models. On the one hand, Kendler and Kendler (1975) demonstrated that classical behavioral theory could not explain the reversal shift phenomenon and that internal mediational processes must consequently be postulated. Meanwhile, constructivists became increasingly dissatisfied with Piagetian theory, particularly the doctrine of stages. The operational structures of serial ordering, classification, transitivity, and conservation were not found to develop synchronously, as would be predicted; even within each domain of operations, different abilities appear to emerge unevenly. Moreover, Piaget's theory of the process of developmental change depends upon abstract concepts (e.g., equilibration), which have proven difficult or impossible to operationalize.

The dominant contemporary model of cognitive development is that of the computer, as embodied in the information-processing approach. Information-processing theory reduces cognition to sets of sequential operations that function separately and combine serially to process information. However, the information-processing paradigm has been criticized in that it emphasizes strategy execution at the expense of strategy selection. The computer is not a satisfactory analog for the self-aware, meaning-seeking, strategy-selecting, execution-monitoring person. The problem appears to reside in the difficulty of encompassing metacognition in a computer model. An active learner in the natural environment owns a problem, analyzes it, selects or designs strategies that fit the problem and environment, and checks the process of problem resolution. A problem is not owned if it is not appreciated as significant or important. Attention, perception, and memory are sets of processes that are part of the broader enterprise of problem identification, analysis, and resolution. Moreover, in contrast to the behaviorist model, information processing lacks a powerful, experimental methodology. Although, as Horowitz (1987) suggests, developmental psychology is still in search of a paradigm, the recent marriage of neuroscience and cognitive psychology points the way to new directions.

References

Acredolo LP: The development of special orientation in infancy. *Dev Psychol* 14:224–234, 1978.

Acredolo LP, Hake JL: Infant perception. In: Wolman BB (ed): *Handbook of Developmental Psychology*. Englewood Cliffs, NJ, Prentice-Hall, 1982.

Anders TF, Chalemian RJ: The effect of circumcision on sleep-wake states in human neonates. *Psychosom Med* 36:174–179, 1974.

Aslin RN, Pisoni DB, Jusczyk PW: Auditory development and speech perception in infancy. In: Mussen PH, Haith MM, Campos JJ (eds): *Handbook of Child Psychology*. Vol 2: *Infancy and Developmental Psychobiology* (4th ed). New York, Wiley, 1983.

Atkinson R, Shiffrin R: Human memory: A proposed system and its control processes. In: Spence KW, Spence JT (eds): *The Psychology of Learning and Motivation* (Vol 2). New York, Academic Press, 1968.

Bach MJ, Underwood BJ: Developmental changes in memory attributes. *J Educ Psychol* 61:292–296, 1970.

Ball W, Tronick E: Infant responses to impending collisions: Optical and real. *Science* 171:818–820, 1971.

Banks MS, Salapatek P: Infant visual perception. In: Mussen PH, Haith MM, Campos JJ (eds): *Handbook of Child Psychology*. Vol 2: *Infancy and Developmental Psychobiology* (4th ed). New York, Wiley, 1983.

Barkley RA: Attention. In: Tramontana MG, Hooper SR (eds): *Assessment Issues in Child Neuropsychology*. New York, Plenum, 1988.

Baudry M, Lynch G: Properties and substrates of mammalian memory systems. In: Meltzer HY (ed): *Psychopharmacology: The Third Generation of Progress*. New York, Raven Press, 1987.

Bench J: The auditory response. In: Steve V (ed): *Perinatal Physiology*. New York, Plenum, 1978.

Benson JB, Uzgiris RC: Effect of self-initiated locomotion on infant search activity. *Dev Psychol* 21:923–931, 1985.

Berg WK, Berg KM: Psychophysiological development in infancy: State, sensory function, and attention. In: Osofsky JD (ed): *Handbook of Infant Development*. New York, Wiley, 1979.

Bornstein MH: Psychological studies of color perception in human infants: Habituation, discrimination and categorization, recognition, and conceptualization. In: Lipsitt LP (ed): *Advances in Infancy Research* (Vol 1). Norwood, NJ, Ablex, 1981.

Bornstein MH: A descriptive taxonomy of psychological categories used by infants. In: Sophian C (ed): *Origins of Cognitive Skills*. Hillsdale, NJ, Erlbaum, 1984.

Bornstein MH: Perceptual development across the life cycle. In: Bornstein MH, Lamb ME (eds): *Developmental Psychology: An Advanced Textbook* (3rd ed). Hillsdale, NJ, Erlbaum, 1992.

Bornstein MH, Kessen W, Weiskopf S: The categories of hue in infancy. *Science* 191:201–202, 1976a.

Bornstein MH, Kessen W, Weiskopf S: Color vision and hue categorization in young human infants. *J Exp Psychol Hum Percept Perform* 2:115–129, 1976b.

Bornstein MH, Stiles Davis J: Discrimination for symmetry in young children. *Dev Psychol* 20:639–649, 1984.

Bower TGR: Slant perception and shape constancy in infants. *Science* 151:832–834, 1966a.

Bower TGR: The visual world of infants. *Sci Am* 215:80–92, 1966b.

Bower TGR: Blind babies see with their ears. *New Sci* 73:256–257, 1977.

Bowlby J: *Attachment and Loss*. Vol 1: *Attachment*. New York, Basic Books, 1969.

Boyd TA: Clinical assessment of memory in children: A developmental framework for practice. In: Tramontana MG, Hooper SR (eds): *Assessment Issues in Child Neuropsychology*. New York, Plenum, 1988.

Brown AL: The development of memory: Knowing, knowing about knowing, and knowing how to know. *Adv Child Dev Behav* 10, 1988.

Bruner JS, Koslowski B: Visually preadapted constituents of manipulatory actions. *Perception* 1:3–14, 1972.

Campos JJ, Langer A, Krowitz A: Cardiac responses on the visual cliff in prelocomotor human infants. *Science* 170:195–196, 1970.

Cantor S, Evans J, Pearce J, et al: Childhood schizophrenia: Present but not accounted for. *Am J Psychiatry* 139:758–762, 1982.

Caron AJ, Caron RF, Carlson VR: Do infants see objects or retinal images? Shape constancy revisited. *Infant Behav Dev* 1:229–243, 1978.

Case R, Kurland D, Goldberg J: Operational efficiency and the growth of short-term memory span. *J Exp Child Psychol* 33:386–404, 1982.

Ceci SJ, Bruck M: Suggestibility of the child witness: A historical review and synthesis. *Psychol Bull* 113:403–439, 1993.

Cohen LB: Our developing knowledge of infant perception. *Am Psychol* 34:894–899, 1979.

Coldren JT, Colombo J: The nature and processes of preverbal learning: Implications from nine-month-old infants' discrimination problem solving. *Monogr Soc Res Child Dev* 59(4):1–93, 1994.

Condon WS, Sander LW: Neonate movement is synchronized with adult speech. *Science* 183:99–100, 1974.

Craik F, Lockhart R: Levels of processing: A framework for memory research. *J Verb Learn Verb Behav Dev* 11:671–684, 1972.

Crook CK: Taste perception in the newborn. *Infant Behav Dev* 1:52–69, 1978.

De Loache JS, Rissman MD, Cohen LB: An investigation of the attention-getting process in infants. *Infant Behav Dev* 1:11–25, 1978.

Douglas VI: Attention and cognitive problems. In: Rutter M (ed): *Developmental Neuropsychiatry*. New York, Guilford Press, 1983.

Eimas PD: Auditory and phonetic coding of the cues for speech: Discrimination of the (r-l) distinction by young infants. *Percept Psychophys* 18:341–347, 1975.

Eisenberg RB: Stimulus significance as a determinant of infant responses to sound. In: Thoman EB (ed): *Origins of the Infant's Social Responsiveness*. Hillsdale, NJ, Erlbaum, 1979.

Emde R, Harmon R, Metcalf D, et al: Stress and neonatal sleep. *Psychosom Med* 33:491–497, 1971.

Engen T, Lipsitt LP: Decrement and recovery of responses to olfactory stimuli in the human neonate. *J Comp Physiol Psychol* 59:312–316, 1965.

Fagan JF: An attention model of infant recognition. *Child Dev* 48:345–359, 1977.

Fantz RL: Pattern vision in young infants. *Psychol Rec* 8:43–49, 1958.

Field J: Coordination of vision and prehension in infants. *Child Dev* 48:97–103, 1977.

Field TM: Visual and cardiac responses to animate and inanimate faces by young term and preterm infants. *Child Dev* 50:188–194, 1979.

Fitzgerald JM: A developmental account of early childhood amnesia. *J Genet Psychol* 152:159–171, 1991.

Fivush R, Hudson JA: *Knowing and Remembering in Young Children*. Cambridge, Cambridge University Press, 1990.

Flavell JH, Miller PH, Miller SA: *Cognitive Development* (3rd ed). Englewood Cliffs, NJ, Prentice-Hall, 1993.

Freud S: Three essays on the theory of sexuality: In: Strachey J (ed): *The Standard Edition of the Complete Works of Freud* (Vol 7). London, Hogarth Press, 1963.

Gibson EJ: *Principles of Perceptual Learning and Development*. New York, Appleton-Century-Crofts, 1969.

Gibson EJ, Gibson JJ, Pick AD, et al: A developmental study of the discrimination of letter-like forms. *J Comp Physiol Psychol* 55:897–906, 1962.

Gibson EJ, Walk R: The "visual cliff." *Sci Am* 202:64–71, 1960.

Girton M: Infants' attention to intrastimulus motions. *J Exp Child Psychol* 28:416–423, 1979.

Goodman GS, Bottoms BC (eds): *Child Victims, Child Witnesses: Understanding and Improving Testimony*. New York, Guilford Press, 1993.

Graham FK, Clifton RK: Heart rate change as a component of the orienting response. *Psychol Bull* 65:305–320, 1966.

Harris PL: Infant cognition. In: Mussen PH, Haith MM, Campos JJ (eds): *Handbook of Child Psychology*. Vol 2: *Infancy and Developmental Psychobiology* (4th ed). New York, Wiley, 1983.

Hayes LA, Watson JS: Facial orientation of parents and elicited smiling by infants. *Infant Behav Dev* 4:333–340, 1981.

Hirschman R, Melamed LE, Oliver CM: The psychophysiology of infancy. In: Wolman BB (ed): *Handbook of Developmental Psychology.* Englewood Cliffs, NJ, Prentice-Hall, 1982.

Hoffman RF: Developmental changes in human infant visual evoked potentials to patterned stimuli recorded at different scalp locations. *Child Dev* 49:110–118, 1978.

Horowitz FD: *Exploring Developmental Theories: Toward a Structural/Behavioral Model of Development.* Hillsdale, NJ, Erlbaum, 1987.

Hunt RD, Cohen DJ, Anderson G, et al: Noradrenergic mechanisms in ADDH. In: Bloomindale L (ed): *Attention Deficit Disorder and Hyperactivity* (Vol 3). New York, Spectrum, 1987.

Hutt S, Hutt C, Lenard H, et al: Auditory responsitivity in the human neonate. *Nature* 218:888–890, 1968.

Jenkins JJ: Four points to remember: A tetrahedral model of memory experiments. In: Cermak LS, Graik F (eds): *Levels of Processing in Human Memory.* Hillsdale, NJ, Erlbaum, 1979.

Johnson MK: Reflection, reality monitoring and the self. In: Kunzendorf RG (ed): *Mental Imagery.* New York, Plenum, 1991.

Kagan J, Lewis M: Studies of attention in the human infant. *Merrill-Palmer Q* 11:95–127, 1965.

Kail R, Hagen JW: Memory in childhood. In: Wolman BB (ed): *Handbook of Developmental Psychology.* Englewood Cliffs, NJ, Prentice-Hall, 1982.

Kendler H, Kendler T: From discrimination learning to cognitive development. A neobehavioristic odyssey. In: Estes WK (ed): *Handbook of Learning and Cognitive Processes* (Vol 1). Hillsdale, NJ, Erlbaum, 1975.

Kuhn D: Cognitive development. In: Bornstein MH, Lamb ME (eds): *Developmental Psychology: An Advanced Textbook* (2nd ed). Hillsdale, NJ, Erlbaum, 1981.

Levy F: Developmental Hyperkinesis. Unpublished doctoral thesis, University of New South Wales, Sydney, 1979.

Lewis M: Memory and psychoanalysis: A new look at infantile amnesia and transference. J Am Acad Child Adolesc Psychiatry 34:405–417, 1995.

Lewis TL, Mauer D, Kay D: Newborns' central vision: Whole or hole? *J Exp Child Psychol* 26:193–203, 1978.

Lewkowicz DJ, Turkewitz G: Cross-modal equivalence in early infancy: Auditory-visual intensity matching. *Dev Psychol* 16:597–607, 1980.

Lipsitt LP, Reilly BM, Butcher MJ, et al: The stability and interrelationships of newborn sucking and heart rate. *Dev Psychobiol* 9:305–310, 1976.

Ludwig AM: *Principles of Clinical Psychiatry.* New York, Free Press, 1980.

Lynch MP, Eilers RE, Bornstein MH: Speech, vision, and music perception: Windows on the ontogeny of mind. *Psychol Music* 20:3–14, 1992.

MacFarlane A: Olfaction in the development of social preferences in the human neonate. In: *Parent-Infant Interaction.* Amsterdam, Ciba Foundation Symposium, Number 33, New Series, 1975.

Main M: Metacognitive knowledge, metacognitive monitoring, and singular (coherent) vs. multiple (incoherent) model of attachment: Findings and directions for future research. In: Parkes CM, Stevenson Hinde J, Marris P (eds): *Attachment across the Life Cycle.* London, Routledge, 1991.

Margulies DM: Selective attention and the brain. A hypothesis concerning the hippocampal-ventral striatal axis, the mediation of selective attention, and the pathogenesis of attentional disorders. *Med Hypotheses* 18:221–264, 1985.

Mauer D, Salapatek P: Developmental changes in the scanning of faces by young infants. *Child Dev* 47:523–527, 1976.

McCall RB, Kagan J: Stimulus schema discrepancy and attention in the infant. *J Exp Child Psychol* 5:381–390, 1967.

Mednick SA, Schulsinger F, Teasdale TW, et al: Schizophrenia in high-risk children: Sex differences in predisposing factors. In: Serban G (ed): *Cognitive Development of Mental Illness.* New York, Brunner/Mazel, 1978.

Meltzoff AN, Borton RW: Intermodel matching by human neonates. *Nature* 282:403–404, 1979.

Mendelson MJ, Haith M: The relation between audition and vision in the human newborn. *Monogr Soc Res Child Dev* 41(167):1–131, 1976.

Mirsky AF, Anthony BJ, Duncan CC, et al: Analysis of the elements of attention: A neuropsychological approach. *Neuropsychol Rev* 2:109–145, 1991.

Molfese DL, Molfese VJ: Hemisphere and stimulus differences as reflected in the cortical responses of new born infants to speech stimuli. *Dev Psychol* 15:505–511, 1979.

Muir D, Field J: Newborn infants' orientation to sound. *Child Dev* 50:431–436, 1979.

Myers NA, Perlmutter M: Memory in the years from two to five. In: Ornstein P (ed): *Memory Development in Children.* Hillsdale, NJ, Erlbaum, 1978.

Olson GM, Sherman T: Attention, learning, and memory in infants. In: Mussen PH, Haith MM, Campos JJ (eds): *Handbook of Child Psychology.* Vol 2: *Infancy and Developmental Psychobiology* (4th ed). New York, Wiley, 1983.

Owings RA, Peterson GA, Bransford JD, et al: Spontaneous monitoring and regulation of learning: A comparison of successful and less successful fifth graders. *J Educ Psychol* 72:250–256, 1980.

Paris SG, Myers M: Comprehension monitoring memory and study strategies of good and poor readers. *J Reading Behav* 13:5–22, 1981.

Pascual-Leone J: A mathematical model for the transition rule in Piaget's developmental stages. *Acta Psychol* 32:301–345, 1970.

Perlmutter M, Myers NA: Development of recall in 2–4 year old children. *Dev Psychol* 15:73–83, 1979.

Petty L, Ornitz EM, Michelman JD, et al: Autistic children who become schizophrenic. *Arch Gen Psychiatry* 41:129–135, 1984.

Piaget J: *The Construction of Reality in the Child.* New York, Ballantine, 1971.

Pillemer DB, White SH: Childhood events recalled by children and adults. In: Reese HW (ed): *Adv Child Dev Behav* 21:297–340, 1989.

Rose SA, Gottfried AW, Bridger WH: Cross-modal transfer in infants: Relationship to prematurity and SES background. *Dev Psychol* 14:643–652, 1978.

Ruff HA: Individual differences in sustained attention during infancy. In: Colombo J, Fagan J (eds). *Individual Differences in Infancy: Reliability, Stability, Prediction.* Hillsdale, NJ, Erlbaum, 1990.

Rutter M: Behavioral studies, questions and findings on the concept of a distinctive syndrome. In: Rutter M (ed): *Developmental Neuropsychiatry.* New York, Guilford Press, 1983.

Ryan EB: Identifying and remediating failures in reading comprehension: Toward an instructional approach for poor comprehenders. In: Waller TG, MacKinnon GE (eds): *Advances in Reading Research.* New York, Academic Press, 1979.

Salapatek P: Pattern perception in early infancy. In: Cohen LB, Salapatek P (eds): *Infant Perception: From Sensation to Cognition: Basic Visual Processes* (Vol 1). New York, Academic Press, 1975.

Salapatek P, Kessen W: Visual scanning of triangles by the human newborn. *J Exp Child Psychol* 3:155–167, 1966.

Salkind NJ, Nelson CF: A note on the developmental nature of reflection-impulsivity. *Dev Psychol* 3:237–238, 1980.

Sameroff AJ, Cashmore TF, Dykes AC: Heart rate deceleration during visual fixation in human newborns. *Dev Psychol* 8:117–119, 1973.

Schachter J, Williams TA, Khachaturian Z, et al: Heart rate responses to auditory clicks in neonates. *Psychophysiology* 8:163–179, 1971.

Scibetta JJ, Rosen MG, Hochberg CJ, et al: Human fetal brain response to sound during labor. *Am J Obstet Gynecol* 109:82–85, 1971.

Schore A: *Affect Regulation and the Origin of the Self.* New York, Erlbaum, 1994.

Siegel DJ: Perception and cognition. In: Kaplan HI, Sadock BJ (eds): *Comprehensive Textbook of Psychiatry* (6th ed). Baltimore, Williams & Wilkins, 1995a, pp. 277–291.

Siegel DJ: Memory, trauma, and psychotherapy: A cognitive sciences view. *J Psychother Practice Res* 4, 1995b, pp. 93–122.

Sohlberg MM, Mateer CA: *Introduction to Cognitive Rehabilitation: Theory and Practice.* New York, Guilford, 1989.

Sokolov EN: *Perception and Conditioned Reflex.* London, Pergamon, 1963.

Spelke E: Exploring audible and visible events in infancy. In: Pick AD (ed): *Perception and Its Development: A Tribute to Eleanor J. Gibson.* Hillsdale, NJ, Erlbaum, 1979a.

Spelke E: Perceiving bimodally specified events in infancy. *Dev Psychol* 15:626–636, 1979b. Spelke ES, Owsley CJ: Intermodal exploration and knowledge in infancy. *Infant Behav Dev* 2:13–27, 1979.

Squire LR: Memory and the hippocampus: A synthesis from findings with rats, monkeys and humans. *Psychol Rev* 99:195–231, 1992.

Steiner JE: Human facial expressions in response to taste and smell stimulation. In: Reese H, Lipsitt LP (eds): *Adv Child Dev Behav* 13:55–71, 1979.

Steiner JE, Finnegan L: Innate discriminative facial expressions to food-related odorants in the neonate infant. *Isr J Med Sci* 11:858, 1985.

Taylor E: Development of attention. In: Rutter M (ed): *Scientific Foundations of Developmental Psychiatry.* Baltimore, University Park Press, 1980.

Taylor E: Attention deficit and conduct disorder syndromes. In: Rutter M, Tuma AH, Lann IS (eds): *Assessment and Diagnosis in Child Psychopathology.* New York, Guilford Press, 1988.

Trehub SE, Schneider BA, Morrongiello BA, et al: Developmental changes in high-frequency sensitivity. *Audiology* 28:241–249, 1989.

Vygotsky LS: *Mind in Society: The Development of Higher Psychological Processes.* Cambridge, MA, Harvard University Press, 1978.

Wetzler SE, Sweeney JA: Childhood amnesia: A conceptualization in cognitive psychological terms. *J Am Psychoanal Assoc* 34:663–685, 1986.

Zametkin AJ, Rapoport JL: Noradrenergic hypothesis of attention deficit disorder with hyperactivity: A critical review. In: Meltzer HY (ed): *Psychopharmacology: The Third Generation of Progress.* New York, Raven Press, 1987.

Zelniker T, Jeffrey WE: Attention and cognitive style in children. In: Hale G, Lewis M (eds): *Attention and Cognitive Development.* New York, Plenum, 1979.

15 DEVELOPMENT OF COMMUNICATION

Rhea Paul, Ph.D., Lorian Baker, Ph.D., and Dennis P. Cantwell, M.D.

This chapter provides a brief outline of the normal developmental processes involved in the acquisition of communicative skills. We examine the acquisition of these skills within several broad stages, looking first at prelinguistic communication during the first year of life, then describing the acquisition of basic language skills during the preschool years. More advanced communicative abilities acquired during middle childhood and adolescence are also outlined. In each of these developmental periods, four major components of language are addressed: the processing or comprehension of language, the acquisition of speech sounds, the expression of words and sentences, and the pragmatic or social and contextual aspects of communication.

Readers should be aware that this organizational scheme is not the only way to conceptualize language development. Because there is no consensus as to the best model to describe language processing or acquisition, there is no universally accepted categorization method for analyzing the richly integrated system of communication in which we all take part. Lahey's (1978) *content/form/use* model (Fig. 15.1) is often used. This divides language into aspects of *semantics* (content), or meaning; *syntax/phonology* (form), the generative rules that govern the formation of words and sentences; and *pragmatics* (use), the way language is used in context to accomplish social communication. This model is useful for understanding normal development, but it does not correspond as closely as the one employed here to the disorders of language learning that are typically seen in children. DSM-IV classifies disorders of language learning along the speech sound/production/comprehension/pragmatics dimensions, and using this categorical scheme will make it easier to discuss these disorders when we look at them in Chapter 47.

A second caveat readers should bear in mind is that, although the various components of speech and language are described in terms of disparate stages, in reality, there is often a good deal of overlap among the stages. These stages of language development are not necessarily discontinuous steps marked by clear transitions or divisions. Nonetheless, it is usually possible to identify which broad stage of development any given child is in, and consequently, these stages represent a useful method of conceptualizing development for discussion.

Finally, readers should be aware that the normal range of language development is relatively wide, particularly during early childhood. The speech and language milestones that are presented here represent the ages during which the various stages of development generally occur. They are, of course, group averages, which to some extent ignore the possibility of specific (normal) individual differences. There are relatively large standard deviations, or normal variation, around these averages, which decrease somewhat with age. For example, the average vocabulary size for 18 months is 109 words with a standard deviation of 114. At this age, the normal range of variation is over 100% of the mean! By 30 months, though, the standard deviation in vocabulary size declines to 18% of the mean (Stoel-Gammon, 1991). We can see, then, that wide variation in language milestones is very common, especially in the early stages of acquisition. As children grow older, the normal range narrows considerably, which makes the determination of whether a difference represents a disorder much easier in an older child than in a younger one. Generally, the order of acquisition of particular structures, meanings, and uses will be similar across children (with some exceptions), although the rate of acquisition can differ. Clinicians should keep in mind that a specific delay in one or several milestones is not necessarily indicative of disordered acquisition unless the delay persists beyond early childhood or unless there is a general pattern of such delays across several areas of development.

PRELINGUISTIC COMMUNICATION

The production of a "first word" is frequently considered by parents as the first step in communicative development. But actually, long before the first word is said infants engage in a great deal of communication. From the moment of birth, this communication is an active process between child and the social environment. Far from being a passive recipient of adult speech, even the newborn infant engages in behaviors that rivet the adult's attention and elicit social interaction. Let's look at the areas of communicative development that were outlined earlier, and examine how infant communication proceeds in each.

The Newborn's Perceptual Equipment for Processing Language

While, of course, young infants do not understand the literal meaning of language addressed to them, it does appear that newborns begin life with attentional preferences for human, linguistic interaction and with a set of social behaviors that can elicit this stimulation. These abilities would appear, because of their emergence so soon after birth, to be innately programmed, and, as such, provide a great deal of economy in the task of mastering language. Certain propensities present from the first days of life include a preference for sounds in the frequency range of the human voice (Hutt et al., 1968) and a preference for speech over other rhythmic or musical sounds (Butterfield and Siperstein, 1974). Newborns look for the source of a voice they hear, register pleasure with facial expression when they identify the source, and remain quiet, inhibiting their movements, until the voice ceases (Owens, 1984). They do not show this kind of recognition when a nonhuman auditory stimulus is heard. Three-day-old infants have been shown to be able to recognize their own mothers' voices, as opposed to the voices of other women (DeCasper and Fifer, 1980), probably as a result of prenatal experience with the mother's voice heard through the amniotic sac. Newborns are also attracted to and prefer to look at faces (Kagan and Lewis, 1965). Parents, conveniently, interpret this preference as a sign of willingness to interact. The newborn would appear, then, to be biologically organized to attract language input and to attune to the linguistic environment.

There is evidence that speech perception begins at a very early age and may, in fact, be preprogrammed in human infants (Eimas, 1975). For example, infants only weeks old are able to discriminate among a variety of speech sounds, including /pa/ versus /ba/, /ta/ versus /da/, /ba/ versus /ga/, to name a few (Aslin et al., 1983; Eimas et al., 1971; Graham et al., 1983). Even more interestingly, infants make these distinctions along the same categorical boundaries as adults do.

The fact that such distinctions can be made as early as 1 month of age could be interpreted to mean that the ability to make them is innate. Alternatively, it could suggest that this perceptual learning happens very quickly. Researchers have attempted to address this question by looking at sound discriminations that infants could not have learned from their environment because they never heard them made. For example, Werker and Tees (1984) found that infants in English-speaking environments were able to distinguish sounds that are not used in English but are used in Hindi. By 1 year of age, though, this ability to discriminate sounds not heard in the native language had all but disappeared. These findings suggest that the infant does have some ''built-in'' capacity to make discriminations among sounds that are important in speech, but that this ability is modified with experience. Rather than learning to make these distinctions from the language they hear, though, it seems that the infant comes to the task of language with some discriminations ''pre-set.'' Depending on what particular distinctions are used by the ambient language, some of these innately programmed distinctions will be maintained by the child's experience, while others will be extinguished.

Children also acquire a range of differentiated responses to the sounds of language throughout their 1st year. By 4 months they respond to different tones of voice; by 6 months of age they show evidence of selective listening (choosing to respond to some sounds and to ignore others). Toward the last half of the 1st year, babies will inhibit their behavior if told, ''no'' in a loud, sharp voice, but they will do the same if they hear ''yes'' spoken in the same tone (Spitz, 1957). Their response at this stage, then, is not to a specific lexical item, but to an emotional tone in the speech.

Young babies also appear to be able to coordinate acoustic information about speech with visual information about oral posture. Kuhl and Meltzoff (1988) showed that the infants looked for a significantly longer time at the picture of the face whose oral gesture corresponded to the vowel the babies were hearing at the time (retracted lips for /i/; open lips for /a/). This surprising finding suggests a very early ability to integrate visual and auditory cues in perceiving speech and would seem to provide children with an excellent foundation for learning the articulatory movements associated with the speech sounds they will eventually learn to produce.

Although children do not understand words per se until near the end of the 1st year, they appear to begin to develop the bases for the semantic categories with which these words will be associated much earlier. Colombo et al. (1987) showed babies 6–7 months of age slides of various kinds of birds until the children habituated to these stimuli and reduced their visual fixation time. These researchers then showed two new slides simultaneously, one of a parakeet and one of a horse, for example. Babies reliably looked longer at the horse, suggesting that it was more novel to them than the parakeet, which they had also not seen before. Thus, it appears that the children included the parakeet in the category they had formed for the objects viewed previously, i.e., birds. These findings suggest that even at this early age, babies are able to organize their perceptions into conceptual categories that can eventually be mapped onto words.

Recent studies of speech perception in 7-month-old children suggest that they are also sensitive to auditory information that is associated with syntactic boundaries. Hirsh-Pasek et al. (1987) showed that babies of this age preferred to look toward a speaker that played sentences containing pauses at clause or phrase boundaries (''Cinderella lived in a great big house/ but it was sort of dark/ because she had a mean . . .), as opposed to sentences with pauses in the middle of a clause (Cinderella lived in a great big house but it was/ sort of dark because she had/ a

amount of information they will ultimately need to acquire in order to understand sentences.

Although parents have acted as if they believed their child understood speech almost from the 1st day of life, true lexical comprehension does not emerge until about 8 months of age. Around the last quarter of the 1st year, babies begin to respond to certain words that they hear in familiar routines and will, for example, clap hands when mother says, ''Let's play patty-cake.'' This early comprehension is contextually bound, however. If the baby is used to playing patty-cake on the changing table but is told to clap hands in the bathtub, she or he will probably not comply.

Chapman (1978) points out that this contextually bound comprehension often leads parents to believe that babies at 8–12 months understand much more of language than they actually do. Chapman describes a set of strategies for comprehension that are frequently used by infants of this age to comply with parental requests and that give the parent the impression the child is actually understanding language. These are summarized in Table 15.1. For example, babies frequently look at what mother looks at, and this can give the impression that the baby understands what the mother is saying. In fact, though, all the baby has to do is follow the mother's line of regard.

Babies also tend to do something to the objects they notice, and since their repertoire of actions is fairly limited at this stage, parents can, by judiciously choosing their instructions, have a very good chance that the child will comply. For example, a mother might say to the baby, ''See the pretty ball!'' The baby, following her line of gaze, looks at the ball. The baby is very likely, then, to move toward it. If the mother, at the same time says, ''Go get the ball for Mommy,'' the baby can appear to comply with the instruction when, in fact, that was what she or he was going to do anyway.

The function of these strategies is to help the baby participate successfully in an interaction. Mothers are also trying to get the baby to participate and succeed. They unconsciously behave in such a way as to give the baby ample cues, both linguistic and nonlinguistic, as to their meaning. When the baby responds appropriately, two things happen. First, babies experience the pleasure of a positive social interaction. Second, they get another example of the way in which language works to encode what they already know about the world. In this way infants move closer to truly linguistic comprehension.

Table 15.1. Summary of Comprehension Abilities in Children Younger Than 3 Years

Age	Comprehension Ability	Comprehension Strategy
8–12 months	Understands a few single words in routine contexts	1. Look at objects mother looks at 2. Act on objects noticed 3. Imitate ongoing action
12–18 months	Understands single words outside of routine, but still requires some contextual support	1. Attend to object mentioned 2. Give evidence of notice 3. Do what you usually do
18–24 months	Understands words for absent objects, some two-term combinations	1. Locate objects mentioned, give evidence of notice 2. Put objects in containers; on surfaces 3. Act on objects in the way mentioned (child as agent)
24–36 months	Comprehension of three-term sentences, but context or past experience determines meaning; no understanding of word order	1. Probable location/probable event 2. Supply missing information

Adapted from Chapman R: Comprehension strategies in children. In: Kavanagh JF, Strange W (eds): *Speech and Language in Laboratory, School, and Clinic.* Cambridge, MA, MIT Press, 1978, pp. 308–327.

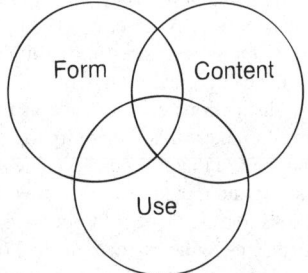

Figure 15.1. Bloom and Lahey's taxonomy of language. (From Bloom L, Lakey M: *Language Development and Language Disorders.* New York, Wiley, 1978.)

Table 15.2. A Summary of Stark's (1979) Stages of Infant Vocalization

Stage	Age Range	Vocalization Types
I	0–2 months	Reflexive cries and vegetative sounds
II	2–5 months	Cooing and laughing
III	4–8 months	Vocal play and beginning babbling
IV	6–9 months	Reduplicated babbling
V	9–18 months	Jargon babbling

Infant Sound Production

Crying is the newborn's principal form of vocal behavior. Beginning in the 1st month after birth, the infant masters the ability to produce cries that differentiate among affective states. Pain versus hunger cries are differentiated within the 1st week of life (Graham et al., 1983). Other noncry vocalizations also emerge early in life. Contentment vocalizations can be distinguished from distress sounds within the 1st month (Ricks, 1975).

The quality of these infant vocalizations changes drastically throughout the 1st year of life. Stark (1979) has presented a framework for describing infant vocal behavior (Table 15.2). According to this framework, the infant from birth to 2 months of age produces primarily reflexive cries and other vegetative sounds. Although the newborn's cries have a profound effect on the adults who hear them, the infant is not using the crying in any intentional way to attract the adult's notice. Rather, the cry is an instinctual response to an internal state such as hunger, cold, or boredom. Vegetative sounds such as burps, coughs, and sneezes are also reflexive, but adults will respond to these noises as if they were communicative. This willingness on the part of the adult to attribute intentionality to the infant's early reflexive sound production may be one of the ways in which infants are "taught" to use sound to communicate.

As the baby grows, the head and neck anatomy changes, resulting in a greater diversity of sounds that can be produced and a more speechlike resonance associated with vocalization. Between 2 and 5 months of age, babies begin two behaviors that are important for the development of speech and communication. One is the pleasant, somewhat speechlike sound that babies produce primarily in response to social interactions, known as *cooing*, or "comfort" sounds. The name arises from the "oo"-like quality of most of the vowels heard during this type of vocalizing and from the fact that most of the consonants produced sound like /k/ and /g/. Again, the reasons for the "coo" quality of these vocalizations are anatomical. As the baby lies in a prone or semiprone position, gravity operates most strongly on the relatively large posterior portion of the tongue, pulling it back toward the roof of the mouth. This oral posture produces the consonants we recognize as /g/ and /k/, as well as the vowel we recognize as "oo."

A second new vocal behavior in this stage is the infant's laugh, which emerges around the same time as cooing. Usually accompanied by a social smile, infant laughing is produced in response to an interaction the infant perceives as pleasurable, very often because it is a known routine whose components are predictable. Thus, babies may laugh when mother plays "peek-a-boo" for them, or when she assumes a posture as if ready to tickle the baby. Crying becomes less frequent during this period of increasingly diverse and speechlike vocalization.

The next stage of vocal development begins at about 4 months of age and extends to about 8 months. Stark refers to this period as "vocal play." In this phase the infant begins to pronounce what sound like single syllables with vowel-like and consonant-like components. Though not approximations of words and not meant to convey any referential meaning, these early forms of babbling continue the infant's progress toward increasingly speechlike sounds. The consonants produced tend to be made more toward the front of the mouth than were those used for cooing.

Vocal play, unlike cooing, does not appear principally in response to social interactions. Although infants do use vocal play as a means of responding to or initiating contact with adults, babies also engage in vocal play when alone. Vocal play may, then, function as a means for the infant to "practice" the new sound production abilities he or she is acquiring.

Lenneberg (1967) was the first to note that it is during this stage that the deaf baby's babbling begins to differ from that of the normal hearing infant, although prior to the vocal play stage, the babbling of deaf babies resembles that of their normal hearing counterparts. More recently, Stoel-Gammon and Otomo (1986) substantiated these observations, showing that hearing-impaired babies at this age level had smaller repertoires of consonants than normal hearing peers and that, in fact, the size of the hearing-impaired babies' inventories decreases between 4 and 18 months, while that of the normal hearing babies increases. Thus, the inability to derive auditory feedback from vocal play appears to be important in the development of the babbling repertoires and their eventual transition to speech.

Stark (1979) reports that a new form of vocal behavior, which she refers to as "reduplicated babbling," appears in the second half of the 1st year of life. This type of vocalization includes consonant-vowel combinations, such as /bababa/ or /nanana/, in which the same syllable is repeated over and over. Consonants most likely to appear include /b/, /p/, /t/, /d/, /m/, /n/ and the glide *y*. Like vocal play, reduplicated babbling often occurs when the baby is alone.

Toward the end of the 1st year of life, many babies begin to use "vocables," or phonetically consistent forms. These are productions that are unique to the child in that they do not closely resemble any adult word, but are used reliably in certain situations. For example, Carter (1979) reported that one child consistently used an /m/ sound along with reaching to indicate that he wanted something. These early consistent forms are sometimes referred to as "protowords."

Infant Interaction and Communication

Infants' early vocalizations appear to constitute protoconversations with parents (Bateson, 1975). Other early forms of interaction include making eye contact with the parents (around 1 month of age), smiling and laughing in response to speech (at 3 months), and vocalizing in response to sounds (at 4 months). Babies may also begin to imitate some of the parent's intonation patterns (Trevarthen, 1979) and by 3 months of age will show more vocal responsiveness to their mothers than to other adults. As the baby gains better motor coordination, more formal interactions occur, such as patty-cake or peek-a-boo games, waving bye-bye, or "following" conversations by looking first at one person then another. However, there is evidence that, even during the prelinguistic stages, infants can detect deviant parental interactions and are disturbed by them. Tronick (1981) found that infants responded to a lack of appropriate maternal reactions by unusual patterns of gaze and finally by self-comforting behaviors.

Babies use gaze extensively to regulate interactions. They look at the parent when they are interested in interacting, and avert their gaze when they become tired or overstimulated (Stern, 1977). Babies can follow their parents' gaze to attend to an object they point at, and later they begin to direct the parents' attention by looking at objects themselves. Parents will follow the infant's line of regard and look at what the baby looks at. Frequently, parents will comment on this object of the baby's gaze. These interactions, in which the parent and child share focus on an object, have been called "joint attention routines" (Bruner, 1977) and are thought to be very important in laying the foundation for the basic topic-comment structure of language in which one speaker directs the other's attention to a focus of interest, on which the conversation then elaborates.

At about 8 months of age, babies begin to develop the representational and intentional skills that allow them to hold goals in mind long enough to pursue them through action. Cognitive development at this time also supports the ability to understand actions as a means to an end, and babies begin to use communication as a means to the outcomes—in parental attention or the acquisition of objects—that they desire. Such communicative acts usually become manifest at about the same time as other forms of intentional behavior emerge—about 8–10 months of age.

Communication at this stage is expressed primarily with gestures, such as holding an object up for the mother to view, or pointing. Acredolo and Goodwyn (1988) reported that the use of idiosyncratic symbolic gestures to communicate is quite common during the last half of the 1st year of life. They found that some children as young as 11 months of age used relatively stable gestures that resembled manual signs to stand for objects or actions for the purpose of communication. For example, a child might bounce up and down to indicate "rabbit" or press on the eyes to indicate "sun." Often these gestures are accompanied by a look at the parent to see that she is attending.

Bates (1976) categorizes these early intentional behaviors into two broad types based on their communicative function: protoimperatives and protodeclaratives. Protoimperative speech acts are those in which the child attempts to get the listener to do something for him, or to stop doing something, and would appear to evolve into linguistic imperatives or commands. Protoimperative speech acts include requests for objects, which the child can indicate by pointing or reaching. Requests for actions, which the child can convey by miming some part of a familiar ritual, also fall into this category. For example, the child might climb on the mother's lap and touch his nose to indicate that he wants his mother to play the "body-part-naming game" that is frequently a part of interactive routines at this stage. Protests or rejections also occur, in which the child communicates, by pushing away or turning away, the desire to turn down some object or activity the mother is attempting to offer.

Protodeclarative speech acts direct the mother's attention to an object of the child's interest by pointing to it, holding it up, showing, or giving it. These acts are thought to lay the basis for the later use of referential language. Protodeclarative speech acts are thought to evolve out of the earlier established joint attentional routines that appear to be very important for later language development. Several studies of language-impaired individuals (Wetherby et al., 1989; Paul and Shiffer, 1991) suggest that protodeclarative speech acts are used with restricted frequency by children with various types of language disorders.

As the babies begin to evidence this intentional communication, parents "up the ante" (Bruner, 1978), requiring a more sophisticated form of response in order for it to "count" as the child's contribution. Whereas we saw earlier that mothers accepted any child behavior, such as a burp or a cough, as a communicative response, when true intentionality does develop, the mother requires the child to do something more communicative in order to fulfill a turn. The child is now expected to imitate the mother, to produce a conventional gesture, and eventually to vocalize. In this way, the baby's communication is "shaped" into language.

LEARNING THE LANGUAGE BASICS

Children's first words usually appear around the 1st birthday. From this time, until they reach the end of the preschool period, their communication develops at an enormous rate. Vocabulary grows from two or three words to over 5000, sentence lengths grow from one word to five or more, and the sophistication of their pragmatic skills often amaze and astound the adults around them. We'll examine the four areas of language development that were outlined earlier, to get a sense of how these changes proceed.

Understanding Language

Comprehension skills begin with the understanding of single words. Before children say their first word, they typically understand the meanings of several (Benedict, 1979). This gap between receptive and expressive vocabulary size continues to exist throughout development. Even adults can often recognize meanings for words that they never use in their own speech. The meanings that children attach to their first words are not identical to the meanings of those words in the adult lexicon. Studies of vocabulary acquisition suggest that children use a "fast mapping" strategy (Carey and Bartlett, 1978) to acquire an incomplete no-

tion of the meaning of a word that allows them to use the word and refine its definition through subsequent feedback. This kind of strategy could help to explain the exponential rate at which words are acquired during this 2nd year.

At first, as we saw, comprehension is context-bound, and children will understand words only within familiar routines. Comprehension begins to be freed from the context around 18 months of age, when children are first able to respond to words for objects that are not immediately visible. When asked to "go get a diaper," at this stage, for example, they can fetch one from another room.

Certain classes of words tend to be acquired in comprehension during this period. By the age of 15–16 months, the child can point to his or her own nose, eyes, mouth, and other body parts on request, and by around 20 months the child can point to these body parts on a doll or on another person. Names of animals the child has toys to represent or sees in picture books, and names of family members tend also to be acquired in receptive vocabulary at this time. By around 2 years of age, children understand the meanings of several prepositions (e.g., in, on, under) (Wiig and Semel, 1980) and action verbs (e.g., run, hit, jump), although comprehension of verbs begins slightly later than the comprehension of nouns.

During the 12- to 24-month period, children's production of sentences is limited to one or two words. Are they able to understand much longer ones? Many parents believe so and will often claim that children as young as 12 months "understand everything" said to them. Linguistic comprehension is still quite limited in this period, however (Chapman, 1978; Paul, 1990). Children manage to convince adults that they understand more than they do by employing a series of strategies or shortcuts for responding to the language that they hear, as they did at the end of the 1st year. Strategies in the 2nd year, however, integrate emerging linguistic knowledge with the understanding of contexts and interactions.

Chapman (1978) characterizes the 12- to 18-month-old child's comprehension as demonstrating the use of "lexical guides to context-determined responses." Here the child pairs his or her newly acquired knowledge of the meaning of single words with knowledge about what usually happens in interactive situations. This integration allows the child to act on objects the mother mentions by name, even if she does not look at them. Knowledge of how objects are conventionally used gives the child access to a "do what you usually do" strategy. This results in the child's using the mentioned object for its intended purpose, without having to understand the full linguistic force of an instruction. Thus, if told to "Brush your hair," the toddler is able to comply without fully understanding the instruction, simply by recognizing the word *brush* and knowing for what brushes are used.

In the latter half of the 2nd year, as the child begins to combine two words in his or her own speech, the ability to understand two-word combinations also emerges, but comprehension is probably limited to not much more than two words per sentence. Understanding two words in a sentence allows the child to respond to apparently complex instructions without having to process their full linguistic form. For example, a child in this stage might successfully comply with the request, "Why don't you go and close that door for me?" not because the child understands the whole question, but because she or he was able to pick out the words *close* and *door* and knows that adults usually ask children to do things (Shatz, 1978).

Around the age of 3 years, there is a considerable expansion in the number of vocabulary and linguistic items (e.g., plurals, present verb tense, adjective comparison forms) that are understood. During the period of rapid growth in expressive language abilities, there is a corresponding rapid growth in the ability to understand language. The 3-year-old child understands much of what is said to him or her, but there are still some sentence types that cause problems, and children continue to use comprehension strategies in responding to these difficult utterances. Again, the child integrates his or her newly acquired linguistic skill with prior knowledge to come up with more sophisticated strategies. Chapman (1978) discusses two strategies that are used in the 3rd year of life: the "probable event" and "supplying missing information" strategies.

The probable event strategy allows children to respond correctly to passive sentences that encode events they know to be likely to happen in the world, even when they do not understand the passive structure. For example, 2-year-old children can correctly act out the sentence, "The baby is fed by the mommy," not because they really understand the syntax of the sentence, but because they know mommies usually feed babies, not the other way around. However, if asked to act out, "The mommy is fed by the baby," or even, "The baby feeds the mommy," 2-year-old children are likely to interpret the sentence according to the probable events, rather than according to its syntactic structure. Similarly, the probable event strategy is used to respond to sentences that contain prepositions the child does not fully understand. Young 2-year-old children, for example, if asked to put a spoon *under* a cup, would be most likely to put the spoon *in* the cup, because they know that containers like cups are usually used to put things *in*.

The strategy of supplying missing information is used to respond to questions that contain question words that the child does not understand. *When*, for example, is not usually comprehended by 2-year-old children because of its temporal features. If asked a *when* question, 2-year-old children are likely to respond as if the question contained some other question word that they do understand. If asked, "When did you have lunch?" for example, a 2-year-old child would be likely to reply, "Hot dogs."

By the age of 4 years, the young child has learned many of the basic grammatical rules of the language, and, unlike the 2-year-old child, can interpret improbable sentences like, "The baby feeds the mommy," correctly. Four-year-olds have learned the basic word order rule of English: the first noun in a sentence is the doer of the action, and the last noun is the receiver. But once this basic rule is learned, it tends to be overgeneralized. Four-year-old children may now misinterpret the same passive sentences they interpreted correctly earlier because of a probable event strategy. If asked to act out, "The baby is fed by the mommy," the 4-year-old child may make the baby feed the mommy doll, operating on the principle that the first noun is the agent of action (Chapman, 1978). Not all children adopt this strategy (Bridges, 1980), but it does at times occur. By 7 years, most children understand that the passive sentence is an exception to normal word order rules (Paul, 1985).

Preschool children also have difficulty understanding complex sentences in which the order of mention of clauses does not correspond to the order of events, such as, "Before you brush your teeth, turn off the water." And they have a hard time understanding sentences with conjunctions such as *unless* and *although*, which involve negative hypothetical propositions (Owens, 1984). A few other specific sentence forms that violate the regular rules for sentence interpretation are also typically misunderstood by preschoolers and young school-aged children (Chomsky, 1969). Although the preschooler sounds much like an adult speaker in terms of the production of grammatical sentences, it is possible to trigger misinterpretations of sentences with forms that violate the general rules of the language.

Speech Sound Production

Typically, children pronounce their first understandable word around 12 months; however, the range of 8–18 months is considered normal (Morley, 1965). Although children begin using real words around their 1st birthday, babbling and nonmeaningful sound play continue to coexist with speech for some time. In both speech and babbling, the same sounds tend to be used. Stark (1979) calls the sound play heard during the 2nd year of life "nonreduplicative babbling" or "expressive jargon." This babbling is more varied than the earlier, reduplicated form. It involves new types of consonants, particularly those known as *fricatives*, that involve constriction rather than complete obstruction of the airway. The /s/ sound is one common early fricative. In addition, more than one consonant may appear within an utterance. So instead of /bababa/a child may produce /pata/. Syllable structures that are produced also become more complex. Reduplicated babbling primarily contains consonant-vowel sequences (/ba/). But jargon babbling may, in addition, contain vowel-consonant-vowel sequences (/aba/), as well as consonant-vowel-consonant productions (/bap/). Still missing from this form of babbling are the liquid

sounds (/l,r/), and any combination of consonants, such as the *pl* in *play*. Sounds made in the front of the mouth, such as /b/, /p/, and /m/, are more frequent than those made in the back, such as /k/ or /g/. Jargon babble begins to take on the intonation contours of the ambient language at this time, so that the child's vocalizations sound as if the child is speaking, but the listener is unable to understand the words.

Regardless of the language being acquired, the first words children say are generated from a limited set of consonants that are similar to those used in jargon babble. These include sounds produced toward the front of the mouth (e.g., /b/, /p/, /m/, /n/, /t/, /d/) (Jakobson, 1968). Although there is some individual variation in the precise order of acquisition of speech sounds, the acquisition of speech sounds does follow certain general patterns across all children (Edwards and Shriberg, 1983; Goad and Ingram, 1987; Sander, 1972; Stoel-Gammon, 1985). The vowel inventory is mastered quickly (by the age of 18 months), whereas acquisition of the full inventory of consonant sounds continues for several more years. The first consonant sounds to be consistently articulated correctly are nasals (/m/, /n/, /ŋ/), stops (/p/, /b/, /t/, /d/, /k/, /g/), and glides (/h/, /w/, *y*). Subsequently, most fricatives (/s/, *sh*, /v/, /f/) are articulated correctly. Liquids (/l/, /r/), affricates (*ch*, *j*), some fricatives (*th*; voiced [thy] and voiceless [thigh]), and consonant clusters (*bl*, *st*, *tr*, *str*) are among the last types of sounds to be consistently articulated correctly.

The first words children say usually have simple syllable shapes, such as consonant-vowel combinations (CV), or reduplicated syllables (CVCV): "ma," "mama." Between 18 and 24 months of age, however, children's repertoire both of sounds and syllable shapes expands with his or her expanding vocabulary. Stoel-Gammon (1987) found that by 24 months of age normal children produce 9–10 different sounds and at least a few words with consonant clusters, like the *pl* in *play*. Paul and Jennings (1992) report that by 24 months normal children produce many syllables that contain two different consonants as well as some multisyllabic words. Stoel-Gammon (1987) also showed that 70% of the consonants produced by normal 24-month-old children were correct according to the adult target word.

Although 2-year-old children are accurate in their production of speech sounds most of the time, they do tend to make some characteristic changes in their pronunciation that serve to simplify the task of articulation. They may leave off the last sounds in words (*ca* for *cat*), delete unstressed syllables in long words (*nana* for *banana*), make the sounds in a word more alike (*doddie* for *doggie*), change certain sounds that are hard to pronounce (*wabbit* for *rabbit*; *sair* for *chair*), or leave out one of the consonants in a consonant blend (*pay* for *play*). These types of errors are very typical of children's speech in the 24- to 36-month period (Shriberg and Kwiatkowski, 1980; Grunwell, 1982).

As we have seen, there is considerable individual variation in normal communicative development. Among the individual variations that have been reported with regard to the production of speech sounds are the avoidance of certain sounds or preference for certain sounds (Farwell, 1977; Vihman, 1981), a tendency toward consistency versus inconsistency of pronunciations (Vihman, 1981), reduplicating the first syllable of a word instead of producing a completely different second syllable (Ferguson, 1978; Schwartz et al., 1980), and using particular modifications of specific sound sequences (Ingram, 1974).

Between ages 2 and 4, though, most of these sound changes, both the typical and the idiosyncratic ones, drop out. Figure 15.2 shows the general order in which these errors, often referred to as *phonological processes*, are resolved. Children older than 4 years who retain use of a significant number of these processes, so that the intelligibility of their speech is affected, would be considered to have an articulation, or phonological, disorder.

By age 4 the normal child is fully intelligible, producing nearly 100% of speech sounds correctly. If errors remain, they are likely to occur on the last sounds to develop: *l*, *r*, *th*, and possibly *s*, as well as on the production of several consonants that occur together within a word, as in *scrape*. Normal preschoolers will also continue to have difficulty with multisyllabic words, such as *spaghetti* or *aluminum*. About 5% of children enter school with phonological deficits (Shriberg, 1980), but most of these involve residual errors on one or two sounds.

During the stage of systematic acquisition of speech sounds, speech dysfluency or stuttering may appear. It appears that approximately 85% of the young children who stutter during this period of time will recover spontaneously within a few months' time (Homzie and Lindsay, 1984). Consequently, intervention is generally not recommended at this age, unless there is evidence of distress, fear of talking, or avoidance of speech.

Producing Words and Sentences

EXPRESSIVE VOCABULARY DEVELOPMENT

The first words of children learning to speak any language share some properties in common. They tend to be words for objects and activities with which the child has direct contact. So, *shoe*, which a child can put on and take off by himself or herself, is more likely to be one of the first words than *shirt*. First words also tend to be those used very frequently in social interactive routines, such as *hi* and *bye-bye*. Although most first words are nouns, or names of things, not all are. *More*, *up*, and *no* are frequent entries in lists of early words.

Children, like adults, understand many more words than they say. What determines which of these comprehended words will be produced? One characteristic that seems to be a factor is the sound structure of the word. Children are more likely to produce words that have at least a beginning sound that is already in their repertoire than they are to produce a word with sounds that are not under their control (Leonard et al., 1979). This active process of selection and avoidance of words based on their sound structure is typical of children in this very early stage of language acquisition (Ferguson and Farwell, 1975).

Children's use of words during this period also may not always conform to adult usage. Two common types of errors seen are *overextension* and *underextension*. Overextension is using a word to mean more than its true meaning (e.g., using "doggie" to mean "animal"), whereas underextension is using a word to mean only part of its true meaning (e.g., using "car" to mean "a car that is moving"). It is important to note, too, that words are overextended in production much more often than in comprehension. Rescorla (1976) reports that children who label both a truck and a plane with the word *car* can very often point to pictures of the correct items when *truck* and *plane* are named for them.

During the period of the first 50 words, children's "sentences" consist of one word at a time. These early one-word sentences are sometimes called "holophrases" because they seem to function as sentences and may convey meanings that are more complex than mere labels. For example, a baby saying "Mama" may actually be trying to convey a more complex message, such as "Mama, come here." First sentences tend to express the same protoimperative and protodeclarative intentions as children expressed during their 1st year with gestures and vocalizations.

Average expressive vocabulary size at 12 months is three words; at 15 months it is ten words (Templin, 1957). By 18 months, most children are producing more than 50 words (Nelson, 1973), and average number of different words produced is about 100 (Fenson et al., 1990). By 20 months, average expressive vocabulary size is about 150 words (Dale et al., 1989). The average 24-month-old child says 300 different words (Dale, 1991). Still, there is a great deal of individual variation in expressive vocabulary size. Fenson et al. (1990) report a standard deviation of 111 at 18 months, larger than the mean of 100 words. Even at 24 months, the standard deviation in vocabulary size is 176, a smaller proportion, but nonetheless nearly half as large as the mean of 300 words (Dale, 1991). Despite this variation, recent studies suggest that children of 24 months of age who produce fewer than 50 words can be considered to be performing below the normal range of expressive language and are at risk for chronic linguistic handicap (Paul, 1991; Rescorla, 1989).

The rate of growth of vocabulary during the 2nd year of life is not linear. Typically, there is slow acquisition of the first 50 words, with points at which new acquisition appears to halt for a time. Some words may temporarily drop out of the vocabulary. But about the time the child acquires the 50th word or so, around 18 months, a spurt in vocabulary acquisition is seen, and vocabulary size increases suddenly and sharply. The failure of a child to undergo this spurt in vocabulary growth during the 2nd year of life may be another warning signal of risk for chronic delay.

Both expressive and receptive vocabulary size continue to grow rapidly during the 3rd year. Smith (1926) estimated expressive vocabulary size at 36 months to be about 900 words, a three-fold increase over this size at 24 months. As children increase their vocabulary, they develop mastery over a range of semantic categories. Spatial terms including *in*, *on*, *under*, *beside*, *next to*, *on*, *off*, *out*, and *over* (Boehm, 1969) are generally mastered by 3 years of age. *Big* and *little* are the first pair of dimensional adjectives to be acquired, with *long* and *short* following soon after, both generally learned by 3 years. Color terms are used occasionally by 2-year-old children. By 36 months, most normal children will be naming two to three colors correctly. Children also learn to produce and understand question words *what* and *where*, and occasionally use *who* and *how* by age 3 (Tyack and Ingram, 1977). Pronouns including *I*, *me*, *my*, *mine*, and *it* are usually used by age 3. *You*, *your*, *she*, *them*, *he*, *yours*, *we*, and *her* are frequently mastered by age 3 as well (Haas and Owens, 1985).

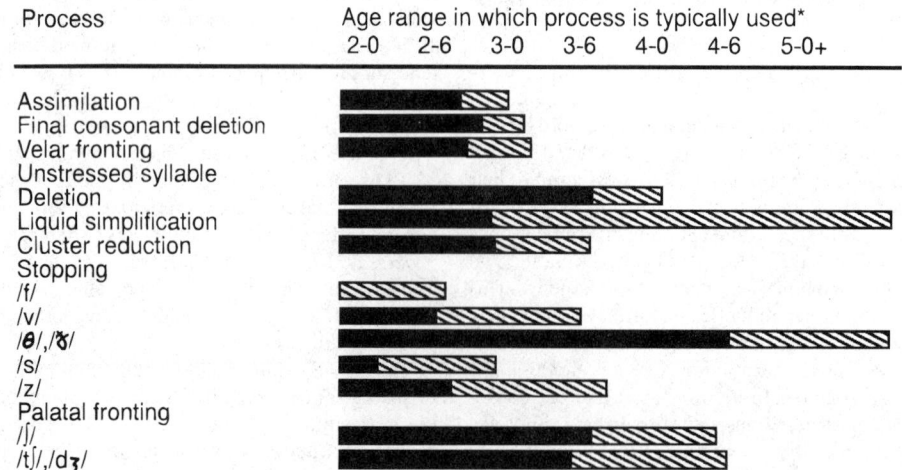

Figure 15.2.   A sequence of phonological processes based on Grunwell (1981). (From Paul R: *Language Disorders from Infancy through Adolescence: Assessment and Intervention.* St. Louis, Mosby-Year Book, 1995.)

The average spoken vocabulary size at age 4 is about 1500 words, and at age 5, about 2100 words (Smith, 1926). Receptive vocabulary size continues to exceed these levels at each age. Children learn to use and understand a great many classes of words during the preschool period. They master the use of most pronouns, with the exception of the reflexives (himself, herself, ourselves, etc.), which are not learned until school age. Kinship terms in addition to *mother* and *father* or their diminutives, which are part of the child's earliest vocabulary, enter the lexicon. Depending on the child's experience, most terms for extended family members will be at least partially understood by age 5 (Haviland and Clark, 1974), but full comprehension is not achieved until age 10 or so. The preschooler, for example, may know that he has a brother, but may not realize that he is a brother to someone.

Temporal terms enter the vocabulary at this time, with *before*, *after*, *since*, and *until* coming in earliest. These are used first as prepositions ("I'll go *after* school."), and only later as subordinating conjunctions ("I'll go *after* I get home from school.") Question words *why*, *how*, and *when* are used with greater frequency during this period, and questions containing these words are answered correctly more often, although the context of the question has an influence on correct responding (James, 1990). Children are more likely to answer most types of wh- questions correctly when they can see the person, object, or event to which the question refers.

Children learn to refine their use of adjectives, adding more precise terms to their vocabulary during the preschool years. While a 3-year-old child may know only *big* and *little*, by 5 years children generally learn *large/small*, *tall/short*, *long/short*, *high/low*, *thick/thin*, *wide/narrow*, and *deep/shallow* (Owens, 1988). The positive member of the pair is usually learned first. *More* and *less* and *same* and *different* are other pairs of dimensional adjectives usually learned during the preschool years. *More* and *less* may be used initially interchangeably. By 5, most children use these terms correctly.

DEVELOPMENT OF SENTENCES

At about the time the child produces the 50th word, usually around 18 months of age, another important language milestone appears. The child begins to combine words into "telegraphic" sentences (Brown, 1973). Structurally, these two-word utterances are not random combinations of words, but follow a "minigrammar," with the positions in which certain words may occur being governed by specific rules (Bloom et al., 1975; Braine, 1963). Two-word utterances may express a variety of different types of meanings (Clark and Clark, 1977) including an agent who performs an action (e.g., "baby cry"), an action that affects an object (e.g., "hit baby"), an entity given a location (e.g., "Daddy home"), or an object or person with a description (e.g., "nice Mommy"). These utterances resemble telegrams in that they include the most important words of the adult sentence, while leaving out the little-function words and word endings.

By the end of the 2nd year of life, most children are beginning to produce some three- and four-word sentences. These early longer forms tend to include the most meaningful elements that were left out of the telegraphic sentences. So while the telegraphic child might say "Daddy ball," to indicate that dad should toss the ball, the slightly older child may say, "Daddy throw ball." Many small, function words and word endings are still omitted (Owens, 1988).

An enormous amount of growth takes place in the child's production of syntax between 2 and 5 years of age. Children learn to elaborate telegraphic utterances through the use of *grammatical morphemes*, the units of meaning that are expressed as inflections on nouns and verbs, or as functor words such as articles (*a*, *an*, and *the*) or *be* verbs. Cazden (1968) studied the acquisition of 14 of these morphemes that seemed to undergo substantial change in children's usage. Her studies and others that followed found that the 14 morphemes were acquired in a relatively consistent order by children learning English. Between 2 and 3 years, children were found to learn to produce the *-ing* ending, plural /s/ and possessive ('s), and the prepositions *in* and *on* in nearly all the contexts in which they were required by the adult grammar. Children learning

other languages, though, do not acquire these morphemes in the same order as English-speaking children do (Kvaal et al., 1988). The differences found across languages in the order of acquisition of grammatical morphemes are thought to reflect the fact that some languages have more difficult or complicated ways of expressing the meaning encoded by these morphemes. For example, in English, articles are learned relatively late, but in Spanish children produce articles as one of their earliest morphemes. The relative ease of acquisition of articles in Spanish is thought to be a result of the fact that the English articles are somewhat harder to hear in running conversation, while the Spanish forms, *el*, *la*, *los*, *las*, etc., are more salient acoustically.

Between 3 and 5 years, children learning English acquire mastery of many grammatical morphemes studied by Cazden (1968), including use of *be* verbs, articles, and third person singular *s* marking on verbs (I run, you run, he run*s*). Children also master the use of past tense markers during this period. Typically, children start out by marking irregularly formed past tense verbs, such as *come/came*, *see/saw*, and *go/went*, correctly, before they begin using the regular past tense marker *-ed*. Between 3 and 5 years, the regular marker is acquired and, when it is, the child very frequently overgeneralizes it, marking incorrectly those irregular forms that were produced right earlier. This overgeneralization of past tense markers results in productions like, "I falled down and got hurted." This replacement of an early correct form by an error that is the result of a process of overgeneralization is often taken as evidence that the child is actually inducing rules from the input language and not merely memorizing the forms heard because, presumably, adults do not produce these overgeneralized forms. The use of overgeneralized past tense forms may persist to age 5 or 6. Some overgeneralized plural forms (foots, mouses) may also appear during this period. Other grammatical morphemes that are mastered during the preschool period include the comparative (small/small*er*) and superlative (small*est*), as well as the agentive *er* marker, used to denote one who performs an action (teach/teach*er*) (Carrow, 1973).

A second aspect of syntactic development includes the expansion of the two basic units of simple sentences: the noun phrase (usually the subject or object of a verb) and the verb phrase, or sentence predicate (Miller, 1981). During the telegraphic period, the noun phrase and verb phrase segments of the sentence generally contain only one word. During the third year, the child learns to elaborate these elements by adding additional words to each. Noun phrase elaboration starts with the addition of a single element, usually an article or a modifier. Modifiers frequently used by 2-year-old children include *this*, *that*, *these*, *those*, *a*, *the*, *some*, *a lot*, *more*, *two*, *my*, and *your* (Miller, 1981). A child just beginning noun phrase elaboration would, for example, be likely to say, "My doggy!" but not "My black doggy." By the end of the 3rd year, children are embedding elaborated noun phrases within sentences. When this occurs, the elaboration is most likely to occur on the object noun phrase at the end of the sentence, rather than on the subject at the beginning (Miller, 1981). So the 3-year-old child is apt to say, "Kitty has black spots," but not "My new kitty has spots."

Verb phrase development begins with the production of single verbs that are unmarked for person, tense, or number. The child may say, "He throw ball" to mean, "Daddy threw the ball to me." *Can* and *will* are the earliest auxiliary verb forms to be used. Forms of the auxiliary verb *be* may also emerge at this time, but will not be used consistently or with correct marking (Miller, 1981). So the child may say, "You am going," or "You going home." Some use of irregular past tense forms (came, saw, went, fell) may appear by age 3, although regular past tense forms, which are marked by *-ed*, may continue to be produced without any marker (Trantham and Pedersen, 1976). The child may use both, "I came home," and "I help Daddy" to refer to events in the past.

Children continue to increase both the elaboration of basic noun and verb phrases as well as the complexity of sentence types produced during the preschool years. Young 3-year-old children consistently include a subject noun phrase in sentences, no longer omitting it as 2-year-old children do. Noun phrase elaboration becomes richer and more flexible throughout the preschool years by means of the ability to mark either the subject or the object noun phrase with a broader range and greater number of modifiers. Toward the end of the preschool period, children begin using clauses rather than single words or phrases to modify nouns. These relative clauses, again, usually are used first to modify nouns in object position ("They're boys *that I know*."). Modification of subject nouns with relative clauses ("The boys *that I know* are big.") is seen in children's speech very infrequently until school age.

Verb phrase elaboration during the preschool period consists of the mastery of the verb inflections for past and third singular marking, as we saw. In addition, new auxiliary verbs are acquired, including *could*, *would*, *should*, *must*, *might*, and *shall* and past tense forms of the verb *to be*, i.e., *was* and *were*. Auxiliary verbs *have*, *had*, and *has* are used very infrequently during the preschool period (Miller, 1981). When preschoolers do use auxiliary verbs, they use only one at a time. They rarely produce sentences with multiple auxiliaries, such as, "I *could have* helped you."

A third area in which syntactic development is seen is the production of the various sentence types available in the language. Two major sentence variants have been found to show significant development between ages 2 and 3 years in children acquiring English: negative sentences and questions. Negative intentions appear very early, as we saw; one of the first preverbal intentions children express is the desire to reject, protest, or deny their interlocutor's utterance. As we saw earlier, *no* is one of the first words almost every child says. Children in the telegraphic period can produce some simple sentence variations. Negative sentences, for example, are produced by putting a *no* or *not* at the beginning or end of a two word phrase (Klima and Bellugi, 1966). So the child may say "No daddy go," meaning "Don't leave, Daddy," or "Go bed no," meaning, "I don't want to go to bed."

Between 2 and 3 years of age, the child learns some new negative markers. These include *can't* and *don't*. It is interesting to note that these early negative forms appear before their positive correlates *can* and *do* are used (Brown, 1973). When *can't* and *don't* are added to the repertoire of negative markers, the child also modifies the rule for placing them in sentences. Although negative markers were first placed at the beginning of the sentence, between 2 and 3 years of age, the child begins to move them inside, generally putting them between the noun and the verb. So the 2-year-old may say, "Daddy, no eat my candy," or "I can't find it."

Negative sentences are generally produced correctly by age 3. Forms such as *isn't*, *aren't*, *doesn't*, *didn't*, and *won't* are added to the repertoire. By age 4, children are also using past tense negative markers such as *wasn't*, *wouldn't*, *couldn't*, and *shouldn't*. By 4½, children use indefinite negative markers such as *nobody*, *no one*, *none*, and *nothing*, but may err by producing these forms in double negatives ("Nobody didn't come.") (Miller, 1981).

Children also ask questions early in their language development, although these tend to be routines that are limited to a few memorized forms such as, "Whazzat?" and "Where (X) going?" A rising intonation contour is used to express questions that require a yes/no answer ("Have cookie?"), as it sometimes is by adults (Klima and Bellugi, 1966). Between 2 and 3 years, the child moves beyond the first routine questions to produce *what* and *where* questions that are novel, and not the result of a learned formula. They can now, for example, not only ask, "Whazzat?" but also, "What you eating?" Similarly, they can not only ask, "Where daddy going?" but also, "Where my glass of milk?" Still, these questions usually leave out auxiliary and *be* verbs. Yes/no questions continue to be marked only by rising intonation in this period (Klima and Bellugi, 1966).

Auxiliary verbs begin to appear in both the yes/no and *wh-* questions of young 3-year-old children. Yes/no questions are produced with auxiliaries that are appropriately inverted, or placed before the subject, at this time ("We *can* go."/"*Can* we go?"). Rising intonation also remains an option for asking this type of question. Shortly after they begin using and inverting auxiliaries in yes/no questions, children begin to use auxiliaries in *wh-* questions as well. At first, these questions are often produced without inverting the auxiliary (Tyack and Ingram, 1977). Instead of asking, "Why *can't* I have a cookie?" preschoolers may say, "Why I *can't* have a cookie?" They leave the auxiliary between the subject and the verb, as it would be placed in a declarative sentence, rather than moving it before the subject, as the rule for forming questions in English requires. Not all preschoolers make this mistake (Klee, 1985), although it is quite common. By age 5, most children will be producing all questions and negatives with auxiliary verbs appropriately placed.

A major addition to the child's repertoire of sentence forms appears at about age 3: Children begin producing complex sentences (Limber, 1973). These forms involve either joining two sentences together by means of a conjunction such as *and*, *if*, or *because* ("I like ice cream because it tastes good"), or embedding one sentence within another ("I think *I'll have an ice cream cone*"). The sentences are important not only because they allow the child to make his or her utterances longer, but also because they allow the combination of ideas within an utterance to produce a more condensed, elaborated statement. At 3 years, 5–10% of the normal child's sentences will contain these conjoined or embedded clauses. This proportion increases to 20–30% by age 6 (Paul, 1981). The proportion of complex sentences continues to increase throughout the school years, although the most dramatic increases are seen not in children's speech, but in their writing (Loban, 1976).

Pragmatic Development

LEARNING TO CONVERSE

By the time the first word is uttered, the child has already learned to express affect vocally and to attend to adults (Dore, 1975). Still, conversations with 1-year-old children are very erratic and disjointed; the child typically uses sequences of utterances that are not directed toward the listener. Throughout the one- and two-word utterance stages, egocentric language is mixed with language being used to ask for needs and to make observations about the environment. It is not abnormal during this period for the child to talk perseveratively about a single topic or to indiscriminantly echo utterances (Fay and Anderson, 1981; Trantham and Pedersen, 1976).

Although young toddlers can respond to adult speech with the communicative means they have available—gestures, vocalizations, or words—they are not very reliable about doing so and often need coaxing to speak when spoken to. Chapman (1981) reports that at 18–24 months children begin to answer questions more reliably, at first responding to primarily routine questions, such as "What does a doggy say?" and "Where is your nose?" In addition, toddlers show their compliance with the conversational obligation to speak when spoken to by acknowledging their partner's comments, often by imitating a portion of the partner's utterance.

A new communicative function emerges in the second half of the 2nd year. Halliday (1975) refers to this as the "mathetic" or heuristic function of language. Although children at 12–18 months of age generally talk about the here and now, making comments on objects and events that are obvious in the immediate context and add little new information to the listener's knowledge base, the older toddler begins to use language both to learn about the world and to provide the listener with new information. One of the first heuristic uses of language is the asking questions. "Whazzat?" is a frequent early question, with which the toddler requests the names of objects. The use of this function is a manifestation of the child's developing understanding that language can be used to learn about the world.

The child's ability to stick to a topic improves in the 3rd year, although by 36 months still only 50% of child utterances continue the topic of the previous utterance (Bloom et al., 1976). Children of this age have difficulty sustaining a topic for more than one or two turns, particularly if the topic is one they did not initiate (Owens, 1988).

Two-year-old children also begin to learn how to deal with conversational breakdowns. If an adult signals such a breakdown, by asking, "What?," the 2-year-old child typically responds by either repeating the utterance, usually with some phonetic change (C: I kit ball. M: What? C: I kick ball.) or by deleting an element (C: I kick big ball. M: What? C: I kick ball.). Children of this age rarely request another speaker to clarify an utterance, however.

Even at age 2, children realize that we talk differently to different people. A 2-year-old child frequently talks differently to his or her mother than to the father, for example, often using more polite language to the father. Two-year-olds will frequently speak to babies in a high-pitched voice, as adults do. Another determiner of how we choose to say things is the level of knowledge we believe the listener possess. Two-year-old children are not very good at making such judgments. They frequently make the assumption that adults know everything and fail to provide necessary information. This tendency can lead, for example, to a 2-year-old child telling his grandmother over the phone, "See, I got this for my birthday!"

Two-year-old children are still in the process of learning the obligation to say things, particularly to make requests, politely. Frequent parent reminders help facilitate this development, and politeness is one of the few aspects of language development that is explicitly taught. Two-year-old children have little flexibility in their range of politeness markers, and if told to "ask more nicely" will either add *please* to their request or produce it with a whining intonation (Bates, 1976). They may also produce problem or need statements, such as "I'm hungry," or "I can't reach it," as forms of requests. Two-year-old children do understand some of the social parameters of polite requesting and are more likely to include *please* in their request if the listener is bigger, less familiar, or in possession of something they want (Ervin-Tripp and Gordon, 1986).

Another way in which the child's communicative skill advances in the 3rd year of life is through the expansion of purposes to which language can be put. Children learn to use language to convey new information, to talk about past events, and to imagine or pretend (Chapman, 1981), as well as to combine more than one intention within an utterance. Similarly, 2-year-old children learn to use a variety of forms to express their intentions. They may say either, "I want cookie," or "I hungry," for example.

By the age of 3, pragmatic development becomes more sophisticated and interactional. Egocentric speech and echolalia gradually disappear, while the range of language functions increases. The child's language is now used to announce intentions and to describe ongoing events. There is a growing awareness of the conversational function of language, with the child being more likely to await responses and less likely to ignore interruptions (Garvey and Berninger, 1981).

Between the ages of 3 and 5 years, there is rapid development of pragmatic skills. Language is still used to announce intentions and to describe ongoing events, but there is also increasing use of language to describe events and incidents from the past and to relate incidents from the past to present events. The child's conversations show increasing sensitivity to the listener (Van Kleeck, 1984) (in allowing turn-taking, in responding appropriately to the other person, in self-correcting speech, in recognizing taboo words, and in providing clarification when requested). Language play occurs in the form of rhymes, jokes, and exaggerations.

In the preschool period, language begins to be put to use for the purpose of reasoning, solving problems, monitoring thought and actions, relating events, and constructing complex imaginative play (Tough, 1977). Language now becomes an instrument of thought, rather than just a system for mapping what one sees and does into words, as it is primarily used by toddlers. This new function of language is, of course, made possible by increasing cognitive development. But it also, in and of itself, contributes to the child's intellectual skill, so that the growth of language and cognition become more closely entwined during the preschool years.

Preschoolers learn a broader range of devices for making requests politely during this time. Rather than merely adding *please*, they begin to use permission requests ("Can I . . .?"), question requests with modals ("Would you . . .?," "Could you . . .?"), and indirect requests such as "Why don't you . . .?" and "Don't forget to . . ." (Garvey, 1975). By 5 years, children are using hints and other forms in which the real object of the request is never mentioned explicitly at all. So they might request a snack by saying, "Gee, Mom, those cookies you made sure smell good. You make the best cookies in the world." In addition, in playing with peers, preschoolers demonstrate knowledge that requests must fulfill certain conditions, such as that the speaker must have some reason for making the request rather than doing the action himself or herself. Garvey (1975) shows that preschoolers often make adjuncts in their requests to each other, in order to establish that these conditions have been met. They might say, for example, "Get that hammer for me. *I can't reach it.*" Despite this demonstration of the forms and conditions necessary for successful requests, preschool children still have much to learn about using verbal means to regulate others' behavior. They are not very efficient at getting others' attention when it is not already directed to them or in persuading others to do something the listener is reluctant about. During the preschool years, children learn to increase the degree to which they can elaborate on a single topic of conversation. By age 5, children spend an average of five utterances on a single topic (Brinton and Fujiki, 1984), increasing the degree to which each utterance maintains the topic and adds new information.

Around 3 or 4 years of age, children begin to use linguistic devices to provide links between the ideas they talk about in the conversations. One of these *cohesion devices* is the use of pronouns to link referents, as in "I have a *friend* at school. *He* builds blocks with me." Use of definite/indefinite articles (a, the) is another cohesive device that emerges during this time. The indefinite article *a* is used to signal that a referent is being introduced into the conversation for the first time ("Alice saw *a* large cake."). When the same referent is mentioned again, the definite article *the* is used to signal the listener to retrieve the original referent from memory ("Alice ate *the* cake."). The ability to build these cohesive units or *texts* is one of the ways the child's discourse skills are advancing during the preschool years.

Children between 3 and 5 years also become more adept at repairing conversational breakdowns. They are able to respond to requests for clarification of specific information, such as "You went *where* for dinner?" and can reply with just the piece being requested (Gallagher, 1981). Still, they rarely request clarification themselves when they misunderstand and cannot reformulate their message or provide missing background information when the listener looks confused.

With increasing linguistic competence, the child is able to take advantage of many more communicative situations during the preschool years than she or he was as a toddler. Not only can the child engage in a carefully scaffolded conversation with mother, but now the preschooler can talk also with peers, older children, and adults outside the family. Less conversational management is needed for the child's talk to succeed. But parent-child conversations at this time still play a very important role in structuring the child's social world, and much social learning goes on through the medium of language (Cook-Gumperz, 1979). Parents tell preschoolers what to do in different situations, how to behave, and what to expect, and interpret situations verbally for the child, providing reasons and explanations. Language itself becomes part of the experience of social relations, and the preschool child is socialized linguistically as well as behaviorally into the community in which he or she will expected to operate. Talk with peers, too, particularly in the context of cooperative play, teaches the child how language can be used to initiate and construct social relations. Much preschool interactive play is done primarily through the medium of language, and by using language in this interactive fashion, the child learns to exploit its flexibility.

NARRATIVE DEVELOPMENT

While conversation is one form of discourse acquired during the preschool period, narrative is another. Narratives are extended monologues that involve the reporting of the actions of people or animals or objects that take on human characteristics. Stories have particular structures that dictate their form and content; these are often referred to as "story grammars" (Stein and Glenn, 1979). Children as young as 2 can tell stories, although their narratives do not adhere to the typical story grammar structure. They are usually collections of tangentially related events without any discernible plot. Their narrations consist of elements "heaped" together and not organized in causal or thematic ways (Applebee, 1978). As children progress through the preschool years, their stories gradually move closer to the conventional form used by adults in their culture. By age 6, most children can relate a more or less coherent narrative that follows a simple story grammar format.

METALINGUISTIC DEVELOPMENT

One new area of language use that arises during the preschool years is the ability to use language to talk about language itself. This capacity is called *metalinguistic awareness*. One way in which preschoolers manifest this ability is in their play with language. Children begin to use words just for the fun of it, in interchanges like this one described by Garvey (1975):

Child 1: It's snaky because it has snakes.
Child 2: And it's hatty because it has hats.

Interest in rhyme is another manifestation of metalinguistic awareness. Here children show that they are attending not only to what a word means, but to other properties, independent of meaning, such as the word's sound and its similarity to the sounds of other words.

Use of language in role playing also demonstrates the child's metalinguistic skills. For example, preschoolers often correct each other's usage in role play, commenting on its appropriateness. A child might tell another, "You can't call me 'Willy.' You're the baby. The baby has to call the father 'Daddy!'" These emerging metalinguistic abilities help to lay the foundation for the acquisition of literacy during the school years.

LANGUAGE DEVELOPMENT AFTER AGE 5

Comprehension

The comprehension abilities that are acquired after the age of 5 years include the ability to decode syntactic structures that constitute exceptions to the usual rules of the language. By age 7 or 8, most children have gone beyond the use of comprehension strategies in processing these sentences and can decipher the intended meaning of sentences such as "The doll is easy to see" (versus "The doll can easily see"), "John asked Mary where to go" (deciphering who it is that is confused about where to go), and "John promised Bill to leave" (versus "John promised that Bill would leave") (Chomsky, 1969). In addition, the child's growing ability to recognize the deep structures of language permits the recognition of different levels of meaning and the understanding that ambiguous sentences have more than one meaning.

Similarly, after the age of 5, the child begins to understand discrepancies between meaning and form in utterances (Ortony et al., 1978). For example, the child gradually learns to move away from literal interpretations (e.g., of metaphoric language, proverbs) to understand connotations, to "read between the lines," and to make inferences (Livingston, 1982; Nippold, 1988; Resnick, 1982). This is a slow process; although the basic comprehension of figurative language is present at the age of 9 years, major improvements in the understanding of idioms, metaphors, and proverbs continue after this age (Nippold, 1988a). And it is not until the teen years that discrepancies between voice and message (e.g., the sarcastic tone of voice) are fully understood.

In addition, a wider understanding develops of the concepts of temporal relations, spatial relations, number markers, emotional expressions, and abstract ideas. This development involves more than simply adding new vocabulary items; it includes refining the child's entire stored lexical network of interrelated meanings. These refinements in vocabulary comprehension are also a slow process that continues until college age (Nippold, 1988c).

Speech Sound Production

By age 7, most children can produce all sounds of their language correctly. Sound errors that persist past this age are no longer developmental; instead they represent a disorder of speech sound development. During the years from 6 to 16, it appears that children add subtle skills to their knowledge of their sound system. These skills may include full use of appropriate morphological derivative forms (e.g., vowel changes in the pronunciation of differing forms, such as *divide/division* (Moskowitz, 1973), the use of contrastive stress (e.g., to distinguish between *greenhouse* and *green house*) (Myers and Myers, 1983), intonational contrasts, such as *pre'sent* versus *present'* (Cruttenden, 1985), use of dialectal variants (Grunwell, 1986), and, ultimately, representations of the sound system in the form of spelling skills.

Producing Words and Sentences

By age 5, the child's basic knowledge of the rules of his or her language is complete, and the child's expressive development takes the form of more subtle refinements to this essential knowledge. Grammatical errors become less common, although they may still occur in noun-verb agreement (e.g., "He haves the toy"), mass-count distinction (e.g., "I want more macaronis"), pronoun case forms (e.g., "Him and her went"), and irregular verb formations ("The candy had been aten"). Much learning about other morphological markers, particularly about prefixes and suffixes, which augment the meaning or modify the part of speech of a word, goes on during the school years (Wiig and Semel, 1984). Vocabulary growth continues throughout the school years, at an estimated nine words per day (Carey, 1978). Both these developments, as well as the acquisition of more formal, literary types of syntactic structures, depend heavily on exposure to literate language forms used in written expression. Children who do not acquire good reading skills will be limited in their access to these more mature forms of expression, and their language development will being to lag behind that of their peers.

By the age of 6 years, grammatical differences between the child's language and adult language are not apparent in general conversations. The formations and concepts that have still not been learned at this stage consist not so much of new structures, but of the ability to combine a greater number of complex structures within one utterance to produce language that is denser. In addition, children exhibit more frequent usage of complex structures more common to literary forms of language than to everyday conversation, but these changes are more likely to be seen in writing than in speech (Barrie-Blackley, 1973; Chomsky, 1969; Scott, 1988). The increase in the use of these low-frequency literary forms and in the propositional density of utterances in written expression continues throughout adolescence.

Pragmatic Development

Pragmatic development continues through the school years, with language being used in a more diverse range of social interactions (Barnes and Todd, 1978; Stephens, 1988), including telling stories, engaging in holiday rituals, sharing ideas, providing examples, taking perspectives, discussing problems, and appraising alternatives. The child's knowledge of rules for language usage expands to include "code-switching" (how to adapt language forms to specific environments) (Gleason, 1973), politeness markers (e.g., "please," "sorry") (Leonard et al., 1978), how to make indirect requests, and how to anticipate and repair breakdowns in conversations.

Gradually, the child's ability to narrate stories becomes more sophisticated, moving from a temporal chain approach toward the ability to link elements logically and develop a central theme (Applebee, 1978). Narrative skills continue improving up until college age (Johnson, 1983), and there is an increasing ability to embed multiple episodes within stories, to understand and express the motivations of characters, and to imply and infer information in narratives.

Metalinguistic abilities continue to improve throughout the school years, serving as both a cause and a consequence of the acquisition of literacy. For example, children learn what a "word" is, that it can be thought of as apart from the concept it stands for, and that it can be identified as a printed symbol. They learn that words can be broken down into smaller units of sounds, and these sounds can be represented as letters that can be decoded into spoken words. Another metalinguistic skill acquired during the school years involves the ability to define words using synonymous or categorical terms instead of by simply stating a function or by giving an idiosyncratic response. The ability to discuss the structure of language is also included in metalinguistic skill. School-age children learn to identify parts of words—such as syllables, first and last sounds—and parts of speech. They learn to discuss similarities and differences in meaning among words and sentences and to talk about ambiguities in meaning and figurative uses of language. Unlike the other areas of language acquisition we have been discussing, though, the acquisition of these metalinguistic skills is highly dependent on instruction. They are not part of the "natural" progression of language, and children not "taught" these skills, through exposure or direct instruction, will not necessarily learn them on their own.

SUMMARY

The developmental pathway from infancy to young adulthood is characterized by increasing complexity in decoding and comprehension of words and structures, speech sound production, encoding and production of words and structures, and finally in the use of language in interactions. Although there is evidence of certain individual differences, speech and language acquisition follows general patterns in which more and more complex structures are acquired, permitting more and more subtle distinctions in meaning and greater flexibility in form.

The enormity of the speech and language acquisition task and the speed with which it is normally accomplished helps us to understand the relatively high frequency of delays and disorders in this area of development. An intact linguistic system is crucial not only for fluid communication, but also for the acquisition of literacy skills that are so necessary to academic success. For this reason, children who demonstrate delays in the development of language are at risk not only for communicative disorders, but for learning difficulties in school. These disabilities, in turn, may result in problems with behavior, social development, and self-esteem that can accompany learning disorders. For these reasons, early identification and remediation of language learning problems is especially important.

References

Applebee AN: *The Child's Concept of Story.* Chicago, University of Chicago Press, 1978.

Baker L, Cantwell DP: The association between emotional/behavioral disorders and learning disorders in children with speech/language disorders. *Adv Learning Behav Disord* 6:27–46, 1990.

Barnes D, Todd F: *Communication and Learning in Small Groups.* London, Routledge & Kegan Paul, 1978.

Barrie-Blackley S: Six-year-old children's understanding of sentences conjoined with time adverbs. *J Psycholinguist Res* 2:153–165, 1973.

Bates E: *Language and Context: The Acquisition of Pragmatics.* New York, Academic Press, 1976.

Bateson MC: Mother-infant exchanges: The epigenesis of conversational interaction. *Ann NY Acad Sci* 263:101–113, 1975.

Benedict H: Early lexical development: Comprehension and production. *J Child Lang* 6:183–200, 1979.

Bever TG: The cognitive basis for linguistic structures. In: Hayes JR (ed): *Cognition and the Development of Language.* New York, Wiley, 1970, pp. 279–372.

Bloom L, Lahey M: *Language Development and Language Disorders.* New York, Wiley, 1978.

Bloom L, Lightbown P, Hood L: Structure and variation in child language. *Monogr Soc Res Child Dev* 40 (serial no. 160), 1975.

Bloom L, Miller P, Hood L: Variation and reduction as aspects of competence in language development. In: Pick AD, (ed): *Minnesota Symposia on Child Psychiatry* (Vol 9). Minneapolis, University of Minnesota Press, 1975, pp. 3–55.

Boehm A: *Boehm Test of Basic Concepts.* New York, Psychological Corp., 1969.

Braine MDS: The ontogeny of English phrase structure: The first phrase. *Language* 39:1–13, 1963.

Bridges A: SVD comprehension strategies reconsidered: The evidence of individual patterns of response. *J Child Lang* 7:89–104, 1980.

Brinton B, Fujiki M: Development of topic manipulation skills in discourse. *J Speech Hear Res* 27:350–358, 1984.

Brown R: *A first language, the early stages.* Cambridge, MA, Harvard University Press, 1973.

Bruner J: Early social interaction and language acquisition. In: Schaffer R (ed): *Studies in Mother-Infant Interaction.* New York, Academic Press, 1977.

Butterfield E, Siperstein G: Influence of contingent auditory stimulation upon non-nutritional suckle. *Proceedings of the Third Symposium on Oral Sensation and Perception: The Mouth of the Infant* Springfield, IL: Charles C Thomas, 1974, pp. 313–334.

Cantwell DP, Baker L: *Developmental Speech and Language Disorders.* New York, Guilford Press, 1987.

Carey S: The child as word learner. In: Halle M, Bresnan J, Miller GA (eds): *Linguistic Theory and Psychological Reality.* Cambridge, MA, MIT Press, 1978.

Cazden C: The acquisition of noun and verb inflections. *Child Dev* 39:433–438, 1968.

Chapman R: Comprehension strategies in children. In: Kavanagh JF, Strange W (eds): *Speech and Language in the Laboratory, School, and Clinic.* Cambridge, MA, MIT Press, 1978, pp. 308–327.

Chomsky C: *The Acquisition of Language from Five to Ten.* Cambridge, MA, MIT Press, 1969.

Clark H, Clark E: *Psychology and Language: An Introduction to Linguistics.* New York, Harcourt Brace Jovanovich, 1977.

Cook-Gumperz J: Communicating with young children in the home. *Theory Pract* 18:207–212, 1979.

Coplan J, Gleason JR: Unclear speech: Recognition and significance of unintelligible speech in preschool children. *Pediatrics* 82:447–452, 1988.

Cruttenden A: Intonation comprehension in ten-year-olds. *J Child Lang* 12:643–661, 1985.

Dale P: The validity of a parent report measure of vocabulary and syntax at 24 months. *J Speech Hear Res* 34:565–571, 1991.

Dale P, Bates E, Reznick J, et al: The validity of a parent report instrument of child language at twenty months. *J Child Lang* 16(2):239–249, 1989.

Dore J: Holophrase, speech acts and language universals. *J Child Lang* 2:21–40, 1975.

Edwards ML, Shriberg LD: *Phonology: Applications in Communicative Disorders.* San Diego, College-Hill Press, 1983.

Eimas PD: Auditory and phonetic coding of the cues for speech: Discrimination of the [r-l] distinction by young infants. *Percept & Psychophys* 18:341–347, 1975.

Ervin-Tripp S, Gordon D: The development of requests. In: Schiefelbusch R (ed): *Language Competence: Assessment and Intervention.* San Diego, College-Hill Press, 1986.

Farwell CB: Some strategies in the early production of fricatives. *Pap Rep Child Lang Dev* 12:97–104, 1977.

Fay W, Anderson D: Children's echo-reactions as a function of increasing lexical difficulty: A developmental study. *J Genet Psychol* 138:259–267, 1981.

Fenson L, Dale P, Reznick S, et al: *Norms for the MacArthur Communicative Development Inventories.* Poster presented at the International Conference on Infant Studies, Montreal, Quebec, 1990.

Ferguson CA: Learning to pronounce: The earliest stages of phonological development in the child. In: Minifie FD, Lloyd LL (eds): *Communicative and Cognitive Abilities: Early Behavioral Assessment.* Baltimore, University Park Press, 1978, pp. 273–297.

Ferguson C, Farwell C: Words and sounds in early language acquisition: English initial consonants in the first fifty words. *Language* 51:419–439, 1975.

Gallagher T: Contingent query sequences within adult-child discourse. *J Child Lang* 8:51–62, 1981.

Garvey C: Requests and responses in children's speech. *J Child Lang* 2:41–63, 1975.

Garvey C, Berninger G: Timing and turn taking in children's conversations. *Discourse Processes* 4:27–58, 1981.

Gleason JB: Code switching in children's language. In: Moore TE (ed): *Cognitive Development and the Acquisition of Language.* New York, Academic Press, 1973.

Goad H, Ingram D: Individual variation and its relevance to a theory of phonological acquisition. *J Child Lang* 14:419–432, 1987.

Graham JM Jr, Bashir AS, Stark RE: Communicative disorders. In: Levine MD, Carey WB, Crocker AC, et al (eds): *Developmental-Behavioral Pediatrics.* Philadelphia, Saunders, 1983, pp. 847–864.

Greenfield P, Smith J: *The Structure of Communication in Early Language Development.* New York, Academic Press, 1976.

Grunwell P: *Clinical Phonology.* Rockville, MD, Aspen System Corp., 1982.

Grunwell P: Aspects of phonological development in later childhood. In: Durkin K (ed): *Language Development in the School Years.* London, Croom Helm, 1986, pp. 34–56.

Haas A, Owens R: Preschoolers' pronoun strategies: You and me make us. Paper presented at the American Speech, Hearing, and Language Association Annual General Conference, 1985.

Haelsig P, Madison C: A study of phonological process exhibited by 3-, 4-, and 5-year-old children. *Lang Speech Hear Services in Schools* 17:107–114, 1986.

Halliday M: *Learing How to Mean: Explorations in the Development of Language.* New York, Arnold, 1975.

Haviland S, Clark E: "This man's father is my father's son": A study of the acquisition of English kin terms. *J Child Lang* 1:23–47, 1974.

Hirsh-Pasek K, Golinkoff R, Cauley K: *The verb's the thing: Therein to catch the origins of grammar.* Paper presented to Society for Research in Child Development, Baltimore, 1987.

Homzie MJ, Lindsay JS: Language and the young stutterer. *Brain Lang* 22:232–252, 1984.

Hutt S, Hutt C, Leonard H, et al: Auditory responsivity in the human newborn. *Nature* 218:888–890, 1968.

Ingram D: Phonological rules in young children. *J Child Lang* 1:49–64, 1974.

Ingram D: Current issues in child phonology. In: Morehead DM, Morehead A (eds): *Normal and Deficient Child Language.* Baltimore, University Park Press, 1976, pp. 3–27.

Jakobson R: *Child language: Aphasia and Phonological Universals.* Hague, Netherlands, Mouton Press, 1968.

Johnson NS: What do you do when you can't tell the whole story: The development of summarization skills. In: Nelson KE (ed): *Children's Language* (Vol 4). Hillsdale, NJ, Erlbaum, 1983, pp. 315–383.

Kagan J, Lewis M: Studies of attention. *Merrill-Palmer Quarterly* 11:92–127, 1965.

Khan L: A review of 16 major phonological processes. *Lang Speech Hear Services in Schools* 132:77–85, 1982.

Kuhl P, Meltzoff A: Speech as an intermodal object of perception. In: Yonas A (ed): *Perceptual Development in Infancy* Hillsdale, NJ, Lawrence Erlbaum, 1988, pp. 235–266.

Kvaal J, Shipstead-Cox N, Nevitt S, et al: The acquisition of 90 Spanish morphemes by Spanish-speaking children. *Lang Speech Hear Serv Schools* 19:384–394, 1988.

Lenneberg E: *Biological Foundations of Language.* New York, Wiley, 1967.

Leonard LB, Schwartz RG, Folger MK, et al: Some aspects of child phonology in imitative and spontaneous speech. *J Child Lang* 5:403–415, 1978.

Limber J: The genesis of complex sentences. In: Moore T (ed): *Cognitive Development and the Acquisition of Language.* New York, Academic Press, 1973.

Livingston KR: Beyond the definition given: On the growth of connotation. In: Kuczaj SA (ed): *Language Development* (Vol 1). Hillsdale, NJ, Erlbaum, 1982.

Loban W: *Language Development: Kindergarten through Grade Twelve.* Urbana, IL, National Council of Teachers of English, 1976.

Miller J: *Assessing Language Production in Children: Experimental Procedures.* Baltimore, University Park Press, 1981.

Morley ME: *The Development and Disorders of Speech in Childhood* (2nd ed). Edinburgh, E & S Livingstone, 1965.

Moskowitz BA: On the status of vowel shift in English. In: Moore TE (ed): *Cognitive Development and the Acquisition of Language.* New York: Academic Press, 1973.

Myers FL, Myers RW: Perception of stress contrasts in semantic and non-semantic contexts by children. *J Psycholinguist Res* 12:327–340, 1973.

Nelson K: Structure and strategy in learning to talk. *Monogr Soc Res Child Dev* 38 (serial no. 149):1–2, 1973.

Nippold MA (ed): Figurative language. In: *Later Language Development: Ages Nine through Nineteen.* Boston, Little, Brown, 1988a, pp. 1979–209.

Nippold MA (ed): Linguistic ambiguity. In: *Later Language Development: Ages Nine through Nineteen.* Boston, Little, Brown, 1988b, pp. 211–223.

Nippold MA (ed): The literate lexicon. In: *Later Language Development: Ages Nine through Nineteen.* Boston, Little, Brown, 1988c, pp. 29–47.

Ortony A, Reynolds RE, Arter JA: Metaphor: Theoretical and empirical research. *Psychol Bull* 85:919–943, 1978.

Patterson CJ, Kister MC: The development of listener skills for referential communication. In: Dickson WP (ed): *Children's Oral Communication Skills*. New York, Academic Press, 1981, pp. 143–166.

Paul R: The emergence of pragmatic comprehension: A study of children's understanding of sentence-structure cues to given/new information. *J Child Lang* 12(1):145–160, 1985.

Paul R: Comprehension strategies: Interactions between world knowledge and the development of sentence comprehension. *Top Lang Disord* 10(3):63–75, 1990.

Paul R: Profiles of toddlers with slow expressive language development. *Top Lang Disord* 11(4):1–13, 1991.

Paul R, Jennings P: Phonological behavior in toddlers with slow expressive language development. *J Speech Hear Res* 35:99–107, 1992.

Paul R, Shiffer M: Communicative initiations in normal and late-talking toddlers. *Applied Psycholinguistics* 1991.

Preisser DA, Hodson BW, Paden EP: Developmental phonology: 18–29 months. *J Speech Hear Disord* 53: 125–130, 1988.

Rescorla L: (1976) Concept formation in word learning. Unpublished doctoral dissertation. Yale University.

Rescorla L: *The Language Development Survey. J Speech Hear Disord* 54:585–599, 1989.

Resnick DA: A developmental study of proverb comprehension. *J Psycholinguist Res* 11:521–538, 1982.

Ricks DM: Vocal communication in preverbal, normal, and autistic children. In: O'Connor N (ed): *Language, Cognitive Deficits, and Retardation*. London, Butterworth, 1975, pp. 75–80.

Sander EK: When are speech sounds learned? *J Speech Hear Disord* 37:55–63, 1972.

Schwartz RG, Leonard LB, Wilcox MJ, et al: Again and again: Reduplication in child phonology. *J Child Lang* 7: 75–87, 1980.

Scott C: Spoken and written syntax. In: Nippold MA (ed): *Later Language Development: Ages Nine through Nineteen*. Boston, Little, Brown, 1988, pp. 49–95.

Shatz M: Children's comprehension of their mother's question-directives. *J Child Lang* 5:39–46, 1978.

Shriberg L: Developmental phonological disorders. In: Hixon T, Shriber L, Saxman J (eds): *Introduction to Communication Disorders*. Englewood Cliffs, NJ, Prentice-Hall, 1980.

Shriberg L, Kwiatkowski J: *Natural process analysis: A procedure for phonological analysis of continuous speech samples*. New York, Wiley, 1980.

Smith M: An investigation of the development of the sentence and the extent of vocabulary in young children. *University of Iowa Studies in Child Welfare*, 3(5), 1926.

Snow C, Fergusen C: *Talking to Children*. Cambridge, Cambridge University Press, 1978.

Spitz R: *No and Yes: On the Genesis of Human Communication*. New York, International Press, 1957.

Stark R: Prespeech segmental feature development. In: Fletcher P, Garman M (eds): *Language Acquisition*. New York, Cambridge University Press, 1979.

Stein N, Glenn C: An analysis of story comprehension in elementary school children. In: Freedle R (ed): *New Directions in Discourse Processing*. (Vol 2) Norwood, NJ, Ablex, 1979, pp. 53–120.

Stephens M: Pragmatics. In: Nippold MA (ed): *Later Language Development: Ages Nine through Nineteen*. Boston, Little, Brown, 1988, pp. 247–262.

Stern D: *The First Relationship*. Cambridge, Harvard University Press, 1977.

Stoel-Gammon C: Phonetic inventories, 15–24 months: A longitudinal study. *J Speech Hear Res* 28:505–512, 1985.

Stoel-Gammon C: Normal and disordered phonology in two year olds. *Top Lang Disord* 11:21–32 1991.

Stoel-Gammon C, Otomo K: Babbling development of hearing-impaired and normally hearing subjects. *J Speech Hear Disord* 51:33–41, 1986.

Sugarman S: Discussion: Empirical versus logical issues in the transition from prelinguistic to linguistic communication. In: Golinkoff R (ed): *The Transition from Prelinguistic to Linguistic Communication*. Hillsdale, NJ, Erlbaum, 1983, pp. 133–145.

Templin M: *Certain language skills in children: Their development and inter-relationships*. Minneapolis, University of Minnesota Press, 1957.

Tough J: *The Development of Meaning*. New York, Halsted Press, 1977.

Trantham CR, Pedersen JK: *Normal Language Development: The Key to Diagnosis and Therapy for Language Disordered Children*. Baltimore, William & Wilkins, 1976.

Tronick EZ: Infant communicative intent: The infant's reference to social interaction. In: Stark R (ed): *Language Behavior in Infancy and Early Childhood*. New York, Elsevier, 1981.

Tyack D, Ingram D: Children's production and comprehension of questions. *J Child Lang* 4:211–224, 1977.

Van Kleeck A: Metalinguistic skills: Cutting across spoken and written language and problem-solving abilities. In: Wallach G, Butler K (eds): *Language Learning Disabilities in School-Age Children*. Baltimore, Williams & Wilkins, 1984, pp. 128–153.

Vihman M: Phonology and the development of the lexicon: Evidence from children's errors. *J Child Lang* 8: 239–264, 1981.

Wallach GP: Later language learning: Syntactic structures and strategies. In: Wallach G, Butler K (eds): *Language Learning Disabilities in School-Age Children*. Baltimore, Williams & Wilkins, 1984, pp. 82–102.

Wetherby A, Yonclas D, Bryan A: Communicative profiles of pre-school children with handicaps: Implications for early identification. *J Speech Hear Disord* 54:148–158, 1989.

Wiig E, Semel E: *Language Assessment and Intervention for the Learning Disabled*. Columbus, OH, Merrill, 1980.

Wiig E, Semel E: *Language Assessment and Intervention for the Learning Disabled*. Columbus, OH, Charles E. Merrill, 1984.

16 COGNITIVE AND AFFECTIVE IMPLICATIONS OF IMAGINATIVE PLAY IN CHILDHOOD

Jerome L. Singer, Ph.D.

I dwell in Possibility
A fairer house than Prose
More numerous of windows, —
Superior of doors.
Emily Dickinson

Why do children play? This issue has intrigued poets as well as behavioral scientists from the days when Friedrich Schiller first proposed his theory of *surplus energy*, which explained that the boisterous play behavior of boys was a necessary preparation for later work activities. Adopting a more clearly evolutionary orientation, the first major researcher on play, Karl Groos (1901), proposed that play emerges out of natural selection as a form of necessary practice on the part of animals or children. The playful fighting of animals or the rough-and-tumble play of children and many of the playful courtship behaviors of animals and children are essentially the practice of skills that will later aid their survival. This adaptive viewpoint is further amplified in the conception of the Viennese psychologist Karl Bühler (1930), who in his concept of *Funktionlust* pointed to the inherently pleasurable nature of play activity as a feature of children's growing skills and abilities.

The psychoanalytic conceptions of play originated in Freud's proposals that play itself emerged under conditions of deprivation of initial gratifications in the child, which caused it to "hallucinate" the image of a satisfying object such as the mother's breast. This hallucinated image later could become a source of at least partial drive satisfaction and permit the child to delay or control random, restless movements and cries of distress. The brief interval of delay becomes a central foundation in psychoanalytic theory for the later formation of the ego (Freud, 1908/1958; Singer, 1955).

Later Freud (1920/1962) modified the theory from its initial purely sensual, instinctual aspect to include the concept of mastery, which he exemplified in a much-cited example of his grandson's playing a kind of hide-and-seek game. Even here Freud continued to emphasize that the game involved an attempt on the part of the child to deal with a conflict over maternal attachment and resentment of the mother's leaving through repetitive efforts at mastery. Psychoanalytic theories of play continued to emphasize the libidinal and drive satisfaction features of play, but there was increasing emphasis in work such as that of Peller (1959) and Waelder (1932) on the mastery elements, which in some respects formed the groundwork for a more cognitive as well as drive-oriented approach. With the important observations of Erikson (1963), this early notion of play was broadened considerably. Erikson suggested that a psychoanalytic theory of play move beyond the satisfaction of early childhood psychosexuality toward incorporating broader features of social development that were "modeled" within the play format. Play thus becomes not just a form of vicarious gratification but provides a way in which complex difficulties and problems experienced by the child can be addressed and even possibly "healed" through the creation of a miniature and manageable world.

Perhaps the most thoroughly worked out theory of the origins of play, one with a much stronger cognitive focus, has been that proposed by Jean Piaget (1962), who believed that play emerges in the context of children's enactment of the two fundamental characteristics of their mode of experience and development, accommodation and assimilation. The former provides an opportunity to imitate and interact physically with the environment, while the latter represents the attempt to integrate externally derived percepts or motor actions into a relatively limited number of schemas or differentiated motor and cognitive skills already available to the child at this age. Physical mastery games, with their repetitious and practice qualities, are more associated with the accommodation feature, while the symbolic play of the child is associated more with assimilation. Piaget used the two notions to argue that play is therefore critical in early childhood for the eventual emergence of concrete operational thought in the child, and he tended to minimize the role of play for children in the older age groups of 7 and up.

For Piaget, play is at least analogous to the fantasy life of the adult, but he does not devote much time in his extensive writings to elaborating this notion. By contrast, Brian Sutton-Smith (1966), while accepting the importance of Piaget's emphasis on early childhood development, has proposed that play continues through adolescence as a means by which preschool and older children can create miniature environments in which they gain a sense of power through elaborating and reconstructing those complexities, emotional and cognitive, that they confront in the adult world that surrounds them.

It is important at the outset to be clear about a definition of play. The term has been widely extended to range from children's activity to more complex forms of adult ritual and competition (for the latter, see Caillois, 1958; Huizinga, 1950; and Geertz, 1976). Indeed, the emphasis on all forms of play and their role in learning elaborated by Bruner et al. (1976) has moved the notion perhaps too far afield from the focus of this chapter. The definition we shall entertain was proposed by Klinger (1971): Play is behavior that is neither consummatory, instrumental, nor competitive; it involves behavior that is neither socially prescribed, as in ritual, nor constrained in some way by social expectations and conventions. More concretely, then, play is behavior that is not obviously associated with direct satisfaction of biological needs such as eating, drinking, overt sexual gratification, or the overcoming of immediate obstacles in one's life situation. It is also relatively free of any effort to meet standards set up by society. At least the standards of play, one might say, are established by the players themselves within a context that may not be the same as those ordinarily observable in society.

Piaget confronted this issue more clearly in his organization of play into games that involve simple sensory pleasure and exploration, games that involve mastery and expression of physical skills, symbolic play (with which this chapter deals), and games with rules that are manifest in activities, such as the structured play of athletic contests or board or card games. The focus of this chapter is specifically on the nature of symbolic play as exemplified by games of pretend and make-believe. Such play seems of special importance not only for the child's mental development but also for the gradual emergence of the capacity for fantasy and imagination in the older child and in the adult. The theories we have mentioned have in many ways gradually been integrated into a cognitive-affective approach that will serve as the organizing focus of the present chapter.

It is becoming increasingly clear to those of us who study both adult and children's imagination that the make-believe or pretending of early childhood is fundamental for the development of all competent adult cognition and emotional functioning. Piaget (1962) emphasized the role of symbolic play as a precursor for those processes of logic and orderly sequence whose epistemology was his main concern. Increasingly, we can also recognize that all mature human thought and information processing is not limited only to scientific or mathematical sequences that are sequential in nature and characterized strongly by verbal expression and grammatical structure. The seminal analyses of Jerome Bruner (1986) have made it evident that effective thought takes on a narrative or subjunctive form as well. In our processing of information we must not only organize it into logical structures but also examine the alterna-

tive and future possibilities or even consider the darker alternatives that appear in any new human experience. Indeed, we store information, as is increasingly clear in memory research, by organized verbal schemas, on the one hand, and through narrative episodes or possibilities in the form of fantasies and daydreams, on the other (Singer, 1985; Singer and Salovey, 1990). Narrative thought and subjunctive structure reflect the human capacity for what the great neurologist Kurt Goldstein (1940) called "taking an attitude toward the possible." He believed this capacity reflected the optimal functioning of both a healthy and intact brain. Through this orientation to the possible one becomes capable of exploring a range of potential futures or, in effect, traveling through time and space to a different or better childhood or maturity (D. Singer and J. Singer, 1990). Sigmund Freud (1911/1962) too used the term *trial*, or *experimental action*, to characterize thought and the emergence of his concept of the ego.

This capacity for reconstructing one's past or for planning for one's daily activities through mental rehearsal or simply daydreaming about future vacations, sexual opportunities, or fantastic space adventures also serves a broader function. Our imagination liberates us from the tyranny of *this* place, of *these* particular duties and obligations, of *these* particular people in our social milieu. We accomplish this restructuring not only through the abstraction of high-level logical or mathematical processes but also through our capacity for creating narrative and for using our skills at imagery to provide us with alternative temporary environments that we can manipulate for self-help and ultimately put into the service of orderly living or simply sustaining hope and effort (Singer, 1974; Singer and Bonanno, 1990; Taylor, 1989). As Bruner has proposed, the object of narrative thought is not "truth" but verisimilitude or "lifelikeness." He writes: "Efforts to reduce one mode [the narrative] to the other [the paradigmatic or logical] or to ignore one at the expense of the other inevitably fail to capture the rich diversity of thought" (Bruner, 1986, p. 11).

Viewed from this perspective, the simple make-believe play of the child (pretending early on that a stick is an airplane, that a soft toy can talk or respond to nurturance or admonition, that a few blocks or dolls can become the basis of an imagined city in which a relatively lengthy story unfolds) can be regarded as a fundamental precursor of the full-blown adult imagination. This chapter proposes that we accord the imaginative play of childhood its full weight as a fundamental and significant development of competency in the child. Without an adequate development of this narrative, subjunctive, or imaginative dimension, the child is subsequently handicapped in both cognitive and emotional development. Indeed, without sufficient practice in the skill of generating fantasy for self-regulation, the child not only will experience difficulties in school adjustment but also, if psychotherapy is required at some future point, may not move ahead effectively into the process. Play therapists actually find that some encouragement and even training efforts are necessary to aid young children to engage in symbolic play as part of an ongoing treatment process (D. Singer, 1993; D. Singer and J. Singer, 1990).

A COGNITIVE-AFFECTIVE PERSPECTIVE ON PRETENDING

Information Processing and Emotion

In the so-called cognitive revolution that has dominated psychology since about 1960, we perceive a new model of the human being. We now look on babies and children as information-seeking organisms striving to organize and to integrate novelty and complexity, curious and exploratory but also more likely to feel comfortable and to smile (as the research by Papousek on infants has shown) once they can experience control over novelty and assimilate new information into prior concepts and scripts about the sequence of events. The "smile of predictive pleasure" in babies, described by Papousek (1987) and his collaborators, and other signs of positive emotion (smiling and laughter associated with familiarity in adults) suggest that while cognition and emotion may be different systems in terms of bodily structure, they are closely related in actual human response (Izard, 1977; Kreitler and Kreitler, 1976; Mandler, 1984; Tomkins, 1962, 1963).

Theoretical analyses initiated by Silvan Tomkins have contributed greatly to the paradigm shift toward the cognitive-affective view of the human organism. Tomkins's work has succeeded in putting emotions back at the center of active research in personality and in social psychology. He led the way in demonstrating that a cognitive perspective that involved an emphasis on the fact that human beings are continuously assigning meanings and organizing their experience in schemas and scripts does not preclude a significant motivational role for affect or emotion. With the support of increasing empirical research carried out on both children and adults by investigators such as Carroll Izard (1977) and Paul Ekman (Ekman, 1973; Ekman et al., 1982) and many others, we can now regard human beings as showing differentiated emotional response patterns that are closely intertwined with responses to the novelty, complexity, and other structural properties of information confronted from moment to moment (Shapiro and Emde, 1992; D. Singer and J. Singer, 1990).

This cognitive-affective perspective broadens our conception of human motivation considerably. Rather than reducing all human motivation to some symbolic reflection of infantile sexuality or aggression, one can propose that the basic emotions that have now been shown to exist across human species in the research of Ekman and of Izard are motivating human beings in dozens of different situations independent of presumed drive pressures. Human beings seek, as Tomkins has proposed, to reconstruct in life or in thought situations that evoke the positive emotions of interest-excitement or joy; they seek to avoid in action or thought those situations that have evoked specific negative emotions of anger, fear-terror, sadness-distress (weeping), or the complex of shame-humiliation-guilt. Human beings are further "wired up" to express emotions as fully as possible and finally to control emotional expression where social experience suggests such control is necessary either for safety or to avoid humiliation. Situations that permit experience and expression of positive emotions or that will allow for appropriate control of negative emotions are intrinsically positively reinforcing. Those situations that are more likely to evoke negative emotions, such as fear, anger, distress, or shame, or that have blocked the expression of socially adaptive control of emotions may be experienced as inherently punishing or negatively reinforcing (Singer, 1974, 1984; Tomkins, 1962, 1981).

Memory and anticipation become central features related to emotional experience. This is accomplished by identifying, labeling, and gradually organizing new information into mental representations that are technically labeled as schemas. These structures include schemas about persons or physical objects, schemas about self and others, and also scripts about action sequences or prototypes that become means for encapsulating a variety of common features of situations and persons into one fuzzy concept (J. Mandler, 1984, 1988; Singer and Kolligian, 1987; Singer and Salovey, 1990).

The Child's Task in Information Processing

The problem for the child becomes, in effect, one of making sense of a complex world through the gradual formation of schemas and scripts and through the assimilation of new situations into established organized mental structures or, as language increases, into lexical categories as well. Confronted with extreme novelty that cannot at once be easily assimilated into established structures, a child may respond with fear or terror. Once a match can be made between new information and some well-known schema, and the novelty or ambiguity of the environmental situation can be assimilated, the child may respond with a smile of pleasure. When the new situation is only moderately complex and some overriding schema is still available, the child may move to explore the moderate amount of novelty in the situation, and this evokes the positive affects of interest and excitement. Children and adults live in a situation of a perennially delicate balance between the potential for fear or anxiety evoked by new situations and the excitement of exploring such situa-

tions. By such exploration one can assimilate incongruity into established schemas, enrich such schemas, or start to form new ones. The persistence over time of large amounts of unexpected or ambiguous information evokes the negative affects of anger or of distress and sadness (D. Singer and J. Singer, 1990; Tomkins, 1962). We all learn to bring to each new situation sets of expectations of what may occur. We practice such expectations through brief anticipatory fantasies, some more realistic than others, depending on our maturity, the complexity of our schema structure, and our social development. Our task in each new situation is then to examine new information and determine whether it confirms or disconfirms some of our anticipations. George Mandler (1984) has particularly developed the implications of interrupted sequences of action and thought and of confirmations and disconfirmations of anticipations as the basis for emotional response.

If identifying and organizing new information becomes the fundamental, overarching demand placed on the child, then we can begin to understand the evolutionary function of imaginative play and the thought processes that seem to grow out of such play. As Piaget has shown, the efforts of children to master the environment and their own motor activities involve to some extent an accommodation to the physical characteristics of the environment and also to the speech, gestures, and other physical actions of adults or older children. In these efforts children succeed through some form of successive approximation, but at the same time they need to be able to assimilate such new actions into organized mental structures. This assimilation process is at first expressed by children through repetitive actions and talking aloud. What seems like the intrinsic unmotivated character of play to an adult represents the child's continuing effort to create new meaning structures and to provide itself with a sense of control and power by reducing large-scale settings, persons, or social interactions to meaningful structures that can be assimilated into the as yet limited number of schemas the child has at its command. The startle responses or terror evoked in a toddler by the size and noise of a huge passing truck may be gradually transformed into curiosity and interest as the child attempts to reproduce the noises and movements of the truck through creating its own sound effects and through manipulating blocks or toy trucks. Imaginative play may thus be understood as a means by which the uncontrollable qualities and complexity of one's physical and social environment can be gradually miniaturized and manipulated. In effect, we can see that much of adult human thought involves a similar effort to create at least temporarily a world one can control through replaying memories or through anticipation and fantasy. Indeed, it can be argued that the very act of rehearsal and anticipation or even of elaborating possible future events into somewhat more bizarre fantasies may gradually approximate possible situations we do encounter. Such mental rehearsal may leave us better prepared to handle these or, at least, to be less frightened by them when they do occur (D. Singer and J. Singer, 1990).

Attachment and Individuation: a Persistent Human Dilemma

Beyond the cognitive demand for meaning assignment and organization and its link to the arousal of emotion, human beings also must confront a persisting dialectic tension in their general motivation throughout their life span. This tension becomes evident in some of the very earliest months of childhood. On the one hand there is the need to feel close to others, to be attached to or encompassed by parents, older siblings, or other caregivers and, later, by friends, or by a group by means of some symbolic group participation (e.g., a religious, ethnic, or nationalistic association). On the other hand, we all experience to varying degrees the need to preserve some areas of personal autonomy, some sense of privacy, personal competence, and individualized skill development. We must move through life in effect struggling to preserve a balance between affiliation with others or with groups, thereby gaining a sense of community, while we also strive to maintain a sense of individuality and personal power (Angyal, 1965; Bakan, 1966; Jung, 1971; Rank, 1945; Schachtel, 1959).

More recently in the framework of an object relations psychoanalytic analysis, Sidney Blatt (1990) has sought to show how the early childhood struggle between attachment and individuation may, if one pole or the other is overemphasized, become a focal area of conflict and eventuate in particular forms of psychopathology. Bonanno and Singer (1990) have further extended this polarity to identify a series of personality dimensions that recur in the literature along with particular affective tendencies, defensive patterns, variations in physical illness proneness, and emotional disorders that had already been identified along such dimensions by Blatt.

This conceptualization, while still largely speculative, is built around some available research evidence that suggests that optimal personality functioning and a hardy physical health status necessitate a reasonable balance between one's needs or strivings for affiliation and one's abilities to experience autonomy or individuation (Bonanno and Singer, 1990).

Within this conceptual framework, the child's make-believe world is one that represents a continuous working out of the dialectical tension between the need for closeness and affiliation and the need for privacy with its concomitant experience of personal power and individuality. Indeed, the very act of beginning to form individualized images, memories, and anticipatory fantasies becomes, in our crowded and sensory-bombarded world, the last refuge for an experience of individuality and personal privacy. For the developing child seeking on the one hand to sustain relationships with parents and others and to feel the warmth of what Schachtel (1959) called embeddedness-affect, the ability on the other hand to create private games and to engage in floor play or to sustain a relationship with a personally possessed stuffed animal or invisible playmate provides that experience of individuation that also seems so necessary in our human condition.

In view of this persistent human attachment-individuation tension, the emergence of an increasingly complex imaginative dimension subject to reasonable control (a kind of cognitive skill in itself) sustains the need for self-definition, for a sense of uniqueness and private power. The child must learn gradually to establish priorities in the direction of attention, whether toward the environment or toward material recurring from memory or forming itself into fantasies. Our practical survival may well demand that we assign a somewhat higher priority to the processing of externally generated stimulation, what David Rapaport (1960) wrote of as the "permanent gradient toward the external attention-cathexis." As we will see, our affective development also must involve reflection, introspection, the capacity to enjoy private experiences, to gradually shape and direct them, to plan, and also to create stories and to manipulate mentally the range of future possibilities. For young children with limited motor and linguistic capacities and a smaller and less differentiated range of stored schemas and scripts, the balancing of such priorities may be reflected in the varying amounts of physical, rule-oriented, or social and imaginative play in which they engage.

Of course this very dilemma of attachment versus individuation is not only reflected structurally in the degree of priorities assigned by children to social interaction or to imaginative experience. It is also the basis for the content of the play behavior. The themes of play in the child often reflect the continuing tension between the desire for closeness and the desire for assertions of personal power, importance, or the need for privacy. Such manifestations are readily identifiable in play therapy observations. For the purposes of this chapter, however, we focus more on the structural features of imaginative play and how make-believe and the gradual internalization of such make-believe into childhood fantasy serve the cognitive and affective interests of the developing organism.

EMERGENCE OF IMAGINATIVE PLAY

Forms of Play

The generally accepted definition of play has focused on its intrinsic, nonmotivated nature. Eric Klinger (1971) has perhaps expressed this most clearly by defining play as behavior free of consummatory, competitive, religious, or social motives or constraints.

In his review of the available literature, Philip Smith (1982) raises the issue of whether play in animals serves any intrinsic evolutionary function. He argues that there is little evidence of the benefits of play for later social and cognitive skills, except in a few instances for the most humanoid primates. However, he does make it clear that with respect to human children, where language, imagery, or symbolic functions are involved, play, especially imaginative games, may turn out to have more broadly useful roles.

One need not argue that pretend play serves ultimate survival or reproductive functions from an evolutionary standpoint, however. Most careful observers of childhood and adult play behavior, such as Brian Vandenberg (1986), Brian Sutton-Smith (1982), Michael Lewis (1982), and Mihalyi Csikszentmihalyi (1982), point out that play is just an enjoyable activity in its own right. From the position already presented above, one can argue that most forms of play involve situations of moderate challenge, novelty, or incongruity. The playful interactions between self and others or between self and objects or, in the case of pure fantasy play, between self and symbolic others usually result in a further reduction of novelty or incongruity, thereby invoking the emotions of joy and the smiling response. What follows from such activities may be a further learned recognition (conscious or increasingly automatic) that within the defined structure of such play one can in the future experience moderate challenge and also some reduction of incongruity. I would propose that such a conception seems more specific than Freud's (1920/1962) proposal of a "repetition-compulsion" to explain why children repeat games again and again. As Ernst Schachtel (1959) has also pointed out, the repetitive nature of play in children may reflect not so much a compulsion as a continuing discovery of novelty in what for adults may seem commonplace but for children still provides puzzling material that must be assimilated into a previously limited range of schemas. The repetition thus is characterized by a sustained affect of interest in the elements that are still novel in even a simple story like "The Three Bears."

Jean Piaget (1962) has proposed that play follows a particular sequence in its emergence and in the service of the development of more concrete operational thought. The child begins with more purely sensorimotor play, gradually evolves the capacity for symbolic or pretend play, and then goes on to more structured and orderly games with rules. These rule games range from simple examples such as "Ring around the Rosy" (with hand holding, circling, singing, and the dominant rule, dropping down on the signal "all fall down!") and evolve into more complex games often played outdoors, such as "Red Light," or into parlor games such as "Statues" or "Charades" and board games such as *Chutes and Ladders* or checkers. Such games are critical for mastery of orderly thought, moral judgment, and other phases of concrete operations for mature thought in Piaget's scheme.

It is important to note, however, that for Piaget the functions of play were largely delineated in relation to their role in the emergence of orderly, formal logical thought processes. Piaget has been criticized by other researchers such as Inge Bretherton (1984) and Brian Sutton-Smith (1966) because they feel he tended to devalue the importance of play as a source of mature adult imagery and as the foundation for the playfulness that characterizes all human thought. Bretherton has also pointed out that Piaget tended to think of imaginative play as declining after the age of 4 or 5 rather than recognizing the importance of play as a forerunner for Bruner's narrative thought.

The research of the author and his colleagues with large numbers of children from diverse backgrounds who were observed during spontaneous play has made it clear that pretend play goes on well into the early school years and continues either "underground" in private thought or in the more sanctioned group forms of make-believe that are observable through the life cycle (D. Singer and J. Singer, 1990; J. Singer and D. Singer, 1981). Even games with rules, which are certainly an important step in the child's development of orderly and regulatory processing and self-control, often include elements of pretending or evoke private or shared fantasies well into adult life. If one watches adults and children playing relatively structured games like *Monopoly*, one can frequently observe the tendency for the players to introduce make-believe components, sometimes even taking on particular make-believe roles for themselves as they participate in this otherwise rule-organized game. The reordering of the "given" realities is just as much a fundamental feature of human thought as is the attempt at faithful accommodation to the environment through coherent schemas, which Piaget emphasized in his epistemology. Indeed it was only in his posthumously published work that he finally addressed the question of the origins of possibility (Piaget, 1980).

The balance of this chapter examines some of the potential advantages for cognitive development and emotional expressiveness and control of imaginative play. To assert that imaginative play has a variety of short- and long-term benefits may reflect some cultural bias, as Brian Sutton-Smith has argued in some of his papers (Sutton-Smith and Kelley-Byrne, 1984). But even the subversive quality of *Mad Magazine* cartoon humor, of cards such as the *Garbage Pail Kids*, or of the punning and teasing of adults by children may serve an important balancing function for the developing child in a world in which children are powerless. In the face of life tragedies, parental neglect or abuse, parental poverty or humiliation, abandonment, illness, or death, the ability to step back from the situation and to create playful narrative offers at least some solace if not a complete way out of the distress. Those children who do not experience encouragement through storytelling or pretending that fosters the development of a symbolic dimension or through repetitive sensory or physical play or games with rules may find themselves condemned either to impetuous instrumental activity or to the apathy of a sense of isolation or extreme dependence on conventional rituals (D. Singer and J. Singer, 1990; D. Singer, 1993).

Beginnings of Imaginative Play

It is rare for adults to observe any clear evidence of what might be called pretending or make-believe play before at least the age of $2\frac{1}{2}$ in children. One can observe that such play gradually emerges from parent-child interactions, the beginnings of games of peek-a-boo.

Make-believe play or early pretending takes on two general forms in the preschool child. One involves the overt floor play or monologue of the child, often using limited props and evolving eventually into very elaborate play with a mixture of structured toys, such as Barbie dolls or robot soldiers, mingled with less clearly defined objects such as blocks or cloths and bits of string, that become employed in the more general service of storytelling. Another form of imaginative play emerges from the so-called transitional object of Winnicott (1953), the soft cloth or furry teddy that becomes either a subject of feigned conversation between child and teddy or eventually an invisible playmate assigned a name and personality. I will first deal with the role of floor play and turn a little later to the issue of imaginary playmates and their role in the child's development.

The following criteria, proposed by Greta Fein (1981), represent symbolic or pretend play:

1. Familiar activities may be performed even in the absence of necessary material or social context (e.g., a child pretends to drink from an empty cup or puts a doll to bed on the floor rather than in a doll bed or even on the couch).
2. Activities may not be carried out to their logical outcomes (e.g., a toy presumably imprisoned in a doll house escapes quite magically through the roof).
3. A child may treat an inanimate object as animate (e.g., a furry animal is offered food or a cup of tea).
4. An object or gesture may be substituted for another (e.g., a block is transformed into a spaceship).
5. A child may carry out an activity usually performed by another person or especially by an adult (e.g., pretending to be a doctor, a pilot, a teacher).

Of special importance is the conception of transformation, or the emergence through play of what Alan Leslie (1987) in a fine paper has called a metarepresentational mode of thought. Leslie has proposed the challenging question,

> [How] is it possible that young children can disregard or distort reality (as in using a banana as a telephone). . . .Why does pretending not undermine their representational system and bring it crashing down? (Leslie, 1987, p. 412)

Leslie's argument is that a major step in development involves the "decoupling" of the direct representations that we sustain of objects, persons, or situations from their perceptual images into a new set of metarepresentations that are symbolic or mental representations of the same original set of objects but now treated as part of an entire system of thought that one can modify, manipulate, analogize, or transform to metaphor. With the help to some extent of adults but also on the basis of an inherent capacity in the child, the ability emerges to create a frame in which otherwise very stable objects can be transformed into representations that bear only a tenuous link with their original shapes. When we walk into a room and perhaps unexpectedly see an elongated object on the floor, we may jump because we think it is a snake until we recognize with relief that it is a telephone extension cord. This is an "error" because we had no reason initially to treat the objects of the room as other than percepts. When on another occasion we say to a child playing "Explorer" with us in the same room, "Look! There's a dangerous snake!" the telephone cord is already being treated in this metarepresentational mode, as cued by our remark. Its only casual resemblance to a snake suffices to permit an abuse of what ordinarily might be a fixed representational and semantic structure.

Leslie's conception of the theory of mind implies that human beings have available a domain of metarepresentations that they can manipulate to make inferences about causes and predictions about future events, recognize the consequences of ignorance, distinguish reality from fantasy, acquire a language of words and phrases depicting mental experiences or states, and infer motivations. Such a development begins perhaps in the middle of the 2nd year but does not really reach its peak until the 3rd and 4th years, although some children may use words liked *know, remember, pretend*, and *dream* by the end of the 2nd year. As Leslie puts it,

> Pretend play is thus one of the earliest manifestations of the ability to characterize and manipulate one's own and others' cognitive relations to information (Leslie, 1987, p. 422).

Pretend play and the beginnings of the use of this metarepresentational system can be identified by the end of the 2nd year. Greta Fein (1981) in her research has shown that mothers who interact with their daughters foster the likelihood of an earlier emergence of transformation, such as the child's pretending to drink from an empty cup or at the next stage pretending to feed milk from the empty cup to a toy plastic horse, which is itself treated not as a horse but as a baby. Even with an early manifestation of pretending, such as in the case of a 2-year-old with only a limited vocabulary of perhaps a half-dozen words pretending to read a book by babbling along and pointing at pictures, turning pages, and only occasionally saying a clear word, the more advanced forms of make-believe require a higher level of cognitive development (D. Singer and J. Singer, 1990). The emergence of an ability to move beyond what Piaget called egocentricity to the ability to decenter experience and identify that others may think differently from oneself is necessary for more complex symbolic play.

This is exemplified best in the so-called false belief experiment. A child (the target participant in the study) watches as another person hides a piece of candy in a box (A) and then leaves the room. Someone else then moves the candy from box A to another box (B). The child is then asked where the candy is now and correctly points to box B. The original person who had hidden the candy now returns to the room. At this point the child is asked where this person will look for the candy. Research evidence clearly indicates that only by age 4 do children regularly begin predicting that the deceived original hider of the candy will look in A rather than in B (Wimmer and Perner, 1983).

Leslie and others have actually demonstrated that this fundamental ability to penetrate the ''mind'' of another is demonstrable in older children who are quite severely retarded but rarely is manifest in autistic children who may actually show higher IQs than the retarded participants. The autistic children, as Leslie argues, seem to have a special deficit in such perspective taking and perhaps more generally in their ability to develop the metarepresentational world decoupled from primary representations. Indeed, one of the special difficulties observed in our own and in other studies has been that autistic children show very little capacity for spontaneous or encouraged make-believe play (Leslie, 1987; Nahme-Huang et al., 1977). Recent observations in babies and toddlers born of crack cocaine-addicted mothers seem also to indicate findings comparable to those for autistic children. These children, despite apparently average general intelligence, seem deficient in play skills (Blakeslee, 1989).

It may well be the case that preschool children practicing imaginative play may also be more likely to move naturally into adopting a metarepresentational orientation. They may show an ability to demonstrate a ''theory of mind,'' that is, an ability to be aware of their own thoughts as distinct from others (Harris and Kavanaugh, 1993; Wellman, 1990; Wimmer and Perner, 1983). In a series of as yet unpublished studies under my direction, it has been possible to demonstrate that preschool children who play more imaginatively (on observation by raters on several occasions) may actually perform better on the reality-fantasy and false-belief measures used as estimates of theory of mind. As a matter of fact, even when age and other factors are partialled out in multiple regression analyses, the scores on make-believe play still predict ''reality-fantasy distinction'' results.

What I am proposing, then, is that imaginative play in childhood emerges almost necessarily as the child's cognitive capacities unfold through heightened brain capacity and inevitable social experiences. At the same time this metarepresentational mode makes it possible for increasing complexity of play to occur, and such play provides pleasure for the children by allowing them to miniaturize complex events and objects as well as to gain power over the objects and people around them through manipulating them in original story lines.

This practice of narrative and make-believe play further crystallizes and defines the metarepresentational ability of the child. The child reduces extreme incongruity or the initial shock of unexpectedness to more controllable dimensions. These miniaturized forms still may have many elements of sufficient novelty to excite and interest the child until gradually by play and replay they become assimilated into previous schemas or integrated into new organized schemas about a variety of social situations. The schemas formed may be ''erroneous'' if examined by an adult; depending on what further opportunities the child has to reshape the schemas and scripts formed in this fashion and to what extent experiences of humiliation around play or fear and terror in connection with some social setting preclude their exposure, they may persist as ''neurotic beliefs.'' What Sullivan (1953) might call parataxic distortions or the transference phenomena that are manifest in the psychoanalytic situation may have been formed in the schemas of children that have not been played out openly enough to be corrected by other children or adults (Singer, 1985).

The compensatory or psychologically adaptive role of imaginative play and the adoption of a metarepresentational schema system is exemplified by an example provided by Piaget (1962). His daughter, just a little less than 4 years old, was told that she could not go into the kitchen because pails of hot water were being prepared for her bath. The little girl then said, ''I'll go into the pretend kitchen then. I once saw a little boy who went into the kitchen, and when Odette went past with the hot water, he got out of the way.''

There is good evidence that play between parents and children is a universal experience that has a mutually reinforcing impact (D. Singer and J. Singer, 1990). In a study by Van Hoorn (1987), observations of a diverse mixture of Chinese, Filipino, Mexican, and North American mothers of European descent were made during play interactions with their infants. Despite some cultural variations in games played, there was considerable evidence of mutual enjoyment. Games were characterized by the range of interactive behaviors that promoted cooperation and successive attainments. The positive emotions of joy and surprise and laughter were consistently in evidence.

Imaginative Play in the 3- to 5-year-old: Research Approaches

In studies conducted from our research center at Yale, we followed children from eight nursery schools or day care centers over a year's time. Observations were made by pairs of independently recording raters who watched a given child for a period of time on 2 successive weeks and then returned a few months later to repeat this pattern. Altogether there were eight observations spread across the year's time. In this sample of 141 3- and 4-year-olds the children were rated for variables such as specific positive emotions (e.g., liveliness, excitement, elation and joy, or sadness, anger) as well as behaviors such as imaginativeness, cooperation with peers, and overt aggression. The data clearly indicated that positive emotions such as joy and liveliness were consistently positively correlated with imaginative play. The children who showed various make-believe transformations during play emerged across the year's time as those who engaged in a good deal of smiling and laughter and who were motorically active. Imaginativeness was negatively correlated with evidence of fearfulness, sadness, or fatigue. These relationships could not be attributed solely to language usage, for when there was statistical control for numbers of words employed, the relationship between imaginative play and positive affect still remained statistically reliable (D. Singer and J. Singer, 1980; J Singer and D. Singer, 1981).

As Greta Fein (1981) has stated, ''pretense provides an unusual opportunity for children to control their own emotional arousal and to maintain a level that is both comfortable and stimulating.'' In our own research as well as in reports by Fein and others, it is rare that we have observed pretend play among children who are very angry, anxious, in conflict, or who are hyperactive. We did see children who used their toys as mock weapons or who played fantasy games that involved simulated aggressive acts, but the children were generally in control and used metacommunicative statements such as ''This is my bad guy. . . .Make believe he is chasing your good guy.'' Other studies supporting this generally positive nature of imaginative play as occurring in spontaneous settings confirm this general finding (Stoneman et al., 1984).

In two separate studies, one carried out with a more clearly middle-class sample and one with children from a blue-collar background, we observed 3- and 4-year-olds over a year's time. Samples of play behavior were obtained. From the larger sample of children, 40 children who scored well above or well below the group mean over the year on both imaginativeness of play and frequency of television viewing were identified. Four groups were delineated: high imaginative/high television viewers; high imaginative/low television viewers; low imaginative/high television viewers; low imaginative/low television viewers. Each group was composed of 6 boys and 4 girls. Observers who recorded all of the children's actions for a 10-minute period and who were ''blind'' to the television-viewing patterns of the children recorded in detail both the verbalizations of the children and their actions during play. The data were then scored for categories such as where the play took place, the social structure of the play, the major themes (e.g., adventure, families, school, doctor), the roles assumed (e.g., mother, father, baby, superhero, victim), the type of play (e.g., sensorimotor, mastery, rules, pretending, or symbolic play), evidence of psychodynamic themes (e.g., orality, anality, cleanliness, separation, rejection, sibling rivalry), and finally the references made to television in play. A play protocol analysis chart was developed, listing all of the kinds of play and the scoring procedure. Our data yielded seven statistical factors of play. These included (a) adventurous fantasy play, (b) domestic fantasy play, (c) gross physical activity (running, jumping) versus artistic play, (d) a more general emphasis on make-believe pervading all forms of play, (e) involvement with ritual games or dancing and singing, (f) play with pet animals, and (g) games with rules.

Those children who were highly and consistently imaginative also engaged in more social play; they also participated more in ritual games and singing and were less likely to play alone. The imaginative children tended to be those who initiated games and were rarely solitary, withdrawn, or defensive. They could occasionally play alone, but they did not carve out a limited territory in their course of activities, nor did they play in more bounded space. Over the year we observed that the children tended to decrease their larger motor activity and to increase their art, ritual, or singing and dancing play and in general showed increased social interaction. There was, interestingly, an increasing role of themes of danger, disaster, and physical mutilation. It may well be that these developing preschoolers had become increasingly aware of the real-life dangers and could now express these fears more verbally and work them into their play. It is, of course, also possible that the children chose such plot lines because these themes seemed to be interesting in themselves and more varied than the standard "putting the baby to sleep" and "going to the doctor" games, which they had by now assimilated into organized schemas (D. Singer and J. Singer, 1980, 1990; J. Singer and D. Singer, 1981).

The role of television viewing in play was evident in some of the content of themes. The children who were heavy television viewers and showed in general low fantasy play tendencies were more likely simply to mention television superheroes or heroines and then, in imitation, bound around the room in a rather destructive fashion, knocking over others' toys or occasionally hitting other children. While television may well provide a rich source of thematic content for imaginative play, it is evident from our own and others' research that heavy-viewing children are often less spontaneously imaginative in their play. Symbolic play practice may be displaced by the ease of flicking on a television set to provide entertainment. Moreover, the heavy doses of violent content and the rapid pacing and much-interrupted format of commercial television may generate influences on the heavier viewer that work against imaginative and reflective thought. In one of the few longitudinal studies of imagination in children, we found that early heavy television viewing predicted less imagination in children several years later, even when family life factors were also accounted for (Singer et al., 1984; D. Singer and J. Singer, 1990).

Transitional Objects and Imaginary Playmates

A special form of imaginative play essentially reflecting the same tendency toward the development of a metarepresentational symbol system can be found in the development of an imaginary playmate. Winnicott (1953) identified an early stage in such a development. From about 1 year of age many children show a tendency to carry a soft cloth about with them and often to take it to bed. Often the soft cloth may be a blanket from the crib; it may also be a spare diaper or some other item among the child's assortment of play materials to which the child has become especially attached. In its earliest forms children, especially when sleepy or hungry, may be seen sucking their thumbs and fingering a soft cloth. In later stages of early childhood the soft cloth may simply become a kind of fetish that is sustained even as it becomes more and more ragged; eventually it may simply end up as a bit of cloth, to be tucked under one's pillow or into a purse.

Winnicott's perception was that these cloths serve the purpose of providing a concrete reminder in the absence of the mother's warmth and physical presence. Such a tendency can also be carried over to soft toys such as teddy bears. The term *transitional object* implies that the child is gradually giving up the physical clinging to the parent but sustaining some concrete and palpable feature of that experience.

The function of this soft toy is not only one of reminiscence but also one of possession. That is, while the child cannot possess indefinitely the warmth and closeness of the parent, it can possess the soft cloth or soft toy. Indeed, one can even argue that the emerging sense of individuality and personal entitlement that characterizes all of us even to the point of, as adults, insisting upon our rights for pensions and medical care or "respect" are traceable to these humble beginnings. The child clings to its teddy bear, fights to retain possession, and begins to delineate a sense of self through being able to assert "This is mine."

Tolpin (1971) in an extensive analysis of the phenomenon of the transitional object has gone beyond Winnicott in demonstrating that the transition also involves the child's awareness that thought and fantasy can substitute for the palpable presence of the object. When such blankets or cloths are destroyed, accidentally thrown out by parents, or simply pulled to pieces, children gradually learn they can sustain the experience through their increasing capacity for imagery. Indeed, Metcalf and Spitz (1978) proposed that such transitional objects are sustained during the period when the child's cognitive capacities primarily involve recognition memory and can be gradually given up as the child develops increasing skill of voluntary recall or mental retrieval of desired objects. The extensive research of Litt (1986) has indicated that after 18 months and between the ages of 2 and 5 almost three quarters of American children sampled showed evidence of play with a transitional object. While data from other countries reveal somewhat lower levels of such play, cultural differences may in part reflect differences in forms of inquiry, availability of soft toys, and so forth. Of special relevance is the fact that the child introduces elements of make-believe with the soft toy and begins to treat this teddy as a companion who can be talked to, admonished, and who can also serve as a potential helper.

Litt's research also indicated that transitional objects serve a functional role and are not in themselves indications of emotional distress, poor attachment, or neurotic tendencies. On the contrary, the evidence seems clear from her data that children who have transitional objects report fewer sleep disturbances and are more attractable, self-confident, independent, and affectionate. Such children did not show any evidence of disturbance on personality test measures and, if anything, tended to be less impulsive, aggressive, or antisocial than children who had not played with transitional objects.

Studies with children who report invisible imaginary friends indicate that the phenomenon is relatively common (Manosevitz et al., 1973; Masih, 1978; Somers and Yawkey, 1984). Generally the data indicate that at least a third of various child samples report the phenomenon. In one study comparing blind and sighted children, all of the blind children recorded a sighted imaginary friend (Singer and Streiner, 1966).

In some of the research carried out by the author and his colleagues, with 111 3- to 5-year-old children, the parents of 55% reported that the children had shown indications to some degree of an imaginary playmate—an invisible child or animal for whom a place had to be set at the table on occasion. Actually, in this study as many as 65% of the children reported such an experience. The children were rated for the degree of frequency of imaginary playmates and the extent of such reported play. The score generated by these data proved to be predictive of the children's spontaneous play over a year's time in day care centers and nurseries. Children who had more imaginary playmate experience were rated by "blind" observers as more imaginative in free play, showing especially more positive emotionality, more cooperation with adults, and a more extended language usage. When the imaginary playmate variable was entered as a predictor in multiple regression analyses to predict overt behavior, it proved an especially powerful variable in predicting not only imaginative play or positive affect but also greater persistence in play, less aggression, and less anxiety and fearfulness. There was also considerable evidence that boys who had no imaginary playmates showed more television watching and less vivid language.

In effect, then, the imaginary playmate phenomenon may be understood as a form of imaginative play that emerges as the child gradually acquires the capacity for heightened mental imagery. It has the adaptive function of allowing the child a means of resolving the tension described early in this chapter between the need for affiliation and for a sense of privacy and individuality. The phenomenon is somewhat greater among children without siblings and, as such, reflects, as in the study of the blind children mentioned above, a means of peopling one's world, maintaining some sense of control, and at the same time sustaining the experience of personal possession and privacy, since most children are well aware of the inherent unreality of an invisible imaginary friend.

THE ADAPTIVE ROLE OF IMAGINATIVE PLAY

Specific Functional Correlates of Imaginative Play

GENERAL POSITIVE EMOTIONALITY

A number of studies, some already cited, consistently point to the fact that the use of make-believe in the nursery school or in a variety of other settings or in the form of imaginary playmates is associated with more positive affective states in children. This consistent finding, as well as the tendency for there to be an inverse relationship between imaginative play skills on the part of the child and overt manifestations of anger and aggression, suggests the value of the use of play in a variety of therapeutic efforts with disturbed children. Thus, play therapists confronted with children who show limitations in their ability to engage in make-believe may have to find ways of subtly incorporating these skills in the child, perhaps by example or by gradual training exercises. Without some experience of enjoyment in the psychotherapy sessions, children are unlikely to want to sustain a treatment relationship (D. Singer and J. Singer, 1990).

ENHANCED LANGUAGE SKILL

As already indicated, our own research as well as other findings in the literature make it clear that one feature of imaginary play is that the children are verbalizing aloud increasingly complex situations. While some of their statements may reflect misunderstandings of adult remarks (as in the case of a boy lining up his toy soldiers to rescue Daddy, who was "all tied up at work"), such verbalization provides feedback to the child and may also evoke correcting responses from overhearing adults or peers. In addition, the inherent nature of make-believe play involves the development of plot sequences. This requires increased use of adjectives, future verbs and extended utterance lengths (D. Singer and J. Singer, 1990; J. Singer and D. Singer, 1981).

PERSISTENCE

Imaginative play, because it requires, in effect, a story line, tends to provide the child with focus and direction and then sustains concentration for longer periods. Children who have shown no tendency for imaginative play often are captives of the momentary changes of objects or toys in their environment. They seize at new things and often are embroiled in struggles for possession with other children or flit from group to group. The child engaged in symbolic play has, by virtue of entering into this domain, developed a sense of sequence, is moving in a privately defined direction, and needs less sustenance from concrete external objects.

DISTINGUISHING REALITY FROM FANTASY

There is at least some research evidence to suggest that children who have experience in make-believe games are better able to discriminate real from unreal situations and have learned to identify within their own thoughts that metarepresentational realm described by Leslie (1987). For example, in one study with somewhat older children those who had scored higher on indications of imaginativeness were better able to recall details of a story and then could discriminate real instances from those that were pure fantasy (Tucker, 1975). It may well be that, even in those rare instances of multiple personality, the affected adults may have grown up without a clear sense of the extent to which fantasized alternative selves are natural occurrences as part of a general dimension of make-believe or metarepresentation. Since there is some evidence of early child abuse as a forerunner for such multiple personality developments as well as for certain extremely hypnotizable or fantasy-prone individuals, it could well be that the same brutalizing family atmosphere that necessitated the child's escape to an alternative self also precluded a natural unfolding of make-believe play (Lynn and Rhue, 1988). The abused child has had less opportunity to engage in many different sequences of fantasy play and thus fails to perceive the escapist alternative self as a natural part of a range of make-believe activities. Instead, dissociations may occur that are outside the control of the child.

EMPATHY

One of the consequences of solitary and group make-believe play is that the child often learns to take on different roles. One can be the doctor examining the real or imaginary doll, and then one can reverse roles and pretend that the doll or another child is the doctor. Often in the make-believe play of two or three children, one observes brief struggles over who will be the "good guy" or the "bad guy," the hero or the victim. In such instances these disputes are often resolved by reversing roles either later in the game or on other days. Gradually the child engaged in such play learns what it is to be a victim, to experience others' dilemmas or pain. While we do not have extensive data on this issue, careful clinical studies have supported this finding (Gould, 1972).

COOPERATION

Observational studies of children at play such as those cited above consistently demonstrate that children prone to symbolic play are more likely to prove cooperative both with adults and with peers. Indeed, the very necessity of negotiating roles and plots with other children in order to sustain make-believe provides useful practice in this important social skill. One can observe children who show very little spontaneous imaginative play or who have been heavy television viewers and have not been practicing any make-believe at home dashing madly about the room, disrupting others' play, and in general bringing down upon themselves the wrath of the adults and children (J. Singer and D. Singer, 1981).

LEADERSHIP

While studies have generally not focused on early leadership tendencies at the preschool and early school ages, there are some data to suggest that children who are active in make-believe often are the first to initiate new games. The very practice of creating a series of plots may foster the ability to introduce a new group of children into some game. The experienced make-believe player thus gets "first crack" at assigning roles and plot lines. As imaginative play becomes more internalized and children move into reading and storytelling, there are clinical indications that children who have such storytelling capacities may win the respect of others in a play group (D. Singer and J. Singer, 1980, 1990).

TOLERATION OF DELAY

Of extreme importance for the developing child is the ability to defer immediate gratification in the interest of a longer-term goal or simply to tolerate naturally occurring delays. Make-believe play, whether it is sustained by the use of just few primitive toys or as it gradually becomes internalized in the form of imagery, has been shown in quite a number of studies to be associated with the ability to deal with delay (J. Singer and D. Singer, 1976). For example, in a study with somewhat older children, those who had shown patterns of imaginary play and other signs of imaginativeness were able to sit still longer when asked to do so or could tolerate waiting in an interview situation until the reviewer was ready to speak with them (D. Singer and J. Singer, 1990; J. Singer, 1961). The importance of this capacity cannot be minimized. Indeed, one might argue that the entire conception of the ego in psychoanalysis is built around the notion of deferred gratification and the capacity for delay and self-control in response. Imaginative play may be an important contributor to the development of the experience of self-regulation in this sense (Singer, 1955).

NEW IMAGERY COMBINATIONS

One of the important features of imaginary play is that it provides a child with a general opportunity to practice imagery, that is, to try out mental representations of concrete objects or of transforming such concrete objects. I have already suggested this in connection with Leslie's (1987) more general notion of the metarepresentational system and of the decoupling. But skill in producing images is something that develops in its own right and can be advanced by the ongoing imagined play sequence (Lewis, 1973; Singer, 1973; Tower, 1983).

TAKING TURNS

The careful observations of Catherine Garvey (1974) demonstrate that one of the important features of pretend play in children is the manner in which it is associated with turn taking and a form of social interaction that has long-term socialization potential. Observations of children in various kinds of make-believe indicate that exigencies of the plot in any initially agreed upon make-believe activity impose forms of self-control on the child. As in the case of cooperation more generally, turn taking provides a valuable delineation of orderliness and sequence that has special meaning for the child.

TRYING OUT DIFFERENT ROLES

A special feature of make-believe that goes beyond empathy is the opportunity for children to try different roles and to gradually identify the special qualities of the different kinds of individuals in their environment. When children play ''Bus Trip,'' one of the children becomes a driver, others become passengers, and others become traffic police. Each game reduces to miniature size a variety of adults in the child's real world who are often not well understood. In their efforts to formulate a plot, children again and again try out these roles and can gradually assimilate them into structured schemas that will serve them better as they move on in life and encounter such individuals. The notion of role taking is also a critical one for the development of an awareness of gender and sex role differences. There are indications from research that children who are more experienced in make-believe may also be able to develop a more androgynous orientation and are freer of very traditional and often limiting sex role attitudes or expectations for the future (Repetti, 1984). In the psychotherapeutic situation, one important function of play therapy may be to have the child begin to try out new kinds of roles and interactions, beginning with the therapist but extending to imagined persons with whom the child may come into contact later on (D. Singer and J. Singer, 1990).

ORDERING AND SEQUENCE

I have already emphasized the important role that the inherent plot line of a make-believe game plays in encouraging persistence over time by the children and also in encouraging cooperation or turn taking. The very nature of make-believe play calls for a certain logic, a sense of beginning, middle, and end that gradually becomes the basis for the formation of differentiated scripts that are important forms of action schemas in the child's memory system. Extensive research in cognitive science has pointed to the importance of the ability to sustain a variety of systematic scripts about hundreds of social situations that individuals encounter, from birthday parties to restaurants to attendance at sporting events and, ultimately, to marriage or specific vocational activities. The make-believe play sequence for children provides them with opportuni-

ties to learn the necessity for sustaining and organizing miniature scripts and allows them to be free of purely impulsive associative responding to some degree (Bretherton, 1984; Nelson and Seidman, 1984).

ANTICIPATING CONSEQUENCES

A further extension of the nature of plotting and the emergence of narrative sequences as part of thought fostered by pretend play is the awareness that actions have specific consequences. Thus the beginnings of social cause-and-effect thinking in the child are developed in the course of imaginative play (Bretherton, 1984).

Factors Conducive to Imaginative Play

If pretending and make-believe are so useful in the development of the child, what features of babies' or toddlers' milieux generate, sustain, and enhance the predisposition to such play? Space does not permit an extensive review of this topic, but there are clear indications from research that particular parental or caregiver activities are critical. An early optimal attachment to at least one parent or consistent adult caregiver predicts later emergence of imaginative play. Parental willingness to initiate games of fantasy or to suggest plots or the use of toys and then to step back so that the children experience the games as *their own* is also an important correlate of children's pretending capacities. Parental storytelling or bedtime story reading are also regularly found to be associated with evidence of greater resort to imaginative play in children. A family atmosphere of tolerance for floor play, a physical setting that allows children to find at least some private areas for uninterrupted pretend games, and adult attitudes of acceptance rather than of humiliation of the preschoolers' talking aloud or role playing all contribute. An overall sense of playfulness in the home setting opens the way for the imagination, humor, and even that sense of illusory control that are so crucial for normal coping capacities (D. Singer and J. Singer, 1990).

Imaginative Play, Psychopathology, and Psychotherapy

A fuller exploration of the implications of children's make-believe play for psychopathology and psychotherapy would take us far beyond the scope of this chapter. The general thrust of this presentation suggests that pretend play, the capacity to create miniature, possible worlds, is a critical feature of the healthy development of a child. The available evidence as reviewed by Dorothy Singer and myself elsewhere has suggested that emotional disturbance and cognitive and affective difficulties are often associated with an inability to sustain imaginative play in middle and early childhood (D. Singer and J. Singer, 1990; J. Singer, 1973; J. Singer and D. Singer, 1976). Some classic cases in which children's play revealed elaborate, unrealistic fantasies reflecting their troubled life experiences demonstrate that those children who could sustain such play had better prognoses once play therapy was initiated (D. Singer, 1993; J. Singer, 1973; J. Singer and D. Singer, 1976).

A critical role for the psychotherapist with children is to help them to find ways of miniaturizing their private fears, brutal experiences of abuse, or exposure to parental quarrels or neglect into manageable chunks. The therapist's encouragement of play by the provision of an appropriate setting of toys or (for middle childhood) of games conducive to symbolic representations of children's troubles casts the therapist in the role of the needed mediating parental figure. Delineating in play form key life issues, significant adults or siblings, and conflicts helps the child to develop new schemas and scripts and new knowledge structures that can later reduce the ambiguity, confusion, or affects of fear and terror that new situations may present.

I believe that a key feature of the play therapist's role is to provide a model for the child of a zestful, curious, lively approach to one's experience. While the therapist must often avoid moralizing about the child's hatreds or about presumed parental or sibling cruelties or neglects reflected in play, this does not preclude an emotional response. The therapist's own professional curiosity and willingness to share thoughts and play possibilities, conveyed in a spirit of liveliness and humor, can open the troubled child to the joys of the world of introspection and fantasy. By such an approach one can change the fearful, despairing, or angry child, trapped in a mental world of limited constructs, schemas, or scripts, into one who can savor the excitement of reshaping what had seemed like the given world of recent experiences into a domain of innumerable possibilities. By replaying and thus reshaping schemas, the child can gain at least some sense of control and power within a small region of a vast, seemingly impenetrable universe. The skilled play therapist, whether psychoanalytic or cognitive-behavioral in orientation, not only provides the child an opportunity to identify and work through specific problems but also enhances the child's development of the capacity for play, a powerful cognitive tool for further enhancement of a sense of self and individuation as well as a continuing private theater for developing new scripts of affiliation and attachment. The medium of make-believe in childhood, internalized by middle childhood into a richly elaborated fantasy capacity, becomes eventually a major functional system through which all of us can entertain opportunities and possibilities for warmth, closeness, and communion with others while still sustaining our sense of individuality and privacy.

References

Angyal A: *Neurosis and Treatment: A Holistic Theory.* New York, Wiley, 1965.

Bakan D: *The Duality of Human Existence.* Chicago, Rand McNally, 1966.

Blakeslee S: Crack's toll among babies: A joyless view even of toys. *New York Times,* September 12, 1989, pp. 1, 24.

Blatt SJ: Interpersonal relatedness and self-definition: Two personality configurations and their implications for psychopathology and psychotherapy. In: Singer JL (ed): *Repression and Dissociation.* Chicago, University of Chicago Press, 1990.

Bonanno G, Singer JL: Repressive personality style: Theoretical and methodological implications for health and pathology. In: Singer JL (ed): *Repression and Dissociation.* Chicago, University of Chicago Press, 1990.

Bretherton I: Representing the social world. In: Bretherton I (ed): *Symbolic Play: Reality and Fantasy.* New York, Academic Press, 1984, p. 3.

Bruner J: *Actual Minds, Possible Worlds.* Cambridge, MA, Harvard University Press, 1986.

Bruner J, Jolly A, Sylva K (eds): *Play.* New York, Basic Books, 1976.

Bühler K: *The Mental Development of the Child.* New York, Harcourt, 1930.

Caillois R: *Les Jeux et les Hommes.* Paris, Gallimard, 1958.

Csikszentmihalyi M: Does being human matter? On some interpretative problems of comparative ludology. *Behav Brain Sci* 5:160, 1982.

Ekman P: *Darwin and Facial Expression: A Century of Research in Review.* New York, Academic Press, 1973.

Ekman P, Friesen WV, Ellsworth PC: *Emotion in the Human Face: Guidelines for Research and an Integration of Findings* (rev ed). Cambridge, Cambridge University Press, 1982.

Erikson E: *Childhood and Society.* New York, Norton, 1963.

Fein G: Pretend play in childhood: An integrative review. *Child Dev* 52:1095, 1981.

Freud S: Creative writers and daydreaming. In: Strachey J (ed): *The Standard Edition of the Complete Psychological Works of Sigmund Freud* (Vol 9). London, Hogarth Press, 1958. (Originally published 1908.)

Freud S: Formulations on the two principles of mental functioning. In: Strachey J (ed): *The Standard Edition of the Complete Psychological Works of Sigmund Freud* (Vol 12). London, Hogarth Press, 1958. (Originally published 1911.)

Freud S: Beyond the pleasure principle. In: Strachey I (ed): *The Complete Psychological Works of Sigmund Freud* (Vol 18). London, Hogarth Press, 1962. (Originally published 1920.)

Garvey C: *Play.* Cambridge, MA, Harvard University Press, 1974.

Geertz C: Deep play: A description of the Balinese cockfight. In: Bruner J, Jolly A, Sylva K (eds): *Play.* New York, Basic Books, 1976.

Goldstein K: *Human Nature in the Light of Psychopathology.* Cambridge, MA, Harvard University Press, 1940.

Gould R: *Child Studies through Fantasy.* New York, Quadrangle Books, 1972, p. 34.

Groos K: *The Play of Man.* New York, Appleton, 1901.

Harris P, Kavanaugh RD: Young children's understanding of pretense. *Monograph of the Society for Child Development.* Chicago, Chicago University Press, 1993.

Huizinga J: *Homo Ludens.* Boston, Beacon Press, 1950.

Izard CE: *Human Emotions.* New York, Plenum, 1977.

Jung CG: *Psychological Types.* New York, Pantheon, 1971.

Klinger E: *Structure and Functions of Fantasy.* New York, Wiley, 1971.

Kreitler H, Kreitler S: *Cognitive Orientation and Behavior.* New York, Springer, 1976.

Leslie AM: Pretense and representation: The origins of ''theory of mind.'' *Psychol Rev* 94:412, 1987.

Lewis M: Play as whimsy. *Behav Brain Sci* 5:166, 1982.

Lewis PH: *The Relationship of Sociodramatic Play to Various Cognitive Abilities in Kindergarten.* Unpublished doctoral dissertation, Ohio State University, 1973.

Litt CJ: Theories of transitional object attachment: An overview. *International J Behav Dev* 9:383, 1986.

Lynn SJ, Rhue JW: Fantasy proneness: Hypnosis, developmental antecedents, and psychopathology. *Am Psychol* 43:35, 1988.

Mandler G: *Mind and Body.* New York, Norton, 1984.

Mandler JM: *Stories, Scripts and Scenes: Aspects of Schema Theory.* Hillsdale, NJ, Erlbaum, 1984.

Mandler JM: How to build a baby: On the development of an accessible representational system. *Cognit Dev* 3:113, 1988.

Manosevitz M, Prentice NM, Wilson F: Individual and family correlates of imaginary companions in preschool children. *Dev Psychol* 8:72, 1973.

Masih VK: Imaginary play companions of children. In: Weizman R, Brown R, Levinson P, et al (eds): *Piagetian Theory and the Helping Professions* (Vol 1). Los Angeles, University of Southern California, 1978.

Metcalf DR, Spitz R: The transitional object: Critical developmental period and organizer of the psyche. In: Grolnick SA, Barkin L, Muensterberger W (eds): *Between Reality and Fantasy.* New York, Aronson, 1978.

Nahme-Huang L, Singer DG, Singer JL, et al: Imaginative play training and perceptual-motor interventions with emotionally disturbed hospitalized children. *Am J Orthopsychiatry* 47:238, 1977.

Nelson K, Seidman S: Playing with scripts. In: Bretherton I (ed): *Symbolic Play.* Orlando, Academic Press, 1984.

Papousek M, Papousek H, Harris B: The emergence of play in parent-infant interactions. In: Gorlitz D, Wohlwill J (eds): *Curiosity, Imagination, and Play.* Hillsdale, NJ, Erlbaum, 1987.

Peller L: Libidinal phases, ego development and play. *Psychoanal Study Child* 9:178–198, 1959.

Piaget J: *Play, Dreams and Imitation in Childhood.* New York, Norton, 1962.

Piaget J: *Possibility and Necessity.* Minneapolis, University of Minnesota Press, 1980.

Rank O: *Will Therapy and Truth and Reality.* New York, Knopf, 1945.

Rapaport D: On the psychoanalytic theory of motivation. In: Jones MR (ed): *Nebraska Symposium on Motivation* (Vol 3). Lincoln, NE, University of Nebraska Press, 1960.

Repetti RL: Determinants of children's sex stereotyping: Parental sex-role traits and television viewing. *Pers Soc Psychol Bull* 10:457, 1984.

Schachtel EG: *Metamorphosis.* New York, Basic Books, 1959.

Shapiro T, Emde R: *Affect: Psychoanalytic Perspectives.* New York, International Universities Press, 1992.

Singer DG: *Playing for Their Lives: Helping Troubled Children Through Play Therapy.* New York, Free Press, 1993.

Singer DG, Singer JL: Television viewing and aggressive behavior in preschool children: A field study. *Forensic Psychol Psychiatry Ann NY Acad Sci* 347:292, 1980.

Singer DG, Singer JL: *The House of Make-believe: Children's Play and the Developing Imagination.* Cambridge, MA, Harvard University Press, 1990.

Singer JL: Delayed gratification and ego-development: Implications for clinical and experimental research. *J Consult Clin Psychol* 19:259, 1955.

Singer JL: Imagination and waiting ability in young children. *J Pers* 29:396, 1961.

Singer JL (ed): *The Child's World of Make-Believe.* New York, Academic Press, 1973.

Singer JL: *Imagery and Daydreaming Methods in Psychotherapy and Behavior Modification.* New York, Academic Press, 1974.

Singer JL: *The Human Personality.* New York, Harcourt Brace Jovanovich, 1984.

Singer JL: Transference and the human condition: A cognitive-affective perspective. *Psychoanal Psychol* 2:189, 1985.

Singer JL, Bonanno GA: Personality and private experience: Individual variations in consciousness and in attention to subjective phenomena. In: Pervin L (ed): *Handbook of Personality.* New York, Guilford Press, 1990.

Singer JL, Kolligian J Jr: Personality: Developments in the study of private experience. *Annu Rev Psychol* 38:533–574, 1987.

Singer JL, Salovey P: Organized knowledge structures in personality: Schemas, self-schemas, prototypes and scripts. In: Horowitz MJ (ed): *Person*

Schemas and Recurrent Maladaptive Patterns. Chicago, University of Chicago Press, 1991.

Singer JL, Singer DG: Imaginative play and pretending in early childhood: Some experimental approaches. In: Davids A (ed): *Child Personality and Psychopathology: Current Topics.* New York, Wiley, 1976, p. 69.

Singer JL, Singer DG: *Television, Imagination and Aggression: A Study of Preschoolers.* Hillsdale, NJ, Erlbaum, 1981.

Singer JL, Streiner B: Imaginative content in the dream and fantasy play of blind and sighted children. *Percept Mot Skills* 22:475, 1966.

Singer JL, Singer DG, Rapaczynski W: Children's imagination as predicted by family patterns and television viewing: A longitudinal study. *Genet Psychol Monogr* 110:43, 1984.

Smith PK: Does play matter? Functional and evolutionary aspects of animal and human play. *Behav Brain Sci* 5:139, 1982.

Somers JU, Yawkey TD: Imaginary play companions: Contributions of creative and intellectual abilities of young children. *J Creative Behav* 18:77, 1984.

Stoneman Z, Brady J, et al: Naturalistic observation of children's activities and roles while playing with their siblings and friends. *Child Dev* 55:617, 1984.

Sullivan HS: *The Interpersonal Theory of Psychiatry.* New York, Norton, 1953.

Sutton-Smith B: Piaget on play: A critique. *Psychol Rev* 73:104, 1966.

Sutton-Smith B: The epistemology of the play theorist. *Behav Brain Sci* 5:170, 1982.

Sutton-Smith B, Kelley-Byrne D: The idealization of play. In: Smith PK (ed): *Play in Animals and Humans.* London, Basil Blackwell, 1984, p. 305.

Taylor S: *Positive Delusions: Creative Self-Deceptions and the Healthy Mind.* New York, Basic Books, 1989.

Tolpin M: On the beginnings of a cohesive self. *Psychoanal Study Child* 26:316, 1971.

Tomkins SS: *Affect, Imagery and Consciousness* (Vol 1). New York, Springer, 1962.

Tomkins SS: *Affect, Imagery, and Consciousness* (Vol 2). New York, Springer, 1963.

Tomkins SS: The quest for primary motives: Biography and autobiography of an idea. *J Pers Soc Psychol* 41:306, 1981.

Tower RB: Imagery: Its role in development. In: Sheikh A (ed): *Imagery: Current Theory Research and Application.* New York, Wiley, 1983.

Tucker J: *The Role of Fantasy in Cognitive-Affective Functioning: Does Reality Make a Difference in Remembering?* Unpublished doctoral dissertation, Teachers College, Columbia University, 1975.

Vandenberg B: Play, myth and hope. In: Vanderkooij R, Hellendoorn J (eds): *Play, Play Therapy, Play Research.* Lisse, Swets & Zeitlinger, 1986.

Van Hoorn J: Games that babies and mothers play. In: Monighan-Novrot P, Scales B, Van Hoorn J, et al (eds): *Looking at Children's Play.* New York, Teachers College Press, 1987, p. 38.

Waelder R: The psychoanalytic theory of play. *Psychoanal Q* 2:208, 1932.

Wellman H: *The Child's Theory of Mind.* Cambridge, MA, MIT Press, 1990.

Wimmer H, Perner J: Beliefs about beliefs: Representation and constraining function of wrong beliefs in young children's understanding of deception. *Cognition* 13:103, 1983.

Winnicott D: Transitional objects and transitional phenomena. *Int J Psychoanal* 34:89, 1953.

17   MORAL DEVELOPMENT

Sula Wolff, F.R.C.P., F.R.C.Psych.

The childhood origins of moral behavior and moral judgment have until recently attracted far less research interest than the development of attachment and early affectional relationships (Bowlby, 1982). In 1984, Martin Hoffman could still write that guilt was a relatively neglected topic for research. Both systems of behavioral interactions, cognitions, and emotions share certain features. They represent universal phenomena, present in all human beings unless exceptional individual pathology or environmental privation or distortion intervene; they are biologically adaptive, promoting the survival of the person and the social group within a common human environment; their manifestations form a regular developmental sequence; and deviations in their developmental path can have serious consequences for the individual's later life.

The last 10 years have seen much progress in the exploration of the development of empathy, shame, and guilt, of prosocial behavior and moral judgment. The context within which young children become socialized and acquire moral standards and beliefs and the vicissitudes of this developmental process have become clearer; a start has been made in the elucidation of psychopathological factors; and the stage is set for a more rational treatment approach to early childhood manifestations of antisocial conduct.

This chapter focuses, in turn, on the classical contributions to our understanding of moral development that derive from psychoanalytic theories and from the cognitive-developmental studies of Jean Piaget and his followers, especially Kohlberg. It then deals with Hoffman's discoveries about empathy in childhood; Kagan's observations of the development of self-appraisal and inner standards in the 2nd year; Turiel's explorations of children's discrimination between morality and convention; and with work on the emotions related to morality. Finally, the more recent observational and experimental studies of the context within which children develop moral behavior and form their ideas about moral issues is described, as well as studies relating to social learning and to psychopathological developments.

PSYCHOANALYSIS AND THE MORAL SELF

Freud

Freud (1930/1961a, 1923/1961b) saw the origins of ethical tendencies in the emotional attachments of young children to their caregivers and considered the long period of helpless dependency of the human baby to be the biological basis for the development of conscience. Dependency on parents fosters fear that their love may be lost. Anything that threatens such loss is perceived as bad and to be avoided. Fear is the main emotion in this first stage of moral development, equivalent in adult life to social anxiety: the fear of being found out. Only in the next stage, when parental authority is internalized with the formation of a superego, do conscience and a sense of guilt arise, while at the same time the fear of being found out wanes. Freud commented on the lack of distinction between doing something bad and wishing to do it, that is, between the act and the impulse, during the formation of the superego. He thought this was because the superego, being a part of oneself, is as aware of bad thoughts as of bad deeds.

While in the first stage of moral development parental criticism instills fear that parents will withdraw their love, that the objects of attachment will be lost, in the next stage the objects of attachment become internalized images, and the child now judges itself critically. In order to recover from a sense of a flawed self, he or she develops a fantasy or ego-ideal and strives toward its attainment (Graham, 1972). Failure to meet the standards of this ideal self then results in a sense of guilt. The functions of the ideal self in the development of moral consciousness were first described by that extraordinary developmental psychologist, James Baldwin (1897). He saw the ideal self as submissive to the exhortations of adults, whom the child perceives as superior and to be both obeyed and imitated.

Freud's most original and most controversial contribution to ideas about moral development has been his theory of the Oedipus complex and its attendant anxieties, which he held to be a prerequisite for identification with parents and the formation of an ego-ideal. Children identify with both parents, but become erotically most attached to the parent of the opposite sex. The rivalries, jealousies, and ambivalences toward the same-sex parent then, in turn, engender fears of retribution: castration anxiety, with resulting defensive repression of erotic urges and strengthening of parent identifications, especially with the same-sex parent. Freud emphasized that the introjection of the father's authority in particular lays the foundation for the superego or conscience, the basis for guilt, when one falls short of the demands of one's ideal self (Graham, 1972). He thought that castration anxiety was more severe in boys than in girls. The threat for girls was less because the damage seemed already to have been done. Boys, in contrast, tend to develop a harsher conscience, and paradoxically, this puts them at greater risk of antisocial conduct. Like subsequent analytical writers (e.g., Klein, 1934/1948c), he held that an overharsh conscience, instead of protecting the individual from antisocial acts, at times fosters "criminality from a sense of guilt." He also developed the contrary notion that the more virtuous a person is, the more severe his or her superego—that saints reproach themselves the most for being sinners (Freud, 1930/1961a). An exceptionally punitive superego is thus to be found both among some criminals and in the excessively good.

Anna Freud

Anna Freud (1966) emphasized the importance of language for superego development and for ego control, and she stressed the role of empathy in the development of children's ideas, e.g., about the property rights of others. She too saw the superego as an incorporation of parental strictures—"identification with the aggressor"—but also held that the acceptance of one's own culpability played an essential part. Repression and sublimation, or the displacement of instinctual aims in conformity to social values, are part of this developmental process (Freud, 1961). While defensive processes of projection, introjection, and regression develop very early in life, as soon as the child can distinguish between himself or herself and the outside world, the ego defense mechanisms of repression, sublimation, and reaction formation, essential for subduing childish greed, demands, and the impulse to kill rivals and other frustrating persons, develop later.

Melanie Klein

Melanie Klein (1927/1948a), in contrast, thought the superego was at work much earlier, in the 2nd year of life, and she placed the occurrence of the Oedipus complex at the end of the 1st and the beginning of the 2nd year. Her timing of this last developmental process does not tally with what we now know about children's cognitive capacities, but her descriptions of the harshness of the infantile conscience, much harsher than the real parents had ever been, and the origins of this harshness in the child's own aggressive instincts projected onto the parents have been illuminating (Klein, 1933/1948b), as have her descriptions of how a sadistic superego arousing overwhelming anxiety can lead to compulsive seeking of punishment through criminal activity, with transient relief of guilt (Klein, 1934/1948c).

Erik Erikson

Like Freud (1961a), Erik Erikson, in his scheme of personality development in childhood (Erikson, 1968; see also Wolff, 1989), divides the growth of the moral self into two distinct phases: from about 18 months to 2½ years, the "anal" stage of primary socialization, and from about 2½ to 5 years, the "genital" stage of primary identifications.

During the "anal" stage, toilet training and the acquisition of bowel and bladder control are symbolic of the parents' first attempts to teach the child some of the basic rules of the society in which they live and, on the child's part, of the earliest efforts at self-discipline for the sake of approval. The toddler, now on his feet, his arms freed, is ready for action and, though he still has poor impulse control, he has a choice: whether to throw, to grab, to defecate, or whether, in response to parental

admonition, to desist. He needs the parents to be there in actuality to back his efforts toward success but also, firmly and without animosity, to step in when disaster threatens. For the first time the child now gets pleasure from cooperation with others and gains pride from achievements, but also, and again for the first time, a sense of shame is felt at failure. In contrast to the concerns of previous analytical writers with the young child's fantasies, Erikson gave due weight to actual life experiences in this stage as determinants of future self-esteem, in particular whether one will grow up with a sense of autonomy and self-confidence in relation to cooperative enterprises, or with a sense of shame and self-doubt.

Many parents, especially the socioeconomically deprived, themselves with limited occupational autonomy and without a firm sense of control over their destiny, find this stage of child rearing difficult. While offering good nurturing care to the baby, they have unrealistic expectations of their toddler's capacity for self-restraint. Instead of physically taking over control for their offspring, they exhort and admonish verbally and from a distance, allow accidents and disasters to occur, and then reprimand, threaten, and punish, sometimes aggressively. The anxiety engendered by such child rearing reinforces the toddler's fears of what could happen if he or she were to lose control and, in line with the idea of "criminality through guilt," induces him or her to act ever more outrageously. The actual consequences are never as bad as those feared; anxiety is temporarily assuaged, only to return as the cycle of interactions repeats itself.

The next Eriksonian stage of moral development, the "genital" stage, is the "play age" of childhood, when language transforms both children's social interactions and their inner life, and a sense of the future is born. It is the stage of curiosity and make-believe, of storytelling and identification with adult role models, especially parents. It is also the stage in which children engage in their first triadic and group relationships: with both parents, with mother and sibling, with an adult and other children in a play group. New emotional experiences now arise, which must be mastered, especially rivalry and jealousy. The child has more self-control and can compensate for present frustrations of wishes in play, in imagination, and especially, in hopes for the future.

Erikson considered the development of girls to be the more hazardous because, as they imagine themselves in the future as wife and mother and develop erotic longings for their father, their jealousy of their mother is the more frightening because she becomes a potentially hostile rival and is lost as a haven of security. Boys, in contrast, while now attached to their mother in a new way, still have her as a safe source of comfort. On the other hand, the role models parents provide for their children at this stage are more secure for girls than for boys. Far fewer mothers than fathers are lost from the family, and the status of mothers within the home is universally high, while that of fathers, especially in socioeconomically deprived sections of society, is often low.

As children identify with and incorporate their parents' standards of conduct, a powerful new source of anxiety—guilt or the pangs of conscience—arises together with a division between the self in action and the moral self (ego and superego). Erikson believed that actual life experiences at this stage determine whether the person will emerge with his or her initiative for affectionate intimate and sexual relationships strengthened or will instead become constrained and inhibited.

We shall see that children's cognitive development during these years fosters misinterpretations of their experiences and magnifies the possible anxieties that arise. The harshness of conscience and the strength of guilt in early childhood are more comprehensible when we appreciate the nature of children's logic at this time of life.

PSYCHOANALYTICAL THEORIES AND DEVELOPMENTAL RESEARCH ARE NO LONGER APART

Developmental psychologists now take note of children's cognitions and emotions, that is, of their inner worlds and, as the work on attachment has shown, are prepared to explore psychoanalytical concepts experimentally. Likewise, psychoanalysts are ready to amend their theories in the light of observations. Buchsbaum and Emde (1990) have recently questioned the notion that moral development depends on the resolution of the Oedipus conflict at the end of the genital stage and is therefore deferred until the 4th or 5th year of life. Using a play narrative technique, they found children as young as 36 months capable of articulating coherent stories about rules, reciprocity, empathy, and internalized prohibitions. Even at this early age, children could deal with alternative outcomes to resolve a moral dilemma. In this important paper the authors stress the dual origins of moral development: biological preparedness and early caregiving relationships.

THE CONTRIBUTION OF JEAN PIAGET

The objective study of moral development in childhood got its impetus from Piaget's systematic observations (Piaget, 1932; Piaget and Inhelder, 1969; for a summary, see also Wolff, 1989). Before summarizing his specific studies of moral judgment in childhood, it needs to be said that Piaget's general discoveries about children's immature logic and reasoning between the ages of about 2 and 7 years have shed much light on early childhood fears and on some of the psychoanalytical postulates about early emotional experiences. During the precausal, animistic stage, children cannot yet detach thoughts from the events and objects thought about. They do not yet identify themselves as thinkers about the world. They cannot, for example, explain how it comes about that they are both in their bed asleep at night and yet also in the dream they have while sleeping. Their explanations of events and circumstances tend to be psychological rather than rational, and the notion of chance events cannot yet be grasped. Moreover, while aware of their own viewpoint, they find it hard to conceive that this is not also uppermost in the minds of others. Piaget's ideas about the child's early egocentrism have been criticized by researchers who found children much more capable of logical inferences when problems are embedded in a child-centered context (Donaldson, 1978/1992). The fact remains, however, that children spend much of their lives in an adult world, and the distortions and misperceptions that Piaget's work so vividly revealed are common experiences for everyone in touch with young children.

Like psychoanalytical writers in relation to emotional and behavioral development, Piaget held to a stage theory of cognitive development. Each stage differs qualitatively from the next, and teaching of logical operations is ineffective until the child has reached the necessary level of understanding.

The Rules of Games

Piaget concerned himself with children's perceptions of the rules of games and with their views about morality. He did not, as did later workers (e.g., Turiel, 1983), focus particularly on the distinction between convention and morality, being concerned rather to identify in both spheres changing but parallel developmental sequences in how children perceive and respond to rules.

The game of marbles is played the world over. Piaget watched how children of different ages played this game and questioned them systematically about their understanding of the rules and how these had originated. He found that under about 7 years of age, in the precausal, animistic stage of development, children grasp rules imperfectly, make errors in their application, and are content to play alongside others. Yet they think of rules as obligatory, inviolate, sacrosanct, and inherent in the game. When asked who made them, they said the rules had always been there, and if pressed, they resorted to ''God.'' Older children, in contrast, played competently, knew what the rules were, but viewed them as conventions devised by ''children long ago.'' If everyone agrees, the rules can be changed and the game played differently. Piaget saw this shift at between 6 and 8 years of age as a move from an authoritarian to a democratic viewpoint, from a position of unilateral respect for sacred laws and duties to one of mutual respect and reciprocity.

Ethical Beliefs

This paralleled the shift Piaget observed also in his systematic questioning of children about their ethical beliefs, from an authoritarian morality in which obedience is equated with goodness and all adults are seen to be right, to a view of morality where concepts of justice and a more detached evaluation both of adults and of ethical standards are paramount. Piaget explored children's ideas about culpability at different ages by giving them pairs of stories to evaluate, for example, one in which a child's clumsiness led to a big accidental breakage paired with one where a lesser mishap followed the pursuit of a forbidden goal (taking jam off a high shelf); stealing to help a poor and hungry child contrasted with stealing for oneself alone; inaccurate reporting of a frightening event paired with telling a deliberate but lesser untruth. Again he found a shift of moral attitude. Although there was much overlap, younger children tended to judge actions according to their material consequences, older children, according to their underlying intentions. Children's views of naughtiness and punishment also underwent a change with age. Younger children operated with the notion of *immanent justice*—that the crime begets the punishment and that, if you are punished, you must have done something bad to deserve it. They also held to notions of *retributive justice* (the *jus talionis*)—that the punishment must fit the crime irrespective of circumstances and motivation. *Moral realism* is the term Piaget applied to these immature ideas of morality, and he linked this to adult constraints on young children and to the children's sense of unilateral respect or duty. In contrast, older children operated with a different morality based on autonomous judgments, on reciprocity and cooperation, on the internalization of rules, and on ideas of justice and mutual service.

Piaget saw in the children he studied the development of a morality of good, deriving from affection, and a morality of rights and duties (ideas later taken up by Turiel (1983) in his distinction between morality and convention), and he thought that some people operated only with the latter.

Although his critics have accused him of ignoring the influence of the child's social environment in fostering developmental changes (Haste, 1987), Piaget in fact made very clear his belief that social interactions with other children in middle childhood were essential for the transformation of an authoritarian to a democratic view of morality, from a position in which obedience to adults and avoidance of punishments are primary to one in which conformity to social rules and, later still, participation in rule making for the sake of universal, ethical principles predominate.

The biological advantage of the young child's gullibility has been discussed by Butterworth (1987). He suggests that cognitive/social immaturity is itself biologically adaptive, that in the process of socialization, unquestioning acceptance of adult rules has to come before the doubting and self-judging phase, and that for the culture to be maintained, it must make indelible impressions on the very young. This view parallels the notion that small stature and physical immaturity too contribute to the acculturation of the young of many species, ensuring that they are relatively docile and sexually noncompetitive during their early years of socialization (Tanner, 1984).

An Important Proviso

We must be clear that Piaget, and even more so Kohlberg as we shall see, was concerned with moral reasoning, that is, with what children and older people *say* about their ideas and beliefs about moral dilemmas, often concerning not themselves but other people. This requires greater cognitive, linguistic, and social skills and is quite different from the way in which young children grapple with moral issues in their everyday lives and in play, when they themselves are the central characters. As Margaret Donaldson (1978/1992) made clear (see also Buchsbaum and Emde, 1992), when moral dilemmas are embedded in real-life or in age-appropriate, child-centered play settings and are tied to the here-and-now or to concrete events in the past or the future, moral sophistication is apparent at a much younger age.

KOHLBERG'S STUDIES

Lawrence Kohlberg and his colleagues (Colby and Kohlberg, 1987; Colby et al., 1983, 1987) made two major research contributions in this field. Some 25 years ago they embarked on a long-term longitudinal study of the development of moral judgment and, in the course of this, devised two sets of interviews, tested for reliability and consisting of standard questions about stories involving people faced with conflicts about moral issues. A detailed scoring manual exists (Colby et al., 1987) in which the liveliness of the stories and their sensible scoring are evident. The stories include one about Heinz, whose dying wife needs a drug for which the druggist is proposing an exorbitant charge that Heinz cannot afford. Would it be right for him to steal the drug, and if so, why? Others concern a boy who has saved his pocket money for camp when his father demands the money instead; a doctor faced with a mercy killing; and a mother who had promised to let her daughter go to a rock concert and then changed her mind. Piaget's work and theories were the starting point for these studies, but unlike Piaget himself, this group of workers did not study very young children.

Eighty-four boys aged 10, 13, and 16 years at the outset, equally distributed by social class, IQ, and sociometric status, were individually interviewed, 58 at least twice (most of these four times), out of six planned occasions over the course of 20 years. The sophisticated interviews and their scoring are complex, but the standard stories tap nine hypothetical but true-to-life moral dilemmas about which a series of questions are asked relating to the values and reasons underlying the subjects' judgments.

Kohlberg described six stages of moral judgment. Longitudinal stage reversals occurred less often than test-retest unreliability; that is, the sequence was always forward. No subject reached a stage without passing through the previous one; that is, the sequence was invariable. Most youngsters scored within a single or two adjacent stages at any one time, only a few in three stages, so that there was internal consistency in moral judgments. No differences were found between the three age cohorts. Relative developmental delays were modestly associated with low socioeconomic status at 10 years and with intelligence and, especially, educational level at 24 and 23 years, when both tended to have reached their ceiling. Upper levels of moral development were generally reached in the mid-20s or 30s, but in a sizeable proportion of individuals not even then.

In very abbreviated summary form, Kohlberg's six stages, grouped into three levels, are as follows (Colby et al., 1983; Graham, 1972):

Level I—Premoral: The child is responsive to cultural rules but sees these in terms of pleasant or unpleasant consequences of behavior and relates them to the power of authority figures. He follows the rules for the sake of self-interest.
Stage 1: The child is oriented to obedience and punishment, with egocentric deference to authority figures and avoidance of unpleasantness for himself or herself.
Stage 2: There is a naively egoistic orientation, with concern for one's own needs but with some awareness of the needs of others, a wish for egalitarianism, and an orientation toward exchange and reciprocity.
Level II—Conventional Role Conformity: The child is now oriented toward maintaining the expectations of others close to him or her, as a value in its own right.
Stage 3: The orientation is to be a good person in the eyes of others and in one's own eyes, with a wish to please and help. Intentions of behavior are taken note of and the moral perspective includes interactions with others.
Stage 4: The orientation is toward the social order and its maintenance for its own sake and to fulfilling agreed duties in conformity to authority.
Level III—Self-Accepted Moral Principles: The individual is now concerned with defining moral values and principles apart from the supporting authority.

Stage 5: The orientation is contractual and legalistic, with a sense of obligation to the law, but also an acceptance that people can have a variety of different values and that their individual rights take precedence over the social contract.
Stage 6: The orientation has become a sociomoral one, with the recognition of valid universal ethical principles to which the person can choose to commit himself or herself.

The interview methods devised by Kohlberg's group for young people in the United States have been applied also in researches in other parts of the world with similar results. A study in which attempts were made to induce stage skipping in 11- to 13-year-olds by having them listen to adults reasoning at different levels about the solutions to moral dilemma stories of the Kohlberg type found all changes to be to the next higher stage to the subject's own (Walker, 1982).

Kohlberg's major study involved only boys. His colleague, Carol Gilligan (1982), developed the idea of fundamental sex differences in orientation toward moral issues, with men giving priority to justice and rights, women to care and responsibility in human relationships. She also held that hypothetical and real-life moral dilemmas elicit different types of responses. Her arguments are based on three studies. In the first, 25 male and female college students taking a course on moral and political choice were interviewed as senior students and again 5 years after graduation about their own experiences of moral conflict and their thinking about morality. In the second, 25 women undergoing counseling before a possible abortion were, both at that time and a year later, asked about their experiences of moral conflict. In the third, very small numbers of male and female subjects, ages 6–60, were questioned about their own and about hypothetical moral dilemmas. While the narrative descriptions and quotations from the responses elicited are convincing, illuminating, and often moving, no account of systematic analyses of the data is either given or referred to.

A subsequent replication of Kohlberg's and Gilligan's work, with a bigger sample of both male and female subjects between 5 and 63 years old, confirmed that there are few violations of stage sequence over time. In contrast to Gilligan's study, no significant sex differences were found, but the types of responses to real-life and hypothetical dilemmas did differ, although not systematically, in the direction of care and responsibility for real-life problems, justice, and rights for hypothetical issues (Walker, 1989). More recent studies have, however, as we shall see, revealed sex differences in early socialization and in early prosocial behavior (Hay, 1994; Lewis et al., 1992).

The causes of variations in moral judgments have recently been explored. Cultural transmission is likely to play a part, as are individual life experience and accommodation to the environment; different developmental stages as outlined by Kohlberg; different domains of social judgment, e.g., moral or conventional (see below); and the need to judge multifaceted situations. But there is a further, very important cause: the information available. Wainryb (1991) studied children's moral judgments of events before and after being given information that challenged their initial judgments. All children, for example, thought it was wrong for an irritable adult to spank a child who had not erred. But some thought it was right to spank a repeatedly misbehaving child because they thought this taught children to behave better. If the responders were told that spanking was not an effective way to socialize children, most of them changed their mind. In this study, manipulation of information profoundly affected the moral judgments of young people 11–21 years old. The finding has implications for education but also for the information presented in the media to the general public.

THE ROLE OF EMPATHY IN THE DEVELOPMENT OF PROSOCIAL BEHAVIOR

Anna Freud and Piaget had already, as we saw, referred to the importance of empathy for the feelings and thoughts of others in the development of morality. Martin Hoffman (1975, 1984), however, was the first to give due emphasis to this important human faculty. He saw guilt and other emotional aspects of morality as springing from the capacity for empathy with the suffering of others, evident from the 1st year of life but becoming differentiated only with the advent of the ability to take roles in the 3rd year.

Emotional responses to the feelings of others occur even in the newborn: When one baby in a nursery begins to cry, all the others follow suit. This "reflexive emotional resonance" (Campos et al., 1983) manifests before the infant can distinguish between himself or herself and others, between his or her own emotions and those of other people. Only at around 9 months are babies thought to be capable of locating feelings in others. Hoffman too (1984) noted that in their 1st year children respond to distress in others as if it were happening to themselves. But in the 2nd year they are capable of sympathy, that is, of offering comfort to others. Toddlers, for example, whose mothers suffer from depression make active attempts to offer solace when their mothers weep (Radke-Yarrow et al., 1985). Such activity is at first often inappropriate. When one toddler cries, another will call upon her own mother for help even if the crying child's mother is there too, or she will offer her own comforter rather than that of the toddler in distress. By the 3rd year, however, when role taking occurs in play and children begin to model themselves on others, they are capable of realizing that the feelings of other people are different from their own, and in the 4th year empathic distress prompts the offering of help geared to the needs of the other person.

Hoffman (1975) regarded empathic responsiveness together with a cognitive sense of the other person as the basis for altruism, and this he thought to be a biological motive to help others in distress, independent of egoism and the prospects of reward or punishment. People tend to help others in need even when there are no witnesses to give social approval. Moreover, popular children, emotionally secure and much loved at home and hence less in need of approval from others, are more inclined to help than children who receive little affection. Hoffman speculated that children exposed to frequent, severe distress and frustration are likely to develop egoistic self-absorption, which interferes with their sensitivity and openness to the needs of others.

He suggested also (Hoffman, 1984) that in middle childhood empathic responses are further differentiated. When the distress of others is overwhelming, children tend to withdraw. They now empathize more with others like themselves, offering less help to outsiders. They also now concern themselves with the more enduring sufferings of other people, even when far away or unknown, such as the victims of war or famine in other countries.

In summary, four stages of empathic development have been described (Hoffman, 1987): global empathy in the 1st year; "egocentric" empathy in the 2nd year, when differentiation of self from others and object permanence have been attained; empathy for another's feelings, depending on role and perspective-taking capacities, at between 2 and 3 years of age; and in later childhood, empathy for the experiences of others beyond the immediate situation, associated with the development of a sense of personal identity.

Hoffman believes that children are best socialized to act in accordance with an inner principle of altruism if, once capable of empathic understanding of others, parents consistently point out the possibly harmful effects on others of antisocial conduct. His important ideas about affective and cognitive aspects of the development of altruism in childhood have stimulated much later research.

Zahn-Waxler and Radke-Yarrow (1982) trained 24 middle-class mothers to record observations of their young children in response to emotional distress in others (natural and simulated, caused and not caused by the child) over a 9-month period. Somewhere between 12 and 18 months, most children's behavior changed from a few interactive and merely diffuse affective responses to positive forms of reaching out toward and caring for another person in need. By 18 to 24 months, verbal expressions of sympathy accompanied such behaviors. The authors' findings contradict psychoanalytic postulates about egocentric

narcissism since it is unlikely that at this very early age the children's reactions could all be due to the learning of cultural norms and values. Empathic distress together with subsequent observation learning, the authors hold, promote prosocial development. In their own samples this was linked to maternal disciplinary techniques, in particular to the mothers' use of affective and moralistic explanations of the harmful effects on others of the children's hurtful actions.

Further insights into young children's understanding of feelings, especially in relation to conflict, and into the earliest teaching and understanding of rules have come from Judy Dunn's detailed observations of siblings and their mothers. Even at 24 months, in pretend play between siblings social rules were explored and feeling states simulated. Some 18-month-old children, with an affectionate older sibling, could already take part in a shared fantasy involving the feelings of others. These very young children were clearly practicing, in play, how to conform to rules and engage in other prosocial behaviors (Dunn, 1987).

Brothers (1989) has argued for a biological, evolutionary, basis for empathy: primate survival depends on the capacity for rapid and accurate evaluation of the motivations of others. He instances the absence of empathy in some pathological states such as autism and is seeking its neurological substrate. There is also now some evidence for a genetic basis for individual differences in empathy and other forms of prosocial behavior (Hay, 1994).

THE ORIGINS OF EVALUATIVE BEHAVIOR AND SELF-AWARENESS

A critical study of the early development of morality, supporting a biological basis for the acquisition of inner standards of behavior and self-evaluation and a readiness to learn the morality and conventions of the culture is Kagan's short-term longitudinal investigation of American and Fijian children in the course of their 2nd year (Kagan, 1981). Although reluctant to give credence to psychoanalytic theories about the development of a sense of shame in the 2nd year and of conscience and guilt from about 2½ years onward, Kagan was led through his observations to identify a second stage in the biological maturation of children, following the stage of specific attachments to their caregivers, a stage in which the capacity for the development of inner standards first shows itself.

He observed children together with their mothers at monthly intervals in a variety of standard play settings. In one he presented the child with three types of play material: 10 unflawed toys, 10 damaged toys (such as a doll with a missing eye or a car with chipped body work), and two undamaged meaningless objects. No 14-month-old child discriminated between damaged and undamaged toys, but thereafter, and increasingly as the second birthday drew near, children began to show unambiguous concern about the damaged objects, commenting "broke," "fix it," "yucky," or taking the broken toy to the mother. In another experiment, an adult demonstrated skilled play with toys. All 13- and 14-month-old children watched calmly or seemed bored. But from 15 months onward more and more began to fret, protest, wish to leave the room, or indicate "It's mommy's turn to play." These older children seemed to feel under an obligation to copy what the adult did, realized it was beyond their capacity, and became distressed. These changes occurred just before the use of "evaluative language." Between 19 and 26 months the first references to "dirty," "can't," and "hard do" appeared, and at 20 months most children used words like "good," "bad," "dirty," and "nice."

Because American and Fijian children responded similarly, Kagan concluded that the acquisition of this set of new functions centered on children's sensitivity to adult standards and their own capacity to meet these, that is, on an awareness of what they can and cannot do. This development, in the second half of the 2nd year of life, represented a maturational shift rather than the influence of the specific culture. The standards now acquired relate to cleanliness, integrity of property, toileting behavior, and harm to others.

Work on this important early milestone of self-evaluation has been taken further by the experimental studies of Stipek et al. (1992). They identified three stages in its development in young children: (*a*) in the first half of the 2nd year, pleasure at mastery, that is, joy in causality, with anger and distress, but no shame, at failure and no anticipation of the reactions of others to their performance; (*b*) from 21 months onward, pride in accomplishment, that is, an anticipation of the reactions of adults, and active seeking of positive responses to success and avoidance of negative reactions to failure; and (*c*) a gradual internalization of these external reactions with children beginning to evaluate their own performance and reacting emotionally to success and failure independently of their expectations of adult responses. The authors stress that they investigated only the domain of achievement, not morality, and they point out that praise is always commoner than disapproval *except* in the moral domain.

These workers made one further observation: Winning or losing in a competitive task was not understood by children younger than 33 months of age, but thereafter, pleasure in completing a task was increased by winning. The timing of this development, we must note, is in line with psychoanalytic ideas about the "genital" stage, when competition was thought to enters the child's range of experiences for the first time.

MORALITY AND CONVENTION

Turiel (1983) helpfully defined the distinction between morality and convention and charted children's understanding of these from the age of 6 to 17 years. Even young children were able to differentiate between them. Conventions are behavioral uniformities that serve to harmonize social interactions and form, and are themselves determined by, the specific social system. Morality, in contrast, concerns prescriptive judgments of justice, rights, welfare, and the avoidance of harm to others and is inherent in interpersonal relationships, not tied to the social context. It is a convention, for example, that in most schools children address the teacher by his or her second, not first, name. In themselves such rules are arbitrary and could be changed by consensus. Turiel asked children of different ages if it would be wrong to call teachers by their first names if there were no rule about that. Even quite young children thought not. Turiel also questioned children about the rights and wrongs of a playground situation in which all swings are occupied, and a little girl eager for a turn comes along and pushes another child off a swing. All children agreed that this was wrong and would be wrong even if there were no rule about it. Most children thought that, if everyone agreed, the rules of games and social conventions could be changed, but not such inherent moral dictates as that it is wrong to hurt other people or to steal.

Younger children regarded rules as more fixed, and older ones had a better understanding of their underlying purpose. But all children, from 6 upward, distinguished between conventional rules and morality, and in an earlier study, even preschool children could do so (Nucci and Turiel, 1978). But very young children respond more often to moral rather than to social conventional events, and even in middle childhood, children are more responsive to moral events and moral injustice than to conventional transgressions, although these acquire increasing salience with age (Nucci and Nucci, 1982).

THE CONTEXT OF MORAL DEVELOPMENT

Stipek et al. (1992) found that children's behavior in relation to success and failure was far more mature than their expressed ideas, although the sequence, from the pleasure of success, to pleasure from the approval from others, to satisfaction from meeting inner standards, was the same in both spheres. Implicit knowledge long precedes explicit understanding. This point is made also by Judy Dunn (1988) in her major contributions to unravelling the origins of social and moral under-

standing in early childhood. Detailed home observations were made of children during their 2nd and 3rd years in the company of their mothers and younger siblings. Dunn takes issue with the relentless seriousness with which moral development is usually discussed and with the "bleak emphasis" on anxiety, guilt, and fear. What she found instead in the natural settings of children's own homes was that, even before they use many words, children are amused by rules, roles, and the relationships in their world and share jokes about these with others. Just as they play with the rules of language, so they joke about what is expected, allowed, or punishable. They find it funny to distort or exaggerate rules, make scatological jokes, and teasingly misname things and make false assertions.

From 18 months onward, children understand how to hurt and comfort others, what the consequences of their own hurtful actions are, what is allowed or disapproved of within their own family, and what the responses of adults are likely to be to their own misdeeds and to those of others.

Dunn stresses four features:

1. *Understanding the feelings of others* grows in the 2nd year from the "affective resonance" in the 1st year to empathic responsiveness to the distress of others in the 2nd year: "...the foundations for the moral virtues of caring, considerateness, and kindness are well laid by three years" (p. 170).
2. *Understanding of the goals of others* develops during the 2nd year, as shown in children's behavior during conflicts and cooperative endeavors, and in the 3rd year, as shown in pretend games, narratives, and questions about other people.
3. *Understanding of social rules* is manifested by children's discussion and jokes about transgressions and rules and of their differential application. By 2½–3 years children have a practical knowledge of the idea of responsibility and of excuses on the basis of intent and incapacity. They know that rules can apply differently to different family members, that rules can be questioned, and transgressions justified. They understand something about authority relations within their family and comment on the behavior of others in moral terms.
4. *Understanding other minds* represents a new stage in social understanding and also begins in the 3rd year. Children now talk about mental states such as remembering and forgetting both in themselves and others. Although capable of feeling embarrassment, guilt, and shame, they are probably not yet able to recognize these more sophisticated emotions in themselves or others.

Dunn comments on differences in parents' disciplinary strategies and on the effects on these of children's growing cognitive and communicative skills. She recognizes cultural differences in how parents react to their children's anger and aggression. Parents are also likely to respond differently to their sons than they do to their daughters. Three-year-old girls, for example, show more shame than do boys when they fail at both simple and more complex experimental tasks (Lewis et al., 1992). This was attributed to their lower expectations of success, but also, although more speculatively, to the probability that they themselves and their parents tend to emphasize their overall value rather than their specific achievements.

Emotion plays a large part in interactions in which moral and social rules are discussed. Children in their 3rd year are most likely to reason during disputes that earlier caused them the most distress. But they also learn from calm reflective discourse. Dunn takes issue with Kagan and Hoffman's views and holds instead that the child's part in the power relationships within the family, rather than the urge to conform or allay guilt, is the main motive toward understanding of social and moral rules. In her view, it is the child's need to assert his or her own place, for example, vis-à-vis a sibling, and the active enjoyment of rule breaking, teasing, and exerting power within the family, but also happy cooperative play, rather than socialization pressures, which foster moral behavior.

THE MORAL EMOTIONS

Exploration of the development of the moral emotions requires accurate descriptions of the emotions of self-assessment—pride, shame, and guilt. The philosopher Gabriele Taylor (1985) makes clear that shame and embarrassment depend on an awareness of being observed and relate to all wrongdoing and to one's standing in society. Guilt, on the other hand, appearing later in development, relates to law breaking and, specifically, to doing something morally wrong rather than to breaking a convention. The sense of an authority to be obeyed plays the major role in conscience, while an awareness of a watchful audience is a major factor in shame. Both guilt and punishment concentrate on the bad deed or the omission and are linked with a sense of responsibility for one's own actions, but shame concerns the kind of person one is. Taylor considers that neither shame nor guilt is related to empathic feelings for others, but that remorse, the "emotion of salvation," is. Remorse is also the precursor of self-forgiveness, essential if the destructive forces of guilt are to be assuaged.

Harris (1989), in a number of imaginative experiments, explored the development of children's emotional understanding. He tested 3- to 5-year-olds on a perspective-taking task and found those who were good at it to be much more attentive to their distressed younger siblings when temporarily separated from their mother. The mothers, in turn, more often asked these more empathically competent older children to "look after your brother." Whether these maternal responses were causes or consequences of the older child's empathic skills is not known.

Children's recognition of emotions and their understanding of what brings them about develops in a similar age sequence in quite different cultures. Children are born with a capacity to experience the basic emotions of happiness, sadness, anger, and fear, which are associated with facial expressions. They come to understand that other people have them too. They learn to differentiate between morality and convention on the emotional basis of the distress that moral, but not social, rule infringements induce in the victim. This, Harris believes, is learned from other children rather than from adults.

Under about 8 years children find it difficult to identify the emotions of pride, shame, and guilt in others because they are not accompanied by characteristic facial expressions. Understanding of these more complex emotions depends on the ability to imagine the mental state (in terms of these more complex emotions) of another person in a given situation. It depends also on the availability of concepts of personal responsibility and on normative standards of morality and propriety. Children experience a shift of awareness from believing that a person's feelings about his behavior depend on its consequences, to attributing them to the approval or disapproval he expects from other people in the light of social norms. Only at about 8 years of age do children feel proud or ashamed "of themselves" without reference to an external audience. *The developmental sequence* Harris (1989) detects is congruent with both Turiel's and Kohlberg's findings. Even 3- to 4-year-olds know that harming others causes distress and is therefore wrong. Four- to 5-year-olds know that people are happy if they get and do what they want. By 7–8 years children know that people are happy if others approve of them and they act to gain approval. Only after the age of 8 can children work out that they and other people get satisfaction from doing what they think is right.

There is other evidence too that the comprehension of emotional accompaniments of immorality, as the development of empathy itself, changes with age and begins to be accurate only at about 7 or 8 years (Arsenio, 1988). In an illuminating experiment (Nunner-Winkler and Sodian, 1988), 4- to 8-year-olds were told a series of stories of moral transgressions and had to judge how the wrongdoer was likely to feel. Most 4-year-olds thought that the story person who violated a moral injunction, got away with it, and succeeded would be happy, while 8-year-olds attributed negative emotions to this person because he or she would feel bad about what they had done. There was also a shift between 4 and 8 years in the attribution of emotions to a story character who

had resisted temptation. Very young children judged according to the material outcome, older children, according to the character's sense of virtue. When asked to judge the degree of badness of story figures, 6-year-olds already thought that a happy wrongdoer was worse than one who felt sorry for what he or she had done.

When we compare these findings about children's expressed ideas about their understanding, with the observational studies, for example, of Stipek et al. (1992), of children's behavior in relation to success and failure, we see again the large age gap between the attainment of behavioral accomplishments on the one hand and children's expressed ideas on the other. Yet there is a similar sequence: from the satisfaction of success, to pleasure from approval of others, to satisfaction from meeting inner standards.

An experimental study of 7- to 12-year-old children's understanding of the "self-conscious" emotions of guilt and shame (Ferguson et al., 1991) showed that shame resulted both from moral transgressions and from social blunders and led younger children to feel embarrassed and older ones to feel they could not do things right. Guilt, in contrast, was aroused by moral norm violations and involved a conflict between approach toward and withdrawal from the victim as well as self-criticism, remorse, a desire to make amends, and fear of punishment.

Harris (1994) believes that the child's own emotional experiences influence age-related cognitive changes as well as behavior. When parents, instead of punishing, reason with children about the possible effects of their misdeeds on others, they induce anticipatory guilt and increase their children's understanding of social emotions. When children witness parental quarrels, they become more physically aggressive with their peers. This may not be due merely to modelling, because verbal quarrels between parents with no physical violence have the same effect. It is more likely that the children's state of arousal caused by the quarrels they witness leads them to attribute more malign intent to their peers and to react accordingly (Dodge et al., 1990).

Harris (1994) also draws the important distinction, quite insufficiently appreciated by legal experts and by the general public, between knowing what is right and wrong and abiding by moral rules. The impulse to tease or hurt often overrides the moral code: A knowledge of right and wrong is not closely related to action.

SOCIAL LEARNING AND ROLE MODELING

Learning theorists (whose work is referred to in Chapter 9) have also contributed to our understanding of the genesis of prosocial and antisocial behavior in childhood, although they have not generally taken a developmental viewpoint and although the early stimulus-response, or reward and punishment, theories of behavioral change have not been very helpful. Bandura (Bandura, 1977; Bandura and Walters, 1963) adopted a more sophisticated approach, which included the cognitive accompaniments of behavior, and his experimental studies of how and under what conditions children copy the behavior of others have been illuminating both for understanding social development and in the treatment of childhood behavior disorders. We now know that the capacity for role modeling starts toward the end of the 2nd and the beginning of the 3rd year of life (Meltzoff, 1988) and that young children, after watching films of other children playing aggressively, are susceptible, especially when frustrated, to develop similar play patterns.

In what remains a classical study, Patterson and his colleagues (1967) found that in the setting of an unstructured nursery, with little active intervention from their teachers, 4-year-old middle-class boys learn to become ever-more aggressive in imitation of other assertive children when they see assertiveness rewarded with success (as it always is without adult intervention). Only passive children with low rates of interaction with others are spared this development.

That aggressive parents tend to have aggressive children has been documented repeatedly and has often been associated with the norms of a working-class culture (Newson and Newson, 1976), in which parents smack even 1-year-old infants and are more physically punitive, especially to their boys, throughout their children's early years than are middle-class parents. But the precise family interactions that mediate between aggressive conduct in parents and in children have until recently been explored only in later childhood, and the processes underlying early identification with aggressive family role models have not yet been extensively studied.

THE PSYCHOPATHOLOGY OF MORAL DEVELOPMENT

With the early work of Patterson and that of the Newsons, we have already moved from consideration of universal aspects of moral development to its psychopathology. This is of the greatest relevance in our understanding of the origins of that most important group of child psychiatric disorders: the conduct disorders, with their high risk of adult antisocial personality disorder, but also of the affective disorders of later life. Boys are always at greater risk of the first, girls of the second type of disorder.

The psychopathology of moral development is likely to be as important for child psychiatry as that of attachment behavior. While we now know about the affectional needs of young children and the hazards of early separations from parents, of deprivation of continuous parenting, and of distortions of early maternal care, our knowledge about the necessary ingredients in early childhood for promoting the healthy development of empathic feelings for others, of inner standards of self-appraisal and morality, of the capacity to feel shame and guilt, of impulse control, and of sympathetic prosocial behavior through learning from and identifying with role models, is as yet less firm. Studies of the moral development of deviant children and of children exposed to different kinds of adversity are just beginning. But a start has been made. For an excellent review of the correlates of serious and persistent externalizing problems in preschool children, see Campbell, 1995.

COERCIVE CHILD REARING

Patterson's later work (1982, 1986) has been unique in analyzing the mutually reinforcing processes by which coercive, punitive parents evoke counteraggression from their children with escalation of domestic violence. Contributing factors are the parents' own past experiences of coercive rearing, their failure to monitor their children's behavior, the aggressive role models they provide, and maternal depression, and, on the children's part, a difficult temperament, including impulsivity. Social and educational failure at school and low self-esteem often follow such domestic interactions, with further reinforcement of the children's antisocial conduct. Stealing too Patterson regards as a form of noncompliance to unskilled parents. He found the parents of children who steal more often themselves to be delinquent and, unlike the parents of aggressive children, inadequately attached to their offspring. The work of Dodge (Dodge, 1986; Dodge et al., 1990) has similarly illuminated the mutually reinforcing processes that engender aggression between peers.

HOSTILE COGNITIVE ATTRIBUTIONS

Dodge (1986) reminded us that aggressive behavior correlates with deficits in a variety of cognitive skills: self-rehearsal of responses, inhibition of premature social impulses, interpersonal problem solving, referential communication, and role taking. Socially and verbally unskilled people have limited means for handling discord and become physically aggressive with very little provocation. His own studies of children's cognitive attributions have shown that aggressive boys tend to interpret the motivations of their peers as hostile, even when they are not, and to react aggressively, thereby stimulating dislike and hostility in these previously nonhostile peers. This then reinforces the aggressive boys' view of other children's hostile intent. A vicious circle of hostile attributions and aggressive behavior with peers results, similar to the coercive interactions between parents and children described by Patterson (1982/ 1986). The long-term outcomes are academic failure, school dropout, and delinquency. Dodge has shown that children, especially boys, who

have been abused are predisposed to develop hostile attribution and aggressive behavior (Dodge et al., 1990) and that the effect of harsh child rearing is in part mediated by hostile attributions, that is, by maladaptive social information processing, which such child rearing methods induce (Weiss et al., 1992). While these developments are commoner in families living in poverty and marital conflict, such factors alone do not account for the findings.

These studies have been concerned with children from middle childhood onward. But the capacity for empathy, for developing inner standards, and for learning prosocial behavior from adult role models begins, as we saw, much earlier—in the 2nd and 3rd years of life. What goes on in families then is likely to have important consequences for later life.

THE EFFECTS OF EARLY PARENTING STYLES AND CHILDREN'S TEMPERAMENT

Dienstbier's (1984) experimental studies focused on both cognition and affect and suggest that when children are coerced by means of parental punishments, they attribute their resistance to temptation to external forces. They feel bad if they succumb because of the punishment that follows and, if they believe their transgressions will not be discovered, they capitulate. Noncoerced children, in contrast, attribute resistance to temptation to their own choice and to their inner judgment that one course of action is better than another. If they succumb to temptation, they feel bad because of the transgression itself rather than its consequences and are less likely to repeat it even if unobserved. Dienstbier's findings agree with those of Koshanska (see below), that children with high levels of emotional tension learn better to make internal attributions about transgression and to feel appropriate guilt. Children with low levels of emotional tension learn poorly, evoke ever more coercion from parents, and have their external attributions reinforced every time they transgress and "get away with it" without feeling bad. This is in line also with the view that children are best socialized when parents use inductive, that is, reasoning methods, but do so with an emotional charge.

The effects of differences in mothers' early socializing styles on their children's later development of guilt and conscience have been meticulously investigated by Koshanska (1991) in the important longitudinal study of children of depressed and well mothers (see Radke-Yarrow et al., 1985). She also studied the influence on these processes of the child's temperament. Self-reported and observed parental rearing styles when children were 18–42 months old, in terms of coercive/ noncoercive methods, were compared with children's contemporaneously observed compliance to maternal demands and with their affective/ moral orientation when 8–10 years old. The latter was assessed on the basis of narrative responses to semiprojective stories. The main finding was that noncoercive child rearing was associated with evidence for internalized conscience in later years, but only for children prone to fearful arousal. Early compliance to maternal demands predicted later internalized conscience. The author concludes that anxious children are well socialized by noncoercive methods and that their conscience development may be interfered with by coercive methods. Less anxious children are more heterogeneous and their later conscience acquisition was not related to coercive or noncoercive child rearing styles.

In this same study (quoted by Hay, 1994), daughters and sons of healthy mothers did not differ in their advocacy of aggressive solutions to conflict. But sons of depressed mothers, while more prosocial and empathic than other boys, were also the most likely to advocate aggression. Daughters of depressed mothers, who also had high rates of empathy and prosocial behavior, almost never did so, even to defend their own property, seeming to wish at all costs to avoid conflict.

In a comprehensive review of moral development, Koshanska (1993) proposes a new framework for the study of early conscience formation that integrates parental socialization methods with the temperamental characteristics of their children. She suggests two components of conscience that contribute significantly to moral conduct: a child's affective discomfort brought about by actual or potential wrong doing and the capacity for behavioral self-control. The first was salient in psychoanalytical models, the second in social learning and cognitive models of moral development. Both have temperamental underpinnings, which may account for the differential effects of parental socialization methods. Fearfulness and social inhibition interact with high levels of moral motivation to reduce immoral behavior in situations of temptation (Asendorpf and Nunner-Winkler, 1992). Impulsivity versus behavioral control, Koshanska suggests, is a more complex temperamental dimension, and precisely how it interacts with parents' socialization efforts is less well established. Reasoning may be less effective in encouraging the internalization of standards for impulsive children. Shaw and Bell (1993) suggest that irritable, hyperactive, demanding infants can increase maternal unresponsiveness and that the resulting auxious, avoidant attachment leads to later noncompliance and hostility. Securely attached infants, by contrast, become compliant in later years, eager to please their parents.

THE IMPACT OF MATERNAL DEPRESSION

In an earlier study, Dowdney et al. (1985) had already observed differences in the disciplinary behavior in interaction with their toddlers of mothers who were either depressed or had, as children, been in care (i.e., in children's homes), compared with a control group. Koshanska (1991), as we saw, explored the long-term effects on children's conscience of exposure to different child-rearing patterns in early life. Zahn-Waxler et al. (1990) in the same controlled longitudinal study documented the relationship between maternal depression in children's toddler years and their later distorted and exaggerated expressions of guilt. Young children, highly aroused, overinvolved, and causally implicated in the distress of their mothers, before they have the cognitive and emotional maturity to cope with this, are at risk of later excessive guilt and of distortions of their capacity for empathy and concern with others. Such overinvolved young children are also often deprived of normal opportunities for play with peers, experiences that are vital for social competence and moral development.

OTHER FACTORS

A recent longitudinal study established that aspects of their parenting, assessed when children were 5 years old, correlated with measures of their empathic concern for others at the age of 31 (Koestner et al., 1990). In particular, high levels of empathic concern in adult life were related to paternal involvement in child care, maternal tolerance of the child's dependent behavior, maternal control (inhibition) of the child's aggression, and the mother's satisfaction with her maternal role.

These studies are still in their infancy, as are studies of the effects of constitutional deviations in children on their moral development. A low potential for anxiety arousal, poor impulse control, and a difficult temperament are potential obstacles (Asendorpf et al., 1992; Koshanska, 1993). In addition, the lack of empathy that characterizes not only autistic children but children with schizoid/Asperger disorders is likely to contribute in an important way to the failure of early socialization and the genesis of some forms of later conduct disorder and adult sociopathy (Wolff, 1992).

SUMMARY

The last 10 years have seen much progress in the exploration of the development of morality and prosocial behavior. Throughout early and middle childhood, emotions and cognitions are intimately connected in all aspects of development (Donaldson, 1992) including moral development, and the basis for developmental changes with age and for individual differences in moral behavior and beliefs is both constitutional and experiential.

Prosocial impulses arise in the 1st year of life with manifestations of empathic responsiveness. In the 2nd and 3rd years children become aware of norms of behavior and of their own achievements and shortcomings. Within the context of family life, even 2- to 3-year-old children display surprising knowledge about moral and conventional rules and do so with enjoyment and humor. It is at this stage that parental behavior and parents' beliefs and expectations about their children's moral development and their own contributions to this are likely to be crucial. Parents' behavior is influenced by many factors: their socioeconomic and cultural milieu, their marriage, their health, and by their children's gender and temperamental responsiveness in family interactions.

Only at 7 or 8 years of age can children reason about moral issues. Concepts of guilt and shame are now articulated. Children develop notions of morality independent of external approval and begin to be able to reason about principles not tied to concrete events. Abstract ideas of justice and welfare arise later still. Children's cognitions, especially their attributions of hostile intent, their peer relationships, and prosocial behavior remain crucially influenced by their experiences, now both within their families and at school.

Research into therapeutic interventions for families with young children, guided by the discoveries of how parental disability and different methods of child rearing interact with children's different temperamental styles in the genesis of conscience and prosocial behavior, is likely to contribute in a major way to the more effective treatment of antisocial conduct in children and its prevention in later life.

References

Arsenio WF: Children's conceptions of the situational affective consequences of socio-moral events. *Child Dev* 59:1611, 1988.

Asendorpf JB, Nunner-Winkler G: Children's moral motive strength and temperamental inhibition reduce their immoral behavior in real moral conflicts. *Child Dev* 63:1223, 1992.

Bandura A: *Social Learning Theory*. Englewood Cliffs, NJ, Prentice-Hall, 1977.

Bandura A, Walters RH: *Social Learning and Personality Development*. New York, Holt, Rinehart & Winston, 1963.

Baldwin JM: *Social and Ethical Interpretations of Mental Development: A Study in Social Psychology* (4th ed). New York, Macmillan, 1897.

Bowlby J: *Attachment and Loss. Vol I: Attachment* (2nd ed). London, The Tavistock Institute of Human Relations and the Hogarth Press, 1982.

Brothers L: A biological perspective on empathy. *Am J Psychiatry* 146:10, 1989.

Buchsbaum HK, Emde RN: Play narratives in 36-month-old children: Early moral development and family relationships. *Psychoanal Study Child* 45:129, 1990.

Butterworth G: Some benefits of egocentrism. In: Bruner J, Haste H (eds): *Making Sense: The Child's Construction of the World*. London, Methuen, 1987, p. 62.

Campbell SB: Behavior problems in preschool children: A review of recent research. *J Child Psychol Psychiatry* 36:113, 1995.

Campos JJ, Barrett KC, Lamb ME, et al: Socioemotional development. In: Haith MM, Campos II (eds): *Developmental Psychobiology*. New York, Wiley, 1983, p. 783.

Colby A, Kohlberg L: *The Measurement of Moral Judgement. Vol 1: Theoretical Foundations and Research Validation*. Cambridge, Cambridge University Press, 1987.

Colby A, Kohlberg L, Gibbs J, et al: A longitudinal study of moral judgement. *Monogr Soc Res Child Dev* 48(20), 1983.

Colby A, Kohlberg L, Speicher B, et al: *The Measurement of Moral Judgement. Vol 2: Standard Issue Scoring Manual*. Cambridge, Cambridge University Press, 1987.

Dienstbier RA: The role of emotion in moral socialization. In: Izard CE, Kagan J, Zajonc RB (eds): *Emotion Cognition and Behavior*. Cambridge, Cambridge University Press, 1984, p. 484.

Dodge KA: Social information-processing variables in the development of aggression and altruism in children. In: Zahn-Waxler C, Cummings EM, Iannotti RJ (eds): *Altruism and Aggression: Biological and Social Origins*. Cambridge, Cambridge University Press, 1986, p. 280.

Dodge KA, Bates JE, Pettit GS: Mechanisms in the cycle of violence. *Science* 250:1678, 1990.

Donaldson M: *Children's Minds*. Glasgow, Fontana/Collins, 1978.

Donaldson M: *Human Minds: An Exploration*. London, Penguin, 1992.

Dowdney L, Skuse D, Rutter M, et al: Parenting qualities: Concepts, measures and origins. In: Stevenson JE (ed): *Recent Research in Developmental Psychopathology*. Oxford, Pergamon, 1985, p. 19.

Dunn J: Understanding feelings: The early stages. In: Bruner J, Haste H (eds): *Making Sense: The Child's Construction of the World*. London, Methuen, 1987, p. 26.

Dunn J: *The Beginnings of Social Understanding*. Oxford, Basil Blackwell, 1988.

Erikson EH: *Identity, Youth and Crisis*. London, Faber & Faber, 1968.

Ferguson TJ, Stegge H, Damhuis I: Children's

understanding of guilt and shame. *Child Dev* 62:827, 1991.

Freud A: *The Ego and the Mechanisms of Defence.* London, Hogarth Press and the Institute of Psycho-Analysis, 1961.

Freud A: *Normality and Pathology in Childhood.* London, Hogarth Press and the Institute of Psycho-Analysis, 1966.

Freud S: *Civilization and Its Discontents.* In: Strachey J (ed): *The Standard Edition of the Complete Psychological Works of Sigmund Freud* (Vol 21). London, Hogarth, 1961a. (Originally published 1930.)

Freud S: *The Ego and the Id.* In: Strachey J (ed): *The Standard Edition of the Complete Psychological Works of Sigmund Freud* (Vol 19). London, Hogarth, 1961b. (Originally published 1923.)

Gilligan C: *In a Different Voice: Psychological Theory and Women's Development.* Cambridge, MA, Harvard University Press, 1982.

Graham D: *Moral Learning and Development: Theory and Research.* New York, Wiley, 1972.

Harris P: *Children and Emotion: The Development of Psychosocial Understanding.* Oxford, Basil Blackwell, 1989.

Harris P: The child's understanding of emotion: Developmental change and the family environment. *Annu Res Rev J Child Psychol Psychiatry* 35:3, 1994.

Haste H: Growing into rules. In: Bruner I, Haste H (eds): *Making Sense: The Child's Construction of the World.* London, Methuen, 1987, p. 163.

Hay DF: Prosocial development. *Annu Res Rev J Child Psychol Psychiatry* 35:29, 1994.

Hoffman ML: Developmental synthesis of affect and cognition and its implications for altruistic motivation. *Dev Psychol* 11:607, 1975.

Hoffman ML: Moral development. In: Bornstein MH, Lamb ME (eds): *Developmental Psychology: An Advanced Textbook.* Hillsdale, NJ, Erlbaum, 1984, p. 279.

Hoffman ML: The contribution of empathy to justice and moral judgment. In: Eisenberg N, Strayer I (eds): *Empathy and Its Development.* New York, Cambridge University Press, 1987, p. 47.

Kagan I: *The Second Year: The Emergence of Self-Awareness.* Cambridge, MA, Harvard University Press, 1981.

Klein M: Criminal tendencies in normal children. In: *Contributions to Psycho-Analysis 1921–1945.* London, Hogarth Press and the Institute of Psycho-Analysis, 1948a, p. 185. (Originally published 1927.)

Klein M: The early development of conscience in the child. In: *Contributions to Psycho-Analysis 1921–1945.* London, Hogarth Press and the Institute of Psycho-Analysis, 1948b, p. 267. (Originally published 1933.)

Klein M: On criminality. In: *Contributions to Psycho-Analysis 1921–1945.* London, Hogarth Press and the Institute of Psycho-Analysis, 1948c, p. 278. (Originally published 1934.)

Koestner R, Weinberger J, Franz C: The family origins of empathic concern: A 26-year longitudinal study. *J Pers Soc Psychol* 58:709, 1990.

Koshanska G: Socialization and temperament in the development of guilt and conscience. *Child Dev* 62:1379, 1991.

Koshanska G: Towards a synthesis of parental socialization and child temperament in early development of conscience. *Child Dev* 64:325, 1993.

Lewis M, Alessandri SM, Sullivan MW: Differences in shame and pride as a function of children's gender and task difficulty. *Child Dev* 63:630, 1992.

Meltzoff AN: Imitation of television models by infants. *Child Dev* 59:1221, 1988.

Newson E, Newson J: *Seven Years Old in the Home Environment.* London, Allen and Unwin, 1976.

Nucci LP, Nucci MS: Children's social interactions in the context of moral and conventional transgressions. *Child Dev* 53:403, 1982.

Nucci LP, Turiel E: Social interactions and the development of social concepts in preschool children. *Child Dev* 49:400, 1978.

Nunner-Winkler G, Sodian B: Children's understanding of moral emotions. *Child Dev* 59:1323, 1988.

Patterson GR: *Coercive Family Process.* Eugene, OR, Castalia, 1982.

Patterson GR: Performance models for antisocial boys. *Am Psychol* 41:432, 1986.

Patterson GR, Littman RA, Bricker W: Assertive behavior in children: A step towards a theory of aggression. *Monogr Soc Res Child Dev* 32 (no. 5), 1967.

Piaget J: *The Moral Judgement of the Child.* London, Routledge & Kegan Paul, 1932.

Piaget J, Inhelder B: *The Psychology of the Child.* London, Routledge & Kegan Paul, 1969.

Radke-Yarrow M, Cummings EM, Kuczynski L, et al: Patterns of attachment in two- and three-year-olds in normal families and families with parental depression. *Child Dev* 56:884, 1985.

Shaw DS, Bell RQ: Developmental theories of parental contributors to antisocial behavior. *J. Abnorm Child Psychol* 21:493, 1993.

Stipek D, Recchia S, McClintic S: Self-evaluation in young children. *Monogr Soc Res Child Dev* 57(226), 1992.

Tanner JM: Physical growth and development. In: Forfar JO, Arneil GC (eds): *Textbook of Paediatrics* (Vol 1, 3rd ed). Edinburgh, Churchill Livingstone, 1984, p. 278.

Taylor G: *Pride, Shame and Guilt.* Oxford, Clarendon Press, 1985.

Turiel E: *The Development of Social Knowledge: Morality and Convention.* Cambridge, Cambridge University Press, 1983.

Walker LI: The sequentiality of Kohlberg's stages of moral development. *Child Dev* 53:1330, 1982.

Walker LI: A longitudinal study of moral reasoning. *Child Dev* 60:157, 1989.

Wainryb C: Understanding differences in moral judgements: The role of informational assumptions. *Child Dev* 62:840, 1991.

Weiss B, Dodge KA, Bates JE, et al: Some consequences of early harsh discipline: Child aggression and a maladaptive social information processing style. *Child Dev* 63:1321, 1992.

Wolff S: *Childhood and Human Nature: The Development of Personality.* London, Methuen, 1989.

Wolff S: Psychiatric morbidity and criminality in "schizoid" children grown-up. *Eur Child Adolesc Psychiatry* 1:214, 1992.

Zahn-Waxler C, Radke-Yarrow M: The development of altruism. In: Eisenberg N (ed): *The Development of Prosocial Behavior* (2nd ed). New York, Academic Press, 1982.

Zahn-Waxler C, Koshanska G, Krupnick J, et al: Patterns of guilt in children of depressed and well mothers. *Dev Psychol* 26:51, 1990.

18 CHILDHOOD SEXUALITY

Alayne Yates, M.D.

Human sexuality is surely as old as the human race. Although sexual activity is based on instinct, the sexual act is influenced by political, economic, medical, social, and religious concerns. In the United States, sexual expression is influenced by assumptions about sex handed down through generations, depictions of sexuality currently in the media, fear of venereal disease (especially AIDS), the changing status and role of women, and medical achievements such as effective birth control and in vitro fertilization.

HISTORY

Prior to the 16th century, families in Britain and Western Europe did not enjoy privacy as we know it today (Jackson, 1993). Family members, employees, and servants worked, ate, and slept under one roof, usually in the same room. Children were seen as small, socially inferior, adults. They were expected to contribute to the family economy and were held legally responsible for their actions. They freely observed the sexual acts of adults and heard open discussion of licit and illicit acts. They engaged in masturbation and sex play with other youngsters. Sexual crimes involving children did occur, but the effect on children's emotional well-being was not an issue. Sexual development was not regarded as problematic.

From the 16th to the 19th century, families began to live apart from the workplace. The single, great room had been divided by walls so that sleeping rooms were apart from eating and work areas. Sexual relations occurred behind closed doors. Servants had their own quarters. With the advent of Puritanism, sexuality was identified with sinfulness, except in the narrow context of procreation. Sexual relations became more and more secretive. Conversation was sanitized and sexual matters were discussed only in private. Parents tried to raise modest, notably asexual children. Children were told to cover the body at all times and not to look at or touch other potentially sexual objects (Elias, 1978). Children became ashamed of the body and of such common behaviors as blowing the nose without a handkerchief, burping, and toileting (Whitehurst,

1971). Children could not refer to "legs" or to "bellies" but were to use the correct terms, which were "nether limbs" and "lower portion." The dinner table stood on "limbs" rather than "legs," and children could never ask for slices from the "breast" of the chicken. Girls and women were told to avoid strong foods such as corned beef and blood pudding, but boys and men could eat anything they wished (Lockwood, 1978).

In the 19th century, Victorian parents were tormented by the fear that their children would masturbate, as "self-abuse" was thought to cause insanity, lethargy, tuberculosis, syphilis, eventual impotence or sterility, deformed children, and epilepsy. Spike-lined rings that fit around the penis; steel and leather jackets that enveloped the entire torso; electric shocks; and tight bandages were used to prevent children from pleasuring themselves. Some parents would tie their children's extremities to each post of a four-poster bed at night. Children who masturbated in spite of these measures might have the nerves to the penis severed or the clitoris cauterized with a white-hot iron. Clitorectomy by scalpel or by scissor was a common treatment for recalcitrant masturbation in young girls (Schwartz, 1973). Among the many civilizations that practice clitorectomy, ours is the only one that has used the excision of the clitoris as a cure for masturbation (Huelsman, 1976).

In the mid-19th century, under the influence of literary romanticism, attitudes toward children and sexuality started to soften. Liberal, well-educated parents began to regard children as innocent, asexual, and in need of protection (Jackson, 1993). This idea slowly spread throughout society, although it has never completely replaced the concept of the demonic child among fundamentalist groups. Because children were vulnerable, the family's responsibility was to protect them against danger, especially threats to their "natural" state of innocence.

20th Century

Relatively ineffective forms of contraception, such as silk handkerchiefs and pig's intestines, have been employed throughout recorded history. In the 18th and 19th centuries, the use of contraceptives was highly suspect, as this was thought to indicate immoral intent (Jackson, 1993). The only acceptable form of contraception was abstention. Indeed, many women avoided intercourse because of their fear of pregnancy. It was not until the early part of the 20th century that truly effective contraceptive devices, such as the latex condom, became available. The early 20th century also marked the end of territorial expansion, the closing of the frontiers, lower infant mortality rates, a longer life span, and the demise of the need for a large family. For the first time in several centuries, intercourse assumed recreational, as well as procreational, significance.

Effective birth control has been the single strongest force in the emancipation of women (Pickett, 1971). Women could explore roles other than that of servant or childbearer. As women became less committed to the home and to child rearing, the structure of the family began to change. As in the 16th century, women once again were gainfully employed, but this time the employment removed them from the home.

At the same time that birth control was increasing in popularity and acceptance, the automobile became the common mode of transportation. Young people could attend a titillating, if nonexplicit, movie and then "neck" or "pet" in the privacy of the car. The advent of the automobile was credited with the decline of the brothel (Pickett, 1971). Adolescents also began to use the home, as well as the car, for sexual experimentation.

The decades from 1930 to 1950 witnessed a marked decline in the severity of the sanctions against sex play and masturbation in childhood (Wolfenstein, 1953). Parents began to caution, dissuade, or distract rather than punish or scold youngsters for sexual activities or interests (Finkelhor, 1980). In the 1950s a new theme emerged: Parents were told not to worry about children's sexual interest. It was perfectly normal for children to explore the body, and once they learned about the body, they would no longer be curious. Some parents could accept sex play as "probably not abnormal." Upper socioeconomic (SES) parents began to name the boy's penis but continued to avoid naming the girl's genitals.

Current Status

From the 1970s into the 1990s, child sexuality was seen as increasingly problematic because of political and social concern about child sexual abuse, molestation, unintended adolescent pregnancy, homosexuality, and AIDS. These concerns intensified the need to protect innocent children from danger. Children were cautioned about disease, "stranger danger," and "bad touch." Any positive reference to sexual activity was omitted and there was no sexual activity defined as healthy or acceptable for children. At present, children who display sexual interest continue to be judged deviant or abnormal. There is little doubt but that the culture will persist in protecting children against sex. How this will effect sexual function and dysfunction in the future is yet to be determined.

At the same time that children are told that sex is dangerous, they are exposed to increasingly explicit, sophisticated television productions in which sexual events are often depicted as delightful or intriguing. Sexual exploitation and rape are also portrayed. Cable and satellite television bring hard-core films into many a living room, and "soaps" are readily available in the daytime. Children might well be confused by these messages and by their variance from the messages of their parents.

Children's sexual development should be directly assessed and tracked, as are other facets of development. Unfortunately, this is not possible in today's climate. Most parents do not want their children to be asked questions about sex. Concerned about parents' reactions, schools are not willing to grant permission to conduct research (Yates, 1993). There is little understanding of children's anxiety about sex, the degree of confusion they experience, or the effect of sex abuse prevention programs. Research studies are largely limited to parents' observations of children's sexual behavior and adult retrospective recall of early sexual experience. Conclusions drawn from this material can be misleading. For instance, Friedrich et al. (1991) collected data from parents about children's sexual behavior and concluded that sexual activity gradually declined from age 4 to age 12. Yet this could simply reflect older children's greater awareness of sanctions and greater skill in concealing their sexual activity.

Dissonance

At present, our culture is dissonant in its standards for sexual conduct in that children are not reared in ways that would facilitate the assumption of the adult sexual role (Benedict, 1950). Most periods in history presented a greater degree of consonance than is currently the case. For example, in Victorian times, prescribed standards for children closely matched those for adults. "Good" asexual girls grew to be "good" women who tolerated intercourse in order to bear children. They did not seek or expect to have orgasms. "Good" little boys grew to become "good" men who engaged in sex because they needed to make babies. They equated the loss of semen with the loss of strength. Today's inhibited children may experience difficulty in becoming fully sexual adults (Yates, 1993).

CULTURAL PERSPECTIVES

Civilizations have devoted considerable time and effort to curbing and redirecting the sexual interests and activities of children and adolescents. Sanctions against sexual activity are usually more stringent for the female. Various rationales for restricting sexual activity include the protection and stability of the family unit, the value placed on work or spirituality in contradistinction to pleasure, and the need for men to possess women for their economic, aesthetic, and procreational worth. However, as society also protects its institutions in nonsexual ways, the restrictiveness of a given culture is not necessarily related to the stability of the family, sexual constancy in marriage, or the industry of the people (Elwin, 1968).

Perspective on sexual development can best be gained through a knowledge of the sexual customs and methods of child rearing used in a wide range of societies (Ford and Beach, 1951; Marshall and Suggs, 1971). Currier (1981) describes four general approaches to sexuality found in various cultures: (*a*) repressive, (*b*) restrictive, (*c*) permissive, and (*d*) supportive.

Sexually repressive cultures include Victorian England and, until recently, the United States. The rural Irish island of Ibis Beag and the Cheyenne Plains Indians are examples of other sexually repressive societies. Cultures such as these believe that sexual activity is dangerous. Celibacy is the ideal. Sexual expression is narrowly defined, and sexual pleasure has little value. Breast-feeding is shunned or concealed, and physical contact with children may be avoided. Children's sexual interests and activities are prohibited, and formal sex education does not exist, as sexual topics are viewed as dangerous or dirty. Boys are separated from girls from earliest childhood and erotic interests or activities are severely punished. Across cultures, punishment for sexual activity in childhood is related to restrictions and concerns over sexual matters in adult life (Munroe and Munroe, 1975)

Sexually restrictive cultures are frequently found among developed nations. The United States is now a sexually restrictive culture rather than a sexually repressive culture. In cultures such as this, sex is valued but tends to be feared because of the problems that can result from sexual activity. There is often a double standard by which women are viewed as property, and sexual access becomes a property right. Various practices, such as the segregation of sexes and the high value placed on virginity, ensure the male sole sexual rights to the woman or women whom he marries. Although children may not be punished for sexual interests, they are inhibited in other ways, and parents view children's sexual activities as problematic. Sex education emphasizes the danger of venereal disease, molestation, and unintended pregnancy.

Sexually permissive cultures tolerate or condone a good deal of sexual interest and behavior. Cultures such as these are common in Africa and Oceania. Sex is considered a normal, natural, and valuable aspect of human existence. However, the culture does not actively encourage sexual activity. Adults expect that children engage in sex play and that adolescents are likely to become sexually active. Latency does not exist in the form found in repressive and restrictive cultures. Premarital sex is common.

Sexually supportive cultures cultivate early sexual experience as a necessary part of growing up. These cultures are found in equatorial Africa, Southern Asia, and the South Pacific. There children are actively introduced into situations where they will experience sexual feelings and learn sexual activities. This is the only group of cultures in which there is intergenerational involvement in the teaching of sexual practices. Sexual pleasure is highly valued and is demanded or expected by both sexes. Relationships, including marriage, may be terminated because of insufficient sexual gratification.

In sexually permissive or supportive cultures, infant genitals are usually bare, and there is ample skin-to-skin contact with adults. There is direct genital stimulation as the children are held or carried astride the hip. When the infants are cross or restless, adults, usually women, may stimulate the genitals in order to soothe them. This is done manually or orally and is a relatively common practice. Infants of any age have ready access to the mother's breast, and sometimes the breasts of other adult women.

Davenport (1976) states that "every society shapes, structures, and constrains the development and expression of sexuality in all its members. This is universally achieved by social training from infancy and by constant social reward and punishment throughout life." Children reared in a sexually permissive society would have their sexual learning promoted by the customs of the culture. Although this is commonly associated with sound adult sexual function, this is not invariably the case (Frayser, 1993). Other factors such as sibling rivalry and conflicts in the mother-child relationship influence the outcome.

In his original cross-cultural analysis of 250 societies, Murdock (1960) placed ours among the three most sexually restrictive. Our culture presents an extremely high incidence of adult sexual dysfunction. Seventy-five percent of male and female patients in a family practice clinic report problems with sexual desire, arousal, or orgasm (Schein et al., 1988). In a sample of apparently healthy, young, upper SES adults, 40% of the males and 50% of the females indicated that they suffered from a sexual dysfunction (Frank et al., 1978). In the same sample, 50% of the males and 77% of females complained of lesser problems, such as lack of interest or inability to relax. Disorders of desire are becoming extremely common in the sex therapy clinic. Complaints of inhibited desire increased from 32 to 50% over a span of only 6 years (Schover and LoPiccolo, 1982). After age 46, a substantial number of adults have given up intercourse entirely (Gagnon and Simon, 1973). In sexually permissive cultures, individuals report relatively few sexual dysfunctions, 100% of the women may be orgasmic, and individuals usually remain sexually active into old age (Marshall and Suggs, 1971).

A few well-respected researchers suggest that some positively perceived early learning about sexuality must occur in childhood in order to preserve or permit sexual enjoyment in adult life. Gadpaille (1978) wonders if childhood is not the optimal time for sexual development. If children have not had the opportunity to engage in sex play, they may not be emotionally ready for sexual experiences later on. Money and Ehrhardt (1972) describe juvenile copulatory rehearsal play as necessary for adult erotic proficiency among primates. They are concerned about the consequences of the prohibition and punishment of such play in this society. They note that more permissive cultures do not have the adult paraphilias and deviations found in sexually restrictive Western cultures.

A common adult concern is that if children engage in sex play, this will lead to more and more inappropriate kinds of sexual activity. Yet in the sexually permissive kibbutzim, sex play follows a predictable course. Masturbatory and peer play begins in infancy, becomes very intense in early childhood, but becomes less intense in the early school years (Shepher, 1971). Sexual shame appears at about age 9 or 10, and at that time the relations between sexes become strained. This tension disappears at ages 13 to 14, when a warm and friendly, but completely asexual, relationship ensues. Individuals from the same peer group do not become sexually active with one another in adolescence, and they do not marry one another later on. This avoidance is completely voluntary.

The early experience of being held and loved is a significant factor in the development of sexual responsiveness in adult life. When infants are more often held or carried by caregivers, they are more likely to be interested in and open to sexual interchange later on (Broude, 1976). Broude and Prescott (1975) have shown that a low level of physical affection expressed toward children is associated with a high level of violence in the culture. The physical contact between infants and caregivers in the United States is quite variable, but it is probably much less than in nonindustrialized nations. In U.S. society, more women have been breast-feeding their infants in recent years, suggesting that there is more physical contact. On the other hand, there is an increase in the number of mothers who are working outside of the home, often leaving their very young children with relatively impersonal and often changing baby sitters. These same mothers continue to be largely responsible for household duties and may be overly stressed even when they are not at work. Because of this, they may have less time or interest in maintaining physical and affectionate contact with their children.

RECENT CULTURAL CHANGE

Recent changes within our culture have affected the sexual development of children. One important change is the trend toward smaller families. Upper SES, mobile parents often place inordinately high expectations on the shoulders of their children, especially the eldest or only child. Parents can become quite intrusive and restrictive in their attempts to enhance accomplishment. The early use of flash cards, computer projects, elitist nursery schools, and school readiness programs are current cultural phenomena designed to foster industriousness and self-control in children so that they will be "worth something" when they grow up. However, an overemphasis on achievement can impair the child's ability to establish a separate identity apart from the parents' projected wishes. In effect, the child becomes the extension of the parents' dreams and aspirations and, as such, functions as the parents' narcissistic projection. When the goals are impossible to attain, depression, substance abuse, or an eating disorder can result. When parents overemphasize achievement, they often undercut sexual aspects of the child's development, assuming that the child who is properly occupied in learning should not have time for reflection, sexual yearning, or other forms of receptive pleasure (Yates, 1978).

A second change within the culture is the stronger emphasis on being independent (Yates, 1991a). People of the United States rank independence as the number-one value, giving it a higher ranking than do people in other developed countries. The emphasis on independence commences at an early age as the majority of infants and toddlers are placed at preschools or with sitters where they must learn to exist independently of both parents. Even at home, they are often encouraged to play by themselves so that the parents can have time to catch up on household duties or other pursuits. There are no longitudinal studies that examine the long range effect of these practices, but the extreme value placed on self-sufficiency could be expected to engender increased anxiety about dependence and difficulty in establishing mutuality. The high divorce rate, the incidence of sexual dysfunction, and the increased number of adults who choose to live alone may, in part, reflect an overemphasis on independence.

SEX EDUCATION

Sex abuse prevention programs often begin in kindergarten, while sex education programs rarely begin before the 5th grade. The sex education curriculum almost always omits controversial topics such as sexual pleasure, masturbation, and homosexuality. Many parents think that these topics are harmful or overstimulating for children. The curriculum must focus on "safe" topics, especially the dangers of sexually transmitted disease. In grade school, analogies may be used to make the material more palatable. Analogies can mislead or confuse children: eggs are seen as brittle, encased objects produced by hens, geese, and ducks; seeds are seen as the beginnings of plants growing in soil attached to the wall of the mother's stomach, watered occasionally by the father's semen (Goldman and Goldman, 1981).

Campbell (1986) reviewed more than 400 sex advice books for young people, published over the past 100 years. These volumes uniformly emphasized the danger of sex, the consequences of unintended pregnancy, the ravages of sexually transmitted disease, and problematic aspects of sexual deviance and dysfunction. Discussion of sensual pleasure was conspicuously absent. In the past decade, sex advice books have been joined by sex abuse prevention books and pamphlets. They focus on the threat of sexual abuse without normalizing masturbation, body exploration, or sex play. Frayser (1993) warns that these programs can traumatize children who have engaged in normal sex play. Prescott (1975) suggests that a literal translation of "bad touch" messages could cause children to cut themselves off from the sensual pleasures of being touched and hugged by parents. Fortunately, a few, more positive sex education programs are now available (Krivacska, 1990; Siecus, 1991), but there is some question as to how widely used they will be, given school administrators' concern about parent protest.

NORMAL SEXUAL DEVELOPMENT

The Infant

Anyone who has the opportunity to observe a suckling infant soon becomes aware that the infant's first sexual experience is with the nipple and the broader extension of the nipple, the primary caregiver. As feeding time approaches and the infant appreciates the nearness of the breast or bottle, his or her activities suddenly become organized, predictable, and goal directed: The infant inhibits crying, closes the fists, opens the mouth, searches and thrusts toward the nipple, seizes it, and sucks

vigorously. The infant's face is red, and his or her mood might best be described as anxious. When the milk comes down, the fists relax, the eyes turn up and close, and the infant's body melts to conform with the curves of the mother. Within a few moments, the anxious mood has become a peaceful, pleasurable state. The infant continues to suck, even when satiated, repetitively touching the nipple with the tongue although apparently asleep. The mother's scent, warmth, and closeness are part of this first, highly erotic experience.

As infants grow, they develop erotic interests apart from the breast and the larger dimension of mother. These interests mark the commencement of the separation individuation process. After the 12th week of life, the infant may employ the thumb as an autoerotic object. As thumb sucking does not occur in cultures where the breast is readily available to the infant, it would seem that this early diversion of sexual interest from the nipple to the thumb is precipitated by the relative unavailability of the primary caregiver in this culture (Sarlin, 1975). Although in the past, thumb sucking was thought to be associated with psychopathology, this is not the case.

Within the first 4 months of life, infants of both sexes learn to appreciate the sensations associated with diapering and the cleansing of the genitals. They adopt an anticipatory stance and demonstrate obvious enjoyment in the caregiver's touch. It is not unusual for infants to begin to play with their genitals, occasionally to the point of orgasm in the 1st year of life. Infant girls are more likely to stimulate themselves at this time (Galenson, 1993), while boys are more likely to do so in the 2nd and 3rd years of life. Infants may begin touching to explore the body and determine body boundaries, but pleasure soon becomes the primary motive (Spitz and Wolf, 1949). Self-pleasuring is under the child's direction, an autonomous activity. This confers a sense of independent identity, aiding the process of separation and individuation (Sarlin, 1975).

Anatomical differences between the male and female genitals must have far-reaching import for children's psychosexual development (Gadpaille, 1976; Kestenberg, 1968). Boys can easily identify a tangible, predictably pleasurable focus in the erect penis. The penis is visible, often has a name, and has a readily observable function. Because of this, little boys are easily able to integrate their genitals within the body concept. Boys' ability to "make it happen" is thought to foster the development of an active, acquisitive stance, task orientation, pragmatism, goal directedness, and logical thought, all of which are attributes often associated with maleness.

Girls may have difficulty in differentiating the clitoris from "dirty" areas associated with odor and excrement, especially in a culture that tends to emphasize cleanliness and control and that hides the genitals of both sexes (Yates, 1978). Kestenberg (1968) describes ordinary infant care as providing direct and indirect stimulation to the genitals via nervous and vascular connections. This prepares children for adult genitality. Because girls' genitals are hidden, their sexual experience is inwardly oriented and permeated more by purely visceral sensations than by sensations from the exterior of the body. In contrast, boys' sexual experience is outwardly oriented and focused on phallic sensations. In the absence of easy, external, male genital eroticism, females become more inwardly attentive and aware, more intuitive, expressive, and patient, but with less of the "male" pragmatism and goal directedness (Galenson, 1974; Kestenberg, 1968).

An early interest in the genitals is associated with emotional health and a positive caregiver-child relationship. Problematic infant-caregiver relationships are more likely to produce troubled infants who ruminate, rock, head bang, or evidence unusual eating behaviors such as pica. Spitz's original study of 248 infants (Spitz and Wolf, 1949) determined that genital play was completely absent in the foundling home where infants were severely deprived, was uncommon in the prison nursery where the infants received problematic care, but was generally present in the control group where the parenting was advantageous. Galenson (1974) noted the same association in her longitudinal study. Seven of the 70 mother-infant pairs demonstrated a problematic relationship. Infants in problematic relationships did not stimulate themselves, whereas the well-nurtured infants did. However, self-stimulation is not a prerequisite for healthy development as there are well-nurtured infants who have never masturbated (Kleeman, 1975) and many others who began to masturbate but were discouraged from doing so by the caregivers.

In children who are not unduly inhibited, one might expect to note a developmental progression toward adult erotic responsiveness, commencing with the highly pleasurable sensations generated by the infant-mother transaction. The developmental line would continue through the differentiation and appreciation of the genitals; incorporation of the sexual parts in the body concept; exhibitionism to "test" adult reactions; mastery of a variety of self-elicited sensations; the expansion of erotic interest to include parents, siblings, and peers; and the final integration of the genitals and genital function within the concept of the self. A developmental line such as this would be independent of, but related to, that of psychosexual development, which includes object relatedness. A separate developmental line for eroticism would explain the heightened eroticism of children who have been involved in long-term molestation (Johnson, 1993; Yates, 1982, 1991b) and the well-developed object relationships of many sexually dysfunctional adults.

The Toddler

Infant observation studies (Galenson, 1993; Galenson and Roiphe, 1976; Kleeman, 1975) indicate that infants become interested in toilets, in observing others defecate, and in sensing their own bowel movements toward the beginning of the 2nd year. This is called "anal eroticism." At the same time, youngsters become more opinionated, stubborn, and negativistic. All of these traits intensify if caregivers try to exert control. Urinary eroticism surfaces a bit later, between 12 and 14 months. At that time, children become intensely interested in faucets, hoses, and squirt balloons. In girls this may be fueled by the realization that they do not have a penis. By 15 months, most children know the difference between the sexes. This process is facilitated if the child has the opportunity to view the genitals of the other sex. Genital pride and exhibitionism are often noted (Galenson, 1974; Kleeman, 1976). Girls commonly begin to behave erotically toward their fathers at about 18 months of age. This may indicate an early identification with the mother's gender role. An admiring response from adults gives little girls confidence and pride in their femininity.

The change from genital play to intentional masturbation is a gradual, discontinuous process that extends into the 2nd year of life. Between 15 and 24 months, infants become increasingly aware of their genitals, especially during bathing and diapering (Galenson, 1974, 1993). Now, there are fewer girls than boys who self-stimulate, and they do so less vigorously, less often, and less intensely (Kleeman, 1975). Self-stimulation is accompanied by flushing, rapid breathing, and increased perspiration. At first, infants try to maintain affectionate contact with the caregiver while they self-stimulate. Adults in the United States are uncomfortable with this and tend to discourage further contact. Those children who continue to pleasure themselves do so by distancing from the parents, with glazed eyes and an inner-directed gaze. Galenson (1993) suggests that this marks the beginning of masturbatory fantasy (Galenson, 1993).

The pattern of masturbatory activity established in the 2nd year of life tends to remain constant among boys, while it undergoes a further evolution among girls (Galenson, 1973; Galenson and Roiphe, 1976). Girls more often learn to employ indirect techniques, using legs, thighs, toes, or rocking horses to self-stimulate. Girls may cease masturbation completely or they may continue to masturbate without pleasure. Frustration reactions are almost universal and sometimes severe among girls in the second half of the 2nd year. A few boys display a similar pattern. Psychoanalysts call this a preoedipal castration reaction (Roiphe and Galenson, 1973). Reactions include regression, fearfulness, loss of enthusiasm, sadness, and the displacement of masturbatory interests to other parts of the body and to inanimate objects such as dolls and fuzzy toys. Some girls become erotically interested in the father, while others

show an increase in hostile dependence on the mother. Frustration reactions seem to enhance girls' symbolic thought and internal complexity. However, the girls most severely affected may constrict their imagination and retreat emotionally. Boys show far less overt disturbance, often displacing their anxiety in physical activity.

Some 2- to 3-year-old girls show signs of penis envy. They insist that they have a penis and try to urinate standing up or hold sticks or toys in the genital area. These reactions may stem from their observations of incompleteness at a time when the genitals have a distinct narcissistic importance (Galenson and Roiphe, 1976). Boys may express the wish to grow breasts or to have babies (Edgcumbe, 1976).

In Western cultures the sexual socialization of 2-year-old children mixes issues of autonomy, separation and individuation, covering the body, toilet training, cleaning the genitals, and the avoidance of feces (Newson and Newson, 1962). Youngsters identify sexual interests as bad or dirty, just like feces. Sexual activity assumes a distinctly anal cast with superimposed concerns about control and concealment. Girls are apt to be more affected than boys because of the lack of genital differentiation. Early negative sexual attributions may be the reason why Conn (1948) could find no North American child under age 9 who thought that people had intercourse because it was pleasurable.

The Preschool Child

As children grow, their erotic interests come to include siblings and peers. Many 4-year-old children play games such as "Mommy and Daddy" or "Doctor." One-half of all preschoolers engage in sex games or masturbation (Clower, 1976; Newson and Newson, 1962). Sexual activities commonly observed in 4- to 6-year-old children include exposing and scratching the crotch, touching the genitals and exhibiting them to others, touching breasts of women (Friedrich et al., 1991), liking to be nude and look at others in the nude, and trying to put objects in the vagina or rectum (Johnson, 1993). These behaviors are more common when there is nudity in the home. After age 4, fewer girls are involved in these activities than boys (Sears et al., 1957). Children's concepts of sexuality remain primitive; many believe that the infant is born by cutting the mother's stomach open, or that the infant exits through the mother's anus (Goldman and Goldman, 1981).

The years that have been tagged as the oedipal period are marked by increased erotic interest, often focused on the parent of the opposite sex. Preschoolers have avid imaginations and they ask many questions about anatomical differences, intercourse, and reproduction (Robinson et al., 1991). Boys may wish to marry and sleep with their mothers. They may ask the mother to rub the penis because it "feels good." Three- to 5-year-old girls become highly erotic in the context of the relationship to the father. However, they are less likely to try to make genital contact and instead may attempt to achieve a sense of completion and specialness through the relationship (Roiphe and Galenson, 1973).

FATHERS' ROLE

While fathers participate less in caregiving, they participate more in playing with young children than do mothers (Flerx et al., 1976). The play patterns of fathers are far more stimulating and unconventional than the play patterns of mothers (Ablin, 1971; Lamb, 1980). When child care is shared by both parents, the children acquire more balanced and realistic images of both parents. Unfortunately, child care remains the mother's prime responsibility in the great majority of homes, whether or not she is employed outside of the home (Hochschild, 1989).

Fathers who are nurturant, dominant, and actively involved in child care are most likely to produce masculine sons and feminine daughters (Spieler, 1984). Paternal absence seems to lower the masculinity scores of sons (Mead and Rekers, 1979) and males from fatherless homes display a less successful heterosexual adjustment in adult life (Cinch, 1949). In general, the earlier the paternal deprivation, the more profound the debilitating impact on the psychosexual development of boys (Hetherington, 1971).

Girls learn to be feminine through a positive relationship with a masculine father. When fathers reject daughters, perhaps because they would prefer a son, this is a blow to girls' self-esteem and ability to relate to others (Spieler, 1984). Fathers who validate their daughters' sexual attractiveness enable them to accept themselves as sexual beings even though the concept of the genitals remains amorphous. Confirmation of sexual attractiveness, when enhanced by a firm identification with mother, can lead to a more integrated sense of self.

Fathers who are firm but supportive help daughters separate emotionally from the mother by providing an alternative role model. Girls can have trouble forming a separate sense of self if they are infantilized, overprotected, idealized, or depended upon by the mother, or if the environment appears threatening. Girls reared without fathers can have difficulty learning the feminine role. Adolescent girls reared without a father (or who have had a poor relationship with their father) become sexually active earlier and tend to have more partners (Hetherington, 1971/2). Also, girls who have known much family conflict or who are not close to their mothers are more likely to become promiscuous. Yet father absence appears less damaging to the psychosexual development of girls than it does for boys.

The School-aged Child

There is a relative decline in sexual activity at the time of entrance into grade school (Kinsey et al., 1948; Ramsey, 1943). This is the beginning of what has been called "latency," a period from 6 until puberty, when children demonstrate little overt sexual interest. Yet in the Kinsey et al. (1953) sample, 57% of males and 48% of females recalled sex play prior to puberty, with most of it occurring between ages 8 and 13. When boys are interviewed prior to puberty, 70% of them report sex play. This suggests that early sex play is often forgotten or repressed (Kinsey et al., 1948). The expression of "latency" appears to be weak at best and largely culturally determined (Kinsey et al., 1948). Even in our sexually restrictive society, children steadily increase their sexual activity from age 6 to 12 (Rutter, 1971). Five- to 15-year-old children from England, Australia, Sweden, and the United States never lose an interest in sex (Goldman and Goldman, 1982). They are keen observers and creative theoreticians.

School-aged children no longer try to touch breasts or show off the genitals but they add sexual activities such as drawing breasts or genitals on human figures, touching or comparing genitals with friends, telling dirty jokes, and watching animals breed (Johnson, 1993). The concept of "sex is dirty" is joined by "sex feels good." By age 9, a third of boys (but no girls) see enjoyment as a reason why adults engage in sexual activity (Conn, 1948).

By the time they enter grade school, youngsters know that sex play is a very bad thing to do. If caught, they are acutely embarrassed. In spite of this, many children continue to invent sex games, finding them to be both fascinating and pleasurable. The games validate the attractiveness of the body and the existence of sexual interests and activities in others (Langfeld, 1990; Yates, 1978). The games progress from brief, dyadic formats in the preschool years to more organized group games, like "Truth, Dare, or Consequences" and strip poker, among older school-aged children. Boys usually initiate these games, recruiting one or more of the less-inhibited girls.

Girls become modest about being seen naked sometime between age 4 and 6, while boys show a similar trend between 5 and 8 (Rosenfeld et al., 1984; Rosenfeld and Wasserman, 1993). Children with older siblings become modest sooner, perhaps because of role modeling or because they are more likely to be teased for being naked. Soon after they enter school, children learn to toilet separately and not to be seen naked by the other sex. By 4th or 5th grade, children are extremely embarrassed if their underwear shows at all.

Parents become more modest as their children grow older. It is uncommon for mothers to bathe with sons who are older than 8 years of age or for fathers to bathe or shower with daughters older than 9 years

of age (Rosenfeld et al., 1987). Children interpret parents' modesty as a message that there is something intrinsically bad or dirty about the body. This concept persists indefinitely, affecting how they parent their own children when they grow up (Rosenfeld et al., 1984; Wake, 1969).

Parents

Most upper SES parents respond to children's sexual activities by warning, chastising, scolding, and employing nonverbal persuaders such as averting the eyes, closing doors, and avoiding sexual topics (Finkelhor, 1980). They often mislabel or do not label children's sexual activities. Fathers seldom participate in sexual training. Discussions about sex are most likely to occur between mothers and daughters, and these discussions center on menstruation or the negative aspects of premarital intercourse (Gagnon and Simon, 1973). Sixty-four percent of adolescent boys and 33% of adolescent girls report that neither parent has spoken to them about any aspect of sex and even fewer talk about intercourse or masturbation. Eighty-five to 95% of parents state that they have *never* mentioned any aspect of erotic behavior to their children (Gagnon and Simon, 1973).

Children are most likely to learn about sex from same-sex peers (Gebhard, 1977). They are more likely to learn about sex from reading materials and teachers than they are from their parents (Thornberg, 1972). However, the situation is improving in that they are learning sooner than did their parents and grandparents. This seems to be because mothers are trying harder to sex educate, because there is more sex education in the schools, and because more sexual material is presented in the media.

In a survey of more than 1000 parents, Gagnon (Gagnon and Simon, 1973) found that not one parent had named the little girl's clitoris. Parents postponed discussions about sex again and again. When they did occur, they were limited to safe topics such as love, pregnancy, and the physical differences between males and females. Risky topics such as masturbation, intercourse, and homosexuality were almost never mentioned. Parents (and others) communicate strong nonverbal sanctions against male homosexuality to children. Boys are systematically discouraged from touching, kissing, or hugging other males (Gagnon and Simon, 1973). On the playground and in the schoolyard, "queer" and "fag" are common taunts. Youngsters may not fully comprehend the meaning but understand that the words mean something dirty, bad, and sexual.

There are class differences in the way in which parents rear their children. Professional and upper SES parents are relatively open and accepting of their children's sexuality (Sears et al., 1957). Upper SES mothers are more apt to neutralize their children's sexual interest by bringing the issues out into the open, while working-class mothers simply suppress these interests and try to keep the children ignorant. Upper SES parents may watch children closely and distract them from sexual interests, whereas working-class parents will punish children for sexual curiosity, as if it were a powerful force that needed to be controlled. Upper SES mothers view guilt as unhealthy, whereas working-class mothers try to instill guilt in their children as a form of control (Newson and Newson, 1962).

Despite increasing flexibility in roles and activities considered permissible for adults of both sexes, there is evidence that traditional sex role stereotypes are intact (Flerx et al., 1976). Most children's books continue to portray males and females in the traditional manner and children in therapy continue to choose toys according to their gender. The stability of children's sex roles may be related to the stability of parental roles within the home, with mothers continuing to assume major responsibility for cooking and cleaning.

The Adolescent

At age 6–8, adrenal androgen secretion increases, reaching a peak in midadolescence (Nottelman et al., 1990). This paves the way for a sharp rise in gonadotropin-induced hormone production between 9 and 13 years of age (Fitschen and Clayton, 1965; McCandless, 1960). The testosterone level reached by male adolescents is 8 times that reached by females (Udry et al., 1986). The higher level of androgens in males triggers a striking increase in eroticism (Money, 1961). The free testosterone index becomes the single strongest predictor of sexual motivation and behavior (Udry et al., 1985; Udry and Billy, 1987). Boys become intensely embarrassed due to the persistence and recurrence of sexual thoughts and penile erections.

Girls enter puberty approximately 2 years earlier than boys. They complete their changes in 3 or 4 years, while boys take 4 or 5 years. Menarche in girls is marked by an increase in estradiol, which reaches adult levels by age 19. There is a lag in progesterone secretion, so that anovulatory cycles are common in the 1st 2 years after menarche. Adrenal androgens increase around the time of puberty and they are erotogenic in the female, but the levels are lower than in the male. In pubescent girls, hormones exert only a weak effect on sexual behavior, but a stronger effect on motivation (Smith et al., 1985).

Boys who reach puberty late tend to be less popular, less assertive, and less confident, but eager, talkative, and attention seeking (McCandless, 1960; Sorensen, 1973). They tend to have problems with self-esteem because of associated deficiencies in muscle mass, athletic prowess, and sexual striving, all of which are highly regarded for males in Western culture. Girls are more variable in their response to the signs of maturation. Some early-maturing girls are embarrassed by breast enlargement and some late-maturing girls are relieved not to have begun to menstruate sooner (McCandless, 1960). In any case, the commencement of menstruation is an important marker in the life of a girl, establishing her identification with her mother and her maturity. If girls insert tampons, this may be the first time they are aware of, or touch, the inside of the vagina (Whisnant et al., 1979).

A real crisis occurs with the biological changes of adolescence. Incestuous and bisexual conflicts are revived and sexual orientation becomes a central issue. Many boys and girls engage in homosexual behavior even though they are heterosexually oriented. Same sex peer contacts are readily available while heterosexual contacts are not. Homosexual activities are even more common at boarding schools, at camp, and in other circumstances in which same-sex individuals live together.

The average age of first intercourse is 16.2 for girls and 15.7 for boys in the United States at present (Wyatt, 1990; Zelnik and Shah, 1983). Twice as many black adolescents have intercourse before age 15 as white adolescents, and 61% of low income black males report initiating intercourse prior to puberty (Zabin et al., 1986). Among whites, girls tend to look for a romantic relationship, while boys seek a sexual adventure. Most first sexual liaisons are spur of the moment events that take place at the home of the girl or her partner. The two usually have known each other for some time and are going steady. Girls are serious about the relationship while boys tend to see it as casual (Whatley et al., 1989). After initiating intercourse, girls commonly avoid coitus for an extended period of time. Males, also, tend to have few partners and long periods of abstinence (Sonnenstein et al., 1991).

The number of sexually active girls increased from 1971 through 1979 but decreased in 1982 (Hofferth, 1990). In 1988, adolescent boys were having intercourse less frequently and with fewer partners than they had in 1979 (Sonnenstein et al., 1991). In the 1980s, more adolescents identified promiscuity as immoral than had done so in the 1960s or 1970s (Robinson et al., 1991; Sugar, 1993). Most girls who have had sex think that it was wrong, and they wish that they had remained a virgin until they were married (Coles and Stokes, 1985). Two-thirds of the boys and girls who masturbate feel guilty and ashamed about doing so. They view it as bad, dirty, and a sign of moral weakness. They are actively trying to restrain themselves (Yates, 1993).

Adolescents who feel close to their parents and share the parents' values are less likely to have sex at an early age (Fox, 1981; Jessor and Jessor, 1975; Shah and Zelnik, 1981). When parents control dating, adolescents are less likely to initiate intercourse or become pregnant (Hogan and Kitigawa, 1985). This reflects the fact that early and frequent dating commonly precedes the first sexual experience (Thorton, 1990). Adolescents who view their parents as "moderately strict" are less likely to have sexual experience (Miller et al., 1986)

Adolescent contraceptive use has improved over the past two decades, but many youth never or rarely use it (Santelli and Beilenson, 1992). In the United States, adolescents initiate intercourse at about the same age as teens in Western Europe and Canada, but they are more likely to become pregnant (Jones et al., 1985). Compared with Sweden, Australia, and England, North American 15-year-olds, especially girls, develop their contraceptive knowledge late (Goldman and Goldman, 1981). There are many reasons why adolescents do not use contraception: for boys this is commonly related to the drive to prove themselves or "to score" quickly when the opportunity presents. In the heat of passion, contraceptive measures seem irrelevant. Boys often view contraception as the girl's responsibility. Both sexes are highly unrealistic about the girl's chances of becoming pregnant. No contraceptive use in girls is related to a lack of planning to have sex. Having sex is something that happens to them because they are overtaken or persuaded by the male or because they are in love and powerless to resist. To plan to have sex makes the sexual act seem immoral for many teenage girls. Unfortunately, girls who don't plan to have sex are much less likely to use contraception at first intercourse (Zelnik and Shah, 1983).

Adolescents who have low self-expectations for achievement, lesser ability, and poorer grades in school are more likely to have sex at an early age (Abrahamse et al., 1988; Hofferth, 1987; Robbins et al., 1985). These students are more tolerant of deviance and tend to have friends who role model deviance. These results are stronger at the high school than at the college level and stronger for females than for males (Jessor and Jessor, 1975). Early sexual activity has also been linked to other risk taking behaviors such as delinquency, smoking, and drug or alcohol abuse (Rosenbaum and Kandel, 1990; Orr et al., 1991). On the other hand, Gadpaille (1975) notes that a significant number of sexually active adolescents are emotionally mature by the most well-accepted criteria.

One third of all abortions are performed on adolescents (Santelli and Beilenson, 1992). Girls are more likely to opt for an abortion if they are younger, doing well in school, and planning for the future, and have better educated parents, less religious involvement, and friends with negative attitudes toward pregnancy (Hofferth, 1987). When an adolescent girl becomes pregnant and does not have an abortion, this may be related to her need to remain close to her own mother, rebellion against the parents, self-destructive or self-defeating tendencies, guilt and religious convictions, the need to be loved by an infant, and/or the fear of entering dating, vocational, or educational arenas. Unfortunately, the culture tends to view the unmarried pregnant teen as "getting what she deserved" (for having had sex).

ADOLESCENT EROTICISM

Lower SES males view masturbation as unmanly and they are less likely than upper SES males to fantasize during masturbation (Gagnon and Simon, 1973). Although masturbation is more acceptable for upper SES males, it is commonly accompanied by guilt and anxiety (Kinsey et al., 1948). In adolescence, boys are much more open about genital masturbation than are girls. Prior to age 15, 80% of the boys and 20% of the girls have masturbated (Kinsey et al., 1948, 1953). More recent data indicate that 24% of adolescent girls masturbate (Coles and Stokes, 1985).

Because masturbation acts as a self-regulator for sexual and aggressive tensions, genital excitation is commonly accompanied by fantasy. The content of the fantasy may remain unconscious or be expressed in disguised form through daydreams, games, or patterns of relatedness (Freud, 1965). The fantasy often reflects the wish to remain a child and the desire to assume the adult role (Moore, 1975). Healthy adolescents have a masturbation fantasy that includes the seeking of a sexual partner. In the fantasy they are, at least partially, in control. The less-healthy adolescent, who is incapable of warding off the regressive pull of pregenital wishes, may experience the central masturbation fantasy as overwhelming. The fantasy may give rise to a feeling of deadlock, followed by a sense of giving in and then surrender (Laufer, 1968).

Male adolescent fantasies are usually explicit and aggressive; they tend to focus sexual desire on the genitals. In girls, autoerotic activities are much less open and less likely to be accompanied by conscious fantasy. Girls often feel that they are living two lives, one of which is secret and little recognized. Unlike boys, girls do not accord the genitals a central position; genital priority occurs at a far later date if at all (Lamb, 1980). Even girls who have masturbated to orgasm do not describe the genitalia themselves as sources of pleasure. If orgasm occurs, it is something that happens ''down there'' (Gagnon and Simon, 1973). The girl's masturbation fantasy emphasizes romantic and affectionate aspects and often contains pregenital exhibitionistic, sadomasochistic, and narcissistic themes (Moore, 1975).

In both sexes, fantasies become more realistic and more explicit with age. Sixty percent of adolescent females report being different from their real selves in their fantasies, as opposed to 32% of males. Women's responses indicate a deep preoccupation with appearance-related concerns. Half report that they are prettier in their fantasies and 23% imagine themselves thinner (Kirkendall and McBride, 1990). A majority of adult women report that concerns about their physical appearance interfere with their sexual response.

Sexually active university students struggle with sexual dysfunctions, inhibitions, lack of desire, guilt, and fear (Darling and Davidson, 1986; Yates, 1993). Sexually active women students are unlikely to experience orgasm. Only 28% say they are satisfied. Eleven percent of male students experience erectile dysfunction and 20% have premature ejaculation (Miller and Cirone, 1978). Fifty-five percent of students say that they are afraid to have intercourse, and 44% doubt if there is such a thing as safe sex. Eleven percent indicate that they have an ''abnormal'' fear of sex (Katz et al., 1989). Women students are more anxious about the social consequences of having sex while men are more worried about disease (Darling and Davidson, 1986). Students are disturbed by these problems but rarely seek help because of shame and embarrassment.

Conclusion

In this culture, sexual development is clearly problematic. The prevailing assumption, that children are innocent and need to be protected against sexual knowledge and activity, has far-reaching implications. Consequences may include the embarrassment of 6-year-old children who inadvertently show their underwear; the guilt experienced by adolescents who masturbate; the anorgasmia of adolescent girls; the fear, sexual anxiety, and frustration of adolescent boys; and the reluctance of all adolescents to ask for help.

Accurate information is essential, if we are to deal constructively with something as basic as sexuality. Children's erotic development should be directly assessed, by explicit question and objective measurement. Data must be analyzed in terms of culture, social class, family, identification, and socialization. This information should be used to generate clinically based standards of expectable sexual interests, attitudes, and behaviors. Then, subjects should be periodically reassessed through adolescence and into maturity. The data should yield correlates and predictors of adult sexual function and dysfunction. Information such as this would finally allow us to move beyond the concept of childhood innocence toward programs of primary prevention.

THEORIES OF SEXUAL DEVELOPMENT

Desire

Since Freud's early emphasis on the libido, there has been little further development of the concept of sexual energy or desire. In part, this is because of defects in the libido theory (Freud, 1947, 1961), in particular the postulate that each individual is born with a finite amount

of sexual energy available. Once the energy is discharged, the motivation or readiness to act again is minimal. This theory fails to explain a great many phenomena, such as the fact that penile erection is not dependent upon the expectation of ejaculation or orgasm (Whalen, 1966) or that many individuals are more likely to engage in sex if they have been so engaged the day before and are less likely to have coitus if they have been abstinent (Barnett, 1963).

With a few exceptions (Greenacre, 1950; Kestenberg, 1968), analytic writers since Freud have not emphasized the sensual or erotic component of development. The libido has usually been characterized as a facilitator of identification. Even the concept of narcissism has largely lost its erotic connotation. Recently, however, there have been reports by Kleeman (1976), Galenson (1993), and Roiphe and Galenson (1973) that emphasize the erotic component in psychosexual development. In contrast to many analytic writers, the sex therapists Masters and Johnson (1966) and Kaplan (1979) emphasize desire as a critical factor in sexual function; however, they do not address the interrelationships of desire and personality development. A further integration of the two disciplines could lead to a better understanding of the development of eroticism in childhood and, eventually, to methods of primary prevention of adult sexual dysfunction.

The concept of an inherent drive or desire is important; it may be that some individuals have more sexual energy, or energy in general, available from the time of birth. Sexual energy may be simply one component of the overall activity level. Activity level is largely genetically determined (Plomin, 1986). Some infants are extremely active and some are passive and inhibited from the very beginning. Kagan et al. (1984) have described a group of behaviorally inhibited children who seem to be at risk to develop an anxiety disorder later on. Inactive and/or inhibited children might demonstrate lower levels of desire, in which case they would be more likely to suffer from an inhibited sexual desire disorder later on.

Clearly, the vast majority of individuals experience ample sexual desire and ability if they are reared in social, cultural, and family circumstances conducive to the expression of sexuality. The regulation of the drive in the human being is complex. Arousal depends on factors such as the context in which arousal is experienced, the quality of the object relatedness, the individual's intrapsychic state, and prior experiences that may have enhanced, inhibited, or distorted his or her sexual expression (Rutter, 1971). Desire also may be inhibited by depression, stress, drugs, and medical illness.

Theoretical Bases

The four major schools—cognitive-developmental, social learning, analytic, and biologic—sometimes seem to contradict one another. However, they become remarkably synergistic when used to understand the interplay of forces in a given individual. Each theory contributes a unique understanding of the development of human behavior (Maier, 1965). Analytic theory ascribes behavior to a struggle between internal forces; cognitive-developmental theory ascribes behavior to an encounter between the individual's cognitive world and the reality of the outside environments; learning theory ascribes behavior to the interplay of stimulus and response as the child progresses through a series of dyadic interactions (Bennett, 1976); biologic theory addresses the relationship between genetic givens and environmental influences. Clearly, these are all fundamental aspects of human development. It would require all four theoretical approaches, for instance, to explain why sex education makes a difference for some individuals and not for others, why a long-term sexual molestation in the formative years can lead some individuals to prostitution while others become responsible and productive community members, or why children raised by homosexuals or transsexuals overwhelmingly choose a heterosexual, conventional life-style for themselves (Green, 1978b).

A boy reared in this culture by a puritanical father and a liberal mother, who watches the Playboy channel at a friend's house but who is beaten at home for having a copy of *Hustler* under the mattress, who is urged by his friends to score as soon as possible, who is called a "fag" when he disagrees, who learns in school about the inevitability of death from AIDS, and who sees his sister struggling to rear an out-of-wedlock child after having been expelled from home for her sinfulness, must indeed be confused about sexuality. No one theory can explain this child's ability or inability to function sexually when he becomes an adult.

COGNITIVE-DEVELOPMENTAL THEORY

Piaget (1950; Piaget and Inhelder, 1950) traced the learning process from egocentric reasoning to socialized thought. This process is fueled by the child's delight in mastery and pleasure in repeating the process. Repetitive behavioral sequences lead to learning and then to internal change. Development is intrinsically motivated and interactive from birth onward.

According to cognitive-developmental theory (Kohlberg, 1966; Piaget, 1950; Piaget and Inhelder, 1958), the child first learns to discriminate between the male and female genders through the formation of sexual schemas. This leads to the establishment of a cognitive self-categorization of male or female at around age 5. The child then identifies with certain stereotypic aspects of the prescribed gender role. These sex-typed interests, attitudes, and values expand because of the spontaneous tendency to value "like self" entities, including the same-sex parent. However, at age 5 the child thinks dichotomously, is relatively rigid in approach, and is unable to consider individual differences. Therefore, the child's initial adoption of sex-role tends to be simplistic and exaggerated. At about age 8, the child is able to selectively internalize properties of the parent. When this occurs, the child can form a more flexible and individualized identification, selecting from role models those qualities that seem to fit existing schemata. A number of studies (Meyer, 1980) tend to support this progression from a rigid, stereotypic view of gender role to a more flexible, individualized approach. An interesting facet of this is that television seems to transmit sex role stereotypes to younger children, whereas older children grow away from these overly restrictive characterizations (Beuf, 1974; Freud and McGhee, 1975).

Adolescents gain the ability to think abstractly. Now, they are able to reevaluate their gender role in the context of individual and cultural values and a reappraisal of significant role models. A notable modification can ensue. Sometimes a process called counter-modeling (Simmons and Turner, 1976) occurs, whereby the adolescent may drastically change attitudes and goals in the opposite direction. For instance, an adolescent girl with a low opinion of her mother, who happens to be a housewife, may decide to become a career woman (Callagan, 1981).

SOCIAL LEARNING THEORY

The social learning theory of Sears (Sears et al., 1957) and Mischel (1966) views the developmental process as one in which children relate sequentially to the social environment, increasing the ability to communicate with others and to obtain gratification for socialized behavior. Each new acquisition builds upon a previous one. The additive process gradually shapes children's future. Progress depends on the character of the dyadic interactions between children and their caregivers, as child development is the visible product of the parents' child-rearing efforts (Maier, 1965). Presumably adults could mold children in whatever direction they wished by providing specific social experiences.

Learning theory regards sexual differences as important only to the extent that they affect children's immediate environment, which will in turn affect the child. Parents respond differently to male and to female infants as they reinforce sex-typed behavior. Later on, children learn that they are boys or girls and that various characteristics are assigned to each sex. Children choose models with whom to identify, based on the satisfactions derived from previously positive experiences. Identification with the parent of the same sex occurs in the preschool years. The process of identification becomes the basis for the adoption of sex

role stereotypes. Role stereotypes are then reinforced by the appropriate behavior of powerful and respected adults. Parents, as social agents, should model the kind of behavior that reflects competency and that will be rewarded as children grow. Each successful identification provides the potential for renewed and improved identifications on a higher social level. Thus, identification is the product of children's search for continuing satisfaction in keeping with their past experiences. Learning theory views gender identity and sex role stereotypes as outcomes rather than as integral parts of a process.

Social learning theory allows for continuing flexibility in identification and sex role orientation. If social reinforcements or contingencies change, the identification could change also. Spontaneous changes in identification have been described in adolescence, especially when there has not been a good relationship with the same-sex parent (Callagan, 1981).

ANALYTIC THEORY

Freud did not distinguish between sex and gender. In his writings, the two concepts were so closely interrelated as to be indistinguishable. Freud described the libido as the genetically based foundation of personality development, a driving force that was apparent in infancy and at every subsequent stage of development, existing regardless of environmental influences (Kohlberg, 1966).

Oral Phase

Libido or drive is first directed toward the mother's breast but then toward other aspects of the relationship with mother as she teaches the child to love. This becomes the prototype of all later object relationships. The relationship to the mother enables the infant to begin the pleasurable process of defining body boundaries and establishing genital awareness (Tyson, 1982). Thus, the concept of an oral stage refers to many more and various transactions than those involving the mouth. The term *oral stage* is somewhat misleading in suggesting that oral behaviors are the only or even the most important focus of this stage of life (Rutter, 1971).

Narcissism was originally defined as a perversion in which the individual withdrew from relationships, investing all libidinal energies in the self (Freud, 1957). Autoerotic activities were indicative of narcissism. It now seems clear that high self-regard does not preclude a high regard for objects (Dare and Holder, 1981). In fact, narcissism seems to be a prerequisite for sexual enjoyment and (to a lesser extent) the sexual response. Narcissism is now defined as the positive affect associated with self-experience that subsequently becomes part of the self-representation (Kohut, 1971). If children have good feelings about the self, including the genitals, and have been able to integrate these feelings into the emerging ego, they will approach sexual encounters in later life expecting to be valued and expecting to be gratified.

Anal Phase

According to analytic theory, the 2nd and 3rd years of life comprise the anal stage, during which libidinal energies are directed toward anal and urinary functions. Ambivalence and aggression, struggle for autonomy and control, are hallmarks of this phase. Children do not want to obey Mother but are terrified of losing her. They derive enormous pleasure and a sense of power from retaining the stool and from expelling it. Urination is regularly associated with genital arousal. It is at this juncture that toilet training often begins; this sets up potential conflicts and the possibility of fixation at the anal stage. There may be diarrhea or constipation, resistance to diaper changing, considerable interest in the stool, and concern about what happens when it is flushed down the toilet.

Phallic Phase

According to Freudian analytic theory, the phallic stage extends from age 4 to age 6. Because boys and girls become intensely interested in the genitals as a source of pleasure and excitement in this phase, it might be more correctly termed the ''genital'' phase. Little boys may approach little girls to play ''Mommy and Daddy,'' and little girls enjoy rubbing the genitals against knees, bedposts, and rocking horses. Freud was correct in describing an increase in genital interest during the preschool years.

Freud may not have been correct about the timing of the phallic or genital phase. Galenson and Roiphe (1976) have directly observed the emergence of earlier genital awareness, following anal and urinary awareness, sometime between the 15th and 19th month of life. This begins with repetitive genital self-stimulation and the visual and tactual exploration of the genitals. This is followed by the emergence of genital derivative behavior. In girls this consists of undressing dolls, examining the crotch, and sometimes using the dolls for masturbation or placement at the genital area. Boys begin to use ''phallic'' toys such as cars and trucks. Boys strut and appear proud of their genitals, while girls become flirtatious and lift their skirts. However, the exhibitionism is in order to gain approval and admiration rather than to seduce the parent. This stage seems to usher in the awareness of genital differences.

Freud's (1961) view of penis envy was essentially a deficiency theory by which girls envied the male organ and sought, in one way or another, to gain masculine power for themselves. Freud witnessed the beginning of the women's movement, which he saw as one example of this phenomenon. Galenson and Roiphe (1976) believe that Freud's original position regarding women was correct in that penis envy and the castration complex critically influence development. More recent extensions of analytic theory tend to see penis envy more as a function of the little girl's hostility toward the mother, with whom she is identified, and an attempt to regain a sense of bodily integrity. If the mother-child relationship is poor, the lack of a penis may come to represent the child's inadequacy and vulnerability (Tyson, 1982).

Oedipus Complex

The Oedipus complex refers to the child's attachment to the parent of the opposite sex and hostility to the parent of the same sex. The Oedipus complex is resolved when the child identifies with the parent of the same sex. Boys traverse the Oedipus complex differently from girls. The boy's hostile rivalry with his father is a natural outcome of his earlier erotic attachment to his mother. The boy sees himself as his father's competitor and begins to project his own hostility on his father. This frightens the boy and leads to castration anxiety. He then chooses safety and the narcissistic cathexis of his penis over the libidinal cathexis to his mother. Renouncing his mother, he identifies with his father, thus resolving the oedipal conflict. This eventuates in superego formation, the internalization of paternal authority, and the repression of sexual impulses. According to Freud, masculinity is an innate, instinctual striving, that is not dependent upon the boy's identification with his father.

In classic analytic theory, the girl also enters the oedipal period upon discovering the anatomical distinction between boys and girls. On observing her genitalia, she assumes that she has been castrated and that she is inferior. For the rest of her life she will suffer from penis envy. She holds her mother responsible for the inadequacies of her equipment and turns to her father in an attempt to acquire a penis. Later she learns that this is impossible and wishes instead to have her father's baby as a form of compensation. According to Freud, the girl's inevitable sense of inferiority leads to such traits as passivity, masochism, and narcissism. Freud was unable to formulate the final solution to the Oedipus complex for women. He thought that the conscience was formed differently in women, not out of castration anxiety but from the fear of loss of love. He thought that penis envy would remain at the center of the female psyche, whereas castration anxiety would be the central determinant for the male.

The negative Oedipus complex exists when a child, more often a girl, retreats from the oedipal conflict rather than resolving it. In this case, her drive development and object relationships resemble in all

respects those of the boy in his (positive) oedipal phase (Edgcumbe, 1976). This may occur if the child is bound too closely to one parent or is frightened of either parent, when the father is unresponsive, or when the mother is not a suitable model. For instance, a girl may take tentative steps toward her father but then become terrified of her mother's wrath. The mother may be enraged at her daughter's apparent independence, or the daughter may perceive her as angry because of her own dependence and inability to separate. In this case the girl must negotiate her relationship with the mother in order to continue to develop.

Freud failed to consider the preoedipal importance of the father (Spieler, 1984). If the little girl finds that her father is reliable, available, attuned, and nurturant, she is likely to acquire a predominantly favorable mental representation (Jacobson, 1964), which can provide her with the incentive to relinquish her preoedipal attachments. If she is frightened by the father, she may not express her emerging oedipal eroticism toward him. She may feel abandoned by him on the one hand while clinging desperately to his idealized image on the other.

Projective techniques have produced age-specific findings that tend to support Freud's oedipal theory (Freidman, 1952). However, some children present an oedipal pattern of relationships at age 5 and some do not. The existence of the Oedipal complex depends upon family relationships characteristic of that particular culture (Honigman, 1957). Thus the Oedipus complex does seem to exist, but it is far from universal and it is not due to any innate predisposition (Rutter, 1971).

Latency

According to Freudian theory, the latency period exists from age 6 until puberty. Castration anxiety, the resolution of the Oedipus complex, and the formation of the superego cause children to repress their sexual interests. Freud's assumption that latency was biologically based has been proven false (Money, 1961).

Numerous sociological studies have contradicted the existence of latency in this and in other cultures. In this culture there is a steady increase in children's sexual interests and covert activities between ages 6 and 12 (Bennett, 1976). Children reared in more liberal cultures remain sexually interested and active throughout childhood (Honigman, 1957).

Adolescence. According to traditional psychoanalytic theory, adolescence is ushered in by a period of regression in which youths relive the oedipal conflict. Anna Freud (1958) viewed almost all youngsters as developmentally disturbed at this time. They were said to experience increased egocentricity and concern about sexual urges and the developing body parts. While in the throes of ''adolescent turmoil,'' they might qualify as conduct disordered, neurotic, or even psychotic. Early adolescence was regarded as a transitory, necessary phase that paved the way for a more mature organization in later adolescence. Through the loosening of inner structures, adolescents were able to redefine the self so that they could begin to face the basic life tasks of loving and working.

Early adolescents do regress, and they do have many sexual concerns. However, most adolescents do not reach a level of disturbance that would qualify as ''adolescent turmoil.'' Several longitudinal studies of normal adolescents indicate that about two-thirds of adolescent males do not demonstrate any significant psychopathology during the adolescent years, although in early adolescence they may break rules and bicker with their parents (Offer and Offer, 1975; Rutter et al., 1976). In middle and late adolescence, they are able to relate to their parents and they hold ideologically similar views. In addition, studies by Masterson (1967, 1968) indicate that when adolescents present with significant psychopathology, they are likely to continue to manifest the same pathologies in early adult life, but at that time they tend to fall into certain well-defined disorders that are apt to persist into later adult life (Strober et al., 1981).

Blos (1967) views adolescence as a process of disengagement from the internalized representations of the parents so that other relationships can be formed. In order to do this, youths must distance themselves and abandon their belief in parental omnipotence. They may vigorously test parental authority and search frantically for substitute attachment figures. The search, and the inevitable disillusionments that follow, pave the way for fresh internalizations and further maturation. However, adolescents also experience a persistent need to be cared for by the parents. This triggers fear of regressive engulfment, leading to a renewed quest for autonomy.

Establishing independence in adolescence means far more than moving out of the parents' house. It means gaining autonomy from inordinate control from within by internalized objects. Attitudes and standards assimilated in the early years remain potent determinants of self-esteem and the ego ideal. This causes some adolescents to strive for perfection and to be harshly self-critical. If they are unable to measure up, they feel defeated and inadequate (Blos, 1954). Others externalize conflicts, making the environment responsible. They may attack the value systems of the parents or the culture. This can result in heightened idealism and patriotism as well as promiscuity, delinquency, and attacks on authority (Lustman, 1971).

Males and females follow a somewhat different developmental path in adolescence. Girls are more likely to become eating disordered or depressed and boys are more likely to drink or be delinquent. Girls are thought to have a more difficult process of separation and individuation from the mother because of blurring of boundaries between mothers and daughters or because mothers may project their hopes and dreams on daughters (Blos, 1983). As adolescent girls attempt to resist the profound regressive need for the mother, they may turn passionately to the other sex.

Biologic Theory

Gender identity is the primary identification an individual establishes with one sex. *Gender role*, on the other hand, describes culturally underwritten behavior that differentiates males from females, such as game and work preferences, social aggression, and courtship and sexual behavior. *Sexual orientation* describes the individual's erotic preference for a particular sex. Individuals are not necessarily consonant in all three dimensions; any variation from all maleness or all femaleness does not necessarily connote pathology.

GENDER IDENTITY

The human infant is born with a bias toward a certain gender identity, one that usually matches the genital or anatomical sex. The differentiation of the external genitalia depends on the presence or absence of systemic androgen, more specifically dihydrotestosterone, the 5-α-reduced metabolite of testosterone (Wilson et al., 1981). The emergence of male gender differentiation appears to be related to the organizing influence of fetal gonadal androgens on the hypothalamus, the preoptic area, and the amygdala during the 6th to the 12th week of fetal development. This depends upon the presence of the embryonic testis. If the gonads are removed before the 8th week of fetal development, the embryo will develop as a female (Jost, 1953). At birth, testosterone levels are elevated in boys, and estradiol levels are elevated in both boys and girls. Estradiol levels drop quickly after birth. In boys, testosterone begins to decline after 6 months to the prepubertal range.

The development of gender identity in humans is primarily influenced by the environment: the assignment of sex by the parents and the differential responses accorded to male and to female children in the first years of life (Money and Tucker, 1975). Core gender identity is set before the end of the 2nd year of life, in that sex reassignment after age 3 is associated with serious psychological disturbance. Gender role typically crystallizes at age 4–5 and, compared to gender identity, remains somewhat malleable. Contradictory behavioral manifestations due to prenatal hormonal influences can be accommodated within the male or the female gender identity as long as the child's physical appearance is gender appropriate and the parents are not unduly confused or conflicted in their approach to the gender chosen for the child. Decisions concerning assignment need to be based on the presence and adequacy of

the genitals, the expected social and sexual functioning, and the parent's preferences. The assignment should avoid, as far as possible, the development of a gender-incongruent physique. An important consideration in choosing a female gender for a child with ambiguous genitalia is that it is far easier for the surgeon to construct a vagina than to construct a functional phallus.

When individuals change their gender identity, this seems to be precipitated by the individual's appreciation of a difference between his or her physical appearance, including the genitals, and the already assigned and accepted gender (Sagarin, 1975). Changes in gender identity are more likely when the child rearing has been ambiguous and when there have been conflicts about gender identity and role. As this society now permits androgenous behavior in both sexes, there probably will be more individuals who change their gender identity in the future.

Gender Role

Biological factors play a role in the existence and persistence of sex-specific traits (Gadpaille, 1983). These traits contribute to typical or atypical gender role behaviors. Across almost all cultures, men are more aggressive and more likely to fight one another than women (Piacente, 1986; Symons, 1979). Men have the highest status and are the best hunters. Men almost always are dominant: in a great many cultures men can have more than one spouse, but it is rare for women to be able to do so (Harlow and Harlow, 1962). Men are more likely to be jealous and possessive. Women's sex-specific traits include wanting to care for and teach children. Women are more likely to be modest and to cover their genitals (Ford and Beach, 1951).

Men and women perceive their environment in a different manner and they process information by different modes. Women's mode tends to be expressive or emotional while men's mode is instrumental or goal oriented. This may have to do with women's greater propensity for verbal and affective communication and men's logical, analytic, and spatial abilities. This could be related to male fetal development. Higher testosterone levels in the male fetus foster a delay in right hemisphere development with greater left hemispheric specialization (Geschwind, 1983).

The expression of gender role may be influenced by prenatal hormones. In a study based on the blind ratings of teachers of boys who had or had not been prenatally exposed to female hormones, the exposed 6-year-olds were found to be significantly more assertive and athletically coordinated (Yalom et al., 1971). Girls with congenital adrenal hyperplasia or progestin-induced hermaphroditism expend higher levels of energy in rough outdoor play and are less interested in doll play and infant care (Ehrhardt and Baker, 1974). Boys' sex role expression may be similarly influenced by a prenatal androgen deficiency (Ehrhardt and Meyer-Bahlberg, 1981). Boys exposed to antiandrogens early in their fetal existence seem to display lower energy levels, less aggression, and less heterosexual activity in adolescence. Girls exposed to antiandrogens prenatally appear more traditionally feminine than normal controls. However, in spite of these positive findings, there is a vast literature that is not only confusing but also reveals many negative findings about the effects of prenatal exposure to hormones. It would seem, except in the most unusual cases, that the influence prenatal hormones exert on the developing organism is much less than the influence of the environment, whether this is translated to the child by social learning or through dynamic, intrapsychic forces.

Sexual Orientation

Sexual orientation refers to an individual's overall sexual responsiveness to men and/or women (Meyer-Bahlberg, 1993). Sexual orientation has four components: (*a*) imagery (daydreams, masturbation fantasies, etc.); (*b*) use of erotica, such as magazines; (*c*) erotic attraction; and (*d*) actual partner experience. Homosexuality is not a disorder of gender identity. Homosexuality is an orientation that is usually, but not always, constant throughout life, although various degrees of bisexuality are common. However, there are societies where virtually all males are at first exclusively homosexual and then convert to become primarily heterosexual (Herdt, 1981). This attests to the plasticity of sexual orientation and the enormous adaptability of the human organism.

Homosexual adult men describe themselves as having felt different from their same sex peers in early childhood. Often accused of being sissies, they were relatively uninterested in sports. Lesbian women report having felt less feminine and less beautiful. Two-thirds of homosexuals give a history of gender atypical behavior such as a preference for female toys or cross-dressing from early childhood (Bell et al., 1981; Whitam and Zent, 1984). Boys in treatment because of gender atypical behavior often grow up to become homosexual (Green, 1987). Homosexual males usually become aware of homoerotic fantasies in early adolescence, when they are likely to experience considerable conflict and confusion (Cass, 1984; Yates, 1983). Seventy-five percent experience a mixture of heterosexual and homosexual arousal (Bell et al., 1981). It is not until early adult life that most of them identify themselves as homosexual (Troiden, 1989). That this is indeed a difficult transition is shown by the fact that gay youth account for almost a third of all adolescent suicides. Homosexual youth also are more likely than heterosexual youth to drop out of school (Remafedi, 1987).

Some researchers have speculated that homosexuality in males could be due to lower plasma testosterone levels. Genetic males who are insensitive to androgen are attracted to men, but they have usually been raised as girls and have feminine appearing genitals (Masica et al., 1971). Investigations in this area have yielded largely negative results; sexual orientation in males is not correlated with the androgen/estrogen balance in adolescence or adulthood (Green, 1978a). This area is less clear-cut in regard to female homosexuals; about one-third of lesbians show elevated levels of testosterone (Gartrell et al., 1977), although the levels are well below the male range (Meyer-Bahlberg, 1982). Dorner et al. (1991) suggest that these findings are due to predisposing factors of prenatal stress and a deficiency of enzymes involved in steroid synthesis. They found that in homosexual men and women, compared with nonhomosexual subjects, adrenocorticotropic hormone (ACTH) administration significantly increased production of the cortisol precursor, 21-deoxycortisol. A similar increase was demonstrated in the mothers of the homosexual men.

Prenatal exposure to estrogenic or androgenic hormones seems to influence, but certainly not determine, sexual orientation. However, changes in prenatal hormones could influence attitudes, thoughts, and behaviors without necessarily influencing sexual orientation (Money, 1988). Women with congenital adrenal hyperplasia who were not treated until age 8 present a feminine gender identity in consonance with the sex of assignment but a masculine pattern of arousal in that they quickly respond to visual and narrative erotic stimuli, experiencing a strong sexual appetite that is localized in the genitals and that leads to masturbation or the pursuit of intercourse with a casual partner (Ehrhardt et al., 1968; Money, 1965). They do not demonstrate an exclusively homosexual preference, but 48% have homosexual dreams or fantasies, and 18% have had homosexual experiences. They report fewer than expected fantasies of marriage, pregnancy, or motherhood. Women who were treated earlier in childhood demonstrate an increased likelihood of being bisexual (Money and Schwartz, 1977).

Recently, there have been neuromorphologic differences identified in brains of homosexuals, compared with those of heterosexuals. These include an increase in the size of the suprachiasmatic nucleus of the

hypothalamus (Swaab and Hofman, 1990); diminished size of one of the sex dimorphic interstitial nuclei of the anterior hypothalamus (Le Vay, 1991); and an increase in the size of the anterior commissure (Allen and Gorski, 1992). So far, the evidence relating brain structure to sexual orientation is very limited and inconsistent. Methodological problems abound: samples are small and, in most studies, the homosexual subjects have died of AIDs. Findings that do exist demand replication.

Genetic influences are the best established biologic explanation for the occurrence of homosexuality. Pillard and Weinrich (1986) found that 22% of the brothers of homosexual or bisexual men were either homosexual or bisexual, compared with 4% of the brothers of heterosexual men. Another study shows a concordance for homosexuality rate of 52% among monozygotic twins, compared with 22% among dizygotic twins (Bailey and Pillard, 1991). Genetic influences have also been shown in lesbianism. Monozygotic female twins demonstrate 48% concordance while dizygotic twins demonstrate only 16% concordance for homosexuality (Bailey et al., 1993).

A family pedigree study by Hamer et al. (1993) demonstrated that nonsibling increases in homosexual orientation occur mainly in male relatives on the mother's side of the family. This suggests transmission via the sex chromosome. Indeed, Hamer et al. were able to correlate the existence of homosexuality with the inheritance of polymorphous markers on the long arm of the X chromosome. This is convincing evidence that genetic factors do influence sexual orientation. However, a single gene is not likely to predict sexual orientation (Bancroft, 1994). That more than one gene is involved is suggested by the highly variable nonconcordance rate found in different studies (Meyer-Bahlburg, 1993).

If homosexuality were indeed genetically determined, this could lessen social sanctions against gay persons who would be seen as unfortunate recipients of the "wrong" genes rather than as choosing to be gay. However, since psychosocial as well as biologic factors determine homosexuality, moral and political issues should be resolved on some other basis (Bancroft, 1994). Genetic transmission theory could actually promote antihomosexual bias by fostering the development of techniques to weed out fetuses that carry the "wrong" genetic material.

Cross-cultural studies support the importance of biological forces in the genesis of homosexuality. Behavioral prodromata of male homosexuality (interest in girls' toys, cross-dressing, etc.) exist in several other cultures regardless of how the culture views homosexuality. These prodromata first occur at approximately the same age and are remarkably persistent thereafter (Green, 1978a). However, biological factors are certainly not the only, or perhaps the most important, determinant. Bancroft (1994) states that if an exclusive homosexual orientation were decided solely by biological forces, counterparts should be readily found in other species. Yet, in other species, homosexual behavior appears to be more the result of learned behavior than of an innate predisposition. Homosexuality must be determined by psychosocial, as well as biologic, factors.

CONCLUSION

Although there is reason to believe that biological factors influence and are inextricably intertwined with environmental factors in determining gender identity, role, and preference, it would seem that social learning and psychodynamic issues are the decisive determinants in all but the rarest of cases.

References

Ablin EL: The role of the father in the separation-individuation phase. In: Devitt JV, Settlage CF (eds): *Separation Individuation: Essays in Honor of Margaret S. Mahler*. New York, International University Press, 1971.

Abrahamse AF, Morrison PA, Waite LJ: Teenagers willing to consider single parenthood: Who is at greatest risk? *Fam Plann Perspect* 20:13–18, 1988.

Allen LS, Gorski RA: Sexual orientation and the

size of the anterior commissure in the human brain. *Proc Natl Acad Sci USA* 89:7199–7202, 1992.

Bailey JM, Pillard RC: A genetic study of male sexual orientation. *Arch Gen Psychiatry* 48:1089–1096, 1991.

Bailey JM, Pillard RC, Neale MC, et al: Heritable factors influence sexual orientation in women. *Arch Gen Psychiatry* 50:217, 1993.

Bancroft J: Homosexual orientation. *Br J Psychiatry* 164:437–440, 1994.

Barnett SA: *A Study of Behavior*. London, Methuen, 1963.

Bell AP, Weinberg MS, Hammersmith SK: *Sexual Preference. Its Development in Men and Women*. Bloomington, IN, Indiana University Press, 1981.

Benedict TR: Continuities and discontinuities in cultural conditioning. In: Mullahy P (ed): *A Study of Interpersonal Relations*. New York, Hermitage Press, 1950.

Bennett SL: Infant-caretaker interactions. In: Rexford EN, Sander LW, Shapiro P (eds): *Infant Psychiatry: A New Synthesis*. New Haven, CT, Yale University Press, 1976.

Beuf A: Doctor, lawyer, household grudge. *J Commun* 24:142– 145, 1974.

Blos P: Prolonged adolescence: The formulation of a syndrome and its therapeutic implications. *Am J Orthopsychiatry* 24:733– 742, 1954.

Blos P: Second individuation process of adolescence. *Psychoanal Study Child* 22:162–186, 1967.

Blos P: The contribution of psychoanalysis to the psychotherapy of adolescents. *Psychoanal Study Child* 38:577–600, 1983.

Broude GJ: Cross-cultural patterning of some sexual attitudes and practices. *Behav Sci Res* 11: 227–262, 1976.

Callagan AR: Gender role and family relationships in adolescent children of chronic schizophrenic mothers: Findings from a longitudinal study of whole families. *Am J Orthopsychiatry* 51:521–535, 1981.

Campbell PJ: *Sex Guides: Books and Films about Sexuality for Young Adults*. New York, Garland, 1986.

Cass VC: Homosexual identity formation: Testing a theoretical model. *J Sex Res* 20:143–167, 1984.

Cinch RF: The relation between the loss of a parent and progress in courtship. *J Soc Psychol* 29: 55–56, 1949.

Clower VL: Theoretical implications in current views of masturbation in latency aged girls. *J Am Psychoanal Assoc* 24:109–125, 1976.

Coles R, Stokes G: *Sex and the American Teenager*. New York, Harper & Row, 1985.

Conn J: Children's awareness of the origin of babies. *J Child Psych* 1:140–176, 1948.

Currier RL: Juvenile sexuality in global perspective. In: Constantine LL, Martinson FM (eds): *Children and Sex: New Findings New Perspectives*. Boston, Little, Brown, 1981.

Dare C, Holder A: Developmental aspects of the interaction between narcissism, self-esteem and object relations. *Int J Psychoanal* 62:323–337, 1981.

Darling CA, Davidson JK: Coitally active university students: Sexual behaviors, concerns, and challenges. *Adolescence* 21:403–419, 1986.

Davenport WH: Sex in cross-cultural perspective. In: *Human Sexuality in Four Perspectives*. Baltimore, Johns Hopkins University Press, 1976.

Dorner G, Poppe I, Stahl F, et al: Gene- and environment-dependent neuroendocrine etiogenesis of homosexuality and transsexualism. *Exp Clin Endocrinol* 98:141–150, 1991.

Edgcumbe R: Some comments on the concept of the negative oedipal phase in girls. *Psychoanal Study Child* 31:35–61, 1976.

Ehrhardt AA, Baker SW: Fetal androgens, human central nervous system differentiation, and behavior sex differences. In: Friedman RC, Richart RM, Vande Wiele RL (eds): *Sex Differences in Behavior*. New York, Wiley, 1974.

Ehrhardt AA, Meyer-Bahlberg HFL: Effects of prenatal sex hormones on gender related behavior. *Science* 211:1312–1318, 1981.

Ehrhardt AA, Evers K, Money J: Influence of androgen and some aspects of sexually dimorphic behavior in women with the late treated adrenogenital syndrome. *Johns Hopkins Med J* 123:115–122, 1968.

Elias N: *The Civilizing Process*. New York, Urizen Books, 1978.

Elwin V: *The Kingdom of the Young*. London, Oxford University Press, 1968.

Finkelhor D: The sexual climate in families. Paper presented at the International Conference on Family Sexuality, Minneapolis, MN, June 1980.

Fitschen W, Clayton BE: Urinary excretion of gonadotrophins with particular reference to children. *Arch Dis Child* 40:16–26, 1965.

Flerx VC, Fidlerd S, Rogers RW: Sex roles stereotypes: Developmental aspects and early intervention. *Child Dev* 47:998–1007, 1976.

Ford CS, Beach F: *Patterns of Sexual Behavior*. New York, Harper & Row, 1951.

Fox GL: The family's role in adolescent sexual behavior. In: Ooms T (ed): *Teenage Pregnancy in a Family Context*. Philadelphia, Temple University Press, 1981.

Frank E, Anderson C, Rubenstein D: Frequency of sexual dysfunction in "normal" couples. *N Engl J Med* 229:111–115, 1978.

Frayser SC: Anthropologic perspective. In: Yates A (ed): *Sexual and Gender Identity Disorders. Child and Adolescent Psychiatric Clinics of North America*. Philadelphia, Saunders, 1993.

Friedman SM: An empirical study of the castration and Oedipus complexes. *Genet Psychol Monogr* 46:61–130, 1952.

Friedrich W, Grambsch P, Broughton, et al: Normative sexual behavior in children. *Pediatrics* 88: 456–464, 1991.

Freud A: Adolescence. *Psychoanal Study Child* 13:255–278, 1958.

Freud A: Normality and pathology in childhood. In: *The Writings of Anna Freud*. New York, International Universities Press, 1965.

Freud S: *The Ego and the Id*. London, Hogarth Press, 1947.

Freud S: On narcissism: An introduction. In: Strachey J (ed): *The Standard Edition of the Complete Psychological Works of Sigmund Freud* (Vol 14). London, Hogarth Press, 1957. (Originally published 1914.)

Freud S: Three essays on the theory of sexuality. In: Strachey J (ed): *The Standard Edition of the Complete Psychological Works of Sigmund Freud* (Vol 7). London, Hogarth Press, 1961. (Originally published 1905.)

Freud T, McGhee P: Traditional sex role development and amount of time watching television. *Dev Psychol* 11:109, 1975.

Gadpaille WJ: Adolescent sexuality—A challenge to psychiatrists. *J Am Acad Psychoanal* 3: 163–177, 1975.

Gadpaille WJ: A consideration of two concepts of normality as it applies to adolescent sexuality. *J Am Acad Child Psychiatry* 15:679–692, 1976.

Gadpaille WJ: Psychosexual developmental tasks imposed by pathologically delayed childhood: A cultural dilemma. In: Feinstein SC, Gioracehini PL (eds): *Adolescent Psychiatry* (Vol 4). Chicago, University of Chicago Press, 1978.

Gadpaille WJ: Innate masculine/feminine traits: Their contributions to conflict. *J Am Acad Psychoanal* 11:401–424, 1983.

Gagnon IN, Simon W: *Sexual Conduct*. Chicago, Aldine Publishing, 1973.

Galenson E: The emergence of genital awareness during the second year of life. In: Friedman KC (ed): *Sex Differences in Behavior*. New York, Wiley, 1974.

Galenson E: Sexuality in infancy and preschool aged children. In: Yates A (ed): *Sexual and Gender Identity Disorders. Child and Adolescent Psychiatric Clinics of North America*. Philadelphia, Saunders, 1993.

Galenson E, Roiphe H: Some suggested revisions concerning early female development. *J Am Psychoanal Assoc* 24:29–57, 1976.

Gartrell NK, Loriaux DL, Chase TN: Plasma testosterone in homosexual and heterosexual women. *Am J Psychiatry* 134:1117– 1119, 1977.

Gebhard P: The acquisition of basic sex information. *J Sex Res* 13:148–169, 1977.

Geschwind N: Biological foundations of cerebral dominance. *Trends Neurosci* 6:354–359, 1983.

Goldman RI, Goldman JDG: *Children's Sexual Thinking*. London, Routledge & Kegan Paul, 1981.

Green R: *Sexual Identity Conflict in Children and Adults*. New York, Basic Books, 1978a.

Green R: Sexual identity of 37 children raised by homosexual or transsexual parents. *Am J Psychiatry* 135:692–697, 1978b.

Green R: *The "Sissy Boy Syndrome" and the Development of Homosexuality*. New Haven, CT, Yale University Press, 1987.

Greenacre P: Special problems of early female sexual development. *Psychoanal Study Child* 5: 122–138, 1950.

Hamer DH, Hu S, Magnuson VL, et al: A linkage between DNA markers on the X chromosome and male sexual orientation. *Science* 261:321–327, 1993.

Harlow HF, Harlow MK: Social deprivation in monkeys. *Sci Am* 207:136–146, 1962.

Herdt GH: *Guardians of the Flutes: Idioms of Masculinity*. New York, McGraw-Hill, 1981.

Hetherington EM: Effects of father absence on child development. *Young Children* 26:233–248, 1971.

Hetherington EM: Effects of father absence on personality development in adolescent daughters. *Dev Psychol* 7:313–326, 1972.

Hochschild A: *The Second Shift*. New York, Viking Press, 1989.

Hofferth SL: Factors affecting initiation of sexual intercourse. In: Hayes CD (ed): *Risking the Future: Adolescent Sexuality, Pregnancy, and Childbearing* (Vol 2). Washington, DC, National Academy Press, 1987.

Hofferth SL: Trends in adolescent sexual activity, contraception, and pregnancy in the United States. In: Bancroft J, Reinisch JM (eds): *Adolescence and Puberty*. New York, Oxford University Press, 1990.

Hogan DP, Kitagawa EM: The impact of social status, family structure, and neighborhood on the fertility of black adolescents. *Am J Sociol* 90:825–855, 1985.

Honigmann JJ: *Culture and Personality*. New York, Harper and Brothers, 1957.

Huelsman BR: An anthropological view of clitoral and other female genital mutilations. In: Lowry TP, Lowry TS (eds): *The Clitoris*. St. Louis, Warren H Green Publishers, 1976.

Jackson S: Childhood and sexuality in historical perspective. In: Yates A (ed): *Sexual and Gender Identity Disorders. Child and Adolescent Psychiatric Clinics of North America*. Philadelphia, Saunders, 1993.

Jacobson E: *The Self and the Object World*. New York, International Universities Press, 1964.

Jessor SL, Jessor R: Transition from virginity to nonvirginity among youth: A social-psychological study over time. *Dev Psychol* 11:473–484, 1975.

Johnson TC: Assessment of sexual behavior problems in pre-school aged and latency-aged children. In: Yates A (ed): *Sexual and Gender Identity Disorders. Child and Adolescent Psychiatric Clinics of North America*. Philadelphia, Saunders, 1993.

Jones EF, Forrest JD, Goldman N, et al: Teenage pregnancy in developed countries: Determinants and policy implications. *Fam Plann Perspect* 17:53–63, 1985.

Jost A: Problems of fetal endocrinology: The gonadal and hypophyseal hormones. *Recent Prog Horm Res* 8:379–386, 1953.

Kagan J, Reznick JS, Clarke C, et al: Behavioral inhibition to the unfamiliar. *Child Dev* 55: 2212–2225, 1984.

Kaplan HS: *Disorders of Sexual Desire*. New York, Brunner/Mazel, 1979.

Katz RC, Gipson, MT, Kearl A, et al: Assessing sexual aversion in college students: The sexual aversion scale. *J Sex Marital Ther* 15:135–140, 1989.

Kestenberg JS: Outside and inside: Male and female. *J Am Psychoanal Assoc* 16:457–520, 1968.

Kinsey AC, Pomeroy WG, Martin CE: *Sexual Behavior in the Human Male*. Philadelphia, Saunders, 1948.

Kinsey AC, Pomeroy WG, Martin CE, et al: *Sexual Behavior in the Human Female*. Philadelphia, Saunders, 1953.

Kirkendall LA, McBride LG: Preadolescent and adolescent imagery fantasies; beliefs and experiences. In: Perry ME (ed): *Handbook of Sexology*. Vol 7: *Childhood and Adolescent Sexology*. Amsterdam, Elsevier Science Publishers, 1990.

Kleeman J: Genital self-stimulation in girls: In: Marcus IM, Francis JJ (eds): *Masturbation: From Infancy to Senescence*. New York: International Universities Press, 1975.

Kleeman J: Freud's views on early female sexuality in the light of direct child observation. *J Am Psychoanal Assoc* 24:29–57, 1976.

Kohlberg L: A cognitive-developmental analysis of children's sex role concepts and attitudes. In: Maccoby EE (ed): *The Development of Sex Differences*. Stanford, CA, Stanford University Press, 1966.

Kohut H: *The Analysis of the Self*. New York, International Universities Press, 1971.

Krivacska JJ: *Designing Child Sexual Abuse Prevention Programs: Current Approaches and a Proposal for the Prevention, Reduction, and Identification of Sexual Misuse*. Springfield, IL, Charles C Thomas, 1990.

Lamb ME: The development of parent-infant attachments in the first two years of life. In: Pedersen FA (ed): *The Father Infant Relationship*. New York, Praeger, 1980.

Langfeld T: Early childhood and juvenile sexuality, its development and problems. In: Perry ME (ed): *Handbook of Sexology*. Vol 7: *Childhood and Adolescent Sexology*. Amsterdam, Elsevier Science Publishers, 1990.

Laufer M: The body image, the function of masturbation, and adolescence. *Psychoanal Study Child* 23:114–137, 1968.

Le Vay S: A difference in hypothalamic structure between heterosexual and homosexual men. *Science* 253:1034–1037, 1991.

Lockwood C: Growing up Victorian. *California Living Magazine* Aug. 13, 1978.

Lustman SL: Yale's year of confrontation: A view from the master's house. *Psychoanal Study Child* 27:57–73, 1971.

Maier HW: *Three Theories of Child Development*. New York, Harper & Row, 1965.

Marshall DS, Suggs R: *Human Sexual Behavior*. New York, Basic Books, 1971.

Masica DN, Money J, Ehrhardt AA: Fetal feminization and female gender identity in the testicular feminizing syndrome of androgen insensitivity. *Arch Sex Behav* 1:131–142, 1971.

Masters WH, Johnson VE: *Human Sexual Response*. Boston, Little, Brown, 1966.

Masterson J: The symptomatic adolescent five years later: He didn't grow out of it. *Am J Psychiatry* 123:1338–1345, 1967.

Masterson J: The psychiatric significance of adolescent turmoil. *Am J Psychiatry* 124:1549–1554, 1968.

McCandless BR: Rate of development, body build and personality. In: Shagass C, Pasamanick B (eds): *Child Development and Child Psychiatry* (Vol 88). Washington, DC, American Psychiatric Press, 1960.

Mead SL, Rekers GA: Role of the father in normal psychosexual development. *Psychol Rep* 45: 923–931, 1979.

Meyer B: The development of girls' sex role attitude. *Child Dev* 51:508–514, 1980.

Meyer-Bahlberg HFL: Hormones and psychosexual differentiation: Implications for the management of intersexuality, homosexuality and transsexuality. In: *Clinics in Endocrinology and Metabolism* (Vol 2). New York, Saunders, 1982.

Meyer-Bahlberg HFL: Psychobiologic research on homosexuality. In: Yates A (ed): *Sexual and Gender Identity Disorders. Child and Adolescent Psychiatric Clinics of North America*. Philadelphia, Saunders, 1993.

Miller BC, McCoy JK, Olson TD, et al: Parental discipline and control attempts in relation to adolescent sexual attitudes and behavior. *J Marriage Fam* 48:503–512, 1986.

Miller GD, Cirone J: Sexual dysfunction in college sexuality course attenders and course treatment benefits. *J Am Coll Health Assoc* 27:107–108, 1978.

Mischel W: A social learning view of sex differences and behavior. In: Maccoby EE (ed): *The Development of Sex Differences*. Stanford, CA, Stanford University Press, 1966.

Money J: Sex hormones and other variables in human eroticism. In: Young WC, Corner GW (eds): *Sex and Internal Secretions* (Vol 2, 3rd ed). Baltimore, Williams & Wilkins, 1961.

Money J: Influence of hormones on sexual behavior. *Annu Rev Med* 16:67–82, 1965.

Money J, Ehrhardt AA: *Man and Woman: Boy and Girl*. Baltimore, Johns Hopkins University Press, 1972.

Money J, Schwartz M: Dating, romantic and non-romantic friendships and sexuality in 17 early treated adrenogenital females. In: Lee PA, Plotnik LP, Kowarski AA, et al (eds): *Congenital Adrenal Hyperplasia*. Baltimore, University Park Press, 1977.

Money J, Tucker P: *Sexual Signatures: On Being a Man or a Woman*. Boston, Little, Brown, 1975.

Moore WT: Masturbation in adolescence. In: Marcus IM, Francis JJ (eds): *Masturbation: From Infancy to Senescence*. New York, International Universities Press, 1975.

Munroe RL, Munroe RH: *Crosscultural Human Development*. Monterey, CA, Brooks/Cole, 1975, p. 107.

Murdock G: *Social Structure*. New York, Macmillan, 1960.

Newson J, Newson E: *Four Years Old in an Urban Community*. London, Allen and Vawin, 1962.

Nottelman ED, Inoff-Germain G, Sussman, EJ, et al: Hormones and behavior at puberty. In: Bancroft J, Reinsich JM (eds): *Adolescence and Puberty*. New York, Oxford University Press, 1990.

Offer D, Offer J: Three developmental routes through normal adolescence. *Adolesc Psych* 4: 121–141, 1975.

Orr DP, Beiter M, Ingersoll G: Premature sexual activity as an indicator of psychosocial risk. *Pediatrics* 87:141–147, 1991.

Piacente GJ: Aggression. *Psychiatr Clin North Am* 9:329–339, 1986.

Piaget J: *The Psychology of Intelligence*. London, Routledge & Kegan Paul, 1950.

Piaget J, Inhelder B: *The Growth of Logical Thinking from Childhood to Adolescence*. New York, Basic Books, 1958.

Pickett RS: Sanger to the seventies. Paper presented at the 4th annual meeting of the American Association of Sex Educators and Counselors, St. Louis, April 1971.

Pillard RC, Weinrich JD: Evidence of familial nature of male homosexuality. *Arch Gen Psychiatry* 43:808–812, 1986.

Prescott JW: Body pleasure and the origins of violence. *The Futurist* 9:64–74, 1975.

Prescott JW: Affectional bonding for the prevention of violent behaviors: Neurobiological, psychological and religious/spiritual determinants.

Hertzberg LJ, Ostrum GF, Field JR (eds): *Violent Behavior*. Vol. 1: *Assessment and Intervention*. Costa Mesa, CA, PMA Publishing, 1990, pp. 339.

Ramsey CV: The sexual development of boys. *Am J Psychol* 56:217–233, 1943.

Remafedi GJ: Adolescent homosexuality: Psychosocial and medical implications. *Pediatrics* 79: 331–337, 1987.

Robbins C, Kaplan HB, Martin SS: Antecedents of pregnancy among unmarried adolescents. *J Marriage Fam* 47:567–583, 1985.

Robinson I, Ziss K, Ganza B: Twenty years of the sexual revolution. *J Marriage Fam* 53:216–220, 1991.

Roiphe H, Galenson E: Some observations on transitional object and infantile fetish. *Psychoanal Q* 42:73–90, 1973.

Rosenbaum E, Kandel DB: Warly onset of adolescent sexual behavior and drug involvement. *J Marriage Fam* 52:783–798, 1990.

Rosenfeld A, Wasserman S: Sexual development in the early school-aged child. In: Yates A (ed): *Sexual and Gender Identity Disorders. Child and Adolescent Psychiatric Clinics of North America*. Philadelphia, Saunders, 1993.

Rosenfeld A, Siegel-Gorelick B, Haavik D, et al: Parental perceptions of children's modesty: A cross-sectional survey of ages two to ten years. *Psychiatry* 47:351–365, 1984.

Rosenfeld A, Siegel B, Bailey R: Familial bathing patterns: Implications for cases of alleged molestation and for pediatric practice. *Pediatrics* 79: 224–229, 1987.

Rutter M: Normal psychosexual development. *J Child Psychol Psychiatry* 11:259–283, 1971.

Rutter M, Graham P, Chadwick OF, et al: Adolescent turmoil: Fact or fiction? *J Child Psychol Psychiatry* 17:35–56, 1976.

Sagarin E: Sex rearing and sexual orientation: The reconciliation of apparently contradictory data. *J Sex Res* 11:329–334, 1975.

Santelli JS, Beilenson P: Risk factors for adolescent sexual behavior, fertility, and sexually transmitted diseases. *J Sch Health* 62:271–279, 1992.

Sarlin CN: Culture and psychosexual development. In: Marcus IM, Francis JJ (eds): *Masturbation: From Infancy to Senescence*. New York, International Universities Press, 1975.

Schein M, Zyzanski SJ, Levine S, et al: The frequency of sexual problems among family practice patients. *Fam Pract Res J* 7:122–134, 1988.

Schover LR, LoPiccolo J: Treatment effectiveness for dysfunctions of sexual desire. *J Sex Marital Ther* 8:179–184, 1982.

Schwartz G: Devices to prevent masturbation. *Med Aspects Hum Sex* 7:141–153, 1973.

Sears R, Maccoby E, Levin H: *Patterns of Child Rearing*. New York, Harper & Row, 1957.

Shah FK, Zelnik M: Parent and peer influence on sexual behavior, contraceptive use and pregnancy experience of young women. *J Marriage Fam* 43: 339–348, 1981.

Shepher J: Mate selection among second generation kibbutz adolescents and adults; incest avoidance and negative imprinting. *Arch Sex Behav* 1:293–307, 1971.

Siecus National Guidelines Task Force: *Guidelines for Comprehensive Sex Education, Grades Kindergarten—12th Grade*. New York, SIECUS, 1991.

Simmons A, Turner J: The socialization of sex roles and fertility ideals: A study of two generations in Toronto. *J Comp Studies* 7:255–271, 1976.

Smith EA, Udry JR, Morris NM: Pubertal development and friends: A biosocial explanation of adolescent sexual behavior. *J Health Soc Behav* 26: 183–192, 1985.

Sonnenstein FL, Pleck JH, Kuo LC: Levels of

sexual activity among adolescent males in the United States. *Fam Plann Perspect* 23:162–167, 1991.

Sorensen RC: *Adolescent Sexuality in Contemporary America*. Mountain View, CA, World Publications, 1973.

Spieler S: Preoedipal girls need fathers. *Psychoanal Rev* 71:63–80, 1984.

Spitz RA, Wolf KM: Autoeroticism: Some empirical findings and hypotheses on three of its manifestations in the first year of life. *Psychoanal Study Child* 3/4:85–120, 1949.

Strober M, Green J, Carlson G: Reliability of psychiatric diagnosis in hospitalized adolescents. *Arch Gen Psychiatry* 38:141–145, 1981.

Sugar M: Adolescent sexuality. In: Yates A (ed): *Sexual and Gender Identity Disorders. Child and Adolescent Psychiatric Clinics of North America*. Philadelphia, Saunders, 1993.

Swaab DF, Hoffman MA: An enlarged suprachiasmatic nucleus in homosexual men. *Brain Res* 537: 141–148, 1990.

Symons D: *The Evolution of Human Sexuality*. Oxford, Oxford University Press, 1979.

Thornberg H: A comparative study of sex education sources. *J School Health* 62:88–91, 1972.

Thorton A: The courtship process and adolescent sexuality. *J Fam Issues* 11:239–273, 1990.

Troiden RR: The formation of homosexual identities. *J Homosex* 17:43–73, 1989.

Tyson P: A developmental line of gender identity, gender role, and choice of love object. *J Am Psychoanal Assoc* 30:59–84, 1982.

Udry JR, Billy JOG: Initiation of coitus in early adolescence. *Am Sociol Rev* 52:841–855, 1987.

Udry JR, Billy JOG, Morris NM, et al: Serum androgenic hormones motivate sexual behavior in adolescent boys. *Fertil Steril* 43:90–94, 1985.

Udry JR, Talbert LM, Morris NM: Biosocial foundations for adolescent female sexuality. *Demography* 23:217–230, 1986.

Wake FR: Attitudes of parents toward the premarital sexual behavior of their children and themselves. *J Sex Res* 5:170–182, 1969.

Whalen RE: Sexual motivation. *Psychol Rev* 73: 151–163, 1966.

Whatley J, Thin N, Reynolds B, et al: Problems of adolescent's sexuality. *J R Soc Med* 82:732–734, 1989.

Whisnant L, Brett E, Zegans L: Adolescent girls and menstruation. *Adol Psychiatry* 7:157–171, 1979.

Whitam FL, Zent M: A crosscultural assessment of early cross gender behavior and familial factors in male homosexuality. *Arch Sex Behav* 13:427–441, 1984.

Whitehurst RN: American sexophobia. In: Kirkendall LA, Whitehurst RN (eds): *The New Sexual Revolution*. New York, Donald Brown, 1971.

Wilson JD, George FW, Griffin JE: The hormonal control of sexual development. *Science* 211: 1278–1284, 1981.

Wolfenstein M: Trends in infant care. *Am J Orthopsychiatry* 23:290, 1953.

Wyatt GE: Changing influences on adolescent sexuality over the past 40 years. In: Bancroft J,

Reinisch JM (eds): *Adolescence and Puberty*. New York, Oxford University Press, 1990, pp. 782.

Yalom ID, Green R, Fisk N: Prenatal exposure to female hormones. *Arch Gen Psychiatry* 28:554–561, 1971.

Yates A: *Sex without Shame: Encouraging the Child's Healthy Sexual Development*. New York, William Morrow, 1978.

Yates A: Children eroticized by incest. *Am J Psychiatry* 139:482–485, 1982.

Yates A: Gender identity assessment and initial intervention. In: Nadelson C, Marcotte D (eds): *Treatment Intervention in Human Sexuality*. New York, Plenum, 1983.

Yates A: *Compulsive Exercise and the Eating Disorders: Toward an Integrated Theory of Activity*. New York, Brunner/Mazel, 1991a.

Yates A: Differentiating hypererotic states in the evaluation of sexual abuse. *J Am Acad Child Adolesc Psychiatry* 30:791–795, 1991b.

Yates A: Sexually inhibited children. In: Yates A (ed): *Sexual and Gender Identity Disorders. Child and Adolescent Psychiatric Clinics of North America*. Philadelphia, Saunders, 1993.

Zabin LS, Smith EA, Hirsch MB, et al: Ages of physical maturation and first intercourse in black teenage males and females. *Demography* 23: 295–605, 1986.

Zelnik M, Shah FK: First intercourse among young Americans. *Fam Plann Perspect* 15:64–70, 1983.

19 FAMILY DEVELOPMENT AND THE ROLES OF MOTHERS AND FATHERS IN CHILD REARING

Kyle D. Pruett, M.D.

Families render humans human. Certainly endowment and maturational forces strongly predispose to the attachments and intimacies that draw the infant into the human race, relationship by relationship. But it is the family that ultimately embraces that child's maturational promise and, through powerful reciprocal, interactive forces, converts tissue and instinct into human development. In this chapter we examine the unfolding of that process through the exploration of the basic unit of all emotional development, the family.

Although families vary enormously, they tend to share certain processes as they go about the life cycle of birth and burial. At first glance, it would appear that family processes would be easy to delineate because they seem linear (i.e., birth to growth to death). Family process itself, however, is more cyclical than linear. Family content is determined by the whole family emotional system, including at least three generations. Those three generations, although they have rarely lived together in large numbers in our culture, are accommodating to their own unique life cycle agendas simultaneously. At every given moment in its life, the family exists at the intersection of two distinctly different linear axes. The family moves along these axes like a vehicle moving down two separate paths simultaneously. One path is the trail of generational myths, expectations, attributes, memories, and secrets—the family's "givens." This is the family's narrative about itself, so articulately described by Pincus and Dare in *Secrets in the Family* (1978) and Vangelisti (1994). The narrative is passed on at times like folk songs in the oral tradition and at others, more subtly, through children being taught who and what their family is now, has been, and is hoped (if not expected) to be.

The other path is the vector formed by the family's movement forward through the dimension of time of its own life cycle. This encompasses both the usual stresses and opportunities of the family's children's developmental requirements and the intrusion of "fateful events." Whether or not a family gets into trouble is determined in part by whether these two axes intersect at strong or weak points, since they perpetually cross and recross each other. Real trouble seems most likely when a vulnerable stretch on the transgenerational axis intersects with an equally vulnerable stretch on the developmental axis. For example: The family narrative trail carries forward a myth/expectation that "Jones boys always marry wild women" at a time when, on the developmental track, the Jones' first-born son is beginning his adolescence by easing up on his academic discipline and starting to push against behavioral boundaries. He tells his parents less and less about his life and whereabouts, especially where girls are concerned, and his and his family's fantasies about "wild women" collide with his own unique developmental course. A boiling point can be reached quickly here, depending on how all the principal players perceive this collision.

Family development as a phenomenon is hard to embrace in all its complexity, precisely because the clinician tends to encounter families, normal or not, at just one nodal point in time, depriving him or her of the critical longitudinal perspective. Research hints that we have significantly underestimated the life cycle connections between early loss, trauma, or disturbance and later interpersonal dysfunction (Ainsworth and Eichberg, 1991; Bowen, 1978; Thomas and Duszynski, 1974).

Within the past two decades, the cycles of family life have undergone significant change. Lower birth rates, increasing divorce and remarriage rates, and longer life expectancies have reduced childbearing from being the major occupation of parents to what is now less than 50% of parents' lifelong commitment.

Historians urge caution in referring to "unprecedented change." Through careful research, Demos (1970) and Laslette and Wall (1972) have largely dispelled the myth of the ideal three-generational family holding sway in preindustrial family life. A process was begun then, however, that did affect major change in overall family functioning, coming to fruition now. Hareven (1982) summarizes: "Through a process of differentiation, the family gradually surrendered functions previously concentrated within it to other social institutions. During the pre-Industrial period, the family not only reared children, but also served as a workshop, a school, a church and an asylum" (p. 460).

Today the difficulties faced by families are rooted in this legacy, with a loss of diversity in households (especially combined with smaller numbers), the weakening of the family's capacity to adapt and cope (partly because of the small numbers), and further decline in the variety of the family's functions.

The declining maternal and child death rates of the 1950s combined with a higher marriage rate and longer life span to create a higher percentage of children growing up in stable, two-parent families than had ever occurred in America. Beginning with the next decade, however, trends began to erode both the ideal and real traditional nuclear family. The sexual revolution uncoupled the association of sexual and reproduction behavior. From 1971 to 1992, the percentage of unmarried teenage girls in American who engaged in premarital sexual intercourse between 15 and 19 rose from 28 to 51%. Curiously, figures are unavailable for boys, as though only female sexual activity is related to family formation. Second, the movement into the paid work force of married women with children saw an increase from the 1960 level of 19% of married women with children under 6 in the labor force to a 58% real figure in 1993 of married women with children under 6. Fertility and fecundity too declined in the United States beginning in the 1960s. We are now at levels lower than those necessary for the replacement of the population, having moved from an average of 3.7 children per woman in 1990 to now 1.76. This may well reflect a dissatisfaction with parenthood, in association with a significant decline in the stigma associated with being childless.

Finally, the divorce rate in American brought us past a landmark in 1974, when for the first time in our history, more marriages concluded in divorce than in the death of a spouse. Nine divorces per 1000 marriages in 1960 became 22 per 1000 in 1992. Single-parent families, unmarried and homosexual couples, and serial and stepfamilies have all increased their percentage of childrearing formats at the expense of nuclear units.

It is the opinion of many clinicians and researchers that the quality of life for children in the past 25 years has not improved at the same rate as the quality of life has improved for adults. Also, rates of distress seem to be on the rise. Achenbach (1993) studied the changes over 13 years of the prevalence of children with behavioral/emotional problems. He found more untreated children who needed psychological intervention in the 1989 sample than in the 1976 sample. Every child needs and longs for two biological parents in and for his or her life. Simply stated, childrearing is most successful when it does involve both biological parents who are committed emotionally and affectively to the job. This is not to say that this is the only way to bring child development to fruition. However, it is to say that, as a group, nurturing forms other than the biological family are not as likely to be as successful in the job. The value of such a family is that it not only promotes development most efficiently but also buffers, cushions, and protects young children while they are learning new ways to cope with the world about them. Patterson (1983) strongly suggests that the relation between stress and developmental outcome for isolated individuals is different from that for children who are part of a social group, the former being at more risk.

Some of the statistics stated above illustrate an important, irreducible fact about change in the American family. Women are in the labor force to stay. Families have changed, yet the institutions the families rely upon most heavily, schools and the workplace, have been much slower not only to change but also to respond to the changes in the family system (Galinsky, 1986). The family structure that is most influential in the child's development, however, is the one perceived by the child as *his* or *her* family, not the one perceived by the Census Bureau. As Robert Coles reminds us (1985), we must listen to the individual always and resist the hegemony of irrelevant, ultimately sterile theoretical oversimplifications.

Each child who enters the family changes it permanently and irreversibly, rendering the child's perception of the family unique to his or her own perceptual apparatus, and not to that of the family as a whole. Sameroff (1993) has helped us move away from the restrictions of the linear, even interactional, model of child development, and toward one more encompassing of the progressive, dynamic, reciprocal forces that have helped children change families and vice versa. His is a "transactional model" that emphasizes the need for incorporating social and economic as well as biological forces. Proposing a "continuum of caretaking causality," such increased emphasis on the qualitative aspects of the nurturing domain has encouraged clinicians and researchers to think anew about who in the family is doing what with the children, and not simply how long they are doing it.

The Berkeley Adult Attachment Interview (George et al., 1985) and its application to family development (Main et al., 1985) are examples of growing interest and skill in our capacity to assess the adult's state of mind (and not simply his or her behavior) with regard to attachment to one's children and vice versa. The interview of the Adult Attachment Classification System is used separately with mother and father. This is an example of how we are returning to the exploration of the overriding significance of the quality and intent of the nurturing interaction, and not merely the biological predispositions of the interactors.

Mothers, fathers, grandparents, siblings—all form unique attachments to children that, in formative settings, are welcomed and easily integrated by the child into a mosaic of consistent, predictable, comforting internalizations of the nurturing experience. Therefore, it is not merely one adult attachment that leads to one internalization of the nurturing experience, be it positive or negative. Much clinical literature, however, falls short in its attempts to clarify distinct maternal and paternal antecedents to psychological syndromes. Bezirganian et al. (1993) found that maternal overinvolvement paired with maternal inappropriateness combined to form pathogenic predispositions toward Borderline Personality Disorder in children. Although paternal means were included, they were not commented upon in the discussion.

Optimal child development is fostered by optimal family development. This occurs by translating the recognizable maturational stages of child development into the interactional modalities and developmental dynamics of the family. Optimal family development, as perceived by the child, begins with a secure individual attachment, which the baby must make with its primary caregiver, typically the mother, although fathers as primary caregivers certainly have the capacity to rear their children without placing them at developmental risk (Pruett, 1983, 1987). In fact, Radin (1989) cites the advantages to young children of paternal involvement, almost regardless of the reasons for the father's presence. The other optimal phenomenon for promoting development within the family network consists of the capacity of mothers and fathers to form reciprocal, empathic relationships with the child, aided by a broad and complete range of affective expression. One must be ready to accept developmental progression and change, as it comes rapidly in the 1st year in particular. It is best if the children are appreciated for their unique and idiosyncratic traits, temperaments, skills, and weaknesses.

Despite the dramatic increase in the number of publications on fathering that has occurred over the last decade and a half, fathers continue to be so underrepresented in the literature compared with mothers that one sees a staggering deficit. Phares and Compass (1992) reviewed research papers in the major journals dealing with clinical child development published from 1984 to 1991, finding that nearly half of all studies involved mothers only. Nearly one quarter of the remaining studies did include father-related material, but did not bother to differentiate its effects. The final quarter did measure father-child effects and found them consistently present. So when researchers bother to look for father effects, they always find them. The authors suggested that the overreliance on mothers as research participants has fostered not only an incomplete data set with regard to child development, but also one that is heavily gender biased because "relations cannot be found among variables that are not investigated" (p. 406).

Before beginning a chronological view of family development across the life cycle, clarification of certain phenomena that guide family function is in order. Understanding the family as a system, we are accustomed to conceptualizing change in one segment of the family as resonating throughout that system, and any negative or positive change in one segment of the system as either promoting or discouraging development in others. Homeostasis is the way that families conserve their energy and socialize their young. Yet the demands of rapidly evolving maturational forces in the child offer continual perturbations to that homeostasis. Therefore, it is important for us to understand how to view a family's potential success in preparing its children for adulthood.

Skinner (1983) created the Family Assessment Measure, consisting of a general and dyadic scale to distinguish reliably between normal and problem families. Fleck (1984, 1989) has offered an efficient, five-factor system for assessing the system's capacity to support the development of its children, consisting of (a) leadership, (b) boundaries, (c) emotional climate, (d) communication, and (e) the establishment and accomplishment of goals and tasks throughout the life cycle. As we begin to examine the family's development across the life cycle, it is critical to remain conscious of these five factors.

Leadership is defined as the decision-making, facilitating source of power and discipline within the biological, adoptive, or serial parents who lead the family unit. It is shaped by the presence or absence of mutual support and esteem and by the effectiveness of the communication between the leaders of the family unit.

Family boundaries refers to (a) boundaries within the individual that define the self, (b) boundaries between generations, and (c) boundaries between the family and the community. It is important that these boundaries be semipermeable, permitting contact and discourse with others outside the family boundary. Self- and generational boundaries remain relatively stable throughout the life cycle, while family/community boundaries must become increasingly permeable as children cross them more frequently to participate in the community about them.

The emotional climate or affectivity of the family unit is the connective tissue that binds the family together into a functioning body. The affective climate is the lifeblood of the family's capacity to care for and support one another, especially since the family has ceased to be such an essential economic unit. Chronic scapegoating of a family member, child abuse, and neglect are classic signs of failure in the family's emotional climate.

Communication within families is both verbal and nonverbal. Certainly communicative language and its use for deepening relationships are learned best within the family. Experiences and feelings are shared through the medium of language, while values and culture are differentiated and reinforced by consistency of communication within the family.

Finally, the expectation that families will nurture and socialize their young so that they develop into contributory members of society is the burden placed upon the above functions. The fulfillment of this expectation is determined by the way the family achieves its goals for individual members and sets the members' tasks toward reaching those goals. Goals and tasks throughout the life cycle change and evolve in complex ways and, unlike communication or boundaries, seem not to diminish in significance. Family development is usually arbitrarily divided into stages for better understanding of its predictable develop-

mental phenomena. This cookbook approach does not obviate the enormous complexity of the relationship systems implied therein, which expand, contract, and realign in order to support the entrance, development, and exit of family members in a profoundly meaningful way, emotionally, culturally, and historically. We tour these stages with an eye to the contributions made by the nurturers and the nurturants, examining the unique and differing roles of mothers and fathers as participants and facilitators of normal development across the life cycle.

COUPLING AND FAMILY FORMATION

Family formation begins anew as a heterosexual pair bonds sexually and, one hopes, psychologically. Both members of this relationship bring conscious and unconscious motivations, both libidinal and aggressive, to their coalition. The choice of mate is governed by a web of intrinsic and experiential factors and tempered by the degree of separation from the family of origin. Contemporary family formation is frequently characterized by a period of joint cohabitation, which is now lasting longer than ever before in the history of family formation. Making a deliberate, conscious decision about family formation strongly predisposes toward health, in the same way that an unconscious, nonjoint decision predisposes to risk. One of the strongest unconscious motivations toward coupling is the wish to acquire in one's spouse a longed for or incomplete aspect of oneself. When the choice is well made, this can strongly predispose toward stability in the marriage. There is evidence to suggest in fact that this may have an ameliorating effect on eventual family formation despite previous negative experiences, particularly on the part of the mother in her own childhood nurturing interactions. Eichberg (1987) has found in her research using the Adult Attachment Inventory that the father's role is positively ameliorative of a mother's previously negative parental experience.

When the coupling results in marriage, it is a joining of two enormously complex historical, interpersonal, emotional, and financial systems. Couples are marrying later and postponing birthing their children more than ever before: The average age of marriage for women in 1994 was 22.6 and for men 24.5 and the birth of their first child came on average 1 year and 10 months later. This implies there is a relatively short period of time given to adjusting to this phase in the life cycle. Sociologists show us there does seem to be a relatively narrow window for the timing of this phase. Women are twice as likely to divorce if they marry before the age of 20 than if they marry during their 20s. They are half again as likely to divorce if they marry after 30 than if they marry during their 20s (Glick and Norton, 1978). A variety of other factors can also contribute to difficulty at this life cycle transition: (a) the couple resides at either great distance or great proximity to either family of origin; (b) the couple either meets or marries in close proximity to a significant loss; (c) the couple marries after knowing each other for fewer than 6 months or after an engagement lasting over 3 years; (d) the wedding is performed without family or friends; (e) the wife becomes pregnant before or within the 1st year of marriage (Bacon, 1974; Becker, 1987). Although no one can possibly predict its ultimate resolution, it does seem that the rise in women's status is correlated with marital instability and with the increasing, although not absolute, marital dissatisfaction of their husbands. We are clearly in a successful transition toward more equal coupledom in our era, and the educational and occupational equality of the sexes is a perturbation to couple formation as we currently know it (Burke and Weir, 1976).

FIRST CONCEPTION, BIRTH, AND NURTURANCE

This era begins with conception and ends at the end of the 1st year. There is a good deal of psychological work to be done by both mother and father in preparing for and dealing with conception. There is also enormous variability in the amount of conscious deliberation devoted to the decision to conceive a child. Once conception does take place, whether planned or not, a series of complex psychological responses occurs in both the wife and husband. The mother begins by struggling with the profound changes occurring within her body during pregnancy and after delivery. Much of the psychological work is fueled by a conscious reassessment of the couple's own family experience. A new identity begins to come to fruition, that of *being* a parent, not just having one. What makes this so interesting is that both maternal and paternal identifications are deeply rooted within each individual. The mother prepares herself psychologically for the coming attachment to her infant by drawing her attention to her own inner experience and her growing fetus, and her preoccupation with the outside world decreases.

Fathers are involved in psychological work of a different sort, albeit active and equally important in terms of preparation. Food cravings, somatic preoccupations such as vague gastrointestinal disorders, and nutritional changes are widely reported. Concern about his adequacy as a provider and protector may erode an expectant father's self-esteem. Mood changes, frequently expected in mothers, also occur within fathers. "Even before the birth of his child, the father's life, his body, and his mind are busy making ready in ways of which he may only have a passing awareness" (Pruett, 1987, p. 28). Birth preparation classes may be helpful and supportive to both mothers and fathers in promoting a sense of mutual commitment and in explaining the universal pleasures and fears during the pregnancy and birth phase. Both mothers and fathers have complex mental images of their children long before the child sees the light of day.

But nothing is more powerful than the parental experience of the birth in terms of its long-term impact. First impressions are enormously powerful for both mothers and fathers. Attachment and bonding research have clearly articulated for us the importance of both the mother-baby haptic and tactile involvement within the hours after birth. Fathers who are present at the birth are more verbal about their babies, more accurate in describing them, and more intimately attached to them at follow-up.

The newborn's job is every bit as complex as that of his or her parents. The neonate must first stabilize and regulate his or her internal life to the point where he or she is able to perceive and respond to events in the external world by processing sensory, vestibular, and human interactional input. Next, the newborn must use his or her repertoire of skills and intrinsic reflexes to elicit pleasurable experiences from the human world, which will make it possible for the newborn to fall in love and establish an intimate attachment to the main caregiver.

Finally, the infant must make use of pleasurable experiences to communicate with the important objects in the world around in a meaningful and personable way in order to be entertained, stimulated, fed, and to have his or her bodily functions attended to. Both mothers and fathers with or without experience learn, via on-the-job training, to read as well as anticipate their infant's signals. Empathic connections and the capacity to comfort, soothe, woo, and entertain are tasks common to both mothering and fathering. Qualitative differences are present, however, in the idiosyncratic ways in which mothers and fathers respond. Mothers tend to respond to their babies on a more intimate scale, facilitating fine motor development and affective differentiation. Fathers tend to be more active and gross-motor involved. Nevertheless, as shown by Parke and Sawin (1975), fathers were able to feed their babies as effectively and efficiently, although somewhat differently stylistically, as their spouses.

Babies appear quite interested and responsive to the differences between paternal and maternal interactive styles. Yogman (1982) noted that by the time babies were 8 weeks old, they were responding differently to their fathers and mothers. At 6 weeks, babies hunched their shoulders and lifted their eyebrows when their fathers appeared in their visual field. The same infants, when they saw or heard their mothers, seemed to expect more routine functional handling such as feeding or diapering and became settled rather than animated.

The involvement in the 1st year of life of two caring and competent adults appears to have a positive effect on overall cognitive development. Pedersen et al. (1979) found that the more actively involved a 6-month-old baby had been with his or her father, the higher the baby's scores on the Bailey test of mental and motor development. Also, Parke (1979), in examining children over the first 8 weeks of life, found that

the more fathers were involved in everyday, repetitive, boring aspects of care, such as bathing, feeding, dressing, and diapering, the more socially responsive the babies were. It is in the mutual pleasures of this early experience that the adults, who have now moved up a generation and become caretakers to the younger generation, feel their own personal development frequently propelled forward to new levels of empathic—even altruistic—connections, not only with their children but also with other important objects in their lives.

TODDLERHOOD AND INDIVIDUATION WITHIN THE FAMILY

The child's astounding increase in mental and physical resources propels him or her out of the omnipotence of the 1st year of life into a much more social context, in which new skills permit more active shaping of the need-satisfying environment. The development of language, increasing sophistication in cognitive structures, mastery over motility and sphincters, and the incorporation of gender identity and gender role expectations all prepare the child for the complex sequences of the vital separation-individuation process. Parents are alternately challenged through intense clinging and contentious interchange, giving this era ambivalence as its quarterboard. Aggression, caretaking, love, anger, and sensuous intimacy are now part of the toddler's repertoire. This makes limit setting a vital companion to the toddler's adventurous experimentation with challenging, aggressive, and seductive behaviors. At the same time, the parent is wise to be led by the toddler, rather than attempt to lead the toddler. By now, fathering styles are quite differentiated from mothering styles of interaction, with fathers initiating more rough-and-tumble, unusual, unpredictable, physical, and stimulating forms of play. Biller and Meredith (1974) noted that mothers tended to engage in more conventional, toy-mediated play, picking up their children to engage in caretaking and nurturing activities more than fathers. Since the child has increased his or her level of mastery over the internal environment, he or she has a good deal more energy available to explore the boundaries of the external environment, giving separation tasks a much higher valence during waking life. Adjustments to the toddler's new, if clumsy, drive for autonomy are necessary to avoid prolonging the child's functional dependency. Since separation from the mother is sometimes the fuel for the sleep disturbances that are common during the 2nd year of life, the father can help decrease the virulence of nighttime disruption by being the one who goes in to soothe and settle the child, spelling the child from another separation from the mother, while helping the child feel safe and secure.

Clearly, the child's unique temperament and style interact with parental values and experience with regard to personal autonomy, separateness from family of origin, and impulse and bodily control. The unique contributions of the father during these years have been increasingly recognized as vital to the success of this developmental era (Greenspan, 1982).

THE PRESCHOOLER AND THE OEDIPAL CONSTELLATION

The preschool child's appropriate use of personal pronouns, ability to say no, and increasingly adaptive capacities all draw the family as a whole further and further into a new domain that will be characterized by the time the stage is complete by three-party rather than two-party relationships. Curiosity, assertiveness, and the capacity to begin to delay gratification help the child regulate and moderate intense instinctual feelings and affects. Cognitive growth, meanwhile, assists the child in learning and remembering what the important objects in his or her life will or will not tolerate. By the beginning of this phase, parents should have largely discarded baby talk, since both the child and the parents can have a more satisfactory communicative interaction. Reasonably adept parents are able to respond with affection, empathy, and a minimum of rejection to the preschool child's bid for intimate, controlling attention from the parent of the opposite sex. Appropriate, predictable limit setting and humor play important roles in helping the heterosexual relationships between child and parent withstand the heavy weather of strong rivalrous feelings. Latent oedipal issues, especially incomplete or conflictual ones, are often resolved with surprising force in the parent metapsychologically. By now parents are able to yield most control over bodily functions to the child, relinquishing him or her as a physical possession, and admiring and encouraging his or her attributes as a separate, gender-specific human being who is beginning to understand the joys of the delay of gratification.

During these preschool years, fathers interact with their children mainly through play and productivity. Through role modeling, the father provides opportunities for children of both sexes to build increasingly positive self-esteem (Sarnoff, 1982).

The press of developmental needs during this period, highlighted in research, shows us a critical relationship between marital satisfaction and parental involvement. There is much research that indicates marital satisfaction to be at its lowest ebb during the childbearing years (Glenn and McLanahan, 1982). Waldron and Routh (1981) note that marital satisfaction follows a U-shaped graph, with high levels of marital comfort before children are born and again after they leave home. Frequently children place such significant demands on the couple that there is often little energy left to fuel the marital relationship, although it is not suggested that children destroy marriages (even though in some instances they may be permitted or even encouraged to do so). Rapoport et al. (1977) report that marriage is often experienced by fathers as better than by mothers during this nadir of marital satisfaction, because it is mothers who usually have more negative experiences with their children, feel more isolated, and are more vulnerable to psychosomatic stress ailments, including fatigue.

Although the discrepancies between maternal and paternal experience during this phase of the life cycle can be problematic, including occasional envy and jealousy on the part of the parent who is having the more difficult and challenging time with the preschool child, the long-term effects of having both parents involved intimately during this phase are strongly positive. One of the most dramatic findings in the father-infant care research is the relationship between early involvement and subsequent sexual abuse. If a man is involved in the physical care of his child before the age of 3, there is a dramatic drop in the probability that that man will be involved later on in life with sexual abuse of his own or anyone else's children (Parker and Parker, 1984).

SCHOOL, LATENCY, AND FAMILY UNITY

The timely desexualization of the child-parent relationship allows the child to make libidinal investments in adults other than his or her own parents, initiating the first disillusionment in one's parents as omnipotent. Just as the child's body is relinquished from parental control, so is the child's mind released. The family now helps the child separate for most of his or her waking hours in order to attend school and make use of the social and cognitive challenges contained therein. Large amounts of energy are made available for relating to other children and adults, as well as for learning and problem solving. License must be granted for further exploration; at the same time, limits are placed in a reasonable, comfortable manner. The integration of family and tradition, as guided by societal mythology, serves as the hallmark of this period of development. Themes of internal control begin to compete with the pursuit of pleasure as the integrated 7- or 8-year-old strives for balance. During this period it is often easier for a family to spend prolonged, uninterrupted segments of time with one another for travel, leisure activities, and neighborhood projects. Interestingly, girls may have only one or two friends they would call ''best,'' while boys may name six or seven friends, who usually turn out to be somewhat more casual acquaintances. It is acknowledged that, as children age, the disciplinary role of the father must increase. But during the school-age and latency period, a father may serve as a confidant, a pal, even a friend or teacher

(Benson, 1968). The opportunity for shared activities and mastery experiences with adults of the same sex is extremely important in terms of the solidification of gender role behavior and gender identity itself. Father absence, however (Pearson, 1994), leads teachers to rate both boys and girls as more aggressive relative to mother-father families. Especially poignant was the finding that the protective factors for mother-father families were not apparent among low-income families.

ADOLESCENCE AND GENERATIONAL REDEFINITION

Families containing adolescents must utilize boundaries that are qualitatively different from those in families with younger children. The boundaries must now assist the children in managing their own impulses, as parents no longer have or can practice complete authority. The boundaries between the family and the outside world must become more permeable without being destroyed. There is a normal careening between independence and dependence. A sense of self is beginning to be consolidated and shaped by values, the search for pleasure, and particular goals and tasks. The primary object relationship between the parents and the teenager now must be retooled for the transition from childhood to adulthood. The teenager is involved in a regular, normative struggle between independence and dependence. The adolescent is also becoming intensely interested in his or her constantly changing body. Values and ''do unto others as they would have you do unto them'' beliefs are subject to greater scrutiny. Developmental stress does not necessarily doom the family to turmoil during this phase, but profound physical and psychological changes threaten the previous level of homeostasis within the family. An adolescent will notice weaknesses and unusual vulnerabilities in the family, as well as in his or her own psychological functioning, but these may also be seen as possible points of departure for new adaptive functioning. But adolescent observations are notoriously selective. Bulimic teenagers and young adults rated their fathers as showing less affection and more control toward them than their nonbulimic siblings, suggesting that the paternal relationship may be a source of nonshared environmental experience associated with bulimia nervosa (Wunderlich et al., 1994).

Adolescence is often a period of significant stress in the family because both the adolescents and their parents are often experiencing significant physiologic and mental changes at the same time. Both generations may be scrutinizing their primary attachments anew and questioning their value and trustworthiness. Just as the adolescent is beginning to make choices regarding values and career goals at the beginning of his or her work life, the parents are needing to accept that certain cherished goals may never be achieved, and they may become quite preoccupied by the limited time left in their lives.

As the adolescent begins to pull further away from the nurturing domain through going to college or taking a full-time job, the parental response can be one of either pride in their capacity to cope with life's new challenges or sadness over what appears to be the permanent loss of one's own progeny.

The family as a whole can have its homeostatic behavior deeply challenged by an adolescent's need to extract his or her autonomy from the parental nurturing domain.

Young adulthood and emancipation, the marriage of offspring (the middle family), and, finally, aging and senescence are the last three phases of normal family development. The kind of influence parents now have on their children is largely encompassed in their availability for discussion and advice and by witnessing to their children's integrity while being careful to plan and sustain their own autonomy. Grandchildren come next, providing a rejuvenation of spirit and body, not to mention occasions of joy.

The developmental tasks faced by the child and the child's caregivers are the same whether the structure of the family is nuclear or reconstituted. The energy and resources, both emotional and physical, to attend to those tasks is strongly influenced, however, by a particular family's structural limits and flexibility. Adoptive, single-parent, foster, and recombined family groupings are all subject to the same leadership, boundary, affectivity, communicative, and task and goal requirements. The issues of attachment, separation, emancipation, loss, and response to change are by and large the same. Each has its own special spin on normal development, but none, however, is by dint of structure alone doomed to trouble.

Adoptive families do not have the same biological preparation time, although given some luck they can follow a similar psychological preparation sequence. The separate biological parents' narrative must be integrated into the family's mental history of itself in some fashion. Single-parent families, whether male or female headed, face depletion and isolation early and often and work best when social support systems are early and flexible enough to supplement parental and child care. Even oedipal phase resolution need not be impossible, given the child's regular access to familiar and caring adults of the opposite sex.

Recombined and reconstituted families, when a divorced, widowed, or never-married single parent forms a household with a new partner who may or may not be a parent, also are increasing exponentially. These families do face special risks. Depending on the mechanism of parental singleness (death, divorce, abandonment), the new parent may be seen as a threat or solution to intimacy between parent and child. Rivalry and jealousy frequently stimulate guilt and anxiety, especially when the same-sex parent has been displaced or replaced. Interestingly, Black and Pedro-Carroll (1993) have shown that the effects of interparental conflict on the psychological well-being of children were mediated more by the overall quality of parent-child relationships, than by interadult conflict itself. Stepparents are frequently in risk situations, being tested by their "new children" while simultaneously feeling special loyalty to their "old children" and trying to sustain a new spousal relationship. Time (measured in years), patience, and liberal, frequent communication (sometimes new to everyone as a process) plus permission to parent are all essential. Society's myths do not help either. *Stepmother* in English conjures up Cinderella's stepmother, and *stepfather* in Spanish is *padrastro*, which also means *hangnail*.

On a smaller scale, all families face some of the same issues because families are always reconstituting, biologically and psychologically. Because of the relentless push of developmental and maturational forces in the individuals of our species, like the river, one can never step into one family in the same place twice.

References

Achenbach T, Howell C: Are American children's problems getting worse? A 13-year comparison. *J Am Acad Child Adolesc Psychiatry* 32: 1145–1154, 1993.

Ainsworth M, Eichberg C: Effects on infant-mother attachment of mother's unresolved loss of an attachment figure or other traumatic experience. In: Morris P, Parks C, Hinde R (eds): *Attachment Through the Lifespan*. New York, Routledge Press, 1991.

Bacon L: Early motherhood, accelerated role transition and social pathologies. *Soc Forces* 52: 333–341, 1974.

Becker G: Economics of marital instability. *J Polit Econ* 85:1141–1187, 1978.

Benson L: *Fatherhood: A Sociological Perspective*. New York, Random House, 1968.

Bezirganian S, Cohen P, Brook J: The impact of mother-child interaction on the development of Borderline Personality Disorder. *Am J Psychiatry* 150:1836–1842, 1993.

Biller H, Meredith D: *Father Power*. New York, David McKay, 1974.

Black A, Pedro-Carroll J: Role of parent-child relationship in mediating the effects of marital disruption. *J Am Acad Child Adolesc Psychiatry* 32: 1019–1027, 1993.

Bowen M: *Family Therapy in Clinical Practice*. New York, Aronson, 1978.

Burke R, Weir T: The relationships of wives' employment status to husband, wife and peer satisfaction. *J Marriage Fam* 2:279–287, 1976.

Coles R: *The Moral Life of Children*. Boston, Atlantic Monthly Press, 1985.

Demos J: *A Little Commonwealth: Family Life in Plymouth Colony*. New York, Oxford University Press, 1970.

Eichberg C: Quality of infant-parent attachment: Related to mother's representation of her own relationship history. Presented at Society for Research in Child Development, Baltimore, 1987.

Fleck S: The family and psychiatry. In: Kaplan HI, Sadock BJ (eds): *Comprehensive Textbook of Psychiatry* (6th ed). Baltimore, Williams & Wilkins, in press.

Fleck S (ed): *Psychiatric Prevention and the Family Life Cycle*. New York, Brunner/Mazel, 1989.

Galinsky E: Family life and corporate policies. In: Yogman M, Brazelton B (eds): *In Support of Families*. Cambridge, MA, Harvard University Press, 1986.

George C, Kaplan N, Main M: *The Berkeley Adult Attachment Interview*. Berkeley, CA, University of California, Department of Psychology, 1985.

Glenn G, McLanahan S: Children and marital happiness: A further specification of the relationship. *J Marriage Fam* 44:63–72, 1982.

Glick P, Norton A: Marrying, divorcing, and living together in the US today. *Pop Bull* 38:3–38, 1978.

Greenspan S: The second other: The role of the father in early personality formation and the dyadic-phallic phase of development. In: Cath S, Gurwitt A, Ross JM (eds): *Father and Child*. Boston, Little, Brown, 1982.

Hareven T: American families in transition: Historical perspectives on change. In: Walsh F (ed): *Normal Family Processes*. New York, Guilford, 1982.

Laslette P, Wall R (eds): *Household and Family in Past Time*. Cambridge, Cambridge University Press, 1972.

Main M, Goldwyn R: Adult attachment classification system. In: Main M (ed): *A Typology of Human Attachment Organization: Assessed in Discourse, Drawings and Interviews*. New York, Cambridge University Press, 1992.

Main M, Kaplan N, Cassidy J: Security in infancy, childhood and adulthood: A move to the level of representation. *Monogr Soc Res Child Dev* 50, 1985.

Parke R: Perspectives on father-infant interactions. In: Osofsky J (ed): *The Handbook of Infant Development*. New York, Wiley, 1979.

Parke R, Sawin D: Infant characteristics and behavior as elicitors of maternal and paternal responsiveness in the newborn period. Paper presented at Society for Research in Child Development, Denver, 1975.

Parker H, Parker S: Cultural roles, rituals and behavior regulation. *Am Anthropol* 86:584–600, 1984.

Patterson GR: Stress: A change agent for family process. In: Garmazy N, Rutter M (eds): *Stress, Coping and Development in Children*. New York, McGraw-Hill, 1983.

Pearson JL, Ialongo NS, Hunter AG, et al: Family structure and aggressive behavior in a population of urban elementary school children. *J Am Acad Child Adolesc Psychiatry* 33:540–548, 1994.

Pedersen F, Rubinstein J, Yarrow L: Infant development in father-absent families. *J Genet Psychol* 135:51–61, 1979.

Phares V, Compas BE: The role of fathers in child and adolescent psychopathology: Make room for daddy. *Psychol Bull* 111:387–412, 1992.

Pincus L, Dare C: *Secrets in the Family*. New York, Pantheon, 1978.

Pruett K: Infants of primary nurturing fathers. *Psychoanal Study Child* 40:257–277, 1983.

Pruett K: *The Nurturing Father*. New York, Warner, 1987.

Radin N, Harold-Goldsmith R: The involvement of selected unemployed and employed men with their children. *Child Dev* 60:454–459, 1989.

Rapoport R, Rapoport R, Strelitz Z: *Fathers, Mothers and Society*. New York, Basic Books, 1977.

Sameroff A: Models of development and developmental risk. In: Zeanah C (ed): *Handbook of Infant Mental Health*. New York, Guilford, 1993.

Sarnoff C: The father's role in latency. In: Cath S, Gurwitt A, Ross J (eds): *Father and Child: Developmental and Clinical Perspectives*. Boston, Little, Brown, 1982.

Skinner HA, Steinhauer PD, Santa-Barbara J: The Family Assessment Measure. *Can J Ment Health* 2:91–105, 1983.

Thomas C, Duszynski D: Closeness to parents and the family constellation in a prospective study of five diseased states: Suicide, mental illness, malignant tumor, hypertension, and coronary heart disease. *Johns Hopkins Med J* 134:251–270, 1974.

Vangelisti AL: Family secrets: Forms, functions, and correlates. *J Soc Pers Relationships* 11:113–135, 1994.

Waldron H, Routh D: The effect of the first child on the marital relationship. *J Marriage Fam* 43: 785–788, 1981.

Wonderlich S, Ukestad L, Perzacki R: Perceptions of nonshared childhood environment in bulimia nervosa. *J Am Acad Child Adolesc Psychiatry* 33: 740–747, 1994.

Yogman M: Development of the father-infant relationship. In: Fitzgerald G, Lester F, Yogman M (eds): *Theory and Research in Behavioral Pediatrics* (Vol 1). New York, Plenum, 1982, pp. 221–297.

D/ Developmental Phases

20 INFANCY

*Michael E. Lamb, Ph.D., Alison Nash, Ph.D., Douglas M. Teti, Ph.D.,
and Marc H. Bornstein, Ph.D.*

By definition, infancy is the period of life between birth and the emergence of language, 1½–2 years later. Despite its brevity, this phase of development has long attracted a disproportionate amount of attention and interest, but infancy as we know it was not considered a distinctive and important stage of life until late in the 18th century (Aries, 1962; Plumb, 1972), and it was not until the 1960s that a variety of scientific, social, medical, and political trends converged to generate professional interest in human infancy (Bornstein and Lamb, 1993; Kessen et al., 1970; Lamb and Bornstein, 1987). In the three decades of intensive theorizing and research since then, a number of core issues have emerged, and these issues constitute the centerpiece of this chapter. Among the most important of these issues are the following: To what extent do "innate" as opposed to experiential factors influence infant behavior and development? How great an impact do early experiences have on later development?

THE NATURE-NURTURE DEBATE

Although the nature-nurture debate is now centuries old, the issues at its core remain central to the study of infancy. Historically, the study of development—especially cognitive and perceptual development—was driven by the nature-nurture debate. Extreme views were put forward by the empiricists on the one hand and the nativists on the other. Empiricists like John Locke and William James asserted that there is no endowed knowledge at birth, that all knowledge comes through the senses, and that perceptual development reflects learned associations. They argued that external stimuli naturally provoke bodily "sensation" and that, through association, separate raw sensations can fuse into meaningful perceptions.

The belief that humans begin life "empty headed" was considered both philosophically intolerable and logically indefensible by nativists like Rene Descartes and Immanuel Kant, who proposed that humans were endowed at birth with ideas or "categories of knowledge" that assist early perception and cognition. They postulated that human beings possess innate perceptual abilities to tell size, form, position, and motion, as well as more abstract conceptions, such as knowledge of space and time.

Historically, a gradual shift in orientation can be discerned in the debates between nativists and empiricists. Initially, a so-called main effects model applied: Either environment or constitution was considered to be important. In the middle of the 20th century, however, an interactional model achieved popularity (Anastasi, 1958). Unlike proponents of the main effect model, interactionists offered an additive view, in which nature and nurture were believed to interact *together* to shape development. Twenty years later, the transactional model was articulated by Sameroff and Chandler (1975); they argued that inherent characteristics are shaped by experience and vice versa and that a constant process of mutual influence continues throughout the life span.

Although developmental psychologists now generally agree that neither experience nor biology alone determines behavior, the 1990s has seen a renewed, transformed nature-nurture debate. Advances in ge-

netics have led to renewed interest in behavioral genetics, and researchers with diverse interests are now collaborating on large-scale longitudinal studies designed to partition variance into genetic and environmental components (such as the MacArthur Longitudinal Twin Study; Emde et al., 1992; Plomin et al., 1993). Scarr (1993) has taken the extreme position of stating that, within the range of normal environments, behavioral variability among individuals can be accounted for by genetic influences. Others argue that the range of normal environments is too imprecise a term and that in fact it is just these details of socialization patterns that are crucial to an understanding of development (e.g., Baumrind, 1993).

In this paper, we take the view that biological adaptation and experience codetermine the course of development; infants are born with simple yet important behavioral proclivities that both constrain and direct development by delimiting the potential for experientially driven change. A baby who is congenitally distractible, for example, is likely to learn slowly about the objects seen or heard because he or she is unable to attend to or concentrate on them for long periods. Biological factors also determine which events may reinforce infant behavior, because certain events inherently complement certain experiences. A bad taste, for example, will make a baby stop eating a certain type of food much more rapidly than would a loud noise that repeatedly accompanied ingestion of that food (cf. Garcia and Koelling, 1966).

Two kinds of biologically based tendencies exist. Species-typical tendencies are those that all humans share. These include predispositions to cry when distressed, to respond to others' cries so as to alleviate them, and to attend to novel sounds, smells, or sights and to ignore those that have become boringly familiar. By contrast, heritable influences are those that distinguish one person's tendencies from those of another and are the basis of genetically rooted individual differences. Both species-typical and heritable tendencies have important influences on development.

As far as experiential or environmental influences are concerned, Gilbert Gottlieb (1983) suggests a useful distinction among inductive, facilitative, and maintenance functions. Induction is the most dramatic form of influence. It occurs when a particular experience or set of experiences completely determines whether or not a capacity, behavior, or tendency will emerge. Facilitation occurs when certain experiences speed up or slow down the emergence of capacities, behaviors, or tendencies. Finally, maintenance describes a situation in which experiences preserve already developed capacities, behaviors, or tendencies.

We view both experiential and environmental influences as functioning together so that it is impossible to assess the extent of their involvement. This chapter repeatedly notes the ways in which biology (in the form of predispositions and innate propensities) constrains or facilitates experience and learning.

THE CONTINUITY DEBATE

The continuity debate focuses on the importance of early experiences. Some view the experiences and behavior patterns developed in infancy of crucial importance to later life. Social orientations, motivations, and intellectual predilections established in infancy set lifelong patterns. Others argue that infancy is not of overriding importance because experiences in infancy have little (if any) long-term predictive significance.

Proponents of Continuity

Early-experience proponents arrived at this position from a diverse array of theoretical starting points. Sigmund Freud (1940/1968) was the first major theorist to focus attention on infancy, justifying this focus by suggesting that the ways babies are treated establish lifelong orientations and personality traits. Freud proposed that there are critical phases in development when certain sorts of experience—affecting specific types of traits—are of special significance. Infancy falls within Freud's oral phase of development, during which feeding experiences and other activities centered on the mouth are particularly relevant. Toward the end of infancy, Freud continued, the oral phase yields to the anal phase. During this period caretaker-infant interactions center on toilet training and are likely to have long-term consequences as well. However smoothly development unfolds in this phase, though, it is never possible to override any oral problems established earlier; difficulties can be overcome only by "reliving" earlier experiences through lengthy psychotherapy.

Erik Erikson (1963) portrayed early experiences and their effects rather differently. From the early feeding experiences, he suggested, children develop a degree of trust or mistrust in the caretaker rather than concrete oral traits. He also believed that the quality of early interactions (i.e., how much "basic trust" the infant develops) has implications for the way the infant will negotiate the next stage of development, in which the key issue is establishing autonomy or shame. With respect to toilet training, therefore, Erikson emphasized not the anal organs but the status of toilet training as a battleground of wills as the child tries to exert initial control (by determining when to give the caretaker the prize the caretaker seeks). Erikson described eight developmental stages, each marked by a crucial issue: Basic trust/mistrust is at issue in the first stage; autonomy/shame is at issue in the second.

Erikson's view of how early experiences affect the child's later personality substantially improved on Freud's in two major ways. First, Erikson portrayed the lessons learned in each phase in more abstract, general terms (e.g., trust, autonomy) than did Freud (e.g., orality, anality), and the psychological issues described indeed seem pertinent to the stages concerned. Second, Erikson explicitly proposed that the ways in which different stages are resolved are somewhat interrelated. From Erikson's perspective, how much the infant trusts the caretaker may affect the infant's willingness to cooperate in toilet training and other matters. This initial mistrust may yield not only a mistrustful adult but one plagued by unsuccessful resolution of later developmental issues as well.

Unfortunately, the ideas of Freud and his followers, including Erikson, were phrased in mentalistic terms that rarely evoked respect from research scientists. Behaviorists and learning theorists like John B. Watson, Clark Hull, and Neal Miller dominated developmental psychology from the second to the sixth decade of this century. Like the psychoanalysts, these theorists emphasized the importance of infant experiences, and Miller even attempted to rephrase many of Freud's ideas in terms compatible with behaviorism (Dollard and Miller, 1950). Learning theorists treated early experience in a fashion very different from that of Freud and Erikson, however. Behaviorists eschewed the notions of stages and phases of development. For the learning theorists, early experiences are important because they are first, have no competing propensities to replace, and thus yield easy and rapid learning. Moreover, early behavior patterns are believed to serve as foundations for more complex behavior patterns, such as personality traits.

A third group of theorists, most of them ethologists and students of animal behavior, adopted a notion of "critical periods" that also emphasized early experiences (Bornstein, 1987). The ethologists argue that there are predetermined periods in the maturation of organisms during which development is maximally susceptible to influence by specific types of experiences. Just as Freud spoke of an oral phase during which feeding experiences make the greatest impact on the developing personality, the ethologists spoke of a critical period for imprinting and for various other behavioral tendencies. During critical periods, lessons are learned more easily and demonstrate greater endurance than hitherto or later possible. This notion accorded biological and scientific support to Freud's own and was later integrated into Bowlby's (1969) theory of attachment (see below) and Lenneberg's (1967) theory of language development (see below). The critical periods concept, and its modern "sensitive periods" emendation, assigned great importance to early experiences because it held that once a particular critical period had passed, it was no longer possible for specific experiences to exert formative influences on the developing organism.

Although this diverse group of theorists underscored the formative importance of early experiences, popular commitment to the proposition developed as a result of some dramatic empirical observations published between 1930 and 1950. At that time, reports that children who were reared in impersonal institutions were psychologically stunted led to widespread belief that children needed close relationships in infancy and that, if they were denied such relationships, they would not develop into psychologically healthy individuals (Bowlby, 1951).

An additional perspective on the continuing importance of infancy was offered by students of cognitive and intellectual development. Jean Piaget (1936/1953, 1937/1954) theorized that all intellectual capacities are built on the simple developments that take place very early in life, and thus by the early 1960s hardly anyone doubted that early experiences were especially important. Two trends resulted: a massive increase in the amount of research on infancy and the first attempts to engineer enriching experiences for deprived children in the form of such programs as Head Start. By capitalizing on the special sensitivity of the very young, politicians hoped to "immunize" children against the debilitating effects of later deprivation. More than anything else, the apparent failure of these interventions triggered a decline of confidence in the notion that early experiences were especially influential.

Proponents of Discontinuity

One of the most vocal opponents of the overemphasis on early experiences is Jerome Kagan (1971, 1980; Kagan et al., 1978). Kagan argued that maturation—the unfolding of genetically determined capacities and individual differences—has been undervalued, and he pointed to research indicating that major differences in rearing environments have little apparent effect on the way children behave. For example, he argued that day care and home care have remarkably similar effects on developing infants (Kagan et al., 1978) and that even the extreme impoverishment of the rural Guatemalan environment does not retard intellectual development (Kagan and Klein, 1973).

Kagan's arguments have been roundly criticized by researchers who argue that his measures may not be sensitive and that the problem therefore lies in the assessment, not in the concept, of experiential influence. Nevertheless, claims that there is little continuity in development have attracted a great deal of attention. Such conclusions were inevitable because of earlier oversimplified notions about how infant experiences influenced later development. The difficulty lies in overreliance on the main effects models of development (like Freud's), holding that early experiences have obvious and direct short- and long-term effects. Unfortunately, simple linear relations are almost never empirically substantiated (M.H. Bornstein, unpublished manuscript, 1986; Caldwell, 1964; Lamb et al., 1985; Sameroff, 1975; Sameroff and Chandler, 1975).

The "Transactional" View

As with the nature-nurture controversy, Sameroff's transactional model now replaces the linear or main effects model. Both child and parent are believed to bring distinctive characteristics to every interaction. The child's characteristics affect how the child behaves, how parents treat the child, and how the parents' behaviors affect the child. The parents' characteristics have the same consequences. During each interaction, both parent and child are psychologically changed, and so they enter the next round of interaction as different individuals. From this perspective, it is naive to expect any single experience to have direct long-term effects, for its impact will be diffuse, triggering multiple indirect effects (e.g., also changing the adult's behavior). Nevertheless, events in infancy are important because they initiate such multiple processes of development.

Using this model, Sameroff and Chandler (1975) were able to explain why prematurity, like other types of perinatal risk (Siegel, 1981), does not always have ill effects. Parents cope with atypical babies in different ways, some providing deprived environments that do not afford the types of experiences that prematurely born children need to offset their potential for developmental delay. Premature infants would be at risk over the long term only if reared in such environments. Thus, in order to make long-term predictions, one has to consider at least characteristics of the child, of the parents, and of the family's physical and social environment. Since linear models typically focus on only one of these factors, it is not surprising that their predictive power is poor. One implication of the transactional perspective is that continuity from infancy may be carried *indirectly*, through continuity in the supporting environment, or continuity from infancy may be carried *directly*, through continuity in the infant, *or* it may be that both are important (Lamb et al., 1984, 1985; Nash and Hay, 1993). Grossmann and Grossmann (1986), for example, found that there was a significant level of stability in neonatal performance from day to day on the Brazelton Scales (Brazelton, 1973) and that it was possible to divide their sample into "good" and "bad" orienters. Subsequent observations of the mothers and infants at home allowed the Grossmanns to assess the mothers' behavioral sensitivity. *All* six of the babies who were good orienters *and* had sensitive mothers developed "secure" attachment relationships at 12 months; however, poor orienters with tender and sensitive mothers did so only about one-third of the time. Good orienters with sober-talking and less sensitive mothers had only a 38% chance of being "securely attached," whereas only one of the eight babies (13%) who were poor orienters and whose mothers were insensitive developed "secure" attachments. Viewed together, these data suggest that the characteristics of the baby and the characteristics of the mother jointly determined what sort of attachment they form—just as Sameroff and Chandler predicted. Of course, the Grossmanns' small sample made it imperative to replicate these findings independently, but they do constitute an elegant confirmation of the transactional model. In this chapter the ways in which genetically determined tendencies interact with both early and later experiences to shape development are repeatedly described; consistent with the transactional theorists, the authors see development as a continuing process of consolidation and change.

The focus now shifts, however, from overarching issues to specific aspects of development, beginning with perception.

PERCEPTUAL DEVELOPMENT

Perception constitutes a necessary first step in experiencing and interpreting the world, and for this reason philosophers, psychologists, physiologists, and physicists alike have been attracted to the study of perception. In fact, the study of perception was initiated by philosophers who were interested in the nature-nurture debate, but it also provides information about the quality, limits, and capacities of the sensory systems at the start of life. In this section, we selectively review research on visual and auditory perception, the modalities that have been studied most extensively.

Visual Perception

PATTERN PERCEPTION

In the 1960s William Kessen (1967) reasoned that it ought to be possible to assess infant vision, even at birth, simply by "looking at looking." He and his colleagues photographed the reflection of a stimulus on infants' corneas and found that, even in the 1st hours after birth, infants looked selectively at parts of stimuli where there was information—usually high-contrast features—instead of scanning the background or central parts of figures randomly.

Subsequent research using this corneal reflection technique has asked not only what the baby looks at but also how scan patterns develop and how babies scan different visual shapes, such as faces and geometric forms (Haith, 1979, 1980; Salapatek, 1975). Younger babies scan in a limited fashion, whereas older babies scan patterns more widely, although the size (Hainline, 1978; Hainline and Lemerise, 1982) and nature of the stimulus (Maurer, 1983, 1985) affect their looking too. Haith et al. (1977), for example, found that infants spend increasing amounts of time looking at faces as they age from 1 to 3 months and that infants also scan different features of the face as they get older. One-month-olds scan the edges and contrasts of the head and background more than the eyes and central features of the face, whereas 2- to 3-month-olds scan the eyes and central features more than the outer contours. Babies at all three ages look at their mothers as much as at strangers, they look at still and moving faces equally, but they look at faces that talk more than at faces that are silent. Haith et al. concluded that perception develops over the first 2 months of life from mere concentration on components to appreciation of the face as a whole.

From such research on infant scanning, Haith (1980) determined that newborn infants actively seek visual stimulation and input, scanning the environment in order to find things to inspect. Newborns also focus most of their attention on the boundaries of figures, where the greatest amount of information is contained. Studies of organized scanning do not tell us *how well* infants see or *what* they see, however. To examine visual acuity in infants, Fantz et al. (1962) capitalized on the observation that infants prefer heterogeneous to homogeneous patterns, posting pairs of patterns for babies to look at; one member of the pair was always gray and the other a set of black and white stripes that varied systematically in width. (The two stimuli were always matched in overall brightness.) The stripe width that failed to evoke a preference was viewed as the one delimiting the baby's ability to tell stripes from the solid gray. By this measure, 2-week-olds showed 20/800 vision (in Snellen notation), whereas 5½-month-olds showed 20/70 vision. In the 30 years since Fantz's original study, techniques for measuring infant visual acuity have grown in sophistication, but the results agree well with Fantz's findings (Banks and Dannemiller, 1987; Gwiazda et al., 1989). Acuity improves steadily from infancy until adult (20/20) levels are reached at about 5 years (Atkinson and Braddock, 1989).

Several studies suggest that young infants can perceive some patterns as whole forms (Bertenthal et al., 1980; Bornstein, 1981b, 1982; Bornstein and Krinsky, 1985). For example, Van Giffen and Haith (1984) followed the eye movements of 1- and 3-month-olds presented with stimuli such as circles composed of interrupted arcs. They found that 3-month-olds scanned irregularities in patterns much more than regularities, implying some rudimentary sensitivity to what constitutes a "good form"; 1-month-olds gave only equivocal data. Further, Philip Kellman (1984; Kellman and Spelke, 1983) studied infants' knowledge of two- and three-dimensional objects when habituated to partly occluded versions of the objects or to multiple perspectives; 4-month-olds who experienced objects moving under these conditions treated them as wholes. Even newborns are attracted by movement (Haith, 1966): Infants fixate dynamic patterns and faces longer than static ones (Carpenter, 1974; Kaufmann and Kaufmann, 1980), and they lock onto moving heads and blinking eyes (Samuels, 1985). The infant's perception of motion is actually quite sophisticated: Ruff (1982a, 1985) demonstrated that 3½- to 5-month-olds discriminated translation from translation plus rotation, and by 5 months infants discriminated translation from rotation alone, rotation from oscillation around the vertical, and left versus right rotation.

Babies also seem to discriminate orientation well: They discriminate vertical from horizontal (Bornstein et al., 1978; Fisher et al., 1981;

McKenzie and Day, 1971; Moffett, 1969) and will even adjust a reaching hand properly to match the orientation of a target (Von Hofsten and Fazel-Zandy, 1984). Five-month-olds discriminate horizontal from 35° off horizontal (Weiner and Kagan, 1976), 4-month-olds vertical from 45° off vertical (Bornstein et al., 1978), and 5- to 6-month-olds a vertical face from the same face at a 45° diagonal (Bornstein et al., 1978). Patterns that are aligned vertically or horizontally are detected more readily than those aligned obliquely (Held, 1989), with vertical stimuli appearing to be the most preferred, perhaps because infants visually scan predominantly along the horizontal (Haith, 1991).

DEPTH PERCEPTION

Depth perception is crucial to determining the spatial layout of the environment, to recognizing objects, and to guiding motor action. The study of depth perception also addresses an interesting psychophysical question, namely, how we perceive the three-dimensional information. Depth perception has served as a kind of battleground between nativists and empiricists. Debate on this question exemplifies the typical historical course: It began with hotly contested disputes between nativists and empiricists that spanned the 17th to 19th centuries and ended only with experimentation in the 20th century.

In the early 1960s, Gibson and Walk (1960) began to investigate depth perception in infants experimentally, using a "visual cliff." One side of the cliff shows the baby an illusory drop, but the other side does not. Gibson and Walk found that almost all infants they tested between 6 and 14 months of age crawled over the glass continuation of the center board on the shallow side when their mothers called them, whereas only a very small minority of infants crawled across the "deep" side. From these results, Gibson and Walk concluded that depth perception must be present in infants as young as 6 months of age. By 6 months, however, children have had plenty of experience perceiving depth. Campos and his colleagues (1970) therefore studied precrawling babies by monitoring heart rate when the babies were exposed to shallow and deep sides of the visual cliff. They found that babies as young as 2 months of age showed defensive changes in heart rate when exposed to the deep side. These differences suggest that babies may perceive depth long before they crawl.

The visual cliff experiments represent one way investigators have sought to explore the capacity to perceive depth. Another mode of study involves "looming." Two-week-olds show an "integrated avoidance response" to impending collision—throwing back their heads, shielding their faces with their hands, and even crying when an object moves at them along a hit path—but do not show these defensive reactions when the same object moves along a "miss path" or recedes in space (Ball and Tronick, 1971; Bower et al., 1970). Yonas (1981; Yonas and Granrud, 1985) pointed out, however, that an object's upper contour naturally moves upward in the field of view as the object advances. In "throwing their heads back," therefore, infants might simply be tracking the upper contour of the advancing image, thereby giving only the impression of "avoiding." Yonas conducted a series of experiments involving babies of different ages in conditions where an object's image remained on a hit path but its upper contour either remained at a constant visual level or rose. The babies appeared to track upper contours, and the "looming response" could not be demonstrated reliably until babies reached approximately 4 months of age. However, Yonas found that babies as young as 1 month show a reasonably consistent eye blink to approaching objects.

A third strategy for investigating depth involves studying sensitivities to isolated visual cues that typically signal depth. Convergence, for example, depends on an organism's capacities to fixate an object binocularly and to fuse the two disparate retinal images into one. If infants rely on convergence of the eyes to cue depth, as Descartes (1638/1824) and Berkeley (1709/1901) proposed, theorists need to show that the eyes indeed converge. We have all noted, however, that babies often seem unable to fix both eyes on an object (called strabismus). Studies of

infants' tracking of moving targets have revealed only minimal convergence of the two eyes at 1 month but regular convergence by 2–3 months (Aslin, 1977; Maurer, 1975). It is at this time that infants also first display sensitivity to the deep side of the visual cliff (Campos et al., 1970).

In sum, studies of the visual cliff, of looming, and of monocular and binocular sensitivity in human babies converge to suggest that depth perception may be relatively poor until about 2 months after birth. The development of depth perception is not complete by 4–6 months of age, however, although infants have the capacity for *relative* distance perception by this age. Because binocularity can provide information about absolute distance only if interocular distance is known, *absolute* distance calibration may depend on nonvisual sources of information. Theorists such as Jean Piaget (1937/1954) have argued that infants can tell the absolute distance of objects in near space only after they have had experience reaching, and the distance of objects in far space (i.e., beyond reach) only after having experienced crawling.

We know that young babies can *locate* stimuli in space, in part from studies of reaching for objects. Recording following motions, goal-directed behaviors, and types of reaches to objects located at different distances and moving at different velocities, Von Hofsten (1984) reported that infants as young as 4½ months will reach and contact an object, even if it is moving (Von Hofsten and Lindhagen, 1979), and that their reaching is accomplished in a way that indicates good predictive targeting of location (Von Hofsten, 1980). Until recently, it was believed that such reaching and grasping of objects resulted from visual guidance of the hand toward the object. However, Ashmead et al. (1993) found that it is not until about 9 months of age that the opportunity to *see* the hand helps infants make adjustments to a change in target locations. Similarly, Clifton et al. (1993), tested very young infants' (up to 6 months of age) abilities to reach for objects in the dark (only the targets were illuminated), and found that sight of their own hands was not necessary for reaching and grasping.

Locomotion also affects depth perception: Infants who crawl or have experience in a "walker" extract form from a fluctuating display (Campos et al., 1980) and avoid the deep side of the visual cliff (Campos et al., 1981) earlier than those without comparable experience. Benson and Uzgiris (1985) demonstrated that infants who searched after crawling to the search location found hidden objects more frequently than did infants who were carried to the search location.

COLOR

Babies are nearly as acute as adults when the task is to compare brightness differences between stimuli presented simultaneously (Teller and Bornstein, 1986), although they are much poorer if the comparison is separated in space or time (Kessen and Bornstein, 1978). Thus, in studies where the task is wavelength discrimination per se, it is possible to unconfound hue and brightness either (*a*) by matching colors in brightness using an adult standard in regions of the spectrum where infants and adults are known to match or in conditions testing successive discrimination (as Chase, 1937, and Bornstein, 1975, did) or (*b*) by varying brightness against hue so that brightness differences are irrelevant (as Peeples and Teller, 1975, and Schaller, 1975, did). In each case, babies of 2–4 months of age were shown to perceive color.

So-called color blind people make identifiable color discrimination errors, and they also confuse certain wavelengths with white. Bornstein (1976) found that 3-month-old infants could discriminate blue-green from white and could discriminate between yellow and green, suggesting that infants are not green-blind. Teller et al. later confirmed these findings and extended them to infants as young as 1 month (Hamer et al., 1982; Packer et al., 1985; Teller et al., 1978), while Adams et al. (1986) showed the same capacity in neonates only hours old. Teller has also found that even 1-month-olds give some evidence that they are not blue-blind, a rare third kind of color blindness (Varner et al., 1984). Additionally, the red/green and yellow/blue sensitivity of 1- to 3-month-olds was found to be similar to that of adults (Maurer et al., 1989; Teller and Lindsey, 1989). The development of color vision right after birth has not been studied so well, and its nature during the 1st month is still undetermined (Clavadetscher et al., 1988). Although 1- and 2-month-olds clearly have largely normal color vision, many questions still remain about infant sensitivity to brightness (Brown, 1990).

Adults do not just see colors; they perceive the color spectrum as organized qualitatively into categories of hue, and the infant's color perceptions seems to be similarly organized. Infants as young as 4 months of age perceive the hues blue, green, yellow, and red categorically and in ways similar to those of adults (Bornstein, 1981a; Bornstein et al., 1976). We do not know whether newborns also perceive color categorically since the phenomenon has not yet been studied at that age. However, after reviewing the physiological, anthropological, and psychological literatures, Bornstein (1981a, 1984) concluded that the ability to perceive color categorically is probably both universal and early appearing, reflecting the normal physiological function of the visual system. Furthermore, there is evidence for a preference for chromatic over achromatic stimuli from birth, although preferences for particular colors do not emerge until the 3rd month; unlike adults, 3-month-olds prefer red and yellow to blue and green (Adams, 1987).

Auditory Perception

Even though audition is of major importance to the infant, much less is known about audition than about vision in early life (Eilers and Oller, 1988; Morrongiello, 1990). Newborns can hear sounds: Make a sudden loud noise, and a neonate will startle. Further, acuity of hearing improves rapidly over the first few days after birth as amniotic fluid drains from the ear.

BASIC AUDITORY PROCESSES

Sound is specified principally by two variables: frequency, the rate at which sound waves vibrate; and amplitude, the intensity of sound waves. Humans hear sounds in the frequency range of approximately 20–20,000 cycles per second, or Hertz (Hz). For adults, auditory threshold varies with the frequency of the sound: Both low and high frequencies (above or below 1000 Hz) require more energy than middle frequencies (around 1000 Hz) to be heard. Schneider (Schneider et al., 1980; Trehub et al., 1980) found that infant thresholds for complex octave-band noises (as opposed to pure tones) vary substantially with frequency, that they are higher than those of adults for low frequencies (200 Hz), approach adult levels for middle frequencies (1000 Hz), are again higher than those of adults at high frequencies (10,000 Hz), and are again nearly equivalent at very high frequencies (19,000 Hz). Olsho et al. (1982a, 1982b; Olsho, 1984) found that infants could discriminate tones differing by only about 2% in frequency in the 1000–3000-Hz range (where adult frequency discrimination is about 1%) and that infant thresholds were twice those of adults at low frequencies (250–1000 Hz), whereas their discrimination was virtually the same as adults' at high frequencies (2000–8000 Hz). Nearly continuous developmental improvements in hearing at low and high frequencies occur during the first 2 years (Schneider et al., 1980; Trehub et al., 1980). Changes in ear structure or nervous system maturation could account for this increasing developmental sensitivity.

In addition, even though infants have smaller heads than do adults, and the locations of sound depends on the distance between the ears, infants are remarkably good at finding the sources of sounds in their environments. By 1 year of age, localization responses are comparable to those of adults (Schneider et al., 1988).

SPEECH PERCEPTION

Infants' excellent hearing abilities (Aslin et al., 1983; Trehub and Schneider, 1985) are applied almost immediately to the highly complex task of perceiving speech. In general, human speech is centered at relatively low frequencies, and numerous investigators have suggested that human speech is special for babies, who seem to be especially "tuned" to the speech register (Eisenberg, 1976; Fernald, 1984). Berg and Smith (1983) found that even 6-month-olds are more sensitive to 500- and 2000-Hz tones than to 8000-Hz tones. The topic that has intrigued researchers most, however, has to do with the infant's ability to perceive special aspects of speech.

Adults perceive differences in voicing more or less *categorically*; that is, although we can distinguish fine differences in the onset times of low- and high-frequency sounds, we tend to classify different examples of the same voiced (/b/) or voiceless (/p/) sounds as similar, but easily discriminate between voiced and voiceless sounds. Of course, different people say /b/ and /p/ in different ways, yet adult listeners seldom misidentify speech sounds, as they employ implicit category definitions to determine whether a sound falls within the /b/ or /p/ categories. Many people have assumed that phenomena so ubiquitous and significant as the categorical perception of speech sounds might have a biological foundation. To test this assumption, Eimas et al. (1971) asked whether preverbal infants perceive voicing categorically and found that they did: 1- and 4-month-olds distinguished between variants of /b/ and variants of /p/.

Not all languages use all voicing categories. Eimas et al. tested an English category distinction in American babies, but if categorical perception is innate, it ought to be universal, and infants from communities where different patterns of voicing prevail should all make the same categorical distinctions. Spanish has a voiced-voiceless distinction that is not in the same frequency location as the English one, yet Spanish 4- and 6-month-olds discriminate the English voiced-voiceless sound contrast rather than the Spanish one (Lasky et al., 1975). Likewise, Kikuyu (Kenyan) 2-month-olds categorize both an English voicing contrast not present in Kikuyu as well as an idiosyncratic Kikuyu prevoiced-voiced contrast not present in English (Streeter, 1976). Interestingly, Spanish and Kikuyu adults perceive (although they do not use) the English voicing contrast, but they perceive it only weakly; between infancy and maturity, therefore, a perceptual discrimination that is present at birth atrophies (but is not lost) if not utilized. The literature on categorical speech perception is replete with numerous examples of this (Aslin et al., 1983; Trehub and Schneider, 1985). Kuhl et al. (1992) have recently found that, by 6 months of age, infants are screening out categorical variations that are meaningless in their native language. Thus, certain perceptions seem to be universal and developed at birth; they are maintained by linguistic experiences, but may decay if absent from the language heard by the child, whereas other perceptions can be induced or altered in infants and children by exposure to certain speech sounds.

The existence of innate capacities to perceive speech sounds and color categorically underscores the perceptual competence of newborn infants. Together with tendencies to seek out stimulation and rapid developmental increases in perceptual acuity, they show that infants are designed for the efficient extraction of information about the environment. Acuity in the other perceptual modalities—the tactile and chemical (olfaction and gustation) senses—is also impressively good. Unfortunately these modalities have received little attention. The next section examines the ways in which infants build upon their perceptual experiences by learning.

CONDITIONING, HABITUATION, AND NOVELTY PREFERENCE

Learning "refers to a more or less permanent change in behavior which occurs as a result of practice" (Kimble, 1961, p. 2), and there has been considerable debate concerning the process and content of infant learning. Mechanistic theorists like Watson and Skinner believed that cognitive and emotional development depended on the infant's ability to learn associations between contiguous actions or events. Moreover, they argued that any environmental stimulus could be associated with any response, given a sufficient amount of practice. By contrast, organismic theorists like Jean Piaget argued that learning could be understood only in light of the organism's phylogenetic and experiential history. As is shown in this section, infants can and do form stimulus-response associations, but not between any stimulus and response. First, classical and operant conditioning and the conditions under which they have been demonstrated in human infants are discussed, then habituation and novelty preference and their use in investigating detection/discrimination, categorization, and concept formation.

Classical Conditioning

The classical conditioning paradigm was developed by Ivan Pavlov (1927), who reported that the salivation response could be elicited in dogs by a ringing bell alone after several trials in which the bell was followed by placement of food in the dogs' mouths. In this paradigm, salivation was the unconditioned response (UCR), which was reliably elicited by food powder, the unconditioned stimulus (UCS). The ringing bell initially had no effects on salivation and was said to be a neutral stimulus. However, the bell acquired the power to elicit salivation after being repeatedly paired with the presentation of food. The bell was then termed the conditioned stimulus (CS), and salivation became the conditioned response (CR).

Classical conditioning deals exclusively with reflexive and autonomic response systems over which the organism apparently has little control. Pavlov and his followers theorized about the importance of classical conditioning for the acquisition of language, culturally prescribed behaviors, normal and neurotic habits, and cognitive processes like thought and problem solving, but few today believe that classical conditioning plays a central role in the development of thought and language. However, many believe that it can help explain how specific emotions become associated with specific stimuli (such as in the development of phobias). Moreover, classical conditioning has provided important information about the types of stimulus-response associations newborns and older infants are "prepared" to make, allowing insights into how the infant mind is organized.

Classical conditioning is not easily demonstrated in newborns, but researchers have successfully conditioned sucking (Blass et al., 1984; Lipsitt and Kaye, 1964), heart rate (Clifton, 1974; Stamps and Porges, 1975), the Babkin reflex (Cantor et al., 1983; Kaye, 1965), pupillary reflexes (Brackbill, 1967), and head turning (Clifton et al., 1972; Siqueland and Lipsitt, 1966). The difficulty in establishing conditioned responses in newborns is probably due in part to the rapidity with which newborns pass through different arousal states; state may influence the likelihood of response elicitation, latency, and magnitude (Fitzgerald and Brackbill, 1976; Sameroff and Cavanagh, 1979). Clifton and Nelson (1976) indicated that most periods of alertness in neonates last less than 10 minutes.

Questioning the traditional assumption that any stimulus could be associated with any response, Seligman (1970) suggested that organisms are prepared, unprepared, or contraprepared to associate specific stimuli and responses. Prepared associations are those that apparently require little learning and that are directly related to an organism's survival (linking certain stimuli with feeding or food seeking). Unprepared stimulus-response combinations become associated only through learning, whereas contraprepared stimulus-response (S-R) combinations are hard to associate no matter how extensive the attempts to condition them. Sameroff and Cavanagh (1979) argued that the most direct means of empirically distinguishing learned from prepared S-R combinations is by examining the speed of association: Prepared associations, like those demonstrated in newborns, should occur rapidly, whereas learned associations should take more time. They concluded that newborns were not capable of learning by conditioning.

Rovee-Collier and Lipsitt (1982) argued in response that the ability to form S-R associations rapidly is biologically adaptive for newborns, and thus that rapidity of association is not a sufficient criterion to judge whether or not learning has taken place. To bolster their argument, they

noted that duration of sucking increases when followed by bursts of music of similar duration (Cairns and Butterfield, 1975), demonstrating that changes in a biological response system can be effected by nonbiological events. According to Rovee-Collier (1987), all infants are capable of conditioning, but the economics of the response demanded of the infants may sometimes require too great an expenditure of effort to be worthwhile.

After 3 months of age, classical conditioning is more easily demonstrated than in the newborn period, although the concepts of preparedness and biological constraints continue to be relevant. Instead of being able to associate any neutral stimulus with any response, infants appear predisposed to associate temporal CSs (i.e., a specified interval of time) with autonomic responses (e.g., pupillary reflexes) and to associate tactile, auditory, and visual CSs with somatic reflexes (e.g., eye blinks, sucking) (Fitzgerald and Brackbill, 1976). Thus, specific classes of stimuli are most readily associated with specific classes of responses.

Operant Conditioning

Unlike classical conditioning, in which a neutral signal comes to elicit an autonomic or reflexive response through repeated pairings with an unconditioned stimulus, operant conditioning increases or decreases the probability of a voluntary, nonreflexive "operant" response by controlling its consequences (Skinner, 1932). The underlying principle is the "Law of Effect," which states that actions followed by positive consequences (reinforcement) are more likely to be repeated, whereas actions followed by negative consequences (punishment) are less likely to be repeated.

Interestingly, operant conditioning is more easily demonstrated in newborns than is classical conditioning, although here again the associations that have survival value are learned most readily. Among newborns, operant conditioning experiments typically involve sucking (DeCasper and Fifer, 1980; Lipsitt and Kaye, 1965; Lipsitt et al., 1966; Sameroff, 1968) or head turning (Siqueland, 1968), two systems that are critical for newborn survival. After obtaining baseline measures of sucking rate for each 3-day-old infant, for example, DeCasper and Fifer (1980) divided their subjects into two groups. Infants in one group were presented with the sound of their mothers' voice whenever the interval between successive sucking bursts was greater than the infant's own average interval, and with the voice of another infant's mother when the interburst interval was less than average. Infants in the second group heard their mothers' voice when the intersucking interval was less than average, and the voice of another mother when the intersucking interval was greater than average. Eight of the 10 infants modified their sucking pattern to produce their own mother's voice more often.

A basic principle of operant conditioning in infancy appears to be that neonatally conditionable responses are those that produce maximum gain for the infant at relative low energy cost (Rovee-Collier and Lipsitt, 1982). Higher energy responses, such as foot kicking, do not appear to be conditionable until after the infant becomes capable of homeostatic thermoregulation, which occurs during the 2nd month. Rovee-Collier and Gekoski (1979) point out that organisms tend not only to learn associations that are adaptive in a biological sense but also to "perform cost-benefit analyses. . . . They cannot afford to exceed their budget for one activity as this will reduce the time and/or energy available for other critical activities" (p. 198).

The propensity to learn associations that have functional significance and require minimal energy expenditure is illustrated by conjugate reinforcement, which involves making the frequency and intensity of reinforcement (e.g., the movement of a mobile) contingent upon the frequency and intensity of a particular response (e.g., kicking) (Rovee and Rovee, 1969; Rovee-Collier and Gekoski, 1979). Learning is easy under conjugate reinforcement, suggest Rovee-Collier and Gekoski (1979), because the contingencies are similar to those that infants encounter most frequently in the real world. For example, intense infant cries are more likely to elicit responses than weak cries are, whereas intense sucking produces more milk than weak sucking. In addition, the behaviors lending themselves most readily to conjugate reinforcement impose low energy costs on the infant while providing information about the parameters that guide the infant's manipulation of and control over the environment.

Habituation and Novelty Preference

Habituation refers to the progressive decline in responding to repeated presentations of a stimulus. The habituation task begins with the presentation of a stimulus, usually visual or auditory, to which the infant's attention is measured. Infants typically respond with longer attention spans during the initial presentations, presumably because the stimulus is novel, but attention declines over subsequent presentations. Sokolov's (1958/1963) theory of orienting and habituation, which stimulated a great deal of work on habituation, postulates that the degree of orientation to a stimulus is a direct function of whatever traces of that stimulus are in memory. The weaker the trace, the stronger the orienting reflex.

Few studies of habituation were conducted in humans prior to the 1960s, perhaps because it was viewed as a very primitive kind of learning, essentially unrelated to the association process considered central to perceptual, cognitive, and emotional development. In the 1950s and 1960s, however, research suggested that habituation depended upon cortical processes that were actually more complicated than those involved in either classical or operant conditioning. For example, Briullova (cited in Lynn, 1966) found that habituation was severely disrupted in humans who had sustained cortical damage, and Jouvet (cited in Lynn, 1966) reported the complete absence of habituation in cats without a neocortex. The role of cortical processes in habituation is not yet clear, however. Research on an anencephalic infant, for example, revealed substantial habituation of heart-rate responses, suggesting that subcortical brain structures can mediate habituation in at least some instances (Graham et al., 1978). Other work on the habituation of visual attention in infants (Cohen, 1973; Jeffrey, 1976; Lewis and Baldini, 1979; McCall, 1971; Olson, 1976) suggests that habituation is a kind of "exposure" learning that reflects underlying brain plasticity. The habituation of visual attention, for example, seems to require some sort of mental representation, memory, internal comparison, and a variety of related perceptual and cognitive activities.

Novelty preference involves a straightforward adaptation of the habituation paradigm. In this procedure, the infant is familiarized with two simultaneously presented exemplars of one stimulus for a fixed time period and is then tested with a novel stimulus that is paired with the familiar stimulus. The proportion of time that the infant looks at the novel stimulus during the test trial is taken as a measure of novelty preference. Greater attention to the novel stimulus is believed to indicate a memory for the familiar stimulus.

Generally speaking, habituation and novelty preference are easily demonstrable in newborns and have been used more extensively than operant and classical paradigms to document individual differences and developmental changes in infant learning abilities. Slater et al. (1984) found habituation and recovery in infants as young as 3 days of age using both simple black and white and complexly colored stimuli. By 3 months of age, nervous system maturation and improved state organization (Parmelee and Stern, 1972) permit longer periods of alertness and improvements in learning ability and memory. These improvements continue with increasing age, along with concomitant developments in infants' information-processing abilities and motor coordination.

Habituation, novelty preference, and procedural variations thereof have been used with infants to investigate the processes of detection and discrimination, categorization, and concept formation. Detection and discrimination are denoted by dishabituation when a novel stimulus is presented following habituation to the familiar stimulus. As described earlier, infants in the first few months of life successfully discriminate among various geometric forms (Cornell, 1975; McCall et al., 1977; Saayman et al. 1964), colors (Bornstein, 1981a), faces (Barrera and Maurer, 1981a, 1981b), sounds (Bartoshuk, 1962; Bridger, 1961), odors (Engen and Lipsitt, 1965), and phonemes (Eimas, 1975). Categorization and concept formation (i.e., clustering a group of perceptually unrelated stimuli according to some underlying function, theme, or construct) are usually explored by habituating infants to several exemplars of a concept or category. The formation of a concept or category is assumed when infants display habituation to familiar exemplars of the "old" concept or category, generalize habituation to novel exemplars of the old concept or category, and dishabituate to exemplars of an unrelated concept. Using this procedure, infants have been shown to form concepts for chromaticity (Bornstein, 1979), numerosity (Strauss and Curtis, 1981), gender invariance (Cohen and Strauss, 1979), facial expression (Caron and Caron, 1981), and letters or furniture (G.S. Ross, 1980).

Overall, then, we see that infants are born with the ability not only to perceive objects and events but also to remember and associate them as well (see Chapter 14). Initially, memory span is quite limited, but improvements take place throughout the 1st year; within the first trimester, infants can remember an association for as long as 2 weeks, especially when prompted (Rovee-Collier et al., 1980). The easiest associations for infants to learn are those that are biologically prepared, and while these may comprise the limits of learning capacity in the neonatal period, older infants are capable of learning unprepared associations, especially when the energetic costs of responding are low. Perception and learning are the basic building blocks of cognitive development, the topic to which we now turn.

INFANT INTELLIGENCE

Interest in the definition and assessment of infant intelligence stems from three conceptually distinct perspectives on the nature of intelligence. The Piagetians believe that intelligence exists on the "plane of action" for much of the infant's life, with true thought emerging only by the end of the 2nd year. In the sensorimotor period of intelligence (0–24 months), six qualitatively different substages are distinguished (see Chapter 11). The psychometric perspective is most closely associated with the assessment of infant intelligence, guiding the construction of such measures as the Gesell and Bayley Scales (see Chapter 38). The following section selectively reviews research identifying environmental predictors of individual differences in infant intelligence and discusses the relation between effectance motivation and infant intelligence. The information-processing perspective on infant intelligence has evolved more recently and is concerned with how efficiently infants encode and store environmental stimuli in memory (see Chapter 11). It has been useful in sharpening our understanding of infant intelligence and its relation to intelligence measured at later developmental periods.

Piaget's View of Infant Intelligence

Born in Switzerland in 1896, Jean Piaget was formally trained in biology and philosophy and was interested in the processes by which children acquire knowledge about the world. Piaget's interest in cognition stemmed from his early work in the Binet laboratory in Paris, where the first intelligence test was developed. Piaget found the general orientation and methodology of psychometric testing deficient in several respects. First, he found incorrect responses to be just as interesting as correct responses. Children of the same age frequently produced the same type of error; moreover, there seemed to be reliable age-related variations in the types of errors children made, variations that were qualitative, not quantitative, in nature. Second, the inflexible methodology used in administering these tests did not allow examiners to probe the "inner workings" of a child's mind. Piaget was interested in the thinking that guided children's answers and in how these processes changed with age.

Frustrated by psychometric procedures, Piaget developed a less structured means of questioning children and learned to tap thought processes by observing how children experiment with and solve simple problems. The latter approach was used extensively to probe for and document changes in intelligence during the first 2 years, using his own children as subjects. Piaget's observations and theoretical notions regarding the sensorimotor period appeared in three extremely influential books: *The Origins of Intelligence in the Child* (1936/1953), *The Construction of Reality in the Child* (1937/1954), and *Play, Dreams, and Imitation in Childhood* (1946/1962).

Piaget viewed development as a continuous process of adaptation to an environment in which the infant plays an active role. Piaget conceived of maturation as a primary driving force behind development. In Piaget's view, behavior is guided and organized around sets of psychological structures or "schemes" that become intercoordinated gradually. For example, the initially uncoordinated schemes of "looking" and "grasping" eventually become coordinated into a higher-order scheme of "visually guided reaching." According to Piaget, all infant schemes are action oriented; he considered infants incapable of true thought (imagery and the mental manipulation of symbols) until late in the 2nd year. By contrast, older children and adults possess schemes that are thought oriented as well as action oriented.

In the view of Piagetians, adaptation to environmental demands depends on the complementary processes of assimilation and accommodation. Assimilation involves the application of an existing scheme to a novel external stimulus. By contrast, accommodation involves the modification of an existing structure to permit its application to a new, unfamiliar stimulus. For example, accommodation of the grasping scheme occurs when the infant attempts to grasp a novel object and has to modify the width of the grasp and the tightness of the grip. Of course, grasping the new object also involves some assimilation, since a generalized grasping scheme has already been established. All actions are believed to involve both assimilation and accommodation.

Piaget believed that all infants passed through the six substages of the sensorimotor phase (0–24 months) in an invariant sequence, although there could be substantial individual differences in the rate at which infants negotiate each stage. The progression through the six substages is associated with a decline in sensorimotor egocentrism, as the infant becomes increasingly aware that he or she is a unique entity, separate and distinct from other people and objects in the environment. Despite the fact that Piaget may have underestimated the age at which some abilities emerged (e.g., the intercoordination of perceptual schemes like looking and hearing appears to exist at birth), subsequent research has generally confirmed the developmental sequence he proposed. In addition, there is now widespread acceptance of the view that children are active participants in their development, not passive reactors to environmental stimuli. Key features of the six substages are provided in Table 20.1.

The Piagetian perspective is not commonly associated with formal assessments of infant intelligence, because Piaget was not concerned with assessing individual differences in intelligence or in identifying the conditions that speed up cognitive development. Of the few Piagetian tests that have developed, the Uzgiris and Hunt (1975) Ordinal Scales of Psychological Development have been most widely used (see Chapter 38).

Table 20.1. Sequence of Some Important Sensorimotor Developments in Piagetian Theory

Sensorimotor Stage	Means-End Behavior	Object Permanence	Space	Imitation
1	Reflex schemes	No special behavior toward absent objects	Practical groups Separate spaces for each scheme (buccal space, visual space, tactile space, etc.)	"Reflexive contagion": stimulus in environment elicits a response in baby, which happens to match the stimulus that elicited the infant's reaction, e.g., contagion of crying in newborn nursery
2	Intercoordination of reflex schemes Primary circular reaction Absence of means-end behavior	Same as 1	Intercoordination of schemes and of separate spaces Baby can look at what he or she hears, hear what he or she says, etc. ending with what he or she grasps	"Pseudoimitation": only certain types of actions are "imitated"—those that continue a movement of accommodation even after the stimulus is no longer preceived. Can imitate an action the infant can produce readily and that is directly available to the senses (e.g., cooing), imitation here "paced" by the parent or model (the parent directly elicits the modeled action, e.g., smiling)
3	Primitive, chance discovered, means-end relationships Secondary circular reaction	Beginnings of search for objects (a) when object is only partially hidden, or (b) when object is systematically transformed	Objects in space understood only in relationship to the infant's body and actions, but are not related to one another	Systematic imitation of models, but only with movements the infant has already made and noticed self doing Cannot imitate new, unfamiliar actions or stimuli
4	Deliberate means-end relationships Means, however, must be familiar	Objects searched for successfully after being seen hidden, but only in place where previously found	Relationships of objects to one another begin to be understood Far-space comprehension Size and shape constancy improve	Imitation of actions whose performance is not visible to baby. However, the actions must already be within the repertoire. Begins to imitate new sounds and sights
5	Use of new means (discovered by chance) to obtain new ends Deliberate variation of means to an end	Object searched for after being visibly displaced from one hiding place to another, but not when invisibly displaced	Understanding of relationship of objects to one another is complete, except for absence of inclusion of self as one of the objects in space, and absence of mental representation of objects in space	Systematic imitation of new models. Infants can imitate actions even though they cannot see themselves make the action
6	Insightful problem solving New means discovered to attain a new end, even in absence of chance discovery Internalized "trial and error"	Correct, systematic search for object after multiple invisible displacements	Infant relats self to other objects in space Representation and imagination of relative position of objects	Deferred imitation

Environmental Correlates of Infant Intelligence

Interest in the links between infant intelligence and environmental quality stemmed from early studies demonstrating that older children from middle class environments score significantly higher on IQ tests than do children from lower class environments (Deutsch and Brown, 1964; Hertzig et al., 1968; Kennedy et al., 1963; Weiner et al., 1963; Willerman et al., 1970). Of course, socioeconomic status (SES) is a marker variable based on parental income, education, and occupation and reveals little about the types of experiences enjoyed by infants of different social classes. Compared with lower class parents, middle class parents experience qualitatively different family life stresses (Hunt, 1969; Ramey et al., 1976), put greater emphasis upon their children's motives, feelings, and self-direction (Kohn, 1963), are more aware of their influence on their children's intellectual development (Tulkin and Kagan, 1975), provide more verbal and object-mediated stimulation contingent on infant behavior (Hunt, 1969; Kagan and Tulkin, 1971; Klaus and Gray, 1968; Tulkin, 1977; Tulkin and Kagan, 1975; Wachs et al., 1971), and provide a greater variety of daily experiences (Kagan et al., 1978). Interestingly, reliable SES differences in standardized measures of infant intelligence are more easily demonstrated after rather than before 12 months of age (Ramey et al., 1982), suggesting that these tests are not as sensitive to variations in environmental stimulation during the 1st year as during the 2nd. Infant intelligence tests during the 1st year tap sensory and motor functions whose development may be more influenced by maturational rather than by environmental factors, whereas environmental quality may have more readily observable effects on functions like language, symbolic play, and problem solving, which emerge during the 2nd year. We do not mean to imply that environmental quality during the 1st year is unimportant, however. Indeed, there is strong evidence that *enduring* environmental influences have the most pervasive and lasting impact on intellectual development (Bond, 1982; Kagan et al., 1978; Lamb and Bornstein, 1987).

By the 2nd year, SES differences in parental behavior and in infant intelligence suggest that cognitive performance is in part associated with the quality of infant-parent interaction. However, there is also considerable variability in the cognitive outcomes of infants of lower SES, highlighting the importance of identifying specific social experiences that reliably predict intellectual performance within and across social class. Global measures of maternal involvement, verbal responsivity, organization of the physical environment, variety in daily stimulation, and provision of play materials at 6 months predict 3-year intellectual performance (Bradley and Caldwell, 1976; Elardo et al., 1975), and intellectual performance after the 1st year is predicted by earlier measures of mothers' verbal stimulation, positive toy play, and contingent responsiveness to infant social cues (Carew, 1980; Clarke-Stewart, 1973; Clarke-Stewart et al., 1979; Cohen and Beckwith, 1979; Olson et al., 1984; Ramey et al., 1979). Restating Piaget's belief that infants are active participants in their own development, Carew (1980) hypothesized that verbal stimulation may develop the ability to "become self-stimulating in a verbal mode" (p. 70). Belsky et al. (1980) speculated that dyadic play with toys may foster the ability to engage in competent, self-directed explorations, and Lewis and Goldberg (1969) suggested that positive social experiences that are contingent upon infant behavior facilitate cognitive growth by fostering the sense of control over and motivation to master the environment. White (1959) suggested that, when infants can perceive the relationship between their own actions and environmental events, feelings of efficacy arise that function to sustain and intensify "effectance motivation." Eight-week-olds who perceived a contingency between their head movements and the movement of an overhead mobile not only increased the frequency of their head movements but showed a much higher frequency of smiling and cooing, an apparent indication of the pleasure derived from perception of the contingency (Watson, 1972). Conversely, infants may show displeasure and distress when their efforts to elicit contingent feedback are violated, as when mothers respond noncontingently to distress and positive social bids (Lamb and

Malkin, 1986; Trevarthen, 1977). Competent infants, therefore, are those who have learned from past experiences of contingency to explore, adapt to, and control their environments (Goldberg, 1977).

Recent studies by Bornstein and his colleagues revealed that the types of activities and experiences provided by parents influence specific areas of mental growth, such as visual, tactual, and perceptual-cognitive competence in infants younger than 6 months, and language and play in 13-month-olds (Bornstein and Tamis-LeMonda, 1990; Tamis-LaMonda and Bornstein, 1989).

Continuity of Infant Intelligence

Despite the environmental correlates of intelligence in the 2nd year, the relation between measures of intelligence in infancy and in later life is not at all straightforward. With few exceptions (Siegel, 1981), correlations between measures of intelligence during the 1st year and IQ scores in later childhood are very low (Fagan and Singer, 1983; Kopp and McCall, 1980). Prediction from scores obtained in the 2nd year of life is somewhat better (Reich et al., 1984; Wilson, 1983), perhaps because by that time scales like the Bayley Mental Development Index tap verbal, symbolic, and problem-solving skills that are similar to the abilities assessed by childhood intelligence tests.

The lack of relation between infant and later intelligence has spurred a heated debate about the nature of intelligence across the life span. Some theorists argued that there was no general intelligence factor, *g*, whereas others argued that if *g* exists, it is not fixed or stable across the life span. Still others argued that *g* may exist but that infant intelligence, with its basis in sensory and motor activity, differs from later intelligence. In any case, being highly intelligent in infancy would not ensure high intelligence later (see Eysenck and Kamin, 1981; Kopp and McCall, 1980; Lewis, 1983; Vernon, 1980, for discussions of these issues). A third perspective on intelligence, the information-processing view, demonstrates that the apparent discontinuity in intelligence from infancy to later periods is due in part to the conceptual dissimilarity between the abilities tapped by standardized tests administered to infants and older children. When conceptually similar abilities are assessed on both occasions, the degree of prediction improves.

Information Processing and Infant Intelligence

The information-processing view of intelligence holds that attention is an important aspect of infant cognitive functioning, conceptually related to measures of intelligence across the life span. Recall from our earlier discussion of habituation and novelty preference that infant attention to a stimulus event has traditionally been indexed in two ways: decrement of attention to repeated presentations of the same stimulus (habituation) and recovery of attention to a novel stimulus after habituation (novelty preference). Efficient information processing is assumed when habituation is rapid and/or when novelty preference is especially marked.

Individual differences in habituation rates in infants younger than 6 months have been reported using such stimulus configurations as geometric shapes, multicolored drawings, and social patterns (Bornstein and Benasich, 1986; DeLoache, 1976; McCall, 1979). Further, McCall (1979) and later Bornstein and Benasich (1986) identified three basic habituation patterns in 5-month-olds: babies who habituated rapidly, babies who first increased looking and subsequently habituated, and babies who showed idiosyncratic and highly individualized looking patterns. These individual differences covary with various other measures of infant cognition. For example, rapid habituation in infancy and childhood is positively associated with preference for complex patterns (Greenberg et al., 1973), advanced sensorimotor development (Johnson and Brody, 1977), rapid exploration of the environment (Fenson et al., 1974; Messer et al., 1970; Pecheux and Lecuyer, 1983), sophisticated play (Kagan, 1971; Riksen-Walraven, 1978), and rapid problem solving (Lewis et al., 1969). In addition, perinatal risk adversely affects decrement of attention (Friedman, 1975; Sigman et al., 1977) and recovery

(Caron and Caron, 1981; Rose, 1980; Rose SA et al., 1979; Sigman and Parmelee, 1974; Siqueland, 1981), just as Down's syndrome adversely affects decrement (Barnet et al., 1971) and recovery (Cohen, 1981; Miranda and Fantz, 1974).

Of course, infants also show individual differences in standardized test performance prior to 12 months of age, but the predictive validity of the attentional measures is better than that for the more traditional infant measures. Several recent studies document that infants who show efficient decrement or recovery of attention in the first 6 months of life perform significantly better on traditional assessments of cognitive and linguistic competence in early to middle childhood (Bornstein, 1989; Caron et al., 1983; DiLalla et al., 1990; Fagan and McGrath, 1981; Lewis and Brooks-Gunn, 1981; Rose and Wallace, 1985; Sigman et al., 1989; Slater et al., 1989). There is also evidence to suggest that infant novelty responsiveness across modalities, such as being familiarized with a stimulus tactually and then distinguishing a novel stimulus from the familiar one visually, is also predictive of later cognitive competence (Rose, 1989).

In their comprehensive review, Bornstein and Sigman (1986) note that the median percent variance shared between infant attentional measures and childhood intelligence is 21% (a correlation of about .44). Although the predictive validity of attentional measures is far from perfect, it is certainly better than that of traditional tests. Moreover, it indicates that, when researchers choose measures of early intelligence that tap the same processes as the measures used to assess intelligence later, some continuity is found.

COGNITIVE CONTINUITY AND THE NATURE-NURTURE ISSUE

It is virtually impossible to demonstrate either an environmental or a genetic basis for any characteristic in children reared by their biological parents because genetic endowment and environmental influences are so closely intertwined (Scarr and Weinberg, 1983). The significant correlations between parental IQ and infant intelligence (Rose et al., 1979, 1980) could be due to a shared gene pool or to parental behavior. There is some evidence, however, that there are inherent individual differences in infant attention. Newborns show individual differences in habituation (Field et al., 1982; Friedman, 1975; Siqueland, 1981; Slater et al., 1984), and identical twins are more alike in the developmental pattern of scores on standardized tests from 3 months to 6 years than are fraternal twins (Wilson, 1983). In addition, Hardy-Brown et al. (1981) found that the linguistic and communicative competence of adopted infants at 12 months of age related more strongly to the cognitive abilities of their biological mothers than to the cognitive abilities of the adoptive parents or to measures of the adoptive parents' communicative styles.

The fact that individual differences exist in relatively homogeneous samples, however, suggests that at least some variation is not accounted for by heredity, and several investigators have found concurrent associations between parental behavior and infant attention. For example, Bornstein (1985) found that mothers' tendency to encourage infants to attend to properties, objects, and events in the environment was related to habituation efficiency in 4-month-olds. Sigman and Beckwith (1980) reported relations between fixation time in 4-month-old preterm females and concurrent measures of verbal and social interaction. Of course, correlations between contemporaneous variables preclude conclusions about causal influences, but studies designed to help identify causal patterns suggest that the direction of influence is from parent to child, not the reverse. Belsky et al. (1980), for example, showed experimentally that parents who focus their infants' attention on objects promote infant competence. In addition, Riksen-Walraven (1978) demonstrated that infants of mothers who participated in a stimulation program habituated more efficiently than babies of control mothers.

It appears, then, that both genetic and environmental factors influence information-processing capacities. Of course, no direct measures of "genetic quality" exist, rendering moot questions about how much of an individual contribution genetics and environment actually make to intel-

ligence. As Yeates et al. (1983) point out, however, questions about the relative contributions of genetics and environment to a developmental process can be asked using measures such as parental IQ, which presumably reflects some genetic variation. Yeates et al. (1983) examined the relative contributions of maternal IQ and measures of environmental quality of the home (e.g., maternal involvement, provision of play materials) to child IQ from 2 to 4 years of age, statistically controlling for the effects of one while assessing the effects of the other at various age points. They found that environmental quality became a more important predictor and maternal IQ a less important predictor over the 2-year period. Although infant cognitive capacities were not assessed, the results suggest that early variation in cognitive abilities may be more attributable to genetic than to environmental factors, with environmental factors playing an increasing role with age.

Although the predictive validity of infant attention to childhood intelligence is better than that of more traditional tests, Bornstein and Sigman (1986) reported predictive correlations ranging in absolute magnitude from .28 to .77. Some of this variation may be due to differences among the techniques used to measure attention, the measures employed to assess childhood intelligence, the intervals between the ages at which infant attention and later intelligence were assessed, and measurement error. However, a potentially important source of variance that has not yet been addressed systematically is the degree of stability in children's environments from infancy to the later assessment. Lewis and Goldberg (1969) have argued that effectance motivation, and hence cognitive development, is facilitated by social environments that are emotionally warm, sensitive, and contingently responsive to children's needs. Further, Bond (1982) has noted that pervasive effects on cognitive development seem to occur when environmental influences are also enduring and long lasting. Thus, the predictive validity of infant attention measures should be relatively high when environmental stability over time is also high, whereas weaker predictive validity should be found when there are fluctuations in environmental quality (e.g., variations in the quality of the parent-child relationship).

Overall, the qualitative (Piagetian) and quantitative (information-processing and psychometric) perspectives on intelligence are complementary, addressing different questions about infant cognition. Although the Piagetian approach has proven useful for normative descriptions of infant cognitions, the information-processing approach is clearly in the ascendancy today, while the psychometric approach remains useful for assessing the current developmental status of individual infants. Except at the extremes, however, these scores have no predictive validity, whereas measures of information processing are predictive of performance on later measures of symbolic and analytic functioning. Perhaps the most dramatic aspect of symbolic function is represented by language, the topic of the next section (for a general overview of the development of communication, see Chapter 15).

LANGUAGE DEVELOPMENT

As mentioned earlier, very young infants seem to be especially tuned to frequencies within the range of human speech sounds. Infants like to listen to voices and will perform some act in order to do so: When speech (but not other sound) is contingent upon nonnutritive sucking, the amount of sucking increases (Trehub and Chang, 1977). In addition, 4- to 16-week-old infants are able to perceive categorically many of the acoustic cues that underlie speech (Aslin et al., 1983; Eimas et al., 1971). Thus, it appears that young infants are primed for hearing the components of language. These perceptual capacities presumably play a role in shaping the infant's vocal output, facilitating the development of language.

Vocal Production

During the 1st month of life, infants make reflexive cries, fusses, and vegetative sounds (Lenneberg, 1967; Oller, 1980; Tal and Bornstein,

1992). As early as 5 weeks to 3 months of age, cooing and laughter emerge, typically in response to the voices and faces of others (Lenneberg, 1967). These cooing sounds involve repeating the same vowel or velar consonant ("g," "k"), sounds in which tongue movements are relatively undifferentiated (Kent, 1981). Between 4 and 6 months of age, infants explore a variety of vocalizations, such as squeals, yells, growls, and vowel-like sounds. Thereafter (7–10 months of age), canonical or reduplicated babbling occurs, with infants producing syllables and reduplicating the same consonant and vowel (e.g., "da, da, da"). Between 11 and 12 months, nonreduplicated babbling (also termed "jargon" or "protowords") emerges; at this stage infants produce a variety of sounds in which syllables, consonants, and vowels may vary, such as "dakee," "babee." Finally, at approximately 12 months, infants produce referential words.

Changes in these vocal abilities are paralleled by changes in the anatomy and physiology of the vocal apparatus, which suggests that the developmental changes in vocal behavior are related to structural changes in oropharyngeal anatomy (Kent, 1981; Lester and Bourkydis, 1991), as does evidence that initial sound production follows a universal pattern (Jakobson, 1941/1968, 1971; Vihman, 1991). Babies brought up in Spanish-, Japanese-, Arabic-, or English-speaking homes show no great differences in their basic sound production repertoire, suggesting that very different linguistic experiences do not affect the elements of babbling very much (Nakazima, 1975; Oller and Eilers, 1982; Vihman, 1993). Additionally, infants with little language experience (e.g., infants with deaf parents) vocalize much like infants in sound-rich environments until the babies are about 6 months old (Lenneberg, 1969;). Thus, infants appear to use a universal core of sounds.

This does not mean that sound production is unaffected by environmental input: Infants eventually do produce the sounds they commonly hear, and they correctly mimic the rhythm and intonation of their native language long before they know what the words mean (Crystal, 1979; de Boysson-Bardies et al., 1984; Weir, 1962). Routh (in Oller, 1981) stimulated 2- to 7-month-olds with either consonant- or vowel-like sounds and thereby selectively increased the number of consonants or vowels the infants produced. By contrast, Webster (1969) found that when 6-month-olds were stimulated with vowel sounds, they increased the proportion of consonants produced, and vice versa. Taken together, these studies suggest that infants can modify their own vocalizations in response to the vocalizations of others, by either matching or contrasting the sounds that they hear (Oller, 1981).

The amount and patterning of babbling is affected by environmental factors as well. Infants vocalize substantially more when they are socially stimulated by others than when they are not, regardless of whether or not the stimulation is contingent on the infants' own vocalizations (Bloom, 1979; Rheingold et al., 1959). Additionally, when adult vocalizations or adult silences are contingent upon infant vocalizations, infants suppress their own vocalizations just after the contingent stimulation or silence, as though listening for something. Responding contingently to infant vocalizations thus allows infants to learn the basic conversational pattern: Talk then listen (Bloom, 1979; Bloom and Esposito, 1975).

The influence of social input on sound production is highlighted in studies contrasting the vocalizations of deaf infants with those of normal-hearing babies; the former appear to fall behind the latter (Gilbert, 1982; Oller, 1981; Stoel-Gammon and Cooper, 1984). Hearing-impaired infants produce fewer consonant types, show a decrease in types over time, and use a lower proportion of multisyllabic utterances than normal-hearing infants (Oller and Eilers, 1988). It thus appears that in the first half-year of life, infants do not require acoustical information in order to produce common precanonical sounds, but that the acoustic environment does influence vocalizations, such as babbling, later. It should be noted, however, that babbling is not restricted to vocalizations. When deaf infants are exposed to sign language from birth, they babble manually in much the same way that hearing infants do through speech (Petitto and Marentette, 1991).

First Words

Gesell (Gesell and Armatruda, 1962) observed that babies regularly say their first words about the time they celebrate their 1st birthday. At this age, children are interested in movements and actions they can perform, both with and without objects, and their first words typically reflect their sensorimotor schema; often they refer to objects that move or can be held rather than to equally common words on which infants seldom act (e.g., diaper, crib, shoe) (Nelson, 1973). In addition, early words (e.g., bye-bye, bang) often express and are accompanied by actions (e.g., waving, hitting) (Corrigan, 1979).

Although many early words refer to objects (Benedict, 1979; Bowerman, 1976; Leopold, 1949), infants also use "expressive" words to engage in social interactions. Nelson (1981) found that infants' early vocabularies consisted of both kinds of words and that infants could be categorized according to the proportion of each in their repertoires. For most children, early vocabularies contain a large proportion of object names, with some verbs, proper names, and adjectives; Nelson termed this style of early word use "referential." A large minority of children, however, have a more diverse vocabulary, with a large number of social routines, such as "stop it" and "what's that" included among the nouns, verbs, and adjectives; Nelson called this style of early word use "expressive." Although children may use one style more than the other, only rarely do they exclusively use either one (Bretherton et al., 1983).

In addition to individual differences in the style of first words used, individual differences in the timing of early word acquisition are common. Bayley (1969), in her assessment of 1200 infants, found that the most advanced imitated a word by 9 months of age, and the least advanced by 18 months of age. Similar variation was found in the number of words in the vocabularies of 13-month-olds; production ranged from 0 to 45 words, and comprehension varied from 11 to 97 words (Snyder et al., 1981). In general, comprehension of words precedes their production.

Sharing a Referent: Development of Gestural Communication

Producing and comprehending words necessitates an understanding of shared referents. Prior to language, such shared reference to objects and events first comes about through gestural communication. During the second half of the 1st year, infants begin to use and understand various communicative signals to potentiate mutual attention to external topics (Bakeman and Adamson, 1984). Joint attention and external reference are the bases of symbolic communication, be it gestural or vocal (Bates, 1979; Schaffer, 1984). There is some evidence indicating that infants who experience more of these joint attention experiences tend to talk earlier and show faster vocabulary development (Dunham and Dunham, 1992; Tomasello, 1990).

Toward the end of the 1st year, infants begin to share objects and events with others by using conventional gestures such as pointing, offering, and showing objects (Hay and Rheingold, 1983). Leung and Rheingold (1981) note that pointing and reaching function to direct another's attention to objects that arouse the infant's interest. Reaching is characteristic of 9- to 10-month-olds, entering the repertoire before pointing, which is first displayed by a majority of children at 12.5 months and is a common gesture at 16.5 months of age (Leung and Rheingold, 1981). Because pointing is modeled and reinforced by adults, it replaces reaching as a referential gesture (Leung and Rheingold, 1981; Murphy and Messer, 1977), gradually being refined until it assumes the conventional form. Language acquisition involves a similar process of learning the conventional means by which to refer to phenomena (Acredolo and Goodwyn, 1990). As with language, the ability to comprehend or to follow another's points precedes the infant's own pointing. By the start of the 2nd year of life, infants frequently use conventional gestures (such as showing and offering objects) with mothers and fathers as well as with unfamiliar men and women (Hay, 1979; Rheingold et al., 1976) and with peers (Bakeman and Adamson, 1986; Eckerman et al., 1975; Nash, 1985).

Conventional gestures and language follow a parallel developmental course. Infants begin to use shared referents, both gestural and verbal, at about 1 year of age, the age at which Piaget suggests that the capacity for symbolic representation first emerges. Other forms of symbolic representation, such as play, also emerge at about this time (Nicholich, 1981). In addition, social gestures (such as pointing) and speech both pass through an initial noncommunicative phase (E. Bates et al., 1982; Leung and Rheingold, 1981; Schaffer, 1984). Both are first tied to specific routines or "action formats" (routines between adult and infant such as peek-a-boo, "So Big," reading, etc.) and occur only in these contexts (Acredolo and Goodwyn, 1985, 1992; Bakeman and Adamson, 1984; Bates, 1979; Ratner and Bruner, 1978). Later they are used in other contexts to stand for objects and events that are not present, thus serving a symbolic communicative function.

Prelinguistic Conversations and Behavioral Dialogues

Besides helping infants understand semantics, interactive routines also help infants learn the pragmatics of language and the rules of conversation, such as mutual attention, sharing a topic, and taking turns (Bruner, 1977; Schaffer, 1984). Dialogues between infants and caretakers begin in the newborn period: The communicative exchanges between parents and 3-day-old infants are smooth, with a high degree of turn taking (Bakeman and Brown, 1977). At this stage, however, adults more frequently initiate, follow through, and complete behavioral sequences.

At 2 months of age, infants regularly respond to attentive, talking adults by orienting to their faces, focusing on their eyes, smiling, becoming more active, and vocalizing, then shifting their gaze to the adults' mouths or away from their faces (Rheingold, 1961; Trevarthen, 1977). Infants thus seem to alternate between attending and expressing themselves. During the expressive phase, they make mouth movements, often accompanied by sounds and gestures. Mothers frequently respond to such prespeech with talk of their own. By 3 months of age, infants and parents tend to alternate their vocalizations, taking turns (Bloom, 1988). Mothers are primarily responsible for initiating exchanges and attempting to elicit responses from infants, but infants at this age sometimes vocalize after silences, as if attempting to keep the "conversations" going. Turn taking becomes more and more refined and predominates in the vocal exchanges of 6- to 16-month-olds and their mothers (Davis, 1978). Similarly, Schaffer et al. (1977) found that turn taking occurs equally often in the vocal exchanges of 12- and 24-month-old children. At both ages, overlaps were rare and brief.

During the first 6 months, conversations and dialogues are sustained mainly by adults, but after this, infants begin to take more responsibility. Rogoff et al. (1984) observed 7-month-olds reaching toward an adult's arm while looking at the handle of a jack-in-the-box, as though attempting to make the adult wind the handle and thus continue the game. The role of infants in the management of joint activities was shown to increase rapidly from 6 to 13 months (Mosier and Rogoff, 1994). H.S. Ross (1980) reported that, when an adult stopped a game by not taking her turn, 12-month-olds reacted as though they had some understanding of the rules of turn taking; for example, they guided the adult's hand to the appropriate object, thus helping the adult to take her turn. The infant's role in taking turns is illuminated by behavior with peers from the start of the 2nd year, when "games" may include turn taking (Goldman and Ross, 1978; Nash, 1986).

Snow (1977) suggests that 1-year-olds understand the rules of conversational turn taking as well, and Schaffer (1984) proposed a mechanism by which even very young infants help sustain a vocal dialogue: They suppress their own vocalizations when stimulated by the sounds of others. Webster et al. (1972) found that infants vocalize less when presented with other sounds and increase them when the sounds stop. Furthermore, infants reduce their own vocalizations, particularly when they hear preferred voices (Barrett-Goldfarb and Whitehurst, 1973).

Although 12-month-olds understand some rules of social exchange and take an active role in keeping exchanges going, adults still take the major responsibility. Schaffer et al. (1977) examined speaker-switch pauses in vocal interchanges between mothers and 1-year-olds and found that child-mother switches were characterized by shorter pauses than mother-child switches, thus highlighting the mothers' greater competence in responding. In addition, by keeping their own vocalizations very brief and pausing often, parents give infants a chance to join in (Schaffer, 1984).

That vocal and behavioral interactive routines follow the same developmental course is illustrated by Bruner's (1977) descriptions of "Give and Take" games and Snow's (1977) examinations of vocal conversations. At 3 months Bruner found the game of "Give and Take" to be one sided, with mothers offering objects to their infants most frequently. At 6 months the infants played a more active role, accepting the objects. By 12 months children both gave and took objects. The number of exchanges and offers of objects initiated by the children increased from 0 to 50% so that "Give and Take" became a game involving reciprocal roles. Similarly, Snow found that mothers took the major responsibility for maintaining conversations by responding to their 3-month-olds' smiles and vocalizations as if they were intending to communicate. When infants did not respond, mothers often filled in. By the end of the 1st year, children more often initiated turns, actively assuming the roles of speaker and listener.

Early interactive routines may thus teach the basic pragmatics of speech. In addition, Bruner (1977, 1983) suggested that they also provide a strong foundation upon which infants build syntax, while learning the sequence of agent, action, object, and recipient. Thus, Bruner argues that, before actually speaking, infants, with adult guidance, have learned language formats. This language support system may thus provide a stepping stone to Chomsky's (1965, 1986) notion of a language acquisition device, an innate mechanism that provides toddlers and preschoolers with an understanding of grammar.

Gestures, nonverbal sounds, and words are important means whereby infants communicate with others. Emotional expressions, discussed in the next section, also serve important communicative functions. Whether the signals are gestural, verbal, or emotional, furthermore, their prevalence and universality underscores the intrinsically social nature of human infants.

SOCIAL AND EMOTIONAL DEVELOPMENT

Emotional Development

Many theorists consider the ability to produce and respond appropriately to emotional expressions to be innate and cite four types of evidence to support this view (Campos et al., 1983; Darwin, 1872; Eibl-Eibesfeldt, 1970; Ekman and Oster, 1979; Izard, 1971, 1979). First, facial expressions are indeed quite similar in different cultures (Eibl-Eibesfeldt, 1970), and expressions posed by Westerners are correctly identified by people in other cultures, including preliterate societies that have had little or no exposure to Westerners (Ekman, 1972). Second, the development of emotional expressiveness seems to be under maturational control; blind infants begin full smiling at the same age as sighted infants (Fraiberg, 1979), and premature infants begin to smile at environmental stimuli at the same conceptional age as full-term infants (Dittrichova, cited in Bower, 1977). Third, monozygotic twins are more alike than dizygotic twins with respect to fear of strangers and smiling over the 1st 4 months (Freedman, 1974; Plomin and Rowe, 1978), suggesting a genetic component to these emotions. Finally, the ability to recognize certain expressive displays has an innate basis in nonhuman primates. Sackett (1966) found that rhesus monkeys raised in total isolation responded with fear to pictures of monkeys making threats and showed positive reactions to pictures of infant monkeys. Mason (1985) found that experience has little influence on several facial and vocal emotional displays in rhesus monkeys.

In order to study the development of emotions, one must decide whether to focus on internal state or on outward expression, as there may not be a direct correspondence between the two. Some theorists assume a correspondence (Darwin, 1872; Ekman 1972; Izard, 1979; Malatesta, 1985), and there is some physiological evidence to support this assumption. Correlations have been found between various facial expressions and distinct patterns of autonomic nervous system activity in adults (Ekman et al., 1983), and between the amount of separation distress (Tennes, 1982) and distress to inoculations (Lewis et al., 1993) and levels of infants' cortisol production. Other researchers have emphasized the lack of synchrony between infant expressions and internal states, however. Citing examples of early asynchrony in relation to infant smiling (Emde and Koenig, 1969; Wolff, 1963), Lewis and Michalson (1985) argue that the relation between internal state and outward expression during infancy is in fact U-shaped, with no synchrony at first, a high degree of synchrony later in infancy, and then less correspondence as infants get old enough to use expressions to communicate intentionally or withhold them to mask certain states. This concern about the correspondence between emotional state and expression is important not only to theorists but also to parents and caretakers, who must understand infant signals and act appropriately, deciding whether such signals necessarily correspond to particular emotional states.

To clarify the relation between expressions and underlying emotions, it is helpful to ask about the likely function of a correspondence between feelings and expressions. Campos and his colleagues (1983) argue that emotions play a primary role in organizing the individual's behavior and signaling others about the individual's tendencies. They assume that the communicative functions of emotions are evident from birth and that there is, as a result, a direct although imperfect correspondence between emotional expressions and internal states.

DEVELOPMENT OF FACIAL AND VOCAL EXPRESSIONS

By responding "appropriately" to infants' facial and vocal expressions, parents indicate that infants are able to communicate effectively with others. The same facial movements used to express distinct emotions in adults are used by infants (Ekman and Friesen, 1976, 1978; C.E. Izard, unpublished manuscript, 1979; Izard and Dougherty, 1982). As a result, even untrained observers can accurately identify the emotion displayed by photographed infants (Emde et al., 1978, 1985; Izard et al. (1980) and show differentiated psychophysiological responses to infant smiles and cries, as well as to cries with different characteristics (Frodi et al., 1978a, 1978b). As infancy proceeds, expressions change from basically reflexive signals to more flexible, graded, instrumental signals, which may be used intentionally as well as unintentionally in social communication. Indeed, one of the tasks of infancy is to modify expressions in light of societal expectations and rules. The frequency of facial expressions also changes, with decreases over the first 6 months (Malatesta and Haviland, 1982) and increases in the next 2 months (Malatesta et al., 1986).

The first emotional expressions involve crying. Brazelton (1962) and Rebelsky and Black (1972) have charted the developmental course of crying, noting an increase over the 1st 6 weeks and then a decrease, with maximum crying initially in the evening, but later near feeding times. Both researchers also noted much variability within and between infants. The communicative function of crying is indicated by the ability of others to identify different kinds of cries. Adults are able to distinguish between the pain and hunger cries of newborns (Zeskind et al., 1985), and Berry (1975) showed that even 7-year-olds could distinguish cry types. It is also possible to distinguish spectrographically among the cries of newborn infants suffering malnutrition, asphyxiation, neurological abnormalities, and chromosomal deviations (Hollien, 1980; Lester and Boukydis, 1985; Zeskind, 1981).

Newborns can communicate emotions through facial expressions as well. Rosenstein and Oster (1988) recorded the facial expressions of 2-hour-old infants who were given sour, sweet, salty, and bitter substances

to taste. They responded to pleasant tastes with apparently positive facial expressions and to unpleasant tastes with negative expressions. Field (1982) reported that facial expressions of surprise were elicited from newborns by some items in the Brazelton Neonatal Behavioral Assessment Scale examination. And of course, newborns are able to smile, although unlike later smiling, which involves both ocular and lower face muscles, neonatal reflex smiling involves only the lower face muscles (Korner, 1969; Wolff, 1963). Newborns smile quite readily, but only during rapid eye movement states in sleep (Emde and Harmon, 1972). According to Sroufe and Waters (1976), who charted the ontogeny of smiling and laughter, smiling progresses from internal to external stimulation. At first it occurs during sleep, later in drowsiness, and finally in attentive states. Sounds are initially the most effective external stimuli, but by the 5th week visual stimuli become more effective. Six- to 12-week-old infants smile at faces as well as at a wide range of nonsocial stimuli, such as bull's-eye patterns and bells (Emde and Harmon, 1972). Gradually, smiling becomes more selective, progressing from any human face, to particular faces, to particular expressions. Newborns do not laugh; the development of laughter trails the developmental course of elicited smiling by about 1 month (Rothbart, 1973). Sroufe and Wunsch (1972) reported that tactile and kinesthetic cues were the strongest elicitors of laughter, that 7- to 9-month-olds laughed more and to a greater variety of stimuli than did 4- to 6-month-olds, and that the frequency of laughing at visual and social stimuli (such as during a peek-a-boo game) increased with age.

One- to 9-month-old infants display all the facial expressions displayed by adults—interest, joy, surprise, sadness, anger, disgust, contempt, and fear (Izard et al., 1980; Malatesta and Haviland, 1982)—although the initial expressions are not always complete or used appropriately. Stenberg and coworkers (Stenberg et al., 1983; Stenberg and Campos, 1990) took a closer look at the development of anger expressions by examining infants' responses to the removal of teething biscuits and to restraints of their arm movements. They found the 1-month-olds showed few clear expressions of anger, but 4- to 7-month-olds showed clear expressions of anger. The oldest infants directed their anger expressions toward the person who was restraining their arms or removing the biscuit. Additionally, anger in response to inoculations increases with age (Izard et al., 1983).

The last emotional expression to occur appropriately is fear. Between 6 and 9 months, infants begin to display fear to a variety of social (e.g., separation from a parent, approach of a stranger) and nonsocial (e.g., heights, looming stimuli) stimuli (Campos and Stenberg, 1981; Cicchetti and Hesse, 1983). Not all infants display fear in response to each of these stimuli, however. In particular, fearful reactions to strangers, once thought of as a developmental milestone (Bronson, 1972; Freedman, 1974; Hess, 1970; Spitz, 1950a), vary depending on the particular stranger involved, his or her behavior, and the context in which infant and stranger meet (Clarke-Stewart, 1978; Rheingold and Eckerman, 1973; Thompson and Limber, 1991). Nevertheless, although fear of strangers is not universal, it emerges during the second half of the 1st year if it does occur (Bronson, 1972; Haith and Campos, 1977).

Nonhuman primates go through the same developmental sequence, with positive expressions toward social stimuli being used appropriately before negative ones. In this way, sociability is fostered; nonhuman and human infants form ties with fellow conspecifics before they begin to fear particular individuals. Additionally, as young infants do not have the motor skills to protect themselves from potentially dangerous situations, fear is not adaptive for protection until later (Izard and Malatesta, 1987). Indeed, although infants can distinguish the two sides of a visual cliff (a shallow and deep side) by 2 months of age (Campos et al., 1970), they show no fear of the deep side until the 3rd quarter-year of life; that is, they begin to show fear of heights at about the same time they are beginning to locomote and are thus able to flee (Campos and Bertenthal, 1989).

In summary, infants are able to express all the primary emotions at or soon after birth; during the next 6–12 months, infants learn to express these emotions fully and appropriately, so as to communicate successfully with others. Next, the ability to respond to the emotional expressions of others is considered.

INFANTS' RESPONSES TO THE EMOTIONAL EXPRESSIONS OF OTHERS

As members of a social species, humans must constantly modulate their emotions in response to the emotions of others (Nelson, 1987). Newborns are able to discriminate among happy, sad, and surprised faces (Field et al., 1982), and at 3–5 months of age they are able to discriminate among expressions of joy, surprise, anger, and sadness (Barrera and Maurer, 1981a; LaBarbera et al., 1976; Young-Browne et al., 1977), as well as degrees of such expressions (Kuchuk et al., 1986). Between $5\frac{1}{2}$ and 7 months of age, infants can discriminate happy and surprised expressions (Caron et al., 1982), and at 7 months, infants also show generalized discrimination (across several models) of happy and frightened faces and prefer looking at frightened rather than happy faces (Nelson and Dolgin, 1985). Interestingly, this preference for looking at frightened faces emerges at about the age when infants themselves begin to express fear appropriately.

Emotional contagion occurs in a variety of social species (Hinde, 1970), and human newborns may be capable of some such modulation; they appear to match (''imitate'') both facial expressions (Field et al., 1982; Meltzoff and Moore, 1977, 1983) and vocal expressions (crying; Martin and Clarke, 1982; Sagi and Hoffman, 1976; Simner, 1971). In addition, 3-month-olds become inactive when their mothers act depressed (Cohn and Tronick, 1983; Lamb and Malkin, 1986). As infancy proceeds, this immediate response to the emotion of others becomes less automatic. Although newborns readily cry when they hear other newborns crying (Martin and Clark, 1982; Sagi and Hoffman, 1976; Simner, 1971), 6-month-olds do not cry so rapidly in response to the cries of their peers. Hay et al. (1981) found that the probability of a 6-month-old's crying in response to the distress of a peer increased the longer the peer cried; if the peer cried for $2\frac{1}{2}$ minutes, the listening infant was sure to cry. Further demonstrating that automatic responding decreases as infants age, Nelson and Horowitz (1983) found that 2-month-olds respond to expression changes in holograms of faces, whereas 5-month-olds do not.

Older infants use more deliberate means to match the emotions of others than do younger infants. By 12 months of age, infants in ambiguous situations use other peoples' emotional expressions as cues for their own, a phenomenon termed ''social referencing'' (see Feinman, 1992). Infants are more likely to cross a visual cliff of ambiguous height when their mothers look happy than when they look afraid (Sorce et al., 1985) and are more likely to approach and explore novel toys and animals when an adult signals joy and to seek reassurance from the adult when she or he signals fear (Hornik et al., 1987; Hornik and Gunnar, 1988; Klinnert et al., 1983; Zarbatany and Lamb, 1985). By 18 months of age, infants are able to respond with recognizable empathy to the distress of their companions, offering teddies or restoring desired toys to distressed peers (Hoffman, 1978).

Responses to particular auditory displays are more difficult to document, although most theorists agree that emotions are reflected in vocalizations (Darwin, 1872; Scherer et al., 1972; Zahavi, 1982). Newborns cry in response to the distress of others, whereas exposure to recordings of their own cries calm newborns, indicating that they can discriminate their own cries from those of others and do not merely become distressed because they find crying irritating (Martin and Clarke, 1982). This differential responding may be an early precursor of empathy. Twelve-month-olds avoid crossing a visual cliff of ambiguous depth when their mothers' vocal tone is negative (angry or fearful) but cross immediately when the mothers speak positively (Svejda and Campos, 1982). Such social referencing in response to vocal expressions of emotion has been found in other situations as well (Walden and Baxter, 1989). Recent studies have indicated that infants begin to coordinate vocal and facial features

of emotional expression early in infancy—between 4 and 9 months of age (Caron et al., 1988).

SOCIALIZATION OF EMOTIONS

The fact that the production and recognition of emotional expression is innate does not mean that experience plays no role in emotional development. As Fraiberg (1979) reported, social smiling in response to familiar voices first emerges at about the same age for blind and sighted infants, but smiling by blind infants subsequently becomes less frequent and more muted. Unlike sighted infants, furthermore, blind infants do not initiate interaction by smiling. Similarly, Ambrose (1969) reported that smiling to external stimuli occurred later in institution-reared infants, who receive little social feedback, than in home-reared infants.

Experimental studies indicate that emotional expressions can be modified by conditioning and social learning (reviewed by Campos et al., 1983), processes that also occur during face-to-face interactions between mothers and their 3- to 6-month-old infants (Malatesta and Haviland, 1982, 1985; Malatesta et al., 1986). According to Malatesta, maternal expressions typically changed less than a half second after the infants' expressions changed, the optimal delay for instrumental conditioning. Mothers contingently responded to their infants' positive expressions more than to their negative expressions, thus producing an increase in positive emotional expressions and a decrease in negative expressions. Contingent maternal responses also led to increases in the overall rate of infants' facial expression changes.

Malatesta's studies also implicate observational learning in the modification of infants' emotional expressiveness. Malatesta and Haviland (1985) reported that mothers on average changed their expressions 8 times per minute. From this they estimated that mothers change their expression 362 times per day in face-to-face play, and 32,580 times over the 3-month period of peak face-to-face play. As these investigators remarked, ''This is not a trivial learning opportunity for the infant'' (p. 104). The amount of joy and interest modeled by mothers at 5 months predicted increases in the amount of joy and interest expressed by infants at $7\frac{1}{2}$ months (Malatesta et al., 1986).

The infant's role in the socialization of emotions is underscored by comparing the face-to-face interactions of preterm and full-term infants. Mothers of preterm infants matched their infants' facial expressions less and ignored their anger expressions more than did mothers of full-term infants. The former also responded randomly rather than contingently to their infants' sad expressions. These differences in maternal behavior were attributed to the fact that preterm infants expressed more negative emotions and gazed at their mothers less than full-term infants did (Malatesta et al., 1986).

In addition to being an arena in which instrumental and social learning can take place, early face-to-face play reflects cultural values concerning emotional expression (Super and Harkness, 1982). Among the Gusii of Kenya, for example, social interaction is characterized by bland countenances. Face-to-face play is rare, and when it does occur eye contact is avoided (as it is between adults). When infants become excited, mothers respond with a variety of strategies to dampen the infants' emotional displays, looking away or blinking rapidly to break visual contact. The cultural norm of avoiding emotional displays is thus taught in the earliest social interactions (Dixon et al., 1981).

During early face-to-face interactions, North Americans instill cultural norms concerning the greater acceptability of emotional displays by girls (Malatesta, 1985). Malatesta and Haviland (1982) found that, although female and male infants display similar facial expressions, American mothers respond differently to them. As infants grow older, mothers smile increasingly in response to their sons' smiles and decreasingly in response to their daughters' smiles. Similarly, Lewis and Michalson (1985) found that after 6 months mothers responded less to boys' crying than to girls', were more likely to imitate their sons' expressions, and were more likely to show a wider range of expressions, both imitative and dissimilar, to their daughters. Girls were reinforced for a wider range of emotional expressions than were boys, which may explain why girls are better at decoding emotional expressions than are boys at all ages (Hall, 1978).

In summary, infants' abilities to communicate emotionally are well-documented. These abilities allow for the formation of close, special, relationships. Such attachments to particular individuals typically emerge during the second half of the first year of life. We next discuss the development of such attachments.

Development of Attachment

The most popular explanation of attachment formation was provided by Bowlby (1969, 1988), a psychoanalyst who was much impressed by the capacity of ethological theorists to explain early emotional communication between nonhuman infants and their parents. Bowlby's influential theory consequently emphasizes the infant's innate capacity to emit signals to which adults are biologically predisposed to respond. Adults' responses to these signals may account for the development of attachments, as we show shortly.

Bowlby began with the assumption that the behavioral propensities of infants and parents are most profitably considered in the context of the environment in which our species evolved. In that ''environment of evolutionary adaptedness,'' the survival of infants would have depended on their ability to maintain proximity to protective adults. Unlike the young of many other species, however, human infants are unable to move closer to or to follow adults for several months, and they are even incapable of clinging to adults. Instead, human infants rely on signals to entice adults to approach them. In order for these signals to be effective, adults must be predisposed to respond to them. The best example of such a prepotent signal is the infant cry, which very effectively entices adults to approach, pick up, and soothe the infant (Bell and Ainsworth, 1972; Frodi et al., 1978b; Korner and Thoman, 1970, 1972; Murray, 1979). As they grow older, infants develop a variety of means of achieving proximity or contact, including independent locomotion. Throughout infancy, babies seek proximity to protective adults in order to obtain nourishment, comfort, and security. Gradually, infants come to focus their bids on those people with whom they are familiar and on whom they can count, and this is one crucial aspect of the process called attachment formation.

BASIC PHASES OF SOCIAL DEVELOPMENT

Bowlby (1969) described four phases in the development of infant-parent attachments. The first phase in the attachment process (indiscriminate social responsiveness, 1–2 months) is marked by the development of a repertoire of signals, labeled attachment behaviors. The defining or common characteristic of these behaviors is that they all help achieve comfort and security by bringing the baby close to protective, caretaking adults.

From the time of birth, there is one very effective signal at the baby's disposal—the cry. A second potent attachment behavior enters the baby's repertoire in the 2nd month of life—smiling. Like crying, smiling is a signal that powerfully affects adult behavior. However, smiles are effective because they encourage adults to stay near and continue interacting with the baby because adults find the interaction pleasant, whereas cries encourage adults to approach the baby in order to terminate a signal that they find aversive (Ambrose, 1969; Frodi et al., 1978b).

From birth, therefore, babies are capable of affecting the people around them, but in this phase babies use proximity-promoting signals indiscriminately. They are satisfied when anyone responds to their attachment behaviors.

Frequent encounters with caretakers at times when infants are alert may also facilitate infants' capacities to recognize caretakers, and Bowlby suggested that acquisition of the ability to recognize specific people marks the transition to the second phase of attachment development (discriminating sociability, 2–7 months). In fact, infants seem able to recognize their parents much earlier than Bowlby believed. Macfarlane

(1975) provided anecdotal evidence that infants could distinguish between their mothers' smell and that of other nursing mothers within the first 2 weeks of life. After teaching infants to suck in one way to turn on a tape recording of their mothers' voices and in another way to produce the voice of another woman, DeCasper and Fifer (1980) found that 2-day-old infants could not only discriminate between two voices but worked harder (i.e., sucked in a special way) to hear their own mothers' voices.

Presumably because significant others (such as parents) have been associated with pleasurable experiences (e.g., cuddling and play) and with the relief of distress from early in life, familiar people become persons with whom babies prefer to interact. Initially, these preferences evidence themselves in fairly subtle ways: Certain people will be able to soothe the baby more easily and to elicit smiles and coos more readily, broadly, and frequently. According to Bowlby, these preferences are initially based on recognition only: Babies do not even have a primitive conception of the permanent existence of their parents. Following various psychoanalytic theorists (Freud, 1965; Spitz 1950b, 1965), Bowlby (1969) and Ainsworth (1973) believe that infants cannot be said to love parents until they understand that their parents exist even when they are neither interacting with nor visible or audible to the infants. Consequently, Bowlby argued, we cannot claim that 3- or 4-month-olds have formed attachments, although they have taken another step toward this achievement.

The third of Bowlby's phases (attachment, 6–7 to 24–30 months) is marked by the emergence of intentional and focused attachment behavior. Seven-month-olds clearly understand and respect the rule of reciprocity in their interactions. Their confidence in others reinforced, 7-month-olds enjoy the newly acquired ability to creep around and to take responsibility for getting close to their parents at will, instead of waiting for others to come in response to their cries or coos. Intentional social behavior is now possible (Lamb, 1981a), and 6- to 12-month-olds are increasingly likely to initiate interaction using directed social behaviors, whereas mothers more frequently initiate games, terminate or redirect their infants' activities, and issue verbal requests (Green et al., 1980). Caretaking becomes less prominent. One sign of the increased intentionality of infant behavior is that 7-month-olds begin to protest more reliably when parents leave. Wariness of strange adults may also become more prominent around this time.

Especially from the parents' point of view, the transition between phase 2 and phase 3 is not abrupt, since babies have been showing preferences for parents over others for several months. Nevertheless, the beginning of phase 3 is marked by two major behavioral changes. First, when babies protest when left by an attachment figure, they are no longer satisfied by the appearance of substitute interactive partners (Stayton et al., 1973). According to Bowlby, separation protest should be viewed as a signal aimed at making attachment figures come back to the baby, and its emergence can be linked to the attainment of some primitive conception of person permanence—the notion that people have a permanent existence independent of the infant (Ainsworth, 1973). Second, the emergent ability to crawl permits exploration of the environment on a scale hitherto inconceivable, affording babies the capacity to move toward attachment figures when they want to be near them. From this point on, infants assume an increasingly active role in their relationships with attachment figures.

Of course, major changes in social relationships occur between 6 and 7 months (the beginning of phase 3) and about 24–30 months (the end of this phase): Infants become increasingly sophisticated in their abilities to behave intentionally, to communicate linguistically, and to respond appropriately in a variety of different contexts. As infants grow older, they initiate an increasing proportion of their interactions. They can tolerate a growing distance from attachment figures as they grow older (Anderson, 1972; Rheingold and Eckerman, 1970).

According to Bowlby (1969), the next major transition occurs at the beginning of the 3rd year of life, when children become able to take their parents' needs into account when interacting with them (phase 4, goal-corrected partnerships). For example, they are now able to respect others' differing perspectives and appear to recognize for the first time that parents must sometimes give priority to other activities, while the child's needs or wants wait (Marvin, 1977; Mossler et al., 1976).

The beginning of phase 3 is thus the time at which the first infant-adult attachments are formed. Most theorists define attachment as a specific, enduring, emotional bond whose existence is of major importance in the process of sociopersonality development.

To whom do attachments form? In many places in the world, infants are cared for primarily by their mothers. The universality of traditional parental roles has led psychologists to assume that the first persons to whom infants become attached are their mothers. Until very recently in fact, most theorists assumed that the infant-mother relationship was not simply most important but uniquely important (Ainsworth, 1973; Bowlby, 1969; Maccoby and Masters, 1970), thus accepting Freud's (1940/1968, p. 48) dictum that the mother-infant relationship is "unique, without parallel, established unalterably as the prototype of all later love relations . . . for both sexes." Fathers were not considered important until the oedipal period began, around 3 years of age.

In fact, most babies become attached to their fathers at around 7 months of age, the same age at which they form attachments to their mothers (Lamb, 1976b, 1977, 1981b), although many U.S. mothers are the primary or preferred attachment figures in the sense that infants prefer mothers at times of stress (Lamb, 1976a, 1976c). In many parts of the world, infants may have several caregivers who are emotionally involved in their lives, and thus may form several attachments (Dunn, 1993; Nash and Hay, 1993).

In the United States, infant-mother and infant-father relationships offer different sorts of experiences for young infants. A detailed analysis of face-to-face play between parents and very young infants (2- to 6-month-olds) shows that fathers provide more unpredictable, less rhythmic, and more exciting (rather than calming) physical and vocal stimulation than do mothers (Yogman, 1982). Naturalistic home observations of older infants and their parents yield similar findings (Lamb, 1976b). In addition, mothers hold their babies most often for caretaking purposes; fathers hold their babies most often to play with them (Lamb, 1976b, 1977).

These differences are significant because they show parental roles being translated into distinctive styles of interaction. Children learn to expect playful stimulating interactions with their fathers and thus come to prefer playing with them (Clarke-Stewart, 1980; Lamb, 1977; Lynn and Cross, 1974).

SECURITY OF INFANT-PARENT ATTACHMENTS

Attachment theory was developed by clinically oriented scholars primarily interested in how early attachment relationships might affect subsequent development. Much research on this issue involves use of the "Strange Situation" for assessing "the security of attachment" (Ainsworth and Wittig, 1969; Ainsworth et al., 1978). Ainsworth et al. (1978; Ainsworth and Bowlby, 1991) also provided an elegant and persuasive account of the relation among prior infant-mother interaction, security of infant attachment, and subsequent child development.

The Strange Situation can be used only when infants are old enough to have formed attachments and be mobile (say, older than 10 months), yet are young enough to be stressed by strangers and brief separations from their parents (say, younger than 24 months). The procedure has seven episodes, which are outlined in Table 20.2, and is designed to expose infants to increasing amounts of stress in order to observe how they organize their attachment behaviors around their parents when distressed. Stress is stimulated by the unfamiliar environment, by the entrance of an unfamiliar adult, and by two brief separations from the parent.

A Typology of Infants

According to Bowlby and Ainsworth, infants in the Strange Situation should be able to use their attachment figures as secure bases from

which to explore the novel environment. The stranger's entrance should lead infants to inhibit exploration and draw a little closer to their parents, at least temporarily. The parents' departure should lead to attempts to bring them back by crying or searching, and to less exploration and affiliation. Following the parents' return, infants should seek to reengage in interaction and, if distressed, may wish to be cuddled and comforted. The same responses should occur, with somewhat greater intensity, following the second separation and reunion. In fact, this is how about 65% of the infants studied in the United States in the Strange Situation behave. Following the practices of Ainsworth and her colleagues, these "securely attached" infants are designated type B.

By contrast, some infants seem unable to use their parents as secure bases from which to explore. Furthermore, although they are distressed by their parents' absence, they behave ambivalently upon reunion, both seeking contact and interaction and angrily rejecting it when it is offered. These infants are conventionally labeled type C and typically account for about 15% of the infants in American research samples. Another group of infants seem little concerned by their parents' absence. Instead of greeting their parents upon reunion, they actively avoid interaction and ignore the parents' bids. These infants are said to exhibit type A attachments; they typically constitute about 20% of the infants in American samples.

Although the behavior of most infants allows them to be classified into one of these categories, it has been noted that some infants are difficult to classify (Main and Solomon, 1986). Main and Solomon (1986) observed such infants and found that, rather than using different patterns of behavioral organization, these infants appear disorganized. They have designated a new category, type D attachment, to reflect infants who show behavioral indices of disorganization and disorientation in the Strange Situation. Main and Solomon have compiled a list of behaviors that reflect such disorganization and disorientation, thought to reflect a conflict between behavioral systems (e.g., "cries while moving away from parent" or "falls prone on reunion").

Determinants of Strange Situation Behavior

According to ethological attachment theorists, infants count on attachment figures to protect them and to be accessible when needed and so use them as secure bases from which to explore and interact with other people. However, not all infants trust their attachment figures equally, and these differences in security of attachment might affect how willingly infants use their attachment figures as bases of security. In fact, Ainsworth has argued that the A, B, and C patterns of attachment behavior in the Strange Situation indeed reflect individual differences in attachment security. Moreover, Ainsworth has developed hypotheses concerning the ontogeny of these individual differences.

Almost from birth, infants learn about people from their interactions with them (Lamb, 1981a; Watson, 1985). The extent to which their behaviors—particularly their cries—are answered depends, of course, on the responsiveness of the babies' caretakers. When caretakers hear

Table 20.2. The Strange Situation

Episode[a]	Persons Present	Change
1	Parent, infant	Enter room
2	Parent, infant, stranger	Unfamiliar adult joins the dyad
3	Infant, stranger	Parent leaves
4	Parent, infant	Parent returns Stranger leaves
5	Infant	Parent leaves
6	Infant, stranger	Stranger returns
7	Parent, infant	Parent returns Stranger leaves

Adapted from Ainsworth MD, Wittig BA, Attachment and the exploratory behavior of one-year-olds in a strange situation. In: Foss BM (ed): Determinants of infant behavior (Vol. 4) London, Methuen, 1969, pp. 113–136.
[a] All episodes are usually 3 minutes long, but episodes 3, 5, and 6 can be curtailed if the infant becomes too distressed, and episodes 4 and 7 are sometimes extended.

the babies' signals, interpret them correctly, and make consistently appropriate responses, infants will develop confidence in their own "effectance" (ability to act upon the environment successfully) and trust in the reliability or predictability of the persons concerned. Evidence gathered in an exploratory longitudinal study (Ainsworth and Bell, 1974; Blehar et al., 1977) led Ainsworth to propose that caretakers' sensitivity is important from the first months of life—the months during which infants come to understand what it means to be social. Since adults differ in their sensitivity, there would be differences among infants in the extent to which infants had confidence in their own effectance and in the reliability of others. Ainsworth equates these with differences in the security of attachment (Ainsworth et al., 1974; Ainsworth and Bowlby, 1991).

Since Ainsworth's hypotheses were proposed, many other researchers have attempted to test them in independent longitudinal studies (Bates, Maslin et al., 1985; Belsky et al., 1984; Egeland and Faber, 1984; Erickson et al., 1985; Grossmann et al., 1985; Miyake et al., 1985; Sagi et al., 1985; reviewed by Belsky and Cassidy, 1994). After reviewing the complicated results of these many studies, Lamb and his coauthors (1985) concluded that there was general support for the notion that more socially desirable parental behavior, that is, nurturant, attentive, nonrestrictive parental care, was associated with type B infant behavior in the Strange Situation, at least when studies were conducted in the United States. The mothers of infants who behave in type A or type C fashion (often called "insecurely attached") manifest less socially desirable patterns of behavior: They may overstimulate or understimulate, fail to make their behaviors contingent on infant behavior, appear cold or rejecting, and sometimes appear inept to observers. Unfortunately, there is too much variability in the results to identify precisely what aspects of parental behavior are formatively important. Some studies identify warmth but not sensitivity; some identify level of stimulation; some, patterning of stimulation but not warmth or amount of stimulation, and so forth.

Stability and Prediction

Stability. The notion that Strange Situation behavior reflects something meaningful is supported by findings showing stability over time in patterns of infant behavior. Both Waters (1978) and Connell (1976) reported remarkable stability between 12 and 18 months of age in the way infants behave in the Strange Situation when observed twice with the same parent. According to Waters, 48 of 50 infants—96%—obtained the same classification on both occasions! However, test-retest reliability is not always so high. Vaughn et al. (1979) showed that, in an economically disadvantaged sample, many infants changed from one mode of behavior to another between 12 and 18 months of age. Changes were systematic: When the families had experienced considerable social stress during the 6-month period, type B attachments often changed to types A or C, although when families experienced a low degree of stress, types A or C attachments did not necessarily become type B. Later, Thompson et al. (1982) found equivalent instability in a middle-class sample. In this study, major changes in family circumstances or caretaking arrangements (e.g., the onset of maternal employment) led to changes in Strange Situation behavior, but they did not necessarily engender change from the more desirable type B to the less desirable types A and C any more often than the reverse. Since parents' sensitivity to the infants' signals appears to influence Strange Situation behavior (Ainsworth et al., 1974, 1978), these data might mean that changes in the amount of stress to which the mothers were subjected affected the manner in which they interacted with their infants. No one has yet shown, however, that this is how changing life events affect infants' Strange Situation behavior.

Predictive Validity. Another reason why attachment classifications intrigue developmentalists is that they sometimes predict aspects of the child's future behavior. Attachment theorists believe that when babies encounter people for the first time, they tend to assume that those persons will treat them in the same way that others have treated them in the past. Thus, babies who have developed trust in their attachment figures will tend to regard new people they encounter as trustworthy too. As babies get to know each individual, of course, they develop a set of expectations about that specific individual.

The relation between Strange Situation behavior and styles of interaction with unfamiliar adults has been well documented. Main (1983), for example, showed that babies who had type B attachments to their mothers were later more cooperatively playful when interacting with a friendly stranger than were type A or C infants. Type A infants (who were avoidant of their mothers) later avoided the stranger, whereas type C infants were later resistant with the stranger. Main and Weston (1981) as well as Thompson and Lamb (1983) confirmed that type B infants were more sociable with unfamiliar adults than type A or C infants were. Similarly, Lieberman (1977), Easterbrooks and Lamb (1979), and Pastor (1981) showed that Strange Situation behavior was associated with social behavior in initial encounters with peers as well as over longer periods of time in preschool play groups (Booth et al., 1991; Sroufe, 1983; Waters et al., 1979) and summer camp at age 11 (Elicker et al., 1992). Type B infants engaged in more frequent and more mature forms of interaction with their peers, sharing more and showing a greater capacity to initiate and maintain interactions, for example. For reasons that are not clear, however, Jacobson and his colleagues (Jacobson and Wille, 1984; Jacobson et al., 1983, 1986) have reported contrasting results, suggesting that the relation between attachment classification and peer competence is neither direct nor powerful (see Lamb and Nash, 1989, for a review of the studies and issues concerning the influence of attachment relationships in infancy on later peer relationships).

Other research (Arend et al., 1979; Frankel and Bates, 1990; Matas et al., 1978; Seuss et al., 1992; Sroufe, 1983) addresses the relation between Strange Situation classifications and aspects of achievement motivation. These researchers found that Strange Situation behavior at 12 or 18 months predicts cognitive performance in problem-solving situations and in a variety of stressful and challenging contexts, at least until kindergarten age. Placed in cognitively challenging situations, children who, as infants, had type B attachments to their mothers persisted longer and more enthusiastically than did children who had type A or C attachments. Type B infants also seemed to be more resilient and robust when stressed or challenged (Block and Block, 1980). In addition, type B infants appeared more socially competent and independent when they later entered preschool (Sroufe, 1983; Sroufe et al., 1984) and also showed fewer behavior problems (Bates, Maslin, et al., 1985: Erickson et al., 1985; Lewis et al., 1984). In general, although some researchers have found that insecure attachments may be associated with severe behavior and adjustment problems, others have not (Belsky and Cassidy, 1994; Belsky and Nezworski, 1988; Fagot and Kavanaugh, 1990; Lyons-Ruth et al., 1993).

Evidence concerning the temporal stability of Strange Situation behavior and its relation to measures of earlier infant-mother interaction and later child achievement and personality suggests that the Strange Situation measures some meaningful aspect of mother-infant attachment and has important implications for understanding and predicting development. Presumably, Strange Situation behavior with fathers affects development in analogous ways. However, the recent attention given to multiple attachment figures for many infants—mothers, fathers (Lamb, 1981, in press), siblings (Teti and Ablard, 1989), grandparents (Myers et al., 1987), day care providers (Howes et al., 1988)—highlights the need for a model of such combined influences (Nash and Hay, 1993; Tavecchio and Van IJzendorn, 1987; Thompson, 1990). Are these influences additive, such that a secure attachment to one parent and an insecure attachment to the other leads to intermediary levels of functioning later on (Easterbrooks and Goldberg, 1990; Pipp et al., 1992)? Or are these influences compensatory, such that a secure relationship with a day care provider, for example, can compensate for an insecure attachment to a parent (Goossens and Van IJzendoorn, 1990)? (See Nash and Hay, 1993, for a fuller discussion of the issue of combining influences from several early close relationships.)

Even for the relatively simpler infant-mother predictions, Lamb et al. (1985) have pointed out that the predictive validity of longitudinal associations is far from perfect. Rather, the relation between Strange Situation behavior and subsequent child behavior is found only when there is stability in the caretaking arrangements and family circumstances, which (as we noted previously) seems to maintain stability in patterns of parent-child interaction. Thus, the question first encountered when considering the stability of cognition in infancy arises again: Is the prediction over time attributable to individual differences in the quality of early parent-child interaction, or is it attributable to the continuing quality of child-parent interactions? If the latter were true, it would imply that the quality of early relationships was predictively valuable, not because it caused later differences directly, but because it presaged later differences in the quality of relationships, which in turn, would cause differences in the child's behavior. Such a pattern of findings would place the locus of stability in the continuing quality of parent-child interactions rather than in some aspect of the child's personality. Surprisingly, no researchers have actually tested this possibility, although it has major relevance for long-standing assumptions concerning the critical importance of early experiences.

Although Strange Situation behavior, measures of prior infant-parent interaction, and measures of the child's later behavior are all interrelated, the relations are not very strong. This suggests that factors other than quality of attachment, such as temperament or familiarity with strangers and brief separations, influence children's Strange Situation behavior. In turn, this means that researchers and clinicians need to rely on multiple convergent methods to assess constructs as complex and as important as the quality of infant attachments, rather than relying on a single measure like the Strange Situation in which behavior is influenced by factors other than quality of attachment.

Cross-Cultural Research

Some of the most provocatively informative recent work on Strange Situation behavior has been conducted outside the United States. The distribution of infants across the A, B, and C categories in many other countries differs from that typically found in American samples (Lamb et al., 1985). One could interpret these results by concluding that parents in the cultures are either much more or much less sensitive than American parents, but that ethnocentric interpretation seems improbable. Rather, these results may demonstrate the importance of factors *other than* the quality of parental behavior in explaining Strange Situation behavior (Campos et al., 1983; Lamb et al., 1985). For example, the high degrees of stress manifested by Japanese and Israeli babies leads to increases in the proportion of infants classified as type C. It may be that Japanese infants appear inordinately distressed because they have much less experience with separations from their mothers than American infants typically have; thus, the situation is not psychologically similar for Japanese and American babies. For infants growing up on Israeli kibbutzim, encounters with strangers are unusual and may thus elicit great distress. Again, therefore, even though the procedure was structurally the same for Japanese, Israeli, and American infants, the psychological experiences or meanings for infants from each culture might be very different. In addition, Miyake et al. (1985) reported that the Japanese infants who were later classified as type C were temperamentally more irritable than type B infants from birth. Thus, it appears that culture-specific rearing practices and/or temperamental differences account for at least some of the variance in Strange Situation classifications across cultures.

The picture emerging from the many studies in which Strange Situation behavior was assessed is a complicated one. Strange Situation behavior appears to reflect individual differences in patterns of infant-parent interaction, with type B attachments potentiated by warm, sensitive, and supportive parental behavior. However, other factors seem to be important as well, notably culture-specific rearing practices and (perhaps) infant temperament. To understand the formative importance of infant-parent attachment, we need to obtain multiple measures of attachment, rather than rely exclusively on the observation of Strange Situation behavior. Additionally, we need to better understand how several early attachment relationships together may affect later functioning (Nash and Hay, 1993).

The next two sections take into account such a diverse social milieu, which for many infants involves not only parents but also grandparents and other adults, siblings, and peers. We now discuss infants' relationships with nonparental figures and illustrate similarities and differences among the infant-adult, infant-sibling, and infant-peer systems.

Sibling Relationships

Siblings in many nonindustrialized countries assume a major responsibility for infant caretaking (Dunn, 1988; Rogoff, 1990; Weisner, 1982; Werner, 1984; Zukow, 1989). These siblings may spend relatively little time playing with the infants; most of their interactions, like those of Western parents, involve protection or caretaking. In our society, by contrast, siblings seldom assume any responsibility for infant caretaking, and sibling relationships appear to incorporate features of both the infant-adult and infant-peer systems (Pepler et al., 1982). On the one hand, sibling dyads share common interests and have more similar behavioral repertoires than do infant-adult dyads. On the other hand, sibling pairs resemble infant-adult pairs to the extent that they differ with respect to amount of experience and levels of both cognitive and social ability. These discrepancies often lead to differences in the ways younger and older siblings relate to each other, differences that distinguish them from the infant-peer system (see below). In two observational studies of sibling interaction in a laboratory playroom, Lamb (1978a, 1978b) found consistent asymmetries between the roles assumed by older and younger children. Older siblings "led" the interaction: They engaged in more dominant, assertive, and directive behaviors than their younger siblings did. The infants, meanwhile, appeared inordinately interested in what their siblings were doing; they followed them around, attempting to imitate or at least explore the toys just abandoned by the older children. This is, of course, a strategy that maximizes the amount the baby can learn about the environment from the older child. As Zajonc (1983) suggests, older siblings offer young children cognitive models, albeit less sophisticated ones than do adults. In a home observational study, Abramovitch and her colleagues (1979) reported patterns of interaction similar to those reported by Lamb (1978b), although siblings at home engaged in much more interaction than in the laboratory. In a longitudinal study, Lamb (1978a) found remarkable stability across time in the amount of interaction engaged in by siblings. The pattern of correlations, furthermore, suggested that the sociability of the younger babies determined the amount of attention they later received from their siblings, rather than the reverse.

Individual differences in the quality of sibling relationships were also the focus of a longitudinal study conducted in England by Dunn and Kendrick (1980, 1981a, 1981b, 1982a, 1982b). Dunn found that same-sex siblings got along better than different-sex siblings. In addition, siblings interacted more poorly when mothers and first-born girls had very positive relationships before and immediately after the birth of the second child and when there was frequent interaction and play between the siblings and their mothers. These findings suggest that parents exert an important influence on the mutual affective involvement of siblings, who may compete for parental attention.

In a variety of studies, researchers have found that older siblings spend at least some of their time teaching object-related and social skills to their younger siblings (including infants) and that the amount of teaching increases with the age of the older child (Cicirelli, 1973, 1974; Minnett et al., 1983; Pepler, 1981; Stewart, 1983). These studies, along with the finding that infants monitor and imitate their older siblings (Lamb, 1978a, 1978b), confirm that older siblings may influence the cognitive and social skills of infants through some combination of teaching and modeling (Zajonc, 1983). Dunn (1988) very richly documents the enhanced arena for the development of social understanding provided by siblings, and infants' considerable practical understanding of the feelings and intentions of other family members, siblings and parents alike. There is also evidence to suggest that infants form attachment relationships with their older siblings, as assessed by the Strange Situation (Teti and Ablard, 1989) and other means (Dunn, 1993).

It should be noted that not only do older siblings influence infants, but the reverse also occurs. For example, Howe and Ross (1990) found that friendly interactions between preschoolers and their infant siblings increased the older children's perspective-taking abilities.

The effects of age spacing on the patterns of interactions between infants and their preschool-aged older siblings are unclear; Abramovitch and her colleagues (1979), like Dunn and Kendrick (1981b, 1982a), found no age-spacing differences in amounts of positive, negative, and imitative sibling behaviors. Suggesting that broad summary measures may not have been sensitive enough to detect actual differences, Teti et al. (1986) used a more fine-grained coding scheme and found that older preschool-aged first-borns indeed created more "intellectual" (e.g., language mastery) and "social" (e.g., game) experiences for their infant siblings than did younger preschool-aged first-borns. In addition, Gibbs et al. (1985) found that widely spaced siblings were more interactive and responsive to one another than closely spaced siblings were. In neither of these investigations, however, did the researchers uncover relations between measures of infant cognitive or linguistic level and either sibling age or measures of sibling interaction. Thus, the net impact of siblings on infant development remains unclear, partly because such influences depend on sex of the siblings, birth order, and family size (Wagner et al., 1993).

Infants' Interactions with New People

Prior to the 1970s, it was commonly believed that infants were uninterested in their peers and afraid of strangers. Studies conducted since then, considered alongside earlier studies, indicate otherwise (Bridges, 1933; Buhler, 1933; Maudry and Nekula, 1939; Ross and Goldman, 1977). In fact, infants are both interested and competent in their interactions with strangers, whether peers or adults.

INFANT-PEER INTERACTIONS

Even newborns are responsive to their peers. As described above, they respond to the distress of their peers by becoming distressed themselves (Martin and Clark, 1982; Sagi and Hoffman, 1976). Two- and 3-month-olds attend to the activities of their peers (Bridges, 1933) and increase their own activity level in a peer's presence (Field, 1979; Fogel, 1979). By 6 months of age, peers do not simply elicit responses in infants; infants respond to one another in socially complex ways. They initiate interactions by touching, vocalizing, and/or smiling at peers (Hay et al., 1983; Vandell, 1980; Vandell et al., 1980), and their increased sensitivity to social cues is indicated by tendencies to continue interactions when peers are responsive and to stop when they are not (Hay et al., 1983). In addition, 6-month-olds do not automatically cry in response to their peers' cries but instead attend to a peer's distress, becoming distressed themselves only if the other's distress is prolonged (Hay et al., 1981).

Between 6 and 12 months of age, infants direct increasing numbers of social behaviors toward peers (Jacobson, 1981; Maudry and Nekula, 1939; Vandell, 1980), although the amount of physical contact decreases (Vandell, 1980; Vandell et al., 1980). Perhaps this reflects an increasing reliance on distal rather than proximal modes of interaction, for during the second half of the 1st year infants begin to use conventional acts (gestures and words) to communicate with their peers (Bakeman and Adamson, 1986). The structural complexity of peer-directed acts also increases with age so that by 9 months infants can synchronize several social behaviors (Becker, 1977; Vandell et al., 1980) and can attend simultaneously to objects and peers and thus engage in joint play (Adamson and Bakeman, 1985). Infants at this age also express more affect

during periods of joint engagement with peers than when alone (Adamson and Bakeman, 1985) and begin to distinguish between familiar and unfamiliar peers (Dontas et al., 1985; Jacobson, 1981).

At the start of the 2nd year of life, both cooperation and conflict begin to occur in interactions between peers (Eckerman and Whatley, 1977; Goldman and Ross, 1978; Hay, Caplan, et al., 1991; Howes, 1988; Nash, 1985, 1986). The ability to engage in conflicts over toys and personal space, not present among 6-month-olds (Hay et al., 1983), is found at the start of the 2nd year of life (Nash, 1986; Caplan et al., 1991). The social nature of such early conflicts is suggested by Hay and Ross (1982), who found that 21-month-olds did not simply grab toys from one another but used gestures and vocalizations to resolve disputes. Additionally, when children yielded possession of objects to peers, the winners often turned their attention elsewhere, as though the interaction itself, and not obtaining the object, was important. These infants spent only 5% of their time with one another in conflicts.

Studies comparing interactions with peers and mothers indicate that infants demonstrate similar social competencies in their interactions with peers and mothers (Adamson and Bakeman, 1985; Bakeman and Adamson, 1984, 1986; Nash, 1985, 1986; Vandell and Wilson, 1982). Additionally, several studies of 10- to 19-month-olds revealed that interactions with peers were more frequent than those with mothers when both were present (Eckerman and Whatley, 1977; Eckerman et al., 1975; Nash, 1986; Rubenstein and Howes, 1976; Rubenstein et al., 1982), even though mothers of 13- to 15-month-olds initiate more interactions with their infants than vice versa and initiate as many interactions as peers do (Nash, 1986). Novelty is not the issue either: When given the opportunity to interact with peers, mothers, and unfamiliar adults, infants interact more frequently with peers than with unfamiliar adults (Eckerman and Whatley, 1977; Lewis et al., 1975).

INFANT-ADULT INTERACTIONS

The fact that infants prefer to socialize with peers rather than with adults does not mean that they are uninterested in, or wary of, unfamiliar adults. Indeed, they are quite adept in their social relations with new adults as well. When infants are about 8 months of age, they begin to distinguish between unfamiliar and familiar adults by showing signs of apprehension about the former (Bronson, 1972; Emde et al., 1976). This wariness was at one time termed stranger anxiety and was treated as a developmental milestone. More recent studies have shown that in many situations infants do not always behave anxiously and that infants' responses to strangers depend to a large extent on the strangers' behavior. When an unfamiliar adult approaches an infant in a warm, friendly manner, the infant usually responds in kind (Bretherton, 1978; Bretherton et al., 1981; Clarke-Stewart, 1978; Rheingold and Eckerman, 1973). The parent's behavior, too, can affect the infant's response: Infants whose mothers talked to them in a happy tone about a stranger were friendlier toward the stranger than infants whose mothers talked about the stranger in a neutral tone (Feinman et al., 1986). Thus, when placed in a situation conducive to socializing, i.e., when those present act in a friendly manner, infants respond accordingly.

A variety of studies have indicated that infants are quite interested in and able to interact with new people. Rheingold and Eckerman (1973) found that nearly all the 8- to 12-month-olds in their study looked and smiled at strangers and appeared comfortable in their presence. Many let the stranger pick them up while their mothers were out of the room. With both their mothers and a friendly, interactive stranger present, 12-month-olds approached the stranger and spent more time with her than with their mothers (Ross and Goldman, 1977). Furthermore, 9- to 12-month-old infants were as likely to follow an unfamiliar woman as their mothers into another room (Hay, 1977) and also actively interacted with strangers, willingly sharing objects with them (Hay and Murray, 1982; Rheingold et al., 1976; Ross and Goldman, 1977). One-year-olds engaged in cooperative play (Bretherton, 1978) and games (Ross and Goldman, 1977) with unfamiliar adults, while 18-month-olds imitated unfamiliar adults as much as they imitate their mothers (Hay et al., 1985), and will help unfamiliar adults to shelve groceries (Rheingold, 1982). Infants can also request help from unfamiliar adults effectively (Mosier and Rogoff, 1994; Rogoff et al., 1984) and in one study used social referencing with adults they had known for only 10 minutes when confronted with a mildly frightening toy (Klinnert et al., 1986).

Infants' interest in and abilities to interact with people other than their parents can set the stage for the formation of relationships with others. Thus, 10- to 14-month-olds who were cared for by an unfamiliar adult for 2½ hours during each of 3 consecutive days formed bonds to the caretaker: They consistently approached her and cried when she left them with a person they had seen for only a few minutes (Fleener, 1973). One-year-olds who had interacted with a stranger for 8 minutes either did not cry when left alone with the stranger or were more effectively soothed by her than were infants who had interacted with a stranger for only 1 minute (Bretherton, 1978). Furthermore, infants cried when a stranger whom they had only recently met departed, leaving them alone in an unfamiliar room (Ipsa, 1981). Not surprisingly, infants can feel secure with people in addition to their parents. Thus, infants formed attachments to care providers both in day care centers (Ainslie and Anderson, 1984; Goossens and Van IJzendoorn, 1990; Ricciuti, 1974) and in Israeli kibbutzim (Fox, 1977; Sagi et al., 1985). As with parents, the type of attachments infants formed with major care providers affected aspects of their personality several years later (Howes, 1990; Howes et al., 1988; Oppenheim et al., 1988, reviewed by Nash and Hay, 1993).

Findings like these highlight the roles played by social interaction in shaping development in infancy. Born with the ability to express emotions, infants effectively engage adults from the start. Over time, the infant's expressive and social skills improve as a result of social experiences; the interactions between infants and their care providers establish dispositions that, when maintained by a stable social environment, may predict aspects of the children's functioning years later.

We began this chapter with a discussion of the transactional model; its portrayal of development as a joint function of infant and exogenous influences improves on the more static main effects and interactional models. It is fitting, then, to conclude the chapter with a discussion of infant temperament. From a transactional perspective, temperament appears to be an early emerging and direct way in which infants affect other individuals and, thereby, their own development.

INFANT TEMPERAMENT

Interestingly, developmentalists traditionally believed that individual differences in infant behavior were determined by differences in infant-mother interactions, with genetic/constitutional factors playing a minor role, such as in explaining susceptibility to separation distress. Today, however, theorists and researchers agree that individual differences may play a far more important role than this, and consequently issues concerning the definition, measurement, and origins of temperament have moved to the forefront of infant research (Bates, 1986; Bornstein et al., 1986; Goldsmith et al., 1987). Temperament is generally viewed as having a genetic/constitutional base and as being somewhat stable over time, although theorists disagree over the stability and modifiability of temperament and the relation between infant temperament and later personality (Buss and Plomin, 1975; Thomas and Chess, 1977) (see Chapter 13 for a general historical account of the concept of temperament.)

Conceptualizations of Infant Temperament

Temperament can be thought of as a constitutionally based source of individual variation in personality functioning, emerging early in life. Most measures of temperament sample aspects of infant affect, attention, and activity, attending to temporal (e.g., latency of response) and intensive (e.g., strength and sensitivity of response) characteristics of certain behaviors.

Although Gesell and Ames (1937) first suggested research on infant temperament, it was not until Thomas and Chess began the New York Longitudinal Study (NYLS) in the 1950s that research on infant temperament began in earnest (Thomas and Chess, 1977; Thomas et al., 1963, 1968). The subjects of the NYLS were followed at regular intervals from infancy through adolescence and adulthood. Mothers were first interviewed when the infants were 2–3 months of age, and from these interviews Thomas and Chess derived nine dimensions of infant temperament: activity level, rhythmicity, approach/withdrawal, adaptability, intensity of reaction, attention span and persistence, distractibility, quality of mood, and threshold of responsiveness. Four behavior styles were ultimately identified. "Easy babies" were positive in mood, regular in body functions, and adaptable; these babies (comprising about 40% of the entire sample) approached new situations positively and reacted with low to moderate intensity. By contrast, "difficult babies" (10%) were negative in mood, irregular, and slow to adapt; they withdrew from new situations and reacted with high intensity. "Slow-to-warm-up babies" (15%) were negative in mood and slow to adapt; they withdrew from new situations, reacted with low to moderate intensity, and were low in activity. "Average babies" (35%) were not rated highly on any dimension.

Thomas and Chess reported that individual differences in infant temperament were fairly stable over time. However, one of their most important and provocative findings was that a child's behavioral style was not always predictable from knowledge of behavioral style in infancy. Thomas et al. (1968) reported that about 70% of infants characterized as "difficult" eventually developed behavior problems. Not surprisingly, these "difficult" children created special challenges for parents, who were described as behaviorally and emotionally inconsistent with their children; they frequently blamed themselves for their children's problems. Parents of those "difficult" infants who had no significant problems in later childhood adapted much more successfully to their children's difficult behavior, however; they were tolerant, patient, and consistent. Rather than blaming themselves, these parents accepted their children's temperamental difficulties with good humor. The major differences between these two groups of "difficult" children suggested that temperamental characteristics early in life can be modified by environmental experience. Thomas et al. (1968) argued that the "goodness of fit" between the child's temperament and the demands of the environment determined whether outcomes would be favorable or unfavorable.

Like many pioneering studies, the NYLS has been the target of much criticism. One major question concerns the close contact the investigators maintained with their subjects, raising the possibility that knowledge of the child's temperament at one point may have inadvertently influenced investigators' judgments of the same child's later behavior. Second, most of the information about temperament and behavior was obtained from parental interviews, raising questions concerning the extent to which data were influenced by parental perceptions. A third criticism arose from the conception of temperament as a behavioral "style," which implies a kind of pervasiveness that seldom occurs in human behavior. Fourth, other researchers have failed to find evidence of the nine NYLS divisions (Buss and Plomin, 1984; Hagekull et al., 1980).

Despite these criticisms, however, the growing recognition of constitutional differences at birth led Brazelton (1973) to develop an objectively administered Neonatal Behavioral Assessment Scale (NBAS). This scale was originally designed to assess neonatal behaviors having clear social significance to parents. Thus, it has many of the features of a measure of temperament, although the scale was not specifically designed as such. NBAS items assess states of alertness, capacities to self-soothe, responses to adult ministrations, and the abilities to respond and cease responding to animate and inanimate stimuli of various types. The NBAS also assesses motor abilities, muscle tone, and some neurological reflexes. Early reports suggested that NBAS scores tended to correlate with later parental reports of temperamental traits, such as distractibility (Sostek and Anders, 1977).

During the 1970s, the NBAS became popular for documenting individual differences in the social capacities of neonates. Unfortunately, however, researchers failed to find significant reliability in neonatal performance on the NBAS, even from day to day (Sameroff, 1978). This could have a variety of explanations. First, infant social capacities may be genuinely unstable. Second, these social capacities may be stable, but fluctuations in infant state may mask stability. Third, the type and dosage of medication administered to mothers during childbirth, as well as the time elapsed between birth and testing, may also affect the temporal stability of the NBAS. Despite these limitations, the NBAS has become popular as an intervention tool for demonstrating infant capacities to parents (Nugent et al., 1986; Nurcombe et al., 1984; Rauh et al., 1986).

From the original interview responses obtained by Thomas and Chess, Carey (1970) developed the Infant Temperament Questionnaire (ITQ), which was later refined by Carey and McDevitt (RITQ; 1978a, 1978b). The ITQ and RITQ measure the nine dimensions derived by Thomas and Chess and also allow summary characterizations of infants as easy, slow to warm up, difficult, intermediate low, and intermediate high. Bates et al. (1979) have also developed a parent-report measure, the Infant Characteristics Questionnaire (ICQ), measuring the dimensions of "fussiness-difficult" (upon which they place greatest emphasis), "unadaptable," "dull," and "unpredictable." Rothbart (1981; Rothbart and Derryberry, 1981) has developed a third parent questionnaire, the Infant Behavior Questionnaire (IBQ), which measures the dimensions of activity level, soothability, fear, distress to limitations, smiling and laughter, and duration of orienting. Finally, Buss and Plomin (1975, 1984) have developed a parent questionnaire measuring the dimensions of emotionality, activity, sociability, and impulsiveness. Three additional temperament measures involve more objective home or laboratory assessments. Bornstein et al. (1986) have developed a measure that couples home observations and parent reports, which is built around infants' spontaneous activity and infant responsivity in structured vignettes. This measure assesses the dimensions of positive affect, negative affect, persistence, and motor activity. Matheny and Wilson (1984; Matheny, 1980, 1983) have created a laboratory-based assessment of temperament, measuring the dimensions of test extraversion, activity level, and task orientation. Finally, Goldsmith and Campos (1982, 1986) have developed a laboratory observation technique, tapping 10 task-specific dimensions.

Clearly, little consensus exists regarding the prominent characteristics of infant temperament. Moreover, in a review of the psychometric properties and convergent validity of temperament measures, Hubert et al. (1982) pointed out that "convergence between different temperament instruments, supposedly measuring the same dimensions at the same point in time, have yielded generally low correlations" (p. 575). Most instruments also show only moderate temporal stability, low interparent and parent-observer agreement, and inconsistent relations to observed interaction patterns. Nevertheless, it may be desirable to obtain information from both parents and observers, even if scores on the two measures differ, because temperament is so complex a construct. Both may measure valid aspects of infant temperament, and although parental ratings may be colored by idiosyncratic perceptions and parental personality (Goldsmith and Campos, 1982; Sameroff et al., 1982), these perceptions may be more important predictors of infant-parent relationships than "objective" measures of the infant's temperament would be (Bates, 1980, 1983).

During the 1990s, investigators began focusing on physiological measures of temperament, after its successful use in studies of toddlers and preschoolers during the 1980s (see Kagan et al., 1987, for a review). Individual differences in positive and negative emotionality are thought to reflect difference in temperament. Thus, measures of neural and endocrine processes (related to genetic differences) should correlate with other measures of emotionality. In support of this, Gunnar and Nelson (1994) have found that differences in event-related potentials were associated with differences in emotionality and cortisol levels. Higher cortisol levels have been reported for behaviorally inhibited infants, compared to uninhibited infants in several studies by Gunnar and her

associates (Gunnar et al., 1992; Larson et al., 1991). Stifter and Fox (1990; Fox and Stifter, 1989) included measurements of vagal tone in their longitudinal study of emotional reactivity in infants and found that at 5 months infants with high vagal tone were emotionally more reactive to negative events, and at 14 months they were quicker to positively approach a stranger and a new toy than were infants with lower vagal tone. They concluded that individual differences in parasympathetic control (as indexed by vagal tone) affect socioemotional organization, such that infants with higher parasympathetic control (higher vagal tone) are better organized socioemotionally and more behaviorally responsive to others.

Stability of Infant Temperament

Given the expected relation between infant temperament and later personality, temporal stability was initially seen as a necessary component of temperament (Buss and Plomin, 1984). However, the age-to-age correlations for different dimensions of temperament are variable and may be especially low in the 1st years of life. This apparent instability was first attributed to measurement error or to environmental flux, but most recently researchers have begun to ascribe the fluctuations to the discontinuous actions of genes over time (Matheny, 1980, 1983; Plomin, 1983; Scarr and McCartney, 1983; Wilson, 1983, 1984). In fact, temperament seems to follow a complex fluctuating course in the earliest years, as befits characteristics regulated in part by "on again, off again" gene programs (Plomin, 1983, 1993). The patterns of developmental acceleration and lag also appear to be more synchronous in more genetically similar organisms, suggesting that the fluctuations are meaningful, not random (Matheny, 1983; Wilson, 1978, 1983, 1984). Most likely, certain dimensions of temperament show considerable longitudinal stability, whereas others fluctuate.

Temperament and Infant-Parent Interaction

It was widely assumed for many years that individual differences in parent-infant interaction were determined by prior parental behaviors, but parental behavior may itself be influenced by the infant's temperament and behavior (Bell, 1968, 1971). Parents are extremely sensitive to their infants' temperaments, and different temperaments can be expected to elicit different behaviors from caretakers. Difficult babies demand and receive more attention than easy babies in the United States (Bates et al., 1982; Petit and Bates, 1984), Israel (Klein, 1984), and Kenya (deVries, 1984). Moreover, the perception of difficultness in early infancy increases the likelihood of later maltreatment (Sherrod et al., 1984; Vietze et al., 1980).

Temperament is also constructive. An infant's temperament affects those around the infant, who in turn are likely to treat the infant in consistent ways that help construct the infant's own personality. A temperamentally active infant might be considered "inquisitive"; a temperamentally inactive baby, by contrast, might be seen as "thoughtful" or "passive." Insofar as parents believe that their infants' temperaments fit a particular mold, they may mold their infant's environment to suit these expectations. In this sense, parental perceptions are important regardless of their relationship to objectively defined characteristics.

More than any other investigators, J. Bates and his colleagues (1980, 1983, 1986b; Bates, Maslin, et al., 1985; Bates, Petit, et al. 1985; Petit and Bates, 1984) have explored the assessment and clinical implications of infant "difficultness." Difficultness has at its core frequent and intense expressions of negative emotion that are part of the child's disposition. If difficultness is dispositional in nature, it ought to appear early, have a biological basis, and endure. Bates has confirmed that difficultness manifests itself in infant crying, and Lounsbury and Bates (1982) found that hunger cries of difficult infants are higher pitched and are perceived as aversive and demanding even by unrelated adults. Bates et al. (1984) believe that the excessive demands for social interaction made by difficult infants also lie at the root of their mothers' attributions of difficulty, because mothers interpret this "coercive control" negatively. Further, difficultness is relatively stable between 6 and 24 months (Fish and Crockenberg, 1981; Lee and Bates, 1985; Snow et al., 1980). Finally, difficultness assessed by maternal report at 6 months predicted maternal perceptions of aggressiveness and anxiety at 3–5 years (Bates, Maslin, et al., 1985; Bates, Petit, et al., 1985). Therefore, it is possible that difficult infants have troublesome dispositions that endure, or it could be that, as infants, they behave in ways that encourage their parents to treat them so that they act out, years later, as a result.

In addition, difficultness can have distinctly positive connotations in some circumstances. DeVries (1984) studied 4-month-old Masai infants in Kenya, where drought and malnutrition take the lives of many babies. In an admittedly small sample, difficult babies—those who were intense, irregular, unadaptable, and fussy—tended to survive, whereas easy babies tended not to survive. DeVries hypothesized that the demandingness of difficult babies is an advantage in the Masai society. The moral here is that temperamental concepts like difficultness must be understood in context; in our culture, difficulty may be associated with behavior problems, but in the Masai environment it may promote survival and health.

Of course, difficultness is not the only infant characteristic that may predict later behavior problems. Activity level could be associated with a propensity to childhood accidents, whereas many psychiatric syndromes, including manic-depression and anxiety neurosis, could involve premorbid characteristics even in infancy. Perhaps the study of infant temperament, in conjunction with a certain parental personality and/or disciplinary styles, will lead to the identification of significant early indicators of risk, and, more generally, of the diverse ways infants contribute to their development.

References

Abramovitch R, Corter C, Lando B: Sibling interaction in the home. *Child Dev* 50:997–1003, 1979.

Acredolo LP, Goodwyn SW: Symbolic gesturing in language development. *Hum Dev* 28:40–49, 1985.

Acredolo LP, Goodwyn SW: Sign language in babies: The significance of symbolic gestures for understanding language development. In: Vasta R (ed): *Annals of Child Development* (Vol 7). Greenwich, CT, JAI Press, 1990.

Adams PI, Maurer A, Davis M: Newborns' discrimination of chromatic from achromatic stimuli. *J Exp Child Psychol* 41:267–281, 1986.

Adams RJ: An evaluation of color preference in early infancy. *Infant Behavior and Development* 10:143–150, 1987.

Adamson LB, Bakeman R: Affect and attention: Infants observed with mothers and peers. *Child Dev* 56:582–593, 1985.

Ainslie R, Anderson C: Daycare children's relationships to their mothers and caregivers. In: Ainslie RC (ed): *Quality Variations in Daycare*. New York, Praeger, 1984.

Ainsworth MDS: The development of infant-mother attachment. In: Caldwell BM, Ricciuti HN (eds): *Review of Child Development Research* (Vol 3). Chicago, University of Chicago Press, 1973.

Ainsworth MDS, Bell SM: Mother-infant interaction and the development of competence. In: Connolly KJ, Bruner J (eds): *The Growth of Competence*. New York, Academic Press, 1974.

Ainsworth MDS, Bowlby J: An ethological approach to personality development. *Am Psychol* 46:333–341, 1991.

Ainsworth MDS, Wittig BA: Attachment and the exploratory behavior of one-year-olds in a strange situation. In: Foss BM (ed): *Determinants of Infant Behavior* (Vol 4). London, Methuen, 1969, pp. 113–136.

Ainsworth MDS, Bell SM, Stayton DJ: Infant-mother attachment and social development: "Socialization" as a product of reciprocal responsiveness to signals. In: Richards MPM (ed): *The Integration of a Child into a Social World*. London, Cambridge University Press, 1974.

Ainsworth MDS, Blehar MC, Waters E, et al: *Patterns of Attachment: A Psychological Study of the Strange Situation*. Hillsdale, NJ, Erlbaum, 1978.

Ambrose A (ed): *Stimulation in Early Infancy*. New York, Academic Press, 1969.

Anastasi A: Heredity, environment, and the question, "how?" *Psychol Rev* 65:197–208, 1958.

Anderson JW: Attachment behavior out of doors. In: Blurton Jones N (ed): *Ethological Studies of Child Behaviour*. Cambridge, United Kingdom, Cambridge University Press, 1972.

Arend R, Clove F, Sroufe LA: Continuity of individual adaptation from infancy to kindergarten: A predictive study of ego-resiliency and curiosity in preschoolers. *Child Dev* 50:950–959, 1979.

Aries P: *Centuries of Childhood*. New York, Vintage, 1962. (Originally published 1960.)

Ashmead DH, McCarty ME, Lucas LS, et al: Visual guidance in infants' reaching toward suddenly displaced targets. *Child Dev* 64:1111–1127, 1993.

Aslin RN: Development of binocular fixation in human infants. *J Exp Child Psychol* 23:133–150, 1977.

Aslin RN, Pisoni DB, Jusczyk PW: Auditory development and speech perception in infancy. In: Haith MM, Campos JJ (eds): *Handbook of Child Psychology*. Vol 2: *Infancy and Developmental Psychobiology*. New York, Wiley, 1983.

Atkinson J, Braddock O: Development of basic visual functions. In: Slater A, Bremner G (eds): *Infant Development*. Hillsdale, NJ, Erlbaum, 1989.

Bakeman R, Adamson LB: Coordinating attention to people and objects in mother-infant and peer-infant interaction. *Child Dev* 55:1278–1289, 1984.

Bakeman R, Adamson LB: Infants' conventionalized acts: Gestures and words with mothers and peers. *Infant Behav Dev* 9:215–230, 1986.

Bakeman R, Brown IV: Behavioral dialogues: An approach to the assessments of mother-infant interaction. *Child Dev* 48:195–203, 1977.

Ball W, Tronick E: Infant responses to impending collision: Optical and real. *Science* 171:818–820, 1971.

Banks MS, Dannemiller JL: Infant visual psychophysics. In: Salapatek P, Cohen L (eds): *Handbook of Infant Perception: From Sensation to Perception* (Vol 1). New York, Academic Press, 1987, pp. 115–184.

Barnet AB, Ohlrich ES, Shanks BL: EEG evoked responses to repetitive auditory stimulation in normal and Down's syndrome infants. *Dev Med Child Neurol* 13:321–329, 1971.

Barrera ME, Maurer D: The perception of facial expressions by the three-month-old. *Child Dev* 52:203–206, 1981a.

Barrera ME, Maurer D: Recognition of mother's photographed face by the three-month-old infant. *Child Dev* 52:714–716, 1981b.

Barrett-Goldfarb MS, Whitehurst GJ: Infant vocalizations as a function of parental voice selection. *Dev Psychol* 8:273–276, 1973.

Bartoshuk AK: Human neonatal cardiac acceleration to sound: Habituation and dishabituation. *Percept Mot Skills* 15:15–27, 1962.

Bates E: *The Emergence of Symbols: Cognition and Communication in Infancy*. New York, Academic Press, 1979.

Bates E, Bretherton I, Beeghly-Smith M, et al: Social bases of language development: A reassessment. In: Reese H, Lipsitt LP (eds): *Advances in Child Development and Behavior* (Vol 16). New York, Academic Press, 1982, pp. 7–75.

Bates JE: The concept of difficult temperament. *Merrill-Palmer Q* 26:299–319, 1980.

Bates JE: Issues in the assessment of difficult temperament: A reply to Thomas, Chess, and Korn. *Merrill-Palmer Q* 29:89–97, 1983.

Bates JE: Temperament in infancy. In: Osofsky JD (ed): *Handbook of Infant Development*. New York, Wiley, 1986.

Bates JE, Freeland CA, Lounsbury ML: Measurement of infant difficultness. *Child Dev* 50:794–803, 1979.

Bates JE, Maslin CA, Frankel KA: Attachment security, mother-child interaction, and temperament as predictors of behavior problem ratings at age three years. *Monogr Soc Res Child Dev* 50 (serial no. 209), 1985.

Bates JE, Miller E, Bayles K: Understanding the link between difficult temperament and behavior problems: Toward identifying subtypes of difficultness. Paper presented at the International Conference on Infant Studies, New York, 1984.

Bates JE, Olson SL, Petit GS, et al: Dimensions of individuality in the mother-infant relationship at 6 months of age. *Child Dev* 53:446–461, 1982.

Bates JE, Petit GS, Bayles K: Infancy and preschool antecedents of behavior problems at 5 years. Paper presented at the meeting of the Society for Research in Child Development, Toronto, Canada, 1985.

Baumrind D: The average expectable environment is not good enough: A response to Scarr. *Child Dev* 63:1299–1317, 1992.

Bayley N: *Bayley Scales of Infant Development*. New York, Psychological Corp., 1969.

Becker JMT: A learning analysis of the development of peer-oriented behavior in 9-month-old infants. *Dev Psychol* 13:481–491, 1977.

Bell RQ: A reinterpretation of the direction of effects in studies of socialization. *Psychol Rev* 75:81–95, 1968.

Bell RQ: Stimulus control of parent or caretaker behavior by offspring. *Dev Psychol* 4:63–72, 1971.

Bell SMV, Ainsworth MDS: Infant crying and maternal responsiveness. *Child Dev* 43:1171–1190, 1972.

Belsky J, Cassidy J: Attachment: Theory and evidence. In: Rutter M, Hay DF, Baron-Cohen S (eds): *Developmental Principles and Clinical Issues in Psychology and Psychiatry*. Oxford, United Kingdom, Blackwell, 1994.

Belsky J, Nezworski T (eds): *Clinical Implications of Attachment*. Hillsdale, NJ, Erlbaum, 1988.

Belsky J, Goode MK, Most RK: Maternal stimulation and infant exploratory competence: Cross-sectional, correlational, and experimental analyses. *Child Dev* 51:1163–1178, 1980.

Belsky J, Rovine M, Taylor D: The Pennsylvania Infant and Family Development Project. III: The origins of individual differences in infant mother attachment: Maternal and infant contributions. *Child Dev* 55:718–728, 1984.

Benedict H: Early lexical development: Comprehension and production. *J Child Lang* 6:183–200, 1979.

Benson JB, Uzgiris IC: Effect of self-initiated locomotion on infant search activity. *Dev Psychol* 21:923–931, 1985.

Berg K, Smith M: Behavioral thresholds for tones during infancy. *J Exp Child Psychol* 35:409–415, 1983.

Berkeley G: *An Essay toward a New Theory of Vision.* Oxford: Claredon Press, 1901. (Originally published 1709.)

Berry KK: Developmental study of recognition of antecedents of infant vocalization. *Percept Mot Skills* 41:400–402, 1975.

Bertenthal B, Campos J, Haith M: Development of visual organization: Perception of subjective contours. *Child Dev* 51:1072–1080, 1980.

Blass EM, Ganchrow JR, Steiner JE: Classical conditioning in newborn humans 2–48 hours of age. *Infant Behav Dev* 7:223–235, 1984.

Blehar MC, Lieberman AF, Ainsworth MDS: Early face-to-face interaction and its relation to later infant-mother attachment. *Child Dev* 48:182–194, 1977.

Block JH, Block J: The role of ego-control and ego-resiliency in the organization of behavior. In: Collins WA (ed): *Minnesota Symposia on Child Psychology* (Vol 13). Hillsdale, NJ, Erlbaum, 1980.

Bloom K: Evaluation of infant vocal conditioning. *J Exp Child Psychol* 27:60–70, 1979.

Bloom K, Esposito A: Social conditioning and its proper control procedures. *J Exp Child Psychol* 19:209–222, 1975.

Bond LA: From prevention to promotion: Optimizing infant development. In: Bond LA, Joffe JM (eds): *Facilitating Infant and Early Childhood Development.* Hanover, NH, University Press of New England, 1982.

Booth CL, Rose-Krasnor L, Rubin K: Relating preschoolers' social competence and their mothers' parenting behaviors to early attachment security and high-risk status. *J Soc Personal Relationships* 8: 363–382, 1991.

Bornstein MH: Qualities of color vision in infancy. *J Exp Child Psychol* 19:401–419, 1975.

Bornstein MH: Infants are trichromats. *J Exp Child Psychol* 21:425–445, 1976.

Bornstein MH: Effects of habituation experience on posthabituation behavior in young infants: Discrimination and generalization among colors. *Dev Psychol* 15:348–349, 1979.

Bornstein MH: Psychological studies of color perception in human infants: Habituation, discrimination and categorization, recognition, and conceptualization. In: Lipsitt LP (ed): *Advances in Infancy Research* (Vol 1). Norwood, NJ, Ablex, 1981a.

Bornstein MH: Two kinds of perceptual organization near the beginning of life. In: Collins WA (ed): *Minnesota Symposia on Child Psychology* (Vol 14). Hillsdale, NJ, Erlbaum, 1981b.

Bornstein MH: A descriptive taxonomy of psychological categories used by infants. In: Sophian C (ed): *Origins of Cognitive Skills.* Hillsdale, NJ, Erlbaum, 1984.

Bornstein MH: How infant and mother jointly contribute to developing cognitive competence in the child. *Proc Natl Acad Sci USA* 82:7470–7473, 1985.

Bornstein MH (ed): *Sensitive Periods in Development: Interdisciplinary Perspectives.* Hillsdale, NJ, Erlbaum, 1987.

Bornstein MH, Benasich AA: Infant habituation: Assessments of individual differences and short-term reliability at 5 months. *Child Dev* 57:87–99, 1986.

Bornstein MH, Krinsky SJ: Perception of symmetry in infancy: The salience of vertical symmetry and the perception of pattern wholes. *J Exp Child Psychol* 39:1–19, 1985.

Bornstein MH, Lamb ME: *Development in infancy* (3rd ed). New York, McGraw-Hill, 1993.

Bornstein MH, Sigman MD: Continuity in mental development from infancy. *Child Dev* 57: 251–274, 1986.

Bornstein MH, Tamis-LeMonda CS: Activities and interactions of mothers and their firstborn infants in the first six months of life: Covariation, stability, continuity, correspondence, and prediction. *Child Dev* 61:1206–1217, 1990.

Bornstein MH, Gaughran J, Homel P: Infant temperament: Tradition, critique, new assessments, and prolegomena to future studies. In: Izard CE, Read PB (eds): *Measurement of Emotions in Infants and Children* (Vol 2). New York, Cambridge University Press, 1986.

Bornstein MH, Gross CG, Wolf JZ: Perceptual similarity of mirror images in infancy. *Cognition* 6: 89–116, 1978.

Bornstein MH, Kessen W, Weiskopf S: Color vision and hue categorization in young human infants. *J Exp Psychol* 2:115–129, 1976.

Bowlby J: *A Secure Base.* New York, Basic Books, 1988.

Bower TGR: *A Primer of Infant Development.* San Francisco, Freeman, 1977.

Bower TGR, Broughton JM, Moore M: Infant response to approaching objects: An indication of response to distal variables. *Percept Psychophys* 9: 193–196, 1970.

Bowerman M: Semantic factors in the acquisition of rules for word use and sentence construction. In: Morehead DM, Morehead AE (eds): *Normal and Deficient Child Language.* Baltimore, University Park Press, 1976.

Bowlby J: *Maternal Care and Mental Health.* Geneva, World Health Organization, 1951.

Bowlby J: *Attachment and Loss.* Vol 1: *Attachment.* New York, Basic Books, 1969.

Brackbill Y, Fitzgerald HE, Lintz LM: A developmental study of classical conditioning. *Monogr Soc Res Child Dev* 32 (serial no. 16), 1967.

Bradley RH, Caldwell BM: Early home environment and changes in mental test performance in children 6 to 36 months. *Dev Psychol* 12:93–97, 1976.

Brazelton TB: Crying in infancy. *Pediatrics* 29: 579–588, 1962.

Brazelton TB: *Neonatal Behavioral Assessment Scale* (Clinics in Developmental Medicine, no. 50). Philadelphia, Lippincott, 1973.

Bretherton I: Making friends with one-year-olds: An experimental study of infant-stranger interaction. *Merrill-Palmer Q* 24:29–51, 1978.

Bretherton I, McNew S, Snyder L, et al: Individual differences at 20 months: Analytic and holistic strategies in language acquisition. *J Child Lang* 10: 293–320, 1983.

Bretherton I, Stolberg U, Kreye M: Engaging strangers in proximal interaction: Infants' social initiative. *Dev Psychol* 17:746–755, 1981.

Bridger WH: Sensory habituation and discrimination in the human neonate. *Am J Psychiatry* 117: 991–996, 1961.

Bridges KMB: A study of social development in early infancy. *Child Dev* 4:36–49, 1933.

Bronson G: Infants' reactions to unfamiliar persons and novel objects. *Monogr Soc Res Child Dev* 32 (serial no. 112), 1972.

Brown AM: Development of visual sensitivity to light and color vision in human infants: A critical review. *Vision Res* 30:1159–1188, 1990.

Bruner JS: The organization of early skilled action. *Child Dev* 44:1–11, 1977.

Bruner JS: *Child's Talk: Learning to Use Language.* New York, Norton, 1983.

Buhler C: The social behavior of children. In: Murchison CA (ed): *Handbook of Child Psychology.* New York, Russell & Russell, 1933, pp. 374–416.

Buss AH, Plomin R: *A Temperament Theory of Personality.* New York, Wiley, 1975.

Buss AH, Plomin R: *Temperament: Early Developing Personality Traits.* Hillsdale, NJ, Erlbaum, 1984.

Cairns GF, Butterfield EC: Assessing infants' auditory functioning. In: Friedlander BZG, Sterritt M, Kirk GE (eds): *Exceptional Infant.* Vol 3: *Assessment and Intervention.* New York, Brunner/Mazel, 1975, pp. 84–108.

Caldwell B: The effects of infant care. In: Hoffman M, Hoffman L (eds): *Review of Child Development Research* (Vol 1). New York, Russell Sage Foundation, 1964.

Campos JJ, Bertenthal B: Locomotion and psychological development. In: Morrison F, Lord K, Keating D (eds): *Applied Developmental Psychology* (Vol 3). New York: Academic Press, 1989.

Campos JJ, Stenberg C: Perception, appraisal, and emotions: The onset of social referencing. In: Lamb ME, Sherrod LR (eds): *Infant Social Cognition: Empirical and Theoretical Considerations.* Hillsdale, NJ, Erlbaum, 1981.

Campos JJ, Barrett KC, Lamb ME, et al: Socioemotional development. In: Haith MM, Campos JJ (eds): *Handbook of Child Psychobiology.* Vol 2: *Infancy and Developmental Psychobiology.* New York, Wiley, 1983.

Campos JJ, Bertenthal B, Benson N: Self-produced locomotion and the extraction of form invariance. Paper presented at the International Conference on Infant Studies, New Haven, CT, 1980.

Campos JJ, Langer A, Krowitz A: Cardiac responses on the visual cliff in prelocomotor human infants. *Science* 170:196–197, 1970.

Cantor DS, Fischel JE, Kaye N: Neonatal conditionability: A new paradigm for exploring the use of interceptive cues. *Infant Behav Dev* 6:403–413, 1983.

Caplan M, Vespo J, Pedersen J, et al: Conflict and its resolution in small groups of one- and two-year-olds. *Child Dev* 62:1513–1524, 1991.

Carew JV: Experience and the development of intelligence in young children in home and in day care. *Monogr Soc Res Child Dev* 45 (serial no. 187), 1980.

Carey WB: A simplified method for measuring infant temperament. *J Pediatr* 77:188–194, 1970.

Carey WB, McDevitt SC: Revision of the Infant Temperament Questionnaire. *Pediatrics* 62: 735–739, 1978a.

Carey WB, McDevitt SC: Stability and change in individual temperamental diagnoses from infancy to early childhood. *J Am Acad Child Psychiatry* 17: 331–337, 1978b.

Caron AJ, Caron RF: Processing of relational information as an index of infant risk. In: Friedman SL, Sigman M (eds): *Preterm Birth and Psychological Development.* New York, Academic Press, 1981.

Caron AJ, Caron RF, Glass P: Responsiveness to relational information as a measure of cognitive functioning in nonsuspect infants. In: Field T, Sostek A (eds): *Infants Born at Risk.* New York, Grune & Stratton, 1983.

Caron AJ, Caron RF, MacLean DJ: Infant discrimination of naturalistic emotional expressions: The role of face and voice. *Child Dev* 59:604–616, 1988.

Caron RF, Caron AJ, Myers RS: Abstraction of invariant face expressions in infancy. *Child Dev* 53: 1008–1015, 1982.

Carpenter GC: Visual regard of moving and stationary faces in early infancy. *Merrill-Palmer Q* 20: 181–194, 1974.

Chase W: Color vision in infants. *Psychology* 20: 203–222, 1937.

Chomsky N: *Aspects of the Theory of Syntax.* Cambridge, MA, MIT Press, 1965.

Chomsky N: *Knowledge of Language: Its Nature, Origin, and Use.* New York, Praeger, 1986.

Cicchetti D, Nesse P: Affect and intellect: Piaget's contributions to the study of infant emotional development. In: Plutchik R, Kellerman N (eds): *Emotions: Theory, Research and Experience* (Vol 2). New York, Academic Press, 1983.

Cicirelli VG: Effects of sibling structure and interaction on children's categorization style. *Dev Psychol* 9:132–139, 1973.

Cicirelli VG: Relationship of sibling structuring and interaction on younger sib's conceptual style. *J Gen Psychol* 125:36–49, 1974.

Clarke-Stewart KA: Interactions between mothers and their young children: Characteristics and consequences. *Monogr Soc Res Child Dev* 38 (serial no. 153), 1973.

Clarke-Stewart KA: Recasting the lone stranger. In: Glick J, Clarke-Stewart KA (eds): *The Development of Social Understanding.* New York, Gardner Press, 1978, pp. 109–176.

Clarke-Stewart KA: The father's contribution to children's cognitive and social development in early childhood. In: Pedersen FA (ed): *The Father-Infant Relationship: Observational Studies in a Family Setting.* New York, Praeger Special Publications, 1980.

Clarke-Stewart KA, Vanderstoep LP, Killian GA: Analysis and replication of mother-child relations at two years of age. *Child Dev* 50:779–793, 1979.

Clavadetscher JE, Brown AM, Ankrum C, et al: Spectral sensitivity and chromatic discriminations in 3- and 7-week-old human infants. *J Opt Soc Am* 5: 2093–2105, 1988.

Clifton RK: Heart rate conditioning in the newborn infant. *J Exp Child Psychol* 18:9–21, 1974.

Clifton RK, Nelson MN: Developmental study of habituation in infants: The importance of paradigm, response system, and state. In: Tighe TJ, Leaton RN (eds): *Habituation: Perspectives from Child Development, Animal Behavior, and Neuropsychology.* Hillsdale, NJ, Erlbaum, 1976.

Clifton RK, Muir DW, Ashmead DH, et al: Is visually guided reaching in infancy a myth? *Child Dev* 64:1099–1110, 1993.

Clifton RK, Siqueland ER, Lipsitt LP: Conditioned head turning in human newborns as a function of conditioned response requirements and states of wakefulness. *J Exp Child Psychol* 13:43–57, 1972.

Cohen LB: A two-process model of infant visual attachment. *Merrill-Palmer Q* 19:157–180, 1973.

Cohen LB: Examination of habituation as a measure of aberrant infant development. In: Friedman SL, Sigman M (eds): *Preterm Birth and Psychological Development.* New York, Academic Press, 1981.

Cohen LB, Strauss MS: Concept acquisition in the human infant. *Child Dev* 50:419–424, 1979.

Cohen SE, Beckwith L: Preterm infant interaction with the caregiver in the first year of life and competence at age two. *Child Dev* 50:767–776, 1979.

Cohn JE, Tronick EZ: Communicative rules and the sequential structure of infant behavior during normal and depressed interaction. In: Tronick E (ed): *The Development of Human Communication and the Joint Regulation of Behavior.* Baltimore, University Park Press, 1983.

Connell DB: *Individual Differences in Attachment: An Investigation into Stability, Implications, and Relationships to Structure of Early Language Development.* Unpublished doctoral dissertation, Syracuse University, Syracuse, NY, 1976.

Cornell EH: Infants' visual attention to pattern arrangement and orientation. *Child Dev* 46:229–232, 1975.

Corrigan R: Cognitive correlates of language: Differential criteria yield differential results. *Child Dev* 50:617–631, 1979.

Crystal D: Prosaic development. In: Fletcher P, Garman M (eds): *Language Acquisition.* Cambridge, United Kingdom, Cambridge University Press, 1979.

Darwin C: *The Expression of the Emotions in Man and Animals.* London, Murray, 1872.

Davis HA: A description of aspects of mother-infant vocal interaction. *J Child Psychol Psychiatry* 19:379–386, 1978.

de Boysson-Bardies B, Sagant L, Durand C: Discernible differences in the babbling of infants according to target language. *J Child Lang* 11:1–15, 1984.

DeCasper AJ, Fifer WP: Of human bonding: Newborns prefer their mothers' voices. *Science* 208: 1174–1176, 1980.

DeLoache JS: Rate of habituation and visual memory in infants. *Child Dev* 47:145–154, 1976.

DeVries MW: Temperament and infant mortality among the Masai of East Africa. *Am J Psychiatry* 141:1189–1194, 1984.

Descartes R: La dioptrique. In: Coursin V (ed): *Oeuvres de Descartes* (Boring MD, trans). Paris, 1824. (Originally published 1638.)

Deutsch M, Brown B: Social influences in Negro-white intelligence differences. *J Soc Influence* 20:24–35, 1964.

Dixon S, Tronick E, Keefer C, et al: Mother-infant interaction among the Gusii of Kenya. In: Field TM, Sostek AM, Vietze P, et al (eds): *Culture and Early Interaction.* Hillsdale, NJ, Erlbaum, 1981.

Dollard J, Miller N: *Personality and Psychotherapy.* New York, McGraw-Hill, 1950.

Dontas C, Maratos O, Fafoutis M, et al: Early social development in institutionally reared Greek infants: Attachment and peer interaction. *Monogr Soc Res Child Dev* 50 (serial no. 209), 1985.

Dunham P, Dunham F: Lexical development during middle infancy: A mutually driven infant-caregiver process. *Dev Psychol* 28:414–420, 1992.

Dunn J: *The Beginnings of Social Understanding.* Cambridge, MA, Harvard University Press, 1988.

Dunn J: *Young Children's Close Relationships.* Newbury Park, CA, Sage Publications, 1993.

Dunn J, Kendrick C: The arrival of a sibling: Changes in patterns of interaction between mother and first-born child. *J Child Psychol Psychiatry* 21: 119–132, 1980.

Dunn J, Kendrick C: Interaction between young siblings: Associations with the interactions between mothers and first-born. *Dev Psychol* 17:336–343, 1981a.

Dunn J, Kendrick C: Social behavior of young siblings in the family context: Differences between same-sex and different-sex dyads. *Child Dev* 52: 1265–1273, 1981b.

Dunn J, Kendrick C: *Siblings: Love, Envy, and Understanding.* Cambridge, MA, Harvard University Press, 1982a.

Dunn J, Kendrick C: Siblings and their mothers: Developing relationships in the family. In: Lamb ME, Sutton-Smith B (eds): *Sibling Relationships: Their Nature and Significance across the Life Span.* Hillsdale, NJ, Erlbaum, 1982b.

Easterbrooks MA, Goldberg WA: Security of toddler-parent attachments: Relation to children's socio-personality functioning during kindergarten. In: Greenberg M, Cicchetti D, Cummings M (eds): *Attachment in the Preschool Years: Theory, Research, and Intervention.* Chicago, University of Chicago Press, 1990.

Easterbrooks MA, Lamb ME: The relationship between quality of infant-mother attachment and infant competence in initial encounters with peers. *Child Dev* 50:380–387, 1979.

Eckerman CO, Whatley JL: Toys and social interaction between infant peers. *Child Dev* 48: 1645–1656, 1977.

Eckerman CO, Whatley JL, Kutz SL: Growth of social play with peers during the second year of life. *Dev Psychol* 11:42–49, 1975.

Egeland B, Farber EA: Infant-mother attachment: Factors related to its development and changes over time. *Child Dev* 55:753–771, 1984.

Eibl-Eibesfeldt I: *Ethology.* New York, Holt, Rinehart & Winston, 1970.

Eilers RE, Oller DK: Precursors to speech: What is innate and what is acquired? *Ann Child Dev* 5: 1–32, 1988.

Eimas PD: Speech perception in early infancy. In: Cohen LB, Salapatek P (eds): *Infant Perception: From Sensation to Cognition* (Vol 2). New York, Academic Press, 1975.

Eimas PD, Siqueland ER, Jusczyk P, et al: Speech perception in infants. *Science* 171:303–306, 1971.

Eisenberg RB: *Auditory Competence in Early Life: The Roots of Communicative Behavior.* Baltimore, University Park Press, 1976.

Ekman P: Universal and cultural differences in facial expressions of emotion. In: Cole JK (ed): *Nebraska Symposium on Motivation 1971* (Vol 19). Lincoln, NE, University of Nebraska Press, 1972.

Ekman P, Friesen WV: Measuring facial movement. *Environ Psychol Nonverbal Behav* 1:56–75, 1976.

Ekman P, Friesen WV: *Facial Action Coding System.* Palo Alto, CA, Consulting Psychologists Press, 1978.

Ekman P, Oster H: Facial expressions of emotion. In: Rosenzweig MR, Porter LW (eds): *Annual Review of Psychology.* Palo Alto, CA, Annual Reviews, 1979.

Ekman P, Levenson RW, Friesen WV: Autonomic nervous system activity distinguishes among emotions. *Science* 221:1208–1210, 1983.

Elardo R, Bradley R, Caldwell BM: The relation of infants' home environments to mental test performance from six to thirty-six months: A longitudinal analysis. *Child Dev* 46:71–76, 1975.

Elicker J, Englund M, Sroufe LA: Predicting peer competence and peer relationships in childhood from early parent-child relationships. In: Parke RD, Ladd GW (eds): *Family-Peer Relationships: Modes of Linkage.* Hillsdale, NJ, Erlbaum, 1992.

Emde RN, Harmon R: Endogenous and exogenous smiling systems in early infancy. *J Am Acad Child Psychiatry* 11:177–200, 1972.

Emde RN, Koenig KL: Neonatal smiling and rapid eye-movement states. *J Am Acad Child Psychiatry* 8:57–67, 1969.

Emde RN, Gaensbauer TG, Harmon RJ: Emotional expression in infancy: A biobehavioral study. *Psychol Issues Monogr Ser* 10 (no. 1), 1976.

Emde RN, Izard C, Huebner R, et al: Adult judgments of infant emotions: Replication studies within and across laboratories. *Infant Behav Dev* 8:79–88, 1985.

Emde RN, Kligman D, Reich J, et al: Emotional expression in infancy. I: Initial studies of social signaling and an emergent model. In: Lewis M, Rosenblum LA (eds): *The Development of Affect.* New York, Plenum, 1978.

Emde RN, Plomin R, Robinson J, et al: Temperament, emotion, and cognition at 14 months: The MacArthur Longitudinal Twin Study. *Child Dev* 63: 1437–1455, 1992.

Engen T, Lipsitt LP: Decrement and recovery of responses to olfactory stimuli in the human neonate. *J Comp Physiol Psychol* 59:312–316, 1965.

Erickson MF, Sroufe LA, Egeland B: The relationship between quality of attachment and behavior problems in preschool in a high risk sample. *Monogr Soc Res Child Dev* 50 (serial no. 209), 1985.

Erikson E: *Childhood and Society*. New York, Norton, 1963.

Eysenck HJ, Kamin L: *Intelligence: The Battle for the Mind*. London, Pan Books, 1981.

Fagan JF, McGrath SK: Infant recognition memory and later intelligence. *Intelligence* 5:121–130, 1981.

Fagan JF, Singer LT: Infant recognition memory as a measure of intelligence. In: Lipsitt LP (ed): *Advances in Infancy Research* (Vol 2). Norwood, NJ, Ablex, 1983.

Fagot BI, Kavanaugh K: The prediction of antisocial behavior from avoidant attachment classifications. *Child Dev* 61:864–873, 1990.

Fantz RL, Ordy JM, Udelf MS: Maturation of pattern vision in infants during the first six months. *J Comp Physiol Psychol* 55:907–917, 1962.

Feinman S (ed): *Social Referencing and the Social Construction of Reality in Infancy*. New York, Plenum, 1992.

Feinman S, Roberts D, Morissette L: The effect of social referencing on 12-month-olds' responses to a stranger's attempts to "make friends." Paper presented at the Fifth International Conference on Infant Studies, Los Angeles, 1986.

Fenson L, Sapper V, Milner DG: Attention and manipulative play in the 1-year-old child. *Child Dev* 45:757–764, 1974.

Fernald A: The perceptual and affective salience of mothers' speech to infants. In: Feagans LC, Garvey R, Golinkoff MT, et al (eds): *The Origins and Growth of Communication*. Norwood, NJ, Ablex, 1984.

Field T: Differential behavioral and cardiac responses of 3-month-old infants to a mirror and a peer. *Infant Behav Dev* 2:179–184, 1979.

Field TM: Individual differences in the expressivity of neonates and young infants. In: Feldman R (ed): *Development of Nonverbal Behavior in Children*. New York, Springer-Verlag, 1982.

Field TM, Woodson R, Greenberg R, et al: Discrimination and imitation of facial expressions by neonates. *Science* 218:179–181, 1982.

Fish M, Crockenberg S: Correlates and antecedents of nine-month infant behavior and mother-infant interaction. *Infant Behav Dev* 4:69–81, 1981.

Fisher CB, Ferdinandsen K, Bornstein MN: The role of symmetry in infant form perception. *Child Dev* 52:457–462, 1981.

Fitzgerald HE, Brackbill Y: Classical conditioning in infancy: Development and constraints. *Psychol Bull* 83:353–376, 1976.

Fleener DE: Experimental production of infant-maternal attachment behaviors. Paper presented to the American Psychological Association, Montreal, Canada, 1973.

Fogel A: Peer- vs. mother directed behavior in 1- to 3-month-old infants. *Infant Behav Dev* 2:215–226, 1979.

Fox N: Attachment of kibbutz infants to mother and metapelet. *Child Dev* 48:1228–1239, 1977.

Fox NA, Stifter CA: Biological and behavioral differences in infant reactivity. In: Kohnstamm CA, Bates J, Rothbart MK (eds): *Handbook of Temperament in Childhood*. New York, Wiley, 1989.

Fraiberg S: Blind infants and their mothers: An examination of the sign system. In: Bullowa M (ed): *Before Speech*. Cambridge, Cambridge University Press, 1979, pp. 149–169.

Frankel KA, Bates JE: Mother-toddler problem solving: Antecedents in attachment, home behavior, and temperament. *Child Dev* 61:810–819, 1990.

Freedman D: *Human Infancy: An Evolutionary Perspective*. Hillsdale, NJ, Erlbaum, 1974.

Freud A: *Normality and Pathology in Childhood*. New York, International Universities Press, 1965.

Freud S: An outline of psychoanalysis. In: Strachey J (ed): *The Standard Edition of the Complete Psychological Works of Sigmund Freud* (Vol 23). London, Hogarth Press, 1968. (Originally published 1940.)

Friedman S: Infant habituation: Process, problems and possibilities. In: Ellis N (ed): *Aberrant Development in Infancy: Human and Animal Studies*. New York, Halstead Press, 1975.

Frodi AM, Lamb ME, Leavitt LA, et al: Fathers' and mothers' responses to the faces and cries of normal and premature infants. *Dev Psychol* 14:490–498, 1978a.

Frodi AM, Lamb ME, Leavitt LA, et al: Fathers' and mothers' responses to infant smiles and cries. *Infant Behav Dev* 1:187–198, 1978b.

Garcia J, Koelling R: Relation of cue to consequence in avoidance learning. *Psychon Sci* 4:123–124, 1966.

Gardner RA, Gardner BT: Teaching sign language to a chimpanzee. *Science* 165:664–672, 1969.

Gesell A, Ames LB: Early evidences of individuality. *Hum Infant Sci Monthly* 45:217–225, 1937.

Gesell A, Armatruda CS: *Developmental Diagnosis: Normal and Abnormal Child Development, Clinical Methods, and Practical Applications* (3rd ed). New York, Harper & Row, 1962.

Gibbs ED, Teti DM, Bond LA: Infant-sibling communication as a function of age-spacing. Paper presented to the Society for Research in Child Development, Toronto, Canada, 1985.

Gibson EJ, Walk RD: The "visual cliff." *Sci Am* 202:64–71, 1960.

Goldberg S: Social competence in infancy: A model of parent-infant interaction. *Merrill-Palmer Q* 23:163–177, 1977.

Gilbert JHV: Babbling and deaf children: A commentary on Lenneberg et al. (1965) and Lenneberg (1967). *J Child Lang* 9:511–515, 1982.

Goldman BD, Ross HS: Social skills in action: An analysis of early peer games. In: Glick J, Clarke-Stewart KA (eds): *The Development of Social Understanding*. New York, Gardner Press, 1978, pp. 177–212.

Goldsmith HH, Campos JJ: Toward a theory of infant temperament. In: Emde RN, Harmon RJ (eds): *The Development of Attachment and Affiliative Systems*. New York, Plenum, 1982.

Goldsmith HH, Campos JJ: Fundamental issues in the study of early temperament: The Denver twin temperament study. In: Lamb ME, Brown A, Rogoff B (eds): *Advances in Developmental Psychology* (Vol 4). Hillsdale, NJ, Erlbaum, 1986.

Goldsmith HH, Buss AH, Plomin R, et al: Roundtable: What is temperament? Four approaches. *Child Dev* 58:505–529, 1987.

Goossens FA, van IJzendoorn MH: Quality of infants' attachments to professional caregivers: Relation to infant-parent attachment and daycare characteristics. *Child Dev* 61:832–837, 1990.

Gottlieb G: The psychobiological approach to developmental issues. In: Haith MM, Campos JJ (eds): *Handbook of Child Psychology*. Vol 2: *Infancy and Developmental Psychobiology*. New York, Wiley, 1983.

Graham FK, Leavitt LA, Strock BD, et al: Precocious cardiac orienting in a human anencephalic infant. *Science* 199:322–324, 1978.

Green JA, Gustafson GE, West MJ: Effects of infant development on mother-infant interactions. *Child Dev* 51:199–207, 1980.

Greenberg DJ, O'Donnell WJ, Crawford D: Complexity levels, habituation, and individual differences in early infancy. *Child Dev* 44:569–574, 1973.

Grossmann K, Grossmann KE: Newborn behavior, early parenting quality and later toddler-parent relationships in a group of German infants. In: Nugent JK, Lester BM, Brazelton TB (eds): *The Cultural Context of Infancy* (Vol 2). Norwood, NJ, Ablex, 1986.

Grossmann K, Grossmann KE, Spangler G, et al: Maternal sensitivity and newborns' orientation responses as related to quality of attachment in northern Germany. *Monogr Soc Res Child Dev* 50 (serial no. 209), 1985.

Gwiazda J, Bauer J, Held R: Binocular function in human infants: Correlation of stereotropic and fusion-rivalry discriminations. *J Pediatr Ophthalmol Strabismus* 26:128–132, 1989.

Hagekull B, Lindhagen K, Bohlin G: Behavioral dimensions in one-year-olds and dimensional stability in infancy. *Int J Behav Dev* 3:351–364, 1980.

Hainline L: Developmental changes in visual scanning of face and nonface patterns by infants. *J Exp Child Psychol* 25:90–115, 1978.

Hainline L, Lemerise E: Infants' scanning of geometric forms varying in size. *J Exp Child Psychol* 33:235–256, 1982.

Haith MM: The response of the human newborn to visual movement. *J Exp Child Psychol* 3:235–243, 1966.

Haith MM: Visual competence in early infancy. In: Held R, Leibowitz H, Teuber H-L (eds): *Handbook of Sensory Physiology* (Vol 8). Berlin, Springer-Verlag, 1979.

Haith MM: *Rules That Babies Look By*. Hillsdale, NJ, Erlbaum, 1980.

Haith MM: Gratuity, perception-action integration and future orientation in infant vision. In: Kessel F, Sameroff A, Bornstein M (eds): *Contemporary Construction of the Child: Essays in Honor of William Kessen*. Hillsdale, NJ, Erlbaum, 1991.

Haith MM, Campos JJ: Human infancy. *Annu Rev Psychol* 28:251–294, 1977.

Haith MM, Bergman T, Moore M: Eye contact and face scanning in early infancy. *Science* 198:853–855, 1977.

Hall JA: Gender effects in decoding nonverbal cues. *Psychol Bull* 85:845–857, 1978.

Hamer RD, Alexander K, Teller DY: Rayleigh discriminations in young human infants. *Vision Res* 20:575–584, 1982.

Hardy-Brown K, Plomin R, DeFries JC: Genetic and environmental influences on rate of communicative development in the first year of life. *Dev Psychol* 17:704–717, 1981.

Hay DF: Following their companions as a form of exploration for human infants. *Child Dev* 48:1624–1632, 1977.

Hay DF: Cooperative interactions and sharing between very young children and their parents. *Dev Psychol* 15:647–653, 1979.

Hay DF, Murray P: Giving and requesting: Social facilitation of infants' offers to adults. *Infant Behav Dev* 5:301–310, 1982.

Hay DF, Rheingold HL: The early appearance of some valued social behaviors. In: Bridgemen DL (ed): *The Nature of Prosocial Development: Interdisciplinary Theories and Strategies*. New York, Academic Press, 1983.

Hay DF, Ross HS: The social nature of early conflict. *Child Dev* 53:105–113, 1982.

Hay DF, Caplan M, Castle J, et al: Does sharing become increasingly "rational" in the second year of life? *Dev Psychol* 27:987–999, 1991.

Hay DF, Murray P, Cecire S, et al: Social learning of social behavior in early life. *Child Dev* 56:43–57, 1985.

Hay DF, Nash A, Pedersen J: Responses of six-month-olds to the distress of their peers. *Child Dev* 52:1071–1075, 1981.

Hay DF, Nash A, Pedersen J: Interaction between six-month-old peers. *Child Dev* 54:557–562, 1983.

Held R: Perception and its neuronal mechanisms. *Cognition* 33:139–154, 1989.

Hertzig ME, Birch HG, Thomas A, et al: Class and ethnic differences in the responsiveness of preschool children to cognitive demands. *Monogr Soc Res Child Dev* 33 (serial no. 117), 1968.

Hess E: Ethology and developmental psychology. In: Mussen P (ed): *Carmichael's Manual of Child Psychology*. New York, Wiley, 1970, pp. 1–38.

Hinde RA: *Animal Behavior: A Synthesis of Ethology and Comparative Psychology*. New York, McGraw-Hill, 1970.

Hoffman ML: The arousal and development of empathy. In: Lewis M, Rosenblum LA (ed): *The Development of Affect*. New York, Plenum, 1978.

Hollien H: Developmental aspects of neonatal vocalizations. In: Murry T, Murry J (eds): *Infant Communication: Cry to Early Speech*. Houston, College Hill Press, 1980.

Hornik R, Gunnar M: A descriptive analysis of infant social referencing. *Child Dev* 59:626–634, 1988.

Hornik R, Risenhoover N, Gunnar M: The effects of maternal positive, neutral, and negative affective communications on infant responses to new toys. *Child Dev* 58:937–944, 1987.

Howe N, Ross HS: Socialization, perspective-taking, and the sibling relationship. *Dev Psychol* 26:160–165, 1990.

Howes C: Peer interaction of young children. *Monogr Soc Res Child Dev* 53(1), 1988.

Howes C: Can the age of entry into child care and the quality of child care predict adjustment in kindergarten? *Dev Psychol* 26:292–303, 1990.

Howes C, Rodning C, Galluzzo DC, et al: Attachment and child care: Relationships with mother and caregiver. *Early Childhood Res Q* 3:403–416, 1988.

Hubert NC, Wachs TD, Peters-Martin P, et al: The study of early temperament: Measurement and conceptual ideas. *Child Dev* 53:571–600, 1982.

Hunt JMcV: *The Challenge of Incompetence and Poverty: Parents and the Role of Early Education*. Urbana, IL, University of Illinois Press, 1969.

Ipsa J: Peer support among Soviet day care toddlers. *Int J Behav Dev* 4:255–269, 1981.

Izard CE: *The Face of Emotion*. New York, Appleton-Century-Crofts, 1971.

Izard CE: Emotions as motivations. In: Howe HE Jr (ed): *Nebraska Symposium on Motivation*. Lincoln, NE, University on Nebraska Press, 1979, pp. 163–200.

Izard CE, Dougherty LM: Two systems for measuring facial expressions. In: Izard CE (ed): *Measuring Emotions in Infants and Children*. New York, Cambridge University Press, 1982.

Izard CE, Malatesta CZ: Perspectives on emotional development. I: Differential emotions theory of early emotional development. In: Osofsky JD (ed): *Handbook of Infant Development* (2nd ed). New York, Wiley, 1987.

Izard CE, Hembree E, Dougherty L, et al: Changes in facial expressions of two- to nineteen-month-old infants' facial expressions following acute pain. *Dev Psychol* 19:418–426, 1983.

Izard CE, Huebner R, Risser D, et al: The young infant's ability to produce discrete expressions. *Dev Psychol* 16:132–140, 1980.

Jacobson JL: The role of inanimate objects in early peer interaction. *Child Dev* 52:618–626, 1981.

Jacobson JL, Wille DE: The influence of attachment pattern on peer interaction at 2 and 3 years. Paper presented to the International Conference on Infant Studies, New York, 1984.

Jacobson JL, Tianen RL, Wille DE, et al: Episode-based rating scales: Assessing the influence of parental attachment on early peer relations. In: Mueller E, Cooper C (eds): *Process and Outcome in Peer Relationships*. New York, Academic Press, 1986.

Jacobson JL, Wille DE, Tianen RL, et al: The influence of infant-mother attachment on toddler sociability with peers. Paper presented to the Society for Research in Child Development, Detroit, 1983.

Jakobson R: *Child Language, Aphasia and Phonological Universals*. New York, Humanities Press, 1968. (Originally published 1941.)

Jakobson R: Why "Mama" and "Papa"? In: Bar-Adon A, Leopold WF (eds): *Child Language*. Englewood Cliffs, NJ, Prentice-Hall, 1971.

Jeffrey WE: Habituation as a mechanism of perceptual development. In: Tighe TJ, Leaton RN (eds): *Habituation: Perspectives from Child Development, Animal Behavior, and Neurophysiology*. Hillsdale, NJ, Erlbaum, 1976.

Kagan J: *Change and Continuity in Infancy*. New York, Wiley, 1971.

Kagan J: Perspectives on continuity. In: Brim OF Jr, Kagan J (eds): *Continuity and Change in Human Development*. Cambridge, MA, Harvard University Press, 1980.

Kagan J, Klein R: Cross-cultural perspectives on early development. *Am Psychol* 28:947–961, 1973.

Kagan J, Tulkin SR: Social class differences in child rearing during the first year. In: Schaeffer HR (ed): *The Origins of Human Social Relations*. New York, Academic Press, 1971, pp. 165–183.

Kagan J, Kearsley P, Zelazo P: *Infancy: Its Place in Human Development*. Cambridge, MA, Harvard University Press, 1978.

Kagan J, Reznick JS, Snidman N: The physiology and psychology of behavioral inhibition in children. *Child Dev* 58:1459–1473, 1987.

Kaufmann R, Kaufmann F: The face schema in 3- and 4-month-old infants: The role of dynamic properties of the face. *Infant Behav Dev* 3:331–339, 1980.

Kaye H: The conditioned Babkin reflex in human newborns. *Psychon Sci* 2:287–288, 1965.

Kellman PJ: Perception of three-dimensional form by human infants. *Percept Psychophys* 36:353–358, 1984.

Kellman PJ, Spelke ES: Perception of partly occluded objects in infancy. *Cogn Psychol* 15:483–524, 1983.

Kennedy WA, Van der Riet, White JC: A normative sample of intelligence and achievement of Negro elementary school children in the southeastern United States. *Monogr Soc Res Child Dev* 28 (serial no. 90), 1963.

Kent RD: Articulatory and acoustic perspectives on speech development. In: Stark RE (ed): *Language Behavior in Infancy and Early Childhood*. New York, Elsevier, 1981, pp. 105–126.

Kessen W: Sucking and looking: Two organized congenital patterns of behavior in the human newborn. In: Stevenson HW, Hess EH, Rheingold HL (eds): *Early Behavior: Comparative and Developmental Approaches*. New York, Wiley, 1967.

Kessen W, Bornstein MH: Discriminability of brightness change for infants. *J Exp Child Psychol* 25:526–530, 1978.

Kessen W, Haith MM, Salapatek PH: Human infancy: A bibliography and guide. In: Mussen P (ed): *Carmichael's Manual of Child Psychology*. New York, Wiley, 1970.

Kimble GA: *Hilgard and Marguis' Conditioning and Learning*. New York, Appleton-Century-Crofts, 1961.

Klaus RA, Gray SW: The early training project for disadvantaged children: A report after five years. *Monogr Soc Res Child Dev* 33 (serial no. 120), 1968.

Klein PS: Behavior of Israeli mothers toward infants in relation to infants' perceived temperament. *Child Dev* 55:1212–1218, 1984.

Klinnert M, Campos JJ, Sorce J, et al: Emotions as behavior regulators: Social referencing in infancy. In: Plutchik R, Kellerman H (eds): *Emotions in Early Development*. Vol 2: *The Emotions*. New York, Academic Press, 1983.

Klinnert MD, Emde RN, Butterfield P, et al: Social referencing: The infant's use of emotional signals from a friendly adult with mother present. *Dev Psychol* 22:427–432, 1986.

Kohn ML: Social class and parent-child relationships: An interpretation. *Am J Sociol* 68:471–480, 1963.

Kopp CB, McCall RB: Stability and instability in mental test performance among normal, at-risk, and handicapped infants and children. In: Baltes PB, Brim OG Jr (eds): *Life-Span Development and Behavior* (Vol 4). New York, Academic Press, 1980.

Korner AF: Neonatal startles, smiles, erections, and reflex sucks as related to state, sex, and individuality. *Child Dev* 40:1039–1053, 1969.

Korner AF, Thoman EB: Visual alertness in neonates as evoked by maternal care. *J Exp Child Psychol* 10:67–78, 1970.

Korner AF, Thoman EB: The relative efficacy of contact and vestibular-proprioceptive stimulation in soothing neonates. *Child Dev* 43:443–453, 1972.

Kuchuk A, Vibbert M, Bornstein MH: The perception of smiling and its experiential correlates in three-month-old infants. *Child Dev* 57:1054–1061, 1986.

Kuhl PK, Williams KA, Lacerda F, et al: Linguistic experience alters phonetic perception in infants by 6 months of age. *Science* 255:606–608, 1992.

LaBarbera JD, Izard CE, Vietze P, et al: Four- and six-month-old infants' visual responses to joy, anger, and neutral expressions. *Child Dev* 47:535–538, 1976.

Lamb ME: Effects of stress and cohort on mother- and father-infant interaction. *Dev Psychol* 12:435–443, 1976a.

Lamb ME: Interactions between eight-month-old children and their fathers and mothers. In: Lamb ME (ed): *The Role of the Father in Child Development*. New York, Wiley, 1976b.

Lamb ME: Twelve-month-olds and their parents: Interaction in a laboratory playroom. *Dev Psychol* 12:237–244, 1976c.

Lamb ME: Father-infant and mother-infant interaction in the first year of life. *Child Dev* 48:167–181, 1977.

Lamb ME: The development of sibling relationships in infancy: A short-term longitudinal study. *Child Dev* 49:1189–1196, 1978a.

Lamb ME: Interactions between 18-month-olds and their preschool-aged siblings. *Child Dev* 49:51–59, 1978b.

Lamb ME: Developing trust and perceived effectance in infancy. In: Lipsitt LP (ed): *Advances in Infancy Research* (Vol 1). Norwood, NJ, Ablex, 1981a.

Lamb ME: The development of father-infant relationships. In: Lamb ME (ed): *The Role of the Father in Child Development* (rev ed). New York, Wiley, 1981b.

Lamb ME: The development of father-infant relationships. In: Lamb ME (ed): *The Role of the Father in Child Development* (3rd ed). New York, Wiley, in press.

Lamb ME, Bornstein M: *Development in Infancy* (2nd ed). New York, Random House, 1987.

Lamb ME, Malkin CM: The development of social expectations in distress-relief sequences: A longitudinal study. *Int J Behav Dev* 9:235–249, 1986.

Lamb ME, Nash A: Infant-mother attachment, sociability, and peer competence. In: Berndt TJ, Ladd GW (eds): *Peer Relationships in Child Development*. New York, Wiley, 1989.

Lamb ME, Thompson RA, Gardner W, et al: Security of infantile attachment as assessed in the

"Strange Situation": Its study and biological interpretation. *Behav Brain Sci* 7:127–171, 1984.

Lamb ME, Thompson RA, Gardner W, et al: *Infant-Mother Attachment: The Origins and Developmental Significance of Individual Differences in Strange Situation Behavior.* Hillsdale, NJ, Erlbaum, 1985.

Lasky RE, Syrdal-Lasky A, Klein RE: VOT discrimination by four to six and a half month old infants from Spanish environments. *J Exp Child Psychol* 20: 215–225, 1975.

Lee CL, Bates JE: Mother-child interaction at age two years and perceived difficult temperament. *Child Dev* 56:1314–1325, 1985.

Lenneberg EH: *The Biological Foundations of Language.* New York, Wiley, 1967.

Lenneberg EH: On explaining language. *Science* 164:635–643, 1969.

Leopold WF: *Speech Development of a Bilingual Child: A Linguist's Record* (Vol 3). Evanston, IL, Northwestern University Press, 1949.

Lester BM, Boukydis CFZ (eds): *Infant Crying: Theoretical and Research Perspectives.* New York, Plenum, 1985.

Lester BM, Boukydis CFZ: No language but a cry. In: Papousek H, Jurgens U, Papousek M (eds): *Nonverbal Vocal Communication: Comparative and Developmental Approaches.* Cambridge, England, Cambridge University Press, 1991.

Leung E, Rheingold H: Development of pointing as a social gesture. *Dev Psychol* 17:215–220, 1981.

Lewis M (ed): *Origins of Intelligence: Infancy and Early Childhood* (2nd ed). New York, Plenum, 1983.

Lewis M, Baldini N: Attentional processes and individual differences. In: Hale GA, Lewis M (eds): *Attention and Cognitive Development.* New York, Plenum, 1979.

Lewis M, Brooks-Gunn J: Visual attention at three months as a predictor of cognitive functioning at two years of age. *Intelligence* 5:131–140, 1981.

Lewis M, Goldberg S: Perceptual-cognitive development in infancy: A generalized expectancy model as a function of mother-infant interaction. *Merrill-Palmer Q* 15:81–100, 1969.

Lewis M, Michalson L: Faces as signs and symbols. In: Zivin G (ed): *The Development of Expressive Behavior: Biology-Environment Interactions.* Orlando, Academic Press, 1985, pp. 153–180.

Lewis M, Feiring G, Mcguffog C, et al: Predicting psychopathology in six-year-olds from early social relations. *Child Dev* 55:123–136, 1984.

Lewis M, Goldberg S, Campbell H: A developmental study of learning within the first three years of life: Response decrement to a redundant signal. *Monogr Soc Res Child Dev* 34 (serial no. 133), 1969.

Lewis M, Ramsay DS, Kawakami K: Differences between Japanese infants and Caucasian infants in behavioral and cortisol response to inoculation. *Child Dev* 64:1722–1731, 1993.

Lewis M, Young G, Brooks J, et al: The beginning of friendship. In: Lewis M, Rosenblum L (eds): *Friendship and Peer Relations.* New York, Wiley, 1975.

Lieberman AF: Preschoolers' competence with a peer: Relations with attachment and peer experience. *Child Dev* 48:1277–1287, 1977.

Lipsitt LP, Kaye H: Conditioned sucking in the human newborn. *Psychon Sci* 1:29–30, 1964.

Lipsitt LP, Kaye H: Change in neonatal response to optimizing and nonoptimizing sucking stimulation. *Psychon Sci* 2:221–222, 1965.

Lounsbury ML, Bates JE: The cries of infants and different levels of perceived temperamental difficultness: Acoustic properties and effects on listeners. *Child Dev* 53:677–686, 1982.

Lynn DB, Cross AR: Parent preferences of preschool children. *J Marriage Fam* 36:555–559, 1974.

Lynn R: *Attention, Arousal and the Orientation Reaction.* Oxford, United Kingdom, Pergamon, 1966.

Lyons-Ruth K, Alpern L, Repacholi B: Disorganized infant attachment classification and maternal psychosocial problems as predictors of hostile-aggressive behavior in the preschool classroom. *Child Dev* 64:572–585, 1993.

Maccoby EE, Masters JC: Attachment and dependency. In: Mussen PH (ed): *Carmichael's Manual of Child Psychology* (Vol 2, 3rd ed). New York, Wiley, 1970.

Macfarlane A: Olfaction in the development of social preferences in the human neonate. In: *Parent-Infant Interaction.* Amsterdam, CIBA Foundation, 1975.

Main M: Exploration, play, and cognitive functioning related to infant-mother attachment. *Infant Behav Dev* 6:167–174, 1983.

Main M, Solomon J: Discovery of an insecure disorganized/disoriented attachment pattern. In: Brazelton TB (ed): *Affective Development in Infancy.* Norwood, NJ, Ablex, 1986, pp. 95–124.

Main M, Weston D: Security of attachment to mother and father: Related to conflict behavior and the readiness to establish new relationships. *Child Dev* 52:932–940, 1981.

Malatesta CZ: Developmental course of emotional expression in the human infant. In: Zivin G (ed): *The Development of Expressive Behavior: Biology-Environment Interactions.* Orlando, Academic Press, 1985, pp. 183–219.

Malatesta CZ, Haviland JM: Learning display rules: The socialization of emotion expression in infancy. *Child Dev* 53:991–1003, 1982.

Malatesta CZ, Haviland JM: Signals, symbols, and socialization: The modification of emotional expression in human development. In: Lewis M, Saarni C (ed): *The Socialization of Emotions.* New York, Plenum, 1985, pp. 89–116.

Malatesta CZ, Grigoryev P, Lamb C, et al: Emotion socialization and expressive development in preterm and fullterm infants. *Child Dev* 57:316–330, 1986.

Martin G, Clarke R: Distress crying in neonates: Species and peer specificity. *Dev Psychol* 18:3–10, 1982.

Marvin RS: An ethological-cognitive model for the attenuation of mother-child attachment behavior. In: Alloway TM, Krames L, Pliner P (eds): *Advances in the Study of Communication and Affect.* Vol 3: *The Development of Social Attachment.* New York, Plenum, 1977.

Mason WA: Experiential influences on the development of expressive behaviors in rhesus monkeys. In: Zivin G (ed): *The Development of Expressive Behavior: Biology-Environment Interactions.* Orlando, Academic Press, 1985, pp. 117–152.

Matas L, Arend R, Sroufe LA: Continuity of adaptation in the second year: The relationship between quality of attachment and later competence. *Child Dev* 49:547–556, 1978.

Matheny AP: Bayley's Infant Behavior Record: Behavioral components and twin analyses. *Child Dev* 51:1157–1167, 1980.

Matheny AP: A longitudinal twin study of stability of components from Bayley's Infant Behavior Record. *Child Dev* 84:356–360, 1983.

Matheny AP, Wilson RS: Stability and transformation of toddler temperament across settings and ages. Paper presented at the International Conference on Infant Studies, New York, 1984.

Maudry M, Nekula M: Social relations between children of the same age during the first two years of life. *J Gen Psychol* 54:193–215, 1939.

Maurer D: Infant visual perception: Methods of study. In: Cohen LB, Salapatek P (eds): *Infant Perception: From Sensation to Cognition.* Vol 1: *Basic Visual Processes.* New York, Academic Press, 1975.

Maurer D: The scanning of compound figures by young infants. *J Exp Child Psychol* 35:437–448, 1983.

Maurer D: Infant's perception of facedness. In: Field TM, Fox NA (eds): *Social Perception in Infants.* Norwood, NJ, Ablex, 1985.

Maurer D, Lewis T, Cavanaugh P, et al: A new test of luminous efficiency for babies. *Invest Ophthalmol Vis Sci* 30:297–303, 1989.

McCall RB: Attention in the infant: Avenue to the study of cognitive development. In: Walcher DN, Peters DL (eds): *Early Childhood: The Development of Self Regulatory Mechanisms.* New York, Academic Press, 1971.

McCall RB: Individual differences in the pattern of habituation at 5 and 10 months of age. *Dev Psychol* 15:559–569, 1979.

McCall RB, Eichorn DH, Hogarty PS: Transitions in early mental development. *Monogr Soc Res Child Dev* 42 (serial no. 171), 1977.

McKenzie B, Day RH: Orientation discrimination in infants: A comparison of visual fixation and operant training methods. *J Exp Child Psychol* 11: 366–375, 1971.

Meltzoff AN, Moore MK: Imitation of facial and manual gestures by human neonates. *Science* 198: 75–78, 1977.

Meltzoff AN, Moore MK: Newborn infants imitate adult facial gestures. *Child Dev* 54:702–709, 1983.

Messer SB, Kagan J, McCall RB: Fixation time and tempo of play in infants. *Dev Psychol* 3:406, 1970.

Minnett AM, Vandell DL, Sandrock JW: The effects of sibling status in sibling interaction: Influence of birth order, age spacing, sex of child, and sex of sibling. *Child Dev* 54:1064–1072, 1983.

Miranda SB, Fantz RL: Recognition memory in Down's syndrome and normal infants. *Child Dev* 45: 651–660, 1974.

Miyake K, Chen SJ, Campos JJ: Infant temperament, mother's mode of interaction, and attachment in Japan: An interim report. *Monogr Soc Res Child Dev* 50 (serial no. 209), 1985.

Moffett A: Stimulus complexity as a determinant of visual attention in infants. *J Exp Child Psychol* 8: 173–179, 1969.

Morrongiello BA: The study of individual differences in infants: Auditory processing measures. In: Colombo J, Fagan J (eds): *Individual Differences in Infancy: Reliability, Stability, Prediction.* Hillsdale, NJ, Erlbaum, 1990.

Mosier CE, Rogoff B: Infants' instrumental use of their mothers to achieve their goals. *Child Dev* 65:70–79, 1994.

Mossler DG, Marvin RS, Greenberg MT: Conceptual perspective taking in 2- to 6-year-old children. *Dev Psychol* 12:85–86, 1976.

Murphy CM, Messer DJ: Mothers, infants, and pointing: A study of a gesture. In: Schaffer HR (ed): *Studies in Mother-Infant Interaction.* London, Academic Press, 1977, pp. 325–354.

Murray A: Infant crying as an elicitor of parental behavior: An examination of two models. *Psychol Bull* 86:191–215, 1979.

Myers RJ, Jarvis PA, Creasey GL: Infants' behavior with their mothers and their grandmothers. *Infant Behav Dev* 10:245–259, 1987.

Nakazima S: Phonemicization and symbolization in language development. In: Lenneberg EH, Lenneberg E (eds): *Foundations of Language Development: A Multidisciplinary Approach* (Vol 1). New York, Academic Press, 1975.

Nash A: *Infants' Social Competence with Their Mothers and a Peer.* Doctoral dissertation, State University of New York at Stony Brook, 1985.

Nash A: A comparison of infants' social competence with mother and peer. Paper presented to the American Psychological Association, Washington, DC, 1986.

Nash A, Hay DF: Relationships in infancy as precursors and causes of later relationships and psychopathology. In: Hay DF, Angold A (eds): *Precursors and Causes in Development and Psychopathology*. Chichester, United Kingdom, Wiley, 1993.

Nelson CA: The recognition of facial expressions in the first two years of life: Mechanisms of development. *Child Dev* 58, 1987.

Nelson CA, Dolgin KG: The generalized discrimination of facial expressions by 7-month-olds. *Child Dev* 56:58–61, 1985.

Nelson CA, Horowitz FD: The perception of facial expressions and stimulus motion by two- and five-month-old infants using holographic stimuli. *Child Dev* 54:868–877, 1983.

Nelson K: Some evidence for the cognitive primacy of categorization and its functional basis. *Merrill-Palmer Q* 19:21–39, 1973.

Nelson K: Individual differences in language development: Implications for development and language. *Dev Psychol* 17:170–187, 1981.

Nicholich LM: Toward symbolic functioning: Structure of early pretend games and potential parallels with language. *Child Dev* 52:785–797, 1981.

Nugent JK, Hoffman J, Brazelton TB: An NBAS-based intervention with fullterm low-birth-weight infants. Paper presented at the International Conference on Infant Studies, Los Angeles, 1986.

Nurcombe B, Howell DC, Rauh VA, et al: An intervention program for mothers of low-birth-weight infants: Preliminary results. *J Am Acad Child Psychiatry* 23:319–325, 1984.

Oller DK: The emergence of the sounds of speech in infancy. In: Yeni-Komshian G, Ferguson CA, Kavanagh J (eds): *Child Phonology*. Vol 1: *Production*. New York, Academic Press, 1980.

Oller DK: Infant vocalizations: Exploration and reflexivity. In: Stark RE (ed): *Language Behavior in Infancy and Early Childhood*. New York, Elsevier, 1981, pp. 85–103.

Oller DK, Eilers RE: Similarity of babbling in Spanish- and English-learning babies. *J Child Lang* 9:565–577, 1982.

Oller DK, Eilers RE: The role of audition in infant babbling. *Child Dev* 59:441–449, 1988.

Olsho LW: Infant frequency discrimination. *Infant Behav Dev* 7:27–35, 1984.

Olsho LW, Schoon C, Sakai R, et al: Preliminary data on frequency discrimination. *J Acoust Soc Am* 71:509–511, 1982a.

Olsho LW, Schoon C, Sakai R, et al: Auditory frequency discrimination in infancy. *Dev Psychol* 18:721–726, 1982b.

Olson GM: An information processing analysis of visual memory and habituation in infants. In: Tighe TJ, Leaton RN (eds): *Habituation: Perspectives from Child Development, Animal Behavior, and Neurophysiology*. Hillsdale, NJ, Erlbaum, 1976.

Olson SL, Bates JE, Bayles K: Mother-infant interaction and the development of individual differences in children's cognitive competence. *Dev Psychol* 20:166–179, 1984.

Oppenheim D, Sagi A, Lamb ME: Infant-adult attachments on the kibbutz and their relation to socioemotional development 4 years later. *Dev Psychol* 24:427–433, 1988.

Packer O, Hartmann EE, Teller DY: Infant-color vision: The effect of test field size on Rayleigh discriminations. *Vision Res* 24:1247–1260, 1985.

Parmelee AH, Stern E: Development of states in infants. In: Clements C, Purpura D, Meyer F (eds): *Sleep and the Maturing Nervous System*. New York, Academic Press, 1972, pp. 199–228.

Pastor DL: The quality of mother-infant attachment and its relationship to toddlers' initial sociability with peers. *Dev Psychol* 17:326–335, 1981.

Pavlov I: *Conditioned Reflexes*. London, Oxford University Press, 1927.

Pêcheux MG, Lecuyer R: Habituation rate and free exploration tempo in 4-month-old infants. *Int J Behav Dev* 6:37–50, 1983.

Peeples DR, Teller DY: Color vision and brightness discrimination in two-month-old human infants. *Science* 189:1102–1103, 1975.

Pepler D: Naturalistic observations of teaching and modeling between siblings. Paper presented at the Biennial Meeting of the Society for Research in Child Development, Boston, April 1981.

Pepler D, Corter C, Abramovitch R: Social relations among children: Comparison of sibling and peer interaction. In: Rubin KH, Ross HS (eds): *Peer Relationships and Social Skills in Childhood*. New York, Springer-Verlag, 1982.

Petit GS, Bates JE: Continuity of individual differences in the mother-infant relationship from 6 to 13 months. *Child Dev* 55:729–739, 1984.

Petitto LA, Marentette PF: Babbling in the manual mode: Evidence for the ontogeny of language. *Science* 251:1493–1496, 1991.

Piaget J: *The Origins of Intelligence in the Child*. London, Routledge & Kegan Paul, 1953. (Originally published 1936.)

Piaget J: *The Construction of Reality in the Child*. New York, Basic Books, 1954. (Originally published 1937.)

Piaget J: *Play, Dreams and Imitation in Childhood*. New York, Norton, 1962. (Originally published 1946.)

Pipp S, Easterbrooks MA, Harmon RJ: The relation between attachment and knowledge of self and mother in one- to three-year-old infants. *Child Dev* 63:738–750, 1992.

Plomin R: Developmental behavioral genetics. *Child Dev* 54:253–259, 1983.

Plomin R, Rowe D: Genes, environment, and development of temperament in young human twins. In: Gurghardt GM, Bekoff M (eds): *The Development of Behavior: Comparative and Evolutionary Aspects*. New York, Garland Press, 1978.

Plomin R, Emde RN, Braungart JM, et al: Genetic change and continuity from fourteen to twenty months: The MacArthur Longitudinal Twin Study. *Child Dev* 64:1354–1376, 1993.

Plumb JH: *In the Light of History*. Harmondsworth, United Kingdom, Penguin, 1972.

Ramey CT, Collier AM, Sparling JJ, et al: The Carolina Abecedarian project: A longitudinal and multidisciplinary approach to the prevention of developmental retardation. In: Tjossem TD (ed): *Intervention Strategies for High Risk Infants and Young Children*. Baltimore, University Park Press, 1976.

Ramey CT, Farran DC, Campbell FA: Predicting IQ from mother-infant interactions. *Child Dev* 50:804–814, 1979.

Ramey CT, MacPhee D, Yeates KO: Preventing developmental retardation: A general systems model. In: Bond LA, Joffe JM (eds): *Facilitating Infant and Early Childhood Development*. Hanover, NH, University Press of New England, 1982.

Ratner N, Bruner JS: Games, social exchange, and the acquisition of language. *J Child Lang* 5:391–401, 1978.

Rauh V, Nurcombe B, Achenbach T: Three-year follow-up of an intervention for LBW infants. Paper presented at the International Conference on Infant Studies, Los Angeles, 1986.

Rebelsky F, Black R: Crying in infancy. *J Gen Psychol* 121:49–57, 1972.

Reich JN, Holmes DL, Slaymaker FL, et al: Infant assessments as predictors of 3-year IQ. Paper presented at the International Conference on Infant Studies, New York, 1984.

Rheingold HL: The effect of environmental stimulation upon social and exploratory behavior in the human infant. In: Foss BM (ed): *Determinants of Infant Behavior* (Vol 1). London, Methuen, 1961.

Rheingold HL: Little children's participation in the work of adults, a nascent prosocial behavior. *Child Dev* 53:114–125, 1982.

Rheingold HL, Eckerman CD: The infant separates himself from his mother. *Science* 168:78–83, 1970.

Rheingold HL, Eckerman CO: Fear of stranger: A critical examination. In: Reese HW (ed): *Advances in Child Development and Behavior* (Vol 8). New York, Academic Press, 1973, pp. 185–222.

Rheingold HL, Gewirtz J, Ross H: Social conditioning of vocalizations in the infant. *J Comp Physiol Psychol* 52:68–73, 1959.

Rheingold HL, Hay DF, West MJ: Sharing in the second year of life. *Child Dev* 47:1148–1158, 1976.

Ricciuti H: Fear and the development of social attachments in the first year of life. In: Lewis M, Rosenblum L (eds): *The Origins of Human Behavior: Fear*. New York, Wiley, 1974, pp. 73–106.

Riksen-Walraven JM: Effects of caregiver behavior on habituation rate and self-efficacy in infants. *Int J Behav Dev* 1:105–130, 1978.

Rogoff B: *Apprenticeship in Thinking*. New York, Oxford University Press, 1990.

Rogoff B, Malkin CM, Gilbride K: Interaction with babies as guidance in development. *New Dir Child Dev* 23:41–43, 1984.

Rose RJ, Boughman JA, Corey LA, et al: Data from kinships of monozygotic twins indicate maternal effects on verbal intelligence. *Nature* 283:375–377, 1980.

Rose RJ, Harris EL, Christian JC, et al: Genetic variance in nonverbal intelligence: Data from the kinships of identical twins. *Science* 205:1153–1155, 1979.

Rose S: Enhancing visual recognition memory in preterm infants. *Dev Psychol* 16:85–92, 1980.

Rose SA, Wallace IF: Visual recognition memory: A predictor of later cognitive functioning in preterms. *Child Dev* 56:843–852, 1985.

Rose SA, Gottfried AW, Bridger WG: Effects of haptic cues on visual recognition memory in fullterm and preterm infants. *Infant Behav Dev* 2:55–67, 1979.

Rosenstein D, Oster H: Differential facial responses to four basic tastes in newborns. *Child Dev* 59:1555–1568, 1988.

Ross GS: Categorization in 1- to 2-year-olds. *Dev Psychol* 16:391–396, 1980.

Ross HS: Infants' use of turn-alternation signals in games. Paper presented at the International Conference on Infant Studies, New Haven, CT, 1980.

Ross MS, Goldman BD: Establishing new social relations in infancy. In: Alloway T, Pliner P, Krames L (eds): *Advances in the Study of Communication and Affect*. Vol 3: *Attachment Behavior*. New York, Plenum, 1977.

Rothbart MK: Laughter in young children. *Psychol Bull* 80:247–256, 1973.

Rothbart MK: Measurement of temperament in infancy. *Child Dev* 52:569–578, 1981.

Rothbart MK, Derryberry P: Development of individual differences in temperament. In: Lamb ME, Brown AL (eds): *Advances in Developmental Psychology* (Vol 1). Hillsdale, NJ, Erlbaum, 1981.

Rovee CK, Rovee DT: Conjugate reinforcement of infant exploratory behavior. *J Exp Child Psychol* 8:33–39, 1969.

Rovee-Collier CK: Learning and memory in infancy. In: Osofsky JD (ed): *Handbook of Infant Development* (2nd ed). New York, Wiley, 1987.

Rovee-Collier CK, Gekoski MJ: The economics of infancy: A review of conjugate reinforcement. In: Reese HW, Lipsitt LP (eds): *Advances in Child Development and Behavior* (Vol 13). New York, Academic Press, 1979.

Rovee-Collier CK, Lipsitt LP: Learning, adaptation, and memory. In: Stratton PM (ed): *Psychobiology of the Human Newborn*. New York, Wiley, 1982.

Rovee-Collier CK, Sullivan MK, Enright M, et al: Reactivation of infant memory. *Science* 208:1159–1161, 1980.

Rubenstein J, Howes C: The effects of peers on toddler interaction with mothers and toys. *Child Dev* 47:597–605, 1976.

Rubenstein J, Howes C, Pedersen FA: Second order effects of peers on mother-toddler interaction. *Infant Behav Dev* 5:185–194, 1982.

Ruff H: Infants' exploration of objects. *Infant Behav Dev* 5:207, 1982a (Abstract).

Ruff H: The role of manipulation in infants' responses to invariant properties of objects. *Dev Psychol* 18:682–691, 1982b.

Ruff H: Detection of information specifying the motion of objects by 3- and 5-month-old infants. *Dev Psychol* 21:295–305, 1985.

Saayman G, Ames EW, Moffett A: Response to novelty as an indicator of visual discrimination in the human infant. *J Exp Child Psychol* 1:189–198, 1964.

Sackett GP: Monkeys reared in isolation with pictures as visual input: Evidence for an innate releasing mechanism. *Science* 154:1468–1473, 1966.

Sagi A, Hoffman M: Empathic distress in the newborn. *Dev Psychol* 12:175–176, 1976.

Sagi A, Lamb ME, Lewkowicz K, et al: Security of infant-mother, -father, and -metapelet attachments among kibbutz-reared Israeli children. *Monogr Soc Res Child Dev* 50 (serial no. 209), 1985.

Salapatek P: Pattern perception in early infancy. In: Cohen LB, Salapatek P (eds): *Infant Perception: From Sensation to Cognition* (Vol 1). New York, Academic Press, 1975.

Sameroff A, Chandler MJ: Reproductive risk and the continuum of caretaking casualty. In: Horowitz FD (ed): *Review of Child Development Research* (Vol 4). Chicago, University of Chicago Press, 1975.

Sameroff A, Seifer R, Elias P: Sociocultural variability in infant temperament ratings. *Child Dev* 53:164–173, 1982.

Sameroff AJ: The components of sucking in the human newborn. *J Exp Child Psychol* 6:607–623, 1968.

Sameroff AJ: Early influences on development: Fact or fancy? *Merrill-Palmer Q* 21:267–294, 1975.

Sameroff AJ: Organization and stability of newborn behavior: A commentary on the Brazelton Neonatal Behavior Assessment Scale. *Monogr Soc Res Child Dev* 43 (serial no. 177), 1978.

Sameroff AJ, Cavanaugh P: Learning in infancy: A developmental perspective. In: Osofsky JD (ed): *Handbook of Infant Development*. New York, Wiley, 1979.

Samuels CA: Attention to eye contact opportunity and facial motion by three-month-old infants. *J Exp Child Psychol* 40:105–114, 1985.

Scarr S, McCartney K: How people make their own environments: A theory of genotype-environment effects. *Child Dev* 54:424–435, 1983.

Scarr S, Weinberg FA: The Minnesota adoption studies: Genetic differences and malleability. *Child Dev* 54:260–268, 1983.

Schaffer HR: *The Child's Entry into a Social World*. London, Academic Press, 1984.

Schaffer HR, Collis GM, Parsons G: Vocal interchange and visual regard in verbal and pre-verbal children. In: Schaffer MR (ed): *Studies in Mother-Infant Interaction*. London, Academic Press, 1977.

Schaller J: Chromatic vision in human infants: Conditioned operant fixation to "hues" of varying intensity. *Bull Psychon Soc* 6:39–42, 1975.

Scherer KR, Koivumaki J, Rosenthal R: Minimal cues in the vocal communication of affect: Judging emotions from content masked speech. *J Psycholinguist Res* 1:269–285, 1972.

Schneider BA, Bull D, Trehub SE: Binaural unmasking in infants. *J Acoust Soc Am* 83:1124–1132, 1988.

Schneider BA, Trehub SE, Bull D: High-frequency sensitivity in infants. *Science* 207:1003–1004, 1980.

Seligman MEP: On the generality of the laws of learning. *Psychol Rev* 77:406–418, 1970.

Sherrod KB, Altemeier WA, O'Connor L, et al: Early prediction of child maltreatment. *Early Child Dev Care* 13:335–350, 1984.

Siegel LS: Infant tests as predictors of cognitive and language development at two years. *Child Dev* 52:545–557, 1981.

Sigman MD, Beckwith L: Infant visual attentiveness in relation to caregiver-infant interaction and developmental outcome. *Infant Behav Dev* 3:141–154, 1980.

Sigman MD, Parmelee AM: Visual preferences of four-month-old premature and full-term infants. *Child Dev* 45:959–965, 1974.

Sigman MD, Kopp CB, Littman B, et al: Infant visual attentiveness in relation to birth condition. *Dev Psychol* 13:431–437, 1977.

Simner M: Newborn's response to the cry of another infant. *Dev Psychol* 5:136–150, 1971.

Siqueland ER: Reinforcement patterns and extinction in human newborns. *J Exp Child Psychol* 6:431–442, 1968.

Siqueland ER: Studies of visual recognition memory in preterm infants: Differences in development as a function of perinatal morbidity factors. In: Friedman SL, Sigman M (eds): *Preterm Birth and Psychological Development*. New York, Academic Press, 1981.

Siqueland ER, Lipsitt LP: Conditioned head-turning behavior in newborns. *J Exp Child Psychol* 3:356–376, 1966.

Skinner BF: On the rate of formation of a conditioned reflex. *J Gen Psychol* 7:274–286, 1932.

Slater A, Morison V, Rose D: Habituation in the newborn. *Infant Behav Dev* 7:183–200, 1984.

Snow CE: The development of conversations between mothers and babies. *J Child Lang* 4:1–22, 1977.

Snow ME, Jacklin CN, Maccoby EE: Crying episodes and sleep-wakefulness transitions in the first 26 months of life. *Infant Behav Dev* 3:387–394, 1980.

Snyder LS, Bates E, Bretherton I: Content and context in early lexical development. *J Child Lang* 8:565–582, 1981.

Sokolov YN: *Perception and the Conditioned Reflex* (Waydenfeld SW, trans). New York, Macmillan, 1963. (Originally published 1958.)

Sorce JF, Emde RN, Campos JJ, et al: Maternal emotional signaling: Its effect on the visual cliff behavior of 1-year-olds. *Dev Psychol* 21:195–200, 1985.

Sostek AM, Anders TF: Relationships among the Brazelton Neonatal Scale, Bayley Infant Scales, and early temperament. *Child Dev* 48:320–323, 1977.

Spitz RA: Anxiety in infancy: A study of its manifestations in the first year of life. *Int J Psychoanal* 31:138–143, 1950a.

Spitz RA: Possible infantile precursors of psychopathology. *Am J Orthopsychiatry* 20:240–248, 1950b.

Spitz RA: *The First Year of Life*. New York, International Universities Press, 1965.

Sroufe LA: Individual patterns of adaptation from infancy to preschool. In: Perlmutter M (ed): *Minnesota Symposium on Child Psychology* (Vol 16). Hillsdale, NJ, Erlbaum, 1983.

Sroufe LA, Waters E: The ontogenesis of smiling and laughter: A perspective of the organization of development in infancy. *Psychol Rev* 83:173–189, 1976.

Sroufe LA, Wunsch JP: The development of laughter in the first year of life. *Child Dev* 43:1326–1344, 1972.

Sroufe LA, Schork E, Motti F, et al: The role of affect in social competence. In: Izard CE, Kagan J, Zajonc R (eds): *Affect, Cognition, and Behavior*. New York, Plenum, 1984.

Stamps LE, Porges SW: Heart rate conditioning in newborn infants: Relationships among conditionability, heart rate variability, and sex. *Dev Psychol* 11:424–431, 1975.

Stark RE: Prespeech sequential feature development. In: Fletcher P, Garman M (eds): *Language Acquisition*. Cambridge, United Kingdom, Cambridge University Press, 1980.

Stayton DJ, Ainsworth MDS, Main M: The development of separation behavior in the first year of life: Protest, following, and greeting. *Dev Psychol* 9:213–225, 1973.

Stenberg C, Campos JJ: The development of anger expressions in infancy. In: Stein NL, Leventahl B, Trabasso T (eds): *Psychological and Biological Approaches to Emotion*. Hillsdale, NJ, Erlbaum, 1990.

Stenberg C, Campos JJ, Emde RN: The facial expression of anger in seven-month-old infants. *Child Dev* 54:178–184, 1983.

Stewart RB: Sibling interaction: The role of the older child as teacher for the younger. *Merrill-Palmer Q* 29:47–68, 1983.

Stifter CA, Fox NA: Infant reactivity: Physiological correlates of newborn and 5-month temperament. *Dev Psych* 26:582–588, 1990.

Stoel-Gammon C, Cooper JA: Patterns of early lexical phonological development. *J Child Language* 11:247–271, 1984.

Strauss MS, Curtis LE: Infant perception of numerosity. *Child Dev* 52:1146–1152, 1981.

Suess GJ, Grossman KE, Sroufe LA: Effects of infant attachment to mother and father on quality of adaptation in preschool: From dyadic to individual organisation of self. *Int J Behav Dev* 15:43–65, 1992.

Super CM, Harkness S: The development of affect in infancy and early childhood. In: Wagner DA, Stevenson HW (eds): *Cultural Perspectives on Child Development*. San Francisco, Freeman, 1982.

Tal J, Bornstein MH: Infant vocal distress: Conceptual structure, responsiveness, and sampling in mother and independent observer. In: Lester BM, Newman JD, Pedersen F (eds): *Social and Biological Aspects of Infant Crying*. New York, Plenum, 1992.

Tamis-LeMonda CS, Bornstein MH: Habituation and maternal encouragement of attention in infancy as predictors of toddler language, play, and representational competence. *Child Dev* 60:738–751, 1989.

Tavecchio LWC, van IJzendoorn MH: *Attachment in Social Networks*. Amsterdam, Elsevier, 1987.

Teller DY, Bornstein MH: Infant color vision and color perception. In: Salapatek P, Cohen LB (eds): *Handbook of Infant Perception*. New York, Academic Press, 1986.

Teller DY, Lindsey DT: Motion nulls for white versus isochromatic gratings in infants and adults. *J Opt Soc Am* 1945–1954, 1989.

Teller DY, Peeples DR, Sekel M: Discrimination of chromatic from white light by two-month-old infants. *Vision Res* 18:41–48, 1978.

Tennes K: The role of hormones in mother-infant transaction. In: Emde RN, Harmon RJ (eds): *The Development of Attachment and Affiliative Systems*. New York, Plenum Press, 1982, pp. 75–80.

Teti DM, Ablard KE: Security of attachment and infant-sibling relationships: A laboratory study. *Child Dev* 60:1519–1528, 1989.

Teti DM, Bond LA, Gibbs ED: Sibling-created experiences: Relationships to birth-spacing and infant cognitive development. *Infant Behav Dev* 9:27–42, 1986.

Thomas A, Chess S: *Temperament and Development*. New York, Brunner/Mazel, 1977.

Thomas A, Chess S, Birch H, et al: *Behavioral Individuality in Childhood*. New York, New York University Press, 1963.

Thomas A, Chess S, Birch HG: *Temperament and Behavior Disorders in Children*. New York, New York University Press, 1968.

Thompson RA: Construction and reconstruction of early attachments: Taking perspective on attachment theory and research. In: Keating D, Rosen H (eds): *Constructivist Perspectives on Atypical Development and Developmental Psychopathology*. Hillsdale, NJ, Erlbaum, 1990.

Thompson RA, Lamb ME: Security of attachment and stranger sociability in infancy. *Dev Psychol* 19:184–191, 1983.

Thompson RA, Limber S: "Social anxiety" in infancy: Stranger wariness and separation distress. In: Leitenberg H (ed): *Handbook of Social Evaluation Anxiety*. New York, Plenum, 1991.

Thompson RA, Lamb ME, Estes D: Stability of infant-mother attachment and its relationship to changing life circumstances in an unselected middle class sample. *Child Dev* 53:144–148, 1982.

Tomasello M: The role of joint attentional processes in early language development. *Lang Sci* 10:68–88, 1990.

Trehub SE, Chang H: Speech as reinforcing stimulation for infants. *Dev Psychol* 13:121–124, 1977.

Trehub SE, Schneider B (eds): *Auditory Development in Infancy*. New York, Plenum Press, 1985.

Trehub SE, Schneider BA, Endman M: Developmental changes in infants' sensitivity to octave-band noises. *Exp Child Psychol* 29:282–293, 1980.

Trevarthen C: Descriptive analyses of infant communicative behavior. In: Schaffer HR (ed): *Studies in Mother-Infant Interaction*. London, Academic Press, 1977, pp. 227–270.

Tulkin SR: Social class differences in maternal and infant behavior. In: Leiderman PH, Tulkin SR, Rosenfeld A (eds): *Culture and Infancy*. New York, Academic Press, 1977.

Tulkin SR, Kagan J: Mother-child interaction in the first year of life. In: Bronfenbrenner U, Mahoney MA (eds): *Influences on Human Development*. Hinsdale, IL, Dryden, 1975.

Uzgiris ID, Hunt JM: *Assessment in Infancy: Ordinal Scales of Psychological Development*. Urbana, IL, University of Illinois Press, 1975.

Vandell DL: Sociability of peer and mother during the first year. *Dev Psychol* 16:335–361, 1980.

Vandell DL, Wilson KS: Social interaction in the first year: Infants' social skills with peers versus mother. In: Rubin KH, Ross HS (eds): *Peer Relationships and Social Skills in Childhood*. New York, Springer-Verlag, 1982, pp. 187–208.

Vandell DL, Wilson KS, Buchanan NR: Peer interaction in the first year of life: An examination of its structure, content, and sensitivity to toys. *Child Dev* 51:481–488, 1980.

Van Giffen K, Haith MH: Infant visual response to Gestalt geometric forms. *Infant Behav Dev* 7:335–346, 1984.

Varner D, Cook JE, Schneck ME, et al: Tritan discriminations by 1- and 2-month-old human infants. *Vision Res* 25:821–832, 1984.

Vaughn B, Egeland B, Sroufe LA, et al: Individual differences in infant-mother attachment at twelve and eighteen months: Stability and chance in families under stress. *Child Dev* 50:971–975, 1979.

Vernon PE: *Intelligence: Heredity and Environment*. San Francisco, Freeman, 1980.

Vietze P, Falsey S, Sandler J, et al: Transactional approach to prediction of child maltreatment. *Infant Ment Health J* 1:248–261, 1980.

Vihman M: Phonological development. In: Bernthal JE, Bankson N (eds): *Articulation Disorders*. Englewood Cliffs, NJ, Prentice-Hall, 1993.

Von Hofsten C: Predictive reaching for moving objects by human infants. *J Exp Child Psychol* 30:369–382, 1980.

Von Hofsten C: Developmental changes in the organization of pre-reaching movements. *Dev Psychol* 20:378–388, 1984.

Von Hofsten C, Fazel-Zandy S: Development of visually guided hand orientation in reaching. *J Exp Child Psychol* 38:208–219, 1984.

Von Hofsten C, Lindhagen K: Observations on the development of reaching for moving objects. *J Exp Child Psychol* 28:158–173, 1979.

Wachs TD, Uzgiris IC, Hunt JM: Cognitive development in infants of different age levels and from different environmental backgrounds: An exploratory investigation. *Merrill-Palmer Q* 17:283–317, 1971.

Wagner ME, Schubert HJP, Schumbert DSP: Sex-of-sibling effects. Part 1: Gender role, intelligence, achievement, and creativity. *Adv Child Dev Behav* 24:181–214, 1993.

Walden TA, Baxter A: The effect of context and age on social referencing. *Child Dev* 60:1511–1518, 1989.

Waters E: The reliability and stability of individual differences in infant-mother attachment. *Child Dev* 49:483–494, 1978.

Waters E, Wippman J, Sroufe LA: Attachment, positive affect, and competence in the peer group: Two studies in construct validation. *Child Dev* 50:821–829, 1979.

Watson JS: Smiling, cooing, and "the game." *Merrill-Palmer Q* 18:323–340, 1972.

Watson JS: Contingency perception in early social development. In: Field TM, Fox NA (eds): *Social Perception in Infants*. Norwood, NJ, Ablex, 1985.

Webster RL: Selective suppression of infant's vocal responses by classes of phonemic stimulation. *Dev Psychol* 1:410–414, 1969.

Webster RL, Steinhardt MH, Senter MG: Changes in infants' vocalizations as a function of differential acoustic stimulation. *Dev Psychol* 7:39–43, 1972.

Weiner G, Rider RV, Oppel W: Some correlates of IQ changes in children. *Child Dev* 34:61–67, 1963.

Weiner K, Kagan J: Infants' reaction to changes in orientation of figure and frame. *Perception* 5:25–28, 1976.

Weir RH: *Language in the Crib*. The Hague, Mouton, 1962.

Weisner T: Sibling interdependence and child caretaking: A cross-cultural view. In: Lamb ME, Sutton-Smith B (eds): *Sibling Relationships*. Hillsdale, NJ, Erlbaum, 1982.

Werner EE: *Kith, Kin, and Hired Hands*. Baltimore, University Park Press, 1984.

White RW: Motivation reconsidered: The concept of competence. *Psychol Rev* 66:297–333, 1959.

Willerman L, Broman SH, Fiedler M: Infant development, preschool IQ, and social class. *Child Dev* 41:69–77, 1970.

Wilson RS: Synchronies in mental development: An epigenetic perspective. *Science* 202:939–948, 1978.

Wilson RS: The Louisville twin study: Developmental synchronies in behavior. *Child Dev* 54:298–316, 1983.

Wilson RS: Twins and chronogenetics: Correlated pathways of development. *Acta Genet Med Gemellol* 33:149–157, 1984.

Wolff PH: Observations on the early development of smiling. In: Foss BM (ed): *Determinants of Infant Behavior* (Vol 2). New York, Wiley, 1963.

Yeates KO, MacPhee D, Campbell FA, et al: Maternal IQ and home environment as determinants of early childhood intellectual competence: A developmental analysis. *Dev Psychol* 19:731–739, 1983.

Yogman MW: Development of the father-infant relationship. In: Fitzgerald HE, Lester BM, Yogman MW (eds): *Theory and Research in Behavioral Pediatrics*. New York, Plenum, 1982.

Yonas A: Infants' responses to optical information for collision. In: Aslin RN, Alberts JR, Peterson MR (eds): *Development of Perception: Psychobiological Perspectives* (Vol 2). New York, Academic Press, 1981.

Yonas A, Granrud CE: Development of visual space perception in young infants. In: Mehler J, Fox R (eds): *Neonate Cognition: Beyond the Blooming, Buzzing Confusion*. Hillsdale, NJ, Erlbaum, 1985.

Young-Browne G, Rosenfeld HM, Horowitz FD: Infant discrimination of facial expressions. *Child Dev* 48:555–562, 1977.

Zahavi A: The pattern of vocal signals and the information they convey. *Behavior* 80:1–8, 1982.

Zajonc RB: Validating the confluence model. *Psychol Bull* 93:457–480, 1983.

Zarbatany L, Lamb ME: Social referencing as a function of information source: Mothers versus strangers. *Infant Behav Dev* 8:25–33, 1985.

Zeskind P: Behavioral dimensions and cry sounds of infants of differential fetal growth. *Infant Behav Dev* 4:297–306, 1981.

Zeskind PS, Sale J, Mais ML, et al: Adult perceptions of pain and hunger cries: A synchrony of arousal. *Child Dev* 56:549–554, 1985.

Zukow PG: *Sibling Interaction across Cultures: Theoretical and Methodological Issues*. New York, Springer-Verlag, 1989.

21 DEVELOPMENT OF SCHOOL-AGE CHILDREN
Lee Combrinck-Graham, M.D.

BACKGROUND: WHAT IS THE SCHOOL-AGE PERIOD?

School-age is just one name for that period of childhood that begins when a child enters elementary school and ends at the beginning of junior high school. The name, though not specific, because both younger children and adolescents attend school, conveys the central focus of emotional and psychological development of children ranging in age from 5 to 12 years old.

The terms latency and middle childhood imply that not much goes on in this transitional era between the more psychologically active preschool and adolescent periods. The term ''latency'' is derived from the psychoanalytic perception of biphasic sexual development, with peaks in this developmental area hypothesized to occur in the preschool and adolescent periods. The sexually quiet latent period was thought to be entered with the mastery of oedipal strivings and the establishment of the superego. Freud likened the period to the glacial epoch in the earth's history, romanticizing that the ice-covered period was necessary for the birth of civilization (Buxbaum, 1980). Nowadays lines of development other than libidinal usually command more attention when studying the evolution of an individual's psyche, but Freud's metaphor was both aesthetic and accurate in recognizing the importance of this developmental era to the children's becoming civilized and acculturated members of their societies.

There has been significant progress in developmental study since these early efforts to grasp, characterize, and produce a framework for describing evolving issues and accomplishments in childhood. In particular, there has been increasing attention to observing and describing how each individual child's development is an ongoing transaction between the child and numerous dynamic systems around him or her. Early theorists and observers studied children as if they were the containers of their own development, mastering and defending themselves against internal strivings that were built into the organism. Neo-Freudians (e.g., Horney, Thompson, Sullivan) shifted the focus considerably from the internal life of the child to the interaction between the child and key persons in his or her life—the parents. Now it is widely accepted that the model of a child as the container of his or her own development does not adequately represent the complex activities of and differences in children's development.

Moving away from individualism, which makes the child the basic unit of study, many contemporary developmental psychologists have observed that development is largely a social construction (Kessen, 1979). Contemporary psychological concepts include Vygotsky's ''mind in society'' and Bateson's ''ecology of the mind,'' requiring an active consideration of interpersonal interaction; school and social experience as a system of developing self-view, mastery, and morality; and sociocultural variables such as gender, ethnicity, and social, economic, and occupational status as critical ingredients in development.

These ecological facets are influential throughout the life cycle, but many have focused on the school-age period as a most exciting vantage for studying these exquisite interactions. Erik Erikson (1950) introduced a psychosocial modification of psychosexual stages and observed that across cultures this was the time when the child set out to master the industry of his or her society. Harry Stack Sullivan (1953) put it in even more social terms when he described what he called the ''juvenile era'' as the first opportunity that society has to correct the influence of the family. Robert White's (1959, 1960) postulation of ''competence moti-

vation'' provided a new lens for observing the activity of the school-age child. Perhaps because the management of sexuality is not so distracting to observers of children of this era, it has become a time to examine cognitive development as it relates to the acquisition of learning, the mastery of the industry of one's society, the development of the concept of oneself as a person who can make contributions through industry, and, what is perhaps more important, development of personal values, standards, affection, morality, loyalty, and trust. In short, it is an era when children actively involve themselves with the fundamentals of civilization that Freud envisioned emerging out of the glacial epoch.

It is not surprising to note that in this contemporary view of development the school-age period is more actively defined by social institutions, the school, and laws regulating schooling, than by the particular accomplishments of all children prior to and during this developmental epoch. Remember, schooling has been timed to reflect the readiness for school of the majority of children. Since schooling is now required for all 6-year-olds, regardless of whether they are majority children or whether or not they are ready for school, there are now substantial variations in the developmental levels of the children entering school, and there will undoubtedly be further redefinitions of the demarcation of the period as well as the meaning of the educational system into which such a diversity of 6-year-olds enter.

To expand further on this point, it is useful to review the four definitions of normality articulated by Offer (1980): normal as utopia, normal as average, normal as the absence of illness or pathology, and normal as transaction. The last definition, normal as transaction, is most useful in examining school-age children's development.

The transactional conundrum for normal development has been tackled by many, but a particularly articulate explorer has been Jerome Kagan. Through many studies, Kagan has attempted to tease out the ''nature'' of the child from the experiences that envelop him or her. One particular cross-cultural study (Kagan and Klein, 1973) illustrates distinctions between the actual unfolding of abilities, which he argues are latent in all individuals, and the effect of environment on the timing of this unfolding. Kagan raises a need to reexamine developmental continuity (meaning that early experiences determine and predict later ones) when he describes rural Guatemalan Indian infants and preschoolers who by all culturally relevant measures are ''retarded'' but who at 11 perform at the same level as American children in tests of cognitive functioning. While concentrating data on the contrasts in rate of development, he also suggests processes and influences. The Guatemalan infant is unstimulated and left alone; only basic physical needs are attended to. Thus, Guatemalan infants do not have the assertive interaction with environment that is so prized in American infants and preschoolers. Kagan suggests that in the school-age period, where the relative neglect of these children by adults leaves them to form their own social groupings, Guatemalan youngsters begin to practice and learn assertiveness through jockeying for social position. In contrast, he proposes, American children have already been identified as assertive or passive or as successful or failing by the time they enter the school-age period. Many American children in the school-age period may become involved in patterns that further confirm who they have already been described or ascribed to be. The successes of assertive majority children will be reinforced; the failures of poorly prepared minority children will also be reinforced. Developmental events are built into the organism, but the timing of their appearance as well as the degree to which they are fully mastered are intricately interwoven with interpersonal-social factors.

FROM PRESCHOOL TO ADOLESCENCE

A general overview of the movement through the school-age period can be achieved by reviewing where most youngsters seem to be when they enter the period and when they move on to the next developmental era.

End of Preschool

Physically the American 5-year-old child is already quite agile, having mastered running, jumping, skipping, and cartwheels, and is beginning activities that involve more sensory-physical coordination, such as catching and throwing with accuracy. In the fine motor area, the late preschool child has the ability to draw and copy circles, squares, triangles, and crosses and can draw a person with separate head, body, and limbs. Cognitively, the late preschooler's concepts are dominated by "centration," meaning allowing material to be defined by only one of several possible dimensions. This is manifested in conservation tasks by a child's concentrating on either length or density, either height or width, and not grasping how changes in these dimensions may compensate each other. In classification exercises, the child may choose an idiosyncratic characteristic by which to classify, and/or the classification scheme may be a personal association.

Personally meaningful but unconventional rationales also characterize the preschool child's moral judgment, where decisions about right and wrong are made in the very personal terms of the child's experience, both past punishment and current likelihood of being punished.

In the social arena the child ending the preschool era has usually made some significant inroads with peers and adults outside the family, since most young children have substantial experience outside the home from toddlerhood or before. The late preschool child has formed friendships, has some empathy, and enjoys the company of other children (Grunebaum and Solomon, 1982). Most observers have agreed that the preschooler's gender identity is well formed, and young children already prefer to play with same-sex age-mates.

Entering Adolescence

The child leaving the school-age era is undergoing a growth spurt, is experiencing the upsurge of both androgen and estrogen production stimulated by increase in gonadotrophic hormone activity, and is beginning to observe major changes in body habitus as well as the development of secondary sex characteristics. This child has achieved physical coordination, permitting not only accuracy, fine tuning, strength, and endurance but also coordination of physical activity into teamwork.

In the fine motor area, the youngster leaving the school-age period can write in cursive and do so within prescribed lines, can organize written material on a piece of paper, and can execute the fine detail of visual-motor planning and integration required in many hobbies, such as elaborate Lego constructions, knitting, weaving, building, woodworking, and the like.

The early adolescent may begin to perform cognitive operations in his or her head, and this permits planning and predicting the outcome of a series of experiments without having to actually carry them out. Furthermore, this independence of substance, or abstracting ability, permits the youngster to imagine activity and to prejudge whether a particular course of action is advisable or not, leading to the potential moral developments of the adolescent which at once express the individual and the individual's acknowledgment of accountability to others.

School-age Accomplishments

Something extraordinary happens during the 5- to 7-year period that transforms a preschooler into an early adolescent. The early psychoanalytic developmental theorists may have thought that sexual drives were latent, but there is certainly no time for latency. What is ideally achieved during the school-age period might best be summarized as "interpersonally accountable, independent competence." It differs from adult maturity in that it does not involve sexuality nor does it involve self-sufficiency or the ability to assume complete responsibility for the care of others. It represents a major change from the preschool position of having to ask "why" in order to receive an explanatory framework for almost every domain of experience. The child at the end of successful school-age years can apply his or her own system for satisfying curiosity. He or she is prepared for the achievements of the next era by setting the stage for intimate and sexual relationships with nonfamiliars, by being a person who is equipped with a sense of competent self, but also a sense of interdependence.

The rate and quality of the movement from preschool to adolescence is facilitated by many factors. There are physiological developments that occur within the child. There is the preparation the child has received in the early years. There are the interactions of the child with the environment. Both the child's interactions and the environment with which he or she interacts increase in complexity. More independent relationships with adults and children outside the family are developed, as are ideas and interpersonal organizational structures that both broaden the child's experience and challenge his or her evaluation of the views learned in and represented by the family.

What the child brings to school-age from earlier experience is one important area of influence. How competent and mature the child is affects how ready he or she will be for formal schooling. In addition, as the Kagan work, just described, suggests, how successful the child has already been sets a tone for the character of further success or failure in the school-age period, even in the face of adequate biological maturation.

The family environment is an important influence on how the child moves into the school society. It is important for the school-age child to move back and forth from family to school and peer milieu, to bring back commentary and criticism from the outside, which may modify his or her view of her family members while they are still held in esteem. Combrinck-Graham (1985) has characterized this period of the family life cycle as a time of opening up from the centripetal energy state of the family of infants and young children, an opening up that involves all generations. The children go out of the family to school; caretaking parents develop activities other than those involved with the children and emerge into the society of their children's friends' parents; working parents are often in parallel stages of settling in and establishing themselves in their careers. Ideally, then, the family environment of the school-age child is characterized by multiple levels of active involvement with social institutions and peers, which both enrich and modify the central family interaction and encourage further explorations outside as the family system spirals to the centrifugal period of its children's adolescence.

Finally, the school environment is crucial to the successful accomplishment of school-age development. How the school functions to support each child's development may be conceptualized as a complex matter of fit between child, family, and school. Aspects of fit include whether there is congruence between the expectations of the child and the child's ability, between goals for education of the school and of the dominant culture of the family, between the standards for excellence of the school system and gender expectations, and between the dominant social morality and experienced rewards of child and family.

In sum, the ideal accomplishments of the school-age child are increasing diversity of abilities and activities—branching out and expanding his or her personal world view, and in doing so, expanding that of the family. Clearly there are important conditions within and outside the child that will influence how successful the entire enterprise is.

SCHOOL-AGE CHILDREN

Maturation

One can assume that maturation of the brain is common to children cross-culturally, though we know that rates of maturation vary from individual to individual. Nevertheless, generally the brain undergoes a period of rapid growth to age 2 and grows at a much slower rate until puberty. At birth the brain is estimated to be about 10% of adult volume: it grows to 90% of adult volume by age 5 and completes its growth slowly over the next 9 years. What is more significant than actual volume, however, is the modification of anatomical structures and myelinization, which is almost completed around the age of 7 (Shapiro and Perry, 1976).

Some data on neurotransmitter development may further sharpen our view of the intrinsic maturational schedule of the child and elucidate the emergence of the abilities of school-age children. In contrast to noradrenergic systems, which develop early and early exert influence on the formation of the cortex, dopaminergic systems, associated with attention regulation, and serotoninergic systems, associated with mood and aggression, have a much more gradual establishment of crucial connections between brainstem nuclei and cortical structures. Cholinergic systems, which are associated with memory and higher cortical functions, develop relatively late. Most of the studies of neurotransmitter development have been in rats and primates, but it is likely that these systems are elaborated in humans during the school-age period (Coyle and Harris, 1987).

These refinements in brain structure result in the maturation of higher cortical functions, with the expressed abilities in motor coordination, increased attention and focus, and expanded consideration for others being related to increased self-regulation.

As an example of how these changes may be reflected in modifications of cognitive style, it has been observed that children asked to solve problems increase the amount of time they take to consider their answers (latency) as they grow older. Generally, 5-year-olds answer quickly and make many errors, while older children have longer latencies and make fewer errors. This trend must be an outcome of refinements of brain function, but one study of children in diverse cultures such as Japan, the United States, Israel, and the Netherlands, while marking the trend to increase latency and decrease errors through the early school-age period, found that the Japanese children began with a longer latency and lower error rate than the others at the same age, and as they grew older, the latency changed little but the error rate decreased even more than that of the others. Two things are of importance about these findings: (a) there is a general observed trend to increase latency, which is associated with self-regulation; and (b) there are differences in style in different cultures. Japanese children learn to reflect early; then they seem to learn that there is a maximum beneficial amount of reflection time needed to get the correct answer, while other children, particularly Americans, may become inefficient, increasing reflection time and not increasing accuracy proportionately, becoming obsessive or lacking in self-confidence about their responses (Smith and Caplan, 1988).

Psychosexual and Gender Development

Psychoanalytic developmentalists regarded sexual development as biphasic, with a "latent" period during the school-age years. Freud felt that latency was a distinguishing feature of humans over animals and hoped to discover anatomical evidence of this through then-promising studies of changes in the interstitial portions of the "sex glands" (Buxbaum, 1980). Contemporary studies of sex hormones do not support the biphasic theory, however. Infants have relatively high but varying proportions of sex hormones in cord blood. The levels of sex hormones fall after birth and begin to rise, due to endogenous production, during the school-age period (ages 7–8 in girls, and about 2 years later in boys). Some have postulated that school-age children's greater sexual awareness may be related to their expressed feelings of disgust and shame and the strong sense of modesty that develops during the school years. Others have reported that sex play among school children is a natural extension of that of preschoolers (Rutter, 1971). Infants and preschool children have the physical capacity to respond in a sexual manner, but it is difficult to know whether or not these responses are simply reflexive and associated with self-exploration and at what point the child becomes conscious of erotic pleasure and desire (Green, 1988).

It was posited that sexual strivings in the oedipal child were overcome with the development of a variety of defense mechanisms, which in the first part of the school-age period were relatively harsh and primitive: introjection, projection, and turning passive into active to avoid guilt feelings. In the second part of the period, more sophisticated defense mechanisms free the ego for somewhat more autonomous assessments of self and others (Bornstein, 1951). Themes of the fantasies of school-age children include power, weakness, skill, and competence. Toward the later school years, fantasies become more complex, exploratory, and extensive (Minuchin, 1977, p. 41). Girls' attraction to movie stars and rock idols seems to have more a group interactional than a sexual meaning. Most significant in the child's internal life is the development of a relationship with the outer world in which with the increase in self-regulation come the rewards of a broader range of cognitive, behavioral, emotional, and social competence.

It is well established that children adopt a firm gender identity by age 3. This expression of their maleness or femaleness is manifested early by choices of role models and friends. With gender differences, as with so many of the other issues discussed in this chapter, the question of what is innate and what is the outcome of socialization is very intriguing.

Money's studies of infants with ambiguous genitalia established that gender identity was primarily determined through socialization. But explorations of differences in sexual preference and transsexual behaviors have raised questions about the roles of sex hormones in determining gendered behaviors. Carol Jacklin (1989) reviewed a number of purported relationships of hormones to behavior. For example, androgens in cord blood were negatively correlated with girls' spatial abilities at age 6; a relationship has been found between neonatal hormones and fear and timidity in boys but not in girls; and hormones are associated with positive moods for boys and girls, but the associated ratio of androgens to estrogens is different for boys and girls. Many of these studies compare behavior of children at school-age with hormone levels of cord blood without concurrent hormone levels. The daily variation in hormone levels makes it difficult to draw conclusions about absolute levels, but Jacklin suggests that it is the pattern of variability that is stable within individuals and that is important to behavioral outcomes.

Jacklin proposes that gender is represented internally by schemata, which are changing and evolving networks of associations used to filter and organize information. Gender schemata evolve out of diverse information, including modes of behavior, properties of objects, attitudes, and feeling states. One can observe how information is processed differently for boys and girls. For example, Jacklin notes, it is rare to see someone compliment a girl on how strong she is getting, or a boy on how nurturant he is. Gender schemata and their expressions are evolved and maintained in gendered society where it is most likely that girls will keep the company of women and other girls, and boys will do likewise with men. Cross-cultural studies do show male and female characteristic distinctions, but it appears that association with children and adults of the same sex is a powerful influence. We become the company we keep.

There is a number of characteristics associated with being male or female in the school-age period. Carol Gilligan (1982, p. 9) cites Janet Lever's studies of 181 5th-grade children at play. She observed that boys play outdoors in large and heterogeneous groups, and they play competitive games that last longer than those of girls. The games played by boys are more complex and consequently less boring, but full of disputes that seem to add interest to the interaction and do not derail the game. Similar observations of children playing led Piaget to conclude that boys were more advanced in moral development because of their fascination with legal procedures and experience at generating fair arbitration of disputes. Many other developmentalists concluded similarly that in the area of moral development and the development of the capacity to exert effective leadership in complex groups, boys preceded girls; few girls ever caught up.

In proposing that women listen to the demands of socialization and morality "in a different voice," Gilligan (1982) added new value to the "instrumental-expressive" gender dichotomy. Her own studies detail separate lines of moral development for boys and girls, with boys progressing along the steps described by Kohlberg (1969) and Piaget (1948) and girls following a different but equally sophisticated path. The moral stage described by Piaget through which school-age children pass was called the "interpretation of rules stage," in which the child became more aware of the spirit of a rule and would be able to make subjective moral judgments. In Kohlberg's schema, the school-age child went through the "conventional stage," of which there were two substages: "interpersonal concordance," in which a child would evaluate behavior on whether it pleases others, and the "orientation toward authority," in which the child learns to value duty, respect, and law and order. Gilligan's studies of girls' and women's moral development led her to emphasize the importance of relationship and, in contrast to an almost mathematical system for evaluating moral choices, a kind of narrative that evolves solutions within conversations and interpersonal action. Thus, Gilligan interprets the 5th-grade girls' play observed by Lever not as poorly developed or socially immature but as valuing different aspects of the social experience.

Recognizing that as a generalization boys develop instrumental functions and girls develop expressive ones has provided explanations for other observed differences between boys and girls. In academic achievement, for example, girls tend to do better in verbal areas, while boys have done better in math and science. Even as the causes of these differences are being explored, they are also being denied and recharacterized. Feminism apparently has had its effects on gender identity and gender role behaviors in both girls and their mothers. For example, the widely held view that boys are more mathematically capable than girls has been demonstrated to be more an effect of socialization than innate capability; it was found that math anxiety was related to gender-stereotyped beliefs of parents, the mothers being most influential (Eccles and Jacobs, 1986). Furthermore, gender differences in academic skills that had been previously noted are now not found on many tests of academic competence (Jacklin, 1989). It is likely that other so-called innate gender differences will be similarly reviewed in the future.

Cognitive Development and Learning

The standard by which school-age children's cognitive competence has been evaluated has been the achievement of what Piaget termed "concrete operations." The preschooler's cognitive schemas were creative efforts to grasp causality and make meaning of experience, but they were idiosyncratic and egocentric, while the school-age child masters important operations that increase his or her objectivity and brings his or her thinking into line with that of others. Classification and conservation are the two crucial achievements of concrete operational thinking. Classification is the ability to group objects or concepts; conservation is the ability to recognize constant qualities/quantities of material even when the material undergoes changes in morphology. The concrete logical operations are (a) composition—combining elements leads to another class (e.g., red triangles and blue triangles leads to another group, i.e., triangles); (b) associativity—combinations may be made in different orders with the same result; and (c) reversibility—being able to return mentally to an earlier point in the process. They enable the child to deal systematically with hierarchies and categories, series and sequences, alternative and equivalent ways of getting to the same place, and reciprocal relationships (Minuchin, 1977, p. 14).

Logical operations are crucial to mastering basic reading and mathematics skills, and they are also necessary for conducting social interaction, with its increasing complexity of groups, games, and rules. Acquisition of the ability to do conventional and objective mental operations is associated with an interest in the birth process, which has a more scientific basis than the preschooler's fantasies of incorporation and radical surgery, though it is not until late in the school-age period that an understanding of the role of the father is fully grasped (Rutter, 1971). Also associated with objective mental operations comes the grasp of the finality, universality, and inevitability of death.

There is general agreement that the achievement of concrete operations is accumulated through the school-age period and represents a discrete advance over preschool logic. There is some evidence that preschoolers do have abilities to classify and conserve, but the wording of the questions has to be just right to elicit responses that reveal it. For example, Kagan reports the "sleeping cow" test, where young children are shown four cows lying on their sides, three black and one white. They are asked, "Are there more black cows or more cows?" The preschool children generally say there are more black cows. However, if the question is asked, "Are there more black cows or more sleeping cows," the children will quickly observe that there are more sleeping cows (1984, p. 234).

Careful attention to wording also makes a difference in evaluating children with different cultural backgrounds. Kagan again notes that inner city Baltimore children could not respond to the question, "What should you do to make water boil?" But if asked, "What do you do to make water boil?" they gave complete answers (1984, p. 34).

Thus, it appears that a child's evaluated cognitive capacity is very much a product of his or her experience and the nature of the interaction between child and evaluator. There are several important points to be derived from this observation. The first is that children obviously arrive at the school-age era with diverse experiences. Most dramatically different are the experiences of children from middle-class, educated families and those from poor, minority, inner city families. The former are more likely to have attended educationally oriented preschools, have traveled at least in their own communities, have visited libraries and museums, and have been read to by their parents and teachers, while the latter have more likely been involved with complex family and "adoptive" family relationships ("play" mamas and many "aunts" and "uncles"), have experienced many comings and goings of people in their daily worlds, and have been exposed to situations of danger and hardship with little sense of control over these situations. Some of the latter group of youngsters may not ever have seen a book or a piece of paper or a crayon by the time they enter school, but many of them may have been assuming responsibilities in the household, such as caring for younger children, getting meals, and caring for themselves while adults are away. The former group has been prepared to enter school since toddlerhood, while the latter group is prepared to manage an entirely different set of experiences, which may not be compatible with what is expected in school (Heath, 1989; Miller-Jones, 1989; Wilson, 1989) (see Chapter 109).

Studies of the effects of model preschool programs and general application of Head Start programs for poor and minority children demonstrate that there is some advantage to having had a preschool experience, and this advantage is more dramatic and more lasting if the experience was in a model preschool program (Haskins, 1989). In follow-up throughout the remainder of their school lives, children from model preschools were significantly less likely to be placed in special education programs than controls (13% of children in preschool versus 31% of controls). But most often effects were not significant or disappeared in 3–6 years after the children entered formal public school. Reactions to the disappearing effect of Head Start programs have ranged from dismissing the effort as costly and ineffective to observing that the investment in these children's reacculturation into the school environment is not sustained through their public school experience. It is important to note that the most effective early education programs involved the parents in the school effort, so that the fit between home culture and school culture was enhanced.

Reading comprehension, at one time associated with psychosexual development and commonly experienced as a logical, sequential relationship with the words as they are deciphered and understood, is now largely thought to be text-based and interactional. It is increasingly evident that reading success depends upon the preparation of the reader, who brings to the task his or her expectations, prior knowledge of the content and structure of the material, and cultural background (Hall, 1989). Studies of problem readers and experiments with preparing young children for eventual reading further support the notion that preparation is a critical ingredient to academic success. Gerald Coles (1987) cites several examples to support this. One study reported that a group of 4-

year-olds given simple instructions in segmenting and blending words of two and three syllables 10 minutes a day for 13 weeks resulted in dramatically higher reading scores than those of children involved in nonspecific reading-related activities (1987, p. 52). Coles further reports on observations of the families of children with reading disabilities, finding a significant lack of preparation of these children for reading. In some families, messages about expectations of failure were transmitted; in others there were failures to provide exposure to preparatory material; in still others there was obvious evidence of "communication deviance" whereby the explanatory frameworks of language were so odd or idiosyncratic to the family that the child had unusual difficulty adapting to a school learning program (Ditton et al., 1987).

What develops specifically in successful school-age children may be not only the ability to perform the specific concrete operations themselves (this may have been accomplished some time earlier, as the "sleeping cows" example suggests) but also the ability to communicate about them consistently in conventional ways. Indeed, with cognition, as with almost every other aspect of the school-age youngster's development, joining society and sharing conventions is the theme. And, of course, the conventions to be shared, which differentiate the successful from the unsuccessful children, will be those established by the majority culture.

Schooling

Schooling refers to the ecological setting in which children learn. It refers to the environment, the size, the philosophy, the characteristic transactions between teachers and students, and the culture of the school. Patterns that reflect these aspects of schooling have been termed social regularities (Linney and Seidman, 1989). Schooling has a major effect on whether children succeed in adopting the conventions that will enable them to progress as contributing citizens. Remembering Erikson's articulated task for the school-age period, to master the industry of the society, attention must be directed to the larger ecological processes of schooling, the assessment of the developmental and cultural appropriateness of the environment, and the ways in which the school environment fosters participation, identity, and satisfaction.

Four aspects of schooling are discussed in this chapter. The first is the congruence of school environment with family culture and expectations, which is called "fit." The second is the social regularities within the school and their impact on the students. The third is the learning interaction; and the fourth is the involvement and effect of peers.

Two facets of congruence between the style of school and family as interfacing systems have been studied. The first involves expectations in the areas of educational goals, what is expected of the child, rules, and areas of permissiveness. Since the education system has been established by the majority culture, generally goals are congruent between school and majority families. Parents expect their children to attend school regularly, to be respectful, to be motivated, and to achieve. Problems come up when children can't or don't fulfill these expectations, which are ordinarily shared by family and school systems. They also come up, however, when these expectations are not shared by family and school systems. Then the all-too-common complaint that the child misbehaves at school but is fine at home, or, less commonly, the reverse, is brought to the attention of a counselor or mental health professional. This type of problem is most likely to be found in children from ethnic and cultural minority families (Phinney and Rotheram, 1986) and can be ameliorated when parents are intimately involved in school life, as James Comer has so elegantly demonstrated (see Chapter 109). The second facet concerns the congruence of the way school and family systems are organized. In general systems terms, interpersonal systems can be open and relatively closed, referring to characteristics of freedom of exchange with other systems, definition of system boundaries, and amount of variety that is encouraged or tolerated within the system. Some schools formed around specific religions are examples of closed systems, and these often serve a specific population with shared rules and values, constituting a good fit. Rules about conduct, limits, and

privacy are consistent across school and family and may differentiate each from the rest of society. Some schools have a more closed system than many of the families of children attending. The school personnel tends to see the families as irresponsible and incompetent, themselves as more capable caretakers. Open school systems allow for variability and have the potential of being flexible. But in many instances, open school systems interfacing with open family systems may have such a lack of definition that the children have no clear framework within which to define themselves. This kind of "congruence" between open family and open school systems often results in the involvement of the child with more systems, such as welfare, juvenile justice, or mental health (Rotheram, 1989).

A list of characteristics of effective schools includes strong leadership, an atmosphere that is orderly and not oppressive, teachers who participate in decision-making, school staff that has high expectations of students, and frequent monitoring of student progress (Linney and Seidman, 1989). A specific aspect of school environment that has been studied is school size. It has been shown that large schools are often "overmanned," meaning that there are more students than role opportunities; whereas in "undermanned" schools there are more opportunities for students to be involved in activities and to take more initiative. In these latter settings, the environmental role demands on the students increase the levels of student participation so that students can contribute to the school community, develop identified roles in this community, and become known to themselves and each other as distinctive individuals. In large schools there is the danger of anonymity and ultimately a high rate of dropping out and involvement in antisocial behavior and substance abuse. The movement to consolidate schools thus increases the chances that students will not have a positive experience in school, unless the student population is broken down into smaller units within which students experience a manageable-size community (Linney and Seidman, 1989).

The third aspect of schooling involves the interaction around learning. I have already discussed cognitive development and the importance of preparation and experiential congruence for the school-age child's success in mastering the academic material to be presented in primary school. Increasingly researchers in children's learning are informed by Vygotsky's ideas about the evolving mind in society. Children's accomplishments are evaluated not so much in terms of their individually self-contained abilities as in terms of their aggregate experiences, both historically and those presenting current challenges for mastery. In this framework, learning represents the transfer of responsibility for reaching a particular goal (Belmont, 1989). This transfer takes place in the zone of proximal development, which is defined as "the distance between the actual developmental level as determined by independent problem solving and the level of potential development as determined through problem solving under adult guidance or in collaboration with more capable peers" (Vygotsky, cited in Slavin, 1987, p. 1162). Some have proposed that the zone of proximal development (ZPD) might present a more useful measure of learning potential than IQ, since it realistically includes the instructional context as indispensable to the measured achievement. Evaluating the outcomes of strategy instruction (i.e., whether children adopt a presented strategy and apply it to other, similar situations without further instruction) leads to the observation that strategies presented in the lower area of the ZPD are readily generalized, in the midrange are adopted and gradually generalized, and toward the higher end of the zone may not be adopted at all (Belmont, 1989). Regarding learning as a transfer of responsibility and including the instructor in the measure of learning success puts the focus on areas of a particular child's readiness to advance as well as the particular teaching approach that is most likely to assist with those advances.

Fellow students as well as teachers provide assistance with developing more sophisticated problem solving, as is stated in Vygotsky's definition of the ZPD. Beyond the peer atmosphere, which is in itself dependent upon other aspects of schooling already discussed, there are specific methods of peer involvement in learning that have come to be known as "cooperative learning." Cooperative learning refers to any number of types of student groupings for learning but differs from peer tutoring in that the material is presented by the teacher rather than by the peers. Students may be given problems to solve or projects to complete, and the incentive to work together is encouraged by either rewarding the group's efforts, rewarding each individual child on the basis of the group's efforts, or rewarding the group on the basis of each child's achievement. Children can and will positively influence one another's progress. This is particularly true when some children in the group are more advanced than others, but it is also true when children are struggling to solve a new challenge. For example, using the Piagetian accomplishment of conservation, nonconserving children learn from peers who have mastered conservation, but they also progress in conservation skills when struggling with conservation problems with other nonconserving children (Slavin, 1987). When the process of working together is not specifically supervised and rewarded, often the more competent children take most of the responsibility for accomplishing the objectives or completing the project, while the less competent children do not contribute. But properly conceived, the value of cooperative teaching extends beyond the opportunities it creates for learning. It also provides a framework for learning about others, valuing differences, observing and utilizing the strengths of others, helping one another, and making a contribution to a community goal.

Self in Society

The school-age period is the first developmental epoch in which all children spend most of their waking hours in the company of children and adults who are not their family members; thus, this is a critical period for the formation of friendships, the evaluation of self in relation to others, and becoming a friend.

As with other developmental tasks, each child brings a particular pattern of prior experience to the task of developing a social self. Traditionally this has been in sharp focus in the psychological arena of the oedipal struggle and the child's own mastery of his or her drives. Further, this view explains the school-age child's interest in peers as in some ways compensating for the expulsion from the Eden of the relationship with the opposite-sex parent. There is considerable evidence that peers themselves have their own attractions, that a substantial if not primary influence over a child's social self development comes from the outside, predominantly through peer culture and its particular draw on the child's drives for mastery and competence. Robert White's (1959, 1960) description of the growth of competence drive in the school-age period emphasizes how to get along with others in the sense of competing, compromising, learning the rules of the game, and protecting oneself from injury. He points out that other children afford an opportunity to do something interesting with the environment and that gradually the world of contemporaries competes with the family circle. Bemporad (1984) describes the juvenile era as a period between separation and procreation in which peers are the intermediaries. He compares school child peer development with chimpanzee juveniles who learn without being taught, through imitation of adults. Bemporad suggests that Erikson's ideas about mastering industry place too much emphasis on personal development, encouraging competition and overlooking cooperation. In his earlier-cited cross-cultural comparisons, Kagan (Kagan and Klein, 1973) credits the society of peers for advancing the development of children in San Marcos from relative retardation in cognitive and interpersonal functioning. Several stages of peer development have been identified and described, and the ways in which peers distinguish and characterize one another become increasingly sophisticated over the course of the school-age period. Grunebaum and Solomon (1980) refer to Harlow's studies, concluding that young rhesus monkeys leave their mothers because peer relationships are interesting, not because they are rejected by their mothers (to this might be added that with humans, the mother's peers may also draw her away to a less-involved relationship with her child). Furthermore, the rhesus monkey studies indicate that affection and friendship between peers precedes aggressive behavior. In discussing cooperative learning, we have already seen how peer involvement shapes the intellectual and cognitive output of school-age children.

Sullivan (1953) was the first to emphasize the social influence on development. He described a series of internal processes that occur in the juvenile era, by which the child gradually substitutes his or her own standards of evaluation for those of family members. Sullivan proposed that, stimulated by the availability of adult and child models other than relatives, these processes unfold throughout the early school period. The first is *social subordination*, which reflects a change in the child's acceptance of authority from the specifics of personal caretakers to general categories such as the principal, police, crossing guards, and teachers. The child first evaluates peers in terms of how they are regarded by these authority figures. Next comes *social accommodation*, a process of acknowledging that there are differences between people. In young juvenile society, Sullivan points out, children are intolerant of differences and cruel, but gradually differences come to be respected. The child moves to *differentiation of authority figures*, comparing them, and even comparing parents to school-based authorities. *Control of focal awareness* refers to the child's response to social pressure to abandon some of his or her egocentric ideas and adopt a more conventional stance. *Sublimatory reformation* refers to the reorientation of focal awareness to the group-approved satisfactory behavior. And, finally, *supervisory patterns* reflect an awareness of one's behavior in groups. The supervisory patterns are almost like imaginary characters that develop in order to monitor oneself and eventually become internalized. Sullivan referred to his own ''editor,'' a critic of his writing who persisted into adulthood. (Sullivan's works were collected by his colleagues from lecture notes; his ''editor'' never allowed him to write anything that satisfied him.)

Sullivan's distinctive contribution provided a framework for study of social development. Grunebaum and Solomon (1982) proposed the following stages in the development of peer relationships from preschool through school-age: (*a*) unilateral partners and one-way assistance—the preschool child; (*b*) bilateral partners and fair-weather cooperation—middle childhood; and (*c*) chumship and consensual exchange—preadolescence (pp. 288–291). The late preschooler seeks out preferred friends for sustained periods of interactional play, but friendships are based on the playmate's ability and willingness to play in the way the child wishes. The first school-age phase is characterized by membership in peer groups, which offers a sense of belonging and an opportunity to manage aggressive impulses. ''Best friends'' are selected (and rejected) on a more abstract basis than in the preschool period. The second school-age stage (from about age 9) advances friendship to a closeness that Sullivan referred to as ''chumship'' with a peer of the same sex with whom an intimacy is formed, which paves the way for heterosexual intimacy and caring beginning in adolescence. Buhrmester and Furman's study of movement away from family into the peer culture confirm these hypothetical stages to some degree (1987). They examined children's attitudes and choices for companionship and intimacy by having children in the 2nd, 5th, and 8th grades rate the importance of companionship and intimate disclosure in different types of relationships, including those with parents, teachers, and peers. Family members were the most important sources for companionship for both 2nd and 5th graders, and same-sex peers were important throughout but were increasingly important as the subjects grew older. Only for 8th graders did opposite-sex peers become at all interesting. Girls tended to report intimate disclosure to peers earlier than boys, and this is probably a reflection of the fact that girls may value intimacy more than boys.

As peer interaction and the view of self in relation to others is vital to cognitive and intellectual development, so cognitive operations are vital to a child's emerging social self in the school-age period. Minuchin (1977) points out that children move from games such as ''Simon Says,'' ''Mother May I,'' and ''Follow the Leader,'' in which the children in groups follow the directions of a leader, to games in which the rules are set and governed by the players themselves, to games that involve contributions to the efforts of a team. This evolution involves shifts in the ways in which others are evaluated. Children begin the period by deeming others good if they give them things and bad if they take things away and move to recognizing skills and personal attributes, to finally acknowledging and valuing social attributes, such as fairness. This shift, in turn, requires the expansion of perspective, which permits a child to see a situation from another's point of view. The mountain range experiment illustrates the development of perspective. Here the child is shown the silhouettes of an irregular mountain range and is asked to draw how it looks to the examiner, who is behind them. The ability to imagine the other's perspective in the three-mountain test seems to correlate with the ability to imagine another's point of view about social and emotional issues as well. This may be seen as a cognitive component to empathy.

With social development, as with intellectual development, preparation and prior experience are substantial influences. Some patterns of interpersonal behavior are established very early, and some patterns may be more stable than others. For example, it has been observed that aggressiveness is established early, and generalized aggressive disposition and the tendency to exhibit aggression in the context of specific relationships are quite stable (Cummings et al., 1989). Aggressiveness is also associated with social rejection in the school-age period (Boivin and Begin, 1989; Rogosch and Newcomb, 1989). One view of the stability of aggression is that it is, indeed, constitutionally determined. An interactional pattern view of aggression is also supported by a number of observations. For example, Hartup (1989) reports that "early-timing" mothers, those whose first children are born when they are in their 20s, have more difficulty setting limits on their children than "late-timing" mothers do. Children of early-timing mothers are more likely to be aggressive, and in the absence of good limit setting within the family, the aggression becomes less amenable to social intervention.

Sociometric studies of school-age children yield up to five groups: popular, average, rejected, neglected, and controversial. Boivin and Begin (1989) found that there were two subgroups of rejected children, those who undervalued themselves and had low self-esteem, even in comparison to their teachers' evaluations of them, and those who had a positive view of themselves but were seen as defensive and aggressive. Rogosch and Newcomb (1989) asked children in different sociometric groups to evaluate themselves and one another and found that while they had anticipated that aggressive children would show attributional biases not shown by nonaggressive children, in fact these children's evaluations of others were not out of line, even though other children clearly identified the reputation of rejected children. They also found that negative reputation increasingly separates the rejected group at older ages.

In sum, the school-age child's development of self and self-concept is dependent upon the interaction with people outside the family, most particularly peers. Self-evaluation and evaluation of others, attachment and loyalty, and attribution of qualities evolve primarily through the peer culture. Effects of and on successful peer relationships resonate with cognitive development and academic success as well as with interpersonal patterns established in the family.

Clinical Syndromes Emerging in the School-age Period

There are a number of clinical syndromes that may make their first appearance or become pronounced in the school-age period because of the exposure of the child to social and experiential influences outside of his/her family.

Separation-anxiety disorder ("school phobia") may become apparent at this time, even though a child may have had a relatively successful adjustment to kindergarten.

Various developmental and learning disorders may also be noticed for the first time as youngsters face the formal learning environment. These include borderline or mild mental retardation and specific learning disorders.

While the activity level of youngsters with attention deficit hyperactivity disorder may have been noted during preschool, the difficulties such children have with organization, following, and conforming to the expectations of a classroom may emerge only in the first classroom experience. Similarly, these youngsters' problems with social coordination will become more apparent in the social environment of the early school-age period.

Encopresis and enuresis may become obvious first during the school-age period, because while excuses may be made for the preschooler, few would judge that a school-aged child who wets or soils is just a "late bloomer."

Finally, affective disorders, particularly depression, and anxiety disorders may make their appearance at this time in the context of the child's having to evaluate himself or herself in relation to other children and as viewed by adults who are not parents. Issues of self-esteem and worry about performance are just some of the stimuli for depression or anxiety in a vulnerable youngster.

CLINICAL IMPLICATIONS

This chapter has discussed the importance of socializing influences in the major developmental accomplishments in the school-age period. Developmental success is the outcome of intricate interactions between each child's individual developmental schedule, biological or constitutional endowments, and early life experience and the social and intellectual environment of school and life around school. Of the factors brought by the child into the school-age years, only extremes of biological or constitutional functioning are difficult to modify in the intensely socializing environment of schooling. This has been observed for social behavior, such as inhibition and extroversion (Kagan et al., 1989) and aggression (Cummings et al., 1989), and learning potential (Coles, 1987). What all of these authors note is that the child whose constitutional predisposition to inhibition, aggression, or learning disabilities presents serious obstacles to mastery of school-age tasks is rare. Kagan et al. (1989) maintain that a very shy child born with a low threshold for the generation of limbic arousal and psychological uncertainty about unfamiliar events, is qualitatively different from a child of average shyness. They propose that the long-term stability of such characteristics may hold for extremes but not for the entire group of children.

This means that most children are amenable to the socializing experiences of the school-age period, and when they experience difficulties, as so many do, it is necessary to consider the nature of their interactions in the important developmental areas that have been discussed. These include the fit between the child's prior and current experience, cognitive level, and the teaching received, the fit between schooling and the child's cultural expectations, and the child's integration into society outside of the family, particularly the peer group.

Patterns of fit are crucial to evaluate and modify, because there is considerable evidence that they have stability or a tendency to amplify deviance. In an assessment of home environment and school performance over the first 10 years of a child's life, Bradley et al. (1988) examined three models of environmental action: the early development effect, the prominence of contemporary environment, and the stability of environments over time. They found that there is a generally high correlation between early environment and later environments in terms of patterns and attitudes interacting with the child. If a child is regarded as academically less able in early school years and is placed in special education settings, the differences between his or her achievement and that of regular children are likely to increase over time. Similarly, a child who is socially rejected is likely to be further rejected as school life proceeds. The attitudes and ways peers behave toward socially rejected or vulnerable children can exacerbate early difficulties and increase the probability of later problems with adjustment (Cowen et al., 1973).

Indeed, most of the children designated as severely emotionally disturbed are dysfunctional in these very ways. They are failing academically, are socially rejected, and have a poor evaluation of themselves and their potential contribution to their present society. In addition, they frequently come from environments where there are impoverished resources, both financial and emotional. The influences of bad fit, social rejection, and academic failure have lasting consequences for these youngsters, not just because of their constitutional vulnerability but because of the recursiveness of interactional patterns, which perpetuate and accelerate bad fit, social rejection, and academic failure. These children become delinquent under the desperate influence of more competent peers; they drop out; they experience depression and hopelessness. They are prime targets for substance abuse, homelessness, and, if they survive, chronic involvement with institutional systems: criminal justice for males; protective services for females.

The task for the clinician assessing the development of school-age children, then, is to include with the careful evaluation of neurophysiological status an equally careful evaluation of child-in-society status. Together these complete the picture of the ongoing match between this child and the context in which he or she is to achieve mastery of the industry of society and entry into full participation into civilization.

References

Belmont JM: Cognitive strategies and strategic learning: The socio-instructional approach. *Am Psychol* 44:142–148, 1989.

Bemporad JR: From attachment to affiliation. *Am J Psychoanal* 44:792–799, 1984.

Boivin M, Begin G: Peer status and self-perception among early elementary school children: The case of the rejected children. *Child Dev* 60:591–596, 1989.

Bornstein B: On latency. *Psychoanal Study Child* 6:279–285, 1951.

Bradley RH, Caldwell BM, Rock SL: Home environment and school performance: A ten year follow-up and examination of three models of environmental action. *Child Dev* 69:852–867, 1988.

Buhrmester D, Furman W: The development of companionship and intimacy. *Child Dev* 58:1101–1113, 1987.

Buxbaum E: Between the Oedipus complex and adolescence: The "quiet" time. In: Greenspan SI, Pollock GH (eds): *Psychoanalytic Contributions Toward Understanding Personality Development*. Vol 2: *Latency, Adolescence, and Youth*. Rockville, MD, National Institute of Mental Health, 1980, pp. 121–136.

Coles G: *The Learning Mystique*. New York, Pantheon, 1987.

Combrinck-Graham L: A developmental model for family systems. *Fam Proc* 24:139–150, 1985.

Cowen EL, Pederson A, Babigian H, et al: Long term follow-up of early detected vulnerable children. *J Consult Clin Psychol* 41:438–445, 1973.

Coyle JT, Harris JC: The development of neurotransmitters and neuropeptides. In: Noshpitz J (ed): *Textbook of Child Psychiatry* (Vol 7). New York, Basic Books, 1987, pp. 14–25.

Cummings EM, Iannotti RJ, Zahn-Waxler C: Aggression between peers in early childhood: Individual continuity and developmental change. *Child Dev* 60:887–895, 1989.

Ditton P, Green RJ, Singer MT: Communication deviances: A comparison between parents of learning-disabled and normally achieving students. *Fam Process* 26:75–87, 1987.

Eccles JS, Jacobs JE: Social forces shape math attitudes and performance. *Signs* 11:367–389, 1986.

Erikson E: *Childhood in Society*. New York, Norton, 1950.

Gilligan C: *In a Different Voice: Psychological Theory and Women Development*. Cambridge, MA, Harvard University Press, 1982.

Green AH: Overview of normal psychosexual development. In: Schetky DH, Green AH (eds): *Child Sexual Abuse: A Handbook for Health Care and Legal Professionals*. New York, Brunner/Mazel, 1988, pp. 5–18.

Grunebaum H, Solomon L: Toward a peer theory of group psychotherapy. I: On the developmental significance of peers and play. *Int J Group Psychother* 30:23–49, 1980.

Grunebaum H, Solomon L: Toward a theory of peer relationships. II: On the stages of social development and their relationship to group psychotherapy. *Int J Group Psychother* 32:283–307, 1982.

Hall WS: Reading comprehension. *Am Psychol* 44:157–161, 1989.

Hartup WW: Social relationships and their developmental significance. *Am Psychol* 44:120–126, 1989.

Haskins R: Beyond metaphor: The efficacy of early childhood education. *Am Psychol* 44:274–282, 1989.

Heath SB: Oral and literate traditions among black Americans living in poverty. *Am Psychol* 44:367–373, 1989.

Jacklin CN: Female and male: Issues of gender. *Am Psychol* 44:127–133, 1989.

Kagan J: *The Nature of the Child*. New York, Basic Books, 1984.

Kagan J, Klein RE: Cross-cultural perspectives on early development. *Am Psychol* 28:947–961, 1973.

Kagan J, Resnick JS, Gibbons J: Inhibited and uninhibited types of children. *Child Dev* 60:838–845, 1989.

Kessen W: The American child and other cultural inventions. *Am Psychol* 34:815–820, 1979.

Kohlberg L: Stage and sequence: The cognitive-development approach to socialization. In: Goslin DA (ed): *Handbook of Socialization Theory and Research*. Chicago, Rand-McNally, 1969.

Linney JA, Siedman E: The future of schooling. *Am Psychol* 44:336–340, 1989.

Miller-Jones D: Culture and testing. *Am Psychol* 44:360–366, 1989.

Minuchin P: *The Middle Years of Childhood*. Belmont, CA, Brooks-Cole, 1977.

Offer D: Adolescent development: A normative perspective. In: Greenspan SI, Pollock GH (eds): *Psychoanalytic Contributions Toward Understanding Personality Development*. Vol 2: *Latency, Adolescence, and Youth*. Rockville, MD, National Institute of Mental Health, 1980, pp. 357–372.

Phinney J, Rotheram MJ: *Children's Ethnic Socialization: Pluralism and Development*. New York, Sage, 1986.

Piaget J: *The Moral Judgement of the Child*. New York, Free Press, 1948.

Rogosch FA, Newcomb AF: Children's perceptions of peer reputations and their social reputations among peers. *Child Dev* 60:597–610, 1989.

Rotheram MJ: The family and the school. In: Combrinck-Graham L (ed): *Children in Family Contexts*. New York, Guilford, 1989, pp. 347–368.

Rutter M: Normal psychosexual development. *J Child Psychol Psychiatry* 11:259–283, 1971.

Shapiro T, Perry R: Latency revisited: The age of 7 plus or minus 1. *Psychoanal Study Child* 31:79–105, 1976.

Slavin R: Developmental and motivational perspectives on cooperative learnings: A reconciliation. *Child Dev* 58:1161–1167, 1987.

Smith JD, Caplan J: Cultural differences in cognitive style development. *Dev Psychol* 24:46–52, 1988.

Sullivan HS: *The Interpersonal Theory of Psychiatry*. New York, Norton, 1953.

White RW: Motivation reconsidered: The concept of competence. *Psychol Rev* 66:297–333, 1959.

White RW: *Competence and the Psychosexual Stages of Development* (Nebraska Symposium on Motivation), 1960, pp. 97–141.

Wilson MN: Child development in the context of the black extended family. *Am Psychol* 44:380–385, 1989.

22 NORMAL ADOLESCENT DEVELOPMENT: EMPIRICAL RESEARCH FINDINGS

Daniel Offer, M.D., Kimberly A. Schonert-Reichl, Ph.D., and Andrew M. Boxer, Ph.D.

Recent years have witnessed a heightened interest in the scientific study of adolescence (e.g., Dornbusch et al., 1991; for reviews see Feldman and Elliott, 1990a; Offer and Schonert-Reichl; 1992; Takanishi, 1993). Adolescence is, perhaps more than ever before, regarded as a critical phase of the life course, deserving of attention and study. This increased attention to this phase in the life cycle has emerged, in part, due to the growing realization that youth today face more difficult problems and pressures than did youth a decade or two ago (Dryfoos, 1990; Hamburg, 1986; Phelan et al., 1994). Higher divorce rates, increases in the number of unwed mothers, competition for jobs, and continuing geographic mobility have all been cited as issues that render adolescents more vulnerable today than in the past (Cote and Allahar, 1994; Feldman and Elliott, 1990b). One of the current trends among adolescent researchers is to conduct studies that will provide beneficial information for those individuals involved in determining social policy (e.g., Dougherty, 1993). Thus, it is not surprising that the accumulating body of research findings on adolescence has been particularly useful in addressing national concerns regarding youth, such as teen pregnancy and parenting, substance abuse, school failure, and mental and physical health.

While adolescence is often described as an emergent life phase of the 20th century (for a review, see Aries, 1962; Petersen, 1988), reference to stereotypic behavior of adolescents can be found in the writings of both Plato and Aristotle. Rousseau is typically identified as having written about life cycle concepts, earlier described by Plato and Aristotle, describing two phases similar to what we now identify as adolescence (Rousseau, 1969). Adolescence is a socially defined phase of life in contemporary society (Demos and Demos, 1969; Kett, 1977; Modell et al., 1976; Petersen and Epstein, 1991) and may be differentiated from puberty. Puberty is frequently considered to mark the beginning of adolescence and is usually completed before adolescence has ended; however, the transition to adulthood, as a terminus to adolescence, is a more gradual process (Arnett and Taber, 1994; Greene and Boxer, 1986; Petersen and Taylor, 1980).

Within our own society, the course of life is understood as progression through a series of "life stations" (Neugarten and Hagestad, 1976; Riley et al., 1972), or socially defined tasks, stages, or strata, each of which is accompanied by a set of expectations regarding performance as well as sanctions for non-performance. The early part of the life cycle is more clearly age-graded now than was the case in the 19th century (Hagestad and Neugarten, 1984; Hogan, 1982; Neugarten and Hagestad, 1976). Age-grading is the system by which a society allocates role responsibilities and behaviors (Boxer and Petersen, 1986). In complex societies there are multiple systems of age-grading, both formal and informal, in relation to particular social institutions. For example, one is an adult in the American political system at age 18, but not in the economic system until one becomes a full-time worker (Neugarten and Hagestad, 1976).

The way in which adolescents are perceived at any given time is often a reflection of the needs of the society in which the adolescent is growing toward adulthood. For example, research conducted by Enright et al. (1987) demonstrated that even psychological theories of adolescence change in response to larger societal and economic conditions. Specifically, these researchers found that during times of economic depression theoretical writings about adolescents tended to emphasize characteristics such as immaturity and the need for prolonged schooling. Such writings would most likely reflect the society's need to deter youth's entrance into the labor force. In contrast, during times of war, theorists characterized adolescents as competent and adultlike—qualities necessary for success in warfare. Thus, it is important to recognize that the opportunities, demands, and constraints that adolescents face can change in response to the sociopolitical climate in which they are developing.

During adolescence a great deal of age-grading occurs, for example, in the ascription of social maturity related to such behaviors as alcohol consumption, driving, and voting. This age-gradedness increases the usefulness of chronological age (or grade in school) as a marker of social status and thereby accentuates the distinctiveness of subgroups of adolescents. Traditionally, adolescence has been viewed as a single, undifferentiated transition en route to adulthood. The predominant emphasis was on a set of age-related changes as they were thought to characterize the phase in its entirety (see Greene and Boxer, 1986). More recently, some investigators have begun to conceptualize adolescence as a *course* of events and experiences, with the impact of distinct life events having differential implications for early, middle, and late adolescence. Therefore, many researchers who now study adolescent development often differentiate divisions of that stage into early, middle, and late adolescence because of age-associated differences in the biological, social, and cognitive behaviors of adolescents (Hamburg, 1974; Kagan, 1971; Thornburg, 1983). The individual's lifetime is further shaped by the superimposition of a biological clock. It is possible, for example, for a young person of 9 years to be labeled adolescent because of a biological status in the early stages of puberty. Conversely, another young person may not begin puberty until age 15 or 16 years. Typically, however, for most individuals, puberty is a phenomenon characteristic of early adolescence.

Puberty involves a rather dramatic set of changes in which a child's body gradually comes to approximate that of an adult. Physical maturation presages many other changes for a developing adolescent. For example, one of the outcomes of puberty is the attainment of mature reproductive potential. This potential affects the adolescent's self-image, as well as assumptions and expectations regarding sexual behavior and social interactions. The new physical status of the postpubertal adolescent, in terms of size, shape, and appearance, is accompanied by a variety of social and psychological expectations. Significant others, such as friends, teachers, and family members, may begin to react differently to a young adolescent, effecting a shift in the socially shared definitions of the self (Tobin-Richards et al., 1983).

From the standpoint of many adults, including a surprisingly large number of mental health professionals, adolescence is perceived as a particularly tumultuous phase of development (see, for example, Blos, 1962; Erikson, 1959; Freud, 1946, 1958; Offer et al., 1981a; Rabichow and Sklansky, 1980). Indeed, from the perspective of several noted theorists and clinicians, if an adolescent does not go through a serious and prolonged identity crisis, something will be very much disturbed about the adolescent's psychological adjustment. The term *adolescent turmoil* has been used freely by mental health professionals to describe both disturbed adolescents and processes of normal development (Offer, 1987). During the last two decades, Offer and his colleagues have examined normal adolescent development (Offer, 1969; Offer and Offer, 1975; Offer et al., 1981b, 1988) across many diverse populations of teenagers both within the United States and around the world. The findings from these studies indicate that the majority of teenagers (approximately 80%) do not experience turmoil or psychological disturbance. These teenagers portray themselves in ways that bear little resemblance to the stressed, stormy, and rebellious youths described originally by G. Stanley Hall (1904), Anna Freud (1946), and other psychoanalytic theorists. Those who study representative samples of normal teenagers have come to the conclusion that good coping and a smooth transition into adulthood are more typical than the opposite (e.g., Csikszentmihalyi and Larson, 1984; Douvan and Adelson, 1966).

In this chapter we review empirical research on normative adolescent development. We first consider the biological and psychosocial changes associated with puberty, followed by a discussion of the general social and psychological changes that occur during adolescence. Next we consider the definitions of normality within the adolescent phase of life. We then provide results of empirical research on the self-image of representative samples of adolescents and describe gender and age differences in self-image during this phase of life. Finally, we present information regarding adolescent development and clinical services, with particular focus on mental health professionals' conceptions of normal adolescent and adolescent help-seeking behavior. Our purpose is to highlight some of the recent empirical research on adolescence in order to convey a general sense of adolescents in today's society. It should be noted that this review is not meant to be exhaustive because of the plethora of recent adolescent research that has emerged in the last 10 years. For the current review, we provide just a sampling of important work in this area. For further information concerning research on adolescent development not covered in the present chapter, the reader is referred to several excellent recent works (e.g., Feldman and Elliott, 1990a; Lerner et al., 1991; Takanishi, 1993).

PUBERTY

Puberty is actually the culmination of a lengthy and complex maturational process that begins before birth (Brooks-Gunn and Reiter, 1990; Petersen and Taylor, 1980) and may be indexed by a set of physical changes. We shall not review in depth the biology of puberty but draw attention to the contours of this process, which have implications for the psychological development of youth. The hormonal systems that mature during puberty have been established since birth but are then suppressed for several years. When compared to other biological changes that occur over the course of a lifetime, the changes of the phase we call puberty are dramatic both in their rate and in the magnitude of change that occurs. The rate of growth and development during puberty is second only to that which occurs in infancy (Petersen and Taylor, 1980).

In the 1970s, endocrine studies documented the rise in pubertal hormones that is generally parallel to the emergence of secondary sex characteristics. Some of the most important work on puberty has examined mechanisms that control pubertal processes (Comite et al., 1987; Grumbach et al., 1974; see also Petersen, 1988).

The most observable changes of puberty emerge over an average of 4 years. They begin and end approximately 2 years earlier for girls than for boys (Tanner, 1962, 1971, 1974); however, depending upon the indicators being examined, the variability between boys and girls is different. For example, while pubic hair development is about 2 years later for males than for females, breast and genital development differ by approximately only 6 months (Petersen and Taylor, 1980). The lag between pubic hair and breast development is greater in girls than is the time difference between genital and pubic hair development in boys. These variations seem to be due, in part, to the different hormones responsible for these changes. While androgens influence pubic hair and genital development, estrogens are primarily responsible for mammary development.

During puberty, as levels of particular hormones increase sharply, secondary sex characteristics emerge with increases in body size. Secondary sex characteristics refer to any of various anatomical characteristics that first emerge at puberty and differentiate between the sexes but do not have a direct reproductive function. These characteristics include body and facial hair, breast development, and voice change. Primary sex characteristics, also transformed during puberty, refer to those differentiating anatomical and physiological characteristics, internal and external, that bear directly on reproductive functioning (e.g., genitalia). Although the physically apparent changes are dramatic, the underlying hormonal process itself is very gradual and lasts much longer, with hormone increases starting between the ages of 5 and 8 years in both sexes (Brook, 1981).

The hormonal systems were established prenatally but become activated with puberty. Some investigators believe that the system is suppressed to maintain low levels of hormones during childhood (Grumbach et al., 1974). With puberty, the suppression is gradually released, and hormones in the brain stimulate the production of gonadal hormones such as testosterone in the testes and estrogen in the ovaries. It has also been observed that reaching a critical "metabolic level" or fat-to-lean ratio, roughly represented by weight, appears to be correlated with the beginning of puberty in both boys and girls (Frisch, 1980a, 1980b, 1983a, 1983b; Frisch and McArthur, 1974; Frisch et al., 1980).

Timing of Puberty

The implications of pubertal change for mental health seem to be related to two aspects of puberty: pubertal status and pubertal timing (Petersen, 1988). The timing of pubertal changes is likely to be important for an adolescent's peer group status and for the social stimulus value that may produce particular psychological and social responses from the adolescent and others around him or her. Timing effects may also have particular consequences for growth. For example, some evidence suggests that late developers have longer limbs, resulting from a longer prepubertal period of growth (Tanner, 1974).

The physical changes of puberty have been divided into stages by the pediatrician J. Tanner (1962, 1974). Pubertal stages are described in terms of genital development (boys), breast development (girls), and pubic hair development (both sexes). The stages have enabled researchers interested in the pubertal process to make ratings of these visual changes as an index of biological status. Because they do not reflect measurement of precise levels of circulating hormones, these stages can be regarded as a rough index of an underlying biological process resulting in physiological change. Studies have found predicted endocrine changes for groups of individuals at each pubertal stage (see, for example, Gupta et al., 1975).

The changes of puberty follow a characteristic or typical sequence. In a small number of individuals, a step may be skipped or, infrequently, when there is a serious illness during puberty, an individual may return to an earlier stage of development. The timing of changes in characteristics also shows typical patterns.

For girls, beginning breast development is one of the first signs of puberty. The onset of menstruation (menarche) occurs later in the pubertal sequence. Two earlier visible changes are the appearance of pubic hair and growth spurt; further development of both of these characteristics continues across the pubertal phase. For boys, pubic hair growth and penis growth frequently initiate the visible pubertal changes. Axillary (underarm) hair then appears, and pubic hair distribution is extended, while voice changes and facial hair generally occur somewhat later (Brook, 1981; Petersen and Taylor, 1980).

In contrast to these normative patterns for both boys and girls, the timing of each physical characteristic relative to the others can vary considerably from individual to individual (Eichorn, 1975). Indeed, a great deal of variation occurs interindividually. Of course, the variation that occurs is not readily apparent when examining the average patterns of pubertal changes across groups of individuals. How fast a child proceeds through puberty does not seem to be related to whether puberty is occurring early or late (Tanner, 1971). Although for girls puberty begins and ends, on the average, about 1½–2 years before it does for boys, depending on which characteristic is compared, timing of pubertal onset and its completion varies by as much as 6 years for both boys and girls (Hagg and Taranger, 1982). When examining the range of variation possible, puberty for girls normally occurs between the ages of 8 and 18. For boys puberty normally occurs between the ages of 9 and 19.

Most data suggest that puberty has been beginning earlier and earlier for at least the last century. For example, there has been a trend to an earlier menarche of approximately 3–4 months per decade in Europe during the last 100 years (Frisch, 1983b; Tanner, 1991). Data reported in Britain during the 19th century on age-specific fertility, the ages of reproductive events, and nutrition and growth showed that undernourished males and females completed their growth 4–5 years later than well-nourished contemporary males and females (Frisch, 1978, 1980b, 1983b, 1978). The existence of this secular trend toward earlier puberty has raised concern, particularly among educators and service providers, as to the limits at which this trend will stop. However, the onset of puberty appears to be associated with a critical "metabolic level" roughly represented by weight. Gradually over several generations, nutrition and health care have improved, resulting in taller and heavier people, probably coming closer to their optimal genetic potentials (Tanner, 1981). Thus, improvements in nutrition and health are likely to be the main cause of earlier pubertal onset. Given an adequate environment, including sufficient nutrition, good medical care, and generally good health, people will grow no taller than they are genetically programmed to grow. Nutrition and health status for many in America today have reached this level; therefore, both final height attained and timing of pubertal onset appear to have reached stable plateaus (Petersen, 1988).

Gender Differences in Pubertal Development

Particular physical sex differences emerge, and others are enhanced during puberty. Body shape changes during puberty, with girls developing broader hips and boys broader shoulders (Faust, 1977; Petersen, 1979). Sex differences also appear in the amount of body hair that emerges during puberty, with boys developing more hair than girls. After the adolescent growth spurt, boys are taller and heavier than girls, primarily because of the growth-limiting effect of the earlier onset of puberty in girls (Petersen and Taylor, 1980). The prepubertal, or childhood, growth period involves especially the growth of the long bones in the arms and legs; thus, an earlier puberty terminates this sort of growth sooner (Garn, 1980). Boys, on the average, grow for 2 more years than girls before they begin the adolescent growth spurt. This results in shorter stature for girls by the conclusion of the growth spurt. Although the amount of growth that occurs during puberty is somewhat greater for boys than girls, most of the sex difference in adult height is caused by the longer period of prepubertal growth in males (Bock et al., 1973; Hagg and Taranger, 1982). While some of the hormones that control the adolescent growth spurt are different from those that control prepubertal growth, the amount of height added during the adolescent growth spurt is highly related to the amount of growth attained prior to it (Tanner, 1974). Someone who is tall prior to puberty will generally, though not always, be tall after puberty.

In addition to the sex difference in height, a sex difference in the ratio of muscle to fat is seen postpubertally. At the conclusion of puberty, boys generally have greater strength and musculature. Succumbing to the strong sociocultural pressure to cease what is considered to be a masculine activity, many girls tend to exercise less than boys, especially from puberty onward. This may contribute to the sex difference in strength. Cross-cultural research as well as research with women athletes in this country has shown that when girls engage in strenuous and vigorous exercise through childhood, they develop a magnitude of strength similar to that of boys (Buchbinder, 1976; see also Warren, 1983). Although many of the physical sex differences are related to the differential levels of hormones active in male and female bodies, the extent of development of the biological potential of a physical characteristic in an individual is due to cultural values, expectations, practices, opportunities, and activities.

Social-Psychological Influences on Puberty

It often has been assumed that biological processes influence an individual's psychological state in a unidirectional manner. More recently, however, research has indicated that psychological, social, and physical events also influence biological systems, at times synergistically. The fact that an adolescent is conscious of and can attribute meaning to pubertal changes contributes to the potential for influencing biological development (Boxer and Petersen, 1986). Therefore, not only does a child respond psychologically to biological change, but a child's psychological state may, in turn, influence biological systems. In addition, both the timing and final outcome of the pubertal process can be affected by psychosocial factors. These influences may also have indirect effects on the growth process.

For example, in an earlier onset of puberty, the duration of the prepubertal or childhood period is reduced, and therefore the time available for prepubertal height growth is affected. Correspondingly, it has been reported that the onset of menarche can be delayed by maintaining a low fat-to-muscle ratio, thereby affecting metabolic level. In regard to physical events that contribute to this outcome, extensive exercise (at least 5 hours of training per day) in combination with a restricted diet, a routine maintained by some serious dancers and runners, typically leads to amenorrhea, if menstruation had begun, or to postponement of menarche (Frisch, 1980a, 1980b; Frisch et al., 1980). Also related to this is the idea that an individual's psychological state (including such aspects as motivation) may influence whether he or she chooses to engage in particular behaviors, such as exercise or other forms of physical training (Gargiulo et al., 1987).

Under extreme stress the menstrual cycle may be interrupted or cease completely for a time, as is the case for many women with anorexia nervosa. If anorexia starts early enough and continues long enough during important periods of growth, it approximates a state of near starvation, resulting in stunted growth (Crisp, 1969; Garfinkel and Garner, 1982). While there may be a physical deprivation component involved

that affects biological systems (e.g., lack of food leading to weight loss), the precipitant that may lead some girls to believe that they need to lose weight may be psychological in origin. Additionally, there are documented cases of girls with diagnosed anorexia who had reached a near ideal weight but who were still suffering from various psychological difficulties (Katz et al., 1977). The young women in this study were demonstrated (in detailed endocrine analyses) to have immature patterns of particular hormone secretions. These abnormalities were present despite the minor weight deficit but with the presence of active psychological symptoms. The authors advanced the explanation of the possible role of psychological factors in influencing hormone functioning.

The hormone behavior literature is replete with examples of the ways in which psychological states can affect biological systems. Recently, researchers have suggested that the timing of puberty may be affected by the degree to which adolescents experience stressful interpersonal relationships within the family (Belsky et al., 1991). They suggest that adolescents may be likely to respond to family discord by maturing as quickly as possible in order to leave an unhappy family situation and find other relationships outside the home. This is a sociobiological argument because it emphasizes that members of a species are likely to have evolved behaviors that enable them to successfully adapt to different environmental situations. Extrapolating from research on animals suggesting that continued close association with parents or other dominant adults delays physical maturation while forceful removal from the family unit leads to the earlier onset of puberty, Belsky et al. (1991) argue that adolescents with a family history of conflict and stress may experience puberty earlier than their same-age peers. Some research exists that supports Belsky et al.'s contention. For example, Moffitt et al. (1992), in a longitudinal study examining the association of childhood family experiences and the time of menarche, found that girls with unhappy family experiences at age 7 experienced puberty earlier than those girls who experienced happier family experiences. Although much more research is needed in order to offer a firm conclusion that stressful family circumstances lead to earlier onset of puberty among some adolescents, Belsky et al. have raised some interesting questions concerning the links between puberty and psychosocial experiences in human development.

Another example is found in cases of pseudocyesis (false pregnancy) (Yen et al., 1976). In one detailed case study (Yen et al., 1976), a 16-year-old female with no previous history of physical or psychological difficulties believed she was pregnant (after a pregnancy test revealed what later turned out to be a false positive); she manifested all the visual signs of pregnancy (including cessation of the menses, as well as a distended stomach). After what she believed was 38 weeks of gestation, the young woman went to a hospital where it was determined, through physical examination, that she was not pregnant. Endocrine studies of this young woman revealed that she had significantly elevated levels of particular hormones related to the reproductive system (luteinizing hormone and prolactin). When she was told of her actual condition (no pregnancy), these hormone levels dropped significantly and her distended stomach deflated within 30 minutes (after the discharge of large amounts of flatus). This study provided evidence of actual hormonal changes resulting from pseudocyesis.

From these examples it should be clear that biological development is difficult to separate neatly from psychological or social dimensions of change. In addition, many other factors also interact with biological systems, including nutritional intake, physical activity level, and even such environmental conditions as season of the year or time of the day (Halberg, 1980). Therefore, there is a complex interplay among biological, social, and psychological domains of development, an interaction that has been termed *biopsychosocial*.

Psychological Significance of Pubertal Change

Research that has examined pubertal development in relation to psychological functioning has found some evidence for an association between pubertal effects and psychological adjustment. Many researchers measure pubertal effects indirectly, rather than through the direct measurement of hormones. For example, congruent with other research conducted to date, Crockett and Petersen (1987) found, controlling for age, that advancing pubertal status was related to improved moods and increased body image for boys but decreased feelings of attractiveness for girls. Other research, examining the association between pubertal development and the daily subjective states of young adolescents, found that, for both boys and girls, pubertal development was associated with the specific emotional experience of the feeling of being in love (Richards and Larson, 1993). In accord with previous findings, Richards and Larson also found no association between average mood state and emotional variability to puberty for girls and an association between physical maturity and positive mood states to puberty in boys.

Some researchers have hypothesized that pubertal change is most stressful when it puts the young adolescent in a different or "deviant" status from his or her peers (Simmons et al., 1983). It has been suggested that pubertal events noticeable by others (e.g., height, weight, breast development) are more likely to affect psychological states than nonpublic changes (Petersen, 1985, 1988).

Pubertal timing is one area of research that has received widespread attention in the last several years. Pubertal timing refers to whether or not the adolescent's physiological maturation is occurring on time, early, or late relative to his or her same-sex peers. Several researchers have noted effects of early and late maturation on boys' and girls' psychological and academic adjustment. Research conducted by Dubas et al. (1991) found that late maturing boys displayed the lowest academic achievement and late maturing girls displayed the highest. In general, it appears that early maturing boys seem to have an advantage over late maturing boys in many aspects of both psychosocial and academic functioning. However, the effects of early maturation on girls' psychological development and academic achievement is more variable (Brooks-Gunn and Reiter, 1990). For example, in a study conducted by Simmons and Blyth (1987), early-maturing girls experienced more popularity with boys but poorer academic achievement. The grade in which adjustment was assessed also seemed to be a factor. In the sixth grade, early-maturing girls possessed more positive body images than did late-maturing girls, whereas in the tenth grade the opposite pattern emerged. That is, by grade ten, late-maturing girls were more satisfied with their bodies than were early-maturing girls. One reason offered for this finding concerns the relationship between physical development and pubertal timing. Specifically, by late adolescence, early-maturing females tend to be shorter and stockier due to the early occurrence of their growth spurt. In contrast, late-maturing females tend to be taller and thinner by late adolescence, thereby more closely approximating North America's ideal of feminine beauty.

Fewer studies have employed direct measurement of pubertal change (e.g., examining hormone levels) in relation to psychological development. Nottelmann et al. (1987) have found some associations between adjustment problems, particularly for boys, and a profile of later physical maturation. Since adrenal androgen level is responsive to environmental stressors, lower levels of sex steroids and higher levels of both adrenal androgen and adjustment were interpreted as indexing a stress-related process.

While pubertal hormones may affect sexual interest and aggression (Meyer-Bahlburg et al., 1985; Susman et al., 1987; Udry et al., 1985, 1986), the discernible effects are mediated by and interact with social and psychological factors (Petersen, 1988). The social stimulus value of puberty (Petersen and Taylor, 1980) is likely to be as important as the biological changes of puberty themselves. Future research on puberty may find particular effects on specific subgroups of adolescents (see Petersen, 1988). Newer and more sophisticated methods of endocrine assay may be able to further specify the relations between hormones and behavior.

During adolescence, cognitive abilities increase, particularly with regard to abstract thinking (Keating and Clark, 1980; Petersen, 1983). While some investigators have demonstrated pubertal timing effects

(e.g., early maturers manifest higher IQ test performance) on aspects of cognition (Newcombe and Dubas, 1987), there is no evidence that links changes in cognition to pubertal processes (Petersen, 1985, 1988).

Adolescence has typically been identified as the phase during which abstract thinking first emerges. Piaget's stages of formal operations, for example, have been assessed in many different ways and along many different dimensions (Martorano, 1977). In consequence there appear to be many variations in the extent to which youth develop these capacities (Keating, 1990). Most adolescents develop some capacity to take account of the perspectives or viewpoints of others (Keating and Clark, 1980). The sensitivity many adolescents manifest in response to evaluation by parents, teachers, and peers is also likely to be a result of egocentric thinking (Dornbusch, 1989). Elkind (1975) described a heightened egocentrism emerging during early adolescence. Such egocentricity may lead to increased introspection and a propensity for youth to feel themselves the center of attention by others. Many youth often believe their thoughts and feelings are unique to them. These tendencies have been shown to decrease from early to late adolescence (Lapsley, 1990). Newer research on cognition is focused on investigating situation-specific and context-related influences that are likely to be partially responsible for the variations found in adolescent cognitive changes.

The role of puberty in adolescent development has thus been attributed a more powerful influence than appears to be justified. Existing evidence does not suggest a "raging hormone" theory regarding the impact of puberty on adolescents' behavior (for a review of research on the direct effects of pubertal hormones on behavior, see Buchanan et al., 1992). It is quite clear, however, that puberty culminates in a dramatic and visually apparent set of changes. The sociocultural meanings of these changes are an important social-psychological component to understanding the significance of puberty for adolescents and their behavior (Boxer et al., 1989; Petersen, 1985).

Biopsychosocial Development: the Sample Case of Sexuality

We have been discussing adolescence as a unique phase of life because of the simultaneous occurrence of a set of developmental changes in physical maturation, psychological adjustment, and social relations. Adolescence is also generally regarded as a critical period for the emergence of adult forms of sexual behavior (Boxer et al., 1989; Petersen and Boxer, 1982). However, the development of sexual behavior differs in some important respects from other aspects of development at adolescence. There is some expectation that individuals will learn behavior that facilitates reproduction. However, sexuality is not simply the result of biological factors; sociocultural and psychological determinants of development are interwoven in a way that is usually synergistic. Psychological aspects include sexual identity and the desire or motivation for sexual involvement, subjective perceptions of invulnerability (and other health-related beliefs relating to risk taking), and self-image (including body image), as well as more personal meanings that sexuality may hold for the individual. Sociocultural factors include cultural values and beliefs and the implicit and explicit sexual socialization influences of one's social context (e.g., community and peer group). Importantly, AIDS as a life-threatening illness and as a historical event is changing the meanings and context of sexuality in general, and in particular for adolescents. While there are few existing data on human immunodeficiency virus (HIV) seroprevalence rates among adolescent populations, the number of reported AIDS cases (approximately 1% of all reported AIDS cases are adolescents between 13 and 21), although currently low, is doubling each year (Brooks-Gunn et al., 1988; Hein, 1989).

In order to understand the development of sexual behavior, a life course perspective is necessary, in which earlier and later phases of adolescence are considered, as well as the sociocultural context of these phases of development. This includes important groups in which youth spend time and are socialized (Csikszentmihalyi and Larson, 1984). Traditionally, adolescence has been viewed as a single, undifferentiated transition en route to adulthood (A.L. Greene and A.M. Boxer, unpublished manuscript, 1990). The predominant emphasis was on a set of age-related changes as they were thought to characterize the phase in its entirety. More recently, some investigators have begun to conceptualize adolescence as a course of events and experiences, with the impact of distinct life events having differential implications for early, middle, and late adolescence (Hamburg, 1974; Kagan, 1971; Lerner and Foch, 1987; Thornburg, 1983). The timing of first intercourse, for example, has been found to be an important predictor of psychosexual adjustment in young adulthood (Jessor and Jessor, 1975, 1977; Jessor et al., 1983). Ethnic differences in the timing and structure of sexual experiences are also apparent. For example, white youth, more than black youth, have been found to engage in a predictable series of noncoital behaviors for a period of time before their first intercourse experience (Smith and Udry, 1985). First-time heterosexual intercourse among youth has been found typically to be an unplanned and unprotected event (Alan Guttmacher Institute, 1981; Zelnik and Kantner, 1977, 1980; Zelnik et al., 1981). In a survey conducted in the early 1980s, Zelnik and Shah (1983) found that only 17% of young women and 25% of the men had planned their first act of sexual intercourse. Not surprisingly, then, increases in teen pregnancy have been attributed to teenagers who become sexually active before the age of 15 (Alan Guttmacher Institute, 1981). Taken together, the available data suggest that, while teens become more sexually active over time, their first and/or earliest sexual experiences may carry the greatest risk for pregnancy, sexually transmitted diseases (STDs), and HIV infection and may carry other psychosocial consequences.

Studies conducted in the 1970s suggest that adolescents generally are engaging in a greater range of sexual behaviors at earlier ages. Over the past 30 years fundamental changes in adolescent sexual development have lowered the mean age of first sexual intercourse. However, there is little current information on specific sexual behaviors outside of genital intercourse. Although the best studies of contemporary adolescent sexual behavior are now dated, Zelnick and Kantner's work demonstrated changes during the 1970s that also carry implications for the changing context of adolescent development as well as for the transmission of HIV infection and STDs. They found that in metropolitan areas of the United States in 1979, 50% of all 15- to 19-year-old females reported having engaged in premarital intercourse, compared with 43% in 1976 and 30% in 1971 (Zelnik and Kantner, 1980). While large increases have been documented between 1971 and 1979, subsequently the percentage of sexually active girls appears to be more stable (Brooks-Gunn and Furstenberg, 1989; Hayes, 1987; Hofferth and Hayes, 1987). Data on males comparable to that reported on females are nonexistent, largely because fertility has been considered a female issue (Brooks-Gunn and Furstenberg, 1989).

Historical changes have also been demonstrated in recent cohort analyses of young adult samples. Gebhard's (Gebhard, 1977; Gebhard and Johnson, 1979) comparison of Kinsey data and more contemporary data on college youth shows that most aspects of sexual knowledge are being learned earlier than they had been 30 years ago. Wyatt's recent studies (Wyatt et al., 1988a; see also Wyatt et al., 1988b) also reveal many fundamental changes in sexuality among groups of women, with three-quarters of the respondents reporting coitus by age 18. The relationship of gender and ethnicity to these sexual behaviors appears to be changing. While boys tend to begin practicing sexual behaviors at younger ages than girls, some evidence suggests the differences between boys' and girls' sexual experiences are narrowing (Brooks-Gunn and Furstenberg, 1989; Dreyer, 1982).

There is a paucity of studies of black adolescents, but existing data suggest that black youth begin sexual activity earlier than white youth (Dreyer, 1982). Data from the National Longitudinal Survey of youth demonstrate that 60% of white boys had intercourse by 18, and 60% of white girls by age 19. For black boys, 60% had intercourse by age 16, and 60% of black girls by age 18 (Hofferth and Hayes, 1987).

A conservative estimate places the number of Americans living ex-

clusively as "homosexual" at 12 million adults; teenagers comprise some 3 million homosexually inclined youth (Sladkin, 1983). Transient homosexual contact between heterosexually active adolescent males is typically not defined as "homosexuality" and does not necessarily lead to the sexual identity "gay" or "homosexual" (Gagnon and Simon, 1973). Homosexual contacts are most frequent before age 15 and are more likely to be experienced by boys than by girls (Kinsey et al., 1948, 1953). The label "gay" or "lesbian" adolescent appears to represent a unique cultural category in history. This category is manifested in a newly emerging generation of gay-/lesbian-identified adolescents who should be distinguished from other youth who may experience homosexual desires or engage in homosexual behavior (but who may not identify as being "gay" or "lesbian"). Where earlier generations of same-sex attracted persons lived less openly, many of today's gay youth, by contrast, assume the possibility of striving for and achieving unprecedented life goals and open social relationships at home, school, and work, unknown to most persons of the earlier generations (Gerstel et al., 1989). Empirical studies across the past 20 years show that the mean age of self-identification as gay/lesbian has been decreasing across age cohorts. Most findings have been reported retrospectively but are consistent. For example, in their study conducted in the late 1960s, Saghir and Robins (1973) report a mean age of 21 for males and 22 for females. In their San Francisco study of gays and lesbians conducted in 1970, Bell and Weinberg (1978) report mean ages of 18 for males and 23 for females, and they also demonstrated significant minority differences, blacks having developmentally earlier homosexual experiences than whites. A recent investigation conducted in Chicago examined developmental and cultural dimensions of the "coming out" process as they occurred among 202 self-identified gay and lesbian youth (ages 14–21) (Boxer and Cohler, 1989; Gerstel et al., 1989). The mean age of gay/lesbian self-identification among this culturally diverse sample is 16.7 years for males and 16.0 for females (Boxer, 1988). These studies suggest that, as cultural barriers against homosexuality have lessened, the age of self-definition as gay or lesbian is lowering among both sexes and generally occurs after subjects have engaged in some homosexual behavior.

With the threat of AIDS, prevention research on the impact of adolescent sex education and decision-making has taken on a new significance and importance. There is little conclusive evidence that demonstrates that sex education improves adolescents' responsible sexual behavior (e.g., using contraceptives, including condoms, when sexually active, or abstaining from sexual behavior when unprotected, etc.) (Boxer et al., 1989). A national evaluation of sex education programs (Kirby, 1983, 1984; Kirby et al., 1979) indicates that most nonclinic sex education courses increase knowledge; however, they have no significant impact on sexual behavior or contraceptive use. In a recent short-term longitudinal study of sexually active adolescents in the San Francisco area, perceptions that condoms prevent STDs were high, but only 2.1% of the females and 8.2% of the males reported condom use every time they had intercourse during the year of the study (Kegeles et al., 1988). The only programs that had a clear impact on behavior were those that provided a directly relevant experiential component. In addition, when health clinics were included within high schools, there was an increase in contraceptive use, decreased teen pregnancy rates, and no demonstrable increase in sexual behaviors (Kirby, 1984; Zabin et al., 1986).

Engaging adolescents in successful sexuality prevention/intervention programs necessitates the discussion of sexual desire and the pleasurable aspects of sex, because typically youth experience sex in this manner and are likely to ignore interventions that do not acknowledge this (Fine, 1988; Levinson, 1986). Students appear to be unlikely to relate to a model who treats sexual decision-making as only an informational process. The most effective intervention strategies may need to include helping teens recognize, accept, and plan for sexual feelings (Levinson, 1984, 1986). Youths can gain mastery of their sexual feelings by correctly attributing their physical and emotional states to sexual arousal rather than to other kinds of external forces (e.g., persuasion, drugs, etc.).

Social Change

Adolescence is a time in development in which individuals are expanding their relationships beyond the family and into the larger social world. One of the most salient change that takes place concerns the shift from parents to peers as providers of companionship and intimacy (Buhrmester and Furman, 1987). Indeed, adolescents spend twice as much time with their peers than do children (Csikszentmihalyi and Larson, 1984), and such peer experiences serve a developmental need that cannot be fulfilled by parents (Youniss and Smollar, 1985). Moreover, adolescents begin to place greater importance on their peers' approval and advice (Brown, 1990). The salience of the peer group in adolescence also appears to differ across the various stages of adolescence. Gavin and Furman (1989) found that early and middle adolescents reported placing more value on being a member of a popular peer group and perceived more group conformity among peer group members than did preadolescents and late adolescents. In addition, they found that more antagonist interactions and fewer positive interactions were characteristic of early and middle adolescent peer groups than they were of the preadolescent or late adolescent peer groups. The authors suggest that "The sense of belonging gained by membership in a popular group may allow teens to feel secure in the social arena, bolstering their sense of identity as they seek to separate from the family unit" (p. 832).

Adolescents' relationships with peers are qualitatively different from those of children. Take, for example, the way in which friendships are defined. Whereas childhood conceptualizations of friendship emphasize concrete and quantitative dimensions (e.g., sharing toys, frequency of contact), it is during adolescence that more abstract dimensions, such as self-disclosure (e.g., "I can tell my friend anything about myself") are emphasized (Selman, 1980). Empathy (i.e., an individual's responsiveness to the emotional experiences of another) is considered to develop during adolescence and play a significant role in the adolescent's ability to develop and maintain important quality relationships (Schonert-Reichl, 1993). Moreover, empathy is believed to be an important component of social competent behavior (Ford, 1982). These changes in the manner in which friendships are defined and maintained occur, in part, due to adolescents' more sophisticated social cognitive abilities that allow them to recognize that their particular point of view may be unique and that others also have unique perspectives (Selman, 1980). Indeed, adolescents, more so than children, have more complex concepts of themselves in relation to other people.

Individuals' relationships with parents also undergo marked changes as they enter adolescence. In accordance with Blos' (1962) description of the "second individuation process," recent research indicates that early adolescents attempt to increase their emotional distance from parents as they seek to raise their level of independence (Glenn, 1995). In fact, a converging body of evidence has demonstrated that early adolescents distance themselves somewhat from their parents as they seek to develop a sense of autonomy and identity. It appears, however, that the common portrayal of adolescent-parent relationships as inevitably conflictual has not received empirical support. Instead, the majority of adolescents report being quite satisfied with their relationships with their parents and report that they continue to rely on them for help and advice, particularly when they are confronted with important life decisions, such as career choice (Brown, 1990).

Psychological Change

There is an increasing body of research that suggests that during early adolescence one's sense of self (self-concept, self-image) is more negative and less stable than in later adolescence (e.g., Abramowitz et al., 1984), with one study also finding that it is more negative than it is earlier in childhood (Simmons et al., 1973). In particular, feelings about the body or body image differ for young adolescent boys and girls, with girls seeming to feel less satisfied with their bodies at this stage of life (Casper and Offer, 1990). Feeling attractive may become overly important to girls in the traditional female role, with perceptions that an attractive body may enhance dating opportunities.

The phase of early adolescence has received much attention in the last two decades (see, e.g., Hamburg, 1974; Lipsitz, 1977; Montemayor et al., 1990; Simmons and Blyth, 1987). The results of this research are mixed. Some research suggests that early adolescence is characterized by few major difficulties. Petersen and her colleagues (Petersen and Ebata, 1987) report that 11% of young adolescents have serious chronic difficulties, 32% have more situational and intermittent difficulties, and 57% have positive healthy development during the first phase of adolescence.

In contrast, other research suggests that the early adolescent years are characterized by a number of problems and changes that can eventually lead to academic failure and school dropout. Drops in school grades along with declines in such motivational constructs as intrinsic motivation, interest in school, and confidence in one's intellectual abilities, especially following failure, have been cited as factors that render early adolescents as particularly at risk for successful adult adjustment (see Eccles et al., 1993).

Gender differences in mental health appear to emerge as important during early adolescence. Adolescent girls appear to manifest increases in depressive affect (Allgood-Merton et al., 1990; Lewinsohn et al., 1994; Petersen et al., 1993; Rutter, 1986) across adolescence. The causes of these different developmental patterns are likely to be multidetermined and include genetic, hormonal, and environmental influences (see Rutter, 1986). Some recent work in this area has suggested that girls' proclivity to depression may be due, in part, to increases in self-consciousness that occur in adolescence (Schonert-Reichl, 1994). Other research has suggested that adolescent girls are more reactive to stressful experiences involving others than are boys and therefore are more likely to become depressed (for a review, see Leadbeater et al., 1995).

Cultural definitions of what is desirable and expectable play an important part in mediating the psychological experience of puberty (Boxer et al., 1990; Petersen and Taylor, 1980; Tobin-Richards et al., 1983). The normal increment in weight associated with pubertal development, which leads to a heavier but normal body weight, has been found to be a significant contributor to girls' lowered satisfaction with their bodies (e.g., Blyth et al., 1985). Previous research suggests that adolescents' perceptions of and satisfaction with their weight are more important for girls' body image than for boys' (Tobin-Richards et al., 1983). As a girl progresses through the pubertal stages, satisfaction with her weight decreases, rendering her at significantly greater risk for lowered self-image (Blyth et al., 1985; Duke-Duncan et al., 1985; Tobin-Richards et al., 1983). These developmental changes may contribute to other mental health concerns as well; for example, postpubertal girls have been found to manifest a higher prevalence of depression (Hodges and Siegel, 1985).

Weight has been found to become a particularly salient component of how a girl feels about her body. A strong cultural pressure to be tall and slim may contribute to the finding that the heavier a girl is, or the heavier she thinks she is, the more dissatisfied she is with both her weight and figure (Faust, 1983; Richards et al., 1990; Simmons et al., 1983; Tobin-Richards et al., 1983). Increments in weight appear to be an important aspect of the negative feelings that early maturing girls experience about their bodies. In a recent study of 497 randomly selected high school seniors, Offer (*A Manual for the Offer Self-Image Questionnaire for Parents of Adolescents.* Chicago, in preparation) found that, while most students reported feeling physically healthy, two-thirds of female adolescents were preoccupied with weight and dieting, as opposed to only a small group (about 15%) of males. Youth who manifested weight and dieting concerns were more likely to demonstrate greater body and self-image dissatisfaction, with a depressed mood and greater symptomatic distress. However, ethnic differences were also apparent, and black adolescent females were found to be less weight- and diet-conscious than the white females.

A study conducted by Richards et al. (1990) examined a random sample of 284 young adolescent males and females in two different communities matched for social class. Predictable sex differences were found, with girls manifesting a poorer body image and less satisfaction with weight; for girls these feelings about their perceptions of weight were associated with advanced pubertal development. However, negative feelings associated with pubertal changes were differentially diminished in one community and enhanced in the other. Boys' feelings were similar in both communities; they demonstrated more positive body image and satisfaction with weight and perceived themselves to be more average in weight than did the girls. Context-related variables appeared to partially explain these community differences. Community differences were identified in girls' participation in school-related activities, satisfaction with athletic strength, and degree of perceived school cliquishness. The differences were reflected in community values, probably transmitted through school policies and practices as well as attitudes of the youths, families, and their peers. Thus, cultural and contextual factors may exert important influences on the experience of adolescents across different social groups within the same society.

NORMALITY AND HUMAN DEVELOPMENT

Normality has been a controversial subject since the beginning of psychiatry and psychology. The interpretation of how normality should be defined, however, has many implications for mental health policies today. During the last two decades, Offer and his colleagues have examined various constructs of normality in relation to human development and mental health (Offer and Sabshin, 1974, 1984b, 1991). The definitions of normality have been encompassed in four perspectives, which, while overlapping somewhat, can help investigators organize and interpret their data.

The first perspective is *normality as health* and includes the traditional medical-psychiatric approach, which equates normality with health and views health as an almost universal phenomenon. In this perspective, health is defined by the absence of symptoms and refers to a reasonable rather than an optimal state of functioning. The second perspective defines *normality as utopia*, which is the most widely held definition by psychoanalysts. In this definition, normality is a harmonious and optimal blending of diverse elements of the mental apparatus that culminates in optimal functioning or self-actualization. In this perspective, normality is a state rarely achieved by most individuals. The third perspective defines *normality as average*. This approach is based on the mathematical principle of the bell-shaped curve and its applicability to physical, psychological, and sociological data. In this definition, then, normality is the average, middle range, and both extremes of a bell-shaped distribution are deviant. The fourth perspective defines *normality as a transactional system* and emphasizes that normal behavior is the end result of interacting systems that change over time.

In contrast to the other three perspectives, normality as a transactional process is viewed in temporal progress. This means that individuals are in a continual state of change, as are the world and social contexts in which an individual lives. From this perspective, development is viewed in terms of individual differences, including those determined by temperament and unique life experiences, together with socially defined patterns of wishes and intents, including those that are historically determined (see Cohler and Boxer, 1984). Particular patterns of adjustment and disturbance are understood in terms of transactions between person and social system over time, a view consistent with Grinker's (1967) emphasis on a systems approach in psychiatry.

SELF-IMAGE OF ADOLESCENTS

Adolescence is a critical period with respect to psychological development of the self (Offer and Sabshin, 1984a). An increased ability to think logically and abstractly ensures a more articulated view of the self, while more varied social experience and greater knowledge ensure a more complex social construction of the adolescent's own reality. At the same time, adolescence is a stage of life rich in a variety of issues, such as emerging sexuality, increasing autonomy from family, increased motility, and striving for vocational identity and independence. Aspects of the self will emerge most clearly in this developmental stage, as self-feelings are tested in the interaction of physiological, psychological, and social changes. To learn about adolescents, the authors' approach is data oriented and epidemiologic. Adolescents are as competent as other observers to provide such data (Offer and Offer, 1975). Generalizing from the experiences of a highly select group of teenagers who come for or are brought for psychiatric treatment would be inappropriate. Nor are the retrospections of adolescence presented by adults likely to be valid for an understanding of adolescent experience, although they may tell us much about the adults (Cohler and Boxer, 1984).

In order to gather systematic psychological information, Offer constructed in 1962 the Offer Self-Image Questionnaire for Adolescents (OSIQ). The OSIQ is a self-descriptive personality test whose goal is to assess the adjustment of teenage boys and girls between the ages of 13 and 19. It measures the teenagers' feelings about their own psychological world in 11 content areas, or scales: impulse control, mood, body image, social relations, morals, sexual attitudes and behavior, family relations, mastery of the external world, vocational and educational goals, psychopathology, and superior adjustment (coping). The 11 scales are made up of 130 individual items, with 10–20 items in each scale. The scales are combined to cover five major psychosocial areas of adolescence: the psychological world (scales 1, 2, 3), the social world (scales 4, 5, 9), the sexual self (scale 6), the family (scale 7), and the ability to cope (scales 8, 10, 11). Since 1962 the questionnaire has been administered to over 30,000 teenagers in more than 11 countries. The populations include males and females; younger and older teenagers; normal, delinquent, psychiatrically disturbed, and physically ill adolescents; and urban, suburban, and rural adolescents in the United States as well as in Canada, Australia, Israel, Ireland, Africa, New Guinea, Hungary, West Germany, Italy, Turkey, Japan, Taiwan, and Russia.

This particular approach is necessary to evaluate adolescents' functioning in multiple areas, since they can master one aspect of their world while failing to adjust in another. Second, adolescents' psychological sensitivity is sufficiently acute to allow us to utilize their self-descriptions as a basis for reliable selection of subgroups. Empirical work with the questionnaire has validated these assumptions. In general the larger goal has been to study a group of adolescents not previously studied by psychiatric researchers: the mentally healthy or normal adolescent. The authors collected data directly from adolescents, with the aim of discovering what their world was like and how they perceived it.

The focus of this section is to summarize the results of several recent studies utilizing the OSIQ. As the findings correlated well with data collected from other sources, the large number of studies available will not be detailed. Results have been previously compared with other survey studies (Douvan and Adelson, 1966; Rosenberg, 1979), with clinical studies of normal adolescents (Block, 1971; Offer and Offer, 1975), with family studies (Lewis and Looney, 1983), and with a study of adolescent self-image (Dusek and Flaherty, 1981).

The Psychological Self of the Normal Adolescent

Our results clearly indicate that it is normal for young people in our culture to enjoy life and to be happy with themselves most of the time. The adolescents studied did not feel that others treated them adversely. Normal adolescents also reported that they were relaxed under usual circumstances. They believed that they could control themselves in ordinary life situations. Anxiety was embedded in a generally strong and positive psychological picture.

In another area, body image, the data indicated that normal adolescents felt proud of their physical development and that the vast majority believed that they were strong and healthy. The implication here is that a positive psychological self complements a feeling of physical health.

The Social Self of the Normal Adolescent

The item that received the highest endorsement in the test, ''A job well done gives me pleasure,'' showed the work ethic in its purest form. Judging by the adolescents' responses, that ethic is a universal value in our culture. The adolescents were unreservedly work oriented. They said that they would be proud of their future profession. It is as if they believed that there were jobs out there waiting to be taken when they were ready to take them. They also stated that they did not wish to be supported for the rest of their lives. As a group, the adolescents in our study saw themselves as making friends easily, and they believed that they would be successful both socially and vocationally in the future.

The Sexual Self of the Normal Adolescent

In general, our findings showed that normal adolescents were not afraid of their sexuality. Seven of 10 adolescents stated that they liked the recent changes in their body. Both boys and girls strongly rejected the statement that their bodies were poorly developed. Both boys and girls indicated that they had made a relatively smooth transition to more active sexuality. Nine of 10 subjects said no to the statement ''The opposite sex finds me a bore.'' A majority of the subjects stated that it was important for them to have a friend of the opposite sex.

The Familial Self of the Normal Adolescent

Normal adolescents did not perceive any major problems between themselves and their parents. No evidence was presented for major intergenerational conflict. The generation gap, so often written about, was not in evidence among the vast majority of the teenagers studied. Not only did they have positive feelings toward their parents in the present, they also felt that these good feelings had been true in the past. In addition, they expected that the positive feelings would persist into the future. The most impressive finding in this scale was that 18 of 19 items strongly indicated that adolescents had positive feelings toward their families.

The Coping Self of the Normal Adolescent

Normal adolescents were hopeful about their future, and they believed that they could participate actively in activities that would lead to success. They seemed to have the skills and confidence that they would need for adult life. They were optimistic, and they enjoyed challenges; they tried to learn in advance about novel situations. Normal adolescents had the willingness to do the work necessary to achieve. They liked to put things in order. Moreover, even if they failed, they believed that they could learn from experience.

Normal adolescents denied having the psychopathological symptoms listed in the psychopathology scales. On the whole, they saw themselves as having no major problems. This does not mean that they all said that they did not have problems. A significant minority did not feel secure about their coping abilities. About one in five normal adolescents, data indicated, felt empty emotionally; these adolescents felt that life was an endless series of problems without a solution in sight. A similar number of adolescents stated that they were confused most of the time. In other words, although most subjects stated that they were ''doers'' and that they got pleasure from challenges, some were uncertain about what was going on around them and about their capacity to affect the world.

Gender, Age, and Self-Image of the Normal Adolescent

Using two-way analyses of variance (as mentioned above), the authors assessed the effects of gender and age on the five selves. Only the major differences are discussed here. There were no age differences with respect to the psychological self. Gender effects showed that, in general, adolescent girls had significantly more moods than the adolescent boys. Adolescent girls described themselves as sadder, lonelier,

and easier to hurt. They were more sensitive to their internal world than were the boys. These findings held both for younger and older groups. Other items indicated that girls more often felt ashamed of their bodies, ugly, unattractive, and less good about recent changes in their bodies than did boys. In the area of self-control, more girls than boys stated that they had fits of crying that they could not control. Adolescent girls affirmed social values much more strongly than the adolescent boys. For example, girls were more concerned with the other person, and they would not hurt another person ''just for the heck of it.'' Girls denied more strongly than boys that telling the truth meant nothing to them. Although most normal adolescents preferred to work, girls affirmed this value even more strongly than boys did. Boys showed a more autonomous, less other-directed attitude and were less concerned than girls. Fewer boys than girls agreed with the statement ''If others disapproved of me, I get terribly upset.'' In the same vein, more boys than girls said that they felt like leaders. Adolescent girls reported that they were more empathic than adolescent boys. Similarly, adolescent girls felt more attached to their relatives and friends.

Adolescent boys appeared to be more open to their sexual feelings than did girls. There were no significant age differences. There were no significant differences by age or gender with regard to the familial self. In the coping self, the only age differences that were observed concerned younger adolescent girls describing themselves as having more symptoms than older girls. In general, girls showed more confusion, shame, and fears than adolescent boys. Girls' faith in their coping abilities was strong but not as strong as that of the boys.

As adolescents move through the years of transitions, they have to accomplish three psychological tasks. These are building blocks for their adult personality, which they will need and utilize throughout their lives. First, during the early adolescent years (12–14), the adolescent has to accept his or her growing and changing body. This includes an understanding of the self. The adolescent realizes that one is theoretically, if not practically, an adult. During the second adolescent phase (14–16 years), the adolescent has to separate from the internalized figure of the parent and venture out of his or her own family world. Included in this world is an erotically tinged playfulness with the parent of the opposite sex. Thus, a good experience with parents will go a long way toward helping the adolescent's confidence in his or her self. The idea that one's parent can let one go, still love the adolescent, and allow him or her to experiment with different relationships is most important for healthy development. Third, during the late adolescent years (16–19), the internal problems that adolescents have to learn how to handle are organized around the issue of identity. The tasks of crystallizing one's own sexual identity and vocational identity (i.e., plans for school, work) need to be addressed during the third phase of adolescence. It is now that the final issues of dependency left over from childhood get resolved. It is, according to Blos (1962), a time when a person gets a second chance to resolve the psychological conflicts left over from childhood. That is why Blos calls adolescence the ''second individuation stage.'' Most of these processes take place internally. We see only their behavioral sequelae when the adolescent has failed in his or her attempt to resolve them.

DEVELOPMENTAL RESEARCH ON ADOLESCENCE AND THE PROVISION OF CLINICAL SERVICES

Developmental research has generally had a profound impact on the delivery of services to adolescents. Since Anna Freud's (1958) comment that adolescence was the ''stepchild of developmental theory,'' more sophisticated and comprehensive understandings of adolescence have emerged in research, theory, and clinical services. Accompanying the recognition of adolescence as being distinctly different from both childhood and adulthood is the emerging idea that what is ''normal'' or expectable for an adolescent is different from what is normal or expectable for an adult (Offer, 1987; Offer and Sabshin, 1984a). Longitudinal research on adolescence has had particularly important implications for mental health practitioners and service providers in providing a baseline in terms of which the origin, course, and treatment of psychological distress and disturbances may be evaluated. This perspective has been particularly useful in informing diagnosis and assessment of psychopathology during the adolescent years. Nevertheless, much more research is needed in the area of adolescent developmental psychopathology (Kazdin, 1993). For the most part, it appears that the investigation of adolescent disturbance has been circumvented by strongly held beliefs that adolescent problems are temporary and something they will simply "grow out of" with time.

The tendency among clinicians has been to base their understanding of problems characteristic of adolescents upon generalizations derived from small psychopathological samples. For example, Offer et al. (1981a) conducted a study in which they asked mental health professionals to complete the OSIQ the way they believed a normal, mentally healthy adolescent (of the same sex as the respondent) would complete it. Their results indicated that the mental health professional described normal adolescents as significantly more disturbed than adolescents saw themselves. A similar study was completed by Swedo and Offer (1990), in which pediatricians were asked to complete the OSIQ as they believed a mentally healthy adolescent would. The results of this study were in accord with the results of Offer et al.'s previous research with clinicians. That is, pediatricians also saw normal adolescents as more disturbed than adolescents saw themselves.

However, more recent research indicates that psychiatrists today have a more accurate concept of normal adolescent development than in previous decades. Specifically, Stoller et al. (1994) investigated 145 psychiatrists' perceptions of the self-images of both mentally healthy and mentally disturbed adolescents. Eighty-four psychiatrists completed a modified version of the OSIQ, and their responses were compared to those of 140 nonpatient 15-year-olds. In turn, 61 psychiatrists completed the same measure as they believed a mentally disturbed adolescent would respond and their responses were compared to those of 70 psychiatric inpatients of the same gender. Results indicated that psychiatrists' perceptions of normal adolescents was more in sync with adolescents' themselves than were those perceptions of psychiatrists in the 1981 sample. Thus, it appears that psychiatrists' concepts of normal adolescents' self-images has become more accurate over the past decade. This improvement may be due, in part, to the widespread dissemination of the empirical data that have emerged during the past decade refuting the "turmoil theory" of adolescence.

Stoller et al. (1994), however, did find that psychiatrists' perceptions of the self-images of disturbed adolescents were more negative than the disturbed adolescents reported themselves. Indeed, the psychiatrists reported lower than average self-images for disturbed adolescents on all 10 subscales of the OSIQ. The disturbed adolescents reported lower than average self-images on only 6 of the 10 subscales. Disturbed adolescents did not see themselves differently from nondisturbed adolescents with regard to their self-perceptions of their body image, social functioning, vocational goals, and sexuality. According to Stoller et al., one possible interpretation for their finding draws from theoretical work in the area of social psychology. They believe that the concept of the "illusory correlation" (Fiske and Taylor, 1984) may shed light on the finding that psychiatrists' generalize disturbed functioning to all aspects of the disturbed adolescents' self-image. That is, psychiatrists may see psychopathology in adolescence as an all or nothing event.

Although the common portrayal of adolescence as a time of "storm and stress" or psychological upheaval has been debunked in recent years, recent research indicates that adolescents report higher levels of distress and more negative and stressful life events than do children (Larson and Ham, 1993). Moreover, findings from epidemiological studies indicate that about one in five, or 20%, of individuals under the age of 18 suffer from developmental, emotional, or behavioral difficulties (Costello, 1989). Because the adolescent period is a time in the life cycle in which individuals must acquire important skills and accomplish a multitude of developmental tasks (e.g., career and vocational choices, interpersonal relationships), understanding the manner in which adolescents cope with stress is very important.

Several recent investigations have been conducted investigating how adolescents cope with stress (e.g., Ebata and Moos, 1994; Windle et al., 1991). For example, Williams et al. (1993) found that adolescents more often utilize avoidant coping strategies (e.g., listening to music, playing sports, sleeping, drinking alcohol) than approach-oriented coping strategies (e.g., trying to directly solve the problem, seeking help and guidance from someone about the problem) to deal with negative affective experiences. Schonert-Reichl (1995) most recently found that adolescents' preferred source of help were best friends (75%), followed by mothers (57%), other family members (52%) (e.g., siblings, aunt, uncle), professionals (42%), and fathers (35%). Also evidenced in the study was a relationship between social cognitive ability and help-seeking. In particular, the relation of perspective-taking to help-seeking varied by age and the source from whom help was sought. For example, whereas during early adolescence more sophisticated perspective-taking abilities were associated with seeking help from fathers, during middle adolescence the opposite pattern emerged. That is, those middle adolescents who did not seek help from their fathers possessed higher perspective-taking abilities than those adolescents who did seek help from their fathers. It may be that older adolescents with more sophisticated abilities to think about the perspectives of others, are more "discriminate consumers" of the various sources of help available to them in their social support network.

Other research by Offer et al., 1991 has shown that, when normal adolescents have an emotional problem, they almost never discuss it with a teacher ($<10\%$), often discuss it with their parents ($>60\%$), and very often discuss it with a friend ($>75\%$). The rates for disturbed adolescents were the same for teachers and for friends. However, less than 35% of the teens would discuss an emotional problem with a parent. Approximately one-third of the disturbed group (20% of the total sample) had consulted mental health professionals. Two-thirds had never seen either a psychiatrist, a psychologist, or a social worker. This current research demonstrates that adolescents, their parents, and mental health professionals are not yet able to reach out and help most adolescents in need. Parents, the first line of defense, seem to be helping their healthy children more than they are helping their disturbed ones.

What are the differences between those adolescents who seek help only from parents and friends versus those adolescents who seek help from both informal and formal sources of support? This was the question asked by Schonert-Reichl et al. (1995) in their study investigating the sociodemographic and psychological correlates of help-seeking in adolescence. Altogether 497 adolescents completed measures regarding demographics (e.g., age, gender, family compositions, socioeconomic status (SES)), self-image, symptomatology, delinquency, and help-seeking behaviors with reference to parents, friends, and mental health professionals. The findings indicated that those adolescents who sought help from both informal and formal helping resources were more likely to be younger, white, and female with lower self-images and higher rates of symptomatology and delinquency than those adolescents who sought help from just parents and friends. Interestingly, African American, Asian, and Hispanic adolescents were more likely than Caucasian youth to report seeking help from school counselors. Such findings lend support to the contention that a developmental approach that takes into account both gender and race must be considered when devising effective treatments and interventions (see Noam, 1992).

In conclusion, it is important to keep in mind that adolescence is an in-between transitional stage. The person is no longer a dependent, biologically immature, socially inept, and psychologically weak child. He or she is also not yet an independent, mature, resolute, strong young adult. The adolescent is really both part child and part adult, and hence it is often difficult to describe him or her extremely accurately. We believe that for adolescents the physical changes associated with puberty are the fastest occurring during the life cycle, with the exception of the 1st year of life. That demands considerable coping abilities and psychological flexibility for the adolescent, since major psychosocial reactions to puberty are set into motion. We have, therefore, focused in detail on puberty, as well as on the psychosocial aspects of development.

We have also stated that, based on data presented above, we need to better understand the normal teenager in order for us to make more accurate diagnoses on those adolescents requiring professional help. The needs of adolescents can be addressed only when service providers are informed by a broad understanding of development across the adolescent decade, including the complex interplay between maturational and personality processes and the reciprocal impact of increasingly complex socially defined expectations regarding major roles upon self-conceptions and individual well-being. (For psychoneuroendocrinological aspects of child and adolescent development, see Chapter 6; for a psychoanalytic viewpoint, see Chapter 12.)

References

Abramowitz RH, Petersen AC, Schulenberg JE: Changes in self-image during early adolescence. In: Offer D, Ostrov E, Howard K (eds): *Patterns of Adolescent Self-Image*. San Francisco, Jossey-Bass, 1984.

Alan Guttmacher Institute: *Teenage Pregnancy: The Problem That Hasn't Gone Away*. New York, Alan Guttmacher Institute, 1981.

Allgood-Merton B, Lewinsohn PM, Hops H: Sex differences and adolescent depression. *J Abnorm Psychol* 99:55–63, 1990.

Aries P: *Centuries of Childhood: A Social History on Family Life* (Baldick R, trans). New York, Random House, 1962.

Arnett JJ, Taber S: Adolescence terminable and interminable: When does adolescence end. *J Youth Adolesc* 23:517–537, 1994.

Bell A, Weinberg M: *Homosexualities: A Study of Diversity among Men and Women*. New York, Simon & Schuster, 1978.

Belsky J, Steinberg L, Draper P: Childhood experience, interpersonal development, and reproductive strategy: An evolutionary theory of socialization. *Child Dev* 62:647–670, 1991.

Block J, with Haan N: *Lives through Time*. Berkeley, CA, Bancroft Books, 1971.

Blos P: *On Adolescence*. New York, Free Press, 1962.

Blyth D, Simmons RG, Zakin D: Satisfaction with body image for early adolescent females: The impact of pubertal timing within different school environments. *J Youth Adolesc* 14:207–225, 1985.

Bock RD, Wainer H, Petersen AC, et al: A parameterization for individual human growth curves. *Hum Biol* 45:63–80, 1973.

Boxer AM: Betwixt and between: Developmental discontinuities among gay and lesbian youth. Paper presented in the symposium, Coming of Age as Gay and Lesbian Youth: Interdisciplinary Perspectives on Homosexuality and the Adolescent Life Course, at the biennial meetings of the Society for Research on Adolescence, Alexandria, VA, March 27, 1988.

Boxer AM, Cohler BJ: The life course of gay and lesbian youth: An immodest proposal for the study of lives. *J Homosex* 17:315–355, 1989.

Boxer AM, Petersen AC: Pubertal change in a family context. In: Leigh GK, Peterson GW (eds): *Adolescents in Families*. Cincinnati, South-Western Publishing, 1986.

Boxer AM, Levinson R, Petersen AC: Adolescent sexuality. In: Worrell J, Danner F (eds): *The Adolescent as Decision-Maker: Issues for Education*. New York, Academic Press, 1989.

Brook CG: Endocrinological control of growth at puberty. *Br Med Bull* 37:281–285, 1981.

Brooks-Gunn J, Furstenberg FF Jr: Adolescent sexual behavior. *Am Psychol* 44:249–257, 1989.

Brooks-Gunn J, Reiter EO: The role of pubertal processes. In: Feldman SS, Elliott GR (eds): *At the Threshold: The Developing Adolescent*. Cambridge, MA, Harvard University Press, 1990.

Brooks-Gunn J, Boyer C, Hein K: Preventing HIV infection and AIDS in children and adolescents. *Am Psychol* 43:958–964, 1988.

Brown BB: Peer groups and peer cultures. In: Feldman SS, Elliott GR (eds): *At the Threshold: The Developing Adolescent*. Cambridge, MA, Harvard University Press, 1990.

Buchanan CM, Eccles JS, Becker JB: Are adolescents the victims of raging hormones? Evidence for the activational effects of hormones on moods and behavior at adolescence. *Psychol Bull* 111:62–107, 1992.

Buchbinder G: *Man and Woman in the New Guinea Highlands*. Washington, DC, American Anthropological Association, 1976.

Buhrmester D, Furman W: The development of companionship and intimacy. *Child Dev* 58:1101–1113, 1987.

Casper RC, Offer D: Weight and dieting concerns in adolescents, fashion or symptom? *Pediatrics* 86:384–390, 1990.

Cohler BJ, Boxer AM: Middle adulthood: Settling into the world—Person, time, and context. In: Offer D, Sabshin M (eds): *Normality and the Life Cycle*. New York, Basic Books, 1984.

Comite F, Prescovitz OH, Sonia WA, et al: Premature adolescence: Neuroendocrine and psychosocial studies. In: Lerner RM, Foch TT (eds): *Biological-Psychosocial Interactions in Early Adolescence: A Life-Span Perspective*. Hillsdale, NJ, Erlbaum, 1987.

Costello EJ: Developments in child psychiatric epidemiology. *J Am Acad Child Adolesc Psychiatry* 28:836–841, 1989.

Cote JE, Allahar AL: *Generation on Hold: Coming of Age in the Late Twentieth Century*. Toronto, Stoddart, 1994.

Crisp AH: Some skeletal measurements in patients with primary anorexia nervosa. *J Psychosom Res* 13:125–242, 1969.

Crockett L, Petersen AC: Pubertal status and psychosocial development: Findings from the Early Adolescence Study. In: Lerner R, Foch T (eds): *Biological Psychosocial Interactions in Early Adolescence: A Life-Span Perspective*. Hillsdale, NJ, Erlbaum, 1987.

Csikzsentmihalyi M, Larson R: *Being Adolescent: Conflict and Growth in the Teenage Years*. New York, Basic Books, 1984.

Demos J, Demos V: Adolescence in historical perspective. *J Marriage Fam* 31:632–638, 1969.

Dornbusch SM: The sociology of adolescence. *Annu Rev Sociol* 15:233–259, 1989.

Dornbusch SM, Petersen AC, Heterhington EM: Projecting the future of research on adolescence. *J Res Adolesc* 1:7–17, 1991.

Dougherty DM: Adolescent health: Reflections on a report to the U.S. Congress. *Am Psychol* 48:193–201, 1993.

Douvan E, Adelson J: *The Adolescent Experience*. New York, Wiley, 1966.

Dreyer P: Sexuality during adolescence. In: Wolman B (ed): *Handbook of Developmental Psychology*. Englewood Cliffs, NJ, Prentice-Hall, 1982.

Dryfoos J: *Adolescents at Risk*. New York, Oxford University Press, 1990.

Dubas JS, Graber JA, Petersen AC: The effects of pubertal development on achievement during adolescence. *Am J Educ* 99:444–460, 1991.

Duke-Duncan P, Ritter P, Dornbusch S, et al: The effects of pubertal timing on body image, school behavior and deviance. *J Youth Adolesc* 14:227–236, 1985.

Dusek JB, Flaherty JF: The development of the self-concept during the adolescent years. *Monogr Soc Child Dev* 46:1–191, 1981.

Ebata AT, Moos RH: Personal, situational, and contextual correlates of coping in adolescence. *J Res Adolesc* 4:99–125, 1994.

Eccles JS, Midgley C, Wigfield A, et al: Development during adolescence: The impact of stage-environment fit on young adolescents' experiences in schools and in families. *Am Psychol* 48:90–101, 1993.

Eichorn D: Asynchronizations in adolescent development. In: Dragastin SE, Elder GH Jr (eds): *Adolescence in the Life Cycle*. Washington, DC, Hemisphere, 1975.

Elkind D: Recent research on cognitive development in adolescence. In: Dragastin SE, Elder GH Jr (eds): *Adolescence in the Life Cycle*. Washington, DC, Hemisphere, 1975.

Enright RD, Lapsley DK, Shukla DG: Adolescent egocentrism in early and late adolescence. *Adolescence* 14:687–696, 1979.

Enright RD, Levy VM Jr, Harris D, et al: Do economic conditions influence how theorists view adolescents? *J Youth Adolesc* 16:541–559, 1987.

Erikson EN: Identity and the life cycle. *Psychol Issues* 1:1–171, 1959.

Faust MS: Somatic development of adolescent girls. *Monogr Soc Res Child Dev* 42:1, 1977.

Faust MS: Alternative constructions of adolescent growth. In: Brooks-Gunn J, Petersen AC (eds): *Girls at Puberty: Biological and Psychosocial Perspectives*. New York, Plenum, 1983.

Feldman SS, Elliott GR (eds): *At the Threshold: The Developing Adolescent*. Cambridge, MA, Harvard University Press, 1990a.

Feldman SS, Elliott GR: Progress and promise of research on adolescence. In: Feldman SS, Elliott SR (eds): *At the Threshold: The Developing Adolescent*. Cambridge, MA, Harvard University Press, 1990b.

Fine M: Sexuality, schooling, and adolescent females: The missing discourse of desire. *Harvard Educ Rev* 58:29–53, 1988.

Fiske S, Taylor S: *Social Cognition*. Reading, MA, Addison-Wesley, 1984.

Ford ME: Social cognition and social competence in adolescence. *Dev Psychol* 18:323–340, 1982.

Freud A: *The Ego and the Mechanisms of Defense*. New York, International Universities Press, 1946.

Freud A: Adolescence. *Psychoanal Study Child* 16:225–278, 1958.

Frisch RE: Population, food intake, and fertility. *Science* 199:22–30, 1978.

Frisch RE: Fatness, puberty, and fertility. *Nat History* 89:16, 1980a.

Frisch RE: Pubertal adipose tissue: Is it necessary for normal sexual maturation? Evidence from the rat and human female. *Fed Proc* 39:2395–3400, 1980b.

Frisch RE: Fatness, menarche, and fertility. In: Golub S (ed): *Menarche.* New York, DC Health, 1983a.

Frisch RE: Fatness, puberty, and fertility: The effects of nutrition and physical training on menarche and ovulation. In: Brooks-Gunn J, Petersen AC (eds): *Girls at Puberty: Biological and Psychosocial Perspectives.* New York, Plenum, 1983b.

Frisch RE, McArthur J: Menstrual cycles: Fatness as a determinant of minimum weight for height necessary for their maintenance or onset. *Science* 195:949–951, 1974.

Frisch RE, Wyshak G, Vincent L: Delayed menarche and amenorrhea in ballet dancers. *N Engl J Med* 303:17–19, 1980.

Gagnon J, Simon W: *Sexual Conduct: The Social Sources of Human Sexuality.* Chicago, Aldine, 1973.

Garfinkel PE, Garner DM: *Anorexia Nervosa: A Multidimensional Perspective.* New York, Brunner/Mazel, 1982.

Gargiulo J, Attie I, Brooks-Gunn J, et al: Girls' dating behaviors as a function of social context and maturation. *Dev Psychol* 23:730–737, 1987.

Garn SM: Continuities and change in maturational timing. In: Brim OG Jr, Kagan J (eds): *Constancy and Change in Human Development.* Cambridge, MA, Harvard University Press, 1980.

Gavin LA, Furman W: Age differences in adolescents' perceptions of their peer groups. *Dev Psychol* 25:827–834, 1989.

Gebhard PH: The acquisition of basic sex information. *J Sex Res* 13:148–149, 1977.

Gebhard PH, Johnson AB: *The Kinsey Data: Marginal Tabulations of the 1938–1963 Interviews Conducted by the Institute for Sex Research.* Philadelphia, Saunders, 1979.

Gerstel C, Feraios AJ, Herdt G: Widening circles: An ethnographic profile of a youth group. *J Homosex* 17:75–92, 1989.

Glenn MD: Gender and developmental differences in adolescents' perceptions and standards of their relationships with their parents. Paper presented at the biennial meeting of the Society for Research in Child Development, March, 1995.

Greene AL, Boxer AM: Daughters and sons as young adults: Restructuring the ties that bind. In: Datan N, Greene AL, Reese H (eds): *Life-Span Developmental Psychology: Intergenerational Relations.* Hillsdale, NJ, Erlbaum, 1986.

Grinker R: Normality viewed as a system. *Arch Gen Psychiatry* 17:320–324, 1967.

Grumbach MM, Grave GD, Mayer FE (eds): *Control of the Onset of Puberty.* New York, Wiley, 1974.

Gupta DA, Attanasio A, Raaf S: Plasma estrogen and androgen concentrations in children during adolescence. *J Clin Endocrinol Metab* 40:636–643, 1975.

Hagestad GO, Neugarten BL: Age and the life course. In: Shanas E, Binstock R (eds): *Handbook of Aging and the Social Sciences* (2nd ed). New York, Van Nostrand Reinhold, 1984.

Hagg U, Taranger J: Maturation indicators and the pubertal growth spurt. *Am J Orthod* 82:299–309, 1985.

Halberg F: Implications of biologic rhythms for clinical practice. In: Krieger DT, Hughes JC (eds): *Neuroendocrinology.* Sunderland, MA, Sinauer Associates, 1980.

Hall GS: *Adolescence: Its Psychology and Its Relations to Physiology, Anthropology, Sociology, Sex, Crime, Religion, and Education.* New York, Appleton, 1904.

Hamburg B: Early adolescence: A specific and stressful stage of the life cycle. In: Coelho G, Hamburg DA, Adams JE (eds): *Coping and Adaptation.* New York, Basic Books, 1974.

Hamburg D: Preparing for life: The critical transition of adolescence. In: *1986 Annual Report of the Carnegie Corporation of New York.* New York, The Carnegie Corporation, 1986.

Hayes CD (ed): *Risking the Future: Adolescent Sexuality, Pregnancy, and Childbearing* (Vol 1). Washington, DC, National Academy Press, 1987.

Hein K: AIDS in adolescence: Exploring the challenge. *J Adolesc Health Care* 10:105–355, 1989.

Hodges KK, Siegel LJ: Depression in children and adolescents. In: Beckham EE, Leber WR (eds): *Handbook of Depression: Treatment, Assessment and Research.* Homewood, IL, Dorsey Press, 1985.

Hofferth SL, Hayes CD: *Risking the Future: Adolescent Sexuality, Pregnancy, and Childbearing.* Vol 2: *Working Papers and Statistical Reports.* Washington, DC, National Academy Press, 1987.

Hogan DP: Subgroup variations in early life transitions. In: Riley MW, Abeles RP, Teitelbaum M (eds): *Aging from Birth to Death.* Vol 2: *Sociotemporal Perspectives.* Boulder, CO, Westview Press, 1982.

Jessor SL, Jessor R: Transition from virginity to nonvirginity among youth: A social-psychological study over time. *Dev Psychol* 11:473–484, 1975.

Jessor R, Jessor SL: *Problem Behavior and Psychological Development.* New York, Academic Press, 1977.

Jessor R, Costa F, Jessor L, et al: Time of first intercourse: A prospective study. *J Pers Soc Psychol* 44:608–626, 1983.

Kagan J: A conception of early adolescence. *Daedalus* 100:997–1012, 1971.

Katz IL, Boyar RM, Roffwar H, et al: LHRH responsiveness in anorexia nervosa: Intactness despite prepubertal circadian LH pattern. *Psychosom Med* 39:241–251, 1977.

Kazdin AE: Psychotherapy for children and adolescents: Current progress and future research directions. *Am Psychol* 48:644–657, 1993.

Keating DP: Adolescent thinking. In: Feldman SS, Elliott GR (eds): *At the Threshold: The Developing Adolescent.* Cambridge, MA, Harvard University Press, 1990.

Keating DP, Clark LV: Development of physical and social reasoning in adolescence. *Dev Psychol* 23:23–30, 1980.

Kegeles SM, Adler NE, Irwin CE: Sexually active adolescents and condoms: Changes over one year in knowledge, attitudes and use. *Am J Public Health* 78:460–461, 1988.

Kett J: *Rites of Passage: Adolescence in America, 1790 to the Present.* New York, Basic Books, 1977.

Kinsey AC, Pomeroy WB, Martin CE: *Sexual Behavior in the Human Male.* Philadelphia, Saunders, 1948.

Kinsey AC, Pomeroy WB, Martin CE, et al: *Sexual Behavior in the Human Female.* Philadelphia, Saunders, 1953.

Kirby D: The mathtech research on adolescent sexuality education programs. *SIECUS Rep* 12:11–22, 1983.

Kirby D: A summary of the national study of selected sexuality programs. *Fam Life Educ* 2:24–26, 1984.

Kirby D, Alter J, Scales P: *An Analysis of US Sex Education Programs and Evaluation Methods.* Bethesda, MD, Mathtech, 1979.

Lapsley D: Continuity and discontinuity in adolescent social cognitive development. In:

Montemayor R, Adams GR, Gullotta TP (eds): *From Childhood to Adolescence: A Transitional Period?* Newbury Park, Sage, 1990.

Larson R, Ham M: Stress and "storm and stress" in early adolescence: The relationship of negative events with dysphoric affect. *Dev Psychol* 29:130–140, 1993.

Larson R, Richards M: Daily companionship in late childhood and early adolescence: Changing developmental contexts. *Child Dev* 62:284–300.

Leadbeater BJ, Blatt SJ, Quinlan DM: Gender-linked vulnerabilities to depressive symptoms, stress, and problem behaviors in adolescence. *J Res Adolesc* 5:1–29, 1995.

Lerner RM, Foch TT (eds): *Biological-Psychosocial Interactions in Early Adolescence: A Life-Span Perspective.* Hillsdale, NJ, Erlbaum, 1987.

Lerner RM, Petersen AC, Brooks-Gunn J (eds): *Encyclopedia of Adolescence* (Vol 1–2). New York, Garland, 1991.

Levinson RA: Contraceptive self-efficacy: Primary prevention. *J Soc Work Hum Sex* 3:1–15, 1984.

Levinson RA: Contraceptive self-efficacy: A perspective on teenage girls' contraceptive behavior. *J Sex Res* 22:347–369, 1986.

Lewinsohn PM, Roberts RE, Seeley JR, et al: Adolescent psychopathology. II: Psychosocial risk factors for depression. *J Abnormal Psychol* 103:302–315, 1994.

Lewis JM, Looney JG: *The Long Struggle.* New York, Brunner/Mazel, 1983.

Lipsitz J: *Growing Up Forgotten: A Review of Research and Programs Concerning Early Adolescence.* Lexington, MA, DC Heath, 1977.

Martorano SC: A developmental analysis of performance on Piaget's formal operations tasks. *Dev Psychol* 13:666–672, 1977.

Meyer-Bahlburg HFL, Ehrhardt AA, Bell JJ, et al: Idiopathic precocious puberty in girls: Psychosexual development. *J Youth Adolesc* 14:339–353, 1985.

Modell J, Furstenberg F, Hershberg TR: Social change and transitions to adulthood in historical perspective. *J Fam Hist* 1:7–32, 1976.

Moffitt TE, Caspi A, Belsky J, et al: Childhood experience and the onset of menarche: A test of a sociobiological model. *Child Dev* 63:47–58, 1992.

Montemayor R, Adams GR, Gullotta TP: *From Childhood to Adolescence: A Transitional Period?* Newbury Park, Sage, 1990.

Neugarten BL, Hagestad GO: Age and the life course. In: Binstock RL, Shanas E: *Handbook of Aging and the Social Sciences.* New York, Van Nostrand Reinhold, 1976.

Newcombe N, Dubas IS: Individual differences in cognitive ability: Are they related to timing of puberty. In: Lerner R, Foch T (eds): *Biological-Psychosocial Interactions in Early Adolescence: A Life-Span Perspective.* Hillsdale, NJ, Erlbaum, 1987.

Noam GG: Development as the aim of clinical intervention. *Dev Psychopathol* 4:679–696, 1992.

Nottelmann ED, Susman EJ, Blue JH, et al: Developmental processes in early adolescence: Relations between adolescent adjustment problems and chronological age, pubertal stage, and puberty-related serum hormone levels. *J Pediatr* 110:473–480, 1987.

Offer D: *The Psychological World of the Teenager: A Study of Normal Adolescent Boys.* New York, Basic Books, 1969.

Offer D: In defense of adolescents. *JAMA* 257:3407, 1987.

Offer D, Offer JB: *From Teenage to Young Manhood: A Psychological Study.* New York, Basic Books, 1975.

Offer D, Sabshin M: *Normality: Theoretical and*

Clinical Concepts of Mental Health (2nd ed). New York, Basic Books, 1974.

Offer D, Sabshin M: Adolescence: Empirical perspectives. In: Offer D, Sabshin M (eds): *Normality and the Life Cycle.* New York, Basic Books, 1984a.

Offer D, Sabshin M: Patterns of normal development. In: Offer D, Sabshin M (eds): *Normality and the Life Cycle.* New York, Basic Books, 1984b.

Offer D, Sabshin M (eds): *The Diversity of Normal Behavior: Further Contributions to Normatology.* New York, Basic Books, 1991.

Offer D, Schonert-Reichl KA: Debunking the myths of adolescence. *J Am Acad Child Adolesc Psychiatry* 31:1003–1014, 1992.

Offer D, Howard KI, Schonert KA, et al: To whom do adolescents turn for help? Differences between disturbed and non-disturbed adolescents. *J Am Acad Child Adolesc Psychiatry* 30:623–630, 1991.

Offer D, Ostrov E, Howard KI: The mental health professional's concept of the normal adolescent. *Arch Gen Psychiatry* 38:149–153, 1981a.

Offer D, Ostrov E, Howard KI: *The Adolescent: A Psychological Self-Portrait.* New York, Basic Books, 1981b.

Offer D, Ostrov E, Howard KI, et al: *The Teenage World: Adolescents' Self-Image in Ten Countries.* New York, Plenum, 1988.

Petersen AC: Female pubertal development. In: Sugar M (ed): *Female Adolescent Development.* New York, Brunner/Mazel, 1979.

Petersen AC: The development of self-concept in adolescence. In: Lynch MD, Norem-Heibeisen A, Gergen K (eds): *The Self-Concept.* New York, Ballinger, 1981.

Petersen AC: Pubertal development and cognition. In: Brooks-Gunn J, Petersen AC (eds): *Girls at Puberty: Biological and Psychosocial Perspectives.* New York, Plenum, 1983.

Petersen AC: Pubertal development as a cause of disturbance: Myths, realities, and unanswered questions. *Genet Soc Gen Psychol Monogr* 111:205–232, 1985.

Petersen AC: Adolescent development. *Ann Rev Psychol* 39:583–607, 1988.

Petersen AC, Boxer AM: Adolescent sexuality. In: Coates TJ, Petersen AC, Perry C (eds): *Promoting Adolescent Health: A Dialog on Research and Practice.* New York, Academic Press, 1982.

Petersen AC, Ebata AT: Developmental transitions and adolescent problem behavior: Implications for prevention and intervention. In: Hurrelmann K (ed): *Social Prevention and Intervention.* New York, Aldine de Gruyter, 1987.

Petersen AC, Epstein JL: Development and education across adolescence: An introduction. *Am J Ed* 99:373–398, 1991.

Petersen AC, Taylor B: The biological approach to adolescence. In: Adelson J (ed): *Handbook of Adolescent Psychology.* New York, Wiley, 1980.

Petersen AC, Compas BE, Brooks-Gunn J, et al: Depression in adolescence. *Am Psychol* 48:155–168, 1993.

Phelan P, Yu HC, Davidson AL: Navigating the psychosocial pressures of adolescence: The voices and experiences of high school youth. *Am Ed Res J* 31:415–447, 1994.

Rabichow HG, Sklansky MA: *Effective Counseling of Adolescents.* Chicago, Follett, 1980.

Richards M, Larson R: Pubertal development and the daily subjective states of young adolescents. *J Res Adolesc* 3:145–168, 1993.

Richards M, Boxer A, Petersen A, et al: Relation of weight to body image in pubertal girls and boys from two communities. *Dev Psychol* 26:313–321, 1990.

Riley MW, Johnson M, Foner A: *Aging and Society.* Vol 3: *A Sociology of Age Stratification.* New York, Russell Sage, 1972.

Rosenberg M: *Conceiving the Self.* New York, Basic Books, 1979.

Rousseau JJ: *Emile.* London, Dent-Everyman's, 1969.

Rutter M: The developmental psychopathology of depression: Issues and perspectives. In: Rutter M, Izard C, Read P (eds): *Depression in Young People: Developmental and Clinical Perspectives.* New York, Guilford Press, 1986.

Saghir MT, Robins E: *Male and Female Homosexuality.* Baltimore, Williams & Wilkins, 1973.

Schonert-Reichl KA: Gender differences in depressive symptomatology and egocentrism in adolescence. *J Early Adolesc* 14:49–65, 1994.

Schonert-Reich, KA: The relation of social cognition to help-seeking behaviors during adolescence. Paper presented at the annual meeting of the American Educational Research Association, San Francisco, 1995.

Schonert-Reichl KA, Offer D, Howard KI: Seeking help from informal and formal resources during adolescence: Sociodemographic and psychological correlates. *Adolesc Psychiatry* 20:165–178, 1995.

Simmons RG, Blyth DA: *Moving into Adolescence: The Impact of Pubertal Change and School Context.* New York, Aldine de Gruyter, 1987.

Simmons RG, Blyth DA, McKinney KL: The social and psychological effects of puberty on white females. In: Brooks-Gunn J, Petersen AC (eds): *Girls at Puberty: Biological and Psychosocial Perspectives.* New York, Plenum, 1983.

Simmons RG, Rosenberg MF, Rosenberg MC: Disturbance in the self-image at adolescence. *Am Sociol Rev* 38:553–568, 1973.

Sladkin K: Section on American Health, American Academy of Pediatrics. *Pediatr News* December: 34, 1983.

Smith EA, Udry JR: Coital and non-coital sexual behaviors of white and black adolescents. *Am J Public Health* 75:1200–1203, 1985.

Stoller CL, Offer D, Howard KI, et al: Psychiatrist's concept of adolescent self-image. Paper presented at the annual meeting of the American Psychiatric Association, 1994.

Susman EJ, Inoff-Germain G, Nottelmann ED, et al: Hormones, emotional dispositions, and aggressive attributes in young adolescents. *Child Dev* 58: 1114–1134, 1987.

Swedo SE, Offer D: The pediatrician's concept of the normal adolescent. *J Adolesc Health Care* 12: 6–10, 1991.

Takanishi R: The opportunities of adolescence: Research, interventions, and policy. Special Issue: Adolescence. *Am Psychol* 48:85–87, 1993.

Tanner JM: *Growth at Adolescence.* Springfield, IL, Charles C Thomas, 1962.

Tanner JM: Sequence, tempo, and individual variation in the growth and development of boys and girls aged twelve to sixteen. *Daedalus* 100:907–930, 1971.

Tanner JM: Sequence and tempo in the somatic changes in puberty. In: Grumbach MM, Grave GD, Mayer FE (eds): *Control of the Onset of Puberty.* New York, Wiley, 1974.

Tanner JM: *A History of the Study of Human Growth.* Cambridge, MA, Harvard University Press, 1981.

Tanner JM: Menarche, secular trend in age of. In: Lerner RM, Petersen AC, Brooks-Gunn J (eds): *Encyclopedia of Adolescence.* New York, Garland, 1991.

Thornburg H: Is early adolescence really a stage of development? *Theor Prac* 22:79–84, 1983.

Tobin-Richards M, Boxer AM, Petersen AC: The psychological significance of pubertal change: Sex differences in perceptions of self during early adolescence. In: Brooks-Gunn J, Petersen AC (eds): *Girls at Puberty: Biological and Psychosocial Perspectives.* New York, Plenum, 1983.

Udry JR, Billy JOG, Morris N, et al: Serum androgenic hormones motivate sexual behavior in adolescent boys. *Fertil Steril* 43:90–94, 1985.

Udry JR, Talbert LM, Morris N: Biosocial foundations for adolescent female sexuality. *Demography* 23:217–230, 1986.

Warren MP: Physical and biological aspects of puberty. In: Brooks-Gunn J, Petersen AC (eds): *Girls at Puberty: Biological and Psychosocial Perspectives.* New York, Plenum, 1983.

Williams S, Offer D, Howard KI, et al: How do adolescents regulate affect? Differences between disturbed and normal teenagers. Paper presented at the American Psychiatric Association, San Francisco, CA, 1993.

Windle M, Miller-Tutzauer C, Barnes GM, et al: Adolescent perceptions of help-seeking resources for substance abuse. *Child Dev* 62:179–189, 1991.

Wyatt GE, Peters SD, Guthrie D: Kinsey revisited. Part I: Comparisons of the sexual socialization and sexual behavior of white women over 33 years. *Arch Sex Behav* 17:201–239, 1988a.

Wyatt GE, Peters S, Guthrie D: Kinsey revisited. Part 2: Comparisons of the sexual socialization and sexual behavior of black women over 33 years. *Arch Sex Behav* 17:289–332, 1988b.

Yen SSC, Rebar RW, Quesenberry W: Pituitary function in pseudocyesis. *J Clin Endocrinol Metab* 43:132–136, 1976.

Youniss J, Smollar J: *Adolescent Relations with Mothers, Fathers, and Friends.* Chicago, University of Chicago Press, 1985.

Zabin LS, Hirsch MB, Smith EA, et al: Evaluation of a pregnancy prevention program for urban teenagers. *Fam Plann Perspect* 18:119–126, 1986.

Zelnik M, Kantner JF: Sexual and contraceptive experience of young unmarried women in the US, 1976 and 1971. *Fam Plann Perspect* 9:55–71, 1977.

Zelnik M, Kantner JF: Sexual activity, contraceptive use and pregnancy among metropolitan teenagers: 1971–1979. *Fam Plann Perspect* 12:230–243, 1980.

Zelnik M, Shah FK: First intercourse among young Americans. *Fam Plann Perspect* 15:64–70, 1983.

Zelnik M, Kantner JF, Ford K: *Sex and Pregnancy in Adolescence.* Beverly Hills, CA, Sage, 1981.

23 ANXIETY

Cynthia G. Last, Ph.D., Deborah C. Beidel, Ph.D., and Sean Perrin, Ph.D.

Although during the past two decades we have witnessed a dramatic increase in attention paid to adult anxiety disorders, it is only recently that a similar trend has begun to emerge for the childhood anxiety disorders. It is probable that the major classification changes appearing in the third edition of DSM-III (1980) were responsible, at least in part, for spurring research on anxious children and adolescents. In DSM-III a new diagnostic category was introduced that specifically focused on anxiety disorders that usually first arise during childhood or adolescence ("Anxiety Disorders of Childhood or Adolescence").

Prior to DSM-III, anxiety disorders were rarely identified in children, with symptoms of fear and worry being attributed to "normal" developmental phases. Although clinical experience and empirical research indicate that certain fears are common to different developmental stages during infancy, childhood, and adolescence ("age or stage specific"), age appropriateness in and of itself does not negate the presence of an anxiety disorder. If an age-appropriate fear is found to be excessive (i.e., over and above what would be expected in a normal child of that age) and causes impairment in functioning or high levels of subjective distress, a psychiatric diagnosis (and intervention) should be considered. In addition to cases such as these, specific fears or patterns of worry that are not appropriate for a particular developmental period (e.g., separation anxiety in a 13-year-old boy or excessive worries about family finances and college in a 10-year-old girl) are equally likely to be manifestations of early anxiety disorder.

The prevalence of anxiety disorders in childhood and adolescence really should not be surprising, in light of the large amount of follow-back data that has suggested that adult anxiety disorders often can be traced back to childhood. Indeed, currently there are a number of outpatient clinics throughout the United States that focus exclusively on the assessment and treatment of youngsters with anxiety disorder, and data on the phenomenology of anxiety in this population have begun to emerge.

In this chapter, we focus on the development of anxiety disorders in children and adolescents, examining a number of factors hypothesized to play a role in the pathogenesis of childhood-onset anxiety disorders. More specifically, we review the literature in regard to ethological considerations, temperament, familial/genetic factors, physiological variables, stressful life events, and vicarious conditioning, in order to attempt to tease apart which of these, if any, may be of etiological significance.

FAMILY STUDIES

Family studies generally are considered to be important means for establishing whether specific psychiatric disorders run in families. In addition to theoretical significance, the investigation of familial aggregation of psychiatric disorders provides information that may be useful for early detection and intervention, and, ultimately, prevention. Of course, the fact that specific types of psychiatric illnesses run in families does not in and of itself address the issue of genetic versus environmental mode of transmission. However, information obtained from family studies is an important first step in understanding whether familial genetic and/or environmental factors may play a role in the development of psychiatric disorders.

Information concerning familial prevalence of psychiatric disorders may be obtained by either the family history method or the family study method (Andreasen et al., 1977; Mendlewicz et al., 1975; Thompson et al., 1982). The family history method consists of obtaining information from the patient or other relatives about all family members. The family study method, on the other hand, involves direct interviewing of all available relatives concerning their own present and/or past psychiatric illnesses and symptomatology.

The family study method has been noted to be the preferred technique for studying familial prevalence, since this method yields data that are more precise and accurate than that obtained through use of the family history method. However, the family history method remains widely used because it is often difficult or impossible to directly interview relatives. This is especially true in family research that examines close relatives of adult probands. In these cases, relatives of adult probands often are inaccessible because of geographic location or death. These factors usually do not constitute major problems for family studies of child probands. This is especially true for first-degree relatives, that is, the parents and siblings of child probands, who usually will be residing in the same household as the proband. In addition, because of the younger age of child and adolescent probands, one may anticipate that a higher percentage of first-degree relatives will still be living and available for interview.

Review of the Literature

Whether there is a familial factor involved in the development of childhood anxiety disorders has been addressed by a number of investigations. One approach for studying this question has been referred to as the "top down" method, where the children of adult patients diagnosed as having an anxiety disorder are studied. The second approach has been referred to as the "bottom up" method, where parents and other relatives of children diagnosed as having anxiety disorders are studied. Investigations using both of these methods and their results will be described.

TOP DOWN STUDIES

Four studies have used the top down method to assess anxiety disorders in children. Berg (1976) investigated the prevalence of school phobia in the children of agoraphobic women via a questionnaire survey. School phobia was assumed to have been present when mothers answered yes to this question: "Has the child ever completely refused to go to school for longer than 1 or 2 days since starting junior school at 7?" (p. 86). Results for children 7–15 years old showed a prevalence rate of 7%. However, when children of secondary school age (11–15 years) were considered separately, the prevalence rate rose to 15%. Berg states that these rates (particularly for children 11–15 years) are higher than what would be expected in the general population.

Interpretation of findings for this study is hampered by several methodological problems: (a) The criterion for identifying cases of school phobia is overinclusive, as cases of depression, medical illness, and truancy may meet the criterion and result in misclassification as "school phobia,'' although it is less likely for truancy to be misclassified as school phobia since truants do not resist going to school (they leave for school willingly but never get there); (*b*) lack of a psychopathological control group renders one unable to determine whether the rates of school phobia observed are due to psychopathology per se, rather than agoraphobia specifically; and (*c*) lack of a matched normal control group precludes comparison of obtained rates with ''base rates'' for the general population.

In a similar but smaller study, Buglass et al. (1977) compared the offspring of 30 agoraphobic women with the offspring of 30 matched nonpsychiatrically disturbed women. Information on the children was obtained through interviewing of the mothers and a symptom checklist. Results indicated that the two groups did not differ in the rate of psychiatric illness in general, or school phobia in particular. In fact, contrary to expectation, none of the agoraphobics' children showed agoraphobia or school refusal.

Unfortunately, the investigation did not report the number of offspring in different age brackets. Since school phobia has been shown to yield a higher prevalence rate in preadolescence and adolescence, rather than in early or middle childhood (e.g., Berg, 1976; Last et al. 1987a), such information is of importance. As noted by Gittelman (1986), it is possible for no case of school phobia to occur in a very small sample if the expected rate is relatively low (e.g., 10% to 15%) (p. 114). Moreover, the use of the family history method, where the children themselves are not interviewed directly, most probably resulted in an underestimate of psychiatric illness in this study.

Weissman and colleagues (Weissman et al., 1984) compared children of women with major depression with or without a history of anxiety disorders and a group of matched control subjects. The family history method was used, where information on the children's psychiatric status was obtained from the proband, spouse, and other first-degree relatives. The depressed probands with concurrent anxiety disorders were divided into three groups: (*a*) depression and agoraphobia, (*b*) depression and panic disorder, and (*c*) depression and generalized anxiety disorder. The anxiety groups then were compared with women who had depression but no anxiety disorder and normals.

An increased risk of anxiety disorders, specifically separation anxiety disorder, was present in the children of women with depression and panic disorder, with 11 of 19 (36.8%) offspring meeting DSM-III criteria for the diagnosis. None of the offspring of normal or depressed-only probands met criteria for separation anxiety disorder. In the other two depression plus anxiety disorder groups, relatively low rates were obtained for separation anxiety disorder, with 2 of 18 (11.1%) children of agoraphobic probands and 2 of 32 (6.3%) children of generalized anxiety disorder women meeting diagnostic criteria. When the offspring of agoraphobic and panic disorder women are combined, the risk of separation anxiety disorder decreased to 24.3%, a rate still greater than seen in the other groups.

Although these data are important, it should be noted that use of the family history method, where the offspring are not interviewed directly, most probably resulted in an underestimation of the rate of psychopathology. Therefore, the study addresses the *relative* rate of separation anxiety disorder in the children of the groups studied, but not the expected rates. The possible effect of comorbid major depression in the mothers cannot be evaluated since the children of patients with anxiety disorders only were not included in the study (such studies are ongoing in several centers). It should be emphasized that an increased rate of anxiety disorders *only* was obtained in the children of patients with panic disorder. Agoraphobia and generalized anxiety disorder did not result in a higher morbid risk for offspring. The reason for this is unclear, at least for agoraphobia, given previous research findings supporting a relationship between panic disorder and agoraphobia. Indeed, both DSM-III-R and DSM-IV consider the two illnesses to be variants of the same disorder (American Psychiatric Association, 1987, 1994). However, the number of mothers with agoraphobia was small and was probably insufficient to yield firm results.

Turner et al. (1987) directly assessed children of patients with anxiety-disorder. These children were compared with children of patients with dysthymic disorder, children of normal parents, and normal schoolchildren. All children were assessed with a semistructured interview schedule and diagnosed according to DSM-III. Results indicated that of 16 children of probands with anxiety-disorder, 6 (38%) received a diagnosis of an anxiety disorder. Four of the children met criteria for separation anxiety disorder, and 2 met criteria for overanxious disorder. By comparison, 3 of the 14 offspring (21%) of patients with dysthymic disorder met diagnostic criteria for an anxiety disorder, including 1 child with separation anxiety disorder, 1 with overanxious disorder, and 1 with social phobia. Only 1 child of the normal parents and none of the normal schoolchildren met criteria for an anxiety disorder diagnosis. Statistical analysis of the data indicated that the anxiety disorders group significantly differed from both normal control groups but not from the dysthymic disorder group.

The above results were obtained by the inclusion of multiple offspring of the same parents. Turner et al. reanalyzed their data with a reduced sample, randomly selecting only one child from each of the families with multiple children. Reanalysis with the reduced sample replicated the full sample results, with 6 of 13 offspring (46%) in the anxiety disorders group meeting criteria for an anxiety disorder (4 with separation anxiety and 2 with overanxious disorder), 3 of 11 dysthymic offspring (27%) meeting diagnostic criteria for an anxiety disorder (1 with overanxious disorder, 1 with separation anxiety disorder, and 1 with social phobia), and no children in the solicited normal or school normal groups meeting diagnostic criteria.

Although Turner et al. were able to demonstrate an increased risk of anxiety disorders in the children of patients with anxiety disorder compared with the two nonpatient groups, they were not able to demonstrate differences between the two patient groups. The selection of dysthymic disorder probands as the psychopathological control group for the study may be problematic, in that a relationship between affective and anxiety disorders has been suggested by previous research. Therefore, studies with more power (i.e., larger samples) are necessary to investigate the issue.

BOTTOM UP STUDIES

A number of bottom up studies have been conducted, where the relatives of child patients with anxiety disorders have been evaluated. Berg et al. (1974) evaluated maternal psychiatric illness in school-phobic adolescents admitted to an inpatient psychiatric unit. The maternal psychiatric histories of 100 school-phobic youngsters were compared with maternal histories of 113 hospitalized non-school-phobic patients. Maternal psychiatric illness was evaluated by examining hospital and medical records. One-fifth of the mothers in both groups had a history of some type of psychiatric disturbance. Of these, approximately one-half were diagnosed as having an affective disorder, which was defined in this study as anxiety, depression, or phobias. Thus, maternal psychiatric illness in the two patient groups did not significantly differ. Obviously, the use of record review as opposed to direct interviews severely hampers the conclusions that can be drawn from this investigation. Moreover, the lumping together of affective and anxiety disorders under the category of ''affective disorders'' limits interpretation of findings.

Gittelman-Klein (1975) interviewed the parents of 42 school-phobic and 42 hyperactive children to determine their psychiatric histories. Results were analyzed for three specific diagnostic categories: major depression, specific phobias, and separation anxiety disorder. No differences appeared between the two groups of parents for major depression or specific phobias. However, the parents of school-phobic youngsters were found to have a significantly higher rate of separation anxiety disorder than parents of hyperactive children (19 versus 2%, respectively).

In addition to the above, parents reported on siblings' histories of psychiatric illness, particularly school phobia. Among 67 siblings of the school-phobic children, 11 (16%) had a clear-cut history of school phobia. By contrast, none of 66 siblings of hyperactive probands were reported to have a history of school phobia. These differences between the two groups were statistically significant. Interestingly, when the relationship between parental separation anxiety disorder and school phobia in siblings was examined, it was found that separation anxiety in the parents was not correlated with the presence of school phobia in the siblings. Interpretation of findings from this investigation is hampered by several ambiguities. First, the diagnostic criteria for school phobia and separation anxiety disorder are not reported. Second, it is unclear why separation anxiety disorder was examined in the parents while school phobia was examined in the siblings. Finally, although interviewers were unaware of the questions investigated, they were not blind to the children's diagnostic status, which potentially could seriously bias results.

Last, Phillips et al. (1987) examined the prevalence of two childhood anxiety disorders, separation anxiety and overanxious disorders, in the mothers of children diagnosed as having one or both of these disorders and in a control group of mothers of children who were psychiatrically disturbed but did not have an anxiety or affective disorder. DSM-III diagnostic criteria were used to diagnose both the children and their mothers, and the diagnosis of the mothers' childhood disorders was conducted blindly through the use of a structured diagnostic questionnaire (''Childhood History Questionnaire'') by raters who were unaware of the children's disorders. The study was designed to determine whether there was a relationship between mothers and their children for childhood anxiety disorders and whether the nature of this relationship was general or specific. It was hypothesized that a specific relationship would exist, that is, (a) mothers of children with separation anxiety disorder had separation anxiety disorder as children, and (b) mothers of overanxious children had overanxious disorder as children.

Results indicated that only one of the two hypotheses was supported. For separation anxiety disorder, no differences were found in the rates for the three groups of mothers. By contrast, the rate of overanxious disorder was significantly higher in mothers of overanxious children than in mothers of either separation-anxious children or control children. More specifically, in the overanxious disorder group, 18 of 43 mothers (42%) reported a childhood history of overanxious disorder, compared to 2 of 21 mothers (9.5%) in the separation anxiety disorder group and 5 of 33 mothers (15%) in the control group.

While data from this study supported a specific relationship between overanxious disorder in mothers and their children, such a relationship was not shown for separation anxiety disorder. These findings are in contrast to those reported above from Gittelman-Klein. It is possible that the method of assessment utilized in the Last et al. study obscured a relationship for separation anxiety disorder. Separation anxiety disorder symptoms, as compared to those present in overanxious disorder, generally are more specific and of a shorter duration, with DSM-III requiring only a 2-week duration for the diagnosis. Direct interviews with the mothers, rather than a symptom checklist, might have helped to probe for the more specific and relatively transient symptoms of separation anxiety disorder.

In a recent bottom up study conducted by Livingston et al. (1985), the relatives of 12 anxious and 11 depressed children were examined using the family history method. Relatives primarily included mothers, fathers, and grandparents, yielding a sample size of 69 in the anxiety disorder group and 58 in the depressed group. Results indicated that in most respects the family histories of the two groups did not differ. Strikingly, only one relative in each of the groups was diagnosed as having an anxiety disorder. As the investigators themselves note, their study must be considered in light of methodological limitations, including the small number of probands included and use of the family history method to diagnose psychiatric illness. In concluding their paper, they state that large-scale family studies utilizing instruments sensitive to anxiety disorders are needed.

Another small study (Bernstein and Garfinkel, 1988) examined psychopathology in the first-degree relatives of 6 children with school phobia using the family study method. Familial psychopathology in the school-phobic families was compared to rates obtained in five families of children with other psychiatric disorders. Results indicated that 7 of 12 (58%) parents of school-phobic children showed an anxiety disorder, as compared to 3 of 10 (30%) parents of psychiatric controls. For siblings, 5 of 10 (50%) met criteria for an anxiety disorder in the school-phobic group, compared to none of 5 (0%) siblings in the control group. Unfortunately, the findings from this study may be regarded as only preliminary, given the very small number of probands included in the school-phobic and control groups (6 and 5, respectively).

Last, Hersen et al. (1987) utilized the family study method to compare maternal psychiatric illness for children with separation anxiety disorder and/or overanxious disorder (n = 58) and for children who were psychiatrically disturbed but did not manifest an anxiety or affective disorder (n = 15). Mothers were interviewed directly about lifetime psychiatric illness with a semistructured diagnostic interview and diagnosed according to DSM-III criteria. Interviewers were blind to children's diagnoses, and diagnostic agreement was evaluated by having a second clinician, also blind to children's diagnoses, independently score audiotapes of the interviews. Children in the control group were diagnosed as having behavior disorders, including conduct disorder, attention deficit disorder, and/or oppositional disorder.

Results indicated that mothers of children with anxiety disorders had a significantly higher lifetime rate of anxiety disorders than mothers of control children (83 versus 40%, respectively). Moreover, when current rates of anxiety disorders were examined, the mothers of children with anxiety disorder once again showed a significantly higher rate than the mothers of control children (57 versus 20%, respectively).

Findings from the study are striking in that the vast majority of mothers of this clinic sample of children with anxiety disorder showed a lifetime history of anxiety disorder. Moreover, approximately one-half of these mothers presented with an anxiety disorder at the same time at which their children were seen for similar problems. However, since mothers alone were interviewed, it is unclear whether the relationship for anxiety disorders was specific to the mother-child dyad or was indicative of a more general pattern of familial aggregation. The authors call for large-scale family studies of this population in order to address this question.

Lenane et al. (1990) present data on the prevalence of psychiatric disorder in the first-degree relatives of children and adolescents with obsessive compulsive disorder (OCD). Probands included 46 clinically referred children with severe primary OCD who were participants in a drug treatment trial for OCD. Proband diagnoses were based on direct semistructured interviews and DSM-III criteria. There were 145 first-degree relatives (parents and siblings) in the OCD group. Interviews with the relatives also were conducted with semistructured interview and based on DSM-III criteria. While interviews with the parents were conducted by raters blind to the proband's diagnosis, the same was not true for sibling interviews. A small sample of age-matched children with conduct disorder (n = 34) and their parents were included in the study, but complete diagnostic information on this group was not provided.

Overall, 30% of the OCD probands had at least one family member with OCD. By contrast, only 1.5% of the parents of children with conduct disorder received a diagnosis of OCD. For the parents of OCD probands, OCD occurred in fathers more frequently than in mothers (25 versus 9%). Moreover, there was a 2:1 ratio of males to females with OCD in the study, with the most common parent-child combination being father and son with OCD. The age-corrected rate of OCD in siblings was 35%. Almost half (45%) of the fathers and two-thirds of the mothers were diagnosed with an Axis I disorder other than OCD. Thirty-six percent of the siblings were diagnosed with a non-OCD Axis I disorder. The most frequent psychiatric disorders diagnosed in relatives were mood disorders (mothers, 59%; fathers, 36%; and siblings, 45%). Anxiety disorders other than OCD were found in 11% of the fathers, 17% of the mothers, and 7% of the siblings of probands with OCD.

Generalized anxiety disorder was the most frequently diagnosed non-OCD anxiety disorder in parents (12%), while separation anxiety disorder and phobias were the most common (2% each) in siblings. The authors note that, in families of OCD probands where either a parent or older sibling also was diagnosed with OCD, no clear pattern emerged in terms of similar ages-at-onset or symptom profiles. Based on these findings, they conclude that children with OCD did not appear to "learn" their disorder from parents or older siblings with the disorder. However, the absence of a clearly defined control group, and the severity of this clinically referred sample, may limit the generalizability of these findings.

Last and colleagues (Last et al., 1991) have conducted a large-scale family study of childhood anxiety disorders. Lifetime psychiatric illness was assessed in the first- and second-degree relatives of child probands diagnosed as having an anxiety disorder. Probands included 94 children with an anxiety disorder, a psychopathological control group of 58 children with attention deficit hyperactivity disorder (ADHD), and a normal control group of 87 children who never had been psychiatrically ill (NPI). Probands in the NPI group were matched for age (within 1 year) and sex to the anxiety disorder probands. All children in the study were administered a modified version of the Schedule for Affective Disorders and Schizophrenia for School-Age Children (present episode) (K-SADS-P). First-degree relatives (mothers, fathers, and full siblings 5 years or older) were interviewed directly using the family study method. Adult first-degree relatives (18 years or older) were interviewed for current and past psychiatric illness with the Structured Clinical Interview for DSM-III-R (SCID) (R.L. Spitzer, J.B.W. Williams, M. Gibbon, unpublished manuscript, 1986). Screenings for childhood disorders not contained in the SCID (i.e., separation anxiety disorder, overanxious disorder, avoidant disorder, and ADHD) also were administered to the adult relatives using sections from the modified K-SADS-P. Child and adolescent siblings of the probands were interviewed for current and past psychiatric illness with the modified K-SADS-P. Information on second-degree relatives (maternal and paternal grandparents, aunts, and uncles) was obtained from the parents using the family history method. The number of first-degree relatives included in the study was as follows: 274 in the anxiety disorder group, 152 in the ADHD group, and 240 in the NPI group. Second-degree relatives included 812 in the anxiety disorder group, 484 in the ADHD group, and 718 in the never psychiatrically ill group. All family interviews were conducted blindly.

The rate of anxiety disorders found in first-degree relatives of probands with anxiety disorder (34.6%) was significantly greater than that found in first-degree relatives of probands with ADHD (23.5%) and NPI controls (16.3%). The differences among the three groups were due in large part to differences obtained for first-degree male relatives. Male relatives of anxious children were two times more likely to have an anxiety disorder than the male relatives of either control group (anxiety, 23.9%; ADHD, 10.5%; and NPI, 8.0%). Although the risk for female relatives did not differ for the families of anxiety and ADHD probands, both groups showed significantly higher morbidity risks for first-degree female relatives compared with risks for normal controls (anxiety, 45.5%, and ADHD, 37.0% versus NPI, 24.2%). The increased rate of anxiety disorders in relatives of anxious children were concentrated in the parents. Male and female siblings of probands in the three groups did not differ significantly for the rate of anxiety disorder. Finally, comparison of all second-degree relatives did not show differences between the anxiety (11.5%) and ADHD (11.0%) groups, but both differed significantly from the NPI group (7.3%).

Morbidity risks for specific anxiety disorders in first-degree relatives were compared for the three proband groups. Only two anxiety disorders were more prevalent in the relatives of anxious children than of ADHD children: overanxious disorder (anxiety, 18.9%, versus ADHD, 10.3%) and simple phobias (anxiety, 11.7%, versus ADHD, 4.7%). In comparison with the NPI group, the first-degree relatives of anxious children had a higher frequency of panic disorder, social phobia, simple phobia, OCD, overanxious disorder, and avoidant disorder. Although rates were

in the predicted direction, the anxiety and NPI groups did not differ in their rates of generalized anxiety disorder, posttraumatic stress disorder, or separation anxiety disorder among first-degree relatives.

Rates for the specific anxiety disorders also were compared, separately, for male and female first-degree relatives of probands in the three groups. Simple phobias, overanxious disorder, and separation anxiety disorder were more prevalent in male relatives of probands with anxiety disorder than in male relatives of children in the two control groups. By contrast, first-degree female relatives of anxious and ADHD probands did not differ for any of the specific anxiety disorders. However, each of the anxiety disorder subtypes, except for generalized anxiety disorder, posttraumatic stress disorder, and separation anxiety disorder, were more prevalent in the female relatives of anxious probands than of normal controls. Finally, the female relatives of children with ADHD showed significantly higher rates of posttraumatic stress disorder and avoidant disorder than female relatives of normal controls.

The relationship between proband's and relatives' anxiety disorders were examined in this study. Interestingly, children with separation anxiety disorder were no more likely to have a relative with separation anxiety disorder or panic disorder than were any other anxiety disorder group of children. By contrast, children with overanxious disorder were significantly more likely than children with anxiety disorder without overanxious disorder to have a relative with overanxious disorder (29.8 versus 11.0%), panic disorder (11.5 versus 0%), and separation anxiety disorder (18.8 versus 3.4%). There was a trend toward significance in the rate of OCD in the relatives of children with this disorder compared with those without OCD (6.7 versus 1.4%, respectively). A similar trend was observed for panic disorder in children with and without panic disorder (10.8 versus 3.9%, respectively). No other specific relationships were observed for phobic disorders, posttraumatic stress disorder, or avoidant disorder.

Although morbidity risks provide useful information, they give little indication about how anxiety disorders may segregate within families. To examine this factor, Last et al. used individual families as the unit of analysis and compared the three groups on the following: (a) number (percentage) of families containing a first-degree relative with an anxiety disorder, (b) number (percentage) of families containing a parent with an anxiety disorder, and (c) number (percentage) of families containing a sibling with an anxiety disorder.

A significantly higher percentage of families in the anxiety group had at least one first-degree relative with an anxiety disorder when compared with the two control groups (anxiety, 69.9%; ADHD, 50.0%; and NPI, 40.5%). In terms of the percentage of families with at least one parent with anxiety disorder, the anxiety group differed significantly from the NPI control group (65.6 versus 35.7%, respectively), but showed only a statistical trend ($P = .10$) toward difference with the ADHD group (50.0%). The percentage of families with at least one sibling with an anxiety disorder were in the expected direction but did not statistically differ for the three groups (anxiety, 26.3%; ADHD, 20.7%; and NPI, 13.6%).

Overall, findings from this family study showed a very high morbidity risk for anxiety disorders in the relatives of children with anxiety disorder. Differences for the male relatives of this group compared with both the psychopathological and NPI control groups were particularly striking. Female relatives of probands with anxiety disorder showed a greatly increased risk for anxiety disorder only when compared with female relatives of NPI children. In terms of the specific types of anxiety disorders found in the families of the three proband groups, relatives of probands with anxiety disorder were more likely to receive diagnoses of simple phobia and overanxious disorder than were the ADHD group. Significant differences were found in the rates of panic disorder, phobias, OCD, and overanxious disorder. Finally, the segregation of anxiety disorders within individual families occurred most frequently in the anxiety disorder proband group.

Recently, Fyer and colleagues (Fyer et al., 1993) conducted a bottom up study of psychopathology in the first-degree relatives of socially phobic adults. Probands included 30 adults (mean age, 33 years) with a lifetime history of social phobia but no other anxiety disorder. A control group of 77 probands (mean age, 42 years) without a lifetime history of any psychiatric disorder was included in the study. The number of first-degree relatives in the two probands groups were social phobia, 83, and NPI, 231. All diagnoses were obtained from direct semi-structured interviews with the proband and first-degree relatives and based on DSM-III-R criteria. Relative and control interviews were conducted by raters blind to proband diagnosis.

First-degree relatives of socially phobic probands (SP) were almost two times more likely (risk ratio = 1.73, $P < .05$) to have an anxiety disorder (including social phobia) than were relatives of NPI controls (25 versus 16%, respectively). Social phobia occurred three times as often (risk ratio = 3.12, $P < .01$) in the relatives of the SP group than in the relatives of the NPI group (16 versus 5%, respectively). No significant differences were found between the two probands groups for any other anxiety disorders in their relatives. The findings of this study are notable because of the absence of comorbid anxiety disorders in the social phobia proband group. Thus, familial risk attributable to social phobia, specifically (as opposed to other anxiety disorders), could be examined.

In summary, both top down and bottom up studies suggest that anxiety disorders tend to run in families. Evidence for the transmission of specific disorders were extremely limited. Still, there appears to be a strong familial link in the development of OCD and social phobia. However, the studies reviewed above rely primarily on diagnostic data collected from the families of clinically referred probands. It is possible that the observed rates of anxiety disorder in the relatives of these treatment-seeking probands are higher than what would be found in the relatives of nonreferred probands, who presumably are less disturbed. Family studies of nonreferred, anxiety disorder probands are needed to help clarify this issue. Also, treatment-seeking, anxiety disorder individuals frequently present with more than one psychiatric disorder (Brown and Barlow, 1992; Last et al., 1992). Findings suggesting an increased risk of anxiety disorders in families are obscured by the presence of multiple psychiatric disorders in the probands. Additional studies, with larger samples of pure anxiety disorder probands would be helpful in determining if anxiety disorder, or psychopathology in general, runs in families.

Genetic Versus Environmental Transmission

Obviously, the studies reviewed above do not address the issue of mode of transmission, that is, environmental or genetic transmission. The top down and bottom up studies indicate that anxiety disorders tend to run in families, but only investigations utilizing methodologies common to genetic research (twin studies, adoption studies) can assess whether a hereditary component is present. What family studies can accomplish, in this regard, is to generate "negative proof," that is, if a higher frequency of a disorder is not observed among biological relatives, then genetic factors cannot be involved.

In a review of genetic factors in the transmission of anxiety disorders, Torgersen (1988) concluded that panic disorder, phobic disorders, and OCD seemed to be influenced by genetic factors. By contrast, generalized anxiety disorder and posttraumatic stress disorder did not appear to be mediated through genetic transmission.

Two interesting questions emerge in regard to the mode of transmission of childhood anxiety disorders. If transmission is genetic, what, specifically, is inherited? Conversely, if transmission is environmental, how, specifically, is it accomplished?

From a hereditary perspective, individual differences in infants' temperaments (e.g., Kagan, 1988: Thomas et al., 1963) and/or in arousal level and habituation to stimuli (Johnson and Melamed, 1979) may be related to the acquisition of fear and anxiety disorders in childhood. This may be referred to as "anxiety proneness" or "vulnerability," but in either case denotes an inherited "disposition" toward developing anxiety disorders. This is discussed in further detail elsewhere in this chapter.

Such an inherited disposition may interact adversely with certain environmental events, such as stressful life events (see below) or family interaction patterns and child-rearing practices. In this regard, the mother-child relationship has repeatedly been implicated, on both theoretical and empirical grounds, as an etiologic factor in the development of separation anxiety disorder and school phobia (e.g., Berg and McGuire, 1974; Eisenberg, 1958; Hersov, 1960). Generally, mothers are described as overprotective, having separation anxiety issues of their own, and reinforcing dependency and lack of autonomy in their children. The notion that maternal psychopathology plays a causal and/or maintenance role in children's anxiety disorders is of considerable importance since inferences have been drawn regarding intervention (Eisenberg, 1958). Considerably more research is needed regarding the relative roles (alone and in combination) of hereditary and family interaction variables.

At a more basic level, children may inherit certain physiological predispositions to develop anxiety disorders. Recent developments in brain-imaging technologies and psychopharmacology have spurred research interest into the neuronal bases of anxiety disorder. While this area of research is relatively new and beyond the scope of this chapter, a few general comments can be made. First, noradrenergic agents have been found to produce the autonomic symptoms associated with anxiety (Wamboldt and Insel, 1988). Charney et al. (1990) and Pohl et al. (1990) have conducted a series of studies that provide limited support for the hypothesis relating development of panic disorder, and anxiety in general, to hyperactivity in the noradrenergic pathways of the brain. Second, anxiogenic agents acting through a receptor complex involving benzodiazepines, γ-aminobutyric acid (GABA), and chloride ionophore, concentrated in the neocortex and limbic structures, have been shown to produce the cognitive aspects of anxiety (Wamboldt and Insel, 1988). Increased receptor sensitivity in this complex may be related to the development of anxiety (Wamboldt and Insel, 1988). Third, there is evidence, albeit limited, linking dysfunction in the serotonergic pathways connecting the frontal lobe and basal ganglia in the development of OCD (see Rapoport, 1989). However, additional research is needed to establish the specific neuronal pathways that mediate anxiety, as well as the heritability of these biological mechanisms.

STRESSFUL LIFE EVENTS

In a recent review of the adult literature, Monroe and Wade (1988) concluded that the available evidence suggests a relationship between life events and the development of anxiety disorders. Unfortunately, at least to our knowledge, almost no data exist pertaining to an association between life events and the onset of anxiety disorders in childhood.

From our clinical experience, it is clear that the onset and exacerbation of childhood anxiety disorders often are precipitated by stressful life occurrences. This particularly appears to be the case for separation anxiety disorder and school phobia, which may develop (or exacerbate) following a loss, such as illness or death of a significant other or a move to a new neighborhood or school. In this regard, Gittelman-Klein and Klein (1980) have reported that in their experience approximately 80% of school refusers show an onset associated with one of the aforementioned events.

Interestingly, early studies that were conducted following major traumatic events (e.g., cyclone, war zone, desegregation) consistently showed negative results (Gordon, 1977; Martinez-Monfort and Dreger, 1972; Ziv and Israeli, 1973). A methodological problem common to each of these investigations, however, was exclusive reliance on children's self-ratings of their affective state. By contrast, subsequent studies using more rigorous methodological approaches have shown adverse reactions in children exposed to massive traumas and natural disasters (Galante and Foa, 1986; Handford et al., 1986; Kinzie et al., 1986: Malmquist, 1986; Terr, 1981).

Certainly there is a major difference between children who have a pattern of attachment disrupted and those who experience a major traumatic or life-threatening event. It may be that children who already are vulnerable or predisposed to developing anxiety disorders may be affected significantly by seemingly more innocuous events. In any event, more research is needed on evaluating the association between life events and anxiety disorders in children before conclusions can be drawn.

ETHOLOGICAL CONSIDERATIONS

Those who ascribe to an ethological perspective consider that much of behavior is biologically or genetically based, that some behavioral patterns are species specific and necessary to the survival of the organism, and indeed to the ultimate survival of the species. In humans, some of the clearest examples of survival-dependent behaviors are apparent at birth, including activities such as crying and clinging, which function to keep the helpless infant in close contact with nurturing adults upon whom they are dependent for sustenance and protection (Ainsworth, 1969; Bowlby, 1969; Campbell, 1986). From this vantage point, many of the "normal" fears displayed by infants and young children also may be conceptualized as possessing species survival value.

Infants are frightened by loud noises, heights, darkness, and strangers. These fears are easily elicited and predictably appear during certain developmental stages. As noted by Campbell (1986), some fears, including loud noises or looming objects, are present at birth, while others, such as stranger anxiety, hinge upon the infant's cognitive development. Although superficially the objects or events that the infant fears may appear quite random, from an ethological perspective they form a coherent group of stimuli, all of which contain a core element of danger that may threaten the organism's ultimate survival. While a specific object or event may not be inherently fearful, its survival value may be that it serves as a signal of impending danger, thus allowing the individual time for withdrawal or protection (Bowlby, 1973; Campbell, 1986). The predictable expression of these fear responses among young children is less consistent with traumatic conditioning theories of fear acquisition but quite consistent with the view that the fears may be an expression of genetic programming (Bowlby, 1973). In addition, the consistency of the developmental stage when certain fears are expressed lends credence to their conceptualization as biologically determined, species-specific behavioral patterns, which at least in the past functioned to promote the organism's survival.

The "preparedness" hypothesis proposed by Seligman (1971) also stems from a survival perspective. An examination of the most common fears in the adult population, which include heights and snakes (Agras et al., 1969), combined with the absence of traumatic conditioning events to explain the prevalence of these fears, contributed to Seligman's proposal that certain fears had species survival value. Using the Darwinian notion of survival of the fittest, Seligman proposed that long ago, individuals who reacted fearfully to situations such as heights or snakes were more likely to avoid the associated danger than other persons and thus more likely to survive and pass on these traits to future generations. In contrast, those who were nonfearful were more likely to engage in risky behaviors and have an increased likelihood of premature death, and thus were less likely to significantly affect the gene pool. An advantage of Seligman's theory is that empirically testable hypotheses can be derived from it, and studies by Ohman and his colleagues (e.g., Ohman, 1986; Ohman et al., 1975, 1976) provide some empirical support. Based on skin conductance responses during classical conditioning trials, responses to fear-relevant stimuli such as spiders and snakes could be more easily conditioned and were more resistant to extinction than were responses to fear-irrelevant stimuli such as flowers and mushrooms. While other researchers also have provided partial evidence for a preparedness model based on heart rate conditioning (Cook et al., 1986), many others have failed to replicate these findings. (The interested reader is referred to an excellent review of this area by McNally, 1987.)

As noted in another section of this chapter, one variable that could intervene in the attempt to condition fears in the laboratory is the individual's prior experience with the object serving as the conditioned stimulus. For example, it may be more difficult to condition fear in subjects who have prior positive or neutral experiences with a stimulus. While it is difficult to control prior experience with human subjects, this can be accomplished using animal models. Recent studies with nonhuman primates, where prior experience can be controlled, have rekindled interest in preparedness theory. Cook and Mineka (1989) have demonstrated that fearful reactions are more easily acquired when laboratory-reared monkeys observe other monkeys behaving fearfully in the presence of fear-relevant stimuli such as snakes or lizards than when they behave fearfully in the presence of rabbits or flowers. In each case, videotapes of a monkey behaving fearfully in the presence of a live snake were spliced and edited so that it appeared to the observer monkey that this fearful reaction was elicited by a toy snake, toy lizard, toy rabbit, or a flower. Despite the identical reaction of the model, superior observational conditioning and demonstration of fear responses occurred consistently and significantly more often in the monkeys who viewed the videotapes that included the lizard or snake, objects known to elicit fear in wild-bred rhesus monkeys. The authors interpreted these findings as supporting the predisposition of these monkeys to develop fearful reactions to objects representing danger in the natural environment.

In summary, the contribution of both ethological perspectives (Bowlby, 1973; Seligman, 1971) is that they are useful in understanding "normal" developmental fears as well as the unequal distribution of simple fears among the general population. The theories are less useful, however, in explaining the onset of specific anxiety disorders such as panic disorder or OCD. In addition, a simple ethological perspective cannot account for why some children outgrow these developmental fears whereas others do not. Finally, while contributing much to our understanding of normal development, these theories alone are insufficient to fully explain childhood psychopathology.

TEMPERAMENT AND SHYNESS

The search for etiological factors contributing to the onset of anxiety leads to the concept of temperament. Although generally defined as personality traits found in young children, there is little agreement about the specific nature of this construct (Garrison and Earls, 1987). Thus, while some view temperament as a consistent characteristic of the individual (Buss and Plomin, 1975), others focus on an interactional style, giving equal emphasis to the organism and the psychosocial context (Thomas and Chess, 1977). Although a discussion of temperament research is beyond the scope of this chapter, specific temperamental dimensions such as "sociability" (Buss and Plomin, 1975), "approach-withdrawal" (Thomas and Chess, 1977), and "shyness" (Daniels and Plomin, 1985) are often used as behavioral indicators of anxious emotion. Thus, a brief description of these traits may be useful in understanding their importance for childhood anxiety.

All of these dimensions attempt to characterize the child's social behavior, and at least some infer that negative social behavior stems from anxiety. For example, approach-withdrawal refers to the valence (positive or negative) of the organism's response to new objects, situations, and individuals (Thomas and Chess, 1977). Shyness describes inhibition, withdrawal, and fear displayed by infants in response to novel social situations, while sociability is the tendency to prefer to be with others rather than alone (Daniels and Plomin, 1985). The relationship of these characteristics to distinct psychopathological states such as anxiety disorders is unknown, since, to date, much of the literature pertaining to these constructs has focused on examining the heritability of the factors. This research does suggest, however, that certain temperamental characteristics appear to run in families. Furthermore, research with infants and toddlers (to be discussed below) and nonhuman primates reveals that shyness, or the tendency to become anxious in novel social settings, may have a biological component.

Similar to human primates, rhesus monkeys behave differently when placed in strange social situations. Some will play or explore the new setting, while others will withdraw, cling, grimace, or emit "coo" vocalizations indicative of distress (Suomi et al., 1981). These behaviors have been termed "anxiety like" (Suomi, 1986), and repeated assessments throughout development indicate that for any monkey such behaviors are consistent and persist into the animal's adulthood. Furthermore, those with closer genetic backgrounds tend to display more similar adrenocortical and behavioral fear responses (Suomi, 1986). Thus, when introduced into an unfamiliar social group, biological siblings who were separated at birth and reared apart from their biological mother and from one another showed less variability in their cortisol levels and greater similarity in the fearful behaviors described above than did nongenetically related monkeys who were reared as adopted siblings. Together, these studies suggest that the tendency of some nonhuman primates to respond anxiously to challenging situations may be constitutionally based and unremitting without appropriate intervention.

While the study of nonhuman primates allows for an examination of biological tendencies under strict environmental controls, research with human subjects necessitates an examination of the interplay between somatic and environmental factors. In the case of temperamental characteristics that may be related to specific anxiety disorders, longitudinal studies of monozygotic and dizygotic twins find that, with increasing maturation, higher heritability correlations are maintained for social introversion-extroversion (a combination of shyness, low sociability, and lack of impulsivity) than for general fearfulness (cf. Garrison and Earls, 1987). The relative importance of genetics and the environment is further illustrated by a study of adopted-away infants and their biological and adoptive mothers (Daniels and Plomin, 1985). Adopted parents rated their infant using the Colorado Childhood Temperament Inventory (Rowe and Plomin, 1977), while both biological and adoptive mothers completed the 16 Personality Factor Questionnaire (Cattell et al., 1970) and the Emotionality, Activity, Sociability, and Impulsivity Questionnaire (Buss and Plomin, 1975). At 24 months of age, infant shyness was significantly related to shyness and sociability in the biological mother, and also to low sociability in the adopted mothers. The relationship was quite complex in that the heritability of infant shyness appeared to involve both adult sociability and shyness and to be related to both genetic and environmental influences. As noted by Daniels and Plomin (1985) and corroborated by data from Kagan and colleagues (discussed below), one important environmental variable affecting an individual's degree of shyness may be the amount of experience with novel social situations. Mothers who are shy and unsociable may not expose themselves or their infants to novel social events. However, with increasing maturation, other life events such as entry into school or establishment of peer relationships may function to mediate or alter biological predispositions.

Identifying components of shyness or behavioral introversion, and the stability of this construct, has been the focus of research by Kagan and his colleagues. Kagan (1982) identified 60 children, from an initial pool of 300, who were consistently inhibited or uninhibited in their behavior when exposed to novel situations (see Kagan, 1982, for the specific behaviors used to define these categories). When placed in these situations, the inhibited children had higher heart rates and less heart rate variability than the noninhibited children. Heart rate patterns were stable across several years of follow-up, with individual differences in response to challenging tasks preserved in one cohort from 21 months to 7.5 years ($r = .62$ and $r = .54$, P's $< .001$) and in a second cohort from 31 months to 5.5 years ($r = .59$ and $r = .61$, P's $< .001$; Kagan et al., 1987, 1988). More recent investigations also assessed the children's home and laboratory salivary cortisol levels, an endocrinological measure that has been associated with the presence of negative emotional states (Reznick et al., 1986). At both sites, cortisol levels were higher in the inhibited children than in the noninhibited group. In addition, 6 of the 9 inhibited children with consistently high cortisol levels exhibited somatic and behavioral signs often associated with anxiety states, including gastrointestinal distress, nightmares, and separation fears. The specific symptoms varied across the children, and clinical interviews were not conducted, yet the complaints are consistent with the clinical pictures

of overanxious disorder, separation anxiety, or generalized anxiety disorder. Thus, this particular subgroup of inhibited children may be manifesting the precursors of an anxiety disorder, if not the full clinical syndrome.

Although the somatic parameters of inhibition appeared relatively stable, there was less behavioral consistency. First, the original index of behavioral inhibition at 14 and 20 months was not predictive of scores at age 4. When the subject sample was reduced to those children who fell in the top and bottom 20% of behavioral inhibition at *both* 14 and 20 months (n = 26, or 13 per group), there was a statistically significant difference between the behavioral inhibition scores at age 4. However, this reduces the sample to only 3.25% of the original group, thus limiting the generalizability of the findings. In addition, a statistically significant difference still does not address behavioral stability, and the correlation between behavioral inhibition scores at 14 months and 4 years was not reported. In examining some possible reasons for the limited consistency in overt behavior, both environmental and somatic factors appeared to play a role. For example, preservation of the original behavioral index was apparent for inhibited children whose heart rates were most stable. Inhibited children whose heart rates were highly variable during the original assessments were more likely to change classification. On the environmental side, those children whose mothers, recognizing their child's fearfulness, made special efforts to expose them often to interactions with their peers also moved from inhibited to uninhibited status. In all, approximately 33% of the original sample changed classification, with most of this group becoming less inhibited (Kagan et al., 1988).

Davidson (1993) has suggested that asymmetries in anterior cerebral cortex activity may serve as a biological marker of childhood temperament, specifically behavioral inhibition. In this model, the left frontal lobe is seen to mediate "approach-related" positive emotions and behaviors, while the right frontal lobe is associated with "withdrawal-related" negative emotions and behaviors. Evidence of this asymmetry in frontal lobe activity in behaviorally inhibited children was reported by Davidson et al. (1992, cited in Davidson, 1993) in a recent study. Using procedures developed by Kagan and colleagues, toddlers (31 months of age) were placed into groups based on their level of behavioral inhibition, and their brain electrical activity was measured during presentations of novel stimuli. Behaviorally inhibited children showed much less electrical activity in their left frontal lobes when presented with novel stimuli than did uninhibited children. Moreover, this pattern of lower activity was stable over a 7-month period. Based on these findings, the authors concluded that behavioral inhibition may be associated with deficits in this frontal-lobe-mediated approach system. However, this is a relatively new area of research, and the influence of heritable and environmental factors on this system and their relationship to childhood psychopathology remains to be seen (Davidson, 1993).

As noted earlier, although currently there are few data examining the correlation between temperament and anxiety-based psychopathology, these variables may indeed be related. The descriptors of shyness or behavioral inhibition include increased anxiety and social avoidance designed to decrease the individual's distress (Buss and Plomin, 1985) and appear strikingly similar to the diagnostic criteria of social phobia or avoidant disorder of childhood. Yet it is unclear if temperament is a qualitatively distinct state that predisposes the individual to the onset of these disorders or if the characteristics called temperament actually represent the initial stages of the disorder's onset. In addition, as noted by Garrison and Earls (1987), all of the temperament literature is confounded by methodological difficulties. First, the items that comprise temperament instruments and child behavior problem checklists are virtually identical. Second, all of the measures are administered at the same time. Thus, these data cannot be used to examine etiology. This is particularly true in the most recent studies reported by Kagan, where a biological basis for the inhibited behavior has been implied. Yet despite the stability of the biological correlates, none of the extant data presented by temperament researchers allow for the conclusion that the physiological differences preceded the onset of the overt behavioral characteristics.

In other words, while behavioral and physiological abnormalities coexist, to date there are no data by which to infer causality.

A second criticism concerns the idea of biological determinism. As noted earlier, the lack of exposure to novel social situations may have a significant effect on infant shyness. Longitudinal studies of twins suggest only limited stability for the construct of fearfulness, and the difference between monozygotic and dizygotic twins diminishes with increasing age and increasing socialization opportunities. Similarly, the mothers of the behaviorally inhibited children in Kagan's studies who made an effort to expose their children to other peers and encouraged them to interact with others appeared to have been effective in diminishing the children's behavioral inhibition. Taken together, these data suggest that environmental influences play a significant role in mediating the biological factors that may contribute to the concept of temperament.

In summary, although aspects of temperament such as introversion and shyness may be predispositional states preceding the development of anxiety states or disorders, studies that directly assess the relationship of temperament to child psychopathology have yet to be conducted. In addition, the course does not appear to be invariably determined by biological factors alone, inasmuch as environmental events, particularly in the form of repeated exposure, may exert significant influence to change overt behavior, and perhaps with ever-increasing exposure, physiology as well.

PSYCHOPHYSIOLOGICAL ASSESSMENT

Despite the limitations of the current temperament models, physiological factors are often cited as predisposing an individual to the development of anxiety. Maturation plays a significant role in physiological response characteristics, and therefore assessment in children requires careful attention to the physical and cognitive developmental stage of the organism (Beidel and Stanley, 1993). While recent data indicate that children with DSM-III anxiety disorders and related anxiety states such as test anxiety do exhibit higher heart rates than their nonanxious peers when engaged in social-evaluative situations (Beidel, 1988), as noted above, neither these data nor those of other researchers address etiological issues. Research designs that employ normal or high-risk samples would be necessary for this type of investigation.

In a pilot study designed to determine somatic variables that might be useful in determining the constitutional basis of individuals at risk for anxiety disorders, Turner et al. conducted a series of habituation trials using children diagnosed with anxiety disorders, as well as a group of normal controls (S.M. Turner, D.C. Beidel, L.E. Epstein, unpublished manuscript, 1988). Children were repeatedly exposed (20 trials) to a 100-dB tone or a picture of a snake while electrodermal, electromyographic, and cardiovascular variables were assessed. These particular stimuli were chosen due to their prior use in conditioning and habituation trials with adult populations. The failure to habituate when a stimulus is repeatedly presented has been suggested as one mechanism for the development of anxiety disorders (Lader and Mathews, 1968). The results of the Turner et al. (1988) study indicated that, while the majority of the normal children had a pattern of decreasing skin conductance level and, in fact, habituated to repeated presentations of the tone or snake, few of the anxious children did so. In addition to their failure to habituate, the anxious children had a significantly greater number of spontaneous fluctuations, another indication of their greater autonomic arousal. Furthermore, while the normal children evidenced an electromyographic pattern commonly attributed to the presentation of negative emotional states (significantly greater tension in the corrugator or "frown" muscle compared with the zygomatic or "smile" muscle (Ekman and Oster, 1979)), the anxious children demonstrated equally high levels of tension at both muscle sites. While their greater level of overall distress may have been reflected in undifferentiated muscle tension, a second and equally compelling explanation draws from the primate literature, where grimacing behavior is a common expression of fearfulness. Further investigations are needed to determine which of these two hypotheses might be more appropriate.

The most interesting findings from this investigation is that while there were highly significant differences between these two groups based on their autonomic response to these events, the groups did not differ in their subjective distress level during the habituation trials. All of the children rated their anxiety as very minimal. Thus, while repeated presentations of these stimuli produced heightened autonomic arousal in the anxious children, it would appear that these responses were undetected, indicating that the autonomic responses were not a response to the child's cognitive perception of these stimuli as something that they find frightening. However, it should be noted that these data still do not allow for the determination of these autonomic responses as a trait or constitutional variable that may predispose one to the onset of a frank anxiety disorder. Studies that examine groups perceived to be at high risk, yet not currently experiencing anxiety disorders, will be necessary to address this issue. However, by eliciting a pattern of autonomic arousal in anxious children that occurs undetected by the individual and by demonstrating the feasibility of conducting such trials with young children, the stage has been set for these future investigations.

VICARIOUS CONDITIONING

Although learning theories, including vicarious conditioning, have often been considered a mechanism for the acquisition of fears (e.g., Bandura and Rosenthal, 1966), recent reviews have highlighted several deficiencies for classic behavioral models. As noted by Delprato and McGlynn (1984), these include the failure of some individuals to acquire fear when placed in a traumatic situation, human subject constraints that preclude researchers from attempting to experimentally condition strong fears, and the inability of conditioning studies with human subjects to be able to control for prior experience with the "fearful" stimulus. Recently, a series of studies with nonhuman primates has served to rekindle interest in vicarious conditioning models (Cook et al., 1985; Mineka et al., 1984). Briefly, while rhesus monkeys reared in the wild show strong fears of snakes (even toy snakes), this fear is absent in monkeys reared in a laboratory environment. However, after only 8 minutes of observing nonrelated wild-reared monkeys behaving fearfully in the presence of a snake (and nonfearfully in the presence of neutral stimuli), most of the laboratory-reared monkeys demonstrated a level of snake fear that was almost identical to that of the models and that was still evident 3 months later, although there had been no further opportunity for observation or direct exposure. Another study by these investigators (Mineka and Cook, 1986) highlights the importance of prior information in the acquisition of fear. In this experiment, laboratory-bred monkeys first observed other monkeys behaving nonfearfully in the presence of toy snakes. Later, they observed wild-reared monkeys behaving fearfully in the presence of the same stimulus. However, those that had first observed the nonfearful models did not acquire the fear but continued to display nonfearful behaviors. The authors discussed this phenomenon in terms of immunization, in that prior observational learning appeared to be important in preventing the acquisition of the fear, despite the previously demonstrated power of this form of learning. Thus, similar prior environmental experiences might be an important factor in explanations of why some children become fearful after experiencing a traumatic event, while others do not.

In summary, these studies illustrate that vicarious conditioning is a powerful mechanism for the acquisition of fear. Observational learning occurred within a very brief period of time (8 minutes) and led to the acquisition of a strong emotional response that was readily observable and approximately equal in intensity to that of the model. Furthermore, the fear was still very apparent 3 months after it had been acquired, although there had been no opportunity for further learning. These data provide important support for conditioning models as a method of fear acquisition. Observation of a parent's anxious behaviors may increase the likelihood that similar behaviors or fears may be expressed by the children. Extant family studies of anxiety disorders have often rushed to attribute increased prevalence rates among first-degree family members to biological and genetic factors. Studies such as those of Mineka and Cook, which allow for stricter experimental controls than is possible with human subjects, and also allow for the conditioning of strong emotional responses, illustrate that vicarious conditioning may play an important role in the etiology of anxiety. Similarly, the opportunity to observe alternative nonfearful behaviors by one parent may serve to immunize some children from the acquisition of fear responses, which may be modeled by a second parent or another individual in the child's social network. However, as has been noted for biological models, invoking a pure conditioning model to explain the etiology of anxiety disorders in children is overly simplistic. For example, even under the strictest environmental controls, not all of Mineka and Cook's subjects acquired a fear of snakes, and the reasons for this remain unclear. It is likely that multiple factors are important, and the search for a comprehensive model must continue.

PSYCHOANALYTIC THEORIES

Freud's first (1894/1962b) psychoanalytic theory, that anxiety arose from undischarged sexual excitation and that intercourse might relieve that anxiety (Freud, 1895/1962a, p. 104), was largely a mechanical, hydraulics-like theory and was found to be inadequate. It was subsequently discarded in favor of his second theory.

Freud's second (1926/1959) theory was formulated in the light of his structural theory, particularly the construct of ego, whereby the ego initially was thought to respond with a signal of anxiety to an external or internal threat or anticipated threat (e.g., a danger situation) against which the individual felt helpless. The signal anxiety might never reach consciousness, but the unconscious ego presumably would recognize the danger, regulate the anxiety, and mobilize defenses. If this first major response to the signal anxiety (i.e., the mobilization of various defense mechanisms) failed to inhibit or sufficiently control the anxiety, panic would ensue. The typical danger situations were viewed developmentally and consisted of loss of the mothering person, loss of that person's love, fear of bodily harm, and fear of guilt, punishment, or abandonment.

The original data used by psychoanalysts to support this second, more psychological theory were and are derived mostly from the psychoanalytic treatment situation. These data, as presented, do not contradict the theory. However, the reliability of the data has been questioned. Since the validity of the theory rests essentially on this body of published psychoanalytic data, the status of the theory has remained essentially unchanged since it was put forward in 1926 (see Moore and Fine, 1990).

FUTURE DIRECTIONS

On the previous pages we have highlighted areas of current research into childhood anxiety. Although the knowledge base has expanded considerably over the past 10 years, there is much more that remains to be addressed. These studies illustrate the complexity of the psychopathology and demonstrate that an understanding of etiology requires a broader view, one that will include developmental as well as clinical perspectives, and attention to the interaction of biological, psychological, and psychosocial factors.

One fruitful area of future research is an examination of the boundaries between temperament and child psychopathology. For example, is behavioral inhibition in children a precursor of anxiety states and thus a specific indicator for children at risk for these disorders? Alternatively, behavioral inhibition may be an analogue of adult shyness, which is a term applied to a heterogeneous group of individuals who refrain from social contact yet only some of whom would meet criteria for an anxiety disorder (S.M. Turner, D.C. Beidel, unpublished manuscript prepared for the DSM-IV Task Force, 1989). Although a recent study has documented that adults with anxiety disorders are more likely to have children who are behaviorally inhibited when compared to depressed parents or psychiatric controls (Rosenbaum et al., 1988), the rates of inhibition for all three groups were quite high, suggesting that these behaviors may be a nonspecific indicator of children at risk for future psychopathology. Research investigations where behaviorally inhibited children are interviewed by clinicians utilizing standardized interview schedules and followed across time will be necessary to untangle these issues.

The hypothesis that behavioral inhibition may be a precursor for a range of psychopathology and not specifically anxiety illustrates the need for a broader view of this emotional state. Recent research by Kovacs and her colleagues (Kovacs et al., 1989) indicates that some types of depressive disorders can be preceded by anxiety states. If these findings are replicated by other investigators, childhood anxiety, like behavioral inhibition, may be indicative of the potential for the development of a range of psychopathological conditions. The need to assess a broader range of variables is also apparent in the areas of familial and high-risk studies. Now that studies such as those of Last et al. (unpublished manuscript, 1988) and Turner et al. (1987) have documented increased familial rates for these disorders, attention now must turn toward identifying the mode of transmission. Psychophysiological assessment directed at factors theoretically related to anxiety-proneness, such as those assessed by Turner et al., for example, may illuminate the constitutional basis for these concepts (unpublished manuscript, 1988). Similarly, genetic studies must turn attention toward isolation of a specific gene or location.

Research with nonhuman primates has been extremely important in clarifying issues such as the biological underpinnings for anxiety-like disorders (Suomi, 1986); the potency of environmental modes of transmission, such as vicarious conditioning (Cook et al., 1985; Mineka et al., 1984); and mechanisms of prevention, such as immunization (Mineka and Cook, 1986). Again, the use of high-risk groups may prove fruitful in determining the role of these factors in human subjects. In summary, while extant data document that both biological and environmental factors may play a role in the etiology and expression of anxiety disorders in children, it is likely that the mechanisms responsible are interdependent, complex, and synergistic.

References

Agras WS, Sylvester D, Oliveau D: The epidemiology of common fears and phobias. *Comp Psychiatry* 10:151–156, 1969.

Ainsworth MDS: Object relations, dependency and attachment: A theoretical review of the infant-mother relationship. *Child Dev* 40:969–1025, 1969.

American Psychiatric Association: *Diagnostic and Statistical Manual for Mental Disorders* (3rd ed, rev). Washington, DC, American Psychiatric Association, 1987.

American Psychiatric Association: *Diagnostic and Statistical Manual for Mental Disorders* (4th ed). Washington, DC, American Psychiatric Association, 1994.

Andreasen NC, Endicott J, Spitzer RL, et al: The family history method using diagnostic criteria. *Arch Gen Psychiatry* 34:1229–1235, 1977.

Bandura A, Rosenthal TL: Vicarious classical conditioning as a function of arousal level. *J Pers Soc Psychol* 3:54–62, 1966.

Beidel DC: Psychophysiological assessment of anxious emotional states in children. *J Abnorm Psychol* 97:80–82, 1988.

Beidel DC, Stanley MA: Developmental issues in the measurement of anxiety. In: Last CG (ed): *Anxiety across the Lifespan: A Developmental Perspective on Anxiety and the Anxiety Disorders*. New York, Springer, 1993, pp. 167–203.

Berg I: School phobia in children of agoraphobic women. *Br J Psychiatry* 128:86–89, 1976.

Berg I, McGuire R: Are mothers of school-phobic adolescents overprotective? *Br J Psychiatry* 124: 10–13, 1974.

Berg I, Butler A, Pritchard J: Psychiatric illness in the mothers of school-phobic adolescents. *Br J Psychiatry* 125:466–467, 1974.

Bernstein GA, Garfinkel BD: Pedigrees, functioning, and psychopathology in families of school phobic children. *Am J Psychiatry* 145:70–74, 1988.

Bowlby J: *Attachment and Loss*. Vol 1: *Attachment*. New York, Basic Books, 1969.

Bowlby J: *Attachment and Loss*. Vol 2: *Separation*. New York, Basic Books, 1973.

Brown TA, Barlow DH: Comorbidity among anxiety disorders: Implications for treatment and DSM-IV. *J Consult Clin Psychol* 60:835–844, 1992.

Buglass D, Clarke J, Henderson AS, et al: A study of agoraphobic housewives. *Psychol Med* 7:73–86, 1977.

Buss AH: A theory of shyness. In: Jones WH, Check JM, Briggs SR (eds): *Shyness: Perspectives on Research and Treatment*. New York, Plenum, 1985, pp. 39–46.

Buss AH, Plomin R: *A Temperament Theory of Personality Development*. New York, Wiley, 1975.

Campbell SB: Developmental issues in childhood anxiety. In: Gittelman R (ed): *Anxiety Disorders of Childhood*. New York, Guilford, 1986, pp. 24–57.

Cattell RB, Eber HW, Tatsuoka MM: *Handbook for the Sixteen Personality Factor Questionnaire*. Champaign, IL, Institute for Personality and Ability Testing, 1970.

Charney DS, Woods SW, Price LH, et al: Noradrenergic dysregulation in panic disorder. In: Ballenger JC (ed): *Neurobiology of Panic Disorder*. New York, Wiley-Liss, 1990, pp. 91–105.

Cook M, Mineka S: Observational conditioning of fear to fear relevant versus fear irrelevant stimuli in rhesus monkeys. *J Abnorm Psychol* 98:448–459, 1989.

Cook M, Hodes R, Lang P: Preparedness and phobia: Effects of stimulus content on human visceral conditioning. *J Abnorm Psychol* 95:195–207, 1986.

Cook M, Mineka S, Wolkenstein B, et al: Observational conditioning of snake fear in unrelated rhesus monkeys. *J Abnorm Psychol* 94:591–610, 1985.

Daniels D, Plomin R: Origins of individual differences in infant shyness. *Dev Psychol* 21:118–121, 1985.

Davidson RJ: Childhood temperament and cerebral asymmetry: A neurobiological substrate of behavioral inhibition. In: Rubin KH, Asendorpf JB (eds): *Social Withdrawal, Inhibition, and Shyness in Childhood*. New Jersey, Erlbaum, 1993, pp. 31–48.

Delprato DJ, McGlynn FD: Behavioral theories of anxiety disorders. In: Turner SM (ed): *Behavioral Theories of Anxiety Disorders*. New York, Plenum, 1984, pp. 1–39. Eisenberg L: School phobia: A study in the communication of anxiety. *Am J Psychiatry* 114:712–718, 1958.

Ekman P, Oster H: Facial expressions of emotion. *Ann Rev Psychol* 30:527–574, 1979.

Feyer AJ, Manuzza S, Chapman TF, et al: A direct family interview study of social phobia. *Arch Gen Psychiatry* 50:286–293, 1993.

Freud S: Inhibitions, symptoms and anxiety. In: Strachey J (ed): *The Standard Edition of the Complete Psychological Works of Sigmund Freud* (Vol 20). London, Hogarth Press, 1959, pp. 75–174. (Originally published 1926.)

Freud S: On the grounds for detaching a particular syndrome from neurasthenia under the description "anxiety neurosis." In: Strachey J (ed): *The Standard Edition of the Complete Psychological Works of Sigmund Freud* (Vol 3). London, Hogarth Press, 1962a, pp. 87–115. (Originally published 1895.)

Freud S: The neuro-psychoses of defense. In: Strachey J (ed): *The Standard Edition of the Complete Psychological Works of Sigmund Freud* (Vol 3). London, Hogarth Press, 1962b, pp. 43–61. (Originally published 1894.)

Galante R, Foa D: An epidemiological study of psychic trauma and treatment effectiveness for children after a natural disaster. *J Am Acad Child Adolesc Psychiatry* 25:357–363, 1986.

Garrison WT, Earls FJ: *Temperament and Child Psychopathology*. Newbury Park, CA, Sage, 1987.

Gittelman R: Childhood anxiety disorders: Correlates and outcomes. In: Gittelman R (ed): *Anxiety Disorders of Childhood*. New York, Guilford, 1986, pp. 101–125.

Gittelman-Klein R: Psychiatric characteristics of the relatives of school phobic children. In: Sankar DVS (ed): *Mental Health in Children* (Vol 1). Wesbury, NJ, PJD Publications, 1975, pp. 325–334.

Gittelman-Klein R, Klein DF: Separation anxiety in school phobic children. In: Hersov L, Berg I (eds): *Out of School*. London, Wiley, 1980, pp. 321–341.

Gordon M: Cyclone Tracey II: The effects on Darwin. *Aust Psychol* 12:55–82, 1977.

Handford HA, Mayes SD, Mattison RE, et al: Child and parent reaction to the Three Mile Island nuclear accident. *J Am Acad Child Adolesc Psychiatry* 25:346–356, 1986.

Hersov LA: Persistent non-attendance at school. *J Child Psychol Psychiatry* 1:130–136, 1960.

Johnson SB, Melamed BG: Assessment and treatment of children's fears. In: Lahey BB, Kazdin AE (eds): *Advances in Clinical Child Psychology* (Vol 2). New York, Plenum, 1979.

Kagan J: Heart rate and heart rate variability as signs of a temperamental dimension in infants. In: Izard CE (ed): *Measuring Emotions in Infants and Children*. Cambridge, Cambridge University Press, 1982, pp. 38–66.

Kagan J: Biological bases of childhood shyness. *Science* 240:167–171, 1988.

Kagan J, Reznick JS, Snidman N: The physiology and psychology of behavioral inhibition in children. *Child Dev* 58:1459–1473, 1987.

Kagan J, Reznick JS, Snidman N: Biological bases of childhood shyness. *Science* 240:167–171, 1988.

Kinzie JD, Sack WH, Angell RN, et al: The psychiatric effects of massive trauma on Cambodian children. I: The children. *J Am Acad Child Adolesc Psychiatry* 25:370–376, 1986.

Kovacs M, Gatsonis C, Paulauskas SL, et al: Depressive disorders in childhood. *Arch Gen Psychiatry* 46:776–782, 1989.

Lader MN, Mathews AM: A physiological model of phobic anxiety and desensitization. *Behav Res Ther* 6:411–421, 1968.

Last CG, Francis G, Hersen M, et al: Separation anxiety and school phobia: A comparison using DSM-III criteria. *Am J Psychiatry* 144:653–657, 1987a.

Last CG, Hersen M, Kazdin AE, et al: Psychiatric illness in the mothers of anxious children. *Am J Psychiatry* 144:1580–1583, 1987b.

Last CG, Hersen M, Kazdin AE, et al: Anxiety disorders in children and their families. *Arch Gen Psychiatry* 48:928–934, 1991.

Last CG, Perrin S, Hersen M, et al: DSM-III-R anxiety disorders in children and adolescents: Sociodemographics and clinical characteristics. *J Am Acad Child Adolesc Psychiatry* 31:1070–1076, 1992.

Last CG, Phillips JE, Statfeld A: Childhood anxiety disorders in mothers and their children. *Child Psychiatry Hum Dev* 18:103–112, 1987c.

Lenane MC, Swedo SE, Lenonard H, et al: Psychiatric disorders in first degree relatives of children and adolescents with obsessive compulsive disorder. *J Am Acad Child Adolesc Psychiatry* 29:407–412, 1990.

Livingston R, Nugent H, Rader L: Family histories of depressed and severely anxious children. *Am J Psychiatry* 142:1497–1499, 1985.

Malmquist CP: Children who witness parental murder. *J Am Acad Child Adolesc Psychiatry* 25:320–325, 1986.

Martinez-Monfort A, Dreger RM: Reactions of high school students in school desegregation in a Southern metropolitan area. *Psychol Rep* 30:543–565, 1972.

McNally R: Preparedness and phobias: A review. *Psychol Bull* 101:283–303, 1987.

Mendlewicz J, Fleiss JL, Cataldo M, et al: Accuracy of the family history method in affective illness. *Arch Gen Psychiatry* 32:309–314, 1975.

Mineka S, Cook M: Immunization against the observational conditioning of snake fear in rhesus monkeys. *J Abnorm Psychol* 95:307–318, 1986.

Mineka S, Davidson M, Cook M: Observational conditioning of snake fear in rhesus monkeys. *J Abnorm Psychol* 93:355–372, 1984.

Monroe SM, Wade SL: Life events. In: Last CG, Hersen M (eds): *Handbook of Anxiety Disorders*. New York, Pergamon, 1988.

Moore BE, Fine BD (eds): *Psychoanalytic Terms and Concepts*. New Haven, CT, The American Psychoanalytic Association Press and Yale University Press, 1990.

Ohman A: Face the beast and fear the face: Animal and social fears as prototypes for evolutionary analyses of emotion. *Psychophysiology* 23:123–145, 1986.

Ohman A, Erikson A, Olafsson C: One-trial learning and superior resistance to extinction of autonomic responses conditioned to potentially phobic stimuli. *J Comp Physiol Psychol* 88:619–627, 1975.

Ohman A, Fredrickson M, Nygdahl K, et al: The premise of equipotentiality in human classical conditioning: Conditioned stimuli. *J Exp Psychol Gen* 105:313–337, 1976.

Pohl R, Yeragani V, Balon R, et al: Isoproterenol-induced panic: A beta-adrenergic model of panic anxiety. In: Ballenger JC (ed): *Neurobiology of Panic Disorder*. New York, Wiley-Liss, 1990, pp. 107–120.

Rapoport JL: The biology of obsessions and compulsions. *Sci Am* 3:83–89, 1989.

Reznick JS, Kagan J, Sniderman N, et al: Inhibited and uninhibited children: A follow-up study. *Child Dev* 57:660–680, 1986.

Rosenbaum JR, Biederman J, Gersten M, et al: Behavioral inhibition in children of parents with panic disorder and agoraphobia. *Arch Gen Psychiatry* 45:463–470, 1988.

Rowe DC, Plomin R: Temperament in early childhood. *J Pers Assess* 41:150–156, 1977.

Seligman M: Phobias and preparedness. *Behav Ther* 2:307–320, 1971.

Suomi SJ: Anxiety in young nonhuman primates. In: Gittelman R (ed): *Anxiety Disorders of Childhood*. New York, Guilford, 1986, pp. 1–23.

Suomi SJ, Kraemer GW, Baysinger CM, et al: Inherited and experiential factors associated with individual differences in anxious behavior displayed by rhesus monkeys. In: Klein DF, Rabkin J (eds): *Anxiety: New Research and Changing Concepts*. New York, Raven Press, 1981, pp. 179–199.

Terr LC: Psychic trauma in children: Observations following the Chowchilla school bus kidnapping. *Am J Psychiatry* 138:14–19, 1981.

Thomas A, Chess S: *Temperament and Development*. New York, Brunner/Mazel, 1977.

Thomas A, Chess S, Birch NG, et al: *Behavioral Individuality in Early Childhood*. New York, University Press, 1963.

Thompson WD, Orvashel N, Kidd JR: An evaluation of the family history method for ascertaining psychiatric disorders. *Arch Gen Psychiatry* 39:53–58, 1982.

Torgersen S: Genetics. In: Last CG, Hersen M (eds): *Handbook of Anxiety Disorders*. New York, Pergamon, 1988, pp. 159–170.

Turner SM, Beidel DC, Costello A: Psychopathology in the offspring of anxiety disorders patients. *J Consult Clin Psychol* 55:229–235, 1987.

Wamboldt MZ, Insel TR: Pharmacologic models. In: Last CG, Hersen M (eds): *Handbook of Anxiety Disorders*. New York, Pergamon, 1988, pp. 181–216.

Weissman MM, Leckman JF, Merikangas KR, et al: Depression and anxiety disorders in parents and children: Results from the Yale Family Study. *Arch Gen Psychiatry* 41:845–852, 1984.

Ziv A, Israeli R: Effects of bombardment on the manifest anxiety level of children living in kibbutzim. *J Consult Clin Psychol* 40:287–291, 1973.

24 DEVELOPMENT OF THE SYMPTOM OF DEPRESSION

Judy Garber, Ph.D., and Javad H. Kashani, M.D.

The term *depression* has been used to refer to either a symptom, a syndrome, or a nosological disorder. The symptom of depression is a mood characterized by feelings of sadness, gloom, misery, dysphoria, or despair. It typically is a transient state that is experienced by most people at various points in their lives and by itself is not necessarily pathological. However, when the symptom of sadness is intense, persistent, and occurs in combination with the full symptom complex, or syndrome of depression, then it is considered to be clinically significant. The other symptoms that comprise the syndrome of depression are sleep disturbance, loss of appetite, anhedonia, difficulty concentrating, low self-esteem, guilt, low energy, psychomotor changes, and suicidal ideation. When this particular symptom picture is accompanied by a specifiable etiology, course, duration, prognosis, and treatment response, then it is referred to as a discrete nosological disorder.

Although depressed affect is a normal part of life, it also tends to be a concomitant of many childhood psychiatric disorders. Achenbach and Edelbrock (1981, 1986) reported that, according to both parents' and teachers' report on the Child Behavior Checklist, of all 117 items the item "unhappy, sad, or depressed" was the strongest discriminator between clinically referred and nonreferred children ages 4–16. This was especially true for young adolescent females. Thus, although sadness is a fairly common and universally experienced affect, it also may indicate more severe problems, particularly when it is accompanied by other symptoms.

There is some question concerning whether there is continuity between the "normal" symptom of sadness and the depressed affect experienced by individuals who manifest the full syndrome of depression (Bowlby, 1980; Eisenberg, 1986; Izard and Schwartz, 1986; Rutter, 1983, 1986). Izard and Schwartz (1986), for example, found some support for the continuity between normal sadness and clinical states of depressed affect, although this varied depending upon the level of depression, age, and gender of the subjects.

Whereas much has been written over the last two decades concerning the causes of depressive disorder (e.g., Abramson et al., 1989; Akiskal and McKinney, 1975; Beck, 1967; Brown and Harris, 1978; Gershon et al., 1976; Jacobson, 1971; Paykel, 1979; Schildkraut, 1965), there has been less attention to the causes of the *symptom* of depression. The purpose of the present chapter is to specifically address the question of the potential causes of sadness. The focus will be on depression as a symptom, mood, or affect. Other terms that are used somewhat interchangeably with depression are sadness, blue, "down in the dumps," and misery. Physical distress, discomfort, or pain, however, are not synonymous with sadness (Boucher, 1969; Ekman and Friesen, 1975), although emotional distress has been used by some (e.g., Izard, 1977) as a broader term that incorporates sadness.

Emotions generally are considered to be multidimensional (Hesse and Cicchetti, 1982; Izard, 1972, 1977) and include verbal and nonverbal expression, neurophysiological/biochemical processes, cognitive appraisal, and behavioral activation. There is still some debate among emotion researchers (e.g., Izard, 1977; Kagan, 1984; Lazarus, 1982; Zajonc, 1980, 1984), however, concerning which of these components is most central. The current discussion presents the evidence concerning the interaction among these various components with regard to the affect of sadness. We particularly focus on the cognitive and biological processes that are associated with verbal and nonverbal expressions of sad affect.

In order to understand the potential causes of sadness, it first is necessary to describe the extent to which the experience and expression of the symptom of depression change with age. Therefore, the first section of the chapter highlights several important developmental issues with respect to the affect of sadness. Next, we make a distinction between the content, processes, and mechanisms that are associated with the causes of sadness. Content here refers to the types of experiences or themes that are correlated with depression, including such things as loss, rejection, and failure. The processes by which an individual may become sad can be experiential, cognitive, or vicarious. Finally, several mechanisms by which such contents and processes might produce sadness are suggested, including evolutionary, biological, and social learning.

DEVELOPMENT OF SADNESS

Emotional development theorists (e.g., Demos, 1986; Izard et al., 1987; Oster, 1978, 1984; Stenberg et al., 1983) generally agree that emotional expressions change with age. Whereas certain emotional expressions are present at birth, others are not apparent until later in development (Izard and Malatesta, 1987). Moreover, emotional expression becomes more graded, subtle, and complex over the first years of life (Demos, 1986), and through the processes of socialization children eventually learn to control the expression of their emotions (Cassidy and Kobak, 1989; Cole, 1985; Saarni, 1979).

In one of the first studies of emotional development, Bridges (1932) suggested that infants' earliest emotional reactions are poorly organized and generally undifferentiated. It is only over the course of development that there occurs a process of differentiation of the various emotions. Bridges suggested that excitement and distress were the original emotions and that other distinct emotions were derivatives of these. The emotions of fear, disgust, and anger were considered subcategories of the more general emotion of distress. It is noteworthy that Bridges did not include the affect of sadness among these derivatives of distress.

In contrast, discrete emotions theorists (e.g., Ekman, 1973; Ekman and Friesen, 1971; Ekman et al., 1983; Izard, 1971, 1977; Tomkins, 1962, 1963) have suggested that sadness is one of the basic, fundamental emotions that can be observed universally. Izard and colleagues (1980) found that infants were able to produce eight reliably identifiable expressions, and sadness was among them. This was the first empirical demonstration that the facial expressions of distress and sadness could be distinguished in infants. Moreover, Johnson et al. (1982) found that 34% of mothers interviewed reported that their 1-month-old babies expressed sadness; even more mothers reported that their babies expressed several other distinct emotions as well (e.g., interest, anger, fear). Finally, sadness has been observed in young infants in a form that is basically isomorphic with that observed in adulthood (Gaensbauer, 1980, 1982).

Thus, there is evidence that sadness is one of the earliest emotions to be expressed. It still is unclear, however, whether these early expressions of distress that are labeled as sadness by adult observers are actually early forms or precursors (Sroufe, 1979) of the sadness and depression observed later in development and whether the underlying causes of sadness are the same over the course of development. There are several additional, important developmental questions concerning the symptom of sadness. For example, to what extent does the manifestation of sadness change as a function of development? Are there developmental differences in children's ability to recognize sadness in others, or to control their own expression of sadness? At what point are children capable of discriminating degrees of intensity of sadness? What is the prevalence of sadness at different ages? Do the factors that are associated with sadness change with development? The following sections briefly address these developmental questions.

Manifestation, Control, and Recognition of Sadness

Infants' expressions of sadness have been reported to be basically similar to those of adults (Gaensbauer, 1982), although there is some debate as to whether infants experience emotions in the same way as adults do (e.g., Campos et al., 1983; Lewis and Brooks, 1978; Saarni, 1978). The prototype manifestation of distress and sadness is crying (Izard, 1977; Tomkins, 1963). Nevertheless, there are changes with age in the predominant manner in which sadness is expressed. Whereas toddlers and young children are more likely to cry or to use other nonverbal forms of expression, older children and adolescents increasingly tend to verbalize their sadness or express it through a different kind of nonverbal expression (e.g., absence of smiling, decreased eye contact) (Kazdin et al., 1985; Poznanski et al., 1985).

Tomkins (1963) observed that individuals learn to attenuate or modify their facial expressions and cries of distress. For example, during late childhood, cries tend to become abbreviated and lower in volume. Adults cry less than children, and men cry less than women. Factors such as the development of language (e.g., Bretherington et al., 1986; Dunn and Brown, 1991; Dunn and Kendrick, 1982), the processes of socialization (Lewis and Michalson, 1982; Lewis and Saarni, 1985; Saarni, 1985), and cultural forces (Harkness and Super, 1983; Izard, 1977; Lutz, 1985) influence these changing expressions of emotions.

Saarni (1984), for example, found that by the age of 10, children (especially girls) were more likely to inhibit the facial display of disappointment than were 4- to 6-year-olds. Saarni (1979) used the concept of display rules to describe children's intentional attempt to control their expression of their real emotion. Children learn over time that sometimes it is not appropriate to express emotions such as disappointment or sadness. Indeed, Glasburg and Aboud (1981) argued that children as young as 5 have acquired the belief that there is a stigma associated with the expression of sadness (although see Garber et al., 1987, for an alternative perspective). Moreover, Barden et al. (1980) reported that children were more likely to attribute sadness to others than to themselves in affect-producing situations. Thus, children may be reluctant to describe themselves as sad due either to a presumed stigma or to the expected consequences associated with the expression of sadness.

Finally, young babies are able to recognize and distinguish different emotional expressions as indexed by their reaction to them, although there is some debate concerning the age at which this ability develops (Klinnert et al., 1983). Field and Walden (1982), for example, found that 1-day-old "neonates can discriminate among at least three basic expressions—happy, sad, and surprised" (p. 189). Barrera and Maurer (1978) noted that 3-month-olds can discriminate smiling from frowning expressions. Haviland and Lelwica (1987) reported that, in response to their mothers' expressions of happiness, 10-week-old infants looked happy, whereas in response to the mothers' sadness, the babies often engaged in mouthing, chewing, and sucking. Finally, Cohn and Tronick (1983; Cohn et al., 1986) have shown that 3-month-old infants become disorganized and distressed in response to their mother's expression of sadness.

Others (e.g., Caron et al., 1982; Klinnert et al., 1983; Termine and Izard, 1988) have argued that infants do not consistently discriminate emotional expressions and respond differently to them until the second half of the 1st year of life. Young-Browne et al. (1977), for example, found that, although 3-month-old infants could discriminate surprised-looking faces from happy and sad ones, they could not discriminate happy and sad faces. Termine and Izard (1988) found that, by 9 months of age, babies respond differently to their mothers' expressions of sadness versus happiness as evidenced by their looking less when their mothers express sadness. In fact, the babies themselves expressed more

anger and occasional sadness in response to their mothers' sad displays. Klinnert et al. (1983) suggested that infants' increased responsiveness to facial configurations may be related to their increasingly improving perceptual abilities.

Children become even more adept at discriminating emotions as they develop language. The emotion labels of *happy* and *sad* are acquired the earliest, and by 4 years of age, children are using affect terms that include happy, sad, angry, and scared (Amen, 1941; Michalson and Lewis, 1985). Moreover, children produce verbal labels for emotional behaviors such as crying and laughter even earlier (Zahn-Waxler et al., 1979).

As children grow older, they are not only able to recognize sad affect in others but they also can respond to it in empathic and sympathetic ways (Hoffman, 1977, 1978). Dunn and colleagues (Dunn and Kendrick, 1979; Dunn et al., 1981) reported that toddlers will make active attempts to comfort siblings in distress. Similarly, Borke (1971) found that 2-year-olds displayed comforting behavior toward their fathers when they expressed sadness. Zahn-Waxler et al. (1979) have detailed how children's reactions to another's distress changes from 10 to 30 months. At 10–12 months, children reacted to a stranger's distress with signs of distress themselves and typically would not make an effort to comfort the person in distress. Between 12 and 18 months, children showed less distress themselves, although they still did little to comfort the other person. By 18 months, however, children began to make active verbal and nonverbal attempts to comfort the distressed other. Finally, by 20–24 months, most children responded when they saw another person in distress, although there were significant individual differences in the frequency and extent of their reactions.

Thus, there are clear developmental changes in how children express their own sadness, and in when and under what circumstances they attempt to control their expression of sadness. There also are developmental trends and individual differences in children's ability to recognize distress in others and to make an effort to comfort the other person once they become aware of the distress.

Discriminating Degrees of Intensity of Sadness

Harris and colleagues (Harris, 1983; Harris et al., 1985; Taylor and Harris, 1983) have demonstrated that children can distinguish different intensities of sadness. Harris et al. (1985) asked children about the degree of unhappiness that one would experience immediately following a negative event, such as the loss of a pet or important possession, as well as the expected emotional reaction at a later point in time. In general, children reported that the reaction of sadness would be intense initially but that the intensity would wane over time, eventually returning to a neutral state. Harris et al. (1985) found this to be true for 6- and 10-year-olds in both the West and in China and for both hypothetical events and actual experiences. The results were somewhat less consistent for 4-year-olds, although when the rating scale was made clearly understandable for them (faces showing varying degrees of sadness), the 4-year-olds also reported that the intensity of sadness wanes over time.

Thus, children as young as preschoolers can discriminate different intensities of sadness and recognize that the intensity of sadness will lessen with time. Harris (1989) suggested that these results have two important implications. First, children who are experiencing sadness should be able to anticipate that the intensity eventually will decrease with time. It remains to be tested, however, whether children who are currently experiencing sadness are able to maintain such a hopeful cognition, or if the sadness itself blocks their accessibility to this knowledge.

Second, children's knowledge of differences in intensity of sad affect may be helpful in the assessment process. That is, they may be able to recognize and acknowledge when their level of sadness is beyond what they typically experience, and that it represents something unusual or deviant. The development of such emotional insight needs to be studied further in children who are currently experiencing different intensities of sad affect at the time of the assessment.

Prevalence of Sadness

Do the actual rates of the symptom of sad affect change with development? Rutter (1986, 1991) has highlighted both the importance of studying age changes in depressive feelings as well as the methodological problems associated with the assessment of such feelings. Rutter further suggested that there are age changes in the manifestation of sadness, the manner in which it can be assessed, and in the potential causes of sadness over the course of development.

Epidemiological studies indicate that there are developmental changes in the frequency of sadness in the general population, although the nature of these developmental changes may vary depending upon whether the symptom or disorder is the focus and what index of depression is used to assess it. Whereas it is fairly rare to see the full syndrome of depression in young children (Kashani and Ray, 1983), it is not unusual to see transient expressions of sadness in children as young as 6 months (Emde et al., 1965; Harmon et al., 1982).

Shepherd et al. (1971) reported that the incidence of crying declined with age; at age 6, approximately 18% of the children cried two to three times per week, whereas by puberty, the rate had dropped to about 2%. In contrast, using indices of persistent sad feelings rather than the overt behavioral index of crying, Rutter et al. (1970) found a different developmental picture. In a survey of the general population, Rutter et al. reported that among 10- to 11-year-old children, 13% showed depressed mood, 17% failed to smile, and 9% were preoccupied with depressive topics. Consistent with the children's report, parents and teachers described approximately 10–12% of the children as feeling "miserable." When the same children were reassessed at ages 14–15 years, over 40% of the adolescents reported depressive feelings and 7–8% reported suicidal feelings. Parents and teachers, however, apparently were less aware of the adolescents' level of depressive feelings (Rutter et al., 1976).

In a review of the literature concerning developmental differences in the symptoms of major depressive disorder, Weiss and Garber (1995) found that there was a tendency for nonverbal expressions of sad affect to decrease with age (Carlson and Kashani, 1988; Friedman et al., 1983; Ryan et al., 1987), whereas verbal expressions of sad mood either showed no age trends or tended to increase with age (Achenbach and Edelbrock, 1981, 1983; Carlson and Kashani, 1988; Garber, 1984). Thus, there may be some validity to the notion currently endorsed by DSM-IV that sad and tearful appearance may be the likely manner in which young children express their dysphoria, although the reliability of this observation needs to be studied further.

Moreover, DSM-IV accepts irritability as an index of dysphoric mood in children and adolescents. Clinical experience, especially with preschoolers and young teens, supports this notion. Many times the same circumstance that makes children sad also makes them angry (Blumberg and Izard, 1985), and it is this anger that is often likely to be expressed in the form of irritability. This is an important distinction in DSM-IV that is given to child and adolescent depression in recognition of developmental differences in symptom expression.

What are the implications of these apparent differences in the manifestation and prevalence of sad affect at different ages? One possibility is that there really aren't differences in the rate of sadness at different ages, but that it simply is more difficult to assess the symptom of sadness in young children. That is, the apparent increased frequency of depression with increasing age could be the result of older children's growing linguistic ability to express their distress verbally rather than any real age difference in the rate at which children experience sadness.

A related assessment issue is that how sadness is defined and measured needs to vary depending on the age of the child. In order to obtain an accurate evaluation of the prevalence of sad affect in children at different ages, it is necessary to assess the symptom in the most developmentally appropriate way. This perspective is consistent with DSM-IV, Poznanski et al. (1985), and others who have suggested that nonverbal indices of sadness should be used, especially with young children.

One final issue concerning age changes in the prevalence of the symptom of sadness is the nature of the population (i.e., community, clinic, diagnosed depressed) being studied (Weiss and Garber, 1995). It could be that the rates of sad affect increase with age in the general population of children, but that among children with a diagnosis of major depressive disorder, there might be no difference in the rates of the symptom of sadness at different ages. In fact, it would almost be surprising to find differences in the rate of sadness among children with the diagnosis of major depressive disorder, since this symptom is one of the criteria that define the disorder in the first place.

It also is theoretically possible that there could be age changes in the rate of reported sadness among depressed children, but not among children in the general population. This finding would support the view that there are real differences in the manifestation of the disorder at different ages. Finally, it is possible that there could be age differences in the rate of reported sadness in both the community and depressed samples. Such a finding would suggest that these observed differences are probably a function of normal developmental processes rather than a reflection of differences in the manifestation of the syndrome per se.

Although existing data do not allow us to decide which of these alternatives accurately describes the observed age differences in reported rates of sad affect, these various explanations should be considered in future investigations of developmental differences with respect to any of the symptoms of depressive disorders. Moreover, investigations of the question of developmental differences in depressive symptomatology should include both community and clinical samples.

CONTENT: ELICITORS ASSOCIATED WITH SADNESS

Not only does the spectrum of sources of distress grow wider with development, but there are many sources of distress which so much depend on environmental vicissitudes as to be essentially independent of personality and personality development. (Tomkins, 1963, p. 53)

Children as young as 2 and 3 years old are aware of the emotional consequences for themselves and others of different categories of experiences (Barden et al., 1980; Borke, 1971; Bretherington and Beeghly, 1982; Harris et al., 1985; Michalson and Lewis, 1985; Stein and Jewett, 1985). Young children reliably (although not invariably) judge that losing a significant person, pet, or treasured possession; experiencing failure; or receiving punishment will provoke sadness. Interestingly, as children grow older, although they continue to acknowledge such situation-response relations, they also begin to recognize that mental processes accompany and even engender emotional reactions (Harris, 1985; Harris et al., 1985).

A variety of life events have been found to be associated with sadness and depression (e.g., Billings et al., 1983; Finlay-Jones and Brown, 1981; Paykel, 1979). This literature has a number of difficulties, however, including the issues of specificity, causality, and universality (Monroe et al., 1983). That is, to what extent do particular negative life events specifically produce sadness rather than other emotions? Second, to what extent are certain life events a sufficient cause of sadness and depression? Third, do certain life events produce sadness in all individuals? If not, how are individual differences in response to life events explained?

There are several specific life events that reliably produce sadness in most individuals, such as loss, separation, and failure. However, these events also may produce a variety of other emotions as well, such as anger, guilt, and anxiety. Several theorists (e.g., Bowlby, 1961; Klinger, 1975; Shontz, 1975; Wortman and Brehm, 1975) have suggested that individuals progress through a particular sequence of stages in reaction to undesirable life events that typically includes shock, anger, and depression. Moreover, it also is possible for individuals to experience several different emotions at the same time (Harter, 1983). Thus, it is difficult to identify an event that is *uniquely* associated with sadness. Even separation, which is considered by most to be a primary cause of sadness, is actually known to initially produce fear in infants (Izard, 1977). Similarly, various other negative life events, such as the death of a significant other (Glick et al., 1974; Parkes, 1975), life-threatening illness (Chesser and Anderson, 1975; Hinton, 1963; Maguire, 1978), and rape (Burgess and Holmstrom, 1974; McCombie, 1975), have been found to be characterized by intense anxiety in addition to sadness.

Another important issue is whether any events universally and necessarily lead to sadness. The one situation that may fulfill this requirement is the loss of a loved one. This event seems to be unquestionably tied with sadness and grief and such sadness may play an important adaptive function for the species (Averill, 1968). However, sadness is not necessarily reported in 100% of individuals who experience loss (Clayton et al., 1968; Glick et al., 1974). There also is great variability with respect to the intensity, duration, and timing of the sadness that is experienced as a result of loss of a loved one (Clayton et al., 1968), and again, grief may be accompanied by other emotions, such as anger ("How could he have died now?") and guilt ("If only I had taken better care of him").

Thus, there may not be any one life event that causes sadness in all individuals at all times (universality) or that does not also produce other affects as well (specificity). Nevertheless, there are some life events that are likely to be associated with sadness and depression. We suggest that *circumstances characterized by either the lack or loss of a highly desirable and formerly believed to be (but no longer) obtainable goal or the presence of a highly undesirable and believed to be inescapable event will produce sadness.* We briefly highlight five broad categories of life events that are likely to fit this characterization: interpersonal losses, achievement/competence concerns, material deprivation, physical illness or injury, and victimization. These categories are somewhat similar to Freud's (1950) distinction between "Arbeit und Liebe" and Connell's (Connell and Wellborn, 1991) motivational model that emphasizes competence, interpersonal relatedness, and autonomy. Finally, although we focus here on the association between sadness and major life events, we recognize that minor daily hassles and chronic stressors also may be significantly correlated with sadness as well (e.g., Kanner et al., 1980; Monroe, 1983).

Interpersonal Loss and Separation

The prototypical sadness-inducing situation is the separation from or total loss of a loved one (Bowlby, 1969, 1980; Izard, 1977; Mineka and Suomi, 1978; Spitz, 1946). Interpersonal losses, disruptions, and disappointments as well as illnesses and/or injuries to loved ones appear to be the events that are most closely associated with depression in adults (e.g., Brown and Harris, 1978; Crook and Eliot, 1980; Tennant et al., 1982). Somewhat less is known, however, about the particular relation of such events to sadness and depression in children (Garmezy, 1986; Rutter, 1966).

There is considerable evidence that depression is a very common response to the loss of a loved one (Clayton et al., 1972; Glick et al., 1974). There also is evidence in human infants (Field, 1985; Freud and Burlingham, 1974; Robertson and Robertson, 1971; Spitz, 1946) and toddlers (Bowlby, 1969, 1980; Maccoby and Feldman, 1972), as well as in primates (Mineka and Suomi, 1978; Suomi et al., 1975), that separation from significant others, particularly caretakers, leads to a sequence of emotional reactions ranging from initial protest, to despair, to eventual detachment.

In addition to these themes of loss and separation, there are several other interpersonal situations that are likely to be associated with sadness. These include being rejected by a significant other, being left out or unaccepted by important others, loneliness or the absence of significant relationships, and conflict in one's important interpersonal interactions (Weissman and Paykel, 1974). Thus, either the absence of a desired relationship or a disruption in an ongoing significant relationship is one of the most likely conditions to produce sadness.

Intrapersonal Incompetence or Failure

The second type of event that is likely to produce sadness is anything that is associated with the lowering of self-esteem. Most representative of this category is failure at important tasks such as one's job or school. Failure can be defined according to objective, external standards that are imposed upon the individual or in terms of not meeting one's own self-imposed standards. Basically, situations that highlight one's incompetence or weaknesses are likely to produce lowered self-esteem and a sense of worthlessness that then result in sad affect. The focus of the perceived incompetence typically includes areas in which the individual defines his or her identity, such as vocation, role (e.g., being a "good" mother), or avocation (e.g., sports or art).

Either the loss of self-esteem or the lack of achievement of one's desired goals is likely to produce sadness (e.g., Metalsky et al., 1987; Weiner, 1985). The desired goals that are most relevant here include status, prestige, power, personal or public achievement and recognition, or anything else that gives one a sense of identity and a feeling of self-worth.

Deprivation

In addition to the loss of significant relationships and one's self-esteem, the loss or lack of material possessions also has been found to be associated with depression (Belle, 1982; McLoyd, 1989). Situations involving extreme poverty and the absence of the basic needs of food, shelter, and clothing are likely to produce sadness and a sense of despair. A decline in the amount of material possessions through the loss of a job, business failure, natural disaster, or war also is likely to be associated with sadness (Buss and Redburn, 1983; Galambus and Silbereisen, 1987; Garmezy and Rutter, 1985).

Physical Incapacitation

The loss of physical functioning through illness or injury also is associated with increased sadness. For example, depression occurs in spinal cord injury patients (e.g., McDaniel and Sexton, 1970; Siller, 1969), burn victims (e.g., Campbell et al., 1987; Stoddard et al., 1989), cancer patients (e.g., Peck, 1972; Plumb and Holland, 1977), and heart patients (e.g., Kimball, 1969). The intensity and duration of the sadness experienced by these individuals and the adequacy of their subsequent adjustment depends, in part, upon the extent of social support available, their premorbid personality, and their capacity for coping (Barron, 1955; Cobb, 1976; Pearlin and Schooler, 1978; Silver and Wortman, 1980; Ward et al., 1987).

Injuries and illnesses that result in permanent changes in one's physical abilities, appearance, or intellectual capacities also are going to require some change in the individual's identity. Therefore, in some sense this category of events overlaps with the second category noted above that was concerned with the lowering of self-esteem. It does not necessarily follow that physical incapacitation always will result in lower self-esteem (e.g., Orr et al., 1989), but there is a period of transition that is required that may be associated with sadness until the individual has established a new sense of himself or herself and what he or she is now capable of achieving.

Victimization

Finally, the experience of being a victim of a crime or abuse also is associated with sadness and depression, although feelings of fear and anger may be even more prevalent (Brown and Finkelhor, 1986; Burgess and Holmstrom, 1974; McCombie, 1975; Sutherland and Scherl, 1970). Apart from the physical pain and discomfort that accompanies being physically attacked, there also often is a sense of humiliation, anger, and possibly self-blame and guilt (Silver and Wortman, 1980). Also particularly salient here is the sense of having been violated and having lost control over one's body or possessions. This sense of helplessness and loss of control also has been proposed as a cause of emotional distress and sadness (Seligman, 1975).

Thus, there are several different categories of events that have been found to be associated with sadness. None of these events necessarily or universally produces sadness all the time in all people, however. There also might be situations other than those mentioned here that at times and for some people are associated with depressed mood. What these various circumstances have in common is that they are either the absence of something highly desirable or the presence of something highly undesirable. Moreover, we suggest that individual variability in the intensity and duration of sadness is a function of the type of life event, individual (e.g., motivation, personality), and contextual (e.g., social support and resource) factors.

DEVELOPMENTAL DIFFERENCES IN RESPONSE TO LIFE EVENTS

Are there developmental differences in children's reactions to the same negative life event? Do the circumstances that are associated with sadness change as a function of development? Garmezy and Rutter (1985; Garmezy, 1986; Rutter, 1981, 1986) have noted that children's reactions to the same events vary with development. Rutter (1981, 1986), for example, suggested that the well-documented protest-despair-detachment sequence associated with separation (Bowlby, 1969, 1980) is most evident from ages 6 months until about 4 years. Prior to 6 months, infants tend not to show such reactions to separations, presumably because they have not yet developed a sense of object permanence or established selective attachments. After about age 4, children are less affected by separations because they have the cognitive ability to understand that separations can be temporary and that they are not being abandoned.

There also are age changes in children's grief reactions to the death of a loved one (Bowlby, 1980; Furman, 1974; Kliman, 1968; Rutter, 1966, 1986; van Eerdewegh et al., 1982). Often to the surprise and dismay of observing adults, young children do not seem to experience the loss of a loved one with as much intensity or for as long a duration as do older children, adolescents, and adults. This probably is the result of their limited cognitive ability to understand that the loss is irreversible (White et al., 1978) and to anticipate its consequences. As time passes, however, and they become more aware of the reality or implications of the death, the young child may show a delayed reaction of sadness as well as other accompanying affective and behavioral symptoms (Rutter, 1966). These delayed reactions, however, may be as much a reaction to the consequences of the death as to the death itself (Furman, 1974; Rutter, 1966, 1986).

There also is evidence from the work of Hetherington and Wallerstein and colleagues (Hetherington et al., 1979a, 1979b, 1981; Wallerstein, 1983; Wallerstein and Kelly, 1980) that children's reactions to divorce vary as a function of their gender, temperament, and developmental status. (See also Chapter 112.) In general, these researchers have found that younger children are particularly affected by divorce because of their more limited social and cognitive competencies that thereby make it more difficult for them to cope with the additional stressors that accompany divorce. There also is evidence that the nature of the reaction differs with age and that, although sadness is part of it, other affects such as anxiety, guilt, and anger also are present (Wallerstein and Kelly, 1980).

Children's reactions to physical illness and disability also tend to vary with age. Sawyer et al. (1983), for example, found that adolescent burn victims showed markedly poorer psychosocial adjustment than did younger burn victims.

Finally, there are important developmental factors in response to failure. Kagan (1983) demonstrated in the laboratory that children's sense of social comparison and self-evaluation develops as early as 18–24 months. Kagan found that the discrepancy between demand and ability in this situation tended to evoke distress in many, although not all, of these young children.

Heckhausen (1982), however, suggested that children under the age of about 3.5 years do not attribute success and failure to personal characteristics, nor do they engage in much self-evaluation. Young children tend to be overly optimistic in their self-evaluations and expectations of success, although this optimism can be reduced if the failure experiences are made more salient (Dweck and Elliott, 1983). These young children also tend to deny their failures, make excuses, or avoid the failure-producing situation (Heckhausen, 1982). As children grow older and acquire greater cognitive and social maturity, they learn to evaluate themselves and the situations more realistically (Garmezy, 1986), and therefore failures become more salient and more distressing over the course of development.

In sum, there are a variety of negative life events that have a high probability of being associated with the symptom as well as the full syndrome of depression. Other factors such as the individual's age, cognitive maturity, social supports, and preexisting personality can influence the intensity and duration of the sadness and the adequacy of the subsequent adjustment. Some of the potential mechanisms by which negative life events produce sad affect are discussed in a subsequent section.

PROCESSES THAT INDUCE SAD AFFECT

There are at least three processes by which individuals may become sad: experiential, cognitive, and vicarious. That is, the various undesirable events described in the previous section can produce sadness if one actually experiences them, imagines them, or observes another experience them. (It also is possible to combine the cognitive and vicarious methods by imagining someone else experiencing the situation.)

Behavioral (e.g., Ferster, 1973: Lewinsohn, 1974) and environmental (e.g., Billings and Moos, 1982; Paykel, 1979) models of depression emphasize the experiential process. Thus, the actual experience of negative life events or of receiving low rates of positive reinforcement are the hypothesized processes by which sad affect as well as the other symptoms of depressive disorder are produced. According to these experiential views, no further processes are necessary in order to mediate the link between experience and affect.

In contrast, both cognitive perspectives (Abramson et al., 1978; Beck, 1967) and psychoanalytical views (Bibring, 1968; Freud, 1968) assert that depression can result from either real or imagined negative life events. The cognitive processes that involve remembering a previously sad event, imagining or currently experiencing an undesirable situation, or anticipating a future bad circumstance can all produce sad affect. According to this perspective, it is not necessary to have ever actually experienced the event; the cognitive processes are hypothesized to be sufficient. Moreover, cognitive theorists (e.g., Abramson et al., 1989; Beck, 1967) argue that negative life events might produce transient feelings of sadness, although cognitions regarding the meaning of the event to the individual's sense of self, security, and future will lead to more enduring sad affect and associated depressive symptoms.

Finally, sad affect also can be produced vicariously. This can occur through actual observation, imagination, or the media (e.g., newspapers, books, movies). The process underlying the vicarious production of sadness is empathy (Hoffman, 1977, 1978). Hoffman (1978) defined empathy as the vicarious arousal of affect in an observer "that is not a reaction to his own situation but a vicarious response to another person's situation" (p. 229). According to Hoffman (1977, 1978), empathic arousal occurs as a result of reflexive action, motor mimicry, conditioning, and imagining oneself in the other's place. Hoffman also proposed that empathy undergoes developmental changes that are associated with a growing cognitive sense of the delineation of the self from others. Nevertheless, certain forms of reflexive emotional resonance such as empathic crying have been noted as early as the neonatal period (Martin and Clarke, 1982; Sagi and Hoffman, 1976; Simner, 1971).

Harris (1989) suggested that empathy is particularly likely to be triggered when the other person's situation is especially vivid (e.g., in a very descriptive novel or well-acted movie) or when the observer has a close personal history or shared characteristics with the target, so that it is easy for the observer to put himself or herself in the other's place.

Experimental studies with both children (Terwogt et al., 1986) and adults (Koriat et al., 1972; Lerner and Simmons, 1966) have found that having the observer pretend as if he or she were in the situation is more likely to lead to the empathic arousal of distress than having subjects take a detached view of the victim.

In a laboratory study comparing three different methods of inducing negative affect, Barden et al. (1985) induced sad affect experientially, cognitively, and vicariously in 2nd-grade children using the same negative event (rejection by a peer). They found that subjects in all three conditions showed the same degree of sadness according to ratings of their facial expressions. Moreover, in all three methods of negative affect induction, the children performed worse on a learning task and were significantly less altruistic than were children who had not received any affect induction.

Thus, all three processes are capable of producing significant levels of sad affect. What are the possible mechanisms through which these various processes operate? Do the processes differ for each method, or can they be reduced to a single mechanism? For example, is it possible that both the experiential and the vicarious methods require cognitions, particularly regarding the meaning of the event for the self and one's future? Alternatively, do all three processes set off some common biological process that then produces sad affect (e.g., Akiskal and McKinney, 1975)? Do such cognitive or biological mechanisms explain the observed individual differences in peoples' responses to the same negative event? The final section of this paper addresses the issue of mechanisms.

Underlying Mechanisms

Several mechanisms have been proposed to explain the onset of emotions in general, and sadness in particular. The nativist perspective, for example, asserts that emotions are innate and that many emotions are present and functional at birth. Discrete emotions theories (Ekman, 1984; Izard, 1971, 1977; Plutchik, 1980; Tomkins, 1962, 1963) are most representative of this view. In contrast, the constructivist orientation (e.g., Kagan, 1978, 1984; Lewis and Michalson, 1983; Sroufe, 1979) emphasizes the role of cognitions in the development of emotional expression. Cognitions are hypothesized to be the central mechanism in the growth and differentiation of emotions over the course of development.

We focus here on three mechanisms: evolutionary, biological, and cognitive/social learning. Although each is discussed separately, we recognize that more than one mechanism can explain the onset and maintenance of sadness and that these mechanisms can be interrelated.

EVOLUTIONARY PERSPECTIVE

His nurse pretended to cry, and I saw that his face instantly assumed a melancholy expression, with the corners of the mouth strongly depressed; now this child could rarely have seen any other child crying, and never a grown-up person crying, and I doubt whether at so early an age he could have reasoned on the subject. Therefore it seems to me that an innate feeling must have told him that the pretended crying of his nurse expressed grief; and this through the instinct of sympathy excited grief in him. (Darwin, 1872, p. 368)

Darwin (1872) observed that there was a basic similarity of facial expressions of people from different cultures and nations, and he therefore argued that there was an innate, universal basis for emotional expressions. He further argued that the ability to recognize the facial expression of emotions of others and the reactions to such expressions in infants also were innate.

The empirical work of Ekman and Friesen (1971) and Izard (1971, 1977; Izard et al., 1980) has provided some support for Darwin's claims regarding the universality of facial expressions of emotion. Ekman and Friesen (1971), for example, found that a group of adults as well as children from New Guinea who had had no contact with Western culture could correctly match certain emotion-arousing situations with the photographed facial expressions that would be expected in that situation.

In particular, they correctly identified sadness 79% of the time. They also showed good accuracy for the affects of happiness, anger, and disgust, but were somewhat less accurate discriminating surprise and fear. These findings were seen as supporting the case for the universality of at least some facial expressions.

In addition, studies by Izard et al. (1980) and Ganchrow et al. (1983) in which very young infants were found to produce discriminably different facial expressions, including sadness, are further support for Darwin's view that there is a direct, unlearned link between particular emotional states and particular facial expressions. Although the universality of facial expressions of emotions does not necessarily establish its innateness, since it is possible that children learn to copy the expression of discrete emotions, the fact that infants as young as a few days or weeks old can produce such discriminable expressions does cast some doubt on the imitation hypothesis (Harris, 1989).

Adaptive Function of Sadness

The evolutionary perspective also suggests that emotions are adaptive. In particular, several adaptive functions have been ascribed to the expression of sadness and distress (Averill, 1968; Darwin, 1872; Tomkins, 1963). Darwin suggested that tears help to prevent the mucous membranes of the eyes and nose from drying and assist in flushing out unhealthy bacteria. Tomkins (1963) proposed that distress serves a communicative, motivational, and cohesive function. The expression of distress communicates to others that something is wrong and that help is needed (Ellsworth and Smith, 1988). A distressed face, particularly in a child, typically elicits sympathy and empathy from others. Savitsky and Sim (1974), for example, found that judges were more lenient in their proposed punishments for juvenile offenders who looked distressed as opposed to those who appeared angry or happy (all of the offenders had supposedly committed equally serious crimes). The extent to which sadness elicits help versus rejection from others, however, has been found to vary across different cultures (Stearns, 1993).

Second, sadness and distress serve to focus persons inwardly so they can solve their problems and engage in coping behaviors in order to reduce the distress (Cunningham, 1988). During periods of sadness individuals have an opportunity to "work through" difficult situations and to adjust to them. They may engage in such coping responses as altering the stress-inducing situation or its consequences, altering their own cognitions about the situation, and/or seeking social support.

Third, distress, particularly grief over the loss of a loved one, can facilitate the cohesiveness of the family, community, or species. Averill (1968) asserted that "grief is a biological reaction, the evolutionary function of which is to insure group cohesiveness in species where a social form of existence is necessary for survival" (p. 729). Averill further asserted that group cohesiveness is maintained because separation from the group or particular members can be an extremely stressful event, both psychologically and physiologically. Thus, the anticipation or actual experience of distress associated with separation causes us to stay close to our loved ones and friends and thereby perpetuates the survival of the species.

Maladaptive Responses Associated with Sadness

Despite these various adaptive functions of sadness, there also are several consequences of sadness that are maladaptive. Sad affect has been found to be associated with decreases in cognitive performance and learning (Barden et al., 1985; Masters et al., 1979), impaired attention to tasks (Potts et al., 1989), less altruism (Barden et al., 1981; Cialdini and Kendrick, 1976; Isen et al., 1973), less resistance to temptation (Fry, 1975; Mischel et al., 1972), negative reactions from others (e.g., Coyne, 1976), and increases in memory for other sad events, which may prolong the negative state (Bower, 1981). Moreover, contrary to the view that sadness motivates the individual to cope with negative events, Garber et al. (1991) found that depressed children reported that they were more likely to withdraw and less likely to engage in behavioral or problem-focused coping strategies than were nondepressed children. Thus, although sadness and grief may serve some broad evolutionary function for the species as a whole, it is less clear that sadness is adaptive at the individual level. It may be that brief expressions of normal sadness can elicit help from others, whereas prolonged and more intense depression can result in rejection from others (Swallow and Kuiper, 1987).

BIOLOGICAL PERSPECTIVE

The image that comes to mind in considering the biological view is that of a sudden automatic reflex syndrome, Darwin's instant snarl expression, Freud's tension discharge and a given breaking point of tension overload, James and Lang's notion of an instantaneously unmediated visceral reaction to perceived stimulus. (Hochschild, 1979, pp. 553–554)

Cannon (1927, 1931) proposed that emotions are produced by brain mechanisms. In several experiments, Cannon (1929) removed parts of the brain in cats and showed that visceral activity would not account for the expression of emotion. Cannon's work highlighted the significance of subcortical structures as they relate to emotions. Cannon considered the thalamus to be the source of emotion, and he hypothesized that the *experience of emotion* is related to neural impulses originating from the thalamus and relayed to the cortex. He further suggested that the *expression of emotion*, however, has to do with neural impulses that the thalamus sends to the motor center in the body.

Bard's (1928) research focused on another anatomical structure (the hypothalamus), which was reported to be the major structure in emotional reactions. Years later, the research conducted by Pribram (1967, 1984) confirmed the fact that indeed both the thalamus and hypothalamus are involved in emotions. In 1937 Papez extended the center of emotion to the limbic forebrain. He suggested that the mechanism of emotions is not located in one particular focus of the brain; rather, it is handled through various cortical structures.

Over the years, MacLean's (1949, 1954, 1970) findings have suggested that the limbic system organizes the integration of emotional experiences, and he viewed the hypothalamus as the center for connecting the periphery to the cortex. He believed that all limbic system structures are involved in emotion, but that there are no specific mechanisms responsible for particular emotional patterns.

Pribram (1967, 1970, 1984) integrated several theories and studies and proposed that the entire brain is very much involved in regulating emotions. Each specific part of the brain, however, has a particular role in the overall regulation. Pribram's emphasis on the importance of the total brain structure and the coordination of several systems in the brain as well as specific patterns within each system has been widely accepted in recent years.

Tomkins (1962) proposed that emotions are elicited by neural activation, and the specific quality of the emotion is determined by the direction and gradient of such activation. For example, fear supposedly results when the gradient of neural activation is steep and positive, whereas joy results when the gradient is positive but more gradual. In contrast to fear, distress appears to be based not on an increase in density of stimulation but rather on an absolute level of density of stimulation or neural firing. Tomkin's theory has been criticized, however, because he did not propose an operationalization of neural activation, and it does not specify how real-life events are mapped onto gradients of neural firing (Campos et al., 1983).

Much of the work concerning the psychophysiology of emotions has focused on emotions in general (e.g., Izard and Schwartz, 1986; Lewis and Michalson, 1983). Since sadness is one of the most prominent emotions, we suggest that the above perspectives apply to sadness as well as to other emotions. Although there are an increasing number of studies that report biological aspects of childhood depression, such as hypothalamic-pituitary-adrenal axis dysfunction (as elevated through dexamethasone suppression tests (e.g., Weller et al., 1985), growth hormones (Puig-Antich et al., 1984), and sleep EEGs (Puig-Antich, 1985), these studies generally deal with the syndrome rather than the symptom of depression. Less is known about the specific psychophysiology of sad affect in children, and thus this needs to be studied further. Another important question for future study is whether the various biological correlates of depressive disorder are associated with the symptom of sadness or only with the full syndrome of depression.

COGNITIVE/SOCIAL LEARNING PERSPECTIVE

Whereas biological and evolutionary perspectives emphasize the constant and universal aspects of emotion, the social learning perspective focuses on individual differences in emotion experience and expression. Although the socialization approach recognizes the importance of organismic factors, it particularly emphasizes the equally important role of learning in emotional development. The fact that there is variability in response to common elicitors suggests that although biological pressures may partially influence emotions, socialization exerts a powerful influence as well (Michalson and Lewis, 1985). How does socialization explain individual differences in emotions? What aspects of emotions are socialized, and what are the processes by which such socialization takes place? It is beyond the scope of this chapter to review all of the relevant literature to answer these questions (see Campos et al., 1983; Lewis and Saarni, 1985). Rather, we highlight here the cognitive and socialization processes that may be particularly relevant to the development of sad affect.

What Aspects of Emotion Are Socialized?

There are various components of emotion that are differentially accessible to socialization. Buck (1983) defined accessibility as "the degree to which a response is normally perceivable and apparent to the responder and to others around the responder via sensory cues" (p. 270). According to Buck, overt, goal-directed, instrumental behavior and expressive behavior are particularly accessible to socialization pressures, whereas subjective experience and physiological responding are relatively less accessible to, although not totally independent of, learning. For example, individuals can learn to label their subjective experiences through the process of associating private arousal experiences with interpretations provided by others (Schachter, 1964).

Lewis and Saarni (1985) described the extent to which socialization influences the developmental course of each of five components of emotion (emotional elicitors, emotional receptors, emotional states, emotional expression, and emotional experience). Although socialization clearly can affect each of these components, emotional expression and the elicitor-emotion relation probably are the most accessible to learning. Lewis and Michalson (1982) and Hochschild (1979) similarly have suggested that socialization affects individuals' judgments about the circumstances under which and the targets toward whom emotions may be expressed, the labels given emotional states, and how emotions are regulated.

The growing literature concerning emotion display rules (e.g., Cole, 1986; Gnepp and Hess, 1986; Saarni, 1979, 1984) suggests that children learn over the course of development how, when, and with whom to intentionally control their emotional expressions such that the external representation of their affect differs from their internal affective state. Izard (1971) speculated that "as the individual moves into later childhood, peers and parents begin to discourage the ready display of strong emotions on the face" (p. 192). Saarni (1979) asserted that "with increasing cognitive complexity and socialization, children learn to monitor and regulate their expressive-affective behavioral displays according to social conventions" (p. 424). Indeed, older children have been found to conceal expressions of disappointment significantly more than do younger children (Saarni, 1979), although children as young as 3 or 4 years old also have been found to monitor their emotional expressions (Cole, 1986).

Several authors (e.g., Reichenbach and Masters, 1983; Yarczower et al., 1979) have suggested that strong negative emotions are particularly likely to be influenced by socialization, although most laboratory studies of display rules have focused on the somewhat less intense emotion of disappointment. In one study that explicitly examined the conditions that influence the expression of sadness, Fuchs and Thelen (1988) found that socialization practices are particularly likely to be directed at the suppression of sadness in males and the suppression of anger in females. According to the children's report, fathers especially discouraged the expression of sadness in their sons, whereas parents were perceived as encouraging the expression of sadness and discouraging the expression of anger in girls. Thus, the display of the emotional expression of sadness appears to be particularly vulnerable to socialization pressures.

The regulation of affect also is susceptible to social learning influences. Emotion regulation is the process of making a coordinated response to aversive environmental stimuli across and between three response systems: neurophysiological-biochemical, motor-expressive, and experiential-cognitive (Dodge, 1989). Recently, there has been increasing attention paid to the development of emotion regulation, which has highlighted the important role of experience, social support, and developing cognitive sophistication in coordination with prewired action tendencies and neural and motor processes (Campos et al., 1989; Dodge, 1989; Garber and Dodge, 1991; Kopp, 1989). Gottman and Katz (1989), for example, showed how young children acquire emotion-regulating behaviors through interaction with parents and how such learning is disrupted by marital discord in the home.

Garber et al. (1991) described how children learn to regulate sad affect, in particular in the context of parent-child interactions, and how such learning may be affected when one of the parents is depressed. They found that both depressed mothers and their offspring reported using less effective strategies to regulate their sadness than did nondepressed mothers and their children. Moreover, depressed mothers were significantly less responsive and less supportive of their children's expressions of negative affect than were nondepressed mothers. Garber et al. concluded that parents play a central role in the socialization of affect regulation through direct modeling as well as contingent responding to children's own expressions of emotional distress.

Socialization also has an important influence on whether an individual reacts emotionally to a particular elicitor. Although some elicitors, such as loud noises and falling, seem to have a strong immediate biological consequence, most elicitors are associated with large individual variability in emotional responding due to maturation, cognitive development, and socialization experiences (Lewis and Saarni, 1985). As discussed earlier, there are certain types of negative life experiences that have a high, although not inevitable, likelihood of being associated with sadness (e.g., separations, loss, failure). How does social learning theory explain individual differences in response to life events? Why are there some people who seem "to have everything" yet feel sad, whereas others who seem "to have nothing" manage to remain content (Beck, 1976)? What is it that is learned with regard to potential elicitors by some individuals but not others?

A classical behaviorist perspective (Skinner, 1953, 1971; Watson, 1930; Wolpe, 1969) uses a stimulus-response model to explain emotional reactions and suggests that emotions are learned like any other behavior. The association between stimulus events and emotional responses is established as the result of previous conditioning. Thus, individuals respond differently to stimulus events because they have had different learning histories with them. For example, whereas some individuals may have been conditioned to fear certain places (e.g., heights, elevators), others may not have been exposed to such conditioning.

Social learning theorists (e.g., Bandura, 1977) expanded this strict behaviorist perspective by including cognitive factors as well. According to the cognitive/socialization model (Michalson and Lewis, 1985), an elicitor produces an emotional expression through the mediation of a cognitive connection. Various forms of this cognitive perspective have been proposed by numerous theorists (e.g., Abramson et al., 1978, 1989; Arnold, 1960; Beck, 1967, 1976; Ellis, 1962; Kagan, 1984; Klinger, 1975; R.S. Lazarus, 1968; Lazarus et al., 1980; Mandler, 1975; Roseman, 1979; Schachter and Singer, 1962; Seligman, 1975; Sroufe, 1979; Weiner, 1985), though it has not been without its critics (see Zajonc, 1980). Although the cognitive theories emphasize different intervening cognitive processes (e.g., attributions, appraisal, schema, expectancies, meaning) and a variety of motivational constructs (e.g., importance, commitment, current concerns, goals, values), they generally agree that how individuals think about events influences the type, intensity, and duration of the affect experienced.

Arnold (1960) asserted that stimuli that are appraised as detrimental to one's personal domain lead to negative emotions. Lazarus and colleagues (Folkman and Lazarus, 1986, 1988; Lazarus et al., 1980) similarly have suggested that "emotions depend on cognitive appraisals of the significance of the person-environment relationship for the individual's well-being and the available options for coping" (Folkman and Lazarus, 1988, p. 466). Indeed, Folkman and Lazarus (1986) found that individuals reporting higher levels of depressive symptomatology appraised various situations as having much greater significance to their general well-being (e.g., self-esteem, finances) than did individuals low in depressive symptoms.

Beck (1967, 1976) has stated that the same stimulus event can produce different emotions in different people or within the same individual at different points in time, depending upon the specific content of the cognitions or meaning of the event. Beck proposed, for example, that anxiety occurs when an individual perceives threat (real or imagined) to his or her own or a significant other's health or safety; anger follows when others assault, transgress, or breach a code of behavior or standards; sadness results from the interpretations that "something of value has been lost" (1976, p. 58). According to Beck (1976), sadness is characterized by a sense of irreversible and significant loss that has implications for one's sense of self-efficacy and future well-being. Using a sample of depressed and anxious outpatients, Beck and colleagues (Beck et al., 1987) found support for the cognitive content-specificity hypothesis in that depression was more highly correlated with themes of loss, failure, and worthlessness, whereas anxiety was more highly correlated with anticipated physical threat and harm.

Elsewhere (Garber et al., 1980; Hollon and Garber, 1980) we have suggested that sadness results when individuals believe that the probability of obtaining a highly desired, and formerly presumed to be attainable goal (e.g., an interpersonal relationship, occupational status, self-esteem), is zero, or the probability that a highly undesirable outcome (e.g., loss of a loved one, loss of a job, imprisonment) will occur is 1.0. This formulation is similar to those of several of the leading cognitive theories (e.g., Abramson et al., 1989; Beck, 1967, 1976; Lazarus et al., 1980) and emphasizes the constructs of expectations, importance or desirability, and certainty.

Interestingly, although eliciting events are likely to trigger a set of depressogenic cognitions, such events are not necessary for sadness to occur. Rather, cognitions alone (i.e., one's expectations about important events) are critical for the experience of sadness. Thus, real as well as imagined negative outcomes can produce sad mood if they are accompanied by the relevant cognitions. The intensity and duration of the sadness depends on how important the outcome is to the individual, how certain he or she is that nothing can be done to alter the outcome (the concept of secondary appraisal and coping (Lazarus et al., 1980)), and how many other aspects of one's life are affected. *The more important the goal and the more certain that the outcome and its associated consequences are irreversible, the more severe the depressed mood.*

One criticism of the various cognitive perspectives is that the processing of information about events appears to be cold, calculated, conscious, and deliberate (Campos et al., 1983; Zajonc, 1980). Cognitive theorists (e.g., Beck, 1967; Dodge, 1986) have argued, however, that affect-relevant information processing can occur quite automatically and is not necessarily within immediate awareness. It is likely that earlier in the individual's development he or she learned to make the kinds of interpretations and value judgments that later appear to be automatic and outside of conscious awareness. Thus, the belief systems or schema that guide current interpretations and the associated affective responses developed as a function of earlier socialization experiences with significant adults and peers.

There is a growing conceptual and empirical literature describing social influences on the development of such cognitive processes as attributions, expectations, schema, and values (e.g., Costanza and Dix, 1983; Grusec and Dix, 1986; Higgins et al., 1983; Shantz, 1983). In general, this literature has shown that children learn about attributions, beliefs, morals, and values through much of the same processes of direct instruction, modeling, and reinforcement by which other behaviors are acquired. More research is needed, however, concerning the specific socialization conditions that are likely to lead to the negative cognitive schema that are associated with the development of sadness in particular. That is, what kinds of parent-child interactions produce the tendency to make internal, stable, and global attributions for negative events (Abramson et al., 1978) or to develop negative beliefs about the self, the world, and the future (Beck, 1967)?

One other criticism of the cognitive perspective is that certain emotions appear to be present even before infants are capable of having the kinds of cognitions that presumably are associated with sadness. That is, sadness is considered to be one of the basic emotions that can be observed very early in infancy (e.g., Ekman, 1984; Izard, 1971). According to the cognitive perspective (e.g., Bowlby, 1951; Sroufe, 1979), however, sadness emerges only after the child has a sufficiently elaborated cognitive representation of the mother and a differentiated sense of the self (i.e., at about 6–9 months of age). Either such cognitive maturation is not necessary for sadness or the early forms of distress that are labeled as sadness may not be the same as the sadness seen later. Indeed, the fact that the facial expression in infancy *looks like* sadness does not necessarily mean that it is experienced as sadness. Moreover, the fact that the expression of sadness can be observed in infants before the development of the kinds of cognitions posited to be associated with sadness (e.g., expectations about the future, concept of self) does not mean that such cognitions do not play an important role in the experience and expression of sadness at a later point in development. It also is possible, as suggested by Sroufe (1979), that the noncognitive display of distress seen in infancy may be a precursor or prototype of the more mature form of sadness. Although this earlier form of distress may not be accompanied by the relevant cognitions, later expressions of sadness may.

Thus, according to the cognitive/socialization perspective, cognitions play an important role in whether, when, and how sadness is expressed and regulated in association with certain life events. Interactions with important others (e.g., parents, teachers, peers) are considered to be the primary contexts in which learning about salient cognitions takes place.

How Do Children Learn about Emotions?

What are the processes by which children learn about emotions in general and sadness in particular? Basically, emotions are learned according to the same principles as are other behaviors, including such direct methods as classical conditioning, instrumental learning, and didactic teaching, and such indirect methods as observational learning, imitation, and the media (e.g., books, television, movies) (Dorr, 1985; Lewis and Saarni, 1985). Watson (1919, 1930), for example, classically conditioned fear in a young child by pairing a formerly neutral stimulus with an unconditioned stimulus. There are few, if any, examples, however, of classical conditioning being used to produce sadness. Wolpe (1971) has come the closest to suggesting that depression may be classically associated with severe states of anxiety.

Instrumental conditioning also plays a role in the socialization of emotion and its expression. Expressions of emotional distress can be both punished (e.g., scolded) or rewarded (e.g., comforted) (Izard, 1977; Tomkins, 1963). Smiling in infants, for example, has been found to be responsive to both operant conditioning and extinction (Brackbill, 1958; Brossard and Decarie, 1968).

Malatesta and colleagues (Malatesta and Haviland, 1985; Malatesta et al., 1989) have suggested that caregivers have many opportunities for shaping via instrumental conditioning infants' affect because infants have a wide range of emotional expressions and high lability. Malatesta and Haviland (1985) reported that observed differences in the emotional expression of male versus female babies was the result of differential reinforcement. Mothers showed a significant increase, with increasing infant age, in contingent responding (especially contingent smiling) to the smiles of infant males and a decrease for females. Moreover, they found that, although mothers displayed and reinforced positive affect in both sexes, they displayed a wider range of contingent emotional expressivity with females.

Behaviorists (e.g., Ferster, 1973; A. Lazarus, 1968; Lewinsohn, 1974; Lewinsohn et al., 1976) have suggested that depressed affect, in particular, results from a reduction in the rate of response-contingent positive reinforcement. "Dysphoria is assumed to occur when there is either little reinforcement or when available reinforcers are not contingent on the person's behavior" (Lewinsohn et al., 1973, p. 103). Lewinsohn and colleagues (Lewinsohn and Graf, 1973; MacPhillamy and Lewinsohn, 1974) have found a positive association between depressed mood and low rates of positive reinforcement. In addition, Lewinsohn (1974; Lewinsohn et al., 1976) also has suggested that depressed affect is maintained by the social attention of others.

Didactic teaching and instruction by significant others (e.g., parents and teachers) also are direct processes used in the socialization of emotion. For example, a parent may communicate such affect rules as "Big boys don't cry," "When you look that way, I know that you are feeling angry," or "It helps to talk about your feelings when you are upset." Thus, children can learn the rules of emotion expression, emotion labeling, and emotion regulation through direct instruction.

The more indirect methods of social learning typically involve the observation of others. Such observation might include being the direct target of another's emotional display, being a common target of an emotion-eliciting situation (e.g., social referencing), or being an uninvolved observer of others (e.g., watching an argument between parents or reading a book) (Dorr, 1985). By observing the emotions of others, children learn about the conditions that elicit emotions, the methods for expressing and regulating emotion, and the consequences of such emotion expression. Children may or may not choose to imitate the expressions of others, depending on the observed consequences to the model of expressing emotion, or the direct consequences to themselves of such imitation.

There is some debate concerning whether and when young infants actually are capable of imitating modeled emotional expressions. Whereas some investigators have suggested that 2- and 3-day-old infants can imitate facial expressions (e.g., Field et al., 1982; Field and Walden, 1982), others have questioned this finding (e.g., Campos et al., 1983; Kaitz et al., 1988). Based upon a review of the relevant literature, Malatesta and Izard (1984) concluded that there was more support for the case than against it. Malatesta and Haviland (1985) asserted that young infants are capable of matching part or whole facial expressions of others with similar expressions of their own, although older infants appear to engage in such matching more than do younger ones.

Harris (1989) has argued that imitation can explain how infants come to copy a particular facial expression at some point in time, but that it cannot explain how infants come to produce that expression in particular circumstances. Harris further suggested that a more parsimonious explanation is that certain elicitors more or less automatically produce specific emotional expressions. Harris notes, however, that for the facial expressions of sadness, surprise, and fear, there still is a lack of evidence for their connection to particular elicitors.

Do babies imitate their mother's expressions of sadness? The burgeoning literature concerning the interactions of depressed mothers and their infants suggests that although infants might not necessarily show the same sad facial expressions as their sad mother, they clearly react negatively to their mother's sad displays (Cohn and Tronick, 1983; Field, 1984; Termine and Izard, 1988). In a study in which mothers were instructed to simulate sad expressions in face-to-face interactions with their babies, Cohn and Tronick (1983) found that infants frequently looked wary, averted their gaze, protested, and attempted to elicit responses from the mother. Studies that have observed clinically depressed mothers interacting with their children (Cohn et al., 1986; Field, 1984) also have reported that the children tended to withdraw, look away, play less, and protest more, and seldom showed positive affect. Field (1984), however, found that the offspring of depressed mothers did not react any differently when their mothers were instructed to "look depressed," whereas the offspring of the nondepressed mothers showed the same kinds of disorganization and distress as had been reported by Cohn and Tronick (1983) in their study of mothers simulating depression.

Tronick and Gianino (1986) have proposed a mutual regulation model in order to explain infants' disturbed reactions to their mother's depression. According to this model, a depressed mother's failure to respond to her infant's emotion-regulating signals results in poorly coordinated interactions that cause the infant to experience further distress. Although infants initially persist in trying to obtain their mother's help, they soon turn to self-regulatory behaviors (e.g., gaze aversion) in order to deal with the negative interaction. Tronick and Gianino concluded that the affective disturbance of infants of depressed mothers does not result from imitation or the mother's somehow "feeding" her affect to her infant. "Rather, it is the result of the infant's normal regulatory capacities becoming increasingly narrowly deployed . . . in the face of the mother's failure to play her normal external regulatory role" (1986, p. 9). Field (1987; Field et al., 1990) similarly has suggested that depressed mother-infant dyads are less likely to have behavior-state matching and synchrony than are nondepressed mothers and their infants. Thus, although infants may at times imitate the sad expressions of their parents, the distress observed in the infant offspring of depressed mothers seems to involve a more complex failure in mutual regulation and affect matching.

Do older children learn about sadness through observation and imitation of sad adults? Although there is a growing literature showing that the offspring of depressed parents are significantly more likely to be depressed themselves than are the offspring of nondepressed parents (e.g., Beardslee et al., 1983; Weissman et al., 1984), less is known about the processes that produce this depression. Several mechanisms have been suggested, including problem parenting, parental emotional unavailability and insensitivity, modeling of depressive symptoms, shared stresses and strains, child abuse and neglect, and marital discord (e.g., Goodman and Brumley, 1990; Hammen et al., 1987; Rutter, 1990; Rutter and Quinton, 1984). Rutter (1990) recently has noted, however, that it is difficult to specify the mechanisms by which parental depression produces problems in offspring because of the difficulty of disentangling the effects of the parents' depression per se from the associated risk factors.

It also is difficult to determine how the various components of the parent's depression differentially influence their children's outcomes. For example, what is the impact on children of a parent's expression of sad affect? Do children learn to be sad through the social learning processes of observing and imitating a depressed parent? Unfortunately, there have been few studies that have examined specifically the question of affect imitation per se in depressed parents and their children.

Garber et al. (1991) observed the affective expressions of depressed versus nondepressed mothers and their children while they engaged in a mildly stressful laboratory interaction task. They found that whereas the depressed mothers showed significantly more negative affect than did nondepressed mothers, the offspring of the depressed mothers showed significantly *less* negative affect than the offspring of the nondepressed mothers. Garber et al. speculated that the children of the depressed mothers might have been reluctant to display negative emotions to their depressed mothers either because they did not want to cause her further distress or because they have learned that their own expressions of distress typically are met with either punishment (e.g., rejection) or nonresponsiveness by their depressed mothers. Further research is needed to identify the factors that might influence whether and under what conditions children imitate the expressions of sad affect of depressed and nondepressed parents.

Finally, the phenomenon of social referencing has been used to describe the process by which individuals seek out and use the facial, vocal, and gestural emotional expressions of others to help clarify an uncertain situation (Campos and Stenberg, 1981; Klinnert et al., 1983). The behavior of the referencing individual has been found to differ as a function of the emotional information provided by the other person (Campos et al., 1983). For example, when mothers display negative expressions, their infants tend to avoid crossing visual cliffs (Sorce et al., 1985), inhibit playing with toys (Gunnar and Stone, 1984; Walden and Ogan, 1988), and are less friendly toward strangers (Feinman and Lewis, 1983).

In only one study thus far (Sorce et al., 1985) have maternal expressions of sadness been studied using the social-referencing paradigm. Sorce et al. found that infants were more likely to cross a visual cliff in response to their mother's expressions of sadness versus either fear or anger. This study, however, was not an adequate test of the social referencing of sadness since the visual cliff was not really an appropriate context for the expression of sad affect. Studies are needed that use a more sadness-appropriate setting in order to examine the extent to which social referencing of maternal expressions of sad affect influences children's behaviors and emotions.

In sum, various aspects of emotion, including its expression, labeling, regulation, and associated elicitors, can be learned through socialization. The particular social learning processes by which this learning occurs include both direct conditioning and indirect observational methods. There is some empirical evidence that the affect of sadness in particular is responsive to such socialization experiences.

CONCLUSIONS AND FUTURE DIRECTIONS

The present chapter outlined various issues that influence the development of the symptom of sadness. There clearly are significant age changes in the prevalence, manifestation, expression, and recognition of sadness over the course of development. There also is important variability with regard to processes that produce sadness (e.g., experiential, cognitive, vicarious) and whether a particular life event will elicit sadness. Although several categories of potential elicitors were outlined, none universally, inevitably, or specifically is known to produce sadness. Various mechanisms to explain the developmental and individual differences in sadness were discussed, including evolutionary, biological, and cognitive/socialization processes.

Using this chapter as a base, we suggest that there are several interesting questions with regard to continuity, development, and mechanisms that should be the focus of future investigations. Do the same underlying mechanisms explain normal sadness as the sadness seen among clinically depressed individuals? Are the processes that produce the symptom of sadness different from those that produce the other symptoms or full syndrome of depression? Is there continuity over the course of development from the early expressions of sadness seen in infancy to those observed in older children and adults? Finally, how do biological, cognitive, and social processes interact to produce both the symptom of sadness and the full syndrome of depression, and how do these factors change over the course of development?

References

Abramson LY, Metalsky GI, Alloy LB: Hopelessness depression: A theory-based subtyped of depression. *Psychol Rev* 96:358–372, 1989.

Abramson LY, Seligman MEP, Teasdale JD: Learned helplessness in humans: Critique and reformulation. *J Abnorm Psychol* 87:49–74, 1978.

Achenbach TM, Edelbrock CS: Behavioral problems and competencies reported by parents of normal and disturbed children ages four to sixteen. *Monogr Child Dev* 46(188), 1981.

Achenbach TM, Edelbrock CS: *Manual for the Teachers Report Form and Teacher Version of the Child Behavior Profile*. Burlington, VT, Department of Psychiatry, University of Vermont, 1986.

Akiskal H, McKinney W: Overview of recent research in depression: Integration of ten conceptual models into a comprehensive clinical framework. *Arch Gen Psychiatry* 32:285–305, 1975.

Amen E: Individual differences in apperceptive reaction: A study of the responses of preschool children to pictures. *Genet Psychol Mongr* 23:319–385, 1941.

Arnold M: *Emotion and Personality* (Vol 1). New York, Columbia University Press, 1960.

Averill JR: Grief: Its nature and significance. *Psychol Bull* 70:721–748, 1968.

Bandura A: *Social Learning Theory*. Englewood Cliffs, NJ, Prentice-Hall, 1977.

Bard PA: A diencephalic mechanism for the expression of rage with special reference to the sympathetic nervous system. *Am J Physiol* 84:490–515, 1928.

Barden RC, Garber J, Duncan SW, et al: Cumulative effects of induced affective states: Accentuation, inoculation, and remediation. *J Pers Soc Psychol* 40:750–760, 1981.

Barden RC, Garber J, Leiman B, et al: Factors governing the effective remediation of negative affect and its cognitive and behavioral consequences. *J Pers Soc Psychol* 49:1040–1053, 1985.

Barden RC, Zelko FA, Duncan SW, et al: Children's consensual knowledge about the experiential determinants of emotion. *J Pers Soc Psychol* 39:962–976, 1980.

Barrera M, Maurer D: Recognition of mother's photographed face by three-month-old infants. Paper presented at the meeting of the International Conference on Infant Studies, Providence, RI, April 1978.

Barron J: Physical handicap and personality: Study of the seen versus the unseen disabilities. *Arch Phys Med Rehabil* 36:639–643, 1955.

Beardslee WR, Bemporad J, Keller MB, et al: Children of parents with major affective disorder: A review. *Am J Psychiatry* 140:825–832, 1983.

Beck AT: *Depression: Clinical, Experimental, and Theoretical Aspects*. New York, Harper & Row, 1967.

Beck AT: *Cognitive Therapy and the Emotional Disorders*. New York, International Universities Press, 1976.

Beck AT, Brown G, Steer RA, et al: Differentiating anxiety and depression: A test of the cognitive content-specificity hypothesis. *J Abnorm Psychol* 96:179–183, 1987.

Belle D: *Lives in Stress: Women and Depression*. Beverly Hills, CA, Sage, 1982.

Bibring E: The mechanism of depression. In: Gaylin W (ed): *The Meaning of Despair*. New York, Science House, 1968, pp. 154–181.

Billings AG, Moos RH: Psychosocial theory and research on depression: An integrative framework and review. *Clin Psychol Rev* 2:213–237, 1982.

Billings AG, Cronkite RC, Moos RH: Social-environmental factors in unipolar depression: Comparisons of depressed patients and nondepressed controls. *J Abnorm Psychol* 92:129–133, 1983.

Blumberg SH, Izard CE: Affective and cognitive characteristics of depression in 10- and 11-year old children. *J Pers Soc Psychol* 49:194–202, 1985.

Borke H: Interpersonal perceptions of young children: Egocentrism or empathy. *Dev Psychol* 5:263–269, 1971.

Boucher JD: Facial displays of fear, sadness, and pain. *Percept Mot Skill* 28:239–242, 1969.

Bower GH: Mood and memory. *Am Psychol* 36:129–148, 1981.

Bowlby J: *Maternal Care and Mental Health*. Geneva, World Health Organization, 1951.

Bowlby J: Processes of mourning. *Int J Psychoanal* 42:317–340, 1961.

Bowlby J: *Attachment and Loss. Vol 2: Attachment*. London, Hogarth Press, 1969.

Bowlby J: *Attachment and Loss. Vol 3: Loss, Sadness and Depression*. New York, Basic Books, 1980.

Brackbill Y: Extinction of the smiling response in infants as a function of reinforcement. *Child Dev* 29:115–124, 1958.

Bretherington I, Beeghly M: Talking about internal states: The acquisition of an explicit theory of mind. *Dev Psychol* 18:906–921, 1982.

Bretherington I, Fritz J, Zahn-Waxler C, et al: Learning to talk about emotions: A functionalist perspective. *Child Dev* 57:529–548, 1986.

Bridges KMB: Emotional development in early infancy. *Child Dev* 3:324–341, 1932.

Brossard L, Decarie T: Comparative reinforcing effects of eight stimulations on the smiling responses of infants. *J Child Psychol Psychiatry* 9:51–60, 1968.

Brown A, Finkelhor D: Impact of child sexual abuse: A review of the research. *Psychol Bull* 99:66–77, 1986.

Brown GW, Harris TO: *Social Origins of Depression*. London, Tavistock, 1978.

Buck R: Emotional development and emotional education. In: Plutchik R, Kellerman H (eds): *Emotion: Theory, Research, and Experience*. New York, Academic Press, 1983, pp. 259–292.

Burgess AW, Holmstrom LL: Rape trauma syndrome. *Am J Psychiatry* 131:981–986, 1974.

Buss T, Redburn FS: *Mass Unemployment: Plant Closings and Community Mental Health*. Beverly Hills, CA, Sage, 1983.

Campbell JL, La Clave LJ, Black G: Clinical depression in paediatric burn patients. *Burns* 13:213–217, 1987.

Campos JJ, Sternberg C: Perception, appraisal, and emotion: The onset of social referencing. In: Lamb M, Sherrod L (eds): *Infant Social Cognition*. Hillsdale, NJ, Erlbaum, 1981, pp. 273–314.

Campos JJ, Barrett KC, Lamb ME, et al: Socioemotional development. In: Campos JJ, Haith MH (eds): *Handbook of Child Psychology. Vol 2: Infancy and Developmental Psychobiology*. New York, Wiley, 1983, pp. 783–915.

Campos JJ, Campos RG, Barrett KC: Emergent themes in the study of emotional development and emotion regulation. *Dev Psychol* 25:394–402, 1989.

Cannon WB: The James-Lange theory of emotion: A critical examination and an alternative theory. *Am J Psychol* 39:106–124, 1927.

Cannon WB: *Bodily Changes in Pain, Hunger, Fear, and Rage*. New York, Appleton, 1929.

Cannon WB: Again the James-Lange and the thalamic theories of emotion. *Psychol Rev* 38:281–295, 1931.

Carlson GA, Kashani JN: Phenomenology of major depression from childhood through adulthood: Analyses of three studies. *Am J Psychiatry* 145:1222–1225, 1988.

Caron RF, Caron AJ, Myers RS: Abstraction of invariant face expressions in infancy. *Child Dev* 53:1008–1015, 1982.

Cassidy J, Kobak R: Avoidance and its relation to other defensive processes. In: Belsky J, Nezworski T (eds): *Clinical Implications of Attachment*. Hillsdale, NJ, Erlbaum, 1989, pp. 300–323.

Chesser ES, Anderson JL: Psychological considerations in cancer of the breast. *Proc R Soc Med* 68:793–795, 1975.

Cialdini RB, Kendrick DT: Altruism as hedonism: A social developmental perspective on the relation of mood states and helping. *J Pers Soc Psychol* 34:907–914, 1976.

Clayton PJ, Desmarais L, Winokur G: A study of normal bereavement. *Am J Psychiatry* 125:168–178, 1968.

Clayton PJ, Halikas JA, Maurice WL: The depression of widowhood. *Br J Psychiatry* 120:71–78, 1972.

Cobb S: Social support as a moderator of life stress. *Psychosom Med* 38:300–312, 1976.

Cohn JF, Tronick EZ: Three-month-old infants' reactions to simulated maternal depression. *Child Dev* 54:185–193, 1983.

Cohn JF, Matias R, Tronick EZ, et al: Face-to-face interactions of depressed mothers and their infants. In: Tronick EZ, Field T (eds): *Maternal Depression and Infant Disturbance* (New Directions for Child Development, no. 34). San Francisco, Jossey-Bass, 1986, pp. 31–44.

Cole PM: Display rules and the socialization of affective displays. In: Zivin G (ed): *The Development of Expressive Behavior: Biology-Environment Interactions*. New York, Academic Press, 1985, pp. 269–290.

Cole PM: Children's spontaneous control of facial expression. *Child Dev* 57:1309–1321, 1986.

Connell JP, Wellborn J: Competence, autonomy, and relatedness: Self-system processes for a motivational perspective. In: Gunnar M, Sroufe A (eds): *Self Processes and Development*. (Minnesota Symposium on Child Psychology, Vol 23). Hillsdale, NJ, Erlbaum, 1991, pp. 43–77.

Costanza PR, Dix TN: Beyond the information processed: Socialization in the development of attributional processes. In: Higgins ET, Ruble DN, Hartup WW (eds): *Social Cognition and Social Development: A Sociocultural Perspective*. London, Cambridge University Press, 1983, pp. 63–81.

Coyne JC: Depression and the response of others. *J Abnorm Psychol* 85:186–193, 1976.

Crook T, Eliot J: Parental death during childhood and adult depression: A critical review of the literature. *Psychol Bull* 87:252–259, 1980.

Cunningham MR: What do you do when you're happy or blue? Mood, expectancies, and behavioral interest. *Motiv Emotion* 12:309–331, 1988.

Darwin C: *The Expression of the Emotions in Man and Animals*. London, Murray, 1872.

Demos V: Crying in early infancy: An illustration of the motivational function of affect. In: Brazelton TB, Yogman M (eds): *Affect and Early Infancy*. New York, Ablex, 1986, pp. 39–73.

Dodge KA: A social-information processing model of social competence in children. In: Perlmutter M (ed): *Minnesota Symposium in Child Psychology* (Vol 18). Hillsdale, NJ, Erlbaum, 1986, pp. 77–125.

Dodge KA: Coordinating responses to aversive stimuli: Introduction to a special section on the development of emotion regulation. *Dev Psychol* 25:339–342, 1989.

Dorr A: Contexts for experience with emotion, with special attention to television. In: Lewis M, Saarni C (eds): *The Socialization of Emotions*. New York, Plenum, 1985, pp. 55–85.

Dunn J, Brown J: Relationships, talk about feelings, and the development of affect regulation in early childhood. In: Garber J, Dodge K (eds): *The

Development of Emotion Regulation and Dysregulation. Cambridge, Cambridge University Press, 1991, pp. 84–108.

Dunn J, Kendrick C: Interaction between young siblings in the context of family relationships. In: Lewis M, Rosenblum LA (eds): *The Child and Its Family.* New York, Plenum, 1979, pp. 143–168.

Dunn J, Kendrick C: *Siblings: Love, Envy and Understanding.* Cambridge, MA, Harvard University Press, 1982.

Dunn J, Kendrick C, MacNamee R: The reaction of first-born children to the birth of a sibling: Mother's reports. *J Child Psychol Psychiatry* 22:1–18, 1981.

Dweck CS, Elliott ES: Achievement motivation. In: Hetherington EM (ed): *Handbook of Child Psychology. Vol 4: Socialization, Personality and Social Development* (4th ed). New York, Wiley, 1983, pp. 643–691.

Eisenberg L: When is a case a case? In: Rutter M, Izard CE, Read PB (eds): *Depression in Young People: Clinical and Developmental Perspectives.* New York, Guilford, 1986, pp. 469–478.

Ekman P: Cross-cultural studies of facial expression. In: Ekman P (ed): *Darwin and Facial Expression.* New York, Academic Press, 1973, pp. 169–222.

Ekman P: Expression and the nature of emotion. In: Scherer K, Ekman P (eds): *Approaches to Emotion.* Hillsdale, NJ, Erlbaum, 1984, pp. 329–343.

Ekman P, Friesen WV: Constants across culture in the face and emotion. *J Pers Soc Psychol* 17:124–129, 1971.

Ekman P, Friesen WV: *Unmasking the Face: A Guide to Recognizing Emotions from Facial Clues.* Englewood Cliffs, NJ, Prentice-Hall, 1975.

Ekman P, Levenson RW, Friesen WV: Autonomic nervous system activity distinguishes among emotions. *Science* 221:1208–1210, 1983.

Ellis A: *Reason and Emotion in Psychotherapy.* New York, Lyle Stuart, 1962.

Ellsworth PC, Smith CA: From appraisal to emotion: Differences among unpleasant feelings. *Motiv Emotion* 12:271–302, 1988.

Emde RN, Plak PR, Spitz RA: Anaclitic depression in an infant raised in an institution. *J Am Acad Child Psychiatry* 4:545–553, 1965.

Feinman S, Lewis M: Social referencing at ten months: A second-order effect on infants' responses to strangers. *Child Dev* 54:878–887, 1983.

Ferster CB: A functional analysis of depression. *Am Psychol* 28:857–871, 1973.

Field TM: Early interactions between infants and their postpartum depressed mothers. *Infant Behav Dev* 7:527–532, 1984.

Field TM: Affective response to separation. In: Brazelton TB, Yogman MW (eds): *Affective Development in Infancy.* Norwood, NJ, Ablex, 1985.

Field TM: Interaction and attachment in normal and atypical infants. *J Consult Clin Psychol* 55:853–859, 1987.

Field TM, Walden T: Perception and production of facial expression in infancy and early childhood. In: Reese HW, Lipsitt LP (eds): *Advances in Child Development and Behavior.* New York, Academic Press, 1982, pp. 169–211.

Field TM, Healy B, Goldstin S: Behavior-state matching and synchrony in mother-infant interactions of nondepressed versus depressed dyads. *Dev Psychol* 26:7–14, 1990.

Field TM, Woodson R, Greenberg R, et al: Discrimination and imitation of facial expression of neonates. *Science* 218:179–181, 1982.

Finlay-Jones R, Brown GW: Types of stressful life events and the onset of anxiety and depressive disorders. *Psychol Med* 11:803–815, 1981.

Folkman S, Lazarus RS: Stress processes and depressive symptomatology. *J Abnorm Psychol* 95:107–113, 1986.

Folkman S, Lazarus RS: Coping as a mediator of emotion. *J Pers Soc Psychol* 54:466–475, 1988.

Freud A, Burlingham D: *Infants without Families and Reports on the Hampstead Nurseries, 1939–1945.* London, Hogarth Press, 1974.

Freud S: *Collected Papers* (Vol 2). London, Hogarth Press and the Institute of Psychoanalysis.

Freud S: Mourning and melancholia. In: Strachey J (ed): *The Standard Edition of the Complete Works of Sigmund Freud* (Vol 14). London, Hogarth Press, 1968. (Originally published 1917.)

Friedman RC, Hurt SE, Clarkin JF, et al: Symptoms of depression among adolescents and young adults. *J Affect Disord* 5:37–43, 1983.

Fry PS: Affect and resistance to temptation. *Dev Psychol* 2:466–472, 1975.

Fuchs D, Thelen MN: Children's expected interpersonal consequences of communicating their affective state and reported likelihood of expression. *Child Dev* 59:1314–1322, 1988.

Furman E: *A Child's Parent Dies: Studies in Childhood Bereavement.* New Haven, CT, Yale University Press, 1974.

Gaensbauer TJ: Anaclitic depression in a three-and-a-half-month-old child. *Am J Psychiatry* 137:841–842, 1980.

Gaensbauer TJ: Regulation of emotional expression in infants from two contrasting caretaking environments. *J Am Acad Child Psychiatry* 21:163–170, 1982.

Galambus NL, Silbereisen RK: Income change, parental life outlook, and adolescent expectations for job success. *J Marriage Fam* 49:141–149, 1987.

Ganchrow JR, Steiner JE, Daher M: Neonatal facial expressions in response to different qualities and intensities of gustatory stimuli. *Infant Behav Dev* 6:473–484, 1983.

Garber J: The developmental progression of depression in female children. In: Cicchetti D, Schneider-Rosen K (eds): *Childhood Depression* (New Directions in Child Development, no. 26). San Francisco, Jossey-Bass, 1984, pp. 29–58.

Garber J, Dodge HA (eds): *The Development of Emotion Regulation and Dysregulation.* New York, Cambridge University Press, 1991.

Garber J, Braafladt N, Zeman J: The regulation of sad affect: An information processing perspective. In: Garber J, Dodge KA (eds): *The Development of Emotion Regulation and Dysregulation.* New York, Cambridge University Press, 1991, pp. 208–240.

Garber J, Miller SM, Abramson LY: On the distinction between anxiety and depression: Perceived control, certainty, and probability of goal attainment. In: Garber J, Seligman MEP (eds): *Human Helplessness: Theory and Application.* New York, Academic Press, 1980, pp. 131–169.

Garber J, Quiggle N, Panak W: Children's liking for self and others: Affect and situational cues. Paper presented at the annual meeting of the American Psychological Association, New York, 1987.

Garmezy N: Developmental aspects of children's responses to the stress of separation and loss. In: Rutter M, Izard CE, Read FB (eds): *Depression in Young People: Developmental and Clinical Perspectives.* New York, Guilford, 1986, pp. 297–323.

Garmezy N, Rutter M: Acute reactions to stress in children. In: Rutter M, Hersov I (eds): *Child and Adolescent Psychiatry: Modern Approaches* (2nd ed). Oxford, Blackwell Scientific Publications, 1985, pp. 152–176.

Gershon ES, Bunney WE, Leckman JF, et al: The inheritance of affective disorders: A review of data and of hypotheses. *Behav Genet* 6:227–261, 1976.

Glasberg R, Aboud F: A developmental perspective on the study of depression: Children's evaluative response to sadness. *Dev Psychol* 17:195–202, 1981.

Glick IO, Weiss RS, Parkes CM: *The First Year of Bereavement.* New York, Wiley, 1974.

Gnepp J, Hess DLR: Children's understanding of display rules for expressive behavior. *Dev Psychol* 22:103–108, 1986.

Goodman SH, Brumley HE: Schizophrenic and depressed mothers: Relational deficits in parenting. *Dev Psychol* 26:31–39, 1990.

Gottman JM, Katz LF: Effects of marital discord on young children's peer interaction and health. *Dev Psychol* 25:373–381, 1989.

Grusec JE, Dix T: The socialization of prosocial behavior: Theory and reality. In: Zahn-Waxler C, Cummings EM, Iannotti R (eds): *Altruism and Aggression: Biological and Social Origins.* London, Cambridge University Press, 1986, pp. 218–237.

Gunnar M, Stone C: The effects of positive maternal affect on infant responses to pleasant, ambiguous, and fear-provoking toys. *Child Dev* 55:1231–1236, 1984.

Hammen C, Gordon D, Burge D, et al: Maternal affective disorders, illness and stress: Risk for children's psychopathology. *Am J Psychiatry* 144:736–741, 1987.

Harkness S, Super C: The cultural construction of child development: A framework for the socialization of affect. *Ethos* 11:221–231, 1983.

Harmon RJ, Wagonfeld S, Emde RN: Anaclitic depression: A follow-up from infancy to puberty. *Psychoanal Study Child* 37:67–94, 1982.

Harris PL: Children's understanding of the link between situation and emotion. *J Exp Child Psychol* 36:490–509, 1983.

Harris PL: What children know about the situations that provoke emotions. In: Lewis M, Saarni C (eds): *The Socialization of Emotions.* New York, Plenum, 1985, pp. 161–186.

Harris PL: *Children and Emotion: The Development of Psychological Understanding.* Oxford, Basil Blackwell, 1989.

Harris PL, Gus GR, Lipian MS, et al: Insight into the time-course of emotion among Western and Chinese children. *Child Dev* 56:972–988, 1985.

Harter S: Children's understanding of multiple emotions: A cognitive-developmental approach. In: Overton WF (ed): *The Relationship Between Social and Cognitive Development.* Hillsdale, NJ, Erlbaum, 1983, pp. 147–194.

Haviland JM, Lelwica M: The induced affect response: 10-week-old infants' responses to three emotional expressions. *Dev Psychol* 23:97–104, 1987.

Heckhausen H: The development of achievement motivation. In: Hartup WW (ed): *Review of Child Development Research* (Vol 6). Chicago, University of Chicago Press, 1982, pp. 600–668.

Hesse P, Cicchetti D: Perspectives on an integrated theory of emotional development. In: Cicchetti D, Hesse P (eds): *Emotional Development* (New Directions for Child Development, no. 16). San Francisco, Jossey-Bass, 1982, pp. 3–48.

Hetherington EM, Cox EM, Cox R: Family interaction and the social-emotional and cognitive development of children following divorce. In: Vaughn V, Brazelton TB (eds): *The Family: Setting Priorities.* New York, Science and Medicine, 1979a, pp. 71–87.

Hetherington EM, Cox EM, Cox R: Play and social interaction in children following divorce. *J Social Issues* 35:26–49, 1979b.

Hetherington EM, Cox EM, Cox R: Effects of divorce on parents and children. In: Lamb M (ed): *Non-traditional Families.* Hillsdale, NJ, Erlbaum, 1981, pp. 233–288.

Higgins ET, Ruble DN, Hartup WW: *Social cognition and social development: A sociocultural perspective*. London, Cambridge University Press, 1983.

Hinton JM: The physical and mental distress of the dying. *Q J Med* 32:1–21, 1963.

Hochschild AR: Emotion work, feeling rules, and social structure. *Am J Sociol* 85:551–575, 1979.

Hoffman ML: Empathy, its development and prosocial implications. In: Keasy CB (ed): *Nebraska Symposium on Motivation* (Vol 26). Lincoln, NE, University of Nebraska Press, 1977, pp. 169–217.

Hoffman ML: Toward a theory of empathic arousal and development. In: Lewis M, Rosenblum LA (eds): *The Development of Affect*. New York, Plenum, 1978, pp. 227–257.

Hollon SD, Garber J: A cognitive-expectancy theory of therapy for helplessness and depression. In: Garber J, Seligman MEP (eds): *Human Helplessness: Theory and Applications*. New York, Academic Press, 1980, pp. 173–194.

Isen AM, Horn H, Rosenhan DL: Effects of success and failure on children's generosity. *J Pers Soc Psychol* 27:239–247, 1973.

Izard CE: *The Face of Emotion*. New York, Appleton-Century-Crofts, 1971.

Izard CE: *Patterns of Emotion: A New Analysis of Anxiety and Depression*. New York, Academic Press, 1972.

Izard CE: *Human Emotions*. New York, Plenum, 1977.

Izard CE, Malatesta CZ: Perspectives on emotional development: I. Differential emotions theory of early emotional development. In: Osofsky JD (ed): *Handbook of Infant Development* (2nd ed). New York, Wiley, 1987, pp. 494–554.

Izard CE, Schwartz GM: Patterns of emotion in depression. In: Rutter M, Izard CE, Read PB (eds): *Depression in Young People: Clinical and Developmental Perspectives*. New York, Guilford, 1986, pp. 33–70.

Izard CE, Hembree EA, Huebner RR: Infants' emotion expression to acute pain: Developmental changes and stability in individual differences. *Dev Psychol* 23:105–113, 1987.

Izard CE, Huebner RR, Risser D, et al: The young infant's ability to produce discrete emotion expressions. *Dev Psychol* 16:132–140, 1980.

Jacobson E: *Depression: Comparative Studies of Normal, Neurotic, and Psychotic Conditions*. New York, International Universities Press, 1971.

Johnson W, Emde RN, Pannabecker B, et al: Maternal perception of infant emotion from birth through 18 months. *Infant Behav Dev* 5:313–322, 1982.

Kagan J: *The Growth of the Child*. New York, Norton, 1978.

Kagan J: Stress and coping in early development. In: Garmezy N, Rutter M (eds): *Stress, Coping, and Development in Children*. New York, McGraw-Hill, 1983, pp. 191–216.

Kagan J: The idea of emotion in human development. In: Izard CE, Kagan J, Zajonc R (eds): *Emotions, Cognition, and Behavior*. London, Cambridge University Press, 1984, pp. 38–72.

Kaitz M, Meschulach-Sarfaty O, Auerbach J, et al: A reexamination of newborns' ability to imitate facial expressions. *Dev Psychol* 24:3–7, 1988.

Kanner A, Coyne J, Schaefer C, et al: Comparison of two modes of stress measurement: Daily hassles and uplifts versus major life events. *J Behav Med* 4:1–39, 1980.

Kashani JN, Ray JS: Depressive related symptoms among preschool-age children. *Child Psychiatry Hum Dev* 13:233–238, 1983.

Kazdin AE, Sherick BA, Esveldt-Dawson K, et al: Nonverbal behavior and childhood depressions. *J Am Acad Child Psychiatry* 24:303–309, 1985.

Kimball CP: Psychological responses to the experience of open-heart surgery. *Am J Psychiatry* 126:96–107, 1969.

Kliman GW: *Psychological Emergencies of Childhood*. New York, Grune & Stratton, 1968.

Klinger E: Consequences of commitment to and disengagement from incentives. *Psychol Rev* 82:1–25, 1975.

Klinnert MD, Campos JJ, Sorce JF, et al: Emotions as behavior regulators: Social referencing in infancy. In: Plutchik R, Kellerman H (eds): *Emotion: Theory, Research, and Experience* (Vol 2), New York, Academic, 1983, pp. 57–86.

Kopp CB: Regulation of distress and negative emotions: A developmental view. *Dev Psychol* 25:343–354, 1989.

Koriat A, Melkman R, Averill JR, et al: The self-control of emotional reactions to a stressful film. *J Pers* 40:601–619, 1972.

Lazarus AA: Learning theory and the treatment of depression. *Behav Res Ther* 6:83–89, 1968.

Lazarus RS: Emotions and adaptation: Conceptual and empirical relations. In: Arnold WJ (ed): *Nebraska Symposium on Motivation*. Lincoln, NE, University of Nebraska Press, 1968, pp. 175–266.

Lazarus RS: Thoughts on the relations between emotion and cognition. *Am Psychol* 37:1019–1024, 1982.

Lazarus RS, Kanner AD, Folkman S: Emotions: A cognitive-phenomenological analysis. In: Plutchik R, Kellerman H (eds): *Theories of Emotion*. New York, Academic Press, 1980, pp. 189–217.

Lerner MJ, Simmons C: Observer's reaction to the innocent victim: Compassion or rejection? *J Pers Soc Psychol* 4:203–210, 1966.

Lewinsohn PM: A behavioral approach to depression. In: Friedman RJ, Katz MM (eds): *The Psychology of Depression: Contemporary Theory and Research*. Washington, DC, Winston, 1974, pp. 157–185.

Lewinsohn PM, Graf M: Pleasant activities and depression. *J Consult Clin Psychol* 41:261–268, 1973.

Lewinsohn PM, Biglan A, Zeiss AM: Behavioral treatment of depression. In: Davidson PO (ed): *The Behavioral Management of Anxiety, Depression, and Pain*. New York, Brunner/Mazel, 1976, pp. 91–146.

Lewis M, Brooks J: Self-knowledge and emotional development. In: Lewis M, Rosenblum LA (eds): *The Development of Affect*. New York, Plenum, 1978, p. 205–226.

Lewis M, Michalson L: The socialization of emotions. In: Field TM, Fogel A (eds): *Emotion and Early Interaction: Normal and High Risk Infants*. Hillsdale, NJ, Erlbaum, 1982, pp. 189–212.

Lewis M, Michalson L: *Children's Emotions and Moods*. New York, Plenum, 1983.

Lewis M, Saarni C: *The Socialization of Emotions*. New York, Plenum, 1985.

Lutz C: Cultural patterns and individual differences in the child's emotional meaning system. In: Lewis M, Saarni C (eds): *The Socialization of Emotions*. New York, Plenum, 1985, pp. 37–54.

Maccoby EE, Feldman SS: Mother-attachment and stranger-reactions in the third year of life. *Monogr Soc Res Child Dev* 37 (1, serial no. 146), 1972.

MacLean PD: Psychosomatic disease and the visceral brain. *Psychosom Med* 3:338–353, 1949.

MacLean PD: The limbic system and its hippocampal formation: Studies in animals and their possible application to man. *J Neurosurg* 2:29–445, 1954.

MacLean PD: The limbic brain in relation to the psychoses. In: Black PD (ed): *Physiological Correlates of Emotion*. New York, Academic Press, 1970, pp. 129–146.

MacPhillamy DJ, Lewinsohn PM: Depression as a function of levels of desired and obtained pleasure. *J Abnorm Psychol* 83:651–657, 1974.

Maguire GP: Psychiatric problems after mastectomy. In: Brand PC, vanKeep OA (eds): *Breast Cancer: Psycho-Social Aspects of Early Detection and Treatment*. Baltimore, University Park Press, 1978.

Malatesta CZ, Haviland JM: Signals, symbols, and socialization: The modification of emotional expression in human development. In: Lewis M, Saarni C (eds): *The Socialization of Emotions*. New York, Plenum, 1985, pp. 89–116.

Malatesta CZ, Izard CE: The ontogenesis of human social signals: From biological imperative to symbol utilization. In: Fox N, Davidson RJ (eds): *The Psychobiology of Affective Development*. Hillsdale, NJ, Erlbaum, 1984, pp. 161–206.

Malatesta CZ, Culver C, Tesman JR, et al: The development of emotion expression during the first two years of life. *Monogr Soc Res Child Dev* 54(219), 1989.

Mandler G: *Mind and Emotions*. New York, Wiley, 1975.

Martin G, Clarke R: Distress crying in neonates: Species and peer specificity. *Dev Psychol* 18:3–10, 1982.

Masters JC, Barden RC, Ford ME: Affective states, expressive behavior and learning in children. *J Pers Soc Psychol* 37:380–390, 1979.

McCombie SL: Characteristics of rape victims seen in crisis interviewing. *Smith Coll Stud Soc Work* 46:137–158, 1975.

McDaniel JW, Sexton AW: Psychoendocrine studies of patients with spinal cord lesions. *J Abnorm Psychol* 76:117–122, 1970.

McLoyd VC: Socialization and development in a changing economy. *Am Psychol* 44:293–308, 1989.

Metalsky GI, Nalberstadt LJ, Abramson LY: Vulnerability and invulnerability to depressive mood reactions. *J Pers Soc Psychol* 52:386–393, 1987.

Michalson L, Lewis M: What do children know about emotions and when do they know it? In: Lewis M, Saarni C (eds): *The Socialization of Emotion*. New York, Plenum, 1985, pp. 117–139.

Mineka S, Suomi SJ: Social separation in monkeys. *Psychol Bull* 85:1376–1400, 1978.

Mischel W, Ebbersen EB, Zeiss AR: Cognitive and attentional mechanisms in delay of gratification. *J Pers Soc Psychol* 21:204–218, 1972.

Monroe SM: Major and minor life events as predictors of psychological distress: Further issues and findings. *J Behav Med* 6:189–205, 1983.

Monroe SM, Imhoff DR, Wise BD, et al: Life events, symptom course, and treatment outcome in unipolar depressed women. *J Consult Clin Psychol* 51:604–615, 1983.

Orr DA, Reznikoff M, Smith GM: Body image, self-esteem, and depression in burn-injured adolescents and young adults. *J Burn Care Rehabil* 10:454–461, 1989.

Oster H: Facial expression and affect development. In: Lewis M, Rosenblum LA (eds): *The Development of Affect*. New York, Plenum, 1978, pp. 43–76.

Oster H: Signal value of smiling and brow knitting in infants. Paper presented at the International Conference on Infant Studies, New York, 1984.

Papez JW: A proposed mechanism of emotion. *Arch Neurol Psychiatry* 38:725–743, 1937.

Parkes CM: The emotional impact of cancer on patients and their families. *J Laryngol Otol* 89:1271–1279, 1975.

Paykel ES: Causal relationships between clinical depression and life events. In: Barrett JE (ed): *Stress and Mental Disorder*. New York, Raven Press, 1979, pp. 71–86.

Pearlin LR, Schooler C: The structure of coping. *J Health Soc Behav* 19:2–21, 1978.

Peck A: Emotional reactions to having cancer. *AJR* 114:591–599, 1972.

Plumb MM, Holland J: Comparative studies of psychological function in patients with advanced cancer. I: Self-reported depressive symptoms. *Psychosom Med* 4:264–275, 1977.

Plutchik R: *Emotion: A Psychoevolutionary Emphasis*. New York, Harper & Row, 1980.

Potts R, Camp C, Coyne C: The relationship between naturally occurring dysphoric moods, elaborative coding, and recall performance. *Cognition Emotion* 3:197–205, 1989.

Poznanski EO, Mokros HB, Grossman J, et al: Diagnostic criteria in childhood depressions. *Am J Psychiatry* 142:1168–1173, 1985.

Pribram KH: The new neurology and the biology of emotion. A structural approach. *Am Psychol* 22:830–838, 1967.

Pribram KH: Feelings as monitors. In: Arnold MB (ed): *Feelings and Emotions*. New York, Academic Press, 1970, pp. 41–53.

Pribram KH: Emotion: A neurobehavioral analysis. In: Scherer KR, Ekman P (eds): *Approaches to Emotion*. Hillsdale, NJ, Erlbaum, 1984, pp. 13–38.

Puig-Antich J: Affective disorders. In: Kaplan HI, Sadock BJ (eds): *Comprehensive Textbook of Psychiatry* (Vol 2, 4th ed). Baltimore, Williams & Wilkins, 1985, pp. 1850–1861.

Puig-Antich J, Novacenko H, Davies M, et al: Growth hormone secretion in prepubertal children with major depression. *Arch Gen Psychiatry* 41:455–460, 1984.

Reichenbach L, Masters JC: Children's use of expressive and contextual cues in judgments of emotion. *Child Dev* 54:993–1004, 1983.

Robertson J, Robertson J: Young children in brief separation: A fresh look. *Psychoanal Study Child* 26:264–315, 1971.

Roseman I: Cognitive aspects of emotion and emotional behavior. Paper presented at the annual meeting of the American Psychological Association, New York, September 1979.

Rutter M: *Children of Sick Parents: An Environmental and Psychiatric Study*. London, Oxford University Press, 1966.

Rutter M: Stress, coping and development: Some issues and some questions. *J Child Psychol Psychiatry* 22:323–356, 1981.

Rutter M: Continuities and discontinuities in socio-emotional development: Empirical and conceptual perspective. In: Emde R, Harmon R (eds): *Continuities and Discontinuities in Development*. New York, Plenum, 1983, pp. 41–68.

Rutter M: The developmental psychopathology of depression: Issues and perspectives. In: Rutter M, Izard CE, Read PB (eds): *Depression in Young People: Clinical and Developmental Perspectives*. New York, Guilford, 1986, pp. 3–30.

Rutter M: Commentary: Some focus and process considerations regarding effects of parental depression on children. *Dev Psychol* 26:60–67, 1990.

Rutter M: Age changes in depressive disorders: Some developmental considerations. In: Garber J, Dodge KA (eds): *The Development of Emotion Regulation and Dysregulation*. New York, Cambridge University Press, 1991, pp. 273–300.

Rutter M, Quinton D: Parental psychiatric disorder: Effects on children. *Psychol Med* 14:853–880, 1984.

Rutter M, Graham P, Chadwick O, et al: Adolescent turmoil: Fact or fiction? *J Child Psychol Psychiatry* 17:35–56, 1976.

Rutter M, Tizard J, Whitmore K: *Education, Health, and Behavior*. London, Longmans, 1970. Reprint: Huntington, NY, Krieger, 1981.

Ryan ND, Puig-Antich J, Ambrosini P, et al: The clinical picture of major depression in children and adolescents. *Arch Gen Psychiatry* 44:854–861, 1987.

Saarni C: Cognitive and communicative features of emotional experience: Do you show what you think you feel? In: Lewis M, Rosenblum LA (eds): *The Development of Affect*. New York, Plenum, 1978, pp. 361–376.

Saarni C: Children's understanding of display rules for expressive behavior. *Dev Psychol* 15:424–429, 1979.

Saarni C: An observational study of children's attempts to monitor their expressive behavior. *Child Dev* 55:1504–1513, 1984.

Saarni C: Indirect processes in affect socialization. In: Lewis M, Saarni C (eds): *The Socialization of Emotions*. New York, Plenum, 1985, pp. 187–209.

Sagi A, Hoffman M: Empathic distress in the newborn. *Dev Psychol* 12:175–176, 1976.

Savitsky JC, Sim M: Trading emotions: Equity theory of reward and punishment. *J Community* 24:140–146, 1974.

Sawyer MG, Minde K, Zuker R: The burned child—Scarred for life?: A study of the psychosocial impact of a burn injury at different developmental stages. *Burns* 9:205–213, 1983.

Schachter S: The interaction of cognitive and physiological determinants of emotional state. In: Berkowitz L (ed): *Advances in Experimental Social Psychology* (Vol 1). New York, Academic Press, 1964.

Schachter S, Singer J: Cognitive, social, and physiological determinants of emotional state. *Psychol Rev* 69:379–399, 1962.

Schildkraut JJ: The catecholamine hypothesis of affective disorders: A review of supporting evidence. *Am J Psychiatry* 122:509–522, 1965.

Seligman MEP: *Helplessness: On Depression, Development, and Death*. San Francisco, Freeman, 1975.

Shantz CU: Social cognition. In: Flavell JH, Markman EM (eds): *Handbook of Child Psychology. Vol 3: Cognitive Development* (4th ed). New York, Wiley, 1983.

Shepherd M, Oppenheim B, Mitchell S: *Childhood Behavior and Mental Health*. London, University of London Press, 1971.

Shontz FC: *The Psychological Aspects of Physical illness and Disability*. New York, Macmillan, 1975.

Siller J: Psychological situation of the disabled with spinal cord injuries. *Rehabil Lit* 30:290–296, 1969.

Silver RL, Wortman CB: Coping with undesirable life events. In: Garber J, Seligman MEP (eds): *Human Helplessness: Theory and Applications*. New York, Academic, 1980, pp. 279–340.

Simner M: Newborn's response to the cry of another infant. *Dev Psychol* 5:136–150, 1971.

Skinner BF: *Science and Human Behavior*. Glencoe, IL, Free Press, 1953.

Skinner BF: *Beyond Freedom and Dignity*. New York, Knopf, 1971.

Sorce JF, Emde RN, Campos J, et al: Maternal emotional signaling: Its effect on the visual cliff behavior of 1-year-olds. *Dev Psychol* 21:195–200, 1985.

Spitz R: Anaclitic depression. *Psychoanal Study Child* 2:313–342, 1946.

Sroufe LA: Socioemotional development. In: Osofsky J (ed): *Handbook of Infant Development*. New York, Wiley, 1979, pp. 462–515.

Stearns CZ: Sadness. In: Lewis M, Haviland JM (eds): *Handbook of Emotions*. New York, Guilford, 1993, pp. 547–561.

Stein NL, Jewett JL: A conceptual analysis of the meaning of negative: Implications for a theory of development. In: Izard CE, Read P (eds): *Measuring Emotion*. Cambridge, UK, Cambridge University Press, 1985.

Stenberg C, Campos J, Emde R: The facial expression of anger in seven-month-old infants. *Child Dev* 54:178–184, 1983.

Stoddard FJ, Norman DK, Murphy JM, et al: Psychiatric outcome of burned children and adolescents. *J Am Acad Child Adolesc Psychiatry* 28:589–595, 1989.

Suomi SJ, Eisele CJ, Grady SA, et al: Depression in adult monkeys following separation from nuclear family environment. *J Abnorm Psychol* 84:576–578, 1975.

Sutherland S, Scherl D: Patterns of response among victims of rape. *Am J Orthopsychiatry* 40:503–511, 1970.

Swallow SR, Kuiper NA: The effects of depression and cognitive vulnerability to depression on judgments of similarity between self and other. *Motiv Emotion* 11:157–167, 1987.

Taylor DA, Harris PL: Knowledge of the link between emotion and memory among normal and maladjusted boys. *Dev Psychol* 19:832–838, 1983.

Tennant C, Hurry J, Bebbington P: The relation of childhood separation experiences to adult depressive and anxiety states. *Br J Psychiatry* 141:475–582, 1982.

Termine NT, Izard CE: Infants' responses to their mothers' expression of joy and sadness. *Dev Psychol* 24:223–229, 1988.

Terwogt M, Schene J, Harris PL: Self-control of emotional reactions by young children. *J Child Psychol Psychiatry* 27:357–366, 1986.

Tomkins SS: *Affect, Imagery and Consciousness* (Vol 1). New York, Springer, 1962.

Tomkins SS: *Affect, Imagery and Consciousness* (Vol 2). New York, Springer, 1963.

Tronick EZ, Gianino AF: The transmission of maternal disturbance to the infant. In: Tronick EZ, Field T (eds): *Maternal Depression and Infant Disturbance*. (New Directions for Child Development, vol 34). San Francisco, Jossey-Bass, 1986, pp. 5–11.

van Eerdewegh MM, Bieti MD, Parilla RH, et al: The bereaved child. *J Psychiatry* 140:23–29, 1982.

Walden TA, Ogan TA: The development of social referencing. *Child Dev* 59:1230–1240, 1988.

Wallerstein JS: Children of divorce: Stress and developmental tasks. In: Garmezy N, Rutter M (eds): *Stress, Coping and Development in Children*. New York, McGraw-Hill, 1983, pp. 265–302.

Wallerstein JS, Kelly JB: *Surviving the Breakup: How Children and Parents Cope with Divorce*. New York, Basic Books, 1980.

Ward HW, Moss RL, Darko DF, et al: Prevalence of postburn depression following burn injury. *J Burn Care Rehabil* 8:294–298, 1987.

Watson JB: *Psychology from the Standpoint of a Behaviorist*. Philadelphia, Lippincott, 1919.

Watson JB: *Behaviorism*. Chicago, University of Chicago Press, 1930.

Weiner B: An attributional theory of achievement motivation and emotion. *Psychol Rev* 92:548–573, 1985.

Weiss B, Garber J: *Developmental differences in symptoms of depression: A meta-analysis*. Manuscript under review, 1995.

Weissman MM, Paykel ES: *The Depressed Woman: A Study of Social Relationships*. Chicago, University of Chicago Press, 1974.

Weissman MM, Prusoff BA, Gammon GC, et al: Psychopathology in the children (ages 6–18) of depressed and normal parents. *J Am Acad Child Adolesc Psychiatry* 23:78–84, 1984.

Weller RA, Weller EB, Fristad MA, et al: A comparison of the cortisol suppression index and the dexamethasone suppression test in pre-pubertal children. *Am J Psychiatry* 142:1370–1372, 1985.

White E, Elsom B, Prawat R: Children's conception of death. *Child Dev* 49:307–310, 1978.

Wolpe J: *The Practice of Behavior Therapy*. New York, Pergamon, 1969.

Wolpe J: Neurotic depression: Experimental analog, clinical syndromes, and treatment. *Am J Psychother* 25:362–368, 1971.

Wortman CB, Brehm JW: Responses to uncontrollable outcomes: An integration of reactance theory and the learned helplessness model. In: Berkowitz L (ed): *Advances in Experimental Social Psychology* (Vol 8). New York, Academic Press, 1975, pp. 277–336.

Yarczower M, Kilbride JE, Hill LA: Imitation and inhibition of facial expression. *Dev Psychol* 15: 453–454, 1979.

Young-Browne G, Rosenfeld NM, Horowitz F: Infant discrimination of facial expressions. *Child Dev* 48:555–562, 1977.

Zahn-Waxler C, Radke-Yarrow M, King RA: Child rearing and children's prosocial dispositions towards victims of distress. *Child Dev* 50:319–330, 1979.

Zajonc RB: Feeling and thinking: Preferences need no inferences. *Am Psychol* 35:151–175, 1980.

Zajonc RB: On the primacy of affect. *Am Psychol* 39:151–175, 1984.

25 Development of Psychotic Thinking in Children

Rochelle Caplan, M.D., and Peter E. Tanguay, M.D.

HISTORICAL OVERVIEW

Impaired thinking or thought disorder has been regarded as the hallmark of schizophrenia since the first descriptions of this illness by Bleuler (1951). Bleuler regarded loosening of associations as a fundamental sign that represents the pathology of schizophrenia. In contrast, he regarded hallucinations and delusions as accessory signs that were secondary to the pathology of schizophrenia.

From the clinical perspective, earlier theories on thought disorder were all-encompassing and tried to explain thought disorder as a unitary concept (Holzman et al., 1986). In contrast, the extensive research that has been conducted during the last 15 years has highlighted that thought disorder is not a unitary concept and does not occur specifically in schizophrenia (Andreasen and Grove, 1986; Butler and Braff, 1990; Harrow and Marengo, 1986; Holzman et al., 1986).

During this period, the introduction of the DSM-III (American Psychiatric Association, 1978) and DSM-III-R (American Psychiatric Association, 1987) provided further clarification of terms by clearly differentiating between disturbances in the form and content of thought. Thus, formal thought disorder describes the clinical manifestations of the manner in which patients present their thoughts to the listener (F.J. Fish, 1962) and the organization, control, and processing of thoughts (Holzman, 1986). Delusions, a thought content disturbance, describe firmly held personal beliefs that are based on incorrect inference about external reality in spite of obvious proof or evidence to the contrary (Butler and Braff, 1991).

Unlike earlier studies, the clinical studies that have been conducted since the late 1970s have used reliable and valid instruments for the assessment of well-defined aspects of thought disorder (Andreasen et al., 1986; Harrow and Marengo, 1986; Holzman et al., 1986). These studies have characterized the positive and negative dimensions of formal thought disorder in schizophrenic adults, as well as their relationship with clinical symptoms (Andreasen et al., 1990; Pogue-Geile et al., 1984), cognitive/attentional deficits (Braff et al., 1991; Cornblatt et al., 1985; Gruzelier et al., 1988; Nuechterlein et al., 1986), treatment responses (Angrist et al., 1980; Spohn et al., 1986), and biological measures (Andreasen et al., 1990; Liddle et al., 1990; Marks et al., 1990; Paulman et al., 1990; Weinberger et al., 1988).

In contrast, very few studies were conducted on thought disorder in childhood prior to the DSM-III. The DSM-III made two important contributions to this field of research. First, it put an end to the historical debate on the relationship between infantile autism and schizophrenia (Bender, 1947; Eisenberg et al., 1956; Fish and Ritvo, 1978; Kanner, 1957; Kolvin, 1971a; Makita, 1966; Rutter et al., 1967a and 1967b;

Rutter, 1972). Second, the DSM-III provided well-defined inclusionary and exclusionary criteria of schizophrenia. Use of these criteria stopped the practice of labeling a variety of clinical manifestations, such as impaired social relationships, language deviance, disturbed reality testing, delusions, as well as abnormal stream and form of thought as thought disorder. In addition, investigators have become cognizant of the impact of developmental factors on the methods for eliciting and coding thought disorder in childhood (Arboleda and Holzman, 1985; Caplan et al., 1989, 1990). As a result, research on DSM-III and DSM-III-R diagnosed schizophrenic children began to follow a similar trajectory to that of schizophrenic adults, albeit at a slower pace.

This chapter includes three sections that describe three aspects of psychotic thinking in children: formal thought disorder, hallucinations, and delusions. Each of the chapter's three sections reviews studies on the clinical assessment, underlying mechanisms, and differential diagnosis of formal thought disorder, delusions, and hallucinations, respectively, in childhood onset schizophrenia.

FORMAL THOUGHT DISORDER

Definition

Formal thought disorder represents clinical measures of the form or manner in which the patient presents his or her thoughts to the listener. Numerous clinical signs have been used to describe these communicative characteristics, such as illogical thinking, incoherence, loose associations, digressive speech, circumstantiality, tangentiality, vague speech, overelaborate speech, clanging, neologisms, poverty of speech, poverty of content of speech, echolalia speech, and others (Andreasen, 1979a).

The DSM-IV (American Medical Association, 1994) uses the term disorganized speech (e.g., frequent derailment or incoherence) rather than formal thought disorder. The DSM-III-R (American Medical Association, 1987) required the presence of loose associations or incoherence to diagnose formal thought disorder. The DSM-III (American Medical Association, 1980) included four formal thought disorder signs: illogical thinking, loose associations, incoherence, and poverty of content of speech.

Clinical Assessment Studies of Formal Thought Disorder in Childhood

A review of the literature demonstrates a dearth of studies on formal thought disorder in childhood. Seven studies have been conducted on formal thought disorder in schizophrenic and schizotypal children (Arboleda et al., 1985; Cantor et al., 1982; Caplan et al., 1989, 1990a; Green et al., 1984; Kolvin et al., 1971; Russell et al., 1989; Tompson et al., 1990) and one study on children at risk for schizophrenia (Arboleda and Holzman, 1985). Only three of these childhood studies, however, have used reliable and valid instruments for the clinical assessment of formal thought disorder (Arboleda and Holzman, 1985; Caplan et al., 1989, 1990a; Tompson et al., 1990).

Kolvin et al. (1971) reported that 60% of children with late-onset psychosis had disorder of association, 45% had derailment of thought, and 51% had talking past the point as described by F.J. Fish (1962). The criteria for assessing formal thought disorder, however, were not operationalized for use with children. Cantor identified formal thought disorder signs, such as loose associations, neologisms, illogicality, clanging, poverty of speech, and poverty of content of speech, in both the early-onset and adolescent-onset groups of children with schizophrenia (Cantor et al., 1982). Like Kolvin, Cantor did not use a reliable and valid instrument for assessing formal thought disorder in these children. In addition, she did not clarify how she operationalized these formal thought disorder signs for the younger group.

Green et al. (1984) reported that all the schizophrenic children in their sample fulfilled the DSM-III schizophrenic inclusionary criterion for formal thought disorder signs. Since the clinical characteristics of the schizophrenic children in this study were retrospectively obtained from medical charts, it is not clear how the DSM-III formal thought disorder signs were operationalized in this 6.7- to 11.11-year-old sample.

Russell et al. (1989) made reliable global clinical ratings of the DSM-III criteria of formal thought disorder from the Interview for Childhood Disorders and Schizophrenia. These investigators reported that 40% of their schizophrenic sample exhibited incoherence or marked loosening of associations, illogical thinking, or poverty of content of speech accompanied by affect disturbance, delusions, hallucinations, or disorganized behavior (Russell et al., 1989).

From the developmental perspective, normal children learn to present the listener with their thoughts in a logical and coherent fashion from the toddler period through adolescence (Shatz, 1982). Formal thought disorder, a clinical measure of the way the child presents his or her thoughts to the listener, involves the maturation of cognitive, linguistic, and pragmatic skills (Caplan, 1994). Two studies have addressed the relationship between age and formal thought disorder in childhood.

Using the Thought Disorder Index (TDI), Arboleda and Holzman (1985) conducted the first study that demonstrated the importance of controlling for the level of cognitive development when assessing thought disorder in normal children under 10 years of age. This was also the first study to use a formal psychological test with suitable control groups to assess thought disorder in psychotic and high-risk children.

The TDI has demonstrated reliability and validity in schizophrenic, manic, and depressed adults and in their first-degree relatives (Holzman et al., 1986). It codes 22 categories of verbal responses to the standardized percepts on the Rorschach cards as associative, combinatory, disorganized, and unconventional verbalizations (Holzman et al., 1986). The TDI, therefore, examines a broader range of thought disturbance categories than the DSM-IV (i.e., derailment and incoherence), DSM-III-R (i.e., loosening of associations and incoherence), and DSM-III formal thought disorder signs (i.e., loose associations, illogical thinking, incoherence, and poverty of content of speech). Arboleda and Holzman (1985) found that children with psychosis, psychotic spectrum disorders, and children at risk for schizophrenia and affective disorder had more severe TDI levels than normal children and children with nonpsychotic psychiatric diagnoses. Using the TDI and the Family Consensus Rorschach Task (Loveland et al., 1963), Tompson and Asarnow (1990) demonstrated that schizophrenic and schizotypal children had significantly more thought disorder and disturbed attention than depressed children.

In an earlier study, Asarnow et al. (1988) also described a relationship between low Weschler Intelligence Scale for Children-Revised (WISC-R) distractibility factor scores and communication deviance in the par-

ents of children with schizophrenia and schizotypal personality disorder, but not with depression and dysthymia. From the developmental perspective, the findings of Asarnow and her colleagues (1988, 1990) suggest that the thought disorder of schizophrenic children might also reflect an attentional impairment in both the parents and child with difficulty establishing a shared focus of attention.

Caplan et al. (1989) developed a play procedure, the Story Game, and a coding system, the Kiddie Formal Thought Disorder Rating Scale (K-FTDS), for the assessment of formal thought disorder in middle childhood. Compared with a structured psychiatric interview, the Story Game elicited adequate speech samples that could be reliably rated for formal thought disorder in children (Caplan et al., 1989). The K-FTDS operationalized the four DSM-III signs of formal thought disorder—illogical thinking, loose associations, incoherence, and poverty of content of speech—so that they could be coded even if children spoke in small paragraphs of one to two utterances.

Studies conducted on 31 schizophrenic, 14 schizotypal, and 71 normal children demonstrated that illogical thinking and loose associations were reliable, valid, sensitive, and specific measures (Caplan et al., 1989, 1990a; Caplan, 1994). Loose associations occurred almost specifically in the schizophrenic and schizotypal (Caplan et al., 1989, 1990a; Caplan, 1994). There were no significant differences in the illogical thinking and loose associations scores of the schizophrenic and schizotypal children (Caplan et al., 1990a; Caplan, 1994).

From the developmental perspective, the normal children under age 7 years had illogical thinking and loose associations (Caplan et al., 1990a; Caplan, 1994). The young schizophrenic, schizotypal, and normal children have significantly higher illogical thinking and loose associations scores than the older children with these respective diagnoses (Caplan et al., 1990a; Caplan, 1994).

Studies on the relationship of these two formal thought disorder signs with attention/information processing (Caplan et al., 1990b, 1990c) and discourse measures (Caplan et al., 1992a; Caplan, 1994) in schizophrenic children indicate that illogical thinking might be a negative and loose associations a positive sign of formal thought disorder in childhood-onset schizophrenia.

Etiology and Pathogenesis

Examination of the relationship of well-defined clinical measures of thought disorder with attention/information processing, linguistic/pragmatic, and biological measures has been an important step in defining and delineating the components of thought disorder in schizophrenic adults (Caplan et al., 1994). The pathogenesis of formal thought disorder in adult schizophrenia is, nevertheless, still unclear.

In terms of attention/information processing, negative signs of formal thought disorder are associated with poor performance on cognitive tasks that demand effortful recruitment of information processing (Nuechterlein et al., 1986). Positive signs of formal thought disorder, however, are related to distractibility (Cornblatt et al., 1985; Harvey et al., 1986; Oltmanns et al., 1979).

From the linguistic/pragmatic perspective, schizophrenic adults with formal thought disorder underutilize some discourse devices that link clauses (sentences) and overutilize others (Harvey et al., 1986; Rochester and Martin, 1979). Both positive and negative signs of formal thought disorder are related to reference failure (i.e., underutilization or inappropriate use of pronouns, demonstrative, and the article to refer to people, objects, or events during conversation and distraction) (Harvey et al., 1986).

From the biological perspective, there is evidence that the temporal lobe and prefrontal-limbic network are involved in the impaired thought processing of schizophrenic adults (Liddle et al., 1992; Shenton et al., 1992). Andreasen and Grove (1986) proposed that negative formal thought disorder signs of schizophrenic adults, such as poverty of content of speech, are akin to the alogia (i.e., difficulty generating organized speech) found in patients with frontal lobe disease.

Similar to the recent research on thought disorder in adult schizophrenia, research on the etiology and pathogenesis of formal thought disorder in childhood schizophrenia has included studies on attention/information processing (R. Asarnow and Sherman, 1984; R. Asarnow et al., 1986; Schneider et al., 1987; Strandburg et al., 1992; Watkins and R. Asarnow, 1992), linguistic/pragmatic deficits (Caplan et al., 1992a), and possible biological correlates of thought disorder (Caplan et al., 1992b, 1993, 1994) in DSM-III (American Psychiatric Association, 1978) and DSM-III-R (American Psychiatric Association, 1987) diagnosed schizophrenic children.

From the *cognitive* perspective, Caplan et al. (1990) found that illogical thinking and loose associations are related to different aspects of impaired attention/information processing in children with schizophrenic spectrum disorder. Illogical thinking appears to be related to a deficit in momentary processing capacity, measured by the partial report span of apprehension task and to the schizophrenic child's difficulty screening out extraneous stimuli and focussing on the task at hand (Caplan et al., 1990c). The requirement to present the listener with logical reasoning might tax these cognitive skills in the schizophrenic child (Caplan, 1994).

In the case of loose associations, the child unpredictably changes the topic of conversation without preparing the listener for the topic change. Loose associations is associated with distractibility (Caplan et al., 1990b) and difficulty using linguistic devices for topic maintenance (Caplan, 1994). Thus, the cognitive demands of this situation appear to be different from those eliciting illogical thinking (Caplan, 1994).

From the *linguistic/pragmatic* perspective, as demonstrated in schizophrenic adults (Harvey, 1983; Rochester and Martin, 1979), schizophrenic children underutilize discourse devices that link clauses (sentences) and establish coreference. The listener, therefore, has difficulty following who and what the child is talking about (Caplan et al., 1992a). Schizophrenic children also repeatedly disrupt the ongoing conversation to refer to the immediate surroundings (exophoria). This difficulty in focusing on the ongoing conversation is associated with severity of illogical thinking (Caplan, 1994). In contrast, the schizophrenic child with high loose associations scores underutilizes conjunctions that provide the listener with the link between ideas presented in contiguous clauses (Caplan, 1994).

Finally, from the *biological* perspective, as demonstrated in adults with complex partial seizure disorder (Csernansky et al., 1990; Perez et al., 1985; Slater and Beard, 1963; Taylor and Marsh, 1979), a schizophrenia-like psychosis is found in children with this form of epilepsy (Caplan et al., 1991, 1992b; Lindsay et al., 1979). In search of a possible biological model of formal thought disorder in childhood-onset schizophrenia (Caplan et al., 1992b, 1993, 1994), this association has led to several studies of thought disorder (i.e., formal thought disorder and discourse deficits) in children with complex partial seizure disorder.

Although preliminary, the following findings suggest that illogical thinking in middle childhood might reflect frontal lobe dysfunction (Caplan et al., 1993). First, children with complex partial seizure disorder and EEG evidence for frontotemporal involvement had significantly higher illogical thinking than those without frontal involvement (Caplan et al., 1992b). Second, follow-up of 7 children who attained seizure control after temporal lobectomy for intractable complex partial seizures revealed postoperative normalization of their high illogical thinking scores (Caplan et al., 1993). Seizure control following temporal lobectomy might, therefore, stop frontal lobe dysfunction and reduce the illogical thinking found in these children. This hypothesis is based on the propagation patterns of temporal lobe seizures with spread first to the ipsilateral and contralateral frontal lobes and then to the contralateral temporal lobe (Lieb et al., 1991). It is also based on Mizrahi et al.'s (1990) intraoperative electrocorticography evidence for functional frontal abnormalities in more than half the patients who underwent temporal lobectomy for intractable complex partial seizures.

In summary, illogical thinking and loose associations represent different attentional and linguistic impairments in childhood-onset schizophrenia. Preliminary evidence suggests that illogical thinking might reflect frontal dysfunction in the child.

Differential Diagnosis

Formal thought disorder in children occurs in three main nosological categories: psychotic disorders, personality disorders, and developmental disorders. The *psychotic* disorders are subdivided into those with and without clinical, laboratory, and ancillary evidence for organic disease. The nonorganic psychoses include schizophrenia, affective disorders, dissociative disorder, and psychotic disorders not classified elsewhere.

I. PSYCHOTIC DISORDERS

Schizophrenia. Schizophrenic adolescents have both positive (loose associations) and negative formal (i.e., poverty of content of speech, illogical thinking) thought disorder signs. Although infrequent, incoherence is found in the severely ill adolescent patient. As previously mentioned, schizophrenic children have illogical thinking and loose associations.

Affective Disorder, Mania. It is important to note that formal thought disorder occurs in the manic patient with and without psychoses (Marengo and Harrow, 1985). The formal thought disorder manifestations of adolescent manic patients are similar to those of adults. Manic adolescents demonstrate positive formal thought disorder signs (i.e., loose associations, distractibility, tangentiality, and digressiveness), together with pressure of speech. Mania in middle childhood is rare and sometimes thought to be comorbid with attention deficit hyperactivity disorder (ADHD) (see Carlson 1990 for review).

Affective Disorder, Depression. Formal thought disorder is relatively infrequent in adult patients with depressive disorder (Andreasen, 1979b; Oltmanns et al., 1985) and has not been described in depressed children and adolescents.

Dissociative Disorder. With the exception of brief episodes of disorganized thinking, children with dissociative disorder have no formal thought disorder (Hornstein and Putnam, 1992).

Psychotic Disorders, Not Otherwise Specified. There have been no studies to date on thought disorder in these children.

Organic Psychoses. The severity of formal thought disorder is related to the severity of global cognitive impairment in the child with organic psychosis (Caplan et al., 1987, 1992b). Severe incoherence and fragmentation of utterances are usually indicative of "organic" formal thought disorder. Whereas the clinical manifestations of formal thought disorder wax and wane in the child with nonorganic psychosis, they tend to be pervasive in the child with organic psychosis (Caplan et al., 1987).

II. PERSONALITY DISORDERS

Schizotypal Personality Disorder. Inclusion of children with this disorder in the differential diagnosis of formal thought disorder might appear controversial. First, to make a diagnosis of a personality disorder in childhood and adolescence, one needs to demonstrate stable, maladaptive personality traits. J. Asarnow et al. (1988) have shown that children who meet criteria for schizotypal personality disorder have long-standing maladaptive traits. Second, according to the DSM-III-R, patients with a diagnosis of schizotypal personality disorder meet criteria for odd speech but not for such formal thought disorder signs as loose associations and incoherence. However, Caplan et al. (1990a) demonstrated that a sensitive and specific instrument, such as the K-FTDS, can detect formal thought disorder not otherwise identified by structured psychiatric interviews in schizotypal children. Although the schizotypal children had lower illogical thinking and loose associations scores than did the schizophrenic children, these differences were not significant (Caplan et al., 1990a).

III. DEVELOPMENTAL DISORDERS

These disorders are included in the differential diagnosis of formal thought disorder because these children might have formal thought disorder secondary to their cognitive and/or language delay.

Mental Retardation. Since normal children with a mental age below 7 have illogical thinking and loose associations (Caplan et al., 1989, 1990a, in press a), children with mental retardation might exhibit illogical or loose disorder by virtue of their low mental age. Evidence for generalized cognitive and developmental delay and the absence of signs of psychosis or schizotypal personality disorder would suggest a diagnosis of mental retardation.

Developmental Language Disorder. Children with specific expressive language disorders and with developmental aphasia have deficits in the social use of language (i.e., pragmatics). Clinically, therefore, their speech could meet criteria for formal thought disorder. The presence of a specific language disorder without signs of psychosis and schizotypal personality disorder would support a diagnosis of a specific expressive disorder.

Pervasive Developmental Disorder. Due to their impaired communication skills, children with pervasive developmental disorder not otherwise specified could also meet criteria for formal thought disorder (van der Gaag, 1993). The presence of a qualitative impairment in reciprocal social interaction and verbal and nonverbal communication, as well as a restricted repertoire of activities and interests will guide the clinician toward the pervasive developmental disorder diagnosis.

Conclusions

Illogical thinking and loose associations are reliable and valid measures of formal thought disorder in middle childhood schizophrenia and schizotypal personality disorder. Reliable clinical assessment of formal thought disorder involves the use of specific instruments for eliciting speech samples from children (e.g., Rorschach cards, the Story Game) and for measuring formal thought disorder (e.g., the TDI, the K-FTDS). Developmental norms are needed to differentiate between immature forms of speech and formal thought disorder in middle childhood. Age 7 is the cutoff point for normal developmental changes in these measures. Different attention/information processing and linguistic/pragmatic deficits underlie illogical thinking and loose associations in schizophrenic children. Underlying pathogenetic mechanisms might involve the frontal lobe.

HALLUCINATIONS

Definition

The hallucinatory experience has been defined variously as a "false sensory perception not associated with real external stimuli" (Kanner, 1957; Kaplan and Sadock, 1985) and as "an apparent perception of an external object when no such object is present" (Hinsie and Campbell, 1970). Hallucinations may involve any of the senses and are to be distinguished from vivid eidetic imagery, intensified images or sensory impressions, fantasy productions, and imaginary companions. Hallucinations that occur while falling asleep or waking (hypnagogic and hypnopompic hallucinations) are often categorized as distinct from hallucinations that occur in the fully awake state. Hallucinations may be more or less vivid. Less vivid hallucinations include hearing nonverbal noises, such as footsteps or knocking, seeing shadows or fleeting images, or experiencing unusual olfactory or haptic sensations. These may be difficult to distinguish from illusions, vivid imaginings, or dissociative states. More vivid hallucinations include hearing commands, voices commenting on one's actions or one's thoughts or feelings, persecutory voices, or, in the visual mode, three-dimensional persons and objects present for 10 seconds or longer in one's visual field.

Clinical Studies of Hallucinations in Children

OCCURRENCE

Earlier psychoanalytic theorists postulated that young children might experience infantile hallucinations that could serve to gratify instinctual wishes in the absence of actual gratification (Freud, 1975). Some authors (Wilking and Paoli, 1966) have even suggested that all young children hallucinate as part of their normal development, because of their difficulty in distinguishing between external and internal reality. More recent empirical work does not support this idea. Objective studies of young infants and their mothers (Tanguay, in press) demonstrate that, under conditions of optimal arousal, infants are alert, in full emotional contact with their caretakers, and carefully watchful of events around them. They show no evidence of preoccupation with internal stimuli or social disconnection that might suggest hallucination. There is also no hard evidence to suggest that infants hallucinate when they are in less optimal states of arousal.

Despert reported that by 3 years of age a child of normal intelligence should be able to distinguish between fantasy and reality (Despert, 1948). She found no evidence for true hallucinations in her normal nursery population of 106 children. Some children reported what might be more correctly understood as representations from dreams or misinterpretations of sensory stimuli, particularly in a hypnagogic state. Eisenberg (1962) concurred that young children can distinguish between reality and imagination.

Hallucinations, even organic ones, appear to be rare in children less than 6 or 7 years of age. Even though it might be expected that young children with high fevers and severe medical illnesses might suffer more often than older children from delirium with hallucinations, common experience on pediatric units indicates that this is not so.

Rothstein (1981) reviewed 21 studies published between 1931 and 1975 of children who experienced auditory or visual hallucinations. The definition of hallucinations and the quality of the behavioral observations varied across these studies. Rothstein (1981) concluded that hallucinations in children were not pathognomonic of psychosis. They were found in normal children suffering from anxiety states, in transient situational responses, in deprived children with personality disorders, and in schizophrenic children. The definition of "schizophrenia" in a number of the studies reviewed by Rothstein (1981) differed from that found in the DSM-III, DSM-III-R, and DSM-IV.

Four more recent studies of the prevalence of hallucinations in children treated in child and adolescent psychiatry services confirm that hallucinations are not pathognomonic for schizophrenia and that they are infrequent in the young child. Garralda (1984) reviewed the case records for 4767 children seen at the Children's Department of the Maudsley Hospital between 1954 and 1966. None of the 1.1% of the children noted to have hallucinations on admission were under 8 years of age.

Kemph (1987) examined the hospital records of 331 children admitted to a public psychiatric hospital and diagnosed psychotic. Of the 171 children with hallucinations, 3 were under 8 years of age and none of the children were under age 6. It is unclear if age 6 years was the cutoff age for admission to the hospital in this study.

Egdell and Kolvin (1972) reported hallucinations in only 2 of 40 inpatients between 5 and 15 years of age who were suffering from a variety of psychiatric disorders, excluding psychosomatic conditions. The ages of the 2 patients were not given. Kotsopoulos et al. (1987) also studied the nature of hallucinations in a population of child psychiatry outpatients. Eleven children (of an approximate sample of 100) were reported to hallucinate, all of them above age 7.

Kolvin et al. (1971), Green et al. (1984), and Russell et al. (1989) have all reported finding hallucinations in substantial portions of children having "late-onset psychosis" or DSM-III schizophrenia. Even in this highly selected sample, very few children younger than 8 years could be identified as having hallucinations.

TYPES OF HALLUCINATIONS

Hallucinations in children resemble hallucinations in adults. Kemph (1987) described children as reporting voices "ordering me to kill my sister," "telling me to run away," "calling my name," "telling me to do bad things," "telling me to steal," "telling me to destroy." He also described children who heard voices calling them "faggot," "punk," and "prostitute." One child heard a voice telling him to do good things. Sometimes the voice was identified as that of a relative; sometimes it was not identifiable. The context of the visual hallucinations comprised people, but most children reported seeing monsters.

Kotsopoulos et al. (1987) described a child who believed he had "a bunch of kids in the head" or who heard voices talking of murder or lurking monsters, "a friendly man talking from the closet," or "the voice of a man urging disobedience."

Burke et al. (1985) reported mumbling voices and voices telling the child to hurt himself or others, for example, "a voice telling him to stab his sister" and "the voice of a man and a woman, one telling him to hurt other children, one telling him not to." Visual hallucinations varied from menacing figures to shapes and scenes.

FOLLOW-UP

Few studies have provided diagnostic outcome data. Garralda (1984) followed up 20 subjects who had been identified in childhood as having hallucinations and compared them with a control group. After a mean follow-up period of 17 years, Garralda retested 16 of the 20 subjects whose mean age was then 30 years. Sixty-seven percent of the index subjects continued to have hallucinatory experiences. Garralda's findings indicate that continued hallucinations was not associated with an increased risk for later psychosis, depressive illness, organic brain damage, or other psychiatric disorder.

Like Garralda (1984), Del Beccaro et al. (1988) reported hallucinations in 50% of their adolescent sample (mean age 17 years) following a 4-year follow-up. Eighty percent of these subjects had required further psychiatric care during the 4 years.

Etiology and Pathogenesis

NEUROBIOLOGICAL MECHANISMS

An early neurobiological hypothesis for hallucinations was proposed by West (1962). His "perceptual release" theory, in part derived from studies of sensory deprivation, proposed that the brain continuously receives sensory input of many kinds from the external environment as well as from within the body. The brain selectively excludes much of this information from consciousness, and according to the theory, it can do so only if there is a constant flow of sensory impulses. If sensory input is disturbed or absent, the censorship mechanism is impaired, and earlier traces may emerge as hallucinations. Increased cortical arousal, induced by diminution of sensory input, is essential for the process to take place.

More recently, additional hypotheses have arisen based upon research in sleep and dreams, schizophrenia, and epilepsy. The phenomenological similarity between dreams during rapid eye movement (REM) sleep and hallucinations has been noted by many philosophers and scientists for many years (Evarts, 1962). Studies of persons with narcolepsy provide some support for this relationship. These patients precipitously fall into REM sleep during the day (Rechtschaffen and Dement, 1969), at which time they frequently have vivid hypnagogic and hypnopompic hallucinations, with vivid and sensory images of a frightening type. This can occur in both adults and children (Wittig et al., 1983). It has been shown that during REM sleep the forebrain is periodically and widely stimulated by activity emanating from the brainstem. Hobson and McCarely (1977) have postulated, on the basis of previous neurophysiological studies, the existence of a "dream state

generator" in the pontine reticular formation. Activity of this generator has been linked to ponto-geniculate-occipital (PGO) waves in the EEG during REM sleep. They propose that this center is responsible both for the bursts of rapid eye movements in REM sleep and the intrusion of new subject matter into ongoing dreams. Because PGO waves seem to coincide with hallucinatory behavior in awake animals, Fishman (1975) has proposed a similar relationship between dreams and hallucinations. Such a mechanism, if not suppressed during the waking state or if activated by toxic substances, might lead to hallucinations of various types.

Recent controlled postmortem studies of brain tissue in persons having a diagnosis of schizophrenia have found nonspecific anatomic pathology in the periventricular limbic and diencephalic areas and in the prefrontal cortex (Kirch and Weinberger, 1986). Numerous investigations of living patients by computed tomography have found evidence for brain pathology in the form of enlarged third ventricles (Shelton and Weinberger, 1986), which may be consistent with periventricular limbic and diencephalic pathology. Depth-electrode studies of these regions in humans indicate that hallucinations, perceptual distortions, and irrational fears can result from electrical discharges in either the temporal cortex, amygdala, or hippocampus (Gloor et al., 1982; Halgren et al., 1978; Wieser, 1983). A recent study using single-photon emission computed tomography (SPECT) has demonstrated increased blood flow in Broca's area while schizophrenic adults were hallucinating (McGuire et al., 1993). Hallucinations appear to reflect dysfunction in circuits that involve the amygdala, the limbic system, and cortical areas associated with language.

PSYCHOLOGICAL MODELS

At an empirical level, nonpsychotic forms of hallucinations would appear to be associated with states of extreme stress and altered consciousness. Illusions and fleeting pseudohallucinations have been reported in posttraumatic stress disorder in adults, though the phenomena have not been especially marked or vivid, even in severe cases (Horowitz, 1987). Terr (1985) has reported that, after a traumatic event that contributes to the death of someone close, a survivor may see or hear the dead friend or family member. Hallucinations of a more vivid type have also been reported in children who have lost close relatives (Andrade and Srinath, 1986; Yates and Bannard, 1988). Such effects might be mediated through increased cortical arousal secondary to emotional activation, though this is speculative. Auditory and visual hallucinations are phenomena associated with shamanistic altered states of consciousness, although in many instances the latter phenomena may have been induced by ingestion of various psychotomimetic substances (LaBarre, 1975).

Earlier psychoanalytic writers have suggested that hallucinations could be viewed as the breakthrough of preconscious or unconscious material into consciousness in response to psychological stress and conflict. As such, the material would be projected onto the world and then perceived as coming from outside. Censuring voices might represent critical superego contents (Modell, 1958). While somewhat metaphorical in nature, these suggestions allow a bridging between the biological events that underlie hallucinations and the nature of the hallucinatory experience, reflecting as it must a person's prior experiences, current unconscious, and preconscious fears, conflicts, defenses, and general mental state.

Differential Diagnoses of Hallucinations in Children

Not all of the studies of hallucinations in children have given the children's diagnoses. Of the 11 nonpsychotic children studied by Kotsopoulos et al. (1987), many were suffering from anxiety and/or depression, but, it would appear, of no great severity, since most were described as having an adjustment disorder. As noted above, children may experience brief hallucinatory episodes following bereavement (Yates and

Bannard, 1988). The authors have personally observed similar brief episodes of auditory hallucinations in children who had been sexually or physically abused prior to entering the psychiatric hospital. Only 20% of Burke and colleagues' (1985) 25 hallucinating children were diagnosed as psychotic (2 as manic, 2 as schizophreniform, 1 with reactive psychosis). The remainder were diagnosed as schizotypal personality disorder, undersocialized aggressive disorder, or depressive disorder. Some children who hallucinate do have more serious illnesses. Egdell and Kolvin's (1972) cases (2 who hallucinated of a group of 49 inpatients) were diagnosed as having a nonpsychotic behavior disorder and a "late-onset psychosis." Green et al. (1984) and Russell et al. (1989) have described hallucinations in children who meet DSM-III criteria for schizophrenia, and Chambers et al. (1982) have found hallucinations to be often present in prepubertal children with major depressive disorder.

Hallucinations in children have been reported as a side effect of medication. Those medications reported to induce hallucinations include promethazine hydrochloride (Zametkin et al., 1986), decongestants, such as pseudoephedrine and triprolidine (Sills et al., 1984), and methylphenidate (Bloom et al., 1988).

Conclusions

Hallucinations do occur in children, though they appear to be rare prior to 8 years of age. They may be associated with a wide variety of diagnoses, ranging from response to stress and bereavement to more serious disorders having some of the features of schizophrenia and depressive disorders. Clinicians should be aware that hallucinations may occur as a side effect of medications, though this appears to be relatively rare. Hallucinations often persist, suggesting that some persons may have a propensity to hallucinate. Whether these same individuals might also have a propensity to develop more serious psychiatric disorders remains to be elucidated.

DELUSIONS

Definition

A delusion is a belief that appears quite false (and sometimes bizarre) to others of the person's same cultural, social, and religious group and that cannot be charged by logical argument or evidence against it. Mullen (1979) has suggested that the characteristics of a delusion include that the belief (a) is held with total conviction, (b) may have great personal significance to the individual, and (c) is not amenable to reason or modifiable by experience. In adults, delusions are often of a persecutory or a grandiose nature. Persecutory delusions include the idea that one is threatened with personal harm, that one is being systematically robbed, or that one's spouse is unfaithful. They may be simple beliefs or complex ideas with multiple false inferences.

Manifestations in Children

In contrast to studies of hallucinations, few studies have objectively studied the phenomenon of delusions in children. Delusions are occasionally mentioned as concomitants to the symptom of hallucination in several of the papers cited in the section on hallucinations. It is interesting that none of the studies that dealt with milder hallucinations or with hallucinations in "nonpsychotic" children mention delusions (Andrade and Srinath, 1986; Burke et al., 1985; Egdell and Kolvin, 1972; Kotsopolous et al., 1987; Yates and Bannard, 1988). Those authors who describe more psychotic populations of children all mention the presence of delu-

sions in their results. Garralda (1984) found that paranoid and persecutory delusions were common in her 20 "late-onset" psychotic children. The children complained that they were being poisoned or that someone was following them. One boy claimed that people were shooting at him from under the floor. Both Green et al. (1984) and Russell et al. (1989) reported that prepubertal children with DSM-III schizophrenia had hallucinations similar to those seen in adult schizophrenia. Chambers et al. (1982) reported delusions of control, persecution, or sin in children suffering from major depressive disorder. Ideas of reference or thought insertion were not noted in these samples.

Bettes and Walker (1987) examined the records of a sample of 11,478 children between the ages of 5 and 18 years who had been admitted to a New York State Department of Mental Hygiene facility. They found that the prevalence of delusions was relatively low in childhood and early adolescence (approximately half the recorded rate of hallucinations). It rose precipitously after age 17, when, presumably, schizophrenia was diagnosed with increasing frequency.

Etiology and Pathogenesis

NEUROBIOLOGICAL FACTORS

In contrast to the literature on hallucinations, few hypotheses have been advanced to explain the neurobiological origin of delusions or to specify what brain mechanisms might be at their root. When such ideas are discussed, they are almost always in the context of the positive symptoms of schizophrenia, which have been attributed by some to limbic and diencephalic pathology (Weinberger, 1987). Delusions are seen in 50% of patients with Alzheimer's disease (Cummings et al., 1987), again suggesting the possibility of their being related to reticular and limbic pathology. Delusions may be found in many types of metabolic disorders, in deficiency states, and in drug intoxication (Cummings, 1985).

The paucity of speculation regarding the biology of delusions may reflect the much more complex cognitive and emotional factors that may underlie a delusion. Given our lack of knowledge about the neurobiology of thought and emotion, it is not surprising that we cannot begin to conceptualize what mechanisms might be involved.

PSYCHOLOGICAL FACTORS

A search of *Psychoanalytic Study of the Child* between 1978 and 1989 revealed only one article on delusions in children (Cummings, 1985). This was a case study of a 7-year-old boy who told others, including his therapist, that he was a cat. Occasionally he pretended to be a cat when he was with his parents, in school, or with his therapist. It is not clear from this account if he really believed his claim or whether he was using it as a metaphor to express his need for greater parental comforting and nurturance. Following treatment, the child no longer thought he was a cat.

Conclusions

In the absence of a more serious disorder such as schizophrenia or major depressive disorder, young children develop delusions infrequently. From a cognitive viewpoint, children continue to develop their understanding of the world and of others well into their early school years. Although they may have many "erroneous" notions about events, causes, and relationships between phenomena in their world, children rarely develop fixed delusions.

References

American Psychiatric Association: *Diagnostic and Statistical Manual of Mental Disorders* (3rd ed). Washington, DC, American Psychiatric Association Press, 1980.

American Psychiatric Association: *Diagnostic and Statistical Manual of Mental Disorders* (3rd ed, rev). Washington, DC, American Psychiatric Association Press, 1987.

American Psychiatric Association: *Diagnostic and Statistical Manual of Mental Disorders* (4th ed).

Washington, DC, American Psychiatric Association Press, 1994.

Andrade C, Srinath S: True auditory hallucinations as a conversion syndrome. *Br J Psychiatry* 148: 100–102, 1986.

Andreasen NC: Thought, language, and communication disorders. I: Clinical assessment, definition of terms and evaluation of their reliability. *Arch Gen Psychiatry* 36:1315–1323, 1979a.

Andreasen NC: Thought, language, and communication disorders. II: Diagnostic significance. *Arch Gen Psychiatry* 36:1325–1330, 1979b.

Andreasen NC, Grove WM: Thought, language, and communication in schizophrenia: Diagnosis and prognosis. *Schizophr Bull* 12:348–359, 1986.

Andreasen N, Nasrallah HA, Dunn V, et al: Structural abnormalities in the frontal system of schizophrenia. *Arch Gen Psychiatry* 43:136–144, 1986.

Andreasen NC, Flaum M, Swayze VW, et al: Positive and negative symptoms in schizophrenia. *Arch Gen Psychiatry* 47:615–621, 1990.

Angrist B, Rotrosen J, Gershon S: Differential effects of amphetamine and neuroleptics on negative vs. positive symptoms in schizophrenia. *Psychopharmacology* 72:17–19, 1980.

Arboleda C, Holzman PS: Thought disorder in children at risk for psychosis. *Arch Gen Psychiatry* 42:1004–1013, 1985.

Asarnow JR, Goldstein MJ, Carlson GA, et al: Childhood-onset depressive disorders: A follow-up study of rates of rehospitalization and out-of-home placement among child psychiatric inpatients. *J Affect Disord* 15:245–248, 1988.

Asarnow RF, MacCrimmon DJ: Span of apprehension deficits during postpsychotic stages of schizophrenia: A replication and extension. *Arch Gen Psychiatry* 38:1001–1006, 1981.

Asarnow RF, Sherman T: Studies of visual information processing in schizophrenic children. *Child Dev* 55:249–261, 1984.

Asarnow RF, Sherman TL, Strandburg R: The search for the psychobiological substrate of childhood onset schizophrenia. *J Am Acad Child Adolesc Psychiatry* 26:601–604, 1986.

Bettes BA, Walker E: Positive and negative symptoms in psychotic and other psychiatrically disturbed children. *J Child Psychol Psychiatry* 28:555–568, 1987.

Bleuler E: *Dementia Praecox of the Group of Schizophrenia*. Monograph series on Schizophrenia. no. 1. (Zinkin J, trans.). New York, International Universities Press, 1951.

Bloom AS, Russell LJ, Weisskopf N, et al: Methylphenidate-induced delusional disorder in a child with attention deficit disorder with hyperactivity. *J Am Acad Child Adolesc Psychiatry* 27:88–89, 1988.

Braff DL, Heaton R, Kuck J, et al: The generalized pattern of neuropsychological deficits in outpatients with chronic schizophrenia with heterogenous Wisconsin card sorting test results. *Arch Gen Psychiatry* 48:891–898, 1991.

Burke P, Del Beccaro M, McCauley E, et al: Hallucinations in children. *J Am Acad Child Psychiatry* 24:71–75, 1985.

Butler RW, Braff DL: Delusions: A review and integration. *Schizophr Bull* 17:633–647, 1991.

Cantor S, Evans J, Pearce J, et al: Childhood schizophrenia: Present but not accounted for. *Am J Psychiatry* 139:758–763, 1982.

Caplan R: Thought disorder in middle childhood. *J Am Acad Child Adolesc Psychiatry* 33:605–615, 1994.

Caplan R: Communication deficits in childhood schizophrenia spectrum disorder. *Schizophr Bull* 20:671–684, 1994.

Caplan R, Foy JG, Asarnow AF, et al: Information processing deficits of schizophrenic children with formal thought disorder. *Psychiatry Res* 31:169–177, 1990b.

Caplan R, Foy JG, Sigman M, et al: Conservation and focused thought disorder. *Dev Psychopathol* 2:183–192, 1990c.

Caplan R, Guthrie D, Fish B, et al: The Kiddie Formal Thought Disorder Scale (K-FTDS). Clinical assessment, reliability, and validity. *J Am Acad Child Adolesc Psychiatry* 28:408–416, 1989.

Caplan R, Guthrie D, Foy JG: Communication deficits and formal thought disorder in schizophrenic children. *J Am Acad Child Adolesc Psychiatry* 31:151–159, 1992a.

Caplan R, Guthrie D, Shields WD, et al: Formal thought disorder in pediatric complex partial seizure disorder. *J Child Psychol Psychiatry* 33:1399–1412, 1992b.

Caplan R, Guthrie D, Shields WD, et al: Communication deficits in children undergoing temporal lobectomy. *J Am Acad Child Adolesc Psychiatry* 32:604–611, 1993.

Caplan R, Guthrie D, Shields WD, et al: Discourse deficits in pediatric complex partial seizure disorder and schizophrenia. *Dev Psychopathol* 6:499–517, 1994.

Caplan R, Perdue S, Tanguay PE, et al: Formal thought disorder in childhood onset schizophrenia and schizotypal personality disorder. *J Child Psychol Psychiatry* 31:1103–1114, 1990a.

Caplan R, Shields WD, Mori L, et al: Middle childhood onset of interictal psychoses: Case studies. *J Am Acad Child Adolesc Psychiatry* 30:893–896, 1991.

Caplan R, Tanguay PE, Szekely AG: Subacute sclerosing panencephalitis presenting as childhood psychosis: A case study. *J Am Acad Child Adolesc Psychiatry* 26:440–443, 1987.

Carlson GA: Annotation: Child and adolescent mania—Diagnostic considerations. *J Child Psychol Psychiatry* 31:331–341, 1990.

Chambers WJ, Puig-Antich J, Tabrizi MA, et al: Psychotic symptoms in prepubertal major depressive disorder. *Arch Gen Psychiatry* 39:921–927, 1982.

Cornblatt BA, Lenzenweger MF, Dworkin RH, et al: Positive and negative schizophrenia symptoms, attention, and information processing. *Schizophr Bull* 11:397–407, 1985.

Csernansky JG, Mellentin J, Beauclair L, Lombrozo L: Mesolimbic dopaminergic supersensitivity following electrical kindling of the amygdala. *Biol Psychiatry* 23:285–294, 1988.

Cummings JL: Organic delusions: Phenomenology, anatomical correlations, and review. *Br J Psychiatry* 146:184–197, 1985.

Cummings JL, Miller B, Hill MA, et al: Neuropsychiatric aspects of multi-infarct dementia and dementia of the Alzheimer type. *Arch Neurol* 44:389–392, 1987.

Del Beccaro M, Burke P, McCauley E: Hallucinations in children: A follow-up study. *J Am Acad Child Adolesc Psychiatry* 27:462–465, 1988.

Despert IL: Delusional and hallucinatory experiences in children. *Am J Psychiatry* 104:528–537, 1948.

Egdell HG, Kolvin I: Childhood hallucinations. *J Child Psychol Psychiatry* 13:279–287, 1972.

Eisenberg L: Hallucinations in children. In: West LJ (ed): *Hallucinations*. New York, Grune & Stratton, 1962.

Eisenberg L, Kanner L: Childhood schizophrenia. *Am J Orthopsychiatry* 26:556–564, 1956.

Evarts EV: A neurophysiological theory of hallucinations. In: West LJ (ed): *Hallucinations*. New York, Grune & Stratton, 1962.

Fish B, Ritvo ER: Psychoses of childhood. In: Noshpitz JD (ed): *Basic Handbook of Child Psychiatry* (Vol 2). New York, Basic Books, 1978, pp. 249–304.

Fish FJ: *Schizophrenia*. London, John Wright & Sons, 1962.

Fishman LC: Dreams and other hallucinations: An approach to the underlying mechanism. In: Siegal RK, West LI (eds): *Hallucinations, Behavior, Experience, and Theory*. New York, Wiley, 1975.

Flor-Henry P: Determinants of psychosis in epilepsy: Laterality and forced normalization. *Biol Psychiatry* 18:1045–1057, 1983.

Freud S: Metapsychological supplement to the theory of dreams. In: Strachey J (ed): *The Standard Edition of the Complete Psychological Works of Sigmund Freud*. London, Hogarth Press, 1975.

Garralda ME: Hallucinations in children with conduct and emotional disorders. I: The clinical phenomena. *Psychol Med* 14:589–596, 1984.

Gloor P, Olivier A, Quesney LF, et al: The role of the limbic system in experiential phenomena of temporal lobe epilepsy. *Ann Neurol* 12:129–144, 1982.

Green WH, Campbell M, Hardesty AS, et al: A comparison of schizophrenic and autistic children. *J Am Acad Child Psychiatry* 4:399–409, 1984.

Gruzelier J, Seymour K, Wilson L, et al: Impairments on neuropsychological tests of temporohippocampal and frontohippocampal functions and word fluency in remitting schizophrenia and affective disorders. *Arch Gen Psychiatry* 45:623–629, 1988.

Gur RE, Gur RC, Skolnick B, et al: Brain function in psychiatric disorders. III: Regional cerebral blood flow in unmedicated schizophrenics. *Arch Gen Psychiatry* 42:329–334, 1985.

Halgren E, Walter RD, Cherlow DG, et al: Mental phenomena evoked by electrical stimulation of the human hippocampal formation and amygdala. *Brain* 101:83–117, 1978.

Harrow M, Marengo JT: Schizophrenic thought disorder at followup: Its persistence and prognostic significance. *Schizophr Bull* 12:373–393, 1986.

Harvey PD: Speech competence in manic and schizophrenic psychoses: The association between clinically rated thought disorder and performance. *J Abnorm Psychol* 92:368–377, 1983.

Harvey PD, Earie-Boyer EA, Levinson JC: Distractibility and discourse failure. Their association in mania and schizophrenia. *J Nerv Ment Dis* 174:274–279, 1986.

Hinsie LE, Campbell AJ: *Psychiatric Dictionary* (4th ed). New York, Oxford University Press, 1970, p. 333.

Hobson JA, McCarley RW: The brain as a dream-state generator: An activation-synthesis hypothesis of the dream process. *Am J Psychiatry* 134:1335–1348, 1977.

Holzman PS, Shenton ME, Solovay MR: Quality of thought disorder in differential diagnosis. *Schizophr Bull* 12:360–372, 1986.

Horowitz M: Stress-response syndromes: Posttraumatic and adjustment disorders. In: Michels R, Cavenar I (eds): *Psychiatry* (Vol I). Chapter 41, pp. 1–16, New York, Lippincott, 1987.

Hornstein NL, Putnam FW: Clinical phenomenology of child and adolescent dissociative disorders. *J Am Acad Child Adolesc Psychiatry* 31:1077–1085, 1992.

Ingvar DH: Mental illness and regional brain metabolism. *Trends Neurosci* 5:199–202, 1985.

Kanner L: *Child Psychiatry*. Springfield, IL, Charles C Thomas, 1957.

Kaplan HI, Sadock BJ: *Comprehensive Textbook of Psychiatry* (4th ed). Baltimore, Williams & Wilkins, 1985, p. 501.

Kaufman AS: *Intelligence Testing with the WISC-R*. New York, Wiley, 1979.

Kelsoe JR Jr, Cadet JL, Pickar D, et al: Quantitative neuroanatomy in schizophrenia. *Arch Gen Psychiatry* 45:533–541, 1988.

Kemph JP: Hallucinations in psychotic children. *J Am Acad Child Adolesc Psychiatry* 26:556–559, 1987.

Kirch DG, Weinberger DR: Anatomical neuropathology in schizophrenia: Post-mortem findings. In: Nasrallah HA, Weinberger DR (eds): *The Neurology of Schizophrenia*. New York, Elsevier, 1986.

Kolvin I, Ounsted C, Humphrey M, et al: Studies in the childhood psychoses. I: The phenomenology of childhood psychoses. *Br J Psychiatry* 118:385–395, 1971.

Kotsopoulos S, Kanigsberg I, Cote A, et al: Hallucinatory experiences in nonpsychotic children. *J Am Acad Child Adolesc Psychiatry* 26:375–380, 1987.

LaBarre W: Anthropological perspectives on hallucination and hallucinogens. In: Siegal RK, West LI (eds): *Hallucinations, Behavior, Experience, and Theory*. New York, Wiley, 1975.

Lieb JP, Rausch R, Engel J Jr, et al: Changes in intelligence following temporal lobectomy: Relationship to EEG activity, seizure relief, and pathology. *Epilepsia* 23:1–13, 1982.

Liddle PF, Friston SR, Hirsch SR: Regional cerebral metabolic activity in chronic schizophrenia. *Schizophr Res* 3:23–24, 1990 (Abstract).

Liddle PF, Friston KJ, Hirsch SR, et al: Patterns of cerebral blood flow in schizophrenia. *Br J Psychiatry* 160:179–186, 1992.

Lindsay J, Ounsted C, Richards P: Long-term outcome in children with temporal lobe seizures. III: Psychiatric aspects in childhood and adult life. *Dev Med Child Neurol* 21:630–636, 1979.

Loveland NT, Wynne LC, Singer MT: The family Rorschach: A new method for studying family interaction. *Fam Process* 2:187–215, 1963.

Makita K: The age of onset of childhood schizophrenia. *Folia Psychiatr Neurol Jpn* 20:111–121, 1966.

Marengo I, Harrow M: Thought disorder. A function of schizophrenia, mania, or psychosis? *J Nerv Ment Dis* 173:35–41, 1985.

Marks RC, Luchins DJ: Relationship between brain image findings in schizophrenia and psychopathology: A review of the literature relating positive and negative symptoms. In: Andreasen NC (ed): *Modern Problems of Pharmacopsychiatry: Positive and Negative Symptoms and Syndromes*. Basel: Karger, 1990, pp. 89–123.

McGuire PK, Shah GM, Murray RM: Increased blood flow in Broca's area during auditory hallucinations in schizophrenia. *Lancet* 342(8873):703–706, 1993.

Mizrahi EM, Kellaway P, Grossman RG, et al: Anterior temporal lobectomy and medically refractory temporal lobe epilepsy of childhood. *Epilepsia* 31:302–312, 1990.

Modell A: The theoretical implication of hallucinations in schizophrenia. *J Am Psychoanal Assoc* 6:422–480, 1958.

Mullen P: Phenomenology of disordered mental function. In: Hill P, Murray R, Thorley A (eds): *Essentials of Postgraduate Psychiatry*. London, Academic Press, 1979.

Nuechterlein KH, Edell WS, Norris M, et al: Attentional vulnerability indicators, thought disorder, and negative symptoms. *Schizophr Bull* 12:408–426, 1986.

Oltmanns TF, Murphy R, Berenbau H, et al: Rating verbal communication impairment in schizophrenia and affective disorders. *Schizophr Bull* 11:292–299, 1985.

Oltmanns TF, Ohayon J, Neale JM: The effect of antipsychotic medication and diagnostic criteria on distractibility in schizophrenia. *J Psychiatr Res* 14:81–91, 1979.

Paulman RG, Devous MD Sr, Gregory RR, et al: Hypofrontality and cognitive impairment in schizophrenia: Dynamic single-photon tomography and neuropsychological assessment of schizophrenic brain function. *Biol Psychiatry* 27:377–399, 1990.

Perez M, Trimble MR, Murray NMK, et al: Epileptic psychoses: An evaluation of PSE profiles. *Br J Psychiatry* 146:155–163, 1985.

Pogue-Geile MF, Harrow M: Negative and positive symptoms in schizophrenia and depression: A follow-up. *Schizophr Bull* 10:371–381, 1984.

Rechtschaffen AM, Dement WC: Narcolepsy and hypersomnia. In: Kales A (ed): *Sleep: Physiology and Pathology*. Philadelphia, Lippincott, 1969.

Rochester SR, Martin JR: *Crazy Talk: A Study of the Discourse of Schizophrenic Speakers*. New York, Plenum, 1979.

Rothstein A: Hallucinatory phenomena in childhood. *J Am Acad Child Psychiatry* 20:623–635, 1981.

Russell AT, Bott L, Sammons C: The phenomenology of schizophrenia occurring in childhood. *J Am Acad Child Adolesc Psychiatry* 28:399–407, 1989.

Rutter M: Childhood schizophrenia reconsidered. *J Autism Child Schizophr* 2:315–337, 1972.

Rutter M, Lockeyer L: A five to fifteen year follow-up study of infantile psychosis. I: Description of sample. *Br J Psychiatry* 113:1169–1182, 1967a.

Rutter M, Greenfield D, Lockeyer L: Five to fifteen years follow-up study of infantile psychosis. II: Social behavioral outcome. *Br J Psychiatry* 113:1183–1199, 1967b.

Schneider SG, Asarnow RF: A comparison of cognitive/neuropsychological impairments of nonretarded autistic and schizophrenic children. *J Abnorm Child Psychol* 15:29–46, 1987.

Shatz M: Communication. In: Musson P (ed): *Carmichael's Manual of Child Psychology*. New York, Wiley, 1982, pp. 841–889.

Shelton RC, Weinberger DR: X-ray computerized tomography studies of schizophrenia. In: Nasrallah HA, Weinberger DR (eds): *The Neurology of Schizophrenia*. New York, Elsevier, 1986.

Shenton ME, Kikinis R, Jolesz FA, et al: Abnormalities of the left temporal lobe and thought disorder in schizophrenia. *N Engl J Med* 327:604–612, 1992.

Sills JA, Nunn AJ, Sankey RJ: Visual hallucinations in children receiving decongestants. *Br Med J* 288:1912–1913, 1984.

Slater E, Beard AW: The schizophrenia-like psychoses of epilepsy. *Br J Psychiatry* 109:95–150, 1963.

Spohn HE, Lolafaye C, Larson J, et al: Episodic and residual thought pathology in chronic schizophrenics: Effect of neuroleptics. *Schizophr Bull* 12:394–407, 1986.

Strandburg RJ, Marsh JT, Brown WS, et al: EEG abnormalities support continuity in information processing deficits across childhood and adult onset schizophrenia. *Schizophr Bull* (in press).

Tanguay PE: Child and adolescent psychiatry: Building the data base. In: Kales A, Pierce C, Greenblatt M (eds): *The Mosaic of Contemporary Psychiatry in Perspective*. New York, Springer-Verlag, 1992.

Taylor DC, Marsh SM: The influence of sex and side of operation on personality questionnaire responses after temporal lobectomy. In: Gruzelier H, Flor-Henry, P (eds): *Hemisphere Asymmetries of Function in Psychopathology. Development and Psychiatry Series*. Amsterdam, Elsevier, 1979, pp. 391–400.

Terr LC: Remembered images and trauma. *Psychoanal Study Child* 40:493–533, 1985.

Tompson M, Asarnow J, Goldstein M, et al: Thought disorder and communication problems in schizophrenia and depressed children and their parents. *J Child Psychol Psychiatry* 2:159–168, 1990.

van der Gaag RJ: Multiplex Development Disorder: An Exploration of Borderlines on the Autistic Spectrum (pp. 81–98). Unpublished Thesis University of Utrecht, the Netherlands, 1993.

Watkins JM, Asarnow RF, Tanguay PE: Symptom development in childhood onset schizophrenia. *J Child Psychol Psychiatry* 29:865–878, 1988.

Weinberger DR: Implications of normal brain development for the pathogenesis of schizophrenia. *Arch Gen Psychiatry* 44:660–669, 1987.

Weinberger DR, Berman KF, Illowsky BP: Physiological dysfunction of dorsolateral prefrontal cortex in schizophrenia. *Arch Gen Psychiatry* 45:609–615, 1988.

Weinberger DR, Berman KF, Zec RF: Physiological dysfunction of dorsolateral prefrontal cortex in schizophrenia. I: Regional cerebral blood flow evidence. *Arch Gen Psychiatry* 43:114–124, 1986.

West LJ: A general theory of hallucinations and dreams. In: West LJ (ed): *Hallucinations*. New York, Grune & Stratton, 1962.

Wieser HG: Depth recorded limbic seizures and psychopathology. *Neurosci Biobehav Rev* 7:427–440, 1983.

Wilking V, Paoli C: The hallucinatory experience. *J Am Acad Child Psychiatry* 5:431–440, 1966.

Wittig R, Zorick F, Roehrs T, et al: Narcolepsy in a 7-year-old. *J Pediatr* 102:725–727, 1983.

Yates T, Bannard IR: The "haunted" child: Grief, hallucinations, and family dynamics. *J Am Acad Child Adolesc Psychiatry* 27:573–581, 1988.

Zametkin AJ, Reeves JC, Webster L, et al: Promethazine treatment of children with attention deficit disorder with hyperactivity—Ineffective and unpleasant. *J Am Acad Child Adolesc Psychiatry* 25:854–856, 1986.

26 DEVELOPMENTAL, NEUROBIOLOGICAL, AND PSYCHOSOCIAL ASPECTS OF HYPERACTIVITY, IMPULSIVITY, AND ATTENTION

Lily Hechtman, M.D., F.R.C.P.(C)

In this chapter we examine the developmental, neurobiological, and psychosocial aspects of hyperactivity, impulsivity, and attention. These three symptoms are grouped together because, although they are distinct in many ways, there is a great deal of overlap among them. It is thus difficult, particularly in young children, to determine if the behavior one observes is purely a problem of attention, hyperactivity, or impulsivity or a conglomerate of all three. This chapter presents a brief developmental description of how these symptoms can be expressed at various ages. This is followed by a summary of key neurobiological aspects that may underlie these symptoms, and finally, psychosocial factors that may contribute or complicate the symptoms are discussed.

DEVELOPMENTAL ASPECTS OF HYPERACTIVITY, IMPULSIVITY, AND ATTENTION

General Considerations

TEMPERAMENT

One cannot discuss the developmental aspects of symptoms such as hyperactivity, impulsivity, and attention without an appreciation of the role of temperament in these behavioral characteristics. One of the first researchers to investigate temperamental differences in young children was Gesell (1937). Using films and direct observation, he identified some 15 behavioral characteristics that could be identified in the 1st year and remained relatively stable till the 5th year. The work on temperament by Thomas and Chess and their coworkers (Thomas et al., 1968) is well known. They interviewed and observed parents and their infants periodically, beginning when the children were approximately 3 months of age, and delineated various behavioral or temperamental profiles. These profiles were composed of the following behavioral aspects: activity level, rhythmicity of biological functions, approach or withdrawal to new situations, intensity of emotional reactions, threshold of sensory responsiveness, adaptability, quality of mood, distractibility, attention span, and persistence. We thus see that activity and attention are key elements in the temperamental profiles. It was further shown that children, even in the 1st few months, differ greatly on the above temperamental characteristics. In discussing the symptoms of hyperactivity, impulsivity, and attention, one needs to be aware of normal temperamental variability in these behaviors.

The individual variability of temperamental characteristics may have a number of different origins. Hereditary factors certainly play an important role. Several twin studies (Freedman and Keller, 1963; Rutter et al., 1963; Torgersen and Kringlen, 1976; Vandenberg, 1969) have all shown that monozygotic twins were significantly more alike than dizygotic twins on various behavioral and temperamental characteristics including those delineated by Thomas and colleagues (1968). As Dobzhansky (1967) suggested, these behavioral aspects are probably polygenetically inherited and constitute patterns of growth and ways of responding to the environment rather than specific traits. There is also a suggestion that some minor congenital physical anomalies may be associated with behavioral differences, e.g., impulsivity and hyperactiv-

ity in boys (Quinn and Rapoport, 1974; Waldrop et al., 1968, 1978).

Organic brain damage either prenatally, perinatally, or postnatally has a significant effect on behavioral development and may influence temperamental characteristics. The marked irritability, low frustration tolerance, and short attention of the brain-injured child has been well documented.

Psychosocial factors such as parenting style, family and environmental stressors, and psychological intervention may influence and modify behavioral, developmental, and temperamental characteristics. This dynamic interplay among genetic, biological, and psychosocial influences on behavioral and temperamental profiles results in the individual variability one sees. An extreme expression of this variability gives rise to symptoms that prove problematic to the child and his or her family. A description of how the symptoms of hyperactivity, impulsivity, and inattention can be expressed at various ages now follows.

Hyperactivity, Impulsivity, and Inattention in Infancy

In infancy the above symptoms are often expressed by sleep disturbance, feeding problems, increased fidgetness (not cuddly), excessive irritability, and crying.

Sleep disturbance may take the form of sleeping very little or for very short periods of time with the result that the infant is awake and demanding. Sleep, when it does occur, is often very restless. The infant may also wake with a startle reaction followed by screaming.

Feeding problems may include poor sucking or crying during feedings, needing to be fed for brief periods of time fairly often, and not being able to settle into a workable sucking or feeding rhythm. The infant may be irregular in his or her wish for food or easily distracted from feeding. Infants sometimes become picky eaters and these problems may give rise to problems in the mother-infant relationship. The increased irritability, fidgetness, crying, and/or colic makes it difficult to soothe or cuddle the child or have him or her settle down for any length of time. Sometimes the child may develop self-soothing or -stimulating behaviors such as excessive thumb sucking, head rolling, head banging, or rocking. Once the infant begins to crawl he or she may be in constant motion with relative disregard to mother's presence or absence or other dangers. This makes the child extremely accident prone, requiring constant close supervision.

The infant may be hypertonic or may not enjoy being held. All these behaviors make it difficult to establish a harmony with the child and feel effective as a parent.

The constant activity, which is forever changing and often dangerous, is evident, but at this stage it is difficult to delineate what the relative contributions of impulsivity and inattention may be to the behavior one sees.

Symptoms in the Toddler and Preschooler

It must be recognized that normal preschoolers are very active, have short attention spans, and are fairly impulsive. It is therefore often difficult to identify children whose behavior in these areas constitutes symptoms as opposed to normal variability. Two researchers who have looked at these problems in this age group in great detail are Weiss (Schleifer et al., 1975) and Campbell (Campbell et al., 1982).

HYPERACTIVITY

Interestingly, direct observations (Schleifer et al., 1975) or actometer measures (Campbell et al., 1982) did not show "hyperactive" preschoolers to be more active than normal controls in the free play situations. However, the two groups were significantly different in more structured settings. Generally, in this age group, hyperactivity presents with the child always running, never walking, always being on the go, changing the focus of his or her activity frequently so it appears to be without purpose or goal. The child may have difficulty sitting still for any length of time. For example, he or she frequently leaves the table during meals, cannot sit through the reading of a story or is in constant state of motion, even when watching television. This inappropriate activity is particularly more evident in structured situations.

Despite the marked gross motor activity, which is sometimes developmentally precocious, fine motor coordination and language are often delayed. The marked hyperactivity and inattention may contribute to these delays. The child may thus be very active but poorly coordinated and clumsy, making him or her quite accident prone. Sleep disturbances may continue, with children sleeping little, restlessly, or for short periods of time.

IMPULSIVITY

In this age group, impulsivity (often referred to as cognitive impulsivity) has been measured directly by various laboratory tests and described by careful observations (Campbell et al., 1982; Schleifer et al., 1975). Tests of impulsivity in this age group have included the Early Childhood Matching Familiar Figures Test (ECMFFT), which measures dimensions of reflectivity–impulsivity, Draw A Line Slowly Test (DALS), which measures motor impulsivity, and the Cookie Delay Test, which measures more global impulsive responses. All these tests have shown that some preschoolers are much more impulsive than others. Observational (Schleifer et al., 1975) and descriptive data show that children with this symptom will shift their activities unpredictably: They will dash out into the street for no apparent reason, grab toys, or hit other children without any discernible provocation. The impulsivity makes their behavior unpredictable, very disruptive, and often dangerous. It also presents problems in behavioral management, limit setting, and discipline. Parents frequently complain that children with these symptoms "do not listen," do not learn from their mistakes, as they seem to be unresponsive to praise or punishment, and continue to repeat behaviors parents try to curtail.

PROBLEMS OF ATTENTION

Attention has also been studied by laboratory means, e.g., Auditory Continuous Performance Test (Schleifer et al., 1975) and direct observations (Campbell et al., 1982; Schleifer et al., 1975). Children in this age group with attention problems shift their activities frequently, are inattentive during structured tasks, do not complete activities they begin, cannot play alone, and are easily distracted.

Symptoms in the Elementary School-Age Child

HYPERACTIVITY

Hyperactivity in this age group is measured by parents' and teachers' rating scales, direct observational measures, or direct mechanical measures via actometers, stabilimeter, electrical mats, wrist microcomputers, or ultrasonic or photoelectric systems. Generally these measures can identify some children who are significantly more active than age-matched controls. Perhaps the longest and most naturalistic study that focused on measuring activity in this age group was carried out by

Porrino and coworkers (Porrino et al., 1983). Children in this study wore an actometer with a memory continuously 24 hours a day for 7 days. The authors showed that hyperactive children were in fact more active in all situations, structured or free, even during sleep than were matched controls.

However, overall activity levels tell only part of the story. The activity is often "off task," disruptive, and random with no apparent goal or purpose. Much of it may be fidgetiness and restlessness, which take the form of leaving one's seat in the classroom, walking around, or engaging in some other somewhat inappropriate activity.

Hyperactivity may also be expressed in being unable to sit through a meal, a story, a game, or a television program. The marked disruptive nature of the activity (Klein and Young, 1979) is what is often disturbing to parents and teachers and what distinguishes it from high normal activity, frequently resulting in referrals for professional help. In a free play environment the increased activity may be expressed by disruptive physical contact with other children (running into them, pushing, hitting, disrupting their play). This may be done without any particular anger, hostility, or malicious intent, but often results in quarrels and fights with other children.

IMPULSIVITY

As the child matures, there is the general expectation that he or she will develop greater inhibiting control over his or her behavior and become progressively less impulsive. Impulsivity in this age group can again be divided into an impulsive, cognitive, or problem-solving style (Kagan et al., 1964) and general behavioral impulsivity. The Matching Familiar Figures Test (Kagan et al., 1964) is a frequently used measure for assessing an impulsive cognitive style. As Weiss (Weiss and Hechtman, 1993) has pointed out, any test (e.g., Continuous Performance Test) that requires some inhibition or delay in response may also measure an element of impulsivity. This impulsive cognitive style may be seen in poor, incomplete, or error-ridden school work, as the child rarely follows a careful systematic stepwise approach. It may also express itself in a variety of games, particularly those requiring some strategy and ones where moves that are impulsive and not well thought out result in failure (e.g., chess).

However, it is the impulsive behavior that often proves the most difficult and dangerous. The impulsivity is often characterized by uncontrolled behavior with no thought as to the consequences. It may be dangerous, such as walking on a high ledge or leaning from a balcony, or not socially accepted, such as taking another child's toy or stealing a candy bar or comic on the spur of the moment. As the child matures, his or her impulsive behavior can become more dangerous and problematic. Some authors have linked this characteristic to adult antisocial personality characteristics (Clouston, 1982; Lewis, 1974; Weiss and Hechtman, 1993).

PROBLEMS OF ATTENTION

Attention is not a uniform dimension or a single cognitive process. As Taylor has pointed out, the many different functions involved in attention include "the ability to resist distraction; to maintain one's performance on a long task; to focus intensely on specific stimuli; and to explore complex stimuli in a planned and efficient way" (Taylor, 1985, p. 427). The school-age child who has attentional problems may have difficulty in some or all of the above aspects of attention.

Distractibility is often described in children with attentional problems, but several investigators (Davidson and Prior, 1978; Taylor, 1982) have been unable to document this difficulty in a laboratory setting. However, Radosh and Gittelman (1981) found that a very distracting stimulus affected performance on a very boring arithmetic task in children with attentional problems.

It has been argued that the apparent distractibility of these children is really a problem of *sustained attention*. They cannot focus on anything for any extended period of time and so appear easily distractible. Developmentally as the child matures his or her attention span should lengthen and he or she should be able to concentrate for progressively longer periods of time. This developmental task is not readily achieved in children with attentional problems. Their short attention span results in not completing tasks, games, or projects, frequently shifting from one activity to another, and generally doing poorly on any task requiring sustained attention, e.g., Continuous Performance Test (CPT).

Children with attentional problems are often very disorganized in problem-solving activities and cannot deal with complex stimuli and/ or tasks in a planned and efficient way. Tests such as the embedded figures test clearly show the deficits that exist in this area. Attempts to teach children with attentional difficulties more organized and effective cognitive strategies have met with limited success (Abikoff, 1987).

Symptoms in the Adolescent

In adolescence, symptoms such as hyperactivity, impulsivity, and inattention may change in presentation because of the child's developmental stage and because of psychosocial aspects of the child's life, e.g., school failure, social ostracism, which also affects how symptoms are expressed.

HYPERACTIVITY

There is clearly a decrease in gross motor hyperactivity. The adolescent can usually sit through a meal and is not grossly running around all over the place like the younger child. However, he or she is still very restless and fidgety. Hyperactivity takes the form of a lot of small muscle versus large muscle movements, e.g., tapping one's fingers, shaking one's leg, shifting positions in one's chair, as opposed to getting up and running around. This change in gross motor hyperactivity has led some authors (Eisenberg, 1966; Laufer and Denhoff, 1957) to suggest that the symptoms are limited to childhood and that, by adolescence, the child may "outgrow" the problem. This became a common belief perpetuated by clinicians to parents.

However, recent prospective follow-up studies of hyperactive adolescents by Gittelman-Klein (1987) and Lambert et al. (1987) suggest that 20–30% of adolescents may no longer have problems. However, most (<70%) continue to have difficulties. Their hyperactivity merely takes another form. In addition to the restlessness and fidgetiness already described, they may become involved in many sports activities (if coordination problems are not too severe) or ride their bikes for long periods of time. They seem always on the go, going to and from places and rarely staying put for any extended period of time. They may listen to music but are in almost constant motion while doing so. Thus, the hyperactivity persists, but may have found more acceptable channels (e.g., sports) and by and large more often involves small muscle movement expressed as restlessness or fidgetiness.

IMPULSIVITY

As the child enters adolescence, persistent impulsivity may result in ever increasingly dangerous impulsive acts, leading to ever greater problems for the adolescent and his or her family. Again, for 20–30% of adolescents who had problems with impulsivity in childhood, this difficulty is no longer significant (Gittelman-Klein, 1987; Lambert et al., 1987). However, for the vast majority of children, the continued impulsivity makes these children appear very immature and leads to ever greater problems. The impulsivity may be expressed in dangerous and at times socially maladaptive ways. For example, playing the class clown and impulsively calling out, making jokes, or otherwise disrupting the class is not uncommon.

The adolescent may impulsively take a car and go on a joy ride. He may blow up at teachers, peers, or parents. Sometimes these blowups may be physical. Impulsive, excessive drug and/or alcohol use may occur from time to time. It should be noted that some of these impulsive behaviors are affected by the child's poor self-esteem arising from chronic school failure and social ostracism by parents, teachers, and peers. The impulsive cognitive style also persists into adolescence, with the result of decreased organized problem-solving capabilities and continuing poor academic achievement.

ATTENTIONAL PROBLEMS

Attentional problems often persist into adolescence and are expressed in easy distractibility, failure to complete tasks, short attention span for particular activity, and frequent shifts from one activity to another. Continued difficulties with tasks requiring sustained attention or organized problem-solving and planning capacities are often seen. Thus, the attentional problems continue to be experienced in adolescence, causing the same deficits as they did earlier. However, the continued difficulties and failures may lead to poor self-esteem and poor motivation with a sense of hopelessness and helplessness. An adolescent may then give up and make few attempts to tackle difficult tasks. This giving up in turn contributes to the adolescent falling further behind and experiencing a greater sense of failure.

Symptoms in Adulthood

Symptoms of hyperactivity, impulsivity, and inattention in adulthood may present in a form different from that seen in previous age groups because of the person's developmental state, their life circumstances, and psychosocial factors influencing their previous and current situation.

Our knowledge regarding the adult picture of these symptoms comes from very different data sources. These sources include (a) controlled prospective follow-up studies, which follow children with these symptoms prospectively into adult life; (b) retrospective studies, which look at old records, try to reconstruct childhood diagnoses from them, and then attempt to contact these adults; (c) studies that look at adults with these or similar symptoms; and (d) family studies of parents and relatives of children with these symptoms.

Space does not permit a detailed description of the above studies, but a brief mention of some key ones in each category is made here.

CONTROLLED PROSPECTIVE STUDIES

Drs. Weiss and Hechtman (1993; Weiss et al., 1985) conducted controlled prospective 10-, 12-, and 15-year follow-up studies on 75 young adults who had symptoms of hyperactivity, impulsivity, and inattention during childhood and 45 matched normal control subjects (mean age 19 at 10-year follow-up, mean age 25 at 15-year follow-up). The evaluations were comprehensive, assessing academic, work, psychiatric, social, physiological, and psychological parameters. The psychological parameters addressed key symptoms of hyperactivity, impulsivity, and attention. In addition to interviews with subjects and parents, reports were obtained from schools, employers, and the court system.

Gittelman and colleagues (1985) also conducted a controlled prospective study of 101 subjects who had these symptoms in childhood and 100 matched normal control subjects (mean age at follow-up 18.3 and 26 years). Comprehensive evaluations included interviews with subjects and parents and various rating scales. Forty percent of the subjects continued to have two or more symptoms of hyperactivity, impulsivity, or inattention. It also appeared that those subjects who continued to have the above symptoms were more likely to have conduct disorder and substance abuse.

RETROSPECTIVE STUDIES

Retrospective studies, e.g., Borland and Heckman (1976), Feldman et al. (1979), have usually not focused on the key symptoms of hyperactivity, impulsivity, and inattention but have focused on overall educational, employment, social, and emotional outcome of adults who had these symptoms in childhood.

STUDIES OF ADULTS WITH THESE AND SIMILAR SYMPTOMS

Wood and coworkers (1976) selected 15 adults from a psychiatric outpatient clinic whose main presenting complaints were impulsivity, restlessness, irritability, inattentiveness, and emotional lability. Some of these patients also had childhood histories of these symptoms, and these subjects tended to respond to stimulant treatment for the symptoms outline in adulthood.

Similarly, Mattes and colleagues (1984) selected 66 patients from an outpatient psychiatry clinic with symptoms of restlessness, excitability, impulsivity, and irritability. Twenty-nine of these subjects had similar symptoms in childhood, but unlike the Wender study (Wender et al., 1981), this fact did not predict responsiveness to stimulant medication.

FAMILY STUDIES

Generally, studies of parents and other relatives of children with symptoms of hyperactivity, impulsivity, and inattention have looked at various diagnostic categories as opposed to these specific symptoms in the adult relatives under study. These family studies were comprehensively reviewed by Hechtman (Weiss and Hechtman, 1993). As they did not focus particularly on the symptoms under discussion, they are not detailed here.

HYPERACTIVITY

Generally, the significant gross motor hyperactivity described at younger ages is much less frequent and pronounced in adulthood. Prospective studies by Weiss et al. (1985) and Gittelman et al. (1985) that have followed subjects into adulthood have shown that 35 to 40% no longer have these symptoms as adults. The symptoms of hyperactivity that are expressed usually take the form of restlessness and fidgetiness and always being on the go. Adults with these symptoms tend to gravitate toward jobs which require a good deal of physical activity (Weiss et al., 1985) (e.g., sales, construction, mechanics) as opposed to sitting at a desk. Their leisure time is also spent actively doing various sports or going from one place to another. These subjects have difficulty with any endeavor requiring long periods of inactivity, e.g., reading a long novel. During interviews adults who continued to be hyperactive were observed to be more restless and fidgety with many small muscle movements or frequent changes in their sitting positions (Weiss et al., 1985).

IMPULSIVITY

In adulthood, impulsivity is expressed socially and cognitively. Socially, it may take the form of frequent sudden changes of job or place of residence. The sudden job changes often follow some dispute with colleagues or supervisors where the subject simply suddenly quits without warning. Changes of residence similarly are frequent and sudden, often following some dispute with family or roommates.

It is difficult to pinpoint if the increased number of car accidents reflects problems of impulsivity, inattention, or both. Characteristically it is coupled with some aspects of poor judgment. Other perhaps less significant examples of impulsive actions these subjects are likely to engage in include suddenly leaving an interview, work, a movie, or a party for no apparent reason. Restlessness may be associated with this behavior, but impulsivity is a key factor. Cognitive impulsivity is reflected in a continuing cognitive style that is impulsive and somewhat disorganized. This affects problem-solving capabilities, which may then affect work performance.

The impulsivity in this age group has serious social and work consequences, as it may result in changing unstable social relationships and a poorer work record.

PROBLEMS OF ATTENTION

In adulthood, attentional problems can be seen in leisure and work activities. In terms of leisure activity, these subjects do not enjoy any-thing that requires sustained concentration or attention, e.g., reading long novels, playing chess. In the work setting, activities requiring sustained attention are often difficult, and/or boring for these individuals. They can be easily distracted, and completing such tasks quickly and accurately may present problems. At university, subjects tend to study for short periods with frequent breaks to cope with the difficulties of sustained attention.

Generally, these symptoms in adulthood continue to affect the person's work, social, and emotional adjustment. The problems result in poor self-esteem, hopelessness, depression, and anxiety and are at times accompanied by excess drug and/or alcohol use. This causes the situation to deteriorate still further. Unraveling this complex picture of pain and problems to detect the key underlying symptoms is often difficult and so these basic handicaps are frequently not thought of and remain undetected in adulthood.

NEUROBIOLOGICAL ASPECTS OF HYPERACTIVITY, IMPULSIVITY, AND INATTENTION

Generally speaking, the neurobiological aspects of the symptoms outlined have not been comprehensively worked out. Several excellent recent reviews on the subject (Jensen and Garfinkel, 1988; Mirsky, 1987; Zametkin and Rapoport, 1986, 1987) clearly illustrate the complexity of the area, the divergent findings, and the many questions yet to be resolved. The symptoms are not unidimensional and probably involve various interrelated neuroanatomic and neurochemical systems. This complexity and interrelatedness makes it unlikely that any one area or neurochemical system will be found to be solely or primarily involved in any particular symptom. What follows is a brief summary of the current evidence suggesting involvement of various neuroanatomical and neurochemical systems in different aspects of these symptoms.

The neurobiological aspects of the symptoms outlined include the following areas:

1. Neuroanatomical aspects
2. Neurochemical aspects that will address:
   Neuroanatomical aspects of neurotransmitters
   Nonpharmacological studies of neurotransmitters
   Psychopharmacological studies of neurotransmitters
   Neurotransmitter theories and neuroendocrine studies
3. Neurophysiological aspects dealing with CT, magnetic resonance imaging (MRI), positron-emission tomography (PET) scans, EEG, and evoked potential data.

Neuroanatomical Aspects

The complexity of trying to pinpoint particular neuroanatomical areas that might be involved in symptoms such as hyperactivity, impulsivity, and inattention can be best illustrated in the following example. Mirsky (1987) in his review entitled "Behavioral and Psychophysiological Markers of Disordered Attention" makes the case that attention is not a single function but has various distinct and separate aspects such as focusing, executing, sustaining, and shifting attention. He further suggests that these different functions involve different brain regions that are interconnected and organized into a system. This attentional system is so widespread that it is very vulnerable to damage and dysfunction. Depending on where the damage or dysfunction occurs, different aspects of attention may be affected (Fig. 26.1).

Specifically, Mirsky suggests that "the functions of focusing on environmental events are shared by superior temporal and inferior parietal cortices, as well as by structures that comprise the corpus striatum, including caudate, putamen, and globus pallidus. The inferior parietal and corpus striatal regions have strong motor executive functions. Considerable amounts of encoding of stimuli are accomplished by the hippocampus, an essential mnemonic function that seems to be required for some aspects of attention. The capacity to shift from one salient aspect of the environment to another is supported by the prefrontal cortex.

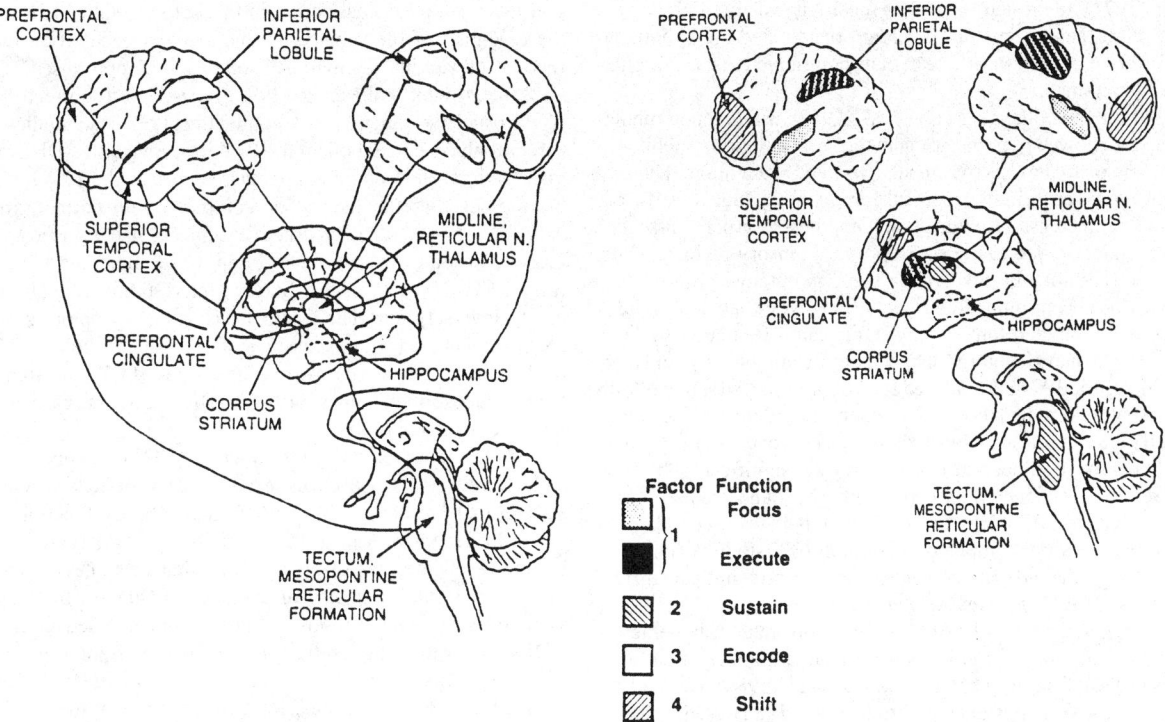

Figure 26.1. Semischematic representation of brain regions involved in attention. *Left,* Some interconnections among the regions are shown. The connections are conceivably sufficient to support the concept of an attention system. *Right,* Tentative assignment of functional specializations. (From Mirsky A: Behavioral and psychophysiological markers of disordered attention. *Environ Health Perspect* 74: 191–199, 1987.)

Sustaining a focus on some environmental event is the major responsibility of rostra structures, including the tectum, mesopontine reticular formation and midline, and reticular thalamic nuclei'' (Mirsky, 1987, p. 197). It is therefore not surprising that, in his review of the literature, Zametkin (Zametkin and Rapoport, 1987) showed that over the years a wide variety of brain areas have been implicated in these symptoms by various authors (Table 26.1).

Thus, Laufer et al. (1957), in an early description of children with symptoms of hyperactivity, impulsivity, and inattention, suggested a ''diencephalic dysfunction.'' However, as the diencephalon includes the thalamus, the hypothalamus, subthalamus and the epithalamus, it is not a very specific anatomic hypothesis. Nonetheless, the thalamus and the subthalamic nuclei are part of the basal ganglia and are important in the transmission of information regarding the initiation of motion between the basal ganglia and the motor cortex. The area is thus implicated in symptoms of hyperactivity and possibly impulsivity.

Satterfield and Dawson (1971) suggested that the hyperactivity was caused by a lower level of reticular activating system excitation. This led to the underarousal hypothesis. However, various studies addressing this hypothesis have been inconclusive.

Table 26.1. Neuroanatomical Hypotheses of Dysfunction in Attention Deficit Disorder with Hyperactivity

Investigator	Hypothesis	Test
Laufer, 1957	Diencephalic dysfunction (thalamus, hypothalamus)	Hyperactives have lower photometrazol seizure
Knobel et al., 1959	Cortical ''overfunctioning''	
Satterfield and Dawson, 1971	Decreased levels of reticular activating system excitation	See text
Wender, 1971, 1972	Decreased sensitivity in limbic areas of positive reinforcement, (medial forebrain bundle) (hypothalamus) (norepinephrine)	Multiple medication trials
Conners and Eisenberg, 1964	Lack of ''cortical inhibitory capacity''	
Dykman et al., 1971	Defect in forebrain inhibitory system over ventral formation + diencephalon	
Hunt et al., 1985	Locus ceruleus dysfunction (hypersensitive α-postsynaptic receptor)	Clonidine growth hormone response
Lou et al., 1984	Central frontal lobes, anterolateral, posterolateral Caudate region	Cerebral blood flow
Gorenstein and Newman, 1980	Dysfunction of medial septum, hippocampus orbito-frontal cortex	Animal lesion studies
Porrino et al., 1984	Nucleus acumbens	Animal studies 2-D-G studies with low-dose stimulants
Mattes, 1980	Frontal lobe	Speculation
Gualtieri and Hicks, 1985	Frontal lobe	Speculation
Arnold et al., 1977	Nigrostriatal tract	Amphetamine therapy
Chelune et al., 1986	Frontal lobe	Neuropsychiatric testing

From Zametkin A, Rapoport J: The pathophysiology of attention deficit disorder with hyperactivity: A review. *Adv Clin Child Psychol* 9:177–216, 1986.

Wender (1971) suggested decreased sensitivity of the limbic areas of positive reinforcement (medial forebrain bundle and the hypothalamus). He further proposed that these deficits contributed to the perpetuation of the symptoms.

Recently Lou and colleagues (Lou et al., 1989), using xenon inhalation techniques, showed hypoperfusion in the striatal regions of children with symptoms of hyperactivity, impulsivity, and inattention. The primary sensory and sensorimotor cortical regions were highly perfused. Methylphenidate increased flow to striatal and posterior periventricular regions and tended to decrease flow to primary sensory regions. Thus, low striatal activity may be involved in these symptoms.

The cortex has been implicated in a study by Nasrallah et al. (1986) who carried out computed tomography (CT) scans of 24 adult subjects (mean age 23) who had symptoms of hyperactivity, impulsivity, and inattention as children and 27 male matched control subjects. All subjects with the childhood symptoms had received stimulants in childhood. These subjects showed mild cerebral atrophy in adulthood. However, a large proportion of the hyperactive subjects also had a history of significant substance abuse. Therefore, it is unclear if the cortical atrophy found was associated with hyperactivity or stimulant medication or if it was secondary to chronic drug use. Previous computed tomography (CT) studies of children with similar symptoms and matched controls showed no significant differences (Caparulo et al., 1981; Shaywitz et al., 1983).

Suggestions that there may be frontal lobe involvement in hyperactivity, impulsivity, and inattention have come from a number of authors, e.g., Mattes (1980), Chelune et al. (1986), Lou et al. (1984), and Zametkin et al. (1990, 1993). For example, Lou et al. (1984) used a xenon inhalation technique in studies of cerebral blood flow in 11 children (6½–15 years) with symptoms of hyperactivity, impulsivity, and inattention and 9 normal sibling controls. All 11 children with these symptoms had central hypoperfusion in the frontal lobes, while 7 of the 11 children also had hypoperfusion of the caudate nuclei. The decreased blood flow was usually seen in areas between major arterial territories and is possibly linked to early ischemic episodes. Methylphenidate increased flow to mesencephalon and basal ganglia and decreased perfusion of motor and primary cortical areas.

Chelune et al. (1986) pointed out that the prefrontal regions of the frontal lobes had reciprocal pathways with the reticular formation and the diencephalic structures, which regulate arousal and the ability to suppress responses to task-irrelevant stimuli. Lesions in this area decrease goal-directed activity and the modulation of impulsive behavior. Thus, frontal lobe lesions result in hyperactivity and disturbed higher level cortical inhibition, with the resulting failure to inhibit inappropriate responses. The authors found partial support for this frontal lobe dysfunction hypothesis by comparing normal controls and children with symptoms of hyperactivity, impulsivity, and inattention on a comprehensive neuropsychological test battery designed to assess the above functions.

Data supporting possible frontal lobe involvement in inattention, hyperactivity, and impulsivity have also been presented by Zametkin and colleagues (1990). The authors evaluated glucose metabolism via positron emission tomography in 25 biological parents of hyperactive children. The parents had retrospective histories of childhood hyperactivity and met Utah criteria for adult attention deficit hyperactivity disorder (ADHD) but had not received any stimulant medication in childhood. The control group consisted of 50 normal subjects of similar age, sex, and IQ. Glucose brain metabolism tests were performed during a 35-minute auditory attention task. Zametkin reported that global glucose metabolism was decreased by 8.1% in the hyperactive adults versus that in controls. Specifically, in the hyperactive subjects, absolute rates of glucose metabolism were significantly low in 30 of 60 brain regions examined, including lateral, frontal, and parietal cortex (bilaterally), medial frontal cortex (including the cingulate), and some subcortical structures (the striatum and the thalamus). When the rates of glucose metabolism were normalized (i.e., regional rate of glucose metabolism was divided by global glucose metabolism rate to minimize the effect of individual variation in global glucose metabolism on regional metabolism), the only regions with significantly reduced metabolism were the

premotor and prefrontal cortex in the left hemisphere. However, since the diagnosis of the subjects in this study was based on retrospective reports, its validity is obviously somewhat compromised.

Zametkin and colleagues (1993) have tried to correct this problem of retrospective diagnosis by conducting PET scan studies measuring cerebral glucose metabolism in 10 adolescents with ADHD and 10 normal controls. He found that hyperactive girls had a 17% lower absolute brain glucose metabolism when compared with normal girls. Specifically, he showed that hyperactive subjects had significantly reduced glucose metabolism in 6 of 60 brain areas, including the left anterior frontal lobe ($P < .05$). This finding, interestingly enough, was significantly inversely correlated with measures of symptom severity ($P < .001$). Global or absolute measures of glucose metabolism did not statistically differ between the two groups. These PET scan studies suggest lower glucose metabolism in hyperactive subjects, particularly in the left anterior frontal lobe.

Other authors, e.g., Gorenstein et al. (1989), Tannock et al. (1989), and Everett et al. (1991), have also shown deficits in children with ADHD that are compatible with frontal lobe dysfunction. Recent reviews by Heilman et al. (1991) and Benson (1991), which explore a number of syndromes of abnormal mental awareness associated with prefrontal, frontal, and striatal dysfunction, suggest that abnormalities seen in these patients resemble deficits documented in children with ADHD. They thus suggest that these areas—prefrontal and right frontal-striatal systems—may be affected in children with ADHD.

We thus see that a number of different areas of the brain have been implicated in these symptoms. It is likely that different areas may be associated with different aspects of a symptom, as Mirksy (1987) has suggested for attention, and that many of the areas mentioned may be interconnected into a reciprocal modulated system, which further complicates the picture. Unravelling which areas may be affected and how these interconnections function is being explored with new neuroimaging tools, such as CT scans, MRI, and PET scans.

Neurochemical Aspects

Our understanding of the neurochemical aspects of the symptoms of hyperactivity, impulsivity, and inattention came from three general types of studies, e.g., neuroanatomical studies, nonpharmacological biochemical studies of neurotransmitters and their metabolites, and psychopharmacological studies of neurotransmitters.

NEUROANATOMICAL STUDIES OF NEUROTRANSMITTERS

Even though some areas of the brain have been clearly associated with certain neurotransmitters, e.g., caudate nucleus and corpus striatum with dopamine (Mattes, 1980) and median raphe area with serotonin (Wirtshafter et al., 1986), neuroanatomical studies of neurotransmitters have proven very complex. The complexity comes from the fact that any particular area can be involved with several different neurotransmitters or receive projections from various neurotransmitter pathways or nuclei. Thus, there is rarely a one to one correspondence between a particular area and a sole neurotransmitter that exerts exclusive influence on this area.

NONPHARMACOLOGICAL STUDIES OF NEUROTRANSMITTERS AND THEIR METABOLITES

These types of studies have compared subjects with symptoms of hyperactivity, impulsivity, and inattention and normal controls with respect to monoamines and their metabolites in urine, plasma, platelets, and rarely cerebral spinal fluid. The limitations of such peripheral measures in reflecting an accurate central nervous system neurotransmitter picture are well outlined by Zametkin and Rapoport (1986). A comprehensive review and outline of these types of studies was carried out by Zametkin and Rapoport (1987) and is summarized in Table 26.2. Generally, no consistent differences in any of the peripheral measures

Table 26.2.   Blood, Urine, and CSF Comparisons of Control and ADDH Children

Investigation	ADDH	Control	Fluid	Metabolic	Findings
Shetty and Chase, 1976	24	6	CSF	HVA, 5HIAA[a]	No difference in HVA, 5HIAA
Shaywitz et al., 1977[b]	6	16	CSF	5HIAA[a]	No difference in 5HIAA
Mikkelson et al., 1981	15	18	Serum	AO, DBH	No difference in AO, DBH
Shekim et al., 1982	8	18	Platelets	MAO	Decreased MAO in ADDH
Brown et al., 1984	18	15	Platelets	AO, MAO	Decreased AO in ADDH, no difference in MAO
Rapoport et al., 1974	35	19	Serum	NE	No difference in NE
Bhaganan et al., 1975	11	11	Serum	5HT	Decreased 5HT in ADDH
Ferguson et al., 1981	49	11	Serum	NE	No difference in NE
Coleman et al., 1971	25	—[b]	Whole blood	5HT	Decreased 5HT in ADDH
Irwin et al., 1981	55	38[c]	Platelets	5HT	No difference in 5HT
Rapoport et al., 1974	17	75	Platelets	5HIAA	No difference in 5HIAA
Wender et al., 1971	9	6	Urine	HVA	No difference
Shekim et al., 1977	7	12	Urine	HVA	No difference
Shekim et al., 1983	9	9	Urine	HVA	No difference
Shekim et al., 1983	9	9	Urine	MHPG	Decreased MHPG in ADDH
Yu-cun and Yu-feng, 1984	73	51	Urine	MHPG	Decreased MHPG in ADDH
Shekim et al., 1977	7	12	Urine	MHPG	Decreased MHPG in ADDH
Shekim et al., 1979	15	13	Urine	MHPG	Decreased MHPG in ADDH
Khan and DeKirmenjian, 1981	10	10	Urine	MHPG	Increased MHPG in ADDH
Wender et al., 1971	9	6	Urine	MHPG	No difference in ADDH
Rapoport et al., 1978	13	14	Urine	MHPG	No difference in ADDH
Rapoport et al., 1978	13	14	Urine	Dopamine	No difference in ADDH
Rapoport et al., 1978	13	14	Urine	Norepinephrine	Increased in ADDH
Shekim et al., 1977	7	12	Urine	Normetanephrine	Increased in ADDH
Zametkin et al., 1984	23	28	Urine	Phenylacetic acid	No difference in ADDH
Zametkin et al., 1984	23	28	Urine	Phenylalanine	No difference in ADDH
Zametkin et al., 1984	23	28	Urine	Tyrosine	No difference in ADDH
Zametkin et al., 1984	23	28	Urine	Phenylethylamine	Decreased ADDH

From Zametkin A, Rapoport J: Neurobiology of attention deficit disorder with hyperactivity: Where have we come from in 50 years? *J Am Acad Child Adolesc Psychiatry* 26:676–686, 1987.
[a] HVA, homovanillic acid dopamine metabolite; 5HIAA, 5-hydroxyindoleacetic acid serotonin metabolite; AO, amine oxidase; MAO. monoamine oxidase; NE, norepinephrine; 5HT, hydroxytryptamine (serotonin); HPG, 3-methoxy-4-hydroxyphenylglycol (norepinephrine metabolite).
[b] Normal values.
[c] Young adults.

of monoamines and their metabolites were found between children with these symptoms and normal control subjects.

PSYCHOPHARMACOLOGICAL STUDIES OF NEUROTRANSMITTERS

These types of studies look at the particular psychopharmacological agent, its possible relationship to one or more neurotransmitters, and its clinical effect. From such analysis it is then postulated how the drug may work and what the possible underlying problem in the neurotransmitter systems may be.

Again Zametkin and Rapoport (1987) provide an excellent review and summary of these studies (Table 26.3).

Dopamine Hypothesis

Shaywitz et al. (1977) first suggested that children with symptoms of hyperactivity, impulsivity, and inattention may have an abnormality in the brain dopamine system. The same authors (Shaywitz et al., 1976) proposed an animal model of hyperactivity in rats whose brains were dopamine depleted by injection of hydroxydopamine (6-OHDA).

Dopamine agonists, which stimulate postsynaptic dopamine receptors, e.g., piribedil, amantadine, L-dopa, have been ineffective in children with these symptoms, and dopamine blocking agents, e.g., antipsychotics, have not been particularly detrimental. However, stimulants (dextroamphetamine, methylphenidate, and pemoline) affect both the dopamine and norepinephrine systems and are very effective in ameliorating these symptoms.

It has been suggested (Lou et al., 1989) that methylphenidate activates dopamine neurons by decreasing the reuptake of dopamine. Thus, some dopamine involvement can be hypothesized.

Noradrenergic Hypothesis

The noradrenergic system has been implicated in a number of ways. Stimulants, particularly dextroamphetamine have reduced the urinary excretion of 3-methoxy-4-hydroxyphenylglycol (MHPG), a metabolite of norepinephrine (Brown et al., 1981).

A norepinephrine agonist, clonidine (an α-adrenergic agonist), has been somewhat effective in treating symptoms of hyperactivity, impulsivity, and inattention (Hunt et al., 1984). Hunt and colleagues (1984) have suggested that the effectiveness of clonidine is mediated by direct stimulation of presynaptic sites to decrease production or release of norepinephrine and corresponding increase in postsynaptic noradrenergic sensitivity. Because chronic methylphenidate treatment decreases receptor response to clonidine, the authors (Hunt et al., 1984) believe that the drug may normalize neurotransmitter production and receptor sensitivity. Furthermore, the moderate effectiveness of some antidepressants, e.g., desipramine (Donnelly et al., 1986), and some monoamine oxidase inhibitors also suggest drug-induced changes in noradrenergic metabolism.

Serotonergic Hypothesis

Suggestions for this hypothesis come from the fact that serotonin-depleted animals show increased aggression and hyperactivity. In addition, hyperactive subjects have shown inconsistent changes in platelet and blood 5-hydroxytryptophan (serotonin). The hypothesis was supported by results of drug studies involving tricyclic antidepressants and monoamine oxidase inhibitors, which affect serotonin metabolism and are moderately effective with the symptoms of hyperactivity, impulsivity, and inattention. However, pharmacological studies involving L-tryptophan, a serotonin precursor (Nemzer et al., 1986), and fenfluramine, which acutely increases and then depletes brain serotonin, showed no consistent results.

Nonspecific Catecholamine Hypothesis

It is clear from the foregoing discussion on specific neurotransmitter systems that not one but several neurotransmitter systems are involved. Currently, the norepinephrine system seems most involved, followed

Table 26.3. Pharmacologic Probes of Attention Deficit Disorder with Hyperactivity

	Very Effective[a]		Moderately Effective		Minimally Effective	
Dopamine						
Agonist			L-dopa (Langer ry sl. (1982)	N = 8	Piribidel (Brown et al., 1979a)	N = 8
Antagonist			Haloperidol (Winsberg and Yepes, 1978)		Amantadine (Mattes and Gittelman, 1979)	N = 9
			Thioridazine (Werry, 1970)	N > 50 N = 39		
			Chlorpromazine (Werry et al., 1966)	N = 39		(41)
Norepinephrine			Desipramine (Garfinkle et al., 1983; Donnelly et al., 1986)	N = 28 N =	Mianserin (Langer et al., 1984)	N = 5 (54)
			Imipramine (Rapoport et al., 1974; Winsberg and Yepes, 1978)	N = 29 N = 29		
			Clomipramine (Garfinkle et al., 1983)	N = 11		
Both NE and DA[b]	Dextroamphetamine Pemoline Methylphenidate (Cantwell and Carlson, 1978)	N > 100 N > 75 N > 100				
NE and DA MAO A-I	Clorgyline (Zametkin et al., 1985c)	N = 6				
MAOI B	Tranylcypromine (Zametkin et al., 1985c)	N = 8				
MAOI A + B					Deprenyl[a] (Donnelly, personal communication)	N = 14
Serotonin					Fenfluramine[a] (Donnelly, personal communication)	N = 9
					L-Tryptophan[a] (Brown et al., personal communication)	N = 13
					L-Tryptophan (Nemzer et al., 1986)	N = 15

From Zametkin A, Rapoport J: The pathophysiology of attention deficit disorder with hyperactivity: A review. *Adv Clin Child Psychol* 9:177–216, 1986.
[a] On measures of behavior.

by the dopaminergic system, with the serotonergic system being less involved. Stimulants, which are the most effective treatment, promote catecholamine utilization in the synapse by facilitating synthesis and release of the catecholamines and by blocking their reuptake. Furthermore, stimulants appear to inhibit the catabolic monoamine oxidase enzyme. A summary of various neurotransmitter systems and how they may be affected by various drugs was presented by Zametkin and Rapoport (1986) and is seen in Figure 26.2.

The interrelationship of the various neurotransmitter systems further supports the unlikelihood of a single neurotransmitter hypothesis.

Enzymatic regulation of neurotransmitter production and metabolism have also been investigated. Children with these symptoms and normal children have shown no significant differences in levels of dopamine β-hydroxylase (DBH), monoamine oxidase (MAO), and catechol-*o*-methyltransferase (COMT) (Brown et al., 1985).

Other Neurotransmitters

One should note that other neurotransmitters such as γ-aminobutyric acid (GABA), which is thought to be predominantly an inhibiting neurotransmitter in the central nervous system, and histamine, which acts centrally and peripherally, have not been studied in relation to the symptoms outlined, but may be implicated in the future.

Neuroendocrine Aspects

The interest in neuroendocrine aspects in children with symptoms of hyperactivity, impulsivity, and inattention comes from two main but interrelated areas. The preceding discussion suggested that norepinephrine dopamine and serotonin may be involved in the symptoms described. However, these same neurotransmitters are known to affect hormone production and release in the anterior pituitary and thus affect the hypothalamic-pituitary-adrenal axis, the hypothalamic pituitary-thyroid axis, and the hypothalamic pituitary growth hormone axis. Reports of possible growth suppression in children given stimulants to treat symptoms of hyperactivity, impulsivity, and inattention has resulted in considerable interest in the growth hormone axis in these children. A number of studies looked at growth hormone levels in children with these symptoms on and off stimulant medication and matched normal control subjects. In a series of studies, Greenhill and colleagues (1981) showed no change in sleep-related pattern of human growth hormone secretion before or after treatment with *d*-amphetamine. An insulin tolerance test also showed no differences in growth hormone response. However, boys who received long-term methylphenidate treatment for their symptoms showed elevations of sleep-related growth hormone when compared to normal controls (Greenhill et al., 1984). Shaywitz et al. (1982) looked at hyperactive children treated with methylphenidate and found that growth hormone levels increased with plasma levels of methylphenidate, both peaking at the same time. Garfinkel, exploring the effect of *d*-amphetamine in hyperactive adolescents, found that growth hormone response in these subjects was greater than that of normal controls and that it peaked at the point of maximal absorption and clinical effect of the amphetamine (Garfinkel et al., 1986). Weizman et al. (1987) studied the effects of acute and chronic methylphenidate administration on β-endorphin, growth hormone, prolactin, and cortisol levels in children with these symptoms. They found that, with chronic use of methylphenidate, growth hormone challenge tests were augmented. Hunt and colleagues (1984) demonstrated growth hormone response to clonidine administration in similar children.

The complexity of the neuroendocrine issue has been well illustrated by Jensen and Garfinkel (1988), who looked at prepubescent and pubertal hyperactive and control children and measured their growth hormone response to L-dopa and clonidine challenges. They found that the growth hormone response was lower in the prepubescent children and also less to the L-dopa than the clonidine challenge. In addition, the response in the hyperactive children was lower than that in controls. This clearly suggests that both the dopamine and norepinephrine systems are involved in growth hormone release and that this process is affected by pubertal development and stimulant medication.

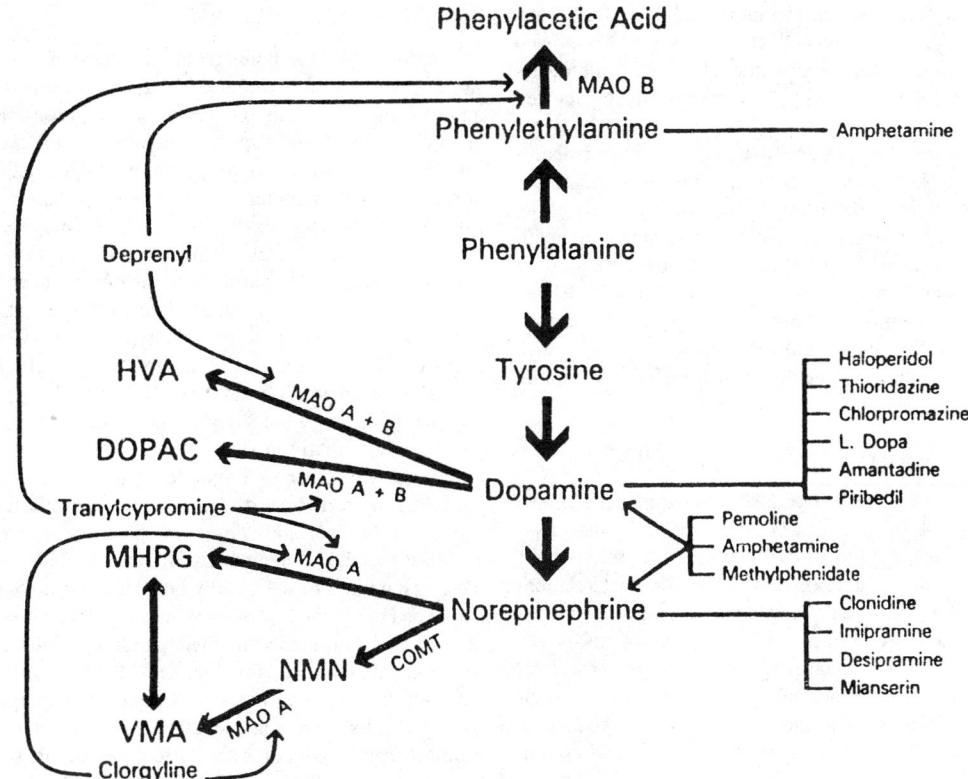

Figure 26.2. Presumed effect of drugs that have been studied with hyperactive children. *HVA*, homovanillic acid; *DOPAC*, 3,4-dihydroxyphenylacetic acid; *MHPG*, 3-methoxy-4-hydroxyphenylglycol; *VMA*, vanillylmandelic acid; *COMT*, catechol-*o*-methyl transferase; *MAO*, monoamine oxidase. (From Zametkin A, Rapoport J: The pathophysiology of attention-deficit disorder with hyperactivity: A review. *Adv Clin Child Psychol* 9:179, 1986.)

Neurophysiological Aspects

In an effort to determine whether neuronal responses differ significantly in children with symptoms of hyperactivity, impulsivity, and inattention, researchers have examined the central and peripheral neural conducting responses in children with these symptoms. Centrally, these studies have involved electroencephalograms and evoked potential recordings, and peripherally they have focused on motoneuron excitability. In reviewing many of these neurophysiological studies (Weiss and Hechtman, 1993), one is struck by the variability of the findings and the difficulty in coming to firm conclusions.

It has been estimated (Cantwell, 1980) that 35–50% of children with the symptoms outlined may have abnormal EEGs. The most common abnormality reported involves diffuse nonspecific changes and extensive slow EEG activity (Grunwald-Zuberbier et al., 1975; Satterfield et al., 1974). Shetty (1973) indicated that, in his series of 75 hyperactive subjects, the most consistent abnormality was the absence of an appropriate amount of well-organized alpha waves for age.

Another EEG abnormality that has been described in hyperactive children involves difficulties with attenuation of alpha waves, which presumably reflect the decreased capacity of these children to stop attending to redundant events (Fuller, 1977).

All of the above abnormalities have been described as immature patterns and interpreted as representing delayed CNS maturation in these children. Some support for this hypothesis was provided by Hechtman and colleagues (1978) when they compared sequential EEG of hyperactive children, adolescents, and young adults and found increasing normalization of EEGs of subjects with increasing age, particularly in late adolescence.

Evoked potential studies have been inconclusive, giving conflicting results. Thus, Satterfield (1973) reported that the auditory evoked potentials in hyperactive subjects had longer latencies and lower amplitudes compared with age-matched controls. On the other hand Buchsbaum and Wender (1973), studying visual and auditory average evoked responses, showed increased latencies and higher amplitudes with increases in intensity of visual stimuli. Age- and sex-matched control subjects showed lesser increases in amplitude and decreases in latency. Hall et al. (1976), recording evoked potentials in response to four stimulus intensities under conditions of attention and inattention, found no differences in stability, amplitude, or latency between hyperactive children and control children. Most of these studies recorded evoked potentials at one or, at most, a few electrode sites.

Recently, Satterfield et al. (1988) conducted a study on 20 6-year-old children with attentional problems and 20 matched normal control subjects, using 19 recording sites and two choice discrimination tasks. They concluded that the children with attentional problems had abnormalities in the mismatch process, resulting in poor discrimination of salient stimuli. This is an automatic process not under voluntary control. It is thought to be a component of a basic orienting response that is mediated via the reticular activating system of the norepinephrine system in unanesthetized animals (Aston-Jones, 1985). A second abnormality found by Satterfield involved frontal processing negativity, reflecting additional processing (e.g., rehearsing of the standard in memory) of the attended stimulus. This activity is thought to be under voluntary control. Thus, the multisite recording studies illustrate the greater complexity of these functions.

Halliday and colleagues (1983) investigated the effect of methylphenidate on visual evoked potential in hyperactive children and concluded that the evoked response potential measures were more sensitive to age and attention conditions and less to methylphenidate dose.

Peripheral studies that have looked at motoneural excitability also give conflicting results. Thus, Pivik and colleagues (1986) showed that some hyperactive children had significantly elevated, while others had significantly depressed, responses when compared to matched controls.

The divergent inconsistent and inconclusive findings of these neurophysiological events may be related to the fact that one is attempting to understand complex, multifaceted central processes via fairly gross and perhaps nonspecific peripheral measures. Recent technological advances, which include measures of cerebral blood flow and glucose utilization, and positron emitting liquids that can quantitate and label specific neurotransmitter receptors will enable researchers to examine the functions of hyperactivity, impulsivity, and inattention with much greater precision centrally and peripherally and hopefully will more fully illuminate the many questions that still remain.

CONTRIBUTING PSYCHOSOCIAL FACTORS

In this section we discuss possible psychosocial factors that can give rise to or complicate symptoms of hyperactivity, impulsivity, and inattention. Furthermore, these symptoms can significantly affect one's emotional, social, and academic development. It is clear that relationships with parents, teachers, and peers, academic success, and self-esteem are all directly or indirectly influenced by these symptoms. Needless to say, these social and emotional parameters may in turn affect self-esteem and motivation and further augment the handicaps associated with the primary symptoms. Thus, the biological, social, academic, and emotional spheres are all interrelated and significantly and continually influence each other.

Environmental Factors

PHYSICAL ENVIRONMENT

It has been suggested that the physical environment may significantly contribute to the development and/or worsening of symptoms of hyperactivity, impulsivity, and inattention. Some authors (Needleman, 1983) have suggested that children living in environments where they are exposed to high lead levels are more likely to develop such symptoms. Some food additives may contribute to the development of these symptoms in a small subgroup of children who have an idiosyncratic reaction to these substances (Conners, 1980; Feingold, 1975). It is unclear how significant a physically chaotic environment may be in contributing to the development of these symptoms, though such an environment is certainly important in maintaining and augmenting these difficulties.

The prevalence of children with hyperactivity, impulsivity, and inattention is greater in disadvantaged, large inner city environments. However, such settings also have more poverty, malnutrition, poor prenatal, paranatal, and neonatal health care, and more family disturbance and disruption, including drug and alcohol abuse and family violence. Any one or any combination of these factors may also play a significant contributory role in the development and perpetuation of these symptoms.

Similarly, a school or classroom setting that is very unstructured and/or disorganized has a detrimental effect on children with these symptoms, causing their behavior to deteriorate and their learning and academic achievement to be significantly impaired.

EMOTIONAL-SOCIAL ENVIRONMENT

Taylor (1985) has pointed out the importance of cultural, social, and family variables in learning to focus attention and control impulsivity and hyperactivity. This process of socialization may be influenced by characteristics of the parents, the child, and the reciprocal interactions that develop between them. Increased psychopathology has been reported in parents of children with hyperactivity, impulsivity, and inattention (Morrison 1980; Stewart et al., 1980). This may suggest the genetic vulnerability of these children, but it may also result in problematic parenting, which can contribute to the development and/or perpetuation of these symptoms in the child. Parenting styles of parents whose children have symptoms of hyperactivity, impulsivity, and inattention have been looked at by number of authors (Campbell, 1973; Humphries et al., 1978; Mash and Johnston, 1982). Generally these researchers found that parenting styles tended to be more intrusive, controlling, and disapproving (particularly in structured tasks as opposed to free play) when compared with parents of age-matched normal controls. This negative parenting style improved significantly when the child's behavior improved because of stimulant medication treatment (Humphries et al., 1978). It was thus concluded by Humphries et al. (1978) that the parents were responding ot the child's behavior and not causing it. Mash and Johnston (1983) showed that having a child with these difficulties affects the parents' confidence in their parenting skills and results in more reported stress, social isolation, self-blame, and depression in the parents. We can thus clearly see the effects of this negative parenting style on the child's emotional development, competence, and self-esteem. Similarly, the child's problems affect the parents sense of effectiveness and emotional well being, which in turn reverberates in their interactions and relationship with their child. The same vicious cycle of negative interactions, stress, and sense of failure for both child and teacher can get set up in the school with similar detrimental effects.

It has been suggested that the symptoms of hyperactivity, impulsivity, and inattention may be expressions of underlying anxiety and/or depression. Tizard and Hodges (1978) showed that overactivity and inattention were prominent in children growing up in institutions. It is thus hypothesized that the underlying anxiety resulting from lack of secure and stable relationships is expressed via these symptoms. Similarly, children raised in a disturbed family environment may experience similar insecurities and anxieties and express these feelings in a similar way. Children can show symptoms of hyperactivity, impulsivity, and inattention during acute periods of stress. However, these periods are usually of short duration (a few days or weeks), and the stress is usually readily identifiable, e.g., parental separation, a new sibling.

For children who live in chronically stressful multiproblem circumstances, it becomes difficult to delineate whether the symptoms reflect expression of underlying anxiety and/or depression, a problem in parenting and socialization, a genetically influenced biological problem, or some interaction of a number of these factors.

Relatively little research has addressed the psychosocial versus the biological aspects of these symptoms. The combination and interrelationship of both of these aspects has received even less attention. It is hoped that with current technological advances and our greater ability to look at such problems in a more multifaceted way, we will gain a clearer, more comprehensive understanding of the possible etiology, development, and treatment of symptoms of hyperactivity, impulsivity, and inattention.

References

Abikoff H: An evaluation of cognitive behavior therapy for hyperactive children. In: Lahey BB, Kazdin AE (eds): *Advances in Clinical Child Psychology*. New York, Plenum, 10:171–216, 1987.

Aston-Jones G: Behavioral functions of locus ceruleus derived from cellular attributes. *Physiol Psychol* 13:118–126, 1985.

Benson F: Role of frontal dysfunction in attention deficit hyperactivity disorder. *J Child Neurol* (Suppl) 6:S9–S12, 1991.

Borland B, Heckman H: Hyperactive boys and their brothers: A 25 year follow up study. *Arch Gen Psychiatry* 33:669–679, 1976.

Brown GL, Ebert MH, Hunt RD, et al: Urinary 3-methoxy-4-hydroxyphenyl glycol and homovanillic acid response to *d*-amphetamine in hyperactive children. *Biol Psychiatry* 16:779–787, 1981.

Brown GL, Ebert MH, Minichiello MD: Bio-

chemical and pharmacological aspects of attention deficit disorder. In: Bloomingdale LM (ed): *Attention Deficit Disorder Identification, Course and Treatment Rationale*. New York, Spectrum, 1985, pp. 93–130.

Buchsbaum M, Wender PH: Average evoked response in normal and minimally brain dysfunctioned children treated with amphetamine: A preliminary report. *Arch Gen Psychiatry* 29:764–770, 1973.

Campbell SB: Mother-infant interaction in reflective, impulsive and hyperactive children. *Dev Psychol* 8:341–349, 1973.

Campbell SB, Szumowski EK, Ewingh JM, et al: A multidimensional assessment of parent-identified behavior problem toddlers. *J Abnorm Child Psychol* 10:569–592, 1982.

Cantwell DP: Drug and medical intervention. In: Rie HE, Rie ED (eds): *Handbook of Minimal Brain Dysfunction. A Critical Review.* New York, Wiley, 1980.

Caparulo B, Cohen D, Rothman S, et al: Computed tomographic brain scanning in children with developmental neuropsychiatric disorders. *J Am Acad Child Psychiatry* 20:339, 1981.

Chelune GJ, Ferguson W, Koon R, et al: Frontal lobe disinhibition in attention deficit disorder. *Child Psychiatry Hum Dev* 16:221–232, 1986.

Clouston TS: *Clinical Lectures on Mental Health* (3rd ed). London, Churchill, 1982.

Conners CK: *Food Additives and Hyperactive Children.* New York, Plenum, 1980.

Davidson EM, Prior MR: Laterality and selective attention in hyperactive children. *J Abnorm Child Psychol* 6:475–481, 1978.

Dobzhansky T: On types, genotypes and the genetic diversity in populations. In: Spuhler JN (ed): *Genetic Diversity and Human Behavior.* Chicago, Aldine, 1967.

Donnelly M, Zametkin AJ, Rapoport JL, et al: Treatment of hyperactivity with desipramine: Plasma drug concentration, cardiovascular effects, plasma and urinary catecholamine levels, and clinical response. *Clin Pharmacol Ther* 39:72–81, 1986.

Eisenberg L: The management of the hyperkinetic child. *Dev Med Child Neurol* 8:593–632, 1966.

Everett J, Thomas J, Cote F, et al: Cognitive effects of psychostimulant medication in hyperactive children. *Child Psychiatr Hum Dev* 22:79–87, 1991.

Feingold BF: Hyperkinesis and learning disabilities linked to artificial food flavors and colors. *Am J Nurs* 75:797–803, 1975.

Feldman S, Denhoff E, Denhoff E: The attention disorders and related syndromes outcome in adolescence and young adult life. In: Denhoff E, Shenker L (eds): *Minimal Brain Dysfunction: A Developmental Approach.* New York, Masson, 1979, pp. 133–148.

Freedman DG, Keller B: Inheritance of behavior in infants. *Science* 140:196–198, 1963.

Fuller PW: Computer estimated alpha attenuation during problem solving in children and learning disabilities. *Electroencephalogr Clin Neurophysiol* 42:148–156, 1977.

Garfinkel BD, Brown WA, Klee SH, et al: Neuroendocrine and cognitive response to amphetamine in adolescents with a history of attention deficit disorder. *J Am Acad Child Adolesc Psychiatry* 25:503–508, 1986.

Gesell A: Early evidence of individuality in human infant. *Sci Monthly* 45:217–225, 1937.

Gittelman R, Mannuzza S, Shenker R, et al: Hyperactive boys almost grown up: Psychiatric status. *Arch Gen Psychiatry* 42:937–947, 1985.

Gittelman-Klein R: Prognosis of attention deficit disorder and its management in adolescence. *Pediatr Rev* 8:216–223, 1987.

Gorenstein EE, Mammato CA, Sandy JM: Performance of inattentive-overactive children on selected measures of prefrontal-type function. *J Clin Psychol* 45:619–632, 1989.

Greenhill LL, Puig-Antich J, Chambers W, et al: Growth hormone prolactin and growth responses in hyperkinetic males: Treatment with d-amphetamine. *J Am Acad Child Psychiatry* 20:84–103, 1981.

Greenhill LL, Puig-Antich J, Novacenko H, et al: Prolactin growth hormone and growth responses in boys with attention deficit disorder and hyperac-

tivity treatment with methylphenidate. *J Am Acad Child Psychiatry* 23:58–67, 1984.

Grunwald-Zuberbier E, Grunewald G, Rasche A: Hyperactive behavior and EEG arousal reactions in children. *Electroencephalogr Clin Neurophysiol* 38:149–159, 1975.

Hall RA, Griffin RB, Moyer DL, et al: Evoked potential stimulus intensity and drug treatment in hyperkinesis. *Psychophysiology* 13:405–418, 1976.

Halliday R, Callaway E, Naylor H: Visual evoked potential changes induced by methylphenidate in hyperactive children: Dose/response effects. *Electroencephalogr Clin Neurophysiol* 55:258–267, 1983.

Hechtman L, Weiss G, Metrakos K: Hyperactive individuals as young adults. Current and longitudinal electroencephalographic evaluation and its relationship to outcome. *Can Med Assoc J* 118:919–923, 1978.

Heilman KM, Voeller KS, Nadeau SE: A possible pathophysiologic substrate of attention deficit hyperactivity disorder. *J Child Neurol* (Suppl) 6:S76–S81, 1991.

Humphries T, Kinsbourne M, Swanson J: Stimulant effects on cooperation and social interaction between hyperactive children and their mothers. *J Child Psychol Psychiatry* 19:13–22, 1978.

Hunt RD, Cohen DJ, Anderson G, et al: Possible changes in noradrenergic receptor sensitivity following methylphenidate treatment. Growth hormone and MHIG response to clonidine challenge in children with attention deficit disorder and hyperactivity. *Life Sci* 35:885–897, 1984.

Jensen JB, Garfinkel BD: Neuroendocrine aspects of attention deficit hyperactivity disorder. *Endocrinol Metab Clin North Am* 17:111–129, 1988.

Kagan J, Rasman BL, Day D, et al: Information processing in the child: Significance of analytic and reflective attitudes. *Psychol Monogr* 78:1 (whole no. 578), 1964.

Klein AR, Young RD: Hyperactive boys in their classroom: Assessment of teacher and peer perceptions, interactions and classroom behavior. *J Abnorm Child Psychol* 7:425–442, 1979.

Lambert N, Hartsaugh C, Sassone D, et al: Persistence of hyperactivity symptoms from childhood to adolescence and associated outcomes. *Am J Orthopsychiatry* 57:22–31, 1987.

Laufer MW, Denhoff E: Hyperkinetic behavior syndrome in children. *J Pediatr* 50:463–474, 1957.

Laufer NW, Denhoff E, Solomon G: Hyperkinetic impulse disorder in children's behavior problems. *Psychosom Med* 19:38–49, 1957.

Lewis AJ: Psychopathic personality: A most elusive category. *Psychol Med* 4:133–140, 1974.

Lou HC, Henriken L, Bruhn P: Focal cerebral hyperperfusion in children with dysphasia and/or attention deficit disorder. *Arch Neurol* 41:825–829, 1984.

Lou HC, Henriksen L, Bruhn P, et al: Striatal dysfunction in attention deficit and hyperkinetic disorder. *Arch Neurol* 46:48–52, 1989.

Mash EJ, Johnston C: A comparison of the mother-child interactions of younger and older hyperactive and normal children. *Child Dev* 53:1371–1381, 1982.

Mash EJ, Johnston C: Parental perceptions of child behavior problems, parenting, self-esteem and mother's reported stress in younger and older hyperactives and normal children. *J Consult Clin Psychol* 51:86–99, 1983.

Mattes JA: The role of frontal lobe dysfunction in childhood hyperkinesis. *Compr Psychiatry* 21:358–369, 1980.

Mattes J, Boswell L, Oliver H: Methylphenidate effects on symptoms of attention deficit disorder in adults. *Arch Gen Psychiatry* 41:1059–1063, 1984.

Mirsky A: Behavioral and psychophysiological markers of disordered attention. *Environ Health Perspect* 74:191–199, 1987.

Morrison JR: Adult psychiatric disorders in parents of hyperactive children. *Am J Psychiatry* 137:825–827, 1980.

Nasrallah HA, Loney J, Olsen SC, et al: Cortical atrophy in young adults. *Psychiatry Res* 17:241–243, 1986.

Needleman H: The neuropsychological consequences of low level exposure to lead in childhood. In: Rutter M, Russell Jones R (eds): *Lead versus Health; Sources and Effects of Low Level Lead Exposure.* England, Chichester, Wiley, 1983, pp. 229–248.

Nemzer ED, Arnold LE, Votolato NA, et al: Amino acid supplementation as therapy for attention deficit disorder. *J Am Acad Child Adolesc Psychiatry* 25:509–513, 1986.

Pivik RT, Bylsma FW, Margithai K: Abnormal motoneural excitability in hyperkinetic children. *Psychophysiology* 23:146–155, 1986.

Porrino CJ, Rapoport JL, Behar D, et al: A naturalistic assessment of the motor activity of hyperactive boys in comparison with normal boys. *Arch Gen Psychiatry* 40:681–687, 1983.

Quinn PO, Rapoport JL: Minor physical anomalies and neurological status in hyperactive boys. *Pediatrics* 53:742–747, 1974.

Radosh A, Gittelman R: The effect of appealing distractors on the performance of hyperactive children. *J Abnorm Child Psychol* 9:179–189, 1981.

Rutter M, Korn S, Birch H: Genetic and environmental factors in development of primary reaction patterns. *Br J Clin Psychol* 2:161–173, 1963.

Satterfield JH: EEG issues in children with minimal brain dysfunction. *Semin Psychiatry* 5:35–46, 1973.

Satterfield JH, Dawson ME: Electrodermal correlates of hyperactivity in children. *Psychophysiology* 18:191–197, 1971.

Satterfield JH, Cantwell DP, Saul RE, et al: Intelligence, academic achievement and EEG abnormalities in hyperactive children. *Am J Psychiatry* 133:391–395, 1974.

Satterfield JH, Schell AM, Nicholas T, et al: Topographic study of auditory event-related potentials in normal boys and boys with attention deficit disorder and hyperactivity. *Psychophysiology* 25:591–606, 1988.

Schleifer M, Weiss G, Cohen NJ, et al: Hyperactivity in the preschooler and the effect of methylphenidate. *Am J Orthopsychiatry* 45:38–50, 1975.

Shaywitz BA, Cohen DJ, Bower MB: CSF monoamine metabolites in children with minimal brain dysfunction: Evidence of alteration of brain dopamine, a preliminary report. J Pediatr 90:671–677, 1977.

Shaywitz BA, Shaywitz SE, Byrne T, et al: Attention deficit disorder—Quantitative analysis of CT. *Neurology* 33:1500, 1983.

Shaywitz BA, Yager RD, Klopper JH: Selective brain dopamine depletion in developing rats. *Science* 191:305–308, 1976.

Shaywitz SE, Hunt RD, Jatlow P, et al: Psychopharmacology of attention deficit disorder. Pharmacokinetic, neuroendocrine and behavioral measures following acute and chronic treatment with methylphenidate. *Pediatrics* 96:688–694, 1982.

Shetty T: Some neurologic, electrophysiologic and biochemical correlates of the hyperactive syndrome. *Pediatr Ann* 29:29–38, 1973.

Stewart MA, de Blois CS, Cummings C: Psychiatric disorder in parents of hyperactive boys and those with conduct disorder. *J Child Psychol Psychiatry* 21:283–292, 1980.

Tannock R, Schachar RJ, Carr RP, et al: Effects of methylphenidate on inhibitory control in hyperactive children. *J Abnorm Child Psychol* 17:473–491, 1989.

Taylor E: *Attention Deficit in Primary School Children*. Paper presented at 10th Congress of International Association of Child and Adolescent Psychiatry and Allied Professions, Dublin, 1982.

Taylor E: Syndromes of overactivity and attention deficit. In: Rutter M, Hersow L (eds): *Child and Adolescent Psychiatry*. London, Blackwell, 1985, pp. 424–443.

Thomas A, Chess S, Birch HG: *Temperament and Behavior Disorders in Children*. New York, New York University Press, 1968.

Tizard B, Hodges J: The effect of early institutional rearing on the development of 8 year old children. *J Child Psychol Psychiatry* 19:99–118, 1978.

Torgersen AM, Kringlen E: Genetic aspects of temperamental differences in infants: Their causes as shown through twin studies. *J Am Acad Child Adolesc Psychiatry* 17:433–444, 1978.

Vandenberg SG: Contributions of twin research to psychology. In: Manosevitz M, Lindzey G, Thiessen DD (eds): *Behavioral Genetics, Century Psychology Series*. New York, Appleton-Century-Croft, 1969.

Waldrop MF, Bell RQ, McLaughlin B, et al: Newborn minor physical anomalies predict short attention span, peer aggression and impulsivity at age 3. *Science* 199:563–565, 1978.

Waldrop M, Pederson FA, Bell RQ: Minor physical anomalies and behavior in preschool children. *Child Dev* 39:391–400, 1968.

Weiss G, Hechtman L: *Hyperactive Children Grown Up* (2nd ed). New York, Guilford Press, 1993.

Weiss G, Hechtman L, Milroy T, et al: Psychiatric status of hyperactives as adults: A controlled prospective 15 year follow up of 65 hyperactive children. *J Am Acad Child Psychiatry* 23:211–220, 1985.

Weizman R, Dick J, Gil-Ad I, et al: Effects of acute and chronic methylphenidate administration on B-endorphin, growth hormone, prolactin and cortisol in children with attention deficit and hyperactivity. *Life Sci* 40:2247–2252, 1987.

Wender P: *The Minimal Brain Dysfunction Syndrome in Children*. New York, Wiley, 1971, pp. 163–191.

Wender P, Reimher F, Wood D: Attention deficit disorder in adults. *Arch Gen Psychiatry* 38:449–456, 1981.

Wirtshafter D, Montana W, Asin KE: Behavioral and biochemical studies of the substrates of median raphe lesion induced hyperactivity. *Physiol Behav* 38:751–759, 1986.

Wood D, Reimher F, Wender P, et al: Diagnosis and treatment of MBD in adults. *Arch Gen Psychiatry* 33:1453–1460, 1976.

Zametkin A, Rapoport J: The pathophysiology of attention deficit disorder with hyperactivity: A review. *Adv Clin Child Psychol* 9:177–216, 1986.

Zametkin AJ, Rapoport J: Neurobiology of attention deficit disorder with hyperactivity: Where have we come in 50 years? *J Am Acad Child Adolesc Psychiatry* 26:676–686, 1987.

Zametkin AJ, Liebenauer LI, Fitzgerald GA, et al: Brain metabolism in teenagers with ADHD. *Arch Gen Psychiatry* 50:333–340, 1993.

Zametkin AJ, Nordahl TE, Gross M, et al: Cerebral glucose metabolism in adults with hyperactivity of childhood onset. *N Engl J Med* 323:1361–1366, 1990.

27 DEVELOPMENT OF THE SYMPTOM OF VIOLENCE

Dorothy Otnow Lewis, M.D.

What sort of animal are we? For millennia, priests, poets, philosophers, and scientists have grappled with this question. Are we born sinful or do we come into the world in a state of innocence, "trailing clouds of glory" (Wordsworth, 1802–1804)? Are we then corrupted by society (Rousseau, 1754)? Is our aggression simply a response to frustration (Dollard et al., 1939) or is it an inherent characteristic, a basic drive that will find expression one way or another (Freud, 1922; Lorenz, 1966)? Or do we arrive on the planet a blank slate on which different experiences will make their mark and thereby chart our course for better or for worse (Locke, 1690)? Are we all "created equal," or are some of us inherently more aggressive than others? How does one begin to answer these kinds of questions from a psychobiological rather than a religious or philosophical perspective?

Human behaviors and motivations are extremely complex. Animal behaviors, however, are more stereotyped and thus easier to classify and study. For example, Moyer (1971) has categorized animal aggressive behaviors as follows: predatory, intramale, fear induced, irritable, territorial, maternal, and instrumental. Flynn and colleagues (1970) condensed these 7 types of aggression into two categories, affective and predatory. Affective aggression, which includes, intramale, fear induced, irritable, territorial, and maternal, involves intense activation of the sympathetic nervous system. There is an increase in blood pressure, piloerection, pupillary dilation, and threatening behaviors. Predatory aggression, on the other hand, evokes little autonomic activation. The predatory animal silently stalks its prey, then expediently subdues it in the interest of securing fast food. Others have divided animal behaviors into offensive and defensive (Blanchard and Blanchard, 1977) and spontaneous versus conditioned (Thompson, 1969).

Human behaviors are so complex that we cannot even agree on what we mean when we speak of human aggression. Are we referring to the kinds of activities that led to the takeover of RCA by Mitsubishi? Or are we talking about behaviors of the Hutu and Tutsi in Rwanda? The Serbs and Moslems in Bosnia? Are we discussing the behaviors of John D. Rockefeller or Jack the Ripper? Leona Helmsley or Lizzie Borden? Whether considering the acts of moguls or murderers, human aggressive behavior defies simple categorization.

For purposes of this chapter, the term *human aggression* is used simply to denote behaviors by one person intended to cause physical pain, damage, or destruction to another. It is not used as a synonym for assertiveness or ambitiousness.

INTRINSIC OR BIOLOGICAL CONTRIBUTIONS TO AGGRESSIVE BEHAVIOR

We know that each human being enters the world with his or her unique temperamental characteristics (Chess and Thomas, 1984). A word of caution: Intrinsic does not necessarily mean genetic. Much occurs during the 9 months preceding birth that may affect our abilities to adapt peacefully to our environment. Some infants are calm, relaxed, at ease; some are tense, irritable, and hard to comfort. Whereas some infants are relatively unfazed by major vicissitudes in their surroundings, others are reduced to temper tantrums by minor changes. Clearly, we are not initially identical blank slates; the same squeaky chalk will feel more abrasive to some of us than to others.

However, early temperament does not necessarily presage later aggressiveness. Frequent temper tantrums prior to 3 years of age are thought not to be predictive of a life of violent crime. However, some studies suggest that frequent aggressive behaviors that occur after 3 years of age are often associated with ongoing behavior problems and interpersonal difficulties (Farrington, 1978; Kagan and Moss, 1962). Others have reported that a sizeable minority of children manifesting problems with aggression at 8 years of age will have similar problems in adolescence and adulthood (Farrington, 1978; Lefkowitz et al., 1977; McFarlane et al., 1954; West and Farrington, 1973.) Thus, there is some evidence of a continuity of aggressive behavior over time. Nevertheless, the fact that the earliest manifestations of aggression (e.g. infantile temper tantrums) are not predictive of later behaviors, and the fact that the majority of aggressive young children adapt normally, suggest that our behavioral styles are not fixed at birth or even in early childhood. Much depends on the ways in which our behaviors impinge on our environments and the ways in which our environments respond to our individual needs throughout our lives.

Genetic Contributions

Are any of us predestined to act violently by virtue of our genetic inheritance? Experiments with rodents have shown that it is possible to create a strain of violent animals by mating aggressive males with aggressive females (Ebert, 1983; Lagerspetz and Lagerspetz, 1971). In humans, however, no particular racial or ethnic group has distinguished itself as being innately or enduringly more violent than any other. Some researchers have reported greater concordance for aggressiveness in monozygotic than dizogotic twins; however, even in these kinds of studies, the relative contributions of environmental factors to aggression remain unclear (Tellegen et al., 1988; Young et al., 1994).

Studies during the 1960s and 1970s, suggesting the association of certain chromosomal abnormalities with antisocial violent behaviors (i.e., XYY and XXY) (Casey et al., 1966; Forssman and Hambert, 1967; Hook, 1973; Nielson, 1968; Owen, 1972; Telfer, 1968; Witkin, 1976), have been called into question (Baker et al., 1970; Gerald, 1976; Jacobs et al., 1971; Schiavi et al., 1984). It seems unlikely that these chromosomal anomalies impart a specific tendency toward violence. Like many other conditions, they probably predispose an individual to a variety of different kinds of adaptational problems that may or may not be expressed by aggression, depending on the individual's upbringing and environmental stressors.

Nielson and colleagues (1994) recently reported an association between an individual's tryptophan hydroxylase genotype and his or her levels of cerebrospinal fluid 5-hydroxyindoleacetic acid (5-HIAA). Since 5-HIAA is the metabolite of serotonin, and diminished levels of serotonin have been associated with impulsivity and irritability, this finding suggests that there may indeed be a genetic component to the way in which a person tends to react to particular stressors. However, impulsivity and irritability are not synonymous with violence.

One of the most fascinating reports regarding genetics and aggression comes from the Netherlands. Brunner and colleagues (1993) described a Dutch family in which several males had similar histories of erratic, assaultive, and even criminal behaviors. Rape, arson, and other socially inappropriate behaviors were also characteristic of these males. Chromosome studies revealed that five of the behaviorally disturbed males had a point mutation in the gene controlling the production of monoamine oxidase-A (MAO-A), the enzyme responsible for the breakdown of certain neurotransmitters (e.g. dopamine, norepinephrine). Aggressive males with this genetic anomaly had reduced MAO-A activity compared with their more peaceful male relatives. This gene was found to be located on the X chromosome. Females, with the mutation, who had two X chromosomes, were spared the behavioral manifestations of the anomaly, although they were found to be carriers. Even in this documented instance of an association between a specific genetic characteristic and certain aberrant behaviors, the influence of the anomaly on aggression itself remains to be clarified.

Two recent studies have reported an association between the biochemical characteristics of a portion of the gene that influences the structure of particular dopamine receptors in the brain and a specific aspect of temperament. Ebstein and colleagues (1996) and Benjamin and colleagues (1996) have found a relationship between the structure of a locus on the D4 dopamine receptor gene and the tendency toward novelty seeking as measured on personality inventories. D4 dopamine receptors are found in parts of the limbic system associated with cognition and emotion (Benjamin et al., 1996; Meador-Woodruff et al., 1994). The Ebstein and Benjamin papers are the first to report a relationship between a normal personality trait and the structure of a gene segment. Attempts will undoubtedly be made to ascertain whether genetic characteristics like these are related to daredevil, antisocial behaviors. However, it is important to keep in mind that this genetic characteristic is thought to account for but 10% of the genetic influences on novelty seeking. Furthermore, genetic factors are estimated to account for between 30 and 60% of temperament (Bouchard, 1994). Family practices, societal expectations, and individual experiences interact with inherent temperamental predispositions and strongly influence temperament and behavior.

At this time the consensus regarding genetics and violence is that no single gene or known constellation of genes accounts for violence and that psychological and social factors strongly influence the ways in which biological vulnerabilities may express themselves (Reiss and Roth, 1993).

Although there is no known genetically transmitted abnormality that predisposes a person specifically to violence, there is a genetically transmitted normal condition, inherited by 50% of the human population, that is associated with aggressiveness: the XY syndrome, better known as being male.

Hormones and Sexual and Aggressive Behaviors

In almost all species of animals, including humans, the male is more aggressive than the female. Whether measured during childhood in terms of roughness of play (Maccoby and Jacklin, 1974) or in adulthood in terms of violent crime (Federal Bureau of Investigation, 1993), the human male behaves in demonstrably more aggressive ways than the female. This difference between the sexes is not peculiar to a particular society but has been observed cross-culturally in societies as different and distant from each other as Ethiopia and Switzerland (Omark et al., 1973; Whiting and Edwards 1973).

There is ample evidence from animal studies that gonadal hormones affect behavior. If animals are to respond in adulthood with aggressive behaviors, it is essential that they have had early (probably in utero) exposure to testosterone (Brain, 1979; Gandelman, 1980). Hormones affect the structure and physiology of the developing brain in mammals. "Testosterone and estradiol reaching the nuclei of hormonally sensitive nerve cells during critical periods for sexual differentiation activate some genes and suppress others" (Brain and Haug, 1992). Hormones influence synapse formation and enzyme systems. The importance of androgens for the development of fighting behaviors and/or dominance has been demonstrated in such diverse species as fish, lizards, birds, and chimpanzees (Floody and Pfaff, 1972). However, even castrated animals have been able to fight fiercely if sufficiently threatened (Barfield, 1984).

Estrogens have been observed to have varying behavioral effects, depending on the developmental stage of the animal. For example, estrogens suppress fighting in intact adult males of many species (Floody and Pfaff, 1972). On the other hand, in some species, when given prenatally, estrogen has been associated with masculine brain development and aggressive behavior (Paup et al., 1972; Ruppert and Clemens, 1981). Androgens such as testosterone are metabolized in the brain to form estrogens (Reddy et al., 1974). Thus, although numerous studies attest to the masculinizing effects of androgens on developing animals, their effects, at least in some animals, may come about as a result of their metabolism to estrogens such as estradiol (Reddy et al., 1974).

Gonadal hormones are not the only hormones that affect and are affected by conflict. In monkeys, defeat causes circulating corticosteroids to rise (Christian, 1955, 1959). When an animal has been repeatedly exposed to defeat, even exposure to a potential aggressor will cause a surge of corticosteroids (Bronson and Eleftheriou, 1965a, 1965b). Similarly, the administration of high doses of corticosteroids to a dominant male will induce submissive behavior (Flannelly et al., 1984). On the other hand, acutely administered dexamethasone and adrenocorticotropic hormone (ACTH) increased social conflict in rodents, ACTH by stimulating secretion of corticosterone, dexamethasone ostensibly by its intrinsic glucocorticoid properties (Brain and Haug, 1992).

In animals, adult sexual behaviors as well as aggressive behaviors depend on modifications of the brain in utero in response to gonadal hormones (Brain, 1979; Gandelman, 1980). Evidence of the association of sexual and aggressive behaviors in animals is voluminous. For example, aggression between males of the same species increases appreciably during mating season, probably in response to increases in luteinizing hormone (LH) and/or androgens (Flannelly et al., 1984). Studies of male rats have shown that simply living in the presence of estrous females increases gonadal hormone functioning (Herz et al., 1969). Likewise, cohabitation with females increases the number and intensity of aggressive attacks on male littermates (Barr, 1981; Flannelly and Lore, 1975). Just the smell of an estrous female can increase aggression among sexually experienced male rats. Male rats that have coupled with females are far more aggressive than male rats that have lived alone or in the company of other males only. Their previous sexual experience does not result in a continuous high level of circulating androgens. Instead, it seems to enable the animal to respond quickly with a surge of testosterone when next exposed to a female (Kamel et al., 1975). In laboratory mice there is also a high correlation between sexual and aggressive behaviors. Just a few intromissions with females are sufficient to increase aggressive behavior in male mice.

The effects of gonadal hormones on human sexual and aggressive behaviors are difficult to study. Obviously one cannot simply administer hormones and observe their effects. Therefore, by and large, information must be gleaned from experiments in nature. For example, girls with congenital adrenal hyperplasia, who were exposed to high levels of androgens in utero, have been reported to be labeled tomboys (Ehrhardt et al., 1968), to be athletic and energetic, and to be relatively uninterested in hairstyles, jewelry, and other more traditionally feminine concerns (Ehrhardt and Baker, 1974). Girls exposed in utero to exogenous masculinizing progestins administered to their mothers were reported to have masculine attributes similar to girls with congenital adrenal hyperplasia (Ehrhardt and Money, 1967). Putnam (personal communication) has described the premature onset of puberty in sexually abused girls, a finding which would suggest an effect in humans of postnatal experience on physiology and sexuality.

Several studies of aggressive males have suggested a possible association between testosterone levels and aggression, but the findings are equivocal (Ehrenkranz et al., 1974; Kreuz and Rose, 1972; Meyer-Bahlberg, 1974; Monti et al., 1977; Rada et al., 1976). Dabbs et al. (1991), in a study of concentrations of testosterone and cortisol in the saliva of adolescent offenders, reported that subjects high in salivary testosterone committed more violent acts than subjects with low levels. They found that this relationship of testosterone to aggression was strongest when salivary cortisol levels were low. Virrkunen (1985) reported that in humans low concentrations of circulating corticosteroids as reflected in urinary free cortisol were correlated with habitual violence.

One cannot necessarily extrapolate from adult or adolescent humans to children. Constantino and colleagues (1993), in a study comparing serum androgen levels of aggressive and nonaggressive prepubertal boys, found absolutely no differences between the groups. They concluded, ''Testosterone does not appear to be a useful biological marker for aggressivity in children.'' Our own studies of sexually assaultive juveniles (Lewis et al., 1979; Rubinstein et al., 1994), as well as the work of others, suggest that sexually abused boys are more likely to become sexually assaultive than are their nonabused peers. It may be that early sexually abusive experiences set up physiological response patterns as well as psychological response patterns that make sexually abused males more likely than nonabused males to become perpetrators, given certain stressors or stimuli. The failure of investigators to find consistent differences in testosterone levels between offenders and nonoffenders may be because measurements are taken when subjects are confined. The rates and degrees of hormonal responses to sexual or aggressive stimuli might reveal differences between offenders and nonoffenders that are not evident in resting states.

Exactly how hormones influence behavior remains to be understood. In animals, ''evidence for hormonal involvement in perception has been obtained for all the major sensory systems'' (Brain and Haug, 1992). Suffice it to say that the effects of hormones on the brain and on behavior are ''complex, subtle and wide ranging'' (Brain and Haug, 1992). Clearly, many factors in addition to gonadal hormone levels influence the expression of aggression.

Neurotransmitters and Aggression

An ever-growing literature attests to the role of neurotransmitters in the genesis as well as the suppression of aggression. Norepinephrine, acetylcholine, dopamine, serotonin, and γ-aminobutyric acid (GABA) have been associated with levels of affective aggression in animals, and data are slowly accumulating regarding their role in human violence.

Increases in the turnover of norepinephrine have been demonstrated in the brains of animals in which aggression was induced by isolation or by other stressors (Kety et al., 1967; Welch and Welch, 1971). Aggressive behaviors have also been induced by administering precursors of norepinephrine and by administering noradrenergic-mimetic drugs (Lal et al., 1968, 1970; Randrup and Munkvad, 1966; Reis, 1972). Drugs that increase noradrenergic activity in the brain, such as MAO inhibitors and tricyclic antidepressants, have been reported to increase aggression in rats, whereas those like clonidine or propranolol that reduce noradrenergic activity have been reported to decrease such aggression (Eichelman, 1988).

We do not yet understand the ways in which norepinephrine is associated with the initiation and intensification of aggression. However, it has been suggested that part of its effect results from its inhibition of certain brainstem neurons known to suppress aggression (Reis, 1972). Of note, norepinephrine, while facilitating affective aggression in rats, inhibits predatory aggression.

Acetylcholine has also been found to increase both predatory and affective aggression in animals. The injection of acetylcholine into the hypothalamus of cats has been reported to stimulate predatory biting (Bear, 1991). These kinds of findings may shed light on some of the calming effects of certain pharmacologic agents with anticholinergic side effects such as amitriptyline.

Dopamine is also thought to play a role in facilitating affective aggression in animals and, possibly, in humans. For example, dopamine agonists, such as apomorphine, have been demonstrated to increase aggressive behavior in rats (McKenzie, 1971). Mice that have become aggressive as a result of herpes simplex encephalitis have been shown to have an increased synthesis of dopamine and a decreased synthesis of serotonin in their brains. What is more, when these animals are given methylparatyrosine, an inhibitor of dopamine synthesis, their aggressiveness diminishes (Lycke et al., 1969). Blackburn and colleagues (1992) have hypothesized that the stimulation of dopamine in the brain creates an emotional state in which an animal's ability to respond quickly to environmental stimuli is enhanced.

Numerous studies have suggested the importance of serotonin in the modulation of aggression in animals. For example, Sahakian (1981) reported low concentrations of serotonin in the cerebrospinal fluid of hyperaggressive rats. Others have demonstrated increased aggression in mice and rats depleted of serotonin (Alpert et al., 1981). Conversely, substances that potentiate serotonin have been demonstrated to diminish aggression (Alpert et al., 1981).

Experiences can affect neurotransmitter levels in the brain. For example, the isolation of mice at critical developmental stages will diminish levels of serotonin in the brain. What is more, these serotonin-depleted mice will behave in more aggressive ways than their nonisolated peers (Garatinni et al., 1969; Valzelli, 1974).

In humans there is a growing body of literature suggesting a relationship between diminished levels of brain serotonin and self-injury (Asberg et al., 1976, 1987) as well as outwardly aggressive behaviors (Brown et al., 1979). Based on studies of violent offenders and impulsive firesetters, Linnoila and colleagues (1983) have suggested that low cerebral serotonin concentration (as reflected in low cerebrospinal fluid 5-HIAA) may be associated with impulsive behaviors in general rather than with aggressiveness or violence in particular. In a follow-up of these subjects, Virrkunen and his colleagues (1989) reported diminished concentrations of both 5-HIAA and homovanillic acid (HVA) (metabolites of serotonin and dopamine) in recidivists compared with concentrations in nonrecidivists. Coccaro and colleagues (1989) demonstrated diminished prolactin responses to fenfluramine, (a serotonin-releasing agent) in impulsive, aggressive patients diagnosed as having personality disorders, and in depressed suicidal patients, compared with control subjects. They hypothesized the existence of a psychobiological susceptibility to impulsive aggressive behavior, secondary to insufficient serotonin in the brain.

Virrkunen and colleagues (1994) recently reported especially low concentrations of cerebrospinal fluid 5-HIAA in alcoholic, impulsive, violent offenders. In a recent study of serotonin and norepinephrine precursors, Candito et al. (1993) reported low levels of circulating tryptophan in a small sample of impulsive adolescents. In short, there is an ever-growing body of research indicating a relationship between suicidal, impulsive, or aggressive behaviors and dysfunction of the serotonergic system (Coccaro et al., 1992; Van Praag, 1991).

Clinicians and researchers are becoming increasingly aware of the importance of GABA in the regulation of aggressive behaviors. Studies on rats suggest that low concentrations of GABA in the brains of certain rats is associated with aggressiveness. Aggressiveness in mice has been shown to subside in response to increases in brain GABA activity (Eichelman, 1988).

In human beings, the benzodiazepines, which are thought to enhance GABA activity at receptor sites, usually have a calming effect (Young et al., 1994).

Interactions of Hormones and Neurotransmitters

The effects on behavior of hormones and neurotransmitters cannot really be studied separately. A few examples of their interactions are offered:

1. In vitro studies of the effects of hormones on the embryonic rat brain show that both estrogen and progesterone enhance the growth of mesencephalic dopamine neurons (Reisert et al., 1987). Thus, hormones actually affect brain structure and function.
2. Studies of rats and hamsters reveal that hormones associated with aggression, such as estradiol and testosterone, concentrate in specific limbic system nuclei (Floody and Pfaff, 1972).
3. The introduction of testosterone into particular hypothalamic nuclei of castrated rats causes them to resume those aggressive behaviors that had previously been suppressed by castration (Herbert, 1989). In this study, testosterone was thought to act as a neurotransmitter.
4. In vitro studies of the effect of neurotransmitters on testicular tissue in hamsters reveal the role of catecholamines in the production of testosterone (Mayerhofer et al., 1989).
5. Serotonin agonists, releasers, precursors, and uptake inhibitors have been found to elevate corticosterone levels in rats (Fuller, 1981).

Clearly, the actions of hormones cannot be studied without considering their interactions with neurotransmitters and vice versa.

Neuroanatomy and Violence

Where in the brain do the neurophysiological interactions related to aggression occur? Clinical data and data from experimentation with animals have shown that three areas of the brain are especially important in terms of the modulation of violent behaviors. MacLean (1985) and Weiger and Bear (1988) have conceptualized a hierarchy of neural controls that involves particularly the hypothalamus, amygdala, and orbital prefrontal cortex. The hypothalamus, which receives input from osmoreceptors and chemoreceptors and from the amygdala, affects endocrine responses through its influence on the pituitary. For example, damage to the anterior hypothalamus of male rats reduces sexual and aggressive behaviors (Floody and Pfaff, 1972).

In addition, hypothalamic projections to the brainstem control allegedly stereotyped behaviors, a phenomenon illustrated by what has been called sham rage in decorticate cats (Bard, 1928). Aggressive behaviors can be elicited or suppressed, depending on which parts of the hypothalamus are stimulated or ablated. Acetylcholine has been shown to be an important neurotransmitter in this area of the brain (Bandler, 1970; Bear et al., 1986; Smith et al., 1970). In humans, lesions in the hypothalamus have been associated with unplanned animal-like attacking behaviors (Ovsview and Yudofsky, 1993). Although clinical cases of aggression in humans caused by hypothalamic abnormalities are relatively rare, several cases have been reported. Reeves and Plum (1969) reported intermittent aggressive behavior in a woman with a medial hypothalamic

tumor. Similar cases were reported by Killefer and Stern (1970), Haugh and Markesbery (1983), and Ovsview and Yudofsky (1993).

In contrast with the hypothalamus, the amygdala, receives input from all sensory modalities. It has projections to the hypothalamus and plays a role in the association of particular sensory stimuli with aggressive responses (Downer, 1961; Weiger and Bear, 1988). Lesions in the amygdala have been shown to impair an animal's ability to distinguish between appropriate and inappropriate objects for satisfying hunger and sexual drives (Keating, 1971; Kluver and Bucy, 1939). Experiments on animals suggest that stimulation of the amygdala, located deep within the temporal lobe, is involved in the kind of aggression that occurs in response to fear (Egger and Flynn, 1963; Siegel and Flynn, 1968). On the other hand, damage to the amygdala has been reported to result in a diminution of aggressive behaviors in response to novel stimuli.

In humans, lesions in the amygdaloid area have been associated with apathy and hyposexuality, whereas abnormal electrical activity in this area has been associated with aggression. Insight into the functions of the amygdala can be gleaned from the recent case report of a woman whose amygdala was destroyed bilaterally as a result of calcification. This woman was found to be utterly incapable of feeling fear or of appreciating its expression in others (Adolph et al., 1994). The finding that a particular part of the brain known to be involved in aggression is especially sensitive to stimuli that elicit fear is important because fearfulness, hypervigilance, and an unwarranted sense of being threatened (i.e., paranoid feelings and misperceptions) play such an important role in the etiology of violent behavior in some human beings.

The frontal cortex, that part of the brain so essential for abstract thought, planning, and judgment, interacts with the rest of the neocortex as well as the amygdala and hypothalamus. Lesions of the frontal cortex have been associated with apathy, impulsivity, and irritability, depending on their location. Damage to the dorsolateral convexity has been linked with apathetic, irresponsible behaviors, whereas damage to the orbital area is more commonly linked with impulsive, inappropriate behaviors (Blumer and Benson, 1975; Luria, 1980). There have been several reports of episodic violence in patients with frontal lobe injuries (Eslinger and Damasio, 1985; Macmillan, 1986; Ovsview and Yudofsky, 1993). Miller (1987) has suggested that frontal dysfunction plays a role in the aggressive behaviors of many individuals who are diagnosed "antisocial personality." More recently, Blake and colleagues (in press) have reported evidence of frontal lobe abnormalities in a series of adult murderers.

In spite of the clinical and experimental data presented above, only rarely can specific kinds of criminally aggressive behaviors be explained in terms of the anatomical location of brain lesions. The above examples of brain function and dysfunction are, in fact, gross oversimplifications. No part of the brain works in isolation, and, as noted, the structures involved in aggression have widespread connections to other parts of the brain. The essential principle to keep in mind is that in real life the expression of violence is not simply the outcome of localized stimulation. Different parts of the brain are continuously interacting with each other in response to internal and external stimuli.

Neurotransmitters, Hormones, and Moral Behavior

Morality or the ability to behave altruistically toward others would seem to be a quintessentially human trait, a manifestation of rationality, uninfluenced by biological drives or needs. Such is probably not the case.

Behaviors that are characteristic of almost all members of a species, regardless of their experiences or cultures, are considered to be strongly predisposed. "Across cultures humans are strongly predisposed to assess the behaviors of others as just or unjust and to respond with anger when the behavior of others is perceived as unjust" (McGuire, 1992). In his elegant chapter on moralistic aggression and brain mechanisms, McGuire (1992) points out that individuals ultimately tend to act in their own self-interest. Behaviors that appear altruistic often reflect a person's assessment of the long-term cost-benefit ratio of a particular act. What is surprising is that, according to McGuire, these kinds of assessments are not uniquely human.

McGuire postulates in humans and in nonhuman primates "a mechanism for calculating the physiological, psychological and/or resource costs of granting a helping request, as well as the probability that the requested help will be reciprocated." He provides as an example of these kinds of assessments in nonhuman primates the fact that vervet monkeys will respond about 50% of the time to the requests of other vervets to be groomed. He reports that the longer the interval between grooming another animal and a request for reciprocation, the more likely an animal will respond positively to the request. He cites as another example of the tendency of animals to assess the likelihood of reciprocity, the delay between the time when an animal enters a new group and the time others in the group will share food with the newcomer. McGuire believes that the delay provides group members enough time to size up the chances that the new animal will reciprocate helping behaviors.

Whether or not reciprocal behaviors in nonhuman primates reflect cost-benefit assessments is not a certainty. However, certain neurotransmitters and hormones have been shown to influence benevolent interactions in animals. They affect the ways that animals perceive, interpret, and respond to each other. For example, Olson and colleagues (1979) reported that increased concentrations of certain endorphins was associated with increases in cognitive flexibility in monkeys and with a greater likelihood that the neutral behaviors of others would be interpreted as beneficial. Adult nonhuman primates with high levels of serotonin activity have been found to be especially generous; they are more tolerant of juveniles, more sociable with other adult animals, and more likely to defend an injured animal (McGuire et al., 1983; Raleigh et al., 1984). In contrast, diminished serotonin activity has been found to be associated with the opposite kinds of perceptions and behaviors (McGuire and Troisi, 1987). Animals with low levels of serotonin activity tend to view neutral behaviors as threatening. Decreased norepinephrine and dopamine activity have also been associated with hostile interactions (McGuire, 1992; Redmond, 1983). Primate hostile misinterpretation of environment may have its human counterpart in the common symptom of paranoia. Paranoid feelings and misperceptions are characteristic of so many mental illnesses that are recognized as having strong biological components.

It would seem from the studies cited that physiology plays as important a role in positive social interactions as it does in interpersonal aggression. Because of physiological differences, given the same upbringing, it may be harder for some of us to behave decently to each other than for others.

Alcohol, Drugs and Violence

There is solid evidence that over half of violent crimes are committed when perpetrators are under the influence of alcohol (Pihl and Peterson, 1993). In a review of 26 studies from 11 different countries, Murdoch and colleagues (1990) reported that 62% of violent offenders were under the influence of alcohol at the time of their offenses. Moreover, the Murdoch review noted that 45% of the victims of these acts were also intoxicated. Thus, alcohol seems to embolden provocateurs as well as perpetrators.

Given the important role played by alcohol in the genesis of violence, surprisingly little is known about exactly how the substance affects brain function and consequent behavior. Pihl and Peterson describe the current state of our knowledge as follows:

> It has proved difficult to determine precisely how the central nervous system is affected by ethanol. Alcohol flows through the body like water, and easily penetrates the blood-brain barrier. It bathes all of the body's tissues. Ethanol's effects are dependent upon dose, rate of administration, time passed postconsumption, and subject characteristics that are determined by genetic factors and by previous drinking experience. (Pihl and Peterson, 1993, p. 266)

The effects of ethanol also depend on the individual's upbringing (i.e., family, medical, and social history) and on the immediate circumstances surrounding alcohol consumption. The same amount of gin may loosen control of one's fists when gulped from a flask while ringside at a boxing match and merely loosen the tongue when sipped (with a twist of lemon) from a long stemmed glass at a cocktail party.

Experiments, using as a measure of aggression a subject's willingness to inflict pain on another subject (e.g., willingness to shock a victim), have been interpreted as revealing the following (Gustafson, 1986; Pihl and Peterson, 1993):

1. Alcohol in subanesthetic doses seems to increase pain sensitivity (a counterintuitive finding).
2. Alcohol reduces an individual's fear or anxiety in response to threat or frustration.
3. Alcohol impairs the person's judgment and ability to respond flexibly to dangerous or novel situations.
4. The behavioral effects of alcohol are influenced by genetic factors.

Findings obtained under laboratory conditions cannot necessarily be extrapolated to phenomena occurring in the real world. For example, the commonly observed touchiness and paranoid misperceptions of some inebriates are inconsistent with the laboratory finding that alcohol diminishes a person's response to pain or threat. Whatever the physiological and psychological mechanisms may be, a recent review of 30 experimental studies concluded that "alcohol does indeed cause aggression" (Bushman and Cooper, 1990).

Clinical reports have linked a variety of different drugs to aggressive behaviors. However, it is extremely difficult to gauge the contribution of specific drugs per se to the aggressive acts of drug abusers. The psychological and physiological condition of the user/abuser prior to drug ingestion undoubtedly influences the drug's behavioral effects. Nevertheless, certain substances, such as crack cocaine (Honer et al., 1987; Taylor, 1990), phencyclidine (Fauman and Fauman, 1982), and amphetamines (King and Ellinwood, 1992) have been associated with violent behaviors. Paradoxically, amphetamine is used widely to calm certain extremely aggressive, so-called hyperactive children. Nicotine (Cherek, 1981) and caffeine (Cherek et al., 1983, 1984) have also been found to have calming properties. The effects of the benzodiazepines and barbiturates are reported to be dose dependent: Low doses tend to decrease aggression (Cherek, 1990), whereas moderate and high doses may increase aggression (Taylor, 1990).

Ironically, drugs such as heroin, which themselves have calming effects, may, nevertheless, be associated with violence. The kinds of crimes (e.g., armed robbery) associated with their use occur as a result of addicts' attempts to generate money to support their habits (Nurco, 1984; Tinkenberg, 1973). A flourishing drug trade in our inner cities has affected youth and even child violence. Young children are frequently used as messengers (sometimes armed messengers) by teenaged drug dealers. Thus, drugs have a potent indirect effect on the genesis of violence in children. The drug trade, coupled with the ready availability of handguns, accounts to some extent for the increasing rate of homicide by young juveniles.

EXPERIENTIAL CONTRIBUTIONS TO AGGRESSIVE BEHAVIOR

This chapter has focused so far almost exclusively on the neurophysiological, biochemical, and neuroanatomical underpinnings of aggression. However, without question, the most important influences on aggressive behaviors are environmental or experiential. Whether we consider animal studies or studies of human beings, all evidence indicates that the ways in which living creatures are treated in utero, in infancy, and in childhood affect their subsequent behaviors toward others. In mice, maternal stress has been shown to affect the size, the hormone levels, and the behaviors of newborns (Vom Saal, 1984).

The quality of early nurturing also affects temperament. Animals bred to have an especially gentle nature, if cross-fostered by adult females of a violent strain, will become more aggressive than is their usual nature (Southwick, 1968). There is evidence that mice reared in the company of their fathers as well as their mothers grow up to be more aggressive than those raised only by mothers (Mugford and Nowell, 1972). The effects of cross-fostering aggressive mice by less aggressive females are more variable. Certain strains retain their aggressiveness (Southwick, 1968), while others become less aggressive (McCarty and Southwick, 1979). In another study, mice from an aggressive strain reared by males and females of their own strain were more aggressive than those raised either by two females or by a male and female of a less aggressive strain (Smith and Simmel, 1977). Thus, there is evidence from animal studies that innate temperament can be modified to some extent environmentally and that the nature of early parenting influences subsequent behaviors.

Very early experiences have an especially powerful and enduring effect on physiological and psychological development and, therefore, on behavior. In animals, qualities of parenting during the very first days and weeks of life are particularly important to subsequent social adaptation. Although many reptiles are equipped to defend themselves shortly after birth, most mammals require parental protection for varying periods of time. It is not always clear, however, whether the ability of offspring to protect themselves develops as their mothers lose interest in them, or whether parental protection declines in response to signals from their more self-sufficient offspring (Archer, 1988).

We do know that isolation during critical developmental periods can engender aggression in otherwise gentle animals (Brain and Nowell, 1971; Goldsmith et al., 1976; Luciano and Lore, 1976). Similarly, overheating, crowding, and uncomfortable living conditions promote aggression (Griffitt, 1970; Hutchinson, 1972) in animals. The repeated infliction of pain will also engender aggression (Berkowitz, 1984). So strong is this tendency in animals that a conventional experimental method for inducing aggression in mice and rats involves administering painful shocks to their feet (an ethically questionable practice). Similarly, the training of fighting dogs (e.g., pit bulls) involves physical torment.

The reactions of animals to maltreatment resembles in many respects the response of human infants and children to similar treatment. There is a vast literature suggesting that early maltreatment of children is associated with the development of aggressive, maladaptive behaviors (Cicchetti and Carlson, 1989). Whereas complete emotional deprivation of infants leads to severe depression and even to death (Bowlby, 1969, 1975; Spitz, 1946), lesser degrees of neglect have been associated with poor peer relationships and aggressive behaviors (Mueller and Silverman, 1989). Severe physical abuse has been associated with subsequent extremely violent behaviors (Lewis et al., 1986, 1988; Feldman et al., 1986).

Early repeated sexual abuse seems to have especially unfortunate consequences. There is evidence that a disproportionate percentage of sexually assaultive adults have histories of having been sexually abused as children (Groth, 1979). In the author's experience, the most grotesque sexual crimes have been committed by men who, as children, experienced extraordinary sexual abuse.

How does severe abuse and neglect engender aggression in human beings? The answer is not simple and must be inferred from a variety of different kinds of studies and observations. What is clear is that the human organism is so constructed that maltreatment affects every aspect of functioning—cognitive, emotional, and physiological.

We know that aggression can be learned, and there is sound experimental evidence that modeling plays an important role in the development of aggressive behaviors in animals (Hamburg, 1971) as well as children (Bandura, 1973). We also know that aggressive behaviors (like more adaptive behaviors) can be learned through reinforcement. One of the most important contributions to our understanding of the role of reinforcement in the genesis of aggression is Patterson's (1977) observation that when children's aggressive behaviors are punished severely by parents, they tend to persist. Farrington (1978) also found severe physical punishment to be a major antecedent of aggressive delinquency. On the other hand, when positive, nonviolent behaviors are reinforced and aggressive behaviors given less attention, aggressive behaviors diminish (Patterson, 1979).

Important as these influences may be, there is strong evidence that children do not develop aggressive behaviors simply as a result of modeling or as a result of the reinforcement of learned behaviors. Maltreatment actually changes the way in which the environment is perceived. Studies of animals as well as children have shown that one of the consequences of maltreatment is the development of hypervigilance. It has been demonstrated that defeat increases defensiveness in laboratory mice (Flannelly et al., 1984). What is more, this conditioned defensiveness is generalized to other situations and other opponents (Leshner, 1981; Seward, 1946). Likewise, abused children seem to become hypervigilant, repeatedly misinterpret their surroundings, and perceive ambiguous stimuli as threatening (Dodge et al., 1984; Rieder and Cicchetti, 1989). These observations regarding young children are consistent with the author's own clinical findings regarding violent juvenile delinquents. In fact, the psychiatric symptom that we have found most clearly distinguishes violent delinquents from their less aggressive peers is episodic paranoid ideation and paranoid misperceptions (Lewis et al., 1989).

Exactly how maltreatment heightens vigilance and enhances the likelihood of responding aggressively to unfamiliar or unexpected stimuli remains to be elucidated. Of note, testosterone, a prerequisite for aggression in animals, also has been reported to heighten animals' awareness of their surroundings (Andrew, 1972; Andrew and Rogers, 1972; Archer, 1974; Thompson and Wright, 1979; Thor, 1980). We do know that, in animals, once a physiological response to certain stimuli has been established (e.g., a hormonal response to sexual or aggressive stimuli), it is easily reevoked by exposure to similar stimuli. Thus, one cannot help but wonder whether a similar recurrent maladaptive physiological response also plays a role in the hypervigilance and retaliatory aggression of many abused children who become repeatedly violent. It is possible that early severe maltreatment establishes neural circuits and patterns of physiological responsiveness that make abused children fearful and more likely than nonabused children to retaliate violently when confronted with ambiguous stimuli that are misperceived as potentially harmful. Of note, any physical or psychological condition that enhances paranoia (e.g. schizophrenia, mania, depression, toxic psychosis) also increases the likelihood of aggression. There is a growing recognition that severe mental illness, such as the disorders currently categorized as schizophrenia, is often associated with violent criminality (Hodgins, 1993).

Child maltreatment also contributes to violence by diminishing certain kinds of expressive skills. Emotionally neglected, understimulated infants suffer from a variety of motor and cognitive developmental delays (Provence and Lipton, 1962). Severely abused children manifest specific kinds of deficits in verbalization. For example, toddlers who have been abused are less able than normal children to use words that reflect their inner states or feelings (Cicchetti and Beeghly, 1987). Ironically, these truly tortured souls speak less about their negative feelings than do children from nonabusive backgrounds.

Cicchetti has hypothesized that maltreated children refrain from speaking about unhappiness because they have developed an overcontrolled style of coping. In our own experience at a clinic for children with dissociative disorders, we have found that the most severely abused children repress and even totally deny brutal experiences. This phenomenon is illustrated most dramatically in the dissociative phenomena characteristic of Dissociative Identity Disorder/Multiple Personality Disorder. In these kinds of cases, the child is sometimes totally unaware of having ever been abused. What is more, when the child is in the personality state that is ignorant of the abuse, the child is not violent. On the other hand, those alternate personalities that experienced and remember the maltreatment may be extraordinarily aggressive.

The inability of abused children to identify, much less verbalize, their own feelings of distress is related to their apparent difficulty appreciating the distress of others. They block out and thus cannot see what is too painful for them to see. Even toddlers who have been physically abused have been said to show less empathy than their peers for the distress of other children (Main and George, 1985). The problem is that they feel too much, not too little. But it does not look that way.

Another common result of abuse and/or neglect is injury to the central nervous system. Almost any central nervous system trauma may be associated with hyperactivity, emotional lability, diminished intelligence, poor judgment, and impulsiveness. Children with these kinds of deficits and vulnerabilities are less able to think ahead and understand the consequences of their behavior. They are more likely than normal children to respond aggressively to provocative stimuli, be these stimuli violent television programs or interpersonal challenges.

The capacity of abused children to repress or deny their own painful feelings as well as the pain of others, their inability to articulate emotions, their emotional lability and impulsivity, their distortions of reality, their perceptions of threat where no threat exists, and their resultant tendency to put angry feelings into actions rather than words can become a relatively enduring adaptational style. This constellation of unlovable characteristics accounts in great measure for the tendency of clinicians to dismiss severely abused, aggressive children and adolescents as simply conduct disordered or sociopathic.

In summary, abusive experiences contribute to aggression in the following ways: They provide a model for violence; they teach aggression through reinforcement; they inflict pain; they cause the kinds of central nervous system injuries that are associated with impulsivity, emotional lability, and impaired judgment; in animals, and most probably in humans, they affect neurotransmitters and brain physiology; they create a sense of being endangered and thus increase paranoid feelings and misperceptions; and they diminish the child's ability to recognize feelings and to put feelings into words not actions. The earlier, the more pervasive, and the more enduring the abuse, the more likely violent behaviors will ensue. The more neuropsychiatrically impaired the child is to begin with, the more likely abuse will result in a violent adaptational style (Lewis et al., 1989, 1994).

The Media and Violence

It has been estimated that "the average child will watch 100,000 acts of simulated violence before graduating from elementary school. And studies have shown that poor children see even more" (Kolbert, 1994). A survey conducted by the Center for Media and Public Affairs found that, on a single day in April 1994, in Washington, DC, between the hours of 6 AM and midnight, 2,065 acts of violence were depicted on television (Kolbert, 1994). Children in our society imbibe a media cocktail laced with extraordinary amounts of aggression. The very quality of aggression depicted in the media has changed over the past several years, becoming increasingly graphic. So-called "gangsta rap" extols the pleasures of rape and even murder.

To what extent does exposure to violent materials in the media engender violence? Evidence regarding the influence of violent entertainment on children's behaviors is not yet conclusive. However, enough studies have been completed to suggest that the viewing of violent material, especially by vulnerable children, contributes to aggressive behaviors (Lagerspetz, 1989). Youth makes an individual especially vulnerable to the effects of exposure to violence. Small children seem to react differently from older children to observing the effects of aggression on others. For example, small children will often continue to act aggressively in spite of a victim's expressions of pain; older children and adults are more likely to be inhibited by a victim's suffering (Patterson et al., 1967). In an experiment in which children of different ages were shown the beginnings of a series of aggressive films and asked to choose among endings for them, younger children tended to choose violent outcomes for violent films, whereas older children, when choosing an outcome, were more likely to take into consideration whether or not the violence they had observed at the beginning of the film was justified or unjustified (Leifer and Roberts, 1972). Emotional and cognitive maturity modulate the behavioral consequences of exposure to violence in the media. However, there is also evidence that children who are aggressive to begin with tend to gravitate toward aggressive films and television programs (Lagerspetz, 1989). Hence, studies that indicate that children who watch violent programs become violent adolescents and adults should be interpreted with caution. The relationship of early viewing to later violence may not be causal (Kolbert, 1994).

The extent to which the media contribute to violence not only by producing violent films but also by transmitting news of violence from all over the globe deserves attention. Phillips (1979) documented an increase in suicides and single vehicle fatal accidents following well-publicized suicides. The more space devoted to the reportage of the suicides, the greater the number of apparent copycat behaviors in areas exposed to the news coverage. Phillips also found an increase in homicides following well-publicized heavyweight boxing matches (Phillips, 1983). Most ironic were his findings regarding the effects of publicized executions. In theory, capital punishment is meted out in murder cases, not just as retribution, but also as a deterrent to other potential murderers. And indeed, in his study of homicides in London between 1858 and 1921, Phillips found a decline by one-third in homicides immediately after a publicized execution. Unfortunately, by the end of 2 weeks, the deterrent effects had worn off and, over the next 3 weeks, marked increases in homicide rates occurred (Phillips, 1980, 1983).

Groebel and Hinde (1989) capture the interaction among biological and psychological vulnerabilities and the influence of the media in their statement, "The most likely link between the media and aggression is a reciprocal one. News media reflect societal aggressiveness but also create the image of a violent world. Viewers with aggressive predispositions prefer violent programs which in turn reinforce their aggressive tendencies" (p. 139). Thus, in a free society, in which there are few restrictions on the aggressive content of programming, and in which all individuals can have unlimited access to information, we accept the risks inherent in exposing more vulnerable individuals, the young and the emotionally unstable, to violent stimuli.

SOCIAL AND CULTURAL CONTRIBUTIONS TO AGGRESSIVE BEHAVIOR

It is obvious from the differences in the rates of violent crime in different societies and in different sectors within societies that social factors influence aggressive behaviors. Numerous theories have been proffered to explain why one nation or one group within a given nation behaves more violently than another. The answers are not simple.

One of the most convincing and thought-provoking theories was proposed by Landau (1984), who hypothesized that violence and aggression would increase in societies when social support systems malfunctioned or totally failed. Using inflation rates and the ratio between marriage rates and divorce rates as measures of social stress and family instability, Landau found an association to exist between these indices of societal malfunction and rates of violent crime in 11 of 12 countries studied in the 1960s and 1970s. The only country in which this association was not found was Japan, a country, as Landau noted, in which there are strong behavioral controls outside the family (e.g., in schools and places of work). The Japanese culture itself instills strong feelings of shame for moral transgressions. Thus, the societal stressors associated with violence in other countries are associated with suicide rates in Japan.

In most of the societies studied to date, the majority of violent individuals are males between the ages of 15 and 30 years, living in impoverished urban areas and belonging to ethnic or racial groups that are low in the social hierarchy of the country (Naroll, 1983; Newman, 1979). Clearly, something about being young, male, and raised under adverse conditions is conducive to violence. Given the fact that these characteristics transcend individual societies and are common to different ethnic and racial groups, it is doubtful that violence results primarily from cultural or subcultural values. It is more likely that the kinds of external stressors and intrinsic vulnerabilities that we have identified above as contributing to individual violence (e.g., physical pain, discomfort, central nervous system dysfunction, abusive upbringing, rates of mental illness) are more pervasive in these disadvantaged communities and contribute significantly to the disproportional rate of violence found there.

Data regarding the interaction of neurophysiology and aggression may shed light on the apparent increase in the occurrence and degree of violence in our society, especially in our crowded, bustling urban centers. Is it possible that the extraordinary stresses imposed on more and more of us in order to survive in our ever more complex and demanding technological society not only cause emotional distress but also have physiological consequences? Do we deplete our central nervous systems of sufficient concentrations of the kinds of substances that we require in order to sustain civilized interactions with each other? Is the popularity of jogging and Prozac the reflection of a struggle to compensate artificially for the maladaptive physiologic and emotional consequences of our stressful way of life? If so, would it not make sense to reassess some of our values and life styles in light of what we know is and is not physiologically conducive to peaceful interactions?

CONCLUSION

We do not enter the world as perfectly blank slates. Our individual temperaments result in part from our genetic makeup and in part from the uterine environment in which we grew. However, by far the most important influences on our behaviors are experiential. Whether or not we become violent depends for the most part on how we are treated. Some of the factors that influence aggression are the timing, duration, and intensity of negative stimuli, early stimuli having an especially strong impact. These influences cannot really be separated into psychological and biological, environmental and intrinsic, because, as we have seen, there is a constantly changing dynamic interaction between the two. We know from animal studies as well as clinical studies of human behavior that intrinsic vulnerabilities and environmental stressors interact to generate violence.

A useful way to conceptualize the development of aggression is as follows: Anything that increases irritability, discomfort, fearfulness, suspiciousness, and impulsivity lowers the threshold for aggression. Furthermore, anything that impairs reality testing, judgment, self-esteem, self-control, and the ability to verbalize feelings rather than act on them will also lower this threshold and increase the likelihood of violent behavior.

On the other hand, those programs that enhance emotional stability, encourage self-control, improve judgment, promote self-esteem, reinforce a sense of security, develop the ability to recognize one's own feelings and the feelings of others, and increase the ability to express these feelings verbally will raise the threshold for aggression and diminish the likelihood of violent behavior. The obvious settings in which to begin to attempt to promote these enhancers of civilized interaction are homes and schools. The data on animal and human development are unequivocal. Harsh parenting is inimical to peaceful behavior. Punitive institutions foster violence.

Can aggression be prevented? Once set in motion, what are the possibilities of reversing or inhibiting aggressive patterns of behavior? Are there particular treatment modalities for particular kinds of aggression? These are the kinds of questions that remain to be answered. However, although we do not yet have cures for violence, we have excellent indicators of what does not work. As this review of violence illustrates, we know that isolation and neglect often lead to aggressive behaviors. We know that responding punitively to aggressive behaviors reinforces them. We know that pain and frustration increase violence. We know that physical brutality engenders similar behavior. And we know that living in close proximity to violent individuals, witnessing their aggressive behaviors, is conducive to the development of a violent adaptational style.

Given all that we know about how to create aggressive individuals (and how not to), it is ironic that our correctional systems for children as well as for adults reproduce all of the conditions that are documented to promote violence. Surely with a little ingenuity we could make use of our knowledge of the causes of violence to create systems that would have the opposite effect. We also are gaining insight into some of the physiological as well as psychological conditions that enhance mutually supportive behaviors as opposed to violent ones. Our knowledge about the psychophysiologic correlates of civilized behaviors could have important implications for reducing violence by modifying the ways in which we organize our everyday lives.

References

Adolph R, Tranel D, Damasio H, et al: Impaired recognition of emotion in facial expressions following bilateral damage to the human amygdala. *Nature* 372(15):669–672, 1994.

Alpert JE, Cohen DJ, Shaywitz BA, et al: Neurochemical and behavioral organization: Disorders of attention, activity, and aggression. In: Lewis DO (ed): *Vulnerabilities to Delinquency*. New York, Spectrum, 1981, pp. 109–171.

Andrew RJ: Recognition processes and behavior with special reference to effects of testosterone on persistence. In: Lehrman DS, Hinde RA, Shaw E (eds): *Advances in the Study of Behavior* (Vol 4). New York, Academic, 1972, pp. 175–208.

Andrew RJ, Rogers L: Testosterone, search behaviour, and persistence. *Nature* 237:343–346, 1972.

Archer J: The effects of testosterone on the distractibility of chicks by irrelevant and relevant novel stimuli. *Anim Behav* 22:397–404, 1974.

Archer J: *The Behavioural Biology of Aggression*. Cambridge, Cambridge University Press, 1988.

Asberg A, Traskman L, Thoren P: 5HIAA in cerebrospinal fluid: A biochemical suicide predictor? *Arch Gen Psychiatry* 33:1193–1196, 1976.

Asberg M, Schalling D, Traksman-Bendz L, et al: Psychobiology of suicide, impulsivity, and related phenomena. In: Meltzer HY (ed): *Psychopharmacology: Third Generation of Progress*. New York, Raven Press, 1987, pp. 655–688.

Baker D, Telfer MA, Richardson CE, et al: Chromosome errors in men with antisocial behavior: Comparison of selected men with "Klinefelter's syndrome" and XYY chromosome pattern. *JAMA* 214: 869–878, 1970.

Bandler RJ: Cholinergic synapses in the lateral

hypothalamus for the control of predatory aggression in the rat. *Brain Res* 20:409–424, 1970.

Bandura A: *Aggression: A Social Learning Analysis*. Englewood Cliffs, NJ, Prentice-Hall, 1973.

Bard P: A diencephalic mechanism for the expression of rage with special reference to the sympathetic nervous system. *Am J Physiol* 84:490–515, 1928.

Barfield R: Reproductive hormones and aggressive behavior. In: Flannelly KJ, Blanchard RJ, Blanchard DC (eds): *Biological Perspectives on Aggression*. New York, Liss, 1984, pp. 105–134.

Barr GA: Effects of different housing conditions on intraspecies fighting between male Long-Evans hooded rats. *Physiol Behav* 27:1041, 1981.

Bear DM: Neurological perspectives on aggressive behavior. *J Neuropsychiatry* 3:S3–S8, 1991.

Bear DM, Fulop M: The neurology of emotion. In: Hobson A (ed): *Behavioral Biology in Medicine*. South Norwalk, CT, Meduration, Inc., 1987.

Bear DM, Rosenbaum JF, Norman R: Aggression in cat and man precipitated by a cholinesterase inhibitor. *Psychosomatics* 26:535–536, 1986.

Benjamin J, Li L, Patterson C, et al: Population and familial association between the D4 dopamine receptor gene and measures of novelty seeking. *Nature Genet* 12(1):81–84, 1996.

Berkowitz L: Physical pain and the inclination to aggression. In: Flannelly KJ, Blanchard RJ, Blanchard DC (eds): *Biological Perspectives on Aggression*. New York, Liss, 1984, pp. 27–47.

Blackburn JR, Pfaus JG, Phillips AG: Dopamine functions in appetitive and defensive behaviours. *Prog Neurobiol* 39:247–279, 1992.

Blake PY, Pincus JH, Buckner C: Neurological abnormalities in murderers. *Neurology*, in press.

Blanchard RJ, Blanchard DC: Aggressive behavior in the rat. *Behav Biol* 21:197, 1977.

Blumer D, Benson DF: Personality changes with frontal and temporal lobe lesions. In: Benson DF, Blumer D (eds): *Psychiatric Aspects of Neurologic Disease*. New York, Grune & Stratton, 1975, pp. 151–170.

Bouchard TJJ: Genes, environment, and personality. *Science* 264:1700–1701, 1994.

Bowlby J: *Attachment and Loss* (Vol 1). New York, Basic Books, 1969.

Bowlby J: *Attachment and Loss* (Vol 2). Harmondsworth, Middlesex, UK, Penguin, 1975.

Brain PF: *Hormones and Aggression* (Vol 2). Montreal, Eden Press, 1979.

Brain PF, Haug M: Hormonal and neurochemical correlates of various forms of animal "aggression." *Psychoneuroendocrinology* 17(6):537–551, 1992.

Brain PF, Nowell NW: Isolation versus grouping effects on adrenal and gonadal function in albino mice. I: The male. *Gen Comp Endocrinol* 16:149, 1971.

Bronson FH, Eleftheriou BE: Adrenal response to fighting in mice: Separation of physical and psychological causes. *Science* 147:627, 1965a.

Bronson FH, Eleftheriou BE: Relative effects of fighting on bound and unbound corticosterone. *Proc Soc Exp Biol Med* 118:146, 1965b.

Brown GL, Goodwin FK, Ballenger JC, et al: Aggression in humans correlates with cerebrospinal fluid amine metabolites. *Psychiatry Res* 1:131–139, 1979.

Brunner HG, Nelen M, Breakefield XO, et al: Abnormal behavior associated with a point mutation in the structural gene for monoamine oxidase A. *Science* 262:578–580, 1993.

Bushman BJ, Cooper HM: Effects of alcohol on human aggression: An integrative research review. *Psychol Bull* 107:341–354, 1990.

Candito M, Askenazy F, Myquel M, et al: Tryptophanemia and tyrosinemia in adolescents with impulsive behavior. *Int Clin Psychopharmacol* 8(2):129–132, 1993.

Casey LJ, Segall DR, Street K, et al: Sex chromosome abnormalities in two state hospitals for patients requiring special security. *Nature* 209:641–642, 1966.

Cherek DR: Effects of smoking different doses of nicotine on human aggressive behavior. *Psychopharmacology* 7:339–345, 1981.

Cherek DR: Laboratory studies of aggression and drugs: Variations in behavioral effects. Paper presented at the annual meeting of the American Psychological Association, Boston, 1990.

Cherek DR, Steinberg JL, Brauchi JT: Effects of caffeine on human aggressive behavior. *Psychiatry Res* 8:137–145, 1983.

Cherek DR, Steinberg JL, Brauchi JT: Regular or decaffeined coffee and subsequent human aggressive behavior. *Psychiatry Res* 11:251–258, 1984.

Chess SE, Thomas A: *Origins and Evolution of Behavior Disorders*. New York, Brunner/Mazel, 1984.

Christian JJ: Effect of population size on the adrenal glands and reproductive organs of male mice in populations of fixed size. *J Physiol* 182:292, 1955.

Christian JJ: Lack of correlation between adrenal weight and injury from fighting in grouped male albino mice. *Proc Soc Exp Biol Med* 101:166, 1959.

Cicchetti D, Beeghly M: Symbolic development in maltreatment youngsters: An organizational perspective. In: Cicchetti D, Beeghly M (eds): *Atypical Symbolic Development*. San Francisco, Jossey-Bass, 1987.

Cicchetti D, Carlson V: *Child Maltreatment: Theory and Research on the Causes and Consequences of Child Abuse and Neglect*. New York, Cambridge University Press, 1989.

Coccaro EF, Kavoussi RJ, Lesser JC: Self- and other-directed human aggression: The role of the central serotonergic system. *Int Clin Psychopharmacol* 6(6):70–83, 1992.

Coccaro EF, Siever LJ, Klar HM, et al: Serotonergic studies in patients with affective and personality disorders. *Arch Gen Psychiatry* 587–588, 1989.

Constantino JN, Grosz D, Saenger P, et al: Testosterone and Aggression in Children. *J Am Acad Child Adolesc Psychiatry* 32(6):1217–1222, 1993.

Dabbs JM, Jurkovic GJ, Frady RL: Salivary testosterone and cortisol among late adolescent male offenders. *J Abnorm Child Psychol* 19(4):469–478, 1991.

Dodge K, Murphy R, Buchsbaum KC: The assessment of intention-cue detection skills in children: Implications for developmental psychopathology. *Child Dev* 55:163–173, 1984.

Dollard JE, Doob AL, Miller N: *Frustration and Aggression*. New Haven, CT, Yale University Press, 1939.

Downer JL: Changes in visual gnostic functions and emotional behaviour following unilateral temporal pole damage in the ''split-brain'' monkey. *Nature* 191:50–51, 1961.

Ebert PD: Selection for aggression in a natural population. In: Himmel EC, Hahn ME, Walters JK (eds): *Aggressive Behavior: Genetic and Neural Approaches*. Hillsdale, NJ, Erlbaum, 1983, pp. 103–127.

Ebstein RP, Novick O, Umansky R, et al: Dopamine D4 receptor (D4DR) exon III polymorphism associated with the human personality trait of novelty seeking. *Nature Genet* 12(1):78–80, 1996.

Egger MD, Flynn JP: Effects of electrical stimulation of the amygdala on hypothalamically elicited attack behavior in cats. *J Neurophysiol* 26:705–720, 1963.

Ehrenkranz J, Bliss E, Sheard MH: Plasma testosterone: Correlation with aggressive behavior and social dominance in man. *Psychosom Med* 36:469–475, 1974.

Ehrhardt AA, Baker SW: Fetal androgens, human central nervous system differentiation and behavior sex differences. In: Friedman RC, Richart RM, Vande Wiele RL (eds): *Sex Differences in Behavior*. New York, Wiley, 1974.

Ehrhardt AA, Money J: Progestin-induced hermaphroditism: IQ and psychosexual identity in a sample of ten girls. *J Sex Res* 3:83–100, 1967.

Ehrhardt AA, Epstein R, Money J: Fetal androgens and female gender identity in the early treated adrenogenital syndrome. *Johns Hopkins Med J* 122:160–167, 1968.

Eichelman B: Toward a rational pharmacotherapy for aggressive and violent behavior. *Hosp Community Psychiatry* 39:31–39, 1988.

Eslinger PJ, Damasio A: Severe disturbance of higher cognition after bilateral frontal lobe ablation: Patient EVR. *Neurology* 35(12):1731–1741, 1985.

Farrington DP: The family backgrounds of aggressive youths. In: Hersov LA, Berger M, Shaffer D (eds): *Aggression and Antisocial Behavior in Childhood and Adolescence*. Oxford, Pergamon, 1978, pp. 73–93.

Fauman BJ, Fauman MA: Phencyclidine, abuse and crime: A psychiatric perspective. *Bull Am Acad Psychiatry Law* 10:171–176, 1982.

Federal Bureau of Investigation. *Uniform Crime Report*. Washington, DC, 1993.

Feldman M, Mallouh C, Lewis DO: Filicidal abuse in the histories of 15 condemned murderers. *Bull Am Acad Psychiatry Law* 14(4):345–352, 1986.

Flannelly K, Lore R: Dominance-subordinance in cohabiting pairs of adult rats: Effects on aggressive behavior. *Aggress Behav* 1:331, 1975.

Flannelly KJ, Flannelly L, Blanchard RJ: Adult experience and the expression of aggression: A comparative analysis. In: Flannelly KJ, Blanchard RJ, Blanchard DC (eds): *Biological Perspectives on Aggression*. New York, Liss, 1984, pp. 207–259.

Floody OR, Pfaff DW: Steroid hormones and aggressive behavior: Approaches to the study of hormone-sensitive brain mechanisms for behavior. In: Frazier SH (ed): *Aggression: Proceedings of the Association*. (Research Publication Association for Nervous and Mental Disease, Vol 52). Baltimore, Williams & Wilkins, 1972, pp. 149–185.

Flynn JP, Vanegas H, Foote W, et al: Neural mechanisms involved in a cat's attack on a rat. In: Whalen RE, Thompson RF, Verzeano M, et al (eds): *Neural Control of Behavior*. New York, Academic Press, 1970.

Forssman H, Hambert G: Chromosomes and antisocial behavior. *Excerpta Criminologica* 7:113–117, 1967.

Freud S: *Beyond the Pleasure Principle*. In: Strachey J (ed): *The Standard Edition of the Complete Psychological Works of Sigmund Freud* (Vol 23). London, Hogarth Press, 1962. (Original edition published 1922.)

Fuller RW: Serotonergic stimulation of pituitary-adrenocortical functions in rats. *Neuroendocrinology* 32:118–127, 1981.

Gandelman R: Gonadal hormones and the induction of intraspecific fighting in mice. *Neurosci Biobehav Rev* 4:133, 1980.

Garattini S, Giacolone E, Valzelli L: Biochemical changes during isolation-induced aggressiveness in mice. In: Garattini S, Sigg E (eds): *Aggressive Behavior*. New York, Wiley, 1969.

Gerald PS: Current concepts in genetics: Sex chromosome disorders. *N Engl J Med* 294:706, 1976.

Goldsmith JF, Brain PF, Benton D: Effects of age at differential housing and the duration of individual housing/grouping on intermale fighting behavior and adrenocortical activity in TO strain mice. *Aggress Behav* 2:307–323, 1976.

Griffitt W: Environmental effects on interpersonal affective behavior: Ambient effective temperature and attraction. *J Pers Soc Psychol* 15:240, 1970.

Groebel J, Hinde RA: *Aggression and War: Their Biological and Social Bases*. New York, Cambridge University Press, 1989.

Groth AN: Sexual trauma in the life histories of rapists and child molesters. *Victimology: An International Journal* 4(1):10–16, 1979.

Gustafson R: Threat as a determinant of alcohol-related aggression. *Psychol Rep* 58:287–297, 1986.

Hamburg DA: Psychobiological studies of aggressive behaviour. *Nature* 230:19–23, 1971.

Haugh RM, Marksbery WR: Hypothalamic astrocytoma: Syndrome of hyperphagia, obesity, and disturbances of behavior and endocrine and autonomic function. *Arch Neurol* 40(9):560–563, 1983.

Herbert J: The physiology of aggression. In: Groebel J, Hinde RA (eds): *Aggression and War: Their Biological and Social Bases*. New York, Cambridge University Press, 1989, pp. 58–71.

Herz Z, Floman Y, Drori D: The testosterone content of the testes of mated and unmated rats. *J Endocrinol* 44:127, 1969.

Hodgins S: *Mental Disorder and Crime*. Newbury Park, CA, Sage Publications, 1993.

Honer WG, Gewertz G, Turey M: Psychosis and violence in cocaine smokers. *Lancet* 8556:451, 1987.

Hook EB: Behavioral implications of the human XYY genotype. *Science* 179(4069):139–150, 1973.

Hutchinson RR: The environmental causes of aggression. In: Cole JK, Jensen DD (eds): *Nebraska Symposium on Motivation*. Lincoln, NE, University of Nebraska Press, 1972.

Jacobs PA, Prince WH, Richmond S, et al: Chromosome surveys in penal institutions and approved schools. *J Med Genet* 8:49–58, 1971.

Kagan J, Moss H: *From Birth to Maturity*. New York, Wiley, 1962.

Kamel F, Mock EJ, Wright WW, et al: Alterations of plasma concentrations of testosterone, LH, and prolactin associated with mating in the male rat. *Horm Behav* 6:277, 1975.

Keating EG: Somatosensory deficit produced by parieto-temporal disconnection. *Anat Rec* 169:353–354, 1971.

Kety SS, Javoy F, Thierry AM, et al: A sustained effect of electroconvulsive shock on the turnover of norepinephrine in the central nervous system of rat. *Proc Natl Acad Sci USA* 58:1249, 1967.

Killefer FA, Stern WE: Chronic effects of hypothalamic injury. *Arch Neurol* 22(5):419–429, 1970.

King GR, Ellinwood EH: Amphetamines and other stimulants. In: Lowinson JH, Ruiz P, Millman RB, et al (eds): *Substance Abuse: A Comprehensive Textbook*. Baltimore, Williams & Wilkins, 1992, pp. 247–270.

Kluver H, Bucy PC: Preliminary analysis of functions of the temporal lobes in monkeys. *Arch Neurol Psychiatry* 42:979–1000, 1939.

Kolbert E: Television gets closer look as a factor in real violence. *The New York Times* December 14, 1994.

Kreuz LE, Rose RM: Assessment of aggressive behavior and plasma testosterone in a young criminal population. *Psychosom Med* 34:321–332, 1972.

Lagerspetz K: Media and the social environment. In: Groebel J, Hinde RA (eds): *Aggression and War: Their Biological and Social Bases*. New York, Cambridge University Press, 1989, pp. 164–172.

Lagerspetz KMJ, Lagerspetz KYH: Changes in the aggressiveness of mice resulting from selective breeding, learning, and social isolation. *Scand J Psychol* 12:241–248, 1971.

Lal H, De Feo JJ, Thut P: Effect of amphetamine

on pain-induced aggression. *Commun Behav Biol* 1: 333, 1968.

Lal H, Nesson B, Smith N: Amphetamine-induced aggression in mice pretreated with dihydroxyphenylalanine (DOPA) and/or reserpine. *Biol Psychiatry* 2:299, 1970.

Landau SF: Trends in violence and aggression: A cross-cultural analysis. *Int J Comp Sociol* 24: 133–158, 1984.

Lefkowitz MM, Eron LD, Walder LO, et al: *Growing Up to Be Violent: A Longitudinal Study of Aggression*. Oxford, Pergamon, 1977.

Leifer AP, Roberts DF: Children's response to television violence. In: Murray JP, Rubenstein EA, Comstock GA (eds): *Television and Social Behavior. Vol 2: Television and Social Learning*. Washington, DC, Government Printing Office, 1972.

Leshner AI: The role of hormones in the control of submissiveness. In: Brain PF, Benton D (eds): *Multidisciplinary Approaches to Aggression Research*. Amsterdam, Elsevier/North-Holland Press, 1981, p. 309.

Lewis DO, Lovely R, Yeager CA, et al: Intrinsic and environmental characteristics of juvenile murders. *J Am Acad Child Adolesc Psychiatry* 27(5): 582–587, 1988.

Lewis DO, Lovely R, Yeager C, et al: Toward a theory of the genesis of violence: A follow-up study of delinquents. *J Am Acad Child Adolesc Psychiatry* 28(3):431–436, 1989.

Lewis DO, Pincus J, Feldman M, et al: Psychiatric, neurological, and psychoeducational characteristics of 15 death row inmates in the United States. *Am J Psychiatry* 143:838–845, 1986.

Lewis DO, Shanok S, Pincus JH: Juvenile male sexual assaulters. *Am J Psychiatry* 136:1194–1196, 1979.

Lewis DO, Yeager CA, Stein A, et al: A clinical follow-up of delinquent males: Ignored vulnerabilities, unmet needs, and the perpetuation of violence. *J Am Acad Child Adolesc Psychiatry* 33(4):518–528, 1994.

Linnoila M, Virkkunen M, Scheinin M, et al: Low cerebrospinal fluid 5-hydroxyindoleacetic acid concentration differentiates impulsive from nonimpulsive violent behavior. *Life Sci* 33:2609–2614, 1983.

Locke J: *An Essay Concerning Human Understanding*. 1690.

Lorenz K: *On Aggression*. New York, Harcourt, Brace & World, 1966.

Luciano D, Lore R: Aggression and social experience in domesticated rats. *J Comp Physiol* 88:917, 1976.

Luria AR: *Higher Cortical Functions in Man*. New York, Basic Books, 1980.

Lycke E, Modigh K, Roos BE: Aggression in mice associated with changes in the monoamine-metabolism of the brain. *Experientia* 25:951, 1969.

Maccoby EE, Jacklin CN: *The Psychology of Sex Differences*. London, Oxford University Press, 1974.

MacLean P: Brain evolution relating to family, play and the separation call. *Arch Gen Psychiatry* 42:405–417, 1985.

Main M, George C: Response of abused and disadvantaged toddlers to distress in agitates: A study in the day care setting. *Dev Psychol* 21:407–412, 1985.

Mayerhofer A, Bartke A, Steger RW: Catecholamine effects on testicular testosterone production in the gonadally active and the gonadally regressed adult golden hamster. *Biol Reprod* 40(4):752–761, 1989.

McCarty R, Southwick CH: Parental environment: Effects on survival, growth and aggressive behaviors of two rodent species. *Dev Psychobiol* 12: 269–279, 1979.

McFarlane JW, Allen L, Honzik MP: *A Developmental Study of the Behavior Problems of Normal Children Between 21 Months and 14 Years*. Berkeley, University of California, 1954.

McGlone J: Sex differences in human brain asymmetry: A critical survey. *Behav Brain Sci* 3: 215–263, 1980.

McGuire MT: Moralistic aggression, processing mechanisms, and the brain: The biological foundations of the sense of justice. In: Roger DM, Margaret G (eds): *The Sense of Justice: Biological Foundations of Law* (Vol 136). Sage Focus Editions. Newbury Park, CA, Sage Publications, 1992, pp. 31–46.

McGuire MT, Troisie A: Physiological regulation-deregulation and psychiatric disorders. In: Fejerman J (ed): *The Ethology of Psychiatric Populations*. [Special issue]. *Ethology and Sociobiology* 8: 95–125, 1987.

McGuire MT, Raleigh MJ, Johnson C: Social dominance in adult male vervet monkeys. I: General considerations. *Soc Sci Information-Behav Biol* 22: 89–121, 1983.

McKenzie GM: Apomorphine-induced aggression in the rat. *Brain Res* 34:323, 1971.

McMillan MB: A wonderful journey through skull and brains: The travels of Mr. Gage's tamping iron. *Brain Cogn* 5:67–107, 1986.

Meador-Woodruff JH et al: Dopamine receptor-gene expression in the human medial temporal lobe. *Neuropsychopharmacology* 10:239–248, 1994.

Meyer-Bahlburg HFL, Boon DA, Sharma M, et al: Aggressiveness and testosterone measures in man. *Psychosom Med* 36:269–274, 1971.

Miller L: Neuropsychology of the aggressive psychopath: An integrative review. *Aggress Behav* 13:119–140, 1987.

Monti PM, Brown WA, Corriveau MA: Testosterone and components of aggressive and sexual behavior in man. *Am J Psychiatry* 134:692–694, 1977.

Moyer KE: *The Physiology of Hostility*. Chicago, Markhans Publishing, 1971.

Mueller E, Silverman N: Peer relations in maltreated children. In: Cicchetti D, Carlson V (eds): *Child Matreatment: Theory and Research on the Causes and Consequences of Child Abuse and Neglect*. New York, Cambridge University Press, 1989, pp. 529–578.

Mugford RA, Nowell NW: Paternal stimulation during infancy: Effects upon aggression and open-field performance of mice. *J Comp Physiol Psychol* 79:30–36, 1972.

Murdoch D, Pilh RO, Ross D: Alcohol and crimes of violence: Present issues. *Int J Addict* 25: 1065–1081, 1990.

Naroll R: *The Moral Order: An Introduction to the Human Situation*. Beverly Hills, CA, Sage, 1983.

Newman G: *Understanding Violence*. New York, Lippincott, 1979.

Nielsen DA, Goldman D, Virkkunen M, et al: Suicidality and 5-hydroxyindoleacetic acid concentration associated with a tryptophan hydroxylase polymorphism. *Arch Gen Psychiatry* 51:34–38, 1994.

Nielson J: The XXY syndrome in a mental hospital. *Br J Criminol* 8:186–203, 1968.

Nurco DN, Shaffer JW, Ball JC, et al: Trends in the commission of crime among narcotics addicts over successive periods of addiction and non-addiction. *Am J Drug Alcohol Abuse* 10:481–489, 1984.

Olson GA, Olson RD, Kastin AJ: Effects of an enkephalin analog on complex learning in the rhesus monkey. *Pharmacol Biochem Behav* 11:341–345, 1979.

Omark DR, Omark M, Edelman M: Dominance hierarchies in young children. Paper presented at International Congress of Anthropological and Ethnological Sciences, Chicago, 1973. Abstract in: Maccoby EE, Jacklin, CN (eds): *The Psychology of Sex Differences*. London, Oxford University Press, 1974.

Ovsview F, Yudofsky S: Aggression: A neuropsychiatric perspective. In: Glick RA, Roose SP (eds): *Rage, Power and Aggression. The Role of Affect in Motivation Development, and Adaptation* (Vol 2). New Haven, CT, Yale University Press, 1993, pp. 213–230.

Owen DR: The 47XYY male: A review. *Psychol Bull* 79:209–233, 1972.

Patterson GR: Accelerating stimuli for two classes of coercive behaviors. *J Abnorm Child Psychol* 5:335–350, 1977.

Patterson GR: A performance theory for coercive family interaction. In: Cairns RB (eds): *The Analysis of Social Interactions: Methods, Issues, and Illustrations*. Hillsdale, NJ, Erlbaum, 1979.

Patterson GR, Littman RA, Bricker W: Assertive behavior in children: A step toward a theory of aggression. *Monogr Soc Res Child Dev* 32:1–43, 1967.

Paup DC, Coniglio LP, Clemens LG: Masculinization of the female golden hamster by neonatal treatment with androgen or estrogen. *Horm Behav* 3: 123–131, 1972.

Phillips DP: Suicide, motor vehicle fatalities, and the mass media: Evidence toward a theory of suggestion. *Am J Sociol* 84:1150–1174, 1979.

Phillips DP: The deterrent effect of capital punishment: New evidence on an old controversy. *Am J Sociol* 86:139–148, 1980.

Phillips DP: The impact of mass media violence on U.S. homicides. *Am Sociol Rev* 48:560–568, 1983.

Pihl RO, Peterson JB: Alcohol/drug use and aggressive behavior. In: Hodgins S (ed): *Mental Disorder and Crime*. Newbury Park, CA, Sage, 1993, pp. 263–283.

Provence S, Lipton R: *Infants in Institutions*. New York, International Universities, 1962.

Rada RT, Laws DR, Kellner R: Plasma testosterone levels in the rapist. *Psychosom Med* 38:257–268, 1976.

Raleigh MJ, McGuire MT, Brammer GL, et al: Social and environmental influences on blood serotonin concentrations in monkeys. *Arch Gen Psychiatry* 41:405–410, 1984.

Randrup A, Munkvad I: DOPA and other naturally occurring substances as causes of stereotype and rage in rats. *Acta Psychiatry Scand Suppl* 191: 193, 1966.

Reddy VVR, Naftolin F, Ryan KJ: Conversion of androstenedione to estrone by neural tissues from fetal and neonatal rats. *Endocrinology* 94:117–121, 1974.

Redmond DE Jr: Social effects of alterations in brain noradrenergic function on untreated group members. In: Steklis H, Kling AS (eds): *Neuroendocrine Regulation and Altered Behavior*. New York, SP Medical and Scientific Books, 1983, pp. 207–219.

Reeves AG, Plum F: Hyperphagia, rage and dementia accompanying a ventromedial hypothalamic neoplasm. *Arch Neurol* 20(6):61–124, 1969.

Reis DJ: Central neurotransmitters in aggression. In: Frazier SF (ed): *Aggression: Proceedings of the Association* (Research Publication Association for Nervous and Mental Disease, Vol 52). Baltimore, Williams & Wilkins, 1972, pp. 119–147.

Reisert I, Han V, Lieth E, et al: Steroids promote neurite growth in mesencephalic tyrosine hydroxylase immunoreactive neuron in vitro. *J Dev Neurosci* 5(2):91–98, 1987.

Reiss AJ Jr, Roth JA (eds): *Understanding and Preventing Violence*. Washington, DC, National Academy Press, 1993.

Rieder C, Cicchetti D: An organizational perspective on cognitive control functioning and cognitive-affective balance in maltreated children. *Dev Psychol* 25(3):382–393, 1989.

Rousseau JJ: *Discourse on Inequality*. 1754.

Rubinstein M, Yeager CA, Goodstein C, et al: Sexually assaultive male juveniles: A follow-up. *Am J Psychiatry* 150:262–265, 1993.

Ruppert PH, Clemens LG: The role of aromatization in the development of sexual behavior of the female hamster. *Horm Behav* 15:68–76, 1981.

Sahakian BJ: The neurochemical basis of hyperactivity and aggression induced by social deprivation. In: Lewis DO (ed): *Vulnerabilities to Delinquency.* New York, Spectrum, 1981, pp. 173–186.

Schiavi R, Theilgaard A, Owen D, et al: Sex chromosome anomalies, hormones and aggressivity. *Arch Gen Psychiatry* 41:93–99, 1984.

Seward JP: Aggressive behavior in the rat. IV: Submission determined by conditioning, extinction and disuse. *J Comp Psychol* 39:51, 1946.

Siegel A, Flynn JP: Differential effects of electrical stimulation and lesions of the hippocampus and adjacent regions upon attack behavior of cats. *Brain Res* 7:252–267, 1968.

Smith DE, King MD, Hoebel BG: Lateral hypothalamic control of killing: Evidence for a cholinoceptive mechanism. *Science* 167:900–901, 1970.

Smith ML, Simmel EC: Paternal effects on the development of social behavior in *Mus musculus. Dev Psychobiol* 10:151, 1977.

Southwick CH: Effect of maternal environment on aggressive behavior of inbred mice. *Commun Behav Biol* 1:129, 1968.

Spitz RA: Anaclitic depression. *Psychoanal Study Child* 2:313–342, 1946.

Taylor SP: Alcohol, drugs and human aggressive behavior. Paper presented at the 98th American Psychological Association Convention, Boston, 1990.

Telfer MA: Are some criminals born that way? *Think* 34:24–28, 1968.

Tellegen A, Lykken DT, Bouchard TJ Jr, et al: Personality similarity in twins reared apart and together. *J Pers Soc Psychol* 54:1031–1039, 1988.

Tinkenberg J: *Drugs and Crime in Drug Use in America.* Vol 1: *Patterns and Consequence of Drug Use.* Washington, DC, Government Printing Office, 1973.

Thompson T: Aggressive behaviour of Siamese fighting fish. In: Garattini S, Sigg EB (eds): *Aggressive Behaviour.* Amsterdam, Excerpta Medica Foundation, 1969, pp. 15–31.

Thompson WR, Wright JS: Persistence in rats: Effect of testosterone. *Physiol Psychol* 7:291–294, 1979.

Thor DH: Testosterone and persistence of social investigation in laboratory rats. *J Comp Physiol Psychol* 94:970–976, 1980.

Valzelli L: 5-Hydroxytryptamine in aggressiveness. In: Costa E, Gessa G, Sandler M (eds): *Advances in Biochemical Psychopharmacology.* New York, Raven Press, 1974.

van Praag HM, Brown SL, Asnis GM, et al: Beyond serotonin: A multiaminergic perspective on abnormal behavior. In: Serena-Lynn B, Herman MVP (eds): *The Role of Serotonin in Psychiatric Disorders.* Clinical and experimental psychiatry monograph, No. 4, 1991, pp. 302–332.

Virkkunen M: Urinary free cortisol secretion in habitually violent offenders. *Acta Psychiatr Scand* 72:40–44, 1985.

Virkkunen M: Personality profiles and state aggressiveness in Finnish alcoholic, violent offenders, fire setters, and healthy volunteers. *Arch Gen Psychiatry* 51:28–33, 1994.

Virkkunen M, DeJong J, Bartko J, et al: Relationship of psychobiological variables to recidivism in violent offenders and impulsive fire setters. *Arch Gen Psychiatry* 600–603, 1989.

Vom Saal FS: The intrauterine position phenomenon: Effects on physiology, aggressive behavior and population dynamics in house mice. In: Flannelly KJ, Blanchard RJ, Blanchard DC (eds): *Biological Perspectives on Aggression.* New York, Liss, 1984, pp. 135–179.

Weiger WA, Bear DM: An approach to the neurology of aggression. *J Psychiatry Res* 22(2):85–98, 1988.

Welch A, Welch B: Isolation, reactivity and aggression: Evidence for an involvement of brain catecholamines and serotonin. In: Eleftheriou B, Scott J (eds): *The Physiology of Aggression and Defeat.* New York, Plenum, 1971.

West DJ, Farrington DP: *Who Becomes Delinquent?* London, Heinemann, 1973.

Whiting B, Edwards CP: A cross-cultural analysis of sex differences in the behavior of children aged three through 11. *J Soc Psychol* 91:171–188, 1973.

Witkin HA, Mednick SA, Schulsinger F, et al: Criminality in XYY and XXY men. *Science* 193:547–555, 1976.

Wordsworth W: Ode: Intimations of Immortality from *Recollections of Early Childhood.* Boston, D Lothrop & Co, 1804.

Young JG, Brasic JR, Sheitman B, et al: Brain mechanisms mediating aggression and violence. In: Colette C, Gerald H (eds): *Children and Violence.* Vol 11: *The Child in the Family.* The Monograph Series of the International Association for Child and Adolescent Psychiatry and Allied Professions. Northvale, NJ, Aronson, 1994, pp. 13–48.

28 Neuropsychiatric Signs, Symptoms, and Syndromes

Daniel T. Williams, M.D.

In recent years, psychiatrists have been rediscovering the clinical importance of their historical roots in medicine in general and in neurology in particular. The proliferating volume of clinical research data has generated a growing awareness of important biological influences in psychiatric disorders, which for some time had been viewed almost exclusively in terms of their psychological and environmental determinants. The reactivation of a neuropsychiatric perspective is reflected in several recent publications on the subject (Pincus and Tucker, 1985; Yudofsky and Hales, 1989, 1992). This reintegrated perspective has, in turn, been associated with an increased concern by psychiatrists with the psychiatric manifestations of and complications of primary neurologic disorders.

In this context, clinicians evaluating children and adolescents with neurologic dysfunction must be additionally prepared to integrate developmental considerations in evaluating and treating these patients (Cook and Leventhal, 1992; Williams et al., 1987). Syndromes that affect the CNS tend to have particularly augmented cognitive, emotional, and behavioral effects if beginning and persisting during these early periods of development. In this regard, a syndrome that is static in its neurologic sequelae (e.g., cerebral palsy) is quite different in its psychiatric implications from a progressive disorder, such as one of the neurodegenerative disorders, commonly diagnosed initially in childhood. Furthermore, the area and extent of neurological involvement is crucial to determining the impact on development. Thus, a CNS lesion that generates intellectual impairment in the form of learning disabilities or frank mental retardation will make a substantial difference in the patient's coping capacities, quite apart from other focal neurologic or psychiatric impairments.

The Isle of Wight study demonstrated that children with brain injury suffer a significantly greater rate of psychiatric impairment than children with comparable degrees of physical disability not involving the CNS (Goodman, 1994; Rutter, 1989). Beyond the psychological sequelae of impaired physical functioning, the clinician must consider the potential direct neurophysiologic impact of CNS dysfunction on emotional, cognitive, and behavioral capacities (Howe et al., 1993; Pine et al., 1993).

Not all CNS dysfunction meriting differential diagnostic consideration by child psychiatrists is as evident as that following a well-documented brain injury. Indeed, one of the crucial tasks of the clinician in evaluating a youngster manifesting signs or symptoms of dysfunctional behavior or emotion is to assess the patient multidimensionally. This precludes the simplistic assumption that the dysfunction can be understood as deriving exclusively from either neurogenic or psychogenic origins. The multiaxial diagnostic format of DSM-IV encourages clinician consideration of psychopathology in this multidimensional manner.

With a growing level of sophistication in recent years, we have come to appreciate important neurogenic substrates of the CNS dysfunction central to a growing number of traditional psychiatric disorders, including the schizophrenias, pervasive developmental disorders, tic and Tourette disorders, attention deficit hyperactivity disorder, affective dis-

Table 28.1. Neuropsychiatric Signs and Symptoms Important to the Diagnosis of Psychiatric Syndromes

Diagnostic Parameter	Signs and Symptoms
Consciousness and arousal	Is there a reduced clarity of awareness, clouding? Is there a disturbance or reversal of the sleep-wake cycle? Is there a marked change in psychomotor activity level?
Attention	Is the capacity to shift, focus, and sustain attention impaired?
Perception	Are there any misinterpretations, illusions, hallucinations?
Cognitive processing	Is the ability to process information reduced? Is there an impairment of abstract thinking (i.e., concrete proverbs, poor similarities, poor concept-forming ability)?
Cognitive content	Is there a loss of general intellectual content? Are there any delusions or overvalued ideas, suspiciousness?
High cortical functions	Is there evidence of aphasia (fluent or nonfluent) or incoherent speech, apraxia or constructional difficulty, agnosia?
Memory	Is there ability to learn new information and to transfer it from short- to long-term memory? Is there ability to remember information known in the past? Is there difficulty with recall or recognition? Is there difficulty with verbal or visual memory? Is the patient oriented to time, place, person?
Mood	Is the mood prominently depressed, anxious, irritable, aggressive, or jocular? Is there an affective instability, marked shifts of mood, outbursts, or rage? Is the mood shallow, apathetic, indifferent?
Judgment	Is social judgment impaired? Is there any insight or foresight?
Time course	Do the symptoms fluctuate? Do the symptoms progress abruptly in a stepwise manner? Is there a steady decline in capacities or a steady increase in symptoms?

From Horvath T et al. Organic mental syndromes and disorders. In: Kaplan HI, Sadock BJ, eds. *Comprehensive Textbook of Psychiatry* (Vol 1). Baltimore, Williams & Wilkins, 1989, pp. 599–641.

orders, and anxiety disorders, to name just a few. Since we now recognize that every behavior and subjective experience has a neurophysiologic correlate (which most often is currently not identifiable), the neurogenic versus psychogenic distinction is ultimately a semantic one, determined by our current level of neurophysiologic sophistication or lack thereof.

For purposes of this chapter, the neuropsychiatric signs, symptoms, and syndromes considered will be those relevant to definable or presumed brain lesions. *Signs* are objective, observable deviations from normal behavior, performance, or neurophysiology. The mental status examination and more formal psychological testing assess both spontaneous behaviors and responses to standard cognitive queries. These are often usefully supplemented by formal neurologic evaluation, with its associated assessment of other areas of CNS function. *Symptoms* are the subjective observations by the patient of some deviation of experience or behavior from the norm. It is important in the case of children and adolescents to ascertain independently, from parents, to what extent such subjective complaints by the patient represent a change from the youngster's preexisting state and over what time frame.

Table 28.1 delineates a variety of diagnostic parameters, together with relevant signs and symptoms important to the diagnosis of neuropsychiatric syndromes (Horvath et al., 1989). It must be emphasized that, in assessing children and adolescents, the clinician needs to have a sense of the relative range of normal vis-à-vis an individual patient's age. This makes more complicated an assessment that, for adults, by contrast, can be gauged against a relatively unimodal standard normal range.

This chapter follows the DSM-IV format of replacing the DSM-III-R category of "Organic Mental Syndromes and Disorders" because this designation incorrectly implies that "nonorganic" mental disorders do not have a biological basis (American Psychiatric Association, 1994). Instead, DSM-IV utilizes two categories for what have traditionally been regarded as neuropsychiatric syndromes: (*a*) Delirium, Dementia, and Amnestic and Other Cognitive Disorders; and (*b*) Mental Disorders Due to a General Medical Condition.

The essential ingredient in both of these broad diagnostic groups is an experiential or behavioral abnormality associated with transient or permanent documentable dysfunction of the brain. In this chapter, several of the above-noted DSM-IV categories of mental disorder are addressed as they pertain to children and adolescents. Mental disorders associated with intoxication and withdrawal are discussed in Chapter 69. Mental disorders associated with acquired brain injury are addressed in Chapter 30. Mental disorders associated with brain tumors, neurodegenerative disorders, epilepsy, and cerebral palsy are addressed in Chapter 59.

DELIRIUM

Delirium may be defined as a transient and usually reversible dysfunction in cerebral metabolism that has an acute or subacute onset and is manifest clinically by a wide array of neuropsychiatric abnormalities (Wise and Brandt, 1992). Although the term has been used with differing connotations over the years and has many synonyms in the neurologic and psychiatric literature, it seems best for current purposes to define delirium as outlined in DSM-IV. Since, as noted above, disorders associated with intoxication and withdrawal are discussed in another chapter, Table 28.2 outlines diagnostic criteria for delirium due to general medical conditions.

Predisposing Factors and Clinical Features

Aside from the factor of age (children and the elderly reportedly have a higher risk), the following factors predispose to the development of delirium: postcardiotomy status, severe burns, preexisting brain damage, drug addiction, and acquired immune deficiency syndrome (AIDS). Although formal epidemiological studies are lacking, there is a consensus of reported clinical impressions regarding the vulnerability of children to delirium (Amit, 1988; Prugh et al., 1980). Because of the general acceptance of a tendency for children to regress under stressful circumstances, milder forms of delirium may be mistaken for simply regressive or provocative behavior. As with adults, however, undetected delirium may proceed to the point of self-injury and/or serious interference with medical treatment.

Paradoxically, children have an apparently reduced risk of postcardiotomy delirium compared with the risk for adults. Kornfeld et al. (1965) reported on a sample of 119 unselected open heart patients that included 20 children who had surgical procedures for repair of congenital lesions. One of the children developed delirium, whereas 30% of the adults operated on for congenital repairs experienced delirium. It is noteworthy that preoperative psychiatric interviews may reduce postoperative delirium and psychosis by 50% (Kornfeld et al., 1974).

Table 28.2. Diagnostic Criteria for Delirium Due to . . . (Indicate the General Medical Condition)

A. Disturbance of consciousness (i.e., reduced clarity of awareness of the environment) with reduced ability to focus, sustain, or shift attention.

B. A change in cognition (such as memory deficit, disorientation, language disturbance) or the development of a perceptual disturbance that is not better accounted for by a preexisting, established, or evolving dementia.

C. The disturbance develops over a short period of time (usually hours to days) and tends to fluctuate during the course of the day.

D. There is evidence from the history, physical examination, or laboratory findings that the disturbance is caused by the direct physiological consequences of a general medical condition.

Reprinted with permission from American Psychiatric Association: *Diagnostic and Statistical Manual of Mental Disorders* (4th ed). Washington, DC, American Psychiatric Association, 1994.

A clinical consensus suggests that, as the severity of a pathophysiologic stress increases, so does the probability of developing a delirium (Wise and Brandt, 1992). This is particularly true for burn patients, as well as for postoperative patients. Additional factors that are considered to foster the development of delirium include sleep deprivation, sensory deprivation, and sensory overload.

In addition to those clinical features outlined in Table 28.2, one should also note the possible presence of a prodromal period, characterized by restlessness, anxiety, sleep disturbance, and irritability. Also noteworthy and frequently present is a rapidly fluctuating and usually reversible course, which may include either hypoactivity and/or hyperactivity. Emotional lability is often observed, as is disorientation, dysgraphia (difficulty writing), constructional apraxia (difficulty drawing), and dysnomic aphasia (difficulty naming objects). Motor abnormalities that may be observed include tremor, asterixis (hand flap on extension), myoclonus (clonic muscle spasm), and symmetric reflex and muscle tone changes (Lipowski, 1990).

Differential Diagnosis

Insofar as the basic etiology of delirium is conceptualized as a derangement in the functional metabolism of the brain, it is clear that a vast array of medical conditions originating within as well as outside the CNS can engender such a derangement. Since these numerous medical conditions cannot be reviewed here, an outline of more common causes is presented in Table 28.3. As Wise and Brandt (1992) note, the catchy mnemonic "I WATCH DEATH" serves to remind the clinician of the potentially severe morbidity and mortality that can ensue from untreated or undertreated delirium.

Ordinarily, a psychiatrist confronted by a delirious patient will promptly involve a neurologic colleague in clarifying the differential diagnosis. It behooves the child psychiatrist, nevertheless, to be familiar with the neuropsychiatric evaluation of the patient with delirium. A summary of this process is outlined in Table 28.4.

The prognosis for a given patient with delirium will vary with the etiology and, most important, with whether irreversible damage to the CNS is sustained. Hence, the outcome, depending on the timeliness and effectiveness of treatment, may vary from full recovery through progression to stupor and coma, to seizures, to chronic brain syndromes, or to death.

Treatment

If one's differential diagnostic assessment has elucidated an etiology for the delirium, then often specific treatments that can lead to resolution of the delirium may be initiated. Specific treatments for identified causes of delirium are beyond the scope of this chapter and would be dictated by the tenets of accepted medical practice. In those situations where the etiology is unknown, even after a thorough initial evaluation, some interim supportive measures may well be helpful while diagnostic efforts continue. These are outlined under the following headings.

Table 28.3.   Causes of Delirium ("I WATCH DEATH")

Infectious	Encephalitis, meningitis, syphilis, AIDS
Withdrawal	Alcohol, barbiturates, sedatives-hypnotics
Acute metabolic	Acidosis, alkalosis, electrolyte disturbance, hepatic failure, renal failure
Trauma	Heat stroke, postoperative, severe burns
CNS pathology	Abscesses, hemorrhage, normal pressure hydrocephalus, seizures, stroke, tumors, vasculitis
Hypoxia	Anemia, carbon monoxide poisoning, hypotension, pulmonary/cardiac failure
Deficiences	B_{12}, hypovitaminosis, niacin, thiamine
Endocrinopathies	Hyper-/hypo- adrenalcorticism hyper-/hypo- glycemia
Acute vascular	Hypertensive encephalopathy, shock, migraine
Toxins/drugs	Medications, pesticides, solvents
Heavy metals	Lead, manganese, mercury

Adapted from Wise MG, Brandt GT: Delirium. In: Yudofsky SC, Hales RE (eds): *The American Psychiatric Press Textbook of Neuropsychiatry* (2nd ed). Washington, DC, American Psychiatric Press, 1992, pp. 291–310.

Table 28.4.   Neuropsychiatric Evaluation of the Patient

1. Mental status
   Interview (assess level of consciousness, psychomotor activity, appearance, affect, mood, intellect, thought processes)
   Performance tests (memory, concentration, reasoning, motor and constructional apraxia, dysgraphia, dysnomia)
2. Physical status
   Brief neurologic exam (reflexes; limb strength, Babinski's, cranial nerves, meningeal signs, gait)
   Review past and present vital signs (pulse, temperature, blood pressure, respiration rate)
   Review chart (labs, abnormal behavior noted and if so when it began, medical diagnoses, VDRL or FTA, HIV)[a]
   Review medication records (correlate abnormal behavior with starting or stopping medications)
3. Laboratory exam: basic
   Blood chemistries (electrolytes, glucose, Ca^{2+}, albumin, blood urea nitrogen, NH_4^+, liver functions)
   Blood count (hematocrit, white count and differential, MCV, sedimentation rate)
   Drug levels (need toxic screen? medication blood levels?)
   Arterial blood gases
   Urinalysis
   Electrocardiogram
   Chest x-ray
4. Laboratory: based on clinical judgment
   Electroencephalogram (seizures? focal lesion? confirm delirium by noting slowing or low-voltage fast activity)
   Computed tomography (normal pressure hydrocephalus, stroke, space-occupying lesion)
   Additional blood chemistries (heavy metals, thiamine and folate levels, thyroid battery, LE prep, ANA, urinary porphobilinogen)
   Lumbar puncture (if indication of infection or intracranial bleed)

Adapted from Wise MG, Brandt GT: Delirium. In: Yudofsky SC, Hales RE (eds): *The American Psychiatric Press Textbook of Neuropsychiatry* (2nd ed). Washington, DC, American Psychiatric Press, 1992, pp. 291–310.
[a] VDRL, Venereal Disease Research Laboratory; FTA, fluorescent treponemal antibody; HIV, human immunodeficiency virus; MCV, mean corpuscular volume; LE, lupus erythematosus; ANA, antinuclear antigens.

MEDICAL MEASURES

A patient with delirium should not only be in a hospital setting, but should also be under close observation by nursing staff who are familiar with the management of delirium. This should involve frequent monitoring of not only vital signs but also mental status, especially with a view to preventing self-injurious behavior.

PHARMACOLOGIC MEASURES

In the absence of double-blind trials, clinical experience has led to the advocacy of haloperidol administration in such situations because of its negligble anticholinergic and hypotensive properties and because it can be given parenterally (Lipowski, 1990). While adjustments of dosage are needed based on the size and age of the patient, general guidelines may be delineated. In children 6–12 years old, regardless of the route of administration, the advisable initial dosage would be 0.5 mg for mild agitation, 1 mg for moderate agitation, and 2 mg for severe agitation. For larger, older adolescents, reasonable dosages for the three categories above would be 2, 5, and 10 mg, respectively. The dose may be repeated every 30–60 minutes until the patient is calm, but this process requires close monitoring.

Benzodiazepines have the disadvantage of engendering sedation, which may further impair the delirious patient's cognition and may exacerbate the delirium. Small doses of intravenous lorazepam have been reported to be of some benefit, however, for patients who have not responded to high doses of haloperidol alone (Adams, 1984; Lipowski, 1990).

PSYCHOSOCIAL MEASURES

The presence of a calm family member or nursing attendant to provide reality testing, orientation, and reassurance can be very helpful in diminishing anxiety and allaying fears.

DEMENTIA

Dementia is a disorder of significant decline in multiple cognitive functions from the individual's previous intellectual level (McHugh and Folstein, 1991). In terms of the DSM-IV definition, the essential feature of dementia is impairment of memory, associated with at least one of the following cognitive disturbances: (a) aphasia (language disturbance); (b) apraxia (impaired ability to carry out motor activities despite intact motor function); (c) agnosia (failure to recognize or identify objects despite intact sensory function); and (d) disturbance in executive functioning (i.e., planning, organizing, sequencing, abstracting) (American Psychiatric Association, 1994). The disturbance is severe enough to interfere with work and school, usual social activities, and relationships with others. The diagnosis of dementia is not made if these symptoms occur only in the presence of reduced ability to maintain or shift attention to external stimuli, as in delirium; however, delirium and dementia may coexist.

Although dementia is found predominantly in the elderly, some neuropsychiatric disorders described later in this volume (Chapters 30 and 59) may cause dementia in childhood and adolescence. In terms of DSM-IV criteria, the diagnosis of dementia may be made at any time after the IQ is fairly stable (usually by age 4–6 years). Examples of medical conditions that may induce dementia in children or adolescents would include head injury, brain tumors, HIV infection, cerebrovascular accidents, or neurodegenerative disorders. Dementia in children may present as a deterioration in functioning, such as in school performance, or as a significant delay or deviation in normal development.

The mode of onset, subsequent course, and clinical management of dementia depend substantially on the underlying etiology. For this reason, such clinical features are addressed with reference to both dementia and other organic mental syndromes in the subsequent chapters of this volume dealing with acquired brain disorders and neurologic syndromes (Chapters 30 and 59).

AMNESTIC DISORDERS

Amnestic disorders are characterized by an impairment of memory that is attributable to a specific organic factor, such as a general medical condition (e.g., brain injury, vitamin deficiency), a substance of abuse, a toxin, or a medication side effect. The diagnosis requires the absence of the clouded sensorium associated with delirium or the more pervasive cognitive impairments associated with dementia. The syndrome, more commonly encountered as the Wernicke-Korsakoff syndrome among adult chronic alcoholics and attributed to thiamine deficiency, is relatively uncommon in children. It may be associated in children, however, with head trauma, hypoxia, lead or carbon monoxide poisoning, and herpes simplex encephalitis (Mikkelsen, 1991). Temporal lobectomy for intractable complex partial seizures may result in memory deficits, but this is usually of major significance only when surgery is bilateral (Shimanura and Gershberg, 1992).

OTHER ALTERED STATES OF CONSCIOUSNESS

Not all altered states of consciousness encountered clinically by child psychiatrists are subsumed by the neuropsychiatric syndromes outlined above. Indeed, on a broad basis, most of the diagnostic categories encountered clinically, ranging from anxiety disorders and affective disorders to the schizophrenias, involve subtle or not so subtle alterations of attention, perception, cognitive processing, consciousness, and the like, subsuming all the diagnostic parameters delineated in Table 28.1. A critical diagnostic task, therefore, is that of distinguishing those constellations of signs and symptoms associated with "traditional" psychiatric disorders from those associated with neuropsychiatric syndromes. The general current presumption is that the traditional psychiatric disorders are by-products of particular constitutional or genetically based vulnerabilities, interacting with the individual's life experiences. In neuropsychiatric disorders, by contrast, the CNS abnormality is viewed as the overriding determinant of the presenting psychopathology. As reflected in our previous discussion, there are may instances where such distinctions are not absolute, for example, when a de novo organic brain injury generates new psychopathology that interacts with a patient's preexisting vulnerabilities and personality structure. Alternatively, for example, a patient with a long-standing epileptic seizure disorder may develop secondary psychogenic seizures as a result of developmental adversities and/or intervening life stresses. The clinician's task, therefore, is to draw upon all available sources of information so as to formulate as comprehensive a diagnostic assessment as possible, as the prerequisite for an effective treatment plan. Implicit in the above is the premise of the multivariate etiology of any psychopathologic picture and an intent to give adequate consideration to both psychogenic and neurogenic factors. With these considerations in mind, three additional syndromes presenting as altered states of consciousness and presenting potential challenges to neuropsychiatric assessment are briefly noted; one other is discussed in some detail.

Altered states of consciousness associated with alcohol and drug use are addressed in Chapter 69, those associated with dissociative disorders are addressed in Chapter 64, and those associated with seizure disorders are addressed in Chapter 59.

STUPOR AND CATATONIA

Stupor has been defined differently by different authors. For most neurologists, stupor connotes a condition of behavioral nonresponsiveness, including loss of speech (mutism), markedly reduced movement (hypokinesis), and a reduced level of consciousness, from which the subject can be aroused only by vigorous and repeated stimulation. Stuporous patients are thus seen by most neurologists as having diffuse organic cerebral dysfunction of greater severity than that encountered in delirium, representing usually the next stage along a neurophysiologic continuum between clear consciousness and coma (Cutting, 1992; Plum and Posner, 1980). For many psychiatrists, on the other hand, stupor descriptively has connoted a relative preservation of consciousness in conjunction with mutism and hypokinesis (Roberts, 1984; Rogers, 1991). As such, stupor has been associated in the psychiatric literature with traditional psychiatric conditions characterized by catatonia.

One of the most reasonable ways of reconciling the above disparity in perspectives regarding stupor is to observe that both neurologists and psychiatrists see patients to whom they apply the symptomatic designation of stupor, but that the samples of patients they see, while overlapping somewhat, are significantly divergent. This becomes important in the differential diagnosis of stupor, regarding the need to separate organic from psychogenic stupors. Thus, Plum and Posner (1980) found psychogenic unresponsiveness to occur in only 4 of 386 unresponsive patients they saw on a neurology service. The predominant "psychogenic" diagnoses in their series of patients were catatonic schizophrenia and hysterical conversion, the latter generally associated with depression. By contrast, Joyston-Bechal (1966) found that in a psychiatric population, 69% of 100 "stuporous" patients had nonorganic disorders only. Of these 100 patients, 25% had depression, 34% schizophrenia, 23% organic disorders (mainly dementia), and 10% hysterical features. The vast majority of patients in both of the above and other studies (Cutting, 1992) have been adults, with no comparable series being available for children and adolescents.

It is noteworthy that Cutting, in The American Psychiatric Press Textbook of Neuropsychiatry (1992), proposes a classification in which catatonia is designated as a subtype of stupor, referring primarily to psychiatric symptoms traditionally associated with mood disorders, schizophrenia, and less commonly, somatoform disorder. By contrast, the DSM-IV manual (American Psychiatric Association, 1994), in addition to the above-noted traditional categories for catatonia, has added the category of "catatonic disorder due to a general medical condition," presumably as a way of reminding the psychiatrist to consider possible underlying organic factors rather than jumping to a premature diagnostic conclusion, premised on the more familiar, traditional psychiatric diagnoses. In this regard, DSM-IV defines catatonia as being characterized by any of the following: motoric immobility (hypokinesia or akinesia), excessive motor activity, extreme negativism or mutism, peculiarities of voluntary movement (e.g., waxy flexibility), echolalia, or echopraxia. The diagnosis of catatonic disorder due to a general medical condition is not given if the catatonia occurs exclusively during the course of a delirium.

Clarification of the cause of stupor or catatonia is clearly crucial, in light of the potentially serious morbidity and mortality involved if the underlying condition is not effectively treated. Furthermore, inappropriate treatment, such as the use of additional neuroleptics in patients with neuroleptic-induced catatonic stupor (Weinberger and Wyatt, 1978) or other mismanagement of organic stupor, can cause further deterioration. Since by definition the patient will be unable to give a history, securing other reliable informants becomes important. The history may disclose previous physical or mental illness or recent insults that may help clarify etiology.

On physical examination, a psychogenic disorder is suggested by closed eyes that resist opening and that close rapidly when the force used to open them is released. Although fixation of the eyes on objects in the patient's field of vision suggests alertness and awareness of the environment, this also may be seen in some organic disorders. Random roving eye movements, however, strongly suggest an organic disorder. On the other hand, voluntary deviation of eyes to the ground, no matter which side the patient is lying on, points to a psychogenic stupor (Henry and Woodruff, 1978).

The alert patient in psychogenic stupor will usually attempt to protect himself or herself from injury (Roberts, 1984). Thus, if the physician lifts the patient's arm and allows it to fall toward the patient's face, the patient will usually modify its path to avoid it's striking him or her. Alertness is also suggested by a blink response to visual threat and purposeful, directed attempts by the patient to deflect a painful stimulus. Autonomic hyperarousal is usually present, with tachycardia, hypertension, and pupils that are equal, dilated, and responsive briskly and symmetrically to light.

The oculocephalic reflex (doll's head eye phenomenon) is a simple test that can be used in the unresponsive patient, provided there are no indications that a cervical injury is present. The reflex involves conjugate deviation of both eyes to one side when the head is turned quickly to the other side. If the reflex is consistently positive, this strongly suggests the presence of organic brain disease, probably involving the area of the frontal eye fields (Plum and Posner, 1980).

Another useful diagnostic sign is the oculovestibular reflex. This involves instillation of cold water into the patient's external auditory canal, with care taken beforehand to ensure that the canal is patent and the tympanic membrane intact. The normal ocular response is a regular rhythmic nystagmus, with the slow component directed toward the irrigated ear. When present, this "firmly indicates that the patient is physiologically awake and that the unresponsive state cannot be caused by structural or metabolic disease of the nervous system" (Plum and Posner, 1980).

The use of intravenous Amytal Sodium may be helpful when there is a strong index of suspicion that a patient's stupor or catatonia may be of psychogenic etiology (Roberts, 1984). Careful neurologic evaluation of the patient should precede the use of this procedure, however, as the drug may confuse the monitoring of the patient's level of consciousness, which is vital when a progressive neurologic lesion is suspected. Similarly, it may interfere with interpretation of the EEG tracing. In organic brain disorders, Amytal Sodium tends to cause cognitive deterioration: If this occurs, its use must be immediately stopped and the patient examined for any neurologic signs that may have been revealed. In the psychogenic patient, underlying psychopathology, such as positive symptoms of psychosis, may be revealed. The unresponsiveness of psychogenic patients tends to diminish with Amytal Sodium, but this may require a high dose of the drug. This is in contrast with the relatively low dose that will often cause sedation and confusion in patients with organic brain disorders (Perry and Jacobs, 1982; Rogers, 1991).

Further aspects of differential diagnosis and treatment would follow similar channels of consideration as those outlined under "Delirium" above. Certainly involvement of a neurologic colleague in the assessment to rule out pertinent neurologic etiology is essential before proceeding to treatment intervention for presumed psychogenic etiology. Furthermore, positive evidence for an underlying psychiatric diagnosis should be delineated before a specific treatment plan can reasonably be initiated.

CONCLUSIONS

Being cognizant of the diagnostic significance of neuropsychiatric signs, symptoms, and syndromes is essential for the well-trained child and adolescent psychiatrist. Implicit in this is the psychiatrist's developing a multidimensional perspective that carefully attends to both the neurogenic and psychogenic influences that each patient brings to his or her interactions with the outside world. Only with such an adequately broad-based perspective of diagnosis can effective treatment planning for patients ensue.

References

Adams F: Neuropsychiatric evaluation and treatment of delirium in the critically ill cancer patient. *Cancer Bull* 36:156–160, 1984.

American Psychiatric Association: *Diagnostic and Statistical Manual of Mental Disorders* (4th ed). Washington, DC, American Psychiatric Press, 1994.

Amit R: Acute confusional state in childhood. *Childs Nerv Syst* 4:255–258, 1988.

Cook EH, Leventhal BL: Neuropsychiatric disorders of childhood and adolescence. In: Yudofsky SC, Hales RE (eds): *The American Psychiatric Press Textbook of Neuropsychiatry* (2nd ed). Washington, DC, American Psychiatric Press, 1992, pp. 639–661.

Cutting J: Neuropsychiatric aspects of attention and consciousness: Stupor and coma. In: Yudofsky SC, Hales RE (eds): *The American Psychiatric Press Textbook of Neuropsychiatry* (2nd ed). Washington, DC, American Psychiatric Press, 1992, pp. 277–290.

Goodman R: Brain disorders. In: Rutter M, Taylor E, Hersov L (eds): *Child and Adolescent Psychiatry: Modern Approaches* (3rd ed). Oxford, Blackwell, 1994, pp. 129–151.

Henry JH, Woodruff GH: A diagnostic sign in states of apparent unconsciousness. *Lancet* 2: 920–921, 1978.

Horvath TB, Siever LJ, Mohs TC, et al: Organic mental syndromes and disorders. In: Kaplan EH, Sadock BJ (eds): *Comprehensive Textbook of Psychiatry* (5th ed). Baltimore, Williams & Wilkins, 1989, pp. 599–641.

Howe GW, Feinstein C, Reiss D, et al: Adolescent adjustment to chronic physical disorders. I: Comparing neurological and non-neurological conditions. *J Child Psychol Psychiatry* 34:1153–1171, 1993.

Joyston-Bechal MP: The clinical features and outcome of stupor. *Br J Psychiatry* 112:967–981, 1966.

Kornfeld DS, Heller SS, Frank KA, et al: Personality and psychological factors in postcardiotomy delirium. *Arch Gen Psychiatry* 31:249–253, 1974.

Kornfeld DS, Zimberg S, Malm JR: Psychiatric complications of open-heart surgery. *N Engl J Med* 273:287–292, 1965.

Lipowski ZJ: *Delirium: Acute Confusional States*. New York, Oxford University Press, 1990.

McHugh PR, Folstein MF: Organic mental disorders. In: Cavenar JO (ed): *Psychiatry* (Vol 1). Philadelphia, Lippincott, 1991, pp. 1–21.

Mikkelsen EJ: Organic mental disorders. In: Cavenar JO (ed): *Psychiatry* (Vol 2). Philadelphia, Lippincott, 1991, pp. 1–13.

Perry JC, Jacobs D: Overview of clinical applications of the amytal interview in psychiatric emergency settings. *Am J Psychiatry* 139:552–559, 1982.

Pincus JH, Tucker GJ: *Behavioral Neurology* (3rd ed). New York, Oxford University Press, 1985.

Pine D, Shaffer D, Schonfeld IS: Persistent emotional disorder in children with neurological soft signs. *J Am Acad Child Adolesc Psychiatry* 32: 1229–1236, 1993.

Plum F, Posner JB: *The Diagnosis of Stupor and Coma*. Philadelphia, FA Davis, 1980.

Prugh DG, Wagonfeld S, Metcalf D, et al: A clinical study of delirium in children and adolescents. *Psychosom Med* 42(suppl):177–197, 1980.

Roberts JK: *Differential Diagnosis in Neuropsychiatry*. New York, Wiley, 1984.

Rogers D: Catatonia: A contemporary approach. *J Neuropsychiatry Clin Neurosci* 3:334–340, 1991.

Rutter M: Isle of Wight revisited: Twenty-five

years of child psychiatry epidemiology. *J Am Acad Child Adolesc Psychiatry* 28:633–653, 1989.

Shimanura AP, Gershberg FB: Neuropsychiatric aspects of memory and amnesia. In: Yudofsky SC, Hales RE (eds): *The American Psychiatric Press Textbook of Neuropsychiatry* (2nd ed). Washington, DC, American Psychiatric Press, 1992.

Weinberger DR, Wyatt RJ: Catatonic stupor and neuroleptic drugs. *JAMA* 239:1846, 1978.

Williams DT, Pleak RR, Hanesian H: Neuropsychiatric disorders of childhood and adolescence. In: Hales RE, Yudofsky SC (eds): *The American Psychiatric Press Textbook of Neuropsychiatry*. Washington, DC, American Psychiatric Press, 1987, pp. 365–383.

Wise MG, Brandt GT: Delirium. In: Yudofsky SC, Hales RE (eds): *The American Psychiatric Press Textbook of Neuropsychiatry* (2nd ed). Washington, DC, American Psychiatric Press, 1992, pp. 291–310.

Yudofsky SC, Hales RE: The reemergence of neuropsychiatry: Definition and direction. *J Neuropsychiatry Clin Sci* 1:1–6, 1989.

Yudofsky SC, Hales RE (eds): *The American Psychiatric Press Textbook of Neuropsychiatry* (2nd ed). Washington, DC, American Psychiatric Press, 1992.

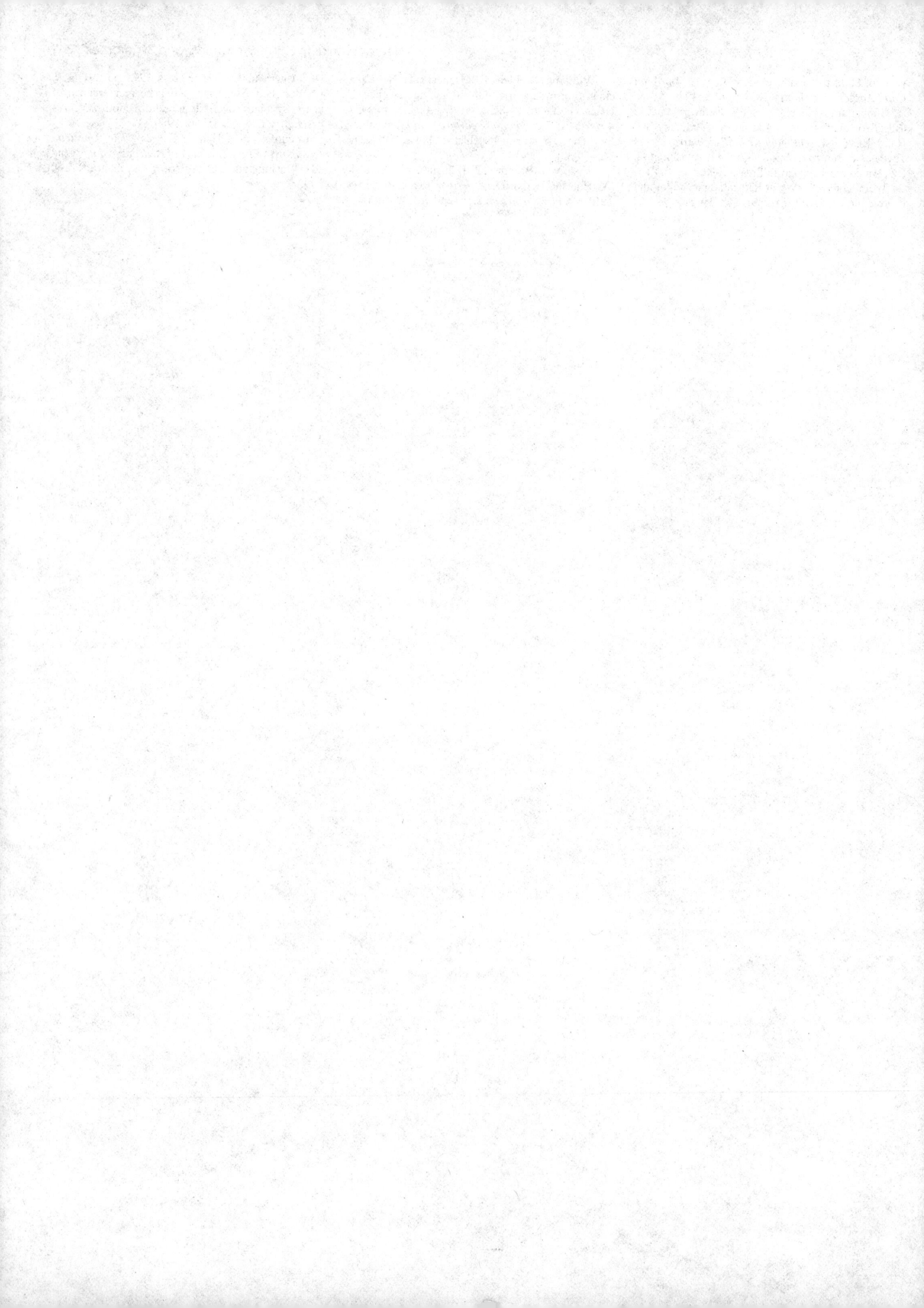

29 GENETIC INFLUENCES ON CHILD PSYCHIATRIC CONDITIONS

John P. Alsobrook II, M. Phil., Dorothy Grice, M.D., and David L. Pauls, Ph.D.

In child psychiatry, interest in genetic factors is high. Psychiatric disorders often run in families, and research has implicated genetic factors in a variety of mental, developmental, and behavioral disorders of childhood onset (Lombroso et al., 1994). Specific genetic mutations have been characterized in some developmental neuropsychiatric disorders (e.g., fragile X syndrome and Prader-Willi syndrome), although thus far identification of etiological gene mutations in psychiatric illness has been unsuccessful.

Psychiatric disorders are examples of complex traits. As such, the transmission within families does not follow classic mendelian inheritance patterns, and it is presumed that a number of factors contribute to the ultimate expression of clinical psychiatric symptoms. These factors may include environmental variables, such as gestational and psychosocial conditions, and biological variables, such as comorbid medical conditions and genetic factors. The genetic factors could be single loci or, as is more likely to be the case, psychiatric disorders could result from the expression of more than one gene (oligogenic or polygenic) in a larger context of potentially numerous environmental influences. It is quite likely that none of these etiologic factors are both necessary and sufficient for the expression of any psychiatric disorder.

While vital contributions come from research on environmental influences in psychiatric disorders, genetic study of disease yields evidence about the underlying biology and transmission of the illness, two important areas related to treatment and prevention. It is expected that early identification of vulnerability to psychiatric illness would allow for the development of early intervention and prevention strategies.

Considerable work has been done over the last decade to develop valid and reliable assessment instruments for the diagnosis and measurement of child psychiatric disorders. These instruments have made it more feasible to undertake genetic studies of childhood disorders. Concurrently the development of more sophisticated genetic methods and successful genetic studies of other complex human diseases (e.g., colon cancer, diabetes, hypercholesterolemia) has led to an overall increased interest in the importance of genetic factors for the manifestation and expression of human disease.

Interest in the genetics of child psychiatric disorders is a part of a substantial increase in basic research in child psychiatry over the last two decades. The purpose of this chapter is to summarize the methods suitable for the genetic study of child psychiatric conditions and to provide a brief review of the current understanding of the genetics of several of these disorders.

METHODS SUITABLE FOR THE GENETIC STUDY OF CHILDHOOD DISORDERS

Historically, the approach taken in human genetics to determine whether an illness has a genetic basis is to search for an aberrant or missing protein that would result in some observable structural or biochemical change. While this approach has been successful for many human diseases, it has not been effective in the study of psychiatric/behavioral disorders of childhood. In the absence of such data, other methods are useful to help establish the importance of genetic factors in the expression of an illness. Those methods include (*a*) studies of twins, (*b*) studies of adopted children, and (*c*) studies of families.

Twin Studies

Twin studies are quite useful in establishing that genetic factors are important in the manifestation and expression of a disorder (LaBuda et al., 1994). Historically, this approach came into use to estimate the relative contribution of genetic and environmental influences. The underlying genetic theory is straightforward. Monozygotic (MZ) twins are genetically identical. If a trait is completely determined by genetic factors, then MZ twins should have exactly the same phenotype. In contrast to MZ twins, dizygotic (DZ) twins share, on average, only 50% of their genetic material. Thus, if there is no unique contribution of twin environments, DZ twins should be no more similar than singleton siblings. For example, if a trait is determined by a fully penetrant autosomal-dominant gene, then the concordance rate for DZ twins should be 0.50 compared with 1.0 for MZ twins. If a trait is determined by an autosomal recessive gene, then the expected concordance for DZ twins would be 0.25.

When the inheritance is complex, mendelian patterns are not observed, and the concordance rates for MZ and DZ twins are not expected to approximate Mendelian segregation ratios. In these circumstances, a significantly greater concordance for MZ twins when compared to the concordance for DZ twins is taken as evidence for the involvement of genetic factors in the phenotype being studied.

One of the advantages of the twin methodology is that it is possible to study the contribution of genetic factors to traits that may not present a stable phenotype throughout the course of development. A major complication of research designs that require assessment of children and adults in families is the determination of the "childhood affected status" of adults within the family units under study. Although various attempts have been made both to establish methods to assess adult phenotypes of childhood disorders and to develop methods to make retrospective diagnoses of childhood conditions, major questions remain concerning their reliability and validity. Twin studies can surmount these difficulties because twin pairs can be studied within the appropriate development epoch so that reliable assessments can be made.

As has been pointed out (Pauls, 1985), one of the most interesting applications of the twin study paradigm is the examination of discordant MZ twin pairs. Assuming a genetic etiology for a behavioral disturbance, MZ twins should show full concordance rates. The fact that they do not implies that environmental factors are also of etiological importance. A closer examination of discordant twins should help to identify important nonheritable factors that mediate the expression of the underlying genetic vulnerability.

Another potentially important use of twin studies has been illustrated by Plomin and Daniels (1987). These investigators have demonstrated the ability for twin studies to estimate the nonshared environmental variance important for the manifestation of a phenotype. As these investigators have pointed out, nonshared environment may be the most influential factor in contributing to the phenotypes of children within families.

The greatest weakness mentioned by critics of the twin studies is the assumption that the environments for MZ and DZ twins are comparable. The assumption has been examined (Cohen et al., 1975), and no relevant differences have been found. In addition, as Rowe (1983) has indicated, it is not enough to show that DZ twins differ from MZ twins or that singletons differ from twins and use this to condemn twin studies in general. It must be demonstrated that such differences in biology or environment are etiologically important for the particular disturbance under investigation.

Adoption/Separation Studies

If there is a substantial environmental component important for the manifestation of a disorder, the twin study design will not be able to completely separate out its effect from the genetic factors that may also influence the trait. Adoption or separation studies provide a method to examine more closely the extent to which environmental factors influence the phenotype being studied. If a trait is genetic, then children should resemble their biological relatives to a greater degree than they resemble their adoptive relatives. Thus, the extent to which adopted children resemble their biological parents is taken as evidence of a genetic contribution. If children resemble their unrelated adoptive relatives to any degree, then that resemblance is, at least in theory, due to shared environments. Thus, separation studies provide a potentially powerful method for separating the effects of genes and environment.

Although quite useful, adoption studies have some significant drawbacks in the study of childhood disorders. In fact, it is noteworthy that few adoption studies of childhood psychiatric disorders have been reported. One reason for this could be that it is critical to obtain reliable diagnostic assessments of the parents as children. Since much of the information about the biological parents comes from obstetric records, it is often impossible to retrieve the necessary information for reliable and valid assessment of the parents. A further complication is that data about the biological father are often completely missing, so to the extent that the father may also have behavioral difficulties, it is not possible to evaluate the phenotype of the child in light of the phenotype of the father. As pointed out (Pauls, 1985; Rutter et al., 1990), having missing or incomplete data regarding one or both biological parents can seriously compromise the usefulness of adoption studies. One way to overcome this limitation is through the use of prospective longitudinal study designs (Plomin and DeFries, 1985; Plomin et al., 1988).

Family Studies

As discussed, twin and adoption studies provide data useful in establishing that genetic factors are important for the expression of a disorder. However, both approaches are limited in that it is not possible to test hypotheses about specific genetic mechanisms of transmission. Studies of biological families yield data that will allow examination of specific genetic hypotheses. However, as with twin studies, if there is a major environmental component important for the manifestation of the phenotype under investigation, data from family studies will not prove the existence of genetic factors. Genetic and family environmental factors can interact in determining similarities and differences among relatives and cannot be unambiguously quantified without prior specific identification. Thus, it is important to distinguish between shared and nonshared familial and nonfamilial environmental factors. It is also important to keep in mind the possibility of confounding familial environmental similarity and genetic similarity within a given family.

Family studies have been quite helpful in establishing that most major adult psychiatric disorders are inherited. A major limitation of family studies for childhood psychiatric disorders is related to assessment and diagnosis. It is the same limitation as was discussed for adoption studies. It is essential that all relatives in a family study be reliably and validly assessed. Since there will always be at least two adults (i.e., the parents) in every nuclear family, it is essential that methods be available to obtain the necessary information to assess the childhood phenotype of those adults. Retrospective data may be unreliable or unavailable. Information regarding current symptomatology is useful only if there is a one-to-one correspondence between the childhood phenotype and adult phenotype. Clearly, more longitudinal studies need to be completed to learn more about the adult phenotypic outcomes of child psychiatric disorders.

Molecular Genetic Studies

While results from twin, adoption, and family studies can provide convincing evidence that genetic factors contribute significantly to the expression of childhood psychiatric disorders, none of these methods can prove the existence of specific genetic etiologic factors. One of the strongest forms of evidence for a genetic etiology is the demonstration of a molecular abnormality or the existence of a linked genetic marker. The search for specific molecular abnormalities and/or biochemical markers has not been fruitful in child psychiatry. A potentially more promising approach is the use of genetic linkage information.

Genetic linkage occurs when two different loci are located sufficiently close on the same chromosome, so that they are transmitted together from parent to child. The demonstration of linkage in humans requires family studies to establish that alleles at the two loci cosegregate within families. Family data are used to estimate how frequently alleles at two loci are transmitted in combinations different from those occurring in the parents. If new combinations occur with equal frequency to parental combinations, then the two loci are not linked. If the frequency of parental combinations is relatively greater than that of new recombinants, the two loci are linked, and the frequency of new recombinants can be used to estimate the strength of linkage. The degree of linkage is measured as the recombination fraction and can range from 0.0 (complete linkage) to 0.5 (independent assortment). The minimum recombination frequency of 0.0 is found when alleles at two separate loci are always transmitted together. The maximum recombination frequency of 0.5 is found for alleles that have the same likelihood of being transmitted in new combinations as in the old combinations, from generation to generation. The maximum recombination occurs for loci far apart on the same chromosome and for loci on different chromosomes.

The statistical significance for a particular recombination fraction is determined by measuring the difference in the probability of observing linkage and comparing it to the probability of observing independent assortment in a given family. Finding statistically significant deviation from independent assortment for alleles at a known marker locus and at a hypothesized locus for a complex trait provides convincing evidence that there is a major gene contributing to the expression of the disorder. It is highly unlikely that any other explanation could mimic linkage with a marker locus.

Some problems in detecting linkage in human data include small family size, the inability to control matings, and the small prior probability that two loci are linked. The linkage method has had limited applicability until recently because of the paucity of available marker loci in humans. With the advent of recombinant DNA technology, this has changed dramatically. As part of the advance in genetics brought about by recombinant DNA techniques, two of the many recently discovered classes of polymorphisms have proven to be most useful in linkage studies.

The first class of these polymorphisms is known as restriction fragment length polymorphisms (RFLP); RFLPs exist as inherited variations in the length of fragments of DNA (Botstein et al., 1980). The length of these fragments is defined by the distance between specific short sequences of DNA ("restriction sites"), which are recognized and cleaved enzymatically by restriction endonucleases. Alterations in the nucleotide sequence of a restriction site may render it unrecognizable to an endonuclease (eliminating the site) or they may transform a normally unrecognized sequence into a new restriction site, in either case altering the lengths of the fragments produced by the enzymatic cleavage. The results of such "restriction digests" yield precise DNA fragments whose lengths are defined by the position of the restriction sites contained in a subject's intact DNA. The resulting fragments can then be separated according to their lengths by subjecting them to an electric field while inside a supporting matrix (gel electrophoresis); smaller fragments migrate through the matrix more rapidly than larger fragments, and thus a size gradient of fragments is produced.

A second critical component of the RFLP method is the ability to identify a piece or pieces of DNA that contain the unique marker sequence under study. When DNA from the entire genome is restriction-digested and electrophoresed, the resulting fragment sizes range from tens of bases to hundreds of thousands of bases. This produces a smear of DNA along the gel, representing a continuum of all possible sizes of fragments. What is then needed is a way to identify the position of a particular marker sequence in that smear, differentiating the desired marker "signal" from the background "noise" of all other fragments. Recombinant DNA techniques allow us to accomplish this by labeling or tagging the marker DNA, which is referred to as the "probe." The classic labeling method incorporates nucleotides containing radioactive isotopes into the probe DNA, but the use of radioactivity is now being supplanted by the use of fluorescent dyes. The labeled probe can then be used to locate the position of the marker sequence of interest within the gel smear.

The second class of commonly used polymorphisms also relies on variations in the length of specific nucleotide sequences known as tandem nucleotide repeats. The analysis of these repeats relies on the polymerase chain reaction (PCR), a method of exponentially amplifying the number of copies of a specific DNA sequence between two flanking primer sequences (Mullis et al., 1986; the importance of PCR is evidenced by the award of the 1993 Nobel Prize in chemistry to its inventor, Kary Mullis).

Tandem repeats are islands of DNA consisting of multiple units of a very short sequence motif; the first to be described as polymorphisms were repeats of the dinucleotide sequence C-A (Weber and May, 1989). The number of repeated dinucleotide units at a given $(CA)_n$ repeat site has been shown to vary among individuals within a species; this number directly determines the discrete variations in length of the $(CA)_n$ segment (in increments of 2 base pairs). Since these repeat segments are typically flanked by unique genomic DNA sequences, it is possible to use PCR to produce millions of copies of the DNA fragment containing the tandem repeats, at the same time incorporating a radioactive or fluorescent label into the newly synthesized copies. When the amplification products are electrophoresed in a gel system that resolves single base pair length differences (a denaturing polyacrylamide gel) and subsequently exposed to x-ray film (in the case of radioactive labels) or read by fluorometrically scanning the gel (in the case of fluorescent labels), the allelic variation in the lengths of the $(CA)_n$ repeat segments is revealed, and typings can be assigned. Subsequent investigation has revealed the presence of additional trinucleotide and tetranucleotide tandem repeats throughout the human genome.

The current inventory of marker loci now spans the entire human genome at a moderately fine level. A large number of $(CA)_n$ repeat segments and RFLP probes have been catalogued, and more are being developed each week. These new marker technologies have made linkage studies in humans feasible, and in addition have led to the initiation of work necessary to map and sequence the entire human genome. Thus, in the very near future, there will be a significant number of genetic markers available to identify genetic linkages to loci of etiologic importance for child psychiatric conditions.

Much work needs to be done before that time, however. One of the most difficult problems with linkage studies of psychiatric disorders relates to the phenotype. All mental disorders have variable expression,

and the data from twin studies demonstrate reduced penetrance. The presence of reduced penetrance and a variable age of onset reduces the power of the statistical methods available for the detection of linkage. Methods have been developed to incorporate the possibility of reduced penetrance into the analyses (Hodge et al., 1979; Lathrop et al., 1985); however, it is not clearly understood what the impact of misspecification of penetrance will have on the results of the analyses.

In the absence of a well-understood etiology, demonstration of the presence of genetic factors usually does not resolve questions about the nature of the genes involved and how they interact with environmental factors. Is a particular gene necessary for the disease to develop? Will a certain genotype always lead to illness? Are there ameliorating environments that prevent illness in persons otherwise genetically susceptible? Answers to these questions need to be addressed. The full scope of gene-environment interactions can be understood only after the full disease process is understood.

Establishing that a disease locus is linked to a specific marker will be a major step in understanding the pathophysiology for child psychiatric disorders. However, before this methodology can be used successfully, there needs to be fairly strong evidence that at least some forms of a specific illness have an underlying genetic mechanism that is relatively simple (i.e., one or two major genes contributing significantly to the expression of the phenotype). As is discussed in the section to follow, there is some evidence that childhood psychiatric/behavioral disorders are influenced by genetic factors. However, the specific mode of transmission is not understood for most disorders of childhood; thus at this time, the pursuit of genetic linkages needs to be in the context of other studies that are examining specific genetic hypotheses of transmission.

REVIEW OF THE GENETICS OF CHILDHOOD NEUROPSYCHIATRIC DISORDERS

In this section the evidence that genetic factors are important for some of the more extensively studied childhood disorders is reviewed. A comprehensive review of all childhood disorders is beyond the scope of this chapter. Thus for the purposes of the current presentation, disorders were chosen that provide examples of the application of the approaches discussed above.

Attention Deficit Hyperactivity Disorder

Attention deficit hyperactivity disorder (ADHD) is a common neuropsychiatric and behavioral disorder of childhood onset. The prevalence of ADHD is high—it is the most frequently observed neurobehavioral problem in the pediatric age group. Prevalence rates have been estimated to range between 2 and 15% (Rutter, 1983), and males are affected approximately four times as often as females (Shaywitz et al., 1983). While a variety of etiologies (infections (Shaywitz and Shaywitz, 1982), head trauma (Rutter, 1981), and intrauterine exposure to toxins (Shaywitz et al., 1983)) have been identified for some cases, in the majority of individuals no single etiologic factor is evident.

Cumulative results from several lines of investigation yield evidence that genetic factors play an important etiologic role in the expression of hyperactive and inattentive behaviors and ADHD. Results of several twin studies suggest that genetic factors are important for the expression of normal activity levels (Scarr, 1966; Vandenberg, 1962; Willerman, 1973). However, many studies are weakened by uncertain validity of diagnosis and rating scales, small sample sizes, and ascertainment bias.

In an early study, Lopez (1965) examined 10 twin pairs (4 MZ, 6 DZ) in which one twin had "clinical hyperactivity." He found 100% concordance in the MZ pairs, compared with 17% concordance in the DZ pairs. However, in light of several methodological weaknesses in this study (four of the DZ twins were opposite-sex pairs), these results could not be considered definitive. In a large study of 13-year-old twin pairs (102 MZ and 111 same-sex DZ twin pairs), Goodman and Stevenson (1989) found that MZ twins had higher concordance on objective measures of inattentiveness and hyperactivity than same-sex DZ twins. Family environment measures and perinatal adversity did not significantly relate to hyperactivity measures. The researchers concluded that the heritability accounted for 30–50% of the explainable variance in inattention and hyperactivity in this twin population. The common environment effects accounted for less than 30% of the variance. Stevenson (1992) also performed a multiple regression analysis on data from a sample of 91 MZ twins and 105 same-sex DZ twins. These results also showed a significant genetic contribution to individual differences in activity levels (those measured through maternal ratings but not teacher ratings) and attention abilities.

Family history studies also provide support for the hypothesis that hyperactivity (and by implication, ADHD) is familial. Morrison and Stewart (1971) surveyed first- and second-degree relatives of 59 hyperactive children and 41 control children. Twenty per cent of parents of ADHD children were retrospectively diagnosed as hyperactive compared with 5% of parents of the control group. When data from first- and second-degree relatives were combined, the rates of hyperactivity were significantly higher in the relatives of the hyperactive children. Cantwell (1972) also showed that the frequency of hyperactivity was higher among relatives of hyperactive children than among relatives of control children. In a clinic sample of children (N = 72), Pauls et al. (1983) demonstrated that ADHD is familial and that it is vertically transmitted within families. Logistic regression analyses of family history data incorporating sex of the proband, parental affected status, and family history most adequately explained the patterns of ADHD in these families.

Separation studies also suggest a genetic component in ADHD. Morrison and Stewart (1973) compiled self-report data from the adoptive parents of 35 hyperactive children. The adoptive parents reported lower levels of childhood hyperactivity among their biological relatives than the control group of biological parents raising their own hyperactive children. Because no information was obtained from the biological parents of the adopted children, no direct comparisons could be made between the adoptive and biological parents of the 35 adopted hyperactive children. In a separate study of adopted children, Cantwell (1975) reported similar results to those of Morrison and Stewart (1973). A weakness of both studies is bias resulting from the selection process used to permit families to adopt and the inability to compare the families of the biological parents of adopted hyperactive children with the families of the adoptive parents of these same children. Nevertheless, these studies show that children may more closely resemble the families of their biological parents than those of their adoptive parents. Hence these results suggest that some genetic component is important for the manifestation of hyperactivity.

Another line of evidence for a genetic component of ADHD comes from a study comparing full- and half-sibling pairs (Safer, 1973). In a comparison of the concordance of such sibling pairs for the diagnosis of minimal brain dysfunction (MBD), significantly higher concordance levels were found among the full-sibling pairs than among the half-sibling pairs.

In more recent family studies of patients with ADHD, Biederman and co-workers (Biederman et al., 1986, 1987a, 1987b) reported a higher frequency of ADHD among first-degree relatives of affected probands. These investigators interviewed all family members of 22 male ADHD subjects and 20 unaffected controls. The morbidity ratio for ADHD was 31.5% among relatives of ADHD subjects, compared with 5.7% for relatives of controls. In addition, rates of major affective disorder, conduct disorder, and oppositional disorder were significantly increased in the relatives of the ADHD probands. This study was the first to directly assess all first-degree relatives using structured interviews. The results give strong support to the hypothesis that ADHD is familial. However, due to comorbidity in the probands it is not clear whether ADHD is a primary or secondary phenomenon. It appears that the increased rates of conduct and oppositional disorders occurred in only those families where the ADHD proband also had conduct disorder (Biederman et al.,

1987a). While this suggests some specificity of transmission, the sample was too small to obtain definitive results. Additionally, the considerable comorbidity (affective disorders and anxiety disorders) in first-degree relatives of ADHD children complicates genetic interpretations of these findings (Biederman et al., 1991a, 1991b). More recent analyses of ADHD probands (N = 140) and first-degree relatives explores the validity of subgrouping probands with ADHD by comorbid status and determines evidence for family-genetic risk factors in ADHD (Biederman et al., 1992).

While all of these studies lend support to a hypothesis that some heritable component is important in the expression of ADHD, no clear mode of transmission has been determined. Because of the preponderance of males, Omenn (1973) examined a sex-linked hypothesis. He concluded that it was unlikely because of the frequency of father-to-son transmission. Morrison and Stewart (1974) suggested a polygenic mode of transmission, but the report was based on a small number of families of hyperactive children. In a genetic latent structure analysis of dysmorphology in children with ADHD, an autosomal dominant model emerged when dysmorphology and ADHD were compiled into a single factor (Deutsch et al., 1990). However, the validity of this model has not yet been tested.

In an interesting new study of 18 families by Hauser et al. (1993), ADHD was strongly associated with a generalized resistance to thyroid hormone. This thyroid disorder is caused by mutations in the thyroid receptor β gene and characterized by reduced responsiveness of peripheral and pituitary tissues to the actions of thyroid hormone. This study showed that among the affected children 70% met criteria for ADHD while 20% of those who were unaffected met ADHD criteria. Among the affected adults, 50% met criteria for ADHD as children compared with 2% of the unaffected subjects. Although there is no (converse) increased incidence of resistance to thyroid hormone (a rare disorder) in children with ADHD (Weiss et al., 1993), this finding should help guide future genetic and biological/hormonal studies of ADHD.

Thus far, no clear understanding of the genetics or the pattern of transmission of ADHD has emerged. Previous studies have been limited because either (a) only families of males were examined, (b) only parents of subjects were included, or (c) sample sizes were too small. Larger family studies of ADHD that assess all relatives with valid diagnostic instruments are needed. Additionally, the phenotype of ADHD needs to be clearly defined and scientific unification of our nosological classification of ADHD (e.g., inattention and hyperactivity-impulsivity subtypes) and exploration of the effect of comorbid illness on ADHD classification need to occur.

Affective Disorders

Although considerable work has been published on the genetic basis of affective illness, relatively little has been reported concerning the inheritance of the major affective disorders in childhood. Several studies have examined children of depressed parents and found an elevated rate of affective disorders when compared with offspring of normal controls (Kashani et al., 1985; Orvaschel et al., 1988; Weissman et al., 1984). However, there is a paucity of studies that have investigated families ascertained through childhood probands.

At least two studies examined the relatives of childhood subjects. Strober et al. (1988) compared families of 50 adolescent probands with a diagnosis of bipolar affective disorder to families of 30 adolescent schizophrenic probands. All first-degree relatives were personally interviewed with the schedule for Affective Disorders and Schizophrenia—Lifetime Version (SADS-L). These investigators found a significantly higher rate of bipolar (BP) affective disorders (15%) among relatives of the BP I probands when compared with the relatives of schizophrenics (0%). For all major affective disorders, the recurrence risks were 30 and 4%, respectively, for relatives of bipolar and schizophrenic probands. The rate of affective disorders among relatives of BP I probands whose first psychiatric symptoms occurred prior to 12 years was 44%, compared with 24% among relatives of probands whose onset occurred during adolescence. It is noteworthy that the early symptoms observed in prepubertal onset probands usually involved hyperactivity and/or conduct difficulties.

In a family history study of childhood-onset major affective disorders, Puig-Antich et al. (1989) examined the first- and second-degree adult relatives of prepubertal children with major depression (N = 48), nonaffective psychiatric disorders (N = 20), and no psychiatric disorder (N = 27). All relatives were assessed by the Family History-Research Diagnostic Criteria (FH-RDC) method. A single adult informant (usually the mother of the proband) was directly interviewed. Relatives of the prepubertal children with major depressive disorder (MDD) had significantly higher rates of psychiatric disorders when compared with the relatives of normal control children. Specifically, age-corrected rates of MDD and alcoholism among first-degree relatives of MDD probands were 0.53 and 0.31, respectively, compared with 0.28 and 0.15, respectively, for relatives of normal children. The rate (0.27) of "other" (mostly anxiety) psychiatric disorders among relatives of MDD children was also significantly higher than the rate (0.06) among relatives of normal controls. Rates of MDD and alcoholism were not significantly elevated among relatives of the nonaffective psychiatrically ill children when compared with relatives of normal control subjects, whereas the rates of "other" psychiatric disorders and suicide attempts were considerably higher.

Results of this study support the validity of prepubertal-onset MDD. The rates of illness reported are consistent with the high rates of MDD and other psychiatric disorders observed in families of early-onset affective disorder probands and suggest that prepubertal-onset MDD is etiologically related to other forms of MDD. This does not, however, suggest that all affective disorders in childhood are related to adult forms of MDD, nor, for that matter, that they represent an etiologically homogeneous disorder.

Prepubertal-onset MDD may indeed be the key to increasing our understanding of the genetics of affective disorders. A prospective family study by Todd et al. (1993) ascertained 79 MDD-affected children aged 6–12 years; diagnostic information about them and their families was used to test for differences in prevalence and/or severity of affective disorder among relatives of the probands and controls. The probands were followed up between 2 and 5 years after ascertainment; eight had changed diagnosis from MDD to BP I, and 14 had changed diagnosis to BP II. The rate of MDD among first-degree relatives of all probands was 42.8%, greatly elevated over the control subjects (7.9%); increased rates were also seen in the second- and third-degree relatives (25.1 versus 17.1% and 15.5 versus 3.5%, respectively). Additionally, the affected family members also had an early age of onset; the median age of onset of first psychiatric disorder was 14 years for MDD affected relatives, compared with 27.5 years in the control group. Among the relatives of BP or MDD probands, little difference was found in the frequency or severity of affective disorder diagnoses; essentially, whether the child had BP or MDD, the type, frequency, and severity of affective disorder in the relatives remained the same. Using the same family data, Todd et al. performed segregation analyses, which allowed them to reject a purely environmental model of transmission for affective disorder. While this study has several caveats (only family history information was obtained for extended family members, controls were "super-normals" with unaffected first-degree relatives), it underscores the need for homogeneity in the sampling of nuclear families when attempting to answer genetic questions.

Depressive symptoms are common in childhood disorders, and there is need for considerable work to more completely understand affective difficulties in childhood psychiatric disorders.

Autism

The evidence for a genetic contribution to the syndrome of autism comes from twin studies and family studies. Several reports of twins appeared in the literature prior to 1977. Rutter (1967) reviewed all twin studies reported before 1967 and concluded that no valid inferences about a genetic contribution to autism could be drawn from them. Additional reports appeared during the next 10 years (Kean, 1975; Kotsopoulos, 1976; McQuaid, 1975), but the conclusion remained unchanged (Hanson and Gottesman, 1976).

The results of another twin study were reported by Ritvo et al. (1985a). Their sample included 40 twin pairs ascertained through a registry established to identify high-density families and twin pairs. Individuals were included in the registry as a result of response to an advertisement published in a newsletter of the National Society for Autistic Children. The sample thus does not represent a random ascertainment of twin pairs. There were 23 MZ and 17 DZ twin pairs. The concordance rate was 95.7% for the MZ twins, compared with 23.5% for the DZ twins. These rates were significantly different and seem to give striking evidence for genetic factors. It is difficult to interpret these results, however, because the sample relied on voluntary participation. It also included opposite-sex twins in the DZ sample, which, as explained below, skews results. Thus, although the concordance rate evidence is impressive, it is of limited value because it is not clear what biases were operating in the selection of the sample.

The twin studies reported prior to 1977 and the Ritvo et al. (1985a) study are difficult to interpret because of the way that all were ascertained. Most of the studies prior to 1977 appeared as case reports in the literature and, as such, represented a biased sample of twins. Folstein and Rutter (1977), summarizing the reports of 32 twin pairs that appeared prior to 1977, suggested two problems in interpretation of the existing data. First, the sample of 32 pairs contained approximately two times as many MZ twin pairs as DZ twin pairs (22 versus 10). DZ twins are approximately twice as frequent in the general population as MZ twins, and therefore, these 32 pairs are not a representative sample of twins. The same can be said for the Ritvo et al. sample (1985a), which contained 23 MZ and 17 DZ twin pairs. Second, in all of these studies, many of the twin pairs were opposite-sex pairs. With the reported sex difference in the frequency of autism, these twin pairs are of limited value since their inclusions would tend to decrease the DZ concordance rate. In addition, few reports of same-sex twin pairs contained adequate clinical description and evidence of zygosity to allow confident interpretation of the data.

In response to the problems of ascertainment bias, Folstein and Rutter (1977) sought to obtain a complete and unbiased sample of same-sex twin pairs that included at least one autistic child. They reported on a study of 21 pairs of same-sex twins that were systematically collected through schools, hospital twin registries, and the National Society for Autistic Children in England. Of the 21 pairs, 11 were MZ twins. The diagnosis of autism was based on the criteria developed by Kanner (1943) and Rutter (1971). In all, the 21 twin pairs gave rise to 25 autistic children. Four of the MZ co-twins were diagnosed as having autism, whereas none of the DZ co-twins met the criteria for the syndrome. This difference is significant (P = .055).

Another twin study using a similar ascertainment strategy was recently reported (Steffenburg et al., 1989). These investigators screened all Nordic countries for the occurrence of cases of autism with a same-sex twin under the age of 25. Twenty-one pairs (11 MZ and 10 DZ) of twins and one set of MZ triplets were ascertained. Zygosity testing was completed for 18 of the twin pairs. In the remaining 4 pairs, zygosity was determined on the basis of placental evidence and physical appearance. The pairwise concordance for autism was 91% for MZ twins and 0% for DZ twins.

Both of these studies suggest that genetic factors are of importance in the expression of autism. However, because the MZ twins were not always fully concordant, they also suggest that nongenetic factors exist that may be of etiologic importance. Discordance for autism among twins could be due to the fact that autism represents only the most severe expression of some other cognitive disorder. Presumably, several factors could interact to produce the severe phenotype, but the underlying genetic liability would be for a milder cognitive impairment. Folstein and

Rutter (1977) developed this hypothesis. They proposed that, if it was correct, the co-twins might exhibit some cognitive impairment without necessarily manifesting the full syndrome of autism. When Folstein and Rutter examined the co-twins in their study for some cognitive deficit, they found that, in addition to the 4 autistic MZ co-twins, 5 other MZ co-twins showed some cognitive impairment. Hence, 9 of 11 MZ twin pairs were concordant for a cognitive deficit, whereas only 1 of 10 DZ twin pairs was concordant for a cognitive impairment. This difference is highly significant ($P = .0015$). Further evidence for this hypothesis comes from a subsequent twin study (Bailey et al., 1994), which found 60% of MZ twins concordant for autism versus 0% for DZ pairs. The majority of the nonautistic MZ twins were beset by social difficulties when examined at follow-up; using a combined broad phenotype of cognitive/social difficulties, the concordance rate in MZ pairs was 92% versus 10% in DZ pairs.

These results suggest that there are genetic factors that may contribute to the expression of autism in some individuals. In addition, they support the hypothesis that these genetic factors may also be responsible for a different, possibly milder, manifestation in the relatives of autistic individuals. If this hypothesis is true, then there should be a higher-than-expected frequency of this milder disorder in the relatives of autistic patients compared with the frequency of this disorder in the general population.

August et al. (1981) attempted to test the hypothesis proposed by Folstein and Rutter (1977) by examining the siblings of autistic children. They used a case-control study design. The experimental group consisted of the siblings of 41 autistic individuals ascertained from the records of the autism program at the University of Iowa child psychiatry service. These 41 probands had a total of 71 siblings. The control group consisted of the 38 siblings of 15 Down's syndrome individuals. Only Down's syndrome with the standard trisomy 21 was included in the study, to ensure that this type of cognitive deficit would not be transmitted within these families. The families of Down's patients were chosen because August and co-workers wanted to compare the rates of cognitive impairment in two types of families in which at least one individual was impaired. The rationale was that if having an impaired child in the family was detrimental for nongenetic reasons, the rates of cognitive impairment should be similar in the two types of families. If, on the other hand, there were some factors specific to autism that could cause other cognitive deficits, the rates of disabilities should be higher in the siblings of autistic individuals. The Down's subjects were selected so that the ages of the siblings were in the same range as the ages of the siblings of the autistic children.

Only two (2.8%) siblings of autistic children in this study (August et al., 1981) met Rutter's (1971) criteria for autism. None of the siblings of the Down's probands was autistic. This rate is similar to that reported by Rutter (1968) (2%) for siblings of autistic individuals and by Folstein and Rutter (1977) (2.8%) for the siblings of twins. Although this is a very small recurrence risk, Rutter has pointed out that it represents at least a 50-fold increase over the general population prevalence.

Additional evidence for the familiality of autism comes from a recent report by Ritvo et al. (1989b), in which the authors reported recurrence risk estimates obtained from families identified through an epidemiologic study of autism in Utah. Two hundred and seven families of autistic individuals were ascertained. The recurrence risk for autism in these families was estimated to be 8.6%. There was a suggestion of a sex difference in that if the first autistic child was male, the rate among siblings was 7% compared with 14.5% when the first autistic child was female, although these differences were not significantly different. The overall risk of 8.6% represents a 215-fold increase over the population prevalence estimate in the state (Ritvo et al., 1989a).

While these findings considerably strengthen the evidence that autism is inherited, the data for the familial character of autism are even more convincing when the information on cognitive impairment is examined. In the study of August and coworkers discussed above, a separate diagnosis of cognitive disability was made if at least one of the following criteria was met: (a) delay in spoken language persisting beyond the age of 30 months; (b) gross abnormality in language (either expressive or receptive); (c) verbal, or full-scale IQ score less than 80; (d) specific learning disability in the areas of reading, spelling, or arithmetic as assessed by a standard score of less than 80 on the Wide Range Achievement Test; and (e) scholastic performance deficits of such severity as to require special educational remediation. One criterion omitted by August and co-workers, but included in the Folstein and Rutter twin study, was the symptom of grossly abnormal articulation persisting to age 5. Thus, although the two sets of criteria were not exactly the same, there was substantial overlap, so a meaningful comparison could be made.

August and colleagues showed that the rate of cognitive impairment in the siblings of autistic children was considerably higher than the rate among the siblings of Down's patients. Of the siblings of autistic patients, 11 (15.5%) showed some cognitive impairment, whereas only 1 (2.6%) of the siblings of Down's patients was cognitively impaired. The difference is statistically significant. These results are consistent with those of Folstein and Rutter (1977) and suggest that autism may be etiologically related to these disorders of cognition, at least within families of autistic individuals. Autism thus may be the most severe expression of a disorder of cognition, and there may be genetic factors important for the manifestation of this spectrum of disabilities.

In a more recent study, Freeman et al. (1989) present data that they conclude do not support this hypothesis. Weschsler Intelligence Scales, Wide-Range Achievement Tests, and the Shipley-Hartford Tests were administered to 122 parents and 153 siblings of 62 autistic probands who were part of the Utah study discussed earlier (Ritvo et al., 1989a, 1989b). All of these studies of cognitive difficulties need to be interpreted with care. In all studies, learning problems were defined as being below some score on some cognitive or achievement test. Learning problems are usually defined as a discrepancy between IQ and achievement, so it is difficult to determine just what the frequency of learning problems was in the families of autistic probands.

While the bulk of the studies of autism presented suggest the importance of genetic factors, most of the data do not allow specific genetic hypotheses about mode of inheritance to be tested. Genetic hypotheses were examined in a study by Ritvo et al. (1985b). The authors limited themselves to families in which at least two children met DSM-III criteria for autism. The families were ascertained through several sources, including medical records, referral from other clinicians, and response to an advertisement for "high-density" families. After attempting to correct for the bias introduced by this ascertainment scheme, the researchers employed two methods to test several genetic hypotheses. Using a method developed by Gladstein et al. (1978), they tested the multifactorial-polygenic hypothesis and were able to reject it. They also tested the autosomal-dominant and autosomal-recessive hypotheses with classical segregation analysis. They were able to reject the dominant hypothesis but not the recessive hypothesis.

These results need to be interpreted with caution. First, as Ritvo and colleagues point out, their findings do not generalize to all patients with autism. These multiple incidence families are a highly selected group and are not representative of all families. Second, the particular ascertainment scheme employed makes it difficult to estimate accurately the ascertainment probability. As the authors point out, the estimates of the segregation frequency are fairly robust if the estimate of the ascertainment probability is reasonably close. However, it is not clear how misspecification of the ascertainment probability affected the estimate of the segregation ratio in these families. Thus, these results should be viewed as preliminary. Additional work is needed with a sample selected through conventional ascertainment procedures.

An important point to keep in mind when studying the genetics of autism is that it is likely to be a heterogeneous disorder. It is known that the syndrome has multiple etiologies (Rutter, 1974). It can develop in association with (and presumably as a result of) conditions as pathologically diverse as congenital rubella (Chess et al., 1971) and infantile spasms (Taft and Cohen, 1971). In addition, Folstein and Rutter (1977) suggested other possible nongenetic etiologic factors. They found that the autistic twin in a discordant twin pair was more likely to have experienced events that could have resulted in brain damage than were the autistic twins in a concordant twin pair. In all of the concordant MZ twin pairs, neither twin had experienced any trauma that could be interpreted as contributing to the development of their autistic behavior. These findings suggest etiologic heterogeneity.

Certainly autism can (and does) develop after an environmental insult. However, it can also develop in the absence of any identifiable environmental agents. Any genetic factors that might exist for autism will almost certainly be more easily identifiable in the group of patients who do not experience any major environmental trauma. Thus, in future studies a sufficient number of patients should be included so that the data can be divided into groups based on presumed environmental insult to the proband. If the recurrence risks differ between the groups, this would provide additional evidence for specific etiologic subtypes and would suggest which types were most likely to be genetic.

However, even the subset of patients with no known environmental risk factors could be heterogeneous. Nearly all inherited disorders in which the genetic mechanism is clearly understood have been shown to be genetically heterogeneous. The mucopolysaccharide storage diseases provide an excellent example. Initially, all affected children were considered to have "gargoylism." The clinical characteristics were quite uniform, and it was thought to represent a single disorder that showed a familial tendency. It has been shown subsequently that the mucopolysaccharidoses encompass defects of many different enzymes, each with a different underlying genetic mechanism.

Often the multiple etiologies of a "single disease" become easily identifiable as new phenotypic levels are defined: What is apparently homogeneous at the level of gross symptomatology becomes obviously heterogeneous as physiological and/or biochemical aberrations are used to redefine the phenotype. In future studies of the genetics of autism, care needs to be taken to obtain a homogeneous sample of autistic patients. A level of homogeneity can be achieved by using very strict diagnostic rules or by studying only those patients with a specific biochemical abnormality or genetic marker. For example, it has been shown that some autistic individuals also have the marker X syndrome (August, 1983; Brown et al., 1982; Gillberg, 1983; Meryash et al., 1982). Certainly not all autistic patients have the mar(X) chromosome (Watson et al., 1984), but those who do may represent a subtype of autism with unique etiologic factors. By studying the families of a group of patients positive for the mar(X) chromosome, it might be possible to identify unique factors associated with this subset of autistic patients.

Although the results from these types of studies will not generalize to all autistic individuals, this should not be a deterrent for special ascertainment strategies. If it is possible to identify a specific etiology for a homogeneous group selected with a unique ascertainment, the residual cases will then be more homogeneous than the original population. Thus, the chances of determining the important etiologic factors for them are enhanced.

Specific Reading Disability

Specific reading disability (RD) or dyslexia is characterized by the presence of a discrepancy between predicted reading ability and actual reading achievement. Poor reading skills are present despite conventional instruction and adequate intelligence and sociocultural opportunity. The prevalence of RD among school-age children has been estimated to be between 6 and 9% (Shaywitz et al., 1990). These investigators found an equal gender ratio for RD in their sample. This is in contrast to many other identified samples, in which the rates of RD are 2–4 times higher in males than in females. These differences could be due to differing ascertainment strategies or possibly different diagnostic criteria for RD.

Over the years the definition and diagnosis of RD has not been uniform. It is not always clear that the results from various studies can be easily compared. Attempts have been made to identify more homogenous subtypes. Johnson and Myklebust (1967) and Boder (1971) observed that the spelling errors made by dyslexic persons could be categorized into several types: (a) auditory-predominant, (b) visual-predominant, and (c) a mixed subtype. Mattis et al. (1975) also suggested three distinct subtypes of RD. They used neuropsychological tests to define each of the three categories: (a) language disorder, (b) articulatory and graphomotor dyscoordination, and (c) visual-spatial perceptual disorder. The Colorado Family Reading Study (CFRS) (Decker and DeFries, 1980; DeFries and Decker, 1981; DeFries et al., 1978; Foch et al., 1977; Lewitter et al., 1980) identified four dyslexia subtypes in probands: (a) a spatial/reasoning deficit; (b) a coding/speed deficit; (c) a relatively specific reading disability subtype, with a deficit only in reading; and (d) a mixed or global subtype. These subtypes accounted for 91% of the CFRS proband sample. It is difficult to say whether the relatively specific reading-disabled subtype found by these investigators has been identified by others. Unfortunately most classifications used slightly different diagnostic schemes for patient identification, and few attempts have been made at cross-validation.

RD is familial. As early as 1905, studies were reported where children with dyslexia often had affected relatives (Fisher, 1905; Hinshelwood, 1907, 1911; Stephenson, 1907; Thomas, 1905). Later, Orton (1937) and Eustis (1947) also reported the familial nature of RD and, in addition, noted that affected individuals usually had normal intelligence. In 1950 Hallgren published the results of one of the largest family studies of RD with 116 probands and 391 first-degree relatives. Hallgren reported an excess of males among affected probands and affected first-degree relatives. Overall, 160 of the 391 (41%) first-degree relatives were affected with RD. Hallgren calculated segregation ratios based on several mendelian models and proposed that RD was an autosomal-dominant trait with sex-modified expression. Other studies confirm the familial nature of RD and that males have higher prevalence rates than females, but no specific genetic models were tested (DeFries et al., 1978; Finucci et al., 1976; McGlannon, 1968; Owen et al., 171; Walker and Cole, 1965).

Further attempts to examine specific genetic hypotheses have resulted in inconsistent findings. Symmes and Rapaport (1972) proposed sex-linked recessive inheritance after studying the families of 54 RD children. Zahalkova and co-workers (1972) studied the families of 65 dyslexic children, calculated a segregation ratio of 0.42 + 0.06, and concluded that inheritance was autosomal-dominant, with partial sex limitation. Lewitter et al. (1980) performed segregation analyses on families collected through 133 RD children to test the hypotheses proposed by previous investigators. They also analyzed three subsets of the total data: families of male probands, families of female probands, and families of severely affected probands. No one hypothesis was supported in all the analyses. The researchers concluded that the results suggested that RD was genetically heterogeneous; however, when the analysis was restricted to children only, they were unable to reject the hypothesis of a single major locus. In 1991 Pennington et al. examined four independently ascertained samples (204 RD families) and found evidence for the hypothesis of major locus transmission in three samples and polygenic transmission in one sample.

Although RD clusters in families and appears to be transmitted, the data do not prove that the transmission is genetic. Additional evidence for a genetic contribution to the manifestation of RD has come from at least two other sources. The first is twin studies. In a 1967 literature review, Zerbin-Rudin found that of 17 MZ twin pairs 100% were concordant for RD, compared with 35% (12/34) of the DZ twin pairs. Bakwin (1973) examined 338 pairs of same-sex twins and found 14% (97/676) affected with RD. In the MZ twin pairs in which at least one twin had RD, 84% of the co-twins were also affected. In contrast, only 29% of the DZ twin pairs were concordant.

More recent twin studies continue to support a genetic hypothesis for RD. DeFries et al. (1987) estimated heritability for RD to be 30%.

Stevenson et al. (1987) also found a low heritability for reading accuracy, but a substantially higher estimate (73%) for spelling. Ho et al. (1988), using a small sample of twins with the Bannatyne cognitive profile, reported that the MZ concordance for the profile was 67% compared with 30% for DZ twins. However, these results may be compromised by the fact that reading problems are significantly more common in twins than in singletons (Hay et al., 1984). This finding suggests that there may be a major environmental component important for the expression of RD in twins, and therefore, the estimates of heritabilities from twin data could be grossly inaccurate.

A second source of evidence for a genetic contribution to RD comes from linkage studies. As discussed earlier, the demonstration of linkage of a purported locus for a trait with a known genetic marker locus is strong evidence that a genetic component is important in the etiology of the trait. Smith et al. (1983) performed the first linkage analysis of RD families with multiple affected individuals (in order to minimize heterogeneity). Their results supported linkage of RD to a heteromorphic section of chromosome 15. However, there was also evidence for heterogeneity. One kindred gave less evidence for linkage, suggesting that the form of RD in this family was not linked to the marker on chromosome 15. And although tests for heterogeneity were not significant, the sample size was too small for that test (Morton, 1956). Attempts to confirm and extend this finding have not yet been fruitful (e.g., Bisgaard et al., 1987). In 1990 Smith and colleagues studied 21 families with RD. Data were insufficient to establish linkage between RD and chromosome 15, although questions about the genetic heterogeneity of RD remain.

Recent work suggests that RD is likely to be genetically heterogeneous. Cardon and colleagues (in press) examined 114 sib-pairs and 50 dizygotic twins and found significant evidence for linkage to markers in the human lymphocyte antigen (HLA) complex. While these findings must be replicated in an independent sample, it is noteworthy that similar results were obtained in both the sib-pair and twin samples. Furthermore, when analyses were limited to the most severely affected individuals, the findings were even more statistically significant, even with a reduced sample size.

RD is a complex disorder that is clinically heterogenous and probably heterogenous in etiology and pathogenesis. As noted above, several attempts have been made to identify different subtypes. Two studies (Omenn and Weber, 1978; Pennington and Smith, 1983) have used the classification schemes of Boder (1971) to determine if the defined subtypes would "breed true" within families.

Omenn and Weber (1978) studied 21 families with multiple members with RD. Following criteria proposed by Boder (1971), individuals were classified as auditory-predominant subtypes if their history and test results showed dysphonetic spelling errors, striking mispronunciation, and greater difficulty in learning from oral presentation; individuals were classified as visual-predominant subtypes if their history and test results showed phonetic spelling errors, no mispronunciation, and greater difficulty in learning from written or visually presented material. Individuals were classified as mixed if they had characteristics of both previous subtypes. Eleven probands were classified visual-predominant, 7 as auditory-predominant, and 3 as mixed. Most of the affected relatives who could be diagnosed had the same subtype as the proband, giving "support for the hypothesis that the phenotypic subtypes reflect independent familial predispositions" (Boder, 1971, p. 339).

Of the four groups identified by Decker and DeFries (1980), the relatively specific reading-disabled subtype showed the most significant concordance between probands and other family members, specifically siblings. Thus, this subtype gave strong evidence for genetic factors contributing to a specific form of RD. However, as indicated above, it is difficult to know whether this group identifies the same group as the Boder scheme.

Pennington and Smith (1983) indicated that there appears to be some evidence for specific subtypes to cluster in the same families in the study reported by Smith and colleagues (1983). The families giving evidence for linkage tended to have dyslexia due to subtle language-

processing deficits, but appeared to have good visual-spatial skills. However, individuals in the family that did not give evidence for linkage appeared to have a visual-spatial dyslexia.

It is interesting to note that although all of the above reports suggest some specificity, there have been no reports of specific tests of genetic hypotheses for these subtypes. The analyses done by Lewitter et al. (1980) divided the sample into age- and sex-defined groups but not into groups of clinically defined subtypes.

As noted above, many studies show a preponderance of males affected with RD. Using these data, several authors have suggested that RD may be a trait with a sex-modified threshold important for its expression (Childs and Finucci, 1979; Herschel, 1978). If the genetic mechanism for the trait is also related to its differential expression in the sexes, then the risk to relatives should differ depending on the sex of the proband. That is, since females are less frequently affected, the risk to the relatives of female probands should be greater than the risk to relatives of male probands. This is not the case for RD. Childs and Finucci (1979) state that the risk to the relatives of females is not significantly greater than the risk to the relatives of males. Omenn and Weber (1978) show that the risk is greater for relatives of females but not significantly so. When the data presented by Finucci et al. (1976) are separated by sex of proband, the risks are not different for the two classes of relatives (Pauls and Kidd, 1981). These results could mean that (a) in each of these studies the sample size is too small to obtain significance or (b) the sex difference observed is not related to the transmission of the trait. These ideas are supported by the work of Shaywitz and colleagues (1990) that distinguishes between school-identified RD sex ratios and research-identified sex ratios.

If the sex difference is not related to the transmission of RD, then it could be explained in several ways. First, the social and/or educational environment could be sufficiently different—favorable to girls so that females would express the trait less often, even when they were genetically predisposed. If that were the case, one would expect a slightly different concordance rate for male and female MZ twins. If, in fact, males were more apt to experience RD or be identified as having RD because of a detrimental, and biased, social and/or educational environment, then their concordance rate should be somewhat lower than that for females. Bakwin (1973) reported concordance rates for male and female MZ twins to be 84 and 83%, respectively.

Another explanation for the observed difference could be that the developmental processes of males and females interact differently with the genetic predisposition for RD and that the interaction produces more severe effects in males than it does in females. If that is the case, one would also expect males to be more severely affected than females.

In summary, it is clear that much work remains to be done to gain a better understanding of RD and its etiology. It is known that RD is familial and that part of the reason for the familial clustering is an underlying genetic mechanism. At the present time, it is not known what that genetic mechanism is. A variety of models have been proposed. The most frequently mentioned one is an autosomal-dominant mode of inheritance, with reduced and sex-modified penetrance. Few, if any, of the alternative hypotheses have been rigorously excluded. Diagnostic uncertainty and probable etiologic and phenotypic heterogeneity cloud the picture. Work is needed to establish useful and unified criteria for all age ranges and to determine if there are phenotypic differences that tend to cluster within families.

Gilles de la Tourette's Syndrome

Gilles de la Tourette's syndrome (TS) is a familial neuropsychiatric disorder with onset in childhood, characterized by chronic intermittent motor and vocal tics. The familial nature of TS was first described by Gilles de la Tourette in 1885. However, it was not until the 1970s (Eldridge et al., 1977: Shapiro et al., 1978) that studies demonstrated an increased frequency of positive family history for tics in families of TS patients. The family history study of Kidd et al. (1980) was the first to present frequencies of TS and chronic tics (CTs) among relatives. That early study combined TS and CTs into a single category and showed that the risk to relatives was significantly elevated over what would be expected by chance. In 1981, Pauls and colleagues analyzed the data collected by Kidd and co-workers as well as family history data collected from TS clinic patients to demonstrate that (a) the increased risk for TS and CTs was consistent across the two samples and higher than expected by chance, (b) CT appeared to represent a variant expression of the syndrome, and (c) the patterns of occurrence of TS and CTs were consistent with vertical transmission within families.

Subsequent to these studies, six groups (Baron et al., 1981; Comings et al., 1984; Curtis et al., 1992; Devor, 1984; Kidd and Pauls, 1982; Price et al., 1987) reported results of genetic analyses of family history data in which specific transmission hypotheses were examined. All groups concluded that the pattern of transmission within families was consistent with a genetic hypothesis that postulated a single major locus to be responsible for susceptibility to TS and/or CTs. However, this was not the only hypothesis supported. Kidd and Pauls (1982) were unable to reject the hypothesis that transmission of the syndrome was consistent with the contribution of many genes, each with equal and additive effect to the expression of the disorder (the so-called multifactorial-polygenic (MFP) model). Likewise, Comings et al. (1984) could not reject the MFP model unless extended relatives were included and the population prevalence for TS and CTs was restricted to be less than 0.0075. However, the consistent conclusion of authors in all of the studies was that the mode of inheritance that gave the best fit to the data was one that postulated an underlying single major locus with two alleles. While all studies supported a single-locus model, not all studies suggested an identical mode of inheritance. Three of the studies (Baron et al., 1981; Comings et al., 1984; Price et al., 1987) concluded that the most likely mode of inheritance for TS and/or CTs was autosomal-dominant with sex-specific penetrances. Curtis et al. (1992) did not detect the excess of male cases of TS that is commonly described. Results from the remaining two studies suggested an additive model.

As indicated above, all of these studies relied on family history data for the analyses. That is, the diagnoses of relatives were based on information given by one or at most two informants per family. It has been demonstrated in studies of other neuropsychiatric disorders that family history data underestimate the "true" rates of illness as determined by direct assessment (Andreason et al., 1977; Orvaschel et al., 1982). This was demonstrated to be true for TS and CT as well (Pauls et al., 1984). Thus, the results of the genetic analyses summarized above should be interpreted with caution. This is particularly true if the underestimation of rates does not occur uniformly across all classes of relatives. For example, if the rate of illness is consistently underestimated in the parents of the patients, then the pattern of illness will more closely resemble the pattern for a recessive or partially dominant condition. Or, if there is a consistent underestimate of the illness in the relatives of a particular kind of proband (e.g., relatives of male probands), the resulting patterns could lead to spurious conclusions.

Pauls and co-workers (1984) demonstrated that there appeared to be consistent underestimation of rates in the parents of TS probands in the family history studies of Kidd et al. (1980) and Pauls et al. (1981). Thus, the penetrances reported by Kidd and Pauls (1982) would be expected to be underestimates. This could also be true for the results reported by Devor (1984) since he analyzed only pedigrees reported in the literature.

Biases resulting from consistent underreporting of illness in relatives of a specific type of proband could also occur when it is generally believed by the informant that the illness is more common in one type of relative than it is in another. This appears to have happened in the data collected by Kidd et al. (1980) and Pauls et al. (1981). These investigators reported an apparent increased risk to relatives of female probands in the family history they collected. However, data collected in the Yale Family Study of TS (Pauls and Leckman, 1988) suggest that the sex of the proband has no effect on the rates among relatives.

Thus, the analyses of Kidd and Pauls that incorporated a sex difference need to be reevaluated.

The results presented by Baron et al. (1981), while appearing to be consistent with a dominant mode of inheritance, predicted that approximately 70% of males and 50% of females would be phenocopies (individuals with the disorder but without the gene.) This high phenocopy rate could have resulted from a combination of underreporting for parents and/or underreporting for female relatives. Since fewer parents and female relatives would have been identified as affected, there would have been more families with isolated cases and thus a higher estimate of phenocopies.

Due to a variety of reporting biases, each of the studies discussed above has some potential difficulties. Since these reporting biases can affect patterns within pedigrees, it is not surprising that the specific estimates of gene frequency and penetrances vary considerably from study to study. Accurate estimates of genetic model parameters are critical for genetic counseling and for genetic linkage analyses.

A twin study completed in the Child Study Center and Department of Human Genetics at Yale also demonstrates the effect of relying on family history data for diagnostic purposes. Price et al. (1985) reported the concordance rate for TS to be 0.53 for MZ twin pairs and 0.08 for DZ twin pairs. The data for this study were obtained by questionnaires sent to the mothers of twins and from follow-up telephone interviews with those mothers.

The results from the twin study are quite comparable to those reported in some of the studies discussed earlier. Concordance rates for MZ twins can be interpreted as an estimate of penetrance if the underlying genetic mechanism is a single locus. Thus, the concordance rate of 0.77, when co-twins with either TS or CTs are considered to be affected, can be thought of as a penetrance of 0.77. The estimate compares favorably with the estimates of penetrance reported by Baron et al. (1981), Comings et al. (1984), and Price et al. (1987). However, just as a number of possible reporting biases could affect the results of genetic analyses based on family history data, reporting biases could also affect the results in a twin study.

As a follow-up to the Price et al. study, investigators at the Yale Child Study Center contacted all twin pairs and conducted personal interviews with each twin. The resulting estimates of concordance indicate that, even for twins, the rates of illness can be underestimated if the investigator relies on historical data provided by an informant rather than on data collected by direct personal interview of the subject. The concordance rates estimated from personal interview data increased to 1.0 for MZ twins when co-twins with either TS or CTs were included as affected (Walkup et al., 1987).

Another major focus of the TS family studies has been the delineation of the behavioral phenotype associated with the underlying genetic diathesis. Although a number of psychiatric and behavioral disorders have been hypothesized (Comings and Comings, 1987), the strongest data concern obsessive compulsive disorder (OCD). Evidence in support of this association comes from uncontrolled clinical studies (Cummings and Frankel, 1985; Fernando, 1967; Jagger et al., 1982; Kelman, 1965; Montgomery et al., 1982; Morphew and Sim, 1969; Nee et al., 1980, 1982; Stefl, 1984; Yaryura-Tobias et al., 1981). In addition, family study data indicate that OCD alone (no current or past history of tics) could represent a variant expression of the disorder (Pauls et al., 1986). Recently, results from several studies have supported these earlier findings (Curtis et al., 1992; Frankel et al., 1986; Green and Pitman, 1986; Robertson et al., 1988; Walkup et al., 1987), and it is generally accepted that within families of TS individuals the two disorders are etiologically related. In addition, Pauls and Leckman (1986) reported that in relatives of TS probands, females were at greater risk for developing OCD without TS or CTs than were males. These data suggest that rather than a sex-specific frequency of the illness (limited to only TS or CTs), there could be a sex-specific expression of the illness, with OCD representing the part of the TS spectrum more frequently expressed in females.

To determine whether the occurrence of OCD within these families was consistent with genetic transmission of TS, CT, and/or OCD together, Pauls and Leckman (1986) performed segregation analyses to test specific genetic hypotheses. They concluded that the syndrome is inherited as an autosomal-dominant condition. What is noteworthy is that, regardless of who was included as affected, whether (a) only relatives with TS, (b) relatives with TS or CTs, or (c) relatives with TS, CTs, or OCD, the results were all consistent with an autosomal-dominant hypothesis. The fact that the inclusion of OCD resulted in a significantly better fit to the observed data within families suggests that OCD is part of a genetically mediated TS spectrum. Penetrances estimated when relatives with OCD are included suggest that there may not be a large difference in the probability of expression of some form of the illness, but that the expression may be more specific to a particular sex.

These findings have been replicated in two independent samples (Eapen et al., 1993; van de Wetering, 1993). Eapen and co-workers studied the families of 40 consecutive TS probands seen in a London clinic, and van de Wetering and colleagues studied the families of approximately 45 TS patients seen in Rotterdam. Both studies found strong statistical evidence that the pattern of transmission of TS, CTs with OCD, and OCD without tics was consistent with autosomal dominant inheritance. The penetrances obtained for these two samples were remarkably similar to those reported above, ranging from 0.5 to 0.9 for males and 0.2 to 0.8 for females depending on the diagnostic scheme used in the analyses. These consistent findings provide a strong rationale for the ongoing linkage studies.

Since all published reports of genetic analyses suggest that the TS spectrum is inherited as a single gene, genetic linkage studies are warranted as the next step in our understanding of the inheritance of this syndrome. A linkage study of TS is under way. A large multigenerational kindred has been ascertained (Kurlan et al., 1986), and genetic typing is ongoing. Pauls et al. (1990) reported the results of linkage analyses of the first 180 markers typed. No significant evidence for linkage was obtained. However, a substantial proportion of the gene has been excluded as the site of the susceptibility gene for the TS spectrum. At the present time, over 600 marker loci have been typed. No strong positive evidence for linkage with TS has been obtained. At least 75% of the autosomal genetic map has been excluded if it is assumed that chronic tics are part of the inherited spectrum of TS. The exact calculation of the proportion excluded cannot be carried out due to imprecision of the total length of the autosomal map, because some of the genetic markers are not localized precisely and because the exclusion region is dependent upon the specific genetic model used in the linkage analyses. Pakstis and colleagues (1991) point out that an important assumption of these analyses is that the major locus for TS is the same in different pedigrees under study. Genetic heterogeneity could obscure a positive finding and needs to be considered.

Obsessive Compulsive Disorder

Obsessive compulsive disorder (OCD) has a lifetime prevalence of approximately 2% in the United States (Robins et al., 1984). Previously thought to be a rare disorder, it is now estimated that OCD affects nearly 5 million U.S. citizens. OCD is characterized by the presence of distressful, time-consuming obsessions and/or compulsions (Committee on Nomenclature and Statistics, American Psychiatric Association, 1994). Evidence for a genetic basis of OCD is found in family-genetic studies of OCD and Gilles de la Tourette's syndrome and in twin studies of OCD.

The notion that OCD has a familial form is well supported by the current literature. Recent family-genetic studies (Bellodi et al., 1992; Black et al., 1992; Lenane et al., 1990; Leonard et al., 1992) report an increased prevalence of OCD and related obsessional traits among first-degree relatives of OCD-affected probands. Lenane et al. show 30% of probands with at least one first-degree relative affected with OCD.

Including a diagnosis of subclinical OCD as affected, they find an overall rate of 22% among all first-degree relatives, 10-fold greater than either the control group or the general population prevalence (subclinical OCD was defined as meeting all DSM-III-R criteria except one of the following: symptoms occur less than 1 hour per day, lack of ego dystonicity/insight, or lack of interference/distress). In a similar study, Black et al. found that the risk of broadly defined OCD was increased in parents of probands but not in controls (16 versus 3%). A study by Leonard et al. showed the age-corrected risk of OCD in all first-degree relatives of 54 childhood-onset OCD probands to be 17%, compared with the population prevalence of 2%; similarly, Bellodi et al. found an OCD rate of 9% among first-degree relatives of 21 childhood onset probands. Few of the OCD family studies reported in the literature have failed to find an increased risk of OCD among first-degree relatives of probands; in those cases, methodologic questions concerning data collection techniques (e.g., reliance on family history information obtained from only one informant in each family) and diagnostic categories (e.g., subclinical OCD classified as an anxiety disorder rather than a form of OCD) may have contributed to an underestimation of the rate of OCD in relatives.

The most recent OCD family study has addressed these shortcomings by combining a large sample size with a control group, use of sensitive family history methods, and blind best-estimate diagnoses (Pauls et al., 1995). Results from that study show the rate of OCD is significantly higher in the relatives of OCD probands when compared with controls (10.3 versus 1.9%). This is also true for subclinical OCD, 7.9% of the first-degree relatives of OCD probands are affected compared with only 2.0% of the controls. The overall rate of OCD and subclinical OCD among relatives of OCD probands was 18.2% compared with 4.0% among controls. The rate of tics (TS and CTs) among relatives of OCD probands was 4.6%, significantly higher than that among controls (1%). The gender effect seen in previous studies of families of TS probands (with female relatives being more likely to have OCD without tics) was marginally supported in these data. There is a trend for a higher rate of tics among relatives of female probands when compared with relatives of male probands. Interestingly, these data also suggest that not all OCD is related to TS, since it is more likely that a relative will have tics if the proband also has tics: if all OCD was related to TS, the rate of TS and CT should be the same among relatives of OCD probands with and without tics. An important effect of the proband's age at OCD onset on the rates of illness among the first-degree relatives was also seen. If a child's onset is between the ages of 5 and 9, the risk to relatives increases until it is twice that of relatives of probands whose onset is between ages 9 and 18.

Twin studies of OCD also reveal a strong hereditary component. Inouye (Inouye, 1965) reported 80% concordance between MZ twins and 25% between DZ twins for obsessional neuroses, and 15 years later Carey and Gottesman (1981) report 87% concordance between MZ twins and 47% between DZ twins. Both studies indicate a large heritability for OCD, although they are constrained by small sample sizes and diagnostic categories that are no longer used.

The only published segregation analysis using OCD probands (Nicolini et al., 1991) is a preliminary report indicating autosomal mendelian inheritance, but the authors could not differentiate between recessive or dominant modes; their data also show a similarly high penetrance for OCD.

Family-genetic studies of Gilles de la Tourette's syndrome (see the previous section on TS) provide another line of evidence for a genetic basis of some form of OCD. Interestingly, in the study by Leonard et al. of OCD probands, TS was an exclusionary criterion for participation in the study; at follow-up 2–7 years later, 12% of probands had onset with TS.

SUMMARY

While the notion that genetic factors may be important for the manifestation of childhood psychiatric disorders is not new, most of the work done to examine hypotheses about the importance of genetics is relatively recent. The evidence reviewed in this chapter suggests that genetic factors are important in the expression of some of more serious neuropsychiatric disorders of childhood. Given the speed with which new methods are being developed to study the inheritance of human disorders and the advances being made in learning more about the nosology of child psychiatric conditions, it should be possible to make major strides in our understanding of the underlying genetic and biological mechanisms important for the manifestation of childhood psychiatric disorders.

Acknowledgments. *This work was supported in part by Grants NS-16448, MH-00508 (a National Institute of Mental Health Research Scientist Development Award), MH28287, MH18268, and MH49351-03.*

References

American Psychiatric Association, Committee on Nomenclature and Statistics: *Diagnostic and Statistical Manual of Mental Disorders* (4th ed). Washington, DC, American Psychiatric Press, 1993.

Andreason NC, Endicott J, Spitzer RL, et al: The family history method using diagnostic criteria: Reliability and validity. *Arch Gen Psychiatry* 34: 1229–1235, 1977.

August GJ: A genetic marker associated with infantile autism. *Am J Psychiatry* 140:813, 1983.

August GJ, Stewart MA, Tsai L: The incidence of cognitive disabilities in the siblings of autistic children. *Br J Psychiatry* 138:416–422, 1981.

Bailey A, Le Couteur A, Gottesman I, et al: Autism as a strongly genetic disorder: Evidence from a British twin study. *Psychol Med* 25:63–77, 1995.

Bakwin H: Reading disability in twins. *Dev Med Child Neurol* 15:184–187, 1973.

Baron M, Shapiro E, Shapiro A, et al: Genetic analysis of Tourette syndrome suggesting a major gene effect. *Am J Hum Genet* 33:767–775, 1981.

Bellodi L, Sciuto G, Diaferia G, et al: Psychiatric disorders in the families of patients with obsessive-compulsive disorder. *Psychiatry Res* 42:111–120, 1992.

Biederman J, Faraone SV, Keenan K, et al: Familial association between attention deficit disorder and anxiety disorders. *Am J Psychiatry* 148: 251–256, 1991a.

Biederman J, Faraone SV, Keenan K, et al: Evidence of familial association between attention deficit disorder and major affective disorders. *Arch Gen Psychiatry* 48:633–642, 1991b.

Biederman J, Faraone SV, Keenan K, et al: Further evidence for family-genetic risk factors in attention deficit hyperactivity disorder. *Arch Gen Psychiatry* 49:728–738, 1992.

Biederman J, Munir K, Knee D, et al: A family study of patients with attention deficit disorder and normal controls. *J Psychiatr Res* 20:263–274, 1986.

Biederman J, Munir K, Knee D: Conduct and oppositional disorder in clinically referred children with attention deficit disorder: A controlled family study. *J Am Acad Child Adolesc Psychiatry* 26: 724–727, 1987a.

Biederman J, Munir K, Knee D, et al: High rate of affective disorders in probands with attention deficit disorder and in their relatives: A controlled family study. *Am J Psychiatry* 144:330–333, 1987b.

Bisgaard ML, Eiberg H, Moller N, et al: Dyslexia and chromosome 15 heteromorphism: Negative lod score in a Danish study. *Clin Genet* 32:118–119, 1987.

Black DW, Noyes R Jr, Goldstein RB, et al: A family study of obsessive-compulsive disorder. *Arch Gen Psychiatry* 49:362–368, 1992.

Boder E: Developmental dyslexia—Prevailing diagnostic concepts and a new diagnostic approach. In: Myklebust RH (ed): *Progress in Learning Disabilities* (Vol 2). New York, Grune & Stratton, 1971.

Botstein D, White RL, Skolnick M, et al: Construction of a genetic linkage map in man using restriction fragment length polymorphisms. *Am J Hum Genet* 32:314–331, 1980.

Brown WT, Friedman E, Jenkens EC, et al: Association of fragile X syndrome with autism. *Lancet* 1: 100, 1982.

Cantwell D: Psychiatric illness in the families of hyperactive children. *Arch Gen Psychiatry* 27: 414–417, 1972.

Cantwell D: Genetic studies on hyperactive children. Psychiatric illness in biologic and adoptive parents. In: Fieve R, Rosenthal D, Brill H (eds): *Genetic Research in Psychiatry*. Baltimore, Johns Hopkins University Press, 1975.

Cardon LR, DeFries JC, Fulker DW, et al: Quantitative trait locus on chromosome 6 predisposing to reading disability. *Science*, 1994.

Carey G, Gottesman II: Twin and family studies of anxiety, phobic, and obsessive disorders. In: Klein DF, Rabkin JG (eds): *Anxiety: New Research and Changing Concepts*. New York, Raven Press, 1981.

Chess S, Korn SJ, Fernandez PB: *Psychiatric Disorders of Children with Congenital Rubella*. New York, Brunner/Mazel, 1971.

Childs B, Finucci JM: The genetics of learning disabilities. *Ciba Found Symp* 66:359–376, 1979.

Cohen D, Dibble E, Grawe JM, et al: Reliably separating identical from fraternal twins. *Arch Gen Psychiatry* 32:1371–1378, 1975.

Comings DE, Comings BG: A controlled study of Tourette syndrome. *Am J Hum Genet* 41:701–838, 1987.

Comings DE, Comings BG, Devor EJ, et al: Detection of a major gene for Gilles de la Tourette syndrome. *Am J Hum Genet* 36:586–600, 1984.

Cummings IL, Frankel M: Gilles de la Tourette syndrome and the neurological basis of obsessions and compulsions. *Biol Psychiatry* 20:1117–1126, 1985.

Curtis D, Robertson MM, Gurling HM: Autosomal dominant gene transmission in a large kindred with Gilles de la Tourette syndrome. *Br J Psychiatry* 160:845–849, 1992.

Decker SN, DeFries JC: Cognitive abilities in families with reading disabled children. *J Learn Disabil* 13:53–58, 1980.

DeFries JC, Decker SN: Genetic aspects of reading disability: The Colorado Family Reading Study. In: Aaron PG, Malatesha M (eds): *Neuropsychological and Neuropsycholinguistic Aspects of Reading Disability*. New York, Academic Press, 1981.

DeFries JC, Fulker DW, LaBuda MC: Evidence for a genetic etiology in reading disability of twins. *Nature* 329:537–539, 1987.

DeFries JC, Singer SM, Foch TT, et al: Familial nature of reading disability. *Br J Psychiatry* 132: 361–367, 1978.

Deutsch CK, Matthysse S, Swanson JM, et al: Genetic latent structure analysis of dysmorphology in attention deficit disorder. *J Am Acad Child Adolesc Psychiatry* 29:189–194, 1990.

Devor EJ: Complex segregation analysis of Gilles de la Tourette syndrome: Further evidence for a major locus mode of transmission. *Am J Hum Genet* 36:704–709, 1984.

Eapen V, Pauls DL, Robertson MM: Evidence for autosomal dominant transmission in Gilles de la Tourette syndrome: United Kingdom Cohort Study. *Br J Psychiatry* 162:593–596, 1993.

Eldridge R, Sweet R, Lake CR, et al: Gilles de la Tourette's syndrome: Clinical, genetic, psychologic, and biochemical aspects in 21 selected families. *Neurology* 27:115–124, 1977.

Eustis RS: Specific reading disability. *N Engl J Med* 237:243–249, 1947.

Fernando SJM: Gilles de la Tourette's syndrome. *Br J Psychiatry* 113:607–617, 1967.

Finucci JM, Guthrie JT, Child AL, et al: The genetics of specific reading disability. *Ann Hum Genet* 40:1–23, 1976.

Fisher JH: A case of congenital word-blindness (inability to learn to read). *Ophthalmic Rev* 24: 315–318, 1905.

Foch TT, DeFries JC, McClearn GE, et al: Familial patterns of impairment in reading disability. *J Educ Psychol* 69:316–329, 1977.

Folstein S, Rutter M: Infantile autism: A genetic study of 21 twin pairs. *J Child Psychol Psychiatry* 18:297–321, 1977.

Frankel M, Cummings JL, Robertson MM, et al: Obsessions and compulsions in the Gilles de la Tourette syndrome. *Neurology* 36:379–382, 1986.

Freeman BJ, Ritvo ER, Mason-Brothers A, et al: Psychometric assessment of first-degree relatives of 62 autistic probands in Utah. *Am J Psychiatry* 146: 361–364, 1989.

Gillberg C: Identical triplets with infantile autism and the fragile-X syndrome. *Br J Psychiatry* 143: 256–260, 1983.

Gladstein K, Lange K, Spence MA: A goodness of fit test for the polygenic threshold model: Application to pyloric stenosis. *Am J Med Genet* 2:7–13, 1978.

Goodman R, Stevenson J: A twin study of hyperactivity. II: The aetiological role of genes, family relationships and perinatal adversity. *J Child Psychol Psychiatry* 30:691–709, 1989.

Green RC, Pitman RK: Tourette syndrome and obsessive compulsive disorder. In: Jenike MA, Baer L, Minicheillo WE (eds): *Obsessive Compulsive Disorders, Theory and Management*. Littleton, MA, PSG Publishing, 1986.

Hallgren B: Specific dyslexia. *Acta Psychiatr Neurol Scand Suppl* 65:1–287, 1950.

Hauser P, Zametkin AJ, Martinez P, et al: Attention deficit-hyperactivity disorder in people with generalized resistance to thyroid hormone. *N Engl J Med* 328:997–1001, 1993.

Hanson DR, Gottesman II: The genetics, if any, of infantile autism and childhood schizophrenia. *J Autism Child Schizophr* 6:209–234, 1976.

Hay DA, O'Brien PJ, Johnston CJ, et al: The high incidence of reading disability in twin boys and its implication for genetic analyses. *Acta Genet Med Gemellol* 33:223–236, 1984.

Herschel M: Dyslexia revisited. *Hum Genet* 40: 115–134, 1978.

Hinshelwood J: Four cases of congenital word-blindness occurring in the same family. *Br Med J* 2: 1229–1232, 1907.

Hinshelwood J: Two cases of hereditary word-blindness. *Br Med J* 1:608–609, 1911.

Ho HZ, Gillger JW, Decker SN: A twin study of Bannatyne's "genetic dyslexia" sub-type. *J Child Psychol Psychiatry* 29:63–72, 1988.

Hodge SE, Morton LA, Tideman S, et al: Age-of-onset correction available for linkage analysis (LIPED). *Am J Hum Genet* 31:761–762, 1979.

Inouye E: Similar and dissimilar manifestations of obsessive-compulsive neurosis in monozygotic twins. *Am J Psychiatry* 121:1171–1175, 1965.

Jagger J, Prusoff BA, Cohen DJ, et al: The epidemiology of Tourette's syndrome: A pilot study. *Schizophr Bull* 8:267–278, 1982.

Johnson D, Myklebust H: *Learning Disabilities: Educational Principles and Practices.* New York, Grune & Stratton, 1967.

Kanner L: Autistic disturbances of affective contact. *Nerv Child* 2:217–250, 1943.

Kashani JH, Burk JP, Horwitz B, et al: Differential effect of subtype of parental major affective disorder on children. *Psychiatr Res* 15:195–204, 1985.

Kean JM: The development of social skills in autistic twins. *NZ Med J* 81:204–207, 1975.

Kelman DH: Gilles de la Tourette's disease in children: A review of the literature. *J Child Psychol Psychiatry* 6:219–226, 1965.

Kidd KK, Pauls DL: Genetic hypotheses for Tourette syndrome. In: Friedhoff AJ, Chase TN (eds): *Gilles de la Tourette Syndrome.* New York, Raven Press, 1982.

Kidd KK, Prusoff BA, Cohen DJ: The familial pattern of Tourette syndrome. *Arch Gen Psychiatry* 37:1336–1339, 1980.

Kotsopoulos S: Infantile autism in DZ twins: A case report. *J Autism Child Schizophr* 6:133–138, 1976.

Kurlan R, Behr J, Medved L, et al: Familial Tourette syndrome: Report of a large pedigree and potential for linkage analysis. *Neurology* 36:772–776, 1986.

Lathrop GM, Lalouel JM, Julier C, et al: Multilocus linkage analysis in humans: Detection of linkage and estimation of recombination. *Am J Hum Genet* 37:482–498, 1985.

Lenane MC, Swedo SE, Leonard H, et al: Psychiatric disorders in first degree relatives of children and adolescents with obsessive-compulsive disorder. *J Am Acad Child Adolesc Psychiatry* 3:407–412, 1990.

Leonard HL, Lenane MC, Swedo SE, et al: Tics and Tourette's disorder: A 2- to 7-year follow-up of 54 obsessive-compulsive children. *Am J Psychiatry* 149:1244–1251, 1992.

Lewitter FI, DeFries JC, Elston RC: Genetic models of reading disabilities. *Behav Genet* 10:9–30, 1980.

Lombroso PJ, Pauls DL, Leckman JF: Genetic mechanisms in childhood psychiatric disorders. *J Am Acad Child Adolesc Psychiatry* 33:921–938, 1994.

Lopez RE: Hyperactivity in twins. *Can Psychiatr Assoc J* 10:421–426, 1965.

Mattis S, French JH, Rapin I: Dyslexia in children and young adults: Three independent neuropsychological syndromes. *Dev Med Child Neurol* 17:281–300, 1975.

McGlannon FK: Familial characteristics of genetic dyslexia: Preliminary report of a pilot study. *J Learn Disabil* 1:185–191, 1968.

McQuaid PE: Infantile autism in twins. *Br J Psychiatry* 127:530–534, 1975.

Meryash DL, Szymanski LS, Gerald PS: Infantile autism associated with the fragile-X syndrome. *J Autism Dev Disord* 12:295–301, 1982.

Montgomery MA, Clayton PJ, Friedhoff AJ: Psychiatric illness in Tourette syndrome patients and first-degree relatives. In: Friedhoff AJ, Chase TN (eds): *Gilles de la Tourette Syndrome.* New York, Raven Press, 1982.

Morphew JA, Sim M: Gilles de la Tourette's syndrome: A clinical and psychopathological study. *Br J Med Psychol* 42:293–301, 1969.

Morrison J, Stewart M: A family study of hyperactive child syndrome. *Biol Psychiatry* 3:189–195, 1971.

Morrison JR, Stewart M: The psychiatric status of the legal families of adopted hyperactive children. *Arch Gen Psychiatry* 28:888–891, 1973.

Morrison JR, Stewart M: Bilateral inheritance as evidence for polygenicity in the hyperactive child syndrome. *J Nerv Ment Dis* 158:226–228, 1974.

Morton NE: The detection and estimation of linkage between the genes of elliptocytosis and the Rh blood groups. *Am J Hum Genet* 26:489–503, 1956.

Mullis K, Faloona F, Scharf S, et al: Specific enzymatic amplification of DNA in vitro: The polymerase chain reaction. *Cold Spring Harbor Symp Quant Biol* 51:263, 1986.

Nee LE, Caine ED, Polinsky RJ, et al: Gilles de la Tourette syndrome: Clinical and family study of 50 cases. *Ann Neurol* 7:41–49, 1980.

Nee LE, Polinsky RJ, Ebert MH: Tourette syndrome: Clinical and family studies. In: Friedhoff AJ, Chase TN (eds): *Gilles de la Tourette Syndrome.* New York, Raven Press, 1982.

Nicolini H, Hanna G, Baxter L, et al: Segregation analysis of obsessive compulsive and associated disorders. Preliminary results. *Ursus Medicus* 1:25–28, 1991.

Omenn GS: Genetic issues in the syndrome of minimal brain dysfunction. *Semin Psychiatry* 5:5–17, 1973.

Omenn GS, Weber BA: Dyslexia: Search for phenotypic and genetic heterogeneity. *Am J Med Genet* 1:333–342, 1978.

Orton ST: *Reading, Writing and Speech Problems in Children.* New York, Norton, 1937.

Orvaschel H, Thompson WD, Belanger A, et al: Comparison of the family history method to direct interview: Factors affecting the diagnosis of depression. *J Affective Disord* 4:49–59, 1982.

Orvaschel H, Walsh-Allis G, Ye W: Psychopathology in children of parents with recurrent depression. *J Abnorm Child Psychol* 16:17–28, 1988.

Owen FW, Adams PA, Forrest T, et al: Learning disorders in children: Sibling studies. *Monogr Soc Res Child Dev* 36:1–77, 1971.

Pakstis AJ, Heutink P, Pauls DL, et al: Progress in the search for genetic linkage with Tourette syndrome: A exclusion map covering more than 50% of the autosomal genome. *Am J Hum Genet* 48:281–294, 1991.

Pauls DL: Strategies for the genetic study of child psychiatric disorders. In: Michels R, Cavenar J, Brodie H, et al (eds): *Psychiatry* (Vol 2). Philadelphia, Lippincott, 1985.

Pauls DL, Kidd KK: Genetics of childhood behavioral disorders. In: Lahey BB, Kazdin AE (eds): *Advances in Clinical Child Psychiatry.* New York, Plenum, 1981.

Pauls DL, Leckman JF: The inheritance of Gilles de la Tourette's syndrome and associated behaviors. *N Engl J Med* 315:993–997, 1986.

Pauls DL, Leckman JF: The genetics of Tourette's syndrome. In: Cohen DJ, Bruun RD, Leckman JK (eds): *Tourette's Syndrome & Tic Disorders: Clinical Understanding and Treatment.* New York, Wiley, 1988.

Pauls DL, Alsobrook JP II, Goodman W, et al: A family study of obsessive compulsive disorder. *Am J Psych* 152:76–84, 1995.

Pauls DL, Cohen DJ, Heimbuch R, et al: Familial pattern and transmission of Gilles de la Tourette syndrome and multiple tics. *Arch Gen Psychiatry* 38:1091–1093, 1981.

Pauls DL, Kruger SD, Leckman JF, et al: The risk of Tourette's syndrome and chronic multiple tics among relatives of Tourette's syndrome patients obtained by direct interview. *J Am Acad Child Psychiatry* 23:134–137, 1984.

Pauls DL, Pakstis AJ, Kurlan R, et al: Segregation and linkage analyses of Tourette's syndrome and related disorders. *J Am Acad Child Adolesc Psychiatry* 29:195–203, 1990.

Pauls DL, Shaywitz S, Kramer P, et al: Demonstration of vertical transmission of attention deficit disorder. *Ann Neurol* 14:363, 1983.

Pauls DL, Towbin KE, Leckman JF, et al: Gilles de La Tourette's syndrome and obsessive compulsive disorder: Evidence supporting a genetic relationship. *Arch Gen Psychiatry* 43:1180–1182, 1986.

Pennington DF, Smith SD: Genetic influences on learning disabilities and speech and language disorders. *Child Dev* 54:369–387, 1983.

Pennington DF, Gilger JW, Pauls D, et al: Evidence for major gene transmission of developmental dyslexia. *JAMA* 266:1527–1534, 1991.

Plomin R, Daniels D: Why are children in the same family so different from one another? *Behav Brain Sci* 10:1–15, 1987.

Plomin R, DeFries JC: *Origins of Individual Differences in Infancy: The Colorado Adoption Project.* New York, Academic Press, 1985.

Plomin R, DeFries JC, Fulker DW: *Nature and Nurture during Infancy and Early Childhood.* New York, Cambridge University Press, 1988.

Price RA, Kidd KK, Pauls DL, et al: A twin study of Tourette's syndrome. *Arch Gen Psychiatry* 42:815–820, 1985.

Price RA, Pauls DL, Kruger SD, et al: Family data support a dominant major gene for Tourette syndrome. *Psychiatry Res* 24:251–261, 1987.

Puig-Antich J, Goetz D, Davies M, et al: A controlled family history study of prepubertal major depressive disorder. *Arch Gen Psychiatry* 46:406–418, 1989.

Ritvo ER, Freeman BJ, Mason-Brothers A, et al: Concordance for the syndrome of autism in 40 pairs of afflicted twins. *Am J Psychiatry* 142:74–77, 1985a.

Ritvo ER, Freeman BJ, Pingree C, et al: The UCLA-University of Utah epidemiologic survey of autism: Prevalence. *Am J Psychiatry* 146:194–199, 1989a.

Ritvo ER, Jorde L, Mason-Brothers A, et al: The UCLA-University of Utah epidemiologic survey of autism: Recurrence risk estimates and genetic counseling. *Am J Psychiatry* 146:1032–1036, 1989b.

Ritvo ER, Spence MA, Freeman BJ, et al: Evidence for autosomal recessive inheritance in 46 families with multiple incidences of autism. *Am J Psychiatry* 142:187–192, 1985b.

Robertson MM, Trimble MR, Lees AJ: The psychopathology of the Gilles de la Tourette: A phenomenological analysis. *Br J Psychiatry* 152:383–390, 1988.

Robins LN, Helzer JE, Weissman MM, et al: Lifetime prevalence of specific psychiatric disorders in three sites. *Arch Gen Psychiatry* 41:949–958, 1984.

Rowe D: Biometrical genetic models of self-reported delinquent behavior: A twin study. *Behav Genet* 13:473–489, 1983.

Rutter M: Psychotic disorders in early childhood. *Br J Psychiatry*, Special Publication No. 1, 1967.

Rutter M: Concepts of autism: A review of research. *J Child Psychol Psychiatry* 9:1–25, 1968.

Rutter M: The description and classification of infantile autism. In: Churchill DW, Alpern GD, DeMyer MK (eds): *Infantile Autism.* Springfield, IL, Charles C Thomas, 1971.

Rutter M: The development of infantile autism. *Psychol Med* 4:147–163, 1974.

Rutter M: Psychological sequelae of brain damage in children. *Am J Psychiatry* 138:1533–1544, 1981.

Rutter M: Behavioral studies: Questions and findings on the concept of a distinctive syndrome. In: Rutter M (ed): *Developmental Neuropsychiatry.* New York, Guilford Press, 1983.

Rutter M, Macdonald H, Le Couteur A, et al: Genetic factors in child psychiatric disorders. II: Empirical findings. *J Child Psychol Psychiatry* 31:39–83, 1990.

Safer D: A familial factor in minimal brain dysfunction. *Behav Genet* 3:175–186, 1973.

Scarr S: Genetic factors in activity motivation. *Child Dev* 37:663–673, 1966.

Shapiro AK, Shapiro ES, Bruun RD, et al: *Gilles de la Tourette Syndrome*. New York, Raven Press, 1978.

Shaywitz SE, Shaywitz BA: Biologic influences in attention deficit disorders. In: Levine MD, Carey WB, Crocker AC, et al (eds): *Developmental-Behavioral Pediatrics*. Philadelphia, Saunders, 1982.

Shaywitz SE, Cohen DJ, Shaywitz BA: Pharmacotherapy of attention deficit disorder. In: Swaiman K (ed): *Pediatric Update*. New York, Elsevier, 1983.

Shaywitz SE, Shaywitz BA, Fletcher JM, et al: Prevalence of reading disability in boys and girls. *JAMA* 264:998–1002, 1990.

Smith SD, Kimberling WJ, Pennington BF, et al: Specific reading disability: Identification of an inherited form through linkage analysis. *Science* 219:1345–1347, 1983.

Smith SD, Pennington BF, Kimberling WJ, et al: Familial dyslexia: Use of genetic linkage data to define subtypes. *J Am Acad Child Adolesc Psychiatry* 29:204–213, 1990.

Stefl ME: Mental health needs associated with Tourette syndrome. *Am J Public Health* 74:1310–1313, 1984.

Steffenburg S, Gillberg C, Hellgren L, et al: A twin study of autism in Denmark, Finland, Iceland, Norway and Sweden. *J Child Psychol Psychiatry* 30:405–416, 1989.

Stephenson S: Six cases of congenital word-blindness affecting three generations of one family. *Ophthalmoscope* 5:482–484, 1907.

Stevenson J: Evidence for a genetic etiology in hyperactivity in children. *Behav Genet* 22:337–344, 1992.

Stevenson J, Graham P, Fredman G, et al: A twin study of genetic influences on reading and spelling ability and disability. *J Child Psychol Psychiatry* 28:229–247, 1987.

Strober M, Morrell W, Burroughs J, et al: A family study of bipolar I disorder in adolescence: Early onset of symptoms linked to increased familial loading and lithium resistance. *J Affective Disord* 15:255–268, 1988.

Symmes JS, Rapaport IL: Unexpected reading failure. *Am J Orthopsychiatry* 42:82–91, 1972.

Taft LT, Cohen HI: Hypsarrhythmia and infantile autism: A clinical report. *J Autism Child Schizophr* 1:327–336, 1971.

Thomas CJ: Congenital "word blindness" and its treatment. *Ophthalmoscope* 3:380–385, 1905.

Todd RD, Neuman R, Geller B, et al: Genetic studies of affective disorders: Should we be starting with childhood onset probands? *J Am Acad Child Adolesc Psychiatry* 32:1164–1171, 1993.

Vandenberg SG: The hereditary abilities study: Hereditary components in a psychological test battery. *Am J Hum Genet* 14:220–237, 1962.

Vandenberg SG, Singer SM, Pauls DL: *The Heredity of Behavior Disorders in Adults and Children*. New York, Plenum Medical, 1986.

van de Wetering BJM: *The Gilles de la Tourette Syndrome: A Psychiatric-Genetic Study*. Doctoral thesis, Rotterdam, The Netherlands, Erasmus University, 1993.

Walker L, Cole EM: Familial patterns of expression of specific reading disability in a population sample. *Bull Orton Soc* 15:12–24, 1965.

Walkup JT, Leckman JF, Price RA, et al: Nongenetic factors associated with the expression of Tourette syndrome. Unpublished paper presented at the 34th annual meeting of the American Academy of Child and Adolescent Psychiatry, 1987.

Watson MS, Leckman JF, Annex B, et al: Fragile X in a survey of 75 autistic males. *N Engl J Med* 310:1462, 1984.

Weber JL, May PE: Abundant class of human DNA polymorphisms which can be typed using the polymerase chain reaction. *Am J Hum Genet* 44:388, 1989.

Weiss RE, Stein MA, Trommer BA, et al: Attention-deficit hyperactivity disorder and thyroid function. *J Pediatr* 123:539–545, 1993.

Weissman MM, Prusoff BA, Gammon GD, et al: Psychopathology in the children (ages 6–18) of depressed and normal parents. *J Am Acad Child Psychiatry* 23:78–84, 1984.

Willerman L: Activity level and hyperactivity in twins. *Child Dev* 44:288–293, 1973.

Yaryura-Tobias JA, Neziroglu F, Howard S, et al: Clinical aspects of Gilles de la Tourette syndrome. *Orthomolecular Psychiatry* 10:263–268, 1981.

Zahalkova M, Vrzal V, Kloboukova E: Genetical investigations in dyslexia. *J Med Genet* 9:48–52, 1972.

Zerbin-Rudin E: Congenital word-blindness. *Bull Orton Soc* 17:47–54, 1967.

30 ACQUIRED BRAIN DISORDERS

Boris Birmaher, M.D., and Daniel T. Williams, M.D.

Any acquired brain disorder carries with it a high probability of associated psychiatric disturbance. In this chapter we review the psychiatric complications of CNS infections and traumatic brain injury in children and adolescents. Neuropsychiatric signs, symptoms, and syndromes are addressed in Chapter 28. Other CNS disorders are discussed in Chapter 59.

The common feature in all acquired CNS disorders is brain damage. As reviewed below, brain damage during childhood or adolescence by itself increases the likelihood of psychiatric disorders, after controlling for other variables such as IQ, socioeconomic status, premorbid psychiatric symptoms, physical handicaps, and visible physical deformities. The implications of this common feature is therefore addressed before discussing specific etiologies of acquired brain disorders.

Rutter et al. (1970) compared the psychiatric status of all school-age children living on the Isle of Wight and known to have epilepsy or unequivocal brain damage with children in the general population and with children suffering from chronic physical illness and/or handicap not involving the CNS. As assessed on both a teacher's questionnaire and a clinical psychiatric interview, children of *normal intelligence* with an organic brain condition were twice as likely as children with other physical handicaps (such as asthma, diabetes, or heart disease) to show behavioral deviance or disorder. The difference between these two groups suggested that it was the brain injury that increased the psychiatric risk. This increased risk for psychiatric disorders was unlikely to be due to the nonspecific effects of chronic illness or to social and family adversity. However, in this study children with neurological disorders were more likely to have visible crippling than children with other physi-

cal handicaps, and this may explain the difference in psychopathology between the two groups.

Seidel et al. (1975) addressed this issue. He compared 33 *normally intelligent* school-age children with brain disorders (mostly cerebral palsy) and 42 children with handicapping conditions originating below the brainstem (e.g., polio, muscular dystrophy). Both groups were comparable in terms of visible crippling, but psychiatric disorder was found to be twice as frequent in the group with brain damage. In the same line, Breslau et al. (1985) compared 304 children with cystic fibrosis, cerebral palsy, myelodysplasia, and multiple physical handicaps with 360 normal children. In comparison with the normal group, children with chronic physical disabilities were at increased risk for nonspecific psychiatric disturbances. Those with brain pathology were associated with more severe psychiatric impairment. This impairment, however, varied with the level of mental retardation. The severity of physical disability was found to have little relationship to psychiatric disturbance, when type of condition and mental retardation were controlled.

As reviewed by Rutter (1981) and Shaffer (1985), brain damage is associated with increased risk not only for psychiatric disorder, but for intellectual impairment. The intellectual impairment is directly associated with the severity of brain damage, especially with bilateral damage (Rutter, 1981). The psychiatric disorder is more likely to occur after severe damage, although it does not follow a clear "dose-response" pattern described for the intellectual impairment. The intellectual impairment per se may increase the risk for psychiatric disorder. Other mechanisms, however, are involved in the development of psychiatric disorder. In the Isle of Wight study, the highest rate of psychiatric disorder was found in children with structural disorders of the brain accompanied by functional disorders, as evidenced by seizures or abnormalities in the EEG. Psychiatric disturbances were influenced also by the child's preinjury behavior and psychosocial factors such as social disadvantage, broken homes, and their mother's having had an emotional disturbance (Rutter, 1981; Shaffer, 1985). The types of psychiatric disturbances encountered among brain-injured children were found to cover a broad spectrum and hence were not specific to this group, with the exception of an increased incidence of social isolation (Breslau, 1985) and disinhibited social behavior (Rutter, 1981). Brain-damaged children were markedly outspoken, with general lack of regard for social convention (e.g., they asked embarrassing questions and undressed in social situations). In addition, they showed forgetfulness, overtalkativeness, poor hygiene, and impulsive behavior. Retrospectively, the composite of these symptoms is most compatible with the DSM-III-R diagnosis of organic personality disorder (APA, 1987) and with the DSM-IV diagnosis of personality change due to a general medical condition, disinhibited type (APA, 1994).

CENTRAL NERVOUS SYSTEM INFECTIONS

Despite the prevalent use and growing sophistication of antibiotic treatments, children and adolescents still die or suffer permanent neurological and/or psychological sequelae as a result of CNS infections. This section briefly discusses several CNS infectious diseases, their acute symptoms, and their known neuropsychiatric sequelae.

The CNS responds to injury in a limited number of ways, regardless of the nature of the infecting organism. Infectious diseases share a number of clinical and pathological features, with the extent of various ensuing neuropsychiatric symptoms being determined by the virulence of the invading organism, the site and the extension of the infection, and the immunological response of the individual (Menkes, 1990). It is difficult to distinguish among chronic granulomatous, viral bacterial, fungal, spirochetal, or protozoan infections solely from the history and physical examination of the patient. The diagnosis requires laboratory studies, including the isolation and, if possible, propagation of the suspected organisms.

For the purpose of this section we will use the following definitions: *Meningitis* denotes inflammation of the meninges and is identified by an abnormal number of white blood cells (WBCs) in the cerebrospinal fluid (CSF). *Bacterial meningitis* denotes meningitis with evidence of a bacterial pathogen in the CSF. *Aseptic meningitis* denotes meningitis with no evidence of a bacterial pathogen detectable in the CSF by usual laboratory techniques. Most cases of aseptic meningitis have a viral etiology but can also be caused by rickettsia, spirochetes, and other nonbacterial infections, as well as noninfectious diseases such as lupus, multiple sclerosis, malignancies, and others. *Encephalitis* denotes inflammation of the brain. *Meningoencephalitis* denotes inflammation of the brain accompanied by meningitis (Klein et al., 1986).

Epidemiology

The incidence of bacterial meningitis and the causative organisms are closely related to age. During the 1st month of life, the age-specific incidence in the United States is nearly 100 cases per 100,000 live births. The incidence falls to 45 per 100,000 during the 2nd month of life but reaches a second peak at 6–8 months with an incidence of nearly 80 per 100,000. At 1 year of age, the incidence is approximately 20 per 100,000. At 5 years of age the incidence is 2 per 100,000, and between 10 and 19 years it decreases to 0.9 per 100,000 (Centers for Disease Control (CDC), 1979).

Meningitis caused by *Mycobacterium tuberculosis* has gradually diminished in frequency over the past few decades and now, at least in economically developed countries, is unusual. However, due to the increased incidence of pulmonary tuberculosis in the United States, it will not be surprising to see a surge in the prevalence of meningitis by tuberculosis.

The incidence of viral meningitis ranges, in different years, from 1.5 to 4 cases per 100,000 population. The incidence in children is actually much higher because aseptic meningitis is also a disease of the young (CDC, 1977).

Bacterial Meningitis

The pathogenesis, microbiology, diagnosis, and management of bacterial meningitis varies in the different periods of childhood. In the newborn infant (0–28 days), meningitis in most cases is the result of infection by organisms acquired at delivery, and to a lesser extent by organisms acquired in the nursery or household. The major pathogens are Group B streptococcus and *Escherichia coli*.

The highest age-specific attack rates for bacterial meningitis (other than the newborn period) occur between 3 and 8 months of age. *Haemophilus influenzae* type B, *Neisseria meningitidis*, and *Streptococcus pneumoniae* are responsible for most of the infections in this age group. The incidence decreases after 2 years of age and is sharply reduced in older children and adolescents, the bacteria responsible being the same as those in the youngest children (Klein et al., 1986).

PATHOGENESIS OF BACTERIAL MENINGITIS

Most of the cases progress through four stages: (*a*) infection of the upper respiratory tract, (*b*) invasion of the blood from the respiratory focus, (*c*) seeding of the meninges by the blood-borne organism, and (*d*) inflammation of the meninges and brain. Most children with an upper respiratory infection by an organism that causes meningitis are asymptomatic or have mild symptoms. Some of them have bacteremia, but the organisms are cleared from the bloodstream by an immune system or antimicrobial agents. However, in a few children, treated or untreated infection progresses to seeding of the CNS and meningitis. Why some children develop this progression is unknown (Evans, 1987; Klein et al., 1986; Menkes, 1990).

In newborns, meningitis most commonly follows or is associated with septicemia. The blood is invaded from a colonized site, usually the respiratory tract or umbilical cord. The same bacteria generally can be recovered from the maternal vaginal tract (Klein et al., 1986). Uncommonly, infection may spread to the meninges via the hematogenous route in children with endocarditis, pneumonia, or thrombophlebitis, or by direct extension in children with sinusitis, otitis media, and mastoiditis or osteomyelitis of the skull. Meningitis also may follow head trauma or neurosurgical procedures or may develop in individuals with sinus tracts or a meningomyelocele (Evans, 1987; Klein et al., 1986; Menkes, 1990).

Once the bacteria seed the meninges, they produce an inflammation whose subsequent exudate enters the subarachnoid space, leading to arteritis, arterial or venous thrombosis, and perineuritis. When the exudate is abundant, it may obstruct the subarachnoid space around the midbrain or pons or over the cerebral convexity, producing a communicating hydrocephalus or obstructing the foramina of Luschka and Magendie and as a result produce a noncommunicating hydrocephalus (Evans, 1987; Klein et al., 1986; Menkes, 1990).

Changes in cerebral function may occur because of occlusion of the meningeal or cerebral vessels, direct interference with cerebral metabolism by the bacteria and its toxins, or cerebral edema. The increased intracranial pressure or the acute hydrocephalus may decrease the perfusion of blood to the brain. The ensuing changes in neuronal metabolism may cause edema or predispose to seizures. If the edema progresses rapidly, it can induce cerebral herniation and death. If the process continues more slowly, for several days, glial proliferation occurs. The changes in nerve cells may be slight, or there may be widespread destruction of cortical cells and myelinated fibers.

The disorder of the cortical neurons, with change in mental status or seizures, occurs as much as several days before microscopic alterations; this is the result not of bacteria within the substance of brain but of a metabolic or toxic encephalopathy (Evans, 1987; Klein et al., 1986; Menkes, 1990).

Susceptibility to bacterial meningitis is affected by age and congenital or acquired deficiencies in host defense mechanisms. Thus, the risk of meningitis is increased in very young children, after splenectomy, in children with sickle cell anemia or other hemoglobinopathies, in deficiency of the terminal components of the complement system, and in children with malignancies. Also, some studies have indicated the possibility of genetic predisposition (Evans, 1987; Menkes, 1990).

CLINICAL DIAGNOSIS

No one clinical sign is pathognomonic of meningitis. Symptoms and signs of meningitis are variable and depend in part on the age of the patient, the duration of the illness before examination, and the child's response to the infection. As a rule, findings in neonates and young infants are minimal and often subtle, making early diagnosis difficult to establish clinically (Klein et al., 1986). Infants may present with fever (50%), lethargy, respiratory distress, jaundice, disinterest in feeding, vomiting, diarrhea, irritability (30%), poor muscle tone, alterations in consciousness, convulsions (40%), and a bulging fontanel (30%) (Klein et al., 1986).

In children, fever, headache, photophobia, nausea, vomiting, mental confusion, lethargy, and irritability are the usual initial complaints. These manifestations are nonspecific and are like those of nonmeningeal viral infections or other febrile illnesses. A change in the child's affect or alertness is one of the most important signs of meningitis (Klein et al., 1986). Stiff neck and other meningeal signs, seizures, and coma occur less commonly and usually later in the illness. However, when encountered, these are sufficiently characteristic of meningitis to prompt physicians to perform an immediate diagnostic lumbar puncture. Papilledema is uncommon early in the course of acute meningitis and, when present, prompts the need to rule out venous sinus thrombosis, subdural effusions, or brain abscess (Klein et al., 1986; Menkes, 1990).

The definitive diagnostic test of meningitis is the examination of the CSF by spinal tap. The routine CSF analyses are bacterial cultures, protein and glucose determinations, cell count, and differential Gram stain. If available, detection of capsular antigens using counterimmune electrophoresis or other techniques can also be helpful (Klein et al., 1986; Menkes, 1990).

COMPLICATIONS AND PROGNOSIS

Neurological Sequelae

The mortality rate for bacterial meningitis in the neonate remains high, varying between 15 and 20%. The mortality rate for bacterial meningitis in children who are beyond the neonatal period has been reduced by antibiotic therapy to less than 10%. Nevertheless, as many as 50% of the survivors of meningitis have some sequelae of their disease (Evans, 1987; Klein et al., 1986; Menkes, 1990).

Specific sequelae or complications of bacterial meningitis that have been observed include cranial nerve involvement, which often improves with the time. But 10% remain with hearing loss, hemiparesis or quadriparesis, muscular hypertonia, ataxia, mental retardation, permanent seizure disorders, or hydrocephalus. Thirty percent develop the syndrome of inappropriate antidiuretic hormone secretion, but this is rarely persistent or clinically significant. Approximately 40% develop subdural effusions, and they are so frequent in young children that they can be considered as part of the general disease process rather than as a complication. Brain abscess following meningitis is rare; when present, one must rule out other infections such as endocarditis (Evans, 1987; Klein et al., 1986; Menkes, 1990).

The following factors have been associated with worse prognosis in case of bacterial meningitis: highly infectious agent and severe initial process, young age of the patient (less than 2 years, worse prognosis), significant delay between onset of symptoms and diagnosis and therapy,

seizures after the 3rd or 4th day of therapy, focal seizures, neurological focal signs, a low CSF glucose, and a high amount of WBCs. However, not all investigations agree with regard to all these prognostic parameters, so that no one alone should become the basis of an overly definite prognostic projection (Dodge and Swartz, 1965; Klein et al., 1986; Menkes, 1990; Sell, 1983; Sell et al., 1972a, 1972b; Swartz and Dodge, 1965; Taylor et al., 1984; Tejani et al., 1982; Wald et al., 1986).

Psychiatric Sequelae

Behavior and learning problems constitute frequent but variably reported sequelae of bacterial meningitis. More specifically, mild to severe mental retardation, learning difficulties, perceptual and attention deficits, and nonspecific disturbances in behavior or adjustment have been reported. However, as pointed out by Taylor et al. (1984), there are deficiencies in the methodology of most of the studies. Sample selection procedures are often unspecified, and appropriate control groups are seldom included. Sometimes follow-up intervals between the meningitis and the evaluation are too short, and raters are nonblind. School performance, language deficits, and behavior problems are vaguely defined or measured, and formal achievement tasks are rarely carried out.

Noncontrolled studies had reported that neuropsychiatric sequelae develop in 10–50% of children after *H. influenza* meningitis (Feigin et al., 1976; Sell, 1983; Sell et al., 1972a, 1972b; Taylor et al., 1984; Tejani et al., 1982) and 4–50% after Group B streptococcus meningitis (Chin and Fitzhardinge, 1985; Edwards et al., 1985; Wald et al., 1986). Taylor et al. (1984) studied 24 schoolchildren 6–8 years after recovery from *H. influenzae* meningitis and compared them with a similar group of school-age siblings. Evaluations were blind and consisted of test of IQ, academic achievement, neuropsychological skills, and behavior ratings. Results showed that postmeningitis children scored significantly lower on full-scale and performance IQ. Also, they performed poorly on several neuropsychiatric tasks. They did not differ in verbal IQ, performed comparably on all academic measures, and did not differ on behavior measurements. Twenty-one percent of the postmeningitis children had neurological sequelae, and they comprised the bulk of those with the lowest IQ and/or academic scores. The authors defined children with mild handicap as those with neurological residua and an IQ or academic score that fell at least 1 SD below age standard. They found that 46% of postmeningitis children and 29% of the sibling group were in the mild handicap group, suggesting that, although meningitis may produce neuropsychiatric sequelae, this is not the only factor involved in the outcome.

Sell et al. (1972b) followed 50 infants and children who recovered from *H. influenzae* meningitis. Of this group, 50% were normal, 9% had nonspecific behavior problems, and 28% had significant handicaps (hearing loss, language disorders, impaired vision, mental retardation, motor abnormalities, and seizures). Twenty-one postmeningitis children were paired with a sibling and tested by means of IQ tests. The mean IQ of the postmeningitis children was significant lower than that of their own siblings (86 versus 97). Comparison of results for individual pairs revealed that 29% of postmeningitis children scored 1 SD below their siblings; no survivor of meningitis had a score 1 SD higher than their sibling.

Feigin et al. (unpublished data, cited in Klein et al., 1986) followed a group of 235 postmeningitis children. Their mean IQ was 94, with a range of 33–150. Twenty-nine children (17.3%) had IQ scores less than 70. A comparison of these patients with their own siblings and with other control children revealed no significant differences in mean IQ. However, a significantly greater proportion of children who recovered from meningitis had IQ scores less than 80.

Tejani et al. (1982) compared a group of 15 children who had recovered 1–5 years previously from *H. influenzae* meningitis with 15 siblings. Five postmeningitis children had IQs between 70 and 90, but in all but one case the siblings had similar IQs. Wald et al. (1986) compared a group of 34 children who had recovered 3–18 years previously from Group B streptococcus meningitis with 21 siblings. They found that those children without major neurological sequelae (spastic quadriplegia, profound mental retardation, hemiparesis, deafness, or blindness) were functioning normally or comparably with their siblings in intellectual, academic, social, and behavioral matters. Wald et al. also concluded that children who had recovered from meningitis may have mild retardation or behavior problems, attributable not to the previous infection but rather to environmental or genetic factors.

Recently, Taylor et al. (1992) compared two groups of children with normal IQ who had recovered from complicated and noncomplicated *Haemophilus influenzae* type B meningitis. The two groups had similar normal hearing and similar verbal IQs. The complicated group, however, had lower mean performance IQ and performed less well on perceptual neurological tests. Parent and teachers ratings of behavior and frequencies of grade repetitions and special education placement failed to distinguish the two groups.

Reviewing these studies suggests that bacterial meningitis may constitute a risk factor for a significant minority of children affected but should not by itself be presumed to negatively affect the behavioral or cognitive development of any individual child so exposed. It seems that sequelae after bacterial meningitis are mainly seen in those cases with neurological complications during the acute phase of the illness (Taylor et al., 1990, 1992).

Viral Central Nervous System Infections

The incidence of viral meningoencephalitis is greater than that of bacterial meningitis in children, though the morbidity is generally less than that of bacterial meningitis. The major exception is infection due to herpesvirus, whose morbidity and mortality are very high (Evans, 1987; Menkes, 1990). The most common mode of viral CNS infection is hematogenous. The virus enters the CNS through the choroid plexus and then enters the CSF by replication in the capillary endothelium of the brain. The other route of CNS inoculation is contiguous spread through the peripheral nervous system, as in the case of herpesvirus or rabies. Injury occurs by the process of viral replication and by vascular injury, which causes destruction of neurons and glial cells. The pathology of viral encephalitis shows perivascular mononuclear cells and neuronal destruction. In approximately 60% of cases, a specific virus can be identified by either culture or serology (Evans, 1987; Menkes, 1990).

The clinical spectrum of viral CNS infections ranges from aseptic meningitis to encephalitis to chronic infections and postinfectious neural illnesses. The clinical picture of aseptic meningitis is similar to that of bacterial meningitis. Chronic infections are discussed below, and postinfectious diseases (e.g., Guillain-Barré syndrome) are described in Chapter 59.

Neurological and Psychiatric Sequelae

Enteroviral meningitis accounts for at least 50% of cases of viral meningitis occurring in the United States. Most of the patients are infants younger than 1 year of age, and most of the infections are mild (Evans, 1987; Menkes, 1990). Enteroviral meningitis had been reported to produce a low frequency of adverse neurological, cognitive, or language sequelae (Bergman et al., 1987; Sells et al., 1975). Bergman et al. (1987) followed 33 8-year-old survivors of enteroviral meningitis that occurred when the children were between the ages of 4 months and 1 year and compared them with 31 siblings. None of the survivors had a major neurological sequela, and they performed as well as the controls on the cognitive and behavior tests administered.

Similarly, Farmer et al. (1975) followed for 6 years 15 infants with meningoencephalitis due to Coxsackievirus B5 and compared them with 15 controls matched by age, sex, socioeconomic status, birth weight, and gestational age. There was no difference in the IQ and visual perception test between both groups.

Some studies followed children for various periods of time after the California arbovirus encephalitis (Chun et al., 1960; Gunderman and

Stamler, 1973; Matthews et al., 1968; Rie et al., 1973; Sabatino and Cramblet, 1968) and found an incidence rate of between 0 and 40% for such neurological complications as soft signs, seizures, or hemiparesis, some nonspecific behavior difficulties, and nonsignificant depressed IQs. By contrast, other studies (Earnets et al., 1971; Finley et al., 1953) have reported high rates of neurological morbidity (up to 69%) and mortality in children who suffered Western equine encephalitis, especially in those children younger than 1 year old.

As in the morbidity studies after bacterial meningitis, studies of morbidity after viral infections are flawed by methodological problems that limit the generalization of their findings.

Acquired Immunodeficiency Syndrome and Related Disorders

Acquired immunodeficiency syndrome (AIDS) is defined by the CDC (1986a) as "a disease, at least moderately predictive of a defect in cell-mediated immunity, occurring in a person with no known cause for diminished resistance. Diseases diagnostic for AIDS include Kaposi's sarcoma, *Pneumocystis carinii* pneumonia and other opportunistic infections." AIDS is caused by a retrovirus (human immunodeficiency virus (HIV)) (Coffin et al., 1986) that infects the T-helper lymphocytes. The virus is characterized as a member of the HIV family of retroviruses, but recent studies indicate that the genome of HIV is more closely related to visna virus, a lente virus that causes a chronic degenerative neurological disease in sheep (Gonda et al., 1985).

The virus alters the immune system of its host by infecting the T4-helper/inducer lymphocyte. By depleting the number and adversely affecting the function of the T4 cell, the action of other cells, including antibody-producing B lymphocytes, is compromised. This results in vulnerability to infection to opportunistic agents such as fungi, protozoa, parasites, and bacteria, as well as to the development of uncommon neoplasms such as Kaposi's sarcoma and non-Hodgkin's lymphoma (Goodman, 1988).

In addition to presenting as AIDS, infection by the HIV retrovirus may manifest in two milder forms: (*a*) persistent generalized lymphadenopathy (PGL), which occurs in absence of concurrent infection other than HIV infection, and (*b*) AIDS-related complex (ARC), which is characterized by lethargy, fatigue, weight loss, generalized lymphadenopathy, and fever or night sweats (CDC, 1986a, 1986b, 1987). While PGL initially appeared to have a benign prognosis, recent estimates indicate that approximately one-third of HIV-positive individuals and one-fourth of patients with ARC will have AIDS within approximately 5 years (CDC, 1986a, 1986b, 1987). Clinical AIDS thus appears currently to be the invariable, fatal outcome of an HIV infection, with 80% mortality within 2 years of diagnosis (CDC, 1986a, 1986b, 1987).

The World Health Organization estimates that currently a total of 8–10 million persons worldwide are infected with HIV. The total number of infected persons in the United States by 1989 was estimated to be 1 million, or about 1 in 250 persons (CDC, 1993). AIDS has become the sixth leading cause of death among youths ages 15–24 (CDC, 1993).

Homosexual/bisexual men and intravenous drug users comprise 90% of AIDS patients. The remainder consists of heterosexual contacts, children of infected mothers, and persons who received contaminated blood via transfusion. It is important to mention, however, that from 1990 to 1991, the percentage of AIDS cases attributed to heterosexual contact has increased by 21%. Also, the rate of reported AIDS cases in nonmetropolitan areas is increasing faster than in urban areas (CDC, 1993). Transmission occurs primarily through the exchange of contaminated blood or blood products and via sexual activity through transfer of and exposure to semen and perhaps cervical secretions (Goodman, 1988).

Neurological and Psychiatric Sequelae

AIDS is frequently complicated by CNS dysfunction (Helweg-Larson et al., 1986; Hollander and Levy, 1987; Navia et al., 1986a, 1986b;

Price et al., 1987; Snider et al., 1983). In some patients, this is due to well-defined focal lesions in the brain, such as those resulting from toxoplasmosis, cryptococcal meningitis, multifocal leukoencephalopathy, or lymphoma. However, far more common than these focal disturbances is the development of more generalized encephalopathy (Ho et al., 1987; Navia et al., 1986a, 1986b; Navia and Price, 1987; Price et al., 1987; Shaw et al., 1985; Snider et al., 1983) characterized by progressive motor, cognitive, and behavioral disturbances in at least two-thirds of patients with AIDS. This syndrome has been variously referred to as subacute encephalitis, subacute encephalopathy, or AIDS dementia complex (ADC). The syndrome may result from direct brain infection by HIV (Goudsmit et al., 1986; Ho et al., 1987; Hollander and Levy 1987; Navia et al., 1986a, 1986b; Navia and Price, 1987; Shaw et al., 1985), which may occur early in the course of systemic virus infection. Many adult AIDS patients eventually develop this encephalopathy, which characteristically begins with impaired concentration and mild memory loss and progresses to severe global cognitive impairment. Motor signs, including generalized hyperreflexia and increased tone, may accompany the dementia. These neurological symptoms and signs usually progress over a course of several weeks and months. Behavioral disturbances are common, and among the early features are apathy, loss of spontaneity, and social withdrawal. Rarely, agitated psychosis with paranoia and hallucinations may ensue (Navia et al., 1986a, 1986b). Pathological evidence of subacute encephalitis is found in 90% of these patients at autopsy (Gabuzda et al., 1986). It affects primarily the white matter and subcortical structures of the brain and is characterized by diffuse pallor, focal vacuolization, and multifocal perivascular rarefaction (Navia et al., 1986a; Navia and Price, 1987).

Positive CSF findings offer little diagnostic and prognostic assistance, since their significance has not yet been determined (Navia and Price, 1987; Price et al., 1987). Computed tomography (CT) and magnetic resonance imaging (MRI) remain the most sensitive tools. Both reveal cerebral atrophy, with enlargement of the ventricles and/or sulci, even early in the disease (Price et al., 1987).

HIV is also the etiological agent in aseptic meningitis associated with a disease, AIDS dementia, that may occur at the time of seroconversion. Other neurological disorders frequently associated with HIV include peripheral neuropathies and vascular myelopathy (Britton and Miller, 1984; Helweg-Larsen et al., 1986; Snider et al., 1983). Thus, HIV is neurotropic and may enter the CNS early in the course of the infection. Neurological disease may be the only clinical manifestation of HIV infection (Navia et al., 1986a, 1986b; Navia and Price, 1987).

Further evidence that HIV virus directly affects the brain and may cause neurological disease early in the course of infection is demonstrated by the following findings: Intrathecal synthesis of antibodies to HIV has been seen in asymptomatic seropositive persons (Goudsmit et al., 1986); HIV has been isolated from the CSF of patients with HIV-associated lymphadenopathy without neurological symptoms (Hollander and Levy, 1987); changes in CSF have been detected early in infection (McArthur et al., 1987); abnormalities have been seen early in infection on brain CT scan, MRI (Levy et al., 1986; Sze et al., 1987), and EEGs (Smith et al., 1988); and the nature of the neuropathological findings in the white matter and subcortical structures suggests a chronic, insidious process (Cummings and Benson, 1984; De La Monte et al., 1987; Navia et al., 1986a, 1986b; Navia and Price, 1987).

Marotta and Perry (1989) reviewed all the studies so far published regarding the early neuropsychological dysfunction caused by HIV. Several studies find that patients with AIDS and ARC who do not have opportunistic infections or tumor within the CNS nevertheless have abnormal neuropsychological tests that suggest cortical or subcortical impairment. Systematic studies comparing asymptomatic seropositive and seronegative HIV subjects have reported neuropsychological deficits in those subjects with positive HIV (Marotta and Perry, 1989; Perry et al., 1989). Recently, Borenstein et al. (1992) reported that a small subgroup of HIV asymptomatic patients showed mild neurological impairments that may influence their daily lives. However, other studies have not found differences between these two groups of subjects (Marotta and Perry, 1989).

AIDS-related psychopathology can be nonorganic (reactive) and/or organic (Vomvooras, 1989). As described above, organic psychopathology includes psychiatric manifestations secondary to malignancies, opportunistic infections, metabolic derangements of the CNS, and/or the primary encephalopathic action of HIV. Reactive psychopathology includes stress shock, guilt, denial, fear, anger, sadness, bargaining, and resignation (Deuchar, 1984). These symptoms are similar to those described in other terminal illnesses. Holland and Tross (1985) found the most common psychiatric symptoms in patients with AIDS to be anxiety ("uncertainty about disease and treatment; anxiety about any new physical symptom") and depression (sadness, hopelessness, anticipatory grief, suicidal ideation). Most of the diagnoses found in AIDS patients were adjustment disorders and major depression.

AIDS-related psychopathology is modified and complicated by behavioral and psychological factors that characterize the individual's premorbid level of functioning by the previous personality and by the presence or lack of social support systems, including acceptance or rejection by friends and family (Vomvooras, 1989). Because the disease strikes primarily homosexual men and intravenous drug abusers, it often compounds previous social alienation and stigmatization (Vomvooras, 1989).

Appropriate psychiatric assessment must consider the presence of underlying psychopathology, such as personality disorders and affective disorders, frequently associated with substance abuse (Bukstein et al., 1989). Long-term drug or alcohol abuse may contribute to the development of independent organic mental disorders (Buckstein et al., 1989). Superimposed psychological symptoms and maladaptive reactions, when combined with the distress of the diagnosis of AIDS (Holland and Tross, 1985) and with prior psychopathology, are more likely to result in severe psychiatric illness.

AIDS IN CHILDREN AND ADOLESCENTS

Approximately 2% of the AIDS cases so far reported to the CDC (March, 1993) are children and adolescents under 18 years, and 64% of these are younger than 5 years. A mortality rate of 65% has been reported in those children who have developed opportunistic infections. Children who have a history of a risk factor associated with AIDS, isolation of AIDS virus, or detection of the antibody to the virus and laboratory evidence of immunodeficiency probably number two to three times those reported to the CDC. The percentage of those who will ultimately develop CDC-defined AIDS is unknown.

Most of the children are infected by transplacental exposure (approximately 80%), the rest through blood products, sexual contact, or sexual abuse. Sixty-five percent of babies of infected mothers may develop the disease (CDC, 1986b). The triad of chronic interstitial pneumonitis, hepatosplenomegaly, and failure to thrive is present in almost all these cases. Clinical abnormalities are often present by age 3 months, and many of these infants die within 2–4 years (Shannon and Ammann, 1985).

Almost all children diagnosed as having AIDS had multiple symptoms before and at the time of the diagnosis. Patients present with fever, diarrhea, malaise, weight loss, recurrent or chronic infections (including those by opportunistic organisms), lymphadenopathy, hepatosplenomegaly, chronic parotitis, lymphoid interstitial pneumonitis, fever, failure to thrive, hypertonicity, and irritability (Belman et al., 1985; Epstein et al., 1985; Minkoff et al., 1987; Pahwa et al., 1986; Shannon and Ammann, 1985). Approximately 50% of the children develop progressive loss of developmental milestones (in the younger child) and loss of higher cortical function (in the older child) (CDC, 1986b). All subjects have shown evidence of impaired brain growth, sometimes accompanied by distinct secondary microcephaly occurring as a consequence of CNS infection.

Congenital HIV in children is associated with microcephaly and neurological dysfunction in children (Belman et al., 1985; Epstein et al.,

1987). Static or progressive encephalopathy occurs in at least 75% of children with HIV infection. The presence of antigens in the CSF may be correlated with a progressive course (Epstein et al., 1987). The most common clinical manifestations of HIV involvement of the CNS in children include microcephaly, cognitive deficits, weakness associated with diparesis or quadriparesis, hypotonia or hypertonia, developmental delay, and loss of milestones (Belman et al., 1985; Epstein et al., 1985). The course can be static or progressive. In some patients, deterioration occurs in a stepwise fashion, interrupted by plateaus (Belman et al., 1985). The CT scan frequently shows prominent basal ganglia calcifications, white matter abnormalities, and atrophy (Belman et al., 1985). The pathological features are otherwise similar to those found in adults with subacute HIV encephalitis.

Besides the above medical and neurological complications, children and adolescents with AIDS may be at risk for emotional problems because of parents' psychiatric problems, parents' history of drug abuse, the active presence of AIDS in the parents, or parental death (Belfer et al., 1988). The clinical picture is often even more complicated because the population more likely to be infected with HIV is also likely to be affected by other disadvantageous psychological, economic, and sociocultural conditions (Belfer et al., 1988).

Slow Virus Infections

Slow virus infections of the CNS may be classified into those caused by unconventional agents (kuru, Jakob-Creutzfeldt disease) and those caused by conventional agents (subacute sclerosing panencephalitis (SSPE) due to measles virus, progressive rubeola encephalitis, progressive multifocal leukoencephalitis (herpes simplex)). Characteristically, slow viruses multiply in the host for prolonged periods without producing clinical symptoms. These viruses are not recognized as "foreign" by the host, and the immune response is either very late or absent. Therefore, the disease produced by a slow virus may be the result of either gradual destruction or an autoimmune response caused by termination of tolerance (Menkes, 1990). All of these infections are characterized by progressive dementia and neurological symptoms such as ataxia, involuntary movements, and seizures.

SSPE is more likely to occur in children who had measles early in childhood. Its incidence ranges from 0.475 per million in urban populations to 1.4–1.8 per million in rural or suburban areas. It affects more boys than girls, in a ratio of 5:1.

Initial symptoms appear after a latency period of 4–15 years and are manifested by personality changes and deterioration in school performance, followed by myoclonic seizures, involuntary movements, dementia, and ataxia. The alterations within the brain consist of subacute encephalitis that is accompanied by demyelinization lesions that generally involve the cerebral cortex, hippocampus, thalamus, brainstem, and cerebellar cortex. Characteristic EEG abnormalities may be seen as early as 4 years prior to the clinical appearance of myoclonus and are manifested by generalized paroxysmal bursts of high activity, with spike discharges followed by a short period of flattened activity-suppression burst pattern (Evans, 1987; Menkes, 1990).

Rubella panencephalitis has been described in children with congenital rubella. It has an earlier onset than SSPE but has similar clinical features. Children with immunological disorders may develop chronic enteroviral encephalitis or progressive multifocal leukoencephalitis, manifested also by dementia and movement disorders.

Kuru is a progressive degenerative disease of the CNS with predominantly cerebellar features; it is limited to a population in New Guinea that, until recently, practiced cannibalism (Evans, 1987; Menkes, 1990).

Granulomatous Meningitis

TUBERCULOUS MENINGITIS

In children, tuberculous meningitis usually occurs within 3–6 months of primary pulmonary tuberculosis (TB) from hematogenous spread dur-

ing the miliary phase. The clinical picture is similar to that of bacterial meningitis, and the course of the disease may be fulminant or slowly progressive. The granulomatous reaction is more intense in the basal subarachnoid space. Progressive strokes, cranial nerve palsies, and communicating hydrocephalus are the major pathogenic mechanisms of the neurological disease. If untreated, tuberculous meningitis is fatal; even with appropriate antituberculosis treatment, the mortality is 20%, and morbidity is between 20 and 30% (Evans, 1987; Menkes, 1990).

Intellectual deficits occur in about 20% of the survivors of tuberculous meningitis. These patients have a high incidence of EEG abnormalities, which correlate with the persistence of sequelae such as convulsions and mental retardation. The most important prognostic factor is the stage of the disease when therapy is started. Children younger than 3 years old have a poorer prognosis for survival than do older children (Lorber, 1961; Sumaya, 1975).

FUNGAL MENINGITIS

Several fungi are capable of producing neurological disease (*Cryptococcus, Histoplasma, Candida, Actinomyces,* etc.) Fungal infections may present first as a primary pulmonary infection, with hematogeneous spread to the CNS similar to what occurs in TB. Often this is associated with disseminated disease of many organs. Most common fungal infections are associated with an immunocompromised host in which an old infection is reactivated or an unusual organism causes opportunistic infection. The clinical presentation of CNS fungal infections consists most commonly of chronic meningitis and focal infections of the brain. Rarely, fulminant meningitis occurs, particularly in the immunosuppressed child (Evans, 1987; Menkes, 1990).

Spirochetal Meningitis

SYPHILIS

Syphilis is caused by the spirochete *Treponema pallidum*, and the infection is usually classified as primary, secondary, latent, or tertiary syphilis. Children may get the infection through sexual contact or abuse but are infected most often by transplacental inoculation from the mother. If the mother has primary or secondary syphilis during the pregnancy, stillbirth or fetal death usually occurs. If the mother has latent or tertiary syphilis, the fetus may survive and develop congenital syphilis. Of the children of syphilitic parents, 25–80% develop syphilis. The manifestations of congenital syphilis can be divided into: (a) early manifestations, which appear within the first 2 months of life, often between 2 and 10 weeks of age, are infectious, and resemble secondary syphilis of the adult; (b) late manifestations, which appear after 2 years and are noninfectious; and (c) the residual cases of congenital syphilis.

The earliest sign of congenital syphilis is usually rhinitis ("snuffles"), which is soon followed by mucocutaneous lesions, osteochondritis and osteitis (particularly involving the metaphyses of long bones), hepatosplenomegaly, jaundice, and anemia. Later, it manifests by interstitial keratitis, chorioretinitis, bilateral knee effusions (Clutton's joints), and neurosyphilis. Symptoms of neurosyphilis occur in 2–16% of those infected and may develop into tertiary or neurovascular syphilis anywhere from 5 to 15 years after birth, which manifests in diverse vascular syndromes because of arteritis and thrombosis of cerebral vessels. Residual cases of congenital syphilis may be manifested by one or more of the following stigmata: defective teeth (mulberry molars centrally notched, widely spaced, peg-shaped upper central incisors), abnormal facies (frontal bossing, saddle nose, and a poorly developed maxilla), anterior tibial bowing (saber shins), rhagades (linear scars at the angles of the mouth, nose, or anus), nerve deafness, long-standing chorioretinitis, optic atrophy, and corneal opacities.

Mental retardation and nonspecific behavior disorders are more common in subjects with congenital syphilis than in the general population. However, it seems that this is not due only to the infection but to other hereditary and environmental factors as well.

As stated before, neurosyphilis is a late complication, and although rare in children, it should be considered in any child with a degenerative neurological disease. It has four major clinical presentations: meningovascular, tabes dorsalis, general paresis, and focal neurological symptoms secondary to gumma formation.

Meningovascular syphilis presents as a chronic meningitis without fever, recurrent cerebrovascular disease, and dementia. General paresis denotes a dementia associated with predominantly psychiatric disturbances ranging from organic personality changes to florid psychosis and dementia. Tabes dorsalis, rare in children, may be manifested as failing vision, urinary incontinence mainly during the night, and, in 50% of cases, cranial palsies. Lightning pains, ataxia, and arthropathies are rare in childhood and adolescence. Gumma formation is rare at any age but can present as a space-occupying mass, with the associated neurological and neuropsychiatric complications ensuing therefrom (Evans, 1987; Menkes, 1990).

OTHER SPIROCHETAL CENTRAL NERVOUS SYSTEM INFECTIONS

Leptospirosis and Lyme disease are produced by spirochetes and may manifest as acute meningitis or encephalitis with delirium. Lyme disease may also cause postinfectious complications including irritability, anxiety, and mood and memory disturbances that may be misdiagnosed as primary psychiatric disease (Evans, 1987; Menkes, 1990).

Congenital Infections of the Central Nervous System

Infections of the fetal CNS may cause significant damage and multiple defects. The extent and type of induction of congenital anomalies in the infected embryo depends on the time of action of the teratogen. After the second trimester, congenital malformations pursuant to congenital infections become increasingly uncommon. The main pathway of transmission of infection to the fetus is the transplacental route. Most of these congenital infections remain subclinical during the neonatal period (Menkes, 1990; Starr et al., 1970).

RUBELLA

The frequency of congenital rubella after maternal infection with rash is more than 80% during the first 12 weeks of pregnancy, 54% at 13–14 weeks, and 25% at the end of the second trimester. When the CNS is involved during prenatal life, congenital malformations including microcephaly, hydrocephalus, and spina bifida may develop but may not be recognized until delayed motor development or speech retardation becomes obvious. Retarded language development may be due to peripheral hearing loss, focal CNS damage, or mental retardation. Most long-term survivors are deaf and have cataracts and chorioretinopathy. Severe mental retardation may occur in 24%, and spasticity is frequent, but most patients who have sustained severe neurological damage die during the early years of life. Among the survivors, some children develop limitations of language, cognition, and social relatedness similar to those found in autistic children (Chess, 1977; Desmond et al., 1969; Evans, 1987).

CYTOMEGALOVIRUS

Cytomegalovirus (CMV) infection of the fetus is typically manifested at birth by persistent jaundice, hepatosplenomegaly, thrombocytopenia, anemia, and neurological abnormalities. CMV frequently reaches the developing fetus when the mother is infected and may have important CNS sequelae. It has become clear that the majority of newborns with CMV infections are asymptomatic at birth and remain so throughout infancy. However, Hanshaw et al. (1976) found that 10% of infected neonates had delayed psychomotor development and observed that impaired hearing may increase the number of those at subsequent neuropsychiatric risk. Reynolds et al. (1974) followed 18 asymptomatic CMV-infected children for 38 months and compared them blindly through IQ tests with normal control subjects. The mean IQ was 92 for the CMV

carriers (7 had IQs less than 90 and 1 less than 32) and 100 for the control subjects. Hanshaw et al. (1976) followed 44 asymptomatic children with positive CMV titers in blood and compared them with a similar group of control subjects and a random sample of normal siblings. The children had psychometrics, school evaluations, and physical examinations at the ages of 3.5–7 years. The CMV group mean IQ was significantly lower, and they experienced failure at school 2.7 times more frequently than the matched control subjects and 8 times more frequently than the randomly selected siblings. Bilateral hearing loss was present in 1% of the CMV group. All children with IQs below 80 were positive for CMV and belonged to a low socioeconomic class. There was no school failure among the CMV-positive children of higher socioeconomic status. The authors concluded that a child born with serologic evidence of congenital cytomegalovirus infection is at higher risk for school failure if he or she is born into a family of a lower socioeconomic group.

TOXOPLASMOSIS

Toxoplasmosis is caused by the protozoan *Toxoplasma gondii*, which is infectious to a wide range of birds and mammals. Pregnant women may acquire the infection by ingestion of oocyst in uncooked meat or from cat feces. As in the case for other congenital infections, chorioretinitis and neurological symptoms may not be present at birth but may appear late in infancy or childhood. Rarely, toxoplasmosis may be responsible for seizures or psychomotor retardation. However, a 4-year follow-up of toxoplasmosis-infected children with apparent neurological disease in infancy disclosed mental retardation in 89% and seizures in 83% of the cases (Menkes, 1990). Saxon et al. (1973) followed 8 children ages 2–4 who were identified at birth as having subclinical congenital toxoplasmosis and compared them blindly with 8 normal children. There was no difference in assessments of behavior or motor development. The mean IQ for the untreated cases was 93, whereas for the control subjects and three children who were treated for toxoplasmosis, the mean IQ was 110.

Treatment

A detailed description of the treatment of CNS infectious diseases is beyond the scope of this chapter. Briefly noted, the therapy depends on the child's age and the pathogen (Evans, 1987; Klein et al., 1986; Menkes, 1990). For bacterial meningitis of unknown etiology in newborns, a penicillin, usually ampicillin, and an aminoglycoside, such as gentamicin, are recommended. For children older than 1 month, the combination of ampicillin and chloramphenicol has been used, and recently fourth-generation cephalosporins have been advocated as a single treatment in initial management until culture sensitivities are obtained. TB meningitis is treated with isoniazid and, at the beginning of the infection, also with rifampicin and streptomycin. Fungal infections are generally treated with amphotericin B or sulfonamides in the case of *Nocardia* infection, and penicillin for actinomycosis. Syphilis is treated with penicillin, and rickettsial infections with tetracyclines or chloramphenicol. Acyclovir has been shown to reduce the mortality and serious morbidity of herpes encephalitis if instituted early in the course of the disease (Evans, 1987; Menkes, 1990). Some reports suggest that zidovudine (AZT) may reverse or delay the development of HIV-caused mental changes (Schmitt et al., 1988; Yachoan et al., 1987), and children with AIDS dementia have shown recovery of motor skills and IQ levels after continuous infusions of AZT (Brouwers et al., 1990; DeCarli et al., 1991; McKinney et al., 1991).

Aside from pharmacotherapy for the infectious pathogen, children must be carefully evaluated for the development of neuropsychiatric complications of these CNS infections in order to implement prompt remedial treatment and appropriate school placement. As was shown by several studies reviewed above, the prognosis depends not only on the illness per se but also on associated hereditary and environmental factors.

In the acute phase of treatment, children and their families may require supportive psychiatric intervention to help them deal with the traumatic experiences of being admitted to the hospital with a CNS infection, invasive procedures, and sometimes confusion and delirium (see Chapter 28).

Children with chronic neuropsychiatric residua of CNS infections and their families need frequent reassurance and support from both primary treating physicians and mental health professionals familiar with chronic diseases. As discussed above, children with mental retardation or brain injury require psychiatric follow-up because it has been shown that these children are at higher risk of developing a variety of psychiatric disorders (Rutter et al., 1970: Shaffer, 1985).

Patients with AIDS and their families need special support in order to cope with the initial crisis induced by the knowledge that the child is suffering from an illness with a fatal outcome. Mental health workers need to help them cope with maladaptive behaviors, such as suicidal inclinations, and need to support and counsel them for the additional stress created by discrimination emanating from families, caregivers, friends, and even health professionals. Mental health workers should follow up patients for the development of any psychiatric disturbances and should help families to cope with anticipatory guilt and retrospective guilt after the death of the child. A multidisciplinary team approach should be used to help children who already come from families with social and psychiatric problems and in which often several members suffer or have already died from AIDS (Adler, 1987).

Conclusions

Children may develop permanent neuropsychiatric sequelae as a result of diverse congenital and acquired CNS infections. Children who were infected at an early age, did not receive prompt or appropriate treatment, were infected by certain virulent pathogens, or had focal seizures or residual neurological deficits are at risk of remaining with greater degrees of mental retardation, school failure, and nonspecific behavior problems. This is especially so if they are from lower socioeconomic backgrounds, have independently inherited a predisposition for low-level intellectual functioning, or have a previous history of psychiatric disorder.

The neuropsychiatric problems emerging after CNS infections have not yet been adequately studied. Emerging emotional problems may be secondary to the CNS injury itself but may also involve mental retardation, deafness, language disorders, environmental or hereditary factors, or a combination of these.

A multidisciplinary professional approach is recommended for the follow-up, remediation, and prevention of CNS infections and their neuropsychiatric complications.

TRAUMATIC BRAIN INJURY

Trauma is the leading cause of death in the young, and head injuries account for a large proportion of these deaths. The spectrum of head injury, however, ranges from minor scalp laceration to devastating brain injury resulting in permanent and severe neurological disability. The initial evaluation and treatment of patients who have sustained head injury is clearly the neurologist's responsibility. Yet a significant proportion of these patients experience subtle or substantial neuropsychological and/or neuropsychiatric deficits that may bring them to psychiatric attention. Some of these deficits will be phenomenologically quite similar to the features of static encephalopathy described for cerebral palsy (see Chapter 59). Yet there are some special considerations that merit separate discussion here. Of particular note, many traumatic brain injuries, in contrast to most neuropsychiatric disorders, are potentially preventable. This is discussed below.

Epidemiology

Trauma is the leading cause of death in persons younger than 35 in the United States, with motor vehicle accidents being the most common cause of this trauma (Silver et al., 1992).

Because the term *head injury* is used to describe patients with a wide range of severity and type of injury, statistics in this area vary greatly among reported studies. The National Head and Spinal Cord Injury Survey recently estimated the rate of occurrence of new cases of head injury (defined as an injury to the head severe enough to require hospitalization) as 200 per 100,000 population per year (Kalsbeeck et al., 1980). Head injury was found to occur most often in the 15- to 24-year-old age group, and to occur twice as often in males as in females.

Children are highly vulnerable to motor vehicle accidents (as passengers and as pedestrians), to falls, to being struck by moving objects, and to sports injuries. It has been estimated that as many as 5 million children sustain head injuries each year; of this group, 200,000 children are hospitalized (Raphael et al., 1980). Almost one-sixth of all pediatric hospital admissions in one series was for observation and treatment of head injury, making this the most frequent reason for pediatric hospital admissions. Prolonged hospitalization is required for 15,000 children per year, with 2–5% of these remaining severely handicapped. Four thousand children per year die as a result of head trauma.

Etiology

Although traumatic brain injury may arise from many causes, the neuropsychiatric consequences relate primarily to the site, extent, and type of injury to the brain. A direct blow to the skull, as during battery, a fall, or a vehicular accident, may injure practically any portion of the brain. Shearing forces caused by deceleration in automobile accidents frequently result in injury to the frontal or temporal lobes. Falls may produce acute or chronic subdural hematomas, often without indications of an initial focal neurological deficit. Gunshot wounds and other penetrating injuries frequently cause both focal damage and residual epileptiform irritability. Detailed discussions of the pathology, pathophysiology, neurological evaluation, and treatment of traumatic brain injuries may be found in Dacey and Jane (1988).

Implicitly, the issue of risk-taking behavior as an etiological contributor to traumatic brain injury among children and adolescents is an important consideration. In this regard, a number of studies (Rimel et al., 1982) point to the elevated incidence of documented alcohol-use, preexisting cognitive deficits, preexisting deviant behavior, and diminished parental emotional stability among youngsters suffering traumatic brain injury.

Clinical Features

With the exception of those patients seen in liaison consultation in the acute phases of recovery from traumatic brain injury, where considerations of delirium may apply (see Chapter 28), most such patients seen by psychiatrists have been neurologically stabilized. In such circumstances, pertinent neuropsychiatric considerations may include those subsumed under the headings of either static encephalopathy, where focal brain injury has ensued, or epilepsy, if it has developed as a sequela of brain injury. These are discussed in Chapter 59. Some additional considerations are outlined below.

Postconcussional Syndrome

This refers to a constellation of somatic and psychological symptoms, including headache, dizziness, fatigue, diminished concentration, memory deficit, irritability, anxiety, insomnia, hypochondriacal concern, hypersensitivity to noise, and photophobia (Levin et al., 1982). Implicit in the term *postconcussional*, these symptoms are frequently reported in patients with brief periods of coma or otherwise disturbed consciousness following head trauma.

The concept of concussion as a fully reversible injury with no structural alteration of the brain has been challenged on the basis of several studies using both CT scanning and MRI (Levin et al., 1987a). These studies have demonstrated occult intracranial lesions (cerebral contusions, intracranial hematomas, and subarachnoid hemorrhage) in a significant number of patients designated as having "minor head injury" (initial loss of consciousness of 20 minutes or less).

Further complicating the assessment of minor head injury and the postconcussional syndrome are individual patient variables, including preexisting neuropsychiatric disorder, nonspecific effects of hospitalization after trauma, and secondary emotional factors, including the possible effects of potential litigation. Each of these factors may contribute disproportionately to the apparent sequelae of a head injury, quite apart from actual neurological and neuropsychiatric sequelae.

It seems reasonable to suggest that, when a patient presents after minor head injury with persistent symptoms associated with the postcussional syndrome, a full reassessment addressing the above-enumerated differential diagnostic possibilities should be pursued. In addition to neurological reassessment and a repeat EEG, neuroradiological reassessment is often advisable. Thus, Levin et al. (1987) reported that, of 16 consecutive admissions with minor or moderate closed head injury, 14 had abnormalities on MRI, although their prior CT scans were normal or showed fewer abnormalities. Similarly, an apparent decline in academic performance, emotional responsiveness, or behavioral appropriateness should prompt formal neuropsychological and psychiatric consultation, with the above-outlined considerations in mind. If a patient shows no objective evidence of neurological or cognitive impairment on the various diagnostic parameters enumerated, a supportive psychotherapeutic strategy geared to reassuring both the patient and family regarding a generally favorable prognosis and avoiding the secondary gains of invalidism is most judicious. Advising prompt settlement of any outstanding legal claims is helpful in this regard.

Characteristics of Children Experiencing Head Injury

Children experiencing head injury are not a random sample of the general population (Rutter et al., 1983). Consequently, since most studies showing intellectual impairment and behavioral difficulties following head injury lack a control group, it is impossible to discern to what extent the problems derived from cerebral trauma, from nonneurological consequences of the injury, or from preexisting difficulties that antedated the injury. Studies comparing children who have experienced accidental head injuries with control groups have consistently shown differences in both the children and their families (Brown et al., 1981; Chadwick et al., 1981a, 1981b; Rutter et al., 1970; Shaffer et al., 1975). By studying head-injured children and their families in a retrospective manner immediately after the trauma, a picture of their premorbid functioning unconfounded by the sequelae of the head injury can be elicited. Children with head injuries have tended to be impulsive, aggressive, attention-seeking, and behaviorally disturbed, engendering a greater probability of being in dangerous situations likely to result in accidents. The families of children experiencing accidents also show more parental illness and mental disorder, more social disadvantages of various kinds, and less adequate supervision of children's play activities than is found for the general population (Brown et al., 1981; Chadwick et al., 1981a, 1981b; Rutter et al., 1970; Shaffer et al., 1975). Clearly, these other risk variables must be taken into account in any assessment of the neuropsychiatric sequelae of traumatic head injury.

COGNITIVE SEQUELAE

Several studies have demonstrated a direct correlation between duration of coma and postinjury IQ level (Brink et al., 1970; Levin and Eisenberg, 1979) or between duration of posttraumatic amnesia (PTA) and subsequent intellectual impairment (Brown et al., 1981). The consistent dose-response relationship in these studies provides a strong indication that intellectual deficits seen in children with severe head injuries are indeed due to brain injury. Also of note, however, based on the work of Chadwick et al. (1981a, 1981b), is the finding that substantial intellectual improvement continues in children throughout the 1st year after brain trauma. Smaller relative gains may continue to accrue during the 2nd year, perhaps particularly in those children with the most severe injuries.

Recently, Jaffe et al. (1992) studied 98 children ages 6–15 years old with mild, moderate, and severe closed head injuries and compared them with control subjects matched for age, gender, school grade, and academic performance. In agreement with above studies, Jaffe et al. (1992) found a strong dose-response relationship between the severity of the brain injury and the degree of impairment on almost all neurobehavioral measures. Mildly injured subjects did not differ from the normal controls.

PSYCHIATRIC SEQUELAE

In studies by Brown et al. (1981) and Rutter et al. (1983), a comparison of children with accidental orthopaedic and head injuries who were evaluated immediately after the accident and then reassessed over time was informative. The rate of newly appearing psychiatric disorders was much increased in the severe head injury group, whereas new psychiatric disturbance in the mild head injury group was no different from that seen in the orthopaedic controls. This was true at 4 months, 1 year, and $2\frac{1}{4}$ years after the accident. Mild head injuries' sequelae tend to be transient and resolve within months after the injury (Farmer et al., 1987; Levin et al., 1987a, 1987b). Those children with persistent behavior problems after the head injury usually had pretrauma psychiatric disturbances (Chadwick et al., 1981a; Rutter et al., 1981). They frequently come from broken homes and families with marital disturbances, psychiatric problems, or social disadvantage, or have parents who overreact to the child's head injury (Brown et al., 1981; Casey et al., 1986; Chadwick et al., 1981a, 1981b; Rutter et al., 1981; Shaffer et al., 1981).

A natural point of inquiry here is the *threshold* of injury above which neuropsychiatric sequelae can be found. Chadwick et al. (1981a, 1981b) determined that both cognitive and behavioral sequelae could be identified only with injuries of sufficient severity to give rise to a posttraumatic amnesia of at least 1 week. Also noteworthy in that study, although psychiatric disorder was most frequent among the children showing persistent neurological abnormalities at the $2\frac{1}{4}$-year follow-up, the rate of new psychiatric disorder was still substantially raised in those head trauma children with no demonstrable abnormalities on thorough and systematic neurological examinations, hence the need for clinical sensitivity in considering traumatic head injury as a potential source of psychiatric morbidity, even in the absence of abnormal neurological findings.

Generally, the patterns of psychiatric disorder found in head-injured children are similar to that found in the general population of children coming to a child psychiatrist's attention (Brown et al., 1981). One difference, however, was an increased incidence of socially disinhibited behavior, particularly after severe head injuries. In addition to the problems caused by the injury per se, as with other handicapping conditions, many families and patients with brain injury face a variety of limitations and developmental challenges (e.g., autonomy issues of adolescents) which may induce severe behavioral problems (Bragg et al., 1992).

The question of whether the *locus of brain injury* influences the type of psychiatric symptomatology in childhood was examined by Shaffer et al. (1985) in a study of 98 children with localized head injuries. Although the site of injury was not associated with the overall psychiatric diagnosis, examination of individual symptom clusters disclosed a significant association between depression and lesions in the right frontal and left posterior regions. Several cases of mania have been reported following head injury, especially in those cases with damage in the right hemisphere or limbic system (Robinson et al., 1988; Salle and Kindlon, 1987; Starkstein et al., 1987, 1988). While further studies are needed in this area, it seems reasonable to postulate, as has been suggested by studies involving adult brain injury (Robinson et al., 1988), that psychopathological features in brain-injured patients are likely to be the product of an interaction among the extent and location of brain injury, genetic factors, and other predisposing influences such as preaccident behavior, intellectual level, and socioeconomic status (Brown et al., 1981; Chadwick et al., 1981; Eide and Tysnes, 1992; Rutter et al., 1981; Shaffer et al., 1985).

Recently, MRI and CT have been used to follow up patients with head injury. Wilson et al. (1988) followed 25 patients with closed head injury and found that deep lesions visualized by MRI at the end of 18 months were correlated with poor neuropsychological test performance. Neither CT at the beginning or at the end of the follow-up period nor MRI at the beginning of the follow-up period correlated with the neuropsychological testing.

Kriel et al. (1988) followed 26 children who remained unconscious longer than 90 days after traumatic brain injury. Children with the best recovery (defined as having an IQ greater or equal to 70) were predicted by minimal cerebral atrophy demonstrated by CT performed 2 months after the injury. In subjects over 12 years old, minimal atrophy predicted a good outcome with 89% accuracy.

Treatment

In the absence of controlled studies demonstrating clear-cut efficacy for specific treatment interventions, a broad-based, multidisciplinary approach seems most reasonable, based on accumulated clinical experience to date (Silver et al., 1992). Insofar as the range of child psychopathology encountered in the wake of brain injury is representative of the spectrum of child psychopathology generally, those treatment strategies that would ordinarily apply would still pertain to specific psychopathology encountered in the wake of brain injury. Only a few additional considerations particularly pertinent to the brain-injured child are addressed here.

In the psychopharmacological domain, the greater sensitivity of brain-injured patients to the sedative and anticholinergic effects of various psychotropic medications leads to the advisory of starting with lower doses and raising them in small increments over time. Similarly, because of the greater incidence of disinhibited, impulsive, and aggressive behavior documented in children with brain injury, it is important to avoid indiscriminate use of neuroleptic drugs in such patients, in the absence of documented psychosis (Silver et al., 1992). This is true not only because of potential sedative and anticholinergic side effects and the dangers of tardive dyskinesia but also because neuroleptics may lower the threshold for seizures, to which brain-injured patients are particularly vulnerable (see Chapter 59's section on epilepsy).

Carbamazepine has been used in increasing numbers of pediatric patients with a variety of neuropsychiatric disorders (Evans et al., 1987). There is some anecdotal support for the use of carbamazepine in children with disinhibited aggression, affective lability, and other psychopathological states, in the wake of brain injury (Lewin and Sumners, 1992). This would be particularly justified if the patient's EEG demonstrated epileptiform abnormalities despite the absence of clinical seizures. It should be noted, however, that clinical experience has expanded our awareness of potentially untoward effects of carbamazepine, including the possible worsening of irritability and aggressive behavior, as well as precipitation of mania (Pleak et al., 1988).

There have been a number of reports regarding the potential merits of using β-adrenergic blocking medications for the treatment of uncontrolled aggressive outbursts in patients with organic brain impairment (Connor, 1993; Williams et al., 1982). This can be done in conjunction with or independent of any concomitant anticonvulsant medication. Clinical experience to date, which requires controlled replication, suggests that some patients demonstrate improved behavioral control of aggressivity and irritability after appropriate dose titration. Knowledge of appropriate monitoring and titration procedures is important and easily mastered.

Probably of equal importance to any psychopharmacological intervention are behavioral and psychosocial measures that are widely utilized and of apparent benefit to a significant proportion of brain-injured youngsters, though again the results have not thus far been systematically evaluated. These measures include parental counseling, individual and family education and supportive psychotherapy, speech therapy, associated rehabilitative therapies, and academic tutoring. Also, it has been suggested that it is possible to improve the performance from head injury subjects by slowing down the pace at which information is presented, reducing background distractions or noise, or allowing additional time to complete tasks (Ponsbord and Kinsella, 1992). While systematic studies are undoubtedly desirable in this area, the many clinical variations within the broad spectrum of brain-injured youngsters will continue to require individual tailoring of treatment plans to meet the unique needs of individual patients.

Prevention

Children less than 4 years old who are not restrained in safety seats are 11 times more likely to be killed in motor vehicle accidents (Silver et al., 1992). Conversely, child safety seats have been found to be 80–90% effective in the prevention of serious injuries to children. All 50 states in the United States and the District of Columbia have mandatory laws for child safety seats. Public education to encourage compliance with these laws would contribute to primary prevention of a large proportion of pediatric traumatic brain injuries. More effective public health measures to curb child abuse, alcoholism (especially drunk driving), and preventable accidental injuries would similarly be desirable.

References

Adler MAC: Psychiatric aspects of AIDS. A biopsychosocial approach. In: Wormser GP, Stahl RE, Bottone EJ (eds): *AIDS-Acquired Immunodeficiency Syndrome and Other Manifestations of HIV Infection.* New Jersey, Noyes Publications, 1987.

American Psychiatric Association: *Diagnostic and Statistical Manual of Mental Disorders* (3rd ed, rev). Washington, DC, American Psychiatric Association, 1987.

American Psychiatric Association: *Diagnostic and Statistical Manual of Mental Disorders* (4th ed, rev). Washington, DC, American Psychiatric Association, 1994.

Belfer M, Penelope K, Miller F: AIDS in children and adolescents. *J Am Acad Child Adolesc Psychiatry* 2:147–151, 1988.

Belman AL, Ultman MH, Horoupian D, et al: Neurological complications in infants with acquired immune deficiency syndrome. *Ann Neurol* 18:560–566, 1985.

Bergman I, Painter M, Wald E, et al: Outcome in children with enteroviral meningitis during the first year of life. *J Pediatr* 110:705–709, 1987.

Bornstein RA, Nasrallah HA, Para MF, et al: Neuropsychological performance in asymptomatic HIV infection. *J Neuropsych Clin Neurosci* 4:386–394, 1992.

Bragg RM, Klockars AJ, Berninger VW: Comparison of families with and without adolescents with traumatic brain injury. *J Head Trauma Rehabil* 7:94–108, 1992.

Breslau N: Psychiatric disorder in children with physical disabilities. *J Am Acad Child Psychiatry* 1:87–94, 1985.

Brink JD, Garrett AL, Hale WR, et al: Recovery of motor and intellectual function in children sustaining severe head injuries. *Dev Med Child Neurol* 12:565–571, 1970.

Britton CB, Miller JR: Neurological complications in AIDS. *Neurol Clin* 2:315–339, 1984.

Brouwers P, Moss H, Wolters P, et al: Effect of continuous infusion zidovudine therapy on neuropsychologic functioning in children with symptomatic human immunodeficiency virus infection. *J Pediatr* 4:585–592, 1991.

Brown G, Chadwick O, Shaffer D, et al: A prospective study of children with head injuries. III: Psychiatric sequelae. *Psychol Med* 11:63–78, 1981.

Bukstein O, Brent D, Kaminer Y: Comorbidity of substance abuse and other psychiatric disorders in adolescents. *Am J Psychiatry* 146:1131–1141, 1989.

Casey R, Ludwing S, McCormick MC: Morbidity following minor head trauma in children. *Pediatrics* 78:497–502, 1986.

Centers for Disease Control: *Aseptic Meningitis Surveillance* (Annual Summary). Atlanta, Centers for Disease Control, 1977.

Centers for Disease Control: Bacterial meningitis and meningococcemia in the United States. *MMWR* 28:277, 1979.

Centers for Disease Control: Classification system for human T-lymphotropic virus type III/lymphadenopathy-associated virus infections. *MMWR* 35:334–339, 1986a.

Centers for Disease Control: Update: Acquired immunodeficiency syndrome—United States. *MMWR* 35:17–21, 1986b.

Centers for Disease Control: AIDS information. *Statistical Projections/Trends.* April 21, 1993.

Chadwick O, Rutter M, Brown G, et al: A prospective study of children with head injuries. II: Cognitive sequelae. *Psychol Med* 11:49–61, 1981a.

Chadwick O, Rutter M, Shaffer D, et al: A prospective study of children with head injuries. IV: Specific cognitive deficits. *J Clin Neuropsychol* 3: 101–120, 1981b.

Chess S: A follow-up report of autism in children with congenital rubella. *J Autism Child Schizophr* 7: 69–81, 1977.

Chin K, Fitzhardinge P: Sequelae of early onset group B streptococcal neonatal meningitis. *J Pediatr* 106:819–822, 1985.

Chun RW, Thompson WG, Grabow ID, et al: California arbovirus encephalopathy in children. *Neurology* 18:369–375, 1960.

Coffin I, Haase A, Levy JA, et al: Human immunodeficiency viruses. *Science* 232:697, 1986.

Connor DF: Beta blockers for aggression: A review of pediatric experience. *J Child Adolesc Psychopharmacol* 4:99–114, 1993.

Cummings IL, Benson DF: Subcortical dementia. Review of an emerging concept. *Arch Neurol* 41: 874–879, 1984.

Dacey RG, Jane IA: Craniocerebral trauma. In: Baker AB, Joynt RI (eds): *Clinical Neurology* (Vol 3). Philadelphia, Harper & Row, 1988, pp. 1–61.

De Carli C, Fugate L, Faloon J, et al: Brain growth and cognitive improvement in children with human immunodeficiency virus induced encephalopathy after 6 months of continuous infusion zidovudine therapy. *J Acquir Immune Defic Syndr* 4: 585–592, 1991.

De la Monte WM, Ho DD, Schooley RT, et al: Subacute encephalomyelitis of AIDS and its relation to HTLV-III infection. *Neurology* 37:562–569, 1987.

Desmond M, Montgomery J, Melnick J, et al: Congenital rubella encephalitis: Effects on growth and early development. *Am J Dis Child* 118:30–31, 1969.

Deuchar N: AIDS in New York City with particular reference to the psychosocial aspects. *Br J Psychiatry* 145:612–619, 1984.

Dodge PR, Schartz MN: Bacterial meningitis: A review of selected aspects II. *N Engl J Med* 272: 954–1003, 1965.

Earnets MP, Goolishian HA; Calverley JR, et al: Neurological, intellectual and psychological sequelae follow Western encephalitis. *Neurology* 21: 969–974, 1971.

Edwards MS, Rench MA, Haffar AA, et al: Long term sequelae of group B streptococcal meningitis in infants. *J Pediatr* 106:717–722, 1985.

Eide PK, Tysnes OB: Early and late outcome in head injury patients with radiological evidence of brain damage. *Acta Neurol Scand* 86:194–198, 1992.

Epstein LG, Gouldsmit J, Paul DA, et al: Expression of human immunodeficiency virus in cerebrospinal fluid of children with progressive encephalopathy. *Ann Neurol* 21:397–401, 1987.

Epstein LG, Sharer LR, Joshi VV, et al: Progressive encephalopathy in children with acquired immune deficiency. *Ann Neurol* 17:488–496, 1985.

Evans OB: *Manual of Child Neurology* (1st ed). New York, Churchill Livingstone, 1987, pp. 320–350.

Evans RW, Clay TH, Gualtieri CT: Carbamazepine in pediatric psychiatry. *J Am Acad Child Adolesc Psychiatry* 26:2–8, 1987.

Farmer K, McArthur BA, Clay MM: A follow-up study of 15 cases of neonatal meningoencephalitis due to Coxsackievirus B5. *J Pediatr* 87:568–571, 1975.

Farmer MY, Singer HS, Mellits ED, et al: Neurobehavioral sequelae of minor head injuries in children. *Pediatr Neurosci* 13:304–308, 1987.

Feigin RD, Stechenberg B, Chang W, et al: Prospective evaluation and treatment of *Hemophilus influenzae*. *J Pediatr* 88:542–548, 1976.

Finley KH, Langshore W, Palmer R, et al: Western equine and St. Louis encephalitis: A preliminary report of clinical follow-up study in California. *Neurology (Minn)* 5:233, 1953.

Gabuzda DH, Ho DD, de la Monte SM, et al: Immunohistochemical identification of HTLV-III in brains of patients with AIDS. *Ann Neurol* 20: 289–295, 1986.

Gonda MA, Wong-Stall F, Gallo RC, et al: Sequence homology and morphologic similarity of HTLV-III and Visna virus, a pathogenic lente virus. *Science* 227:173–177, 1985.

Goodman J: AIDS. In: Wyngaarden JB, Smith LH (eds): *Cecil Textbook of Medicine*. Philadelphia, Saunders, 1988, pp. 1799–1808.

Goudsmit J, Wolters EC, Bakker M, et al: Intrathecal synthesis of antibodies to HTLV-III in patients without AIDS or AIDS related complex. *Br Med J* 292:1231–1234, 1986.

Gunderman JR, Stamler R: Neuropsychological residuals, after acute encephalitis. Results of a 7 year follow up study of 21 children. *Clin Pediatr* 12: 228–230, 1973.

Hanshaw J, Scheimer A, Maxley A, et al: School failure and deafness after "silent" congenital cytomegalovirus infection. *N Engl J Med* 295:468–470, 1976.

Helweg-Larsen S, Jakobsen J, Boesen F, et al: Neurological complications of AIDS. *Acta Neurol Scand* 74:467–474, 1986.

Ho DD, Rota TR, Scholley RT, et al: Isolation of HTLV III from CSF and neural tissue of patients with AIDS-related neurological syndromes. In: Gluckman JC, Vilmer E (eds): *Acquired Immunodeficiency Syndrome*. Paris, Elsevier, 1987, pp. 211–219.

Holland IC, Tross S: The psychosocial and neuropsychiatric sequelae of the acquired immunodeficiency syndrome and related disorders. *Ann Intern Med* 103:760–764, 1985.

Hollander HR, Levy IA: Neurological abnormalities and recovery of human immunodeficiency virus from cerebrospinal fluid. *Ann Intern Med* 106: 692–695, 1987.

Jaffe KM, Fay GL, Polissar NL, et al: Severity of pediatric traumatic brain injury and early neurobehavioral outcome: A cohort study. *Arch Phys Med Rehabil* 73:540–547, 1992.

Kalsbreeck WD, McLaurin RL, Harris BS, et al: National head and spinal cord injury survey: Major findings. *J Neurosurg* Nov (Suppl): 519–531, 1980.

Klein J, Feigin R, McCracken GH: Report of the task force on diagnosis and management of meningitis. *Pediatrics* 78:956–982, 1986.

Kriel RL, Krach LE, Sheean M: Pediatric closed head injury: Outcome following prolonged unconsciousness. *Arch Phys Med Rehabil* 69:678–681, 1988.

Levin HS, Eisenberg HM: Neuropsychological outcome of closed head injury in children and adolescents. *Child's Brain* 5:281–292, 1979.

Levin HS, Benton AL, Grossman RG: *Neurobehavioral Consequences of Closed Head Injury*. New York, Oxford University Press, 1982, pp. 181–184.

Levin HS, Gary HE, High WM, et al: Minor head injury and the post concussion syndrome: Methodological issues in outcome studies. In: Levin HS, Grafruan J, Eisenberg HM (eds): *Neurobehavioral Recovery from Head Injury*. New York, Oxford University Press, 1987a, pp. 262–276.

Levin HS, Mattis S, Ruff RM, et al: Neurobehavioral outcome following minor head injury: A three-center study. *J Neurosurg* 147:977–983, 1987b.

Levy RM, Rosenbloom S, Perrett LV: Neuroradiologic findings in AIDS: A review of 200 cases. *AJR* 147:977–983, 1986.

Lewin J, Sumners D: Successful treatment of episodic dyscontrol with carbamazepine. *Br J Psychiatry* 261–2, 1992.

Lorber J: Long term follow up of 100 children who recovered from tuberculous meningitis. *Pediatrics* 28:778–884, 1961.

Marotta R, Perry S: Early, neuropsychological dysfunction caused by human immunodeficiency virus. *J Neuropsychiatry* 1:225–235, 1989.

Matthews CG, Chun RW, Grabow ID, et al: Psychological sequelae in children with California arbovirus encephalitis. *Neurology* 18:1023–1030, 1968.

McArthur IC, Farzadegan H, Cornblatt DR, et al: Cerebrospinal fluid abnormalities in homosexual/bisexual men with and without neuropsychiatric symptoms. Paper presented at the Third International Conference on AIDS, Washington, DC, Abstract No. MP66: 21, 1987.

McKinney RE, Maha MA, Connor EM, et al: A multicenter trail of oral zidovudine in children with advanced human immunodeficiency virus disease. *N Engl J Med* 324:1018–1025, 1991.

Menkes JH: *Textbook of Child Neurology* (3rd ed). Philadelphia, Lea & Febiger, 1990, pp. 316–431.

Minkoff H, Nanda D, Menez R, et al: Pregnancies resulting in infants with acquired immunodeficiency syndrome or AIDS-related complex: Follow-up of mothers, children, and subsequently born siblings. *Obstet Gynecol* 69:288–291, 1987.

Navia BA, Price R: The acquired immunodeficiency syndrome dementia complex as presenting or sole manifestation of human immunodeficiency virus infection. *Arch Neurol* 44:65–69, 1987.

Navia BA, Cho E-S, Petito CK, et al: The AIDS dementia complex. II: Neuropathology. *Ann Neurol* 19:525–535, 1986a.

Navia BA, Jordan BD, Price RW: The AIDS dementia complex. I: Clinical features. *Ann Neurol* 19: 517–524, 1986b.

Pahwa P, Kaplan M, Fikrig S, et al: Spectrum of human T cell lymphotropic virus type III infection in children. *JAMA* 255:2299–2305, 1986.

Perry S, Belsky-Barr D, Barr W, et al: Neuropsychological function in physically asymptomatic, HIV-seropositive men. *J Neuropsychiatry* 1: 296–302, 1989.

Pleak R, Birmaher B, Gavrelescu A, et al: Mania neuropsychiatric excitation following carbamazepine. *J Am Acad Child Adolesc Psychiatry* 27: 500–503, 1988.

Ponsford J, Kinsella G: Attentional deficits following closed head injury. *J Exp Neuropsychol* 14: 822–838, 1992.

Price RW, Navia BA, Pumarola-Sune T, et al: The AIDS dementia complex: Answers and questions. In: Gluckman JC, Vilmer E (eds): *Acquired Immunodeficiency Syndrome*. Paris, Elsevier, 1987, pp. 205–210.

Raphael RL, Swedlow DB, Downes II, et al: Management of severe pediatric head trauma. *Pediatr Clin North Am* 27:715–727, 1980.

Reynolds D, Stangnos S, Stubs G, et al: Inapparent congenital cytomegalovirus infection with elevated cord IGM levels. *N Engl J Med* 290:291–296, 1974.

Rie HE, Hilty MD, Cramblett HG: Intelligence and coordination following California encephalitis. *Am J Dis Child* 125:824–827, 1973.

Rimel RW, Giodani B, Barth JT, et al: Moderate head injury: Completing the clinical spectrum of brain trauma. *Neurosurgery* 11:344–354, 1982.

Robinson RG, Boston ID, Starkstein SE, et al: Comparison of mania and depression after brain injury: Causal factors. *Am J Psychiatry* 145:172–178, 1988.

Rutter M: Psychological sequelae of brain damage in children. *Am J Psychiatry* 138:1533–1544, 1981.

Rutter M, Chadwick O, Shaffer D: Head injury. In: Rutter M (ed): *Developmental Neuropsychiatry*. New York, Guilford, 1983, pp. 83–111.

Rutter M, Graham P, Yule W: *A Neuropsychiatric Study in Childhood* (Clinics in Developmental Medicine 35/36). London, William Heinemann Medical Books/SIMP, 1970.

Sabatino DA, Cramblet HG: Behavior sequelae of California encephalitis virus infection in children. *Dev Med Child Neurol* 10:331–337, 1968.

Salle ND, Kindlon DJ: Lateralized brain injury and behavior problems in children. *J Abnorm Child Psychol* 15:479–491, 1987.

Saxon S, Knight W, Reynolds D, et al: Intellectual deficits in children born with subclinical congenital toxoplasmosis: A preliminary report. *J Pediatr* 82:792–797, 1973.

Schmitt FA, Bigley IW, McKinnis R, et al: Neuropsychological outcome of zidovudine (AZT) treatment of patients with AIDS and AIDS related complex. *N Engl J Med* 319:1573–1578, 1988.

Seidel VP, Chadwick OFD, Rutter M: Psychological disorders in crippled children: A comparative study of children with and without brain damage. *Dev Med Child Neurol* 17:563–573, 1975.

Sell SH: Long term sequelae of bacterial meningitis in children. *Pediatr Infect Dis J* 2:90–93, 1983.

Sell SH, Merril RE, Doyne EO, et al: Long term sequelae of *Hemophilus influenzae* meningitis. *Pediatrics* 49:206–211, 1972a.

Sell SH, Webb WW, Pate JE, et al: Psychological sequelae of bacterial meningitis. Two controlled studies. *Pediatrics* 49:212–221, 1972b.

Sells CJ, Carpenter RL, Ray CG: Sequelae of central nervous system enterovirus infections. *N Engl J Med* 293:1–4, 1975.

Shaffer D: Brain damage. In: Rutter M, Hersov L (eds): *Child and Adolescent Psychiatry: Modern Approaches* (2nd ed). London, Blackwell, 1985, pp. 129–151.

Shaffer D, Chadwick O, Rutter M: Psychiatric outcome of localized head injury to children. In: Porter R, Fitzsimons DW (eds): *Outcome of Severe Damage to the Central Nervous System* (CIBA Foundation Symposium, no. 34). Amsterdam, Elsevier Excerpta Medica, 1975, pp. 191–214.

Shannon K, Ammann A: Acquired immune deficiency syndrome in childhood. *J Pediatr* 106:332–342, 1985.

Shaw GM, Harper HC, Hahn BH, et al: HTLV III infection in brains of children and adults with AIDS encephalopathy. *Science* 227:177–182, 1985.

Silver JM, Yudofsky SC, Hales RE: Neuropsychiatric aspects of traumatic brain injury. In: Hales RE, Yudofsky SC (eds): *The American Psychiatric Press Textbook of Neuropsychiatry* (2nd ed). Washington, DC, American Psychiatric Press, 1992, pp. 363–396.

Smith T, Jacobsen J, Gaub J: Clinical and electrophysiological studies of human immunodeficiency virus—Seropositive men without AIDS. *Ann Neurol* 23:295–297, 1988.

Snider WD, Simpson DM, Nielesen S, et al: Neurological complications of AIDS: Analysis of 50 patients. *Ann Neurol* 14:403–418, 1983.

Starkstein SE, Boston JD, Robinson RG: Mechanisms of mania after brain injury: 12 case reports and review of the literature. *J Nerv Ment Dis* 176:87–100, 1988.

Starkstein SE, Pearlson GD, Boston J, et al: Mania after brain injury: A controlled study of causative factors. *Arch Neurol* 44:1069–1073, 1987.

Starr J, Bart R, Gold E: Inapparent congenital cytomegalovirus infection. *N Engl J Med* 282:1075–1077, 1970.

Sumaya CV: Tuberculous meningitis in children during the isoniazid era. *J Pediatr* 87:43–49, 1975.

Swartz MN, Dodge PR: Bacterial meningitis. A review of selected aspects. I. *N Engl J Med* 272:725–730, 1965.

Sze G, Brant-Zanadski MN, Norman D, et al: The neuroradiology of AIDS. *Semin Roentgenol* 22:42–43, 1987.

Taylor HG, Michaels RH, Mazur PM, et al: Intellectual, neuropsychological and achievement outcomes in children six to eight years after recovery from *Hemophilus influenzae* meningitis. *Pediatrics* 74:198–205, 1984.

Taylor HG, Mills EL, Ciampi A, et al: The sequelae of *Haemophilus influenzae* for school-age children. *N Engl J Med* 323:1657–1663, 1990.

Taylor HG, Schat S, Schneider C: Academic achievement following childhood brain disease: Implications for the concept of learning disabilities. *J Learn Disabil* 25:630–638, 1992.

Tejani A, Dobias B, Sambursky I: Long term prognosis after *Hemophilus influenzae* meningitis: Prospective evaluations. *Dev Med Child Neurol* 24:338–343, 1982.

Vomvooras S: Psychiatric manifestations of AIDS spectrum disorders. *South Med J* 82:352–357, 1989.

Wald E, Bergman I, Taylor HG, et al: Long term outcome of group B streptococcal meningitis. *Pediatrics* 77:217–221, 1986.

Williams D, Mehl R, Yudofsky S, et al: The effect of propranolol on uncontrolled rage outbursts in children and adolescents with organic brain dysfunction. *J Am Acad Child Psychiatry* 21:129–135, 1982.

Wilson JT, Weidman KD, Hadley DM, et al: Early and late magnetic resonance imaging and neuropsychological outcome after head injury. *J Neurol Neurosurg Psychiatry* 51:391–396, 1988.

Yachoan R, Brouwer P, Spitzer AR: Response of human immunodeficiency virus-associated neurological disease to 3'-azio-3'-deoxythymidine. *Lancet* 1:132–135, 1987.

31 TERATOLOGIC AND DEVELOPMENTAL EFFECTS OF PRENATAL DRUG EXPOSURE: ALCOHOL, HEROIN, MARIJUANA, AND COCAINE

Linda C. Mayes, M.D., and Richard H. Granger, M.D.

The study of behavioral teratology has a long-standing tradition beginning as early as Hippocrates' warning about "uterine suffocation" with maternal opiate use (Hans, 1992; Zagon and McLaughlin, 1984) and the Old Testament advice to a pregnant woman to "drink not wine nor any strong drink" (Judg. 13:7, cited in Heath, 1991). These traditional and deep-seated cautions woven into the fabric of each culture's protection and valuing of a pregnancy have also fueled a long-standing scientific tradition—the investigation of the potential physical, acute, and long-term physiologic and immediate and long-term neurodevelopmental effects of prenatal exposure to drugs and other environmental substances. To date, more than 20 agents have been shown to have demonstrated teratogenic and postnatal toxic effects (Levy and Koren, 1992), while for many others, concern persists but data are inconclusive. In many instances, science takes its initial cue from the prevailing public belief and fear about how a given drug or substance affects its adult user and thus how detrimental it may be to the fetus. Because of this, commonly the first reports about the effects of prenatal exposure to a given drug or substance describe far more deleterious and severe outcomes than are true once larger and more heterogeneous samples are examined. That the first probands of any epidemic or new illness are often the most severe, most obvious, and least representative of the natural history of a condition is an observation not limited to behavioral teratology, but nonetheless particularly relevant to considerations of drugs such as alcohol, opiates, or cocaine (Day and Richardson, 1992).

The thalidomide tragedy notwithstanding, in most instances, demonstrated links in humans between prenatal drug exposure and immediate physical, neurological, or later developmental and psychological outcomes are fraught with problems such as determining frequency, dose, and duration of exposure, associated conditions (e.g., poor nutrition, polydrug use, parental stress, and psychiatric illness) that also impact on development, and the developmentally toxic effects of a postnatal substance-abusing environment. Animal models provide some basis for comparison, particularly about physical effects, but are less useful for studies of complex developmental capacities found only in higher order primates and humans (e.g., language, complex problem-solving tasks, and neuropsychological functions such as certain domains of memory) (see Stanton and Spear, 1990, for a comparison of findings in studies of animal models and prenatal cocaine exposure with findings in infants). Also, although there is an increasing literature for each drug about physical and behavioral teratologic effects in the infant and child related to maternal substance abuse during pregnancy (see below; also see Day, 1992; Hans, 1992; Mayes, 1992; Streissguth, 1992; Zuckerman and Frank, 1992), far less systematic information is available about the effects of any one drug on parental or family functioning or the interaction between the effects of prenatal drug exposure on development and the effects of drug abuse on parenting. In the next section, we review what is known about the effects of alcohol, heroin, marijuana, and cocaine on fetal development and later behavior and developmental outcome. Following that overview, we also discuss how substance abuse influences the caregiving environment.

NEUROTOXICOLOGY OF PRENATAL SUBSTANCE ABUSE

More information is available about short- and long-term outcomes of prenatal alcohol, heroin, or marijuana exposure than for cocaine, but it is important to note that abuse of each of these agents is often associated with other factors that contribute to poor fetal health and infant outcome apart from the specific teratologic effects of any one agent. Women who are chronic alcohol, heroin, marijuana, or cocaine abusers often fail to seek prenatal care and are themselves in sufficiently poor health to compromise the growth and well-being of the fetus. Thus, among pregnant women who are substance abusers, associated complications include preterm deliveries and infants who are intrauterine growth retarded or small for gestational age (SGA). The difficulties of caring for preterm or SGA infants are well documented since these infants often have labile states and are difficult to interact with (Watt, 1990; Watt and Strongman, 1985), problems that will likely be compounded if the substance-abusing environment is chaotic and inconsistent. Additionally, substance abuse often defines a postnatal environment that affords a number of serious risks to infants' and children's development. These factors include severe poverty, virtual homelessness, early histories of abuse and neglect, chronic and acute violence, and multigenerational substance abuse with the resulting parental isolation and lack of family support systems.

Prenatal Alcohol Exposure

Studies of the teratologic effects of prenatal alcohol exposure have been ongoing for many years since the initial reports of fetal alcohol syndrome (FAS) (Jones and Smith, 1973; Jones et al., 1973). Alcohol acts as a direct neuroteratogen affecting not only fetal facial morphology and growth but also brain growth, structure, and function through mechanisms not yet elucidated (Goodlett and West, 1992; Schenker et al., 1990). In infancy, FAS is characterized by (a) intrauterine growth retardation with persistent postnatal poor growth in weight and/or height; (b) a pattern of specific minor physical anomalies that include a characteristic facial appearance; and (c) central nervous system deficits including microcephaly, delayed development, hyperactivity, attention deficits, intellectual delays, learning disabilities, and in some cases, seizures (Claren and Smith, 1978; Smith, 1982). The characteristic facial features include microphthalmia, short palpebral fissures, a thin upper lip, midface hypoplasia, and a smooth and/or long philtrum. Children with a history of in utero alcohol exposure who have either the characteristic physical appearance and/or central nervous system dysfunction are given the diagnostic label of having fetal alcohol effects (Claren and Smith, 1978). Even in the absence of FAS, infants born to *alcoholic* mothers show an increased incidence of intellectual impairment, congenital anomalies, and decreased birth weight (Aronson et al., 1985; Day, 1992; Sokol et al., 1980). Partial expression of FAS and the issue of fetal alcohol effects have led to a number of studies relating amount of exposure to the presence or absence of diagnostic criteria and to the severity of the central nervous system manifestations.

In the general population, the syndrome occurs in approximately 1 or 2 live births per 1000, and the incidence of FAS among alcoholic women is between 2.5 and 10% (Sokol et al., 1980). Although in general the more severe effects on physical growth are associated with more severe intellectual impairments (Streissguth, 1992) and heavier alcohol use is associated with more severe physical effects, the relationships are not entirely consistent, and dose-response and duration of exposure questions remain significant issues in the study of prenatal alcohol exposure (Day, 1992; Streissguth et al., 1990). For example, in one study of newborn behavior (Smith et al., 1986), differences in orientation responses on the Brazelton Neonatal Behavioral Assessment Scale (NBAS) were related to differences in the duration of prenatal alcohol exposure, while differences in autonomic regulation were related to both duration and amount of exposure. Others, however, have failed to find similar relations between prenatal alcohol exposure and NBAS performance (e.g., Ernhart et al., 1985).

Hundreds of reports of children with FAS are now available detailing the delayed development in the first 2–3 years of life of children exposed to alcohol prenatally (e.g., Coles et al., 1987; Gusella and Fried, 1984; O'Connor et al., 1986). However, significantly fewer studies describe follow-up findings through school age and adolescence (Streissguth, 1992). Coles and colleagues (1991), studying children at age 70 months who were exposed to alcohol throughout gestation, reported deficits in sequential processing and on some measures of academic skills including reading and mathematics. Streissguth (1976) reported on a 7-year follow-up of 23 children of alcoholic mothers compared with 46 children of nonalcoholic mothers matched for socioeconomic status, age, education, race parity, and marital status. At 7 years of age, children of the alcoholic mothers had significantly lower IQ scores and poorer performance on tests of reading, spelling, and arithmetic, and 44% of the children of alcoholic mothers compared with 9% in the control group had IQ scores in the borderline to retarded range. Significant differences in height, weight, and head circumference were also apparent. In a study of 21 children of alcoholic mothers again compared with a matched control sample, Aronson and colleagues (1985) described significantly greater problems with distractibility, hyperactivity, and short attention spans in the alcohol-exposed group. Similar behavior problems have been described for other cohorts (e.g., Steinhausen et al., 1982), and impairments in concentration and attention, social withdrawal, and conduct problems continue to be described for adolescents and young adults (Streissguth et al., 1991).

Prenatal Opiate Exposure

In contrast to those exposed to alcohol, newborns who have been exposed prenatally to opiates (heroin or methadone) are born passively addicted to the drug and exhibit withdrawal symptoms in the first days to weeks after delivery (Desmond and Wilson, 1975). Numerous studies have now also replicated the finding that prenatal opioid exposure reduces birth weight and head circumference (Finnegan, 1976; Hans, 1992; Jeremy and Hans, 1985; Kaltenbach and Finnegan, 1987; Wilson et al., 1981). Similar findings in animal models that control for exposure to other drugs such as alcohol or tobacco and for poor maternal health support the finding of an opiate effect on fetal growth (Zagon and McLaughlin, 1984). Prenatal exposure to opiates also contributes significantly to an increased incidence of sudden infant death syndrome (SIDS). In some studies, the incidence of SIDS is eight times that reported for non-opiate-exposed infants (Finnegan, 1979; Hans, 1992; Rosen and Johnson, 1988; Wilson et al., 1981).

On neurobehavioral assessments in the newborn period, opiate-exposed infants are more easily aroused and more irritable (Jeremy and Hans, 1985; Marcus and Hans, 1982; Strauss et al., 1976). They exhibit proportionately less quiet compared with active sleep and show increased muscle tone and poor motor control (e.g, tremulousness and jerky movements). Opiate-exposed infants are less often in alert states and are more difficult to bring to an alert state. The dramatic neurobehavioral abnormalities seen in the newborn period generally diminish over the 1st month of life (Jeremy and Hans, 1985) for the majority of infants and are thus assumed to reflect the transitory symptoms of narcotic withdrawal rather than evidence of permanent neurological dysfunction (Hans, 1992).

Past the neonatal period, a number of studies have documented small, and not usually statistically significant, delays in the acquisition of developmental skills as measured by Bayley's Scale of Infant Development (1969; Hans, 1989; Hans and Jeremy, 1984; Rosen and Johnson, 1982; Wilson et al., 1981). However, much more consistent and significant across studies have been the findings of persistent problems in poor motor coordination, high activity level, and poor attention among opiate-exposed infants in the 1st year of life (Hans and Marcus, 1983; Hans et al., 1984). These state and motor regulatory difficulties make it hard for even a well-functioning adult in a relatively nonstressed environment to care for the infant and present significant problems for an opiate-addicted adult experiencing his or her own state and attentional regulatory problems (Hans, 1992).

Follow-up studies through early childhood of opiate-exposed compared with non-opiate-exposed children have continued to report few to no differences in cognitive performance (Kaltenbach and Finnegan, 1987; Strauss et al., 1976; Wilson et al., 1979). However, opiate-exposed school-age children show higher activity levels, are often impulsive with poor self-control, show poor motor coordination, and have more difficulty with tasks requiring focused attention (Olofsson et al., 1983). There is also an increased incidence of attention deficit disorder among opiate-exposed school-age children (Hans, 1992). Most recently, two studies have described altered sex-dimorphic behavior in opiate-exposed males (Sandberg et al., 1990; Ward et al., 1989). Opiate-exposed boys showed more stereotypically feminine behavior than nonexposed boys, but there were no differences between exposed and nonexposed girls. These findings are consistent with similar observations of male rats exposed to opioid drugs in utero (Ward et al., 1983).

Past the years of early childhood, there are few studies of the long-term effects of prenatal opiate exposure, and those available usually lack a nonexposed control group or are not based on a longitudinal design (Hans, 1992). The data from these studies suggest that, by adolescence, opiate-exposed children exhibit an increased incidence of behavior and conduct problems including impulsivity, involvement in criminal activities or in early substance abuse, more antisocial behavior, and increased school dropout (Bauman and Levine, 1986; Sowder and Burt, 1980; Wilson, 1989). It is not altogether clear how much these problems in conduct and impulse regulation are attributable to persistent effects of prenatal opiate exposure and how much they are the consequence of cumulative exposure to the discord and dysfunction often characterizing substance-abusing households.

Prenatal Marijuana Exposure

After alcohol, marijuana is the most commonly abused drug in the United States, and like alcohol, marijuana abuse cuts across different socioeconomic groups and strata. Marijuana, also known an cannabis, is obtained from the flowering tops of the hemp plant from which more than 300 natural compounds including at least 61 different cannabinoids are extracted. Of these, tetrahydrocannabinol (THC), or marijuana, is the most potently psychoactive (Levy and Koren, 1992). THC readily crosses the placenta and, among heavy users, is also concentrated in breast milk (Blackard and Tennes, 1984; Perez-Reyes and Wall, 1982). THC has a strong affinity for lipids and is stored in fatty tissue throughout the body (Kruez and Axelrod, 1973). Thus, a single dose of THC in humans has a half-life of 7 days but may take up to 30 days to be excreted completely and accumulates throughout the body with chronic use (Nahas, 1976).

The rate of women reporting marijuana use during pregnancy varies from 5 to 34% (Zuckerman, 1988). During pregnancy, THC has documented effects in animals and humans on pituitary ovarian function,

prolactin secretion, and uterine contractility (Harclerode, 1980). However, no relation has been documented between marijuana use and length of gestation or birth weight (Fried et al., 1983). It should be noted that birth weight reductions associated with marijuana use have been described by others studying higher risk, lower income families (Hingson et al., 1989) and the results are conflicting (Zuckerman et al., 1989). Marijuana has an indirect effect on fetal oxygenation through the high levels of carbon monoxide found in marijuana smoke (higher than that in cigarette smoke (Wu et al., 1988)), which in turn results in fetal hypoxia. This type of effect may influence fetal growth, particularly in instances of heavy use (Zuckerman and Frank, 1992).

Few physical anomalies have been reported with marijuana exposure (O'Connel and Fried, 1984; Rose et al., 1982), although several studies have suggested a link between prenatal marijuana exposure and features similar to those of FAS (Hingson et al., 1989; Qazi et al., 1982). In one study, the incidence of fetal alcohol-like features was estimated to be five times higher in users of THC. It is quite likely, however, that heavy marijuana users are also abusing alcohol, and thus, the similarity to fetal alcohol effects is more likely to reflect the accompanying alcohol use (Fried et al., 1984). Several neurobehavioral findings in the newborn period point to decreased responsiveness on the Brazelton NBAS, particularly in visual, but not auditory, responsiveness to both animate and inanimate stimulation (Fried, 1980, 1982) and a higher pitched cry (Fried and Makin, 1987). Another characteristic of newborns exposed to heavy maternal THC use are tremors and increased startle in the first 7–14 days of life (Levy and Koren, 1992). Changes in sleep patterns have also been reported including a decrease in the amount of trace alternans quiet sleep (Scher et al., 1988) and lower sleep efficiency and maintenance as measured by sleep EEG by as late as 3 years of age (Day and Richardson, 1991).

Postnatally, marijuana has been identified in the urine of breast-fed infants whose mothers continue to use after delivery (Perez-Reyes and Walls, 1982). However, no acute toxic effects have been identified with this level of passive exposure though a few studies suggest possible developmental effects related to heavy postpartum exposure via breast milk (Zuckerman and Frank, 1992). In one study, marijuana exposure via breast milk in the 1st postpartum month was related to decreased motor development at 1 year, and there appeared to be a dose-related pattern to the level of association between exposure and motor delay (Astley and Little, 1990). Longer term studies of the outcome of prenatal marijuana exposure are few in number. In one study, no association was found between prenatal marijuana use and developmental scores at 12 and 24 months (Fried and Watkinson, 1988). When these children were 4 years of age, heavy prenatal use (more than six joints per week) was associated with lower scores on memory and verbal subscales of standard preschool intelligence tests. These findings pertained in comparison with the scores of children whose mothers had not used marijuana and after controlling for factors such as the home environment (Fried and Watkinson, 1990). A second study (Streissguth et al., 1989) has found no correlation with IQ scores at age 4 years. The paucity of long-term follow-up studies and the few findings make it difficult to conclude whether or not prenatal marijuana exposure has a direct effect on later developmental functions such as memory.

Prenatal Cocaine Exposure

In many inner city populations, nearly 50% of women giving birth report or test positive for cocaine use at the time of delivery (Amaro et al., 1990; Osterloh and Lee, 1989). A recent study of consecutively recruited women in routine prenatal care reported that 17% used cocaine during pregnancy (Frank et al., 1988), and national estimates across all socioeconomic groups suggest that 10–20% of all infants are exposed to cocaine prenatally (Chasnoff et al., 1990). Most often, infants exposed prenatally to cocaine are also exposed to a number of other risk factors that may also contribute to impaired development (Mayes, 1992). These include exposure to other substances of abuse including alcohol and tobacco as well as opiates, marijuana, and amphetamines. Mothers who abuse cocaine often have associated health problems including a higher incidence of HIV-positive titers with or without AIDS-related illnesses, and they have pregnancies more often complicated by preterm delivery and intrauterine growth retardation. Postnatally, infants exposed to cocaine continue to be exposed to ongoing parental substance abuse, they are more often neglected and abused, and they have parents with more frequent depression and higher overall stress and anxiety (Mayes, 1995). Any one of these factors may also influence the development of early attentional and arousal regulatory functions, later language, and potentially overall developmental competency.

An increasing number of studies in both human and animal models has reported potential cocaine-related teratologic effects on the developing fetal brain (Dow-Edwards, 1991; Mayes, 1992; Zuckerman and Frank, 1992). While the reports to date have been essentially inconclusive as to the presence of one or more cocaine-specific effects or to critical issues such as the timing or dose of exposure, there is some evidence that cocaine may have an effect on attention and arousal regulation. Cocaine and crack are CNS stimulants that act through the monoaminergic neurotransmitter systems including dopamine, norepinephrine, and serotonin (5-HT) (Gawin and Ellinwood, 1988; Wise, 1984). The primary CNS action of cocaine occurs at the level of neurotransmitter release, reuptake, and recognition at the synaptic junction. Cocaine blocks the reuptake of dopamine, norepinephrine, and 5-HT by the presynaptic neuron (Swann, 1990), a process that is primarily responsible for the inactivation of neurotransmitters. Blocking reuptake leaves more dopamine, norepinephrine, and 5-HT available within the synaptic space (and thus, in the peripheral blood as well) and results in enhanced activity of these agents in the CNS (Goeders and Smith, 1983) with associated physiologic reactions (e.g., tachycardia and vasoconstriction with hypertension (see Richie and Greene, 1985)) and behaviors (e.g., euphoria and increased motor activity). Within the various dopamine-rich areas of the brain, certain areas of the prefrontal cortex (mesocortical system) are somewhat insensitive to the effects of cocaine on dopamine reuptake, whereas the corpus striatum (nigrostriatal system) is 100% sensitive to the effect (Hadfield and Nugent, 1983). The dopamine-rich nigrostriatal system projects from cell bodies in the substantia nigra to the corpus striatum and innervates the prefrontal cortex, nucleus accumbens, amygdala, and septum (Goeders and Smith, 1983; Shepherd, 1988). Each of these areas is involved in a number of basic neuropsychological functions including arousal and attentional modulation, the regulation of anxiety and other emotional states, and in the reinforcing properties basic to stimulant addiction in adults.

In fetal brain development, dopamine, serotonin, and norepinephrine play critical roles in defining brain structure and neuronal formation by influencing cell proliferation, neural outgrowth, and synaptogenesis (Lauder, 1988; Mattson, 1988). Cocaine readily crosses the placenta as well as the blood-brain barrier, and brain concentrations of cocaine have been reported as high as four times that of peak plasma levels (Farrar and Kearns, 1989). Thus, cocaine may affect the formation and remodeling of brain structures through this effect on the release and metabolism of monoamines. Additionally, cocaine may influence the actual ontogeny of the neurotransmitter systems and thus again modify a number of critical processes in brain development. In prenatally cocaine-exposed animal models, several structures associated with mesocortical dopamine activity, including the cingulate cortex and the ventral tegmental area, as well as the ventral thalamic nucleus, show significant changes in dopaminergic activity compared with that in controls (Dow-Edwards, 1989; Dow-Edwards et al., 1988). Effects on developing monoaminergic neurotransmitter systems have wide-reaching implications, for they may lead to mistimed neurogenesis between the affected and unaffected areas of the brain with resultant changes in synaptic connections (Lauder, 1991). By altering monoaminergic neurotransmitter control of morphogenesis, chronic exposure to cocaine in utero may adversely affect autonomic function, state regulation, and regulation of attention in the developing nervous system.

The effect of cocaine on fetal development may also be expressed through the norepinephrine-related effects of cocaine on vascular tone. These consist of decreased uteroplacental blood flow, severe uteroplacental insufficiency (acute and chronic), maternal hypertension, and fetal vasoconstriction (Moore et al., 1986; Woods et al., 1987), in turn, resulting in a relative state of fetal hypoxia. Moreover, in humans, cocaine use has been associated with spontaneous abortion, premature labor, and abruptions (Bingol et al., 1987; Cherukuri et al., 1988; Lindenberg et al., 1991). The effect of cocaine use on placental blood flow probably contributes to the relation between cocaine and fetal growth (low birth weight and microcephaly) reported now by several investigators (Fulroth et al., 1989; Hadeed and Siegel, 1989; MacGregor et al., 1987; Mayes et al., 1993a; Oro and Dixon, 1987; Ryan et al., 1987). One report showed that crack-exposed infants were 3.6 times more likely to have intrauterine growth retardation than were infants born to non-drug-using women matched for age, socioeconomic status, and alcohol use (Cherukuri et al., 1988). Additionally, because of the effect of cocaine on overall adult nutrition, compliance with prenatal care, and the usual association between cocaine use and use of other drugs such as alcohol, tobacco, and opiates (Amaro et al., 1989; Frank et al., 1988), women using cocaine while pregnant are in an overall poorer state of health, which in turn increases the risk of impaired fetal outcome and fetal growth retardation. Intrauterine growth-retarded, small for gestational age infants show persistent problems with irritability and distractibility well into the 1st year of life (Watt, 1990; Watt and Strongman, 1985). A higher rate of congenital malformations in infants exposed to cocaine has also been reported (Chasnoff et al., 1988; Isenberg et al., 1987; Teske and Trese, 1987), but when various confounding factors are taken into account, only the relation between genitourinary malformations or spontaneous abortions and gestational cocaine remains significant (Lutiger et al., 1991).

Behavioral and cognitive outcome measures beyond the neonatal period in studies of children exposed to cocaine prenatally have, for the most part, utilized general measures of developmental competency (Mayes, in press), and few studies have examined more specific neuropsychological functions such as attention, information processing, or state regulation. On general measures of developmental competency such as the Bayley Scales of Infant Development (1969) that index information processing and indirectly attention, few differences are apparent between cocaine-exposed and non-cocaine-exposed infants (Chasnoff et al., 1992). The developmental profiles of a group of 106 cocaine/alcohol-exposed 24 month olds followed from birth were compared with the performance of 45 toddlers exposed to marijuana and/or alcohol but no cocaine and 77 non-drug-exposed children (Chasnoff et al., 1992). Mothers of infants in the two comparison groups were similar to the cocaine-using mothers on socioeconomic status, age, marital status, and tobacco use during pregnancy. On repeated developmental assessments using the Bayley Scales (1969) at 3, 6, 12, 18, and 24 months, albeit with a high rate of attrition from the original cohort, there were no mean differences in either the mental or motor domains. However, the investigators cautioned that a higher percentage of cocaine-exposed infants scored 2 S.D. below the mean (Chasnoff et al., 1992). Three other investigative groups have reported similar failures to find differences among cocaine-exposed groups on general measures of developmental competency in the 1st, 2nd, and 3rd years of life (e.g., Anisfeld et al., 1991; Arendt et al., 1993; Billman et al., 1991).

Findings such as these have required a reevaluation of earlier concerns about global developmental delay in cocaine-exposed children. Conversely, as more children who were prenatally exposed have been evaluated in a variety of research and clinical contexts, more evidence is beginning to accumulate about impairments in specific functions such as neonatal habituation, attentional or arousal regulation, reactivity to novelty, and conditioned learning (Alessandri et al., 1993; Eisen et al., 1990; Mayes et al., 1993, 1994; Struthers and Hansen, 1992). Although these findings are reported presently in only one or two studies for each function, impairments in these domains would potentially make the normal parenting activities of contingent responsiveness and structuring attention more important for those prenatally cocaine-exposed infants who are more reactive and easily overaroused (Mayes et al., 1994).

In studies of newborns and 3- to 6-month-old cocaine-exposed infants, impairments have been reported in startle responsivity, habituation, recognition memory, and reactivity to novelty. Anday and colleagues (1989) reported that cocaine-exposed newborns were more reactive to reflex-eliciting stimuli as well as to specific auditory stimuli. In the neonatal period, findings of neurobehavioral impairments as measured by the Brazelton Neonatal Behavioral Assessment Scales (NBAS) have been inconsistent. Chasnoff and colleagues (1989) found impairments of orientation, motor, and state regulatory behaviors on the NBAS. In contrast, Coles (1992) reported that NBAS scores for all infants fell within a clinically normal range regardless of cocaine or alcohol exposure, but did not examine the habituation cluster for all infants. Eisen and colleagues (1990), studying neonates who were urine screen positive only for cocaine at birth and whose mothers denied opiate use, and Mayes et al. (1993) found significant deficits in cocaine-exposed infants in habituation performance as assessed by the NBAS. No other aspects of neonatal performance were affected.

Links between the dopaminergic system and attentional mechanisms that are likely to involve the habituation process (Coles and Robbins, 1989) make it plausible to hypothesize that prenatal cocaine exposure could affect the infant's early habituation performance. Struthers and Hansen (1992) reported impaired recognition memory among cocaine or amphetamine-exposed infants compared with a non-drug-exposed group between 7 and 8 months of age. Similarly, Alessandri and colleagues (1993) reported delays in novelty responsiveness and conditioned learning well into the second half of the 1st year of life. Recognition memory tasks rely in part on habituation processes and, while measuring infant responsiveness to novel versus familiar stimuli rather than decrement of attention over time, nevertheless require an integrated capacity to attend selectively to novel information.

Mayes and colleagues (1993) have found that, compared to the non-drug-exposed group, infants exposed prenatally to cocaine are significantly more likely to fail to begin a habituation procedure and significantly more likely to react with irritability early in the procedure. However, the majority of infants reached the habituation criterion, and among those who did not, significant differences emerged between cocaine-exposed and non-cocaine-exposed infants in habituation or in recovery to a novel stimulus. Thus, for at least a subgroup of cocaine-exposed infants, initial reactivity and selectivity toward novel stimuli appears impaired. As a similar finding, in older children it has been reported that, despite no apparent differences on either motor or mental indices on the Bayley Scales (1969), cocaine-exposed 24 month olds appear to have more difficulty attending to several objects at the same time and in structuring an approach to a nonfamiliar task on their own in the context of the developmental assessment (Hawley and Disney, 1992). Longer term follow-up of cocaine-exposed children into school age is necessary in order to explore the implications of impairments in reactivity and attention and state regulation for later learning.

However, as a caveat, it is important to note that establishing cause-effect relations between prenatal cocaine exposure and attentional deficits is problematic given the number of additional variables that might affect vulnerability for such neurodevelopmental outcomes. In addition to a direct effect on developing monoaminergic neurotransmitter systems in fetal brain, prenatal cocaine exposure may potentially affect attentional and state regulation indirectly because of effects on fetal growth, and in humans, cocaine use is usually accompanied by at least alcohol use. Also, continued maternal postnatal use of cocaine affects the child's caregiving environment at two levels, which may contribute to attention regulation. Adults who are under the influence of cocaine are less able to respond adequately to their children at any given time (Bauman and Dougherty, 1983; Mayes, 1995). The effects of cocaine on memory and attention impair the adult's ability to care for a child. More generally, because of the lifestyle adjustments necessary with co-

caine use—including, for example, prostitution, crime, exposure to violence, and the overwhelming power of the addiction—the overall environment for these children is often chaotic, violent, and neglectful (Black and Mayer, 1980; Regan et al., 1982). Specific outcomes in children such as attentional regulation are also influenced by maternal interactive style (Bornstein, 1985; Bornstein and Tamis-LeMonda, 1990; Tamis-LeMonda and Bornstein, 1989). Similarly, the psychological/personality factors that lead an adult to substance abuse may have genetic as well as experiential implications for the fetus. For example, attention deficits or chronic affective disorders in the adult, both of which may be partially medicated by cocaine (Khantzian, 1983; Khantzian and Khantzian, 1984; Rounsaville et al., 1982), are associated with genetic risks for similar disorders in the child, and these disorders, particularly depression, also impinge on the adult's capacity to care adequately for the child (Fendrick et al., 1990; Field, 1995).

Thus, prenatal exposure to alcohol, heroin, marijuana, or cocaine may contribute to specific short- and long-term impairments or vulnerabilities in arousal modulation, activity level, or attentional regulation, which may make it more difficult for an adult to parent the child. Moreover, when that adult is involved in substance abuse, his or her addiction and the associated environmental, psychiatric, and neuropsychological effects may further impair the interactions between the child and parent, as assessed through both indirect measures of the incidence of abuse and neglect and direct observational measures of parenting attitudes and behaviors.

POSTNATAL SUBSTANCE-ABUSING ENVIRONMENT

Each of these presumed effects relating prenatal drug exposure to neurobehavioral and developmental dysfunctions must be viewed in the context of the postnatal substance-abusing environment in which many prenatally drug-exposed children remain. As already alluded to, the postnatal drug-using world carries a number of risks to children's development. These include exposure to extreme, often chronic violence, virtual homelessness, poverty, parental neglect and abuse, and parental depression and associated psychopathology. Each of these factors, in turn, influences the parenting behaviors of adults who are also substance abusers.

Addiction to any substance (or condition) points to personality characteristics, disabilities, or impairments, each of which may have significant implications for an adult's ability to parent a child. Moreover, all substances of abuse alter in varying degree an individual's state of consciousness, memory, affect regulation, and impulse control and may become so addictive that the adult's primary goal is to be able to supply his or her addiction to the exclusion of all else and all others in his or her life. These alterations likely influence markedly at any given moment the adult's capacity to sustain contingent, responsive interactions with an infant and young child. For example, neuropsychological impairments in concentration and memory associated with chronic cocaine abuse (O'Malley et al., 1992) might be expected to influence certain parenting behaviors such as the capacity to sustain an interaction.

There are differences in the behavioral and personality characteristics of substance-abusing adults according to the specific substance of abuse. Systematic studies of psychopathology among substance abusers find, for example, that abuse of cocaine versus opiates is associated with a different spectrum of psychological disorders (Khantzian, 1985). Heroin addicts are generally considered a more psychiatrically deviant group than cocaine abusers (Rounsaville et al., 1991), but there are higher incidences of drug abuse and alcoholism among the relatives of cocaine abusers than among the relatives of heroin addicts (Rounsaville and Luthar, 1992). These factors influence treatment issues according to the specified drug of abuse and probably also affect the adult's parenting capacities. Moreover, abused drugs differ markedly in their psychological and physiological effects on the user, and these effects, in turn, differentially influence the adult's capacity to respond to a child. Agents such as alcohol, marijuana, heroin, or antianxiety drugs such as Valium tend to depress mood, whereas stimulants such as cocaine or amphetamines increase activity and contribute to a sense of euphoria and elation. In either case, the adult's moment-to-moment responsiveness to children's needs is impaired, but in one case the impairment is toward depression and withdrawal and in the other toward unpredictable activity and impulsivity. Although the distinctions are not absolute, because, for example, chronic cocaine abusers often experience depression and alcoholics may be quite agitated, the child's experience will differ depending on whether or not the parent is predominantly withdrawn or unpredictably agitated. Moreover, as cited earlier, for a proportion of substance-abusing adults, the individual's drug of choice may also in part indirectly reflect different preexisting conditions that the drug use may be intended to self-medicate (Khantzian, 1985; Khantzian and Khantzian, 1984). These conditions such as depression or anxiety disorders not only carry potential genetic risks for the child but will also surely influence parenting in the domains of affective availability, capacity to foster the child's independence, and the parent's tolerance for the child's aggression.

The social context of the particular abused substance varies markedly, and these factors also indirectly influence parenting. Alcohol, when abused, poses major health and psychological problems, but it is legally available, and its use is more socially acceptable for women and men than cocaine, heroin, or even marijuana abuse, all of which are illegal. Abuse of cocaine far more often involves the user directly or indirectly in criminal activities such as prostitution, theft, or drug dealing (Boyd and Mieczkowski, 1990) and exposes the user, as well as his or her children, to personal and property violence. Because of these activities, cocaine-abusing adults are more likely to be arrested and incarcerated repeatedly, exposing their children to multiple episodes of parental separation and placements usually with different foster families or with other (often substance-abusing) neighbors or relatives (Lawson and Wilson, 1980). Additionally, substance-abusing parents often report feeling more isolated and lonely with few friends or relatives in their neighborhoods or immediate communities whom they identify as supportive and helpful (Tucker, 1979). Feelings of isolation and self-denigration may reflect both premorbid and postmorbid states related to the adult's substance abuse, but in any case, parents who experience isolation and separateness may be at greater risk for problems in caring for their children, especially when their isolation is compounded by the psychological effects of their addiction. Multiple studies from substance abuse treatment programs also document the high incidence of unemployment and less than a high school education among participating substance-abusing women (Hawley and Disney, 1992). Among this population, the rate of unemployment has been shown as high as 96% (Suffet and Brotman, 1976). The level of violence in substance-abusing families, particularly between women and their spouses or male friends, is markedly high and exposes children to a considerable amount of witnessed violence (Regan et al., 1982). Studies have repeatedly documented the markedly increased occurrence of severe, often multigenerational, impairments in parenting among substance-abusing families as measured by the incidences of physical and sexual abuse, neglect, abandonment, and foster placement (Black and Mayer, 1980; Lawson and Wilson, 1980; Wasserman and Leventhal, 1993). Neglect and out-of-home placement are extremely common among the children of opiate-using adults. In a sample of heroin-exposed children followed through school age (Wilson, 1989), only 12% were living with their biological mother, 60% lived with extended family or friends, and 25% had been adopted. By their first birthday, nearly half (48%) of these children as infants were living away from their biological mothers.

There are surprisingly few direct observational studies of parent-child interactions among substance-abusing mothers and their children, and most of these have involved adults addicted to alcohol or opiates (Mayes, 1995). In 1985, Lief presented a series of clinical descriptions of interactions between mothers in treatment and their infants and toddlers. Described as points for intervention were the impoverished use of language between substance-abusing mothers and their infants, restriction of exploration that was seen as the infant's "getting into things" (Lief, 1985, p. 76), and a diminished responsiveness to the infant's bids for social interaction. Few studies have systematically investigated the interactive behaviors between substance-abusing mothers and their infants. The measures employed have been quite variable both in the amount of interactive detail studied and in the aspects of interaction considered potentially impaired by substance abuse.

Most studies have reported impairments in a number of interactive domains, although these differences have not always been attributed to substance abuse only. Householder (1980, cited in Hans, 1992), reporting on the interactions between opioid-using mothers and their 3-month-old infants, described more physical activity, less emotional involvement with the infant, and less direct gaze toward the infant than non-opioid-using mothers. Opiate-addicted mothers tended either to withdraw completely from the interaction or to be persistently physically intrusive. In a study of 15 mothers in a methadone maintenance clinic compared to 15 non-opiate-addicted women interacting with 2- to 6-year-old children (Bauman and Dougherty, 1983), addicted women were more likely to use a threatening, commanding, or provoking approach to discipline and "to reinforce a disruptive method of attention seeking" (Bauman and Dougherty, 1983, p. 301) in comparison with nonaddicted mothers who relied more on positive reinforcement. The 2- to 6-year-old children of the substance-abusing mothers in that study also were significantly more provocative and complaining with their mothers.

Studies of attachment profiles among prenatally and postnatally substance-exposed children are, to date, few. Goodman (1990, cited in Hans, 1992) studied attachment patterns in 35 methadone-exposed and 46 non-exposed 1-year-old infants. Methadone-exposed infants more often showed disorganized (group D; Main and Solomon, 1986) or mixed insecure attachment patterns. Similarly, Roach and colleagues (1989, 1991), studying 18 13-month-old children prenatally exposed to cocaine, phencyclidine (PCP), heroin, and/or methadone compared with 41 socioeconomic status (SES)-matched preterm children, showed that drug-exposed toddlers were more likely to be insecurely attached to their mothers, whereas most of the non-drug-exposed premature infants were securely attached. In addition, the drug-exposed children showed higher rates of disorganized attachment behaviors. In a similar study of maternal alcohol use (O'Connor et al., 1990, reported in Griffith and Freier, 1992), maternal interactions and maternal prenatal alcohol use significantly predicted infant attachment behaviors at 1 year of age.

Importantly, several studies have emphasized that, although the substance-abusing mothers had apparently more impaired interactions than comparison groups, a number of associated (e.g., comorbid) factors in addition to, or instead of, their substance abuse seemed to predict poor parenting. Jeremy and Bernstein (1984), reporting on the dyadic interactions of a cohort of 17 methadone-maintained women and their 4-month-old infants compared to 23 non-opiate-using mothers (Bernstein et al., 1984, 1986), found that drug use status alone did not significantly predict maternal interactive behavior. Instead, maternal psychological and psychosocial resources, as measured by assessments of maternal IQ and semistructured, diagnostic psychiatric interviews, were more predictive of the quality of the maternal-infant interaction than was drug-use status. Indeed, maternal drug-use when analyzed together with other maternal variables was not a significant predictor of mothers' interactive performance. However, coexisting maternal psychopathology contributes to greater impairments in parenting interactions among substance-abusing adults compared with nonsubstance abusers and with those substance abusers with no coexisting psychiatric disturbance. Hans and colleagues (Hans et al., 1990, reported in Griffith and Freier, 1992) reported that mothers using methadone who were also diagnosed as having antisocial personality disorders were significantly more dysfunctional in their interactions with their 24-month-olds than were methadone-maintained mothers either having no significant psychopathology or affective disorders alone. Moreover, the latter group did not differ in their interactions from drug-free mothers. Findings such as these, albeit from small cohorts, point to the importance of not considering drug use alone as the single determining variable for observed differences in maternal interactive behaviors, but rather as a marker for several predictor variables that are more often associated with substance abuse (Mayes, 1995).

CONCLUSIONS

The field of behavioral and developmental teratology focuses on identifiable effects of prenatal exposure to substances such as alcohol, heroin, marijuana, and cocaine. Children developing amid the violence, substance abuse, poverty, and discord increasingly common in inner city neighborhoods are at risk for dysfunctional development on a number of accounts. While specific syndromes such as that associated with maternal alcoholism during pregnancy have been clearly identified, controversy and conflicting findings still pertain regarding long-term effects of any one of these agents on cognitive and intellectual development. Suggestive findings, particularly with prenatal cocaine exposure, point to impairments in more basic neurodevelopmental domains of arousal and attentional regulation, functions that underlie learning and information processing. However, the postnatal substance-abusing environment, both in its more general factors of poverty, homelessness, and violence and in the specific dysfunctions of parenting that accompany substance abuse, almost certainly exacerbate the effects of prenatal substance exposure.

References

Alessandri SM, Sullivan MW, Imaizumi S, et al: Learning and emotional responsivity in cocaine-exposed infants. *Dev Psychol* 29:989–997, 1993.

Amaro H, Fried LE, Cabral H, et al: Violence during pregnancy and substance use. *Am J Public Health* 80:575–579, 1990.

Amaro H, Zuckerman B, Cabral H: Drug use among adolescent mothers: Profile of risk. *Pediatrics* 84:144–151, 1989.

Anday EK, Cohen ME, Kelley NE, et al: Effect of in utero cocaine exposure on startle and its modification. *Dev Pharmacol Ther* 12:137–145, 1989.

Anisfeld E, Cunningham N, Ferrari L, et al: *Infant development after prenatal cocaine exposure.* Abstract, Society for Research in Child Development, 1991.

Arendt R, Singer L, Minnes S: *Development of cocaine exposed infants.* Abstract, Society for Research in Child Development, 1993.

Aronson M, Kyllerman M, Sabel KG, et al: Children of alcoholic mothers: Developmental, perceptual, and behavioral characteristics as compared to matched controls. *Acta Paediatr Scand* 74:27–35, 1985.

Astley SJ, Little RE: Maternal marijuana use during lactation and infant development at one year. *Neurotoxicol Teratol* 12:161–168, 1990.

Bauman P, Levine SA: The development of children of drug addicts. *Int J Addict* 21:849–863, 1986.

Bauman PS, Dougherty FE: Drug-addicted mothers' parenting and their children's development. *Int J Addict* 18:291–302, 1983.

Bayley N: *Manual for the Bayley Scales of Infant Development.* New York, Psychological Corp., 1969.

Bernstein V, Jeremy RJ, Hans S, et al: A longitudinal study of offspring born to methadone-maintained women. II: Dyadic interaction and infant behavior at four months. *Am J Drug Alcohol Abuse* 10: 161–193, 1984.

Bernstein V, Jeremy RJ, Marcus J: Mother-infant interaction in multiproblem families: Finding those at risk. *J Am Acad Child Adolesc Psychiatry* 25: 631–640, 1986.

Billman D, Nemeth P, Heimler R, et al: Prenatal cocaine exposure: Advanced Bayley Psychomotor Scores. *Clin Res* 39:697A, 1991.

Bingol N, Fuchs M, Diaz V, et al: Teratogenicity of cocaine in humans. *J Pediatr* 110:93–96, 1987.

Black R, Mayer J: Parents with special problems: Alcoholism and opiate addiction. *Child Abuse Negl* 4:45–54, 1980.

Blackard C, Tennes K: Human placental transfer of cannabinoids. *N Engl J Med* 311:797, 1984.

Bornstein MH: How infant and mother jointly contribute to developing cognitive competence in the child. *Proc Natl Acad Sci USA* 85:7470–7473, 1985.

Bornstein MH, Tamis-LeMonda CS: Activities and interactions of mothers and their firstborn infants in the first six months of life: Covariation, stability, continuity, correspondence, and prediction. *Child Dev* 61:1206–1217, 1990.

Boyd CJ, Miecskowski T: Drug use, health, family, and social support in "crack" cocaine users. *Addict Behav* 15:481–485, 1990.

Chasnoff I, Griffith DR, MacGregor S, et al: Temporal patterns of cocaine use in pregnancy. *JAMA* 261:1741–1744, 1989.

Chasnoff IJ, Chisum GM, Kaplan WE: Maternal cocaine use and genitourinary tract malformations. *Teratology* 37:201–204, 1988.

Chasnoff IJ, Griffith DR, Freier C, et al: Cocaine/polydrug use in pregnancy: Two-year follow-up. *Pediatrics* 89:284–289, 1992.

Chasnoff IJ, Landress HJ, Barrett ME: Prevalence of illicit drugs or alcohol abuse during pregnancy and discrepancies in mandatory reporting in Pinellas County, Florida. *N Engl J Med* 322: 102–106, 1990.

Cherukuri R, Minkoff H, Feldman J, et al: A cohort study of alkaloidal cocaine ("crack") in pregnancy. *Obstet Gynecol* 72:147–151, 1988.

Claren SK, Smith DW: The fetal alcohol syndrome. *N Engl J Med* 298:1063–1067, 1978.

Coles BJ, Robbins TW: Effects of 6-hydroxydopamine lesions of the nucleus accumbens septi on performance of a 5-choice serial reaction time task in rats: Implications for theories of selective attention and arousal. *Behav Brain Res* 33:165–179, 1989.

Coles C, Brown R, Smith I, et al: Effects of prenatal alcohol exposure at school age. I: Physical and cognitive development. *Neurotoxicol Teratol* 13: 357–367, 1991.

Coles CD, Platzman KA, Smith I, et al: Effects of cocaine and alcohol use in pregnancy on neonatal growth and neurobehavioral status. *Neurotoxicol Teratol* 14:23–33, 1992.

Coles CD, Smith IE, Lancaster JS, et al: Persistence over the first months of neurobehavioral differences in infants exposed to alcohol prenatally. *Infant Behav Dev* 10:23–37, 1987.

Day NL: Effects of prenatal alcohol exposure. In: Zagon IS, Slotkin TA (eds): *Maternal Substance Abuse and the Developing Nervous System.* Boston, Academic Press, 1992, pp. 27–44.

Day NL, Richardson GA: Prenatal marijuana use: Epidemiology, methodologic issues, and infant outcome. *Clin Perinatol* 18:77, 1991.

Day NL, Richardson GA: Cocaine use and crack babies: Science, the media, and miscommunication. *Neurobehav Toxicol* 16:293–294, 1993.

Desmond MM, Wilson GS: Neonatal abstinence syndrome: Recognition and diagnosis. *Addict Dis* 2: 113–121, 1975.

Dow-Edwards D: Long-term neurochemical and neurobehavioral consequences of cocaine use during pregnancy. *Ann NY Acad Sci* 562:280–289, 1989.

Dow-Edwards D: Cocaine effects on fetal development: A comparison of clinical and animal research findings. *Neurotoxicol Teratol* 13:347–352, 1991.

Dow-Edwards D, Freed LA, Milhorat TH: Stimulation of brain metabolism by perinatal cocaine exposure. *Brain Res* 470:137–141, 1988.

Eisen LN, Field TM, Bandstra ES, et al: Perinatal cocaine effects on neonatal stress behavior and performance on the Brazelton Scale. *Pediatrics* 88: 477–480, 1990.

Farrar HC, Kearns GL: Cocaine: Clinical pharmacology and toxicology. *J Pediatr* 115:665–675, 1989.

Fendrick M, Warner V, Weissman M: Family risk factors, parental depression, and psychopathology in offspring. *Dev Psychol* 26:40–50, 1990.

Field TM: Psychologically depressed parents. In: Bornstein MH (ed): *Handbook of Parenting.* Vol III: *Status and Social Conditions of Parenting.* Hillsdale, NJ, Erlbaum, 1995.

Finnegan LP: Clinical effects of pharmacologic agents on pregnancy, the fetus, and the neonate. *Ann NY Acad Sci* 281:74–89, 1976.

Finnegan LP: In utero opiate dependence and sudden infant death syndrome. *Clin Perinatol* 6: 163–180, 1979.

Frank DA, Zuckerman BS, Amaro H, et al: Cocaine use during pregnancy: Prevalence and correlates. *Pediatrics* 82:888–895, 1988.

Fried PA: Marijuana use by pregnant women: Neurobehavioral effects in neonates. *Drug Alcohol Depend* 6:415–424, 1980.

Fried PA: Marijuana use by pregnant women and effects on offspring: An update. *Neurobehav Toxicol Teratol* 4:451–454, 1982.

Fried PA, Makin JE: Neonatal behavioral correlates of prenatal exposure to marijuana, cigarettes, and alcohol in a low-risk population. *Neurobehav Toxicol Teratol* 9:1–7, 1987.

Fried PA, Watkinson B: 12- and 24-month neurobehavioral follow-up of children prenatally exposed to marijuana, cigarettes, and alcohol. *Neurotoxicol Teratol* 10:305–313, 1988.

Fried PA, Watkinson B: 36- and 48-month neurobehavioral follow-up of children prenatally exposed to marijuana, cigarettes, and alcohol. *J Dev Behav Pediatr* 11:49–58, 1990.

Fried PA, Buckingham M, Von Kulmitz P: Marijuana use during pregnancy and perinatal risk factor. *Am J Obstet Gynecol* 144:922–924, 1983.

Fried PA, Innes KS, Barnes MV: Soft use prior to and during pregnancy: A comparison of samples over a four year period. *Drug Alcohol Depend* 13: 161–176, 1984.

Fulroth R, Phillips B, Durand DJ: Perinatal outcome of infants exposed to cocaine and/or heroin in utero. *Am J Dis Child* 143:905–910, 1989.

Gawin FH, Ellinwood FH: Cocaine and other stimulants. *N Engl J Med* 318:1173–1182, 1988.

Goeders NE, Smith JE: Cortical dopaminergic involvement in cocaine reinforcement. *Science* 221: 773–775, 1983.

Goodlet CR, West JR: Alcohol exposure during brain growth spurt. In: Zagon IS, Slotkin TA (eds): *Maternal Substance Abuse and the Developing Nervous System.* Boston, Academic Press, 1992, pp. 45–75.

Goodman G: Identifying attachment patterns and their antecedents among opioid-exposed 12-month-old infants. Unpublished doctoral dissertation, Northwestern University Medical School, Chicago, Illinois, 1990.

Griffith D, Freier C: Methodological issues in the assessment of the mother-child interactions of substance-abusing women and their children. Natl Inst Drug Abuse Res Monogr 117:228–247, 1992.

Gusella J, Fried P: Effects of maternal social drinking and smoking on offspring at 13 months. Neurobehav Toxicol Teratol 6:13–17, 1984.

Hadeed AJ, Siegel SR: Maternal cocaine use during pregnancy: Effect on the newborn infant. Pediatrics 84:205–210, 1989.

Hadfield MG, Nugent EA: Cocaine: Comparative effect on dopamine uptake in extrapyramidal and limbic systems. Biochem Pharmacol 32:744–746, 1983.

Hans SL: Developmental consequences of prenatal exposure to methadone. Ann NY Acad Sci 562:195–207, 1989.

Hans SL: Maternal opioid use and child development. In: Zagon IS, Slotkin TA (eds): Maternal Substance Abuse and the Developing Nervous System. Boston, Academic Press, 1992, pp. 177–214.

Hans SL, Jeremy RJ: Post-neonatal motoric signs in infants exposed in utero to methadone. Infant Behav Dev 7:158, 1984.

Hans SL, Marcus J: Motor and attentional behavior in infants of methadone maintained women. Natl Inst Drug Abuse Res Monogr 43:287–293, 1983.

Hans SL, Marcus J, Jeremy RJ, et al: Neurobehavioral development of children exposed in utero to opioid drugs. In: Yanai J (ed): Neurobehavioral Teratology. New York, Elsevier, 1984, pp. 249–273.

Harclerode J: The Effect of Marijuana on Reproduction and Development. Monograph No. 31. Bethesda, MD, National Institute on Drug Abuse, 1980.

Hawley TL, Disney ER: Crack's children: The consequences of maternal cocaine abuse. Social Policy Report of the Society for Research in Child Development 6(4):1–22, 1992.

Heath DB: Women and alcohol: Cross-cultural perspectives. J Subst Abuse 3:175–185, 1991.

Hingson R, Alpert JJ, Day N, et al: Effects of maternal drinking and marijuana use on fetal growth and development. Pediatrics 70:539–542, 1989.

Isenberg SJ, Spierer A, Inkelis SH: Ocular signs of cocaine intoxication in neonates. Am J Ophthalmol 103:211–214, 1987.

Jeremy RJ, Bernstein V: Dyads at risk: Methadone-maintained women and their four-month-old infants. Child Dev 55:1141–1154, 1984.

Jeremy RJ, Hans SL: Behavior of neonates exposed in utero to methadone as assessed on the Brazelton scale. Infant Behav Dev 8:323–336, 1985.

Jones KL, Smith DW: Recognition of the fetal alcohol syndrome in early infancy. Lancet 2:999–1001, 1973.

Jones KL, Smith DW, Ulleland CN, et al: Pattern of malformation in the offspring of chronic alcoholic mothers. Lancet 1:1267–1271, 1973.

Kaltenbach K, Leifer B, Finnegan L: Knowledge of child development in drug dependent mothers. Pediatr Res 16:87, 1982.

Khantzian EJ: An extreme case of cocaine dependence and marked improvement with methylphenidate treatment. Am J Psychiatry 140:784–785, 1983.

Khantzian EJ: The self-medication hypothesis of addictive disorders: Focus on heroin and cocaine dependence. Am J Psychiatry 142:1259–1264, 1985.

Khantzian EJ, Khantzian NJ: Cocaine addiction: Is there a psychological predisposition? Psychiatr Ann 14:753–759, 1984.

Kruez D, Axelrod J: Delta-9-tetrahydrocannabinol: Localization in body fat. Science 179:391, 1973.

Lauder JM: Neurotransmitters as morphogens. Prog Brain Res 73:365–387, 1988.

Lauder JM: Neuroteratology of cocaine: Relationship to developing monamine systems. Natl Inst Drug Abuse Res Monogr 114:233–247, 1991.

Lawson M, Wilson G: Parenting among women addicted to narcotics. Child Welfare 59:67–79, 1980.

Levy M, Koren G: Clinical toxicology of the neonate. Semin Perinatol 16:63–75, 1992.

Lief NR: The drug user as parent. Int J Addict 20:63–97, 1985.

Lindenberg CS, Alexander EM, Gendrop SC, et al: A review of the literature on cocaine abuse in pregnancy. Nurs Res 40:69–75, 1991.

MacGregor SN, Keith LG, Chasnoff IJ, et al: Cocaine use during pregnancy: Adverse perinatal outcome. Am J Obstet Gynecol 157:686–690, 1987.

Main M, Solomon J: Discovery of an insecure-disorganized/disoriented attachment pattern. In: Brazelton TB, Yogman M (eds): Affective Development in Infancy. Norwood, NJ, Ablex, 1986.

Marcus J, Hans SL: Electromyographic assessment of neonatal muscle tone. Psychiatr Res 6:31–40, 1982.

Mattson MP: Neurotransmitters in the regulation of neuronal cytoarchitecture. Brain Res Rev 13:179–212, 1988.

Mayes LC: Prenatal cocaine exposure and young children's development. Ann Am Acad Polit Soc Sci 521:11–27, 1992.

Mayes LC: Exposure to cocaine: Behavioral outcomes in preschool aged children. In: Finnegan L (ed): Behaviors of Drug-Exposed Offspring. National Institute on Drug Abuse Technical Symposium, in press.

Mayes LC: Substance abuse and parenting. In: Bornstein MH (ed): The Handbook of Parenting. Hillsdale, NJ, Erlbaum, in press.

Mayes LC, Bornstein M, Chawarska K, et al: Information processing and developmental assessments in three-month-old infants exposed prenatally to cocaine. Pediatrics 95:539–545, 1995.

Mayes LC, Granger RH, Frank MA, et al: Neurobehavioral profiles of infants exposed to cocaine prenatally. Pediatrics 91:778–783, 1993.

Moore TR, Sorg J, Miller L, et al: Hemodynamic effects of intravenous cocaine on the pregnant ewe and fetus. Am J Obstet Gynecol 155:883–888, 1986.

Nahas G: Marijuana: Chemistry, Biochemisty, and Cellular Effects. New York, Springer-Verlag, 1976.

O'Connel CM, Fried PA: An investigation of prenatal cannabis exposure and minor physical anomalies in a low risk population. Neurobehav Toxicol Teratol 6:345–350, 1984.

O'Connor MJ, Brill N, Sigman M: Alcohol use in elderly primips: Relation to infant development. Pediatrics 78:444–450, 1986.

O'Connor MJ, Kasari C, Sigman M: The influence of mother-infant interaction on attachment behavior of infants exposed to alcohol prenatally. Paper presented at the Seventh International Conference on Infant Studies, Montreal, 1990. Cited in Griffith and Frier, 1992.

Oloffson M, Buckley W, Andersen GE, et al: Investigation of 89 children born by drug-dependent mothers: Follow-up 1–19 years after birth. Acta Paediatr Scand 72:407–410, 1983.

O'Malley S, Adamse M, Heaton R, et al: Neuropsychological impairment in chronic cocaine abuse. Am J Drug Alcohol Abuse 18:131–144, 1992.

Oro AS, Dixon SD: Perinatal cocaine and methamphetamine exposure: Maternal and neonatal correlates. J Pediatr 111:571–578, 1987.

Osterloh JD, Lee BL: Urine drug screening in mothers and newborns. Am J Dis Child 143:791–793, 1989.

Perez-Reyes M, Wall ME: Presence of δ^9-tetrahydrocannabinol in human milk. N Engl J Med 307:819–820, 1982.

Qazi QH, Mariano E, Beller E, et al: Is marijuana smoking ferotoxic? Pediatr Res 16:272A, 1982.

Regan D, Leifer B, Finnegan L: Generations at risk: Violence in the lives of pregnant drug abusing women. Pediatr Res 16:91, 1982.

Richie JM, Greene NM: Local anesthetics. In: Gilman AG, Goodman LS, Rall TN, Murad F (eds): The Pharmacologic Basis of Therapeutics (7th ed). New York, Macmillan, 1985, pp. 309–310.

Rodning C, Beckwith L, Howard J: Characteristics of attachment organization and play organization in prenatally drug-exposed toddlers. Dev Psychopathol 1:277–289, 1989.

Rodning C, Beckwith, Howard J: Quality of attachment and home environments in children prenatally exposed to PCP and cocaine. Dev Psychopathol 3:351–366, 1991.

Rose HL, Weiner L, Lee A, et al: Effect of maternal drinking and marijuana use on fetal growth and development. Pediatrics 70:539–546, 1982.

Rosen TS, Johnson HL: Children of methadone-maintained mothers: Follow-up to 18 months of age. J Pediatr 101:192–196, 1982.

Rosen TS, Johnson HL: Drug-addicted mothers, their infants, and SIDS. Ann NY Acad Sci 533:89–95, 1988.

Rounsaville BJ, Luthar SS: Family/genetic studies of cocaine abusers and opioid addicts. In: Kosten TR, Kleber HD (eds): Clinician's Guide to Cocaine Addiction. New York, Guilford, 1992, pp. 206–221.

Rounsaville BJ, Anton SF, Carroll K, et al: Psychiatric disorders of treatment-seeking cocaine abusers. Arch Gen Psychiatry 48:43–51, 1991.

Rounsaville BJ, Weissman MM, Wilber CH, et al: Pathways of opiate addiction: An evaluation of differing antecedents. Br J Psychiatry 141:437–466, 1982.

Ryan L, Ehrlich S, Finnegan L: Cocaine abuse in pregnancy: Effects on the fetus and newborn. Neurotoxicol Teratol 9:295–299, 1987.

Sandberg DE, Meyer-Bahlburg HFL, Rosen TS, et al: Effects of prenatal methadone exposure on sex-dimorphic behavior in early school-age children. Psychoneuroendocrinology 15:77–82, 1990.

Schenker S, Becker HC, Randall CL, et al: Fetal alcohol syndrome: Current status of pathogenesis. Alcohol Clin Exp Res 14:635–647, 1990.

Scher MS, Richardson GA, Coble PA, et al: The effects of prenatal alcohol and marijuana exposure: Disturbances in neonatal sleep cycling and arousal. Pediatr Res 24:101–105, 1988.

Shepherd GM: Neurobiology (2nd ed). New York, Oxford University Press, 1988.

Smith DW: Recognizable Patterns of Human Malformation: Genetic, Embryologic, and Clinical Aspects (3rd ed). Philadelphia, Saunders, 1982.

Smith IE, Coles CD, Lancaster J, et al: The effect of volume and duration of prenatal ethanol exposure on neonatal physical and behavioral development. Neurobehav Toxicol Teratol 8:375–381, 1986.

Sokol RJ, Miller S, Reed G: Alcohol abuse during pregnancy: An epidemiological study. Alcohol Clin Exp Res 4:135–145, 1980.

Sowder BJ, Burt MR: Children of Heroin Addicts: An Assessment of Health, Learning, Behavioral, and Adjustment Problems. New York, Praeger, 1980.

Steinhausen HC, Nestler V, Spohr HL: Development and psychopathology of children with the fetal alcohol syndrome. Dev Behav Pediatr 3:49–54, 1982.

Strauss ME, Starr RH, Ostrea EM Jr, et al: Behavioral concomitants of prenatal addiction to narcotics. J Pediatr 89:842–846, 1976.

Streissguth AP: Psychologic handicaps in children with fetal alcohol syndrome. *Work Prog Alcohol* 273:140–145, 1976.

Streissguth AP: Fetal alcohol syndrome and fetal alcohol effects: A clinical perspective on later developmental consequences. In: Zagon IS, Slotkin TA (eds): *Maternal Substance Abuse and the Developing Nervous System.* Boston, Academic Press, 1992, pp. 5–26.

Streissguth AP, Aase IM, Clarren SK, et al: Fetal alcohol syndrome in adolescents and adults. *JAMA* 265:1961–1967, 1991.

Streissguth AP, Barr HM, Sampson PD, et al: IQ at age 4 in relation to maternal alcohol use and smoking during pregnancy. *Dev Psychol* 25:3–11, 1990.

Struthers JM, Hansen RL: Visual recognition memory in drug-exposed infants. *J Dev Behav Pediatr* 13:108–111, 1992.

Suffet F, Brotman R: Employment and social disability among opiate addicts. *Am J Drug Alcohol Abuse* 3:387–395, 1976.

Swann AC: Cocaine: Synaptic effects and adaptations. In: Volkow ND, Swann AC (eds): *Cocaine in the Brain.* New Brunswick, NJ, Rutgers University Press, 1990, pp. 58–94.

Tamis-LeMonda CS, Bornstein MH: Habituation and maternal encouragement of attention in infancy as predictors of toddler language, play, and representational competence. *Child Dev* 60:738–751, 1989.

Teske MP, Trese MT: Retinopathy of prematurity-like fundus and persistent hyperplastic primary vitreous associated with maternal cocaine use. *Am J Ophthalmol* 103:719–720, 1987.

Tucker MB: A descriptive and comparative analysis of the social support structure of heroin addicted women. *Addicted Women: Family Dynamics, Self-Perceptions, and Support Systems.* Washington, DC, National Institute of Drug Abuse, Superintendent of Documents, US Government Printing Office, 1979, pp. 37–76.

Ward OB, Kopertowski DM, Finnegan LP, et al: Gender-identity variations in boys prenatally exposed to opiates. *Ann NY Acad Sci* 562:365–366, 1989.

Ward OB, Orth TM, Weisz J: A possible role of opiates in modifying sexual differentiation. *Monogr Neural Sci* 9:194–200, 1983.

Wasserman DR, Leventhal JM: Maltreatment of children born to cocaine-abusing mothers. *Am J Dis Child* 147:1324–1328, 1993.

Watt J: Interaction, intervention, and development in small for gestational age infants. *Infant Behav Dev* 13:273–286, 1990.

Watt JE, Strongman KT: The organization and stability of sleep states in fullterm, preterm, and small-for-gestational age infants: A comparative study. *Dev Psychobiol* 18:151–162, 1985.

Wilson GS: Clinical studies of infants and children exposed prenatally to heroin. *Ann NY Acad Sci* 562:183–194, 1989.

Wilson GS, Desmond MM, Wait RB: Follow-up of methadone-treated and untreated narcotic-dependent women and their infants: Health, development, and social implications. *J Pediatr* 98:716–722, 1981.

Wilson GS, McCreary R, Kean J, et al: The development of preschool children of heroin-addicted mothers: A controlled study. *Pediatrics* 63:135–141, 1979.

Wise RA: Neural mechanisms of the reinforcing action of cocaine. *Natl Inst Drug Abuse Res Monogr* 50:15–33, 1984.

Woods JR, Plessinger MA, Clark KE: Effect of cocaine on uterine blood flow and fetal oxygenation. *JAMA* 257:957–961, 1987.

Wu T, Tashkin D, Djahed B, et al: Pulmonary hazards of smoking marijuana as compared to tobacco. *N Engl J Med* 318:347–351, 1988.

Zagon IS, McLaughlin P: An overview of the neurobehavioral sequelae of perinatal opioid exposure. In: Yanai J (ed): *Neurobehavioral Teratology.* Amsterdam, Elsevier, 1984, pp. 197–233.

Zuckerman B: Marijuana and cigarette smoking during pregnancy: Neonatal effects. In: Chasnoff I (ed): *Drugs, Alcohol, Pregnancy, and Parenting.* London, Kluwer, 1988, pp. 73–89.

Zuckerman B, Frank DA: Prenatal cocaine and marijuana exposure: Research and clinical implications. In: Zagon IS, Slotkin TA (eds): *Maternal Substance Abuse and the Developing Nervous System.* Boston, Academic Press, 1992, pp. 125–154.

Zuckerman B, Frank DA, Hingson R, et al: Effects of maternal marijuana and cocaine use on fetal growth. *N Engl J Med* 320:762–768, 1989.

32 SEPARATION AND DEPRIVATION

Sally A. Provence, M.D.,† and Linda C. Mayes, M.D.

The impact of separations from loved ones and the often ensuing deprivation on the developing infant and child have been an issue for child psychiatrists and other children's specialists for many years. The extent to which separations are depriving and traumatic or growth promoting, produce overwhelming anxiety or feelings of bereavement, or evoke adaptive responses resulting in a sense of mastery and well-being are very much a part of understanding an individual child. Such considerations also influence planning and policies about the well-being of children in hospitals, schools, day care centers, and other settings in which they are separated from parents and home. That old questions regularly reappear as new concerns reflects how basic the issues of separation and loss are to the human experience, and for both adults and children, separation experiences often lay at the center of character development.

The clinical questions most basic to understanding separation experiences for children often address how those experiences are handled by adults responsible for the child including both family and professionals. For example, how can separation experiences in the life of the young child be managed by adults so that distress is lessened and adaptive and defensive mechanisms that protect and facilitate development are evoked? How can parents and day care providers best help an infant or young child cope with the stresses inherent in being separated from parents for long hours day after day? How can the impact of separation on handicapped or sick infants be lessened, or similarly, how can hospitalization of a child be made less stressful for child and family? When the separation includes placement of the child outside the family, what can be done to improve outcome for children in the foster care system? How can knowledge of child mental health and development be more effectively communicated in order to influence decision-making in child placement and custody cases? Is it possible to design residential group care programs for infants and young children that foster development and address individuals needs, including therapeutic needs?

To be sure, issues of separation and deprivation are not the only considerations involved in the above questions, but they are of central importance and exert a strong influence on recommendations for the care of children and on choice of therapy for a variety of service settings. The role of child psychiatrists and other child mental health professionals includes a wide range of possibilities, from public policy issues to the more traditional roles of consultant, diagnostician, counselor, and therapist for the individual child and family. Crucial for each of these roles is the understanding of what is the meaning of separation both for an individual child and for the broader study of children's development.

Separation experiences are myriad in the lives of children and are a part of expected development. Allowing a parent to leave for work or saying good-bye at the door to school, sleeping overnight at a friend's house, accepting care from another, less familiar, family member are each examples of the many expected, indeed under optimal circumstances, developmentally promoting, separations for the preschool and school-age child. More potentially disruptive experiences include the loss of a parent through parental divorce or a severe debilitating illness or death. Similarly, separations that occur in the context of child abuse or neglect and subsequent foster placements impose multiple burdens on development in addition to the loss of a parent who may or may not have been the abuser.

Even this altogether too cursory typology illustrates that separation is not a single dimension experience. The field has moved past the time when deprivation could be discussed as though insufficient nutriments, the condition of "not enough," had sufficient explanatory value. Similarly, separation cannot be regarded as an event that has a predictable effect whenever it occurs in the earliest years. Such oversimplification disregards the complexity of brain and psychological development and the influence of developmental change on syndrome expression. It is known that a particular clinical disorder can be the result of multiple factors and that similar insults (e.g., deprivation and traumatic separation) may result in different outcomes. Any one separation experience is given weight by the developmental age and competency of the child, by the previous history of loss and separation for the child and family, and by how the family or responsible adults respond to the particular experience vis-à-vis themselves and the child.

For example, separations occurring in the early preschool years have a potentially greater developmental impact than those that occur later. For children with biologically based vulnerabilities such as a sensitivity to novelty and transitions, even expected separations may impose a greater degree of stress than for another less sensitive child. Similarly, for children with specific or general developmental delays, age-expectable separations (e.g., entry into preschool) may be experienced with a degree of anxiety and developmental stress more like a younger child. From the environmental side, how parents or caring adults help the child mediate the separation experience plays a crucial role in the child's acute and long-term responses. In many circumstances, the adult most responsible for the child is unable due to psychological and functional limitations of, for example, substance abuse, to mediate the experience for the child. Also, if the caring adult caring for the child is also acutely affected, as in the death or illness of a spouse, the child may experience a double loss as his or her remaining parent is less available and more acutely depressed. Situations of extreme family disruption such as occurs when a families are displaced from their homes impose not only the potential loss of cared for persons but also the loss of familiar surroundings and routines. There is also the mediating factor of how well cared for the child has been up to the separation. Children from chronically depriving or abusing environments are at much greater risk for severe developmental sequelae from a separation experience. Thus, separation involves not one experience either for an individual child or family or for any group of children at a given developmental age or life circumstances. On this and related notes of caution, selected currently recognized constructs about effects of deprivation and separation follow.

HISTORICAL NOTE ON CHANGING DEFINITIONS AND CONCEPTS

The condition of deprivation, for many years called "maternal" deprivation, has most often been seen as the lack of adequate physical care and of social and emotional stimulation and interchange. As investigators and clinicians looked more closely at specific components found in the environments of infants who were developing well and, by contrast, what was missing in the experience of those who were not doing well, and as we have become more aware of the impact of sensory defects such as deafness and blindness, "deprivation" is recognized as encompassing other conditions as well. "Experiential" deprivation is a more useful and accurate term than is maternal deprivation to express the variety of "not enough" situations that characterize the lives of many children. In addition, multiple risk factors often operate and are cumulative in their impact. Yarrow (1961), in a landmark paper, outlined more rigorous and productive methodological approaches to the study of maternal deprivation and to a conceptual reevaluation of clinical and research studies on the subject.

Traumatic separation and deprivation often, but not always, go hand in hand. The literature on maternal deprivation has included children residing in institutions for prolonged periods; those only temporarily separated because of illness of child or parent; those cared for by several different persons, enduring multiple separations; and children grossly neglected or mistreated by their families, experiencing not only the lack of adequate nurturance in the positive sense but also the trauma of insensitive, intrusive, or hostile treatment by parental figures.

Complex mixtures of experiential deprivation are encountered. Brain insults and congenital or acquired handicaps, prematurity, and neonatal illness increase the probability that an impoverished environment will have an adverse effect on development (Shonkoff and Marshall, 1990). Sensory defects such as deafness and blindness create a situation of needs requiring special environmental response in aspects of child care and education (Fraiberg, 1977; Freedman, 1981). When sensory defects are multiple or combined with motor handicaps, vulnerability to the influence of deprivation is heightened. When parents are markedly dysfunctional, however, even the most biologically resilient infant will be at risk for later problems.

In respect to *separation*, current concepts include consideration of *separateness*, that is, becoming a separate person, and *separation events*, which occur across the life cycle (Bloom-Feshbach and Bloom-Feshbach, 1987). Coping with experiences of separation is a lifelong challenge, not only inevitable but necessary for healthy development (Provence, 1987, p. 88). In childhood, some separation experiences facilitate psychological growth and personality organization by mobilizing new opportunities for learning and adaptation. Others, especially those involving loss of important persons, precipitate states of confusion, anger, anxiety, and grief and are painful and traumatic. Between these two extremes, there are many separation experiences involving varying degrees of psychological and psychobiological stress; adaptive and defensive mechanisms are called into play with varying degrees of effectiveness; feelings of mastery or helplessness are aspects of these responses.

KEY PARENTING REQUIREMENTS THAT MAY BE INSUFFICIENT

Winnicott (1961) emphasized that the young baby is essentially part of a relationship; that is, if you set about to describe a young infant, you find you are always describing a baby *and someone else*. Synchronous communication begins in the newborn period as the nurturing adult responds and learns the baby's rhythms, attentional behaviors, comfort-discomfort "messages," and affective states (Condon and Sander, 1975; Sander, 1980). The very terms *dialogue* (Brazelton and Cramer, 1990) and *the dance* (Thoman and Browder, 1987) are efforts to capture the reciprocity, mutuality, and transactional nature of the relationship from the beginning. But it is an uneven partnership because the baby's dependency needs are great, and so we define a facilitating environment as one that parent figures have the responsibility, gratification, and fulfillment to provide. That parenthood demands adaptation and growth and that the tasks and responsibilities are, at times, strenuous and worrisome is reality.

A conviction about the central importance of the child's human relationships for his or her growth and development physically, cognitively, and emotionally is shared by several developmental theories. Whether one prefers psychoanalytic formulations regarding object relations, ethological attachment theory, social learning theory, self-psychology, or other perspectives, there is strong consensus about the essential role of relationships with parents and others close to the child for his or her psychological well-being and the damage, short- or long-term, that may occur when relationships are seriously deficient or jeopardized. When infants are deprived of the experiences that go into good nurturance from their caregivers, and when there is significant discontinuity of care through separation events, there can be interferences and distortion in many aspects of development.

Among the important features of the kind of parental care that facilitates development are continuity of care and affection from primary human objects who are predictable and trustworthy; the development of a close relationship between adult and child, initiated by the parents' desire to love and nurture and the infant's responsiveness; specific types of stimulation addressed to physical, social, emotional, language, and intellectual growth; models for the development of controls, self-regulation, and socialization through education and guidance in an atmosphere of loving attention; and transmission of societal and cultural values through influencing the manner in which the child solves the tasks imposed by each phase of his or her epigenetic psychosocial development.

Continuity of affectionate care by one or a small number of caregivers who can give of themselves emotionally, as well as in other ways, originates the development of the child's love relationships. The formation of social bonds, of social and emotional communication, the development of a sense of confidence or trust in others, the perception of the parent as the source of security and protection, and feelings of self-esteem are dependent on such care and its reliability. Affectionate and stable patterns of experience facilitate the baby's ability to organize physiological and psychological processes (Escalona, 1968; Greenspan, 1981; Sander, 1980) from early on, influencing perceptions of the outer world and of his inner sensations, feelings, and thoughts. As one example: Being loved and esteemed by others and perceiving that love is believed to be at the heart of the ability to love oneself, and self-love is a part of the capacity to love another in turn. As another example: Having repeated experiences of being comforted when distressed is a part of developing one's own capacity for self-comfort and self-regulation, and later, the capacity to provide the same for others.

Specific types of experience enhance particular aspects of development. For example, the infant's being talked to by his or her caregivers is very important in speech development. Progress in the ability to communicate verbally occurs when intrinsic maturational events interact with environmental influences that organize and give meaning to the child's utterances. The presence of a speaking, interested social partner is vital. Similarly, motor skills, as opposed to mere motor discharge, are stimulated by an array of tactile-kinesthetic experiences that occur in the process of good care and later by opportunities to practice emerging skills in a safe environment. The growth of intelligence in the early years is enhanced by variety, contrast, and novel stimuli when these occur in the context of essentially stable and developmentally appropriate patterns of experience with the environment. The provision of toys and other inanimate objects to manipulate and explore is important for negotiating the stages of sensorimotor intelligence (Piaget, 1952; Piaget and Inhelder, 1969), which takes place in concert with structuring of the affective life. The parent also has importance as educator and guide, helping the child to identify aspects of reality, that is, both as a source of information and as a reinforcer or modifier of the child's cognitive expectations.

The parental role in the child's coming to interact effectively with the environment is significant in both its learning and its motivational aspects. Hartmann (1958) emphasized the importance of the child's social relationships in the learning that is essential for many of the child's adaptation processes. Robert White (1959) and Lois Murphy (1974) emphasized the beneficial influences of experiences of mastery in adaptation. Coping involves original, imaginative, and innovative behavior and helps the child to manage both his or her inner experience and the demands of the outer environment. Studies of the origins of competence in the child, motivation for mastery, and relationships between motivation and cognition (Harter and Zigler, 1974; White, 1975; Yarrow, 1981; Yarrow and Pederson, 1976) further support the view of the importance of an environment in which adults sensitively respond to the child's needs and provide responsive materials.

Parents, as models for the child in the establishment of controls over impulse and behavior, make a significant contribution to the development of a healthy personality. Whether one regards the process as establishing ego control over the drives or as the socialization process, the influence of good parenting is acknowledged. Through the relationship and with the necessary guidance in an atmosphere of loving attention, the child comes to wish to please those the child loves and is motivated to behave in ways of which they approve. The child imitates, identifies with, and gradually incorporates aspects of their behavior, attitudes, and values, making them his or her own. This condensed statement greatly oversimplifies the process through which the child moves toward ego maturity, control over sexual and aggressive impulses, affect regulation, and superego formation. Here, perhaps, it can only be repeated that

parents as models and guides play a central role, and, in their absence or severe dysfunction, this aspect of personality development suffers.

SENSITIVE FUNCTIONS

Deprivation and traumatic separation endanger the development of healthy attachment relationships with others and the formation of social bonds. If one accepts the idea that the child's sense of security, basic trust, and knowledge of others and of self are anchored in and flow from the care of one or a small number of affectionate, available caregivers, then deprivation of essential nutriments and frequent and long disruptions in the interactions with the person one has come to trust and to love can be identified as threats. Infancy research and clinical experience confirm that a growth-inhibiting environment for an infant in the 1st year exists when caregivers are unavailable, understimulating or overstimulating, emotionally distant, ambivalent, or fail to respond contingently to the infant's communication across multiple sensory and affective systems (Greenspan, 1981). In contrast, a growth-promoting environment is characterized by invested, comforting, guiding caregivers who "woo" the infant, encourage the "dialogue," respond appropriately to the infant's communications, and, in the process, transmit feelings as well as bits of "information" about the human and inanimate world that become vital factors in general learning, as well as in relationships with others. Progression from sensorimotor modes to the organization of internal representations of self and human objects and other symbolic elaborations of mental imagery is also sensitive to severe deprivation in the environment and to multiple changes in the continuity of adequate child care. Thus, there is reason for concern about interferences and distortions, especially in the young child's coming to love himself or herself and others and in relationships with peers and others in his or her social environment.

Language, both speech and nonverbal communication, is particularly sensitive to deprivation and separation. Even though speech and the elaboration of social signals have an inner, biological, and maturational basis, their blossoming as agents of communication is closely related to the releasing and stimulating influence of the environment. Infants and toddlers, for example, who are not talked to by their caregivers in families and elsewhere are delayed in speech development (Provence and Lipton, 1962; Spitz, 1945; Spitz and Wolf, 1946). Many years ago, Lewis (1959) wrote: "When does a child begin to speak? . . .If not at the moment of birth, then certainly during the first day. For as soon as a child cries and someone pays attention to his cry, the first steps are taken; the essentials of language are there" (p. 14). The presence and attention of the primary parent, usually the mother, influence the development of speech in several ways, through reinforcing the baby's vocalization, the development of mutually imitative vocalizations that encourage the use of an expanding repertory of sounds, and the "labeling" of people, toys, actions, feelings, and the like (Bornstein, 1989). The mother's speech is also a carrier of emotions and an organizing influence on the infant's psychological life. The sounds that form the building blocks for speech are believed to gain specific meaning because of the parents' response to them. For example, the Mama and Dada sounds that emerge as a result of maturation at somewhere around 9 months become names for the parents because of their strong affective response and reinforcement. It should be said that speech development is a very complex function, and there is considerable variability in its development within what we consider normal. That being acknowledged, the sensitivity of speech development to disruptions in relationships with the partners in communication and to a verbally impoverished environment is a signal to the clinician to look closely at the child's experiences with his or her caregivers.

CONSEQUENCES OF INSUFFICIENCIES

Clinical experience is replete with examples of consequences of deprivation and traumatic separation, described as delays, syndromes, or disorders. Bowlby's (1960) classical description of the strong emotional reactions seen in young children in response to separation from the mother found wide agreement from clinicians and investigators as to their relevance and possible long-term detrimental effects. His review of several decades of studies of separation from the mother revealed an impressive uniformity of observations of behavior in spite of many differences in the settings, situations, and orientation of the investigators. He described a reaction of infants from about 6 months to 3 years of age in which feelings of grief and mourning are intimately related to separation anxiety. Robertson and Bowlby (1952) first defined the three major phases of response as protest, despair, and detachment. Protest is a phase of angry, loud, tearful behavior during which the child looks for the mother and expects her return. The second phase, despair, is one of acute pain and diminishing hope, when there is usually a subdued manner and little interest in the surroundings. In the third or detachment phase, the child shows renewed interest in the environment and may be quite friendly and outgoing to others, but specific reactions to the mother, when she reappears, such as ignoring and walking away, suggest that detachment serves a defensive function. These agreed upon affective responses are interpreted variously depending on theoretical preferences and appear in more or less distinct expressions for any one child enduring a particular loss.

Developmental Delay

Developmental delays in motor, language, intellectual, social/emotional, and adaptive behavior occur singly or, more often, in combination. The classical example of multiple developmental delays found in infants living in foundling homes and other residential institutions has produced a very extensive literature, of which only a small sample is cited here (Ainsworth, 1972; Bowlby, 1951, 1958; Provence and Lipton, 1962; Yarrow, 1961). Moreover, disturbances in such areas as the quality of social relationships, emotional expressiveness, versatility in coping with challenge or stress, and flexibility in thought and problem-solving also occur. Major improvements in the environment, especially the quality of nurturing, are accompanied by encouraging gains, and yet concern about long-term effects on capacities for mature interpersonal relationships and adequate functioning in the society remain. Less pervasive developmental delays are found in situations that may not immediately be identified as depriving. Infants of mothers with masked depression, for example, may present with delays in discrete areas, such as speech or range and variety of emotional expression, in which developmental findings in the infant are clues to maternal dysfunction (Coleman and Provence, 1953; Fendrick et al., 1990; Field, 1995; Provence, 1983).

Insecure or Disordered Attachments

Insecure, avoidant, and disorganized attachments, as classified by the Ainsworth Strange Situation, have been increasingly reported as characterizing infants whose mothers, for a variety of reasons, have been unable to respond to them sensitively and contingently (Ainsworth et al., 1978; Bretherton, 1985; Easterbrooks et al., 1993). The Strange Situation has a superb performance as a research tool and can be useful to clinicians as a marker suggesting the need for further exploration of the child-rearing environment in that it captures aspects of the mother-infant relationship. But the results of the Strange Situation are not established as valid for clinical work in individual cases, and the data derived must be integrated with other knowledge about the infant from other sources, in order to be useful as a clinical instrument (Ainsworth, 1980; Gaensbauer and Harmon, 1982; Greenspan and Lieberman, 1988; Weitzman and Cook, 1986). Clinicians, utilizing information from a broader context, are accustomed to diagnosing reactive disorders of attachment in infants and young children. These include such phenomena as maladaptive patterns of social interaction with adults and peers, shallow or tenuous adult-child relationships, severe separation problems, and poor impulse control. Multiple separations and depriving environments are common occurrences in the lives of young children designated as having disorders of attachment (Tibbits-Kleber and Howell, 1985).

Object Constancy Delay and Instability

Disturbances in the development of a sense of self and the separation-individuation process occur when the benevolence and reliability of caregivers are grossly inadequate. As already indicated, children who do not feel valued cannot value themselves. Those whose sense of self is not nurtured and reinforced by the affection, protection, and guidance of parent figures have little opportunity to develop the pleasure and confidence in independent functioning that is an integral part of healthy personality development. The attainment of emotional object constancy and a stable sense of self is a main task of the subphase of separation-individuation, occurring, roughly, in the 3rd year of life (Mahler et al., 1975). Disturbances in the separation-individuation process are inferred from the behavior of young children in the 3rd year and beyond, when separation becomes a severe problem and maladaptive "solutions" to the feelings associated with separation are manifest. A large number of empirical studies of children entering nursery school support several clinical impressions. Bloom-Feshbach (1987), in studies of 3-year-olds, found clear distinctions between emotionally healthy children and those with problems. After an initial period of adjustment, including protest at separation, emotionally healthy children were better able to seek and use teachers for help and comfort when needed; they investigated the environment more actively and with greater satisfaction; they interacted more confidently with peers; and they regulated their feelings more adaptively. Their behaviors suggest favorable progress in personality organization, healthy coping with stressful events, and the ability to make use of and enjoy a larger world of experience. In contrast, children with problematic separations were marked by the emergence of symptomatic behavior ranging from severe and prolonged distress, to defiance, to apathy. Symptomatic behavior may reflect internal difficulties in differentiation, self-esteem, and identity formation. According to Mahler, Pine, and Bergman (Settlage, 1974), danger signals during the separation-individuation process during the 2nd and 3rd years include the absence of the normal mood of elation related to a sense of power, expected in early toddlerhood; a proclivity toward a depressive mood; and, in some instances, a marked increase in aggressive behavior. Among the behavioral signs of a tendency toward marked ambivalence toward the parent is a greater than average separation anxiety. Clinging, demandingness, and protest as well as superficial indifference and detachment may occur.

Affect Regulation Dysfunction

Disturbances in modulation and regulation of affect are frequently found in infants and young children who encounter deprivation and traumatic separations. Range, differentiation, intensity, and expression of feelings as reflected in behavior are interfered with. Regulatory mechanisms that favor the infant's capacity (a) to recognize pleasure and joy, and their opposites, in himself and in others, and (b) to tolerate these perceptions, are dependent, at least in part, on the infant's interactions with the environment. Insufficient "supplies" and severe disruptions tend to starve or overwhelm the system. Responses and "solutions" ensue, which may have short-term utility but prove to be maladaptive in the long run. At the mercy of poorly regulated affects, young children manifest a variety of problems, including difficulties in peer relationships, severe anxiety, constriction or wide swings in expressive behavior and mood, and conflicts with parent figures. Outbursts of anger, "giddy" excitement, impulsive actions, and panicky behavior may coexist with excessive compliance, blunted affect, depression, or apathy.

Failure to Thrive and Eating Disorders

Environmentally based failure to thrive, as a syndrome defined as a severe deficit in rate of weight gain in the absence of physical disease, was first described, according to Drotar (1985), in association with compromised nurturing in institutional environments (Chapin, 1908, 1915; Spitz, 1945) and family settings (Patton and Gardner, 1963; Talbot et al., 1947). Reduced human potential, as well as the need for a spectrum of services from pediatric hospital care, to foster homes, to psychiatric treatment of severe emotional disturbance, are associated with it. Recent studies have underscored significant individual differences in etiology, age of onset, severity of growth deficits, developmental and behavioral problems, and family stress (Chatoor and Eagan, 1983; Drotar, 1985; Ferholt and Provence, 1976; Mayes and Volkmar, 1993; Woolston, 1983).

Eating disorders are not uncommon in infants and young children experiencing depriving environments and traumatic separations. They range from anorexia to insatiable appetite, from food refusal to overeating, and from malnutrition to obesity. Deprivation in regard to feeding has several meanings: fewer calories than are required for normal growth; being fed, not according to one's own appetite and rhythms but by the schedules or whims of the caregivers; and missing the physical and social stimulation and connectedness that occur when one is fed by an attentive, attuned feeder. The "stomach love" of the young infant for the mother is a metaphor for a mosaic of sensations, perceptions, emotions, and mutual adjustments. Multiple factors will determine the extent to which unsatisfactory feeding experiences will result in clinical disorders, including, as is true in other respects, antecedent experiences, the phase of development during which they occur, and the child's unique endowment and state of physical health. But it can also be said that, when the positive conditions of a satisfactory feeding experience are in short supply, when the relationship with the feeder is disrupted, when mealtime is a time of turbulence or battle, when the child's cognitive and affective expectations are repeatedly violated, eating problems of one kind or another may ensue. The fact that these disorders are usually not the sole clinical findings or necessarily the most significant ones for emotional health requires the coordinated efforts of pediatric and mental health experts. A developmental approach to feeding disturbances that looks at a number of factors in the child and the environment is likely to lead to improved understanding, treatment, and preventive intervention (Chatoor et al., 1985; Mayes and Volkmar, 1993).

Psychiatric Disorders

Psychiatric diagnosis in the early years of life is fraught with difficulty. Aside from agreement about certain syndromes associated with troubled parent-child relationships, including those in which deprivation and separation play a part, clinicians encounter the problem that currently available systems of classification are far from adequate. Limited data on the outcome of early-onset disorders, how developmental change affects syndrome expression, and the degree of dysfunction that should be labeled as clinical disorder complicate classification. That infants and young children become depressed and develop psychophysiological and psychosomatic symptoms and behavior problems is well known, but there is need for a more systematic developmental approach to the classification of early childhood disorders. Disorders of affect, in the early years, for example, can be defined as those that pose serious risk for distortion of expectable development. For a diagnosis of anxiety disorder, the child should exhibit (a) excessive levels of anxiety and fear, as manifested by multiple or specific fears; (b) excessive separation or stranger anxiety; (c) panic without clear precipitants; or (d) inappropriate absence of expectable anxiety or fear. Mood disorders include (a) prolonged bereavement/grief reactions that interfere with development; that is, normal grief reactions qualify for designation as a disorder if they are excessive; (b) depression of infancy and early childhood, reserved for those who exhibit a pattern of depressed mood with diminished interest and/or pleasure in developmentally appropriate activities; or (c) a diminished repertory of social interactions and initiative. "Deprivation syndrome" might be reserved for those in whom gross parental neglect of basic physical and/or psychological needs or the absence of a stable primary caregiver is evident (Volkmar and Provence, 1990).

Poorness of Fit

Goodness of fit and poorness of fit are terms used to describe the way in which infants and their parents enter into and achieve good adjustment to one another or have great difficulty doing so. Difficult temperamental characteristics (Thomas and Chess, 1977), unusual sensitivities (Bergman and Escalona, 1949), and congenital characteristics of activity and reactivity (Korner, 1974) can make some infants difficult to care for by even the most expert of parents. Other infants may be disappointing to their parents because of their unconscious meaning, which interferes with a beneficial parent-child relationship and becomes a pathogenic influence. Various forms of deprivation and traumatic separation events may result from such situations (Kris, 1962; Provence, 1965, 1983). Among the more significant opportunities for preventive intervention is the early recognition of parent-child interaction that reflects problems in reciprocity and mutual adjustment.

FACTORS ADDING TO INSUFFICIENCIES AND THE RISK OF A LONG-TERM EFFECT OF SEPARATION

In the Mothering Person

Many conditions in the mothering person contribute to or complicate deprivation. Maternal depression, for example, often results in a mother's being psychologically unavailable to the child at times, appropriately and lovingly attentive at times, and intrusive and hostile at others. Her failure to respond contingently results in deprivation experiences for the baby, even when she is physically present. Maternal ambivalence in behavior and attitude toward the child is both confusing and painful, interfering, among other things, with a secure attachment and the orderly progression of separation-individuation, self-esteem formation, and affect regulation. Children who are uncertain of the parent's love, guidance, and protection are especially vulnerable to separation. Mothers with severe psychiatric disorders become dysfunctional in a variety of ways: A mother whose own reality awareness is impaired is unable to represent reality for her infant; if she is unpredictable in her behavior toward her infant, those developmental steps that flow from a sense of trust and security will be impeded; if she is severely disorganized, the baby is likely to suffer from pervasive problems of regulation, both of physiological and psychological functions. If the baby is a part of her delusional system, the baby may be in gross danger (Anthony, 1974).

A mother impaired by drugs or alcohol is unable to provide the kind of care that promotes the child's development, both because of her unavailability in the positive sense and because poor control of aggressive behavior may result in abuse (Mayes, 1995). If she has been a substance abuser during pregnancy, the infant is potentially at both biological and environmental risks (Chasnoff et al., 1984; Howard et al., 1989; Jones and Lopez, 1988). Parental substance abuse presents a continuum of vulnerability and risks for the children involved. Chronic substance abuse (e.g., alcohol, heroin, or cocaine) may impair an adult's psychological functioning in domains basic to parenting (e.g., persistence, concentration, memory). Also, for the most part, substance abuse involves the adult in a number of related environmental conditions including poverty and homelessness, frequent violence and family discord, poor physical health, and unstable, erratic relationships with others. Mothers who are chronic substance abusers most often cite their social isolation and deep loneliness as the states of being that most interfere with their ability to reduce or stop their addiction (Mayes, 1995; Tucker, 1979).

Physical and sexual abuse are acts by parent figures against children that stem from the psychological and social pathology of adults. They may be concomitants of deprivation; traumatic separation experiences may be part of the picture. Abusive acts may also occur in child-rearing environments that contain positive features as well. For such children, careful clinical assessment is the basis for recommendations about whether the dangers to physical and emotional survival outweigh the advantages of remaining with the parent. The presence or absence of family members who can adequately protect the young child will be an important determinant of decision-making. Separation from abusing parents and placement in a nurturing environment may permit emotional healing and restore the young child's chances for adequate development (Goldstein et al., 1979).

In the Child

Factors in the child that heighten his or her vulnerability to deprivation and traumatic separation are referred to throughout this chapter. It should be kept in mind, however, that young children vary in their vulnerability to noxious biological influences as well as to environmental situations associated with poor developmental outcome in others.

Genetic disorders associated with mental subnormality (chromosomal or biochemical), malformations of the central nervous system of obscure etiology, toxic insults, infections, malnutrition, and perinatal insults such as hemorrhage and hypoxic injury make the young child more vulnerable to the adverse effects of separation and deprivation. Sensory deficits such as deafness and blindness and musculoskeletal handicaps, whatever their etiology, delay or disrupt the developmental process. Children deemed vulnerable or in need of particularly skilled parenting, such as those called temperamentally slow to warm up or difficult, those with sensory processing problems, and those with unusual sensitivities, often come to attention because of difficult behavior or delays in aspects of development. Such children will often have difficulty with many phase-specific aspects of early development including the usual day-to-day separations between parent and child.

Child characteristics, congenital or acquired, may underlie clinical disorders for two reasons: Intrinsic factors may complicate the nurturing process, and maladaptive child-rearing styles and attitudes may be evoked in the parent by these specific characteristics. Thus, there is often an interaction between basic biology and patterns of parenting that further exacerbate developmental vulnerabilities and responses to situations such as separations.

The child's developmental level and personality organization at the time of separation and deprivation are of great import in determining their influence. A 10-month-old infant, for example, will have both the perception of loss of the differentiated object and distress and despair if the separation is prolonged and there is no satisfactory surrogate. The infant will have very limited resources for self-comfort and will be largely dependent on others to alleviate his or her distress. The previously well-cared-for and adequately developing 4-year-old, in contrast, can identify and verbalize feelings and ask questions; has enough sense of time (before and after, today and tomorrow) and place to use explanations and reassurance; has play skills that enable him or her to express as well as to work at mastery of the anger and discomfort through action and fantasy; will have available mental representations of those whom the child loves and who are sources of security that can be evoked in time of need; and will have developed coping strategies and defense mechanisms that can be mobilized to deal with the stress of separation.

Situational Events

As indicated, whether deprivation and separation are short- or long-term and occur in a well-functioning or dysfunctional family, will also make a difference in impact on the capacity of the family to respond to a crisis or a planned separation in a way that is protective of the young child. This latter includes, for example, the adequacy of the child-rearing arrangements during the parents' absence. Other factors that precipitate separation, such as illness of child or parent, divorce, natural catastrophe, and social upheaval, are diverse examples of the contexts of separation, each bearing its own set of conditions that affect the child and those closest to him or her.

In summary, it is reemphasized that multiple, interdependent, and interacting factors determine developmental outcome and the mental health of the infant and young child.

Theories of Process and Mechanisms

How does one understand what happens to the young child who experiences deprivation and traumatic separation? There is no unitary theory of psychological development that can be called upon to guide diagnostic, therapeutic, and preventive efforts. Nonetheless, empirical data derived from research and practice and theory from a number of developmental psychologies are organized into sets of constructs. Such systematic efforts permit the kind of interaction between clinical experience, data of observation, and theoretical propositions that leads to the refinement of each.

In the following, aspects of attachment theory, psychoanalytic theory, and cognitive psychology are presented because of their contributions to state-of-the-art thinking about separation and deprivation. The distress of the young child at separation and the adverse effects of deprivation are understood in part by each. Clearly one cannot here do full justice to any one of them, but a guide to the salient outlines of each theory is provided.

Contributions from Attachment Theory

Bowlby's attachment theory employs an evolutionary perspective that draws on ethological principles and animal behavior and combines them with aspects of psychoanalytic theory to understand the formation of human social bonds. The infant's survival mechanisms and the adult's nurturing tendencies "bias" them to behave reciprocally and to form an attachment. Attachment as defined by Bowlby (1969) and as used by Ainsworth and colleagues (Ainsworth, 1964; Ainsworth et al., 1978) is an affectional tie that forms with another specific person, a tie that endures over time and has an inner structural basis.

The "internal working model" (Bowlby, 1969) is defined as the child's psychological representation of repeated transactions with the world, a form of mental representation or structure that guides and regulates human functioning and permits, for example, the mental representations of attachment figures to be accessible and emotionally available in time of need. Bowlby argues that, for the child, the knowledge that an attachment figure is available and responsive provides a strong and pervasive feeling of security, and that separation is a signal of potential danger. Biologically rooted reactions of fear and wariness are evoked most readily when the infant is separated from the person to whom he or she is attached. Separation anxiety is viewed as an adaptive response to the signal of the potential dangers that attend the child in the mother's absence, which has become intrinsic to the behavioral repertoire of the human child over generations and serves survival.

Bowlby (1973) is in basic agreement with Freud's view that anxiety is a response to the danger of loss of a love object; pain or mourning is the response to actual loss, and defenses are mobilized to cope with pain.

Bowlby (1960) used the terms *mourning* to characterize the psychological process set in motion by loss and *grief* to denote the sequences of subjective states that follow loss and accompany mourning and suggested that mourning in the infant differs in no material way from mourning at later ages. Anna Freud (1960), in responding to Bowlby's hypotheses, agreed with the descriptions of behavior and the painfulness of the experience but took issue with his view of mourning. She proposed that the term *bereavement* be used and that the term mourning be reserved for later reactions when development in object relations and ego maturity make it possible for the mourning process, as defined in psychoanalysis, to occur.

Distress at separation from the mother is intensified when the young child is placed in a strange environment and cared for by a succession of strange persons. The typical sequence of protest, despair, and detachment, described earlier, ensues. The phase of *protest*, Bowlby (1973) writes, is found to raise the problem of separation anxiety; *despair*, that of grief and mourning; *detachment*, that of defenses. The three types of responses are seen as phases of a single process. Acute anxiety recurs when there is fear or anticipation of losing the mother again. The onset of psychiatric conditions, in Bowlby's view, is linked to the premature detachment masking "strong residual yearning for and anger at the lost object . . .ready for expression at an unconscious level" (1961, p. 269). This leads Bowlby (1980) to argue that, because there are cumulative effects, strong preventive efforts are called for, and that "the safest dose [of separation] is a zero dose" (p. 3). Such a prescription, while certainly applicable to acute and unanticipated loss or abandonment, does not as easily apply to the vicissitudes and developmentally promoting aspects of expectable, anticipated, and usual separations in early childhood.

Since Bowlby, extensive empirical research (Bretherton, 1985; Easterbrooks et al., 1993; Goldberg, 1991) using the Strange Situation has documented at least four patterns of 12- to 18-month-old children's response to brief separation including secure, avoidant, ambivalent or resistant, and disorganized. The crux of the separation situation designed to elicit these behavior patterns is a standard sequence of separations and reunions during which the infant experiences increasing distress and a greater need for proximity (Goldberg, 1991). The strategies children use to cope with their increasing needs for proximity with the adult are considered indicators of the quality of the attachment. The individual behavioral components that go into an attachment category include seeking and maintaining contact with the adult, avoidance, and resistance to physical contact. Behaviors on reunion appear to be the most salient in distinguishing among these different attachment categories. In the secure category, infants seek their caregiver only when their security is threatened, as when they are left in a novel or frightening place. When the adult returns, these children are able to explore comfortably and securely. Avoidant or dismissing children appear not to notice or be distressed by the caregiver's absence or return, while ambivalent children are often overly distressed and disorganized even when they are not in danger. Children with ambivalent attachment patterns are often unable to resume their usual play even on the adult's return. In Ainsworth's original study (1969), 65% of toddlers exhibited secure patterns of attachment, 21% an avoidant pattern, and the remaining 14% an ambivalent pattern. These patterns and their distribution are consistent in larger series of infants and toddlers from several different cultures (Van Ijzendoorn and Kroonenberg, 1988). Also, under stable environmental conditions, individual attachment patterns are stable both over a short-term period of 6 months and for up to 5 years (Main et al., 1985; Waters, 1978).

A number of studies have shown that securely attached infants are more competent than insecure infants in several later cognitive and social domains (Matas et al., 1978; Sroufe et al., 1983; Waters et al., 1979). In a longitudinal study of children followed from the 1st year through puberty, reports document the positive relation between early attachment behaviors and later social competency (Sroufe et al., 1990). Studies of attachment under at-risk conditions such as prematurity, maternal depression, and maltreatment have shown mixed patterns of attachment emerging from these early stressful situations and led to the creation of a fourth attachment category, the disorganized pattern (Main and Solomon, 1990). Infants who appear disorganized during separations and reunions exhibit confused, often fearful reactions to the adult's return and have few to no strategies for coping with the stress of separation. Disorganized attachment patterns occur more frequently among groups of abused and/or neglected children (Carlson et al., 1989) but may also reflect, in some instances, transient normative reactions to extremely disruptive situations (e.g., parental illness, birth of a sibling) (Goldberg, 1991). The relation between disorganized attachment patterns and later adaptation or subsequent psychopathology has not been adequately studied.

Studies of attachment behaviors beyond the 2nd year of life have also been extended to preschool-age children, 5- to 7-year-olds, and to adults. For children, the procedures again rely on separations and observations of reunions, and for adults, on an extensive interview about the individual's early relationships (Goldberg, 1990). Categories similar to those described in toddlers apply to older children and to adults.

The secure/autonomous pattern describes a child who acknowledges the adult's return, but continues usually to play and finds a way to invite the adult to join his or her activity. For adults, secure attachments are indexed by both a valuing of close relationships and a realistic acceptance of the strengths and weaknesses of those persons. Avoidant preschoolers and older children appear to be more interested in other activities than the adult's return, and though they may greet the adult, show minimal response to overtures for engagement and little effort to include the adult in their play. Avoidant or dismissing adults idealize their childhood experiences and downplay the importance of close, intimate relationships in their lives. Dependent/ambivalent children, like their infant counterparts, are preoccupied with the adult's whereabouts at the expense of all else including their own play and other activities. Similarly, the adult analogue describes an individual caught in old struggles, lacking a sense of their own personal identity, and their own role within relationships. The fourth category, disorganized, as with toddlers, requires more clarification, but in its present form, describes a child who is not so much behaviorally disorganized but rather is controlling of the interaction. The child works hard to keep the parent happy or engaged or is controllingly hostile and demanding. For the adult, this attachment pattern may be inferred from unresolved mourning over losses of important others in which there is continuing cognitive disorganization around discussions of the lost figure.

These techniques for studying attachment patterns in older children and adults have permitted closer study of both the stability of attachment across the life span and the transmission of attachment patterns across generations. There appears to be a high degree of concordance between adult attachment patterns and their relations to their infants (Main and Hesse, 1990). Parents who are secure or autonomous in their view of their own parenting tend to have securely attached infants, while those who are dismissing tend to have avoidant infants, and those who are preoccupied have ambivalent infants. It is important to note that studies of adult attachment do not purport to provide a "historically accurate" picture of an adult's childhood—adults with extremely traumatic early childhood's may nevertheless be securely attached. Rather the studies of adult attachment tap into how the adult views important relationships in his or her life (the internal object world in the language of psychoanalysis), and these views in turn influence how the adult responds to his or her children. An active area of research is the relation between patterns of attachment in infancy, childhood, and adults and behavior and psychiatric problems. For example, Sroufe et al. (1990) have shown a relation between early attachment patterns and later behavior problems in school, and more children with insecure attachment patterns (avoidant or ambivalent) are referred to child guidance clinics (Goldberg, 1991).

Contributions from Psychoanalysis

Lieberman's (1987) discussion of separation in infancy and early childhood presents suggestions for a synthesis of aspects of attachment theory and psychoanalysis. The effort to select relevant propositions from psychoanalysis regarding separation and deprivation is immediately challenged by the complexity of the theory, which emphasizes the uniqueness of the inner life of each child in determining the influence of a reality event, such as separation. The nature of the child's relationships with loved ones are seen as centrally important in determining how he or she will experience, cope with, and defend against separation from them. Antecedent experiences and phases of psychosexual, cognitive, and psychosocial development, with their expectable sources of conflict, anxiety, and satisfaction, as well as the effectiveness of adaptive and defensive mechanisms, play a part in how reality events acquire psychological meaning.

Given this complexity, one can only illustrate by defining a few developmental lines and psychological processes, selected because of their demonstrated usefulness in dealing with separation issues in the very young.

In psychoanalytic developmental theory, the concept of separation involves two related but distinct perspectives: separation as a *process*, through which the child develops an awareness of the physical and mental self as distinct from all others, and separation as an *event*, in which an individual experiences being parted from those to whom he or she is most strongly attached. Separation events occur throughout the life cycle, as Bloom-Feshbach and colleagues (1987) have recently summarized, and their influence is determined by multiple, interacting factors. The landmark studies of Margaret Mahler and her colleagues (Mahler, 1963; Mahler et al., 1975) addressed the separation-individuation process, tracing "the psychological birth" of the human infant. Mahler's theory of separation-individuation emphasizes that, while the process is never finished and reverberates through the life cycle, the principal psychological achievements are placed within the period from the 4th or 5th month of life to the 30th to 36th months. "The normal separation-individuation process . . .involves the child's achievement of separate functioning in the presence of, and with the emotional availability of, the mother. . . .This normal separation-individuation process takes place in the setting of developmental readiness for, and pleasure in, independent functioning" (Mahler, 1963, pp. 3–4).

The development of a sense of awareness of the body and mental self as distinct from all others and the gradual formation of a personal identity are aspects of the individual's view of his or her totality as a person. The self as a cohesive psychological organization is, as Loewald (1980) has emphasized, contingent upon the differentiation between self and other. In the life of the infant, these distinctions develop in myriad day-to-day experiences and transactions with persons, sensations, and actions, in concert and interwoven with other lines of development. The awareness or *sense* of a personal identity is influenced by factors affecting perception of the external world; that is, there are important cognitive elements. Comparisons and contrasts become more clear through intellectual growth. Identity is maintained by continual redefinition (Greenacre, 1971). In this process, the nature of the child's relationships with others is a vital factor. "There is wide agreement . . .that it is those to whom the child is most strongly attached with whom the most important patterns of separation and individuation are played out as part of the process through which awareness of the separate self identity and self-esteem come into being" (Provence, 1987, p. 95).

In psychoanalytic theory, anxiety is a response to the danger, real or imagined, of loss of a love object, but is viewed in much more complex terms than it is in attachment theory. Inherent in the fear of object loss is the mixture of feelings that characterize love relationships: Loving, tender feelings are mingled with hostile feelings. Libidinal and aggressive cathexes of the mental representations of loved persons coexist. Longing for that person and sadness at separation or anticipation of loss, as well as shame or guilt about one's hostile wishes and feelings, stimulate eagerness for reunion.

The studies of Benjamin (1961, 1963) and Spitz (1957, 1965) contributed much to psychoanalytic approaches to understanding developmental aspects of anxiety. Freud's (1959) introduction of the concept of anxiety, psychological pain, and mourning as responses to object loss formed the background of these and other studies. Two overlapping but different anxiety responses occur during the 1st year, defined operationally as infantile stranger anxiety and infantile separation anxiety. Fear of loss of the loved person in reality, fear of loss of that person's love and approval, fear of loss of the loved self, and fear of one's own disapproval in sequence overlap and span the years of infancy and early childhood. Each of these phase-associated anxieties influences the way in which separation or the withdrawal of parental interest is experienced by the child.

The developmental progression in the child's psychological life in regard to separation anxiety begins with reaction to loss of what Benjamin called a *pre-object*, a person or persons who reduce tension and provide security and pleasure, and progresses to fear of loss of a *differentiated* object, a particular person one knows and loves. Benjamin's (1963) hypothesis that fear of loss of the person one loves and depends on is the immediate dynamic determinant of separation anxiety appears

valid. With its later derivative, fear of loss of love, it is universal or nearly universal in our culture in psychologically healthy children, though varying in intensity.

Psychoanalytic developmental theory also brings to bear on separation propositions regarding the stability and permanence of psychic representations. In this connection, the construct of *object constancy* has relevance. It is believed that the child's ability to cope with the stress of separation events leans heavily on the capacity to evoke reassuring mental images of those to whom the child attributes his or her sense of security and well-being. Solnit's (1982) definition is useful: "Object constancy is that state of object relations in which the child has the capability to retain the memory of the emotional ties to parents, . . .and to feel their nurturing, guiding presence even if they are a source of frustration or disappointment or when they are absent" (p. 202).

Fraiberg (1969) did much to clarify issues regarding the development of object constancy, a term that has been used differently by various psychoanalytic theorists and investigators. She supported a view put forward by Nagera (1966) that one may distinguish between the very beginnings of object constancy in the 1st year and its attainment at the end of the 2nd year. Similarly, Mahler (1966) indicated that the achievement of object constancy is a characteristic of the 4th subphase of separation-individuation, when, as Hartmann (1965) suggested, mental representations of the mother become intrapsychically available. Fraiberg reviewed the concept of object constancy in its libidinal and cognitive aspects, distinguishing between the formation of the libidinal tie during the 1st year and the attainment of object constancy, which requires the development of crucial cognitive structures. Evocative memory, demonstrable in the middle of the 2nd year, is probably a necessary, though not sufficient, condition for the child's awareness that the loved figure from whom he or she is separated has not been lost. Object permanence and mental representation in Piaget's sense, occurring at around 18 months, appear to be cognitive predecessors for the development of object constancy in the psychoanalytic sense.

Anxiety at separation, however, is not necessarily traumatic. The concept of anxiety as a signal affect through which adaptive and defensive mechanisms are prepared and mobilized is relevant. If not overwhelming at a given point, anxiety sharpens perception of the self and others and of the ways in which challenges can be met, thus contributing to personality organization and health.

Contributions from Other Developmental Psychologies

Other psychological theorists and investigators have contributed constructs that have heuristic value in views of separation and deprivation. Escalona (1963), in bringing together aspects of ego psychology, and Lewin and Piaget's studies of the development of intelligence, says,

My data suggest the possibility that what Piaget proposes for cognition is true of all adaptive aspects of mental functioning: namely, that the emergence of such functions as communication, modulation of affect, control over excitation, delay and aspects of object relations, and hence identification; all are the result of a developmental sequence in sensory motor terms before they merge as ego functions in the narrower sense.

Deprivation experiences in particular would begin to exert a noxious effect on these adaptive functions from early on. De Carie (1965) demonstrated a significant correlation between stages of affectivity and Piaget's theory of cognitive constructions of the inanimate object. Bell (1970) found that infants develop a concept of a person's independent existence (person permanence) even more quickly than a homologous concept of inanimate objects, findings that reflect Piaget's realization of the emotional importance of the mother. Piaget saw affectivity as the energy source upon which the full functioning of intelligence depends. Neither can exist functionally without the other. Emotional processes can accelerate, delay, or disturb mental acquisitions (De Carie, 1978). Concepts of recognitory versus evocative memory, means-end relationships, time and space, progression from prerepresentational sensorimotor schemes to representational and symbolic thinking, verbal communication, fantasy, and perception of reality are among other cognitive constructs found useful in examining issues of the effect of deprivation and separation experiences.

PREVENTION AND TREATMENT

The rapidly growing literature on early intervention programs addresses effectiveness of treatment, as well as its method, and these programs vary widely in sponsorship, types of problems addressed, and theoretical orientation of those who conduct them. In general, clinically oriented programs can be classified as (*a*) those directed primarily at strengthening or supporting families in their child-rearing functions (i.e., caregiver-focused services), (*b*) those that provide direct services to the child with little or much parent involvement, (*c*) those whose focus is on simultaneous work with parent and child, aimed at facilitating the relationship between them, and (*d*) those that take place in extrafamilial settings. One model of caregiver-focused intervention is the parent as recipient of developmental guidance, a generally educative model, but also conceived as a process in which facts and information are provided in the context of a working relationship and in accordance with what parents are ready to hear and able to use. The assumption is that such guidance will enhance parental ability to function more competently and comfortably as parents for the child in question (Seitz and Provence, 1990). Three models of work with parent and infant simultaneously or conjointly illustrate the use of the child's presence as a catalyst for change primarily in the parent. The child's development, actions, and reactions during the sessions facilitate and shape the direction of the work. For example, the method of parent-infant psychotherapy created by Fraiberg and her colleagues (Fraiberg et al., 1980, 1981; Pawl and Pekarsky, 1983) is directed at alleviation of severe conflict between parent and infant/toddler, in which the infant's development has been adversely affected. Experience with this method shows that it can be used in a broad range of cases. Emotional support, interpretation, nondidactic guidance, and counseling are integral to the process.

The Tripartite Therapeutic Design developed by Mahler (1968), in which parent and therapist join in the treatment of the psychotic child, engages the parent in an emotional-intellectual learning experience that permits her or him to sustain the corrective experiences for the child. This method has more recently been effectively utilized in other kinds of cases, for example, in young children with severe hearing impairments in which there are problems of social and emotional communication between child and parent (Fields et al., in press). Still another is the Parent-Infant Interaction Model (Bromwich, 1981), which focuses on the process of attachment. It is the role of the intervention to assess the nature of the interaction and to enable infant and parent to behave more reciprocally and with mutual enjoyment. The consequences of a positive outcome in the short-term can have long-range benefits, primarily because of an increase in the sensitivity and self-confidence of the parent (Provence and Naylor, 1983).

Preschool children and their parents are also treated in the conventional child psychiatry modes, in which simultaneous work with child and parent is carried out with careful attention to its coordination. Treating toddlers and young children singly or in small groups and mother-toddler groups are other useful and effective methods of treatment. For the very young, psychotherapy has a considerable educational component directed at enhancing autonomous ego functions but with careful attention to its appropriateness in the child's emotional life (Dahl, 1983; Pruett, 1983).

Home Care for Troubled Families in Crisis

Since the mid-1970s efforts have been intensified to prevent the breakup of families and placement of children in foster care and to promote family reunification through around-the-clock response to trou-

bled families. The Tacoma Homebuilders model (Kinney, 1978; Kinney et al., 1977), utilizing teams of professionals, was a successful effort that has been replicated or adapted for use elsewhere, often under public auspices (Schorr, 1988). The advantages of improving family functioning to avoid the many separations experienced by infants and young children in the foster care system is obvious. Paraprofessional home visitors backed up by professionals have also demonstrated success (Adnopoz, 1993). Services for the children that specifically address their psychosocial as well as educational and health needs are essential to the success of such efforts in order that the impact of the deprivation and traumatic experiences that are common in troubled families be minimized. This requires sustained efforts to coordinate community services.

Foster Home Care

Foster care, as part of the child welfare system, is so overburdened that for many children it is perceived by professionals as a sentence to certain emotional damage and disability. That families willing to care for a child not their own would be sought as a next-best choice to the child's own family makes eminently good sense, and there are children who have been well served by marvelous foster parents. What has caused great alarm, however, is the frequency of multiple placements, long periods in limbo awaiting decisions about custody or for rehabilitation of dysfunctional parents, the inability of some foster parents to encourage a close relationship with the foster child, and, in some instances, neglect and abuse of foster children. Separation and deprivation are dangers found in situations leading to foster home placement in children of all ages. One of the most urgent needs is for timely and targeted assistance to families in trouble, to prevent their disintegration as child-rearing environments through a spectrum of family support services. Another is to recognize that the passage of time while an infant or young child is in a "temporary" situation can become a great enemy. Clinics, child welfare, mental health services (unless they define themselves as crisis oriented), and, surely, the judicial system have their own rhythms and calendars, not geared to prompt and constructive response to the compelling needs of the very young, in spite of laudable intentions. Whatever can be done to persuade the various systems involved that the dangers of physical and sexual abuse are not the only situations deserving prompt mobilization of services for children or a particular child will make for improvement in the current scene (Goldstein et al., 1979).

Day Care

The growth of the demand for child day care in recent years is staggering. At least half of the mothers of preschool children are in the labor force, and day care for infants under 1 year of age is the fastest growing segment. Much of day care is informally arranged with relatives or neighbors in family settings and is dependent on the parents' assessments of its appropriateness for their child. Licensed day care centers and registered or licensed family day care homes vary widely in the quality of care they provide. In spite of sound knowledge about the major characteristics of developmentally appropriate day care (Neubauer, 1974; Prescott et al., 1972; Sale and Torres, 1971) and about the training needs of child care providers, many children are in day care of poor quality. States vary widely in their regulations about such things as staff:child ratios and qualifications of providers, and there are as yet no national standards for day care. At its best, day care in center and family settings can be supportive of parents and child in spite of the strain that separation imposes (Bredekamp, 1986; Pawl, 1990; Provence et al., 1977). When the care is not at least reasonably good or, even in good programs, not individualized, there can be substantial interference in healthy development. Because for the infant and toddler in day care separation is a major issue, measures that minimize the stress of separation are very important. To mention just a few, there are the following: commitment to a partnership between parent and day care provider on behalf of the child, which involves good communication and mutual respect and a willingness to exchange information that facilitates the child's use of the program and supports the parent-child relationship; the provision of caregivers and teachers whose qualities encourage the infant to establish the trusting and friendly relationships that enhance social/emotional communication and alleviate the stress of separation; provision of a program of care and education anchored in knowledge of child development, which, among other advantages, enhances general learning and the child's ability to cope with inner and outer demands and stimulates intellectual growth.

Day care research studies support both sides of the question of whether it supports or impedes the young child's development. The reality is that day care is here to stay for the foreseeable future, and the urgent tasks are those of seeing to it that its advantages, on the whole, outweigh the disadvantages. For the mental health professional there is no way to avoid the careful individualization of advice, based on a unique child, his or her unique family, and its situation in the society. In addition, there are opportunities to serve as expert consultants regarding individual day care children with problems and as advisors to staff about program content and working relationships.

Head Start

One of the few early childhood programs that has been valued and supported by successive administrations of the United States government since 1965, Head Start is regarded as an important program for poor children. Through the provision of education, health, and social services, beginning as a component of President Johnson's War on Poverty, it has aimed to enable the child to make a successful start at school. Now deeply embedded, it has demonstrated the advantages of a strong commitment by parents, citizen groups, and a broad array of professionals, and grass-roots enthusiasm. The long-term benefits of Head Start are well documented and are manifested particularly in greater school success (Zigler and Muenchow, 1992; Zigler and Styt, 1993). Improvement in social competence and motivation are regarded as more important than changes in IQ scores, and the involvement with families is as integral to the program's success as the services for the children (Schorr, 1988; Zigler and Valentine, 1979).

Mental health services in Head Start leave much to be desired, in spite of policies and guidelines that made them part of the program. They have been less visible, less valuable, and less adequately funded than other components (Cohen et al., 1979). As a result, Head Start children suffering from emotional or behavioral problems have not always received the service they need. Current efforts to improve this situation through revised guidelines and improved funding are progressing. Most recently, the expansion of Head Start to include more children is under way, as well as the downward extension to include infants and children under age 3 years.

Group Residential Care

There is reason to believe that, in the spectrum of services required to care for vulnerable infants and young children, the group residential setting has a place. As a temporary place for healthy infants without families, a residential setting *of good quality* can be used to avoid "bouncing" from one foster home to another while a permanent placement or restoration to the infant's own family is worked out. In addition, as a therapeutic environment for infants impaired by drugs, repeated traumatic experiences, and other conditions that render them extremely difficult to be effectively cared for in families, a group residential setting may be the treatment of choice.

Such care must be organized as an active therapeutic program which includes carefully designed, individualized treatment, as well as general developmentally appropriate care. The duration of residential care for each child should be determined by the time at which he is judged to be healthy enough and well-organized enough (at whatever level) that home care by parents or foster parents has a good chance of success (Provence, 1989).

That such a position is advocated by one of the authors whose studies of infants in institutions spoke strongly against such care (Provence and Lipton, 1962) is a measure of the growing need for alternative solutions for caring for children who cannot be maintained in their own families. It is also a realization that group residential care, in and of itself, does not have to be damaging. It appears to be a much-needed service at this time, and the knowledge of how to create a facilitating environment for infants and young children is advanced enough to make a strong argument for residential care in the spectrum of clinically sound services.

TREATING OUTCOMES

Treatment outcomes in the short-term are relatively easy to evaluate in infants and young children in terms of improvement across a number of developmental and behavioral domains. Judgments about the extent to which the type of treatment chosen and its specific elements have brought about change is not a simple matter. Long-term outcomes of treatment are even more difficult to evaluate. Nevertheless, the aggregation of individual carefully studied cases as well as epidemiological studies and evaluation of the later status of participants in early intervention programs will continue to inform the mental health field. The effectiveness of early childhood programs for socioeconomically disadvantaged infants and young children is now well established, including their long-term benefits. But long-term outcomes, important in understanding the natural history of syndromes, should not determine the development of treatment programs. It is enough that we can recognize the need of a young child and family for psychotherapeutic and supportive services and have at hand clinically sound rationales and methods of carrying them out.

FUTURE RESEARCH DIRECTIONS

Continuing developmental research, basic and applied, in laboratory and clinical settings, in almost any special field one can imagine, will contribute to further understanding of early development and the impact of separation. A trend of particular importance is in the acknowledgment of complexity in developmental processes and the trend away from isolation of variables and pursuit of linear concepts of causality toward the study of concurrent and interactive effects of multiple variables and the formulation of nonlinear concepts of causality (Sander, 1980). Studies of normal and deviant development in a variety of settings can only benefit from such an approach.

CONCLUSIONS

Studies of children's response to separation and loss inherently involve notions of risk and vulnerability and are fundamentally about the interaction between children's endowment and their parenting environment. To return to the beginning: Werner's (1990) report on protective factors and individual resilience—the positive counterparts of vulnerability and risk—summarizes major studies in this area. In her own longitudinal study of the children of Kauai, protective as well as risk factors were identified. "The majority of resilient boys and girls were characterized by their caregivers as very active, affectionate, cuddly, good-natured, and easy to deal with, when they were infants." All elicited a great deal of warmth from their caregivers. Similar reports regarding resilient children (Murphy, 1987) in middle-class families describe notable responsiveness to people and objects. Secure attachments to another family member were found in alert, responsive infants of abusive mothers (Farber and Egeland, 1987). Resilient infants appear to successfully elicit positive attention, tend to be active, alert, and sociable, and have experienced nurturance and learned to trust its availability (Werner, 1990).

In the contexts of secure, stable, loving relations, infants and children are more able to respond to separations, brief and long, in developmentally adaptive and facilitating ways that lead to adaptive coping, structure formation, and healthy defenses. In these contexts, separations prime the child's psychological immune system, allowing him to accommodate to the experiential viruses of the real world. Persistent distress, as in repeated moves from one foster home to another, predispose to failure in developing the ability to feel safe and secure with others or when alone, to enjoy reciprocity, or to be able to tolerate normal frustra-

tions. Such distress is heightened in the face of biologic impairments, chronic illness, parental discord, psychiatric impairment, and inconsistent care. What constitutes a normal, immunizing dose and what overwhelms the mental adaptive immune system remain crucial questions for understanding the growth promoting and inhibiting factors involved in separation and loss.

References

Adnopoz J: Reaching out: The experience of a family support agency. In: Fenichel E, Provence S (eds): *Development in Jeopardy: Clinical Responses to Infants and Families*. Madison, CT, International Universities Press, 1993.

Ainsworth MDS: Patterns in attachment behavior shown by the infant in interaction with his mother. *Merrill-Palmer Q* 10:51, 1964.

Ainsworth MDS: The effects of maternal deprivation: A review of findings and controversy in the context of research strategy. In: *Deprivation of Maternal Care: A Reassessment of Its Effects* (Public Health Paper no. 14). Geneva, World Health Organization, 1972.

Ainsworth MDS: Attachment and child abuse. In: Gerbner G, Ross C, Zigler E (eds): *Child Abuse: An Agenda for Action*. New York, Oxford University Press, 1980, pp. 35–47.

Ainsworth MDS, Wittig BA: Attachment and exploratory behavior of one-year-olds in a strange situation. In: Foss BM (ed): *Determinants of Infant Behavior*. London, Methuen, 1969.

Ainsworth MDS, Blehar M, Waters E, et al: *Patterns of Attachment: A Psychological Study of the Strange Situation*. Hillsdale, NJ, Erlbaum, 1978.

Anthony EJ: A risk-vulnerability intervention model for children of psychotic parents. In: Anthony EJ, Koupernik C (eds): *The Child in His Family: Children at Psychiatric Risk*. New York, Wiley, 1974, pp. 99–121.

Bell S: The development of the concept of object as related to infant-mother attachment. *Child Dev* 41: 291, 1970.

Benjamin JD: Some developmental observations relating to the theory of anxiety. *J Am Psychoanal Assoc* 9:652, 1961.

Benjamin JD: Further comments on some developmental aspects of anxiety. In: Gaskill H (ed): *Counterpoint: Libidinal Object and Subject*. New York, International Universities Press, 1963, pp. 121–153.

Bergman P, Escalona SK: Unusual sensitivities in very young children. *Psychoanal Study Child* 3: 333, 1949.

Bloom-Feshbach S: From family to classroom: Variations in adjustment to nursery school. In: Bloom-Feshbach J, Bloom-Feshbach S (eds): *The Psychology of Separation and Loss*. San Francisco, Jossey-Bass, 1987, pp. 207–231.

Bloom-Feshbach J, Bloom-Feshbach S (eds): *The Psychology of Separation and Loss*. San Francisco, Jossey-Bass, 1987.

Bornstein MH: Between caregivers and their young: Two modes of interaction and their consequences for cognitive growth. In: Bornstein MH, Bruner JS (ed): *Interaction in Human Development*. Hillsdale, NJ, Erlbaum, 1989, pp. 197–214.

Bowlby J: *Maternal Care and Mental Health* (Monograph no. 2). Geneva, World Health Organization, 1951.

Bowlby J: The nature of the child's tie to his mother. *Int J Psychoanal* 39:350, 1958.

Bowlby J: Grief and mourning in infancy and early childhood. *Psychoanal Study Child* 15:9, 1960.

Bowlby J: Processes of mourning. *Int J Psychoanal* 42:317, 1961.

Bowlby J: *Attachment and Loss*. Vol 1: *Attachment*. New York, Basic Books, 1969.

Bowlby J: *Attachment and Loss*. Vol 2: *Separation, Anxiety and Anger*. New York, Basic Books, 1973.

Bowlby J: *Attachment and Loss*. Vol 3: *Loss, Sadness, and Depression*. New York, Basic Books, 1980.

Brazelton TB, Cramer BG: *The Earliest Relationship: Parents, Infants and the Drama of Early Attachment*. Reading, MA, Addison-Wesley, 1990.

Bredekamp S (ed): *Developmentally Appropriate Practice*. Washington, DC, National Association for the Education of Young Children, 1986.

Bretherton I: Attachment theory: Retrospect and prospect. *Monogr Soc Res Child Dev* serial no. 209, 1985.

Bromwich RM: *Working with Parents and Infants: An Interactional Approach*. Baltimore, University Park Press, 1981.

Carlson V, Cicchetti D, Barnett D, et al: Disorganized/disoriented attachment relationships in maltreated infants. *Dev Psychol* 25:525–531, 1989.

Chapin HD: A plan of dealing with atrophic infants and children. *Arch Pediatr* 25:491, 1908.

Chapin HD: Are institutions for infants necessary? *JAMA* 64:103, 1915.

Chasnoff I, Schnoll S, Burns WI, et al: Maternal non-narcotic abuse during pregnancy: Effects on infant development. *Neurobehav Toxicol Teratol* 6: 277, 1984.

Chatoor I, Eagan J: Nonorganic failure to thrive and dwarfism due to food refusal: A separation disorder. *J Am Acad Child Psychiatry* 22:294, 1983.

Chatoor I, Schaefer S, Dickson L, et al: A developmental approach to feeding disturbances: Failure to thrive and growth disorders in infants and young children. *Zero to Three* 5:3, 1985.

Cohen DJ, Solnit AJ, Wolford P: Mental health services in Head Start. In: Zigler E, Valentine J (eds): *Project Head Start: A Legacy of the War on Poverty*. New York, Free Press, 1979, pp. 259–282.

Coleman RW, Provence S: Environmental retardation (hospitalism) in infants living in families. *Pediatrics* 11:288, 1953.

Condon W, Sander L: Synchrony demonstrated between movements of the neonate and adult speech. *Child Dev* 45:456, 1975.

Dahl EK: The therapist as decoder: Psychotherapy with toddlers. In: Provence S (ed): *Infants and Parents. Clinical Case Reports*. New York, International Universities Press, 1983, pp. 213–245.

De Carie TG: *Intelligence and Affectivity in Early Childhood: An Experimental Study of Jean Piaget's Object Concept and Object Relations*. New York, International Universities Press, 1965.

De Carie TG: Affect development and cognition in a Piagetian context. In: Lewis M, Rosenblum LA (eds): *The Development of Affect*. New York, Plenum, 1978, pp. 183–204.

Drotar D: Research and practice in failure to thrive: The state of the art. *Zero to Three* 3:1, 1985.

Easterbrooks MA, Davidson CE, Chazan R: Psychosocial risk, attachment, and behavior problems among school-aged children. *Dev Psychopathol* 5: 389–402, 1993.

Escalona SK: Patterns of infantile experience and the developmental process. *Psychoanal Study Child* 18:197, 1963.

Escalona SK: *The Roots of Individuality*. Chicago, Aldine, 1968.

Farber EA, Egeland B: Invulnerability among abused and neglected children. In: Anthony EJ, Cohler B (eds): *The Invulnerable Child*. New York, Guilford, 1987, pp. 253–288. Fendrick M, Warner V, Weissman M: Family risk factors, parental depression, and psychopathology in offspring. *Dev Psychol* 26:40–50, 1990.

Ferholt J, Provence S: Diagnosis and treatment of an infant with psychophysiological vomiting. *Psychoanal Study Child* 31:439, 1976.

Field TM: Psychologically depressed parents. In: Bornstein MH (ed): *Handbook of Parenting*. Vol III: *Status and Social Conditions of Parenting*. Hillsdale, NJ, Erlbaum, 1995.

Fields B, Bum E, Scharfman H: Mental health intervention with very young children and their parents: A model based on the infant deal? In: Provence S (ed): *A Stitch in Time: Clinical Responses to Infants and Families*. Madison, CT, International Universities Press, in press.

Fraiberg S: Libidinal object constancy and mental representation. *Psychoanal Study Child* 24:9, 1969.

Fraiberg S: *Insights from the Blind: Comparative Studies of Blind and Sighted Infants*. New York, Basic Books, 1977.

Fraiberg S, Adelson E, Shapiro V: Ghosts in the nursery: A psychoanalytic approach to the problems of impaired infant-mother relationships. In: Fraiberg S (ed): *Clinical Studies in Infant Mental Health*. New York, Basic Books, 1980, pp. 164–196.

Fraiberg S, Lieberman AF, Pekarsky JH, et al: Treatment and outcome in an infant psychiatry program. Part I. *J Prev Psychiatry* 1:89, 1981.

Freedman DA: Speech, language and the vocal-auditory connection. *Psychoanal Study Child* 36:105, 1981.

Freud A: Discussion of Dr. John Bowlby's paper. *Psychoanal Study Child* 15:53, 1960.

Freud S: Inhibition, symptoms, and anxiety. In: Strachey J (ed): *The Standard Edition of the Complete Psychological Works of Sigmund Freud* (Vol 20). London, Hogarth, 1959, pp. 87–174. (Originally published 1926.)

Gaensbauer TJ, Harmon RI: Attachment behavior in abused/neglected and premature infants: Implications for the concept of attachment. In: Emde RN, Harmon RJ (eds): *Attachment and Affiliative Systems*. New York, Plenum, 1982, pp. 245–279.

Goldberg S: Recent developments in attachment theory and research. *Can J Psychiatry* 36:393–400, 1991.

Goldstein J, Freud A, Solnit AJ: *Before the Best Interests of the Child*. New York, Free Press, 1979.

Greenacre P: Early physical determinants in the development of identity. In: Greenacre P (ed): *Emotional Growth: Psychoanalytic Studies of the Gifted and a Variety of Other Individuals* (Vol 1). New York, International Universities Press, 1971, pp. 113–127.

Greenspan SI: *Psychopathology and Adaptation in Infancy and Early Childhood: Principles of Clinical Diagnosis and Prevention Intervention*. New York, International Universities Press, 1981.

Greenspan SI, Lieberman AF: A clinical approach to attachment. In: Belsky J, Nezworski T (eds): *Clinical Implications of Attachment*. Hillsdale, NJ, Erlbaum, 1988.

Harter S, Zigler E: The assessment of effectance motivation in normal and retarded children. *Dev Psychol* 10:169, 1974.

Hartmann H: *Ego Psychology and the Problem of Adaptation*. New York, International Universities Press, 1958.

Hartmann H: The mutual influences in the development of the ego and the id. In: Hartmann H (ed): *Essays in Ego Psychology: Selected Problems in Psychoanalytic Theory*. New York, International Universities Press, 1965. (Originally published 1952.)

Howard J, Beckwith L, Rodning C, et al: The development of young children of substance-abusing parents: Insights from seven years of intervention and research. *Zero to Three* 5:8, 1989.

Jones CL, Lopez R: *Direct and Indirect Effects on the Infant of Maternal Drug Abuse*. Washington, DC, US Department of Health and Human Services, National Institutes of Health, 1988.

Kinney JM: Homebuilders: An in-home crisis intervention program. *Child Today* 7:15, 1978.

Kinney JM, Madsen B, Fleming T, et al: Homebuilders: Keeping families together. *J Consult Clin Psychol* 45:667, 1977.

Korner AF: Individual differences at birth: Implications for child care practices. In: Bergsma D (ed): *The Infant at Risk*. New York, International Medical Book Corporation, 1974, pp. 51–61.

Kris E: Decline and recovery in the life of a three year old. *Psychoanal Study Child* 17:175, 1962.

Lewis MM: *How Children Learn to Speak*. New York, Basic Books, 1959.

Lieberman A: Separation in infancy and early childhood: Contributions of attachment theory and psychoanalysis. In: Bloom-Feshbach J, Bloom-Feshbach S (eds): *The Psychology of Separation and Loss*. San Francisco, Jossey-Bass, 1987, pp. 109–135.

Loewald HW: Book review: Heinz Kohut, The Analysis of the Self. In: *Papers on Psychoanalysis*. New Haven, CT, Yale University Press, 1980.

Mahler MS: Certain aspects of the separation-individuation phase. *Psychoanal Q* 32:1, 1963.

Mahler MS: Notes on the development of basic moods: The depressive affect. In: Loewenstein RM, Newman LM, Schur M, et al (eds): *Psychoanalysis—A General Psychology: Essays in Honor of Heinz Hartmann*. New York, International Universities Press, 1966, pp. 152–168.

Mahler MS: *On Human Symbiosis and the Vicissitudes of Individuation*. Vol 1: *Infantile Psychosis*. New York, International Universities Press, 1968.

Mahler MS, Pine F, Bergmann A: *The Psychological Birth of the Human Infant*. New York, Basic Books, 1975.

Main M, Hesse E: Parents' unresolved traumatic experiences are related to infant disorganized attachment status: Is frightened or frightening behavior the linking mechanism? In: Greenberg M, Cicchetti D, Cummings EM (eds): *Attachment in the Preschool Years: Theory, Research, and Intervention*. Chicago, University of Chicago Press, 1990.

Main M, Solomon J: Procedures for identifying infants as disorganized/disoriented during the Ainsworth Strange Situation. In: Greenberg MT, Cicchetti D, Cummings EM (eds): *Attachment in the Preschool Years*. Chicago, University of Chicago Press, 1990.

Main M, Kaplan N, Cassidy J: Security in infancy, childhood, and adulthood: A move to the level of representation. *Monogr Soc Res Child Dev* 50: 6–104, 1985.

Matas L, Arend RA, Sroufe LA: Continuity and adaptation in the second year: The relationship between quality of attachment and later competence. *Child Dev* 49:549–556, 1978.

Mayes LC: Alcoholic and drug abusing parents. In: Bornstein MH (ed): *The Handbook of Parenting*, in press.

Mayes LC, Volkmar F: Nosology of eating and growth disorders in early childhood. *Child Adolesc Psychiatr Clin North Am* 2:15–35, 1993.

Murphy LB: Coping, vulnerability and resilience in childhood. In: Coehlo GV, Hamburg DA, Adams JE (eds): *Coping and Adaptation*. New York, Basic Books, 1974, pp. 69–100.

Murphy LB: Further reflections on resilience. In: Anthony EJ, Cohler B (eds): *The Vulnerable Child*. New York, Guilford, 1987, pp. 84–105.

Nagera H: Sleep and its disturbances approached developmentally. *Psychoanal Study Child* 21:393, 1966.

Neubauer P (ed): *Early Child Day Care*. New York, Aronson, 1974.

Patton RG, Gardner LI: *Growth Failure in Maternal Deprivation*. Springfield, IL, Charles C Thomas, 1963.

Pawl J: Infants in day care: Reflections on experiences, expectations and relationships. *Zero to Three* 3:1, 1990.

Pawl JH, Pekarsky JH: Infant-parent psychotherapy: A family in crisis. In: Provence S (ed): *Infants and Parents: Clinical Case Reports*. New York, International Universities Press, 1983, pp. 39–84.

Piaget J: *The Origins of Intelligence in Children*. New York, International Universities Press, 1952.

Piaget J, Inhelder B: *The Psychology of the Child*. New York, Basic Books, 1969.

Prescott E, Jones E, Kritchevsky S: *Day Care as a Child Rearing Environment* (Vol 2). Washington, DC, National Association for the Education of Young Children, 1972.

Provence S: Disturbed personality development in infancy: A comparison of two inadequately nurtured infants. *Merrill-Palmer Q* 2:149, 1965.

Provence S: Struggling against deprivation and trauma. *Psychoanal Study Child* 38:233, 1983.

Provence S: Psychoanalytic views of separation in infancy and early childhood. In: Bloom-Feshbach J, Bloom-Feshbach S (eds): *The Psychology of Separation and Loss*. San Francisco, Jossey-Bass, 1987, pp. 87–108.

Provence S: Infants in institutions revisited. *Zero to Three* 9:3, 1989.

Provence S, Lipton R: *Infants in Institutions*. New York, International Universities Press, 1962.

Provence S, Naylor AK: *Working with Disadvantaged Parents and Their Children: Scientific and Practice Issues*. New Haven, CT, Yale University Press, 1983.

Provence S, Naylor AK, Patterson JM: *The Challenge of Daycare*. New Haven, CT, Yale University Press, 1977.

Pruett KD: Babies everywhere: Accessing and tracking a toddler's pervasive developmental disorder. In: Provence S (ed): *Infants and Parents: Clinical Case Reports*. New York, International Universities Press, 1983, pp. 177–212.

Robertson J, Bowlby J: Responses of young children to separation from their mothers. *Courr Centre Int L'Enfance* 2:131, 1952.

Sale JS, Torres YL: *I'm Not Just a Sitter. A Descriptive Report of the Community Family Day Care Project*. Pasadena, CA, Pacific Oaks College, 1971.

Sander L: Investigating the infant and its caregiving environment. In: Greenspan SI, Pollock GA: *The Course of Life: Psychoanalytic Contributions toward Understanding Personality Development*. Vol I: *Infancy and Early Childhood*. Washington, DC, National Institute of Mental Health, 1980, pp. 177–201.

Schorr LB: *Within Our Reach: Breaking the Cycle of Disadvantage*. New York, Anchor Press-Doubleday, 1988.

Seitz V, Provence S: Caregiver-focused models of early intervention. In: Meisels SJ, Shonkoff JP (eds): *Handbook of Early Childhood Intervention*. New York, Cambridge University Press, 1990, pp. 400–427.

Settlage CF: Danger signals in the separation-individuation process: The observations and formulations of Margaret S. Mahler. In: Bergsma D (ed): *The Infant at Risk*. New York, International Medical Book Corp., 1974, pp. 63–75.

Shonkoff JP, Marshall PC: Biological bases of developmental dysfunction. In: Meisels SJ, Shonkoff JP (eds): *Handbook of Early Childhood Intervention*. New York, Cambridge University Press, 1990, pp. 35–52.

Solnit AJ: Developmental perspectives on self and object constancy. *Psychoanal Study Child* 37: 201, 1982.

Spitz R: Hospitalism: An inquiry into the genesis of psychiatric conditions in early childhood. *Psychoanal Study Child* 1:53, 1945.

Spitz RA: *No and Yes: On the Beginnings of Human Communication*. New York, International Universities Press, 1957.

Spitz RA: *The First Year of Life: A Psychoanalytic Study of Normal and Deviant Development of Object Relations*. New York, International Universities Press, 1965.

Spitz R, Wolf KM: Anaclitic depression: An inquiry into the genesis of psychiatric conditions in early childhood. *Psychoanal Study Child* 2:313, 1946.

Sroufe LA, Fox N, Pancake V: Attachment and dependency in the developmental perspective. *Child Dev* 54:1335–1354, 1983.

Sroufe LA, Egeland B, Kreutzer T: The fate of early experience following developmental change: Longitudinal approaches to individual adaptation in childhood. *Child Dev* 61:1363–1373, 1990.

Talbot NB, Sobel EA, Burke BS, et al: Dwarfism in healthy children: Its possible relation to emotional, nutritional and endocrine disturbances. *N Engl J Med* 236:783, 1947.

Thoman EB, Browder S: *Born Dancing: How Intuitive Parents Understand Their Baby's Unspoken Language and Natural Rhythms*. New York, Harper & Row, 1987.

Thomas A, Chess S: *Temperament and Development*. New York, Brunner/Mazel, 1977.

Tibbits-Kleber AL, Howell RJ: Reactive attachment disorder of infancy. *J Clin Child Psychol* 14: 301–310, 1985.

Tucker MB: A descriptive and comparative analysis of the social support structure of heroin addicted women. *Addicted Women: Family Dynamics, Self-Perceptions, and Support Systems*. Washington, DC, National Institute on Drug Abuse, Superintendent of Documents, US Government Printing Office, 1979, pp. 37–76.

Van IJzendoorn MH, Kroonenberg PM: Cross cultural patterns of attachment: A meta-analysis of the strange situation. *Child Dev* 59:147–156, 1988.

Volkmar F, Provence S: *Disorders of Affect* (Yale Child Study Center Working Paper). New Haven, CT, Yale Child Study Center, 1990.

Waters E: The stability of individual differences in infant-mother attachment. *Child Dev* 49:483–494, 1978.

Waters E, Wippman J, Sroufe LA: Attachment, positive affect, and competence in peer group: Two studies in construct validation. *Child Dev* 50: 821–829, 1979.

Weitzman J, Cook RE: Attachment theory and clinical implications for at-risk children. *Child Psychiatry Hum Dev* 17:95, 1986.

Werner EE: Protective factors and individual resilience. In: Meisels SJ, Shonkoff JP (eds): *Handbook of Early Childhood Intervention*. New York, Cambridge University Press, 1990, pp. 97–116.

White B: Critical influences in the origins of competence. *Merrill-Palmer Q* 21:243, 1975.

White RW: Motivation reconsidered: The concept of competence. *Psychol Rev* 66:297, 1959.

Winnicott DW: The theory of the parent-infant relationship. *Int J Psychoanal* 41:585, 1961.

Woolston JL: Eating disorders in infancy and early childhood. *J Am Acad Child Psychiatry* 22:11, 1983.

Yarrow LJ: Maternal deprivation: Toward an empirical and conceptual reevaluation. *Psychol Bull* 58: 459, 1961.

Yarrow LJ: Beyond cognition: The development of mastery motivation. *Zero to Three* 1:3, 1981.

Yarrow LJ, Pederson FA: The interplay between cognition and motivation in infancy. In: Lewis M (ed): *Origins of Intelligence*. New York, Plenum, 1976.

Zigler E, Valentine J (eds): *Project Head Start: A Legacy of the War on Poverty*. New York, Free Press, 1979.

Zigler E, Muenchow S: *Head Start: The Inside Story of America's Most Successful Educational Achievement*. New York, Basic Books, 1992.

Zigler E, Styt S: *Head Start and Beyond: A National Plan for Extended Child Intervention*. New Haven, Yale University Press, 1993.

33 GRIEF

Elizabeth B. Weller, M.D., Ronald A. Weller, M.D., and Julie J. Wiltsie Pugh, B.A.

The death of a close friend or relative is one of the most difficult and stressful events in life. The experience is even more difficult when the bereaved individual is a child who has lost a parent. The child is not only emotionally attached to the parent but also financially dependent upon him or her; thus, both emotional and financial hardships are worked on the growing child when he or she loses a parent.

Bereavement is not uncommon in children. Four percent of children in the United States will lose a parent by age 15, according to *Statistical Abstracts of the United States* (1985). Thus, approximately 1.2 million children are affected. Despite this fact, there are very few methodologically sound prospective studies that examine how grief affects these children and what needs they may have. The factors that may promote their well-being and coping as well as those that may lead to poor outcomes, such as depression, drug or alcohol abuse, or just being inadequate or dysfunctional as adults, have not been fully examined (Osterweis et al., 1984).

In a discussion of grief, several terms should be defined. Usually bereavement is defined as a separation or detachment that leaves one destitute. It refers to the physical separation from the deceased. Grief is the emotional pain or anguish one feels after the loss of a loved one. Anticipatory grief is a similar emotional pain that may occur prior to the impending death. It might be experienced before the expected loss of a loved one from a terminal illness such as cancer. Mourning is somewhat different from grief. According to Bowlby (1961a, 1980), it is defined as the psychological processes that are set in motion by the loss of a loved object that commonly lead to the relinquishment of the object.

DSM-IV

According to DSM-IV (American Psychiatric Association, 1994), normal grief is not considered a psychiatric diagnosis (Table 33.1). Instead it is considered a V Code condition. V Code diagnoses are conditions that may be a focus of clinical attention, but are not attributable to any of the mental disorders. According to DSM-IV, in some instances a thorough evaluation has failed to uncover any mental disorder; in other instances, the scope of the diagnostic evaluation has not been adequate to determine the presence of a mental disorder, but there is a need to note the reason for contact with the mental health care system. The DSM-IV suggests that at times, with further information, the presence of a mental disorder may become apparent. In adults a full depressive syndrome is frequently a normal reaction to the death of a close friend or relative. The most common symptoms are insomnia, poor appetite, and weight loss. Morbid preoccupation with worthlessness, prolonged impairment, and marked psychomotor retardation are uncommon symptoms and if present may suggest that the bereavement is complicated by the development of a major depression. The reaction to the loss rarely occurs after 2 or 3 months, and the duration of "normal" bereavement

varies among different cultures. In a classic bereavement study by Clayton and Darvish (1979), 42% of widows were depressed immediately following the death of a spouse; however, by the end of 1 year, only 16% were clinically depressed.

A prime concern for bereaved children is whether such a loss in childhood leads to adult psychopathology. Several studies address this issue from different perspectives; however, there is as yet no clear answer. In studies of psychiatrically disturbed adult patients, there are two schools of thought. The first believes loss of a parent in childhood has a detrimental effect lasting into adulthood. Psychopathology such as depression, schizophrenia, drug abuse, and alcoholism has been attributed to childhood bereavement. However, others believe parental loss in childhood does not contribute to adult psychopathology if children are taken care of by parental substitutes (Osterweis et al., 1984). Breier et al. (1988) concluded that child care following the loss of a parent was a crucial issue in relation to adult psychopathology.

More recent papers have also examined this problem. Breier (1989) found that depressed adults who had experienced a childhood loss had more neuroendocrine abnormalities than those without a childhood loss. Specifically, he reported increased resting plasma levels of cortisol and β-endorphin as compared with subjects who had early loss and no adult history of psychiatric illness. Moreover, increased hypothalamic pituitary axis activity in adulthood was significantly related to poor childhood adjustment to parental loss.

EPIDEMIOLOGY

As stated earlier, 4% of children (1.2 million) lose a parent by age 15. Overall, 2.8% are orphaned by their fathers' death, 1% are orphaned by their mothers' death, and 0.1% experience the death of both parents. Although childhood bereavement is a fairly common occurrence, it has not been studied as well as some conditions that are far more rare. This is in part due to the fact that many want to avoid the topic of death altogether. It is a subject that is very difficult to be objective about. Some have hypothesized that if adults could come to terms with death themselves, they could handle the emotional reaction of their children to death.

A child's reaction to death depends on his or her emotional and cognitive maturity. The understanding of death differs in children according to their maturation. Based on the evaluation of 378 children, Nagy (1948) was able to categorize a child's concept of death as falling into one of three categories based primarily on age. Three- to 5-year-olds look at death as sleep, or a long journey. Five- to 9-year-olds are able to accept the fact that someone can die; however, they don't believe it happens to everyone and especially not to themselves. Nine- to 10-year-olds are able to think of death as inevitable and know it may happen to them.

Studies on the impact of parental death on children can be divided

Table 33.1. Changes in Nomenclature from DSM-III-R to DSM-IV

DSM-III-R	DSM-IV
Uncomplicated bereavement	Bereavement
Adjustment disorder	Adjustment disorder
	Acute <6 months
	Chronic >6 months

into four categories. The first is retrospective studies of psychiatrically ill adults who lost a parent in childhood; the second, prospective studies of psychiatrically ill children who were in psychiatric treatment prior to their parents' death (Furman, 1974; Wolfenstein, 1966). Often these studies have few subjects, so it is difficult to generalize their findings.

A third group of studies consists of three different research groups who studied the same sample of adolescents at different points in time (Bendickson and Fulton, 1976; Gregory, 1965; Markusen and Fulton, 1971). The adolescents were compared to normal control subjects who were recruited at the same time and also followed up at the same intervals. Initially, in the 10th grade the bereaved group had a higher rate of delinquency; in their early twenties the bereaved had more legal offenses; and when studied in their thirties, bereaved subjects had more serious medical illnesses and had less satisfying lives.

The fourth group of studies is prospective in nature. Elizur and Kaffman (1983) studied children 2–10 years old who lived in a kibbutz and lost a parent in a national war. These children often had sleep disturbance, social withdrawal, and restlessness. When compared with age-matched children who had lost a parent but did not live in the kibbutz, living in a kibbutz did not appear to be a protective factor for developing psychiatric symptomatology.

Van Eerdewegh et al. (1982) reported that 2- to 17-year-old children who had lost a father had depressive symptoms, including dysphoria, social withdrawal, sleep disturbance, and anhedonia, especially in those who also had a depressed mother. The shortcoming of this study was that the information was gathered from parents and teachers; children were not interviewed. The child psychiatric literature emphasizes interviewing children especially in affective symptomatology because underreporting of subjective symptoms in children is common when parents alone are interviewed about the child (Weller and Weller, 1984).

CLINICAL DESCRIPTION

A child psychiatrist may be asked to evaluate a child who has lost a loved one to determine if the child is manifesting normal grief and if some intervention is warranted. Unfortunately, there is limited information available from research studies; thus, it is difficult to clearly delineate normal grief from psychopathology at present. In order to provide systematic data to address this issue, the authors are conducting a project sponsored by the National Institute of Mental Health to describe grief in normal parentally bereaved children. Although this study is not yet completed, preliminary data will be presented in the hope of providing some useful information (Weller and Weller, 1990).

In the bereaved prepubertal children studied to date, the most common presentation is sadness and yearning for the dead parent. Prepubertal children often wish to die, so they can see and visit the missing parent. Yet they clearly say they do not want to be dead in the way that a child with major depression does. Suicide attempts are very rare in bereaved children and should be immediately evaluated if they do occur. Sleeping problems, appetite changes, difficulty with concentration, and not having fun in normal activities are common. Frequently parents are not aware of these difficulties. Schools tend to be sympathetic toward the children and will not send them for treatment unless there is a major problem in their academic and social functioning. At times, bereaved children with headaches and stomachaches are taken to pediatricians for evaluation. In adolescents, problems are similar but tend to be less

frequent than those observed in prepubertal bereaved children. However, it is not yet clear whether adolescents actually have fewer symptoms or merely *report* fewer symptoms, as they may be either more hesitant to disclose their discomfort or unwilling to report symptoms that make them appear different from their peers.

A child's reaction and adjustment to a parent's death often appears to be related to the adjustment of the surviving parent. A study done by Weller et al. (1991) compared symptoms between 38 grieving children and 38 depressed children. DSM-IV suggests that thoughts of death such as, "the survivor feeling that he or she would be better off dead or should have died with the deceased person" are normal. Sixty-one percent of the bereaved children and/or parents reported that the child had suicidal ideations, and none actually attempted suicide. Eighty-nine percent of the depressed children reported suicidal ideations, and 42% of them had attempted suicide. Depression and other psychiatric problems in children were predicted by preexisting psychiatric disorder in the child or family history of psychiatric disorders, most often depression, in the surviving parent. The majority of children have their psychiatric symptoms "peak" at 1 month after the death. However, one-third will have peak symptomatology 6 months after the death, and one-sixth will have peak symptoms 1 year after the death (MA Fristad et al., unpublished manuscript).

It is important to be supportive of a family who has had a major loss. This is especially true in the case of a bereaved family with dependent children. In this situation, the surviving parent often becomes depressed, especially if he or she had a predisposing factor (e.g., past history of depression or family history of depression). Bereaved families experience hardships, both financial and emotional. The socioeconomic status of bereaved families will usually decline. This may lead to a move to a neighborhood of a lower socioeconomic level and a change in schools. Also, the surviving parent may choose to move closer to his or her family of origin in order to gain more support. However, as a result, the child gets uprooted from his or her familiar surroundings and will lose his or her friends in addition to losing a parent.

As a practical matter, a grieving child often loses more than the deceased parent. Surviving parents are often engulfed in their own grief and are unable to provide normal parenting. The surviving parent often is the mother (70% of deaths in people with dependent children involve males). As a result of the death, a mother who had not been previously employed outside the home may now have to go to work outside the home in order to support the family. Children tend to resent this, especially when they are asked to do additional chores in the home or have to stay at home alone before or after school while waiting for the working parent to return home. Children may also resent the surviving parent if he or she shows interest in dating or adult companionship. Children may feel this is a betrayal of the dead parent. As children grow and mature, their grief may change in its manifestation. For example, a child whose grief appears to be resolving may show a resurgence of symptoms with an upcoming birthday or graduation ceremony. Adolescents especially tend to grieve over the importance the dead parent would have had in their life (e.g., the bereaved parent will not be present for special events such as their marriage or birth of a child).

CASE ILLUSTRATION

K.G. was an 8-year-old boy who knew his mother was ill with cancer but didn't expect her to die. Two months after the death, he felt "low down in the dumps" and had started to gain weight excessively (10-pound weight gain in 2 months). He had trouble falling asleep and had dreams about his mother. One night he felt his mother was standing over his bed to protect him. He had also lost his energy and was no longer interested in school activities. His grades were dropping because he could not concentrate on his schoolwork, and because he had missed 27 days of school during and after his mother's death. K.G. also missed his half-brother who had lived with him but now moved to live with his biological father.

He complained he had to do more chores at home and that the food his dad cooked was not good. "Mom was the good cook," and dad "was trying hard but wasn't good." He appeared to be a very caring, responsible child who was worrying about the welfare of his father and little sister.

Six months after the death he appeared quite calm. He denied any problems. His interest in activities had returned to normal, and he was looking forward to participating in baseball and was sleeping and eating well. One year after the death, he appeared shy but warmed up quickly. He said he didn't remember his mother very well. He said he had to stay by himself after school until 6 o'clock when his father came home from work. He no longer complained about having additional responsibilities around the home. K.G. had written and illustrated a book about his mother that won a local award.

CASE ILLUSTRATION

M.S. was 14 years old when her father died of lung cancer. She had been anticipating his death for a year. She was the youngest of seven children and was a good student in advanced English and science classes. She was closer to her father than to her mother. When she knew her father was dying, she refused to leave the hospital for 1 week and stayed by his bedside until he died. One month after the death she had dysphoria, loss of interest, insomnia, loss of energy, recurring nightmares, and trouble concentrating. She was also having repeated stomachaches because of "worrying." Menstrual cramps had become worse since her father's death, and her grades dropped in school. She was not sure if her friends understood her feelings and was trying "to be strong for my mother." She was not pleased with her mother's decision to move out of their home "to get away from the memories." Six months after the death, she was not able to talk about her father without crying. She reported her father's death was "a shock," and she was visiting his grave twice a week. Her mother had begun dating, which was upsetting to her. She had no energy and was becoming a loner. She had thoughts of suicide but reported, "I couldn't do it because it would be painful to my mom." She was staying in bed and not going to school because she was unable to fall asleep and was frequently waking up in the middle of the night. She was referred for counseling and possible medication management.

Differential Diagnoses

The DSM-IV clearly differentiates bereavement, which is a V Code, from adjustment disorder with depressed mood. Adjustment disorder with depressed mood usually does not fulfill the criteria for major depression, but significant depressive symptoms are present over a time period of less than 6 months, or over 6 months. DSM-IV categorizes acute adjustment disorder as symptoms lasting less than 6 months after a disturbance, and chronic adjustment disorder occurs when symptoms last for longer than 6 months after a major stressor that has enduring consequences.

As mentioned earlier, following bereavement, all signs and symptoms of depression may occur. The authors' preliminary study found that 37% of bereaved prepubertal children met criteria for depression 1 month after parental death (Weller et al., 1991).

In major depression, suicidal thoughts and attempts are common. In grief, suicidal thought may be present. However, such thoughts usually focus on wanting to reunite with the dead parent and do not involve self-deprecatory thoughts of wanting to no longer exist. Suicide attempts are uncommon in simple grief. Thus, if they occur, they should be brought to immediate psychiatric attention. Anxiety symptoms may occur, but diagnosable anxiety disorders are uncommon immediately after death (Sanchez et al., 1994). Thus, the presence of an anxiety disorder should not be automatically attributed to the grieving process and should be evaluated. Somatic symptoms should be handled in a fashion similar to that for anxiety disorders because somatization in the

bereaved population of children and adolescents is uncommon. When somatic symptoms occur, the most frequent complaints are of headaches and stomachaches, especially in prepubertal children (Sood et al., 1992).

The possibility that conduct disorder may occur has been suggested by Markusen and Fulton (1971). However, further study is needed before the development of conduct disorder can be considered a sequela of bereavement. Clearly, long-term follow-up of a well-defined sample is necessary to look at the long-term sequelae of bereavement.

TREATMENT

If grief is a normal and necessary reaction to the death of a loved one (Bowlby, 1961b, 1980, 1982; Freud, 1966), then intervention may not be necessary. Most people go through the grief process with a painful sense of growth and responsibility. Being a compassionate listener and lending support to grieving families may be all that is necessary for most bereaved families. One of the first decisions a grieving parent has to make is how to inform the children of their parent's death. Such questions arise as who should tell the children, how it should be explained, and should they be allowed to go to the funeral. Previous studies on the advisability of children's attending their parents' funerals are somewhat contradictory. Some believe this is traumatic to the children (Furman, 1974), while others think children should attend (Weller et al., 1989). To answer such questions, Weller et al. (1988b) studied normal prepubertal children shortly after the death of a parent. Most often the surviving parent told their children about the death. Most children wanted to go to the funeral and participated in making arrangements for the funeral. Most children reported that participating in these activities made it easier for them to accept the loss, and that they were glad they attended the funeral.

In explaining death to children, especially very young children, it is important not to compare death to sleep, as this might increase a child's anxiety about whether he or she too might die upon going to sleep. A good explanation would be to describe death as cessation of bodily activities.

Often grieving parents and children find comfort in reading about the subject. Some, but not all, may benefit from self-help groups. Sometimes these groups will combine bereaved and divorced families; however, this combination should usually be avoided. The issues for the two groups can be quite different, and resentment can occur in such combined groups. For example, grieving children tend to be less angry than children from a divorcing family. The grieving child often yearns for the dead parent and wants to remember good times. A grieving child often knows that the dead parent did not choose to part from the child, while a child from a divorced family almost always blames the parents for wanting to part from him or her. A child from a divorced family will often have friends who are from divorced families, whereas fewer children have friends who have lost a parent through death. Hence, it is harder for a grieving child than for a child from a divorcing family to find a peer with whom to identify. A parent should not be pushed to join adult support groups or to put his or her children in similar groups unless the parent chooses to do so and wants to participate.

Individual therapy can be helpful for those who have complicated grief, that is, grief that has become pathological. Individual therapy may help the bereaved work through their grief and achieve a healthy outcome. Family therapy can be helpful for a dysfunctional family where some members are having difficulty adjusting to their loss.

Sleep disturbance and appetite disturbances in adults are symptoms frequently treated by family physicians. However, these are also symptoms of depression. One should make sure that one is not missing a major depression. Most sleep-inducing medications are not good for people who are depressed. An antidepressant might be helpful in a grieving parent who clinically gets depressed and "can't shake it," especially if he or she had a depression preceding the grief that needed pharmacological intervention.

In children and adolescents, there are few data on how to differentiate normal grief from pathological grief. Also, guidelines on when to intervene are lacking. In cases of pathological grief, depression should always be considered. Further, in such situations, extreme caution should be taken to ensure the child is not suicidal or involved in acts that could put his or her life in danger (e.g., drug/alcohol abuse or reckless driving).

A major depression that interferes with a child's ability to function (scholastic, family, peer group) should be carefully evaluated and treated with individual therapy and medications as indicated. Children who have a history of depression prior to bereavement might be more likely to require antidepressant treatment than those who have no prior history of mood disorder. In considering the use of an antidepressant in children and adolescents, the lethality of such medications should always be considered in a potentially suicidal patient. In children and adolescents, risk of mediation overdose can be minimized by placing a responsible adult (i.e., a parent) in charge of dispensing the pills. In the parent-bereaved family with a clinically depressed child, the surviving parent may also be depressed. Thus, extra care should be taken in selecting the adult to be responsible for the child's medicine. When using medication, a physical examination, electrocardiogram, and liver function tests should always be done. Currently imipramine is a good choice as an antidepressant, as it has been used more than any other antidepressant in children. The dose should not exceed 5 mg/kg. Steady-state plasma levels of 125–225 ng/ml have been correlated with good clinical outcome in depression (Preskorn et al., 1982, 1987). In depressed adolescents with hypersomnia and hyperphagia, monoamine oxidase inhibitors might also be considered. If using such agents, the diet must be carefully monitored because of possible hypertensive crises if foods high in tyramine are ingested. This is especially important in adolescents, who tend to take risks. Foods to be avoided include pepperoni, sausage, chicken livers, and cottage cheese. Fortunately, most children do not enjoy chianti wine or blue cheese, which are also high in tyramine. In case of potential hypertensive crises, some clinicians prescribe a dose of 25–50 mg of Thorazine as needed to take with the child until the child gets to an emergency room.

Baker et al. (1992) believe that treatment following the loss of a child's loved one should be psychoeducational. The parents of the child sometimes need education on the needs of a grieving child. This information can help explain death and mourning to the child and also help with any questions the child may have. If a child needs a new caregiver appointed, developmental needs of the child should be taken into consideration.

BEREAVEMENT AS A RISK FACTOR FOR PSYCHOPATHOLOGY

As mentioned earlier, bereavement in childhood has been considered a potential risk factor for subsequent psychopathology (Breier, 1989). A preliminary analysis of data from the authors' prospective study of normal bereavement in children focused on depression, anxiety disorders, and somatization. Thirty-eight prepubertal children were compared with 38 matched inpatient depressed child psychiatric control subjects. About one-third of the bereaved children met DSM-IV criteria for depression. Each symptom of depression was more common in the clinically depressed children as compared with the bereaved children. Parents of the bereaved children were often unaware of their children's symptoms, as compared with the parents of clinically depressed children. Several children reported they had intentionally concealed symptoms so as not to worry their surviving parent (Weller and Weller, 1990).

In a small sample of bereaved adolescents (N = 24) compared with depressed adolescents, again, depressed adolescents exhibited DSM-IV symptoms more frequently than bereaved adolescents. Overall the par-

ents of the bereaved adolescents were less aware of their children's symptomatology than were the parents of the depressed adolescents. This was especially true of bereaved parents' not being aware of concentration problems and suicidal thoughts in their offspring. When children and adolescents were compared overall, bereaved children reported more depressive symptomatology compared with bereaved adolescents. One should be cautious not to conclude on the basis of these findings that children get more depressed than adolescents. It could be that adolescents are more reluctant to disclose their feelings.

In looking at anxiety symptoms (since separation gives rise to anxiety, and death is the ultimate separation), surprisingly the authors found very few anxiety symptoms in the short-term period (1–3 months) after parental death in children and adolescents. Again, children reported anxiety symptoms more often than adolescents; worrying about their surviving parent as well as worrying about "little things" was significantly more common in children than in adolescents. Comparing bereaved children and adolescents to clinically depressed controls, the depressed population had many more anxiety symptoms; that is, clinically depressed children and adolescents very often had a comorbid diagnosis of anxiety disorder (Sanchez et al., 1994).

Somatic symptoms were hypothesized to be more common in bereaved children since children might use somatic symptoms such as stomachaches and headaches to express their concerns. Bereaved children reported significantly more concern with somatic symptoms than did adolescents. The most common complaints were headaches, stomachaches, and nausea. Overall, the authors did not find overwhelming somatization (Sood et al., 1992).

In general, the most common psychiatric disorder experienced both by children and adolescents in the immediate period after parental death is depression. Interestingly, preliminary analysis indicates that bereaved children with a positive dexamethasone suppression test (DST) have more DSM-IV depressive symptoms than do bereaved children with a negative DST (Weller et al., 1992).

RESEARCH DIRECTIONS

Previous studies of grief in children have suggested a possible link between bereavement and subsequent pathology. However, many early studies suffer from small sample size and methodological weaknesses that hinder their generalizability. Several studies have suggested that a depressive syndrome is a common sequelae of bereavement in adults. Recent studies of bereaved children and adolescents suggest that depressive symptoms are also common soon after the death of the parent. However, long-term prospective studies of larger groups of subjects utilizing standardized assessment techniques are needed to more completely describe the natural course of grief and possible pathological outcomes.

Research on grief in preschoolers has been almost nonexistent and is needed. A few groups are beginning to study this age group, and more information can be expected (E. Kranzler, personal communication, 1988). We need assessment instruments to be able to communicate better with 3- to 6-year-olds. Also, further research needs to be done in children who have lost a sibling, a close friend, or grandparents, to be able to generalize findings. Studies of children who have lost a sibling will also be important in that a child's death may be a greater stressor for a parent than the death of a spouse.

The authors' preliminary reports suggest that the child's adaptation is dependent on the parents' adaptation. It might be anticipated that, if parents are devastated by the loss of a child, the surviving siblings would be at high risk for developing psychiatric symptomatology. However, further work will be needed to establish the validity of such hypotheses.

References

American Psychiatric Association: *Diagnostic and Statistical Manual of Mental Disorders* (4th ed). Washington, DC, American Psychiatric Press, 1994.

Baker KE, Sedney MA, Gross E: Psychological tasks for bereaved children. *Am J Orthopsychiatry* 62:105–116, 1992.

Bendickson R, Fulton R: Death and the child: An anterospective test of the childhood bereavement and

later behavior disorder hypothesis. In: Fulton R (ed): *Death and Identity*. Bowie, MD, Charles Press, 1976.

Bowlby J: Process of mourning. *Int J Psychoanal* 42:317–340, 1961a.

Bowlby J: Childhood mourning and its implications for psychiatry. *Am J Psychiatry* 118:481–498, 1961b.

Bowlby J: *Attachment and Loss. Vol 3: Loss: Sadness and Depression.* London, Hogarth Press, 1980.

Bowlby J: Attachment and loss: Retrospect and prospect. *Am J Orthopsychiatry* 52:664–678, 1982.

Breier A: Experimental approaches to human stress research: Assessment of neurobiological mechanisms of stress in volunteers and psychiatric patients. *Biol Psychiatry* 26:438–462, 1989.

Clayton PJ, Darvish HS: Course of depressive symptoms following the stress of bereavement. In: Barrett JE (ed): *Stress and Mental Disorders.* New York, Raven Press, 1979, pp. 121–135.

Elizur E, Kaffman M: Factors influencing the severity of childhood bereavement reactions. *Am J Orthopsychiatry* 53(4):668–676, 1983.

Furman E: *A Child's Parent Dies.* New Haven, CT, Yale University Press, 1974.

Gregory I: Anterospective data following childhood loss of a parent. I: Delinquency and high school dropout. *Arch Gen Psychiatry* 13:99–109, 1965.

Kranzler E, Shaffer D, Wasserman G, et al: Early childhood bereavement. *J Am Acad Child Adolesc Psychiatry* 29:513–520, 1990.

Markusen E, Fulton R: Childhood bereavement and behavior disorders: A critical review. *Omega* 2: 107–117, 1971.

Nagy M: The child's theories concerning death. *J Genet Psychol* 73:3–27, 1948.

Preskorn SH, Weller EB, Hughes CW, et al: Depression in prepubertal children: Dexamethasone nonsuppression predicts differential response to imipramine vs. placebo. *Psychopharmacol Bull* 23(1): 128–133, 1987.

Preskorn SH, Weller EB, Weller RA: Depression in children: Relationship between plasma imipramine levels and response. *J Clin Psychiatry* 43(11): 450–453, 1982.

Sanchez L, Fristad MA, Weller RA, et al: Anxiety symptoms in acutely bereaved prepubertal children. *Ann Clin Psychiatry* 6(1):39–44, 1994.

Solomon F, Osterweis M, Green M: Bereavement intervention programs. In: Osterweis M, Solomon F, Green M (eds): *Bereavement: Reactions, Consequences, and Care.* Washington, DC, National Academy Press, 1984, pp. 239–279.

Sood B, Weller EB, Weller RA, et al: Somatic complaints in grieving children. *Compr Mental Health Care* 2:17–25, 1992.

Van Eerdewegh MM, Beiri MD, Parrilla RH, et al: The bereaved child. *Br J Psychiatry* 140:23–29, 1982.

Weller EB, Weller RA: Neuroendocrine changes in affectively ill children and adolescents. In: Brown W (ed): *Endocrinology of Neuropsychiatric Disorders.* Philadelphia, Saunders, 1988, pp. 41–54.

Weller EB, Weller RA: Grief in children and adolescents. In: Garfinkel BD, Carlson GA, Weller EB (eds): *Psychiatric Disorders in Children and Adolescents.* Philadelphia, Saunders, 1990, pp. 37–47.

Weller EB, Weller RA, Fristad MA: Historical and theoretical perspectives on childhood depression. In: Weller EB, Weller RA (eds): *Current Perspectives on Major Depressive Disorders in Children.* Washington, DC, American Psychiatric Press, 1984.

Weller EB, Weller RA, Fristad MA, et al: Should children attend their parent's funeral? *J Am Acad Child Adolesc Psychiatry* 27(5):559–562, 1988.

Weller EB, Weller RA, Fristad MA, et al: Dexamethasone suppression test and depressive symptoms in bereaved children: A preliminary report. *J Neuropsychiatry* 2:418–421, 1990.

Weller RA, Weller EB, Fristad MA, et al: Depression in recently bereaved prepubertal children. *Am J Psychiatry* 148(11):1536–1540, 1991.

Wolfenstein M: How is mourning possible? *Psychoanal Study Child* 21:93–123, 1966.

34 EFFECT OF DISORDERED PARENTING ON THE DEVELOPMENT OF CHILDREN

Klaus Minde, M.D., F.R.C.P.(C)

Evolutionary theory suggests that living things should be concerned with the production and rearing of offspring to ensure genetic representation in the next generation (Barash, 1977). In fact, human adults all over the world see children as helpless, needing protection and training, but also as a valuable asset to society (Mead and Wolfenstein, 1955). This explains the common aim of parents everywhere in the world to raise their children to be independent, responsible adults capable of full participation in society (LeVine, 1977) and may also be reflected in the great similarity that has been found in early child-rearing practices all over the world (Ainsworth, 1957).

Given these similarities, evolutionary theory also predicts conflict between parents and offspring (Trivers, 1974). Because children and their parents have different genetic makeups and different needs, parental behaviors will not always be optimal for each infant at all times. The degree to which these conflicts can affect the development of children is examined in this chapter.

THEORETICAL ISSUES PERTAINING TO DISORDERED PARENTING

Textbooks of child and adolescent psychiatry have not traditionally defined what constitutes adequate, optimal, or disordered parenting. The reason for this hesitation is undoubtedly related to the enormous complexity of the caretaking function. In addition to the instrumental task of keeping a child healthy and providing him or her with sufficient clothing and shelter, there are the many psychological factors that make up the parenting role. Parenting also has an important developmental component, since we would all agree that adequate parenting of an infant and a teenager may require some common skills (such as patience) but will also draw on very different parental characteristics. While a newborn needs a mother who can "understand" his or her body language

and help the infant to organize his or her psychological states into predictable rhythms, a teenager will more directly benefit from a parent who can help him or her to explore the range of socially acceptable experiences.

Describing its instrumental and developmental variations is only one way to characterize good and inadequate parenting. Another way of understanding parenting practices is to see them in terms of theoretical models of development. For example, there is a rich literature, based on psychoanalytic theory, that deals with such issues as maternal overprotectiveness (Levy, 1943) or the formation of abnormal defense reactions in children with particular family constellations (Freud, 1937).

On the other hand, we have a large current literature that describes how specific psychiatric or medical conditions may influence the parenting style of an adult individual. For example, we talk about the effects maternal depression (Cox et al., 1987; Puckering, 1989; Weintraub et al., 1986), the one-parent family (Ferri, 1976), or abuse by adults (Cicchetti and Carlson, 1989) has on children, and how children who live with "disordered" parents fare in their overall development. The advantage of this literature is the empirical nature of the presented data. However, many of these studies tend to ignore that the association between parental behavior and child disorders is not unidirectional, and that it is necessary to evaluate possible contributions of genetic or other factors within the child in each case. There is also the ecological perspective to be considered. For example, mothering is usually embedded within the context of a family or a community, with all its stresses and potential support structures (Bronfenbrenner, 1979). Others have called such contexts "distal" factors, indicating degrees of risk and resilience children are exposed to (Luthar, 1993).

Another focus of investigation has been the effect specific rearing practices or "proximal" factors have on the child. Discipline, personal warmth, and the amount and type of interaction or parental regulation of affect are examples of dimensions that have been studied (Emde, 1989; Maccoby and Martin, 1983; Minde et al., 1988; Patterson, 1982).

These latter studies attempt to provide insight into the process of parenting and the possible mechanisms responsible for the transmission of both adaptive and maladaptive behaviors from parent to child. Some of the work on proximal factors has also been used to support theoretical developmental constructs, such as the need for special attachment relationships in infancy (e.g., Ainsworth et al., 1978; Bowlby, 1969, 1973, 1979; Hinde and Stevenson-Hinde,1988) as well as nontheoretical observation, such as mother-infant bonding or parental quarreling (Crockenberg, 1985; Cummings et al., 1989; Klaus and Kennell, 1982).

As can be seen from this brief review, the literature on parenting has been driven by a wide range of theories and empirical data. This has often led to seemingly contradictory popular advice to those interested in the care of children. Yet two things seem to be clear. Theories based on classical psychoanalytic or learning principles have failed to stand up to modern empirical findings, as they do not sufficiently explain important aspects of children's development. On the other hand, there is increasing evidence supporting concepts of parenting based on principles of attachment theory and developmental psychopathology (Bowlby, 1988; Sroufe and Rutter, 1984). Both emphasize the importance that functional factors (e.g., parental emotional support, the role of an intimate confiding relationship) and structural factors (e.g., low socioeconomic status or mental illness in the family) have on the quality of parenting and they conceptualize life as an ongoing developmental process. This is in contrast to classical psychoanalytic theory, which placed undue importance on the very early years of a child's life to determine later mental health.

This chapter first briefly reviews some early work that has linked parenting styles with later problems in children. We then summarize some major characteristics present-day investigators associate with competent caretaking and comment on how specific parental disorders influence these characteristics. As troubled parents communicate their difficulties through their child-rearing activities, we then examine some of the clinical manifestations of disordered parenting skills and how they come about. At that point we also evaluate how children influence the parenting they receive and highlight this with examples of children with developmental disorders. The chapter ends with some thoughts on the efficacy of parent education and a discussion of unresolved issues requiring further study.

HISTORICAL FACTORS

The importance of linking specific caretaking experiences in early life with later psychopathology has long been recognized. John Locke (1632–1704) wrote an essay in 1693 entitled "Some Thoughts Concerning Education," wherein he described the consequences of specific parenting styles. He admonished parents to observe their children carefully in order to understand their "native propensities" and emphasized their role in "weeding out" their faults and "planting good habits" early on in life (see Locke, 1947). Locke's influence was such that he has been called the Dr. Spock of the 18th century (Brant and Cullman, 1980).

One hundred years later, Jean Jacques Rousseau wrote extensively on the consequences specific parenting practices such as coddling and neglect have on the future development of young children. In his book *Emile* (1762/1979) he spoke at length about the need for and style of punishment that should be used to help children in their socialization.

Later, clinicians concentrated on specific child-rearing practices and evaluated them by their effect on a child's alleged later development. For example, Luther Emmett Holt (1855–1924) wrote a book entitled *The Care and Feeding of Children*, which went through 75 printings between 1894 and 1943 (Holt, 1902). Among other things, he emphasized the untoward effects of early swaddling and of the habit of playing with children under 6 months, warning that engaging in these activities was likely to lead to various mental and physical problems.

In the beginning of this century, clinicians from the psychoanalytic school began to label specific parental activities as pathological for the development of children. Examples here are Freud's early concerns about the prohibition of masturbation in young children and the importance of specific psychosexual stages in their relationships with their parents (Freud, 1958). Anna Freud and others later extended these views by discussing how children develop defense mechanisms that compromise development in response to overindulgent and/or rejecting parent attitudes (Freud, 1937; Levy, 1943).

Others wrote about more practical aspects of caretaking. For example, Buxbaum (1959) discussed the need of children to breast-feed so as to obtain sufficient oral pleasure, and Sears et al. (1957) emphasized the need for children to be allowed adequate genital play. These authors also felt that certain activities, such as the type and length of toilet training or breast-feeding a child experienced, carried distinct predictions for the infant's future mental health.

However, in a careful review of the then-available data on child-rearing, Caldwell (1964) concluded that neither the timing of various aspects of child care nor the method of toilet training was of particular psychological consequence. This suggested that parenting could not be explained by studying single dimensions but that it had to be understood as a multifactorial phenomenon, including child factors such as temperament and developmental status as well as parental behaviors.

WHAT CONTRIBUTES TO DEVELOPMENTALLY APPROPRIATE PARENTING?

On the most general level, parenting is a task concerned with the raising of children. Children need an environment that provides them with sufficient material and emotional care to further their physical, cognitive, and social development. At least six aspects of parenting can be identified.

Sensitive Responsiveness

How parents respond to their children's behaviors, demands, and distress (Mrazek et al., 1982) and how they deal with the resolution of interpersonal conflicts (Shure and Spivak, 1978) is a key aspect of the parenting task. Adequate parents are generally sensitive to their children's cues in relation to their developmental needs (Rutter, 1989).

Emde (1989) suggests that it is the parents' sense of protectiveness vis-à-vis their small children that provides a basis for parental sensitivity, i.e., that it is survival-oriented. Parents show this sensitivity when they engage in both the physiological regulation of their infant's needs (e.g., by keeping them warm and well-fed) and in the regulation of affect. The latter is demonstrated in the empathic responsiveness by the caregiver to the child's overall adaptive needs. This means that parents try to avoid having their child experience extremes of excitement, anger, or distress. Empathic responsiveness also facilitates the sharing of feelings and expression of positive social behaviors (Easterbrooks and Emde, 1988).

A further parental activity that needs to be guided by sensitive responsiveness is the function of disciplining. Normal parents encourage self-control in a child by regulating the expression of feelings. This enables the child to be increasingly in charge of his or her activities in the midst of conflicting opportunities and demands. Finally, Emde feels that the ability to engage a youngster in appropriate play activities is also a reflection of parental sensitive responsiveness.

The Parent-Child Dyad

Parenting is always determined by the individual parent-child relationship (Minde, 1986). It therefore has very special qualities that are specific to each particular dyad, although it also forms part of a broader system of relationships involving other family members, neighbors, or friends. Emde (1989), in his previously described treatise, suggests that the initial and enduring tie between parent and child is an important determinant of this relationship. Bowlby and others have convincingly shown that the quality of this tie or attachment plays an important part in the overall social and emotional functioning of a child (Ainsworth et al., 1978; Bowlby, 1969, 1979; Bretherton, 1985).

Given the complexity of human motivation and behavior, it is not surprising that the early mother-child relationship also has an intergenerational component. Main and her group have shown that a mother's understanding of her own early experiences with her caretakers is an important predictor of the internal representations she has of her child and that these representations in turn will determine the quality of the infant's attachment to the mother (Fonagi et al., 1991; Main and Goldwyn, 1984; Main and Hesse, 1990). This means that both the interpretation we as parents make of the behaviors of our children and the way we respond to them is significantly determined by the way we have learned to interpret the world through past experiences with our own caretakers.

Parental Mental Health

The parents' psychosocial functioning is an essential component in the quality of parenting they can provide. As we see later in this chapter, parenting functions can be severely compromised by mental disorders and the associated distorted internal representations of the world. Psychiatrically disturbed parents are generally more preoccupied with themselves. Hence they are also less responsive to their children and regulate and discipline them less effectively.

Parenting Experience

Parenting is a function of experience. Both in monkeys and people we find mothers to be more patient, sensitive, and competent with later born than with first-born children (Rutter, 1981; Suomi et al., 1974). Older mothers have also been shown to interact more sensitively and provide more appropriate stimulation (Jones et al., 1980; Ragozin et al., 1982).

The Extended Family and Social System

Parenting, even though usually practiced within the individual parent-child relationship, is also a reflection of a broader social nexus. Thus, it must be seen as a reflection of the interaction between external stresses and supports (Belsky and Vondra, 1989) and also be placed in the context of family dynamics (Bell and Harper, 1977; Hetherington et al., 1982; Wynne, 1984). Seen from this perspective, the absence or presence of a father, to take just one example, will not only influence the child (Clarke-Stewart, 1978) but also, through its effect on the overall functioning of the family, be an important influence on the parenting process of other caretakers (Steinhauer, 1984).

While the measurement of family functioning is a complex undertaking, there are basically two ways in which families have been conceptualized (Jacob and Tennenbaum, 1988). According to Olson and his colleagues (1979), families can best be assessed on their level of cohesion and adaptability. They suggest that cohesion can range from very high (enmeshed) to very low (disengaged) and is related to the emotional bond people have toward one another and their degree of individual autonomy. Adaptability, in turn, refers to the way a family can adapt to changing developmental demands and ranges from rigidity to disorganization.

Other workers measure family functions by assessing how families deal with specific roles such as task accomplishments, role performance, communication, affective expression, and control of values and norms (Minuchin, 1985; Skinner et al., 1983). However, both groups believe that the disordered functioning of the family in one or more areas (e.g., poor communication, rigid enmeshment) is a primary factor in children's behavioral dysfunction.

Direct Caretaker-Child Interaction

The actual behaviors parents and children show toward each other can vary from supportive and helpful to oppositional or hostile. The interactions are affected by the characteristics of both child and parent (Maccoby and Martin, 1983). As we see later in this chapter, the individual child's temperamental characteristics as well as physical and mental intactness are important contributors to parenting competence.

In summary, parenting cannot be viewed as a unidimensional variable; a multitude of factors are involved. Inadequate parenting may be related to any number of circumstances both within and beyond the parents' control. For example, the lack of social support or other environmental stressors may be translated into unduly harsh discipline or emotional unavailability (Quinton and Rutter, 1985; Rutter and Cox, 1987; Rutter et al., 1983).

PARENTAL PSYCHIATRIC DISORDERS

Empirical studies that examine the effects that specific mental disorders have on the development of children go back to the early part of the century. Janet (1925) concluded that mental disorders of parents had a negative effect on their offspring due to their impact on the social life of others in the family. He based this conclusion on his observations of 3 of 18 families in which the precipitating mental illness occurred in stepparents and, hence, affected children who were not genetically related to their caretakers. He also described cases where children of psychiatrically ill parents had fared well because they had been brought up away from their families. Canavan and Clark (1923a, 1923b) undertook the first controlled study by examining from 1912 to 1921 the 463 children of 136 married patients diagnosed as having dementia praecox, or schizophrenia. The authors compared these youngsters with 581 children of 145 families attending a medical outpatient clinic. They found the incidence of conduct disorders among the children in the study group to be significantly higher (9.5 versus 1.6%) than in the control children.

Other early investigators (e.g., Gardner, 1949; Preston and Antin, 1933; Ramage, 1925) also examined children of psychotic parents. They suggested that overall the offspring of dementia praecox patients showed comparatively few mental peculiarities and virtually no occurrence of the parental psychotic illness (Canavan and Clark, 1936). While this early work suggested a nongenetic intergenerational transmission of psychiatric illness, it was Rutter's monograph of "Children of Sick Parents" (Rutter, 1966) that set a new standard for examining the effect of a parent's emotional or physical handicap on his or her children. From 922 children who had attended the Maudsley Hospital Children's Department in 1955 and 1959, Rutter selected specific subsamples. There was a group who had at least one parent with a mental illness (N = 137), a group who were bereaved (N = 85), and a group who had parents with either a chronic or recurrent physical disease (N = 190). The following are some of the relevant findings of this study:

1. There is a strong association between parental illness and psychiatric disorder in children.
2. This is true for both psychiatric and physical illness in the parent.
3. As parental illness usually precedes the development of the child's disorder, it is reasonable to suggest a parent-to-child effect.
4. Parental disorder is most likely to be followed by behavioral disturbances in children when the parent exhibits a "long-standing abnormality of personality."

A number of later studies involving general population samples (e.g., Richman et al., 1982; Rutter et al., 1975) and case-controlled comparisons of the children of parents with a mental disorder (e.g., Beardslee, 1986; Cytryn et al., 1984) have further extended our knowledge, permitting us to ask some specific questions about the linkage between parental and child psychiatric disorder.

How Close is the Demonstrated Link between Psychiatric Disorder in Parents and Children?

The answer is "significant but not very close." This can be best explained by describing a recent study by Rutter and Quinton (1984b) where 137 newly referred psychiatric patients in London with 292 children under 15 years of age were evaluated and followed prospectively for 4 years (1966–1967, 1970–1981). Patients were initially interviewed at home to obtain their diagnosis and family characteristics. Both patients and their children were followed by means of questionnaires. Twenty-one percent of the boys versus 11% of the girls were seen as persistently abnormal by their teachers over the 4-year period. During the psychiatric interview, figures were very similar, in that about one third of the boys and one quarter of the girls were judged to have currently handicapping problems.

Are there some Parental Psychiatric Disorders that have a more Detrimental Effect on the Development of Children than do Other Psychiatric Disorders?

The evidence here seems to support this notion. Even in 1925, Janet had stated that children of psychiatrically ill parents were most affected if their families showed conflict and disturbances in addition to their mental illness. In the study by Rutter and Quinton, the same findings emerged; the presence of an antisocial personality disorder in one or both parents was the most significant factor in the incidence of childhood psychopathology. Thus, 45% of all children who had one or two parents with an antisocial personality disorder showed a disturbance on the teacher questionnaire, and 48% in the psychiatric interview. This was in contrast to 21% of children whose parents had a psychosis or an affective disorder.

Children who had one parent with a psychosis or an affective disorder and one healthy parent did not show any increased risk for a psychiatric disorder. However, many of the disturbed parents also had a disturbed partner, and in these families children showed a high rate of disorders (20 versus 54%, as determined by the psychiatric interview).

These findings support those from Wynne's project in Rochester (Harder et al., 1980; Kokes et al., 1980), where boys aged 7 and 10 who had nonpsychotically ill parents showed far less overall psychological competence than those with schizophrenic or affectively ill parents.

The Minnesota Study of Garmezy and his group can also be considered here (Garmezy, 1984; Garmezy and Devine, 1984). In that study, children ages 9–11, of schizophrenic and internalizing (primarily depressed) mothers, were studied using peer and teacher ratings and school records. The authors' initial findings suggested that the children of internalizing (i.e., depressed) mothers were most like the control group. Seven years later, however, only 48% of the children of depressed mothers received an overall good outcome score, while 82% of the controls did (Garmezy and Devine, 1984). Rutter and Quinton (1984b), in their previously cited study, evaluated the persistence of abnormalities in their sample and report that continuing psychiatric abnormalities in the children were not related to a particular parental diagnosis but to the associated presence of quite specific types of family interactions. Most important here was the child's exposure to hostile behavior. Thus, 17% of boys with nonhostile fathers and mothers versus 40% of those with hostile mothers and 71% with hostile fathers showed persistent disturbance.

Are there Age Differences in the Susceptibility of Children to the Adversities of having a Mentally Ill Parent?

This question has never been examined directly. However, a number of related findings would suggest that one can expect to see developmental differences. For example, it is well known that repeated hospitalization is especially difficult for children between the ages of 6 months and 5 years (Quinton and Rutter, 1976). This is due to the fact that young children cannot yet "understand" that the separation from the family they experience upon hospitalization is not permanent and has nothing to do with naughty or "bad" things they have done. One would

therefore expect that certain characteristics of a mentally ill mother or father, such as their need to be hospitalized at unpredictable intervals, would be associated with difficulties in young children and that the presence of concrete or overinclusive thinking in some schizophrenic patients may be more traumatic to older children.

These data suggest that some interactive factors, such as hostility, may be pathogenic for a wide age range of children, while others, such as parental sadness, may be especially problematic for older children.

Are there Sex Differences in the Susceptibility of Children to Parental Mental Illness?

The data here are not very clear. In general, it has been documented that boys are more susceptible to psychosocial stressors than are girls (Maccoby and Martin, 1983). However, this may in part be due to the fact that, as we have seen, an ongoing parental personality disorder, especially if associated with hostile interpersonal child-rearing practices, shows the strongest association with the child's persistent emotional or behavioral disturbance. Personality disorders are more common in men, and because disturbances seem to impinge more on the children of the same sex, one would expect boys to be more affected by paternal psychiatric deviance.

Rutter and Quinton's findings confirm that children of the same sex as the mentally ill parent are more profoundly affected. In their study, 40% of the boys versus 23% of the girls were judged disturbed by teachers when the father was mentally ill, while 11% of daughters of mentally ill mothers versus 0% of daughters of mentally ill fathers were seen as abnormal (Rutter and Quinton, 1984b).

To What Extent are Psychiatric Disorders shown by Children of Mentally Ill Parents simply a Reflection of the Common Gene Pool between the Generations?

Both schizophrenia and major depressive illness have a well-established genetic component. In fact, there are some adoption studies in which rates of schizophrenia were found to be equally high for adopted and nonadopted children (Gottesman and Shields, 1982). This has been taken to mean that a genetic predisposition accounts for much of the disorder seen in children. However, other data suggest that the more severe the parental pathology, the more likely a child is to be placed for adoption (Sameroff and Zax, 1978). This would indicate that adopted-away children cannot be readily compared with those who are kept by their original families.

More recent work by Plomin and his group has introduced the concept of shared and nonshared environmental influences (Plomin and Daniels, 1987). Plomin developed this concept in response to his work on adopted children and twins. In particular, he documented that children living in the same family may nevertheless perceive their environment quite differently. For example, one child may have been influenced by the musical activities she shared with her father and report her home to have been a peaceful one. Her brother, in contrast, may have focused on the verbal battles between father and mother and, as a consequence, may have grown up feeling rejected and become a disturbed youngster.

Reitsma-Street et al. (1985) tested this hypothesis by examining 71 antisocial Canadian adolescents with same-sex siblings 2 years younger to 5 years older who had not been involved in antisocial activities. The authors found evidence for differences in the sibling pairs long before one sibling began his or her antisocial activities. For example, siblings had developed significant differences in their relationship with their mothers, and their mothers identified other environmental factors differentiating the proband from his or her nondelinquent sibling. For example, the delinquent child on average was 2 years younger when his or her parents separated from each other and had experienced more medical illnesses. This seems to indicate that some children within the same family are genetically more "at risk" to develop the psychiatric disorder shown by one or both of their parents.

In summary, there is good evidence that children are adversely affected by parents with a psychiatric illness. However, their vulnerability is primarily related to the pervasiveness with which each parental illness affects the actual caretaking practices of the parent and by their genetic risk status. Thus, personality disorders in parents showing a pervasive and chronic course are more difficult for children to cope with than, say, an intermittent psychotic illness in the parent. Age and sex differences in susceptibility also exist but vary in developmentally expected ways.

DEPRESSION

Depression in mothers has long been considered a major stressor for young children (Rutter, 1986). As the incidence of this condition among young women is as high as 9% (Boyd and Weissman, 1981), it potentially affects a large number of children. In fact, there are reports that the rate of depression in nonworking mothers of preschool children may be as high as 40% (Richman et al., 1982). Both Richman and her group and Boyd and Weissman defined depression as a condition where women show symptomatology for depression as defined by ICD-9 that is exclusive of postpartum depression. Thus, this condition is different from "maternal blues," which occurs in more than 80% of women and is usually self-limiting (Stein, 1982). However, it may include individuals who by DSM-IV criteria have a single or recurrent episode of a major depression (296.2 or 296.3), a bipolar disorder, depressed (296.5), as well as dysthymia (300.40), with all the ensuing differences in each condition's genetic vulnerability.

The effects of depression on children have often been described (Beardslee et al., 1993; Cantwell, 1983; Coghill et al., 1986; Cox et al., 1987; Cytryn et al., 1984, 1986; Gershon et al., 1982; L. Murray, unpublished manuscript, 1988; Puckering, 1989). Findings have suggested that these children display a wide range of behavioral management problems. While some children appear depressed, others show conduct disorders or hyperactivity.

More important, data from Richman et al. (1982), Coghill et al. (1986), and Cox et al. (1987) show that a substantial number of children of depressed mothers tend to maintain their abnormal behavior even after remission of the mother's depressive illness. For example, Richman reports that 58% of her 3-year-old youngsters still showed behavior problems at age 8 even though maternal depression had remitted.

What is the mode of transmission of this condition? There is some suggestion that the genetics of the disorder play at least some part. Thus, findings suggest that children of parents with bipolar disorder are at significantly higher risk of showing disturbed behavior than are those whose parents have a unipolar illness (20 versus 43%). Children with one affected parent also show far less morbidity than those with two affected parents (24 versus 74%) (Gershon et al., 1982; Puig-Antich et al., 1985; Weissman et al., 1984, 1987).

However, it is obvious that the children of depressed parents are subject not only to genetic risk but also to an environment that may be highly stressful. Studies examining the parenting style of depressed mothers have primarily reported on direct mother-child interactions. For example, Richman et al. (1982) in a longitudinal prospective study of nearly two hundred children evaluated at age 3, 4, and 8, found a high correlation between maternal depression, the frequency the child was read to at home, and his or her reading age measured at age 8. This was particularly prominent in boys. In another study, children of depressed mothers who at 2 years had received little reciprocal cognitive stimulation, performed poorly on cognitive tasks in school at 5 years (Meadows and Mills, 1987). It is of interest that our knowledge about the impact of depression on parenting older children is still quite limited. Good data are also missing on the degree to which abnormal interactions are specific to a mother who has a lifetime diagnosis of depression (i.e., may have been depressed 5 years ago) or whether they relate only to individuals who show clinical evidence of depression at the time of observation. Nevertheless, the overall findings indicate that depressed mothers are more preoccupied with themselves and consequently less

sensitive to the needs of their children (Billings and Moos, 1983: Cox et al., 1987; Field, 1984; L. Murray, unpublished manuscript, 1988; Zekoski et al., 1986). In particular, there are reports that depressed mothers stimulate their babies less by using fewer questions (L. Murray, unpublished manuscript, 1988), explanations, and suggestions (Cox et al., 1987), and that they have a less consistent attitude toward disciplining. They are also less able to compromise and, as a possible result, were seen to use a more controlling way of speech (Kochanska et al., 1987). Furthermore, recent data by Sameroff and his colleagues suggest that depressed women more often marry or live with depressed or otherwise psychiatrically disturbed men than do women with, e.g., obsessive compulsive disorders (Sameroff et al., 1993). This suggests that assortative mating takes place in this population. The same group of investigators also found that overall functioning in depressed families is compromised only when mothers are symptomatically depressed and not when they are between depressive episodes. Nevertheless, it must be emphasized that depressed mothers overall show a wide variety of interactional patterns, and some of them appear warm and very involved with their children (Cox et al., 1987).

Another important area of research has been the relationship between maternal depression and children's attachment patterns. Findings suggest that an increased number of children of depressed mothers (65 versus 35% in control populations) display an insecure attachment pattern when tested on the Ainsworth Strange Situation Paradigm at 12 or 18 months (Radke-Yarrow et al., 1985). However, this finding must be interpreted with caution since a similarly high rate of insecure attachment patterns have been found among children who live with a wide variety of psychologically compromised parents (Benoit et al., 1989, 1992; Minde et al., 1990). In addition, Jaenicke et al. (1987) found that children at risk for depression had a more negative self-concept, a finding these authors thought to be related to the degree of blame and criticism they received from their mothers. Hammen et al. (1987) suggest that this sort of negative cognition about one's self-worth may well function as a mediator for later experiences, which then seemingly confirm a basically depressive predisposition.

In summary, it appears that parental depression is a significant risk factor for the mental health of children. The abnormal behavior in these youngsters is not limited to depression but can encompass a wide range of both introverted and acting-out behaviors. While genetic factors seem to be important, the children's interpersonal experiences may also affect their self-esteem, attachment patterns, and cognitive style, which in turn may be related to later depressive symptomatology.

OTHER PSYCHOSOCIAL ABNORMALITIES IN PARENTS

In addition to the effects general psychiatric disorders in parents have on parenting skills, there have been two other groups of problematic parents whose behavior toward their children has been thoroughly examined by mental health researchers. These are parents with a criminal history and those who abuse their children. While some parenting characteristics of these two groups are similar to parents who show a personality disorder or other psychiatric disability, and while criminal parents also abuse their children more often than do noncriminal parents, these groups display sufficiently distinct patterns of disordered parenting to warrant a separate review.

Parental Criminality

A large number of investigations have documented that criminality in parents is associated with delinquency as well as conduct disorders in children (Hinde, 1980; Le Blanc and Loeber, 1993; Loeber and Stouthamer-Loeber, 1986; McCord and McCord, 1959; Wadsworth, 1979). This has been true in different ethnic and cultural groups the world over (Minde, 1993; Rohner, 1975; Werner, 1979).

Loeber and Stouthamer-Loeber (1986) have recently published a meta-analysis of parental behaviors in an attempt to understand the difficulties of children living with criminal parents. They found that data can best be clustered around four paradigms: conflict, neglect, deviant values, and marital conflict.

CONFLICT

Antisocial parents of delinquent children differ from parents of normal children in that they issue more commands (Forehand et al., 1975; Lobitz and Johnson, 1975) and get involved in long sequences of coercive interchanges (Patterson, 1982). Typically parents are aware of their child's disobedience but are unable to set adequate limits or employ a manner of discipline that would modify the abnormal behavior of their youngster in a nonaggressive manner. As a consequence, the child's behavior fails to improve, leading to an escalation of parental manipulative efforts. This in turn increases the evasiveness of the child, to a point where parents and youngsters see each other as enemies and may totally reject each other. The basic deficit underlying this paradigm seems to be parental insensitivity to the child's emotional needs, especially in regard to structure and regulation. This makes children feel rejected and, together with the nagging and coercive discipline, is directly related to later delinquent behavior.

NEGLECT

Loeber and Stouthamer-Loeber (1986) in assessing available studies conclude that both the lack of parental supervision and parental involvement with their children is significantly correlated with the development of later conduct disorders. It appears that lack of parental supervision is also strongly associated with delinquency (Wilson, 1980). Inadequate disciplining, in turn, is associated with an absence of house rules and parental monitoring of delinquent children (Patterson, 1982).

DEVIANT VALUES

Parents with a criminal record show a high incidence of condoning abnormal behavior in their children and therefore may serve as a model for deviant problem solving (West and Farrington, 1973). Support for this notion comes from the fact that delinquency in children is more strongly associated with parental criminality in adult life than with parental adolescent delinquency (Robins et al., 1975). Thus children experience their parents' delinquent activities and may model their own behavior accordingly.

MARITAL DISCORD

As in other families in which a parent has a specific psychiatric diagnosis, families with criminal members show a significant amount of family discord (Rutter and Giller, 1983; West, 1982). Thus, there is abundant evidence that children in these families are exposed to frequent and prolonged quarreling among their parents and temporary separations because of arguments and expressed hostility, as well as abuse of alcohol and drugs. In fact, it appears that these variables are the most predictive of recidivism within a delinquent group (Clarke and Cornish, 1978).

It should be stressed that parental criminality and mishandling are very important factors associated with "troublesomeness" in early life, while economic deprivation and poor school functioning frequently lead to later antisocial behavior (Farrington, 1986). Specific parental behaviors or psychosocial stressors are also related to the different duration or onset of various antisocial behaviors. For example, parental mishandling seems particularly relevant for behavior difficulties in children between the ages of 8 and 10, whereas it is more often deviant friends who influence the rate of offending during young adulthood.

Child Abuse

By definition, child maltreatment is the most telling syndrome associated with deviant parenting. As is shown in Chapters 99 and 100, child abuse is a complex problem that cuts across all classes of society, al-

though it is more commonly seen in poor families (Pelton, 1978). Official sources claim that there were more than 1,700,000 cases of suspected child maltreatment in 1984 (American Association for Protecting Children, 1986). Prevalence rates of sexual abuse in the general population are estimated to be as high as 62% for girls and 31% for boys (Dubowitz, 1986).

While these figures appear horrendous, the reader should be aware that there are significant differences in the definitions of abuse. This has to do, among other things, with the preconceptions of individual professional groups and with differing community variables (Barnett et al., 1993).

What, then, are the parental behaviors associated with abuse? Direct answers are difficult to come by because the most frequently used definition of maltreatment of a child states that abuse is usually the result of an interaction between a child and parental behavior, and not just a function of parental deviance (Cicchetti and Rizley, 1981). This suggests that parenting outcomes are determined by a reactive balance of risk and compensating factors experienced by a given family. Parental behaviors seen in abusive parents, in this model, are seen as a consequence of an interaction between parental stresses and available support (Belsky and Vondra, 1989).

One can also argue, as Rutter (1989) does, that child maltreatment reflects primarily a substantially abnormal pattern of parenting that secondarily may lead to such manifestations as failure to thrive, physical or sexual abuse, or even to deliberately created iatrogenic illnesses such as are seen in the Munchausen by proxy syndrome.

Authors who have studied the parental contribution to abuse have described the following abnormalities:

PERSONALITY

There is reasonable evidence that psychological maturity and parental competence are correlated and that it is younger mothers who abuse their children (Ragozin et al., 1982; Wandersman and Unger, 1983).

In a longitudinal study of 267 economically deprived families, those who abused their children early on had lower scores on scales assessing locus of control, aggression, suspicion, and defensiveness (Brunquell et al., 1981). In another investigation of 570 German families with abusing parents who came from diverse social classes, Engfer and Schneewind (1982) found the abusing parents to report very unfavorable socialization experiences in their own past. This in turn was related to a heightened irritability and nervous tension as well as family conflict, leading to frequent angry outbursts and harsh punishments of the children.

PSYCHOLOGICAL DISTURBANCES

There has been a long-held belief in the scientific literature and popular press alike that the majority of abused children will become abusing parents (Friedrich and Wheeler, 1982). Reports emphasizing such continuities are usually retrospective, i.e., based on studies that examined parents who had in fact abused a child and then reported about their own backgrounds (Steele and Pollock, 1968). Investigations that have used an epidemiological and prospective approach found a much lower rate of intergenerational transmission of maltreatment. For example, in one prospective study (Hunter and Kilstrom, 1979), in which 282 parents of newborns admitted to an intensive neonatal care unit were interviewed and followed for 1 year, only 18% of mothers who had reported abuse in their own childhood repeated it with their children. Similar figures have been presented by others (Kaufman and Zigler, 1987; Strauss, 1979).

The mechanism of transmitting maltreatment from one generation to the other has not yet been established (Egeland et al., 1984; Kaufman and Zigler, 1989). Some authors claim abusive parents teach their children that aggression is an appropriate way of dealing with conflict (Burgess and Youngblade, 1990; Hertzberger, 1983). Proponents of attachment theory suggest that children in abusing families develop representational models of the world that are so traumatic that they cannot be remembered in an integrative fashion and therefore cannot serve to prevent a repetition of these behaviors in the next generation (Bowlby, 1980; Sroufe and Fleeson, 1986). There is some support for this by very recent studies that prospectively followed abused children. For example, Dodge and his colleagues found that children physically abused during their preschool years were more disliked than were non-abused control subjects by classmates, teachers, and their mothers during the first 5 years of their schooling (Dodge et al., 1994). This suggests that early maltreatment disrupts attachment relationships with adult caregivers, and these disruptions subsequently impair a child's ability to form positive relationships. Cummings et al. (1994) also found that physically abused boys were more behaviorally reactive to interadult anger than comparison subjects. This implies that greater anger and aggression experienced across various family subsystems (e.g., parent to child, parent to parent) has a cumulative effect and sensitizes rather than habituates children to other's hostility. This means that there are important mediating factors that can increase the likelihood of abuse.

Belsky (1984, 1993; Belsky et al., 1984), who has developed the most comprehensive model of abuse to date, suggests that low self-esteem, poor interpersonal skills, and a low IQ provide a matrix that often leads to marriages to deviant and unsupportive spouses. This in turn creates marital discord, which leads to poorly behaving children whose behavior irritates their parents and causes them to commit abuse. Quinton et al. (1984), Quinton and Rutter (1985), and Dowdney et al. (1985), in a study that assessed parenting capacities of women raised in institutions, also demonstrated that both assortative mating and marital discord provide an important link that continues poor parenting from generation to generation, but also pointed out the ever-present possibility for an individual to move from a deviant life path to a more integrated and positive developmental trajectory.

In summary, there is much evidence pointing to the association between an antisocial parental lifestyle and/or child abuse and later psychopathology in children and adolescents. However, here again we do not find a parenting style that is specific to a particular disorder in the caretaker. Rather, we observe that such parents clearly neglect their children, dismiss their need for sensitive understanding, or use a wide range of other behaviors that compromise their children's overall social and emotional development. As there is now a substantial literature that examines how specific problematic parenting patterns come about and how they are transmitted from one generation to the next, we devote the final segment of this chapter to this discussion.

WHAT ARE THE CLINICAL MANIFESTATIONS OF DISORDERED PARENTING SKILLS, AND HOW DO THEY COME ABOUT?

In a previous section of this chapter, we discussed the skills and attitudes that appear to be associated with successful parenting. In the present section, we examine the question of the degree to which specific parental actions or strategies can be associated with behavioral difficulties in children. We will also attempt to trace the origin of these parenting problems as far as this is possible in order to help in the overall understanding of what parenting is all about and to facilitate remedial efforts.

In looking for meaningful general dimensions of problematic parent-child interactions, two categories have been conceptualized most clearly, one of unemotional detachment and lack of involvement, the other one of control through hostile discipline and overt maltreatment.

The Unemotional Detachment, Lack of Involvement, or Unresponsive, Insensitive Category

Parenting behaviors that fit this category are those that make children feel misunderstood, rejected, or potentially abandoned. Much work supporting this association comes from clinicians and investigators who emphasize the need for a secure attachment for normal social and cognitive development to occur (Ainsworth et al., 1978; Bowlby, 1973; Sroufe, 1983).

However, the association between parental detachment early on in life and later psychological disturbance has also been found in other studies. For example, recent work by Minde and his colleagues shows that a mother's sensitivity to the social cues of premature twins within the first 3 weeks of life will predict which one of the twins will be preferred by mother 4 years later (Minde et al., 1990). Rutter, in his studies on the parenting abilities of women who have been reared in institutions, also showed that among women placed in care before the age of 2, a much higher proportion had a personality disorder than among those whose primary attachments were disrupted after age 2 (32 versus 5%). These authors also assessed the degree to which parental pathology influenced the age of separation and found that children who were placed in early infancy were more likely to have had grossly deviant parents (i.e., parents who took "hard" drugs or alcohol or had a criminal record). Yet their own later parenting competence was not significantly influenced by their parents' deviance but by the age of placement, with placement at a younger age predicting poorer parenting later on. Most importantly, 80% of the girls who were admitted to an institution before age 2 and remained there until at least age 16 were poor mothers, while only 30% of those who returned home before age 16 showed poor parenting skills. This occurred even though many of these girls returned to families that experienced severe social disadvantage and marital discord. Some 45% of the girls who were placed after age 2 also showed significant problems in their parenting skills later on, and here those who returned home did not differ from those who remained in the institution during all their childhood. This was thought to be due to the degree of active hostility, rejection, and punitiveness the children encountered upon returning home (Rutter et al., 1983; Rutter and Quinton, 1984a).

There is one other longitudinal study that highlights the crucial importance of parental sensitivity and care for normal development. Tizard and her group studied a sample of 65 children who had been placed in well-run institutions shortly after birth in Britain. Twenty-four of these children were adopted by the age of 4; others remained in institutions longer. Most had returned to some type of family by age 16. In an early paper (Tizard and Hodges, 1978), the authors emphasized that most of the early-adopted children (before age 4) had developed good, stable, affectionate relationships with their adoptive parents, whereas those adopted between ages 4 and 8 showed poorer relationships with peers and others.

At age 16, we find that the children who were returned to their biological parents (the restored group) sometime after the age of 2 showed a far higher rate of serious psychiatric disorders than did those who had been adopted early on, partly because the former group had lived in a highly disadvantaged environment after their return home (Hodges and Tizard, 1989b). However, even the successfully adopted children 12 years later were more indiscriminately friendly, had fewer close peer relationships, and confided less in others than did the control group. At the same time, their academic performance was not affected (Hodges and Tizard, 1989a). This suggests that a lack of sensitive early caretaking had left a mark on the quality of social relationships these youngsters had in late adolescence but not on their later academic functioning.

The Control through Hostile, Rejecting, Harsh Discipline and Overt Maltreatment Category

The way parents control the behavior of their children has long been seen as an important predictor of children's later social and intellectual competence (Maccoby and Martin, 1983). Recent work has broadened the concept of control, which now includes not only discipline and punishment but also overall parental monitoring of behavior, the handling of conflict, and the emotional style of coping (Dowdney et al., 1984). Thus, control now not only relates to the degree of power a parent uses in disciplining children but also includes a democracy-versus-autocracy dimension.

Empirical studies document that children in autocratic or authoritarian families face severe restrictions in expressing their overall needs and experience much physical punishment and/or verbal anger (Patterson, 1982; Rutter, 1989). Baumrind (1967, 1971, 1989), in an extensive prospective study involving 134 children, documented that children with authoritarian parents were more passively hostile and unhappy than children raised in other families. Other authors have confirmed these results and also shown that authoritarian parenting is associated with low scores on measures of conscience (Hoffman. 1975) and low self-esteem (Loeb et al., 1980). More recent work has extended these concepts to groups of adolescent children. For example, Dornbusch et al. (1987), using a sample of 8000 children from different ethnic regions, found that the association between low self-esteem and authoritarian parenting held true in all social classes and among all ethnic groups and, more importantly, also influenced the academic achievement of these youngsters. Steinberg et al. (1989) confirmed these results and documented that children who live in authoritarian families are not only affected in their emotional development but show academic difficulties up to age 17.

In addition to the authoritarian parenting style, Baumrind also identified a permissive pattern of parenting that was based on the observation that some parents employ a low level of control either because of their ideological orientation (i.e., they have democratic principles and trust their children) or because they are not very interested in taking on child-rearing responsibilities (Lamborn et al., 1991). A third style of parenting, called authoritative, combines parental warmth and acceptance or involvement with an index of parental control or strictness. This seems to give children a feeling that their parents take them seriously and will help them if they need assistance, but that parents also have clear expectations of acceptable behaviors, which will be enforced. In follow-up studies, authoritative parents have children with the best behavioral outcome and highest school achievement, at least up to late adolescence (Steinberg et al., 1989).

Nevertheless, there is evidence that African American parents who use some aspects of authoritarian child-rearing, e.g., are more controlling, more critical, and more inclined to value conformity than independence in their children, have better adjusted youngsters than those exercising permissive or authoritative child-rearing patterns. This confirms the clinical observation that optimal child-rearing techniques may differ among families living in different cultures and socioeconomic circumstances (Baldwin et al., 1989, 1993).

It should be emphasized that the category of control through hostile, rejecting discipline also includes families where parents show disregard for the needs of their children by an intrusive and infantilizing caretaking style. Parents here have difficulties permitting their children to develop personal autonomy, a pattern described as enmeshment by family therapists and those studying attachment patterns (Main and Goldwyn, 1984; Minuchin, 1985). Other parents have inappropriate expectations and use children primarily as a source of support for themselves. This is especially common following divorce or in single-parent families (Hetherington, 1989).

Finally, there is evidence for an association between an authoritarian parenting style and childhood aggression (Patterson, 1982; Yarrow et al., 1968). Patterson's data, for example, show that aggressive children receive more punishment for an aggressive act than do normal controls. However, some children of authoritarian parents also become subdued and passive. The aspects of family interactions that determine whether a child of authoritarian parents will be passive or aggressive have not been precisely identified, although data point to particular modulating factors within the environment and the child. These are discussed in the next section.

INFLUENCES THAT CAN EXACERBATE OR MODERATE THE EFFECTS OF DISORDERED PARENTING ON CHILDREN'S DEVELOPMENT

There are a host of life events that can have a profound effect on the behavior of parents and, through them, on their children. Such events include parental separation, divorce, or the death of a primary caretaker. Each of these topics is discussed in other chapters of this volume (see Chapters 32, 33, and 112).

There is also a rich literature that has examined the effects of the parents' marital relationship on the development of their children. Emery (1982) in a review of this literature points out that despite methodological variations among empirical studies, the connection between interparental conflict and behavior problems in children is solidly established. However, other investigators find evidence for a compensatory process, that is, parents in less satisfied marriages may show especially sensitive and involved caretaking (Brody et al., 1986). Still others find evidence for both facilitating and detrimental effects (Cowan and Cowan, 1983; Goldberg and Easterbrooks, 1984). Cox and her colleagues (1989) hypothesize that the reason for this apparent discrepancy in the data is related to the psychological adjustment of the parents. Thus, disturbed individuals tend to marry partners with a complimentary psychiatric disorder (Merikangas, 1982), which may lead poorly adjusted partners to have an outwardly harmonious marriage and family life, while in fact their children receive compromised parenting.

Looking at some of the empirical studies that support the notion of a connection between marital discord and child behavior, one finds that the behavioral observations on which this assumption is based usually come from laboratory studies. The number of symptoms displayed by children in the laboratory is correlated with specific marital satisfaction scale scores, filled in by the mothers (e.g., Emery and O'Leary, 1984; Jouriles et al., 1988; Weiss and Summers, 1983). Correlations between marital status and child behavior in these studies usually range between .20 and .25. While this is statistically significant, it nevertheless explains only about 5% of the variance and leaves much room for other factors.

Another strategy for looking at the impact parental relationships have on children has been developed by Cummings and his colleagues. In a number of experiments, this group and others exposed pairs of children to an adult couple who, after an initial friendly encounter, engaged in a carefully rehearsed verbal argument, followed by reconciliation. The children would be observed both during and after each episode. Results showed that children as young as 2 years get very upset when they see adults quarrel and that they become more aggressive toward each other after they have witnessed such an argument (Crockenberg, 1985; Cummings et al., 1985, 1989; El Sheikh et al., 1989). It is of special interest that children who come from families with reportedly higher marital discord show more preoccupation and feel more responsible for the arguments they see in the laboratory. This suggests that children living in troubled families get sensitized to parental arguments and are potentially more affected by each recurrent disagreement.

More recent work by other investigators provides important additional information about these relationships. Thus, boys are generally more affected by parental strife than girls are affected, and behavioral consequences to the witnessing of behavioral discord may not be apparent for years (Waughn et al., 1988). More importantly, there is increasing evidence that the negative effect of parental arguments can be significantly modified if the parents can make up after a fight (Cummings et al., 1993). On the other hand, Vuchinich and colleagues (1993) recently documented that parents who invariably unite against their children when problems occur, i.e., present a "parental coalition," prevent their children from learning problem-solving skills, and their children present with more externalizing symptoms, at least in preadolescence. This supports the notion that arguing things out can be a useful process and that it may be the lack of an opportunity to do so that compromises the children's later emotional well-being.

Finally, it appears that marital patterns are fairly stable and predictable. For example, Howes and Markman (1989) found a significant correlation between a mother's premarital relationship with her later husband and their child's later attachment status. Thus, mothers who confided in their husbands and expressed their feelings freely were more sensitive toward their children who, in turn, were more securely attached. This underlines the remarkable intergenerational continuity of good as well as problematic internalized relationships (Sroufe and

Fleeson, 1988), which may well be one important mechanism through which we transmit psychological abnormalities to our children.

These observations support the attachment theory literature, which suggests that children develop specific types of attachment through actual experiences, creating inner working models of the world that are based on these same actual events in their lives (Main and Goldwyn, 1984; Sroufe and Fleeson, 1988).

As stated previously, modulations in the quality of parenting can come both through changing support and stress factors within the environment and from the object of parental caretaking, the child. While many child characteristics have been seen as potential contributors to parenting style, the difficult temperament of a child has been most frequently identified as a potential stress factor for parents. It has been observed that parents who view their children as temperamentally difficult, display more negative affect toward them, are more critical, and punish them more severely (Bates, 1980; Campbell, 1979; Dunn, 1980; Kelley, 1976). Such children, in turn, appear to be less able to cope with negative parental behavior. For example, Dunn and Kendrick (1981) reported that children with a high intensity of emotional expression and a negative mood showed more difficulties coping with a new baby than did children with easy temperaments. On the other hand, Washington et al. (1986) have shown that sensitive and committed mothers of small premature infants will report an improvement of temperament in their infants between 3 and 12 months of age, while mothers who behaved less contingently in the nursery did not report such temperamental changes. This underlines the multifactorial nature of even such allegedly biological constructs as temperament.

There are other aspects of children that contribute to the caretaking they receive. Patterson (1982), in his study of aggressive youngsters, points out that some children react in an unusual way to punishment. When a normal child is punished by a parent, the probability that the child will continue to be aggressive is reduced. With aggressive children, the probability is increased. This suggests that aggressive children, at least by school age, are less responsive than nonaggressive children to social reinforcement. In fact, there is evidence that aggressive children respond less to all types of social stimuli and may therefore indeed be harder to raise (Maccoby and Martin, 1983). Block et al. (1988), in a study of 105 adolescents who were followed between the ages of 3 and 14, were able to make significant predictions of these youngsters' adolescent use of marijuana and hard drugs by examining their early behavior patterns. Thus, children who used marijuana in adolescence had been seen as rebellious, unconventional in their thinking, unable to delay gratification, and without ambition during their preschool years. Those who later used hard drugs in addition were described as emotionally bland, keeping people at a distance, and lacking in personal charm. Whether such behavior patterns are due to a genetic difference or are the result of a parenting style that leads to a general hyporesponsivity or rebelliousness of the child is not known. However, it may be worth noting here that direct genetic effects on juvenile delinquency and conduct disturbances have not yet been established (Rutter et al., 1990).

Finally, there is good evidence that prenatal and perinatal factors may be important contributors to later parental styles. Work by one group (Minde et al., 1983, 1988) has shown that the severity of illness a premature infant suffers in the neonatal unit will significantly affect the type of parenting he or she receives. Parents of sicker babies initially behave in a more intrusive way, but after about 6 months seem to give up, that is, decrease their overall stimulation and contact significantly (Minde et al., 1988). Similar findings were reported by Wasserman and Allen (1985) from an observational study that compared the play, with their mothers, of premature, non-CNS-damaged, physically handicapped children and control children between the ages of 9 and 24 months. They reported that by 2 years of age, the mothers of the handicapped children had withdrawn from interaction, and this was associated with an average IQ drop of up to 20 points. This suggests that the absence of expected events characterizing normal physical or cognitive development can lead to a disruption of mother-child relations through maternal detachment or other parenting disorders (Affleck et al., 1982).

Parents of mentally handicapped children have also been observed while parenting their children. Byrne and Cunningham (1985) in a review paper stress that the problems such parents face in raising their children are multifaceted and complex. It appears that parenting patterns are largely determined by factors such as the age and competencies of the child and the practical needs of each family. There is also evidence that mothers are more flexible when teaching their young mentally handicapped than their nonhandicapped children, but may provide them with insufficient positive feedback (McConachie and Mitchell, 1985). They may also underestimate their children's actual abilities (Banu and Begum, 1991). Finally, in a study that compared the way mothers feed 15- to 39-month-old normal children and children with severe cerebral palsy, Reilly and Skuse (1992) documented that the handicapped children were fed with minimal verbal interactions and in a rather mechanical way. Furthermore, while the duration of feeds for the two groups was almost identical, the handicapped youngsters, because of their severe motor dysfunction and poor overall feeding skills, were offered only 60% and ate only 50% as much food as their nonhandicapped peers. The authors suggest that such feeding practices may be responsible for a significant part of the retarded growth exhibited by mentally handicapped children. This study also confirms the data by Wasserman and Allen (1985) and Minde and his group (1988), which suggested that parents need to be validated in their parenting activities by their children and that one important aspect of this validation is the child's "normal" look and behavior.

PARENT EDUCATION

Recognizing the powerful impact primary caretakers have on the behavior and emotional well-being of their children, also as future adults, has long stimulated educators and clinicians to think about how one might educate parents for the task of raising children and make them more sensitive to their needs (Sunley, 1955). While many different parenting programs have been offered to the public during the past 50 years, only recently has there been an interest in developing specific guidelines for assessing parenting ability and empirically validating parent education programs (Fine and Henry, 1989; Steinhauer, 1988; Steinhauer et al., 1993). An examination of the literature suggests that parent education programs focus on one or more of the following areas:

1. *Information sharing:* This consists of providing knowledge about developmental expectations, legal rights of parents and children, or other factual information. Lectures, printed materials, or group discussions are used to reach parents.
2. *Improving self-awareness:* This aspect stresses the need for parents to reflect on their own behaviors and helps them to understand how their actions may influence their children. Group discussions, specific individual activities, and the use of diaries or logbooks are the most common methods of instruction.
3. *Skill acquisition:* Here parents learn ways to appropriately manage children's behavior. Parents are trained through group discussions, practice assignments, and analysis of videotapes.
4. *Problem-solving:* This relates to the use of more constructive strategies in situations that may previously have led to conflict and arguments. These skills are taught by using feedback from reported actual events at home, direct observations during group sessions, as well as video or audiotapes.
5. *Psychoeducational preventive intervention:* These programs aim to identify etiological factors that may compromise parenting skills (e.g., a parent's mental illness or an infant's high risk condition such as prematurity or hyperactivity) and enhance the strengths of both parents and children. Intervention plans are individually tailored and designed to establish a therapeutic alliance within which information about a psychiatric illness or medical condition and the need for adjusting parenting practices become clinically meaningful (Beardslee and Poderefsky, 1988; Beardslee et al., 1993; Brent et al., 1993; Minde et al., 1980).

Three major conceptual models are used in parent education programs. Each is based on different aspects of developmental or psychotherapeutic theories and, despite common features, addresses different areas of caregiver and child behavior.

1. *Reflective counseling:* These programs are based on Carl Roger's teaching and emphasize the understanding and acceptance of the child's feelings. Parent Effectiveness Training or PET (Gordon, 1975) is a good example of this approach. Reflective counseling also helps parents to become more authoritative in their interactions with their children.
2. *Behavioral management courses:* Managing the actual behavior of children through behavioral analysis is the dominant feature of these parent educations courses, such as the Responsive Parenting Program (Clark-Hall, 1978). These programs emphasize information sharing and skill training and devote less attention to improving parental self-awareness.
3. *Adlerian counseling:* Education programs based on Adler's teaching emphasize that parents must understand the goals and meanings of their children's behavior in order to deal with their children successfully. These programs aim to establish a more cooperative family environment and use logical consequences to control behaviors. The best known proponents of this approach are Dreikurs and Soltz (1964).

Evaluations of individual programs have been questionable. As Medway (1989) observes in a recent chapter on the effectiveness of parent teaching programs, few workers in this area have used clearly defined methodologies, objective measurements, matched samples of control populations, and adequate follow-up evaluations. Furthermore, different programs demand varying degrees of training and sophistication from their respective group leaders and therapists.

Despite these difficulties, there are a number of studies that have attempted to assess the effectiveness of parent education (Beardslee et al., 1993; Minde et al., 1980; Patterson et al., 1983). In addition, the 24 scientifically most acceptable programs have recently been analyzed in a meta-analysis by Medway (1989). This analysis included studies of 12 behavioral training programs, 5 parent effectiveness training (PET) programs, and 7 Adlerian programs. Medway reports that all of them were effective in that children and parents showed an average of 62% improvement over their respective control populations. Those studies that followed their samples for up to 6 months indicated that gains were enduring. While outcome results were similar, data suggest that behavioral management courses improved child behavior more rapidly than did programs using reflective or Adlerian counseling.

Programs using psychoeducational preventive interventions in clinical settings have typically been carefully evaluated (e.g., Beardslee et al., 1993; Minde et al., 1980). However, leading such parenting programs usually requires lengthy training and detailed knowledge about specific medical or psychiatric conditions. This makes it more difficult for others to replicate the initially reported treatment effects.

In summary, there is some evidence that parent training can be helpful to adults who are interested and committed to improving their parenting skills. While parent education programs have been based on various educational models, there are few if any differences in their effectiveness. This suggests that behavioral changes in children can be brought about both by parental insight and through direct behavioral intervention by the parent. However, the long-term effects of such changes as well as their relationship to more global behavioral variables, such as problem-solving or social skills in children, have not yet been established.

CONCLUSIONS AND UNRESOLVED ISSUES

The evidence from the studies cited in this chapter shows the complexity of the factors that constitute the task of parenting. Possible processes of psychological development that underlie the numerous research findings have been outlined. Disorders of parenting are not static single variables but reflect interactions between internal representations within parents and outside stresses and supports, as well as among a range of child-related variables.

While some of the data are strong enough to provide a basis for teaching parents who come for advice, many of the hypotheses still need elaboration and confirmation. For example, little is still known about the degree to which genetic factors determine parenting competence and the compensating influence nonparental caretakers can have on the later behavior of a child.

We also still poorly understand the effect of some child-centered mediating variables. For example, does the possible genetic contribution children make to the parenting they receive operate through temperamental features or overall vulnerability to stress, or through ways in which aspects of the environment are selectively perceived by the child, leading to greater or lesser levels of experienced adversity? The difference that sex or the presence of older and younger siblings makes on the susceptibility of children to abnormal parenting also needs to be further explored. However, the overall recognition in child psychiatry that developmental pathways show both continuities and discontinuities and that there are few experiences that cannot be made up later in life makes the study of parenting competence central to the development of preventive and therapeutic interventions.

References

Affleck G, Allen D, McGrade BJ, et al: Home environments of developmentally disabled infants as a function of parent and infant characteristics. *Am J Ment Defic* 86:445, 1982.

Ainsworth MD: *Infancy in Uganda: Infant Care and Growth of Love.* Baltimore, Johns Hopkins University Press, 1957.

Ainsworth MD, Blehar MC, Waters E, et al: *Patterns of Attachment: A Psychological Study of the Strange Situation.* Hillsdale, NJ, Erlbaum, 1978.

American Association for Protecting Children: *Highlights of Official Child Neglect and Abuse Reporting 1984.* Denver, CO, American Humane Association, 1986.

Baldwin AL, Baldwin C, Kasser T, et al: Contextual risk and resiliency during late adolescence. *Dev Psychopathol* 5:741–761, 1993.

Baldwin AL, Baldwin C, Sameroff AJ, et al: Protective features in adolescent development. Paper presented at the biennial meeting of the Society for Research in Child Development, Kansas City, MO, March 1989.

Banu S, Begum S: Parents beliefs about cognitive abilities of handicapped and non-handicapped children. *Pak J Child Ment Health* 2:102–120, 1991.

Barash D: *Sociobiology and Behavior.* New York, Elsevier, 1977.

Barnett D, Manley JT, Cicchetti D: Defining child maltreatment: The interface between policy and research. In: Cicchetti D, Toth SL (eds): *Child Abuse, Child Development and Social Policy.* Norwood, NJ, Ablex, 1993, pp. 7–73.

Bates J: The concept of difficult temperament. *Merrill-Palmer Q* 26:299, 1980.

Baumrind D: Child care practices anteceding three patterns of preschool behavior. *Genet Psychol Monogr* 75:43, 1967.

Baumrind DH: Harmonious parents and their preschool children. *Dev Psychol* 4:99, 1971.

Baumrind D: Rearing competent children. In: Dounon W (ed): *Child Development Today and Tomorrow.* San Francisco, Jossey-Bass, 1989, pp. 349–378.

Beardslee WR: The need for the study of adaptation in the children of parents with affective disorders. In: Rutter M, Izard CE, Read PB (eds): *Depression in Young People: Developmental and Clinical Perspectives.* New York, Guilford, 1986.

Beardslee WR, Poderesfsky D: Resilient adolescents whose parents have serious affective and other psychiatric disorder: The importance of self-understanding and relationships. *Am J Psychiatry* 145: 63–69, 1988.

Beardslee WR, Keller MB, Lavori PW, et al: The impact of parental affective disorder on depression in offspring: A longitudinal follow-up of a non-referred sample. *J Am Acad Child Adolesc Psychiatry* 32: 723–730, 1993.

Beardslee WR, Salt P, Porterfield K, et al: Comparison of preventive intervention for families with parental affective disorder. *J Am Acad Child Adolesc Psychiatry* 32:254–263, 1993.

Bell RQ, Harper LV: *Child Effects on Adults.* Hillsdale, NJ, Erlbaum, 1977.

Belsky J: The determinants of parenting: A process model. *Child Dev* 55:83, 1984.

Belsky J: Etiology of child maltreatment: A development-ecological analysis. *Psychol Bull* 114: 413–433, 1993.

Belsky J, Vondra J: Lessons from child abuse:

The determinants of parenting. In: Cicchetti D, Carlson V (eds): *Child Maltreatment: Theory and Research on the Causes and Consequences of Child Abuse and Neglect*. Cambridge, Cambridge University Press, 1989.

Belsky J, Gilstrap B, Rovine M: The Pennsylvania Infant and Family Development Project. Stability and change in mother-infant and father-infant interaction in a family setting at one, three, and nine months. *Child Dev* 52:692, 1984.

Benoit D, Zeanah CH, Barton ML: Maternal attachment disturbances in failure to thrive. *Infant Ment Health J* 10:185, 1989.

Benoit D, Zeanah CH, Boucher C, et al: Sleep disorders in early childhood: Association with insecure maternal attachment. *J Am Acad Child Adolesc Psychiatry* 31:86–93, 1992.

Billings AG, Moos RH: Comparisons of children of depressed and nondepressed parents: A social-environmental perspective. *J Abnorm Child Psychol* 11:463, 1983.

Block J, Block JH, Keyes S: Longitudinally foretelling drug usage in adolescence: Early childhood personality and environmental precursors. *Child Dev* 59:336, 1988.

Bowlby J: *Attachment and Loss*. Vol 1: *Attachment*. New York, Basic Books, 1969.

Bowlby J: *Child Care and the Growth of Love*. London, Pelican, 1973.

Bowlby J: *The Making and Breaking of Affectional Bonds*. London, Tavistock, 1979.

Bowlby J: *Attachment and Loss*. Vol 3: *Loss*. New York, Basic Books, 1980.

Bowlby J: *A Secure Base. Clinical Application of Attachment Theory*. London, Routledge, 1988.

Boyd JH, Weissman MM: Epidemiology of affective disorders: A reexamination of future directions. *Arch Gen Psychiatry* 38:1039, 1981.

Brant S, Cullman E: *Small Folk: A Celebration of Childhood in America*. New York, Dutton, 1980.

Brent DA, Poling K, McKain B, et al: A psychoeducational program for families of affectively ill children and adolescents. *J Am Acad Child Adolesc Psychiatry* 32:770–774, 1993.

Bretherton I: Attachment theory: Retrospect and prospect. In: Bretherton I, Waters E (eds): *Growing Points of Attachment Theory and Research* (Monographs of the Society for Research in Child Development, 50, serial no. 209). Chicago, University of Chicago Press, 1985.

Brody G, Pellegrini A, Sigel I: Marital quality and mother-child and father-child interactions with school-aged children. *Dev Psychol* 22:291, 1986.

Bronfenbrenner U: *The Ecology of Human Development: Experiments by Nature and Design*. Cambridge, MA, Harvard University Press, 1979.

Brunquell D, Crichton L, Egeland B: Maternal personality and attitude in disturbances of child rearing. *Am J Orthopsychiatry* 51:680, 1981.

Burgess R, Youngblade L: The intergenerational transmission of abusive parental practices: A social interactional analysis. In: Gelles R, Hotaling G, Finkelhor D, et al (eds): *New Directions in Family Violence Research*. New York, Sage, 1990.

Buxbaum E: Psychosexual development: The oral, anal and phallic phases. In: Levitt D (ed): *Readings in Psychoanalytic Psychology*. New York, Appleton, 1959.

Byrne EA, Cunningham CC: The effects of mentally handicapped children on families—A conceptual review. *J Child Psychol Psychiatry* 26:847–864, 1985.

Caldwell BM: The effects of infant care. In: Hoffman ML, Hoffman LW (eds): *Review of Child Development Research* (Vol 1). New York, Russell Sage Foundation, 1964.

Campbell S: Mother-infant interaction as a function of maternal ratings of temperament. *Child Psychiatry Hum Dev* 10:67, 1979.

Canavan MM, Clark R: The mental health of 463 children from dementia praecox stock (1). *Ment Hyg* 7:137, 1923a.

Canavan MM, Clark R: The mental health of 581 offspring of nonpsychotic parents. *Ment Hyg* 7:770, 1923b.

Canavan MM, Clark R: The mental health of 463 children from dementia praecox stock (2). *Ment Hyg* 20:463, 1936.

Cantwell DP: Depression in childhood: Clinical picture and diagnostic criteria. In: Cantwell DP, Carlson GA (eds): *Affective Disorders in Childhood and Adolescence: An Update*. New York, Spectrum, 1983.

Cicchetti D, Carlson V (eds): *Child Maltreatment: Theory and Research on the Causes and Consequences of Child Abuse and Neglect*. Cambridge, Cambridge University Press, 1989.

Cicchetti D, Risley R: Developmental perspectives on the etiology, intergenerational transmission, and sequelae of child maltreatment. In: Risley R, Cicchetti D (eds): *Developmental Perspectives on Child Maltreatment* (New Directions for Child Development, no. 11). Chicago, University of Chicago Press, 1981.

Clark-Hall M: *Responsive Parenting Manual*. Lawrence, KS, H & H Enterprises, 1978.

Clarke RVG, Cornish DB: The effectiveness of residential treatment. In: Hersov LA, Berger M, Shaffer D (eds): *Aggression and Antisocial Behaviour in Childhood and Adolescence*. Oxford, Pergamon, 1978.

Clarke-Stewart KA: And daddy makes three: The father's impact on mother and the young child. *Child Dev* 50:446, 1978.

Coghill SR, Caplan NH, Alexander H, et al: Impact of maternal postnatal depression on cognitive development of young children. *Br Med J* 292:1165, 1986.

Cowan FP, Cowan P: A preventive intervention for couples during family formation. Paper presented at the meetings for the Society for Research in Child Development, Detroit, April 1983.

Cox AD, Puckering C, Pound A, et al: The impact of maternal depression in young children. *J Child Psychol Psychiatry* 28:917, 1987.

Cox MJ, Owen MT, Lewis JM, et al: Marriage, adult adjustment, and early parenting. *Child Dev* 60:1015, 1989.

Crockenberg S: Toddlers' reactions to maternal anger. *Merrill-Palmer Q* 31:361, 1985.

Cummings EM, Hennessy KD, Rabideau GJ, et al: Responses of physically abused boys to interadult anger involving their mother. *Dev Psychopathol* 6:31–41, 1994.

Cummings EM, Iannotti RJ, Zahn-Waxler C: Influence of conflict between adults on the emotions and aggression of young children. *Dev Psychol* 21:495, 1985.

Cummings JS, Pellegrini DS, Notarius CI, et al: Children's responses to angry adult behavior as a function of marital distress and history of interparent hostility. *Child Dev* 60:1035, 1989.

Cummings EM, Simpson KS, Wilson A: Children's responses to interadult anger as a function of information about resolution. *Dev Psychol* 29:978–985, 1993.

Cytryn L, McKnew DW, Zahn-Waxler C, et al: A developmental view of affective disturbances in the children of affectively ill parents. *Am J Psychiatry* 141:219, 1984.

Cytryn L, McKnew DW, Zahn-Waxler C, et al: Developmental issues in risk research: The offspring of affectively ill parents. In: Rutter M, Izard CE, Read P (eds): *Depression in Children: Developmental Perspectives*. New York, Guilford, 1986.

Dornbusch SM, Ritter PL, Leiderman PH, et al: The relation of parenting style to adolescent school performance. *Child Dev* 58:1244, 1987

Dowdney L, Mrazek DA, Quinton D, et al: Observation of parent-child interaction with two to three-year-olds. *J Child Psychol Psychiatry* 25:379, 1984.

Dowdney L, Skuse D, Rutter M, et al: The nature and qualities of parenting provided by women raised in institutions. *J Child Psychol Psychiatry* 26:599, 1985.

Dreikurs R, Soltz V: *Children: The Challenge*. New York, Hawthorn, 1964.

Dubowitz H: Child malnutrition in the United States: Etiology, impact and prevention. Background paper prepared for the Congress of the United States, Office of Technology Assessment, 1986.

Dunn J: Individual differences in temperament. In: Rutter M (ed): *Scientific Foundations of Developmental Psychiatry*. London, Heinemann, 1980.

Dunn J, Kendrick C: Interaction between young siblings: Association with the interaction between mother and first-born. *Dev Psychol* 17:336, 1981.

Easterbrooks A, Emde R: Marital and parent-child relationships: The role of affect in the family system. In: Hinde R, Stevenson-Hinde J (eds): *Relationships within Families: Mutual Influences*. Oxford, Oxford University Press, 1988.

Egeland B, Jacobvitz D, Papatola K: Intergenerational continuity of abuse. Paper presented at the Social Science Research Council Conference on Child Abuse and Neglect, York, ME, May 20–23, 1984.

El Sheikh M, Cummings EM, Goetsch V: Coping with adults' angry behavior: Behavioral, physiological, and verbal responses in preschoolers. *Dev Psychol* 25:490, 1989.

Emde RN: The infant's relationship experience: Developmental and affective aspects. In: Sameroff A, Emde RN (eds): *Relationship Disturbances in Early Childhood: A Developmental Approach*. New York, Basic Books, 1989.

Emery RE: Interparental conflict and the children of discord and divorce. *Psychol Bull* 92:310, 1982.

Emery RE, O'Leary D: Marital discord and child behavior problems in a nonclinic sample. *J Abnorm Child Psychol* 12:411, 1984.

Engfer A, Schneewind K: Causes and consequences of harsh parental punishment. *Child Abuse Negl* 6:129, 1982.

Farrington DP: Age and crime. In: Toury M, Morris N (eds): *Crime and Justice* (Vol 7). Chicago, University of Chicago Press, 1986.

Ferri E: *Growing Up in a One-Parent Family*. Slough, England, NFER, 1976.

Field T: Early interactions between infants and their postpartum depressed mother. *Infant Behav Dev* 7:527, 1984.

Field T, Healy B, Goldstein S, et al: Infants of depressed mothers show "depressed" behavior even with nondepressed adults. *Child Dev* 59:1569, 1988.

Fine MJ, Henry SA: Professional issues in parent education. In: Fine MJ (ed): *The Second Handbook on Parent Education*. New York, Academic Press, 1989, pp. 3–20.

Fonagi P, Steele H, Steele M: Maternal representations of attachment during pregnancy predict the organization of infant-mother attachment at one year of age. *Child Dev* 62:891–905, 1991.

Forehand R, King H, Peed S, et al: Mother-child interaction: Comparison of a non-compliant clinic group and a non-clinic group. *Behav Res Ther* 13:79, 1975.

Freud A: *The Ego and the Mechanisms of Defense*. London, Hogarth, 1937.

Freud S: Analysis of a phobia in a five-year-old boy. In: Struchey J (ed): *The Standard Edition of the Complete Psychological Works of Sigmund Freud*

(Vol 10). London, Hogarth Press, 1958. (Originally published 1909.)

Friedrich W, Wheeler K: The abusing parent revisited: A decade of psychological research. *J Nerv Ment Dis* 170:577, 1982.

Gardner NH: The later adjustment of children born in mental hospital to psychotic mothers (Thesis Abstract). *Smith Coll Stud Soc Work* 19:137, 1949.

Garmezy N: Stress-resistant children: The search for protective factors. In: Stevenson JE (ed): *Recent Research in Developmental Psychopathology (J Child Psychol Psychiatry* book supplement, no. 4). Oxford, Pergamon, 1984.

Garmezy N, Devine V: Project competence: The Minnesota studies of children vulnerable to psychopathology. In: Watt N, Rolf J, Anthony EJ (eds): *Children at Risk for Schizophrenia*. London, Cambridge University Press, 1984.

Gershon ES, Hamovit J, Guroff J, et al: A family study of schizoaffective, bipolar I, bipolar II, unipolar probands and normal controls. *Arch Gen Psychiatry* 39:1157, 1982.

Giovannoni J: Definitional issues in child maltreatment. In: Cicchetti D, Carlson V: *Child Maltreatment: Theory and Research on the Causes and Consequences of Child Abuse and Neglect*. Cambridge, Cambridge University Press, 1989.

Goldberg WA, Easterbrooks MA: The role of marital quality in toddler development. *Child Dev* 20:504, 1984.

Gordon T: *P.E.T. Parent Effectiveness Training*. New York, American Library, 1975.

Gottesmann I, Shields J: *Schizophrenia the Epigenetic Puzzle*. Cambridge, Cambridge University Press, 1982.

Hammen C, Gordon D, Burge D, et al: Maternal affective disorders, illness and stress: Risk for children's psychopathology. *Am J Psychiatry* 144:736, 1987.

Harder DW, Kokes RF, Fisher L, et al: Child competence and psychiatric risk. IV: Relationship of parent diagnostic classification and parent psychopathology severity to child functioning. *J Nerv Ment Dis* 168:343, 1980.

Hertzberger S: Social cognition and the transmission of abuse. In: Finkelhor D, Gelles R, Hotaling G, et al (eds): *The Dark Side of Families: Current Family Violence Research*. Beverly Hills, Sage, 1983.

Hetherington EM: Coping with family transitions: Winners, losers, and survivors. *Child Dev* 60:1, 1989.

Hetherington EM, Cox M, Cox CR: Effects of divorce on parents and children. In: Lamb M (ed): *Nontraditional Families*. Hillsdale, NJ, Erlbaum, 1982.

Hinde RA: Family influences. In: Rutter M (ed): *Scientific Foundations of Developmental Psychiatry*. London, Heinemann, 1980.

Hinde RA, Stevenson-Hinde J (eds): *Relationships within Families: Mutual Influences*. Oxford, Clarendon, 1988.

Hodges J, Tizard B: IQ and behavioural adjustment of exinstitutional adolescents. *J Child Psychol Psychiatry* 30:53, 1989a.

Hodges J, Tizard B: Social and family relationships of exinstitutional adolescents. *J Child Psychol Psychiatry* 30:77, 1989b.

Hoffman ML: Moral internalization, parental power and the nature of parent-child interaction. *Dev Psychol* 11:228, 1975.

Holt LE: *The Care and Feeding of Children*. New York, Appleton, 1902.

Howes P, Markman HJ: Marital quality and child functioning: A longitudinal investigation. *Child Dev* 60:1044, 1989.

Hunter R, Kilstrom N: Breaking the cycle in abusive families. *Am J Psychiatry* 136:1320, 1979.

Jacob T, Tennenbaum DL: *Family Assessment. Rationale, Methods, and Future Directions*. New York, Plenum, 1988.

Jaenicke C, Hammen C, Zupan B, et al: Cognitive vulnerability in children at risk for depression. *J Abnorm Child Psychol* 15:559, 1987.

Janet P: *Psychological Healing* (Vol 1) (Paul E, Paul C, trans). London, Allen & Unwin, 1925.

Jones TA, Green V, Krauss DR: Maternal responsiveness of primiparous mothers during the postpartum period: Age differences. *Pediatrics* 65:579, 1980.

Jouriles EN, Pfiffner LJ, O'Leary SG: Marital conflict, parenting and toddler conduct problem. *J Abnorm Child Psychol* 16:197, 1988.

Kaufman J, Zigler E: Do abused children become abusive parents? *Am J Orthopsychiatry* 57:186, 1987.

Kaufman J, Zigler E: The intergenerational transmission of child abuse. In: Cicchetti D, Carlson V (eds): *Child Maltreatment: Theory and Research on the Causes and Consequences of Child Abuse and Neglect*. Cambridge, Cambridge University Press, 1989.

Kelley P: The relation of infant's temperament and mother's psychopathology to interactions in early infancy. In: Riegel KF, Meacham JA (eds): *The Developing Individual in a Changing World* (Vol 2). Chicago, Aldine, 1976.

Klaus MH, Kennell JH: *Parent-Infant Bonding* (2nd ed). St. Louis, Mosby, 1982.

Kochanska G, Kuczynski L, Radke-Yarrow M, et al: Resolution of control episodes between well and affectively ill mothers and their young children. *J Abnorm Child Psychol* 15:441, 1987.

Kokes RF, Harder DW, Fisher L, et al: Child competence and psychiatric risk. V: Sex of patient parent and dimensions of psychopathology. *J Nerv Ment Dis* 168:348, 1980.

Lamborn SD, Mounts NS, Steinberg L, et al: Patterns of competence and adjustment among adolescents from authoritative, authoritarian, indulgent, and neglectful families. *Child Dev* 62:1049–1065, 1991.

LeBlanc M, Loeber R: Precursors, causes and the development of clinical offending. In: Hay DF, Angold A (eds): *Precursors and Causes in Development and Psychopathology*. New York, Wiley, 1993, pp. 233–263.

LeVine R: Child rearing as a cultural adaptation. In: Leiderman PH, Tulkin SR, Rosenfeld A (eds): *Culture and Infancy, Variations in the Human Experience*. New York, Academic Press, 1977.

Levy DM: *Maternal Overprotection*. New York, Columbia University Press, 1943.

Lobitz GK, Johnson SM: Parental manipulation of the behavior of normal and deviant children. *Child Dev* 46:719, 1975.

Locke J: Some thoughts concerning education. In: *John Locke on Politics and Education*. New York, Walter Black, 1947.

Loeb RC, Horst L, Horton PJ: Family interaction patterns associated with self-esteem in preadolescent girls and boys. *Merrill-Palmer Q* 26:203, 1980.

Loeber R, Stouthamer-Loeber M: Family factors as correlates and predictors of juvenile conduct problems and delinquency. In: Toury M, Morris N (eds): *Crime and Justice* (Vol 7). Chicago, University of Chicago Press, 1986.

Luthar S: Annotation: Methodological and conceptual issues in research on childhood resilience. *J Child Psychol Psychiatry* 34:441–453, 1993.

Maccoby E, Martin J: Socialization in the context of the family: Parent-child interaction. In: Hetherington EM (ed): *Handbook of Child Psychology. Vol 4: Socialization, Personality, and Social Development*. New York, Wiley, 1983.

Main M, Goldwyn R: Predicting rejection of her infant from mother's representation of her own experience: Implications for the abused-abusing intergenerational cycle. *Child Abuse Negl* 8:203, 1984.

Main M, Hesse E: Lack of resolution of mourning in adulthood and its relation to disorganization in infancy: Speculations regarding causal mechanisms. In: Greenberg M, Cicchetti D, Cummings M (eds): *Attachment in the Preschool Years*. Chicago, University of Chicago Press, 1990.

McConachie H, Mitchell DR: Parents teaching their young mentally handicapped children. *J Child Psychol Psychiatry* 26:389–405, 1985.

McCord W, McCord J: *Origins of Crime: A New Evaluation of the Cambridge-Sommerville Study*. New York, Columbia University Press, 1959.

Mead M, Wolfenstein M (eds): *Childhood in Contemporary Cultures*. Chicago, University of Chicago Press, 1955.

Meadows S, Mills M: Preschool parenting style and children's cognition: Follow-up on starting school. *ESRC Final Report*, July 1987.

Medway FJ: Measuring the effectiveness of parent education. In: Fine MJ (ed): *The Second Handbook on Parent Education*. New York, Academic Press, 1989, pp. 237–255.

Merikangas KR: Assortative mating for psychiatric disorders and psychological traits. *Arch Gen Psychiatry* 39:1173, 1982.

Minde K: Bonding and attachment: Its relevance for the present-day clinician. *Dev Med Child Neurol* 28:803, 1986.

Minde K, Nikapota AD: Child psychiatry and the developing world: Recent developments. *Transcult Psychiatr Res Rev* 30:315–346, 1993.

Minde K, Corter C, Goldberg S, et al: Maternal preference toward premature twins: Stability and effect on behavior over four years. *J Am Acad Child Adolesc Psychiatry* 29:367, 1990.

Minde K, Perrotta M, Corter C: The effect of neonatal complications in same sexed premature twins on their mother's preference. *J Am Acad Child Psychiatry* 21:443–452, 1982.

Minde K, Perrotta M, Hellmann J: The impact of delayed development in premature infants on mother-infant interaction: A prospective investigation. *J Pediatr* 112:136, 1988.

Minde K, Shosenberg N, Marton P, et al: Self-help groups in a premature nursery—A controlled evaluation. *J Pediatr* 96:933–940, 1980.

Minde K, Whitelaw H, Brown J, et al: Effect of neonatal complications in premature infants on early parent-infant interaction. *Dev Med Child Neurol* 25:763, 1983.

Minuchin S: Families and individual development: Provocations from the field of family therapy. *Child Dev* 56:289, 1985.

Mrazek D, Dowdney L, Rutter M, et al: Mother and preschool child interaction: A sequential approach. *J Am Acad Child Psychiatry* 21:453, 1982.

Olson DH, Sprenkle DH, Russel CS: Circumplex model of marital and family systems. I: Cohesion and adaptability dimensions, family types, and clinical applications. *Fam Process* 18:3, 1979.

Patterson GR: *Coercive Family Processes*. Eugene, OR, Castalia, 1982.

Patterson GR, Chamberlain P, Reid JB: A comparative evaluation of a parent-training program. *Behav Ther* 13:638–650, 1983.

Pelton L: Child abuse and neglect: The myth of classlessness. *Am J Orthopsychiatry* 48:608, 1978.

Plomin R, Daniels D: Why are children in the same family so different from one another? *Behav Brain Sci* 10:1, 1987.

Preston G, Antin R: A study of the children of psychotic parents. *Am J Orthopsychiatry* 2:231, 1933.

Puckering C: Maternal depression. *J Child Psychol Psychiatry* 30:807, 1989.

Puig-Antich J, Lukens E, Davis M, et al: Psychosocial functioning in prepubertal major depressive disorders. *Arch Gen Psychiatry* 42:500, 1985.

Quinton D, Rutter M: Early hospital admissions and late disturbances of behavior. *Dev Med Child Neurol* 18:447, 1976.

Quinton D, Rutter M: Parenting behaviour of mothers raised "in care." In: Nicol AR (ed): *Longitudinal Studies in Child Psychology and Psychiatry: Practical Lessons from Research Experience*. Chichester, Sussex, Wiley, 1985.

Quinton D, Rutter M, Liddle C: Institutional rearing, parenting difficulties and marital support. *Psychol Med* 14:107, 1984.

Radke-Yarrow M, Cummings EM, Kuszynski L, et al: Patterns of attachment in two and three year olds in normal families and families with parental depression. *Child Dev* 56:884, 1985.

Ragozin AS, Basham RB, Crnic KA, et al: Effects of maternal age on parenting role. *Dev Psychol* 18:627, 1982.

Ramage M: *Mental Health of Children of Psychotic Mothers*. Unpublished master's thesis, New York, Smith College, 1925.

Reilly S, Skuse D: Characteristics and management of feeding problems of young children with cerebral palsy. *Dev Med Child Neurol* 34:379–388, 1992.

Reitsma-Street M, Offord DR, Finch T: Pairs of same-sexed siblings discordant for antisocial behaviour. *Br J Psychiatry* 146:415, 1985.

Richman N, Stevenson J, Graham PJ: *Preschool to School: A Behavioural Study*. London, Academic Press, 1982.

Robins L, West PA, Herjanic BL: Arrests and delinquency in two generations: A study of black urban families and their children. *J Child Psychol Psychiatry* 16:125, 1975.

Rohner RP: *They Love Me, They Love Me Not: A Worldwide Study of the Effects of Parental Acceptance and Rejection*. New Haven, CT, HRAF Press, 1975.

Rousseau JJ: *Emile*. New York, Basic Books, 1979. (Originally published 1762.)

Rutter M: *Children of Sick Parents: An Environmental and Psychiatric Study* (Institute of Psychiatry Maudsley Monographs no. 16). London, Oxford University Press, 1966.

Rutter M: *Maternal Deprivation Reassessed* (2nd ed). Harmondsworth, UK, Penguin, 1981.

Rutter M: The developmental psychopathology of depression: Issues and perspectives. In: Rutter M, Izard CE, Read PB (eds): *Depression in Young People: Developmental and Clinical Perspectives*. New York, Guilford, 1986.

Rutter M: Intergenerational continuities and discontinuities in serious parenting difficulties. In: Cicchetti D, Carlson V (eds): *Child Maltreatment: Theory and Research on the Causes and Consequences of Child Abuse and Neglect*. Cambridge, Cambridge University Press, 1989.

Rutter M, Cox A: Other family influences. In: Rutter M, Hersov L (eds): *Child and Adolescent Psychiatry* (2nd ed). Oxford, Blackwell, 1987.

Rutter M, Giller H: *Juvenile Delinquency: Trends and Perspectives*. Harmondsworth, UK, Penguin, 1983.

Rutter M, Quinton D: Long-term follow-up of women institutionalized in childhood: Factors promoting good functioning in adult life. *Br J Dev Psychol* 2:191, 1984a.

Rutter M, Quinton D: Parental psychiatric disorder: Effects on children. *Psychol Med* 14:853, 1984b.

Rutter M, Cox A, Tupling C, et al: Attainment and adjustment in two geographical areas. I: The prevalence of psychiatric disorder. *Br J Psychiatry* 126:493, 1975.

Rutter M, Macdonald H, Le Couteur A, et al: Genetic factors in child psychiatric disorders. II: Empirical findings. *J Child Psychol Psychiatry* 31:39, 1990.

Rutter M, Quinton D, Liddle C: Parenting in two generations: Looking backwards and looking forwards. In: Madge N (ed): *Families at Risk*. London, Heinemann Educational, 1983.

Sameroff AJ, Zax M: In search of schizophrenia: Young offspring of schizophrenic women. In: Wynne LC, Cromwell RL, Mathysse S (eds): *The Nature of Schizophrenia: New Approaches to Research and Treatment*. New York, Wiley, 1978.

Sameroff AJ, Dickstein S, Hayden SC, et al: Effects of family process and parental depression on children. Paper presented at 60th meeting of the Society for Research in Child Development, New Orleans, March 1993.

Sears R, Maccoby E, Levin H: *Patterns of Child Rearing*. Evanston, IL, Row, Peterson, 1957.

Shure MB, Spivack G: *Problem-Solving Techniques in Child Rearing*. San Francisco, Jossey-Bass, 1978.

Skinner HA, Steinhauer PD, Santa-Barbara J: The family assessment measure. *Can J Community Ment Health* 2:91, 1983.

Sroufe LA: Infant-caregiver attachment and patterns of adaptation in preschool: The roots of maladaptation and competence. In: Perlmutter M (ed): *The Minnesota Symposium on Child Development* (vol 16). Hillsdale, NJ, Erlbaum, 1983.

Sroufe LA, Fleeson J: Attachment and the construction of relationships. In: Hartup W, Rubin Z (eds): *Relationships and Development*. New York, Cambridge University Press, 1986.

Sroufe LA, Fleeson J: The coherence of family relationships. In: Hinde R, Stevenson-Hinde J (eds): *Relationships within Families*. Oxford, UK, Oxford University Press, 1988.

Sroufe LA, Rutter M: The domain of developmental psychopathology. *Child Dev* 83:173, 1984.

Steele B, Pollock C: A psychiatric study of parents who abuse infants and small children. In: Helfer R, Kempe C (eds): *The Battered Child Syndrome*. Chicago, University of Chicago Press, 1968.

Stein G: The maternity blues. In: Brockington IF, Kumar R (eds): *Motherhood and Mental Illness*. London, Academic Press, 1982.

Steinberg L, Elmen JD, Mounts NS: Authoritative parenting, psychosocial maturity, and academic success among adolescents. *Child Dev* 60:1424, 1989.

Steinhauer PD: Assessing for parenting capacity. *Am J Orthopsychiatry* 53:468–481, 1983.

Steinhauer P: Clinical applications of the process model of family functioning. *Can J Psychiatry* 29:98, 1984.

Steinhauer P, Dymetryczyn R, Goncalves L, et al: The Toronto Parenting Capacity Assessment Project. Unpublished manuscript, Hospital for Sick Children, August 1993.

Strauss M: Family patterns and child abuse in a nationally representative sample. *Int J Child Abuse Negl* 3:23, 1979.

Sunley R: Early nineteenth century American literature on child rearing. In: Mead M, Wolfenstein M (eds): *Childhood in Contemporary Cultures*. Chicago, University of Chicago Press, 1955, pp. 150–176.

Suomi SJ, Harlow HF, Novak MA: Reversal of social deficits produced by isolation rearing in monkeys. *J Hum Evol* 3:527, 1974.

Tizard B, Hodges J: The effect of early institutional rearing on the development of eight-year-old children. *J Child Psychol Psychiatry* 19:99, 1978.

Trivers R: Parent-offspring conflict. *Am Zool* 14:249, 1974.

Vaughn BE, Block JH, Block J: Parental agreement on child rearing during early childhood and the psychological characteristics of adolescents. *Child Dev* 59:1020–1033, 1988.

Vuchinich S, Vuchinich R, Wood B: The interparental relationship and family problem solving with pre-adolescent males. *Child Dev* 64:1389–1400, 1993.

Wadsworth M: *Roots of Delinquency: Infancy, Adolescence and Crime*. Oxford, UK, Martin Robertson, 1979.

Wandersman L, Unger DG: Interaction of infant difficulty and social support in adolescent mothers. Paper presented at the biennial meeting of the Society for Research in Child Development, Detroit, April 1983.

Washington J, Minde K, Goldberg S: Temperament in preterm style and stability. *J Am Acad Child Adolesc Psychiatry* 25:493, 1986.

Wasserman G, Allen R: Maternal withdrawal from handicapped toddlers. *J Child Psychol Psychiatry* 26:381, 1985.

Weintraub S, Winters KC, Neale JM: Competence and vulnerability in children with an affectively disordered parent. In: Rutter M, Izard CE, Reid PB (eds): *Depression in Young People: Developmental and Clinical Perspectives*. New York, Guilford, 1986.

Weiss B, Dodge KA, Bates JE, et al: Some consequences of early harsh discipline: Child aggression and a maladaptive social information processing style. *Child Dev* 63:1321–1335, 1992.

Weiss PL, Summers KJ: Marital interaction coding system—III. In: Filsinger E (ed): *Marriage and Family Assessment*. Beverly Hills, CA, Sage, 1983.

Weissman MM, Gammon D, John K, et al: Children of depressed parents: Increased pathology and early onset of major depression. *Arch Gen Psychiatry* 44:847, 1987.

Weissman MM, Gershon ES, Kidd KK, et al: Psychiatric disorders in the relatives of probands with affective disorders: The Yale-NIMH collaborative family study. *Arch Gen Psychiatry* 41:13, 1984.

Werner EE: *Cross-Cultural Child Development: A View from the Planet Earth*. Monterey, CA, Brooks/Cole, 1979.

West DJ: *Delinquency: Its Roots, Careers and Prospects*. London, Heinemann, 1982.

West DJ, Farrington DP: *Who Becomes Delinquent?* London, Heinemann, 1973.

Wilson H: Parental supervision: A neglected aspect of delinquency. *Br J Criminol* 20:203, 1980.

Wynne C: The epigenesis of relational systems: A model for understanding family development. *Fam Process* 23:297, 1984.

Yarrow MR, Campbell JD, Burton R: *Child Rearing, an Inquiry into Research and Methods*. San Francisco, Jossey-Bass, 1968.

Zekoski E, O'Hara MW, Wills KE: The effects of maternal mood on mother-infant interaction. *J Abnorm Child Psychol* 15:361, 1986.

35 EFFECTS OF ETHNICITY ON CHILD AND ADOLESCENT DEVELOPMENT

John F. McDermott, Jr., M.D.

Culture consists of the variable values, attitudes, beliefs, and behaviors shared by a people and transmitted between generations. They constitute "a way of life" that help shape the developing personality from infancy through adulthood. It is generally accepted, then, that cultural forces imprint the human personality, that part of us that deals with the outside world. But how? Culture is not simply a layer on top of a biological core. Rather, cultural influences are woven into personality like a tapestry. The development of this tapestry can actually be seen by watching the direct influence of child-rearing practices on the evolving personality of the child. In every country across the globe, the world of the infant is seen through the lens of a parenting person or persons. In many cultures, the main parenting person is the mother, with the father an important but secondary influence. In Chinese society, grandparents have an important child-rearing function, so that the refraction of the lens becomes more complex. In African societies, infants and preschool children are managed by older siblings, offering them a very different view of the world (Earls, 1982). But whoever the primary caretaker may be, the infant's world soon grows to include others—first relatives, and then neighbors, who add new perspective. Later the child's world expands to include community influence—peers and other adults such as schoolteachers. As the number of interaction partners expands and changes, the mix of new perspectives forms a more and more complex pattern in the evolving personality tapestry.

The view presented above, of a primary relationship with one individual or a few individuals, to relationships with a growing number of individuals inside and outside the family unit, is the traditional dominant view of social development, sometimes called the continuous care and contact model (Tronick et al., 1987). It was derived from the work of Spitz (1965), Bowlby (1969), and Provence and Lipton (1962) on institutionalized children. More recent work in other parts of the world, however, suggests that early social experiences may be powerfully shaped by others including fathers, siblings, and other children (Morelli and Tronick, 1992; Whiting and Edwards, 1988; Zukow, 1989). A new "strategic" model has emerged—that infant social engagement occurs in an interactive context between infant and caregiver that is heavily influenced by group composition, values, and customs. It is based on studies (Tronick et al., 1992) that show patterns of simultaneous multiple relationships, rather than a single "mothering" person, may be determined by physical and social ecological factors. An intriguing notion has been put forth by these developmentalists that such cultural practices may develop in the child a basic sense of self that incorporates other people, and thus buffers against feelings of insecurity. It is a model that suggests that the enhancement of self-confidence through multiple secure bases in the surrounding world allows children in some societies to more readily explore their social and physical environment.

CULTURAL VARIATIONS IN CHILD REARING

How has the influence of culture on personality been studied? What is the evidence that differing child-rearing practices produce differences in personality traits? An anthropologist, William Caudill, was one of the first to scrutinize the interaction between children and the culture in which they grow. He found consistent cross-cultural differences in behavior that persisted from infancy through early childhood. Caudill studied cohorts of Japanese and American mother-infant dyads at 3

months, 2½ years, and 6 years, to test the degree to which culture transmits personality traits through mother-child interaction and the stability of those cultural variations (Caudill and Schooler, 1973; Caudill and Weinstein, 1969; Tulkin and Leiderman, 1973). All the infants were first-born, equally divided by sex, and living in intact urban middle-class families. Caudill found basic similarities in biologically rooted behaviors, as well as similarities of maternal behavior in time spent feeding, diapering, and dressing the infants. Beyond these similarities there were distinct cultural differences: American infants showed greater amounts of gross bodily activity, play, and happy vocalization. In comparison, Japanese infants were passive, with a greater amount of unhappy vocalization. American mothers encouraged their babies to be more active, while Japanese mothers soothed and quieted their babies. American mothers viewed their babies as separate and autonomous individuals who should learn to think and do things for themselves, perhaps reflecting their own needs for independence. Japanese mothers, on the other hand, appeared to view their babies as extensions of themselves, with the psychological boundaries between them blurred. The responses of the infants in both cultures appeared to be in line with the expectations of that culture. At each subsequent age period, the behavior of the children mirrored that of their mothers. The 3-year-old American children expressed a greater amount of both positive and negative emotional behavior. American mothers encouraged independence in their toddlers, so that by the age of 6, the American children emphasized their own personal possessions and were taking care of their own bodily needs.

Caudill concluded that the mothers in these two cultures engaged in different styles of caretaking and that the children in each culture became habituated to respond appropriately to these different styles. Their differential responses were in line, both with the mothers' expectations and with the general expectations in the two cultures. They reflected the development of a so-called national character. In America, the individual becomes physically and verbally assertive, in Japan, physically and verbally restrained. To summarize studies of socialization in Japan, two aspects—closeness of the mother-child bond, shaping obedience of young children, and the acquisition of a sense of obligation to the family and responsibility to group expectations—are powerful elements in shaping the behavior of the young child (Hess et al., 1987).

Other studies of preschool children in these cultures (Tobin and Davidson, 1989) also contrast the American orientation toward verbal self-expression and personal autonomy with that seen in Japanese children in other cultural settings. American preschool teachers are observed to encourage children to use words instead of physical expression toward one another, while Japanese preschool teachers believe that children should settle their own quarrels—that doing so contributes to group cohesion. Japanese teachers are reluctant to punish or exclude a disruptive child. Only behavior beyond the tolerance of the group is disapproved, and then teachers help the group contain or moderate it. A group orientation is more valued than an individual one.

By the time they are in elementary school, Japanese children are far more disciplined than American counterparts (Bell, 1989), perhaps because they have learned to accommodate to the group. Even disciplinary practices make use of these differences, in which Japanese parents cherish group harmony and American parents emphasize independence. While American mothers threaten to punish children by making them stay home, Japanese mothers threaten to punish by putting them out of the house.

Other cross-national studies (Gannon, 1975) also suggest that American parents emphasize independence to a greater extent than parents in other cultures. They make more demands for task mastery, self-feeding, and self-dressing, and these differences may determine the nature of developmental problems found in different groups of children. For example, among Puerto Rican children, more than a third of 5-year-olds take a bottle to bed with them. Sleep problems are much less prevalent than among the American children, who almost never take a bottle to bed because parents discourage it. On the other hand, Puerto Rican children show more developmental problems around discipline than American children.

Efforts have been devoted to quantitative studies on the social environments of infancy and early childhood. For example, Morelli (1992) suggests that the American middle-class custom of having children go to sleep by themselves and spend the night alone is unusual across the globe. Mayan mothers show shocked disapproval of American sleep practices as contrasted with their own custom of cosleeping that they consider important for the child's psychological development. It is speculated that Mayan parents may favor cosleeping as a way of protecting infants in a culture of high early mortality and for socialization of infants into the group, contrasting with American parents' emphasis on training for independence. Thus, there appear to be immediate parental values and goals related to psychological concerns that support some child-rearing customs.

Epidemiological surveys, one British and the other American (Earls, 1980; Richman et al., 1975; Richman and Tulpin, 1974), also demonstrate developmental differences in children reared in different cultures. A high frequency of fears in children from West Indian families in London and the similar higher frequency of fears in American girls have led to speculation that this higher frequency may be a response to social factors that promote dependency in children. American girls and West Indian children in England were encouraged to assume more dependent roles, and perhaps an increased number of fears was a consequence. While this has been traditionally linked to male dominance over women in the lives of young children, girls today are increasingly encouraged to be independent in American families. (The change in male/female personality type is further considered later in this chapter.)

In any case, we can conclude that human development is not bound to a single cultural model. Some cultures are individual centered, placing emphasis on independence and self-reliance, while others emphasize the interdependence of individuals within larger groups such as the family (Chiu, 1987; Hsu, 1981). In these cultures, when individuals are successful, that success is attributed to the group rather than to the individual.

The effect of this different value system can be seen beyond the individual and small group. It is reflected, for example, at a national (and international) level in the so-called national character that is responsible for Japan's economic success. A national commitment to the success of the group over that of the individual and the relative absence of adversarial relationships in the industrial work force have shifted competition from within the group to another level—with other countries. Cultural values, built in from birth, are considered to be the reason for Japan's rise as the world's leading economic power.

The interaction between different value systems can be seen within a culture as well as between two cultures. The conflict between Chinese youth and the government of their country in the 1980s has brought into focus the Western versus the Eastern value system. For centuries, the traditional organizing principle of Chinese society has depended upon individuals giving up individual freedom and subordinating their own interests to the interest of the group. This traditional societal value has recently come into sharp conflict with Western values oriented toward autonomy and self-expression. The resolution of this conflict poses national as well as international dilemmas. Countries in Eastern Europe have also undergone this shift in recent years—from a collective society to one that is oriented toward Western values of individuality and competition. The symptoms among people who are in conflict over this sudden shift in ego ideal are considered below.

ETHNOCENTRICITY

Western theories of personality development have been oriented toward individuality and autonomy. The ethnocentricity or culture blindness of this "single model" approach is illustrated by the most widely known theories of emotional and cognitive development. The concept most central to psychoanalytic theory, the Oedipus complex, was shaped by the middle-class family roles of Little Hans and his parents in 19th-century Vienna. Piaget's own grandchildren in turn-of-the-century Geneva served as his research subjects, and generalizations were made from their cognitive development to that of others throughout the world. Kohlberg's six-stage hierarchy of morality clearly reflects a narrow cultural ideal, and one that is male oriented. These observations about the cognitive and emotional development of middle-class European children led to narrow conclusions and far-reaching generalizations to other cultures. The broad application of the stereotype American nuclear family model of psychopathology—overinvolved mother, peripheral father, and triangulated child—also suggests a degree of culture blindness. Recent research has described different culturally determined family styles that are equally adaptive, but just different from one another. For example, a comparative study of Japanese and Caucasian families living side by side (McDermott et al., 1983a) in Hawaii suggests that Japanese families emphasize collective action, cognitive approaches, and task orientation, in contrast to the emphasis in Caucasian families on affective expression and individuality. Both styles are quite functional in the same society. Neither is right or wrong. And certainly, no single model can explain the complexity of child and family development across the cultures of the world.

CROSS-NATIONAL STUDIES

Studies of children in cultures whose child-rearing patterns differ from one another teach us not only different models of child development but also what those different models have in common. The Whitings were an anthropological team who conducted the first large-scale international research project to observe children systematically. They studied adult expectations of child behavior in seven different cultures (India, Okinawa, the Philippines, Mexico, Kenya, the United States, and Liberia) (Whiting and Edwards, 1988; Whiting and Whiting, 1975). Their findings led to two major conclusions. First, they found that the traditional stereotype of maternal behavior characterized by nurturance must be revised. Across all the cultures studied, parental efforts to control their children's aggression loomed much larger than nurturance did in the profile of mothers' behaviors. Second, the influence of siblings and peers appeared to occur earlier and be more powerful than previously thought. The influence of children upon children, whether siblings, friends, or day care companions, must be better understood in order to outline a model of personality development.

Reports of child-rearing practices in other cultures featuring group settings with multiple caretakers have also highlighted the factors shaping character. In the kibbutz (Beit-Hallahmi, 1977), the number of significant others interacting with the child is higher than in the traditional family unit. But the relationships with these figures is nonexclusive and often discontinuous. That is, the caretaker is likely to be changed several times during childhood, so the youngster is exposed to a uniform, but less personal, treatment than in the traditional family. Theoretically, this weakens the dependence on a single significant figure, such as a parent, and reduces the intensity of feelings toward specific individuals, spreading it among others (Rabin, 1961, 1964, 1965). A study specifically focusing on multiple caretakers in early life and its affect on personality development has been referred to earlier (Tronick et al., 1992). Indeed, a "kibbutz personality" has been described, one that shows positive but only moderate attachment to others, with a reduction in intimacy as well as rivalry with peers. However, few differences were found between kibbutz and nonkibbutz children within the same culture, since the Israeli culture as a whole is more collectivistic than Western societies.

EFFECTS OF MINORITY STATUS ON PERSONALITY

Let us move from the usual way in which cultural forces are considered—that is, the effects of child-rearing practices on personality formation—to a consideration of the effects of negative sociocultural forces on development. Some of the most important findings about personal identity and self-esteem have emerged from studies of minority children in the United States. Much of this work relates to locus of control. Individuals differ in the extent to which they feel their own efforts can control the environment. This sense of internal control was found to be stronger in white children than in black children living side by side but having very different sociocultural experiences (Karon, 1958). In other words, caste or discrimination situations may result in lowered self-esteem in minority group children. As one might expect, however, the context is an important variable. Other studies have indicated that ethnic minority status per se is not related to lower self-concept (Long and Hamlin, 1988) if readily identifiable models for the self can be found among the minority group (Chang, 1975; Powell, 1985).

Differences in self-concept between majority and minority groups should be viewed with caution because the specific attributes tapped by conventional measures of self-esteem are not equally important for self-concept in different races; therefore, differences in self-esteem may not be representative (Rotenberg and Cranwell, 1989).

The issue is complicated by methodological factors (Scott et al., 1991). Specifically, a study across seven cultures found that the child's self-esteem and emotional well-being depended on its *own* view of parental nurturance and permissiveness, but not on parent's reports of these characteristics. Furthermore, the child's interpersonal competence was favorably affected by its *own* view of parental nurturance, but *negatively* associated with parent-reported nurturance, regardless of culture.

Studies of Native American culture have carried these findings further. Cultural beliefs about the nature of the world affect locus of control and shape personality development. American Plains Indians emphasize a unity with nature. Thus, acceptance of natural events such as life and death, geography and climate, is the norm, rather than action to control or alter them. These values appear to produce accepting attitudes and behaviors in the children, in contrast to the competitive achievement orientation of Caucasian children in the same culture (Long and Hamlin, 1988).

An important value Native American children are taught is to share (Yates, 1987). Allegiance to the family and community is valued more highly than allegiance to the self. Competitive striving is not highly valued. Thus, a particular form of individualism emerges, one that is adaptive in Native American culture but not in the Caucasian world (Wax and Thomas, 1972). Life is considered to be an unhurried natural progression, with disease, death, and disability accepted as part of life's progress. Children progress at their own pace and are responsible for making their own choices. The result is adaptive within the culture but not across cultures. The basic cognitive development of Native American children approximates that of white children, but progress on culture-bound standardized tests declines as the verbal content of the scales become more prominent with increase in age (Cazden and John, 1971).

Some studies have not separated ethnic from socioeconomic variables. A group of children called *disadvantaged* have been noted to demonstrate (*a*) limitations in the ability to use abstract symbols, abstract cognitive processes, and complex language for interpretation and communication, with compensatory overemphasis on motoric modes of problem solving; (*b*) low motivation for academic learning, with difficulty in sustained application to tasks; (*c*) deviance from the perceptual modes commonly employed in school, such as short auditory attention span and predominance of understanding in spatial rather than temporal terms. On the other hand, they may possess certain skills and competencies that are superior to those of middle-class peers, such as (*a*) accuracy of social perceptions, (*b*) resourcefulness in the pursuit of self-selected goals, (*c*) sustained involvement in a self-selected task, (*d*) capacity for independence and self-care and a high capacity for spontaneity of response (LaVietes, 1972).

EFFECTS OF ACCULTURATION ON PERSONALITY

Acculturation (Berry, 1979) is defined as a shift between cultures that forces personality change on the individual. The amount of stress on the developing personality is directly proportional to the distance between the two cultural groups and to the degree of insistence on change. The highest stress is seen in those groups who have been uprooted and geographically transplanted to another culture and have lost traditional social supports. In these cases, youngsters are confronted with a conflict between traditional values from the old country and contemporary values from the new country (Lee, 1988). Differences between conflicting values of the two cultures then become highlighted: group versus individual, extended versus nuclear family, interdependence versus independence, conformity versus competition, past versus future orientation, emphasis on age versus youth, harmony with nature versus conquest of nature, fatalism versus mastery of one's own fate, patience and modesty versus aggression and assertion, suppression versus expression of emotion. In successful acculturation, adaptation can be seen to occur by the formation of various combinations of these personality traits. But conflict in values between the two cultures may delay acculturation (Messer and Rasmussen, 1986; Tobin and Friedman, 1984). For example, many Southeast Asian adolescents who came to the United States had been primary caregivers or breadwinners for their families. Young girls may have been responsible for the care of the younger children; young men may have been heads of households, primary wage earners, or soldiers. To come from a culture in which one becomes an adult at puberty to a culture with the concept of adolescence as a prolonged transition between childhood and adulthood disrupts the developmental process. When a new set of values that reinstitutes dependence is superimposed on an old set in which independence had been achieved, the process of separation and individuation must begin all over again. Other studies of refugee teenagers (Nguyen and Williams, 1989) clearly demonstrate how contrasting values such as obedience to parental authority from the old culture versus freedom of choice regarding marriage and career in the new society are a source of stress to families and adolescents. The difficulty in the shift in values appears to be greater for girls, who experience more distress and resulting disruption of personality organization than do boys.

CULTURE AND BIOLOGICAL ASPECTS OF PERSONALITY

Cross-cultural studies have demonstrated that the pace and timing of the biological developmental process is significantly influenced by child-rearing practices (deVries and Sameroff, 1984; Levine, 1974; Thomas and Chess, 1980; Whiting and Child, 1953). In one study, in which major influences on temperament were measured, cultural affiliation proved to be the strongest predictor of infant temperament in the 1st year of life. It was clearly demonstrated that parental orientation toward child-rearing practice is a major contributor to the development of the child's temperament. In other words, temperament is not a pure biological measure but is exquisitely sensitive to environmental influences. Perhaps temperament can best be viewed as a constellation of traits with a threshold for expression that varies from culture to culture. Temperament traits tend to fall into two clusters, which can be seen as culture related: Rhythmicity, approach, and adaptability form one cluster, while activity, intensity, and distractibility form another. Group differences in neonatal behavior organization have been reported by comparing different cultural groups to American Caucasian infants (Coll et al., 1981). Chinese Americans, Navajo Indians, and Japanese Americans were found to be temperamentally less excitable as evidenced by lower levels of arousal, fewer state changes, and ease of consolability. Mexican Indians scored higher on motor maturity, had smoother transitions from one state to another and maintained quiet, alert states for longer periods of time as did African infants from Kenya, who scored higher on motor maturity and were better able to control increased motor tone.

Brazelton (Lester and Brazelton, 1981) has stated that African babies motor precocity was facilitated by culturally determined child-rearing practices built on the infant's responsiveness to being handled in the neonatal period. Motor excitement of infants may elicit intense social handling from caregivers, which in turn promotes accelerated developmental advance in motoric skills. The conclusion is that child-rearing practices may facilitate early motor development. On the other hand, Camras (1992) presents empirical findings that Japanese and American babies' facial expressions of emotion are similar both in type and proportion of occurrence in spite of differing child-rearing practices. The authors caution that the universality of infant facial expressions may be limited to similar repertoires of expression.

Finally, Super and Harkness (1986) have conceptualized the "developmental niche" (niche is a term borrowed from biological ecology, meaning place in a biosystem) to describe the interface between culture and child development. It consists of three complementary components: (a) the physical and social setting, (b) the customs of child care and child rearing, and (c) the psychology of caregivers. According to the authors, they are coordinated systems that relate to the larger culture and environment. Homeostatic mechanisms keep the three subsystems in harmony with each other and appropriate to the developmental level of the child. While synchronous in developmental thrust, they constitute somewhat independent routes for disequilibrium and change.

CULTURE AND SEXUAL IDENTITY

It is generally accepted that sex is biologically determined. However, gender is a broader term that includes cultural forces that shape that biological substrate. Indeed, there is evidence that gender orientation is determined as much by postnatal socialization influences as by the prenatal influence of sex hormones on brain development (Money, 1987). This is dramatically illustrated in cultures in which bisexuality is sanctioned. Among the peoples of the eastern highlands of New Guinea (Herdt, 1981) a developmental period of homosexuality preceding heterosexual adjustment is institutionalized. Prepubertal boys must leave the society of their mother and sisters and enter the society of men in order to achieve the fierce headhunter's role of manhood. In infancy the boy was fed woman's milk in order to grow. Now, in the secret society of men, he must be fed men's milk—that is, the semen of mature but unmarried young men—in order to become pubertal and mature himself. Such an exchange is not allowed between adult males but is reserved for the adult-youth relationship. When the prepubertal boy reaches marrying age, a marriage is arranged for him, marking the shift to a heterosexual career. He cannot become a complete man on the basis of heterosexual experience alone. Full manhood requires a prior phase that is exclusively homosexual. Thus, homosexual behavior becomes a defining characteristic of masculinity in the culture.

Studies in which traditionally feminine tasks were assigned to boys or in which male/female roles were not differentiated (Whiting and Edwards, 1973) suggest that the nature of the task assigned, rather than the biological sex of the individual, is the best predictor of masculine or feminine behavior. In societies where boys cook, take care of infants, and perform other domestic functions, there are fewer differences between boys and girls. Boys score proportionately lower in aggression, are less dominant, and score higher in responsibility (Harkness and Super, 1985).

On the other hand, other studies find that during certain phases of life such as adolescence, maturational forces weaken the influence of culture on the individual (Hsu et al., 1985; McDermott et al., 1983a, 1983b). In a study of boys and girls from different ethnic groups in the United States, gender differences proved more powerful than cultural affiliation during adolescence. While family loyalty and emotional constraint characterize Japanese American families, compared with affective expression and individual orientation in Caucasian American families, the adolescent sons and daughters from both sets of families grouped themselves by gender rather than cultural affiliation. Girls, whether Japanese or Caucasian, valued close family relationships and emotional expression significantly more than did boys. In following these Caucasian and Japanese teenagers from early to late adolescence, the researchers (McDermott et al., 1987) also found changes in male/female role perception that were gender rather than culture related. Traditional roles (male/power and female/support) were perceived as merging by girls, while sons held to an earlier male/female dichotomy. In other words, young males remained relatively fixed in their male/female role orientation regardless of ethnicity, while young females shifted their role definitions, which earlier had been determined by family and cultural values.

Thus, the powerful influence of culture on personality formation in infancy appears to loosen in adolescence. As we have found, culturally determined parental values indelibly imprint the younger child, but broader social forces lessen the intensity of family forces as adulthood approaches.

CONCLUSIONS

While early work on the interface between culture and development came from anthropological studies, recent research uses tests of statistical significance to separate universal tendencies among different settings from the unique influence that cultural variation imposes. In any case, the link between cultural forces and personality is clear. Culture is a powerful shaper of behavior in infants and young children, determines the age at which serious learning and work begin, and influences the very existence or nonexistence of adolescence as a transition from childhood to adulthood. Culture provides one of the basic organizing principles of human behavior, a set of hidden rules by which individuals operate. The clinician should approach each child or adolescent as a member of a specific culture with its own developmental pathways (and pitfalls), culturally determined symptomatic expressions of dysfunction, and culture-specific pathways of influence.

References

Bell L: Song without words. *Networker*, March-April, 1989, pp. 48–53.

Berry J: Acculturations as varieties of adaptation. In: Padilla AM (ed): *Acculturation: Theory, Models, and Some New Findings.* Boulder, CO, Westview Press, 1979.

Beit-Hallahmi B: The kibbutz as a social experiment and as a child rearing laboratory. *Am Psychol* 32:532–541, 1977.

Bowlby J: *Attachment.* New York, Basic Books, 1969.

Camras L, Oster H, Campos J, et al: Japanese and American infant's responses to arm restraint in developmental psychology. *Dev Psychol* 28:578–583, 1992.

Caudill W, Schooler C: Child behavior and child rearing in Japan and the United States: An interim report. *J Nerv Ment Dis* 157:323–338, 1973.

Caudill W, Weinstein H: Maternal care and infant behavior in Japan and America. *Psychiatry* 32:12–43, 1969.

Cazden C, John V: Learning in American Indian children. In: Wax NL, Diamond S, Gearing F (eds): *Anthropological Perspective on Education.* New York, Basic Books, 1971.

Chang T: The self-concept of children in ethnic groups: Black and American Korean children. *Elementary School J* 76:52–58, 1975.

Chiu L-H: Locus of control differences between American and Chinese adolescents. *J Soc Psychol* 128:411–413, 1987.

Coll C, Sepkoski C, Lester B: Cultural and biomedical correlates of neonatal behavior. *Dev Psychobiol* 14:147–154, 1981.

deVries M, Sameroff A: Culture and temperament: Influences of infant temperament in three East African societies. *Am J Orthopsychiatry* 54:83–96, 1984.

Earls F: Prevalence of behavior in three year old children: A cross-national replication. *Arch Gen Psychiatry* 37:1153–1157, 1980.

Earls F: Cultural and national differences in the epidemiology of behavior problems of preschool children. *Cult Med Psychiatry* 6:45–56, 1982.

Gannon S: *Behavioral Problems and Temperament in Middle-Class and Puerto Rican Five Year Old Boys.* Unpublished master's thesis, New York, Hunter College, 1975.

Harkness S, Super CM: The cultural context of gender segregation in children's peer groups. *Child Dev* 56:219–224, 1985.

Herdt GH: *Guardians of the Flutes: Idioms of Masculinity*. New York, McGraw-Hill, 1981.

Hess R, Azuma H, Kashiwagi K, et al: Cultural variations in socialization for school achievement: Contrasts between Japan and the United States. *J Appl Dev Psychol* 8:421–440, 1987.

Hsu FLK: *Americans and Chinese: Passage to Differences* (3rd ed). Honolulu, University Press of Hawaii, 1981.

Hsu J, Tseng W-S, Ashton GC, et al: Family interaction patterns among Japanese-American and Caucasian families in Hawaii. *Am J Psychiatry* 142:577–581, 1985.

Karon B: *The Negro Personality*. New York, Springer, 1958.

LaVietes R: Psychiatry in the school. In: Freedman A, Kaplan H (eds): *The Child: His Psychological and Cultural Development*. New York, Atheneum, 1972.

Lee E: Cultural factors in working with Southeast Asian refugee adolescents. *J Adolesc* 11:167–179, 1988.

Lester BM, Brazelton TB: Cross-cultural assessment of neonatal behavior. In: Stevenson H, Wagner D (eds): *Cultural Perspectives on Child Development*. San Francisco, Freeman, 1981.

Levine R: Parental goals: A cross-cultural view. *Teachers Coll Rec* 76:226–239, 1974.

Long K, Hamlin C: Use of the Piers-Harris self-concept scale with Indian children: Cultural considerations. *Nurs Res* 37:42–46, 1988.

McDermott J, Char W, Robillard A, et al: Cultural variations in family attitudes and their implications for therapy. *J Am Acad Child Psychiatry* 22:454–458, 1983.

McDermott JF, Robillard A, Char WF, et al: Reexamining the concept of adolescence: Differences between adolescent boys and girls in the context of their families. *Am J Psychiatry* 140:1318–1322, 1983.

McDermott JF, Waldron JA, Char WF, et al: New female perceptions of parental power. *Am J Psychiatry* 144:1086–1087, 1987.

Messer M, Rasmussen N: Southeast Asian children in America: The impact of change. *Pediatrics* 78:323–329, 1986.

Money J: Sin, sickness, or status? Homosexual gender identity and psychoneuroendocrinology. *Am Psychol* 42:384–399, 1987.

Morelli G, Rogoff B, Oppenheim D, et al: Cultural variation in infants' sleeping arrangements: Questions of independence. *Dev Psychol* 28:604–613, 1992.

Morelli GA, Tronick EZ: Efe fathers: One among many? A comparison of forager children's involvement with fathers and other males. *Soc Dev* 1:36–54, 1992.

Nguyen N, Williams H: Transition from east to west: Vietnamese adolescents and their parents. *J Am Acad Child Adolesc Psychiatry* 28:505–515, 1989.

Powell G: Self concepts among Afro-American students in racially isolated minority schools: Some regional differences. *J Am Acad Child Psychiatry* 24:142–149, 1985.

Provence S, Lipton RC: *Infants in Institutions*. New York, International Universities Press, 1962.

Rabin A: Kibbutz adolescents. *Am J Orthopsychiatry* 31:493–504, 1961.

Rabin A: Kibbutz mothers view ''collective education.'' *Am J Orthopsychiatry* 34:140–142, 1964.

Rabin A: *Growing Up in the Kibbutz*. New York, Springer, 1965.

Richman N, Tulpin H: A computerized family register of children under five in a London borough. *Health Trends* 6:19–22, 1974.

Richman N, Stevenson JC, Graham P: Prevalence of behavior problems in three year old children: An epidemiological study in a London borough. *J Child Psychol Psychiatry* 16:277–287, 1975.

Rotenberg K, Cranwell F: Self concept in American Indian and white children: A cross-cultural comparison. *J Cross-Cult Psychol* 20:39–53, 1989.

Scott W, Scott R, Boehnke K, et al: Children's personality as a function of family relation within and between cultures. *J Cross-Cult Psychol* 22:192–208, 1991.

Spitz R: *The First Year of Life*. New York, International Universities Press, 1965.

Super C, Harkness S: The developmental niche: A conceptualization of the interface of child and culture. *Int J Behav Dev* 9:545–569, 1986.

Super CH, Harkness S: The infant's niche in rural Kenya and metropolitan America. In: Adler LL (ed): *Cross-Cultural Research at Issue*. New York, Academic Press, 1982.

Thomas A, Chess S: *The Dynamics of Psychological Development*. New York, Brunner/Mazel, 1980.

Tobin J, Friedman J: Intercultural and developmental stresses confronting Southeast Asian refugee adolescents. *J Operational Psychiatry* 15:39–45, 1984.

Tobin J, Wu D, Davidson D: *Preschool in Three Cultures: Japan, China and the United States*. New Haven, CT, Yale University Press, 1989.

Tronick EZ, Morelli GA, Ivey PK: The Efe forager infant and toddler's pattern of social relationships: Multiple and simultaneous. *Dev Psychol* 28:568–577, 1992.

Tronick EZ, Morelli GA, Winn S: Multiple caretaking of Efe (pygmy) infants. *Am Anthropol* 89:96–106, 1987.

Tulkin S, Leiderman H: Child rearing: Infancy in a cultural context. *J Nerv Ment Dis* 157:320–322, 1973.

Wax R, Thomas R: American Indians and white people. In: Bahr H, Chadwick B, Day R (eds): *Native Americans Today: Sociological Perspectives*. New York, Harper & Row, 1972.

Whiting B, Edwards C: A cross-cultural analysis of sex differences in the behavior of children aged 3 through 11. *J Soc Psychol* 91:171–188, 1973.

Whiting B, Edwards C: *Children of Different Worlds: The Formation of Social Behavior*. Cambridge, MA, Harvard University Press, 1988.

Whiting B, Whiting J: *Children of Six Cultures: A Psychocultural Analysis*. Cambridge, MA, Harvard University Press, 1975.

Whiting J, Child I: *Child Training and Personality*. New Haven, CT, Yale University Press, 1953.

Yates A: Current status and future directions of research on the American Indian child. *Am J Psychiatry* 144:1135–1142, 1987.

Zukow PG: *Sibling Interaction across Cultures*. New York, Springer-Verlag, 1989.

36 CLASSIFICATION IN CHILD AND ADOLESCENT PSYCHIATRY: PRINCIPLES AND ISSUES

Fred R. Volkmar, M.D.

PRINCIPLES OF CLASSIFICATION

The ability and urge to classify is a unique aspect of human experience. It provides us with the capacity to observe, order our observations, and abstract general principles and hypotheses. Classification enables us to make use of information for purposes of communication, prediction, and explanation. At the present time in child and adolescent psychiatry, classification systems have their greatest role in facilitating communication for both clinical and research purposes; their role in prediction is somewhat more limited, and their explanatory value is often quite limited. The process of assigning a label may itself be associated with some sense of relief on the part of the patient or the patient's parents (Werry, 1985). Sometimes this reflects the misconception that having a label implies having an explanation (Jaspers, 1962). Like all human constructions, classification schemes can be abused or ill-used (Hobbs, 1975). This chapter provides an overview of classification in child and adolescent psychiatry. Specific "official" diagnostic systems are discussed in detail in Chapter 37.

Various authors (Blashfield and Draguns, 1976; Hempel, 1961; Jaspers, 1962; Quay, 1986; Rutter, 1965; Rutter et al., 1975; Spitzer and Cantwell, 1980) have discussed criteria for psychiatric classification systems. It is important to note that there is no single "right" way to classify disorders in childhood. Classification systems vary, depending upon the purpose of classification and what is being classified. As is described below, "official" diagnostic systems have tended to adopt, on the whole, a categorical approach, but a dimensional approach would be equally as valid, if perhaps less useful for clinical purposes.

The goals of classification include facilitating communication among professionals, providing information about given disorders that is relevant to treatment and/or to prevention, and providing information useful for research aimed at understanding the pathogenesis of disorders. To achieve these goals, classification schemes must be readily and reliably used by clinicians and researchers, hence the need for phenomenologically based, readily comprehensible, diagnostic terms and descriptions. The disorders should be described so that they can be differentiated from one another; they should differ in important ways, such as associated features and course. The classification system must be applicable over the range of development and must be comprehensive and logically consistent (Rutter and Gould, 1985).

Any number of conditions could be classified without having any clinical relevance. A classification of *disorders* implies that some clinically significant patterns of symptoms/behaviors/signs is observed in individuals and is a source of significant distress or impairment (American Psychiatric Association, 1994). Deviant behavior per se does not necessarily constitute a disorder unless it is a manifestation of dysfunction within the individual (e.g., conflicts over political beliefs do not constitute a mental disorder). Although it is often assumed that mental disorders must have a biological basis, this need not be the case; for example, maladaptive, enduring personality patterns can readily be classified as disorders (Morey, 1988).

Development of a general classification system for psychiatric disorders inevitably involves various tradeoffs. General classification systems must cover the entire range of disorders in a logically consistent fashion; classification systems developed for a highly specific purpose do not share this concern. The need for reasonable parsimony must be balanced with the need for adequate coverage (Rutter, 1965; Werry, 1985). The needs for a clinically relevant system differ somewhat from those for a research system; for example, highly detailed criteria might be useful for research purposes but would be cumbersome in clinical practice. Different diagnostic systems address these issues in different ways. The DSM-III (American Psychiatric Association, 1980), DSM-III-R (American Psychiatric Association, 1987), and DSM-IV (American Psychiatric Association, 1994) are intended to be useful for *both* clinical work and research. The ICD-10 (World Health Association, 1986, 1990) system (see Chapter 37) provides *separate* clinical and research descriptions.

ISSUES IN CLASSIFICATION

Developmental Aspects of Classification

Developmental considerations assume major importance in the provision of a classification scheme for children and adolescents, and, indeed, for adults as well (Zigler and Glick, 1986). Some disorders have their origin in a specific developmental period (e.g., autism; see Chapter 44). In other instances the disorder may be commonly associated with developmental problems (e.g., Tourette's syndrome and attention deficit hyperactivity disorder). At other times the child's overall level of development may have a major impact on the ways in which various disorders can be expressed (e.g., the child with mental retardation who also exhibits conduct problems). Classification systems must be able to encompass such issues without simultaneously making the disorder so developmentally specific that the utility of the category is compromised.

The developmental approach to classification is used whenever disorders are viewed in the context of the unfolding of basic developmental processes. The use of standard, developmentally based assessment instruments such as tests of intelligence or communication skills exemplifies this approach. In contrast, many categorical and dimensional classification systems rely on assessment of deviant behavior. The use of such an approach is often complicated, as issues of how deviant behavior is to be evaluated and how instruments are to be "normed" become quite important, and reliability between examiners can be low. Both the ICD-10 and the DSM-IV systems include some categories in which the definition is fundamentally development in nature (e.g., mental retardation, articulation disorders), while in others the deviant nature of the disorder predominates (autism, schizophrenia of childhood onset).

The Role of Theory

Theoretical models of psychological disturbance have developed from rather diverse historical traditions; they have considerable value for the individual clinician in understanding and treating children with emotional and behavioral problems. For example, Anna Freud (1965) proposed a developmental profile based on and applicable to psychoanalytic assessment of children. Although this profile has been used in some cases (e.g., Nagera, 1981), it is not widely used. More phenomenologically based classification systems can be traced to Kraeplin's delineation of schizophrenia and bipolar disorder (Mattison and Hooper, 1992). In the early "official" classifications, theoretical concerns were variably included, and coverage of disorders specific to the developmental period was inconsistent and spotty. Terms like "schizophrenic reaction of childhood" or "obsessional neurosis" emphasized a particular theoretical perspective.

Classification schemes that are driven by theory are limited in important respects. In the first place, theory-driven classification schemes are, by their nature, based on a set of assumptions and hypotheses that are not generally shared (Stengel, 1959). Often the language used to describe the same phenomena by theoreticians with different orientations is quite different; for example, a learning theorist might invoke principles of conditioning to explain a child's phobia, while a psychoanalytically oriented theorist might be more concerned with the child's level of psychosexual organization. If theoretically laden descriptions are used for classification, communication regarding the same basic clinical phenomena becomes complicated. As a result, classification schemes intended for general use should strive, to the extent possible, to describe phenomena without invoking specific theoretical concepts (Stengel, 1959). Particularly following the work on development of research diagnostic criteria (Feighner et al., 1972), the phenomenological approach to classification has predominated in the various "official" diagnostic systems. It should also be noted that, consistent with the phenomenological approach, diagnostic concepts have generally emerged from clinical experience rather than from theory (Weber and Scharfetter, 1984). In some instances, a theory has been invoked to account for a given set of phenomena, but it is the set of phenomena rather than the theory that has endured. For example, Langdon Down provided a complex theoretical explanation for children with the condition now known as Down's syndrome. His theory, based on obsolete racial stereotypes (mongolism), was incorrect, but his observation of some element of commonality among a large group of children with mental retardation has proved enduring.

The phenomenological approach to classification is often a source of frustration to clinicians with pronounced theoretical views. Sometimes the phenomenological approach is, incorrectly, taken to suggest that such matters as history, course, and outcome and, for that matter, etiology are irrelevant to classification. Information on course and outcome may, for example, provide important data relative to external validation of diagnostic categories, and information on the development of the disorder may be highly relevant to differential diagnosis regardless of how similar, at one point in time, two different disorders appear to be. For example, the syndrome of childhood disintegrative disorder (see Chapter 44) clearly appears to resemble autistic disorder once it is established; however, patterns of early development differ in these conditions as does outcome (Volkmar and Cohen, 1989).

The fact that official diagnostic schemes tend, by their nature, to be atheoretical does not mean that theory is unimportant. Although theoretical views may not be reflected in official classification schemes, they are of considerable value for both clinical work and research since they are more likely to generate truly testable hypotheses.

Etiology and Classification

It is often assumed that classification systems are developed to approximate some ideal diagnostic system in which etiology could be directly related to clinical condition. This is not, in fact, the case, in that there is no single ideal system waiting to be discovered and because etiology need not necessarily be included in classification systems (Rutter and Gould, 1985). Similarly, classification need not necessarily reflect a "disease" model (Rutter and Gould, 1985). Different etiological factors may result in rather similar conditions, and the same etiological factor may be associated with a range of clinical conditions. Aspects of intervention may be more directly related to the clinical condition than to etiology. Remedial services for children with mental retardation are, for example, much more likely to be oriented around aspects of developmental level than the precise etiology of the specific mental retardation syndrome. With a few exceptions (e.g., reactive attachment disorder in the DSM-IV), etiological factors are not generally included in official diagnostic systems.

Contextual Factors

In certain situations and populations, contextual variables such as family, school, or cultural setting pose major complications for application of diagnostic systems. The attentional problems of a child whose difficulties arise only as a result of an inappropriate school placement would not, for example, merit a diagnosis of attention deficit disorder. Contextual variables probably assume their greatest importance in the attempt to define and study disorders of infancy and early childhood. The infant exerts effects on the parents, who in turn exert effects on the child, and attributions of causality may be particularly difficult to make (Bell and Harper, 1977). A few of the traditional categorical disorders can be readily observed in infants and young children (e.g., autism, severe or profound mental retardation). In general, however, clinical complaints in this age group are usually centered around problems that encompass the infant in the context of his or her family or life situation. Although research on disorders of infancy is limited (Zeanah, 1993), it is clear that infants exhibit a tremendous ability to react, even over relatively short periods of time, to their environment, and change, rather than stability, is often the rule (Kagan, 1971). Clinical problems often relate more to issues of "goodness of fit" between parents and the infant than to a disorder in the infant (Chess and Thomas, 1986). As children become slightly older, traditional diagnostic groupings become more applicable (Earls, 1982). Issues of developmental level also become important in specifying inclusion/exclusion criteria for diagnostic categories; for example, a diagnosis of pica might be appropriate for a 12-year-old with profound retardation but is less appropriate for a normally developing 10-month-old.

Cultural differences may also affect diagnostic concepts and practice (Mezzich and von Cranach, 1988). Clearly, certain sociocultural factors are associated with certain types of problems (e.g., economic disadvantage is associated with conduct and attentional problems), but the meanings of such relationships often remain unclear (Farrington, 1986).

What is Classified?

It is particularly important that clinicians and researchers alike bear in mind that it is disorders, rather than children, which are classified. This is a source of considerable confusion. Concerns have been raised about the possible effects of labeling children (Hobbs, 1975), and to some extent these concerns are valid. It is, of course, also the case that having an adequate label for a child's disorder may be helpful—for example, in securing him or her needed services. Thus, a diagnosis of mental retardation or learning disability may be associated with social stigma or other untoward effects, or it may be associated with more realistic expectations on the part of parents and teachers and provision of potentially more appropriate services. These tensions are also exemplified in the debate between those who advocate broad and encompassing definitions (e.g., for service provision) versus those who advocate narrow definitions (e.g., to enhance research). Similar debates arise about aspects of social stigma related to mental illness and behavioral and developmental problems. In this regard it is always important to refer to the child's disorder, *not to the child as the disorder*. The term *diagnosis* refers both to the notion of assigning a label to a given problem and to the act of evaluation. In important respects it is the diagnostic process (Cohen et al., 1988) that is the most important of the two.

Although diagnostic labels have considerable value, they do not provide information about the individual, which is unique and uniquely related to intervention. Diagnostic categories will, and should, change, and children may exhibit a disorder for variable periods of time. The needs of individuals will vary depending on the individual and not simply as a function of whatever disorder(s) he or she has. The unfortunate tendency, particularly in the United States, to relate diagnosis, rather than individual needs, to eligibility for services does present additional complications for the diagnostic process.

Validation and Statistical Issues

As official classification systems have become more complex and probably more sophisticated, various statistical issues and methods have assumed increasing importance in the derivation of diagnostic definitions and their validation. Classification models based on theorizing have been replaced by more empirically, phenomenologically based categories. For example, both the DSM-IV and the ICD-10 utilize results of large national or international field trials in providing definitions of disorders. Categorical and dimensional approaches to classification share certain statistical concerns (Blashfield and Draguns, 1976).

VALIDITY

Validity is the extent to which a classification system does what it purports to do in terms of facilitating communication, intervention, and research. Various types of validity have been identified—for example, face validity (a category description appears to capture the diagnostic construct), predictive validity (some aspect of subsequent course or response to treatment is predicted), and construct validity (the category has meaning in terms of what it purports to assess). Generally such concepts are derived from work on psychometric assessment instruments, and their applicability to classification systems is somewhat different. In general, childhood psychiatric disorders have face validity but not necessarily predictive or construct validity (Spitzer and Cantwell, 1980). The validity of a given diagnostic category can be established on the basis of its association with various features other than those incorporated in the definition (e.g., response to treatment, natural history in the absence of treatment, family pattern, biological correlates, and developmental correlates such as age at onset and IQ). The validity of some categories included in DSM-III-R appeared to be questionable (e.g., identity disorder), whereas for other categories (e.g., autism; see Rutter, 1978), the disorder appears to have considerable validity, but the validity of rating scales and diagnostic criteria is more questionable.

The sensitivity and specificity of a given categorical diagnostic instrument can be assessed relative to the presence/absence of a specific disorder. However, a general problem for both categorical and dimensional classification systems is the nature of the "gold standard" against which a given category or criteria set is to be judged. Given the usual absence of an unequivocal diagnostic "marker" for the various conditions, clinical judgment is often used as the standard against which new instruments or definitions are assessed. The issues of "caseness" and diagnostic thresholds are particularly important in the derivation and validation of diagnostic systems (Swets, 1988; Valliant and Schnurr, 1988) (see Chapter 119).

RELIABILITY

In addition to validity, classification systems should exhibit reliability; that is, users in different locations seeing rather similar disorders should be able to agree on the applicability of a specific category or criterion (Grove et al., 1981). Various kinds of reliability have been identified: interrater, test-retest, internal consistency. If a given disorder is not used reliably, it has little value for purposes of communication. Some disorders, almost by definition, would have limited test-retest reliability over a relatively short period of time, while others would be presumed to be highly stable (e.g., adjustment disorders versus profound mental retardation). Sources of unreliability in psychiatric diagnosis include differences in the kinds of information clinicians collect, theoretical biases on the part of clinicians, and differences in diagnostic thresholds, as well, of course, as the true differences that individuals with disorders will exhibit at various points in time.

It is possible that a disorder could be reliably defined but have little or no validity. Conversely, a disorder might have validity, but criteria and diagnostic instruments designed to detect its presence might have little or no reliability. In providing diagnostic criteria and descriptions, there is often a tradeoff between the preciseness of a definition and its reliability. More detailed definitions, designed for research studies, may, for example, be used reliably in such contexts but may not prove reliable when applied by clinicians less experienced with the disorder. What appear to be relatively minor changes in the wording of a criterion can produce major changes in the way in which a diagnosis or diagnostic criterion is applied.

STATISTICAL ANALYSES

Various statistical techniques have been applied to data derived from assessment methods (Achenbach, 1988; Achenbach and Edelbrock, 1978; Quay, 1986). These techniques are, theoretically, of great interest in that they can provide more rational and empirical approaches in the derivation of diagnostic schemes; results of several studies are described subsequently. The fundamental assumption of such techniques is that the variables of interest lie along some dimension of function/dysfunction that all individuals exhibit to some degree. For many types of problems, this assumption is probably justified, e.g., relative to anxiety or depression. However, the usefulness of such techniques is limited in important ways (Rutter and Gould, 1985). In the first place, these methods are highly dependent on both the sample and the data entered in the analysis; that is, one can only get out what is there to be factor or cluster analyzed. For example, factor analysis of an instrument designed to detect conduct problems would not likely produce a factor related to eating disturbance. Similarly, cluster analysis of even a very large normative sample would not likely produce a cluster that corresponded to autism given its low base rate in the population. For very rare disorders, other statistical approaches may be useful. Other relevant statistical procedures include signal detection analysis (Kraemer, 1988), which can be used to establish which symptoms and symptom combinations are most strongly related to a particular diagnosis. Similarly, latent trait and latent class analyses (e.g., Szatmari et al., 1995; Zoccolilio et al, 1992) provide opportunities to examine aspects of diagnosis relative to multiple "informants."

MODELS OF CLASSIFICATION

Three general approaches to classification of disorders have been identified: categorical, dimensional, and idiographic (Werry, 1985). The categorical approach, sometimes referred to as the medical model of classification, views disorders as either present or absent (e.g., the patient does or doesn't have appendicitis). This approach assumes that cases exhibiting a given disorder display certain similarities, that these similarities outweigh differences, and that this knowledge has certain implications for understanding pathophysiology, course, treatment, and so on. Unlike the categorical approach, which views disorders as dichotomous, the dimensional approach to classification relies on assessment of dimensions of function or dysfunction by reducing phenomena to various dimensions along which a child can be placed. Various sources of data can be used for this approach, such as behavioral ratings, parental reports, yes/no criteria, developmentally based test scores, and the like. Although the dimensional approach is more commonly used in nonmedical settings, many medical phenomena also exhibit continuous (i.e., dimensional) characteristics (e.g., short stature, hypertension). For some purposes categorical diagnoses (e.g., levels of mental retardation) are derived from what is essentially a continuous variable, while some dimensional assessment instruments can similarly be used to generate categorical diagnoses (Werry, 1985). Ideographic classifications reject simple labels and focus on the total context of the child's life in formulating a case; these classifications may be theory driven (e.g., by psychoanalytic or behavioral theories) or may be used eclectically. Ideographic approaches are commonly used in clinical work; that is, the child or adolescent is viewed in the totality of his or her life circumstance, and various disorders, problems, and psychosocial situations may be viewed as worthy of notation and treatment.

Categorical Approaches

The most widely used "official" systems are those proposed by the World Health Organization (ICD-10) and the American Psychiatric Association (DSM-IV). As noted in Chapter 37, both systems have undergone revision and have their historical origins in medicine.

During the 19th century, a considerable number of advances in the taxonomy of adult psychiatric disorders were made. In particular, Kraepelin's attempt (1883) to outline a comprehensive classification system stimulated considerable interest in issues of diagnosis and taxonomy, and his emphasis on phenomenological descriptions was a marked advance. By the mid-20th century, a number of psychiatric disorders were generally recognized. Many of these were included in both the World Health Organization's 1948 International Classification of Diseases Manual (ICD-6) and in the first edition of the DSM, which appeared in 1952. The Group for the Advancement of Psychiatry (1966) also proposed a diagnostic system for children that was in many respects theoretically based but which did prefigure certain subsequent developments in the classification of children in the DSM and the ICD. Both the ICD and the DSM have undergone various revisions.

For example, the DSM-II included only a handful of diagnostic categories specific to children: mental retardation, childhood schizophrenia, adjustment, and other "reactions" (hyperkinetic, withdrawing, overanxious, runaway, unsocialized aggressive, group delinquent, and "other"). The categories included reflected a mixture of psychodynamic theory and Adolf Meyer's notions of reaction types. By the time the DSM-III appeared, the number of disorders first evidenced in infancy, childhood, or adolescence had increased over 4-fold, to include the following major classes of disorder, each of which included a number of specific diagnostic categories: mental retardation, specific developmental disorders, attention deficit disorder, conduct disturbance, eating disorders, stereotyped movement disorders, pervasive developmental disorders, other disorders with physical manifestations, and other disorders of infancy, childhood, or adolescence (see Mattison and Hooper, 1992, for a review). Similar, although not precisely corresponding, changes occurred in the revision of the ICD (Rutter et al., 1975). In the DSM-III, for example, disorders generally specific to childhood were grouped together, and there were many more DSM-III subcategories. The DSM-III and its successor, the DSM-III-R, differ from the ICD-9 in terms of their greater diagnostic reliance on explicit (if not always truly operationalized) diagnostic criteria (Puig-Antich, 1982; Spitzer and Endicott, 1978). Both the DSM-III and the ICD-9 incorporated a multiaxial framework, although the specific systems adopted differed from each other in some respects. Both systems were hierarchically organized, although the DSM-III and the DSM-III-R encourage multiple diagnoses. The complex issue of comorbidity (Rutter and Tuma, 1988) is treated differently in the ICD-10 and the DSM-IV. However, despite obvious points of difference, the ICD and the DSM systems are more alike than different (Werry, 1985). These diagnostic systems are described in detail in Chapter 37.

The proliferation in categories and the development of detailed diagnostic criteria resulted from various developments in the field. These included cross-national studies, the development of the research diagnostic criteria approach, and the development of a number of structured and semistructured rating scales and assessment instruments. The provision of detailed diagnostic criteria for essentially all mental disorders in the DSM-III marked a major advance (Cantwell 1988; Russel et al.,

1983). Development of the various official diagnostic systems became less theoretically based and more empirically derived. For example, field trials were used in the DSM-III to examine aspects of diagnostic reliability (Cantwell et al., 1979); other reliability studies have also appeared (Mezzich et al., 1985). The reliability of the ICD-9 has also been examined (Gould et al., 1988).

Detailed critiques of the various diagnostic approaches have appeared (Achenbach, 1980; Garmezy, 1978; Quay, 1986; Rutter and Shaffer, 1980). Criticisms have been made of both the overarching framework and its specifics. In the DSM-III in particular, a number of categories were introduced on the basis of rather limited data. The reliability and validity of at least some of the various categories proposed (e.g., childhood-onset pervasive developmental disorder) were questionable. Reliability is generally best for the more common and more broadly defined disorders. Information on the stability of the various childhood diagnoses has been limited.

Dimensional Approaches

In contrast to the more clinically oriented (categorical) approach, multivariate (dimensional) approaches to diagnosis offer several potential advantages in that various behaviors and dimensions of behavior are assessed rather than single, presumably pathognomonic, features (Achenbach, 1988; Achenbach and Edelbrock, 1978; Quay, 1986). Similarly, the dimensional approach can encompass symptom coding in other than a dichotomous fashion; for example, "never," "sometimes," "always" could be coded, rather than presence/absence, to rate-specific diagnostic features. Various rating scales, checklists, and so forth can be used for multivariate classification schemes based on self, parent, or teacher report or on direct observation; many such instruments are described in subsequent chapters. As noted previously, various statistical techniques such as factor and cluster analysis may be used to derive relevant clinician patterns or profiles. These patterns may, in turn, be used to derive categorical diagnoses. Given the inherent problems in sample selection and instrument development, issues of replication are particularly important (Rutter and Gould, 1985).

Jenkins and Glickman (1946) and Hewitt and Jenkins (1946) were among the first to examine patterns of relationships (correlations) between variables to derive syndrome groupings. A large series of case records was studied, and the presence/absence of specific behaviors was noted in each case. Clusters of deviant behavior were noted, and broad patterns of disturbance (socialized delinquent, overinhibited, unsocialized aggressive) were identified. Subsequently, more sophisticated methods have been applied to a range of children using a variety of assessment instruments (Achenbach, 1988). Studies done using this approach have generally identified several factors with relative consistency; factors identified have included conduct disturbance, overactivity, and emotional disturbance (Achenbach et al., 1989; Rutter and Gould, 1985). Not surprisingly, the stability of more narrowly defined factors has been less robust. Similarly, as would be expected, such techniques have had limited usefulness in detecting children with disorders of very low prevalence.

Reliability of dimensions derived from multivariate studies has been assessed and is generally satisfactory (Quay, 1986). Stability of dimensions or profiles is somewhat more complex to assess, in that some change is, of course, expected, but short-term stability appears to be within acceptable limits (Quay, 1986). The use of dimensional assessment instruments clearly avoids certain of the pitfalls inherent in the categorical approach—for example, in terms of the loss of information inherent in application of dichotomous categories, in increasing reliability, and in issues of "caseness." These issues are relevant to medicine in general and not just psychiatry.

For some purposes, dimensional assessment instruments are particularly valuable. For such assessments to be clinically useful, their validity must be demonstrated, for example, in terms of some associated features, such as familial pattern or course. The assumption that characteristics have the same meaning throughout their distribution is often questionable (e.g., severe mental retardation differs in a host of ways from normal intelligence) (Rutter and Tuma, 1988). Certain disorders clearly do *not* shade off into normality.

There are major areas of agreement between both the categorical and dimensional approaches; this is particularly true for the more prevalent disorders. Analysis of data from dimensional assessment instruments has proved useful in the development of categorical systems—for example, in supporting division of conduct disorder into various types. Probably the greatest drawback to the use of such assessments in clinical practice arises from the difficulty in using such instruments in a simple way for purposes of communication; for clinical purposes, it is more helpful to know that a child has attention deficit hyperactivity disorder and learning problems than to know his or her factor or profile scores on a dimensional assessment instrument. Dimensional and categorical approaches need not be used in mutually exclusive ways; the multiaxial classification used in the DSM-III-R, for example, employs both approaches in that while disorders are categorically defined, assessments of severity of psychosocial stressors and global assessment of functioning are dimensional.

Ideographic Approaches

Ideographic approaches to diagnosis are common in clinical practice. In the broader sense of diagnosis (i.e., as diagnostic process) (Cohen et al., 1988), most clinicians will target a number of problems or issues for intervention that relate only in part to categorical or even dimensional diagnosis. In some ways such approaches are more practical in certain situations (e.g., family therapy), although again they can be used in conjunction with categorical approaches. They are less useful for certain purposes (e.g., in considering pharmacological intervention) (Werry, 1985). Past the level of the individual cases, the utility of ideographic approaches is limited. Such approaches make it very difficult to communicate information for clinical and research purposes in a concise and readily understood fashion.

Multiaxial Classification

Multiaxial classification offers considerable potential advantages for child and adolescent psychiatric disorder (Cohen et al., 1988; Rutter and Gould, 1985; Rutter et al., 1975). In important ways it parallels the diagnostic process in that different kinds of information are collected and coded independently. Given that the diagnostic picture is often complex and that different conditions and types of conditions are associated with one another, the use of a multiaxial system, at least theoretically, should help clinicians by directing their attention to the major relevant areas of diagnosis. In actual practice clinicians vary considerably in their use of multiple axes, although the use of such a system would be expected, generally, to increase reliability. Putting developmental disorders on a separate axis would, for example, emphasize their developmental, as opposed to "psychiatric," nature and would remind clinicians to look for such disorders in the course of their regular clinical work. On the other hand, the placement of certain disorders within a multiaxial framework is problematic; enuresis, for example, clearly has developmental correlates but is generally included as a psychiatric, as opposed to developmental, disorder.

In the absence of a multiaxial system, certain conditions are particularly likely to be overlooked, such as the developmental learning disorders of a child with conduct disorder. Similarly, coding of medical syndromes is helpful in alerting the clinician to potential problems that either contribute to the mental or developmental disorder, are associated with it, or should be considered in the provision of a remedial plan. Theoretically many different kinds of information could be incorporated within a multiaxial framework (e.g., intellectual level, adequacy of school placement, associated psychosocial problems). Numerous mul-

tiaxial systems have been proposed; aspects of the DSM and the ICD approaches are discussed in Chapter 37. One of the dilemmas, particularly for disorders in adolescence, relates to the problem of comorbidity, i.e., often children have more than one diagnosis. This comorbidity may be more apparent than real or may represent a more substantive problem in which, for example, having one disorder predisposes to the second or where the risk factors for one disorder are also risk factors for the second. Artifactual comorbidity adds little to the classification system, e.g., for a child with autism to also receive a diagnosis of stereotypy-habit disorder seems somewhat pointless since stereotypies are commonly observed in autism and are included as one of the potential defining features of this condition. In other instances, e.g., conduct disorder with depression, the particular comorbid pattern does appear to have some important distinguishing features (Angold and Rutter, 1992). In ICD-10 the general approach is to provide a special code for such conditions, whereas in DSM-IV the usual diagnoses would be made with no special notation of the co-occurrence of the condition(s). Despite this difference, the general difference in approach to clinical and research diagnosis, and some differences around a few categories, these two systems have tended toward convergence.

SUMMARY

Classification in child and adolescent psychiatry has multiple meanings and functions. Complications for classification of child and adolescent disorders are myriad: The child is often not the person complaining; rather different kinds of data may be used in making a diagnosis; developmental factors may have a major impact on the expression of disorders; certain features (e.g., beliefs in fantasy figures) are normative at certain ages but not at others. Additional complications are posed by the unintended, but no less real, uses to which diagnostic concepts are put, such as their inclusion in legislation and their use as mandates for services in educational programs or for purposes of insurance reimbursement for services. Different kinds and levels of classification are needed for different purposes.

The past decade has witnessed tremendous advances in the area of diagnosis and classification of child and adolescent psychopathology (Rutter and Tuma, 1988). These advances are particularly welcome since work in this area had lagged behind that in the adult psychiatric disorders. Various approaches to classification have been employed; each has its advantages and limitations. Issues of reliability and validity remain to be addressed for many categories and classification systems; the attempt to address these issues through empirical data rather than theorizing is, perhaps, the greatest accomplishment of the past 10 years.

Tensions between clinical and research utility will continue to exist. As classification systems become more complex, they are less readily used; on the other hand, overly simplistic systems fail to capture important aspects of clinical experience. The likely ability, over the next decade, to more clearly identify the role of genetic factors for at least a few conditions and the growing sophistication of statistical approaches to aspects of classification and diagnosis represent important areas for future work.

A classification scheme is best used by persons with considerable training who take the task of diagnosis (in its broadest sense) seriously. Although categorical systems increasingly use diagnostic criteria, these are often not truly operationalized, although they are often abstracted and reified for specific purposes (e.g., development of interview schedules administered by lay interviewers, or the use of simple frequency counts or symptom duration that obscures the more central aspects of the underlying clinical construct). Although the various "official" systems present areas of disagreement, the areas of agreement are even more noteworthy. Certain issues, such as classification of comorbid condition versus use of multiple diagnoses, remain to be resolved. Specific issues arise with respect to inclusionary/exclusionary rules and aspects of comorbidity. While much has been accomplished, considerable work remains to be done.

References

Achenbach TM: DSM-III in light of empirical research on the classification of child psychopathology. *J Am Acad Child Psychiatry* 19:395–412, 1980.

Achenbach TM: Integrating assessment and taxonomy. In: Rutter M, Tuma H, Lann IS (eds): *Assessment and Diagnosis in Child Psychopathology*. New York, Guilford, 1988, pp. 300–339.

Achenbach TM, Edelbrock CS: The classification of child psychopathology: A review and analysis of empirical efforts. *Psychol Bull* 85:1275–1301, 1978.

Achenbach TM, Conners CK, Quay HC, et al: Replication of empirically derived syndromes as a basis for taxonomy of child/adolescent psychopathology. *J Abnorm Child Psychol* 17:299–323, 1989.

American Psychiatric Association: *Diagnostic and Statistical Manual* (3rd ed). Washington, DC, American Psychiatric Press, 1980.

American Psychiatric Association: *Diagnostic and Statistical Manual* (3rd ed, rev). Washington, DC, American Psychiatric Press, 1987.

American Psychiatric Association: *Diagnostic and Statistical Manual* (4th ed). Washington, DC, American Psychiatric Press, 1994.

Angold A, Rutter M: Effects of age and pubertal status on depression in a large clinical sample. *Dev Psychopathol* 4:5–28, 1992.

Bell RQ, Harper LV: *Child Effects on Adults*. Hillsdale, NJ, Erlbaum, 1977.

Blashfield RG, Draguns JG: Evaluative criteria for psychiatric classification. *J Abnorm Psychol* 85: 140–150, 1976.

Cantwell DP: DSM-III studies. In: Rutter M, Tuma H, Lann IS (eds): *Assessment and Diagnosis in Child Psychopathology*. New York, Guilford, 1988, pp. 3–36.

Cantwell DP, Russell AT, Mattison R, et al: A comparison of DSM-II and DSM-III in the diagnosis of childhood psychiatric disorders. I: Agreement with expected diagnosis. *Arch Gen Psychiatry* 36: 1208–1213, 1979.

Chess S, Thomas A: *Temperament in Clinical Practice*. New York, Guilford, 1986.

Cohen DJ, Leckman JF, Volkmar FR: The diagnostic process and classification in child psychiatry—Issues and prospects. In: Mezzich JE, von Vranach M (eds): *International Classification in Psychiatric: Unity and Diversity*. Cambridge, Cambridge University Press, 1988, pp. 284–297.

Earls FR: Application of DSM-III in an epidemiological study of preschool children. *Am J Psychiatry* 139:242–243, 1982.

Everitt BS, Gourlay AJ, Kendell RE: An attempt at validation of traditional psychiatric syndromes by cluster analysis. *Br J Psychiatry* 119:399–412, 1971.

Farrington DP: The sociocultural context of childhood disorders. In: Quay HC, Werry JS (eds): *Psychopathological Disorders of Childhood* (3rd ed). New York, Wiley, 1986, pp. 391–422.

Feighner J, Robbins E, Guze DB, et al: Diagnostic criteria for use in psychiatric research. *Arch Gen Psychiatry* 26:57–63, 1972.

Freud A: *Normality and Pathology in Childhood*. New York, International Universities Press, 1965.

Garmezy N: Never mind the psychologists: Is it good for children? *Clin Psychol* 31:1–6, 1978.

Gould MS, Rutter M, Shaffer D, et al: UK/WHO Study of ICD-9. In: Rutter M, Tuma H, Lann IS

(eds): *Assessment and Diagnosis in Child Psychopathology*. New York, Guilford, 1988, pp. 37–65.

Group for the Advancement of Psychiatry: *Psychopathological Disorders in Childhood: Theoretical Considerations and a Proposed Classification* (report no. 62). New York, Group for the Advancement of Psychiatry, 1966.

Grove WM, Andreasen NC, McDonald-Scott P, et al: Group for the Advancement of Psychiatry, 1966. Reliability studies of psychiatric diagnosis: Theory and practice. *Arch Gen Psychiatry* 38: 408–413, 1981.

Hempel CG: Problems of taxonomy. In: Zubin J (ed): *Field Studies in the Mental Disorders*. London, Grune & Stratton, 1961, pp. 3–22.

Hewitt LE, Jenkins RL: *Fundamental Patterns of Maladjustment: The Dynamics of Their Origin*. Springfield, IL, State of Illinois, 1946.

Hobbs N (ed): *Issues in the Classification of Children*. San Francisco, Jossey-Bass, 1975.

Jaspers K: *General Psychopathology* (Hoenig J, Hamilton M, trans). Manchester, University Press, 1962.

Jenkins RL, Glickman S: Common syndromes in child psychiatry. *Am J Orthopsychiatry* 16:244–261, 1946.

Kagan J: *Change and Continuity in Infancy*. New York, Wiley, 1971.

Kraepelin E: *Compendium der Psychiatrie*. Leipzig, Abel, 1983.

Kraemer HC: Assessment of 2×2 associations: Generalization of signal detection methodology. *Am Statist* 42:37–49, 1988.

Mattison RE, Hooper SR: The history of modern classification of child and adolescent psychiatric disorders: An overview. In: Hooper SR, Hynd GW, Mattison RE (eds): *Assessment and Diagnosis of Child and Adolescent Psychiatric Disorders*. Volkmure 1: *Psychiatric Disorders*. Hillsdale, NJ, Erlbaum, 1992.

Mezzich AC, Mezzich JE, Coffman GA: Reliability of DSM-III vs. DSM-II in child psychopathology. *J Am Acad Child Psychiatry* 24:281–285, 1985.

Mezzich JE, von Cranach M: *International Classification in Psychiatry: Unity and Diversity*. Cambridge, Cambridge University Press, 1988.

Morey LC: Personality disorders in DSM-III and DSM-III-R: Convergence, coverage, and internal consistency. *Am J Psychiatry* 145:573–577, 1988.

Nagera H: *The Developmental Approach to Childhood Psychopathology*. New York, Aronson, 1981.

Quay HC: Classification. In: Quay HC, Werry JS (eds): *Psychopathological Disorders of Childhood* (3rd ed). New York, Wiley, 1986, pp. 1–34.

Puig-Antich J: The use of RDC criteria for major depressive disorder in children and adolescents. *J Am Acad Child Psychiatry* 21:291–293, 1982.

Russel AT, Mattison R, Cantwell DP: DSM-III in the clinical practise of child psychiatry. *J Clin Psychiatry* 44:86–90, 1983.

Rutter M: Classification and categorization in child psychiatry. *J Child Psychol Psychiatry* 6: 71–83, 1965.

Rutter M: Diagnosis and definition. In: Rutter M, Scholper E (eds): *Autism: A Reappraisal of Concepts and Treatment*. New York, Plenum, 1978, pp. 1–25.

Rutter M, Gould M: Classification. In: Rutter M, Hersov L (eds): *Child and Adolescent Psychiatry:*

Modern Approaches (2nd ed). Oxford, Blackwell Scientific Publications, 1985, pp. 304–321.

Rutter M, Shaffer D: DSM-III: A step forward or back in terms of the classification of child psychiatric disorder. *J Am Acad Child Psychiatry* 10:371–394, 1980.

Rutter M, Tuma AN: Diagnosis and classification: Some outstanding issues. In: Rutter M, Tuma H, Lann IS (eds): *Assessment and Diagnosis in Child Psychopathology*. New York, Guilford, 1988, pp. 437–445.

Rutter M, Shaffer D, Shepherd M: *A Multiaxial Classification of Child Psychiatric Disorders*. Geneva, World Health Organization, 1975.

Spitzer RL, Cantwell DP: The DSM-III classification of the psychiatric disorders of infancy, childhood, and adolescence. *J Am Acad Child Psychiatry* 19:356–370, 1980.

Spitzer RL, Endicott JE, Robins E: Research diagnostic criteria. *Arch Gen Psychiatry* 35:773–782, 1978.

Stavrakaki C, Vargo B: The relationships of anxiety and depression: A review of the literature. *Br J Psychiatry* 149:7–16, 1986.

Stengel E: Classification of mental disorders. *Bull World Health Org* 21:601–663, 1959.

Swets JA: Measuring the accuracy of diagnostic systems. *Science* 240:1285–1292, 1988.

Szatmari P, Volkmar F, Walter S: Latent class models and the evaluation of diagnostic criteria for autism. *J Am Acad Child Adolesc Psychiatry* 1995

Valliant GE, Schnurr P: What is a case? *Arch Gen Psychiatry* 45:313–319, 1988.

Volkmar FR: Annotation: Diagnostic issues in the pervasive developmental disorders. *J Child Psychol Psychiatry* 28:365–369, 1987.

Volkmar FR, Cohen DJ: Disintegrative disorder or ''late onset'' autism. *J Child Psychol Psychiatry* 30:717–724, 1989.

Volkmar FR, Bregman J, Cohen DJ, et al: DSM III and DSM III-R diagnoses of autism. *Am J Psychiatry* 145:1404–1408, 1988.

Weber AC, Scharfetter C: The syndrome concept: History and statistical operationalizations. *Psychol Med* 14:315–325, 1984.

Werry JS: ICD 9 and DSM III classification for the clinician. *J Child Psychol Psychiatry* 26:1–6, 1985.

World Health Organization: *International Classification of Diseases* (9th ed). Geneva, World Health Organization, 1977.

World Health Organization: Mental and behavioural disorders, diagnostic criteria for research (Draft). In: *International Classification of Diseases* (10th ed). Geneva, World Health Organization, 1990, chap 5.

World Health Organization: Mental and behavioral disorders, clinical descriptions and diagnostic guidelines (Draft). In: *International Classification of Diseases* (10th ed). Geneva, World Health Organization, 1992, chap 5.

Zeanah C (ed): *Handbook of Infant Mental Health*. New York, Guilford, 1993, pp. 236–249.

Zigler E, Glick M: *A Developmental Approach to Psychopathology*. New York, Wiley, 1986.

Zoccolillo M, Pickes A, Quinton D, et al: The outcome of conduct disorder: Implications for defining adult personality disorder and conduct disorder. *Psychol Med* 22:971–986, 1992.

37 SYSTEMS OF PSYCHIATRIC CLASSIFICATION: DSM-IV AND ICD-10

Mary E. Schwab-Stone, M.D., and Elizabeth L. Hart, Ph.D.

During periods of extensive research activity and rapid growth of knowledge in a field, the system used to organize that knowledge will be challenged and at certain points revised. The past decade and a half have seen the publication of three editions of the classification system for psychiatric disorders that is used in the United States, the *Diagnostic and Statistical Manual of Mental Disorders* (DSM) (American Psychiatric Association (APA), 1980, 1987, 1994), and a new version of the system used in most of the rest of the world, the International Classification of Diseases (ICD) (World Health Organization (WHO), 1992). The appearance of a new classification demands accommodation on the part of practitioners and researchers and is frequently surrounded by some controversy. This chapter reviews recent developments in both systems, highlighting areas of change and controversy in each.

HISTORICAL PERSPECTIVE

Advances in psychiatric taxonomy, particularly those of Kraepelin, in the mid to late 19th century, as well as service system needs for describing hospitalized patients, provided impetus for the development of early systems of psychiatric classification both in Europe and the United States (Rutter et al., 1975; Schwab-Stone et al., 1991; Spitzer and Williams, 1980) (see Chapter 36). The recent histories of both systems (see Schwab-Stone et al., 1991, and Chapter 36) reflect the periodic rethinking of the knowledge base that informs the description and delineation of psychiatric disorders. In child and adolescent psychopathology, the development of this knowledge base has trailed its counterpart in adult psychiatry. Not until the appearance of DSM-III in 1980 was a broad range of child-specific disorders represented in the DSM. Changes since then, i.e., in the revision to DSM-III-R (APA, 1987) and then to DSM-IV (APA, 1994), represent less dramatic advances overall but are significant in keeping nosology in step with advances in the understanding of child psychopathology. (More detailed discussion of the historical development of both ICD and DSM systems with reference to child psychiatric disorder can be found in Schwab-Stone et al., 1991, and in Chapter 36.)

FROM DSM-III-R TO DSM-IV: THE REVISION PROCESS

In 1988 work began on the fourth edition of the American Psychiatric Association's *Diagnostic and Statistical Manual of Mental Disorders* (DSM-IV). At that time it was argued that the development of DSM-IV might be premature, as a new manual might disrupt or confuse clinicians and researchers, create unnecessary disagreement about diagnostic categories, lead to excessive minor changes, or might not even be needed (Frances et al., 1989). Nevertheless, the United States is under treaty obligation to maintain a terminology that is compatible with the ICD, and publication of the 10th edition of the World Health Organization's International Classification of Diseases (ICD-10) was scheduled for 1993. Thus, revision of the DSM-III-R was deemed appropriate so that the two major classification systems could be revised with mutual input and maximal coordination of efforts (Frances et al., 1989).

A major goal for the revision of DSM-III-R to DSM-IV was one of process, so that the nosology would be grounded in systematic and thorough documentation, with safeguards against hasty or arbitrary changes (APA, 1994; Frances et al., 1989). In DSM-III and DSM-III-R, categories and criteria had been based in large part on expert group consensus. The absence of systematic literature reviews and of documentation of the empirical basis for changes led to concerns that opinion, rather than research findings, had at times played too heavy a role in guiding such decisions (Frances et al., 1989). However, the inclusion of explicit diagnostic criteria beginning with DSM-III had stimulated a wealth of research that informed the deliberations about changes from DSM-III-R to DSM-IV (Widiger et al., 1991).

In addition to the revision goals of documentation and empirical grounding, emphasis was placed on clinical utility, user-friendliness, and compatibility with ICD-10, but not at the expense of clinical concepts/distinctions (Frances et al., 1989). The requirements for evidence to support change were intended to be higher than for DSM-III and DSM-III-R, but varied across disorders. Overall, the intent of the revision process was to find the optimal balance between the traditions of DSM-III/III-R, evidence from literature reviews, analysis of unpublished data sets, and expert consensus.

The work of this revision was conducted by 13 work groups of experts under the overarching direction of the 27-member task force on DSM-IV. Each group had responsibility for a section of the manual. These work groups related to an extensive list of advisors representing a broad range of theoretical perspectives (APA, 1994). An early task for each work group was to review drafts of the ICD-10 to identify and prioritize areas of disagreement between the two systems (Frances et al., 1989).

The work groups engaged in a three-step process for examining and revising the manual in their respective areas. These steps included: (*a*) systematic literature reviews, (*b*) focused analyses of existing data sets, and (*c*) field trials (APA, 1994). The literature reviews were conducted to obtain evidence to support revisions of criteria, address issues of subtypes, etc., and to support the material in the text of DSM-IV, e.g., associated features, prevalence, course, prognosis, differential diagnosis, demographics, etc. (Frances et al., 1989).

In addition to reviews of published data, over 40 reanalyses of existing data sets were conducted to examine issues that were not adequately addressed in the published literature. These reanalyses were used to evaluate the current lists of criteria and diagnostic algorithms and to generate and pilot new criteria sets (APA, 1994). Where appropriate, field trials were conducted to compare alternative diagnostic options and to examine the possible effects of proposed changes. The field trials relevant to the diagnosis of psychopathology in children and adolescents included those for the disruptive behavior disorders and for autism and related pervasive developmental disorders. Overall, the goal of the revision process was to develop diagnostic criteria that would maximize (*a*) identification of functionally impaired children and adolescents, (*b*) agreement with clinical diagnosis, (*c*) internal consistency of the symptom lists, and (*d*) reliability of the diagnosis (Lahey et al., 1994a). An extensive process of review and discussion took place involving distribution of an "Options Book" and circulation of a near final draft to allow critique and input prior to publication of the DSM-IV in 1994 (APA, 1994).

THE INTERNATIONAL CLASSIFICATION OF DISEASES: FROM ICD-8 TO ICD-10

The International Classification of Diseases has undergone numerous revisions since an early version, the International Classification of

Causes of Death, was adopted by the International Statistical Institute in Paris in 1893 (Kramer, 1968). In the late 1950s, the section covering psychiatric diagnoses in the seventh edition came under scrutiny and was found lacking in its representation of the state of knowledge in psychiatry (Rutter et al., 1975). An international program sponsored by the World Health Organization was initiated to develop a more adequate and acceptable classification for the mental disorders, which appeared with the publication of the eighth edition of the ICD in 1968 (Spitzer and Williams, 1980). Recognized as an important achievement in international collaboration and a major improvement over previous versions, the ICD-8 classification of mental disorders also clearly represented a compromise that would need further revision (Kramer, 1968). A 10-year research plan, initiated in the 1960s, employed case history exercises and extensive seminars to evaluate the functioning of the system in various areas of psychiatric diagnosis, including the child psychiatric disorders. An important product of this effort was a multiaxial system for classifying child psychiatric disorders, which was evaluated for reliability and clinical utility in field trials that yielded good results (Rutter et al., 1975).

In 1978 the ICD-9 was published, with plans for further research and revision that opened the way for a system of comprehensive descriptions for clinical and research diagnosis. The ICD-10, which incorporates these changes, is the last of the series of 10-year revisions. At this point, minor modifications can be made and categories added without a general revision of the entire system (Sartorius, 1988).

Work on the tenth revision of the ICD (WHO, 1992) began even before ICD-9 was completed and involved an extensive rethinking of the structure and presentation of that classification (Bramer, 1988). This process, undertaken as an international collaborative effort, utilized an extensive evaluation process and resulted in a greatly expanded number of categories (Cooper, 1988). In addition, the ICD system was conceptualized as a family of documents written to address the needs of different users, e.g., primary health care providers, specialty-based researchers, and psychiatric practitioners.

The development of the ICD-10 chapter on psychiatric disorders was informed by a large international field trial, which was conducted in 39 countries by 711 clinicians who performed over 15,000 assessments (Sartorius, 1988). The goals of the field trial were to evaluate the applicability of ICD-10 psychiatric diagnoses in different countries, the ease of use of the system, and the level of interrater agreement when the system was applied by clinicians to make diagnoses in clinical contexts. The ICD-10 draft was generally found to be easy to use and the diagnostic descriptions showed good fit with psychiatric conditions as conceptualized in the many participating countries around the world. Interrater reliability was satisfactory for most diagnoses, with the highest levels of agreement for disorders in which symptomatology was most distinct; agreement was less satisfactory for the disorders in which symptomatology was less pronounced, as well as for the personality disorders (Sartorius, 1988). Results from the field trial were used in refining the ICD-10 draft prior to publication in 1992.

SYSTEMS COMPARED

Beginning with the DSM-II, there has been some effort to maintain a level of correspondence between the DSM and ICD systems. Nevertheless, some important differences exist in the approaches to classification and in the specifics of how the childhood disorders are delineated. To some extent, the differing purposes of each system determine the differences in orientation and content.

As part of an international nosology, Chapter V of the ICD-10, which is devoted to the mental disorders, must be serviceable within two important constraints (Cooper, 1988). First, it must fit into the structure of a classification for all medical conditions and be usable with a set of rules that apply to the entire system. Second, it must be internationally acceptable and useful to those who treat and document psychiatric conditions in settings that vary widely with respect to culture, language, and resources for diagnosis and treatment. By contrast, the DSM systems,

developed as they are by the major psychiatric organization in the United States, are less constrained because they are not tied to a larger system and because they address the needs of a smaller group of clinicians, with considerably more homogeneity in language, training, and patterns of practice.

A major difference between ICD-10 and DSM-IV is the degree to which criteria for diagnosis are operationalized or specified. The ICD-10 offers a comprehensive description of the clinical concept underlying the disorder, followed by points of differential diagnosis and diagnostic guidelines indicating the main symptoms that should be present for a diagnosis. Even the diagnostic guidelines read rather like sections from a clinical text in contrast to the operationalized criteria of DSM-IV. Thus, the experience of using the ICD-10 involves matching a patient's clinical presentation to an overall description, rather than determining whether a sufficient number of specified symptoms are present as in the DSM system since DSM-III. Whether this is a more "clinical" approach and whether that is a good thing are issues open for debate, but the ICD-10 system does offer the clinician somewhat more flexibility than the DSM-IV. Such flexibility is necessary for an international system that must be used in diverse settings under a variety of clinical circumstances.

Both systems encourage the recording of all diagnoses relevant to a patient's clinical presentation; however, the ICD-10 retains the possibility of applying a few combination categories (e.g., hyperkinetic conduct disorder, depressive conduct disorder) in which comorbid symptom patterns are indicated as one diagnosis rather than two, as in DSM-IV. The combination categories are used to describe a few commonly co-occurring patterns where there is evidence for some difference in long-term outcome for those with the two-symptom pattern compared to those showing either symptom type alone (Rutter, 1989a). Rutter has noted the research risk of attributing characteristics to one condition when they may in fact be associated with a co-occurring condition that has simply not been considered in the study. Retaining the combination categories was seen as a means of ensuring further study of these comorbid patterns and more accurate diagnostic assignment in research studies (Rutter, 1989a).

A series of meetings between DSM-IV work group chairpersons and WHO advisers involved in the development of ICD-10 has led to considerable congruence in the conceptualization of disorders in the two systems (Cooper, 1995). Appendix H of the DSM-IV contains a diagnostic crosswalk between the systems, which illustrates the good fit that has been achieved through that collaborative process. In reviewing below the major diagnostic categories that are used in child psychiatric diagnosis, some differences in the handling of disorders will be noted, but generally, the differences are slight relative to the substantial areas of similarity.

DISRUPTIVE BEHAVIOR DISORDERS

The publication of DSM-III-R brought significant changes in symptom lists and quantitative criteria for the disruptive behavior disorders (DBDs), i.e., attention-deficit hyperactivity disorder (ADHD), conduct disorder (CD), and oppositional defiant disorder (ODD). After some experience with the DSM-III-R, concerns developed about how well the criteria for these diagnoses were functioning. For the DBDs these concerns focused on the balance between narrow and highly specified as opposed to broader and more conceptual criteria, the developmental appropriateness of criteria (particularly for the very young and also for older adolescents), and on the degree of comorbidity within the DBDs (Shaffer et al., 1989).

The DBD field trials were undertaken to provide data for the revision process and to complement other sources of data, such as reviews of the existing empirical literature (Lahey et al., in press) and reanalyses of existing data sets (August and Garfinkel, 1993; Biederman and Newcorn, 1993). The field trials were conducted as a multisite collaborative study, which recruited 440 clinic-referred children and adolescents (ages

4–17 years) from a range of mental health services. Interviews were conducted with child, parent, and teacher informants using a standard protocol designed to assess the range of emotional and behavioral problems as well as cognitive ability, academic achievement, and functional impairment. Different combinations of symptoms were evaluated to determine which showed the best correspondence to clinical diagnoses, were most reliable, and were associated most strongly with indices of impairment.

DSM-IV Attention-Deficit Hyperactivity Disorder and ICD-10 Hyperkinetic Disorders

Attention-deficit hyperactivity disorder is characterized by developmentally inappropriate levels of inattention, impulsivity, and/or motor hyperactivity, beginning before 7 years of age. The revision of the DSM diagnostic nomenclature has reflected considerable ongoing change in the conceptualization of this disorder. DSM-III (APA, 1980) provided a model of the disorder in which symptoms of inattention, motor hyperactivity, and impulsivity reflected three separate dimensions. According to DSM-III, a child was considered to exhibit attention deficit disorder with hyperactivity (ADD/H) if she or he demonstrated significant difficulties in all three symptom areas. A diagnosis of attention deficit disorder without hyperactivity (ADD/WO) was given if the child exhibited difficulties with sustained attention and impulsivity but did not have motor hyperactivity. Several studies supported the distinction between ADD/H and ADD/WO, showing that children with these two patterns of dysfunction differed with respect to comorbid disorders, social status, school adjustment, and neuropsychological profile (e.g., Carlson, 1986; Edelbrock et al., 1984; Lahey et al., 1984, 1987).

In DSM-III-R, however, this distinction was changed substantially. The DSM-III-R diagnostic category of attention-deficit hyperactivity disorder (ADHD) provided a unidimensional definition according to which diagnostic criteria were met if a child exhibited at least 8 of a list of 14 symptoms related to difficulties in attention, impulsivity, and motor hyperactivity. Symptoms did not need to be shown in all three areas to satisfy the criteria for a diagnosis of ADHD. This change was based largely on the assertion that the constructs of inattention, impulsivity, and hyperactivity could not always be reliably distinguished (Newcorn et al., 1989). However, concerns were raised that this unidimensional DSM-III-R definition of ADHD might result in the identification of a heterogeneous population, including some children who would also meet the DSM-III criteria for ADD/WO. In addition, because of the distribution of different types of symptoms within the list of 14, at least some difficulties with hyperactivity and impulsivity would need to be present if a diagnosis were made, but it was possible to qualify for the diagnosis without showing any symptoms of inattention. This definition represented a significant conceptual change from the DSM-III definition, which identified difficulties with sustained attention as the core feature of the syndrome. The category of undifferentiated attention deficit disorder (UADD) was included in DSM-III-R for disturbances in which symptoms of inattention were the primary feature; however, no specific criteria were included for UADD, and a call was made for future research to validate this diagnostic category.

In preparation for the development of DSM-IV, a review of the relevant literature (Lahey et al., in press) suggested that the symptoms of the attention deficit disorders might be best described using a two-dimensional model, with one dimension comprised of symptoms reflecting inattention and disorganization and a second dimension consisting of symptoms reflecting motor hyperactivity and impulsive responding. This model was consistent with the factor-analytic literature, which suggests that symptoms of inattention are more strongly correlated with one another than with symptoms of hyperactivity-impulsivity and vice versa (Bauermeister et al., 1992; Lahey et al., 1988; Pelham et al., 1992). In addition, findings from longitudinal studies indicate that the symptom dimensions of inattention and hyperactivity-impulsivity follow different developmental courses, with hyperactivity-impulsivity declining with increasing age and symptoms of inattention remaining relatively constant (Hart et al., 1995). The two dimensions also differ in terms of their association with comorbid disorders and indices of functional impairment (Lahey et al., in press), suggesting that they represent distinct patterns of dysfunction. Based on this literature, a two-dimensional model was proposed for DSM-IV.

This two-dimensional model was compared to the unidimensional DSM-III-R model using field trial data. All symptoms of DSM-III ADD/H, DSM-III-R ADHD, and ICD-10 hyperkinetic disorder, as well as additional symptoms found to distinguish the two dimensions in clinical research, were considered for inclusion. Optimal diagnostic thresholds for each of the two symptom dimensions were determined that maximized the identification of impaired cases, test-retest reliability, and agreement with clinician diagnoses. For both the inattention and hyperactivity-impulsivity dimensions, the optimal diagnostic threshold was determined to be six symptoms (Lahey et al., 1994b).

The analyses of the field trial data supported the adoption of a DSM-IV definition of ADHD whereby a diagnosis may be given when either clinically significant numbers of inattention symptoms (≥ 6) or clinically significant numbers of hyperactivity-impulsivity symptoms (≥ 6) "have persisted for at least 6 months to a degree that is maladaptive and inconsistent with developmental level" (APA, 1994). Using this definition, three types of ADHD were identified: those with clinically significant numbers of inattention symptoms only (predominantly inattentive type), those with clinically significant levels of hyperactivity-impulsivity only (predominantly hyperactive-impulsive type), and those with clinically significant numbers of both types of symptoms (combined type). This identification of three DSM-IV subtypes results in a reduction in the heterogeneity that was problematic in the DSM-III-R conceptualization (Waldman et al., manuscript in preparation).

The DSM-IV definition also provides greater specification of criteria on impairment, pervasiveness, and age of onset. It adds the specific requirement of clinically significant impairment in social, academic, or occupational functioning. Unlike DSM-III-R, pervasiveness is required in that some impairment must be present in two or more settings. As in the DSM-III-R definition, the DSM-IV requires an onset of symptoms before 7 years of age. Moreover, by requiring that some symptoms causing impairment be present by age 7, DSM-IV reduces the likelihood that levels of activity, impulsiveness, or inattentiveness that are normal for younger children will be counted as symptoms in documenting the ADHD onset criterion. These added requirements are intended to make the criteria more precise and to minimize the chances of overdiagnosing ADHD.

In the ICD-10, the category of hyperkinetic disorders includes a group of disorders characterized by "overactive, poorly modulated behaviors," in combination with inattentiveness and lack of persistence. This constellation must be early in onset (<6 years), pervasive across situations, and persistent over time. Following long-standing differences in the conceptualization of this disorder in the United States and the United Kingdom, the hyperkinetic disorders have been more narrowly conceptualized in the ICD-10 than in DSM-IV (Rutter, 1989a). While difficulties with attention are thought to be a central feature of the disorder and must co-occur with hyperactivity, it is not possible to receive a diagnosis solely on the basis of symptoms of inattention. In fact, the term attention deficit disorder is not used because it "implies a knowledge of psychological processes that is not yet available, and it suggests the inclusion of anxious, preoccupied, or 'dreamy' apathetic children whose problems are probably different" (WHO, 1992, p. 262).

The presence or absence of CD symptoms provides the basis for the major subdivision within the class of hyperkinetic disorders. When CD criteria are met along with those for hyperkinetic disorder, the latter is given some priority since the combination diagnosis, hyperkinetic conduct disorder, from the hyperkinetic disorders grouping would be applied. Hyperkinetic disorder alone, without CD symptoms, goes by the term "disturbance of activity and attention." Overall, moderate differences remain between the DSM and ICD systems in this area of psychopathology, with the ICD-10 requiring overactivity in addition to inattention and with subtypes determined on the basis of whether CD symptoms are present.

DSM-IV Oppositional Defiant Disorder and Conduct Disorder and ICD-10 Conduct Disorders

The work group faced two major issues in revising these diagnoses for DSM-IV. One involved the changes in diagnostic threshold from DSM-III to DSM-III-R. Specifically, the concern was whether the threshold changes had produced overly stringent diagnostic requirements so that the symptomatology of clearly impaired children failed to meet diagnostic levels (Lahey et al., 1992; Shaffer et al., 1989). The other issue was a more fundamental concern involving the appropriateness of delineating two separate categories, as opposed to one with ODD incorporated as a less severe or developmental form of CD.

DSM-III defined explicit and distinct operational criteria which were intended to capture two constructs involving patterns of problematic behavior. Oppositional disorder (OD) is a pattern of defiant, hostile, negativistic behavior that is more frequent than in other children of the same mental age. Conduct disorder involves the repeated violation of the basic rights of others and of age-appropriate societal norms. The introduction of the two diagnoses in DSM-III stimulated debate about the utility of the new oppositional disorder diagnosis (Loeber et al., 1991), which in DSM-III required the presence of two symptoms from a list of five. In DSM-III-R the syndrome was renamed oppositional defiant disorder; the milder, more prevalent symptoms were eliminated, and the threshold for diagnosis was raised to five symptoms from a list of nine.

The DSM-IV DBD field trials provided data that could be used to examine the optimal symptoms and diagnostic cutpoints for ODD and CD, as well as address the more fundamental issue of one versus two diagnoses. Analyses of data for the nine DSM-III-R symptoms of ODD indicated that the symptom of "frequently swears or uses obscene language" showed weak diagnostic utility and should therefore be dropped from the list of criteria. No additional symptoms were added for DSM-IV, resulting in the adoption of a list of eight symptoms. A diagnostic cutoff of four symptoms within the previous 6 months was found to maximize the identification of impaired youth, agreement with clinician diagnoses, and test-retest reliability (Lahey et al., 1994a). In the field trials, this cutoff of one symptom fewer than the diagnostic threshold of five symptoms used in DSM-III-R resulted in a 23% increase in the prevalence of DSM-IV ODD relative to that for the DSM-III-R form of ODD (Lahey et al., 1994a). This was almost exactly the magnitude of the decrease in prevalence of DSM-III OD that was noted after the more stringent DSM-III-R criteria were introduced (Lahey et al., 1990). Nevertheless, the more inclusive DSM-IV definition appears to capture mostly impaired cases (Lahey et al., 1994a). To clarify further the boundary between age-appropriate and clinically significant behavior, the DSM-IV has added a requirement of clinically significant impairment in social, academic, or occupational functioning.

In the developing the DSM-IV criteria for CD, several issues were addressed. These included not only the establishment of a clinically meaningful cut-score, but also changes to the symptom list, the problem of defining subtypes, and the choice of an optimal time frame during which the symptoms must co-occur.

The DSM-IV symptom list for CD expands that of DSM-III-R by adding two new items: "often bullies, threatens, or intimidates others" and "often stays out late at night despite parental prohibitions, beginning before age 13 years." The addition of these two symptoms was based on field trial analyses indicating that these behaviors were highly predictive of the diagnosis of CD (Frick et al., 1994). In addition, the DSM-III-R symptom "often lies" has been modified to refer to lying that is intended to "con" others, and the DSM-III-R symptom referring to truancy has been limited in DSM-IV to truancy that begins prior to 13 years of age in order to avoid attributing this symptom to normal

adolescents, for whom truancy is not necessarily uncommon. Further, the item list in DSM-IV has been divided into thematic subgroups (aggression to people and animals, destruction of property, deceitfulness or theft, and serious violations of rules) for ease of use.

In the DSM-III definition of CD, a diagnostic threshold of one symptom was implied, but a minimum number of symptoms was not specified. In the revision of the CD criteria from DSM-III to DSM-III-R the threshold was raised to three symptoms, and again the more prevalent and milder symptoms were eliminated, resulting in a substantial decrease in the prevalence of CD. This change was met with some controversy in light of findings indicating that the presence of even 1 or 2 symptoms of CD in childhood predicts poor outcome in adulthood (Robins and Price, 1991). However, other evidence suggests that the change in criteria resulted in improved concurrent validity of the diagnosis, as indicated by correlations with indices of functional impairment such as school suspensions and contacts with law enforcement officials (Lahey et al., 1990). In the DSM-IV field trial data, the likelihood of having had police contact increased markedly when a threshold of three symptoms was required, thus supporting the continued use of this threshold level (Lahey et al., 1994a).

Antisocial behavior in children and adolescents is clearly a heterogeneous phenomenon in terms of behaviors, developmental trajectories, prognosis, biological factors, and presumably, etiology (Farrington, 1987; Loeber, 1988). Several methods for distinguishing subtypes of CD have been proposed and/or utilized in earlier versions of the DSM and ICD systems. These have included subtypes based on the capacity for establishing and maintaining social relationships, the presence or absence of aggression, and the age of onset of symptomatology (Lahey et al., 1992). In DSM-III, a dimension of subtypes was distinguished on the basis of the presence or absence of significant peer relationships, i.e., socialized and unsocialized. DSM-III also further subdivided the socialized and unsocialized subtypes according to the presence of aggression, i.e., aggressive and nonaggressive. The distinction of subtypes based on the presence of aggressive symptomatology is supported by evidence that youths rated as physically aggressive were significantly more likely than nonaggressive delinquent youths to commit serious criminal acts, particularly aggressive acts, in adulthood (Henn et al., 1980; Stattin and Magnusson, 1989).

In DSM-III-R this two-dimensional system of subtyping was simplified somewhat and was designed to emphasize the context, and to some extent the nature, of the antisocial behavior, i.e., antisocial behavior (aggressive or not) with a group of peers versus activity that is specifically aggressive and is undertaken alone. Although a solitary aggressive type was distinguished, a solitary nonaggressive subtype was not included, on the assumption that few such youth would be identified (Lahey et al., 1992).

In DSM-IV two subtypes of CD are identified on the basis of age of onset of the disorder (childhood-onset type and adolescence-onset type). The socialized/unsocialized distinction was dropped since degree of socialization had been difficult to define in operational terms (Lahey et al., 1992). Similarly, aggressive behavior waxes and wanes over time; thus, concerns about the reliability of these dimensions as the bases for subtypes led to the new approach. Results of the field trial analyses indicated that the two groups identified by age of onset differed with respect to specific symptom presentations, gender ratio, developmental course, and prognosis (B.B. Lahey, personal communication, 1995). The childhood-onset subtype is defined by the presence of at least one CD symptom prior to 10 years of age. As compared with their adolescence-onset counterparts, youngsters who meet diagnostic criteria for childhood-onset CD are more likely to be male, to have poor peer relationships, and to exhibit physical aggression. These youngsters often have a history of ODD during their early childhood and typically meet full criteria for CD prior to puberty. The developmental course of childhood-onset CD tends to be more chronic, with many of these individuals developing adult antisocial personality disorder (Robins and Price, 1991).

The DSM-IV diagnostic criteria for CD also reflect a revision in the time frame during which symptoms must co-occur. Whereas the DSM-III-R criteria required the presence of at least three symptoms during a period of 6 months, the DSM-IV criteria require that at least three symptoms have occurred within the past 12 months, with at least one present in the past 6 months. This change was based on analyses of the field trial data, which indicated that clinicians often consider relevant symptoms that have occurred within the preceding year, even if some of these symptoms were not present during the preceding 6 months. The DSM-IV requirement of at least one symptom in the past 6 months assures that the diagnosis of CD is not given to youth who have been free of symptoms for a period of several months.

The results of the field trial analyses also provided strong evidence of a developmental relationship between ODD and CD, in the sense that a significant majority of youth who meet diagnostic criteria for CD before puberty meet criteria for ODD at some earlier age. In addition, ODD and CD appear to have many of the same correlates, including parent antisocial behavior and low socioeconomic status, although CD is more strongly related to these factors (Lahey et al., 1992).

While these findings suggest that ODD may represent a less severe and less mature manifestation of the same disorder as CD, these two syndromes appear to be distinct enough to be conceptualized as separate disorders. For example, evidence suggests that many children with ODD do not go on to meet diagnostic criteria for CD, and many youth who first meet criteria for CD in adolescence did not previously meet criteria for ODD (Lahey et al., 1992; Loeber et al., 1991). Additionally, factor analyses of the symptoms of ODD and CD have yielded two separate factors of intercorrelated behaviors, representing the two clinical symptom lists (Frick et al., 1991).

In the ICD-10 the broad category of conduct disorders includes three specific types of conduct disorder and oppositional defiant disorder. ODD is defined by the presence of defiant, disobedient behavior and the absence of antisocial behaviors that would warrant a diagnosis of conduct disorder. Rutter (1989a) notes some reluctance among British child psychiatrists to include this diagnosis because of the risk that it would be applied too inclusively. However, the weight of research findings supporting its applicability and validity in younger children led to its inclusion with the caveat that it was intended to describe the problematic behaviors of younger children and should be used cautiously with older youth (Rutter, 1989a).

While the ICD-10 and DSM-IV are quite similar in their definitions of ODD and of CD as a broad category, the major differences with respect to this group of disorders reside in how the CD subtypes are specified. ICD-10 retains the socialized-unsocialized distinction that was lessened in the revision of DSM-III to DSM-III-R and then replaced by age of onset in the DSM-IV. Acknowledging the limited evidence available to support the distinction by degree of socialization, Rutter (1989a) notes that poor peer relationships have been associated with poor outcome (citing Henn et al., 1980) and that impaired capacity for social relationships may be at the core of antisocial personality disorder (Rutter, 1989a, citing Rutter, 1987). Thus, the distinction between unsocialized and socialized types of conduct disorder resides in whether the individual is or is not integrated into a peer group. The emphasis that ICD places on the socialized dimension is reflected in the specification that, for the diagnosis of unsocialized conduct disorder, the nature of the behavior is less important than the quality of social relationships. Also requiring further validation is the other conduct disorder subtype, CD confined to the family context, in which the abnormal behavior occurs at home or in the context of relationships with members of the household. As the name implies, the symptomatic behaviors must not occur in other contexts, and social relationships outside the family must be essentially normal. Rutter (1989a) notes that such a highly situational disturbance may not carry the same risk for adult antisocial personality disorder as the other, more pervasive types, but that further work is needed to validate this distinction.

PERVASIVE DEVELOPMENTAL DISORDERS

The pervasive developmental disorders (PDD) are a group of disorders characterized by significant impairment in social, behavioral, and communicative functioning. Autism, the prototype of this group, was first described by Kanner (1943) as primarily a disturbance of affective contact. Although well-recognized as a syndrome for a number of years, it was first specified in the DSM-III, where it was termed infantile autism (with onset before 30 months of age) and was classified along with two other forms of PDD (childhood onset PDD and atypical PDD). In DSM-III the PDDs were coded on Axis I along with mental retardation.

The addition of these diagnostic categories was a major advance over DSM-II, which had not recognized a distinction between this type of disorder and childhood schizophrenia. However, there was extensive concern about the lack of attention to developmental change in symptom expression (Volkmar et al., 1994) and about the validity and utility of the other categories (e.g., Cohen et al., 1986). Extensive revisions of the criteria were undertaken for DSM-III-R that produced more criteria with greater detail and the removal of the DSM-III age-of-onset criterion. The DSM-III-R PDD section restructured the three DSM-III categories into a broad category of autistic disorder and a residual "not otherwise specified" category, which were coded on Axis II with the other developmental disorders, rather than on Axis I.

Although these changes brought a stronger developmental orientation and criteria that were better specified, the diagnostic construct of autism had also been substantially broadened in the process (see Chapter 36). In particular, the DSM-III-R definition overidentified children with severe mental retardation as exhibiting autistic disorder (Volkmar et al., 1988). Another criticism of the DSM-III-R approach was that the elimination of all but the one diagnosis and the "not otherwise specified" category created new difficulties since certain recognized types of disorder, e.g., Rett's syndrome, disintegrative psychosis, Asperger's syndrome, fit poorly into this schema. The draft form of the ICD-10, which appeared shortly after the publication of the DSM-III-R, followed a more fine-grained approach that accommodates these categories (see Volkmar et al., 1994, and Chapter 36).

In preparation for the DSM-IV, literature reviews and data reanalyses were conducted to define issues for consideration in developing the PDD section. This work supported the ICD-10 strategy of specifying three other PDD diagnoses, specifically Rett's disorder, childhood disintegrative disorder, and Asperger's disorder. Rett's disorder, reported exclusively in girls to date, involves loss of acquired hand skills and social capacities, deceleration of head growth between ages 5 and 48 months, impaired language development, and evidence of poor coordination. These appear after a period of normal development in the months following birth. Childhood disintegrative disorder is characterized by normal development for at least the 2 years after birth, with the subsequent loss, before age 10 years, of acquired skills and capacities resulting in a state of impaired functioning in two of the three domains of social interaction, communication and interests/activities. Asperger's disorder (previously termed schizoid disorder of childhood) involves impairments in social interaction and stereotyped patterns of behavior and interests that are similar to those seen in autism, but without significant delay in language development, adaptive behavior (other than social), or cognitive development.

The field trials for DSM-IV autism and other PDDs were undertaken to address patterns of agreement and discrepancy across diagnostic systems, the frequency and nature of "false positives" generated by the application of DSM-III-R criteria for autistic disorder, the use of historical data (i.e., age of onset) in diagnostic formulation, and the validity of the three additional diagnoses within the larger PDD category (Volkmar et al., 1994). In this large multisite field trial, 977 subjects were rated on a range of symptoms for the various PDDs as defined by DSM-III, DSM-III-R, and ICD-10, and by new criteria (see study description in Volkmar et al., 1994). Previously assigned clinical diagnoses served as the standard against which the utility of alternative diagnostic schema were evaluated. Signal detection analyses were used to identify the most efficient sets of criteria and the relationship of the various criteria to subject characteristics.

In the field trials, cases of autistic disorder that were diagnosed according to only one of the diagnostic systems were most likely to be diagnosed according to the DSM-III-R definition (Volkmar et al., 1994). This finding was interpreted in support of earlier indications that the DSM-III-R definition was too broad. Also, many cases with clinician-generated diagnoses of other PDDs met DSM-III-R criteria for autistic disorder, providing further support for the argument that the DSM-III-R definition was too inclusive. Overall, the ICD-10 criteria for autism showed the best correspondence with clinicians' diagnoses; however, some simplification was desired. Further analyses and testing led to the adoption of a streamlined set of those criteria, which nevertheless offered good correspondence with ICD-10-identified cases of autism (Volkmar et al., 1994).

The result of this process was a more highly specified categorization of the PDDs in DSM-IV than in DSM-III-R. In addition to autistic disorder, three PDDs (Rett's disorder, childhood disintegrative disorder, and Asperger's disorder), along with a category termed pervasive developmental disorder not otherwise specified, have been added and are coded as Axis I diagnoses. Overall, the revision process for DSM-IV has led to a convergence with the ICD-10 categorization and to congruent definitions for autism and the other PDDs (Volkmar et al., 1994).

ANXIETY DISORDERS OF CHILDHOOD

Rutter has noted (1989a) that, for the anxiety disorders affecting children and adolescents, the major classification problem is how to distinguish those anxiety disorders that are specific to childhood from those that are precursors to adult anxiety states. The latter could reasonably be classified using criteria that are applied in the diagnosis of these disorders in adults and would not require inclusion in a special "childhood" section. Changes in the classification of children's anxiety disorders from DSM-III-R to DSM-IV reflect this perspective in that two conditions, previously listed in the "childhood onset" section, have been removed and are incorporated in the main section on anxiety disorders. Some allowance is made in the criteria for particular symptom features that reflect children's developmental capacities for expressing anxiety.

In the DSM-III and DSM-III-R, three anxiety disorders were listed in the section for disorders with onset in childhood—separation anxiety disorder, avoidant disorder, and overanxious disorder. Few changes were made in the DSM-III-R version. In DSM-IV, however, concern about the number of categories in the childhood onset section and about their validity led to a reconceptualization of those categories so that only separation anxiety disorder has been retained as a childhood-specific condition. Avoidant disorder has been subsumed under social phobia, with some modification in criteria to accommodate childhood manifestations (e.g., notes in the criteria to indicate that in children anxiety may be manifest in crying, tantrums, freezing, etc. or that children may not recognize the unreasonable nature of the fear). Similarly, overanxious disorder of childhood has been subsumed under generalized anxiety disorder, with some accommodation for childhood in that only one, rather than three, of six physical symptoms of anxiety is required (note: the six physical symptoms represent a substantial reduction from the 18 included in DSM-III-R). Separation anxiety remains in the childhood section, with minimal changes that include the combination of two items into one (DSM-III-R covered distress when separation occurs or when it is anticipated as two items) and the lengthening of the duration requirement from 2 to 4 weeks to achieve compatibility with ICD-10 research criteria.

While DSM-IV has pulled all but separation anxiety disorder into the general section for anxiety disorders, thereby removing the implication that they are somehow specific to childhood, ICD-10 proposes the overarching concept of developmental appropriateness as an "experimental" approach to defining the childhood anxiety disorders (Rutter,

1989a). Thus, exaggerations of developmentally normal anxiety states are considered to be the childhood-specific disorders; these are separation anxiety disorder, phobic disorder of childhood, social sensitivity disorder, and sibling rivalry disorder.

In these conditions, anxiety symptoms must have their onset in a developmentally appropriate period, occur in the absence of a generalized disorder of development or functioning, be severe in intensity (including persistence beyond the usual age), and result in social impairment (Rutter, 1989a). While this admittedly unproven approach to the classification of anxiety disorders in childhood awaits empirical validation, Rutter (1989a) notes that it addresses the need for "some explicit means of defining this group of emotional disorders, and seems worth a try" (Rutter, 1989a, p. 506).

Thus, the DSM-IV and ICD-10 approaches to the classification of childhood anxiety disorders vary conceptually, and to some extent practically. For example, there is no DSM-IV analog to sibling rivalry disorder, and the phobias are handled differently in that ICD-10 has a special category for disorders arising at a developmentally appropriate time (as opposed to those that are not normal at any stage, e.g., agoraphobia). The diagnosis of separation anxiety disorder is similar, although ICD-10 requires onset in the developmentally appropriate age period.

Despite the frequent occurrence of anxiety symptomatology in general population samples (see Rutter, 1989b), limited knowledge exists to help delineate the categories of childhood anxiety disorder and to suggest a coherent approach to classification. For the childhood anxiety disorders—perhaps even more than for the other disorders discussed—the real problem involves lack of knowledge rather than classification issues per se. If an important first step is to distinguish childhood forms from adult-type neurotic disorders (Rutter, 1989a), then identifying those anxiety disturbances that are prognostically (and presumably etiologically) continuous with adult anxiety disorders may leave a group of disorders with features that are unique to childhood. ICD-10 suggests that prognosis is one such distinguishing feature for these disorders and notes some support for the view "that the developmentally appropriate emotional disorders of childhood have a better prognosis" (WHO, 1992). Four specific disorders are included; of these, separation anxiety disorder of childhood is probably the least controversial. The need for the others in this group—sibling rivalry, phobic and social sensitivity disorders—may be less apparent. Certainly they are less well grounded empirically than many other disorders in the child psychiatric section of ICD-10 (Rutter, 1989a). If the disorders in this section receive validation in future research, then the ICD-10 approach is certainly an appealing one that would lend coherence to an otherwise confusing area of phenomenology. On the other hand, there is also the risk that use of this unproven schema will foster inconsistent classification between these categories and those in the adult psychiatric section, thus complicating the picture at a time when research would benefit from a simpler, less theoretically bound set of diagnostic possibilities.

CONCLUSIONS

In the above review of the DSM-IV and ICD-10 approaches to the classification of child psychopathology, it is apparent that these systems have achieved considerable convergence in the current psychiatric nosologies. The differences are greatest in the areas of the anxiety disorders of childhood. While each system has certain relative strengths, the most significant limitations are shared. These stem from deficiencies in our knowledge of childhood psychiatric disorders, their symptom manifestations, presentations at different stages of development, natural histories, and patterns of comorbidity.

A psychiatric nosology designed to accommodate disorders of infancy, childhood, and adolescence must grapple with the challenge of representing developmental processes in psychopathology while also providing descriptions or criteria that are sufficiently fixed so as to capture the key features of the disorder for those who use the system. Both the DSM-IV and ICD-10 were developed with attention to developmental issues; however, neither one fully integrates that perspective into the nosology. This is reflected in the descriptions of specific disorders, which note qualifications for applying criteria for generalized anxiety disorder or dysthymia in childhood, but which rarely trace changes in symptom manifestations over the course of childhood and adolescence. In both systems, little attention is given to childhood manifestations of disorders, such as depression and most anxiety disorders, that are not located in the childhood sections. Conversely, descriptions of adult manifestations of disorders that have their onset in childhood, such as autism, are lacking. At points, this reflects limited knowledge, e.g., typical clinical features of older children who once had reactive attachment disorder. At other points, more knowledge is available than is reflected, e.g., adult manifestations of autism. A developmental orientation is also absent in the area of the personality disorders. Neither system provides adequate descriptions or a framework for capturing temperamental and personality features in youngsters. Thus, both systems do better at providing "snapshots" in the form of clinical descriptions and diagnostic guidelines or criteria than in conveying their order and progression. Certainly providing a stronger developmental basis for the classification of psychopathology is a challenge that cannot be easily met; however, it should remain a goal for research that will inform revisions of both systems.

Another challenge faced by those charged with producing and refining systems of medical classification is that of suiting the differing needs of a wide range of users. The ICD-10 addresses this need through the development of a family of related documents tailored to the varying requirements of psychiatric clinical practice, research, and primary care. This plan recognizes the need for compatibility of categories across clinical and research settings, as well as the somewhat differing resources and purposes of classification in those contexts. The conceptual unity of the ICD-10 approach has a great deal of appeal. Not the least of the advantages of this approach is the comprehensibility of a given set of terms to a broad audience of clinicians and researchers.

By contrast, the DSM system has attempted to cover the range of needs in one document. This approach encourages the uniform application of diagnostic concepts but potentially carries other limitations. The stringency required of a research document may leave the clinician with more unclassifiable cases than is appropriate for a clinical nosology. On the other hand, by bending to a clinical need for some flexibility, limits are set on the rigor of the criteria, which may introduce unwanted heterogeneity into research samples. The process by which the DSM-IV has been developed, including extensive literature reviews, reanalyses of existing data sets, and focused field trials, speaks to the challenge posed by the task of producing a document that combines scientific rigor with firm clinical grounding. The success that has been achieved in gaining acceptance for a criterion-based system in U.S. child psychiatry is evidenced by the level of use and approval of DSM-III-R that was reported through a 1989 survey of 460 child psychiatrists (Setterberg et al., 1991). Ninety-eight percent agreed that a criterion-based system was useful and half to two-thirds reported that they generally assessed all relevant criteria in making a diagnosis. This is particularly noteworthy when one considers that only 9 years had passed since the introduction of DSM-III, with the considerable changes that it brought for diagnostic classification in clinical practice.

The processes by which the two classification schemes have been developed are indeed impressive. For the DSM-IV it was noted early on that possibly "the major innovation of DSM-IV will not be in its having surprising new content but rather will reside in the systematic and explicit method by which DSM-IV will be constructed and documented" (Frances et al., 1989). Certainly this process and its product are worthy of praise, as is the extensive international collaborative effort represented in the development and field testing of the ICD-10. Some level of justifiable criticism has been voiced because the decision to publish a revision of the DSM-III in 1987 put the development of DSM-IV on a timetable that substantially reduced the possibility of mutual influence in the development of DSM-IV and ICD-10, as the latter was already in a fairly advanced state before the task force on DSM-IV ever met (Kendell, 1991). That a considerable degree of convergence has, nevertheless, been achieved is a tribute to the spirit of international collaboration and bodes well for communication in the worldwide psychiatric community. For the future, there remains the important work of using these systems to gain new knowledge through research and of improving clinical care through more efficient and systematic communication. In view of the accomplishments represented in the production of the DSM-IV and ICD-10, one can hope, as Cooper notes, for "a period of classificatory rest and calm, during which experience can be gained and evaluations carried out" (Cooper, 1995). It has been wisely suggested (Cooper, 1995; Kendell, 1991) that we have probably accomplished what is possible in the refining of classificatory schema and that progress at this point lies instead in the challenge to develop new techniques and test new ideas about the fundamental nature of psychiatric disturbance.

Acknowledgments. *The authors gratefully acknowledge Drs. Kenneth Towbin and Gerald Tarnoff who worked closely with the first author in the development of the chapter that appeared in the first edition of this book.*

References

American Psychiatric Association: *Diagnostic and Statistical Manual of Mental Disorders* (3rd ed). Washington, DC, American Psychiatric Association, 1980.

American Psychiatric Association: *Diagnostic and Statistical Manual of Mental Disorders* (3rd ed, rev). Washington, DC, American Psychiatric Association, 1987.

American Psychiatric Association: *Diagnostic and Statistical Manual of Mental Disorders* (4th ed). Washington, DC, American Psychiatric Association, 1994.

August GJ, Garfinkel BD: The nosology of attention-deficit hyperactivity disorder. *J Am Acad Child Adolesc Psychiatry* 32:155–165, 1993.

Bauermeister JJ, Alegría M, Bird HR, et al: Are attentional-hyperactivity deficits unidimensional or multidimensional syndromes? Empirical findings from a community survey. *J Am Acad Child Adolesc Psychiatry* 31:423–431, 1992.

Biederman J, Newcorn J, Sprich SE: Comorbidity of attention deficit hyperactivity disorder with conduct, depressive, anxiety, and other disorders. *Am J Psychiatry* 148:564–577, 1993.

Brämer G: Tenth revision of the International Classification of Diseases—In progress. *Br J Psychiatry* 152(suppl):29–32, 1988.

Carlson CL: Attention deficit disorder without hyperactivity: A review of preliminary experimental evidence. In: Lahey BB, Kazdin AE (eds): *Advances in Clinical Child Psychology* (Vol 9). New York, Plenum, 1986, pp. 153–175.

Cohen DJ, Paul R, Volkmar FR: Issues in the classification of pervasive and other developmental disorders: Toward DSM-IV. *J Am Acad Child Adolesc Psychiatry* 25:213–220, 1986.

Cooper JE: The structure and presentation of contemporary psychiatric classifications with special reference to ICD-9 and 10. *Br J Psychiatry* 152(suppl):21–28, 1988.

Cooper J: On the publication of the *Diagnostic and Statistical Manual of Mental Disorders*: Fourth edition (DSM-IV). *Br J Psychiatry* 166:4–8, 1995.

Edelbrock C, Costello AJ, Kessler MD: Empirical corroboration of attention deficit disorder. *J Am Acad Child Psychiatry* 23:285–290, 1984.

Farrington DP: Epidemiology. In: Quay HC (ed): *Handbook of Juvenile Delinquency*. New York, Wiley, 1987, pp. 33–61.

Frances AJ, Widiger TA, Pincus HA: The development of DSM-IV. *Arch Gen Psychiatry* 46:373–375, 1989.

Frick PJ, Lahey BB, Applegate B, et al: DSM-IV field trials for the disruptive behavior disorders: Symptom utility estimates. *J Am Acad Child Adolesc Psychiatry* 33:529–539, 1994.

Frick PJ, Lahey BB, Loeber R, et al: Oppositional defiant disorder and conduct disorder in boys: Patterns of behavioral covariation. *J Clin Child Psychol* 20:202–208, 1991.

Hart EL, Lahey BB, Loeber R, et al: Developmental change in attention-deficit hyperactivity disorder in boys: A four-year longitudinal study. *J Abnorm Child Psychol*, 23:729–739, 1995.

Henn FA, Bardwell R, Jenkins RL: Juvenile delinquents revisited: Adult criminal activity. *Arch Gen Psychiatry* 37:1160–1163, 1980.

Kanner L: Autistic disturbances of affective contact. *Nerv Child* 2:217–250, 1943.

Kendell RE: Relationship between the DSM-IV and the ICD-10. *J Abnorm Psychiatry* 100:297–301, 1991.

Kramer M: The history of the efforts to agree on an international classification of mental disorders. In: *Diagnostic and Statistical Manual of Mental Disorders* (2nd ed). Washington, DC, American Psychiatric Association, 1968, pp. xi–xx.

Lahey BB, Applegate B, Barkley RA, et al: DSM-IV field trials for oppositional defiant disorder and conduct disorder in children and adolescents. *Am J Psychiatry* 151:1163–1171, 1994a.

Lahey BB, Applegate B, Barkley RA, et al: DSM-IV field trials for attention deficit hyperactivity disorder in children and adolescents. *Am J Psychiatry* 151:1673–1685, 1994b.

Lahey BB, Carlson CL, Frick PJ: Attention deficit disorder without hyperactivity: A review of research relevant to DSM-IV. In: Widiger TA, Frances AJ, Davis W, et al (eds): *DSM Sourcebook* (Vol 1). Washington, DC, American Psychiatric Association, in press.

Lahey BB, Loeber R, Quay HC, et al: Oppositional defiant and conduct disorders: Issues to be resolved for DSM-IV. *J Am Acad Child Adolesc Psychiatry* 31:539–546, 1992.

Lahey BB, Loeber R, Stouthamer-Loeber M, et al: Comparison of DSM-III and DSM-III-R diagnoses for prepubertal children: Changes in prevalence and validity. *J Am Acad Child Adolesc Psychiatry* 29:620–626, 1990.

Lahey BB, Pelham WE, Schaughency EA, et al: Dimensions and types of attention deficit disorder. *J Am Acad Child Adolesc Psychiatry* 27:330–335, 1988.

Lahey BB, Schaughency EA, Hynd GW, et al: Attention deficit disorder with and without hyperactivity: Comparison of behavioral characteristics of clinic-referred children. *J Am Acad Child Adolesc Psychiatry* 26:718–723, 1987.

Lahey BB, Schaughency EA, Strauss CC, et al: Are attention deficit disorders with and without hyperactivity similar or dissimilar disorders? *J Am Acad Child Psychiatry* 23:302–309, 1984.

Loeber R: Natural histories of conduct problems, delinquency, and associated substance use: Evidence for developmental progressions. In: Lahey BB, Kazdin AE (eds): *Advances in Clinical Child Psychology* (Vol 11). New York, Plenum, 1988, pp. 73–124.

Loeber R, Lahey BB, Thomas C: Diagnostic conundrum of oppositional defiant disorder and conduct disorder. *J Abnorm Psychol* 100:379–390, 1991.

Newcorn JH, Halperin JM, Healey JM, et al: Are ADDH and ADHD the same or different? *J Am Acad Child Adolesc Psychiatry* 28:734–738, 1989.

Pelham WE, Gnagy EM, Greenslade KE, et al: Teacher ratings of DSM-III-R symptoms for the disruptive behavior disorders. *J Am Acad Child Adolesc Psychiatry* 31:210–218, 1992.

Robins LN, Price RK: Adult disorders predicted by childhood conduct problems: Results from the NIMH Epidemiologic Catchment Area Project. *Psychiatry* 54:116–132, 1991.

Rutter M: Temperament, personality and personality disorder. *Br J Psychiatry* 150:443–458, 1987.

Rutter M: Annotation: Child psychiatric disorders in ICD-10. *J Child Psychol Psychiatry* 30:499–513, 1989a.

Rutter M: Isle of Wight revisited: Twenty-five years of child psychiatric epidemiology. *J Am Acad Child Adolesc Psychiatry* 28:633–653, 1989b.

Rutter M, Shaffer D, Shepherd M: *A Multi-Axial Classification of Child Psychiatric Disorders.* Geneva, World Health Organization, 1975.

Sartorius N: International perspectives of psychiatric classification. *Br J Psychiatry* 152(suppl):9–14, 1988.

Schwab-Stone M, Towbin KE, Tarnoff GM: Systems of classification: ICD-10, DSM-III-R, and DSM-IV. In: Lewis M (ed): *Child and Adolescent Psychiatry: A Comprehensive Textbook.* Baltimore, Williams & Wilkins, 1991, pp. 422–434.

Setterberg SR, Ernst M, Rao U, et al: Child psychiatrists' views of DSM-III-R: A survey of usage and opinions. *J Am Acad Child Adolesc Psychiatry* 30:652–658, 1991.

Shaffer D, Campbell M, Cantwell D, et al: Child and adolescent psychiatric disorders in DSM-IV: Issues facing the work group. *J Am Acad Child Adolesc Psychiatry* 28:830–835, 1989.

Spitzer R, Williams JBW: Classification in psychiatry. In: Kaplan H, Freedman A, Sadock B (eds): *The Comprehensive Textbook of Psychiatry* (3rd ed). Baltimore, Williams & Wilkins, 1980.

Stattin H, Magnusson D: The role of early aggressive behavior in the frequency, seriousness, and types of later crime. *J Consult Clin Psychol* 57:710–718, 1989.

Volkmar FR, Bregman J, Cohen DJ, et al: DSM-III and DSM-III-R diagnoses of autism. *Am J Psychiatry* 145:1404–1408, 1988.

Volkmar FR, Klin A, Siegel B, et al: Field trial for autistic disorder in DSM-IV. *Am J Psychiatry* 151:1361–1367, 1994.

Widiger TA, Frances AJ, Pincus HA, et al: Toward an empirical classification for the DSM-IV. *J Abnorm Psychol* 100:280–288, 1991.

World Health Organization: *The ICD-10 Classification of Mental and Behavioral Disorders: Clinical Descriptions and Diagnostic Guidelines.* Geneva, 1992.

38 INFANT ASSESSMENT

Linda C. Mayes, M.D.

The developmental assessment of infants involves more than the simple administration of a set of developmental test protocols. Assessments performed in the first 2 years of life require the clinician to function simultaneously as a generalist and a specialist, to blend quiet observation with active probing, to synthesize information from parents with that gathered through direct observation of the child, and to be involved in a curious blend of searching for specifically defined responses from a child with inferences based on behavior. In this chapter on infant assessment, four areas of inquiry implicit in these introductory statements are addressed:

1. What is the history of the field of infant assessment, and what concepts underlie the process of infant assessments?
2. What are the available formal assessment tools?
3. What kinds of information define an assessment of an infant's development? Does such an assessment entail only a simple quantitative charting of emerging skills and capacities, or does it require a more complex qualitative evaluation of the infant's developing social, affective, and cognitive adaptation within the environmental matrix? What are the sources of data for this more complex assessment profile, and does the process itself have a therapeutic effect?
4. Why perform developmental assessments of infants? When are such assessments indicated, what can we learn from the process, and what, if anything, can we predict about the infant's future development?

Most commonly, infancy refers to the time after birth and before the appearance of verbal communicative speech, that is, the first 18 months. Various authors extend the definition to the end of the 2nd year, but whatever the exact chronological time frame, "infancy" encompasses the most rapid neurodevelopmental change of any period in the life span. All assessments of infants are framed by the context of rapidly changing, growing systems that may be in or out of synchrony with one another.

HISTORICAL BACKGROUND

In the late 19th century, the European scientific community was consumed with a fervor and creativity best characterized by the studies of evolution, theories about the unconscious mind, and a growing concern for the mentally deficient and insane. The concept of measuring infant capacities grew out of the concern of scientists of the time to find a metric for human intelligence that would identify the mentally deficient. The French had been the first to distinguish mental deficiency from insanity (Esquirol, 1938) and in so doing had started a controversy about the educability of the former. Schools for the mentally retarded were being opened throughout Europe. The interest in measuring intelligence reflected a practical need to find criteria for mental deficiency in order to develop standards for admission to such schools.

In 1904 the minister of public education in Paris appointed Binet and Simon to be members of a commission studying the question of special education. Binet, an experimental psychologist, had been interested in mental functioning in normal children, and Simon had worked with him on earlier versions of tests to rank intellectual functioning. In response to their charge from the minister, Binet and Simon developed the concept of mental age, which described how an individual child's performance on tasks involving memory and reasoning compared to the chronological age of a large group of children who had succeeded with the tasks. This test, published in 1905, revolutionized the testing movement, and the concepts quickly spread to other scientific and educational communities (Brooks and Weinraub, 1976). In the United States, Terman revised Binet and Simon's mental age concept by creating the intelligence quotient (IQ), a ratio between mental age and chronological age multiplied by 100.

It is not an exaggeration to say that the concept of IQ singularly preoccupied many psychologists for several decades. American psychologists in particular believed that IQ was fixed, and they found it an exciting possibility that one well-administered test would provide stable, predictive information about a child's underlying potential. In the 1920s, a few "infant tests," which were actually revisions of the Binet-Simon Scales, were introduced. These early tests were never adequate measures of the range of infants' capacities, and by the late 1920s the field of infant testing became a serious endeavor in its own right. Though several investigators became interested in infant assessment at the same time, Arnold Gesell was the prime mover.

Gesell's goals were no less pragmatic than Simon and Binet's, for he focused on "infant hygiene" and "infant welfare" and wanted to develop assessments that would identify infants for whom such issues were paramount. He gathered detailed data on normative behavioral development, and he brought an emphasis on growth and change. As early as 1916, Gesell and his colleagues had begun a series of meticulous observations of infants' and preschool children's behavior at home and in the well-child clinic, in order to define norms for behavior (Yang, 1979). An important footnote to this is that the Gesell group was actually the first to develop the procedure of systematically observing the infant's natural responses in a natural setting (Buhler and Hetzer, 1935). As is covered in more detail below, Gesell's careful delineation of behaviors across ages became the main source of material for many other infant tests that would follow in the next two decades (Stott and Ball, 1965). This is not to say that other tests being developed at the same time, such as the Viennese Series of Buhler and Hetzer, have not been influential, but rather that Gesell's conceptual legacy has predominated over most others.

In the 1940s and 1950s, infant assessment techniques were used primarily for diagnosis and categorization purposes, for example, preadoptive screening, testing for admission to special schools, or evaluating physical handicaps (Stott and Ball, 1965). Few used the techniques for longitudinal studies or empirical research. The assessments for diagnosis and categorization were predicated on clinicians' continuing adherence to the belief that intelligence is fixed from infancy. So prevalent was this belief that a fair amount of evidence to the contrary, such as an increase in IQ with nursery school attendance, was dismissed and attributed to poor standardization of the scales (Brooks and Weinraub, 1976).

The 1960s and 1970s brought a new wave of infant tests, more rigorously standardized on larger numbers of infants, with careful testing of interobserver agreement and test-retest reliability. Thoughtful research led to far more caution about the predictive validity of early assessment and to important conceptual revisions, such as recognizing that IQ is not a unitary construct. Moreover, investigators added more global appraisals to their scales (Escalona and Moriarity, 1961) and began to understand that some items, particularly verbal items, had higher predictive validity than the overall scales (Cameron et al., 1967). These and other conceptual shifts led to yet another group of infant tests designed to measure specific types of behavior, such as social competency or language development. Concomitant interest in newborn capacities and the rapidly emerging field of newborn sensory perception also led to the development of a number of scales to measure competency in the newborn (see below).

This brief historical overview serves to make two points that are relevant for a chapter intended primarily to outline the ''how to's'' of infant assessment: (*a*) The field of infant assessment has quite pragmatic origins—categorization and diagnosis for the purpose of intervention and treatment; (*b*) these origins have contributed to a strong and persistent focus on prediction of later capacities. Only relatively recently has the nature of early learning mechanisms attracted investigators' interest. Moreover, only recently have investigators and clinicians acknowledged that early development represents a complex interplay among social/environmental factors, affective experience, motivation, and cognitive capacities. Those entering the field of infant assessment at this point will find such issues active, clinically influential, and always providing a cautionary note to the push to predict later capacities based on earlier measures.

FORMAL ASSESSMENT INSTRUMENTS

A number of assessment instruments are available to evaluate developmental status in infants and newborns, and each is different conceptually, administratively, and psychometrically. Three such instruments will be discussed below: the Bayley Scales, the Uzgiris-Hunt Scales, and the Brazelton Neonatal Behavioral Assessment Scales. These three were chosen partly because they are commonly used in clinical work, but also because each is representative of a dominant conceptual theme in infant assessment. Bayley represents the Gesell tradition, Uzgiris and Hunt reflect a Piagetian focus, and Brazelton's work emphasizes individual differences, newborn competencies, and social regulation. Before the description of each instrument, the major points of these individual conceptual traditions will be outlined.

The Gesell Tradition

For Gesell, diagnosis was the primary objective of measuring infant development. He modeled his approach after the work of Wilhelm His, one of the first investigators of human embryology (Yang, 1974). In 1925, when his observational techniques were well established, Gesell wrote, ''Just as the embryologist gets his basic conceptions of morphogenesis by building up indefatigably, step by step, detailed sectional views of growing organisms . . ., so may genetic psychology build up a continuing series of sections corresponding to the stages and moments of development'' (Gesell, 1925, p. 26). Gesell began his descriptions of infants at 3 months of age and initially included five other assessment points in the first 2 years (6, 9, 12, 18, and 24 months). For Gesell, the scales were descriptive, and specific items were included for normative purposes rather than for measuring intelligence. He did argue, however, that the scales were a measure of a child's capacity and personality characteristics (Honzik, 1976).

For the Gesell Scales, data were collected about several areas of development, including motor development (posture, prehension), language development (comprehension, imitation), adaptive behavior (eye-hand coordination, recovery and manipulation of objects, alertness), and personal-social behaviors (reactions to people, play behavior, independence). The first completed scale, published initially in 1925, consisted of 144 items divided among these four general fields. Some items appeared in more than one subdomain, and motor items predominated at the early ages, while language and personal-social items predominated later. Age placements were determined by the percentage of subjects who passed each item.

The first Gesell Scales were based on a small, normative sample (107 infants from white middle-class families), and subsequent revisions of the 1925 scales were directed toward making finer gradations of responses instead of changing items (e.g., defining by weeks the appearance of the response to the sound of a bell). Gesell and his colleagues did not report any analysis of the reliability or validity of the original schedules. Nevertheless, other investigators liberally borrowed test items from the Gesell schedules, and many items persist unchanged in the scales of other authors (Honzik, 1976). Of these researchers, the most well known is Nancy Bayley.

THE BAYLEY SCALES

Bayley relied heavily on the individual items from the Gesell Scales to develop her own instrument. The Bayley Scales are divided into mental and motor domains. The motor items deal with gross motor movements and body coordination, and the mental items deal with fine motor coordination, tests of sensory acuity, and tests of learning or adaptability. The first versions of the mental and motor scales, published in 1933 and 1935, respectively (Bayley, 1933, 1969), were tested in a normative sample of 61 infants from upper-middle-class families in the Berkeley area. Although test-retest correlations averaged .58 to .63 for the first 3 months and greater than .74 after 3 months, the initial normative sample was not representative of the general population.

The scales were restandardized later using a much larger sample of 1262 infants, all of whom were born at term (Bayley, 1969). No significant differences in the sample were found for sex, birth order, parental education, or geographic location (urban versus rural) stratification variables. However, one racial group difference was reported. Nonwhite infants scored higher than white infants on the motor scale between the 3rd and 14th month. In this 1969 revision, the order of item administration was revised, and new items were added (see Bayley, 1969, for details).

The 1969 version of the scales was revised and restandardized in 1993 with again a larger group of infants (Bayley, 1993). The standardization sample consisted of a national, stratified random sample of children 1–42 months of age. The total sample of 1700 children were divided into 17 age groups of 100 children each. More age groups were sampled in the 1- to 12-month range than in the 13- to 42-month range because of more rapid developmental shifts in the 1st year. For each age group, there was an equal number of males and females, and the proportions of children in different ethnic groups were based on the ethnic distribution of children ages 1–42 months according to the U.S. Bureau of the Census, 1988. The standardization sample was also stratified by region of the country and by parental education level.

While the 1969 version of the scales can be used with children 2–30 months of age, the restandardization extended the applicable age range to 1–42 months. The mental scale contains 178 items and is averaged at 1-month intervals between 1 and 14 months and then every 2 months between 14 and 42 months. The motor scale contains 111 items and is averaged similarly. The mental scale assesses information processing, habituation, memory, language, social skills, and strategies such a generalization and categorization. The motor scale assesses control of gross and fine motor muscle groups. This includes movements such as crawling, sitting, rolling, walking, and then running and jumping. Examples of fine motor capacities include patterns of grasping, imitation of hand movements, and use of writing implements.

Also included in both the 1969 and 1993 revisions is the Infant Behavior Record (IBR-1969) or Behavior Rating Scale (BRS-1993), which contains a set of ratings that are completed at the end of the assessment and that provide qualitative and quantitative information about the infant's social, emotional, and organizational behavior during the assessment in the following domains: quality of motor activity, attention/arousal (for children under 12 months), orientation and engagement, and emotional regulation. Each item on the BRS has a 5-point rating system with descriptors specific to the behavior being rated. Items on the BRS are grouped into three age levels (1–5 months; 6–12 months; 13–42 months). Additionally, in the BRS the clinician asks the parent his or her assessment of the child's behavior and of how representative the child's performance is of his daily capacities.

Although Bayley did not report interobserver reliability for the 1969 revision, others reported reliability estimates for a 1966 version of the scales (Werner and Bayley, 1966). For 59 items on the mental scale and at 8 months, simultaneous observers agreed 89% of the time. For 20 items on the motor scale, agreement was 93%. More specifically, for the mental scales, agreement was highest for those items describing item- or object-oriented behaviors and lowest for items depending on social interaction. For the motor scales, items requiring adult assistance had slightly lower reliability than those pertaining to control of head and extremities. In more extensive studies of observer agreement performed for the 1993 revision (Bayley, 1993), interrater reliabilities for the motor scale were .96 and .75 for the motor scale. For the BRS, interobserver agreement varied, with the lowest agreement being for ratings of attention and arousal in younger children (.57). Agreement among observers for the behavioral ratings improved for children older than 12 months (Bayley, 1993). Test-retest performance was also quite high for sessions separated from 1 to 16 days with a median retest interval of 4 days. For the mental scale, test-retest correlation was .83 and .77 for the motor scale. For the BRS, test-retest performance was more variable, particularly for younger children in the domain of attention and arousal ($r = .48$), but was more stable for children older than 12 months (Bayley, 1993). Because the BRS samples behaviors as observed during a given testing session, it is more subject to state and day-to-day variation than items contributing to either the mental or the motor scales.

The Bayley Scales are administered in an hour or less. After completing the testing, the examiner determines a basal level for the infant by noting the last item passed. The raw score for each scale is the total number of items the child passed, including all items below the basal level. The raw score is converted to a standard score by consulting the norms established for a child of a given age, as derived by Bayley (1969) or from the 1993 standardization sample (Bayley, 1993). The resulting two standard scores are expressed as the Mental Development Index (MDI) and the Psychomotor Development Index (PDI). For a delayed infant, Bayley suggested finding the child's raw score in the normative table in the rows corresponding to an MDI or PDI of 100 and noting the age group column in which the raw score is nearest that obtained by the child. This is the age equivalent or mental age. Bayley reports correlations between the mental and motor scale range from $r = .24$ to .78, with higher correlations at the younger ages. The 1969 version of the Bayley is also well-correlated with the 1993 version: MDI and PDI scores on the most recent standardization are on average 12 and 7 points, respectively, lower than scores from earlier versions. Positive relations also pertain between the behavior ratings and MDI/PDI (Matheny et al., 1974; McGowan et al., 1981). For example, those items most conceptually related to cognition (alertness, sensorimotor skills) were moderately correlated with MDI performance (Matheny et al., 1974). Similarly, there are low to moderate correlations between the domains of the BRS and the PDI/MDI.

It is important to note that Bayley did not interpret either the MDI or the PDI as intelligence quotients or scores. Correlations between Bayley performance and subsequent IQ assessments are variable. In her 1933 sample of 61 infants, Bayley found no relation between the mental scale administered before 24 months and the Stanford-Binet administered from 5 to 13 years of age (Bayley, 1949). For the 24-month mental age scale with another sample of infants, she reported a correlation of .53 with the Stanford-Binet. Others have investigated the relation between performance on the 1969 version of the Bayley Scales and subsequent IQ tests and have found modest correlations between MDI and PDI measures collected through 24 months with 30- to 36-month Stanford-Binet scores (McCall, 1979; Ramey, 1973; Siegel, 1979). In the 1993 version, more robust correlations pertain between the MDI and subscales of both the Wechsler Preschool and Primary Scale of Intelligence and the McCarthy Scales of Children's Abilities (1972), a finding suggesting that items added to the 1993 version may tap constructs similar to earlier and later measures of information processing (Bayley, 1993). However, for the most part, Bayley performance does not consistently predict later cognitive measures, particularly when socioeconomic status and level of functioning are controlled (Rubin and Balow, 1979). Nevertheless, the Bayley Scales have been extremely well standardized, have proven reliable, and both the 1969 and more currently revised 1993 versions are probably the most widely used measure of infant development both in clinical assessments and in research.

The Piagetian Tradition

Piaget presented a view of the child that was quite different from Gesell's and that reflected, at the least, their different theoretical backgrounds (Yang, 1979). Gesell, the essential pragmatist, presented development as the steady march forward of increasingly complex behaviors and capacities that were relatively unaffected by environmental contingencies. Piaget, the essential epistemologist, described development as a hierarchical series of qualitatively different stages that cut across observable behaviors and that are closely linked to environmental influence. For Gesell, children unfolded on a maturational timetable. For Piaget, children grew to understand the world and themselves, and development was the process of "knowing" in ever more complex ways. Maturation of motor skills and other capacities was the vehicle that would lead to such knowing, and progress depended on previous achievements in all functional areas.

As Baldwin (1967) pointed out, it was essentially not until the 1950s that American psychologists became interested in Piaget's work, and this was long after the infant assessment field was well established in the tradition of Gesell and Bayley. Thus, the assessment techniques based on Piagetian theories are even now far less widely used or considered, but two such techniques are available and present a useful contrast to the Bayley Scales. These are the Einstein Scales of sensorimotor intelligence (Corman and Escalona, 1969) and the Uzgiris-Hunt Scales (Uzgiris and Hunt, 1975). Of these two, the latter is used more often.

UZGIRIS-HUNT SCALES

These scales are based on Piaget's sensorimotor period, which encompasses approximately the first 2 years of life. The position of an item in the Uzgiris-Hunt Scales is determined a priori by the theory, not by the chronological age at which most children complete the item, as in the Gesell-based scales. There is also an ordinal assumption in the Piagetian-based scales; that is, success on an item at one level presumes success at all previous levels because of the hierarchical assumptions in the theory.

The Uzgiris-Hunt Scales are divided into six subscales. The first scale, visual pursuit and permanence of objects, deals with infants' increasing awareness of objects outside their immediate perceptual field. Behaviors involving searching for a hidden object fall within this subdomain. The second subscale, development of means for achieving desired ends, covers such activities as using a tool to obtain an object. Development of imitation, the third subscale, is divided into vocal imitation and gestural imitation and includes not only repetition of words but also different sounds for distress and pleasure. The fourth subscale, development of operational causality, includes anticipatory behaviors such as attempting to start a mechanical toy or, in younger infants, watching one's own hand movements. Object relations in space, the fifth subscale, describes the infant's capacity to discriminate dimensionality, to track and locate objects, or to localize perceptual cues. Finally, the sixth subdomain involves the development of schemas for relating to objects (e.g., how the infant's use of toys changes) and how exploratory behaviors with objects become increasingly differentiated and complex.

The Uzgiris-Hunt Scales are administered using a series of situations and materials that elicit children's responses in the various subdomains. The procedures for administering the situations are quite flexible. The six scales are not presented in a specified sequence, nor does the examiner need to cover all the scales. Specific directions for types of items, number of presentations, and types of expected responses are given, but judging success is more flexible because of the more conceptual nature of the tasks. Unlike other infant tests, only a ceiling level of highest performance is available from these scales. There is no level at which all items are passed (basal level). Thus, the scales do not permit deriving an overall mental age equivalent. Also, the patterns of performance among the various subdomains may be quite different; that is, a child can function better in one subdomain than in another.

The scales were tested and revised in three samples of infants drawn exclusively from middle-class families. Observer agreement and test-retest reliability were high in the three original samples, ranging between 92 and 97% and 70 and 85%, respectively, for the six subscales. The subscales were also highly intercorrelated ($r > .80$), and each subscale was highly correlated with age ($r > .88$). Although Uzgiris and Hunt did present mean ages for the achievement of each scale stage, they emphasized that their samples were not selected to provide normative data for different ages. Subsequently, Dunst (1980) has estimated norms for age-equivalent scores based on performance in the various subdomains.

In terms of predictive relations to concurrent and later assessments, there appears to be little correlation with Bayley scores but moderate correlation with later Stanford-Binet scores (King and Seegmiller, 1973; Wachs, 1975). Wachs, followed a sample of infants between 12 and 24 months and correlated their performance with the Stanford-Binet at 31 months. By 24 months, all scales except means for obtaining an end were significantly correlated with Stanford-Binet performance.

Neuroregulation in the Neonate

While the authors of the first infant assessment techniques were interested in neonates, the assessments for infants younger than 1–2 months ultimately developed out of a different conceptual focus. Many of the procedures for assessing the very young infant were developed expressly to describe the range of individual differences in normal newborns and to highlight the areas of newborn competency. Tests such as the Brazelton Neonatal Behavioral Assessment Scale (NBAS) placed a greater emphasis on assessing the infant's social competencies as opposed to assessing only perceptual capacities or behaviors that were presumed related to cognitive functioning (Brooks and Weinraub, 1976).

Another conceptual difference is key. Beginning in the early 1960s, the newborns and young infants were seen as more active participants in their environment (Bullowa, 1979). Not only were they developing intrinsic perceptual-cognitive competencies, but they also brought a repertoire of behaviors, individually variable, that elicited different responses from their environment. The NBAS in particular was developed, as Brazelton (1984) stated, in "an attempt to score the infant's available responses to his environment, and so, indirectly his effect on the environment" (p. 4). Thus, in contrast to Gesell's emphasis on maturation, the NBAS emphasizes individual variability in the infant's organization of early neurological capacities. Although clinicians assessing infants are not often asked to evaluate neonates, the conceptual point inherent in these instruments—combining an assessment of innate capacities with attention to individual variability and responsivity—is relevant to all assessments of infants and young children.

BRAZELTON NEONATAL BEHAVIORAL ASSESSMENT SCALE

The NBAS (Brazelton, 1984) describes the range of behavioral responses to social and nonsocial stimuli, as the neonate moves from sleeping to alert states. The Brazelton assessment evaluates the infant's neurological intactness, behavioral organization (e.g., state regulation and autonomic reactivity), and interactiveness and responsiveness with both animate and inanimate stimuli on the basis of 27 behavioral items and 20 reflexes. The NBAS is begun optimally when the infant is sleeping and completed as the infant is brought to an alert, interactive state. Each behavioral observation is scored along a seven- to nine-point continuum. Approximately 30 minutes are required to administer the scales.

Unlike the Bayley, the NBAS does not yield a single score, although Als et al. (1977) have proposed an a priori four-factor solution for the 27 items. The four-factor scores describe interactiveness, motoric behavior, state control, and physiological response to stress. Lester and others (1982) have summarized the behavioral items into six clusters and use the neurological reflex behaviors to define a seventh cluster. Each of the seven clusters yields a numerical score describing the infant's performance in that area. The six behavioral clusters are habituation, orientation, motor, range of state, regulation of state, and autonomic regulation. A higher score on any one of the six behavioral clusters indicates better, or more mature, newborn performance. The reflex cluster is the total number of deviant reflex scores so that, in the case of the reflex cluster, a higher number indicates more deviant neurological examination results.

With training, interobserver and test-retest reliability for the 27 items has been shown to be adequate (Lancione et al., 1980; Sameroff, 1978), although a considerable degree of judgment is required of the examiner for assigning a rating to the infant's responses. The NBAS has been used in a number of studies of newborns from the first 24 hours to 1 month of age. These studies have examined the effect of general anesthesia on infants, have followed infants withdrawing from methadone, and have used the NBAS as a demonstration technique to teach mothers and fathers about their infants' capacities (Sostek, 1978). There are very weak correlations between scores from a Brazelton assessment in the newborn period and developmental evaluations at 1–2 years (Vaughn, 1980). Of the dimensions assessed by the Brazelton, state control appears the most stable and predictive (Als et al., 1979). This latter finding also speaks to the fundamental importance of early state regulatory capacities for other more complex functions, such as attention and social interactiveness, that emerge in the 1st year.

LEVELS OF INFORMATION IN AN INFANT ASSESSMENT

In this section, we address the clinical aspects of an infant assessment. It would be incomplete to say that a formal development evaluation is the only task involved in an infant assessment. Indeed, in some ways, it is the least critical of the tasks and serves more as a frame for clinicians to guide their observations. It is not sufficient in assessing infants simply to say that the infant is developmentally delayed or age adequate. For very young children, assessing development involves elaborating a more complex view of the child and his or her environment, and at this age, every developmental evaluation must include descriptions of behavior and the qualitative aspects of the child's behavior in the structured setting. For example, *when* the infant turned to a voice or successfully retrieved a toy in a manner appropriate for age may be less important than *how* he or she responded to these tasks—with excitement, positive affect, and energy or slowly, deliberately, and with little affective response?

Such qualitative observations are often the best descriptors of those capacities for which we have few standardized assessment techniques but that are absolutely fundamental for fueling the development of motor, language, and problem-solving skills. Through observing how infants do what they do, the clinician gains information about how infants cope with frustration and how they engage the adult world, as well as about their emotional expressiveness, their capacity for persistence and sustained attention, and the level of investment and psychological energy given to their activities. These areas are the bricks and mortar of development.

Also, as stated in the introduction, in performing the infant assessment the clinician must be both generalist and specialist. More specifically, the clinician must draw upon and synthesize knowledge from child psychiatry, pediatrics, neurology, developmental psychology, and often genetics. Additionally and increasingly, clinicians evaluating young children need also know about early educational programs and laws about child abuse and neglect. Knowledge from these diverse fields allows a clinician to place the results of a developmental assessment in a meaningful context for the individual child. For example, understanding the physiological effects of prolonged malnutrition helps the clinician evaluate the relatively greater gross motor delays of a child with failure to thrive who has no other neurological signs. Similarly, understanding the effects of a parent's affective disorder on a child's responsiveness to the external world adds another dimension to understanding the infant's muted or absent social interactiveness, babbling, and smiling.

In this section, we discuss how the clinician uses interviewing and observation of the infant and the interactions between parent and infant to round out the assessment. We will also cover how information from many different sources may be synthesized. In order to address these issues, we must examine four developmental principles that should underlie the clinician's thinking: (a) the distinction between innate and experiential factors, (b) the role of maturation, (c) the essential place of relationships with others for healthy development; and (d) phases of development. While each of these areas is interrelated, there are points that are unique to each.

Innate and Experiential Factors

The interactive balance between innate and experiential factors is a well-worn, time-honored controversy in developmental science, and even now it is possible to find proponents emphasizing the singular importance of one over the other. Rarely are these issues clearly distinguishable in a clinical evaluation. At the least, infants bring a set of innate capacities that influence how they respond to the environment and how it responds to them. The clinician is always faced with considering how intrinsic and extrinsic factors have interacted to contribute to an infant's developmental difficulties or strengths. Infants are more vulnerable to developmental dysfunction, even with a supportive environment, if there is biological dysfunction, as in genetic disorders or severe prematurity. Conversely, even well-endowed infants are at risk for developmental dysfunction if their environment provides inadequate or inconsistent nurturing. A combination of a poor and dangerous environment with biological risks is a significant one for developmental dysfunction, and the notion of cumulative risks is a familiar topic in the developmental field (Sameroff and Chandler, 1975).

Maturation

Depending on the clinician's frame of mind, maturation, or the progressive unfolding and differentiation of intrinsic capacities, presents either a complication or a challenge in the process of developmental assessment. Infants change rapidly, and the appearance of behaviors and responses can be highly variable despite certain expected sequences. Also, although very young infants begin life in a relatively undifferentiated state, within the first months, perceptual and motor systems differentiate rapidly. Implicitly, we accept Gesell's models by accepting the assumption that sequences of development are based upon orderly maturational steps that have been well described and defined. We take these as norms against which we consider the development of the infant we are evaluating. As Provence (1972) has stated, "Maturation . . .is a necessary construct, an invisible process represented by observable behaviors" (p. 4).

However, maturation and development are often two different concepts, and in general, the maturational process is more regular and predictable than the developmental functions and behaviors that reflect such function. For example, we expect grasping patterns to follow an expectable, regular sequence of neurological maturation but know that the timetable for infants' use of a particular grasp to hold a toy or explore a box is individually variable. Or, although the infant may have the neurological capacity for a responsive smile and the perceptual-motor integration to extend his or her arms toward an adult, experience in interaction with the environment is a necessary factor for such observable behaviors to emerge.

Relationships with Adults

To say human relationships are essential for healthy human development is at this point a given. But, as outlined above, formal infant assessment techniques such as the Bayley Scales grew out of the tradition that presumed that development proceeded often relatively independent of environmental input. Thus, it is important to emphasize that every infant assessment must consider the other individuals in that infant's life. Understanding either normal or deviant development requires some understanding of the infant's experiences with adults. The younger the child, the more central are such individuals to the child's safety and total well-being. Such serious events as traumatic separation, physical abuse, deprivation, object loss, and neglect often have devastating effects on a child's development (Rogeness et al., 1986).

Adequate care and nurturing for an infant involves a balance between gratification, comfort, and support and the frustration inevitable in all developmental phases. Adequacy, difficult as it is to define, generally includes attempts to mediate painful, tension-producing situations and to adjust the balance between comfort and frustration. The appropriate balance varies depending on the child's age. For example, the infant's frustration at not being fed immediately is different from the toddler's frustration at being unable to reach a favorite toy, and each requires a different response from the parents. In one instance, frustration may produce a painful, tense state; in another, it may lead to an adaptive solution that enhances further learning.

Moreover, we are not always dealing with gross parenting deficits or failures, such as in serious abuse and neglect. For many infants and young children, there are crucial experiences that may have adverse effects that are much harder to identify. For example, we are only beginning to understand the critical effect of maternal depression in the 1st month to year, when the mother is psychologically and sometimes physically unavailable to her infant (Garrison and Early, 1986). Parents, however articulate and enlightened, may be unaware of their own difficulties in responding to their infants, or of how their mood states, worries, and frustrations affect their responsiveness. It is at this level that the importance of establishing a working relationship between parents and evaluator is clearest.

Finally, how to assess the "adequacy" of parenting is an issue fraught with difficulty and not altogether free, however hard we try, of value judgment and bias. It is a difficult but necessary part of the young child clinician's own development to acknowledge that parents may have harmed their infant in serious ways, whether intentional or not, and may confess to negative feelings about the child and their own role as parents. Maintaining a view of the infant's family that allows the parents their own psychological adjustments and weaknesses can be one of the more difficult tasks for the clinician.

Developmental Phases

The concept of phases in development is much discussed and involves such notions as the stages of psychosexual development outlined in psychoanalytic theory, Erikson's psychosocial stages, and Piaget's theories of cognition. Clinically, the concept is a valuable one when used to refer to groups of developmental tasks that infants must learn in a given phase. When we speak of critical periods for the optimal development of different functions, we mean certain capabilities are optimally mastered at certain times, and difficulties arise when this optimal period is disrupted. It appears clinically true that when the critical period passes without optimal organization of a given function, mastery is fully achieved with far more difficulty, if ever.

It is also a clinical truism that when a function is newly emerging, it is most vulnerable to environmental stresses. This statement is supported by the common observation that an infant may stop talking if hospitalized just as the first words appear. Similarly, for an infant, chronic environmental stressors may result in a delay of appearance of phase-appropriate skills. For example, a parent's anxiety over a toddler's growing motoric independence may slow the development of motor skills and the elaboration of exploration.

For the 12- to 24-month-old child, a major phase is the development of walking or independent locomotion. This skill, more so than crawling, heralds independence and a broadening world. Use of words and verbal communication represents another critical phase, since with words the child's social world expands markedly. For infants less than 1 year old, Greenspan (1981) has suggested several other stages that are critical points in social-cognitive differentiation. In the first 3 months, infants achieve homeostasis, or the capacity for maintaining physiological equilibrium, in the face of internal and external stimulation. Between 2 and 7 months, infants begin to develop more differentiated social responses and the capacity for social regulation and active interaction.

The particular stage or phase of development influences what issues are uppermost in a child's mind and most vulnerable to stress. During an evaluation session, the valence of a particular stage will influence not only the child's success or failure on individual items, but also how he approaches such items. For example, infants struggling with emerging independence will react differently to an examiner's interventions than will the younger child who is focused on sociability and engaging the world.

Keeping these four issues in mind, we next discuss three general techniques that are central for the clinician doing infant assessments: interviewing skills, observation of children and of parent-child interactions (apart from formal structured testing), and synthesis of the information gathered during the evaluation. While interviewing, observation, and synthesis are the skills of medical diagnosis in general, there are unique aspects to each in the process of evaluating infants.

Interviewing Skills

It is axiomatic that skillful interviewing is central to a complete developmental assessment since much of the data about infants' daily functioning and their relationship with their parents come from interviews with the parents. "Skillful" interviewing techniques include letting parents begin their story wherever they choose; using directed, information-gathering questions in such a way as to clarify but not disrupt the parents' account; and listening for affect as much as content. Importantly, nearly every step of the assessment process requires an alliance between clinician and parent or foster parent since infants usually perform better when they are in the company of familiar adults, and the initial interview between clinician and family is crucial in setting the tone for such an alliance. Moreover, establishing an alliance is central to evaluating infants' interactions with the adults in their world. Indeed, infant assessments are quite compromised when there are no familiar adults available to meet with the clinician and be with the infant. Parenthetically, it is often in cases involving the most severe environmental disturbance that clinicians do not have caretaking adults available to describe the infant's history.

When parents, foster parents, or other caregivers are available, skillful interviewing is also critical in helping parents follow through with the assessment process. Coming for a developmental evaluation or participating in one while their infant is hospitalized is enormously stressful and often frightening for parents. Clinicians working with infants and their families need to understand that, regardless of what parents have been told about the assessment, parents' fears and fantasies about the process are as potent as the facts of the presenting problem. Not uncommonly, parents have begun to see the infant as damaged or defective in ·

some way and are afraid and guilty about the effect of their own behavior on the infant. Their fears of what the infant's problems signify may be expressed in many ways. They may anticipate that their infant is retarded or will have serious emotional difficulties in school, or that they will be, or already are, inadequate parents. It is always a vulnerable time for parents, and clinicians should keep in mind that what seem inconsequential moments and statements to them may be memorable and powerful for parents.

Furthermore, the stress of coming for an assessment affects the parents' abilities to report about the infant's development. The "facts" start to change as the alliance between parent and clinician develops. When first interviewed, parents may be reluctant to be candid or may not themselves be fully aware of their own perceptions and beliefs about the infant. Open-ended questions, allowing parents to begin their story wherever they feel most comfortable, and conveying a nonjudgmental attitude are crucial beginning points in establishing the working alliance with the parents. Also, at the risk of stating the obvious, such "interviews" involve as much listening as active questioning (if not more).

Practically, the purpose of interviews with parents, foster parents, or other caregivers is to gather information about the infant. What we have highlighted above is the affective atmosphere in which such data gathering occurs. The important areas to cover in terms of the infant's development are the medical history and major developmental milestones; the history of the mother's pregnancy, delivery, and immediate perinatal period; the number, ages, and health of family members; and how the infant fits in the family's daily life. Also, the meaning of the individual child for both parents may be an important window on the infant's place in the family.

More specifically, the interviewer should try to get a picture of the parents' perceptions of the infant's level of functioning in several areas. These include motor development and activity level, speech and communication, problem-solving and play, self-regulation (ease of comforting, need for routines), relationships with others, and level of social responsiveness. Questions about whether or not the pregnancy was planned or came at a good time for the family and what expectations the parents had for the infant provide important information about perceptions, disappointments, and stresses. Similarly, at some point asking the parents who the infant reminds them of or what traits they like best and least may be useful avenues for learning about how the parents view both the infant's problem and place within their family.

Provence (1977) has suggested that a productive method of gathering developmental and family data is to ask the parents to describe a day in the life of a child. She outlines how this question can be the framework for learning about daily activities, how the infant and parent interact throughout the day, and about interactions around mealtime, bedtime, or times of distress. When both parents are present for the interview, this question provides a time for each of them to present descriptions of his or her time with, and perceptions of, the child.

Implicit in this overview of interviewing parents as a part of the developmental assessment is the assumption that such assessments require several sessions. Minimally one meeting with parents, two or more with the child and parents together, and another to present the results to the parents are necessary. The sessions with the infant also provide an opportunity to gather more interview information, as other questions will occur in the context of the child's behavior and performance. For example, asking whether the child's response to a particular situation within the evaluation context is usual for him or her may open up another area of information from the parents. As is likely clear from these suggestions, in our view, infant assessment is a process of constantly gathering information, revising impressions, and testing hypotheses, and it requires time.

On the other hand, clinicians asked to evaluate infants and young children will not always have the ideal situation outlined above. At times, consultants, parents, or both may insist that the evaluation be done in one session, or the clinician may have limited access to the child, as with evaluations done in a hospital setting. It is important at these times for the clinician to be clear about what he or she feels certain about and what are the limitations of the evaluation findings. Another situation that occurs increasingly commonly and does not fit the ideal model just outlined is when no parents, family members, or caregiving adults are available. Situations of severe abuse, abandonment, multiple placements, or seriously ill parents are examples of times in which the clinician will not have available certain critical sources of information. In these instances, certain hypotheses suggested by the child's presentation and status may be left unconfirmed. As in situations where the time for the evaluation is brief, it is most important for clinicians to acknowledge what diagnoses they are certain about, which they are not, and what information would likely be clarifying were it available.

Observational Techniques

Observation is the fundamental skill needed for measuring infants' development. After all, most diagnostic evaluations are based on observation of physical signs and/or behavioral responses. However, what distinguishes the observational skill necessary for developmental assessment is that it occurs on many levels simultaneously and is perhaps the area in which the developmentalist's dual role as both generalist and specialist is most evident. Moreover, the observational skills inherent in assessments of infants require a blend of free-floating attention bounded by a structure. In other words, while the clinician must be comfortable enough in the setting to attend to whatever occurs, he or she must also have a mental framework by which to organize the observations collected during the session. Such a framework entails at least four broad areas: (a) predominant affective tone of the participants, (b) involvement in the situation (curiosity and interest), (c) use of others (child's use of the parents or examiner, or parents' of examiner), and (d) reactions to transitions (initial meetings, end of sessions, changes in amount of structure).

Using this framework, the clinician makes observations continuously on at least three levels. Perhaps the most obvious level is the observations of how the child responds to the structured assessment items administered during formal testing. As already stated above, observations during formal testing should not be confined solely to whether or not the child passes or fails a given item but to how the child approaches the task. The second level of observation during an infant assessment is how the child reacts to the situation apart from the formal testing structure. Does the child approach toys, initiate interactions, refer to the examiner or his parents? How does the child react in the beginning of the evaluation and later when the situation and the examiner are familiar?

The third observational level is a specific focus on the interactions between parent and infant. The clinician makes these observations throughout the evaluation process and revises his or her hypotheses as both parent and infant become familiar with the process. How to interpret the behaviors one observes between parent and child in terms of their ongoing relationship is learned partially by experience and requires time to gather many observational points. However, several general areas may provide important descriptive clues. Does the child refer to the parent for both help and reassurance? Similarly, does the child show his successes to the parent, and does the parent respond? Another important observation for toddlers is whether or not the child leaves his parent's immediate company to work with items or explore. For infants, how parents hold, feed, and comfort their baby may be windows in the emerging relationship between the two. A parent' participates with his or her child during such sessions in varying ways, and the clinician will be judging continuously how intrusively involved, withdrawn, or comfortably facilitative a parent is. One of the tasks of learning to observe interactions between parents and their children is to understand that adults may appear very different as individuals in their own right compared to when they are interacting with their children and that the very act of having one's child (and by implication, one's self) observed by another is anxiety provoking in varying degrees for all parents.

Synthesis

The process of synthesizing all the data gathered from the different sources during an assessment is a technique and skill unto itself. Moreover, how this synthesis, with its attendant recommendations, is conveyed to parents (and consultants) is another essential step in the assessment process, and the assessment is not complete until the parental alliance is brought to fruition in a collaborative formulation. Also, infant assessments often involve referring pediatricians and other clinicians, who need to be included individually in the clinician's data-gathering interviews and in the final synthesis.

The synthesis of information from an infant assessment differs from the synthesis involved in other medical diagnostic processes in that there are very few specific diagnostic categories that encapsulate all the findings of an infant assessment. As already stated, assigning a mental age or developmental quotient is often the least important goal of the assessment. The synthesis involved in an infant assessment involves bringing together all the data gathered from interviews, observations, and testing into a qualitative description of that infant's capacities in different functional areas (motor, problem-solving, language and communication, and social) and of the infant's current strengths and weaknesses. It involves integrating the assessment information in the context of the infant's individual environment. For example, an infant who has experienced multiple foster placements may be socially delayed, but such a finding assumes a different significance for an infant who has had a stable home environment.

Finally, it is often during the synthesis process that the therapeutic effect for parents of participating in the assessment is most evident. At the very least, parents often change their perceptions of their infant's capacities. They may see strengths in their infant they had not previously recognized or become deeply and painfully aware of weaknesses and vulnerabilities that they may or may not have feared before the assessment. Any of these changes in perceptions will affect the parents' view of themselves and of their role as parents. Also, infants often change during an assessment process as their parents become more involved in the alliance with the clinician and they experience, at least temporarily, another adult's concern and interest in their family. Emphasizing the potentially therapeutic value of an infant assessment at this point in the discussion underscores that the synthesis process is not simply wrapping up the assessment and conveying information but is also a time to explore with the parents the meaning of the process for them.

OBJECTIVES OF INFANT ASSESSMENTS

Why perform infant assessments? It is perhaps easier to state definitively what infant assessments cannot provide. They do not provide a measure of intelligence, a trajectory for future development, or a window on future adjustment. Questions such as "How much of this infant's delay comes from his environment, and how much from his prematurity?" or "How retarded will this child be?" are not definitively answerable by a developmental assessment. Developmental assessments, however complete and skillfully done, cannot provide sure predictions of long-term outcome or parcel out the complex contributions of endowment, experience, and maturational forces.

Following so broad a disclaimer, it is important to emphasize the limits of prediction in early childhood, based on formal assessment techniques. As noted above, there have been several studies examining the predictive relationship between early infant tests such as the Bayley and later performance on cognitive tests. These studies have produced varying results, though it seems generally fair to say that no one assessment technique provides a robust predictive relation with later IQ. One reason infant tests may show little predictive validity for later IQ is that so many of the items used in the early months require motor skills or essentially test gross and fine motor development and the emergence of perceptual motor coordination (e.g., reaching for a toy or transferring objects between hands). Motor capacities probably have little to do with

Table 38.1.   Clinical Indications for an Infant Assessment

1. Regulatory disturbances
     Sleep disturbances (e.g., frequent waking)
     Excessive crying or irritability
     Eating difficulties (e.g., finicky eating or food refusal)
     Low frustration tolerance
     Self-stimulatory or unusual movements (e.g., rocking or head banging, excessive finger sucking)
2. Social/environmental disturbances
     Failure to discriminate mother
     Apathetic, withdrawn, no expression of affect or interest in social interaction
     Excessive negativism
     No interest in objects or play
     Abuse, neglect, or multiple placements
     Repeated or prolonged separations
3. Psychophysiological disturbances
     Nonorganic failure to thrive
     Recurrent vomiting or chronic diarrhea
     Recurrent dermatitis
     Recurrent wheezing
4. Developmental delays
     Specific delays (e.g., gross motor, language)
     General delays or arrested development

information processing capacities, and few items in the early assessments test directly and independently emerging information-processing skills (Bornstein, 1989). More recently introduced research-based measures of early information-processing capacities in infancy, such as the habituation procedures, seem to show a much stronger predictive relation with measures of cognition as at ages 4–6 years (for a review, see Bornstein, 1986). However, habituation measures are not widely available as clinical assessment techniques.

From a problem-oriented stance, there are at least four general problem areas for which infant assessments may be indicated. These problems are summarized in Table 38.1 and below:

1. Disturbances in self-regulatory capacities, such as sleep or eating disturbances, including food refusal, night terrors, repeated waking, or problems in impulse control such as excessively aggressive behavior: Low frustration tolerance is another mark of regulatory difficulties. Self-stimulatory behaviors, such as rocking or head banging, may indicate a variety of social or regulatory difficulties, may be a manifestation of environmental stress, or may signify more profound difficulties in relatedness, as in pervasive developmental disorder.

2. Disturbances in social development and/or the caregiving environment, including serious and profound problems in differentiating mother or caregiver, such as might be seen in pervasive developmental disorder or infantile autism, and disturbances in predominant mood: Infants who are excessively negative or predominantly withdrawn and apathetic are at great risk for developmental difficulties. In this category are also included environmental conditions such as repeated or prolonged separations or neglect, which place infants at risk for social and affective disturbances.

3. Psychophysiological disturbances, including failure to thrive, recurrent vomiting, wheezing, or chronic skin rashes: The younger the child, the more likely the response to an environmental stress will be a global one involving several organ systems (e.g., failure to grow). Clearly, any one of these problems may have physical causes, but clinicians should be alert to the close connection between physiological and psychological adjustment in young children.

4. Delays in specific areas of development, including motor development and activity, language and communication, awareness of others and degree of relatedness to others (seen often together with language delay), or delays in more than one of these areas. Such delays may be more common among infants with complicated perinatal courses such as those born severely premature or following parental substance abuse and prenatal exposure to alcohol, cocaine, or other drugs. Thus, infants with such histories will more often be referred for assessments early in order to plan for appropriate interventions.

The specific disturbances listed in the four categories in Table 38.1 may be characteristic of more than one general area. For example, failure to thrive may also indicate social and/or environmental disturbances, or general developmental delay may occur with repeated separations or in a withdrawn, apathetic child. A particular developmental profile, such as delayed language skills but age-appropriate motor and problem-solving skills, may occur with different presenting difficulties, and thus it is not possible to specify a characteristic diagnostic developmental pattern for failure to thrive, sleep disturbances, or the other problems listed in the table. However, three general points are important.

First, language and communication skills are the most vulnerable to biological and environmental stresses. Moreover, problems in communication will also affect personal-social development. For most of the problems listed under social/environmental disturbances, the infant will likely show minimally delayed language and personal-social development. Also, any adaptive or motor items that require interaction with the examiner will be affected by disturbances in relatedness, and the child's skills in these areas will appear scattered not necessarily because of motor impairment but rather because of the necessity for social interaction for administering the item.

Second, it is possible for an infant presenting with some of the difficulties outlined in the table to have an age-appropriate developmental profile. In this case, the qualitative observations of how the infant approached the setting are crucial.

Third, one common developmental profile is for an infant to show "scattered" skills in different areas, that is, not to reach a basal level in any domain but to have successes scattered above and below his or her chronological age. Infants with psychophysiological disturbances often show such a pattern. Qualitative observations are again important with this kind of profile, as well as a repeat assessment within a few months.

Generally, the developmental assessment provides a description of the child's functional capacities, the relationships among the various domains such as language and socialization, the child's ability to adapt, and the range of coping strategies. For the very young infant, developmental assessments describe neurodevelopmental functioning and individual regulatory capacities. For parents, the evaluation provides information about both their child and the potential therapeutic value of the alliance established with the clinician. For the referring physician, the assessment information may provide a more integrated view of the infant's psychological as well as physical status. Finally, infant assessments often serve the purpose of facilitating referrals to appropriate educational or rehabilitative services. In such cases, the useful question is not whether or not the infant is delayed or has problems but rather what are the most appropriate services to ameliorate these problems. In cases such as these, the evaluating clinicians will need to be collaborators themselves with individuals directing intervention and educational services for infants. (For a review of the development of early intervention services for infants, see Clarke-Stewart and Fein, 1983, and Meisels and Shonkoff, 1990.)

CONCLUSIONS

Infant assessments are in part clinical explorations involving a fair amount of uncertainty and inference. While the medical diagnostic process always involves some element of uncertainty, the assessments made in infancy require of the clinician a particular comfort with uncertainty and the unknown. Though the latter half of this century has brought a veritable explosion of knowledge about the neonatal period and the first 2 years, the more we learn, the more we see how little we know and how complicated these early years are.

It has been said that the responses of infants are relatively simple, so that infant tests can be based on simple, readily observable behaviors and that infant assessments are straightforward measures of neurodevelopmental status. Such a statement assumes that the behaviors we can observe in infants are a direct measure of the infant's mental activity. The more we understand about the neurobiology of learning in the first months, the clearer it is how simplistic that viewpoint is. The complexities of early information processing and perceptual function have been revealed only by very sophisticated observational and experimental techniques not readily available to clinicians. Moreover, as emphasized throughout this chapter, infant assessment involves far more than the infant and is as much a measure of the infant's environment as it is of his or her functional status. Thus, clinicians assessing infants are always dealing more with what they cannot know than with what they can and with the limits of their predictive capacities, and they must be clear about those distinctions.

References

Als H, Tronick E, Lester BM, et al: The Brazelton Neonatal Behavior Assessment Scale (BNBAS). *J Abnorm Child Psychol* 5:215–231, 1977.

Als H, Tronick E, Lester BM, et al: Specific neonatal measures: The Brazelton Neonatal Behavior Assessment Scale. In: Osofsky J (ed): *Handbook of Infant Development*. New York, Wiley, 1979, pp. 185–215.

Baldwin AL: *Theories of Child Development*. New York, Wiley, 1967.

Bayley N: Mental growth during the first three years. *Genet Psychol Monogr* 14:1–92, 1933.

Bayley N: The development of motor abilities during the first three years. *Monogr Soc Res Child Dev* 1:1–26, 1935.

Bayley N: Consistency and variability in growth and intelligence from birth to eighteen years. *J Genet Psychol* 75:165–196, 1949.

Bayley N: *Bayley Scales of Infant Development*. New York, Psychological Corp., 1969.

Bayley N: *Bayley Scales of Infant Development* (2nd ed). New York, Psychological Corp., 1993.

Bornstein MH: Stability in early mental development: From attention and information processing in infancy to language and cognition in childhood. In: Bornstein MH, Krasnegor NA (eds): *Stability and Continuity in Mental Development: Behavioral and Biological Perspectives*. Hillsdale, NJ, Erlbaum, 1989, pp. 147–170.

Bornstein MH, Sigman MD: Continuity in mental development from infancy. *Child Dev* 57: 251–274, 1986.

Brazelton TB: *Neonatal Behavioral Assessment Scale* (2nd ed). Philadelphia, Lippincott, 1984.

Brooks J, Weinraub M: A history of infant intelligence testing. In: Lewis M (ed): *Origins of Intelligence: Infancy and Early Childhood*. New York, Plenum, 1976, pp. 19–58.

Buhler C, Hetzer H: *Testing Children's Development from Birth to School Age*. New York, Farrar & Rinehart, 1935.

Bullowa M: *Before Speech*. New York, Cambridge University Press, 1979.

Cameron J, Livson N, Bayley N: Infant vocalizations and their relationship to mature intelligence. *Science* 157:331–333, 1967.

Clarke-Stewart K, Fein GG: Early childhood programs. In: Haith MM, Campos JJ (eds): *Handbook of Child Psychology* (Vol 2). New York, Wiley, 1983, pp. 917–999.

Corman HH, Escalona S: Stages of sensorimotor development: A replication study. *Merrill-Palmer Q* 15:351–361, 1969.

Dunst CJ: *A Clinical and Educational Manual for Use with the Uzgiris and Hunt Scales of Infant Psychological Development*. Baltimore, University Park Press, 1980.

Escalona SK, Moriarty A: Prediction of school-age intelligence from infant tests. *Child Dev* 32: 597–605, 1961.

Esquirol JD: *Des maladies mentales considerees sous les rapports medical, hygienique, and medicolegal*. Paris, Bailliere, 1938.

Garrison WT, Earls FT: Epidemiology and perspectives on maternal depression and the young child. In: Tronick E, Field T (eds): *Maternal Depression and Infant Disturbance*. San Francisco, Jossey-Bass New Divisions for Child Development, pp. 13–30, 1986.

Gesell A: *Mental Growth in the Preschool Child*. New York, Macmillan, 1925.

Greenspan S: *Psychopathology and Adaptation in Infancy and Early Childhood*. New York, International Universities Press, 1981.

Honzik MP: Value and limitations of infant tests: An overview. In: Lewis M (ed): *Origins of Intelligence. Infancy and Early Childhood*. New York, Plenum, 1976, pp. 59–96.

King WL, Seegmiller B: Performance of fourteen- to twenty-two- month-old black, firstborn male infants on two tests of cognitive development: The Bayley scales and the infant psychological development scale. *Dev Psychol* 8:317–326, 1973.

Lancione E, Horowitz FD, Sullivan JW: The NBAS-K 1: A study of its stability and structure over the first month of life. *Infant Behav Dev* 3:341–359, 1980.

Lester B, Als H, Brazelton TB: Regional obstetric anesthesia and newborn behavior: A reanalysis toward synergistic effects. *Child Dev* 53:687–692, 1982.

Matheny AP, Dolan AB, Wilson RS: Bayley's infant behavior records: Relations between behaviors and mental test scores. *Dev Psychol* 10:696–702, 1974.

McCall RB: The development of intellectual functioning in infancy and the prediction of later IQ. In: Osofsky J (ed): *Handbook of Infant Development*. New York, Wiley, 1979, pp. 707–741.

McCarthy D: *McCarthy Scales of Children's Abilities*. San Antonio, TX, Psychological Corp., 1972.

McGowan RJ, Johnson DL, Maxwell SE: Relations between infant behavior ratings and concurrent and subsequent mental test scores. *Dev Psychol* 17: 542–553, 1981.

Meisels SJ, Shonkoff JP: Early childhood intervention: The evolution of a concept. In: Meisels S, Shonkoff J (eds): *Handbook of Early Childhood Intervention*. New York, Cambridge University Press, 1990.

Provence S: Developmental assessment: Principles and process. In: *Brennemann's Practice of Pediatrics* (Vol 1). Hagerstown, MD, Harper & Row, 1972, chap 5.

Provence S: Developmental assessment. In: Green M, Haggarty R (eds): *Ambulatory Pediatrics*. Philadelphia, Saunders, 1977, pp. 374–383.

Ramey CT, Campbell FA, Nicholson JE: The predictive power of the Bayley scales of infant development and the Stanford-Binet intelligence test in a relatively constant environment. *Child Dev* 44: 790–795, 1973.

Rogeness GA, Suchakorn A, Amrung SA, et al: Psychopathology in abused children. *J Am Acad Child Adolesc Psychiatry* 25:659–665, 1986.

Rubin RA, Balow B: Measures of infant development and socio-economic status as predictors of later intelligence and school achievement. *Dev Psychol* 5: 225–227, 1979.

Sameroff A (ed): Organization and stability of newborn behavior: A commentary on the Brazelton Neonatal Behavior Assessment Scale. *Monogr Soc Res Child Dev* 43:1–138, 1978.

Sameroff AJ, Chandler MJ: Reproductive risk and the continuum of caretaking causality. In: Horowitz FD, Hetherington M, Scarr-Salapatek S, et al (eds): *Review of Child Development Research* (Vol 4). Chicago, University of Chicago Press, 1975, pp. 187–244.

Siegel LS: Infant perceptual, cognitive, and motor behaviors as predictors of subsequent cognitive and language development. *Can J Psychol* 33: 382–394, 1979.

Sostek AM: Annotated bibliography of research using the neonatal behavior assessment scale. *Monogr Soc Res Child Dev* 43:124–131, 1978.

Stott LH, Ball RS: Evaluation of infant and preschool mental tests. *Monogr Soc Res Child Dev* 30: 1–151, 1965.

Uzgiris IC, Hunt JMcV: *Toward Ordinal Scales of Psychological Development in Infancy*. Champaign, IL, University of Illinois Press, 1975.

Vaughn BE, Traldson B, Crichton L, et al: Relationships between neonatal behavioral organization and infant behavior during the first year of life. *Infant Behav Dev* 3:47–66, 1980.

Wachs TD: Relation of infants' performance on Piaget scales between twelve and twenty-four months and their Stanford-Binet performance at thirty-one months. *Child Dev* 46:929–935, 1975.

Werner EE, Bayley N: The reliability of Bayley's revised scale of mental and motor development during the first year of life. *Child Dev* 37:39–50, 1966.

Yang RK: Early infant assessment: An overview. In: Osofsky J (ed): *Handbook of Infant Development*. New York, Wiley, 1979, pp. 165–184.

39 PSYCHIATRIC ASSESSMENT OF INFANTS, CHILDREN, AND ADOLESCENTS

Melvin Lewis, M.B.B.S, F.R.C.Psych., D.C.H.

The psychiatric assessment of infants, children, and adolescents is both complex and subtle, requiring multiple sources of information, including the child, parents, teachers, pediatricians, hospital records, and previous evaluations, as well as observations of family interactions. The range of assessment instruments includes the clinical interview, standardized structured and semistructured interviews, questionnaires, rating scales (see Chapter 40), standardized tests (including developmental, psychological, neurological, educational, and linguistic tests; see Chapters 38, 41, 43, and 47), and biological studies (see relevant chapters in Section VI on syndromes).

REFERRAL AND GOALS

Before proceeding with a formal psychiatric assessment of the child, it is important to consider the goals and context of the referral. Diagnosis of psychiatric disorder may be just one of many possible reasons for parental referral; other reasons, sometimes covert, may include marital problems, child custody conflicts, problems in the school, and pending juvenile court decisions. Indeed, the impetus for the referral may lie outside the family; for example, the school or court are frequent sources for the referral. When the referral is external, the parent's (or legal custodian's) permission for the evaluation is usually required. In any event, the referral question or questions must be clearly understood by the evaluating clinician.

The parents' questions often need to be clarified in order to be understood: Why are the parents coming at this time with these apparent referral questions? What help is truly being sought? Parents may be seeking (or fearing) a diagnosis, treatment recommendations, relief and respite, safety for the child or adolescent and themselves, or answers to questions for which the presenting symptom is but a "ticket of admission" for some other problem that troubles them, e.g., a marital problem.

A universal set of questions for the clinician concerns the basic goals of every evaluation: Does the child indeed have a psychiatric disorder and, if so, what are the causes of that disorder and what treatment is needed? Sometimes the child's symptoms reflect more a problem of "fit" between parent and child, or between the school and child, rather than a psychiatric disorder. At other times, the presenting problem may represent the child's reaction to an environment that is stressful and adverse for that particular child.

Certain special questions, e.g., custody disputes, will require special arrangements and are discussed elsewhere, e.g., see Chapter 118. At all times, a good diagnostic interview should also be a therapeutic interview. The child's and his or her family's experience of the diagnostic interviews will, at the very least, influence how the diagnosis and recommendations are heard and understood. More than that, the diagnostic interviews may sometimes provide an opportunity to offer a therapeutic intervention.

HISTORY TAKING

The clinician should consider the above questions before proceeding with the first part of the psychiatric assessment of the child, namely, taking the history. At the same time, many of these questions may only emerge or become more sharply focused in the course of taking the history and performing the whole evaluation.

A prerequisite of an informed history taking is a knowledge of normal development and its variations, and of common psychological reactions to various developmental stresses. A knowledge of psychiatric disorders is, of course, essential. In short, the history and evaluation should help one understand in detail how this particular child has arrived at this point in his or her life.

The history is the beginning of an exploration, not only of the child's symptoms, behavior, thought processes, feelings, and environment in its largest sense (e.g., family, school, community, culture), but also of the child's total inner life of fantasies, wishes, fears, hopes, and anxieties, as well as the child's strengths and supports.

CLINICAL INTERVIEWS

History taking and the mental status examination of the child are best performed in the context of clinical interviews. A major advantage of clinical interviewing techniques with children is that their flexibility offers the clinician the opportunity to explore clinical clues in detail. Disadvantages of clinical interviews are that they may not be comprehensive enough for some diagnoses, the data may be unreliable, and often there is a high level of disagreement among clinicians. In addition, the acquisition of the necessary clinical skills requires considerable training. Finally, the initial impression gained by the clinician sometimes overpowers and obscures or discourages the search for other possible diagnoses.

Parents are most often interviewed first, especially in the case of infants. Adolescents may be given the choice of being seen first or of being present during the initial interview with the parents. Each parent should also be interviewed individually. Sometimes, seeing the whole family together is a useful diagnostic approach.

Historical and factual data, such as age, sex, race, legal status, birth history, developmental milestones, and previous illnesses, generally are best gathered by asking specific questions (Cox et al., 1981), whereas data about feelings and relationships are best elicited by an open, indirect approach. Parents, in any case, frequently recall historical dates incorrectly, although they may offer comparisons—for example, "Johnny was much slower in learning to talk than Jane." To offset these shortcomings, data should be gathered from as many objective sources as possible, including hospital records, school reports, previous tests, and multiple observers (child, mother, father).

A comprehensive and detailed pediatric psychiatric history should include a careful description of the problem as seen by the child and his or her parents; the personal history; the developmental history; the history of previous illnesses and accidents; the social history; the family history; the school history; the history of such biological functions as appetite, sleep, bladder and bowel control, and menstruation; a description of the child's relationship within the nuclear and extended family and with peers; a description of significant events, such as separations, losses, illnesses, accidents, abuse, and deaths; and an account of the previous and present psychiatric status of the parents, the marriage, and of both the nuclear and extended family. Parenting skills are also noted.

Each question should have a purpose and should be asked with tact. The clinician listens intently to the reply, not only for its content but also for its tone and affect.

The larger context of the child and family should also be considered; viz., school, community, and culture. Lastly, various administrative aspects of the evaluation process may be clarified. Thus fees, releases for information requests, and an outline or overview of what is entailed in an evaluation should be discussed with the parents. There should also be some discussion of what the parents will tell the child to prepare the child for the forthcoming evaluation.

Infants and Preschool Children

Clinical interviews with infants and preschoolers require special techniques in a suitably designed room (see Chapter 38). A simple screening technique for preschool children is shown in Table 39.1. The parents of infants and preschoolers should be present to share in the observations and to learn; their presence will also allow the examiner to observe the parent-child interactions.

An evaluation of the parents' child-rearing skills is particularly important in the psychiatric assessment of the infant. General characteristics to be assessed include the parents' physical health, self-esteem, competence, flexibility, and ability to provide a safe, nurturing, and appropriately stimulating environment. Specific characteristics to be assessed include the parents' perceptions of and sensitivity to the infant's needs; the "goodness of fit" between parent and child; the parents' ability to respond rapidly on a contingent basis to the infant's expressed needs; the quality of play between parent and infant, and the amount of support, encouragement, and assistance (scaffolding) the parent can provide for the child. The parents should also be able to provide a stimulus shelter, to prevent the child from being overwhelmed.

Infants under the age of 18 months should also subsequently be observed in spontaneous, free play, using such games as peek-a-boo and pat-a-cake.

Children between the ages of 18 months and 3 years can participate more fully in regular unstructured play interviews. The play items should look reasonably realistic, since children at this age have a limited capacity for abstraction and symbolic play.

A more detailed assessment will require the use of such scales as the Gesell Infant Scale, the Bayley Infant Scale of Development, the Uzgiris-Hunt Scales, and the Denver Developmental Screening Test (Table 39.2). See also Chapter 38 for a full discussion of the above scales.

School-Age Children

Clinical interviews with school-age children similarly require sufficient time (a minimum of 45 to 60 minutes for each interview) and suitable space, and the availability of such play items as a ball, crayons and paper, a doll house, rubber dolls, puppets, toy guns, a toy doctor's bag, and toy telephones. These unstructured play sessions allow the clinician to make inferences about the child's psychic life, including the child's wishes, fears, impulses, conflicts, defenses, affects, and relationships.

The interviewer should keep a reasonable physical distance from the child in the waiting room, in order not to loom too large and forbidding. The interviewer should introduce himself or herself to the child and invite the child to come into the office, reassuring the child that his or her parent or parents will be in the waiting room on return. Once inside the office, the interviewer should ask for the child's preferred name and make sure the child knows the interviewer's name. The interviewer should not sit behind a desk. He or she should clarify what is the child's understanding of why the child has come, and then the interviewer should give his or her own understanding. Next, the interviewer should tell the child what will take place: "It's a time set aside to see whether I can help you understand what may be bothering you. We will have 45 minutes together, at the end of which you will return to your parents."

Table 39.1.   Checklist for Assessment by Observation of Developmental Level of Preschool-Age Child

Age	Historical (or Observed) Items	Items to Be Tested
2 years	Runs well Walks up and down stairs—one step at a time Opens doors Climbs on furniture Puts three words together Handles spoon well Helps to undress Listens to stories with pictures	Builds tower of six cubes Circular scribbling Copies horizontal stroke with pencil Folds paper once
2½ years	Jumps Knows full name Refers to self by pronoun "I" Helps put things away	Builds tower of eight cubes Copies horizontal and vertical strokes (not a cross)
3 years	Goes upstairs, alternating feet Rides tricycle Stands momentarily on one foot Knows age and sex Plays simple games Helps in dressing Washes hands	Builds tower of nine cubes Imitates construction of bridge with three cubes Imitates a cross and circle
4 years	Hops on one foot Throws ball overhand Climbs well Uses scissors to cut out pictures Counts four pennies accurately Tells a story Plays with several children Goes to toilet alone	Copies bridges from a model Imitates construction of a gate with five cubes Copies a cross and circle Draws a man with two to four parts—other than head Names longer of two lines
5 years	Skips Names four colors Counts 10 pennies correctly Dresses and undresses Asks questions about meaning of words	Copies a square and triangle Names four colors Names heavier of two weights

From Paine RS, Oppe TE: Neurological examination of children. In: Clinics in developmental medicine. New York, Heinemann, 1966, p. 40.

Table 39.2.   Selected Developmental and Psychological Tests

Test Category	Age Range	Test Description
Developmental assessments		
Bayley Infant Scale of Development-Revised	1 mo–42 mos	Motor, mental and behavior rating scales
Yale Revised Developmental Schedule	4 wk–6 yr	Gross motor, fine motor, adaptive, personal-social language
Mullen Scales of Early Learning (MSEL)	0–39 mos	Infant: gross motor, visual receptive, visual
	24 mos–69 mos	Preschool: expressive, language receptive, language expressive
Individual intelligence tests, Stanford-Binet (ed #4)	2 yr–24 yr	Verbal reasoning, abstract visual reasoning, quantitative reasoning, short-term memory composite score (IQ equivalent)
Wechsler Intelligence Scale for Children III (WISC-III)	6 yr–17 yr	Verbal, performance, and full-scale IQ
McCarthy Scales of Children's Abilities	2 yr–8 yr	General cognitive index (IQ equivalent)
		Score for:
		Verbal
		Quantitative
		Memory
		Motor
		Laterality
Kaufman Adolescent and Adult Intelligence Test (KAIT)	11 yr–90 yr	Crystalized and fluid intelligence, IQ scores
Kaufman Assessment Battery for Children (KABC)	2 yr–12 yr	Sequential processing
		Simultaneous process
		Achievement
		Mental processing
		Composite score (IQ equivalent)
Motor skills		
Bruininks-Oseretsky Test of Motor Proficiency	4 yr–14 yr	Eight subtests
		Gross and fine motor balance
Perceptual and perceptuomotor		
Bender Visual-Motor Gestalt Test	4 yr–12 yr	
Draw-a-Person	All ages	
Benton Visual Retention Test (BVRT)	8 yr–adult	
Beery Test of Visual Motor Inspection (VMI)	2 yr–15 yr	
Speech and language		
Peabody Picture Vocabulary-Revised (PPVT-R)	2 yr–adult	Screening
Test of Early Language Development (TELD)	3 yr–8 yr	
Clinical Evaluation of Language Fundamentals-Revised (CELF-R)	7 yr–15 yr	
Personality		
Rorschach Inkblot Test	3 yr–adult	
Thematic Apperception Test (TAT)	6 yr–adult	
Children's Apperception Test (CAT)	2 yr–adult	
Roberts Apperception	Latency age	
Adaptive and social behavior		
Vineland Adaptive Behavior Scales-Survey Form	0–adult	Interview with parent or caregiver on communication, daily living, socialization, motor and maladaptive behaviors, composite score
Vineland Adaptive Behavior Scales-Expanded Form Classroom Edition	3 yr–12 yr	As above
School grade level skills		
Wide Range Achievement Test-Revised (WRAT-R)	5 yr–adult	Reading, spelling, math
Peabody Individual Achievement Test-Revised (PIAT-R)	5 yr–18 yr	Word identification
		Spelling
		Math
		Reading comprehension
		General information
Kaufman Test of Educational Achievement (K-TEA)	Grades 1–12	Reading decoding
		Spelling
		Reading comprehension
		Math application
		Math computation
Wechsler Individual Achievement Test (WIAT)	5 yr–19 yr	Oral and written expression
		Mathematic reasoning
		Spelling
		Reading comprehension
		Listening comprehension
		Numerical operations
Gray Oral Reading Test 3rd Edition (GORT-III)	Grades 1–12	Oral reading and comprehension

From Lewis M: Psychiatric examination of the infant, child, and adolescent. In: Kaplan HI, Sadock BJ (eds): *Comprehensive Textbook of Psychiatry.* Baltimore, Williams & Wilkins, 1989. With special thanks to Sara Sparrow, Ph.D., and Diane Goudreaux, Ph.D., for helpful suggestions and review of this table.

The interviewer should clarify the extent of the confidentiality: ''I will be meeting with your parents, but I will first discuss with you what I will or will not say to your parents.'' In some circumstances, such as a court-ordered evaluation, there is no confidentiality, and a report must be rendered to the court. The interviewer should inform the child of this fact.

It is probably best not to take notes during the interview. Note taking may inhibit the child, and it will inhibit the interviewer's ability to observe. The interviewer should avoid leading questions or any kind of demanding interrogation, because that, too, is unproductive and may inhibit the play and communication. Open-ended questions (e.g., ''What happened then?'') are better than leading questions and questions that require only a single-word answer.

The clinician interviewing a child or adolescent can also sometimes offer an interpretation of an obvious preconscious feeling or fantasy: It is often eye-opening, clarifying, and interesting for the child or adolescent and sets a model for any subsequent psychotherapy that might be recommended. For example, the child's attention can be directed to the content of his or her actions or verbalizations. Sometimes attention can be drawn to a coincidence that the child has perceived but has not, or professes not to have, registered; more frequently, one can draw attention to certain paradoxes. Thus, in the course of the child's play, the therapist may provide a verbal counterpart to the action being portrayed, an affect that might be present, or the conspicuous absence of certain persons, actions, or affects. (For an example of such an "attention" interpretation, see Chapter 73.)

This kind of interpretation during a diagnostic interview is different from the direct translation of a possible unconscious symbolic representation in the play that may occur in the course of psychodynamic psychotherapy. The play characteristic to which attention is drawn here is in bold relief, capable of being fully recognized and understood by the child.

Adolescents

Clinical interviews with adolescents require an even more explicit approach. The clinician can explain to the adolescent that his or her parents came to see the clinician and spoke of their concerns, but that the clinician would like to learn directly from the adolescent his or her views on what the parents have said, or on what bothers him or her. The clinician should show genuine interest and should not try to be deceptive or phony with the adolescent. He or she should not overidentify with the adolescent's dress or talk, nor should he or she talk down to or belittle the adolescent's views. If the clinician feels bored, rushed, uncertain, or uncomfortable, these feelings should be self-examined, preferably before interviewing the adolescent. The clinician should give the adolescent undivided and uninterrupted attention.

If the adolescent talks in terms of a third person ("I have a friend who . . ." or "Can a person catch herpes from kissing . . ." or "I read that . . ."), the clinician should answer matter-of-factly, in the same third-person way. The adolescent is not fooling the clinician, and the clinician is not fooling the adolescent; the adolescent is being allowed room to move and then will not feel so much on the spot.

Rejection, even outright hostility, on the first few visits with an adolescent is not uncommon. The clinician should be patient and not jump to conclusions. This attitude may turn out to be a test of how much the clinician can be trusted, a defense against anxiety, or a transference phenomenon. The clinician should recognize the anger by saying something such as, "I can see you're pretty angry at being here. What are you particularly angry about? Perhaps there is some way I can be of help to you."

Silences should not be allowed to continue for too long—this may just start a useless power game to see who can last longer. Similarly, it is important not to be rigid about the length of the interview. The 50-minute session is not a sacred rule; the clinician should feel free to vary the time according to the situation at hand. In some instances, an adolescent might feel more comfortable initially if he or she is invited to go for a walk with the clinician rather than asked to sit face-to-face in a confined space.

The clinician must be particularly clear with the adolescent about the extent of confidentiality. When appropriate, the adolescent should be informed that a report will be made to a third party, such as a judge. A sense of trust is infinitely preferable to a feeling of betrayal, even at the expense of some tidbit of knowledge.

In general, it is better not to give advice; however, the clinician should not obsessively deny any opinion or advice. An occasional well-judged opinion (if asked) on, for example, the color of a lipstick, or some well-chosen advice may help an adolescent feel understood and supported.

Eventually, the clinician must inquire about such sensitive areas as suicidal thoughts, hallucinations, drug use, and sexual relationships. This should be done in a matter-of-fact, straightforward manner (see below).

COUNTERTRANSFERENCE

During clinical interviews with children and adolescents, the clinician should be aware of important countertransference, as well as trans-ference, phenomena that may occur. For example, children who are aggressive often tend to mobilize strong defenses in the clinician, mentally retarded children are often overlooked or inadequately served, and deformed children may initially repel some clinicians. Other signs of countertransference include the following:

1. The clinician may fail to recognize the developmental level of the child or adolescent. Expectations will then not be commensurate with the child's or adolescent's maturational and developmental capacities.
2. The regressive pull experienced by the clinician interviewing the child or adolescent may give rise to the temptation to identify or act out with the child or adolescent.
3. A misreading by the clinician of the child's or adolescent's relationship with the clinician may occur, whereby the relationship is regarded as realistic when, in fact, it may be a transference from the child's or adolescent's feelings toward his or her parents. Clinicians are usually well aware of a child's or adolescent's aggressive feelings but may be less aware of their seductiveness toward an adult (parent).
4. When exposed to certain specific behaviors in the child or adolescent, old conflicts may be stirred up within the clinician, and anxiety in the clinician may result. For example, aggressive behavior or disguised masturbation may be upsetting to the clinician.
5. Sometimes clinicians transfer early feelings from their own childhood onto the parents of the child or adolescent. Clinicians may then overidentify with the child or adolescent in their own struggles with their parents. Similarly, residual feelings from the clinician's own childhood relations with brothers and sisters may be an important source of ambivalence toward the child or adolescent.
6. Sometimes the clinician simply cannot understand the meaning of certain behaviors in a child or adolescent. Anyone can occasionally find some item of behavior inexplicable. However, the persistent drawing of a blank in understanding a repeated item of behavior should lead to the suspicion of an interference by one's own conflicts—an emotional blind spot, so to speak.
7. A clinician may feel depressed or uneasy when working with a child or adolescent. Assuming that the clinician is not suffering from a true depression, the possibility exists that emotions from old conflicts have been aroused and are interfering with the clinician's functioning. A clinician may occasionally become aroused and experience great affection for a child or adolescent, which also may interfere with the treatment of the child or adolescent.
8. A clinician may wish to encourage acting out in children or adolescents. For example, a clinician may suggest to them that they must stand up for themselves and hit back. The wish and the suggestion should be carefully examined.
9. A clinician may feel the need for approval from the child or adolescent. Such a desire often represents a need of the clinician and may not be in the best interests of the child or adolescent
10. Conversely, repeated arguing with a child or adolescent may suggest that the clinician has not only become involved but has become enmeshed with that child or adolescent.
11. Recurring countertransference problems commonly arise in relation to specific characteristics of a child or adolescent. For example, a retarded child or adolescent may evoke guilt and defenses against such guilt in the clinician, or the clinician may act out omnipotent rescue fantasies. Passive, hostile children or adolescents may arouse anger in a clinician. Aggressive children and adolescents of either sex may threaten the clinician, leading either to vicarious and excessive exploitation of sexual issues or to denial and avoidance.

The Mental Status Examination

How and what the child plays, says, and does constitute the raw data for the mental status examination. To bring some order to the understanding of what may seem like random play, it is useful to have

Table 39.3. Categories of Psychopathology

Developmental delay
Organic brain dysfunction
Thought disorder
Anxiety
Mood disorder
Temperament and personality (character) problems
Somatoform disorders
Effects of general medical conditions
Mental retardation
Reaction to unfavorable environment

Adapted from Lewis M: Psychiatric examination of the infant, child, and adolescent. In: Kaplan HI, Sadock BJ (eds). *Comprehensive Textbook of Psychiatry.* Baltimore, Williams & Wilkins, 1989.

Table 39.4. Mental Status Examination Outline

1. Physical appearance
2. Separation
3. Manner of relating
4. Orientation to time, place, and person
5. Central nervous system functioning
6. Reading and writing
7. Speech and language
8. Intelligence
9. Memory
10. Quality of thinking and perception
11. Fantasies and inferred conflicts
12. Affects
13. Object relations
14. Drive behavior
15. Defense organization
16. Judgment and insight
17. Self-esteem
18. Adaptive capacities
19. Positive attributes

From Lewis M: Psychiatric examination of the infant, child, and adolescent. In: Kaplan HI, Sadock BJ (eds): *Comprehensive Textbook of Psychiatry.* Baltimore, Williams & Wilkins, 1989.

an outline of points one particularly wants to observe and why. When completed, such an outline constitutes the report of the child's mental status.

Another useful organizing principle is to keep in mind the major categories of psychopathology one wants to be sure to cover. A list of such categories is shown in Table 39.3.

Some of the data emerge spontaneously, some only after questioning. The categories in the mental status examination outline that follows are for convenience only; the behaviors listed usually do not occur in any special sequence and are not isolated items. The child or adolescent acts as a whole and in the context of a given environment, and his or her present behavior is always continuous with past behavior. It is not necessary to elicit the information required in the precise order presented here, and all of these categories need not be covered in equal detail or in one sitting. The presenting symptom and history might indicate important areas for close attention. The clinician should use clinical judgment to determine what to look for and how fast and in what detail to proceed. The clinician should also consider the age and developmental level of the infant, child, or adolescent when assessing a given response. An outline of the mental status examination is shown in Table 39.4. A useful questionnaire that can be used as a checklist in the emergency room is shown in Appendix A.

PHYSICAL APPEARANCE

1. *Small stature* is often associated with a more infantile self-image; the child who is short may be depressed because of his or her size. The cause of shortness must be determined.
2. *Head size* may indicate microcephaly and mental retardation, or hydrocephaly.
3. *Physical stigmata* may indicate the presence of a chromosomal disorder or prenatal toxicity (e.g., Down syndrome, Turner's syndrome, fragile X syndrome, or fetal alcohol syndrome).

4. *Bruising* may indicate child abuse.
5. *Nutritional state* may indicate an eating disorder, ranging from anorexia nervosa to obesity.
6. *Level of anxiety* may be manifested by hyperalertness, tics, nail biting, or hair pulling. The activity may have a driven quality: The child cannot sit still, has motor overflow as he or she moves from one thing to another, is easily distracted, and has a short attention span, a low frustration tolerance, and labile emotions. Some of these symptoms may be found in attention deficit hyperactivity disorder, hypomania, and anxiety disorders.
7. *Momentary lapses of attention* (staring, head nodding, eye blinking) may indicate epilepsy or hallucinatory phenomena. The clinician will subsequently inquire about such seizure phenomena as auras (nausea, vomiting, epigastric sensations), micropsia or macropsia (''Do things seem to get smaller or bigger as you look at them?''), and hallucinations.
8. *Gait* may indicate a particular disorder (e.g., walking on tiptoe may indicate childhood autism; a stiff gait may indicate cerebral palsy).
9. *Dress* gives some idea of the care the child receives and how much the child cares for himself or herself. Sexual orientation and conflicts may be expressed in attitudes, behavior, and dress.
10. *Mannerisms* may provide a clue to a disorder (e.g., smelling everything may be a sign of childhood autism; tics may be a sign of anxiety, Tourette's disorder, or obsessive-compulsive disorder; thumb sucking or repetitive play may be a sign of regression).

SEPARATION

Some caution on the part of the child is usually appropriate. Too much ease in separating from the parents may indicate superficial relationships associated with frequent separations and maternal deprivation. Difficulty in separating may indicate an ambivalent parent-child relationship.

MANNER OF RELATING

The child usually relates to the clinician cautiously at first. However, some children (e.g., deprived or abused children) are indiscriminately friendly and shallow. Children with autism appear to look through people.

ORIENTATION TO TIME, PLACE, AND PERSON

Orientation may be impaired by organic brain factors, low intelligence, anxiety, or a thought disorder.

CENTRAL NERVOUS SYSTEM FUNCTIONING

Child psychiatrists are often particularly interested in the presence of so-called soft neurological signs as a possible indication of organic dysfunction (see also Chapter 42). The term *soft signs* was coined by Paul Schilder and first used by Lauretta Bender in 1956. Soft neurological signs are those signs that do not in themselves signify a definitive, manifest, specific localized neurological lesion but that, taken together, may indicate organicity. Clinically they constitute a statistical association rather than a pathognomonic finding. They are often neurodevelopmental immaturities that have persisted. Clinical findings of soft neurological signs should be followed up with a complete neurological examination (Rutter et al., 1970).

There is no completely satisfactory classification of soft neurological signs. One classification is as follows:

1. *Group A signs:* These consist of developmental delays in relation to chronological and mental age in such functions as speech, motor coordination, right-left discrimination, and perception. They are reli-

ably present and may be associated with mental retardation, specific genetically determined maturational disorders, or brain damage.

2. *Group B signs:* These include singly occurring signs, such as nystagmus or strabismus, that may or may not have determinable neurological causes.

3. *Group C signs:* These include slight, unreliably present signs, such as asymmetry of tone or asymmetry of reflexes, that may be associated with various deprivational states or any of the conditions just mentioned.

Clinical phenomena suggesting soft neurological signs include the following:

Gross Motor Coordination

Awkwardness, clumsiness, motor overflow with extraneous movements, and contralateral minor movements of the opposite limb seen in posture, gait, balance, skill in climbing stairs, and ball throwing and catching.

Fine Motor Coordination (Perceptuomotor Capacities)

The child is asked to copy the designs seen in Figure 39.1.

Peformance on the Bender-Gestalt Test

Clinically, it is useful to ask the child to copy various Bender (1938) designs (Fig. 39.2).

Formal testing is required if the child has difficulty copying the designs. The difficulties may include trouble with angulatiom and juxtaposition, a tendency to verticalize a diagonal, and substitution of loops for dots. It is important to take into account the child's developmental level (Fig. 39.3).

For a further discussion and illustration of the Bender-Gestalt Test, see Chapter 41.

Laterality

Laterality, preference, and dominance are not identical. Laterality is a measurable, specialized, central function of a paired faculty, such as eyes, ears, hands, and feet. Preference is the subjective, self-reported experience of an individual, as opposed to laterality, which may be objectively measured. Preference may be related more to the state of the peripheral organ (e.g., an eye infection) than to anything else. Dominance is the term used for the concept of cerebral hemisphere specialization, such as in language and speech. Clinically, one may merely be testing preference, which in turn may depend more on the peripheral organ than on any central mechanism.

Handedness is usually consolidated by age 5, footedness by about age 7, eye lateralization by about age 7 or 8, and ear lateralization by about age 9 (Towen, 1980). Clinically, these may be tested as follows:

1. *Hand:* Observe while the child is writing.
2. *Foot:* Observe while the child is kicking a ball.
3. *Eye:* The child might be asked to look through a rolled-up piece of paper (a "telescope") or asked to look at an object through a small, fixed aperture with each eye in turn (the object in view persists with the dominant eye but not with the nondominant eye).

Right-Left Discrimination

The child should be asked to put the right hand to the left ear, the left hand to the right knee, and so forth. At the age of 5 years, children can identify right and left hands (i.e., if they have been taught). At age 6, the child has ipsilateral double orientation (i.e., left hand on left ear), and at age 7, contralateral orientation is achieved (i.e., left hand on right ear) (Silver and Hagan, 1982).

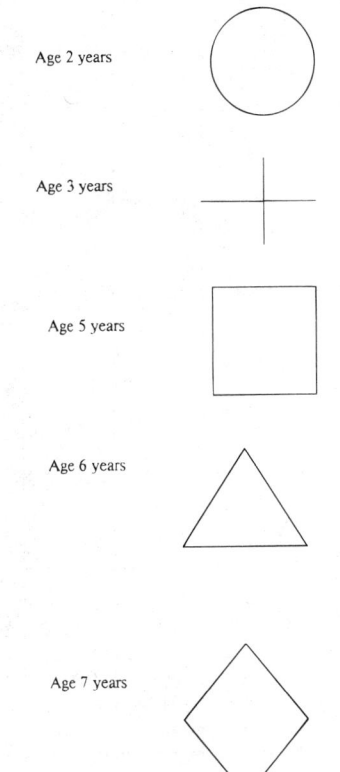

Figure 39.1. Simple designs by age.

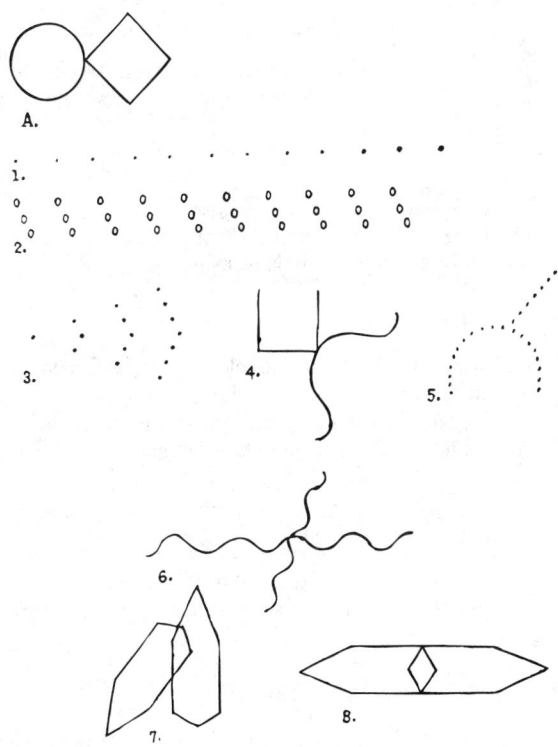

Figure 39.2. The Visual Motor Gestalt Test figures. (From Bender L: *A Visual Motor Gestalt Test and Its Clinical Use.* New York, American Orthopsychiatric Association, 1938.)

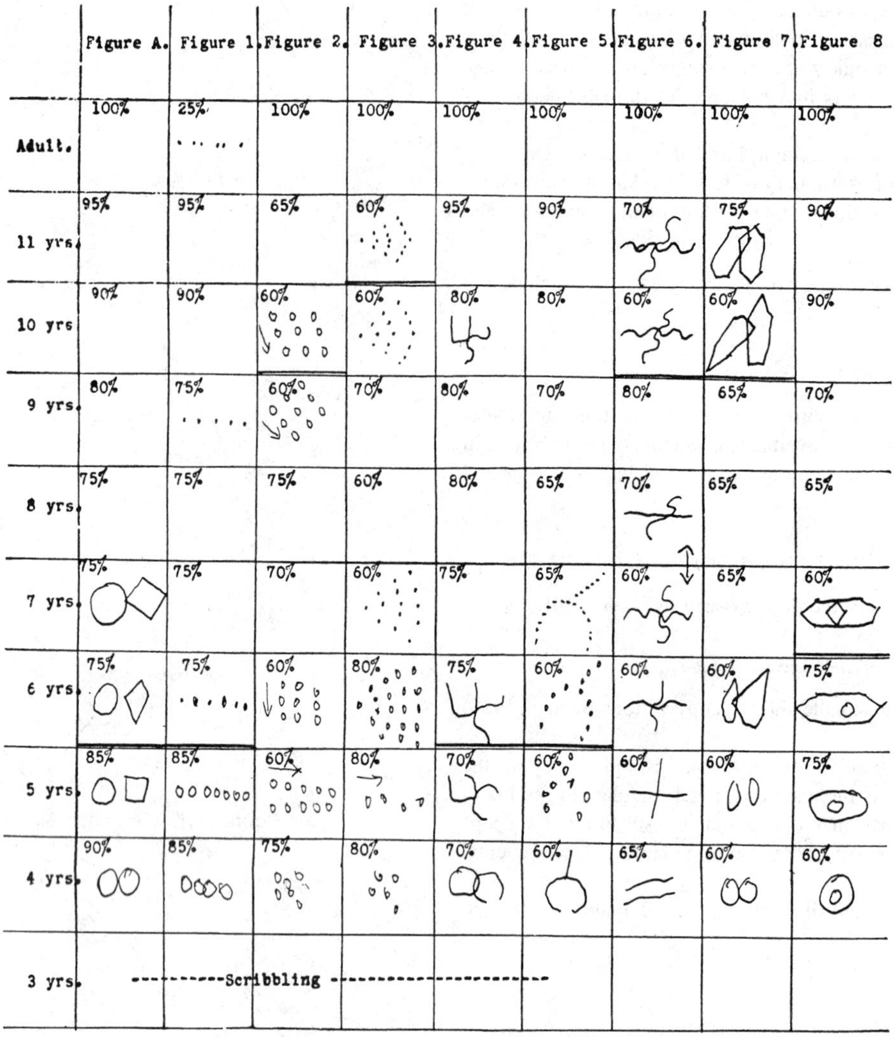

	Figure A.	Figure 1.	Figure 2.	Figure 3.	Figure 4.	Figure 5.	Figure 6.	Figure 7.	Figure 8
Adult.	100%	25%	100%	100%	100%	100%	100%	100%	100%
11 yrs.	95%	95%	65%	60%	95%	90%	70%	75%	90%
10 yrs	90%	90%	60%	60%	80%	80%	60%	60%	90%
9 yrs.	80%	75%	60%	70%	80%	70%	80%	65%	70%
8 yrs.	75%	75%	75%	60%	80%	65%	70%	65%	65%
7 yrs.	75%	75%	70%	60%	75%	65%	60%	65%	60%
6 yrs.	75%	75%	60%	80%	75%	60%	60%	60%	75%
5 yrs.	85%	85%	60%	80%	70%	60%	60%	60%	75%
4 yrs.	90%	85%	75%	80%	70%	60%	65%	60%	60%
3 yrs.	----------Scribbling -------------------								

Figure 39.3. Norms for the Visual Motor Gestalt Test. (From Bender L: *A Visual Motor Gestalt Test and Its Clinical Use.* New York, American Orthopsychiatric Association, 1938.)

Tremors

The child is asked to extend his or her arms and outstretch the hands. The clinician looks for choreiform movements.

Extension Test

The child stands, feet together, eyes closed, arms extended and dorsiflexed, for 20 seconds. In right-handed children from age 5 and up, the right hand is elevated, perhaps reflecting hemispheric dominance. Right-handed children with reading disability tend to elevate the left hand.

Wrist Rotation Movements

These movements include rapid pronation and supination of one hand against the palm of the other hand and can usually be performed well from age 5 up.

Rapid Finger-Tapping Movements

These movements involve patting the back of one hand with the index finger of the other hand and can usually be performed well from age 5 up.

Muscle Strength

The clinician should observe how firmly the child handles toys or crayons.

Eye Tracking

The child should be asked to look right or left at a moving object (e.g., a finger) with eyes only. The clinician should observe whether the child turns his or her entire body.

Heel-to-Toe Walking and Hopping on One Foot

These movements are usually achievable by the age of 7 years.

Reflex Asymmetry

This may be elicited in the major reflexes.

Short Attention Span

There are several possible causes, including a high level of distractibility, poor discrimination of foreground from background, fatigue, anxiety, or a too-difficult task.

Hyperactivity

Pathological hyperactivity frequently is disorganized activity. Such hyperactivity may be more noticeable in the classroom than in one-to-one situations.

Motor Overflow

This phenomenon may be observed when, say, the child is throwing a ball; flailing movements of the unused hand may occur. The phenomenon is more marked when the child is excited.

Visual Difficulties

These include strabismus, nystagmus, convergence difficulties, and delayed or absent light reflexes.

Reading, Writing, Language, and Speech Difficulties

These are discussed below.

Reading and Writing

The child may struggle to read or write and may exhibit poor spelling. Typical reading difficulties include reversals and inversions (e.g., d-b, q-p; was-saw, felt-left), confusions (e.g., f-l, m-n; of-off, me-we), omissions (e.g., *afaid* for *afraid*, *place* for *palace*, and substitutions (e.g., *a* for *the*, *house* for *home*). At the same time, many normal 1st-grade (6-year-old) children show reversals. These reversals usually disappear as reading skill matures. The brief screening test shown in Table 39.5 can be used to approximate the child's reading ability (Kanner and Eisenberg, 1957).

A much more accurate assessment of reading can be obtained through the administration of the Gray Oral Reading Tests-Revised (GORT-R). The GORT-R yields information about (a) oral reading speed and accuracy, (b) oral reading comprehension, (c) total oral reading ability, and (d) oral reading miscues. Grade-equivalent scores are not given because they are virtually useless in assigning students to classroom texts. Instead of grade equivalents, standard scores and percentile ranks are provided.

Children with reading difficulties often come from large families and may have symptoms of attention deficit hyperactivity disorder or of conduct disorder. Children with general reading backwardness usually have a broadly retarded reading level, consistent with their below-average IQ scores. These levels are often 2–2½ years below those of normal-IQ children. Children with specific reading retardation (sometimes called dyslexia or developmental reading disorder and often part of a multifaceted, complex learning disability) are presumed to have some as yet undetermined CNS dysfunction.

If the child shows positive findings in any of these clinical screening tests for reading, writing, and spelling, more systematic evaluation is required using standard tests. (See Chapter 48 for further details.)

Table 39.5. Screening Tests of Reading Ability

First grade	40 seconds; 4 errors A little boy had a cat; she ran away; she said, ``I want some milk.''
Second grade	25 seconds; 2 errors A man took me to see his large barn. There was a horse in the yard; its tail was black.
Third grade	30 seconds; 2 errors One of our favorite birds is the robin. He is a very useful bird. He eats many insects and worms. The robin is less afraid of people than most birds.

Reproduced by permission of *Pediatrics*, 20;155, Copyright 1957.

SPEECH AND LANGUAGE

Children who do not use words by age 18 months or phrases by age 2½–3 years, but who have a history of normal babbling, understand commands, and can use, as well as respond to, nonverbal cues and gestures are probably developing normally. However, delays beyond these ages or disturbances in these and other forms of communication are indicators for further evaluation. The general clinical signs of a language dysfunction include the following:

1. Reduced vocabulary, especially for abstract concepts such as feelings and for question words such as "when" and "where."
2. Overuse of concrete nouns and verbs.
3. Underuse or omission of abstract word classes (e.g., adjectives, adverbs, prepositions, articles, and conjunctions) often giving rise to telegraphic or unintelligible speech. (Some children may then avoid speaking or may have interpreters speak for them.)
4. A tendency to repeat their utterance, or simply nod their head, rather than clarify what they were trying to say.

Specific language difficulties may be due to receptive or expressive problems: Clinically, both commonly occur together.

Receptive language problems include sensory impairment (e.g., deafness, giving rise to delayed and unclear speech), neurological damage (e.g., cerebral mental retardation, and intrinsic developmental delay; Table 39.6).

Expressive language problems involve delays in the development of syntax and semantics and certain abnormal developments. Syntax, the

Table 39.6. Receptive Abilities

	Deafness	Mental Retardation	Infantile Autism	Elective Mutism
Sound discrimination	↓	Normal	Normal	Normal
Attentiveness	↓ Watches face	↓	↓↓	Normal
Understanding complex orders	↓	↓	↓↓	Normal

From Lewis M: *Clinical Aspects of Child Development* (2nd ed). Philadelphia, Lea & Febiger, 1982, p. 357.

Table 39.7. Language and Speech Tests

Analyses of Spontaneous Speech Samples
Developmental Sentence Scoring (Lee)
Assigning Structure Stages (Miller)
Linguistic Analysis and Remediation Procedure (Crystal)
Systematic Analysis of Language Transcripts (Miller and Chapman)

Language
Preschool Language Scale (Zimmerman)
Language Screening Test (Bankson)
Test for Auditory Comprehension of Language (Woolfolk)
Sequenced Inventory of Cummunicative Development (Hedrik, Prather, and Tobin)
Reynell Developmental Language Scales
Miller Yodor Language Comprehension Test
Clinical Evaluation of Language Functions (Seimel-Mintz, Wiig, and Merrill)
Illinois Test of Psycholinguistic Abilities (Kirk)
Detroit Tests of Learning Aptitude

Vocabulary Tests
Peabody Picture Vocabulary Test, Revised Edition (Dunn)
Expressive One Word Picture Vocabulary Test (Gardner)

Articulation Tests
Goldman-Fristoe Test of Articulation
The Assessment of Phonological Processes (Hodson)

Auditory Discrimination
Goldman-Fristoe-Woodcock Test
Wepman Auditory Discrimination Test

From Lewis M: Psychiatric examination of the infant, child, and adolescent. In: Kaplan HI, Sadock BJ (eds): *Comprehensive Textbook of Psychiatry*. Baltimore, Williams & Wilkins, 1989.

term used to categorize the rules for combining words to form sentences, may be delayed. The normal child can make one-word utterances at age 18 months, two- to three-word phrases at age 30 months, and four-word sentences at age 40 months. Semantics, the term used to categorize the meaning of language, may similarly be delayed. Delays in syntax and semantic development may first be encountered in a history of limited or poor babbling. The child may subsequently use gestures instead of verbal language to communicate.

Abnormalities of expressive language include echolalia and delayed echolalia, the persistent use of neologisms, and misuse of pronouns and gender. Such abnormalities are commonly seen in childhood autism and may be associated with a lack of nonverbal communication behavior, including lack of direct eye gaze and lack of facial expression. Some useful language tests are shown in Table 39.7.

Common speech difficulties consist of delays, omissions, or distortions in the normal acquisition of particular sounds, e.g., *wabbit* instead of *rabbit*. Most uncomplicated, common speech acquisition difficulties of this kind resolve by the age of 7 or 8 years. Stuttering (consisting of repetitions, hesitations, or blocks in the production of a speech sound) often begins about the age of 3 years, follows a fluctuating course, and usually ends at adolescence. In some cases (less than 20%) it may persist into adulthood. There is often a family history of stuttering, suggesting a genetic component.

Other dysfunctional speech patterns may reflect the level of integration at which the CNS is affected. Thus aphonia may occur when the neuromuscular level is involved, including such apparatuses as the lips, tongue, palate, nasopharynx, larynx, and medulla oblongata: dysarthria may occur when the cortico-bulbar level is involved; scanning, explosive, and monotone speech may occur when the cerebellar level is affected; and agnosia (failure to understand symbols) and aphasia (failure to understand the spoken word or to speak) may occur when the cerebral level is affected.

Temporary speech problems may occur during regressive episodes (infantile speech patterns may reappear), during drug intoxication (dysarthria and slurred speech may occur), during anxiety (a high-pitched, tight voice may inhibit speech), and when the child refuses to talk (so-called selective mutism).

When one or more of the above clinical findings are present, a full diagnostic evaluation is indicated. This evaluation may include a complete physical examination, neurological examination, hearing assessment, reading assessment, comprehensive language and speech tests, and an educational test battery (see Chapter 47).

INTELLIGENCE

An approximate idea of the child's intelligence may be assessed by an evaluation of the following:

1. General vocabulary, responsiveness, and level of comprehension and curiosity.
2. Ability to identify the parts of the body. For example, at age 5 years, the normal child may be able to identify the jaw, temples, forearms, and shins.
3. Drawing ability; the child is asked to draw a person (see below).
4. Ability to subtract serial 7s or serial 3s.
5. Results on the Wechsler Intelligence Scale for Children-Revised (WISC-R).

MEMORY

At age 8 years, the normal child can count five digits forward and two or three digits backward; at age 10, the child can count six digits forward and four digits backward. Very poor performance on the digit span test may indicate brain damage (particularly left-hemisphere damage) or mental retardation. Minor difficulties may simply reflect anxiety. The child should also be able to repeat three items 5 minutes after they have been presented.

QUALITY OF THINKING AND PERCEPTION

The process of thinking has three major clinical dimensions: actual thought content, speed of thinking, and ease of flow. A variation in any of these dimensions may be of such a degree and duration as to constitute a thought disorder.

Disordered thought content may take the form of neologisms and idiosyncratic logic, including developmentally inappropriate transductive reasoning (things that are related in time or space are believed to be related causally), difficulty in discerning differences and similarities, difficulty in distinguishing the relevant from the irrelevant, and excessive concreteness. Disordered speed of thinking may take the form of retardation or a push of thinking and speaking. Disorder of flow may take the form of blocking, muteness, or excessive repetition of words and sentences. A child may experience any of these manifestations subjectively as being alien, out of his or her control, and sometimes frightening. There may be an associated disorder of mood (depression, elation, inappropriateness, or paranoid rage), of behavior (disorganized, regressive, aggressive, withdrawn, or bizarre), or of perception (delusions or hallucinations).

The causes of a thought disorder may be classified clinically as follows:

1. Genetic (e.g., inborn errors of metabolism, such as Hartnup disease, Kufs' disease, and schizophrenia)
2. Traumatic (e.g., postconcussion syndrome)
3. Infective (e.g., viral encephalitis and brain abscesses)
4. Neoplastic (e.g., brain tumor)
5. Toxic (e.g., amphetamines, corticosteroids, bromism)
6. Deficiencies (e.g., pellagra)
7. Endocrine (e.g., thyrotoxicosis)
8. Metabolic (e.g., electrolyte disturbance and delirium)
9. Multiple (e.g., pervasive developmental disorder, schizophrenia)
10. Psychological (e.g., acute and massive psychological stress reaction)

The symptoms that constitute a thought disorder should lead to a systematic review of the above possible causes. Obviously, some causes will easily be ruled out, and others will immediately appear to be likely possibilities. Once the field has been narrowed in this way, a more detailed study can lead to a further narrowing. For example, the associated presence of hallucinations may give a cross-differential diagnosis of specific syndromes.

Hallucinations

The clinician should ask about auditory and visual hallucinations as though he or she were taking a medical history of the eyes and ears. The clinician might ask, "Do you have any trouble with your ears?" "Do your ears ever hurt you?" "Do your ears ever play tricks on you?" "Do you ever think you hear something, but nothing is there?" A similar sequence can be designed for inquiring about visual hallucinations.

Hallucinations in childhood are frequently pathological, although the literature is confusing. The following major clinical categories should be considered.

Drug Intoxication. Many drugs are potentially hallucinogenic; they include marijuana, mescaline, psilocybin, lysergic acid diethylamide (LSD), amphetamines, barbiturates, bromides, monoamine oxidase inhibitors (MAOIs), antihistamines, and atropine-like drugs. At the same time, children and adolescents who take drugs may have an antecedent psychiatric disturbance. Sometimes, the timing and form of the hallucinations suggest the possibility of drug ingestion. Other symptoms of drug ingestion may be present, including drowsiness, paranoid behavior, confusion, restlessness, excitement, violence, dilated pupils, ataxia, dysmetria, tremor, dysarthria, dyskinesia, akathisia, and hypotensive signs. The clinician must ask about drug ingestion. Urine and blood samples must be tested when drug ingestion is suspected.

Seizure Disorder. Hallucinations, particularly hypnagogic hallucinations, may occur in narcolepsy and other seizure disorders. Hallucinations may be the first symptom of degeneration following previous encephalitic illness. A neurological examination and an EEG are required.

Metabolic Disorders. The metabolic disorders that may give rise to hallucinations include adrenal cortical hypofunction, thyroid and parathyroid disease, hepatolenticular degeneration, porphyria, beriberi, and hypomagnesemia (secondary to prolonged parenteral fluid replacement therapy, diuretic therapy, excess vitamin D intake, or diabetic acidoses). Signs of the primary metabolic disorder are usually present.

Infection. Encephalitis, meningitis, and acute febrile illnesses (especially in young children) may give rise to hallucinations.

Immaturity, Stress, and Anxiety. Acute grief reactions following the death of a parent may give rise to hallucinations. Usually, these hallucinations are auditory and consist of admonitions and prohibitions attributed to the dead parent. Hallucinations following severe anxiety may occur when the anxiety overwhelms the child. Young children who are under severe stress and resort to the defense mechanisms of repression, projection, and displacement may also have hallucinations. The hallucinations appear to be part of a regressive phenomenon, in which the distinction between fantasy and reality is temporarily lost. Often, the stress is sexual, and the child may have been exposed to too much stimulation. The content of the hallucination may suggest the underlying psychological conflict.

CASE ILLUSTRATION

A 4-year-old boy was taken to the emergency room at 4:00 AM in an acutely agitated state. For the previous 4 hours he had said there were spiders under his pajamas and there were shadows inside him. While in the waiting room, he screamed as his aunt attempted to keep a coat over his completely nude body. He refused to wear any clothes at all, and he remained unashamedly naked. He repeatedly attempted to brush off the hallucinated spiders.

On further study, it was found that the boy and his mother slept in the same bed. There was a serious marital difficulty, which included a severe sexual problem and violent behavior between the parents, who slept apart. Later, it was learned that the boy's mother often allowed him to sit on her lap. He would feel her pelvis and ask her why she did not have the same feeling his father had. He would also be allowed to fondle his mother's breasts, and his mother noticed that he got an erection at the slightest touch—her touch. It became clear that this boy's fears about wearing clothes were his way of reassuring himself and allaying his anxiety by keeping his genitals always in sight. For example, in a progressive play sequence the boy first exhibited his fear of spiders crawling on his skin, then he touched his thigh, then his penis, and finally he wanted to look inside his trousers in search of his penis.

In older children, external conflicts rarely, if ever, give rise to hallucinations. However, if the stress is massive and overwhelms the child, it can lead to profound regression. The circumstances in which this occurs include severe and sudden illness.

CASE ILLUSTRATIONS

A previously healthy 15-year-old girl suddenly developed hemolytic uremic syndrome, with acute renal shutdown that necessitated immediate hemodialysis. While undergoing hemodialysis, the girl began to hallucinate.

An active child who was suddenly immobilized for treatment of a fractured limb hallucinated during a moment of acute anxiety.

In some instances, severe cultural deprivation, together with a disturbed parent-child relationship, may result in hallucinations. The hallucinations in this situation are often localized, orderly, and related to reality, and may consist of forbidding voices and overt wish fulfillments.

Often, such hallucinations are consistent with the superstitions of the parents. The child may appear to be well organized in other ways. However, often there is evidence of an associated personality disturbance in the child and psychosis in the parent, suggesting at least the possibility of a genetic or organic component, as well as powerful sociocultural influences. For example, in some fundamentalist sects, a high value is placed on being possessed by the Spirit. Hysterically inclined children and youths may lend themselves to this experience and may hear voices.

Mood Disorders. Here the hallucinations are consistent with the depression (e.g., a voice says that the child is bad and should commit suicide).

Schizophrenia. When hallucinations are more fragmented, incoherent, and bizarre in content, there is a greater likelihood that schizophrenia is present (Bender, 1954). Bodily complaints and paranoid delusions may be associated with the psychosis. The child is often frightened and secretive about the hallucinations, which are often alien and out of the child's control. Other signs of a thought disorder, including disordered, illogical thought processes and inappropriate affect, are usually present. A history of psychiatric disturbance in the family and maternal deprivation during infancy may be obtained. Sometimes the child shows delinquent behavior. Psychological tests, particularly projective tests, are indicated.

The phenomenon of imaginary companions is usually easily distinguished from hallucinations by the following features:

1. The child is normal in all other respects and shows no signs of a thought disorder.
2. The imaginary companion can be imagined at will.
3. The companion is just that—a friendly person who poses no threat to the child and is often a comfort to the child.
4. The imaginary companion, unlike hallucinations, is not ego-alien, and the child can freely talk about the "friend."
5. The imaginary companion is often highly elaborate and can be described in detail.
6. The imaginary companion appears, functions, and disappears at the wish of the child.

The natural history of the imaginary companion and its possible relationship to multiple personality disorder (see Chapter 65) requires further study.

FANTASIES, FEELINGS, AND INFERRED CONFLICTS

The clinician might evaluate the following:

1. The child's spontaneous play.
2. The child's response when asked, "Do you have good dreams or bad dreams? Tell me one of your dreams."
3. The child's response to the question, "If you could have three wishes, what would you wish for?" (Winkley, 1982).
4. The child's productions in the game of squiggles (Berger, 1980; Winnicott, 1971). The squiggles game is a way of getting into contact with the child. The clinician briefly explains to the child that he or she will make a squiggle with a pencil or crayon on a sheet of paper and the child will then turn it into something, and then it will be the child's turn to make a squiggle and the clinician's turn to make it into something. As they take turns, a theme may emerge in the sequence of squiggles and constructions. The clinician uses the drawings, the child's approach to the game, and what the child says about the squiggles to help both of them gain some insight into the child's mind.
5. The child's drawings of a person or whatever he or she wants to draw.

The child's drawings, particularly the child's drawings of a person, are useful in assessing the child's intelligence, (Harris, 1963) fantasies, and feelings (Burns, 1982; DiLeo, 1973; Klepsch and Logie, 1982).

Since human beings are the objects of most intense interest to the child, the child's developing conceptual abilities may be readily seen in his or her drawings of a person. Thus, a general course or line of progression can be seen in children's drawings at different ages. As long ago as 1921, Burt was able to discern the following sequence:

1. Scribbling (2 to 3 years): The circular motor activity itself is pleasurable to the child as the child increasingly adapts his or her hand to the crayon and also tries to imitate the actions of others.
2. Single lines (4 years): The child soon draws a single line and tends to juxtapose parts.
3. Symbolic representation (5 to 6 years): The child can now draw a person consisting mostly of circles and ellipses representing head and body, "stick" lines representing arms and legs (and an indeterminate number of digits), and some curvilinear lines to represent eyes, mouth, and ears (hair arrangement usually distinguishes the sexes) (Fig. 39.4).

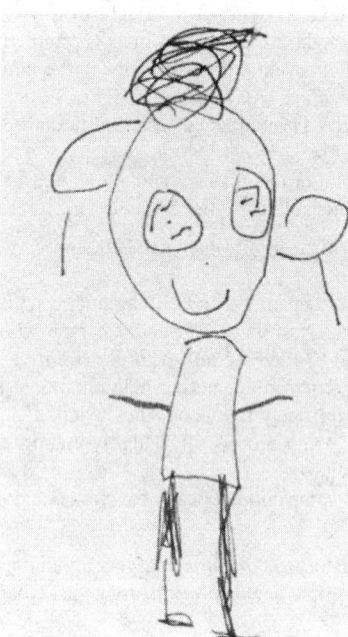

Figure 39.4. Drawing of a person by child aged 4 years.

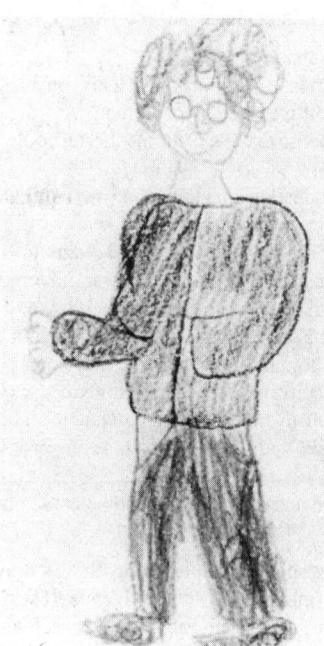

Figure 39.5. Drawing of a person by child aged 8 years.

4. Descriptive drawing (7 to 10 years): The child now pays more attention to detail, and clothing details appear (Fig. 39.5).
5. Visual realism (11 years onward): The child can draw in profile and attempts a realistic visual representation. The child may subsequently show a tendency to inhibition, with a preference for geometric designs, although later a true artistic talent may emerge (Fig. 39.5).

A more precise assessment and measurement of the child's drawings can be obtained through formal psychological testing (see Chapter 41).

The child's drawings may also reveal clinically useful information about his or her feelings and fantasies. However, the scientific reliability and validity of studies of this aspect of children's drawings are modest at best.

Clinically, it is often useful to invite a child to draw a person and then to make up a story about the drawing ("Pretend the boy (girl) has just finished doing something, is doing something now, and is going to do something soon").

In observing the child while he or she is drawing, one might notice the following:

1. *Motivation and self-esteem:* The child may be eager to draw or may be self-effacing ("I'm no good at drawing" or "I can't draw very well").
2. *Motor skill and activity:* Observe how the child holds the crayon and how careful or slapdash is the child's approach. Does the child erase frequently, perseverate, or confine the drawing to a small corner of the paper? Neurological impairment may reveal itself in the execution of the drawing.
3. *Sex of the figure drawn:* In general, children prefer to draw their own sex first and, initially, will identify whether it is a boy or girl "by the hair."
4. *Special features of the child's drawing:*
   a. *Heavy pressure* may suggest tension, assertiveness, aggression, or organicity; light pressure may suggest indecisiveness, timidity, depression, and low self-esteem.
   b. Large drawings may suggest aggressiveness, or perhaps compensatory expansiveness to cover feelings of inadequacy; small drawings may suggest withdrawal, insecurity, or depression.
   c. Drawings placed low or on the edge may suggest insecurity or dependency.
   d. Very enlarged drawings of the head may suggest preoccupation with symptoms related to the head, or possibly concern about intelligence.
   e. Omission of facial features may suggest evasiveness; large eyes may suggest anxiety or suspiciousness; small eyes may suggest guilt or a self-absorbed tendency. Sometimes the size of a part (e.g., ear, nose, or mouth) may be related to a possible handicap. Bared teeth may suggest aggression.

Numerous other inferences have been suggested (DiLeo, 1973; Hammer, 1980; Handler, 1985; Koppitz, 1968; Machover, 1949), but, again, it must be noted that the scientific validity of these inferences is often low.

AFFECTS

The clinician should observe affects, such as anxiety, depression, apathy, guilt, and anger.

Depression is a particularly important affect that must not be overlooked. Depression affect is often accompanied by low self-esteem (e.g., "I can't do that," "I'm no good at drawing") as well as fatigue, loss of interest and pleasure, guilt, difficulty in concentrating, and disturbances in sleep, appetite, and motor activity. These symptoms constitute a diagnosis of major depression.

The child may be asked: "Do you ever feel sad, upset, or bad?" "Do you ever feel unloved or uncared for?" "Do you feel you're not very good?" "Do you cry a lot?" "Do you have trouble making or keeping friends?" "Do you prefer to keep to yourself?" "Do you blame yourself a lot?"

Suicidal risk may be part of a major depressive disorder and should be specifically investigated. When there is overt suicidal ideation or suicidal behavior, one assesses the events and circumstances leading up to the episode, whether the act was planned or impulsive, lethal in the child's mind, an act of desperation or depression, and whether the child's reaction to his or her suicide attempt was one of continuing desperation/depression or abhorrence and fright. One might, for example, ask the following questions:

1. *Present episode*:
   Tell me what happened. And what happened next?
2. *Motivation*:
   Were you feeling sad, or depressed and frustrated?
   Were you angry with someone?
   Had someone important to you left you?
   Did you hope something would change afterward?
   Did you hear voices telling you to hurt yourself?
3. *Previous suicidal thoughts or behavior*:
   Have you ever thought of hurting yourself in the past?
   Have you ever done anything to hurt yourself?
   Have you ever tried to kill yourself? What did you do?
   What was the reason then?
   What happened afterward?
   Did anything change for you then, or did things just stay the same?
4. *Related experiences*:
   Do you know of anyone else, either in the past or more recently, who has thought about or tried to kill himself or herself?

What did you think or feel when you heard about it?
Did it make you upset?
5. *Concepts*:
   When you (e.g., took the pills), did you think you would die?
   Did you hope someone would find you?
6. *Symptoms of depression*:
   How is your appetite?
   Do you have any trouble going to sleep or sleeping through the night?
   Is it hard for you to concentrate on school work?
   Do you feel tired a lot of the time?
   Do you feel no one loves you or cares for you?
   Do you want to cry a lot?
7. *Common stresses*:
   Has anyone close to you left you, or died?
   How are things between your parents?
   Is anyone in the family sad or depressed?
   How are things going in school?
   Do you worry that your parents will be disappointed with you?

A more detailed set of questions to ask in the evaluation of suicidal risk in children (see Table 39.8) has been provided by Pfeffer (1986).

Essentially, the risk is high when the intent is clear, the act is planned with a highly lethal method, and the adolescent is lonely and alone, under stress, has poor family supports, shows marked psychopathology, manifests hopelessness about any change for the better in the future, and has poor judgment and poor impulse control. (For further discussion of the causes and management of attempted suicide, see Chapter 61).

Table 39.8. Questions to Ask in the Evaluation of Suicidal Risk in Children

1. *Suicidal fantasies or actions*:
   Have you ever thought of hurting yourself?.
   Have you ever threatened or attempted to hurt yourself?
   Have you ever wished or tried to kill yourself?
   Have you ever wanted or threatened to commit suicide?
2. *Concepts of what would happen*:
   What did you think would happen if you tried to hurt or kill yourself?
   What did you want to have happen?
   Did you think you would die?
   Did you think you would have severe injuries?
3. *Circumstances at the time of the child's suicidal behavior*:
   What was happening at the time you thought about killing yourself or tried to kill yourself?
   What was happening before you thought about killing yourself?
   Was anyone else with you or near you when you thought about suicide or tried to kill yourself?
4. *Previous experiences with suicidal behavior*:
   Have you ever thought about killing yourself or tried to kill yourself before?
   Do you know of anyone who either thought about, attempted, or committed suicide?
   How did this person carry out his suicidal ideas or action?
   When did this occur?
   Why do you think that this person wanted to kill himself?
   What was happening at the time this person thought about suicide or tried to kill himself?
5. *Motivations for suicidal behaviors*:
   Why do you want to kill yourself?
   Why did you try to kill yourself?
   Did you want to frighten someone?
   Did you want to get even with someone?
   Did you wish someone would rescue you before you tried to hurt yourself?
   Did you feel rejected by someone?
   Were you feeling hopeless?
   Did you hear voices telling you to kill yourself?
   Did you have very frightening thoughts?
   What else was a reason for your wish to kill yourself?
6. *Experiences and concepts of death*:
   What happens when people die?

Can they come back again?
Do they go to a better place?
Do they go to a pleasant place?
Do you often think about people dying?
Do you often think about your own death?
Do you often dream about people or yourself dying?
Do you know anyone who has died?
What was the cause of this person's death?
When did this person die?
When do you think you will die?
What will happen when you die?
7. *Depression and other affects*:
   Do you ever feel sad, upset, angry, bad?
   Do you ever feel that no one cares about you?
   Do you ever feel that you are not a worthwhile person?
   Do you cry a lot?
   Do you get angry often?
   Do you often fight with other people?
   Do you have difficulty sleeping, eating, concentrating on school work?
   Do you have trouble getting along with friends?
   Do you prefer to stay by yourself?
   Do you often feel tired?
   Do you blame yourself for things that happen?
   Do they often feel guilty?
8. *Family and environmental situations*:
   Do you have difficulty in school?
   Do you worry about doing well in school?
   Do you worry that your parents will punish you for doing poorly in school?
   Do you get teased by other children?
   Have you started a new school?
   Did you move to a new home?
   Did anyone leave home?
   Did anyone die?
   Was anyone sick in your family?
   Have you been separated from your parents?
   Are your parents separated or divorced?
   Do you think that your parents treat you harshly?
   Do your parents fight a lot?
   Does anyone get hurt?
   Is anyone in your family sad, depressed, very upset? Who?
   Did anyone in your family talk about suicide or try to kill himself?

From Pfeffer CR: *The Suicidal Child*. New York: Guilford Press, 1986.

RELATIONSHIPS

The clinician may explore the following areas:

1. *With the family:* The clinician might ask the child who is in the family and which family members the child gets along with best and worst.
2. *With peers:* The clinician might ask the child who his or her friends are and whom he or she likes the most and the least.
3. *With teachers:* The clinician might ask the child which teachers he or she likes and dislikes.

DRIVE BEHAVIOR

Basic drive behavior is observed:

1. *Sexual:* Is the child seductive? Autoerotic?
2. *Aggressive:* Is the child provocative, destructive, or violent?

DEFENSE ORGANIZATION

The defense organization is studied. Is the child phobic? (Does he or she show such phobic symptoms as apparent fear of elevators or touch inhibitions?) Is the child obsessive or compulsive? (Are the drawings too neat? Does the child repeatedly erase?) Does the child show denial (saying that there are no problems?)

POSITIVE ATTRIBUTES

The following description of a child who has many positive attributes might help the clinician decide what positive attributes are possessed by the child being examined: The child is attractive looking, well groomed, and has a pleasant smile. He is of normal height and weight and has normal vision and hearing. He separates easily and comes readily to the playroom. He is a likable person and seems to be in a happy mood. He relates well to others and appears to have formed a number of suitable and long-lasting friendships. He is of normal intelligence. He plays well (i.e., the play is imaginative, has themes, is sustained, and is age appropriate). He draws well and is good at ball play. His coordination is good. His emotional responses are appropriate, and he does not have extreme mood swings. The child is in touch with his feelings and fantasies, has a good command of language, and can verbalize his thoughts and feelings. He does not shirk problems and feels good about himself. He does well at school, both academically and socially.

The Formulation

The complete psychiatric assessment of the child or adolescent should enable the clinician to formulate a useful description of how and why the particular child or adolescent presents in the way he or she does (Shapiro, 1989). Thus the formulation is, in essence, an integrated summary of the unique way in which organic factors, environmental stresses, and inner conflicts have interacted over time for a particular child or adolescent. Through the formulation one obtains a full, multidimensional picture of the child or adolescent that goes far beyond the diagnostic label, and this complete and unique picture of the child or adolescent provides a sound basis for devising an appropriate comprehensive treatment plan.

Concluding the Evaluation

In the course of the evaluation of the child, the clinician establishes a trusting relationship with the child and the parents. Consequently, the clinician considers the feelings of the child and the parents during the conclusion phase of the evaluation. For example, the clinician informs the child ahead of time as to when the last session will take place. Then, during the final interview, he or she ensures that the child knows what will take place next by asking the child or adolescent: "Are there any

things you would particularly like me to tell your parents?" "Are there any things you don't want me to say to your parents?" "This is what I plan to say to your parents. How does that sound to you?" "Do you have any questions?" Sometimes a child will express feelings about the ending. These feelings should be recognized, acknowledged, and dealt with sympathetically and realistically.

At the final review meeting with the parents, the clinician may start by asking how the child reacted to coming for his or her interviews. Sometimes information comes to light that may help the clinician in assessing the child's capacity to form a relationship and engage in psychotherapy. The clinician can then give the parents an account of the child's strengths. Every child has some strengths (e.g., the child may be attractive, intelligent, delightful to be with, well coordinated, able to think clearly), and it is important that the clinician tell the parents about such qualities.

Next, the clinician talks with the parents about his or her assessment of the child's difficulties. The assessment should be discussed in clear language and documented with vignettes from the clinical interviews or from any of the special tests that help to illustrate and clarify the nature of the difficulty. If psychological tests have been performed, the psychologist may wish to participate in the review meeting with the parents.

The parents should be given every opportunity to ask questions. Their reactions should be recognized and understood; the parents need the support of the clinician. They need an explanation of the possible causes of their child's condition. They should also be reassured about all the good things they have done to help the child. Finally, treatment options and recommendations should be discussed with the parents. The parents should not be rushed, and they should be invited to telephone or return if they so wish.

Documentation of the basis for the findings is particularly important when a written report has to be submitted—for example, to a court for evidence in a custody dispute (Lewis, 1974). When appropriate, and with the parents' permission, the clinician should also send a report to the referring person. The limits of confidentiality, again, must be clearly understood by the child, the parents, and the clinician, and the clinician must exercise special care to safeguard this confidentiality.

Finally, it is important to remember that the psychiatric evaluation of the child and the child's family goes beyond the diagnosis. Each child and each family member has his or her own private experience of life. In a good psychiatric evaluation, the clinician is privileged to enter that private experience momentarily and to empathize with that person's feelings, hopes, and fears. One tries to capture this aspect of a person's life in the descriptive diagnostic formulation that follows the formal diagnosis.

STRUCTURED INTERVIEWS, QUESTIONNAIRES, AND RATING SCALES

Structured psychiatric interviews, questionnaires, and rating scales for children and parents have been devised to improve the reliability and validity of information and observations regarding psychiatric diagnosis. Currently, the greatest use for these instruments is in research. However, many of these instruments have been used successfully for screening purposes and as diagnostic aids in the clinical situation. In turn, their use has sharpened clinical inquiry in such areas as the assessment of mood disorders, cognitive functions, attention, and thinking processes.

Structured interviews have the advantage of focusing on important areas and therefore do not leave to chance observations of important items that may not come to light in an unstructured interview. Structured interviews provide comparable data and are usually comprehensive with respect to a specific diagnosis. One further advantage is the relatively short training period required in order to be able to administer a structured interview.

Structured interviews are more or less rigid, however, and do not admit much in the way of clinical judgment. Sometimes the conclusions do not correspond to the complexity of the clinical diagnosis. In many instances, a support system is required (e.g., computer technology and staff). Structured interviews for preschool children are generally unreliable. Questionnaires that have long lists of questions—for example, the Diagnostic Interview for Children and Adolescents (DICA), which has 207 items—may exhaust a child. The clustering of items around symptoms may also be a limiting factor as far as rapport is concerned, because the focus on negative behavior may be too exclusive for too long. The lack of normative data in some instances is a handicap. Few structured interviews focus specifically on father-child interactions.

On balance, structured psychiatric interviews for children and adolescents supply a useful safety floor and a reliable screening mechanism. In general, children report better about feelings, whereas parents report better about behavior.

The number of schedules and scales now available is formidable and increasing steadily. See Chapter 40 and the relevant chapters on syndromes for a more detailed description and indications for the use of structured interviews.

STANDARDIZED TESTS

Standardized tests, such as developmental, psychological, neurological, educational, linguistic, and biological studies, are described in the relevant chapters in Sections V, Diagnostic Assessment, and VI, Syndromes.

Acknowledgments. *Copyright © 1994 by Melvin Lewis. Earlier versions of this chapter were published in Kaplan HI, Sadock BJ (eds): Comprehensive Textbook of Psychiatry (5th ed). Baltimore, Williams & Wilkins, 1989, 1716–1727; and in Lewis M, Volkmar F: Clinical Aspects of Child and Adolescent Development (3rd ed). Philadelphia, Lea & Febiger, 1990, pp. 295–321.*

References

Bender L: *A Visual Motor Gestalt and Its Clinical Use*. New York, American Orthopsychiatry Association, 1938.

Bender L: *A Dynamic Psychopathology of Childhood*. Springfield, IL, Charles C Thomas, 1954, pp. 16–79.

Berger LR: Winnicott squiggle game. *Pediatrics* 66:921, 1980.

Burns RC: *Self-Growth in Families. Kinetic Family Drawings (K-F-D). Research and Applications*. New York, Brunner/Mazel, 1982.

Burt C: *Mental and Scholastic Tests*. London, PS King & Son, 1921.

Cox A, Rutter M, Holbrook D: Psychiatric interviewing techniques. V: Experimental study: Eliciting factual information. *Br J Psychiatry* 139:29, 1981.

DiLeo JH: *Children's Drawings as Diagnostic Aids*. New York, Brunner/Mazel, 1973.

Hammer EF: *The Clinical Application of Projective Drawings*. Springfield, IL, Charles C Thomas, 1980.

Handler L: The clinical use of the Draw-a-Person Test (DAP). In: Newmark CS (ed): *Major Psychological Assessment Instruments*. Boston, Allyn & Bacon, 1985, pp. 165–216.

Harris DB: *Children's Drawings as Measures of Intellectual Maturity*. New York, Harcourt, Brace & World, 1963.

Kanner L, Eisenberg L: Childhood problems in relation to the family. *Pediatrics* 20:155, 1957.

Klepsch M, Logie L: *Children Draw and Tell*. New York, Brunner/Mazel, 1982.

Koppitz E: *Psychological Evaluation of Children's Human Figure Drawings*. New York, Grune & Stratton, 1968.

Lewis M: The latency child in a custody conflict. *J Am Acad Child Psychiatry* 13:635, 1974.

Machover K: *Personality Projection in the Drawing of the Human Figure*. Springfield, IL, Charles C Thomas, 1949.

Pfeffer C: *The Suicidal Child*. New York, Guilford Press, 1986.

Rutter M, Graham P, Yule W: *A Neurological Examination: Description*. New York, Heinemann, 1970, pp. 27–39.

Shapiro T: The psychodynamic formulation in child and adolescent psychiatry. *J Am Acad Child Adolesc Psychiatry* 28:675–680, 1989.

Silver AA, Hagan RA: A unifying concept for the neuropsychological organization of children with reading disability. *J Dev Behav Pediatr* 3:127, 1982.

Towen BCL: Laterality. In: Rutter M (ed): *Scientific Foundations of Developmental Psychiatry*. London, Heinemann, 1980, pp. 154–164.

Winkley L: The implication of children's wishes: Research note. *J Child Psychol Psychiatry* 23:477, 1982.

Winnicott DW: *Therapeutic Consultations in Child Psychiatry*. New York, Basic Books, 1971.

Selected Readings

Anthony EJ, Bene E: A technique for the objective assessment of the child's family relationships. *J Ment Sci* 103:541–555, 1957.

Beiser HR: Psychiatric diagnostic interviews with children. *J Am Acad Child Psychiatry* 1:652, 1962.

Beiser HR: Formal games in diagnosis and therapy. *J Am Acad Child Psychiatry* 18:480, 1979.

Bender L: *Child Psychiatric Techniques*. Springfield, IL, Charles C Thomas, 1952, p. 335.

Berger LR: Winnicott squiggle game. *Pediatrics* 66:921, 1980.

Conn JH: The play interview: A method of studying children's attitudes. *Am J Dis Child* 58:1199, 1939.

Cox A, Rutter M: Diagnostic appraisal and interviewing. In: Rutter M, Hersov L (eds): *Child Psychiatry*. Oxford, UK, Blackwell Scientific Publications, 1976.

Despert JL: Technical approaches used in the study and treatment of emotional problems in children. V: The playroom. *Psychiatr Q* 11:677, 1937.

DiLeo JH: *Children's Drawings as Diagnostic Aids*. New York, Brunner/Mazel, 1970a, p. 386.

DiLeo JH: *Young Children and Their Drawings*. New York, Brunner/Mazel, 1970b, p. 386.

Felice M, Friedman SB: The adolescent as a patient. *JCE Pediatr* Oct:15, 1978.

Group for the Advancement of Psychiatry: *The Diagnostic Process in Child Psychiatry* (report no. 38). New York, Group for the Advancement of Psychiatry, 1957, p. 44.

Group for the Advancement of Psychiatry: *From Diagnosis to Treatment: An Approach to Treatment Planning for the Emotionally Disturbed Child* (report no. 87). New York, Group for the Advancement of Psychiatry, 1973, p. 139.

Goodman J, Sours J: *The Child Mental Status Examination*. New York, Basic Books, 1967, p. 134.

Gubbay SS, Ellis E, Walton JN, et al: Clumsy children: A study of apraxic and agnosic defects in 21 children. *Brain* 88:295, 1965.

Levy DM: Use of play technic as experimental procedure. *Am J Orthopsychiatry* 3:266, 1933.

Lowe M: Trends in the development of representational play in infants from one to three years: An observational study. *J Child Psychol Psychiatry* 16:33, 1974.

MacCarthy D: Communication between children and doctors. *Dev Med Child Neurol* 16:279, 1974.

McDonald PF: The psychiatric evaluation of children. *J Am Acad Child Psychiatry* 4:569, 1965.

Paine RS, Oppé TE: Neurological examination of children. *Clin Dev Med* 20/21:40, 1966.

Reisman JM: *Principles of Psychotherapy with Children*. New York, Wiley, 1973.

Rutter M: Clinical assessment of language disorders in the young child. *Clin Dev Med* 43:33–48, 1972.

Rutter M, Graham P, Yule W: *A Neurological Examination: Description*. London, SIMP/Heinemann, 1970, p. 270.

Simmons JE: *Psychiatric Examination of Children* (2nd ed). Philadelphia, Lea & Febiger, 1974, p. 239.

Werkman SC: The psychiatric diagnostic interview with children. *Am J Orthopsychiatry* 35:764, 1965.

Winnicott DW: *Therapeutic Consultations in Child Psychiatry*. New York, Basic Books, 1971.

Yarrow LJ: Interviewing children. In: Mussen PH (ed): *Handbook of Research Methods in Child Development*. New York, Wiley, 1960, pp. 561–602.

Appendix A/Child Psychiatry Emergency Consultation Mental Status Examination Checklist

Patient name: _____   Age: _____   Sex: _____   Examination date: _____

Behavior:	Yes	No	No Info	Comments
Alert	☐	☐	☐	_____
Cooperative	☐	☐	☐	_____
Agitated	☐	☐	☐	_____
Belligerent	☐	☐	☐	_____
Reliable Historian	☐	☐	☐	_____

Speech:				
Slowed	☐	☐	☐	_____
Pressured	☐	☐	☐	_____
Monotone	☐	☐	☐	_____
Ataxic	☐	☐	☐	_____

Mood (Self Report):				
Sad	☐	☐	☐	_____
So-So	☐	☐	☐	_____
Happy	☐	☐	☐	_____
Angry	☐	☐	☐	_____
Nervous	☐	☐	☐	_____

Affect (Observed):				
Congruent	☐	☐	☐	_____
Euthymic	☐	☐	☐	_____
Expansive	☐	☐	☐	_____
Dysphoric	☐	☐	☐	_____
Anxious	☐	☐	☐	_____
Irritable	☐	☐	☐	_____
Angry	☐	☐	☐	_____

Neurovegetative Symptoms:				
Poor Sleep	☐	☐	☐	_____
Poor Appetite	☐	☐	☐	_____
Anhedonic (loss of interests)	☐	☐	☐	_____
Guilty/Worthless Feelings	☐	☐	☐	_____
Decreased Energy	☐	☐	☐	_____
Impaired Concentration	☐	☐	☐	_____
Psychomotor Agitation	☐	☐	☐	_____
Psychomotor Slowing	☐	☐	☐	_____
Recurrent Thoughts of Death (SI is below)	☐	☐	☐	_____

Substance Use:

Tobacco	☐	☐	☐	_____
Alcohol	☐	☐	☐	_____
Marijuana	☐	☐	☐	_____
Stimulants	☐	☐	☐	_____
Narcotics	☐	☐	☐	_____
Hallucinogens	☐	☐	☐	_____
Other	☐	☐	☐	_____

Detail Any "Yes" Responses: _____

Thought Processes:

Circumstantial	☐	☐	☐	_____
Loosened Associations	☐	☐	☐	_____
Paranoid	☐	☐	☐	_____
Delusional	☐	☐	☐	_____
Auditory Hallucinations	☐	☐	☐	_____
Visual Hallucinations	☐	☐	☐	_____
Ideas of Reference	☐	☐	☐	_____
Grandiosity	☐	☐	☐	_____

Suicidality:

Presenting Suicidal Ideation	☐	☐	☐	_____
Previous Suicidal Ideation	☐	☐	☐	_____
Presenting Suicidal Behavior	☐	☐	☐	_____
Previous Suicidal Behavior	☐	☐	☐	(If yes, # of times: _____)

N.B. If "yes" to presenting suicidality questions, then complete the following:

1. Type of Present Episode: specify:
   - None ☐ (0)
   - Ideation without plan ☐ (1) _____
   - Ideation with plan ☐ (2) _____
   - Threat (Verbal) ☐ (3) _____
   - Gesture (e.g., only brandishes, knife or pills) ☐ (4) _____
   - Attempt (deliberate self-injurious) ☐ (5) _____

2. Method of Attempt:
   - Overdose/Ingestion ☐ Type/Amount: _____
   - Cutting/Slashing ☐ _____
   - Firearms ☐ _____
   - Hanging ☐ _____
   - Other ☐ _____

3. Alcohol or drug use prior to episode:
   ☐ No (0) ☐ Yes (2) ☐ Don't Know   ☐ Type/Amount: _____

4. Intent Rating: ☐ No data
   - ☐ Wanted to die   ☐ _____
   - ☐ Did not want to die   ☐ _____
   - ☐ Ambivalent; did not care whether lived or died   ☐ _____

5. Premeditation Rating:
   - ☐ Impulsive act; no premeditation—less than one hour   ☐ _____
   - ☐ Less than 1 day   ☐ _____
   - ☐ Longer than 1 day   ☐ _____

6. Suicide Note: ☐ No data
   ☐ Absence of note   ☐ _____
   ☐ Note written but torn up, or note just thought about   ☐ _____
   ☐ Presence of note   ☐ _____

7. Degree of Planning: ☐ No data
   ☐ No preparation   ☐ _____
   ☐ Minimal/moderate preparation   ☐ _____
   ☐ Extensive preparation   ☐ _____

8. Preparation: (Arrangements made while thinking he/she was going to die; giving things away, etc.)   ☐ No data
   ☐ None   ☐ _____
   ☐ Partial preparation or ideation   ☐ _____
   ☐ Definite plans made   ☐ _____

9. Precautions: ☐ No data
   ☐ No precautions   ☐ _____
   ☐ Passive precautions (such as avoiding others but doing   ☐ _____
      nothing to prevent their intervention,
      e.g., alone in room, door unlocked)
   ☐ Active precautions (e.g., locking doors)   ☐ _____

10. Proximity of other people: ☐ No data
    ☐ Somebody present—Who? _____

    ☐ Somebody nearby or in contact—Who? _____
    ☐ No one nearby or in contact

11. Intervention Rating: ☐ No data
    ☐ Intervention was probable
    ☐ Intervention was not likely, or uncertain
    ☐ Intervention was highly unlikely

12. Notification: Did pt. let anyone know what he/she had done?   ☐ Yes   ☐ No

         Who? _____
              ☐ Key person
              ☐ Professional
              ☐ Passerby

13. Notification Cont.
         How did pt. let them know?
              ☐ Notified potential helper regarding attempt
              ☐ Contacted but did not specifically notify potential helper regarding the attempt
              ☐ Other _____

14. Delay until discovery: ☐ No data
    ☐ Immediate—1 hour
    ☐ Less than 4 hours
    ☐ Greater than 4 hours

15. Did pt. pass out or get confused?
    ☐ No
    ☐ Confusion, semicoma
    ☐ Coma, deep coma

16. Medical Treatment: (if any)   If cutting: ☐ Sutures
    ☐ None   ☐ No sutures
    ☐ First Aid, E. care
    ☐ House admission, routine treatment
    ☐ Intensive care, special treatment

17. Patient's statement of lethality: ☐ No data
    ☐ Thought it would not kill him/her
    ☐ Unsure whether it would kill him/her
    ☐ Believed that it would kill him/her

18. Risk Rating (Medical Estimate):
    ☐ No risk
    ☐ Small risk—probability of only minor injury
    ☐ Medium risk—possibility of significant physical injury, low probability
    ☐ Large risk—significant risk of death or disability

☐ Extreme risk—high probability of death

19. Patient's feelings about episode: ☐ No data
   ☐ Glad he/she recovered
   ☐ Uncertain whether he/she is glad or sorry
   ☐ Sorry he/she recovered

Clinician Signature _____   Date _____

Modified from unpublished working draft. Reprinted with permission from Brad Peterson MD, Melvin Lewis MD and Robert King MD.

40 STRUCTURED INTERVIEWING
Anthony J. Costello, M.D.

Psychiatric interviewing has gone through many phases of development, each reflecting current interest in a different aspect of mental disorder. Early in the century, the interview was typically discursive and indirect, the psychiatrist allowing the patient to set the content and direction of the discussion and only making such interjections as might prompt the patient to elaborate his or her spontaneous narrative. This style was fostered by a deep interest in the phenomena of serious mental illness and reflected the work of such heroes as Emil Kraepelin, Karl Jaspers, and Eugen Bleuler.

Freud's emphasis on the hidden meaning of apparently innocuous conversation or everyday happenings prompted an even more passive interviewing style, carried to the extreme in the techniques of classical psychoanalysis. In his words, "I must ask you to tell me frankly and without any criticism everything that occurs to your mind after you focus your attention, without any particular intention, on the forgotten word" (Freud, 1962). In the passage quoted, Freud goes on to comment on the material his subject produces (in a conversation on a train!) but never asks a direct question except to confirm what he has already deduced. Though this tradition has been much modified over the years, it persists in the preference of some clinicians to observe child behavior and to concentrate on the inferences that can be made from spontaneous remarks. Assessment based on this approach, it is argued, allows one to understand what the child brings to the interview, uncontaminated by the products of any structure that the clinician introduces (Greenspan, 1981).

Against this can be contrasted a goal-oriented approach to interviewing, in which the interviewer structures the questioning to follow his or her own internal model for the information that the interviewer hopes to obtain. The interviewer is much more likely to adopt this style of interviewing if the aim of the interview is to classify the patient's problem within a choice of diagnostic categories. The last 2 decades have seen a resurgence of the "medical model," used here to mean the concept of definable and distinct psychopathological entities, each with a unique pattern of symptoms, and, in theory at least, each with a different etiology and a different course, and each responding to a specific type of treatment. Though this model has been under attack from many directions, it has dominated diagnosis and hence assessment. With the advent of definable criteria for making each diagnosis, first in research procedures such as the Feigner criteria or the Research Diagnostic Criteria for schizophrenia and affective disorders, and now in everyday practice, it is possible to identify more precisely the information needed to make

a diagnosis. In turn, this has influenced the style of psychiatric interviewing.

The notorious unreliability of psychiatric diagnosis has been a weakness of the field for several decades. This unreliability can stem from a variety of reasons. It could be because each psychiatrist has a different concept of diagnosis or is using different criteria. Differences such as these accounted for most of the variation found in international comparisons of diagnostic rates (Cooper et al., 1972; World Health Organization, 1973), and it was the recognition of these problems that prompted the introduction of criterial diagnostic systems. Unreliability might also arise because each interviewer uses different wordings of questions to elicit information from the patient, which unintentionally convey different meanings. Finally, disagreement between psychiatrists might happen because the patient has answered inconsistently in each of the interviews. Reliability, in the sense that two experts can independently assess a patient and reach the same diagnosis, remains hard to achieve, but the diagnoses under such systems as the ICD-10 or the DSM-IV are now defined so well that variation in the information obtained has come to contribute more to the disagreement that is still found.

There has also been an increasing tendency to use "behavioral" concepts in defining a disorder. This is another term that has been used in more than one sense, but in this context it usually means that the definition rests on simple descriptions of behavior. Even though these behaviors may be self-reported, the psychiatrist does not have to infer psychological states, such as anxiety or depression, from the patient's account in order to make a diagnosis, though the diagnosis may imply such states of mind. Though the patient may be asked, for example, if he or she is depressed and miserable, the report of subjective experience is considered a behavioral item. This changes the strategy of assessment—because it then becomes possible to obtain the information needed by asking straightforward questions using terms that adults at least can readily understand—and correspondingly reduces the importance of observational data.

If the content of psychiatric interviewing can be defined by straightforward items of information, all dependent on answers given by the patient, then the path is open to standardized interviews that lay down the content and form of questioning, thus avoiding or at least reducing the variation introduced by differences between interviews. In theory, if the same questions are asked about the same topics in the process of making a psychiatric diagnosis, and standardized procedures are used to make the diagnosis from the information thus obtained, then the only source of variation in diagnosis must come from variation in the patient's answers. This strategy of interviewing is known as "structured" interviewing. Within this broad approach there are several variations. At one extreme, the range of answers to be determined and the concept to be explored are defined, but the wording of the questions is left to the interviewer to determine, depending on his or her judgment of the patient's understanding of the concept. More structure can be introduced if the interviewer is required to ask set questions using the standard wording but is then allowed to ask further probes in his or her own words, to clarify the response. In the most highly structured approach, the questions for the interviewer are completely specified, and probes are written for all probable replies. So far as is possible, the interviewer never has to devise a new question but always has available a standard question or phrase to elucidate the patient's response if necessary.

By convention, structured interviews have been divided into semi-structured and highly structured types. Since the strategies that can be employed lie on a continuum, and many authors of interviews have left the user to judge how rigidly the written format should be followed, this simple classification is often misleading. In subsequent discussions of specific interviews I will attempt to give some indication of where a particular interview lies on this continuum.

Arguments can be offered for preferring more or less structure in the interview, but in child psychiatry other factors also have to be considered. The child's developmental status may limit his or her ability to understand the question. It may be too complex in structure, with too many qualifying clauses, or it may contain concepts unfamiliar to a young child. The time criteria may not match a child's understanding of the passage of time, or a child's memory may be colored by more recent events, even if the interview lays a groundwork of relevant recent events against which symptoms can be timed. A young child may also find it difficult to understand the purpose of an interview, and minimize or deny events or feelings through fear of the consequences of reporting them. All these issues demand a sophisticated understanding on the part of the interview and interviewer.

The changes that have come about in the assessment of adults have had parallels in child psychiatry, though, often, these changes have been prompted by the recognition of the benefits that have ensued for adult practice, rather than by direct prompting from research on childhood disorders. The DSM-III enlarged substantially the range of diagnoses available for children, for not only could many adult diagnoses be applied but also a number of new diagnostic categories were added that were specific to childhood or adolescence. Even before DSM-III, changing views of child psychiatry had spurred the modification of adult structured interviews with the child version of the Interview Schedule for Schizophrenia and the Affective Disorders, the Kiddie Schedule for Affective Disorders and Schizophrenia (K-SADS) (J. Puig-Antich and W. Chambers, unpublished manuscript, 1978), and an exploration of the strategy of structured interviewing directly with children with the Diagnostic Interview for Children and Adolescents (Herjanic et al., 1975).

These pioneering efforts have provided patterns for subsequent developments. The motivation for the use of structured interviewing has been a desire for improved diagnostic accuracy and reliability, either to describe the populations of treatment studies, where homogeneity of diagnosis is important, or in epidemiological and quasi-epidemiological studies, where standard descriptions of diagnostic entities are necessary. In either case, the basic scientific requirement is that the investigator can specify a diagnostic procedure so precisely that another investigator can replicate his or her results. In addition, since such studies are generally expected to have clinical relevance, the diagnostic procedure chosen is usually similar to the clinical process. Most of the problems of diagnostic interviewing can be overcome by alternative procedures, such as the use of self-response checklists, which lend themselves well to statistical procedures of classification and measurement and avoid many of the distortions that potentially are introduced by the interaction between interviewer and interviewee. Unfortunately, checklists and empirically

based classifications still are sufficiently different from the content of clinical practice to limit their application, if established knowledge that is based on clinical experience is not to be discarded.

EVALUATION OF STRUCTURED INTERVIEWS

Though structured interviewing has been applied to child psychiatric diagnosis for over a decade, the criteria for choosing a structured interview or for developing a new interview are still difficult to determine. There are some obvious practical limitations, such as the range of diagnoses the interview is designed to cover or the previous training that an interviewer needs. Another common reason for rejecting any of these interviews may be the time that it takes. Structured interviewing, of course, entails reviewing systematically many possible psychiatric diagnoses, even though what is already known about the child may render some improbable. Inevitably, this makes the interview last longer than many less structured clinical interviews, even though a lot of basic background detail, such as the family structure or the school history, may not be covered. When this material has to be collected as well, the total interview may be dauntingly long. To add to this difficulty, nothing is known about what happens to performance if the interview is modified by omitting unneeded sections. Finally, the prospective user must consider the feasibility of the procedures used to reach diagnoses, the availability of suitable software and data-processing resources, and similar administrative issues.

CHARACTERISTICS OF AN INTERVIEW

Practical issues aside, the user still has to decide how to choose an interview. One test that has often been used to evaluate instruments that are supposed to make psychiatric diagnoses is to compare a group of normal children with a group of children referred for psychiatric treatment. Such a comparison may be weakened by the probability that some children referred to a psychiatrist may be normal, and many children who have not been referred do, in fact, have psychiatric symptoms, but these possibilities will not lead one to believe that the instrument is more effective than is actually the case. Because of the difficulty of obtaining unbiased samples of the normal population, pediatric patients have sometimes been used as normal control subjects, a practice that may further diminish apparent differences between the groups since, among adults at least, heavy users of general medical services tend to have higher rates of psychiatric disorder. The ability to discriminate between normal subjects and psychiatric patients is essential as a minimal requirement, but the evaluation of this property may be misleading, particularly if a diagnostic instrument is very limited in diagnostic range. If, for example, an interview is designed only to diagnose depression, unless the rate of depression in the referred sample is very high, most of these supposed cases would be diagnosed as not depressed, and the discrimination from the normal sample would be poor. Of course, this difficulty does not apply to instruments designed to have comprehensive diagnostic coverage.

However, if the diagnostic system is not comprehensive, it may be impossible to achieve good discrimination. The more specific and circumstantial the criteria for diagnoses are, the greater the probability that it will be difficult to make a diagnosis if the criteria are followed faithfully. Since in DSM-IV the criteria for some of the commonest psychiatric disorders of childhood and adolescence have been made more stringent, it is likely that the number of referred children who do not reach strict diagnostic criteria has risen. Hence, the ability to discriminate between normal and referred populations may be harder to achieve with interviews designed to make DSM-III-R diagnoses. No diagnostic interview can be evaluated independently of the diagnostic system it serves if diagnoses are the only product of the interview. Since the validity of all diagnostic systems remains to be established by systematic research, but such research is very dependent on diagnostic interviews, there is no simple solution to this dilemma.

OTHER APPROACHES TO VALIDATION

Usually, one needs to use an interview not only to detect abnormality but also to discriminate between different types of abnormality. After all, the simple recognition that a child's behavior is abnormal can usually be achieved with sufficient accuracy for screening purposes with a relatively brief symptom checklist, such as Rutter's A scale (Rutter, 1967) or the Child Behavior Checklist (CBCL) (Achenbach and Edelbrock, 1983). To validate a specific diagnosis, a group of children that have been accurately diagnosed is required—an almost impossible task, since the main reason for using structured interviews is that the unreliability of conventional diagnostic procedures sets an unreasonably low upper boundary on the validity of any diagnosis. The usual solution is to merge data from different sources, acquired by several methods, and to try to reach an expert consensus on the diagnosis—the so called lead standard. Though diagnosing a child in this way is the best solution that anyone can offer, the use of so much diverse information, by procedures that are not incorporated into the diagnostic manual, greatly increases the chances that criteria other than those formally defined are being used to make the diagnosis. Only one elaborate study, of a restricted set of diagnoses, has shown that independent experts or expert teams operating in this way are no more able to agree with one another than are individual diagnosticians (Prendergast et al., 1989).

In other fields of psychological measurement, it is possible to compare a new instrument with an established one and, if the performance of the two is similar, to obtain a measure of "concurrent validity." Though there are no established instruments other than interviews that generate standard DSM diagnoses, there are several measures available of such constructs as attentional problems, depression, aggression, anxiety, and so on, which should at least bear some relationship to the relevant diagnostic entity (Edelbrock et al., 1986). To demonstrate such relationships supports validity but does not supplant the need for a more adequate test.

DIAGNOSTIC RELIABILITY

Another criterion of performance that must be considered is reliability. The standards of science demand that it should be possible to replicate a study, and to say that an instrument is reliable implies that at least the performance of the instrument can be replicated. In theory, reliability limits validity, in the sense that a very unreliable test can never achieve adequate validity, but in practice, even an unreliable measure is better than none. Unfortunately, the concept of reliability soon becomes complicated when it is applied to diagnostic interviewing. The least demanding estimate, at least in the experimental design it demands, is so called split-half reliability, which basically is a measure of internal consistency that can be applied to continuous or scalar measures. The statistic estimates the extent to which each part of the scale contributes to the whole. It can only be applied to diagnostic interviews if the interview provides continuous scales of disability, so it is rarely applicable to interviews designed to generate diagnostic categories. However, the necessary data for the Kuder-Richardson alpha can be calculated from a set of single interviews, so this aspect of performance is relatively easy to provide.

If the interview can be filmed or videotaped, the reliability of coding the interview can be evaluated. If the interview is highly structured and the set of responses expected of the informant is confined to simple numerical data or yes/no answers, there should be little room for error. Indeed, highly structured interviews generally perform almost perfectly by this criterion. If the interviewer asks questions that prompt more elaborate and qualified answers, it is necessary to rely on the interviewer's judgment to evaluate and code the reply, and then a measure of interrater agreement is important. With careful training and well-written criteria for coding, interviewers can be expected to have reliabilities of the order of .75 to .9 (Pearson's r), if continuous measures are available. If only categorical decisions are made, a more appropriate statistic is

Cohen's kappa, which is differently distributed. Because κ is sensitive to marginal distributions in an agreement matrix, a desirable range cannot be specified in any simple way. If the majority of cases in a sample are alike, so that only a few can be expected to receive another coding, even a small level of disagreement will produce small values of κ. To test agreement on an item rigorously when the probability of chance agreement is lower, it is better to devise a sample in which the chance of the item's occurring is close to the chance of its not occurring. Then it is reasonable to expect κ values of .7 to .8.

Measures of reliability that depend on designs in which the subject is interviewed twice are the most difficult to evaluate, since so many factors can contribute to variation. However, such a design is the only one that can test the ability of different interviewers to give the interview and obtain the same result. Unfortunately, a different result may be obtained because the subject has changed, or at least changed his or her replies. If the interviews are closely spaced in time, the person interviewed may well remember the answers that he or she gave the first time, so apparently good reliability may be misleading. If the interviews are separated by even as little as 2 weeks, there may still be room for significant change, so a lack of test-retest reliability may not reflect adversely on the interviewing method. A finding common to a wide variety of diagnostic instruments and subject populations is that a second interview detects less pathology than was discovered by the first. There are several possible explanations for this phenomenon (Robins, 1985), but none offered so far are wholly convincing, and the studies that might throw light on the problem have not yet been done.

SPECIFICITY AND SENSITIVITY

The current interest in epidemiology has led to a better understanding of the merits of specificity and sensitivity as measures of interview performance. Sensitivity is the ability of the interview to detect cases. The ratio is calculated by dividing the number of cases identified as abnormal by the number of true cases. A very sensitive interview will identify nearly all the true cases, and the sensitivity will approach 1. Specificity is the ability of the interview to identify only those that are true cases and is calculated by dividing the number of cases assessed as healthy by the actual number of healthy cases in the population. The cases identified by a very specific interview are all likely to be true cases. When an interview is used to find or confirm cases that are to be the subjects of detailed studies (e.g., the evaluation of treatment), it is usually important to be sure that cases are representative and that marginal cases are excluded. Then, a highly specific interview should be selected. For epidemiological studies, it is usually more important to avoid missing cases, and then a very sensitive interview should be used. It is usually the case that interviews that have high sensitivity have low specificity, and vice versa, though with increasing understanding of the technology of interviewing, both qualities may be improved. The assumption in calculating these ratios is, of course, that true cases can be identified, which returns us to the problem of validity.

OTHER ASPECTS OF VALIDITY

The validation of diagnoses generated by any method ultimately must depend on the validation of the diagnostic category itself. For example, there is still much uncertainty on how to combine information provided by the parent with information obtained from the child. The official diagnostic manuals provide no guidance on this point, though it is self-evident that some diagnoses, such as anxiety or depression, involve much subjective experience and so may depend more heavily on the child's report. However, when information is available from the parent about behavioral changes, it may carry more weight. In contrast, diagnoses of disruptive disorders involve behavior that may distress adults but only cause the child discomfort secondarily, through the adults' reactions. There is no satisfactory resolution of the choice of informant until we understand the etiological associations better and have followed the response to treatment and the outcome of diagnoses made both by parent and by child report. If diagnoses based on an interview with one informant offer a better understanding of etiology and prognosis than those based on the other's, then this will give us a better diagnostic definition and a better interviewing strategy. Meanwhile, both method and diagnostic categorization are interdependent and, inevitably, somewhat arbitrary.

EFFECT OF CHANGES IN INTERVIEWS AND DIAGNOSTIC SYSTEMS

Since 1980, when DSM-III was finally published, this system has been revised twice, and ICD, to which DSM can in theory be mapped, has also been revised. In child psychiatry, each revision has added some diagnoses and removed others, and the criteria for many diagnoses have been changed in ways that at least require changes in the diagnostic algorithms, whether performed by clinician or computer. In many instances the changes also require that questions be reworded or added. Though the changes often seem minor, they may alter prevalence rates substantially. Cases diagnosed under one version of a diagnostic system may fail to meet criteria for diagnosis in the next. Conversely, other individuals who were not diagnosable before are so now.

As though these revisions were not anarchy enough to obstruct the would-be researcher who tries to stay up to date, investigators have often modified interviews, expanding, adding, or deleting sections to suit their particular diagnostic interests. Unhappily, an investigator rarely checks the performance of such revisions. Though some changes may be harmless, ample evidence exists to suggest that changes of this type may significantly alter reliability and validity. Just as a few decades ago an interview by an experienced clinician was considered sufficient, so now an interview claiming the same acronym as one used in previously published work may be deemed adequate. Only boring but necessary methodological studies will solve this problem. Regrettably, as Offord (1993) has pointed out, these comparative studies, so sorely needed, have still to be done.

SELECTION OF A STRUCTURED INTERVIEW

It is probably a mistake at this stage of our knowledge to use a structured interview for routine clinical diagnosis. Used properly, this type of interview will take longer than a normal interview and generate less information. Moreover, the diagnosis may be misleadingly invested with an authority that no interview can as yet claim to possess. Equally, it would be a mistake in routine interviewing to ignore the experience derived from structured interviews and to omit systematic screening for common symptoms, whether or not they have featured in the presenting complaints.

For research applications, a simple checklist should help the investigator to select an interview.

1. *The question*: Define the hypothesis to be tested or the question to be asked. Often, when this is done, it becomes evident that a diagnostic interview is not even needed. Assuming that the need is established, proceed to 2.
2. *Coverage*: Does the full range of diagnoses need to be covered? Are there some that will not occur in the sample to be interviewed? Are there diagnoses that are so central to the study that good performance on these is essential? Is it important to use a particular diagnostic framework (DSM-III, DSM-III-R, DSM-IV, ICD9 or 10)?
3. *Choice of interviewer*: What is the scale of the study, and what resources are available? Can you only afford lay interviewers, or is it possible to employ skilled clinicians? Are enough skilled clinicians available?
4. *Products from the interview*: Do you need diagnoses only, or are symptom scores more useful for some projected analyses?
5. *Data-processing capacity*: Do you plan to maintain a large database? Will it contain raw data from interviews or only products? Is there software available to enter data and score the interview? Do you

have the computer resources to process the data if the diagnoses are computer generated, or the personnel to check interviews that are scored manually?
6. *Performance*: Which aspects of performance (internal, interrater, and retest reliability; specificity and sensitivity; concurrent validity) are most important for this study? Are data on all these aspects available for all alternative instruments that you are considering?

The would-be investigator should consider each of these points in turn. Usually there is a trade-off between different aspects of the interviews; the one with the best diagnostic cover may be the one demanding the most data processing, or the one with the best coverage of a symptom area that you wish to study may be the one that demands the most highly trained interviewers. By ranking items 2 to 6 in this checklist in order of priority, it should be possible to make a rational choice.

SPECIFIC INSTRUMENTS

Highly Structured Interviews

Two highly structured interviews have been fairly widely used. The Diagnostic Interview for Children and Adolescents (DICA) was one of the first of its type and employs a modular structure, with questions organized by syndrome. The authors of the Diagnostic Interview Schedule for Children (DISC) attempted to make a more naturally flowing interview by organizing questions by topic, to make it appear that the interviewer was more interested in the child's everyday life and activities.

DIAGNOSTIC INTERVIEW FOR CHILDREN AND ADOLESCENTS

The DICA was developed by Herjanic et al. (Herjanic and Campbell, 1977; Herjanic et al., 1975) at Washington University. This instrument was one of the earlier attempts to develop a highly structured interview and has been revised several times. As with other interviews, it has to be assumed that performance has not been changed by such revisions, since performance data are only available for some of these versions. The DICA is a structured interview that demands no exercise of clinical judgment on the part of the interviewer. It is designed for children aged 6 to 17 and has both parent and child versions. Each version takes approximately 60 to 90 minutes. Questions are to be asked initially as worded, but if the question is not understood, the interviewer is asked to give examples, drawn as far as possible from information the child has already given. However, at several points in the interview the interviewer has to use some judgment in deciding how to follow up the answers the child gives. The interview is organized mainly by syndrome, though some sections have a thematic organization. A skip structure is employed. Items are designed to be coded as present or absent. When the answer is ambiguous, subsidiary questions resolve the question, and the interviewer can go back to recode the root item. Questions generally deal with the present, but when an item is not present, inquiries are made about past symptomatology.

The interview yields information on a wide range of symptoms and gives details of their onset, duration, severity, and associated impairment. Summary scores grouping symptoms together are available, and ICD-9, DSM-III, and DSM-III-R diagnoses can be derived from some versions.

Interrater reliability studies using videotaped interviews show good percentage agreement, but since the rate of occurrence of most symptoms is relatively low, high-percentage agreement can be achieved by the absence of symptomatology (Herjanic and Reich, 1982). Another version of this study had five psychiatrists code the same child interview twice at an interval of 2 to 3 months. Though interview agreement was high, the same objection applies. Parent-child agreement on specific items range from .0 to .87 (κ) (Herjanic and Reich, 1982). Parent and child tended to agree on items that were objective and concrete or serious and to disagree on items that required judgment or were subject to misinterpretation. Parent-child agreement on diagnosis was a little better, but the majority of diagnoses were below .4 (Reich et al., 1982).

The most recently published study on the performance of the DICA examined test-retest reliability between interviews of inpatients by different interviewers 1 to 7 days apart. Diagnoses based on pooled data from parent and child showed very satisfactory reliability (κ ranged from .76 to 1 for anxiety disorders and conduct disorder, respectively) (Welner et al., 1987).

The validity of the DICA was initially supported by a comparison study of samples referred to pediatric or psychiatric clinics. The summary scores for relationship problems and academic problems provided the best discrimination, whereas neurotic and somatic symptoms gave little discrimination (Herjanic and Campbell, 1977). For relationship problems, which provided the best discrimination, the sensitivity was 72% and the specificity 76%. Since data from parent and child were pooled to construct these summary scores, it is possible that this analysis does not do justice to the power of the interview. Interview diagnoses show only modest agreement with discharge diagnoses, a finding that others have repeated. Since clinicians make fewer diagnoses, use other information, and tend to assume hierarchical structures even when DSM does not require these, this result should not be considered discouraging (Herjanic and Campbell, 1977). There are some data suggesting that the DICA may be more sensitive than specific, when compared with a semistructured interview (Carlson et al., 1987).

The DICA can be described as a highly structured interview, but it still allows the interviewer some latitude. Its main strength, judging from published studies that use the DICA, is in the area of attention deficit and conduct disorders. Its dichotomous scoring and inability to measure the severity of symptoms in any extensive way may limit its usefulness, but the interview has been used extensively in many successful studies.

DIAGNOSTIC INTERVIEW SCHEDULE FOR CHILDREN

The DISC was developed for use in epidemiological studies of childhood psychiatric disorder (A. J. Costello et al., unpublished manuscript, 1984a). Though similar in purpose to the Diagnostic Interview Schedule (DIS) developed for epidemiological studies of adult disorder (Robins et al., 1981), it departs from the DIS in several ways. The original content was developed from a review for the National Institute of Mental Health by Kovacs, Connors, Herjanic and Puig-Antich, and some relationship to the instruments devised by these authors can still be detected. The DISC is a highly structured interview in which the exact wording of questions, the order in which they are presented, and the method of recording are all predetermined. There is an explicit skip structure so that when a primary symptom question is negative, no probes are asked. Training takes 2 to 3 days, and the interview is suitable for use by lay interviewers as well as by clinicians. Both parent and child versions have been developed. The child version has 760 items in Costello's most recent revision and takes about 45 to 60 minutes to complete with clinically referred children. Nonsymptomatic children may take a little less time. The parent version includes more items, covering areas on which a child could not be expected to self-report, and takes approximately 60 to 70 minutes. The time frame of the interview is the last year. Interviewers are instructed to use temporal landmarks to identify significant durations, such as 2 weeks, 1 month, or 6 months. The interview is designed for children between the ages of 6 and 18, though data on its performances suggest that the clinical yield for younger children is poor.

The DISC, in its original version, covers a broad range of child behaviors and symptoms and obtains details on the onset, duration, severity, and associated impairment of each. Symptom items are coded 0, 1, or 2. Zero corresponds to no or never; 1 corresponds to somewhat, sometimes, or a little; and 2 corresponds to yes, often, or a lot. Since both children and adults tend to respond unpredictably to questions about psychopathology that are outside their personal experience, for most

main symptom areas that are coded positive, and for some corroborating details, the interviewer is asked to record the respondent's verbatim reply. This makes it possible to check the transcript when a positive diagnosis is made, to confirm that the verbatim responses support the diagnosis. Diagnoses are generated by computer algorithm. Computer programs are also available to administer the interview and perform data entry, and a simple editor is provided for those who wish to modify the interview.

Interrater reliability was examined by comparing symptom scores for 10 videotaped child interviews independently coded by three lay interviewers (Costello et al., 1984). Reliabilities averaged .98 for symptom scores (range, .94 to l). Test-retest reliability was determined on a sample of 242 clinically referred children and their parents (Edelbrock et al., 1985). Parent and child were interviewed separately and were assessed twice at an interval of 7 to 14 days. For the parent interview, test-retest reliability was .9 for total symptom scores (interclass correlation) and averaged .76 for symptom clusters (range .44 to .86). For the child interview, test-retest reliability was closely related to age. It ranged from .43 for children aged 6 to 9, to .71 for children aged 14 to 18. Total symptom score was much more reliable among children aged 14 to 18 (interclass correlation, .81). For those diagnoses that had sufficient prevalence in this sample, the reliability of the parent interview averaged 0.56 (gk) and ranged from 0.35 to 0.81. Reliabilities of diagnoses derived from the child interview alone were much lower, ranging from .12 to .71, with an average of .36.

Parent-child agreement was examined for 299 families (Edelbrock et al., 1986). The average correlation between symptom scores from the two informants was 0.27. Parent-child agreement was highest for disruptive disorder and least for symptoms of depression and anxiety. Agreement was substantially higher between children aged 14 to 18 and their parents than between the younger age groups and their parents. In all age groups, parents tended to report more conduct problems than did their children, whereas the children reported more symptoms of anxiety and depression and of alcohol and drug abuse.

Validity was explored using a pediatric referral control group. Forty of the original clinical sample aged between 7 and 11 were compared with children attending a community-based pediatric clinic. For the DISC-P (parent version), psychiatric referrals scored significantly higher in nearly all symptom areas, with the total symptom score providing the greatest difference between the groups. For the child interviews, psychiatric referrals scored higher in most symptom areas, but the greatest separation between psychiatric and pediatric patients was found in the area of simple fears and phobias.

Using the parent interview, the psychiatric referrals received 51 significant psychiatric disorder diagnoses, whereas in the pediatric group only 2 severe disorders were diagnosed. When symptom scores derived from both parent and child interviews were combined in a multiple discriminatory analysis, a sensitivity of 95% and a specificity of 98% were achieved (Costello et al., 1985). Compared with a semistructured interview such as the K-SADS the DISC tends to be more sensitive and less specific, though the study from which this can be inferred has some technical limitations (Cohen et al., 1987). However, this finding is consistent with similar comparisons of more structured and semistructured interviews. The comparisons with clinicians' diagnoses are generally disappointing (Costello et al., 1984), which is not surprising, given the poor reliability of clinical diagnosis, but they tend to improve if "probable" rather than "possible" diagnoses are used (Weinstein et al., 1989).

Further support for the validity of the DISC comes from comparing data from the interview with data from the parent and teacher versions of the CBCL. Such relationships fall in the expected direction, with very different symptom profiles on the checklist matching different DISC diagnoses, regardless of informant. Moreover, there is a tendency for related scores to be associated in a linear fashion. The higher the checklist score for depression or hyperactivity/inattentiveness, for example, the greater the probability that the corresponding diagnoses will be made by the DISC (Edelbrock and Costello, 1988).

Shaffer (1989) used data drawn both from the original study of the DISC and from epidemiological studies to make revisions which, it was hoped, would improve the performance of this instrument. The effect of the revisions was satisfactory for some diagnoses but not all (Shaffer et al., 1993; Piacentini et al., 1993; Schwab-Stone et al., 1993), though these findings may be obscured by other changes made to accommodate DSM-III-R. Since a later version of the DISC-2 was used to provide data on which some of the revisions of DSM-IV are founded (Frick et al., 1994), it is probably the first interview to be able to make some (though not all) DSM-IV diagnoses with reasonable confidence. The DISC is the only instrument designed specifically and solely for epidemiological studies, and it seems likely that its applications will remain in this field. It is the most highly structured of all instruments currently available and shows clearly both the advantages and disadvantages of this interviewing strategy.

Semistructured Interviews

Three semistructured instruments have been commonly used. The most widely used is the K-SADS. Another notable for the interesting research that has come from its use is the Interview Schedule for Children (ISC). A third, the Child Assessment Schedule (CAS), though less widely used, has some unique features and has the benefit of more studies of concurrent validity than any other instrument.

SCHEDULE FOR AFFECTIVE DISORDERS AND SCHIZOPHRENIA FOR SCHOOL-AGE CHILDREN

The K-SADS is a semistructured diagnostic interview for children aged 6 to 17, developed by Puig-Antich and Chambers after the Schedule for Affective Disorders and Schizophrenia (SADS) designed for adults (Endicott and Spitzer, 1978). The K-SADS has been revised several times. Several versions are now available, including a present episode version and an epidemiological version that also covers past episodes (Orvaschel et al., 1982). The last published revision of the K-SADS was in 1987, by Orvaschel and Puig-Antich, and this version also incorporated revisions for DSM-III-R. The interview is designed to be administered by clinically sophisticated interviewers. The interviewer is given considerable latitude in adapting questions to suit the respondent, and is allowed to make further probes depending on the response. The interviewing plan follows a clinical format. In the first part of the interview, the informant is asked to identify all presenting problems and symptoms so that the interviewer can obtain a history of the present illness and determine current symptoms. The treatment history is then recorded, and the period when symptoms were most severe is identified. The second part includes questions on approximately 200 areas of symptomatology relevant to diagnosis. In the third section there are observational items that are rated by the interviewer, and the interviewer is also required to rate on the children's version of the Global Assessment of Functioning scale. Most items are rated on a 6-point range of severity, with specific criteria for each level. A skip structure is embodied so that probes need not be asked if the response to the initial question for a specific syndromic area is negative. Diagnoses are achieved by the clinician's summary ratings. In order to make diagnoses from the K-SADS, it is essential to be familiar with DSM-III and DSM-III-R (and now DSM-IV) criteria, though the interview itself offers guidelines for using the ratings. Computerized diagnoses are not available.

The K-SADS gives much more emphasis to affective disorders, anxiety, and schizophrenia and schizophreniform disorders than to the disruptive disorders, though items relating to the latter are included. The epidemiological version (K-SADS-E) is somewhat broader in scope. Both interviews are designed to be administered to the parent first. When seeing the child, the interviewer is expected to be familiar with the parent's responses, though their responses are recorded separately. However, when discrepancies between the informants are found, the clinician is encouraged to resolve these differences, if necessary by going back to the first informant. Though this strategy presents some difficulties, it may at times resolve problems of disagreement whose solution is otherwise elusive (Nguyen et al., 1994).

Interrater reliability for individual symptoms of major diagnostic syndromes range from .65 to .96. Short-term (2 to 3 day) test-retest reliability shows moderate consistency on individual symptoms (average interclass correlation, .55; range, .09 to .89) (Chambers et al., 1985). The summary scales showed somewhat higher reliabilities (average interclass correlation, .68; range, .41 to .81). The reliability of diagnoses ranges from .24 to .7. Mother-child agreement for the K-SADS-P and K-SADS-E has shown surprising diversity, with a range from .08 to 1 for symptoms; most items and syndromes have fallen into an acceptable range (Chambers et al., 1985; Orvaschel et al., 1982), though agreement between informants is low if diagnoses are made independently (Ivens and Rehm, 1988). In any case, the emphasis on resolving disagreement in interview makes this aspect of performance less relevant for this interview. The performance of the interview has been most closely studied for depressive disorders, which it was originally designed to identify. Items relating to the diagnosis of affective disorder have test-retest reliabilities between .63 and .81 and have good internal consistency.

The validity of the K-SADS-E was tested by asking former patients about their previous symptoms 6 months to 2 years later. Of 17 patients, 16 obtained the same diagnosis in the K-SADS-E interview, but the range of diagnoses was limited, though this can only be regarded as preliminary support for the usefulness of lifetime diagnoses. Supportive data for the validity of the K-SADS-P comes from drug trials that show the ratings are sensitive to changes as a result of treatment (Puig-Antich, Perel, et al., 1979, 1987) and from studies suggesting that there are biological correlates of K-SADS diagnoses (Puig-Antich, Chambers, et al., 1979, 1984).

The K-SADS was designed primarily to select children who met criteria for a diagnosis of an affective disorder. Though performance details are not available for this aspect, it is likely that the instrument is highly specific but relatively insensitive. In clinical studies requiring very homogeneous groups, these are ideal characteristics. The stringent requirements for interviewers and the more modest performance of the interview on other disorders probably make it unsuitable for epidemiological studies. It should be noted that, like other instruments in the hands of subsequent users, the administration has varied considerably, with some tendency for investigators other than the original developers to use the K-SADS as a more structured interview.

CHILD ASSESSMENT SCHEDULE

The CAS (Hodges et al., 1982, 1987) is a semistructured interview originally designed for children aged 7 to 12. It has now been extended to cover children up to the age of 16, and a parallel form for parents has also been developed. Parents and children are interviewed separately. Each version takes 45 to 60 minutes to complete. There are three parts. Part 1 contains 75 items grouped by topic rather than by diagnostic syndrome. The time frame is within the last 6 months. Each item is rated as positive, negative, ambiguous, not applicable, or no response. The second part allows the interviewer to record onset and duration of selected symptoms; this makes it possible to generate a DSM-III (now DSM-IV) diagnosis, which was not possible in the earliest version as it did not include this section. In the third section, the interviewer is asked to rate a number of observational items. Unlike other semistructured psychiatric interviews, the authors claim that specific training in child mental health and familiarity with child psychopathology are not required, though specific interview training is necessary. Most childhood psychiatric disorders are covered by the interview. Interrater reliability is based on independent ratings and videotapes of 53 interviews, and for the total symptom score it is .9. Content areas average .73, and symptom complexes slightly less. Interrater reliabilities are rather higher for hyperactivity and aggression (average, .8) and for fears, worries, and anxiety (average, .6). The reliability of individual items was .57 (κ). Test-retest reliability is not reported, nor is there any information on parent-child agreement.

Validity is supported in several ways. The total score discriminates significantly between inpatient, outpatient, and normals and correlates significantly ($r = .53$) with the total behavior problem score derived from the CBCL. Scores on the overanxious scale have been shown to correlate well with Spielberger's State-Trait Anxiety Inventory for Children (Spielberger, 1973), and the depression scores correlate significantly with the Child Depression Inventory (Kovacs, 1980). Using referral for inpatient or outpatient psychiatric services as a criterion of psychopathology, the total score discriminated well, achieving a sensitivity of 78% and a specificity of 73.8% (Hodges et al., 1982). Concordance between the CAS and the K-SADS-E was moderate to high, with the surprising exception of overanxious disorder. As might be expected, agreement was better if information from parent and child was pooled, or if only the parent versions of each interview were used. Agreement for conduct disorder, in contrast, is good when either parent or child information is used.

The CAS is a sensitive, well-written interview with a variety of supporting data, including more psychometric data than is available for other semistructured interviews, but it has been less popular, perhaps because it has not been adopted for any major research study so far. It is somewhat more structured than most semistructured interviews and so would probably be easier to use for less experienced clinicians.

INTERVIEW SCHEDULE FOR CHILDREN

The Interview Schedule for Children (ISC) was developed by Kovacs, in 1983, for a longitudinal study of childhood depression (M. Kovacs, unpublished manuscript, 1983). Since then, it has undergone further development and revision and, like other interviews, some caution must be used in assuming that early psychometric data applies to the current version. The ISC is a semistructured interview that requires the interviewer to have considerable clinical skill, extensive specific training on the interview, and to be knowledgeable about the interview content, the rating procedures, and DSM-IV criteria. The interview is designed for children aged 8 to 17. Like the K-SADS, the interview begins with an unstructured section to establish rapport and to determine the nature of the current disorder. The mother is interviewed first, then the child is interviewed by the same clinician. The interview with the parent takes 90 to 120 minutes, the interview with the child, approximately 45 to 60 minutes. A follow-up version is also available, which can be used to assess changes over time (Kovacs, 1985). Forty-three symptoms are recorded, with ratings that cover the presence and severity of each and a global rating of functional impairment. Items are rated on a 0 to 8 scale with criteria along the continuum. The interviewer rates 12 observational items and is required to dictate a clinical summary.

The ISC has several unique features. The order of questions may vary to correspond to those that the respondent mentions spontaneously. A number of confirmation questions are designed to check the child's initial response before making a final rating. The prompt system is standard, which necessitates quite extensive interviewer training but results in a very smooth and flowing interview when the prompts are mastered. Interrater reliability between the interviewer conducting the interview and another observing it and making ratings independently is high, with interclass correlations averaging .89, with a range of .64–1. Mental status items tend to be somewhat more reliable than observational items or clinical impressions. Parent-child agreement on 75 clinic cases ranges from .02 to .95 for symptoms (average, .61) and .32 to .86 for syndromes (M. Kovacs, unpublished manuscript, 1983, 1985). Agreement was highest for overt and observable behaviors and lowest for affective and subjective symptomatology. Validity rests primarily on the content, which is firmly based on a clinical approach and on the instrument's utility in research on childhood depression (Kovacs et al., 1984a, 1984b). Though the ISC has been less widely used than some

other interviews, its thoughtful design and wording makes it a strong contender for studies of childhood depression or anxiety where high specificity and careful description are the goals. On the spectrum of structure it lies at the least-structured end, very close to the K-SADS.

Interviews with More Limited Goals

Though most structured and semistructured interviews have been used as general diagnostic instruments, the same method can be used to construct interviews with more restricted coverage. One example is the Schedule for the Assessment of Conduct, Hyperactivity, Anxiety, Mood, and Psychoactive Substances (CHAMPS) (S. Manuzza and R. Gittelman-Klein, unpublished manuscript, 1987), a semistructured interview for use by trained clinicians in follow-up studies of individuals who had been diagnosed earlier with attention deficit disorder or separation anxiety disorder. Another is the Interview for Childhood Disorders and Schizophrenia (ICDS) (Russell et al., 1989), a semistructured interview for use by trained clinicians in studies of schizophrenic, autistic, or schizophrenic spectrum-disordered children. The same approach can be used to explore aspects of behavior that do not directly relate to diagnosis, as in the Social Adjustment Inventory for Children and Adolescents (SAICA) (John et al., 1987). Performance data for such restricted instruments have to be evaluated carefully, for the reasons outlined earlier, but the general interviewing strategy is as appropriate for these specialized uses as it is for more general applications.

CURRENT PRACTICE

Most psychiatric research is done in clinical settings where highly trained clinicians are available to conduct interviews. The samples tend to be small and clinically selected, so many individuals in the sample are highly symptomatic. Studies carried out with such subjects favor the use of semistructured interviews. In 45 of 110 research articles published in the *Journal of the American Academy of Child and Adolescent Psychiatry* in 1995, a diagnostic interview was used, most commonly the K-SADS or one of its variants. A structured interview was only used 11 times, and sometimes inappropriately, in that high specificity was desirable and clinically trained interviewers could have been available. Given the paucity of comparative data and the many problems related to the assumptions inherent in using a highly structured interview, this distribution reflects a reasonable approach to the choice of interview.

FUTURE DEVELOPMENTS

The distinction between highly structured and semistructured instruments that has been maintained to this date in the relevant literature should probably be abandoned. It is evident from personal accounts of the usage of both types of instruments that these theoretical distinctions have been blurred in practice. Some semistructured instruments have been administered in highly structured fashion, with little variation from the suggested wording, by relatively inexperienced clinicians. On the other hand, some experienced clinicians have varied the wording of highly structured interviews without apparently changing the performance of the interview, and some lay interviewers have proved capable of making judgments about answers that, it was held, could only be made by experienced clinicians. There seems to be merit in merging the two approaches, combining questions that are always asked in the same words with more flexible probes that depend on interviewer judgment, to determine the presence or absence of specific symptoms. Applying the computer programs known as expert systems also seems to be a promising approach; these recently developed programs help to clarify the decision rules that are used by experts but are not always clearly articulated. Such programs might be used to detect those features of a case that deflect an expert diagnostician from conclusions based on simple algorithms.

Other developments may come from using the trade-off between sensitivity and specificity as a dimension that may determine the type of interview to be used. Unfortunately, specificity cannot be adequately measured at the level of specific diagnoses until a satisfactory criterion of validity is available for every diagnosis.

Validation is an area that needs more study, and validation of diagnostic instruments and diagnostic rules cannot proceed independently of the development of the diagnostic system itself. So far, the creation of a diagnostic system, the rules it uses, and the instruments developed to aid diagnosis have all rested heavily on expert opinion. Such data as are available mainly consist of concurrent data on performance, such as reliability, or correlations with other instruments that also lack adequate validation. This type of information strengthens construct validity but is still inadequate. Current research projects are generating enough information to allow us to hope that the validation of diagnoses and diagnostic instruments will be more influenced in the future by longitudinal outcome data, particularly in the areas of depression and the disruptive disorders, where most work of this sort has been concentrated.

Meanwhile, there is a real need for comparative studies of different diagnostic systems, rules, and instruments, to establish the true differences between various approaches and to make choices that are influenced more by scientific theory and knowledge than by considerations of convenience, availability, or feasibility. As this work progresses, perhaps the technology of interviewing will come to be influenced more by data and less by intuition.

References

Achenbach TM, Edelbrock CS: *Manual for the Child Behavior Checklist and Revised Child Behavior Profile*. Burlington, VT, University of Vermont, 1983.

Carlson GA, Kashani JH, Thomas MDF, et al: Comparison of two structured interviews on a psychiatrically hospitalized population of children. *J Am Acad Child Adolesc Psychiatry* 26:645–648, 1987.

Chambers W, Puig-Antich J, Hirsch M, et al: The assessment of affective disorders in children and adolescents by semi-structured interview: Test-retest reliability of the K-SADS-P. *Arch Gen Psychiatry* 42:606–702, 1985.

Cohen P, O'Connor P, Lewis S, et al: Comparison of DISC and K-SADS-P interviews of an epidemiological sample of children. *J Am Acad Child Adolesc Psychiatry* 26:662–667, 1987.

Cooper JE, Kendell RE, Gurland BJ, et al: *Psychiatric Diagnosis in New York and London* (Maudsley Monograph no. 20). London, Oxford University Press, 1972.

Costello EJ, Edelbrock CS, Costello AJ: Validity of the NIMH Diagnostic Interview Schedule for Children: A comparison between psychiatric and pediatric referrals. *J Abnorm Child Psychol* 13:579–595, 1985.

Costello AJ, Edelbrock C, Dulcan MK, et al: *Development and testing of the NIMH Diagnostic Interview Schedule for Children in a Clinic Population*. Final Report (Contract no. RFP-DB-81-0027). Rockville, MD, Center for Epidemiologic Studies, National Institute of Mental Health, 1984.

Edelbrock C, Costello AJ: Convergence between statistically derived behavior problem syndromes and child psychiatric diagnoses. *J Abnorm Child Psychol* 16:219–231, 1988.

Edelbrock C, Costello AJ, Dulcan MK, et al: Age differences in the reliability of the psychiatric interview of the child. *Child Dev* 56:265–275, 1985.

Edelbrock, C, Costello AJ, Dulcan MK, et al: Parent-child agreement on child psychiatric symptoms assessed via structured interview. *J Child Psychol Psychiatry* 27:181–190, 1986.

Endicott J, Spitzer RL: A diagnostic interview: The Schedule for Affective Disorders and Schizophrenia. *Arch Gen Psychiatry* 35:837–844, 1978.

Freud S: Psychopathology of everyday life. In: Strachey J (ed): *The Standard Edition of the Complete Psychological Words of Sigmund Freud* (Vol 6). London, Hogarth Press, 1962. (Originally published 1901).

Frick PJ, Lahey BB, Applegate B, et al: DSM-IV field trials for the disruptive disorders: Symptom utility estimates. *J Am Acad Child Adolesc Psychiatry* 33:529–539, 1994.

Greenspan SI: *The Clinical Interview of the Child*. New York, McGraw-Hill, 1981.

Herjanic B, Campbell W: Differentiating psychiatrically disturbed children on the basis of a structured interview. *J Abnorm Child Psychol* 5:127–134, 1977.

Herjanic B, Herjanic M, Brown F, et al: Are children reliable reporters? *J Abnorm Child Psychol* 3:41–48, 1975.

Herjanic B, Reich W: Development of a structured psychiatric interview for children: Agreement between child and parent on individual symptoms. *J Abnorm Child Psychol* 10:307–324, 1982.

Hodges K, Kline J, Stern L, et al: The development of a child assessment interview for research and clinical use. *J Abnorm Child Psychol* 10:173–189, 1982.

Hodges K, McKnew D, Burbach DJ, et al: Diagnostic concordance between the Child Assessment Schedule (CAS) and the Schedule for Affective Disorders and Schizophrenia for school age children K-SADS-P) in an outpatient sample using lay interviewers. *J Am Acad Child Adolesc Psychiatry* 26:654–661, 1987.

Ivens C, Rehm LP: Assessment of childhood depression: Correspondence between reports by child, mother and father. *J Am Acad Child Adolesc Psychiatry* 27:738–741, 1988.

John K, Gammon GD, Prusoff BA, et al: The Social Adjustment Inventory for Children and Adolescents (SAICA): Testing of a new semistructured interview. *J Am Acad Child Adolesc Psychiatry* 26:898–911, 1987.

Kovacs M: Rating scales to assess depression in school-aged children. *Acta Paedopsychiatr* 46:305–315, 1980.

Kovacs M: The Interview Schedule for Children (ISC). *Psychopharmacol Bull* 21:991–994, 1985.

Kovacs M, Feinberg TL, Crouse-Novak MA, et al: Depressive disorders in childhood I: A longitudinal prospective study of characteristics and recovery. *Arch Gen Psychiatry* 41:229–237, 1984.

Kovacs M, Feinberg TL, Crouse-Novak M, et al: Depressive disorders in childhood II: A longitudinal study of the risk for a subsequent major depression. *Arch Gen Psychiatry* 41:643–649, 1984.

Nguyen N, Whittlesey S, Scimeca K, et al: Parent-child agreement in prepubertal depression: Findings with a modified assessment method. *J Am Acad Child Adolesc Psychiatry* 33:1275–1283, 1994.

Offord, DR: Discussion of "Epidemiology and Mental Health Services" (Costello EJ, Burns BJ, Angold A, and Leaf PJ). *J Am Acad Child Adolesc Psychiatry* 32:1116–1117, 1993.

Orvaschel H, Puig-Antich J, Chambers W, et al: Retrospective assessment of prepubertal major depression with the Kiddie-SADS-E. *J Am Acad Child Adolesc Psychiatry* 21:695–707, 1982.

Piacenti J, Shaffer D, Fisher P, et al: The Diagnostic Interview for Children-Revised Version (DISC-R): III Concurrent criterion validity *J Am Acad Child Adolesc Psychiatry* 32:658–665, 1993.

Prendergast M, Taylor E, Rapoport J, et al: The diagnosis of childhood hyperactivity: A US-UK cross-national study of DSM-III and ICD-9. *J Child Psychol Psychiatry* 29:289–300, 1989.

Puig-Antich J, Chambers W, Halpern F, et al: Cortisol hypersecretion in prepubertal depressive illness: A preliminary study. *Psychoneuroendocrinology* 4:191–197, 1979.

Puig-Antich J, Novacenko MS, Goetz MA, et al: Cortisol and prolactin responses to insulin-induced hypoglycemia in prepubertal major depressives during episode and after recovery. *J Am Acad Child Adolesc Psychiatry* 23:49–57, 1984.

Puig-Antich J, Perel J, Lupatkin W, et al: Plasma levels of imipramine (IMI) and desmethylimipramine (DMI) and clinical response in prepubertal major depressive disorder: A preliminary report. *J Am Acad Child Psychiatry* 18:616–627, 1979.

Puig-Antich J, Perel J, Lupatkin W, et al: Imipramine in prepubertal major depressive disorders. *Arch Gen Psychiatry* 44:81–89, 1987.

Reich W, Herjanic B, Welner Z, et al: Development of a structured interview for children: Agreement on diagnosis comparing parent and child. *J Abnorm Child Psychol* 10:325–336, 1982.

Robins LN: Epidemiology: Reflections on testing the validity of psychiatric interviews. *Arch Gen Psychiatry* 42:918–924, 1985.

Robins L, Helzer JE, Croughan J, et al: National Institute of Health Diagnostic Interview Schedule: Its history, characteristics and validity. *Arch Gen Psychiatry* 38:381–389, 1981.

Russell AT, Bott L, Sammons C: The phenomenology of schizophrenia occurring in childhood. *J Am Acad Child Adolesc Psychiatry* 28:399–407, 1989.

Rutter M: A children's behaviour questionnaire for completion by teachers: Preliminary findings. *J Child Psychol Psychiatry* 8:1–11, 1967.

Shaffer D: *The Diagnostic Interview Schedule for Children (DISC-2): Its development and administration*. Paper presented at the annual meeting of the American Academy of Child and Adolescent Psychiatry, New York, 1989.

Shaffer D, Schwab-Stone M, Fisher P, et al: The Diagnostic Interview for Children-Revised Version (DISC-R): I Preparation, field testing, inter-rater reliability and acceptability. *J Am Acad Child Adolesc Psychiatry* 32:643–650, 1993.

Schwab-Stone M, Fisher P, Piacenti J, et al: The Diagnostic Interview for Children-Revised Version (DISC-R): II Test-retest reliability. *J Am Acad Child Adolesc Psychiatry* 32:651–657, 1993.

Spielberger CD: *Manual for the State-Trait Anxiety Inventory for Children*. Palo Alto, CA, Consulting Psychologists Press, 1973.

Weinstein S, Stone K, Noam GG, et al: Comparison of DISC with clinicians' DSM-III diagnoses in psychiatric inpatients. *J Am Acad Child Adolesc Psychiatry* 28:53–60, 1989.

Welner Z, Reich W, Herjanic B, et al: Reliability, validity and parent-child agreement studies of the Diagnostic Interview for Children and Adolescents. *J Am Acad Child Adolesc Psychiatry* 26:649–653, 1987.

World Health Organization: *The International Pilot Study of Schizophrenia*. Geneva, World Health Organization, 1973.

41 PSYCHOLOGICAL ASSESSMENT OF CHILDREN AND ADOLESCENTS[1]

Gary R. Racusin, Ph.D., and Nancy E. Moss, Ph.D.

Psychological testing conducted by a trained clinical psychologist is a method of obtaining developmentally informed, concrete, and standardized data regarding an individual's capacities and behavior in a wide variety of domains (Allison et al., 1968; Sparrow et al., 1985; Sparrow et al., 1995). The domains that are most pertinent to the assessment of children and adolescents include intellectual ability, educational accomplishment, language skills, visual-motor coordination, adaptive behaviors, and personality functioning (Sparrow et al., 1985).

In clinical practice, psychological assessment constitutes an important type of inpatient or outpatient consultation. Historically, when done as an inpatient procedure, psychological testing has often been part of a comprehensive, multidisciplinary work-up aimed at facilitating long-term treatment. In such circumstances, referral questions may be broad to contribute to the overall understanding of a patient. Test data are typically integrated with findings from other relevant disciplines. While such long-range inpatient treatment is still conducted in some sites, recent developments in national health care practices have reduced dramatically the typical length of inpatient stay. To keep pace with these developments, psychologists in these settings have had to respond with flexible, creative approaches to more time-efficient assessment. Careful choices must be made among the test instruments discussed below to answer highly specific referral questions. More comprehensive psychological assessment often must be deferred until after the patient has been discharged to a less restrictive treatment setting.

While the foundation of inpatient psychological assessment has been modified as noted above, the basic approach to outpatient assessment has remained fairly constant. Therefore, to articulate most clearly the discrete phases of a comprehensive psychological evaluation, this chapter is organized to reflect the typical flow of an outpatient consultation. Accordingly, the chapter first addresses the identification of appropriate referral questions and the preparation of the child or adolescent patient and of the parents. Choice of assessment procedures and instruments along with test administration are then discussed, with emphasis on recent contributions to the test library. This discussion particularly reflects recent activity in the psychoeducational evaluation of Attention Deficit Hyperactivity Disorder and in infant assessment. The chapter then focuses on developments in test interpretation, and concludes with a discussion of issues involved in the communication of findings.

REFERRAL QUESTIONS

To ensure that psychological assessment is most efficacious, the testing should be directed at specific referral questions. Appropriate referral questions facilitate the psychologist's choice of test instruments and, upon analysis of the test data, help to determine which are the relevant issues. When not guided by particular questions, the testing often yields general information that lacks the precision necessary to be of clinical utility. Relevant referral questions are often formulated by the referring clinician. When the referring clinician is uncertain about the focus of the testing, consultation with the psychologist may help to articulate referral questions. For children and adolescents, the referral

questions are also often designated by parents who make direct requests for psychological assessments.

The great variety of suitable referral questions for psychological assessment may be grouped into several areas. First, for the very young child, clinical psychological testing offers answers to pressing questions regarding the progress of development. Many times, parents, pediatricians, educators, and mental health professionals form impressions and concerns about the rate and nature of a youngster's development. Testing compares the individual child to agemates, providing a reliable indicator of developmental level and, thus, permits the substantiation or modification of such assumptions. Such assessment is most useful in the identification of developmental disorders and the sequelae of neurobehavioral insult from sources such as lead poisoning. It also highlights the need for early interventions that may greatly improve an individual's and a family's long-term quality of life.

Second, for the school-age child and adolescent, psychological testing provides a more reliable estimate of intellectual capacity than does clinical impression. Often, a clinical estimate of an individual's intelligence level based on self-presentation can be misleading. Interpersonal behaviors may be confusing or disturbing if they seem discrepant with the individual's apparent level of intelligence. This is particularly true when a youngster's verbal skills are quite different from other intellectual abilities. Intellectual assessment also serves as a foundation on which to base evaluation of other areas of functioning. In this regard, it is important to note that intellectual capacity, as defined by most intelligence measures, is both a global characteristic and the interaction of several specific subdomains. As elaborated upon below in regard to choice of test procedures, each intelligence test is constructed based on a particular characterization of global intelligence and the more specific skills of which it is comprised. While some individuals' intellectual endowment is relatively consistent across these diverse areas, many children display quite striking intellectual strengths and weaknesses. Psychological testing makes a major contribution to clinical care by elucidating the child's strengths and weaknesses and identifying the ways in which they are manifested in behavior.

In clinical work with children and adolescents, it is often most useful to compare and contrast measured intelligence with results of individualized academic achievement testing. Appropriate academic achievement testing samples accomplishments in reading, arithmetic, spelling and written language, and more specialized skill areas as they may pertain to individual patients. Comparison of intellectual with academic test results allows the psychologist to respond to referral questions regarding the presence of learning disabilities. It is to be expected that academic achievement levels will be commensurate with intelligence levels (Kaufman and Kaufman, 1983; Sattler, 1988). When these levels are inconsistent, with academic achievement statistically significantly higher than intellectual levels, it is likely that the individual has expended extreme effort to attain educational goals. It is also possible, although less common, that the individual's true intellectual potential is greater than his/her measured intelligence. In contrast, when academic achievement levels are significantly below intelligence levels, the individual may be considered learning disabled in one or more areas of academic functioning. It is critical to note that diagnosis of a learning disability denotes an inborn information-processing problem requiring particular special

---

[1] See Linda Maye's chapter for further information on developmental assessment.

educational techniques (Kaufman and Kaufman, 1983; Sparrow and Blackman, 1985). In cases of learning disability, psychological test findings form the basis for educational placement and programming recommendations.

Clinical psychological assessment may also respond to questions regarding psychodiagnosis and psychotherapeutic treatment of children and adolescents. Use of projective test materials and projective indicators on other instruments makes it possible to elucidate specific areas of psychopathology to aid in diagnosis. Very specific differential diagnoses can be considered, such as documentation in an adolescent of a thought disorder or affective disorder, or differentiation between psychotic functioning and extreme anxiety in a younger child.

Once diagnosis has been established, psychological assessment can also assist in treatment. Psychological test results can assist in the selection of the type of therapy to be attempted. For example, information regarding the integrity of a child's thought processes would be helpful in determining the appropriate level of the therapist's supportive activity in promoting the child patient's psychological insight (Pine, 1985). For a case in which testing provided assurance of solid, realistic thinking, intensive therapy might be attempted with confidence. In contrast, therapy would best be approached more cautiously and combined with more comprehensive services following testing that indicated frankly compromised reality orientation.

Similarly, test findings may help to predict the course of treatment. Test data about a youngster's degree of relatedness would help to foresee the youngster's likely response to a developing therapeutic alliance. For example, documentation of a youngster's association of intimacy with aggression would prepare a therapist for that youngster's psychological distancing following establishment of a close therapeutic relationship. Test results might also help to address a treatment impasse. Frequently, psychological assessment identifies patient characteristics that were less prominent earlier, attention to which would facilitate progress in an otherwise stalled treatment. Such identification is most helpful in highlighting the severity of disturbances that were previously considered less serious or remained unrecognized.

Psychological testing is also useful to answer very practical questions regarding disposition planning and program eligibility. Many programs designed to meet the special needs of certain children and adolescents, such as classes for the intellectually gifted, services for the retarded, and residential treatment centers, require documentation of need based on psychological assessment results. For children with less unusual needs, psychological test results can also assist with grade placement decisions. With disposition planning in mind, a psychological test battery can be designed efficiently.

PREPARATION OF PATIENT AND PARENTS

For psychological testing to be most useful, the patient should be prepared adequately. With children and adolescents, such preparation typically begins with the parent. When the testing referral comes from another educational or mental health professional, the preparation should be initiated by the referring professional and completed by the psychologist.

The referring professional's preparatory function can be divided into three parts. First, the purpose of the testing should be explained to the parents in a clear, forthright manner. Referral questions should be discussed in nontechnical language so that parents have a good understanding of the need for consultation. Second, the referring clinician should clarify his or her own ongoing relationship with the patient and parents, apart from the work with the testing psychologist. If the referring professional will continue to work with the child and family after the testing, this should be explained. If the testing referral actually constitutes a transfer to the psychologist for care, this, too, should be explained carefully. The usefulness of psychological testing is compromised severely when parents are confused about the psychologist's role in the provision of care. Finally, pragmatic directions should be provided about how to

make contact with the psychologist for the assessment consultation. This sort of direction increases the likelihood that the referral will proceed smoothly.

Preparation of the young patient follows directly from the parent preparation. Parents should be encouraged to share the preparatory information with their youngster (s), presenting information in an honest, open manner appropriate to the child or adolescent's developmental level. In many cases, it is most helpful if the referring clinician assists the parents with this task. Several factors should be emphasized. First, it should be stressed that the testing is being pursued in an effort to provide relevant interpersonal or educational help to the child or adolescent, rather than as a means of being derogatory or punitive. Second, especially with younger children, it is helpful to assure the patient that the psychologist is a "talking doctor" who will not perform any physically invasive procedures. Preparation of the youngster best concludes with assurance that the psychologist will provide complete instructions, guidance, and assistance throughout the assessment.

Even when the patient is well and fully prepared, s/he usually meets the psychologist for the first time with considerable anxiety and asserts that s/he has received no information about the assessment to be completed. As part of establishing the necessary testing rapport, the psychologist should reiterate the preparatory information, instruct the child about testing procedures, and move on to carrying out the assessment. In the great majority of cases, careful preparation and establishment of initial rapport provides sufficient comfort to enable the youngster to cooperate easily in the collection of reliable and valid test data.

TEST ADMINISTRATION

This section reviews salient test procedures, psychometric issues, and examples of commonly utilized assessment instruments for each of the functional domains noted above. While not an exhaustive list, the instruments included are those that the relevant literature and clinical experience have demonstrated to be of value in constructing test batteries that respond to the majority of referral questions for psychological assessment.

Procedures

BATTERY COMPOSITION

Following clarification of the referral question, the child psychologist is faced with the task of making an initial determination as to which instruments will comprise the assessment battery. In rendering this determination, the psychologist must weigh the wish to obtain the most comprehensive possible data with such realistic matters as the need for expeditious completion of the battery, the child's developmental capacity to withstand the rigors of testing, and developmental variables pertaining to the individual child's functioning across domains to be assessed (Goldman et al., 1983; Siegel, 1988). The psychologist then must consider adjusting the battery composition as emerging test data refine the known referral question or suggest new questions (Sattler, 1988). For instance, if a child's performance on screening measures of academic achievement indicate deficits in acquisition of grade-appropriate reading skills, more intensive examination may be required to specify whether the child's deficits are more attributable to problems with reading decoding or reading comprehension.

ADMINISTRATION

The length of time required for a child to complete a test battery depends upon a number of variables, including the complexity of the referral question and the associated number of required test instruments, the child's capacity to sustain work on focused tasks, and the family's cooperativeness in keeping scheduled appointments. As a rule of thumb, experienced psychologists expect that the administration of a comprehensive psychoeducational assessment battery requires from 4–6 sessions of from approximately 60–90 minutes each. Scoring test protocols absorbs an additional 1–2 hours of the psychologist's time.

Because the goal of testing is generally to obtain a picture of the child's maximum capacity, the psychologist must be certain of sufficient rapport to ensure the child's best effort. To accomplish this aim, the examiner employs the clinical skills, used by most clinicians in evaluating children, that serve to allay the child's anxiety and enlist cooperation in completing the tasks at hand. At the same time, however, the psychologist must bear in mind the distinguishing hallmarks of the psychological assessment enterprise, which are the acquisition of data in a structured setting utilizing appropriate standardized measurements (Sparrow et al., 1985). The psychologist must therefore be certain that the establishment of rapport does not violate standardized administration procedures permitting comparison of the child's test performance with those of the normative sample.

Although the principal focus of this chapter is on psychological assessment in outpatient settings, it was noted at the outset that changes in the current health care climate have compelled psychologists working in inpatient settings to address creatively the need for more time-efficient testing that does not sacrifice the integrity of the testing process. In constructing appropriate test batteries in such settings, it is critical to define the limited number of specific questions to be addressed and to confine inferences accordingly. Typically, appropriate questions for testing under these conditions focus on ruling out major intellectual and psychiatric deficits or disorders (e.g., mental retardation and psychosis). A sample battery to fulfill these needs might include five subtests from the Wechsler Intelligence Scale for Children—Third Edition (Wechsler, 1991) (Information, Vocabulary, Similarities, Block Design, and Picture Completion), the Vineland Screener (Sparrow et al., 1994a; Sparrow et al., 1994b), and the Rorschach (Rorschach, 1921). Each of these instruments is discussed below.

Psychometric Issues

An extensive literature exists pertaining to technical and methodological principles associated with psychological assessment (Anastasi, 1988; Sattler, 1988; Sparrow et al., 1984). To judge the utility of assessment instruments, this literature can be distilled to three concepts: validity, reliability, and standardization.

VALIDITY

An instrument's validity concerns the extent to which it measures what it purports to measure. In summarizing the Standards of Educational and Psychological Testing (American Psychological Association, 1985), Anastasi (1988) found that the many methods for determining validity can be organized into three principal groups. An instrument possesses content-related validity to the extent that its item content covers a representative sample of the measured domain, a validation issue typically considered in evaluating achievement tests (Anastasi, 1988). If an instrument is effective in predicting an individual's performance in specified activities, it is said to possess criterion-related validity. This form of validity is determined by checking test performance against a direct and independent criterion measure of that which the test is supposed to measure, for instance by comparing scholastic aptitude test scores with grades obtained in college. Finally, a test's construct-related validity refers to the test's capacity to measure a theoretical construct upon which the test is based. Derived from documented interrelationships among behavioral measures, this form of validation requires the accumulation of a variety of types of information, including correlations with other tests and statistical techniques such as factor analysis and measurements of the test's internal consistency.

RELIABILITY

An instrument's reliability refers to the degree to which results obtained from the instrument can be reproduced within acceptable levels

of agreement. The most commonly required measures of consistency for a psychological test are that its scores can be reproduced over time (test-retest reliability) and across examiners (interrater reliability). An additional estimate of reliability that is frequently reported is "interitem consistency," or the consistency of responses to all items in the test (Anastasi, 1988). This form of reliability provides information about the degree of homogeneity of the domain which the test is purported to sample, and is typically reported in the form of reliability coefficients (either the Kuder-Richardson coefficient for dichotomous responses or Cronbach's coefficient alpha for continuous responses) (Cronbach, 1951; Kuder, 1937; Novick and Lewis, 1967).

STANDARDIZATION

To be well standardized, an instrument should be pretested on a large demographically representative sample of subjects. Comparison of a given child's performance on a test with an appropriate standardization group can occur only if such standardization has been conducted (Sparrow et al., 1985). Such comparisons provide a context for understanding the child's test performance from a developmentally-informed perspective, permitting more powerful inferences about strengths or deficits documented in the child's testing.

Commonly Utilized Assessment Instruments

The tests presented in this section (Table 41.1) are organized according to the functional domain assessed (i.e., intellectual ability, academic achievement, visual-motor functioning, adaptive behavior, attentional capacity, personality organization, neuropsychological functioning, and developmental status). The discussion of each test includes a description of its purpose, format, and appropriate subjects, as well as commentary about the types of scores derived, administration time, psychometric properties and unique features.

MEASURES OF INTELLECTUAL ABILITY

Wechsler Intelligence Scale for Children—Third Edition (WISC-III) (Wechsler, 1991). Like its two predecessors, the original WISC (Wechsler, 1949) and the WISC-R (Wechsler, 1974), the WISC-III is a downward extension of adult intelligence scales. In its new revision published in 1991, it remains the most widely used individually-administered intelligence test for children in the age range for which it was designed, six years to 16 years, 11 months. The WISC-III provides several welcome improvements, including updated and more culturally sensitive test items, more user-friendly materials (such as larger color, as opposed to black-and-white, stimulus cards for the Picture Arrangement subtest), and a restandardization providing more contemporary and psychometrically sound norms and standard scores. The WISC-III consists of 13 subtests divided into a six-subtest Verbal scale and a seven-subtest Performance scale (for a description of the 12 subtests retained from the WISC-R and capacities tapped by each, see Sattler, 1988). The Verbal Scale is comprised of the Information, Similarities, Arithmetic, Vocabulary, Comprehension, and Digit Span subtests, and the Performance Scale includes the Picture Completion, Picture Arrangement, Block Design, Object Assembly, Coding, Symbol Search, and Mazes subtests. Symbol Search is a new subtest developed for the WISC-III and is designed to measure processing speed. Administration time for the total instrument is approximately 60–90 minutes.

The instrument was constructed on the notion that intelligence may be defined as an individual's overall capacity to understand and cope with the world (Wechsler, 1991). The author emphasizes that this definition requires an assessment instrument that appreciates the global nature of intelligence, and that avoids placing undue emphasis on any one ability in assessing overall intellectual capacity. The subtest tasks therefore attempt to challenge a child's abilities in a broad variety of ways so as to provide a fuller estimate of capacity. Tasks require children to answer verbal queries and work several types of visual or visual-motor puzzles.

Table 41.1. Commonly Used Child and Adolescent Psychological Assessment Instruments

Test	Age/Grades	Comments and Data Generated
	Intellectual Ability	
Wechsler Intelligence Scale for Children—Third Edition (WISC-III) (Psychological Corporation)	6–16	Standard scores: verbal, performance and full scale IQ; scaled subtest scores permitting specific skill assessment.
Wechsler Adult Intelligence Scale—Revised (WAIS-R) (Psychological Corporation)	16–adult	Same as WISC-III
Wechsler Preschool and Primary Scale of Intelligence—Revised (WPPSI-R) (Psychological Corporation)	3–7	Same as WISC-III
McCarthy Scales of Children's Abilities (MSCA) (Psychological Corporation)	2.6–8	Scores: General Cognitive Index (IQ equivalent); language, perceptual performance, quantitative memory and motor domain scores; percentiles.
Kaufman Assessment Battery for Children (K-ABC) (American Guidance Service)	2.6–12.6	Well grounded in theories of cognitive psychology and neuropsychology. Allows immediate comparison of intellectual capacity with acquired knowlege. Scores: Mental Processing Composite (IQ equivalent); sequential and simultaneous processing and achievement standard scores; scaled mental processing and achievement subtest scores; age equivalents; percentiles.
Kaufman Adolescent and Adult Intelligence Test (KAIT)	11–85+	Composed of separate Crystallized and Fluid scales. Scores: Composite Intelligence Scale; Crystallized and Fluid IQs; scaled subtest scores; percentiles.
Stanford-Binet, 4th Edition (SB:FE) (Riverside Publishing Company)	2–23	Scores: IQ; verbal, abstract/visual, and quantitative reasoning; short-term memory; standard age.
Peabody Picture Vocabulary Test—Revised (PPVT-R) (American Guidance Service)	4–adult	Measures receptive vocabulary acquisition. Standard scores, percentiles, age equivalents.
	Achievement	
Woodcock-Johnson Psycho-Educational Battery—Revised (W-J) (DLM Teaching Resources)	K–12	Scores: reading and mathematics (mechanics and comprehension), written language, other academic achievement; grade and age scores, standard scores, percentiles
Wide Range Achievement Test—Revised, Levels 1 and 2 (WRAT-R) (Jastak Associates)	Level 1: 5–1 Level 2: 12–75	Permits screening for deficits in reading, spelling and arithmetic; grade levels, percentiles, stanines, standard scores.
Kaufman Test of Educational Achievement, Brief and Comprehensive Forms (K-TEA) (American Guidance Service)	1–12	Standard scores: reading, mathematics and spelling; grade and age equivalents, percentiles, stanines. Brief Form is sufficient for most clinical applications; Comprehensive Form allows error analysis and more detailed curriculum planning.
Wechsler Individual Achievement Test (WIAT) (Psychological Corporation)	K–12	Standard scores: basic reading, mathematics reasoning, spelling (constituting Screener); reading comprehension, numerical operations, listening comprehension, oral expression, written expression. Conormal with WISC-III.
	Adaptive Behavior	
Vineland Adaptive Behaivor Scales (American Guidance Service)	Normal: 0–19 Retarded: All ages	Standard scores: adaptive behavior composite and communication, daily living skills, socialization and motor domains; percentiles, age equivalents, developmental age scores. Separate standardization groups for normal, visually-handicapped, hearing impaired, emotionally disturbed and retarded.
Scales of Independent Behavior (DLM Teaching Resources)	Newborn–adult	Standard Scores: four adaptive (motor, social interaction, communication, personal living, community living) and three maladaptive (internalized, asocial, and externalized) areas; General Maladaptive Index and Broad Independence cluster.
	Attentional Capacity	
Controlled Word Association Test (Benton and Hamsher, 1978)	6–adult	Standard scores, standard deviations, percentiles, descriptive classifications.
Trail Making Test (Reitan, 1971)	8–adult	Standard scores, standard deviations, ranges; corrections for age and education.
Wisconsin Card Sorting Test (Berg, 1948; Grant and Berg, 1948)	6.6–adult	Standard scores, standard deviations, T-scores, percentiles; developmental norms for number of categories achieved, perseverative errors, and failures to maintain set.
Behavior Assessment System for Children (BASC) (American Guidance Service, 1992).	4–18	Teacher and parent rating scales and child self-report of personality permitting multireporter assessment across a variety of domains in home, school and community. Provides validity, clinical, and adaptive scales.
Home Situations Questionnaire-Revised (HSQ-R) (DuPaul, 1990)	6–12	Permits parents to rate child's specific problems with attention or concentration. Scores for number of problem settings, mean severity, and factor scores for compliance and leisure situations.
ADHD Rating Scale (DuPaul, 1990)	6–12	Score for number of symptoms keyed to DSM cutoff for diagnosis of ADHD; standard scores permit derivation of clinical significance for total score and two factors (Inattentive-Hyperactive and Impulsive-Hyperactive).
School Situations Questionnaire (SSQ-R) (DuPaul, 1990)	6–12	Permits teachers to rate a child's specific problems with attention or concentration. Scores for number of problem settings and mean severity.
Child Attention Profile (CAP) (Edelbrock, 1991)	6–12	Brief measure allowing teachers' weekly ratings of presence and degree of child's inattention and overactivity. Normative scores for inattention, overactivity, and total score.

(continued)

Table 41.1.—*(continued)*

Test	Age/Grades	Comments and Data Generated
Projective Tests		
Rorschach Inkblots (Huber, Haus; U.S. Distrib.: Grune and Stratton)	3–adult	Special scoring systems. Most recently developed and increasingly universally accepted is Exner's Comprehensive System (1974). Assesses perceptual accuracy, integration of affective and intellectual functioning, reality testing, and other psychological processes.
Thematic Apperception Test (TAT) (Harvard University Press)	6–adult	Generates stories which are analyzed qualitatively. Assumed to provide especially rich data regarding interpersonal functioning.
Machover Draw-A-Person Test (DAP) (Charles C Thomas)	3–adult	Qualitative analysis and hypothesis generation, especially regarding subject's feelings about self and significant others.
Kinetic Family Drawing (KFD) (Brunner/Mazel)	3–adult	Qualitative analysis and hypothesis generation regarding an individual's perception of family structure and sentient environment. Some objective scoring systems in existence.
Rotter Incomplete Sentences Blank (Psychological Corporation)	Child, adolescent and adult forms	Primarily qualitative analysis, although some objective scoring systems have been developed.
Personality Tests		
Minnesota Multiphasic Personality Inventory-Adolescent (MMPI-A) (U. of Minnesota Press)	14–18	1992 version of widely used personality measure, developed specifically for use with adolescents. Standard scores: 3 validity scales, 14 clinical scales, additonal content and supplementary scales.
Millon Adolescent Personality Inventory (MAPI) (National Computer Systems)	13–18	Standard scores for 20 scales grouped into three categories: Personality Styles, Expressed Concerns, Behavioral Correlates. Normed on adolescent population. Focuses on broad functional spectrum, not just problem areas.
Children's Personality Questionnaire (Institute for Personality and Ability Testing)	8–12	Measures 14 primary personality traits, including emotional stability, self-concept level, excitability, and self-assurance. Generates combined broad trait patterns including extraversion and anxiety.
Neuropsychological Screening Tests and Test Batteries		
Developmental Test of Visual-Motor Integration (VMI) (Modern Currciulum Press)	2–16	Screening instrument for visual motor deficits. Standard scores, age equivalents, percentiles.
Benton Visual Retention Test (Psychological Corporation)	6–adult	Assesses presence of deficits in visual-figure memory. Mean scores by age.
Bender Visual Motor Gestalt Test	5–adult	Assesses visual-motor deficits and visual-figural retention. Age equivalents.
Reitan-Indiana Neuropsychological Test Battery for Children	5–8	Cognitive and perceptual-motor tests for children with suspected brain damage.
Halstead-Reitan Neuropsychological Test Battery for Older Children	9–14	Same as Reitan-Indiana
Luria-Nebraska Neuropsychological Battery: Children's Revision LNNB:C	8–12	Sensory-motor, perceptual, cognitive tests measuring 11 clinical and 2 additional domains of neuropsychological functioning. Provides standard scores.
Developmental Status		
Bayley Scales of Infant Development-Second Edition	16 days–42 months	Mental, motor, and behavior scales measuring infant, development. Provides standard scores.
Mullen Scales of Early Learning	Newborn–5 years	Language and visual scales for receptive and expressive ability. Yields age scores and T scores.

The test generates Full Scale, Verbal and Performance IQ scores, individual subtest scaled scores, and test-age equivalents. Factor analytic research has been conducted and summarized in the manual (Wechsler, 1991) revealing four principal factorial underpinnings of the WISC-III: Verbal Comprehension (Information, Similarities, Vocabulary, and Comprehension), Perceptual Organization (Picture Completion, Picture Arrangement, Block Design, and Object Assembly), Freedom from Distractibility (Arithmetic and Digit Span), and Processing Speed (Coding and Symbol Search). To facilitate scoring and interpretation, the WISC-III provides easy computation of Index Scores for each of these factors.

Interpretation of the test protocol requires several levels of analysis (Kaufman, 1979; Sattler, 1988), including placing of the global IQ scores into ranges of intellectual functioning (Table 41.2), calculating the significance of any difference between Verbal and Performance IQ scores, comparing the Verbal Comprehension, Perceptual Organization, Freedom from Distractibility, and Processing Speed index scores, determining the presence of significant individual relative subtest strengths and weaknesses, conducting comparisons of individual subtest scores, and appreciation of the quality of individual item responses. This approach to profile analysis permits generation of hypotheses about cognitive strengths and weaknesses based on statistically significant differences between scores.

The psychometric properties of the WISC-R have been extensively researched, and this research base provides a foundation for the psychometrics of the WISC-III. Reliability is reportedly outstanding (Sattler, 1988; Wechsler, 1974; Wechsler, 1991), with steadily strong internal consistency reliability coefficients (Sattler, 1988; Wechsler, 1974). Sattler (1988) has also summarized the plethora of research studies which, collectively, document the instrument's satisfactory concurrent, criterion, and construct validities.

Wechsler Adult Intelligence Scale—Revised (WAIS-R) (Wechsler, 1981). As noted above, the WISC-III represents a downward extension

Table 41.2. Commonly Used Intelligence Classification

Standard Score	Level
130+	Very superior
120–129	Superior
110–119	High average
90–109	Average
80–89	Low average
70–79	Borderline
50–69	Mild retardation
40–49	Moderate retardation
20–39	Severe retardation
Below 20	Profound retardation

of Wechsler's theories of assessing adult intelligence. The most recent revision of the adult instrument is the WAIS-R, published in 1981, 26 years after its immediate predecessor, the WAIS (Wechsler, 1955). The theoretical underpinnings and structure of the instrument are virtually identical to that of the WISC-III, with the exception that there are only 11 subtests as opposed to the 13 WISC-III subtests (Mazes and Symbol Search are not included on the WAIS-R). The procedure for analyzing the test profile is identical to that described above for the WISC-III. Similar to the WISC-III, the WAIS-R has been the subject of extensive investigations of its reliability, validity, and standardization, and receives very high marks for its psychometric properties (Anastasi, 1988; Sattler, 1988; Wechsler, 1981).

The WAIS-R is appropriate for use with individuals between the ages of 16 years and 74 years, 11 months. This instrument may therefore be employed in testing adolescents above the age of 15. The age ranges of the WISC-III and WAIS-R overlap between the ages of 16 years and 16 years, 11 months. Sattler (1988) states that a more thorough sampling of ability can be obtained with the children's instrument when it is used with children of below-normal ability in the overlapping age range. For normal and gifted children, however, both instruments provide adequate sampling.

Wechsler Preschool and Primary Scale of Intelligence—Revised (WPPSI-R) (Wechsler, 1987).   Published in 1989, the WPPSI-R is a revision of the original Wechsler Preschool and Primary Scale of Intelligence (WPPSI) (Wechsler, 1967), a further downward extension of the Wechsler scales for use with children between the ages of 3 years and 7 years, 3 months. Several significant improvements have been incorporated in the revision to address concerns and limitations raised about its predecessor. For instance, the WPPSI-R age range represents an extension of approximately 1 year both upward and downward. To provide greater comparability to the WISC-III, the WPPSI-R adds a 12th subtest (Object Assembly) to the WPPSI's 11. Eight of the subtests (Information, Vocabulary, Arithmetic, Similarities, Comprehension, Picture Completion, Mazes, and Block Design) are also found on the WISC-III, while 3 subtests (Sentences, Animal House, and Geometric Design) were developed exclusively for the WPPSI and have been retained in the revision. New items and changes in design intended to enhance interest among young children have made the revision more user-friendly. In the tradition of the other Wechsler scales, the WPPSI and WPPSI-R possess well-documented reliability and validity and were standardized adequately (Anastasi, 1988; Sattler, 1988; Sparrow et al., 1985; Wechsler, 1967; Wechsler, 1987). The interpretation of results follows the same course as noted above.

McCarthy Scales of Children's Abilities (MSCA) (McCarthy, 1972).   As noted by Kaufman and Kaufman (1977), the MSCA is a welcome instrument appropriate for the assessment of children between the ages of 2 years, 6 months and 8 years, 6 months. Its 18 subtests are clustered into 5 domains (Verbal, Perceptual-Performance, Quantitative, Memory, and Motor), and also allow for the calculation of a General Cognitive Index, which serves as the equivalent of the Full Scale IQ on the Wechsler scales. Administration time is approximately 45–60 minutes depending on the subject's age. Particular advantages of the MSCA are its fine standardization and psychometrics, ease and enjoyableness of administration for both examiner and subject, and direct measurement of fine and gross motor skills and acquisition of eye, hand, and leg dominance, which are of particular importance in this age-group (Sparrow et al., 1985; Sattler, 1988). The MSCA does not include tasks tapping social judgment. To compensate for this shortcoming, Kaufman and Kaufman (1977; 1983) encourage administration of the appropriate subtest of the WPPSI-R or WISC-III.

Kaufman Assessment Battery for Children (K-ABC) (Kaufman and Kaufman, 1983).   The K-ABC measures the cognitive abilities of children between the ages of 2 years, 6 months and 12 years, 5 months. The K-ABC differs from other assessment instruments in its purpose and its theoretical basis. The test attempts to distinguish between a child's acquired knowledge (Achievement) and intellectual capacity as understood from the perspective of cognitive processing abilities. The K-ABC is firmly rooted in theories of cognitive psychology and neuropsychology, which posit that intelligence should be understood in terms of a child's relative facility in processing simultaneously- or sequentially-presented information. The processing of these different forms of information is understood to require different cognitive styles and to draw from different lateralized hemispheric brain functions, with sequential processing primarily associated with left-brain functioning and simultaneous processing with activities in the right hemisphere. Reliability levels are highly acceptable and numerous validation studies have appeared in print. The standardization sample closely matched 1980 U.S. census data for age, gender, race, geographic region, community size, and socioeconomic status.

The K-ABC requires approximately 45–75 minutes of administration time. Its 10 mental processing subtests are divided into Sequential Processing (Hand Movements, Number Recall and Word Order) and Simultaneous Processing (Magic Window, Face Recognition, Gestalt Closure, Triangles, Matrix Analogies, Spatial Memory, and Photo Series) Scales. A Mental Processing Composite score can be derived from these subtest scores that is equivalent to a Full Scale IQ score on the Wechsler scales. Six subtests (Expressive Vocabulary, Faces and Places, Arithmetic, Riddles, Reading/Decoding and Reading/Understanding) contribute to the Achievement Scale. The number of subtests administered varies according to the child's age.

Clinical experience indicates that because of its Mental Processing and Achievement scale construction, the K-ABC provides an efficient means of comparing a child's intellectual capacity and level of academic achievement, a comparison at the core of assessment of learning disability. On the other hand, although research has suggested possibilities for richer profile interpretation (Kamphaus and Reynolds, 1987), K-ABC profile interpretation does not possess the same heuristic value as the Wechsler scales to generate hypotheses about the interplay between intrapsychic conflict and selective ego deficits. Additionally, critics have labelled the distinction between mental processing ability and acquired knowledge faulty because of the test's artificial distinction between the ways in which children acquire and process information (Sattler, 1988).

Kaufman Adolescent and Adult Intelligence Test (KAIT) (Kaufman and Kaufman, 1993).   As outlined in an interview with Alan Kaufman presented in Kamphaus' *Clinical Assessment of Children's Intelligence* (Kamphaus, 1993), the KAIT is a recently published instrument that derives its theoretical foundation from three sources: the Cattell-Horn theory of fluid and crystallized intelligence; Piaget's concept of formal operational thinking; and Luria and Golden's articulation of the planning functions of the prefrontal lobes. The Cattell-Horn theory is the primary of these three sources, and guides the test's organization into Fluid and Crystallized scales. These scales measure novel problem-solving skills and knowledge derived from acculturation and education, respectively. This theoretical construction is developmentally informed and has received strong empirical support, as research has consistently demonstrated that crystallized skills are maintained throughout the life span while fluid skills plummet after peaking in young adulthood. As was true of the Kaufmans' other published tests, the KAIT was well standardized and reports very strong reliability coefficients. Additionally, the authors report construct validity through correlations with other commonly used intelligence tests (WISC-R, WAIS-R, K-ABC), and through studies with a variety of adult clinical populations.

The KAIT was designed to be administered efficiently, requiring only 60 minutes for its Core Battery of 6 subtests. An Expanded Battery, including 4 additional subtests, can be used for further clinical or neuropsychological assessment, and customized assessment can be obtained by selecting from among any or all of these additional subtests. The Core Battery's three-subtest Fluid Scale consists of Rebus Learning, Mystery Codes, and Logical Steps, and the Crystallized Scale is comprised of Auditory Comprehension, Double Meanings, and Definitions. The Expanded Battery subtests are Memory For Block Design, Famous

Faces, Rebus Recall, and Auditory Recall. The ten subtests provide age-based scaled scores, and global IQ scores are generated for the Fluid Scale, Crystallized Scale, and Composite Intelligence.

Preliminary clinical experience with the KAIT indicates that the instrument is challenging to both administrator and subject, and should not be administered without substantial practice on the part of the examiner. Test items often prove difficult for adolescents with less intellectual ability, and examiners may wish to administer another instrument in conjunction with the KAIT in order to be most confident of test findings.

Stanford-Binet Intelligence Scale: Fourth Edition (SB:FE) (Thorndike et al., 1986). The SB:FE represents the latest revision of an instrument whose modern history dates back to 1916, and whose roots extend back to at least 1905. This version represents a significant departure from the 1937 Forms L and M and the 1960 Form L-M, for which revised norms were provided in 1972. A three-level theoretical model guided the construction of the instrument, postulating a general intelligence factor (*g*) at the highest level of inference; a second level of factors, including crystallized, fluid, and short-term memory; and a final level comprising more specific factors such as verbal, quantitative, and abstract visual reasoning. Traditionally, a major advantage of the Stanford-Binet has been its broad age range, permitting more accurate assessment of individuals functioning at either extremely low or high cognitive levels. A significant criticism of the SB:FE is its lack of a comparable battery throughout the scale's age range, meaning that scores obtained by children at different ages are based on different subtest combinations (Sattler, 1988).

Administration time for the SB:FE may be quite long, in some cases exceeding 2 hours, because the instrument includes only 1 timed subtest. This is a significant drawback for utilization of the test. The 15 subtests of the SB:FE are divided into 4 larger areas: Verbal Reasoning (consisting of the Vocabulary, Comprehension, Absurdities, and Verbal Relations subtests); Abstract/Visual Reasoning (Pattern Analysis, Copying, Matrices, and Paper Folding and Cutting); Quantitative Reasoning (Quantitative, Number Series, and Equation Building); and Short-Term Memory (Bead Memory, Memory for Sentences, Memory for Digits, and Memory for Objects). Standard scores are generated for the subtests, the 4 areas, and a Composite Score similar to the Wechsler IQ score. Because later factor analytic studies did not support the original factorial structure of the test, Sattler (1988) has suggested an alternate, more valid set of factor scores and means of computation. The psychometric properties of the test are very good, with excellent reported reliability. The SB:FE was well standardized on a population similar to that of the 1980 U.S. census, and weighting procedures were utilized to assure maximum conformity to census data. A large number of validation studies summarized by Sattler (1988) conclude that the SB:FE and the Wechsler scales yield similar scores for subjects in the average range of cognitive functioning, but that the SB:FE may produce lower scores for gifted or mentally retarded subjects. Because of the limitations noted, clinical experience suggests that the employment of other instruments (Wechsler scales, McCarthy Scales and K-ABC) be ruled out before utilizing the SB:FE.

Peabody Picture Vocabulary Test—Revised (PPVT-R) (Dunn and Dunn, 1981). The PPVT-R provides a rapid assessment of receptive vocabulary acquisition in individuals from age 30 months through adulthood. The instrument is very well standardized, reliable, and valid (Sparrow et al., 1985). Two alternate forms (L and M) are available, each consisting of 175 plates that are displayed consecutively to the subject on a small desktop easel. Each plate contains 4 pictures, and the subject is instructed to either point out or announce the number of the picture that portrays the vocabulary word read by the examiner.

When used in conjunction with the WISC-R Vocabulary subtest, which assesses expressive vocabulary skills, the PPVT-R provides a more rounded view of an individual's vocabulary acquisition. Because of its short administration time and high correlation with the WISC-R, it has often been employed for research purposes as a screening measure of children's cognitive abilities (Sparrow et al., 1985). This practice has been discouraged more recently, however (Sattler, 1988), presumably because of the limitations inherent in relying on vocabulary skills as an indicator of overall intellectual capacity, and other instruments (e.g., Kaufman Brief Intelligence Test; Kaufman and Kaufman, 1990) have been developed for such research uses. Similar to the VMI and Bender-Gestalt, the PPVT-R serves as a fine "ice-breaker" in an assessment battery because of the limited demands for responsiveness placed upon the child.

MEASURES OF ACADEMIC ACHIEVEMENT

Woodcock-Johnson Psycho-Educational Battery—Revised (Woodcock and Johnson, 1989). The revised form of the Woodcock-Johnson Battery was published in 1989. The revision offered organizational, procedural, psychometric, and scoring improvements as well as new subtests. Although this revised version, like the original Woodcock-Johnson Battery, was published to provide an estimate of both intellectual capacity and academic achievement, it is not currently viewed as a major competitor with the cognitive assessment instruments listed above (Sattler, 1988). Rather, the Tests of Achievement comprising Part II of the Battery are more commonly utilized to estimate levels of scholastic accomplishment. The Achievement section of the battery measures reading decoding and comprehension skills, math reasoning and calculation skills, written language skills, as well as knowledge of specific subject areas (Science, Social Studies, and Humanities). In clinical practice, most extensive use is made of the Reading, Mathematics, and Written Language Clusters. Although efficient to administer, the instrument is cumbersome to score and, for many psychoeducational purposes, has been supplanted by the Kaufman Test of Educational Achievement and/or the Wechsler Individual Achievement Test (see below).

Wide Range Achievement Test—Revised, Levels 1 and 2 (WRAT-R) (Jastak and Wilkinson, 1984). The WRAT-R and its predecessor, the WRAT, have been used for many years as brief screening instruments for identifying academic skills deficits (Anastasi, 1988; Sattler, 1988). A newer version, the WRAT-III, appeared too late for review in this chapter. The WRAT-R is better standardized than the earlier version, thus addressing a major criticism of the instrument. In the new version, Level 1 is appropriate for children between the ages of 5 and 11, and Level 2 is used with individuals aged 12 through 75. Administration time is approximately 20 minutes. Because of its brevity, however, some academic domains receive shorter shrift (e.g., there is no measure of reading comprehension). The WRAT-R is best used when administration time is a critical factor.

Kaufman Test of Educational Achievement, Brief and Comprehensive Forms (K-TEA) (Kaufman and Kaufman, 1985). The K-TEA is a well-standardized screening instrument for assessing academic achievement in children aged 5 through 18. It is easy to administer and score, and takes approximately 30 minutes to complete. Five subtests are included: Reading Decoding, Reading Comprehension, Mathematics Applications, Mathematics Computation, and Spelling. The Comprehensive Form provides a systematic approach for evaluating errors, which is of potential use to clinicians interested in devising curricular interventions to address skills deficits but which is also cumbersome for most examiners. The Brief Form, with a reduced item sample, is appropriate for most psychoeducational applications. Because it provides data about a child's functioning across domains of most general interest, possesses a reasonable item sample and good psychometric properties, and is easy to administer and score, the K-TEA has proven to be the academic achievement screening instrument of choice for children in its age range, especially when used in conjunction with the MSCA or the appropriate Wechsler scale. Although there is some overlap of items between the K-TEA and the Achievement section of the K-TEA, each test does make a unique contribution to the assessment of a child's level of educational accomplishment. For instance, the K-TEA Reading subtest provides a wide range of item difficulty, permitting a more refined assessment of reading skills. On the other hand, the K-ABC Faces & Places and Riddles subtests assess aspects of acquired knowledge not tapped by the K-TEA.

Wechsler Individual Achievement Test (WIAT) (Wechsler, 1992). A recent addition to the available library for the individual assessment of academic achievement, the WIAT was designed to accompany the Wechsler intelligence scales. The instrument was developed for use with children in kindergarten through grade 12, and aged 5 years through 19 years, 11 months. The test requires approximately 30–60 minutes to administer the comprehensive battery, depending on age, although a briefer core battery can be administered as a screening instrument in approximately 15 minutes. The WIAT is well standardized, and has the advantage of being conormed on the populations used to standardize the Wechsler intelligence scales, thus enhancing the psychologist's confidence in inferring discrepancies between intellectual ability and level of achievement. The Screener comprises 3 subtests: Basic Reading, Mathematics Reasoning, and Spelling. In conjunction with these 3 subtests, 5 additional subtests are included in the Comprehensive Battery: Reading Comprehension, Numerical Operations, Listening Comprehension, Oral Expression, and Written Expression. The latter 3 subtests provide welcome data not typically available in academic achievement tests, permitting a richer sample of a child's receptive, expressive, and written language functioning that may be contributing to academic performance deficits. Because of these unique aspects and its conorming with the most commonly utilized intelligence tests (the Wechsler scales), the WIAT has become a significant alternative to the K-TEA.

MEASURES OF ADAPTIVE BEHAVIOR

Vineland Adaptive Behavior Scales (Sparrow et al., 1984). A revision of the Vineland Social Maturity Scale (Doll, 1965), the Vineland Adaptive Behavior Scales assess an individual's personal and social sufficiency. A semistructured interview is conducted by a trained examiner with a respondent familiar with the subject. Four functional domains are assessed: Communication, Daily Living Skills, Socialization, and Motor Skills (up to age 4 years, 11 months). Domain scores in turn generate an Adaptive Behavior Composite. An additional checklist taps behaviors typically construed as maladaptive. There are 3 forms of the instrument: Survey Form, Expanded Form, and Classroom Edition. The Survey Form contains approximately half the items of the Expanded Form, requires approximately 1 hour to administer, and has proved sufficient for the purposes of most clinicians. The Expanded Form divides many of the skills on the Survey Form into discrete steps to be mastered and thus offers valuable programming assistance for work with low-functioning individuals. The Classroom Edition is designed to be completed by a child's teacher in approximately 20 minutes, and does not require an interview with the teacher. The strongest criticism levelled to date against the Vineland is that there is apparently substantial fluctuation of means and standard deviations across age groups, thus limiting the extent to which the instrument can be used for longitudinal comparisons (Silverstein, 1986). In clinical practice, however, the scales have proved to provide an excellent estimate of adaptive behavior, which is of significant value in developing a fuller picture of a child's psychosocial functioning. As development of the *Diagnostic and Statistical Manual of Mental Disorders* proceeds toward publication of DSM-V, it is anticipated that assessment of adaptive functioning will become even more central in psychiatric diagnosis. Thus, it should be expected that the utility of the Vineland in clinical practice will increase.

With this anticipated increase in demand in mind, and to meet current demands for expedited assessment, the Vineland Screener was developed (Sparrow et al., 1994a; Sparrow et al., 1994b). Although aimed at research needs with large subject pools, the Screener's high correlation with the full Vineland and clinical requirements have led to its increasing use in clinical settings as well. The Screener is administered in the same semistructured interview format as the Survey and Expanded forms of the Vineland. Key items have been selected from the full instrument to allow for speedier administration. Screener raw scores are then equated

with raw scores on a fuller version of the Vineland to serve as the basis for the calculation of derived scores. Although in use for a relatively short period, the Vineland Screener has demonstrated its usefulness both in research and in inpatient treatment settings, where accommodation to shortened hospitalizations has become mandatory.

Scales of Independent Behavior (SIB) (Bruininks et al., 1984). The SIB is an individually-administered measure of the personal and social sufficiency of individuals across a broad age range. As opposed to the Vineland, it is not administered via a semistructured interview and permits estimates of the adaptive behavior functioning of nonretarded adults. In most cases, data is collected from an informant, but the individual being assessed may also serve as the respondent. The SIB was developed to be used in conjunction with the Woodcock-Johnson Broad Cognitive Ability cluster score to provide an efficient estimate of both adaptive ability and intellectual capacity. Research questioning the validity of the Cluster score (Sattler, 1988), however, requires that clinicians proceed with caution in using these two instruments for the purposes advocated by the authors. The SIB consists of 14 subtests that produce 4 adaptive behavior (Motor, Social Interaction and Communication, Personal Living, and Community Living) and 3 maladaptive behavior (Internalized, Asocial, and Externalized) clusters. The adaptive behavior clusters, in turn, generate a Broad Independence summary cluster score. The full SIB requires approximately 1 hour of administration time, but a 15-minute Short Form has also been developed.

MEASURES OF ATTENTION AND CONCENTRATION

Most recently, increased research and clinical attention has been aimed at gaining a more comprehensive understanding of Attention Deficit Hyperactivity Disorder (ADHD). The Fourth Edition of the *Diagnostic and Statistical Manual of Mental Disorders* (American Psychiatric Association, 1994) summarizes much of the current thinking about this multifaceted disorder.

Advancement in knowledge about this disorder has been accompanied by a need for psychological test data to assist with differential diagnosis. Often, clinical psychologists have relied on indicators embedded in a traditional test battery to help confirm or rule out the diagnosis of ADHD. Such indicators have included behavioral observations in the test setting, Hand Movements performance on the K-ABC, Digit Span scores on the WISC-R and, more recently, the Freedom from Distractibility Scale on the WISC-III. More currently, however, a cluster of instruments has been developed that can allow for more direct determination of the accuracy of the ADHD diagnosis. The rationale for administering a variety of instruments is to ascertain the subject's capacity to marshall attention and concentration in response to stimuli presented through different sensory input modes and requiring different forms of response. This cluster should be administered and interpreted as part of a standard, thorough, psychoeducational assessment. Findings of attentional difficulty should be used to place a child accurately in an attentional, behavioral, academic, or emotional diagnostic category, or to make the diagnosis of comorbid difficulties.

Given that ADHD is a difficulty in attending to a focused task on demand amidst competing stimuli, it should not be surprising if ADHD symptoms do not manifest in the controlled atmosphere of the psychologist's office. Accordingly, in addition to direct evaluation of the child or adolescent, data must be gathered from multiple observers in settings where the child encounters situational demands that make the emergence of ADHD symptoms more probable. To accomplish this task, relevant instruments can be administered to parents, teachers, and the identified child or adolescent. These instruments are discussed below, organized according to informant/subject involved.

Child/Adolescent

Controlled Word Association Test (Benton and Hamsher, 1978). This test was designed originally as part of the Benton Battery, and was used for assessment of aphasia. In a 1-minute period, the subject is required to say as many acceptable words as possible beginning with a specified letter, i.e., /F/, /A/, or /S/. Successful completion requires continued attention. Average response scores are tabulated for each of the 3 specified letters and for the test as a whole. Normative data is available for children and adolescents (Gaddes and Crockett, 1975). Percentile scores can be calculated. To make valid interpretations of attentional capacity on this test, accurate information must also be available about the subject's level of knowledge about letter-sound combinations.

Trail Making Test (Reitan, 1971).   Derived from the Army Individual Test Battery (1944) and revised by Reitan (1971), this is a widely used and popular instrument requiring the subject to connect a series of numbered circles in Part A and a series of alternating numbers and letters in Part B under timed conditions. Most pertinent to assessment of ADHD, the test requires sustained concentration for successful completion. Normative information is available in the neuropsychological literature (Spreen and Gaddes, 1969), including means, standard deviations, medians, and score ranges.

Wisconsin Card Sorting Test (Berg, 1948; Grant and Berg, 1948).   Designed originally in the 1940s and modified in the 1980s (Heaton, 1981), this test requires the subject to sort given cards into appropriate piles. The criteria for proper assignment must be determined by the subject using feedback provided either by the examiner directly or by a computer program. Attention to relevant card attributes, sustained concentration, and mental flexibility are all essential for successful task completion. Percentiles, T scores, and standard scores may all be derived from the raw scores.

Computerized Tests.   Assessment of a child's or adolescent's ability to maintain attention and concentration on a somewhat monotonous, continuous performance task is helpful in the diagnosis of ADHD. Such computerized tests as VIGIL (Cegalis and Volin, 1991) and PASAT (Cegalis and Birdsall, 1992) are appropriate choices for this purpose.

Parent

Behavior Assessment System for Children (BASC)—Parent Rating Scales (Reynolds and Kamphaus, 1992).   A relatively new addition to the collection of instruments available for assessment of childhood behavior, the BASC offers a comprehensive, structured assessment of a child's behavioral functioning across a variety of domains. Most salient in this discussion, the BASC contains both an Attention Problems and a Hyperactivity Scale, as well as other clinical scales to help provide greater certainty in differential diagnosis. Test authors assert that the BASC is useful in diagnosing attentional deficit disorders with and without hyperactivity (Reynolds and Kamphaus, 1993). Parents are asked to rate 131 behaviors as occurring never, sometimes, often, or almost always. A full range of derived scores, including standard scores, percentiles, and age equivalents may be derived.

Home Situations Questionnaire—Revised (HSQ-R) (DuPaul, 1991).   One of several behavior checklists popularized by Barkley and his colleagues (Barkley, 1991), the HSQ-R is a 14-item list of behaviors denoting attentional or concentration problems as they might manifest in home activities, such as driving in a car, playtime, social visiting, and attending religious services. Parents are asked to rate each behavior as either present or absent. If the behavior is rated as present, the parent is asked further to rate its severity. The scale yields total scores as well as factor scores differentiating between difficulty in compliance versus leisure situations. Means and standard deviations are provided. Scores more than 1.5 standard deviations above the mean for the age and sex of the child are considered indicative of diagnosable attentional difficulty.

Attention Deficit Hyperactivity Disorder Rating Scale (ADHD) (DuPaul, 1991).   Another of the scales popularized by Barkley and his colleagues (1991), the ADHD scale is comprised of 14 items. Each item refers to a problematic behavior suggestive of attentional problems. The parent is asked to rate the degree to which each behavior noted describes the individual of concern. Rating choices are: not at all, just

a little, pretty much, and very much. Again, the scale yields a total score and factor scores. Factors on this scale are Inattentive-Hyperactive and Impulsive-Hyperactive. Means and standard deviations are provided. These values are interpreted just as they are on the HSQ-R discussed above.

Teacher

Behavior Assessment System for Children (BASC)—Teacher Rating Scales (Kamphaus and Reynolds, 1993).   The teacher form of the BASC is quite similar to the parent form in aim, format, scoring, and psychometric properties. The content of the scales is directed to relevant school-based situations, such as adjustment to new teachers, completion of assigned tasks, and disruptiveness of others.

School Situations Questionnaire—Revised (SSQ-R) (DuPaul, 1991).   Completed by teachers, this test is a parallel instrument to the HSQ-R described above. One of the instruments utilized by Barkley and those working with him (1991), the SSQ-R is an 87-item scale. Items refer to school-based settings, asking the rater to note the presence/absence of attentional difficulty in each setting and to rank the severity of the difficulty from mild to severe. Total scores and mean severity ratings are derived, and these scores are then compared with normative means and standard deviations. As on the other Barkley scales, scores more than 1.5 standard deviations above the mean are considered significant for ADHD.

Attention Deficit Hyperactivity Disorder Scale (ADHD Scale) (DuPaul, 1991).   This instrument is described above and is appropriate for use by teachers as well as parents. Whereas the parent completes the form to describe behaviors witnessed at home, the teacher targets school-based behaviors in completing the form.

Child Attention Profile (CAP) (Edelbrock, 1991).   The CAP is a 10-item scale also popularized by Barkley and his group of colleagues (1991). The items refer to behaviors indicative of problems with attention and concentration relevant to completion of structured work. The rater is asked to designate each behavior as: not true, somewhat or sometimes true, or very or often true of the child in question. The test yields a total score and two factor scores, Inattention and Overactivity. Means and standard deviations are provided. Scores more than 1.5 standard deviations above the mean are understood as clinically significant.

PROJECTIVE TESTS

Rorschach Inkblots (Rorschach, 1921).   The Rorschach enjoys great popularity among clinicians (Erdberg and Exner, 1984). First described in 1921, the Rorschach consists of 10 inkblots each printed on a separate rectangle made of heavy cardboard. Five of the cards are monochromatic, 2 are black and red, and 3 are polychromatic. Standard administration consists of 2 phases: free association, in which the subject simply states what each blot might represent; and inquiry, in which the clinician seeks clarification from the subject as to what aspects of the blot contributed to the percept identified in the free-association phase. Clinicians typically allow approximately 1 hour for administration time. Although a number of administration and scoring systems have been developed for use with the Rorschach (Beck, 1944; Klopfer, 1954), the work of Exner and colleagues (Exner, 1986; Exner and Weiner, 1982; Wiener-Levy and Exner, 1981) represents the most ambitious effort to establish a psychometrically sound basis for scoring this instrument (Anastasi, 1988). The Rorschach is primarily utilized as a clinical device for assessing personality organization and, with children, also provides data regarding the developmental status of such organization (Zlotogorski, 1986). Particularly significant data is generated regarding a child's developmental capacities for reality testing, integration of affect, and maturational level of object relations. The Rorschach has been subjected to extensive research that establishes its satisfactory reliability, particularly since the introduction of Exner's Comprehensive System (Anastasi, 1988; Zlotogorski, 1986).

Thematic Apperception Test (TAT) (Murray et al., 1938).   The TAT consists of 20 picture cards, 1 of which is blank and 19 of which vary in their degree of ambiguity. Cards are presented one at a time and the child is asked to tell a story, as opposed to simply stating what the card portrays. The story is to include a beginning, a middle, and an end, and is to describe something about the thoughts and feelings of the characters. The story is recorded verbatim by the clinician, who may actively request clarification of the story as it is being told. Following administration, the clinician analyzes the story to determine the identification of the story's hero, the hero's attributes, and the conflicts, defenses, and adaptations evidenced in the hero's individual and interpersonal functioning. The underlying assumption of this analysis is that the respondent makes particular use of the hero as the object for unconscious projections and identifications.

According to many authors (e.g., Anastasi, 1988; Siegel, 1987; Siegel, 1988), the TAT is appropriate for use with older children, adolescents, and adults. Others (e.g., Goldman et al., 1983) point out that Murray originally intended his method for use with individuals above 4 years of age. While thematic assessment instruments have been developed for use with younger children, between approximately the ages of 3 and 10 (e.g., Children's Apperception Test, Bellak and Bellak, 1961; Roberts Apperception Test for Children, McArthur and Roberts, 1982), in clinical practice the TAT is generally utilized as the apperception test of choice. This is because the TAT, by virtue of its greater stimulus ambiguity, is considered to elicit more efficiently the subject's projections, and because greater examiner familiarity with the TAT engenders more of an internal frame of reference and face validity. The recent publication of a version of the Children's Apperception Test in which stimulus cards depict human as opposed to animal figures has generated enthusiasm among clinicians. These pictures appear more developmentally appropriate and better preserve the valuable ambiguity that is a hallmark of the TAT.

Typically, clinicians administer 8–10 cards selected for the individual child or adolescent being tested. While this approach reduces the instrument's reliability, it generates a rich lode of clinical data for use in deriving clinical hypotheses that may be confirmed or denied elsewhere in the test battery.

Machover Draw-A-Person Test (DAP) (Machover, 1949).   In this commonly utilized projective test, the subject is provided with a piece of standard-size, 8½″ x 11″ paper and a pencil with an eraser, and is instructed to draw a person. The only constraints placed on the figure are that it portray the entire body and that it not be drawn as a "stick figure." Upon concluding this drawing, the subject is then asked to draw a person of the opposite gender from that of the initial drawing. The examiner notes the subject's behavior, verbalizations and demeanor while drawing, and the sequence in which body parts are drawn. The productions are then subjected to a qualitative analysis, focusing on such variables as figure size, page placement, arm position, clothing, significant omissions and disproportions, shading, and erasures (Anastasi, 1988).

Machover (1949) provided a guide for interpretations of drawings without providing data in support of those interpretations. Research has been conducted that fails to validate Machover's diagnostic inferences (Klopfer and Taulbee, 1976). In clinical practice, the DAP is typically used as a source for generating clinical hypotheses. It may be helpful to conceptualize two broad categories of such hypotheses, which may be derived from qualitative analysis of the DAP: 1) hypotheses pertaining to the subject's perception of and feelings about the self, particularly ego development and bodily integrity; and 2) hypotheses pertaining to the subject's perception of and feelings about interactions with the social environment, particularly with primary nurturing caregivers.

Kinetic Family Drawing (KFD) (Burns, 1982).   The KFD is frequently administered by clinicians to generate hypotheses regarding the subject's perceptions of and feelings about family structure and sentient environment, particularly the subject's own sense of connectedness to individual family members and the family as a whole. Administration

and interpretation are similar to that of the DAP. The subject is provided with paper and pencil and asked to draw a picture of the family doing something. It is important that this latter instruction not specify "doing something *together*," as this instruction would contaminate data regarding perceived family cohesion.

One manual for KFD interpretation (Burns, 1982) cites references for inferences drawn about KFD productions. Machover is one of the most frequent citations, however, reducing the reliability of the citations because of the above-noted research failing to support her diagnostic inferences. KFD interpretation is therefore subject to the same caution as other projective data, and is best used as a source of clinical hypotheses requiring confirmation or denial elsewhere.

Rotter Incomplete Sentences Blank (Rotter and Rafferty, 1950).   The Rotter is one of many sentence completion tasks that are widely used by clinicians and researchers (Goldberg, 1965). The Blank consists of 40 sentence stems, which the subject is instructed to complete so as to express true feelings. A scoring manual permits ratings of each response on a seven-point scale assessing degree of adjustment or maladjustment. Other more recently developed sentence completion instruments (e.g., Incomplete Sentences Task, Lanyon and Lanyon, 1980) provide forms for school- and college-age children.

As with many of the instruments noted above, many clinicians utilize a more clinical approach to sentence analysis. Such clinicians often work from a theoretical position that holds that sentence completion protocols can provide a particularly rich source of heuristic data about a child's level of ego development (Loevinger, 1977).

PERSONALITY TESTS

Minnesota Multiphasic Personality Inventory-Adolescent (MMPI-A) (Butcher et al., 1992).   The MMPI (Hathaway and McKinley, 1940; Hathaway and McKinley, 1943) has been the most widely used personality inventory (Anastasi, 1988). A revision, the MMPI-2, was published in 1989 (Butcher et al., 1989). Like its predecessor, the MMPI-2 is a self-report, criterion-keyed instrument, which means that the instrument's items were selected according to an external criterion, in this case the item's ability to discriminate a group carrying a clinical diagnosis from a normal control group. While the original MMPI and MMPI-2 were designed for use with an older adolescent/adult population, there has always been caution about the validity of MMPI-based clinical inferences as applied to a broad adolescent population. To address this caution and provide more valid data regarding adolescents, the MMPI-A was published in 1992. The MMPI-A was standardized on a school-based national adolescent population. Some possible limitations that persisted in the normative population were its relative weighting toward better-educated, higher socioeconomic status (SES) families.

The MMPI-A consists of 478 forced-choice, true-false items provided in a test booklet. Answers are recorded on a separate answer sheet and then may be hand- or computer-scored. The MMPI-A includes several validity scales (lie, validity, correction, and variability scores) designed to check on such test-taking variables as carelessness, misunderstanding, malingering, and special response sets, 10 original clinical scales (hypochondriasis, depression, hysteria, psychopathic deviance, masculinity-femininity, paranoia, psychasthenia, schizophrenia, hypomania, social introversion), 15 content scales specifically related to adolescent development (anxiety, obsessiveness, depression, health concerns, alienation, bizarre mentation, anger, cynicism, conduct problems, self-esteem, aspiration level, social discomfort, family problems, school problems, and negative treatment indicators), as well as supplementary scales to measure anxiety, repression, alcoholism, and immaturity. A profile is generated in which raw scores are converted to standard Z-scores, and interpretation is based on consulting available references providing descriptions of clinical populations consistent with different MMPI-A profiles.

Millon Adolescent Personality Inventory (MAPI) (Millon et al., 1982).   The MAPI consists of 150 true-false items and was designed to be completed in approximately 20 minutes by adolescents between the ages of 13 and 18. The instrument's two forms (MAPI-C and MAPI-G) are intended for clinical and guidance applications, respectively. Twenty scales are produced, clustering into measures of personality style (introversive, inhibited, cooperative, sociable, confident, forceful, respectful, sensitive), expressed concerns (self-concept, personal esteem, body comfort, sexual acceptance, peer security, social tolerance, family rapport, academic confidence), and behavioral correlates (impulse control, social conformity, scholastic achievement, attendance consistency). The MAPI was intended specifically for use with adolescents and was standardized on relevant normative populations.

Children's Personality Questionnaire (CPQ) (Porter and Cattell, 1972). The CPQ represents one attempt to provide a measure of personality functioning in younger children, in this instance aged 8 through 12. The test is grounded in the theoretical work of Cattell, which led to the development of the Sixteen Personality Factor Questionnaire (16PF) (Cattell and Eber, 1970). Consisting of 140 forced-choice questions that may be broken into short forms of 70 items each, the test's administration time generally does not exceed 45 minutes.

The CPQ generates factor scores tapping 14 hypothesized primary personality traits, including emotional stability, self-concept, excitability, and self-assurance. Consistent with the 16PF, second order, broad trait factors may be derived, including extraversion, anxiety, tough poise, and independence. Critiques support the instrument's research utility, but raise questions regarding its clinical applicability (Goldman et al., 1983). The relative dearth of theory-based instruments for this age group, however, leads many clinicians to include the CPQ in assessment batteries for elementary-school-age children.

NEUROPSYCHOLOGICAL SCREENING TESTS AND TEST BATTERIES

Developmental Test of Visual-Motor Integration (VMI) (Beery, 1989). First introduced in 1964, the VMI has since been renormed twice, in 1981 and again in 1989. The VMI was developed for use in both academic and clinical settings, and can be administered either individually or in groups to children between the ages of 2 and 15, inclusive. The child is presented with a booklet containing 24 geometric designs and is simply instructed to copy each with no erasures permitted. Designs are scored on a pass-fail basis, according to criteria and examples provided in the manual. Testing is discontinued when the child fails to accurately reproduce three consecutive designs. Administration time is approximately 10–15 minutes.

The VMI enjoys satisfactory psychometric properties (Beery, 1989; Polubinski et al., 1986), and is commonly employed by clinicians as a measure of children's perceptual-motor ability. Such a measure is an important component of assessment batteries constructed to rule out the presence of learning disabilities (Jansky, 1988). Because it requires minimal interaction with the examiner, the VMI is often administered early in the assessment battery as a means of introducing children to the task of testing.

Benton Visual Retention Test (Benton, 1974). The Benton Visual Retention Test is used as a measure of visual-figural memory in adults and in children beginning at age 8. The test consists of 10 cards on each of which is reproduced one or more geometric designs. The manual outlines several different administration procedures. In the recommended standard administration, the subject is told that each card will be presented for 10 seconds, after which the card will be removed and the subject will reproduce the figure from memory. Reproductions are scored on both a pass-fail basis (''number correct'' score) and in terms of the total number of errors (''error'' score). Utilizing tables provided in the manual, both of these scores are then compared with the anticipated ''normal'' score for each age and intellectual level (typically determined by the IQ score obtained on the cognitive instrument utilized in the assessment battery). Scores deviating from this expected score by a significant number of points are considered to either ''raise the question'' or ''suggest'' the presence of a visual-figural memory deficit.

Used together, the VMI and the Benton provide well-standardized data about a child's visual-motor and visual-memory functioning. Depending on the data obtained, hypotheses about perceptual, motor, or memory deficits can be further explored by administering additional instruments (e.g., Jordan Left-Right Reversal Test, Jordan, 1973; Motor-Free Visual Perception Test, Colarusso and Hammill, 1972).

Bender Visual Motor Gestalt Test (Bender-Gestalt) (Bender, 1938). Widely used by clinical psychologists to rule out the presence of brain damage (Anastasi, 1988; Sattler, 1988), the 9 Bender-Gestalt cards each present a geometric design which the subject is asked to copy with the card remaining in sight. This Copy phase is typically followed by the Recall phase, in which the child is next asked to reproduce from memory as many of the figures as possible after they have been removed from sight. While Bender did not develop objective and standardized scoring criteria and normative data, a number of such systems have subsequently been developed. The most well-known scoring system for children is that of Koppitz (Koppitz, 1964; Koppitz, 1975), which provides norms for subjects in kindergarten through 4th grade.

Similar to the VMI and the Benton, the Bender-Gestalt provides an efficient screen for detecting brain damage. In the past, clinicians also utilized the Bender-Gestalt as a source of projective test data, a practice which has received little validational support (Sattler, 1988).

Reitan-Indiana Neuropsychological Test Battery for Children (Reitan and Davison, 1974) and Halstead-Reitan Neuropsychological Test Battery for Older Children (Reitan and Wolfson, 1985; Selz, 1981). These two batteries are discussed together because of their conceptual, structural, and clinical similarity. The batteries were designed to assess a broad range of functions, and their content is somewhat flexible, permitting different degrees of emphasis on various aspects of the child's functioning. Most clinicians administer 11 tests including sensorimotor and perceptual tasks as well as an aphasia screening test (Anastasi, 1988). In addition, the complete battery also includes administration of an intelligence test, typically the WISC-III. Administration time for the full battery can therefore be as long as 6 hours.

The utility of these batteries is compromised by virtue of limited available reliability, validity, and normative data (Sattler, 1988). In the hands of sophisticated and well-trained neuropsychologists, the derived data can be employed to differentiate brain-damaged children (Reitan and Herring, 1985; Selz and Reitan, 1979) and specific associated syndromes, and to assist in rehabilitation planning by articulating behavioral deficits related to central nervous system pathology (Anastasi, 1988).

Luria-Nebraska Neuropsychological Battery: Children's Revision (LNNB-C) (Golden, 1987). Similar to the Reitan batteries noted above, the LNNB-C was developed to investigate a wide variety of neuropsychological functions, assess cognitive deficits and provide data to guide rehabilitation in children aged 8–12. This battery differs from the Reitan instruments, however, in its abbreviated administration time (approximately 2½ hours) and greater standardization of content, materials, administration, and scoring (Anastasi, 1988). The battery's 149 items are grouped into 11 clinical and 2 optional scales (assessing sensorimotor, perceptual, and cognitive abilities), 3 summary scales (discriminating brain-damaged from normal children), and 11 factor scales (assessing specific neuropsychological functions and requiring caution in interpretation). All items receive scores of 0, 1, or 2, with higher scores indicating greater evidence of brain dysfunction. A companion 57-category qualitative scoring system permits further evaluation of error items.

The LNNB-C is a downward extension of an adult version of the battery (Sattler, 1988), an approach to neuropsychological assessment which has been the focus of substantial controversy and criticism (Adams, 1980; Delis and Kaplan, 1983; Sattler, 1988; Sparrow et al., 1985; Stambrook, 1983). The manual provides more substantial standardization, reliability, and validity data than is available for the Reitan batteries, but concern has been raised about the adequacy of the battery for each of these psychometric issues (Nolan et al., 1983; Sattler, 1988; Sparrow et al., 1985). Given these concerns, pending completion of further research caution is required in the clinical interpretation of data generated by this battery.

MEASURES OF INFANT AND PRESCHOOL DEVELOPMENT

Bayley Scales of Infant Development, Second Edition (BSID-II) (Bayley, 1993). The BSID-II is a revision of the Bayley Scales of Infant Development (Bayley, 1969). Like its predecessor, the BSID-II assesses the developmental functioning of infants and toddlers with the aim of detecting developmental delay and pointing the way toward appropriate intervention strategies. The revision was undertaken to update the normative data; extend the age range beyond what was covered by the original BSID; improve the content coverage to make the test more useful clinically; enhance the test materials to increase their attractiveness for subjects; improve the psychometric properties of the test; improve the clinical utility of the test by including standardization data on such special populations as those with Down syndrome, prematurity, and prenatal drug exposure; all while preserving the original basic focus of the BSID on deriving sound developmental information from stimulating, standardized interaction with an infant or young child. The test consists of Mental, Motor, and Behavior Rating scales. The Mental scale focuses on the infant's early ability to direct his or her attention to appropriate people and objects in the environment and then on the development of age-appropriate interactive, language, conceptual, and memory skills. The Motor Scale focuses on early development of both fine and gross motor skills, as well as sensory integration and visual-motor coordination. Both the Mental and Motor Scales are completed using a flexible administration format. Test materials are attractive and resemble captivating toys. Test subjects are offered the materials, along with stimulating guidance about the developmentally-adequate way of interacting with the materials. The subject's actual use of the materials is then evaluated. Rather than relying on the type of direct assessment used for administration of the Mental and Motor scales, the Behavior Rating scale is completed based on informal observation of the infant/preschooler during the testing. Styles of interpersonal relating, attunement to others, and accessibility to limit-setting are examples of the types of behaviors assessed. Test sessions are typically fast-paced, in order to maintain the very young child's interest, and require considerable creativity as well as test familiarity from the examiner. For these reasons, the Bayley is often considered a challenging instrument for examiners to master. Once mastered, however, the test can be administered in a smooth, systematic, enjoyable manner. The BSID-II was standardized on a representative national sample that conformed to the 1988 update of the 1980 national census reported by the National Census Bureau. The sample was designed to conform to racial, ethnic, and socioeconomic proportions in the national population. At each age level, there was equal representation of males and females. Reliability and validity data for the BSID-II are provided in the test manual. The data indicate that the test is a reliable and valid instrument that can be used with confidence. It should be noted that the reliability and validity data pertain to documentation of current developmental status. Early developmental data do not serve to predict long-term intellectual ranking. In clinical practice, the Bayley provides very valuable information about the status of the youngest of patients. One drawback, however, is that the Bayley does not provide a discrete measure of language development. Such a measure is often needed in the assessment of potential developmental delay.

Mullen Scales of Early Learning (MSEL) (Mullen, 1981). Developed by Eileen Mullen, an expert in early childhood development and education, the MSEL is a comprehensive measure of early development based on a neurosensory processing model. The MSEL is aimed at diagnosing developmental delay and providing support for developmentally-informed intervention. The MSEL resembles the BSID-II in that it documents the earliest stages of development using a flexible, play-like administration format and attractive, stimulating materials. Like the BSID-II, the MSEL challenges the examiner to develop an intimate familiarity and thorough proficiency with the test materials. There are two forms of the MSEL, one for infants and one for preschoolers. Unlike the BSID-II, the MSEL is comprised of 4 subscales, specifically the Visual Receptive Scale, Visual Expressive Scale, Language

Receptive Scale, and the Language Expressive Scale. The visual scales measure the infant or young child's ability to take in information from the environment and to manipulate concrete materials in a meaningful way. The language scales measure the young subject's capacity to make sense of and respond accurately to verbal communication, along with making himself or herself understood verbally. Thus, whereas the MSEL supplies a direct measure of language, a measure lacking on the BSID-II, it does not contain the sort of clear measures of gross motor skills and behavioral functioning provided by the BSID-II. The examiner should choose between the instruments based on particular case needs. Reasonable reliability and validity data are provided regarding the MSEL, although some characteristics of the standardization sample raise mild questions about the psychometric foundation of the instrument. In 1993, the MSEL was purchased by the American Guidance Service. At the time of this writing, a new, consolidated version of the MSEL was planned for publication within a year. Updated information on improved psychometric properties of the new version of the MSEL was expected. Given a stronger psychometric foundation, the MSEL should continue to be an invaluable addition to the testing library.

PSYCHOLOGICAL TEST RESULTS

As discussed above, psychological testing yields a wealth of data regarding a child's or an adolescent's functioning. It is important to address both the nature of the data gathered and the means by which it is most usefully communicated to young patients and their parents.

Nature of the Data

Consistent with the multifaceted test battery described above, psychological assessment provides data on a youngster's cognitive, behavioral, and personality functioning. For each domain assessed, test findings place the youngster at a particular level of functioning overall. To obtain the most sophisticated benefit of psychological testing, however, it is critical to go beyond a summary analysis of each distinct domain to analyze both the interrelationships among the domains assessed and, further, the profile of individual strengths and weaknesses within each global domain (Novick and Lewis, 1967). This is because an identical performance in one area of functioning by several youngsters may have vastly different implications depending upon how each one of them performs in other areas. For example, projective evidence of highly original, complex, rich, reality-oriented internal mental processes would be reassuringly unremarkable for a child with a high I.Q. The same projective data from a child with a Low Average or Borderline I.Q., though, would raise important questions about the accuracy of measurement of that child's intelligence. Once the individual features of a youngster's test profile have been analyzed, the psychologist provides a formulation that integrates the diverse findings into a comprehensive view of the patient. The data analysis concludes with the offer of recommendations on how best to address the needs noted in the assessment.

Communication of the Findings

To facilitate appropriate interventions on behalf of the child or adolescent assessed, psychological test results must be communicated in understandable language and with interpersonal sensitivity appropriate to the recipient of the information. If the results are communicated in overly technical language or without regard for their impact on parents, clinicians, and others invested in the child or adolescent patient, the test data are likely to be ignored and the benefits of testing negated.

Assessment findings should also be shared in a particular order to facilitate their incorporation into clinical care. The initial step of this sequence depends upon the referral source. If the test referral came from another professional, test data and recommendations should be communicated initially to the referring clinician. By communicating first with this colleague, appropriate primary responsibility for patient care and relationships to the patient are safeguarded. The psychologist and referring clinician can then decide together how best to proceed with further communication of the test findings to those concerned. In some instances, the referring clinician and testing psychologist may elect to present the findings together. The advantage to this presentation mode is that all concerned can develop a shared, multidimensional understanding of the child or adolescent. In other cases, it may be best for the psychologist to present the assessment data alone. The data can then be brought back to the clinical relationship with the referring professional. This method is best when time constraints make a joint meeting difficult. The method also has special advantages for those cases in which the psychological test data may be at odds with clinical expectations. Separate communication of the data by the psychologist allows the referring clinician to maintain better a therapeutic alliance with the patient and family. Together, the clinician and family can then begin to incorporate the data obtained from the testing. Finally, for those cases in which fragile patient functioning highlights the importance of the relationship with the referring clinician, it is often best to have that clinician relay the test findings to those concerned. For these patients and their families, the information may be best accepted and understood in the context of a supportive, therapeutic relationship.

For cases of the type discussed above, findings and recommendations should then be communicated to the parents in the most efficacious presentation style. If the parents themselves initiated the referral, sharing these findings and recommendations with the parents constitutes the first step in the interpretive process. Just as good rapport is necessary in the testing situation to guarantee testing accuracy, so is it necessary in consulting with parents to facilitate their willingness to make good use of the data. Care should be taken to demonstrate some empathy for the parents' understanding of the child or adolescent so that they can feel confident about the veracity of the test results. Findings should be communicated in a forthright but tactful manner, with particular sensitivity to shared family traits and for parental attitudes toward the youngster involved.

With elementary-school-age children and adolescents, it is always important to then consider providing the test findings directly to the patient. The offer of an interpretive meeting for the child or adolescent should be made pending parental approval. If the child or adolescent requests such an interpretive meeting, a careful clinical decision should be made by parents and professionals regarding the best setting and participants for this meeting. Some children prefer to safeguard their self-esteem by hearing the results privately from their parents. Those who have developed an initial attachment to the testing psychologist often want to hear about their test performance from him or her. Still others, who have therapists to whom they are closely attached, request that their therapists communicate the test results. These latter two formats may or may not include the parents. With the patients themselves, test findings should also be shared in a straightforward, honest manner. The child's or adolescent's strengths should be emphasized, his or her weaknesses discussed in an empathetic manner, and hopeful recommendations offered.

At times, other interested parties also need to share in the assessment findings. For children and adolescents, the school is the likeliest other recipient of the information. It may also be helpful to communicate the test findings to programs for young people with special needs as well as to other caregivers. Parents should make informed decisions with the psychologist and, when relevant, the referring clinician about the format in and extent to which the findings are to be shared with outside parties. These decisions should balance protection of family privacy with sufficiently full communication of findings to allow for appropriate interventions on behalf of the child or adolescent.

References

Adams K: In search of Luria's battery: A false start. *J Consult Clin Psychol* 48:511–516, 1980.

Allison J, Blatt SJ, Zimet CN: *The interpretation of psychological tests*. New York, Harper & Row, 1968.

American Psychiatric Association. *Diagnostic and Statistical Manual of Mental Disorders* (4th ed). Washington, DC, American Psychiatric Press, 1994.

American Psychological Association: *Standards for educational and psychological testing*. Washington, DC, American Psychological Association Press, 1985.

Anastasi A: *Psychological testing*. (6th ed). New York, Macmillan, 1988.

Army Individual Test. *Manual of Direction and Scoring*. Washington, DC, War Department, Adjutant General's Office, 1944.

Barkley RA: *Attention-Deficit Hyperactivity Disorder: A Clinical Workbook*. New York, Guilford, 1991.

Bayley N: *Bayley Scales of Infant Development*. New York, Psychological Corporation, 1969.

Bayley N: *Bayley Scales of Infant Development* (2nd ed). San Antonio, Psychological Corporation, 1993.

Beck SJ: *Rorschach's Test*. New York, Grune & Stratton, 1944.

Beery KE: *The Developmental Test of Visual-Motor Integration: Administration, Scoring and Teaching Manual* (3rd ed, rev). Cleveland, Modern Curriculum Press, 1989.

Bellak L, Bellak SS: *Children's Apperception Test (C.A.T.) Manual*. (4th ed). Larchmont, NY, CPS, 1961.

Bender L: *A Visual Motor Gestalt Test and Its Clinical Use*. Albany, NY, American Orthopsychiatric Association, 1938.

Benton AL: *Revised Visual Retention Test: Manual*. San Antonio, Psychological Corporation, 1974.

Benton AL, Hamsher K: *Multilingual Aphasia Examination*. Iowa City, University of Iowa Hospitals, 1978.

Berg EA: A simple objective technique for measuring flexibility in thinking. *J Gen Psychol* 39: 15–22, 1948.

Bruininks RH, Woodcock RW, Westherman RF, et al: Scales of Independent Behavior (SIB). Allen, TX, DLM Teaching Resources, 1984.

Burns RC: *Self-growth in Families: Kinetic Family Drawings (K-F-D) Research and Application*. New York, Brunner/Mazel, 1982.

Butcher JN, Dahlstrom WG, Graham JR, Tellegen A, Kaemmer B: *Minnesota Multiphasic Personality Inventory-2 (MMPI-2): Manual for Administration and Scoring*. Minneapolis, University of Minnesota Press, 1989.

Butcher JN, Williams CL, Graham JR, et al.: *Minnesota Multiphasic Personality Inventory—Adolescent: Manual for Administration, Scoring, and Interpretation*. Minneapolis, The University of Minnesota Press, 1992.

Cattell RB, Eber HW, Tatsuoka MM: *Handbook for the Sixteen Personality Factor Questionnaire*. Champaign, IL, Institute for Personality and Ability Testing, 1970.

Cegalis JA, Birdsall W: PASAT. Nashua, NH, Forethought, 1992.

Cegalis JA, Volin J: VIGIL. Nashua, NH, Forethought, 1991.

Colarusso RP, Hammill DD:*Motor-Free Visual Perception Test: Manual*. San Rafael, CA, Academic Therapy Publications, 1972.

Cronbach LJ: Coefficient alpha and the internal structure of tests. *Psychometrika* 16:297–334, 1951.

Delis DC, Kaplan E: Hazards of a standardized neuropsychological test with low content validity: Comment on the Luria-Nebraska Neuropsychological Battery. *J Consult Clin Psychol* 51:396–398, 1983.

Doll EA: *Vineland Social Maturity Scale: Manual of Directions* (rev. ed). Circle Pines, MN, American Guidance Service, 1965.

Dunn LM, Dunn LM: *Peabody Picture Vocabulary Test—Revised: Manual for Forms L and M*. Circle Pines, MN, American Guidance Service, 1981.

DuPaul GJ: Home situations questionnaire—revised. In Barkley RA, *Attention-Deficit Hyperactivity Disorder: A Clinical Workbook*. New York, Guilford, 1991 (a).

DuPaul GJ: ADHD rating scale. In Barkley RA: *Attention-Deficit Hyperactivity Disorder: A Clinical Workbook*. New York, Guilford, 1991 (b).

DuPaul GJ: School situations questionnaire—revised. In Barkley RA, *Attention-Deficit Hyperactivity Disorder: A Clinical Workbook*. New York, Guilford, 1991 (c).

Edelbrock C: Child attention profile. In Barkley RA, *Attention-Deficit Hyperactivity Disorder: A Clinical Workbook*. New York, Guilford, 1991.

Erdberg P, Exner JE Jr: Rorschach assessment. In: Goldstein G, Hersen M (eds): *Handbook of Psychological Assessment*. New York, Pergamon, 1984, pp. 332–347.

Exner JE Jr: *The Rorschach: A Comprehensive System. Vol 2: Current Research and Advanced Interpretation*. New York, Wiley, 1978.

Exner JE Jr: *The Rorschach: A Comprehensive System. Vol 1: Basic Foundations* (2nd ed). New York, Wiley, 1986.

Exner JE Jr, Weiner IB: *The Rorschach: A Comprehensive System. Vol 3: Assessment of Children and Adolescents*. New York, Wiley, 1982.

Gaddes WH, Crockett DJ: The Spreen-Benton Aphasia Tests: Normative data as a measure of normal language development. *Brain & Language* 3: 257–280, 1975.

Goldberg PA: A review of sentence completion methods in personality assessment. *J Projective Techniques Pers Assess* 29:12–45, 1965.

Golden CJ: *Luria-Nebraska Neuropsychological*

Battery: Children's Revision. Los Angeles, Western Psychological Services, 1987.

Goldman J, Stein CL, Guerry S: *Psychological Methods of Child Assessment.* New York, Brunner/Mazel, 1983.

Grant DA, Berg EA: A behavioral analysis of degree of reinforcement and ease of shifting to new responses in a Weigl-type card-sorting problem. *J Exp Psychol* 38:404–411, 1948.

Hathaway SR, McKinley JC: A multiphasic personality schedule (Minnesota). I: Construction of the schedule. *J Psychol* 10:249–254, 1940.

Hathaway SR, McKinley JC: *The Minnesota Multiphasic Personality Inventory* (rev ed). Minneapolis, University of Minnesota Press, 1943.

Heaton RK: *A Manual for the Wisconsin Card Sorting Test.* The University of Colorado School of Medicine, Department of Psychiatry, 1981.

Jansky JJ: Assessment of learning disabilities. In: Kestenbaum C, Williams DT (eds): *Handbook of Clinical Assessment of Children and Adolescents* (Vol 1). New York, New York University Press, 1988, pp. 296–311.

Jastak S, Wilkinson GS: *Wide Range Achievement Test—Revised.* Wilmington, DE, Jastak Associates, 1984.

Jordan BT: *Left-Right Reversal Test: Manual.* San Rafael, CA, Academic Therapy Publications, 1973.

Kamphaus R: *Clinical assessment of children's intelligence.* Boston: Allyn & Bacon, 1993.

Kamphaus RW, Reynolds CR: *Clinical and Research Applications of the K-ABC.* Circle Pines, MN, American Guidance Service, 1987.

Kaufman AS: *Intelligent Testing with the WISC-R.* New York, Wiley-Interscience, 1979.

Kaufman AS, Kaufman NL: *Clinical Evaluation of Young Children with the McCarthy Scales.* New York, Grune & Stratton, 1977.

Kaufman AS, Kaufman NL: *K-ABC: Kaufman Assessment Battery for Children.* Circle Pines, MN, American Guidance Service, 1983.

Kaufman AS, Kaufman, NL: *Kaufman Test of Educational Achievement.* Circle Pines, MN, American Guidance Service, 1985.

Kaufman AS, Kaufman NL: *Kaufman Brief Intelligence Test: Manual.* Circle Pines: American Guidance Service, 1990.

Kaufman AS, Kaufman NL: *Kaufman Adolescent & Adult Intelligence Test.* Circle Pines: American Guidance Service, 1993.

Klopfer B: *Developments in the Rorschach Technique* (Vol 1). New York, Harcourt, Brace & World, 1954.

Klopfer WG, Taulbee ES: Projective tests. *Annu Rev Psychol* 27: 543–568, 1976.

Koppitz EM: *The Bender Gestalt Test for Young Children.* Orlando, FL, Grune & Stratton, 1964.

Koppitz EM: *The Bender Gestalt Test for Young Children: Research and Application, 1963–1973.* Orlando, FL, Grune & Stratton, 1975.

Kuder GF, Richardson MW: The theory of estimation of test reliability. *Psychometrika* 2:151–160, 1937.

Lanyon BP, Lanyon RI: *Incomplete Sentences Task: Manual.* Chicago: Stoelting, 1980.

Loevinger J: *Ego Development: Conceptions and Theories.* San Francisco, Jossey-Bass, 1977.

Machover K: *Personality Projection in the Drawing of the Human Figure.* Springfield, IL, Charles C Thomas, 1949.

McArthur DS, Roberts GE: *Roberts Apperception Test for Children: Manual.* Los Angeles, Western Psychological Services, 1982.

McCarthy DA: *Manual for the McCarthy Scales of Children's abilities.* San Antonio, The Psychological Corporation, 1972.

Millon T, Green CJ, Meagher RB Jr: *Millon Adolescent Personality Inventory Manual.* Minneapolis, National Computer Systems, 1982.

Mullen EM: *Mullen Scales of Early Learning.* Circle Pines, American Guidance Service, 1981, 1984.

Murray HA, et al: *Explorations in Personality.* New York, Oxford University Press, 1938.

Nolan DR, Hammeke TA, Barkley R: A comparison of the patterns of neuropsychological performance in two groups of learning disabled children. *J Child Clin Psychol* 12:22–27, 1983.

Novick MR, Lewis C: Coefficient alpha and the reliability of composite measurements. *Psychometrika* 32:1–13, 1967.

Pine F: *Developmental Theory and Clinical Process.* New Haven, Yale University Press, 1985.

Polubinski J, Melamed LE, Prinzo OV: Factor structure evidence for developmental levels of perceptual processing on the Developmental Test of Visual-Motor Integration. *Psychol Schools* 23:337–341, 1986.

Porter RB, Cattell RB: *Handbook for the Children's Personality Questionnaire.* Champaign, IL, Institute for Personality and Ability Testing, 1972.

Reitan R: Trail making test results for normal and brain-damaged children. *Percept Mot Skills* 33: 575–581, 1971.

Reitan RM, Davison LA (eds): *Clinical Neuropsychology: Current Status and Applications.* Washington, DC, VH Winston & Sons, 1974.

Reitan RM, Herring S: A short screening device for identification of cerebral dysfunction in children. *J Clin Psychol* 41:643–650, 1985.

Reitan RM, Wolfson D: *The Halstead-Reitan Neuropsychological Test Battery.* Tuscon, AZ, Neuropsychology Press, 1985.

Reynolds CR, Kamphaus RW: *Behavior Assessment System for Children (BASC) Manual.* Circle Pines, American Guidance Service, 1992.

Rorschach H: *Psychodiagnostics: A Diagnostic Test Based on Perception.* Berne, Hans Huber, 1921.

Rotter JB, Rafferty JE: *Manual: The Rotter Incomplete Sentences Blank.* San Antonio, The Psychological Corporation, 1950.

Sattler JM: *Assessment of Children* (3rd ed). San Diego, JM Sattler, 1988.

Selz M: Halstead-Reitan neuropsychological test battery for children. In: Hynd GW, Obrzut JE (eds). *Neuropsychological Assessment and the School-Age Child: Issues and Procedures.* New York, Grune & Stratton, 1981, pp. 195–235.

Selz M, Reitan RM: Neuropsychological test performance of normal, learning-disabled, and brain damaged older children. *J Nerv Ment Dis* 167: 298–302, 1979.

Siegel MG: *Psychological Testing from Early Childhood through Adolescence: A Developmental and Psychodynamic Approach.* Madison, International Universities Press, 1987.

Siegel MG: Cognitive and projective test assessment. In: Kestenbaum CJ, Williams DT (eds). *Handbook of Clinical Assessment of Children and Adolescents* (Vol 1). New York, New York University Press, 1988, pp. 59–84.

Silverstein AB: Nonstandard standard scores on the Vineland Adaptive Behavior Scales: a cautionary note. *Am J Ment Defic* 91:1–4, 1986.

Sparrow SS, Balla DB, Cicchetti DV: *The Vineland Adaptive Behavior Scales.* Circle Pines, MN: American Guidance Service, 1984.

Sparrow SS, Blackman B: Developmental learning disorders. In: Cavenar JO (ed): *Psychiatry* (Vol 2). Philadephia, JB Lippincott, 1985, pp. 1–9.

Sparrow SS, Carter AS, Cicchetti DV: *Vineland screener, Book 1: Overview, Reliability, Validity, Administration and Scoring.* Available from Sara S. Sparrow, Ph.D., Yale Child Study Center, 230 So. Frontage Road, New Haven, CT, 1994a.

Sparrow SS, Carter AS, Cicchetti DV: *Vineland screener, Book 2: Record Booklets, Administration and Scoring.* Available from Sara S. Sparrow, Ph.D., Yale Child Study Center, 230 So. Frontage Road, New Haven, CT, 1994b.

Sparrow SS, Carter AS, Racusin G, et al.: Comprehensive psychological assessment through the lifespan: A developmental approach. In: Cicchetti D, Cohen D (eds): *Manual of Developmental Psychopathology,* New York, Wiley, 1995, pp. 81–105.

Sparrow SS, Fletcher JM, Cicchetti DV: Psychological assessment of children. In: Michels R, Cavenar JO, Brodie HKH et al (eds): *Psychiatry.* Philadelphia, JB Lippincott, 1985, pp. 1–12.

Spreen O, Gaddes WH: Developmental norms for 15 neuropsychological tests age 6 to 15. *Cortex* 5:170–191, 1969.

Stambrook M: The Luria-Nebraska neuropsychological battery: a promise that may be partly fulfilled. *J Clin Neuropsychol* 5:247–269, 1983.

Thorndike RL, Hagen EP, Sattler J.M: *Guide for Administering and Scoring the Stanford-Binet Intelligence Scale* (4th ed). Chicago, Riverside Publishing, 1986.

Wechsler D: *Manual for the Wechsler Intelligence Scale for Children.* San Antonio, Psychological Corporation, 1949.

Wechsler D: *Manual for the Wechsler Adult Intelligence Scale.* San Antonio, Psychological Corporation, 1955.

Wechsler D: *Manual for the Wechsler Preschool and Primary Scale of Intelligence.* San Antonio, Psychological Corporation, 1967.

Wechsler D: *Manual for the Wechsler Intelligence Scale for Children—Revised.* New York, Psychological Corporation, 1974.

Wechsler D: *Manual for the Wechsler Adult Intelligence Scale—Revised.* San Antonio, Psychological Corporation, 1981.

Wechsler D: *Wechsler Preschool and Primary Scale of Intelligence—Revised.* San Antonio, Psychological Corporation, 1987 (a).

Wechsler D: *Wechsler Intelligence Scale for Children* (3rd ed). San Antonio, Psychological Corporation, 1987 (b).

Wechsler D: *Wechsler Individual Achievement Test.* San Antonio, Psychological Corporation, 1992.

Wiener-Levy D, Exner, JE Jr: The Rorschach comprehensive system: an overview. In McReynolds P (ed): *Advances in Psychological Assessment* (Vol 5). San Francisco, Jossey-Bass, 1981, pp. 236–293.

Woodcock RW, Johnson MB: *Woodcock-Johnson Psycho-Educational Battery—Revised.* Allen, TX, DLM Teaching Resources, 1989.

Zlotogorski Z: Recent research on the Rorschach test with children. In: Rabin AI (ed): *Projective Techniques for Adolescents and Children.* New York, Springer, 1986, pp. 154–167.

42 The Neurological Meaning of Soft Signs

Jonathan H. Pincus, M.D.

The term *soft signs* has become a subterfuge for clinicians who are avoiding hard scientific thinking. It is almost a slang expression, like "stroke," which can mean cerebral thrombosis, embolus, hemorrhage, convulsion, or even heart attack. The term *soft signs* has been used to refer both to *historical evidence* of events that can be associated with brain damage and certain kinds of behavior (e.g., hyperactivity, impulsiveness, poor attention span) and to *physical findings* elicited by examination of the patients. A huge variety of different symptoms and signs are subsumed under the title soft signs. Some of these are maturational and probably represent variants of normal. Others relate to hereditary conditions and diseases, and still others to acquired disorders of the brain. Hyperactivity, emotional lability, disorders of attention, and impulsiveness have been considered soft signs by some. Even if these symptoms do sometimes arise in a setting of damage, they are not necessarily the equivalents of such neurological signs as EEG spikes, disorders of hearing and speech, and specific learning disabilities—although all of these have been inappropriately equalized under the heading "soft signs." Yet the idea that children may have minor motor, perceptual, linguistic, adaptive, social, and educational problems of various types as the result of brain abnormality is valid. In order to identify useful evidence of organic brain dysfunction, there must be a search for findings that will reliably reflect brain abnormality. This has only partly been accomplished.

Asymmetrical physical-neurological findings are clearly reliable indicators of pathology. Still, there are a number of "hard" neurological findings, on which neurologists rely daily in the performance of routine examinations, that have not actually been subjected to careful scientific scrutiny. For example, it is not known how often patients who are free of nervous system diseases have Babinski reflexes, especially when tired or stressed. Not only do we not know how many normals manifest this sign, we also do not know exactly how many people with demonstrable brain damage—even those with corticospinal tract damage—fail to manifest this sign.

Despite this failure, there is great and appropriate emphasis placed on the significance of the neurological examination in general and on the Babinski reflex in particular, even though the neurologist may be influenced in his or her interpretation by the fact that patients have been referred because of their failure to conform to some normal behavioral pattern and are, therefore, abnormal almost by definition. It is up to the neurologist to discover independent evidence of abnormality. Therefore, the signs the neurologist elicits are taken as confirming the presence of lesions in the brain.

Exactly the same thing can be said of soft signs. There have been relatively few systematic studies of large populations of children in whom meticulous neurological examinations have been carried out. The Isle of Wight Study (Rutter and Tizard, 1970) suggested that there was not as close an association between the presence of abnormal neurological findings and behavioral abnormalities as might have been assumed from earlier publications. Not only did neurological findings fail to predict behavioral distortions, but behavioral abnormalities also failed to predict physical abnormalities. Some statistical correlation between the two did exist, however. Other studies have confirmed the lack of specificity of soft signs in the neurologically impaired and in normals (Werry and Aman, 1976).

When soft signs are identified as reliably indicating the presence of brain dysfunction, they will no longer be soft. If they reflect brain damage in some patients and can be seen in others who have no evidence of brain dysfunction, then they are soft indeed and probably not very helpful in determining whether or not a patient has brain dysfunction. Signs and symptoms that are found in normals more frequently than in people with brain damage are not soft signs of abnormality but, rather, are within the normal range. To determine which signs are truly soft—that is, those that can be associated with organic damage but need not be—requires correlational statistical studies in patients who are known to be abnormal and in people who are known to be normal, recognizing that the former is easier to establish than the latter. This has not been completed for each of the physical signs that are called soft.

Consistency has been considered important in determining the long-term significance of soft signs in children. Though follow-up studies can provide considerable information, the fact that minor or major neurological abnormalities may disappear in the course of development does not necessarily mean that the findings originally elicited were not significant or should be considered "merely maturational." A mild hemiparesis or diparesis may disappear, hypotonia may become normotonia, seizures may stop, but the importance of these findings as evidence of encephalopathy in the past remains. Such historical encephalopathy may still be relevant to contemporary behavioral disturbances.

One of the commonest clinical settings in which learning and behavioral disturbances turn up is seizures that originate in the temporal lobe. The etiological dilemma of this association has not been fully resolved. Are the learning and behavior problems secondary to the emotional trauma of susceptibility to seizures? Does the uncontrolled seizure disorder, or the medication that is used to control it, lead to a partial functional disruption of the system that is sufficient to cause defects of attention and learning? Are seizures and behavior problems coincident symptoms of the same basic neurological abnormality? If so, can the seizures resolve while the behavior and learning problems remain?

The search for validating correlations among various findings requires a standard against which to compare them. There is a tendency to ascribe certainty to tools that are used by an allied profession. Child psychiatrists may tend to regard the physical examination of a child neurologist with greater respect than do neurologists themselves. Consistency of findings and interrater reliability can be a problem. The EEG may provide borderline or frankly paroxysmal abnormalities in a certain percentage of patients with learning disability who have no clinical seizures. This may be a soft finding to many neurologists but may not be to some psychologists. On the other hand, psychological tests, especially the Wechsler Intelligence Scale for Children (WISC) and Bender tests, may provide evidence that to neurologists is less equivocal than it may be to psychiatrists or even to psychologists. All groups are somewhat in awe of computed tomography (CT) and magnetic resonance images of the brain, though findings such as cerebral atrophy and enlarged ventricles are quite soft because they do not reliably predict behavioral or cognitive dysfunction (Shaywitz et al., 1983). The fact is that we lack an acceptable "gold standard" against which to measure each of the multitudinous symptoms and signs included in the vague expression, "soft signs." This being the case, we have been forced to make correlations among tests of unproven value (Barlow, 1974).

INVESTIGATION OF PARTICULAR SOFT SIGNS—MOTOR AND SENSORY

Prechtl and Stemmer (1962) first pointed out the significance of choreiform movements. This phenomenon consists of random, quick, irregular movements, most prominently seen in the fingers of the supinated outstretched forearms. Prechtl and Stemmer correlated this phenomenon with perinatal distress and neonatal abnormality. Wolf and Hurwitz (1966) reported an overall incidence of the choreiform syndrome of roughly 10% in elementary school children aged 10 to 12, with a significant difference between boys (17%) and girls (5%). The incidence of choreiform signs dropped from 50% at age 10 years to 3% among 12-year-olds. Additional studies documented that boys with choreiform twitches had more reading and spelling difficulties than boys without, but there was no such correlation in girls (Wolff and Hurwitz, 1973).

Development of the ability to appreciate simultaneous touch to face and hand is clearly age related. Most normal children achieve this ability by age 7. This is also the age during which concepts of body image enlarge to include a body under the large head of children's drawings (Bender et al., 1951). Kraft (1968) basically confirmed these findings but found no correlation with the scored Goodenough Draw-a-Man test. Kraft found that 30% of 7-year-old nonreaders gave an immature response to the face-hand test, whereas 20% of normal readers gave an immature response—a difference that is not particularly impressive. When combined with the Draw-a-Man test, however, defects in the combined tests were found in 83% of nonreaders (Kraft, 1968).

In a longitudinal study of 66 prematurely born children from advantaged homes, neurological examinations were performed at 8 years of age. Thirteen of these children had localizing neurological findings, and 20 were found to have two or more nonlocalizing (soft) signs of CNS dysfunction. These included tests of speech, balance, coordination, gait, sequential finger-thumb opposition, muscle tone, graphesthesia, stereognosis, and choreiform movements. These 33 neurologically abnormal children were significantly more likely to have sustained perinatal complications than were children whose neurological examinations were normal. Though children with soft signs were at a consistent disadvantage—in relation to IQ, reading, and arithmetic achievement test score levels—compared to those who were neurologically normal, these differences did not reach conventional levels of significance. However, the children with soft signs were significantly more likely to have received special education and to have been referred for psychiatric consultation than were the neurologically normal children. Almost half of the children with two or more of the physical soft signs elicited by the investigators required special educational intervention to reach the same overall level of academic school performance achieved by the neurologically normal children. Ninety percent of the neurologically normal children made satisfactory progress without any modification of the school program. This finding, coupled with the high frequency of psychiatric consultations and continuing intervention among the soft-signs group, provided support for the view that these children are, indeed, at greater risk for the emergence of behavioral and/or school learning problems (Hertzig, 1981).

Reliability and Stability of Soft Signs

Any conclusion regarding the validity of soft signs assumes a satisfactory interrater reliability, internal consistency, and retest stability of subtle signs. Though this has not been studied extensively, some information is available (Stokman et al., 1986). The Physical and Neurological Examination for Soft Signs (PANESS) has been used with 54 psychiatric patients and 25 normal children aged 5 to 17 years. Acceptable interrater reliability was found for most of the items tested. Test-retest reliability at 2 weeks was not satisfactory for some of the categorically scored items. But continuous items, such as the time needed to perform 20 consecutive movements, remained relatively stable at retest (Vitiello et al., 1989).

To assess the persistence of soft signs outside a referred sample, 159 members of a local birth cohort of the United States National Collaborative Perinatal Project were traced and their performance on six neurological test scales was measured at age 17 by examiners who were unaware

of their status at age 7. A comparison group was also formed that had been sign-free at age 7. On four of the six tests (dysdiadochokinesia, mirror movements, dysgraphesthesia, and motor slowness), index boys did significantly worse than the comparison boys. In contrast, index girls scored significantly worse than comparisons only on motor slowness. The consistency of neurological test performance through the years contradicts the idea, at least in boys, that soft signs are only maturational lags destined to fade with age. The worse the boy's neurological score at age 17, the stronger is the relationship with his status at age 7.

This important study made another observation that was of great significance. Analysis of the data that categorized findings as either absent or present, rather than of varying intensity, would have shown almost no statistically significant relationship in the 7 to 17 year data. If neurological test performance is intrinsically a continuous function, such categorical analysis, which was used in most of the earlier studies, would be likely to underestimate the true strength of relationships (Shafer et al., 1986). Unfortunately, the large population studies that have been interpreted as casting doubt on the usefulness of abnormalities found on neurological examination did use a categorical approach to describing them.

SOFT SIGNS AND ATTENTION DEFICIT HYPERACTIVITY DISORDER

The literature on this subject is contradictory. Wikler et al. (1970) and Camp et al. (1978) have found no difference in the prevalence of signs between children with and without Attention Deficit Hyperactivity Disorder (ADHD). Nichols and Chen (1981) analyzed a large sample drawn from all 7-year-old participants in the National Collaborative Perinatal Project and found only a small excess of overactivity and inattention among children who had neurological soft signs. Shaffer et al. (1985) found no relationship between early soft signs and attention deficit or conduct disorders in 63 male and 27 female adolescents known to have had neurological soft signs at the age of 7 years. However, Lucas et al. (1965), Mikkelsen et al. (1982), and McMahon and Greenberg (1977) all found soft signs to be more common in generally younger groups of children with ADHD than in controls (Wikler et al., 1970).

There is thus considerable evidence that, although soft neurological signs reflect organic brain dysfunction, they are rather inconsistently seen in the syndrome of ADHD, once called minimal brain damage. This does not mean that ADHD is unrelated to brain dysfunction. If a particular psychiatric condition were associated with soft neurological findings, this would presumably constitute evidence in favor of the organic nature of such a psychiatric disturbance. If a psychiatric disturbance were not associated with soft neurological findings, it would not necessarily mean that the psychiatric disturbance arose from some source other than brain dysfunction.

The frontal lobes have increasingly been targeted as the possible source of abnormality in ADHD (Benson, 1991). Quantitative analysis of magnetic resonance images of 18 boys with ADHD and 18 carefully matched controls supports the theory of abnormal frontal lobe disturbance in ADHD (Giedd et al., 1994). Magnetic Resonance Imaging (MRI) studies of the cross-sectional area of the corpus callosum also reveal that the anterior regions were smaller in ADHD boys (Giedd et al., 1994; Hynd et al., 1991). A similar study using positron emission tomography (PET) identified hypometabolism in the left anterior frontal lobe as a significant correlate of ADHD severity in adolescents (Zametkin et al., 1993).

Reports of psychological tests that generally reflect frontal dysfunction have been somewhat conflicting. Deficits in verbal fluency were found in male ADHD inpatients compared with inpatient controls (Koziol and Stout, 1992). Other tests reflecting frontal lobe dysfunction distinguished ADHD children and controls, although general cognitive impairment was not found in the former group (Shue and Douglas, 1992). Some measures of frontal lobe dysfunction did not reliably distinguish ADD with and without hyperactivity but the Continuous Performance

Test and the Stroop Test did distinguish ADD groups from normal (Barkley et al., 1992). Yet others (Loge, et al., 1990) have reported impaired WISC performance in ADHD but no difference from controls in the Wisconsin Card Sorting Test or tests of verbal and design fluency.

Clearly, the preponderance of evidence (MRI, PET, psychological tests) favors the concept that frontal dysfunction explains some of the behavior in ADHD. We must now ask, are there neurological signs that reflect frontal lobe dysfunction? The answer is yes, but none of them are part of the ordinary neurological examination of school-age children and, for the most part, they have not been standardized and validated in these age groups as they have been in adults (Jenkyn et al., 1977). These are the snout reflex (Paulson and Gottlieb, 1968), suck and grasp reflexes (Shahani et al., 1970), paratonia, persistent glabellar (Damasio, 1985), abnormal visual tracking movements (Rodin, 1964), abnormal response in performing reciprocal coordination of the hands, and three-step motor sequences of the hands (Luria, 1962; Ozeretski, 1930). The presence of three frontal signs discriminated between subjects with normal and abnormal MRIs with 93% accuracy, and normal and abnormal neuropsychological testing with 85% accuracy, when applied to 31 murderers whose average age was 32. Half had been diagnosed as ADHD in their youth: Grasp reflex, suck reflex, and paratonia were the best discriminators (Blake et al., unpublished data).

If ADHD is, in fact, a reflection of frontal lobe dysfunction, the neurological signs for its evaluation must be those that reflect frontal lobe dysfunction reliably.

NEUROLOGICAL SOFT SIGNS AND OTHER PSYCHOPATHOLOGY

Neurological soft signs have been described as being overrepresented in patients carrying a diagnosis of childhood autism, Tourette's syndrome, schizophrenia, borderline personality disorder, or anxiety-withdrawal.

Like ADHD, autism is not a disease entity itself but, rather, a behavioral syndrome of childhood that can result from many different disorders of the CNS that cause bilateral dysfunction. Defective speech is a hallmark, but autistic children often have varying deficits in comprehension, symbolic thinking, and the formation of abstract concepts that reflect varying degrees of CNS dysfunction and the diseases that cause it. This is consistent with the variegated pattern of cognitive functioning in autism, which is often uneven in an individual case, with preserved "islets of intelligence." Autism is often seen in children who show strong independent evidence of neurological abnormality. It may be associated with phenylketonuria, tuberous sclerosis, and infantile spasms during the first year of life. Many autistic children have multiple cognitive deficits and perhaps half have, or once had, electroencephalographic abnormalities or a history of seizures or both. The symptoms of autism resemble those of congenital aphasia. It is worth noting that permanent aphasia can only be produced in children by bilateral cerebral lesions. Hardly any information on the neuropathological correlates of autism has been published. It is a nonprogressive, nonfatal syndrome, and brain biopsies cannot usually be justified. Some defects in cerebral myelination and myelination of the cerebellum have been reported, but it seems highly unlikely that these constitute the root of the disturbance, which symptomatically resembles more a problem of the gray matter and cerebral cortex than of the white matter or the cerebellum.

Children with autism have been compared to normals matched for both chronological and mental ages on two tests of motor imitation and on the Herzig Battery for nonfocal neurological signs (Jones and Prior, 1985). The latter includes tests of speech, balance, coordination, double simultaneous stimulation, gait, sequential finger-thumb opposition, muscle tone, graphesthesia, astereognosis, and choreiform movements. Performance was rated as normal, mildly impaired, or markedly impaired. Imitation ability was defective in the children with autism who showed an average of four soft signs. All had two or more such signs, the most frequent of which were choreiform movements (100% markedly

impaired), imbalance (70% markedly, 30% mildly impaired), extinction to double simultaneous stimulation (60% markedly impaired), incoordination (40% markedly, 50% mildly impaired), finger-thumb opposition (40% markedly, 30% mildly impaired), and speech disarticulation (40% markedly, 40% mildly impaired).

The significant prevalence of soft signs in this group of 6–10-year-old children with autism was marked, universal, and excessive, compared to both chronologically and mentally age-matched controls. Yet some of the soft signs were also seen among the controls. The lack of true, normative developmental data makes it difficult to utilize the soft signs to support the theory of the organic pathogenesis of autism. The lack of complete understanding of autism makes it unsound to utilize the supposed organic pathogenesis of autism to validate the meaningfulness of soft signs (Jones and Prior, 1985).

Tourette's syndrome is a familial neuropsychiatric disorder of unknown etiology that is characterized by waxing and waning multiform motor and phonic tics and a range of complex and intriguing behavioral symptoms. Typically, it is a lifelong disorder that can be disabling and that usually begins in the 1st decade. In addition to the motor and phonic symptoms, several behavioral symptoms are often seen in patients with Tourette's syndrome, including diminished ability to concentrate, impulsiveness, impaired regulation of activity, and disabling obsessions and compulsions. As many as half of the children with Tourette's syndrome satisfy the diagnostic criteria for ADHD. Although most do not have primary learning disabilities, their conduct disturbance can substantially impair school performance. Many Tourette's patients do have specific learning disabilities as well, however. Obsessive-compulsive symptoms seen in patients with Tourette's syndrome usually appear late in the developmental course of the syndrome. These include obsessive doubting of decisions, concern about touching objects or persons, and elaborate compulsive rituals.

Family studies and twin data support the notion that Tourette's syndrome and multifocal tics are inherited as an autosomal dominant on a single major gene locus (Shapiro et al., 1978). The genetic evidence strongly implicates brain dysfunction as the source of the symptomatology. The relationship between Tourette's and ADHD is controversial. Some studies suggest that ADHD is etiologically related to Tourette's syndrome, while other reports are more consistent with the hypothesis that ADHD is a comorbid condition and that the high prevalence of ADHD in a clinical population of patients with Tourette's syndrome may result from an ascertainment bias (Cohen, 1982). Increased rates of obsessive-compulsive symptoms in Tourette's patients, and the finding that about 20% of first-degree relatives of Tourette's probands display prominent obsessive-compulsive symptoms, have led to the provocative hypothesis that some forms of obsessive-compulsive disorder may be an alternate phenotypic expression of the Tourette's gene.

Obsessive-compulsive disorder (OCD) has been linked to altered neurological function following head trauma, encephalitis, abnormal birth events, and Tourette's syndrome. Abnormalities in CT scans, EEGs, PET scans, and evoked potentials have been described in this disorder, but are neither consistent nor pathognomonic of OCD. Forty-one medication-free patients with OCD who met DSM III-R criteria, as well as 20 normal controls matched for age, sex, and handedness, were studied on 20 individual tasks that involved fine motor coordination, involuntary movements, and sensory and visuospatial function. There were significantly more signs of CNS dysfunction in the OCD group, as shown by abnormalities in fine motor coordination, involuntary and mirror movements, and visuospatial function. An excess of findings on the left side of the body and abnormalities in drawing cubes may suggest right hemispheric dysfunction in a subgroup of patients with OCD. Soft signs correlated with the severity of obsessions. There was also a correlation between abnormalities in visual memory and recognition on neuropsychological testing, and total soft signs. These findings provided additional evidence for a neurological deficit in some patients with OCD. However, the lack of understanding of the neurological basis of soft signs and OCD makes it difficult to use one to establish the organicity of the other (Hollander et al., 1990).

Minor neurological abnormalities and physical anomalies are commonly found in *schizophrenia*. This is not what one would expect in a "functional" disease and, for this reason, such signs were often overlooked or considered epiphenomena. One only has to walk through the chronic wards of a large state hospital to be impressed by the number of patients who suffer from neurological dysfunction, in terms of impaired equilibrium, gait, and coordination, and even gross mental retardation. The effects of medication, malnutrition, and multiple electrical shock treatments, may have something to do with these abnormalities. Certainly, many of the studies of neurological changes in state hospital populations, for which both the cause for admission and original symptoms often have been long forgotten, are suspect when a high incidence of neurological findings in schizophrenics is cited. The few such studies done on acute patients, however, have documented a significant degree of neurological dysfunction. Abnormalities include minor motor and sensory (soft) neurological signs on physical examination, electroencephalographic abnormalities, and abnormal CT scans.

Rochford et al. (1970) examined 65 hospitalized, untreated psychiatric patients for the presence of the following minor signs: (*a*) motor impersistence; (*b*) stereognosis; (*c*) graphesthesia; (*d*) extinction during bilateral simultaneous stimulation; (*e*) bilateral marked hyperreflexia; (*f*) coordination defects; (*g*) disturbance of balance and gait; (*h*) cortical sensory abnormalities; (*i*) mild movement disorders; (*j*) speech defects; (*k*) abnormal motor activity; (*l*) defective auditory-visual integration; (*m*) choreiform movements and adventitious motor overflow (tremor); (*n*) cranial nerve abnormalities, such as slight anisocoria, esotropia, auditory deficit, and visual field and retinal defects; and (*o*) unequivocally abnormal EEGs. They found neurological abnormalities in 36.8% of the psychiatric patients (all diagnostic groups). This was significantly different from an age-matched, normal control population (5%). Neurological soft signs were found in 65.5% of the schizophrenic patients. By way of comparison, there were no soft signs in patients with primary affective disorders.

Neurological deficits have been included in descriptions of schizophrenia since Kraepelin first defined dementia praecox. One group of studies reported a greater-than-normal overall number of neurological signs in patients with adult and childhood schizophrenia and in the offspring of schizophrenics (Reider and Nichols, 1979). Another group reported more neurological signs in the schizophrenic twin of identical twins discordant for schizophrenia. A third group of studies found deficits in a broad range of specific neurological areas, including psychomotor integration, vestibular reactivity, lateralization, and involuntary muscle coordination and tone (Marcus et al., 1985). In fact, the presence of neurological signs in schizophrenia is so strong a finding that a congenital neurointegrative defect is now believed to be at the base of at least some subtypes of the illness.

Fish et al. (1965) reported in detail on 10 infants, each of whom had a schizophrenic parent. During the neonatal period, these children showed poor muscle tone and an unusually torpid biological state and, later, they showed irregular or uneven rates of physical growth and motoric development.

The original neurological examination for the Israeli study of children of schizophrenics (Marcus et al., 1985) was constructed in 1966 and used child neurology scales. The examination, which contained over 30 items, was constructed to cover a broad group of areas that might reveal minor deficiencies in neural integration. In line with the prevailing opinion at that time, the neurological examination was evaluated by an overall score of nonoptimal functioning, computed by adding the scores of all items on the examination. Results showed a subgroup of offspring of schizophrenic parents with poorer cumulative scores.

Five years after the original data were collected, another neurological assessment was made of the same children using a similar examination. Several statistically significant group differences in neurological functioning were found. In the original assessment, neurological signs were more severe in males than in females. This sex difference is consistent with the higher incidence of many kinds of major and minimal brain

dysfunction and developmental delay observed in boys. A group of children with multiple areas of neurological deficits was identified, consisting almost exclusively of the offspring of schizophrenic patients. Twenty-two of the 50 index cases demonstrated this level of poor functioning during at least one of the testing periods; only 3 of the 50 control cases showed this level of poor functioning at either period. In contrast, children with good neurological functioning were a mixture of index and control cases. This pattern of results is consistent with the model described previously: Only a subgroup of the offspring of schizophrenics would show biological deficits, while others would be indistinguishable from normal children. Forty-four percent of the offspring of schizophrenics in this study had signs of a neurointegrative defect during at least one of the time periods. This result is consistent with the hypothesis that approximately half of the offspring of schizophrenic patients have neurological deficits. These data are intriguing and hint at the possibility of a single dominant gene hypothesis for the genetic transmission of vulnerability to schizophrenia.

The types of neurological signs most typical of the offspring of schizophrenics were perceptual-sensory signs, poor motor coordination, poor right-left orientation, poor balance, and motor overflow (the latter especially at the older ages). Such minor deficits in attention and inhibition suggest a strong resemblance between this subgroup of offspring of schizophrenics and children with ADHD. While many of the offspring of schizophrenics had other neurological signs, such as dyskinesias, abnormal reflexes, and facial asymmetries, it was the above group of motor and sensory signs that best defined the poorly functioning subgroup and probably represents the genetically determined dysfunction.

Yet, in this study, the offspring of schizophrenic patients who showed poor levels of functioning varied considerably across the two assessments: 22 children showed multiple areas of neurological dysfunction during at least one of the two age periods; only 6 showed such dysfunction in both periods. This relative lack of stability of signs is difficult to interpret. Are the signs meaningless and random? Do they represent a fluctuating state of brain abnormality? Again, without knowing the meaning of the signs or the pathogenesis of schizophrenia, it is difficult to use either to shore up theories concerning the organic etiology of the other.

Reports of electroencephalographic abnormality in schizophrenic patients referred at random range from 5% to 80%, with an average of 25%, but the vagaries of EEG interpretation and the variability in diagnosing schizophrenia obscure the meaning of these data. Patients diagnosed as catatonic schizophrenics seem to show consistently higher rates of electroencephalographic abnormality, usually manifested as nonspecific slowing. Since catatonic states are often acute and have a relatively good prognosis, one wonders if all cases so labeled are really catatonic schizophrenia. The higher rate of electroencephalographic abnormality in catatonic schizophrenics raises some question about the diagnosis.

Yet electroencephalographic abnormalities are seen in schizophrenics, especially catatonic schizophrenics, more often than in the general population. This statement seems valid even when allowances are made for an occasional misdiagnosis and the effect of drugs and shock therapy. It is not known whether the schizophrenic process or an underlying or associated brain defect causes these electroencephalographic abnormalities. One possibility is that brain damage, which may be reflected in the EEG, could facilitate the development of schizophrenia in individuals with a genetic tendency toward the disease.

CT and, more recently, PET have opened exciting possibilities for studying the structure and function of the CNS in schizophrenics. Since 1976 there have been persistent reports of ventricular enlargement, hemispheric asymmetry, and cerebellar atrophy in schizophrenic patients. Rider et al. (1983) and Shelton et al. (1983) have shown ventricular changes in schizophrenics and have shown that these ventricular changes correlate with other findings, such as increased neuropsychological impairment, poor response to treatment, and poor premorbid adjustment. The ventricular enlargements demonstrated would not be called abnormal by radiologists but, rather, are subtle variations within the normal range, and even these are not present in all the schizophrenics studied. Other investigations have not confirmed the findings of ventricular enlargement. Almost all the studies in this area, whatever their results, suffer from serious methodological problems, such as the following: (a) The study populations have been disparate, ranging from old to young, chronic to acute, rigidly diagnosed to less rigidly diagnosed; (b) the techniques of measuring ventricular size in each study were not standardized and vary from actual manual measurements to computer measurements, leading to a great variation from study to study in the incidence of abnormal findings and in their comparability; (c) the control populations have varied from none, to reported norms in the literature, normal populations, or neurological patients with headaches who are referred for evaluation. Very few of these studies have compared other chronic psychiatric patients to the schizophrenic patients, and none has utilized a blind technique for reading CT scans.

PET is now being used to study schizophrenia, and this new technique is so sophisticated that we may be able to observe dynamic changes of cerebral function in schizophrenic patients during different psychopathological states and to follow these changes through the course of illness. The PET studies seem to show that there is some decrease of blood flow in the frontal lobes of schizophrenics. Minor asymmetrical hemispheric differences have been noted as well (Berman et al., 1988; Buchsbaum et al. 1984). These studies, however, have involved so few patients with such varying diagnoses and drug regimens that we must await larger studies and more standardization of the research methods to lend them more weight.

Extensive investigation of patients with *borderline personality disorder* (BPD) suggests that underlying organic factors may play a role in this complex disorder that consists of affective, behavioral, and cognitive abnormalities. One area of focus has been neurological and neurophysiological dysfunction. Findings in borderline patients of abnormal EEG results, histories including head trauma, seizures, and learning disabilities, and similarities to patients with episodic dyscontrol syndrome and adult ADHD have led several authors to postulate that a neurophysiological dysfunction of the CNS may be responsible for mediating some of the symptoms experienced by patients with BPD (Gardner et al., 1987).

Patients with BPD were found to have a significantly greater number of soft-sign neurological abnormalities when compared with a group of normal control subjects. The presence of two or more soft signs differentiated the two groups statistically. The authors speculated that the nonfocal, soft-sign neurological abnormalities may reflect underlying CNS dysfunction, which may, in turn, be associated with the development of BPD.

In their study of soft signs, Shaffer et al. (1985) found an odd correlation of early soft signs with *anxiety and withdrawal*. Sixty-three male and 27 female adolescents at 17 years of age, known to have had neurological soft signs at the age of 7 years, were compared with controls with no soft signs at age 7. Adolescents with early soft signs had significantly lower IQs and were more likely to have a psychiatric disorder characterized by anxiety, withdrawal, and depression. All the girls and 80% (12 of 15) of the boys with an anxiety-withdrawal diagnosis showed early soft signs. There was no relationship between early soft signs and attention deficit or conduct disorders. Examination of relative contributions of anxiety at age 7, IQ, and social and family disadvantage to later diagnosis showed that most of the variance was accounted for by soft signs, independently of IQ. Soft signs and anxious, dependent behavior at age 7 were strongly predictive of persistent psychiatric disorder characterized by anxiety and withdrawal.

The origins of soft signs remain obscure. It is widely held that they have a developmental origin, by which it is usually meant that they diminish in prevalence or severity with age. This hypothesis is supported to some extent by cross-sectional studies that find a higher prevalence of individual signs among younger than older children. However, there have been relatively few longitudinal studies. Shaffer et al. (1985) found that a large proportion of children who had soft signs at age 7 continue to show such signs at age 17. Hertzig (1981), who studied a neurologically deviant population, found that although there is a diminution in amplitude and range of signs found in an individual child, children with a sign at one age are likely to show signs, not necessarily the same ones, 5 years later. Further, the notion of signs being ''developmental'' does not elucidate the problem. The study by Nichols and Chen (1981) on the cohort of children aged 7 from the entire National Collaborative Perinatal Project found few prenatal predictors, other than maternal smoking or diabetes and chorionitis, to be related to soft signs. Although the relative risk for having soft signs given one of these maternal factors was significantly increased, it was nevertheless low. Postnatal infections, illnesses, and injuries did not predict soft signs.

Nichols and Chen also studied concordance for signs among the monozygotic and the dizygotic twins in the study population. The difference between them was statistically significant, with greater concordance being found in the monozygotic twins. This finding, coupled with observations on the ratio of concordance between full siblings and first cousins, is compatible with a genetic origin of soft signs.

One is led to the conclusion that soft signs on the neurological examination do reflect brain dysfunction in most cases and are influenced by heredity. They do not reliably predict ADHD, but they are prevalent in other behavioral disorders. The inconsistency with which they are encountered in ADHD gives no clue as to the etiology of ADHD, but this is a subject that is discussed elsewhere (see Chapter 50).

References

Barkley RA, Grodzinsky G, DuPaul GJ: Frontal lobe functions in attention deficit disorder with and without hyperactivity: A review and research report. *J Abnorm Child Psychol* 20:163–168, 1992.

Barlow CF: Soft signs in children with learning disorders. *Am J Dis Child* 128:605–606, 1974.

Bender MB, Fink M, Green M: Patterns in perception on simultaneous tests of face and hand. *Arch Neurol Psychiatry* 66:355–362, 1951.

Benson DF: The role of frontal dysfunction in attention deficit hyperactivity disorder. *J Child Neurol* 6:suppl 9–12, 1991.

Berman KF, Illowsky BP, Weinberger DR: Physiological dysfunction of the dorsolateral prefrontal cortex in schizophrenia. IV: Further evidence for regional and behavioral specificity. *Arch Gen Psychiatry* 45:616–622, 1988.

Buchsbaum MS, DeLisi LE, Holcomb HH, et al: Anteriorposterior gradients in cerebral glucose use in schizophrenia and affective disorders. *Arch Gen Psychiatry* 41:1159–1166, 1984.

Camp JA, Bialer I, Sverd J, et al: Clinical usefulness of the NIMH physical and neurological examination for soft signs. *Am J Psychiatry* 135:362–364, 1978.

Cohen DJ, Detlor J, Shaywitz BA, et al: Interaction of biological and psychological factors in the natural history of Tourette syndrome: A paradigm for childhood neuropsychiatric disorders. *Adv Neurol* 35:31–40, 1982.

Damasio AR: The Frontal Lobes. In: Heilman KM, Valenstein E, (eds.): *Clinical Neuropsychology,* (2nd ed.) New York, Oxford University Press 1985.

Fish B, Shapiro T, Halpern F, et al: The prediction of schizophrenia in infancy. III: A ten year follow-up report of neurological and psychological development. *Am J Psychiatry* 121:768–775, 1965.

Gardner D, Lucas PB, Cowdry RW: soft sign neurological abnormalities in borderline personality disorder and normal control subjects. *J Nerv Ment Dis* 175:177–180,1987.

Giedd JN, Castellanos FX, Casey BJ et al: Quantitative morphology of the corpus callosum in attention deficit hyperactivity disorder. *Am J Psychiatry* 151:665–669, 1994.

Hertzig ME: Neurological soft signs in low birth weight children. *Dev Med Child Neurol* 23:778–791, 1981.

Hollander E, Schiffman E, Cohen B, et al: Signs of central nervous system dysfunction in obsessive-compulsive disorder. *Arch Gen Psychiatry* 47: 37–32, 1990.

Hynd GW, Semrud-Clikeman M, Lorys AR, et al: Corpus callosum morphology in attention deficit hyperactivity disorder: Morphometric analysis of MRI. *J Learn Disabil* 24:141–146, 1991.

Jenkyn LR, Walsh DB, Culvert CM, et al: Clinical signs in diffuse cerebral dysfunction. *J Neurol Neurosurg Psychiatry* 40:956–966, 1977.

Jones V, Prior M: Motor imitation abilities and neurological signs in autistic children. *J Autism Dev Disord* 15:37–46, 1985.

Koziol LF, Stout CE: Use of a verbal fluency measure in understanding and evaluating ADHD as an executive function disorder. *Percept Mot Skills* 75:1187–1192, 1992.

Krail MB: The Face-Hand Test. *Dev Med Child Neurol* 10:214–219, 1968.

Loge DV, Staton RD, Beatty WW: Performance of children with ADHD on tests sensitive to frontal lobe dysfunction. *J Am Acad Child Adolesc Psychiatry* 24 29:540–545, 1990.

Lucas AR, Rodin EA, Simson CB: Neurological assessment of children with early school problems. *Dev Med Child Neurol* 7:145–156, 1965.

Luria AR: *Higher Cortical Functions in Man*, (2nd ed.) New York, Basic Books 1962, pp 415–422.

Marcus J, Hans SL, Lewow E, et al: Neurological findings in high-risk children: Childhood assessment and 5 year follow-up. *Schizophr Bull* 11: 85–100,1985.

McMahon SA, Greenberg LM: Serial neurologic examination of hyperactive children. *Pediatrics* 59: 584–587, 1977.

Mikkelsen EJ, Brown GL, Minichiello MD, et al: Neurologic status in hyperactive, enuretic, encopretic and normal boys. *J Acad Child Psychiatry* 21:75–81, 1982.

Nichols PL, Chen TC: *Minimal Brain Dysfunction: A Prospective Study*. Hillsdale, NJ, Erlbaum, 1981.

Ozeretski NI: Techniques in Investigating Motor Function. In: Gurevich M, Ozeretski N (eds.): *Psychomotor Functions* Moscow, Medzig, 1930.

Paulson G, Gottlieb G: Developmental reflexes: the reappearance of fetal and neonatal reflexes in aged patients. *Brain* 91:37–52, 1968.

Pincus JH, Tucker GJ: *Behavioral Neurology* (3rd ed). New York, Oxford University Press, 1983.

Prechtl HFR, Stemmer CJ: The choreiform syndrome in children. *Dev Med Child Neurol* 4: 119–127, 1962.

Rieder RO, Mann LS, Weinberger DR, et al: Computerized tomographic scans in patients with schizophrenia, schizoaffective and bipolar affective disorder. *Arch Gen Psychiatry* 40:735–739, 1983.

Rieder RO, Nichols PL: Offspring of schizophrenics. III: Hyperactivity and neurological soft signs. *Arch Gen Psychiatry* 36:665–674, 1979.

Rochford JM, Detre T, Tucker GJ, et al: Neuropsychological impairments in functional psychiatric diseases. *Arch Gen Psychiatry* 22:114–122, 1970.

Rutter M, Tizard J, Whitmore K (eds): *Education, Health, and Behavior*. London, Longmans, 1970.

Shaffer D, Schonfeld I, O'Connor P, et al: Neurological soft signs; their relationship to psychiatric disorder and intelligence in childhood and adolescence. *Arch Gen Psychiatry* 42:342–351, 1985.

Shafer SQ, Stokman CJ, Shaffer D, et al: Ten year consistency in neurological test performance of children without focal neurological deficit. *Dev Med Child Neurol* 28:417–427, 1986.

Shahani B, Burrows P, Whitty CWM: The grasp reflex and perseveration. *Brain* 93:181–192, 1970.

Shapiro AK, Shapiro ES, Brunn RD, et al: *Gilles de la Tourette Syndrome*. New York, Raven, 1978.

Shaywitz BA, Byrne T, Shaywitz SE: Attention deficit disorder: Quantitave analysis of CT. *Neurology* 33:1500, 1983.

Shelton RC, Karson CN, Doran AR, et al: Cerebral structural pathology in schizophrenia: Evidence for a selective prefrontal cortical defect. *Am J Psychiatry* 145:154–163. 1988.

Shue KL, Douglas VI: Attention deficit hyperactivity disorder and the frontal lobe syndrome. *Brain Cogn* 20:104–124, 1992.

Stokman CJ, Shafer SQ, Shaffer D, et al: Assessment of neurological soft signs in adolescents: Reliability studies. *Dev Med Child Neurol* 28:428–439, 1986.

Vitiello B, Ricciuti AJ, Stoff DM, et al: Reliability of subtle (soft) neurological signs in children. *J Am Acad Child Adolesc Psychiatry* 5:749–753, 1989.

Werry JS, Aman MG: Reliability and diagnostic validity of the physical and neurological examination for soft signs. *J Autism Child Schizophr* 6:253–262, 1976.

Wikler A, Dixon JF, Parker JB Jr: Brain function in problem children and controls: Psychometric, neurological, intellectual, encephalographic comparisons. *Am J Psychiatry* 127:94–105, 1970.

Wolff TH, Hurwitz J: The choreiform syndrome. *Dev Med Child Neurol* 8:160–165, 1966.

Wolff TH, Hurwitz J: Functional implications of the minimal brain damage syndrome. *Semin Psychiatry* 5:105–115, 1973.

Zametkin AJ, Liebenauer LL, Fitzgerald GA et al: Brain metabolism in teenagers with attention deficit hyperactivity disorder. *Arch Gen Psychiatry* 50: 333–340, 1993.

43 PSYCHOEDUCATIONAL ASSESSMENT

Barbara K. Keogh, Ph.D., and Judith Margolis, Ph.D.

Psychoeducational assessment continues to be a flourishing enterprise and a subject of controversy. Historically, psychoeducational tests were used in schools primarily to determine eligibility for special education services. Thus, the targets of assessment were cognitive competencies and deficits and knowledge in traditional school subjects, such as reading and arithmetic. IQ tests and standardized achievement tests constituted the standard test battery. In the past two decades, both aptitude and achievement tests have been challenged because of possible bias related to ethnic, linguistic, and gender status of the test takers (see Reschley, 1988, for discussion). Questions of appropriateness, validity, and utility have become particularly important, given the demographic changes in school populations and the extension of mandated special services to preschool disabled children.

The adoption of an educational policy of inclusion for disabled learners has also affected assessment practices. The current inclusion movement, widely supported on a policy level, directs placement of *all* children in regular education programs wherever possible, and places major responsibility for their instruction on regular, rather than special, educators (Lipsky and Gartner, 1989; Stainback and Stainback, 1991). Two implications of the inclusion policy are that assessment techniques must be appropriate for a range of disability conditions, and that assessment must provide information relevant to the instruction of problem learners in mainstream educational programs.

An additional issue in assessment is related to both the concern for early identification and intervention with young children and the need to include families in intervention planning. These concerns present serious measurement challenges, as there are relatively few well-developed assessment techniques, especially for assessing families. Many of the techniques now available have only limited evidence of predictive validity, particularly when applied to children with moderate delays or problems in development. Further, although information derived from developmental tests allows inferences about a given child's status relative to a normative group, such information provides little direction for treatment or intervention. Standardized tests that are widely used in schools to assess cognition and achievement have been similarly criticized. In this regard, Campione (1989) distinguishes between assessment for prediction and assessment for prescription. In his terms, prediction refers to the likelihood of success or failure in school programs based on a normative frame of reference. Such test results are used primarily for classification or placement decisions. Prescription refers to assessment information that will " . . . inform the development of instructional programs that can facilitate . . . performance . . ." (Campione, 1989). An examination of the content and methods of many standardized tests suggests that they are predominantly predictive.

Given the limitations of space, in this chapter our emphasis is on assessment approaches that are appropriate for school-age children with minimal/moderate cognitive handicaps. These pupils make up the largest group requiring special services and are usually identified in schools as learning disabled or mildly retarded. Because of the movement for inclusion and the concern for possible bias in normative-based standardized tests, we consider alternative approaches to psychoeducational assessment, specifically, curriculum-based assessment, dynamic-interactional techniques, and portfolio methods. Prior to a more detailed discussion of these approaches, however, we provide a brief discussion of widely-used traditional techniques for assessing aptitude and achievement. The reader is referred to texts by Salvia and Ysseldyke (1991) and

McLoughlin and Lewis (1990), and to the *Ninth Mental Measurements Yearbook* (Mitchell, 1985) for in-depth reviews.

Assessing Aptitude and Achievement

Techniques for assessing aptitude and achievement may be individually or group administered, broad or narrow in content, and for survey or diagnostic purposes. Individually administered tests are considered more valid than group techniques because their administration can be paced to accommodate the tempo of the pupil, there is less chance for errors resulting from misunderstood instructions, and the tester has the opportunity to observe closely the pupil's behavior during testing. For diagnostic purposes, individual administration is clearly preferred. Broad and narrow band tests as well as survey and in-depth techniques all provide useful information. It is important to emphasize, however, that findings from survey techniques are not adequate for diagnostic decisions and should not be the basis for intervention planning. The selection of a specific test or instrument is clearly linked to the purpose(s) of assessment.

Assessing Aptitude

Instruments and approaches for assessing aptitude have been developed mainly from two major perspectives: cognitive/psychometric and neuropsychological. Most are based in the psychometric tradition. Unfortunately, both approaches often provide limited information of direct educational relevance. For example, learning problems have been shown to have associations with many neuropsychological characteristics, e.g., laterality, hemispheric processes, and attentional mechanisms. Yet the causal links between the assessed variables and the expression of specific educational problems have not been well documented. In addition, with a few exceptions, the educational interventions that presumably follow from diagnostic classification have not been specified or tested (see Sandoval and Haapanen, 1981, for discussion of the "brain disability-school disability" notion). The establishment of meaningful links between psychoneurological data and task content, learning processes, and instructional procedures is a high priority if this approach to assessment is to be educationally useful.

Standardized psychometric tests of cognition, such as the Stanford-Binet and the Wechsler scales, are widely used, primarily for classification purposes under the DSM or public law (PL) 94–142 guidelines. They provide normative information that summarizes an individual child's cognitive status relative to his or her chronological peers and the score is expressed as the intelligence quotient or IQ. The Wechsler scales yield both verbal and performance IQs, and also allow the analysis of profiles based on subtest scores within both verbal and performance areas. In addition to the IQ, the fourth edition of the Stanford-Binet has a nonverbal component and yields standard scores for each of 15 subtests (e.g., vocabulary, comprehension, pattern analysis, short-term memory). These tests are well constructed and have impressive statistical support. For the most part, they provide predictive rather than prescriptive information.

A number of tests have been developed specifically to assess the developmental level (and by inference, the aptitude) of young children (see Brown et al., 1992; Gibbs and Teti, 1990; Trad, 1989, for full discussion). Examples of well-known instruments are the Bayley Scales, the Gesell Developmental Schedules, and the Extended Merrill Palmer Scale. It should be noted that, although many of the developmental tests lack the psychometric power characteristic of the Binet or Wechsler scales, they have considerable clinical utility, particularly in documenting development relative to normative expectancies. The systematic assessment of families is still in an infancy stage, but new approaches are emerging in response to the increased recognition of the importance that families have in the cognitive and social development of children with developmental problems (Fewell, 1986). The HOME inventories (Bradley et al., 1992; Caldwell and Bradley, 1984) are examples of a widely used method for describing the stimulating aspects of home environments. The family-focused interview (Winton and Bailey, 1988) is a clinically useful system for identifying family needs, resources, and goals. The assessment of the daily routine of a family, as proposed by Bernheimer and Keogh (1995), provides information that is essential in planning family-based interventions. Given the changes in policy that emphasize family involvement in children's education, methods for assessing families clearly constitute an important topic of research and development.

Although it is often not feasible, practical, or valid to test children with severe cognitive or physical limitations using standardized norm-referenced tests, such as the Binet or Wechsler scales, these tests continue to be used in states requiring IQs for placement in special programs. A few test developers have provided modifications in administrative procedures and in norms for special populations. The Battelle Developmental Inventory is an example of an assessment approach that provides specific adaptations for children with motor, visual, hearing, or emotional problems. The Kaufman Assessment Battery for Children (KABC), based on Luria's distinction between simultaneous and sequential processing, provides global scale and subtest norms for children ranging from seriously retarded to gifted, as well as for children with behavior disorders and hearing impairments; it covers the age range 2.5 through 12 years. The K-ABC yields summarizing IQs and subscale scores. Severely impaired children are also tested using nonverbal tests, such as the Peabody Picture Vocabulary Test, and developmental/adaptive behavior scales, such as the Adaptive Behavior Inventory for Children, the AAMD Adaptive Behavior Scales, and the Vineland Adaptive Behavior Scale.

Assessing Achievement

Achievement tests are widely used in schools to provide information about individual pupils and to assess the relative standings of schools and school districts. Achievement test results may also be used as evidence of teacher effectiveness, a controversial evaluation practice. Achievement measures may focus on a single academic domain, such as reading or spelling, or may tap subject matter from several content areas. Both single and comprehensive subject matter tests may be further classified as survey (screening) or diagnostic measures. Screening batteries typically contain a limited sampling of items from several content areas and are intended to provide a quick estimate of academic functioning level. Commonly used screening tests are the Wide Range Achievement Test (WRAT) and the Basic Achievement Skills Individual Screener (BASIS).

Like the major tests of aptitude, the majority of standardized achievement tests are normatively based, and summary information about a given child or group of children may be expressed as percentiles, standard scores, and/or grade-level equivalents. Examples of widely used norm-referenced tests include the California Achievement Test, the Iowa Test of Basic Skills, the Metropolitan Achievement Tests, the Stanford Achievement Test, and the SRA Achievement Series. Many normative tests, like their cognitive counterparts, have good psychometric properties. Like cognitive tests, however, they often provide limited prescriptive information. For example, a given child may do poorly on an arithmetic test but, from the summary score, it is not possible to determine if the performance was due to limited calculation skills, poor reasoning ability, or both.

Diagnostic tests are more detailed and comprehensive and provide summary information about performance in particular areas or specific subskills, e.g., subsections often tap word recognition, comprehension, and word analysis. The Woodcock Reading Mastery Tests form an example of a widely used, individually administered instrument. This is actually a test battery, composed of five specific subtests, tapping letter and word identification, word attack, and word and passage comprehension. The test provides both reading grade scores (norm referenced) and relative mastery (criterion referenced) information. The Enright Diagnostic Inventory of Basic Arithmetic Skills is an example of an approach for assessing arithmetic computational skills and includes a method of error analysis that pinpoints where and how errors occur.

In summary, there are many standardized and nonstandardized approaches to assessment in specific subject-matter areas. Reynolds and Elliott (1983) identified over 160 published tests of reading, but noted that tests varied in subskills assessed and in technical adequacy. We emphasize also that tests vary in power. In addition to formal testing, reading and arithmetic are frequently assessed with informal techniques, such as checklists or inventories of skills, or through criterion-based measures that may be program specific. Many of these approaches are relatively quick to administer, allow considerable flexibility in administration, and are helpful in specifying areas in need of more in-depth assessment.

Some Limitations of Current Assessment Practices

An increasing number of aptitude and achievement tests are available for use in schools. Their use is based on a number of assumptions: Test items tap relevant intellectual processes; the distribution of intelligence and achievement follows a normal curve; test takers have had similar experiences and similar opportunities for learning. If these assumptions are met, differences in performance on tests are inferred to represent real ''in-person'' differences in intellectual competence and achievement. Standardized norm-based tests vary in content, coverage, administrative procedures, and technical adequacy. Even when psychometrically sound, standardized tests have been challenged about possible bias in content and interpretation. The item content of some tests may not be relevant to assess the skills of individual pupils or to determine the efficacy of particular instructional programs. Normative information provides a picture of a given child's performance at a given time point, but it does not provide information about how the child arrived at that point, nor does it allow reliable inferences about the underlying processes involved in problem resolution or about specific and functional intervention techniques.

Other Assessment Approaches

Recognizing the need to bridge the gap between psychoeducational assessment and educational practice, a number of different approaches to assessment have been proposed. In this chapter we focus on three: curriculum-based assessment, interactive-dynamic assessment, and portfolio assessment.

Curriculum-Based Assessment

Curriculum-based approaches (CBA) may be designed to test commonly taught objectives or may be linked to specific curricula. Pupils are assessed according to their mastery of selected skills or subject matter rather than in terms of normative status. While they are appealing for instructional purposes, CBA measures may lack psychometric adequacy, be narrow in scope, and assess trivial or overly specific skills. They do, however, address the prescriptive aspect of assessment.

Curriculum-based assessment is widely used in special education programs. Broadly defined, CBA is not a particular instrument but a method for assessing a student relative to the curricular requirements of a class or school. The premise is that students' needs are best defined within the context of their local instructional programs (Tucker, 1985). Its adherents suggest that it is a way of linking assessment to instruction, a procedure in which a pupil's performance is evaluated in terms of expected and specific curricular outcomes.

Some types of CBA are relatively informal, with most decisions made by the individual teacher in the classroom. Other versions are more formal, using standardized procedures for developing and administering the assessment. However, all CBA approaches share a common set of principles (Tucker, 1987): Test items are drawn directly from the curriculum, measurement is ongoing, and assessment findings are used as the basis for instructional decisions. Unlike standardized psychoeducational tests, CBA teaches according to the test and tests what it teaches. CBAs measure whether or not a student has mastered a particular skill, and at what level of proficiency. Presumably, therefore, CBAs provide teachers with explicit content for use in instruction. CBA approaches rely heavily on systematic and ongoing monitoring of student performance, as there is evidence that systematic monitoring of student progress is associated with achievement gains (Fuchs et al., 1992). Monitoring is characterized by explicit and frequent measurement and clearly stated, observable goals and decision rules that indicate to teachers when they need to modify instructional programs (Shinn et al., 1989).

A large body of both information and research documents the use of curriculum-based assessment with exceptional children and youths (Bigge, 1988; Howell and Morehead, 1987). Useful applications include identifying students in need of special education intervention, developing Individual Educational Plans (IEPs), monitoring student progress, and evaluating the overall efficacy of special education programs (Fuchs et al., 1984; Fuchs and Fuchs, 1989; Marston, 1987-88). All individuals served in special education programs are required to have a written IEP. In CBA programs, the goals and objectives stated in the IEP become the curriculum for that individual and the content of assessment. Systematic monitoring activities of CBA fit the procedural and substantive evaluation requirements of PL 94–142.

In summary, adherents state that curriculum-based approaches are useful for assessment and analysis of the learning environment, for analysis of the procedures, methods, and approaches used by pupils in problem solution, and for specification of factors associated with the presentation and arrangement of academic tasks. In addition, curriculum-based assessment is frequently the assessment method of choice for pupils who are physically disabled and/or have severe language or cognitive limitations, requiring special assessment and curricular adaptations. Critics argue that the content of CBAs is narrow, that there are unanswered questions about generalization or transfer to new learning, and that the approach is driven by and limited to quantitative data (Heshusius, 1991).

Interactive-Dynamic Assessment

Interactive-dynamic assessment is not a single method but, rather, is an approach that focuses on learners' potential for change and their ability to profit from instruction and experience. Haywood and Wingenfeld (1992) state that ''interactive assessment refers to a group of psychological and psychoeducational procedures that differ from each other but have in common: a) an active role for the examiner, b) a collaborative interaction between examiner and subject, c) a deliberate effort to change what is assessed, and d) the broad goal of assessing *potential* rather than only present performance,'' (p. 254). Lidz (1987; 1991) argues that dynamic-interactive assessment provides a picture of the learners' potential for development, identifies the processes used in problem solving, and yields instructionally useful information (see also Haywood and Tzuriel, 1992).

Interactive-dynamic assessment takes a number of different forms and targets different skills or domains of content. The theoretical underpinnings of the approaches come from the work of Vygotsky, particularly the idea of ''the zone of proximal development'' (ZPD). Vygotsky (1978) defined the ZPD as ''the distance between an individual's actual developmental level as determined by independent problem solving and the level of potential development as determined through problem solving under adult guidance or in collaboration with more capable peers'' (p.86). Consistent with the Vygotskian notion of potential for change, most of the dynamic-assessment approaches seek to provide opportunities for demonstration of maximum performance. Examples of different approaches include Budoff's (1987) learning-potential assessment, Carlson and Weidel's (1992) modification of testing procedures, Campione and Brown's assessment via assisted learning and transfer (Campione, 1989), and Feuerstein's Learning Potential Assessment Device (Feuerstein, 1977; Feuerstein et al., 1979).

Feuerstein (1977), an early proponent of dynamic assessment, developed an essentially clinical and individualized set of procedures known as the Learning Potential Assessment Device (LPAD). The purpose of the LPAD is to determine how and in what ways individuals respond to instruction. Feuerstein argues that change in performance, following instruction, reflects real change in generalized cognitive processes. The LPAD is essentially a clinical intervention. There is no formal pretest or standardized assessment. Learners are provided with a range of materials and problems and assisted in reaching solutions through questions, cuing, and modeling; there is no formal sequence or organization of the assistance, but, rather, assistance is provided as needed. A strong positive affective interaction between learner and examiner is emphasized. In the LPAD, examiners are teachers and clinicians, not evaluators, and the goal is to find how pupils' learning and performance can be modified.

Feuerstein's program is intuitively attractive but there are some serious questions that require consideration. Because the materials used for assessment and instruction are purposefully non-school-subject specific, a major question relates to transfer of results to school-relevant content. A second question has to do with the determination of efficacy when each assessment and intervention is individualized. Feuerstein specifically rejects the use of a test-intervention-retest model because he considers psychometric tests to be invalid and to have a potentially negative impact on problem learners, but this makes it difficult, if not impossible, to document change. Further, the highly individualized, clinical nature of the program makes it difficult to evaluate the program as a whole or to assess the relative effects of particular procedures. The evidence for a positive impact of the program on problem learners' educational performance is equivocal (see critical reviews by Bradley, 1983; Frisby and Braden, 1992). Thus, despite its relatively wide use and its clinical appeal, the LPAD suffers because it is not a comprehensive empirical test.

In contrast to the clinical approach of Feuerstein, Campione and Brown and their associates have defined and implemented a program of research focused on assessment within an assisted learning and transfer model (Campione, 1989; Campione and Brown, 1987). These researchers focus on the efficiency of learning and transfer. They use a test-teach-test method, providing learners with a prearranged sequence of hints or cues for problem solution. Their method yields a quantitative score of learning efficiency (number of hints necessary for problem resolution), and a measure of how much help is needed for learners to make near and far transfers. They underscore the strong relationship between transfer performance and performance on academic tasks. In a series of studies, they have provided evidence of stronger relationships between learning/transfer scores and gains than between standardized test scores and gains (Campione, 1989).

The Campione and Brown work is focused on specific content areas, such as reading or math, rather than on the general cognitive or problem-solving skills targeted by Feuerstein. The model is well documented and well researched, and supports the generalization that the interactive-dynamic approach yields better predictive information than the information derived from norm-referenced standardized tests. It is likely that the assessment process itself helps to define and direct intervention, a missing link in more traditional psychoeducational tests.

In summary, interactive-dynamic assessment approaches differ from traditional assessment approaches in a number of ways. First, while typical assessment procedures place primary emphasis on product (correctness of response), dynamic assessment targets processes and strategies used in learning; i.e., on the how and why in problem solution. Second, the approaches differ in the procedures of test administration and in the role of the examiner. In standardized testing, procedures are specified and the examiner is objective. In interactive-dynamic assessment, the role of the assessor is one of active teacher. Third, whereas most psychoeducational testing provides a picture of the child's abilities at a single time point, interactive-dynamic assessment is based on an ongoing evaluation.

Portfolio Assessment

Portfolio assessment is an example of a recent performance-based approach that resulted from the current movement away from norm-referenced assessment and toward ongoing classroom-based measurement (Black, 1993). Portfolios are best described as a collection of work samples, even as artists use portfolios to display samples of their art. Portfolios for educational assessment became popular several years ago as a way to assess content areas not easily and accurately measured through traditional analog testing (e.g., written language and creative arts). At present, there is strong support for using portfolio assessment in most content areas when assessing special education pupils, as the content of the portfolios can be linked directly to the goals established in the child's IEP. Portfolio assessment is not limited to special education pupils, however, as portfolio systems are used in several states (e.g., Vermont, Rhode Island) for all students. The International Reading Association (IRA) recently issued a position paper advocating wide use of portfolios in reading assessment.

The purpose of portfolio assessment is to show how pupils' competencies develop. In most instances, teachers and pupils identify two or three goals or topics, and materials are collected over time. Pupils choose what is to be included, and portfolios usually contain drafts and revisions of written work, samples of math processes and problems, a list of books read, and art work. In this regard, critics point out that there are no set rules for how much and what kind of work samples to include or criteria for determining what constitutes success or failure in meeting objectives. The reliability of interevaluator agreement is also uncertain. Critics argue that there is little consensus regarding procedures to be followed in setting up portfolios, and no empirical basis for using portfolio assessment to make instructional decisions (Gomez et al., 1991; Nolet, 1992). Advocates point out that portfolios allow true individualization in assessment and provide information on progress made from first attempt to final product

In summary, portfolio assessment is not a single, defined approach to assessment, but it subsumes a group of approaches for collecting and displaying pupils' work over a specified period of time. Students, as well as their teachers, participate in determining which work samples are to be included. Pupils are provided the opportunity to participate in goal setting and in self-evaluation. Although serious questions have been raised concerning possible bias in the selection of materials to be included, as well as teacher bias in rating the portfolio, we see portfolio assessment as a valuable adjunct to curriculum-based measurement. While CBA with its measurement-driven emphasis can demonstrate whether a skill has been mastered or not, the portfolio can show changes from first draft to final copy. Where CBA is curriculum/teacher controlled, decisions concerning the portfolio are primarily those of the pupil.

Conclusions

It is clear from this brief review that there are a number of different tests and approaches that are useful in psychoeducational assessment. It is also clear that particular tests or techniques have different functions or uses. Standardized measures of both aptitude and achievement provide summary, normative information that is useful for diagnostic classification and educational placement. This information often has relatively little direct instructional relevance. In contrast, many of the alternative methods of assessment provide insights that are closely linked to instruction, yet the results are so highly individualized that it is difficult to generalize beyond a given child. We stress that the validity of a particular test or assessment approach must be considered relative to the purposes of testing. In this regard we support Campione's (1989) distinction between prediction and prescription, and we underscore the importance of tying test selection to testing purposes.

References

Bernheimer, LP, Keogh, BK: Weaving interventions into the fabric of everyday life: An approach to family assessment. *Top Early Child Educ* 15(4), 415–433, 1995.

Bigge J: *Curriculum Based Instruction for Special Education Students.* Mountain View, CA, Mayfield, 1988.

Black S: Portfolio assessment. *Executive Educ* 15:28–31, l993.

Bradley TB: Remediation of cognitive deficits: A critical appraisal of the Feuerstein model. *J Ment Defic Res* 27:79–92, 1983.

Bradley RH, Caldwell BM, Brisby J, et al.: The home inventory: A new scale for families of pre- and early adolescent children with disabilities. *Res Dev Disabil* 13:310–333, 1992.

Brown R III, Aylward E, Keogh BK: *Diagnosis and Management of Learning Disabilities—An Interdisciplinary Lifespan Approach.* San Diego, Singular Publishing Group, 1992.

Budoff M: Measures for assessing learning potential. In: Lidz CS (ed): *Dynamic Assessment: An Interactional Approach to Evaluating Learning Potential.* New York, Guilford Press, 1987, pp. 52–81.

Caldwell B, Bradley R: *Home Observation for Measurement of the Environment.* Little Rock, AK, University of Arkansas at Little Rock, 1984.

Campione JC: Assisted assessment: A taxonomy of approaches and an outline of strengths and weaknesses. *J Learn Disabil* 22:151–165, 1989.

Campione JC, Brown AC: Learning ability and transfer propensity as sources of individual differences in intelligence. In: Brooks PH, Sperber RD, McCauley C, (eds), *Learning and Cognition in the Mentally Retarded.* Baltimore, University Park Press, 1984, pp. 265–299.

Campione JC, Brown AC: In: Lidz CS (ed): *Dynamic Assessment: An Interactional Approach to Evaluating Learning Potential.* New York, Guilford Press, 1987, pp. 82–115.

Carlson JS, Weidl KH: The use of testing the limits procedures in the assessment of intellectual capabilities in children with learning difficulties. *Am J Ment Defic* 82:559–564.

Feuerstein R: Mediated learning experience: A theoretical basis for cognitive human modifiability during adolescence. In: Mittler P (ed): *Research to Practice in Mental Retardation: Proceedings of the 4th Congress of IASSMD. Vol 2: Education and training.* Baltimore, University Park Press, 1979, pp. 105–106.

Feuerstein R, Rand Y, Hoffman MB: *The Dynamic Assessment of Retarded Performers: The Learning Potential Assessment Device, Theory, Instruments, and Techniques.* Baltimore, University Park Press, 1979.

Fewell RR: The measurement of family functioning. In: Bickman L, Weatherford DL (eds). *Evaluating Early Intervention Programs for Severely Handicapped Children and Their Families.* Austin, Texas, Pro-Ed, 1986, pp.263–307.

Frisby CL, Braden JP: Feuerstein's dynamic assessment approach: A semantic, logical, and empirical critique. *J Special Educ* 26:281–301, 1992.

Fuchs LS, Deno S, Mirkin P: The effects of frequent curriculum-based measurement and evaluation on pedagogy, student achievement and student awareness of learning. *Am Educ Res J* 2(1), 449–460, 1984.

Fuchs LS, Fuchs D: Curriculum-based assessment. In: Reynolds C, Kamphaus R (eds): *Handbook of Psychological and Educational Assessment of Children. (Vol 1): Intelligence and Achievement.* New York, Guilford Press, 1989.

Fuchs LS, Fuchs D, Bishop N, et al: Classwide decision-making strategies with curriculum-based measurement. *Diagnostique* 18:39–52.

Gibbs Ed, Teti DM: *Interdisciplinary Assessment of Infants: A Guide for Early Intervention Professionals.* Baltimore, Paul Brookes, 1990.

Gomez MI, Grave ME, Black MN: Reassessing portfolio assessment: Rhetoric and reality. *Lang Arts* 68:620–628.

Haywood HC, Tzuriel, D (eds): *Interactive Assessment.* New York, Springer-Verlag, 1992.

Haywood HC, Wingenfeld SA: Interactive assessment as a research tool. *J Special Educ* 26(3): 253–268.

Heshusius L: Curriculum-based assessment and direct instruction: Critical reflections on fundamental assumptions. *Exceptional Child* 57:315–328.

Howell KE, Morehead MK: *Curriculum-Based Evaluation for Special and Remedial Education.* Columbus, OH, Merrill Publishing, 1987.

Lidz CS (ed): *Dynamic Assessment: An Interactional Approach to Evaluating Learning Potential.* New York, Guilford Press, 1987.

Lidz CS: *Practitioner's Guide to Dynamic Assessment.* New York, Guilford Press, 1991.

Lipsky DK, Gartner A: *Beyond Separate Education: Quality for All.* Baltimore, Paul Brookes, 1989.

Marston D: The effectiveness of special education; a time series analysis of reading performance in regular and special education settings. *J Special Educ* 21:13–26, 1987–88.

McLaughlin JA, Lewis RB: *Assessing Special Students* (3rd ed). New York, Merrill, 1990.

Mitchell JV Jr: *The Ninth Mental Measurements Yearbook.* Lincoln, NE, Buros Institute of Mental Measurements, 1985.

Nolet V: Classroom-based measurement and portfolio assessment. *Diagnostique* 18(1), 5–26, 1992.

Reschley DJ: Minority mild mental retardation over- representation. Legal issues, research findings, and reform trends. In: Wang MC, Reynolds MC, Walberg HJ (eds): *Handbook of Special Education: Research and Practice* (Vol 1) Oxford, United Kingdom, Pergamon Press, pp. 23–41, 1988.

Reynolds CR, Elliott SN: Trends in commercial development and publication of educational and psychological tests. *Prof Psychol Res Pract* 14:554–558, 1983.

Salvia J, Ysseldyke JE: *Assessment* (5th ed). Boston, Houghton Mifflin, 1991.

Sandoval J: Haapanen RM: A critical comment on neuropsychology in the schools: Are we ready? *School Psychol Rev* 10:381–388, 1981.

Shinn MR, Tindal G, Stein S: Curriculum based assessment and the identification of mildly handicapped students: A research review. *Prof School Psychol* 3:69–86, 1989.

Stainback W, Stainback S: Rationale for integration and restructuring: A synopsis. In: Lloyed JW, Repp AC, Singh NN (eds): *The Regular Education Initiative: Alternative Perspectives on Concepts, Issues, and Models.* Sycamore, IL, Sycamore, 1991.

Trad PV: *The Preschool Child: Assessment, Diagnosis, and Treatment.* New York, Wiley, 1989.

Tucker JA: Curriculum-based assessment: An introduction. *Exceptional Child* 52:199–204, 1985.

Tucker J: Curriculum-based assessment is no fad. *Collab Educ* 1:4–10, 1987.

Vygotsky LSI: *Mind in Society: Development of Higher Psychological Processes.* (Cole R, John-Steiner V, Scribner E, Sauberman E, eds. and trans.). Cambridge, Harvard University Press, 1978.

Winton PJ, Bailey DB Jr: The family-focused interview: A collaborative mechanism for family assessment and goal setting. *J Div Early Childhood* 12(3), 195–207 1988.

44 AUTISM AND THE PERVASIVE DEVELOPMENTAL DISORDERS

Fred R. Volkmar, M.D.

DEFINITION

The pervasive developmental disorders (PDDs) are a group of neuropsychiatric disorders characterized by specific delays and deviance in social, communicative, and cognitive development, with an onset typically in the first years of life. Although commonly associated with mental retardation, these disorders differ from other developmental disorders in that their developmental and behavioral features are distinctive and do not simply reflect developmental level (Rutter, 1978). Although better definitions of the syndrome of autism continue to be needed, the validity of autism as a diagnostic category is now well established. The validity and definition of other proposed PDDs is more controversial (Volkmar and Cohen, 1988), but several of these conditions are included in DSM-IV (APA, 1994).

Present definitions of the disorder remain profoundly influenced by Leo Kanner's (1943) original and phenomenological description of the disorder as well as its subsequent modification by Rutter (1978). Of the various PDDs, autism has been the most intensively studied. Both categorical and dimensional approaches to diagnosis have been used (Parks, 1983; Volkmar and Cohen, 1988). Categorical approaches have typically emphasized three different areas of disturbance: social dysfunction, communicative deviance, and a number of unusual behavioral features often subsumed under the rubric of ''insistence on sameness.'' Typically, the characteristic social and communicative deficits are believed to be aberrant relative to the individual's developmental level (Volkmar et al., 1993). The development of truly operational definitions has been hindered by various factors: (*a*) issues of continuity with other disorders, such as schizophrenia; (*b*) the broad range of syndrome expression; (*c*) changes in syndrome expression with age; (*d*) the frequency of autistic-like symptoms in individuals with severe mental retardation; and (*e*) the relative infrequency of the disorder (Volkmar and Cohen, 1988). Autism was not accorded official diagnostic status in the American Psychiatric Association's *Diagnostic and Statistical Manual* until 1980, when it was included within a new *class* of disorders—the Pervasive Developmental Disorders.

The DSM-III criteria for infantile autism included pervasive social deficits, gross deficits in language development, unusual speech patterns (when speech was present), bizarre responses to the environment, and an absence of the delusions or hallucinations typical of schizophrenia. By definition, autism was apparent by 30 months of age. A ''residual'' category was included for those individuals who had once met criteria for autism but no longer do. Even in the relatively short period of time between DSM-III's appearance and this revision (American Psychiatric Association, 1987), problems with the DSM-III system were apparent (Volkmar and Cohen, 1988). It lacked a developmental focus, criteria were overly restrictive, and language problems rather than broader *communication* problems were emphasized. In response to the criticism that DSM-III criteria for autism were too ''infantile'' in nature (i.e., most appropriate to younger and more impaired individuals), major revisions were made in DSM-III-R.

The DSM-III-R provided a series of 16 individual criteria for autistic disorder. These 16 criteria were grouped into 3 categories (impaired social interaction, impaired communication, and restricted repertoire of activities). To achieve a diagnosis of autism, an individual had to exhibit at least 8 of the 16 criteria, with a specified distribution across categories. Age of onset was no longer an essential diagnostic feature, although onset (before or after 36 months) could be specified. These changes gave the DSM-III-R a greater developmental orientation, but at the apparent cost of a broadened diagnostic concept, i.e., in comparison to other systems and to the substantial revisions made in DSM-IV (Volkmar et al., 1994).

In the DSM-IV (American Psychiatric Association, 1994) the definition of autism was developed on the basis of a very large, international, multi-site field trial. The final DSM-IV definition (Table 44.1) retains historical continuity with previous definitions of autism, i.e., in relation to the requirements for disturbance in three broad areas of developmental dysfunction. It differs from DSM-III-R in that age of onset is included as a necessary diagnostic feature. More importantly, this definition is conceptually identical to that employed in the International Classification of Diseases (ICD-10) (World Health Organization, 1994) (see Chapters 36 and 37) as are the definitions of other disorders in this class; aspects of the historical development of these diagnostic concepts are discussed subsequently.

In addition to autism, other diagnostic categories are included within the PDD class in DSM-IV. Although research on these conditions is less advanced than that on autism, there appeared to be sufficient justification for their inclusion as specific diagnostic categories.

In childhood disintegrative disorder (also sometimes referred to as Heller's syndrome or disintegrative psychosis) (Table 44.2), children develop a condition that resembles autism but arises only after a relatively prolonged period of clearly normal development (Volkmar, 1994). This condition apparently differs from autism in the pattern of onset, course, and outcome (Volkmar, 1994).

In Rett's disorder (Table 44.3) a very brief period of normal development is followed by a period of decelerated head growth, loss of purposeful hand movements, and development of severe psychomotor retardation (Tsai, 1994). This condition has, to date, been observed only in girls. Although the course of this condition differs markedly from autism, there is a period of time, particularly in the preschool years, when confusion with autism may occur.

Of the various disorders potentially included with the PDD class, the validity of Asperger's disorder as separate from autism has probably been the most controversial. Given the absence of ''official'' definitions, the concept has been used in markedly different ways (Klin, 1994). It would appear that the condition differs from autism in that it is associated with higher levels of cognitive and communicative skills and an absence of signs of CNS dysfunction. Unusual preoccupations (e.g., with train schedules) and high degrees of egocentrism are common, as are motor delays (Klin, 1994). Similar traits are sometimes noted in family mem-

Table 44.1. DSM-IV Criteria for Autistic Disorder (299.0)

A. A total of at least six items from (1), (2), and (3), with at least two from (1), and one each from (2) and (3):
 (1) Qualitative impairment in social interaction, as manifested by at least two of the following:
  (a) marked impairment in the use of multiple nonverbal behaviors such as eye-to-eye gaze, facial expression, body postures, and gestures to regulate social interaction
  (b) failure to develop peer relationships appropriate to developmental level
  (c) a lack of spontaneous seeking to share enjoyment, interests, or achievements with other people (e.g., by a lack of showing, bringing, or pointing out objects of interest to other people)
  (d) lack of social or emotional reciprocity
 (2) Qualitative impairments in communication as manifested by at least one of the following:
  (a) delay in, or total lack of, the development of spoken language (not accompanied by an attempt to compensate through alternative modes of communication, such as gestures or mime)
  (b) in individuals with adequate speech, marked impairment in the ability to initiate or sustain a conversation with others
  (c) stereotyped and repetitive use of language or idiosyncratic language
  (d) lack of varied spontaneous make-believe play or social imitative play appropriate to developmental level
 (3) Restricted repetitive and stereotyped patterns of behavior, interests, and activities, as manifested by at least one of the following:
  (a) encompassing preoccupation with one or more stereotyped and restricted patterns of interest that are abnormal either in intensity or focus
  (b) apparently compulsive adherence to specific, nonfunctional routines or rituals
  (c) stereotyped and repetitive motor mannerisms (e.g., hand or finger flapping or twisting, or complex whole body movements)
  (d) persistent preoccupation with parts of objects
B. Delays or abnormal functioning in at least one of the following areas, with onset prior to age three: (1) social interaction, (2) language as used in social communication, or (3) symbolic or imaginative play.
C. Not better accounted for by Rett's disorder or childhood disintegrative disorder.

Reprinted, with permission, from American Psychiatric Association: *Diagnostic and Statistical Manual* (4th ed). Washington, DC, American Psychiatric Association Press, 1994.

Table 44.2. DSM-IV Criteria for Childhood Disintegrative Disorder (299.10)

A. Apparently normal development for at least the first two years, as manifested by the presence of age-appropriate verbal and nonverbal communication, social relationships, play, and adaptive behavior.
B. Clinically significant loss of previously acquired skills in at least two of the following areas:
 (1) expressive or receptive language
 (2) social skills or receptive language
 (3) bowel or bladder control
 (4) play
 (5) motor skills
C. Abnormalities of functioning in at least two of the following areas:
 (1) qualitative impairment in social interaction (e.g., impairment in nonverbal behaviors, failure to develop peer relationships, lack of social or emotional reciprocity);
 (2) qualitative impairments in communication (e.g., delay or lack of spoken language, inability to initiate or sustain a conversation, stereotyped and repetitive use of language, lack of varied make-believe play);
 (3) restricted repetitive and stereotyped patterns of behavior, interests and activities, including motor stereotypies and mannerisms.
D. Not better accounted for by another specific Pervasive Developmental Disorder or by Schizophrenia

Reprinted, with permission, from American Psychiatric Association: *Diagnostic and Statistical Manual* (4th ed). Washington, DC, American Psychiatric Association Press, 1994.

Table 44.3. DSM-IV Criteria for Rett's Disorder (299.80)

A. All of the following:
 (1) apparently normal prenatal and perinatal development
 (2) apparently normal psychomotor development through the first six months
 (3) normal head circumference at birth
B. Onset of all of the following between 5 and 48 months:
 (1) deceleration of head growth
 (2) loss of previously acquired purposeful hand movements, with the development of stereotyped hand movements (e.g., handwringing or handwashing)
 (3) loss of social engagement early in the course (although often social interaction develops later)
 (4) appearance of poorly coordinated gait or trunk movements
 (5) marked delays and impairment of expressive and receptive language with severe psychomotor retardation

Reprinted, with permission, from American Psychiatric Association: *Diagnostic and Statistical Manual* (4th ed). Washington, DC, American Psychiatric Association Press, 1994.

Table 44.4. DSM-IV Criteria for Asperger's Disorder (299.80)

A. Qualitative impairment in social interaction of the type described for autism (Table 44.1)
B. Restricted, repetitive, and stereotyped patterns of behavior, interests, and activities of the type described for autism (Table 44.1)
C. Lack of any clinically significant general delay in language (e.g., single words used by age two, communicative phrases used by age three).
D. Lack of any clinically significant delay in cognitive development, as manifested by the development of age-appropriate self-help skills, adaptive behavior (other than in social interaction), and curiosity about the environment.
E. Does not meet criteria for another specific Pervasive Developmental Disorder.

Adapted and reprinted, with permission, from American Psychiatric Association: *Diagnostic and Statistical Manual* (4th ed). Washington, DC, American Psychiatric Association Press, 1994.

but full criteria for autism or another explicitly defined PDD are not met. It should be emphasized that this "subthreshold" category is, thus, defined implicitly, i.e., no specific guidelines for diagnosis are provided and the concept has been broadened compared to DSM-III-R. While deficits in peer relations and unusual sensitivities are typically noted, social skills are less impaired than in classical autism. The lack of definition(s) for this relatively heterogeneous group of children presents problems for research on this condition.

In addition to categorical diagnostic systems, various dimensional approaches to diagnosis have also been employed (Parks, 1983). These approaches are based on parent or teacher report or direct observation. Typically deviant behaviors are rated or sampled with attendant issues of standardization and reliability. Changes in syndrome expression over the course of development and the prevalence of high levels of "autistic-like" behaviors in severely retarded individuals also pose problems for the development of such instruments. Recent work (Lord et al., 1991), focused on the development of diagnostic and assessment instruments specifically keyed to diagnostic criteria, offers particular advantages for research studies.

HISTORICAL NOTE

Over the past century, various diagnostic concepts have been proposed to encompass severe psychiatric disturbances of childhood onset. The history of diagnostic concepts illustrates the pitfalls of simple extension of concepts derived from work with psychotic adults; indeed, children's changing conceptions of reality and normative beliefs in fantasy figures suggest the need for considerable caution in such attempts.

Diagnostic concepts proposed for childhood "psychosis" are presented in Table 44.5. Of particular note is the early interest in the extension of Kraepelin's description of dementia praecox to children. Early assumptions of continuity between severe childhood psychiatric disturbance and adult schizophrenia were based, in large part, on the severity

bers. The DSM-IV and ICD-10 definitions of this condition are compatible (Table 44.4).

The term Pervasive Developmental Disorder–Not Otherwise Specified (PDD-NOS) (also referred to as atypical personality development, atypical PDD, or atypical autism) is included in DSM-IV to encompass "subthreshold" cases, e.g., where marked impairment of social interaction, communication, interest, or stereotyped behavior patterns is found

Table 44.5. Development of Diagnostic Concepts: Childhood "Psychosis"

Diagnostic Concept (Current Terminology)	Originator
Dementia praecocissima	DeSanctis, 1906
Dementia infantilis (disintegrative disorder)	Heller, 1908
Early infantile autism (autistic disorder)	Kanner, 1943
Autistic psychopathy (Asperger's syndrome)	Asperger, 1944
Atypical personality development	Rank, 1949
Rett's syndrome	Rett, 1966

of the disorders. The term *childhood schizophrenia* became synonymous with *childhood psychosis*. In 1943, Leo Kanner described 11 cases of "early infantile autism" and noted various ways in which this disorder appeared to be distinctive. These children exhibited an apparently congenital inability to relate to other people (in contrast to an apparent ability to relate to objects); their language (when it developed at all) was remarkable for echolalia, pronoun reversal, and concreteness. Behaviorally, these children engaged in repetitive, apparently purposeless activities (stereotypy), were highly responsive to the inanimate environment, and were intolerant of change. Kanner's use of the term *autism* was meant to convey the unusual, self-centered quality that his cases exhibited, but was also suggestive of the autism associated with schizophrenia. Although Kanner's description has been remarkably enduring, his speculations about certain aspects of the condition (e.g., normal levels of intelligence, lack of association with other medical conditions, unusual levels of parental education) proved incorrect (Cohen et al., 1994). The validity of Kanner's concept as distinct from schizophrenia was established over the next several decades only, as various lines of evidence became available.

Heller proposed the term *dementia infantilis* to account for children who develop normally for some period prior to profound developmental regression (see Heller, 1930). His concept, now known as disintegrative disorder, is now included in DSM-IV. In 1944, Asperger proposed a novel concept, autistic psychopathy, which resembled Kanner's concept in some ways. This disorder, now usually known as Asperger's syndrome to avoid the confusion produced by the word *psychopathy*, has been described particularly in the European literature; in the United States such individuals are more likely to be termed autistic (Cohen et al., 1994). The continuity of Asperger's disorder with autism remains debated; the disorder is of some interest, to the extent that it may establish areas of continuity between autism and other disorders.

PREVALENCE AND EPIDEMIOLOGY

Several major methodologically sound epidemiological studies of autism have been conducted, particularly in Great Britain (see Zahner and Pauls, 1987, for a review). Not surprisingly, results obtained have been very dependent on the methods used and, particularly, on the nature and "stringency" of the diagnostic criteria employed. Several factors pose problems for epidemiological studies. The best-defined disorder, autism, is very uncommon, so that studies must be able to draw on large samples of the population; similarly, because cases can be identified in various treatment settings (psychiatric, educational, etc.), multiple service providers must typically be involved. The particular definition used in epidemiological surveys vary considerably, with consequent problems in interpretation of available results. Early studies suffered from questions regarding the distinctiveness of autism from other forms of childhood "psychosis," and recent changes in the diagnostic criteria for autism pose further obstacles for research studies. The lack of reliable and valid definitions for other PDDs severely limits our knowledge of these conditions.

Given these difficulties, it is noteworthy that available research is in general agreement regarding the prevalence of autism. Studies have generally suggested that the condition is rare. If autism is most strictly defined, prevalence rates of 2 cases per 10,000 are usually reported;

less stringent definitions typically suggest prevalence rates of 4–5 cases per 10,000 (Zahner and Pauls, 1987). Recent work suggests that as many as 10 children per 10,000 may be affected. Although information is limited, it appears that the atypical PDD/PDD-NOS group is much more common than more strictly defined autism, with a prevalence of perhaps as many as one in several hundred school-age children. With the possible exception of Asperger's disorder, the other PDDs are apparently less common than autism. For example, childhood disintegrative disorder is perhaps 10 times less common than more strictly defined autism (Volkmar, 1994) and Rett's syndrome is similarly uncommon (Tsai, 1994). The lack of official and consensus definitions of Asperger's syndrome has meant that prevalence estimates of this condition have varied widely (Klin, 1994).

Epidemiological studies have provided important information about aspects of autism in relation to other subject characteristics. It is clear that autism is much more common in boys than in girls: Typically, ratios of 4:1 or 5:1 are reported (Zahner and Pauls, 1987); and, girls are more severely affected (Lord et al., 1982). Comparisons of various samples suggest that the majority of autistic individuals function within the retarded range. The suggestion of an association of autism with high social class was initially made by Kanner (1943). Although available evidence is somewhat conflicting, it is now clear that the condition is observed in families from all levels of education and that various factors may bias case ascertainment and may account for the initial impression of an unusual social class distribution (Schopler et al., 1980). With the exception of Rett's disorder, where only females have been observed to have the disorder, male predominance has been noted in the other specifically defined PDDs.

CLINICAL DESCRIPTION

Age of Onset

In the majority of cases, the apparent onset of autism is within the 1st or 2nd year of life. Age of onset (more properly termed age of recognition) of the PDDs has been important in differentiating these disorders from others (e.g., childhood schizophrenia) and making distinctions within the PDD class. Studies of large series of cases of "psychotic" children have generally revealed a bimodal distribution of age of onset; children with disorders developing in the 1st or 2nd year of life are more likely to be autistic, while those with disorders developing later in childhood exhibit problems more typical of schizophrenia (see Chapter 58).

Although Kanner (1943) believed that autism was present from, or shortly after, birth, subsequent work has suggested that the disorder can be observed after some period of months, or even a few years, of normal development (Volkmar, 1985). Figure 44.1 illustrates the age of apparent onset (i.e., recognition) of 103 individuals with DSM-III diagnoses of infantile autism or childhood-onset PDD and suggests that most cases are recognized in the 1st or 2nd year of life. Certain factors (e.g., parental denial, bilingual household, relatively high intellectual level in child) might act to delay case detection. For example, Asperger's disorder might be detected somewhat later than more typical autism, given the relatively higher intellectual levels and the relative preservation of communicative skills reported to be associated with the disorder (Klin, 1994). Children with apparent disintegrative disorder develop an autistic-like condition after a long period (2 or more years) of unequivocally normal development (Volkmar, 1994). In contrast, in Rett's syndrome the period of normal development is quite short, usually a few months (Tsai, 1994).

Social Disturbance

Autism was initially described by Kanner as a disturbance of affective contact. Social dysfunction in autism is distinctive and not explicable in terms of mental age delay per se and is a, if not the, central defining feature of the disorder. However, comparatively less research has been conducted on the social aspects of autism. This has reflected

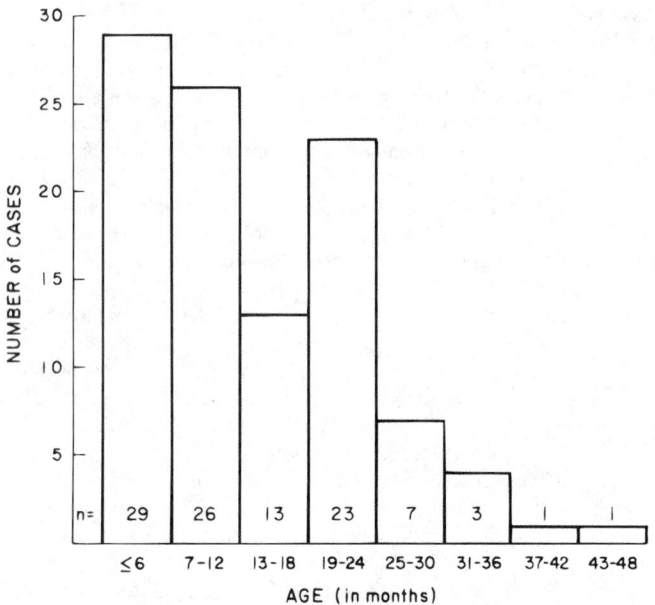

Figure 44.1. Age of recognition of autism/childhood onset PDD. (From Schopler E, Mesibov G. Diagnosis and assessment in autism. New York, Plenum, 1988, p. 80.)

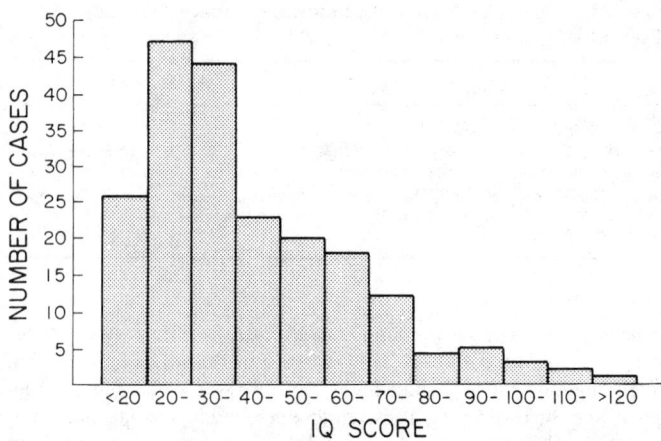

Figure 44.2. Full-scale IQ distribution for 203 autistic individuals, Child Study Center sample. (From Volkmar FR, Cohen DJ. Classification and diagnosis of childhood autism. In: Schopler E, Mesibov G, eds: *Diagnosis and assessment in autism*. New York, Plenum, 1988.)

both an awareness that some social skills do develop over time (Lotter, 1978) and an assumption that other deficits (e.g., cognitive or communicative) are more primary determinants of the disorder (Cohen et al., 1994).

Normally developing infants are remarkably social, even from the 1st weeks of life. They exhibit an apparent predisposition to form social relationships; this predisposition appears to be an important foundation for the development of other skills (Stern, 1987). The social development of autistic individuals is distinctive in many ways. The human face holds little interest for the autistic infant; lack of eye contact, poor or absent attachments, and a general lack of social interest are typical. Deficits in social interaction in autism change somewhat over the course of development but remain an area of great disability even for the highest-functioning, nonretarded autistic adults. The social deficits in childhood disintegrative disorder and Asperger's disorder are similar to those observed in autism.

Communicative Disturbance

Deficits in the development of expressive language are typically the parents' presenting concern about the child's development in cases of autism. Communication problems appear to be a central aspect of the syndrome. About half of autistic individuals never gain useful communicative speech, and those who do speak exhibit language that is distinctive in numerous ways (Paul, 1987). The speech of autistic individuals is remarkable for echolalia, pronoun reversal, failure to use appropriate cadence and intonation, impaired semantic development, extreme literalness, and failure to use language for social interaction. It is important to note that echolalia per se is observed in normally developing children who are acquiring language, and adaptive functions of echolalia in autistic children have been noted. Deficits in pragmatic communication are common. The language and communicative deficits in autism differ from those seen, for example, in the developmentally language-disordered child (Paul, 1987). The communicative development of individuals with apparent Asperger's disorder appears to be less impaired than that observed in more classically autistic individuals and may represent an area of strength, at least in certain respects (Klin, 1994). In Rett's disorder and childhood disintegrative disorder communication skills, particularly expressive language skills, are usually highly limited (Tsai, 1994; Volkmar, 1994).

Cognitive Development

Kanner's initial impression that autistic children exhibited normal levels of intelligence was based on the observation that autistic individuals performed quite well on certain parts of traditional tests of intelligence; this initial impression proved incorrect. Although attempts were made to account for poor test performance on the basis of "negativism" or "untestability," it became clear that, when developmentally appropriate tests were employed, most (approximately three-fourths) autistic individuals scored in the mentally retarded range (Fig. 44.2). IQ scores are relatively stable and predictive of outcome (Klin and Shepard, 1994). Marked scatter in performance on tests of intelligence is common and differs from the usual pattern observed in retarded nonautistic children. Islets of unusual ability (such as rote memory or block design) may be present (Klin and Shepard, 1994). A few autistic individuals exhibit truly remarkable abilities, for example, in musical or drawing ability or in exceptional feats of memory, such as the ability to name days of the week corresponding to dates several years in advance ("calendar calculators"). Autistic persons exhibit persistent deficits in abstract thinking and in sequencing and processing information. Lower levels of intelligence are associated with greater risk for the development of a seizure disorder in adolescence and with a worse outcome. The pattern of verbal vs. nonverbal (performance) IQ appears to differentiate individuals with autism from those with Asperger's disorder. As might be expected, given that relative preservation of early language skills is the major differential feature of the two conditions, cases with Asperger's disorder often have markedly higher verbal IQ scores, whereas even in higher functioning autistic persons, performance on nonverbal IQ usually is higher (Klin, 1994).

Cognitive deficits may be apparent in infancy, and scatter in developmental examination is apparent during the preschool years. In general, autistic children do best with tasks that involve motor and perceptual-motor skills and worst with tasks that involve symbolic information and verbal skills (Klin and Shepard, 1994). Autistic children have difficulty responding to multiple aspects of stimuli (a phenomenon known as stimulus overselectivity).

Behavioral Features

Although unresponsive to aspects of the social environment, autistic children's responsiveness to the inanimate environment is often quite striking. A child may fail to respond differentially to parents but be particularly attached to an unusual object. Although parents may initially be concerned that their autistic child is deaf, often, in fact, the child is exquisitely sensitive to certain nonspeech sounds (e.g., the vacuum cleaner). Interest in nonfunctional aspects of objects (e.g., taste or feel) and stereotyped (purposeless and repetitive) movements are common and include hand flapping, toe walking, spinning objects, and the like. Such activities appear to be preferred modes of behavior and can consume much of the child's time. Bizarre affective responses are also common; a child may become panicked in response to new situations or regularly recurring stimuli. Play skills are typically quite deviant and deficits in imaginative play are typical. It is unclear to what extent these unusual behavioral features are primary aspects of the disorder or are secondary to social or cognitive features, since, for example, many severely retarded children exhibit autistic-like behaviors (Volkmar et al., 1994).

Developmental Changes

As with other children, significant changes occur over the course of development (Rutter, 1970). Typically, preschool autistic children exhibit the more classic syndrome picture previously referred to as infantile autism, with marked and pervasive lack of interest in other people, absent or severely delayed communication, and cognitive delays. Delays in case detection remain, unfortunately, relatively common, as parents are often initially reassured that the child is "just a late talker." Although parents often report earlier concerns about the child's development, usually delayed language development is the cause for referral. By school age, many autistic children do develop some limited attachments to parents and some differential social responsiveness. Communicative skills may emerge, although these are typically quite deviant. Self-stimulatory and other problematic behaviors, such as self-abuse, also become more common and more difficult to manage. In adolescence, a small number of autistic individuals make marked developmental gains; another subgroup will behaviorally deteriorate. The onset of seizures in adolescence is relatively common, particularly in more severely retarded individuals (Rutter, 1970). As adults, many autistic individuals remain severely impaired. Those individuals who are able to achieve personal and occupational self-sufficiency exhibit residual difficulties in interpersonal interaction; typically, these are individuals with the highest levels of cognitive and communicative skills.

In Asperger's disorder, the higher intellectual levels would, in general, suggest a somewhat better long-term prognosis. On the other hand, individuals with this condition have been reported to be at increased risk for other psychiatric disturbance, e.g., psychosis (Klin, 1994). The limited data available suggest that the outcome in childhood disintegrative disorder is even *worse* than that of autism, i.e., minimal levels of developmental recovery are typical, following the developmental regression. In Rett's disorder the course of the condition is quite characteristic. Various unusual behaviors (e.g., breath holding, air swallowing) and motor problems (ataxia, apraxia) are observed and the individual becomes severely or profoundly mentally retarded (Tsai, 1994).

ETIOLOGY AND PATHOGENESIS

Biological Mechanism

As the validity of the autistic syndrome became more firmly established, various lines of evidence converged to suggest the importance of neurobiological factors in the pathogenesis of this, and similar, conditions. While the variety and consistency of this evidence are impressive, neither a specific biological marker for autism nor precise pathogenic mechanisms have been identified. Autistic individuals exhibited an increased frequency of physical anomalies, persistent primitive reflexes, and various neurological "soft" signs, as well as increased abnormalities on EEG (Golden, 1987). Brain-imaging studies have revealed various associated abnormalities. Autistic individuals are at increased risk for the development of seizure disorders (Rutter, 1970). The autistic syndrome has been observed more commonly (although by no means invariably) in an apparently diverse group of medical conditions, such as tuberous sclerosis, phenylketonuria (PKU), and Fragile X syndrome,

but much less commonly with others, such as Down syndrome (Cohen et al., 1994). Autism has also been associated with diverse pre- and perinatal risk factors (Tsai, 1987). Similar, although less extensive, data suggest the importance of neurobiological factors in Rett's disorder and childhood disintegrative disorder. The role of genetic mechanisms is suggested by the observation that siblings of affected individuals are at greater risk for autism and are at higher risk for the development of various language and cognitive problems; studies of monozygotic and dizygotic twins have shown an increased concordance for autism in monozygotic twin pairs (Cohen et al., 1994). The apparent genetic component is likely even more robust in Asperger's disorder (Klin, 1994).

Studies of neuroanatomical and neurochemical correlates of autism have been limited by the lack of knowledge regarding specific neuronal systems and the relative inaccessibility of brain tissue. Studies of biochemical correlates of the disorder have examined various neurotransmitters, hormones, trace elements, and amino acids (Anderson and Hoshino, 1987). Although no specific biochemical marker has been found, it is clear that autistic individuals, as a group, exhibit significant increases in peripheral blood levels of serotonin, a central neurotransmitter involved in various regulatory neuronal systems that is also found in blood platelets and the digestive system. The observation that approximately one-third of autistic individuals exhibit high peripheral serotonin levels has proved to be remarkably robust, but its significance remains unclear, since elevations in peripheral serotonin levels are observed in other disorders—notably mental retardation not associated with autism—and since the relationship of peripheral measures to central activity of the compound remains unclear (Anderson and Hoshino, 1987). Defects have been hypothesized at various levels of the CNS, ranging from the brain stem to the cortex. However, the relatively few neuropathological studies conducted have generally not revealed, in a replicable manner, specific structural defects.

Taken as a whole, the available evidence clearly suggests some degree of CNS involvement, and most researchers now share the view that some factor, or combination of factors, acts through one or more mechanisms to produce the final behavioral syndrome known as autism. It is important to note, however, that associated neurobiological findings vary considerably within the group of autistic individuals and that, unfortunately, methodological problems such as small sample size or failure to include appropriate comparison groups have complicated interpretation of available research. Precise neuropathological mechanisms remain to be established (Cohen et al., 1994).

Psychological Processes

FAMILY FACTORS

Kanner's initial report of the autistic syndrome emphasized the apparently congenital nature of autism but also noted the remarkable degrees of occupational success observed in the parents of these first cases, as well as evident deficits in parent-child interaction. These latter observations were subsequently taken to suggest some role of parental psychopathology in syndrome pathogenesis. During the 1950s and 1960s, considerable efforts were made to remediate the effects of deviant caregiving practices of cold ("refrigerator") parents through, for example, extensive child and parent psychotherapy (Riddle, 1987). Various lines of evidence now make it clear that deviant child-rearing practices do not account for autism. Parents of autistic children resemble parents of children with other developmental problems; they do not exhibit specific deficits in child-rearing practice, nor do they exhibit unusual personality traits (Cohen et al., 1994). In retrospect, it appears that early notation of deviant patterns of parent-child interaction might just as well have reflected deviance contributed by the child rather than by the parent; similarly, early studies showing an association of autism with higher social class appear to be artifacts introduced by ascertainment bias, for example, that more successful and well-educated families would be more likely to seek treatment (Schopler et al., 1980). It is clear that the parents of autistic children may be understandably stressed by the experience of caring for a very impaired child and may suffer from depression and anxiety. In childhood disintegrative disorder it is often the case that parents observe some psychosocial or medical event in association with the onset of the condition, e.g., birth of a sibling, death of a grandparent, hospitalization for elective surgery. It seems likely that such events are simply chance, rather than causal associations, given their frequency in this age group (Volkmar, 1994).

ENVIRONMENTAL AND SOCIAL INFLUENCES

The word autism suggests the self-contained quality exhibited by autistic individuals. Although evocative, this description tends to minimize the significant impact that the environment can have on individuals with autism and related disorders. Early psychodynamic views tended to overemphasize the maladaptive qualities of certain deviant behaviors; for example, poor performance on IQ tests was thought to result from intentional "negativism," and echolalia was seen as a maneuver used by the child to distance himself or herself from social interaction. Experimental and other data have led to a significant revision of this view. It is clear, for example, that autistic children are not unduly negativistic; they may behave oddly in certain situations, but many aspects of behavioral functioning can be understood as adaptive attempts to cope with a confusing environment. Levels of appropriate behavior are, for example, highest in more highly "structured" situations, and treatment programs that emphasize specific educational goals in the context of highly regulated interactions are more commonly associated with behavioral improvement (Lockyer and Rutter, 1969).

LABORATORY STUDIES

Biological

Autism and related conditions have been observed in association with a number of other conditions (Golden, 1987). As part of a comprehensive examination, it is important to conduct a careful medical and family history. Genetic screening for various inherited metabolic disturbances is indicated, since some inherited disorders are associated with autism (e.g., PKU). Chromosome analysis and, possibly, genetic consultation are indicated in the presence of either a positive family history of mental retardation or signs of inherited disorders, such as the Fragile X syndrome. Hearing tests have often been conducted prior to the time a child is referred for specialized evaluation; in instances where usual audiological assessment procedures cannot be employed, brain stem auditory evoked response testing is indicated. Neurological consultation should be obtained if signs suggestive of overt seizure disorder or other evidence of gross neurological dysfunction is evident, or if unusual features are present (e.g., late onset). EEGs may be helpful in such cases. Computed tomography (CT) or magnetic resonance imaging (MRI) scans may be indicated and sometimes reveal disorders like tuberous sclerosis or degenerative CNS disease. A history of pre- or postnatal infections (e.g., congenital rubella) is sometimes elicited. The nature of medical conditions associated with autism and other PDDs remains somewhat controversial. Some investigators suggest a very high frequency of associated medical conditions (e.g., Gillberg, 1990), but such estimates may be artificially inflated by methodological and other problems. It appears that the frequency of autism is probably higher than expected in relation to certain medical conditions, although such instances account for only a small proportion of cases of autism (Bailey et al., 1993). In general, it seems appropriate to conduct a reasonable search for such conditions keeping in mind the relative costs of laboratory and other procedures, i.e., the choice of laboratory tests or consultations should be guided by the history and examination.

Psychological

By definition, individuals with PDDs have developmental problems in multiple areas of functioning. It is particularly important to approach

Table 44.6.   Evaluation Procedures: Autism and Pervasive Developmental Disorders

1. Historical information
   Early development and characteristics of development
   Age and nature of onset
   Medical and family history
2. Psychological/communicative examination
   Estimate(s) of intellectual level (particularly nonverbal IQ)
   Communicative assessment (receptive and expressive language, use of nonverbal communication, pragmatic use of language)
   Adaptive behavior
   Evaluate social and communicative skills relative to nonverbal intellectual abilities
3. Psychiatric examination
   Nature of social relatedness (eye contact, attachment behaviors)
   Behavioral features (stereotypy/self-stimulation, resistance to change, unusual sensitivities to the environment, etc.)
   Play skills (nonfunctional use of play materials, developmental level of play activities)
4. Medical evaluation
   Note associated medical conditions (infectious, genetic, pre- and perinatal risk factors, etc.)
   Genetic screen (chromosome analysis and genetic consultation if indicated)
   Hearing test (if indicated)
   Consultation (neurological/pediatric/occupational or physical therapy) as indicated by history and current examination (e.g., EEG, CT/MRI scan)

aspects of psychological assessment, as broadly defined, in a systematic fashion. Problems in assessment are often posed by the difficulties in engaging affected individuals, the need to employ developmentally appropriate assessment methods, and the degree of developmental scatter commonly associated with these conditions. Commonly, multiple evaluation sessions and the efforts of an interdisciplinary treatment team (including a psychiatrist, a psychologist, and a speech and communication specialist) are needed. Services of neurologists as well as physical and occupational therapists may also be appropriate, e.g., regarding management of seizure disorder or motor problems.

Assessment of intellectual functioning can be accomplished through the administration of various standard tests of intelligence or development (Klin and Shepard, 1994). To the extent possible, it is helpful to obtain estimates of both verbal and nonverbal or performance IQ. Typically, nonverbal skills are less impaired than more abstract verbal skills, which involve sequencing and coding of information. For very low-functioning individuals, administration of tests developed for infants and very young children may be appropriate. Adaptive behavior should be systematically evaluated; this is relevant both in terms of documenting degrees of associated mental retardation and for program planning. Speech and communication assessment, not simply limited to evaluation of expressive language or articulation, should be conducted. Psychiatric assessments should include both direct observation and consultation with parents and schools; careful evaluation of reported autistic-like symptoms is indicated. Various rating scales and checklists may aid the diagnostic process but do not replace the need for careful and thoughtful clinical assessment. Associated behavior problems are best evaluated in light of careful developmental assessments. Table 44.6 summarizes evaluation procedures.

DIFFERENTIAL DIAGNOSIS

Autism and related disorders must be differentiated from other conditions, such as language and other developmental disorders and sensory impairments, particularly deafness. Mental retardation often coexists with autism, and the frequency of autistic-like symptoms increases with more severe retardation (Wing and Gould, 1979). Disagreements around diagnosis are most pronounced at both ends of the IQ distribution, i.e., among very low and high functioning individuals (Volkmar et al., 1994). Due to the multiple areas of impairment, a multiaxial, developmentally based approach is particularly useful. Specific behavioral features are best viewed in the context of measures of both intellectual and communicative capacities (Table 44.6). Individual tests and assessment instruments should be selected as appropriate to the individual; measures of adaptive skills in communication and socialization can be viewed in relation to overall cognitive skills and also serve a valuable function in guiding remedial programs. The degree of any associated mental retardation should be noted. Associated medical conditions should be identified; audiological evaluation is indicated if there are concerns about the child's hearing ability.

Provision of historical information can aid the diagnostic process. The diagnosis of autism is more straightforward in instances where the parents report no history of apparently normal development and in which the behavioral deviation is long-standing. Less commonly, some period of apparently normal development precedes the apparent onset of the illness. Questions about specific developmental skills or about development at times of usually well-remembered events (e.g., the child's first birthday) may help clarify aspects of the early history. Although a minority of autistic children appear to have had some period of reasonably normal development, such a history suggests that elective mutism, Rett's disorder, childhood disintegrative disorder, language disorder, schizophrenia, and degenerative CNS disorder should be considered in addition to autism. Although some children with histories of severe neglect exhibit deficits in attachment, such deficits typically remit with adequate care, and other features of autism are not typically present. The limited available evidence suggests that children with PDD-NOS probably come to professional attention rather later than is the case with autistic children, and that intellectual deficits are less common (Dahl and Cohen, 1986). The pattern of onset in disintegrative psychosis is distinctive, although, behaviorally, such cases may be indistinguishable from more typically autistic ones. Both abrupt and gradual developmental regressions have been noted, and intensive neurological examination does not necessarily reveal a specific etiology. Reports of cases of apparent Asperger's disorder suggest that language skills are relatively more preserved, while motor delays are more common than in autism. Unusual features (e.g., rapid deterioration in an otherwise normally developing child) suggest the need for thorough medical evaluation. The diagnostician's task is particularly complex when dealing with younger and more impaired individuals. In some cases, the exact nature of the disorder becomes most clear only over the course of development.

TREATMENT

Given the severity of these conditions and the relatively poor prognosis, it is not surprising that essentially all possible treatments have been utilized, including various pharmacological treatments, somatic treatments (such as electroshock therapy and "patterning"), behavior modification, educational intervention, psychotherapy, dietary change, and the like (Demyer et al., 1981). Unfortunately, until relatively recently, problems in study design and in sample description or selection have made it difficult to assess many treatments systematically. Short-term changes may reflect nonspecific effects and be neither sustained nor clinically significant; it is just such changes, which may be associated with various novel and unproven treatments, that are reported, on average, approximately every 6 months in the lay press. Sadly, such reports, usually of amazing successes, are almost never rigorously conducted or evaluated. Recent reports, for example, have suggested that very low-functioning persons with autism are able to communicate through a special modality (facilitated communication) in which the hand of another person (the facilitator) guides that of the person with autism to type out messages on a keyboard or letterboard (Cohen et al., 1994). While the utility of various augmentative communication skills in autism is well established, and while some individuals with autism do indeed have particular facility with written (as opposed to oral expression), systematic study generally reveals that the alleged communications are the product of the facilitator rather than the child (Eberlin et al., 1993).

At present, the best available evidence points to the importance of appropriate educational interventions to foster the acquisition of basic social, communicative, and cognitive skills and the relation of such interventions to ultimate outcome. Behavior modification procedures may be helpful in increasing appropriate and decreasing inappropriate behaviors and may facilitate involvement in educational programming. It is clear that early and continuous intervention is highly desirable; some reports have noted sustained improvement following intensive early intervention (Lovass, 1987). Educational interventions are best provided on a year-round basis; the usual pattern of summer school vacations is typically not well tolerated by autistic children. Professionals should work with parents to advocate the availability of appropriate educational placements and ancillary services, such as respite care. Because many professionals are often involved in aspects of an evaluation, it is vital that fragmentation of effort be avoided. It is important to realize that engagement with disordered individuals and their families can be lifelong and will entail attention to educational interventions, group living situations, and involvement in community-based day and vocational programs, as well as to aspects of family support. The efforts of advocacy groups like the Autism Society of America and similar groups in other countries have been helpful in this regard; these groups may offer important sources of support to parents as well. Psychotherapy is not usually indicated for the affected autistic child, although it may be useful in higher-functioning individuals or those with atypical PDD: In such cases, therapy should be carefully focused and supportive in nature (Riddle, 1987).

Although none of the pharmacological agents used in the treatment of autism and related conditions have proven curative, certain medications, particularly the major tranquilizers, have been shown to have an important, limited role in the management of certain cases (Campbell, 1987). Careful double-blind studies using haloperidol have demonstrated enhanced learning and improved behavioral adaption. The major tranquilizers may act to decrease activity levels, increase relatedness and task involvement, and increase accessibility to remediation programs. Individuals who receive major tranquilizers or other pharmacological treatments should be carefully monitored for side effects, and the agents should be used in the lowest effective dose for the shortest possible period of time. Oversedation should particularly be avoided. Recent reports have suggested the potential usefulness in autism and related conditions of other agents, e.g., those used in treatment of compulsive behavior (McDougle et al., 1994). Studies of additional agents, e.g., fenfluramine (Campbell, 1988) or naltrexone (Campbell et al., 1990) have not revealed particular benefit. Although considerable interest has centered on the possibility that dietary or vitamin treatments may produce behavioral change, available studies have been difficult to interpret. The nonspecific increases in activity levels autistic individuals sometimes exhibit may be taken to suggest a trial of stimulant medications. In general, stimulants worsen behavioral functioning; this result is not surprising, given that stimulants can induce stereotypies in animals by facilitating the action of the neurotransmitter dopamine. Various somatic treatments have not proven clinically useful. Pursuit of unproven treatments at the expense of educational interventions should be avoided.

OUTCOME AND FOLLOW-UP DATA

A number of methodologically sound follow-up studies of infantile autism have been conducted (Lotter, 1978; Rutter, 1970). As adults, about two-thirds of autistic individuals remain severely handicapped and unable to meet even minimal basic personal needs; many of these individuals are, and remain, institutionalized. About one-third of individuals with the disorder are able to achieve some level of personal and occupational independence, with perhaps 1% to 2% of all cases becoming able to live fully independently. Important predictors of adult outcome include both intellectual level and communicative competence. Individuals with IQ scores below 50 are more likely to have worse outcomes as adults, to develop seizures during adolescence, and to be mute. The presence of communicative speech by age 5 (i.e., speech truly used for purposes of communication) has been identified to be an important prognostic sign. The best outcomes are observed for individuals with normal nonverbal intellectual skills as well as communicative language, but even the very highest-functioning individuals typically exhibit residual impairments in social interaction. It now seems highly probable that recent advances in case detection and earlier remediation are associated with a better outcome.

In childhood disintegrative disorder and Rett's disorder the outcome appears to be even worse than in autism. In Asperger's disorder and PDD-NOS the outcome is apparently much better—likely reflecting the relative preservation of intellectual skills.

Follow-up studies have illustrated some intriguing aspects of autism that remain poorly understood. It is clear, for example, that autistic individuals are at higher risk for seizures throughout childhood and particularly in adolescence—a pattern quite unlike that of the normal population, in which the risk of seizures decreases with age. A small number of autistic individuals exhibit a pattern of behavioral deterioration during adolescence. Similarly, a small number of adolescent autistic individuals appear to improve during this period of development (Rutter, 1970). About 40% to 50% of autistic individuals gain some degree of useful speech, although even these individuals exhibit unusual language characteristics and problems in the use of speech for social interaction (Paul, 1987). Although some changes in capacity to form social relationships occur over the course of development, it is vanishingly rare for autistic individuals to be capable of achieving sexual relationships or marriage. While levels of retardation are important predictors of adult outcome, capacities for forming social relationships are significantly impaired even when developmental level is taken into account, and adaptive outcome is even worse than that predicted by degree of mental retardation alone. It should be noted that the phenomenon of adult autism, as reflected, for example, in the change from "infantile autism" in DSM-III to "autistic disorder" in DSM-III-R, has yet to be adequately studied.

DIRECTIONS FOR RESEARCH

Considerable progress in understanding the biological basis of autism has occurred over the last 5 decades. The validity of the disorder has now been established and attempts to provide more precise definitions have facilitated research studies. Knowledge regarding the validity and definition of other PDDs remains quite limited, however. Continued research is needed to establish their validity, and the development of truly operational definitions for these disorders and autism remains an important research priority. It is now clear that the term *infantile autism* was, in many ways, a misnomer, since autistic infants grow up to be autistic adults. Studies of adults with PDDs remain relatively uncommon. New diagnostic and other techniques, such as positron emission tomography (PET) or nuclear magnetic resonance (NMR) scanning, may help elucidate underlying pathophysiological mechanisms. The study of conditions such as childhood disintegrative disorder may be particularly appropriate to attempt to clarify underlying pathological mechanisms. At the present time, it appears that the final behavioral syndrome known as autism may well represent the effects of multiple insults on the developing CNS acting through one or more mechanisms. The explication of underlying CNS substrates for social behavior is particularly important. Similarly, the development of testable hypothesized mechanisms of CNS dysfunction will significantly advance our understanding of these complex disorders.

CASE ILLUSTRATION: AUTISM

John was the second of two children born to middle-class parents after normal pregnancy, labor, and delivery. As an infant, John appeared undemanding and relatively placid; motor development proceeded appropriately, but language development was delayed. Although his parents indicated that they were first concerned about his development when he was 18 months of age and still not speaking, in retrospect they noted that, in comparison to their previous child, he had seemed relatively uninterested in social interaction and the social games of infancy. Stranger anxiety had never really developed, and John did not exhibit differential attachment behaviors toward his parents. Their pediatrician initially reassured John's parents that he was a "late talker," but they continued to be concerned. Although John seemed to respond to some unusual sounds, the pediatrician obtained a hearing test when John was 24 months old. Levels of hearing appeared adequate for development of speech, and John was referred for developmental evaluation. At 24 months, motor skills were age appropriate and John exhibited some nonverbal problem-solving skills close to age level. His language and social development, however, were severely delayed, and he was noted to be resistant to changes in routine and unusually sensitive to aspects of the inanimate environment. His play skills were quite limited and he used play materials in unusual and idiosyncratic ways. His older sister had a history of some learning difficulties, but the family history was otherwise negative. A comprehensive medical evaluation revealed a normal EEG and CT scan; genetic screening and chromosome analysis were normal as well.

John was enrolled in a special education program, where he gradually began to speak. His speech was characterized by echolalia, extreme literalness, a monotonic voice quality, and pronoun reversal. He rarely used language in interaction and remained quite isolated. By school age, John had developed some evidence of differential attachments to family members; he also had developed a number of self-stimulatory behaviors and engaged in occasional periods of head banging. Extreme sensitivity to change continued. Intelligence testing revealed marked scatter, with a full-scale IQ in the moderately retarded range. As an adolescent, John's behavioral functioning deteriorated, and he developed a seizure disorder. Now an adult, he lives in a group home and attends a sheltered workshop. He has a rather passive interactional style but exhibits occasional outbursts of aggression and self-abuse.

CASE ILLUSTRATION: ASPERGER'S SYNDROME

Tom was an only child. Birth, medical, and family histories were unremarkable. His motor development was somewhat delayed, but communicative milestones were within normal limits. His parents became concerned about him at age 4 when he was enrolled in a nursery school and was noted to have marked difficulties in peer interaction that were so pronounced that he could not continue in the program. In grade school, he was enrolled in special education classes and was noted to have some learning problems. His greatest difficulties arose in peer interaction; he was viewed as markedly eccentric and had no friends. His preferred activity, watching the weather channel on television, was pursued with great interest and intensity. On examination at age 13, he had markedly circumscribed interests and exhibited pedantic and odd patterns of communication with a monotonic voice quality. Psychological testing revealed an IQ within the normal range with marked scatter evident. Formal communication examination revealed age-appropriate skills in receptive and expressive language, but marked impairment in pragmatic language skills.

CASE ILLUSTRATION: DISINTEGRATIVE DISORDER

Bob's early history was within normal limits. By age 2, he was speaking in sentences and his development appeared to be proceeding appropriately. At age 40 months he was noted to exhibit, abruptly, a period of marked behavioral regression shortly after the birth of a sibling. He lost previously acquired skills in communication and was no longer toilet trained. He became uninterested in social interaction, and various unusual self-stimulatory behaviors became evident. Comprehensive medical examination failed to reveal any conditions that might account for this developmental regression. Behaviorally, he exhibited features of autism. At follow-up at age

12 he still was not speaking, apart from an occasional single word, and was severely retarded.

CASE ILLUSTRATION: RETT'S DISORDER

Darla was born at term after an uncomplicated pregnancy. An amniocentesis had been obtained because of maternal age and was normal. At birth, Darla was in good condition; weight, height, and head circumference were all near the 50th percentile. Her development during the first months of life was within normal limits. At around 8 months of age, her development seemed to stagnate and her interest in the environment, including the social environment, waned. Her developmental milestones then became markedly delayed; she was just starting to walk at her 2nd birthday and had no spoken language. Evaluation at that time revealed that head growth had decelerated. Some self-stimulatory behaviors were present. Marked cognitive and communicative delays were noted on formal testing. Darla began to lose purposeful hand movements and developed unusual ``hand washing'' stereotyped behaviors. By age 6, her EEG was abnormal and purposeful hand movements were markedly impaired. Subsequently, she developed truncal ataxia and breath-holding spells and motor skills deteriorated further.

CASE ILLUSTRATION: ATYPICAL PDD/PDD-NOS

Leslie was the oldest of two children. She was noted to be a difficult baby who was not easy to console but whose motor and communicative development seemed appropriate. She was socially related and sometimes enjoyed social interaction, but was easily overstimulated. She was noted to exhibit some unusual sensitivities to aspects of the environment and, at times of excitement, exhibited some hand flapping. Her parents sought evaluation when she was 4 years of age because of difficulties in nursery school. Leslie was noted to have problems with peer interaction. She was often preoccupied with possible adverse events. At evaluation she was noted to have both communicative and cognitive functions within the normal range. Although differential social relatedness was present, Leslie had difficulty using her parents as sources of support and comfort. Behavioral rigidity was noted, as was a tendency to impose routines on social interaction. Leslie was enrolled in a therapeutic nursery school where she made significant gains in social skills. Subsequently, she was placed in a transitional kindergarten and did well academically, although problems in peer interaction and unusual affective responses persisted. As an adolescent, she describes herself as a ``loner'' who has difficulties with social interaction and who tends to enjoy solitary activities.

References

American Psychiatric Association: *Diagnostic and Statistical Manual* (3rd ed). Washington, DC, American Psychiatric Association Press, 1980.

American Psychiatric Association: *Diagnostic and Statistical Manual* (3rd ed., rev). Washington, DC, American Psychiatric Association Press, 1987.

American Psychiatric Association: *Diagnostic and Statistical Manual* (4th ed). Washington, DC, American Psychiatric Association Press, 1994.

Anderson GM, Hoshino Y: Neurochemical studies of autism. In: Cohen D, Donnellan A (eds): *Handbook of Autism and Pervasive Developmental Disorders*. New York, John Wiley & Sons, 1987, pp. 166–191.

Asperger H: Die ``autistichen Psychopathen'' im Kindersalter. *Arch Psychiatrie Nervenkrankheiten* 117:76–136, 1944.

Bailey A, Bolton P, Butler L, et al.: Prevalence of the Fragile X anomaly amongst autistic twins and singletons. *J Child Psychol Psychiatry* 34:673–688, 1993.

Campbell M: Fenfluramine treatment of autism. *J Child Psychol Psychiatry* 29:1–10, 1988.

Campbell M, Anderson LT, Green WH, et al: Psychopharmacology. In: Cohen D, Donnellan A (eds): *Handbook of Autism and Pervasive Developmental Disorders*. New York, Wiley, 1987, pp. 545–565.

Campbell M, Anderson L, Small A., et al.: Naltrexone in autistic children: A double-blind and placebo-controlled study. *Psychopharmacol Bull* 26: 130–135, 1990.

Cohen DJ, Pauls D, Volkmar FR: Recent research in Autism. *Child Adolesc Psychiatry Clin North Am* 3:161–171, 1994.

Dahl K, Cohen DJ, Provence S: Clinical and multivariate approaches to nosology of the pervasive developmental disorders. *J Am Acad Child Adolesc Psychiatry* 25:170–180, 1986.

Eberlin M, McConnachie G, Ibel S, et al.: Facilitated communication: A failure to replicate the phenomenon. *J Autism Dev Disord* 23:L507–530, 1993.

Gillberg C: Medical work-up in children with autism and Asperger syndrome. *Brain Dysfunction* 3: 249–260, 1990.

Golden G: Neurological functioning. In: Cohen D, Donnellan A (eds): *Handbook of Autism and Pervasive Developmental Disorders*. New York, Wiley, 1987, pp. 133–147.

Heller, T: Uber Dementia infantalis. *Zeitschrift fur Kindeforschung* 37:661–667, 1930. Reprinted in Howells JG (ed): *Modern Perspectives in International Child Psychiatry*. Edinburgh, Oliver and Boyd, 1969.

Kanner L: Autistic disturbances of affective contact. *Nerv Child* 2:217–250, 1943.

Klin A: Asperger Syndrome. *Child Adolesc Psychiatry Clin North Am* 3:131–148, 1994.

Klin A, Shepard, BA: Psychological assessment of autistic children. *Child Adolesc Psychiatry Clin North Am* 3:53–70, 1994.

Lockyer L, Rutter M: A five to fifteen year follow-up study of infantile psychosis. III: Psychological aspects. *Br J Psychiatry* 115:865–882, 1969.

Lord, C., Rutter, M., Goode, S., et al.: Autism diagnostic observation schedule: A standardized observation of communicative and social behavior. *J Autism Dev Disord* 19, 185–212, 1991.

Lord C, Schopler E, Revicki D: Sex differences in autism. *J Autism Dev Disord* 12:317–322. 1982.

Lotter V: Follow-up studies. In: Rutter M, Schopler E (eds): *Autism: A Reappraisal of Concepts and Treatment*. New York, Plenum, 1978, pp. 475–496.

Lovass OI: Behavioral treatment and normal educational and intellectual functioning in young autistic children. *J Consult Clin Psychol* 55:3–9, 1987.

McDougle CJ, Price LH, Volkmar, FR: Recent advances in the Pharmacotherapy of autism and related conditions. *Child Adolesc Psychiatry Clin North Am* 3:53–70, 1994.

Parks SL: The assessment of autistic children: A selective review of available instruments. *J Autism Dev Disord* 13:255–267, 1983.

Paul R: Communication in autism. In: Cohen D, Donnellan A (eds): *Handbook of Autism and Pervasive Developmental Disorders*. New York, Wiley, 1987, pp. 61–84.

Riddle M: Individual and parent psychotherapy in autism. In: Cohen D, Donnellan A (eds): *Handbook of Autism and Pervasive Developmental Disorders*. New York, Wiley, 1987, pp. 528–541.

Rutter M: Autistic children: Infancy to adulthood. *Semin Psychiatric* 2:435–450, 1970.

Rutter M: Diagnosis and definition. In: Rutter M, Schopler E (eds): *Autism: A Reappraisal of Concepts and Treatment*. New York, Plenum, pp. 1–25, 1978.

Schopler E, Andrews CE, Strupp K: Do autistic children come from upper-middle-class parents? *J Autism Dev Disord* 10:91–103, 1980.

Stern D: *The Interpersonal World of the Human Infant*. New York, Basic Books, 1987.

Tsai LY: Pre-, peri-, and neonatal factors in autism. In: Schopler E, Mesibov GB (eds): *Neurobiological Issues in Autism*. New York, Plenum, pp. 180–187, 1987.

Tsai LY: Rett Syndrome. *Child Adolesc Psychiatry Clin North Am* 3:105–118, 1994.

Volkmar FR: Childhood Disintegrative Disorder. *Child Adolesc Psychiatry Clin North Am* 3:119–130, 1994.

Volkmar FR, Bregman J, Cohen DJ, et al: DSM III and DSM III-R Diagnoses of Autism. *Am J Psychiatry* 145:1404–1408, 1988.

Volkmar FR, Cohen DJ: Diagnosis of pervasive developmental disorders. In: Lahey B, Kazdin A (eds): *Advances in Clinical Child Psychology* (Vol II). New York, Plenum, pp. 249–284, 1988.

Volkmar FR, Cohen DJ: Disintegrative disorder or ``late onset'' autism. *J Child Psychol Psychiatry* 30:717–724, 1989.

Volkmar FR, Stier DM. Cohen DJ: Age of recognition of pervasive developmental disorder. *Am J Psychiatry* 142:1450–1452, 1985.

Wing L, Gould J: Severe impairments of social interaction and associated abnormalities in children: Epidemiology and classification. *J Autism Dev Disord* 9:11–30, 1979.

Zahner GEP, Pauls DL: Epidemiological surveys of infantile autism. In: Cohen D, Donnellan A (eds): *Handbook of Autism and Pervasive Developmental Disorders*. New York, Wiley, 1987, pp. 199–210.

45 Reactive Attachment Disorders of Infancy or Early Childhood

Margot Moser Richters, Ph.D., and Fred R. Volkmar, M.D.

DEFINITION

It would be natural for a clinician or researcher to assume that the diagnosis *reactive attachment disorder* (RAD) refers fundamentally to a disturbance in the child-parent attachment relationship. Not only does the diagnostic label juxtapose the terms attachment and disorder but, during the past few decades, the term "attachment" has become virtually synonymous with the infant-caregiver relationship in psychiatry and psychology (Bowlby, 1951; 1969; 1980; 1982, Provence and Lipton, 1962; Spitz, 1946). The reactive attachment disorder diagnosis, however, does not necessarily refer to a child's primary attachment relationship. Rather, it applies more broadly to a child's manifestation of disturbances in social relatedness across individuals and contexts.

The abnormal development of social behaviors is presumed to be in response to (hence, the term "reactive") early and profoundly pathological caregiving operationalized as either "persistent disregard of the child's basic emotional needs for comfort, stimulation and affection," "persistent disregard of the child's basic physical needs," or "repeated changes of primary caregiver that prevent formation of stable attachment" (DSM-IV, APA, 1994). The diagnosis, therefore, is an "attachment disorder" in the sense that disturbances in the early relationship *between* parent and child are thought to give rise to a diathesis for social dysfunction *within* the child. Thus, although the disorder is thought to arise from a relational context, it differs from V codes and other "relational problems" in that the behavioral constellation persists over time, is evident across situations, is manifested in contexts well beyond the confines of the child-caregiver relationship, and is therefore a disorder thought to reside within the child.

In its initial incarnation in DSM-III (APA, 1980), reactive attachment disorder was described in general terms as a disorder marked by lack of developmentally appropriate social responsiveness and delayed physical development. With an age of onset *before* eight months, the diagnostic criteria included detailed descriptions of socially unresponsive behaviors in infants, such as lack of visual tracking, lack of smiling response, lack of alerting and turning toward caregiver's voice, and abnormal physical development such as weak rooting, hypomotility, and failure to gain weight or exhibited weight loss (with no physical explanation).

The diagnosis was essentially a description of failure-to-thrive (FTT) symptoms, but was distinguished from this pediatric syndrome by its psychosocial or "nonorganic" etiology. Locating the origin of the socioemotional disturbances in the context of the primary attachment relationship also served to differentiate reactive attachment disorder from the pervasive developmental disorders. While abnormal social relatedness is the hallmark of children with these disorders, their defects are thought to be neurobiological in nature, resulting in a lack of capacity for normal social development. Moreover, in contrast to the pervasive developmental disorders, marked improvement in the clinical picture subsequent to adequate caregiving was considered a diagnostic confirmation of the disorder.

The inclusion of reactive attachment disorder in DSM-III was a significant step toward defining an important clinical phenomenon, but the criteria proved difficult to apply. Some aspects of the definition seemed overly detailed and applicable only to very young infants (Rutter and Shaffer, 1980). Additionally, the inclusion of failure-to-thrive as an essential feature artificially narrowed the diagnostic concept. In response to these problems, the diagnosis underwent major revisions in DSM-III-R (APA, 1987). The transformation of reactive attachment disorder included a dramatic shift from a diagnosis primarily for infants to a disorder more easily applied to young children and a broadening of the diagnostic concept to incorporate the diversity of clinical presentations. The unusual age of onset—before 8 months—was raised to 5 years of age, and the failure-to-thrive symptoms were converted from defining features to associated features documented on Axis III. Rather than a detailed list of symptomatic characteristics, the criteria incorporated two general descriptions of abnormal social relatedness: *1*) excessively inhibited, ambivalent interactions, and *2*) indiscriminate social behaviors. The psychosocial nature of the disorder was retained through the continued requirement for a history of grossly pathogenic care, diagnostic confirmation via reversed clinical presentation subsequent to exposure to adequate caregiving, and the exclusion criteria of children with infantile autism or mental retardation.

Although the criteria for reactive attachment disorder in DSM-IV have undergone few substantive changes, they do provide a more accurate interpretation of the research findings. Those findings suggest that the relationship between grossly pathological care and reactive attachment disorder is not as direct as presupposed in DSM-III or DSM-III-R, as children's responses to pathological care can be markedly different. The text now clearly states that there are children who, despite experiencing maltreatment, are able to develop selective attachments to caregivers and do not necessarily develop reactive attachment disorder. In addition, the revised definition deemphasizes the importance of *grossly* pathological care (stating in the text that it is usually but not necessarily present) in recognition that less severe environments can also give rise to the clinical syndrome. The criteria now require the presence of pathogenic care, rather than grossly pathogenic care.

Disturbances in social relatedness continue to be defining features of the disorder, but there are now two designated subtypes: *inhibited* type and *disinhibited* type. Children manifesting the *inhibited* type are characterized by "excessively inhibited, hypervigilant, or highly ambivalent and contradictory responses" and may exhibit resistance to comforting and "frozen watchfulness" (DSM-IV, APA, 1994). The child with *disinhibited* type, in contrast, exhibits diffuse attachments "manifest by indiscriminate sociability with marked inability to exhibit appropriate selective attachments" (DSM-IV, APA, 1994). In addition, mental retardation is no longer an exclusionary criterion. These revisions essentially increase the diagnostic similarities between DSM-IV and ICD-10, although ICD-10 still does not require any specific etiology.

HISTORICAL NOTE

The recognition that an appropriately nurturing psychosocial environment is a necessary condition for the development of differential relatedness in infants is, surprisingly, a relatively recent phenomenon. Throughout most of history, the emphasis in the "nature-nurture" debate has been on the "nature" side. The presumption that development was largely unrelated to the quality of the psychosocial environment was reflected in institutional care practices for infants and young children and in early work, in this century, that suggested that "IQ" could be assessed in infancy and was stable into adult life (see Boswell, 1988, and Hunt, 1961, for interesting reviews of these issues). The recognition of the profound impact of disruptions in the processes of attachment, by such factors as maternal deprivation or institutional rearing, signaled a marked shift in the understanding of social developments in infants and young children (Ainsworth, et al., 1985; Bowlby, 1951; Rutter, 1971, 1979). Accordingly, only recently have efforts been made to develop a diagnostic classification that would capture the clinical picture of children who have experienced pathological care, particularly in the form of abuse, neglect, or repeated changes in caregivers. The clinical literature has proffered an array of diagnostic labels for these children, some describing or emphasizing major signs and symptoms—such as nonorganic failure to thrive, psychosocial dwarfism, and anaclitic depression—while others have emphasized the major environmental circumstances of the child—such as hospitalism, maternal deprivation, and maltreatment syndrome. Reactive attachment disorder is the label selected for the DSM in an attempt to capture both the context of the disorder ("reactive" in response to caregiving) and the sequelae of the caregiving (problems in the child's social relatedness).

What has been curious in the development of the diagnostic category is the relative lack of influence from the field of attachment (Zeanah and Emde, 1993). Researchers working in the area of attachment suggest that the name of the disorder is somewhat misleading because the criteria do not directly address attachment as it is defined by developmentalists. It is their suggestion that the diagnosis should also include an assessment of the child-caregiver relationship in terms of comfort seeking, exploratory behavior, secure-base behavior, and responsiveness (Zeanah et al., 1993). The conceptualization of attachment disorders as a characterization of child-caregiver relationships has been formalized in a diagnostic classification system developed by Zero to Three/National Center for Clinical Infant Programs (NCCIP) in their recently published manual, *Diagnostic Classifications of Mental Health and Developmental Disorders of Infancy and Early Childhood* (ZTT/NCCIP, 1994).

Similar to DSM-IV, the NCCIP system provides an Axis I diagnosis, Reactive Attachment Deprivation/Maltreatment Disorder of Infancy and Early Childhood, to be applied when a child has experienced persistently inadequate basic emotional, physical, or psychological care and manifests a disturbance in social relatedness. But the NCCIP diagnostic framework extends beyond DSM-IV by also including a classification system for disordered parent-child relationships. Coded on Axis II, there are nine so-called Relationship Disorders in which the child presents with a disturbance specific to a primary attachment figure, but for which a history of grossly pathogenic basic care is not required; these include relationship problems characterized by over/under involvement, anxiety, hostility, abuse (verbal, physical, or sexual), or mixed types. In contrast to reactive attachment disorder, in which the child necessarily presents with pervasive developmental delays in social relatedness, a child diagnosed with a relationship disorder may manifest symptoms that exist only in the context of the primary caregiving or attachment relationship. Through this classification system, NCCIP has furnished a meaningful way to understand and address disorders specific to the quality of the child-parent relationship.

PREVALENCE AND EPIDEMIOLOGY

To date, extensive literature searches reveal no epidemiological studies of the prevalence and incidence of reactive attachment disorder as it was defined in DSM-III-R. According to DSM-IV, the disorder appears to be "very uncommon," but exactly how uncommon it is and what is the empirical source for this estimate are not specified (APA, 1994). Cases reported in the literature have included children from all socioeconomic levels, although descriptions of children with associated disorders, such as failure to thrive, have reported relationships to variables such as poverty, family dysfunction, and parent psychopathology (Richters and Volkmar, 1994; Skuse, 1984a, 1984b). The paucity of epidemiological data is due, in part, to the repeated changes is the diag-

nostic criteria and the lack of familiarity with the disorder among clinicians. Given the etiological requirements for the disorder, it might seem plausible to derive an estimate of affected children from the statistics on maltreated and institutionalized children. Researchers concede, however, that establishing rates of child abuse and neglect is fraught with difficulties. Such estimates depend not only on "reported cases," the substantiation of reports, and variations in the content, interpretation, and enforcement of reporting laws, but also on our definition of "maltreatment," which shifts with the prevailing cultural and political winds (Barnett et al., 1993). In addition, while the Panel on Research on Child Abuse and Neglect (1993) suggested that 1,000,000 was a *conservative* estimate of the number of children who have been maltreated in the United States, it is not clear what proportion of these children would meet the DSM-IV criteria for experiencing grossly pathogenic care. Clearly, some children who are abused *do* form attachments to their caregivers (Egeland and Sroufe, 1981). Finally, there are no available estimates of the number of children experiencing multiple substitutions in caregivers for reasons such as court-ordered custody changes, prolonged parental absences due to military deployments, and extensive hospitalizations due to illness.

CLINICAL DESCRIPTION

Since the diagnostic category of reactive attachment disorder is relatively new and has undergone considerable revision, the data available to provide a complete clinical description are limited. Some of what follows therefore, has been drawn from related literature on failure to thrive, child maltreatment, institutionalization, and attachment. In this context it should be noted that the large body of literature on the development of attachment and, in particular, on attachment types as assessed in the Ainsworth strange situation (Ainsworth, et al. 1985) has only some relationship to attachment *disorder* as such.

Age of Onset

The literature on maternal deprivation, maltreatment, and institutionalization suggests that children who suffer insults to their early attachment and bonding relationships subsequently exhibit pervasive and persistent defects in their social development. The current diagnostic requirement is that there be marked disturbances in social behavior *before* the age of five (although the diagnosis can be applied as early as the first month of life). The reliability and validity of this specific age of onset have not yet been established, although it seems reasonably clear that, while the task of forming attachments continues throughout life, it is during the first years of life that the process is most prone to fundamental disruption (Volkmar, in press).

Empirical questions aside, from a practical standpoint, determining age of onset can be a remarkably challenging task. A review of the clinical literature suggests that there are two common pathways to treatment for children with reactive attachment disorder: (*a*) pediatric assessments for failure-to-thrive symptoms in infancy and, (*b*) psychiatric evaluations for behavioral and language delays in early childhood (often subsequent to changes in custody or entrance into school settings). Often, it is someone other than the primary caregiver who brings the child in for an evaluation. As a result, ascertaining the quality of early social behaviors becomes almost impossible, because the details of the child's early history are often fragmented and incomplete—particularly for those being assessed only after permanent removal from the home. Further research is needed to establish the distribution of apparent onset ages as well as to determine the sensitivity and specificity that the criterion contributes to the diagnosis (Volkmar, in press).

Social Disturbance

Social dysfunction is the central defining feature of children with reactive attachment disorder. The *inhibited* type is marked by the child's persistent failure to initiate and respond to social interactions in an age-appropriate manner. Instead, the child appears wary and hypervigilant, excessively inhibited, and generally ambivalent in response to caregivers and social interactions. Additionally, caregivers find the child resistant to comforting or prone to exhibit "frozen watchfulness." In the maltreatment and deprivation literature, these children are described as affectively withdrawn, apathetic, and unresponsive. They are often remarkable for their gaze abnormalities and idiosyncratic or atypical responses to social cues.

In this same literature are descriptions of children manifesting the *disinhibited* subtype. While these children seem to be quite interested in interacting with others, they do not appear to make selective attachments. Rather, their relationships are marked by superficiality, "clinginess," and indiscriminate sociability. These children also exhibit excessive aggressiveness and incompetence in their peer relationships (Alessandri, 1991; Erickson et al., 1989; Hoffman-Plotkin and Twentyman, 1984; Main and George, 1985; Salzinger et al., 1993). For either subtype, the clinical picture may vary depending upon chronological age, developmental level, and early caregiving history.

Communication Disturbances

While not included in the diagnostic criteria, indirect evidence from the failure-to-thrive, maltreatment and deprivation literature, and case descriptions of children with reactive attachment disorder suggest that *some* affected children may evidence delays in language development (Cicchetti, 1989; Coster et al., 1989; Harris, 1982; Oates et al., 1985; Richters and Volkmar, 1994; Rutter and Garmezy, 1983; Skuse, 1984; Vondra et al., 1990). The linguistic disturbances, when present, appear to range from poor articulation to mild echolalia. The communication impairments among children with reactive attachment disorder appear to be more similar to those of language-disordered children and less similar to the severe forms often seen in children with autism. In addition, language development in these children appears to improve after intervention. Further research is needed to determine the nature and extent to which language disturbances are present among children with reactive attachment disorder.

Cognitive Development

Since the emphasis of reactive attachment disorder is on abnormal social development, and because mental retardation was an exclusionary criterion prior to DSM-IV, there is a paucity of data concerning cognitive impairments among affected children. Reports on children diagnosed with reactive attachment disorder, and the indirect evidence from research on children raised in depriving and maltreating environments, suggest that intellectual functioning is often below average or delayed at initial assessment. It is, however, clear that children with mental retardation also usually form attachments, albeit at a time commensurate with developmental level (Berry and Gunn, 1980). Again, reactive attachment disorder differs from other disorders by the presence of marked improvements after therapeutic intervention (Crittenden, 1985; Erickson et al., 1989; Hoffman-Plotkin and Twentyman, 1984; Richters and Volkmar, 1994; Tizard and Rees, 1974).

The cognitive deficits exhibited by some children with reactive attachment disorder are most accurately described as an associated feature. Researchers in the field of maltreatment and deprivation have identified multiple pathways to cognitive impairments, ranging from physical abuse to low economic status. More specifically, in these pathogenic environments intellectual deficits may be the result of brain damage from head injuries, neurological insults due to malnutrition, or depressed language development because of inadequate verbal stimulation (Herrenkohl et al., 1984; Kaufman and Cicchetti, 1989; Skuse and Bentovim, 1994; Terwogt et al., 1990).

Behavioral Features

Clearly, the most striking feature of children with reactive attachment disorder is their atypical social presentations. Yet there are other behav-

iors frequently associated with the disorder. Disruptive, disorganized behaviors, along with poor affect regulation and low frustration tolerance, have been noted particularly among the *disinhibited* type. Some of these children also exhibit distractibility and attentional problems. Anecdotal clinical descriptions have also cited underdeveloped self-care skills and self-stimulatory behaviors (Richters and Volkmar, 1994).

Developmental Changes

As a diagnosis in its own infancy, there are as yet no longitudinal data on the developmental trajectory of children with reactive attachment disorder. The reduction and/or resolution of symptoms probably depends in large part on the nature, duration, and severity of pathogenic care experienced by the child, on the child's own constitutional factors, and on the interaction between these two. In general, the prognosis is less hopeful the more severe and prolonged the environmental deprivation and the later adequate caregiving and interventions are introduced. From the clinical descriptions and from studies on children from maltreating and depriving environments, there is a body of evidence suggesting that the symptoms appear to be responsive to therapeutic intervention. Improvements in cognitive functioning, language development, and motor development have been cited (e.g., Hodges and Tizard, 1989a, 1989b). In addition, there are reports of decreases in behavioral problems and increases in age-appropriate self-care skills (Richters and Volkmar, 1994).

Unfortunately, improvements in the quality of social relatedness are more difficult to measure. There are reports of improved social skills, but the concern is that these changes may only be superficial. For some children, atypical gaze patterns, idiosyncratic interactive styles, and poor integration of social-emotional cues appear to persist (Richters and Volkmar, 1994). Many have hypothesized that problems with social development may endure throughout adulthood in the form of difficulty in establishing and/or maintaining meaningful relationships and persistence of idiosyncratic styles of relating. The question remains as to whether or what extent social and emotional development in children with reactive attachment disorder will be systematically different from that in other children.

ETIOLOGY AND PATHOGENESIS
Biological Mechanisms

To date, there are no known primary biological mechanisms underlying the development of the disorder. Evidence for the presence of a biological predisposition may be eventually revealed, given the considerable variation that has been reported among siblings raised together in extremely depriving early environments (Skuse, 1984). In the maltreatment literature, a transactional model has emerged as a way to understand such diversity in outcomes (Cicchetti, 1987). There may, for example, be biological factors, such as physical anomalies, persistent colic, or difficult temperament that influence the likelihood that a child will be victimized by a caregiver. Moreover, certain factors, such as difficult temperament, may also influence the likelihood that a child will react pathogenically to maltreatment. Children with these biological risk factors, who also experience pathogenic infant-caregiver relationships, may consequently experience disruptions in their achievement of, or successful progression along, normal developmental lines. The formation of selective attachment relationships may be one of the normal developmental tasks that falters, thereby setting the stage for the emergence of reactive attachment disorder.

Psychological Processes

FAMILY FACTORS

By definition, reactive attachment disorder arises in the context of pathological caregiving. In fact, it was the growing body of literature on the effects of maternal deprivation, maltreatment, and institutionalization that led to the recognition of reactive attachment disorder as a clinical phenomenon. However, to date, there has been no systematic research published detailing significant family factors among affected children. The omission of *grossly* pathogenic care from the formal DSM-IV criteria (it has been replaced with, simply, "pathogenic care") suggests that there is a continuum of inadequate caregiving that may give rise to the disorder. While it is clear in the maltreatment literature that severe abuse and/or neglect can give rise to disorders of attachment, there is still no definitive evidence on the effects of milder forms of disturbed caregiver-child interaction styles (Zeanah and Zeanah, 1989; Volkmar, in press).

Researchers in the area of nonorganic failure-to-thrive have described some differences between mothers with and without nonorganic failure-to-thrive infants (Drotar et al., 1990). In parent-child interactions, mothers of affected infants were observed to have less adaptive social interactions, less positive affect, and more arbitrary termination of feedings. In addition, researchers have also reported that mothers with nonorganic failure to thrive infants frequently complain of lack of perceived emotional support from family members (Drotar, 1991). No differences have been found, however, on factors such as family size, maternal age, maternal education, parent marital status or sex of child.

ENVIRONMENTAL AND SOCIAL INFLUENCES

As is the case with family factors, there are no empirical data on the effects of environmental and social influences. In cases reported thus far, however, it appears that the symptoms of children with reactive attachment disorder are pervasive, and are typically manifested across situations and across relationships. Our current understanding of the disorder also suggests that environmental and social influences play an essential role in reversing the clinical picture. In fact, it has been the amelioration of symptoms subsequent to the introduction of adequate caregiving that has often been used as a means for confirming the diagnosis.

DIFFERENTIAL DIAGNOSIS

Various conditions or situations may give rise to problems in infant-parent attachment. For example, the separation of a young child from a primary attachment figure may be associated with the sequence of *protest*, *despair*, and *detachment* outlined by Bowlby. In some such instances, particularly with somewhat older children, depressive symptoms may predominate and, if the reaction is prolonged, a diagnosis of depression may be indicated. Sometimes blind or deaf children may, initially, seem to have deficits in attachments but, usually, once the sensory impairment is identified and the appropriate interventions are made, the apparent social deficit improves markedly.

Infants and young children with mental retardation that is not associated with autism or another pervasive developmental disorder develop attachments that are appropriate to their developmental level; such attachments may, however, be more prone to disruption, e.g., as a result of unstable environments, and it is possible that such children are at greater risk for developing reactive attachment disorder. In the pervasive developmental disorders, deficits in reciprocal social interaction are, by definition, present and are usually observed from very early in life. Social deficits may be particularly profound in autistic disorder, especially in very young children. However, over time some selective attachments do develop, although these are usually highly deviant. The presence of other characteristic symptoms (e.g., marked deficits in communication and unusual behavioral responses to the environment, such as stereotypy and resistance to change) will usually alert the clinician to the diagnosis. Because autism and related conditions are usually associated with mental retardation, the child's overall mental age should be taken into consideration. A substantial body of evidence suggests that, in most cases, the psychosocial environment provided by parents of children with autism and related conditions is appropriately stimulating and the failures in social development observed reflect a fundamental disturbance in the child. As would then be expected, changes in the environment do not typically result in major behavioral improvement nor the development of more robust attachments.

As was suggested in the DSM-III (APA, 1980) criteria for this condition, some infants and young children with reactive attachment disorder may also exhibit disturbances in feeding (e.g., feeding disorder of infancy, rumination disorder, or pica) and in growth (e.g., psychosocial dwarfism).

TREATMENT

Intervention should focus on the totality of the child's situation. Efforts should be made to support the child's development, the adequacy and responsiveness of the parents, and the provision of an appropriately stimulating and nurturing psychosocial environment. Although foster placement is best avoided if possible, sometimes removal of the child is mandatory, e.g., because the child has sustained life-threatening injuries or is in immediate danger. While the usual presumption is that reunification of child and parent(s) is the eventual goal, it is important to balance attempts at rehabilitation with the child's need for stability. Provision of appropriate pediatric and early intervention services should be made.

The attempt to produce major changes in the child-caregiver relationship often requires sustained, intensive, and highly structured work with the child, the caregiver, and the dyad. Appropriate additional support services should be made available to the caregiver. Pediatric monitoring is particularly critical if eating or growth problems are present.

Directions for Research

The relative absence of research on this condition is, in some ways, paradoxical, given both the history of work on the effects of maternal deprivation and orphanage rearing and the important social policy problems created by caring for children with reactive attachment disorders. Information on such basic aspects of the condition as clinical phenomenology, course, epidemiology, and response to treatment is lacking. While the distinction, as in DSM-IV, of subtypes of the condition seems generally reasonable, research on the potential importance of this distinction, e.g., for intervention and outcome, remains unclear.

References

Ainsworth MDS, Blehar MS, Waters E, et al.: *Patterns of Attachment: A Psychological Study of the Strange Situation.* Erlbaum, Hillsdale NJ, 1985.

Alessandri SM: Play and social behaviors in maltreated preschoolers. *Dev Psychopathol* 3:191–206, 1991.

American Psychiatric Association. *Diagnostic and Statistical Manual of Mental Disorders* (3rd ed). Washington, DC, 1980.

American Psychiatric Association. *Diagnostic and Statistical Manual of Mental Disorders* (3rd ed, rev). Washington, DC, 1987.

American Psychiatric Association. *Diagnostic and Statistical Manual of Mental Disorders* (4th ed). Washington, DC, 1994.

Barnett D, Manly JT, Cicchetti D: Defining child maltreatment: The interface between policy and research. In D Cicchetti, S Toth (eds) *Child Abuse, Child Development and Social Policy.* Norwood, NJ, Ablex, 1993, pp. 7–74

Berry P, Gunn P, Andrews R: Behavior of Down syndrome infants in a strange situation. *Am J Ment Defic* 85:213, 1980.

Boswell J: *The Kindness of Strangers—The Abandonment of Children in Western Europe from Late Antiquity to the Renaissance.* Pantheon Books, New York, 1988.

Bowlby J: *Maternal Care and Mental Health.* World Health Organization, Geneva, 1951.

Bowlby J: *Attachment and Loss,* (Vols 1–3). Basic Books, New York, 1969, 1982 (2nd ed), 1973, 1980.

Cicchetti D: Developmental psychopathology in infancy: Illustrations from the study of maltreated youngsters. *J Consult Clin Psychol* 55:837–845, 1987.

Coster WJ, Gersten MS, Beeghly M, et al.: Communicative functioning in maltreated toddlers. *Devel Psychopath* 25:1020–1029, 1989.

Crittenden P: Maltreated infants: Vulnerability and resilience. *J Child Psychol Psychiatry* 6:85–96, 1985.

Drotar D: The family context of nonorganic failure to thrive. *Am J Orthopsychiatry* 61:23–34, 1991

Drotar D, Eckerle D, Satola J, et al: Maternal interactional behavior with nonorganic failure to thrive infants: A case comparison study. *Child Abuse Negl* 14:41–51,1990.

Egeland B, Sroufe LA: Attachment and early maltreatment. *Child Dev* 52:44, 1981.

Erickson MF, Egeland B, Pianta R: The effects of maltreatment on the development of young children. In: D Cicchetti, V Carlson (eds): *Child Maltreatment*. Cambridge, Cambridge University Press, 1989, pp. 647–684.

Harris JC: Nonorganic failure-to-thrive syndromes: Reactive attachment disorder of infancy and psychosocial dwarfism in childhood. In: PJ Accardo (ed): *Failure to Thrive in Infancy and Early Childhood*. Baltimore, University Park Press, 1982 pp. 229–242.

Herrenkohl EC, Herrenkohl RC, Toedter L, et al: Parent-child interactions in abusive and nonabusive families. *J Am Acad Child Adolesc Psychiatry* 23,6: 641–648, 1984.

Hodges J, Tizard B: IQ and behavioral adjustment of ex-institutional adolescents. *J Child Psychol Psychiatry* 30:53, 1989(a).

Hodges J, Tizard B: Social and family relationships of ex-institutional adolescents. *J Child Psychol Psychiatry* 30:77, 1989(b).

Hoffman-Plotkin D, Twentyman CT: A multimodal assessment of behavioral and cognitive deficits in abused and neglected preschoolers. *Child Dev* 55:794–802, 1984.

Hunt J McV: *Intelligence and Experience*. Ronald Press, New York, 1961.

Kaufman J, Cicchetti D: Effects of maltreatment on school-age children's socioemotional develop-

ment: Assessments in a day camp setting. *Dev Psychol* 25:516–524, 1989.

Main M, George C: Responses of abused and disadvantaged toddlers to distress in agemates: A study in the day care setting. *Dev Psychol* 21: 407–412, 1985.

Oates RK, Peacock A, Cortes D: Long-term effects of nonorganic failure to thrive. *Pediatrics* 75: 36–40, 1985.

Provence S, Lipton R: *Infants in Institutions*. International Universities Press, New York, 1962.

Richters MM, Volkmar, FR: Reactive attachment disorder in infancy and early childhood. *J Am Acad Child Adolesc Psychiatry* 33:328–332, 1994.

Rutter M: *Maternal Deprivation Reassessed*. Penguin, Harmondsworth, Middlesex, 1972.

Rutter M: Maternal deprivation, 1972–1978: New findings, new concepts, new approaches. *Child Dev* 50:283, 1979.

Rutter M, Garmezy N: Development and Psychopathology. In: P Mussen (ed): *Handbook of Child Psychol*. New York: Wiley, pp. 775–911, 1983.

Rutter M, Shaffer D: DSM-III: A step forward or back in terms of classification of child psychiatric disorders? *J Am Acad Child Psychiatry* 19:371, 1980.

Salzinger S, Feldman RS, Hammer M: The effects of physical abuse on children's social relationships. *Child Dev* 64:169–187, 1993.

Skuse D: Extreme deprivation in early childhood—I. Diverse outcomes for three siblings from an extraordinary family. *J Child Psychol Psychiatry* 25:523, 1984(a).

Skuse D: Extreme deprivation in early childhood—II. Theoretical issues and a comparative review. *J Child Psychol Psychiatry* 25:543, 1984(b).

Skuse D, Bentovim A: Physical and emotional maltreatment. In: M. Rutter, E. Taylor, L Hersov (eds). *Child and Adolescent Psychiatry* (3rd ed). Oxford, Blackwell, 1994, pp. 209–228.

Spitz R: Anaclitic depression. *Psychoanal Study Child* 2:313, 1946.

Terwogt MM, Schene J, Koops W: Concepts of emotion in institutionalized children. *J Child Psychol Psychiatry* 31:1131, 1990.

Tizard B, Rees J: The effect of early institutional rearing on the behavior problems and affectional relationships of four-year-old children. *J Child Psychol Psychiatry* 16:61–73, 1975.

Volkmar, FR: Reactive Attachment Disorder. In: *DSM-IV Source Book*, American Psychiatric Association Press, in press.

Vondra JI, Barnett D, Cicchetti D: Self-concept, motivation, and competence among preschoolers from maltreating and comparison families. *Child Abuse Negl* 14:525–540, 1990.

Zeanah CH, Emde RN: Attachment disorders in infancy and childhood. In: M Rutter, L Hersov, E Taylor (eds): *Child and Adolescent Psychiatry*, (3rd ed), Oxford, Blackwell, 1994.

Zeanah CH, Mammen OK, Lieberman AF: Disorders of attachment. In: CH Zeanah (ed): *Handbook of Infant Mental Health*, New York, Guilford, 1993, pp. 332–349.

Zeanah CH, Zeanah PD: Intergenerational transmission of maltreatment: Insights from attachment theory and research. *Psychiatry* 52:177, 1989.

Zero to Three/National Center for Clinical Infant Programs: *Diagnostic Classification of Mental Health and Developmental Disorders of Infancy and Early Childhood: 0–3*. Arlington, VA 1994.

46 MENTAL RETARDATION

Andrew T. Russell, M.D., and Peter E. Tanguay, M.D.

The work of diagnosing and treating mental and emotional disorders in the retarded, whether they be children, adolescents, or adults, has usually fallen to the child psychiatrist rather than to the general psychiatrist. There may be several advantages to this. The child psychiatrist is usually more familiar with developmental issues and more at home in talking to persons who have not reached full cognitive maturation. Another consideration is that the child psychiatrist, because of his or her training and practice, may be somewhat more accustomed to working in a team setting with other professionals such as psychologists, educators, language specialists, or social service personnel who deal with child abuse, placement, and the courts. Inasmuch as this is true, the child psychiatrist should feel at home in diagnosing and treating mental illnesses in the retarded. As is shown in this chapter, the diagnosis and treatment of mental illness in retarded persons is beginning to be both scientifically informed and data based. New instruments for identification of psychiatric symptoms are being developed and tested. We are coming to recognize that the signs and symptoms of psychiatric disorders are not necessarily different in moderately and mildly retarded persons (those whose IQ is greater than 40). Medication, carefully used, may be effective in treating mental disorders in retarded persons.

These advances are important because it is recognized that mental illness can make it much more difficult for retarded persons to adjust to their living arrangements and to the people with whom they come in contact. Effective treatment of their psychiatric illness may make it

possible for the retarded to take full advantage of existing programs in special education, social skills training, and other forms of sophisticated help with daily living that may be available to them. The psychiatrist is needed as part of the treatment team that cares for retarded persons. The authors have found such teamwork to be rewarding in a variety of hospital and community settings. As long as the psychiatrist knows what he or she can and cannot realistically accomplish, and how the other disciplines on the team can help advance treatment, the task of treating mental illness in retarded persons is not especially daunting, or at least no more so than is treating mental illness in the general population.

This chapter begins with an overview of the subject of mental retardation, reviewing its definition, history, epidemiology, and etiology. The discussion then turns to mental disorders in mentally retarded persons, focusing on the work of the psychiatrist in evaluation, diagnosis, and treatment.

DEFINITION

The definition of mental retardation adopted by DSM-IV involves three components with corresponding diagnostic criteria.

The essential feature of Mental Retardation is significantly subaverage general intellectual functioning (Criterion A) that is accompanied by significant limitations in adaptive functioning in at least two of the following skill areas: communication, self-care, home living, social/interpersonal skills, use of community resources, self-direction, functional academic skills, work, leisure, health, and safety (Criterion B). The onset must occur before 18 years (Criterion C). (From American Psychiatric Association: *Diagnostic and Statistical Manual of Mental Disorders* (4th ed). Washington, DC, American Psychiatric Association, 1994, p. 39)

This definition incorporates features of prior diagnostic criteria developed by the American Association on Mental Retardation (see Grossman, 1983) with some aspects of that organization's latest definitions (Luckasson et al., 1992). The diagnosis is not one to be given lightly to patients, since it can bring social approbation and a lessening of its possessor's opportunities in life. Conversely, for those who are truly intellectually *and* adaptively impaired, the label may open the doors to school and social services that can be not only helpful but also crucial to attaining a high quality of life.

Measuring intellectual functioning is largely done through psychometric tests. Three of the most widely used intelligence tests in the United States are the Wechsler Adult Intelligence Scale-Revised (WAIS), the Wechsler Intelligence Scale for Children III (WISC-III, age range 6–16 years), and the revised Stanford-Binet (age range 2–18 years). The Stanford-Binet yields a single composite IQ score and mental-age score. The Wechsler scales yield a full-scale composite score, a verbal score, a performance score, and component subtest scores. The Stanford-Binet is considered to be somewhat more dependent on language ability in comparison to either of the Wechsler scales.

Intelligence testing may not tell us much about *intelligence*. The tests measure a standard set of skills, without providing information about why a person might have failed to give the expected answer or might have obtained a low score. IQ tests may give misleading results when used with persons from a different culture or whose native language is not English. If they are administered and scored by someone who knows the limits of the tests, however, the risk of misinterpretation is lessened. Standardized test scores are very useful in assessing mental retardation and can be a useful predictor of outcome and developmental course.

Cognitive functioning is a complex matter, not well understood. Its component skills, apart from such basic phenomena as attention, perception, and memory, remain poorly defined, except in global psychological terms. Experimental studies provide some tantalizing glimpses of fundamental processes that may underlie information processing and storage, such as unconscious parallel versus conscious sequential analysis of informative neural input (Kihlstrom, 1987). Piaget, who described himself as a *genetic epistemologist*, developed an elaborate system to conceptualize the nature of thought using logical-deductive algebra (see Flavell, 1973), but the idea did not catch on. Piaget's stage model of cognitive development has been more popular. Continuing work by developmental psychologists has served to modify and extend it (see Flavell and Markman, 1983).

Sternberg and Gardner (1982) have characterized intellectual functioning along several dimensions. In their highly theoretical system, executive components evaluate a problem, consider possible responses, rehearse strategies and their possible outcome, and choose a course of action. Performance components retrieve information items from memory, compare them, note the higher and lower correlations between items (''A'' and ''a'' are physically different but represent the same linguistic symbol), select the correct meaning, compare options, justify a conclusion, and respond accordingly. Additional components add new information to memory after assessing its relevance to present and future needs.

Learning how to problem solve requires not only an intact central nervous system but also the knowledge that others have minds and that others can transmit information both as language and as nonverbal facial expressions, nods, gestures, and changes in tone of voice. From birth to 1 year of age, children spend enormous energy in learning the nonverbal aspects of social communication. Only after they have begun to master social nonverbal communication do they begin to learn semantic and syntactic verbal communication skills. The latter are tested by intelligence and language tests; the former are rarely examined in retarded subjects. Hobson and his colleagues (1989) studied the ability of mildly retarded adolescents to match photographs of sad, angry, happy, surprised, and disgusted faces with vocal expressions of the same emotions. The retarded subjects performed less well than did nonretarded control subjects. To control for the intellectual aspects of the task, the ability of subjects to match nonemotional stimuli was also studied. The retarded subjects were less impaired in this than they were on the emotional task. The nature of the deficits in matching the emotional stimuli remained open to question, however.

The concept of adaptive functioning mentioned in the DSM-IV and in American Association on Mental Retardation (AAMR) definitions is an attempt to encompass important motivational, social, and cultural aspects of human intellectual functioning, above and beyond the narrow confines of the numbers generated by an intelligence test. Adaptive function is a broad concept that in essence refers to ''how effectively individuals cope with common life demands and how well they meet the standards of personal independence expected of someone in their particular age group, sociocultural background, and community setting'' (APA, 1994). The ability of a person with mental retardation to adapt to life demands is of critical importance and may make the difference between living at home or in a residential facility. Overall adaptive functioning may be dramatically affected by numerous factors, for example, the presence of concurrent psychiatric disorder. However, the use of impairment in adaptive functioning as an essential criterion for the *diagnosis* of mental retardation continues to be debated (Greenspan and Granfield, 1992; MacMillan et al., 1993; Scott, 1994; Zigler and Hodapp, 1986). A major problem is that measuring adaptive functioning has not proven easy.

One instrument designed to measure adaptive functioning is the Vineland Adaptive and Maladaptive Behavior Scales (Sparrow et al., 1984). The scales measure social and functional areas of adaptive development and have been revised and standardized for normal and retarded populations. The AAMR Adaptive Behavior Scale for Children and Adults (Nihara et al., 1974) is another instrument for assessing adaptive functioning, albeit one used primarily in rehabilitation and hospital settings, for the more severely retarded. The scales are divided into two parts. The first part measures behavioral domains important in maintaining independent living, and the second focuses on maladaptive behavior. The reliable measurement of adaptive behavior using the current diagnostic criteria may be even more problematic given the necessity to assess 10 individual domains of adaptive functioning (MacMillan et al., 1993).

HISTORICAL NOTE

Severe forms of mental handicap could not have gone unnoticed in early times, perhaps even before there was much recognition of mental illness. The ''village idiot'' and Simple Simon are more gentle reflections about the retarded in medieval times. The tale of the Wolf Boy and stories of feral children are darker versions of the same persona. In reality, life may not have been easy or pleasant for the retarded, though they are not spoken of very often before the late 16th century.

Early religious leaders and sages such as Zoroaster, Confucius, and the early writers of the Koran advocated compassion for the retarded. What programs were established as a result of this concern were custodial, however, given that there were no guiding educational principles upon which intervention could be based. After the Middle Ages, organized attempts to help the handicapped, including the retarded, were begun. Some of the earliest and more successful efforts to help retarded persons began in Paris. About the middle of the 17th century, the religious leader Vincent de Paul gathered into his Conferie de Charite the homeless and the disadvantaged, among whom were persons of subnormal intellect. A place of refuge was created for them at the Bicetre.

The unfolding of interest in the plight of the retarded came from parallel fields: education of the deaf and of the blind. In the 18th century, people had begun to study new approaches to teaching these people and to show that remarkable strides could be made in improving their lives. By the early 1800s a school for the deaf and laloplegic was a striking success in Paris. A school was subsequently established along similar lines for teaching the blind, and not long after, Louis Braille perfected a reading system for the blind today known by his name. Soon a question was asked by others: Why not start a corresponding school for the retarded? It was an exciting idea, but it needed something else to set it into motion.

That event, in 1801, was the finding of a ''wild boy'' in the town of Aveyron, who was brought to Paris for further study. Fantastic stories abounded about him, among which was the notion that he had been raised by wolves. The idea was wrong, but it served greatly to increase public interest in him. A physician, Jean Marie Gaspard Itard, who had been a student at the Bicetre and was now employed as a teacher of the deaf in Paris, heard about the boy and became interested in him. He determined to learn whether the boy, named Victor by his rescuers, could be trained and educated. Itard studied Victor assiduously, applied himself to educating him, and began to enunciate principles upon which such treatment could be guided. Although his efforts with Victor were unsuccessful, he decided to devote his life to studying others with similar handicaps and to training students who could carry on his work. Among his students was Edward Seguin, who would introduce the principles of education of the retarded to America in 1848, when he became associated with the newly created Massachusetts Experimental School for the Teaching and Training of Idiots, later called the Fernald School. Many of the future leaders in special education in America were to come from this school, the first of its kind in this country.

Optimistic views about the rehabilitation of retarded people through special education had begun to give way to pessimism toward the end of the 19th century, and there was once more a move toward building large, impersonal institutions to house the retarded. The eugenics movement, whose proponents demanded that the retarded be segregated and sterilized, rose to considerable prominence and power in 20th-century America. Sterilization laws were passed in many states and remained in force until the early 1960s in some places. Sentiments of a similar nature were voiced in Nazi Germany, where retarded persons were systematically exterminated.

A backlash against eugenics and forced sterilization developed by the 1960s, and people began to be aware that retarded people needed protection if their rights were to be preserved. In 1962 President John F. Kennedy proclaimed that America must better serve the needs of citizens who are mentally retarded. Under Kennedy's leadership, the Congress that year passed the Mental Retardation and Developmental Disabilities Act. This act provided greatly increased funding for the study of mental retardation and for multidisciplinary training of professionals to work with retarded persons. The act also required that local school districts provide adequate educational services to these children. The act was a striking and important milestone in dealing with retarded persons in America.

In the past three decades, there have been several developments that have greatly changed how retarded persons are treated. One development has been the almost complete separation of services for the mentally ill and the mentally retarded in most states. While this may have been useful in allowing a more precise focus upon the special problems of the retarded, it has made it less likely that the psychiatric care of retarded persons will be adequately attended to.

Other developments have been the deinstitutionalization of retarded persons and the move to ''mainstream'' retarded students in the public school system. The first has led to an influx of retarded persons into residential care in the community. More sheltered workshops and community living arrangements have been created, some quite good. Several questions have yet to be answered about this turn of events. Is such care necessarily better for all retarded persons? Because of inadequate funding of some programs, are we in danger of creating a new set of disgraceful ''back wards,'' hidden in our poorest neighborhoods? How large should the ideal residential placement be?

Mainstreaming implies that the retarded student spends at least 50% of his or her day in the regular classroom. There is disagreement among educators about the extent more severely impaired individuals can bene-fit from it. At present less than a third of mentally retarded children are mainstreamed in public schools in America (U.S. Office of Special Education Programs, 1994), and there is concern about its effectiveness (Fuchs and Fuchs, 1994).

Head Start and other special preschool programs were begun in the early 1960s to help poor and disadvantaged children. What they appear to do, and do quite effectively, is decrease the likelihood that children from disadvantaged, low-income, and socially impoverished homes will be misidentified as mentally retarded as they move through the school system. Detailed and sophisticated follow-up studies of the children in 11 of the earliest preschool enrichment programs (Consortium for Longitudinal Studies, 1983) indicate that, while the immediate IQ and learning gains of preschool programs tend to wash out within 3 or 4 years after entry into regular school, the children who participated fared better in their long-range schooling than did children in control groups. In particular, they did better on two very important measures: never placed in special education for the retarded and never held back a grade. Both of these indices were found to be significantly related to whether the children later remained in school or graduated. The effect of the program was deemed to have resulted from higher parental expectations in the experimental group and greater aspirations on the part of the children themselves. Currently there is more emphasis on early and accurate identification of children with learning disorders in the Head Start program (Forness and Finn, 1993).

PREVALENCE AND EPIDEMIOLOGY

Although current diagnostic criteria emphasize that adaptive functioning *and* IQ scores should be considered in making a determination that a person is retarded, in practice the decision is based almost exclusively on IQ scores. This may in part reflect that the determination is often made in the early school years, when the degree to which the person will *adapt* is harder to judge. IQ scores are distributed as a bell curve, but one whose leftward tail, representing the less gifted, is longer than its rightward counterpart, representing those with higher scores. The likely explanation for this set of events is that the leftward tail represents two separate groups: those who by genetic distribution and environmental opportunity fall on the lower end of the bell curve and those who might have fallen elsewhere but who because of prenatal misadventure or other cause of brain damage have been shortchanged and now are handicapped (see Fig. 46.1). Many of the severely to profoundly retarded belong to this latter group.

The prevalence of mental retardation is determined entirely by where we wish to place our cutoff point on the leftward tail of the IQ distribution. At one time the AAMR recommended that the upper cutoff point be 1 S.D. below the mean, and that an additional category of borderline retardation be created above the mild level. This effectively would classify 16% of the American population (40 million people) as retarded. In rethinking this turn of events, the category of borderline was dropped, and the cutoff point was placed at 2 S.D. from the mean (corresponding to a Wechsler IQ of 70), below which 2.28% of the population is found. The current DSM-IV classification system identifies four degrees of severity: mild (IQ level 50–55 to approximately 70), moderate (35–40 to 50–55), severe (20–25 to 35–40), and profound (below 20–25). The flexibility in ranges of IQ scores accounts for error of measurement, which is approximately ± 5 IQ points, depending on the IQ test selected. Based on the above psychometric definitions, the proportion of retarded persons falling in each category is very different. Approximately 85% are in the mild category, 10% in the moderate range, and only 5% in the severe and profound categories combined (APA, 1994).

Epidemiological studies have shown that the prevalence rates of mental retardation in the community may be considerably less than the 2–3% expected using the above psychometric definition. This is especially true if ascertainment is based on the receipt of services and/or as people get beyond school age. Rutter and his colleagues (1970) studied the entire population of 9-, 10-, and 11-year-olds on the Isle of Wight. They

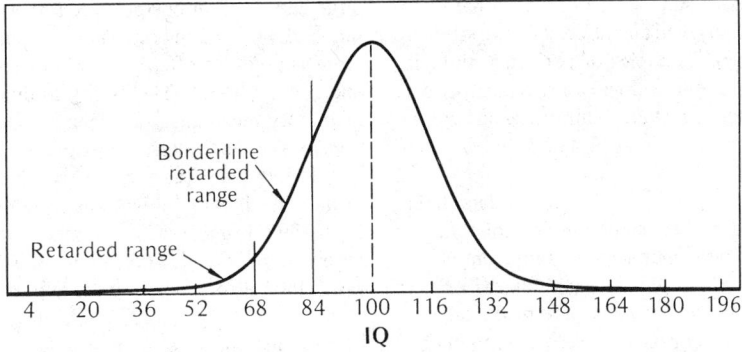

(a) Distribution of Stanford-Binet IQs expected from the normal curve.

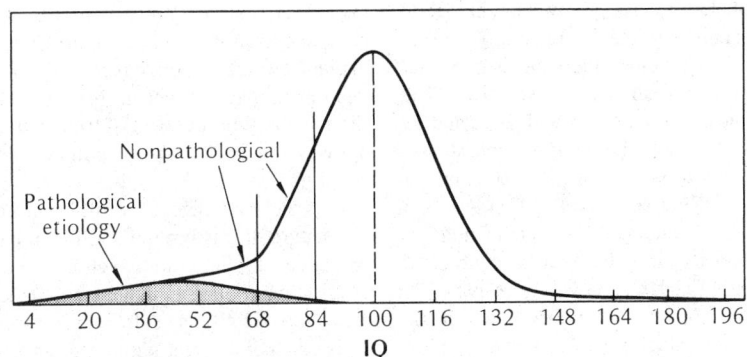

(b) Approximate distribution of IQs actually found, with individuals having signs of pathological etiology separated from those not having signs of pathological etiology.

Figure 46.1. **A,** Distribution of Stanford-Binet IQ expected from the normal curve. **B,** Approximate distribution of IQs actually found, with individuals having signs of pathological etiology separated from those not having signs of pathological etiology. (From Achenbach T: *Developmental Psychopathology* (2nd ed). New York, Wiley, 1974. Reprinted by permission of John Wiley & Sons, Inc. © 1974.)

found that 2.5% of the children were identified as intellectually retarded by IQ score. However, if prevalence rates were based on those children receiving services for mental retardation and/or special school placement, a prevalence rate of 1.3% was obtained. In a series of European and Canadian studies reviewed by Scott (1994), based on regional service registers, prevalence was typically less than 1%. Scott concludes that the lower rate is due to the fact that less than one-half of children and adolescents with mild mental retardation are identified as needing services. In adulthood this proportion drops to less than 25%. This does not necessarily imply that those individuals with mild mental retardation who are not identified are functioning in society without difficulty. A significant proportion continue to have problems in a variety of emotional and adaptive domains (Edgerton, 1984; Granat and Granat, 1978; Scott, 1994).

ETIOLOGY AND PATHOGENESIS

Heritable Factors Versus the Environment

In past years there has been a strong reliance on environmental explanations to account for human traits and behavior. Recent studies (see Holden, 1987) suggest that this may be only partially correct. Many personality traits are heritable, with environmental factors determining the degree to which the traits are expressed or suppressed. Although some have argued that this is not the case for intelligence (Kamin, 1974), numerous twin and adoption studies (see Plomin and DeFries, 1980; Scarr and Carter-Saltzman, 1982) indicate that the heritability of intelligence is between 0.45 and 0.80; that is, 45–80% of the variation in IQ scores is attributable to heritable factors (see Zigler and Hodapp, 1986, for a more detailed discussion of the subject). The heritability factor

appears to be complex and best explained by polygenic models. One such model, proposed by Gottesman (1963), postulated a five-gene explanation to account for IQ scores within the normal distribution of intelligence. In this five-gene model (the actual number of genes is likely to be much greater and their interaction more complicated than this simple model posits, but the model has a certain heuristic value), each gene has two alleles, some of which have a positive effect on IQ, some a negative effect. For each inherited positive allele, the person's IQ would be boosted 10 points above a postulated base of IQ 50, up to IQ 150 if all 10 alleles were positive. Intermediate scores would represent various combinations of positive and negative alleles. Offspring of parents with extremes of IQ would tend to regress toward the mean, while parents with average IQ would tend to have children who also have average IQs.

Organic Factors Leading to Retardation

In the majority of children (estimates range from 60 to 75%) with more severe forms of mental retardation (IQ < 50), a specific organic or genetic etiology can be determined. In milder forms of retardation a specific etiology is found in less than half of the cases (McClaren and Bryson, 1987). It is expected, however, that, as our knowledge of biological factors leading to mental retardation and our ability to detect their presence increases, the proportion of "etiology unknown" cases will diminish. The organic and genetic etiologies can be classified as occurring in the prenatal, perinatal, or postnatal periods. Prenatal etiologies predominate, with perinatal and postnatal etiologies occurring in only about 10–25% of cases of more severe forms of mental retardation (McClaren and Bryson, 1987; Scott, 1994). Examples of causal factors in the prenatal period include chromosomal anomalies and other genetic errors (see below), exposure to toxins such as alcohol, maternal infections (e.g., rubella), and a variety of physical alterations of brain structure or functioning (e.g., hydrocephalus). Examples of perinatal etiologies include fetal distress and anoxia or complications of prematurity. Some postnatal causes of mental retardation include central nervous system infections, hypothyroidism, malnutrition, trauma, and toxin exposure (e.g., lead).

Among the most important nongenetic causes of mental retardation is exposure to alcohol in utero. Maternal consumption of alcohol during pregnancy, especially in large amounts, may lead to significant abnormalities in the newborn known as fetal alcohol syndrome (FAS), or somewhat less severe abnormalities, which have been termed fetal alcohol effects (FAE). The full syndrome consists of prenatal growth deficiency, characteristic dysmorphic facial features, and effects on the central nervous system often manifested as mental retardation. The more characteristic dysmorphic features include microcephaly, short palpebral fissures, a flat midface, an indistinct philtrum, and thin upper lip (Streissguth et al., 1991). Intellectual functioning varies widely, but is generally correlated with the amount of alcohol exposure and the severity of the syndrome. In a recent follow-up study of 27 children with FAS and 13 with FAE, IQ scores were found to be stable through midadolescence. The mean IQ for the FAS adolescents was 67 (range 20–91), and for the FAE group was 82 (range 65–114) (Streissguth et al., 1991). Another important longitudinal study showed similar stability in intellectual impairment and presented other findings of particular importance to child psychiatrists. Steinhausen et al. (1993) found that 63% of a sample of 90 FAS children exhibited psychiatric disorders at follow-up. Hyperkinetic disorders, emotional disorders (anxiety and depression), stereotypies, speech and eating disorders were commonly noted. It was concluded that although the physical stigmata associated with FAS may ameliorate over time, the intellectual and psychopathological sequelae persist. It is hoped that ongoing education and other preventive efforts will help decrease the worldwide prevalence of this disorder.

Genetic Factors Leading to Retardation

Genetic abnormalities account for many of the *known* organic causes of mental retardation. It is beyond the scope of this chapter to provide a detailed overview of the subject (see Baroff, 1986; Bregman and Hodapp, 1991; Lombroso et al., 1994; Trembath, 1994, for reviews), but certain of the more frequently encountered defects need to be understood. The most common autosomal chromosome defect is Down's syndrome, seen in 1 in 700 live births. Three forms of Down's syndrome have been identified: trisomy 21, translocation 18, and mosaicism. The latter may be associated with near-normal IQ. In addition to the well-known cardiac and musculoskeletal abnormalities, there is a high incidence of Alzheimer's disease in people with Down's syndrome after age 30–40.

Sex chromosome abnormalities include Klinefelter's syndrome (XXY males), XYY males, XXX females, and Turner's syndrome (XO females). Although each of these may be associated with various physical anomalies, only XXY males and XXX females are likely to be cognitively impaired, and the retardation will be mild in most instances. In Klinefelter's syndrome, specific learning disabilities are more likely than mental retardation (Mandoki et al., 1992).

The most important recent advance in understanding the genetic basis of mental retardation has been the discovery and elucidation of the genetic mechanism of the fragile X syndrome (Warren and Nelson, 1994). Fragile X is the leading known cause of inherited mental retardation with an incidence approaching 1/1000 (Sherman, 1991). It is second only to Down's syndrome as a genetic cause of mental retardation. Its frequency may in part explain the higher rates of mental retardation found in males as compared with females. The degree of retardation typically ranges from mild to severe, although some males with normal IQ and learning disabilities have been identified (Hagerman, 1992). Anomalies often seen in fragile X syndrome are a large, prominent jaw,

large ears, and, in postpubescent males, enlarged testes. However, the physical stigmata may be subtle, especially in younger children and in females, and are often not apparent to the average clinician (Warren and Nelson, 1994). The ability to diagnose fragile X by more precise laboratory techniques has been available in only the last 3 years and revisions of our understanding of the clinical presentation will undoubtedly follow. For example, the earlier belief that fragile X was common in individuals with autism has recently been questioned (Einfield and Hall, 1992; Fisch, 1992). Symptoms of hyperactivity are reported commonly in individuals with fragile X (see Bregman et al., 1988), but this association also needs to be carefully tested with mental age matched comparison groups. Fragile X is of extraordinary interest to geneticists because it is the first demonstrated example of a new mechanism of genetic disorders involving the abnormal presence and amplification of triplet base repeats in a genome, in this case named FMR1 (fragile X mental retardation-1) (see Warren and Nelson, 1994, for an especially lucid explanation of this complex topic). In normal individuals the particular CGG trinucleotide is repeated 6–52 times. In affected individuals this repeat may number in the hundreds or thousands. Female carriers show increasing numbers of triplets in successive generations, explaining why fragile X tends to be more common and more severe in subsequent generations. Excessive repeats lead to methylation and inactivation of the FMR1 gene, resulting in an absence of the coded protein. The nature of this protein and the impact of the absence of the protein on the developing brain is yet to be elucidated but could potentially be of great importance in understanding the neurobiology of brain development and of intelligence. In only 3 years, seven other neurological conditions (including Huntington's disease) have been identified that may also involve mutations of repeated trinucleotides (Trembath, 1994). The clinical importance of all of this is that the identification of the mechanisms underlying fragile X has led to a variety of laboratory tests that can identify both carriers and affected individuals. Fragile X should be considered in any undiagnosed child with mental retardation. If confirmed, testing of family members and appropriate genetic counseling should follow.

Another important single gene abnormality linked to mental retardation is phenylketonuria (PKU) (found in 1 in 11,500 births). Using molecular techniques, Woo et al. (1983) localized the PKU gene responsible for the deficiency in phenylalanine hydroxylase production to chromosome 12. Dietary therapy from birth can prevent mental retardation in affected individuals; however, females with treated PKU are known to be at risk for giving birth to mentally retarded non-PKU children. This is a result of high phenylalanine levels in the maternal blood, which enters the fetal circulation and adversely affects brain development. If the mothers remain on a strict phenylalanine-free diet during their pregnancy, the risk may be considerably reduced.

Neurofibromatoses (prevalence of 1 in 3000) may result in mild mental retardation and learning disorders. Café au lait spots are often a sign of the disorder. The common form of neurofibromatoses has been localized to chromosome 17 (Watkins, 1988), and a method of prenatal diagnosis can be expected in the future.

MENTAL ILLNESS IN MENTAL RETARDATION

Many studies have concluded that mental and emotional disorders are present to a greater degree in mentally retarded than in nonretarded persons (see Borthwick-Duffy, 1994; Bregman, 1991; Russell, 1988; Tanguay, 1990). In Rutter's Isle of Wight study (Rutter et al., 1970), 30.4% of the children with IQs less than 70 were found to have a psychiatric disorder on the parent questionnaire, and 41.8% on the teacher questionnaire. Comparable rates for nonretarded persons in the population were 7.7 and 9.5%, respectively. An interesting additional finding was that behavioral disturbances of almost all types were inversely correlated with IQ. Gifted children had the least, average children had more, and retarded children the most emotional and behavioral disorders.

Among 30,000 persons receiving developmental disability service in New York State, Jacobson (1982) estimated that 47.7% of the retarded persons displayed some type of problem behavior. In collecting data from this large a sample, the rating instruments were somewhat limited and crude, and many of the problems would not have merited a specific psychiatric diagnosis. Although Rutter used good diagnostic instruments, many other studies have used clinical interviews or nonstandard instruments to identify problems or to determine if the person has a mental disorder. Nonetheless, it is a commonly held belief among those who work with mentally retarded persons that they exhibit high rates of diagnosable mental disorders.

Role of the Child Psychiatrist

The child psychiatrist will occupy one of three roles in terms of diagnosing and treating mental disorders in retarded persons. Often one role will be as an outside consultant to the school program, to the sheltered workshop, to the state agency for developmental disabilities, or to the residential treatment center or hospital. Child psychiatrists with a special interest in mental retardation may join the treatment team itself in the hospital or other setting. Occasionally, the child psychiatrist may be in charge of a hospital for the retarded.

As a consultant, the child psychiatrists should always begin by establishing the reason for the patient's referral for consultation. It is important to sort out the deleterious effects that the patient's behavior may be having on his or her caretakers, as well as to identify the specific psychiatric symptoms the person may have. The former may require that the team as a whole deal with the frustration, anger, helplessness, or fear they feel about dangerous or self-destructive behavior exhibited by their patient or client.

Interviewing the Retarded Person

Before meeting the patient for the first time, it is important to learn about his or her current life situation, living arrangements, and school or work experience. Ask about previous treatment, its nature, and its effects. If the person is living with his or her family, it is important to talk with the person alone, to hear not only any worries or complaints, but also what he or she hopes the visit to the psychiatrist will accomplish. The retarded person may have little idea of why he or she is being brought to you or what you intend to do during the visit. He or she may see it as punishment for bad behavior or failure. Asking about what the person was told about the visit can be helpful, as well as explaining carefully what you will be doing during the session.

Retarded persons will do better when the interview has structure. Toys and games can be used, with the interviewer giving the person permission to play with the toys if necessary. The pace of the interview may be slower than if the patient were not retarded. It is important that the interviewer probe to be sure that the person has understood the question and knows that alternative replies are possible. The interview may begin with the psychiatrist asking the patient about his or her current living conditions and what he or she likes or doesn't like about them. Try to establish what activities the person enjoys and what he or she views as his or her special talents and strengths. Only then is it useful to go on to a careful review of major symptom complexes, trying to establish if a particular diagnosis is present. Information provided by the referring persons can be useful in guiding this latter search. It should be remembered that 89% of retarded persons are only mildly retarded, with IQs above 55. An IQ of 55 is equivalent to a mental age of roughly 8 years. A retarded person with an IQ of 55 may know more in some ways than an average 8-year-old and may be less capable (and probably less self-confident) in some other respects, but he or she should be able to engage in an interview.

Just as in the practice of adult and child psychiatry in general, specific symptom questionnaires and diagnostic instruments can be very helpful in providing a structure for assessing mentally retarded patients. The goal of using such rating scales is 2-fold: to assure that important symptoms are not missed and to establish symptom severity vis-à-vis a clinical standard. Some instruments are designed to be rated by the parents or school or residential care personnel, and some are meant to be used directly with the patient. In the past several years, reports have appeared in which the use of such instruments is described. Some of the instruments are ones previously standardized for use with nonretarded children and adults; others are newly designed for exclusive use with retarded persons.

STANDARD SYMPTOM RATING SCALES

A variety of rating instruments developed for use in nonretarded children and adolescents have been used with retarded children, taking into account the need for changes in administration, e.g., reading items to children and adolescents who are unable to read on their own. Examples of rating scales used in this way include the Child Behavior Checklist, the Beck Depression Inventory (BDI), and the Childhood Depression Inventory (CDI) (Beck et al., 1987; Benavidez and Matson, 1993; Matson et al., 1988). In general, these and similar scales may be useful in mildly or even moderately retarded groups, but are of less utility in more severely retarded individuals. An example of such difficulty is provided by Lindsay and Michie (1988) who rewrote the Zung Self-Rating Anxiety Scale so that its questions could be better understood by retarded persons. In a study of 29 mildly and moderately retarded adults, they found that the scale had good test-retest reliability, but only if the answers were couched as a yes/no dichotomy. When subjects were required to categorize their symptoms along an intensity or duration scale, retarded persons found this difficult, and the test-retest reliability of the inventory fell.

NEWLY DEVELOPED RATING SCALES

Aman (1991) has provided a very useful and wide-ranging review of instruments available for use with mentally retarded individuals. Aman described a variety of problems with many of the instruments. These included a lack of sensitivity and specificity data, absent or insufficient standardization data, and a relative lack of useful instruments for children and severely and profoundly retarded individuals. Examples of some promising instruments are the Psychopathology Instrument for Mentally Retarded Adults (PIMRA) (Watson et al., 1988), the Aberrant Behavior Checklist (Aman et al., 1985), and the Developmentally Delayed Children's Behavior Checklist (Einfield and Tonge, 1991).

Reynolds and Baker (1988) have developed a 32-item Self-Report Depression Questionnaire (SRDQ) designed to be used in persons with mental retardation. Eighty-nine subjects were studied. Subject IQs were estimated to range from borderline to severe. An internal consistency reliability of .90 was obtained for the instrument, and an 11-week test-retest reliability of .63. Validity was demonstrated by a high degree of relationship between the symptoms reported using the instrument and symptoms identified by clinical interview using the Hamilton Depression Rating Scale. The total possible scores on the SRDQ range from 32 to 98. The mean rating of the subjects was 58, though the range of scores extended to 89.

Reiss has pointed out that scales such as the Aberrant Behavior Checklist identify behavior problems but are not necessarily measures of psychopathology and do not yield findings that are directly related to standard classifications of psychiatric disorders such as DSM-IV (Reiss and Valenti-Hein, 1994). In an attempt to meet a need for a screening instrument for children which more directly reflects psychopathological constructs, Reiss has developed the Reiss Scales for Children's Dual Diagnosis. The scales were developed with a total sample of 583 children in a two-stage process. The 60-item instrument produces scores on 10 psychometric scales (e.g., depression, attention deficit, anger/self control), 10 specific behavior items (e.g., hallucinations, pica) and a total score. The instrument has good internal reliability and the total score was a reliable indicator of psychopathology as determined by prior diagnoses on case records. Reiss concludes that the instrument is well suited for screening but not for detailed assessment of specific psychiatric disorders (Reiss and Valenti-Hein, 1994).

The recent use of standard diagnostic tools with retarded children and adolescents and the development of useful new instruments is encouraging. First, it suggests that the symptoms of mental disorders in mild and moderately retarded subjects are not much different from those of nonretarded people and that reliable diagnoses can be made by standard psychiatric interviews (involving child and caretaker) and by using existing or newly developed psychiatric rating scales. Both could prove especially useful in future treatment and epidemiological research.

TREATMENT OF MENTAL DISORDERS IN RETARDED PERSONS

Careful, controlled studies of the effects of various treatments on mental disorders in retarded persons are relatively lacking at present. Even behavioral treatments, which have been the mainstay of programs aimed at helping retarded persons learn the social and personal skills necessary for them to live in the community, have not been extended much into the domain of mental illness in this population.

Because it now appears that many mental disorders in retarded persons resemble the same disorders in the general population, a rational approach to treatment might be to try what works in the general population. These include medications and psychotherapy, the latter modified to take into account the mental level of the patient.

Medication

It is beyond the scope of this chapter to review the growing body of psychopharmacological research with children and adults with mental retardation. The reader is referred to Aman (1991), Aman and Singh (1988), and Bregman (1991) for important, comprehensive reviews. A few general comments and some examples of recent studies are noted here. In general terms, the response of retarded persons to stimulant, psychotropic, and antidepressive medications is similar to that of the nonretarded. Treatment research is complicated by the fact that precise diagnosis using DSM categories is often difficult, and there is a lack of reliable diagnostic instruments, as mentioned above.

Rates of attention-deficit/hyperactivity disorder (ADHD) in mentally retarded children may range from 9 to 18% (Handen et al., 1994). A recent series of pharmacological studies have confirmed that stimulant medications may be as effective in children with mental retardation as in children with normal intelligence (Aman, 1991; Handen et al., 1992, 1994). Overall response rates to stimulant medications are 60–75%. Side effect profiles are similar, but motor tics and emotional withdrawal may be somewhat more common (Handen et al.,1992).

Surveys of the use of neuroleptics in retarded persons, especially those in residential or institutional care (Gadow, 1986), have shown that as many as 50% of retarded patients were on high doses of neuroleptics, while few are on other medications. These findings suggest that in many instances medications have been prescribed primarily for behavioral control, rather than to treat a specific psychiatric illness. This can be avoided if medications are used conservatively. The patient should have a diagnosis for which treatment by medication has been shown to be efficacious, target symptoms should be identified and monitored, side effects should be looked for, and polypharmacy should be avoided. Avoid changing more than one medication at a time, and do not make major medication changes before the patient is due for a vacation or prolonged home visit. Alternatives to neuroleptics in aggressive or self-injurious patients should be carefully considered (see Smith and Perry, 1992, for an important review of alternative medication strategies). One

important complication of neuroleptic treatment may be neuroleptic malignant syndrome, a potentially fatal disorder (Boyd, 1993).

What of the patient who is seriously self-injurious or episodically dangerous and violent? Such a patient is likely to be referred to the psychiatrist after behavioral interventions have been tried and found wanting. There are no easy solutions to the problem, and the child psychiatrist will need to work closely with the treatment team and with its behavioral experts if medication trials are begun. Aman (1993) has reviewed medication strategies.

Psychotherapy

Supportive psychotherapy, and even therapy aimed at helping a patient gain some insight into his or her feelings and actions, can be helpful to mildly and some moderately retarded people. Goals of therapy include helping the patient to (a) identify and capitalize on areas of strength; (b) set realistic goals and plan to reach them; (c) reflect on maladaptive behaviors, especially social ones, and understand them from someone else's viewpoint; (d) find other ways of expressing anger; and (e) separate from an overprotective family or from exploitative peer relationships.

Sigman (1985) reviewed the nature and outcome of psychotherapy with retarded adolescents whose IQs ranged from 45 to 77. In some cases, building rapport was the only goal that could be reached, but in most cases, the therapists felt that the therapy helped the patients make better use of their school, rehabilitative, and vocational opportunities.

Family Interventions

Most parents expect their children to grow up, leave home, and live productive, independent lives. There may be some rough periods during adolescence, but the parents know that they will likely end during the college years. If their child becomes seriously mentally ill during adolescence or young childhood, the family will suffer along with the grown-up child. Retarded children may be identified early in life, and in such instances families face a lifetime of concern. Various parental responses may be seen—denial, anger, sorrow, acceptance—sometimes as successive phases but more likely as responses that wax and wane in less predictable ways. Even after parents have adjusted to the immediate problems of their retarded child, they face additional long-term questions: What will happen to my child after I am gone? Will his or her brothers and sisters be there to help? The spectrum of parental adaptation can vary from very successful to overprotective, or, occasionally, abusive and neglectful.

Parents need more than the guidance of mental health specialists. They need to find special services for their child, beginning in the preschool years. They need to find specialists who are accustomed to providing medical and dental care to retarded persons. They need to find good special education and a place where the child can lead as normal a life as possible in adulthood. All parents should be told early of the existence of special support groups, such as the Association for Retarded Citizens (ARC). The telephone number for the local chapter of the ARC can be found in the telephone directory of any major city. Members of ARC support one another and inform one another of where and how to get needed services for their children. They lobby for services at both the local and state level, and they effectively lobby Congress about the need for more research.

RESEARCH NEEDS

Basic Science

Ultimately, our understanding of the causes and prevention of mental retardation must come from a better understanding of how the brain works. A substantial long-term investment must be made in animal neuroscience research. Almost any type of neuroscience research could ultimately prove crucial to our understanding of retardation, or, for that matter, mental disorders in general.

Clinical Research

The most immediate need is for research into the treatment of mental disorders in the mentally retarded. We are beginning to develop better symptom rating instruments for use with retarded persons, and these can be put to good use in looking at the effects of medication and other treatments. Mental disorders for which this is particularly applicable in the retarded are attention deficit disorder and hyperactivity, depression, anxiety disorder, and psychosis. The National Institute of Mental Health and the National Institutes of Health are interested in funding well-designed projects in this arena and welcome applications of this sort.

References

Aman MG: *Assessing Psychopathology and Behaviour Problems in Persons with Mental Retardation: A Review of Available Instruments*. Rockville, MD, US Department of Health and Human Services, 1991.

Aman MG: Efficacy of psychotropic drugs for reducing self-injurious behavior in the developmental disabilities. *Ann Clin Psychiatry* 5:171–188, 1993.

Aman MG, Singh NN: *Psychopharmacology of the Developmental Disabilities*. New York, Springer-Verlag, 1988.

Aman MG, Singh NN, Stewart AW, et al: The aberrant behavior checklist: A behavior rating scale for the assessment of treatment effects. *Am J Ment Defic* 89:485–491, 1985.

American Psychiatric Association: *DSM-IV: Diagnostic and Statistical Manual of Mental Disorders* (4th ed). Washington, DC, American Psychiatric Association, 1994.

Baroff GS: *Mental Retardation, Nature, Cause and Management* (2nd ed). Washington, DC, Hemisphere, 1986.

Beck DC, Carlson GA, Russell AT, et al: Use of depression rating instruments in developmentally and educationally delayed adolescents. *J Am Acad Child Adolesc Psychiatry* 26:97–100, 1987.

Benavidez DA, Matson JL: Assessment of depression in mentally retarded adolescents. *Res Dev Disabil* 14:179–188, 1993.

Borthwick-Duffy SA: Epidemiology and prevalence of psychopathology in people with mental retardation. *J Consult Clin Psychol* 62(1):17–27, 1994.

Boyd RD: Neuroleptic malignant syndrome and mental retardation: Review and analysis of 29 cases. *Am Assoc Ment Retard* 98(1):143–155, 1993.

Bregman JD: Current developments in the understanding of mental retardation part II: Psychopathology. *J Am Acad Child Adolesc Psychiatry* 30:861–872, 1991.

Bregman JD, Hodapp RM: Current developments in the understanding of mental retardation. Part I: Biological and phenomenological perspectives. *J Am Acad Child Adolesc Psychiatry* 30(5):707–719, 1991.

Bregman JD, Leckman JF, Ort SI: Fragile X syndrome: Genetic predisposition to psychopathy. *J Autism Dev Disord* 18:343–345, 1988.

Chandler M, Gualtieri CT, Fahs II: Other psychotropic drugs: Stimulants, antidepressants, the anxiolytics, and lithium carbide. In: Aman MG, Singh NN (eds): *Psychopharmacology and the Developmental Disabilities*. New York, Springer-Verlag, 1988.

Consortium for Longitudinal Studies: *As the Twig Is Bent . . . Lasting Effects of Preschool Programs*. Hillsdale, NJ, Erlbaum, 1983.

Edgerton RB: *Lives in Process: Mildly Retarded Adults in a Large City*. Washington, DC, American Association on Mental Deficiency, 1984.

Einfield S, Hall W: Invited Editorial Comment: Behaviour phenotype of the Fragile X syndrome. *Am J Med Genet* 43:56–60, 1992.

Einfield S, Tonge BJ: Psychometric and clinical assessment of psychopathy in developmentally disabled children. *Aust NZ J Dev Disabil* 17:147–167, 1991.

Fisch GS: Is autism associated with the fragile X syndrome? *Am J Med Genet* 43:46–55, 1992.

Flavel J: *The Developmental Psychology of Jean Piaget*. New York, Van Nostrand Reinhold, 1973.

Flavell J, Markman EM (eds): *Handbook of Child Psychology*. Vol 3: *Cognitive Development*. New York, Wiley, 1983.

Forness SR, Finn D: Screening children in Head Start for learning disorders. *Monogr Behav Disord* 16:6–14, 1993.

Fuchs D, Fuchs LS: Inclusive schools movement and the radicalization of special reforms. *Except Child* 60:294–309, 1994.

Gadow KD: *Children on Medication* (Vol I). San Diego, College Hill Press, 1986.

Gottesman II: Genetic aspects of intelligent behavior. In: Ellis N (ed): *Handbook of Mental Deficiency*. New York, McGraw-Hill, 1963.

Granat K, Granat S: Adjustment of intellectually below-average men not identified as mentally retarded. *Scand J Psychol* 19:41–51, 1978.

Greenspan S, Granfield JM: Reconsidering the construct of mental retardation: Implications of a model of social competence. *Am J Ment Retard* 96(4):442–453, 1992.

Grossman HJ: *Manual on Terminology and Classification in Mental Retardation*. Washington, DC, American Association on Mental Deficiency, 1983.

Hagerman RJ: Annotation: Fragile X syndrome: Advances and controversy. *J Child Psychol Psychiatry* 33(7):1127–1139, 1992.

Handen BL, Breaux AM, Janosky J: Effects and noneffects of methylphenidate in children with mental retardation and ADHD. *J Am Acad Child Adolesc Psychiatry* 31(3):455–461, 1992.

Handen BL, Janosky J, McAuliffe S, et al: Prediction of response to methylphenidate among children with ADHD and mental retardation. *J Am Acad Child Adolesc Psychiatry* 33(8):1185–1193, 1994.

Hobson RP, Ouston J, Lee A: Recognition of emotion by mentally retarded adolescents and young adults. *Am J Ment Retard* 93:434–443, 1989.

Holden C: The genetics of personality. *Science* 237:598–601, 1987.

Jacobson JW: Problem behavior and psychiatric impairment within a developmentally disabled population: Behavior frequency. *Appl Res Ment Retard* 3:121–139, 1982.

Kamin LG: *The Science and Politics of IQ*. New York, Wiley, 1974.

Kihlstrom JF: The cognitive unconscious. *Science* 237:1445–1452, 1987.

Lindsay WR, Michie AM: Adaptation of the Zung Self-Rating Anxiety Scale for people with mental handicap. *J Ment Defic Res* 32:485–490, 1988.

Lombroso PJ, Pauls DL, Leckman JF: Genetic mechanism in childhood psychiatric disorders. *J Am Acad Child Adolesc Psychiatry* 33(7):921–938, 1994.

Luckasson R, Coulter DL, Polloway EA, et al: Mental retardation: Definition, classification, and systems of supports. American Association on Mental Retardation, 1992.

MacMillan DL, Gresham FM, Siperstein G, et al: Conceptual and psychometric concerns about the 1992 AAMR definition of mental retardation. *Am J Ment Retard* 98:325–335, 1993.

Mandoki MW, Sumner GS, Hoffman RP, et al: A review of Klinefelter's syndrome in children and adolescents. *J Am Acad Child Adolesc Psychiatry* 30:167–172, 1991.

Matson JL, Barrette RP, Halsel WJ: Depression in mentally retarded children. *Res Dev Disabil* 19:39–46, 1988.

McLaren J, Bryson SE: Review of recent epidemiological studies of mental retardation: Prevalence, associated disorders, and etiology. *Am J Ment Retard* 92:243–254, 1987.

Nihara K, Foster R, Shellaus M, et al: *Manual for AAMD Adaptive Behavior Scale, 1974 Edition*. Austin, TX, Pro-Ed Publishers, 1974.

Plomin R, DeFries JC: Genetics and intelligence: Recent data. *Intelligence* 4:15–24, 1980.

Ratey JJ, Mikkelson EJ, Smith GB, et al: β-Blockers in the severely and profoundly retarded. *J Clin Psychopharmacol* 6:103–107, 1986.

Reiss S, Valenti-Hein D: Development of a psychopathology rating scale for children with mental retardation. *J Consult Clin Psychol* 62(1):28–33, 1994.

Reynolds WM, Baker JA: Assessment of depression in persons with mental retardation. *Am J Ment Retard* 93:93–103, 1988.

Russell AT: The association between mental retardation and psychiatric disorder: Epidemiological issues. In: Stark JA, Menolascino FJ, Albarelli MH, Gray (eds): *Mental Retardation and Mental Health: Classification, Diagnosis, Treatment, Services*. New York, Springer-Verlag, 1988.

Rutter M, Graham P, Yule W: *A Neuropsychiatric Study in Childhood*. London, Spastics International Medical Publications and Heinemann, 1970.

Scarr S, Carter-Saltzman L: Genetics and intelligence. In: Sternberg R (ed): *Handbook of Human Intelligence*. Cambridge, Cambridge University Press, 1982.

Scott S: Mental retardation. In: Rutter M, Taylor E, Hersov L (eds): *Child and Adolescent Psychiatry* (3rd ed). Oxford, Blackwell, 1994.

Sherman S: Epidemiology. In: Hagerman J, Cronister AC (eds): *The Fragile X Syndrome Diagnosis, Treatment and Research*. Baltimore, Johns Hopkins University Press, 1991.

Sigman M: Individual and group psychotherapy with mentally retarded adolescents. In: Sigman M (ed): *Children with Emotional Disorders and Developmental Disabilities*. New York, Grune & Stratton, 1985.

Smith DA, Perry PJ: Nonneuroleptic treatment of disruptive behavior in organic mental syndromes. *Ann Pharmacother* 26:1400–1408, 1992.

Sparrow S, Balla D, Cicchetti D: *Vineland Adaptive Behavior Scales (Survey Form)*. Circle Pines, MN, American Guidance Service, 1984.

Steinhausen HC, Willms J, Spohr HL: Long-term psychopathological and cognitive outcome of children with fetal alcohol syndrome. *J Am Acad Child Adolesc Psychiatry* 32(5):990–994, 1993.

Sternberg RJ, Gardner MK: A componential interpretation of the general factor of human intelligence. In: Eysenck HJ (ed): *A Model for Intelligence*. Berlin, Springer-Verlag, 1982.

Streissguth AP, Randels SP, Smith DF: A test-retest study of intelligence in patients with fetal alcohol syndrome: Implications for care. *J Am Acad Child Adolesc Psychiatry* 30(4):584–587, 1991.

Tanguay PE: Mental retardation. In: Garfinkel BD, Carlson GA, Weller EB (eds): *Psychiatric Disorders in Children and Adolescents*. Philadelphia, Harcourt Brace Jovanovich, 1990.

Trembath RC: Genetic mechanisms and mental retardation. *J R Coll Physicians Lond* 28(2): 121–125, 1994.

US Office of Special Education Program: *16th Annual Report to Congress on Individuals with Disabilities Education*. Washington, DC, 1994.

Warren ST, Nelson DL: Advances in molecular analysis of fragile X syndrome. *JAMA* 271(7): 536–542, 1994.

Watkins PC: RFLPs: Applications in human chromosome mapping and genetic disease research. *Biol Tech* 6:310–320, 1988.

Watson JE, Aman MG, Singh NN: The Psychopathology Instrument for Mentally Retarded Adults: Psychometric characteristics, factor structure, and relationship to subject characteristics. *Res Dev Disabil* 9:277–290, 1988.

Williams DT, Mehl R, Yudofsky S, et al: The effect of propranolol on uncontrolled rage outbursts in children and adolescents with organic brain dysfunction. *J Am Acad Child Psychiatry* 21:129–135, 1982.

Woo SLC, Lidsky AS, Gutler F, et al: Cloned human phenylalanine hydroxylase allows prenatal diagnosis and carrier detection of classical phenylketonuria. *Nature* 306:151–155, 1983.

Zigler E, Hodapp RM: *Understanding Mental Retardation*. Cambridge, Cambridge University Press, 1986, pp. 68–89.

47 DISORDERS OF COMMUNICATION

Rhea Paul, Ph.D.

Language, a unique and characteristic capacity of the human mind, is also one of its most vulnerable. Virtually any disruption in cognitive function, particularly during early development, can affect language acquisition. For this reason, disorders of language development typically accompany a variety of other conditions. This chapter first outlines briefly the most common syndromes in which disorders of communication may play a part. Specific disorders of speech and language development, which are not accompanied by deficits in other areas of mental function, are then discussed.

SYNDROMES INVOLVING COMMUNICATION DISORDERS

Mental Retardation

Limitation in communicative skill is often one of the first signs of mental retardation. Children with retardation are often first recognized because of their failure to begin talking at the normal time. The sequence of language acquisition in children with retardation follows, in general, the sequence of normal acquisition, although some differences can be identified. Many children with mental retardation (MR) show communicative skills that are commensurate with their developmental level, but more than half have language skills that are less than what would be expected for mental age (Miller and Chapman, 1984). Productive deficits are common, with some children with MR showing deficits relative to mental age in this area only. Others have both receptive and expressive limitations relative to mental age. Phonological errors are prevalent in children with MR. These children make similar errors to those seen in normal development, but errors are more frequent (Shriberg and Widder, 1990). Pragmatic skills are usually similar to those seen in children at similar developmental levels (Lahey, 1988). The two most prevalent syndromes of MR, Down's syndrome and fragile X syndrome, are both very frequently associated with various problems in language development.

Hearing Impairment

Children with impaired hearing are vulnerable to language disorders because of their lack of access to the linguistic information in the auditory signal. Still, children with hearing impairments vary greatly in their oral language ability, and as Boothroyd (1982) pointed out, an unaided audiogram is not a child's fate. With amplification via hearing aids, children can be moved from greater to lesser levels of severity of hearing loss. Cochlear implants and tactile aids are also used to provide auditory information to children who would otherwise be considered deaf (Roeser, 1988). Language acquisition in children with hearing impairment (HI) follows the same general sequence as it does in children with normal hearing, although it is greatly delayed, and the delays affect all modalities: articulation, receptive and expressive communication, and oral and written language (Quigley et al., 1977). Lahey (1988) concluded, however, that use of language for communication is not a major problem area for children with HI, but that most of their difficulties lie in acquiring the conventional verbal forms of communication. Reading and writing present particular problems, primarily because of the language basis necessary for acquiring these skills. Average reading comprehension levels for adolescents with HI is third to fourth grade (King and Quigley, 1985; Trybus and Karchmer, 1977).

Many children can be taught to bypass the auditory channel through the use of manual sign language. Using this method, children can develop fluency and eloquence in sign that would never be available to them through the modality of speech. There is great controversy within the community of the hearing impaired as to the role of sign language versus oral language instruction for children with severe hearing losses. In general, children taught sign develop higher level language skills than those taught speech, although their communication may be limited to those in the deaf community who use sign as their mode of communication. Oral language training, on the other hand, appears to correlate highly with reading achievement. The decision whether to use an oral or signed mode of communication with a child who has severe HI must be made carefully in consultation with the child's family. Deaf parents of deaf children may feel it is more important for their child to be fluent in sign and comfortable in deaf culture than to achieve the maximum possible reading level. For these families, instruction in sign may make more sense. Deaf children of hearing parents may have families that feel speech and reading achievement are their highest goals. For children in these families, oral instruction may work better. Each family must be presented with all available options in order to make the most informed decision for their child.

Psychiatric Disorders

There is a very high coincidence of sociobehavioral and communicative disorders. Prizant and Meyer (1993) reported that over half of children diagnosed with communication disorders have socioemotional and behavioral problems. Conversely, Prizant et al. (1990) found that two-thirds of children referred to a psychiatric inpatient hospital failed speech and language screening. Giddan (1991) showed that 65% of children in psychiatric outpatient clinics were similarly impaired. Giddan also found that a third of children referred for conduct disorders had concomitant speech and language difficulties, and more than two-thirds of children with some form of attention deficit disorder have language disabilities as well. And, as Prizant et al. (1990) showed, some children with anxiety and affective disorders fail language screenings. It may be impossible to know the source of this connection. Does a communication problem lead to frustration, creating behavioral or emotional disorders? Or is it that a behavioral/socioemotional problem leads to decreased motivation to communicate or to an inability to ''tune in'' to learn the rules of communication or to use language for self- and other-regulation? Is there some other underlying factor affecting both aspects of development? Whatever the answer to these questions, children with language problems are vulnerable to socioemotional difficulties, and children with psychiatric diagnoses show a higher than normal prevalence of language disorders.

The psychiatric disorder most consistently associated with communication deficits is autism, or pervasive developmental disorder (PDD). Communication problems—including severe delays in language, inability to communicate nonverbally, inability to sustain conversation, stereotyped and repetitive use of idiosyncratic language, and abnormal ability to use language for social communication—are included in the diagnostic criteria for autism/PDD. Virtually all children with autism have some form of communication disorder that presents as part of their syndrome. What differentiates autism from a more circumscribed language disorder is the global nature of the child's communication problem. Not only is language affected, but the ability and motivation to send messages by any means, either verbal or nonverbal, is severely impaired. Although sign and other alternative forms of communication are often tried with autistic patients, it is their underlying deficit in communicative skill and motivation that impedes their use of language, so that providing an alternate channel does not usually result in dramatic improvement (see Paul, 1987, 1995, for review).

Acquired Disorders of Communicative Function

Language disorders can be acquired during the developmental period through four types of neurological insults: focal lesions; damage associated with seizure disorders; damage resulting from tumors, infection, or radiation; and traumatic brain injury. Focal lesions affect language in children primarily if they are unilateral on the left side. These kinds of lesions are relatively rare in children, and children younger than 10 years tend to recover from the aphasias that follow these insults nearly completely, although some subtle effects on language and learning abilities can persist (Bishop, 1992).

Landau and Kleffner (1957) identified a syndrome of expressive and receptive language deficits accompanied by seizures that usually has its onset between 4 and 7 years of age after a period of otherwise normal development. The Landau-Kleffner syndrome has no known cause and is, fortunately, quite rare. Unlike aphasias associated with focal lesions, Landau-Kleffner syndrome usually ends in a permanent aphasia. Cognitive functioning is usually impaired, as well. Anticonvulsant medication can help to control the seizures, but will not improve communication. Some behavioral and educational intervention is almost always warranted.

Brain radiation treatment used to treat acute lymphocytic leukemia (ALL) in children has greatly reduced the mortality rate of this disease, but this ''cure'' sometimes has the unfortunate consequence of causing language and learning problems, loss of developmental skills previously acquired, or seizures (Riddle et al., 1991). Brain tumors can also affect communicative functioning. And brain damage that can affect language development may also result from infectious diseases, such as meningitis. The long-term sequelae of these kinds of insults can be subtle and variable, depending on timing, location, size, and area of the brain affected by the damage. Children with these injuries may retain a great deal of language function but have deficits that surface only during complex tasks, like those required for school. They may have expressive skills that are relatively intact, but poor comprehension. This can result in adults' being fooled into thinking comprehension is on par with production and being frustrated when the child ''refuses'' to follow instructions. The range of severity of these effects can extend from almost nonexistent to severe enough to result in a diagnosis of mental retardation.

Traumatic brain injuries (TBIs) can be focal in nature, usually involving open head injuries such as bullet wounds. Closed head injuries, such as those resulting from blows or collisions, tend to involve diffuse damage, affecting larger areas of the brain. Like children with acquired aphasias associated with focal lesions, children with TBIs of both types show a great deal of spontaneous recovery. Russell (1993) reported that outcome is generally predicted by the degree of coma, the length of time a child spends in an impaired state of consciousness following the injury, and the length of the posttraumatic amnesia (PTA) period. PTAs longer than 24 hours are considered signs of severe injury. Age at injury does not appear to affect prognosis, and the onset of deficits may be delayed for long periods of time after the injury has taken place. Although some children retain physical disabilities from TBIs, many do not show obvious physiological damage. But a substantial minority of these children suffer long-term deficits in cognitive and language function (Satz and Bullard-Bates, 1981). Gerring and Carney (1992) reported that, during the acute recovery process, children tend at first to be mute. They may comprehend only simple commands. First language productions often reflect the confused state the child is in and are often dysarthric or dysfluent. Speech may be slow, and prosody may be affected so the speech sounds monotonic and ''flat.'' Swallowing disorders are also common during this phase of recovery.

Disorders with Environmental Components

Communication disorders can be associated with prenatal exposure to substances such as drugs and alcohol or with parental behavior disorders like abuse and neglect. Language disorders are frequently part of the picture seen in fetal alcohol syndrome (FAS) or fetal alcohol effects (FAEs). They include delayed development, poor receptive vocabulary and comprehension, and pragmatic difficulties. The communication disabilities children with FAS and FAE display are related to the level of intellectual impairment. In children with more severe impairments, perseveration and echolalia are often present.

Children with a history of prenatal exposure to cocaine or other street drugs are also described as showing deficits in language development, among other symptoms (Sparks, 1993). But it is important to remember that many women who abuse street drugs during pregnancy take more than one drug and may mix abuse of both drugs and alcohol. Also, the effects of the mother's drug abuse on her caretaking ability are just as important as any biological effects the abuse may have caused before birth. As far as biological effects are concerned, Sparks (1993) pointed out that less than half of children exposed to drugs prenatally experience low birth weight, prematurity, intrauterine growth retardation, or small head circumference. Further, the developmental problems these children exhibit are not much different from those of other children who live in chaotic homes but who did not have prenatal drug exposure. In terms of communicative development, prenatal drug exposure should be considered a *risk* for communication disorder, rather than a cause of it.

Children with communicative and other developmental disorders are, as Knutson and Sullivan (1993) pointed out, more likely than normally developing children to experience maltreatment. Fox et al. (1988) suggested that a child with a communication disorder may be less satisfying for a parent to care for and provide less rewarding interactions. These difficulties might predispose a child to abuse.

Maltreatment itself also constitutes a risk for language disorder. Culp et al. (1991) argued that language development is particularly vulnerable in the maltreatment situation because of the disruption in social interaction it entails. Coster et al. (1989) showed that maltreated toddlers had more limited expressive language during play with their mothers than peers from nonabusing homes. Allen and Oliver (1982) found that maltreated 4-year-olds had significantly lower language scores than peers of similar socioeconomic level. Lynch and Roberts (1982) showed that children with a history of maltreatment scored significantly lower on verbal IQ relative to nonverbal scores. Fox et al. (1988) found that maltreated children had receptive language deficits, with neglected children suffering greater lags than those shown by children who were abused. In general, severe neglect seems to be a greater risk factor for communicative handicap than does abuse (Allen and Oliver, 1982; Culp et al. 1991). Coster and Cicchetti (1993) point out, however, that it is not entirely clear that the language problems seen in these children are greater than what would be expected on the basis of the generally depressed cognitive levels associated with their maltreatment.

SPECIFIC SPEECH AND LANGUAGE DISORDERS

Communication disorders can, as we have seen, be associated with a variety of conditions. They can also occur in relative isolation. These more specific disorders of speech and language development can still, because communication is so central to human interaction, have broad effects on a child's ability to succeed in social and academic pursuits. We examine the two types of specific speech disorders discussed in the DSM-IV (APA, 1994), phonological disorders and stuttering, and the two types of language disorders addressed there, i.e., specific language disorders and selective mutism.

Specific Speech Disorders

STUTTERING

Stuttering involves an impairment in speech fluency characterized by frequent repetitions or prolongations of sounds or syllables. Other types of speech dysfluencies may also be involved, including blocking of sounds, hesitations, and tense pauses (Perkins, 1980). Stuttering usually begins somewhere between 2 and 7 years of age, with a peak between 3 and 4 years. It begins with a fragmentation of syllables and words in the form of easy repetition of single sounds or syllables, prolongations of sounds, hard vocal attacks, and forceful articulatory pressures. In the beginning, the dysfluency fluctuates in severity over time, so that the course is not steady; the dysfluency seems to wax and wane for some time. Despite these fluctuations, children do not continue to be dysfluent in the same way over a long period of time. They either get better or get worse. If dysfluencies continue to be relatively effortless, there is a good chance of recovery. If the child begins to struggle to talk, chances are that the stuttering will get worse. When recovery occurs, it usually does so by adolescence, often around the time of puberty. About 1% of children stutter at some time, but by adolescence, the prevalence drops to 0.8%. The disorder is much more common in boys than in girls, with a male-to-female ratio of about 3:1 (Ham, 1990).

For individuals with chronic stuttering, the severity of the disturbance varies from situation to situation and is more severe when there is pressure to communicate. Stress or anxiety have been shown to exacerbate stuttering, but are not thought to play a role in the etiology. Reducing stress during speaking can reduce stuttering episodes (Van Riper, 1973). General treatments for anxiety, including the use of tranquilizing medication, have not been found to be effective treatments (Ham, 1990).

Although stuttering has at times been thought to be a learned behavior, most researchers today consider stuttering to have a biological component. People who stutter have been found to show laryngeal behavior different from that in normal speakers, even when their speech is apparently fluent (Conture et al., 1985). There also appears to be a familial component in stuttering (Kidd, 1977). The risk of stuttering among first-degree relatives is more than three times the population risk (APA, 1994). Stuttering is believed by most researchers today to have a complex multiplicity of causes that include biological vulnerability, environmental demands and expectations, and temperamental characteristics of the speaker (Adams, 1990)

It is important to distinguish stuttering from normal dysfluencies used commonly by young children. Normal dysfluencies include whole word or phrase repetitions—such as "I want, I want ice cream"—and occur frequently in young children. Only if these dysfluencies persist, become more frequent and severe, or lead the child to struggle with speech or avoid speaking, should a diagnosis of stuttering be considered in a young child.

PHONOLOGICAL DISORDER

Phonological or articulation disorders are characterized by impaired production of developmentally expected speech sounds. To diagnose a specific phonological disorder, it is necessary to ascertain that the problem is not attributable to deficits or abnormalities in intelligence, hearing, or the structure and physiology of the speech mechanism. So a phonological disorder is one in which, although there is no organic reason for the disability, the child's speech is marked by misarticulations, including distortions of sounds (e.g., /s/ is produced with a lisp), omissions of sounds (e.g., *up* is pronounced "uh," *play* is pronounced "pay"), and incorrect substitutions of one sound for another (e.g., *cat* is pronounced "dat"). Many of these misarticulations represent processes that are present in the speech of young normal children (e.g., deletions of final consonants, simplifications of consonant clusters), but in phonological disorders more of them are used, they are used more often, and their use persists beyond the normal developmental period. There may also be idiosyncratic preferences for and/or avoidances of certain sounds or sound simplification processes (Dunn and Davis, 1983; Ingram, 1976; Weiner, 1981) and/or reversals or misordering of sounds in words (Trantham and Pedersen, 1976). The age of recognition/onset of the disorder is related to severity. Typically the disorder becomes apparent around the age of 4 years, when normal children become fully intelligible and eliminate almost all of their normal developmental sound change patterns. Children as young as 3 years can be diagnosed with this disorder, however, if their speech is unintelligible even to family members. Milder cases may not be identified until the child is in school.

Phonological disorders are the most prevalent type of communication problem. Edwards (1984) reported that 80% of speech clinic referrals were for articulation disorder. Hixon et al. (1980) reported that 2% of school-age children have phonological disorders. The prevalence is higher for preschoolers, with estimates ranging from 3 to 15%.

The characteristics of the misarticulated speech are related to the child's age and the severity of the disorder. Younger and/or more severely impaired children may have difficulties involving a wide range of speech sounds, including those like /b/, /p/, and /m/ that are acquired early in the developmental sequence. A variety of sound changes may occur, including dropping syllables ("nana" for *banana*), dropping final sounds (/da/ for *doll*), or leaving sounds out of consonant blends ("bu" for *blue*). These changes, cumulatively, can render the child's speech moderately to severely difficult for others to understand. Older children and/or children who are less severely affected may make only a few kinds of errors, usually substitutions or deletions. Errors in older or more mildly impaired children will occur only on sounds that are acquired later in the developmental sequence (e.g., /s/, /r/, /l/, th). Misarticulations of vowel sounds are rare in this disorder.

Phonological disorders can, of course, occur with many of the syndromes discussed earlier. They can also occur in isolation, but they are commonly associated with specific language disorders. Shriberg and Kwiatkowski (1988) found that 75% of the children with delayed speech development as preschoolers had associated language disorders as well. Shriberg and Kwiatkowski also found that a significant minority of these children, with either speech-only or speech/language delays as preschoolers, required continuing special services throughout their elementary school years. They emphasize the importance of careful assessment and follow-up of both speech-only and speech/language delayed children. Although most of these children do "outgrow" their unintelligible speech, some do continue to require services for other aspects of language and academic development.

Specific Language Disorders

Some kinds of language disorders have no known concomitants. These disorders have been traditionally defined by exclusion, that is, by the absence of the other factors—mental retardation, sensory disorders, neurological damage, emotional problems, or environmental deprivation. The terms *childhood aphasia* or *congenital aphasia* were used in the past to describe these disorders. The use of these terms grew out of the conviction of the early neurologists who studied the problem that difficulties in children's learning language were analogous to the loss of language seen in adults who suffered acquired aphasias. This notion evolved from observations that "aphasic" children often appeared bright in other ways and were clearly not retarded. They seemed also to have normal affective bonds to the people around them and were not emotionally disturbed. Their inability to acquire language normally was attributed to some sort of neurological dysfunction, thought to be comparable to localized brain lesions that resulted in aphasia in adults.

A multitude of studies that attempted to identify these neurological lesions in children with language deficits (see Paul, 1993, for review) were unsuccessful in finding brain structure or function differences that were either common to all the children studied or specific to children with language disorders. This is not to say that children with language disorders do not have neurological involvement, but simply that the CNS involvement they have does not appear to be similar to the localized pathology seen in adults with aphasia—it probably involves more diffuse aspects of the nervous system—and is not readily identifiable, given current technology. Certainly, new diagnostic techniques, such as magnetic resonance imaging (MRI) and positron-emission tomography (PET) scanning, for example, have great promise of discovering some of these neurological markers. But so far no definitive finding has been reported. For these reasons, i.e., because language disorders in children do not seem to have the same root in localized brain lesions as do adult aphasias and because no specific, reliable brain differences have been identified to date, the terms *aphasia* or *dysphasia* seem too weighted toward neurological explanations of dubious value. More descriptive terms are now used to label these disorders. DSM-IV uses *specific language disorder. Specific language impairment*, often abbreviated SLI, is also commonly used to label this diagnostic category.

While biological factors are implicated, if not explicitly identified in specific language disorders, the role of environmental factors in these disorders has long been at issue. While aberrant parental linguistic input has often been suspected as a cause, numerous researchers (e.g., Conti-Ramsden, 1990; Leonard, 1989; Paul and Elwood, 1991; Whitehurst et al., 1988) have concluded that linguistic input to children with language disorders is well-matched to the children's language level. Some environmental factors do appear to be associated with language disorders, however. These include lower socioeconomic status, larger family size, recurrent otitis media, neglectful home environment, and later birth order (Nelson, 1993). It appears that the operative mechanism behind these factors is deprivation of auditory or linguistic input (Bishop, 1987), occurring at a critical stage in language development.

Accurate estimates of prevalence of specific language disorders are difficult to come by, due to methodological differences across studies (e.g., in the subclassifications and definitions; in the cutoffs and inclusionary criteria; and in the age, sex, and other characteristics of the children sampled). The literature provides a wide range of prevalence estimates. Although they are less common than phonological disorders, specific language disorders are among the most prevalent handicapping conditions found in school children, along with learning disabilities (United States Department of Education, 1987). Definitive prevalence data are not available, either for speech/language disorders in general or for specific types of speech/language disorders, although is it clear that expressive-only disorders are more common than mixed expressive-receptive impairments. It is also known that language disorders of both types are more prevalent in males than in females.

There has been a long-running debate in the literature about whether children with language disorders show "deviant" acquisition patterns—patterns unlike those seen in younger normal children—or whether they exhibit a slowed-down version of normal development. Early studies (Lee, 1966; Menyuk, 1964) reported that there were qualitative differences in the linguistic systems of normal and disordered children. But recent research, summarized by Leonard (1989), suggests that children with language disorders do resemble younger normal

speakers in the general nature of their linguistic systems and in most aspects of the order of acquisition. While this pattern holds true when we look at one specific feature of development at a time, Leonard (1991) pointed out that children may be 1 year below age level in one set of features, 1.5 years below in another, 6 months below in a third, and so on. The result will be that the overall profile of language skills in a child with SLI may not resemble that of a normal child at any point in development. This does not mean that language development is deviant, but rather that it is in some ways asynchronous.

How specific are specific language disorders? Children with SLI are at greatly increased risk for attention and activity problems (Cantwell et al., 1979; Tallal, 1988). Other "soft" neurological signs are also frequently present in children with SLI (Benton, 1964; Eisenson, 1972). The involvement of a variety of nonverbal cognitive skills in SLI has also been indicated, including symbolic play, classification, figurative thinking, mental rotation, haptic perception, and hypothesis formation (Johnston and Ramstad, 1978; Johnston and Weismer, 1983; Kamhi, 1981; Kamhi et al., 1984; Rescorla and Goosens, 1992). These findings have led to the hypothesis that children with SLI may have not just a language problem, but a general representational deficit, affecting a variety of kinds of symbolic functioning. Tallal (1988) cautioned, however, that in each of these studies there were children with SLI who could perform the nonverbal cognitive tasks adequately, and that sometimes the differences between groups were not qualitative, but a matter of speed of response. Leonard (1987) pointed out that, although some children with SLI fall below age mates on such tasks, they still do better than younger children with comparable language skills.

Leonard (1991) provided an alternative explanation for SLI. He contended that children who score low on language tests, relative to their scores on other areas of cognition, may no more have a "disorder" than children who cannot learn to play the violin. He argued that some children are just "limited" in their ability to learn language, falling (as someone must) at the low end of the normal distribution of language ability. If this were the case, in his view, it would not be surprising that such children would also be limited in other abilities that related to symbolic function. He referred to Gardner's (1983) notion of "multiple intelligences," which proposes that there are a variety of somewhat independent spheres of intellectual functioning and that some people have greater abilities in some than in others. The tendency to call a language limitation a "handicap" stems, in Leonard's view, from the importance of linguistic skills for academic and vocational success in our society, not from any significant neurological or neuropsychological pathology in people limited in this way. The fact that language problems tend to aggregate in families (Tallal et al., 1989; Tomblin, 1989) could be taken to support the view that some people just have less optimal "language genes," and therefore less talent in language areas, than others.

Many would contest this view, however. They would hold that the frequent co-occurrence of SLI with attention and activity problems and other "soft" neurological signs raises questions about its relation to normal development. Aram (1991) argued that children with nearly age-appropriate comprehension but expression limited to single words could not be seen to be functioning simply at the low end of the normal range, nor could a 3-year-old who can read but cannot produce spontaneous speech (Aram and Healy, 1988). Clearly some children with SLI do have pathological factors involved. The question for researchers and theoreticians is whether these children are the exception or the rule.

In terms of natural history, SLI tends to change shape with age. Children with SLI, particularly those with mild to moderate impairment, often outgrow the most obvious aspects of their linguistic deficits by the end of the preschool period (Paul, 1993b; Scarborough and Dobrich, 1990; Tallal, 1988). Tallal (1988) has suggested that many children with mild to moderate forms of SLI "change diagnoses" when they get to school age, not because the underlying nature of their problem changes, but simply because the demands of the school situation stress recently acquired language skills that they developed so slowly and with such difficulty during the preschool period. The deficits that remain in oral language by school age in these children often surface only in situations requiring complex language skills, such as metalinguistic and narrative tasks. These situations are just the ones, though, that are required for success in learning to read, write, spell, and do mathematical problems. Although not all children with learning disabilities have a history of SLI, a very high proportion of children with SLI also have trouble in school, particularly in learning to read. Again, as Leonard (1991) argued, this progression may reflect language skills that are simply limited relative to those in the general population, rather than reflecting a specific pathology. Tallal (1988) has suggested that language disorders and learning disabilities should not be considered separate problems, but simply different manifestations of the same problem at different ages.

Another controversy in the field of SLI concerns subtypes of the disorder. There has been much debate in the literature on this issue, too, and no definitive subtyping scheme has been established. Several schemes have been proposed, including those of Aram and Nation (1975), Fey (1986), Naremore (1980), and Rapin and Allen (1983). The most common subtyping systems concern the division between disorders restricted to expressive language and those that involve both reception and expression. This is the categorization method used in DSM-IV (APA, 1994). Still, this scheme is not universally accepted. Curtiss and Tallal (1985), for example, reported that patterns of performance on language testing over time in a longitudinal study were the same for children with SLI regardless of the subgroup in which they had been placed. They also found no differences among subgroups on pragmatic measures. More recent work (Craig and Evans, 1993), however, suggested that children with expressive and mixed expressive-receptive language disorders do differ on pragmatic performance.

Some long-term outcome studies suggest differences in prognosis for children with expressive-only language problems, as opposed to those with both expressive and receptive disorders. Both Paul and Cohen (1984) and Whitehurst and Fischel (1994) reported that children with expressive language disorders but intact comprehension skills fare better than those with deficits in both language modalities. For preschoolers with expressive-only language problems, risk for long-term deficits is about 20% (Paul, 1994). For children with both expressive and receptive deficits, risk estimates for persistent problems in oral language and academic skills range from 40 to 80% (Nelson, 1993). More careful research on children with language disorders subtyped in various ways and followed over extensive periods of time needs to be done in order to resolve this issue.

Other prognostic indicators for SLI, besides the presence of receptive difficulties, have been identified. The degree of the impairment is one factor (Bishop and Edmundson, 1987), with more severely affected preschoolers showing less favorable outcomes at school age. Nelson (1993) reported that better prognosis in SLI is associated with few perinatal problems, higher nonverbal IQ, and willingness on the child's part to participate in groups. Certain measures have been shown to be good predictors of school-age outcome in preschoolers with mild to moderate SLI. These include measures of narrative skills and nonverbal cognition (Bishop and Edmundson, 1987).

For children with chronic mild to moderate language disorders, problems in the school years tend to narrow in their focus and to be concentrated in subtle difficulties of language organization and efficiency, rather than in frank errors. Academic problems tend to involve primarily reading and writing. Some mild social deficits may also be seen. Despite their persistent problems, however, most of these children do finish high school, some go on to college, and most live independent lives (Hall and Tomblin, 1978).

For children with severe SLI, prognosis is more guarded. Paul and Cohen (1984) studied long-term outcomes in children diagnosed as SLI as preschoolers who were not speaking in full sentences by the time they were 6. By the time they were adolescents, these subjects with severe impairments were likely to score in the retarded range on IQ tests, even if they had scored in the normal range at the preschool level.

Given intensive intervention, all made steady progress in receptive language skills throughout their school years, and progress in expressive ability was at a rate that exceeded their growth in age. Still, 90% of these subjects were significantly below the normal range in both areas by adolescence, and all required intensive special education, with most in special classrooms, schools, or residential facilities.

SPECIFIC EXPRESSIVE LANGUAGE DISORDER

Children with specific expressive disorders are late to begin talking. They may not say their first word until well into their 2nd year. When they do begin to talk, they add new words slowly. They may continue to use single word or telegraphic utterances into their 3rd year. Although expressive vocabularies tend to reach normal size by age 3 in children with mild to moderate handicaps, problems in various areas of syntax, such as verb endings and pronoun usage, persist throughout the preschool period (Paul, 1993). Grammatical usage may be characterized by omissions of words (e.g., prepositions, indefinite pronouns, or verbal auxiliaries: "He sitting," "Where we going?") or morphemes (e.g., "Dad wear white shoe," "She sleep"), use of a limited selection of grammatical structures (e.g., only the present tense of verbs), incorrect word ordering (e.g., "Car Mummy have"), or the use of inappropriate combinations of words or morphemes ("They was reading," "two foots"). Phonological problems very frequently coexist with slow expressive language development during the preschool years. In children with mild to moderate disorders, many of these problems will resolve by the early school years.

Even during the school age period, however, word usage of a child with expressive language disorder may reveal word retrieval or "word-finding" difficulties, and/or word substitutions. Instead of using correct words (e.g., "chair"), an child with an expressive language disorder may substitute an incorrect word of related meaning (e.g., "table"), may use functional descriptors (e.g., "thing to sit on"), may use vague or general terms (e.g., "thing"), or may use his or her own made-up jargon.

Storytelling and discourse problems often persist and affect both oral and written modes of expression (Bliss, 1985; Tomblin, 1978). These children may lack the ability to elaborate and/or self-correct when needed for clarity in conversation (Graham et al., 1983; Trantham and Pedersen, 1976). There may be tangential or inappropriate responses to questions, a limited range of communicative functions (e.g., requests, imperatives, questions) expressed, difficulty maintaining and/or changing topics, and difficulty initiating interactions. Many of these pragmatic difficulties in children with expressive language disorder are due to a lack of flexibility in language (Lucas, 1980; Zirkelbach and Blakesley, 1985). These children may sound abrupt, rude, or impolite simply because they do not have access to the full and diverse range of linguistic forms used in normal conversation to encode pragmatic nuance and make language sound appropriate to the social context. Generally, the formal aspects of language, such as syntax, are more severely affected than is language usage.

Expressive language disorder can demonstrate a wide range of severity. The more severe the expressive language disorder is, the earlier it will be recognized. Severe forms of the disorder are typically apparent by the age of 3 years, whereas milder forms may remain undetected until school age. Associated neurological, developmental, and psychiatric disorders are common in children with expressive language disorder, but these are less common than with receptive language disorder.

MIXED RECEPTIVE-EXPRESSIVE LANGUAGE DISORDER

Children with developmental language disorders almost never show a circumscribed deficit in comprehension, analogous to a Wernicke's aphasia in adults. If comprehension is affected in a developmental disorder, there is almost always an effect on expressive ability as well. For this reason, DSM-IV describes a more global disorder of language acquisition that is not limited to expressive ability but also involves impairments in language comprehension. This is referred to as a *mixed receptive-expressive (R/E) language disorder*.

The cardinal feature of receptive expressive language disorder is some type of impairment in the understanding of language in conjunction with impaired expressive language ability. The comprehension difficulty in receptive expressive language disorders may be present in any or all aspects of language (e.g., vocabulary, grammatical units, word ordering, and/or language usage). Young children first identified with this disorder tend to resemble those with expressive-only disorders. Because of their intact social skills and their ability to use comprehension strategies, these children may seem to their parents to "understand everything" and have problems only in talking. Since the expressive disorder can so easily mask receptive deficits, careful assessment of both modalities of language is necessary in order to identify the full range of deficits and abilities a child with a language disorder possesses.

Children with mixed R/E disorders manifest expressive language problems very similar to those seen in the expressive-only disorder. Like those in the more circumscribed expressive impairment, these deficits change over time. They narrow in scope from affecting all aspects of expression (semantics, phonology, syntax, and morphology) to centering primarily on phonology, verb and pronoun marking, and sentence elaboration. While this process parallels that seen in expressive-only disorders, it can occur even more slowly in children with R/E impairment so that, even by school age, problems in basic expression of words and sentences persist.

Comprehension deficits can involve the inability to understand single-word utterances, a limited understanding of concepts (e.g., time, space, causality, or relationships), or an inability to recognize multiple meanings of words. Some vocabulary deficits will involve difficulties with only particular types of words (e.g., abstract nouns, spatial prepositions, or complex verbs). Generally, all but the most severely affected children will master a basic knowledge of a core set of vocabulary items.

Comprehension of grammatical units is marked by difficulty in understanding the meanings of various grammatical morphemes (e.g., plurals versus singular, present versus past tense). Comprehension deficits in the area of word-ordering rules (or syntax) are manifested by difficulty understanding sentences whose meaning is indicated to some degree by word order (e.g., "The car was hit by the bus" versus "The car hit the bus"). Deficits in the comprehension of language usage may be manifested by difficulty understanding the significance of polite forms, slang forms, or, in severe cases, paralinguistic aspects of communication (e.g., facial expressions, speech intonation patterns, and tones of voice).

Selective Mutism

Selective mutism is a failure to speak in one or more particular definable communicative environments. Historically, stuttering, phonological disorders, and specific language disorders have been considered the domain of speech pathology and psycholinguistics, whereas selective mutism has been considered the domain of psychiatry and psychology. This division remains, to some extent, today, as exemplified by the placement of selective mutism outside the Communication Disorders section in DSM-IV. Still, selective mutism does involve a form of communication disorder and is important in the differential diagnosis of other forms of communication impairment. Since this is the case, a brief discussion of this disorder is presented here.

As is the case with other communication disorders, accurate estimates of the prevalence of selective mutism are difficult to find, although the condition is known to be rare. DSM-IV estimates the prevalence at less than 1% of children seen in mental health settings, a very small proportion of the population in general. Unlike all the other communication disorders discussed here, selective mutism is thought to be somewhat more common in females than in males. Selective mutism has been found to be associated with the other speech/language disorders at greater than chance rates.

Because the disorder is so rare, the major variations in symptomatology are unclear. It appears, however, that the most common manifestation is a refusal to speak in school and to adults outside the home despite speaking normally within the home to siblings and at least one parent (APA, 1987; Browne et al., 1963).

The child's silence seems to represent a refusal to talk rather than an inability to talk, although, as noted above, language disorders are associated with this syndrome more often than would be expected by chance alone. While these other speech/language impairments are sometimes present (Cantwell and Baker, 1985; Kolvin and Fundudis, 1981), they are not sufficiently severe to account for a lack of speech. Intellectual functioning is generally found to be average or above (Browne et al., 1963; Hayden, 1980; Hesselman, 1983), although one study found slightly lower performance intelligence levels (Kolvin and Fundudis, 1981).

Despite their "refusal to talk," selectively mute children usually appear interested in communication and, in the situations where they will not talk, they may attempt to communicate by using gestures, pantomimes, drawings, nods or shakes of the head, whispers, or monosyllabic utterances (Cantwell and Baker, 1985, 1987; APA, 1987). In those settings where they are not mute, these children may be quite talkative (Hesselman, 1983).

The disorder usually has its onset between 3 and 8 years, although the most frequent point of onset is school entry. However, some cases have been reported with onset after 12 years of age (Kaplan and Escoll, 1973). Among the symptoms reported (APA, 1987; Browne et al., 1963; Hayden, 1980; Hesselman, 1983; Kolvin and Fundudis, 1981) to be associated with selective mutism are excessive shyness, social isolation, immaturity, school refusal, compulsive traits, anxiety, aggression, depression (and suicide attempts), oppositional behavior, and motoric rigidity. The majority of patients with selective mutism recover from their symptoms within months or years (APA, 1994; Kolvin and Fundudis, 1981). Improvements usually occur before the age of 10 years (Kolvin and Fundudis, 1981); the prognosis is poorer for children older than 12 years (Hayden, 1980; Kaplan and Escoll, 1973).

Biological factors are usually not thought to play a significant role in the etiology of selective mutism. Still, it has been found that children with selective mutism are at a somewhat increased risk for other developmental disorders (including speech/language disorders, enuresis, and encopresis) and for EEG immaturity. This suggests that a biologically based maturational disorder may play some role in the etiology of selective mutism (Kolvin and Fundudis, 1981).

Family and interpersonal dynamics have long been suspected to play a major role in the etiology of selective mutism. Some studies have found that selectively mute children have increased rates of psychiatrically ill parents and/or abnormal family dynamics (Browne et al., 1963; Hayden, 1980; Hesselman, 1983; Kaplan and Escoll, 1973: Kolvin and Fundudis, 1981). Anecdotal reports mention isolated family situations; at least one very shy or uncommunicative parent; broken families; hospitalization (Browne et al., 1963); significant separations from family (Kolvin and Fundudis, 1981); physical traumas (Hayden, 1980) such as child abuse, rape, or mouth injuries; and an overly strong attachment to the mother. Still, careful controlled research on this disorder is scarce, and larger studies with appropriate contrast groups are needed before definitive conclusions on the role of family dynamics can be drawn.

DIFFERENTIAL DIAGNOSIS

When seeing children suspected of specific speech and language disorders, the main diagnostic task is to rule out other syndromes with which speech and language problems are frequently associated. These syndromes include the ones discussed in the first section of this chapter, i.e., deafness or significant hearing loss, mental retardation, pervasive developmental disorder, autism, psychiatric disorder, and organically based communication disorders (e.g., cleft palate, apraxia, cerebral palsy, or childhood-acquired aphasia).

The absence of significant hearing impairment or deafness must be established by audiometric testing by a certified audiologist. Since subtle deficits in hearing can affect language acquisition, it is important to get complete and accurate results in order to assure that hearing deficits do not play a role in the disorder. Although chronic middle ear pathology is sometimes associated with speech and language problems, recent research (Gravel and Wallace, 1992; Paul et al., 1993; Roberts et al., 1991) suggests that chronic otitis media alone does not significantly increase the risk of language disorder in otherwise normal children. If parents report chronic otitis in a child who presents with a communication disorder, attributing the problem entirely to the middle ear problem is not justified, and treatment for the otitis will not necessarily alleviate the language disorder.

Mental retardation must be diagnosed by means of an individually administered, standardized test of intelligence, as well as by a standardized measure of adaptive behavior. For children suspected of language disorders, it is necessary to use nonverbal intelligence tests to assess intellectual ability, so as not to penalize the child for the language deficit and to get an estimate of intelligence unbiased by language performance. Table 47.1 provides a sample of nonverbal intelligence assessments that can be used in the determination of cognitive level in children with communication disorders. To be diagnosed with a specific speech or language disorder, a child must score significantly higher on the nonverbal intelligence assessment than on the language measure.

Organic disorders that can affect the speech mechanism, such as dyspraxia, dysarthria, and motor deficits associated with cerebral palsy can be ruled out by physical and functional assessment of the speech mechanism (oral peripheral examination). A speech-language pathologist typically examines the morphology, symmetry, and alignment of the facial features. The functional integrity of the larynx, lips, tongue, and velopharyngeal structures as well as the respiratory support for speech are also assessed. The quality of oral volitional movements may also be examined if an apraxia is suspected. If physical limitations to speech production are identified in this examination, an alternative system of communication—such as a picture board or electronic communicative device—may be indicated.

Pervasive developmental disorder, autism, and other psychiatric disorders can be ruled out by psychiatric/behavioral features. Features associated with autism/PDD include lack of (nonverbal) social interactions, absence of imaginative activity, stereotypic behaviors, self-injurious behaviors, odd responses to sensory input, and mood abnormalities. Language features that characterize these disorders include abnormal use of imitation (echolalia); idiosyncratic use of words or phrases for "private" meaning; pronoun reversals (saying "you" when the speaker means "I"); persistent, obsessive preoccupation with one topic of conversation (such as bus schedules reiterated, elaborated on, and questioned about incessantly); and repetitive, inappropriate use of questions.

The differential diagnosis among stuttering, phonological disorder, expressive language disorder, mixed receptive-expressive language disorder, and selective mutism requires detailed speech/language testing. Some examples of the most commonly used language tests are given in Table 47.2. To diagnose stuttering, a clinician should ascertain, by means of standardized testing, that phonological, receptive, and expressive language skills are age-appropriate. Many children go through periods of developmental dysfluency, and children with language disorders may persist in developmental dysfluency longer than normal because their developmental period is longer than normal. If dysfluency coexists with other speech and language disorders, it may be appropriate to delay making a diagnosis of stuttering until some of the other problems resolve, then reevaluate to determine whether the dysfluency has persisted.

Phonological disorders are diagnosed by means of standardized testing of phonological production, usually using procedures that ask children to name pictures or objects and transcribing the child's rendition of the target word for comparison with adult production standards. Since phonological disorders typically coexist with other language disorders, it is acceptable to confer a concurrent diagnosis of phonological disorder even if other language disorders are present. However, it is necessary to rule out hearing impairment, mental retardation, and speech mechanism limitations before diagnosing a specific speech disorder.

To diagnose a specific expressive language disorder, it is necessary to demonstrate—by means of individually administered, standardized tests—that both nonverbal intelligence and receptive language skills are significantly better than expression. Again, since phonological disorders so frequently coexist with expressive language deficits, both conditions can be diagnosed concurrently.

To make a diagnosis of mixed receptive-expressive language disorder, it is must be shown—again using individually administered, standardized tests—that nonverbal intelligence is significantly higher than *both* expression and comprehension of language. As with expressive disorder, phonological deficits can coexist with R/E disorders and would be diagnosed according to the criteria given earlier.

TREATMENT OF SPEECH AND LANGUAGE DISORDERS

It is important to make a careful differential diagnosis of any communication disorder in order to decide whether the problem is specific to speech and language or is part of a larger syndrome. In the case of communication disorders associated with syndromes like hearing impairment, mental retardation, and autism, treatment must address all aspects of the child's problem, not just those of speech and language.

Still, once a communication problem has been identified and the broad range of interventions necessary to address all the child's needs has been instigated, treatment for the communicative aspect of the disorder is quite similar, regardless of whether the problem is specific to speech and language or part of a bigger picture of developmental disorder.

The treatment of choice for all the disorders discussed here, except

Table 47.1. A Sample of Nonverbal Cognitive Assessments

Instrument	Age Range
Cognitive Behavior Scale. Johnson S. Vero Beach, FL, The Speech Bin, 1987.	24–36 months
Harris-Goodenough Draw-A-Person Test. Harris D. New York, Harcourt, Brace, and World, 1963.	3–12 years
Hiskey-Nebraska Test of Learning Aptitude. Hiskey M. Lincoln, NE, University of Nebraska Press, 1966	3–17 years
Kaufman Assessment Battery for Children—Nonverbal Scale. Kaufman A, Kaufman N. Circle Pines, MN, American Guidance Service, 1983.	30 months to 12 years
Arthur Adaptation of the Leiter International Performance Scale. Arthur G. Washington, DC, Psychological Service Center, 1969.	2–16 years
Merrill-Palmer Scale of Mental Tests. Stutsman R. New York, Harcourt Brace Jovanovich, 1948.	1–6 years
Performance Scale of *Wechsler Intelligence Scale for Children.* Wechsler D. San Antonio, TX, Psychological Corp., 1974.	7–16 years
Performance Scale of *Wechsler Preschool and Primary Scale.* Wechsler D. San Antonio, TX, Psychological Corp., 1967.	4–6 years
Raven's Progressive Matrices. Raven J. San Antonio, TX, Psychological Corp., 1965.	5–11 years (colored) 6–13 years (standard)
Symbolic Play Test. Lowe M, Costello A. (Experimental Ed.) London, NFER-Nelson, 1976.	12–36 months
Test of Nonverbal Intelligence. Brown L, Sherbenou R, Dollar S. Austin, TX, Pro-Ed, 1982.	5–85 years
Uzgiris-Hunt Scales of Infant Development. Dunst C. Austin, TX, Pro-Ed. 1980.	Birth to 24 months

From Paul R: *Language Disorders from Infancy through Adolescence: Assessment and Intervention.* Mosby-Year Book, St. Louis, MO, 1995.

Table 47.2.   A Sample of Language Assessment Tools

Test Name/Author(s) Publisher/Source	Developmental Range	Areas Assessed
Arizona Articulation Proficiency Scale. Fudala J, Reynolds W. Los Angeles, Western Psychological Services, 1989.	1-6 to 14 years	Articulation
Assessment of Children's Language Comprehension (ACLC). Foster R, Giddan J, Stark J. Chicago, Riverside Publishing, 1983.	3-6½ years	Receptive only, auditory comprehension; syntax, concepts, vocabulary
Assessment of Phonological Processes (rev) (APP-R). Hodson B. Austin, Pro-Ed, 1986.	Preschool	Articulation
Bankson Language Test-2 (Bankson-2). Bankson N. Austin, Pro-Ed, 1990.	3-6 years	Receptive/expressive language, auditory memory/discrimination
Bankson-Bernthal Test of Phonology. Bankson N. Bernthal J. Chicago, Riverside Publishing, 1990.	3-9 years	Articulation
Boehm Test of Basic Concepts (rev). Boehm A. San Antonio, Psychological Corp., Harcourt Brace Jovanovich, 1986.	K to 2nd grade	Receptive concepts: space, time, quantity
Carolina Picture Vocabulary Test (CPVT), Layton T, Holmes D. Austin, Pro-Ed, 1985.	4-11½ years	Receptive sign vocabulary
Clark-Madison Test of Oral Language. Clark J, Madison C. Austin, Pro-Ed, 1986.	4-8 years	Expressive syntax, verbs/inflections, pronouns/modifiers, determiners/prepositions
Clinical Evaluation of Language Fundamentals—Preschool (CELF-Preschool). Wiig E, Secord W, Semel E. San Antonio, Psychological Corp., Harcourt, Brace, Jovanovich, 1992.	3-6 years	Concepts, syntax, semantics, morphology
Clinical Evaluation of Language Fundamentsls (rev) (CELF-R). Semel E, Wiig E, Secord W. San Antonio, Psychological Corp., Harcourt Brace Jovanovich, 1987.	5-16 years	Semantics, syntax, memory, receptive/expressive, composite
Communication Abilities Diagnostic Test (CADeT). Johnston E, Johnston A. Chicago, Riverside Publishing, 1990.	3-9 years	Syntax, semantics, pragmatics
Deep Test for Articulation. McDonald E. Pittsburgh, Stanwix House Corp., 1968.	3-12 years	Articulation
Developmental Sentence Score (DSS). Lee L. Evanston, IL, Northwestern University Press, 1974.	2-7 years	Expressive language: indefinite pronouns, personal pronouns, main verbs, secondary verbs, negatives, conjunctions, interrogative reversals, wh- questions
Evaluating Communicative Competence. Simon C. Tucson, Communication Skill Builders, 1986.	9-17 years	Language processing, metalinguistic skills, functional uses of language
Expressive One-Word Picture Vocabulary Test (EOWPVT) (rev). Gardner M. Novato, CA, Academic Therapy, 1990.	2-12 years	Expressive vocabulary
Fisher-Logemann Test of Articulation Competence. Fisher H, Logemann J. Boston, Houghton Mifflin, 1971.	3 years to adult	Articulation
Fullerton Language Test for Adolescents (FLTA). Thorum A. Chicago, Riverside Publishing, 1986.	11 to adult	Auditory synthesis, morphology, oral commands, convergent/divergent production, syllabication, grammar competency, idioms
Goldman-Fristoe Test of Articulation (GFTA). Goldman R, Fristoe M. Circle Pines, MN, American Guidance Service, Inc., 1986.	2-16+ years	Articulation
Let's Talk Inventory for Children (LTI-C). Bray C, Wiig E. San Antonio, Psychological Corp., Harcourt Brace Jovanovich, 1987.	4-8 years	Social-verbal communication
Let's Talk Inventory for Adolescents (LTI-A). Wiig E. San Antonio, Psychological Corp., Harcourt Brace Jovanovich, 1982.	9 to adult	Communicative function
Miller-Yoder Language Comprehension Test. Miller J, Yoder D. Baltimore, University Park Press, 1984.	4-8 years	Receptive grammar and morphology
Patterned Elicitation of Syntax Text (PEST). Young E, Perachio J. Tucson, Communication Skill Builders, 1993.	3-7½ years	Expressive syntax and morphology
Peabody Picture Vocabulary Test (rev) (PPVT-R). Dunn L, Dunn L. Circle Pines, MN, American Guidance Service, 1981.	2-6 to adult	Receptive vocabulary
Photo Articulation Test. Pendergast K, Dickey S, Selman J, Soder A. Danville, IL, The Interstate Printers and Publishers, Inc., 1969.	3-12 years	Articulation
Porch Index of Communicative Ability in Children (PICA-Children). Porch B. Chicago, Riverside Publishing, 1979.	4-12 years	Verbal, gestural, graphic abilities
Preschool Language Scale-3. Zimmerman, I, Steiner V, Pond R. San Antonio, Psychological Corp., Harcourt Brace Jovanovich, 1992.	Birth to 6 years	Language precursors: expressive/receptive semantics, syntax, morphology, integrative thinking, auditory comprehensive
Receptive One-Word Picture Vocabulary Test (ROWPVT). Gardner M. Novato, CA, Academic Therapy, 1985.	2-11 to 12 years	Receptive vocabulary
Rhode Island Test of Language Structure (RITLS). Engen E, Engen T. Austin, Pro-Ed, 1983.	3-20 years	Receptive syntax
Sequenced Inventory of Communication Development (SICD). Hedrick D, Prather E, Tobin A. Seattle, University of Washington Press, 1975.	4 months to 4 years	Receptive language (speech/sound awareness and understanding); expressive language (imitating, initiating, responding)
Structured Photographic Expressive Language Test—Preschool (SPELT-P). Werner E, Krescheck J. Sandwich, IL, Janelle Publications, 1983.	3-6 years	Syntax: declarative, interrogative, negative, embedded sentences
Structured Photographic Language Test II (SPELT-II). Werner E, Kreschek J. Sandwich, IL, Janelle Publications, 1983.	4-9½ years	Syntax and morphology
Templin-Darley Texts of Articulation. Templin M, Darley F. Iowa City, Bureau of Educational Research and Service, University of Iowa, 1969.	3-8 years	Articulation
Test for Auditory Comprehension of Language (rev) (TACL-R). Carrow-Woolfolk E. Chicago, Riverside Publishing, 1985.	3-10 years	Auditory comprehension, word classes/relations, grammatical morphemes, elaborated sentence constructions
Test of Adolescent Language-2 (TOAL-2). Hammill D, Brown VB, Larsen S, Wiederholt J. Austin, Pro-Ed, 1987.	12-18½ years	Receptive/expressive, vocabulary/grammar, reading/writing, auditory comprehension
Test of Early Language Development (TELD-2). Hresko W, Reid K, Hammill D. Austin, Pro-Ed, 1991.	2-8 years	Receptive and expressive syntax, semantics
Test of Language Competence—Expanded Edition (TLC-Expanded). Wiig E, Secord W. San Antonio, Psychological Corp. Harcourt Brace Jovanovic, 1989.	Level 2: 9-19 years	Metalinguistics, multiple meanings, multiple inferences, figurative usage, conversational sentence production

(continued)

Table 47.2.—*continued*

Test Name/Author(s) Publisher/Source	Developmental Range	Areas Assessed
Test of Language Development-2 Primary (TOLD-2). Newcomer P, Hammill D. Austin, Pro-Ed, 1991.	4–9 years	Receptive/expressive semantics and syntax
Test of Language Development—Intermediate (TOLD-I: 2)/Primary (TOLD-P-2). Newcomer P, Hammill D. Austin, Pro-Ed, 1988.	8½–13 years	Receptive/expressive semantics, syntax
Test of Minimal Articulation Competence (TMAC). Secord W. Columbus, OH, Charles E. Merrill Publishing, 1981.	3 to adult	Articulation
Test of Pragmatic Skills (Revised). Shulman B. Tucson, Communication Skill Builders, 1986.	3–8 years	Pragmatics: verbal/nonverbal, naming, labeling, reasoning, denying
Token Test for Children. DiSimoni F. Chicago, Riverside Publishing, 1978.	3–12 years	Auditory comprehension temporal/spatial concepts
Utah Test of Language Development-3 (UTLD-3). Mecham M, Joy J, James J. Austin, Pro-Ed, 1967.	3–11 years	Language comprehension/expression
Woodcock Language Proficiency Battery, English and Spanish Form. Woodcock R Chicago, Riverside Publishing, 1980.	3–80 years	Oral language, vocabulary, antonyms/synonyms

From Paul R: *Language Disorders from Infancy through Adolescence: Assessment and Intervention.* St. Louis, Mosby-Year Book, 1995.

for selective mutism, is individual or small group therapy administered by a certified speech/language pathologist (SLP). Because associated educational and/or psychiatric problems are common with these disorders, educational tutoring, social skills training, and/or psychiatric intervention may also be indicated, even if the disorder is specific to communication.

Methods of intervention are essentially behavioral. Some clinicians use strict operant procedures, while others favor more child-centered approaches such as indirect language stimulation, or "whole language" intervention that involves a rich communicative environment with opportunities for incidental learning. Many SLPs take a middle ground between these extremes, using structured play opportunities and focused stimulation to provide examples of desired forms and elicit language targets. While all these methods have been shown to be effective in small studies (see Fey, 1986, for review), much more research is needed

on the efficacy of particular approaches to intervention and variables that can be used to best match the method to the child.

Because selective mutism is seen more as an anxiety disorder than as a developmental disorder, treatment methods differ somewhat for this syndrome. Although some authors have suggested psychodynamic therapy for selective mutism, the most convincing literature pertains to behavioral modification approaches. Contingency management (positive reinforcement of verbalizations and nonreinforcement for nonverbal responses), stimulus fading (gradually extending the number of people with whom and environments wherein verbalization is rewarded), shaping (rewarding gradual approximations to speech, such as mouthing and whispering), and response cost procedures (losing money or tokens for not speaking) have all been reported to be successful in eliciting and maintaining speech in selectively mute children (Labbe and Williamson, 1984).

References

Adams M: The demands and capacities model I: Theoretical elaborations. *J Fluency Disord* 15:135–141, 1990.

Allen R, Oliver J: The effects of child maltreatment on language development. *Child Abuse Negl* 6:299–305, 1982.

American Psychiatric Association: *Diagnostic and Statistical Manual of Mental Disorders* (3rd ed, rev). Washington, DC, American Psychiatric Press, 1980.

American Psychiatric Association: *DSM-IV Draft Criteria.* Task force on DSM-IV. Washington, DC, American Psychiatric Association, 1994.

Aram D: Comments on specific language impairment as a clinical category. *Lang Speech Hear Serv Schools* 22:84–87, 1991.

Aram D, Healy J: Hyperlexia: A review of extraordinary word recognition. In: Obler LK, Fein D (eds): *The Exceptional Brain: Neuropsychology of Talent and Special Abilities.* New York, Guilford Press, 1988, pp. 70–102.

Baker L, Cantwell D: A prospective psychiatric follow-up of children with speech/language disorders. *J Am Acad Child Adolesc Psychiatry* 26:546–553, 1987.

Beitchman J, Hair R, Clegg M, et al: Prevalence of psychiatric disorders in children with speech and language disorders. *J Am Acad Child Adolesc Psychiatry* 25:528–535, 1986.

Benton A: Developmental aphasia and brain damage. *Cortex* 1:40–52, 1964.

Bishop D: The causes of specific developmental language disorders. *J Child Psychol Psychiatry* 28:1–8, 1987.

Bishop D: Language development after focal brain damage. In: Bishop D, Mogford K (eds): *Language Development in Exceptional Circumstances.* Hillsdale, NJ, Erlbaum, 1992, pp. 203–219.

Bishop D, Edmundson A: Language-impaired 4-year-olds: Distinguishing transient from persistent impairment. *J Speech Hear Disord* 52:156–173, 1987.

Bliss L: A symptom approach to the intervention of childhood language disorders. *J Commun Disord* 18:91–108, 1985.

Boothroyd A: *Hearing Impairments in Young Children.* Englewood Cliffs, NJ, Prentice-Hall, 1982.

Bradley R, Stoudt R Jr: A five-year longitudinal study of development of articulation proficiency in elementary school children. *Lang Speech Hear Serv Schools* 8:176–180, 1977.

Bradley S, Sloman L: Selective mutism in immigrant families. *J Am Acad Child Psychiatry* 14:510–514, 1975.

Brown J, Lloyd H: A controlled study of children not speaking in school. *J Assoc Workers Maladjusted Child* 18:49, 1975.

Browne E, Wilson V, Laybourne P: Diagnosis and treatment of elective mutism in children. *J Am Acad Child Psychiatry* 2:605–617, 1963.

Cantwell D, Baker L: Psychiatric and learning disorders in children with speech and language disorders: A descriptive analysis. *Adv Learn Behav Disabil* 4:29–47, 1985.

Cantwell D, Baker L: *Developmental Speech and Language Disorders.* New York, Guilford Press, 1987.

Cantwell D, Baker L, Mattison R: The prevalence of psychiatric disorder in children with speech and language disorder: An epidemiologic study. *J Am Acad Child Psychiatry* 18:450–461, 1979.

Conti-Ramsden G: Maternal recasts and other contingent replies to language-impaired children. *J Speech Hear Disord* 55:262–274, 1990.

Conture E, Schwartz H, Brewer D: Laryngeal behavior during stuttering: A further study. *J Speech Hear Res* 28:233–240, 1985.

Coster W, Cicchetti D: Research on the communicative development of maltreated children: Clinical implications. *Top Lang Disord* 13(4):25–38, 1993.

Coster W, Gersten M, Beeghly M, et al: Communicative functioning in maltreated toddlers. *Dev Psychol* 25:1020–1029, 1989.

Craig H, Evans J: Pragmatics and SLI: Within-group variations in discourse behaviors. *J Speech Hear Res* 36:777–789, 1993.

Curtiss S, Tallal P: On the question of subgroups in language impaired children: A first report. Paper presented at the Tenth Annual Boston University Conference of Language Development, 1985.

Dunn C, Davis B: Phonological process occurrence in phonologically disordered children. *Appl Psycholinguist* 4:187–207, 1983.

Edwards M: Speech disability in children: Some general considerations. *Int Rehabil Med* 6:114–116, 1984.

Eisenson J: *Aphasia in Children.* New York, Harper & Row, 1972.

Fey M: *Language Intervention with Young Children.* San Diego, College-Hill Press, 1986.

Fox L, Long S, Anglois A: Patterns of language comprehension deficit in abused and neglected children. *J Speech Hear Disord* 53:239–244, 1988.

Freeman F: Stuttering. In: Lass N, McReynolds L, Northern J, et al (eds): *Speech, Language, and Hearing: Pathologies of Speech and Language* (Vol 2). Philadelphia, Saunders, 1982, pp. 673–691.

Fundudis T, Kolvin I, Garside R: *Speech Retarded and Deaf Children: Their Psychological Development.* New York, Academic Press, 1987.

Gardner H: *Frames of Mind: The Theory of Multiple Intelligences.* New York, Basic Books, 1983.

Gerring J, Carney J: *Head Trauma: Strategies for Educational Reintegration* (2nd ed). San Diego, Singular Publishing Group, 1992.

Giddan J: School children with emotional problems and communication deficits: Implications for speech-language pathologists. *Lang Speech Hear Serv Schools* 22:291–295, 1991.

Graham J Jr, Bashir A, Stark R: Communicative disorders. In: Levine M, Carey W, Crocker A, et al (eds): *Developmental-Behavioral Pediatrics*. Philadelphia, Saunders, 1983, pp. 847–864.

Gravel J, Wallace I: Listening and language at 4 years of age: Effects of early otitis media. *J Speech Hear Res* 35:588–595, 1992.

Hall P, Tomblin J: A follow-up study of children with articulation and language disorders. *J Speech Hear Disord* 43: 227–241, 1978.

Ham R: *Therapy of Stuttering: Preschool through Adolescence*. Englewood Cliffs, NJ, Prentice-Hall, 1990.

Hayden T: Classification of elective mutism. *J Am Acad Child Psychiatry* 19:118–133, 1980.

Hesselman S: Elective mutism in children 1877–1981: A literary summary. *Acta Paedopsychiatr* 49:297–310, 1983.

Hixon T, Shriberg L, Saxman J (eds): *Introduction to Communication Disorders*. Englewood Cliffs, NJ, Prentice-Hall, 1980.

Ingram D: *Phonological Disability in Children*. New York, Elsevier, 1976.

Johnston J, Ramstad V: Cognitive development in pre-adolescent language impaired children. In: Burns M, Andrews EJ (eds): *Selected Papers in Language and Phonology*. Evanston, IL, Institute for Continuing Professional Education, 1978.

Johnston J, Weismer S: Mental rotation abilities in language-disordered children. *J Speech Hear Res* 26:397–404, 1983.

Kamhi A: Developmental vs. different theories of mental retardation: A new look. *Am J Ment Defic* 86:1–7, 1981.

Kamhi A, Catts H, Koenig L, et al: Hypothesis testing and nonlinguistic symbolic activities in language impaired children. *J Speech Hear Disord* 49: 169–176, 1984.

Kaplan S, Escoll P: Treatment of two silent adolescent girls. *J Am Acad Child Psychiatry* 12:59–71, 1973.

Kidd K: A genetic perspective on stuttering. *J Fluency Disord* 2:259–269, 1977.

King C, Quigley S: *Reading and Deafness*. San Diego, College-Hill Press, 1985.

Knutson J, Sullivan P: Communicative disorders as a risk factor in abuse. *Top Lang Disord* 13:1–14, 1993.

Kolvin T, Fundudis T: Elective mute children: Psychological development and background factors. *J Child Psychol Psychiatry* 22:219–232, 1981.

Kratochwill T: *Selective Mutism: Implications for Research and Treatment*. Hillsdale, NJ, Erlbaum, 1981.

Labbe E, Williamson D: Behavioral treatment of elective mutism: A review of the literature. *Clin Psychol Rev* 4:273–292, 1984.

Lahey M: *Language Disorders and Language Development*. New York, Macmillan, 1988.

Landau W, Kleffner F: Syndrome of acquired aphasia with convulsive disorder in children. *Neurology* 7:523–530, 1957.

Lee L: Developmental sentence types: A method for comparing normal and deviant syntactic development. *J Speech Hear Disord* 31:311–330, 1966.

Leonard L: What is deviant language? *J Speech Hear Disord* 37:427–446, 1972.

Leonard L: Is specific language impairment a useful construct? In: Rosenberg S (ed): *Advances in Applied Psycholinguistics. Vol 1: Disorders of First Language Acquisition*. New York, Cambridge University Press, 1987, pp. 1–39.

Leonard L: Language learnability and specific language impairment in children. *Appl Psycholinguist* 10:179–202, 1989.

Leonard L: Specific language impairment as a clinical category. *Lang Speech Hear Serv Schools* 22:66–68, 1991.

Lucas E: *Semantic and Pragmatic Language Disorders*. Rockville, MD, Aspen, 1980.

Lynch M, Roberts J: *The Consequences of Child Abuse*. New York, Academic Press, 1982.

Madison C: Spontaneous remission of misarticulations. *Percept Mot Skills* 54:135–142, 1982.

Menyuk P: Comparison of grammar of children with functionally deviant and normal speech. *J Speech Hear Res* 7:109–121, 1964.

Miller J, Chapman R: Disorders of communication: Investigating the development of mentally retarded children. *Am J Ment Defic* 88:536–545, 1984.

Naremore R: Language disorders in children. In: Hixon T, Shriberg L, Saxman J (eds): *Introduction to Communication Disorders*. Englewood Cliffs, NJ, Prentice-Hall, 1980.

Nelson N: *Childhood Language Disorders in Context: Infancy through Adolescence*. Columbus, OH, Merrill, 1993.

Paul R: Communication. In: Cohen D, Donnellan A, Paul R (eds): *Handbook of Autism and Pervasive Developmental Disorders*. New York, Wiley, 1987.

Paul R: Specific developmental language disorders. In: Michels R (ed): *Psychiatry*. New York, Lippincott, 1993.

Paul R: Patterns of development in late talkers: Preschool years. *J Child Commun Disord* 15:7–14, 1993b.

Paul R: Clinical implications of the natural history of slow expressive language development. Miniseminar presented at American Speech, Language, Hearing Association National Convention, New Orleans, 1994.

Paul R, Cohen D: Outcomes of severe disorders of language acquisition. *J Autism Dev Disord* 14:405–421, 1984.

Paul R, Elwood T: Maternal linguistic input to toddlers with slow expressive language development. *J Speech Hear Res* 34:982–988, 1991.

Paul R, Lynn T, Lohr-Flanders M: History of middle ear involvement and speech/language development in late talkers. *J Speech Hear Res* 36:1055–1062, 1993.

Perkins W: Disorders of speech flow. In: Hixon T, Shriberg L, Saxon J (eds): *Introduction to Communication Disorders*. Englewood Cliffs, NJ, Prentice-Hall, 1980, pp. 450–489.

Prizant B, Meyer E: Socioemotional aspects of language and social-communication disorders in young children. *Am J Speech-Lang Pathol J Clin Pract* 2(3):56–71, 1993.

Prizant B, Audet L, Burke G, et al: Communication disorders and emotional/behavioral disorders in children and adolescents. *J Speech Hear Res* 55:179–192, 1990.

Quigley S, Power D, Steinkamp M: The language structure of deaf children. *Volta Rev* 79:73–84, 1977.

Rapin I, Allen D: Developmental language disorders: Nosologic considerations. In: Kirk U (ed): *Neuropsychology of Language, Reading, and Spelling*. New York: Academic, 1983.

Riddle M, Anderson G, Cicchetti D, et al: Increases with whole brain radiation in childhood leukemia [Summary]. Scientific Proceedings of the Annual Meeting of the American Academy of Child and Adolescent Psychiatry, VII, 1991, p. 63.

Roberts J, Burchinal M, Davis B, et al: Otitis media in early childhood and later language. *J Speech Hear Res* 34:1158–1168, 1991.

Roeser R: Cochlear implants and tactile aids for the profoundly deaf student. In: Roeser RJ, Downs MP (eds): *Auditory Disorders in School Children*. New York, Thieme, 1988, pp. 260–280.

Russell N: Educational considerations in traumatic brain injury: The role of the speech-language pathologist. *Lang Speech Hear Serv Schools* 24:67–75, 1993.

Satz P, Bullard-Bates C: Acquired aphasia in children. In: Sarno MT (ed): *Acquired Aphasia*. New York, Academic Press, 1981.

Scarborough H, Dobrich W: Development of children with early language delay. *J Speech Hear Disord* 33:70–83, 1990.

Shriberg L, Kwiatkowski J: A follow-up study of children with phonological disorders of unknown origin. *J Speech Hear Disord* 53:144–155, 1988.

Shriberg L, Widder C: Speech and prosody characteristics of adults with mental retardation. *J Speech Hear Res* 33:627–653, 1990.

Sparks S: *Children of Prenatal Substance Abuse*. San Diego, Singular Publishing Group, 1993.

Tallal P: Developmental language disorders. In: Kavanagh JF, Truss TJ Jr (eds): *Learning Disabilities: Proceedings of the National Conference*. Parkton, MD: York Press, 1988, pp. 181–272.

Tallal P, Ross R, Curtiss S: Familial aggregation in specific language impairment. *J Speech Hear Disord* 54:167–173, 1989.

Tomblin J: Children's language disorders. In: Curtis J (ed): *Processes and Disorders of Human Communication*. New York, Harper & Row, 1978, pp. 246–271.

Trantham C, Pedersen J: *Normal Language Development: The Key to Diagnosis and Therapy for Language Disordered Children*. Baltimore, Williams & Wilkins, 1976.

Trybus R, Karchmer M: School achievement scores of hearing impaired children: National data on achievement status and growth patterns. *Am Ann Deaf Directory Programs Services* 122:62–69, 1977.

United States Department of Education: Ninth Annual Report to Congress: US Department of Education, Washington, DC, 1987.

Van Riper C: *The Treatment of Stuttering*. Englewood Cliffs, NJ, Prentice-Hall, 1973.

Weiner F: Systematic sound preference as a characteristic of phonological disability. *J Speech Hear Disord* 46:281–286, 1981.

Weiner F: Treatment of phonological disability using the method of meaningful minimal contrast: Two case studies. *J Speech Hear Disord* 46:97–103, 1981.

Whitehurst G, Fischel J: Early developmental language delay: What, if anything, should the clinician do about it? *J Child Psychol Psychiatry*, 35: 613–648, 1994.

Whitehurst G, Falco F, Lonigan C, et al: Accelerating language development through picture-book reading. *Dev Psychol* 24:552–558, 1988.

Zirkelbach T, Blakesley K: The language deficient child in the classroom. *Acad Ther* 20:605–612, 1985.

48 Developmental Learning Disorders

Larry B. Silver, M.D.

DEFINITION

Developmental learning disorders are listed in DSM-IV under the Axis II diagnosis of learning disorders. These disorders are characterized by inadequate development of specific academic, language, speech, and motor skills that are not due to demonstrable physical or neurologic disorders, a pervasive developmental disorder, mental retardation, or deficient educational opportunities. These disorders are subgrouped as

1. Learning disorders
   a. Reading disorder
   b. Mathematics disorder
   c. Disorder of written expression
2. Communication disorders
   a. Developmental expressive language disorder
   b. Mixed receptive/expressive language disorder
   c. Phonological disorder (articulation disorder)
   d. Stuttering
3. Motor skills disorder
   a. Developmental coordination disorder

This chapter addresses the learning disorders.

The DSM-IV conforms to the international classification system, thus the above-noted diagnostic categories. The term used by the educational system in the United States is *learning disability.* Thus, clinicians may use DSM-IV codes for third-party forms but refer to the term *learning disability* when interacting with the family or school system.

The DSM-IV definition of a learning disorder relates to the individual's ability in specific areas. An individual has one of the disorders if his or her ability is "substantially below the expected given the person's chronological age, measured intelligence, and age-appropriate education." No clarification is given on the extent of the disability needed to be "substantial." Within the public school system, the definition of a learning disability is based on a specific level of discrepancy. As will be discussed later, the definition of the extent of the discrepancy may vary from school system to school system. It is not uncommon for a child or adolescent to meet the medical criteria for having a learning disorder but not meet the educational criteria for having a learning disability.

The definition of a learning disability is based on Public Law 94-142, Education for Handicapped Children and its revision, Public Law 101-476, Individuals with Disabilities Education Act (IDEA). In this law, learning disability is defined as a disorder in one or more of the basic psychological processes involved in understanding or in using language, spoken or written, which may manifest itself in an imperfect ability to listen, think, speak, read, write, spell, or to do mathematical calculations. The term includes such conditions as perceptual handicaps, brain injury, minimal brain dysfunction, dyslexia, and developmental aphasia. The term does not include children who have learning problems that are primarily the result of visual, hearing, or motor handicaps; mental retardation; emotional disturbance; or environmental, cultural, or economic disadvantage.

The most recent federal guidelines for determining if a student is eligible for special programs for learning disabilities list four criteria (reviewed in Silver and Hagin, 1992): (*a*) documented evidence indicating that general education has been attempted and found to be ineffective in meeting the student's educational needs; (*b*) evidence of a disorder in one or more of the basic psychological processes required for learning

(A psychological process is a set of mental operations that transform, access, or manipulate information. The disorder is relatively enduring and limits ability to perform specific academic or developmental learning tasks. It may be manifested differently at different developmental levels.); (*c*) evidence of academic achievement significantly below the student's level of intellectual function (A difference of 1.5–1.75 S.D. between achievement and intellectual functioning is considered significant.) on basic reading skills, reading comprehension, mathematic calculation, mathematic reasoning, or written expression; and (*d*) evidence that the learning problems are not due primarily to other handicapping conditions, i.e., visual acuity, auditory acuity, physical impairment, emotional handicap, mental retardation, cultural differences, or environmental deprivation.

The presence of a CNS processing deficit is essential for the diagnosis of a learning disability. A child might meet the discrepancy criteria, but without central processing deficits in functions required for learning, he or she is not considered to have a learning disability.

Within public school systems, it is the extent of discrepancy between potential and actual achievement that determines who will be eligible for services and who will not (Chalfant, 1989). Different school systems use different models for determining the extent of discrepancy (reviewed in Silver and Hagin, 1992, 1993).

Historical Background

Prior to the 1940s in the United States, children who had academic difficulties were considered to be mentally retarded, emotionally disturbed, or socially and culturally disadvantaged. During the 1940s a fourth possibility for these difficulties was introduced: Children might have problems with academic performance for neurological reasons. That is, the cause of the difficulty is presumed to be related to brain function. Two different research approaches explored these neurologically based learning disorders.

One group of researchers noted that these children had the same types of learning difficulties as known brain-damaged individuals. They concluded that these children also had brain damage; however, it was so subtle or minimal that it could not be confirmed clinically. The term *minimal brain damage* was introduced (Strauss and Lehtinen, 1947; Werner and Strauss, 1941). Other researchers explored the possibility that the learning difficulties reflected a brain that functioned differently, possibly due to being "wired" differently rather than to being damaged. The term *minimal brain dysfunction* was used to reflect this concept (Clements, 1966). Recent research, discussed later, supports the concept of brain dysfunction rather than of brain damage.

Initially, the types of academic difficulties were described based on the primary skill disorder (reviewed in Farnham-Diggory, 1978). Reading disorders were called dyslexia, writing disorders were called dysgraphia, and arithmetic disorders were called dyscalculia. Later efforts focused on the underlying learning difficulties or learning disabilities that caused the problems with reading, writing, and arithmetic. The term *learning disability* was introduced. At this time the preferred term within education is learning disability.

Prevalence

The true prevalence of learning disabilities is not known. The problem is the many case definitions used over time in different studies. The

Centers for Disease Control (1987) attempted to establish the prevalence of this disorder. These researchers concluded that because the definition and the diagnostic criteria for learning disabilities have not been standardized, consistency in the design of prevalence studies has not been maintained. Thus, accurate analyses of data over time are not possible. In the absence of good prevalence data, they concluded that between 5 and 10% was a reasonable estimate of the percentage of persons affected by learning disabilities. Until a uniform definition and uniform diagnostic criteria are used, more accurate data will not be available.

Studies consistently note an increased prevalence of this disorder in males. The ratio ranges from 3:1 to 5:1 and higher (Ackerman et al., 1983; Finucci and Childs, 1981; Rutter et al., 1976). Recent studies suggest that this increased prevalence in males over females may, in part, be explained by referral bias. Males, because they are more likely to act out, are more likely to be referred for study (Berry et al., 1985). Females, when frustrated, may become anxious or depressed more than disruptive and may not be recognized as quickly as having difficulty. Females appear to tolerate deficits in reading and spelling skills more easily than males, showing less antipathy to reading and less emotional impact (Finucci and Childs, 1981). Johnson and Blalock (1987) found no specific cognitive differences or patterns of problems between the sexes.

Associated Disorders

Individuals with a learning disorder might have an emotional or behavioral problem. Many develop social problems. They might also have a related neurological disorder. The interrelationship and statistical comorbidity between these conditions is still being clarified. It is critical to be aware of these associated disorders. Each disorder should be considered and, if present, diagnosed. The treatment plan must address each disorder present.

EMOTIONAL/BEHAVIORAL PROBLEMS

It is not uncommon for children and adolescents with a learning disorder to have a diagnosable psychiatric disorder. For many, these psychological problems are secondary to the frustrations and failures experienced because the disabilities were not identified or were inadequately treated (Silver LB, 1989, 1993).

For others, these psychological problems may be another reflection of a dysfunctional nervous system. The behavioral or emotional manifestations might be the individual's characteristic style for coping with a dysfunctional nervous system. Studies of youth diagnosed as having a conduct disorder or young adults diagnosed as having a personality disorder, especially the borderline type, show that about one-third have unrecognized or recognized but poorly treated learning disabilities (Forness, 1981; Hunt and Cohen, 1984; Rutter et al., 1970). Similar findings have been observed with adolescent boys in detention centers (Berman and Siegal, 1976; Keilitz, 1979; Lewis et al., 1979; Lewis and Balla, 1980; Mauser, 1974; Robbins et al., 1983).

SOCIAL PROBLEMS

The learning disabilities that result in learning disorders may directly contribute to peer problems by interfering with success in doing activities required to interact with certain age groups (e.g., visual perception and visual motor problems interfering with ability to quickly do such eye-hand activities as catching, hitting, or throwing a ball).

Children and adolescents with learning disabilities may have difficulty learning social skills and being socially competent (reviewed in Hazel and Schumaker, 1988). These individuals do not pick up such social cues as facial expressions, tone of voice, or body language and adapt their behaviors appropriately. Rourke identifies a specific subtype of learning disabilities, called nonverbal learning disabilities, that often appear to be associated with social skill problems (Rourke, 1987, 1988, 1989; Rourke and Fuerst, 1991). With some, he reports a difficulty in social and emotional functioning that includes a predisposition toward adolescent and adult depression and suicide risk (Rourke et al., 1986).

NEUROLOGICAL DISORDERS

The first neurologically based disorder recognized as frequently associated with a learning disability (learning disorder) was attention deficit hyperactivity disorder (Halperin et al., 1984; Silver LB, 1981). Recent studies suggest that there is a continuum of disorders associated with neurological dysfunction that are often found together. Thus, when one is diagnosed, the others must be considered in the diagnostic process.

The related theme appears to be that, if something impacts on the developing brain during pregnancy or during the critical early months of life, the effects will depend on which areas of the brain are involved and when and for how long the impact took place. In approximately 40% of cases, this impact might be based on a familial pattern and be directed by the genetic code or might relate to subtle shifts or changes in specific amino acids at the level of the gnome. In most cases, the cause or type of impact is not known.

The result is that some of the circuits or "wires" are laid down differently. We classify the presenting problems by the areas of faulty "wiring" or dysfunction. If the dysfunctional areas interfere with receiving, processing, and expressing information, the clinical problem is called a learning disability (learning disorder). If the dysfunctional areas result in difficulty receiving, processing, and expressing language, it is referred to as a language disability. If the dysfunctional areas result in hyperactivity, distractibility, and/or impulsivity, the clinical problem is called attention deficit hyperactivity disorder (ADHD). Recent studies and studies in progress suggest that other disorders might be part of this continuum of neurological dysfunctions. Each might reflect the brain's difficulty modulating the many stimulant and inhibitory functions involved with cognitive, language, and motor functioning. For some, the problems relate to integrating and modulating the sensory inputs needed to coordinate body movement and motor planning activities. This clinical problem is called a sensory integrative disorder (SID). If the dysfunctional areas relate to certain modulating tasks, the clinical picture might include motor or vocal tics and the clinical picture is called a chronic motor tic disorder or Tourette's Disorder (TD) or the clinical picture might include obsessive thoughts or compulsive behaviors and be called an obsessive compulsive disorder (OCD).

The early statistical data supporting the concept of a "continuum of neurological dysfunctions" are growing. For individuals with learning disabilities, 20–25% have ADHD (Halperin et al., 1984; Silver, 1981). Depending on the criteria used to define a learning disability, 30–70% of individuals with ADHD have a learning disability (reviewed in Biederman et al., 1992). About 60% of patients with TD have a learning disability (Hagin and Kuler, 1988; Hagin et al., 1982). Further, 50% of individuals with TD have ADHD (Comings, 1990; Comings and Comings, 1987, 1988). Fifty percent of patients with TD have OCD (Frankel et al., 1986; Pauls et al., 1990; Pitman et al., 1987). A study by Silver (in press) attempts to correlate the frequency with which children and adolescents with a learning disability also have a language disability, ADHD, SID, TD, and/or OCD.

SPECIFIC DEVELOPMENTAL LEARNING DISORDERS

Before describing the specific developmental disorders related to reading, writing, and arithmetic, it is helpful to review the concept of specific learning disabilities. The evaluation process focuses on the specific learning disabilities, not just the presenting skill disorders. It is the knowledge of the specific learning disabilities and learning abilities that is useful in explaining the problems to parents, children, and adolescents and is useful in planning the necessary interventions.

The tests used to do psychological and educational evaluations relating to learning and possible learning disorders use an information processing or cybernetics model. Learning is evaluated based on the steps for processing information in the brain. The first task is to receive the information and record it in the brain (input). Once recorded, this information must be handled in such a way that it can be understood (integration). The third process is storage and retrieval (memory). Finally, information must be communicated from the brain (output).

Learning disabilities are defined based on this input-integration-memory-output model. Each area will be described briefly.

Input Disabilities

The central brain process is called perception; a person might have a visual perception disability or an auditory perception disability. Visual perception disabilities might be reflected in distinguishing subtle differences in shapes (misperceiving *d* and *b*, or *p* and *q*, or *6* and *9*). One might have difficulty with figure-ground tasks, that is, not be able to focus on the relevant stimulus in a field of vision. Judging distance or depth is another visual perceptual task. A child or adolescent might misjudge depth, bumping into things or falling off a chair.

Auditory perception disabilities might be in the area of distinguishing subtle differences in sounds, thus misunderstanding what is being said. There are 43 units of sound in the English language, called phonemes. Many words sound similar, such as *hair* and *air*, *ball* and *bell*. Some individuals have difficulty with auditory figure-ground, confusing what sounds to listen to when there is more than one source. Some children and adolescents cannot process sound inputs quickly. They appear to have to think about what is heard briefly, but longer than normal, before understanding what is said. This is called an auditory processing problem or an auditory lag. They appear to be lost or confused when too much is said and may appear to be preoccupied.

Integration Disabilities

At least three steps are needed to understand what is recorded in the brain. The individual incoming stimuli must be placed in the correct order (sequencing), then understood in the context used (abstraction), and finally integrated with all other incoming stimuli plus all relevant memory tracks into a concept (organization). One can have an integrative disability in any of these areas: sequencing, abstraction, or organization. Such a disability might be more for visual or for auditory inputs. Thus, one can have visual-sequencing or auditory-sequencing disabilities, visual-abstraction or auditory-abstraction disabilities, and so forth.

Sequencing disabilities can result in an individual's confusing inputs, for example, writing *21* rather than *12*, *dog* rather than *god*, or mixing up the parts of words and mispronouncing the word. A child might try to explain something but start in the middle, then go to the beginning, and finally to the end. These individuals often have difficulty using sequences. They can memorize the months of the year, for example, but be unable to say what comes after any month without starting with January and working their way up.

The inability to derive the correct meaning of a word based on how it is used can result in an abstraction disability. These individuals may have difficulty generalizing out from specific words or concepts. They might miss the meaning of jokes, puns, idioms, or other plays on words. They may appear to be paranoid because they interpret what others say in a more concrete or literal way than what is intended.

Organizational disabilities can result in difficulty pulling multiple parts of information into a full or complete concept or in difficulty breaking down whole concepts into parts. Such individuals may show this ''disorganization'' in other aspects of their life. Their notebooks or desk or their room may be totally disorganized. Organizing time or making plans might be difficult. They lose things, forget things, or do their homework but forget to turn it in.

Memory Disabilities

Children or adolescents with learning disabilities usually have excellent long-term memory. They can retain information once stored. They might have difficulty, however, in short-term memory, the ability to concentrate on information and store it. They might learn information well while attending to it (spelling list, math concept, etc.), yet they will not retain this information a short time later. These students need many more repetitions to process information into long-term memory than do the average students. They can learn, but they must work on the process

over time. One might have a visual-short-term memory disability or an auditory-short-term memory disability.

Output Disabilities

One may have difficulty getting information out of the brain through oral communication (i.e., a language disability) or through the use of muscles (i.e., a motor disability). The individual may have a disability in one or both of these areas.

Most individuals have little difficulty with spontaneous language. In this situation, the person initiates the conversation. There is the opportunity to organize thoughts and find words before speaking. Some individuals might have difficulty with demand language. If such people are asked to produce language, they must organize their thoughts and find the right words as they speak. They might speak with ease when they initiate the conversation; however, they might not be able to respond when asked a question or requested to speak. In this situation, they might struggle for words, ramble, or say the wrong word and appear to be disorganized.

Some people with learning disabilities will have trouble coordinating the use of groups of large muscles (gross motor disability). Others may have difficulty coordinating groups of small muscles (fine motor disability). Gross motor disabilities will result in the individual's being clumsy or having difficulty with such activities as running, climbing, or swimming. The most frequently found fine motor disability relates to writing. This skill requires the coordination of teams of small muscles. These individuals have difficulty getting their dominant hand to write in a fast and legible way. In addition to having poor handwriting, they may have difficulty with such written language tasks as spelling, grammar, spacing, or punctuation.

Learning Disability Profile

Each individual with a learning disability will have his or her own profile of learning abilities and learning disabilities. Each will have one or more of the above-described disabilities. There is no stereotyped individual; each must be assessed and understood individually. These learning disabilities can result in academic skill, language, or motor skill disorders.

DEVELOPMENTAL READING DISORDER

Definition

In DSM-IV there are three criteria for establishing this disorder: (*a*) Reading achievement, as measured by an individually administered standardized test of reading accuracy or comprehension, is substantially below that expected, given the person's chronological age, measured intelligence, and age-appropriate education; (*b*) the disturbance in achievement significantly interferes with academic achievement or activities of daily living that require reading skills; and (*c*) if a sensory deficit is present, the learning difficulties are in excess of those usually associated with it.

Children who experience problems in reading typically have difficulty in decoding the letter-sound associations involved in phonic analysis (reviewed in Shepherd and Uhry, 1993). As a result, they may read in a disjointed manner, knowing a few words on sight and stumbling across other unfamiliar words. They might guess. If they have difficulty with visual tracking, they might skip words or lines. If comprehension is a problem, they will report that they have to read material repeatedly before they understand.

Etiology

The process of reading involves two tasks, decoding, or word recognition, and reading comprehension. Decoding refers to the act of transcribing a printed word into speech. Comprehension refers to the process of interpreting the message or meaning of the text. Decoding is unique to reading and different from the recognition of words in speech; however, the linguistic skills that subserve reading comprehension are the same for both reading and listening.

Research shows that the primary disabilities are related to verbal or linguistic deficits and not to visual processing disorders (reviewed in Johnson, 1988; Tallal, 1985). Reading disabilities may occur in one of three ways (reviewed in Shepherd and Uhry, 1993): (a) The ability to decode might be impaired but comprehension is intact. Most students with a reading disorder have this problem. (b) Decoding could be intact but comprehension is impaired. This relatively rare problem is the reverse of dyslexia and is called hyperlexia. Students can read almost any text but do not understand the text read. (c) Both decoding and comprehension could be impaired. This double impairment results from a general cognitive impairment and is usually called reading backwardness.

Most students with a reading disorder have difficulty acquiring the knowledge and skills essential for rapid automatic decoding. Because spelling uses the same knowledge as word recognition, it is also frequently impaired. Reading comprehension, thus, is limited by weak decoding skills.

Diagnosis

The cause and specific distinguishing features of this disorder are not known. The diagnosis is made by first establishing a discrepancy between reading skill and intelligence and then systematically eliminating all other explanations for the discrepancy.

Treatment

Direct instruction in reading (and spelling and writing) is considered the essential treatment for a student with a reading disorder. These efforts are provided by a person trained to use appropriate remedial methods. These methods emphasize explicit instruction in letter-sound associations. Instruction is described as multisensory. Children see a letter and hear its name and sound; they trace the letter saying its name and sound; and, then they write the letter repeating its name and sound. Sounds and letters are blended to form words. Reading, spelling, and writing are taught simultaneously. Instruction involves extended practice and is supplemented by speech segmentation training and study skills instructions. Parents are asked to read to their children to enhance appreciation of reading and to give the children access to knowledge normally obtained by reading.

Reading disorders are not cured. Even with appropriate interventions, children and adolescents with this disorder learn to read and spell at a slower rate than normally developing individuals. It is essential for this student to learn compensatory skills and for the classroom teachers to provide essential accommodations.

DEVELOPMENTAL DISORDER OF WRITTEN EXPRESSION

Definition

In DSM-IV there are three essential criteria for establishing this disorder: (a) Writing skills, as measured by an individually administered standardized test (or functional assessment of writing skills), are substantially below that expected given the person's chronological age, measured intelligence, and age-appropriate education; (b) the disturbance in skills significantly interferes with academic achievement or activities of daily living that require the composition of written texts (e.g., writing grammatically correct sentences and organized paragraphs); and (c) if a sensory deficit is present, the learning difficulties are in excess of those usually associated with it.

It is helpful to distinguish between a fine motor problem that results in difficulty with the mechanics of writing and a language-based learning disability that results in problems with the language of writing. Individuals with a disorder of written expression might have a fine motor problem but always have a language-based disorder, resulting in difficulty with spelling, grammar, punctuation, capitalization, and/or composition.

Etiology

For skilled writing, there must be an automatization of most of the lower level mental activities. These lower level mental activities guide handwriting, spelling, word choice, and the construction of sentences that conform to the conventions of written language. Lower-level mental activities also guide the construction of textual connections, specifically connections between sentences. If these activities are functioning, the writer's attention can focus on the content, organization, and clarity of the task. One can shift attention between levels of mental processing without losing control of the text. Difficulties with lower-level mental activities are probably the source of the problem in expressive writing disorder (reviewed in Uhry and Shepherd, 1993).

Research focuses on the relationship between writing disorders and reading disorders (Johnson, 1988). They may be linked in two ways. First, the same linguistic deficits that impede learning to read (phonological awareness) could impede learning to write and spell. Further, slow progress in learning to read might deprive the child of knowledge about writing that is gained by reading (e.g., about sentences, punctuation, spelling).

Diagnosis

The diagnosis is made by first establishing a discrepancy between writing skill and intelligence and then systematically eliminating all other explanations for the discrepancy.

Treatment

Treatment for a writing disorder might involve a skills approach or a holistic approach (reviewed in Uhry and Shepherd, 1993). Skills programs are often used with younger children and focus on letter-sound associations, focusing on reading and spelling. Children might be asked to listen carefully for the sounds in words and then to represent these sounds with written letters, saying each letter aloud as it is written.

The holistic approach to writing begins with the student's ideas. It involves a series of highly structured steps for narrowing ideas to one topic, writing a first draft, reading it aloud to an audience of peers, and then refining organization and language. The final step involves working on mechanics in preparation for ''publishing'' a draft for peers to read.

Most efforts combine these two approaches. Children with a writing disorder need direct, sequential instructions in letter-sound associations and in spelling rules as well as in sentence structure and the connections between sentences and paragraphs that make text cohesive. Even with good remedial interventions, writing requires enormous effort because the disorder is not ''cured'' but compensated for and this compensation must continue into adulthood. Appropriate accommodations, such as using a computer, may be needed throughout the individual's education and career. The use of the computer is an example of using strengths to compensate for weaknesses. Writing requires detailed fine motor planning, using one's dominant hand. Typing requires the use of the lower arm muscles to lower and raise the fingers and, thus, is predominantly a gross motor planning task. Individuals who write slowly and with difficulty might be able to type with great speed and accuracy.

MATHEMATICS DISORDER

Definition

In DSM-IV three criteria are used to establish this diagnosis: (a) Mathematical ability, as measured by an individually administered standardized test, is substantially below the expected, given the person's chronological age, measured intelligence, and age-appropriate education; (b) the disturbance in ability significantly interferes with academic achievement or activities of daily living that require mathematical ability; and (c) if a sensory deficit is present, the learning difficulties are in excess of those usually associated with it.

Children and adolescents with a mathematics disorder may have a wide range of symptoms, including delays in the acquisition of basic spatial and number concepts, problems learning and using number words and number facts or writing numbers correctly (and in correct alignment when doing computations), and difficulty in applying arithmetic skills when solving everyday problems. Because math achievement is highly dependent on the quality of instruction offered students, it may be that a significant number of those students who are coded as having a learning disability by the school system do not have intrinsic math disorders but have not had appropriate instruction.

Etiology

Research suggests that there may be several factors involved in mathematics achievement (Johnson, 1988). In addition, knowing how to use the correct strategy is important (reviewed in Fleischner and Garnett, 1993). Information-processing capabilities research suggests that one area of difficulty might be in visual-spatial processing deficits. Another problem might relate to the ability to use the necessary pattern of strategic behaviors associated with arithmetic learning. Proficiency in mathematics requires more than computational skills. The difficulty might be in an inability to develop a systematic plan for problem solution. Memory is essential to the ability to do mathematics. One must retain basic number facts. In addition, it is necessary to remember specific equations or other steps necessary to solve a problem. Once a problem is started, students must remember where they are in the process as they proceed from step to step.

Diagnosis

The diagnosis is made by first establishing a discrepancy between arithmetic skill and intelligence and then systematically eliminating all other explanations for the discrepancy.

TREATMENT

Treatment involves general concerns and specific interventions (reviewed in Fleischner and Garnett, 1993). Initially, the problem of anxiety, withdrawal, defeatism, or other responses to repeated failure must be addressed. Much of the teaching of math is based on criticism of failure. The emphasis is on getting the right answer rather than in problem-solving. Because of this overfocus on getting the right answer, children may develop performance anxiety or feel they are stupid in math. For some, the premature pressure for speeded answers can short-circuit reasoning and foster impulsivity, resulting in the belief that math has little to do with thinking. Students who have difficulty with math memory may be deprived of compensatory techniques, only adding to the problem. They are told that it is shameful to use their fingers or to mark down intermediate calculations or to use a calculator. These are considered as ''cheating.''

Sometimes the difficulties reflect poor teaching in math. Further, math learning is very instruction bound. Absenteeism, missed lessons, and inconsistency of instruction can leave gaps that result in persistent confusion. Those students with learning disabilities in the areas that result in deficits in short-term memory, language, attention, or spatial perception and students with ADHD are especially susceptible to weak instruction. Appropriately focused and systematic instruction in improving math abilities may be all that is needed.

Specific interventions focus on the underlying difficulties. Some students have problems relating to acquiring the conceptual underpinnings of the subject, and some have problems relating to procedural learning, recall of discrete information, and self-monitoring. These remedial efforts must take into account the student's areas of learning abilities and learning disabilities.

NEUROLOGICAL EXPLANATION FOR DEVELOPMENTAL LEARNING DISORDERS

Research into these developmental disorders has focused primarily on the reading disabilities. Such studies show a higher incidence in males (Ackerman et al., 1983; Finucci and Childs, 1981) and a strong familial pattern (reviewed in Duane, 1989). There is more than suggestive evidence that reading disorders occur more frequently in non-right-handed people (Geschwind and Behan, 1982).

Gross and microscopic studies of the brain as well as newer imaging techniques have focused on finding the proposed biological substrate for reading disorders and other learning disabilities (reviewed in Duane, 1989). Recent studies by Galaburda et al. (1985) on detailed microscopic analysis of the brains of individuals known to have had dyslexia strongly support the concept of ''faulty wiring.'' Each case studied demonstrated the same microscopic findings: (a) neurons in places where they are normally absent (ectopias), (b) cortical cellular disorganizations (dysplasias), and (c) polymicrogyria. These cortical anomalies were located predominantly in the left hemisphere and mainly around the left sylvian fissure. These findings have been interpreted as anomalies of neuronal migration that are most likely to have occurred between the 16th and 24th weeks of gestation. It is suggested that these findings are not due to genetic factors but may be due to the male sex steroid testosterone from the male fetus or from maternal circulation, which may induce the above-described cortical cell migration anomalies (Galaburda et al., 1985).

Several prenatal difficulties have been studied in relation to future motor or cognitive difficulties: bleeding in pregnancy, maternal malnutrition and/or anemia, hypertension, fetomaternal blood incompatibility, prematurity (low birth weight or small for gestation), preeclampsia and eclampsia, placental difficulties, cord compression, and postmaturity. No clear relationships to learning difficulties have been established, although some data are suggestive of a correlation.

Follow-up studies from the Perinatal Collaborative Study in the United States (Nichols and Chen, 1981) and the British National Child Development Study (Butler and Goldstein, 1973) suggest that cigarette use by pregnant women may result in a reduction in birth weight and may be associated with academic difficulties by age 7. Similar studies suggest that the use of alcohol in small quantities throughout the pregnancy might result in learning disabilities (Shaywitz et al., 1980).

The impact on the fetus of various medications taken during pregnancy and at delivery and the possible long-term outcomes are being studied. It is known that many of these medications rapidly cross the placenta and enter the fetal circulation. The ability of the neonate to metabolize many drugs is poorly developed, so that the effects of drugs given during labor may persist after delivery, when elimination through the maternal circulation is no longer possible.

With the newer methodologies for studying brain function and dysfunction, it is hoped that a clearer knowledge of the causes of these learning disorders will become known.

Diagnosis of Developmental Learning Disorders

The DSM-IV and education definitions of learning disorders/learning disabilities were discussed earlier. The use of a discrepancy model for determining who would be eligible for services was also discussed.

Children and adolescents with learning disorders (learning disabilities) are often first referred for an evaluation because of their behavior. When a mental health professional evaluates a child or adolescent with emotional, social, and/or family problems plus academic difficulties, it is essential that one differentiate between cause and symptom (reviewed in Silver LB, 1993). Are the emotional, social, and/or family problems causing the academic difficulties, or are they a consequence of the academic difficulties and the resulting frustrations and failures? The emotional, social, and/or family problems may have started from the unrecognized and untreated learning disabilities and then evolved into established disorders that must be treated. It is essential to understand the total clinical picture in designing the treatment plan.

The clinical history will help to raise the suspicion of a learning disability. The clinician should ask about school performance and ability with each academic skill area (reviewed in Ostrander, 1993). If one hears of difficulty with reading or reading comprehension or with written language or mathematics, further studies are needed.

The diagnostic evaluation to rule in or rule out a learning disability is called a psychoeducational assessment. The first studies assess the individual's intellectual level, as well as potential intellectual ability and cognitive style. Next, the current level of academic skills is measured through standardized achievement tests. Finally, a comprehensive special education diagnostic evaluation is done to clarify areas of learning abilities and learning disabilities. These studies should be done by the individual's school system. If this is not possible, they can be done privately and then presented to the school system.

The psychological assessment may consist of a neuropsychological or a clinical psychological evaluation of the individual's intellectual ability. Of importance will be any discrepancies or scatter within the intelligence test. Other psychological studies may focus on perceptual, cognitive, or language abilities. The educational diagnostician will assess the current level of academic skills using achievement tests, as well as evaluate for the presence of learning disabilities using specific test instruments. A speech and language pathologist might do further studies to clarify areas of auditory perception, expressive language, or other language disabilities. An occupational therapist might do further studies to clarify gross or fine motor disabilities or sensory-motor integration difficulties.

The results of these evaluations should establish the presence or absence of a learning disability. If present, the data will clarify the specific areas of learning disability and learning ability. These results, along with the psychosocial and other developmental evaluations, should clarify the diagnosis. If emotional, social, and/or family problems are noted, it should be possible to integrate these diagnoses into a full treatment plan.

It is critical to identify preschoolers as well as school-age children and adolescents. Early intervention works and avoids the experiences of failure later. The term "at risk" is usually used before the student enters the first grade because of the difficulty saying one has a learning disability before being in a setting requiring learning. Although these children have not failed in school learning, we can predict that they are likely candidates for school failure. Among the characteristics seen in preschoolers that are suggestive of learning disabilities are delayed motor development, language delays, speech disorders, poor cognitive abilities (as might be reflected in the level of play obtained), and poor concept development.

Some of the currently used evaluation tests in the United States include the following:

1. Psychological tests
   a. Stanford-Binet Intelligence Scale (ages 2 to adulthood)
   b. Wechsler Pre-School and Primary Scale of Intelligence (WPPSI) (ages 4–6½)
   c. Wechsler Intelligence Scale for Children (WISC) (ages 6–16)
   d. Wechsler Adult Intelligence Scale (WAIS) (ages 16 and over)

2. Achievement tests
   a. Woodcock-Johnson Psychoeducational Battery
   b. Metropolitan Achievement Tests
   c. Peabody Individual Achievement Test
   d. Stanford Diagnostic Achievement Tests
   e. Wide-Range Achievement Tests

3. Educational diagnostic tests
   a. Woodcock-Johnson Psychoeducational Battery
   b. Detroit Tests of Learning Aptitude
   c. Illinois Test of Psycholinguistic Abilities
   d. McCarthy Scales of Children's Abilities
   e. Slingerland Screening Tests for Identifying Children with Specific Language Disabilities

TREATMENT OF DEVELOPMENTAL LEARNING DISORDERS

The treatment of choice for a learning disorder (learning disability) is special education. The specific approaches to treatment were described for each disorder.

If emotional, social, and/or family problems are present, they must be addressed in a multimodal treatment plan. When doing individual, group, family, or behavioral therapy, it is important to be aware of the impact of the learning disabilities on the individual's life, as well as the impact of the disabilities on the treatment itself (Ostrander and Silver, 1993). For example, auditory perception or demand language disabilities may affect any form of a listening-talking therapy.

It is important to explore if any of the other disorders found in the continuum of neurological dysfunctions are present. If so, those disorders must also be treated.

OUTCOME

For most, the disorder will persist through life. The child with a learning disability will become the adolescent with a learning disability who will become the adult with a learning disability. Thus, treatment planning must be adapted to the demands of each developmental stage.

With early recognition and appropriate special education intervention, most individuals can overcome or learn to compensate for the learning disabilities that cause their developmental learning disorder. This treatment may be needed throughout the individual's education. Today there are such services available in postsecondary training programs, vocational programs, and colleges.

As noted earlier, without recognition or treatment, the outcome can be poor. The current view is that the learning disabilities do not cause these problems. It is the lack of appropriate treatment for the learning disabilities that contributes to the cause of these problems. The best preventive intervention is early recognition of the learning disabilities followed by appropriate treatment.

References

Ackerman P, Dykman R, Oglesby D: Sex and group differences in reading and attention disordered children with and without hyperkinesis. *J Learn Disabil* 16:407–415, 1983.

Berry CA, Shaywitz SE, Shaywitz BA: Girls with attention deficit disorder: A silent minority? A report on behavioral and cognitive characteristics. *Pediatrics* 76:801–809, 1985.

Berman A, Siegal A: Adaptive and learning skills in delinquent boys. *J Learn Disabil* 9:583–590, 1976.

Biederman J, Faraone SV, Lapey K: Comorbidity of diagnosis in attention-deficit hyperactivity disorder. In: Weiss G (ed): *Child and Adolescent Psychiatric Clinics of North America. Attention-Deficit Disorder.* (Vol 1, No. 2) October 1992, pp. 335–360.

Butler NR, Goldstein H: Smoking in pregnancy and subsequent child development. *Br Med J* 4: 573–575, 1973.

Centers for Disease Control: Assessment of the number and characteristics of persons affected by learning disabilities. In: Interagency Committee on Learning Disabilities: *Learning Disabilities. A Report to the U.S. Congress.* Washington, DC, US Department of Health and Human Services, 1987, p. 107.

Chalfant JC: Diagnostic criteria for entry and exit from services: A national problem. In: Silver LB (ed): *The Assessment of Learning Disabilities: Preschool through Adulthood.* Boston, College Hill Publishers, 1989, pp. 1–26.

Clements S: *Minimal Brain Dysfunction in Children* (National Institute of Neurological Diseases and Blindness, Monograph no. 3). Washington, DC, US Department of Health, Education, and Welfare, 1966.

Comings DE: *Tourette Syndrome and Human Behavior.* Durante, CA, Hope Press, 1990.

Comings DE, Comings BG: A controlled study of Tourette syndrome I-VII. *Am J Hum Genet* 41: 701–866, 1987.

Comings DE, Comings BG: Tourette syndrome and attention deficit disorder. In: Cohen DJ, Bruun RD, Leckman JF (eds): *Tourette Syndrome and Tic Disorders.* New York, Wiley, 1988, pp. 19–35.

Duane DD: Neurobiological correlates of learning disorders. *J Am Acad Child Adolesc Psychiatry* 28:314–318, 1989.

Farnham-Diggory S: *Learning Disabilities: A Psychological Perspective.* Cambridge, MA, Harvard University Press, 1978.

Finucci JM, Childs B: Are there really more dyslexic boys than girls? In: Ansara A, Geschwind N, Galaburda A, et al (eds): *Sex Differences in Dyslexia.* Towson, MD, Orton Dyslexia Society, 1981, pp. 1–9.

Fleischner JE, Garnett K: Math disorders. *Child*

Adolesc Psychiatr Clin North Am 2:221–231, 1993.

Forness SB: *Recent Concepts in Dyslexia: Implications for Diagnosis and Remediation.* Reston, Virginia, ERIC Exceptional Child Education Reports, 1981.

Frankel M, Cummings JL, Robertson MM, et al: Obsessions and compulsions in Gilles de la Tourette's syndrome. *Neurology* 36:378–382, 1986.

Galaburda AM, Sherman GF, Rosen GD, et al: Developmental dyslexia: Four consecutive patients with cortical abnormalities. *Ann Neurol* 18:222–233, 1985.

Geschwind N, Behan P: Left handedness: Association with immune disease, migraine and developmental learning disorders. *Proc Natl Acad Sci USA* 79:5097–5100, 1982.

Halperin JM, Gittelman R, Klein DF, et al: Reading-disabled hyperactive children: A distinct subgroup of attention deficit disorder with hyperactivity. *J Abnorm Child Psychol* 12:1–14, 1984.

Hagin RA, Kugler J: School problems associated with Tourette's syndrome. In: Cohen DJ, Bruun RD, Leckman JF (eds): *Tourette's Syndrome and Tic Disorders: Clinical Understanding and Treatment.* New York, Wiley, 1988.

Hagin RA, Beecher R, Pagano G, et al: Effects of Tourette syndrome on learning. In: Friedhoff AJ, Chase TN (eds): *Gilles de la Tourette Syndrome.* New York, Raven Press, 1982.

Hazel JS, Schumaker JB: Social skills and learning disabilities: Current issues and recommendations for future research. In: Kavanagh JF, Truss TJ (eds): *Learning Disabilities: Proceedings of the National Conference.* Parkton, MD, York Press, 1988, pp. 293–344.

Hunt RD, Cohen DJ: Psychiatric aspects of learning difficulties. *Pediatr Clin North Am* 31:471–497, 1984.

Johnson D: Review of research on specific reading, writing, and mathematics disorders. In: Kavanagh JF, Truss TJ Jr (eds): *Learning Disabilities: Proceedings of the National Conference.* Parkton, MD, York Press, 1988, pp. 79–177.

Johnson D, Blalock J (eds): *Adults with Learning Disabilities: Clinical Studies.* New York, Grune & Stratton, 1987.

Keilitz I, Zaremba BA, Broder PK: The link between learning disabilities and juvenile delinquency. *Learn Disabil Q* 2:2–11, 1979.

Lewis D, Balla D: Psychiatric correlates of severe reading disabilities in an incarcerated delinquent population. *J Am Acad Child Psychiatry* 19:611–622, 1980.

Lewis D, Shanok SS, Pincus JH: Juvenile male sexual assaulters. *Am J Psychiatry* 136:1194–1196, 1979.

Mauser AJ: Learning disabilities and delinquent youth. *Acad Ther* 9:389–402, 1974.

Nichols PL, Chen TC: *Minimal Brain Dysfunction: A Prospective Study.* Hillsdale, NJ, Erlbaum, 1981.

Ostrander R: Clinical observations suggesting a learning disability. *Child Adolesc Psychiatr Clin North Am* 2:249–263, 1993.

Ostrander R, Silver LB: Psychological interventions and therapies for children and adolescents with learning disabilities. *Child Adolesc Psychiatr Clin North Am* 2:323–337, 1993.

Pauls DC, Pakstis A, Kurlan R, et al: Segregation and linkage analysis of Tourette's syndrome and related disorders. *J Am Acad Child Adolesc Psychiatry* 29:195–203, 1990.

Pitman RK, Gren RC, Jenicke MA, et al: Clinical comparison of Tourette's disorder and obsessive-compulsive disorder. *Am J Psychiatry* 144:1166–1171, 1987.

Robbins DM, Beck JC, Pries R, et al: Learning disability and neuropsychological impairment in adjudicated, unincarcerated male delinquents. *J Am Acad Child Psychiatry* 22:40–46, 1983.

Rourke BP: Syndrome of nonverbal learning disabilities: The final common pathway of white-matter disease/dysfunction? *Clin Neuropsychol* 1:209–234, 1987.

Rourke BP: Socioemotional disturbances of learning disabled children. *J Consult Clin Psychol* 56:801–810, 1988.

Rourke BP: *Nonverbal Learning Disabilities: The Syndrome and the Model.* New York, Guilford, 1989.

Rourke BP, Furest DR: *Learning Disabilities and Psychosocial Functioning: A Neuropsychological Perspective.* New York, Guilford, 1991.

Rourke PB, Young GC, Stang JD, et al: Adult outcomes of childhood central processing deficiencies. In: Grand I, Adams KM (eds): *Neuropsychological Assessment of Neuropsychiatric Disorders: Clinical Methods and Empirical Findings.* New York, Oxford University Press, 1986, pp. 244–267.

Rutter M, Tizard J, Whitmore K: *Education in Health and Behavior.* London, Longman, 1970.

Rutter M, Tizard J, Yule W, et al: Research report. Isle of Wight studies, 1964–1974. *Psychol Med* 6:313–332, 1976.

Shaywitz SE, Cohen DJ, Shaywitz BA: Behavior and learning difficulties in children of normal intelligence born to alcoholic mothers. *J Pediatr* 96:978–982, 1980.

Shepherd MJ, Uhry JK: Reading disorder. *Child Adolesc Psychiatr Clin North Am* 2:193–208, 1993.

Silver LB: The relationship between learning disabilities, hyperactivity, distractibility, and behavioral problems. *J Am Acad Child Psychiatry* 20:385–397, 1981.

Silver LB: Psychological and family problems associated with learning disabilities: Assessment and intervention. *J Am Acad Child Adolesc Psychiatry* 28:319–325, 1989.

Silver LB: The secondary emotional, social, and family problems found with children and adolescents with learning disabilities. *Child Adolesc Psychiatr Clin North Am* 2:295–308, 1993.

Silver LB: A study of the comorbidity between a continuum of neurologically-based disorders and learning disabilities. *J Am Acad Child Adolesc Psychiatry*, in press.

Silver AA, Hagin RA: *Disorders of Learning in Childhood.* New York, Wiley, 1992, pp. 23–42.

Silver AA, Hagin RA: The educational diagnostic process. *Child Adolesc Psychiatr Clin North Am* 2:265–281, 1993.

Strauss AA, Lehtinen LE: *Psychopathology and Education of the Brain-Injured Child.* New York, Grune & Stratton, 1947.

Tallal P: Neuropsychological foundations of specific developmental disorders (language, reading, articulation). *Psychiatry* 3:1, 1985.

Uhry JK, Shepherd MJ: Writing disorder. *Child Adolesc Psychiatr Clin North Am* 2:209–219, 1993.

Werner H, Strauss AA: Pathology of figure-background relation in the child. *J Abnorm Soc Psychol* 36:236–248, 1941.

49 PSYCHIATRIC EVALUATION OF PERCEPTUALLY IMPAIRED CHILDREN: HEARING AND VISUAL IMPAIRMENTS

Ian Ross Jenkins, M.D., and Stella Chess, M.D.

GENERAL CONSIDERATIONS

Sensory impairments do not per se cause psychiatric illness. Misdiagnosis of psychiatric disorders in sensory-impaired children, particularly a mislabel of mental retardation, may occur if the diagnostician is unaware of the adaptive differences and hence the variability in timing and acquisition of developmental milestones due to the sensory impairment. Troubled behavior may represent psychiatric conditions independent of the sensory impairments or be the summation of acquired mal-adaptive behaviors. In comprehending such maladaptations, the psychiatrist must keep in mind that the sensory impairment will influence the acquisition of skills, the self-concept of the child, and the interaction with the environment. Conversely, the child's environment, in response to the impairment, can shape the sequential acquisition of skills and the developmental process.

Fundamental considerations for the evaluation of a sensory-impaired child are (a) the tremendous range and heterogeneity of the individual impairments, (b) the frequent occurrence of multiple impairments, (c) the complex interdependence of the impairments with the environment and caretaker response, and (d) the differing potentials among children with similar impairments. The nature and extent of the impairment will differ based on etiology, age of onset, and other complicating factors.

Visual or hearing impairments oftentimes do not exist alone. There is a high frequency of additional impairments, especially of the central nervous system. Suchman (1967) evaluated and examined the population of an entire school for deaf children, a sample of 103 children between the ages of 4 and 12.9 years. Sixty (58%) had some degree of visual impairment. Forty-seven of the 54 children whose visual problem was correctable had never received correction.

Professionals who evaluate and work with sensory-impaired children must be alert to their own attitudes. Many professionals lack exposure to profoundly impaired individuals who are leading successful and constructive lives, a fact that is important inasmuch as professional attitudes subtly shape the evaluation, bringing expectations and recommendations that may, in turn, influence parental expectations. Conversely, overidentification with the child's and family's difficulties, the pressures of advocacy groups, or the needs of the parents or schools can shape assessments.

We would recommend that child psychiatrists, when evaluating a sensory-impaired child, use the following definitions to help clarify their own thinking and communication with their patients:

1. *Impairment:* Identifiable defect of the basic functions of an organ system or any part of the body.
2. *Disability:* Limitation, restriction, or disadvantage imposed on an individual's functioning as a result of the impairment (the extent of an impairment can be accommodated or reduced by modifications such as eyeglasses or hearing aids).
3. *Handicap:* Result of placing an individual at an actual or perceived disadvantage in the performance of normal life functions because of personal and/or societal expectations and attitudes toward the impairment (Scholl, 1986).

The special role of the child psychiatrist is the capacity to interface with many professional disciplines and members of a team to assess a variety of contributing factors that can influence or shape the child's behavior. Current educational trends away from centralized state residential schools, with the integration of sensory-impaired children into local schools, increases the probability that more child psychiatrists without specialized experience will be asked to evaluate sensory-impaired youngsters. The child psychiatrist's training permits integrating biological/medical/physiological components, developmental issues, family/environmental influences, and learning/education questions, as well as psychodynamic/psychiatric issues. In both evaluation and treatment or management recommendations, the consulting psychiatrist will need to establish a collegial relationship with the parents and school staff. Frequently, the child will already be known to the schools or rehabilitation services. Respect for and awareness of the specialized knowledge of other disciplines and their accumulated experience with children is essential. Inasmuch as sensory impairments are lifelong challenges, the nature of the initial involvement of the child psychiatrist and cooperation with other professionals will be significant in determining the usefulness of long-range assistance and counseling.

Child and adolescent psychiatrists must also develop and accommodate themselves to specialized and innovative interviewing techniques to evaluate the child. For example, although learning manual sign language is extraordinarily helpful, it is time-consuming and difficult to master. In the evaluation, the use of an interpreter for hearing-impaired children and creative utilization of play therapy with a blind child can be feasible alternatives. The child psychiatrist who is best able to approach the evaluation (a) does not apply preconceived theoretical formulations of personality development established for able-bodied youngsters, (b) is knowledgeable in child development, (c) looks for adaptational, problem-solving, and functional strengths while avoiding

the "deficit assumption," i.e., that a sensory impairment will routinely result in psychological impairment, and (d) appreciates the strengths and weaknesses within the family. The most helpful attitude is to keep in mind the conceptual question, "How does the impairment interface with the developmental process and/or the environment, and what have been the adaptive responses?"

The goals of the examination should include looking for the child's level of independence, cognitive abilities, functional abilities, and social and psychological adjustment/adaptations. Further, the examiner would want to consider (a) why this case has been referred at this time, and who made the referral; (b) what is happening in the home, family, or school (e.g., is the child aging out of the school, or has the child grown physically to the point where previous management techniques are no longer possible and medications are being requested); and (c) whether there is an underlying purpose for the referral, such as expediting removal of the child from the home or school. Further, the examiner would want to assess the child's ability to understand cause and effect relationships to modify his or her behavior. Reviewing various records and looking for the longitudinal patterns in addition to associated impairments will answer some of these questions.

ADDITIONAL CONSIDERATIONS

It is important for the evaluating psychiatrist to ascertain what the parents' expectations are for their child and from what sources they have received advice. Professional direction that is overly optimistic can be as inappropriate as unduly negative predictions. The normal parental wish is for a happy, unimpaired child, and at times parents may disregard or deny the reality of their child's circumstances and pursue unrealistic treatments and goals, thus not appreciating the gains their child has attained. However, the authors have repeatedly seen that the level of the parental involvement and advocacy for their child is an important predicator of the child's success, and the "validity" of the parental expectations in many cases can only be determined after the fact, retrospectively, once the child has grown.

Assessment of the environment and family of the sensory-impaired child should recognize the increased demands in time and energy required of parents. Beyond their own emotional needs and reactions, engendered by having an impaired child, there may be an increased drain of resources from other areas of life. Family structure is often distorted. There are many additional, both obvious and hidden, financial costs, from hearing aids and batteries to special visual assistance devices or simply parking fees when the child is taken frequently for rehabilitation services and public transportation is not possible. Mothers frequently spend a great deal of time attending clinics and rehabilitation services, thereby shortchanging their personal needs and those of their other children and husband. A gulf can grow between mother and father. Nonimpaired siblings often feel excluded, jealous, or cheated while simultaneously ambivalently conflicted with the relief that they themselves are not impaired. On the other hand, many families are able to establish a constructive response wherein the needs of all members are met (Lobato et al., 1988). An area of family life that is insufficiently researched and tends to be underappreciated by mental health professionals is the role of religion as a source of both strength and support and/or conflict for the parents and family (Erin et al., 1991a), and this should be explored. The child psychiatrist evaluating an impaired child and concerned that the family/environment may have contributed to limited development and maladaptive behaviors is cautioned against inadvertently aggravating the parents' emotional strain and intensifying a sense of guilt.

HEARING IMPAIRMENTS

Definition

Hearing-impaired children have been traditionally divided into hard of hearing and profoundly hearing-impaired (deaf) groups. Historically, the distinction was based on those youngsters who could utilize their diminished auditory perceptions for communication and those who could not. The advent of more effective hearing-assistive devices and habilitation services has permitted an increasing number of hearing-impaired children with significant hearing loss to effectively use their residual hearing. There is a growing group of children who have received cochlear implants and will present as yet unknown challenges. Hearing-impaired children are also classified by the age of onset of their hearing loss: prelingual (before the use of spoken language) or postlingual. Generally, a loss of hearing before 2 years of life is considered prelingual. There are significant differences in subsequent language outcome between the prelingual and postlingual child, even with similar levels of hearing loss.

Historical Note

Hearing deprivation has existed throughout history. Western European attitudes and practices have been influenced by educators and religious figures who have taken on the task of instruction of deaf pupils. The ability to inherit property, in some Western European cultures, was dependent on the ability to confess to God, so teaching oral speech took on a special significance. To a large extent, early teaching combined variations of oral and sign communication. The turns in the bitter, and still ongoing, battle between manual communication, oralism, and total communication (sign combined with speech articulation) are detailed graphically by Harlan Lane (1984). Currently, there is a growing political debate surrounding cochlear implants and whether a parent has the right to remove the child from Deaf Culture.

Prevalence and Epidemiology

Epidemiological estimates of the number of hearing-impaired children vary, based on methodology and definitions. The Annual Survey of Hearing Impaired Children and Youth conducted by the Center for Assessment and Demographic Studies at Gallaudet University, states that in 1991–1992 there were 47,822 hearing-impaired children reportedly receiving educational services. The reported number might be a low, since compliance with the survey is voluntary by local schools, and definitions of services might be interpreted differently. Comparison of these numbers with those of the 1984–1985 survey (N = 50,731)

shows that there has been a decline in hearing-impaired children. This is possibly the result of "aging out" of the rubella cohort from the 1963–1964 epidemic. As an etiology of impairment, rubella fell from 11% in 1984–1985 to 2% by 1991–1992. There has also been a slight shift of approximately 6% away from residential schools to local schools. It is uncertain whether this is the result of increased emphasis on mainstreaming or if with the aging out of severe multiply handicapped children a higher percentage of youngsters can be accommodated in the local systems (Schildroth and Hotto, 1993). The broad estimates of children with some level of hearing impairments has been approximately 350,000 (Meadow, 1980). Critics point out that there may be many more children who are struggling in school and social relationships due to undetected mild hearing impairments. It is suggested that children with learning difficulties, educational delays, or disruptive school behavior might benefit from audiological evaluation.

The degree of hearing impairment has been traditionally stated in terms of volume or decibel loss over the speech frequencies (250–8000 Hz). The testing procedure is not actually measuring "loss" but rather the volume threshold at which a youngster perceives a pure single tone at a particular frequency. This form of testing does not determine the usefulness of the auditory input, as it excludes associated frequency harmonics, does not measure the capacity to distinguish meaningfully the subtleties of sounds when frequencies are mixed, and does not distinguish the desired auditory input from competing background noise. A comprehensive audiological evaluation will probe utilization of input in terms of "discrimination." The vowel sounds tend to group in the low- to mid-range frequencies, whereas the consonants and sibilants tend toward the higher ranges. Thus, a child with partial loss might be able to comprehend some words but be required to guess at others, leading to potential errors of communication (Northern and Downs, 1984). The child psychiatrist is encouraged to examine the audiological report and consult with the audiologist to understand the implications of a particular hearing loss. The generally accepted audiological classifications for hearing impairments are given in Table 49.1.

Many states set the criterion of an average 80-dB loss in the better ear for admission to a state school for the deaf. This criterion does not accommodate individual auditory differences among children nor consider the interaction with other impairments. A number of children with a greater than 80-dB loss can, with training and amplification,

Table 49.1. Handicapping Effects of Hearing Loss in Children

Average Hearing Level 500–2000 Hz	Description	Possible Condition	What Can Be Heard without Amplification	Handicapping Effects (If Not Treated in First Year of Life)	Probable Needs
0–15 dB	Normal range	Conductive hearing losses	All speech sounds	None	None
15–25 dB	Slight hearing loss	Conductive hearing losses, some sensorineural hearing losses	Vowel sounds heard clearly; may miss unvoiced consonants sounds	Mild auditory dysfunction in language learning	Consideration of need for hearing aid; speechreading, auditory training, speech therapy, preferential seating
25–30 dB	Mild hearing loss	Conductive or sensorineural hearing loss	Only some of speech sounds, the louder voiced sounds	Auditory learning dysfunction, mild language retardation, mild speech problems, inattention	Hearing aid, speechreading, auditory training, speech therapy
30–50 dB	Moderate hearing loss	Conductive hearing loss from chronic middle ear disorders; sensorineural hearing losses	Almost no speech sounds at normal conversational level	Speech problems, language retardation, learning, dysfunction, inattention	All of the above, plus consideration of special classroom situation
50–70 dB	Severe hearing loss	Sensorineural or mixed losses due to a combination of middle ear disease and sensorineural involvement	No speech sounds at normal conversational level	Severe speech problems, language retardation, learning dysfunction, inattention	All of the above, probable assignment to special classes
70+ dB	Profound hearing loss	Sensorineural or mixed losses due to a combination of middle ear disease and sensorineural involvement	No speech or other sounds	Severe speech problems, language retardation, learning dysfunction, inattention	All of the above, probable assignment to special classes

From Northern JL, Downs MP: *Hearing in Children* (4th ed). Baltimore, Williams & Wilkins, 1991.

utilize their residual hearing and function in a mainstream hearing school, while others with a loss less than 80 dB cannot. A child with intermittent middle ear conductive impairment tested on a bad day would have greater difficulty understanding the instructions, resulting in a lower score than would be achieved on a good day. Further, Northern feels that a loss of more than 15 dB, especially following several episodes of otitis media during critical periods of language acquisition and education, results in diminished attainment, potential, and IQ scores (Northern and Downs, 1984).

Etiology

The relative etiologies of childhood hearing loss have varied historically based on the presence of epidemics, pandemic diseases, and preventive measures available, while genetic inheritance has persisted in stable numbers. Prior to the advent of antibiotics and vaccination, ear infections and systemic diseases frequently included the sequela of deafness. Congenital deafness includes intrauterine etiologies. Boughman reports more than 100 distinct genetic forms of hearing loss interfering with normal conversation, a number of which, however, present only in adult life (Boughman and Shaver, 1982). Deaf children with hearing parents comprise more than 90% of the pediatric deaf population (Meadow, 1980). The child psychiatrist is most likely to encounter the hearing-impaired child as the only audiologically impaired member of the family.

The timing of the etiological event during the child's intrauterine and postnatal life will result in differing presentations and associated complications. Viral infections of the fetus (e.g., rubella) frequently interfere with other organ development, and multiple impairments are found, including visual impairments (e.g., congenital cataracts), cardiac malformations, neurological impairments, seizure disorders, mental retardation, and a rare delayed sequela of panencephalitis. Autism has been seen in disproportionate numbers among youngsters with rubella and several other viral intrauterine etiologies, especially in association with an increased number of impairments (Chess et al., 1971). Prematurity with deafness is often complicated by cerebral palsy, mental retardation, and neurological immaturity (Vernon, 1982). Rh incompatibility hearing impairment is associated with an increase over the normal incidence of aphasic disorders (Vernon, 1967). Postnatal ailments such as meningitis, mumps, measles, middle ear infections, and allergies may be complicated by deafness and a wide range of sequelae due to encephalopathy (Vernon, 1967).

Pathogenesis in Development

Meadow-Orlans (1987) states, "The basic deprivation of profound congenital deafness is not the deprivation of sound; it is the deprivation of language." This is not to imply that hearing-impaired children do not have the innate capacity for language, communication, or symbolic thought. Rather, during the early developing preschool years, when hearing children gain sufficient mastery of spoken language to express needs, desires, and emotions, the hearing-impaired children of hearing families are confronted with tremendous obstacles to learning through language communication. The diverse influence and interrelationship of sound and language to the developmental processes is profound and is the overriding conceptual consideration in the evaluation of the hearing-impaired child.

For discussion, the effects of profound prelingual hearing impairment can be grouped into (a) language development and acquisition, (b) cognitive development and information acquisition, and (c) social development and behavioral difficulties.

LANGUAGE DEVELOPMENT

A deaf baby will babble at the same age as will a hearing baby. However, at about 10 months, when babbling becomes social and infants begin to model the sounds they produce upon the sounds they hear, the deaf baby will cease to babble (Ling and Ling, 1975). Diagnostic features of delayed speech may have been ignored since there are wide variations in the milestones of the onset of speech in hearing children. The child's lack of response to sounds might be rationalized away. For the hearing parents, the delayed and startling diagnosis of deafness requires a massive reorientation of their conceptualization of their child. The parents, struggling with complicated emotions, are faced simultaneously with a major decision as to the type of language acquisition training to follow—sign alone, oral alone, or total communication—often in the face of conflicting professional opinions.

Language, the tool for formulating thoughts, is differentiated from speech (articulation) or communication (which is an interactive exchange). The campaign against the use of manual language in schools for the deaf and in general use was, to a large extent, based on the conceptions that (a) oral language is necessary for abstract thought, (b) oral language is necessary for interacting with the hearing world, and (c) sign language is not a true language. However, Noam Chomsky (1957) has postulated an innate preprogramming for the process of language. Furth (1971), in an authoritative review of language and thought in deaf children, states, "The general conclusion seems abundantly clear that thinking processes of deaf children are similar to hearing children." Lane (1984) lists the main fallacies used by oralists in the effort to ban manual language from school curricula, one of these being its assumed absence of grammar. The linguist Stokoe in his 1960 seminal monograph demonstrated sign language to be a true language through linguistic analysis of American Sign Language (ASL) (Stokoe, 1978) and later published the first dictionary of American Sign Language that was based on linguistic principles (Stokoe et al., 1976).

The hearing child with hearing parents learns spoken language through environmental interaction. The deaf child will have to learn communicative language in a manner that accommodates to the hearing impairment. The oral position is that without spoken communication the deaf child will not be able to interact with the dominant hearing population. Conversely, the manual argument asserts that the vast majority of deaf people, for social and personal needs, will ultimately enter Deaf Culture and that they should therefore feel comfortable with themselves and accomplished in the language of their culture. The potential psychological conflicts in this dichotomy are highly emotionally charged and will confront the consulting psychiatrist.

There is broad agreement on the need for early identification and intervention with hearing-impaired children. Ling and Ling (1978) argue that, with early auditory amplification and training, the natural process of vocalization and babbling can be preserved and the concept of sound for communication and shaping of the vocalizations can be habilitated. Northern and Downs (1984) summarize the data on "critical periods" for language acquisition and conclude that, although early deprivation of communicative language might be partially reversed, there are long-term deficiencies in formal skills.

Oral training is slow and demanding during the preschool years. Schlesinger and Meadow (1972) argue that by the age of 5 most orally taught deaf children will have a significantly limited vocabulary, but that a deaf child of hearing parents who acquires language through sign or a combination of sign and spoken communication, called total communication (TC), will have a vastly greater vocabulary, permitting greater communication and social development. This is contrary to the oral argument, which excludes the use of signs, arguing that signing hinders successful mastery of vocalized communication (Ling and Ling, 1978). A broad survey by Conrad in England (Freeman and Blockberger, 1987) showed generally poor results with pure oral education and found that the introduction of sign did not inhibit the acquisition of speech or speech reading skills when vigorously pursued. There remains great heterogeneity of achievement within both the oral and total communication groups and varying degrees of success in formal language acquisition. The tragedy of this controversy is that, during the time that the parents are facing emotional upheaval, they are required to make a lifelong decision for their child. Further, it is occurring during the child's crucial cognitive and social development period. Child and adolescent psychiatrists evaluating a deaf child's behavioral problems must consider the parent-child communication and how parents teach acceptable behavior, including rules, compromise, and delayed gratification, which are difficult to clarify when the parent is dependent on only a ''yes'' or ''no'' response.

The eventual language preference among deaf young adults appears to vary greatly depending on the nature of the residual hearing, quality of early training, usefulness of a particular method for communication, and cultural orientation of the individual toward either the hearing world or Deaf Culture and social groups. Many adults develop bilingualism in varying degrees. The issue of language and social isolation, however, persists, with consequent psychological stresses. The deaf child in a hearing family, irrespective of communication mode, tends to be isolated. Deaf adolescents who are trying to function within the hearing environment particularly complain about their difficulty at parties and dances, where lowering of lights and background dance music, amplified by their aids, makes communication and flirting almost impossible. To conceptualize such difficulties, one may analyze any number of situations the child may encounter where vision and hearing are used and coordinated simultaneously, such as note taking in class, talking at the dinner table, or honking cars warning of danger. Many children who later prefer to use sign language, but whose parents do not learn to sign, often view the parents' lack of communication skills as evidence that they do not love them or want them, or that the child is ''damaged'' and bad. Some parents will pursue oral training for their children and leave the impression with the child that this is an attempt to disguise or hide the hearing impairment. Adolescents will often try to fake hearing and discard aids, and negative self-concepts are frequent.

COGNITIVE PROCESSES AND THEORIES

The second area of developmental consideration is cognition, which is linked to language acquisition. Areas of exploration, including memory style, visual-motor and perceptual-motor functions, and problem-solving strategies, are being actively researched but much remains unknown (Meadow, 1980). Two concerns for the child psychiatrist, reported IQ scores and academic achievement, deserve note. Levine (1981) found that psychologists evaluating hearing-impaired clients were limited in experience, training, and communication skills. It is very valuable, for later review of results by others, if examiners indicate in reports their personal skill levels and prior experience with impaired children. An additional consideration is the extent of the impairment on the day the tests are administered.

Levine's (1981) comprehensive review traces the history of efforts to establish psychometric testing among deaf children and the many pitfalls encountered. The most commonly used tests among deaf children are the Wechsler Intelligence Scale for Children (WISC), Leiter International Performance Scale, Wechsler Adult Intelligence Scale, Hiskey-Nebraska, and the Goodenough Draw-a-Person Test. The Merrill-Palmer and Ravens Progressive Matrices are also widely reported. Caveats about psychometric testing of hearing-impaired children include the following: (a) The instrument should be nonverbal since a verbal instrument can reflect language limitations rather than cognitive functions; (b) there is a far greater danger that the instrument will report a falsely low score as opposed to a falsely elevated score; (c) there is increased potential error when the test is administered by an examiner not familiar with hearing impairments and unable to communicate instructions in the child's preferred mode; (d) personality tests, because of the communication issues, are difficult to interpret, as the subtlety of instructions might not have been communicated, and consequently the responses may be limited or unintelligible; and (e) testing of preschool children, at whose age communication skills are only beginning to develop, is tremendously vulnerable to error and underestimation of potential (Vernon and Alles, 1986). In an attempt at fairness, many examiners will now only report the Performance Scale of the WISC-R but, as Wechsler

himself reported, even the Digit-Symbol subtest is not culture-fair for the child who has not had experience with pencil and paper (Levine, 1981). The WISC-R Performance Scale has been normed for hearing-impaired children, but, as Vernon comments, the reported IQ may result from and reflect a difference in the communication abilities of examiners, and the IQ numbers for an individual child should be interpreted with caution (Vernon and Alles, 1986). Braden has explored the predictive validity of the nonverbal, WISC-R Performance Scale (PS) IQ to academic achievement using the Stanford Achievement Test–Hearing Impaired Edition and found little correlation. He suggests that the criteria of academic achievement, especially reading, might not be an accurate reflection of the deaf child's innate cognitive abilities. He has found, however, that the widely used WISC-R PS IQ is helpful in the psycho-educational assessment of deaf children to diagnose mental retardation. He concludes that a ''normal'' WISC-R PS IQ in a deaf child with limited academic achievement suggests that the depressed achievement is secondary to auditory and linguistic deprivation (Braden, 1989). Broad surveys of the reading levels of deaf adolescents consistently report mean paragraph comprehension results in the midelementary school level or significantly below grade level (Meadow, 1980). There are suggestions that the child's reading level, which is not necessarily correlated with intelligence, may be linked to the communication modes between parent and child, with children whose parents used manual communication performing better (Meadow, 1980). Currently many schools for the deaf are utilizing a total communication approach in which the teacher articulates and simultaneously signs the communication in an attempt to improve education. It is uncertain at this time what will be the long-range achievement results for deaf children taught by total communication. The psychiatrist, however, will probably be evaluating a child with academic delays.

SOCIAL DEVELOPMENT AND BEHAVIORAL DIFFICULTIES

The third major area where language difficulties intrude is social behavior and psychological difficulties. The Vineland Scale reports tend to show a lower social quotient among deaf children, but Meadow sees this as linked to parent-child communication (Meadow, 1980). Using Erikson's theoretical model of the stages of development, Schlesinger and Meadow (1972) connect the impact of deafness and child development. The development of basic trust is affected when the child, who cannot hear or understand the caretaker, experiences as an unpredictable abandonment being put in the crib while the mother goes to another room. Hearing children can hear mother coo to them and learn that by crying they can attract attention. This experience is not available to the deaf child. Teaching social rules and concepts of right and wrong cannot be done easily by explanations, and limit setting is often perceived by the child as capricious.

The Meadow and Trybus (1979) review of the prevalence of behavioral problems among deaf children concludes that there is a three to six times greater reported rate of behavioral and emotional problems compared with the rate of problems of broad samples of the pediatric population. There are numerous methodological problems in reported studies, but the trends are consistent. Mindel and Vernon (1971) link the differing etiologies of hearing impairment to characteristic behavioral difficulties. Schlesinger and Meadow (1972) utilized a teacher questionnaire, previously administered in a survey of all schoolchildren in Los Angeles County, with the teachers of 516 deaf youngsters at a California school for the deaf. The teachers rated 11.6% of the deaf children as severely disturbed, as compared with 2.4% of the Los Angeles County sample. Further, 19.6% of the deaf children had ''milder behavioral problems,'' compared with 7.3% of the countywide sample.

Meadow (1980), summarizing various reports, states that deaf children are more likely to be described as hyperactive, immature, and impulsive. She is concerned that the literature overemphasizes neurological soft signs that inappropriately direct the consultant to ascribe behavioral problems to brain damage, while overlooking other issues, including parental response and management of the impaired child, language and communication issues between parent and child, lower education expectations for deaf than for hearing children, and the fundamentally different adaptive needs of the deaf child.

There is a general impression that a typical ''deaf personality'' exists. Among these personality features are usually included such characteristics as impulsivity, hyperactivity, rigidity, suspiciousness, and immaturity. Following other investigators who have challenged these suppositions, Chess and Fernandez (1980) used a sample of 248 children with congenital rubella followed longitudinally from age 2.5 to 14 years. From their data they concluded that deafness itself cannot be considered to confer any ''typical personality''; it is the behavioral symptomatology of those with neurological damage that is largely responsible for such a stereotype, at least for the rubella-deaf population.

Adolescent development poses different difficulties. The acquisition of information for the youngster comes primarily from peers and the environment outside of the home, maybe at the mall, in the pizza parlor, or on the street. Most manual communicators, especially in a school for the deaf, by this age have developed a social network within the deaf community. They often obtain from older deaf adolescents information, which unfortunately, is not, or cannot be, accessed from their hearing parents or adults. Charlson et al. have reported on in-depth evaluations of successful deaf teenagers and reported that all of their subjects (N = 23), whether oral or manual, reported some degree of isolation from peers or family that was often associated with communication difficulties. Their sample included several deaf teenagers with deaf parents and 12 of the sample were in residential schools. Most of the students had developed a strategy for coping with the isolation, and the case reports provide an intimate insight into the problems faced by these adolescents (Charlson et al., 1992). Gathering social information is particularly difficult for oral adolescents in a mainstream program. One highly intelligent oral adolescent boy, who was referred for treatment of inappropriate social behavior toward girls, reported to one of us (Jenkins) that trying to learn about girls and sex was '' . . .like looking through a hole in a wall.'' He described himself as ''paranormal'' and not ''abnormal.'' This concept was helpful to the therapist in this and other treatments, viewing parallel developmental tracks, when the motivation is the same as ''normal,'' thus removing the psychopathological implications. Unfortunately, this conceptual approach is vulnerable to subjective judgments by the therapist, and there is a persistent risk of overidentifying with the child, leading to minimizing or excusing real problematic developmental issues (I.R. Jenkins, unpublished observations).

Evaluating a Hearing-Impaired Child or Adolescent

Beyond the general techniques of child psychiatry interviewing, the examiner should focus on the preferred mode of communication for the child and be prepared to function within that modality. The oral child, relying on speech-reading (lip-reading) cues, will be expending great effort concentrating on the examiner's lips, and the examiner should provide a continuous unobstructed view. If the examiner turns away or casually puts a hand over the mouth, the child will lose the flow of a question. To communicate with a deaf child who is looking away, a gentle touch or waving the hand in the child's visual field is an accepted maneuver. The examiner should not sit with the sun or a bright light behind his or her back, as this creates shadows and eyestrain for the patient. If the child's preferred mode of communication is manual language, unless the examiner has sign skills greater than those of the child or adolescent, a certified sign interpreter is required, barring emergency examination. A family member is an unacceptable interpreter, as the child is not free to communicate confidentially, nor is someone who ''knows some signs'' acceptable. An examiner who regularly evaluates manually communicating patients should have a working knowledge of sign language even though an interpreter is used. A knowledge of sign, even if limited, will assist in the assessment of the child's or adolescent's use of language.

The syntax and grammar of ASL, as with other languages, are completely different from those of English; ASL is a distinct language and not a codified form of English. When ASL is translated word for word, or when evaluating the written communications of an ASL communicator, the language form will appear fragmented and disorganized and may incorrectly be confused with psychotic processes (Evans and Elliott, 1987). Formal language defects are often similar in sign language to those found among hearing populations, with changes in rate of production, echolalia, perseveration, and neologisms.

The assessment of language and communication is fundamental to any psychiatric evaluation and is particularly vulnerable to errors when assessing the hearing impaired. The good speech reader is usually able to understand only a limited percentage of the mouth and lip formations without cues (Quigley, 1979), including vocabulary knowledge, context, and other visual cues (Moores, 1982).

Thus, effective communication requires constant concentration, guesses, adequate vocabulary level, quality training, and experience/exposure. English slang and idioms create trouble spots. The common use of idioms and slang in verbal conversations can present problems when working with oral (speech-reading dependent) youngsters. One of us (Jenkins), in a therapy session with an oral deaf adolescent boy who was considered to have excellent speech-reading skills, encountered a rather confusing and inappropriate response to a question that included, ''when push comes to shove.'' After a prolonged effort to understand and explore the bizarre response, it came to light that the youngster had speech read, ''put it on the shelf'' and that his response was congruent to that reading. Proverbs, typically used in the psychiatric examination in an attempt to explore abstracting ability, often lose the implied abstraction when translated into another language and tend to become literal. The patient will give a concrete answer in response to a concrete translation. Many proverbs that are based on experience can have no meaning, e.g., ''The squeaky wheel gets all the grease.''

Many words and phrases routinely used in mental health settings have been adapted from physical medicine and assume a mental health, context-dependent meaning. For example, ''How are you feeling?'' has brought the response ''Nothing'' from a crying deaf adolescent because she had no physical pain. With children and adolescents, it is important to establish a common vocabulary and determine if they know the sign ''emotion'' and its connotations. The examiner might list for the child the signs of happy, sad, and the like, interspersed with some simple nouns (e.g., car), to determine if the patient can distinguish which are emotions.

Deaf individuals have hallucinations, look into space, and even sign into space toward the source, but it is not helpful to pursue the question ''Are you hearing voices?'' Some may report that people or sources such as loudspeakers are talking about them or commenting specifically to them or about them. Care must be taken to distinguish this from the very prevalent belief within Deaf Culture that hearing people talk about the deaf behind their backs. Schneiderian first-rank symptoms can be elicited, but again, ideas of reference must be carefully teased away from cultural belief systems and experience. The psychopathology of paranoia poses similar problems.

Drawings can be a helpful route to gather psychodynamic material. The Draw-a-Person Test scored on the Goodenough Scale can provide an indirect but nonvalidated intelligence level (Heller and Harris, 1987). Such a nonverbal approach can provide a mental age that can be compared with the IQ reported from other examinations. It is best to interpret the drawings based on a story obtained about the drawing, including what is happening and what the subject of the drawing is thinking, feeling, and hopes for the future, rather than using the usual theoretical interpretive formulations of symbolic meanings.

Differential Diagnosis

The main psychiatric differential diagnosis for a deaf child or adolescent with problematic behavior is mental retardation. Pervasive developmental disorder, autism, childhood schizophrenia, conduct disorder, and parent-child conflict are also to be considered. Delays in academics or in simple knowledge about the world, however, may be secondary to environmental restrictions imposed upon an intellectually normal deaf child and may present as immaturity, dependency disorder, or educational delay. Deaf children are accustomed to routine sequences of actions because their parents and mentors have found it difficult to explain changes. They themselves may later insist on sameness, leading inaccurately to a diagnosis of childhood schizophrenia, autism, or obsessive compulsive personality disorder. In a deaf child, these diagnoses must be considered and explored.

Differential diagnosis of behavioral disturbances among sensory-impaired children requires the clinician to consider unusual presentations of conditions that exist in nonimpaired children. The problem of tinnitus among hearing-impaired children is a unique problem. This relatively common and occasional disabling condition among the hearing population is easy to diagnose but difficult to quantify. Drukier, along with others, has reported that, among the 331 children, 6- to 18-years-old enrolled at a state school for the deaf, one-third suffered from tinnitus of varying severity (Drukier, 1989). One of us (Jenkins) has seen several cases of tinnitus referred for psychiatric assessment. In one case a 10-year-old profoundly hearing-impaired boy at a school for the deaf was referred for evaluation of classroom behavioral disruptiveness. History elicited from the teacher showed that just prior to outbursts he would put his hands to his ears. Subsequent follow-up established that severe attacks of tinnitus precipitated the disruptions. An adolescent girl from rural South America was referred for evaluation with the working diagnosis of paranoid schizophrenia with auditory hallucinations. Several interviews in sign language established a tentative diagnosis of tinnitus. She communicated that, since she had never heard the hearing talk, she assumed that the sounds that she heard were ''voices.'' This had become fused and exaggerated with generalized deaf cultural beliefs, specifically suspiciousness of the hearing world, and South American cult beliefs of voodoo to create the clinical picture. Another adolescent girl, struggling with developmental issues and her reality testing, signed, ''I am deaf. How can I hear these noises if I am deaf? Am I really deaf?''

The assessment of multihandicapped deaf children requires a large team of highly specialized evaluators. The position paper on recommended assessment procedures for these youngsters adopted by the Conference of Educational Administrators Serving the Deaf provides a useful and comprehensive listing of all the areas that need to be considered. They do consider deafness to be the primary disability and state that, due to the lack of theoretical knowledge about the interactions of the differing impairments, it is not realistically possible to go beyond that position when generating information (Johnson, 1989). However, we believe if the clinician, evaluating a deaf multihandicapped child, places the impairments in a hierarchy with the sensory impairments as most important, this formulation could lead to underestimation of other impairing conditions that might more accurately dictate outcome, functional capacity, or treatment, e.g., mental retardation, psychosis, etc.

Treatment and Management

Psychiatric treatment oftentimes means that effective prevention might not have been implemented. Establishing an effective communication system, both prelanguage and language based, is a high priority for prevention. The selection of total communication or oral training depends upon a variety of factors beyond the quality of residual hearing. These include parental expectations and capacity to sustain a demanding communication therapy program (either for oral training or to learn sign language), along with the child's intelligence, temperament, and associated impairments. Although the authors know, have met, and have worked with profoundly hearing-impaired children and adults who lead successful lives with purely oral communication, our general recommendation has been a total communication approach. This is a complicated

recommendation that should be made on a case-by-case basis. It must be remembered that, as child psychiatrists, we tend to place a high priority on social and behavioral development, psychosocial group identification and support, and a sense of self-identity, which is the core of Deaf Culture based on sign language. We do recognize that many of the referrals we have seen in practice, among oral children, are older, where problems have developed, and we tend not to see the successful youngsters. Referrals of the manual communicators tend to come from dysfunctional families or they are multihandicapped and their difficulties are frequently attributed to factors other than communication. It is emerging from very preliminary evidence that, for successful use of cochlear implantation, initial oral training is important, both prior to and almost indefinitely after the surgery. Thus, if implantation is planned, then an early oral approach is preferred. The Rubella Longitudinal Study suggests that, if postsecondary education is to be used as a criteria of success, then mainstreaming with oral education is helpful, although not mandatory. There is a tremendous heterogeneity among hearing-impaired children, and the clinician is best advised to remain flexible in his or her recommendations. But, any 2- to 3-year-old child in a purely oral program who is not making prompt and significant progress should be quickly transferred to a total communication program. Delays beyond the 4th birthday leave a child ill-prepared for school. Should the child be brought for treatment of a behavior problem at a later age, the absence of a practical communication mode may have been the largest contributor to the problem. Meadow-Orlans' (1987) review of the effectiveness of intervention programs for hearing-impaired children will be helpful for the consultant.

The treatment of the child focuses on the acquisition of acceptable behaviors for the developmental period, if it has been determined that the behavior problem is not the result of independent psychiatric conditions. Behavior modification has long been used with deaf children (Levine and Naiman, 1970) and has been found to be ''the most viable'' approach, especially in the school setting (Lennan, 1981). Counseling and group work with the hearing impaired (Bonham et al., 1981) emphasize the value of groups for transmitting information and sharing feelings among sensory-impaired adolescents, especially around maturational and adjustment issues.

The efficacy of individual psychotherapy in the language used by the child has not been clearly established, as the availability of therapists for individual work is limited, and reports tend to be single-case studies or highly selected samples. This is not to imply that sensory-impaired clients cannot benefit from individual psychotherapy. Non-sensory-impaired therapists will be most successful if they utilize a transcultural model and acquaint themselves with the cultural beliefs of their clients. Further, the nonimpaired therapist or consultant should not convey to the client ''I know how you feel'' but rather a ''teach me what your experience is like'' attitude. Psychoactive medications, especially neuroleptics, can be used successfully with deaf children for management, but the common anticholinergic side effects of psychoactive medications can be difficult to communicate in sign language. The blurry vision often experienced with these drugs is intolerable for an individual dependent on vision and limits the usefulness of some medications; an adolescent treated by one of the authors had the side effects fully explained but stopped the medications, signing, ''Doctor, I'm deaf, and I was afraid of becoming blind.'' (I.R. Jenkins, personal experience).

Stimulant medications can effectively be used for attention deficit hyperactivity disorder (ADHD) in carefully diagnosed cases. With hearing-impaired children, apparent hyperactivity may be confused with the lack of effective communication or of learning social graces. The determination is complicated by reported impulsivity among deaf children. Cases referred for stimulant medications have often shown overwhelmed parents lacking communication skills who, having had trouble setting limits, have overused physical punishment to establish their authority. Kelly et al. evaluated a state residential school for the deaf and obtained ratings on 238 students using the Conners Parent Rating Scale (answered by the dormitory counselors) and the Attention Deficit Disorder with

Hyperactivity (ADD-H) Comprehensive Teacher Rating Scale. They found that the Conners ratings did not statistically differ from normative numbers for hearing children. Among those youngsters who were considered positive for ADD-H, their hearing loss tended to be acquired, e.g., bacterial meningitis or congenital rubella (Kelly et al., 1993a). Another report by these authors details a wide range of management intervention they developed either prior to and/or including stimulant medications (Kelly et al., 1993b).

The consultant will encounter occasions when neuroleptic medications are requested to contain children with management problems, despite the lack of clear traditional target symptoms, when other techniques have not been successful. The dilemma regarding symptomatic relief versus possible long-term adverse effects, especially for the severely impaired, multihandicapped child, involves the chronic nature of the condition, which often results in a lifetime commitment to medications in an attempt to maintain the child in the least restrictive environment. This clinical and ethical dilemma can be faced by the clinician only on a cautious, case-by-case basis. If a review of previous attempts at management shows a wide range of unsuccessful nonmedication attempts, then one may proceed with medication, following careful baseline medical and laboratory evaluations, clearly stating what the treatment goals are, and setting a time-limited period when a full reassessment will be undertaken. Periodic review of the medications should include a risk/benefit analysis and periodic reduction of the dosages to see if tapering or discontinuing the medications is possible.

Treatment and management of the family should include counseling and supportive measures. The emotional reaction of parents to having a deaf child can interfere and/or limit their capacity to respond to their child's needs. An impaired child's temperament and the concept of goodness of fit should be considered (Chess et al., 1980). Most reports involving counseling parents whose child has been diagnosed as deaf build on the mourning and grief format as popularized with terminal patients and families. One must wonder what covert message the therapist is giving parents about their child when they are told or believe they should mourn and grieve for the loss of their "idealized" child. Further, many parents tend to reexperience painful emotional feelings with each new developmental transition, which brings a new set of problems reminding them of their child's impairment. It is not helpful to parents for the consultant to imply that they have failed to work the steps and "march" successfully through the stages to "acceptance," when they will continue to shudder at the fact that their child is impaired, as they reexperience their emotions. A more helpful goal for parents is successful adaptation to the impairment while loving their child (S. Chess and I.R. Jenkins, professional experience). Kampfe has adapted the House Social Stress Model for transitions into her work with parents whose child has recently been diagnosed as deaf. She refers to conditioning variables of the parents including social status, experiences, personal resources, social support, etc., which interact with the various responses and especially influence the central core of the transition to adaptation, which is the parent's perceptions of deafness. She has found working with these perceptions a helpful supplement to the more simplistic mourning and grief structure (Kampfe, 1989). Family therapy with a hearing family and a deaf child should consider the use and role of interpreters, even if the therapist can sign (Harvey, 1982). Counseling for the parents should include teaching some technical information in terms that can be clearly understood.

The first experimental cochlear implants on adults were performed in the early 1960s, and clinical trials began in 1973. In 1984 the Food and Drug Administration (FDA) gave marketing approval for the devices in adults. The first implant trial on children was initiated in 1980 at the House Ear institute in California. By 1990, over 500 children, ranging in age from 2 to 17 years, had received the device when the FDA gave marketing approval for implantation in children. The Subcommittee on Cochlear Implants of the American Academy of Otolaryngology makes clear that pediatric candidate selection requires more than a failure to benefit from a full trial of appropriately fitted hearing aids and other devices. Medical history must be considered in addition to psychosocial factors. The psychosocial factors for successful selection include 1) no evidence of severe organic brain damage, 2) no evidence of psychosis, 3) no evidence of mental retardation, 4) no behavioral-personality traits that would make completion of the program unlikely, 5) no . . . unrealistic expectations . . . on the part of the family, and 6) parent-child interaction that will permit follow-up rehabilitation (Kveton, 1991). The later requirement is important because long-term speech therapy training is required following surgery, and readjustment of the device is frequently necessary. Kampfe et al. reviews the literature on the impact of parental expectations as a contributing factor to successful procedures and suggests that parents in early stages of either shock or denial surrounding their child's deafness are not in a position for managing successfully implantation for their child. They are either grabbing for any solution or hoping that the professionals will resolve and "take away" the problems, whereas cochlear implantation requires active long-term participation for parents and children (Kampfe et al., 1993). At the present time, there are only a few implant centers around the country where the staff is adequately trained to provide a full range of services. The experience with adult recipients of the device is more extensive. The Cooperative Veterans Implant Study showed that all recipients were able to hear sound with their implants but that there was a varying degree of effective meaningful auditory perceptions, although being able to hear warning sounds, like horns, is considered a benefit to the patient. Their patients were all postlingually deafened and had a working knowledge of spoken language, but only 61% showed improvement in "open-set" speech recognition, i.e., where the listener cannot be aided by speech reading (Cohen et al., 1993).

Waltzman et al. have reported success implanting multichannel implants in prelingually deaf children. Fourteen prelingually profoundly deaf children (ages 2.6–5.1 years) were given implants following intensive screening evaluations. The children had varying means of communication including sign, oral, total communication, and no demonstrable means of communication. Follow-up data on a variety of testing instruments, only partially complete at the time of writing, but extending to 24 months postsurgically for some children, showed benefit in auditory reception and the acquisition of speech and language expressive skills. They found that children who had received only sign language training prior to implantation did not progress as rapidly as the oral youngsters, but that all of the youngsters continue to require habilitation services (Waltzman et al., 1992). It is unclear, at this time, the ultimate level of open-set auditory receptive and expressive communication these youngsters will achieve. Informal observations from clinicians suggest that the youngsters are also expanding their social interactive potential. Initial reports are encouraging; however, the clinician should not view cochlear implants as a "bionic" ear or cure for profound hearing impairments.

Outcome and Follow-up Data

Parental and professional expectations for the deaf child are cited as significant in terms of the eventual success of the child. Prospective studies provide longitudinal data free from retrospective modification. In 1967 Dr. Stella Chess initiated the Congenital Rubella Behavioral Study, at Bellevue Hospital in New York City, to follow youngsters whose mothers had contracted the virus, generally in the first trimester of their pregnancy, during the worldwide epidemic of 1963–1964. The cohort consisted of 243 children, of whom 177 (72%) had some level of hearing impairment and 61 had severe to profound loss. The other three common impairments of rubella—cardiac, visual, and neurological—were also represented in the cohort at varying percentages (Chess et al., 1971). The cohort was initially evaluated at the age of 3.5–5.5 years, again at 8–9 years of age, and then at 13–15 of age by Dr. Chess. A recent follow-up of the cohort was conducted by Drs. Cohen and Kasen. The cohort were young adults, age 22–24 (Kasen et al., 1990; Kasen et al., unpublished data, 1989; additional findings were presented at the American Psychiatric Association (Jenkins, 1991)). Cohort retrieval was approximately 80% for the first two waves of follow-up, but an increasing percentage were lost by young adulthood. Clinical highlights of the psychiatric and behavioral findings of the cohort include a direct inverse correlation between the number of impairing conditions and those youngsters who were free of psychiatric diagnosis, i.e., from zero impairments had the highest rate free of psychiatric diagnosis, but while serologically positive for rubella, compared with those with all four of the frequent impairing complications who had the lowest rate free of psychiatric impairment. Among the deaf, normal IQ youngsters (N = 83), 71% were free of psychiatric diagnosis on initial evaluation, and that percentage remained stable longitudinally into adolescence. Among the deaf with normal IQ there was a drop in reactive behavioral disorders from the initial evaluation into adolescence. There were 30 youngsters who were deaf and mentally retarded, and their preschool temperamental profile showed that they had higher activity levels, were less adaptable, and were more difficult children. At initial evaluation, 18 of the 243 children (7.4%) showed either the full or partial symptoms of autism, giving a prevalence rate of 741/10,000, several hundredfold greater than in the population at large. Early acquisition of oral skills seemed to be partially important for children who were mainstreamed. By adolescence the mainstreamed group was reading nearly three grade levels higher then the nonmainstreamed group but still only on a fifth grade level. Kasen and Cohen reported on 46 of the deaf, normal IQ cohort as young adults and divided them into two groups, those with 1 year or less of postsecondary or vocational education, and those with more. The former group (N = 22) tended to be unemployed or in limited jobs, while the later group (N = 24) were either still in school or holding better jobs. There was a statistically significant difference between the two groups as to whether they had been mainstreamed or not and their employment status. The mainstreamed group tended to be more successful. Due to sample size, neither socioeconomic status of the parents nor ethnicity could be established as a determinate of the length of postsecondary education. But, trends suggest that higher socioeconomic status and the underrepresentation of minorities determined which children were mainstreamed. Other trends among this young adult cohort, awaiting statistical analysis, include, irrespective of whether mainstreamed or not, the youngsters report communication to be a major problem interfering with family closeness. The majority felt most comfortable in the deaf community, with 84% of the mainstreamed group reporting that their best friend was deaf. The mainstreamed young adults remembered greater social problems in elementary school than their parents reported, while the nonmainstreamed group reported more support and respect from friends and family. On self-reporting scales of social adaption, differences between the two groups were not statistically significant but the mainstreamed group seemed to cope better while the nonmainstreamed group were viewing themselves by different standards, i.e., as in a special handicapped community. The parents of the mainstreamed group tended toward the view that the problems their children faced were either manageable or nonextraordinary with a tendency toward denial, while their children remembered greater difficulties. The mothers of the nonmainstreamed group tended to take more of the responsibility for their child onto themselves and placed less on their children. The suggestion is that in mainstreaming families the psychological burden shifts toward the child, whereas in the nonmainstreamed group, the youngster tends to move into the deaf community, feeling less stress about external realities and possibly not as well prepared for adulthood. The New York Longitudinal Rubella Study covered over 22 years, during which time public attitudes and awareness concerning the special needs of impaired children and their families have dramatically changed. Thus, future research, especially in the area of language education or English as a second language, might result in different conclusions on optimal educational methods for hearing-impaired children. The complexities of culture, socioeconomic status, parental education, parental expectations for their children, educational issues, the heterogeneity of hearing capacity and associated other impairments present daunting research challenges.

This complexity and heterogeneity of the population attest to the inadequacies of simplistic approaches, based on a unitary theoretical formulation, or dogmatism, as to the "correct" communication modality for hearing-impaired children.

Data on employment of deaf individuals is sparse. An important report by Vernon and LaFalce-Landers presents some discouraging data. Although this follow-up does not have a rigorous design, the trend is clear. Forty-seven deaf and hard of hearing individuals for whom Vernon had performed psychometric evaluations throughout his career, and for whom test results indicated a gifted IQ score (IQ 130–150), were followed up after a period ranging from several months to 36 years. Generally the clients had been routine school evaluations while two had been done in psychiatric hospitals. Most had attended or graduated from college or graduate schools for the deaf or were in the mainstream, receiving liberal arts or technical/vocational training, but there had been only a 52% graduation rate. Dropouts were generally attributed to (a) a woman's withdrawal as part of marriage plans, (b) the emotional stress of starting college at age 16 or younger because available secondary school education had been completed, and (c) because hearing colleges lacked sufficient deaf support services.

Employment data showed that one-third, at the time of follow-up, were in professional or supervisory work, almost all within the deaf community, while 30% were unemployed. The remainder were underemployed with respect to their training. Forty percent had received psychiatric therapy for emotional problems or mental illness; 9% of these had been hospitalized (Vernon and LaFalce-Landers, 1993).

Research Directions

Research into sign language as a true language has already been done. While most deaf children learn to read and write English as a second language, the pros and cons of the use of Signed Exact English or ASL in schools need further examination. Educational research to improve language and reading skills is most urgent.

CASE ILLUSTRATION

Jason, a 9-year-old profoundly hearing-impaired boy who was a residential student at a state school for the deaf, was referred for "hyperactivity, he needs Ritalin." The etiology of his impairment was unknown. Deafness was his only impairment, diagnosed at the age of 23 months. Prior to that, his parents' concern about delayed speech was dismissed by their pediatrician. Jason's infant temperament was characterized as difficult, with high energy and irregular unpredictable patterns in comparison with his parents' very organized style. When the diagnosis of deafness was made, his parents felt devastated, but emotionally reorganized themselves around the idea that "Jason would be able to talk and be normal." They both threw themselves into a highly respected oral training program. Jason's mother brought him to a speech therapist daily and worked with him each afternoon. These consuming efforts became the central focus of the family, and his mother remembered, "I felt more like a teacher than a mother." By the age of 5, Jason had approximately a 25-word vocabulary that only his parents, grandmother, and speech therapist could regularly understand. The parent-child relationship was characterized by conflict. Jason started the 1st grade in a mainstream school with resource room support, but he could not be contained in the classroom. After this disastrous year, his parents accepted the suggestion that Jason learn sign language, but they saw this as a defeat. As he learned some sign, he made a friend, his first, but his parents learned only a few basic signs after dropping out of sign language classes. The following year Jason was placed in the state residential school on weekdays, coming home on weekends.

Play therapy evaluation using total communication showed an alert child with very limited capacity to express himself beyond well-practiced phrases and constant repetition of the sign "sorry," which had little meaning for him. He was unable to explain why he was at the residential school other than to sign "friends, friends," and he was unable to describe feelings (e.g., happy, sad, angry). He could not explain why there were problems at school except to sign "teacher angry, teacher angry." He did not demonstrate hyperactivity during the evaluation, although his drawings were undisciplined, suggesting agitation. His drawing of a person scored 6 years on the Goodenough scale. The consultant diagnosed a reactive behavioral disorder in the face of limited communication and limited experience with rules. Stimulant medications were not prescribed; it was suggested the school implement a behavior modification program and that the parents learn sign language.

CASE ILLUSTRATION

Fifteen-year-old Marion was referred for evaluation of possible hysterical deafness. Her audiogram showed moderate to severe impairment, worse in the higher frequencies. Past history included repeated episodes of serous otitis media and a variety of allergies. Her parents complained that she could hear "when she wanted to." Frequently, they would test her by making sudden loud noises to see if she would respond. The evaluation was conducted orally, as Marion did not know sign language. In a quiet one-to-one setting, communication was effective, and her formal mental status examination was within normal limits. Once her confidence was obtained, she confided that sometimes she could hear everything. She said, "In the morning I test myself: I go to the window and listen for the birds. If I can hear them, it will be a good day. If I can't, I listen for the cars. If I can hear them, it will be an OK day. If I can't hear the cars, I turn the radio up all the way to see if I can hear anything." Marion described how she never knew from day to day, depending on her allergies, whether she would be able to hear, and as people would not always believe her, it was just safer to always be "deaf." She said, "When people say I won't listen, it's 'cause they think I don't want to do what they tell me to do, but sometimes I'm not sure what they are telling me, but they think I'm being bad."

VISUAL IMPAIRMENT

Definitions and Historical Note

Blindness was legally defined by the American Medical Association in 1934 at the request of the federal government as central vision of 20/200 or less in the better eye with corrective glasses, and a visual field subtending an angular field of no greater than 20 degrees in the better eye (Scholl, 1986). The purpose of the definition was to determine eligibility for federal insurance programs. This definition does not relate to educability, functional potential, or the nature and quality of the residual vision. The legal definition varies worldwide. Alternative definitions have been developed focusing on functional or educational perspectives (Scholl, 1986). Thus, a child who is legally blind may be able to read large-type materials. Approximately 20% of legally blind children receive no visual input and are totally blind, while the remaining 80% have some form of visual stimulus of tremendously varying quality and usefulness (Scholl, 1986). Currently, there is increased interest in low vision, which has generally been associated with the aging process. The World Health Organization (WHO) definition of low vision overlaps with the legal definition of blindness in the United States (Lawrence et al., 1992). Hofstetter evaluated 137 low vision children, ranging in age from 4 to 18 years, who represented approximately 25% of the students classified as visually impaired in Indiana and determined that only 23% were receiving maximum ophthalmic benefits at that time (Hofstetter, 1991). The nature of the visual pathology and quality of vision can result in varying perceptions and often is dependent on lighting conditions. The legal definition is essentially a distance definition, and although there is usually a correlation between near and far vision, this is not consistent. Attempts at a functional definition usually involve a reading task and are most helpful for educational purposes.

The collection of statistics on incidence and etiology of visual impairments is vulnerable to the definitions of blindness. Nelson and Dimitrova, based on data gathered on the Health Interview Survey (HIS) conducted by the National Center for Health Statistics (NCHS) in 1990, state that there are 95,410 "severely visually impaired" children between the ages of 0 and 17 years old in the United States. They point out that the definition of severely visually impaired differs from that of legal blindness and is not based on visual acuity but on perceived vision problems generally based on reading. This number does not include institutionalized individuals (Nelson and Dimitrova, 1993). In 1992 the American Printing House for the Blind in their annual survey reported that 51,813 students in the United States were registered with the Federal government as visually impaired. Of that group, 27% were classified as visual readers, 9% were in residential schools, and 4% were in programs for multihandicapped individuals (American Print House for the Blind, 1992). Children who are legally blind, but either below school age, institutionalized and not receiving educational services, or otherwise unidentified might not have been counted.

Etiology

The etiologies of visual impairments have varied through time, reflecting changing medical ability to treat infections and infective epidemics. Management of premature infants has improved and reduced the incidence of retinopathy of prematurity (ROP), previously referred to as retrolental fibroplasia. Kirchner has noted from her work and others a higher incidence of handicapping conditions and blindness among lower socioeconomic classes. She points to the increasing number of children born into poverty as a possible explanation for the recently noted increase in the incidence of visually impaired children. She points out that there is no nationwide trend data regarding the changing etiologies of visual impairments, but data collected in Virginia show ROP to be alarmingly increased among children under 5 years of age compared to older cohorts, suggesting a possible trend. She also notes that 64% of the children with ROP have multiple handicaps (Kirchner, 1990). Prenatal congenital conditions including genetic etiologies represent approximately 50% of cases (Ward, 1986).

Clinical Description and Developmental Approach

The section "General Considerations" at the start of the chapter should be consulted, inasmuch as it also applies to blind children. It is initially helpful, although not always correct, to assume that developmental delays and maladaptive, troublesome behavior among visually impaired children is most likely to result from failure to learn a correct behavior, or to reflect lacunae in social training. Visually impaired children can also suffer the full range of clinical psychiatric syndromes. Stereotypic rocking movements in a blind youngster are not pathognomonic of autism (Warren, 1984) or mental retardation; passivity and immobility may or may not reflect depression; and late achievement of motor milestones does not necessarily reflect cognitive problems. All these can stem from environmental issues unique to the visually impaired child.

Substantial developmental data on visually impaired children are accumulating, and the interested reader is referred to the comprehensive and thoughtful review of Warren and the edited text by Scholl. Ferrell et al., in an initial report from the Visually Impaired Infants Research Consortium, found there were some delays in acquisition of the 21 developmental milestones studied, but the median was generally within the age range of the nonimpaired norms. They note that within their sample of 82 youngsters there were distinct differences between the 39 children in which visual impairment existed alone versus the 43 with multihandicaps. This latter group was invariably slower. They also note, but as yet are unable to explain differences in, the acquisition sequence of several milestones between the visually impaired group and the published nonimpaired norms (Ferrell et al., 1990). Vision provides the infant and young child with stimulation and observation to permit imitation and modeling and encourage exploration necessary for further developmental milestones beyond those of infancy. This would include motor, cognitive, social, and language skills (O'Donnell and Livingston, 1991). Scholl (1986) considers the limitation on imitative learning as placing the blind child at a particular disadvantage.

Conceptual Approach to the Evaluation

The psychiatric evaluation of the troubled, visually impaired child, is conceptually aided by the observations of Berthold Lowenfeld. Lowenfeld wrote in 1948 that blindness imposes three major effects on the cognitive functions of children: (*a*) in the range and variety of experiences, (*b*) in the ability to get about, and (*c*) in the control of the environment and the self in relation to it (Lowenfeld, 1981). It is instructive to integrate these influences on developmental acquisition with personality development and the potential psychiatric pitfalls for the visually impaired child. It is not, however, correct to assume that these effects represent restrictions on personality development, nor do they create a "blind personality" (Vander Kolk, 1987).

The effect of visual impairment in the range and variety of experiences is primarily a perceptual consideration. Lowenfeld points out that a blind child, using auditory abilities, can locate a bird by its song but cannot describe its shape, size, or flight. While the tactile sense can describe concrete objects that can be held in the hand, it does not help to describe clouds, stars, or colors, nor can the child experience a very large object or a very small one (Lowenfeld, 1981). Language development for the blind and the sighted infant are essentially equivalent through the babbling stages (Warren, 1984). However, early sensorimotor cognitive development, as described by Piaget, is influenced by the visual-perceptual impairment, and early concept development leading to object constancy, object classification, and ideas of size and weight is vulnerable (Scholl, 1986). The visually impaired child must rely on verbal descriptions provided by the sighted, which when repeated by the blind child can seem shallow or meaningless and are referred to as "verbalisms" (Lowenfeld, 1981). Consequently, development of vocabulary can lag (Warren, 1984), as can general information. Intelligence testing, especially the verbal portions of the WISC-R, should be performed with care by an experienced examiner. It is more appropriate to look for problem-solving strategies than to compute the IQ score (Vander Kolk, 1981). Warren argues that it may be inappropriate to compare the IQ scores of sighted versus blind children, as they have differing cognitive abilities that cannot be measured by one interchangeable test or a particular mode of testing. Groenveld and Jan analyzed the subtests of the WISC-R and the Wechsler Preschool and Primary Scale of Intelligence (WPPSI) in a group of 118 visually impaired children between the ages of 3 years, 10 months and 16 years, 11 months. This sample of children was strictly controlled to exclude children with neurological impairments. Their sample, divided into three groups of visual acuity, ranged from low vision impaired though total blindness. The authors considered the essential cognitive task in each subtest in the batteries and conclude that the WISC-R and WPPSI can offer valuable information as long as the subtests are not used to generate a composite IQ score. They state that the nature of the errors can be analyzed and the batteries used as a diagnostic tool, to tease apart whether errors are the result of vision, understanding sequential relationships, or the interpretation of spatial relationships (Groenveld and Jan, 1992). Clearly, unique issues are faced by research psychologists investigating cognitive development of visually impaired children. Hull and Mason (1993) have reviewed the difficulties faced in Great Britain of standardizing a psychometric test. Alternative psychometric approaches are actively under investigation. The group led by Riet Dekker in The Netherlands have been productive. Their several reports, including Dekker et al. (1990), review the literature and conceptual psychometric issues that go beyond the scope of this chapter. A latter report describes the results of a new testing instrument, the Intelligence Test for Visually Impaired Children, that combines verbal and haptic subtests and which they feel has predicative validity for school achievement (Dekker et al., 1991).

The second effect of visual impairment that Lowenfeld described, the ability to get about, he considers a crucial issue for the blind. Mobility has two components: mental orientation and physical locomotion. Mental orientation is the ability of the individual to recognize and orient in a temporal and spatial way within the environment (Lowenfeld, 1981). This capacity will vary tremendously depending on the age of onset of the visual impairment and the quality of the usable perceptions, if any. Early teaching by caretakers and the environment are influential. For many blind children, early movements within the environment can be an endless sequence of bumping into objects, which can discourage exploration. Fearful or overly protective caretakers might discourage exploration and consequently limit development of mental orientation, resulting in environmentally imposed passivity and dependency. Current trends over the past decade are, however, to start introducing the preschool child to long cane mobility instruction. This involves orientation and mobility training by specialists, who when surveyed generally recommended use of the cane in those areas where a sighted child might wander independently (Skellenger and Hill, 1991).

Physical locomotion is the physical capacity of mobility. Evaluation should consider associated impairments, especially neurological and motor, such as those of cerebral palsy. The early motor developmental milestones of the blind infant are similar to those of the sighted child until the age of 4 months (Warren, 1984). After this early period, however, the lack of visual stimulation as a motivator for the child to explore and interact with the environment can lead to delays in crawling, walking, reaching, grasping, and bilateral hand coordination. Langley's summary as adapted by Hill (1986) reveals that in motor tasks where visual stimulation is a motivator, the blind child tends to lag behind the sighted, but when the task is purely neuromuscular (e.g., sitting or standing alone), there is little difference. Adelson and Fraiberg presented detailed motor developmental data on 10 congenitally blind infants and found developmental differences surrounding self-initiated mobility. They warn that a prolonged period of immobility and limited environmental stimulation for the blind infant can result in poor ego development, especially in the areas of initiative and self-confidence (Adelson and Fraiberg, 1974). Ferrell (1986) urges caution in drawing conclusions about the developmental data in the literature, citing methodological problems including small sample size and lack of control for the etiology, age of onset, and differences in reporting techniques. She is concerned about the assumed validity of comparing visually impaired to sighted children and points to the extent to which parental and teacher expectations foster some of the reported lags (Ferrell, 1986).

Lowenfeld's third observation, about control of the environment and the self in relation to it, is described as a subtle but profound influence on the child's development. In the sighted child, seeing overcomes distances and provides a quick way to evaluate new or changing situations or emergencies. Vision provides the means for observing the behavior of others, especially parents or peers, and for learning by imitation while obtaining immediate feedback through observing facial expressions or nonverbal responses. Early face recognition and social smile by the infant along with eye-to-eye contact are important both to the infant and to caretakers in establishing and developing affective bonds. The blind infant's reaction of stillness to the caretaker's approach can detract from parental affective response (Jan et al., 1977). Nonverbal social cues and body language are not available to the visually impaired child, complicating the development of peer and social relationships. The socially isolated child who is around only adults does not have the opportunity to learn age-appropriate social behaviors and may tend to be the central focus of the family. McGuinness (1970) found that blind children in a mixed educational setting with nonvisually impaired children tended to be more socially mature than visually impaired children in a residential setting. However, the visually impaired children in integrated school settings had more usable residual vision and thus greater potential to observe behaviors.

The developmental tasks of adolescence, separation, and individuation are particularly vulnerable to troubled behaviors, especially if the visually impaired child is reluctant to separate from parents and lacks skills for self-sufficiency. Increased passivity and lack of aggression are seen as consequences of being unable to focus aggression and fear of the consequences (Vander Kolk, 1987). Visually impaired adolescents cannot tailor their clothing or appearance to conform with their peer group and may worry about how acceptable they look. Lowenfeld points to the potential residual worry among the blind that the sighted are looking at them, leading to self-consciousness.

The psychiatric implications of these social issues in the development of personality structure are clear.

Personality Development and Psychiatric Issues

There is no typical blind personality (Warren, 1984). Personality research comparing the visually impaired and the sighted have resulted in inconsistent findings (Vander Kolk, 1981). There has been limited research on the early personality development of visually impaired children. Psychoanalytic reports are often speculative, based on only a few cases, and use poorly defined terms (Warren, 1984). Lowenfeld (1981) critiques the psychoanalytic writings as being overly pessimistic, assuming that ego damage is inevitable and, if not irreversible, at best only partly compensated. The child and adolescent psychiatrist is cautioned against using a ''deficit model,'' which assumes that, because there is an impairment of vision, this means there is necessarily a psychiatric impairment.

Cruickshank (1964) found that among 2,236 visually impaired children for whom reports of emotional status were available, 790 were described as having emotional problems. However, the definition of the visual impairment, background reports, and, as Warren (1984) points out, a definition of what constitutes a serious emotional disorder as opposed to emotional maladjustment were not available.

The Vancouver study of 86 visually impaired children reports that 18.6% of these children were mentally retarded, 3.5% psychotic, and 5.8% suffered organic brain syndromes. Although some children carried multiple diagnoses, 43% of the children were considered to be free of psychiatric diagnosis, and the remainder had a range of difficulties, including adjustment reactions and neurotic and behavior disorders (Jan et al., 1977). The report makes note of several significant points for personality development. The totally blind children in the study had averaged 50 days in the hospital during the 1st year of life, as opposed to 20 days for the partially sighted and only 2 days for the unimpaired controls. Many of those days were spent in an incubator. Breast-feeding was markedly reduced, and the parents showed increased worries about their child's health status in comparison with the control group parents. Later, difficulties with clinging and separation problems were noted, as almost 40% of the mothers noted emotional reactions by their children to further hospitalizations. Other areas of difficulty encountered included prolonged bottle-feeding and chewing problems that seemed to be associated with delays in offering solid foods to the children and in teaching self-feeding, since the mess created discouraged the parents. There was an increased use of pacifiers. Activity levels varied: sleep-wake cycles and dreaming were not a problem compared with that in control subjects. Toilet training, although more difficult because imitation was not available as a teaching mode, was, however, essentially on the same time schedule as for the control children. Control data were not available about fears, but 9% of the visually impaired children had a major problem with fears. However, 28% were reported not to be appropriately fearful. Wiemer and Kratochwill provide a helpful review of the literature regarding fears and anxieties among blind children, as they report the findings of their work looking at the content of fears of blind children at a residential school for the blind. They note that the average number of fears among the children was high and differed in content from reports among sighted children. The blind children's most common fear was that someone they loved would be hurt, followed by fears of physical

danger and harmful situations, whereas among sighted children there tends to be a higher percentage of fears about being hurt psychologically. The study also asked the school's counselors to report fears they most frequently encountered among the children. ''Severe'' fears reported by the counselors, but not the children, included getting a shock from electricity, getting lost, snakes, fire, and guns. Whereas, the children reported falling from high places, strangers, walking alone in the night, dying and bombing attacks, and getting or losing a boyfriend or girlfriend, which the counselors did not include in the severe category (Wiemer and Kratochwill, 1991).

Visually impaired children are reported to have restrictive, unimaginative play patterns. Jan et al. (1977) suggest from their findings that play might serve a different function for blind children. The inability to imitate, in addition to a reluctance on the part of caretakers to spend the time teaching a wide variety of toys to the child, contributed to the observed phenomena. Learning social skills is hampered due to the visually impaired child's lack of interactive play experience (Jan et al., 1977). The requirement for adults to intervene actively to promote social contacts leads further to the child's tendency to focus toward the adult, even if other children are present. Lowenfeld also points to this issue in adolescence, when dating is arranged by sighted friends or adults, thus reducing privacy and inhibiting acquisition of social skills (Lowenfeld, 1981). Jan et al. find it not unsurprising that many visually impaired children and adolescents are quite skillful at interpersonal manipulation, especially when caretakers and the environment find it difficult to set appropriate limits.

Lowenfeld describes four major concerns that present difficulty to the visually impaired adolescent: (a) sexual curiosity, (b) dating, (c) mobility, and (d) concern for the future. The inability to gather sexual information from observation or magazines might compel the sexually curious adolescent to touch or behave in a manner that would violate cultural/social taboos. Dating is an important arena in which one develops self-confidence and asserts a gender role, but ability to date is dependent on meeting another person with the often nonverbal rituals of flirtation and personal appearance. The visually impaired must rely on introductions and arrangements that diminish flexibility and self-confidence while invading privacy. Limited mobility and the lack of access to the family car reduce opportunities for the individuation process. Concerns for the future, involving leaving a protective family or school setting, accepting vocational challenges, and worrying about marriage and genetic transmission of the visual impairments, pose significant hurdles.

Interviewing a Visually Impaired Child

Preceding the interview, the interviewer should have knowledge of the child's degree of independence and cognitive level, events in the home, purposes of the referral, as well as the child's ability to modify behavior (see fuller discussion under ''General Considerations'').

The child psychiatrist evaluating a visually impaired child must modify examination techniques and be prepared to touch the child more than he or she would touch sighted children. The patient should be led to the examining room, and the examiner may initially remain in continuous physical contact with the child holding his or her hand or touching the shoulder in this new environment. The examiner needs to describe all of the toys available to the child in the room if any conclusions are to be drawn about what the child chooses to play with. The child will often ask seemingly impertinent personal questions of and about the examiner, including appearance and marital status, all of which a sighted child or adolescent can determine by observation. Whether answered or not, a friendly tone is essential. The child might not have had experience or orientation to the examination's purposes and procedures, and these should be clearly outlined for the child, including where to sit.

The vast majority of legally blind children are better described as low vision, thus lighting in the examining room is important. There are no fixed rules for lighting, but the examiner must be alert to the unique nature of the child's vision and maximize the residual capacities. The examiner should be alert for glare, background light, and shadows, along with placement of objects in the visual field. Sometimes it is helpful to have a gooseneck lamp available on the table, which the child can move around to maximize vision while playing or drawing. Creating nonglare contrast can be helpful to increase visual perceptions. If drawing tasks are to be part of the evaluation, then the table surface should not be white or shiny, which creates glare, and the child might not be able to tell where the edge of the white paper is as he or she draws. A dull light blue-gray table surface works well, contrasting both white and dark drawing paper, but covering a white table with brown wrapping paper is a satisfactory solution. If white paper is used for drawings, the standard number 2 pencil often does not provide sufficient contrast; a black felt-tipped pen or marker would provide the best contrast. Conversely some children respond better to dark drawing paper and a light-colored or white marker.

Play therapy can be used in the evaluation of blind children, but often the child must be taught how to play. The process of learning play through imitation is often not available to the blind child. In the process of teaching a particular type of play, the clinician can make some valuable observations about the child. Blind children respond best to very realistic objects or toys. For example, play is better with utensils that the child routinely uses, such as real forks and spoons, as opposed to small plastic or metal toys, which have no meaning to the child. Similarly, dolls close to life size with molded realistic facial features and hair will elicit a better response as the child fingers the face than would the soft, more stylized, cloth dolls whose facial feature are sewn on as pieces of fabric and do not have realistic hair. Dollhouses with realistic figures of people (not the wooden stylized ones) and furniture can often elicit helpful information about the home life of the child, but again, the clinician might first have to teach the child how these small objects correspond to, or symbolize, real people or furniture. In general the clinician might find the child will play with toys that are for a younger age group than the chronological age of the child. To develop pretend, imaginative play as part of therapy, it is best to start with real props, if possible, before using more stylized symbolic ones. The children will tend to do pretend play verbally by telling stories as opposed to acting out the behaviors. The clinician can elicit psychodynamic material and dreams in a verbal form, but often the content will seem to be lacking in affect. The lack of apparent substance or affective content is often referred to as "verbalisms" with blind children. Verbalism seems to be more related to the language acquisition process than to the potential for affective content, and the alert clinician by listening to the story content can piece together the affective web that binds the meaning for the child (M. Talbot and A. Henry, Perkins School for the Blind, personal communication).

In conducting the mental status examination, it is to be expected that the visually impaired child may be slower to warm up; long silences should be avoided. Echolalic language is relatively common and not pathological. Body posture, activity levels, and various movements differ from those of the sighted child. Self-stimulative behavior and stereotypic movements are frequently seen and not diagnostic of specific psychiatric conditions. The examiner should speak directly to the child and should accept as an indication of relatedness that the child faces him or her with the ear and not the eyes. The examining clinician should be alert to his or her own personal bias and unconscious judgments, especially involving the child's body posture and direction of gaze during the evaluation. Raver-Lampman (1990), in an interesting protocol, asked 50 subjects who were informed about blindness and in contact with the blind, e.g., counselors, parents, rehabilitation staff, and coworkers with the blind, to evaluate videotapes of two children without gaze direction and two with gaze direction as they answered questions from examiners sitting on either side of them. The tapes were presented in a random order and in opposite recording positions. The results revealed that, when a visually impaired child utilized gaze direction toward the questioner, the child was evaluated by the responding subjects as being more

intelligent and more socially competent than when the child did not use gaze direction. The subjects did comment that gaze direction influenced their judgments.

The consultant doing an evaluation of a blind child should hold in abeyance making clinical assessments for a longer period of time than might be common with an unimpaired child. It is helpful when accepting the referral to indicate that several meetings with the child are normally required. The clinician should be ready initially to teach the child tools necessary for psychodynamic evaluation, e.g., pretend play and drawing tasks. In effect, the assessment is often a functional protocol looking at the child's strengths, learning and problem-solving styles, and what, if any, interfering psychiatric processes are present.

Differential Diagnosis

The differential diagnoses most highly to be considered include mental retardation, pervasive developmental disorder, childhood schizophrenia, and conduct and personality disorders, including immaturity, dependency, and obsessiveness. Mannerisms are likely to give the most diagnostic trouble. Repetitive rocking, swaying, or eyeball pressing have been referred to as "blindisms." These stereotypic behaviors are also seen in other child psychiatric entities, especially mental retardation and autism, which might confuse the evaluation of the visually impaired child. When these behaviors are found among blind children, they should not be considered a symptom of other conditions. There is wide speculation and conflicting research data as to the etiology of these behaviors among blind children. Warren (1984) summarized the data and concluded that currently the most compelling notion is that these repetitive behaviors constitute compensatory self-stimulation for the child in the absence of visual stimulation. Brambring and Troster (1992) looked at the stability of stereotyped behaviors in both infants and preschool blind children over 1 year using questionnaires to the parents. The children were divided into two groups, under 24 months of age and those over. Findings showed that age of onset and the frequency of the behaviors influenced the stability of the behaviors. The more frequent the behaviors and later age of onset, the greater was the probability of the behaviors remaining in the child's repertoire. However, the brief follow-up period was limited to only preschool age.

In addition, if not offered educational opportunities in a mode familiar as a tool of communication, blind youngsters may not have had the opportunity to acquire many facts or learning skills. Early social interaction may have been delayed or nonexistent for blind youngsters, and care should be taken when assessing interpersonal affective responses as an indicator of clinical psychiatric conditions. Superficial symptoms suggesting autism in a blind child often abate when meaningful personal interaction is offered. This is particularly true in the differentiating of blind mannerisms and autistic mannerisms. Unless hearing is an associated handicap, if the child has been exposed to a normal speaking environment, the linguistic criteria of autism, including strange pronunciations as well as use of monotones, are reasonably clear signals of the diagnostic probability of autism. For reasons of convenience and safety, many parents and caretakers tend to require unchanging sequences of activity from their charges, a liking and insistence on invariance in activity requires careful scrutiny before being declared pathological rather than an adaptation to visual impairment and past learning.

Treatment

Prevention of psychiatric problems is clearly most desirable through early intervention programs with blind infants and preschoolers by teaching social skills while supporting the family structure. Reactive disorders are found when the individual, enmeshed in a social network, is uncomfortable and conflict arises. Providing some means of communication and socialization is the first consideration for preventing the most elementary causes of conflict. The blind child will learn to speak in the usual manner, but the meanings of words the youngster cannot experience are difficult to convey and may cause frustration. Colors and the contours of large objects or very small ones are most difficult to describe. Checking of self-appearance for neatness and simple rules of social behavior (such as chewing with the lips closed) cannot be learned by imitation and must be demonstrated, or alternate strategies learned, if the blind child is to be welcomed into society; confrontations, tantrums, and shame may thus be avoided.

As with all sensory-deprived children, when treating a blind child or adolescent, the psychiatrist may be involved triply, providing advice on management to parents and family, to the school, and to the child. This has been discussed above under "General Considerations."

Behavior modification has been used for both deaf and blind children. However, Warren comments that behavior modification approaches among blind children have not been as widely used or reported in the literature as might be expected. Ross and Koenig (1991) provide an interesting single case study, where cognitive therapy was successfully used for a highly motivated 11-year-old blind boy with head rocking. The boy, embarrassed by the rocking and seeking social acceptability, learned to diminish the rocking by placing his hand to his chin in different socially acceptable positions. Counseling with the visually impaired has been reviewed by Johnson (1989). It is emphasized that group sharing of feelings, experiences, and problems, especially with regard to maturational and adjustment issues, is highly useful to the participants. Erin et al. (1991b) have provided a helpful review of the literature regarding teaching social skills to blind and visually impaired individuals. They raise several points, including the value of social skills for a visually impaired child to be successful in a mainstream program. Unfortunately, the literature has paid little attention to younger and preadolescent blind children receiving appropriate training. The studies strongly support that social skills can be developed using different approaches, but most of the intervention reports lack empirical findings, outcome measures, and follow-up. There is the interesting question of whether the goal of social skills training should be to teach the blind the behaviors of the sighted or whether there might be other skills more appropriate to the blind.

Individual psychotherapy has been looked upon as a luxury, but can be invaluable. The therapist must constantly keep alert to the possibility of confusion in the use of language. While blind individuals cannot follow a description of color, they do use many vision-related idioms, such as "I see" for "now I understand."

Medications can be employed with the same criteria as for nonhandicapped children and adolescents. Medications with the potential of interfering with residual visual acuity should be avoided, especially when some vision remains. Jan et al. (1977) point out that their findings suggest an overuse of psychoactive medications among visually impaired clients. Stimulant medications can be used for attention deficit disorder, giving both child and caregiver an opportunity for better communication, education, and other interaction. Consideration must be given to the possibility that frustrations may lead to behavior problems. If frustrations can be eliminated, medication may not be indicated.

Outcome Study

The Vancouver, British Columbia, group, led by Drs. Jan and Freeman, in 1973–1974 studied a group of 92 legally blind children. The results of their original work has been noted earlier in this chapter. The cohort was reevaluated by Freeman et al. in 1987–1988. They were able to retrieve 69 of the original 92 subjects. The full paper should be reviewed by the interested clinician, as a number of subtle points are developed that go beyond the scope of this chapter. Of note is that prior to the reevaluation two senior authors reviewed the original information from the first evaluation to clarify their expectations. The expectations were then compared to the follow-up results in terms of exceeding expectation "somewhat" or "much better." There was varying outcome and many of their subjects defied negative predictions. The follow-up in-

volved two lengthy semistructured interviews covering a wide range of material that permitted the formulation of a psychiatric diagnosis. The extent of visual impairment covered a wide range from partially sighted (legally blind) to totally blind. Interestingly, there was a deterioration of vision among 29% of the partially sighted, which created a higher rate of psychiatric disorder (68.7%) than with those with stable vision. Other important findings that would be helpful to the child psychiatrist making recommendations and treatment plans include that the presence of hard neurological signs, in the absence of mental retardation, was a nonpredictor of psychiatric outcome. Of the 34 subjects without hard neurological signs, 67.6% were rated as psychiatrically normal. When one removes the retarded subjects from the group with hard neurological findings (N = 9), 66.7% had a normal psychiatric diagnosis. Of the 40 subjects whose only impairment is vision, 71.1% had a normal psychiatric diagnosis. Of the 29 with other impairments, only 24.1% received a normal psychiatric diagnosis. An interesting finding was that originally the blind children had undergone standardized IQ testing, and although they were not formally retested, the authors found that the original narrative written descriptions by the psychologists were more helpful than the early IQ numbers themselves. About half of the cohort, both men and women, had romantic relationships, and about one-fifth were now partnered in a relationship, but all with sighted partners. An alarming number, especially women, had reported sexual molestation or abuse. Of particular note was that stereotyped mannerisms had almost disappeared, with the exception of a few multihandicapped subjects. Several participants revealed that at home and alone they do perform the mannerisms but understand that they are socially unacceptable and so control them in public. They remembered their mainstreaming school experiences as being very difficult, with 73% being teased in a mean way. Most (73%) traveled independently and only 3 used dogs, but 40% reported having been hit by a car. For the partially sighted, there was a strong tendency to avoid the negative stereotype of blindness and try to "pass." Freeman et al. comment that the perceived stigma of blindness is such that the routine counseling recommendation of "accepting the handicap" before adjustment might be inappropriate. This corresponds with our (Chess and Jenkins) experience in deafness, that you might always hate having the impairment, but you must adapt. Freeman et al. found deplorable levels of unemployment among the subjects who were qualified for competitive jobs (Freeman et al., 1991).

Research Directions

A central issue at this time is the future direction of education for blind children. The passage of Public Law (PL) 99-457 has provided educational services for impaired children, including infants, along with encouraging educational integration of blind with sighted children. There are an increasing number of blind children who are currently mainstreamed. There has been a long-standing concern that the development of social skills among visually impaired children is delayed in a segregated school for the blind. The belief is that these skills are better developed in an integrated environment as preparation for adult roles in the sighted world. Conversely, with the push for mainstreaming, literacy in Braille has declined and other important unique skills are neglected including abacus use, cane travel, etc., along with specialized support and counseling services for a low incidence impairment like blindness. Currently, the tradeoff appears to be between social versus educational skills. Some are concerned that local school boards see mainstreaming as a way to save money compared with supporting a blind child in a residential school for the blind. Clearly, ongoing research into the relative merits of mainstreaming must look at these issues. The consulting child psychiatrist will continually have to remind school boards about the broad heterogeneity of the blind pediatric population, to forestall decisions that are made based on monolithic assumptions about the visually impaired, in order to provide, on a case-by-case basis, for the best interests of each child.

CASE ILLUSTRATION

Lucy, a 14-year-old blind girl, lost her vision at the age of 1 year following bilateral enucleation for retinoblastoma. She was referred for uncontrollable outbursts of crying, screaming, and striking out wildly at people. She had been diagnosed with borderline personality disorder and was started on neuroleptic medications in fairly substantial doses. Both of her parents were professionals with graduate degrees.

Lucy's early developmental milestones were within normal limits, and her infant temperament was remembered as easy, although she tended to be very moody. Following her surgery and numerous prolonged hospitalizations, her development was delayed, and she was remembered as a very "whiny," crying child, clinging to her mother. The family situation was complicated by several geographical moves. When Lucy was 4 years old, a sister was born. Lucy had been enrolled in a special program and later in a school for the blind. She used a Braille typewriter skillfully. She did well academically but was always described as clinging to her mother, who was described by teacher reports as "too protective and overenmeshed." In school she had no friends or social skills and was described as shy and slow to warm up. There were several school changes, all as a result of family relocations, which disrupted her education and friendships. Several years prior to referral, marital strains had increased.

On psychiatric examination Lucy had difficulty separating from her mother but did come into the consulting room alone. She sat with her head looking down and her right ear turned toward the examiner as she gently swayed forward and back. Her speech was clear and her vocabulary age-appropriate, although she spoke loudly with a broadcasting style. Her concepts were immature, and she repeatedly wanted reassurance that her mother would take care of her and wouldn't leave her. She then described how her father didn't love her or want her. She told how he would hit her on the head when she made a mistake, bumped into something, or knocked something over, calling her "dumb." She then said, "I couldn't see him when he hit me, I never knew which way he was hitting me from, I couldn't protect myself or get out of the way."

Following a trial of family therapy, the parents decided to separate. Lucy entered supportive psychotherapy, and although her medications could not be completely discontinued, they were reduced. A behavior management program was introduced to increase her sense of self-sufficiency and independence.

DEAF-BLINDNESS

Definition

Deaf-blindness is defined in PL 94-142 as "concomitant hearing and visual impairments, the combination of which causes such severe communication and other developmental and educational problems that they cannot be accommodated in a special program solely for the deaf or blind child" (U.S. Department of Health, Education and Welfare, 1985). The definition is educational and does not focus on specific clinical measures. It implies that in combination the two concomitant impairments generate specialized educational needs. As with auditory or visual impairments, the child might be classified as deaf-blind while still retaining some usable residual hearing and/or vision sufficient to permit education, self-sufficiency, and in some cases supported or independent living. The term "deaf-blind," although professionally widely used, might not accurately convey the individual client's circumstances. The words "deaf" and "blind" have strong connotations and the combination can be overwhelming. The clinician might find it helpful to think in terms of the client as being dual sensory impaired.

In 1983–1984 the U.S. Department of Education reported 2,492 deaf-blind children enrolled in educational programs under various assistance programs. These numbers would not include those children receiving no services or those remaining at home or institutionalized. There has been ongoing difficulty gathering accurate numbers. In many jurisdictions the deaf-blind children are classified as multihandicapped and not separately identified. More recent data from the 1990 survey has put the number at 7,297; however, the University of Arkansas Rehabilitation group's work suggests that the mean expectation is 9,805, based on statistical data. Their report provides an interesting overview of the identification and demographic issues (Watson and Taff-Watson, 1993). Although the total numbers are relatively small, Vernon's summary of the literature suggests that the incidence is rising. The increase is secondary to changing social/sexual mores, as a major etiology of deaf-blindness is sexually transmitted neonatal diseases, including herpes simplex virus (Vernon, 1982). As noted earlier in the section of this chapter entitled "Visual Impairment," with the increasing number of children born into poverty, improved neonatal ICU success with low birth weight infants, and the increasing number of high risk pregnancies, it can be assumed that the number of dual sensory impaired children will rise.

Compared with research data collected on deafness or blindness, the literature on deaf-blindness is quite limited. There is a tendency for workers in the field of deafness to view the deaf-blind child as being deaf with an associated visual problem, and vice versa for workers in visual impairments (Warren, 1984). Very few centers are equipped to provide the comprehensive assessment that a deaf-blind child requires. The consulting child psychiatrist should approach the diagnostic evaluation carefully, recognizing the expertise of specialized professionals in visual, auditory, rehabilitation, and educational areas. The psychiatric evaluation has three potential pitfalls: (*a*) failure to recognize the presence of an additional diagnosis of either visual or auditory impairment when evaluating a child who is known to be either deaf or blind, but ascribing the behavioral difficulties to a clinical psychiatric illness (e.g., autism); (*b*) diagnosing a child as deaf-blind when only one sensory impairment exists concurrently with a major clinical psychiatric syndrome; and (*c*) diagnosing mental retardation, schizophrenia, autism, or organic brain syndrome in a deaf-blind child, based on an unusual presentation, without being fully aware of the child's potential strengths or problem-solving and adaptive abilities. Tragically, many deaf-blind children have spent years or a lifetime in custodial institutions, based on inaccurate diagnosis.

Clinical Description

The remarkable achievements of Helen Keller are inspiring and instructive. In her autobiography she remembered speaking words by the toddler years; later, unable to hear, she could use a variety of gestures for communication. She also understood that adults were communicating by speaking, as she retained enough vision to observe their mouths. It was not until she was 7 years old that she was finally diagnosed as deaf-blind (Bjorling, 1981). Her case points to the essential issues for evaluating the deaf-blind child: (*a*) age of onset, (*b*) etiology and associated other impairments, (*c*) degree of sensory loss, and (*d*) strengths and adaptive abilities.

Vernon states that if other factors (e.g., intelligence, degree of sensory loss, and associated impairments) are equal, the age of onset of deaf-blindness is the crucial consideration. There are four possible combinations that can result in deaf-blindness, (*a*) congenital deaf-blindness, (*b*) onset after 3 years of age, (*c*) congenital deafness and adventitious loss of vision, and (*d*) congenital blindness and adventitious deafness. Estimates of independent function for deaf-blind individuals vary and depend on definitions of differing multihandicapped clients and the degree of residual vision and hearing available to the individual. Further, the historical evolution in societal attitudes has changed from simply warehousing people in large public institutions, who might have benefited from a less restrictive environment, to actively seeking alternative dispositions. There has been a large public investment in programs but little solid longitudinal follow-up of the efficacy of various programs, and thus predictions and prognosis are uncertain (Watson and Taff-

Watson, 1993). Bjorling (1981) summarizes the findings to estimate that probably no more than 3–5% of deaf-blind individuals are considered to function independently, and the vast majority of this small group come from adventitiously impaired groups. For the congenitally deaf-blind child, Vernon considers the remaining sensory inputs for information to be inadequate for the child to gather the information necessary to master formal language communication. Michael and Paul strongly advocate early infant intervention programs for deaf-blind children. They point to the uniqueness of the dual sensory combination as dynamically and neurologically linked, necessitating a systematic conceptual approach for the child to acquire various skills. They argue that often, in multihandicapped programs, the specialization is not available for appropriate intervention. Their report also includes an interesting analysis of cognitive theory and review of specialized procedures that go beyond the scope of this chapter (Michael and Paul, 1991).

Etiology

Etiologies, especially of adventitious onset, include trauma, infections (including maternal rubella, a major cause), diabetes, tumors, and injudicious use of antibiotic medications (aminoglycosides). Usher's syndrome, a major contributor, is congenital deafness with progressive visual impairment of varying degrees secondary to retinitis pigmentosa, the latter starting usually during adolescence. The incidence is approximately 3 per 100,000 in the general population but is reported to be between 3 and 6% of the congenitally deaf population (Hicks and Hicks, 1981).

The etiology of a case of deaf-blindness will influence the incidence of associated handicapping conditions. Congenital rubella has a 50–71% reported rate of associated neurological complications among deaf-blind children, with a high incidence of mental retardation (Vernon, 1982).

Stein et al. (1982) reported a high frequency of abnormal head size (40%), neuromuscular disorders (40%), and abnormal EEG (55%). Remarkable in their population of 141 "deaf-blind" children referred to their statewide research institute for special evaluation, 38 (27%) proved to have normal or near-normal hearing, and one had normal vision. These children had been misdiagnosed as deaf-blind, in some cases for many years.

The degree of sensory loss is quite variable and will influence outcome. Hearing tends to be more profoundly impaired than vision.

The combination of dual sensory impairment results in a profoundly different environment for the child's development. Language and general information development have been reported to be significantly below expectations for 75% of these children (Stein et al., 1982).

Psychopathology

Difficult as it is for a hearing parent of a deaf child to communicate, teach social skills, and impart learning, it is even more demanding with a deaf-blind child. It is not merely the addition of blindness that adds to the difficulty, but possibly that the environmental experience or the dynamic neurological linkage referred to previously by Michael and Paul, of the deaf-blind child is beyond our comprehension. The techniques for teaching age-appropriate rules of society and for imparting knowledge to a blind child assume common conceptualizations about the environment and society between the teacher and the child. A formal evaluation of adaptive behaviors and functional strengths is helpful (Suess et al., 1981), as are functional activities (Dunlap, 1985), inasmuch as functional strengths as well as limitations must be known in order to formulate recommendations.

All that has been said in the introductory sections on deafness and blindness about the effect of a handicapped child upon family cohesion and disruption, ambivalence of sibs, and strengths in the family and environment is even more pertinent in the case of deaf-blindness.

Psychiatric evaluation of multiply handicapped children reveals a direct correlation between the number of impairments and the incidence of clinical psychiatric syndromes, including autism and organic brain syndromes (Chess et al., 1971). There is an increase in mental retardation associated with dual sensory loss. Limited research data are available on the psychodynamic aspects of deaf-blindness. Smithdas (1980), commenting on his own experience of being deaf-blind since the age of 4 years, describes the world as "shrinking in size and scope." Yoken (1979), summarizing the extensive profiles of nine deaf-blind individuals who had sufficient language for exploratory interviews, found themes of isolation, dependence, anger, and resentment present but not dominating. Isolation was a reality, and societal rejection based on being different was felt. Many reported being teased as children and became increasingly solitary. Adjustment followed the lines of mourning and grief and religious beliefs were important, but Yoken cautions against drawing generalized conclusions. Psychiatric evaluation of adventitiously impaired deaf-blind children might reveal the characteristics associated with the underlying original sensory impairment, and often the reactive feelings of anxiety, progressive isolation, and grief for the loss.

Evaluation of the Deaf-Blind Child

The practicing clinician, unless he or she is associated with a specialized referral center, will probably not receive a referral for a psychiatric evaluation of a deaf-blind child. However, one should remain alert to the dual sensory impairment in general practice. One of the authors was asked to evaluate a deaf child, at a school for the deaf, who was thought to be autistic. When the examiner made physical contact with the 4-year-old girl laying on the floor flicking her fingers in space, she got up, molded to the examiner's leg, and made affective contact. A diagnosis of deaf-blindness without autism was subsequently made; the visual impairment had not been previously appreciated (Jenkins, personal experience). But, conversely, the clinician might encounter a child who is diagnosed deaf-blind and might be deaf-autistic, blind-autistic, or sensory impaired and mentally retarded. The diagnostic process is really a collaborative team effort with psychologists, educators, and rehabilitation specialists, and the clinician should not feel reluctant to defer diagnosis pending further evaluation. The essence of the evaluation is functional, i.e., looking closely at the child's capacity to function on different tasks, etc. and what clinical psychiatric conditions might interfere with learning and acquiring skills.

Techniques for eliciting information, especially physical contact, lighting, and realistic props for toys, are all similar to those described for blind children (P. Ryan, Perkins School for the Blind, personal communication). A system of manual sign language has been developed. For the few who know it, or with the use of an interpreter, an evaluation can be done, but it requires a great deal of time and patience.

Differential Diagnosis

The psychiatric diagnoses to be differentiated in deaf-blind individuals include mental retardation, childhood autism, childhood schizophrenia, organic brain syndrome, and reactive behavior disorder. One of the sensory impairments may be missed when a diagnosis (accurate or not) of schizophrenia or autism has been decided upon early in the evaluation. The converse might also occur if the clinician attributes behavior to only deaf-blindness. One must recall that ritualistic acts resembling blindisms, such as head weaving and eyeball pressing, are common in severe or profound mental retardation as well as in childhood autism, and both rigidity of behavior and perseveration may characterize deafness or blindness, as well as mental retardation or autism. Generally, deaf-blind individuals without additional pathology will easily stop the rituals if offered gentle human contact as a substitute.

Treatment

Data on treatment of deaf-blind individuals with reactive or more serious psychopathology are woefully lacking. The case of Helen Keller is not a good model, since she had acquired a foundation of remembered visual vistas and words before her deafness and blindness occurred. Also, there was a most unusual combination of intelligence and determination in both herself and her mentor, Anne Sullivan. Behavior therapy is useful in deafness, less so in blindness, and no literature reports have been found for it in deaf-blindness. Psychotherapy or counseling, for the reasons given above, may be useful and available for a chosen few. Medications, simply because symptomatic treatment can at least help in daily living, are used sparingly in carefully monitored protocols. One must be most wary of employing the antibiotic aminoglycosides, because of their potential damage to residual hearing, and the anticholinergic side effects of psychotropic medication might diminish visual perception.

Outcome and Follow-up Data

There have been no organized follow-up or longitudinal studies of deaf-blind individuals to study either psychiatric diagnosis or efficacy of interventions. Nevertheless, some individuals who are deaf and blind do fulfill at least part of their potential and lead competent lives. There has been increased recognition of deaf-blind clients who are aging out of the educational system and the lack of appropriate supportive services available. There has been a shift in focus to establish greater independence during the adolescent years and not have the clients abruptly transferred from the more protective educational systems into the adult rehabilitation facilities when they reach 21. The Arkansas Center's Model Program is one of a number of reports in the literature and is a helpful place for the clinician to review developments in community-based approaches to service delivery (Watson and Taff-Watson, 1993).

CASE ILLUSTRATION

D.W. was a large, Afro-American, deaf-blind 18-year-old youth referred for neuroleptic medication and ''sedation'' by the residence where he lived. He was profoundly hearing impaired, although he wore a postauricular aid to obtain warning signals, and was legally blind, although with corrective glasses he could see images in part of his visual field, permitting him to understand simplified and exaggerated sign language. He was unable to use finger spelling or more intricate sign formations and had a usable vocabulary of approximately 50 formal signs. The residency staff was concerned that when he was upset he swung his arms and banged chairs on the floor.

The etiology of his impairments was uncertain, but was possibly rubella; also, early in life he suffered physical abuse from his mother prior to placement in a custodial institution for the mentally retarded at the age of 4. He had been removed from this institution approximately 9 months earlier following a court order.

Mental status examination showed D.W. to be a very large, neatly dressed Afro-American male, looking older than his age. His behavior and communication were characterized by frequently jumping up from his chair and pantomiming his responses, intermixed with exaggerated signs. He would stand up, move closer to and tower over the seated examiner, and rapidly move his arms in excited gesturing as he expressed himself with affect-laden signs and pantomime. Yet when he was asked to stop or sit down, or when the examiner acknowledged that he understood the communication, D.W. would immediately sit down in his chair with a composed smile appearing satisfied that he had communicated with the examiner. His use of language was restricted and at times perseverative, but his response to limit setting was predictable and appropriate. He was alert. There was no evidence observed that he was hallucinating, nor did he at any time sign to himself or into space. The remainder of the formal mental status examination could not be obtained. Close questioning of the counselor who worked with the client and accompanied him to the evaluation revealed that, although he swung his arms around, D.W. had never hit anyone, and that on every occasion when he picked up furniture he had never thrown or broken it, nor threatened anyone. He would, rather, pick up the furniture and bang the floor and then return it to the same position. There were periods when he did become agitated, go to his room, and ''bang around'' a little.

The residency staff responded to the consultant's interpretation of the communicative nature of D.W.'s behavior and how he had never crossed the line to violence while responding to firm limit setting. The staff acknowledged that, because of their difficulty communicating with him and because of his size and race, people were intimidated by him. The staff agreed to a trial period of recording his baseline behaviors, if we were to initiate a full course of medications, and to try to correlate his behavior with precipitating events over a 3-month period. They accepted the plan, and a backup prescription for neuroleptics was provided, as part of the agreement, to be given if necessary by the on-site staff nurse at her discretion. On follow-up D.W. has been successfully maintained in his residency over the past 4 years without any untoward events, and only on three occasions was he given a single dose of medication.

Acknowledgments. *The authors extend their gratitude to Ruth Green, New York League for the Hard of Hearing, and Kenneth Stuckey, Mary Talbot, Ann Henry, and Pam Ryan, all of the Perkins School for the Blind.*

References

Adelson E, Fraiberg S: Gross motor development in infants blind from birth. *Child Dev* 45:114–126, 1974.

American Printing House for the Blind: *Annual Report*, 1992.

Bjorling B: There was only one Helen Keller. *J Visual Impairment Blindness* 7:305–308, 1981.

Bonham H, Armstrong T, Bonham G: Group psychotherapy with deaf adolescents. *Am Ann Deaf* 7: 806–809, 1981.

Boughman J, Shaver K: Genetic aspects of deafness: Understanding the counseling process. *Am Ann Deaf* 4:393–400, 1982.

Braden J: The criterion-related validity of the WISC-R Performance Scale and other nonverbal IQ tests for deaf children. *Am Ann Deaf* 134:329–332, 1989.

Brambring M, Troster H: On the stability of stereotyped behaviors in blind infants and preschoolers. *J Visual Impairment Blindness* 86:105–110, 1992.

Charlson E, Strong M, Gold R: How successful deaf teenagers experience and cope with isolation. *Am Ann Deaf* 137:261–270, 1992.

Chess S, Fernandez P: Do deaf children have a typical personality? *J Am Acad Child Psychiatry* 19: 654–664, 1980.

Chess S, Fernandez P, Korn S: The handicapped child and his family: Consonance and dissonance. *J Am Acad Child Psychiatry* 19:56–67, 1980.

Chess S, Korn S, Fernandez P: *Psychiatric Disorders of Children with Congenital Rubella.* New York, Brunner/Mazel, 1971.

Chomsky N: *Syntactic Structure.* The Hague, Mouton, 1957.

Cohen N, Waltzman S, Fisher S: A prospective, randomized study of cochlear implants. *N Engl J Med* 328:233–237,1993.

Cruickshank W: The multiple-handicapped child and courageous action. *Int J Educ Blind* 14:1964.

Dekker R, Drenth PJD, Zall JN, et al: An intelligence test series for blind and low vision children. *J Visual Impairment Blindness* 84:71–76, 1990.

Dekker R, Drenth PJD, Zaal JN: Results of the Intelligence Test for Visually Impaired Children (ITVIC). *J Visual Impairment Blindness* 85: 261–267, 1991.

Drukier G: The prevalence and characteristics of tinnitus with profound sensori-neural hearing impairment. *Am Ann Deaf* 134:260–263, 1989.

Dunlap W: A functional classification system for the deaf-blind. *Am Ann Deaf* 130:130, 1985.

Erin JN, Dignan K, Brown PA: Are social skills teachable? A review of the literature. *J Visual Impairment Blindness* 85:58–61, 1991b.

Erin JN, Rudin D, Njoroge M: Religious beliefs of parents of children with visual impairments. *J Visual Impairment Blindness* 85:157–162, 1991a.

Evans J, Elliott H: The Mental Status Examination. In: Elliott H, Glass L, Evans J (eds): *Mental Health Assessment of Deaf Clients: A Practical Manual.* Boston, Little, Brown, 1987.

Ferrell K: Infancy and early childhood. In: Scholl G (ed): *Foundations of Education for the Blind and Visually Handicapped Children and Youth.* New York, American Federation for the Blind, 1986.

Ferrell KA, Trief E, Dietz SJ, et al: Visual Impaired Infants Research Consortium (VIIRC): First-year results. *J Visual Impairment Blindness* 84: 404–410, 1990.

Freeman R, Blockberger S: Language development and sensory disorder: Visual and hearing impairments. In: Yule W, Rutter M (eds): *Language Development and Disorders.* Oxford, Blackwell, 1987.

Freeman RD, Goetz E, Richards DP, et al: Defiers of negative prediction: A 14-year follow-up study of legally blind children. *J Visual Impairment Blindness* 85:365–370, 1991.

Furth H: Linguistic deficiency and thinking. *Psychol Bull* 76:58–72, 1971.

Groenveld M, Jan JE: Intelligence profiles of low vision and blind children. *J Visual Impairment Blindness* 86:68–71, 1992.

Harvey M: The influence and utilization of an interpreter for deaf persons in family therapy. *Am Ann Deaf* 127:821–827, 1982.

Heller B, Harris B: Assessment of hearing impaired persons. In: Heller B, Flohr L, Zegans L (eds): *Psychosocial Interventions with Sensorially Disabled Persons*. Orlando, FL, Grune & Stratton, 1987.

Hicks W, Hicks D: The Usher's syndrome adolescent: Programming implications for school administrators, teachers, and residential advisors. *Am Ann Deaf* 126:422–431, 1981.

Hill E: Orientation and mobility. In: Scholl G (ed): *Foundations of Education for Blind and Visually Handicapped Children and Youth*. New York, American Foundation for the Blind, 1986.

Hofstetter H: Efficacy of low vision services for visually impaired children. *J Visual Impairment Blindness* 85:20–22, 1991.

Hull T, Mason H: Issues in standardizing psychometric tests for children who are blind. *J Visual Impairment Blindness* 87:149–150, 1993.

Jan JE, Freeman RD, Scott EP: *Visual Impairments in Children and Adolescents*. New York, Grune & Stratton, 1977.

Johnson C: Group counseling with blind people: A critical review of the literature. *J Visual Impairment Blindness* 83:202–207, 1989.

Johnson W: Assessment of multi-handicapped deaf students. *Am Ann Deaf* 134:79–83, 1989.

Kampfe C: Parental reaction to a child's hearing impairment. *Am Ann Deaf* 134:255–259, 1989.

Kampfe C, Harrison M, Oettinger T, et al: Parental expectations as a factor in evaluating children for the multichannel cochlear implant. *Am Ann Deaf* 138:297–303, 1993.

Kasen S, Ouellette R, Cohen P: Mainstreaming and postsecondary educational and employment status of a rubella cohort. *Am Ann Deaf* 135:22–26, 1990.

Kelly D, Forney J, Parker-Fisher S, et al: The challenge of attention deficit disorder in children who are deaf or hard of hearing. *Am Ann Deaf* 138:343–348, 1993a.

Kelly D, Forney J, Parker-Fisher S, et al: Evaluating and managing attention deficit disorder in children who are deaf or hard of hearing. *Am Ann Deaf* 138:349–357, 1993b.

Kirchner C: Trends in the prevalence rates and numbers of blind and visually impaired schoolchildren. *J Visual Impairment Blindness* 84:478–479, 1990.

Kveton J, Balkany T: Status of cochlear implantation in children. *J Pediatr* 118:1–7, 1991.

Lawrence M, Lovie-Kitchin J, Brohier WG: Low vision: A working paper for the World Health Organization. *J Visual Impairment Blindness* 86:7–9, 1992.

Lane H: *When the Mind Hears*. New York, Random House, 1984.

Lennan R: Behavior-modification model in a residential setting for multihandicapped deaf children. In: Stein L, Mindel E, Jabaley T (eds): *Deafness and Mental Health*. New York, Grune & Stratton, 1981.

Levine E: *The Ecology of Early Deafness*. New York, Columbia University Press, 1981.

Levine E, Naiman D: Seminar on behavior modification methods for psychologists working with the deaf. *Am Ann Deaf* 115:455–491, 1970.

Ling D, Ling A: *Aural Habilitation*. Washington DC, The Alexander Graham Bell Association for the Deaf, 1978.

Lobato D, Faust D, Spirto A: Examining the effects of chronic disease and disability on children's sibling relationships. *J Pediatr Psychol* 13:389–407, 1988.

Lowenfeld B: *Berthold Lowenfeld on Blindness and Blind People, Selected Papers*. New York, American Foundation for the Blind, 1981.

McGuinness R: A descriptive study of blind children educated in the itinerant teacher, resource room, and special school settings. In: Clark L (ed): *The Research Bulletin*. New York, American Foundation for the Blind, 1970, pp. 39–67.

Meadow K: *Deafness and Child Development*. Berkeley, University of California Press, 1980.

Meadow K, Trybus R: Behavioral and emotional problems of deaf children: An overview. In: Bradford L, Hardy W (eds): *Hearing and Hearing Impairment*. New York, Grune & Stratton, 1979.

Meadow-Orlans K: An analysis of the effectiveness of early intervention programs for hearing-impaired children. In: Guralnick M, Bennett F (ed): *The Effectiveness of Early Intervention for At-Risk and Handicapped Children*. New York, Academic Press, 1987.

Michael M, Paul P: Early Intervention for Infants with Deaf-Blindness. *Except Child* 57:200–209, 1991.

Mindel E, Vernon M: *They Grow in Silence*. Silver Spring, MD, National Association of the Deaf, 1971.

Moores D: *Educating the Deaf* (2nd ed). Boston, Houghton Mifflin, 1982.

Nelson KA, Dimitrova E: Severe visual impairment in the United States. *J Visual Impairment Blindness* 87:80–85, 1993.

Northern J, Downs M: *Hearing in Children* (3rd ed). Baltimore, Williams & Wilkins, 1984.

O'Donnell LM, Livingston RL: Active exploration of the environment by young children with low vision: A review of the literature. *J Visual Impairment Blindness* 85:287–291, 1991.

Quigley S: Environment and communication in language development. In: Bradford L, Hardy W (eds): *Hearing and Hearing Impairment*. New York, Grune & Stratton, 1979.

Raver-Lampman SA: Effect of gaze direction on evaluation of visually impaired children by informed respondents. *J Visual Impairment Blindness* 84:67–70, 1990.

Ross DB, Koenig AJ: A cognitive approach to reducing stereotypic head rocking. *J Visual Impairment Blindness* 85:17–19, 1991.

Schildroth A, Hotto S: Annual survey of hearing-impaired children and youth: 1991–92 school year. *Am Ann Deaf* 138:163–175, 1993.

Schlesinger H, Meadow K: *Sound and Sign*. Berkeley, University of California Press, 1972.

Scholl G: What does it mean to be blind? In: Scholl G (ed): *Foundations of Education for Blind and Visually Handicapped Children and Youth*. New York, American Foundation for the Blind, 1986.

Skellenger AC, Hill EW: Current practices and considerations regarding long cane instruction with preschool children. *J Visual Impairment Blindness* 85:101–104, 1991.

Smithdas R: Reflections of a deaf-blind adult. *Am Ann Deaf* 125:1015–1017, 1980.

Stein L, Palmer P, Weinberg B: Characteristics of a young deaf-blind population. *Am Ann Deaf* 127:828–837, 1982.

Stokoe W: *Sign Language Structure* (rev ed). Silver Spring, MD, Linstok Press, 1978.

Stokoe W, Casterline D, Croneberg C: *A Dictionary of American Sign Language on Linguistic Principles* (new ed). Silver Spring, MD, Linstok Press, 1976.

Suchman R: Visual impairment among deaf children. *Arch Ophthalmol* 77:18–21, 1967.

Suess J, Dickson A, Anderson H, et al: The AAMD Adaptive Behavior Scale norm referenced for deaf-blind individuals: Application and implication. *Am Ann Deaf* 126:814–818, 1981.

US Department of Education, Office of Special Education and Rehabilitative Services: Fifth and Seventh Annual Reports to Congress on the Implementation of Public Law 94-142. In: *Summary of Data on Handicapped Children and Youth*. Washington, DC, Human Services Research Institute, 1985.

Vander Kolk C: *Assessment and Planning with the Visually Impaired*. Baltimore, University Park Press, 1981.

Vander Kolk C: Psychosocial assessment of visually impaired persons. In: Heller B, Flohr L, Zegans L (eds): *Psychosocial Interventions with Sensorially Disabled Persons*. Orlando, FL, Grune & Stratton, 1987.

Vernon M: Rh factor and deafness: The problem, its psychological, physical, and educational manifestations. *Except Child* 34:5–12, 1967.

Vernon M: Multihandicapped deaf children: Types and causes. In: Tweedie D, Shroyer E (eds): *The Multihandicapped Hearing Impaired*. Washington, DC, Gallaudet College Press, 1982.

Vernon M, Alles B: Psychoeducational assessment of deaf and hard of hearing children and adolescents. In: Lazarus P, Strichart S (eds): *Psychoeducational Evaluation of Children and Adolescents with Low-Incidence Handicaps*. Orlando, FL, Grune & Stratton, 1986.

Vernon M, LaFalce-Landers E: A longitudinal study of intellectually gifted deaf and hard of hearing people. *Am Ann Deaf* 138:427–434, 1993.

Waltzman S, Cohen N, Shapiro W: Use of a multichannel cochlear implant in the congenitally and prelingually deaf population. *Laryngoscope* 102:395–399, 1992.

Ward M: The visual system. In: Scholl G (ed): *Foundations of Education for Blind and Visually Handicapped Children and Youth*. New York, American Foundation for the Blind, 1986.

Warren D: *Blindness and Early Childhood Development* (2nd ed). New York, American Foundation for the Blind, 1984.

Watson D, Taff-Watson M (eds): *A Model Service Delivery System for Persons Who Are Deaf-Blind*. University of Arkansas Rehabilitation, Research and Training Center, 1993.

Wiemer SA, Kratochwill TR: Fears of visually impaired children. *J Visual Impairment Blindness* 85:118–124, 1991.

Yoken C: *Living with Deaf-Blindness, Nine Profiles*. Washington, DC, The National Academy of Gallaudet College, 1979.

50 ATTENTION DEFICIT HYPERACTIVITY DISORDER

Gabrielle Weiss, M.D., F.R.C.P.(C.)

The characteristics of this disorder were colorfully described in a popular German children's book, written in 1863 by Heinrich Hoffman, entitled Struwel Peter. In the English translation, one verse reads:

Phil stop acting like a worm
the table is no place to squirm
Thus speaks the father to his son
severely say it, not in fun.
Mother frowns and looks around
although she doesn't make a sound.
But Phillip will not take advice
he'll have his way at any price.
He turns and churns
he wriggles and jiggles
here and there on the chair.
Phil these twists I cannot bear.

Struwel Peter's antics were like those of normal children, but worse—he was like that all the time; he was always in trouble. There is something to be learned from this. Most symptoms of the syndrome are at times manifested by all children. One major difference is that in children with attention deficit hyperactivity disorder (ADHD), the symptoms are more severe and pervasive. They cluster together to form a syndrome, and they are present for many years; they are not a temporary reaction to a stressful event.

For convenience in this chapter, the DSM-IV (American Psychiatric Association, 1994) term *attention deficit hyperactivity disorder* will be used interchangeably with the term *hyperactive child*. That there is not one type of hyperactive child but several subsyndromes and overlapping syndromes will become increasingly clear throughout the chapter.

This syndrome has captured the interest of researchers and clinicians for 3 decades. It is now the most intensively studied syndrome in child psychiatry and possibly also the most controversial. For example, between 1957 and 1960, 31 articles were published on hyperactivity in children, and between 1977 and 1980 this figure rose to 7000. The increase in the rate of publication of articles related to the syndrome is continuing and, as a result, it is no longer possible to write a comprehensive chapter on all aspects of the syndrome. Key clinical issues and recent research findings have been selected in this chapter for emphasis. It is of some interest to speculate on the reasons for this degree of research activity on the syndrome:

1. The disorder is prevalent, especially in boys (and there is increasing recognition of its presence also in girls).
2. Children with ADHD are conspicuous, both because of their annoying disruptive behavior and because of their school underachievement. Yet, unlike the more serious disorders, such as pervasive developmental disorders, the children look normal and behave normally at times. This makes them a special challenge to understand better and to treat more effectively.
3. The syndrome is a paradigm for a true biopsychosocial disorder. This generates clinical and research interest for many different professional disciplines.
4. By the 1960s, numerous double-blind placebo-controlled studies were published indicating that stimulants were highly effective in improving most of the symptoms of the syndrome. The therapeutic optimism was heuristic for initiating studies on details of the effects of the stimulants (Gittelman-Klein, 1987), as well as generating testable hypotheses on the underlying neurochemical basis of the disorder (Zametkin and Rapoport, 1987).

5. The results of well-controlled follow-up studies contradicted the earlier optimistic view that children naturally outgrow this disorder by adolescence. It was found that almost half the children did not outgrow the symptoms and that a few were at risk for developing antisocial behavior in adolescence and adulthood (Gittelman et al., 1985; Weiss and Hechtman, 1985). This highlighted the importance of treatment to prevent future academic failure, social isolation, and possible criminal behavior.

DEFINITION

Hyperactive children have a short attention span; difficulties with inhibitory control, manifested by behavioral and cognitive impulsivity; and inappropriate restlessness. They do not reflect, but jump in where angels fear to tread. They have a hard time regulating their activity, attention, and social interactions to conform to the expected norms of the particular situation. These traits lead to their being frequently in trouble with adults and unpopular with peers. They underachieve at school (or do not achieve at the level expected for their intelligence), and most have learning difficulties—due, mostly, to poor attention, poor organization, and impulsive cognitive styles. In addition, a minority have specific learning disabilities, such as reading disorders. Many children have concomitant externalizing disorders, such as conduct disorder or oppositional defiant disorder. A minority have depressive or anxiety disorders as well as the core syndrome.

The condition is seen in all areas of the world and, while it is more common in males, the ratio of male to female decreases when the condition is diagnosed in community samples rather than in clinical samples.

HISTORICAL NOTE

Some of the controversy around this syndrome was generated by the many changes in the terminology of the disorder—changes that reflected historical trends in conceptualizing either various etiologies or cardinal features of the syndrome. The syndrome was described in the medical literature at the end of the 19th century by terms such as "mad idiots," "impulsive insanity," and "defective inhibition" (Thorley, 1984).

In 1902, Still gave a lucid description that sounds similar to present-day definitions. He described the children as being hyperactive, unable to concentrate, and having learning difficulties and conduct problems. He terms the children as having "morbid defects of moral control." He noted that boys were more often affected than girls and postulated both organic and environmental etiologies.

Subsequently, in a historical shift, the syndrome began to be viewed as organic in origin. This was due, in part, to the influenza pandemic following World War I and the epidemic of encephalitis lethargica that occurred as a sequela. Children who survived the latter frequently developed a severe behavior disorder (Hohman, 1922), similar to that described by Still, and were described as being "organically driven" (Kahn and Cohen, 1934). Lewin (1938), in Great Britain, was also influential in that he described a link between severe brain damage and restlessness in retarded children and adults, as well as a similar correlation in laboratory animal studies. Finally, the organic etiology hypothesis was emphasized by Strauss and co-workers (1947), in the United States, who described retarded children who had hyperactivity, distractibility, impulsiveness, perseveration, and cognitive defects. He considered these retarded children to be brain damaged even when the latter could not be demonstrated. Strauss termed these children as having "minimal brain damage syndrome."

Some clinicians at the time recognized the circular reasoning implied and suggested that a child should not be labeled as brain damaged solely because of his or her behavior, unless the damage was demonstrated. In an attempt to compromise between the idea that some disorder not constituting actual damage appeared to be present in the brains of these children, and the idea that there was a purely environmental etiology (which would thus blame parents for their children's difficulties), Clements and Peters (1962) coined the term *minimal brain dysfunction* (MBD). The term achieved widespread popularity and was endorsed, but with a warning, by Ronald MacKeith, M.D., at the conclusion of an international conference held in Oxford in 1962. In an article entitled "Minimal Brain Damage: A Concept Discarded" (1963) MacKeith warned that the new terminology of MBD, while an improvement over the older one, included a heterogeneous group of children who would have to be subclassified in the future. Nevertheless, the term MBD was held onto tenaciously in spite of criticism of overinclusiveness.

Efforts to create a more scientifically valid and reliable classification began with the ICD-9 (World Health Organization, 1965) and the DSM-II (American Psychiatric Association 1968), when the terminology was changed to *hyperkinetic syndrome of childhood*. In Great Britain, this term is still in use (now replaced by ICD-10) and refers to a relatively rare disorder of pervasive overactivity and inattention. Retarded and/or brain-damaged children are included in the diagnosis but, unlike practice in the United States, disorders of conduct, even if they co-occur, exclude children from the diagnosis. This difference in diagnostic criteria between the two countries has made comparisons of many studies meaningless.

In the past decade, the work of Douglas (1983) was influential in postulating that the basic deficit of the disorder lies in a failure to regulate attention arousal and inhibitory control, defects that were more fundamental to the disorder than restlessness. The DSM-III (American Psychiatric Association, 1980 recognized this emerging opinion and renamed the condition *attention deficit disorder* with or without hyperactivity (ADDH or ADD). Three core constituents of the disorder were described and symptoms were listed under them, namely, inattention, impulsiveness, and restlessness. More recently, emphasis is being placed on the lack of inhibitory control—meaning, specifically, the inability to delay response—as being the cardinal difficulty of children with ADHD (Barkley, 1994; Quay, 1988). It was also found in factor analysis studies that this difficulty correlated highly with hyperactivity, and this is reflected in the diagnostic criteria for ADHD in DSM-IV.

The distinction between the three core problems of the syndrome was short-lived, and DSM-III-R (1987) changed the terminology to *attention deficit hyperactivity disorder* (once again making restlessness more primary to the disorder) Porrino et al., 1983, and ADD—without hyperactivity—was omitted. ADHD lists 14 symptoms, of which 8 are required for a diagnosis. The reasons for this change are discussed in a review by Cantwell in 1988 and are beyond the scope of this chapter.

In DSM-IV (1994) the terminology remains the same, *attention deficit/hyperactivity disorder*, and the disorder once again is described under *Disruptive Behaviors*. In this classification, however, a patient would obtain the diagnosis by scoring on 6 out of 9 items related to inattention (that have persisted for at least 6 months to a degree that is maladaptive and inconsistent with developmental norms), or by scoring on 6 out of 9 items related to hyperactivity/impulsivity. When a patient scores on both the inattentive type and the hyperactive-impulsive type he is said to have ADHD combined type. This last classification suggests 2 possible subtypes, one related to inattention and the other to hyperactive/impulsive behaviors, which may well co-exist. It emphasizes the importance of impulsivity, which for some is a very enduring symptom, continuing into adulthood. DSM-IV has grouped hyperactivity-impulsivity together as a single subtype of ADHD because studies confirm that they constitute a single dimension of behavior.

For several reasons DSM-IV, as a diagnostic instrument, results in a larger number of patients receiving a diagnosis of ADHD, and these patients are potential candidates for stimulant therapy. We have seen an increasing number of girls in elementary school and both male and female adolescents who are not hyperactive-impulsive or disruptive, but who present with severe underachievement because of inattention and who fit criteria for ADHD-inattentive type. This, together with making the terminology suitable also for the diagnosis of adults, has resulted in an increase in the number of patients given the diagnosis and for whom stimulants may be prescribed. It has been estimated that DSM-IV has increased the diagnosis of ADHD by 24% (Lahey, 1994), even without counting adults thus diagnosed.

In summary, this historical survey of terminologies of the disorder highlights (*a*) that the disorder was described over 100 years ago, (*b*) that changes in terminology have reflected changing concepts of the etiology and cardinal underlying difficulties of the syndrome, and (*c*) that differences in the criteria used in Great Britain and the United States have made comparison of research studies between the two countries difficult.

PREVALENCE

The prevalence figures given for ADHD vary greatly, not only among countries but also within a given country. In Great Britain, one study showed that 1 of 1000 children had the hyperkinetic reaction of childhood (Rutter et al., 1970), while in the United States a figure of 20% was given (Huessy, 1967). These differences result not from real discrepancies in prevalence rates but from important methodological differences among the various studies, such as the following:

1. Differences in terminologies used, resulting in the inclusion of different kinds of children: This alone accounts in large measure for the above-mentioned variance in prevalence rates.
2. The use, in some studies, of rating scales to determine prevalence: An arbitrary selection of a cut-off point, such as 1, 1.5, or 2 SD above the mean, will obviously affect the results. (In choosing a cut-off point, it should be remembered that we are probably not dealing with a normal distribution curve [Shapiro and Garfinkel, 1986].)
3. Differences in the number of sources of information required in order to make a diagnosis: For example, if parents, teachers, the child, and his or her physician are all required to make the diagnosis, the prevalence figure will be lower (Lambert et al., 1978). In contrast, if a single source of information (e.g., teacher or parent) is required for a single symptom, such as hyperactivity, 58% of boys have been considered deviant (Lapousse and Monks, 1958). (The latter shows that parents and teachers tend to have unrealistic expectations regarding childhood behaviors that they find annoying.)
4. The inclusion, in some prevalence studies, of the requirement that the syndrome of ADHD be pervasive: That is, it has to be present in more than one situation (e.g., at home and at school).
5. Differences in the ages of the children sampled in the various studies.

In the recent comprehensive prevalence study of ADDH from the Ontario Child Health Study by Offord and co-workers (Szatmari et al., 1989a and b), 11 studies are summarized. Table 50.1 shows the differences in age, type of sample, sample size, method of diagnosis, sex ratio, urban versus rural living, and socioeconomic class, all of which may affect prevalence.

Offord's study indicated that the peak prevalence of 8% occurs between 6 and 9 years in a representative community sample and is lower for preschoolers and adolescents. The condition is more common in boys (9%) than in girls (3.3%). (Studies based on clinical samples have found a higher differential prevalence between boys and girls.) In this study, ADDH was the most common diagnosis in children 4–11 years of age, and conduct disorder the most common in adolescents of 12–16 years. Forty percent of ADDH children and adolescents also had a diagnosis of conduct disorder. ADDH was more common in urban than in rural areas. This study has certain unique features. The sample size was large enough to guarantee, with 95% certainty, that the estimated rates

Table 50.1. Prevalence Surveys of ADHD

Authors	N	Age	Sample	Method of Diagnosis	Prevalence Rates (%)	Male/Female Ratio	Socioeconomic Effects	Urban-Rural
Werner et al. (1968)	750	10	Birth cohort	Interview	5.9	2.7/1	No effect	No data
Rutter et al. (1970)	2,199	10–11	Total population	Interview	0.09	Two few cases	No data	No pop.
Miller et al. (1973)	849	Grade 3–6	Schools	Interview	5.5	6.8/1	No data	No data
Nichols and Chen (1977)	29,889	7	Birth cohort	1.0 S.D. on questionnaire	7.9	1.6/1	Slight in low SES	No data
Glow (1980)	256	5–12	School	2 S.D. on Conners	6.6	4.6/1	No data	No data
Lambert et al. (1978)	5,212	K–Grade 5	Schools	Questionnaire	1.19	6–8/1	Slight in low SES	No data
Trites et al. (1979)	14,083	3–12	Schools	1.5 S.D. on Connors	14.3	2.7/1	No data	No data
Schachar et al. (1981)	1,536	10–11	Total population	Score >3 on both Rutter Scales	2.2	2.9/1	Slight in low SES	No data
Holborrow et al. (1984)	1,908	Grade 1–7	Schools	2 S.D. on	5.6	3.7/1	No data	No data
McGee et al. (1985)	951	7	Birth cohort	Score >5 on Rutter B Scale	1.9	8.3/1	No data	No data
Shekim et al. (1985)	114	9	Schools	DISC, and DISC-P interview	1.4 (either parent or child)	2/1	No data	No data

From Szatmari P, Offord DR, Boyle MH, Ontario Child Health Study: Prevalence of attention deficit disorder with hyperactivity. *J Child Psychology Psychiatry* 30:220, 1989.

were within 4% of the population rates. Multiple sources of information were used to make the diagnoses. The sample had a wide age range (4–16 years), and socioeconomic data, including urban versus rural living, were included.

The first investigations (Lambert et al., 1978) to recognize the marked differences in prevalence rates, depending on the number of sources who diagnosed the disorder, found that when three defining systems—parent, teacher, and physician—all diagnosed the disorder, the prevalence for the East Bay area of San Francisco was 1.2%. The rate was five times as high when the condition was diagnosed by one of the three sources. A fairly similar result was obtained when Schachar and co-workers (1981) returned to the Isle of Wight in 1975, 5 years after Rutter's original prevalence study (Rutter et al., 1970). Schachar found that 2.2% of the 1500 children about whom questionnaires were completed were pervasively hyperactive. The 500 children whose parents did not cooperate with the study made up a more deviant subgroup. Hence, his prevalence rate was probably an underestimate.

When all children in grades 2–6 were comprehensively evaluated by the Connors Teachers Rating Scale, a structured interview (Diagnostic Interview for Children and Adults), and an attentional battery of tests, a prevalence rate of 2.3% was found. Another 3% had ADDH and conduct problems, and 3.6% had conduct disorder only (Shapiro and Garfinkel, 1986).

The higher prevalence rate of the Ontario study probably reflects the fact that the diagnosis was based only on rating scales and, in addition, that the majority of children in the Ontario study were situationally hyperactive, with only 15% of those diagnosed being pervasively hyperactive. Whalen and Henker (1991) have suggested that the condition is more common than expected in subgroups assumed to have low rates, such as girls or adolescents.

CLINICAL DESCRIPTION

ADHD is one of three disruptive disorders of childhood that are distressing to adults. It is included, along with oppositional defiant disorder and conduct disorder, in the DSM-III-R and DSM-IV categories of disruptive behavior disorders of childhood and adolescence (Table 50.2).

In DSM-III-R, the 14 behaviors listed were not grouped, as they were in DSM-III, under the three core symptoms of inattention, impulsiveness, and restlessness. Omitting the distinction and assuming, as DSM-III-R did, that the behaviors were part of a unitary dimension has allowed the inclusion of some additional behaviors that are hard to assign to one of the three core symptoms. Furthermore, DSM-III-R and DSM-

IV have an advantage in including degrees of severity of the disorder. In DSM-IV, symptoms are grouped under 2 core problems: The first is related to inattention and the second to hyperactivity-impulsiveness. This new classification allows a category of disorder related to attention deficits alone, without hyperactivity-impulsiveness, as did DSM-III. For details of DSM-IV current classification see Table 50.2 (see DSM-IV published version).

Our understanding of the behavioral differences of children with ADHD from those with other disorders comes from many studies whose results are based on mean group differences between hyperactive and normal children. Information about the specificity of the syndrome thus obtained has some limitations. For example, the inclusion of a more deviant subgroup into the larger group of hyperactive children (such as children who have concomitant conduct disorders or severe specific learning disabilities) could theoretically account for all the difference between the whole group and the matched normal control group. In addition, group means tell us nothing about the sometimes marked individual differences between children within the group. Finally, a comparison of a hyperactive group of children with a normal control group cannot give information about whether any differences found are specific to ADHD.

Core Difficulties of the Syndrome

In spite of the difficulties encountered in interpreting some research findings, there is generally good agreement among clinicians and researchers on the main types of problems shown by hyperactive children. Their most distinguishing feature is that they constantly get into trouble at home, within the family, and at school, with their teachers and peers. They find it very difficult to complete any task and, in spite of generally good intelligence, are unsuccessful at school.

Although the syndrome manifests itself somewhat differently at different ages, the most frequent age of referral for help is between the ages of 6 and 9 years. Most studies have concentrated on this age range and, hence, most of our knowledge is about hyperactive children in elementary school. These children have the following characteristics:

1. Inappropriate or excessive activity unrelated to the task at hand, which generally has an intrusive or annoying quality
2. Poor sustained attention
3. Difficulties in inhibiting impulses in social behavior and on cognitive tasks
4. Difficulties getting along with others

Table 50.2. Diagnostic Criteria for Attention Deficit Hyperactivity Disorder

A. Either (1) or (2):
  (1) six (or more) of the following symptoms of **inattention** have persisted for at least 6 months to a degree that is maladaptive and inconsistent with developmental level:

  Inattention
  (a) often fails to give close attention to details or makes careless mistakes in schoolwork, work, or other activities
  (b) often has difficulty sustaining attention in tasks or play activities
  (c) often does not seem to listen when spoken to directly
  (d) often does not follow through on instructions and fails to finish schoolwork, chores, or duties in the workplace (not due to oppositional behavior or failure to understand instructions)
  (e) often has difficulty organizing tasks and activities
  (f) often avoids, dislikes, or is reluctant to engage in tasks that require sustained mental effort (such as schoolwork or homework)
  (g) often loses things necessary for tasks or activities (e.g., toys, school assignments, pencils, books, or tools)
  (h) is often easily distracted by extraneous stimuli
  (i) is often forgetful in daily activities
  (2) six (or more) of the following symptoms of **hyperactivity-impulsivity** have persisted for at least 6 months to a degree that is maladaptive and inconsistent with developmental level:

  Hyperactivity
  (a) often fidgets with hands or feet or squirms in seat
  (b) often leaves seat in classroom or in other situations in which remaining seated is expected
  (c) often runs about or climbs excessively in situations in which it is inappropriate (in adolescents or adults, may be limited to subjective feelings of restlessness)
  (d) often has difficulty playing or engaging in leisure activities quietly
  (e) is often ``on the go'' or often acts as if ``driven by a motor''
  (f) often talks excessively

  Impulsivity
  (g) often blurts out answers before questions have been completed
  (h) often has difficulty awaiting turn
  (i) often interrupts or intrudes on others (e.g., butts into conversations or games)
B. Some hyperactive-impulsive or inattentive symptoms that caused impairment were present before age 7 years.
C. Some impairment from the symptoms is present in two or more settings (e.g., at school (or work) and at home).
D. There must be clear evidence of clinically significant impairment in social, academic, or occupational functioning.
E. The symptoms do not occur exclusively during the course of a Pervasive Developmental Disorder, Schizophrenia, or other Psychotic Disorder and are not better accounted for by another mental disorder (e.g., Mood Disorder, Anxiety Disorder, Dissociative Disorder, or a Personality Disorder).

Code based on type
314.01 Attention-Deficit/Hyperactivity Disorder, Combined Type: if both Cirteria A1 and A2 are met for the past 6 months.
314.00 Attention-Deficit/Hyperactivity Disorder, Predominantly Inattentive Type: if Criterion A1 is met but Criterion A2 is not met for the past 6 months
314.01 Attention-Deficit/Hyperactivity Disorder, Predominantly Hyperactive-Impulsive Type: if Criterion A2 is met but Criterion A1 is not met for the past 6 months

Coding note: For individuals (especially adolescents and adults) who currently have symptoms that no longer meet full criteria, ``In Partial Remission'' should be specified.

From American Psychiatric Association: *Diagnostic and Statistical Manual of Mental Disorders* (4th ed). Washington, DC, American Psychiatric Association, 1994.

5. School underachievement
6. Poor self-esteem secondary to the above (self-rating scales may give erroneously high results, not borne out once a clinician knows the child well)
7. Other, coexisting externalizing behavior disorders (i.e., oppositional defiant disorder or conduct disorder), concomitant specific learning disabilities, anxiety disorders and depression

INAPPROPRIATE OR EXCESSIVE ACTIVITY

Rutter (1982) has pointed out that hyperactivity as a symptom is not a unitary variable and that the fidgety child is different from the child who runs up and down all the time. This observation is true not only for hyperactivity but also for all the above-mentioned symptoms.

The restlessness of the hyperactive child is not only overactivity (although the latter is generally present even in sleep, Porrino et al., 1983) but, rather, an activity off-task, out of seat, and disruptive to the class as a whole. Klein and Young (1979) hold the view that it is the combination of high activity with high disruptive behavior that distinguishes hyperactive from normal children, or is at least responsible for the referral.

At a first visit to a physician for evaluation of the syndrome, the child may not manifest this restlessness. The unusually good behavior (which does not characterize the first visit of all hyperactive children) may be the result of better inhibition due to anxiety. The syndrome should not be ruled out because of failure to observe symptoms at a first visit.

Restlessness is measured by various well-standardized rating scales, by direct observation, and by actometers. These different gauges measure different facets of activity and do not necessarily correlate well. This lack of correlation is well known. It is not surprising that actometers measure dimensions of activity that are different from those measured by observers. The lack of correlation between different observers, however, is more complex. That teachers and parents may not agree with one another could be related to the condition being present (or more severe) either at school or at home. It could also be related to different levels of tolerance, or the likelihood that children act differently in different situations, so that there may even be poor correlation between two teachers of one child. A child with ADHD may not show his behaviors if he likes a teacher and tries harder or if he likes a particular subject and is good at it. On the other hand, different teachers may have different tolerance for what constitutes a problem. ``Each measure reflects a unique child x perceiver x setting sample,'' as suggested by Whalen and Henker (1991).

Over the course of development, restlessness diminishes and frequently changes from running all the time in preschool years, to not being able to sit quietly in a chair in the early grades of school, to fidgetiness in the adolescent and adult years. Some hyperactive adults ``feel restless'' even when it is not observed (Weiss and Hechtman, 1993).

POOR SUSTAINED ATTENTION

In class, difficulty sustaining attention on a given assignment until it is completed contributes to poor schoolwork. Not paying attention in games and wanting to do something different may contribute to unpopularity with peers.

One puzzling aspect of this cardinal feature of the syndrome of ADHD is its variability. The children are frequently described by their teachers as having an attention span of only a few minutes in school. Report cards over the years are monotonous in comments like ``must learn to listen, must learn to pay more attention.'' Yet these same children are often able to concentrate for hours on an activity they particularly like and at which they are good. One child, for example, could draw excellent cartoons for hours. Another child who could concentrate neither at school nor when doing homework, was able to concentrate for hours on making electronic trains from models with his father. He was so good at this that he competed with adults in racing the trains that he had constructed and often won. A possible explanation of this ``selective inattention'' is related to motivation and pleasure in the task. Hyperactive children are particularly poor at attending to tasks they find boring, repetitive, or difficult, and that give them no satisfaction. However, there is evidence from one study (Tannock, 1993) that they do, in fact, have a poorer attention span than do normal children, even for Nintendo® games.

In the laboratory, difficulties paying sustained attention are commonly measured by the Continuous Performance Test (CPT). For this vigilance task, children are required to respond (by pressing a button) to an auditory or visual stimulus occurring in a background of similar signals (e.g., letters appear on a revolving visual screen, and the child is asked to respond when X appears). The task, which is monotonous and requires constant attention, can be made more complicated by either increasing the speed of the letters appearing or increasing the complexity of the instructions (e.g., press when the letter A follows the letter X). Hyperactive children perform more poorly than normal children, making more errors of omission (missed signals) and errors of commission (pressing the button in error). The latter is considered to reflect impulsivity better and the former poor sustained attention. The reaction time of hyperactive children on the CPT is longer and more variable (Douglas, 1980). A correlation between performance on the CPT and ability to pay attention in the classroom has been demonstrated, but the overlap is far from perfect (Rapport et al., 1986). Some experienced investigators consider that the poor correlation indicates that the CPT is not useful in the clinic for diagnosis and remains a research instrument.

Distractibility (response to irrelevant extraneous stimuli) is present in some hyperactive children. Historically, it was considered to be such an important aspect of their difficulties that many were educated isolated in a cubicle within the classroom. Whalen (1989), in her excellent review of this syndrome, suggests that ''distractibility is more likely to emerge when the distracters are particularly salient and relevant to the child, and when they are embedded in the task . . . than when they are external to it, such as white noise or flashing lights'' (p. 140).

It is well known that attention is not a uniform concept and that it is strongly correlated with motivation. Mirsky (1985) described 4 different processes (which may be regulated in different but interconnected sites in the brain)–focused attention, encoding/manipulating, paying sustained attention to the task at hand, and flexibility. Each of these processes is measured in the laboratory by different tasks. Different children with ADHD may have deficits in one or more of these processes.

DIFFICULTIES IN INHIBITING IMPULSES

Impulsivity in everyday life and in the performance of cognitive tasks is pervasive in hyperactive children. In school, they have impulsive styles in their work, difficulty waiting their turn, they interrupt others, blurt out answers without waiting to hear the complete question, and some may engage in physically dangerous activities without considering the consequences. The latter leads to more self-poisoning and fractures in children with ADHD (Szatmari et al., 1989b) and to more car accidents in adolescents and adults (Weiss and Hechtman, 1985; Barkley, 1993).

In the laboratory, impulsivity may be measured by the errors of commission on the CPT, on the Matching Familiar Figures Test (MFFT), and on the Porteus Maze Test. The MFFT yields an accuracy score that may reflect different cognitive functions and a latency score that reflects impulsivity. It is considered that the Porteus Maze Test measures impulsivity. In general, hyperactive children find it difficult to fulfill any laboratory task that requires an inhibition of response to a designated signal in a task requiring fast and accurate response, e.g., making a choice. Impulsivity in ADHD is not only pervasive, it is likely to be the most enduring symptom as they grow up (Weiss and Hechtman, 1993). It is the symptom that, along with oppositional and aggressive behaviors, is most likely to result in rejection by peers.

In a recent report, (Barkley, 1993) Russell Barkley states, ''I now believe that the manifold deficits witnessed in ADHD can be reduced to a single deficiency in the capacity to delay responding to a signal, event, or stimulus.'' Barkley quotes several studies that indicate that hyperactive children choose task strategies that reduce the need for delay intervals imposed by the task. He then cites Bronowsky's essay (Bronowsky, 1967), which recognizes that this one attribute, i.e., the ability to delay a response, facilitates the complex cognitive abilities that are distinctly human, such as the development of language. Bronowsky states that 4 abilities result from this human development—as opposed

to the development of lower mammals—the separation of affect, prolongation (prolonging the delay to connect the stimulus with memory), internalization of language, and reconstitution. The latter is a consequence of internalization of language that can affect breaking up the stimulus into components and reconstituting these parts to influence the response. Barkley suggests that, possibly through genetic mechanisms, children with ADHD are deficient in delaying a response and are hyper-responsive to their setting and its immediate events—perhaps via under-functioning of the orbital frontal cortex and connections to the limbic system—compared to other children. He feels that poor attention and hyperactivity are secondary to this core deficit.

DIFFICULTIES GETTING ALONG WITH OTHERS

Delineating the specific interactional problems of hyperactive children has been an increasingly important and growing research interest in the past years (Whalen and Henker, 1985). As a result, much information has been gained. Children with ADHD are unpopular with their peers (Pelham and Bender, 1982) and have difficulties with parents, siblings, and teachers. Enduring friendships are rare, and this unpopularity, which in later life may be replaced by social isolation (Weiss and Hechtman, 1993) is another characteristic of hyperactive children that is both pervasive and enduring over time.

In childhood, sometimes the only one willing to play with a hyperactive child is a younger child or a child with some other similar difficulty. Sociometric ratings from peers indicate that hyperactive children cause trouble, get others into trouble, bother others, and are not liked. The negative effect of hyperactive children on others has been observed with respect to their teachers and their participation in both dyads and groups of normal children. When jointly observed completing a given task, parents interact with a hyperactive child in a more negative and intrusive way. This is greatly ameliorated (although not totally normalized) when the hyperactive child improves with medication and becomes more cooperative.

The difficulties with others have been studied via sociometric ratings and by direct observation in dyads with a normal child, with a parent jointly completing a task, and in group situations. The different studies are in solid agreement with one another in describing the nature of the difficulties. It is not as clear, however, whether the cause is a social skill deficit or a performance deficit, or both. (The latter would mean that the child knows how to interact but cannot do it.)

For an excellent recent review of the nature of the social difficulties of children with ADHD, the reader is referred to a chapter by Whalen and Henker (1992).

While it is impossible within the confines of this chapter to do justice to the volume of work by Whalen, Henker, and others on the kinds of social-skills deficits hyperactive children have, among the various possible difficulties is the high intensity of intrusive, undesirable behavior, particularly when it is aggressive. This type of behavior is probably the most salient of their plight that results in rejection. While prosocial behaviors and social-information processing are normal in many children with ADHD, they have more difficulty in fine-tuning their responses to changing situations during an interaction. All the research aimed at better understanding why children with ADHD are so quickly unpopular with peers is extremely important in that it will guide the direction social-skills training will take in the years ahead.

SCHOOL UNDERACHIEVEMENT

It is highly unlikely that a child correctly diagnosed as having ADHD can achieve in school according to his or her intellectual potential. Cantwell (Cantwell et al., 1988) showed that even when intelligence was controlled for, hyperactive children were behind normal children in their grade level in reading, spelling, and arithmetic.

The core symptoms of the syndrome described above impair learning. They are associated in some hyperactive children with the specific learning disabilities already described, but are also frequently associated with poor organizational skills, poor sequential memory, deficits in fine and gross motor skills (affecting handwriting), and inefficient and unproductive cognitive styles. The more unsuccessful hyperactive children become in their schoolwork, the less they are motivated to succeed because their effort does not produce results. All these factors interact to cause school failure and lower final levels of scholastic achievement by adulthood.

LOW SELF-ESTEEM

All studies that have investigated this have found that, at least clinically, hyperactive children have low self-esteem. This is hardly surprising in view of their unpopularity, their being frequently in trouble, and their school failure. While some degree of impaired self-esteem may be inevitable, not enough attention has been paid to how to avoid the cycle of failure and/or criticism to which these children are exposed at school and in the family. Unless these children experience some pleasure, love, and success, chronic feelings of failure can lead to depressive childhood disorders in some ADHD children. In contrast, on some self-rating self-esteem scales, denial results in children with ADHD scoring themselves higher than do normal children. The author considers these results to be an artifact of the measurement.

CO-OCCURRENCE OF OTHER DISORDERS WITH ADHD: COMORBIDITY

The existence of comorbidity and its theoretical and practical implications have been in the forefront of recent literature on ADHD. From a theoretical point of view, the finding that about half or more of the children with ADHD also have other diagnoses poses questions for understanding the disorder. As Biederman and co-workers indicated in their recent update, the fact that so many hyperactive children have other disorders could mean that:

1. Comorbid disorders do not represent distinct entities but are different expressions of the same disorder.
2. Comorbid disorders may each represent distinct disorders.
3. Comorbid disorders share a common vulnerability.
4. Comorbid disorders may represent a subtype in a heterogenous syndrome of ADHD.
5. The ADHD may be an early manifestation of the comorbid disorder.
6. ADHD may put the child at risk for the development of other disorders.

From a practical point of view, it is mandatory to carry out a complete assessment of a child with ADHD to determine the presence or absence of other disorders. In general, the presence of a second or third comorbid disorder indicates a more serious problem with a worse prognosis (Gittelman and Mannuzza, 1988; Weiss and Hechtman, 1993). In making a treatment plan, all the disorders present must be addressed. The exact percentage of children with ADHD who have one or more comorbid disorders is summarized in Table 50.4. The percentage depends on many factors, such as the age of the child, the sex, the socioeconomic status, the morbidity of the parents, and whether the sample is taken from a clinic or from the community.

Oppositional Defiant Disorder and Conduct Disorder

These co-occur with ADHD in about 40% or more of hyperactive children. This high degree of overlap, which has been noted by clinicians and researchers alike, has sparked conceptual controversies. As Loney (1987) has noted, the externalizing disorders may be viewed as "independent, intertwined or interchangeable." Those who consider the disorders to be variations of the same basic disorder postulate that they have the same underlying theoretical construct.

In order for these disorders to be viewed as independent syndromes, each must show postdictive, consensual, and predictive validity. That is, differences should exist in their etiology or antecedent variables (postdictive validity), in the presence of different associated symptoms other than those that define the disorder (consensual validity), in treatment

response, and in outcome (predictive validity). While the evidence from different studies is at times conflicting, several studies have shown antecedent variables (such as more neglect and early separation in conduct disorders) different from those in ADHD. Different associated symptoms exist in ADHD compared to conduct disorder, such as more cognitive impairment, lower IQ, and more developmental disorders (McGee, 1988). There is a different treatment response since symptoms of ADHD respond more sensitively to stimulants than do symptoms of conduct disorder, such as aggression and stealing. Finally, for those with ADHD alone, outcome is more favorable.

It has been shown that children with ADHD who have parents without any mental disorder, such as antisocial personality disorder, alcoholism, or hysteria, generally do not have conduct problems, whereas those whose parents have the above disorders have various degrees of conduct problems as well as ADHD (August and Steward, 1983). This has, in general, been confirmed (Lahey et al., 1988; Taylor et al., 1986).

Nevertheless, the relationship of conduct or oppositional problems to ADHD is not resolved. Diagnoses are made dichotomously, such that one either does or does not have a given disorder; however, this obscures the continuum of these disorders that is so frequently seen. Children with ADHD often have some oppositional behavior, which may be severe enough at various periods to fall into the "disorder" category. It is also not yet certain that the presence of ADHD alone, in the absence of opposition defiant disorder or conduct disorder, independently predicts later antisocial behavior—although evidence suggesting that it does is accumulating. One must conclude that, for a better understanding of the relationship of ADHD and conduct disorder in future studies, children with either ADHD or conduct disorder only and those with both syndromes should be studied separately. Many early studies of ADHD failed to differentiate among the disruptive childhood syndromes, making results more difficult to interpret.

The few studies available on the overlap of ADHD and oppositional defiant disorder (ODD) report a finding of about 35%. Faraone et al. (1991) showed that ODD is also familial; relatives of children with both ADHD and ODD are 3 times more likely to have ODD than relatives of children with ADHD alone, and 10 times more likely to have ODD than the relatives of normal controls.

Mood and Anxiety Disorders

Authors have described that between 15% and 75% of children with ADHD also have mood disorders. However, follow-up studies (Gittelman et al., 1985; Weiss et al., 1985) did not confirm that major depression occurred more frequently in the adolescence and adulthood of ADHD-diagnosed children as compared to normal controls. This discrepancy is likely the result of different criteria for the diagnosis of major depression in adulthood as compared to milder forms, such as mood dysthymia, related to low self-esteem often seen in children with ADHD. In addition, some of the children treated with methylphenidate may have mild dysphoria as a side effect. It has also been noted that some of the children of parents with mood disorders have higher than expected rates of ADHD. Finally, family studies of children with ADHD have shown that their first-degree relatives have higher rates of mood disorder (Biederman et al., 1992).

A comorbid association between ADHD and anxiety disorders of about 25% has been found, and investigators have noted higher rates of ADHD in children of parents with anxiety disorders. The presence of an anxiety disorder in a child with ADHD may result in a poorer response to methylphenidate (Pliszka, 1989); a finding not corroborated by Tannock (1989), who found that clinical efficacy was similar but that there were more side effects.

Specific Learning Disabilities

A recent study (McGee and Shore, 1988) suggested that an overlap between pervasive hyperactivity and a reading lag of 2 years, at age 11 years, existed in 62% of the hyperactive children studies. The academic failure and the behavior disorder were seen as vicious cycles. Another study (August and Garfinkel, 1989) found that 39% of 115 consecutively referred hyperactive children had a concomitant specific reading disorder. For those who had ADHD only, effortful sequential memory was most impaired, whereas in those children who had a specific reading disability without ADHD, the deficit involved the rapid encoding of verbal linguistic stimuli. Those who had both disorders had both types of cognitive deficiency.

Recently, Biederman and his colleagues (1992a) have demonstrated that, if specific learning disabilities are diagnosed by WRAT—reading, and arithmetic scores below 10 standard scores of the full-scale IQ—this cut-off point overdiagnosed specific learning disabilities in children with ADHD. When a standard score discrepancy between reading scores and a full-scale IQ of 15–20 was utilized to define a learning disability, this cut-off clearly distinguished children with ADHD from both psychiatric and normal control children. The comorbidity when specific learning disabilities are defined more stringently is probably about 10–20%.

ETIOLOGY AND PATHOGENESIS

The etiology of the syndrome is not known. The evidence to date suggests that a single etiology is unlikely to account for more than a small subgroup of children with the disorder. For most, the syndrome probably represents a final common pathway for a biological vulnerability and interacting antecedent variables. If there is a uniform underlying CNS dysfunction, its nature has not yet been determined. The expression of this hypothesized dysfunction is seen in difficulties in regulatory control, such as the organizing of information processing, attention, social responses, and appropriate inhibition (Douglas, 1983; Whalen, 1989).

It must be remembered that in the 1920s, the syndrome was described as first appearing in previously normal children following their recovery from encephalitis lethargica. However, brain damage as a result of pre-, peri-, or postnatal events has not been demonstrated to correlate with the appearance of ADHD. The earlier notion that there is a continuum of reproductive casualties (from mental retardation or cerebral palsy to the hyperactive syndrome and learning disabilities) resulting from a large-scale study, has not been borne out.

Genetic Influences

For a recent review of this increasingly important field of study, the reader is referred to the paper by Castellanos and Rapoport (1992).

Many recent studies have documented the importance of genetic transmission of ADHD. A recent study of 570 13-year-old twins concluded that genetic factors account for about 50% of the explainable variance (Goodman and Stevenson, 1989).

Twin studies, while very important, are clouded by the fact that the environment is more similar for monozygotic than for dizygotic twins. Recent adoption studies by Cadoret and Stewart (1991) skirt these problems. Two hundred and eighty-three male adoptees and their adoptive parents were interviewed, and charts containing criminal and psychiatric histories of the biological parents were obtained from adoption agencies. These clearly confirmed a genetic role for ADHD but not for aggression, which was related to socioeconomic status and family factors.

Family studies are the third method of looking at the genetic contribution to etiology by examining first- and second-degree relatives and comparing the incidence of the disorder to relatives of controls; this method has received the most attention recently. Early studies that found an increased incidence of antisocial personality disorder, alcoholism, and drug abuse in fathers and hysteria in mothers failed to distinguish between children with ADHD only and those who also had conduct disorder. The studies (August and Stewart, 1983) suggested that the above parental disorders are more common only in those ADHD children who have comorbid conduct or oppositional defiant disorder.

More recently, Barkley and his colleagues (Barkley, 1990), in their 8-year follow-up studies of hyperactive children, found that the fathers of these children had significantly higher rate of antisocial acts, alcohol abuse, police contacts, and arrests compared to fathers of controls. Their job histories and financial responsibilities were less stable. Barkley concluded that 11% of the fathers of hyperactive children met DSM-III-R criteria for antisocial personality disorder as compared to 1.6% of fathers of normal controls. Fathers of children with ADHD and conduct disorder committed more antisocial acts, but fathers of children who had ADHD only still evidenced significantly more antisocial behavior than normal controls. These studies suggest that genetic and environmental factors act synergistically, as was also shown in the study by Cadoret and Stewart (1991).

The most extensive family studies have been carried out by Biederman and his colleagues (1992b). In their most recent study of 140 children with ADHD, 120 normal controls, and 822 first-degree relatives it was found that 49% of ADHD subjects had no comorbidity, although compared to normal control children they were more likely to have conduct disorder, ODD, major depression, and anxiety disorders. Similarly, 25% of first-degree relatives of the probands had ADHD (versus 8% of the controls), significantly more had antisocial disorder, and 26% (versus 9%) had mood disorders. These authors concluded that ADHD and major depression show common familial vulnerabilities, that ADHD and conduct disorder may be distinct subtypes, and that ADHD and anxiety disorders are transmitted independently.

While the importance of inheritance has been established, the mode of inheritance is still being studied. In the above-mentioned study, the researchers analyzed the family data by applying segregation analysis and using the computer programs POINTER and REGL. They concluded that the familial distribution of ADHD can best be explained by a single gene and not by polygenic transmission, as had been previously suggested.

A rare autosomal disorder, generalized resistance to thyroid hormone (GRTH), is currently being studied at the National Institute of Health. Blinded interviewers using structured questionnaires found that 61% of patients with GRTH had ADHD. It was noted that this represents the first molecular model of ADHD that may lead to new insights into its pathogenesis. Thyroid function was subsequently measured in 53 ADHD children. None was found to have abnormal TSH, T_1 or T_4. It was concluded that thyroid function need not be measured routinely in nonfamilial ADHD (Elia et al., 1994).

In conclusion, 3 aspects of the genetics of the disorder are particularly important from a practical point of view:

1. Only 50% of the variance can be explained by genetic factors, leaving another 50% to be explained by the environment (the latter includes parenting, family functioning, temperament, diet, and gestational and perinatal events).
2. Criminal, antisocial, and drug- or alcohol-abusing parents are significantly higher even in children with ADHD only, and are markedly increased for children with ADHD and conduct disorder.
3. It has become essential to assess parents carefully to determine the possible presence of ADHD, major depression, and antisocial types of problems before a treatment regimen is planned for the child.

Neurochemical Studies

Because of the dramatic therapeutic effect of stimulants on the symptoms of the syndrome, it has been suggested that the disorder is caused by a dysfunction of the adrenergic or serotonergic systems.

The many enthusiastic earlier reports that brain transmitter metabolites, such as MHPG, were lower in the urine of hyperactive children than in normal children's urine have not been replicated. More recent studies measured urinary phenylacetic acid, phenylalanine, and tyrosine and found no differences. It is likely that peripheral measures of neurotransmitter metabolites do not necessarily reflect central values. Furthermore, it is known that stimulants depress the excretion of MHPG for 2 weeks after they are discontinued, which could account for the results of the earlier studies. The measurement of homovanillic acid (HVA) in one study was found to be lower in the spinal fluid of hyperactive children, yet this could not be confirmed in another study. Cerebrospinal fluid (CSF) studies are generally characterized by their small sample size and the unavailability of normal controls, limiting their reliability. Zametkin and Rapoport (1987) conclude that studies comparing ADHD and normal children with respect to monoamines and their metabolism in urine, plasma, CSF, and platelets have been disappointing.

Therapeutic trials have been carried out with various agents known to be agonists of different neurotransmitters. For example, piribidel and amantadine are agonists for dopamine; mianserin and imipramine for noradrenaline; and tryptophan and fenfluramine for serotonin. Therapeutic results were disappointing, working against a theory of disturbed metabolism of one transmitter. Three monoamine oxidase (MAO) inhibitors have been found to improve the behavior of hyperactive children. Clorgyline is a selective MAO A inhibitor, tranylcypromine inhibits both MAO A and MAO B, and deprenyl inhibits MAO B. MAO A inhibitors affect norepinephrine and serotonin, MAO B inhibitors affect B plenylethylamines, and dopamine is affected by both MAO A and B inhibitors. Hence, the positive therapeutic results of these three MAO inhibitors do not allow us to judge the relative importance of one transmitter compared to another.

Zametkin and Rapoport conclude that catecholamine function and its modulation are very probably involved in the pathogenesis and treatment of ADHD, respectively. They suggest that lack of response to one stimulant might predict responsiveness to another. Alteration of noradrenergic function appears necessary, but not essential, for clinical efficacy, since agents such as haloperidol are also efficacious.

While the significance is unclear, a number of studies have found that, in ADHD children, methylphenidate and dextroamphetamine cause a hypersecretion of growth hormone.

McCracken (1991) has reviewed current thinking on the neurobiology of ADHD. He pointed out that all medications shown to be effective for this disorder increase dopamine release and inhibition of the noradrenergic locus ceruleus. Mesocortical dopaminergic cells are linked with the prefrontal cortex, which is involved with attention as well as with circuits that filter out stimuli in the thalamus and may thus influence distractibility. Other researchers have also implicated the role of the locus ceruleus.

One may conclude that recent work has been productive in linking neurochemical differences in children with ADHD with areas in the brain that may be affected and can be controlled by these transmitters.

Diet

LEAD

A study (Thomson et al., 1989) of 501 Edinburgh children reported on a dose-response relationship between high blood levels of lead and ratings on the Rutters Teachers Rating Scale, namely, the total score and the aggressive-antisocial-hyperactive subscores. This study confirms earlier ones reporting that high blood levels of lead produce behavior and cognitive disorders in some children.

On the other hand, the prospective study by Ferguson and co-workers (1988) indicated that the correlation between dentin lead levels and intelligence, school performance, restlessness, and inattention, while statistically significant, accounted for only 1% of the variance, when confounding variables such as socioeconomic status had been controlled for. One might conclude that children of low socioeconomic status are also the ones likely to have high blood levels of lead and may thus form a group at risk.

ALCOHOL

Alcohol that is consumed by pregnant women is concentrated in their foetus's brain and may damage the developing brain (Nanson, 1990).

This has become a major health problem, especially among some subcultures where there is a lack of employment and opportunity, and where the rates of adolescent pregnancy is high and associated with heavy drinking. Fetal Alcoholism Syndrome (FAS) and Fetal Alcoholism Effects (FAE) are conditions currently receiving increasing attention. These syndromes in children, which result from exposure to alcohol while in utero, are very similar to syndromes of ADD or ADHD with many indistinguishable symptoms. It is possible that the known craniofacial features associated with FAS may be one form of the minor physical anomalies known to be associated with ADHD that were studied by Pomeroy et al. (1988).

FOOD ADDITIVES

In the 1970s, the notion that ingestion of food additives was responsible for ADHD gained widespread acceptance on the part of parents. Dr. Ben Feingold had claimed that half of all children with ADHD could be cured by a diet that eliminated all food additives—the "Feingold Diet." A great deal of research funds were subsequently consumed in an attempt to carry out controlled studies to determine the validity of this claim. Connors (1980) summarized both positive uncontrolled studies and mainly negative controlled studies, and concluded that, in general, food additives were not a significant cause of the syndrome, except possibly in an occasional (mainly young) child.

SUGAR

When the enthusiasm of food additives as a cause for ADHD waned, there was a shift to the belief that sugar was a cause of the syndrome. Many parents still limit sugar and foods rich in sugar. A controlled study carried out by Behar et al. (1984) at NIMH was designed to maximize any possible effect of sugar by selecting as probands 28 hyperactive children whose parents claimed they became hyperactive after ingesting an excessive amount of sugar. No differences were found in this study on behavior or attention between sucrose, glucose, or saccharin-flavored placebo. Recent studies have confirmed this.

The Role of the Frontal Lobes

There has been an upsurge of interest in the role played by the frontal lobes in the syndrome. The frontal lobes, by means of adrenergic mediation, exert inhibitory influences on lower striatal structures, which are mediated by dopamine. This could explain why many agents are effective in ameliorating symptoms of the syndrome. The orbital frontal cortex is most likely involved with impulsive and aggressive behavior.

Recent studies using positron emission tomography (PET) have demonstrated developmental changes throughout childhood and adolescence in the density of dopamine receptors. Cerebral blood flow and glucose utilization in the frontal lobes, as measured by PET, have shown differences between hyperactive and normal children in several studies. Furthermore, methylphenidate administration results in increased blood flow to the mesencephalon and basal ganglia, whereas motoric cortical areas show a decrease, which could explain the therapeutic effect of the stimulants on the syndrome.

Lou and colleagues (1984) used Xenon inhalation techniques to show that children with dysphasia and ADD had hypoperfusion in striatal regions. Methylphenidate increased flow to striatal and posterior periventricular regions and decreased flow to primary sensory regions that had shown hyperperfusion.

More recently, Zametkin and colleagues (1990), at the National Institute of Mental Health, studied 25 biological parents of children with ADHD. These parents had childhood histories suggestive of ADHD but had never received methylphenidate. Fifty adults matched for sex, age, and IQ acted as controls. Glucose metabolism was studied while all the subjects were performing an auditory attention task that lasted 35 minutes. PET scans (using updated tomography technology) were performed during the task performance and were analyzed by blinded assistants.

Zametkin found an overall glucose metabolism decrease of 8.1% in the cortical areas of the hyperactive adults, affecting 30 of 60 brain regions. The main regions affected were the premotor and prefrontal cortex in the left hemisphere, areas associated with attention. The direction of this correlation is uncertain. Would poor attention to the task being performed result in decreased glucose metabolism, or vice-versa? Nevertheless, this was an important finding that will require duplication in children with ADHD. While much of this research is in a beginning phase, PET studies may, in the future, provide us with more information on cortical dysfunction in ADHD children.

Psychosocial Influences

Evidence of possible biological determinants has been presented. As the genetic studies indicated, when biological vulnerabilities exist they will interact with psychosocial factors.

There have been reports (Campbell, 1990) of associations of family stress and aspects of lower socioeconomic status with higher ratings and more severe complaints of behavior in referred 3-year-old hyperactive preschoolers. Furthermore, a negative mother-child relationship, which was both reported by the mother and observed, predicted persistence of the problems identified at this young age. This suggests that family factors contribute to the severity of the disorder as well as to its duration. The presence of a biological vulnerability (such as difficulties with inhibitory controls) whose nature is not yet established would render a child diagnosed with ADHD more at risk than a normal child to be adversely affected by any form of family or school stress. Such a child would also be more likely to become a scapegoat for parental or teacher frustrations than a normal child whose temperament is more compliant.

Jacobvitch and Stroufe (1987) carried out a prospective study of 267 at-risk newborns of mothers of low socioeconomic status who enrolled during their pregnancy. Out of these, 34 children were considered hyperactive at age 6 and a significant correlation was found with intrusive or overstimulating mothering. They concluded that for some but not all children with ADHD, abnormal parenting (overarousing or intrusive) may be etiologically important.

In our increasingly technological and competitive society, and the added burden of economic recession, the school underachievement of a boy (whose behavior is also aggravating) is an enormous stress to his parents, generating fear that the boy will not succeed as an adult in obtaining adequate employment. Also, in times of economic difficulty, special school services for troubled children are often reduced. At the same time, with the increase in divorce, single parenting, blended families, and full-time employment of both parents, parents and teachers have less time and fewer emotional resources to deal competently with a child who seems to have good potential but who seems unwilling to try, such as a hyperactive child. A 25-year follow-up of Kauai children who had perinatal complications found that intact, healthy families who provided educational stimulation in the home could fully compensate over time for perinatal risk, except in those children who were severely damaged (e.g., the mentally retarded) (Werner, 1989). In a vulnerable group of children, such as those with ADHD, family stability and quality of parenting interacted with child factors to predict long-term outcome (Weiss and Hechtman, 1993). These interactions and their predictive power are a solidly established finding.

The relationship between family dysfunction, solo parenting, welfare status, and urban living and hyperactivity (even without conduct disorder) was a finding not only of the recent Ontario Child Health Study (Szatmari et al., 1989a) but also of several other studies (Velez et al., 1989).

In conclusion, the specific biological precursor continues to be sought and newer techniques, such as PET, are now available. The biological vulnerability (once it is defined) and psychosocial and economic factors (namely, the child's total environment) interact in a circular manner with respect to cause, severity, and outcome of the disorder.

DIFFERENTIAL DIAGNOSIS

Age-appropriate Overactivity Still within the Norm

Some parents do not know what level of activity, concentration span, and compliance to commands can be expected from a normal child at different ages, particularly in boys.

Specific Learning Disabilities without ADHD

Some learning-disabled children are bored and discouraged at school. They may have restlessness and inattention as a reaction to an inappropriate school situation, where they are not learning and not receiving adequate help for their disability. For example, a child with undiagnosed language delay will not grasp instructions or information in class that are given rapidly in a complex and long-winded manner. For this child, trying to pay attention would be analogous to a normal adult having to remain attentive in a class taught in a foreign language.

Conduct Disorder without ADHD

Conduct disorder may be associated with some degree of restlessness and inattention due to lack of motivation for school. The ADHD symptoms are mild and seem reactive to other core problems of the conduct disorder. The symptoms related to ADHD are too minor to warrant a separate diagnosis, unless an angry parent or teacher exaggerates scores on a rating scale in order to "get help" for the child. School observation is necessary.

Adjustment Disorder

This is a particularly important diagnosis to differentiate from ADHD. Symptoms, particularly in boys, can be quite similar, but usually have a duration of less than 6 months (see DSM-III-R and DSM-IV criteria) and may begin later in life. Most children with ADHD develop their difficulties in the first years of life.

TREATMENT

Bradley, in 1937, was the first to describe the dramatic effect of the stimulant benzedrine (a racemic mixture of dextro- and levoamphetamine) on a group of hospitalized, disturbed children, including some who had the hyperactive syndrome. While this study was not placebo controlled, the accurate and detailed clinical description of the children's improvement in school performance and behavior is remarkable.

In the past 15 years, numerous well-designed, placebo-controlled, acute drug studies established the therapeutic efficacy of the stimulants in treating the symptoms of the hyperactive syndrome (Gittelman-Klein, 1987). The optimism established by the finding of an efficacious medication for a serious disorder, as well as the realization that for many hyperactive children, difficulties continued into adolescence and adulthood, resulted in a continual increase in the United States in the use of methylphenidate. It was recently established, for example, that in Baltimore County (where the prevalence of stimulant therapy for ADHD is higher than the national rate), 5.9% of public school elementary children are being treated with stimulants (Safer and Krager, 1988). The fact that the use of methylphenidate is high and has doubled every 4–7 years since 1971 has generated considerable public criticism of its overuse or misuse. The quotas for stimulants increased 5-fold between 1990 and 1995 (Safer, 1995). The controversy between overprescribing and giving children with a serious disorder the benefit of a useful medication is not easy to resolve. A hopeful result of this controversy would be that the various concerned lay groups, currently organized to fight the use of methylphenidate militantly, could have access to impartial information so that they could evaluate the nature and duration of the disorder, the short-term benefits and side effects of stimulants, and their relative lack of toxicity. Furthermore, physicians clearly require guidelines on when and how they should prescribe medication and on the kind of follow-up they need to carry out. Medication should only be given after careful appraisal. Clear benefit to the child has to be documented, not only when the medication is first prescribed, but also intermittently during the entire time the child remains on medication. Concerned clinicians have recently placed much emphasis on devising and evaluating the efficacy of nonpharmacological treatments as well as medication to be used and, for many children, instead of medication alone.

Use of Stimulants to Treat Children with ADHD

All three stimulants in current use—methylphenidate, dextroamphetamine, and pemoline—have been found to normalize hyperactive children. Methylphenidate has been the most studied drug and has also enjoyed the greatest use in the past 15 years, perhaps because it was shown to have fewer side effects on growth than dextroamphetamine. It will therefore be described in detail, although its therapeutic effects are not superior to those of the other two stimulants.

Dextroamphetamine is the stimulant that has been longest in use, and the dose given is about half that of methylphenidate. It has one advantage that is often forgotten, namely, that its half-life is 3–4 times longer than that of methylphenidate. Pemoline is the most recently available of the three; it differs from the other two in having a delayed therapeutic response of up to 3 weeks. Recently, it was shown that the delayed onset of action may only be 1–2 days and that previous studies had overestimated the time interval before therapeutic results occur. Once the response occurs, about 2 hours after ingestion, the duration of effect of a single dose is longer (e.g., 5–6 hours as compared to 3–4 hours) than that of methylphenidate. This is a definite advantage (Pelham et al., 1990). The average daily dose of pemoline is 1–3 pills daily; each pill contains 37.5 mg. An unusual side effect (seen in about 2%) is liver dysfunction, which on rare occasions may not reverse upon drug discontinuation, requiring liver function tests to be carried out. This side effect, which is unpredictable, has caused clinicians not to use this medication. It is important for a clinician to remember that if one stimulant is clinically ineffective, a second one may be effective and should be tried before using a different group of medications.

The Use of Methylphenidate

Numerous well-controlled studies have established that many symptoms of ADHD are ameliorated by methylphenidate, and the effect can be so global that the children give the impression of being normalized.

These studies have shown that aimless restlessness becomes more goal directed and sustained attention improves, as do measures of inhibitory control. Ratings from parents and teachers indicate improved behavior. Almost all cognitive tasks in the laboratory, such as the CPT, MFFT, Porteus Maze, and Paired Associated Learning, show improvement. The improvement on these laboratory tasks has generally been interpreted as being the result of improved sustained attention, better inhibitory control, and increased motivation. Douglas and co-workers (1988) have questioned this, since they found that both in the classroom and in the laboratory, when children perform complex arithmetic and learning tasks, not only do their output, efficiency, and accuracy improve, but they also show increased learning acquisition. These workers conclude that the organization of information processing is ameliorated. In clinical practice, about 70% of children with ADHD improve on a stimulant regimen. Douglas's studies indicate that all children receiving methylphenidate improve on some cognitive tasks, and that the individual differences between hyperactive children regarding responsiveness on different target behaviors and skills are highly variable.

The increased interest in the difficulties hyperactive children have in their social functioning has led to many recent studies on the effect of methylphenidate on various aspects of social interactions. While it was once believed that children receiving stimulants socialized less, the opposite has been found. In doses of up to 0.6 mg/kg, hyperactive children showed increases in positive social responses and were more frequently nominated as "best friends, cooperative and fun to be with."

However, these medication-related improvements did not normalize the appraisal of hyperactive children as rated by their peers, and there was marked inter-individual variability in medication response (Whalen et al., 1989).

More recently, however, Whalen and co-workers (1992) have reported that, for some children with ADHD, stimulants have a dampening effect on social interactions and, while peers rate them as "better" socially, adult observers noted mild dysphoria. One might conclude from these findings that the annoying qualities (bossiness, intrusiveness, disruptiveness, and immature behaviors) that characterize peer interactions of hyperactive children are improved by stimulants, possibly, for some, at the expense of some degree of social withdrawal and dysphoria.

Many studies have demonstrated a consistent positive methylphenidate effect when a hyperactive child interacts with his or her mother in completing a set task. The child cooperates better with the mother, reducing, in turn, the mother's negative comments and intrusiveness and increasing her positive comments to her child. This improvement in the mother-child interaction, particularly the more constructive interaction of the mother, suggests that parental behavior is not solely responsible for the negative interaction. Improvements in the functioning of families with hyperactive children placed on methylphenidate have recently been noted (Taylor et al., 1987).

DOSAGE OF METHYLPHENIDATE

An early study demonstrated that a dose of 1 mg/kg, optimal for improving social behavior, might impair learning (as measured in the laboratory on a paired associate learning task). This warning generated many studies that attempted to evaluate the effects of increasing dosages on various measures of behavior and cognitive functioning. All these studies have shown a linear dose-response effect regardless of the dependent measure assessed, from doses of 0.1 to 0.6 mg/kg (and for some children, up to 1 mg/kg) (Douglas et al., 1988). While, previously, doses above 1 mg/kg were not recommended because of possible impairment of cognitive skills and more side effects, it was recently shown by Klein (1991) that mean doses of 1.78 mg/kg (mean 50 mg daily, range 20–60 mg daily) did not impair cognitive functioning, as measured on the WRAT reading, arithmetic and spelling tests, the Gray Oral Reading Test, the Porteus Maze, and the Draw-A-Person Test. It was also of interest that no tolerance was found to these doses over a period of 12 weeks. Not all researchers agree. Pelham (1991) described how, for individual children, different target symptoms responded optimally to different doses.

Methylphenidate is frequently given in divided doses, at breakfast and at lunch. The breakfast dose is often double the lunch dose, to avoid insomnia. A third dose is avoided, if possible, to decrease side effects, but it is helpful for some children (e.g., for getting homework done) and it does not increase side effects in all children. While this has not been systematically researched, clinically I have found that some children sleep better when given a bedtime dose.

SIDE EFFECTS

The most common side effects are reduced appetite and difficulty falling asleep. Some children report stomachache or headache. These side effects are generally controllable by reducing the dose, and they frequently wear off over time.

Stimulants have been reported to slow growth (reducing height and weight progress). When children were given drug holidays, a growth rebound was seen. This side effect was found to be dose related and less evident with methylphenidate. Many subsequent studies tried to confirm the possible effect of stimulants on growth but conclusions were inconsistent. Some of the inconsistency may stem from the fact that, since the first report, most of the subsequent studies used lower doses that did not show effects on growth. In many children, high doses of stimulants, given over a long period of time and without drug holidays, would produce some decrement in growth, although the effect is small. Possible growth retardation takes on increasing importance in view of the current practice of keeping adolescents with ADHD on medication during their growth spurt. The treating physician must carefully monitor height and weight on a regular basis.

Stimulants result in small increases in systolic blood pressure and heart rate. It is thought that these effects are not clinically significant. There have been no reports of adults in whom long-term use of stimulants produced cardiovascular difficulties.

The parents of some children may complain about a short-lasting but difficult-to-handle period of 1–2 hours after the last dose of Ritalin given at noon wears off at about 4:00 PM. This "rebound" effect can be handled in different ways.

The effects of stimulants in exacerbating the tics of Tourette's Disorder (TD) or in precipitating the manifestation of TD in children who may be at risk due to a family history of the disorder are not clear. Some studies have indicated that this is a possible side effect and have warned that stimulants should not be given to children with tics or with family histories of TD. It is wise to heed this warning whenever possible. Recently, however, some studies have emphasized the frequent co-occurrence of ADHD with TD and demonstrated that stimulants may be very helpful for these children. In four children who had both syndromes, behavior and frequency of tics were observed and measured in the classroom and in the laboratory during play. No tic exacerbation and an actual reduction of tics were seen at the highest dose used, 15 mg given twice daily (Sverd et al., 1989). Hence the contraindications are individual and relative. A recent review of the use of methylphenidate for ADHD children with tics discusses this treatment dilemma in more detail (Gadow et al., 1995).

Occasional psychotic reactions in children have been reported in the literature. These are very rare and usually take the form of tactile hallucinations, although, recently, there has been a report of delusions. These side effects require discontinuation of the stimulant. In no case did the psychotic reaction persist after medication was stopped.

PLASMA LEVELS OF METHYLPHENIDATE

These have been found to correlate poorly with behavioral or cognitive measures of improvement. Furthermore, the plasma level of one child on a given dose of methylphenidate is quite irregular from day to day. There is some evidence that therapeutic effects may be related to the rate of rise of the plasma level, so that the plasma level itself is not of clinical importance in determining the oral dose.

CAUSAL ATTRIBUTIONS

How children feel about having to take medication is a question that has been asked. Do they attribute their improvement to the pills and feel that they have no influence over their own behavior? This was a warning made by researchers such as Whalen and Henker. However, Hoza (1993) showed that ADHD boys viewed themselves as no worse than control boys, and Pelham and co-workers demonstrated that ADHD boys on methylphenidate showed greater persistence following exposure to insoluble tasks and attributed success to themselves, while blaming failure on external events. Nevertheless, most children with ADHD do not like taking medication. The younger ones complain of the taste, and the older ones explain that taking pills makes them feel different from others. Saliva tests can be taken at intervals, and while they cannot be used as a measure of plasma level, they are useful to determine whether a child is taking his or her prescribed Ritalin.

Long-term Effects of Stimulants

In view of the dramatic short-term therapeutic effect, the inability to demonstrate significant long-term effects on outcome comes as a surprise. Various reasons have been suggested for this discrepancy:

1. Some of the children on long-term stimulant therapy may not have taken their pills.

2. Stimulants are less effective in preventing or reducing aggression and antisocial behavior, which are among the most detrimental aspects of the outcome.
3. The methodologies of the studies are poor and few conclusions can be drawn from them. The use of dependent measures that are not sufficiently sensitive has been noted.
4. The wrong doses were used in the studies.
5. The possibility of tolerance to the effects of stimulants, particularly for some symptoms occurring over years, must be kept in mind. Many clinicians have observed this phenomenon.

All these hypotheses are sound and not exclusive of one another. But they do not totally account for the relatively minor benefits (Hechtman et al., 1989) reported for ADHD children treated over several years with stimulants only. It seems to the author that we have expected too much from medication for a syndrome comprising such diverse and multiple behavioral, social, and cognitive deficits. For example, stimulants have been found not to benefit specific learning disabilities, and they cannot fill in the gaps of knowledge hyperactive children often have because of their inattention. A syndrome as disabling as ADHD is unlikely to be sufficiently improved by medication alone to dramatically affect outcome.

The Decision Whether to Use Stimulants

This is a crucial clinical question for which we have no research to guide us, except the knowledge that stimulants are highly effective in ameliorating symptoms of the disorder, but also that, once discontinued, the symptoms return. The children are not cured and outcome is not affected significantly by treatment with stimulants alone.

Stimulants are used much more frequently in the United States than in Japan, Great Britain, or Canada. Within the United States, child psychiatrists and psychologists might have a wide spectrum of opinion on their use, ranging from those who feel that every child with ADHD deserves a trial with stimulants, to the opposite extreme of those who never, or very rarely, use stimulants. Some are against medicating disturbed children on principle. These professionals frequently know very little about psychoactive agents, including the stimulants in which they "do not believe." Usually, the firm belief held by such professionals is that the symptoms are learned (and hence can be unlearned); fixations of childhood; depressive or manic equivalents (which psychotherapy can alter); or a necessary part of family dysfunction, where the symptoms express important attempts by the family to maintain homeostasis and, hence, are treatable by family therapy alone.

Beliefs aside, the guidelines offered below are based on the experience of following hyperactive children from ages 6–26 and of treating others at various ages in the clinic.

Stimulants are not necessary for all children who have the diagnosis and may be useful for others who have ADHD symptoms, yet do not meet diagnostic criteria, and who may have ODD. The decision to use medication is, therefore, not made on the diagnosis alone. It is based rather on the presence of disabling symptoms that respond to stimulants, including their severity and the degree of incapacity they cause to the child in question. Troubled peer relationships, underachievement at school, and distress in the family as a result of the child's conduct problems must be taken into consideration.

Many clinicians will try simple behavioral measures before using medication. Pelham (personal communication) first institutes the "daily school report card" in which the teachers target work success and behavioral difficulties. The parents then reinforce the goals and institute consequences based on the daily school report. The judgment to use medication should never be made lightly. Once the decision is made to use medication, the best dose has to be ascertained, which ideally involves teachers' and parents' reports and validated rating scales. The child has to be carefully followed to ascertain whether he or she still requires medication and that the dose is optimal. Height and weight have to be measured regularly, to avoid growth suppression. Good supervision of medication is time-consuming and essential. Each year, the child should have a sufficiently long period, e.g., 3–4 weeks, for a trial off medication (unless it is obvious that the child cannot do without medication). If this trial period is too short, it could be a failure because of a complex, not directly drug-related rebound effect.

Since the final outcome is not greatly affected by stimulants (in our present state of knowledge), the purpose of giving them is to help the child function better in school, in the family, and with peers. This has the effect of making the child feel better about himself or herself (Hechtman et al., 1984), especially if it is carefully explained and re-explained that he or she is the one who produces the change; the pills only help the child to improve him or herself.

Hyperactives "grown up" report that as children, they did not like taking pills, which made them feel different from others. In their opinion, what helped them most was an adult (parent, teacher, clinician) who believed in them (Weiss and Hechtman, 1993). Side effects and "feeling different" should be talked about with the child before initiating the medication. A discussion of medication with the child is very important, making him or her an active participant.

FOR PRESCHOOLERS

In general, the efficacy of stimulants is less reliable in children under 6 years, and side effects, such as less positive social behavior and more clinging, have been observed. In addition, an experienced nursery teacher and counseling for the parents of the preschooler are usually effective, unless the condition is very severe. Stimulants are, therefore, rarely required and may be overused until new research findings establish adequate response in the younger age group.

FOR ADOLESCENTS AND ADULTS

It has been common clinical practice to discontinue the use of stimulants during the adolescent growth spurt to avoid growth retardation. This is a relative contraindication if the adolescent's functioning remains impaired by the symptoms of the syndrome and he or she is still responsive to medication. In adulthood, it is useful to continue medication in special circumstances. For example, one young man treated in childhood for ADHD had twice failed out of university. On stimulants, he was able to get his degree and commence postgraduate studies. Once he graduated and obtained a job, the degree of sustained attention required in his work was less than at university, and he no longer required medication.

The Use of Medications Other Than Stimulants

THE ANTIDEPRESSANTS

Many clinicians consider the tricyclics to be the second-line drugs for ADHD if the stimulants are either ineffective or cause side effects that do not disappear. Several double-blind studies have demonstrated the efficacy of various tricyclics (the most studied have been desipramine and imipramine) as compared to placebo. However, it remains controversial whether these drugs significantly improve concentration, and several studies have indicated that tolerance to these drugs may develop after some weeks. Also, when given over long periods, more parents discontinue tricyclic medication than they do stimulants, probably because of side effects and/or development of tolerance. One advantage of tricyclics is that the effect from a single dose is longer lasting so that rebound effects, as are seen with methylphenidate and dextroamphetamine, are not present. When discontinued, tricyclics should be withdrawn slowly.

The mechanism of action of tricyclic medication for symptoms of ADHD is different from their action in depression. Optimal doses are lower and the onset of clinical response is rapid. In theory, it would seem that these drugs would be particularly valuable when ADHD is comorbid with depression; however, because of the different doses required to treat the two disorders, this may not be the case.

The use of tricyclic medication in children with ADHD (or depression) is of major concern because of cardiotoxicity in this age group. About 5% of children are genetically predisposed to metabolize tricyclic antidepressants more slowly, since they are deficient desipramine hydroxylators. When this is the case, a child will have 2–4 times the steady state concentration of desipramine or imipramine per unit dose. In children who were given fixed doses of imipramine, steady state levels varied 22-fold (from 25–553 mg/ml); with desipramine, serum levels from fixed doses varied 16.5-fold. The reason for the cardiotoxicity in children is that they convert tricyclics more efficiently than do adults to 2-OH metabolites, which are cardiotoxic; in addition, children have increased sensitivity to 2-OH metabolites than do adults. If total doses used are over 1 mg/kg/day (in divided doses), children require monitoring with electrocardiograms at baseline. When the child is taking about 3 mg/kg/day, and when maintenance dose is reached subsequently, monitoring should occur regularly at intervals, i.e., at least twice a year. Doses above 5 mg/kg/day should be avoided. It has been pointed out that increasing the frequency ECGs does not necessarily increase the children's safety.

One death occurred in a 6-year-old on high doses of imipramine. More recently, 3 deaths were reported for children receiving various (sometimes unknown) doses of desipramine. While there was no absolute proof that the tricyclics directly caused the deaths, it behooves physicians to use tricyclics with extreme caution in view of their known effect in delaying cardiac conduction. Green (1992) recommends that the "PR interval should not exceed 210 msecs. QRS interval should not widen more than 30% over baseline. QT interval should be less than 450 msecs. Heart rate should be less than 130 beats/min and blood pressure should be below 130/85.

In view of the above, I do not use tricyclics for ADHD, and I have only rarely had any children who do not respond to a carefully monitored dose of one of the stimulants. The development of tics with stimulants is indeed a problem, but is often eliminated by lowering the dose. The use of clonidine is also valuable for children with tics.

New groups of antidepressants, chemically unrelated to the tricyclics or SSRI's, are now on the market for use in adult depression (e.g., Venlafaxine and Tomoxetine). these medications have been reported to be useful for ADHD, but wide-scale, double-blind studies are required to test their efficacy and side effects for ADHD in both children and adults.

CLONIDINE HYDROCHLORIDE

This is one of the α-adrenergic agonists and is a centrally acting antihypertensive agent that acts on presynaptic neurons, inhibiting the release of noradrenaline. In an open, uncontrolled study, Hunt and co-workers (1985) found that, compared to the effect of methylphenidate, clonidine improved frustration tolerance and decreased hyperarousal, while methylphenidate was superior in improving attention span, focusing, and distractibility. The best responders to clonidine seemed to be children with ADHD who were aggressive and had comorbid conduct or oppositional defiant disorders—they became more compliant and cooperative and tried harder. These authors have also reported on a double-blind placebo cross-over study, from which they concluded that clonidine was superior to placebo in treating children with ADHD.

Clonidine is usually started with an initial dose of a $\frac{1}{2}$ tablet (0.05 mg/day) with similar increases every third day until a dose of approximately 0.05 mg tid or qid is achieved (3–5 mg/kg). This drug may also be administered by applying a transdermal patch, obviating the need to take pills, which some children really dislike. In children, the effect of the patch's efficacy lasts about 5 days. It usually takes about 1 month before clonidine's therapeutic effect is optimal, and when this medication is discontinued it should be withdrawn slowly over a few days to avoid hypertensive reactions and withdrawal symptoms of anxiety and agitation. Side effects include headaches and sedation, but often these wear off. Some children develop depression, particularly those with a family history of depression. Blood pressure should be monitored when clonidine is used.

For children with ADHD, clonidine may occasionally be the drug of choice when ADHD co-exists with Tourette's syndrome. It may also be considered for children on stimulants who developed tics that did not disappear when the dosage was lowered. Some physicians have combined clonidine with methylphenidate, enabling a lower dose of the latter to be used, which may be an advantage when methylphenidate results in untoward side effects. For some children, clonidine and Ritalin can be combined. It has been shown, for example, that clonidine 0.05–0.1 mg given 90 minutes before bedtime helped children on Ritalin fall asleep 0.5–1.9 hours earlier.

Recently it was reported that 4 children who were receiving a combination of methylphenidate and clonidine died. The causes of death, including whether they were drug related, are not clear (Walkup, 1995). Nevertheless, in view of this finding, extreme caution is advised when clonidine is combined with Ritalin.

MAJOR TRANQUILIZERS

On the whole, physicians are reluctant to use these for ADHD because of the risk of irreversible tardive dyskinesia and/or dystonic reactions. On the whole, the fears that phenothiazines and butyrophenones (haloperidol) cause sedation to the point of diminished cognitive functioning are not justified for the kinds of doses that are required for children with ADHD. Double-blind studies have been carried out with thioridazine (Mellaril), chlorpromazines (Thorazine) and haloperidol (Haldol). Generally, children benefitted by becoming less frantic, impulsive, and hyperactive; the effect on attention was not clear. This group of medications is useful for some children with developmental delay for whom stimulants may not be effective. For other children with ADHD, they are rarely required. They may be useful for children with Asperger's syndrome when it is comorbid with ADHD and when stimulants for these children exacerbate the more psychotic type of symptoms.

BUPROPION HYDROCHLORIDE (WELLBUTRIN)

This is an antidepressant of the aminoketone class, not related chemically to the tricyclics. It has been found to be useful in adults with ADHD in a recent study by Wender (1990). Clay et al. (1988) and Casat et al. (1989) carried out double-blind studies of bupropion in children who had ADHD, using doses of 3.1–7.1 mg/kg/day to 3–6 mg/kg/day, respectively. Both authors noted an improvement in symptoms compared to placebo. Side effects were allergic skin rash, dry mouth, insomnia, headache, nausea and vomiting, constipation, and tremor. Seizures occur in 0.4% of those treated with doses above 450 mg daily. This drug may be more useful for adults with ADHD than for children.

Nonpharmacological Treatments

Concern about possible overuse of stimulants and disappointment over their lack of sufficient effect on outcome led to a search for nonpharmacological treatments for ADHD used in combination with, or instead of, stimulants. So far, none of these treatment modalities has established its superiority over medication, but the effect of any one of these treatments may enhance the effect of medication. The treatments include behavior therapy, cognitive training, social skills training, parent training, and family and individual therapy. Remedial education may be required. These treatment modalities have been used alone or in combination with one another and with stimulants. Space allows only a brief summary of these various treatments, none of which, as a sole treatment, has as yet demonstrated indisputable efficacy.

BEHAVIOR THERAPY

Most controlled studies that have compared behavior therapy alone, medication alone, and the two combined have found that the combination was the most effective. However, one study found that adding behavior therapy in the classroom did not increase the benefit derived from the medication alone, except regarding classroom aggression.

Initial enthusiasm for this treatment decreased when results were found to be short-lived and difficult to generalize (Rapoport, 1987). The treatment was costly in terms of time and offered only some advantages over medication alone.

As with medication, behavior therapy offered external versus internal control and did not, in the long run, help these children to develop age-appropriate self-regulatory skills to modulate their attentional, motoric, or social behaviors. Nevertheless, clinicians frequently combine behavior modification with stimulants and find that the combination is effective.

COGNITIVE TRAINING

Cognitive training was designed to teach hyperactive children self-control, self-guidance, and reflective, more efficient problem-solving strategies. A comprehensive review of this treatment (Abikoff, 1987) outlined the techniques utilized but was unable to confirm that it was helpful. The possible ceiling effect of medication and the failure to build in generalization into the classroom situation have been suggested as accounting for the negative results. Research on how cognitive training techniques can be modified to be more effective is continuing.

SOCIAL SKILLS TRAINING

As more has been learned about the various difficulties hyperactive children have with parents, teachers, and peers and the negative effects of the children's behavior on the behavior of those significant to them, there have been various attempts to improve the child's behavior through training in social skills. There are many problems to be overcome, some of which apply also to behavior and cognitive therapy, namely, the difficulty of generalization from one situation in which the behavior is learned to other situations in the child's life. Furthermore, the nature of the social difficulties of hyperactive children is still receiving much study; they are not uniform from one child to the next. It is still not clear whether the difficulties are skill deficits or performance deficits, or whether this, too, varies from child to child. Do hyperactive children fail to perceive or wrongly perceive social clues, or do they perceive them correctly but are not able to respond appropriately? One of the difficulties in the interaction between a hyperactive and a normal child was observed to be the failure of the hyperactive child to adjust his or her behavior to the demands of the situation in the game being played. Most children do this intuitively, and it remains to be seen whether and how this can be taught.

Social skills programs generally focus on awareness of and appropriate response to rules, on accurate self-perception and self-monitoring, and on practice with certain content areas, such as being teased, cooperation, effective nonaggressive approaches, and being sensitive to the needs of others. Tokens are used in most programs, often based on accuracy of self-evaluation. So far, social skills training has not been found to be effective as the single treatment. Pelham and co-workers emphasized that combined social skills training, cognitive and operant therapies, and medication offered the best hope (Pelham and Bender, 1982). Pelham has modelled a program providing all these treatments during 2 months of special summer camp (unpublished manuscript, 1993). Whenever possible, an effort is made to facilitate generalization of the improved behavior resulting from the 8-week day-camp program into the home and the school. Parents are asked to attend one evening a week for training, and a counsellor from the program spends time with the child's teacher in the classroom to help implement the token behavior modification program (Pelham, unpublished manuscript, 1993).

A recent review of parent training by Lorne Cousins et al. (1993) emphasizes the role parents play in improving the social skills of their children by participating in their social skills groups and helping them practice what they have learned. For example, the parents may invite a friend of the child's home for a variety of easy-to-handle activities, progressing to more complex ones.

PARENT TRAINING

Barkley (1981) described a detailed training program for groups of parents or for individual parents. The 12-session program provides parents with principles and strategies of behavior management, with emphasis on the particular problems of hyperactive children for which training approaches are most helpful. Parents are assigned homework and keep behavioral and reinforcement charts, reporting on their efforts and experiences. No systematized results are reported, but parents find it helpful to understand better their children's difficulties and deal with the problems more effectively. Some other studies have not found parent training groups to add anything to the children receiving stimulants, although in some of these studies very few sessions were held. Parent satisfaction with this program is an important variable, but further studies are required to document immediate and long-term effects.

Cousins and Weiss (1993) point out that a didactic approach may be less effective than an approach in which parents are active participants in determining what is most effective for their own child in terms of antecedent variables, consequences, and what is "the wrong way" to intervene. Cunningham (1990) has also stressed the importance of active versus passive participation of parents in parent groups.

FAMILY THERAPY

There has been a paucity of research demonstrating the efficacy of parent training groups for hyperactive children, although family difficulties have been documented. After parents have completed a training program as described, it is helpful for them to come as a family, so that what has been learned in the group can be put into practice in the unique and much more emotional context of their family.

Arastopoulos and co-workers (1992) demonstrated what was always known by clinicians, that in families where a child has ADHD, parenting stress is very high. The main predictors of severity of parenting stress were the presence and degree of ODD and maternal psychopathology, the severity of ADHD, and the physical health of both child and mother.

Barkley and co-workers (1992a) showed that adolescents who had ADHD and ODD had more extreme and unreasonable beliefs about their parents. These workers (Barkley, 1992b) randomly assigned 61 adolescents with ADHD into 3 treatment groups: structured family therapy, communication training, and problem solving training. Each of the groups ran for 8–10 sessions. All 3 treatments resulted in a significant reduction of negative communication, conflicts, anger during conflicts, externalizing and internalizing symptoms, and in improved ratings of school adjustment. These results remained stable during 3 months of follow-up. However, no group differences were found between the treatments, and only 5–30% of the adolescents improved.

INDIVIDUAL CHILD THERAPY

The usefulness of this approach with hyperactive children has not been established. Some evidence exists that, in short-term therapy, hyperactive children do less well than children with internalizing disorders. Traditional analytic play therapy is almost impossible to do with hyperactive children, who usually do not play but are restless, inattentive, and easily bored. Techniques for conducting individual therapy with hyperactive children need to be devised and could well have a therapeutic effect on some of their secondary difficulties. Learning to confide in an adult, understanding their own disorder, developing hope at being able to change, and feeling understood would be likely to result in improvement. For further detail, see the review by Greenfield et al. (1992).

REMEDIAL EDUCATION

Space prohibits anything but a token comment on this large area. Hyperactive children may have specific learning disabilities, such as reading disorders or language delay, which require careful diagnosis and a special remedial program. In the absence of these specific disabilities, most hyperactive children have problems with organization and display an inefficient, impulsive cognitive style or approach to problem solving. These deficits have been lessened through training in small groups of children. The results have not been researched.

A COMPREHENSIVE COMBINED TREATMENT PROGRAM (MULTIMODALITY TREATMENT)

Satterfield and co-workers (1987) have demonstrated that when 6–12-year-old hyperactive children receive a comprehensive evaluation of all their specific difficulties, including those of their family, an individualized comprehensive treatment program can be devised, based on the initial assessment. This includes stimulant pharmacotherapy, individual and group therapy for the children, family therapy, and parent groups. At a 3-year follow-up, 36% of the initial 117 children were still receiving treatment. The children who stayed in treatment fewer than 2 years were compared with those who remained in treatment at least 3 years. The children in the longer-treated group did better academically, were better adjusted, and had less antisocial behavior.

This optimistic result is difficult to interpret. The children were not initially randomly assigned into treatment groups. The children and/or their parents in longer treatment are likely to be more motivated for help and for change and more compliant. In spite of these drawbacks, it makes clinical sense that, when children have deficits in emotional, cognitive, and behavioral areas and come from varying degrees of troubled families, all deficits should be targets for treatment. Common sense would suggest (and there is conflicting evidence for this) that even small improvements in one area will synergistically affect other areas of functioning. Hence, the possibility exists that a combination of treatments (even if none of them have proven efficacy when used alone) could be effective. Whether offering a comprehensive treatment program will be more effective than medication alone in affecting outcome, which is the belief of most clinicians, remains to be demonstrated in future studies.

A collaborative treatment study has been completed in Montreal (Dr. Lily Hechtman) and New York (Dr. Howard Abikoff), in which 90 children have been randomly assigned to 3 treatment groups. In one of these, the "multimodality treatment group," children received social skills training, remedial education, and individual psychotherapy, while their parents received parent training, followed by weekly family counselling for one year (all treatments took place once monthly the second year). A second group, the "attention control group," received the same amount of professional attention for two years, in the form of nonspecific treatment, such as a peer activity group, homework help, and relationship therapy. Their parents participate in a parent self-help group led by a professional, followed by supportive family help for each family. In the third group (which is probably what constitutes standard treatment for most children with ADHD), the children were seen monthly for medication monitoring and supportive help. In all 3 groups, the children received methylphenidate titrated up to a dose to achieve maximum benefit, taking side effects into account. The medication was usually taken in 3 doses to a maximum of 50 mg daily, with drug holidays.

The National Institute of Mental Health is initiating a larger and comprehensive collaborative multisite study to evaluate the immediate and long-term efficacy of multimodality treatment for ADHD. Results from these studies are not yet available.

OUTCOME

It was generally believed by pediatricians until the 1970s that children outgrew the "hyperactive child syndrome" sometime during their adolescence. This optimistic picture had to be revised as the results of well-controlled outcome studies became known in the past 10–15 years. The results of these showed good agreement about the chronicity of the initial childhood problems in many, but differed in the percentage of those who, in adolescence and adulthood, had antisocial or criminal behavior, including differences in the severity of the latter problems. These differences are not surprising in that the methodologies of the studies differed in the following ways:

1. The characteristics of the hyperactive children initially included in the study varied in (a) the percentage who had concomitant conduct or oppositional disorders and the severity of these disorders, (b) the IQ, particularly differences in cut-off points at the lower end of the spectrum, (c) the presence and severity of learning disabilities, (d) the presence, absence, and degree of depression and/or anxiety disorders, (e) the pervasiveness of the syndrome, (f) the socioeconomic class of the children, and (g) the amount of treatment received. This aspect may not affect final outcome (Thorley, 1988).
2. Some outcome studies were prospective (i.e., children were followed from the time the diagnosis was made), and others were retrospective catch-up studies (the diagnosis was made by reviewing old charts from previous years and tracing subjects) or retrospective follow-back studies (i.e., a group of deviant adults, such as alcoholics, were evaluated regarding the presence of the hyperactive syndrome in their childhood). Because of the methodological problems in making accurate diagnoses from old charts or obtaining an accurate picture of their childhood from troubled adults, only prospective studies will be summarized. For a review of the various types of studies, the reader is referred to Cantwell (1985) and Hechtman (1992).
3. Studies have varied in the percentage of the initial group lost to follow-up. In general, the longer the study goes on, the more subjects are lost. It has generally been found that those lost to follow-up represent a deviant subgroup (Cox, 1977).
4. Both the duration of the prospective follow-up and the age of hyperactive probands at outcome assessment have varied (e.g., from age 12–30). Hence the studies will be described under adolescent and adult outcomes.
5. The breadth of outcome assessment has varied, with a few studies focusing on one particular measure (e.g., the number of felonies committed) and others carrying out comprehensive evaluation assessments.

Outcome in Adolescence

One of the earliest controlled 5-year follow-up studies assessed 91 hyperactive children (mean age at follow-up, 13.3 years) and compared them to a matched normal control group (Weiss et al., 1971). Hyperactives were found to have improved in the degree of restlessness, impulsivity and inattention they showed compared to levels 5 years previously, but were still worse than normal controls on these symptoms. The hyperactive children had more academic problems and lower self-esteem, and 25% had some antisocial behaviors.

When the outcomes, at age 14, of learning-disabled boys with or without hyperactivity and a group of normal controls were compared, the learning-disabled boys, who were also hyperactive at follow-up, had more antisocial and oppositional behaviors and lower self-esteem and were more impulsive, fidgety, and immature (Ackerman et al., 1977). The learning-disabled boys without hyperactivity differed from the normal controls only in academic performance. This indicates that the presence of hyperactivity associated with learning disabilities predicts poor outcome.

Lambert and co-workers (1987) obtained information on the outcome at age 12 of pervasively hyperactive children, originally followed from an epidemiological sample. Of the total group, 20% were problem free, and 37% had persistent learning disabilities and behavior and emotional problems. By age 14, 19% showed antisocial behaviors. A further report of this cohort followed until ages 18 and 19 (Lambert, 1988) confirmed that the hyperactive group continued to have lower educational status and significantly more antisocial behavior. This study, like many others, found that the interaction of both child variables and family characteristics predicted good or bad outcomes.

The study by Satterfield and co-workers (1982) is frequently cited because of the high percentage and seriousness of the felonies committed. About 50% of 110 hyperactive boys had committed at least one felony by 17 years, compared to 10% of 88 matched controls. The exact percentages of felonies committed depended on the socioeconomic class, with those in the lower socioeconomic class committing a higher percentage of felonies.

When hyperactive children with and without conduct disorder were followed and reassessed at 14 years, those who had both diagnoses showed continuation of the initial symptoms of ADHD but, in addition, had aggressive, noncompliant, and antisocial behaviors, as well as alcohol use. The group that initially had only hyperactive symptoms showed few conduct disorder problems at follow-up. The authors suggest that antisocial behavior in adolescence is related to earlier conduct disorder, rather than to hyperactivity (August et al., 1983).

The most recent prospective study on adolescent outcome was carried out on 123 hyperactive children who were followed for 8 years by Russell Barkley and his co-workers (1990), who compared their results to 60 community control subjects. The average age at follow-up was 15 years and 14 years respectively. At follow-up, 71.5% of the hyperactive adolescents and 3% of the controls met DSM-III-R criteria for ADHD, and 60% of the hyperactives and 11% of the controls also had diagnostic criteria for oppositional disorder, while 40% of the hyperactives and 1.6% of the controls also met criteria for conduct disorder. Conduct-disordered adolescents used more cigarettes and marijuana (though not alcohol) and were expelled from school more frequently. Families of hyperactives were less stable, had higher divorce rates, more frequent moves, and the parents had more job changes. Fathers of hyperactive children showed more antisocial behavior. ADHD adolescents were more likely than controls to have auto crashes and more bodily injuries associated with auto crashes, and to be more frequently at fault for the crashes. They also received more speeding tickets (Barkley, 1993).

Adult Outcome

Weiss and Hechtman (1993) have summarized the findings of their prospective controlled 15-year follow-up of pervasively hyperactive children. This study evaluated 103 children initially and reevaluated them at ages 13.3, 18, and 24. In the final 15-year follow-up assessment, only 64 children of the original 103 were comprehensively evaluated. About half of those lost to follow-up could not be traced and probably represented a more deviant subgroup (Cox et al., 1977). The other half were contacted on the telephone and reported that they were doing well (giving details of their lives) but did not want to come in for reassessment because they did not want to be reminded of past difficulties. These, in contrast, may represent a thriving subgroup.

The results of this study (Weiss et al., 1985) were as follows:

1. Two-thirds of the group continued to be troubled by at least one disabling core symptom of the original syndrome, namely, restlessness, impulsivity, or sustained attention problems.
2. By two different diagnostic criteria, 23% had an antisocial personality disorder; the majority of these fitted into the mild category.
3. The hyperactive adults had more evidence of various kinds of psychopathology. They
   a. made more suicide attempts;
   b. scored lower on self-ratings of self-esteem;
   c. had poorer social skills, with many being socially isolated;
   d. scored worse on self-rating scales of classical psychopathology and on a personality inventory measuring ideals of social living and interaction;
   e. had more psychiatric diagnoses, and had more presenting symptoms.
4. Their work record indicated that, while most were gainfully employed, their job status was inferior and their employers reported

more difficulties with them. They changed jobs more frequently. However, their annual earnings were the same as for normal controls because they more frequently worked at more than one job.

5. Their final level of education was inferior to that of normal controls.

Gittelman-Klein and colleagues (Gittelman et al., 1985) concluded a similar comprehensive controlled follow-up of 101 hyperactive boys and 100 matched controls. The mean age at follow-up was 18 years, and the range was 16–23 years. Hence, these young adults were significantly younger than those in the previous study. Ninety-eight percent of the subjects were able to be followed, thus eliminating possible bias due to subject loss, as occurred in the Weiss and Hechtman study. Results showed that 31% versus 3% of controls continued to have the full syndrome of ADDH at follow-up, 20% versus 8% of controls had a conduct disorder, and 19% versus 7% of controls had a substance use disorder. Many of the subjects who had antisocial problems at follow-up also had continuing symptoms of the syndrome. Drug and alcohol abuse were found in those who had conduct disorders, and usually preceded the conduct disorder.

Subsequent studies (Mannuzza et al., 1988, 1989) by these investigators indicated that probands who did not receive any DSM-III diagnosis at follow-up differed from normals only with respect to lower educational status. The presence of an antisocial personality disorder (APD) at follow-up almost completely accounted for the increased risk of criminal activities. In these studies, it was not possible to determine retrospectively the absence or presence of a coexisting conduct disorder at initial intake. However, questioning parents as to the age of onset of symptoms of APD revealed that 25% of those with the adult disorder had begun to have these problems at the time when they were first diagnosed, that is, at initial intake. The authors concluded that ADDH is a risk factor for later criminality, but that this risk is mediated by the development of APD. It remains unclear from this study whether childhood ADDH presents a risk for the development of APD and criminality in adulthood in the absence of childhood conduct disorder.

The most recent study from this group of investigators (Mannuzza and Klein, 1993) evaluated 91 adults diagnosed as hyperactive in their childhood (88% of the original sample was traced and evaluated). Their mean age at adult follow-up was 25 years. The probands were more likely to have the full syndrome of ADHD as adults than were controls (11% vs. 1%), drug abuse disorder (16% vs. 4%), and APD (18% vs. 2%). In adolescence, APD had been highly correlated with drug abuse, while in adulthood, the correlation was less evident. Probands had completed 2.5 fewer years of school than had controls (12% vs. 34% had completed a bachelor's degree). Their occupational status was lower (3.5% vs. 4.4%) with significantly fewer hyperactive adults holding professional positions.

These results confirm findings from the Weiss and Hechtman study (1993). Differences in how measurements were made in the two studies produced seemingly different results. In Mannuzza's study, only 11% met diagnostic criteria for the full ADHD syndrome in adulthood, while in the Weiss and Hechtman study, 66% of the adults had one disabling core symptom of the syndrome. Besides the difference in what was measured and how it was measured (full adult diagnosis versus one disabling symptom of the original syndrome), the method with which information was obtained also might have resulted in differences. In the Mannuzza and Klein study, all subjects were assessed "blind." In the Weiss and Hechtman study, this was not done. In the latter, subjects were actively *probed* for continuing symptoms and "no complaint" was not accepted without this detailed probe (controls were probed in the same way as probands). In addition, when impaired social skills was a major problem for the subjects, this was included in the "core disabling symptom" if it seemed to be the result of a persistent core symptom (such as impulsivity or short fuse). Finally, the fact that only the subjects' self-reports were used in formulating a diagnosis in the Mannuzza study might account for differences with the Weiss and Hechtman study, where significant others were also used (when this was possible). Find-

ings from the Mannuzza and Klein study confirmed findings from the Weiss and Hechtman study that probands did not show increased risk for major depression, bipolar disorder, schizophrenia, or anxiety disorder.

As the results of the well-known Cambridge study of delinquent development (Farrington, 1990) became known, some light was shed on this vexing question of whether hyperactivity in childhood without concomitant conduct disorder predicts antisocial behavior in adult life. This study followed 411 inner-city London boys from ages 8–30. In their childhood, the boys were classified according to the presence and severity of symptoms of hyperactivity (hyperactivity, impulsivity, and attentional difficulties [HIA]), as well as the presence and severity of conduct and oppositional disorder.

Four groups were studied with respect to differences in the early background, as well as outcome: (a) HIA and conduct problems (N = 59), (b) HIA without conduct problems (N = 34), (c) no HIA but conduct problems (N = 40), and (d) no HIA and no conduct problems (N = 278). If hyperactivity (HIA) and conduct problems are accurate measures of the same theoretical construct, then groups b and c should be similar with respect to their early background and antisocial outcome. If on the other hand, they are measuring different constructs, they should have different antecedent events and outcomes. The latter was found to be the case. HIA was related to low intelligence and to family and socioeconomic factors different from those seen in conduct problems. HIA (only) predicted later criminal behavior in the absence of childhood conduct problems. The two conditions combined had additive effects in predicting the worst prognosis of chronic criminal behavior. The authors concluded that the hyperactive syndrome and conduct disorder should be distinguished as different disorders.

Conclusions about Adolescent and Adult Outcomes

Many hyperactive children (about two-thirds) continue to be disabled into adulthood by one or more initial core symptoms of the syndrome. About one-third are diagnosed as having the full syndrome at 18 years. In one study of subjects with a mean age of 25 years, only 8–11% met full diagnostic criteria for adult ADHD. Hyperactive children are at risk for later development of APD (shown in about 18–23%) and criminal behavior. The higher figures reflect hyperactive children who had concomitant conduct disorder. The risk for a child who has ADHD without a conduct disorder in childhood to develop antisocial behavior in adulthood is much lower but still exists. The development of APD accounts for most of the criminal behavior. Final educational achievement and work record are also inferior to matched normal controls, although most hyperactives are gainfully employed as adults.

Hyperactive children are at risk for having more psychopathology, such as more diagnoses, more suicide attempts, greater social isolation, lower self-esteem, and more presenting symptoms. However, there is, to date, no evidence for an increased risk of developing bipolar disorder, major depressive disorder, or schizophrenia. They have more driving accidents that cause bodily harm.

The presence of hyperactivity in learning-disabled children predicted a worse outcome in adolescence. Prediction of final outcome cannot be made from any single measure at initial assessment. Final good or bad outcome can be predicted only by the interaction of both child factors and family factors.

FUTURE DIRECTIONS

Developmental Psychopathology

It is now known that ADHD can be a life-long disorder for some, even when the full diagnosis is present only during school years. In view of this, too little research has, to date, focused on preschoolers and on adults, most of the studies having been carried out on school-age children.

Screening methods in kindergarten can identify preschoolers at risk. If special services can be provided, it may be possible to reduce the subsequent cycle of school failure, low self-esteem, and poor motivation. This can be systematically researched. The use of medication and psychosocial treatment, including special programs in preschool as prevention for future disability, requires careful study.

Many children with ADHD continue to be disabled in adolescence and in early adulthood. For some, the disorder continues throughout their life. Research is required to study the prevalence in young adulthood of disabling symptoms of the syndrome (without the full diagnosis) as well as the prevalence of the full diagnosis in adulthood. In addition, we require more research on the efficacy of medication for adults whose functioning is disabled by ADHD as well as the efficacy of psychosocial interventions, both individually and in groups.

Clinical experience has shown that interventions in adulthood, such as stimulant medication, psychoeducation, restructuring of daily tasks, and marital therapy can be highly effective. If the parent of a child with ADHD has the adult disorder, treatment of that parent is necessary and correlated, in a circular manner, with the fruitfulness of the child's response to treatment. Treatment resources for adults with ADHD are few and hard to find. Child psychiatrists knowledgeable in this area are likely to become the educators of psychiatrists and family physicians who wish to acquire expertise in diagnosing and treating adults with ADHD symptoms. The whole area of prevalence, diagnosis, and treatment of adult ADHD is ripe for systematic research.

Etiology

Three directions of study have been fruitful and require elaboration and validation:

1. Genetic studies have established the hereditary nature of ADHD for many children. The repercussions of this are that a parent may be affected who needs diagnosis and treatment in addition to the child. The effect of treatment of a parent on the child's disorder requires study. Work on the mode of inheritance also requires further research.
2. Impaired glucose metabolism in select areas of the frontal and prefrontal cortex, as demonstrated by PET scans, needs validation in children with ADHD and in adults whose ADHD was diagnosed in childhood. Finally, brain metabolism differences that have been reported need to be evaluated in terms of specificity for ADHD versus other disorders.
3. Research on family interactions and belief systems in adolescents with ADHD has shown patterns of family difficulties. This kind of research can begin to define differences in families with children who have only ADHD and those who have comorbid conditions.

Evaluation and Assessment of ADHD

It will be interesting to continue studying the correlation between laboratory tasks and real-life situations (e.g., how does the CPT score correlate with teachers' reports?). The tasks that fail to have meaningful correlations can be dropped as part of the psychometric diagnostic battery.

It is of interest that, not infrequently, 2 teachers of one child rate the child very differently on a teachers' rating scale (e.g., the Conners). Studying this could determine if children behave differently with different teachers or in different subjects, or if the discrepancies lie in the differing standards used by teachers, with some being more finely tuned to notice and react negatively to ADHD symptoms while others are more permissive.

Treatment

Multimodality studies are underway and we do not yet have their results. We need to know whether extensive treatment improves both global aspects of functioning as well as specific deficits and, further, how long the improvements last without provision of, at least, "booster" therapy.

Outcome

Because of the known comorbidity of this disorder, we require prospective follow-up studies that separate those with the pure disorder and those with comorbidity. It is still not completely clear if ADHD alone is a risk factor for adult antisocial behavior. Separating comorbid disorders in prospective follow-up studies may also clarify the predictive factors for outcome.

New Conceptualizations

Throughout the 100 years in which ADHD has been described, it has been conceptualized differently at different times. The theoretical framework had to change to take into account and explain new research and clinical findings. Thus, we have the concept of a moral defect (1902), the concept of minimal brain damage (1953), minimal brain dysfunction (1966), attention as the core or cardinal deficit (1983), and, most recently, the idea of poor inhibitory processes (1992). Russell Barkley, using Bronowsky's concepts of how humans differ from other mammals in acquiring complex language as part of evolution, uses the concept of "aversive delayed inhibition." In his view (Barkley, 1993), this concept, namely, that children with ADHD are averse to delaying their inhibitory mechanisms, explains best the sum total of our knowledge, both clinical and from the laboratory, of ADHD. This concept is heuristic for further research to confirm or refute the theory.

CASE ILLUSTRATION

Brought for assessment by a distraught mother, Daniel, at 3 years, was "into everything," "did not listen," did not respond to praise or punishment, and "could not play alone." His mother could not take him to church, to the supermarket, or even to visit her friends. During her visits to friends, unless a house was child-proofed, he touched most of the objects he saw and, although he was not destructive, his impulsive movements and his clumsiness resulted in many things breaking. Also, his mother was embarrassed about his temper tantrums, which occurred anywhere whenever he did not get what he wanted. When they occurred in public, his mother felt others were critical of her as a mother.

During free play periods in a small therapeutic hospital nursery, he was restless and generally changed activities frequently, but he liked to play with water. He was not observed playing cooperatively with other children, although he was not aggressive with them, and he never used any of the toys and play materials constructively. In structured activities, when the children were asked to sit around a table for stories, painting, and so on, Daniel refused to comply and wandered around alone. A nursery teacher trained to work with hyperactive youngsters developed a good relationship with him, and he became more compliant to her instructions. He loved to come to the nursery. The core symptoms of the syndrome did not improve.

At 6 years, Daniel responded to stimulants, which he required to be able to participate and learn in a normal kindergarten (he had not had a good therapeutic response at age 3). For the previous year, his parents had been seen together for weekly behavioral counseling, and he was seen for weekly individual play therapy. While Daniel had not managed much in the way of symbolic play, he had formed a close relationship to the therapist (different from his other troubled relationships). His oppositional behaviors improved, and at his last play visit, he gave his therapist "his most precious thing to keep for him," a mink tail (his transitional object) wrapped in newspaper, done up with much adhesive tape. He thought it was a good present, because he did not need it so much any more.

At 9 years, Daniel showed all the typical difficulties described, but the core symptoms had improved somewhat. He had no specific learning disabilities but was behind in school because of his poor organizational skills, poor handwriting, and poor attention span. He was not aggressive or defiant but was difficult to live with because he did not listen and had become argumentative. He was constantly in his older sister's room, playing with or borrowing her things, which exasperated her. This was the year Daniel was playing outside his house, ran into the street after a ball, and was hit by a car. He suffered a subdural hemorrhage, was hospitalized, treated for epilepsy for 1 subsequent year, and then recovered. In late adolescence (15 to 17 years), Daniel was moving through secondary school but had been expelled from one day school for being a bad influence because he hated school and acted the clown. A second school also asked him to leave because he was not trying hard enough. The third school, a private boarding school, worked out, although he got into drugs (mostly LSD and hashish). He had no special friends, but he mixed with others. Daniel completed his last school year successfully and returned to Montreal. His 1st year back in the city also marked his first, and only, arrest and conviction. He was driving, and he and an unknown other driver began ``playing chicken.'' Finally, Daniel felt the other fellow had gone too far, and they both got out of their cars. Daniel initiated a physical fight, and the other young man sustained a broken nose. Daniel had no other court appearances; he felt ashamed over this foolishness. He avoided a short jail sentence by hiring a good lawyer.

After some very difficult years, during which he had severe conflicts with his father and trouble handling money, resulting in debts, the 25-year-old Daniel went to a private school in the United States for disabled youth and adults, where independent living and work skills were taught. He eventually married one of their best teachers, and the marriage was proceeding well. He came to see his preschool therapist for a follow-up visit at 25 years. At this visit, he asked if he could have his mink tail back since his wife was pregnant. When the therapist returned it to him, he was very pleased and said he

thought that his son or daughter (about to be born) might like it. At age 28 years, Daniel is the manager of a subsidiary of his father's business. His wife organizes his schedule and their social life. He remains restless and has a short fuse. Concentration at work is not complained about, but he does not read. He would probably be diagnosed as ADDH(R) by DSM-III and ADHD combined type-mild by DSM-IV. Without doubt he has severe continuing symptoms of the syndrome.

Comment

This case was chosen because it is typical of many of the children we followed from childhood to adulthood. Daniel, as a preschooler, had severe symptoms of ADHD, which continued into adult life, when, because the core symptoms had diminished and partly because of the contribution of his wife, his adjustment improved. As a child and adolescent, Daniel had, at various times, different degrees of oppositional symptoms and conduct problems. These probably did not at any time reach diagnostic criteria for the disorders. In spite of the absence of specific learning disabilities, he underachieved severely at school, mainly because of his disorganization. Daniel also showed the ability, as a preschooler, of forming a strong, lasting relationship with another adult (the therapist), which, at the time, was different from his other problematic relationships.

Studies (Campbell, 1990) have demonstrated that Daniel's type of difficulties, diagnosed at age 3, have a good chance of improvement by age 8. The degree of improvement depends on the severity of the initial symptoms, their nature, stresses in the family, and the mother-child relationship. At 3, Daniel's symptoms of ADHD were severe, his oppositional behavior was improving with therapy, physical aggression to other children was absent, and his family was relatively stable except for marital problems.

Appendix/Assessment Protocol

The assessment of children or adolescents who present with symptoms of ADHD can be approached as follows:

1. Interview with parents
   a. The child's developmental history.
   b. The age of onset of the symptoms; in what situations they are present, absent, mild, or severe. DSM-IV diagnoses are checked.
   c. The medical history, including vision and hearing.
   d. The learning history; does the child seem to be in an appropriate learning situation?
   e. The presence of family stresses that could affect the child and cause or worsen the behavior (e.g., marital discord).
   f. The type of punishment used: the frequency and severity of punishment.
   g. Does either parent lose control with the child (child abuse must be looked for)?
   h. Does either parent have a diagnosis such as ADHD, antisocial personality disorder, or alcoholism?
   i. Has there been a recent change in the family that could affect the child?
2. Child interview
   a. Target symptoms of ADHD (observed and self-reported).
   b. Can the child relate the origin of the symptoms to any event that occurred at home or at school?
   c. The child's mood, self-esteem, unhappiness, and feelings about his or her role in the family and school.
   d. History of friendships or feelings of isolation or unpopularity.
   e. Ability of child to relate to clinician.
   f. Concurrent disorders such as depression, specific learning disabilities, and conduct problems.

3. Family interview: The family interview invariably gives information not obtained by seeing the parents alone or the child alone. Often, other siblings give information about the roles in the family, which are highly significant for treatment strategies (e.g., the presence of scapegoating or giving all the attention to the referred patient, and the consequent resentment felt by siblings).
4. Standardized rating scales: These may be used to help in the diagnosis and to assess the situational or pervasive nature of the disorder. Standardized scales include the Connors Parent and Teacher Scales and Rutter's Rating Scales. Teachers and parents fill out these forms.
5. Information from the school: In no case should information from the school be omitted. The child's main teacher is often an important part of the treatment team, and his or her input as to progress (and medication effects) is essential. If parents object to the school being involved, it may indicate difficulties in their relationship with the school personnel. The clinician may be able to act as an intermediary to resolve these problems. When this is successful, parents usually agree to let the school be contacted and remain involved.
6. Assessment of cognitive functioning: This is usually carried out by a psychologist or other trained professionals, such as guidance counselors or special education teachers. The child's intelligence and grade levels in reading, arithmetic, and spelling should be ascertained. When learning disabilities are suspected, specialized testing for these is required. The majority of ADHD children require a cognitive assessment.

   In general, information from parents, the child, and the school, as well as specialized cognitive testing are needed to determine the presence, absence, or severity of the diagnosis and other concomitant diagnoses.

References

Abikoff H: An evaluation of cognitive behavior therapy for hyperactive children. In: Lahey BB, Kazdin AE (eds): *Advances in Clinical Child Psychology* (Vol 10). New York, Plenum, 1987, pp. 171–216.

Ackerman P, Dykman R, Peters J: Teenage status of hyperactive and nonhyperactive learning disabled boys. *Am J Orthopsychiatry* 47:577–596, 1977.

American Psychiatric Association: *Diagnostic and Statistical Manual of Mental Disorders* (2nd ed). Washington, DC, American Psychiatric Press, 1968.

American Psychiatric Association: *Diagnostic and Statistical Manual of Mental Disorders* (3rd ed). Washington, DC, American Psychiatric Press, 1980.

American Psychiatric Association: *Diagnostic and Statistical Manual of Mental Disorders* (3rd ed, rev). Washington, DC, American Psychiatric Press, 1987.

American Psychiatric Association: *Diagnostic and Statistical Manual of Mental Disorders* (4th ed). Washington, DC, American Psychiatric Press, in 1994.

Anastopoulos AD, Guevremont DC, Skellon TL, et al: Parenting stress among families of children with attention deficit hyperactivity disorder. *J Abnorm Child Psychol* 20:503–519, 1992.

August GJ, Garfinkel, BD: Comorbidity of ADHD and reading disability among clinic referred children. *J Am Acad Child Adolesc Psychiatry* 28: 739, 1989.

August GJ, Stewart MA: Familial subtypes of childhood hyperactivity. *J Nerv Ment Dis* 171: 362–368, 1983.

August GJ, Stewart MA, Holmes CS: A four-year follow-up of hyperactive boys with and without conduct disorder. *Br J Psychiatry* 143:192–198, 1983.

Barkley RA: *Hyperactive children: A Handbook of Diagnosis and Treatment*. New York, Guilford, 1981, pp. 282–350.

Barkley RA: Impaired delayed responding: A unified theory of attention deficit hyperactivity disorder. *Disruptive Behavior Disorders in Childhood: Essays honoring Herbert Quay*. New York, Plenum, 1994 [Summarized in the ADHD report 1 (5):1–4, 1993].

Barkley RA, Anastopoulos AD, Guevremont DC, et al: Adolescents with attention deficit hyperactivity disorder: Mother-adolescent interactions, family beliefs and conflicts and maternal psychopathology. *J Abnorm Child Psychology* 20:263–288, 1992a.

Barkley RA, Fischer M, Edelbrock CS, et al: The adolescent outcome of hyperactive children diagnosed by research criteria: An 8-year prospective follow-up study. *J Am Acad Child Adolesc Psychiatry* 29:546–557, 1990.

Barkley RA, Guevremont DC, Anastopoulos AD, et al: A comparison of three family therapy programs for treating family conflicts in adolescents with attention deficit hyperactivity disorder. *J Consult Clin Psychol* 3:450–462, 1992b.

Barkley RA, Guevremont DC, Anastopoulos AD, et al: Driving related risks and outcome of attention deficit hyperactivity disorder in adolescents and young adults: A 3–5 year follow-up survey. *Pediatrics* 92:212–218, 1993.

Behar D, Rapoport JL, Adam AJ, et al: Sugar challenge testing with children considered sugar reactive. *Nutr Behav* 1:277–288, 1984.

Biederman J, Faraone SV, Keenan K, et al: Further evidence for family genetic risk factors in ADHD: Patterns of comorbidity in probands and relatives in psychiatrically and paediatrically referred samples. *Arch Gen Psychiatry* 49:728–738, 1992.

Biederman J, Faraone SV, Lapey K: Comorbidity of diagnosis in attention deficit hyperactive disorder.

In: Weiss G (ed): *Child and Adolescent Psychiatric Clinics of North America: Attention Deficit Hyperactivity Disorder*. 1992, pp. 335–360.

Bradley C: The behavior of children receiving benzedrine. *Am J Psychiatry* 94:577–585, 1937.

Campbell SB: *Behavior Problems in Preschoolers: Clinical and Developmental Issues*. New York, Guilford, 1990.

Campbell SB, Breaux AM, Ewing AJ, et al: Correlates and predictors of hyperactivity and aggression: A longitudinal study of parent-referred problem preschoolers. *J Abnorm Psychol* 14:217–234, 1986.

Cantwell D: Hyperactive children have grown up: What have we learned about what happens to them? *Arch Gen Psychiatry* 42:1026–1028, 1985.

Cantwell DP, Baker L: Issues in classification of child and adolescent psychopathology. *J Am Acad Child Adolesc Psychiatry* 27:521–533, 1988.

Carlson CL, Pelham WE, Milich R, et al: Single and combined effects of methylphenidate and behavior therapy on the classroom performance of children with ADD. *J Abnorm Child Psychol* 20:213–232, 1992.

Casat CD, Pleasants DZ, Schroeder DH, et al: Bupropion in children with attention deficit disorder. *Psychopharmacol Bull* 25:198–201, 1987.

Castellanos FX, Rapoport JL: Etiology of ADHD. *Child Adolesc Psychiatr Clin N Am*, Vol 1 (2), 1992.

Clay TH, Gualtieri CT, Evans AW, et al: Clinical and neuropsychological effects of the novel antidepressant bupropion. *Psychopharmacol Bull* 24: 143–148, 1988.

Clements SD, Peters JE: Minimal brain dysfunction in the school-age child. *Arch Gen Psychiatry* 6: 185–197, 1962.

Conners CK: *Food Additives and Hyperactive Children*. New York, Plenum, 1980.

Cousins LS, Weiss G: Parent training and social skills training for children with attention deficit hyperactivity disorder: How can they be combined for greater effectiveness? *Can J Psychiatry* 38:443–448, 1993.

Cox A, Rutter M, Yule B, et al: Bias resulting from missing information: Some epidemiological findings. *Br J Prev Soc Med* 31:131–136, 1977.

Cunningham CE: *A Family Systems Approach to Attention Deficit Hyperactivity Disorder: A Handbook for Diagnosis and Treatment*. New York, Guilford, 1990.

Douglas VI: Attentional and cognitive problems. In: Rutter M (ed): *Developmental Neuropsychiatry*. New York, Guilford, 1983.

Douglas VI, Barr KG, Aman K, et al: Dosage effects and individual responsivity to methylphenidate in attention deficit disorder. *J Child Psychol Psychiatry* 29:453–475, 1988.

Elia E, Gulotta BS, Rose SR, et al: Thyroid function and attention deficit disorder. *J Am Acad Child Adolesc Psychiatry* 35:169–172, 1994.

Faraone SV, Biederman J, Keenan K, et al: Separation of DSM-III ADD and conduct disorder: Evidence from a family genetic study of American child psychiatric patients. *Psychol Med* 21:109, 1991.

Farrington, DP: Long term criminal outcomes of hyperactivity-impulsivity-attention deficit (HIA) and conduct problems in childhood. In: Robins LN, Rutter M (eds): *Straight and Devious Pathways from Childhood to Adulthood*. New York, Cambridge University Press, 1990.

Fergusson DM, Fergusson IE, Howrood LJ, et al: A longitudinal study of dentin lead levels, intelligence, school performance and behavior. *J Child Psychol Psychiatry* 29:811–821, 1988.

Gadow KD, Suerd J, Spratkin J, et al: Efficacy of methylphenidate in Attention Deficit Hyperactivity Disorder in children with Tic Disorder. *Arch Gen Psychiatry* 52:444–555, 1995.

Gittelman, R. Mannuzza S, Shenker R, et al: Hyperactive boys almost grown-up. *Arch Gen Psychiatry* 42:937–947, 1985.

Gittelman-Klein R: Pharmacotherapy in childhood hyperactivity: An update. In: Meltzer HY (ed): *Psychopharmacology: The Third Generation of Progress*. New York, Raven Press, 1987, pp. 1215–1224.

Goodman R, Stevenson J: A twin study of hyperactivity. II: The etiological role of genes, family relationship and perinatal adversity. *J Child Psychol Psychiatry* 30:691–709, 1989.

Green WH: Nonstimulant drugs in the treatment of attention deficit hypeactivity disorder. *Child Adolesc Psychiatr Clin N Am* Vol 1 (2), 1992.

Greenfield B, Gottlieb S, Weiss G: Psychosocial interventions: Individual psychotherapy with the child and family and parent counseling. *Child Adolesc Psychiatr Clin N Am* Vol 1 (2), 1992.

Hechtman L: Long term outcome on attention deficit hyperactivity disorder. *Child Adolesc Psychiatr Clin N Am* Vol 1 (2), 1992.

Hechtman L, Weiss G, Perlman T: Young adult outcome of hyperactive children who received long term stimulant treatment. *J Am Acad Child Psychiatry* 23:261–269, 1984.

Hohman LB: Post-encephalitic behavior disorder in children. *Johns Hopkins Hosp Bull* 33:89–97, 1922.

Hoza B, Pelham WE, Milich R, et al: The self perceptions and attributions of attention deficit disordered and non-referred boys. *J Abnorm Child Psychol* 21:271–286, 1993.

Huessy HR: Study of the prevalence and therapy of the choreiform syndrome of hyperkinesis in rural Vermont. *Acta Paedopsychiatr* 34:130–135, 1967.

Hunt RD, Minderaa RB, Cohen DJ: Clonidine benefits children with attention deficit disorder and hyperactivity: Report of a double-blind placebo-crossover therapeutic trial. *J Am Acad Child Psychiatry* 24:617–629, 1985.

Jacobvitz D, Sroufe LA: The early caregiver—child relationship and attention-deficit disorder with hyperactivity in kindergarten: A prospective study. *Child Dev* 58:1496–1504, 1987.

Kahn E, Cohen L: Organic driveness: A brain stem syndrome and experience. *N Engl J Med* 210: 748–756, 1934.

Klein AR: Effects of high methylphenidate doses on the cognitive performance of hyperactive children. *Bratsl Lak Listy* 92:534–539, 1991.

Klein AR, Young RD: Hyperactive boys in their classroom: Assessment of teacher and peer perceptions, interactions, and classroom behavior. *J Abnorm Child Psychol* 7:425–442, 1979.

Lahey BB, Applegate B, Mc Burne M, et al: DSM-IV field trials for ADHD in children and adolescents. *Am J Psychiatry* 151:1673–1685, 1994.

Lahey BB, Pracentin JC, McBurnett K, et al: Psychopathology in the parents of children with conduct disorder and hyperactivity. *J Am Acad Child Adolesc Psychiatry* 27:163–170, 1988.

Lambert N: Adolescent outcomes of hyperactive children. *Am Psychol* 43:786–799, 1988.

Lambert N, Hartsaugh C, Sassone D: Persistence of hyperactivity symptoms from childhood to adolescence. *Am J Orthopsychiatry* 57:22–31, 1987.

Lambert NM, Sandoval J, Sassone D: Prevalence of hyperactivity in elementary school children as a function of social system definers. *Am J Orthopsychiatry* 48:446–463, 1978.

Lapouse R, Monks M: An epidemiological study of behavior characteristics in children. *Am J Public Health* 48:1134–1144, 1958.

Lewin PM: Restlessness in children. *Arch Neurol Psychiatry* 39:764–770, 1938.

Loney J: Hyperactivity and aggression in the diagnosis of attention deficit disorder. In: Lahey BB, Kazdin AE (eds): *Advances in Clinical Child Psychology*. New York, Raven Press, 1987.

Lou HC, Henrickson L, Bruhn P, et al: Focal cerebral hypoperfusion in children with dysphasia and ADD. *Arch Neurol* 41:825–829, 1984.

MacKeith R: *Minimal Brain Damage: A concept discarded.* Proceedings of the International Study Group of Minimal Brain Dysfunction. Little Club Clinics in Developmental Medicine, (10), London, Heinemann, 1963.

Mannuzza S, Gittelman-Klein R, Bonagura N: Hyperactive boys almost grown-up. II: Status of subjects without a mental disorder. *Arch Gen Psychiatry* 45:13–18, 1988.

Mannuzza S, Gittelman-Klein R, Horowitz-Konig P, et al: Hyperactive boys almost grown-up. IV: Criminality and its relationship to psychiatric status. *Arch Gen Psychiatry* 46:1073–1079, 1989.

Mannuzza S, Klein RG, Bessler A, et al: Adult outcome of hyperactive boys: Educational achievement, occupational rank and psychiatric status. *Arch Gen Psychiatry* 50:565–576, 1993.

McCracken JT: A two-part model of stimulant action on ADHD disorder in children. *J Neuropsychol* 3:201–209, 1991.

McGee R, Share D: Attention deficit disorder—hyperactivity and academic failure: Which comes first and what should be treated? *J Am Acad Child Adolesc Psychiatry* 27:318–325, 1988.

Mirsky AF: The neuropsychology of attention: Elements of a complex behavior. In: Perecman E (ed): *Integrating Theory and Practice in Clinical Neuropsychology*. Hillsdale, NJ, Erlbaum, 1985.

Nanson JL, Hiscock M: Attention deficits in children exposed to alcohol prenatally. *Alcohol Clin Exp Res* 14:656–661, 1990.

Pelham W, Bender M: Peer relations in hyperactive children: Description and treatment. In: Gadow K, Slater I (eds): *Advances in Learning and Behavioral Disabilities* (Vol 1). Greenwich, CT, JAI, 1982.

Pelham WE, Greenslade KE, Vodde-Hamilton M, et al: Relative efficacy of long acting stimulants on ADHD children: A comparison of standard methylphenidate, ritalin, SR-20, dexedrine spansule and pemoline. *Pediatrics* 86:226–237, 1990.

Pelham WE, Milich R: Individual differences in response to ritalin in classwork and social behavior. In: Greenhill L, Osmer BP (eds): *Ritalin: Theory and Patient Management*. New York, Mary Ann Liebert Press, 1991, pp. 203–222.

Pliszka SR: Effect of anxiety on cognition behavior and stimulant response in ADHD. *J Am Acad Child Adolesc Psychiatry* 28:882–887, 1989.

Pomeroy JC, Spralkin J, Gadow FD: Minor physical anomalies as a biological marker for behavior disorders. *J Am Acad Child Adolesc Psychiatry* 27:466–473, 1988.

Porrino L, Rapoport JL, Ismond D, et al: Twenty-four hour motor activity in hyperactive children and controls. *Arch Gen Psychiatry* 40:681–687, 1983.

Quay HC: Attention deficit disorder and the behavioral inhibition system: The relevance of neuropsychological system of Jeffrey A. Quay. In: Bloomingdale L, Sergeant J (eds): *Attention Deficit Disorders: Criteria, Cognition and Intervention*. New York, Pergamon, 1988, pp. 117–120.

Rapport MD: Attention deficit disorder with hyperactivity. In: Hersen M, Van Hassett YB (eds): *Behaviour Therapy with Children and Adolescents*. New York, Wiley-Interscience, 1987, pp. 325–361.

Rapport MD, DuPaul GB, Stone G,. et al: Comparing classroom and clinic measures of attention deficit disorder: Differential idiosyncratic and dose response effects of methylphenidate. *J Consult Clin Psychol* 54:334–341, 1986.

Rutter M: Syndromes attributable to "minimal brain dysfunction" in childhood. *Am J Psychiatry* 139:21–33, 1982.

Rutter M, Graham P, Yule W: *A Neuropsychiatric Study in Childhood* (Clinics in Developmental Medicine). London, Heinemann, 1970.

Safer DJ, Krager JM: A survey of medication treatment for hyperactivity-inattentive students. *JAMA* 260:2256–2258, 1988.

Safer D: Medication Usage for ADD. *Attention* 2(2):11–15, 1995.

Satterfield J, Hoppe C, Schell A: A prospective study of delinquency in 110 adolescent boys with attention deficit disorder and 88 normal boys. *Am J Psychiatry* 139:797–798, 1982.

Satterfield JH, Satterfield BI, Schell AE: Therapeutic interventions to prevent delinquency in hyperactive boys. *J Am Acad Child Adolesc Psychiatry* 26:56–64, 1987.

Schachar R, Logan G: Impulsivity and inhibitory control in normal development and child psychopathology. *Dev Psychol*, in press.

Schachar R, Rutter M, Smith A: The characteristics of situationally and pervasively hyperactive children: Implications of syndrome definition. *J Child Psychol Psychiatry* 23:375–392, 1981.

Semned-Clikeman MS, Biederman J, Sprich-Buchminnsster S, et al: Comorbidity between ADDH and learning disability: A review and report in a clinically referred sample. *J Am Acad Child Adolesc Psychiatry* 31:439, 1992.

Shapiro SK, Garfinkel BD: The occurrence of behavior disorders in children: The interdependence of attention deficit disorder and conduct disorder. *J Am Acad Child Adolesc Psychiatry* 25:809–819, 1986.

Still GF: The Coulston lectures on some abnormal physical conditions in children. *Lancet* 1: 1008–1012, 1902.

Strauss AA, Lehtinen LE: *Psychopathology and Education in the Brain Injured Child*. New York, Grune & Stratton, 1947.

Sverd I, Gadow KD, Paolicelli LM: Methylphenidate treatment of attention-deficit hyperactivity disorder in boys with Tourette's syndrome. *J Am Acad Child Adolesc Psychiatry* 28:574–579, 1989.

Szatmari P, Boyle M, Offord D: Attention Deficit Disorder with hyperactivity and conduct disorder. Degree of diagnostic overlap and differences among correlates. *J Am Acad Child and Adolescent Psychiatry* 28:865–875, 1989a.

Szatmari P, Offord RD, Boyle MN: Correlates, associated impairments and patterns of service utilization of children with attention deficit disorder: Findings from the Ontario Health Study. *J Child Psychol Psychiatry* 30:205–217, 1989a.

Szatmari P, Offord DR, Boyle MN: Ontario Child Health Study: Prevalence of attention deficit disorder with hyperactivity. *J Child Psychol Psychiatry* 30: 205–218, 1989b.

Tannock R, Ickowicz A, Schachar R: Effects of comorbid anxiety disorder on stimulant response in children with ADHD. *Proceedings of the Annual Meeting of the American Academy of Child and Adolescent Psychiatry* 7:56–57, 1991.

Tannock R, Schachar RJ, Carr RP, et al: Dose response effects of methylphenidate on academic performance and overt behavior in hyperactive children. *Pediatrics* 84:648–657, 1989.

Tannock R: Poster presented at the Society for Research in Child and Adolescent Psychopathology, Feb. 1983, Santa Fe, manuscript in preparation.

Taylor E, Schachar R, Thorley G, et al: Conduct disorder and hyperactivity. I: Separation of hyperactivity and antisocial conduct in British child psychiatric patients. *Br J Psychiatry* 149:760–767, 1986.

Taylor E, Wieselberg M, Thorley G, et al: Changes in family functioning and relationships in children who respond to methylphenidate. *J Am Acad Child Adolesc Psychiatry* 26:728–732, 1987.

Thomson G, Raals GM, Hepburn WS, et al: Blood lead levels and children's behavior—results from the Edinburgh lead study. *J Child Psychol Psychiatry* 30:515–528, 1989.

Thorley G: Hyperkinetic syndrome of childhood: Clinical characteristics. *Br J Psychiatry* 144:16–34, 1984.

Thorley G: Adolescent outcome for hyperactive children. *Arch Dis Childhood* 63:1181–1183, 1988.

Velez CN, Johnson J, Cohen P: A longitudinal analysis of selected risk factors for childhood psychopathology. *J Am Acad Child Adolesc Psychiatry* 28:861–864, 1989.

Walkup JT: Methylphenidate and Clonidine Psychopharmacology, AACAP News, Sept-Oct 1995.

Weiss G, Hechtman L: *Hyperactive Children Grown Up: Empirical Findings and Theoretical Considerations* (2nd ed). New York, Guilford, 1993.

Weiss G, Hechtman L, Milroy T, et al: Psychiatric status of hyperactives as adults: A controlled 15-year follow-up of 63 hyperactive children. *J Am Acad Child Psychiatry* 23:211–220, 1985.

Weiss G, Minde K, Werry JS, et al: Studies of the hyperactive child: A five-year follow-up. *Arch Gen Psychiatry* 24:409–414, 1971.

Wender PH, Reimherr F: Bupropion treatment of attention deficit hyperactivity disorder in adults. *Am J Psychiatry* 147:1018–1020, 1990.

Werner EE: Children of the garden island. *Sci Am* 260:106–111,1989.

Whalen C: Attention deficit and hyperactivity disorders. In: Ottendick TH, Nersen M (eds): *Handbook of Child Psychopathology* (2nd ed). New York, Plenum, 1989, pp. 131–169.

Whalen CK, Henker B: The social worlds of hyperactive ADD(H) children. *Clin Psychol Rev* 505: 447–478, 1985.

Whalen CK, Henker B: Therapies for hyperactive children: Comparisons, combinations and compromises. *J Consult Clin Psychol* 91:126–137, 1991.

Whalen CK, Henker B: The social profile of attention deficit hyperactivity disorder: Five fundamental facets. *Child Adolesc Psychiatr Clin N Am* vol 1 (2), 1992.

Whalen C, Henker B, Buhrmester D, et al: Does stimulant medication improve the peer status of hyperactive children? *J Consult Clin Psychol* 57: 545–549, 1989.

World Health Organization: *Manual of the International Statistical Classification of Diseases. Injury and Causes of Death* vols 1 and 2. Geneva, World Health Organization, 1965.

Zametkin AJ, Nordahl TE, Gross M, et al: Cerebral glucose metabolism in adults with hyperactivity of childhood onset. *N Engl J Med* 323:1361–1366, 1990.

Zametkin AJ, Rapoport JL: Neurobiology of attention deficit disorder with hyperactivity: Where have we come in 50 years? *J Am Acad Child Adolesc Psychiatry* 26:676–686, 1987.

51 CONDUCT DISORDER

Dorothy Otnow Lewis, M.D.

The fourth edition of the *Diagnostic and Statistical Manual of Mental Disorders* reads as follows: "Conduct Disorder is one of the most frequently diagnosed conditions in outpatient and inpatient mental health facilities for children" (American Psychiatric Association (APA), 1994, p. 88). This statement should come as no surprise to anyone who works with children. Experienced clinicians know that every other psychiatric diagnosis of childhood and adolescence, ranging from attentional problems to psychoses, may, under certain circumstances, be manifested by disordered, often obnoxious behaviors. Conduct disorder, as currently defined, includes such behaviors as staying out late, firesetting, and sexual assault. By covering such a broad spectrum of behaviors, the diagnosis catches within its net a multitude of sins as well as a multitude of different kinds of neuropsychiatric and psychosocial conditions and combinations thereof. Because of its extraordinary inclusiveness, conduct disorder is a diagnosis that is too easy to make and too difficult to avoid, especially for the inexperienced or hurried clinician. The more sophisticated the clinician, the less frequently will he or she make the diagnosis. Children have a limited verbal capacity as well as a limited repertoire of behaviors with which to express their discomfort, misery, and confusion. Therefore, the very same kinds of behaviors in different children can be indicators of very different kinds of problems. The more knowledgeable and talented the clinician, the more likely he or she will be to make the extra effort necessary to identify underlying, potentially remediable causes of undesirable or antisocial behaviors.

Our current knowledge and diagnostic skills regarding disordered behaviors is analogous in many ways to what our understanding of retardation was 50 years ago. A half century ago, intellectually limited children tended to be lumped together as retarded; however, our increasing understanding of genetics and physiology has enabled us to tease out of the broad category of mental retardation a number of distinct, potentially preventable or treatable syndromes (e.g., Down's syndrome, fragile × syndrome, phenylketonuria). Psychiatrists are now just beginning to appreciate the fact that such potentially treatable conditions as attentional problems, brain damage, mood disorders, psychoses, and dissociative states frequently present with disruptive behaviors that also meet the diagnostic criteria for conduct disorder. Moreover, we are starting to recognize the role played by hidden physical, sexual, and emotional abuse in the genesis of certain kinds of aggressive behaviors and inappropriate sexual behaviors.

The prognosis for children diagnosed as having conduct disorder is considered poor. On the other hand, all of the other conditions listed above, including family violence and abusiveness, have implications for prevention and treatment. For these reasons the clinician must resist the tendency to make a diagnosis with dire prognostic implications based on a potpourri of superficial behaviors. The evaluator must look beneath the obvious for the more subtle indications of potentially remediable biopsychosocial vulnerabilities.

HISTORICAL NOTE

Conduct disorder, listed in DSM-IV under disruptive behavior disorders, is the latest term used to designate children whose signs, symptoms, and behaviors seem to impinge more on others than on the child or adolescent suffering from the condition. Although many of its childhood manifestations are very similar to the behaviors of adults diagnosed antisocial personality, conduct disorder has been separated from the adult diagnosis antisocial personality in order to acknowledge what psychiatrists believe to be a greater potential for change in the young. It represents, in effect, an optimistic attempt to avoid labeling a child with a hard-and-fast personality disorder diagnosis. However, as will be recognized in our exploration of its development, the diagnosis harkens back to a period in the history of psychiatry antedating the very existence of the field of child psychiatry, a time in which adult psychiatrists struggled to understand the behaviors of their recurrently antisocial but not overtly psychotic patients.

In the early 19th century, Pinel (Maughs, 1941) used the term "manie sans delire" (mania without delirium), and Prichard (1837), the term "moral insanity" to designate patients with recurrently antisocial behaviors who were not blatantly psychotic. Subsequently, Kraepelin (1915) suggested that recurrent antisocial behaviors were often manifestations of formes frustes of psychoses.

In 1952 the diagnosis of "Sociopathic Personality: Antisocial Reaction" for adults was codified by the American Psychiatric Association in its first *Diagnostic and Statistical Manual of Mental Disorders.* Individuals so diagnosed were described as always in trouble, immature, disloyal, hedonistic, irresponsible, and unable to benefit from experience or punishment. In short, they were not nice people. In 1967, in Freedman and Kaplan's influential textbook (1967), Stubblefield used the diagnosis "Sociopathic Personality Disorder: Antisocial and Dyssocial Reactions" to describe children "who are always in trouble, who seem not to profit from experience or punishment." To his credit, Stubblefield recognized that such a picture could be caused by a multiplicity of conditions including brain damage and psychosis. In DSM-II, under the category of behavior disorders of childhood and adolescence, the diagnosis became "Unsocialized Aggressive Reaction of Childhood (or Adolescence)." Children with this syndrome were said to have temper tantrums, to lie, to steal, and to tease other children. They were described as having "overt or covert disobedience, quarrelsomeness, physical and verbal aggressiveness, vengefulness, and destructiveness." The adjectives used to delineate this syndrome are more judgmental than scientific and reflect clearly the attitudes of many clinicians toward behaviorally disturbed children and adolescents. Of note, after a brief respite from the use of these kinds of adjectives in DSM-III and DSM-III-R, similar descriptors have reappeared in DSM-IV (e.g., "deceitfulness"; "conning").

In 1980 DSM-III was published, and with it came the new category, conduct disorder. Like its predecessor, unsocialized aggressive reaction, conduct disorder was used to designate children with behaviors ranging from truancy and substance abuse to rape and assault. The work on delinquency of Jenkins and Hewitt (1944), Quay (1964a, 1964b, 1975), and Robins (1966) heavily influenced the division of conduct disorder into four different categories: aggressive and nonaggressive, socialized and undersocialized.

In the 7 years between the publication of DSM-III and DSM-III-R, a revision of the diagnosis took place. The four subtypes of conduct disorder gave way to three other subtypes: (a) solitary aggressive type, (b) group type, and (c) undifferentiated type. In order for a child to qualify for the diagnosis conduct disorder, he or she needed only to have manifested three of 13 types of undesirable behaviors. The severity of the disorder was rated on a 3-point scale.

Little in the definition of conduct disorder has changed between DSM-III-R and DSM-IV. DSM-IV defines conduct disorder as "a repetitive and persistent pattern of behavior in which the basic rights of others or major age-appropriate societal norms or rules are violated as

Table 51.1. Diagnostic Criteria for 312.8 Conduct Disorder

A. A repetitive and persistent pattern of behavior in which the basic rights of others or major age-appropriate societal norms or rules are violated, as manifested by the presence of three (or more) of the following criteria in the past 12 months, with at least one criterion present in the past 6 months:

Aggression to people and animals
  (1) Often bullies, threatens, or intimidates others
  (2) Often initiates physical fights
  (3) Has used a weapon that can cause serious physical harm to others (e.g., a bat, brick, broken bottle, knife, gun)
  (4) Has been physically cruel to people
  (5) Has been physically cruel to animals
  (6) Has stolen while confronting a victim (e.g., mugging, purse snatching, extortion, armed robbery)
  (7) Has forced someone into sexual activity

Destruction of property
  (8) Has deliberately engaged in fire setting with the intention of causing serious damage
  (9) Has deliberately destroyed others' property (other than by fire setting)

Deceitfulness or theft
  (10) Has broken into someone else's house, building, or car
  (11) Often lies to obtain goods or favors or to avoid obligations (i.e., "cons" others)
  (12) Has stolen items of nontrivial value without confronting a victim (e.g., shoplifting, but without breaking and entering; forgery)

Serious violations of rules
  (13) Often stays out at night despite parental prohibitions, beginning before age 13 years
  (14) Has run away from home overnight at least twice while living in parental or parental surrogate home (or once without returning for a lengthy period)
  (15) Is often truant from school, beginning before age 13 years

B. The disturbance in behavior causes clinically significant impairment in social, academic, or occupational functioning.

C. If the individual is age 18 years or older, criteria are not met for antisocial personality disorder.

Specify type based on age at onset:
  Childhood-onset type: onset of at least one criterion characteristic of conduct disorder prior to age 10 years
  Adolescent-onset type: absence of any criteria characteristic of conduct disorder prior to age 10 years

Specify severity:
  Mild: few if any conduct problems in excess of those required to make the diagnosis **and** conduct problems cause only minor harm to others
  Moderate: number of conduct problems and effect on others intermediate between "mild" and "severe"
  Severe: many conduct problems in excess of those required to make the diagnosis **or** conduct problems cause considerable harm to others

From American Psychiatric Association: *Diagnostic and Statistical Manual of Mental Disorders* (4th ed). Washington, DC, American Psychiatric Association, 1994.

manifested by the presence of three (or more) of the following criteria in the past 12 months, with at least one criterion present in the past 6 months." As can be seen in Table 51.1, this statement is followed by a list of 15 widely diverse kinds of behaviors, grouped into four categories: *(a)* aggression to people and animals; *(b)* destruction of property; *(c)* deceitfulness or theft; and *(d)* serious violations of rules. All 13 of the original behaviors listed in DSM-III-R reappear in DSM-IV, sometimes with minor changes of wording. For example, DSM-IV clarifies the concept of lying by adding in parentheses, " 'Con' others." To the original list have been added two behaviors, bullying or intimidating and staying out late in spite of parental prohibitions. In theory, according to DSM-IV, a child who has shoplifted, lied, and stayed out late could receive the same diagnosis as a child who has repeatedly held up banks, pistol whipped guards, and raped toddlers.

DSM-IV distinguishes two kinds of conduct disorder that are based not on behaviors, but rather on age of onset. Childhood-onset type is defined by three or more of the 15 listed behaviors, at least one of which must have occurred before age 10 years. Adolescent-onset type is defined by an absence of any of these behaviors prior to age 10 years. This distinction is made because of the especially poor prognosis for children whose maladaptive behaviors start early in life. As in the case of other diagnostic categories, diagnosticians are required by DSM-IV to specify the severity of the clinical picture by ratings of mild, moderate,

or severe, thus, perhaps, enabling the clinician to distinguish between the recurrent runaway and the rapacious robber. As mentioned, there is a judgmental tone in the DSM-IV definition of this disorder that harkens back to DSM-II. For example, DSM-IV describes "individuals with Conduct Disorder" as having "little empathy," as "callous," and as "lacking remorse." Thus, it seems to stray from its goal of objectivity. Although DSM-IV acknowledges that recurrently aggressive individuals "frequently misperceive the intentions of others as more hostile and threatening than is the case," the manual fails to remind the user that these kinds of misperceptions are paranoid and may indicate the existence of a different disorder all together.

DSM-IV sounds a cautionary note. "Concerns have been raised that the Conduct Disorder diagnosis may at times be misapplied to individuals in settings where patterns of undesirable behavior are sometimes viewed as protective (e.g., threatening, impoverished, high crime)." The clinician is advised to be especially cognizant of "immigrant youth from war ravaged countries" whose aggressive behaviors may have had survival value. Clinicians are advised to make the diagnosis "only when the behavior in question is symptomatic of an underlying dysfunction within the individual and not simply a reaction to the immediate social context." Unfortunately, the evaluator is provided little to help him or her distinguish between these two ostensibly different states of mind. DSM-IV states merely that, "It may be helpful for the clinician to consider the social and economic context in which the undesirable behaviors have occurred." The author of this chapter suggests that one always consider the context in which undesirable behaviors occur before making a diagnosis.

Because all of the behaviors listed are signs, not symptoms, the definition of conduct disorder does not distinguish among assaultive children who are paranoid and retaliate in response to imagined threats, those who fight because they are frequently the butt of teasing, those with episodic manic rages, those with organic conditions that impair impulse control, and those raised under violent conditions who imitate the behaviors of others in their environments. Similarly, no distinctions are made among the runaways who leave in response to command hallucinations, the children who wander off in fugue states, and the children who flee in the course of temper tantrums. It is, therefore, up to the user of DSM-IV to keep in mind that all 15 behaviors listed under conduct disorder, and combinations thereof, occur as part of numerous other diagnoses. The clinician must refrain from using the diagnostic category of conduct disorder in cookbook fashion, ticking off behavioral ingredients and measuring the length of time they have been heating up and rising.

PREVALENCE AND EPIDEMIOLOGY

Because the criteria for the diagnosis of conduct disorder vary widely from time to time and place to place; because its manifestations at different developmental stages differ; and because the databases for different studies are not uniform, it is impossible to determine the prevalence of the condition. These currently daunting issues are reflected in the widely varying prevalence estimates reported in different studies (Bauermeister et al., 1994). For example, Esser and colleagues (1990), using ICD-9 criteria, reported an overall prevalence of conduct disorder of less than 1% in a study of 8-year-olds in Mannheim, Germany. At the other end of the continuum falls the study of Kashani and colleagues (1987) who used DSM-III criteria and who reported a prevalence of 8.7% in a study of Missouri teenagers. DSM-IV reports a prevalence in males of 6–10% and in females of 2–9%.

COURSE

An abundance of data indicates that early severe behavioral problems are often followed by a variety of subsequent adaptational difficulties. Although infantile temper tantrums are common preschool behaviors and are not considered predictive of later severe disturbance (Goodenough, 1931; McFarlane et al., 1954; Shepherd et al., 1971), some studies have reported that high levels of activity and unmanageable behaviors at 4 years of age frequently presage behavioral problems in the later grade school years (Richman et al., 1982). Bauermeister and colleagues (1994), in their elegant literature review, concluded, "Preschool behavior problems are a strong risk factor for antisocial disruptive disorders at preadolescence." Lefkowitz et al. (1977) found that aggressive behavior problems at 8 years of age were good predictors of adolescent aggression. West and Farrington (1973) found that 27% of behaviorally disturbed 8- and 10-year-olds went on to become recidivistic delinquent adolescents. In contrast, fewer than 1% of well-behaved 8- and 10-year-olds demonstrated a similar behavioral course. Three recent follow-up studies of children and adolescents have all reported a greater prevalence of conduct disorder in adolescence compared with preadolescence (Esser et al., 1990; McGee et al., 1992; Offord et al., 1992). Some investigators have reported an increase specifically in nonaggressive behavioral problems (e.g., truancy, substance abuse) in adolescence (McGee et al., 1992). As a result of these findings, DSM-IV distinguishes two types of conduct disorder: one, an aggressive type, starting in early childhood; the other, a nonaggressive type, starting in preadolescence or adolescence. Almost all studies, regardless of time, place, or sample, have found conduct disturbances to be far more common in boys than in girls.

It is important to keep in mind that, despite the above findings, the majority of behaviorally disturbed children do not go on to become antisocial or criminal adults (Robins, 1966; Rutter and Giller, 1984). Even among those children and adolescents whose antisocial behaviors bring them in conflict with the law, there is evidence that only a small proportion become recidivists (Wolfgang et al., 1972). Unfortunately, this recidivistic group commits a disproportionate number of adult criminal acts.

From an epidemiologic perspective, it is essential to keep in mind that conduct disorders, probably because of the diversity of the psychopathology underlying them, are followed by a wide range of psychiatric and adaptational problems other than antisocial or criminal behaviors (Rutter and Giller, 1984). These kinds of psychiatric problems are not trivial. For example, in her 30-year follow-up study, Robins (1966) reported that highly antisocial children who did not appear in juvenile court had a high rate of adult psychosis compared with those antisocial children who did appear in juvenile court (28 versus 8%) (p. 210). In fact, of all the behavior disordered children referred to the child guidance clinic from which Robins drew her sample, only 28% were later diagnosed sociopathic, and "This sociopathic sample averaged over 8 nonsociopathic symptoms each." (p. 119). Consistent with these data were the findings that the subjects who were later diagnosed schizophrenic averaged six sociopathic symptoms; on average they had only three sociopathic symptoms fewer than those subjects dubbed sociopaths. Given these overlapping pictures of psychosis and antisocial behavior in adulthood, one cannot help but wonder whether evidence of psychosis was also present but overlooked in Robins's samples of behaviorally disturbed children who only later were recognized as having psychotic symptoms.

Our own follow-up study of violent, incarcerated delinquent boys revealed that early aggressive offenses alone were not the best predictors of subsequent criminal violence. Rather, the combination of severe neuropsychiatric impairment and a violent, abusive upbringing correlated most significantly with repeated violent adult criminality (Lewis et al., 1989, 1994). Of note, although in our follow-up study of incarcerated female delinquents (Lewis et al., 1991) few went on to lives of violent crime, these young women did tend to couple with violent, abusive men and to give birth to children for whom they were unable to care. Their children, in turn, were placed either in foster homes or with family members whose parenting skills were at best questionable. Thus, society's failure to meet the needs of our sample of female adolescent delinquents was felt by their offspring and, no doubt, will be felt by society at large in years to come. DSM-IV acknowledges that "Individuals with Conduct Disorder are at risk for later Mood or Anxiety Disorders,

Somatoform Disorders, and Substance-Related Disorders." Our own findings and those of Robins (1966) suggest that psychoses and other severe forms of mental illness should also be added to the list of adverse outcomes.

A recently published study of 20,000 adults 18 years of age or older in the United States, which collected data on the relationship of adults' psychiatric status to childhood conduct disorders (Robins, 1991; Robins and Price, 1991; Robins and Regier, 1991) reported that numbers of conduct problems in childhood were predictive of adult antisocial behavior. Numbers of childhood conduct problems were more associated with adult criminality in males and with "internalizing" disorders in adult females. Hechtman and Offord (1994) observe that, "significant conduct problems in childhood predict the same increased rates of psychiatric disorder overall in men and women, but the patterns are different." Our own studies of adult criminals as well as our extensive clinical work with adult offenders suggest that, when males are antisocial, their underlying severe psychopathology, even their psychoses, tend to be overlooked or ignored. Hechtman and Offord (1994) rightly observe that, in addition to criminality and mental illness, early childhood disorders of conduct are predictive also of "widespread social malfunction, as seen in high rates of divorce and separation, poor work history, and unsatisfactory social relationships."

CLINICAL DESCRIPTION

Because disordered conduct can be a manifestation of a wide variety of different neuropsychiatric conditions and/or can coexist with them, a useful way of approaching a child with behavioral problems is to try to identify first his or her intrinsic vulnerabilities to maladaptation. That is, are there any potentially remediable psychiatric, neurologic, or cognitive problems that underly and contribute to the child's undesirable behaviors. Then one must explore the environmental stressors that influence the disruptive ways such vulnerabilities are expressed.

Psychiatric Vulnerabilities

Conduct disordered children present with a wide variety of objectionable behaviors, including disobedience, truancy, repeated physical aggression, firesetting, stealing, running away, cruelty to animals, lying, inappropriate sexual behaviors, and substance abuse. Children with these kinds of behaviors rarely appear to have serious neuropsychiatric problems. The key word in the previous sentence is "appear." The conduct of these youngsters is usually found by others to be so obnoxious that it overshadows any possible underlying symptoms. Unfortunately, these obnoxious behaviors tend to deter clinicians from conducting the kinds of comprehensive evaluations necessary for identifying underlying psychopathology.

It is hard to tap into the inner worlds of conduct disordered children for a variety of reasons. First, they tend to "turn off" their examiners with facades of sullenness or bravado. Unaccustomed to receiving empathy or sympathy from adults, they act as if they don't want it anyway. When apprehended they may denigrate the victim or boast of their own brutality. Alone in their cells or in the company of adults whom they trust, their macho, blasé carapace often dissolves, revealing the distraught child or adolescent underneath. Paradoxically, it is usually the most paranoid or manically grandiose youngsters who maintain their bravado and who continue to boast of their offenses and threaten others with future violence. Consequently, the most impaired, aggressive youngsters are most likely to be dismissed simply as severely conduct disordered and not provided with adequate evaluations. The most violent youths tend also to have been most severely abused. Their tendency to dissociate feelings from actions also makes them seem removed and unempathic. The clinician who is faced with this type of child or adolescent must be especially careful not to allow fear or a negative transference to get in the way of performing a thorough, unbiased evaluation.

Another major reason why the underlying psychopathology of these problematic children is overlooked is because their psychiatric signs and symptoms are rarely flamboyant. Rather, their clinical characteristics place them on the border of many different kinds of diagnoses, ranging from mental retardation and epilepsy to bipolar mood disorder and schizophrenia. When these children's symptoms and signs fail to meet the full set of criteria for other diagnoses, the episodic psychotic, organic, or affective symptoms that do exist are ignored, and the children are categorized simply according to their behaviors.

Few seriously conduct disordered children and adolescents will appear to be psychotic. Many, however, especially those who are most aggressive, will be found to have psychotic first- or second-degree relatives. Investigators who have immersed themselves not only in the study of delinquents and criminals, but also in their care, have been impressed by the severity of psychopathology encountered (Bender, 1959; Healy and Bronner, 1936; Oltman and Freedman, 1941). Heston, recognizing the psychotic core within many behaviorally disordered patients, advocated using the term ''schizoid psychopath'' to describe them.

Similarly, Bender (1959), in her description of behaviorally disturbed, psychiatrically hospitalized adolescents coined the term ''pseudopsychopathic schizophrenia.'' She observed that many children who were recognized as being psychotic in childhood appeared in adolescence to be simply antisocial. It would seem that the very same psychotic aggressive behaviors that were present in childhood became more threatening as the children increased in age and thus in size. It is extremely hard for clinicians to make objective assessments of psychopathology when they feel that their safety is jeopardized. Nevertheless, clinicians should not dismiss repeated, extremely destructive behaviors as simply variants of normal, obstreperous adolescent behavior. Most adolescents, even those from tough neighborhoods, do not indulge in recurrent acts of violence.

Paranoid delusional thinking is often associated with aggressive acts and has been reported to exist and to influence violent behaviors in certain seriously disturbed populations of offenders (Taylor, 1985; Taylor and Gunn, 1984). Our own studies of the psychiatric status of aggressive delinquents (Lewis et al., 1979, 1989) suggest that the more violent the youngster, the more likely is he or she to exhibit psychotic symptoms, particularly paranoid ideation. A prospective study of nine children who subsequent to neuropsychiatric evaluation, went on to commit murder (Lewis et al., 1985b) revealed that all had histories of one or more psychotic symptoms, which included auditory hallucinations, illogical thought processes, and delusions. The most common psychotic symptom was episodic paranoid misperceptions that made them especially likely to harm those individuals from whom they anticipated attack. Of note, every one of these future murderers had a first-degree psychotic relative.

Most adolescents with severe behavior disorders have experienced symptomatology other than just behavior problems, and many have been patients in psychiatric hospitals and residential treatment centers (Lewis and Shanok, 1980). Regardless of underlying psychopathology or previous treatments and diagnoses, the majority of such youngsters, should they wind up in correctional settings, receive the diagnosis conduct disorder (Lewis et al., 1984). Their behavior is so unpleasant, destructive, and frightening that it overshadows other psychopathology.

A major reason why the psychotic symptoms of many delinquent youngsters are not obvious is that they tend to occur sporadically. In spite of their episodic violent, often bizarre behaviors, when they are not under extreme stress, delinquent children and adolescents tend to maintain fairly normal facades. Furthermore, they try to conceal their symptoms, preferring to be considered bad to being considered sick. As a result, they are usually dismissed as simply sociopathic.

Although depressive symptoms are associated more with withdrawal than with aggression, depression can be accompanied by irritability and rage. Furthermore, it is not unusual to encounter a seemingly conduct disordered adolescent whose episodic destructive behaviors or sporadic episodes of robbery and burglary are a reflection, at least in part, of the manic phase of a bipolar disorder. Suicidal ideation and suicide attempts are also characteristic of conduct disordered children and adolescents.

Although the suicidal acts are not necessarily related to depression, they still must be taken seriously. They are often manifestations of extreme frustration, pain, anger, and, of course, impulsiveness. They should not be dismissed as merely manipulative behaviors. Conduct disordered children are notoriously inarticulate and may illustrate their pain with self-destructive behaviors.

Drug and alcohol abuse abounds among conduct disordered children and adolescents. It is not unusual to obtain a history of alcohol abuse starting as early as 11 or 12 years of age. There is a current tendency to send young substance abusers to substance abuse programs and to look no further for the causes of the abuse. Substance abuse is used by different children and adolescents for different reasons, including attempts to self-medicate anxiety, depression, psychosis, dissociative states, and hyperactivity. Alcohol and drugs are often used by abused youngsters to blot out memories, treat insomnia, or face another day in a violent, abusive household. A diagnosis of substance abuse alone in a conduct disordered youngster often reflects a failure to explore underlying symptomatology and family dysfunction. The fact that a parent abuses alcohol does not necessarily mean that the child's substance abuse is a reflection of a genetic predisposition to alcoholism. In the conduct disordered, delinquent population, until proven otherwise, the clinician should suspect that both child and parent have not received the quality of evaluation that would bring to light other kinds of psychiatric problems that frequently give rise to alcoholism or drug abuse.

Most importantly, one cannot diagnose psychiatric disorders that one does not even consider in the differential diagnosis or that one is convinced do not exist. Our own early work is a clear demonstration of this fact. In the 1970s and early 1980s, we rarely considered the contribution of dissociative disorders to disruptive, aggressive behaviors in children; we never even entertained the possibility that dissociative identity disorder (i.e., multiple personality disorder) might account for certain particularly puzzling constellations of undesirable behaviors. The fact that some children do not recall behaviors that occur during dissociative states never even entered our minds. We were ignorant of the fact that during dissociative episodes children may curse, take the belongings of others, or commit aggressive acts that they subsequently cannot remember. When these children disavow their acts, their denials of responsibility come across as lies. In one of our earliest papers, documenting the neuropsychiatric symptoms of delinquents, we did not once make mention of dissociative symptoms (Lewis et al., 1979). In retrospect, many of the symptoms that we saw as psychomotor epileptiform were more likely dissociative in nature.

Since our original studies, and in the light of our greater clinical sophistication, we have had the opportunity to evaluate samples of severely behaviorally disturbed children in residential treatment and samples of normal school children. Although at the time of preparing this chapter all of the data on these subjects have not yet been analyzed, our preliminary findings suggest that, among the abused, behaviorally disturbed children in residential treatment, hidden dissociative symptoms abound. These findings are consistent with what we already know, namely, that many recurrently violent adolescents have been severely abused (Lewis et al., 1979; 1989b). The most extreme forms of abuse are associated with the development of dissociative identity disorder. It is important to appreciate that many of the symptoms considered characteristic of conduct disorder are also associated with dissociative identity disorder. Such symptoms as episodic violence, extreme moodiness, impaired memory for behaviors, wandering off and not returning home for hours or days, finding something in one's possession and denying knowledge of how it got there, and frequent, apparent lying are characteristic of children with dissociative disorders. We recognize now that our failure in the past ever to diagnose severe dissociative disorders in extremely violent children and adolescents was more a reflection of our own diagnostic shortcomings than of the rarity of these conditions.

A reflection of the numerous different kinds of conditions that manifest themselves as conduct disorder is the burgeoning literature on comorbidity. As Newcorn and Halperin (1994) rightly observe, ''Comorbidity among disruptive disorders . . . is the rule rather than the exception'' (p. 227). For example, attention deficit hyperactivity has been reported to coexist in the majority of cases of early onset conduct disorder (Hinshaw et al., 1993). Considering these phenomena from a different perspective, between 50 and 80% of children diagnosed attention deficit hyperactivity disorder also manifest evidence of oppositional defiant disorder or conduct disorder, depending on the sample studied (Newcorn and Halperin, 1994). Conduct disorders have been reported to coexist with depressive disorders (Zoccolillo, 1992), anxiety disorders (Zoccolillo, 1992), borderline and psychotic disorders (Andrulonis et al., 1982; Bellak, 1985; Lewis, 1976), and even Tourette's disorder (Comings and Comings, 1987; Pauls et al., 1986). Newcorn and Halperin summarize the diagnostic confusion regarding the diagnosis conduct disorder when they observe that, ''Comorbidity could also be artifactually increased if a diagnostic category does not include certain information required for accurate differential diagnosis, thereby making it difficult to distinguish between disorders that are related although distinct'' (p. 229).

Neurologic Vulnerabilities

An association between brain damage or brain dysfunction and behavioral problems has long been recognized by clinicians and researchers. Sometimes the cause of these conditions can be identified. For example, Breslau and colleagues (1988) found a relationship between low birth weight and subsequent behavioral problems. Kandel (1992) recently reported an association between perinatal difficulties and the subsequent development of violent behaviors. No association was found between perinatal problems and nonviolent antisocial behaviors.

Three areas of the brain, the hypothalamus, amygdala, and orbital prefrontal cortex, have been conceptualized as especially important in the regulation of aggressive behaviors (Maclean, 1985; Weiger and Bear, 1988). Elliott (1992) has reported episodic violence in patients having small tumors or cysts involving the limbic system, usually in or near the midline.

Experiments on animals have shown that stimulation of the amygdala elicits the kind of aggression that occurs in response to fear (Egger and Flynn, 1963; Siegel and Flynn, 1968), whereas damage to this area has been reported to diminish aggressive behaviors in response to novel stimuli. Similarly, in humans, damage to the amygdaloid area has been associated with apathy and hyposexuality, whereas abnormal electrical activity in the area has been linked to aggressive acts. The association of abnormal electrical activity in specific parts of the brain with fearfulness and aggression is of clinical interest, given the fact that paranoia so frequently contributes to recurrently violent acts.

Damage to parts of the frontal lobes, those parts of the brain essential for abstract thought, planning, and judgment, has also been associated in humans with behavioral abnormalities. Whereas damage to the dorsolateral convexity has been linked to apathy, damage to the orbital area has been associated with impulsive, inappropriate behaviors (Blumer and Benson, 1978; Luria, 1980).

Studies of the medical histories of delinquents indicate that they are more likely than nondelinquents to have adverse medical histories, which include perinatal difficulties and head injuries (Kandel, 1992; Lewis and Shanok, 1977). The kinds of neurologic deficits from which aggressive delinquents often suffer can rarely be localized. However, careful neuropsychological and neurological assessments will often reveal subtle indicators of CNS dysfunction. Similarly, a medical history will frequently bring to light a history of symptoms such as frequent severe headaches, episodes of dizziness, and even of blackouts, unrelated to drug or alcohol ingestion, symptoms which youngsters fail to mention spontaneously.

Few seriously conduct disordered children or adolescents suffer from epilepsy. However, many, perhaps by virtue of their adverse medical histories, will have equivocal or diffusely abnormal EEGs. Psychomotor seizures (complex partial seizures), though uncommon in the conduct disordered population, have been reported to be significantly more common in very violent delinquents than in the general population (Lewis et al., 1982b). More common than actual psychomotor seizures are psychomotor symptoms such as metamorphopsias, impaired memory for behaviors (nonviolent as well as violent), and vivid episodes of déjà vu. These kinds of symptoms suggest that, in some conduct disordered youngsters, abnormal electrical activity in the limbic system may contribute to behavioral problems. Whether or not violent acts can occur during a seizure remains an area of heated debate. However, individuals with these kinds of seizures may be more irritable interictally than persons without the condition.

Attentional problems as well as problems with hyperactivity are also frequent concomitants of behavior problems. Such youngsters often demonstrate a variety of minor neurological problems, such as inability to skip, poor fine motor coordination, and impaired short-term memory. These kinds of nonlocalized indicators of CNS dysfunction are often dismissed by neurological consultants as noncontributory to behavior problems. Their importance rests on the fact that children with such vulnerabilities also often have poor judgment, trouble modulating feelings, and difficulty controlling their actions.

Cognitive Vulnerabilities

Most conduct disordered children are not severely retarded. On the other hand, as a group, they tend to score in the low-normal or borderline ranges of intelligence as measured by standard tests (Hirschi and Hindelang, 1977; Rutter and Giller, 1984; Schonfeld et al., 1988; West, 1982; Wilson and Herrnstein, 1986). This association of behavior problems and IQ has been documented to exist as early as 3 years of age and hence is thought not to be the result of school failure (Richman et al., 1982). Deficits in verbal skills have repeatedly been shown to account predominantly for the diminished IQ in these children (Wilson and Herrnstein, 1986). However, conduct disordered children often are raised in highly dysfunctional households, in which actions frequently speak louder than words. Hence, it would be erroneous to assume the existence of an inherent verbal deficit from these IQ studies. It is likely that the quality of parental stimulation (or lack thereof) has much to do with these verbal deficits. Of note, Schonfeld and colleagues (1988) have found that cognitive deficits tend to precede the onset of behavioral problems.

Regardless of the causes of the conduct disordered child's apparent intellectual deficits, these deficits are rarely severe. Thus, once again, such children find themselves on the border of a diagnosis. In child psychiatry, the border of any condition is a precarious line on which to teeter. With limited funds and resources, only the most obviously handicapped children in our society are likely to receive appropriate individualized attention.

Many conduct disordered youngsters come from impoverished minority backgrounds. Borderline scores on IQ tests or reading tests are more often than not dismissed in these children as reflective simply of cultural deprivation. Such children are often deprived of special educational assistance they may need. Unfortunately, the poor judgment and impaired abstract reasoning that go along with cognitive impairment, whatever the causes, contribute to the genesis of conduct disorder.

Learning disorders are another aspect of the kind of cognitive dysfunction that is characteristic of many conduct disordered children (Poremba, 1975; Tarnapol, 1970; Virkkunen and Nuutila, 1976). Difficulties with reading and language skills contribute to academic difficulties, especially in the higher grades, when success depends so much on understanding the written word. These language deficits may also contribute to an inability to express feelings and attitudes verbally rather than physically. In the past, poor school performance was attributed primarily to truancy and a lack of investment in education. It now seems far more likely that unrecognized and untreated cognitive dysfunction and learning disabilities create intense frustration and make the whole school experience one of defeat and humiliation. When these kinds of recurrent failures become unbearable, children stop going to school, and what was at first simply a conduct disorder often becomes delinquency. Thus, if conduct disordered youngsters are to have a modicum of structure in their lives and remain in school, subtle forms of cognitive dysfunction and learning disabilities must be identified and addressed even in children who appear minimally handicapped.

In summary, the undesirable behaviors of conduct disordered children and adolescents are obvious. Unlike the symptom-based criteria for other disorders (e.g., delusions, hallucinations), the criteria for making a diagnosis of conduct disorder do not even require specialized training or skills. Anyone can tell you whether a child has run away, stolen, hurt others, or lied. These kinds of behaviors are so apparent that they almost invariably overshadow the subtler neuropsychiatric or cognitive vulnerabilities that often underlie and contribute to antisocial behaviors. If clinicians who evaluate disruptive children rely exclusively on the DSM-IV criteria in order to make a diagnosis and look no further, potentially remediable psychiatric, neurologic, and cognitive vulnerabilities will remain hidden.

ETIOLOGY AND PATHOGENESIS

Sociological Theories

For many years the most influential theories regarding the development of antisocial behaviors were sociological. According to one of these theories, socioeconomically disadvantaged youngsters, unable to achieve success through legitimate, socially accepted means, would, of necessity, turn to crime (Merton, 1938, 1957). Closely related to this theory was the assumption that antisocial behaviors were not abnormal; rather, they reflected the values of a delinquent subculture (Cohen, 1955, 1956). Indeed, for many years researchers emphasized the influence of peers on the genesis of socially unacceptable behaviors.

A number of studies that have looked more closely at individual delinquent youngsters have found evidence suggesting that membership in delinquent groups might reflect more the characteristics of the individual youngster attempting to join the group than the influence of the group itself. After all, the onset of antisocial behaviors usually precedes membership in a gang (Wilson and Herrnstein, 1986). In one study (Friedman et al., 1975), the most powerful predictor of gang membership was found to be a youngster's violent behavior prior to joining a gang. There is even some evidence that many delinquent youngsters lack strong attachments to peers, and that the more delinquent the youngster, the less value he or she attaches to the opinions of his friends (Hirschi and Hindelang, 1977). Thus, the sociological theory of a "subculture of delinquency" in which the values of peers preempt those of the rest of society requires reexamination.

Forces within particular communities and cultures, however, cannot be ignored. For example, it is no accident that antisocial behavior abounds in inner city areas that are characterized by family instability, social disorganization, high infant mortality, and a disproportionate amount of severe mental illness (Herrnstein, 1983). However, it is also likely that especially vulnerable people gravitate to these areas or cannot extricate themselves from them. More recently, sociologists have been willing to consider the interplay of individual characteristics and environmental forces (Herrnstein, 1983). The effects on children's socialization of the increased use of "crack" cocaine and other street drugs and the use of children as purveyors and go-betweens remains to be explored. Similarly, over the past decade the increasing availability of firearms has changed the quality of juvenile violence and lowered the age at which lethal acts are committed.

Possible Physiologic and Biochemical Contributions to Conduct Disorder

The past 40 years have witnessed an increasing interest in the possible biochemical underpinnings of aberrant behaviors. The effects of antipsy-

chotic and antidepressant medications have forced a reassessment of the causes of a variety of different conditions previously considered to be exclusively psychodynamic or environmental.

Animal studies have revealed the effects on behavior of such neurotransmitters as dopamine, norepinephrine, and serotonin (Alpert et al., 1981). Most intriguing for the study of human behaviors are the findings that animals such as dogs and rats, raised in social isolation, show increased aggression (Sahakian, 1981; Valzelli, 1974; Welch and Welch, 1971) and that social isolation has been correlated with neurochemical changes in the brain (Melzak, 1968; Morgan, 1973; Sahakian, 1981). Rats raised in social isolation have been reported to experience bouts of hyperactivity and an inability to follow through on directed responses (Sahakian and Robbins, 1977). These kinds of behaviors, as Sahakian has pointed out, are similar to those of many children raised in abusive and neglectful households. They highlight the interactions among psychological trauma, neurochemical function, and behavior.

Studies on humans over the past decade suggest that there may be an association between diminished amounts of serotonin in the CNS and aggressive behaviors (Brown et al., 1979; Coccaro et al., 1989; Virkkunen et al., 1989). In a recent study, Virkkunen and his colleagues (1994) have reported an association of low cerebrospinal concentrations of 5-hydroxyindoleacetic acid (5-HIAA), a serotonin metabolite, and high mean cerebrospinal testosterone levels in alcoholic, impulsive, antisocial offenders compared with levels in normal control subjects. Those subjects with aggressive behaviors characterized by intermittent explosive disorders also were found to have significantly lower mean glucose blood nadirs in response to an oral glucose challenge than did normal, control subjects. Mean CSF corticotropine levels were also reported to have been significantly lower in antisocial than in control subjects. Of note, these investigators failed to find a consistent association between static measures of noradrenergic activity (e.g., CSF levels of monoamine metabolites such as 3-methoxy-4-hydroxyphenylglycol (MHPG) and measures of impulsivity and aggressiveness.

Rogeness (1994), on the other hand, has reported several indicators of decreased noradrenergic activity in undersocialized, conduct disordered subjects. These include lower than normal plasma dopamine-β-hydrozylase activity (an enzyme involved in the transformation of dopamine to norepinephrine) (Rogeness et al., 1988). They also reported higher ratios of MHPG to other metabolites of norepinephrine such as vanillylmandelic acid (VMA), which they interpreted as another indicator of possible diminished efficiency of noradrenergic function (Rogeness et al., 1990). This ratio of MHPG to VMA was also found to correlate with high scores on Conner's Behavior Problem Checklist. Other studies, however, have failed to document a relationship between low dopamine-β-hydroxylase activity and disorders of conduct (Pliszka et al., 1988a, 1988b).

Over the past quarter century, investigators have struggled to find measurable physiologic characteristics with which to identify conduct disordered and antisocial individuals. Gray (1987) and Fowles (1988) have conceptualized behavioral facilitory and behavioral inhibitory systems, the former integrated in the mesolimbic dopaminergic system, the latter in the septohippocampal system. They have theorized that children with less active inhibitory systems would be less likely to learn from negative experiences because of their diminished capacity to be conditioned through negative stimuli (i.e., punishment). Children with overactive behavioral facilitating systems compared with inhibitory systems would also be too responsive to rewarding stimuli and would tend to ignore the potentially negative consequences of acts of immediate gratification. These kinds of theories are consistent with the hypothesis of Mednick (1981) and Hare (1970) that antisocial youngsters share an inherent autonomic hyporeactivity. Their studies comparing the different physiological responses to aversive stimuli of delinquents and nondelinquents have led them to conclude that antisocial individuals are born with an autonomic nervous system that recovers slowly from stressful stimuli. Therefore, they theorize, such delinquency-prone youngsters receive little immediate reinforcement for the inhibition of antisocial acts. Such children, they believe, would be slower than others to learn to inhibit aggressive behaviors.

These findings are both intriguing and puzzling. The wide variety of different kinds of neurological and psychiatric signs, symptoms, and behaviors that are characteristic of aggressive delinquent children raises the question of why youngsters with so many different kinds of vulnerabilities should resemble one another in terms of autonomic responsiveness. If, indeed, such physiological similarities among aggressive individuals exist, and if they are relevant to violent behaviors, one could as easily hypothesize an environmentally induced physiological state secondary to extreme environmental stressors (e.g., an induced tendency to block out feelings and to dissociate) rather than an inborn proclivity toward violence.

Other physiological studies have focused on possible hormonal factors and delinquency. Some studies of girls and boys born with adrenogenital syndrome have suggested that they may be more energetic and physically active than their normal counterparts (Ehrhardt, 1975). Other studies have called these findings into question (Hines, 1982).

Interest has also focused on the relationship of testosterone levels and aggressive behavior in males. Persky and colleagues (1971), in one of the first systematic studies of male aggression and testosterone, reported a positive correlation between self-assessed aggression and plasma levels of testosterone. Others have failed to replicate these findings (Meyer-Bahlberg et al., 1974; Monti et al., 1977). Mattsson and colleagues (1980), in one of the only hormonal studies using juvenile delinquent subjects, found that incarcerated recidivist males had slightly higher testosterone levels than did normal male adolescents. In a unique study of serum androgen levels in aggressive and nonaggressive prepubertal boys, Constantino and colleagues (1993) found no significant differences between their two groups of subjects. They concluded that testosterone was not a good marker for aggressiveness in early childhood. These findings contrast with those of Virkkunen et al. (1994) regarding impulsive, aggressive, antisocial, alcoholic males and elevated CSF testosterone.

Whatever the contribution may be of hormonal changes to violence, it seems unlikely that hormonal factors in and of themselves account for violence in most recurrently aggressive individuals. Nonetheless, it is intriguing to note, if the yearly FBI Uniform Crime Reports can be taken as reflections of the incidence of violent behaviors, that males in our society are approximately nine times as violent as females.

Genetic Perspectives

Modern techniques for visualizing chromosomes have contributed to a renewed interest in the genetics of behavior. Reports in the 1960s and 1970s suggested an association between certain chromosomal anomalies and increased sociopathic tendencies. Several studies indicated a higher than normal prevalence of the 47XYY anomaly in institutionalized populations and in populations of mentally ill offenders (Casey et al., 1966; Forssman and Hambert, 1967; Jacobs et al., 1968; Nielson, 1968; Telfer, 1968). Nonetheless, few prisoners have the 47XYY complement of chromosomes (Baker et al., 1970; Jacobs et al., 1971). Moreover, the overwhelming majority of individuals carrying the XYY complement of chromosomes remain outside prisons and mental hospitals (Gerald, 1976). It is likely, therefore, that a variety of experiential or environmental influences determine which individuals with genetic vulnerabilities will behave antisocially. Certain chromosomal abnormalities may impart a greater vulnerability to a variety of different problems in adaptation which will only manifest themselves as aggressiveness in certain contexts (Owen, 1972). There are studies that indicate that being a member of a dysfunctional household may determine whether or not an individual with a particular genetic anomaly will manifest antisocial behaviors (Nielsen, 1970). This adverse effect on behavior of the interaction of psychological vulnerabilities secondary to intrinsic chromosomal anomalies and environmental stressors is similar to our own findings regarding the interaction of neuropsychiatric vulnerabilities and family

abusiveness in the genesis of violence (Lewis and Shanok, 1979; Lewis et al., 1987, 1989a, 1989b, 1994).

In another approach to issues of heredity, Hutchings and Mednick (1974) studied the records of adopted-away offspring of criminal fathers and found that their children were more likely to become antisocial than were the adopted-away children of noncriminal fathers. The children at greatest risk for antisocial behavior were those with criminal biological fathers and criminal adoptive fathers, a finding suggesting an interplay of genetic and environmental influences.

Studies like these, relying as they do on registered parental criminality, must be interpreted with caution. They do not take into consideration the likelihood that parental criminality, especially in males, may simply be the most obvious manifestation of other, underlying neuropsychiatric disorders, including psychoses and brain damage. There is evidence that the children of parents who suffer from a variety of different psychiatric disorders are more likely than the children of healthy parents to have behavioral problems (Moffitt, 1987; Watt et al., 1984; Wilson and Herrnstein, 1988). That the children of such disordered parents are themselves behaviorally disturbed is not necessarily an indication of a genetic predisposition to antisocial behavior. As Walker (1989) has stressed, mentally ill parents often act in aggressive and neglectful ways and thereby contribute to maladaptation. Regardless of etiology, the adaptational problems of males are especially likely to be manifested through aggressive acts compared with those of females. Unfortunately, behaviorally disruptive males tend to be dismissed simply as delinquent, antisocial, or criminal and to be incarcerated. It makes clinical sense, when thinking about genetic factors, to consider the possibility of an inherent vulnerability to one or another kind of neuropsychiatric condition; these conditions, under certain circumstances, can manifest themselves in antisocial behaviors. To the best of our knowledge, there is no specific inherent predisposition to conduct disorder, antisocial personality, delinquency, criminality, or violence.

Parental Mental Illness and Physical Abuse

The fact that parental attitudes and behaviors influence children's maladaptive behaviors has long been recognized. However, causal explanations are usually vague. For example, from the early studies of the Gluecks (1950) to the more recent studies of Farrington (1978) and others, chaotic home conditions of one sort or another have been associated with delinquency. A consensus today suggests that broken homes per se are not etiologically important in terms of behavior problems. Rather, strife between parents may be even more damaging. Almost half a century ago, Bowlby (1951) described a relationship between maternal deprivation and delinquency or the development of what he called the "affectionless character." Kolvin and colleagues (1988), in their study of a birth cohort of over a thousand babies, documented a relationship between degrees of parenting deprivation and the development of antisocial behaviors. They found that children with one or more of the following environmental vulnerabilities were far more likely than their more fortunate peers to commit offenses in later life: (a) marital disruption, (b) parental illness, (c) defective physical care, (d) social dependence, (e) poor housing conditions (e.g., overcrowding), and (f) poor maternal capacity or coping skills. The researchers demonstrated a clear association between early deprivation, behavior problems at 10 years of age, delinquency at age 15 years, and criminality by age 33 years. Deprivation was less likely to result in these outcomes in girls than in boys.

Many investigators have cited parental psychopathology as an important causal factor in behavior problems (Guze, 1976; Lewis et al., 1978, 1981; Robins, 1966). Parent diagnoses, however, have tended to fall into two overlapping categories, sociopathy and alcoholism. We have found, however, that many of the parents of delinquents suffer from more serious psychopathology, including psychoses, which are often overlooked; their own more obvious antisocial and addictive behaviors, like those of their children, mask other underlying psychopathology (Lewis et al., 1981).

One of the most important characteristics of parents of seriously delinquent, violent juveniles is physical abusiveness toward their children and violence toward each other. The histories of severely behaviorally disturbed aggressive children again and again reveal a picture of physical and or sexual abuse at the hands of adults, usually parents. This abuse is usually sufficient to leave evidence, for example, scars, but is only occasionally obvious enough to elicit protection of the child by the state. In this way, conduct disordered children once again teeter on a border, the border of documented child abuse; and because their precarious situation usually goes unrecognized, nothing is done.

There are several ways in which one might understand how abuse begets violence. First, parental violence becomes a model of behavior; second, it often results in CNS damage, which contributes to a child's adaptational difficulties; third, the stresses of maltreatment may actually alter brain physiology, changing neurotransmitter and hormone levels and diminishing impulse control; and finally, abuse engenders rage that is usually displaced from the abusing parent onto other figures in the child's environment such as teachers and peers.

Medical Histories and Neurological Impairment

Although in the past, delinquent youngsters were considered to be essentially physically healthy (Glueck and Glueck, 1950), more recent studies have demonstrated that delinquents have especially adverse medical histories compared with matched samples of nondelinquents (Lewis and Shanok, 1977). Moreover, trauma of one sort or another to the CNS is extremely common among especially aggressive offenders, juveniles as well as adults (Lewis and Shanok, 1979; Lewis et al., 1984, 1988b). A study comparing black and white delinquents revealed that, whereas white delinquents had far more adverse medical histories than white nondelinquents, the medical histories of black delinquents were only marginally more adverse than those of their black nondelinquent peers (Lewis et al., 1985a). In light of these findings, one cannot help but wonder to what extent severe medical problems, as they affect CNS functioning and thus hyperactivity, mood lability, judgment, and impulsivity, contribute to high rates of conduct disorder and delinquency in socioeconomically disadvantaged populations.

Summary of Etiologies

This review of the intrinsic and extrinsic contributors to disturbances of behavior illustrates that conduct disorder is not a single diagnostic entity. It is, rather, the final common pathway of the interaction of a variety of different kinds of psychobiological vulnerabilities with a variety of different kinds of environmental stressors. Each of these vulnerabilities and stressors must be identified before appropriate interventions can occur.

DIAGNOSTIC EVALUATION

Because the criteria for diagnosing conduct disorder are so broad, and so many different kinds of psychiatric disorders present as behavior problems, it is imperative that the clinician perform a detailed, comprehensive, neuropsychiatric evaluation before dismissing a child as simply having a conduct disorder. A plethora of rating scales has emerged over the years, designed to enable the clinician to obtain information regarding behaviors from children, parents, and teachers. Among the most widely used are the Conners Rating Scales (Rosenberg and Beck, 1986), The Child Behavior Checklist (Achenbach and Edelbrock, 1983, 1986) and the Revised Behavior Problems Checklist (Quay and Peterson, 1987). Unfortunately, these scales focus almost exclusively on conduct, inattention, and hyperactivity; they do not encourage parents or teachers to share other kinds of invaluable observations relevant to diagnosis and treatment.

Some of the semistructured interviews such as the Diagnostic Interview for Children—Revised (DISC-R) (Costello et al., 1984; Schaffer, 1989), Diagnostic Interview for Children and Adolescents (DICA) (Herjanic and Reich, 1982), Schedule for Affective Disorders and Schizophrenia for School-Age Children (K-SADS) (Endicott and Spitzer, 1978), Child Assessment Schedule (CAS) (Hodges et al., 1982), and Interview Schedule for Children (ISC) (Kovacs, 1985) are of potentially greater clinical usefulness because the evaluator is obliged to explore areas other than just behavioral problems. When using these kinds of instruments, the interviewer is well advised to look beyond the question of whether or not the criteria for conduct disorder are met and to explore the diverse symptomatology likely to become evident in the course of a careful interview. Clinicians are obliged to attempt to overcome the negative feelings toward the child that may be aroused by the child's frightening or obnoxious behaviors. One must embark on the evaluation of a behaviorally disturbed child with curiosity and an open mind.

Occasionally the clinician will uncover a distinct diagnostic entity, such as a bipolar mood disorder or paranoid schizophrenia, masquerading as conduct disorder. More often the evaluation will turn into a painstaking search for combinations of biopsychosocial vulnerabilities that affect behavior. Considerations of space preclude a detailed description of the diagnostic process; however, certain aspects of the evaluation should be highlighted.

First of all, the nature of the problematic behaviors must be explored in detail, including the circumstances in which they occur, the precipitants, and the amount of control the child seems to have over them. In the case of aggressive acts, it is essential to learn whether or not the child can tell in advance when the behavior will occur, the extent to which he or she can discontinue it voluntarily, the sequelae of the act (e.g., does the child feel shaky or dizzy or sleepy?), and the child's memory for the act. Many paranoid youngsters will say that they can tell in advance when a fight will begin by the way the other person looks at them or by the way the other person is standing. In the case of complex partial seizures, the child may experience an aura prior to an emotional outburst and may feel confused or sick or sleepy afterwards. After an aggressive act, paranoid or grandiose children often say they feel glad. The victim deserved it. Children with seizure disorders often report sleepiness, and they have trouble recalling what happened. When told what they did, they are often contrite. Children whose violence occurs during dissociative states will also not recall their acts and usually will deny them categorically.

One of the most important aspects of the evaluation is a detailed medical history, obtained from the child as well as the parent. Questions must be asked in ways that avoid yes or no responses, and answers must be pursued to their fullest. For example, after inquiring about the most serious accidents or injuries the child has experienced, the examiner, whether or not a negative response was given, must ask specifically about cars, bicycles, falls from high places, and blows to the head. Dizziness, headaches, and blackouts must be explored. Furthermore, all positive responses should be followed up with such questions as, "And what *other* bicycle accidents have you had?" "And when else did you feel dizzy?" (Hatzitaskos et al., 1994; Stein et al., 1993).

Many conduct disordered youngsters carry evidence of their medical and family histories all over their faces, heads, arms, legs, and bodies in the form of scars. The examiner must take the time not only to inquire about the cause of every visible scar, but also to ask, "Are there any scars I can't see?" These kinds of questions will often bring to light previously ignored evidence of child abuse.

Conduct disordered children, especially those with sexually inappropriate or provocative behaviors, often have histories of having been sexually abused. The examiner must not only develop skill inquiring about sexual abuse (e.g., "We know from TV that many kids have been bothered sexually by other people as they were growing up. What sorts of experiences have you had?") but must also feel comfortable with the follow-up questions, "And who else bothered you? And who else? How about outside the family?" There is an art to enabling a child to reveal the unspeakable without posing unduly leading questions.

We have found the medical history to be a useful device for conducting parts of the mental status examination. Many conduct disordered children affect a tough, challenging facade and are unlikely to admit to hallucinations or delusions when asked about them directly. However, if these issues are integrated into the medical history (e.g., ''How are your ears? Have you ever had an ear infection? Have your ears ever played tricks on you? Have you ever had the experience of thinking someone said something bad about you or your mom, and you turn around to fight, and the person really didn't say anything?''), the tough but paranoid adolescent, who has experienced episodic hallucinations, may reveal them for the first time.

A neurological examination is often valuable, especially to the extent that a detailed neurological history is obtained. The physical parts of the examination will usually simply confirm the existence of nonspecific signs of CNS dysfunction (e.g, choreiform movements, inability to skip). Neuropsychological testing, on the other hand, is often far more valuable than the neurological examination for identifying the specific nature of CNS dysfunction that may be contributing to a child's adaptational problems. Similarly a detailed psychoeducational evaluation may bring to light potentially remediable intellectual or learning problems that, unrecognized and untreated, contribute to academic and behavioral problems at school and ultimately to truancy.

The EEG may confirm the suspicion of a seizure disorder, but a normal EEG does not rule it out. We have found that quantitative EEGs (i.e., computerized) sometimes reveal abnormalities that a conventional EEG has failed to document. It should be emphasized that the existence of a seizure disorder rarely if ever completely explains a disorder of conduct. Finally, the clinician must obtain as detailed a picture of the child's family and social environment as possible in order to appreciate the genetic and experiential factors that influence behavior.

Whatever the individual problems discovered in the course of a careful neuropsychiatric and psychosocial assessment, the clinician must finally determine just how a child's particular vulnerabilities, experiences, and environmental stressors interact to engender his or her particular disruptive behaviors.

DIFFERENTIAL DIAGNOSIS

The differential diagnosis of conduct disorder is almost as broad as the entire field of child and adolescent psychiatry. Learning disorders, attention deficit hyperactivity, mild mental retardation, seizure disorders, schizophrenia, mood disorders, dissociative disorders, and even dissociative identity disorder (multiple personality) may at some time in childhood or adolescence manifest themselves as disorders of conduct. Most often, the conduct disordered child or adolescent will be found to have a variety of different kinds of vulnerabilities, psychiatric, neurological, cognitive, and environmental, which together contribute to maladaptation. Each must therefore be addressed. When these specific vulnerabilities are addressed, the child's conduct almost invariably improves. In the case of maladaptive behaviors, it makes sense to dispense with labels and to identify potentially treatable problems.

A primary diagnosis that reflects the nature of underlying psychotic symptoms or organic impairment is often more useful than the designation conduct disorder. Unfortunately, the diagnosis conduct disorder usually just tells others what they already know; the child behaves badly. Thus, conduct disorder is much like fever; it can have many different causes, and it will resolve only when those causes are identified and treated specifically. Just as, occasionally, in the absence of adequate information, one must make the descriptive diagnosis of fever of unknown origin, so from time to time one may be forced to settle for the purely descriptive designation conduct disorder, or behavior problem of unknown origin. Often conduct disorder proves to be an interim diagnosis on the way to a better understanding of the child's psychopathology and on the way to a more therapeutically useful conceptualization of the clinical picture.

TREATMENT

In his review of treatment modalities for conduct disorder, Kazdin (1987) concludes, ''. . . the diversity of available procedures suggests that no particular approach has been shown to ameliorate antisocial behavior'' (p. 74). This conclusion should come as no surprise, given the fact that conduct disorder is not really a single diagnostic entity. Children and adolescents whose behaviors meet the DSM-IV diagnostic criteria suffer from such a myriad of biopsychosocial vulnerabilities that it would be amazing to find any single effective treatment modality. Nevertheless, single modalities continue to be developed and tested.

One of the modalities that has received special attention in the recent past is parent management training (Reid and Patterson, 1991; Patterson et al., 1982). This treatment method is based on the theory that parents unwittingly encourage undesirable behaviors. They fail to encourage appropriate behaviors and tend to administer excessively harsh punishments for deviant behaviors. Parents of antisocial children are, therefore, taught new ways of interacting with their offspring. They are helped to use positive reinforcement, to make use of mild punishments if necessary, and to develop ways of negotiating with their children (Patterson, 1982). Studies of the effectiveness of this kind of parent training suggest that it can be quite useful, especially in the case of certain aggressive children. Unfortunately, because it depends so heavily on parent participation, it is not useful for multiproblem families in which parents themselves are too disturbed and disorganized to participate consistently.

Another family-focused treatment modality, functional family therapy, is based on a combination of systems theory and behavioral psychology (Kazdin, 1987; Wells and Egan, 1988). Problems are analyzed in terms of the functions they serve for the family as a whole and for individual family members. Based on the observation that families of behaviorally disordered children are especially defensive in their ways of communicating, and that mutual support tends to be lacking, treatment is focused on enhancing direct communication and supportive behaviors among family members. Functional family therapy, like parent management training, tries to increase the positive reinforcement of socially acceptable behaviors and help family members develop new ways of solving their interpersonal problems. Again, this treatment modality relies on a relatively motivated and articulate clientele, which, needless to say, is not usually characteristic of families of severely behaviorally disordered children.

Problem-solving Skills Training is a treatment modality that focuses on the child or adolescent (Spivak and Shure, 1974, 1976, 1978). Based on the theory that conduct disordered youngsters do not make proper use of their potential cognitive abilities, this modality tries to help children identify problems, recognize causation, appreciate consequences, and consider alternative ways of handling difficult situations. As noted, many recurrently aggressive children are oversuspicious, even paranoid. Efforts are made to improve their reality testing by cognitive means (Dodge, 1982, 1983; Dodge and Frame, 1986; Dodge and Tomlin, 1989). Others have focused on improving children's abilities to handle anger (Kendall and Braswell, 1982; Lockman et al., 1991). The effectiveness of these approaches remains to be tested (Hechtman and Offord, 1994).

A variety of school-based treatment approaches are currently in use in different settings around the country. The most commonly employed technique used by teachers is contingency management, in which teachers give consistent verbal and nonverbal feedback in response to children's behaviors. The early outcome findings are somewhat surprising in that the usefulness of praise is unclear, whereas reprimands that focus clearly on the behavior to be discontinued have been reported to be more effective (Abramowitz and Hobbs, Parent and child evaluation of various consequences associated with a daily report card. Unpublished manuscript, 1990). Some investigators have gone as far as to recommend the accompaniment of reprimands with eye contract and ''a firm grasp of the shoulders'' (Abramowitz, 1994). Another common technique is the use of token economies (Kazdin, 1977).

Some have advocated extension of contingency-based reinforcement to the home setting. That is, teachers complete daily ratings, which children are expected to bring home for parental signature. Parents are then encouraged to make use of what Abramowitz (1994) refers to as ''a wider variety of potential reinforcers and other consequences than are available at school'' (p. 34). These kinds of behavior modification techniques, though well-meaning, demonstrate a certain naivete regarding the quality of family life of many of the most severely behaviorally disturbed schoolchildren. Such children tend to come from, at best neglectful, at worst abusive households. In such families, a commonly used ''potential reinforcer'' is a solid beating, the very parental behavior that probably contributed most powerfully to the child's conduct disorder to begin with. The use of peer-mediated reinforcements has also been attempted (Carden and Fowler, 1984; Gresham and Gresham, 1982).

One of the oldest methods of behavioral control is the use of ''time-out'' periods in which the child in one way or another is isolated or separated from the classroom's activities. The procedure harkens back to the ostracism of the ancient Greeks and the dunce cap that was in vogue in the not too distant past (Kubany et al., 1971; MacDonough and Foreheim, 1973; Spitalnik and Drabman, 1976; White et al., 1972). Abramowitz (1994) makes a cogent point with the observation that the effectiveness of all time-out procedures is contingent on the teacher's ability to make the classroom and participation in its ongoing activities a desirable pursuit. Our own clinical observations suggest that, when the classroom is an interesting, creative place to be, behavioral problems diminish in all but the most psychiatrically disturbed children.

A variety of different community-based treatments have been developed in which efforts are made to take advantage of resources within a child's community in order to support prosocial behavior (Hamparian, 1987). Among the more creative community programs are those that make use of college students (Seidman et al., 1980) and adult ''buddies'' (O'Donnell et al., 1979) who act as friends, advocates, and role models.

Since conduct disorder is not really a single entity, it is not surprising that no single medication or type of medication is especially useful. Such medications as stimulants, tricyclic antidepressants, lithium carbonate, monoamine oxidase inhibitors, clonidine, antiepileptics, sedatives, and even β blockers have been tried. Results, except in cases of the use of stimulants for clearly defined attentional problems, have been equivocal at best (Werry, 1994). That is not to say that medication cannot be of enormous help. The choice of which medication or medications to use, however, must rest on the underlying symptoms to be addressed. For those recurrently aggressive youngsters who have paranoid symptoms that cause them to lash out at imagined threats, antipsychotic medications are often helpful. We have found for these children that medications with the fewest extrapyramidal side effects are most acceptable. The high frequency of dystonic reactions to haloperidol in adolescents makes it a more problematic choice than the phenothiazines, when moderate to high doses are needed. Once a behaviorally disturbed, paranoid child has had an adverse reaction, he or she will be extremely wary of taking any other medication.

Youngsters with psychomotor epileptic symptomatology or with other kinds of seizure disorders may be helped with antiepileptic medication. It is common to find conduct disordered children with a clinical picture that includes both psychotic and psychomotor epileptic symptomatology. They may therefore require both antiepileptic and antipsychotic medication if the former fails to improve behavior.

Although bipolar mood disorders are found relatively infrequently in the conduct disordered population, when they do occur, the use of lithium carbonate or some of the mood stabilizers (e.g., carbamazepine, valproate) can be valuable. Depressed, irritable, conduct disordered children often respond well to antidepressant medications.

The point to emphasize is that medication alone is rarely sufficient. Used judiciously and on the basis of the specific clinical findings in each individual case, appropriate medication will enhance the success of other treatment modalities. The treatment of conduct disordered children and adolescents must be multimodal if it is to be helpful. It must address the medical, psychodynamic, cognitive, educational, family, and environmental vulnerabilities of each child.

Unfortunately, each of the vulnerabilities encountered in conduct disordered children is usually chronic. Therefore, any treatment program that hopes to succeed must incorporate a plan for ongoing treatment and support systems. The finest multidisciplinary approach to treatment will fail if it is time-limited to 2–3 years, and then the youngster is returned without support systems to the chaotic environment from which he or she came. Ongoing adequate medical, emotional, educational, and social supports are often required well beyond 18 years of age if severely behaviorally disordered children are to adapt appropriately as adults.

OUTCOME AND FOLLOW-UP

To date, numerous studies have documented the grim outcome for severely behaviorally disordered children (Hechtman and Offord, 1994). DSM-IV highlights the especially poor outcome for children whose behavior problems begin early in life.

Based on her own studies and a review of the findings of others, Robins (1966, 1978, 1986, 1991a, 1991b) concluded that numbers of childhood antisocial behaviors were predictive of adult antisocial behavior; that the variety of childhood behaviors rather than any single type of behavior boded ill for future adaptation; and that family background and social class were less predictive of adult antisocial behavior than were these kinds of childhood behaviors. However, the most important finding of these studies is often overlooked, that is, that most conduct disordered children did not become antisocial, criminal adults.

Several longitudinal studies of children diagnosed with attention deficit hyperactivity disorder have reported high occurrences of adult antisocial behavior compared with that in normal samples (Manuzza et al., 1989; Satterfield et al., 1982; Weiss and Hechtman, 1993). However, other studies suggest that attentional and hyperactive problems alone in childhood are far less ominous prognostic signs than is the combination of attentional problems and behavior problems. For example, August (1983), Barkley (1990), Gitterman et al. (1985), Mannuzza et al. (1989), and Moffitt (1990) have called special attention to the extremely poor outcome for children with combinations of hyperactivity, attentional problems, and disordered conduct.

Our own studies, based on detailed clinical and family evaluations of severely antisocial, violent adolescents, indicate that certain clinical attributes (i.e., the existence of psychiatric, neurologic, and cognitive vulnerabilities) coupled with upbringings in violent abusive households constitute an ominous constellation. This constellation seems to distinguish between conduct disordered children who are likely to go on to a life of violent crime and those who will adapt more appropriately to the constraints of society. The more neuropsychiatrically impaired the child, especially if male, the more likely is he to behave violently if he has been raised in a violent, abusive household. One must keep in mind, however, that all of these dire outcomes do not take into account the potential effects of appropriate early intervention.

EFFECTS OF TREATMENTS AND INTERVENTIONS

No single treatment modality for conduct disorder has proved itself to be especially effective. To date, some of the more promising strategies for the prevention of behavior disorders have been directed at preschool children (Zigler et al., 1992). The most successful interventions will most likely prove to be early, ongoing, and multimodal in nature. Strategies that address the variety of different kinds of vulnerabilities and needs seen in conduct disordered children and their families should lead to sophisticated, individualized treatment plans. Unfortunately, in spite of all that we know about the chronic biopsychosocial vulnerabilities of conduct disordered children, no treatment programs have yet evolved that address this wide variety of underlying biopsychosocial impairments and also take cognizance of their chronicity. Our own follow-up studies of incarcerated delinquents revealed that those returned home after release form juvenile corrections had better adult adjustments than those sent to group homes or punitive settings. Those adolescents sent directly to adult prisons had the most violent outcomes, even when we controlled for early violence and vulnerabilities (Lewis et al., 1994).

RESEARCH DIRECTIONS

The prevention of the development of conduct disordered behavior by improving early health care and diminishing the incidence of abusive parental practices is likely to be more effective than any treatment regimen. Although it is certainly possible that neurochemical or physiological factors related to conduct disorder will be discovered, the fact that so many different kinds of biopsychosocial problems are associated with behavior problems makes it unlikely that a single biological factor peculiar to conduct disorder or its adult counterpart, antisocial personality, will be identified. On the other hand, certain kinds of variations in neurotransmitters may be associated with particular aspects of behavior disorders (e.g., diminished levels of cerebrospinal fluid serotonin and impulsivity). It is also likely that the biochemical and genetic studies of patients and families with psychiatric diagnoses such as schizophrenia and bipolar illness, and the development of laboratory tests for these kinds of disorders, will eventually help identify children whose antisocial behaviors obfuscate underlying, potentially more easily treatable mental illness.

The study of conduct disorder is most fruitful when it is multidisciplinary. To understand it, we must find ways to examine systematically the interactions of intrinsic vulnerabilities, family characteristics, the child's immediate environment (i.e., the community), and the society as a whole in which he or she is raised. That the United States has a murder rate many times that of Canada and Western Europe bears study. To accomplish these kinds of analyses requires the collaboration of many different disciplines, including biochemistry, genetics, medicine, psychology, sociology, epidemiology, public health, and statistics.

Recognition of the biopsychosocial interactions contributing to deviant behavior also raises important ethical and legal questions regarding causality and responsibility. These kinds of questions deserve to be studied in an enlightened society. The attitudes of clinicians toward behaviorally disordered, especially toward violent patients, and the ways these attitudes affect the diagnostic process should also be examined. Our own clinical observations suggest that aggressive patients, children and adults, do not receive as careful, unbiased assessments as do patients with less frightening symptomatology.

A word should be said about the current practice of government funding agencies and foundations of supporting almost exclusively epidemiologic studies of large numbers of subjects. Such studies often have the appearance of being hard science because they permit the use of sophisticated, computer-assisted, statistical analyses. Although these kinds of studies are important in their way, they also have limitations. Research based on questionnaires, structured protocols, administered by relatively clinically inexperienced interviewers, and official records can go only so far in elucidating underlying problems affecting adaptation. For example, epidemiologic studies of the relationship of abuse to later violence, if based only on reported abuse and recorded criminality, overlook the much larger population of abused children whose maltreatment never reaches the attention of authorities; and the numbers of violent offenses reflected in FBI statistics are but a fraction of the violent acts committed by members of society. Furthermore, abused children whose plight is reported to welfare agencies are more likely to receive help than are their ignored, abused counterparts. Hence, outcome studies based on recorded abuse (e.g., those that report a weak association between abuse and violence (Widom, 1989)) are reflective of treated cases and may lead to erroneous conclusions regarding the effects of severe maltreatment. A balance must be struck between systematic, comprehensive clinical studies of small, representative samples of subjects and larger, less detailed, questionnaire- and record-based epidemiologic studies, if we are to understand the different kinds of influences that together breed maladaptive, violent, antisocial behavior.

What is certain is that, as we understand more and more about behaviorally disordered children, the global diagnosis conduct disorder will resolve into more discrete and treatable entities. It may even disappear.

References

Abramowitz AJ: Classroom interventions for disruptive behavior disorders. *Child Adolesc Psychiatry Clin North Am* 3(2):343–360, 1994.

Achenbach TM, Edelbrock CS: *Manual for the Child Behavior Checklist and Revised Child Behavior Profile.* Burlington, VT, Author, 1983.

Achenbach TM, Edelbrock CS: *Manual for the Teacher Version of the Child Behavior Checklist and Child Behavior Profile.* Burlington, VT, Author, 1986.

Alpert JE, Cohen DJ, Shaywitz BA, et al: Neurochemical and behavioral organization: Disorders of attention, activity, and aggression. In: Lewis DO (ed): *Vulnerabilities to Delinquency.* New York, Spectrum, 1981, pp. 109–171.

American Psychiatric Association: *Diagnostic and Statistical Manual of Mental Disorders* (3rd ed). Washington, DC, American Psychiatric Association, 1980.

American Psychiatric Association: *Diagnostic and Statistical Manual of Mental Disorders.* (3rd ed rev). Washington, DC, American Psychiatric Association, 1987.

American Psychiatric Association: *Diagnostic and Statistical Manual of Mental Disorders* (4th ed). Washington, DC, American Psychiatric Association, 1994.

Andrulomnis PA, Glueck BC, Stroebel CR, et al: Borderline personality subcategories. *J Nerv Ment Dis* 170:670, 1982.

August GL, Steward MA, Holmes CS: A four year follow-up of hyperactive boys with and without conduct disorder. *Br J Psychiatry* 143:192–198, 1983.

Baker D, Telfer MA, Richardson CE, et al: Chromosome errors in men with antisocial behavior: Comparison of selected men with "Klinefelter's syndrome" and XYY chromosome pattern. *JAMA* 214: 869–878, 1970.

Barkley RA: *Attention-Deficit Hyperactivity Disorder: A Handbook for Diagnosis and Treatment.* New York, Guiford Press, 1990.

Bauermeister JJ, Canino G, Bird H: Epidemiology of disruptive behavior disorders. *Child Adolesc Psychiatry Clin North Am* 3(2):177–194, 1994.

Bellak L: Psychosis as a separate entity. *Schizophr Bull* 11:523, 1985.

Bender L: The concept of pseudopsychopathic schizophrenia in adolescents. *Am J Orthopsychiatry* 29:491–509, 1959.

Blumer D, Benson DF: Personality changes with frontal and temporal lobe lesions. In: Benson DF, Blumer D (eds): *Psychiatric Aspects of Neurologic Disease.* New York, Grune & Stratton, 1975, pp. 151–170.

Bowlby J: Maternal care and mental health. World Health Organization, Monograph No. 2. Quoted in: Fry M (ed): *Child Care and the Growth of Love.* London, Penguin, 1953.

Breslau N, Klein N, Allan L: Very low birthweight: Behavioral sequelae at nine years of age. *Am Acad Child Adolesc Psychiatry* 27:605–612, 1988.

Brown GL, Goodwin FK, Ballenger JC, et al: Aggression in humans correlates with cerebrospinal fluid amine metabolites. *Psychiatry Res* 1:131–139, 1979.

Carden Smith LK, Fowler SA: Positive peer pressure: The effects of peer monitoring on children's disruptive behavior. *J Appl Behav Anal* 17:213–227, 1984.

Casey LJ, Segall DR, Street K, et al: Sex chromosome abnormalities in two state hospitals for patients requiring special security. *Nature* 209:641–642, 1966.

Coccaro EF, Siever LJ, Klar HM, et al: Serotonergic studies in patients with affective and personality disorders. *Arch Gen Psychiatry* 46:587–598, 1989.

Cohen AK: The origin and nature of the delinquent subculture. In: *Delinquent Boys: The Culture of the Gang.* New York, Free Press, 1955.

Cohen AK: *Delinquent Boys: The Culture of the Gang.* London, Routledge and Kegan Paul, 1956.

Comings DE, Coming BG: A controlled study of Tourette syndrome. I: Attention deficit disorder, learning disorders, and school problems. *Am J Hum Genet* 41:701, 1987.

Constantino JN, Grosz D, Sainger P, et al: Testosterone and aggression in children. *J Am Acad Child Adolesc Psychiatry* 32(6):1217–1222, 1993.

Costello AJ, Edelbrock C, Dulcan MK, et al: *Development and Testing of the NIMH Diagnostic Interview Schedule for Children in a Clinic Population.* Final Report (Contract No. RFP-DB-81-0027). Rockville, MD, Center for Epidemiologic Studies, National Institute of Mental Health, 1984.

Dodge KA: A social information processing model of social competence in children. In: Perlmutter M (ed): *Minnesota Symposia on Child Psychology.* Hillsdale, NJ, Lawrence Erlbaum, 1986, p.77.

Dodge KA: Problems in social relationships. In: Mash EJ, Barkely RA (eds): *Treatment of Childhood Disorders.* New York, Guilford Press, 1989.

Dodge KA, Frame CL: Social cognitive biases and deficits in aggressive boys. *Child Dev* 51: 620–635, 1982.

Dodge KA, Tomlin A: *The role of cue utilization in attributional biases among aggressive children.*

Presented at the Second Invitational Conference on Social Cognition, Nashead, NC, 1983.

Egger MD, Flynn JP: Effects of electrical stimulation of the amygdala on hypothalamically elicited attack behavior in cats. *J Neurophysiol* 26:705–720, 1963.

Ehrhardt AA: Prenatal hormonal exposure and psychosexual differentiation. In: Sachar EJ (ed): *Topics in Psychoendocrinology*. New York, Grune & Stratton, 1975, pp. 67–82.

Elliott FA: Violence: The neurologic contribution: An overview. *Arch Neurol* 49:595–603, 1992.

Endicott J, Spitzer RL: The schedule for affective disorders and schizophrenia. *Arch Gen Psychiatry* 35:837–844, 1978.

Esser G, Schmidt MH, Woermer W: Epidemiology and course of psychiatric disorders in school-age children—results of a longitudinal study. *J Child Psychol Psychiatry* 31:243, 1990.

Farrington DP: The family backgrounds of aggressive youths. In: Hersov LA, Berger M, Shaffer D (eds): *Aggression and Antisocial Behavior in Childhood and Adolescence*. Oxford, Pergamon, 1978, pp. 73–93.

Forssman H, Hambert G: Chromosomes and antisocial behavior. *Excerpta Criminologica* 7:113–117, 1967.

Fowles DC: Psychophysiology and psychopathy: A motivational approach. *Psychophysiology* 25:373–391, 1988.

Friedman CJ, Mann F, Friedman AS: A profile of juvenile street gang members. *Adolescence* 40:563–607, 1975.

Gerald PS: Current concepts in genetics: Sex chromosome disorders. *N Engl J Med* 294:706, 1976.

Gittelman R, Mannuzza S, Shenker R, et al: Hyperactive boys almost grown-up. *Arch Gen Psychiatry* 42:937–947, 1985.

Glueck S, Glueck E: *Unravelling Juvenile Delinquency*. Cambridge, Harvard University Press, 1950.

Goodenough FL: *Anger in Young Children*. Minneapolis, University of Minnesota Press, 1931.

Gray JA: *The Psychology of Fear and Stress*. Cambridge, Cambridge University Press, 1987.

Gresham F, Gresham G: Interdependent, dependent, independent group contingencies for controlling disruptive behavior. *J Special Educ* 16:101–110, 1982.

Guze SB: *Criminality and Psychiatric Disorders*. New York, Oxford University Press, 1976.

Hamparian DM: Control and treatment of juveniles committing violent offenses. In: Roth LH (ed): *Clinical Treatment of the Violent Person*. New York, Guilford Press, 1987, pp. 156–177.

Hare RD: *Psychopathy: Theory and Research*. New York, Wiley, 1970.

Hatzitaskos P, Lewis DO, Yeager CA, et al: The documentation of Central nervous system insults in violent offenders. *Juvenile Fam Court J* 29–37, 1994.

Healy W, Bronner AF: *New Light on Delinquency and Its Treatment*. New Haven, Yale University Press, 1936.

Hechtman L, Offord DR: Long-term outcome of disruptive disorders. *Child Adolesc Psychiatry Clin North Am* 3(2):379–403, 1994.

Herjanic B, Reich W: Development of a structured psychiatric interview of children: Agreement between child and parent on individual symptoms. *J Abnorm Child Psychol* 10:307–324, 1982.

Herrnstein RJ: Some criminogenic traits of offenders. In: Wilson JQ (ed): *Crime and Public Policy*. San Francisco, ICS Press, 1983 p. 31–49.

Hines M: Prenatal gonadal hormones and sex differences in human behavior. *Psychol Bull* 92(1):56–80, 1982.

Hinshaw SP, Lahey BB, Hart EL: Issues of taxonomy and comorbidity in the development of conduct disorder. *Dev Psychopathol* 5:31, 1993.

Hirschi T, Hindelang MJ: Intelligence and delinquency: A revisionist view. *Am Sociol Rev* 42:571–587, 1977.

Hodges K, Kline J, Stern L, et al: The development of a child assessment interview for research and clinical use. *J Abnorm Child Psychol* 10:173–189, 1982.

Hutchings B, Mednick SA: Registered criminality in the adoptive and biological parents of registered male criminal adoptees. In: Mednick SA, Schulsinger F, Higgins J et al (eds): *Genetics, Environment and Psychopathology*. Amsterdam, North Holland/Elsevier, 1974.

Jacobs PA, Price WH, Court Brown WM, et al: Chromosome studies on men in a maximum security hospital. *Ann Hum Genet* 31:339–358, 1968.

Jacobs PA, Price WH, Richmond S, et al: Chromosome surveys in penal institutions and approved schools. *J Med Genet* 8:49–58, 1971.

Jenkins RL, Hewitt L: Types of personality structure encountered in child guidance clinics. *Am J Orthopsychiatry* 14:84–94, 1944.

Kandel E: Biology, violence and antisocial personality. *J Forensic Sci* 37(3):912–918, 1992.

Kashani JH, Beck NC, Hoeper EW, et al: Psychiatric disorders in a community sample of adolescents. *Am J Psychiatry* 144:584, 1987.

Kazdin AE: *The Token Economy: A Review and Evaluation*. New York, Plenum, 1977.

Kazdin AE: Treatment of antisocial behavior in children: Current status and future directions. *Psychol Bull* 102:187–203, 1987.

Kendall PC, Braswell L: Cognitive-behavioral self-control therapy for children: A components analysis. *J Consult Clin Psychol* 50:672–689, 1982.

Kolvin I, Miller FJW, Fleeting M, et al: Social and parenting factors affecting criminal-offence rates: Findings from the Newcastle Thousand Family Study (1947–1980). *Br J Psychiatry* 152:80–90, 1988.

Kovacs M: The Interview Schedule for Children (ISC). *Psychopharmacol Bull* 21:991–994, 1985.

Kraepelin E: *Psychiatric*. Liepzig, Barth, 1915.

Kreusi MJP, Hibbs D, Zahn TP, et al: A 2 year prospective follow-up study of children and adolescents with disruptive behavior disorders. *Arch Gen Psychiatry* 149:429–435, 1992.

Kubany ES, Weiss LD, Sloggett BB: The good behavior clock: A reinforcement/time out procedure for reducing disruptive classroom behavior. *J Behav Ther Exp Psychiatry* 2:173–179, 1971.

Lahey B, Piacentini J, McBurnett M, et al: Psychopathology in the parents of children with conduct disorder and hyperactivity. *J Am Acad Child Adolesc Psychiatry* 27:163–170, 1988.

Lefkowitz MM, Eron LD, Walder LO, et al: *Growing Up to Be Violent: A Longitudinal Study of Aggression*. Oxford, Pergamon, 1977.

Lewis DO: Delinquency, psychomotor epileptic symptoms, and paranoid ideation: A triad. *Am J Psychiatry* 133:12, 1976.

Lewis DO: From abuse to violence: Psychophysiological consequences of maltreatment. *J Am Acad Child Adolesc Psychiatry* 31(3):383–391, 1991a.

Lewis DO: Multiple personality in children and adolescents. In: Lewis M (ed): *Child and Adolescent Psychiatry: A Comprehensive Textbook*, Baltimore, Williams & Wilkins, 1991b.

Lewis DO: Etiology of aggressive conduct disorders: Neuropsychiatric and family contributions. *Child Adolesc Psychiatry Clin North Am* 3(2):303–319, 1994.

Lewis DO, Pincus JH: Epilepsy and violence: Evidence for a neuropsychotic-aggressive syndrome. *J Neuropsychiatry Clin Neurosci* 413–418, 1989.

Lewis DO, Shanok S: Medical histories of delinquent and nondelinquent children: An epidemiological study. *Am J Psychiatry* 134:1020–1025, 1977.

Lewis DO, Shanok S: A comparison of the medical histories of incarcerated delinquent children and a matched sample of nondelinquent children. *Child Psychiatry Hum Dev* 9:210–214, 1979.

Lewis DO, Shanok S: The use of a correctional setting for follow up care of psychiatrically disturbed adolescents. *Am J Psychiatry* 137:953–955, 1980.

Lewis DO, Feldman M, Barrengos A: Race, health, and delinquency. *J Am Acad Child Psychiatry* 24:161–167, 1985a.

Lewis DO, Lewis M, Unger L, et al: Conduct disorder and its synonyms: Diagnoses of dubious validity and usefulness. *Am J Psychiatry* 141:514–519, 1984.

Lewis DO, Lovely R, Yeager C, et al: Intrinsic and environmental characteristics of juvenile murderers. *J Am Acad Child Adolesc Psychiatry* 27(5):582–587, 1988a.

Lewis DO, Lovely R, Yeager C, et al: Toward a theory of the genesis of violence: A follow-up study of delinquents. *J Am Acad Child Adolesc Psychiatry* 28(3):431–436, 1989.

Lewis DO, Mallouh C, Webb V: Child abuse, delinquency, and violent criminality. In: Cicchetti D, Carlson V (eds): *Child Maltreatment: Theory and Research on the Causes and Consequences of Child Abuse and Neglect*. Cambridge, Cambridge University Press, 1989, pp. 707–722.

Lewis DO, Moy E, Jackson L, et al: Biopsychosocial characteristics of children who later murder: A prospective study. *Am J Psychiatry* 142:1161–1167, 1985b.

Lewis DO, Pincus JA, Bard B, et al: Neuropsychiatric, psychoeducational and family characteristics of 14 juveniles condemned to death in the United States. *Am J Psychiatry* 145(5):584–589, 1988b.

Lewis DO, Pincus JH, Feldman M, et al: Psychiatric, neurological, and psychoeducational characteristics of 15 death row inmates in the United States. *Am J Psychiatry* 143:838–845, 1986.

Lewis DO, Pincus JH, Lovely R, et al: Biopsychosocial characteristics of matched samples of delinquents and nondelinquents. *J Am Acad Child Adolesc Psychiatry* 26(5):744–752, 1987.

Lewis DO, Pincus JH, Shanok SS, et al: Psychomotor epilepsy and violence in a group of incarcerated adolescent boys. *Am J Psychiatry* 139(7):882–887, 1982b.

Lewis DO, Shanok S, Balla DA: Toward understanding the fathers of delinquents: Psychodynamic, medical and genetic perspectives. In: Rexford E (ed): *A Developmental Approach of Problems of Acting Out*. New York, International University Press, 1978, 137–152.

Lewis DO, Shanok S, Balla DA: Parents of delinquents. In: Lewis DO (ed): *Vulnerabilities to Delinquency*. New York, Spectrum, 1981, pp. 265–292.

Lewis DO, Shanok S, Pincus J, et al: Violent juvenile delinquents: Psychiatric, neurological, psychological and abuse factors. *J Am Acad Child Adolesc Psychiatry* 18:307–319, 1979.

Lewis DO, Shanok S, Pincus J, et al: The medical assessment of seriously delinquent boys: A comparison of pediatric, psychiatric, neurologic and hospital record data. *J Adolesc Health Care* 3:160–164, 1982a.

Lewis DO, Yeager CA, Cobham-Porterreal CS, et al: A follow-up of female delinquents: Maternal contributions to the perpetuation of deviance. *J Am Acad Child Adolesc Psychiatry* 30(2):197–201, 1991.

Lewis DO, Yeager CA, Lovely R: A clinical follow-up of delinquent males: Ignored vulnerabilities, unmet needs, and the perpetuation of violence. *J Am*

Acad Child Adolesc Psychiatry 33(4):518–528, 1994.

Lochman JE, White KJ, Wayland KJ: Cognitive-behavioral assessment and treatment with aggressive children. In: Kendal PC (ed): *Child and Adolescent Therapy: Cognitive-Behavioral Procedures.* New York, Guilford Press, 1991.

Luria AR: *Higher Cortical Functions in Man.* New York: Basic Books, 1980.

MacDonough TS, Forehand R: Response-contingent time out: Important parameters in behavior modification with children. *J Behav Ther Exp Psychiatry* 4:231–236, 1973.

MacFarlane JW, Allen L, Honzik MP: *A Developmental Study of the Behavior Problems of Normal Children between 21 Months and 14 Years.* Berkeley, University of California Press, 1954.

MacLean P: Brain evolution relating to family, play and the separation call. *Arch Gen Psychiatry* 42:405–417, 1985.

Mannuzza S, Gittelman-Klein R, Horowitz-Konig P, et al: Hyperactive boys almost grown-up. IV: Criminality and its relationship to psychiatric status. *Arch Gen Psychiatry* 46:1073–1079, 1989.

Mark VH, Ervin FR: *Violence and the Brain.* New York, Harper & Row, 1970.

Mattsson A, Schalling D, Olweus D, et al: Plasma testosterone, aggressive behavior and personality dimensions in young male delinquents. *J Am Acad Child Adolesc Psychiatry* 19:476–491, 1980.

Maughs S: Concept of psychopathy and psychopathic personality: Its evolution and historical development. *J Crim Psychopathol* 2:329, 1941.

McGee R, Feehan M, Williams S, et al: DSM-III disorders from age 11 to age 15 years. *J Am Acad Child Adolesc Psychiatry* 31:50, 1992.

Mednick SA: The learning of morality: Biosocial bases. In: *Vulnerabilities to Delinquency.* Lewis DO (ed): New York, Spectrum, 1981, pp. 187–204.

Melzack R: Early experience: A neuropsychological approach to heredity-environment interactions. In: Newton G, Levine S (eds): *Early Experience and Behavior.* Springfield, IL, Charles C Thomas 1968.

Merton RK: Social structure and anomie. *Am Soc Rev* 3:672–682, 1938.

Merton RK: *Social Theory and Social Structure* (rev ed). New York, Free Press, 1957.

Meyer-Bahlburg HFL, Nat R, Boon DA, et al: Aggressiveness and testosterone measures in man. *Psychosom Med* 36:269–274, 1974.

Moffitt T: Parental mental disorders and offspring criminal behavior: An adoption study. *Psychiatry* 50:346–360, 1987.

Moffitt TE: Juvenile delinquency and attention deficit disorder: Boy's developmental trajectories from age 3 to age 15. *Child Dev* 61:893–910, 1990.

Monti PM, Brown WA, Corriveau MA: Testosterone and components of aggressive and sexual behavior in man. *Am J Psychiatry* 134:692–694, 1977.

Morgan M: Effects of post-weaning environment on learning in the rat. *Anim Behav* 21:429, 1973.

Moyer KE: *The Physiology of Hostility.* Chicago, Markhans Publishing, 1971.

Newcorn JH, Halperin JM: Comorbidity among disruptive behavior disorder: Impact on severity, impairment, and response to treatment. *Child Adolesc Psychiatry Clin North Am* 3(2):227–252, 1994.

Nielson J: The XXY syndrome in a mental hospital. *Br J Criminol* 8:186–203, 1968.

O'Donnell CR, Lydgate T, Fo WS: The buddy system: Review and follow-up. *Child Behav Ther* 1:161–169, 1979.

Offord DR, Boyle MH, Racine YA, et al: Outcome, prognosis, and risk in a longitudinal follow-up study. *J Am Acad Child Adolesc Psychiatry* 31:916, 1992.

Oltman JE, Freedman S: A psychiatric study of 100 criminals with particular reference to psychological determinants of crime. *J Nerv Ment Dis* 93:16–41, 1941.

Owen DR: The 47XYY male: A review. *Psychol Bull* 79:209–233, 1972.

Patterson GR: *Coercive Family Processes.* Eugene, OR, Castalia, 1982.

Patterson GR, Chamberlain P, Reid JB: A comparative evaluation of parent training program. *Behav Ther* 13:638–650, 1982.

Pauls DL, Hurst CR, Kruger SD, et al: Gilles de la Tourette's syndrome and attention deficit disorder with hyperactivity: Evidence against a genetic relationship. *Arch Gen Psychiatry* 43:1177, 1986.

Persky H, Smith KD, Basu GK: Relation of psychologic measures of aggression and hostility to testosterone production in man. *Psychosom Med* 33:265–277, 1971.

Pliska SR, Rogeness GA, Medrano MA: DbH, MHP, and MAO in children with depressive, anxiety and conduct disorders: Relationship to diagnosis and symptom ratings. *Psychiatry Res* 24:35–44, 1988a.

Pliska SR, Rogeness GA, Renner P, et al: Plasma neurochemistry in juvenile offenders. *J Am Acad Child Adolesc Psychiatry* 27:588–594, 1988b.

Poremba C: Learning disabilities, youth and delinquency: Programs for intervention. In: Myklebust HR (ed): *Progress in Learning Disabilities* (Vol III). New York, Grune & Stratton, 1975, pp. 123–149.

Prichard JC: *A Treatise on Insanity and Other Disorders Affecting the Mind.* Philadelphia, Haswell, Barrington and Haswell, 1837.

Quay HC: Dimensions of personality in delinquent boys as inferred from the factor analysis of case history data. *Child Dev* 35:479–484, 1964a.

Quay HC: Personality dimensions in delinquent males as inferred from the factor analysis of behavior ratings. *J Res Crime Delinquency* 1:33–37, 1964b.

Quay HC: Classification in the treatment of delinquency and antisocial behavior. In: Hobbs N (ed): *Issues on the Classification of Children* (Vol I). San Francisco, Jossey-Bass, 1975, pp. 377–392.

Quay HC, Peterson DR: *Manual for the Revised Behavior Problem Checklist.* Coral Gables, FL: Author, 1987.

Reid JB, Patterson GR: Early prevention and intervention with conduct problems: A social interaction model for the integration of research and practice. In: Stoner G, Shinn MR, Walker HM (eds): *Interventions for Achievement and Behaviour Problems.* Silver Springs, MD, The National Association of School Psychologists, 1991, p. 715.

Richman N, Stevenson J, Graham PJ: *Pre-school to School: A Behavioural Study.* London: Academic Press, 1982.

Robins LN: *Deviant Children Grown-Up.* Baltimore, Williams & Wilkins, 1966.

Robins LN: Sturdy childhood predictors of adult antisocial behavior: Replications from longitudinal studies. *Psychol Med* 8:611–622, 1978.

Robins LN: The consequences of conduct disorder in girls. In: Olweus D, Block J, Radke-Yarrow M (eds): *Development of Antisocial and Prosocial Behavior: Research, Theories and Issues.* New York, Academic Press, 1986, p. 385.

Robins LN: Conduct disorder. *J Child Psychol Psychiatry* 32:193, 1991.

Robins LN, Price RK: Adult disorders predicted by childhood conduct problems: Results from the NIMH Epidemiologic Catchment Area Project. *Psychiatry* 54:116–132, 1991a.

Robins LN, Regier DA: *Psychiatric Disorders in America: The Epidemiologic Catchment Area Study.* Regier DA (ed): New York, Free Press, 1991b.

Rogeness GA: Biologic findings in conduct disorder. *Child Adolesc Psychiatry Clin North Am* 3(2):271–284, 1994.

Rogeness GA, Javors MA, Maas JW, et al: Catecholamines and diagnosis in children. *J Am Acad Child Adolesc Psychiatry* 29:234–241, 1990.

Rogeness GA, Maas JW, Javors MA, et al: Diagnoses, catecholamine metabolism, and plasma dopamine-β-hydroxylase. *J Am Acad Child Adolesc Psychiatry* 27:121–125, 1988.

Rosenberg RP, Beck S: Preferred assessment methods and treatment modalities for hyperactive children among clinical child and school psychologists. *J Clin Child Psychology* 15:142–147, 1986.

Rutter M, Giller H: *Juvenile Delinquency: Trends and Perspectives.* New York, Guilford Press, 1984.

Sahakian BJ: The neurochemical basis of hyperactivity and aggression induced by social deprivation. In: Lewis DO (ed): *Vulnerabilities to Delinquency.* New York, Spectrum, 1981, pp. 173–186.

Sahakian B, Robbins T: Isolation-rearing enhances tail pinch-induced oral behavior in rats. *Physiol Behav* 18:53, 1977.

Satterfield J, Hoppe C, Schell A: Prospective study of delinquency in 110 adolescent boys with attention deficit disorder and 88 normal adolescent boys. *Am J Psychiatry* 139:797–798, 1982.

Spivak G, Shure MB: *Social Adjustment of Young Children: A Cognitive Approach to Solving Real-Life Problems.* San Francisco, Jossey-Bass, 1974.

Schaffer D: *The Diagnostic Interview Schedule for Children (DISC-2): Its Development and Administration.* Paper presented at the annual meetings of the American Academy of Child and Adolescent Psychiatry, New York, 1989.

Schonfeld IS, Shaffer D, O'Connor P, et al: Conduct disorder and cognitive functioning: Testing three causal hypotheses. *Child Dev* 59:993–1007, 1988.

Seidman E, Rappaport J, Davidson WS: Adolescents in legal jeopardy: Initial success and replication of an alternative to the criminal justice system. In: Ross RR, Gendreau P (eds): *Effective Correctional Treatment.* Toronto, Butterworth, 1980, pp. 101–123.

Shepherd M, Oppenheim B, Mitchell S: (eds) *Childhood Behaviour and Mental Health.* London, University of London Press, 1971.

Siegel A, Flynn JP: Differential effects of electrical stimulaton and lesions of the hippocampus and adjacent regions upon attack behavior of cats. *Brain Res* 7:252–267, 1968.

Spitalnik R, Drabman R: A classroom time out procedure for retarded children. *J Behav Ther Exp Psychiatry* 7:17–21, 1976.

Spivak G, Shure MB: *Social Adjustment of Young Children: A Cognitive Approach to Solving Real-Life Problems.* San Francisco, Jossey-Bass, 1974.

Spivak G, Shure MB: *The Problem-Solving Approach to Adjustment.* San Francisco, Jossey-Bass, 1976.

Spivak G, Shure MB: *Problem Solving Techniques in Child-Rearing.* San Francisco, Jossey-Bass, 1978.

Stein A, Lewis DO, Yeager CA: The Juvenile Justice Assessment Instrument. *Juvenile Fam Court J,* 44(3):91–102, 1993.

Tarnapol L: Delinquency and minimal brain dysfunction. *J Learn Dis* 3:200–207, 1970.

Taylor PJ: Motives for offending among violent and psychotic men. *Br J Psychiatry* 147:491–498, 1985.

Taylor PJ, Gunn J: Violence and psychosis. I: Risk of violence among psychotic men. *Br Med J (Clin Res ed)* 288:1945–1949, 1984.

Telfer MA: Are some criminals born that way? *Think* 34 (Nov–Dec):24–28, 1968.

Valzelli L: 5-Hydroxytryptamine in aggressiveness. In: Costa E, Gessa G, Sandler M (eds): *Advances in Biochemical Psychopharmacology*. New York: Raven Press, 1974.

Virkkunen M, DeJong J, Bartko J, et al: Relationship of psychobiological variables to recidivism in violent offenders and impulsive fire setters. *Arch Gen Psychiatry* 46:600–603, 1989.

Virkkunen M, Rawlings R, Tokola R, et al: CSF biochemistries, glucose metabolism and diurnal activity rhythms in alcoholic, violent offenders, fire setters, and healthy volunteers. *Arch Gen Psychiatry* 50: 20–27, 1994.

Virkkunen N, Nuutila A: Specific reading retardation, hyperactive child syndrome and juvenile delinquency. *Acta Psychiatr Scand* 54:25–28, 1976.

Walker E, Downey F, Bergman A: The effects of parental psychopathology and maltreatment in child behavior: A test of the deathesis-stress model. *Child Dev* 60:15–24, 1989.

Watt N, Anthony EJ, Wymi E, et al: (eds) *Children at Risk for Schizophrenia*. New York, Cambridge University Press, 1984.

Weiger WA, Bear DM: An approach to the neurology of aggression. *J Psychiatr Res* 22(2):85–98, 1988.

Weiss G, Hechtman L: *Hyperactive Children Grown Up*. New York, Guilford Press, 1993.

Welch A, Welch B: Isolation, reactivity and aggression: Evidence for an involvement of brain catecholamines and serotonin. In: Eleftheriou B, Scott J (eds): *The Physiology of Aggression and Defeat*. New York, Plenum, 1971.

Wells KC, Egan J: Social learning and systems family therapy for childhood opposition disorder: Comparative treatment outcome. *Compr Psychiatry* 296:138–146, 1988.

Werry JS: Pharmacotherapy of disruptive behavior disorders. *Child Adolesc Psychiatry Clin North Am* 3(2):321–341, 1994.

West DJ: *Delinquency: Its Roots, Careers and Prospects*. Cambridge, MA, Harvard University Press, 1982.

West DJ, Farrington DP: *Who Becomes Delinquent?* London, Heinemann, 1973.

White GD, Nielsen G, Johnson SM: Timeout duration and the suppression of deviant behavior in children. *J Appl Behav Anal* 5:111–120, 1972.

Widom CS: The cycle of violence. *Science* 244: 160–166, 1989.

Williams DT: Neural factors related to habitual aggression. *Brain* 92:503, 1969.

Wilson J, Herrnstein RJ: *Crime & Human Nature*. New York, Simon & Schuster, 1986.

Wilson JQ, Herrnstein RJ: Constitutional factors in criminal behavior. In: *Crime and Human Nature*. New York, Simon & Schuster, 1988, pp. 69–103.

Wolfgang ME, Figlio RM, Sellin T: *Delinquency in a Birth Cohort*. Chicago, University of Chicago Press, 1972.

Zigler E, Taussig C, Black K: Early childhood intervention: A promising preventive for juvenile delinquency. *Ann Psychol* 47:997–1006, 1992.

Zoccolillo M: Co-occurrence of conduct disorder and its adult outcomes with depressive and anxiety disorders: A review. *J Am Acad Child Adolesc Psychiatry* 31:547, 1992.

52 EATING AND GROWTH DISORDERS IN INFANTS AND CHILDREN

Joseph L. Woolston, M.D.

Although eating disorders are frequently assumed to be synonymous with adolescent-onset anorexia and bulimia nervosa, a panoply of eating and growth disorders occurs earlier in life. This clinical myopia is reflected in DSM-IV (American Psychiatric Association, 1994), which recognizes only three eating disorders of early childhood: pica, rumination, and feeding disorder of infancy or early childhood. The lack of official diagnostic recognition of many eating disorders is reflective of their extraordinary complexity and resulting problems in nosological definition. Eating and growth disorders are unique in medicine and psychiatry in their position at the dynamic interface of the somatopsychic boundary of developmental neuropsychiatric disorders, emotional/behavioral disturbances, and physical changes, which all interact in a complex fashion over time. Unfortunately this complex interaction has not been recognized. For example, the two most common eating and growth disorders of infancy and childhood, failure to thrive syndrome and obesity, are both currently categorized as medical conditions in DSM-IV and ICD-10 (World Health Organization, 1990). The rationale for this approach is that both syndromes are defined by caloric nutritional status regardless of etiology. Therefore, some infants and children may have failure to thrive or obesity but not actually have an eating disorder.

Until recently, understanding, and even categorization of such disorders, has been hampered by a reductionistic approach relying on deterministic, linear causality (Woolston, 1988) in which each disorder or developmental disturbance was viewed as having a single cause. This approach has gradually been replaced by the concept of a multifactorial, transactional model of development (Sameroff and Chandler, 1975; Sameroff and Fiese, 1989; Woolston, 1989). Despite this more sophisticated theoretical approach of developmental psychopathology, advancement in the understanding of early growth disorders has been hampered by a variety of controversies that actually arise from the complexity of the phenomena. Two such controversies are in phenomenology and etiology. The phenomenology of eating disorders has been plagued by a paucity of data and by persistent diagnostic confusion. For example, failure to thrive and psychosocial dwarfism are frequently used synonymously (e.g., Green et al., 1984; Moslen and O'Connor 1989); the distinctions among rumination, gastroesophageal reflux, and psychophysiological vomiting are rarely delineated; and subtypes of such disorders as failure to thrive (Egan et al., 1980; Woolston, 1983), obesity (Woolston, 1987), and rumination (Mayes et al., 1988) have proliferated. Futhermore, controversy about etiology has frequently focused upon a rigid dichotomy between an intrinsic, organic cause ("sick baby") versus an external, environmental disturbance ("bad mother") (Woolston, 1991). The counterproductive effect of such a dichotomous approach has been best demonstrated by the research in failure to thrive syndrome in which the organic/nonorganic differentiation has not held up to scrutiny (Bell and Woolston, 1985; Polan et al., 1991a).

PICA

Pica would appear to be without the nosological problems that beset other eating and growth disorders of infants and children. In fact DSM-IV, which lists pica as the first feeding/eating disorder, defines it as the persistent eating of nonnutritive substances for at least 1 month in such a fashion that such eating is inappropriate to developmental level and is not part of culturally sanctioned practice. The two dependent clauses in this definition disqualify the two largest populations described in the centuries' old literature about pica: toddlers who ingest paint chips and young pregnant women who eat starch and clay (Lacy, 1993). This artificial clarity in definition attempts to solve the confusion that bedevils all aspects of the understanding of this disorder. Rather than being a narrowly homogenous phenomenon, pica represents an eating disorder of enormously differing populations including normally developing toddlers mouthing lead paint chips, rural pregnant women eating clay or starch, severely retarded adults eating feces, and normally developed adults chewing pencil erasers, fingernails, ice, and burnt matches. As if to create an aura of scientific understanding, pica as defined in literature before DSM-IV is subtyped according to the substance ingested. These terms include geophagia (eating clay), pagophagia (eating ice), plambo-phagia (eating lead), amylophagia (eating starch), coprophagia (eating feces), cautopyreiophagia (eating burnt matches), tricophagia (eating hair), lithophagia (eating stones), geomelophagia (eating raw potatoes). Aside from a review of Latin root words, such subtyping is most useful at documenting the extraordinary range of substances that people may ingest.

In many ways, the heterogeneity of pica precludes a coherent state-ment about age of onset, developmental outcome, etiology, or treatment. Because the pediatric literature has paid great attention to the phenome-nology of lead poisoning, pica has become synonymous with children eating paint chips. For these children, pica has been reported to be more common in situations of relative environmental deprivation (Madden et al., 1980) or parental psychopathology. In this population, pica begins in the 2nd and 3rd year of life and may continue into childhood. In a second population, young pregnant women, the onset of pica begins with the first pregnancy in late adolescence or early adulthood and may continue intermittently for several decades. Pica in mentally retarded individuals begins in childhood and may diminish after middle age (McAlpine and Singh, 1986). In this population, the risk of pica appears to be related to the degree of retardation so that the most severely re-tarded are most likely to have the disorder (Danforth and Huber, 1982). Pica in chronically anxious children or adults has never been studied or described in the literature. In this last group, a possible relationship between pica, trichotillomania, and other compulsive behavior disorders has never been investigated.

Incidence and prevalence figures for such a heterogenous disorder are difficult to interpret. However, among specific at-risk populations, pica has been reported to be quite common. Halstead (1968) summarized findings from research studies that indicated that pica occurred in 25–33% of young children and 40–50% of poor black pregnant women. Pica among institutionalized retarded adults has been reported to range from 9% (McAlpine and Singh, 1986) to 25% (Danforth and Huber, 1982).

Numerous studies have documented that the eating of specific sub-stances such as clay and starch has been strongly influenced by cultural and family factors (Lacey, 1990) because various social groups, espe-cially poor and rural people, regard the eating of certain nonnutritive substances as acceptable. In addition, toddlers who are poorly supervised and understimulated are at high risk for ingesting inappropriate materials like paint chips.

Except as mediated by mental retardation, there are no known genetic factors in the etiology of pica. Boredom, anxiety, and depression may exacerbate pica, but little has been reported about such associated psy-chopathology. Iron deficiency is sometimes associated with pica, but the direction of the causal association is unclear (Vyas and Chandra, 1984).

While the extraordinary diversity of this disorder makes any useful classification schema unlikely, the remarkable prevalence and serious-ness of its medical complications require a thoughtful, vigorous ap-proach. These medical complications include heavy metal poisoning, mineral/vitamin deficiency, parasite ingestion, and intestinal obstruc-tion. For toddlers and young children with a history of pica, a careful evaluation of the home environment and family functioning is required. In addition, these children should be evaluated for cognitive and psychi-atric impairments. Pregnant women with pica presumably have more voluntary control over their eating. A careful assessment of their cultural and nutritional beliefs is essential so that nutritional counseling can be helpful. Severely retarded individuals presenting with pica should be assessed for access to noxious materials and provided with sufficient supervision to prevent pica.

RUMINATION DISORDER

Similar to pica, rumination disorder has the superficial appearance of a homogenous, unitary disorder. DSM-IV defines rumination as (a) repeated regurgitation and rechewing of food (in the absence of associ-ated gastrointestinal illness) for a period of at least 1 month following a period of normal functioning and (b) not due to an associated gastroin-testinal or other general medical condition (e.g., esophageal reflux). Unfortunately the clinical reality of this phenomenon is more complex than portrayed by DSM-IV. Some infants and retarded adults may vomit the stomach contents rather than rechewing and reswallowing it. Al-though this phenomenon is called psychophysiological (Ferholt and Provence, 1976) or operant (Johnston, 1993) vomiting, its differentiation from rumination is problematic. Furthermore, the requirement that rumi-nation not be associated with gastrointestinal disorders such as gastro-esophageal reflux is overly restrictive since it implies that rumination has no underlying physiological contributions. Indeed the relationship, if any, between gastroesophageal reflux, rumination, and operant vomit-ing has not been investigated.

Because rumination is apparently a relatively rare disorder, virtually all of the information about the phenomenology must be derived from single case reports or small case series (e.g., Mayes et al., 1988; Sauvage et al., 1985; Winton and Singh, 1983) without comparison groups. In otherwise normally developing infants, the age of onset is in the 1st year of life, whereas in mentally retarded individuals, the age of onset can extend into adulthood (Mayes et al., 1988). In some unknown pro-portion of cases, the disorder remits spontaneously, while in others, the course may be malignant, marked by aspiration, severe malnutrition, growth failure, developmental delay, and death. Some authors (Mayes et al., 1988) have proposed two diagnostic subgroups, psychogenic and self-stimulatory, to capture the difference in the course of retarded and nonretarded individuals. However, the relatively small sample size ap-pears to make diagnostic subtyping premature.

Very little is known about the incidence and prevalence of rumination although the most severely affected cases, which are the ones that have been reported, are rare. The sex ratio of the disorder is also unclear, although one case series (Mayes et al., 1988) reported a male predomi-nance.

Several authors have proposed that an adverse psychosocial environ-ment is central to the development of rumination in otherwise normal infants (e.g., Hollowell and Gardner, 1965; Mayes et al., 1988; Rich-mond et al., 1958). The most common environmental factor cited in the genesis of rumination is an unsatisfactory mother-infant relationship that causes the infant to seek an internal source of gratification. This turning inward by the infant has been proposed to occur because the environment is more stimulating than the infant can tolerate, or because the environment is not gratifying enough (Richmond et al., 1958), or because the environment is too stimulating with negative effects (Ferholt and Provence, 1976; Hollowell and Gardner, 1965). Aside from these proposed contradictory environmental factors, no information has been reported about more general sociodemographic features. Similarly, the role of genetic factors is unknown.

Learning theorists have explained rumination in terms of the reinforc-ing response that it elicits (Johnston, 1993). These proposed feedback mechanisms include positive reinforcement when a desired event such as pleasure or attention follows rumination and negative reinforcement when an undesired event such as anxiety is reduced or removed. A more sophisticated theory involves combining the concept of positive and negative reinforcement by proposing a change in the valence of the behavioral consequences. For example, consequences that are normally behavior suppressing may acquire behavior reinforcing characteristics if other, more usually positive, consequences are lacking (Winton and Singh, 1983). These concepts of the operant conditioning psychogenic factors in rumination are useful as the theoretical underpinnings of cer-tain behavioral treatments of rumination.

The role of organic factors in rumination remains obscure, but some authors have argued that rumination is totally the result of physical disorders including hiatal hernia and other esophageal abnormalities (Herbst et al., 1971). The relationship between the syndromes of rumina-tion and gastroesophageal reflux (GER) is unknown although high rates of association have been reported (Shepherd et al., 1987). GER, or chalasia, is the syndrome of regurgitation of the stomach contents into the mouth and esophagus, apparently as a result of hypomotility of the gastric fundus and delayed gastric emptying rather than a weakened esophageal sphincter (Papaila et al., 1989). A possible but untested hypothesis is that GER is the physiological substrate upon which various psychosocial disruptions or deviant operant conditioning act so that rumination develops.

Rumination appears to require three factors: an impaired ability of the infant or retarded person to regulate his or her internal state of satisfaction, a physical propensity to regurgitate food, and a learned association that regurgitation helps relieve the internal state of dissatisfaction. The assessment of the child must include an evaluation of each of these factors as well as the medical sequelae of rumination such as malnutrition and aspiration. Obviously, these medical sequelae will influence the vigor of the intervention as well as serving as a baseline by which to measure the child's response to treatment.

The assessment of the infant's capacity to regulate his or her internal state must include a general developmental assessment to evaluate for serious developmental delay as well as hyperirritability states. In addition, the mother-infant relationship must be carefully examined for clues to stimuli that are noxious or disruptive to the infant.

The child's propensity to regurgitate can be best evaluated by procedures developed for GER, including esophageal pH monitoring, scintigraphic gastroesophageal reflux scan, endoscopy, and gastric emptying studies. In addition, various radiological procedures that evaluate esophageal abnormalities should be considered.

The learned aspect of rumination, especially in retarded individuals, may be crucial. After careful evaluation of this factor, various behavioral interventions must be considered, especially if there are serious medical complications. These interventions include aversive techniques in which a noxious stimulus is paired with rumination (Glasscock et al., 1986) and nonaversive techniques such as differential reinforcement of other incompatible responses and holding.

FEEDING DISORDER OF INFANCY OR EARLY CHILDHOOD

DSM-IV addressed the complex and controversial issues associated with failure to thrive (FTT) syndrome by creating a new diagnostic category, feeding disorder in infancy or early childhood. DSM-IV defined this disorder as (a) a feeding disturbance as manifested by persistent failure to eat adequately with a significant failure to gain weight or significant loss of weight over at least 1 month; (b) not due to an associated gastrointestinal or other general medical condition (e.g., esophageal reflux); (c) not better accounted for by another mental disorder or lack of available food; and (d) onset before age 6. DSM-IV did not quantify ''significant'' failure to gain weight. In addition, DSM-IV ignored the proven lack of validity of the organic/nonorganic dichotomy implied by the criteria of the absence of a general medical condition (Bell and Woolston, 1985; Polan et al., 1991a, 1991b). Although creating a new diagnostic category has the advantage of freeing it from a long history of misconception and controversy, it has the disadvantage of losing a long, rich history of research. Since there are no publications or data about this new diagnostic category, its closet clinical entity, FTT syndrome, will be discussed.

FAILURE TO THRIVE

FTT is a disorder of infancy and early childhood characterized by a marked deceleration of weight gain and a slowing or disruption of acquisition of emotional and social developmental milestones. Deceleration of linear growth and head circumference growth are associated but not primary phenomena. FTT is a common disorder, occurring at a rate of 1–5% of pediatric hospital admissions (Berwick, 1980). Surveys of low income children in primary care suggest that nearly 10% show weight or length below the 5th percentile for age (Koumjian and Marks, 1985). This common condition is of great concern because FTT is associated with increased risk for lasting deficits in growth, cognition, and socioeconomic functioning (e.g. Oates et al., 1985).

Despite a 45-year history of study, the understanding of FTT has been marked by confusion and controversy about such basic issues as the definition and the name of the disorder. The plethora of syndromic names provides a glimpse into the confused literature: hospitalism, anaclitic depression, institutionalism, environmental retardation, maternal deprivation syndrome, psychosocial deprivation dwarfism, deprivational dwarfism, deprivation syndrome, failure to thrive, environmental failure to thrive, and nonorganic failure to thrive syndrome. This blizzard of interchangeably used but nonsynonomous terms, which frequently represented the mistaken or oversimplified underlying conceptions of the investigators, has created a major obstacle to the course of research. These misconceptions arose out of the multifaceted nature of the syndrome. At different times the three components of FTT, weight gain deceleration, linear growth delay and developmental delays, were separated apart so that each was perceived as the central aspect to the exclusion of other parts. In fact, depending upon the focus of the definition, FTT has been reported as consisting of only one component rather than a triad. For example, when the diagnosis of FTT is made on the basis of primary weight gain deceleration, developmental deficits are less evident (Field, 1986), and indeed, in one study using age-matched controls, there were no differences in development test scores between FTT and normally growing infants (Mitchell et al., 1980).

A second aspect of this confusion in the understanding of FTT has been the controversy between the contribution of emotional deprivation and that of malnutrition. From the earliest observers to present-day clinicians, the correlation between emotional misery and growth problems has been obvious. Perhaps too simplistically, some investigators argued that such disorders were directly caused by misery, mediated by some effect on the mind acting directly upon the body, without requiring such external factors as altered caloric intake.

The starkest presentation of the argument has been the theoretical debate of the importance of love versus food in the etiology of FTT (Widdowson, 1951). Early clinical experience indicated that some infants with FTT who were given a normal caloric intake did not gain weight at their expected rate. These observations were used to bolster the argument that calories alone were not sufficient for weight gain. However, studies of malnourished children have demonstrated that they have supracaloric requirements before catch-up growth is possible (Casey and Arnold, 1985). In addition, Whitten et al. (1969) reported that even grossly understimulated infants with FTT gained weight rapidly if given enough food.

The persistence of this debate about love versus food has several origins. First, FTT is a syndrome with physical (weight gain and growth deceleration) and behavioral/emotional (developmental delays) components. The overwhelming evidence indicates that inadequate caloric intake is the primary cause of growth deceleration while emotional and socioeconomic deprivation is the primary cause of the developmental delays (Casey et al., 1984). However, the depression-like symptoms associated with FTT probably reduce the infant's interest in feeding, rendering the infant harder to feed. Similarly, the significant malnutrition associated with FTT can produce a state of apathetic withdrawal. To further complicate matters, a small group of severely deprived and abused young children have a disruption of pituitary function even in the presence of adequate nutrition. Although these children represent a clearly defined and distinct diagnostic syndrome of psychosocial dwarfism (PSD) (Powell et al., 1967), their conditions are persistently confused with FTT.

FTT is a disorder with an onset in the first 3 years of life. Typically, infants who have the onset of FTT before the end of 1 year of life are more likely to have been actively deprived of food or to have primary physiological disorders that interfere with caloric intake. When the initial onset of FTT occurs in older infants and toddlers, there is more likely to be active interactional difficulties between the child and primary caregiver, which manifest as an eating disorder. Frequently, a young infant who presents with FTT will respond rapidly to adequate feeding. However, the same social/familial conditions that are associated with such acute malnutrition may also be associated with chronic emotional and physical deprivation and poor infant-caregiver relationships. Therefore, infants whose initial episode of FTT is rapidly ameliorated by refeeding may develop a second episode of FTT that is characterized by a more chronic and internalized eating disorder. These toddlers and young children resist ingestion of adequate caloric intake and show secondary stunting of linear growth and head circumference as a result of chronic malnutrition.

The developmental outcome of children with FTT is remarkably heterogenous, perhaps because of the heterogeneity of the syndrome. Significant variables that influence outcome include general factors such as socioeconomic status, maternal education, parental mental illness, and family social functioning. Since these factors are both risk factors for FTT and for poor developmental outcome, they probably mediate their influence somewhat independently of FTT per se. Risk factors that are more directly linked to FTT include degree and chronicity of malnutrition, degree and chronicity of developmental delay, severity and duration of the dysfunction in infant-caretaker relationship, and severity of major medical disorder. Problems associated with FTT such as physical abuse, medical neglect, educational neglect, and social isolation interact with the general and specific risk factors to influence developmental outcome.

As indicated in the introduction, FTT is a common disorder ranging from 1–3% of inpatient pediatric admissions to 10–15% of some outpatient populations. Few data exist on historical trends for shifting prevalence of FTT. Sex ratio is reported to be approximately equal, although studies of older infants indicate a slighter preponderance of boys.

Although FTT occurs in children of all social strata, it is more common in families where functioning is compromised by poverty, unemployment, social dislocation and isolation, and parental mental illness. As with any complex, multifactorial disorder, most infants develop relatively normally in conditions characterized by many of these risk factors while a minority develop an eating/growth disorder such as FTT. On the other hand, some infants develop FTT despite the apparent absence of any of these risk factors. Thus, social and family risk factors are just that: risk factors rather than specific etiological agents.

Virtually nothing is known about what, if any, genetic factors exist in various forms of FTT. Obviously, there are important genetic contributions to various mental disorders that can influence caretaker adequacy.

Since the etiology of FTT is a multifactorial process, virtually any temperament or psychological factor that interferes with somatic homeostasis and/or attunement between infant and caretaker may well disrupt feeding and cause inadequate caloric intake. In young infants, the two most common such difficulties are marked irritability and apathy. Both of these states are themselves the result of multiple underlying factors including basic psychophysiological temperament, nutritional state, physical health, and affective interaction with the primary caregiver. This last factor has been the focus of considerable research as the major etiological factor in the development of FTT. Investigators have postulated that any emotional and/or behavioral disturbance in the primary caretaker that causes her or him to be physically and/or emotionally absent will result in the state of apathetic depression in the infant. Alternatively, emotional disturbance in the caregiver that results in the infant's experiencing constant anger, rejection, irritability, or hatred will cause the infant to be irritable, difficult to soothe, and/or withdrawn.

Clinicians in the past have sometimes overemphasized the importance of the search for occult organic factors, as has been demonstrated by the low yield from exhaustive testing (Sills, 1978). A major impetus for this excessive use of laboratory testing has been the misconception of the organic/nonorganic dichotomy. To be sure, the number of primary medical illnesses that can be associated with FTT is extensive. However, a thorough pediatric history, physical examination, and minimal screening laboratory tests usually identify physical illnesses that are contributing to FTT. These screening tests include complete blood count, lead level and free erythrocyte protoporphyrin, tuberculosis skin test (PPD), urinalysis and urine culture, and a sweat test in populations predisposed to cystic fibrosis (Frank and Zeisel, 1988).

Some organic factors may be caused by the malnutrition associated with FTT as well as aggravating its course. Malnutrition suppresses immune functions so that children with FTT are at risk for chronic respiratory and gastrointestinal infections. The illnesses that these infections produce interfere with the infant's ability to ingest adequate calories, which exacerbates the infant's state of malnutrition. Similarly, infants with FTT are at risk for vitamin and mineral deficiencies, especially of calcium, iron, and zinc. These deficiencies result in blood dyscrasias and metabolic disturbances, which worsen the infant's clinical state. In addition, the mineral deficiencies and malnutrition increase the risk of lead toxicity since lead absorption is significantly increased in these deficiency states. Perhaps most important in evaluation of organic factors is the concept that illnesses that coexist with FTT belong in a continuum, from those that actually cause malnutrition (e.g., malabsorption) at one end to those that are caused by malnutrition (e.g., immunosuppression) (Woolston, 1985) at the other.

The crucial axes on which to evaluate an infant with FTT include age of onset and duration of FTT, degree of malnutrition, degree of linear growth and head circumference stunting, presence of other physical illness, developmental delay, and level of family functioning.

Age of onset is important both in understanding the genesis of the FTT as well as in its prognosis. FTT with onset in the first 12 months of life in the absence of any concurrent medical illness is almost always a feeding disturbance resulting from either the infant's being deprived of adequate caloric intake or being so fussy and irritable that feeding is nearly impossible. In the former situation, the infant will rapidly gain weight when offered enough food. Thus, if the factors that contributed to the inadequate caloric intake can be ameliorated, infants with this pattern of FTT have an excellent prognosis. Similarly, most infants who have severe problems with establishment of basic physiological homeostasis will develop more effective state regulation by the 2nd and 3rd year of life. However, the presence of other risk factors on the multiaxial approach to FTT put such infants at high risk for poor developmental outcome.

Calculation of degree of malnutrition is crucial in all aspects of the clinical management of FTT including diagnosis, prognosis, and treatment. Frequently the severity of the malnutrition is associated with the severity of the other risk factors that are influencing the FTT. The degree of malnutrition affects the severity of medical complications associated with FTT, ranging from acute immunosuppression to permanent interference with brain growth. Calculation of degree of malnutrition is essential for the correct nutritional treatment required for compensatory catch-up growth.

The degree of height and head circumference growth stunting provides important data about the chronicity and severity of malnutrition (McLaren and Reed, 1972). Generally such stunting is associated with a poorer growth prognosis, because such growth arrest is both difficult to overcome as well as is strongly associated with long-standing psychosocial deprivation. Stunting of head circumference growth is especially ominous because it reflects structural alterations in brain size. If nutritional interventions are delayed or inadequate, deficits in head circumference may be lifelong, even if weight and length deficits may be largely restored.

An important caveat in the calculation of growth stunting is the consideration of intrauterine growth retardation (IUGR) and prematurity. IUGR is defined as both weight and height less than the 10th percentile for gestational age (Frank and Zeisel, 1981). The growth prognosis for children with a history of IUGR varies with the nature of the prenatal insult. Infants with IUGR who are underweight as compared with their length or head circumference have the best prognosis for later growth.

Presumably such infants have been poorly nourished during the end of gestation and can regain adequate weight for height by appropriate caloric intake. In contrast, infants with IUGR whose weight and length are equally delayed frequently remain small despite intervention. These infants have often suffered a variety of systemic intrauterine pathological events, including exposure to teratogens, infections, and chromosomal abnormalities (Frank and Zeisel, 1988).

Infants who were born prematurely may appear to be growth delayed simply because they are being evaluated by chronological age of birth rather than by gestational age. The age used to evaluate height and weight should be calculated by subtracting the number of weeks since birth (Frank and Zeisel, 1988). Such corrections should be made for head circumference until 18 months after birth, for weight until 24 months, and for height until 40 months. Obviously children with IUGR and prematurity may develop FTT in addition to their preexisting conditions. In fact, since both conditions are commonly associated with such risk factors for FTT as maternal substance and alcohol abuse, family dysfunction, and maternal mental illness or poor competence, infants with prematurity or IUGR are at higher risk for developing FTT than are full term, normally developed neonates. Thus, while the diagnosis of either of these conditions by no means precludes the diagnosis of FTT, prematurity and IUGR must be taken into account when assessing the infant's degree of growth delay.

The presence of other medical disorders associated with FTT is a complex phenomenon that covers the continuum from illnesses like malabsorption, which directly cause malnutrition, to recurring infections secondary to malnutrition-induced immunosuppression (Frank and Zeisel, 1988). At one time, researchers and clinicians alike attempted rigidly to dichotomize children who were "only" malnourished (so-called nonorganic failure to thrive) and children who had a presumably etiological medical illness (organic failure to thrive). This rigid dichotomy served to obscure both evaluation and treatment (Frank and Zeisel, 1988). Rather than focusing only on a disorder that causes the malnutrition, the clinician must evaluate a child with FTT as being at high risk for chronic infectious illnesses, elevated blood levels of heavy metals, and mineral deficiencies.

As with the other factors in the multiaxial approach to diagnosis and assessment of FTT, developmental delay is an important, multiply determined, and transactional risk factor. Both malnutrition and emotional deprivation are independently associated with developmental delay (Frank and Zeisel, 1988). Obviously, when they are combined, they are potent risk factors. In addition, developmental delays themselves may contribute to the infant's feeding problems.

Level of family functioning is a crucial variable in assessment and treatment of FTT. The clinician must come to understand which of a myriad of family dysfunctions is contributing to the infant's failure to ingest adequate caloric intake. Earlier researchers had wondered about a specific type of family and especially maternal problem. No such specific dysfunctions have been found for children with FTT as a group. However, many reports have described specific family-related problems that appear to be directly related to specific infants with FTT. Thus, the absence of a prototypical family dysfunction that is related to most cases of FTT should not discourage the clinician from the search for sources of family problems for a specific child with FTT. Such an exploration is crucial because the ongoing nutritional supplementation and emotional stimulation must be done in the context of the child's family. Frequently the family problems that contributed to the infant's FTT will serve as roadblocks to effective treatment.

PSYCHOSOCIAL DWARFISM

PSD, also called a variety of other terms, including deprivational dwarfism, is a syndrome of deceleration of linear growth combined with characteristic behavior disturbances (sleep disorder and bizarre eating habits), both of which are reversible by a change in the psychosocial environment (Green et al., 1984; Powell et al., 1967). The deceleration of linear growth is remarkable in that it occurs in the absence of weight gain deceleration. In this way, PSD is quite distinct from growth stunting secondary to malnutrition (FTT), but rather resembles primary hypopituitarism (Blizzard, 1973; Powell et al., 1967). The most common, characteristic abnormal eating behaviors include polyphagia, gorging, vomiting, stealing and hoarding food, and eating from garbage pails and animal food dishes. Other behaviors reported include polydipsia including drinking stagnant water, toilet bowl water, and dishwater. Various sleep disorders have been described such as initial onset insomnia and night wandering. These sleep disturbances may be related to growth delay since they interfere with the major nocturnal pulsatile release of growth hormone. Children with PSD may exhibit a variety of unusual patterns of relatedness and problems with behavior including aggressiveness and impulsivity. Both specific language delays and delays in general intellectual development have been reported (Drash et al., 1986).

PSD apparently is a rare disorder so that virtually all of the available literature consists of case reports or small case series. Incidence, prevalence, sex ratio, and sociodemographic features are unknown. The age of onset is unclear but reportedly occurs between 18 and 48 months. Blizzard (1973) argued that the onset must occur after 24 months in order to reliably distinguish it from FTT.

Developmental outcome appears to be highly variable, although limited outcome data are available. Outcome appears to be highly contingent upon the adequacy of the child's psychosocial environment. Hospitalization or removal to a less noxious home environment is presumed to be ameliorative since it is associated with reversal of some of the neuroendocrine, growth, and behavioral concomitants of the disorder (Powell et al., 1967). If the child is returned to the noxious home environment, the various gains that have been achieved may be arrested or reversed. Behavioral disturbance, developmental delays, and short stature are possible long-term sequelae. In addition, delayed puberty may occur (Howse et al., 1977).

The literature is virtually unanimous in describing parental psychopathology that results in maltreatment of the child (e.g., Powell et al., 1967) including overt abuse and/or neglect (Drash et al., 1968). Several reports have indicated that both the parental psychopathology and maltreatment of the child may be obscured in initial interviews. The parents have been reported to withhold clinical information and be uncooperative with treatment. The frequent association of parental psychopathology and the reversal of the associated features with change in environment appear to be quite convincing. However, since no studies have been reported that control for such basic variables as socioeconomic class, the validity of these findings should be viewed as preliminary.

Much of the research on PSD has focused on neuroendocrine abnormalities found in the syndrome in an attempt to unravel the relationship between growth rate and neuroendocrine changes. Unfortunately, these investigations have led to the discovery of no pathognomonic or consistently abnormal findings, with the possible exception of depressed somatomedin levels (Green et al., 1984). The abnormalities in hormonal levels and hypothalamic functioning have been found to normalize partially or completely following the subjects's removal from the inimical environment. This normalization may occur in several weeks or require as long as 2 years, depending on the specific endocrine disturbance and the type of specific medical, hormonal, or psychiatric treatment (Green et al., 1984). In addition to this great variability in the normalization of endocrine abnormalities, none of the abnormal hormonal findings correlate specifically with growth failure. Growth failure has occurred with normal endocrine values, and catch-up growth has occurred with subnormal values (Green et al., 1984). The mechanisms causing the growth failure in PSD are thus, as yet, unknown.

The explanation for the rarity of PSD, even among children exposed to severe maltreatment, is a mystery. Possible factors may include genetic vulnerability to a disruption in the rate or rhythm of growth hormone production or some specific type of psychosocial deprivation that causes such neuroendocrine dysfunction. However, the unraveling of these mysteries awaits better designed studies that have larger sample sizes and matched controls.

The treatment and evaluation of PSD must include the three cardinal factors associated with the disorder: a reversible neuroendocrine and growth dysfunction, behavioral disturbances and developmental delays, and presumably a noxious psychosocial environment. The evaluation of the neuroendocrine and growth dysfunction is important in the differential diagnosis of other disorders that are associated with short stature as well as in monitoring the response to treatment. These other disorders involving short stature include primordial dwarfism, IUGR with persistent small size, hypopituitarism from a variety of etiologies, constitutional delayed growth, Turner's syndrome (XO chromosomal pattern), osteochondrodystrophies, and growth stunting secondary to chronic malnutrition with or without chronic disease. PSD is virtually unique in being reversible with a change in living situations and in the absence of any signs of physical illness except growth delay.

The behavioral disturbances and developmental delays found in PSD serve as important factors to help monitor response to treatment as well as to represent serious aspects of the disorder that must be addressed. A careful psychiatric evaluation of the child is required that assesses for the presence of bizarre and disruptive behaviors as well as for problems in normal social relatedness. A developmental assessment must evaluate for both specific delays, especially in language, and general developmental delays. In older children, psychoeducational testing is helpful to assess specific intellectual, academic, and adaptive functioning. Psychotherapeutic and educational interventions should be guided by these findings.

The evaluation and intervention to ameliorate the psychosocial adversity is both the most important as well as most difficult task. According to all reports, caretakers of a child with PSD may be actively uncooperative in the assessment and treatment phases. Ideally, the caretakers can be engaged in the appropriate individual and family psychotherapies. In addition, they can use various social supports such as home aides and support groups. In the event of active treatment refusal, which may result in permanent damage to the child, the treaters must consider removal of the child from the home.

CHILDHOOD OBESITY

Considerable attention in the literature has been focused on the eating disorders of early childhood that result in growth failure, such as FTT, PSD, and rumination. In contrast, the eating disorders that result in excessive weight gain have been virtually ignored. DSM-IV has reinforced this prejudice by refusing to classify any form of obesity as an eating disorder (American Psychiatric Association, 1993). Instead, it relegates obesity to Axis III as a physical disorder. In conjunction with this lack of interest in obesity in the psychiatric literature, there are many widely held misconceptions about its etiology, course, and even heterogeneity of subtypes. This state of clinical indifference about the fundamentals of obesity in general, and childhood obesity in particular, makes a scientific strategy for intervention difficult.

The first step in the elucidation of any new field of study is an operational definition that is phenomenologically reliable and valid. In the study of obesity, there needs to be an easy, accurate, reliable method of defining the clinical condition. Since obesity denotes being excessively fat, the operational definition must differentiate the condition of having excessive adipose tissue for chronological age from simply being heavy for chronological age as a result of large muscle mass or skeletal frame. Triceps skin-fold thickness (Garn and Clark, 1976) and an obesity index using weight gain, suprailiac skin fold, and waist circumference (Crawford et al., 1974) are two well-standardized measurements that appear to satisfy the requirements for a useful, operational definition of obesity. A simpler, if slightly less valid, measure of obesity is defined by exceeding 120% of ideal body weight (IBW) for height for a given age and sex. Specifically, IBW is calculated by dividing actual weight by the expected weight for a given age and sex and height percentile.

The study of the natural history of obesity in infancy and childhood is in its beginning stages. Data about the typical course of this disorder

are contradictory. The most widely held belief is that obesity of early onset is a chronic and steadily progressive disorder with very few remissions (Charney et al., 1976; Eid, 1970). However, more recent workers (Poskitt, 1980; Shapiro et al., 1984) have reported that obesity in infancy is a poorer predictor of later childhood obesity than was believed previously.

This rather poor correlation between obesity in infancy and obesity in later childhood calls into question the notion of relentlessly progressive obesity that is triggered by fat cell proliferation in infancy. Rather than there being a critical phase in infancy for fat cell proliferation, it is more likely that the degree and duration of obesity are the major determinants of total adipose cell number in humans.

The incidence and prevalence of obesity in childhood is not nearly as well studied as obesity in adulthood. The few studies indicate that the prevalence rate of obesity is 5–10% of preschool-age children (Maloney and Klykylo, 1980). Occasionally, "epidemics" of infantile obesity have been reported with prevalence rates of 16.7% of infants under 12 months of age (Shukla et al., 1972). These epidemics appear to be caused by culturally determined misinformation or fads about infant feeding practices (Shukla et al., 1972).

Obesity in females is nine times more common in working class families than in middle and upper social class families (Stunkard et al., 1972). The prevalence of obesity is linked to the socioeconomic status of the parents almost as strongly as it is to the subject's own social class (Goldblatt et al., 1965). This finding argues that socioeconomic status is linked to obesity in a causal rather than a simple associative manner, perhaps mediated through culturally determined eating habits and dietary misconceptions.

A family-line analysis of obesity indicates that there is a strong correlation between the fatness of parents and their children. For example, by age 17, the children of obese parents have three times the chance of being obese as the children of lean parents. If one sibling is fat, there is a 40% chance that a second sibling will be fat (Garn and Clark, 1976). If two siblings are fat, there is an 80% chance that the third sibling will be fat. While these data seem to support a genetic basis for obesity, one must keep other nongenetic, but family-related, factors in mind. The same study that reported the sibling data indicates that, if one spouse is fat, there is a 30% chance that the other spouse also will be fat (Garn and Clark, 1976). Obviously this finding cannot be explained by genetic factors. However, well-designed genetic studies involving monozygotic/dizygotic concordance (Stunkard et al., 1986a) and adoption samples (Stunkard et al., 1986b) support a strong genetic contribution to all forms of body habitus ranging from fatness to thinness.

Studies of overt psychopathology in obese adults have been as contradictory as studies of other aspects of obesity. Silverstone (1969) attempted to reconcile these discrepant reports by differentiating between late-onset adult obesity secondary to a gradual accumulation of fat and early-onset adult obesity characterized by a sudden increase in fatness that was the result of anxiety-driven overeating. Indeed, psychogenic obesity of infancy and early childhood has been reported to occur only in the context of a disorganized family in which the child's needs are poorly perceived and even more poorly differentiated (Kahn, 1973; Woolston, 1987; Woolston and Forsyth, 1989).

In the differential diagnosis of infantile or childhood-onset obesity, clinicians frequently search for the discovery of discrete genetic, endocrinological, or neurological syndromes associated with obesity, including Prader-Willi, Klinefelter's, Fröhlich's, Laurence-Moon-Biedl, Kleine-Levin, and Mauriac's syndromes.

Although these syndromes associated with obesity are frequently searched for as an etiology for obesity in childhood, they are quite rare. In addition, a clinical rule of thumb distinguishes between obesity associated with a developmental syndrome and that associated with otherwise normal development. Children with a developmental syndrome are usually below the 25th percentile in height and have delayed bone age, whereas children with normal development are above the 50th percentile in height and have an advanced bone age.

One of the most obvious explanations for the contradictory results of various studies in regard to developmental course and etiology is that obesity in childhood is a heterogeneous syndrome. Many authors (e.g., Maloney and Klykylo, 1983; Stunkard, 1980) have identified multiple factors that contribute to the development of obesity, including emotional, socioeconomic, genetic, developmental, and neurological.

Although preliminary attempts have been made to subdivide forms of juvenile-onset obesity into phenomenologically homogeneous groupings (Woolston, 1988; Woolston and Forsyth, 1989), such attempts are probably premature. Many of the same issues related to diagnostic classification of FTT apply to obesity. Fundamentally all forms of obesity have the same organic basis: caloric intake that exceeds caloric expenditure. Like FTT, there are a multitude of primary medical illnesses that are associated with obesity. However, since it is the excess caloric intake that actually mediates the obesity, there are frequently psychosocial/emotional factors that complicate all forms of obesity including those associated with developmental syndromes. The database of obesity of early childhood is too small to permit construction of clinically useful categorization. Instead, like FTT, a multiaxial list of major risk factors is more helpful. These should include age of onset and duration, degree of obesity, family history of obesity, presence of a medical illness or syndrome associated with obesity, and type of family functioning.

In a similar fashion to FTT, obesity that is associated with an acute onset in the first 12 months has an excellent prognosis since the treatment is simply a matter of reducing the infant's caloric intake to the recommended level for height and age. However, this benign condition can become much more problematic if there are other risk factors such as severe family dysfunction, a strong family history for obesity, or a medical syndrome associated with obesity. The longer the obesity persists beyond infancy and the later is its onset in childhood, the more persistent it is likely to be.

The degree of obesity, expressed either as a percentile of ideal body weight for height and age or as a Z score, predicts prognosis in that the degree of obesity may reflect the seriousness of the underlying risk factors. More importantly, the degree of obesity helps guide the clinician regarding the likelihood of serious medical sequelae of obesity such as slipped femoral head epiphysis, sleep apnea, Pickwickian syndrome, hypercholesterolemia, and diabetes mellitus. In addition, the degree of obesity must guide the nutritional intervention. Caloric restriction below the recommended amounts for height, age, and sex is rarely indicated. Instead, the primary goal is to arrest continued weight gain until the child's height and weight are proportional.

Family history of obesity is important for both genetic and family-cultural reasons. Regardless of the mode of action, obesity that is related to the influence of family history alone has a slow, gradual onset in middle childhood and is frequently persistent into adulthood. Preliminary data indicate that children with a positive family history for being overweight as their only risk factor may have a relatively good response to brief, family-based behavioral intervention. Using a prospective, randomized controlled experimental design, Epstein et al. (1990) reported that an 8-week behavioral intervention program for both the obese child and his or her parents significantly reduced the obesity in the child at the end of the 10-year follow-up. Unfortunately, this study has not been replicated in the absence of other risk factors. Children with this pattern of obesity rarely become morbidly obese, and so, rarely develop the major medical complications of severe obesity. As indicated earlier, children with obesity as part of a primary developmental syndrome are usually below the 25th percentile in height and are frequently cognitively impaired.

Level of family functioning may be crucial in both the genesis of obesity as well as its treatment. Severely dysfunctional families provide the child with an environment of emotional neglect, a sense of abandonment, and no limit setting around the use of food. A small number of children who grow up in such environments develop a pattern of enormous caloric intake and a rapid onset of severe obesity, usually beginning between age 3 and 5 years. These children are at high risk for poor developmental outcome because the constellation of risk factors conspire to produce a powerfully negative synergistic spiral. These children usually have low self-esteem, which is exacerbated by their obesity. They are like to suffer the most serious medical complication of obesity. Most importantly, they are at high risk because the only effective intervention for treatment of obesity is mediated through the family system. This intervention includes the orchestration of appropriate medical and mental health services, effective limit setting, and the development of more positive self-esteem and emotional security. Unfortunately, the very risk factor that contributed so heavily to the genesis of the disorder, family dysfunction, makes intervention difficult (Woolston and Forsyth, 1989).

Obesity in infancy and childhood is a heterogeneous syndrome that has been relatively neglected in the eating disorder literature. The development of obesity is influenced by the interplay of social, familial, emotional, and physical factors. Analogous to FTT, obesity has been subtyped according to the presence or absence of physical disorders that are associated with obesity. Much less attention has been given to the different roles of genetics, cultural eating habits, and psychogenic factors.

BENIGN NUTRITIONAL DWARFING

Benign nutritional dwarfing (BND) is a disorder of school-age children and young adolescents in which maladaptive eating patterns unaccompanied by psychiatric or medical disorders result in a marked slowing of weight gain for at least 1 year followed by a deceleration of linear growth. Delayed puberty may be associated with this disorder. Because the subnormal weight gain in such children is accompanied by a proportionate decline in growth velocity, body weight for height deficits are frequently not evident. Therefore, children with BND do not present with emaciation, as is commonly observed in cases of severe malnutrition. Although dwarfing secondary to chronic malnutrition in childhood is as old as humankind, BND is a relatively newly described disorder (Apley et al., 1971; Davis et al., 1978; Lifshitz et al., 1987; Pugliese et al., 1983; Sanberg et al., 1991). While various authors report various different motivations for the inadequate caloric intake, all reports have been consistent in describing an absence of weight loss (as opposed to a slowing of weight gain) and an absence of body image distortion. A recent, well-controlled study found virtually no differences in various measures of psychological functioning between children with BND and matched constitutionally growth delayed or familial short stature children (Sanberg et al., 1991).

Typically the age of onset of BND is middle childhood to early adolescence (8–14 years) although some authors have included children as young as 2 years (Davis et al., 1978) and as old as 15 (Lifshitz et al., 1971). Although the consequences of chronic insufficient caloric intake can include delayed puberty and permanent short stature, children with BND frequently respond to relatively straightforward nutritional counseling by a sufficient enough increase in caloric intake to reinitiate normal growth. There are no reports of associated development or psychiatric disorders either during the course of BND or as its sequelae.

Because of the relatively recent reporting of BND, satisfactory data on its incidence and prevalence do not exist. In most reports of BND, there is a slight predominance of boys to girls.

BND is characterized by the absence of social or familial dysfunction that typify other eating and growth disorders. There are no reports that indicate any particular parental psychopathology or genetic factors. Some reports have described special nutritional concerns (Pugliese et al., 1983) and chronic nonspecific feeding disturbances (Davis et al., 1978).

The only psychogenic factors reported to be related to BND are inaccurate nutritional beliefs about weight gain or special dietary needs.

As indicated earlier, inadequate caloric intake to maintain normal weight gain is the only known organic factor. Various mineral and vitamin deficiencies may complicate the inadequate caloric intake (Lifshitz et al., 1971).

BND is characterized by chronic inadequate caloric intake as a result of mistaken nutritional beliefs. While a variety of medical and psychiatric disorders may result in chronic malnutrition, children with BND have a normal physical and psychiatric examination except for a history of weight velocity deceleration, followed by growth velocity deceleration. A careful history of growth and of dietary beliefs and eating habits is crucial to establish the diagnosis and guide the intervention. The treatment of BND should focus on nutritional counseling of the child and parents. Follow-up visits should be scheduled to ascertain weight gain.

PREPUBERTAL ANOREXIA NERVOSA

Prepubertal anorexia nervosa has all of the essential features of typical adolescent-onset anorexia, including intense fear of becoming fat, disturbance of body image, significant and defined weight loss, and a refusal to maintain a minimum normal body weight. The only modifications of the standard diagnostic criteria are those required by the physical characteristics of prepubertal children. Obviously, since these children are prepubertal, amenorrhea is not a meaningful criteria. In addition, since prepubertal children have a smaller percentage of body fat than adolescents, a smaller percentage of weight loss will have a greater physiological impact. This relatively greater deleterious effect of weight loss is sometimes compounded by the fact that prepubertal children are more concrete in their thinking, so that they more frequently generalize their pathological eating to include their fluid intake (Irwin, 1984).

Although prepubertal anorexia nervosa was reported in the same year (Collins, 1894) that adolescent-onset anorexia nervosa was first described, substantial case reports did not occur until nearly 70 years later. Indeed, full recognition of the special characteristics of prepubertal anorexia nervosa awaited reports in the 1980s to establish this as a relatively rare but bona fide form of anorexia nervosa (Growers et al., 1991; Irwin, 1984; Jacobs and Isaacs, 1986; Lask and Bryant-Waugh, 1992; Russell, 1985).

Because relatively few cases of prepubertal anorexia nervosa have been reported, conclusions about any aspect of natural history remain tentative. However, existing reports support the notion that prepubertal anorexia carries all of the possible negative sequelae of adolescent anorexia nervosa. In addition, the experience of an episode of acute malnutrition severe enough to cause significant weight loss in a prepubertal child will likely have a deleterious effect on growth (Russell, 1985).

Although anorexia nervosa is a relatively rare disorder, prepubertal anorexia is considerably rarer. The sex ratio and sociodemographics appear to be similar to the more typical anorexia nervosa. Current published reports indicate that the same types of social and family factors are implicated in the genesis of prepubertal anorexia nervosa as with more typical anorexia nervosa. These factors include middle or upper middle class and an enmeshed, intrusive family communication style. Like social and family factors, genetic factors may play an important role in anorexia nervosa regardless of the age of onset (Garfinkel and Garner, 1982; Morgan and Russell, 1975).

Although numerous theories exist about various psychogenic factors related to anorexia nervosa, all remain relatively speculative. Children with prepubertal onset anorexia express fewer concerns about sexual maturity (Jacobs and Isaacs, 1986) than those with older age onset anorexia. In addition, prepubertal children with anorexia nervosa have less cognitive ability to understand various concepts of nutritional counseling. Some of the emotional and social goals in the treatment of adolescent anorexia related to differentiation from the family may be inappropriate for a prepubertal child.

As with other forms of anorexia nervosa, there are no known organic factors related to etiology. Acute malnutrition has a variety of important consequences for neuroendocrine functioning and growth.

Prepubertal anorexia nervosa is a primary psychiatric eating disorder with well-described physical, genetic, psychological, behavioral, and family characteristics. The prepubertal age of onset in this typically adolescent and adult disorder is the main stumbling block to accurate diagnosis and treatment. Generally, clinicians who typically treat anorexia nervosa have little knowledge about the special cognitive, emotional, or physical needs of prepubertal children. Analogously, clinicians who treat prepubertal children have little experience in the diagnosis or treatment of anorexia nervosa. Once these obstacles have been overcome, the diagnosis and treatment is at once as straightforward and as difficult as in more typical anorexia.

CASE ILLUSTRATION: CHRONIC FAILURE TO THRIVE WITH SECONDARY DWARFING

George M. was a 5-year, 8-month-old child who was admitted to a children's psychiatric inpatient service because of his protective service case worker's "concern about his not picking up weight" and because of evidence of depression as indicated by statements such as "I want to be nothing. If I don't eat, I will be nothing."

George had been diagnosed as suffering from FTT at age 3 years, 2 months when he was admitted to a pediatric unit of a community hospital for evaluation of his poor weight gain and linear growth. The workup for an organic etiology of his FTT was negative except that he was noted to consume inadequate calories. His mother was charged with medical neglect and he was committed to the state, which placed him in a series of foster homes with continued visitation with his mother. Finally, at age 4 years, he was placed in a permanent foster home, which allowed ongoing visitation with his mother. His growth failure continued so that he was evaluated on an outpatient basis at a children's hospital. Again the pediatric workup was negative for an organic etiology except for his inadequate caloric intake. The evaluators were concerned by the unresponsive and apathetic styles of interaction with his biological mother and recommended termination of parental rights. However, George's biological mother appeared to improve her parenting style after she was informed of the intention to terminate her parental rights. Because of his apparent improvement, the protective service agency dropped the termination petition.

In the several months prior to admission, the protective service agency had attempted to reunite George with both his biological mother and father. However, this proved difficult especially because George's parents had separated as a result of his father's alcohol abuse and violent temper. George was observed to have a picky and poor appetite in general but especially during and after visits with his parents. At these times, he ate very little and vomited what he did eat.

On admission, George presented as a small, thin 5-year, 8-month-old boy with a flat affect and a depressed mood. He engaged easily with the interviewer and occasionally his affect brightened somewhat. He was unable to describe any wishes because he felt wishes were pointless since they would never come true. He had a realistic assessment of his body image stating he was too skinny and needed to gain weight. George was quite articulate about his concerns about his future placement since he knew that his mother and his foster parents were vying for his custody.

George's developmental history was characterized by a full-term gestation, normal vaginal delivery, and normal early developmental milestones. By age 4 years, he was noted to have mild delays in language and in fine, gross, and visual motor skills.

His admission physical examination was remarkable only for his small stature with a weight of 13.7 kg and height of 102.9 cm. These measurements represent a height age of 3 years, 2 months, a weight age of 2 years, 8 months and a percentage of ideal body weight of 85%. His admission laboratory evaluations including CBC, sedimentation rate, electrolytes, thyroid functions, urinalysis, somatomedin-C, head CT, and bone age were all within normal limits.

During the course of his 3-month hospitalization, George went through three phases in his process of developing greater trust and reliance in close attachments: first was avoidance and rejection of caregivers, second was testing the stability of these relationships, and the third was his realization that he was indeed cared for. Despite ongoing visitation by George's biological mother, she continued her highly ambivalent and highly volatile relationship with George. Although she was sometimes warm and affectionate, at other times she was harsh and overtly rejecting. She persistently maintained that, ``George needed to learn that you can't always be the center of attention.'' She interpreted his slow and picky eating as a personal attack on her parenting skills. Her overall personality structure was so fragile that the stress of a difficult visit with George and her taxi not arriving led her to develop a transient episode of a gross thought process disorder.

The treatment team and protective service agency decided that George could not return to live with his mother. Before discharge, a legal risk adoptive mother was identified and introduced to George. By the time of discharge, he had gained only 1 kg but had progressed considerably in his self-esteem and ability to verbalize his feelings. For the next 1½ years, George continued to improve emotionally and developmentally but remained a picky eater. However, within several months of termination of his mother's parental rights and finalization of his adoption, he began to eat with gusto. His rate of weight gain increased so that he moved from below the 5th percentile to above the 25th. Several months later, his linear growth followed suit.

References

American Psychiatric Association: *Diagnostic and Statistical Manual of Mental Disorders* (3rd ed, rev). Washington, DC, American Psychiatric Association, 1987.

American Psychiatric Association: *Diagnostic and Statistical Manual* (4th ed). Washington, DC, American Psychiatric Association, 1994.

Apley J, Davies J, Davis DR, et al: Dwarfism without apparent physical cause. *Proc R Soc Med* 64:135–138, 1971.

Bell LS, Woolston JL: The relationship of weight gain and caloric intake in infants with organic and non-organic failure to thrive syndrome. *J Am Acad Child Psychiatry* 24:447–452, 1985.

Berwick DM: Nonorganic failure to thrive. *Pediatr Rev* 1:265–270, 1980.

Berwick DM, Levy JC, Kleinerman R: Failure to thrive: Diagnostic yield of hospitalization. *Arch Dis Child* 57:347–351, 1982.

Blizzard RM: Discussion: Plasma somatomedin activity in children with growth disturbances. In: Raiti S (ed): *Advances in Human Growth Hormone Research.* Washington, DC, Department of Health Education and Welfare Publication, NIH, No. 74-612, 1973, pp. 124–125.

Casey PH, Arnold WC: Compensatory growth in infants with severe failure to thrive. *South Med J* 78:1057–1060, 1985.

Casey PH, Bradley R, Worthham B: Social and nonsocial home environment of infants with organic failure to thrive. *Pediatrics* 73:348–353, 1984.

Charney E, Chamblee H, McBride M, et al: The childhood antecedents of adult obesity: Do chubby infants become obese adults? *N Engl J Med* 295:6–9, 1976.

Collins WJ: Anorexia nervosa. *Lancet* 1:202–203, 1894.

Crawford PB, Keller CA, Hampton MC, et al: An obesity index for six month old children. *Am J Clin Nutr* 27:706–711, 1974.

Danforth DE, Huber AM: Pica among mentally retarded adults. *Am J Ment Defic* 87:141–146, 1982.

Davis R, Apley J, Fill G, Grimaldi C: Diet and retarded growth. *Br Med J* 1:539–542, 1978.

Drash PW, Greenberg NE, Mooney J: Intelligence and personality in four syndromes of dwarfism. In: Cheek DB (ed): *Human Growth: Body Composition, Cell Growth, Energy and Intelligence.* Philadelphia, Lea & Febiger, 1986.

Egan J, Chatoor I, Rosen G: Nonorganic failure to thrive: Pathogenesis and classification. *Clin Proc Child Hosp Natl Med Cent* 34:173–182, 1980.

Eid EE: Follow-up study of physical growth of children who had excessive weight gain in the first six months of life. *Br Med J* 2:72–76, 1970.

Epstein LH, Valoski A, Wing RR, et al: Ten-year follow-up of behavioral, family-based treatment for obese children. *JAMA* 264:2519–2523, 1990.

Ferholt J, Provence S: Diagnosis and treatment of an infant with psychophysiological vomiting. *Psychoanal Study Child* 31:439–461, 1976.

Field T: Follow-up developmental status of infant hospitalized for nonorganic failure to thrive. *J Pediatr Psychol* 9:241–256, 1984.

Fischoff J, Whitten CF, Pettit MD: A psychiatric study of mothers of infants with growth failure secondary to maternal deprivation. *J Pediatr* 79:209–215, 1971.

Frank DA, Zeisel SA: Failure to thrive. *Pediatr Clin North Am* 35:1187–1206, 1988.

Garfinkel PE, Garner DM: *Anorexia Nervosa: A Multidimensional Perspective.* New York, Brunner/Mazel, 1982.

Garn SM, Clark DC, Ad Hoc Committee to Review the Ten-State Nutrition Survey: Trends in fatness and the origins of obesity. *Pediatrics* 57:443–456, 1976.

Glasscock SG, Friman PC, O'Brien S, et al: Varied citrus treatment of ruminant gagging in a teenager with Batten's disease. *J Behav Ther Exp Psychiatry* 17:129–133, 1986.

Goldblatt PB, Moore ME, Stunkard AJ: Social factors in obesity. *JAMA* 192:1039–1044, 1965.

Green WH, Campbell M, David R: Psychosocial dwarfism: A critical review of the evidence. *J Am Acad Child Psychiatry* 23:39–48, 1984.

Growers SG, Crisp AH, Jourghin N, et al: Premenarchal anorexia nervosa. *J Child Psychol Psychiatry* 32:515–524, 1991.

Halstead JA: Geophagia in man: Its nature and nutritional effects. *Am J Chem Nutr* 21:1384–1393, 1968.

Herbst J, Friedland GW, Zboralske FF: Hiatal hernia and rumination in infants and children. *J Pediatr* 78:261–265, 1971.

Hollowell JG, Gardner LI: Rumination and growth failure in male fraternal twin: Association with disturbed family environment. *Pediatrics* 36:565–571, 1965.

Howse PM, Rayner, PH, Williams JW, et al: Secretion of growth hormone in normal children of short stature and in children with hypopituitarism and intrauterine growth retardation. *Clin Endocrinol* 6:347–359, 1977.

Irwin M: Early onset anorexia nervosa. *South Med J* 77:611–614, 1984.

Jacobs BW, Isaacs S: Prepubertal anorexia nervosa: A retrospective controlled study. *J Child Psychol Psychiatry* 27:237–250, 1986.

Johnston JM: Phenomenology and treatment of rumination. In: Woolston JL (ed): *Child and Adolescent Psychiatric Clinics of America, Vol 2: Eating and Growth Disorders.* Philadelphia, Saunders, 1993, pp. 93–107.

Kahn EJ: Obesity in children. In: Kiell N (ed): *The Psychology of Obesity: Dynamics and Treatment.* Springfield, IL, Charles C Thomas, 1973.

Koumjian LL, Marks R: *Catching up! Annual Report for Failure to Thrive Program in Massachusetts, 1985.* Boston, Massachusetts Department of Public Health, Division of Family Health Services, Statistics and Evaluation Unit, 1985.

Lacey EP: Broadening the perspective of pica: Literature review. *Public Health Rep* 105:29–35, 1990.

Lacey EP: Phenomenology of pica. In: Woolston JL (ed): *Child and Adolescent Psychiatric Clinics of North America. Vol 2: Eating and Growth Disorders.* Philadelphia, Saunders, 1993, pp. 75–91.

Lask B, Bryant-Waugh R: Early-onset anorexia nervosa and related eating disorders. *J Child Psychol Psychiatry* 33:281–300, 1992.

Lifshitz F, Moses N, Cervantes C, et al: Nutritional dwarfing in adolescents. *Semin Adolesc Med* 3:255–266, 1971.

McAlpine C, Singh NW: Pica in institutionalized mentally retarded persons. *J Ment Defic Res* 30:171–178, 1986.

McLaren DS, Reed WE: Classification of nutritional status in early childhood. *Lancet* 2:146–148, 1972.

Madden NA, Russo DC, Cataldo MF: Environmental influences on mouthing in children with lead intoxication. *J Pediatr Psychol* 5:207–216, 1980.

Maloney MJ, Klykylo WM: An overview of anorexia nervosa, bulimia and obesity in children and adolescents. *J Am Acad Child Psychiatry* 22:99–107, 1983.

Mayes SD, Humphrey FJ, Handford HA, et al: Rumination disorder: Differential diagnosis. *J Am Acad Child Adolesc Psychiatry* 27:300–302, 1988.

Mitchell WG, Gorrell RW, Greenberg RA: Failure to thrive: A study in a primary care setting: Epidemiology and follow-up. *Pediatrics* 65:971–976, 1980.

Morgan HG, Russell GFM: Value of family background and clinical features as predictors of long-term outcome in anorexia nervosa: Four-year follow-up study of 41 patients. *Psychol Med* 5:355–372, 1975.

Oates RK, Peacock A, Forrest D: Long-term effects of nonorganic failure to thrive. *Pediatrics* 75:36–40, 1985.

Papaila JG, Wilmont D, Grosfeld JL, et al: Increased incidence of delayed gastric emptying in children with gastroesophageal reflux. *Arch Surg* 128:933–936, 1989.

Polan HJ, Kaplan MD, Kessler DB, et al: Psychopathology in mothers of children with failure to thrive. *Infant Mental Health J* 12:55–64, 1991a.

Polan HJ, Leon A, Kaplan M, et al: Disturbances of affect expression in failure to thrive. *J Am Acad Child Adolesc Psychiatry* 30:897–903, 1991b.

Poskitt EME: Obese from infancy: A re-evaluation. *Top Pediatr* 1:81–89, 1980.

Powell R, Brasel JA, Raiti S, et al: Emotional deprivation and growth retardation simulating idiopathic hypopituitarism: I. Clinical evaluation of the syndrome. II. Endocrinological evaluation of the syndrome. *N Engl J Med* 276:1271–1283, 1967.

Pugliese MT, Lifshitz F, Grad G, et al: Fear of obesity: A cause of short stature and delayed puberty. *N Engl J Med* 309:513–518, 1983.

Richmond JB, Eddy E, Green M: Rumination: A psychosomatic syndrome of infancy. *Pediatrics* 22:49–55, 1958.

Russell GFM: Premenarchal anorexia nervosa and its sequelae. *J Psychiatr Res* 19:363–369, 1985.

Sameroff AJ, Chandler M: Reproductive risk and the continuum of caretaking causality. In: Horowitz F (ed): *Review of Child Development Research* (Vol 4). Chicago, University of Chicago Press, 1975, pp. 197–244.

Sameroff AJ, Fiese BH: Conceptual issues in prevention. In: Shaffer D, Philips I, Enzer N (eds): *Prevention of Mental Disorders, Alcohol and Other Drug Use in Children and Adolescents*. Rockville, MD, US Department of Health and Human Services, Public Health, Alcohol, Drug Abuse and Mental Health Administration, 1989, pp. 23–53.

Sanberg DE, Smith MM, Fornai V, et al: Nutritional dwarfing: Is it a consequence of disturbed psychosocial functioning? *Pediatrics* 88:926–933, 1991.

Sauvage D, Leddet L, Hameur L, et al: Infantile rumination: Diagnosis and follow-up of twenty cases. *J Am Acad Child Psychiatry* 24:97–203, 1985.

Shapiro LR, Crawford PB, Clark MJ: Obesity prognosis: A longitudinal study of children from age six months to nine years. *Am J Public Health* 74:968–972, 1984.

Shepherd RW, Wren J, Evans S, et al: Gastroesophageal reflux in children: Clinical profile, course, and outcome with active therapy in 126 cases. *Clin Pediatr* 26:55–60, 1987.

Shukla A, Forsyth AA, Anderson CM, et al: Infantile overnutrition in the first year of life: A field study in Dudley, Worcestershire. *Br Med J* 4:507–515, 1972.

Sills RH: Failure to thrive: The role of clinical and laboratory evaluation. *Am J Dis Child* 132:967–969, 1978.

Silverstone JT: Psychological factors in obesity. In: Baird IM, Howard AN (eds): *Obesity: Medical and Scientific Aspects*. London, E & S Livingston, 1969, pp. 45–55.

Stunkard AJ: Obesity. In: Kaplan HI, Sadock BJ, Freedman AM (eds): *Comprehensive Textbook of Psychiatry* (3rd ed). Baltimore, Williams & Wilkins, 1980, pp. 1872–1881.

Stunkard AJ, D'Aquill E, Fox S, et al: Influence of social class on obesity and thinness in children. *JAMA* 221:579–584, 1972.

Stunkard AJ, Foch TT, Hrubec Z: A twin study of human obesity. *JAMA* 256:51–54, 1986a.

Stunkard AJ, Sorenson TIA, Hanis C, et al: An adoption study of human obesity. *N Engl J Med* 314:193–198, 1986b.

Vyas D, Chandra RK: Functional implications of iron deficiency. In: Stekel A, Nestle V (eds): *Iron Nutrition in Infancy and Childhood*. New York, Raven Press, 1984, pp. 45–59.

Whitten CF, Pettit MG, Fischoff J: Evidence that growth failure from maternal deprivation is secondary to undereating. *JAMA* 209:1675–1682, 1969.

Widdowson EM: Mental contentment and physical growth. *Lancet* 1:1316–1318, 1951.

Wilson RS, Mathany AP: Behavioral-genetics in infant temperament: The Louisville twin study. In: Plomin R, Dunn J (eds): *The Study of Temperament: Changes, Continuities and Challenges*. Hillsdale, NJ, Erlbaum, 1986, pp. 81–97.

Winton ASW, Singh NN: Rumination in pediatric populations: A behavioral analysis. *J Am Acad Child Psychiatry* 22:269–275, 1983.

Woolston JL: Eating disorders in infancy and early childhood. *J Am Acad Child Psychiatry* 22:114–121, 1983.

Woolston JL: Diagnostic classification: The current challenge in failure to thrive syndrome research. In: Drotar D (ed): *New Directions in Failure to Thrive: Implications for Research and Practice*. New York, Plenum, 1985, pp. 225–233.

Woolston JL: Obesity of infancy and early childhood. *J Am Acad Child Adolesc Psychiatry* 26:123–126, 1987.

Woolston JL: Theoretical considerations of the adjustment disorders. *J Am Acad Child Adolesc Psychiatry* 27:280–287, 1988.

Woolston JL: Transactional risk model for short and intermediate term psychiatric inpatient treatment of children. *J Am Acad Child Adolesc Psychiatry* 28:38–41, 1989.

Woolston JL: Eating and growth disorder in infants and children. In: Kazdin AE (ed): *Developmental Clinical Pathology* (Vol 24). Newbury Park, CA, Sage Publication, 1991.

Woolston JL, Forsyth DL: Obesity of infancy and early childhood: A diagnostic schema. In: Lahey BB, Kazdin AE (eds): *Advances in Clinical Child Psychology* (Vol 12). New York, Plenum, 1989, pp. 179–192.

World Health Organization: *International Classification of Diseases* (10th ed). Criteria for Research (Draft). Geneva, World Health Organization, 1990.

53 ANOREXIA NERVOSA AND BULIMIA NERVOSA

Alexander R. Lucas, M.D.

DEFINITION

Anorexia nervosa typically occurs in girls shortly after puberty or later in adolescence, although early-onset anorexia nervosa in children between 8 and 14 years old has been well described (Bryant-Waugh, 1988). The disorder is characterized by self-imposed weight loss, amenorrhea, and a characteristic distorted psychopathologic attitude toward eating and weight. Patients with anorexia nervosa are hungry but willfully refuse to eat (Halmi, 1988). A premenarchal form occurring early in puberty is recognized. Onset of the disorder can occur in adulthood. Rarely, the condition occurs in boys.

There are three major diagnostic criteria for anorexia nervosa: (*a*) marked weight loss that is self-induced, (*b*) specific psychopathology characterized by fear of fatness, and (*c*) endocrine changes manifested by amenorrhea in females and loss of sexual interest and potency in males (Russell, 1985). In premenarchal anorexia nervosa there need not be actual weight loss, but there is failure to gain weight during the phase of active growth. The endocrine disorder results in delay of pubertal development and growth. Atypical or partial forms of anorexia nervosa are common. They are diagnosed in individuals who lack one or more of the criteria.

Current diagnostic criteria for anorexia nervosa from DSM-IV (American Psychiatric Association, 1994) are shown in Table 53.1. These criteria suggest that the disorder includes two subtypes, the restricting type and the binge-eating/purging type, depending on whether or not the patient engages in binge-eating or purging behaviors. In practice, clinical characteristics often overlap, with patients starting with one group of symptoms and later moving on to others. Garner et al. (1993) showed that the symptoms of binge-eating, purging, and restrictive dieting develop at different body weights. In anorexia nervosa they occur at an abnormally low weight.

There is still much confusion about the definition of bulimia. The specific meaning of the term is "ravenous appetite." It can be a *symptom* of conditions in which there is overingestion of food. As a *syndrome*, the term loosely has come to mean binge-eating, vomiting, and purging. Bulimia nervosa, as the prototype of this syndrome, is often a sequel of anorexia nervosa. It is characterized by episodes of overeating followed by self-induced vomiting or purging, associated with excessive body preoccupation and concern about weight.

The diagnostic criteria for bulimia nervosa have evolved and have been refined to their present form as outlined in Table 53.2. Purging and nonpurging types have been defined on the basis of whether or not the person engages in vomiting and/or the misuse of laxatives or diuretics or uses other compensatory behaviors, such as fasting or excessive exercise.

When the criteria for anorexia nervosa or bulimia nervosa are not fully met, the diagnosis of eating disorder not otherwise specified may be used, as suggested by DSM-IV. A variant identified as binge-eating disorder has been proposed for those individuals who have recurrent episodes of binge-eating in the absence of the compensatory behaviors characteristic of bulimia nervosa. There continues to be controversy about whether this constitutes a disorder. Such behavior is quite common among males as well as among females and is problematic only when it is carried to excess, such as when obesity ensues. Among adolescents

Table 53.1. Diagnostic Criteria for Anorexia Nervosa

A. Refusal to maintain body weight at or above a minimally normal weight for age and height (e.g., weight loss leading to maintenance of body weight less than 85% of that expected; or failure to make expected weight gain during period of growth, leading to body weight less than 85% of that expected).
B. Intense fear of gaining weight or becoming fat, even though underweight.
C. Disturbance in the way in which one's body weight or shape is experienced, undue influence of body weight or shape on self-evaluation, or denial of the seriousness of the current low body weight.
D. In postmenarcheal females, amenorrhea, i.e., the absence of at least three consecutive menstrual cycles.

From American Psychiatric Association: *Diagnostic and Statistical Manual of Mental Disorders* (4th ed). Washington, DC, American Psychiatric Association, 1994.

Table 53.2. Diagnostic Criteria for Bulimia Nervosa

A. Recurrent episodes of binge eating. An episode of binge eating is characterized by both of the following:
　1. Eating, in a discrete period of time (e.g., within any 2-hour period), an amount of food that is definitely larger than most people would eat during a similar period of time and under similar circumstances
　2. A sense of lack of control over eating during the episode (e.g., a feeling that one cannot stop eating or control what or how much one is eating)
B. Recurrent inappropriate compensatory behavior in order to prevent weight gain, such as self-induced vomiting; misuse of laxatives, diuretics, enemas, or other medications; fasting; or excessive exercise.
C. The binge eating and inappropriate compensatory behaviors both occur, on average, at least twice a week for 3 months.
D. Self-evaluation is unduly influenced by body shape and weight.
E. The disturbance does not occur exclusively during episodes of anorexia nervosa.

From American Psychiatric Association: *Diagnostic and Statistical Manual of Mental Disorders* (4th ed). Washington, DC, American Psychiatric Association, 1994.

and preadolescents, anorexia nervosa and its variants are the most common eating disorder. Bulimic disorders are more prevalent in older adolescents and in adults.

HISTORICAL NOTE

Medical descriptions of anorexia nervosa can be found from several centuries ago (Lucas, 1981). It was formally identified by Gull and Lasègue in the latter part of the 19th century as a consequence of self-starvation due to psychologic causes. Subsequently, however, there was confusion as to whether pituitary failure or psychopathologic factors were responsible for the disorder. Psychoanalytic interpretation of food refusal focused on the inhibition of drives. Child psychiatrists became interested in the disorder in the 1960s, when Lesser and coworkers (1960) and Blitzer and coworkers (1961) reported series of cases. They concluded that diverse psychopathologies led to the disorder. The view that there is a specific psychopathology was espoused by Bruch (1973), Crisp (1965), and Russell (1970). Bruch was instrumental in bringing the disorder from obscurity to the status of a treatable psychiatric condition.

In a historical review of the emergence of bulimia nervosa as a syndrome, Casper (1983) indicated that one of Gull's patients displayed intermittently voracious appetite. Osler (cited by Casper, 1983) had recognized bulimia as a symptom occurring in diabetes mellitus. In the early literature on anorexia nervosa the occurrence of vomiting was occasionally mentioned. After 1930, there were frequent observations of episodes of overeating and self-induced vomiting among patients with anorexia nervosa. Binswanger's case of Ellen West (cited by Casper, 1983) demonstrated severe bulimia, vomiting, and laxative abuse. In 1979 Russell identified bulimia nervosa as a distinct syndrome and noted its close relationship to anorexia nervosa. Shortly thereafter, the differentiation of subtypes among patients with anorexia nervosa—those who restrict and those who binge-eat and purge—was emphasized. It became apparent that many high school girls and college-

age women engaged in binge-eating and purging behaviors without developing the full syndrome of bulimia nervosa and without a history of anorexia nervosa. Binge-eating, although thought to be a new behavior characteristic of the modern lifestyle and social pressure, was observed as early as the end of the 19th century among girls in boarding schools who regularly took something to eat to bed with them (Casper, 1983).

PREVALENCE AND EPIDEMIOLOGY

Anorexia nervosa occurs 8 to 12 times more frequently in females than in males. Among females, more than half of the cases begin before age 20 and about three-quarters occur before age 25. Fewer than 10% have premenarchal onset. Lucas and coworkers (1991) found the prevalence in Rochester, Minnesota, to be 0.3% for females and 0.02% for males in 1985. Among 15- through 19-year-old girls, the prevalence was 0.5%. In vulnerable populations of English schoolgirls, prevalence rates of 0.5–1% were observed. Particularly vulnerable groups, such as female ballet dancers and gymnasts, are subject to even higher rates. Contrary to popular opinion, anorexia nervosa occurs across the socioeconomic and rural/urban spectrum, rather than being confined to upper social classes (Garner, 1993).

Estimates of the annual incidence (newly diagnosed cases) in Western Europe and the United States, based on hospitalized cases and psychiatric case registers, have shown an apparent increase from 0.5 per 100,000 population in 1950 to 5 per 100,000 in the 1980s. The only population-based study covering a 50-year span showed a higher incidence rate of 8.2 per 100,000 (14.6 for females and 1.8 for males). This study showed no change in the rates for females 20 years and older. Among 10- through 19-year-old girls, the incidence rates increased substantially from 1950 to 1984 (Lucas et al., 1991).

Using strict criteria for bulimia nervosa, Timmerman et al. (1990) set the prevalence figure at 2% in high school girls and at almost none in boys. Among female college students, Drewnowski et al. (1988) determined the point prevalence rate to be 3% during both the fall and spring semesters of the freshman year. However, different individuals were identified among the bulimic group at those two times, indicating that untreated remitted cases were replaced by new ones. The full syndrome is extremely rare among boys, but vomiting and purging occur in special groups of boys, such as wrestlers.

Faiburn and Beglin (1990), in a review of more than 50 prevalence studies of bulimia nervosa, noted that the disorder consistently (but not necessarily accurately) appears to have a prevalence rate of about 1% among female adolescents and young adult women. They also suggest that comparisons of clinic and community-based cases are now needed, particularly studies that focus on the nature, course, and etiology of the full spectrum of disturbances that exist in the community.

Soundy et al. (1995) found the community-based incidence of bulimia nervosa to rise sharply from 1980 to 1983 and then to remain relatively constant through 1990. The incidence rates for residents of Rochester, Minnesota, during that decade were 26.5 per 100,000 population for females and 0.8 per 100,000 population for males. The mean age for females was 23 years. Among 15- through 24-year-old adolescent girls and young women, it had become at least twice as common as anorexia nervosa.

CLINICAL DESCRIPTION

Typically anorexia nervosa begins after puberty in a girl whose growth and development have previously been normal. Onset may be early in adolescence shortly after menarche, or later when the girl prepares to leave home, or on entering college. Often these girls have shown no signs of prior psychopathology, and parents frequently describe that daughter as the best adjusted of their children. Typically they have been highly conforming to their parents' expectations, ambitious, and achievement oriented. Although considerable variation in temperament and social interaction exists, more often than not they have been serious-minded and socially involved. They have high standards for their own behavior, have shown concern for others, and have wanted to please.

The history is one of progressive self-starvation. Dieting may begin after a seemingly innocent comment about a girl's figure or weight. Pubertal changes in body shape, with increasing size of thighs, buttocks, and abdomen, give rise to concerns about body image. Often she begins to skip desserts and sweets, then entire meals—usually breakfast and lunch—or eats small quantities at these meals. She eliminates foods considered to be fattening and continues to restrict the amounts of food consumed. Along with increasing food restriction, she begins to exercise more and more, becoming compulsive about it. She feels the need to increase the amount of time spent in doing calisthenics and in running or bicycling. Many accomplish considerable weight loss entirely by restricting intake and by exercising, but some resort to vomiting and taking laxatives as further means of losing weight.

At first parents may not be aware of the weight loss or they may compliment their daughter for losing a moderate amount of weight. Later on they may be startled when they see her partially undressed and note an advanced degree of emaciation. Although menstruation may stop before much weight loss has occurred, it usually ceases only after a significant amount of weight loss, when the proportion of body fat has fallen below the critical level. Behavioral changes ensue, including social withdrawal, irritability, moodiness, and depression. Academic achievement continues to be at a high level but requires increasing hours of application and study. Many patients continue to be active in sports and other extracurricular activities, such as music lessons and dramatics. They may work at several part-time jobs. Less and less time is spent sleeping.

On physical examination, emaciation is seen as the result of the loss of much of the body fat. The patient appears alert and incongruously healthy, considering her degree of emaciation. The cheek bones are prominent, and the eyes are sunken. The upper torso appears particularly thin, with ribs, clavicles, and scapulae highly visible. The breasts are relatively well maintained. The hands and feet are blue and cold, the skin is dry, and the hair is dry. When undernutrition is advanced, fine downy hair (lanugo) appears on the face, trunk, and extremities. The pulse rate is slow and the blood pressure low.

Despite severe wasting, the patient may deny that anything is wrong. She may insist that she is fine and wants to be left alone and suggest that her parents are unnecessarily concerned. She lacks spontaneity, and at first she is guarded and uncommunicative. She may answer specific questions with "yes" or "no" but does not volunteer information or elaborate on emotional content. Further questioning may reveal that she is fearful of becoming fat or believes that she actually is fat.

In premenarchal anorexia nervosa there may be little or no actual weight loss, but the patient fails to gain weight commensurate with developmental expectations. There may be actual weight loss that alarms the parents, but the onset is often insidious. In contrast to the postpubertal form, growth retardation with lack of sexual development often accompanies the poor weight gain. Puberty is delayed or arrested. The psychopathology in premenarchal anorexia nervosa is similar to that in the postpubertal form. There is an overwhelming fear of becoming fat. The youngest age at which patients present with this form of the disorder is 9 or 10 years. Food refusal in younger children usually represents overt rejection of parental wishes to have them eat and results in open conflict over eating. Body image concerns and fear of fatness are not the issues. Jaffe and Singer (1989) described such a group of 5- to 11-year-old children who differed from patients with anorexia nervosa and who presented with diverse family psychopathology. "Infantile anorexia nervosa" has been described but is a misnomer because the psychopathology differs from that of anorexia nervosa (Chatoor et al., 1988). It is as common in boys as in girls and is more appropriately classified as a form of failure to thrive.

Anorexia nervosa in boys is rare. When it occurs early in the process of puberty, retardation of pubertal development and failure to grow in height result. Later in adolescence there is delay or arrest in the develop-

ment of masculine physique and musculature. As in girls, there is an overwhelming aversion to becoming fat and often the incongruous idea equating increasing weight with weakness. Exercise and preoccupation with body building are carried to unusual extremes.

Bulimia as a symptom is recognized in numerous conditions. Individuals with ravenous appetite may be normal weight, overweight, or underweight. Often their weight fluctuates markedly. Some individuals of either sex ingest great quantities of food regularly or intermittently, leading to obesity. Organic brain conditions with appetite dyscontrol are associated with bulimia as a symptom. In Prader-Willi syndrome, bulimia, or voracious appetite, is a prominent feature, along with obesity, hypogonadism, short stature, mental retardation, and a history of floppiness at birth. An abnormality of the long arm of chromosome 15 has been reported in about half the cases, and hypothalamic dysfunction seems to be the central disturbance.

Bulimia nervosa occurs particularly in individuals who have a history of anorexia nervosa. After prolonged periods of semistarvation, they eventually yield to their hunger and secretly gorge themselves. Subsequently they vomit and purge out of guilt. They have in the past been significantly underweight, and their histories may show dramatic weight fluctuations.

Another group of patients whose weight has always been within the normal range engage in binge-eating and vomiting or purging as a means of weight control. Known as the bulimia syndrome in normal-weight individuals, it has become a common affliction among teenage girls and young adult women. They do not have a history of anorexia nervosa, and often there is an absence of significant psychopathology. Overeating may happen occasionally or on a frequent basis. It is likely that a high proportion of teenage girls have engaged in occasional vomiting under these circumstances. The seriousness of the condition depends on the frequency of vomiting and on whether or not a metabolic disturbance is the result of laxative or diuretic use. The condition ranges from a mild one in which the individual eats normally, has never experienced much weight change, and induces vomiting occasionally after a very large meal or snack, to the severe condition alternating between fasting and binge-eating, with vomiting after every meal.

In bulimia nervosa the face has a characteristic appearance, with round, swollen cheeks. In contrast, body shape is relatively thin. Facial swelling is due in part to enlarged salivary glands, chiefly the parotids, but also the submandibular and sublingual glands. Fluid retention adds to the puffy appearance. The patient looks unwell. The skin tends to be dry and marked with cuts and abrasions, particularly over the knuckles of the hands, which may be callused (Russell's sign) from repeated trauma against the teeth associated with putting the fingers down the throat. The dental enamel becomes eroded from repeated vomiting. In contrast to the anorexic patient, who is superficial and quiet about her symptoms, the bulimic young woman may seek help herself and is much more willing to talk about her symptoms and to acknowledge that she is distressed by her behavior. Inquiries into the composition of her diet, quantity of food consumed during binges, frequency of vomiting, and quantity of laxatives consumed, however, meet with less than candid answers. Chronic dysphoria, dissatisfaction with herself, and lability of mood may be prominent.

ETIOLOGY AND PATHOGENESIS

The cause of anorexia nervosa is not known, but evidence strongly suggests an interaction of biopsychosocial factors. Precipitating factors, including environmental and developmental stressors, but often simply the act of dieting, trigger the onset of the illness. Psychosocial influences reinforced by starvation effects then perpetuate the illness. Bulimic syndromes similarly involve a complex interaction of etiologic factors.

Biologic Mechanisms and Hypotheses

Some evidence exists to support a genetic predisposition in anorexia nervosa. Twin studies confirm a higher concordance rate among monozygotic twins (56%) than among dizygotic twins (7%) (Holland et al., 1984). What is inherited that establishes vulnerability for anorexia nervosa, however, is not clear (Garner, 1993). It has also been shown that there is family aggregation of anorexia nervosa with female first-degree relatives having a significantly higher risk of developing an eating disorder than control subjects (Strober et al., 1990). It is well established that there is disturbance in the hypothalamic-anterior pituitary-gonadal axis. Undernutrition results in an endocrinologically mediated hypometabolic state. Elevated plasma cortisol, diminished cortisol metabolism, elevated corticotropin-releasing hormone, elevated endogenous opiates, and lowered serotonin appear to be secondary to malnutrition (Yates, 1989). Amenorrhea occurs when weight and proportion of body fat drop below the critical level. However, amenorrhea may begin before the onset of weight loss. This has led to the hypothesis that a hypothalamic disorder is primary in the origin of the disorder. Depression, athleticism, and menstrual irregularities may occur, along with dysfunction in the hypothalamic-pituitary-adrenalovarian axis and decreased levels of norepinephrine and 3-methoxy-4-hydroxyphenylglycol (MHPG) (Yates, 1989). (See also Chapters 5 and 6). Abnormal hypothalamic-pituitary-adrenal function has been well documented in anorexia nervosa (Gold et al., 1986). Psychologic influences also are thought to contribute to the cessation of menstruation. These act on the hypothalamus through neurohormonal mechanisms that have not yet been thoroughly elucidated (Fava et al., 1989; Lucas and Callaway, 1985).

Recently, altered cerebrospinal neuropeptide Y and peptide YY immunoreactivity has been found to be associated with important symptoms in both anorexia and bulimia nervosa (Kaye et al., 1990).

Another organ system implicated in predisposing to anorexia nervosa is the gastrointestinal tract. A history of feeding disturbances in infancy and early childhood is not unusual. Recent evidence points to gastrointestinal disturbances that heighten patients' awareness of gastric fullness and discomfort (Abell et al., 1987).

A pattern of seasonal onset of anorexia nervosa has been described for anorexia nervosa, with the highest incidence in May (Nielsen, 1992). This should cause renewed interest in the study of the interrelationship between eating disorders and depression (Råstam, 1992).

Bulimic disorders have been much less extensively studied than anorexia nervosa. Some etiologic hypotheses have been formulated, but few biologic studies have been done to elucidate the pathogenesis and pathophysiology. A depressive diathesis has been suggested because of favorable response to antidepressant medication in some patients. One study showed that an impairment in cholecystokinin metabolism reduced satiety (Fava et al., 1989). The clinical heterogeneity of the conditions makes it likely that diverse etiologic factors are operative.

Psychologic Processes and Theories

Pre-illness personality in anorexia nervosa varies considerably. However, starvation affects the individual in characteristic ways. Often there is increased seclusiveness and secretiveness, with alienation from family members. Mood changes with marked lability occur, associated with increased irritability. These manifestations are superimposed on the personality structure and result in the clinical presentation.

Early psychoanalytic concepts, reviewed by Bemis (1978), interpreted the genesis of anorexia nervosa on the basis of inhibition of sexual drives, equating eating behavior with the sexual instinct. It was postulated that adolescents who are unable to meet the demands of mature genitality regress to a primitive level at which oral gratification is associated with sexual pleasure or fertility. Refusal to eat was seen as a defense against oral impregnation fantasies. Later psychoanalytic writers shifted the focus from drive disturbances to disorders in the mother-child relationship, resulting in ego defects that left anorexic individuals unprepared to cope with the demands of adulthood. Bruch (1973) and Selvini Palazzoli (1978) described a mother-child relationship in which the individual needs of the child are subverted to the mother's sense of what is appropriate. This results in an adolescent who is slavishly compliant and who has no clear conception of herself as an individual. The anorexic symptoms are seen as part of a desperate struggle for a self-respecting identity.

Bruch (1973) described three disturbances of psychologic function among patients with anorexia nervosa: (a) a disturbance in body image of delusional proportions; (b) a disturbance in the accuracy of perception or cognitive interpretation of stimuli arising within the body, with failure to recognize signs of nutritional need; and (c) a paralyzing sense of ineffectiveness pervading all thinking and activities. This overall sense of ineffectiveness she viewed as being central to the psychopathology of the disorder. She noted that patients with anorexia nervosa experienced themselves as acting only in response to demands coming from other people and situations, and as not doing anything because they wanted to. She attributed the origins of this core disturbance to early experiences in the mother-child relationship.

Anterospective studies are more likely to shed light on vulnerability and risk for eating disorders than retrospective reconstruction. Some promising research in that direction is being done by Leon et al. (1993) and suggests that body dissatisfaction, negative emotionality, and lack of interoceptive awareness, but not early puberty, increase the risk for eating disorder in adolescent girls.

Much speculation exists about the genesis of the symptoms seen in bulimic syndromes. Family conflicts, history of sexual abuse, issues about femininity, and underlying depression all have been implicated in the cause. The fact that so many causes have been implicated underscores the fact that there is no simple relationship that exists and that the real cause is not well understood. Johnson et al. (1984), in reviewing the personality and psychologic characteristics of normal-weight bulimic patients, indicated that bulimic patients tend to have difficulties with impulse control, chronic depression, exaggerated sense of guilt, intolerance for frustration, and recurrent anxiety. They tend to be troubled by feelings of helplessness and inadequacy and are anxious, depressed, self-critical, impulsive, and concerned with issues related to food and body dissatisfaction (Johnson et al., 1984). The common denominator is that binge-eating usually occurs as a response to semistarvation and that purging is motivated by the desire to avoid gaining weight. Beyond these facts, the preexisting personality structure, environmental experience, and family situation vary widely among persons who engage in this behavior. The sheer frequency of the behavior in the population makes it obvious that individuals who binge and purge are different one from another in genetic background and environmental experience.

Family and Interpersonal Dynamics

Crisp et al. (1974) suggested that family psychopathology in anorexia nervosa is displaced on the patient, with the precarious balance achieved through this distortion being overthrown when the patient regains normal weight. Minuchin and coworkers (1978) suggested that pathologic organization of the family around the symptom provides a mechanism through which family members can avoid interpersonal conflicts. They observed that the families of children who suffer from a number of psychosomatic disorders share general patterns of interaction, such as enmeshment (or overinvolvement), overprotectiveness, rigidity, and poor conflict resolution. They suggested that disordered eating behavior should be viewed as an interpersonal rather than an individual problem.

Strober (1981) studied teenage anorexia nervosa patients, comparing those with and without the syndrome of bulimia. The bulimic patients were more likely to show affective disturbance and alcohol use. Bulimia was more strongly associated with affective instability and other signs of behavioral deviance during childhood. Family environments were characterized by significantly greater conflict and negativity, less cohesion, and less structure than in the nonbulimic anorexic families, and bulimics experienced more stressful life changes prior to illness onset than did nonbulimic patients. Parents of bulimic anorexic patients also reported significantly higher levels of marital discord, were rated as more emotionally distant from their daughters, and exhibited greater psychiatric morbidity and physical health problems (Strober, 1981).

Few studies have investigated the nature of the family environment among bulimic individuals at normal weight. Bulimic patients tend to be older than anorexic patients and thus more often have left their families. Johnson et al. (1984) reported that families of bulimic patients were more disorganized and more conflicted, yet had a higher achievement orientation than normal control families.

Environmental and Social Influences

Social influences and expectations set a climate conducive to the development of eating disorders. The cultural obsession with thinness and emphasis on low-fat diets and exercise reinforce the psychologic motivation of vulnerable individuals in their relentless pursuit of thinness. Johnson and associates (1984) suggested that shifts in the cultural norms for contemporary women have forced them to face multiple, ambiguous, and often contradictory role expectations. In this high-achievement orientation, the pursuit of thinness has emerged in the culture as a way by which young women can compete among themselves and demonstrate that they have self-control (Johnson et al., 1984).

Contemporary family eating patterns that focus on fast food rather than on organized leisurely family meals; the ready availability of snack foods high in fat, carbohydrate, and sodium; and the habit of eating while watching television and eating on the run all have contributed to the frequency of irregular and erratic diet patterns among teenagers. Such habits tend to predispose to binge-eating. Even though boys and girls both adopt irregular eating habits, girls are much more often affected by pathologic eating disorders. This may be due partly to the fact that boys are more often guided by their natural hunger and satiety, whereas girls are guided by their body perceptions and body consciousness. Girls are more apt to deny hunger in order to lose weight and consequently to develop overwhelming hunger after fasting and prolonged semistarvation.

A high frequency of childhood sexual experience is reported in patients with anorexia nervosa and some believe that there is an even higher frequency of sexual abuse history in those with bulimia nervosa. However, this occurrence seems to be no greater than in women with other mental disorders (Palmer and Oppenheimer, 1992).

LABORATORY STUDIES

There are no specific findings that lead to the diagnosis of anorexia nervosa. Laboratory studies reflect undernutrition (Kaplan and Woodside, 1987), indicate a hypometabolic state, and demonstrate diminished levels of pituitary gonadotropic hormones (Tables 53.3 and 53.4). Abnormal findings may reveal complications such as electrolyte and acid-base balance abnormalities, as well as confirm laxative and diuretic abuse (Silverman, 1983). They may signal the presence of another illness that has caused weight loss.

Psychologic testing shows a wide range of intellectual functioning, even though academic performance is usually at a high level.

DIFFERENTIAL DIAGNOSIS

Both physical and psychiatric disorders associated with weight loss are to be differentiated from anorexia nervosa. When there is a history of progressive intentional dieting and weight loss, there should be little doubt about the diagnosis of anorexia nervosa. The chief disorders to be differentiated from anorexia nervosa are major affective disorder (Hudson et al., 1983) and gastrointestinal diseases involving malabsorption. Bizarre eating patterns resembling anorexia nervosa or bulimia nervosa may be seen in schizophrenia, conversion disorder, and hypomania.

Medical disorders that may have presenting symptoms similar to those found in anorexia nervosa include neurological disorders (brain tumors), hormonal disorders (anterior pituitary dysfunction, hyperparathyroidism, diabetes mellitus, and adrenal disease), and gastrointestinal disorders (malabsorption syndromes, gastrointestinal ulcers, and regional enteritis).

Table 53.3. Common Laboratory Findings in Anorexia Nervosa

1. Hematologic
   Anemia
   Leukopenia
2. Chemistry studies
   Hypercarotenemia
   Hypoproteinemia
   Hypercholesterolemia
3. Endocrine
   Decreased estrogens
   Decreased testosterone (in males)
   Immature luteinizing hormone
   Blunted luteinizing hormone-releasing hormone
   Decreased triiodothyronine
   Increased corticoids
   Increased growth hormone
   Increased response to vasopressin
   Low basal metabolic rate
4. Urine
   Increased or decreased osmolality
   Proteinuria

Table 53.4. Common Laboratory Findings in Bulimia Nervosa

1. Hematologic
   Anemia
2. Chemistry studies
   Hypokalemic hypochloremic alkalosis
   Hypoproteinemia
   Elevated amylase
3. Endocrine
   Low thyroid-stimulating hormone
   Low basal metabolic rate
4. Urine
   Increased or decreased osmolality
5. Muscle wasting

Table 53.5. Complications of Bulimia Nervosa

1. Dental problems
2. Subconjunctival hemorrhage
3. Esophageal or gastric rupture
4. Cardiomyopathy
5. Cardiac arrhythmias
6. Heart failure
7. Kidney failure
8. Seizures

Medical complications following some of the symptoms of anorexia nervosa and bulimia nervosa may involve almost every system in the body and add to the complexity of the clinical picture. Thus, cardiac arrhythmias, electrolyte imbalance, anemia, hormonal changes, parotitis, dental caries, and skin changes are some of the results of starvation, dehydration, vomiting, purging, and physical trauma (Table 53.5).

TREATMENT

Treatment has the 2-fold aim of restoring normal nutrition and eating habits and of dealing with psychologic and family issues associated with the eating problem. The nutritional problems, both in anorexia nervosa and in bulimic syndromes, have typical features that can be corrected through nutritional rehabilitation. Psychologic and family problems, however, are quite variable. Thus, they must be addressed in an individualized manner. Principles appropriate to good psychotherapy apply. Programs that use a predetermined protocol for all patients may seem rational, and they provide multidisciplinary staff members with reassuring guidelines. However, they are ineffective and counterproductive for patients who do not accept them and for whom they are inappropriate. Thus, it is necessary for the physician to establish rapport and to gain the patient's confidence before treatment can proceed. One or more lengthy outpatient interviews are needed to begin this process. Some patients will be ready to begin treatment, even though skeptical about its need, whereas others will continue to be resistant and require firm support from their parents that it is necessary. Parents who themselves are ambivalent about their daughter's need for treatment will require considerable guidance from the physician.

In most instances, when the illness is relatively mild or moderately severe, outpatient treatment is preferred. There is an educational component to treatment, a component aimed to correct the nutritional disturbance (weight restoration, regulation of eating pattern, elimination of binge-eating and purging), psychotherapy geared to the patient's individual conflicts, and work with the family.

The relationship established with the therapist is of crucial importance and is one in which a positive influence toward healthier adaptation is exerted. Although the techniques of therapy may vary, with some therapists emphasizing a psychodynamically oriented approach, some utilizing cognitive-behavioral approaches, and some emphasizing conjoint family techniques, all require active rather than passive participation by the therapist, with the therapist conveying a sense of confident competence without being domineering and coercive. Issues of body image and body concept, growth and development, and family and peer interaction need to be addressed. Initially there may be hostile rejection and resistance to therapy. Once a positive relationship is established, the patient may become quite dependent on the therapist. The patient should move gradually from this state of dependence to increasing levels of autonomy and self-reliance. Continuity with one therapist is important. Anorexic patients react with regression to separations and to changes of therapists. The importance of the relationship established in therapy, regardless of the specific techniques used, cannot be overestimated and constitutes part of the art of treatment.

Specific psychotherapeutic approaches have been described more explicitly by Bruch (1978), Garner and Bemis (1982), and Lucas et al. (1976). Beumont et al. (1993) reviewed the principles and techniques both of outpatient and of hospital treatment. Practice guidelines for eating disorders now have been delineated by the American Psychiatric Association (1993) and hopefully will support physicians' treatment recommendations when challenged in the managed care climate of medical practice.

Hospital treatment is required when the medical condition is precarious because of severe undernutrition, dehydration, electrolyte imbalance, or other complications; when there is suicide risk or psychotic decompensation; when the family situation is unworkable on an outpatient basis; when there is poor motivation; and when there has been failure to respond to outpatient treatment. Hospital treatment in another community may also be indicated when outpatient treatment is not locally available.

In the hospital, responsibility for decisions about eating is given to the staff. The patient may be both resistant and relieved by this. The expectation is that the patient will eat regular food, starting with relatively small quantities that are increased gradually in order to achieve continuing weight gain at a rate the patient is able to tolerate. Hiding food and secret exercise must be prevented. Crucial to the success of the treatment approach are the skill and attitude of the nursing staff. Food supplementation, nasogastric feeding, or intravenous nutritional support is rarely necessary. Psychotherapy and appropriate family therapy continue in the hospital setting. The patient is discharged after the weight has stabilized at a satisfactory level, when she is able to eat spontaneously and relatively comfortably, and when psychologic functioning is sufficiently improved. Outpatient follow-up usually is indicated for a considerable time.

There continues to be controversy about how rapidly caloric intake should be increased in order to achieve optimal rate of weight gain. Although some patients tolerate high calorie diets and rapid weight gain, many others become unduly terrified by it and become even more resistant to treatment. They may accede to demands to gain weight rapidly to a level they deem unacceptable in order to be dismissed from

the hospital, but they promptly will lose that weight once they are dismissed. Therefore, engaging the patient's cooperation in the process is more important than achieving a predetermined rate of weight gain. An ultimate weight goal should not be determined arbitrarily or by using tables based on actuarial data. It should be individualized and reflect not only developmental norms, but the patient's weight history and physiologic functioning.

Treatment techniques for bulimic syndromes are still evolving. The principles of treatment are much the same as those for anorexia nervosa. In relatively mild forms of the disorder, when weight is normal, educational discussion about the effects of binge-eating and purging, nutritional advice, encouragement of regular meals, and supportive psychotherapy can be effective in reversing the disorder. When eating behavior and purging are out of control and when there are great weight fluctuations, the patient is seriously underweight, or serious electrolyte imbalance has occurred, hospitalization becomes necessary. Whether a patient with bulimia nervosa can be treated on an outpatient basis or requires hospitalization depends on the patient's motivation for treatment, her degree of control over her eating behavior, and her metabolic status.

Eating disorders per se are not specific indications for pharmacotherapy. Usually lability of mood and depressive symptoms seen in the acute phase respond to improved nutrition. However, when anxiety or obsessive-compulsive symptoms are severe or psychotic symptoms are present, antianxiety or neuroleptic medications may be indicated. Likewise, when depression does not improve, appropriate antidepressant medication may be needed. Studies with adult patients have established the short-term efficacy of antidepressant medication in decreasing the severity of binge-eating. However, recurrence of symptomatic behavior is common.

OUTCOME AND FOLLOW-UP DATA

Herzog et al. (1988) reviewed 40 follow-up studies of anorexia nervosa and bulimia nervosa and concluded that both conditions have substantial associated morbidity and that anorexia nervosa in particular has a significant mortality rate. They found that, while anorexia nervosa tends to be chronic and unremitting and bulimia nervosa tends to be episodic with remissions and relapses, at least one-third of patients with either illness are still ill after several years. There are, however, very few long-term follow-up studies of adolescents with anorexia nervosa. Variability in outcome appears to be great. While spontaneous remission is possible among individuals who have never received formal treatment, the illness can last for many years, even for a lifetime. Follow-up studies, in order to be meaningful, must span many years. Short-term follow-up studies, considering only weight as the criterion for improvement, are meaningless. Although restoration of normal weight is a prerequisite to recovery, the return of menstrual function and satisfactory psychologic and social functioning are perhaps more important criteria of recovery.

The longest follow-up studies, by Theander (1985) in Sweden and Tolstrup et al. (1985) in Denmark, underscore the extreme variability in outcome. These studies followed large numbers of patients who had first been hospitalized for treatment of anorexia nervosa. The Danish study of 151 cases included patients treated in a child psychiatry department. Reexamination 4–22 years after first contact revealed a range of outcomes. One-half had recovered from their disorder, one-fourth had chronic anorexia nervosa, and one-fourth had other psychiatric illness. Six percent of patients had died of suicide or complications from malnutrition. The deaths occurred an average of 7 years after first evaluation (Tolstrup et al., 1985).

Theander's (1985) study in Sweden of 94 female patients is of particular interest because they have been followed for several decades. After 6 years of illness, about half of the patients had recovered, as in the Danish study. As the observation time extended, more patients recovered, but there were also more who died. Twelve years after the onset of the illness, three-quarters had recovered. The remainder developed chronic illness, some with bulimic forms, and death from complications of anorexia nervosa or suicide continued to occur. Recovery after more than 12 years of illness was uncommon. After a mean observation time of 33 years, 6% had poor outcome, and 18% had died. These figures are grim reminders that for a significant proportion of patients with severe anorexia nervosa the illness will be long-lasting or will lead to death. On the other hand, recovery is possible even after many years of illness. In milder nonhospitalized cases, there is a greater likelihood of recovery. Early onset, however, does not necessarily result in better outcome. Mortality figures cited by other writers are extremely variable and must be understood in the context of the characteristics of the patient group studied and the length of follow-up.

The extreme variability in outcome indicates that there are both relatively benign and malignant forms of the disorder. Whether these variations represent distinct illnesses or are due to severity of malnutrition or to other factors is not known. The effect of treatment on outcome is not well understood. It stands to reason that early treatment and prevention of severe starvation should prevent chronicity. Anecdotal observations of experienced clinicians support this. Nonetheless, long-term documentation of treatment outcome is not yet available, nor are there studies comparing the long-term outcome of different treatments focusing on the nutritional or psychologic aspects of the illness.

A significant number of patients with anorexia nervosa develop depressive illnesses later in life. There are as yet no reliable means of predicting this outcome.

The outcome of bulimic syndromes is less well understood than the outcome of anorexia nervosa because of the recent identification of these syndromes. Few patients have been followed for long. Undoubtedly there is much variability, depending on the symptomatology and on psychopathologic variables.

RESEARCH DIRECTIONS

Research studies in recent years have furthered the understanding of the pathophysiology of anorexia nervosa. Epidemiologic and long-term follow-up studies have begun to provide a clearer picture of the incidence and prevalence of the disorder and of its natural history. The effects of treatment still are poorly understood because of the chronicity of the disorder. Studies comparing treatment modalities are necessary in order better to understand their effects on long-term outcome. More effective short-term treatments must be developed. Most important, attention should focus on the identification of vulnerable individuals and on the prevention of the disorder.

Bulimic syndromes require better diagnostic definition and understanding in order to distinguish benign from serious disorders. More effective treatments need to be developed, and the long-term outcome needs to be described.

CASE ILLUSTRATION: TYPICAL ANOREXIA NERVOSA

Laura was 13½ years old when she presented with weight loss of 9.1 kg over a 9-month period from her previous weight of 43 kg. Her height was 160.3 cm. She had become increasingly withdrawn, spending much of her time alone in her room. Her parents noted that she was skipping breakfast and eating little of her school lunch. They stated that "she has never given us a moment of grief—she has been a perfect child." An A student, she spent her time study-

ing, playing her flute, and cleaning her room. In addition, she devoted 2 hours a day to exercise. She had her first menstrual period shortly before the onset of weight loss and had had none since. She did not want to see a physician, insisting that nothing was wrong. She stated the problem was with her parents wanting her to do less homework and to watch television with the rest of the family, but she had set goals for herself. When asked about her weight, she expressed the fear of becoming fat and claimed to be as "big" as her mother and her 18-year-old sister.

She was seen several times in outpatient psychotherapy but continued to lose weight. She was then briefly hospitalized on a pediatric unit with the expectation that longer hospitalization on a psychiatric unit would be needed. Her weight dropped further to 32 kg (loss of 26% of weight). Reluctantly she began eating more in order to avoid psychiatric hospitalization. She was again seen in outpatient psychotherapy over a 6-month period and given a diet plan aimed at gradually increasing her intake and her weight. Although she continued to protest about the need for treatment, she was willing to make changes in her eating habits. At follow-up when she was 14½ years old, she had grown to 163 cm and her weight had increased to 55 kg, normal for her age. Menstrual periods had resumed 3 months earlier. She had become more spontaneous, was maturing physically, and was blossoming socially. She no longer was worried about her weight.

Comment

Many patients with anorexia nervosa can successfully be treated on an outpatient basis despite considerable weight loss and resistance to treatment. Involving the patient in her treatment by letting her monitor her own food intake allowed her to maintain control over her eating. Despite her resistance to treatment, she was able to meet expectations for weight gain, perhaps only to remain out of the hospital. Psychotherapy dealt with issues of peer relationships and her intense commitment to goals for herself.

CASE ILLUSTRATION: ATYPICAL EATING DISORDER

Sabina, age 17, was brought for evaluation by her parents because they noted she was skipping breakfast and lunch. She avoided eating with her family and was seen to eat only salads. Although she had not lost weight, her parents were sensitized to eating problems as her older sister had had severe anorexia nervosa and subsequently became obese. Sabina's height was 156 cm and always had been between the 5th and 10th percentile for age. Her weight history showed her to have been consistently near the 5th percentile. She was attractive and slender but not underweight. Menstrual periods were normal. Socially she was well adjusted. She ran 10 km three times a week and had vowed never to weigh more than 45 kg, her present weight. She admitted to inducing vomiting occasionally when she overate.

Comment

Injudicious dieting, not unusual in teenagers, had not led to actual weight loss. Educational discussion about the hazards of vomiting and meeting with a dietitian to learn about her nutritional requirements allowed Sabina to adopt a more rational pattern of eating. She was able to accept the dietary recommendations and to stop vomiting. Early brief intervention can be effective in preventing a more severe eating disorder.

References

Abell TL, Malagelada J-R, Lucas AR, et al: Gastric electromechanical and neurohormonal function in anorexia nervosa. *Gastroenterology* 93:958–965, 1987.

American Psychiatric Association: Practice guidelines for eating disorders. *Am J Psychiatry* 150: 207–228, 1993.

American Psychiatric Association: *Diagnostic and Statistical Manual of Mental Disorders* (4th ed). Washington, DC, American Psychiatric Association, 1994.

Bemis KM: Current approaches to the etiology and treatment of anorexia nervosa. *Psychol Bull* 85: 593–617, 1978.

Beumont PJV, Russell JD, Touyz SW: Treatment of anorexia nervosa. *Lancet* 341:1635–1640, 1993.

Blitzer JR, Rollins N, Blackwell A: Children who starve themselves: Anorexia nervosa. *Psychosom Med* 23:369–383, 1961.

Bruch H: *Eating Disorders: Obesity and Anorexia Nervosa.* New York, Basic Books, 1973.

Bruch H: *The Golden Cage: The Enigma of Anorexia Nervosa.* Cambridge, MA, Harvard University Press, 1978.

Bryant-Waugh R: Dealing with children and

young adolescents: Special considerations. In: Scott D (ed): *Anorexia and Bulimia Nervosa. Practical Approaches.* New York, New York University Press, 1988, pp. 192–203.

Casper RC: On the emergence of bulimia nervosa as a syndrome: A historical view. *Int J Eating Disord* 2:3–16, 1983.

Chatoor I, Egan J, Getson P, et al: Mother-infant interactions in infantile anorexia nervosa. *J Am Acad Child Adolesc Psychiatry* 27:535–540, 1988.

Crisp AH: Clinical and therapeutic aspects of anorexia nervosa—A study of 30 cases. *J Psychosom Res* 9:67–78, 1965.

Crisp AH, Harding B, McGuinness B: Anorexia nervosa: Psychoneurotic characteristics of parents: Relationship to prognosis; a quantitative study. *J Psychosom Res* 18:167–173, 1974.

Drewnowski A, Yee DK, Krahn DD: Bulimia in college women: Incidence and recovery rates. *Am J Psychiatry* 145:753–755, 1988.

Faiburn CG, Beglin SJ: Studies in the epidemiology of bulimia nervosa. *Am J Psychiatry* 147:401–408, 1990.

Fava M, Copeland PM, Schweiger U, et al: Neurochemical abnormalities of anorexia nervosa and bulimia nervosa. *Am J Psychiatry* 146:963–971, 1989.

Garner DM: Pathogenesis of anorexia nervosa. *Lancet* 341:1631–1635, 1993.

Garner DM, Bemis KM: A cognitive-behavioral approach to anorexia nervosa. *Cognit Ther Res* 6:123–150, 1982.

Garner DM, Garner MV, Rosen LR: Anorexia nervosa "restricters" who purge: Implications for subtyping anorexia nervosa. *Int J Eating Disord* 13:171–185, 1993.

Gold PW, Gwirtsman H, Avgerinos PC, et al: Abnormal hypothalamic-pituitary-adrenal function in anorexia nervosa. *N Engl J Med* 314:1335–1342, 1986.

Halmi AK: Appetite regulation in anorexia nervosa. In: Winick M (ed): *Control of Appetite.* New York, Wiley, 1988, pp. 125–135.

Herzog DB, Keller MB, Lavori PW: Outcome in anorexia nervosa and bulimia nervosa. *J Nerv Ment Dis* 176:131–143, 1988.

Holland AJ, Hall A, Murray R, et al: Anorexia nervosa: A study of 34 twin pairs and one set of triplets. *Br J Psychiatry* 145:414–419, 1984.

Holland AJ, Sicotte N, Treasure J: Anorexia nervosa: Evidence for a genetic basis. *J Psychosom Res* 32:561–571, 1988.

Hsu LKG: *Eating Disorders.* New York, Guilford, 1990.

Hudson JI, Pope HG, Jonas JM, et al: Pharmacologic relationship of eating disorders to major affective disorders. *Psychiatr Res* 9:345–354, 1983.

Jaffe AC, Singer LT: Atypical eating disorders in young children. *Int J Eating Disord* 8:575–582, 1989.

Johnson C, Lewis C, Hagman J: The syndrome of bulimia: Review and synthesis. *Psychiatr Clin North Am* 7:247–273, 1984.

Kaplan AS, Woodside DB: Biological aspects of anorexia nervosa and bulimia nervosa. *J Consult Psychol* 55:645–653, 1987.

Kaye WH, Berrettini W, Gwirtsman H, et al: Altered cerebrospinal neuropeptide Y and peptide YY immunoreactivity in anorexia and bulimia nervosa. *Arch Gen Psychiatry* 47:548–556, 1990.

Leon GR, Fulkerson JA, Perry CL, et al: Personality and behavioral vulnerabilities associated with risk status for eating disorders in adolescent girls. *J Abnorm Psychol* 102:438–444, 1993.

Lesser LI, Ashenden BJ, Debuskey M, et al: Anorexia nervosa in children. *Am J Orthopsychiatry* 30:572–580, 1960.

Lucas AR: Toward the understanding of anorexia nervosa as a disease entity. *Mayo Clin Proc* 56:254–264, 1981.

Lucas AR, Callaway CW: Anorexia nervosa and bulimia. In: Berk JE, Haubrich WS, Kaiser MH, et al (eds): *Bockus Gastroenterology* (Vol 7, 4th ed). Philadelphia, Saunders, 1985, pp. 4416–4434.

Lucas AR, Duncan JW, Piens V: The treatment of anorexia nervosa. *Am J Psychiatry* 133:1034–1038, 1976.

Lucas AR, Beard CM, O'Fallon WM, et al: 50-year trends in the incidence of anorexia nervosa in Rochester, Minn.: A population-based study. *Am J Psychiatry* 148:917–922, 1991.

Minuchin S, Rosman BL, Baker L: *Psychosomatic Families: Anorexia Nervosa in Context.* Cambridge, MA, Harvard University Press, 1978.

Nielsen S: Seasonal variation in anorexia nervosa? Some preliminary findings from a neglected area of research. *Int J Eating Disord* 11:25–35, 1992.

Palmer RL, Oppenheimer R: Childhood sexual experiences with adults: A comparison of women with eating disorders and those with other diagnoses. *Int J Eating Disord* 12:359–364, 1992.

Råstam M: Anorexia nervosa in 51 Swedish adolescents: Premorbid problems and comorbidity. *J Am Acad Child Adolesc Psychiatry* 31:819–829, 1992.

Russell G: Bulimia nervosa: An ominous variant of anorexia nervosa. *Psychol Med* 9:429–448, 1979.

Russell GFM: Anorexia nervosa: Its identity as an illness and its treatment. In: Price JH (ed): *Modern Trends in Psychological Medicine* (Vol 2). London, Butterworth, 1970, pp. 131–164.

Russell GFM: Anorexia and bulimia nervosa. In: Rutter M, Hersov L (eds): *Child and Adolescent Psychiatry: Modern Approaches* (2nd ed). Oxford, Blackwell, 1985, pp. 625–637.

Selvini Palazzoli M: *Self-starvation: From Individual to Family Therapy in the Treatment of Anorexia Nervosa.* (Pomerans A, trans). New York, Aronson, 1978.

Silverman JA: Medical consequences of starvation: The malnutrition of anorexia nervosa: Caveat medicus. In: Darby PL, Garfinkel PE, Garner DM, et al (eds): *Anorexia Nervosa: Recent Developments in Research.* New York, Liss, 1983, pp. 293–299.

Soundy TJ, Lucas AR, Suman VJ, et al: Bulimia nervosa in Rochester, Minnesota, 1980 to 1990. *Psychol Med* 25:1065–1071, 1995.

Strober M: The significance of bulimia in juvenile anorexia nervosa: An exploration of possible etiologic factors. *Int J Eating Disord* 1:28–43, 1981.

Strober M, Lampert C, Morrell W, et al: A controlled family study of anorexia nervosa: Evidence of familial aggregation and lack of shared transmission with affective disorders. *Int J Eating Disord* 9:239–253, 1990.

Theander S: Outcome and prognosis in anorexia nervosa and bulimia: Some results of previous investigations, compared with those of a Swedish long-term study. *J Psychiatr Res* 19:493–508, 1985.

Timmerman MG, Wells LA, Chen S: Bulimia nervosa and associated alcohol abuse among secondary school students. *J Am Acad Child Adolesc Psychiatry* 29:118–122, 1990.

Tolstrup K, Brinch M, Isager T, et al: Long-term outcome of 151 cases of anorexia nervosa: The Copenhagen Anorexia Nervosa Follow-up Study. *Acta Psychiatr Scand* 71:380–387, 1985.

Yates A: Current perspectives in the eating disorders. I: History, psychological and biological aspects. *J Am Acad Child Adolesc Psychiatry* 28:813–828, 1989.

54 MODERN APPROACHES TO ENURESIS AND ENCOPRESIS

Edwin J. Mikkelsen, M.D.

ENURESIS

Definition and Historical Note

Enuresis is subclassified into two subtypes, primary and secondary. *Primary enuresis* encompasses children who have never achieved continence, while the term *secondary enuresis* refers to those children who maintain continence for at least 1 year, only to lose it at some point after that. The term itself is derived from the Greek *enourein*, "to void urine," and has come to imply nocturnal events, although that connotation is not inherent in the derivation of the word itself.

There is a rich literature concerning enuresis and its treatment over the centuries. In retrospect, many of these treatment approaches now appear to have been quite sadistic. This history has been summarized in an excellent review by Glicklich, which covers material dating back to the Papyrus Ebers of 1550 B.C. (Glicklich, 1951).

Prevalence and Epidemiology

Statistics concerning the prevalence of enuresis also must take into account the severity of the disorder. For example, in the Isle of Wight Study, Rutter found that 15.2% of boys were wet less often than once a week, while only 6.7% wet at least once a week. The corresponding figures for girls were 12.2 and 3.3%. By age 14 only 1.9% of boys were wet less often than once a week, and 1.1% were wetting at least once a week, with the corresponding figures for girls being 1.2 and 0.5% (Rutter et al., 1973). Longitudinal data from the Isle of Wight Study have illustrated that many children develop wetting between the ages of 5 and 7. Enuresis was also found in greater frequency in children who were undergoing psychosocial stress and in those living in socially disadvantaged circumstances (Rutter, 1989).

A Scandinavian study of 3206 7-year-old children found an overall prevalence of 9.8%; 6.4% of this group was accounted for by children with night wetting, 1.8% by day wetters, and 1.6% by those with mixed day and night wetting. This study also showed a strong genetic influence in that the risk of a child's having enuresis was 7.1 times greater if the father manifested enuresis after 4 and 5.2 times greater if the mother did (Jarvelin et al., 1988).

An 8-year longitudinal study in New Zealand found a prevalence of 7.4% for nocturnal enuresis in 8-year-olds. This figure was accounted for by 3.3% with primary enuresis and 4.1% with secondary enuresis (Fergusson et al., 1986).

Clinical Description

As noted above, the term *enuresis* itself denotes only the voiding of urine. Over the years the term has acquired both a pathological and a nocturnal connotation. Daytime wetting is correctly referred to as diurnal enuresis, while nighttime wetting is referred to as nocturnal enuresis.

The DSM-IV (1994) defines functional enuresis as "repeated voiding of urine during the day or at night into bed or clothes." DSM-IV goes on to note that "to qualify for a diagnosis of enuresis, the voiding of urine must occur at least twice per week for at least 3 months or else must cause clinically significant distress or impairment in social, academic (occupational) or other important areas of functioning." The child must also have reached an age at which continence could definitively be expected. DSM-IV utilizes a chronological age of 5 as a cutoff or a mental age of 5 for those children with developmental delays. DSM-IV also stipulates that the wetting not be the result of "the direct physiological effects of a substance (e.g., diuretics) or a general medical condition (e.g., diabetes, spina bifida, a seizure disorder)." Three subtypes of enuresis are defined: nocturnal only (nighttime wetting), diurnal only (daytime wetting), and nocturnal and diurnal (mixed day and night wetting). A distinction is also made between "primary" and "secondary" enuresis. Primary enuresis refers to those children who have never achieved urinary continence while secondary enuresis refers to those children who have achieved continence and then lost it. The period of continence necessary to differentiate between primary and secondary enuresis had variously been thought to be 6 months to 1 year. DSM-IV does not put forward a precise period of time for the distinction but instead makes reference to "a secondary type in which the disturbance develops after a period of established urinary continence." A child is not considered to have primary functional enuresis until age 5. Secondary enuresis can begin at any time, once the criterion of initial continence has been fulfilled, but the usual onset is between ages 5 and 7 (Rutter, 1989).

Etiology and Pathogenesis

The physiological manifestations of this disorder have led to a wide range of etiological theories. A primary focus of these studies has naturally been the anatomy of the bladder and urinary tract. Shaffer et al. (1984) elegantly combined an investigation of bladder anatomy and physiology with the covariable of behavioral disturbance. One might intuitively expect that children with dysfunctional or abnormal bladders would be those without a concomitant behavioral disorder to explain their enuresis, and that those whose enuresis could be explained on the basis of psychopathology would have normal bladders. The results were

counterintuitive in that those children who were behaviorally disturbed also had significantly lower functional bladder volumes and more developmental delays (Shaffer et al., 1987). Thus, while not providing a parsimonious explanation to differentiate the etiology of enuretic events between psychiatrically disturbed and nondisturbed children with enuresis, the study did lend further support to a theory of general developmental delay, which would explain both the enuresis and the high frequency of behavioral disturbance. Children with enuresis were found to have developmental delays twice as often as those without in a large longitudinal population study (Essen and Peckham, 1976). A study that compared 35 otherwise healthy children with enuresis with a control group found that the bone age of the children with enuresis displayed a significant lag behind chronological age, leading the authors to speculate about delayed maturation of central nervous system regulatory functions (Mimouni et al., 1985).

There is an obvious relationship between enuresis and bladder infection (Hansson, 1992); thus, an infection of the urogenital tract should be ruled out before a diagnosis of functional enuresis is made. This is especially important for girls, who are more prone to urinary tract infections (Hjalmas, 1992).

The possibility of urinary tract obstruction as a widespread cause of enuresis has been reported (Mahony, 1971) but has been criticized, as such a hypothesis can lead to unnecessary surgery (Smith, 1969). After extensively reviewing the literature on this subject, Shaffer (1985) concluded, "There is no evidence that urethral dilatation or bladder neck repair are effective treatment for enuresis." The only exception to this would be if there are very specific pathophysiological findings.

The nature of the enuretic phenomenon has naturally led to speculation concerning a psychodynamic etiology. These hypotheses have in general evolved from case reports or have been derived from theoretical considerations. There has been one rigorous attempt to define the generalizations derived from the literature regarding enuresis and encopresis and then to determine with what frequency these generalizations were born out by an analysis of the clinical material. This elegant study by Achenbach and Lewis (1971) revealed that "only two of the twenty-four generalizations derived from the literature regarding encopresis and enuresis received support at the conventional level (probability = .05) of statistical significance."

Epidemiological studies have, however, shown a correlation between psychological disturbance and enuresis, which is more pronounced in older children (Rutter, 1989). This observation then raises the question of the nature of the relationship: Is it a causal, incidental, or secondary relationship? The aforementioned link between enuresis and developmental delays, which are also linked to psychopathology, would suggest that there is a common underlying maturational factor that predisposes vulnerable children to manifest both behavioral disturbances and enuresis. In further support of this hypothesis are the observations that the nature of the behavioral disturbance in children with enuresis is nonspecific (Mikkelsen et al., 1980) and that no physiological marker can be found that reliably differentiates psychologically disturbed from nondisturbed children with enuresis (Mikkelsen and Rapoport, 1980; Shaffer et al., 1984). When children with enuresis have been compared to other children attending a child psychiatric clinic, the only discernible differences were an increased frequency of developmental delays and a lesser frequency of eating disorders and specific neurotic patterns (Steinhausen and Gobel, 1989). The association with behavioral disturbance is greater for secondary enuresis (Feehan et al., 1990; McGee et al., 1984).

One study that specifically evaluated risk factors for developing secondary enuresis found that delayed attainment of initial nocturnal continence and exposure to four or more stressful life events in a year were significantly related to the development of secondary enuresis (Fergusson et al., 1990).

The occurrence of the enuretic episodes during sleep naturally led to a series of studies investigating the relationship between sleep states and the occurrence of enuretic events. The earliest of these studies suggested that the enuretic events occurred in "deep sleep" and led to a theory that enuretic events were dream equivalents (Pierce et al., 1961). This theory was subsequently supplanted by Broughton's (1968; Gastaut and Broughton, 1964) view that enuresis was a disorder of arousal. This research suggested that enuretic episodes were preceded by arousal signals and originated in delta sleep. A further elaboration of this theory held that psychiatrically disturbed children with enuresis received normal arousal signals but did not respond to them, while those without psychiatric disturbance did not generate arousal signals (Ritvo et al., 1969). The largest and most convincing sleep studies indicate that enuretic episodes occur in each sleep stage in proportion to the time spent in that stage, when time of night is also considered (Kales et al., 1977; Mikkelsen et al., 1980). Recent research in this area has focused on combining sleep studies with cystometry (Norgaard et al., 1989). This work may lead to the identification of subtypes of children with enuresis (Watanabe and Azuma, 1989).

The development of desmopressin acetate as a treatment for enuresis (see below) has led to the observation that some children with enuresis do not have the ability to concentrate the urine they produce during the night and reduce urine volume (Miller et al., 1992). In a further investigation of this hypothesis, Rittig et al. (1991) compared the circadian variation of plasma atrial natriuretic peptide (ANP) and in relation to the clearance of creatinine and the excretion of sodium and potassium. Subjects in the study consisted of 15 children with nocturnal enuresis and 11 control subjects matched for age, sex, and weight. The children with enuresis did not differ from control subjects with regard to ANP, but during the first hours of sleep they did manifest significantly more polyuria, natriuresis, and kaliuresis despite normal levels of ANP. The authors concluded that children with enuresis display abnormal diurnal rhythmicity in the urinary excretion of potassium and sodium that is not correlated with plasma levels of ANP. They speculate that the abnormalities in sodium and potassium may be related to abnormal tubular handling. Steffens et al. (1993) have used a radioimmunoassay to evaluate the circadian rhythmicity of plasma arginine vasopressin (AVP) in 55 children with enuresis and 15 control subjects. The AVP levels were measured under conditions of controlled water intake three times per day for 72 hours. Only 14 of the 55 children with enuresis had a significant decrease in AVP when compared with control subjects. Nine of these 14 AVP-deficient children were subsequently found to be totally dry with desmopressin acetate (DDAVP) treatment.

Laboratory Studies

The fact that urinary tract infections can precipitate enuretic events in children means that a urinalysis should be performed to rule out this readily treatable cause of enuresis.

The use of more invasive and painful studies remains controversial. While it is certainly possible that altered bladder physiology may lead to primary enuresis, the yield from these studies does not appear to be of sufficient magnitude to warrant subjecting all children with enuresis to these studies. A thorough review of this subject has been performed by Cohen (1975) who found the incidence of obstructive lesions in children with enuresis to be 3.7% in a primary care pediatric setting. Accordingly, he suggested that "contrast studies are indicated only when there is significant evidence of anatomical or functional pathology by history or exam." Subsequent studies have supported this general position (Blickman and Schimmelpenninck-Scheiffers, 1984), while suggesting that those children with daytime wetting and overt symptoms of voiding disturbance are more apt to have urinary tract abnormalities than those who wet solely at night (Jarvelin et al., 1990).

Differential Diagnosis

The differential diagnosis includes the possibility of urinary tract infection and altered bladder physiology. There are scattered case reports of enuresis being secondary to other primary medical problems, such as hyperthyroidism (Stoffer, 1988), constipation (Oregari et al., 1986), and central hormonal abnormalities (Kikuchi et al., 1989). While such reports are infrequent, the clinician should do a thorough physical examination and consider the possibility of underlying organic illness. Psychological testing in conjunction with structured interviews may provide further insight into the coexistence of psychopathology. However, the studies reviewed above would suggest that any coexisting psychological disorder should be viewed as an accompanying finding rather than as a causal effect.

The distinction between primary and secondary enuresis can be made by history.

Treatment

While psychotherapy may be helpful for managing the behavioral disorders that accompany enuresis, it appears to have little effect on primary enuresis itself, with recent studies showing a success rate of 20%, which may largely be accounted for by spontaneous remission (Cohen, 1975). Psychotherapy may be more useful for those children with secondary enuresis, especially those whose episodes begin after a traumatic event or parental divorce.

The two primary means of treating children with enuresis fall into the categories of behavioral methods and psychopharmacological methods.

Behavioral treatment should be attempted first because it is generally more innocuous than pharmacological intervention. This assumes that the underlying assumption of the behavioral strategy is that it is helping children with enuresis and their families master an affliction rather than tacitly implying that the children are either consciously or unconsciously causing the wetting themselves. One unfortunate consequence of various reward-punishment strategies is that they can subtly imply to children and their families that the disorder is quasi-volitional. The bell and pad method of conditioning is a reasonable first approach. In reviewing the results of several studies involving over 1000 children, Werry (1966) found a success rate of 75%. Recent studies are consistent with this (Berg et al., 1982; Devlin, 1990). Psychiatric disorder in the child and family stress appear to be negative prognostic factors when predicating outcome with this modality (Devlin, 1990). An investigation into the effectiveness of a simple bell and pad method as opposed to two variations that had more behavioral embellishments found no statistical difference between the modalities. However, one variation that included reward contingencies tended to have a slightly lower rate of relapse than the bell and pad alone (Kaplan et al., 1989). As noted above, whenever reward-punishment contingencies are considered, it is extremely important to ensure that one is not communicating to the parents and child that the disorder is quasi-volitional. Although their frequency has decreased with improved bell and pad technology, reports of "buzzer ulcers" do continue to appear, and parents should be alerted to this (Diez and Berger, 1988).

An attempt has been made to investigate the relationship between bladder capacity and response to behavioral treatment. A study involving 50 children who were wet at least two nights a week found that children with small pretreatment maximal functional bladder capacities did better with the bell and pad method in conjunction with retention-control training, while the children with larger bladder capacities responded to the bell and pad method alone. However, it should be noted that this was a qualitative difference in response, as 92.5% of the 40 children who completed the study met the outcome criteria of 14 consecutive dry nights, regardless of which group they were in (Geffken et al., 1986). A similar study that examined the impact of bladder capacity on response to the bell and pad system found no association with outcome (Berg et at., 1982). Interestingly, both of these investigations indicated that behavioral disturbance was related to failure to respond to conditioning techniques (Berg et al., 1982; Geffken et al., 1986).

The Australian psychiatrist, MacLean, first described the efficacy of imipramine for nocturnal enuresis in 1960. Since that time, there have been over 40 double-blind studies confirming the efficacy of imipramine for nocturnal enuresis, while results with other classes of psychotropic agents have generally been equivocal or negative (Blackwell and Currah, 1973). Lack of response to imipramine can often be traced to the reluctance of primary care physicians to exceed dosages of 25–50 mg. Nevertheless, it is reasonable to begin at a dose of 25 mg and to titrate up slowly, since some children will respond to the lower dosages. Allowing 4–7 days between dosage increments will make it possible to detect these low-dose responders. Most children will respond in the 75- to 125-mg range. The upper range of dosage is determined by the child's weight, with the standard upper limit being 5 mg/kg. A baseline ECG should be obtained before instituting treatment with imipramine, and monitoring is advised above 3.5 mg/kg (Mikkelsen and Rapoport, 1980). A case of sudden death has been reported in a girl receiving 14.7 mg/kg for school phobia (Robinson and Barker, 1976).

The relatively high rate of spontaneous remission in enuresis mitigates against keeping children on medication for long periods of time. A practical approach is to slowly taper and discontinue the imipramine every 3 months. If wetting resumes as the dosage is tapered or after it is discontinued, then the dosage can simply be titrated back up to the effective dose for another 3-month period. It has been the author's impression that more children will not experience a reactivation of the enuresis after a 3-month period of imipramine treatment than can be accounted for by spontaneous remission alone, but this has not been statistically proven.

There have been tragic reports of children who reasoned that if three pills would stop the wetting for a night, then taking the whole bottle should stop it permanently. Thus, it is important to warn parents about the magical thinking of children in this regard and the importance of controlling the medication. Younger siblings are also at risk of overdosing with the medication if it is not controlled. In cases of mild to moderate overdose, supportive measures, including the symptomatic management of seizures and cardiac arrhythmias, may be sufficient. Physostigmine may also be useful in more severe overdoses (Greene, 1981).

There have been five studies investigating the relationship between blood level of imipramine and clinical response. One study found no correlation between improvement in enuresis and the blood level of imipramine either alone or in conjunction with its metabolites (DeVane et al., 1984). However, three studies have now demonstrated a significant correlation between the diminution of enuretic events and the steady-state concentrations of imipramine plus its metabolite desipramine (de Gatta et al., 1984, 1990; Jorgensen et al., 1980; Rapoport et al., 1980). One of these studies found an optimal effect when the combined steady-state imipramine plus desipramine concentrations were above 60 mg/liter (Jorgensen et al., 1980), and another reported favorable outcome when steady-state combined levels were greater than 80 ng/ml (de Gatta et al., 1984). The most recent study in this line of investigation (Fritz et al., 1994) evaluated the blood level-efficacy equation in 18 children who after baseline and placebo received increasing dosages of imipramine at 2-week intervals. The specific dosages utilized were 1.0, 1.5, 2.0, and 2.5 mg/kg. They found that efficacy was "moderately but significantly" related to increasing dose. However, there was tremendous (700%) variation in serum levels between the individual children at every dosage level. There is a good correlation between side effects and blood level, especially dry mouth (Rapoport et al., 1980). This may prove clinically useful in monitoring children who are extremely phobic about having their blood drawn.

As noted previously, the efficacy of imipramine for enuresis does not imply that it should be the first intervention attempted. Nonpunitive behavioral techniques should definitely be the first approach considered, with pharmacotherapy being reserved for those who do not respond to behavioral interventions. Survey studies, however, tend to indicate that in clinical practice medication is more apt to be used than behavioral interventions (Devlin, 1991). A large population-based study found that only 38% of children with enuresis had seen a physician. Over one-third of this physician-treated group had been prescribed some form of

pharmacotherapy, and only 3% had been advised to utilize the bell and pad conditioning technique. This study also revealed that over half of the children were psychologically distressed by the enuresis, and two-thirds of the parents expressed concern (Foxman et al., 1986). Fortunately, effective treatment of the enuresis does improve the child's self-concept (Moffat et al., 1987). Throughout the literature there are also reports of novel treatment approaches such as acupuncture (Capozza et al., 1991; Minni et al., 1990; Roje-Starcevic, 1990), a prostaglandin synthesis inhibitor (Metin and Aykol, 1992), an anticholinergic calcium antagonist (Elmer et al., 1991), the oral synthetic androgen mesterolone (el-Sadr et al., 1990), and hypnosis (Banerjee et al., 1993). Although many of these studies are controlled, the use of these approaches in enuresis should still be considered experimental.

The newest research into pharmacotherapy for enuresis involves the use of DDAVP. Moffat et al. (1993) have reviewed all of the existing controlled studies concerning the use of DDAVP for enuresis. In the process, they located 18 randomized controlled trials (eleven crossover and seven parallel), which included a total of 689 subjects, most of whom had been refractory to prior treatment. The decreased frequency of enuretic events in the study ranged from 10 to 91%. In general, wetting resumes once the medication is discontinued. Those studies that reported long-term follow-up indicated that 5.7% remained dry after stopping the medication. The most common side effects were nasal stuffiness, headache, epistaxis, and mild abdominal pain. Positive prognostic factors appear to be fewer initial (pretreatment) wet nights and age greater than 9 years. A recent study has suggested that positive family history may also be a favorable prognostic sign. Hogg and Husmann (1993) and Terho (1991) particularly looked at the efficacy of DDVAP for children who had been refractory to conditioning treatment and imipramine, using a randomized double-blind placebo controlled crossover study. Of the 52 children studied (age range 5–13), 53% had a complete cessation of wetting, 19% were partial responders, and 28% had no or minimal response. The dosages used ranged from 20 to 40 μg (intranasal), and response did not persist after termination of treatment. In a 5-year retrospective review of 59 children, Key et al. (1992) have suggested that lower doses may be just as effective. In their series 5 μg at bedtime was the initial starting dose and 81% improved on less than 10 μg. A single-blind study did reveal a dose response phenomenon (Fjellestad-Paulsen et al., 1987).

A study investigating the differential response of children with enuresis to DDAVP and the bell and pad method of conditioning found that 70% improved with the DDAVP and 86% improved with the alarm method, yielding nonsignificant differences (Wille, 1986). A similar experiment that compared the therapeutic benefits of desmopressin in combination with the bell and pad to placebo found that the combination of desmopressin and the alarm resulted in significantly more dry nights (Sukhai et al., 1989). A follow-up study of children receiving long-term treatment (mean, 13 months) with DDAVP revealed no hormonal or hematological side effects, and it was concluded that treatment of this duration was safe (Rew and Rundle, 1989). However, there have been recent reports of hyponatremia (Kallio et al., 1993) and hyponatremic seizures (Beach et al., 1992; Yaouyanc et al., 1992) with intranasal use of DDAVP.

In general, these studies indicate that older children are more apt to respond to desmopressin and that relapse usually occurs after cessation of treatment. Nevertheless, DDAVP should be considered for those children who have been refractory to other approaches.

Outcome and Follow-up

The natural history of primary enuresis must be taken into account in any treatment plan, whether it be primarily behavioral or pharmacological. There is a high rate of spontaneous remission between the ages of 5 and 7 and again after age 12. Accordingly, one might want to wait until after age 7 before instituting pharmacological treatment, unless other factors indicate otherwise. Similarly, the strong possibility of spontaneous remission should be considered in any positive treatment response after age 10 or 11.

Pharmacological studies have indicated that treatment with imipramine can result in three subtypes of response. There are true responders who have a sustained response, and there are also true nonresponders. There is also a surprisingly large group of transient responders. These children have an initial response to imipramine and then lose it over 2–3 weeks. When the dosage is increased by another 25 mg, they again respond for another 2–3 weeks. Eventually, the dosage required to maintain a response becomes prohibitive. While long-term treatment with imipramine is not an option for these children, imipramine can still be used for brief socially important periods, such as camp, as the initial response can be recaptured after a medication-free period of time (Rapoport et al., 1980).

Behavioral approaches assume that learning takes place to produce the cessation of wetting and thus should theoretically be a self-limited intervention.

Areas for Future Research

The phenomenon of enuresis has been actively studied for years. The sleep research reviewed above indicates that the episodes occur relatively randomly throughout the night. Recent investigations have attempted to correlate sleep studies with ongoing assessment of bladder physiology (Norgaard et al., 1989; Robert et al., 1993; Watanabe and Azuma, 1989). While psychopathology is related to enuresis, it is not specifically so and certainly is not causal. Thus, further research into this area may prove fruitful. Investigations into bladder physiology and anatomy in conjunction with other variables has shown some promise (Ringertz, 1984) and would appear worthy of further investigation. Central nervous system (Ambrosini, 1984; Ambrosini and Fried, 1984) and neuroendocrine (Norgaard et al., 1985; Rittig et al., 1989) factors remain the frontiers of research in this area. The exciting new research with DDAVP and the related physiological studies described above would seem to point to a multifactorial pathogenesis (Djurhuus et al., 1992) and/or the existence of subtypes that have similar clinical presentations but differing etiologies.

CASE ILLUSTRATION

John is an 8-year-old boy with primary enuresis. He wets the bed an average of three to four nights per week. At age 5 his pediatrician found no psychological explanation for the enuresis. The family elected to wait on treatment for a few years to see if John would spontaneously remit. The family handled the wetting in a matter-of-fact manner, with John changing the bed each morning. However, the wetting was now beginning to become a social problem for John, as it interfered with his plans to sleep overnight with friends and was an embarrassment at summer camp. Accordingly, the family sought treatment, and their pediatrician recommended the bell and pad method of conditioning. John did not rapidly respond to the bell and pad, and it was quite disruptive for the family as they lived in a small house and John shared a room with his younger brother. At this point the pediatrician decided that medication might be warranted, and he referred the family to a child psychiatrist with whom he was familiar. After receiving medical clearance from the pediatrician and discussing side effects with the family, the child psychiatrist prescribed imipramine 25 mg at night and titrated the dosage up by 25 mg every 4–5 days. John responded at 75 mg with a complete cessation of wetting. The child psychiatrist would taper and discontinue the imipramine every 3 months. During the first such tapering process, John developed breakthrough wetting at 25 mg, and the dosage was returned to 75 mg with good results. Three months later the imipramine was again tapered. On this occasion there was no resumption of wetting as the imipramine was decreased, and it appeared that John's enuresis had now spontaneously resolved.

Comment

Was John's remission spontaneous or due to the imipramine treatment? There is no firm indication that a period of treatment with imipramine will lead to cessation of enuresis after the medication is removed; thus, John most likely had a spontaneous remission.

If John had been a transient responder to imipramine, could it still have been of benefit to him? Yes. Transient responders will usually respond for 2–3 weeks after medication is started, and this response can be recaptured after a period of time off the medication. The enuresis was particularly embarrassing for John when he attended summer camp, and imipramine may have been beneficial to him for those discrete periods of time.

If John had not responded to imipramine, what would have been the next step? The family could have been asked to try the bell and pad method for a longer period of time. Alternatively, the child psychiatrist could discuss with the pediatrician a possible trial of desmopressin.

ENCOPRESIS

Definition

Encopresis is defined by DSM-IV (1994) as the "repeated passage of feces into inappropriate places." The manual goes on to note that the soiling must occur at least once a month for at least 3 months and that the mental and/or chronological age of the child must be at least 4 years. Physical disorders must, of course, be ruled out. If there has been a period of fecal continence preceding the recurrence of soiling, it is classified as secondary encopresis.

DSM-IV also denotes two subtypes of encopresis, which it labels as "with constipation and overflow incontinence" and "without constipation and overflow incontinence." The former category roughly corresponds to what has been referred to in the literature as retentive encopresis while the latter would correspond to what has been known as nonretentive encopresis.

Prevalence and Epidemiology

A study involving 8863 children found a frequency of 1.5% among children between 7 and 8 years of age, with a male:female ratio of over 3:1 (Bellman, 1966). In the Isle of Wight Study, Rudder found that 1.3% of boys between the ages of 10 to 12 soiled at least once a month, with the corresponding figure for girls being 0.3%. That study also found a significant relationship between enuresis and encopresis (Rutter et al., 1981).

Clinical Description

Encopresis has been classified in different ways. As noted above, DSM-IV makes a distinction between primary and secondary encopresis and has added subtypes that denote the distinction between retentive and nonretentive encopresis. Retentive encopresis is characterized by a cycle of several days of retention, a painful expulsion, and another period of retention. While the fecal mass is growing, there may be leakage around the mass. The category of nonretentive encopresis applies to those children who simply do not control the expulsion of feces on either a psychological, physiological, or combined basis.

Hersov (1985) has proposed three categories: (*a*) children who have adequate bowel control and volitionally deposit feces in inappropriate places; (*b*) children who either are unaware that they are soiling or are aware but unable to control the process; and (*c*) situations where the soiling is due to excessive fluid, which may be caused by diarrhea, anxiety, or the retentive overflow process described above. The last mechanism is responsible for approximately 75% of this category.

Etiology and Pathogenesis

There have been extensive investigations into the physiological basis for encopresis. Loening-Baucke (1987) found that 56% of children with retentive encopresis were unable to defecate rectal balloons, and most of these children had abnormal contractions of the external anal sphincter. This study also had prognostic significance in that only 14% of those who were unable to defecate the rectal balloons had responded to treatment after 1 year, whereas 64% of those who could defecate the balloons recovered after 1 year. Similarly, only 13% of patients who were unable to relax the anal sphincter at initial evaluation were improved 1 year later, while the corresponding figure for those who could relax the sphincter was 70%. Interestingly, none of the patients who presented with an abdominal fecal mass at the time of the initial evaluation showed improvement 1 year later, regardless of ability to defecate the rectal balloons. Constipated children were subsequently compared to control subjects on a wide range of physiological measures during the act of bearing down (Loening-Baucke et al., 1986). These studies revealed that the act of bearing down led to decreased anal sphincter activity in 100% of control children, 58% of constipated children who were able to defecate a rectal balloon, and 7% of those constipated children who were unable to defecate the balloon. The latter group were significantly less likely to respond to conventional laxative treatment, and the authors concluded that the increased external sphincter activity could relate to their chronic fecal retention and encopresis. A companion study (Loening-Baucke et al., 1987) investigated the social competence and behavioral profiles of 38 children with encopresis and correlated these variables with the physiological variables of anal-rectal manometric and electromyographic evaluations as they related to treatment outcome. The study found that social competence and behavioral rating scores were not significantly different between those boys who were or were not able to defecate the balloons. The behavioral problem ratings were also similar in both physiological subgroups of girls. Interestingly, the social competence score of the girls who could not defecate the balloons was lower than that of those who could. The follow-up data indicated that the behavioral and social competence scores did not correlate with successful outcome at 6-month and 1-year follow-up, but there was a significant negative correlation between positive outcome in the inability to defecate the balloon and the inability to relax the sphincter. Thus, the physiological variables were predictive of outcome, and the psychological variables were not.

A similar study at a different center concluded that a significant number of boys with encopresis have abnormalities of the anal-rectal expulsion dynamics but the researchers could not find abnormalities of anal-rectal sensory or motor function (Wald et al., 1986).

The dramatic nature of the soiling incident has naturally led to psychodynamic speculation. Bemporad and Hallowell (1987) have identified a "small number" of children with intractable encopresis for which they have proposed the term *chronic neurotic encopresis*. The characteristics of these children were (*a*) history of neurological delay, (*b*) early or harsh bowel training, and (*c*) a distant father and a neurotic mother.

Environmental factors have been noted for some time and include the observations of Freud and Burlingham (1943), who noted a high frequency of soiling and wetting in children separated from their parents during World War II.

At least two studies revealed no correlation between social class and soiling (Rutter et al., 1981; Stein and Susser, 1967).

Laboratory Studies

The physiological studies described above must be considered research investigations and not the representation of a usual and customary workup. However, they do suggest that a more detailed physiological investigation than is usually done may be warranted. Usually, once the more obvious physiological problems, such as Hirschsprung's disease, are ruled out, the problem is considered to be psychogenic.

One of the most important investigations may well be a thorough history that documents the frequency, nature, and circumstances of the soiling events in great detail. This history should be elicited both from the parents and from the child.

Psychological testing and evaluation will be important in providing a thorough picture of the child, but it remains difficult to know if concomitant psychological problems are associated, causal, or secondary.

Differential Diagnosis

The differential diagnosis of encopresis must take into account that the soiling can be either a symptom of another problem or the primary problem itself. For example, historically encopresis and enuresis have been reported to occur under stress in normal children and to remit when the stressor is removed. Similarly, in children who are retarded or significantly developmentally delayed, the encopresis may be only one expression of the primary problem. Children who are impulsive and hyperactive may have occasional episodes of encopresis simply because they do not attend to the stimuli until it is too late. Thus, the symptom of encopresis must be viewed within the context of the child's larger psychological and environmental profile. Strictly medical causes, such as Hirschsprung's disease, stenosis of the rectum or anus, smooth muscle disease, and endocrine abnormalities, should also be ruled out.

Treatment

The most accepted first line of treatment is one that encompasses educational, psychological, and behavioral approaches. As outlined by Levine (1982), this approach entails an initial meeting that is designed to educate both the parents and child about bowel function and to diffuse the psychological tension that may have developed in the family around the encopresis. This educational and psychological intervention is then followed by an initial bowel catharsis, after which the child receives daily doses of laxatives or mineral oil. There is also a behavioral component to the treatment, which consists of daily timed intervals on the toilet with rewards for success. A 78% success rate has been reported for this approach, without symptom substitution (Levine and Bakow, 1976; Levine et al., 1980).

Stark et al. (1990) studied the efficacy of group treatment with an educational and behavioral focus in 18 children (ages 4–11) who had not responded to medical management. The groups were composed of three to five families and met for six sessions. The results indicated that posttreatment fiber consummation was increased 40%, appropriate toileting increased by 116%, and the frequency of soiling accidents decreased by 83%. The improvements were sustained at 6-month follow-up.

The adjunctive use of oral laxatives and conditional rectal cathartics has also been investigated (Sprague-McRae et al., 1993). Specifically, the authors compared the results obtained with children who were all treated with a high fiber diet, initial bowel evacuation, behavior modification program, and random assignment to either oral laxatives (N = 24) or conditioning rectal cathartics (N = 37). Only 61 of 136 patients evaluated completed treatment and thus there was a high dropout rate. No significant outcome difference was found between the two groups and 87% continued in remission at 6- to 12-month follow-up. Nolan et al. (1990) used a random allocation design to compare combined treatment with laxatives and behavior modification (N = 83) to behavior modification alone (N = 86). At 12-month follow-up, 51% of the combined therapy group had at least one 4-week period without an encopretic episode as compared with 36% of the behavior modification group. After the authors excluded children with poor compliance, there was no statistical difference between groups although the authors maintain that from a clinical perspective use of laxatives combined with behavior modification was superior to behavior modification alone.

Loening-Baucke (1990) has expanded on the pathophysiological studies described above by exploring the utility of biofeedback training in children with abnormal defecation dynamics. Specifically, patients (ages 5–16) were randomly assigned to traditional medical treatment alone (N = 19) or conventional treatment plus up to six biofeedback sessions. Eighty-six percent of the biofeedback group had learned normal defecation dynamics at the conclusion of biofeedback treatment. At 7-month follow-up, 77% of the biofeedback group had normal defecation dynamics as opposed to only 13% of the conventionally treated ($P < .01$). The improvement in defecation dynamics was correlated with clinical improvement at 12 months (16% with conventional treatment and 50% with biofeedback, $P < .05$). Similar successful results were reported in a European study (Benninga et al., 1993).

More intensive psychotherapeutic intervention may be required for those children with intractable encopresis who appear to fit the psychological profile described by Bemporad and Hallowell, where it seems clear that interpersonal-psychodynamic factors are perpetuating the problem.

Pharmacological treatment with imipramine has also been reported as useful for encopresis. There have been 15 reported cases of children with encopresis responding to imipramine, which have been described in six papers (Abrahams, 1963; Connell, 1972; Gavanski, 1971; Geormaneanu and Voiculescu, 1980; Siomopoulos, 1976; White, 1977). All but three of the reported subjects are male. In general, the therapeutic effect occurred within a few days to 2 weeks. The dosages of imipramine reported are relatively low, in the 25- to 75-mg range. There is one open study with metoclopramide (cisapride), a new prokinetic-propulsive agent, which has recently become commercially available. At the time of study, the agent was still investigational. The open study investigated the agent's efficacy in eight males and four females ages 2–13 with diagnoses of functional encopresis. Treatment with cisapride lasted for 26–72 weeks with a dosage range of 0.14–0.3 mg/kg/dose. The authors report that encopresis ceased in eight patients and decreased substantially in two others. Side effects were primarily limited to nausea, vomiting, anorexia, headaches, and cramping. In general, the side effects were of mild intensity and tended to occur early in treatment (Murray et al., 1990).

Outcome and Follow-up Data

The 78% success rate described by Levine would suggest that most children will respond to a relatively innocuous approach that involves educational, behavioral, and physiological components. The epidemiological data also indicate that the effects of maturation will provide a significant number of spontaneous remissions from year to year. The evaluation of any long-term intervention such as psychotherapy should take this factor into account. All but a few children will have either responded to treatment or spontaneously remitted by age 16, and persistence beyond that age is quite unusual (Rex et al., 1992).

Areas for Future Research

This review suggests that encopresis is an excellent paradigm for assessing the relative impacts of biological, psychological, and social factors. For example, do the physiological findings described above represent a constitutional vulnerability or are they the result of the effects of chronic constipation on the bowel? The symptom of encopresis in its various presentations can be a fruitful area of research for those interested in elucidating the interrelationship between mind, body, and culture in children.

CASE ILLUSTRATION

Peter is a 10-year-old boy with a 2-year history of encopresis occurring at a frequency of once to twice per week. The feces are formed, and the episodes usually occur at home after school. Frequently he will hide the soiled underclothes, only to have his parents find them around the house a few days later.

Peter's biological parents divorced 3 years ago. His father was awarded custody of Peter and his younger brother and sister. His father remarried 2 years ago. Peter and his stepmother have been at odds since she moved in.

Treatment with the conventional catharsis and bowel training regimen was not successful. The family sought treatment with a child psychiatrist. It was apparent that there was considerable tension between Peter's father and stepmother. His father tended to be removed and distant, which greatly angered his stepmother. The couple tended to blame all of their problems on Peter's encopresis. Peter was treated with once weekly individual and family psychotherapy. As an adjunctive measure, imipramine was prescribed for the encopresis, as it was felt that removing the symptom would help to clarify the other significant family issues. Baseline data on the frequency of encopresis were collected for 1 month. Following this, imipramine was begun at a dosage of 25 mg and titrated up to a dosage of 75 mg. Imipramine was effective, and the frequency of encopresis declined from five times per week to two times per week. However, approximately 6 weeks later the frequency of soiling began to escalate back to its pretreatment levels. In the family sessions it emerged that Peter's stepmother had become very inconsistent in giving him the imipramine. An attempt was made to have his father administer the medication, but he refused.

Even though the encopresis did recur, the response to medication coupled with the parents' apparent sabotaging of the treatment led to a fuller clarification of the family dynamics. The stepmother became more forceful in expressing her hatred of Peter and eventually took the position that either Peter would leave or she would. The father capitulated on this demand, and Peter went to live with his paternal uncle's family. One month after the move, the encopresis completely remitted. As the family lived nearby, Peter was able to maintain close contact with his father and siblings.

Comment

Given the relatively high success rate with the bowel training approach, why did Peter not respond? The literature clearly shows that children who have more psychological disturbance and/or are from more troubled families are less apt to respond to this intervention.

What can be inferred from Peter's positive response to imipramine? This would suggest that imipramine's efficacy in encopresis could be a nonpsychotropic effect. Alternately, it could be argued that Peter was concomitantly depressed and that the therapeutic effect on the encopresis was secondary to an antidepressant effect. It is also quite likely that the response was a placebo effect, as there have not been large placebo-controlled double-blind studies of imipramine's efficacy for encopresis.

References

Abrahams D: Treatment of encopresis with imipramine. *Am J Psychiatry* 119:891–892, 1963.

Achenbach TM, Lewis M: A proposed model for clinical research and its application to encopresis and enuresis. *J Am Acad Child Psychiatry* 10(3):535–554, 1971.

Ambrosini PI: A pharmacological paradigm for urinary incontinence and enuresis. *J Clin Psychopharmacol* 4:247–253, 1984.

Ambrosini PI, Fried J: Preliminary report: Amantadine hydrochloride in childhood enuresis. *J Clin Psychopharmacol* 4:223–253, 1984.

American Psychiatric Association: *Diagnostic and Statistical Manual of Mental Disorders* (4th ed, rev). Washington, DC, American Psychiatric Association, 1994, pp. 106–110.

Banerjee S, Srivastav A, Palan BM: Hypnosis and self-hypnosis in the management of nocturnal enuresis: A comparative study with imipramine therapy. *Am J Clin Hypn* 36(2):113–119, 1993.

Beach PS, Beach RE, Smith LR: Hyponatremic seizures in a child treated with desmopressin to control enuresis. A rational approach to fluid intake. *Clin Pediatr* 31(9):566–569, 1992.

Bellman M: Studies on encopresis. *Acta Paediatr Scand* suppl 170, 1966.

Bemporad JR, Hallowell E: Advances in the treatment of disorders of elimination. In: Noshpitz ID, Call JD, Cohen RL, et al (eds): *Basic Handbook of Child Psychiatry* (Vol 5). New York, Basic Books, 1987, pp. 479–483.

Benninga MA, Buller HA, Iaminiau JA: Biofeedback training in chronic constipation. *Arch Dis Child* 68(1):126–129, 1993.

Berg I, Forsythe I, McGuire R: Response of bed wetting to the enuresis alarm. Influence of psychiatric disturbance and maximum functional bladder capacity. *Arch Dis Child* 57:394–396, 1982.

Blackwell B, Currah J: The psychopharmacology of nocturnal enuresis. In: Kolvin I, MacKeith R,

Meadows S (eds): *Bladder Control and Enuresis.* London, Spastics International Medical Publications in association with Heinemann, 1973.

Blickman JG, Schimmelpenninck-Scheiffers ML: Intravenous urography in children: Is routine tomography useful? *J Can Assoc Radiol* 35: 363–364, 1984.

Broughton RF: Sleep disorders: Disorders of arousal? *Science* 159:1070–1078, 1968.

Capozza N, Creti G, De Gennaro M, et al: The treatment of nocturnal enuresis. A comparative study between desmopressin and acupuncture used along or in combination. *Minerva Pediatr* 43(9):577–582, 1991.

Cohen M: Enuresis. *Pediatr Clin North Am* 22: 545–560, 1975.

Connell HM: The practical management of enco-presis. *Aust Paediatr J* 8:279–281, 1972.

Devlin JB: Prevalence and risk factors for child-hood nocturnal enuresis. *Irish Med J* 84(4):118–120, 1991.

Devlin JB, O'Cathain C: Predicting treatment outcome in nocturnal enuresis. *Arch Dis Child* 65(10):1158–1161, 1990.

Devane CL, Walker RD III, Sawyer WP, et al: Concentrations of imipramine and its metabolites during enuresis therapy. *Pediatr Pharmacol* 4: 245–251, 1984.

de Gatta MF, Galindo P, Rey F, et al: The influ-ence of clinical and pharmacological factors on enu-resis treatment with imipramine. *Br J Clin Pharma-col* 30(5):693–698, 1990.

de Gatta MF, Garcia MJ, Acosta A, et al: Moni-toring of serum levels of imipramine and desipramine and individualization of dose in enuretic children. *Ther Drug Monit* 6:438–443, 1984.

Diez F Jr, Berger TG: Scarring due to an enuresis blanket. *Pediatr Dermatol* 5:58–60, 1988.

Djurhuus JC, Norgaard JP, Rittig S: Monosymp-tomatic bedwetting. *Scand J Urol Nephrol* 141:7–17, 1992.

Elmer M, Adolfsson T, Norgaard JP, et al: Diur-nal enuresis in childhood is effectively treated with terodiline. *Lakartidningen* 6:88(10):850–851, 1991.

el-Sadr A, Sabry AA, Abdel-Rahman M, et al: Treatment of primary nocturnal enuresis by oral an-drogen mesterolone. A clinical and cystometric study. *Urology* 36(4):331–335, 1990.

Essen J, Peckham C: Nocturnal enuresis in child-hood. *Dev Med Child Neurol* 18:577–589, 1976.

Feehan M, McGee R, Stanton W, et al: A 6 year follow-up of childhood enuresis: Prevalence in ado-lescence and consequences for mental health. *J Pae-diatr Child Health* 26(2):75–79, 1990.

Fergusson DM, Horwood LJ, Shannon FT: Fac-tors related to the age of attainment of nocturnal blad-der control: An 8-year longitudinal study. *Pediatrics* 78:884–890, 1986.

Fergusson DM, Horwood LJ, Shannon FT: Sec-ondary enuresis in a birth cohort of New Zealand children. *Paediatr Perinatal Epidemiol* 4(1):53–63, 1990.

Fjellestad-Paulsen A, Wille S, Harris AS: Com-parison of intranasal and oral desmopressin for noc-turnal enuresis. *Arch Dis Child* 62:674–677, 1987.

Foxman B, Valdez RB, Brook RH: Childhood enuresis: Prevalence, perceived impact, and pre-scribed treatments. *Pediatrics* 77:482–487, 1986.

Freud A, Burlingham DT: *War and Children.* New York, Medical War Books, 1943.

Fritz GK, Rockney RM, Yeung AS: Plasma lev-els and efficacy of imipramine treatment for enuresis. *J Am Acad Child Adolesc Psychiatry* 33:60–64, 1994.

Gastaut H, Broughton R: A clinical and poly-graphic study of episodic phenomena during sleep.

In: Wortis J (ed): *Recent Advances in Biological Psy-chiatry.* New York, Plenum, 1964, pp. 196–221.

Gavanski M: Treatment of non-retentive second-ary encopresis with imipramine and psychotherapy. *Can Med Assoc J* 104:46–48, 1971.

Geffken G, Johnson SB, Walker D: Behavioral interventions for childhood nocturnal enuresis: The differential effect of bladder capacity on treatment progress and outcome. *Health Psychol* 5:261–272, 1986.

Geormaneanu M, Voiculescu VP: Treatment of encopresis with imipramine. *Rev Roum Med Neurol Psychiatr* 18:209–210, 1980.

Glicklich LB: An historical account of enuresis. *Pediatrics* 8:859–876, 1951.

Greene AS, Cromie WJ: Treatment of imipra-mine overdose in children. *Urology* 18:314–315, 1981.

Hansson S: Urinary incontinence in children and associated problems. *Scand J Urol Nephrol* 141: 47–55, 1992.

Hersov L: Faecal soiling. In: Rutter M, Hersov L (eds): *Child and Adolescent Psychiatry: Modern Approaches* (2nd ed). London, Blackwell Scientific Publications, 1985, pp. 482–489.

Hjalmas K: Functional daytime incontinence: Definitions and epidemiology. *Scand J Urol Nephrol* 141:39–44.

Hogg RJ, Husmann D: The role of family history in predicting response to desmopressin in nocturnal enuresis. *J Urol* 150:444–445, 1993.

Jarveline MR, Huttunen NP, Seppanen J, et al: Screening of urinary tract abnormalities among day and nightwetting children. *Scand J Urol Nephrol* 24(3):181–189, 1990.

Jarvelin MR, Vikevainen-Tervonen L, Moilanen I, et al: Enuresis in seven-year-old children. *Acta Paediatr Scand* 77:148–153, 1988.

Jorgensen OS, Lober M, Christiansen J, et al: Plasma concentration and clinical effect in imipra-mine treatment of childhood enuresis. *Clin Pharma-cokinet* 5:386–393, 1980.

Kales A, Kales J, Jacobson A, et al: Effects of imipramine on enuretic frequency and sleep stages. *Pediatrics* 60:431–436, 1977.

Kallio J, Rautava P, Huupponen R, et al: Severe hyponatremia caused by intranasal desmopressin for nocturnal enuresis. *Acta Paediatr* 82(10):881–882, 1993.

Kaplan SL, Breit M, Gauthier B, et al: A compari-son of three nocturnal enuresis treatment methods. *J Am Acad Child Adolesc Psychiatry* 28:282–286, 1989.

Key DW, Bloom DA, Sanvordenker J: Low-dose DDAVP in nocturnal enuresis. *Clin Pediatr* 31(5): 299–301, 1992.

Kikuchi K, Fujisawa I, Ohie T, et al: Ectopic posterior lobe of the pituitary gland and intractable nocturnal enuresis in a case with pituitary dwarfism. *Acta Paediatr Scand* 78:479–481.

Levine MD: Encopresis: Its Potentiation, evalua-tion and alleviation. *Pediatr Clin North Am* 29: 315–330, 1982.

Levine MD, Bakow H: Children with encopresis: A study of treatment outcome. *Pediatrics* 58: 845–852, 1976.

Levine MD, Mazonson P, Bakow H: Behavioral symptom substitution in children cured of enco-presis. *Am J Dis Child* 134:663–667, 1980.

Loening-Baucke VA: Factors responsible for persistence of childhood constipation. *J Pediatr Gas-troenterol Nutr* 6:915–922, 1987.

Loening-Baucke V: Modulation of abnormal def-ecation dynamics by biofeedback treatment in chron-ically constipated children with encopresis. *J Pediatr* 116(2):214–222, 1990.

Loening-Baucke VA, Cruikshank BM: Abnor-mal defecation dynamics in chronically constipated children with encopresis. *J Pediatr* 108:562–566, 1986.

Loening-Baucke V, Cruikshank B, Savage C: Defecation dynamics and behavior profiles in enco-pretic children. *Pediatrics* 80:672–679, 1987.

MacLean RE: Imipramine hydrochloride (To-franil) and enuresis. *Am J Psychiatry* 117:551, 1960.

Mahony DT: Studies of enuresis. I: The incidence of obstructive lesions and pathophysiology of enu-resis. *J Urol* 106:951–958, 1971.

McGee R, Makinson T, Williams S, et al: A lon-gitudinal study of enuresis from five to nine years. *Aust Paediatr J* 20:39–42, 1984.

Metin A, Aykol N: Diclofenac sodium supposi-tory in the treatment of primary nocturnal enuresis. *Int Urol Nephrol* 24(2):113–117, 1992.

Mikkelsen EJ, Rapoport JL: Enuresis: Psycho-pathology, sleep stage, and drug response. *Urol Clin North Am* 7:361–377, 1980.

Mikkelsen EJ, Rapoport JL, Nee L, et al: Child-hood enuresis. I: Sleep patterns and psychopathol-ogy. *Arch Gen Psychiatry* 37:1139–1144, 1980.

Miller K, Atkin B, Moody ML: Drug therapy for nocturnal enuresis. Current treatment recommenda-tions. *Drugs* 44(1):47–56, 1992.

Mimouni M, Shuper A, Mimouni F, et al: Re-tarded skeletal maturation in children with primary enuresis. *Eur J Pediatr* 144:234–235, 1985.

Minni B, Capozza N, Creti G, et al: Bladder insta-bility and enuresis treated by acupuncture and elec-tro-therapeutics: Early urodynamic observations. *Acupuncture Electro-Therapeutics Res* 15(1):19–25, 1990.

Moffatt ME, Kato C, Pless IB: Improvements in self-concept after treatment of nocturnal enuresis: Randomized controlled trial. *J Pediatr* 110:647–652, 1987.

Moffatt ME, Harlos S, Kirshen AJ, et al: Desmo-pressin acetate and nocturnal enuresis: How much do we know? *Pediatrics* 92(3):420–425, 1993.

Murray RD, Li BU, McClunk HD, et al: *J Pediatr Gastroenterol Nutr* 11(4):503–508, 1990.

Nolan T, Debelle G, Oberkland F, et al: Random-ized trial of laxatives in treatment of childhood enco-presis. *Lancet* 31:523–527, 1991.

Norgaard JP, Hansen JH, Wildschitz G, et al: Sleep cystometries in children with nocturnal enu-resis. *J Urol* 141:1156–1159, 1989.

Norgaard JP, Pedersen EB, Djurhuus JC: Diurnal anti-diuretic-hormone level in enuretics. *J Urol* 134: 1029–1031, 1985.

Oregan S, Yazbeck S, Hamberger B, et al: Con-stipation a commonly unrecognized cause of enu-resis. *Am J Dis Child* 140:260–261, 1986.

Pierce CM, Whitman RM, Mass JW, et al: Enu-resis and dreaming: Experimental studies. *Arch Gen Psychiatry* 4:116–170, 1961.

Rapoport JL, Mikkelsen EJ, Zavadil A, et al: Childhood enuresis. II: T+ieneretic effect. *Arch Gen Psychiatry* 37:1146–1152, 1980.

Rex DK, Fitzgerald JF, Goulet RJ: Chronic con-stipation with encopresis persisting beyond 15 years of age. *Dis Colon Rectum* 35(3):242–244, 1992.

Rew DA, Rundle JS: Assessment of the safety of regular DDAVP therapy in primary nocturnal enu-resis. *Br J Urol* 63:352–353, 1989.

Ringertz H: Bladder capacity, urethral sensation and lumbosacral anomalies in children with enuresis. *Acta Radiol Diagn* 25:45–48, 1984.

Rittig S, Knudsen UB, Norgaard JP, et al: Abnor-mal diurnal rhythm of plasma vasopressin and uri-nary output in patients with enuresis. *Am J Physiol* 256 (issue 4, pt 2):F664–F671, 1989.

Rittig S, Knudsen UB, Norgaard JP, et al: Diurnal variation of plasma atrial natriuretic peptide in normals and patients with enuresis nocturna. *Scand J Clin Lab Invest* 51(2):209–217, 1991.

Ritvo ER, Ornitz EM, Gottlieb F, et al: Arousal and nonarousal enuretic events. *Am J Psychiatry* 126: 77–84, 1969.

Robert M, Averous M, Besset A, et al: Sleep polygraphic studies using cystomanometry in twenty patients with enuresis. *Eur Urol* 24(1):97–102, 1993.

Robertson D, Barker E: Tricyclic antidepressant cardiotoxicity. *JAMA* 236:2089–2090, 1976.

Roje-Starcevic M: The treatment of nocturnal enuresis by acupuncture. *Neurologija* 39(3):179–184, 1990.

Rutter M: Isle of Wight revisited: Twenty-five years of child psychiatric epidemiology. *J Am Acad Child Adolesc Psychiatry* 28:633–653, 1989.

Rutter M, Tizard J, Whitmore K (eds): *Education, Health and Behavior*. New York, Krieger, Huntington, 1981.

Rutter ML, Yule W, Graham PJ: Enuresis and behavioural deviance: Some epidemiological considerations. In: Kolvin I, MacKeith R, Meadow SR (eds): *Bladder Control and Enuresis (Clinics in Developmental Medicine, nos. 48, 49)*. London, Spastics International Medical Publications in association with Heinemann, 1973, pp. 137–147.

Shaffer D: Enuresis. In: Rutter M, Hersov L (eds): *Child and Adolescent Psychiatry: Modern Approaches* (2nd ed). London, Blackwell Scientific Publication, 1985, pp. 465–481.

Shaffer D, Gardner A, Hedge B: Behavior and bladder disturbance of enuretic children: A rational classification of a common disorder. *Dev Med Child Neurol* 26:781–792, 1984.

Siomopoulos V: Psychogenic encopresis treated with imipramine. *JAMA* 235:1842, 1976.

Smith DR: Critique on the concept of vesical neck obstruction in children. *JAMA* 207:1686–1692, 1969.

Sprague-McRae JM, Lamb W, Homer D: Encopresis: A study of treatment alternatives and historical and behavioral characteristics. *Nurse Pract* 18(10):52–53, 56–63, 1993.

Stark LJ, Owens-Stively J, Spirito A, et al: *J Pediatr Psychol* 15(5):659–671, 1990.

Steffens J, Netzer M, Isenberg E, et al: Vasopressin deficiency in primary nocturnal enuresis. Results of a controlled prospective study. *Eur Urol* 24(3): 366–370, 1993.

Stein Z, Susser M: Social factors in the development of sphincter control. *Dev Med Child Neurol* 9: 692–706, 1967.

Steinhausen HC, Gobel D: Enuresis in child psychiatric clinic patients. *J Am Acad Child Adolesc Psychiatry* 28:279–281, 1989.

Stoffer SS: Loss of bladder control in hyperthyroidism. *Postgrad Med* 84:117–118, 1988.

Sukhai RN, Mol J, Harris AS: Combined therapy of enuresis alarm and desmopressin in the treatment of nocturnal enuresis. *Eur J Paediatr* 148:465–467, 1989.

Terho P: Desmopressin in nocturnal enuresis. *J Urol* 145(4):818–820, 1991.

Wald A, Chandra R, Chiponis D, et al: Anorectal function and continence mechanisms in childhood encopresis. *J Pediatr Gastroenterol Nutr* 5:346–351, 1986.

Watanabe H, Azuma Y: A proposal for a classification system of enuresis based on overnight simultaneous monitoring of electroencephalography and cystometry. *Sleep* 12:257–264, 1989.

Werry J: The conditioning treatment of enuresis. *Am J Psychiatry* 123:226–229, 1966.

White JH: *Pediatric Psychopharmacology*. Baltimore, Williams & Wilkins, 1977, pp. 109–114.

Wille S: Comparison of desmopressin and enuresis alarm for nocturnal enuresis. *Arch Dis Child* 61:30–33, 1986.

Yaouyanc G, Jonville AP, Yaouyanc-Lapalle H: Seizure with hyponatremia in a child prescribed desmopressin for nocturnal enuresis. *J Toxicol* 30(4): 637–641, 1992.

55 FIRESETTING

Jessica Gaynor, Ph.D.

Firesetting behavior in youngsters is the result of a complex interaction of individual, social, and environmental factors. There is a wide range of firesetting activities representing increasingly severe levels of psychopathology. Although current epidemiologic information is somewhat thin, there are studies suggesting that youngsters ages 18 and under represent a significant proportion of individuals involved in firesetting and arson-related behaviors. Several theoretical perspectives present hypotheses regarding the causative factors of firesetting. Research supporting these theories suggests that there is a common group of clinical features describing pathological firesetting. Swift diagnosis of firesetting behavior can result in successful intervention and remediation. There are many clinical reports suggesting the availability of a wide variety of therapeutic methods that are effective in abating pathological firesetting behavior in youngsters.

DEFINITION OF TERMS

The development of fire behavior in youngsters can be viewed as following a naturally occurring sequence of psychosocial phases (Gaynor and Hatcher, 1987; Kafry et al., 1980). There are at least three sequential phases of fire behavior: fire interest, fireplay, and firesetting. These categories of fire behavior represent increasing levels of involvement with fire. By experiencing each of these sequential phases, most children learn age-appropriate, fire-safe behaviors. However, for a percentage of youngsters, the influence of psychosocial determinants, such as deficits in emotional functioning, difficulties in the family environment, or frequent occurrences of significant stressors, impact on their development and produce such fire-risk behaviors as unsupervised fireplay; repeated, intentional firesetting; and malicious firestarts.

Fire interest is experienced by the majority of children between the ages of 3 to 5 years (Gaynor and Hatcher, 1987; Jackson et al., 1987). There are several ways in which youngsters express their interest in fire.

For example, they may ask questions such as, "How hot is fire?" and "What makes fire burn?" Or, they may incorporate fire into their play by wearing fire hats, playing with toy fire trucks, and cooking food on their toy stoves. Fire interest represents one of the many curiosities youngsters have about the physical properties of their natural environment.

Fireplay occurs when children experiment with matches or other firestarting materials. This type of behavior emerges in children between the ages of 5 to 9, and it is observed predominantly in young boys (Gaynor and Hatcher, 1987; Showers and Pickrell, 1987). When this experimentation takes place under controlled and supervised conditions, the result is the development of competent, fire-safe behaviors. For example, if youngsters request and are given permission to light the candles on their birthday cake, they are learning the conditions under which it is safe to strike a match and light candles. Teaching children the importance of fire in their environment and helping them to gain mastery and control over it are benefits of participating in supervised fire-related activities.

Unfortunately, a greater majority of youngsters participate in unsupervised fireplay activities. Studies estimate that over 60% of children interested in fire engage in at least one unsupervised fireplay incident (Cole et al., 1986; Gaynor and Hatcher, 1987). In addition, many youngsters will not admit to having participated in these fireplay activities unless specifically questioned about them (Kafry et al., 1980). Most unsupervised fireplay is a single-episode firestart primarily motivated by curiosity. The resulting fires are either accidental or unintentional, and if a fire becomes out of control, youngsters will make serious attempts to either extinguish the fire themselves or go for help (Cole et al., 1986; Gaynor and Hatcher, 1987; Kafry et al., 1980). Although unsupervised fireplay incidents are unplanned and occur only once or twice for most youngsters, it is estimated that, while the probability is fairly low that first-time fireplay incidents will result in a significant fire, this probability increases significantly for subsequent fireplay activities

Table 55.1. Factors Distinguishing Fireplay and Pathological Firesetting

Factor	Fireplay	Firesetting
History	Single episode	Recurrent
Method	Unplanned	Planned
Motive	Accidental	Intentional
Ignition	Available	Acquired
Target	Nonspecific	Specific
Behavior	Extinguish fire	Run away

(Lewis and Yarnell, 1951). Hence, while fireplay can be the result of innocent curiosity or accidental behavior, the risks of starting a significant fire and the resulting consequences exceed the benefits of the learning that may result from the youngster's experimentation.

By the age of 10, most children have learned the rules of fire safety and prevention and are capable of engaging in age-appropriate firesetting activities such as helping to light the family barbecue or building a campfire (Cole et al., 1986; Gaynor and Hatcher, 1987). If adequate fire-related experiential and educational efforts have occurred at home and in school, youngsters will have achieved a sense of competence and mastery over a powerful and fascinating aspect of their physical environment. However, for a number of children, what begins as one or two unsupervised fireplay incidents leads to repeated, intentional firestarting behavior. Hypothesized explanations for the development of pathological firesetting follow in a subsequent section. Table 55.1 presents a description of the factors distinguishing unsupervised fireplay from pathological firesetting.

Pathological firesetting is characterized by a history of multiple firestarts taking place over at least a 6-month period (Gaynor and Hatcher, 1987). The nature and extent of these firestarts may vary, ranging from parents finding burned candles concealed in their youngsters' rooms to fires requiring fire department suppression. The firestarts are usually planned as opposed to being a spur of the moment, impulsive activity (Gaynor and Hatcher, 1987; Icove and Estepp, 1987). Ignition sources, such as matches and lighters, are often searched for, acquired, and concealed until they are needed (Benians, 1981; Gaynor and Hatcher, 1987; Icove and Estepp, 1987). The firestarting activity will usually take place in a concealed or isolated area in or near the home, where there is little possibility of immediate detection by an adult or authority figure (Icove and Estepp, 1987). When a fire is set, there is often an attempt to gather flammable and combustible materials, such as old newspapers and rags, or chemicals, such as paints and alcohol, to use as aids in spreading the fire (Gaynor and Hatcher, 1987; Icove and Estepp, 1987). These fires can be motivated by a variety of reasons including revenge and anger, attention, malicious mischief, watching the fire burn, and in a small number of older adolescent cases, profit (Benians, 1981; Gaynor and Hatcher, 1987). The target of the firestart often has significant meaning for the firesetter because of the emotional importance of the fire (Gaynor and Hatcher, 1987). For example, if a youngster has set fire to the cushions of his mother's favorite chair, then it is likely that one of the primary motivations for the firesetting lies in the nature of the relationship between the mother and her child. After the firestart, youngsters rarely will voluntarily admit to their involvement in the ignition (Gaynor and Hatcher, 1987). If the fire is out of control, rather than calling for help, they are likely to run away to a safe spot, sometimes to watch the fire burn and await for the arrival of the fire department (Gaynor and Hatcher, 1987; Icove and Estepp, 1987). Although individual case reports reveal variations in patterns of firestarting, these are the predominant characteristics that represent pathological firesetting behavior.

EPIDEMIOLOGY

Information on the prevalence of firesetting behavior in youngsters is derived from four general areas of study. The first resource is the annual fire cause and origin rates in the United States. Fire departments

voluntarily report this data to the National Fire Incidence Reporting System (Hall, 1991). From this database, the National Fire Protection Agency aggregated data from 1980 to 1991 on the category of children playing with fire (Hall, 1991). In 1991, children started 103,260 fires, causing 457 deaths, 1,846 injuries, and $310 million in direct property damage (Hall, 1991). The death rate due to child fireplay rose by 30% from 1990 to 1991, resuming the upward trend observed in the 1980s (Hall, 1991). Children 5 years and younger were responsible for 73% of the fire deaths caused by child-set fires (Hall, 1991). While firesetting is the second leading cause of death (second to automobile accidents) for children and adolescents ages 6–14, it is the number one cause of death (accounting for 33% of the total) for preschoolers (Hall, 1991). Hence, very young children are not only likely to start fires, but they are also most likely to be their victims.

The second source of information relates to the prevalence of unsupervised fireplay and firesetting in populations of school-age children. One study interviewing kindergarten and second and fourth grade children and their parents (N = 139) from three randomly selected schools reveals that 60% of the children admitted to engaging in unsupervised fireplay and 77% of them reported to be present when their friends participated in the same play (Gaynor and Hatcher, 1987). Of the unsupervised fireplay group (N = 83), 37% of the children admitted to one incident, 40% said they played with fire two times, and 23% disclosed that they had participated in unsupervised fireplay more than twice (Gaynor and Hatcher 1987). Of the group reporting to play with fire more than once (N = 52), 55% of the children admitted to purposely burning items such as grass, leaves, rugs, clothes, and paper products (Gaynor and Hatcher, 1987). Of these children, 23 were boys and 15 were girls; boys were more likely to burn items and to set fires outside the home, while girls were more likely to do it indoors. None of these fires required firefighting suppression (Gaynor and Hatcher, 1987). In addition, 47% of the parents reported that they had engaged in unsupervised fireplay during their childhood (Gaynor and Hatcher, 1987). Another study surveying school-age youngsters in grades one through eight (N = 77) indicated that 75% of their sample reported knowing someone who had played with matches or lighters, 58% of the youngsters had actually witnessed unsupervised fireplay, and 38% admitted to engaging in at least one unsupervised fireplay incident (Cole et al., 1986). Of this sample, 3% of the fireplay incidents resulted in fires requiring fire department intervention. Hence, these studies offer preliminary findings suggesting that the greater majority of school children may be exposed to or participate in unsupervised fireplay and firesetting activities, with fortunately few of these incidents resulting in major fires.

The third type of epidemiologic data examines the prevalence of firesetting behavior among psychiatric populations. An early study indicated that 2% of the evaluations in an outpatient child psychiatry clinic of a large voluntary hospital presented with firesetting as the primary complaint, and 3% of the evaluations conducted in a suburban private practice were firesetting cases (Vandersall and Weiner, 1970). A later study confirms these estimates, reporting that between 1973 and 1981 2.45% of their outpatient clinic population (104 of 4242 children) presented with definite or marked firesetting behavior (Jacobson, 1985a). This study also characterized firesetting as a subgroup of conduct disorder diagnosis. Firesetters differed significantly from a matched group of youngsters with conduct disorder in that they demonstrated more antisocial, aggressive, and destructive behaviors. A more recent study examined the frequency with which five categories of fire behavior—match play, participation in at least one unsupervised firestart, setting fire more than twice, setting a fire causing serious damage, and setting a fire requiring firefighter suppression—occurred within psychiatric outpatient and inpatient populations (Kolko and Kazdin, 1988). The results indicate that the prevalence rates for match play and participation in at least one unsupervised firestart were 24 and 19%, respectively, for outpatients and 52 and 35%, respectively, for inpatients (Kolko and Kazdin, 1988). Although these outpatient rates are somewhat lower than previously cited rates in a sample of school children (60% for match play and 37% for firestarting) (Kafry et al., 1980), the rates for inpatients are more closely aligned (Kafry et al., 1980; Kolko and Kazdin, 1988). However, a further comparison of the fire involvement rates from these two studies indicates that more youngsters in the outpatient and inpatient groups were involved in recurrent firesetting (outpatients, 11/21; inpatients, 18/25) than those children sampled from the school population (19/83) (Kafry et al., 1980; Kolko and Kazdin, 1988). In addition, while none of the firestarts in the school sample resulted in significant fires, 13 of 22 fires started by outpatients resulted in serious damage, and 9 of 24 fires started by inpatients resulted in serious damage (Kafry et al., 1980; Kolko and Kazdin, 1988). Therefore, these studies suggest that, while the proportion of psychiatric cases presenting with the primary complaint of firesetting remains at approximately 2%, the frequencies with which outpatient and inpatient populations engage in recurrent fire behaviors, some of which lead to serious and damaging fires, may be remarkably higher.

The final type of epidemiologic information on firesetting comes from the arson arrest records of juveniles. Youngsters starting fires that warrant firefighting suppression and that result in significant property damage, loss, or personal injury are at risk for being investigated by law enforcement for the crime of arson. If probable cause can be demonstrated, that is, if existing evidence indicates that firestarting is the result of a malicious and willful intent to destroy by fire, and youngsters have reached the age of accountability, then they can be arrested for arson. During the last decade, juveniles have accounted for 35–49% of all arson arrestees (Federal Bureau of Investigation, 1985–1995). Arson has the youngest and highest rate of juvenile involvement of all crimes indexed by the Federal Bureau of Investigation (Federal Bureau of Investigation, 1985–1995; Hall, 1989). It has been suggested that this juvenile arrest rate may be artificially inflated because youngsters are less skilled at concealing their firesetting than older, more seasoned arsonists, and therefore are more likely to be apprehended (Karchmer, 1983). Demographic information indicates that the greater majority of these arrested juveniles are white males (in 1993 86% were white males and 13% were African Americans) (Federal Bureau of Investigation, 1985–1995). In addition, most of these youngsters are between the ages of 15 and 18 (in 1995 63% were over 15 years) (Federal Bureau of Investigation, 1985–1995; Hall, 1989). Hence, youngsters involved in firesetting not only pose significant problems for the mental health community, but they also represent a major burden for the law enforcement and juvenile justice systems.

CLINICAL DESCRIPTION

Information on the clinical features of firesetting youngsters primarily comes from descriptive studies with a smaller proportion of data emerging from empirical investigations that meet rigorous scientific standards of acceptability. Therefore, the essential clinical features reportedly associated with firesetting must be viewed as representing emerging trends rather than empirically verified patterns of behavior.

It has been proposed that the clinical features of firesetting can be organized into three major categories: individual characteristics, social circumstances, and environmental conditions (Fineman, 1980; Gaynor and Hatcher, 1987). Each of these categories is comprised of specific dimensions that describe the essential features of firesetting youngsters. In addition, there is a growing amount of research supporting the notion that firesetting youngsters can be divided into two major age groups, younger children averaging 8 years and adolescents 13 years and older (Jacobson, 1985a, 1985b). It is hypothesized that the bimodal nature of this age distribution distinguishes two different classes of firesetters, a younger group whose clinical features and motives for firesetting differ significantly from those of the older group (Jacobson, 1985a, 1985b; Kolko, 1988). Given these general assumptions, Tables 55.2 and 55.3 outline the essential clinical features describing these two age groups of firesetting youngsters.

Firesetting Children

Demographic information indicates that young firesetting children averaging age 8 are predominantly young boys coming from a mixed

Table 55.2. Clinical Features of Pathological Firesetters, Children 12 and Younger

Features	Description
Individual characteristics	
Demographic	Predominantly young boys ranging in age from 3 to 13, but averaging 8 years old and coming from a mixed socioeconomic background.
Intelligence	Normal intelligence levels, but higher than average incidences of learning disabilities.
Experiential	A greater number of reported physical illnesses and alleged histories of sexual abuse.
Emotion	Overwhelming feelings of anger and aggression coupled with an inability to appropriately express these emotions.
Behavior	General behavior patterns are characterized as overactive, impulsive, mischievous, and prone to temper outbursts, resulting in destroying toys and other personal objects.
Social circumstances	
Family	Single-parent homes with an absent father are typical. If both parents are present, there is a higher than average degree of marital discord; an overprotective mother; a father who administers overly harsh methods of punishment; and one or more parents carrying a psychiatric history. Violent patterns of family interaction also are common.
Peers	Socially isolated, detached, and alone. Difficulty establishing and maintaining interpersonal relationships. Poor judgment in social situations.
School	Poor academic performance, evidence of learning disabilities, and histories of behavior and conduct problems.
Environmental conditions	
Antecedent stressors	Specific stressful events occurring, which trigger emotional reactions.
Accompanying behavior	The act of firestarting represents the emotional release of displaced anger, revenge, and aggression.
Consequences	Firesetting has both immediately positive reinforcing properties of attention and effect, with the potentially negative outcomes of property loss, injury, and punishment.

socioeconomic background (Kolko et al., 1985; Showers and Pickrell, 1987). The majority of studies suggest that these youngsters are of average intelligence (Kolko et al., 1985; Ritvo et al., 1982). However, there are widespread reports indicating that firesetting children typically do not perform well in elementary school, and this finding may be related to a handful of studies suggesting that these youngsters have a higher than average incidence of learning disabilities (Kuhnley et al., 1982; Vandersall and Weiner, 1970).

There are scattered studies in the literature pointing to certain types of experiences that occur in the lives of these children that may have a relationship to their firesetting behavior. For example, one study suggests that firesetting children between the ages of 6 and 10 have a greater number of physical illnesses, including allergies and respiratory problems, than their nonfiresetting counterparts (Siegelman and Folkman, 1971). No attempts have been made to replicate these findings. Also, another study found a significant relationship between sexual abuse and firesetting behavior in children under the age of 10 (Wooden and Berkey, 1984). The specific nature of the relationship between experienced sexual abuse and firesetting behavior remains to be explained both clinically as well as empirically.

The emotional style of these children has been described by clinical studies as one in which there appears to be marked difficulty in modulating feelings of anger and revenge (Bumpass et al., 1983, 1985; Sakheim et al., 1991). It has been suggested that not only are these children unable to recognize or understand these types of feelings when they occur, but

Table 55.3. Clinical Features of Pathological Firesetters, Adolescents 13 and Older

Features	Description
Individual characteristics	
Demographic	The majority are young, white males coming from mixed socioeconomic backgrounds.
Intelligence	Normal levels of intelligence, but long histories of academic failure in school.
Experiential	A higher than average number of accidents resulting in physical injuries, higher levels of sexual arousal, fantasy excitement, conflicts, gender confusion, and sexual misbehavior.
Emotion	There is a lack of emotional depth and a restricted capacity of expression. Firestarting represents a display of anger, revenge, and aggression. Feelings of excitement and defiance just prior to the firestart are common. Also, there is difficulty experiencing remorse or guilt after firesetting.
Behavior	Restless, impulsive, mischievous, and defiant are typical behaviors coupled with higher than average levels of risk-taking.
Social circumstances	
Family	Single-parent homes where an absent adult male is most common. If both parents are present, there is a high degree of marital discord, uneven discipline and supervision, poor communication, and one or more parents carrying a psychiatric diagnosis. Physical abuse and other violent patterns of family interaction also are observed.
Peers	Firestarting is influenced by the need for attention, acceptance, and recognition from the peer group.
School	Consistent patterns of poor academic achievement, failure to advance in school grades, and conduct and behavior problems with frequent school suspensions or expulsions.
Environmental conditions	
Antecedent stressors	The peer group supports and encourages firesetting, which often is the result of emotional or impulsive behavior resulting from the occurrence of a stressful event or circumstance.
Accompanying behaviors	Other antisocial and delinquent behaviors such as alcohol consumption, petty theft, and vandalism typically occur at the same time or just prior to firestarting in the company of at least one or two friends.
Consequences	The immediately reinforcing properties of firesetting include the resulting attention from family, friends, and the fire department. There is relatively little fear of punishment or consideration of the negative outcomes of property loss or physical injury.

they do not have the experience nor skill to express them in socially acceptable ways (Bumpass et al., 1983, 1985). Consequently, they engage in firesetting as a means of expressing accumulated feelings of displaced anger, revenge, and aggression (Bumpass et al., 1983, 1985). This is partially substantiated by clinical work suggesting that the targets of young children's firestarts are often the objects and possessions of those to whom their anger is directed (Gaynor and Hatcher, 1987). For example, there have been clinical reports of youngsters who admit to setting their mother's bed on fire because they were angry with her (Minuchin, 1974). It must be noted that the primary justification of this emotional style comes only from clinical observations, and further empirical work needs to be pursued to verify these findings.

The behavior pattern of firesetting children has been characterized as overactive, impulsive, and mischievous (Jacobson, 1985a; Sakheim et al., 1991; Wooden and Berkey, 1984). The early documentation of the relationship between the behavioral triad of enuresis, cruelty to animals, and firesetting has failed to hold up under more recent scrutiny (Fine and Louie, 1979; Heller et al., 1984; Jacobson, 1985a; Showers

and Pickrell, 1987). There have been clinical reports of young firesetters who have difficulty controlling their tempers and have histories of destroying their toys and other personal objects in fits of anger and rage (Gaynor and Hatcher, 1987). This behavioral pattern is fairly consistent with the previously described emotional style of accumulated anger and aggression typically being discharged in a socially inappropriate and unacceptable manner. Clearly, there remains a great deal of work to be done at arriving at a detailed description of the general behavioral style of firesetting children.

There is a growing amount of literature indicating that young firesetting children come either from single-parent homes or from families where one of the two parents, typically the father, is absent for long periods of time (Fine and Louie, 1979; Gruber et al., 1981; Stewert and Culver, 1982; Vandersall and Weiner, 1970). Recent work suggests that, when the family is intact, there appears to be a higher than average amount of marital discord (Kazdin and Kolko, 1986). Patterns of family interaction for firesetting children have been characterized by a greater use of overly harsh methods of discipline, including corporal punishment, and an unaffectionate, distant, negative, and conflicted environment (Jacobson, 1985a; Siegelman and Folkman, 1971; Vandersall and Weiner, 1970). In addition, there have been reports that families of firesetting children tend to exhibit more verbally and physically aggressive patterns of family interaction than families of nonfiresetting children (Patterson, 1975). Finally, there are a number of studies suggesting that parents of firesetting children have significant psychiatric histories including one or more family members carrying a diagnosis of antisocial personality, alcoholism, or depression (Gruber et al., 1981; Kazdin and Kolko, 1986; Stewert and Culver, 1982). Although much of this information on family patterns comes from clinical impressions, it represents a strong starting point for further empirical work.

There is very little information on the behavior of firesetting children in social situations. Preliminary work suggests that these children have a great deal of trouble establishing and sustaining meaningful interpersonal relationships (Heath et al., 1985; Vandersall and Weiner, 1970). In addition, a recent study showed that these youngsters exhibit poor social judgment in that they have an inability to plan and anticipate outcomes in social situations (Sakheim et al., 1991; Sakheim and Osborn, 1994). The degree to which these youngsters feel detached, alone, and isolated may have an effect on their need to gain attention and recognition through firesetting. This is somewhat verified by the finding that young children typically firestart alone rather than in the company of friends (Benians, 1981). These observations regarding behavior in social relationships are of a speculative nature, and until more systematic work is undertaken, they are presented only as possible clues for further investigation.

There is evidence indicating that elementary school children with histories of firesetting experience significant academic and behavior problems in school (Gruber et al., 1981; Kuhnley et al., 1982; Showers and Pickrell, 1987; Vandersall and Weiner, 1970). The higher proportion of learning disabilities experienced by firesetting children may account partially for this poor academic showing (Showers and Pickrell, 1987). In addition, because some firesetting children carry a diagnosis of hyperactivity, which is sometimes accompanied by the feature of shortened attention spans, they may have difficulty concentrating on and completing their assigned work (Gruber et al., 1981). As a result of their academic failures, these children may feel frustrated and angry and they may act out their feelings, thereby becoming conduct and behavior problems in school. Hence, these studies suggest that, for a variety of reasons, firesetting children are not likely to have successful and rewarding experiences in school.

It has been hypothesized that there are immediate environmental conditions that set the stage for firesetting behavior in young children and reinforce the behavior once it has occurred. It has been suggested that there are antecedent stressors that take place in the lives of these youngsters and that trigger particular emotional reactions (Fineman, 1980; Gaynor and Hatcher, 1987). Specifically these antecedent stressors trigger accumulated feelings of anger and revenge experienced by these children. The act of firesetting is motivated by the emotional release of displaced anger and aggression or by feelings of revenge.

Firesetting holds both the positively reinforcing properties of attention and effect, as well as the negative outcomes of property loss, injury, and punishment. Although intuitively interesting, these assumptions have yet to be examined in any systematic fashion, either through clinical observation or empirical investigation.

The following case example is presented for the purpose of illustrating the clinical features of children exhibiting pathological firesetting behavior.

CASE ILLUSTRATION

Frank is 10 years old and lives with his mother and his 11-year-old sister in a lower-middle income urban area. Frank's mom and dad have been divorced for 8 years. Frank's mom had been living with a man whom, she says, was very generous to her family. He liked to spend time with her children, but he could be extremely rigid and overly punitive, particularly when Frank did something that displeased him. Recently the mother separated from him because he physically abused her. Frank had witnessed this abuse several times and also may have been a victim. However, when asked, both mom and Frank deny that any of the physical abuse was directed at Frank.

During the time of the separation, Frank's mom began to notice some behavior problems in her son. His ability to concentrate dramatically decreased, and reports came from school that he was involved in fights with his peers. At home, Frank had frequent temper outbursts during which he would become so angry that he would destroy his toys. Also, Frank was verbally aggressive and belligerent toward his sister. He was being generally disruptive both at school and at home. His mom reported that this was unusual behavior for Frank and that she was very concerned for his well-being.

Frank's mom noted that he had been curious about fire since the age of 3, when she found him playing with matches in their kitchen. At that time she taught him how to correctly strike a match. Together they would practice striking matches, blowing them out, and throwing them in the fireplace. Frank was told never to play with matches. He also was encouraged to come to his mom if he ever felt the urge to strike a match, and they would do it together. Despite these rules about firestarting, during the past few weeks Frank's mom found some scrapes of burned newspaper in their fireplace. One afternoon she arrived home early from work in time to see Frank rolling up pages of newspaper, lighting them, and throwing them into the fireplace. She became angry, describing the possible consequences of what could happen if the flaming newspaper accidentally caught the house on fire.

Frank's most recent fire episode involved igniting his model airplane on the kitchen stove and running with it to the living room fireplace. Unfortunately, he did not reach the fireplace in time, and the burning airplane fell on the carpet, starting a small fire. Frightened and confused, Frank ran out of the house screaming for help. Luckily his mother was nearby and heard his screams. She and Frank ran back to the house and together they were able to extinguish the fire.

Comment

Frank's firesetting episodes are typical of this age group in that his unsupervised firestarts occur alone and in his home. Despite his mother's attempts to be firm and constructive in teaching him fire safety rules, he continues to engage in repeated and intentional firesetting behavior. The question becomes why now has the frequency of his firestarting increased and intensified? There may be several reasons for Frank's apparent preoccupation with firesetting. First, there could be a relationship between his fire behavior and the discord and separation in his family. Children with family histories of divorce, neglect, or physical or sexual abuse may fireset to express their distress. Frank's firestarting may be his way of expressing his inner turmoil about his family situation. Second, he could be testing the limits of his mother's authority. Third, firesetting may be Frank's way of asking for more attention from his mother. Finally, Frank's fire behavior may represent a ``cry for help.'' Frank may be experiencing general psychological distress and he may not have the capa-

bility of understanding or expressing his pain and conflict. Firesetting becomes his method for calling attention to his emotional difficulties and his way of asking for help.

Firesetting Adolescents

There are far fewer systematic studies focused on describing the clinical characteristics of firesetting adolescents than there are studies describing firesetting children. Demographic information indicates that it is 10 times more common for adolescent boys than girls to firestart (Heath et al., 1985). The majority of these young boys are white and typically fall into the age range of 16–18 years (Federal Bureau of Investigation, 1985–1995; Hall, 1989). There is some work indicating that these youngsters are of average intelligence; however, they have long histories of academic and behavior difficulties in school (Kolko et al., 1985; Kuhnley et al., 1982; Ritvo et al., 1982).

There are some preliminary studies suggesting that firesetting adolescents are more likely to have certain types of experiences and conflicts than their nonfiresetting counterparts. For example, one study suggests that adolescents with histories of firesetting have a higher than average number of accidents resulting in physical injuries (Jackson et al., 1987). There have been no attempts to replicate this finding. Also, a series of studies shows that firesetting adolescents may experience a higher level of sexual arousal and fantasy excitement than nonfiresetters (Lewis and Yarnell, 1951; Sakheim and Osborn, 1994; Sakheim et al., 1991; Yarnell, 1940). There also is some work reporting that firesetting adolescents experienced more sexual conflicts and gender conflicts (Bumpass et al., 1985; Sakheim and Osborn, 1986, 1994; Sakheim et al., 1985, 1991). One study indicates that adolescent firesetters are more frequently involved in sexual misbehavior (Jacobson, 1985a). It must be emphasized that this information emerges from a limited number of investigations that rely heavily on clinical impressions rather than on controlled empirical observation.

There is very little work examining the emotional style of adolescent firesetters. Clinical studies characterize them as angry, aggressive youngsters who have little regard for social rules and norms (Gaynor and Hatcher, 1987). They may feel excitement and defiance prior to the actual firestart. Once the fire is set, they often do not feel guilt or remorse for their actions (Gaynor and Karchmer, 1988). These youngsters are unable to experience a depth of emotional feeling and their resulting behavior reflects a restricted capacity of expression. This pattern of emotional functioning is similar to that found in antisocial and delinquent personality patterns (American Psychiatric Association, 1993; Sakheim and Osborn, 1994; Sakheim et al., 1991).

The behavior of firesetting adolescents is characterized as restless, impulsive, mischievous, and defiant (Gaynor and Hatcher, 1987; Wooden and Berkey, 1984). In addition, there is some work indicating that these adolescents demonstrate higher levels of risk-taking behavior (Kafry et al., 1980). These somewhat preliminary findings suggest that, if these youngsters are in a situation where ignition sources or fire materials are readily available, they will be less likely to control their impulse or urge to firestart and more likely to follow through with their aggressive and defiant firesetting behavior.

There is a dearth of studies examining the family patterns of adolescent firesetters. Clinical reports suggest that the characteristics distinguishing the families of firesetting children also may describe the families of adolescent firesetters (Gaynor and Hatcher, 1987). That is, firesetting adolescents come from single-parent households in which patterns of inconsistent supervision and discipline are typical (Gaynor and Karchmer, 1988). There are some studies suggesting that firesetting adolescents are likely to have histories of physical abuse and other violent patterns of interaction within their family (Jayaprakash et al., 1984; Ritvo et al., 1982; Showers and Pickrell, 1987). A recent dissertation demonstrated that families of adolescent firesetters showed significantly more pathological functioning in the areas of problem solving, communication, responsiveness, and involvement than did families of nonproblem adolescents (Reis, 1993). There is a great need for the systematic study of how specific family factors relate to the development of adolescent firesetting.

Just as with the behavior of normal adolescents, there is some work indicating that peer group participation greatly influences the behavior of firesetting adolescents (Gaynor and Hatcher, 1987; Gaynor and Karchmer, 1988). While most children firestart alone, most adolescents firestart with one or two friends (Jackson et al., 1987). There are some clinical cases indicating that the peer group supports, encourages, and condones firesetting, and to some extent provides a safe environment into which adolescents can retreat once they have intentionally set a destructive fire (Gaynor J: Unpublished reports from clinical case files. San Francisco, 1989). Regardless of who leads the group, there may be an agreement among the members that firesetting is an acceptable behavior. In addition, one clinical case report suggests that adolescents who firestart may believe that their behavior will gain them a certain degree of attention and recognition within the peer group (Gaynor J: Unpublished reports from clinical case files. San Francisco, 1989.). It is hypothesized that peer group support of firesetting behavior may be one of the most influential social factors in reinforcing the likelihood that the behavior will recur as long as the firestarting goes undetected and no immediate nor long-term consequences are experienced.

The academic achievement of firesetting adolescents is significantly below the average (Kaufman et al., 1961; Yarnell, 1940). These youngsters have long histories of academic failures in school, and they may be one or more grades behind their class by the time they enter high school (Kaufman et al., 1961). Conduct reports also are less than favorable. One study indicates that firesetting adolescents often are disruptive in class and they frequently engage in fights with their peers (Wooden and Berkey, 1984). Many of them either have been suspended several times or have been expelled from more than one school (Kaufman et al., 1961). In addition, statistical studies indicate that approximately 75% of middle and high school fires are caused by adolescents (National Fire Protection Agency, 1978). Hence, not only do these youngsters fail to achieve or adjust to their school environment, but there is evidence indicating that schools may be one of the primary targets of their firesetting.

There is some preliminary work suggesting that certain environmental conditions may be directly related to adolescent firesetting. There are a few studies indicating that specific stressors may trigger firesetting in adolescents (Fineman, 1980). Such stressors are likely to include sudden alterations in family relationships due to separation, divorce, or death (Fineman, 1980; Strachan, 1981; Vandersall and Weiner, 1970). In one study parents of firesetting youngsters indicated more than twice the number of family disruptions than their nonfiresetting family counterparts (Wooden and Berkey, 1984). These parents also reported that their youngsters experienced a greater degree of stress in their lives 6 months before their firestart than at other times in their lives (Wooden and Berkey, 1984). Clinical reports suggest that, at least in some instances, immediately prior to firesetting, adolescents may engage in alcohol or drug consumption (Gaynor J: Unpublished reports from clinical case files. San Francisco, 1989). In addition, there are clinical cases in which firesetting also was accompanied by other delinquent acts including petty theft and vandalism (Gaynor J: Unpublished reports from clinical case files. San Francisco, 1989). It has been reported that, immediately after firesetting, adolescents may leave the fire scene and move to a safe spot to watch the fire burn. They are not likely to call for help to extinguish the fire. This is somewhat consistent with the notion that these youngsters also are unlikely to experience guilt or remorse once they have set the fire. Perhaps, if they did experience these feelings, they would take the appropriate actions to help suppress the fire. The attention and recognition that they may get from their peer group is likely to reinforce the firesetting behavior, especially if it goes undetected. It appears as if these adolescents experience relatively little fear of punishment for their delinquent activity nor do they consider the potential negative outcomes of property loss or personal injury.

The following case describes one example of pathological firesetting behavior in an adolescent.

CASE ILLUSTRATION

Sixteen-year-old Carl lives with his father and younger brother in an upper-class urban neighborhood. His mother and father divorced when Carl was 12, and his mother recently remarried. Carl's father, a prominent attorney, leaves for work early, comes home late, and does a great deal of traveling. While Carl's father is absent much of the time, a loving, elderly aunt as well as a housekeeper share the responsibility for the two boys. Carl's mother lives in another city a few hundred miles away and visits the two boys on an irregular basis.

Carl's father describes his son as "basically a good kid," but wishes he were more obedient and respectful. His mother says he is hard to talk to and never takes her seriously. Carl's aunt describes him as a charming boy who always seems to get into trouble. Although Carl is very bright, he has been expelled from several private schools because of his inability to follow the rules. These schools characterize him as the class bully and ringleader, and he always seems to be responsible for major class disruptions. Carl currently is attending a private day school, where his grades are average and his conduct marginally acceptable.

Carl has a history of antisocial and delinquent behavior, which began around puberty. Shortly after his mother and father separated, Carl began missing several days of school for unexplained reasons. He would leave home early in the morning and return by dinner, offering no explanation of where he had been or what he had been doing while not attending school. After talking with the school staff, it was decided to move Carl to another educational environment. Several months later Carl's father received a late night telephone call from the local police reporting that they had caught Carl and a few friends slashing car tires at a nearby shopping mall. Carl's father was able to convince the police not to press charges. There have been two additional incidents of shoplifting, one from a local drugstore and one from a large sporting goods store. On both occasions apologies were accepted, and no punishment or retribution was implemented. Carl has an apparent knack for getting into trouble and an ability to avoid experiencing the consequences of his behavior.

Carl's firestarting emerged at age 9 when he was caught setting trash can fires at school. Both his father and the school authorities admonished him, and he was suspended from school for 2 days. The latest known firestart occurred 6 years later. Carl had been invited to spend the night at the house of his friend Kevin. Kevin's parents went out for the evening, and the two boys decided to drink the beer that they found in the refrigerator. Both of the boys together consumed about two six-packs of beer. They then left the house and rode their bikes down to the local park and recreation area. They thought it would be easy and fun to break into the building and steal the petty cash from the park director's desk. Once they had entered the building through an open window, they worked for several minutes to break into the desk where the petty cash was kept. Unsuccessful and frustrated by their attempt to obtain the money, they spotted a lighter on a nearby counter and ignited the papers in the trash can. They fled from the building on their bikes without attempting to extinguish the fire. On their way home they heard the sound of fire engines and assumed that they were responding to the fire.

Comment

Carl has a long-standing history of aggressive and antisocial behavior. It appears as if he seizes every opportunity to get into trouble. Lacking the appropriate attention and supervision at home, he pursues recognition in socially unacceptable ways. Attempts by school authorities to control his disruptive behavior have been unsuccessful. In fact, there does not seem to be any individuals effective in guiding or shaping Carl's behavior. Carl apparently felt no guilt or remorse over having set the fire at the park and recreation building. In addition, neither he nor his friend made any attempt to extinguish the fire or call for help. Hence, together these boys successfully started a significant fire and escaped immediate detection. Unless they are caught, they are unlikely to experience any consequences of their firestarting behavior. Their perceived success in this episode may encourage them to pursue more illegal and dangerous firesetting activities in the future.

THEORY

There are four major theoretical frameworks that present explanations of the development of firesetting behavior in youngsters: psychoanalytic theory, social learning theory, dynamic-behavioral theory, and functional analysis theory. Although they offer intuitively interesting explanations of firesetting behavior, there is remarkably little empirical work either confirming or repudiating these theories. Therefore, until efforts are made to systematically investigate these explanations, the current value of these theories primarily lies in their attempt to provide insights into the psychological dynamics of firesetting behavior.

Freud was the first to examine the psychological meaning of fire (Freud, 1932). His psychoanalytic theory hypothesized a relationship between sexual desires and fire. He wrote that fire symbolically represented the expression of libidinal and strong phallic-urethral drives. That is, men attempt to extinguish fires with their own urine, thereby symbolically engaging in a homosexual struggle with another phallus. Therefore, it is the relationship between sexual arousal and urination that is the underlying motive associated with the thrill of igniting and extinguishing fires. The act of firesetting represents a regression to the urethral-phallic phase of psychosexual development, and setting fire substitutes for forbidden masturbatory or sexual desires (Freud, 1932).

Given this hypothesized relationship between sexual arousal, urination, and firesetting, it is expected that firesetting youngsters might display one or more conflicts with respect to these areas of psychological functioning. There is some clinical as well as empirical work suggesting that various groups of firesetting youngsters have a higher than average incidence of sexual conflicts (Sakheim et al., 1985, 1991; Sakheim and Osborn, 1986, 1994; Yarnell, 1940), abnormal sexual behavior (Jacobson, 1985a), and sexual dysfunction (Yarnell, 1940; Stekel, 1924). However, there is substantial evidence indicating that earlier clinical work showing a relationship between enuresis, firesetting, and general patterns of delinquent behavior (Hellman and Blackman, 1966) is not confirmed by more recent empirical studies (Heller et al., 1984; Prentky and Carter, 1984). Therefore, the major tenets of psychoanalytic theory explaining the development of firesetting behavior in youngsters remains open to verification until further empirical work can substantiate or disclaim these hypothesized relationships.

Social learning theory offers a significantly different explanation of the development of firesetting behavior. Whereas psychoanalytic theory emphasizes the relationship between instincts, specifically sexual drive and firesetting behavior, social learning theory emphasizes the relationship between patterns of family and peer interaction and firesetting behavior. Social learning theory postulates that behavior is learned from the social environment, particularly from families and friends (Patterson et al, 1989). Firesetting occurs because youngsters learn the behavior, that is, they may observe it, imitate it, model it, and perhaps even be rewarded for it. Firesetting is a form of learned aggression, which may first surface in the patterns of family interaction (McKerracher and Dacre, 1966; Vreeland and Waller, 1979). Later firesetting activities may be reinforced by the peer group. Undetected firesetting episodes in which no significant behavioral or social consequences are experienced also reinforce the likelihood that firestarting will recur. Hence, utilizing a developmental framework, initially firesetting behavior emerges and may be learned within the family system; however, it is later reinforced by the peer group, and it recurs because of the lack of socially applied sanctions prohibiting or punishing the behavior (Patterson et al., 1989).

There is very little work investigating the application of social learning theory to the development of firesetting behavior. One clinical study reported that fathers of adolescent firesetters all had significant fire-related employment (fireman, furnace stoker, automobile burner at a junkyard), with one youngster not only watching but participating with his father in the burning of automobiles (Macht and Mack, 1968). There have been no empirical attempts to confirm or disclaim these clinical observations. Another clinical study reported that in a small percentage of firesetting cases (3 of 27) parents admitted to using fire to punish their children, obviously conveying the message that fire is an acceptable form of retaliation (Ritvo et al., 1982). While these clinical studies represent thin evidence in support of a social learning theory explanation of firesetting behavior, there is a long history of empirical studies that have identified family variables as consistent covariates for early forms of antisocial behavior and for later delinquency (Loeber and Dishion, 1983). These covariates, such as harsh and inconsistent discipline, little positive parental involvement with the child, and poor monitoring and supervision are strikingly similar to those family variables characterizing the families of firesetting youngsters. Hence, what remains to be accomplished is the identification of the specific linkages between social learning theory and those family variables characteristic of firesetting youngsters.

Dynamic-behavioral theory is a broad-based conceptual framework designed specifically to explain firesetting behavior. This theory identifies a number of psychosocial determinants related to the development of firesetting behavior in youngsters. Although there have been various attempts to categorize these determinants (Fineman, 1980; Gaynor and Hatcher, 1987; Heath et al., 1985), there is consensus on at least three major dimensions related to the development of firesetting behavior: (a) personality and individual characteristics, (b) family and social circumstances, and (c) immediate environmental conditions. Each of these three dimensions is comprised of specific factors or variables. For example, personality and individual characteristics can include demographics, intelligence, emotional style, and experiential and behavioral factors. Social circumstances can include family variables, peer relationships, and school performance. Environmental conditions are those antecedent events that trigger firesetting and the consequences that may or may not be experienced as a result of the behavior. Regardless of how the specific variables are defined, their common underlying feature is that they can be observed and measured to confirm or reject their hypothesized relationship to firesetting. In addition, dynamic-behavior theory begins to define levels of firesetting behavior. These levels are based on age and severity of the firesetting behavior. It is hypothesized that there is a younger group of firesetting children who primarily firestart out of curiosity and an older group whose firesetting represents psychopathological behavior (Fineman, 1980).

The major contribution of dynamic-behavioral theory is that research related to describing the psychosocial characteristics of firesetting youngsters can be organized and classified utilizing this conceptual framework. It presents the first predictive model of firesetting behavior by trying to define the domain of independent variables, such as personality and social and environmental factors, that will predict the occurrence of the dependent variable, firesetting behavior. Unlike psychoanalytic or social learning theory, it is broad-based in that it does not assume that one major factor, such as instincts or the social environment alone, predicts firesetting. Rather it presents a multivariate approach to predicting levels of firesetting behavior. As research emerges describing the various characteristics of firesetting youngsters, dynamic-behavioral theorists must empirically identify those personality, social, and environmental factors that significantly predict firesetting behavior. The result will be a quantifiable description of various types of youngsters involved in various levels of firesetting behavior.

There is one final theoretical framework that represents the latest attempt to explain firesetting behavior. Functional analysis offers a model for predicting the occurrence of arson and recidivistic fire behavior (Jackson et al., 1980). The application of this framework will be more useful in explaining the firesetting behavior of older children and adolescents, who are more likely to be involved in recurrent firestarting. This paradigm hypothesizes that certain psychosocial stimuli, in the context of major environmental conditions, predispose individuals toward firesetting, which in turn is either positively or negatively reinforced. The psychosocial stimuli and environmental conditions that influence firesetting are not unlike those identified by dynamic-behavioral theory. They include psychosocial disadvantage, dissatisfaction with life, ineffective social interaction, previous experience with fire, the occurrence of emotionally significant events, and opportunities to set fire. Firesetting is viewed as an attempt by firestarters to exert some type of change in their environment, where alternative behaviors motivated by the need to change have proven ineffective. Firesetters are characterized as basically ineffective individuals who have been unable to develop the behaviors necessary to express and satisfy their emotional and social needs. Consequently, they firestart as one way to assert a sense of mastery and control over their environment. This description of recurrent firesetting behavior and the general underlying assumptions are consistent with clinical case reports of adolescent firesetting in which social ineffectiveness coupled with the need to express aggressive behavior have been the primary motivating factors for firestarting (Gaynor, 1980). Hence, a preliminary application of the tenets of functional analysis theory appear to be useful in understanding the clinical dynamics of recurrent firesetting.

DIFFERENTIAL DIAGNOSIS

Current empirical work consistently reports that the most frequently occurring psychiatric diagnosis associated with pathological firesetting is conduct disorder (Jacobson, 1985a; Sakheim et al., 1985, 1991; Showers and Pickrell, 1987). The essential clinical features describing this disturbance, such as behavioral difficulties at home or at school, low self-esteem, low frustration tolerance resulting in irritability or temper outbursts, and poor academic achievement, closely match the observed behavior patterns of pathological firesetters (Gaynor and Hatcher, 1987). In addition, recent studies suggest that the occurrence of firesetting behavior is a significant predictor of the persistence of aggressive and antisocial behavior in youngsters diagnosed with conduct disorder (Kelso and Stewert, 1986; Kazdin, 1987). Therefore, the probability is high that firesetting youngsters diagnosed with conduct disorder will have poor outcomes and will continue to be involved in broader antisocial and delinquent behavior.

A handful of studies report that youngsters diagnosed with hyperactivity and attention deficit disorder have histories of firesetting behavior (Broling and Brotman, 1980; Gruber et al., 1981). Conversely, it has been observed that a proportion of firesetting youngsters display general learning disabilities, which may be related to their below average levels of achievement in school (Wooden and Berkey, 1984). It is unclear from this research whether these learning disabilities are related to diagnosed hyperactivity and accompanying shortened attention span. While preliminary information suggests a relationship between hyperactivity, attention deficit, and firesetting, obviously more empirical investigation is necessary to determine the exact extent and nature of this connection.

There are some studies indicating that a relatively small number of firesetting youngsters are diagnosed with severe mental disturbances such as schizophrenia, organic brain dysfunction, or mental retardation (Wooden and Berkey, 1984; Yarnell, 1940). Those studies suggest that firesetting occurred in psychotic youngsters in response to hallucinations involving themes of persecution, self-abuse, and control. Although in some cases of severe mental disturbance firesetting may be observed, it is likely that the firestarting represents a reactive behavior, rather than a major or essential aspect of the disturbance.

Although pyromania, the only DSM-IV diagnosis related specifically to the behavior of firestarting, was initially reported in children in the classic treatise by Lewis and Yarnell (1951), subsequent empirical work shows that it is not used in diagnosing firesetting youngsters (Gaynor and Hatcher, 1987; Rider, 1980). The diagnosis of pyromania typically is reserved for adults (American Psychiatric Association, 1993). However, according to clinical and empirical observations, pyromania, described by the essential features of a recurrent failure to resist the impulse to set fires, an increased sense of tension before setting fires, and an experience of intense pleasure, gratification, or release at the time of ignition, occurs infrequently in adult populations and is rarely a psychiatric diagnosis attributed to adult firesetters (Zeegers, 1984). More than likely, adult firesetters, when detected, are legally apprehended and become the responsibility of the criminal justice system. Therefore, even if pyromania were an appropriate diagnosis, most criminally incarcerated arsonists do not receive psychiatric evaluations and diagnostic classifications.

TREATMENT

The goals of an effective treatment strategy are to abate firesetting behavior and sustain significant changes in the underlying psychopathology. Specific psychotherapies have been developed to work with youngsters presenting with firesetting as the primary behavior problem. Outpatient treatment is the method-of-choice; however, there are some inpatient settings that have programs designed exclusively for firesetting youngsters (Gaynor and Hatcher, 1987). Because these treatment approaches are recently developed, there is an obvious absence of controlled empirical studies demonstrating their relative effectiveness. Nevertheless, preliminary clinical evaluations of these methods suggest that, at least in the short term, they are highly successful in eliminating firesetting behavior in youngsters. What is less clear is the relative impact these treatment strategies have on sustaining desirable changes in the underlying psychopathology.

Individual and family psychotherapy are the two predominant modalities utilized in the outpatient treatment of firesetting youngsters. The primary focus of individual psychotherapy is on the immediate elimination of firesetting behavior, with a secondary emphasis on adjusting or changing the underlying psychopathology (Gaynor and Hatcher, 1987). Cognitive-emotion and behavior therapy are the two most highly developed outpatient treatment approaches. The major goals of cognitive-emotion psychotherapy is to teach youngsters how to recognize the urge to firestart, interrupt the behavior before it starts, and substitute socially appropriate types of behaviors to express their underlying emotions (Bumpass et al., 1983, 1985).

The primary therapeutic mechanism of the cognitive-emotion approach is the construction of a written graph by youngsters with help from their parents and the therapist. Figure 55.1 represents an example of a graph constructed by a firesetting youngster. Both the feelings and specific events leading up to and following the most recent firestart are graphed. The *vertical axis* of the graph represents the time period before, during, and after firesetting. The *horizontal axis* represents the intensity of the various emotions experienced during this time period. The firestarting episode is graphed in the *center* of the *vertical axis*. Youngsters are asked to list on the *vertical axis* in order of occurrence the significant events leading up to and following the firestart. For example, Johnny came home after school and no one else was home. He wanted to play with some friends, but after calling around, he found that they were all busy. He turned on the television, but there wasn't anything on that he wanted to watch. He decided to make a trip to the corner store to get some candy. He bought his favorite snack and picked up the free book of matches lying on the counter. On his way home he began striking matches and extinguishing them. He passed a vacant lot, which he entered. When no one was looking he set a small plant on fire and ran home. When he got home he turned on the television and watched cartoons for the rest of the afternoon. In the early evening his grandmother arrived to make his dinner. After dinner, Johnny and some of his friends walked over to see the damage that occurred as a result of the fire at the vacant lot.

Once these events are graphed, youngsters are asked to describe their feelings associated with this time period. Each type of feeling, such as loneliness, anger, excitement, fear, and guilt, is graphed separately and represented by an individual line. Because specific feelings will wax and wane during this time period, their various intensity levels will be represented by the relative amplitude of the "feeling" lines on the graph. For example, when Johnny arrived home after school to an empty house, initially he might have felt lonely. After calling around to his friends and finding them all busy, these feelings might have increased. Once he discovered that the television was not going to satisfy him, his feeling of loneliness again may have intensified. However, once he decided on a trip to the store, some of his lonely feelings subsided and were replaced by other types of emotions. Hence, the amplitude of the "loneliness" feeling line would gradually increase once Johnny arrived home from

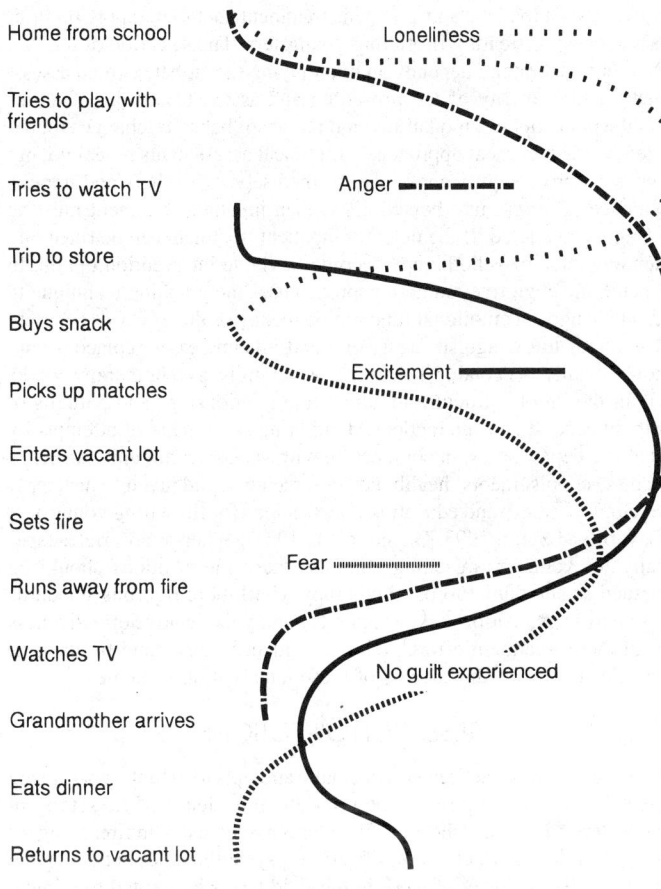

Home from school

Tries to play with friends

Tries to watch TV

Trip to store

Buys snack

Picks up matches

Enters vacant lot

Sets fire

Runs away from fire

Watches TV

Grandmother arrives

Eats dinner

Returns to vacant lot

Loneliness

Anger

Excitement

Fear

No guilt experienced

Figure 55.1. Graphing firesetting behavior.

school; it stays elevated during his struggle to find some form of entertainment, and then it begins to decrease once his trip to the store was underway. In this way, one or more feelings and their relative patterns of experienced intensity are graphically represented in relation to the significant firestarting incident.

A typical or usual graph is expected for the majority of youngsters involved in pathological firesetting. A major assumption of this graphing technique is that, while the specific events surrounding firestarting may vary, the particular pattern of feelings connected with firestarting episodes is expected to be somewhat similar (Bumpass et al., 1983, 1985). It is the role of the therapist, through the process of constructing the graph with the youngsters, to bring to their awareness the usual feeling states associated with the impulse of firesetting. A typical graph indicates that one or more significant events trigger a sequence of sad, lonely feelings. These feelings are replaced by intense, angry feelings, which are in turn controlled by a destructive urge that is significantly relieved by firestarting. A feeling of fear usually emerges before the firesetting and continues for a brief period of time after the fire is set. Feelings of guilt, if experienced, will follow the firesetting. The therapist emphasizes the importance of the relationship between these experienced feelings and the desire to firestart. This pattern of feelings, the associated significant events, and firesetting are the focus of this particular method of cognitive-emotion psychotherapy.

The graphing technique is used as the starting point to help youngsters learn that they can prevent themselves from setting more fires. Once the graph is complete, usually by the second or third session, it is used as a teaching tool for the remainder of the psychotherapy. Youngsters are taught that the feelings they experience early in the typical pattern leading to firesetting, such as loneliness or sadness, are a signal that the impulse to firestart may be imminent. They are reminded that they do not always have to act on their feelings, especially if they firestart. They are told that

they have a choice of what to do about their feelings. They are asked what constructive behaviors they can pursue when they are feeling lonely and sad. These alternative behaviors are listed on the graph. Youngsters are told that they probably will not set anymore fires, but if they have the urge to firestart, they should pay attention to their feelings so that they can talk about them with their therapist. If they become overwhelmed with their feelings and want to set a fire, they are asked to first telephone and talk with their therapist. If subsequent firestarts occur, then these firesetting episodes are graphed and become the focus for future sessions. If youngsters are successful in redirecting their urge to firestart, they are supported and praised by their therapist and their family. This form of cognitive-emotion therapy averages six to eight sessions and can be considered a form of brief psychotherapy.

A follow-up clinical assessment was conducted, with 26 of 29 firesetting youngsters participating in this type of cognitive-emotion therapy (Bumpass et al., 1983, 1985). Only two of the 26 youngsters exhibited single episodes of firesetting behavior subsequent to the termination of their treatment. For six youngsters, additional psychotherapy was recommended once the graphing technique had been successful in abating their firesetting behavior. Unfortunately, these recommendations were not pursued; these youngsters became involved in other acting-out and antisocial behaviors, such as petty theft and vandalism, and were subsequently treated in inpatient and residential treatment facilities. While there was no control group included in this follow-up evaluation, this preliminary assessment indicates that this method shows some promise in eliminating firestarting behavior. It remains unclear how successful this approach is in addressing the underlying psychopathology that frequently occurs in the lives of firesetting youngsters and their families.

There are a number of behavior therapy approaches that have been reported as successful in abating firesetting behavior. The predominant behavior therapy methods employed either alone or in combination are punishment, reinforcement, negative practice or satiation, and operantly structured fantasies. Two case studies report the successful application of various methods of punishment that includes the use of threats, such as work penalties (Carstens, 1982). Sometimes the use of punishment is coupled with positively reinforcing youngsters when they find and return to their parents conspicuously hidden empty matchbooks (Holland, 1969). Negative practice procedures, coupled with the use of positive reinforcement to encourage more socially appropriate behaviors, also have been reported as successful in stopping severe and recurrent firestarting behavior (Kolko, 1988; Kolko, 1983). One behavior therapy case study avoided the application of punishment methods or negative fire experiences by utilizing a positive reinforcement program coupled with the implementation of operantly structured fantasies (Stawar, 1976).

All of the reported behavior therapy techniques—punishment, positive reinforcement programs, negative practice and satiation procedures, and operantly structured fantasies—are successful in stopping pathological firesetting behavior in single case applications. In addition, these methods are short-term interventions that can be employed within an average of six to 12 sessions. However, questions remain regarding the effectiveness of the techniques with more than one or two cases. Also, while these methods appear to be successful in stopping the specific firesetting behavior, there is little evidence indicating that these or other behavioral techniques can change or adjust accompanying psychopathology. Measuring the relative success of behavior therapy is a challenge for the future.

There are only three cases reported in the literature utilizing brief (three to six sessions) family psychotherapy to successfully treat firesetting youngsters (Eisler, 1974; Madanes, 1981; Minuchin, 1974). Two of the three cases employed the use of teaching family members how to safely ignite and extinguish matches in a controlled setting within the therapist's office (Eisler, 1974; Minuchin, 1974). This controlled firestarting task was used as a vehicle to restructure the existing patterns of family communication and interaction. In particular, attention was focused on restoring the appropriate amount of parenting authority and reestablishing communication between youngsters and their parents regarding household rules designed for the safety and protection of the family. In the third case, the youngster's firesetting was viewed as the overt symptom of a dysfunctional family system (Madanes, 1981). Family therapy sessions were focused on a recognition of the underlying distress and helping family members to identify the changes that needed to happen to reshape the nature of their interactions. In all three cases, follow-up studies indicated the successful elimination of firesetting behavior and a higher level of satisfaction among family members regarding patterns of communication and interaction. While these clinical reports are encouraging, the success of family psychotherapy in treating firesetting cases deserves more systematic and widespread application and evaluation.

Inpatient treatment programs for firesetting youngsters have been influenced by two major types of therapeutic philosophies (Gaynor and Hatcher, 1987). The first is a more traditional, psychodynamic approach where the treatment emphasis is on the nature of the therapeutic alliance formed between youngsters and program staff. Both individual and family psychotherapy are the techniques employed and the treatment program is long-term (ranging from 6 months to 2 years). The second theoretical approach is behavioral, where specific behaviors are identified for change and discrete interventions are designed to adjust these behaviors. The firesetting youngsters are the primary focus of the behavior therapy methods, with parents and family members included in the therapeutic endeavor once the firesetting behavior has been eliminated. Behavior therapy programs tend to be relatively short-term (4–8 weeks) and are currently the most widely offered inpatient approach to the treatment of firesetting youngsters.

The most recently developed inpatient program designed specifically for firesetting youngsters and their families is comprised of three major phases (Gaynor and Hatcher, 1987). In the first phase, youngsters enter a hospital setting for a 4-week stay. During this time, they participate in a series of behavioral exercises in which a choice must be made between toys and firestarting materials. These exercises are observed by therapists out of the view of the youngsters. If they choose matches and lighters as opposed to non-fire-related toys, the therapist intervenes and conducts a debriefing. The debriefing focuses on helping youngsters to realize the experienced emotions associated with choosing firestarting materials. The result of these exercises is that children are left with a mild aversion to firestarting materials. During the second phase, while youngsters are still hospitalized, intensive family psychotherapy is employed to adjust those environmental conditions within the family that are associated with the emergence of firesetting behavior. The third phase focuses on reentry into the family and community. Outpatient family psychotherapy is used, and an intensive effort is made to provide special community support services such as schooling and structured activities. At the end of the third phase, it is expected that youngsters will return to the family and social environment, not participate in firestarting activities, and function adequately within their interpersonal and social milieu. No formal clinical or empirical studies have been reported regarding the efficacy of this inpatient treatment program; however, one source indicates that there have been no relapses in 100 cases treated in a 2-year period (Birchill, 1984).

Several outpatient and inpatient treatment methods report preliminary success in treating firesetting youngsters. The selection of the best intervention strategy depends on maximizing the fit between an assessment of the severity of the firesetting and associated clinical features and the philosophies, modalities, and targets of behavior change emphasized by the treatment approaches. If clinical assessments reveal youngsters who are a significant danger to themselves or others and there is evidence of severe psychopathology, then inpatient treatment must be strongly considered. If the need for inpatient treatment can be ruled out, then outpatient psychotherapy becomes a viable intervention option. In general, the cognitive-emotion approach uses the graphing technique to effect changes in emotional functioning, behavior therapy uses a variety of methods to extinguish firestarting and in some cases replace it with more socially acceptable behaviors, and family psychotherapy works within the family structure to adjust role relationships and patterns of communication and interaction. Mention must be made of attempts by local fire departments, in conjunction with various community agencies such as schools, mental health, law enforcement, and juvenile justice, to develop fire safety and education interventions for firesetting youngsters (Gaynor and Stern, 1993; Gaynor et al., 1991). When appropriate, especially for younger firesetting children, these interventions should be pursued as an adjunct to psychotherapy. Until more rigorous standards of scientific evaluation can be applied to study the relative effectiveness of all these treatment efforts, clinical evidence must stand by itself as the sole support of the success of these intervention strategies.

RESEARCH DIRECTIONS

To date there have been no systematic attempts to mount an organized research effort to empirically describe the prevalence of firesetting in youngsters, to quantify the clinical features associated with firesetting, or to test the relative effectiveness of various psychotherapies in treating the problem. The majority of work in the field has been limited to clinical studies with little or no attention paid to rigorous standards of scientific evaluation. The state-of-the art with respect to research is, at best, qualitative in nature. There is a desperate need for an organized effort to empirically quantify the clinical data from which emerges the bulk of our information on firesetting youngsters. The major priorities for future research include: prospective epidemiologic studies focused on the prevalence of unsupervised firestarting behavior in normal populations of children and an estimate of the proportion of these children who later become involved in pathological firesetting; an empirical comparison of the clinical features of firesetting youngsters compared with those youngsters diagnosed with other specific delinquent or antisocial behaviors; and a randomized clinical trial comparing the relative effectiveness of two or more psychotherapy approaches in not only eliminating firesetting behavior but in alleviating the associated psychopathology that accompanies this destructive behavior. If these research goals are achieved, then significant steps will have been taken to prevent the occurrence of pathological firesetting behavior in future generations of our children.

References

American Psychiatric Association: *Diagnostic and Statistical Manual of Mental Disorders IV Draft Criteria*. Washington, DC, American Psychiatric Press, 1993.

Benians RC: Conspicuous firesetting in children. *Br J Psychiatry* 139:366, 1981.

Birchill LE: Portland's firesetter program involves both child and family. *Am Fire J* 23:15–16, 1984.

Broling L, Brotman C: A firesetting epidemic in a state mental health care center. *Am J Psychiatry* 132:946–950, 1975.

Bumpass ER, Brix RJ, Preston D: A community-based program for juvenile firesetters. *Hosp Community Psychiatry* 36(5):529–532, 1985.

Bumpass ER, Fagelman FD, Brix RJ: Intervention with children who set fires. *Am J Psychother* 37:328–345, 1983.

Carstens C: Application of a work penalty threat in the treatment of juvenile fire setting. *J Behav Ther Exp Psychiatry* 13:159–161, 1982.

Cole RE, Grolnick WS, Laurentis LL, et al: Children and fire. Rochester fire related youth project. Second report. New York, Department of State Office of Fire Prevention and Control, 1986.

Eisler EM: Crisis intervention in the family of a firesetter. *Psychother Theory Res Pract* 9:76–79, 1974.

Federal Bureau of Investigation: *Uniform Crime Reports*. Washington, DC, US Government Printing Office, 1985–1995.

Fine S, Louie D: Juvenile firesetters? Do agencies help? *Am J Psychiatry* 136:433–435, 1979.

Fineman KR: Firesetting in childhood and adolescents. *Psychiatr Clin North Am* 3:483–500, 1980.

Freud S: The acquisition of power over fire. *Int J Psychoanal* 13:404–410, 1932.

Gaynor J, Hatcher C: *The Psychology of Child Firesetting*. Detection and intervention. New York, Brunner/Mazel, 1987.

Gaynor J, Hersch R, Cook R, et al: *Juvenile Firesetter/Arson Control and Prevention Program* (Vol I and II). Washington, DC, Juvenile Justice Clearinghouse, 1991.

Gaynor J, Karchmer C: *Adolescent Firesetter Handbook. Ages 14–18*. Washington, DC, US Government Printing Office, 1988.

Gaynor J, Stern D: Juvenile firesetters. Part II: Effective intervention. *Firehouse* 52:69, 1993.

Gruber AR, Heck ET, Mintzer E: Children who set fires: Some background and behavioral characteristics. *Am J Orthopsychiatry* 51:484–488, 1981.

Hall JR: Juvenile firesetting and fireplay. *Fire J* March/April:27–30, 1989.

Hall JR: *Children Playing with Fire: U.S. Experience, 1980–1991*. Quincy, MA, National Fire Protection Agency, 1993.

Heath GA, Hardesty VA, Goldfine PE, et al: Diagnosis and childhood firesetting. *J Clin Psychol* 41(4):571–575, 1985.

Heller MS, Ehrlich SM, Lester D: Childhood cruelty to animals, firesetting and enuresis as correlates of competency to stand trial. *J Gen Psychiatry* 110(2):151–153, 1984.

Hellman DS, Blackman N: Enuresis, firesetting and cruelty to animals: A triad predictive of adult crime. *Am J Psychiatry* 221:1431–1435, 1966.

Holland CJ: Elimination by the parents of firesetting behavior in a 7-year old boy. *Behav Res Ther* 7:135–137, 1969.

Icove DJ, Estepp MH: Motive-based offender profiles of arson and fire-related crimes. *FBI Law Enforcement Bull* April:17–23, 1987.

Jackson H, Glass C, Hope S: A functional analysis of recidivistic arson. *Br J Clin Psychol* 26(3):175–185, 1987.

Jacobson R: Child firesetters: A clinical investigation. *J Child Psychol Psychiatry Allied Discip* 26(5):759–768, 1985a.

Jacobson R: The subclassification of child firesetters. *J Child Psychol Psychiatry Allied Discip* 26(5):769–775, 1985b.

Jayaprakash S, Jung J, Panitch D: Multifactorial assessment of hospitalized children who set fires. *Child Welfare* 63:74–78, 1984.

Kafry D, Block JH, Block J: Children's survival skills: A basis for functioning in society. Final report prepared for the Maternal and Child Health and Crippled Services Research Program. Bureau of Community Health Services, Rockville, MD, 1980.

Karchmer C: Juvenile firesetter and school arson prevention programs. Hartford, CT, Aetna Life Insurance Co., 1983.

Kaufman I, Heins L, Reiser D: A re-evaluation of the psychodynamics of firesetting. *Am J Orthopsychiatry* 31:123–136, 1961.

Kazdin A: Treatment of antisocial behavior in children: Current status and future directions. *Psychol Bull* 102(2):187–203, 1987.

Kazdin AE, Kolko DJ: Parent psychopathology and family functioning among childhood firesetters. *J Abnorm Child Psychol* 14(2):315–329, 1986.

Kelso J, Stewart MA: Factors which predict the persistence of aggressive conduct disorder. *J Child Psychol Psychiatry Allied Discip* 27(1):77–86, 1986.

Kolko DJ: Multicomponent parental treatment of firesetting in a developmentally disabled boy. *J Behav Ther Exp Psychiatry* 14:349–353, 1983.

Kolko DJ: Firesetting and pyromania. In: Last CG, Herson M (eds): *Handbook of Child Psychiatry Diagnosis*. New York, Wiley, 1988, pp. 443–459.

Kolko DJ, Kazdin AE: Prevalence of firesetting and related behaviors among child psychiatric patients. *J Consult Clin Psychol* 56(4):628–630, 1988.

Kolko DJ, Kazdin AE, Meyer EC: Aggression and psychopathology in childhood firesetters: A controlled study of parent and child reports. *J Consult Clin Psychol* 53:377–385, 1985.

Kuhnley EJ, Hendren RL, Quinlan DM: Firesetting by children. *J Am Acad Psychiatry* 21:560–563, 1982.

Lewis NDC, Yarnell H: Pathological firesetting (pyromania). Nervous and Mental Disease Monographs 1951:82.

Loeber R, Dishion TJ: Early predictors of male delinquency: A review. *Psychol Bull* 94:68–99, 1983.

Macht LB, Mack JE: The firesetter syndrome. *Am J Orthopsychiatry* 31:277–288, 1968.

Madanes C: *Strategic Family Therapy*. San Francisco, Jossey-Bass, 1981.

McCord W, McCord J, Howard A: Familial correlates of aggression in nondelinquent male children. *J Abnorm Soc Psychol* 62:79–93, 1963.

McKerracher DW, Dacre JL: A study of arsonists in a special security hospital. *Br J Psychiatry* 112:1151–1154, 1966.

Minuchin S: *Families and Family Therapy*. Cambridge, MA, Harvard University Press, 1974.

National Fire Protection Agency: Fires and fire losses classified. *Fire J* September 1978–1988.

Patterson GR: *A Social Learning Approach to Family Intervention. Vol I: Families with Aggressive Children*. Eugene, OR, Castalia Publishing Co., 1975.

Patterson GR, DeBaryshe BD, Ramsey E: A developmental perspective on antisocial behavior. *Am Psychol* 44(2):329–335, 1989.

Prentky RA, Carter DL: The predictive value of the triad for sex offenders. *Behav Sci Law* 2(3):341–354, 1984.

Reis L: Family functioning of firesetters, antisocial nonfiresetters, and nonproblem adolescents. A dissertation submitted in partial fulfillment of the requirements for the degree of doctor of philosophy in the graduate school of the Texas Woman's University. Denton, TX: College of Education and Human Ecology, 1993.

Rider AO: The firesetter: A psychological profile. Arson. *Resource Exchange Bulletin*. Washington, DC, US Fire Administration, 1980.

Ritvo E, Shanok SS, Lewis DO: Firesetting and nonfiresetting delinquents: A comparison of neuropsychiatric, psychoeducational, experiential and behavioral characteristics. *Child Psychiatry Hum Dev* 13:259–267, 1982.

Sakheim GA, Osborn E: A psychological profile of juvenile firesetters in residential treatment: A replication study. *Child Welfare* 65(5):495–503, 1986.

Sakheim GA, Osborn E: *Firesetting children: Risk assessment and treatment*. Washington, DC, Child Welfare League of America, 1994.

Sakheim GA, Osborn E, Abrams D: Toward a clearer differentiation of high-risk from low-risk firesetters. *Child Welfare League of America* 60(4):489–503, 1991.

Sakheim GA, Vigdor MG, Gordon M, et al: A psychological profile of juvenile firesetters in residential treatment. *Child Welfare* 64:453–476, 1985.

Showers J, Pickrell E: Child firesetters. A study of three populations. *Hosp Community Psychiatry* 38:495–501, 1987.

Siegelman EY, Folkman WS: *Youthful Firesetters: An Exploratory Study in Personality and Background*. Springfield, VA, USDA Forest Service, 1971.

Stawar TL: Fable mod: Operantly structured fantasies as an adjunct in the modification of fire-setting behavior. *J Behav Ther Exp Psychiatry* 7:285–287, 1976.

Stekel W: *Peculiarities of Behavior* (Vol II). New York, Boni and Liveright, 1924.

Stewert MA, Culver KW: Children who set fires: The clinical picture and a follow-up. *Br J Psychiatry* 140:357–363, 1982.

Strachan JG: Conspicuous firesetting in children. *Br J Psychiatry* 138:26–29, 1981.

Vandersall TA, Weiner JM: Children who set fires. *Arch Gen Psychiatry* 22:63–71, 1970.

Vreeland RG, Waller MB: *The Psychology of Firesetting. A Review and Appraisal*. Washington, DC, US Department of Commerce, National Bureau of Standards, 1979.

Wooden WS, Berkey ML: *Children and Arson: America's Middle Class Nightmare*. New York, Plenum, 1984.

Yarnell H: Firesetting in children. *Am J Orthopsychiatry* 10:272–286, 1940.

Zeegers M: Criminal fire-setting: A review and some case studies. *Med Law* 3:171–176, 1984.

56 GENDER IDENTITY DISORDERS

Kenneth J. Zucker, Ph.D., and Richard Green, M.D., J.D.

DEFINITION

At a nascent cognitive level, gender identity has been defined as a child's recognition that he or she is a member of one sex but not of the other sex. Three decades ago, Stoller (1964) coined the term *core gender identity* to refer to the development of a "fundamental sense of belonging to one sex," the "awareness" that one is a male or a female. At an affective level, this sense of belonging is emotionally valued, so that a child experiences a sense of comfort or security from being a boy or a girl. Gender identity can often be inferred from the sex-dimorphic play of young children, in which they express their identification with the male or female sex through culturally sanctioned markers of masculinity or femininity (gender roles).

Utilizing these features of normal or conventional gender identity, what features does one observe in children and adolescents who are said to have gender identity disorder (GID)? The most common feature is a strong identification with, and preference for, the gender role characteristics of the other sex. This can be inferred from various age-related behavioral manifestations of gender identification, such as toy interests, fantasy role and activity preferences, peer affiliation preferences, and personality traits. Cross-gender identification is also expressed through verbal statements that one is, or would like to be, a member of the other sex. Moreover, children with GID often have few positive things to say about their own sex and appear to experience a sense of *gender dysphoria*, or unease, about being of the sex that they are. By adolescence, when the clinical picture can be described by age-appropriate criteria and with the DSM-IV diagnosis *gender identity disorder* (American Psychiatric Association, 1994), the pervasive sense of gender dysphoria is difficult to ignore or dismiss.

HISTORICAL NOTE

In the 1950s, two clinical developments led to an increased interest in the study of children with potential problems in their gender identity development. First, Money et al.'s (1957) research on children with various forms of intersex conditions showed that key milestones in gender identity formation occurred sometime between 18 and 36 months of age, if not earlier. It was observed that, despite the ambiguous sexual biology of hermaphroditic children, they could develop a stable gender identity if they were reared unambiguously as members of one sex or the other. Second, retrospective clinical reports on the adult syndrome of GID, commonly known as *transsexualism* (Benjamin, 1954), led to the recognition that the behavioral markers of this condition could be observed as early as the child's first few years of life.

More than 30 years ago, Green and Money (1960) reported on a series of five boys without detectable physical or biological abnormality who displayed what was described as ''incongruous'' gender role behavior, a pattern that was incorporated 20 years later into the DSM-III diagnosis *gender identity disorder of childhood*. Since this initial report, a number of studies of such children have been conducted, directed at, among other things, developing accurate diagnostic and assessment procedures, evaluating etiological hypotheses, examining the effects of treatment, and tracking long-term development (see, e.g., Green, 1974, 1987; Zucker and Bradley, 1995; Zucker and Green, 1992).

By the 1970s, thinking about children with gender identity problems was being influenced by a third development. A series of studies on adult homosexuality, perhaps peaking with the volume by Bell et al. (1981), indicated that the presence of patterns of childhood cross-gender behavior was a strong developmental predictor of later homosexuality (see also Bailey and Zucker, 1995). Although efforts to treat homosexuality have declined substantially since 1973, when homosexuality was deleted from the DSM as a mental disorder, interest in the determinants of sexual orientation has continued.

EPIDEMIOLOGY

Prevalence

No studies have formally assessed the prevalence of GID in children. It has been suggested, however, that conservative estimates of prevalence can be inferred from data regarding the prevalence of GID (transsexualism) in adults. Such data are based on the number of persons attending clinics that serve as gateways for surgical and hormonal sex reassignment. Since not all gender dysphoric adults make themselves known, this method may underestimate the prevalence of GID; in any case, the number of adult transsexuals is small—one recent estimate from The Netherlands suggests a prevalence of 1 in 11,000 men and 1 in 30,400 women (Bakker et al., 1993).

The prevalence of GID might also be derived from the literature on the epidemiology of homosexuality. Unfortunately, this literature presents two main problems. First, the true prevalence of exclusive, or near-exclusive, preferential homosexuality remains a source of debate (see, e.g., Billy et al., 1993; Diamond, 1993; Fay et al., 1989; Wellings et al., 1994); second, the retrospective literature on childhood cross-gender behavior in homosexual men and women often does not specify how to determine a cutoff score to dichotomize cases as cross-gendered versus not cross-gendered. In addition, cases classified as cross-gendered would not necessarily meet the complete diagnostic criteria for GID in DSM-IV (Friedman, 1988).

More liberal estimates of prevalence can be judged from studies of children in whom specific cross-gender behaviors have been assessed. For example, the standardization study of the Child Behavior Checklist (Achenbach and Edelbrock, 1981), a widely used parent-report questionnaire of childhood behavioral psychopathology, included information on the percentage of mothers of both clinic-referred and nonreferred

boys and girls who endorsed two items pertaining to cross-gender identification: ''behaves like opposite sex'' and ''wishes to be of opposite sex.'' Table 56.1 shows that the endorsement of both items was more common for girls than for boys, regardless of age and clinical status, and ''behaves like opposite sex'' was endorsed more often than ''wishes to be of opposite sex.'' Among referred boys, the desire to be of the opposite sex was quite high for the 4- to 5-year-olds (15.5%) but dropped off sharply thereafter. Among referred girls, the desire to be of the opposite sex seemed more stable (range, 4.2–8.3%) and was consistently higher than for the nonreferred girls. The main problem with such data is that they do not differentiate enduring patterns of cross-gender behavior from transient phenomena (Zucker, 1985). Accordingly, data of this kind would probably overestimate cases of GID, although the methods of data collection may be reasonable screening devices for more intensive evaluation (cf. Linday, 1994; Pleak et al., 1989; Sandberg et al., 1993).

Incidence

Has the incidence of GID changed since it was first described in children over 30 years ago? Unfortunately, the types of child epidemiological data required to answer this question do not exist. Indirect sources of information are available, but they are difficult to employ. Consider, for example, the contemporary debate regarding the incidence of preferential homosexuality. Some authors maintain that this incidence is rather stable, whereas others hold that it has increased (Fay et al., 1989). If the former view is correct, then one might also expect a stable incidence of GID, of which some unspecified percentage of homosexual adults probably experienced in childhood (at least in muted form). If the latter view is correct, then one might expect to find a greater number of children experiencing symptoms of GID. Changes in patterns of child rearing with regard to sex role behavior are another indirect source of information on changes in the incidence of GID. Lothstein (1983) reported his clinical experience that mothers who had attempted to ''masculinize'' their daughters or ''feminize'' their sons in order to prepare them for ''radically new social roles'' did not produce ''androgynous'' children, as they had hoped, but rather children who evidenced a ''stereotypical cross-gender role which was frightening to their parents'' (p. 248). Whether parental efforts to shape children's gender role behavior in less conventional ways is inadvertently inducing GID has, in fact, not been well studied, so no firm conclusions can be drawn as of yet.

Referral Rates

Apart from issues of prevalence and incidence, there has been a consistent observation that boys are more often referred than girls for concerns regarding gender identity. The first author's clinic in Toronto, Canada, has the most systematic data on this point, with a referral ratio of 6.3:1 (N = 249) of boys to girls. The second author was able to generate a research sample of very feminine boys through professional channels but found it necessary to generate a research sample of masculine girls (''tomboys'') by means of newspaper advertisement.

The true prevalence of GID may well be greater in boys than in girls, but social factors also appear to influence the higher referral rate for boys, since there are data suggesting that both peers and adults are more likely to tolerate cross-gender behavior in girls than in boys. In addition, adults are less likely to predict atypical outcomes, such as homosexuality, in masculine girls than in feminine boys (Zucker, 1985) and are therefore less likely to be concerned about cross-gender behavior in girls. Thus, cases of GID in girls may be underreferred due to greater social acceptance of girlhood masculinity. On the other hand, there may be more false-positive referrals of boys than of girls because of overconcern about boyhood femininity. However, clinical experience suggests that the latter possibility is uncommon.

CLINICAL DESCRIPTION

The initial behavioral signs of GID most typically appear during the toddler and preschool years (Green, 1974, 1987), the years in which more conventional patterns of sex-typed behavior can also first be observed. In some cases, however, parents will recall that such behaviors as cross-dressing began prior to the 2nd birthday. The central clinical issue concerns the degree to which a pattern of behavioral signs is present, since this pattern is the basis for inference on the extent to which a child is cross-gender-identified.

In boys, the clinical picture, in its full form, includes at least eight characteristics: (*a*) an occasional or frequently stated desire to be a girl or an insistence that he is a girl; (*b*) verbal or behavioral expressions of ''anatomic dysphoria'' (e.g., saying that he does not like his penis and would prefer a vagina or vulva; urinating in the seated position to enhance the fantasy of having female genitalia); (*c*) frequent cross-dressing in girls' or women's clothing or use of other apparel (e.g., towels) to simulate feminine attire; (*d*) a preference for female roles in fantasy play and an avoidance of male roles in fantasy play; (*e*) a preference for stereotypical feminine toys and activities and an avoidance of stereotypical masculine toys and activities; (*f*) recurrent display of stereotypical feminine or effeminate mannerisms; (*g*) a preference for girls as playmates and an avoidance or dislike of boys as playmates; and (*h*) an avoidance of rough-and-tumble play and/or participation in group sports with males.

In girls, the clinical picture is similar. It includes (*a*) an occasional or frequently stated desire to be a boy or an insistence that she is a boy; (*b*) verbal or behavioral expressions of anatomic dysphoria (e.g., stating a desire to have a penis; urinating in the standing position in order to enhance the fantasy of having male genitalia); (*c*) an intense aversion to wearing stereotypical feminine clothing and an insistence on wearing stereotypical masculine clothing; (*d*) a preference for male roles in fantasy play and an avoidance of female roles in fantasy play; (*e*) a preference for stereotypical masculine toys and activities and an avoidance of stereotypical feminine toys and activities: (*f*) recurrent display of stereotypical masculine mannerisms; (*g*) a preference for boys as playmates and an avoidance or dislike of girls as playmates; and (*h*) a strong interest in rough-and-tumble play and participation in group sports with boys.

During childhood, several developmental issues should be considered. One of these issues concerns the child's remarks about wanting to be of the other sex or insisting that he or she is a member of the other sex. Stoller (1968) argued that boys who literally believed that they were girls constituted an etiologically distinct subgroup within the universe of feminine boys and were most at risk for development as transsexuals. Subsequent clinical observations and empirical data suggest that Stoller's view is not entirely accurate. Relatively young boys who show multiple signs of cross-gender behavior, as was the case in Stoller's (1968) sample, are the ones most likely to misclassify themselves as girls (Zucker et al., 1993b). It is not clear whether this subgroup is etiologically distinct. Developmentally, one would expect younger children to have more difficulty with regard to correct gender self-labeling, and this has been verified by empirical studies of normal children. Among children with GID, then, one would expect more difficulties with correct gender self-labeling to occur during the preschool years when the overall clinical picture is extreme and, perhaps, when there are rather severe problems in general psychosocial functioning. The most common clinical presentation is that of a child who knows what his or her sex is but desires to be the other sex (see Zucker et al., 1993b).

A second developmental issue concerns variation in age-related markers of cross-gender identification. Some behaviors, such as cross-sex peer affiliation preference, appear to remain stable throughout childhood; however, other behaviors, such as activity and role interests, may show important changes. Young boys, for example, who show a preoccupation with female dolls and role play as a mother are much less likely to play with female dolls (or, for that matter, with any dolls) or to role play female characters as they approach adolescence but may well continue to manifest feminine preoccupations, such as an intense interest in feminine fashion and idealization of female actresses or rock stars. The effeminate mannerisms of such boys may become more prominent. In addition, older children are less likely than younger children to verbalize the desire to change sex (Zucker et al., 1984, in press),

although the persistence of gender dysphoria in these children may be expressed in other ways, such as devaluation of their own sex and idealization of the other sex.

A final developmental issue concerns the meaning of the desire to change sex during the childhood and adolescent years. In early childhood, that desire may be related to several factors. For example, a child might reason that because he or she prefers cross-sex activities, it would make sense to become a person of the other sex. Or, a child might believe that engaging in cross-sex activities actually changes his or her sex, a manifestation of the preoperational thinking that takes place prior to the achievement of *gender constancy*. Familial factors may also be important for young children who perceive that a parent would actually like them to be of the other sex (or some subtle variation of this communication). Thus, it is highly unlikely that young children conceptualize the wish to change sex in the same manner as adolescents.

ETIOLOGY AND PATHOGENESIS

Biological Mechanisms and Hypotheses

The search for biological correlates or determinants of gender identity, gender role, and sexual orientation development in humans has been a slow and complex process, with many leads coming to dead ends. There is disagreement about the degree to which biological factors exert fixed versus predisposing influences on the components of psychosexual development.

At present, no specific biological anomaly has been identified in children or adolescents with GID; however, there is evidence that certain behavioral traits associated with biological variables may characterize at least some children with GID. The current state of the art regarding biological factors relies heavily on data from ''allied'' populations, from which tentative generalizations might be drawn. This section reviews the most promising and interesting lines of research.

GENETICS

Over the past several years, a number of studies have reported that homosexuality runs in families (Pillard and Weinrich, 1986). Other studies have reported a greater concordance for homosexuality in monozygotic twins than in dizygotic twins (Bailey and Pillard, 1991; Bailey et al., 1993). Although these studies are not beyond methodological reproach (Bynes and Parson, 1993), the pattern of results is consistent with, though not proof of, a genetic influence. Moreover, it should be noted that the concordance rates for homosexuality in monozygotic twins was far from perfect—about 50% in the methodologically strongest studies. Little is known, however, about familiality in either children (e.g., Zuger, 1989) or adults with GID (e.g., Hoenig, 1985).

Hamer et al. (1993) conducted the first molecular genetic study of sexual orientation in males. Hamer et al. focused a DNA linkage analysis on the X chromosome, since there was independent evidence of increased rates of homosexuality in maternal male relatives. Forty families that contained two homosexual brothers were studied. DNA was typed for 22 markers that spanned the X chromosome. Markers judged specific to sexual orientation were found on the distal portion of Xq28, the subtelomeric region of the long arm of the X chromosome. Of the 40 pairs of brothers, 33 were concordant for all markers and 7 were discordant at one or more loci. Risch et al. (1993) offered some preliminary methodological criticisms of this study, but, in our view, the key issue, like in other molecular genetic studies of behavior, will be whether or not the findings can be replicated by other research teams. The relevance of this work to the origins of GID is not yet clear.

PRENATAL SEX HORMONES

There is substantial evidence from animal and human studies that variations in the prenatal hormonal environment affect sex-dimorphic gender role behaviors and, possibly, the development of gender identity and sexual orientation.

Consider, for example, a recent study (Goy et al., 1988) of the rhesus macaque (*Macaca mulatta*) in which pseudohermaphroditism was induced in genetic females by administration of exogenous androgen to the mother during specific periods of gestation. In this study, certain empirically determined sex-dimorphic behavior patterns (e.g., rough play with peers, foot-clasp mounts, grooming) were examined during the 3rd year of life. The female pseudohermaphrodites showed sex-dimorphic behavior patterns between those of their normal female and male counterparts. The study was particularly intriguing, first, because it showed that the timing of the exogenous hormone manipulation differentially affected specific sex-dimorphic behaviors, suggesting that hormonal treatments exert their influence during more than one "sensitive period," and second, because even female pseudohermaphrodites who did not show genital masculinization as a result of the hormonal treatment exhibited the sex-dimorphic behavioral pattern.

This type of study has generated considerable excitement because it implicates prenatal sex hormones in the "organizing" and shaping of postnatal sex-dimorphic behavior, while leaving the external configuration of the genitalia intact. Other studies of nonhuman primates have attempted to understand how social factors modify or modulate the predisposition induced by hormonal factors and thus represent the type of interactionist perspective advocated by many theorists.

Prenatal sex hormones also appear to exert some effects on human psychosexual development. Such effects have been observed in girls with congenital adrenal hyperplasia (CAH), a particularly illuminating form of pseudohermaphroditism from a theoretical perspective. Treatment of this condition with corticosteroids essentially restricts the effects of the hormonal anomaly to the prenatal period. Empirical studies of girls with CAH have shown that, on average, their behavior is more masculine and/or less feminine than that of unaffected controls (Berenbaum and Hines, 1992; Ehrhardt and Baker, 1974). The evidence regarding the effects of CAH on gender identity is less clear, although the percentage who express some ambivalence about being female or who have been reared as boys (in part because the condition went untreated) is probably higher among girls with CAH than among girls in the general population (Berenbaum, 1990; Zucker et al., 1987). Recent adult follow-up studies of girls with CAH suggest higher rates of bisexuality or homosexuality, particularly in fantasy, and lower rates of marriage and sociosexual experiences than would be expected otherwise (Dittmann et al., 1992; Money et al., 1984; Mulaikal et al., 1987; Zucker et al., 1992).

Although studies of females with CAH implicate the potential role of prenatal hormones on postnatal psychosexual behavior, individual differences in outcome have not been adequately explained. It is not clear, for example, whether such differences result from the severity of the disorder; from biomedical sequelae of the condition, such as the success of surgical correction and cosmesis; or from social factors (e.g., how parents contribute to their daughters' socialization).

In any case, these studies require serious thought by those working with children with GID. Paradoxically, however, no identifiable hormonal anomaly seems to characterize the vast majority of the children with this disorder. Nevertheless, there has been speculation that less pronounced variations in prenatal hormonal influences account, in part, for intrasex differences in the expression of sex-dimorphic behavior. Consider, for example, rough-and-tumble play and activity level in boys. Boys with GID usually dislike rough-and-tumble play (Green, 1974, 1987) and appear to have a relatively low activity level (Zucker and Green, 1993). Both of these behaviors show a strong sex dimorphism (Eaton and Enns, 1986). It is likely that the two behaviors, which are probably closely related, are at least partly determined by biological factors. The high energy level of both boys and girls with CAH lends some support to this suggestion (Berenbaum, 1990).

Boys with GID also seem more prone to internalizing traits or disorders than they are to externalizing traits or disorders (Coates and Person, 1985; Zucker, 1985; Zucker and Bradley, 1995). These boys also appear to be quite shy or behaviorally inhibited (Coates et al., 1994). A very anxious boy is likely to be timid and thus avoidant of rough-and-tumble play. Such a boy may shy away from other boys as playmates, feel more comfortable in the presence of girls, and identify more with his mother

than with his father. Reactions to his anxiety and timidity may exacerbate or attenuate the situation; for example, exposure to less-active boys may accustom the anxious boy to male peers, whereas exposure to only female peers and their conventionally feminine activities may increase a predisposition to cross-gender identification. Thus, the boy may eventually decide that it is better to be a girl than a boy (Green, 1974, 1987).

SEX-RELATED COGNITIVE ABILITIES, NEUROPSYCHOLOGICAL FUNCTION, AND NEUROANATOMIC STRUCTURES

A great deal of research has focused on sex differences (and similarities) in cognitive abilities, neuropsychological functioning, and neuroanatomic structures, which has guided studies of persons with atypical psychosexual differentiation. Over the past several years, a number of studies have suggested sexual orientation differences in these domains, including sex-dimorphic cognitive abilities (Gladue et al., 1990; McCormick and Witelson, 1991; Sanders and Ross-Field, 1986a), handedness (e.g., Becker et al., 1992; McCormick et al., 1990), neuropsychological tests (e.g., Sanders and Ross-Field, 1986b), EEG patterns (Alexander and Sufka, 1993), dermatoglyphic asymmetry (Hall and Kimura, 1994), and neuroanatomic structures (Allen and Gorski, 1992; LeVay, 1991). Although the data suggest an influence of predisposing biological events for sexual orientation development, there are many reasons to treat these studies with caution and to not succumb to the lure of biological reductionism: much of the data are preliminary, consisting of only one study; some of the findings have not been replicated; and there are a host of methodological issues that need to be explored and worked out (for detailed reviews, see Byne and Parsons, 1993; Friedman and Downey, 1993; Meyer-Bahlburg, 1993; Zucker and Bradley, 1995). Moreover, the relevance of these studies for understanding the origins of GID is indirect. Very little work has explored these variables with children and some approaches are likely to be impossible (e.g., assessment of neuroanatomic structures).

SIBLING SEX RATIO AND BIRTH ORDER

Unlike some of the other biological markers of putative causal relevance for psychosexual differentiation, sibling sex ratio and birth order are easy to measure. Sibling sex ratio is the ratio of brothers to sisters collectively reported by a given group of probands. In white populations, the ratio of male live births to female live births is close to 106:100 (Chahnazarian, 1988). The ratio of brothers to sisters reported by any group of men drawn at random from the general population should therefore approach 106 (brothers per 100 sisters). Birth order has been commonly calculated with Slater's (1958) index—a proband's number of older siblings divided by his or her total number of siblings—which expresses birth order as a quantity between 0 (first-born) and 1 (last-born). Observed birth orders can be compared between groups or with the theoretical mean of Slater's index for samples drawn at random from the general population (.50).

Sibling sex ratio with regard to sexual orientation, particularly in males, was first studied by several investigators in the 1930s. Blanchard and Sheridan (1992) recently reviewed this literature and noted that homosexual men had been shown to come from sibships with an excess of brothers to sisters. Earlier summaries of this literature had also identified this pattern (e.g., Money, 1970), but interest in the phenomenon seemed to wane, perhaps because the initial attention given to it had been guided by biological theories that fell into disfavor.

Over the last few years, however, several studies have taken another look at this forgotten biodemographic variable. Blanchard and Zucker (1994) reanalyzed the data from the Kinsey Institute's large-scale study of homosexual and heterosexual men (Bell et al., 1981) and found a sibling sex ratio of 104:100 for the homosexual men, which did not differ significantly from the known proportion of male live births in the general population. The sibling sex ratio of the heterosexual men was 105:100, which was also a nonsignificant difference. Zucker and Blanchard (1994) reanalyzed the data from the Bieber et al. (1962) study of homosexual and heterosexual men in psychoanalytic therapy and found no sibling sex ratio effects; however, the sample sizes were small, and thus one would not have expected to detect a significant effect unless the sibling sex ratio was markedly skewed. Lastly, Blanchard and Bogaert (in press) reanalyzed the original Kinsey et al. (1948) sample of homosexual and heterosexual men and also found no unusual sibling sex ratio.

Blanchard and Sheridan (1992) studied the sibling sex ratio among homosexual men with GID (transsexualism). The sibling sex ratio of 131:100 differed significantly from that of the general population; in contrast, the sibling sex ratio of nonhomosexual men with GID (117:100) was not significantly different from that of the general population. Blanchard et al. (in press) have replicated these findings in another sample of homosexual and nonhomosexual men with GID from The Netherlands.

Blanchard et al. (1995) studied sibling sex ratio in a sample of prepubertal feminine boys (many of whom met the DSM criteria for GID) and male homosexual and/or gender-dysphoric adolescents assessed in the first author's clinic. The feminine boy/homosexual adolescent group had a sibling sex ratio that favored brothers to sisters (141:100), which was significantly greater than the sibling sex ratio of a clinical control group of boys (matched to the probands for age at assessment, number of full siblings, and approximate year of birth) (104:100) and that of the general population.

Regarding the birth order of homosexual men, which was also studied by some of the earlier investigators interested in sibling sex ratio, the two largest older studies found birth order indexes significantly greater than the theoretical mean, indicating that homosexual men were born later than members of the general population (see Blanchard and Sheridan, 1992). In Blanchard and Zucker's (1994) reanalysis of the Kinsey Institute data set, the homosexual men were found to have been born significantly later than the heterosexual men. Zucker and Blanchard (1994) reanalyzed the birth order data from the Bieber et al. (1962) study and Blanchard and Bogaert (in press) reanalyzed the birth order data from Kinsey et al. (1948) and found similar effects.

Blanchard and Sheridan (1992) found that homosexual men with GID had a later birth order than nonhomosexual men with GID. This finding was replicated by Blanchard et al. (in press). Blanchard et al. (1995) found that the birth order of the feminine boy/homosexual adolescent group (.58) was also significantly later than that of the clinical control group (.45) and the theoretical mean of .50.

Taken together, then, the evidence cited suggests that sibling sex ratio and birth order are biodemographic variables that distinguish homosexual men with GID and boys with GID from control subjects. A later birth order, but not an excess of brothers, has been most consistently observed in samples of ordinary homosexual men.

The observed sibling sex ratio and birth order effects are amenable to at least two biological explanations that have been discussed in the literature on psychosexual differentiation. Blanchard and Sheridan (1992) and Blanchard et al. (1995) noted that both explanations, which will be described, are variations on the prenatal hormonal theory implicating incomplete androgenization of the fetal brain in predisposing a male to homosexuality or gender dysphoria (see above). MacCulloch and Waddington (1981) and Ellis and Ames (1987) proposed that antibodies to testosterone produced by a mother pregnant with a male fetus could suppress the hormone's biological activity and thus affect sexual differentiation of the brain. Because such a reaction might develop over several pregnancies, it would be expected to occur more often in later-born males. However, this hypothesized mechanism has never been demonstrated empirically.

The second explanation is related to maternal stress. Because there is some evidence that stressed mothers give birth to a predominance of male offspring (Chahnazarian, 1988), maternal stress might explain the excess in the number of brothers in sibships containing at least one homosexual male, given the possibility that mothers of homosexual men are more likely than mothers of heterosexual men to be stress-prone in general, as judged by personality tests (Bailey et al., 1991). There are,

however, two problems with this reasoning. First, the maternal stress hypothesis, as applied to the period of pregnancy, for human male homosexuality does not have strong empirical support (Bailey et al., 1991; Zucker and Green, 1992); second, the recent analyses of ordinary samples of homosexual men have shown that they do not contain an excess number of brothers—the finding has been limited to extremely feminine men and boys (i.e., those with GID). The latter finding leaves open the possibility of prenatal maternal stress as an operative mechanism for extreme cross-gender behavior and subsequent homosexuality, but this remains to be shown empirically.

PHYSICAL APPEARANCE

The influence of physical appearance, including attractiveness, on social perception and interaction has been widely studied by social psychologists. In a clinical study of several very feminine boys, Stoller (1975) made this serendipitous observation about their physical appearance: ''We have noticed that they often have pretty faces, with fine hair, lovely complexions, graceful movements, and—especially—big, piercing, liquid eyes'' (p. 43).

Green (1987; Green et al., 1985; Roberts et al., 1987) systematically studied physical attractiveness in a sample of cross-gender-identified boys and a male control group. At the time of assessment, the parents of both the cross-gender-identified boys and the control boys were asked to describe the faces of their infant sons. Blind ratings of audiotaped interviews showed that the parents of the feminine boys were more likely than the parents of the controls to describe their sons during infancy as ''beautiful'' and ''feminine.'' The parents of the feminine boys were also more likely to recall that strangers commented, ''He would make a beautiful girl.'' ''Retrospective distortion'' could, however, have operated in this situation. Zucker et al. (1993c) provided some data that were consistent with these parental recollections. University students, masked to group status, rated the attractiveness of boys with GID and clinical control boys from photographs taken at the time of clinical assessment. Boys with GID were judged to be significantly more attractive, beautiful, cute, handsome, and pretty than were the control subjects. In a subsequent study (Fridell et al., 1996), girls with GID were judged to be significantly less attractive, beautiful, cute, and pretty than were clinical and normal control girls.

It should be noted that attractiveness need not be conceptualized as a fixed biophysical trait—social shaping of physical appearance is clearly possible. Clinical observations suggest that some parents subtly alter the physical appearance of children with GID so as to induce a ''feminine'' look in boys and a ''masculine'' look in girls. Moreover, some of the children themselves insist on altering their physical appearance. For example, some gender-disturbed girls insist on cutting their hair short and on wearing clothing that will enable them to pass successfully as boys. Physical appearance, then, may be a predisposing factor in the development of GID, may serve to perpetuate the disorder, or may simply be one of the disorder's clinical signs.

Psychosocial Mechanisms and Hypotheses

Many psychosocial factors have been hypothesized to play a role in either the genesis or the maintenance of GID; most of these factors have been better studied in boys than in girls, and some of them have been viewed as applying to only one of the sexes. This section considers a few of the more prominent hypotheses.

PRENATAL SEX PREFERENCE

It is not unusual for parents to express a prenatal sex preference. Witness, for example, the recent explosion in ''sex selection'' clinics. Other things being equal, parents will have a child of the nonpreferred sex about 50% of the time. One might ask, then, whether parents of children with GID had desired a child of the other sex? Although several clinical case reports of boys with GID noted that their mothers had desired daughters, only two controlled studies have investigated this question systematically. Zuger (1974) reported that of 21 feminine boys (including some who were first assessed in adolescence), 38% of their mothers had wanted a girl (four other mothers simply reported that they had not wanted to have a child). A comparable percentage of clinical control mothers had also wanted a girl, but the specific percentage was not reported. Roberts et al. (1987) found that mothers of feminine boys (N = 52) had not expressed a prenatal wish for a daughter significantly more than had mothers of control boys (N = 52). In fact, the percentage of mothers who had wished for a girl was low in both groups, 26.9 and 19.2%, respectively. In a third sample of 103 boys with GID seen in the first author's clinic, 43.7% of the mothers had wished for a daughter (Zucker et al., 1994b). This percentage was significantly higher than the percentage reported by Roberts et al. (1987); however, a comparison group was not available.

Further analyses of Roberts et al.'s data and the first author's data showed that the maternal wish for a girl was significantly associated with the sex composition and birth order of the sibship (Zucker et al., 1994b). Among the probands with older siblings who were only male, the percentage of mothers who recalled a desire for a daughter was significantly higher than among the probands with other kinds of sibship combinations (e.g., the probands who had at least one older sister). This pattern was also observed in Roberts et al.'s control group. Thus, the maternal wish for a daughter appears to be strongly influenced by the sex composition and birth order of the sibship.

Although the wish for a daughter per se is probably not of etiological importance in explaining the genesis of GID, maternal reactions to bearing a child of the nonpreferred sex may be. In our clinical experience, we have observed several quite striking examples of maternal disappointment. One mother cross-dressed her second-born son in infancy and took photographs of him in hair curlers and ''pink'' baby clothes. Another mother took 2 months to name her second-born son and then chose a variant of the preselected girl's name (Zucker et al., 1993c). During her teenage years, a third mother had given up an infant daughter for adoption. She was very disappointed when her second-born son was not a girl. She commented wistfully that she still ''hoped'' to ''get a daughter'' someday, and she was quite jealous of friends who had had girls. A fourth mother wondered whether her feminine son was the ''reincarnation'' of a daughter who had died in infancy from multiple congenital abnormalities. Because she longed for a daughter when pregnant with the proband, this mother reported that she was severely depressed after her son was born. The depression continued unabated until around her son's 3rd month, when a ''look'' in his eyes suggested to her that he understood what she was feeling. Based on considerable clinical work with this mother, it seemed that she interpreted her infant son's ''gaze'' as meaning that he now understood her need for a daughter. Lastly, a fifth mother kept a detailed diary during her pregnancy with her third-born son, which included repeated entries of prayer to God for a daughter. Similar entries occurred during her pregnancy with her fourth-born son. At this time, the third-born son began to show signs of cross-gender behavior, which increased notably after the birth of the baby. The parents then registered at an adoption agency, requesting a 3-year old girl.

These reactions appear extreme, perhaps representing a form of pathological mourning (Parkes, 1975). They point to the importance of exploring with parents the possible meanings that underlie their gender preferences. In our clinical experience, the most common psychological trait that underlies the strong wish for a daughter is the need to nurture and be nurtured by a female child, which often reflects compensatory needs originating in childhood. For example, one mother commented that she wanted very much to dress a daughter in ''frilly'' clothes and to brush a daughter's long hair in ways that she had never experienced from her own mother. For complex psychological and cultural reasons, it is unlikely that such compensatory fantasies can be acted out with a male child. Unfortunately, no empirical study has formally assessed the reactions of mothers of boys with GID to see whether they differ in any systematic way from mothers of control boys. It would be particularly important to see whether these two groups of mothers react differently to the birth of a child of the nonpreferred sex.

SOCIAL SHAPING AND REINFORCEMENT

A simple, perhaps elegant, explanation of GID posits that parents or significant others socialize a child into the gender role more commonly associated with the opposite sex. This might include cross-dressing the child, providing sex-typed toys typical of the opposite sex, and encouraging cross-gender social role play. Verbal commentary would indicate a greater valuing of the opposite sex.

The actual situation does not appear to be this simple. Active cross-dressing of a child is relatively rare (Green, 1974); the emergence of the behavioral markers of GID appears to be more insidious, although in some cases parents can recall events that seemed to abruptly precipitate or exacerbate the disorder (Coates and Person, 1985). The gradual appearance of the behavioral markers requires a more careful assessment of parental reactions. At present, there is reasonable evidence that tolerance, or nonresponsiveness, is the most common parental reaction to the initial appearance of cross-gender behavior (Green, 1974, 1987; Mitchell, 1991; Roberts et al., 1987); actual encouragement of such behavior is a close second; negative or discouraging reactions seem to be the least common. Green (1987) provided some evidence that the degree of approval of initial cross-gender behavior in boys correlated with a composite index of cross-gender behavior at the time of the initial assessment.

Initial parental tolerance or reinforcement of cross-gender behavior, then, may well be of etiological significance. Such toleration or reinforcement appears to result from many factors, including parental attitudes and values regarding psychosexual ideals, feedback from professionals that the behavior is normative or ''just a phase,'' and parental psychopathology and discord, which render the parents less available to cope with their children's developmental needs.

PARENT-CHILD RELATIONSHIPS

Apart from attempts to examine the specific interactions that occur during the initial display of sex-dimorphic behavior, attempts have been made to examine the general quality of the relationships between gender-disturbed children and their parents.

In the case of boys, Stoller (1968, 1975, 1985) observed clinically an overly close relationship between mother and son and a distant, peripheral father-son relationship. He presented his hypothesis simply: ''The more mother and the less father, the more femininity'' (1985, p. 25). Stoller argued that GID in boys is a kind of ''developmental arrest . . . in which an excessively close and gratifying mother-infant symbiosis, undisturbed by father's presence, prevents a boy from adequately separating himself psychically from his mother's female body and feminine behavior'' (1985, p. 25). In several respects, Stoller's notions point to the crucial role of preoedipal events in the development of GID, a view that is shared by many other contemporary psychoanalytic clinicians and theorists.

Green (1987; Green et al., 1985; Roberts et al., 1987) had the parents of feminine boys and control boys rate the amount of ''shared time'' with their sons during the first 5 years of life. Contrary to prediction, the mothers of feminine boys recalled spending less time with their sons compared with the amount of time the mothers of control subjects remembered spending. Consistent with prediction, the fathers of feminine boys recalled spending less time with their sons from the 2nd to 5th year compared with the amount of time the fathers of control subjects remembered and the father's shared time with masculine male siblings. Thus, this method of assessing parent-son relationships confirmed the paternal side of the equation but yielded results opposite from prediction for the maternal side. Thus, at least with regard to the mother, the quality of the mother-child interaction may have been more important than the sheer amount of time that mother and child spent together.

Table 56.1. Percentage of Children Whose Mothers Endorsed Child Behavior Checklist Items Relevant to Cross-Gender Identification

Group	Age[a]				
	4–5	6–7	8–9	10–11	12–13
	Behaves Like Opposite Sex				
Boys					
Referred	16.3	11.2	9.5	10.7	3.7
Nonreferred	6.0	5.9	2.7	4.9	0.7
Girls					
Referred	18.6	9.1	14.5	13.1	16.5
Nonreferred	11.8	9.6	11.0	12.5	12.9
	Wishes to Be of Opposite Sex				
Boys					
Referred	15.5	2.7	5.1	1.1	2.4
Nonreferred	1.3	0.0	0.0	2.3	0.0
Girls					
Referred	6.5	5.8	8.3	7.4	4.2
Nonreferred	5.0	2.6	2.7	1.9	2.7

Derived from data in Achenbach TM, Edelbrock CS: Behavioral problems and competencies reported by parents of normal and disturbed children aged four through sixteen. *Monogr Soc Res Child Dev* 46 (serial no. 188), 1981. Exact percentages from TM Achenbach, personal communication, December 7, 1982.
[a] N = 100 per cell. Percentages are not exact in some cases due to missing data.

Despite Green's (1974, 1987) finding regarding shared time, there is little question that boys with GID feel closer to their mothers than to their fathers. In part, this may be a function of a boy's perception of similarity to the mother, but it also evolves from the day-to-day subtleties of parent-child interaction.

Unfortunately, no systematic studies on parent-child relationships have been conducted for girls with GID. Preliminary clinical studies suggest that for such girls the mother-daughter relationship is often impaired, leading to what might be described as a "disidentification" from the mother (Green, 1974; Stoller, 1975; Zucker and Bradley, 1995). During the early years of these girls, a variety of factors appear to impair the development of a close mother-daughter relationship; as a result, there is a devaluing of femininity and an overvaluing of masculinity, outcomes that the parents seem to encourage. These preliminary clinical studies suggest, therefore, that the quality of parent-child relationships in gender-disturbed boys is quite different from that in gender-disturbed girls.

MATERNAL PSYCHOSEXUAL DEVELOPMENT

Stoller (1968) reported that the mothers of extremely feminine boys had had gender identity conflicts as children, implicating some type of generational transmission. He stated that these women were initially feminine as girls but that following a rupture in the father-daughter relationship "a degree of masculinity beyond what usually [would] be called tomboyishness" (p. 298) occurred. Although they relinquished their desire to be male at puberty, as adults they seemed somewhat uncomfortable with their femininity: "While these women have a feminine quality, inextricably woven in is this other, difficult to describe but easy to observe use of certain boyish or 'neuter' external features" (1968, p. 298).

Green (1987; Green et al., 1985; Roberts et al., 1987) reported some support for Stoller's contentions. The mothers of the feminine boys were more likely than the mothers of the control boys to describe themselves as tomboys (Green et al., 1985), but they did not differ from those mothers in their recalled display of specific "early girlhood sex-typed behaviors" (Green, 1987, p. 68). The two groups of mothers also did not differ in the extent of their sociosexual experiences during adolescence and young adulthood, although a within-groups analysis showed that the degree of cross-gender behavior in the group of feminine boys correlated negatively with the extent of the mothers' sociosexual experience. Regarding recalled childhood gender identity, Mitchell (1991) also found no differences among mothers of boys with GID, clinical control boys, and normal controls boys.

Extensive clinical experience indicates that the majority of the mothers of cross-gender-identified boys did not have formal childhood histories of GID. The studies by Green (1987) and Mitchell (1991) did not provide strong support for the possibility that less severe signs of cross-gender behavior were present, although clinical experience continues to point to important individual differences in the psychosexual life histories of the mothers. It may well be the case that developmental psychosexual factors interact with other maternal variables, such as global psychopathology, to influence the psychosexual functioning of children.

GENERAL PSYCHOPATHOLOGY

Clinical and empirical studies have reported that the parents of children referred for gender identity problems show levels of psychopathology and marital discord comparable to those of the parents of other clinic-referred children (Coates, 1985; Marantz and Coates, 1991; Zucker and Bradley, 1995). The precise mechanisms by which such general psychopathology exerts its effect on the development of GID remain unclear. Consider, for example, maternal depression and personality disorder. Marantz and Coates (1991) reported that the mothers of feminine boys had higher levels of depression and more borderline personality traits than did the mothers of normal boys. The issue of specificity remains unclear, however, since a clinical control group was not utilized. Assuming that a clinical control group would yield equal levels of maternal psychopathology, it needs to be explained how maternal dysfunction affects the development of specific childhood disorders. It is possible that risk factors act additively or synergistically; for example, it may be that degree of maternal impairment correlates with degree of tolerance of cross-gender behavior, perhaps because the more impaired mother is less able to respond to her child's behavior. Zucker and Bradley (1995) have provided tentative support for this conjecture.

SEPARATION ANXIETY

The finding that clinic-referred gender-problem boys display more internalizing psychopathological traits than externalizing psychopathological traits and that dysfunction is common in the families of such boys has led to efforts to explain the interrelation between associated psychopathology and GID (Zucker and Green, 1992).

Coates and Person (1985) studied 25 boys with GID and reported that 15 (60%) also met DSM-III criteria for separation anxiety disorder (SAD). In general, the boys showed high levels of behavioral disturbance on the Child Behavior Checklist (Achenbach and Edelbrock, 1981) and on personality testing. It was also noted that the family matrix was often dysfunctional; for example, 85% of the boys did not have fathers living in the home (Coates, 1985), and, as noted earlier, the mothers were often depressed and dysfunctional (Marantz and Coates, 1991). It was reasoned, however, that SAD played a specific etiological role in the development of GID. In the context of chronic disruption in the mother-son relationship, severe separation anxiety occurs. Cross-gender behavior then emerges "to restore a fantasy tie to the physically or emotionally absent mother. In imitating 'Mommy' [the boy] confuse[s] 'being Mommy' with 'having Mommy.' [Cross-gender behavior] appears to allay, in part, the anxiety generated by the loss of the mother" (Coates and Person, 1985, p. 708). Although Coates and Person disagree with Stoller's (1968, 1975) claims about the general functioning of the boys themselves, it is readily apparent that preoedipal object relations play a central role in this account of the genesis of GID.

Several methodological issues call for some caution in accepting uncritically the causal link between SAD and GID. The procedure used to assess SAD was not described, and information on interrater reliability was not given. The diagnoses of SAD and GID were made concurrently at the time of assessment, so it is not clear whether SAD actually preceded GID, as the above interpretation would imply. Finally, it remains unclear why cross-gender behavior would follow the emergence of separation anxiety, since not all boys with SAD develop GID and not all boys with GID develop SAD. Zucker et al. (1996a, in press) have, however, provided evidence that, at least at the time of the assessment, gender-referred boys (N = 73) who met the complete criteria for GID were more likely to meet the criteria for a ''liberal'' definition of SAD, using a psychometrically sound interview schedule, than were gender-referred boys (N = 42) who did not meet the complete criteria for GID (44 versus 38.1%).

Despite these problems, the observations of Coates and her colleagues (Coates, 1985; Coates and Person, 1985; Coates et al., 1991; Marantz and Coates, 1991) point to the complexity of the psychopathology that is often observed in clinic-referred boys with GID and in their families.

LABORATORY STUDIES

Biological Assessment

There are no known biological markers that identify children with GID. For such children, the parameters of biological sex, such as the sex chromosomes and the appearance of the external genitalia, are invariably normal (Green, 1976). As noted in the section on differential diagnosis, children with certain intersex conditions may be at some risk for gender dysphoria. Money and Lewis (1982), for example, found that, of 10 boys with idiopathic adolescent gynecomastia, three were homosexual in adolescence. Interestingly, all three showed some features of cross-gender identification during childhood. Subsequently, Money (1988) briefly noted that of 41 idiopathic adolescent gynecomastic males, 8 had ''homosexual (or bisexual) imagery and ideation.'' In these and other instances, pediatric endocrinological evaluations are warranted, since certain biomedical treatments may be required.

Psychological Assessment

Various psychological assessment procedures have been developed for use with cross-gender-identified children (Green, 1974; Zucker, 1992). These procedures include structured parent interviews regarding specific sex-typed behaviors, parent report on questionnaires, measurement of overt and covert sex-typed play in standardized situations, and assessment of sex-typed motoric behavior and sex-typed indices on projective tests, such as the Draw-a-Person, the It Scale for Children, and the Rorschach.

As noted in detail elsewhere (Zucker, 1992), these procedures have been effective in discriminating index groups of gender-referred children from comparison groups, which have included sibling, psychiatric, and normal control subjects. Green (1987), for example, found that a discriminant function analysis of parent interview data required 6 of 16 sex-typed behaviors to classify correctly all boys as members of either the feminine boy group or the male control group.

In general, it is important to note that tests utilized in isolation are particularly likely to yield both false-positive and false-negative diagnoses. For these and other reasons, psychological assessment procedures should be used to identify patterns of cross-gender behavior rather than isolated elements (Zucker, 1992), much as is done in a clinical assessment.

DIFFERENTIAL DIAGNOSIS

Childhood Diagnostic Issues

During childhood, several differential diagnostic issues should be considered in relation to GID. There is a type of cross-dressing in boys that appears to be qualitatively different from the type of cross-dressing that characterizes GID. In the latter, cross-dressing typically involves outerwear, such as dresses, shoes, and jewelry, that helps enhance the fantasy of being like the other sex. In the former, cross-dressing involves the use of undergarments (e.g., panties and nylons). Clinical data show that such cross-dressing is not accompanied by other signs of cross-

gender identification; in fact, the appearance and behavior of boys who engage in it are conventionally masculine. Clinical experience suggests that this type of cross-dressing has some sort of self-soothing function. Many male adolescents and adults who display transvestic fetishism recall such cross-dressing during childhood. It should be noted, however, that prospective study has not verified the assumption that this behavior pattern is contiguous with later transvestism.

When all the clinical signs of GID are present, it is not difficult to make the diagnosis. But the clinician who accepts the notion that there is a spectrum of cross-gender identification must be prepared to identify what Meyer-Bahlburg (1985) described as the ''zone of transition between clinically significant cross-gender behavior and mere statistical deviations from the gender norm'' (p. 682). Clinical experience suggests that boys who fall into this ambiguous zone do poorly in male peer groups, avoid rough-and-tumble play, are disinclined toward athletics and other conventionally masculine activities, and feel somewhat uncomfortable about being male; however, these boys do not wish to be girls and do not show an intense preoccupation with femininity. Friedman (1988) coined the term *juvenile unmasculinity* to describe such boys, who, he argued, suffer from a ''persistent, profound feeling of masculine inadequacy which leads to negative valuing of the self'' (p. 199). It is not clear whether this behavior pattern actually constitutes a distinct syndrome or is simply a mild form of GID; in any case, the residual diagnosis gender identity disorder not otherwise specified (GIDNOS) could be employed in such cases.

In girls, the primary differential diagnostic issue concerns the distinction between GID and tomboyism. The study of a community sample of tomboys by Green et al. (1982) showed that these girls shared a number of the cross-gender traits observed in clinic-referred gender-disturbed girls (Zucker and Bradley, 1995). In part, the DSM-III-R criteria for GID in girls were modified in the hope of better differentiating these two groups of girls (Zucker, 1989). At least three characteristics may be most useful in making the differential diagnosis: (a) By definition, girls with GID indicate an intense unhappiness with their status as females, whereas this should not be the case for tomboys; (b) girls with GID display an intense aversion to the wearing of culturally defined feminine clothing under any circumstances, whereas tomboys do not manifest this reaction, though they may prefer to wear casual clothing, such as jeans; and (c) girls with GID, unlike tomboys, manifest a verbalized or acted-out discomfort with sexual anatomy.

The final differential diagnostic issue concerns children with intersex conditions. In DSM-III an intersex condition was an exclusion criterion for the adult diagnosis of transsexualism, but this criterion was eliminated in DSM-III-R. The DSM-III-R did not formally address the issue of whether children who display significant cross-gender identification and have an intersex condition should be given a diagnosis such as GID. Consider, for example, girls with CAH. As noted earlier, these girls display more masculine behavior than do nonaffected girls. A small percentage of these girls also appear to be gender dysphoric. The phenomenology in these cases appears similar to that observed in physically normal girls with GID, but the etiology may well be different (Meyer-Bahlburg, 1994). Thus, there may be a risk in applying the same diagnosis as that used with physically normal children. On the other hand, the risk is reduced if it is recognized that a particular diagnosis does not dictate identical treatment across cases. These issues were debated by the DSM-IV Subcommittee on Gender Identity Disorders (Bradley et al., 1991; Meyer-Bahlburg, 1994). The final decision was to not diagnose GID in children or adults with nonpsychiatric conditions such as physical hermaphroditism.

Adolescent Diagnostic Issues

During adolescence, the clinician is likely to encounter at least four types of psychosexual problems (Sullivan et al., 1995; Zucker and Bradley, 1995). Children with an unresolved GID are at risk for seeking hormonal and surgical solutions to their distress. The DSM-IV criteria for GID for adolescents or adults emphasize the persistence of cross-gender identification and discomfort with one's assigned sex, including the desire for hormonal or surgical sex-reassignment. Diagnostically, it is important to assess the fixedness of the desire to change sex, since clinical management decisions will be influenced by the relative intractability of the condition. The residual diagnosis GIDNOS can be used for clinically gender dysphoric individuals who do not meet the complete diagnostic criteria for GID.

A second type of psychosexual problem occurs among adolescents who have had a history of GID or a variation of it. These adolescents continue to show signs of cross-gender identification but do not acknowledge a homosexual orientation or profess a desire to change sex. They are often referred because of continued social ostracism. The degree of felt distress varies with regard to the continued cross-gender identification. It is unlikely that any formal DSM-IV diagnosis would apply in such cases, although the residual diagnosis GIDNOS could be employed to indicate that the adolescent continues to struggle with gender identity issues.

A third type of psychosexual problem characterizes adolescents who have been referred by either themselves or by significant others because of homosexual behavior or orientation. Many of these youngsters have a history of GID or a variation of it. The reason for referral varies, but from a differential diagnostic standpoint it is important to rule out continuing problems that center on gender identity. For those youngsters who are distressed about their sexual orientation, the diagnosis of sexual disorder NOS can be given.

The last type of psychosexual problem concerns adolescent boys who cross-dress, in part, for the purpose of sexual arousal. The extent of the cross-dressing varies. In its full form, the diagnosis transvestic fetishism can be applied. These boys appear to have a nascent heterosexual orientation and appear unremarkably masculine in their demeanor. A history of GID is not part of the clinical picture, but some of these boys think about sex-reassignment surgery and are at risk for transsexualism. In DSM-IV, adolescents who meet the criteria for GID with this type of developmental history typically have a heterosexual sexual orientation.

TREATMENT

Several therapeutic approaches have been employed to treat children with GID, including behavior therapy, psychotherapy, family therapy, parental counseling, group therapy, and eclectic combinations of these strategies (Green, 1974, 1987; Zucker, 1985, 1990; Zucker and Green, 1989). As reviewed elsewhere (Zucker, 1985; Zucker and Green, 1989), all of these strategies appear to have clinical utility; unfortunately, formal comparative studies have not been conducted, so the most efficacious types of treatment remain unclear (for specific references to the case report literature, see Zucker and Bradley, 1995).

Three general comments about treatment of GID will be made. First, clinical experience suggests that intervention can more readily reduce gender identity conflict during childhood than during adolescence. The prognosis for reducing severe gender dysphoria after puberty is rather poor. Accordingly, the earlier treatment begins, the better. Second, the importance of working with the parents of children with GID has been much discussed in the literature. When there is a great deal of marital discord and parental psychopathology, treatment of these problems will greatly facilitate more specific work on gender identity issues. Management of the child's gender behavior in his or her daily environment requires that the parents have clear goals and a forum in which to discuss difficulties. Because parental dynamics and parental ambivalence about treatment may contribute to the perpetuation of GID (Newman, 1976), it is important for the therapist to have an appropriate relationship with the parents in order to address and work through these issues. Lastly, the therapist needs to consider closely the goals of treatment (Coates and Zucker, 1988; Green, 1974, 1987; Zucker, 1985, 1990; Zucker and

Green, 1989). In part, this issue will be conceptualized within the therapist's theoretical framework, but it will also be a function of the parents' concern and, to some extent, of the child's concerns. Two short-term goals have been discussed in the clinical literature: The reduction or elimination of social ostracism and conflict and the alleviation of underlying or associated psychopathology. Longer-term goals have focused on the prevention of postpubertal gender dysphoria and homosexuality. Little disagreement about the advisability of preventing gender dysphoria in adolescence or adulthood has been expressed in the clinical literature. Contemporary and secular-minded clinicians are, however, sensitive to the importance of helping people integrate a homosexual sexual orientation into their sense of identity (Friedman, 1988; Green, 1987, 1994). Not surprisingly, however, the development of a heterosexual orientation is probably preferred by most parents of children with GID. It is, therefore, important that clinicians point out to such parents that, as of yet, there is no strong evidence that treatment affects later sexual orientation. Both authors, as well as other experienced clinicians in the field, have preferred to emphasize the merit of reducing childhood gender identity conflict per se and, when it is present, associated behavioral problems, and to orient the parents of children with GID to the short-term goals of intervention.

OUTCOME AND FOLLOW-UP DATA

Green (1987) has conducted the most comprehensive long-term follow-up study of cross-gender-identified boys. An original sample of 66 feminine and 56 control boys was assessed initially at a mean age of 7.1 years (range, 4–12), and about two-thirds of the boys in each of these groups were reevaluated at a follow-up mean age of 18.9 years (range, 14–24). A semistructured interview was employed to assess sexual orientation in fantasy and behavior, using Kinsey scale criteria (Green, 1987). All 35 control boys were heterosexual in fantasy at follow-up; of the 25 control boys who had had overt sexual experiences, one was classified as bisexual and the remainder were classified as heterosexual. In contrast, 75% (33 of 44) of the cross-gender-identified boys were classified as either bisexual or homosexual in fantasy; of those who had had overt sexual experiences, 80% (24 of 30) were classified as either bisexual or homosexual. The remaining boys were classified as heterosexual. One of the cross-gender-identified boys, who was erotically attracted to males, was seriously entertaining the notion of sex-reassignment surgery.

Green's (1987) controlled follow-up study has shown that the most common long-term outcome of GID is homosexuality, a finding that has been reported in other studies, albeit without comparison groups (Zucker, 1985). As discussed in more detail elsewhere (Green, 1987; Zucker, 1985, 1990), these data converge neatly with the retrospective studies of adult male homosexuals that have evaluated the presence of childhood cross-gender behavior (Bailey and Zucker, 1995).

Adults with GID, particularly those with a homosexual orientation (that is, erotic attraction to persons of the same biological sex), invariably recall a childhood cross-gender history. Prospective studies of cross-gender-identified children, mainly of boys, have found that only a very small proportion persist in their wish to change sex after puberty, although the percentage does appear considerably higher than what one would expect based on general population rates for transsexualism. Why is this? As noted elsewhere (Zucker, 1985), there are two main possibilities. One possibility is that the low base rate of adult GID, even within the population of cross-gender-identified children, would require a large sample size to identify the few cases of gender dysphoria; the other possibility is that the assessment process and, when it occurs, therapeutic intervention alter the natural history of cross-gender identification. It should be noted that these two explanations are not mutually exclusive.

Clearly, childhood cross-gender identification is a behavioral marker for either later homosexuality or unresolved adult GID. Can more fine-grained predictions be made (e.g., predicting later homosexuality versus GID; homosexuality versus heterosexuality)? Clinical experience has suggested that children who do not move away from extreme cross-gender identification as they enter adolescence may be at greater risk for later gender dysphoria. Zucker et al. (1986) found that the persistence of gender dysphoria, including the desire to change sex, was considerably higher among patients who were first assessed during adolescence and followed up later, compared with patients who were first assessed during childhood and followed up later. This suggests that the clinical situation at or near the transition from childhood to adolescence may be crucial in differentiating a gender dysphoric outcome from other outcomes.

Green (1987; Green et al., 1987) compared on a number of childhood variables the feminine boys who were subsequently classified as bisexual or homosexual with the feminine boys who were subsequently classified as heterosexual. Although some feminine behaviors distinguished the two subgroups, a composite childhood femininity score only approached conventional levels of significance and only for the rating of sexual orientation in fantasy, not behavior. The lack of a stronger correlation is somewhat surprising, since one might have expected that the degree of cross-gender identification would be related to long-term outcome. However, Green did find that the continuation of certain feminine behaviors throughout childhood was associated with later homosexuality. Thus, it may be that the persistence of the feminine behavior is more important than its extent during the early childhood years.

Less father-son shared time in the first 2 years of life was also associated with later homosexuality, but the amount of mother-son shared time was not. Involvement in treatment also did not distinguish the two subgroups. It should be noted, however, that Green's study was not formally designed to assess the effects of therapy. Cases were not randomly assigned to receive or not receive treatment, and the therapy that occurred was quite variable with regard to length, type, experience of the therapist, and so on.

RESEARCH DIRECTIONS

Over the past 30 years, considerable progress has been made in demarcating the phenomenology of GID. Assessment procedures for a proper diagnostic workup are now widely available (Zucker, 1992). The strong connection between GID and later homosexuality has been verified by prospective study. Some progress has been made in understanding etiological and perpetuating factors. Treatment appears to be capable of interrupting the natural progression toward adult GID, but it is far less clear whether treatment can (or should) influence later sexual orientation.

The biology of gender identity, gender role, and sexual orientation remains an area of intense inquiry. Continued study of the role of prenatal sex hormones on postnatal sex-dimorphic behavior should help clarify the boundaries of their predisposing influence (Gladue, 1988; Gooren, 1988; Hines and Collaer, 1993; Meyer-Bahlburg, 1984). Other biological variables, such as genetic factors, will also likely be subject to vigorous empirical enquiry. More attention to the role of anxiety in boys with GID should help clarify the contribution of internalizing disorders to the development and perpetuation of GID.

Psychosocial influences on GIDs also remain the focus of much study. More work is needed to understand the interconnection, if any, between general and gender-specific psychopathology. The relation between GID and sexual orientation calls for a better understanding of the development of eroticism in its own right, including its development during the years prior to puberty. How do children eroticize stimuli? How is meaning given to the state of sexual arousal? How fixed or flexible is sexual orientation? Over the past few decades, and even in the short time since the first edition of this volume (Lewis, 1991), important advances have occurred in our understanding of psychosexual development. There will be more to come.

References

Achenbach TM, Edelbrock CS: Behavioral problems and competencies reported by parents of normal and disturbed children aged four through sixteen. *Monogr Soc Res Child Dev* 46(1, serial no. 188), 1981.

Alexander JE, Sufka KJ: Cerebral lateralization in homosexual males: A preliminary EEG investigation. *Int J Psychophysiol* 15:269–274, 1993.

Allen LS, Gorski RA: Sexual orientation and the size of the anterior commissure in the human brain. *Proc Natl Acad Sci USA* 89:7199–7202, 1992.

American Psychiatric Association: *Diagnostic and Statistical Manual of Mental Disorders* (4th ed). Washington, DC, American Psychiatric Association, 1994.

Bailey JM, Pillard RC: A genetic study of male sexual orientation. *Arch Gen Psychiatry* 48:1089–1096, 1991.

Bailey JM, Pillard RC, Neale MC, et al: Heritable factors influence sexual orientation in women. *Arch Gen Psychiatry* 50:217–223, 1993.

Bailey JM, Willerman L, Parks C: A test of the maternal stress theory of human male homosexuality. *Arch Sex Behav* 20:277–293, 1991.

Bailey JM, Zucker KJ: Childhood sex-typed behavior and sexual orientation: A conceptual analysis and quantitative review. *Dev Psychol*, 31:43–55, 1995.

Bakker A, van Kesteren PJM, Gooren LJG, et al: The prevalence of transsexualism in the Netherlands. *Acta Psychiatr Scand* 87:237–238, 1993.

Becker JT, Bass SM, Dew MA, et al: Hand preference, immune system disorder and cognitive function among gay/bisexual men: The multicenter AIDS cohort study (MACS). *Neuropsychologia* 30:229–235, 1992.

Bell AP, Weinberg MS, Hammersmith SK: *Sexual Preference: Its Development in Men and Women*. Bloomington, IN, Indiana University Press, 1981, pp. 74–81, 145–151.

Benjamin H: Transsexualism and transvestism as psychosomatic somato-psychic syndromes. *Am J Psychother* 8:219–230, 1954.

Berenbaum SA: Congenital adrenal hyperplasia: Intellectual and psychosexual functioning. In: Holmes CS (ed): *Psychoneuroendocrinology: Brain, Behavior, and Hormonal Interactions*. New York, Springer-Verlag, 1990, pp. 227–260.

Berenbaum SA, Hines M: Early androgens are related to childhood sex-typed toy preferences. *Psychol Sci* 3:203–206, 1992.

Bieber I, Dain HJ, Dince PR, et al: *Homosexuality: A Psychoanalytic Study*. New York, Basic Books, 1962.

Billy JOG, Tanfer K, Grady WR, et al: The sexual behavior of men in the United States. *Fam Plann Perspect* 25:52–60, 1993.

Blanchard R, Bogaert AF: Biodemographic comparisons of homosexual and heterosexual men in the Kinsey interview data. *Arch Sex Behav*, in press.

Blanchard R, Sheridan PM: Sibship size, sibling sex ratio, birth order, and parental age in homosexual and nonhomosexual gender dysphorics. *J Nerv Ment Dis* 180:40–47, 1992.

Blanchard R, Zucker KJ: Reanalysis of Bell, Weinberg, and Hammersmith's data on birth order, sibling sex ratio, and parental age in homosexual men. *Am J Psychiatry* 151:1375–1376, 1994.

Blanchard R, Zucker KJ, Bradley SJ, et al: Birth order and sibling sex ratio in homosexual male adolescents and probably prehomosexual feminine boys. *Dev Psychol*, 31:22–30, 1995.

Blanchard R, Zucker KJ, Cohen-Kettenis PT, et al: Birth order and sibling sex ratio in two samples of Dutch gender-dysphoric homosexual males. *Arch Sex Behav*, in press.

Bradley SJ, Blanchard R, Coates S, et al: Interim report of the DSM-IV subcommittee for gender identity disorders. *Arch Sex Behav* 20:333–343, 1991.

Byne W, Parsons B: Human sexual orientation: The biologic theories reappraised. *Arch Gen Psychiatry* 50:228–239, 1993.

Chahnazarian A: Determinants of the sex ratio at birth: Review of recent literature. *Soc Biol* 35:214–235, 1988.

Coates S: Extreme boyhood femininity: Overview and new research findings. In: DeFries Z, Friedman RC, Corn R (eds): *Sexuality: New Perspectives*. Westport, CT, Greenwood Publishing, 1985, pp. 101–124.

Coates S, Person ES: Extreme boyhood femininity: Isolated behavior or pervasive disorder? *J Am Acad Child Psychiatry* 24:702–709, 1985.

Coates S, Zucker KJ: Gender identity disorders in children. In: Kestenbaum CJ, Williams DT (eds): *Handbook of Clinical Assessment of Children and Adolescents* (Vol 2). New York, New York University Press, 1988, pp. 893–914.

Coates S, Friedman RC, Wolfe S: The etiology of boyhood gender identity disorder: A model for integrating temperament, development, and psychodynamics. *Psychoanal Dialogues* 1:341–383, 1991.

Coates S, Wolfe S, Hahn-Burke S: Do boys with gender identity disorder have a shy, inhibited temperament? Poster presented at the meeting of the International Academy of Sex Research, Edinburgh, Scotland, 1994.

Diamond M: Homosexuality and bisexuality in different populations. *Arch Sex Behav* 22:291–310, 1993.

Dittmann RW, Kappes ME, Kappes MH: Sexual behavior in adolescent and adult females with congenital adrenal hyperplasia. *Psychoneuroendocrinology* 17:153–170, 1992.

Eaton WO, Enns LR: Sex differences in human motor activity level. *Psychol Bull* 100:19–28, 1986.

Ehrhardt AA, Baker SW: Fetal androgens, human central nervous system differentiation, and behavior sex differences. In: Friedman RC, Richart RM, Vande Wiele RL (eds): *Sex Differences in Behavior*. New York, Wiley, 1974, pp. 33–51.

Ellis L, Ames MA: Neurohormonal functioning and sexual orientation: A theory of homosexuality-heterosexuality. *Psychol Bull* 101:233–258, 1987.

Fay RE, Turner C, Klassen AD, et al: Prevalence and patterns of same-gender sexual contact among men. *Science* 243:338–348, 1989.

Fridell SR, Zucker KJ, Bradley SJ, et al: Physical attractiveness of girls with gender identity disorder. *Arch Sex Behav* 25:17–31, 1996.

Friedman RC: *Male Homosexuality: A Contemporary Psychoanalytic Perspective*. New Haven, CT, Yale University Press, 1988.

Friedman RC, Downey J: Neurobiology and sexual orientation: Current relationships. *J Neuropsychiatry Clin Neurosci* 5:131–153, 1993.

Gladue BA: Hormones in relationship to homosexual/bisexual/heterosexual gender orientation. In: Sitsen JMA (ed): *Handbook of Sexology*. Vol 6: *The Pharmacology and Endocrinology of Sexual Function*. Amsterdam, Elsevier, 1988, pp. 388–409.

Gladue BA, Beatty WW, Larson J, et al: Sexual orientation and spatial ability in men and women. *Psychobiology* 18:101–108, 1990.

Gooren LJG: An appraisal of endocrine theories of homosexuality and gender dysphoria. In: Sitsen JMA (ed): *Handbook of Sexology*. Vol 6: *The Pharmacology and Endocrinology of Sexual Function*. Amsterdam, Elsevier, 1988, pp. 410–424.

Goy RW, Bercovitch FB, McBrair MC: Behavioral masculinization is independent of genital masculinization in prenatally androgenized female rhesus macaques. *Horm Behav* 22:552–571, 1988.

Green R: *Sexual Identity Conflict in Children and Adults*. New York, Basic Books, 1974.

Green R: One-hundred ten feminine and masculine boys: Behavioral contrasts and demographic similarities. *Arch Sex Behav* 5:425–446, 1976.

Green R: *The ''Sissy Boy Syndrome'' and the Development of Homosexuality*. New Haven, CT, Yale University Press, 1987.

Green R: Sexual problems and therapies: A quarter century of developments and changes. In: Rossi AS (ed): *Sexuality Across the Life Course*. Chicago, University of Chicago Press, 1994, pp. 341–361.

Green R, Money J: Incongruous gender role: Nongenital manifestations in prepubertal boys. *J Nerv Ment Dis* 131:160–168, 1960.

Green R, Roberts C, Williams K, et al: Specific cross-gender behaviours in boyhood and later sexual orientation. *Br J Psychiatry* 151:84–88, 1987.

Green R, Williams K, Goodman M: Ninety-nine ''tomboys'' and ''nontomboys'': Behavioral contrasts and demographic similarities. *Arch Sex Behav* 11:247–266, 1982.

Green R, Williams K, Goodman M: Masculine or feminine gender identity in boys: Developmental differences between two diverse family groups. *Sex Roles* 12:1155–1162, 1985.

Hall JAY, Kimura D: Dermatoglyphic asymmetry and sexual orientation in men. *Behav Neurosci* 108:1203–1206, 1994.

Hamer DH, Hu S, Magnuson VL, et al: A linkage between DNA markers on the X chromosome and male sexual orientation. *Science* 261:321–327, 1993.

Hines M, Collaer ML: Gonadal hormones and sexual differentiation of human behavior: Developments from research on endocrine syndromes and studies of brain structure. *Annu Rev Sex Res* 4:1–48, 1993.

Hoenig J: Etiology of transsexualism. In: Steiner BW (ed): *Gender Dysphoria: Development, Research, Management*. New York, Plenum, 1985, pp. 33–73.

Kinsey AC, Pomeroy WB, Martin CE: *Sexual Behavior in the Human Male*. Philadelphia, Saunders, 1948.

LeVay S: A difference in hypothalamic structure between heterosexual and homosexual men. *Science* 253:1034–1037, 1991.

Lewis M (ed): *Child and Adolescent Psychiatry: A Comprehensive Textbook*. Baltimore, Williams & Wilkins, 1991.

Linday LA: Maternal reports of pregnancy, genital, and related fantasies in preschool and kindergarten children. *J Am Acad Child Adolesc Psychiatry* 33:416–423, 1994.

Lothstein LM: *Female-to-Male Transsexualism: Historical, Clinical, and Theoretical Issues*. Boston, Routledge & Kegan Paul, 1983.

MacCulloch MJ, Waddington JL: Neuroendocrine mechanisms and the aetiology of male and female homosexuality. *Br J Psychiatry* 139:341–345, 1981.

Marantz S, Coates S: Mothers of boys with gender identity disorder: A comparison of matched controls. *J Am Acad Child Adolesc Psychiatry* 30:310–315, 1991.

McCormick CM, Witelson SF: A cognitive profile of homosexual men compared to heterosexual men and women. *Psychoneuroendocrinology* 16:459–473, 1991.

McCormick CM, Witelson SF, Kingstone E: Left-handedness in homosexual men and women: Neuroendocrine implications. *Psychoneuroendocrinology* 15:69–76, 1990.

Meyer-Bahlburg HFL: Psychoendocrine research on sexual orientation: Current status and future options. *Prog Brain Res* 61:375–398, 1984.

Meyer-Bahlburg HFL: Gender identity disorder of childhood: Introduction. *J Am Acad Child Psychiatry* 24:681–683, 1985.

Meyer-Bahlburg HFL: Psychobiologic research on homosexuality. *Child Adolesc Psychiatr Clin North Am* 2:489–500, 1993.

Meyer-Bahlburg HFL: Intersexuality and the diagnosis of gender identity disorder. *Arch Sex Behav* 23:21–40, 1994.

Mitchell JN: *Maternal Influences on Gender Identity Disorder in Boys: Searching for Specificity*. Unpublished doctoral dissertation, York University, Downsview, Ontario.

Money J: Sexual dimorphism and homosexual gender identity. *Psychol Bull* 74:425–440, 1970.

Money J: *Gay, Straight, and In-Between: The Sexology of Erotic Orientation*. New York, Oxford University Press, 1988, pp. 37–38.

Money J, Lewis V: Homosexual/heterosexual status in boys at puberty: Idiopathic adolescent gynecomastia and congenital virilizing adrenocorticism. *Psychoneuroendocrinology* 7:339–346, 1982.

Money J, Hampson JG, Hampson JL: Imprinting and the establishment of gender role. *Arch Neurol Psychiatry* 77:333–336, 1957.

Money J, Schwartz M, Lewis VG: Adult erotosexual status and fetal hormonal masculinization and demasculinization: 46,XX congenital virilizing adrenal hyperplasia and 46,XY androgen-insensitivity syndrome compared. *Psychoneuroendocrinology* 9:405–414, 1984.

Mulaikal RM, Migeon CJ, Rock JA: Fertility rates in female patients with congenital adrenal hyperplasia due to 21-hydroxylase deficiency. *N Engl J Med* 316:178–182, 1987.

Newman LE: Treatment for the parents of feminine boys. *Am J Psychiatry* 133:683–687, 1976.

Parkes CM: *Bereavement: Studies of Grief in Adult Life*. Middlesex, England, Penguin Books, 1975.

Pillard RC, Weinrich JD: Evidence of familial nature of male homosexuality. *Arch Gen Psychiatry* 43:808–812, 1986.

Pleak RR, Meyer-Bahlburg HFL, O'Brien JD, et al: Cross-gender behavior and psychopathology in boy psychiatric outpatients. *J Am Acad Child Adolesc Psychiatry* 28:385–393, 1989.

Risch N, Squires-Wheeler E, Keats BJB: Male sexual orientation and genetic evidence. *Science* 262:2063–2065, 1993.

Roberts CW, Green R, Williams K, et al: Boyhood gender identity development: A statistical contrast of two family groups. *Dev Psychol* 23:544–557, 1987.

Sandberg DE, Meyer-Bahlburg HFL, Ehrhardt AA, et al: The prevalence of gender-atypical behavior in elementary school children. *J Am Acad Child Adolesc Psychiatry* 32:306–314, 1993.

Sanders G, Ross-Field L: Sexual orientation and visuo-spatial ability. *Brain Cogn* 5:280–290, 1986a.

Sanders G, Ross-Field L: Sexual orientation, cognitive abilities and cerebral asymmetry: A review and a hypothesis tested. *Ital J Zool* 20:459–470, 1986b.

Slater E: The sibs and children of homosexuals. In: Smith DR, Davidson WM (eds): *Symposium on Nuclear Sex*. London, Heinemann, 1958, pp. 79–83.

Sullivan CBL, Bradley SJ, Zucker KJ: Gender identity disorder (transsexualism) and transvestic fetishism. In: Van Hasselt VB, Hersen M (eds): *Handbook of Adolescent Psychopathology: A Guide to Diagnosis and Treatment*. New York, Lexington Books, 1995, pp. 525–558.

Stoller RJ: The hermaphroditic identity of hermaphrodites. *J Nerv Ment Dis* 139:453–457, 1964.

Stoller RJ: *Sex and Gender*. Vol 1: *The Development of Masculinity and Femininity*. New York, Aronson, 1968.

Stoller RJ: *Sex and Gender*. Vol 2: *The Transsexual Experiment*. London, Hogarth Press, 1975.

Stoller RJ: *Presentations of Gender*. New Haven, CT, Yale University Press, 1985.

Wellings K, Field J, Johnson AM, et al: *Sexual Behaviour in Britain: The National Survey of Sexual Attitudes and Lifestyles*. London, Penguin, 1994.

Zucker KJ: Cross-gender-identified children. In: Steiner BW (ed): *Gender Dysphoria: Development, Research, Management*. New York, Plenum, 1985, pp. 75–174.

Zucker KJ: Gender identity disorders. In: Last CG, Hersen M (eds): *Handbook of Child Psychiatric Diagnosis*. New York, Wiley, 1989, pp. 388–406.

Zucker KJ: Treatment of gender identity disorders in children. In: Blanchard R, Steiner BW (eds): *Clinical Management of Gender Identity Disorders in Children and Adults*. Washington, DC, American Psychiatric Press, 1990, pp. 1–23.

Zucker KJ: Gender identity disorder. In: Hooper SR, Hynd GW, Mattison RE (eds): *Child Psychopathology: Diagnostic Criteria and Clinical Assessment*. Hillsdale, NJ, Erlbaum, 1992, pp. 305–342.

Zucker KJ, Blanchard R: Re-analysis of Bieber et al.'s 1962 data on sibling sex ratio and birth order in male homosexuals. *J Nerv Ment Dis* 182:528–530, 1994.

Zucker KJ, Bradley SJ: *Gender Identity Disorder and Psychosexual Problems in Children and Adolescents*. New York, Guilford, 1995.

Zucker KJ, Green R: Gender identity disorder of childhood. In: Karasu TB (ed): *Treatments of Psychiatric Disorders* (Vol 1). Washington, DC, American Psychiatric Press, 1989, pp. 661–670.

Zucker KJ, Green R: Psychosexual disorders in children and adolescents. *J Child Psychol Psychiatry* 33:107–151, 1992.

Zucker KJ, Green R: Psychological and familial aspects of gender identity disorder. *Child Adolesc Psychiatric Clin North Am* 2:513–542, 1993.

Zucker KJ, Bradley SJ, Gladding JA: A follow-up study of transsexual, transvestitic, homosexual, and ''undifferentiated'' adolescents. Poster presented at the meeting of the International Academy of Sex Research, Amsterdam, September 1986.

Zucker KJ, Bradley SJ, Hughes HE: Gender dysphoria in a child with true hermaphroditism. *Can J*

Psychiatry 32:602–609, 1987.

Zucker KJ, Bradley SJ, Ipp M: Delayed naming of a newborn boy: Relationship to the mother's wish for a girl and subsequent cross-gender identity in the child by the age of two. *J Psychol Human Sex* 6: 57–68, 1993a.

Zucker KJ, Bradley SJ, Sullivan CBL: Traits of separation anxiety in boys with gender identity disorder. *J Am Acad Child Adolesc Psychiatry*, 1996a, in press.

Zucker KJ, Bradley SJ, Lowry Sullivan CB, et al: A gender identity interview for children. *J Pers Assess* 61:443–456, 1993b.

Zucker KJ, Bradley SJ, Oliver G, et al: Psychosexual assessment of women with congenital adrenal hyperplasia: Preliminary analyses. Poster presented at the meeting of the International Academy of Sex Research, Prague, Czechoslovakia, 1992.

Zucker KJ, Finegan JK, Doering RW, et al: Two subgroups of gender-problem children. *Arch Sex Behav* 13:27–39, 1984.

Zucker KJ, Green R, Bradley SJ, et al: Gender identity disorder of childhood: Diagnostic issues. In: Widiger TA, Frances AJ, Pincus HA, et al (eds): *DSM-IV Sourcebook*. Washington, DC, American Psychiatric Press, 1996b, in press.

Zucker KJ, Green R, Garofano C, et al: Prenatal gender preference of mothers of feminine and masculine boys: Relation to sibling sex composition and birth order. *J Abnorm Child Psychol* 22:1–13, 1994b.

Zucker KJ, Wild J, Bradley SJ, et al: Physical attractiveness of boys with gender identity disorder. *Arch Sex Behav* 22:23–34, 1993c.

Zuger B: Effeminate behavior in boys: Parental age and other factors. *Arch Gen Psychiatry* 30: 173–177, 1974.

Zuger B: Homosexuality in families of boys with early effeminate behavior: An epidemiological study. *Arch Sex Behav* 18:155–166, 1989.

57 TIC DISORDERS

James F. Leckman, M.D., and Donald J. Cohen, M.D.

DEFINITION

A tic is a sudden, repetitive movement, gesture, or utterance that typically mimics some aspect of normal behavior. Usually of brief duration, individual tics rarely last more than a second. They tend to occur in bouts and at times have a paroxysmal character. Individual tics can occur singly or together in an orchestrated collage. They can vary in their frequency and forcefulness. Although many tics can be temporarily suppressed, they are often experienced as being involuntary. They may be associated with somatosensory "urges" that are relieved with the performance of the tic (Leckman et al., 1993). Motor tics vary from simple, abrupt movements, such as eye-blinking, head jerks, or shoulder shrugs, to more complex, purposeful-appearing behaviors, such as facial expressions or gestures of the arms or head. In extreme cases, these movements can be obscene (copropraxia) or self-injurious (e.g., hitting or biting). Phonic or vocal tics can range from simple throat-clearing sounds to more complex vocalizations and speech. In severe cases coprolalia (obscene speech) is present.

Tic disorders are transient or chronic conditions associated with difficulties in self-esteem, family life, social acceptance, or school or job performance that are directly related to the presence of motor and/or phonic tics. Individuals with tic disorders may manifest a broad array of behavioral difficulties, including uninhibited speech or conduct, impulsivity, distractibility, motoric hyperactivity, and obsessive-compulsive symptoms. Some of these associated "non-tic" symptoms may be a major source of impairment.

Historically, tic disorders have been the province of both neurologists and psychiatrists. They are remarkable disorders that provide a glimpse into some of the processes that govern the interface between mind and body. The psychological dimension is offered not only by the associated behavioral difficulties, but also by the "choice" and timing of the tic behaviors themselves.

Although tic symptoms have been reported since antiquity, systematic study dates only from the 19th century, with the reports of Itard (1825) and Gilles de la Tourette (1885). Gilles de la Tourette, in his classic study of 1885, described nine cases of tic disorder characterized by motor "incoordinations" or tics, and "inarticulate shouts accompanied by articulated words with echolalia and coprolalia." This report also hinted at the hereditary nature of the syndrome and the association between tic disorders and obsessive-compulsive symptoms.

The current classification of tic disorders in DSM-IV includes Tourette's disorder, chronic motor or vocal tic disorder, transient tic disorder, and tic disorder not otherwise specified (American Psychiatric Association, 1994). The diagnostic criteria for these conditions are presented in Table 57.1. These criteria focus on the phenomenology and natural history of the disorder and are readily applied in clinical settings. They also serve as the basis for the diagnostic descriptions contained in the World Health Organization's ICD-l0 (1988).

PREVALENCE AND EPIDEMIOLOGY

Tic behaviors are commonplace among children. Community surveys indicate that 1–13% of boys and 1–11% of girls manifest "frequent" "tics, twitches, mannerisms, or habit spasms" (Zahner et al., 1988). The instability of these estimates is in part due to the wording of items on symptom inventories, the identity of the informant, and the demographic characteristics of the sample studied. Children between the ages of 7 and 11 years appear to have the highest rates. Although boys are more commonly affected with tic behaviors than are girls, the male-female ratio in most community surveys is less than 2:1. Urban living may be associated with elevated rates (Zahner et al., 1988). Race and socioeconomic status have not been shown to influence the point prevalence of tics.

Much less is known concerning the prevalence of tic disorders. Once thought to be rare, current estimates from registers of clinically diagnosed subjects suggest that 1–2% of the general population may be affected (Shapiro et al., 1988). Unfortunately, these estimates are not robust, as only a few rigorous population-based studies have been performed. For example, Apter et al. (1993) screened 28,037 individuals, aged 16–17, prior to their induction into the Israeli army, and reported a point prevalence of 4.3 per 10,000 for Tourette's disorder. Although the rate of any tic disorder was not reported, their data would suggest that this figure would be approximately an order of magnitude higher—in the range of 4.7 per 1,000. In a younger group of 3,034 children, aged 5–15, Comings et al. (1990) reported a prevalence of 3.6 per 10,000 for definite Tourette's disorder and a rate of 1.25 per 100 for any tic disorder. These figures are consistent with the view that children are 5–12 times more likely to be identified as having a tic disorder than adults, and that males are more commonly affected than females (with male-female ratios of 9:1 and 3:1 for children and adults, respectively) (Burd et al., 1986a, 1986b). Although other demographic characteristics have not been systematically investigated, some authors have suggested than tic disorders may be more common among Caucasian and Oriental racial groups.

CLINICAL DESCRIPTIONS

With the exception of Tourette's syndrome (Brunn, 1988; Shapiro et al., 1988), relatively few cross-sectional or longitudinal studies of tic disorders have been performed. Thus, most of the information provided below is based on clinical experience and anecdotal reports.

Table 57.1. DSM-IV Tic Disorder Classification

Diagnostic criteria for Tourette's Syndrome (307.23):
1. Both multiple motor and one or more vocal tics have been present at some time during the illness, although not necessarily concurrently.
2. The tics occur many times a day (usually in bouts), nearly every day or intermittently throughout a period of more than a year; and during this period, there is never a tic-free period of more than 3 consecutive months.
3. The anatomic location, number, frequency, complexity, and severity of the tics change over time.
4. Onset before age 18
5. Not due to the direct physiological effects of a substance (e.g., stimulants) or a general medical condition (e.g., Huntington's chorea or postviral encephalitis).

Diagnostic Criteria for Chronic Motor or Vocal Tic Disorder (307.22):
1. Single or multiple motor or vocal tics, but not both, have been present at some time during the illness.
2. The tics occur many times a day, nearly every day, or intermittently throughout a period of more than a year; and during this period there is never a tic-free interval of more than 3 months.
3. Onset before age 18.
4. Not due to the direct physiological effects of a substance (e.g., stimulants) or a general medical condition (e.g., Huntington's chorea or postviral ecephalitis).
5. Has never met the criteria for Tourette's disorder.

Diagnostic Criteria for Transient Tic Disorder (307.21):
1. Single or multiple motor and/or vocal tics.
2. The tics may occur many times a day, nearly every day for at least 4 weeks, but for no longer than 12 consecutive months.
3. Onset before age 18.
4. Not due to the direct physiological effects of a substance (e.g., stimulants) or a general medical condition (e.g., Hungtington's chorea or postviral encephalitis).
5. Has never met the criteria for Tourette's or chronic motor or vocal disorder.

Diagnostic Criteria for Tic Disorder Not Otherwise Specified (307.20):
This category is for a tic disorder that does not meet criteria for a specific tic disorder. Examples include tics lasting less than 4 weeks or tics with an onset after age 18.

From American Psychiatric Association: *Diagnostic and Statistical Manual of Mental Disorders.* (4th ed). Washington, DC, American Psychiatric Association, 1994.

Transient Tic Disorder

Almost invariably a disorder of childhood, transient tic disorder is usually characterized by one or more simple motor tics that wax and wane in severity over weeks to months. The anatomical distribution of these tics is usually confined to the head, neck, or upper extremities. Transient phonic tics, in the absence of motor tics, can also occur, though more rarely. The age of onset is typically 3–10 years. Boys are at greater risk. The initial presentation may be unnoticed. If medical consultation is sought, family practitioners, pediatricians, allergists, and ophthalmologists are typically the first to see the child. Missed diagnoses are common, particularly as the symptoms may have completely disappeared by the time of the consultation. As prescribed by the prevailing diagnostic criteria, the subsequent natural history of this condition is limited to fewer than 12 consecutive months of active symptomatology. As such, this is often a retrospective diagnosis, as the clinician is unable to know with certainty which children will show progression of their symptoms and which children will display a self-limiting course.

CASE ILLUSTRATION

Todd is a 6-year-old boy with a history of intense eye-blinking of 2 weeks' duration. The symptom was noticeable to others and interfered with his ability to maintain visual attention. The symptoms began toward the end of a family vacation, shortly before Todd was to enter 1st grade. By the time a visit to the family pediatrician was arranged, the symptoms had diminished considerably. In light of a positive family history of tic disorder in the father and an older sibling, the pediatrician tempered his reassurance but indicated to the family that the condition might well be transient in nature. The family was counseled to avoid CNS stimulants, decongestants, and other sympathomimetics.

Comment

Although the value of avoiding CNS stimulants has not been convincingly demonstrated in prospective studies, such recommendations are commonplace and may have merit in light of the available anecdotal literature. Recently, systematic studies of the use of stimulants in children with Tourette's disorder have rekindled this controversy (Sverd et al., 1992) and have shown that short term treatment with stimulants is not associated with increased tic symptoms. Definitive longer term studies have not been reported.

Chronic Motor or Vocal Tic Disorder

This chronic condition can be observed among children and adults. As with other tic disorders, it is characterized by a waxing and waning course and a broad range of severity. Chronic simple and complex motor tics are the most common manifestations. A majority of tics involve the head, neck, and upper extremities. Although some children may display other developmental difficulties, such as attention deficit hyperactivity disorder, the disorder is not incompatible with an otherwise normal course of development. This condition can also appear as a residual state, particularly in adulthood. In such instances, a predictable repertoire of tic symptoms may only be seen during periods of heightened stress or fatigue.

Chronic vocal tic disorder, by all accounts, is a rare condition. Some authors exclude "chronic cough of adolescence" from this category (Shapiro et al., 1988).

CASE ILLUSTRATION

Richard is 16-year-old sophomore in high school. Chronic motor tics were observed by his coach during baseball practice. These included a mouth stretching movement and a head tilt that at times occurred together. The coach was impressed by how little awareness Richard seemed to have concerning these movements despite their disfiguring character and the occasional teasing that they prompted by his teammates. When approached, Richard's mother indicated that tic symptoms had been present off and on since he was 7 years old and that the family had noticed that they had been more frequent as he approached the end of the school term. She mentioned that they were in regular contact with a clinic and that thus far no medications had been used to control the symptoms.

Comment

Given the potential unwanted physical effects of many of the medications used to treat tic disorders, a conservative approach (as illustrated in this vignette) is often indicated.

TOURETTE'S SYNDROME (CHRONIC MOTOR AND PHONIC TIC DISORDER)

The most severe tic disorder is best known by the eponym "Gilles de la Tourette's syndrome." Typically the disorder begins in early childhood with transient bouts of simple motor tics such as eye-blinking or head jerks. These tics may initially come and go but, eventually, they become persistent and begin to have adverse effects on the child and his or her family. The repertoire of motor tics can be vast, incorporating virtually any voluntary movement by any portion of the body. Although some authors have drawn attention to a "rostral-caudal" progression of motor tics (head, neck, shoulders, arms, torso), this course is not predictable. As the syndrome develops, complex motor tics may appear. Often they have a "camouflaged" appearance (e.g., brushing hair away from the face with an arm) and can only be distinguished as tics by their repetitive character. Rarely, complex motor tics can be self-injurious and further complicate management (e.g., punching one side of the face or biting a wrist).

On average, phonic tics begin 1–2 years after the onset of motor symptoms and are usually simple in character (e.g., throat clearing, grunting, squeaks). More complex vocal symptoms, such as echolalia, palilalia, and coprolalia occur in a minority of cases. Other complex phonic symptoms include dramatic and abrupt changes in rhythm, rate, and volume.

Motor and phonic tics tend to occur in bouts. Their frequency ranges from nonstop bursts that are virtually uncountable to rare events that occur only a few times a week. Single tics may occur in isolation, or there may be well-orchestrated combinations of motor and phonic tics that involve multiple muscle groups.

The forcefulness of motor tics and the volume of phonic tics can also vary tremendously, from behaviors that are not noticeable (a slight shrug or a hushed guttural noise) to strenuous displays (arm thrusts or loud barking) that are frightening and exhausting.

Consistent with available epidemiological data, tic disorders tend to improve in late adolescence and early adulthood. In many instances, the phonic symptoms become increasingly rare or may disappear altogether, and the motor tics may be reduced in number and frequency. Complete remission of both motor and phonic symptoms has also been reported (Brunn, 1988; Shapiro et al., 1988). In contrast, adulthood is also the period when the most severe and debilitating forms of tic disorder can be seen.

In addition to the tic behaviors, associated behavioral and emotional problems frequently complicate Tourette's syndrome. These difficulties range from impulsive, "disinhibited," and immature behavior to compulsive touching or sniffing. There is no clear dividing line between these abrupt and disruptive behaviors and complex tics on the one hand and comorbid conditions of attention deficit hyperactivity disorder and obsessive-compulsive disorder on the other.

CASE ILLUSTRATION

Arthur is an 11-year-old prepubertal boy who was referred for psychiatric evaluation and possible placement in a residential treatment facility. His past psychiatric history included symptoms suggestive of attention deficit hyperactivity disorder from an early age and the presence of motor and phonic tics that had increased steadily over the past 2 years. The immediate reason for referral was the emergence of loud coprolalic utterances of "fuc . . ." that would interrupt class and reverberate through the house. His parents reported that, initially, his tic symptoms were seen as intentional and deliberate by both his teachers and his parents. He was teased by his peers and regularly provoked the anger of his parents. Six months earlier, during the course of an educational evaluation, the school psychologist suggested that a medical consultation was needed because of the probable attention deficit disorder and possible Tourette's syndrome. Shortly thereafter, he was seen by a pediatric neurologist who diagnosed Tourette's syndrome and placed him on 2 mg/day of haloperidol. Within a week, the tics had diminished considerably. However, he continued to do poorly in school and began to put on weight. Over the Christmas vacation the tics again worsened despite increasing the haloperidol to 6 mg/day. On return to school, his tic symptoms were severe, and he was unable to concentrate on his school work. His parents became increasingly alarmed at his dazed appearance and weight gain and abruptly took him off the haloperidol. Initially he appeared to do better but, within two weeks, the situation had completely deteriorated, with a marked exacerbation of his motor and phonic tics. A day before the evaluation, the parents had been told that Arthur could no longer remain in school.

Comment

The waxing and waning character of tic symptoms frequently continues despite the use of medications. "Chasing" the symptoms with increases in the medication is often not an effective strategy. Reassurance and educational interventions with both the family and the school often are sufficient to help a child over a period of tic exacerbation. Withdrawal symptoms from neuroleptics are frequently observed in this situation and are usually self-limiting over a period of 4–8 weeks.

ETIOLOGY AND PATHOGENESIS

Genetic Factors

Twin and family studies provide evidence that genetic factors are involved in the vertical transmission within families of a vulnerability to Tourette's syndrome and related disorders (Pauls and Leckman, 1986). The concordance rate for Tourette's syndrome among monozygotic twin pairs is greater than 50%, while the concordance of dizygotic twin pairs approaches 10% (Hyde et al., 1992; Price et al., 1986). If co-twins with chronic motor tic disorder are included, these concordance figures approach 90% for monozygotic and 30% for dizygotic twin pairs. Differences in the concordance of monozygotic and dizygotic twin pairs indicate that genetic factors play an important role in the etiology of Tourette's syndrome and related conditions. These figures also suggest that nongenetic factors are critical in determining the nature and severity of the clinical syndrome.

Other studies indicate that first-degree family members of Tourette's syndrome probands are at substantially higher risk for developing Tourette's syndrome, chronic motor tic disorder, and obsessive-compulsive disorder than are unrelated individuals (Pauls and Leckman, 1986). Overall, the risk to male first-degree family members approximates 50% (18% Tourette's syndrome, 31% chronic motor tics, and 7% obsessive-compulsive disorder), while the overall risk to females is less (5% Tourette's syndrome, 9% chronic motor tics, and 17% obsessive-compulsive disorder) (Pauls et al., 1991).

The pattern of vertical transmission among family members has led several groups of investigators to test whether or not mathematical models of specific genetic hypotheses could account for these data. The bulk of this work favors models of autosomal-dominant transmission (Pauls and Leckman, 1986). These studies have also led directly to the identification of large multigenerational families with the disorder, to facilitate genetic linkage studies (Kurlan et al., 1986). Thus far, linkage studies have not been successful in determining the chromosomal location of the putative Tourette's syndrome gene or genes (Pakstis et al., 1991).

Neuroanatomical Substrates

The basal ganglia and related structures in the midbrain and cortex are likely to serve as the neuroanatomical substrates for Tourette's syndrome and related disorders (Leckman et al., 1991b). These speculations are based on an emerging appreciation of the functional interrelationships among these structures and their regulation of sensorimotor activities. They are also based on preliminary neuropathological and neuroimaging studies, and a large body of neurochemical and neuropharmacological data that implicate some of the neurotransmitter and neuromodulatory systems found in these brain regions.

The basal ganglia have long been recognized as providing a critical way station in corticothalamic circuits involved with motor control and sensorimotor integration (Marsden, 1982). The identification of interrelated corticothalamic circuits that link thalamic sites with areas in the prefrontal and limbic cortex (Alexander and DeLong, 1985a, 1985b) has intensified speculation concerning the role of these structures in the pathobiology of Tourette's syndrome (Leckman et al., 1991b) and obsessive-compulsive disorder (Rapoport, 1989).

Few neuropathological studies have been performed. Balthasar (1956) reported hypoplasia of the corpus striatum (caudate and putamen), with a loss of the interneuronal neuropile. These findings, however, were based on a single case and were not consistent with an earlier report that found no distinctive histological pattern (Dewulf and van

Bogeart, 1940). The case reported by Dewulf and van Bogeart was atypical with regard to age of onset (18 years) and the unremitting progress of this individual's neurological symptoms. Laplane and co-workers (1981) described two intriguing case reports of individuals with basal ganglia lesions that were associated with tics, obsessive-compulsive symptoms, and deficits in motivation. More recently, neuroimaging studies have provided limited support for the involvement of the basal ganglia and related cortical structures in Tourette's syndrome (Peterson et al., 1993; 1994; Singer et al., 1993; Braun et al., 1993).

Neurochemical Systems and Neuropharmacological Data

The functional status of a number of neurotransmitter and neuromodulator systems has been evaluated in Tourette's syndrome. The most compelling evidence has focused attention on nigrostriatal and nigrocortical dopaminergic projections; serotonergic projections from the dorsal raphe to the substantia nigra, globus pallidus, and striatum; and peptidergic projections from the striatum to the pallidum and substantia nigra (Leckman et al., 1995).

Based largely on parallels between the tics, vocalizations, and obsessive-compulsive behaviors seen in some patients with encephalitis lethargica, Devinsky (1983) has suggested that Tourette's syndrome is the result of altered dopaminergic function in the midbrain. The substantia nigra and the ventral tegmental area (VTA) are adjacent midbrain sites that contain large numbers of dopaminergic neurons. The dopamine cell bodies in the substantia nigra give rise to the ascending nigrostriatal pathway. The dopamine neurons of the VTA send ascending projections to various cortical regions, including the anterior cingulate gyrus and other limbic structures. The dopamine neurons in the substantia nigra and those in the VTA also give rise to descending pathways projecting to the dorsal pontine tegmentum in the region of the noradrenergic locus coeruleus.

Other data implicating central dopaminergic mechanisms include clinical trials in which haloperidol and other neuroleptics that preferentially block dopaminergic D2 receptors have been found to be effective in the partial suppression of tics in a majority of Tourette's syndrome patients (Shapiro and Shapiro, 1988). Friedhoff (1986) has suggested that the relationship between D2 and D1 dopamine systems may be of interest in Tourette's syndrome in that a blockade of the D2 receptors by relatively selective agents such as haloperidol and pimozide disinhibits the D1 system.

Tic suppression has also been reported following administration of alpha-methyl-para-tyrosine and following trials of tetrabenazine (Leckman et al., in press; Shapiro and Shapiro, 1988). In contrast, Tourette's-like syndromes have appeared following withdrawal of neuroleptics, and tics are often exacerbated following exposure to agents that increase central dopaminergic activity, such as L-dopa and CNS stimulants, including cocaine.

These pharmacological data, taken together with reports of altered baseline and post-probenecid mean CSF levels of homovanillic acid (HVA) (a major metabolite of brain dopamine) in Tourette's syndrome patients compared to available contrast groups (Butler et al., 1979; Cohen et al., 1978; Leckman et al., 1988a; Singer et al., 1982), have led several groups of investigators to suggest that Tourette's syndrome is a disorder in which postsynaptic dopaminergic D2 receptors are hypersensitive. Recent preliminary positron emission tomography studies (PET) of brain dopamine receptors, however, do not support the view that there are increased numbers of these receptors (Brooks et al., 1992; Singer et al., 1992). Postmortem studies in a very small number of Tourette's syndrome patients have suggested that there is an increased number of dopamine transporter sites in the basal ganglia of patients with Tourette's syndrome (Singer et al., 1991). This work has recently been extended to in vivo single photon emission computerized tomography (SPECT) studies of dopamine transporter sites, which appear to confirm the earlier postmortem data (Malison et al., 1995). Additional imaging and neuropathological studies are needed to address fully the

potential abnormalities of receptor number, affinity, and distribution. If confirmed, the increased number of dopamine transporter sites in the striatum may reflect a dopaminergic hyperinnervation. Given the role of dopaminergic projections in mediating the output of the basal ganglia and the balance of D1 vs. D2 dopamine receptor stimulation (Filion and Tremblay, 1991; Filion et al., 1991), it is possible that Tourette's syndrome may, in part, be mediated by a dopaminergic hyperinnervation of the striatum and a resulting disinhibition of thalamo-cortical projections.

Although serotonergic mechanisms have been repeatedly invoked as potentially playing an important role in the pathophysiology of Tourette's syndrome, there is very little hard evidence to support this connection. Serotonergic inputs from the dorsal raphe to both the substantia nigra and the striatum have been identified and partially characterized, but there are no direct neuropathological data implicating them in Tourette's syndrome. Medications that act by increasing or decreasing serotonergic activity do not consistently alter tic symptoms. Studies of CSF 5-hydroxyindoleacetic acid (5-HIAA), the principal central metabolite of serotonin, have reported a range of low and normal levels in Tourette's syndrome patients compared to contrast groups (Butler et al., 1979; Cohen et al., 1978; Leckman et al., 1988a; Singer et al., 1982). Despite this lack of evidence, serotonergic hypotheses continue to be attractive. Circumstantial evidence includes their neuroanatomical projections and their likely involvement in the pathophysiology of obsessive-compulsive disorder.

Endogenous opiates, including dynorphin and met-enkephalin, are highly concentrated in structures of the extrapyramidal system, known to interact with central dopaminergic neurons, and may play an important role in the control of motor functions (Buck and Yamamura, 1982). These systems have also been directly implicated in the pathophysiology of Parkinson's disease, Huntington's disease and, most recently, in Tourette's syndrome. The neuropathological study of Haber et al. (1986) reported decreased levels of dynorphin A [1-17] immunoreactivity in striatal fibers projecting to the globus pallidus in the brain of a patient with severe Gilles de la Tourette's syndrome. This observation, taken with the finding of elevated levels of CSF dynorphin A [1-8] (Leckman et al., 1988), the neuroanatomical distribution of dynorphin, and its broad-range motor and behavioral effects have lead to speculation concerning its role in the pathobiology of Tourette's syndrome. Additional evidence supporting the role of endogenous opiates comes from dramatic, but poorly documented, effects of opiate antagonists in Tourette's syndrome (Sandyk, 1985; Chappell et al., 1992).

Neuroendocrine Factors

Twin and family studies support the role of nongenetic factors in the expression of Tourette's syndrome. Endogenously active neuroendocrine factors related to gender and stress may be important mediators in this regard. The increased prevalence of Tourette's syndrome and other tic disorders among males may be related to exposure of the developing male CNS to elevated levels of dihydrotestosterone and/or other gender-related factors (Leckman et al., 1984; Peterson et al., 1992). This hypothesis is based in part on the observation that, although Tourette's syndrome is more prevalent among males, it does not appear to be transmitted as a sex-linked trait (Pauls and Leckman, 1986), where higher rates among males would be expected. A second line of evidence comes from the observation that the onset and course of tic symptomatology does not appear to be related to activation during puberty of the hypothalamic-pituitary-gonadal axis, as the tic symptoms usually commence well before this period. It is also intriguing to note that some of the neurochemical and peptidergic systems implicated in the pathophysiology of tic disorders appear to be regulated early in development by gender-specific factors (Freidhoff, 1986; Leckman, 1995; Molineaux et al., 1986). Although the precise mechanism for this action has not been established, it is likely that it is due to altered rates of transcription of androgen-sensitive genes.

Perinatal Factors

The search for nongenetic factors that mediate the expression of a genetic vulnerability to Tourette's syndrome and related disorders has also focused on the role of adverse perinatal events (Leckman and Peterson, 1993). This interest dates from the report of Pasamanick and Kawi (1956), who found that mothers of children with tics were 1.5 times more likely to have experienced a complication during pregnancy than the mothers of children without tics. Other investigators have reported that, among monozygotic twins discordant for Tourette's syndrome, the index twin with Tourette's syndrome uniformly had a lower birth weight than the unaffected co-twin (Hyde et al., 1992; Leckman et al., 1987). Severity of maternal life stress during pregnancy and severe nausea and/or vomiting during the first trimester have also been implicated as potential risk factors in the development of tic disorders (Leckman et al., 1990). Some of these factors may alter dopamine levels on the developing CNS, and this, in turn, may have an enduring effect on the number of striatal D2 receptors in adulthood (Friedhoff, 1986). In contrast, two studies have failed to document any association between adverse perinatal events and manifestations of Tourette's syndrome (see review by Shapiro et al., 1988).

Psychological Factors

Tic disorders have long been identified as "stress-sensitive" conditions (Chappell et al., 1994; Jagger et al., 1982; Shapiro and Shapiro, 1988). Typically, symptom exacerbations follow in the wake of stressful life events. As noted by Shapiro, these events need not be adverse in character to produce this effect (Shapiro and Shapiro, 1988). Clinical experience suggests that, in some unfortunate instances, a vicious cycle can be initiated in which tic symptoms are misunderstood by the family and teachers, leading to active attempts to suppress the symptoms by punishment and humiliation. These efforts can lead to a further exacerbation of symptoms and a further increase in stress in the child's interpersonal environment. Unchecked, this vicious cycle can lead to the most severe manifestations of Tourette's syndrome and dysthymia, as well as maladaptive characterological traits. Although psychoanalytic and dynamic formulations of Tourette's syndrome have been largely discredited (Mahler and Rangell, 1943), the intimate association of the content and timing of tic behaviors with dynamically important events in the lives of children make it difficult to overlook their contribution to the intramorbid course of these disorders (Cohen and Leckman, 1994).

In addition to the intramorbid effects of stress and anxiety, which have been well characterized, some authors have suggested that premorbid stress may play an important role as a sensitizing agent in the pathogenesis of Tourette's syndrome among vulnerable individuals (Leckman et al., 1986).

DIFFERENTIAL DIAGNOSIS

The differential diagnosis of simple motor tics includes a variety of hyperkinetic movements: myoclonus, tremors, chorea, athetosis, dystonias, akathitic movements, paroxysmal dyskinesias, ballistic movements, and hyperekplexia (Jankovic, 1992). These movements may be associated with genetic conditions, such as Huntington's chorea or Wilson's disease; structural lesions, as in hemiballismus (associated with lesions to the contralateral subthalamic nucleus); infectious processes, as in Sydenham's chorea (Swedo et al., 1989); idiopathic functional instability of neuronal circuits, as in myoclonic epilepsy; and pharmacological treatments, such as acute akathisia and dystonias that are associated with the use of neuroleptic agents. Differentiation between these conditions and tic disorders is usually accomplished on clinical grounds and is based on the presentation of the disorder and its natural history. For example, although aspects of tics, such as their abruptness, their paroxysmal timing, or their suppressible nature, may be similar to symptoms seen in other conditions, it is rare for all of these features to be combined in the absence of a bona fide tic disorder. Occasionally, diagnostic tests are needed to exclude alternative diagnoses.

Complex motor tics can be confused with other complex repetitive behaviors, such as stereotypies or compulsive rituals. Differentiation among these behaviors may be difficult, particularly among retarded individuals with limited verbal skills. In other settings, where these symptoms are closely intertwined, as in individuals with both Tourette's syndrome and obsessive-compulsive disorder, efforts to distinguish between complex motor tics and compulsive behaviors may be futile.

Involuntary vocal utterances, in the absence of a tic disorder, are uncommon neurological signs. Huntington's disease may be associated with sniffing and brief sounds. Involuntary moaning can be heard in Parkinson's disease, particularly as a result of l-dopa toxicity. Complex phonic tics, characterized by articulate speech, can be distinguished from other conditions, including voluntary coprolalia. Because of their rarity in other syndromes, phonic tics can play an important role in differential diagnosis.

Anamnesis, family history, observation, and neurologic examination are usually sufficient to establish the diagnosis of a tic disorder. There are no confirmatory diagnostic tests. Neuroimaging studies, EEG-based studies, and laboratory tests are usually noncontributory, except in atypical cases.

Inventories such as the Tourette's Syndrome Questionnaire (Jagger et al., 1982), completed by the family prior to their initial consultation, can be valuable ancillary tools to gain a long-term perspective of the child's developmental course and the natural history of the tic disorder. In addition, several valid and reliable clinical rating instruments have been developed to inventory and quantify recent tic symptoms, including the Yale Global Tic Severity Scale (Leckman et al.,1989), the Shapiro Tourette Syndrome Severity Scale (Shapiro et al., 1988), and the Hopkins Motor and Vocal Tic Scale (Walkup et al., 1992). Some clinicians also make regular use of standardized video-tape protocols to assess current tic severity (Chappell et al., 1994; Shapiro et al., 1988; Tanner et al., 1982).

ASSESSMENT

Table 57.2 presents an outline of clinically relevant areas that should be assessed in patients presenting with a tic disorder. Once the diagnosis has been established, care should be taken to focus on the overall course of an individual's development, not simply on his or her symptoms. This may be a particular problem in the case of Tourette's syndrome, where the symptoms can be dramatic and the temptation to organize all of an individual's behavioral and emotional difficulties under a single all-encompassing rubric is relatively great.

The principal goal of an initial assessment is to determine the individual's overall level of adaptive functioning and to identify areas of impairment and distress. Close attention to the strengths and weaknesses of the individual and his or her family is crucial. Relevant aspects include the presence of comorbid mental, behavioral, developmental, or physical disorders; family history of psychiatric and/or neurological disease; relationships with family and peers; school and/or occupational performance; and the history of important life events.

Medication history is important, particularly if the disorder is longstanding or if medications have been prescribed for physical disorders. It may be necessary to evaluate the adequacy of prior trials with pharmacological agents used to treat tic disorders.

TREATMENT

Tic disorders are frequently chronic, if not lifelong, conditions. Continuity of care is desirable and should be considered before embarking on a course of treatment. Major approaches include education, supportive interventions, and treatment with neuropsychopharmacological agents. Typically, patients with chronic motor tics alone do not require drug treatment. Psychoanalytically oriented psychotherapy can be a useful adjunct in selected cases. Behavioral and dietary treatments have not yet provided consistent positive effects.

Educational and Supportive Interventions

Although the efficacy of educational and supportive interventions has not been rigorously assessed, they can have profoundly positive

Table 57.2. Clinical Evaluation of Tic Disorders

1. *Tics:* Anatomic location, number, frequency, intensity, complexity, degree of interference
   a. *Onset:* Age, characteristics (sudden, gradual, associated with stressful life events)
   b. *Course:* Waxing or waning, suppressibility, rostal-caudal progression, increasing complexity of tics, duration, intramorbid factors associated with worsening or improvement
   c. *Associated mental phenomena:* Premonitory sensory urges, mental tics
   d. *Impairment:* Impact on self-esteem, family function, social adaption, educational or job performance, risk of physical injury
2. *Obsessive-compulsive symptoms and behaviors:* Obsessive worries and thoughts (tics need to be done ''just right,'' simple compulsive rituals (''evening-up,'' ordering behaviors), full-fledged obsessive-compulsive disorder (recurrent ego-dystonic obsessive thoughts and compulsive rituals that are ''resisted'' and interfere with normal cognitive function)
   a. *Onset:* Age, characteristics (associated with puberty)
   b. *Course:* Waxing and waning, progression from ego-neutral to ego-dystonic compulsions
   c. *Impairment:* Impact on self-esteem, family function, social adaption, educational or job performance, risk of physical injury
3. *Past medical and developmental history:* Prenatal events, birth history, developmental delays, medication exposures, injuries, asthma, migraine, other disorders of arousal, allergies, history of streptococcal infections
4. *Other developmental, behavioral, or emotional problems:* Attentional problems, mood lability and increased irritability, major depression, and anxiety disorders
5. *Relationship with family and peers:* Premorbid history, period from onset to diagnosis, current social adjustment, marital status
6. *Life events:* Relationship of life events to onset and exacerbations of tics, stability of family life, coping skills, social supports
7. *History of developmental, behavioral, and emotional disorders in the extended family:* Tics, attentional problems, hyperactivity, learning problems, obsessive-compulsive behaviors, major depression, alcoholism, anxiety disorders
8. *School status:* Cognitive level, specific learning problems, adequacy of placement
9. *Employment status:* Job difficulties associated with tic behaviors or related phenomena, adequacy of placement given patient's native abilities
10. *Physical and neurological examination:* ''Soft,'' nonlocalizing neurological signs; minor EEG abnormalities; CAT scan usually negative
11. *Medication status:* Response to medications, adequacy of trials

Adapted from Leckman JF, Cohen DJ: Descriptive and diagnostic classification of tic disorders. In: Cohen DJ, Bruun RD, Leckman JF (eds): *Tourette's Syndrome and Tic Disorders.* New York, Wiley, 1988.

effects by reshaping negative expectations (Cohen et al., 1988). This is particularly true when the tic behaviors have been misconstrued by the family and others as voluntary and intentionally provocative. Families also find descriptions of the natural history comforting, in that the disorders tend not to be relentlessly progressive and usually improve during adulthood. This information often contradicts the impressions gained from the available lay literature on Tourette's syndrome, which typically focuses on the most extreme cases. In addition, the presentation of Tourette's syndrome as a neuropsychiatric disorder determined by a neurobiological vulnerability and influenced by psychosocial factors can help families fend off the stigmatizing effects of a purely mental disorder. For children, contact with their teachers can be enormously valuable. By educating the educators, clinicians can make significant progress toward securing for the child a positive and supportive environment in the classroom. Self-help organizations such as the Tourette syndrome Association can also be of assistance in providing audiovisual aides as well as peer support and counselling.

Neuropsychopharmacological Treatment

For individuals who are experiencing significant impairment as a result of their tic behaviors, treatment with drugs can provide a source of relief. Although virtually every agent in the *vademecum psychopharmacologium* has been used in the treatment of Tourette's syndrome, only the relatively selective D2 receptor antagonists, haloperidol and pimozide, have proven to be effective during the course of rigorous double-blind clinical trials.

Approximately 70% of Tourette's syndrome patients respond favorably to either haloperidol or pimozide (Shapiro et al., 1989). The mean reduction of symptom severity is also in the 70–80% range. In general, it is useful to start treatment with low doses of medication and to make any necessary increases gradually. Typically, treatment is initiated with a low dose (0.25 mg of haloperidol or 1 mg of pimozide) given before bedtime. Further increments (0.5 mg of haloperidol or 1 mg of pimozide) may be added at 7–14-day intervals if the tic behaviors remain severe. In most instances, 0.5–6 mg/day of haloperidol or 1–10 mg/day of pimozide administered over a period of 4–8 weeks is usually sufficient to suppress tic symptoms.

Tic symptoms often continue to wax and wane, at a much reduced level, even during periods of neuroleptic treatment. Generally, it is not a good idea to ''chase'' the tic symptoms with adjustments in medication dosage. Such adjustments generally are not beneficial and may expose the subjects to additional unwanted physical effects of the medication, many of which appear to be dose related.

The major limiting factor in the use of neuroleptics is the emergence of side effects, including acute dystonias, akathisia, akinesia, cognitive impairment, and weight gain (Shapiro and Shapiro, 1988). A majority of subjects will experience one or more of these effects, and a significant proportion of these subjects elect to discontinue treatment if the side effects are not controlled. In addition to these consequences, pimozide may have an adverse effect on cardiac conduction in some Tourette's syndrome subjects, particularly at doses above 10–12 mg/day. Tardive dyskinesia has also been reported in Tourette's syndrome patients with chronic exposure to neuroleptics. Given the short-term and long-term hazards of neuroleptic medication, many clinicians elect to use these medications only in severe cases. The development of newer neuroleptic agents with reportedly fewer side effects, such as risperidone, leave room for optimism in this regard (Lombroso et al., 1995).

Clonidine, a selective α_2 adrenergic receptor agonist, may be effective for a smaller proportion of Tourette's syndrome subjects (Cohen et al., 1979; Leckman et al., 1991). Clinical trials indicate that subjects can expect on average a 20–30% reduction in their symptoms over an 8–12-week period. The usual starting dose is 0.05 mg on arising. Further 0.05 mg increments at 3–5-hour intervals are added weekly until a dosage of 5 μg/kg is reached or the total daily dose exceeds 0.25 mg.

Although clonidine is clearly less effective than both haloperidol and pimozide, it is considerably safer. The principal side effect associated with its use is sedation, which occurs in 10–20% of subjects and which usually abates with continued use. Related compounds, such as guanfacine, may also prove to be useful, especially in Tourette's syndrome with comorbid attention deficit hyperactivity disorder (Chappell et al., 1995)

PROGNOSIS

The prognosis for tic disorders is generally good, with most subjects experiencing their worst tic symptoms during the ages of 10–15. The course in adulthood is variable, but most subjects report a more or less stable repertoire of tic symptoms that wax and wane over a reduced range of severity.

Poorer prognoses are associated with comorbid developmental and mental disorders, chronic physical illness, unstable and unsupportive family environments, and exposure to psychoactive drugs, such as cocaine. Potential complications include the emergence of obsessive-compulsive disorder, character pathology associated with a chronic stigmatizing disorder, and physical injuries secondary to self-abusive motor tics.

RESEARCH DIRECTIONS

As outlined throughout this chapter, a broad array of research opportunities is now being actively pursued. Based largely on advances in related fields of science, genetic and neurobiological studies show particular promise. Progress in these areas may herald significant advances in early detection and diagnosis as well as in treatment.

References

Alexander GE, DeLong MR: Microstimulation of the primate neostriatum. I: Physiological properties of striatal microexcitable zones. *J Neurophysiol* 53:1401–1416, 1985a.

Alexander GE, DeLong MR: Microstimulation of the primate neostriatum. II: Somatotropic organization of striatal microexcitable zones and their relation to neuronal response properties. *J Neurophysiol* 53:1417–1430, 1985b.

American Psychiatric Association: *Diagnostic and Statistical Manual of Mental Disorders* (4th ed). Washington, DC, American Psychiatric Association Press, 1994.

Apter A, Pauls DL, Bleich A, et al: An epidemiological study of Gilles de la Tourette's syndrome in Israel. *Arch Gen Psychiatry* 50:734–738, 1993.

Balthasar K: Über das anatomishe Substrat der generalisierten Tic-Krankeit (maladie des tics, Gilles de la Tourette): Entwicklungshemmung des Corpus Striatum. *Arch Psychiatr Nervenkr* 195:531–549, 1956.

Braun AR, Stoetter B, Randolph C, et al: The functional neuroanatomy of Tourette's syndrome: An FDG-PET study. I. Regional changes in cerebral glucose metabolism differentiating patients and controls. *Neuropsychopharmacology* 9:277–291, 1993.

Brooks DJ, Turjanski N, Sawle GV, et al: PET studies on the integrity of the pre and postsynaptic dopaminergic system in Tourette syndrome. In: TN Chase, AJ Friedhoff, DJ Cohen (eds): *Advances in Neurology* (Vol. 58). New York, Raven Press, Ltd., 1992, pp. 227–231.

Bruun RD: The natural history of Tourette's syndrome. In: Cohen DJ, Bruun RD, Leckman JF (eds): *Tourette's Syndrome and Tic Disorders.* New York, Wiley, pp. 21–39, 1988.

Buck SH, Yamamura HI: Neuropeptides in normal and pathological basal ganglia. In: Friedhoff AJ, Chase TN (eds): *Advances in Neurology Vol 35: Gilles de la Tourette Syndrome.* New York, Raven Press. 1982, pp. 121–132.

Burd L, Kerbeshian L, Wikenheiser M, et al: Prevalence of Gilles de la Tourette's syndrome in North Dakota adults. *Am J Psychiatry* 143:787–788, 1986a.

Burd L, Kerbeshian L, Wikenheiser M, et al: A prevalence study of Gilles de la Tourette syndrome in North Dakota school-age children. *J Am Acad Child Psychiatry* 25:552–553, 1986b.

Butler IJ, Koslow SH, Seifert WE Jr, et al: Biogenic amine metabolism in Tourette syndrome. *Ann Neurol* 6:37–39, 1979.

Chappell PB, Leckman JF, Riddle MA, et al: Neuroendocrine and behavioral effects of naloxone in Tourette syndrome. In: TN Chase, AJ Friedhoff, DJ Cohen (eds): *Advances in Neurology* Vol. 58. New York, Raven Press, Ltd., 1992, p. 253–262.

Chappell PB, McSwiggan-Hardin M, Scahill L, et al: Videotape tic counts in the assessment of Tourette's syndrome: stability, reliability, and validity. *J Am Acad Child Adolesc Psychiatry,* 33: 386–393, 1994.

Chappell PB, Riddle MA, Anderson GM, et al: Enhanced stress responsivity of Tourette syndrome patients undergoing lumbar puncture. *Biol Psychiatry,* 36:35–43, 1994.

Chappell PB, Riddle MA, Scahill L, et al: Guanfacine treatment of comorbid attention deficit disorder and Tourette's syndrome: Preliminary clinical experience. *J Am Acad Child Adolesc Psychiatry* 34: 1140–1146, 1995.

Cohen DJ, Leckman JF: Developmental psychopathology and neurobiology of Tourette's syndrome. *J Am Acad Child Adolesc Psychiatry* 33, 1:2–15, 1994.

Cohen DJ, Ort SI, Leckman JF, et al: Family functioning and Tourette's syndrome. In: Cohen DJ, Bruun RD, Leckman IF (eds): *Tourette's Syndrome*

and Tic Disorders. New York, Wiley, 1988, pp. 179–196.

Cohen DJ, Shaywitz BA, Caparulo B, et al: Chronic, multiple tics of Gilles de la Tourette's disease: CSF acid monoamine metabolites after probenecid administration. *Arch Gen Psychiatry* 35: 245–250, 1978.

Cohen DJ, Young JG, Nathanson JA, et al: Clonidine in Tourette's syndrome. *Lancet* 2:551–553, 1979.

Commings DE, Himes JA, Commings BG: An epidemiological study of Tourette's syndrome in a single school district. *J Clin Psychiatry* 51:463–469, 1990.

Devinsky O: Neuroanatomy of Gilles de la Tourette's syndrome: Possible midbrain involvement. *Arch Neurol* 40:508–514, 1983.

Dewulf A, van Bogaert L: Etudes anatomo-cliniques de syndromes hypercinétiques complexes. *Mschr Psychiatr Neurol* 104:53–61, 1940.

Fahn S, Erenberg G: Differential diagnosis of tic phenomena: A neurologic perspective. In: Cohen DJ, Bruun RD, Leckman JF (eds): *Tourettes Syndrome and Tic Disorders.* New York, Wiley, 1988, pp. 41–54.

Filion M, Tremblay L: Abnormal spontaneous activity of the globus pallidus neurons in monkeys with MPTP-induced parkinsonism. *Brain Res* 547: 147–151, 1991.

Filion M, Tremblay L, Bédard PJ: Effects of dopamine agonists on the spontaneous activity of the globus pallidus neurons in monkeys with MPTP-induced parkinsonism. *Brain Res* 547:152–161, 1991.

Friedhoff AJ: Insights into the pathophysiology and pathogenesis of Gilles de la Tourette syndrome. *Rev Neurol* 142:860, 1986.

Gilles de la Tourette G: Etude sur une affection nerveuse caractérisée par de l'incoordination motrice accompagnée d'echolalie et de copralalie. *Arch Neurol* 9:19–42, 158, 1885.

Haber SN, Kowall NW, Vonsattel JP, et al: Gilles de la Tourette's syndrome: A postmortem neuropathological and immunohistochemical study. *J Neurol Sci* 75:225–241, 1986.

Hyde TM, Aaronson RA, Randolph C, et al: Relationships of birth weight to the phenotypic expression of Gilles de la Tourette's syndrome in monozygotic twins. *Neurology* 42:652–658, 1992.

Itard JMG: Mémoire sur quelques fonctions involontaires des appareils de la locomotion de la préhension et de la voix. *Arch Gen Med* 8:385–407, 1825.

Jagger J, Prusoff BA, Cohen DJ, et al: The epidemiology of Tourette's syndrome: A pilot study. *Schizophr Bull* 8:267–277, 1982.

Jankovic J: Diagnosis and classification of Tics and Tourette syndrome. In: TN Chase, AJ Friedhoff, DJ Cohen (eds): *Advances in Neurology* (Vol. 58). New York, Raven Press, Ltd., 1992, pg. 7–14.

Kurlan R, Behr J, Medved L, et al: Familial Tourette's syndrome: Report of a large pedigree and potential for linkage analysis. *Neurology* 36: 772–776, 1986.

Laplane D, Widlocher D, Pillon B, et al: Comportement compulsif d'allure obsessionnelle par necrose circonscrite bilatérale pallidostriatale. Encephalopathie par piqûre de guêpe. *Rev Neurol* 137: 269–276, 1981.

Leckman JF: The pathogenesis of Tourette's syndrome: Role of biogenic amines and sexually dimorphic systems active in early CNS development. In: Segawa N, Nomura Y (eds). Age-related dopamine-dependent disorders. Basel, Karger, 1995, pp. 41–49.

Leckman JF, Cohen DJ: Descriptive and diagnostic classification of tic disorders. In: Cohen DJ, Bruun RD, Leckman JF (eds): *Tourettes Syndrome and Tic Disorders.* New York, Wiley, 1988, pp. 3–21.

Leckman JF, Cohen DJ, Price RA, et al: The pathogenesis of Gilles de la Tourette's syndrome: A review of data and hypothesis. In: Shah AB, Shah NS,

Donald AG (eds): *Movement Disorders.* New York, Plenum, 1984, pp. 257–272.

Leckman JF, Dolnansky ES, Hardin MT, et al: Perinatal factors in the expression of Tourette's syndrome: An exploratory study. *J Am Acad Child Adolesc Psychiatry* 29:220–226, 1990.

Leckman JF, Hardin MT, Riddle MA, et al: Clonidine treatment of Tourette's syndrome. *Arch Gen Psychiatry,* 48:324–328, 1991a.

Leckman JF, Knorr A, Rasmusson A, et al: Another frontier for basal ganglia research: Tourette's syndrome and related disorders. *Trends Neurosci* 3: 207–211, 1991b.

Leckman JF, Pauls DL, Cohen DJ: Tic Disorders: In: Bloom FE, Kuper D (eds): *Psychopharmacology: The Fourth Generation of Progress,* 1995, pp. 1665–1674.

Leckman JF, Peterson BD: The pathogenesis of Tourette's syndrome: Epigenetic factors active in early CNS development. *Biol Psychiatry,* 34: 425–427, 1993.

Leckman JF. Price RA. Walkup IT, et al: Letter to the editor: Nongenetic factors in Gilles de la Tourette's syndrome. *Arch Gen Psychiatry* 44:100, 1987.

Leckman JF. Riddle MA, Berrettini WH, et al: Elevated CSF dynorphin A [1–8] in Tourette's syndrome. *Life Sci* 43:2015–2023, 1988.

Leckman JF, Riddle MA, Hardin MT, et al: The Yale Global Tic Severity Scale: Initial testing of a clinician-rated scale of tic severity. *J Am Acad Child Adolesc Psychiatry* 28:566–573, 1989.

Leckman JF, Walker DE, Cohen DJ: Premonitory urges in Tourette syndrome. *Am J Psychiatry* 150: 98–102, 1993.

Leckman JF, Walkup JT, Riddle MA, et al: Tic disorders. In: Meltzer HY (ed): *Psychopharmacology: The Third Generation of Progress.* New York, Raven Press, 1987, pp. 1239–1246.

Lombroso PJ, Scahill l, King RA, et al: Rispendone treatment of children and adolescents with chronic tic disorders: A preliminary reportt. *J Am Acad Child Adolesc Psychiatry* 39:1147–1152, 1995.

Mahler MS, Rangell L: A psychosomatic study of *maladie des tics* (Gilles de la Tourette's disease). *Psychiatr Q* 17: 579–603. 1943.

Malison RT, McDougle CJ, van Dyck CH, et al: [1123] β- CIT SPECT imaging demonstrates increased striatal dopamine transporter binding in Tourette's syndrome. *Am J Psychiatry* 152:1359–1361, 1995.

Marsden CD: The mysterious motor function of the basal ganglia: The Robert Wartenberg lecture. *Neurology* 32:514–539, 1982.

Molineaux CJ, Hassen AN, Rosenberger JG et al: Response of rat pituitary anterior lobe prodynorphin products to changes in gonadal steroid environment. *Endocrinology* 119:2297–2305. 1986.

Pakstis A, Heutink P, Pauls DL, et al: Progress in the search for genetic linkage with Tourette Syndrome: an exclusion map covering more than 50% of the autosomal genome. *Am J Hum Genet* 48: 281–294, 1991.

Pasamanick B, Kawi A: A study of the association of prenatal and paranatal factors in the development of tics in children. *J Pediatr* 48:596–601, 1956.

Pauls DL, Leckman JF: The inheritance of Gilles de la Tourette syndrome and associated behaviors: Evidence for autosomal dominant transmission. *N Engl J Med* 315:993–997. 1986.

Pauls DL, Raymond CL, Stevenson J, et al: A family study of Gilles de la Tourette. *Am J Hum Genet,* 48:154–163, 1991.

Peterson BS, Leckman JF, Duncan JF, et al: Corpus callosum morphology from MR images in Tourette's syndrome. *Psychiatry Res* 55:85–99, 1994.

Peterson BS, Leckman JF, Scahill L, et al: Hypothesis: steroid hormones and CNS sexual dimorphisms modulate symptom expression in Tourette's syndrome. *Psychoneuroendocrinology* 17:553–563, 1992.

Peterson BS, Riddle MA, Cohen DJ, et al: Reduced basal ganglia volumes in Tourette's syndrome using 3-dimensional reconstruction techniques from magnetic resonance images. *Neurology* 43:941–949, 1993.

Price AR, Leckman JF, Paints DL, et al: Tics and central nervous system stimulants in twins and nontwins with Tourette syndrome. *Neurology* 36:232–237, 1986.

Rapoport JL ed: *Obsessive-Compulsive Disorder in Children and Adolescents*. Washington, DC, American Psychiatric Association Press, 1989.

Sandyk R: The endogenous opioid system in neurological disorders of the basal ganglia. *Life Sci* 37:1655–1663, 1985.

Shapiro AK, Shapiro ES: Treatment of Tic disorders with haloperidol. In: Cohen DJ, Bruun RD, Leckman JF (eds): *Tourette's Syndrome and Tic Disorders*. New York, Wiley, 1988, pp. 267–289.

Shapiro AK, Shapiro ES, Young JG, et al. (eds): *Gilles de la Tourette Syndrome* (2nd ed). New York, Raven Press, 1988.

Shapiro ES, Shapiro AK, Fulop G, et al: Controlled study of haloperidol, pimozide, and placebo for the treatment of Gilles de la Tourette's syndrome. *Arch Gen Psychiatry* 46:722–730. 1989.

Singer HS, Hahn IH, Moran TH: Abnormal dopamine uptake sites in postmortem striatum from patients with Tourette's syndrome. *Ann Neurol* 30:558–562, 1991.

Singer HS, Reiss AL, Brown JE, et al: Volumetric MRI changes in basal ganglia of children with Tourette's syndrome. *Neurology* 43:950–956, 1993.

Singer HS, Tune LE, Butler IJ. et al: Clinical symptomatology, CSF neurotransmitter metabolites, and serum haloperidol levels in Tourette syndrome. In: Friedhoff AJ, Chase TN (eds): *Advances in Neurology, Vol 35: Gilles de la Tourette Syndrome*. New York. Raven Press, 1982, pp. 177–183.

Sverd J, Gadow KD, Nolan EE, et al: Methylphenidate in hyperactive boys with comorbid Tic disorder. I. Clinic evaluations. In: Chase TN, Friedhoff AJ, Cohen DJ (eds): *Advances in Neurology, Vol. 58*. New York, Raven Press, Ltd., 1992, pp. 271–281.

Swedo SE, Rapoport JL, Cheslow DL, et al: High prevalence of obsessive-compulsive symptoms in patients with Sydenham's chorea. *Am J Psychiatry* 146:246–249, 1989.

Tanner CM, Goetz CG, Klawans HL: Cholinergic mechanisms in Tourette syndrome. *Neurology* 32:1315–1317, 1982.

Walkup JT, Rosenberg LA, Brown J, et al: The validity of instruments measuring tic severity in Tourette's syndrome. *J Am Acad Child Adolesc Psychiatry* 30, 3:472–477, 1992.

World Health Organization: ICD-10 1988, Draft of Chapter V, Mental, Behavioral, and Developmental Disorders. *Clinical Descriptions and Diagnostic Guidelines*. Geneva, World Health Organization, 1988.

Zahner GEP, Clubb MM, Leckman JF, et al: The epidemiology of Tourette's syndrome. In: Cohen DJ, Bruun RD, Leckman JF (eds): *Tourette's Syndrome and Tic Disorders* New York, Wiley, 1988, pp. 79–90.

58 CHILDHOOD SCHIZOPHRENIA

Fred R. Volkmar, M.D.

DEFINITION

The definition of schizophrenic disorders in childhood has been the topic of considerable debate. While available evidence suggests that the symptoms are rather similar in both childhood and adult schizophrenia, controversies have surrounded the stringency of diagnostic criteria and assumptions about the nature of the disorder. DSM-IV (American Psychiatric Association, 1994) criteria for the condition are presented in Table 58.1. Given the available evidence, which supports a fundamental continuity between childhood, adolescent, and adult schizophrenia, the criteria apply to all age groups.

Relative to the DSM-III-R (American Psychiatric Association, 1987), criteria for schizophrenia have been simplified and the disorder is defined on the basis of characteristic psychotic symptoms, deficits in adaptive functioning, and duration of at least 6 months. The criteria for the characteristic psychotic symptoms have been streamlined with examples moved out of criteria into text; these characteristic psychotic symptoms include delusions, hallucinations, disorganized speech, grossly disorganized or catatonic behavior, and negative symptoms such as flattened affect. As indicated in Criterion B some consideration of age should be made relative to social/occupational dysfunction. Signs of disturbance must be present for at least 6 months with at least 1 month during which active symptoms are present. The disorder cannot be diagnosed in the presence of schizoaffective disorder or mood disorder with psychotic features, nor can it be due to the direct effects of substance abuse or a general medical condition.

Unfortunately the attempt to produce a more concise and efficient criterion set may complicate the tasks of diagnosis of childhood schizophrenia; certain symptoms such as disorganized speech and behavior are relatively common in nonpsychotic children, and the lowered threshold for Criterion A may similarly produce overdiagnosis (see Werry, 1996, for a discussion). On the other hand, particularly in adolescents who develop schizophrenia and where there is a history of substance abuse, Criterion E may tend to produce underdiagnosis of the condition. The reworking of the criterion related to comorbid diagnosis of schizophrenia and autism (Criterion F) reflects recent work suggesting no greater than a chance association of these conditions (Volkmar and Cohen, 1991). Given the lack of familiarity of many clinicians with

schizophrenia in childhood, the condition maybe misdiagnosed in both directions, i.e., both false-positive and false-negative diagnoses are common (e.g., McKenna et al., 1994). The DSM-IV text indicates a differences in symptomatology in children and addresses some aspects of differential diagnosis relevant to children. Review of both text and criteria is indicated relative to a diagnosis of schizophrenia in children and adolescents. The approach to diagnosis of the disorder in ICD-10 is roughly similar (World Health Organization, 1990), although that definition is even less developmentally oriented than DSM-IV (Werry, 1996).

Although DSM-IV and its predecessor, DSM-III-R, represent, in some respects, substantial advances in the classification of schizophrenic disorders, certain problems with respect to diagnosis of the disorder in childhood remain. Problems arise both in applying concepts like psychosis to children and in the specification of criteria applicable to disordered children.

The concept of psychosis, as applied to children, is problematic in several respects. It is clear from the work of Piaget (1954) and others that children's conceptions of reality change over the course of normal development and that fully adult conceptualizations of reality are achieved only in adolescence. Many children have normatively appropriate beliefs in fantasy figures, which would not of themselves suggest psychosis. Finally, since many of these severe disorders have important deleterious effects on development, it is important to note that comorbid associations with conditions like mental retardation or other developmental disorders might pose additional problems in assessing psychotic thinking in children. Issues of the definition of psychosis or thought disorder become extremely complex in relationship, for example, to children who don't talk and are likely never to do so (Caplan, 1994). These observations suggest the importance of incorporating a truly developmental point of view in conceptualizing the nature of psychosis in childhood.

Changes in diagnostic practice and the relative infrequency of the disorder have complicated the development of better definitions of childhood schizophrenia. The relatively small number of studies evaluating DSM-III criteria (American Psychiatric Association, 1980) for schizophrenia in childhood have provided mixed and somewhat conflicting results.

Table 58.1. DSM-IV Diagnostic Criteria: Schizophrenia

A. *Characteristic symptoms:* Two (or more) of the following, each present for a significant portion of time during a 1-month period (or less if successfully treated):
1. Delusions
2. Hallucinations
3. Disorganized speech (e.g., frequent derailment or incoherence)
4. Grossly disorganized or catatonic behavior
5. Negative symptoms, i.e., affective flattening, alogia, or avolition
Note: Only one A symptom is required if delusions are bizarre or hallucinations consist of a voice keeping up a running commentary on the person's behavior or thoughts, or two or more voices conversing with each other.

B. *Social/occupational dysfunction:* For a significant portion of the time since the onset of the disturbance, one or more major areas of functioning such as work, interpersonal relations, or self-care are markedly below the level achieved prior to the onset (or, when the onset is in childhood or adolescence, failure to achieve expected level of interpersonal, academic, or occupational achievement).

C. *Duration:* Continuous signs of the disturbance persist for at least 6 months. This 6-month period must include at least 1 month of symptoms (or less if successfully treated) that meet Criterion A (i.e., active-phase symptoms) and may include periods of prodromal or residual symptoms. During these prodromal or residual periods, signs of the disturbance may be manifested by only negative symptoms or two or more symptoms listed in Criterion A present in an attenuated form (e.g., odd beliefs, unusual perceptual experiences).

D. *Schizoaffective and mood disorder exclusion:* Schizoaffective disorder and mood disorder with psychotic features have been ruled out because either: (1) no major depressive, manic, or mixed episodes have occurred concurrently with the active phase symptoms; or (2) if mood episodes have occurred during active phase symptoms, their total duration has been brief relative to the duration of the active and residual periods.

E. *Substance/general medical condition exclusion:* The disturbance is not due to the direct physiological effects of a substance (e.g., a drug of abuse, a medication) or a general medical condition.

F. If there is a history of autistic disorder or another pervasive developmental disorder, the additional diagnosis of schizophrenia is made only if prominent delusions or hallucinations are also present for at least a month (or less if successfully treated).

From American Psychiatric Association: *Diagnostic and Statistical Manual* (4th ed.) Washington, DC, American Psychiatric Association, 1994.

In DSM-III the term *childhood schizophrenia* was discarded as a separate diagnostic concept, while the validity of infantile autism as a diagnostic concept was recognized; this major change in classification reflected the consensus of most investigators that the term *childhood schizophrenia* had been used too broadly (Rutter, 1972). Cantor and her coworkers (1982) noted problems with this approach since several subjects they believed exhibited schizophrenia had evidenced signs of the disturbance relatively early in life; important developmental correlates of psychotic symptoms were noted. This report suggested that it is more difficult to apply DSM-III criteria for schizophrenia to younger children. In a study comparing schizophrenic and autistic children, Green et al. (1984) suggested that DSM-III criteria for schizophrenia could be meaningfully applied to younger children. In a review of 228 children with childhood "psychosis" using DSM-III criteria, Volkmar et al. (1988) noted difficulties in applying DSM-III criteria for schizophrenia, particularly in relation to documenting a period of deterioration associated with the illness or, in younger children, in relation to the stringency of criteria for hallucinations and delusions. At present the extent to which adult criteria for schizophrenia can be applied to children remains unclear. Some children clearly do meet such criteria, but the classification of children, particularly younger or developmentally delayed individuals, with schizophrenic-like disorders remains problematic. It is hoped that these issues will be addressed in future editions of DSM.

HISTORICAL NOTE

There have been marked changes in the way childhood schizophrenia is both conceptualized and diagnosed. These changes reflect both the recognition of similarities to adolescent and adult forms of schizophrenia and the difficulties inherent in simplistic extensions to children of concepts derived largely from work with adults. In the 19th century considerable interest centered on the role of experience versus endowment; by the mid-19th century Maudsley proposed an extension of concepts of "insanity" to childhood. By the late 19th century Kraeplin had proposed the term dementia praecox to describe a severe disorder with an onset in late adolescence or early adulthood and with characteristic features. This concept, now termed *schizophrenia*, proved particularly influential. Kraeplin (1919) noted that some cases appeared to have an onset in childhood; De Sanctis (1906) proposed the term *dementia praecossima* for children who developed the disorder in childhood. Although Potter (1933) attempted to define childhood schizophrenia on the basis of specific features (e.g., loss of interest in the environment, disturbances in thinking or affect, changes in behavior), the term became synonymous with childhood psychosis despite the fact that the disorder in children appeared less common than in adults and was more difficult to characterize.

It is important to note that disagreements regarding the nature of the adult schizophrenic syndrome resulted in rather different diagnostic approaches to the disorder. Different clinical features, such as a deteriorating course, disturbances in thinking, or specific pathognomonic symptoms, are variously emphasized (American Psychiatric Association, 1987). These controversies have been reflected in the apparent relative overdiagnosis of schizophrenia in adults in the United States compared with that in Britain (Cooper et al., 1972). Similarly, some investigators' approaches to childhood schizophrenia are narrower and more conservative (American Psychiatric Association, 1987; Potter, 1933; Rutter, 1972), while others, particularly those of Bender (1947) and her students, have argued for a very broad and inclusive definition. Early attempts to propose definitions (e.g., by the British Working Party on Childhood Psychosis) (Creak, 1963) were overinclusive, and schizophrenia was broadly defined so as to include all "psychotic" children. Although the narrow view currently predominates, it should be noted that this is a relatively recent historical phenomenon and that, for example, until DSM-III (American Psychiatric Association, 1980), childhood schizophrenia was the only "official" diagnostic term available to describe all psychotic children.

In important respects the modern controversy over the relationship of childhood psychosis to adult schizophrenia can be traced to Kanner's (1943) description of the syndrome of early infantile autism. Kanner's initial report of autism noted various ways in which his proposed disorder appeared to differ from schizophrenia; at the same time, his use of the term *autism* suggested some point of phenomenological similarity. The continuity or discontinuity of autism with schizophrenia became the topic of considerable debate. In retrospect it appears that a central aspect of this controversy related to an assumption of continuity based on severity; that is, since autism is a severe psychiatric disorder with a very early onset, must it not be the case that it represents the earliest manifestation of a similarly severe psychiatric disorder in adults? By the 1970s various lines of evidence began to suggest that infantile autism and childhood schizophrenia differed in important ways; the work of Kolvin (1971) and others (Rutter, 1972) suggested that differentiations could be made within the broad group of "psychotic" children on the basis of various features, for example, age of onset, clinical characteristics, family history, and evidence of CNS dysfunction. In particular it was apparent that almost all cases of childhood psychosis fell into one of two groups on the basis of age at onset of the disorder, and this is true for series of cases collected at different centers in various countries (Fig. 58.1). The early-onset group exhibited difficulties in the 1st years of life more consistent with Kanner's description of autism, while the late-onset group exhibited the delusions, hallucinations, and clinical features more commonly associated with schizophrenia (Kolvin, 1971). It was also clear that family members of the late-onset cases were more likely to exhibit histories of schizophrenia. These various lines of evidence convinced most investigators that autism and schizophrenia were unrelated; this was reflected in the 1980 edition of DSM (American Psychiatric Association, 1980). It should be noted that, while most investigators, including the author of this chapter, have adopted this view, a small number continue to advocate the earlier, broader diagnostic conceptualizations (Cantor, 1988).

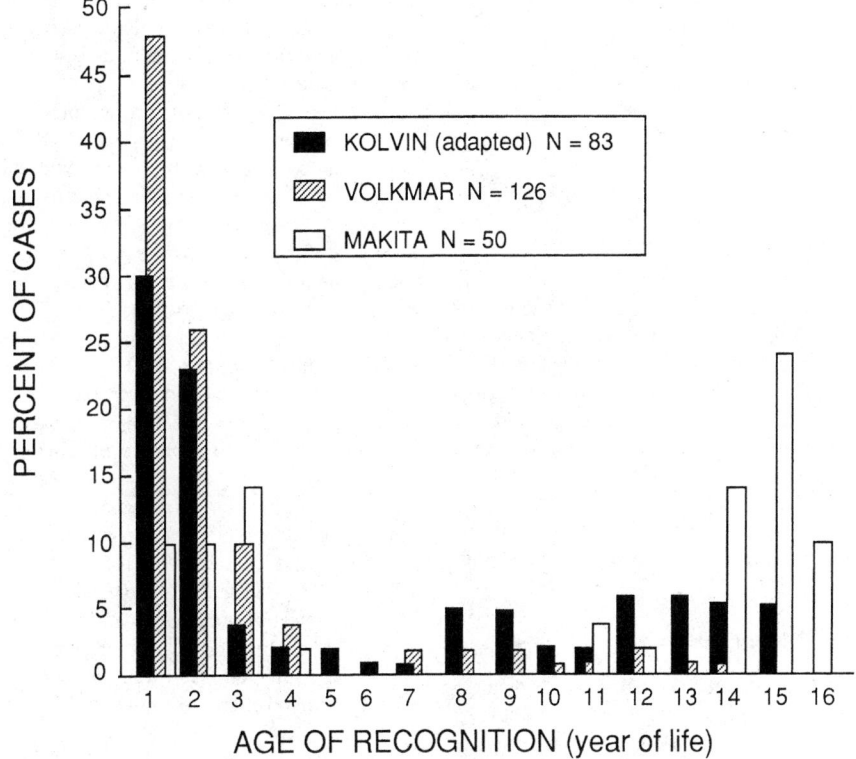

Figure 58.1. Reported age of onset of childhood psychosis. (From Volkmar FR, Cohen DJ, Hoshino Y, et al: Phenomenology and classification of the childhood psychoses. *Psychol Med* 18:191–201, 1988.)

PREVALENCE AND EPIDEMIOLOGY

Given the marked changes in the diagnostic concept over the past decade, it is not surprising that information on the prevalence and epidemiology of the disorder, as strictly defined, is quite limited. Few studies conducted prior to 1980 are readily interpretable, and major epidemiological studies have yet to be conducted. Accordingly, information is limited to estimates provided from case series and comparisons of the frequency of schizophrenia in relation to diagnoses of autism. Available research does, however, indicate that the disorder is probably less common than autism. For example, in Kolvin's (1971) series of cases, autism was noted to be 1.4 times as common as childhood schizophrenia. Similarly, using DSM-III criteria, a prevalence study in North Dakota of schizophrenia presenting in childhood revealed that the disorder appeared to be far less common than autism (Burd and Kerbeshian, 1987).

Characteristics of four samples of schizophrenic children from four studies using rigorous diagnostic criteria are presented in Table 58.2. Reported sex ratios of the disorder have varied across studies. Both a slight male predominance, on the order of 1.5 or 2 males:1 female (Green et al., 1984; Kolvin, 1971; Volkmar et al., 1988), and essentially equal sex ratios (Eggers, 1978) have been reported. In contrast to early reports of a high-socioeconomic-class association with autism (see Chapter 44), there is some evidence that suggests that schizophrenic children may more commonly be observed in less educated and professionally successful families (Table 58.2). It appears that most schizophrenic children function in the low-average to average range of intelligence (Table 58.2).

CLINICAL DESCRIPTION

Precursors of Childhood Schizophrenia

Various attempts have been made to identify possible childhood precursors of adult schizophrenia; both follow-back and prospective studies have been employed. Follow-back studies of the childhood histories of adult schizophrenic patients have suggested some early patterns of

Table 58.2. Sample Characteristics: Childhood Schizophrenia

	Study			
	Kolvin, 1971	Green et al., 1984	Volkmar et al., 1988	Russel et al., 1989
N	33	24	14	35
Male/female	24/9	15/9	10/4	24/11
Sex ratio (M:F)	2.66:1	1.67:1	2.5:1	2.2:1
Mean IQ	86	88 (± 16.0)	82 (± 12.5)	94 (± 10.5)
Social class				
I and II	16%	0	25%	54%
III	37%	17%	33%	23%
IV and V	47%	83%	42%	14%

developmental difference from children who did not become schizophrenic (Goldstein, 1980). Similarly, prospective studies that follow children presumably at greater risk for developing adult schizophrenia have attempted to identify various factors that may contribute to adult schizophrenia. Follow-up studies of children with psychiatric disorders have not shown a clear-cut pattern among children who go on to develop adult schizophrenia; although some differences are noted, it does not appear that shy, withdrawn children are particularly likely to develop adult schizophrenia. The applicability of both types of studies to childhood schizophrenia is somewhat questionable; the limited available data arise from case series. Children who subsequently develop the disorder have been noted to demonstrate various premorbid patterns, such as attentional and/or conduct problems (Russel et al., 1989), or earlier patterns of inhibition, withdrawal, and sensitivity (Kolvin, 1971).

Onset of the Disorder

To a considerable extent, the age at which a diagnosis of childhood schizophrenia is made will vary in association with the criteria used. However, most studies that employ reasonably stringent criteria suggest

Table 58.3. Characteristics of Thought Disturbance in Childhood Schizophrenia Hallucinations

Study	Thought Disorder	Delusions	Hallucinations	
			Auditory	Visual
Kolvin, 1971	60%	58%	82%	30%
Green et al., 1984	100%	54%	79%	46%
Volkmar et al., 1988	93%	86%	79%	28%
Russel et al., 1989	40%	63%	80%	13%

that the disorder is very rarely observed before age 5. The onset of disturbance appears to follow at least three general patterns (Green et al., 1984; Kolvin, 1971). In some instances the onset appears to be acute, without apparent premorbid signs of incipient disturbance. Most commonly the onset appears to be insidious, with a gradual deterioration in functioning. Finally, some cases appear to have an insidious onset with an acute exacerbation of disturbance. As with adult schizophrenia, males appear to be more likely to have an onset of their disorder earlier in childhood (Green et al., 1984). Distinctions between "early onset" and "very early onset" in childhood and adolescence have been suggested (see Werry, 1996).

Thought Disturbance

Available research data on the phenomenology of thought disturbance in childhood schizophrenia are limited. Only a handful of studies have been conducted using reasonably stringent diagnostic criteria (see Caplan, 1994, for a review). Additional problems are posed by the lack, at least until recently, of valid and reasonably standardized assessment instruments, as well as by the difficulties inherent in clinical assessment. However, the results of the few available studies are surprisingly similar (Green et al., 1984; Kolvin, 1971; Russel et al., 1989). Table 58.3 summarizes the results from several series of cases. Auditory hallucinations are consistently the most frequently reported symptoms, usually exhibited by about 80% of cases. Auditory hallucinations may include persecutory or command hallucinations, voices conversing, voices commenting about the child, and the like (Russel et al., 1989). Visual and somatic hallucinations are reported less frequently. Although delusional beliefs can be difficult to assess, available studies suggest that these are exhibited in approximately 50% of cases. Delusional beliefs can involve persecution, somatic concerns, ideas of reference, or grandiose or religious ideas (Russel et al., 1989). The reported presence of formal thought disorder varies considerably from study to study, reflecting the nature of specific definitions used. Magical or irrational thinking and loosening of associations are often observed, but it sometimes is the case that children, particularly in the early phases of the illness, may not clearly exhibit a degree of thought disturbance sufficient to satisfy strict diagnostic criteria; assessment of thought disturbance can be particularly problematic in younger or developmentally delayed children (Caplan, 1994; Russel et al., 1989; Volkmar et al., 1988). The content of hallucinations and delusions varies with age; younger children typically express less complicated hallucinations or delusional beliefs, and the content of the delusions or hallucinations may center around parents, fantasy figures, and animals (Arboleda and Holzman, 1985; Russel et al., 1989).

ETIOLOGY AND PATHOGENESIS

Biological Mechanisms

Although various lines of evidence suggest the involvement of biological processes in syndrome pathogenesis, no specific biological marker for the disorder has been identified. The work of Bender (1947) suggested that childhood schizophrenia, broadly defined, is commonly associated with signs of neurological immaturity, such as delays in motor development and neurological "soft" signs. Similarly, Cantor (1988) suggested that a constellation of hypotonia and hyporeflexia characterizes at least some schizophrenic children. Studies of adult schizophrenic individuals suggest that complications in pregnancy, labor, and delivery may be more frequent, but definitive studies in this regard have yet to be conducted (Werry, 1996). Studies of electrophysiological activity have also provided some general, although nonspecific, evidence of CNS dysfunction. Differences have been noted in the EEGs of schizophrenic children as compared with children with various disorders (Waldo et al., 1978), and abnormalities in event-related potentials have also been noted (Strandburg et al., 1984). Neuropsychological studies have revealed deficits in attentional capacities and the processing of information. Studies of neurotransmitter systems have been uncommon and have not produced consistent results (Werry, 1996); some investigators have suggested a possible role for the cholinergic system in syndrome pathogenesis (Cantor, 1988).

Genetic and family studies provide what is probably the most convincing evidence of some biological basis for the disorder. Rates of schizophrenia among the parents of schizophrenic children are substantially elevated in comparison to those observed in the normal population, apparently in much the same way that rates are noted to be elevated in relatives of adult schizophrenic patients; typically approximately 10% of parents exhibit a schizophrenic disorder (Kallman and Prugh, 1971; Kolvin, 1971). The nature of underlying mechanisms that might account for earlier onset of the disorder in some individuals remains unclear; it might, for example, reflect higher genetic loading or be a function of complicated interactions of various factors in combination with some genetic predisposition (Asarnow et al., 1986; Werry, 1996).

Psychological Processes

The interpretation of studies of children at high risk for schizophrenia is complicated since the disorder is low in frequency, even among those children presumed to be at greatest risk, and other factors may complicate the interpretation of results. As noted previously, no single personality pattern or pattern of premorbid adjustment appears to uniformly characterize preschizophrenic children. Various studies have reported an increased incidence of signs of neurosensory and neuromotor deficits in schizophrenic children and those presumably at risk for the disorder (Bender, 1947; Cantor, 1988; Fish, 1986). Disturbances in attentional capacities have been noted in schizophrenic children; these problems may precede the emergence of frank psychosis and may account, in part, for observed associations with various learning problems. Compared to autistic children, those with schizophrenia are much less likely to exhibit mental retardation (Green et al., 1984; Russel et al., 1989; Volkmar et al., 1988); however, problems in the assessment of retarded individuals may make it more difficult to establish the diagnosis with certainty in such cases.

Family and Interpersonal Dynamics

Various studies have examined patterns of family interaction in the families of individuals with schizophrenia. The available research is primarily concerned with adult patients. The few studies available regarding family dynamics in childhood schizophrenia are difficult to interpret since fairly stringent diagnostic criteria were not used and many early reports were really about autism rather than schizophrenia. Available studies have emphasized disturbances in patterns of communication (e.g., in relation to inconsistent communications or communications with unusual patterns of affective expression, such as high levels of expressed emotion). Various unusual personality profiles have been noted in family members (Kolvin, 1971; Singer and Wynne, 1963), and it clearly is the case that family members are at greater risk for the disorder themselves (Kolvin, 1971). Unfortunately, most theoretical models have not been empirically tested, and the significance of reports of unusual patterns of familial interaction is unclear. In addition to the obvious possibility that unusual patterns of interaction cause schizophrenia in children, it is also quite possible that these abnormalities are reactions to the child's disorder or, alternatively, that they reflect the same underlying vulnerability exhibited more directly by the affected child. At the present time the role of family dynamics in syndrome pathogenesis remains to be established.

Environmental and Social Influences

There is evidence that stressful life events may play a role in precipitating psychotic episodes in children (Birley and Brown, 1970); study of cases in which the onset of the disorder follows a clear environmental precipitant are of some interest since they may clarify how psychological processes interact with biological predispositions for the disorder. Available data suggest that schizophrenic children are more likely to come from lower socioeconomic status families. It is not clear to what extent socioeconomic status (SES) suggests a role for the environment in pathogenesis since lower SES might also be the result of parental psychopathology with a resultant downward drift in occupational status. Also, with adults, exposure to certain pharmacological agents (e.g., stimulants) may produce hallucinations and a schizophrenic-like psychosis.

LABORATORY STUDIES

Biological Studies

To date, no single biological marker for schizophrenia in childhood has been found. Because overt psychosis can be observed in association with organic mental disorders, it is important to conduct a careful medical history and examination, particularly if there are unusual or atypical features. If substance abuse, particularly of stimulants or phencyclidine, is suggested by history or physical signs, appropriate toxicological screening should be obtained. Given the infrequency of the condition, a complete neurological examination including an EEG is indicated.

Psychological Studies

Schizophrenic disorders in childhood are not typically associated with mental retardation, although various developmental and learning problems may be associated with the disorder. Psychological testing is helpful both in documenting current levels of intellectual and adaptive functioning and in pointing out areas of specific strength or weakness important for educational programming (see Chapter 44). In addition to information provided by formal intellectual assessment, projective tests should be administered and may provide important information about the severity of the thought disorder and psychotic thinking, supplementing information obtained from other sources. Several assessment instruments have been developed explicitly for the assessment of psychosis or thought disorder in childhood (Caplan, 1994; Caplan et al., 1989; Puig-Antich and Chambers, 1983). Communication assessments should be obtained, particularly in cases where communication problems are prominent.

DIFFERENTIAL DIAGNOSIS

The diagnosis of schizophrenia in childhood is probably most readily made in older children and adolescents. For children less than 10 years of age or for children with developmental disabilities, difficulties in communication, changes in conceptions of reality, and the nature of symptom expression may complicate the diagnostic picture. The diagnosis should be made only after careful evaluation and only after it is clear that the symptoms do not reflect the presence of an organic process (e.g., the effects of substance abuse, or seizure disorder). Generally multiple informants must be interviewed to obtain an adequate history, and usually several sessions with the child will be required to obtain an adequate mental status examination. The differentiation of schizophrenia from affective disorders can be difficult since, to some degree, mood disturbance can be observed in schizophrenia. Prominent mood disturbance that is prolonged and that is not brief relative to the total duration

Table 58.4. Evaluation Procedures: Childhood Schizophrenia

1. Historical information
    Early development and characteristics of development
    Age and nature of onset
    Medical and family history
2. Psychological/communicative examination
    Assessment of intellectual level (IQ)
    Assessment of adaptive behavior
    Projective testing
    Assessment of communication skills (particularly if communication problems are evident)
3. Psychiatric examination
    Evaluate thought disturbance, hallucinations, delusions, etc.
    Evaluate associated affective problems
    Note unusual features of course/presentation
4. Medical evaluation
    Physical examination for signs of associated medical conditions
    Evaluate for possible substance abuse
    Neurological consultation (including EEG)
    Toxicology screen if indicated

of the apparent schizophrenic illness suggests the need to consider the various affective disorders and schizoaffective disorder in the differential diagnosis (American Psychiatric Association, 1994). Occasionally patients with an obsessive compulsive disorder may exhibit ideas that are difficult to distinguish from delusions, although usually the individual recognizes the irrational nature of such ideas. Hallucinations are occasionally reported as an isolated symptom: A diagnosis of childhood schizophrenia should not be made in such cases. Sometimes only the subsequent course will clarify the diagnosis. Assessment procedures are summarized in Table 58.4.

Schizophrenia can be observed in association with various other psychiatric and developmental problems, for example, conduct disorder, learning disabilities, mental retardation, and even autism; comorbid conditions should be noted when present (Russel et al., 1989). Adherence to a multiaxial approach aids in this process. In individuals with mental retardation, autism, or developmental language disorders, a diagnosis of schizophrenia should be made only if it is clear that the apparent disturbance in thinking does not reflect communication impairments. While the bulk of available evidence has suggested that childhood schizophrenia and autism are unrelated, a few investigators have speculated on possible continuities between autism and schizophrenia, and DSM-III-R and DSM-IV, in contrast to DSM-III, did allow both diagnoses to be made (American Psychiatric Association, 1987, 1994). The change in DSM-III-R reflects an awareness that presumably autism does not protect an individual from also developing schizophrenia; however, individuals with both conditions do not seem to be common (Volkmar et al., 1988). The diagnosis of pervasive developmental disorder not otherwise specified (PDD-NOS) should not be made concurrently with a diagnosis of schizophrenia.

TREATMENT

As with other aspects of the disorder, studies of treatment are few in number and limited in various respects. Apparent variations in the natural history of the disorder (Eggers, 1978) pose further problems for assessing treatment studies. Practice parameters for assessment and treatment have recently been published (McCellan and Werry, 1994). To a considerable extent, treatment programs should attempt to address the specific patterns of strength and weakness exhibited by the individual child; treatment modalities will also depend on the stage of illness (i.e., the presence of active psychotic symptomatology). Typically, multiple treatment modalities will be needed, including medications, educational and family interventions, and supportive psychotherapy; depending on the clinical situation, inpatient treatment may be indicated.

The few available reports suggest that major tranquilizers have a role in treatment and may diminish the positive symptoms of the disorder (e.g., hallucinations and delusions) (Kydd and Werry, 1982). However, concerns about the possible long-term side effects of these medications suggest the need for informed consent, careful monitoring, and periodic reevaluation (McClellan and Werry, 1994). In general no specific major tranquilizer is clearly superior, and the choice of medication should be guided by the particular constellation of problems exhibited. Particularly for children and adolescents whose disturbance does not respond to more usual agents, the "atypical" antipsychotic clozapine may be considered; although considerable interest has centered on this agent in adult "nonresponders," data in children are more limited (Frazier et al., 1994; Jacobsen et al., 1994; McCellan and Werry, 1994). Evidence regarding the use of other classes of medications is even more limited; given the potential for stimulant medications to induce a psychotic illness, their use is probably contraindicated.

Studies of psychotherapy with this population are difficult to interpret given changes in diagnostic practice. It does appear that supportive psychotherapy may be of benefit to some children (Cantor and Kestenbaum, 1986). The usefulness of intensive, insight-oriented therapy is much less clear. Family interventions should aim to increase levels of appropriate family involvement and interaction to support the child's development and enhance communication among family members. Behavior modification procedures may be useful in reducing levels of maladaptive behaviors and increasing the availability of the child for educational and other interventions.

Many schizophrenic children exhibit associated problems in development and learning, which must be addressed through the provision of a comprehensive educational program. The disorder can have a deleterious impact on the acquisition of basic developmental and adaptive skills. Special education should be provided to address associated learning and developmental problems. It is important that the treatment program provided be integrated and that all the various professionals involved be aware of the need for close communication and the provision of a consistent program.

OUTCOME AND FOLLOW-UP DATA

As with other aspects of the disorder, only limited data are available regarding the course and outcome of childhood schizophrenia, if the disorder is strictly defined. Bennett and Klein (1966) reported a follow-up of Potter's (1933) series of rather well-documented schizophrenic children. In these cases the outcome of a 30-year follow-up was quite poor; only one case had made a satisfactory readjustment, although the histories of prolonged treatment in institutional settings may have worsened ultimate outcome.

Eggers (1978) conducted a 20-year follow-up of 57 children who exhibited schizophrenia before age 14. Unfortunately the study is somewhat limited since the accuracy of early diagnosis and clinical information is questionable in these cases. About 20% of cases had apparently experienced complete remission, about 30% had improved, and the remaining 50% had had moderate or poor outcomes. The worst prognostic feature was an early onset (before age 10) in children with premorbid personality difficulties; all such cases had a poor outcome at follow-up. Kydd and Werry (1982) reported a follow-up of 15 children originally diagnosed as schizophrenic between 1971 and 1981. At follow-up all cases were rediagnosed using DSM-III. Of the 15 cases, 11 appeared unequivocally to exhibit schizophrenia, with the remaining four cases exhibiting a schizophreniform disorder. Earlier onset was associated with poorer prognosis, with about half of the more strictly diagnosed schizophrenic cases exhibiting chronic difficulties. As with adults, the use of psychotropic medications appears to be of particular benefit in relation to the "positive" symptoms of the disorder, although the dearth of studies in this area makes this observation only tentative at best. McKenna and colleagues (McKenna et al., 1994) reviewed 71 cases of children and adolescents referred for evaluation of what was presumed to be schizophrenia; only 19 children appeared to meet stringent criteria for the condition. As with adult schizophrenia, "negative" symptoms in

childhood schizophrenia appear to be less responsive to pharmacological intervention. There is some suggestion that the presence of more affective symptoms or a more schizoaffective clinical picture is associated with a more favorable course (Eggers, 1989). In general it would appear that better outcome is related to acute onset, older age at onset, better premorbid adjustment, and well-differentiated symptomatology.

RESEARCH DIRECTIONS

Research on essentially all aspects of the disorder is critically needed. Given the apparent wealth of information on childhood schizophrenia, as broadly defined during the 1950s and 1960s, it is somewhat paradoxical that the available information on this disorder is nevertheless clearly less than that regarding autism. The relationship of childhood schizophrenia to adult forms of the illness remains an important topic for research; although important points of phenomenological similarity are apparent, the relative infrequency of the condition in childhood and the apparent relationship of subsequent outcome to early onset suggest areas of possible difference as well. The study of childhood schizophrenia would appear to be of considerable interest in the extent to which it may clarify aspects of syndrome etiology and pathogenesis. Studies of clinical populations are important for illuminating aspects of the disorder's natural history, neurobiology, treatment, and diagnosis. The applicability of current criteria for schizophrenia to children remains controversial; younger children may not as readily fulfill adult diagnostic criteria for the disorder, when rigidly applied. Misdiagnosis of the condition remains common (e.g., McKenna et al., 1994). The development of more precise and developmentally appropriate diagnostic criteria should facilitate research. Limited efforts to subtype affected individuals have been made (Cantor, 1988); the reliability and utility of such schemes remain to be established. Apart from some studies of information processing using event-related potentials, neurobiological studies have been few in number; explication of underlying biological substrates of the disorder remains an extremely important area for future research (Caplan, 1994; Werry, 1994). Carefully designed follow-up studies are needed to identify those factors most strongly related to ultimate outcome.

CASE ILLUSTRATION

Kristine was the second of two children born to upper-middle-class parents after a term pregnancy complicated by maternal viral illness and a prolonged labor. At birth she was noted to be in good condition. She was a somewhat fussy baby whose motor and communicative development appeared to proceed appropriately. She appeared to be normally related and enjoyed social interaction with her parents and older sister. She was enrolled in a nursery school program at age 4 and subsequently in regular kindergarten and 1st grade classes; although she was noted to be somewhat shy, no other concerns were expressed about her cognitive or emotional development. At age 6 years 11 months she exhibited an episode of acute hallucinations and delusions. This episode had been preceded by a period of several weeks during which she had seemed increasingly withdrawn and was observed talking to herself. The hallucinations were predominately auditory in nature, but were not well described, and apparently consisted of hearing single words; delusions revolved around fears of being kidnapped. Kristine became markedly anxious and developed complex rituals and compulsive behaviors apparently involving some aspect of her delusional fears. She was hospitalized, but extensive medical investigation failed to reveal a specific medical explanation for her difficulties. A positive family history of schizophrenia in a maternal aunt was noted, and a presumptive diagnosis of schizophrenia was made. Low doses of neuroleptics led to partial remission of the hallucinations and delusions, although she remained quite withdrawn. After her hospitalization she began twice weekly psychotherapy and was transferred to a private school where she received extensive special education.

She was seen for comprehensive reevaluation at age 10. At that time psychological testing revealed a full-scale IQ in the borderline retarded range with associated deficits in adaptive behavior. Projective testing revealed marked thought problems. Communication assessment revealed significant difficulties in communication, with marked difficulties in social interaction, use of irrelevant language, and neologisms. On psychiatric examination Kristine was an attractive girl with a generally bland affect. Her initial comment on meeting the examiner was to say "love you." Associations were loose, with marked tangential thinking and irrelevant associations. She denied auditory hallucinations but did admit to seeing "monsters" on occasions; a relatively elaborate delusional system was present. Some obsessional thinking was also in evidence, as were a few peculiar mannerisms.

In adolescence Kristine continued to have marked difficulties. Although she received a comprehensive educational intervention program, deficits in academic performance and cognitive skills increased in severity. In late adolescence the onset of marked behavior problems led to another hospitalization and subsequent placement in a residential institution.

Comment

The case illustrates various points at which childhood schizophrenia differs from autism: The onset in this case was after some years of apparently normal development, the disorder was characterized by prominent delusions and hallucinations, and there was a family history of schizophrenia. Children with an onset of schizophrenia in childhood have a less favorable prognosis than those with onset in adolescence.

References

American Psychiatric Association: *Diagnostic and Statistical Manual of Mental Disorders* (3rd ed, rev). Washington, DC, American Psychiatric Press, 1987.

American Psychiatric Association: *Diagnostic and Statistical Manual of Mental Disorders* (4th ed). Washington, DC, American Psychiatric Press, 1994.

Arboleda C, Holzman PS: Thought disorder in children at risk for psychosis. *Arch Gen Psychiatry* 42:1004–1013, 1985.

Asarnow R, Sherman T, Strandburg T: The search for the psychobiological substrate of childhood onset schizophrenia. *J Am Acad Child Adolesc Psychiatry* 25:601–604, 1986.

Bender L: Childhood schizophrenia. *Am J Orthopsychiatry* 17:40–56, 1947.

Bennett S, Klein HR: Childhood schizophrenia: 30 years later. *Am J Psychiatry* 122:1121–1124, 1966.

Birley JL, Brown GW: Crisis and life changes preceding the onset or relapse of acute schizophrenia: Clinical aspects. *Br J Psychiatry* 116:327–333, 1970.

Burd L, Kerbeshian I: A North Dakota prevalence study of schizophrenia presenting in childhood. *J Am Acad Child Adolesc Psychiatry* 26:347–350, 1987.

Cantor S: *Childhood Schizophrenia*. New York, Guilford, 1988.

Cantor S, Kestenbaum C: Psychotherapy with schizophrenic children. *J Am Acad Child Adolesc Psychiatry* 25:623–630, 1986.

Cantor S, Evans I, Pezzot-Pearce T: Childhood schizophrenia: Present but not accounted for. *Am J Psychiatry* 139:758–762, 1982.

Caplan R: Thought disorder in childhood. *J Am Acad Child Adolesc Psychiatry* 33:605–615, 1994.

Caplan R, Guthrie D, Fish B, et al: The Kiddie formal thought disorder rating scale: Clinical assessment, reliability, and validity. *J Am Acad Child Adolesc Psychiatry* 28:408–416, 1989.

Cooper HE, Kendell RE, Gurland BJ, et al: *Psychiatric Diagnosis in New York and London* (Institute of Psychiatry, Maudsley Monograph no. 20). London, Oxford University Press, 1972.

Creak M: Schizophrenic syndrome in childhood: Further progress of a working party. *Dev Med Child Neurol* 6:530–535, 1963.

De Sanctis S: Sopra alcune varieta della demenzi precoce. *Revista Sperimentale De Feniatria E. Di Medicina Legale* 32:141–165, 1906.

Eggers C: Course and prognosis of childhood schizophrenia. *J Autism Child Schizophr* 8:21–36, 1978.

Eggers C: Schizo-affective psychosis in childhood: A follow-up study. *J Autism Dev Disord* 19:327–342, 1989.

Fish B: Antecedents of an acute schizophrenic break. *J Am Acad Child Adolesc Psychiatry* 25:595–600, 1986.

Frazier JA, Gordon CT, McKenna K, et al: An open trial of clozapine in 11 adolescents with childhood-onset schizophrenia. *J Am Acad Child Adolesc Psychiatry* 33:658–663, 1994.

Goldstein MJ: The course of schizophrenic psychosis. In: Brim O, Kagan I (eds): *Constancy and Change in Human Development*. Cambridge, MA, Harvard University Press, 1980, pp. 325–358.

Green WH, Campbell M, Hardesty AS, et al: A comparison of schizophrenic and autistic children. *J Am Acad Child Psychiatry* 23:399–409, 1984.

Jacobsen LK, Walker MC, Edward JE, et al: Clozapine in the treatment of a young adolescent with schizophrenia. *J Am Acad Child Adolesc Psychiatry* 33:645–650, 1994.

Kallman FJ, Prugh DG: Genetic aspects of preadolescent schizophrenia. *Am J Psychiatry* 112:599–606, 1971.

Kanner L: Autistic disturbances of affective contact. *Nerv Child* 2:217–250, 1943.

Kolvin I: Studies in childhood psychoses. I: Diagnostic criteria and classification. *Br J Psychiatry* 118:381–384, 1971.

Kraeplin E: *Dementia Praecox and Paraphrenia* (Barclay RM, trans). Edinburgh, Livingston, 1919.

Kydd RR, Werry IS: Schizophrenia in children under 16 years. *J Autism Dev Disord* 12:343–357, 1982.

McKenna KM, Gordon CT, Lenane M, et al: Looking for childhood-onset schizophrenia: The first 71 cases screened. *J Am Acad Child Adolesc Psychiatry* 33:636–644, 1994.

McClellan J, Werry J: Practice parameters for the assessment and treatment of children and adolescents with schizophrenia. *J Am Acad Child Adolesc Psychiatry* 33:616–635, 1994.

Piaget J: *The Construction of Reality in the Child* (Cook M, trans). New York, Basic Books, 1954.

Potter HW: Schizophrenia in children. *Am J Psychiatry* 89:1253–1270, 1933.

Puig-Antich J, Chambers W: *The Schedule for Affective Disorders and Schizophrenia for School-age Children (Kiddie-SADS)*. New York, New York State Psychiatric Institute, 1983.

Russel AT, Bott L, Sammons C: The phenomenology of schizophrenia occurring in childhood. *J Am Acad Child Adolesc Psychiatry* 28:399–407, 1989.

Rutter M: Childhood schizophrenia reconsidered. *J Autism Child Schizophr* 2:315–338, 1972.

Singer MT, Wynne LC: Differentiating characteristics of parents of childhood schizophrenics, childhood neurotics, and young adult schizophrenics. *Am J Psychiatry* 120:234–243, 1963.

Strandburg RJ, Marsh JT, Brown WS, et al: Event-related potential concomitants of information processing dysfunction in schizophrenic children. *Electroencephalogr Clin Neurophysiol* 57:236–253, 1984.

Volkmar FR, Cohen DJ: Co-morbid association of autism and schizophrenia. *Am J Psychiatry* 148:1705–1707, 1991.

Volkmar FR, Cohen DJ, Hoshino Y, et al: Phenomenology and classification of the childhood psychoses. *Psychol Med* 18:191–201, 1988.

Waldo M, Cohen DJ, Caparulo BK, et al: EEG profiles of neuropsychiatrically disturbed children. *J Am Acad Child Psychiatry* 17:656–670, 1978.

Werry J: Childhood schizophrenia. In: Volkmar F (ed): *Psychoses and Pervasive Developmental Disorders in Childhood and Adolescence*. Washington, DC, American Psychiatric Press, 1996.

World Health Organization: *International Classification of Diseases* (10th rev). Geneva, World Health Organization, 1990.

59 NEUROLOGICAL DISORDERS

Daniel T. Williams, M.D., Richard R. Pleak, M.D., and Helen Hanesian, Ed.D.

Child psychiatrists and neurologists can benefit from a shared neuropsychiatric perspective that connotes sufficient familiarity with each other's field so as to enable each to optimally meet their patients' needs and to foster appropriate interdisciplinary communication.

A major requirement for the psychiatrist is to be sensitive and responsive to indications of neurogenic substrates that may underlie what may at first appear to be purely psychological or psychopathological phenomena. The psychiatrist should also be prepared to diagnose and formulate treatment plans for psychiatric complications of primary neurological disorders. (For information on neuropsychiatric signs, symptoms, and syndromes, see Chapter 28, and for information on acquired brain disorders, see Chapter 30.)

This chapter deals with psychiatric aspects of the following representative neurological disorders: epilepsy, cerebral palsy, brain tumors, and neurodegenerative and neuromuscular disorders. It is hoped that the perspective developed herein will be of value to the contemporary child and adolescent psychiatrist, who, in the face of accumulating clinical and research data, is called upon to marshal greater sophistication regarding diagnostic and therapeutic challenges at the neuropsychiatric interface.

EPILEPSY

Epilepsy is a condition characterized by sudden, recurrent, and transient disturbances of mental functions or body movements that result from excessive discharging of groups of brain cells (Forster and Booker, 1988). As such, epilepsy does not refer to a specific disease but rather to a group of symptoms that have many different causes in different individuals. In some individuals the underlying causes are static, and in some they are progressive. All of the underlying causes of epilepsy have in common the quality of causing cerebral neurons to become excessively excited. The statistically more common causes of this neuronal hyperexcitability generally involve either structural abnormality of the brain or biochemical aberrations of a metabolic, infectious, or other physical etiology. This broad spectrum of etiologies clearly includes both genetically based and acquired varieties of brain pathology, as well as potential combinations of these.

Reviews of the literature on the psychogenic precipitants of epileptic seizures (Williams, 1982; Williams et al., 1987, 1993) clarify that numerous studies in both experimental animals and patients have substantiated the capacity of emotional stress to precipitate epileptic seizures in neurologically vulnerable individuals. Hence there is an important role for the psychiatrist not only in helping patients and their families to cope with the troubling psychiatric consequences of epilepsy but also in potentially intervening in some cases with regard to influencing the pathogenesis of seizures.

The signs and symptoms of epilepsy are manifold. Among the most common manifestations are episodes of partial or complete loss of consciousness, localized or generalized muscular spasms or jerks, or apparently purposeful behavior performed while awareness is depressed. The multifaceted modes of clinical manifestation of epilepsy and the fact that EEG recordings are not always diagnostic lead to another major diagnostic and therapeutic challenge at the neuropsychiatric interface: recognizing and treating psychogenic nonepileptic seizures.

Epidemiology

Estimates based on epidemiologic studies indicate that up to 1% of the population in the United States has epilepsy and that new cases appear at an annual rate of 40 per 100,000 (Hauser et al., 1983). Furthermore, the rate is highest in children younger than 5, with another peak of incidence at the age of puberty. Thus, it is clear that children and adolescents merit special consideration with regard to developmental issues that interact with the psychiatric complications of epilepsy.

There is evidence that socioeconomic factors play an important role in the development of epilepsy. For example, the incidence was found to be higher in black children (1.96%) than in white children (0.95%) living in New Haven, Connecticut (Hauser et al., 1983). Yet the cause of this difference is uncertain; the relative importance of perinatal factors, trauma, nutrition, other environmental influences, or genetics is unknown.

The relative role of inheritance in epilepsy is controversial. It is often difficult to distinguish social and economic factors from primary genetic predisposition, since poor nutrition and inadequate perinatal care frequently run in families. However, several studies indicate that, in patients with generalized epilepsy, close relatives have a 2- to 4-fold increase in incidence of convulsive disorders, strongly suggesting a genetic component of vulnerability.

Classification of Epileptic Seizures

A revised International Classification of Seizures based on a more contemporary understanding of seizure pathophysiology, which has served to improve professional communication, is summarized as follows (Forster and Booker, 1988):

I. Partial seizures (seizures beginning locally)
  A. Simple partial seizures (consciousness not impaired)
    1. With motor symptoms
    2. With somatosensory or special sensory symptoms
    3. With autonomic symptoms
    4. Compound forms
  B. Complex partial seizures (with impairment of consciousness; temporal lobe or psychomotor seizures)
    1. With impairment of consciousness only
    2. With cognitive symptomatology
    3. With affective symptomatology
    4. With "psychosensory" symptomatology
    5. With "psychomotor" symptomatology (automatisms)
    6. Compound forms
  C. Partial seizures secondarily generalized
II. Generalized seizures (bilaterally symmetric and without local onset)
  A. Absence seizures
  B. Myoclonic seizures
  C. Infantile spasms
  D. Clonic seizures
  E. Tonic seizures
  F. Tonic-clonic seizures
  G. Atonic seizures
  H. Akinetic seizures
III. Unilateral seizures
IV. Unclassified epileptic seizures (due to incomplete data)

Space limitations preclude more detailed consideration of these clinical subtypes here, but it clearly behooves the psychiatrist working with a seizure patient to be cognizant of the specific seizure manifestations, associated clinical and prognostic features, and specific medication requirements as determined by the patient's specific seizure type.

Psychological and Psychiatric Assessment

COGNITIVE FUNCTIONING

A review of several studies in this area (Stores, 1981) indicates that, although many children with epilepsy function normally at school, proportionately more of them have learning problems as compared with nonepileptic children. In the Isle of Wight study, for example, which concentrated on 9- to 11-year-old children, over twice as many of those with epilepsy showed serious specific reading retardation when compared with nonepileptic children.

Developmental considerations are important. O'Leary et al. (1981) administered a neuropsychological test battery to 48 children age 9–12 with tonic-clonic seizures. The children with seizures of early onset (before age 5) were significantly impaired compared with the children with seizures of later onset on 8 of the 14 measures in the battery. The deficits were seen on tasks whose requirements included attention and concentration, memory, complex problem solving, and motor coordination.

Seizure type, duration, and degree of seizure control are also pertinent. Farwell et al. (1985) did detailed neuropsychological testing of 118 epileptic children, age 6–15, and a control group of 100 children without seizures. The Wechsler full-scale IQ of seizure patients was significantly lower than that of control subjects and was related to seizure type. Children with minor motor or atypical absence seizures had the lowest average full-scale I.Q. All seizure types except classic absence alone were associated with below-control intelligence. Intelligence was also correlated with degree of seizure control. A highly significant inverse correlation between years with seizures and intelligence was found. Finally, children with seizures had been placed in special education or had repeated a grade in school almost twice as frequently as control subjects, and their academic achievement was behind grade placement more often than that in the control group.

Essential features of the above study were supported by Seidenberg et al. (1986), who examined the academic achievement scores of 122 children with epilepsy. As a group, these children were making less progress than expected for their age and IQ level. Academic deficiencies were greatest in arithmetic, followed by spelling, reading comprehension, and word recognition. Here also, clinically relevant variables included age of seizure onset, lifetime total seizure frequency, and the presence of multiple seizures.

Lest one fall prey, however, to the erroneous assumption that childhood epilepsy necessarily engenders intellectual deterioration, the study by Ellenberg et al. (1986) is illuminating. They compared the full-scale IQs at 7 years of age of children who had experienced one or more nonfebrile seizures with the IQs of their seizure-free siblings who were tested at the same age in a large longitudinal study. Among 98 children with seizures, the mean score on IQ tests at 7 years was not significantly different from the mean score of their siblings. Mental retardation was more common among the children with seizures, but the excess was accounted for by children who had had neurological abnormalities before the first seizure. It seems likely that sampling difference account for the differences in findings between this and previously cited studies, with the study by Ellenberg et al. drawing a larger proportion of "mild" cases (i.e., better controlled) than the previous studies.

Anticonvulsant drugs, especially in combination, have been shown in recent years to interfere in significant ways with cognitive function, including attention, concentration, memory, motor and mental speed, and mental processing (Reynolds, 1985). These sometimes subtle effects are easily overlooked but may accrue to the point of substantial impairment, particularly for children in learning situations.

Recent studies have shown that most epileptic patients can be controlled on single-drug therapy and that there is little difference in antiepileptic efficacy between the major antiepileptic drugs within designated seizure categories (Corbet et al., 1985; Trimble, 1987; Voorhies, 1988). Consequently, the relative influence of each drug on cognitive function may prove to be a most important factor in the choice of an anticonvulsant drug. In this regard, it should be noted that several studies have shown significant associations between long-term use of phenytoin and phenobarbital and cognitive deterioration in children. By contrast, carbamazepine has been noted in some studies to be less prone to contribute to cognitive impairments in both short- and long-term use in both normal volunteers and seizure patients. This finding needs to be qualified, however. Forsythe et al. (1991) found, in a controlled, prospective study of newly diagnosed childhood epilepsy, that carbamazepine in moderate dosage adversely affected memory, but phenytoin and sodium valproate did not. Valproate had the fewest side effects. Clearly, further studies are indicated.

Despite the above observations, one should not assume that all cognitive impairment of youngsters with epilepsy is due to either static cerebral pathology or the side effects of anticonvulsant medication. Siebelink et al. (1988) studied 21 children with epilepsy having subclinical epileptiform EEG discharges in the waking state, using telemetered EEG studies during psychological testing. The authors found a total IQ below that of control populations, which was accounted for by that subgroup of children who exhibited discharges during the test; those who did not show discharges at that time were unimpaired. These findings need to be replicated and amplified but have implications both for the interpretation of neuropsychological studies in persons with epilepsy and also for the drug treatment of those who continue to exhibit subclinical EEG discharges when overt seizures have been controlled.

From the above, it can readily be discerned that primary attention should be given to periodic formal monitoring of the cognitive functioning of seizure patients, with particular view to picking up signs of progressive cognitive impairment that might otherwise be overlooked. It is certainly within the purview of a psychiatrist treating such a patient to ascertain that such monitoring has occurred, to ascertain that therapeutic serum anticonvulsant levels have been documented, and to discuss with the treating neurologist the possible need for a change in anticonvulsant regimen when indicated by the patient's level of cognitive functioning (Alvarez, 1989).

BEHAVIOR AND PERSONALITY

The literature on personality changes in epilepsy has been prolific, long-standing, and controversial. According to some estimates, for example, 30–40% of patients with temporal lobe epilepsy (complex partial seizures) experience persistent psychiatric symptoms that, more frequently than uncontrolled seizures, become the most incapacitating aspect of the illness (Baer et al., 1984). Multiple clinical reports in adult temporal lobe seizure patients have delineated characteristic features, including deepened emotions, changes in sexual function, aggressivity, development of intense religious or philosophic interests, circumstantiality, and interpersonal viscosity (Baer et al., 1985). One fascinating neuropsychiatric correlate in this regard was the finding in adults of a different constellation of personality features in right versus left temporal lobe seizure patients (Baer and Fedio, 1977).

A study of this issue in children with unilateral temporal lobe seizure foci failed to disclose characteristic differences in cognitive or personality features between right and left temporal lobe seizure patients (Camfield et al., 1984). Yet when the two groups of unilateral seizure patients were combined, 10 of 27 patients (5 with left focus, 5 with right focus) were seen to have personality maladjustment on formal assessment. Furthermore, the group as a whole showed significantly lower neuropsychological test functioning than normally adjusted children.

In support of the contention that increased levels of temporal lobe discharge may have relevance to personality characteristics, the study of Persinger (1987) is of interest. Comparisons were made between personality profiles (MMPI) of 26 university students who scored in the upper and 29 students who scored in the lower one-quarter of the range on a scale that measures temporal lobe signs in the normal population. Compared to the reference group, the subjects who displayed more temporal lobe signs showed significant elevations on the MMPI scales for schizophrenia and hypomania. In addition, in a related study, positive correlations occurred between temporal lobe EEG measures and numbers of temporal lobe signs (Makarec and Persinger, 1987).

Developmental considerations may help understand the evolution of certain psychopathological correlates of the seizure state over time. Thus Flor-Henry (1983) has studied severe psychopathological syndromes (psychosis) seen in adult seizure patients. He found that schizophreniform psychosis in these patients was related to pathology in the dominant hemisphere, whereas depressive psychosis (and neurosis) was related to pathology of the nondominant hemisphere. In relation to this, Lindsay et al. (1979) did a long-term outcome study of 100 children with temporal lobe seizures. In childhood, mental deficiency, the hyperkinetic syndrome, and cataclysmic rage outbursts were prominent. Indeed, only 15 of the 100 probands were wholly free from psychological problems in childhood. Yet follow-up indicated that the occurrence of overt psychiatric disorder in adult life was relatively low: Of those survivors who were not gravely mentally retarded, 70% were regarded as psychiatrically healthy. Overt schizophreniform psychoses developed in 10% of the survivors. Males with continuing epilepsy and left-sided foci were at special risk: 30% of such patients became psychotic. In consonance with the above-noted findings of Flor-Henry and others, no patient coded as having a right-sided focus in childhood became psychotic by the time of follow-up 13 years later. Lindsay et al. emphasize the surprising and hopeful change from the overwhelming presence of psychopathology in the childhood sample to the predominance of relative psychological intactness by adulthood. They note that the majority of their patients received psychiatric intervention in their early years and emphasize the importance of providing such service in the appropriate management of epileptic children.

Further indications of the probably primary role of CNS dysfunction in the psychiatric vulnerabilities of patients with epilepsy are reflected in a study by Hoare (1984b). Two groups of epileptic children, one newly diagnosed and one with chronic epilepsy, were contrasted with two comparable groups of diabetic children and with a nonpatient sample in order to evaluate the development of psychiatric disorder. The results confirm previous findings that children with chronic epilepsy are significantly more disturbed than children with chronic physical illness not involving the CNS and than children in the general population. Children with newly diagnosed epilepsy were also significantly more disturbed than those with newly diagnosed diabetes, and than children in the general population. In both groups of epileptic children, those with focal EEG abnormalities and/or complex partial seizures were particularly vulnerable to psychiatric disturbance. The development of inappropriate dependency was also greater in the two epileptic groups of children than in the comparison groups (Hoare, 1984a).

In addition to the previously noted capacity of anticonvulsants to engender untoward cognitive side effects, these medications also can cause behavioral and emotional symptoms. The capacity of phenobarbital to generate or exacerbate attention deficit hyperactivity symptoms in children is well documented (Voorhies, 1988). Additionally, Brent et al. (1987), in a study comparing 15 epileptic children on phenobarbital to 24 treated with carbamazepine, found a much higher prevalence of major depressive disorder in those on phenobarbital (40 versus 4%, $P = .02$) and suicidal ideation (47 versus 4%, $P = .005$), as determined by semistructured psychiatric interviews. The differential prevalence of depression between medication groups was only noted in those with a family history of a major affective disorder among first-degree relatives.

It should be noted that not all studies of psychopathology among children and adolescents find an increased incidence in these youngsters as compared with control groups (Kaminer et al, 1988). Yet the preponderance of studies suggest that youngsters with epilepsy are at increased risk with regard to the development of psychiatric disturbance. Certainly not every youngster with epilepsy requires psychiatric attention, but a substantial proportion do stand to benefit therefrom. A psychiatrically sophisticated neurologist who routinely follows these youngsters and can make appropriate early referral for psychiatric assessment when needed is probably the best conduit for such intervention. Once this has been done, assessment should follow a standard age-appropriate format for the patient and family, with special focus on those areas of vulnerability that have been noted above. As noted below, these considerations may also apply at times to the issue of seizure control.

A recently developed resource in helping the clinician or researcher to objectively assess psychosocial problems in adolescents with epilepsy is the Adolescent Psychosocial Seizure Inventory (Batzel et al., 1991).

Psychogenically Precipitated Epileptic Seizures and Psychogenic Nonepileptic Seizures

Based on the substantial evidence pointing to the enhanced cognitive and emotional vulnerability of youngsters with epilepsy, it is not surprising that one manifestation of this vulnerability would be a worsening of their presenting seizure symptoms under circumstances of emotional stress. It is important, however, for the clinician to be thoughtful and sensitive in exploring this area because of the many complexities that abound in the areas of differential diagnosis and treatment.

Williams (1982) and Williams et al. (1987, 1993) reviewed several studies pointing to the role of environmental stress and emotional experiences as precipitants of true epileptic seizures. These included reports of the emotional activation of EEG abnormalities in patients with convulsive disorder, particularly those with sensory (simple partial) and complex partial seizures, when exposed to stress interviews. Furthermore, the direct emotional activation of seizures has been documented in several animal species when seizure-prone animals were exposed to various forms of environmental stress. These seizures are designated here as psychogenically precipitated epileptic seizures.

In contrast to the above, the term *psychogenic nonepileptic seizures* has been used to designate seizurelike phenomena of purely psychological origin that are produced by patients with varying degrees of conscious or unconscious intentionality and for a vast array of psychological motivations. While reviewed in detail elsewhere (Williams and Hirsh, 1988; Williams and Mostofsky, 1982; Williams et al., 1993), brief notation is made here of the general categories of diagnostic classification to be considered in the process of assessment. These include somatoform disorders, factitious disorders, and malingering.

It may sometimes be extremely difficult for the clinician (neurologist, psychiatrist, or other), even after a thorough review of the history, physical examination, and laboratory findings, to be certain about the distinction between epileptic seizures, whether psychogenically precipitated or not, and psychogenic nonepileptic seizures. This is not only because of the protean manifestations of epileptic phenomena but also because many patients frequently possess an artful capacity to mimic epileptic seizures on a conscious or unconscious basis.

Simultaneous videotape and EEG recording has been a significant aid in the differential diagnosis of epilepsy and pseudoseizures (Aminoff et al., 1988; Duchowney et al., 1988; Feldman et al., 1982). The procedure focuses one camera on the patient, who is wired with electrodes connected to an electroencephalograph, while a second camera is focused on the EEG write-out. The picture of the patient and the simultaneous EEG tracing appear on a split-screen video monitor. This combined recording is stored on the videotape for future analysis and interpretation. Studies using this technique have helped clarify that, even patients with clearly documented psychogenic nonepileptic seizures, there may be a coexisting neurogenic seizure disorder in from 10% (Lesser et al., 1983) to 37% (Krumholz and Niedermeyer, 1983) of patients.

One limiting factor with the differential diagnostic capacity of video-EEG monitoring, despite its allowing a much longer observational period than a routine EEG, is that the patient may not experience a typical seizure event during the monitoring period. To augment the diagnostic yield of this valuable monitoring technique, a variety of suggestive procedures, including intravenous placebo infusion and hypnosis have been used (Walczac et al., 1994). Placebo infusion elicits typical psychogenic events in most patients with psychogenic seizures. However, atypical events or epileptic seizures may occur in a minority of patients. This points to the need for an adequate monitoring period, corroboration with family or other observers that the elicited events are typical, and close collaboration between the evaluating neurologist and psychiatrist in conducting a comprehensive evaluation of both these overlapping areas.

Some brief guidelines may be outlined for psychiatric intervention in such situations. First, if the diagnosis is not entirely clear at the time of initial psychiatric consultation, as is most often the case in these circumstances, it is best to approach the patient and family with a candid acknowledgment of this. The role of the psychiatrist is explained as that of exploring the possibility that emotional factors may play a role in symptom formation, as they can with virtually any physical symptom (e.g., headache, peptic ulcer, hypertension, etc.). Second, a traditional psychiatric assessment of the patient and parents, separately and together, is then pursued, with particular focus on possible sources of stress or conflict that might contribute to symptom formation. It is best to conceive and discuss any psychodynamic or other formulation deriving from such an exploration in tentative, hypothetical terms, with due regard to the patient's self-esteem and especially avoiding any confrontational or accusatory stance with the patient or family. Third, if the combined outcome of neurological and psychiatric assessments points to the probability that emotional factors do contribute to symptom genesis, then a treatment plan tailored to the individual circumstances of the child and family needs to be formulated (Williams and Hirsch, 1988; Williams et al., 1993).

Epilepsy and Aggressive Behavior

There is controversy in the literature regarding the association between epilepsy on the one hand and aggression and violence on the other (Herzberg and Fenwick, 1988). One well-controlled study of 83 children with epilepsy found an association between the presence of anterior temporal lobe epileptiform spike activity and increased aggression scores on the Achenbach Child Behavior Checklist (Whitman et al., 1982). The authors note, however, that such biological variables predictive of behavioral disorder accounted for only small amounts of the variance in their comparison of children with temporal lobe and generalized epilepsies. In this regard, they recommend that more consideration be given to delineating the "situation-centered" variables predictive of behavioral disorder in children with epilepsy.

Using a different research strategy, clinical studies of violent incarcerated adolescents by Lewis and coworkers (Lewis, 1983; Lewis et al., 1982) have suggested that epilepsy, especially psychomotor (complex partial, temporal lobe) epilepsy, is more prevalent in young offenders than in the general population. Furthermore, psychomotor epilepsy in this population was particularly associated with violence. In a clinical study of 97 incarcerated boys, 11 had psychomotor seizures, and an additional 8 were thought most probably to have psychomotor seizures. Of the 11 boys with definite seizure disorders, all had been seriously assaultive, and 5 had committed acts of violence during seizures, as well as at other times. The authors review some of the diagnostic difficulties inherent in establishing the diagnosis of psychomotor seizures in an individual where such a clinical diagnosis may interact with the perception of legal responsibility for a violent act. Despite some of the imprecision inherent in diagnosing psychomotor seizures, however, added circumstantial support of the diagnosis was lent by the very frequent history of severe CNS trauma, due to such factors as perinatal difficulty, CNS infection, head injury, or a history of frank grand mal seizures. Of note also was the frequent association of reports of severe physical abuse in the histories of these youngsters. The latter association in particular certainly addresses the probable role of situational variables in fostering violence in youngsters biologically at risk by virtue of a greater predisposition to impulsivity and aggression. Most important, the authors emphasize that a clinician called on to evaluate a violent delinquent may render a valuable service in identifying potentially treatable neuropsychopathology so that appropriate intervention can occur (Lewis et al., 1985).

Treatment

In view of the generally acknowledged enhanced psychological vulnerability of epileptic patients, particularly to the effects of anxiety and depression (Betts, 1981), it is clearly advisable to provide appropriate intervention when such symptoms are in evidence. In this regard, the elevated risk of suicide in epileptic patients is noteworthy (Barraclough, 1981). Psychiatric interventions with such patients should be geared to the nature of the presenting symptomatology, while taking note of the relevance of the patient's epileptic condition. Consideration of psychopharmacologic agents requires attention to their potential impact of seizure threshold, as noted below.

PSYCHOTHERAPEUTIC INTERVENTION

A somewhat unique psychotherapeutic challenge in this population is that of treating psychogenically precipitated epileptic seizures and psychogenic nonepileptic seizures. There are many reports of successful psychotherapeutic or psychobiological treatment interventions for purposes of seizure control (Hanesian et al., 1988; Mostofsky and Balaschak, 1977; Williams et al., 1978, 1979, 1993). It should be emphasized that appropriate differential diagnostic assessment is a prerequisite to appropriate treatment planning in this area. The various treatment approaches utilized may be summarized under the following broad headings: conditioning techniques, psychodynamic approaches, relaxation and hypnosis, and biofeedback. Often several such approaches may be usefully integrated in the service of maximizing therapeutic impact to facilitate symptom relinquishment and foster improved adaptation by the patient.

It should be noted that, for patients with refractory epileptic seizures, seizure surgery, with recent improvements in technique and technology, has been offering some very promising results. Thus, Meyer et al. (1986) report that of 50 child and adolescent patients receiving temporal lobectomy for medically refractory seizures, 78% became essentially seizure-free, and 88% benefited significantly from the operation in terms of improved seizure control. The importance of careful and extended presurgical seizure monitoring cannot be overemphasized, however. Our own recent experience includes a patient who illustrates this point.

CASE ILLUSTRATION

R., a 9-year-old girl with an IQ of 117 and a history of gelastic (complex partial) seizures dating from the 1st year of life, was referred for seizure surgery because of a progressive worsening of her seizures despite numerous anticonvulsant medication trials. Seizure surgery was not performed, despite a diffusely abnormal EEG, because a circumscribed seizure focus accessible to surgical removal could not be delineated. While in the hospital, her histrionic and manipulative style was observed, as was the fact that her seizures were more numerous when her parents were present, reaching a peak of more than 300 a day. In light of no further deterioration in her previously abnormal EEG, a hypothesis of either psychogenically precipitated epileptic seizures or psychogenic nonepileptic seizures, or both, superimposed on a preexisting epileptic seizure substrate, was postulated by the consulting psychiatrist. After conferring with the neurologist, an intervention of intensive psychotherapy was initiated, including individual, parental, and family sessions, behavior modification, and hypnosis. With evidence of improvement in seizure control, anticonvulsant medication was gradually tapered. Within 2 weeks, seizure frequency had diminished to zero, and R. was discharged from the hospital. She immediately returned to school and continued to be seizure-free as she was followed over 6 months in supportive outpatient psychotherapy. Her anticonvulsant medication was gradually tapered and she continues seizure-free off all anticonvulsant medication for a 5-year period. In retrospect, the hypothesis of superimposed psychogenic seizures has been confirmed by the patient's clinical response to treatment.

PSYCHOPHARMACOLOGICAL CONSIDERATIONS

Special psychopharmacologic considerations are also noteworthy in this area. Already noted has been the need for the clinician to be aware of potentially cognition-impairing effects of various anticonvulsants, particularly phenytoin and phenobarbital. Additionally, the frequently observed capacity of phenobarbital to generate hyperactivity, irritability, and aggressivity in children should be borne in mind (American Academy of Pediatrics, 1985). Consequently, it is clearly important to advocate the lowest reasonable dose of the least toxic anticonvulsant consonant with good seizure control. Carbamazepine has been reported in a number of studies to manifest mood-stabilizing as well as anticonvulsant properties (Evans et al., 1987). It may thus be advisable in a patient being treated with another anticonvulsant who is experiencing disturbance of ongoing behavior to consider switching to carbamazepine if anticonvulsant efficacy is comparable. More recently, however, it has been recognized that negative psychiatric consequences of carbamazepine may also be encountered (Pleak et al., 1988). Therefore, careful clinical monitoring is in order.

Another developmentally important consideration in children and adolescents is their different rates of metabolizing anticonvulsants. Children generally require higher milligram per kilogram doses of anticonvulsant than do adults by virtue of their metabolizing the drugs more efficiently. In early adolescence there is a shift toward the adult rate. Consequently, an anticonvulsant dose that yielded therapeutic blood levels in late childhood may insidiously be transformed into a toxic dose in early adolescence, if not monitored closely. An associated consideration is the advisability of immediately checking a youngster's serum anticonvulsant level if there is any sudden change in cognitive, emotional, or behavioral functioning, or a worsening of seizure control. Questions of compliance in taking anticonvulsant medication should always be considered (Shope, 1988).

In many epileptic patients, even when the anticonvulsant regimen is optimized, there may still be indications for the additional use of psychotropic medication. Benzodiazepines have a valid place in this regard when minor tranquilization is needed. The value of intravenous diazepam in status epilepticus is well known, so there is clearly no danger of its lowering the seizure threshold, but the capacity to enhance sedation by interaction with a coexisting anticonvulsant should be noted (Stewart et al., 1990).

Although there is a theoretical basis of concern about stimulants lowering the seizure threshold based on animal studies involving high dosages, clinical experience suggests that methylphenidate may be a safe and effective treatment for certain children with seizures and concurrent attention-deficit disorder (Feldman et al., 1989).

Major tranquilizers do have a place in the treatment of interictal psychoses in patients with epilepsy (Trimble, 1985). It should be noted, however, that several neuroleptics, particularly chlorpromazine and clozapine, have a significant capacity to lower the seizure threshold and induce seizures. Of the neuroleptics currently available, molindone appears to be the safest in this regard, followed by haloperidol.

Most antidepressants also have the capacity to lower the seizure threshold and induce seizures (Luchins et al., 1984; Wroblewski et al., 1990). However, this is not necessarily a clinical concern with all patients with epilepsy, particularly if the antidepressant is introduced cautiously and the patient is on an effective anticonvulsant regimen. Clinically, one must balance the significance of depressive symptoms against the potential significance of a possibly lower seizure threshold.

In epileptic patients with uncontrolled aggressive outbursts that have not been controlled by optimal anticonvulsant medication adjustment, there is clinical evidence of the potential benefit of adding propranolol to their medication regimen (Koplewicz and Williams, 1988; Williams et al., 1982). Although this has not yet been subjected to controlled study, open clinical experience to date suggests that a significant proportion of such patients demonstrate improved behavioral control of aggressive behavior and irritability. As long as titration is gradual, with appropriate monitoring of ECG, pulse, and blood pressure and with cognizance of the relevant contraindications to using β-adrenergic blocking medication, side effects are minimal and well tolerated.

An important consideration in treating any child or adolescent with epilepsy and an associated psychiatric problem is the need to take into account family dynamics pertinent to the genesis of the problem, as well as family resources that can be mobilized in the service of effective treatment. This is particularly relevant in light of the frequently encountered problem of heightened dependency needs in such patients, noted above. Finally, the importance of maintaining open lines of communication between the neurologist and mental health practitioner to ensure appropriate psychobiological treatment integration cannot be overemphasized.

Prevention

Efforts at prevention of epilepsy itself are best addressed to the most common and remediable etiologies. These would include improved perinatal care, genetic counseling of individuals with family histories of epilepsy, and early intervention with those infectious, traumatic, or metabolic aberrations known to predispose to epilepsy. Efforts at prevention of the psychiatric complications of epilepsy include judicious use of anticonvulsant medications to minimize adverse side effects, as well as appropriate education of the patient and family to enable early recognition and appropriate early treatment of psychiatric complications should they arise. Finally, educating the public about epilepsy is important to minimize the unwarranted stereotypic stigmatization and discrimination that have long burdened these patients and their families.

CEREBRAL PALSY (STATIC ENCEPHALOPATHY)

The complexity of the problem of cerebral palsy leads to confusion regarding the meaning of the term, for it is comprised of medical, psychological, and social concerns. More than 100 years ago, Little (1882) studied approximately 200 cases of the disorder, and he attributed "spastic rigidity" to "abnormal parturition and asphyxia at birth." He described a number of concomitant traits observed, such as impaired intellect, problems of speech, convulsions, irritability, and impulsive nervous condition. The term *Little's disease* applied to cerebral palsy until the latter term became popular in the United States early in the 1940s. Currently, *cerebral palsy* is not a favored term among pediatric neurologists due to its lack of specificity; for purposes of clarity, pediatric neurologists prefer the general term *static encephalopathy*, followed by delineation of specific motor and other deficits. Nevertheless, *cerebral palsy* continues to appear in medical literature and is used widely by the general community.

A survey of the literature reveals a wide range of definitions for cerebral palsy, from a restricted focus on physical components to a more useful definition of cerebral palsy as a nonprogressive CNS motor deficit with associated handicaps. The motor deficit is one component of a broader brain damage syndrome that may include not only neuromotor dysfunction but also psychological dysfunction, convulsions, and behavioral disorders of organic origin (Scherzer and Tscharnuter, 1982).

Epidemiology

In an international review of population studies since 1950, data on the prevalence of cerebral palsy indicated an estimate of 2 per 1000 school-age children. Only 10% of these cases were estimated to be of postnatal origin (Paneth and Kiely, 1984). Earlier research had reported that perinatal insults were a predominant cause of cerebral palsy. For example, Cruickshank (1976) cited a 1951 survey which reported that factors related to birth injury and developmental problems of a postnatal nature comprised more than 50% of the 1105 cases. Other studies of that period also contended that perinatal insults were a predominant cause of cerebral palsy (Crothers and Paine, 1959). Investigations that followed, however, have allocated less importance to the factor of birth injury and have implicated prematurity, as well as prenatal factors, more prominently (Holm, 1982; O'Reilly, 1981). These findings are summarized by a report based on a review of 681 cases in Sweden, which concluded, ''The factors associated with the greatest risk of developing cerebral palsy are to be born too soon and too small'' (Hagberg and Hagberg, 1984). The relative risk of cerebral palsy for infants weighing 2000–2499 g is 9.2%, and for those weighing less, it is 26% (Golden, 1987). Children of birth weights less than 1251 g had a higher incidence of all major disabilities, including more severe, quadriplegic cerebral palsy (Marlow and D'Souza, 1987). This trend was also seen in a follow-up study conducted at the mean age of 8.3 years for 88 surviving children with birth weights of 500–999 g born in Victoria, Australia in 1979–1980. Severe disability in 18% of these children was related to cerebral palsy, bilateral blindness, and low IQ (Victorian Infant Collaborative Study Group, 1991).

Etiology

The underlying static encephalopathy of cerebral palsy has many possible causes that should be considered in a differential diagnosis. Denhoff (1976) proposed an etiologic classification based on time of onset and cause of the cerebral malformation or injury:

1. *Prenatal:* Heredity, chromosomal abnormality, and congenital (acquired in utero); maternal illnesses or disorders affecting the fetus;
2. *Perinatal:* Asphyxia, trauma, consequences of ''small for date'' babies, isoimmunization hemolytic disorders, obstetrical complications;
3. *Postnatal/early infancy:* Trauma, infections, toxins, nutritional and metabolic factors.

Cerebral palsy may have its origin exclusively in any one of the periods listed above or may be secondary to a combination of factors occurring in more than one period.

Clinical Features and Classification

Classification of cerebral palsy is difficult because there is no single cause of the disorder, nor a characteristic course. More important, the description of the motor disability may not give any insight into associated cognitive and emotional dysfunction.

The basic classification of clinical motor dysfunction in cerebral palsy adopted by the American Academy of Cerebral Palsy includes the following (Minear, 1956):

1. *Spasticity:* Characterized by stiffness of the musculature and slow movement. There is a tendency toward greater involvement and contractures affecting antigravity muscles.
2. *Athetosis:* Characterized by an abnormal amount and type of involuntary motion. It is further differentiated into several subgroups.
3. *Rigidity:* Characterized by decreased motion. The muscles are partially contracted all of the time. The antagonists to the antigravity muscles are predominantly involved.
4. *Ataxia:* Characterized by incoordination due to disturbance in the sense of balance.
5. *Tremor:* Characterized by involuntary motions of a rhythmical manner due to agonist and antagonist contractions.
6. *Atonia:* Characterized by lack of tone and failure of muscles to respond to stimulation.

These types are followed by the topographical involvement of monoplegia, paraplegia, hemiplegia, triplegia, quadriplegia, diplegia, and double hemiplegia. Along with the neuromuscular deficit, there are often other disabilities present. Although investigators differ as to the prevalence of related disabilities, Scherzer and Tscharnuter (1982) note that associated dysfunctions appear frequently:

> These include abnormalities of vision (25 percent), hearing and speech (greater than 50 percent), seizure disorders (one-third), mental retardation (50 to 75 percent, depending on motor severity), learning disabilities among the vast majority, and frequently social, emotional, and intrafamily problems. In every sense, therefore, the term conveys the concept of a multiply handicapping condition.

Assessment

The multiple dysfunctions of children with cerebral palsy require comprehensive assessment of a transdisciplinary nature. Various specialties of medicine are frequently required, including pediatrics, neurology, physiatry, orthopaedics, ophthalmology, dentistry, and psychiatry. In addition, physical, occupational, and speech therapists as well as psychologists, social workers, and teachers are frequently integral contributors to an effective evaluation.

While the motor deficit is often the most obvious disability, it may not be the predominant handicap; a high frequency of associated dysfunctions has been established. Shapiro et al. (1983) reported that 88% of cerebral palsy youngsters have three or more disabilities. The more frequently associated dysfunctions are cognitive deficits, communication disorders, visual dysfunction, seizures, emotional and behavioral disorders, sensory impairments, and orthopaedic deformities. Results of another study (Sillanpaa, 1987), which compared children with various medical impairments to a matched sample of healthy children, found that more than one handicap was associated most frequently with cerebral palsy, and that neurological impairments were more disabling than nonneurological medical handicaps. It is therefore clear that for a thorough understanding of cerebral palsy, it is necessary to identify not only the individual disabilities but also the interaction of these disabilities as they affect the patient and family.

COGNITIVE FUNCTIONING

The most common associated deficit of cerebral palsy is cognitive dysfunction. Mental retardation occurs in approximately 50–75% of patients, while more subtle problems such as learning disabilities are also frequently present (Scherzer and Tscharnuter, 1982). Results from the Isle of Wight studies (Rutter et al., 1976) indicated that children with cerebral palsy tended to be retarded readers even when their intelligence was average. In another study (Rothman, 1987), using an order of movement task designed by Piaget to measure spatial concepts, children with cerebral palsy were significantly delayed in their understanding of the order of movement. It appears that the fact that children with cerebral palsy are restricted motorically by their physical handicap in turn affects their cognitive development and their spatial perception.

Cognitive abilities are difficult to assess in the cerebral palsy child who may, for example, have a quadriplegic motor handicap and be nonvocal due to neuromuscular involvement. Because of the multiple deficits, such a youngster is at a serious disadvantage in a standard psychological evaluation, which would probably and perhaps incorrectly place his or her functioning within the profound range of mental retardation. Such severe deficits may further result in a child's being labeled ''untestable.'' It is understandable, therefore, that a solely quantitative, standard psychometric approach for children with cerebral palsy is inappropriate. Two primary principles guiding the psychological evaluation of such multiply handicapped children are (a) understanding and adaptation of standardized measurement for evaluation of the child's strengths and weaknesses and (b) a systematic/naturalistic observation of the child in the classroom environment.

SOCIAL/EMOTIONAL DEVELOPMENT

Children with cerebral palsy are at high risk for development of emotional and behavioral disturbances. Because of their motor disability, they are readily identified by others, and as children they see themselves as "different" by age 4. Any negative effects on self-esteem are most commonly crystallized during the primary grades at school (Templin et al., 1981). Nielsen (1966) compared cerebral palsy children of normal intelligence with a control group matched for age, sex, IQ, and socioeconomic status and having no evidence of brain damage and found that three times as many cerebral palsy children displayed signs of moderate or severe personality disorders. Although the kinds of disturbances varied greatly, the cerebral palsy youngsters showed some common features, such as difficulties in interpersonal relations, expectation of hostility and rejection from others, and low tolerance for frustration. When they felt frustrated, they revealed tendencies to defiance and aggression.

Based on a study derived from several years of clinical experience, Freeman (1970) concluded that, while individuals with brain damage may show a higher incidence of perceptual disorders and problems with emotional control, there is no typical psychiatric category that can be considered characteristic of adolescents with cerebral palsy. This view is echoed in a review by Rubinstein and Shaffer (1985). Emotional disturbance in the adolescent with cerebral palsy is seen frequently, manifesting the full range of disorders found in the nonhandicapped population.

In a systematic, extensive study of brain-injured children (including children with cerebral palsy) on the Isle of Wight, Rutter et al. (1970) reported psychiatric disorder to be five times higher in children with cerebral palsy than in the general population and three times higher than in children who had physical disorders not involving the brain. The variable of organic brain dysfunction rather than visible disability was seen as the major factor leading to deficient social perceptions (Rutter et al., 1976). Rutter et al. (1970) also examined the association of organic brain dysfunction with specific types of psychiatric problems. The varieties of the psychiatric problems were similar to those found in any group of young people with psychiatric disorder and no known organic brain dysfunction. The majority of these cases showed neurotic or antisocial behaviors. When the variable of psychiatric disorder was controlled, there were few features of behavior, emotions, or relationships that were characteristic of youth with organic brain dysfunction. There was a tendency, however, for children with organic brain dysfunction without psychiatric disorder to show poor concentration more frequently than those in the general population. There was also a weak but significant relationship between hypoactivity and organic brain dysfunction. Using the same measures, in a 3-year longitudinal study of physically handicapped 15-year-olds (approximately 75% with cerebral palsy), Anderson et al. (1982) found a preponderance of neurotic types as compared with antisocial types. The main psychological problems shown were depression, fearfulness, lack of self-confidence, and worry, with anxiety being related to school and the effects of the disability. Emotional problems were also manifested by general irritability, with some cerebral palsy adolescents showing tantrums or rages.

In addition to the direct psychiatric effects of brain injury, factors that may lead to development of secondary emotional disorders in cerebral palsy children range from physical and cognitive limitations to environmental and societal circumstances. In the course of growing up, the child, due to restricted movement and disturbances in perception and ability to react, may fail to engage in normal interactions with objects in the environment, with resultant delays in cognitive development (Shere and Kastenbaum, 1966). Social interactions may also be less frequent and meaningful than those of other children, due to factors such as parental overprotection and sporadic school attendance (Barker et al., 1953). This may result in diminished and distorted interpersonal feedback (Richardson, 1964) such that the child's social development is impoverished, superficial, and immature. A pattern of passivity may have been unwittingly imposed on the child from his or her earliest years.

For the adolescent with cerebral palsy, emotional problems are usually greater and more serious than they are in childhood. Normal devel-

opmental concerns of peer-group acceptance, relationships with the opposite sex, and striving for independence are compounded by the multiple disabilities. This is further complicated by conflicts deriving from parental inclination toward overprotection, on the one hand, and their concern for the disabled youngster's potential for independence in adult life, on the other. In a study that examined mothers' expectations and their children's performance on social, vocational, and intellectual measures, it was found that mothers underestimated the youngsters' level of functioning. The adolescents' own predictions were even lower (Nussbaum, 1966). In a teenage sample of British students, not only the parents but also the school and medical services failed to encourage independence. Sixty percent of the cerebral palsy adolescents did not know the name of their condition and had little accurate information about it (Anderson et al., 1982). Similarly, Minde (1978), in a follow-up study of 34 adolescents with cerebral palsy, also found that poor communication, emotional withdrawal, and distancing existed among parents, siblings, and the cerebral palsy youngsters regarding the nature of the disability. The development of these children, age 10–14, was highlighted by increased awareness that their handicap was permanent and by their consequent search for personal and occupational identity, which in general did not extend beyond a hope to finish school. They showed low self-esteem and the beginning of general passivity. The interrelationship between specific impairments and psychosocial disability was the focus of a study (Hirst, 1989) involving 119 adolescents. Poor psychological adjustment and extreme isolation were not seen as a direct consequence of any one impairment but rather as the combined effect of those disabilities. It is the particular configuration of impairments that determines the extent of functional loss, which is related to limitations of dependency, restricted choices, physical barriers, and adverse reactions from others.

Later, in adult life, 25% of cerebral palsy individuals are socially isolated, and less than 10% marry (Klapper and Birch, 1966). Approximately 90% of youths with cerebral palsy reside in their parents' home, have little responsibility, and develop an orientation toward sedentary activity. In regard to heterosexual relationships, there was a lack of discussion with parents about sexuality, and heterosexual social contacts were either nonexistent or infrequent (Blum et al., 1991). These findings are in accord with a study of 52 disabled adults whose social status was compared with age-matched control subjects. Leaving home and sexual experience were delayed for the disabled group. Half of them received disability benefits and they experienced twice as much unemployment as their age-matched normal peers (Kokknen et al., 1991).

Treatment and Prevention

The most effective treatment for cerebral palsy is primary prevention through improved prenatal care, clinical genetics, and health education. Discussion of these is beyond the scope of this chapter. The understanding of cerebral palsy as a multiply handicapping condition in need of a transdisciplinary approach has led to legislation for provision of services. These laws, which grant rights to handicapped persons and their families, not only mandate services but also, and equally important, reflect public acceptance of responsibility for the disabled. Early intervention programs beginning with children as early as 2 months of age are increasingly available. For the school-age child, 3–21 years old, the 1975 Education for All Handicapped Children Act, Public Law 94-142, requires that every child with a handicapping condition receive an appropriate education. Under these regulations the child, in addition to special education, is entitled to related services. Within this orientation, psychotherapeutic intervention is an integral part of treatment. Appropriate psychopharmacologic intervention, where indicated, is often effective and must also be considered (Wiener, 1985).

Family stress related to the handicapped youth may be expected during periods of transition such as time of diagnosis, entrance to school, change in school placement, puberty, graduation, and transition to adult life (Anderson et al., 1982). The problems were found to be even greater for those mothers from a lower socioeconomic background (Breslau, 1983). In order to meet the complex psychosocial needs of young people with cerebral palsy, many schools and medical facilities offer a variety of services that include individual and peer group therapy, family counseling, and group work for siblings and parents. It has been shown that brothers and sisters of children with cerebral palsy who were taught to be involved in the plan of care served as positive role models and agents of change for their siblings (Craft et al., 1990). Other interventions that have been helpful are behavior modification, hypnotic imagery, and provision of respite care, which allows parents time away from their handicapped child (Botuck and Winsberg, 1991).

BRAIN TUMORS

The incidence of intracranial tumors in youth below the age of 15 years ranges from 2 to 5 in 100,000 per year, which ranks these tumors second only to leukemias as neoplasms in children. Brain tumors make up roughly half of all solid tumors in children. While supratentorial tumors constitute the majority of brain neoplasms in adults, infratentorial tumors predominate in children. Generally, infratentorial or posterior fossa tumors (i.e., those of the cerebellum and brainstem) are more silent than supratentorial tumors, and psychiatric symptoms such as personality change are less common. Instead, children with brain tumors tend to show more signs and symptoms of increased intracranial pressure, often with insidious onset and without localizing signs (Herskowitz and Rosman, 1982). The majority of intracranial neoplasms in children are primary tumors of glial origin, whereas metastatic tumors and meningiomas are quite rare. Thus, the location, presenting symptoms, and representation of the various types of brain tumors in youth differ from those of adults.

The etiology of most nonmetastatic intracranial tumors is unknown, and hence prevention is not possible. Craniopharyngiomas and teratomas are of congenital origin, arising from developmental malformations. Intracranial sarcomas are increased by cranial irradiation. Some tumors are associated with certain systemic conditions (e.g., Wiskott-Aldrich syndrome, renal transplantation, and leukemia) and with neurocutaneous syndromes (e.g., ataxia-telangiectasia, neurofibromatosis, and tuberous sclerosis) (Evans, 1987).

Clinical Features

The presenting symptomatology of brain tumors is largely dependent on tumor location and rate of growth. Because of the predominance of infratentorial and midline locations, most brain tumors in children tend to lead to obstruction of cerebrospinal fluid circulation, resulting in increased intracranial pressure. The symptoms and signs of increased intracranial pressure (IICP) are somewhat variable and are presented in Table 59.1. It should be noted that IICP has multiple etiologies (such as metabolic encephalopathy, intracranial infection, pseudotumor cerebri, and trauma) and is not pathognomonic for brain tumor. Headache is rarely localizing and is not qualitatively different in these brain tumors from that seen with other conditions. Transient accommodation of the brain and skull to IICP is thought to account for the remitting and exacerbating nature of the headache, which is often worse after periods of recumbency or with straining. Similarly, vomiting is often mild, variable, and intermittent.

Personality changes can be seen, such as quietness and decreased motoric activity (in an attempt to lessen headache), restlessness and irritability (often due to headache as well), and diminished levels of consciousness, leading to coma. Presenting symptoms other than those due to IICP are discussed for each tumor type.

Besides the neurological and psychiatric history and examination, intracranial tumors are diagnosed by skull radiography and especially by computed tomography (CT) and nuclear magnetic resonance imaging (MRI) of the brain.

Characteristics of various brain tumors are presented in Table 59.2.

Table 59.1. Signs and Symptoms of Increased Intracranial Pressure in Children, in Approximate Order of Presentation

1. Headache: Bifrontal or occipital; often mild; worse in the morning, after recumbency, and with coughing or Valsava; progressively persistent.
2. Vomiting: Often mild, not usually projectile; intermittent; occurs on rising; with or without headache; progressively more frequent.
3. Personality changes: Restlessness and irritability, memory loss, academic impairment; later, lethargy, apathy, depression, somnolence, and altered consciousness.
4. Papilledema (more common in children after suture fusion).
5. Diplopia, strabismus (cranial nerve VI palsy), impaired upward gaze and proptosis ("setting sun" sign), cranial nerve III palsy.
6. Bulging fontanelle and delayed fontanelle closure (infancy).
7. Widened sutures on x-ray and increased head circumference (0–2 years).
8. Altered vital signs: Increased blood pressure, increased or decreased pulse, decreased and irregular respirations.
9. Diffuse slowing on EEG.
10. Generalized seizures.

Classifications of childhood brain tumors are arbitrary and have undergone change in recent years (Becker, 1985; Swaiman, 1994). The classifications are still rather controversial, partly due to the unusual patterns of growth seen in these tumors, which are comprised of embryonic or poorly differentiated cells (Rorke, 1985). Further details concerning these tumors are discussed below, especially the psychiatric symptomatology and the effect of treatment on neuropsychological functioning.

Infratentorial Tumors

Infratentorial tumors are those of the cerebellum, fourth ventricle, and brainstem. For all of these tumors, IICP is a prominent feature and may be the only cause of symptoms early on. Other presenting symptoms are due to compression of brainstem structures and include progressive cranial neuropathies, often involving ocular and facial muscles; nystagmus, which is nonlateralizing; spasticity; ataxia; cervical pain; and head tilt.

Astrocytomas and medulloblastomas are the two tumor types of the cerebellum and have approximately equal incidences. Cerebellar astrocytomas (primarily pilocytic) are slow growing and mostly noninvasive. The onset of symptoms is insidious, usually beginning many months prior to diagnosis with mild vomiting and/or headache. IICP is due to compression of the fourth ventricle and cerebellar-pontine angle cisterns (Laurent and Cheek, 1986). Nystagmus, ataxia, unilateral hypotonia, and intention tremor may also be present. The course is usually benign. Treatment consists of resection; cerebrospinal fluid (CSF) shunting, if required; and radiation therapy, depending on malignancy and extent of the resection. Medulloblastoma, in contrast, is rapid growing and highly malignant. This tumor arises from the midline cerebellar vermis and may seed into the fourth ventricle and other structures. The onset of symptoms is acute, with vomiting, headache, and axial ataxia presenting several weeks to 2 months prior to diagnosis. Involvement of the reticular activating system may lead to an altered state of consciousness known as a coma vigil or akinetic mutism (Daly and Love, 1958). Treatment consists of excision and chemoradiotherapy (due to universal recurrence and inability to resect the entire tumor). The prognosis is not good; the 5-year survival rate is about 40% (Laurent and Cheek, 1986).

Fourth ventricle tumors include ependymomas and choroid plexus papillomas. Ependymomas, which may arise in any ventricle, predominate in the fourth ventricle in children and may lead to early CSF flow obstruction. IICP is the presenting condition and, when the tumor is infratentorial, may be accompanied by nystagmus, head tilt, and ataxia. Following excision and irradiation, survival rates range from 15 to 100%, depending on the malignancy of the ependymoma and whether seeding has occurred (Laurent and Cheek, 1986). Choroid plexus papillomas arise primarily in the fourth or lateral ventricles, are highly vascularized, and produce CSF, which results in IICP. Additional symptoms reported in one 12-year-old boy by Blackman and Wheeler (1987) consisted of somatic complaints, separation anxiety, school refusal, fearfulness, and crying episodes for a year. This child also had mild ataxia and impaired coordination since the age of 2 and had a head circumference at the 98th percentile. Diagnosis was made by CT scan during the second psychiatric hospitalization. Tumor resection resulted in amelioration of the depressive and anxiety symptoms.

Brainstem tumors are primarily gliomas of the pons. IICP may not be present. Common symptoms are cranial nerve deficits, ataxia, spasticity, and gait disturbance and a classic triad of progressive cranial neuropathies, pyramidal tract signs (hemiparesis), and cerebellar pathway signs (truncal and extremity ataxia and nystagmus) has been described (Chutorian, 1974). Although the duration of symptoms is usually brief, one case with a 6-month history of headaches precipitated by postural change has been reported (Novak and Moshe, 1985). Radiation is the treatment of choice, as surgery does not alter the course (Laurent and Cheek, 1986). Even with irradiation and chemotherapy, prognosis is very poor.

Supratentorial Tumors

Supratentorial tumors include cerebral and parasellar or midline neoplasms.

Cerebral hemisphere tumors can be in any lobe, the basal ganglia, and/or the lateral ventricles and can be of various types, such as those listed in Table 59.2. IICP is not usually found until late in the course, unless the tumor is rapidly growing and malignant (e.g., glioblastomas, in which the duration of symptoms is only about 6 weeks) (Dropcho et al., 1987). With low-grade tumors such as pilocytic and anaplastic astrocytomas, the duration of symptoms is often several years. Personality changes may be some of the earliest manifestations but may be subtle and difficult to ascertain in young children. Hence these tumors may grow quite large before detection. These personality changes may include intermittent irritability, listlessness, depression, and decrements in school performance, memory, attention, social awareness, and personal hygiene, although these are less well documented in children than in adults. In the child with academic or behavioral deterioration, funduscopic examination is important, as it may show papilledema if a brain tumor is the underlying cause (Herskowitz and Rosman, 1982). Headache is also an early complaint. Aggression is sometimes seen with temporal lobe tumors. Seizures (which can be generalized tonic-clonic, complex partial, and/or focal motor) and focal neurological deficits such as motoric weakness, hemiparesis, aphasia, alexia, agraphia, and hemianopsia tend to be later signs that result in diagnosis. In most cases of cerebral tumor, total resection is not possible, and excision is followed by irradiation. Prognosis varies with tumor type: For low-grade astrocytomas, 5-year survival after excision and irradiation is 50% (Laurent and Cheek, 1986).

Parasellar tumors are those arising in proximity to the sella turcica. Craniopharyngioma is the most common of these, arising from remnants of the pharyngeal duct near the pituitary stalk. This leads to endocrine dysfunction, and infiltration of the hypothalamus leads to hypothalamic dysfunction. Growth retardation and delayed sexual maturation are frequent but are difficult to appraise early on. Obesity, somnolence, visual and olfactory hallucinations, and alterations in body temperature and blood pressure may occur. Later signs may be those of IICP and visual disturbances due to optic chiasm compression. Treatment is by resection, with irradiation if resection is subtotal. The prognosis is good; however, these patients have both transient and permanent endocrinological abnormalities requiring treatment. Pituitary adenomas are rare in children and are manifested by growth retardation and visual loss. Optic nerve

Table 59.2. Characteristics of Brain Tumors in Children

Brain Tumor Location and Classification	Approximate % of All Brain Tumors	Peak Ages and Sex of Incidence	Common Presenting and Associated Symptoms and Signs
Infratentorial	50–60	—	IICP, cranial nerve palsies, ataxia, head tilt
Posterior fossa			
Cerebellum			
astrocytoma	15–25	5–8 yrs	Insidious onset: vomiting, headache
medulloblastoma	15–25	3–9 yrs, M > F	Acute onset: vomiting, headache, ataxia
4th ventricle			
ependymoma	5–10	3–8 yrs. M > F	IICP, ataxia
choroid plexus papilloma	Rare	0–3 yrs	IICP, ataxis, ?anxiety
Brainstem pontine glioma	10–20	5–7 yrs	Cranial nerve defects, spasticity (IICP)
Supratentorial	40–50		
Cerebral hemispheres	20–25	7–11 yrs	Personality change, motor weakness, IICP, seizures, focal neurological deficits, language disturbance
All lobes and basal ganglia			
astrocytoma	5–15		
glioblastoma	5–10		
oligodendroglioma	1–5		
ependymoma	1–5		
ganglioglioma	2		
sarcoma	Rare		
malignant teratoma	Rare		
metastatic neuroblastoma	Rare		
choroid plexus papilloma	1	0–3 yrs	IICP
Parasellar/midline	20–25		Often, growth disturbance
Craniopharyngioma	5–15	7–12 yrs	IICP, endocrine disturbance, visual field defects
Pituitary adenomas	Rare		Growth retardation, visual loss
Optic nerve and chiasm gliomas (astrocytomas)	5–10	1–6 yrs M > F	Visual field defects
Third ventricle pinealoma	1–5	10–11 yrs, M > F	Paralysis of upward gaze and ptosis, IICP, precocious puberty
colloid cyst	Rare	—	Sudden and intermittent headache, vomiting
Hypothalamic glioma	Rare	2–5 mos to 4 yrs	Diencephalic syndrome: alert and euphoric despite emaciation
Thalamus	Rare	<20 yrs	IICP, rhythmic alternation of extremity
Miscellaneous			
Meningioma	0–2	—	Usually same as cerebral tumors
Metastases (extraneuronal)	Rare	—	Depends on location
Skull tumors	Rare	—	Cranial lumps and bulges

Compiled primarily from Amador (1983). Chutorian (1974), Cohen and Duffner (1984), Evans (1987), Laurent and Cheek (1986), and Menkes (1990).

and chiasm gliomas are not uncommonly associated with neurofibromatosis. Visual defects are the primary presentation. Treatment is irradiation and possible chemotherapy. In infants, optic gliomas are usually aggressive, and the prognosis is poor, whereas in older children the glioma is often benign and self-limited (Kanamori et al., 1985).

Midline tumors are those in the third ventricle, hypothalamus, or thalamus, in addition to the parasellar region. Pinealoma is the only brain tumor in children with a marked sex difference, having a male: female ratio of about 3–4:1. Pinealomas may be in the pineal region or in the posterior third ventricle (Laurent and Cheek, 1986). Symptoms include those of IICP, endocrine disturbance, and visual defects. Diabetes insipidus, growth retardation, delayed puberty, or precocious puberty may be present. Parinaud syndrome (paralysis of upward gaze with bilateral ptosis due to pressure on the superior colliculi) is characteristic but may also be a sign of IICP (Chutorian, 1974). Other nonspecific signs—ataxia, nuchal rigidity, central deafness, and nystagmus—may be seen. Resection and/or irradiation is the recommended treatment. Colloid cysts of the third ventricle are rare. Movement of the tumor by flexion of the head results in intermittent obstruction of CSF flow, leading to intermittent symptoms of sudden headache, vomiting, and somnolence. Many of these tumors, although occurring in childhood, are not diagnosed until adulthood. Hypothalamic gliomas are rare and cause a characteristic diencephalic syndrome in infants. The infant appears alert and euphoric but becomes markedly emaciated. It is differentiated from failure to thrive by the activated state of the child. Hypothalamic gliomas in later childhood may present with accelerated growth and precocious puberty. Radiation therapy is the only treatment possible. Thalamic tumors are also rare. These often mimic cerebellar tumors but may have more characteristic signs, such as rhythmic alternation of extremities, athetosis, and posturing (Chutorian, 1974).

Psychiatric Sequelae of Brain Tumors and Brain Irradiation

Consideration must not only be given to the presenting neuropsychiatric symptoms of brain tumors but also to those symptoms secondary to the sequelae of the tumor after treatment and to the treatment itself. Standard neurological examinations have little prognostic value for quality of life in children with brain tumors (Milstein et al., 1985). Until recently, as survival rates have increased, very few studies had been done to assess functioning after treatment by means other than neurological examinations. Several studies, using global and specific measurements, have shown many surviving children functioning at near normal and some achieving high levels of education, although substantial proportions of this population, ranging from 40 to 60%, have intellectual and emotional disturbances (Bamford et al., 1982). Emotional disorders that have been reported include psychotic symptoms, immaturity, depression, anxiety, and oppositional and antisocial behavior (Danoff et al., 1982). Many early investigations that reported functional deterioration did not or were not able to separate important variables, including tumor characteristics, age of the child, and treatment modalities (Mulhern et al., 1983). Tumor location is often divided grossly into infratentorial or supratentorial locations for these studies. Impairments from infratentorial tumors are variable, with predominant visual-motor problems and about a 30–60% incidence of neuropsychiatric deficits, behavior disturbance, and need for special education (Mulhern et al., 1983). These latter types of impairments are much more common with supratentorial tumors, with about a 50–85% incidence (Gjerris, 1976; Kun et al., 1983). In five children with temporal lobe tumors, Mulhern et al. (1983) found impulse control problems and special education needs in all, with more severe deficits than in adults with temporal lobe tumors. Further subdivision on the basis of location yields sample sizes too small for generalization.

Age at diagnosis and treatment appears to be positively correlated with better functioning if diffuse CNS damage has occurred, whereas younger children with focal injuries have better recovery than do older children (Eiser, 1981; Mulhern et al., 1983).

IICP has been postulated to be responsible for some of the long-term intellectual deficits with brain tumors; however, it does not seem to have a lasting impact after treatment (Mulhern et al., 1983).

The treatment modality of cranial irradiation has been shown to adversely affect intellectual functioning. Children with acute lymphocytic leukemia (ALL) provide a useful comparison group for investigating the effects of CNS irradiation in children with brain tumors, allowing separation of irradiation effects from those of the tumor and neurosurgery. Cranial irradiation is a standard treatment for ALL, and many children with ALL develop a postirradiation syndrome within 4–8 weeks of treatment (somnolence, anorexia, and lethargy). Longer-term changes consist of cerebral atrophy, distractibility, memory and attention deficits, and declining IQ and achievement test scores, all of which are greater with higher radiation dose and combined irradiation-chemotherapy in the younger child (Cohen and Duffner, 1984; Halberg et al., 1992; Mulhern et al., 1983). Children with brain tumors are thought to be at greater risk for these effects, as radiation dosages for brain tumors are much higher than those for ALL. Indeed, more severe sequelae have been demonstrated, with either pervasive intellectual deterioration or more selective performance and mathematic deficits (Duffner et al., 1985; Kun et al., 1983). These effects have become more noticeable and problematic as rates of survival have increased, especially since these adverse consequences are more prone to occur in younger children, tend to worsen over time, and may take 2–5 years to be fully noted, despite initial improvement in the first 6 months after treatment for older children (Duffner et al., 1985; Mulhern and Kun, 1985; Packer et al., 1989). Irradiation also poses the additional adverse effects of long-term growth hormone suppression with resulting decelerated growth, hypothyroidism, hearing deficits, leukoencephalopathy, and oncogenesis (especially of sarcomas) (Cohen and Duffner, 1984; Duffner and Cohen, 1985).

The diagnosis of brain tumor in a child is clearly devastating to the family. Often there is little time to optimally adjust to this news before the operation and treatment are begun. With increased survival, the family frequently must cope with a "changed" child, and joy over the child's survival can be challenged and tempered by the sorrow over his or her cognitive, behavioral, and emotional deterioration. This may occur even in the child with an IQ in the normal range (Cohen and Duffner, 1984). As with other chronic disease, the parents tend to become unrealistic and overprotective (Danoff et al., 1982). They may infantilize their child and avoid discussion of such issues as tumor recurrence and death. Marital and intrafamilial stress is not uncommon. Long-term psychiatric sequelae of brain tumors in childhood include cognitive deficits, school failure, and unemployment and appear more severe with supratentorial tumors and with cranial irradiation (Glauser and Packer, 1991; Mostow et al., 1991). Educational and psychological services, such as special education, psychotherapy, and national or local brain tumor groups provide much-needed support for the child and family.

Conclusions

Brain tumors in youth are primarily infratentorial, and initially presenting psychiatric symptoms are not as common or as obvious as in adults. When present, these changes are often subtle and include irritability, declining school performance, memory impairment, decreased attention, depression, and changes in sleep (somnolence). Symptoms of IICP are often the primary presentation. Children with academic and behavioral deterioration deserve a neurological examination, and the index of suspicion for intracranial mass should be high if headache, vomiting, alterations in consciousness, visual disturbances, cerebellar signs, or neurological deficits are present. With recent increases in survival rates, long-term sequelae of intellectual, emotional, and behavioral deterioration have been noted. In general, these neuropsychiatric deficits are worse for supratentorial tumors, in younger ages at diagnosis and treatment, and after cranial irradiation. IQ, achievement, and memory testing should be done before and after treatment and followed for several years thereafter to assess long-term sequelae of cranial irradiation. Educational

Table 59.3.   Selected Childhood Neurodegenerative and Neuromuscular Disorders

Neurodegenerative disorders
  Metabolic encephalopathies
    Hypothyroidism
    Hyperphenylalaninemia
    Phenylketonuria
    Galactosemia
  Cerebral storage diseases
    GM$_1$ and GM$_2$ gangliosidoses (including Tay-Sachs)
    Niemann-Pick disease
    Gaucher's disease
    Fabry's disease
    Farber's lipogranulomatosis
    Krabbe's disease (globoid cell leukodystrophy)
  Leukodystrophies and demyelinating scleroses
    Krabbe's disease
    Metachromatic leukodystrophy
    Multiple sclerosis
    Schilder's disease
  System degeneration
    Basal ganglia degenerations
      Juvenile Parkinson's disease
      Huntington's chorea
      Dystonia musculorum deformans
      Wilson's disease (hepatolenticular degeneration)
    Cerebellar degenerations
      Friedreich's ataxia
      Ataxia-telangiectasia
    Brainstem and spinal cord degenerations
      Werdnig-Hoffmann disease (progressive infantile spinal atrophy)
      Familial juvenile amyotrophic lateral sclerosis
  Neurocutaneous diseases
    Neurofibromatosis
    Tuberous sclerosis
    Sturge-Webber syndrome
    von Hippel-Lindau disease
    Ataxia-telangiectasia
Neuromuscular disorders
  Guillain-Barré syndrome
  Juvenile myasthenia gravis
  Muscular dystrophies

and emotional support services for the child and family can have a beneficial impact on adjustment after treatment.

NEURODEGENERATIVE AND NEUROMUSCULAR DISORDERS

For convenience, this section covers the neurodegenerative and neuromuscular disorders together. As with brain tumors, the classification of these disorders is controversial, and neurocutaneous disorders are sometimes considered under nervous system tumors rather than under degenerative diseases (Menkes, 1990). Table 59.3 lists major categories of these disorders and selected diseases for each. Metabolic encephalopathies and cerebral storage diseases are discussed elsewhere in this text (Chapter 96). Of the remaining disorders, only certain diseases—those that have reported psychiatric manifestations—are discussed here.

Neurodegenerative Disorders

The neurodegenerative disorders constitute a wide range of diseases characterized by degeneration of the nervous system diffusely or in part. The neuropathogenesis has been postulated to be caused by abnormal production and accumulation of excitotoxins, neuroexcitant amino acids that produce axon-sparing lesions (Schwarcz et al., 1984).

Leukodystrophies and Demyelinating Scleroses

These disorders have in common demyelination of cerebral and spinal white matter. The etiologies include known or suspected hereditary enzyme defects and possible autoimmune disorders and/or slow virus infections. Varying degrees of intellectual impairment are present, and spasticity, optic atrophy, ataxia, weakness, and seizures are common. In most cases, treatment is purely symptomatic and supportive.

Krabbe's disease (globoid cell leukodystrophy) is a cerebral storage disease resulting in demyelination. It usually begins suddenly at 4–6 months of age and rapidly progresses to death, although later onset and slower progression have been observed (Menkes, 1990). Restlessness, irritability, stiffness, seizures, and peripheral neuropathy are seen.

Metachromatic leukodystrophy (MLD) has different forms with different enzyme defects and different ages of onset, from infancy to adulthood. In the late infant or young child, early hypotonia gives way to spasticity; impairment of speech and intellectual deterioration gradually develop, accompanied by gait disorders, coarse tremor, athetoid movements, decreased deep tendon reflexes, and later, seizures (Drew, 1974). Death ensues within several months of diagnosis. In the juvenile form of MLD, onset begins between 5 and 7 years with ataxia and movement disorders and progresses slowly to spasticity.

Multiple sclerosis (MS) usually begins in the young adult; however, rare cases of MS have occurred in children. Few children have symptoms before 10 years of age; most occur after puberty. As with adults, the course is unpredictable and characterized by waxing and waning symptoms, and the symptoms are similar: ataxia, weakness, blurred vision, paresthesias, dizziness, headache, mood lability, and incontinence can occur (Menkes, 1990). Diagnosis is made retrospectively and is bolstered by CSF abnormalities (especially pleocytosis and elevated gamma globulins), abnormal evoked potentials, and visualization of demyelinated lesions on CT or MRI. The etiology remains unknown, but MS is thought to be autoimmune in nature, perhaps due to a slow virus infection in early life. We have encountered cyclothymia as the presenting feature of this disorder in a 10-year-old girl who was admitted to our child psychiatry inpatient service with an initial diagnosis of bipolar affective disorder. The patient's complaints of visual disturbances were originally interpreted as probable conversion symptoms until funduscopic examination yielded evidence of optic neuritis and led to the appropriate underlying neurological diagnosis.

Schilder's disease (diffuse cerebral sclerosis) is an acute and progressive demyelinating disorder similar to MS, with onset often between ages 5 and 12. Intellectual impairment, emotional lability, gait disturbance, and seizures are early manifestations. Late signs include visual complaints, aphasia, deafness, and cranial nerve palsies, followed by death within 1–2 years (Menkes, 1990).

System Degenerations

These disorders involve progressive degeneration, primarily of one neurological system (Evans, 1987).

BASAL GANGLIA

Parkinson's disease has a rare juvenile form, with the onset around age 10–15 years of resting (pill-rolling) tremor, bradykinesia, rigidity, and intellectual deterioration. Treatment is the same as the adult form, but death usually occurs by the 3rd decade.

Huntington's disease can begin as early as age 3, although only 1–3% of cases have their onset in childhood (Drew, 1974; Hecht, 1987). The inheritance is autosomal dominant, and the juvenile form is usually inherited from the father (Hecht, 1987). Commonly, the disease presents with dementia, personality change, and seizures between ages 5 and 10, followed by marked rigidity and hypokinesia. Choreoathetosis may be absent (Evans, 1987; Hecht, 1987). Death occurs within 3–10 years after onset.

Dystonia musculorum deformans is a genetic disorder marked by increased muscle tone with gait disturbance and abnormal foot positioning, torticollis, and/or dystonic movements, without intellectual impairment. Onset may occur around age 5. The limbs become distorted but relax during sleep. Fixation and incapacitation may ensue. These cases are not infrequently misdiagnosed as conversion disorder or hysteria, but the reverse can happen as well, with psychogenic dystonia sometimes resulting in inappropriate medical therapy or operations (such as insertion of straightening rods or thalamotomy) (Fahn and Williams, 1988).

Wilson's disease is an inborn error of copper metabolism resulting in degeneration of the basal ganglia and hepatic cirrhosis. Initial presentation is with hepatitis and/or dystonia and gait disturbance in midchildhood (Evans, 1987). Intellectual impairment, affective lability, anxiety, and psychotic symptoms are common, as are tremor, dystonia, dysarthria, ataxia, and choreoathetosis. Oral chelating agents and restriction of dietary copper lead to only partial recovery.

CEREBELLAR

Friedreich's ataxia presents with gait disturbance, with peak onset between ages 10 and 13. By age 20, most cases are nonambulatory. Dysarthria and hearing loss can occur, but cognitive deficits are unusual. Hart et al. (1986) reported on two children with Friedreich's ataxia who had deficits in information-processing speed, sustained attention, and memory, which occurred early in the disease course and progressively worsened.

BRAINSTEM AND SPINAL CORD

Degenerations in these structures, such as Werdnig-Hoffmann disease and familial juvenile amyotrophic lateral sclerosis, have no characteristic psychiatric symptoms.

Neurocutaneous Diseases

These diseases, sometimes referred to as phakomatoses, involve both skin and nervous system, which have a common embryonic ectodermal origin. The etiologies are of hereditary enzyme and metabolic defects.

Neurofibromatosis (von Recklinghausen's disease) is characterized by café au lait spots and numerous Schwann cell tumors along nerves and nerve trunks. Giant neurofibromas may cause overgrowth, of the limbs, trunk, and face ("elephantiasis") (Evans, 1987). Intracranial tumors are seen, with optic gliomas being common in children, and acoustic neuromas, ependymomas, and meningiomas being frequent. Mental retardation is often present to varying degrees, visual-spatial integration deficits may be present, and hyperactivity and learning disorders are common (Riccardi, 1982; Varnhagen et al., 1988). The inheritance is autosomal dominant, but about half of the cases represent new mutations of a gene on chromosome 17 (Martin, 1987).

Tuberous sclerosis may present with infantile spasms as early as 6 months, depigmented nevi (ash-leaf spots), adenoma sebaceum, shagreen patches (large, raised, leathery areas of the skin), subungual fibromas, and retinal tumors. There are cardiac, renal, and pulmonary lesions. Sclerotic nodules are found in the brain, which are responsible for developmental delay or arrest, hypsarrhythmia on the EEG, and mixed seizures. Psychiatric symptoms vary; some children will have little or no cognitive impairment, whereas others will be autistic. Hunt and Dennis (1987) have shown that normal intelligence is associated with the absence of infantile spasms, while the majority of cases with a history of infantile spasms show mental retardation and/or classic symptoms of autism. Aggression, obsessions, hyperactivity, psychotic symptoms, and impaired social behavior and communication are prominent, and these behavioral features are often the most pressing concern of the parents (Hunt and Dennis, 1987). The inheritance of tuberous sclerosis is autosomal dominant with variable penetrance (Menkes, 1990).

Sturge-Weber syndrome is manifested by a facial port-wine nevus in the distribution of the trigeminal nerve. Intracranial angiomatous malformations may give rise to focal seizures and hemiplegia, beginning by age 1. Symptoms progress relentlessly, with seizures becoming intractable. Most children are mentally retarded, and dementia becomes severe.

Von Hippel-Lindau disease occasionally presents in children as ataxia and spasticity, with hemangioblastomas of the cerebellum, kidney, liver, pancreas, and epididymis. Symptoms of posterior fossa tumor occur.

Ataxia-telangiectasia is a cerebellar degenerative disorder with characteristic telangiectasiae of the conjunctivae and, less commonly, of the ears, face, and chest. These appear around age 4 and are usually preceded by ocular motor apraxia (difficulty breaking visual fixation without turning the head), ataxia, and intention tremor; later, dysarthria, choreoathetosis, and intellectual deterioration are seen (Evans, 1987). Many of these children have immune dysfunction with recurrent infections and a tendency to develop leukemias and lymphomas. Incapacitation occurs in adolescence, and death is in the early 20s.

Neuromuscular Disorders

The predominant feature of the neuromuscular disorders is weakness, with a variety of manifestations. The child psychiatrist should have familiarity with these disorders, as they may have associated psychopathology or may be misdiagnosed as psychosomatic disorders. Two types of neuromuscular disorders will be considered here: the polyneuropathies and the muscular dystrophies.

POLYNEUROPATHIES

Gullain-Barré syndrome, juvenile myasthenia gravis, and most other polyneuropathies do not have characteristic psychiatric symptoms. However, because of their presenting symptoms, they are not uncommonly discounted as being conversion disorders. Gullain-Barré syndrome is a postinfectious inflammatory neuropathy, usually preceded by a viral infection or immunization. Within a few weeks of an upper respiratory or other infection, the child will typically begin to complain of paresthesias in the extremities, which can have a glove-and-stocking distribution. Difficulty in walking and ataxia follow, and weakness rapidly ascends from the lower to the upper extremities. Maximum deficits occur over several weeks to a month, followed by a plateau phase, then rapid recovery over several months (Evans, 1987). Early in the course, the child may be seen as malingering to avoid school or other responsibilities. In many cases, respiratory insufficiency can occur, necessitating ventilatory support. Most cases recover with no sequelae.

Juvenile myasthenia gravis may also be misdiagnosed as psychosomatic. The symptoms are generally the same as in adults and usually occur after the age of 10 years. Ptosis and diplopia are hallmark signs, with waxing and waning fatigue that may be worse at certain times of day (Evans, 1987).

MUSCULAR DYSTROPHIES

The muscular dystrophies are inherited diseases characterized by progressive, symmetrical muscle weakness and atrophy of unknown etiology. Duchenne muscular dystrophy and Becker type are both X-linked recessive conditions, with about one-third of the Duchenne cases representing new mutations (Martin, 1987). The gene whose dysfunction is responsible for Duchenne muscular dystrophy has been located and its protein product, dystrophin, identified (Hoffman et al., 1987). Dystrophin is absent from the muscle tissue of boys with Duchenne muscular dystrophy (Hoffman et al., 1987). Duchenne-type dystrophy appears between 2 and 4 years of age, with delayed motor milestones, while the Becker type has its onset between 5 and 11 years of age (Williams et al., 1987). Although the Becker type has a slower progression, both lead to wheelchair confinement and a decreased life span. Fascioscapulohumeral and myotonic muscular dystrophies are autosomal dominant disorders. The fascioscapulohumeral type occurs between 6 and 20 years of age and primarily affects the shoulder girdle and face. The myotonic type occurs from infancy to adulthood and involves distal and facial muscles, cataract development, gonadal atrophy, and myotonia.

Varying degrees of mental retardation of unknown pathogenesis have been reported in Duchenne, myotonic, and congenital muscular dystrophies, but less so in the Becker and fascioscapulohumeral types (Williams et al., 1987). With increasing age and physical disabilities, increasing, decreasing, and static intellectual impairment have all been observed. Whelen (1987) reported average IQ but significantly lower verbal fluency and immediate verbal and nonverbal memory. Sollee et al. (1985) noted that IQ deficits in young Duchenne patients are primarily in language and attentional-organizational tasks, not in visual-motor tasks; these impairments improved to average with age. Similar findings have been reported in the Becker and fascioscapulohumeral types (Karagan and Sorensen, 1981). Schorer (1964) suggested that the language defect may represent both the muscle disease and failure in social development. The controversy over the extent of existence of cognitive impairment and the possibility of CNS involvement remains. It is unknown whether the absence of dystrophin in Duchenne patients affects the brain.

Fitzpatrick et al. (1986) found frequent diagnoses of dysthymic disorder and major depressive disorder in Duchenne boys, especially in older boys. Social isolation, depression, and prolonged grief reactions are common; parents exhibit denial, preoccupation with the child, difficulty responding to death issues, guilt over the genetic transmission of the disease, and marital difficulties (Buchanan et al., 1979; Witte, 1985). The parents' initial expectations of a rapid course are greeted with false hope, as the disease progresses slowly; however, as walking becomes more difficult, the parents's grief and conflicts rematerialize (Carroll, 1985). Communication within families about muscular dystrophy presents difficulties for both parents and the child, and the child is often the silent partner in decision-making (Fitzpatrick and Barry, 1986). Proper management includes education, genetic counseling, facilitation of communication, involvement of the child in making decisions, and social and emotional support such as that provided by the Muscular Dystrophy Association.

Conclusions

The neurodegenerative and neuromuscular disorders encompass many diverse diseases with an array of neuropsychiatric effects. There may be no specific neuropsychiatric symptoms (e.g., Becker-type muscular dystrophy), mild intellectual impairment (e.g., neurofibromatosis), depression (e.g., Duchenne muscular dystrophy), severe cognitive disability (e.g., Huntington's chorea), or autism (e.g., tuberous sclerosis). The etiology and pathogenesis for many of these disorders are insufficiently understood, and often treatment is only supportive. For those disorders for which specific treatment is available (e.g., Wilson's disease), the treatment may not reverse some of the neuropsychiatric deficits. As most of these diseases are inherited, genetic counseling is an essential part of treatment. Education about the disorder, enhancement of family communication, and provision of social/emotional supports are beneficial and necessary components of management. Psychotropic medication may be considered for clearly defined symptom alleviation.

References

Alvarez N: Discontinuance of antiepileptic medications in patients with developmental disability and diagnosis of epilepsy. Am J Ment Retard 93:593, 1989.

Amador LV (ed): Brain Tumors in the Young. Springfield, IL, Charles C Thomas, 1983.

American Academy of Pediatrics, Committee on Drugs: Behavioral and cognitive effect of anticonvulsant therapy. Pediatrics 76:644, 1985.

Aminoff M, Goodin D, Berg B, et al: Ambulatory EEG recordings in epileptic and nonepileptic children. Neurology 38:558, 1988.

Anderson EM, Clarke L, Spain B: Disability in Adolescence. London, Methuen, 1982.

Baer D, Fedio P: Quantitative analysis of interictal behavior in temporal lobe epilepsy. Arch Neurol 34:454, 1977.

Baer D, Freeman R, Greenberg M: Behavior alterations in patients with temporal lobe epilepsy. In: Blumer D (ed): Psychiatric Aspects of Epilepsy. Washington, DC, American Psychiatric Press, 1984, p. 197.

Baer D, Freeman R, Schiff D, et al: Interictal behavior changes in patients with temporal lobe epilepsy. In: Hales R, Frances A (eds): Psychiatric Update (American Psychiatric Association Annual Review, Vol 4). Washington, DC, American Psychiatric Press, 1985, p. 190.

Bamford FN, Jones PM, Pearson D, et al: Residual disabilities in children treated for intracranial space occupying lesions. Cancer 49:1580, 1982.

Barker RG, Wright B, Myerson L, et al: Adjustment to Physical Handicap and Illness: A Survey of the Social Psychology of Physique and Disability (Bulletin no. 55, rev ed). New York, Social Science Research Council, 1953.

Barraclough B: Suicide and epilepsy. In: Reynolds E, Trimble M (eds): Epilepsy and Psychiatry. Edinburgh, Churchill Livingstone, 1981, p. 72.

Batzel LW, Dodrill CB, Dubinsky BL, et al: An objective method for the assessment of psychosocial problems in adolescents with epilepsy. Epilepsia 32(2):202–211, 1991.

Becker LE: An appraisal of the World Health Organization classification of tumors of the central nervous system. Cancer 56:1858, 1985.

Betts T: Depression, anxiety and epilepsy. In:

Reynolds E, Trimble M (eds): Epilepsy and Psychiatry. Edinburgh, Churchill Livingstone, 1981, p. 60.

Blackman M, Wheler GHT: A case of mistaken identity: A fourth ventricle tumor presenting as school phobia in a 12 year old boy. Can J Psychiatry 32:584, 1987.

Blum RW, Resnick MD, Nelson R, et al: Family and peer issues among adolescents with spina bifida and cerebral palsy. Pediatrics 88(2):280–285, 1991.

Botuck S, Winsberg BG: Effects of respite on mothers of school-age and adult children with severe disabilities. Ment Retard 29(1):43–47, 1991.

Brent D, Crumrine P, Varma R, et al: Phenobarbital treatment and major depressive disorder in children with epilepsy. Pediatrics 80:909, 1987.

Breslau N: Family care: Effects on siblings and mothers. In: Thompson J, Rubin IL, Bilenker RM (eds): Comprehensive Management of Cerebral Palsy. New York, Grune & Stratton, 1983.

Buchanan DC, LaBarbera CJ, Roelofs R, et al: Reactions of families to children with Duchenne muscular dystrophy. Gen Hosp Psychiatry 1:262, 1979.

Camfield P, Gates R, Rowen G, et al: Comparison of cognitive ability, personality profile, and school success in epileptic children with pure right versus left temporal lobe EEG foci. Ann Neurol 15:222, 1984.

Carroll JE: Diagnosis and management of Duchenne muscular dystrophy. Pediatr Rev 6:195, 1985.

Chutorian AM: Tumors of the central nervous system. In: Carter S, Gold AP (eds): Neurology of Infancy and Childhood. New York, Appleton-Century-Crofts, 1974.

Cohen ME, Duffner PK: Brain Tumors in Children: Principles of Diagnosis and Treatment. New York, Raven Press, 1984.

Corbet J, Trimble M, Nicol T: Behavioral and cognitive impairment in children with epilepsy: The long term effects of anti-convulsant therapy. J Am Acad Child Psychiatry 24:17, 1985.

Craft MJ, Lakin JA, Oppliger RA, et al: Siblings as change agents for promoting the functional status of children with cerebral palsy. Dev Med Child Neurol 32(12):1049–1057, 1990.

Crothers B, Paine RS: The Natural History of Cerebral Palsy. Cambridge, MA, Harvard University Press, 1959.

Cruickshank WM: The problem and its scope. In: Cruickshank WM (ed): Cerebral Palsy: A Developmental Disability (3rd ed). Syracuse, NY, Syracuse University, 1976.

Daly DD, Love JG: Akinetic mutism. Neurology 8:238, 1958.

Danoff BF, Cowchock FS, Marquette C, et al: Assessment of long-term effects of primary radiation therapy for brain tumors in children. Cancer 49:1580, 1982.

Denhoff E: Medical aspects. In: Cruickshank WM (ed): Cerebral Palsy: A Developmental Disability (3rd ed). Syracuse, NY, Syracuse University Press, 1976.

Drew AL: The degenerative and demyelinating diseases of the nervous system. In: Carter S, Gold AP (eds): Neurology of Infancy and childhood. New York, Appleton-Century-Crofts, 1974.

Dropcho EJ, Wisoff JH, Walker RW, et al: Supratentorial malignant gliomas in childhood: A review of fifty cases. Ann Neurol 22:355, 1987.

Duchowney M, Resnick T, Deray M, et al: Video EEG diagnosis of repetitive behavior in early childhood and its relationship to seizures. Pediatr Neurol 4:162, 1988.

Duffner PK, Cohen ME, Thomas PRM, et al: The long-term effects of cranial irradiation on the central nervous system. Cancer 56:1841, 1985.

Eiser C: Psychological sequelae of brain tumors in childhood: A retrospective study. Br J Clin Psychol 20:35, 1981.

Ellenberg JH, Hirts DG, Nelson KB: Do seizures in children cause intellectual deterioration? N Engl J Med 314:1085, 1986.

Evans OB: Manual of Child Neurology. New York, Churchill Livingstone, 1987.

Evans R, Clay T, Gualtieri C: Carbamazepine in pediatric psychiatry. J Am Acad Child Adolesc Psychiatry 26:2, 1987.

Fahn S, Williams DT: Psychogenic dystonia. In: Fahn S, Marsden C, Caine D (eds): Advances in Neurology. Vol 50: Dystonia (Vol 2). New York, Raven Press, 1988, p. 431.

Farwell J, Dodrill D, Batsel L: Neuropsychological abilities of children with epilepsy. Epilepsia 26:395, 1985.

Feldman H, Crumrine P, Handen BL, et al: Am J Dis Child 143(9):1081–1086, 1989.

Feldman R, Paul N, Cummins-Cucharine J:

Video-tape recording in epilepsy and pseudoseizures. In: Riley T, Roy A (eds): *Pseudo-seizures*. Baltimore, Williams & Wilkins, 1982, p. 122.

Fitzpatrick C, Barry C: Communication within families about Duchenne muscular dystrophy. *Dev Med Child Neurol* 28:589, 1986.

Fitzpatrick C, Barry C, Garvey C: Psychiatric disorder among boys with Duchenne muscular dystrophy. *Dev Med Child Neurol* 28:589, 1986.

Flor-Henry P: *Cerebral Basis of Psychopathology*. Boston, John Wright-PSG, 1983.

Forster F, Booker H: The epilepsies and convulsive disorders. In: Baker A, Joynt R (eds): *Clinical Neurology* (Vol 3). Philadelphia, Harper & Row, 1988, 31-1.

Forsythe I, Butler R, Berg I, et al: Cognitive impairment in new cases of epilepsy randomly assigned to carbamazepine, phenytoin and sodium valproate. *Dev Med Child Neurol* 33:524–534, 1991.

Freeman RD: Psychiatric problems in adolescents with cerebral palsy. *Dev Med Child Neurol* 2:64, 1970.

Gjerris F: Clinical aspects and long-term prognosis of intracranial tumors in infancy and childhood. *Dev Med Child Neurol* 18:145, 1976.

Glauser TA, Packer RJ: Cognitive deficits in long-term survivors of childhood brain tumors. *Child's Nerv Syst* 7:2, 1991.

Golden GS: *Textbook of Pediatric Neurology*. New York, Plenum, 1987.

Hagberg B, Hagberg G: Prenatal and perinatal risk factor in a survey of 681 Swedish cases. In: Stanley F, Alberman E (eds): *The Epidemiology of the Cerebral Palsies (Clinics in Developmental Medicine 87)*. Philadelphia, Lippincott, 1984.

Halberg EE, Kramer JH, Moore IM, et al: Prophylactic cranial irradiation dose effects on late cognitive function in children treated for acute lymphoblastic leukemia. *Int J Radiat Oncol Biol Phys* 22:13, 1992.

Hanesian H, Paez P, Williams D: The neurologically impaired child and adolescent. In: Kestenbaum C, Williams D (eds): *Handbook of Clinical Assessment of Children & Adolescents* (Vol 1). New York, New York University Press, 1988, p. 415.

Hart RP, Henry GK, Kwentus JA, et al: Information processing speed of children with Friedreich's ataxia. *Dev Med Child Neurol* 28:310, 1986.

Hauser W, Annegers J, Anderson V: Epidemiology and genetics of epilepsy. *Res Public Assoc Res Nerv Ment Dis* 61:267, 1983.

Hecht F: Advances in medical genetics: Huntington disease. *Pediatr Rev* 9:13, 1987.

Herskowitz J, Rosman NP: *Pediatrics, Neurology, and Psychiatry—Common Ground*. New York, Macmillan, 1982.

Herzberg J, Fenwick P: The etiology of aggression in temporal lobe epilepsy. *Br J Psychiatry* 1153:50, 1988.

Hirst M: Patterns of impairment and disability related to social handicap in young people with cerebral palsy and spina bifida. *J Biosoc Sci* 21:1, 1987.

Hoare P: The development of psychiatric disorder among school children with epilepsy. *Dev Med Child Neurol* 26:3, 1984á.

Hoare P: Does illness foster dependency? A study of epileptic and diabetic children. *Dev Med Child Neurol* 26:20, 1984b.

Hoffman EP, Brown RH, Kunkel LM: Dystrophin: The protein product of the Duchenne muscular dystrophy locus. *Cell* 51:919, 1987.

Holm VA: The causes of cerebral palsy: A contemporary perspective. *JAMA* 247:1473, 1982.

Hunt A, Dennis J: Psychiatric disorder among children with tuberous sclerosis. *Dev Med Child Neurol* 29:190, 1987.

Kaminer Y, Apter A, Aviv A, et al: Psychopath-

ology and temporal lobe epilepsy in adolescents. *Acta Psychiatr Scand* 77:640, 1988.

Kanamori M, Shibuya M, Yoshida J, et al: Long term follow-up of patients with optic glioma. *Child's Nerv Syst* 1:272, 1985.

Karagan NJ, Sorensen JP: Intellectual functioning in non-Duchenne muscular dystrophy. *Neurology* 31:448, 1981.

Klapper Z, Birch H: The relation of childhood characteristics to outcome in young adults with cerebral palsy. *Dev Med Child Neurol* 8:645, 1966.

Kokkonen J, Saukkonen AL, Timonen E, et al: Social outcome of handicapped children as adults. *Dev Med Child Neurol* 33(12):1095–1100, 1991.

Koplewicz H, Williams D: Psychopharmacological treatment. In: Kestenbaum C, Williams D (eds): *Handbook of Clinical Assessment of Children & Adolescents* (Vol 2). New York, New York University Press, 1988, p. 1084.

Krumholz A, Niedermeyer E: Psychogenic seizures: A clinical study with follow-up data. *Neurology* 33:498, 1983.

Kun LE, Mulhern RK, Crisco JJ: Quality of life in children treated for brain tumors: Intellectual, emotional, and academic function. *J Neurosurg* 58:1, 1983.

Laurent JP, Cheek WR: Brain tumors in children. In: Fishman MA (ed): *Pediatric Neurology*. New York, Grune & Stratton, 1986.

Lesser R, Leuders H, Dinner D: Evidence for epilepsy is rare in patients with psychogenic seizures. *Neurology* 33:502, 1983.

Lewis DO: Neuropsychiatric vulnerabilities and violent juvenile delinquency. *Psychiatr Clin North Am* 6:707, 1983.

Lewis DO, Moy E, Jackson LD, et al: Biopsychosocial characteristics of children who later murder: A prospective study. *Am J Psychiatry* 142:1161, 1985.

Lewis DO, Pincus J, Shanok S, et al: Psychomotor epilepsy and violence in a group of incarcerated adolescent boys. *Am J Psychiatry* 139:882, 1982.

Lindsay J, Ounsted C, Richards P: Long-term outcome in children with temporal lobe seizures. III: Psychiatric aspects in childhood and adult life. *Dev Med Child Neurol* 21:630, 1979.

Little WJ: On the influence of abnormal parturition, difficult labors, premature birth, and asphyxia neonatorum, on the mental and physical condition of the child, especially in relation to deformities. *Trans Obstet Soc* 3:293, 1882.

Luchins D, Oliver P, Wyatt R: Seizures with antidepressants: An in vitro technique to assess relative risk. *Epilepsia* 25:25, 1984.

Makarec K, Persinger MA: Electroencephalographic correlates of temporal lobe signs and imagings. *Percept Mot Skills* 64:1124, 1987.

Marlow N, D'Souza SW, Chiswick ML: Neurodevelopmental outcome in babies weighing less than 2001 g at birth. *Br Med J Clin Res* 294:1582, 1987.

Martin JB: Molecular genetics: Applications to the clinical neurosciences. *Science* 238:765, 1987.

Menkes JH: *Textbook of Child Neurology* (4th ed). Philadelphia, Lea & Febiger, 1990.

Meyer FB, Marsh WR, Laws ER Jr, et al: Temporal lobectomy in children with epilepsy. *J Neurosurg* 64:371, 1986.

Milstein JM, Cohen ME, Sinks LF: The influence and reliability of neurologic assessment and Karnofsky performance score on prognosis. *Cancer* 56:1834, 1985.

Minde KK: Coping styles of 34 adolescents with cerebral palsy. *Am J Psychiatry* 135:1344, 1978.

Minear W: A classification of cerebral palsy. *Pediatrics* 18:841, 1956.

Mostow EN, Byrne J, Connelly RR, et al: Quality of life in long-term survivors of CNS tumors of childhood and adolescence. *J Clin Oncol* 9:592, 1991.

Motofsky D, Balaschak B: Psychological control of seizures. *Psychol Bull* 843:723, 1977.

Mulhern RK, Kun LE: Neuropsychologic function in children with brain tumors. III: Interval changes in the six months following treatment. *Med Pediatr Oncol* 13:318, 1985.

Mulhern RK, Crisco JJ, Kun LE: Neuropsychological sequelae of childhood brain tumors: A review. *J Clin Child Psychol* 12:66, 1983.

Nielsen HH: *A Psychological Study of Cerebral Palsied Children*. Copenhagen, Munksgaard, 1966.

Novak GP, Moshe SL: Brainstem glioma presenting as paroxysmal headache. *Dev Med Child Neurol* 27:379, 1985.

Nussbaum J: Self concept of adolescents with cerebral palsy: The relationship between self concept, mothers' concept and reality orientation. *Cereb Palsy J* 27:5, 1966.

O'Leary D, Seidenberg M, Boll T: Effects of age of onset of tonic-clonic seizures on neuropsychological performance in children. *Epilepsia* 22:197, 1981.

O'Reilly D, Walentynowicz JE: Etiological factors in cerebral palsy: An historical review. *Dev Med Child Neurol* 23:633, 1981.

Packer RJ, Sutton LN, Atkins TE, et al: A prospective study of cognitive function in children receiving whole-brain radiotherapy and chemotherapy: 2-years results. *J Neurosurg* 70:707, 1989.

Paneth N, Kiely J: The frequency of cerebral palsy: A review of population studies in industrialized nations since 1950. In: Stanley F, Alberman E (eds): *The Epidemiology of the Cerebral Palsies*. Philadelphia, Lippincott, 1984.

Persinger MA: MMPI profiles of normal people who display frequent temporal lobe signs. *Percept Mot Skills* 64:1112, 1987.

Pleak R, Birmaher B, Gavrilescu A, et al: Case study: Mania & neuropsychiatric excitation following carbamazepine. *J Am Acad Child Adolesc Psychiatry* 27:500, 1988.

Reynolds E: Antiepileptic drugs and psychopathology. In: Trimble M (ed): *The Psychopharmacology of Epilepsy*. New York, Wiley, 1985, p. 490.

Riccardi VM: The multiple forms of childhood neurofibromatosis. *Pediatr Rev* 3:293, 1982.

Richardson SA: The social environment and individual functioning. In: Birch HG (ed): *Brain Damage in Children: The Biological and Social Aspects*. Baltimore, Williams & Wilkins, 1964, p. 100.

Rorke LB: Classification and grading of childhood brain tumors: Overview and statement of the problem. *Cancer* 56:1848, 1985.

Rothman JG: Understanding order of movement in youngsters with cerebral palsy. *Percept Mot Skills* 65:391, 1987.

Rubinstein B, Shaffer D: Organicity in child psychiatry: Signs, symptoms and syndromes. *Psychiatr Clin North Am* 8:755, 1985.

Rutter M, Graham P, Yule W: *A Neuropsychiatric Study in Childhood (Clinics in Developmental Medicine, nos. 35/36)*. London, Spastics International Medical Publications, 1970.

Rutter M, Tizard J, Yule W, et al: Research report: Isle of Wight studies, 1964–1974. *Psychol Med* 6:313, 1976.

Scherzer AL, Tscharnuter I: *Early Diagnosis and Therapy in Cerebral Palsy: A Primer on Infant Developmental Problems*. New York, Marcel Dekker, 1982.

Schorer CE: Muscular dystrophy and the mind. *Psychosom Med* 26:5, 1964.

Schwarcz R, Foster AC, French ED, et al: Excitotoxic models for neurodegenerative disorders. *Life Sci* 35:19, 1984.

Seidenberg M, Beck N, Geisser M, et al: Academic achievement of children with epilepsy. *Epilepsia* 27:753, 1986.

Shapiro BK, Wachtel RC, Palmer FB, et al: Associated dysfunctions. In: Thompson GH, Rubin IL, Bilenker RM (eds): *Comprehensive Management of Cerebral Palsy*, New York, Grune & Stratton, 1983.

Shere E, Kastenbaum R: Mother-child interaction in cerebral palsy: Environmental and psychological obstacles to cognitive development. *Genet Psychol Monogr* 73:255, 1966.

Shope J: Compliance in children and adults: Review of studies. *Epilepsy Res Suppl* 1:23, 1988.

Siebelink BM, Bakker D, Binnie D, et al: Psychological effects of subclinical epileptiform EEG discharge in children. II: General intelligence tests. *Epilepsy Res* 2:117, 1988.

Sillanpaa M: Social adjustment and functioning of chronically ill and impaired children and adolescents. *Acta Pediatr Scand Suppl* 340:1, 1987.

Sollee ND, Latham EE, Kinden DJ, et al: Neuropsychological impairment in Duchenne muscular dystrophy. *J Exp Neuropsychol* 7:486, 1985.

Stewart JT, Myers WC, Burket RC, et al: A review of the pharmacotherapy of aggression in children and adolescents. *J Am Acad Child Adolesc Psychiatry* 29(2):269–277, 1990.

Stores G: Problems of learning and behavior in children with epilepsy. In: Reynolds E, Trimble M (eds): *Epilepsy and Psychiatry*. Edinburgh, Churchill Livingstone, 1981, p. 33.

Swaiman KF: *Pediatric Neurology: Principles and Practice* (2nd ed). St. Louis, Mosby, 1994.

Templin SW, Howard JA, O'Connor MJ: Self concept of young children with cerebral palsy. *Dev Med Child Neurol* 23:730, 1981.

Trimble M: The psychoses of epilepsy and their treatment. In: Trimble M (ed): *The Psychopharmacology of Epilepsy*. New York, Wiley, 1985.

Trimble M: Anticonvulsant drugs and cognitive function: A review of the literature. *Epilepsia* 28 (suppl 3):37, 1987.

Varnhagen CK, Lewin S, Das JP, et al: Neurofibromatosis and psychological processes. *J Dev Behav Pediatr* 9:257, 1988.

Victorian Infant Collaborative Study Group: Eight-year outcome in infants with birth weight of 500–999 grams: Continuing regional study of 1979 and 1980 births. *J Pediatr* 118(5):761–767, 1991.

Voorhies TM: Cognitive and behavioral effects of antiepileptic drugs. *Semin Neurol* 8:35, 1988.

Walczak TS, Williams DT, Berten W: Utility and reliability of placebo infusion in the evaluation of patients with seizures. *Neurology* 44:394–399, 1994.

Whelen TB: Neuropsychological performance of children with Duchenne muscular dystrophy and spinal muscle atrophy. *Dev Med Child Neurol* 29: 212, 1987.

Whitman S, Hermann B, Black R: Psychopathology and seizure type in children with epilepsy. *Psychol Med* 12:843, 1982.

Wiener JW (ed): *Diagnosis and Psychopharmacology of Childhood and Adolescent Disorders*. New York, Wiley, 1985.

Williams DT: The treatment of seizures: Special psychotherapeutic and psychobiological techniques. In: Sands H (ed): *Epilepsy: A Handbook for the Mental Health Professional*. New York, Brunner/Mazel, 1982, p. 58.

Williams DT, Hirsch G: The somatizing disorders: Somatoform disorders, factitious disorders and malingering. In: Kestenbaum C, Williams D (eds): *Handbook of Clinical Assessment of Children Ado-*

lescents (Vol 2). New York, New York University Press, 1988, p. 743.

Williams DT, Mostofsky D: Psychogenic seizures in childhood and adolescence. In: Riley T, Roy A (eds): *Pseudoseizures*. Baltimore, Williams & Wilkins, 1982, p. 169.

Williams DT, Gold AK, Shrout P, et al: The impact of psychiatric intervention on patients with uncontrolled seizures. *J Nerv Ment Dis* 167:626, 1979.

Williams DT, Mehl R, Yudofsky S, et al: The effect of propranolol on uncontrolled rage outbursts in children and adolescents with organic brain dysfunction. *J Am Acad Child Psychiatry* 21:129, 1982.

Williams DT, Pleak R, Hanesian H: Neuropsychiatric disorders of childhood and adolescence. In: Hales R, Yudofsky S (eds): *The American Psychiatric Press Textbook of Neuropsychiatry*. Washington, DC, American Psychiatric Press, 1987, p. 365.

Williams DT, Spiegel H, Mostofsky D: Neurogenic and hysterical seizures in children and adolescents. *Am J Psychiatry* 135:82, 1978.

Williams DT, Walczak TS, Berten W, et al: Psychogenic seizures. In: Mostofsky D, Loyning Y (eds): *The Neurobehavioral Treatment of Epilepsy*. Hillsdale, NJ, Erlbaum, 1993, p. 83.

Witte RA: The psychological impact of a progressive physical handicap and terminal illness (Duchenne muscular dystrophy) on adolescents and their families. *Br J Med Psychol* 58:179, 1985.

Woroblewski BA, McColgan K, Smith K, et al: The incidence of seizures during tricyclic antidepressant drug treatment in a brain-injured population. *J Clin Psychopharmacol* 10:124–128, 1980.

60 MOOD DISORDERS

Elizabeth B. Weller, M.D., Ronald A. Weller, M.D., and Hratch Svadjian, M.D.

Depression and mania have been reported in children and adolescents for many years (Weller and Weller, 1984). However, many doubted their existence because it was felt that children, for theoretical reasons such as "immature personality structures," could not experience extremes of mood (Schulterbrandt and Raskin, 1977).

Mood disorders can be classified into two major types: unipolar depressive disorders and bipolar disorders. Each in turn may be further subclassified (Table 60.1). In DSM-IV the diagnostic criteria for these disorders are similar for children, adolescents, and adults. In this chapter bipolar disorders and unipolar disorders are discussed separately.

BIPOLAR DISORDERS

Definition

According to DSM-IV, the essential feature of a manic episode is an elevated, expansive, or irritable mood, lasting at least 1 week (or any duration if hospitalization is required). This mood is also accompanied by at least three (or four when the mood is only irritable) of the following:

1. Inflated self-esteem or grandiosity;
2. Decreased need for sleep;
3. Increased talkativeness or pressure to keep talking;
4. Racing thoughts or flight of ideas;
5. Distractibility;
6. Increased activity or psychomotor agitation;

7. Excessive involvement in pleasurable activities that have high potential for painful consequences.

To diagnose mania, two additional factors must be considered. First, the disturbance should be severe enough to cause impairment in school or occupational functioning or in peer or family relations or necessitate hospitalization to avoid harming self or others. Second, a manic episode should not be diagnosed if it results from the use of a substance (e.g., a drug of abuse), medication (e.g., antidepressant), electroconvulsive therapy, or is secondary to a general medical condition. A manic episode can be rated mild, moderate, or severe. The presence or absence of psychotic symptoms should be specified. It should also be noted if the patient is in complete or partial remission. In DSM-IV, a hypomanic episode meets all the criteria of a manic episode, except marked impairment necessitating hospitalization. However, the episode should be associated with a clear change in functioning and, together with the change in mood, should be observable by others. In addition, the symptoms should last at least 4 days.

When the clinical presentation is a mixture of both mania and depression, a mixed episode can be diagnosed. Symptom criteria for both manic episode and major depressive episode should be met for a duration of at least 1 week. Bipolar disorders are subclassified as follows (Table 60.1).

Bipolar I Disorder, Single Manic Episode

This disorder presents with a current manic episode and the absence of past manic or major depressive episodes.

Table 60.1. Mood Disorders in Children and Adolescents per DSM-IV

Bipolar Disorders	Depressive Disorders
Bipolar I disorder	Major depressive disorder
Single manic episode	Single episode
Most recent episode hypomanic	Recurrent episode
Most recent episode manic	Dysthymic disorder
Most recent episode mixed	Early onset
Most recent episode depressed	Late onset
Most recent episode unspecified	
Bipolar II disorder	Depressive disorder not otherwise
Most recent episode hypomanic	specified
Most recent episode depressed	
Cyclothymic disorder	
Bipolar disorder not otherwise	
specified	

Specify for manic and depressive episodes

Mild, moderate

Severe with or without psychotic features { Mood congruent / Mood incongruent }

In partial or full remission
Unspecified

Course specifiers for above categories
Chronic (applies to major depressive episode in depressive and bipolar disorders)
With rapid cycling (applies to bipolar disorders)
With seasonal pattern (applies to bipolar and major depressive disorders)
With postpartum onset

Symptom features
With melancholic features (applies to depressive episodes in depressive or bipolar disorders)
With atypical features (applies to depressive episodes in depressive or bipolar disorders)
With catatonic features (applies to manic or major depressive episodes)

Bipolar I Disorder, Most Recent Episode Manic

In this subtype, there should be a current manic episode and at least one manic episode, major depressive episode, or mixed episode in the past.

Bipolar I Disorder, Most Recent Episode Hypomanic

This disorder represents a current episode of hypomania with at least one previous manic episode or mixed episode.

Bipolar I Disorder, Most Recent Episode Depressed

This subtype is diagnosed when a patient presents with a current episode of depression, but has a history of one or more manic or mixed episodes.

Bipolar I Disorder, Most Recent Episode Mixed

To diagnose this subtype, a current mixed episode is required in addition to at least one previous major depressive disorder, manic episode, or mixed episode.

Bipolar II Disorder

Requirements for the diagnosis of this subclass include one or more current or past hypomanic and major depressive episodes with symptoms severe enough to cause significant distress or impairment in important areas of functioning. Additionally, no history of manic or mixed episodes should be present.

Cyclothymic Disorder

In cyclothymic disorder, numerous hypomanic episodes occur over a period of at least 1 year. These hypomanic episodes meet all criteria for mania, except marked impairment is not present. Additionally, numerous periods of depressed mood or loss of interest or pleasure that did not

meet all the criteria for a major depressive episode occur over the same time period. Also, the absence of a major depressive episode, a mixed episode, or a manic episode during the first year of the disturbance is required. Klein et al. (1986) reported that 24% of the offspring of bipolar patients and 0% of the offspring of control subjects had cyclothymia as detected by the General Behavioral Inventory (GBI), which had excellent correlation with the interview-derived diagnosis.

Bipolar Disorder Not Otherwise Specified

In DSM-IV this diagnostic classification includes disorders that have manic features or hypomanic features that do not meet the criteria for any specific bipolar disorder as described above. Examples of these disorders would include a manic episode that was superimposed on schizophrenia or a delusional disorder, or recurrent hypomanic episodes, but no intercurrent depression.

For all the above categories, the diagnoses should not be made if the disturbance can be explained by schizoaffective disorder or (excepting bipolar disorder, not otherwise specified) superimposed on schizophrenia, schizophreniform disorder, delusional disorder or psychotic disorder not otherwise specified. Further information and explanation of the diagnostic criteria for bipolar disorders and details regarding diagnostic subtypes can be obtained from DSM-IV.

Historical Note

Reports of mania in children have been made by several prominent psychiatrists over the years, including Esquirol (1845), Kraepelin (1921), Bleuler (1934), and Kasanin (1931). Kraepelin felt that mania was rare in children but that the incidence increased by adolescence. He reported that approximately 0.5% of his manic patients had their first episode at age 10 or younger. However, some child and adolescent psychiatrists, such as Kanner (1960) and Anthony and Scott (1960), doubted its existence. Anthony and Scott developed and applied very stringent criteria to diagnose mania in a study of psychiatrically ill children. They concluded mania was very rare in children. However, they described a patient who appeared manic as a child who subsequently had his mania confirmed when followed as a young adult.

Davis (1979) developed criteria to diagnose mania in children. However, these criteria were very nonspecific, including minimal brain dysfunction, enuresis, and EEG anomalies. He called this syndrome "manic depressive variant syndrome."

More recently, others have diagnosed bipolar disorders in children and adolescents using adult-type criteria slightly adjusted to children's different maturational levels (Carlson and Strober, 1978; Weinberg and Brumback, 1976; Weller et al., 1986c). Weller et al. (1986c) conducted an extensive review of all available case reports of psychotic or severely disturbed children by blindly reviewing cases to determine how many, if any, met DSM-III criteria for mania. From 1809 to 1982, 157 case reports were reviewed independently by the authors. In doing so they noted that 50% of children who satisfied DSM-III criteria for mania had been previously reported as having conduct disorder, attention deficit hyperactivity disorder, or schizophrenia. This finding suggests that mania may have been previously underdiagnosed in children and adolescents.

Prevalence and Epidemiology

Bipolar disorder occurs in 1% of adults. Males and females are equally afflicted. The epidemiological catchment area studies done on 10,000 young adults 18–24 years old in New Haven, Baltimore, and St. Louis reported a prevalence of 0.6–1% for manic episode (Robins et al., 1984).

Carlson and Kashani (1988a) studied a community sample of 150 adolescents, 14–16 years old, from Columbia, Missouri, using structured diagnostic interviews to ascertain a diagnosis of mania. They reported that 14% satisfied criteria for mania if duration was not taken into account; 7.5% of adolescents met criteria for mania if severity was not taken into account. However, when severity and duration were both taken into account, only 0.6% were diagnosed manic.

As yet there are no published epidemiologic studies of mania in prepubertal children. Since World War II the prevalence of mood disorders, including mania and depression as well as schizoaffective disorders, has been increasing (Gershon et al., 1987; Klerman et al., 1985). This observation has come to be known as the cohort effect. A recent study describes a parallel increase of affective disorders in children and adolescents (Ryan et al., 1992). If this trend continues, it can be anticipated that more children and adolescents will manifest mania in the years to come.

Clinical Description

Manic adolescents often have a clinical presentation similar to that of adults. Symptoms such as elated mood or irritability, push of speech, flight of ideas, grandiosity, sleeplessness, and bizarre behavior including bizarre attire are typically observed.

Carlson (1983) analyzed in detail how symptom patterns vary by age. She concluded that younger manic children (less than 9 years) present with irritability and emotional lability, while older children present with euphoria, elation, paranoia, and grandiose delusions. Hyperactivity, push of speech, and distractibility were present in both age groups. Similarly, DeLong and Aldershof (1987) suggest prepubertal bipolar children begin their illness with cycles in which dysphoria, hypomania, and agitation are commonly intermixed. The extremes of depression and manic excitement become more common with the onset of puberty.

There is also evidence that psychotic symptoms are more common in manics whose age of onset is in adolescence than in those whose age of onset is after age 30 (Ballenger et al., 1982).

CASE ILLUSTRATION

J.R. was 6 years old when he was referred for inpatient treatment by a physician in a day hospital program because J.R.'s behavior could no longer be tolerated. He presented with extreme hyperactivity and push of speech (including profanities and sexual comments in which he invited the female staff to have sex with him). After a careful evaluation, sexual abuse was ruled out. Previous treatment with Mellaril, Thorazine, Navane, Ritalin, Cylert, Dexedrine, and clonidine had been unsuccessful. He was silly and giggly. He made up songs and punned and had clang associations. He spoke so fast it was hard to follow his thoughts. He thought he was Superman and could fly. He ran in front of cars, thinking he could stop them. An interview with his parents revealed that this child's father had been involved in legal trouble and had been jailed on several occasions. The father had been diagnosed as bipolar by the referring physician, who felt the father was medicating himself with psychoactive drugs. The father had stopped abusing drugs and had started on lithium, with dramatic improvement. His early history was very similar to J.R.'s current clinical presentation. J.R. was given a trial of lithium carbonate, and he responded fairly well. He was easier to manage and direct and was able to attend school.

CASE ILLUSTRATION

B.J. was 13 years old when he presented to the emergency room of a pediatric hospital. His chief complaint was "I wanted to take the dog for a walk last night and went to Six Flags (an amusement park) to go to the bathroom!" His speech was very difficult to interrupt. He had paranoid thoughts that his friend and classmates were after him and making fun of him. He also talked about "pumping up my BB gun 10 times before pulling the trigger and slashing my wrists because I want to die." He talked about "wanting to be born over and over again." He was calling his female classmates and asking them to have sex with him and also "wanted to go to the desert to hunt lions." He was refusing to eat and had slept only 2–3 hours per night for 3 days. He paced constantly and made fun of the resident in the emergency room. His maternal grandmother had

depression, and a maternal uncle had been put in detention for behavior similar to this when he was an adolescent.

He reported he came to the hospital to make a death movie, and he was hearing male and female voices telling him to grow up and "to cut it off." When asked what "to cut it off" meant, he replied, "My penis." He had been involved in oral sex for the last month, and he thought this was a punishment. He thought he could fly and make people blind by staring at them. Drug use was denied, and a drug screen was negative. Treatment with Mellaril 200 mg subdued him somewhat. The family refused a trial of lithium carbonate, as their pediatrician was worried about its possible long-term side effects.

Etiology and Pathogenesis

Numerous etiologies have been considered in mania. The major hypotheses are briefly discussed.

PSYCHOANALYTIC THEORY

In psychoanalytic theory, mania is a reaction formation to depression. It is described as a defense against depression that involves a defensive projection where the patient focuses on the weaknesses of others to avoid thinking of his or her own weaknesses.

BIOLOGICAL THEORIES

Genetics

There are three lines of evidence from adult studies that point to the genetic nature of mania. Nurnberger and Gershon (1982) reported the concordance of mania in monozygotic twins to be 65%, whereas concordance is 14% in dizygotic twins. Mendlewicz and Rainer (1977) found that 31% of biological parents of adopted manic probands were affected, whereas only 2% of adoptive parents manifested the illness. Finally, a study of the relatives of bipolar subjects by Rice et al. (1987) showed a 1.5–10.2% incidence of bipolar disorder compared with an incidence of 0.2–1.8% in relatives of normal control subjects. Recently (1993) a multicenter pilot study done by the National Institute of Mental Health Molecular Genetics of Psychiatric Disorders Initiative Group found an increase in lifetime probability of developing affective disorders (bipolar, major depression, or dysthymia) with the number of affected parents who had high density of affective disorder in extended families. The corresponding percentages were 16.7, 23.5, and 100% for 0, 1, and 2 affected parents, respectively. Although such studies are suggestive, methodological issues limit their generalizability, and further studies are needed to further clarify the role of genetics in the etiology of mania.

In studying the parents of bipolar children and adolescents, several investigators reported an increased incidence of both unipolar and bipolar disorders (DeLong and Aldershof, 1987; Strober et al., 1988; Varanka et al., 1988). Further, if onset of illness is in the prepubertal years, the rate of bipolar disorder in family members is three times that of those with an onset after puberty (Strober et al., 1988).

Chromosomal studies in bipolar adults have suggested a possible affliction of X chromosomes, a shortened arm on chromosome 11, and other genetic defects (Carlson, 1990). However, such studies must be regarded as preliminary, and confirmation of their findings is needed. Detailed chromosomal studies of well-defined bipolar children and adolescents are lacking.

Neuroendocrine Changes

Although neuroendocrine changes in depression have been well documented, studies of neuroendocrine changes in bipolar disorder are lacking by comparison. Perhaps this is due in part to the increased difficulty in obtaining the patient's cooperation with such studies. In some adult studies neuroendocrine abnormalities have been documented (Baldessarini, 1983). As yet there are no published studies of neuroendocrine changes in children and adolescents with mania.

FAMILIAL, ENVIRONMENTAL, AND SOCIAL INFLUENCES

As demonstrated earlier, mania tends to run in families. In examining child-rearing practices of manic parents, many have poor parenting techniques (Cytryn et al., 1986). The episodic nature of the unreasonable behavior of these parents may be deleterious to the normal development of these children.

Individuals born after 1940 seem to be at an increased risk for developing both unipolar and bipolar mood disorders and schizoaffective disorders (Gershon et al., 1987; Klerman et al., 1985) (the cohort effect). The reasons for this observed increase in affective disorders in this group is not yet known. It has been postulated that environment and genes interact in some fashion to produce this cohort effect.

Laboratory Studies

There are no specific laboratory studies that will diagnose bipolar disorder in children and adolescents.

Psychoeducational Tests

Paper and pencil tests are currently being developed for use in diagnosing manic disorders. The Structured Diagnostic Interview for Children and Adolescents, Revised (DICA-R) (W. Reich and Z. Welner, unpublished manuscript, 1988), as well as the Schedule of Affective Disorders and Schizophrenia–Child Version (KSADS) (Chambers et al., 1985) have sections devoted to assessing bipolar disorders.

Unfortunately, rating scales to assess the severity of bipolar disorders are quite underdeveloped at the present time. Strober et al. (1987) used the Beigel Murphy Scale (Beigel et al., 1971) in assessing severity of mania in a adolescents and reported the instrument to be quite helpful. Fristad et al. (1988) modified the Mania Rating Scale (Young et al., 1978) for use in prepubertal manic children. A preliminary study found it was helpful in differentiating manic children from hyperactive children on the total score as well as on most individual items.

Differential Diagnosis

In diagnosing a manic episode, other psychiatric and medical illnesses should be excluded. Medical conditions (Table 60.2) may mimic mania, and patients with several other psychiatric illnesses can at times appear manic.

MEDICAL CONDITION

Drugs

One should not make the diagnosis of mania until the child and/or adolescent is observed in a drug-free state. Some of the drugs that have been reported to induce manic states include amphetamines, corticosteroids, sympathomimetics, isoniazid, and antidepressants.

Endocrine Disorders

Hyperthyroidism may present with a manic-like state.

Neurologic Conditions

Mania has been associated with head trauma, multiple sclerosis, stroke (especially with lesions involving the right hemisphere and the thalamus), and seizure disorders with a left temporal focus. Also, space-occupying lesions such as meningiomas, gliomas, and metastatic lesions in the thalamus have been implicated (Wise and Rundell, 1988).

PSYCHIATRIC CONDITIONS

Attention Deficit Disorder with Hyperactivity

Cross-sectionally, children with attention deficit disorder with hyperactivity (ADHD) may appear to resemble those with mania, especially in the prepubertal age range. However, manic children have more affect and are euphoric or irritable. Children with ADHD often have low self-esteem and a much longer duration of symptoms. Psychotic symptoms are common in prepubertal manic children (Varanka et al., 1988) but should not be part of ADHD. Age of onset for mania is usually after 7, while age of onset for ADHD is usually in the toddler years.

Conduct Disorder

Conduct disorder is frequently a comorbid condition with bipolar disorder. Many children with mania have unruly, disruptive behavior suggestive of a conduct disorder. However, children with a ''pure'' conduct disorder do not have push of speech, flight of ideas, or delusions of grandeur. Also, the duration of symptoms is more chronic and less suggestive of an abrupt onset or clearly episodic course. A study done by Weller et al. (1986c) found that children who clearly satisfied criteria for mania were sometimes diagnosed as having conduct disorder. Special attention should be paid to rule out mania in prepubertal children presenting with drug abuse.

Drug and Alcohol Abuse or Dependency

Children and adolescents with mood disorders sometimes become involved with the use of alcohol or drugs in an attempt to treat symptoms attributable to their mood disorder. Most adolescents have easy access to drugs and alcohol.

Schizophrenia

Symptoms such as hallucinations and delusions are common in both mania and schizophrenia. Usually the onset of schizophrenia is insidious, while mania is more sudden in onset. Both schizophrenic and manic adolescents can be delusional, and at times it may be difficult to differentiate paranoid schizophrenia from mania. Assessment of premorbid personality may be helpful in differentiating the two disorders. In schizophrenia there may be either schizoid traits or bizarre conduct disorder, while in mania there may be symptoms suggestive of ADHD or conduct disorder with significant affective symptomatology. A positive family history for bipolar disorder is more common in manic adolescents than in schizophrenic adolescents (Strober et al., 1988).

Treatment

After a diagnosis of mania has been established following a thorough assessment, treatment must be planned and implemented. Psychotherapeutic and pharmacological intervention may be required in children. It is difficult to treat a full-blown manic episode on an outpatient basis.

Table 60.2. Medical Conditions Mimicking Mania in Children and Adolescents

Infections	Endocrine	Neurologic	Tumors	Medications	Others
Encephalitis	Hyperthyroidism	Seizures	Thalamic	Steroids	Alcohol abuse
Influenza		Head trauma	Gliomas	Isoniazid	Drug abuse
Syphilis		Multiple sclerosis	Meningiomas	Sympathomimetics	Amphetamines
AIDS		Stroke			Hallucinogens
		Wilson's disease			Anemia
					Hemodialysis

Adapted from Wise MG, Rundell JR: *Concise Guide to Consultation Psychiatry*. Washington, DC, American Psychiatric Press, 1988.

Table 60.3.   Pretreatment Screen for Mood Disorders in Children and Adolescents

Name: _____ Date: _____ Ht _____ (cm)
DOB: _____ Age: _____ Sex: _____ (0 = Male; 1 = Female) Wt _____ (kg)
Ordered by: _____ Unit: _____ (1 = Child; 2 = Adol; 3 = Out pt.)
CBC w/Diff: WBC _____ HMG _____ HCT _____ RBC _____ HMC _____ MCV _____ MCH _____ MCHC _____
RDW _____ Total Neutrophil _____ SEG _____ LYM _____ MON _____ EO _____ BASO _____ PLTS _____
Electrolytes: Na _____ K _____ Cl _____ CO_2 _____ Ca _____ Mg _____
BUN _____ Cr _____ Glucose _____
ALT(SGPT) _____ AST(SGOT) _____ LD(LDH) _____ Bilirubin: Dir _____ Indir _____ Total _____
Alk Phosphatase (B) _____ Alk Phosphatase _____ CPK _____
Triglycerides _____ Cholesterol _____
Total Protein _____ Albumin _____
T_3RU _____ T_4(RIA) _____ T_3(RIA) _____ TSH _____
Lead _____

For Affective Disorders
Cortisol: Baseline 8am _____ 4pm _____ Dex dose _____ (mg) Post-dex 8am _____ 4pm _____
When Indicated
ECG: H-R _____ P-R _____ QRS _____ Axis _____ Normal (Y/N) _____ If abnormal, note: _____

EEG: Normal (Y/N) _____ If abnormal, note: _____

URINE: Pre-LiCO$_3$
Creatinine Clearance _____ Urine Osmolality _____

Hospitalization is often essential to ensure patient safety. In the hospital, firm limits must be set with the patient. Arguments, challenges, or questions regarding a patient's delusional system should be avoided until the medications take effect and the patient is more amenable to other therapeutic interventions. It is essential to educate parents and children about bipolar illness. Support groups organized through the Association of the Mentally Ill (AMI) are available in certain communities and can be of help to some patients and their families.

Several baseline laboratory studies need to be done prior to starting a child on lithium carbonate or any other psychotropic medication that can affect many organ systems. For example, lithium affects the neuroendocrine, central nervous, reproductive, and gastrointestinal systems.

A good pre-lithium workup should include a complete blood count (CBC) with a differential (Table 60.3), because lithium can cause neutrophilia, and carbamazepine, a mood-stabilizing medication sometimes used in lithium nonresponders or rapid cyclers, may cause suppression of white blood cells.

Electrolytes, blood urea nitrogen (BUN), creatinine, creatinine clearance, urine osmolality, and liver function tests should be performed. Lithium is known to affect serum electrolytes, especially sodium. Also, lithium may affect kidney function tests; hence a baseline creatinine clearance as well as urine osmolality should be determined and repeated periodically if lithium treatment will last more than 6 months. Liver function tests should be done in cases where lithium will be augmented with Tegretol.

Thyroid function tests are required since lithium can alter thyroid function. Hypothyroidism is the most common abnormality. Since a hypothyroid person may also look depressed, baseline measurements of thyroid stimulating hormone (TSH) (most sensitive) and thyroxine (T_4) _and_ triiodothyronine resin uptake (T_3RU) should be measured prior to lithium initiation and should be repeated periodically throughout treatment.

A pregnancy test and serologic tests (for syphilis and AIDS) should be performed, especially in sexually active adolescents. Hypomanic and manic persons are known for their hypersexuality; they may engage in multiple sexual partnerships in an indiscriminate manner. Pregnancy must be ruled out, as lithium has been associated with some teratogenic effects, particularly involving the development of the heart and blood vessels.

Before treating a manic child or adolescent with lithium or other medication, consent from the family and assent from the patient should be obtained and known side effects should be explained. The most common side effects of lithium are gastrointestinal upset, nausea, overeating,

Table 60.4.   Lithium Protocol

A. Administer dosage according to chart below.
B. Take blood levels 12 hours after last dose (8:00 AM _before_ morning dose) every other day (M, W, F) until _two consecutive_ levels appear in the therapeutic range (0.6–1.2 mEq/liter). If no clinical improvement is seen, increase dose to reach 1.4 mEq/liter.
C. Administer Slide Effects Rating Sclae and Mania Rating Scale weekly.

wt (kg)	8 AM	Dosage (mg)		
		12 noon	8 PM	Total Daily
15–25	150	150	300	600
25–40	300	300	300	900
40–50	300	300	600 *	1200
50–60	600	300	600	1500

*_CAUTION:_ In dealing with organic or retarded children, go with lower doses.

Adapted from Weller EB, Weller RA, Fristad MA: Lithium dosage guide for prepubertal children: A preliminary report. _J Am Acad Child Psychiatry_ 25:92–95, 1986.

weight gain, enuresis, tremor, and acne. Diarrhea is sometimes an early sign of toxicity. Seizures may occur with lithium overdose. Children and adolescents often tolerate lithium carbonate better than adults do. Lithium levels of 0.6–1.2 mEq/liter are well tolerated. If there is no response at that level, the level might be increased up to 1.4 mEq/liter with careful monitoring and in the absence of significant side effects (Table 60.4). Weller et al. (1986a, 1986b) have developed a dosing schedule based on weight so that a child can be started on lithium and reach a therapeutic level quickly. Children who have CNS impairment or mental retardation may be particularly sensitive to side effects from lithium and may have difficulty achieving a therapeutic effect.

Other medications have been less well studied in manic children and adolescents (Table 60.5). Carbamazepine (Tegretol) has been used in bipolar adults who are rapid cyclers or who have not responded to therapeutic levels of lithium. Tegretol must be used carefully, as it is known to cause bone marrow suppression with clinically significant neutropenia. Often sore throat and fever are the first warning signs of a seriously low neutrophil count. Usually Tegretol is started at 200 mg twice daily (15–30 mg/kg) and increased every 4th day. Therapeutic plasma levels are 5–11 mEq/liter. Biweekly blood counts to evaluate possible bone marrow suppression should be obtained for 3 months, watching for bone marrow suppression. There are no double-blind placebo-controlled studies of manic children or adolescents on Tegretol.

Valproic acid has been used in patients not responding to lithium or

Table 60.5. Mood-Stabilizing Drugs in Children and Adolescents

	Dose (mg/kg/day)	Blood Levels (mEq/liter)	Side Effects
Lithium	30 (see outline)	0.6–1.4	CNS Gastrointestinal Endocrine Genitourinary
Carbamazepine	15–30	3–11	CNS Gastrointestinal Bone marrow suppression
Valproic acid	25–60	50–120	Gastrointestinal Hepatotoxicity
Clonazepam	0.03–0.1	0.02–0.07	CNS Behavior problems

Adapted from Carlson G: Treatment of mania in children and adolescents. Paper presented at the Midwinter Institute of the Academy of Child and Adolescent Psychiatry, Orlando, FL, 1989.

Tegretol. A starting dose of 250 mg twice daily may be used and increased gradually to a dose not to exceed 25–60 mg/kg/day. Blood levels between 50 and 120 mg/liter are advocated in adults. However, no controlled studies in children or adolescents have been published. The most common side effects are nausea, vomiting, and anorexia. Since hepatotoxicity has been reported, periodic liver function tests are necessary.

Clonazepam has also been reported to be useful in treating adult manics. Dosage is typically 0.03–0.1 mg/kg/day. Irritability, sedation, and behavioral problems may occur. As Clonazepam is potentially addictive, lengthy treatment may require gradual withdrawal of the medication over a period of as long as 3 months (G.A. Carlson, unpublished data presented at the Midyear Institute of the Academy of Child and Adolescent Psychiatry, Orlando, FL, 1989).

Electroconvulsive therapy (ECT) has been reported to treat severe bipolar disorder in children and adolescents. In a literature review, Bertangoli and Borchardt (1990) report that the few systematic studies were done before the early 1950s and that since that time only individual cases have been reported. Data concerning safety and efficacy of ECT in children are sparse. ECT can be considered when other modalities have failed or are unsafe. The American Psychiatric Association (1990) has published specific guidelines regarding indications for, procedures of obtaining consent for, and administration of ECT treatments. Before referring children for ECT, two psychiatrists experienced in treating children and who are not otherwise involved with the case should agree with the recommendation for ECT.

Outcome and Follow-up Data

Several studies have been reported on follow-up data involving adolescent-onset mania. Landolt (1957) reported after 18 years of follow-up that 17% of patients with adolescent onset of mania had recovered, while 50% had had a poor outcome. Data on the rest were inadequate to make a decision as to outcome. Olsen (1961) reported on 28 adolescents with a mean age of onset of 15–16 years. He divided his group into those who had had an acute onset and those with childhood psychopathology. A 25-year follow-up revealed a good outcome for 33% of the first group, whereas only 15% in the second group had a good outcome. Hudgens (1974) and Weiner et al. (1979) reported the outcomes for their adolescent patients with mania to be social disability, substance abuse, multiple suicide attempts, and completed suicide. Carlson et al. (1977) have reported that 60% of subjects studied had a good social outcome, 20% had significant impairment, and 25% were chronically ill, in a 20-year follow-up of adolescents with mania.

Another study that has reported good outcome in adolescents with mania was by McGlashen (1988), who reported on 35 subjects. He divided this sample into two groups: those with onset prior to and those with onset after age 20. Patients with the earlier age of onset had more psychiatric symptoms and trouble with the law, and 70% had "psychotic

assaultiveness." However, there was no difference in the suicide rate or frequency of hospitalizations between the two groups. Also, those with earlier onset performed significantly better regarding work and frequency of social contacts.

Strober et al. (1990) in a naturalistic follow-up study found that adolescents who continued their lithium carbonate treatment had fewer relapses than those who stopped the treatment, which suggests that lithium has a role to play in preventing relapses.

Research Directions

The 1990s should see continued increased interest in studying bipolar disorder in children and adolescents. Emphasis should be on refining existing instruments, such as the DICA and the KSADS, to avoid the high false-positive rates they give for mania. New instruments should be developed, such as the Mania Rating Scale (MRS) by Fristad et al. (1992), which may differentiate mania from other psychiatric disorders. If age-appropriate assessment of mania can lead to more accurate diagnosis, then double-blind placebo-controlled medication trials can be more successfully carried out. Newer therapies based on appropriate biological and psychological theories should also be better evaluated. Studies of children and adolescents at high risk for bipolar disorder (i.e., the offspring of mood-disordered adults) may provide useful information in the prevention of these disorders.

Implementation and completion of such studies should shed more light on the etiology, presentation, and treatment of bipolar children and adolescents.

DEPRESSIVE DISORDERS

The DSM-IV defines a major depressive episode as a syndrome in which at least five of the following symptoms have been present during the same 2-week period:

1. Depressed or irritable mood;
2. Diminished interest or loss of pleasure in almost all activities;
3. Sleep disturbance;
4. Weight change or appetite disturbance (failure to achieve expected weight gain in children or 5% loss of body weight in month);
5. Decreased concentration or indecisiveness;
6. Suicidal ideation or thoughts of death;
7. Psychomotor agitation or retardation;
8. Fatigue or loss of energy;
9. Feelings of worthlessness or inappropriate guilt.

At least one of the symptoms must be diminished interest/pleasure or depressed mood. The symptoms must cause significant distress or impairment of functioning in social, occupational, or other important areas. The syndrome should not have been precipitated by the direct action of a substance or the result of a medical condition and should not be better explained by bereavement or schizoaffective disorder. Also, a major depressive episode should not be superimposed on schizophrenia, schizophreniform disorder, delusional disorder, or a psychotic disorder not otherwise specified (Table 60.1).

The disorder can be rated as mild, moderate, or severe, and with or without psychotic symptoms that can be mood congruent or incongruent. It can also be noted to be in full or partial remission. When the episode has lasted 2 consecutive years, the depression should be diagnosed as chronic.

A depression may also be determined to have melancholic features. Either a loss of pleasure in almost all activities or a lack of reactivity to usually pleasurable stimuli should be present.

Additionally at least three of the following are required:

1. A quality of depressed mood that is distinctly different from the kind felt when a loved one is deceased;
2. Depression worse in the morning;
3. Waking up 2 hours earlier than usual;
4. Observable psychomotor retardation or agitation;

5. Significant weight loss or anorexia;
6. Excessive or inappropriate guilt.

Depressive or manic episodes can also present with catatonic features requiring at least two of the following as delineated in DSM-IV.

1. Motoric immobility in the form of catalepsy or stupor;
2. Motor overactivity that seems purposeless and not in response to external stimuli;
3. Extreme negativism or mutism;
4. Voluntary movement peculiarities such as posturing, grimacing, stereotypy, and mannerisms;
5. Echolalia or echopraxia.

The seasonality of mood disorders can also be specified. To diagnose a seasonal mood disorder, there should be a regular temporal relationship between depression, mania, and a particular period of the year. A full remission or switching from depression to mania should occur within that characteristic time of the year. An individual should manifest at least two episodes of mood disturbance in the last 2 years. Finally, seasonal episodes should substantially outnumber nonseasonal episodes.

It is difficult to diagnose seasonal affective disorder in children, as they experience a recurring universal stressor of starting school every fall. Also, a young child might present with an apparent seasonal depressive disorder picture but not yet have had any prior episodes. In this situation a seasonal mood disorder could not be diagnosed because the required three episodes would be lacking. Manic or depressive episodes can also be considered as postpartum if the onset is within 4 weeks of the delivery according to DSM-IV Criteria.

Dysthymic Disorder

Dysthymic disorder can be diagnosed when there is a depressed or irritable mood that lasts *a year* or longer and the affected individual is never symptom free more than 2 months.

In addition to a mood disturbance, to diagnose dysthymia at least *two* of the following symptoms must be present:

1. Appetite change;
2. Sleep change;
3. Decreased energy;
4. Low self-esteem;
5. Difficulty making decisions or poor concentration;
6. Feelings of hopelessness.

Dysthymia should not be diagnosed if there is a major depressive episode during the first year of the disturbance; if there is a history of manic, hypomanic, or mixed episode; if the disorder is during the course of a psychotic disorder such as schizophrenia; or if it is secondary to a substance or general medical condition.

As dysthymia often starts in childhood, adolescence, or early adult life, it is often referred to as depressive personality. The condition is chronic. If it coexists with anorexia nervosa, anxiety disorder, rheumatoid arthritis, somatization disorder, or psychoactive substance dependence, it is called secondary dysthymia. If the age of onset is prior to 21, it is called early onset. In children and adolescents, predisposing factors include ADHD, conduct disorder, specific developmental disorder, and a chaotic home environment. Children who have dysthymia and subsequently develop a major depressive episode have a so-called double depression. Kovacs et al. (1984) report dysthymic children to be at risk for developing depression and mania on follow-up.

ATYPICAL FEATURES

A depression may also be identified as having atypical features. Characteristics of this subtype are mood reactivity, exclusion of melancholic and catatonic subtypes, in addition to two or more of the following for a period of at least 2 weeks:

1. Increase in appetite or significant weight gain;
2. Increased sleep;

3. Feelings of heaviness in arms or legs;
4. A pattern of long-standing rejection sensitivity that extends far beyond the mood disturbance episodes and results in significant social or occupational impairment.

Depressive Disorder Not Otherwise Specified

In the DSM-IV this category includes disorders with features of depression that do not meet the criteria for a specific mood disorder or adjustment disorder with depressed mood. Examples include depressive episode superimposed on residual schizophrenia, a recurrent, mild depressive disturbance that does not meet criteria for dysthymia, or nonstress-related episodes that do not meet the criteria for a major depressive episode. DSM-IV should be consulted for further details as to the diagnostic criteria for these depressive disorders.

Historical Perspective

Case reports on despondency and depression in children and adolescents date to the early 17th century. Melancholia was reported in the middle of the 19th century. In general, prior to the 1960s, the existence of depression in children was doubted because it was felt children's immature superego would not permit the development of depression (Weller and Weller, 1984a, 1984b). However, this thinking changed following the 1970 meeting of the Fourth Congress of the Union of European Pedopsychiatrists in Stockholm. The theme of this meeting was "Depressive States in Childhood and Adolescence." As a direct result of this meeting, the Union of European Pedopsychiatrists concluded that depression in childhood comprised a significant portion of mental disorders in children and adolescents (Akiskal and Weller, 1989).

Subsequently, the publication of the book *Depression in Childhood: Diagnosis, Treatment and Conceptual Models* by Schulterbrandt and Raskin (1977) increased the awareness of depression in childhood in North America. This book was based on findings by a group of clinicians, researchers, and scientists who were sponsored by the National Institute of Mental Health. They reviewed the existing literature on affective disorders in childhood and came to the conclusion that depression in children and adolescents can be diagnosed using adult criteria if adjusted to assess symptoms in an age-appropriate manner.

The DSM-III, DSM-III-R, and DSM-IV have used the same criteria to diagnose depression in adults and children. A few minor adjustments were made in the criteria to account for differences in age and stage of development between adults and children. For example, in the criteria for depression, *failure to gain expected weight* can substitute for significant weight loss in children. Also, the duration of symptoms required to diagnose dysthymia is 1 year in children and adolescents instead of the 2-year period required for adults.

Prevalence and Epidemiology

Varying prevalence rates have been reported for depression. Such differences may be due to different populations sampled—community, ambulatory psychiatry patients, pediatric outpatients (nonpsychiatric), or pediatric or psychiatric inpatients. Also, the refining of structured and semistructured instruments for use in diagnosing child and adolescent psychiatric disorders that occurred in the 1980s made assessment more accurate (Weller and Weller, 1986; Weller et al., 1984a).

Epidemiologic studies done in the United States have reported the incidence of depression to be 0.9% in preschoolers, 1.90% in school-age children, and 4.7% in adolescents (Kashani and Sherman, 1988).

Studies have also been done in specialized pediatric populations. For example, 40% of patients on a neurology ward with unexplained headaches suffered from depression (Ling et al., 1970), and 7% of general pediatric inpatients (Kashani et al., 1981) had depression. In samples drawn from psychiatric settings, 28% of patients in a child psychiatry clinic (Carlson and Cantwell, 1980), 59% of psychiatric inpatients (Petti, 1978), and 27% of adolescent inpatients (Robbins et al., 1982) could be diagnosed as depressed. Thus, the occurrence of depression, as these studies indicate, is not rare, and it is commonly encountered in psychiatric practice.

Clinical Description

The age of a child and his or her psychological sophistication can play a major role in the child's clinical presentation. Most children do not use language to effectively communicate information until age 7. Thus, it can be more difficult to diagnose depression prior to this age. However, attention to nonverbal communication such as facial expression and body posture can assist in making the diagnosis in the younger children in whom verbal communication is not well developed (Poznanski, 1982). Spitz (1946) and Bowlby (1960) have described anaclitic depression in institutionalized children who were separated from their primary caretakers. The children had listlessness, withdrawal, weepiness, refusal to eat, and sleep disturbances. Unfortunately, there is a paucity of well-designed studies of depression in preschool-age children (Akiskal and Weller, 1989).

As children attend school and begin to better utilize language as a vehicle for exchanging information, they are better able to describe their feelings. Also, the school is another source of information on the child's functioning. As children are in school 6–7 hours a day, teachers can observe the child's behavior as well as compare it to that of their peer group.

As discussed earlier, depression runs in families. Very often at least one of the parents of a depressed child is also depressed. This can present a problem in evaluating a child. The concern is that depressed parents may tend to overreport problems in their children because they tend to view everything in a negative fashion (Weller and Weller, 1990a). Conversely, they may also underreport symptoms in their children when their own symptoms make them more preoccupied with themselves and less aware of things going on around them. School-age children are able to be interviewed and give detailed information as to their emotions and behaviors. Often the child reports sadness, suicidal thoughts, and sleep disturbances that his or her parents are not aware of (Weller and Weller, 1990b).

However, parents may be more likely to report behavioral changes such as irritability, moodiness, "whininess," and loss of interest. Also, parents are often more aware of duration of symptoms. Thus, it is important to interview both parent and child (Weller et al., 1984a, 1984b).

Clinically depressed children look sad, are tearful, have slow movements and a monotone voice, and speak in a hopeless and despairing manner. They describe themselves in negative terms, such as "I'm dumb," "I'm stupid," "I'm a bad girl," and "Nobody loves me." Their school performance deteriorates, and they tend to drop out of favorite extracurricular activities such as baseball, soccer, and Scouting. Somatic symptoms often occur, the most common being stomachaches and headaches (Weller and Weller, 1989). McCauley et al. (1991) reported a direct correlation between the frequency of somatic complaints and severity of depression. In late childhood, depression will more often include low self-esteem. The child may report disappointment with self, apathy, irritability, anxiety, and inability to concentrate. Self-endangering behavior and suicide attempts are quite common.

Carlson and Kashani (1988b) studied the frequency of different symptoms at different ages. Depressed mood, lack of concentration, insomnia, and suicidal ideation occurred equally in all groups. With increasing age, there was decreasing occurrence of depressed appearance and somatic complaints and increasing occurrence of anhedonia, diurnal variation, hopelessness, psychomotor retardation, and delusions. Ryan et al. (1987) reported that depressed appearance, somatic complaints, psychomotor agitation, separation anxiety, and phobias were most common in depressed children; anhedonia, hypersomnia, hopelessness, weight change, and drug abuse were increased in adolescents as compared to children.

In adolescence, the clinical picture comes to resemble more that of the adult. Hopelessness and feeling that things will never change are reflected in the increased prevalence of suicide. At times adolescents attempt to treat themselves with alcohol or drugs, which can complicate the clinical picture. There is a dramatic increase of suicide attempts and completion of suicide with puberty (Akiskal and Weller, 1989). Also, the prevalence of depression among females increases at puberty in comparison with males.

CASE ILLUSTRATION: PREPUBERTAL CHILD

B.J. was an 11-year-old who was admitted to the children's inpatient unit with a chief complaint of "Nothing is working out for me." For the last year he had been failing in school, although he had previously been a B student. He complained of trouble sleeping (middle insomnia). His parents had not bought new clothes for him for the last 2 years "because he had not outgrown his old ones." He looked very sad, cried easily, and thought his peers were making fun of him because he was "ugly and stupid." He had started refusing to go to school, as he felt very tired in the morning and wanted to sleep more. By the afternoon his mood usually improved. His mother had found a note that B.J. had written that said he was planning to jump in front of a car on a busy street "to end my misery" and that listed to whom his belongings should be given after his death. Neither B.J. nor his parents could identify any stressors.

His mother gave a history of numerous depressive episodes in herself, which had responded to antidepressants. Her first episode of depression occurred at age 10 when she was hospitalized on a general pediatric service for aches and pains and being tired all of the time. J.R.'s maternal grandmother had received ECT for a depression that occurred after J.R.'s mother was born.

Initially J.R. was treated with individual and family therapy. However, because of his severe vegetative symptoms, he was given imipramine, to which he responded within 10 days.

CASE ILLUSTRATION: ADOLESCENT

Shelly was a 14-year-old girl hospitalized because she was refusing to take a bath, had no energy, was sleeping 16 hours a day, and had dropped out of school. She had made multiple suicide attempts. These attempts involved taking her mother's antidepressants, overdosing with alcohol and drugs, and trying to jump off the roof of a five-story building. She was quite annoyed that people would not let her die. She saw no hope for the future because "life is a bummer." During a 3-day observation period she rarely interacted with anyone on the unit.

Her parents gave a three-generation history of bipolar illness in their family. As this child was thought to be at high risk for suicide and to develop mania, lithium was recommended. However, her physician refused to give lithium to the child as "it deposits in the bones." She was started on a tricyclic antidepressant and Navane 1 mg twice daily and discharged. A week after discharge, she was found in another state trying to "conduct business." She was admitted to a psychiatric hospital and treated with lithium carbonate and had a fairly good response. Her physician was now willing to consider lithium because Shelly had push of speech and flight of ideas and was very grandiose and hypersexual.

Etiology and Pathogenesis

There are several theories about the etiology of depressive disorders in children and adolescents. Major etiologic theories will be discussed briefly.

BIOLOGICAL MECHANISMS AND HYPOTHESIS

Neuroendocrine Abnormalities

In depressed adults, neuroendocrine abnormalities have been observed. Several such abnormalities have been studied to determine if they are biological markers of depression. Theoretically, there are two major types of markers, state and trait. A state marker is present or "positive" during an episode of illness and becomes absent or "negative" as the illness remits. A positive dexamethasone suppression test (DST) is considered a state marker (Carroll, 1985); the DST is positive in 50% of well-diagnosed endogenously depressed adults. Usually the marker normalizes with response to treatment (Greden et al., 1983; Leckman, 1983).

Cortisol hypersecretion as well as dexamethasone nonsuppression are reported in both prepubertal children and adolescents. Weller and Weller (1988) have reviewed the use of the DST in children and adolescents. Overall, 54% of depressed children and adolescents studied have abnormal DSTs; the abnormality seems more robust in prepubertal children (sensitivity 70%) compared with that in adolescents (43%). Possible explanations for this finding include the possibility that prepubertal-onset depression is more severe than adolescent-onset depression, and the neuroendocrine systems of prepubertal children are more intact, as they have not yet been influenced by drug abuse or the surge of sex hormones. Weller et al. (1985) have also shown that clinical outcome in some prepubertal depressed children is associated with DST results. Children who have normalized their DST at 5 months tended to be clinically well, while those with an abnormal DST at 5 months tended to be depressed.

Other biological markers that have been studied in adults, such as growth hormone, only recently have begun to be studied in children. Published reports are preliminary and need replication. These early results show that depressed children have hyposecretion of growth hormone in response to an insulin challenge; there is also hypersecretion of growth hormone during sleep (Puig-Antich et al., 1987). In a review Brent (1992) reports that similar growth hormone responses can be found in nondepressed children of depressed biological parents, suggesting that these may be related to biological traits predisposing to depression.

The catecholamine theory of depression hypothesizes that norepinephrine levels are decreased in depressed patients. This has been studied by McKnew and Cytryn (1979), who reported urinary 3-methoxy-4-hydroxyphenylethyl glycol (MHPG) was decreased in depressed children. Replication with larger samples is needed.

Sleep Studies

Studies of depressed adults have found shortened rapid eye movement (REM) latency, increased REM density, abnormal slow waves, and a decrease in sleep efficiency (Kupfer et al., 1985). In children and adolescents, preliminary studies are contradictory (Emslie et al., 1990; Puig-Antich, 1987), and additional studies from other centers may be necessary to clearly determine what abnormalities of sleep architecture are present in depressed children and adolescents.

Genetic Studies

Several studies of depressed adult probands suggest a genetic compound in the etiology of affective disorders. Such studies can be grouped in three general categories:

1. Twin studies have found that concordance for affective disorders in monozygotic twins is 76% compared with 19% in dizygotic twins. When monozygotic twins are reared apart, the concordance rate drops to 67%, possibly indicating that environmental factors may play a role in the expression of genetic factors (Akiskal and Weller, 1989).
2. In studying children of depressed adults, there is increased occurrence of affective disorders compared to other psychiatric disorders (Weissman et al., 1984).
3. Studies of parents and other relatives of affectively ill children and adolescents have found an increased age-adjusted morbidity risk for affective disorders, compared with the risk to the relatives of affectively ill adults (Puig-Antich et al., 1988; Strober et al., 1987).

PARENT-CHILD RELATION MODEL

In this model, depression has been conceptualized as resulting from poor parent-child interaction. Depressed adults report low paternal involvement and high maternal overprotection during their early childhood. As children's well-being is dependent on the well-being of the significant adults in their lives, the importance of environmental influences on affectively ill children cannot be ignored. Poor relationships with parents, siblings, and peers are common in affectively ill children and adolescents. An affectively ill child often has an affectively ill parent. In an ongoing study by Weller et al., affectively ill children have reported abuse or neglect by their affectively ill parent(s). Thus, in evaluating an affectively ill parent, it may be advisable to inquire about the well-being of their children (Weller and Weller, 1990a). Hammen et al. (1991) reported a significant temporal association between depression in mother and child. According to their findings, children with substantial stress exposure who concurrently had symptomatic mothers were significantly more depressed than those who were exposed to comparable levels of stress only.

In a review of children of depressed adults, Beardslee et al. (1983) found that, as infants and preschoolers, these children had higher rates of perinatal complications and cognitive and emotional delays and an inability to separate from their parents. As school-age children, they had depression, hyperactivity, school problems, enuresis, and excessive rivalry with peers and siblings for attention. During adolescence, problems with defiance, rebellion, withdrawal, and conflicts and disagreements with parents were reported.

Weissman et al. (1984) reported a 3-fold increased risk for manifesting any DSM-III diagnosis in children (6–18 years of age) of depressed adults. The most commonly observed diagnoses were depression (13%), ADHD (10%), and separation anxiety (10%). Risk factors included both parents being depressed, early onset of illness in the parent, and divorce, separation, or widowhood of the parents.

Keller et al. (1986) studied children of unipolar depressed parents. Severity and chronicity of parental depression was associated with current impaired adaptation in the child, presence of a DSM-III diagnosis in the child, and marital discord associated with a maladaptive child. In addition, depression in the mother was more strongly associated with psychopathology in children than was depression in the father.

Breslau et al. (1987) studied 333 mother-child dyads. Depressed mothers tended to view their children as more symptomatic and reported increased risk for all psychiatric syndromes. Thus, information obtained from depressed parents about their children may be systematically biased. Again, this indicates the importance of directly interviewing a child and not relying on parents as the sole source of information about the child. Only one study (Beardslee and Podorefsky, 1988) has reported an optimistic view of children of depressed parents. In this study, 15 of 18 adolescents who were followed for 2.5 years were doing well. Those doing well at follow-up were characterized by self-understanding, problem-solving ability, commitment to relationships, being action-oriented, and having the ability to think and act separately from their parents. Many of these adolescents were caring for their affectively ill parents.

As described earlier, the findings of a multicenter pilot study done by the NIMH Molecular Genetics of Psychiatric Disorders Initiative Group indicate that the lifetime probability of developing depression correlates with the number of depressed parents having high frequency of depression in extended families.

COHORT EFFECT

The cohort effect discussed earlier in regard to bipolar illness also applies to depressive illness. Thus, an increase in the incidence of depression in children can be expected in the future due to this cohort effect.

Klerman et al. (1985) and Gershon et al. (1987) have reported a progressive increase in the lifetime cases of major depression over the last 70 years. They report high rates of disorders among relatives, with a younger age of onset and decreased age of onset in successive recent cohorts. The implications are that somehow genetics and environment have intermingled to produce an increased incidence as well as an increase in the severity of mood disorders in succeeding generations.

SOCIOLOGICAL MODEL

According to this model, depression is seen as the result of social structures that deprive people of desirable roles. The inability of our social institutions to cope with current social stressors leads to the development of depression in some individuals (Klerman, 1976).

PSYCHOLOGICAL THEORIES OF DEPRESSION

There are numerous theories that have tried to explain why depression occurs.

Psychoanalytic Theory

Freud (1917/1966) and Abraham (1911/1966) theorized that depression was due to the real or imaginary loss of a loved object. As it is difficult to objectively study the loss of an imagined loved object, there is little research to substantiate these theories. (For the impact of real loss on children, see Chapter 33.)

Life Stress Model

This model assumes life stressors or changes in the environment that necessitate readjustments cause depression. Some have theorized that depressive symptoms in children are often a reaction to family turmoil (Lefkowitz and Burton, 1978). Poznanski and Zrull (1970) reported a high incidence of parental aggression, punitive discipline, marital discord, and scapegoating or rejection in the families of depressed children.

It is often difficult to know whether the stressor produced the illness or the illness contributed to the manifestation of the stressor. For example, in a depressed child who also has a learning disability, it is incorrect to always assume that one caused the other. Often a biopsychosocial approach in treating the depression alleviates both the depression and coexisting problems.

Behavioral Reinforcement Model

In this model it is theorized that depressive behaviors and feelings are caused by inadequate or insufficient positive reinforcers. Diminished reinforcers produce crying, irritability, and latency of response in young children (Ferster, 1973). Limited social skills in depressed children may lead to positive reinforcers being unavailable to them. Social skills training may help alleviate this problem (Puig-Antich, 1987b).

Learned Helplessness Model

In this theory a depressed person perceives his or her behavior as independent of reinforcers. This perception leads to a sense of hopelessness and subsequently to "giving up" (Seligman, 1975). The helplessness is due to motivational, cognitive, and emotional deficits.

Cognitive Distortion Model

In this model a negative view of self, the world, and the future (the cognitive triad) are the basic cause of depression. However, it is not clear whether these distorted cognitions are the root or the result of depression. Negative view of self (low self-esteem) is very common in children with all types of psychiatric disorders and is not unique to depression. A negative view of the future has been reported in a group of outpatient depressed children. Although this theory is provocative, well-designed studies to assess its validity are needed.

Self-Control Model

This model assumes that depressed people have deficits in self-reinforcement, self-evaluation, and self-monitoring. Often they focus on the short-term rather than long-term consequences of their actions. They often misattribute personal success to external forces and personal failure to themselves.

Laboratory Studies

A child should always have a medical evaluation as part of a complete psychiatric evaluation. Organic etiologies that might mimic a depressive disorder must be ruled out (Table 60.6). Conditions thought to mimic depressive disorders fall into several general major categories: infections, medications, endocrine disorders, tumors, neurologic disorders, and miscellaneous disorders.

Initial workup should include a CBC with differential, to look for infections and anemia. Electrolytes, BUN, creatinine clearance, creatinine, and urine osmolality should be assayed to rule out kidney disorders. Liver function tests should be performed. Thyroid function tests (T_3, T_4, and TSH) are necessary to rule out thyroid disease and are also a necessary part of a lithium workup. Electroencephalographic (EEG) evaluation may be needed for patients with a history or presentation suggestive of seizure disorder or episodic behavior. Also, an ECG must be done prior to starting a tricyclic antidepressant (Table 60.3).

A properly performed DST (Table 60.7) can be helpful in confirming a clinical diagnosis of depression and also may prove useful in monitoring treatment response during follow-up. The overall sensitivity of the DST is 70% in prepubertal children and 47% in adolescents. Weller et al. (1986a, 1986b) reported that DST results correlated with clinical outcome at 5 months but not at 6 weeks following remission of depression. However, this needs to be replicated. Preskorn et al. (1987) reported that depressed children with a positive DST responded better to therapeutic levels of imipramine than to placebo. Depressed children with a negative DST showed an equal response rate when treated with imipramine or placebo.

In the prepubertal children (Tanner Stage I), the DST is performed by giving 0.5 mg dexamethasone at 11:00 PM and then measuring blood

Table 60.6. Conditions Mimicking Depression in Children and Adolescents

Infections	Neurological Disorders/Tumors	Endocrine	Medications	Others
Infectious mononucleosis	Epilepsy	Diabetes	Antihypertensives	Alcohol abuse
Influenza	Postconcussion	Cushing's disease	Barbiturates	Drug abuse and withdrawal
Encephalitis	Subarachnoid hemorrhage	Addison's disease	Benzodiazepines	Cocaine
Subacute bacterial endocarditis	Cerebrovascular accident	Hypothyroidism	Corticosteroids	Amphetamine
Pneumonia	Multiple sclerosis	Hyperthyroidism	Oral contraceptives	Opiates
Tuberculosis	Huntington's disease	Hyperparathyroidism	Cimetidine	Electrolyte abnormality
Hepatitis		Hypopituitarism	Aminophylline	Hypokalemia
Syphilis (CNS)			Anticonvulsants	Hyponatremia
AIDS			Clonidine	Failure to thrive
			Digitalis	Anemia
			Thiazide diuretics	Lupus
				Wilson's disease
				Porphyria
				Uremia

Adapted from Wise MG, Rundell JR: *Concise Guide to Consultation Psychiatry*. Washington, DC, American Psychiatric Press, 1988.

Table 60.7. Conditions That Can Produce a False-Positive or False-Negative DST

Medical	Psychiatric	Medications
Protein-calorie malnutrition	Anorexia nervosa (DST+)[a]	Phenytoin
Obesity	Alcoholism	Barbiturates (DST+)
Malignancies (e.g., small cell bronchogenic carcinoma)	Acute withdrawal from alcohol (DST+)	Meprobamate
Renovascular hypertension		Reserpine
Chronic hemodialysis		Narcotics
Cushing's disease		Steroids
Uncontrolled diabetes		Benzodiazepines (DST−)
Severe weight loss		
Trauma		(>25 mg/day)
Fever (DST+)		Cyproheptadine/hydrochloride
Dehydration		Spironolactone (?DST−)
Temporal lobe epilepsy		
Pregnancy		
Addison's disease		
Hypopituitarism (DST−)		
Endocrine disorders		

Adapted from Carroll BG: A specific laboratory test for the diagnosis of melancholia. *Arch Gen Psychiatry* 38:16, 1981.
[a] DST+, false positive; DST−, false negative.

cortisol levels the next day at 8:00 AM and 4:00 PM. Weller et al. (1985) emphasize the importance of doing the DST in a standardized fashion. For example, conditions that can affect the neuroendocrine system can invalidate the DST and must be ruled out before the test can be interpreted (Table 60.7 describes such exclusion criteria). Also, the laboratory should be checked for its accuracy and reliability. Radioimmunoassay is currently considered to be the assay method that provides the best results. In general, a cortisol level of 5 μg/liter has been indicative of a positive (nonsuppressed) DST. Ideally, each laboratory should determine its own cutoff value.

When using tricyclic antidepressants or lithium carbonate, plasma levels should be determined to confirm compliance and help avoid toxicity. Urine osmolality and creatinine clearance should be periodically performed in lithium treatment.

Psychoeducational Testing

Diagnostic interviews can be useful in performing a psychiatric evaluation. Structured interviews such as the DICA (W. Reich and Z. Welner, unpublished manuscript, 1988) and semistructured interviews such as the KSADS (Chambers et al., 1985) can be used at baseline and follow-up to obtain additional information in a standardized fashion. The Childhood Depression Rating Scale-Revised (CDRS-R) of Poznanski et al. (1984) is a modified version of the Hamilton Depression Rating Scale that rates severity of depression based on information obtained from child, parent, teacher, and clinician. The Childhood Depression Inventory (CDI) (Kovacs, 1981), a self-report scale similar to the Beck Scale, is not a diagnostic instrument and should not be used to diagnose depression, as its face validity is poor (i.e., children easily identify appropriate or inappropriate responses). The CDI rates severity of depression.

In a study where the CDI and a DST were performed concurrently, 62% of depressed children had both a positive DST and CDI scores indicative of depression. Only 7% of psychiatric controls and 0% of normal subjects had both tests positive (Fristad et al., 1988). Perhaps the use of both measures simultaneously yields more useful information than either test alone.

Differential Diagnosis

As a general guideline in making a psychiatric diagnosis, specific symptoms should be considered less important than symptom clusters. An attempt should be made to rule in or rule out specific disorders. It is also important to consider medical conditions that may produce psychiatric symptoms. Such medical diagnoses should also be evaluated and ruled out before making a definitive psychiatric diagnosis. Collaboration with a pediatrician may be necessary. For a listing of medical mimics, see Table 60.6.

Another factor that must be considered is the developmental stage of children. In determining if a behavior or symptom is abnormal, what is developmentally normal must be known. For example, in preschoolers with depressed mood, one should consider neglect, abuse, failure to thrive, separation anxiety disorder, and adjustment disorder with depressed mood.

In a school-age child with depressed mood, adjustment disorder with depressed mood is a possibility. For this diagnosis, several depressive symptoms are present but not in sufficient number to fulfill criteria for depression, and duration is less than 6 months. Anxiety disorders (especially separation anxiety and overanxious disorder) may also present with depressed mood.

In adolescents, drug/alcohol abuse, anxiety disorders, and early schizophrenia should be ruled out. Frequently, determining the presence or absence of early schizophrenia is difficult. Often, affective prodromal symptoms are common before schizophrenia becomes florid. Sometimes there is a history of insidious onset, or there can be a premorbid history of being schizoid, schizotypal, or having a strange conduct disorder. Occasionally, the family history may be helpful in establishing a diagnosis. When the clinical picture is unclear or in the absence of a positive family history of schizophrenia, the authors suggest diagnosing a mood disorder. There are two reasons for this: (a) The prognosis for affective disorder is better, and (b) when affectively ill patients are treated with neuroleptics, they seem to be at a higher risk for developing tardive dyskinesia, which can be irreversible.

Treatment

A biopsychosocial approach should be used in treating a depressed child or adolescent. Such an approach will include psychotherapy (individual, family, or group, depending on the issues involved), medication management, educational assessment and planning, evaluation of school placement, and social skills training. Before initiating any treatment plan, the treatment setting must be determined. As suicide is a significant problem in depressed children, its risk must be carefully assessed. If a child or adolescent is obsessed with suicide or has definite plans, the patient should be hospitalized. Other factors such as ability to function or family stability might also influence the decision of whether to hospitalize the child.

Psychotherapies

In depressed children, cognitive and emotional development must be taken into account in developing a psychotherapeutic intervention. Several different approaches have been utilized or proposed for depressed children.

INDIVIDUAL PSYCHOTHERAPY

Individual therapy tends to focus on depressive symptoms rather than on the syndrome. Often the therapist's theoretical framework determines which specific symptoms receive attention.

A major role of the psychotherapist is to assess the child's self-perception of competence. If low competence is perceived, the extent to which this perception reflects reality should be assessed. If the perception of low competence is accurate, therapy can focus on skills training to improve competence and enhance the child's self-perception. If the perception of low competence is not true, therapy can enhance realism in self-perception.

Play Therapy

In younger children or children who are developmentally delayed (specifically, speech delayed), play therapy can provide a route of nonverbal communication with the child. Particular attention should be paid to repetitive, reckless activity and issues of loss and retrieval. Play therapy also provides a way of discharging stress via motor activity. Displaced aggression with toys and the acting out of omnipotent fantasies through sadistic or dangerous superhero themes may also be observed in play therapy. Play therapy can be done individually or with a group. It provides the children an opportunity for success. The child is allowed to express feelings and eventually deal with them. The therapist also provides a healthy model for identification.

Insight-Oriented Therapies

The prepubertal child (6–12 years) usually is resistant to the lifting of defenses, does not understand the concept of "going back in order to go forward," and often prefers outside solutions rather than intrapsychic solutions. However, insight-oriented therapies might be successfully employed in older children. Indications for insight-oriented psychotherapy include nonpsychotic depression, behavior problems due to intrapsychic conflict rather than conduct disorder, at least average intelligence, and achievement of formal operational thinking.

Therapy typically starts with a supportive phase, progresses to empathy, and eventually goes to a collaboration/self-observing phase. The therapist gives verbal interpretations of anxiety and affect as well as of impulsive acts. During the course of therapy, the focus goes from current relationships with significant others to transference relationships.

In prepubertal children, play therapy or talk therapy may be chosen. If play therapy is to be used, the child is assigned his or her own cubicle to keep play materials that are not to be shared with others. Paper, pencil, crayons, scissors, string, tape, doll family, animals, fences, and two or three cars are useful play items.

The onset of puberty may be traumatic to depressed children. Usually there is a feeling of increased internal and external pressures. Often there is anxiety about distorted body image and complaints of loneliness and isolation. The therapist needs to be more flexible with adolescents, as frequent cancellations are common. Adolescents often prefer same-sex therapists, and it is important for the therapist to avoid being perceived as a peer. The therapist needs to be active, frank, and able to express self on values if asked. Limits must be set on dangerous behaviors. In late adolescence the therapist can be less active and more of an observer.

BEHAVIORAL THERAPY

In this therapy the necessity of response-contingent positive reinforcement is emphasized. With children, therapy often focuses on skills, especially interpersonal skills, so that reinforcement can be elicited.

LIFE STRESS MODEL

The focus of therapy is either resolving or accepting life stressors that have led to depression. An example might be a child who has an adjustment disorder with depressed mood in response to the separation or divorce of the parents. In this model, the therapist will help the child to accept the decision of the parents to separate or divorce.

COGNITIVE PSYCHOTHERAPY

It is assumed that irrational beliefs and distorted cognitions are the essence of the depression. Thus, the therapist challenges the distorted cognitions and encourages the patient to practice alternate behavior.

Depressive cognitions include a negative view of self, the world, and the future. Usually the depressed child or adolescent personalizes failure, magnifies negative events, and minimizes positive events and attributes. Possible predisposing factors include early parental loss, a parent with negative cognitions (e.g., a depressed parent), or a parent with rigid rules. The therapist focuses on identifying and correcting cognitive distortions and helps the patient reevaluate his or her thinking. Therapy is active and time limited. Initially, the goal is symptom relief, but eventually the goal is to alter depressive beliefs.

This therapy may be most useful in mildly depressed children. Normal intelligence and at least the beginning of formal operational thinking are necessary. Therefore, cognitive therapy is of limited use in preadolescents.

Younger children often have cognitive deficits rather than errors. However, 7- to 12-year-old children can misinterpret, distort, self-blame, feel guilty, and feel angry at themselves.

A diary may be helpful in cognitive therapy. In younger children, parents can serve as "checkpoints." A 10-point scale, where 10 is the best you ever feel and 1 is the worst you ever feel, can be used by children. Pictures of sad and happy faces to identify feelings can be used to self-monitor. Parents can be involved in planning the activities that will occur as part of the therapy. However, children should be given choices as to the activities, and contingent reinforcers should be used. Assignments should be graded in difficulty and should progress from an easy task to a difficult task, to allow success. "Think aloud" is a technique that can be used with the parents' prompting. The strategies employed by the therapist may include persuasion, challenging cognition, examining evidence, exploring alternative explanations, and determining consequences.

Children and adolescents may need shorter sessions than adults. Noncompliance should be tolerated. Therapists should maintain ongoing family contact and be sure not to assign complex homework to those who are learning disabled.

Trautman and Rotheram (1986) have described a modified format for cognitive therapy to be used in adolescents. Formal operational thinking is associated with the ability to conceive of contradictory explanations for a given event. Thus, the first step is to identify feelings, measure their intensity, and compare one feeling experience with others. An antecedent affect leads to a belief that may lead to consequences for the child. The therapist must be very active in engaging the adolescent, emphasize "collaborating" with the patient, involve the family, develop a problem list, and use the subjective units of distress scale (SUDS). "The feeling thermometer" may be used with adolescents; the adolescent identifies best and worst things that have happened to him or her. Homework is assigned concerning three problems that the adolescent had in 1 week, and eventually the therapist helps the adolescent come up with alternative thoughts. Adolescents are taught to be assertive and to use self-instructed thoughts. A list of instructions is developed to be used for crisis situations.

An advantage of cognitive therapy for adolescents is that it is flexible and allows the therapist to move readily between the roles of teacher, confidant, role model, collaborator, and expert. However, cognitive therapy works best in mildly depressed adolescents. It is less effective in severely depressed adolescents, who may need adjunctive medication management.

OTHER THERAPIES

Group Therapy

Group therapy is useful in developing social skills in depressed children. It allows the children to express feelings in a safe and supportive environment. It requires an energetic and empathic therapist.

Parent Training

The purpose of parent training is to teach parents to manage specific problem behaviors and to appropriately use positive or negative reinforcers. Parents are also taught to communicate with their children in an age-appropriate manner. In particular, parents learn how to talk and listen to their children.

Family Therapy

Poznanski and Zrull (1970) described lack of generational boundaries, severe marital conflict, projection of parental feelings onto the child, rigid or chaotic rules, and disengaged or enmeshed relationships in the families of depressed children. The family therapist discourages rejection and encourages increased affection and communication among family members. Also, other family members who are concurrently depressed and require treatment may be identified.

Remedial Education

Depression is frequently associated with decreased academic performance. The aim of remedial education is to increase interaction with teacher and peers. Paper and pencil tasks (passive tasks) are discouraged, and more oral and manipulation tasks (active tasks) are encouraged. Rapid academic gains occur as depression lifts (Quay and Werry, 1979).

Out-of-Home Placement

Removal from the home sometimes is necessary for short periods of time if home is chaotic, especially when a parent is concurrently depressed. Possible placements include a foster home for the less disturbed children, a group home for moderately disturbed children, and a residential home for the most disturbed children.

Psychopharmacological Intervention

To date, most treatment studies of depressed children have focused on pharmacological intervention. To date there is limited evidence that medication management is superior to other kinds of therapies. Double-blind placebo-controlled studies are needed to clearly establish the efficacy of antidepressants. However, individual patients may dramatically respond to medication treatment. Thus, most moderately to severely depressed children and adolescents may be considered for pharmacologic therapy. Before starting medication, side effects as well as anticipated beneficial effects should be explained to the child and parent. Parents should also be informed that the Food and Drug Administration (FDA) has not approved the use of these medications in depressed children, before obtaining informed consent.

Tricyclic antidepressants (TCAs) have been the medications most commonly used to treat depression in children. Imipramine has been available for many years and has been frequently prescribed to children for the treatment of enuresis. This information is reassuring to most parents who are considering the use of imipramine in their depressed child. Weller and Weller (1984b) reviewed the use of TCAs in depressed children. At that time, well-designed open trial studies of TCAs were examined. When data from all the open trials were combined, the overall response was 75%, ranging between 46 and 100%. Noting this wide variance in response rate, the authors suggested that future studies include plasma drug monitoring to determine equivalency of treatment (Table 60.8).

To date, there are two published double-blind placebo-controlled studies of imipramine in depressed children. The first study was done by Puig-Antich et al. (1987). Subjects were 38 children; 22 received a placebo, and 16 received imipramine. Both inpatients and outpatients were included. Imipramine was started at 1.5 mg/kg/day and increased to 5 mg/kg/day; the mean dose was 136 mg (4.35 mg/kg). Response rate was 56% in the imipramine-treated group and 68% in the placebo-treated group. Those who responded to imipramine had higher plasma levels (284 ng/ml) than those who did not respond (145 ng/ml).

A second study by Preskorn and colleagues (1987) used plasma level monitoring as well as DST results to study response to imipramine in 22 moderately to severely depressed prepubertal inpatients. The plasma imipramine levels were adjusted by the laboratory physician to be between 125 and 250 ng/ml. Children responded to imipramine better than to placebo. When DST results were examined, depressed children with a positive DST responded better to imipramine than to placebo, but those with a negative DST responded equally well to imipramine and placebo.

A child's ECG should be monitored throughout treatment with a TCA. Prolongation of the P-R interval should not exceed 0.21, and QRS changes should not exceed 30% of baseline. Other limits that should not be exceeded include a heart rate of 130 beats per minute, a systolic blood pressure of 130 mm Hg, and a diastolic blood pressure of 85 mm Hg (Ryan, 1990). If these parameters are exceeded, dosage adjustment with plasma monitoring may be needed to ensure compliance and avoid toxicity. Preskorn et al. (1988) reported increased neurotoxicity in children who had plasma levels higher than 500 ng/ml.

There are no published placebo-controlled studies of TCAs in adolescents. An open study by Ryan et al. (1986) found a 44% response rate to TCAs. In general, response rates in adolescents tend to be lower than those in prepubertal children. It has been hypothesized that the surge of sex hormones that occurs during adolescence may account in part for poor antidepressant response in children. Although TCAs can be given in a single dose or in divided doses, divided doses might be useful in children who have depression and concomitant ADHD. However, most children do not like taking medications, as they don't want to appear different from their peers. Thus, giving medicine as a single

---

Table 60.8.   Treatment Response to Tricyclic Antidepressants in Depressed Prepubertal Children

Author	Drug	Dose (mg/day)	N	% Improvement	Duration of Treatment (Weeks)
Lucas et al., 1965	Ami[a]	30–50	10	60	6
Ling et al., 1970	Ami/Imi	—	10	90	—
Kuhn and Kuhn, 1972	Imi/Imi +	—	100	72	—
Weinberg et al., 1973	Ami/Imi	25–125	19	95	3
Puig-Antich et al., 1979	Imi	105	13	46	5
Staten et al., 1981	Ami/Dmi	—	11	100	12
Conners and Petti, 1983	Imi	25–200	21	67	9
Geller et al., 1983	Nor	—	8	100	16
Weller et al., 1982	Imi	50–150	16	75	6
Overall Total or Average			208	75	

[a] Ami, amitriptyline; Imi, imipramine; Dmi, desmethylimipramine; Nor, nortriptyline; IMI + 1, 1 imipramine and another psychotropic.

bedtime dose (not to exceed 100 mg) can solve this problem. If additional medicine is required, it can be given at 4:00 PM, after school. The total daily dose should not exceed 5 mg/kg/day.

Monoamine oxidase inhibitors (MAOIs) have been suggested as helpful in treating the so-called atypical depression in adults. To date, MAOIs have been used sparingly in children and adolescents. However, they have occasionally been used in children and adolescents who have not responded to tricyclics.

The major problem with MAOIs is that a tyramine-free diet is necessary. Abstinence from chocolate, chicken livers, chianti wine, pepperoni, bologna, sausage, and aged cheese is required. Many adolescents are too impulsive or lack the discipline to comply with these dietary restrictions. Ryan et al. (1988b) treated 23 adolescents who had not responded to TCAs with an MAOI; 74% responded. Of these, 57% had good response and were able to comply with the diet.

Lithium may be added to a TCA to enhance response in TCA-refractory patients. Ryan et al. (1988a) studied 14 nonbipolar adolescents who had not responded to TCAs alone; patients had a good response when lithium was added. The authors suggested that, as a substantial number of depressed adolescents may become bipolar, this combination of lithium and TCA treatment should be studied further.

Lithium carbonate has been used in children and adolescents to treat aggression, mania, depression, and behavioral problems in children of lithium-responsive parents (Campbell et al., 1984; Youngerman and Canino, 1978). However, there is a lack of double-blind placebo-controlled studies. Lithium carbonate may be most useful in children or adolescents who are at risk for bipolarity. Depressed adolescents presenting with psychomotor retardation, oversleeping, or overeating during a depressive episode or those who have a definite family history of bipolar disorder may be candidates for lithium therapy (Strober et al., 1990).

As mentioned earlier, a thorough workup should be done prior to initiating lithium treatment. Such a workup should include BUN, creatinine, creatinine clearance, and urine osmolality levels. Plasma lithium levels should be followed carefully and should be in the range of 0.6–1.4 mEq/liter (see Table 60.4 for lithium dosage guide).

Recently, selective serotonin uptake inhibitors have been used in adults, with comparable results. In an open trial, Boulos et al. (1992) used fluoxetine in 15 patients, ages 16–24 years, who had previously failed to respond to tricyclic antidepressants. Sixty-four percent of the 11 patients who completed the study displayed greater than 50% improvement in the Hamilton depression rating scale.

Riddle et al. (1991) described behavioral side effects of fluoxetine in 24 children, ages 8–16 years, with doses of 20–40 mg/day. Reported side effects were motor restlessness (N = 11), sleep disturbance (N = 11), social disinhibition (N = 6), and a subjective feeling of excitation (N = 3). These side effects resolved by discontinuation (N = 5) or reducing the dose by half (N = 7). These 7 patients whose doses were reduced maintained their previously achieved improvement. Preliminary data from a multicenter, double-blind placebo-controlled study of fluoxetine in adolescents revealed no advantage over placebo in the treatment of depression. In addition the rate of switching to mania in the fluoxetine group exceeded that of the placebo group (Reported at the Consortium of Mood Disorders in Children and Adolescents, Toronto, 1993). The clinician should be cautious when using fluoxetine in adolescents, especially in those with a personal or family history of mania or hypomania. To date, open studies of a variety of medications have indicated they may be useful in the treatment of depression. However, it is clear that more treatment studies with a double-blind placebo-controlled design are needed to clearly establish the efficacy of such medications in the pharmacotherapy of depressed children and adolescents.

When other measures fail in severe depression, electroconvulsive therapy (ECT) can be effective (Bertangoli and Borchardt, 1990).

However, the data concerning safety and efficacy in children and adolescents are sparse. As stated earlier, specific guidelines for obtaining consent and for the indications and administration of ECT have been published by the APA (1990). Two psychiatrists who are experienced in treating children and who are not otherwise involved with the case should concur with the recommendation for ECT prior to the initiation of treatment.

Outcome and Follow-up Data

The outcome of mood disorders in children and adolescents currently appears poor. The response rate to medication treatment is less than ideal. The efficacy of psychotherapy in depressed children has not yet been established.

A complicating factor in the assessment and treatment of this disorder in children and adolescents is the frequent occurrence of comorbidity. Kovacs et al. (1984, 1988) reported that 79% of depressed prepubertal children had at least one other Axis I diagnosis: 38% had dysthymia, 33% anxiety disorder, and 7% had conduct disorder. A follow-up study of depressed children found that 36% developed conduct disorder as a complication of depression (Kovacs et al., 1988). Kashani and Sherman (1988) studied depressed adolescents. In this report 75% had comorbid anxiety, 50% oppositional disorder, 33% conduct disorder, 25% alcohol abuse, and 25% drug abuse. Those with onset of depression in childhood or adolescence are at risk to develop multiple episodes on follow-up (Kovacs et al., 1984) and often require rehospitalization (Asarnow et al., 1988). Harrington et al. (1991) reported that for depressed children to have comorbid conduct disorder was prognostically favorable for the outcome of depression in adulthood but not for conduct disorder. These patients had a similar likelihood of developing antisocial personality as adults when compared with patients who had conduct disorder without depression, but were much less likely to have depression as adults when compared with a group of patients who were depressed but did not suffer from conduct disorder. These findings suggested that depression may represent an early feature of conduct disorder rather than a separate comorbid illness. In a prospective longitudinal study of the course of depression in children and adolescents, McCauley et al. (1993) reported poorer overall outcome to be associated with increased levels of stress in the family environment.

Research Directions

Although there has been a dramatic surge in studies of depressed children and adolescents, more research is clearly needed. Studies are needed to assess risk factors that may predict depression. Such studies must be done in a longitudinal manner and should focus on children of affectively ill parents, children who have lost a parent through death, and children of divorced parents. In regard to treatment, additional studies are needed not only to determine if pharmacological treatment is helpful but also to identify subgroups who may be most responsive to pharmacological intervention. Controlled studies assessing the helpfulness of the psychotherapies in childhood depression are also critically needed. Studies examining neuroendocrine factors and sleep architecture need to be expanded and replicated. Finally, studies of the brains of depressed children and adolescents who have committed suicide could provide invaluable information about changes in structure and function that occur in childhood depression.

If the cohort effect continues to be manifest, the number of children and adolescents with an affective disorder should continue to increase. If early-onset affective illness is more malignant in its course and outcome, early identification and proper treatment will be essential. With the changes in FDA regulations, an increase in double-blind and placebo-controlled studies is expected for new medications to determine their efficacy and safety in children and adolescents.

References

Abraham K: Notes on the psychoanalytical investigation and treatment of manic-depressive insanity and allied conditions. In: *On Character and Libido Development*. New York, Norton, 1966, pp. 15–34. (Originally published 1911.)

Akiskal HS, Weller EB: Mood disorders and suicide in children and adolescents. In: Kaplan HI, Sadock BJ (eds): *Comprehensive Textbook of Psychiatry* (Vol 2, 5th ed). Baltimore, Williams & Wilkins, 1989.

American Psychiatric Association: *The Practice of Electroconvulsive Therapy: Recommendations for Treatment, Training and Privileging* (A Task Force Report of the APA), Washington, DC, American Psychiatric Association, 1990.

Anthony J, Scott P: Manic-depressive psychosis in childhood. *J Child Psychol Psychiatry* 4:53–72, 1960.

Asarnow JR, Goldstein MJ, Carlson GA, et al: Childhood-onset depressive disorders: A follow-up study of rates of rehospitalization and out-of-home placement among child psychiatric inpatients. *J Affect Disord* 5:245–253, 1988.

Baldessarini RH: *Biomedical Aspects of Depression*. Washington, DC, American Psychiatric Press, 1983.

Ballenger JC, Reus VI, Post RM: The "atypical" presentation of adolescent mania. *Am J Psychiatry* 139:602–606, 1982.

Beardslee WR, Podorefsky D: Resilient adolescents whose parents have serious affective and other psychiatric disorder: The importance of self understanding and relationships. *Am J Psychiatry* 145:63–69, 1988.

Beardslee WR, Bemporad J, Keller M, et al: Children of parents with major affective disorder: A review. *Am J Psychiatry* 140:825–832, 1983.

Beigel A, Murphy DL, Bunney WE Jr: The manic-state rating scale. *Arch Gen Psychiatry* 25:256–262, 1971.

Bertangoli MW, Borchardt CM: A review of ECT for children and adolescents. *J Am Acad Child Adolesc Psychiatry* 29:302–307, 1990.

Bleuler E: *Textbook of Psychiatry*. New York, Macmillan, 1934.

Boulos C, Kutcher S, Gardner D, et al: An open naturalistic trial of fluoxetine in adolescents and young adults with treatment-resistant major depression. *J Child Adolesc Psychopharmacol* 2:103–111, 1992.

Bowlby J: Grief and mourning in infancy and early childhood. *Psychoanal Study Child* 15:9–52, 1960.

Brent DA: Major depressive disorder. *New Dir Ment Health Serv* Summer:39–44, 1992.

Breslau N, Davis GC, Prabucki K: Depressed mothers as informants in family history research—Are they accurate? *Psychiatry Res* 24:345–359, 1987.

Campbell M, Perry R, Green WH: Use of lithium in children and adolescents. *Psychosomatics* 25:95–106, 1984.

Carlson GA: Bipolar affective disorders in childhood and adolescence. In: Cantwell DP, Carlson GA (eds): *Affective Disorders in Childhood and Adolescence, an Update*. New York, Spectrum, 1983, pp. 61–84.

Carlson GA: Bipolar disorders in children and adolescents. In: Garfinkel B, Carson G, Weller EB (eds): *Psychiatric Disorders in Children and Adolescents*. Philadelphia, Saunders, 1990, pp. 21–36.

Carlson GA, Cantwell DP: A survey of depressive symptoms, syndrome and disorder in a child psychiatric population. *J Child Psychol Psychiatry* 21:19–25, 1980.

Carlson GA, Kashani JH: Manic symptoms in a non-referred adolescent population. *J Affect Disord* 15:219–226, 1988a.

Carlson GA, Kashani JH: Phenomenology of major depression from childhood through adulthood: Analysis of three studies. *Am J Psychiatry* 145:1222–1225, 1988b.

Carlson GA, Strober M: Manic-depressive illness in early adolescence. *J Am Acad Child Psychiatry* 17:138–153, 1978.

Carlson GA, Davenport YB, Jamison K: A comparison of outcome in adolescent and late-onset bipolar manic-depressive illness. *Am J Psychiatry* 134:919–922, 1977.

Carroll BJ: Dexamethasone suppression test: A review of contemporary confusion. *J Clin Psychiatry* 46:13–24, 1985.

Chambers WJ, Puig-Antich J, Hirsch M, et al: The assessment of affective disorders in children and adolescents by semistructured interview. *Arch Gen Psychiatry* 42:696–702, 1985.

Connors CK, Petti T: Imipramine therapy of depressed children: Methodologic considerations. *Psychopharmacol Bull* 19:65–68, 1983.

Cytryn L, McKnew DH, Zahn-Waxler C, et al: Developmental issues in risk research: The offspring of affectively ill parents. In: Rutter M, Izard CE, Read PB (eds): *Depression in Young People: Clinical and Developmental Perspectives*. New York, Guilford, 1986.

Davis RE: Manic-depressive variant syndrome in childhood: A preliminary report. *Am J Psychiatry* 136:702–706, 1979.

DeLong GR, Aldershof AL: Long-term experience with lithium treatment in childhood: Correlation with clinical diagnoses. *J Am Acad Child Adolesc Psychiatry* 26:389–394, 1987.

Emslie GJ, Rush AJ, Weinberg WA, et al: Children with major depression show reduced rapid eye movement latencies. *Arch Gen Psychiatry* 47:119–124, 1990.

Esquirol E: *Mental Maladies* (Hunt EK, trans). Philadelphia, Lea & Blanchard, 1845, p. 33.

Ferster CB: A functional analysis of depression. *Am Psychol* 28:857–869, 1973.

Freud S: Mourning and melancholia. In: Strachey J (ed): *The Standard Edition of the Complete Psychological Works of Sigmund Freud* (Vol 14). London, Hogarth Press, 1966. (Originally published 1917.)

Fristad MA, Weller EB, Weller RA, et al: Self-report versus biological markers in assessment of childhood depression. *J Affect Disord* 15:339–345, 1988.

Fristad MA, Weller EB, Weller RA: The Mania Rating Scale: Can it be used in children? A preliminary report. *J Am Acad Child Adolesc Psychiatry* 31:252–257, 1992.

Geller B, Perel JM, Knitter EF, et al: Nortriptyline in major depressive disorders in children: Response, steady-state plasma levels, predictive kinetics, and pharmacokinetics. *Psychopharmacol Bull* 19:62–64, 1983.

Gershon ES, Hamovit JH, Guroff JJ, et al: Birth cohort changes in manic and depressive disorders in relatives of bipolar and schizoaffective patients. *Arch Gen Psychiatry* 44:314–319, 1987.

Greden JF, Gardner R, Kind D, et al: Dexamethasone suppression test in antidepressant treatment of melancholia. *Arch Gen Psychiatry* 40:493–500, 1983.

Hammen C, Burge D, Adrian C: Timing of mother and child depression in a longitudinal study of children at risk. *J Consult Clin Psychol* 59:341–345, 1991.

Harrington R, Fudge H, Rutter M, et al: Adult outcomes of childhood and adolescent depression. II: Links with antisocial disorders. *J Am Acad Child Adolesc Psychiatry* 30:434–439, 1991.

Hudgens RW: *Psychiatric Disorders in Adolescence*. Baltimore, Williams & Wilkins, 1974.

Kanner L: Do behavioral symptoms always indicate psychopathology? *J Child Psychol Psychiatry* 1:17–25, 1960.

Kasanin J: The affective psychoses in children. *Am J Psychiatry* 10:897–924, 1931.

Kashani JH, Sherman DD: Childhood depression: Epidemiology, etiological models, and treatment implications. *Integr Psychiatry* 6:1–8, 1988.

Kashani JH, Barbero GJ, Bolander FD: Depression in hospitalized pediatric patients. *J Am Acad Child Psychiatry* 20:123–134, 1981.

Keller MD, Beardslee WR, Dorer DJ, et al: Impact of severity and chronicity of parental affective illness on adaptive functioning and psychopathology in children. *Arch Gen Psychiatry* 43:930–937, 1986.

Klein DN, Depue RA, Slater JF: Inventory identification of cyclothymia. IX: Validation in offspring of bipolar I patients. *Arch Gen Psychiatry* 43:441–445, 1986.

Klerman GL: Age and clinical depression: Today's youth in the twenty-first century. *J Gerontol* 31:318–323, 1976.

Klerman GL, Lavori PW, Rice J, et al: Birth-cohort trends in rates of major depressive disorder among relatives of patients with affective disorder. *Arch Gen Psychiatry* 42:689–693, 1985.

Kovacs M: Rating scales to assess depression in school-aged children. *Acta Paedopsychiatr* 46:305–315, 1981.

Kovacs M, Feinberg TL, Crouse-Novak M, et al: Depressive disorders in childhood. II: A longitudinal study of the risk for a subsequent major depression. *Arch Gen Psychiatry* 41:643–649, 1984.

Kovacs M, Paulauskas S, Gatsonis C, et al: Depressive disorders in childhood. II: A longitudinal study of comorbidity with and risk for conduct disorders. *J Affect Disord* 15:205–217, 1988.

Kraepelin E: *Manic Depressive Insanity and Paranoia*. Edinburgh, Livingstone, 1921.

Kuhn V, Kuhn R: *Drug Therapy for Depression in Children, in Depressive States in Childhood and Adolescence*. New York, Wiley, 1972.

Kupfer DJ, Ulrich RF, Coble PA, et al: Electroencephalographic sleep of young depressives. *Arch Gen Psychiatry* 42:806–810, 1985.

Landolt AD: Follow-up studies on circular manic depressive reactions occurring in the young. *Bull NY Acad Med* 33:65–73, 1957.

Leckman JF: The dexamethasone suppression test. *J Am Acad Child Psychiatry* 22:477–479, 1983.

Lefkowitz MM, Burton N: Childhood depression: A critique of the concept. *Psychol Bull* 85:716–726, 1978.

Ling W, Oftedal G, Weinberg W: Depressive illness in childhood presenting as severe headache. *Am J Dis Child* 120:122–124, 1970.

Lucas AR, Lockett HJ, Grimm F: Amitriptyline in childhood depression. *Dis Nerv Syst* 26:105–110, 1965.

McCauley E, Carlson GA, Calderon R: The role of somatic complaints in the diagnosis of depression in children and adolescents. *J Am Acad Child Adolesc Psychiatry* 30:631–635, 1991.

McCauley E, Myers K, et al: Depression in young people: Initial presentation and clinical course. *J Am Acad Child Adolesc Psychiatry* 32:714–722, 1993.

McGlashen TH: Adolescent versus adult onset mania. *Am J Psychiatry* 145:221–224, 1988.

McKnew DH, Cytryn L: Urinary metabolites in chronically depressed children. *J Am Acad Child Psychiatry* 18:608–615, 1979.

Mendlewicz J, Rainer JD: Adoption study supporting genetic transmission in manic-depressive illness. *Nature* 265:327–329, 1977.

NIMH Molecular Genetics of Psychiatry Disorders Initiative Child Study Group: Aggression in children/adolescents during treatment with antidepressants. *Biol Psychiatry* 33:37A–162A, 1993.

Nurnberger JI, Gershon E: Genetics. In: Paykel ES (ed): *Handbook of Affective Disorders*. Edinburgh, Churchill-Livingstone, 1982.

Olsen T: Follow-up study of manic-depressive patients whose first attack occurred before the age of 19. *Acta Psychiatr Scand Suppl* 162:45–51, 1961.

Petti TA: Depression in hospitalized child psychiatry patients: Approaches to measuring depression. *J Am Acad Child Psychiatry* 17:49–59, 1978.

Poznanski EO: The clinical phenomenology of childhood depression. *Am J Orthopsychiatry* 52:308, 1982.

Poznanski EO, Zrull JP: Childhood depression: Clinical characteristics of overtly depressed children. *Arch Gen Psychiatry* 23:8–15, 1970.

Poznanski EO, Grossman JA, Buchsbaum Y, et al: Preliminary studies of the reliability and validity of the Children's Depression Rating Scale. *J Am Acad Child Psychiatry* 23:191–197, 1984.

Preskorn SH, Bupp ST, Weller EB, et al: Relationship of plasma imipramine levels to CNS toxicity in children (Letter to the Editor). *Am J Psychiatry* 145:897, 1988.

Preskorn SH, Weller EB, Hughes CW, et al: Depression in prepubertal children: Dexamethasone nonsuppression predicts differential response to imipramine vs. placebo. *Psychopharmacol Bull* 23:128, 1987.

Puig-Antich J: Affective disorders in children and adolescents: Diagnostic validity and psychobiology. In: Meltzer HY (ed): *Psychopharmacology—The Third Generation of Progress*. New York, Raven Press, 1987.

Puig-Antich J, Goetz D, Davies M, et al: A controlled family history study of prepubertal major depressive disorder. *Arch Gen Psychiatry* 46:406–420, 1988.

Puig-Antich J, Perel JM, Lupatkin WM, et al: Imipramine in prepubertal major depressive disorders. *Arch Gen Psychiatry* 44:81–89, 1987.

Quay HC, Werry JS: *Psychopathological Disorders of Childhood* (2nd ed). New York, Wiley, 1979.

Ray JM, Morris-Yates A: Adolescent depression and the child behavior checklist. *J Am Acad Child Adolesc Psychiatry* 31:252–257, 1992.

Rice J, Reich T, Andreasen NC, et al: The familial transmission of bipolar illness. *Arch Gen Psychiatry* 44:441–447, 1987.

Riddle MA, King RA, et al: Behavioral side effects of fluoxetine in children and adolescents. *J Child Adolesc Psychopharmacol* 1:193–198, 1991.

Robbins DR, Alessi NE, Cook SC, et al: The use of the research diagnostic criteria (RDC) for depression in adolescent psychiatric inpatients. *J Am Acad Child Psychiatry* 21:251–255, 1982.

Robins LN, Helzer JE, Weissman MM, et al: Lifetime prevalence of specific psychiatric disorders in three sites. *Arch Gen Psychiatry* 41:949–958, 1984.

Ryan N: Heterocyclic antidepressants in children and adolescents. *J Child Adolesc Psychopharmacol* 1:21–23, 1990.

Ryan ND, Meyer V, Dachille S, et al: Lithium antidepressant augmentation in TCA-refractory depression in adolescents. *J Am Acad Child Adolesc Psychiatry* 27:371–376, 1988a.

Ryan ND, Puig-Antich J, Ambrosini P, et al: The clinical picture of major depression in children and adolescents. *Arch Gen Psychiatry* 44:854–861, 1987.

Ryan ND, Puig-Antich J, Cooper T, et al: Imipramine in adolescent major depression: Plasma level and clinical response. *Acta Psychiatr Scand* 73:289–294, 1986.

Ryan ND, Puig-Antich J, Rabinovich H, et al: MAOIs in adolescent major depression unresponsive to tricyclic antidepressants. *J Am Acad Child Adolesc Psychiatry* 27:755–758, 1988b.

Ryan ND, Williamson DE, Iyengar S, et al: A secular increase in child and adolescent onset affective disorder. *J Am Acad Child Adolesc Psychiatry* 31:600–605, 1992.

Schulterbrandt JG, Raskin A (eds): *Depression in Childhood: Diagnosis, Treatment, and Conceptual Models*. New York, Raven Press, 1977.

Seligman ME: *Helplessness: On Depression, Development, and Death*. San Francisco, Freeman, 1975.

Spitz RA, Wolf KM: Anaclitic depression. An inquiry into the genesis of psychiatric conditions in early childhood, II. *Psychoanal Study Child* 2:312–342, 1946.

Staten RD, Wilson H, Brumback RA: Cognitive improvement associated with tricyclic antidepressant treatment of childhood major depressive illness. *Percept Mot Skills* 53:219–234, 1981.

Strober M, Carlson G, Ryan N, et al: Advances in the psychopharmacology of childhood and adolescent affective disorders. Paper presented at the Scientific Proceedings of the Annual Meeting of the American Academy of Child and Adolescent Psychiatry, Washington, DC, 1987.

Strober M, Morrell W, Burroughs J, et al: A family study of bipolar I in adolescence: Early onset of symptoms linked to increased familial loading and lithium resistance. *J Affect Disord* 15:255–268, 1988.

Strober M, Morrell W, Lampert C, et al: Relapse following discontinuation of lithium maintenance therapy in adolescents with bipolar I illness: A naturalistic study. *Am J Psychiatry* 147:457–461, 1990.

Trautman P, Rotheram MJ: Cognitive behavioral therapy with adolescent suicide attempts, Part I. Paper presented at Taboroff Child Psychiatry Conference, Park City, UT, 1986.

Varanka TM, Weller RA, Weller EB, et al: Lithium treatment of manic episodes with psychotic features in prepubertal children. *Am J Psychiatry* 145:1557–1559, 1988.

Weinberg WA, Brumback RP: Mania in childhood. *Am J Dis Child* 130:380–385, 1976.

Weissman MM, Gershon ES, Kidd KK: Psychiatric disorders in the relatives of probands with affective disorders: The Yale-NIMH collaborative family study. *Arch Gen Psychiatry* 41:13, 1984.

Weller EB, Weller RA: Clinical aspects of childhood depression. *Pediatr Ann* 15:843–847, 1986.

Weller EB, Weller RA: Neuroendocrine changes in affectively ill children and adolescents. *Psychiatr Clin North Am* 6:41–54, 1988.

Weller EB, Weller RA: Pediatric management of depression. *Pediatr Ann* 18:104–113, 1989.

Weller EB, Weller RA: Depressive disorders in children and adolescents. In: Garfinkel B, Carlson G, Weller EB (eds): *Psychiatric Disorders in Children and Adolescents*. Philadelphia, Saunders, 1990a, pp. 3–20.

Weller EB, Weller RA: Grief in children and adolescents. In: Garfinkel B, Carlson G, Weller EB (eds): *Psychiatric Disorders in Children and Adolescents*. Philadelphia, Saunders, 1990b, pp. 37–47.

Weller EB, Weller RA, Fristad MA: Assessment and treatment of childhood depression. In: Weller EB, Weller RA (eds): *Current Perspectives on Major Depressive Disorders in Children*. Washington, DC, American Psychiatric Press, 1984a, pp. 1–18.

Weller EB, Weller RA, Fristad MA: Historical and theoretical perspectives on childhood depression. In: Weller EB, Weller RA (eds): *Current Perspectives on Major Depressive Disorders in Children*. Washington, DC, American Psychiatric Press, 1984b, pp. 1–18.

Weller EB, Weller RA, Fristad MA, et al: The dexamethasone suppression test in prepubertal depressed children. *J Clin Psychiatry* 46:511–513, 1985.

Weller EB, Weller RA, Fristad MA: Lithium dosage guide for prepubertal children: A preliminary report. *J Am Acad Child Adolesc Psychiatry* 25:92–95, 1986a.

Weller EB, Weller RA, Fristad MA, et al: Dexamethasone suppression test and clinical outcome in prepubertal depressed children. *Am J Psychiatry* 143:1469–1470, 1986b.

Weller EB, Weller RA, Preskorn SH, et al: Steady-state plasma imipramine levels in prepubertal depressed children. *Am J Psychiatry* 139:506–508, 1982.

Weller RA, Weller EB: Use of tricyclic antidepressant in prepubertal depressed children. In: Weller EB, Weller RA (eds): *Current Perspectives on Major Depressive Disorders in Children*. Washington, DC, American Psychiatric Press, 1984, pp. 50–63.

Weller RA, Weller EB, Tucker SG, et al: Mania in prepubertal children: Has it been underdiagnosed? *J Affect Disord* 11:151–154, 1986c.

Weiner A, Weiner Z, Fishman R: Psychiatric adolescent inpatients. Eight- to ten-year follow-up. *Arch Gen Psychiatry* 36:698–700, 1979.

Wise MG, Rundell JR: *Concise Guide to Consultation Psychiatry*. Washington, DC, American Psychiatric Press, 1988.

Young RC, Biggs JT, Ziegler VE, et al: A rating scale for mania: Reliability, validity and sensitivity. *Br J Psychiatry* 133:429–435, 1978.

Youngerman J, Canino IA: Lithium carbonate use in children and adolescents. *Arch Gen Psychiatry* 35:216–224, 1978.

61 SUICIDAL BEHAVIOR IN CHILDREN AND ADOLESCENTS: CAUSES AND MANAGEMENT

Cynthia R. Pfeffer, M.D.

Suicidal behavior in children and adolescents is an important mental health problem in the United States. Recognition of the high degree of psychiatric and social morbidity and the increased incidence of mortality associated with suicidal acts among youth were strong stimuli for conducting empirical investigations to identify risk factors for youth suicidal behavior. In the 1980s, new research methods especially involving epidemiological, cross-sectional, psychological autopsy, and longitudinal approaches have been applied to understand aspects important for developing prevention strategies for youth suicidal behavior. This chapter highlights recent knowledge about suicidal behavior among children and adolescents that is derived from these recent innovative studies.

The concept of suicidal behavior in preadolescents and adolescents includes thoughts about causing intentional self-injury or death (suicidal ideas) and acts that cause intentional self-injury (suicide attempt) or death (suicide). Some researchers believe that suicidal behavior involves a continuum that includes nonsuicidal behavior, suicidal ideas, suicide attempts, and suicide. This premise is based on research (Brent et al., 1986, 1988; Pfeffer, 1986; Pfeffer et al., 1982) suggesting that the severity of certain factors, such as depression, death preoccupations, and general psychopathology are directly proportional to the severity of suicidal behavior. However, others (Carlson and Cantwell, 1982; Hawton et al., 1982) suggest that suicidal ideation and acts are discontinuous and that there are no direct correlations between certain factors such as depression and suicidal ideation and acts. The complexity of these concepts requires more research, especially with respect to potential differences in various phases of child and adolescent development.

In this chapter, suicidal behavior is conceptualized along a spectrum that includes nonsuicidal behavior, suicidal ideation, suicide attempts, and suicide. The chapter focuses predominantly on fatal and nonfatal suicidal acts, such as suicide and suicide attempts.

HISTORICAL NOTE

Episodic epidemics of child and adolescent suicidal behavior have stimulated extensive efforts to learn more about the characteristics of youth suicidal behavior and relevant preventive methods to decrease its mortality and morbidity. In the 19th century when the classic book, *The Sorrows of Young Werther*, by Goethe was published, an epidemic of youth suicide occurred. This epidemic was attributed to imitation of the book's hero, who shot himself after the breakup of a love relationship. Subsequently, the book was banned in Europe.

In 1910, the Vienna Psychoanalytic Society convened a special meeting to evaluate risk factors for youth suicidal behavior (Pfeffer, 1986). The impetus for this historic meeting was the significant rise in youth suicide and the anxiety that ensued about how to prevent suicide. Among the participants at this meeting were Drs. Federn, Freud, Rank, Steckel, and Tausk. Sigmund Freud, for example, was concerned that the most significant influence on youth suicide was conflict with loved persons. He recommended that intensive study of specific suicidal individuals will elucidate dynamic aspects of childhood suicidal behavior. Others offered suggestions about how to decrease stresses, such as school pressure, that may enhance risk of youth suicidal behavior. Many advocated the need to develop systematic techniques to study youth suicidal behavior.

In recent decades, there has been a rapid rise in suicide among 15- to 24-year-old males in the United States, which began in the late 1960s and peaked in 1977. Clusters of youth suicide were recognized in the 1980s. As a result, extensive public attention was directed toward developing suicide prevention methods, particularly within schools. Research efforts were stimulated. The importance of developing a well-conceptualized approach to decreasing youth suicide was highlighted in the 1986 Health and Human Services–National Institute of Mental Health Task Force Conferences on Youth Suicidal Behavior. Participants at these conferences included international research experts on youth suicidal behavior. Recommendations made at the close of these conferences (Alcohol, Drug Abuse, and Mental Health Administration, 1989) included the need to:

1. Define suicide and report suicide in national and local databases more consistently.
2. Develop research to identify the multifaceted elements of youth suicidal behavior.
3. Evaluate the efficacy of treatments for suicidal youth and those at risk.
4. Support and plan appropriate suicide prevention methods.
5. Educate those providing health care about identification, treatment, and prevention of youth suicidal behavior.
6. Collaborate within the public and private sectors to prevent youth suicide.

EPIDEMIOLOGY

In 1991, the most recent year for complete records of United States Vital Statistics (National Center for Health Statistics, 1993), the age-specific rate of suicide for 15- to 24-year-olds was 13.1 per 100,000, a rate greater than the rate of 12.2 per 100,000 for all ages. Approximately 13% of all deaths of 15- to 24-year-olds were suicides in that year. In marked contrast is the age-specific suicide rate of 0.7 per 100,000 for 5- to 14-year-olds. Although this rate has more than doubled in the last several decades, this increase is significantly lower than the increase for 15- to 24-year-olds.

Suicide rates of 15- to 24-year-olds began to increase in the late 1960s. In 1960, the youth suicide rate was 5.2 per 100,000, in contrast to the more than 2.5-fold increase in 1991. Suicide rates in the United States in 1991 are highest among white males of all age groups (21.7 per 100,000). These age-specific rates for suicidal death of white males are followed by those for nonwhite males (11.8 per 100,000), white females (5.2 per 100,000) and nonwhite females (2.3 per 100,000). In fact the increase in suicide among 15- to 24-year-olds is mostly due to the rates among white males (13.9 per 100,000 in 1991) and not other groups (for example, in 1991, rates were: black males, 9.0 per 100,000; white females, 4.2 per 100,000; black females, 1.6 per 100,000) (National Center for Health Statistics, 1993).

Birth cohort effects have been identified for youth suicide in several countries (Klerman, 1988). A birth cohort is defined as a group of people born within a specific time period. For example, a birth cohort consists of individuals born between 1940 and 1945. Another birth cohort can be individuals born between 1946 and 1950. Reports from Canada, the United States, and Australia suggest that each successive birth cohort has a higher youth suicide rate than previous birth cohorts. In addition, these reports suggest that suicide rates increase as individuals in a cohort get older.

Period effects have also been identified for youth suicide rates. Period effects represent trends that are associated with phenomena occurring within specific time periods. Notably, there has been a marked increase in suicide rates of 15- to 24-year-olds, specifically among individuals born after World War II (Klerman, 1988). These individuals became known as the Baby Boom Cohort. Other psychological problems, such as violence, substance abuse, and severe depression, were also documented as being significantly higher in these individuals.

Reliable national data exist for suicide. However, the epidemiology of suicide attempts among children and adolescents is gradually being elucidated, especially with the development of systematic methods of surveying youth populations. Among adolescents in the general community, surveys (Friedman et al., 1987) estimate that approximately 9% of adolescents report a suicide attempt at least once in their lifetime. Approximately 1% of preadolescents in the general community report suicide attempts (Pfeffer et al., 1986). The ratio of attempted suicide to suicide in children and adolescents has been estimated to be 50:1 (Andrus et al., 1991).

The rates of suicide attempt for community samples are significantly lower than those found among psychiatric patients. For example, approximately one-third of preadolescent and young adolescent psychiatric inpatients attempted suicide prior to hospitalization (Pfeffer, 1986). Furthermore, suicide rates of children and adolescents in the general community are significantly lower than those of child and adolescent psychiatric patients. Suicide among children and adolescents who had a history of psychiatric hospitalization occurs approximately nine times more often than among children and adolescents in the community (Kuperman et al., 1988).

CLINICAL DESCRIPTION

Suicidal ideation and acts are episodic events that can be clearly defined and characterized to have a discrete onset and duration (Pfeffer, 1986). In cases where repeat suicidal events occur, a youngster, who appears to be chronically suicidal, may be understood as exhibiting multiple suicidal events. By defining suicidal behavior as a distinct event, a clinician can focus interventions to reduce the likelihood for subsequent suicidal acts.

Intent to cause harm to oneself is an essential ingredient in defining suicidal behavior. Suicidal intent may be explicit and strong or it may be ambiguous or not well defined. Evaluating intentionality is often a difficult clinical task, especially among preadolescents. For example, a 9-year-old boy, who was seriously despondent after his dog died, threatened to stab himself with a knife during an argument with his mother. He denied that he had thoughts of wanting to kill himself but stated that he wanted to upset his mother. In this case, the intent was not clear but the overt behavior was potentially life-threatening. In contrast, a 15-year-old girl ingested 127 aspirin tablets after she broke up with her boyfriend. She wanted to kill herself because she felt she "had nothing to live for." In this case, suicidal intent was clearly stated.

Because intentionality is often difficult to define in children and adolescents, it is helpful for a clinician to consider that self-injurious acts in children and adolescents are potentially suicidal. This will enhance the possibility that a clinician will more readily plan appropriate life-sparing interventions.

Suicidal behavior involves a wish to cause death. However, understanding the concept that death is final is not an essential ingredient in considering a child or adolescent as suicidal. Development of concepts of death is a slow process (Pfeffer, 1986). Although appreciation of the finality of death may not occur until adolescence, some suicidal adolescents do not have mature concepts of death. Furthermore, there may be variations in a youngster's concepts of death, especially in how a child evaluates personal death or death of others. For example, a 7-year-old may understand that because his pet bird has died, it will no longer be alive. However, this youngster may not understand that if he dies he will never be alive again. Fluctuations in a child's understanding of death may also occur. A child may realize that death is final at one time but when severely stressed, for example, by the divorce and arguments of his parents, such a child may believe that death is reversible.

Most clinicians and researchers agree that the essential goal in carrying out suicidal acts is to achieve death. However, developmental aspects must be considered with regard to youth suicidal behavior. Specifically, it is not essential that a youngster understand that death is final. Death is the goal of suicidal behavior regardless of how death is conceptualized. Utilizing these concepts, it is evident that very young children, such as preschoolers who do not appreciate the finality of death, can be considered to be suicidal if they wish to carry out a self-destructive act with the goal of causing death.

Children and adolescents plan and carry out suicidal acts using a variety of potentially lethal methods. These include shooting, hanging, ingestion, suffocation, stabbing, running into traffic, burning, and drowning. Within the last few decades, use of firearms is the most common method for youth suicide (Brent et al., 1987). Compared to other suicide methods, the increase in incidence of self-inflicted gunshot wounds has paralleled the rapid increase in youth suicide. Furthermore, females attempt suicide more frequently than do males. Females predominantly use methods that involve ingestion of lethal substances to attempt suicide while males use firearms to commit suicide. These differences in prevalence of suicidal methods used by males and females may account for why suicide is higher among men than among women.

CASE ILLUSTRATION

The following case exemplifies some of the characteristics of a teenage suicidal episode. Sam, a 16-year-old boy, attempted to hang himself in his bedroom but was discovered by his father, who untied the noose. Sam left an extensive note on his desk describing how depressed he felt in the past few months. He had failed two school midterm exams and was not accepted on the varsity swim team. He was very disappointed about these events. In addition, he had had arguments with his girlfriend who wanted to date other boys. The night of his suicide attempt, Sam attended a party and drank excessively. He became loud and argumentative. His girlfriend reprimanded him about his behavior. She told him that she was ashamed to be with him and returned a bracelet he had given her for her birthday. Sam was in despair about the tensions with his girlfriend. He returned home at 3:00 AM and wrote a long note explaining why he wanted to kill himself. After he completed the note, he tried to fall asleep but continued to be very upset. Gradually, he formulated a plan to hang himself Sunday morning while his family was at church. However, that morning Sam's father did not go to church and discovered Sam in the process of attempting suicide.

CASE ILLUSTRATION

The following vignette highlights suicidal behavior in a preadolescent. Susan was 9 years old when she took a dose of her mother's antidepressant medication. That day she was with her father who was drinking heavily. He became angry because she was playing the radio too loudly. He hit Susan with a belt and demanded that she stay in her room. She felt devastated by the harsh discipline of her father and thought that it would be best for her to die. She remembered that she had heard her mother talk about wanting to kill herself, especially after arguments with her father. Susan knew that her mother was depressed and identified with her mother's sadness. She quietly left her room, hoping that her father would not hear her, and went to the medicine cabinet where her mother's medication was kept. She took the 10 pills that were in the bottle and returned to her room.

Approximately 1 hour later, her mother returned. She was told by her husband how poorly Susan had behaved and how he had sent her to her room. Susan's mother felt concerned and went to speak with Susan. She found Susan in her bed and very drowsy. After attempts to arouse Susan, her mother called the pediatrician who advised bringing Susan to the emergency room. On the way to the hospital, Susan told her mother that she had taken her mother's medication and felt that she wanted to die. She was admitted to the pediatric intensive care unit for treatment of the overdose.

Both illustrations depict serious suicide attempts in children and adolescents. Both youngsters wanted to die and carried out their planned suicide attempts after experiencing intense stresses, depression, anger, rejection, and criticism. Each youngster could have died if he or she had not been discovered in the process of carrying out the act.

ETIOLOGY AND PATHOGENESIS

Suicidal behavior is a complex symptom that is markedly influenced by sociocultural factors and on a more microscopic level by presence of psychiatric disorders, other psychiatric symptoms, stressful life events, and poor social adjustment. To better conceptualize the components of youth suicidal behavior, a multiaxial approach, similar to that of the DSM-IV classification for psychiatric disorders, may be utilized as a model of integrating the multifocal attributes associated with suicidal behavior in children and adolescents. Notwithstanding the fact that suicidal behavior is a symptom and not a psychiatric disorder, the factors involved with the incidence and prevalence of youth suicidal behavior can be outlined in accordance with five axes: (*a*) primary psychiatric disorders, (*b*) developmental and personality disorders, (*c*) biological factors, (*d*) stress, and (*e*) social functioning.

Primary Psychiatric Disorders

Studies utilizing psychological autopsy methodology to study factors associated with youth suicide and cross-sectional research designs of children and adolescents who report suicidal ideation and acts validate the significant correlations of suicidal behavior with mood disorders and disruptive disorders among prepubertal children and adolescents and the significant relationship of alcohol and substance abuse disorders with suicidal acts in adolescents. The San Diego Suicide Study (Fowler et al., 1986; Rich et al., 1986) highlighted the comparison of 150 individuals who committed suicide when older than 30 years and 133 who committed suicide when younger. The youth suicide victims had a higher prevalence of drug abuse, noted by the finding that 53% of the younger suicides abused substances. Substance abuse was chronic and prevalent for approximately 9 years among these younger suicide victims. The most frequently abused substances were alcohol, marijuana, and cocaine. The younger suicide victims had a lower prevalence of mood and organic mental disorders.

While the San Diego Suicide Study pointed out important developmental differences for suicide between youth and middle age and older adults, the New York Psychological Autopsy Study (Shaffer, 1988) described psychiatric factors associated with gender differences for 173 youth suicide victims. Utilizing odds ratios, a statistic that defines the likelihood that a given factor will have a specific effect to increase risk for suicide, this study reported that among males, a history of a suicide attempt (odds ratio = 22.5), presence of major depression (odds ratio = 8.6), and presence of substance abuse (odds ratio = 7.1) were the strongest correlates for adolescent male suicide. The strongest correlates for adolescent female suicide were presence of major depression (odds ratio = 49.0) and a history of a suicide attempt (odds ratio = 8.6).

A recent case-control study (Brent et al., 1993) comparing 67 adolescents who committed suicide with 67 demographically matched adolescents in the community reported that the presence of major depressive disorder increased risk for suicide by 27 times. Risk was increased 9 times by presence of bipolar disorder, 8.5 times by presence of substance abuse, and 6 times by presence of conduct disorder. Most (82%) of the suicide victims had a mood disorder, and it was notable that, when substance abuse was co-occurring with a mood disorder, there was 17 times greater risk for suicide. History of previous suicidal thinking or suicide attempts were associated with suicide in this study. Although the suicide rate for young children is low, it has been reported (Hoberman and Garfinkel, 1989) that in a sample of suicide victims involving 21 (3.2%) youth younger than 15 years, 208 (31.7%) adolescents, age 15–19 years, and 427 (65.1%) young adults, age 20–24 years, the youngest group had the highest rates of antisocial behavior, and the adolescents and young adults had higher rates of mood disorders.

Although studies of children and adolescents who report nonfatal suicidal behavior suggest that mood disorders, particularly major depressive disorder are significant correlates of suicidal behavior, clear differences between suicidal depressed youth and nonsuicidal depressed youth have not been identified (De-Wilde et al., 1993). This issue requires further study. Nevertheless, in an effort to identify which aspects of major depressive disorder were associated with elements of suicidal behavior, Robbins and Alessi (1985) reported that, for 64 adolescent psychiatric inpatients, suicidal tendencies, identified with semistructured interviews using The Schedule for Affective Disorders and Schizophrenia, were significantly associated with severity of depressed mood, intensity of negative self-evaluation, increased level of hopelessness, poor concentration, and high levels of anhedonia. Furthermore, the number of suicide attempts reported were related to intensity of depressed mood, presence of alcohol abuse, heightened negative self-evaluation, and presence of substance abuse. The seriousness of suicidal intent was documented to be associated with increased degree of depressed mood and elevated degrees of negative self-evaluation. Finally, the lethality of suicide attempts was found to be correlated with increased level of depressed mood, elevated negative self-evaluation, intense states of anhedonia, presence of psychomotor agitation, and presence of alcohol and/or substance abuse.

The findings from another study of 200 adolescent psychiatric inpatients supported the significant correlations of mood disorders and alcohol abuse disorder with suicidal acts. Specifically, in this study, Pfeffer and colleagues (1988) identified that adolescent males who have histories of a suicide attempt and alcohol abuse are most likely to report a recent suicide attempt. In contrast, adolescent females who are most likely to report a recent suicide attempt have histories of a mood disorder, alcohol abuse, and aggressive behavior.

Research with psychiatric patient and community samples of youth has provided validating information about the significant association of mood disorders with youth suicidal behavior. It has been noted (Myers et al., 1991) that, among child and adolescent psychiatric outpatients with a diagnosis of major depressive disorder, more than 70% reported suicidal ideation or attempts and, although these suicidal tendencies were recurrent, they did not increase in severity over a 3-year period of follow-up. Future suicidal tendencies were best predicted by irritability or anger, past history of suicidal thinking or behavior, and older age.

Several studies have investigated suicidal ideation and suicidal behavior in community samples of adolescents, an important endeavor to provide validating data about aspects of suicidal behavior that have been reported among clinical samples of adolescents. Garrison and colleagues (1991) employed a two-stage approach using self-report surveys and research interviews of 1542 adolescents, age 12–14 years. Prevalence of moderate to severe suicidal ideation was 4.0% in males and 8.7% in females. Prevalence of suicide attempts was 1.9% in males and 1.5% in females. Presence of major depressive disorder imparted an almost seven times greater risk for suicidal ideation and an almost 10 times greater risk for suicide attempts. Lewinsohn et al. (1993) interviewed 1710 older adolescents and reported the significant relation of depression to suicide attempts. Furthermore, when the effects of depression were controlled, the greater the number of other risk factors such as externalizing and internalizing behaviors, lifetime history of psychiatric disorders, school problems, health problems, and gender were associated with a greater likelihood of reporting a suicide attempt. The role of aggression, substance abuse, and cigarette smoking were high risk behaviors noted in community samples. It is notable that most studies of community samples utilize adolescents who attend school. In contrast, Rotheram-Borus (1993) interviewed 576 runaway youths, a group representing a type of deviant adolescent that is usually accessible to most community studies of suicidal youth. Thirty-seven percent of these runaways reported a history of a suicide attempt. Although females were more likely to have attempted suicide, depression was significantly associated with suicide attempts in males and females. These reports substantiate the effects of similar risk factors for suicidal behavior in community samples that have been reported for adolescents in psychiatric patient samples.

Developmental and Personality Disorders

The relations between suicidal behavior in prepubertal children and adolescents and disorders on Axis II of DSM-IV need to be clarified. Although there is evidence that youth who are afflicted with specific developmental disorders that impair their learning skills are at heightened risk for suicidal behavior, research suggests that intelligence quotient is not a predictor of youth suicidal behavior.

In recent years, with attention focused on understanding the effects of comorbid psychiatric disorders, it has become apparent that elements related to personality disorders may be significant correlates of youth suicidal behavior. For example, psychiatric symptoms such as impulsivity and intense aggression, which may be indicators for the future development of adult personality disorders such as narcissistic, antisocial, and histrionic personality disorders, have been reported to be positively associated with suicidal behavior in prepubertal children and adolescents.

A recent psychological autopsy study conducted in Finland (1991) of 53 adolescents who were 13–19 years when they committed suicide highlighted the prevalence of personality disorders. In this study, Marttunen and colleagues (Marttunen et al., 1991) noted that 94% were afflicted with a mental disorder. The most prevalent disorders were mood (51%), alcohol abuse (26%), and personality disorder (32%), especially antisocial personality disorder. A reanalysis of the San Diego Suicide Study (Rich and Runeson, 1992) suggested strong evidence for high prevalence of comorbidity on Axis I with depression and substance abuse and Axis II comorbidity with antisocial personality disorder. Furthermore, 41% of the 133 adolescents in the San Diego Suicide Study (Rich and Runeson, 1992) had symptoms of a borderline personality disorder. The investigators raise the important question about whether Axis I and Axis II psychiatric disorders are independent in relation to youth suicide.

An important report (Apter et al., 1993) of 453 consecutive Israeli male suicides, age 18–21 years, suggested that an appreciable number (18.6%) had no DSM-III-R Axis I disorders and that approximately 9% had no DSM-III-R Axis II psychopathology. The most prevalent diagnosis (53.5%) among these suicide victims was major depressive disorder. Notable were the findings that narcissistic and/or schizoid traits were quite prevalent among youth suicide victims. This report also suggests the importance of focusing on aspects of personality in understanding youth suicidal behavior.

In one of the first reports to identify an association between personality disorder and adolescent suicide attempts, Friedman and coworkers (1983) noted that, among 53 adolescent psychiatric inpatients, those with borderline personality disorder had the most frequent and severe suicide attempts. In another report (Apter et al., 1988) impulsivity and aggression were noted to be associated with suicidal behavior among adolescent psychiatric inpatients. Higher scores on the subscale of The Kiddie Schedule for Affective Disorders and Schizophrenia that indicate degree of suicidal tendencies were found for adolescents with conduct disorder than for adolescents with major depressive disorder. It may be inferred that features of conduct disorder that may predict adult personal-

ity disorder may be important links to youth suicidal behavior. Pfeffer and colleagues (1988), in their study of a large sample of adolescent psychiatric inpatients, reported that borderline personality disorder was associated with suicidal behavior among the females but not among the males.

An important clinical study conducted by Brent and colleagues (1993) evaluated the prevalence and severity of assaultive behavior, impulsivity, and personality disorders in 37 adolescent psychiatric inpatients who attempted suicide and adolescent psychiatric inpatients without a history of suicidal behavior. Significantly more suicide attempters than nonsuicidal adolescents had symptoms of personality disorder, especially borderline personality disorder. However, no discernible differences were found in prevalence or severity of assaultiveness or impulsivity among the two groups of adolescents.

Although reports of prepubertal suicidal children have not focused on disturbances in personality traits, subgroups of suicidal children have been identified. For example, Pfeffer (1986) described that prepubertal children who report both suicidal and violent behavior have significant deficits in impulse control. These features, that is, violence, suicidal behavior, and impulsivity, may be ingredients for future development of personality disorders. In contrast, a group of prepubertal children were described who were suicidal and not violent. These children were predominantly depressed and had good impulse control. The relationship of indicators of personality disorders is still to be identified in this type of subgroup of suicidal children.

Biological Factors

Elucidation of biological correlates of suicidal behavior in prepubertal children and adolescents is emerging and appears, in general, to concur with features described for suicidal adults. For example, although there are diverse research results about the relations between suicidal behavior in adults and hypothalamic-pituitary-adrenal (HPA) axis functioning, elevated levels of plasma cortisol have been noted for suicidal adults. Some reports for youth indicate a possible role for excessive HPA functioning among suicidal youth. Pfeffer and colleagues (1991) reported an elevated level of plasma cortisol during the dexamethasone suppression text for suicidal compared with nonsuicidal prepubertal child psychiatric inpatients. Dahl and collaborators (1990) described that adolescents who reported suicide attempts while in an episode of major depressive disorder had elevated levels of plasma cortisol prior to sleep onset. This was not observed for adolescents with major depressive disorder who did not have a history of a recent suicide attempt. The role of HPA activity, especially as a potential indicator of a response to stress, for risk of youth suicidal behavior requires additional research.

Strong research evidence has been presented for the positive relations between suicidal and violent behavior, impulsivity, and aberrations in neurotransmitter systems, especially those involved with serotonin metabolism and regulation. Asberg was the first to report low levels of 5-hydroxyindoleacetic acid (5-HIAA) in cerebrospinal fluid of violent suicidal adults. Suicide occurred more frequently among those individuals than among those with higher 5-HIAA in their spinal fluid. These results were validated in numerous other studies, suggesting associations between aberrant serotonin system functioning and α_2-adrenoceptors in postmortem brain samples, especially frontal-cortical regions, and low levels of 5-HIAA in cerebrospinal fluid samples of suicidal adults. In addition, some studies of suicidal adults report lower levels of homovanillic acid, a dopamine neurotransmitter metabolite, in the cerebrospinal fluid of suicidal compared with nonsuicidal adults.

Research using similar complex methods to study youth is underway. Greenhill reported at the 1993 Annual Meeting of the Society for Biological Psychiatry preliminary results of suicidal adolescent psychiatric inpatients with a diagnosis of conduct disorder in which these adolescents had low levels of 5-HIAA in their cerebrospinal fluid. A new report (Ambrosini et al., 1992) of peripheral plasma markers suggested that platelet imipramine binding may be lower in depressed prepubertal children and adolescents with a history of suicidal behavior than among youth with no history of suicidal behavior.

Finally, approaches with chronobiological methods (Dahl et al., 1990) suggest that, unlike prepubertal children, adolescents with major depressive disorder who report a recent suicide attempt have aberrations in sleep architecture before the onset of sleep, compared to no aberrations in these chronobiological parameters among depressed adolescents with no history of suicidal behavior. Pursuit of other research into biological factors associated with youth suicidal behavior will elucidate developmental characteristics associated with potential etiologic aspects of suicidal behavior.

Stress

Extensive research results suggest the significant relations between youth suicidal behavior and stressful life events. Prepubertal children who report suicidal ideation or suicide attempts have higher rates of cumulative stressful life events than nonsuicidal prepubertal children. The varied types of stressful events include deaths and separations of relatives, births of siblings, illness, hospitalization, multiple family moves. Similarly, adolescent suicide attempters, compared with depressed nonsuicidal adolescents and normal adolescents, have more lifetime and recent stressful life events.

Family disruptions and discord stemming from excessive arguments and overt violence, loss of relatives due to marital separations and/or divorce, and problems in family interpersonal relations derived from parental psychiatric illness are important aspects of stressful circumstances experienced by suicidal children and adolescents. Shaffi and associates (1985), in a comparative psychological autopsy study, reported that adolescent suicidal victims, compared with nonsuicidal adolescents, had more exposure to suicidal behavior among relatives or friends. For example, 60% of the suicide victims, compared to 12% of the nonsuicidal adolescents, had parents or adult relatives with suicidal tendencies. The parents of these suicide victims had more emotional problems and absence from home, and they abused their children more than did parents of nonsuicidal adolescents.

The New York Psychological Autopsy Study (Shaffer, 1988) reported that a family history of suicide imparted a five times greater risk of suicide on adolescent males and an almost three times greater risk for suicide on adolescent females. Brent and collaborators (1988) reported that, among adolescents who committed suicide and adolescents who reported suicidal ideation or suicide attempts, there was a significantly high prevalence of mood disorders, antisocial personality disorders, and suicide among relatives. In one of the first available systematic controlled family studies of prepubertal suicidal children, Pfeffer et al. (1994) reported high rates of suicidal acts, violence, substance abuse, and antisocial personality disorders among first-degree relatives of prepubertal children who reported suicidal ideation or suicide attempts. Family discord was also marked among these suicidal children.

Violence, especially physical abuse, has been described as a strong risk factor for youth suicidal behavior. Deykin and colleagues (1985) reported that 159 adolescent suicide attempters evaluated in an urban hospital emergency service, compared with a similar number of nonsuicidal adolescents evaluated in the same emergency service, were three to six times more likely to have had contact with the Department of Social Service Registry for suspicion of physical abuse. The estimated proportion of suicide attempts that could be explained by a history of involvement with the Social Service Department was 12%. This study lends support to the idea that physical abuse is a significant risk factor for youth suicidal behavior.

Sequelae of the suicidal death of an adolescent friend or acquaintance, although not likely to increase the incidence of suicidal acts among adolescent peers of the adolescent suicide victim, are characterized by an increased incidence of mood disorders within 6 months after the suicidal death (Brent et al., 1992; Hazell et al., 1993). Future follow-up studies of longer duration are needed to identify if friends or acquaint-

ances of an adolescent who commits suicide are at increased risk for suicidal acts. Similarly, empirical studies are needed to characterize the short- and long-term psychiatric and social sequelae of a suicide of a relative on prepubertal children and adolescents.

Another facet of family disturbance was reported by Salk and colleagues (1985) using a follow-back research design to study the relation between prenatal and perinatal factors and youth suicidal behavior. Fifty-six factors in the prenatal, birth, and neonatal records of 52 adolescents who committed suicide and records of a similar number of two matched nonsuicidal controls were studied. Respiratory distress for more than 1 hour after birth, no antenatal care before 20 weeks of pregnancy, and chronic physical disease of the mother differentiated those who committed suicide from those who did not. An implication of this study is that early stress may enhance vulnerability to suicide, especially among adolescents who have a history of severe stress or psychopathology during adolescence. However, the mechanisms leading to such vulnerability are not known.

Social Functioning

Problems with social adjustment are an important characteristic of suicidal children and adolescents (Pfeffer, 1986). These problems tend to be chronic and similar to the characteristics of depressed children. Poor social adjustment among suicidal youth is apparent even after a child or adolescent no longer reports suicidal tendencies. This feature, in large measure, accounts for the long-term vulnerability of children and adolescents to suicidal acts. For prepubertal suicidal children, interpersonal relations are problematic between parents, siblings, and the suicidal youngster. Added to these problems are difficult relations with peers, which are especially prominent as social adjustment difficulties among suicidal adolescents.

Social adjustment in children and adolescents is influenced by presence of adequate social supports and predictability of the environmental milieu, especially regarding relationships with parents, siblings, and other helpful adults and peers. Suicidal children and adolescents frequently experience a lack of available empathic individuals who are useful to offer guidance and avenues for an adolescent to ventilate distressing ideas and feelings. An unpredictable social support network combined with a suicidal youth's perceptions of inadequacies in mobilizing social support intensify the suicidal youngster's sense of isolation, anxiety, poor self-esteem, rejection, and hopelessness. Perceived hopelessness are among the significant factors that intensify suicidal risk for youth. Hopeless feelings frequently impair a suicidal youngster's ability to remain motivated to solve problems and to cope with adversity.

Specific styles of coping among suicidal children and adolescents limit their flexibility and resourcefulness in coping with intense emotions and in problem solving (Pfeffer, 1986). It is notable that when prepubertal suicidal children encounter ambiguities or difficulties in interpersonal situations, they lack skills to respond with beneficial actions that solve their dilemmas. Rather, suicidal children and adolescents characteristically respond either impulsively or tend to withdraw into states of paralytic rumination or fantasy. Ego mechanisms of defense, empirically studied among suicidal children and adolescents, involve denial of affects or acknowledgment of events (Pfeffer, 1986). This may account for observations suggesting that suicidal youths' reality testing may be impaired. Other ego mechanisms of defense are reaction formation, which operates to modify painful affects and distressing thoughts by turning their perceptions into opposite perceptions. Compensation, another ego mechanism of defense among suicidal children, involves risk-taking behavior or overt exaggeration of one's skills. This defense defuses a youngster's sense of inadequacy. Suicidal adolescents also cope by involving specific ego mechanisms that are similar to those observed for suicidal preadolescents. In general, suicidal adolescents turn feelings against themselves, especially aggressive impulses. They also utilize aspects of reaction formation. These styles of coping are among the important factors that compromise suicidal children and adolescents in maintaining adequate levels of social relatedness. Combined with this, social functioning of suicidal children and adolescents is also impaired by life within an inadequate or unpredictable social milieu.

LABORATORY STUDIES

Biological Assessment

At present, there is no distinct biological test to measure risk for youth suicidal behavior. The most fruitful areas of clinical investigation are in understanding the relation between alterations in serotonin metabolites and neuroendocrine functions and risk for suicidal behavior. However, practical application has not been determined.

Psychological Assessments

Assessment of youth suicidal behavior involves comprehensive interviews with a suicidal youngster and his or her parents and gathering information from other individuals who know the youngster. These assessments are complicated, especially when interviewing prepubertal children about their suicidal ideation and acts (Jacobsen et al., 1994). Some of the aspects that influence the information obtained in a clinical interview are the child's cognitive and emotional state and the degree of psychopathology of parents. It is important that clinical interviews be conducted at the time of maximum suicidal risk and repeated subsequently within close proximity until risk of suicidal behavior is diminished. Table 61.1 lists parameters that suggest high or low risk for youth suicidal behavior.

The most important aspect of the assessment is to determine the degree of immediate danger for a youngster. If a youngster's situation is unpredictable, consideration of emergency psychiatric hospitalization is warranted.

The main ingredients of an evaluation involve determining the circumstances surrounding suicidal ideation or an act, the intent to die or cause injury, the degree of planning involved in carrying out a suicidal act, and the degree that rescue from the act is possible. Accessibility to lethal suicidal methods must be evaluated.

Essential to the evaluation is to determine the current psychological status of a youngster with respect to type and degree of psychopathology and degree and quality of coping mechanisms such as adequacy of judgment, degree of impulse control, intensity of hopelessness and helplessness, and ability to communicate. A youngster may be at lower risk for suicidal acts if he or she has good judgment, high impulse control, low levels of hopelessness and helplessness, and ability to communicate openly and honestly about feelings, worries, and thoughts of suicide. However, it must be appreciated that the status of these variables may change rapidly so that repeated, comprehensive discussion with a suicidal youngster is necessary.

Assessment of family and environmental conditions is essential. It is important to determine whether a family can provide a consistent,

stable environment or whether there is high intensity of stress, violence, psychopathology, and unavailability of relatives. Positive social supports are critical in diminishing suicidal risk among children and adolescents. If an environment does not provide sufficient beneficial social supports, a potentially suicidal child or adolescent will need to be removed from such an environment and placed in a situation, such as a psychiatric hospital, that will promote psychological growth and deter suicidal tendencies.

DIFFERENTIAL DIAGNOSIS

The two most significant issues in a differential diagnosis of youth suicidal behavior is to identify whether the destructive act is self-intended rather than accidental and to identify whether there is a high or low level of risk that an injury will occur. The first issue is a qualitative issue and involves a systematic assessment of intent and the specific circumstances in which a self-destructive act occurred. The second issue is a quantitative one and involves a comprehensive evaluation of the intensity and interactions among risk factors. Since both issues are often difficult to define distinctly, it is more helpful, in situations where a definite conclusion cannot be made, to consider a youngster to be suicidal and at significant risk rather than to minimize the clinical condition. By utilizing this approach, a plan for treatment may be conceptualized and implemented rapidly.

TREATMENT

There are no controlled studies of treatment of suicidal children and adolescents, although beginning efforts are now underway to develop and study controlled treatment conditions for suicidal youth. Currently available reports of treatment describe approaches based on clinical experience.

The most salient acute issue in treatment is to decrease the likelihood that self-inflicted injury or death could occur. Psychiatric hospitalization may be recommended if observation and intensive therapeutic intervention are needed. The hospital offers an environment with structure and a consistent, high availability of staff to provide immediate round-the-clock interventions. Hospitalization is also a way of removing a youngster from an environment that may be too stressful or disorganized.

Psychotherapeutic intervention involves developing a trustful atmosphere for truthful communication. It is essential that a therapist maintain an empathic but objective concept of a suicidal youngster. A therapist's collusion with the perceptions of despair, misery, or hostility of a suicidal child or adolescent will impair treatment progress. Discussion that may elucidate the operation of new and effective coping strategies is essential. This can be achieved by incorporating cognitive orientation to the treatment process.

Delineation of the motivations for a suicidal act is an important feature of treatment. Such motivations may be conscious or out of immediate awareness of a suicidal youth. Common motives for enacting suicidal behavior involve despair over loss of a special person such as a breakup with a boyfriend or girlfriend or the separation of parents. These situations often involve intense guilt that a youngster may have caused the loss. Other motivations involve anger or feelings of revenge in response to frustrations, deprivations, or perceived wrongdoing. Often a youngster will impulsively threaten suicide as an effort to instill guilt in those who are closely involved in a youngster's life situation. Another motivation is based on psychotic functioning. Some psychotic youngsters feel so demoralized and in such psychic pain that they wish to relieve themselves of psychic pain by committing suicide. Such a response may be impulsive and without warning.

Treatment of suicidal children and adolescents is complex and requires simultaneous utilization of multiple modalities. In addition to dynamic, supportive, and cognitive psychotherapy, psychopharmacologic modalities may be indicated. At present, there is no medication specific to suicidal behavior. However, if a biological basis for suicidal behavior is identified, specific psychopharmacological methods of inter-

Table 61.1. High and Low Risk Parameters for Youth Suicidal Behavior

Parameter	High Risk	Low Risk
Predictability of youngster	Low	High
Circumstances of suicidal behavior	Alone	Near someone
	Planned	Less carefully planned
	Lethal methods	Low lethality methods
Intent to die	High	Low
Psychopathology	Present and severe	Absent or mild
Coping mechanisms	Poor judgment	Good judgment
	Impulse control	Good impulse control
	High hopelessness	Low hopelessness
	High helplessness	Low helplessness
Communication	Poor or ambivalent	Good, clear
Family support	Inconsistent	Consistent
Environmental stress	High	Low

vention may be developed. At present, medications useful to decrease suicidal behavior are those used to decrease symptoms of specific psychiatric disorders. Antidepressants and/or lithium may be useful for mood disorders. Major tranquilizers may be useful for psychotic disorders, and psychostimulants may be helpful for attention deficit disorders. By decreasing the symptoms of a psychiatric disorder, suicidal symptoms may also be lessened.

Treatment of parents and other relatives may be indicated, especially if such people have a direct influence on a suicidal youngster, and if they have impairing symptoms of psychopathology that contribute to the adverse family milieu. Parental marriage counselling, individual psychotherapy, or focused psychopharmacotherapy may be required for certain relatives. Detailed assessment and decrease of psychiatric symptoms and psychiatric disorders of family members are necessary, especially in order to promote a stable atmosphere for the youngster.

Collaborative efforts with other professionals who are involved with a youngster must be organized. For example, it may be essential to consult with the school psychologist or guidance counsellor who may speak with a youngster during school hours. Collaboration with the school may help stabilize a youngster within the school and community environment.

The overall strategy for treatment of suicidal children and adolescents requires a flexible and multimodal approach that aims to stabilize the psychological state of the youngster and the social atmosphere of the environment so that risk for suicidal action may be decreased.

APPROACHES FOR PREVENTION OF YOUTH SUICIDAL BEHAVIOR

Although rates of suicide among youth in the United States are high and have not appreciably diminished in the last few years, avenues for developing suicide prevention strategies can be inferred by the recent studies of youth suicidal behavior. For example, it is evident from prospective research that prepubertal children and adolescents who report suicide attempts are at significant risk for recurrent suicidal acts (Pfeffer et al., 1991, 1993). Prepubertal psychiatric inpatients who attempted suicide are six times more likely to attempt suicide in adolescence than are children in the general community. Prepubertal psychiatric inpatients who report thoughts of suicide are at four times higher risk for attempting suicide within less than 10 years than children in the general community. Adolescent psychiatric inpatients who attempt suicide are at significant risk for a repeat suicide attempt within 6 months of follow-up (Brent et al., 1993) and for suicide in less than 10 years (Pfeffer, 1986). The data about suicidal children and adolescents are supported also by studies showing that prepubertal children who have a major depressive disorder are at risk for suicide attempts in adolescence (Kovacs et al., 1993) and suicide in young adulthood (Rao et al., 1993). Suicide prevention efforts should focus on identifying such high risk children and adolescents and monitoring them repeatedly for early signs of risk for a suicidal act.

Consistent with the United States Secretary's Task Force for Youth Suicidal Behavior Report (Alcohol, Drug Abuse, and Mental Health Administration, 1989), efforts to prevent youth suicidal behavior require public health model strategies. Among those are school-based suicide prevention curricula aimed to educate adolescents about the prevalence and warning signs of suicidal behavior. This may, thereby, encourage adolescents to seek help if they recognize symptoms of suicidal risk. A basic premise for the development of such school programs was that all adolescents, especially if they experience severe stress, are at risk for suicidal behavior. Therefore, all adolescents attending school were involved in these special suicide prevention curricula. Reports of evaluations of some of these programs concluded that their efficacy was not adequate to prevent suicide, to change adolescents' attitudes about suicide, or to enhance help-seeking behavior. Some reports (Shaffer et al., 1991) suggested that adolescents who had a history of suicidal behavior were especially upset by these curricula and that those students had negative feelings about these educational programs. Insights gained by evaluating these programs lead to conceptualizing the need to focus on

high risk samples of youth rather than on the general population of youth.

Clusters of youth suicide, notable during the early 1980s in the United States, became phenomena of intensive research investigation (Gould and Shaffer, 1986; Hafner and Schmidtke, 1989; Phillips and Carstensen, 1986). It became apparent that factors promoting youth suicide clusters involved imitation of suicidal acts. Clusters were defined as incidents of youth suicide that occurred either within the same defined time period and/or the same defined location. Complex research methods determined that there was a significant increase in adolescent suicide within 2 weeks after media presentations of stories of actual or fictional youth suicide. An aspect of suicide prevention was proposed to educate media professionals about the importance of less sensational presentations and the complementary inclusion of suicide prevention guidelines with these media reports. In general, media reports have adhered to these suicide prevention techniques.

Another aspect of the problem of imitation of youth suicide involved developing methods for communities to respond to a youth suicidal death so that risk for other youth suicidal acts is lessened. Guidelines were established that included organizing community networks consisting of school professionals, mental health professionals, police, religious leaders, and parents to be available to respond to the community crises of a youth suicide. Organized liaison approaches with the media are essential to promote helpful media coverage of the event and to prevent confusion, fear, and risk for other youth suicidal acts stimulated by the presence of news reporters and presentations of the story of a youth suicide. Focus on other vulnerable youngsters is another aspect of responding to the crisis of a youth suicide. Discussions are helpful with friends and acquaintances of the adolescent who committed suicide. Recent research (Brent et al., 1992; Hazel et al., 1993) suggests that risk for suicidal behavior may be low among friends and acquaintances of an adolescent suicide victim within 6 months of the suicidal death. However, risk for developing a major depressive disorder is high among such friends and acquaintances. Additional research is needed to validate these research results and to determine whether there is risk for suicidal behavior of such friends and acquaintances over longer periods of follow-up.

Suicidal behavior involves a legacy that runs in families. Prepubertal children who report suicidal ideation and suicide attempts have higher rates of suicidal acts among first-degree relatives than nonsuicidal children (Pfeffer et al., 1994). Research is necessary to identify the degree of psychiatric and social morbidity involved with children and adolescents who experience the suicidal death of a parent or sibling. From a clinical perspective, such youth may be vulnerable and are in need of follow-up monitoring.

Finally, strong evidence suggests that availability of guns and firearms is significantly associated with youth suicide risk. Intense efforts to prevent youth suicide require a national focus to advocate for better restriction of availability of guns and firearms, especially to children and adolescents. Furthermore, clinical assessments of suicidal risk among children and adolescents should incorporate inquiry about the presence of such lethal weapons in the home or whether there are other avenues for access to a gun or firearm. Decreasing such accessibility is an important suicide prevention action.

CONCLUSION

Although important and useful knowledge has been acquired in the last decade about suicidal behavior among children and adolescents, future research is necessary to focus on identifying etiologically relevant mechanisms for suicidal behavior and for developing effective treatment strategies to lower risk for youth suicidal behavior. Research is needed to develop large population models for understanding relevant sociocultural phenomena, such as social transitions, that may involve risk and protective factors for youth suicidal behavior. Such research when combined with research that focuses on more microscopic aspects of youth suicidal behavior, such as biological factors or psychiatric phenomenology, may be helpful in reducing rates of suicidal behavior among youth.

References

Alcohol, Drug Abuse, and Mental Health Administration: *Report of The Secretary's Task Force on Youth Suicide*, DHHS Pub. No. (ADM)89-1621. Washington, DC, US Government Printing Office, 1989.

Ambrosini PJ, Metz C, Arora RC, et al: Platelet imipramine binding in depressed children. *J Am Acad Child Adolesc Psychiatry* 31:298–305, 1992.

Andrus JK, Fleming DW, Heumann MA, et al: Surveillance of attempted suicide among adolescents in Oregon, 1988. *Am J Public Health* 81:1067–1069, 1991.

Apter A, Bleich A, King RA, et al: Death without warning? A clinical postmortem study of suicide in 43 Israeli adolescent males. *Arch Gen Psychiatry* 50:138–142, 1993.

Apter A, Bleich A, Plutchik R, et al: Suicidal behavior, depression, and conduct disorder in hospitalized adolescents. *J Am Acad Child Adolesc Psychiatry* 27:696–699, 1988.

Brent DA, Johnson B, Bartle S, et al: Personality disorder, tendency to impulsive violence and suicidal behavior in adolescents. *J Am Acad Child Adolesc Psychiatry* 32:69–75, 1993.

Brent DA, Kalas R, Edelbrock C, et al: Psychopathology and its relationship to suicidal ideation in childhood and adolescence. *J Am Acad Child Adolesc Psychiatry* 25:666–673, 1986.

Brent DA, Kolko DJ, Wartella ME, et al: Adolescent psychiatric inpatients' risk of suicide attempt at 6 month follow-up. *J Am Acad Child Adolesc Psychiatry* 32:95–105, 1993.

Brent DA, Perper JA, Allman CJ: Alcohol, firearms, and suicide among youth: Temporal trends in Allegheny County, Pennsylvania, 1960–1983. *JAMA* 257:3369–3372, 1987.

Brent DA, Perper JA, Goldstein CE, et al: Risk factors for adolescent suicide: A comparison of adolescent suicide victims with suicidal inpatients. *Arch Gen Psychiatry* 45:581–588, 1988.

Brent DA, Perper J, Moritz G, et al: Psychiatric effects of exposure to suicide among friends and acquaintances of adolescent suicide victims. *J Am Acad Child Adolesc Psychiatry* 31:629–639, 1992.

Brent DA, Perper JA, Moritz G, et al: Psychiatric risk factors for adolescent suicide: A case-control study. *J Am Acad Child Adolesc Psychiatry* 32:521–529, 1993.

Carlson GA, Cantwell DP: Suicidal behavior and depression in children and adolescents. *J Am Acad Child Psychiatry* 21:361–368, 1982.

Dahl RE, Puig-Antich J, Ryan ND, et al: EEG sleep in adolescents with major depression: The role of suicidality and inpatient status. *J Affect Disord* 19:63–75, 1990.

De-Wilde EJ, Kienhorst IC, Diekstra RF, et al: The specificity of psychological characteristics of adolescent suicide attempters. *J Am Acad Child Adolesc Psychiatry* 32:51–59, 1993.

Deykin EY, Alpert JJ, McNamarra JJ: A pilot study of the effect of exposure to child abuse or neglect on adolescent suicidal behavior. *Am J Psychiatry* 142:1299–1303, 1985.

Friedman JM, Asnis GM, Boeck M, et al: Prevalence of specific suicidal behaviors in a high school sample. *Am J Psychiatry* 144:1203–1206, 1987.

Friedman RC, Aronoff MS, Clarkin JF, et al: History of suicidal behavior in depressed borderline inpatients. *Am J Psychiatry* 140:1023–1026, 1983.

Fowler RC, Rich CL, Young D: San Diego Suicide Study: Substance abuse in young cases. *Arch Gen Psychiatry* 43:962–965, 1986.

Garrison CZ, Jackson KL, Addy CL, et al: Suicidal behaviors in young adolescents. *Am J Epidemiol* 133:1005–1014, 1991.

Gould MS, Shaffer D: The impact of suicide in television movies: Evidence of imitation. *N Engl J Med* 315:690–694, 1986.

Hafner H, Schmidtke A: Do televised fictional suicide models produce suicides? In: Pfeffer CR (ed): *Suicide among Youth: Perspectives on Risk and Prevention*. Washington, DC, American Psychiatric Press, 1989, pp. 117–141.

Hazell P, Lewin T: Friends of adolescent suicide attempters and completers. *J Am Acad Child Adolesc Psychiatry* 32:76–81, 1993.

Hawton K, Osborn M, O'Grady J, et al: Classification of adolescents who take overdoses. *Br J Psychiatry* 140:124–131, 1982.

Hoberman HM, Garfinkel BD: Completed suicide in youth. In: Pfeffer CR (ed): *Suicide among Youth: Perspectives on Risk and Prevention*. Washington, DC, American Psychiatric Press, 1989, pp. 21–40.

Jacobsen LK, Rabinowitz I, Popper MS, et al: Interviewing prepubertal children about suicidal ideation and behavior. *J Am Acad Child Adolesc Psychiatry* 33:439–452, 1994.

Klerman GL: The current age of youthful melancholia: Evidence for increase in depression among adolescents and young adults. *Br J Psychiatry* 152:4–14, 1988.

Kovacs M, Goldston D, Gatsonis C: Suicidal behaviors and childhood-onset depressive disorders: A longitudinal investigation. *J Am Acad Child Adolesc Psychiatry* 32:8–20, 1993.

Kuperman S, Black DW, Burns TL: Excess mortality among formerly hospitalized child psychiatric patients. *Arch Gen Psychiatry* 45:277–282, 1988.

Lewinsohn PM, Rohde P, Seeley JR: Psychosocial characteristics of adolescents with a history of suicide attempt. *J Am Acad Child Adolesc Psychiatry* 32:60–68, 1993.

Marttunen MJ, Aro HM, Henriksson MM, et al: Mental disorders in adolescent suicide: DSM-III-R axis I and II diagnoses in suicides among 13 to 19 year olds in Finland. *Arch Gen Psychiatry* 48:834–839, 1991.

Myers K, McCauley E, Calderon R, et al: The 3-year longitudinal course of suicidality and predictive factors for subsequent suicidality in youths with major depressive disorder. *J Am Acad Child Adolesc Psychiatry* 30:804–810, 1991.

National Center for Health Statistics: Advance report of final mortality statistics, 1991. In: *Monthly Vital Statistics* Report 42, No. 2 suppl. Hyattsville, MD, Public Health Service, 1993.

Pfeffer CR: *The Suicidal Child*. New York, Guilford Press, 1986.

Pfeffer CR, Klerman GL, Hurt SW, et al: Suicidal children grow up: Demographic and clinical risk factors for adolescent suicide attempts. *J Am Acad Child Adolesc Psychiatry* 30:609–616, 1991.

Pfeffer CR, Klerman GL, Hurt SW, et al: Suicidal children grow up: Rates and psychosocial risk factors for suicide attempts during follow-up. *J Am Acad Child Adolesc Psychiatry* 32:106–113, 1993.

Pfeffer CR, Newcorn J, Kaplan G, et al: Suicidal behavior in adolescent psychiatric inpatients. *J Am Acad Child Adolesc Psychiatry* 27:357–361, 1988.

Pfeffer CR, Normandin L, Kakuma T: Suicidal children grow up: Suicidal behavior and psychiatric disorders among relatives. *J Am Acad Child Adolesc Psychiatry* 33:1087–1097, 1994.

Pfeffer CR, Plutchik R, Mizruchi MS, et al: Suicidal behavior in child psychiatric inpatients and outpatients and in nonpatients. *Am J Psychiatry* 143:733–738, 1986.

Pfeffer CR, Solomon G, Plutchik R, et al: Suicidal behavior in latency-age psychiatric inpatients: A replication and cross validation. *J Am Acad Child Psychiatry* 21:564–569, 1982.

Pfeffer CR, Stokes P, Shindledecker R: Suicidal behavior and hypothalamic-pituitary-adrenocortical axis indices in child psychiatric inpatients. *Biol Psychiatry* 29:909–917, 1991.

Phillips DP, Carstensen L: Clustering of teenage suicides after television news stories about suicide. *N Engl J Med* 315:685–689, 1986.

Rao U, Weissman MM, Martin JA, et al: Childhood depression and risk of suicide: A preliminary report of a longitudinal study. *J Am Acad Child Adolesc Psychiatry* 32:21–27, 1993.

Rich CL, Runeson BS: Similarities in diagnostic comorbidity between suicide among young people in Sweden and the United States. *Acta Psychiatr Scand* 86:335–339, 1992.

Rich CL, Young D, Fowler RC: San Diego Suicide Study: Young versus old subjects. *Arch Gen Psychiatry* 43:577–582, 1986.

Robbins DR, Alessi NE: Depressive symptoms and suicidal behavior in adolescents. *Am J Psychiatry* 142:588–592, 1985.

Rotheram-Borus MJ: Suicidal behaviors and risk factors among run away youths. *Am J Psychiatry* 150:103–107, 1993.

Salk L, Lipsitt LP, Sturner WQ, et al: Relationship of maternal and perinatal conditions to eventual adolescent suicide. *Lancet* March 16, 1985.

Shaffer D: The epidemiology of teen suicide: An examination of risk factors. *J Clin Psychiatry* 49:36–41, 1988.

Shaffer P, Garland A, Vieland V, et al: The impact of curriculum-based suicide prevention programs for teenagers. *J Am Acad Child Adolesc Psychiatry* 30:588–596, 1991.

Shafii M, Carrigan S, Whittinghill JR, et al: Psychological autopsy of completed suicide in children and adolescents. *Am J Psychiatry* 142:1061–1064, 1985.

62 ANXIETY DISORDERS

Richard Livingston, M.D.

"Anxiety is something everybody has, only some of us have the rotten luck to be sick with it." Thus 16-year-old Leslie, who is being treated for panic disorder, capsulizes the subject of this chapter. This group of disorders includes those with primary clinical phenomena of excessive fears and worries, phobic avoidance, generalized vigilance and anticipatory anxiety, and panic attacks in which autonomic symptoms are coupled with a subjective sense of overwhelming dread.

Diagnostically, these clinical phenomena are categorized in both adults and children as phobias when the primary manifestation is a specific fear coupled with avoidance behavior; social inhibitions may be symptoms of social phobia, or a more ego-syntonic personality trait. The disorders in which panic-type attacks and anticipatory distress are major components include panic disorder (in both adults and children) and separation anxiety disorder in children. The more chronic and generalized anxiety state is called generalized anxiety disorder in adults and young people. Nonphobic anxiety reactions to specific stressors may be manifested in children and adolescents as adjustment disorder with anxious mood, in the very young as reactive attachment disorder of infancy, and in extreme cases as posttraumatic stress disorder.

In both adults and children there is considerable overlap among the manifestations of these disorders and significant comorbidity with other psychiatric disorders and probably certain medical disorders as well. Multiple diagnoses should be considered and made when appropriate, but in most cases it will be evident that one form of anxiety is primary and should be so identified; other clinical manifestations that do not reach criterion level should not be ignored, however, and should be duly noted, followed, and treated when necessary.

Although these disorders can cause significant distress and disability while an individual is afflicted, it would appear that the overall prognosis for anxiety disorders that occur in childhood or adolescence is good, and that most neurotic children become normal adults, while most neurotic adults develop their neuroses as adults (Robins, 1971). Exceptions to this may include people with the more severe cases of separation anxiety disorder, up to half of whom may have longer-lasting problems, and chronically anxious children of affectively ill parents (Keller et al., 1992).

In this chapter some general comments are made about definitions, developmental issues, classification, epidemiology, etiology and pathogenesis, assessment, and treatment of anxiety and the anxiety disorders of youth. This is followed by discussions of specific disorders, beginning with separation anxiety disorder, highlighting what is known (and not known) and what is unique about the particular conditions.

DEFINITION

Anxiety may be broadly defined as the emotional uneasiness associated with the anticipation of danger. It is usually distinguished from fear, the emotional response to objective danger, although the physiologic manifestations are the same. (Some definitions limit anxiety to dangers that are not within conscious awareness.)

Such a broad definition suggests that anxiety not only is a common human experience but also is present in many psychiatric and other medical disorders. Anxiety disorders are diagnosed when anxiety symptoms predominate and cause significant distress or impairment.

The manifestations of anxiety are numerous and varied; some common signs and symptoms are listed in Table 62.1.

DEVELOPMENTAL PERSPECTIVE

Before a child is able to verbalize, affects are communicated behaviorally; as verbal ability increases, the young person is able to express—and perhaps to experience—increasingly differentiated affects. The developmental relationship between language and experience is complex and beyond the scope of this discussion, but it is reasonable to assume there is a progression of affective experiences from undifferentiated distress to more discrete forms of distress. Older preschool children can usually identify broad emotions (scared, mad, sad, happy) when experienced singly and can distinguish between, for example, "just a little bit scared" and "very scared," but mixed emotions and subtle qualitative differences are beyond their vocabulary if not their experience.

It is clear that certain fears and anxieties are more common at certain ages than at others (Silver, 1979). In early infancy a generalized kind of distress is displayed, which becomes more differentiated in later infancy, with qualitatively different distress cries; colic may be a manifestation of anxiety. From about 9 months, obvious fear or anger when the parents depart and the need for tangible comforts such as transitional objects may be indicators of a normal and predictable type of separation anxiety. For the later preschool child, specific fears of bodily harm are likely to be the most common manifestation of anxiety, and in the school-age child the fear of disapproval by one's own superego, important adults, and social peers is thought to be the most common form of anxiety. Identity issues, social acceptance, and independence conflicts are sources of "normal" anxiety in adolescence.

Diagnostically, animal phobias characteristically begin in childhood, while serious social phobias do not usually begin before puberty. Specific situational phobias have no characteristic time of onset (Rutter, 1970). The fears that are most common in childhood and adolescence are the ones most likely to diminish with increasing age.

Finally, it should be noted that some investigators interpret available data (especially from factor analytic studies) as showing that anxious

---

Table 62.1. Signs and Symptoms of Anxiety

1. Cardiovascular:
   Palpitations, tachycardia, transient mild to moderate increase in blood pressure, flushing or pallor.
2. Respiratory:
   Subjective shortness of breath, increased respiratory rate.
3. Skin:
   Blotching, "rash," variations in skin temperature, increased perspiration, paresthesias.
4. Musculoskeletal:
   Tremor, tremulousness, muscle tension, muscle cramps.
5. Gastrointestinal:
   Diarrhea, nausea, abdominal pain.
6. Other Physical:
   Headache, chest pain, overalertness, startles easily, insomnia, nightmares, dizziness, fainting, urinary frequency.
7. Psychological-internal:
   Verbalized fears. Feels scared, tense, nervous, upset, stressed, fretful, restless; ruminates. In panic, feels like dying, has derealization, can't think. Described by others as nervous or high-strung. Nightmares, scary fantasies. Feels "different" and left out if avoidant behavior limits activity.
8. Social-behavioral:
   Appears clingy, needy, dependent, and/or shy, withdrawn, uneasy in social situations. Underreacts or overreacts. Often reluctant to engage in activities with any possible danger (e.g., tree-climbing) or may engage in excessive risk-taking (counterphobically).

and depressed affects are not readily or validly distinguished in children or adolescents, but should be considered more globally as "negative affectivity."

HISTORICAL NOTE

From Aristotle to Darwin, emotions were most often viewed, when they were considered at all, as intrinsic and biologically derived, functioning separately from "mind" and "soul." It was recognized that emotions follow events or perceptions, but issues of causality and attribution were widely debated and discussed from the late 19th century on. In the mid-20th century, particularly in the United States, the psychiatric community was more or less in the psychoanalytic camp accepting Freud's emphasis on the importance of mastering the anxieties generated by inevitable and characteristic conflicts at identifiable stages of psychosexual development and attributing psychopathology in general to failure to resolve these conflicts and master the associated anxieties, a failure usually attributed to something wrong in the environment of the developing individual.

Thus, DSM-I (American Psychiatric Association, 1952) listed virtually all the "disorders of psychogenic origin or without clearly defined physical cause" as "reactions": schizophrenic reaction, antisocial reaction, and so on. The "psychoneurotic reactions" included "anxiety reaction," "dissociative reaction," "conversion reaction," "phobic reaction," "obsessive-compulsive reaction," and "depressive reaction." It was implied if not explicit that anxiety was at the core of all these diagnoses, which were manifested differently according to the predominant defenses and coping mechanisms of the afflicted individuals. The DSM-II included brief descriptions of characteristic signs and symptoms of the disorders but no criteria as such. Following the development of diagnostic criteria for research from several centers, with demonstrably better interrater reliability and evidence of predictive validity for several disorders, the authors of DSM-III adopted a similar approach.

A group of disorders was identified as "usually first evident in infancy, childhood or adolescence" in DSM-III, including several with anxiety as a primary manifestation: reactive attachment disorder, separation anxiety disorder, overanxious disorder, and avoidant disorder. Additionally, the anxiety disorder diagnoses applicable to adults were also available for diagnosing children and adolescents, when applicable: agoraphobia with or without panic attacks, panic disorder, simple and social phobias, generalized anxiety disorder, obsessive-compulsive disorder, and posttraumatic stress disorder.

This approach was criticized by some researchers, particularly in regard to childhood diagnoses for which there was limited evidence of validity, but it was lauded by others as a means to test validity and reliability of childhood diagnoses. A number of clinicians, particularly from the psychodynamic tradition, objected to the atheoretical approach of DSM-III and to the elimination of the term *neurosis*. The overall response was positive enough that the same approach was adopted, with relatively minor changes, in the 1987 revision (DSM-III-R) (American Psychiatric Association, 1987). The most recent version, DSM-IV (American Psychiatric Association, 1994), has only minor variations from its predecessor but notably does not include avoidant disorder, and subsumes overanxious disorder under generalized anxiety disorder.

Other classification schemes exist, of course, and the International Classification of Diseases, developed by the World Health Organization, is currently in its ninth edition and is noteworthy not only because of its international use but also because it has been widely used for indexing medical records. Under "neurotic disorders," the ICD-9 included anxiety states, hysteria, phobic states, obsessive-compulsive disorder, neurotic depression, neurasthenia, depersonalization syndrome, and hypochondriasis. Childhood "disturbances of emotions" include that "with anxiety and fearfulness" and "with sensitivity, shyness and social withdrawal." An explicit goal in the formulation of the DSM-IV was a closer correspondence with the ICD-10, as well as a firmer empirical foundation.

PREVALENCE AND EPIDEMIOLOGY

Anxiety disorders are certainly common among children and adolescents, but it is unclear how common. Prevalence estimates from studies that varied significantly in method and in case definition have reported rates of 5–50% (Links, 1989). Currently there are little data from which to generalize about differences among cultures in the prevalence of syndromes or of specific fears or anxieties. African-American children appear to have more "medical" fears than Anglo-Caucasian children (Neal et al., 1993), while Chinese children have "heightened levels of social-evaluative fears" (Dong et al., 1994). Overall comparisons of anxiety symptoms, disorders, and fears among Anglo-Caucasian, African-American, Native American, and Hispanic-American children and adolescents are lacking.

Information about sex ratio is also limited and may reflect referral patterns as much as actual prevalence; but it appears that social phobia is more common among males, while simple phobia, avoidant disorder, and agoraphobia are diagnosed more in females. Separation anxiety, overanxious disorder (as previously defined), panic disorder (without agoraphobia), and generalized anxiety disorder seem to be equally common in the sexes. Sex differences vary with age; Reinherz and colleagues (1993) reported that by later adolescence, phobias were equally distributed by gender, while posttraumatic stress disorder (PTSD) was significantly more common among girls.

Socioeconomic status (SES) also affects distribution of anxiety disorders and symptoms. Reinherz (1993) reported an inverse relationship between SES and prevalence of phobias. Possible differences by ethnicity with adequate controls of SES are being explored currently; data available now suggest that Caucasian youth may have more anxiety symptoms than African-American youth (Fabrega et al., 1993). One environmental variable clearly associated with increased anxiety in African-American children is exposure to violence (Fitzpatrick and Boldizar, 1993).

ETIOLOGY AND PATHOGENESIS

Biologic Factors

There is some evidence that panic anxiety is a phenomenon of the brainstem, especially the pons, while anticipatory anxiety is primarily generated within the cingulate portion of the limbic system and phobic avoidance chiefly within prefrontal cortex (Gorman, 1989). γ-Aminobutyric acid, serotonin, and norepinephrine appear to be the neurotransmitters most closely associated with anxiety phenomena in the central nervous system; epinephrine release, dysfunctional autonomic regulation, variations in response to respiratory carbon dioxide levels, and the generalized stress response are some of the peripheral physiologic mechanisms associated with anxiety.

Kandel (1983) has developed an animal model for a molecular-genetic mechanism by which experiences invoke morphologic changes, that is, increased numbers of active zones at synaptic varicosities, resulting in increased physiologic sensitization; anxiety may become chronic because of such structural changes. Current efforts to extend this line of research include exploration of the differentiation of gene expression required, the biochemical relation to memory, and development of molecular models for other forms of anxiety.

Research with adults has illuminated some of the physiology of panic, which may be induced experimentally, for example, in some subjects with intravenous lactate or by alteration of the proportion of carbon dioxide in breathed air. Ethical and technical problems have limited such research in children.

Genetic predispositions to anxiety disorders are well established for some "adult" disorders, and there is some evidence that this holds true for childhood anxiety disorders as well (Last et al., 1987). Risk for anxiety disorders in childhood or adolescence may be increased not only by familial anxiety disorders but also by familial affective illness, alcoholism, and somatization disorder (Livingston, 1993; Livingston et al., 1985).

Psychosocial Factors

The biological events that produce anxiety symptoms can be precipitated, perpetuated, and modified by both external and internal events and influences. These influences have been studied and considered from a variety of perspectives. The psychoanalytic perspective on anxiety has already been oversimplified and outlined in the historical note. Learning and behavior theorists have demonstrated that anxiety symptoms can come, through conditioning, to be provoked by stimuli that are not ordinarily anxiogenic, and they have also shown that what has become conditioned often can be deconditioned. Cognitive psychologists have studied the mental events between the stimulus and the response and have begun to develop techniques to alter therapeutically the mental events in order to modify responses that are undesirable (i.e., symptoms).

Each of these approaches has clinical value, but a clinician whose repertoire of techniques for treatment is not limited to a single approach is probably at some advantage. There is beginning to be evidence of differing efficacy among treatment approaches for some anxiety disorders; for example, phobias may be best treated by desensitization, and separation anxiety by a combination of medication, behavioral interventions, and psychotherapy.

FUNDAMENTALS OF ASSESSMENT AND TREATMENT

Inquiry about anxiety symptoms should be a standard part of the psychiatric interview regardless of the presenting problem; it is not uncommon for anxiety symptoms to be present that will be elicited only if specifically asked for. Parents or caretakers should be asked about the child's verbal expressions of fear or worry and about signs of anxiety that are ordinarily apparent to others, such as vigilance, sweating, and hyperventilation. The patient should always be asked about these and also about the more internal and private symptoms of anxiety, since young children lack a frame of reference that would lead them to conclude that their feelings are unusual or excessive, and children of any age are under certain circumstances inclined to keep their feelings to themselves.

Children can usually identify their feelings accurately, but young historians will frequently be unable to give precise or reliable answers to open-ended, time-oriented questions about duration and frequency. With younger children, this information can sometimes be approximated by reference to landmark events of which most children are aware; for example, ''Did you start feeling that way during summer vacation, or was it after school started?'' ''Was it before or after Christmas?''

Careful attention must be given, in obtaining the family history of the anxious child, to the whole range of anxiety and mood disorders, as well as to the more general psychiatric family history. A medical family history is important not only because of the heritable medical diseases such as diabetes that may be in the child's differential diagnosis but also because of the potential for illness in the family to make a child anxious.

Often the differential diagnosis of anxiety disorders includes specific medical illnesses, so a thorough medical history is essential. Specific historical factors should always include use of caffeine, tobacco products, sympathomimetic and other medications, and street drugs. Anxiety disorders are associated with physical complaints and are common in somatization and other somatoform disorders, and these possibilities must be explored through a thorough review of systems.

The development and social histories must be sufficiently detailed to give the examiner a sense of the child's usual style of coping with stressors in general and anxiety-provoking situations in particular: it is also important to get a sense of how the family as a unit and the parents individually cope with anxiety and stress.

Physical and mental status examinations should be performed and followed by any laboratory work or psychological evaluations that are suggested by findings in the history, mental status, or physical examinations.

After this evaluation a differential diagnosis and/or provisional diagnosis can be identified and plans made for obtaining further information needed to clarify diagnosis. A case formulation can be devised summarizing the pertinent findings and identifying contributing factors and psychodynamic hypotheses. Biological, psychological, and social influences and conditions that might predispose the individual to anxiety disorder, precipitate the symptoms, or act to perpetuate the pathology should be included. Finally, a prioritized problem list should be generated. The diagnosis, formulation, and problem list provide the foundation upon which a treatment plan is based.

The broad goals of medical treatment are (a) to reduce symptoms and relieve distress, (b) to prevent the complications associated with a disorder, and (c) to minimize the disability associated with the disorder. In child and adolescent psychiatry we have the additional goal of enhancing developmental potential, or, put another way, of helping young people become liberated from internal and external forces and influences that impede their development. Within the broad outline of these four common goals, individualized treatment goals are determined based upon the symptoms presented, complications and disability associated with particular diagnoses, and the clinician's sense (as summarized in the formulation) of the patient's potential, current developmental status, and family and social context. Immediate treatment goals will usually be identified in the general area of symptom reduction and prevention of complications; issues related to minimizing disability and maximizing developmental potential will usually be emphasized more in the long-term treatment plan.

Regarding treatment methods, the literature to date suggests that overall efficacy in childhood anxiety has best been demonstrated for behavioral techniques, with more limited evidence for efficacy of psychotherapies and medications. Specifics are discussed below.

SEPARATION ANXIETY DISORDER

Definition and Clinical Description

Separation anxiety disorder is characterized by anxiety symptoms that range from anticipatory uneasiness to full-blown panic about separation from parents or other loved ones. Affected children are most likely to be brought to the physician's attention when their separation anxiety results in refusal or reluctance to attend school or when it is manifest in somatic symptoms such as recurrent abdominal pain. Other symptoms and signs may include unrealistic and recurrent worries about harm befalling loved ones (particularly if the child is away from the loved ones), reluctance to go to sleep without the attachment figure near, nightmares with separation themes, excessive distress upon anticipation of separation (for example, tantrums or pleading), and the desire to return home or to make contact with the parents frequently when the child is away. By the DSM-IV definition, the disorder is diagnosed only if the symptoms have been present for at least 2 weeks, the age of onset is less than 18, and the symptoms are not limited to the course of schizophrenia, pervasive developmental disorder, or another psychotic disorder.

In addition to the psychological and behavioral manifestations, these children frequently experience physical symptoms. Abdominal pain and palpitations are particularly common, and in one study children with separation anxiety had an average of eight somatic complaints, more than for any other emotional disorder (Livingston et al., 1988).

Possible associated neuroendocrine abnormalities that can be measured in the clinical laboratory have been studied only in the most preliminary way. It appears, for example, that children with severe separation anxiety are nearly as likely as severely depressed children to have an abnormal dexamethasone suppression test; it is not know whether this is true for adolescents (Livingston and Martin-Cannici, 1987). In younger children this test is done by administering an oral dose of dexamethasone (0.5 mg for a child under 40 kg weight, 1 mg for a child over 40 kg) at 11:00 PM and measuring serum cortisol at 8:00 AM and

4:00 PM (or at 4:00 PM only) the following day. A cortisol value at either of these times greater than or equal to 5 mg/dl is suggestive of either failure to suppress cortisol production or early escape from suppression. It is interesting that adults with anxiety disorders are not likely to have this kind of neuroendocrine abnormality. Whether this test will prove to be clinically useful is uncertain.

Developmental Perspective

Separation anxiety is of course a normal developmental phenomenon of late infancy and is frequently seen in a mild form that does not cause much impairment early in kindergarten or 1st grade. Clingy behavior and mild separation distress may also occur as appropriate and adaptive responses to distressing events throughout childhood. Separation anxiety is judged to be clinically significant when the symptoms are severe, exceeding ordinary development events and causing serious distress or functional impairment.

Epidemiology

This disorder appears to be equally common among boys and girls, and the peak incidence is around age 11. Compared to other anxiety disorders, children with separation anxiety tend to come from a slightly lower socioeconomic class (Last et al., 1987). Costello (1989), summarizing several recent studies, reports a prevalence of 3.5–5.4%.

Differential Diagnosis

There is a significant overlap of both symptoms and diagnoses between separation anxiety disorder and *depression* (Bernstein and Garfinkel, 1986a; Puig-Antich and Robinovich, 1986) (Table 62.2). The disorders may in fact overlap in a third or more of cases. The significance of this is unclear at the present; both disorders should be diagnosed if the manifestations of both are present to sufficient degree.

Another important distinction to make is that between school refusal secondary to separation anxiety and simple truancy. In separation anxiety the goal of the school refusal is to avoid separation from the parent; in truancy no such goal is evident. The child with separation anxiety will want to be home or wherever the loved one is; the truant is much more likely to roam if he or she is able. Truancy, if present, should lead to an investigation for possible diagnosis of conduct disorder.

Separation anxiety disorder must be distinguished from generalized anxiety disorder. Young people with separation anxiety are less likely than those with generalized anxiety disorder to have multiple sources or precipitants of anxiety. Symptoms of separation anxiety may also be evident during the course of pervasive developmental disorders or early in the course of schizophrenia; these disorders will usually, however, also present their other, more characteristic manifestations.

Panic disorder can also occur in children with or without separation anxiety (Hayward et al., 1989; Morean et al., 1989). In the few studies currently available it appears that before puberty panic disorder may accompany depression or separation anxiety but rarely occurs alone.

When the presenting symptom is physical (e.g., recurrent abdominal pain), medical causes for the pain should be considered and evaluated with a physical examination, and any laboratory tests suggested by history or examination findings should be done. When the characteristic symptoms of separation anxiety are present and the physical symptom fits into the pattern, as with stomachaches that occur mainly on Sunday night and on school mornings, it is reasonable to consider the pain a symptom of anxiety and to avoid expensive, invasive, and risky evaluative procedures.

Finally, phobic avoidance of school due to fears other than separation will occasionally be seen. Often this is purely situational, as when a child has been threatened by a bully or is fearful of a particular teacher.

Course and Outcome

In general, cases of separation anxiety that have their onset at younger ages and that present in milder forms can be expected to resolve satisfactorily. More intelligent children may have a worse outcome. Older onset and greater severity appear also to be associated with a somewhat worse prognosis. Overall, up to half of these individuals may experience chronic anxiety and persistent school attendance problems; a significant minority may go on to develop agoraphobia. A widely accepted bit of clinical lore based upon case reports that suggested that onset of separation anxiety in late childhood or adolescence is an early manifestation of schizophrenia has not been explored using current diagnostic methodology or criteria.

Etiology and Pathogenesis

There is evidence that some children are at particular risk for the development of significant separation anxiety. These include children who have recently experienced a serious illness or death in the family or a disruptive change of home or school, children with malignant neoplasms, diabetes, Tourette's syndrome, and the combination of attention deficit disorder and reading disability (American Psychiatric Association, 1987; Livingston, 1990). Children whose family histories are positive for panic disorder, agoraphobia, depression, somatization disorder, and alcoholism also appear to be at increased risk (Last et al., 1987a, 1987b; Livingston, 1993; Livingston et al., 1985; Morean et al., 1989).

Another significant factor in the pathogenesis of many cases of separation anxiety appears to be the communication or contagion of anxiety within the family (Eisenberg, 1958). The pathogenesis of the disorder is somewhat variable. In a composite "classical" case, the symptoms will develop gradually and insidiously in a young person who has a parent or grandparent who has recently experienced a life-threatening illness or who has experienced some major life change. This child will begin to experience mild distress upon being away from one or both parents and will begin to appear clingy and reluctant to separate. The parents typically will be uncertain how to handle the child's distress and will themselves be distressed by the child's emotional pain, then a vicious cycle ensues in which the parent's anxiety makes the child more anxious, which makes the parents more anxious, and so forth. During this phase the symptom severity escalates, and new symptoms develop. Often the family will struggle with this situation until the child's refusal to go to school or refusal to sleep alone leads them to seek help, or until the child is taken to the doctor for physical symptoms.

Table 62.2. Comparison of Separation Anxiety, Overanxious, and Major Depressive Disorders

	Separation Anxiety Disorders	Overanxious Disorder	Major Depressive Disorder
Course	Brief episodes usual in younger children Chronicity more likely in older children	Variable	Usually episodic
Family history	Anxiety, mood disorders, alcoholism	Anxiety disorders, depression	Mood disorders, alcoholism
Panic symptoms	Common when separation anticipated	Uncommon	Probably common
Psychosis (hallucinations, delusions)	Rare	Absent	Not rare
Somatic complaints	Abdominal pain and multiple complaints very common	Usually monosymptomatic headache or abdominal pain, if present	Fairly common, especially if psychotic
Delinquent behavior and serious aggression	Rare	Rare	Probably common

Treatment

When the child is young, the severity of the case is mild to moderate, and the symptoms have not been present very long, treatment may be fairly simple and straightforward. The diagnosis and the nature of the disorder are carefully explained to the parents and to the child. This explanation should explicitly include the manner in which anxiety is contagious within the family. The family is told that the key to successful resolution of symptoms is for the child to experience separation until the child discovers that the catastrophic fears are unfounded and the child becomes accustomed enough to separation that he or she can go to school regularly or sleep alone without excessive distress. (A more severely afflicted child may also need relaxation training prior to exposures to separation.) After these explanations, separations are enforced at the natural and usual times; the child is made to go to school by whatever means necessary and is expected to sleep in his or her own room, and so forth. The child should be given lavish praise and appreciation for his or her courage for getting through a school day or a night in the child's own bed. These measures alone will often be sufficient and will be recognized as constituting a course of systematic desensitization.

In cases in which a reasonable trial of these simpler measures is not effective, medication in addition to the supportive and behavioral measures may make a significant difference (Gittleman and Koplewicz, 1986; Gittleman-Klein and Klein, 1971). Imipramine has been found in many cases to reduce school nonattendance, separation difficulties, and physical symptoms. This may require fairly large doses (3–5 mg/kg/day) over several months, so the physician should obtain a baseline electrocardiogram and follow the ECG during treatment, in order to avoid potentially serious cardiotoxicity. In general, a single bedtime dose is satisfactory, but divided doses may be desirable in some cases to ameliorate anticholinergic or other side effects. It is usually considered wise to begin with a daily dose that is approximately one-fourth to one-third of the anticipated total daily dose and increase gradually to the anticipated dose over a period of days or weeks, depending upon the child's tolerance of the medication. It is also considered wiser to taper off the medication than to stop it abruptly, not only to allow time to detect a recurrence of symptoms but also to avoid the sleep disturbances and flulike symptoms that are sometimes encountered upon stopping tricyclics abruptly.

Studies of other tricyclics have been even less consistent in their demonstration of positive effect. Although the clinical lore has long suggested that thioridazine has a place in the treatment of anxiety states, there are no rigorous studies demonstrating its efficacy for any anxiety disorder of childhood. Only one controlled study of antihistamines' effect on children's anxiety has appeared, in which diphenhydramine was reported to be helpful in a mixed population. Small studies do suggest, however, that there may be a role for alprazolam in the treatment of separation anxiety disorder in children, in divided doses of up to a total of 1 mg/day; and preliminary clinical experience with buspirone has been positive, although beneficial effects may not be evident for several weeks.

If serious symptoms persist and function remains impaired even after an adequate trial of medication, it may become necessary to hospitalize the child for up to several weeks, during which the enforced separation (equivalent to prolonged exposure or "flooding") and multimodal treatment will usually bring about a satisfactory degree of symptom control. This measure often requires excellent rapport with the parents and a full appreciation that the hospitalization may be nearly as difficult for them as it is for the child. After an initial forced separation of several days, during which the parents may be seen alone as frequently as necessary to provide them support, the child and parents are brought back together for a series of repeated reunions and separations that will usually help further to desensitize the child to separation. Occasionally a parent will have separation anxiety to such an extreme degree that the parent will haunt the hospital and subvert treatment. It may be necessary in some cases, when there is a legal issue such as school nonattendance upon which to base such a maneuver, to ask a court to order the child's treatment and the parent's cooperation. Even in these extreme cases the outcome will often be satisfactory if the professionals involved maintain a strongly empathic and supportive position with the child and the parents until their anxiety wanes.

Comorbid diagnoses and other identified problems should be included in the long-term treatment plan, but the separation anxiety will usually be the source of the more immediate impairment and warrant a higher priority in the short-term treatment plan. The potential for a poor outcome suggests that, in the majority of more severe cases, long-term treatment will be required.

GENERALIZED ANXIETY DISORDER (OVERANXIOUS DISORDER)

Definition and Clinical Description

The child or adolescent with generalized anxiety disorder (DSM-III-R, overanxious disorder) is afflicted with excessive and unrealistic worries about competence, approval, appropriateness of past behavior, and the future. These individuals show extreme self-consciousness, excessive needs for reassurance, inability to relax, and often have somatic complaints, such as headaches and abdominal pain, with no physical basis. DSM-IV criteria include persistent worrying and at least three of the following, with at least some symptoms present on a majority of days: restlessness or feeling keyed up; being easily fatigued; trouble concentrating; irritability; muscle tension; and sleep disturbance. Symptoms must persist for at least 6 months and be associated with significant distress or functional impairment. The diagnosis is not made if the symptoms or worries are limited to the course of another Axis I disorder or a medical condition.

This diagnosis has only recently been applied to children, but there is some evidence that generalized anxiety disorder (GAD)/overanxious disorder can be reliably and validly discriminated from other anxiety disorders and from other psychiatric disorders (Last et al., 1987c; Mattison and Bagnato, 1987).

To date, there are no laboratory or psychological tests that have specific diagnostic value for GAD. There are indications that children with this condition are likely to score higher on the schizoid and anxious scales of the Child Behavior Checklist and to have elevated scores on the Children's Manifest Anxiety Scale (Mattison and Bagnato, 1987). Also, these children are more likely than children with pure behavior disorder (but less likely than children with major depression or separation anxiety) to have an abnormal dexamethasone suppression test result (Livingston and Martin-Cannici, 1987).

Developmental Perspective

It is during later elementary school age (later latency) that normal developmental concerns include self-comparisons with peers in achievement and status, competitiveness, a solidifying self-image, and emerging superego. Any of these concerns can be a source of transient normal anxieties, and it is in this developmental context that most cases of childhood GAD arise.

A minority of cases, usually in younger children (4–7 years) but occasionally in an adolescent, arise in a developmental circumstance in which omnipotence and control issues have not been resolved.

Epidemiology

Childhood GAD is about equally common in males and females until adolescence, at which time female predominance begins (Werry, 1991). At greatest risk may be first-born children, children from small families, and children from upper-class, achievement-oriented families; it should be noted, however, that cultural differences have not been adequately explored. Prevalence estimates range from 2.7–4.6% (Costello, 1989).

Course and Outcome

Although the natural history of this disorder is not well documented, clinical experience suggests that the onset may be either acute or insidious and that the symptoms wax and wane in severity over time, with a trend toward gradual improvement.

Little is known about predisposing biological factors, but there is some evidence that a family history of anxiety disorder, affective disorder, or alcoholism may be associated (Last et al., 1991; Livingston et al., 1985). There is also evidence that the presence of neurological soft signs in early school age is associated with the development of anxiety and social withdrawal in adolescence (Shaffer et al., 1983). It has been suggested by Kendler (1992) that a common gene predisposes to both GAD and major depression, with environmental factors determining the vector of expression. Finally, inhibition (as a dimension of temperament) is associated with development of social anxieties.

Clinical experience and the little literature that is available suggest that there are two social contexts in which GAD is particularly likely to develop. One is the family in which parental expectations for achievement in sports, academics, or some other area are very high (Adler et al., 1982). The other is the situation in which parents or other caretakers have consistently yielded to a child's demands and the child develops multiple and overwhelming fears and anxieties as well as escalating tyrannical behavior (Barcai and Rosenthal, 1974).

CASE ILLUSTRATION

Sandy, a 10-year-old boy from an achievement-oriented middle-class home, presented for psychiatric consultation after his pediatrician noticed the child to be extremely anxious. Sandy's parents took him to the pediatrician when, in the 4th grade, after being a straight A student for 3 years, he began to make primarily C's and D's; they were interested in ensuring that he did not have a learning disability. Sandy was apparently immensely popular at school and was an excellent pianist and champion gymnast in his age group. He acknowledged being worried all the time since this school year had started about his grades and school performance and was very concerned that his parents and his teachers might have a bad opinion of him. The physical examination was unremarkable, but psychological testing revealed that Sandy had a full-scale IQ of 85; except for a slightly above-average score on the subtest that measures general information, his scores on other parts were very consistent. The parents were given the results and were told that in the consultant's opinion Sandy's current average grades reflected satisfactory achievement. They denied that the test results could possibly be correct and left in anger. At a later date they called back for an appointment, having obtained another evaluation independently with essentially the same results. After a short course of individual and family therapy, Sandy was free of anxiety, and the parents were demonstrating more realistic expectations for academic performance and continued to be fully appreciative of his abilities in other areas.

Comment

This case illustrates one of the common presentations of GAD and underscores two other principles: the necessity of a complete evaluation of every child and the importance of leaving the door open for patients and families to engage in treatment when they are ready.

Differential Diagnosis

Medical causes must be ruled out, particularly when motor tension and autonomic symptoms predominate and psychological symptoms are relatively lacking or are atypical. The most common of these, especially in adolescence, is probably excessive use of caffeine or other stimulants. Hyperthyroidism, hypoglycemia, lupus, and pheochromocytoma should be considered if suggested by the history or physical examination. As with separation anxiety, when the chief complaint is a physical symptom such as recurrent abdominal pain, medical causes should be considered and searched for insofar as the history and examination indicate.

About half of children with GAD also have another anxiety disorder comorbidly (Last et al., 1987c); this presents a problem not so much in differential diagnosis as in setting priorities for treatment. The most common additional diagnosis is simple phobia.

Children with GAD also appear to be at significant risk for comorbid major depression but not for dysthymia or bipolar disorder. When the symptoms develop along with tyrannical behavior, an additional diagnosis of oppositional-defiant disorder may be warranted.

When the symptoms are relatively mild, less than 6 months in duration, and follow shortly the onset of a stressor, the diagnosis of adjustment disorder with anxious mood may be more appropriate.

Treatment

As yet, there is little research to establish that there is or is not a role for medication in the treatment of overanxious disorder. It is possible that buspirone and diazepam or other benzodiazepines will prove to be beneficial, but at present the primary treatment modalities for this disorder are psychotherapeutic (American Academy of Child and Adolescent Psychiatry, 1993; American Psychiatric Association, 1989).

First the patient and family should have the diagnosis and treatment recommendations explained. In the two common contexts described above and frequently in other situations, family therapy will be essential. When high parental expectations have been identified as a source of anxiety and distress, an attempt should be made to deal with this issue directly through advice, negotiation, and support. Even with some initial success in modifying parental expectations, however, old habits die hard, and it must be recognized that the parents' expectations may be reflections of strong psychological needs that will require further therapeutic intervention. If the patient has been living with high expectations and feeling unable to meet those expectations for any period of time, some degree of internalization is probable, and individual psychotherapy will be required to help rebuild self-esteem and a more realistic set of expectations for the self. There is no evidence that any one psychotherapeutic approach is superior to others in accomplishing this goal.

For the special case in which the overanxious symptoms accompany tyrannical behavior, the psychodynamic hypothesis is that having too much power makes children anxious. There is some evidence that getting the parents back into control and diminishing the tyrannical behavior will in and of itself result in significantly diminished fearfulness and anxiety in this situation (Barcai and Rosenthal, 1974).

In other situations in which the dynamics are less clear-cut, the therapist is obliged to consider the range of situational, developmental, and cognitive factors within the individual and within the family system and develop a formulation from which working hypotheses can be developed to explain the origin and perpetuation of the symptoms. A treatment plan is then devised, which may include one or several modalities, such as relaxation training to decrease general tension, cognitive therapies that will help the child replace anxiety-increasing thoughts with more reasonable and less anxiogenic ones, group therapy to reduce social discomfort, family therapy to address sources of anxiety and anxiety-producing behaviors and interactions within the family system, rehearsals through play therapy or role playing in which anxiety-producing situations can be practiced and mastered, and psychodynamic psychotherapy to address long-standing states of conflict or failures to develop adequate mechanisms to cope with the normal developmental issues in previous stages of development.

Regardless of the therapeutic approach, a satisfactory therapeutic relationship is essential. It is also important to remember that external changes precede internalization and that impressive and thoroughly internalized improvement can be seen without any verbalization of insight having occurred.

Even in the presence of clear-cut individual issues that are obvious fodder for psychotherapy, the family must be assessed for the kinds of interactional patterns that are thought to be anxiogenic, such as a lack of role clarity and continuous failure to resolve conflicts (Minuchin et al., 1978). If these factors are present to any significant degree, family therapy should be part of the treatment plan.

REACTIVE ATTACHMENT DISORDER

Definition and Clinical Description

Reactive attachment disorder is the current conceptualization for the emotional disturbance that develops in infants and very young children who have received grossly inadequate emotional nurturing (American Psychiatric Association, 1994). These disturbances were initially described in hospital and institutional settings as "hospitalism" and anaclitic depression, but it was recognized soon afterward that parents could provide as abnormal an attachment in the home as institutions could. The emotional disorder described does not fit entirely well into the affective disorders or anxiety disorders, having elements of both. The characteristic pattern as described by Bowlby (1979) is an initial picture of anxiety and protest followed by depression and detachment.

In DSM-IV, the core features of the diagnosis are a disturbance of social relatedness on the part of the child (which may be expressed as either a lack of appropriate relatedness in the *inhibited type* or indiscriminate and excessive relatedness in the *disinhibited type*), grossly pathogenic care on the part of the parents or other caretakers, and a presumption that the poor care is responsible for the disturbed behavior. Abnormal social relatedness that is a symptom of autism, other pervasive developmental disorders, or mental retardation excludes the diagnosis. If the child also has failure to thrive, this is coded on Axis III.

Because the diagnostic criteria are still relatively new and because the bulk of the research data available is either ethological or focused on failure to thrive (which has a significant but not absolute overlap with reactive attachment disorder), most of our knowledge is based upon case description and indirect scientific evidence (see Chapter 45).

Developmental Perspective

There is growing sense that the development of affectional bonds is more a gradual process than an event that occurs within the early hours of life (Chess and Thomas, 1982), but there is no doubt that under ordinary circumstances the development of such bonds is essential to normal growth and development and perhaps to survival. Without intervention, infants with reactive attachment disorder are at risk for physical failure to thrive, frequent illnesses, and eventual death from the complications of malnutrition or infection.

Epidemiology

The prevalence remains unknown. A number of factors have been found to identify children at risk, including such child characteristics as low birth weight, sickliness, and prematurity, and maternal characteristics such as extreme youth, social isolation, deprived living conditions, postpartum depression, histories of behavioral and relational difficulties, and low self-esteem.

Etiology and Pathogenesis

A history of "grossly pathogenic care," associated with abnormal attachment behaviors, has provided a presumption that this is primarily a disorder of attachment; recently, Richters and Volkmar (1994) have suggested that it is more properly considered a syndrome of abnormal development.

Observations of mother-child interaction in these families shows that, although these mothers generally believe they are caring for their infants as they should, there is little eye contact, lack of responsiveness to the baby's vocalizations and to behavioral indications that suggest the child's needs or wants, inconsistent responses, and general insensitivity to the infant's communication. It is certainly reasonable to assume that this type of caretaking behavior is likely to leave a child most anxious and frustrated. The parent frequently then misinterprets expressions of this distress by assuming the child is physically ill; these infants and children therefore present commonly for "colic," regurgitation of food, poor eating, or various irregularities of body habit. Later in the course of this disorder, failure to grow and gain weight may be the presenting complaint.

Differential Diagnosis

The possibility of explaining the child's behavior as normal developmental variations must sometimes be considered. Indiscriminate acceptance of strangers is common until the age of about 8 months. Some children will make a social connection eventually that is qualitatively quite satisfactory but that develops slowly. Similarly, not every mother whose interactions with her child fail to impress us is launching a case of reactive attachment disorder; there appears to be a great deal of individual variation in how much attachment is enough.

Children with autism and more severely retarded children with autistic characteristics are quite likely to display the kind of disturbed social relatedness that marks this disorder; their parents may appear insensitive and detached in response to the unresponsiveness of the child, so it is important when possible to attempt to ascertain which came first.

A minority of cases of failure to thrive will be found to have a direct medical cause; these can be associated with states of malnutrition and metabolic disturbance that compromise mood and social relatedness.

Treatment

Direct treatment of the baby, which consists primarily of establishing adequate feeding and weight gain, treatment of the complications of malnutrition, and the provision of adequate stimulation and interaction, can in mild cases be undertaken in the outpatient setting or in the patient's home.

The mother or other caretaker is involved in this process in the beginning with instruction and encouragement in appropriate interactions and feeding and appropriate expectations for the infant's behavior. When these mothers feel alienated or socially isolated, a course of group therapy or membership in a support group may be indicated. If the mother is experiencing clinically significant depression, her depression must be treated aggressively. In some places the bulk of the work done with the mothers is done by trained volunteers.

In severe cases a period of hospitalization may be necessary at the beginning of treatment; at times this will require obtaining a court order for the hospitalization or a temporary removal of the child from the parents' custody. Severe reactive attachment disorder can be life-threatening, and safety should be given priority over everything else. By and large, these children will respond to the improved nutrition and tender loving care provided in hospital; a plan then must be devised to see that the child's health and safety will be attended to after discharge as well.

Course and Outcome

Without treatment, reactive attachment disorder will often progress as previously described, and those children who are not devastated by malnutrition or infections are at risk of continued serious impairment in their social and affective as well as physical development. With both good initial treatment and adequate continuity of care, though, many patients will do very well.

PHOBIAS

Definition and Clinical Description

As has been discussed previously, fears are very common in childhood. When a specific fear is associated with avoidance behavior and results in functional or social impairment, a diagnosis of phobia is war-

Table 62.3. Common Phobias of Childhood

Fear	Technical Name
Animals in general	Zoophobia
Blood	Hematophobia
Cats	Ailurophobia
Dark	Nyctophobia
Dogs	Cynophobia
Fire	Pyrophobia
Germs, dirt	Mysophobia
Heights	Acrophobia
Insects	Entomophobia
Small or closed spaces	Claustrophobia
Snakes	Ophidophobia
Spiders	Arachnophobia
Strangers	Xenophobia
Thunder	Brontophobia

ranted. Simple or specific phobias are persistent fears of a specific object or situation that the afflicted individual either avoids or endures with great anxiety. The fear is recognized by the individual to be irrational or excessive. When the stimulus that causes anxiety is a social situation and the fear is that the individual will be humiliated or embarrassed, the diagnosis is social phobia. Table 62.3 lists some common phobias of children with their "technical" names.

DSM-IV excludes fears that are part of, or "better accounted for by," panic disorder or agoraphobia, separation anxiety, obsessive-compulsive disorder, and posttraumatic stress disorder.

Epidemiology

In clinical populations the diagnosis of social phobia is more likely to be made in boys and simple phobias in girls; phobias are, however, common in the general population, and the sex ratio in nonclinical populations is not known. Prevalence estimates for simple phobia vary from 2.3 to 9.2% (Costello, 1989).

Etiology and Pathogenesis

A number of etiological mechanisms have been suggested; these have been reviewed extensively elsewhere (Barrios and O'Dell, 1989; Schwartz and Johnson, 1985). Psychoanalytic hypotheses have emphasized the role of defense mechanisms such as symbolic displacement of intolerable primary fears onto other objects. Classical conditioning of particular fears has been demonstrated, and the possibility of operant conditioning of phobic avoidance has also been discussed. At present, there is simply insufficient evidence upon which to base an estimate of the relative contributions of these or other psychosocial etiological factors. The possibility of a genetic predisposition is raised by the demonstration that phobic behavior can be bred in dogs (Newton and Lucas, 1982).

Differential Diagnosis

Phobias must first be distinguished from developmentally normal fears and from the other anxiety disorders. In schizophrenia and other psychotic disorders, fear and avoidant behavior may be noted, but psychotic individuals do not recognize their fears as unreasonable or excessive. When a patient seems to avoid most social situations, schizophrenia spectrum disorders, avoidant personality traits or disorder, and schizoid disorder must be considered. Anxiety and withdrawal associated with depressive disorders may appear, especially in early stages, as phobic or avoidant behavior.

CASE ILLUSTRATION

J.S. was admitted to the hospital at age 8 for treatment of encopresis and "odd behavior" at school. She started 1st grade at age 8 because her mother had until recently held her out of school due to encopresis; she had simply never registered the child for school. The family lived in an extremely rural area and had no indoor plumbing. The specific behavior that brought the child to the attention of school officials was that the child would scream in panic whenever the bathroom was even mentioned. Careful history taking revealed that the child had become extremely fearful of spiders almost 2 years previously and had developed encopresis secondary to fecal retention; she would not go to the outdoor toilet because there were always spiders there. She had panicked over the possibility of having to go the bathroom at school because she assumed it would be like the one at home. With a combination of medical treatment of her encopresis, bowel retraining, and desensitization and positive reinforcement for resolution of her phobia, she was able to return home and to her school without further difficulty.

Comment

A medical student was the third person to interview and examine this child, but the first whose history taking was thorough enough to discover that the outhouse was the key to understanding this case.

Course and Outcome

Social phobia is likely to be chronic and may occasionally exacerbate in a vicious cycle when anxiety impairs performance, leading to increased anxiety, and so on. This disorder is not usually incapacitating but has considerable potential to interfere with social activities and possibly with occupational functioning. In more severe cases, dropping out of school may result. Secondary depression and secondary substance abuse disorders should be checked for periodically during the course of treatment. Simple phobias that begin early in life usually disappear whether or not the individual is treated. Clinical experience suggests that unusually long persistence of simple phobia is more likely in individuals who have other psychiatric disorders in addition to their phobias.

Treatment

There is little empirical information regarding the pharmacological treatment of phobic disorders. If there is a place for drug therapy of phobic disorders, it is probably as a component of the treatment of severe social phobia. Although benzodiazepines may be effective in reducing stage fright and similar conditions, the individual with social phobia may be at increased risk for becoming dependent upon the medication. Some of these individuals may benefit from propranolol taken either regularly or in anticipation of frightening situations, in doses ranging from 10 to 80 mg up to four times a day. Monoamine oxidase inhibitors or serotonin-specific reuptake inhibitors may be helpful, but their safety and efficacy have yet to be demonstrated systematically for young people.

The assessment process may reveal issues and concerns for which individual or family psychotherapy is indicated. In severely phobic individuals, supportive group therapy can be extremely beneficial. Overall, however, the best evidence of treatment efficacy is for behavioral therapies (Barrios and O'Dell, 1989). These include systematic desensitization, prolonged exposure to the fear stimulus, modeling, contingency management procedures, "self-management," and combinations of these treatments.

In systematic desensitization the child is first trained to relax thoroughly and then practices imagining feared situations, beginning with the least distressing and progressing to the most distressing, while in the relaxed state. In some cases the actual feared object is presented instead of images of the object. Prolonged exposure (also called flooding) likewise may be done in the imagination or in vivo. In modeling, the child observes another person interacting without fear with the feared object, either symbolically or in reality, and then may be asked to participate. Contingency management techniques, which are often done in addition to other methods, most often consist of providing positive reinforcements for interacting with the feared object or stimulation, or the withholding of reinforcement for failure to do so.

Little is known about the comparative efficacy of these behavioral treatments, but some principles are useful in selecting among them. Prolonged exposure will work more rapidly but with increased discomfort to the child. Systematic desensitization may be the best choice when in vivo exposure is easily available or, conversely, when the feared object or situation is conceptual or imaginary (e.g., monsters). Modeling would appear to be a more appropriate choice for an older child and in the situation in which the child admires or identifies with the therapist. Contingency management techniques may be particularly useful when the patient appears unmotivated or overly discouraged. The combination of relaxation training, problem-solving, cognitive rehearsal, and other techniques, collectively referred to as self-management, may offer certain psychological advantages, but its use may be limited to older children who are otherwise well adapted.

ANXIETY ASSOCIATED WITH SPECIFIC STRESSORS

Anxiety symptoms are common after exposure to stressors in individuals of all ages. This occurs in a continuum from mild and very transient symptoms to severe and chronic impairment. When anxiety symptoms such as nervousness and worry begin shortly after the onset or appearance of the stressor, a diagnosis of adjustment disorder with anxious mood (ADAM) may be warranted. The diagnosis is limited to conditions that do not satisfy the criteria for any other psychiatric disorder and in which there is some degree of functional impairment and symptoms beyond what would ordinarily be expected. DSM-IV specifies ADAM as *acute type* if the duration is less than 6 months, or *chronic type* otherwise.

Clinical experience suggests that the most common stressors associated with adjustment disorder with anxious mood in childhood and adolescence are witnessed violence, parental separation or divorce, a family move, and changing schools. Identification of a stressor that precedes the development of symptoms does *not* mandate an adjustment disorder diagnosis; if the symptom picture fits better with another clinical diagnosis, then that diagnosis should be used. When anxiety symptoms are present in adjustment disorder but other symptoms are predominant, adjustment disorder with mixed emotion features, adjustment disorder with mixed disturbance of emotional and conduct, or adjustment disorder with physical complaints may be more descriptively accurate.

The course of adjustment disorder is ordinarily relatively brief. The continuing presence of stressors may, however, perpetuate the symptoms.

Children and adolescents who experience more severe stressors that are outside the usual range of human experience may develop a syndrome in which they continue to reexperience the trauma, and show avoidance behavior, emotional numbness, and the other characteristic symptoms (insomnia, irritability, hypervigilance) of PTSD (Table 62.4). When the duration of symptoms is 2 days to 4 weeks and anxiety symptoms are prominent, a diagnosis of *acute stress disorder* may be more appropriate.

PTSD has been described in children who have experienced natural disasters, witnessed extreme violence, and been victims of sexual and physical abuse. Once again, there is evidence that these more extreme stressors put children at risk for a wide range of psychiatric symptoms and syndromes including all of the anxiety disorders, not just PTSD (Burke et al., 1982; Livingston, 1987).

Treatment

Regardless of the diagnosis, children with anxiety disorders that develop following a stressful event or circumstance should receive a treatment plan that includes the specific issues related not only to the principal stressor but to other stressors as well. Livingston et al. recently

Table 62.4.   Signs and Symptoms of Posttraumatic Stress Disorder in Children

Reexperiencing the traumatic event
  Nightmares, especially of event[a]
  Repetitive play with event-related themes[a]
  Sudden catastrophic anxiety
Avoidance or emotional numbness
  Objects to discussing the event or denies it happened[a]
  Avoids places, people, or things that trigger memory of the trauma[a]
  Developmental regression
  Social withdrawal or detachment
  Blunted affect
Increased arousal
  Insomnia, objects to going to bed, wakes during night
  Irritability, aggression, overreactiveness
  Vigilance and scanning
  Tactile defensiveness, startles easily
  Autonomic overactivity

[a] Signs and symptoms relatively specific to posttraumatic stress disorder, less common in other syndromes.

reported (1993) that development of PTSD in abused children is predicted by the total number of stressors reported by the child and suggested that stressor-specific interventions may therefore help prevent PTSD in that population.

These interventions may include attempts to reduce the stress load, alter the child's response to stressors, or both. The spectrum of environmental measures may range from social casework to assisting family members to behave in less anxiogenic ways. The young person's response to stressors can be addressed, depending on the specific nature and severity of the presenting problems, with pharmacological, behavioral, and psychotherapeutic treatments directed at identified target symptoms.

OTHER ANXIETY DISORDERS OF CHILDHOOD AND ADOLESCENCE

Avoidant disorder of childhood or adolescence has been omitted in DSM-IV, presumably subsumed under *avoidant personality disorder*, which is also characterized by extreme avoidance of contact with unfamiliar people, in an individual who desires social involvement and relates well to those with whom he or she is familiar. The affected individual becomes very anxious when social contact with unfamiliar people is anticipated or experienced. This syndrome has only recently been defined and appears to be relatively uncommon; empirical information to validate it in early life is therefore lacking. It appears to be more common in girls.

Although *panic disorder* most commonly begins in early to middle adulthood, it appears that adolescent onset of the disorder is not rare and that symptoms suggestive of panic disorder appear before adolescence in children who have separation anxiety or depression (Hayward et al., 1989; Morean et al., 1989). Research data are scarce, but experience suggests that in younger children treatment of the primary depression or separation anxiety results in improvement or remission in panic symptoms in most, if not all, cases.

CASE ILLUSTRATION

Leslie was seen at age 16 by a consulting psychiatrist at the request of the cardiologist who was treating her for chest pain of unknown etiology. She had had two echocardiograms, the first of which had been interpreted as suggestive of mitral valve prolapse, and the second as within normal limits. She had no history of maladjustment or previous psychological difficulty and no evidence of other mood or anxiety symptoms. Her episodes of chest pain presented with additional symptoms of palpitations, terror of dying, feelings of dread, and tingling in her fingers and were identified by the psychiatrist as classic panic attacks. Treatment with imipramine and supportive psychotherapy resulted after a few weeks in complete resolution of her symptoms.

Comment

Had her panic symptoms been less typical, particularly if the peripheral symptoms had not been accompanied by psychological anxiety, a more aggressive cardiac workup might have been recommended, and a β-blocker such as propranolol would have been a better first choice for medication of the mitral valve prolapse and limited symptom attacks.

Adolescents with panic disorder seem to respond well to a combination of pharmacological treatment and psychotherapy. Imipramine and desipramine are commonly used; the dose initially should be low (25–50 mg/day), but doses in the adult range may ultimately be required. At higher doses serial electrocardiograms and measurement of blood levels may help to avoid cardiotoxicity. Alprazolam may prove to be useful in some cases for reducing frequency and intensity of attacks, and there may be a place for diazepam or other long-acting benzodiazepines for severe anticipatory anxiety between attacks. The possible contribution of psychological issues that are particularly likely in adolescence, such as identity, social standing, romantic relationships, and family conflict, should be explored and addressed when indicated.

CURRENT KNOWLEDGE AND RESEARCH NEEDS

Despite significant recent advances, much remains unknown about anxiety disorders in childhood and adolescence. We probably know more about separation anxiety and phobias than about any of the other conditions discussed in this chapter, and even these are far from being exhaustively studied. Refined structured diagnostic criteria can be expected to increase further the reliability and ultimately the validity of diagnostic categories and continue to provide a common language and foundation upon which to build. It is especially important, beginning with the common ground of DSM-IV with the International Classification of Diseases (ICD), to build up cross-cultural and international research.

Taxonomy and syndrome validation were identified as key issues at the 1990 research conference on child and adolescent anxiety at the National Institute of Mental Health. In this area there are significant methodological issues that need exploration. Structured diagnostic interviews and rating scales are available to identify anxiety symptoms and syndromes, but they yield significantly different results depending upon the informant. The relative value of the information provided by different informants must be established before a summary or consensus

method that will have adequate validity can be developed. Unfortunately, however, there is still no "gold standard" by which to judge the value of information. There does appear to be a growing consensus in this field that in younger children parents provide more complete information about behavior problems, and the children are likely to report emotional symptoms of which their parents may be unaware. The growing interest in panic disorder in children raises another methodological problem: Several developmental considerations make it improbable that young children will be able to provide accurate information about symptoms, onset, and duration and frequency of panic states. Some objective physiologic means of monitoring panic symptoms would therefore be desirable, and cumulative physiologic data may eventually provide the "gold standard" we need.

Some of the most productive and instructive studies of panic disorder in adults have involved deliberate precipitation of attacks with lactate, carbon dioxide, and various medications; to attempt similar studies in young children may be ethically at least questionable, so naturalistic methods must be sought to study these phenomena when possible. Perhaps the exposure situations used in behavioral treatments will provide some of these data.

For several of the anxiety disorders, there is much yet to establish in the area of basic descriptive pathology. We simply do not know enough about the course and complications of these disorders, which can be established only by longitudinal studies, and we are only beginning to explore issues of comorbidity and other clinical correlates such as family history, laboratory findings, and psychometric findings. Only when the basic descriptive psychopathology has been adequately explored, at least in its fundamentals, can we delve as much as we would like into hypotheses about the etiology and pathogenesis of the syndromes.

Ultimately, the predictive validity and natural history of the disorders will have to be more firmly established before treatment research will tell us whether we are altering the natural history of the disorders and answer important questions of comparative safety and efficacy of our interventions and their effectiveness in various real-world settings. More immediately, it is both possible and desirable to ascertain through well-controlled studies the effects of different interventions on selected target symptoms in appropriately homogeneous populations.

Meanwhile, clinicians are faced daily with the necessity to treat young people with anxiety disorders. Fortunately, the treatment of these children and adolescents often seems to be successful and therefore rewarding and enjoyable. As a firm scientific basis is developed in this field and as evidence develops about the ultimate benefits of treatment, we have every reason to hope that treatment of these disorders will grow to be even more successful and rewarding.

References

Adler R, Bongar B, Katz ER: Psychogenic abdominal pain and parental pressure in childhood athletics. *Psychosomatics* 23:1185–1186, 1982.

Allen AJ, Rapoport JL, Swedo SE: Psychopharmacologic treatment of childhood anxiety disorders. *Child Adolesc Psychiatr Clin North Am* 2:1–23, 1993.

American Academy of Child and Adolescent Psychiatry: Practice parameters for the assessment and treatment of anxiety disorders. *J Am Acad Child Adolesc Psychiatry* 32:1089–1098, 1993.

American Psychiatric Association: *Diagnostic and Statistical Manual of Mental Disorders* (3rd ed). Washington, DC, American Psychiatric Association Press, 1980.

American Psychiatric Association: *Diagnostic and Statistical Manual of Mental Disorders* (3rd ed, rev). Washington, DC, American Psychiatric Association Press, 1987.

American Psychiatric Association: *Treatment of Psychiatric Disorders*. Washington, DC, American Psychiatric Association Press, 1989, pp. 401–412, 734–746.

Barcai A, Rosenthal MK: Fears and tyranny; observations on the tyrannical child. *Arch Gen Psychiatry* 30:392–395, 1974.

Barrios B, O'Dell S: Fears and anxieties. In: Mash EJ, Barkley RA (eds): *Treatment of Childhood Disorders*. New York, Guilford, 1989.

Bernstein GA, Garfinkel B: School phobia, the overlap of affective and anxiety disorders. *J Am Acad Child Adolesc Psychiatry* 25:235–241, 1986a.

Bernstein GA, Garfinkel B: Visual Analogue Scale for Anxiety, Revised. *Scientific Proceedings*, American Academy of Child and Adolescent Psychiatry, 1986b.

Bowlby J: *The Making and Breaking of Affectional Bonds*. London, Tavistock, 1979.

Burke JD, Borus JF, Buras, BJ, et al: Changes in children's behavior after a natural disaster. *Am J Psychiatry* 139:1010–1014, 1982.

Clark DB, Donovan JE: Reliability and validity of the Hamilton Anxiety Rating Scale in an adolescent sample. *J Am Acad Child Adolesc Psychiatry* 33:354–360, 1994.

Chess S, Thomas A: Infant bonding—Mystique and reality. *Am J Orthopsychiatry* 213:222, 1982.

Costello EJ: Developments in child psychiatric epidemiology. *J Am Acad Child Adolesc Psychiatry* 28:836–841, 1989.

Dong Q, Yang B, Ollendick TH: Fears in Chinese children and adolescents and their relations to anxiety and depression. *J Child Psychol Psychiatry* 35: 351–363, 1994.

Eisenberg L: School phobia, a study in communication of anxiety. *Am J Psychiatry* 114:172–178, 1958.

Fabrega H, Ulrich R, Mezzich JE: Do caucasian and black adolescents differ at psychiatric intake? *J Am Acad Child Adolesc Psychiatry* 32:407–413, 1993.

Fitzpatrick KM, Boldizar JP: The prevalence and consequences of exposure to violence among African-American youth. *J Am Acad Child Adolesc Psychiatry* 32:424–430, 1993.

Gittleman R, Koplewics HS: In: Gittleman R (ed): *Anxiety Disorders of Childhood*. New York, Guilford, 1986, pp. 188–203.

Gittleman-Klein R, Klein DF: Controlled imipramine treatment of school phobia. *Arch Gen Psychiatry* 25:204–207, 1971.

Gorman JM, Liebowitz MR, Fyer AJ, et al: A neuroanatomical hypothesis for panic disorder. *Am J Psychiatry* 146:148–161, 1989.

Graae F, Milner J, Rizzotto L, et al: Clonazepam in childhood anxiety disorders. *J Am Acad Child Adolesc Psychiatry* 33:372–376, 1994.

Hayward C, Killen ID, Taylor CB: Panic attacks in young adolescents. *Am J Psychiatry* 146:1061–1062, 1989.

Jolly JB, Aruffo JF, Wherry JN, et al: The utility of the Beck Anxiety Inventory with inpatient adolescents. *J Anxiety Disord* 7:95–106, 1993.

Kandel ER: From metapsychology to molecular biology: Explorations into the nature of anxiety. *Am J Psychiatry* 140:1277–1293, 1983.

Kendall PC: *Anxiety Disorders in Youth, Cognitive-Behavioral Interventions*. Boston, Allyn & Bacon, 1992.

Last CG, Francis R, Hersen M, et al: Separation anxiety and school phobia; a comparison using DSM-III criteria. *Am J Psychiatry* 144:653–657, 1987a.

Last CG, Hersen M, Francis R, et al: Psychiatric illness in the mothers of anxious children. *Am J Psychiatry* 144:1580–1583, 1987b.

Last CG, Hersen M, Kazdin AE, et al: Comparison of DSM-III separation anxiety and overanxious disorders; demographic characteristics and patterns of co-morbidity. *J Am Acad Child Adolesc Psychiatry* 4:527–431, 1987c.

Last CG, Hersen M, Kazdin A, et al: Anxiety disorders in children and their families. *Arch Gen Psychiatry* 48:928–934, 1991.

Links PS, Boyer MH, Offord DB: The prevalence of emotional disorder in children. *J Nerv Ment Dis* 177:85–91, 1989.

Livingston R: Sexually and physically abused children. *J Am Acad Child Adolesc Psychiatry* 3:413–415, 1987.

Livingston R: Psychiatric comorbidity with reading disorder. *Adv Learn Behav Disabil* 6:143–155, 1990.

Livingston R: Children of people with somatization disorder. *J Am Acad Child Adolesc Psychiatry* 32:536–544, 1993.

Livingston R, Martin-Cannici C: Depression, anxiety and the dexamethasone suppression test in hospitalized prepubertal children. *Hillside J Clin Psychiatry* 9:55–63, 1987.

Livingston R, Nugent H, Rader L, et al: The family histories of depressed and severely anxious children. *Am J Psychiatry* 142:1497–1499, 1985.

Livingston R, Lawson L, Jones JG: Predictors of self-reported psychopathology in children abused repeatedly by a parent. *J Am Acad Child Adolesc Psychiatry* 32:948–953, 1993.

Livingston R, Taylor IL, Crawford SL: A study of somatic complaints and psychiatric diagnosis in children. *J Am Acad Child Adolesc Psychiatry* 27:185–187, 1988.

Mattison RE, Bagnato SJ: Empirical measurement of overanxious disorder in boys 8–12 years old. *J Am Acad Child Adolesc Psychiatry* 26:536–540, 1987.

Minuchin S, Baker L, Rosman BL: *Psychosomatic Families*. Cambridge, MA, Harvard University Press, 1978.

Morean DL, Weissman M, Warner V: Panic disorder in children at high risk for depression. *Am J Psychiatry* 146:1059–1060, 1989.

Neal AM, Lilly RS, Zakis S: What are African American children afraid of? A preliminary study. *J Anxiety Disord* 7:129–139, 1993.

Newton JEO, Lucas LA: Differential heart-rate responses to persons in nervous and normal pointer dogs. *Behav Genet* 12:379–393, 1982.

Ollendick TH, Mattis SG, King NJ: Panic in children and adolescents: A review. *J Child Psychol Psychiatry* 35:113–134, 1994.

Puig-Antich J, Rabinovich H: Affective and anxiety disorders. In: Gittleman R (ed): *Anxiety Disorders of Childhood*. New York, Guilford, 1986, pp. 136–156.

Reiter S, Kutcher SP: Disinhibition and anger outbursts in adolescents treated with clonazepam. *J Clin Psychopharmacol* 11:268, 1991.

Richters MM, Volkmar FR: Reactive attachment disorder of infancy or early childhood (Case Study). *J Am Acad Child Adolesc Psychiatry* 33:328–332, 1994.

Robins LN: Followup studies investigating childhood disorders. In: Hareeh A, Wing JK (eds): *Psychiatric Epidemiology*. London, Oxford University Press, 1971.

Rutter M, Tizard J, Whitmore K: *Education, Health and Behavior*. London, Longman, 1970.

Schwartz S, Johnson HJ: *Psychopathology of Childhood*. New York, Pergamon, 1985, pp. 187–198.

Shaffer D, O'Connor P, Shafer S, et al: Neurologic soft signs. In: Rutter M (ed): *Developmental Neuropsychiatry*. New York, Guilford, 1983.

Silver LB: Recognition and treatment of anxiety in children and adolescents. In: Fann WE, Karacan I, Porkory AD, et al (eds): *Phenomenology and Treatment of Anxiety*. New York, Spectrum, 1979, pp. 93–109.

Strauss CC, Last CG: Social and simple phobias in children. *J Anxiety Disord* 7:141–152, 1993.

Werry JS: Overanxious disorder: A review of its taxonomic properties. *J Am Acad Child Adolesc Psychiatry* 30:533–544, 1991.

63 OBSESSIVE-COMPULSIVE DISORDER

Kenneth E. Towbin, M.D., and Mark A. Riddle, M.D.

Although obsessions and compulsions are among the oldest mental symptoms for which we have detailed descriptions, they are also among the most active topics of contemporary psychiatric investigation. Obsessions and compulsions are depicted as possession by the devil in *Malleus Malficarum* (Kramer and Sprenger, 1928) from 1467, described in the "Obsessi" of Paracelsus, and known as religious doubts and excessive devotion—scrupulosity—in the 1600's (Hunter and MacAlpine, 1963). Pioneers of psychiatry like Esquirol (1838), Maudsley (1895), Freud (1953b), and Janet (Pittman, 1987), took up this troubling and fascinating disorder. The surge of research in the last decade has deepened our understanding of the course and etiology of these symptoms and expanded our knowledge of basic brain functions.

DEFINITIONS

Obsessions are unwanted thoughts, images, or impulses that the individual realizes are senseless or unnecessary, intrude into his or her consciousness involuntarily, and cause functional impairment and distress. Despite this lack of control, the sufferer still recognizes that these thoughts originate in his or her own mental process. Since they arise in the mind, obsessions can take the form of any mental event—simple repetitive words, thoughts, fears, memories, pictures, or elaborate dramatic scenes.

Compulsions are actions that are responses to a perceived internal obligation to follow certain rituals or rules; they also cause functional impairment. Compulsions may be motivated directly by obsessions or efforts to ward off certain thoughts, impulses, or fears. Occasionally, children report compulsions without the perception of a mental component. Like obsessions, compulsions are often viewed as being unnecessary, excessive or senseless, and involuntary or forced. Individuals suffering from compulsions will often elaborate a variety of precise rules for the chronology, rate, order, duration, and number of repetitions of their acts.

These definitions reflect three critical concepts with relevance to the differential diagnosis. A most essential criterion is functional impairment as a consequence of symptoms. Two others carry from classic definitions [Jaspers (1963); Maudsley (1895)]: Individuals feel that they are being forced or invaded by the symptoms, and they possess insight into the senselessness or excessiveness of their thoughts or acts. The validity of requiring patients to view their acts as unnecessary or their thoughts as senseless has been challenged, following observations that this objectivity may be inconstant. Insel and Akiskal (1986) and Lelliott and co-workers (1988) reported on severely impaired patients who at times doubted the need to perform their rituals or thought their behaviors were senseless and, at others, were convinced of their necessity to the point of near or actual psychotic proportions. DSM-IV criteria (Table 63.1) for obsessive-compulsive disorder (OCD) have been modified such that awareness of the senselessness or excess of the symptoms

Table 63.1. DSM-IV Criteria for OCD

A. Either obsessions or compulsions:
  Obsessions: as defined by (1), (2), (3), and (4):
   (1) Recurrent and persistent ideas, thoughts, impulses, or images that are experienced at some time during the disturbance as intrusive and inappropriate and cause marked anxiety or distress.
   (2) The thoughts, impulses, or images are not simply excessive worries about real-life problems.
   (3) The person attempts to ignore or suppress such thoughts, impulses, or images to neutralize them with some other thought or action.
   (4) The person recognizes that the obsessional thoughts are the product of his or her own mind (not imposed from without, as in thought insertion).
  Compulsions: as defined by (1) and (2):
   (1) Repetitive behaviors or mental acts that the person feels driven to perform in response to an obsession, or according to rules that must be applied rigidly.
   (2) The behaviors or mental acts are aimed at preventing or reducing distress or preventing some dreaded event or situation; however, these behaviors or mental acts either are not connected in a realistic way with what they are designed to neutralize or prevent or are clearly excessive.
B. At some point, the person has recognized that the obsessions or compulsions are excessive or unreasonable. Note: this does not apply to children.
C. The obsessions or compulsions cause marked distress, are time consuming (take more than 1 hour a day), or significantly interfere with the person's normal routine, occupational (or academic) functioning, or usual social activities or relationships.
D. If another Axis I disorder is present, the content of the obsessions or compulsions is not restricted to it (e.g., preoccupation with food in the presence of an eating disorder; hair pulling in trichotillomania; concern with appearance in the presence of body dysmorphic disorder; preoccupations with having a serious illness in the presence of hypochondriasis; or guilty ruminations in the presence of a major depressive disorder).
E. Not due to the direct effects of a substance (e.g., a drug of abuse, a medication) or a general medical condition.

Adapted from American Psychiatric Association: *Diagnostic and Statistical Manual of Mental Disorders* (4th ed). Washington, DC, American Psychiatric Association, 1994.

only must be present at *some* phase of the illness. For children this criterion is dismissed altogether.

Few studies differentiate between childhood- and adolescent-onset OCD subjects. Therefore, in this chapter, "child," "childhood," or "children" will be used to signify children *and adolescents*. There are studies that have sampled adolescent subjects only. When this is so, the more exclusive term will be employed.

PREVALENCE AND EPIDEMIOLOGY

A review of studies that seek a reliable prevalence for OCD reveals significant disparities and varied methods. Since longitudinal studies suggest that child and adult OCD are the same disorder, adult epidemiologic reports are relevant. Initial reports (Rudin, 1953) gave prevalence rates of 0.05% for adult OCD. This was sustained until the Epidemiologic Catchment Area (ECA) survey produced surprisingly greater lifetime adult prevalences from 1.2–2.4% (Robins et al., 1984). Subsequent examination of these high ECA values showed validity concordances for OCD were among the poorest of all the diagnoses, with κ values in the range of 0.12–0.05 (Anthony et al, 1985; Helzer et al., 1985). The Diagnostic Interview Schedule method of relying on simple "yes" or "no" responses to queries about the presence of broadly defined obsessions or compulsions did not yield reliable measures for actual *clinical cases* of obsessive-compulsive *disorder*. Helzer and co-workers (1985) proposed that in community surveys where many subjects cluster at the "threshold of the diagnostic definition," results will be unreliable, since the response to a single probe carries so much weight. When Karno and co-workers (1988) reanalyzed the ECA data, the prevalence rates were sustained despite the flawed methodology. Although rates derived from clinician interviews were close to those using the original lay interviews, the clinician's records suggested that lay interviews led to many false-negative and false-positive diagnoses. Karno and co-workers (1988) believed that future prevalence studies could attain improved reliability by including open-ended questions and separating symptoms (e.g. washing and checking).

Prevalence rates among clinical populations of children were reported by Berman (1942) (0.2%), Judd (1965) (1.2%) and Hollingsworth and co-workers (1980) (0.2%). Subsequently, Flament and co-workers (1988) examined prevalences in a general adolescent population by screening with a modified Leyton Obsessional Inventory (LOI) and pursuing direct clinical interviews of high-scoring subjects. This yielded a point prevalence of 0.35% and a lifetime prevalence of 0.40%. Weightings, such as those used in the ECA study, gave hypothetical point and lifetime prevalence rates of 1% and 1.9%, respectively (Flament et al., 1988). Of the 18 adolescents diagnosed with OCD, 12 (67%) reported that symptoms resulted in high subjective interference, yet global assessment scores averaged 67 ("generally functioning pretty well") and ranged from 50–90. To ascertain a non-clinical population, Zohar and co-workers (1992) performed detailed clinician-rated evaluations of 562 consecutive 16- to 17-year-old male and female inductees to the Israeli army. OCD prevalence rates were 3.6%; 50% of cases were identified as having "obsessions only." This latter figure was substantially higher than that reported from clinical populations. The authors found support for the validity of their findings in that their rates for compulsions compared so favorably to those of Flament and co-workers (1988).

Overall, it appears that OCD may be relatively prevalent, particularly among adolescents. There are still important methodological problems that must be overcome. There is no consensus over where the line demarcating sub-clinical obsessional-compulsive features and clinical OCD should be drawn. Study designs that employ structured or non-clinician interviews exclusively may be unreliable.

CLINICAL DESCRIPTION

An unlimited variety of obsessions and compulsions can be expressed by the human mind and body. The typical pattern is for the patient to experience both obsessions and compulsions. It has been presumed that few individuals have only one or the other (Riddle et al., 1990; Swedo et al., 1989) but, as noted above, having only obsessions may be more common (Zohar et al., 1992). At any moment, most patients experience multiple obsessions or compulsions; over time, changes in the objects and contents of symptoms develop (Rettew et al, 1992). Although the repertoire of obsessions can range widely, certain contents are reported more frequently and development may influence content. Reports of adolescents suggest that the most common categories of obsessions are concern over dirt and germs, fears of an ill fate befalling loved ones, exactness or symmetry, and religious scrupulousness (Swedo et. al., 1989). Bodily functions, lucky numbers, sexual or aggressive preoccupations, and fear of harm to oneself are less common. In adults, the frequency of these categories is similar, except that aggressive and sexual obsessions are more common (Dowson, 1977; Rachman and Hodgson, 1980; Rasmussen and Tsuang, 1986).

Although a compulsion can be created from any action, only a few are common. An adolescent clinical cohort (Swedo et al., 1989) displayed (in descending order of frequency) cleaning rituals, repeating actions (doing and undoing), and checking rituals most commonly. Many fewer subjects reported rituals to protect themselves from illness or injury, ordering maneuvers, and counting behaviors. In adults, the most common compulsions are checking and cleaning (Rachman and Hodgson, 1980; Rasmussen and Tsuang, 1986; Welner et al., 1976). Slowness (Rachman and Hodgson, 1980), counting (Rasmussen and Tsuang, 1986), or doing things by numbers (Welner et al., 1976) each have been reported as third most common.

Longitudinal clinical data are scanty. Outcome data are discussed below. Retracing the onset of symptoms in adult patients, Black (1974) reported that 40% had onset before age 20, with an average age of onset in the early 20s. The ECA data supported this, with mean onset at 20.9–25.4 years of age (Karno et al., 1988). There is evidence that onset is earlier in men (Swedo et al., 1989; Rasmussen and Tsuang, 1986). Noshirvani and coworkers (1991) reported that males and females were equally represented in their sample, but 35% of male subjects had their onset between ages 5–15 compared to 20% of cohort females. Generally, symptoms exist an average of 7–8 years before reaching clinical attention (Flament et al., 1988). Noshirvani and co-workers (1991) suggested that males tend to have a longer duration of illness prior to seeking treatment, yet the ECA study (Karno et al., 1988) showed that subjects with OCD had rates of medical and mental health service utilization that are roughly identical to those of other disorders. This implies that subjects with OCD seek care as readily as those with other DSM-III-diagnosed disorders.

In other areas of function, children with OCD are more selectively impaired than the general clinical population. Academic achievement and extra-curricular functioning are often preserved, although the quality of peer relationships may be variable (Riddle et al., 1990). Clinical studies of children entering treatment programs have consistently demonstrated average intellectual quotients, although the selection bias of these cohorts must be considered in interpreting these data.

Severe symptoms can envelop the patient and his or her family completely. It is common to learn of washing rituals that consume 4 hours of scrubbing daily, dissolve an entire bar of soap each session, leave the patient's hands worn raw and macerated, and raise monthly water bills dramatically. Counting or ordering compulsions can waste half a day and lead to complete obstruction. Rituals repetitively executed from night to early morning may curtail sleep to a few hours. Checking or cleansing rituals can produce physical injury such as skin lacerations, ulcers, and chemical burns.

The family's reaction to the patient's symptoms is crucial. Several common response patterns may produce delays in evaluation and treatment of childhood OCD. Although patients are embarrassed and secretive about the content of, and the limitations imposed by their symptoms, serious impairments rarely elude family members. Parents may delay obtaining treatment as a result of a false hope that symptoms will extinguish if everyone acquiesces and aids in performing the activities. This kind of family assistance does not relieve the child's anxiety. Many parents have difficulty extricating themselves from aiding in rituals. Children may extort, implore, or otherwise compel their parents to collaborate; the patient and parent become pathologically entwined in rituals. Parents may not understand that their child suffers from a serious disorder despite adequate development in other domains. In addition, the child's claims that the thoughts or acts are ridiculous or unnecessary may instill false security in parents who think that "its just a phase." This may be furthered by parents with subclinical obsession- or compulsion-like behaviors who cannot recognize symptoms in their child. Reassurance from clinicians and pediatricians who are unfamiliar with the disorder may result in mistaking severe symptoms for "normal" reactions. It is a frightening and painful moment when parents recognize that their child is ill and has lost control of his or her thoughts and actions.

ETIOLOGY AND PATHOGENESIS

Since the discovery that medication could improve this condition (Thoren et al., 1980) a great deal of effort has been directed toward identifying relevant biological mechanisms that precipitate or maintain OCD.

Genetic Studies

Current evidence suggests genetic transmission of a vulnerability to OCD in many cases. This stems from increased concordance rates among monozygotic compared to dizygotic twins (Carey and Gottesman, 1981; Rasmussen and Tsuang, 1986) and increased rates among first-degree relatives of clinical probands. Hoover and Insel (1984) discovered increased rates for subclinical obsessive-compulsive *symptoms* among first-degree relatives, but rates of OCD in relatives did not reach statistical significance. Lenane and co-workers (1990) reported that 30% of 46 adolescent probands had a first-degree relative with OCD. OCD

was reported in 17% of parents and the age-corrected rate for siblings was 35%. Riddle and co-workers (1990) reported that 10% of parents from a cohort of 21 clinic patients with OCD were diagnosed with OCD. Twenty-five percent had sub-threshold symptoms of obsessions or compulsions.

McKeon and Murray (1987) performed a family study using a matched control group; of 145 first-degree relatives, only one (0.6%) met Research Diagnostic Criteria (RDC) for OCD. Black and co-workers (1992) conducted a detailed, controlled family study of 166 OCD relatives and 182 control subject relatives using raters who were blind to proband status. Rates of OCD in first-degree relatives of OCD probands were comparable to control relatives (2.5% vs. 2.3%) and the ECA general population prevalence. However the rate of anxiety disorders in relatives was nearly twice that of control relatives.

Reports of elevated rates of OCD among patients with Tourette's syndrome (Pauls et al., 1986) and of tics and a family history of tics among OCD probands (Green and Pittman, 1986; Leonard et al, 1992) suggest that some OCD may arise from the same genetic etiology as Tourette's syndrome (Pauls and Leckman, 1986). Reevaluation of the National Institute of Mental Health (NIMH) cohort and their relatives in a 2–7 year follow-up lends support to this hypothesis (Leonard et al, 1993). Fifty-seven percent of 54 probands had a lifetime history of tics, 15% met criteria for Tourette's syndrome, and 22% had chronic multiple tics. Among their relatives, 14% had lifetime diagnoses of tics. These findings suggest that future investigations of course of illness or treatment efficacy should analyze data according to whether subjects do or do not possess tics and have or do not have a family history of tics (Towbin, 1988).

Electrophysiologic Studies

EEG studies of adult and child OCD subjects have yielded significant variations across subjects (Behar et al., 1984; Flor-Henry et al., 1979; Insel et al., 1983). OCD subjects reportedly exhibit decreased Rapid Eye Movement (REM) latencies but normal REM density (Insel et al., 1982). This pattern is distinct from the one seen in persons with depression, in which there is decreased REM latency and *decreased* REM density. Towey and co-workers (1990) performed event-related potentials in adults with OCD. Reduced P300 and N200 latencies were observed suggesting increased cortical processing speeds. More negativity in the N200 region, greater over the left than right, implied relatively increased responsiveness in the left hemisphere.

Imaging Studies

COMPUTERIZED TOMOGRAPHY (CT) AND MAGNETIC RESONANCE IMAGING (MRI)

CT views of adolescents with OCD or OCD subjects whose onset was in adolescence suggested ventricular enlargement independent of sex, age, duration, and types of symptoms (Behar et al, 1984). Luxenberg and co-workers (1988) employed quantitative scanning in males with adolescent onset OCD and a never-ill control group. In the OCD cohort, decreased mean volumes were seen in caudate nuclei bilaterally. Values of normals and OCD subjects overlapped considerably, but pooled mean differences were consistent with a hypothesis of basal ganglia changes in OCD.

When Garber and co-workers compared MRI scans of adults with OCD and healthy controls, abnormalities in frontal cortex, cingulate gyrus, and lenticular nuclei were seen (Garber et al., 1989). Past medication treatment or family history did not significantly influence findings. Kellner and co-workers did not discover significant structural differences between OCD subjects and normal controls (1991) but Calabrese and co-workers (1993) reported increases in the size of the caudate nuclei. A subsequent study reported left caudate nuclei volumes exceeded those on the right (Calabrese et al., 1993).

CEREBRAL BLOOD FLOW AND SINGLE PHOTON EMISSION TOMOGRAPHY (SPECT)

Zohar and coworkers (1989) observed changes in regional cerebral blood flow (rCBF) with [^{133}Xe]xenon inhalation. Subjects who were stressed specifically to increase anxiety displayed *decreased* temporal rCBF. This pattern was sustained as the stressful stimuli were changed to induce higher levels of anxiety.

There are no published studies of SPECT in children with OCD, but two adult studies reported increases in medial-frontal rCBF (Hoehn-Saric, et al., 1991; Machlin et al., 1991). Rubin and co-workers examined regional cerebral blood flow with xenon inhalation and technetium uptake (1992). Xenon studies did not reveal differences between OCD adults and normal controls, but with technetium uptake increased activity in the orbito-frontal cortex was observed with significantly decreased bilateral activity in the head of the caudate (Rubin et al, 1992)—a phenomenon previously noted by others (Machlin, et al., 1991).

POSITRON EMISSION TOMOGRAPHY (PET)

Over the last five years, PET has become a powerful tool to extend the understanding of OCD. Initial comparisons of OCD and depressed adults suggested bilateral increased metabolism in the orbital gyri (Baxter et al., 1987, 1988; Nordahl et al., 1989) and the head of the caudate nuclei (Baxter et al., 1988). Baxter and colleagues proposed that the orbital gyri might be specific for tension and anxiety in OCD. Swedo and co-workers (1989) scanned adults with both current OCD and documented adolescent onset. Increased bilateral prefrontal and anterior cingulate gyri activity was reported. The data were interpreted as consistent with a "frontal lobe-limbic-basal ganglia loop" mechanism. Other observations of elevated caudate nuclei activity (Baxter et al., 1988) were not confirmed. Increased metabolism in premotor and mid-frontal regions were reported in patients with obsessional slowness (Sawle et al., 1991).

Subsequent work examined regional brain metabolic changes following behavioral or pharmacological treatment. Baxter and co-workers (1992) studied adults before and after treatment with fluoxetine or behavior therapy. Responders displayed decreased right caudate nucleus glucose metabolism; no changes appeared in treatment non-responders and never-ill controls. Change of another kind was reported in a one year medication follow-up study (Swedo et al., 1992). Adults with childhood onset OCD exhibited decreased fronto-orbital metabolism associated with medication-related or spontaneous improvement in OCD severity ratings.

Serotonin, Norepinephrine, and Dopamine

Several lines of evidence lend support to the importance of serotonin (5-HT) in the pathophysiology of OCD. These include: (*a*) Serotonin reuptake inhibitors (SRIs) have been the most effective in the treatment of patients with OCD; (*b*) decreased cerebrospinal fluid concentrations of 5-hydroxyindoleacetic acid (5-HIAA) have correlated with clinical response to SRIs; and (*c*) substances that increase serotonergic transmission, such as L-tryptophan and lithium, have been successful in augmenting serotonergic medication in unresponsive patients.

Yet studies of serotonin in patients with OCD have produced equivocal findings. Adolescents with OCD were found to have normal 5-HT platelet levels when compared to healthy volunteers (Flament et al., 1987), and adults with OCD showed tritiated imipramine binding and 5-HT uptake similar to normals (Insel et al., 1985). A cohort composed of adolescents and adults with OCD displayed a substantial decrease in tritiated imipramine binding but no differences in 5-HT uptake (Weizman et al.,1986). Also, when patients with depression or OCD successfully treated with SRIs undergo tryptophan depletion, depression reemerges in depressed patients but OC symptoms do not in those with OCD (Barr et al., 1994).

"Pharmacologic probes" that are putatively specific for 5-HT, such as metachlorophenylpiperazine (MCPP), tryptophan, and metergoline yield contradictory results. MCPP elevated temperature, obsessive-compulsive symptoms, and anxiety in one study (Zohar and Insel, 1987) and did not affect OCD symptoms or create physiologic responses in another (Charney et al., 1988). In yet another study (Hollander et al., 1992) oral MCPP reportedly increased symptoms in 55% of subjects. Symptom exacerbation with MCPP predicted non-response to a selective serotonin reuptake inhibitor (Hollander et al, 1992). MCPP administered after 3 months of clomipramine treatment did not evoke acute elevations in obsessive-compulsive symptoms that initially were seen in the untreated OCD subjects (Zohar et al., 1988). Metergoline, a specific 5-HT agonist, decreased symptoms only slightly (Zohar and Insel, 1987).

Unresponsiveness to tryptophan depletion, MCPP, and metergoline administration implies that other transmitter systems are relevant in OCD (Charney et al., 1988). Hypotheses of combination noradrenergic-serotonergic activity or effects on calcium channels have been proposed in this vein (Hollander et al, 1991; Insel et al., 1985).

A contributing role also has been proposed for dopamine (Rapoport and Wise, 1988). Support for this includes increased metabolism of basal ganglia regions on PET scanning in persons with OCD, the appearance of OCD symptoms in disorders affecting basal ganglia (e.g. Syndenham's chorea, toxic agents, trauma), the efficacy of dopaminergic blocking agents (such as pimozide and haloperidol) to augment unsuccessful responses to SRIs in some OCD patients (McDougle et al., 1994), and evidence that fluoxetine and clomipramine exert dopaminergic *and* serotonergic activity (Baldessarini and Marsh, 1990; Austin, et al., 1991).

Neuroendocrine Studies

When compared to a matched sample of normal controls and subjects with Tourette's syndrome (TS), a cohort of adults with OCD, who did not have a personal or family history of tic disorders, displayed significantly elevated CSF levels of oxytocin (OT). This is all the more interesting in view of findings of low CSF OT in TS subjects who exhibit OCD. Leckman and co-workers (1994) point out that the cognitive and behavioral symptoms of OCD are similar to the behavioral effects of OT (e.g. cognitive, grooming, affiliative, and reproductive behaviors) that have been observed in animals.

Integration of Biological Studies

Much of these data have been subsumed in a hypothesis of OCD that integrates neuropsychological, anatomical, neurochemical, and electrophysiological findings (Baxter et al, 1992; Insel, 1992). It posits the existence of neuroanatomical lesions in the etiology of OCD. Scanning studies suggest that changes in basal ganglia and frontal lobes are associated with OCD symptoms (Baxter et al., 1987; Luxenberg et al., 1988; Nordahl et al., 1989; Swedo et al., 1989). When linked to reports of acquired OCD following specific brain lesions in the same regions (Laplane et al., 1989) supportive evidence increases. Swedo and colleagues published reports of OCD following Syndenham's chorea and speculated on the correlation of Syndenham's symptoms with changes in cortical and striatal regions, including the caudate nuclei (Swedo et al., 1993). Reports of improvement in OCD following frontal lobe injury, and of increased metabolic activity in frontal regions with habituation and extinction, further support this concept. The physical proximity of the frontal and cingulate gyri to the caudate nuclei and reports of clinical improvement following cingulotomy form additional links.

As early as 1990, Alexander and co-workers (1990) proposed the existence of "basal ganglia-thalamocortical circuits." They suggested that a "lateral orbito-frontal circuit" projecting to ventromedial sectors of the caudate, the substantia nigra, and the globus pallidus might, according to PET and neurophysiologic findings, be active in OCD.

PET findings led Baxter and co-workers (1992) to propose an "orbital-basal ganglia-thalamic circuit" similar to Alexander's. Baxter and colleagues hypothesized that the orbital gyri drive the caudate nucleus which, in turn, inhibits the globus pallidus. Weakened activity in the globus pallidus fails to inhibit the thalamus which, in turn, is more excitatory to the orbital gyri. Their hypothesis proposes that, with treatment, inhibitory activity from the caudate is weakened. With treatment, the globus pallidus inhibits the thalamus and decreases excitatory input to orbital gyri. The hypothetical result of treatment is an increase in the patient's capacity to suppress orbito-frontal output.

An additional attraction of this hypothesis is that it is more compatible with the variety of neurochemical findings. The relationship between serotonin and dopamine is not clear, but there are suggestions that serotonergic neurons regulate some dopaminergic sites via inhibitory effects.

Neuropsychological Processes

Neuropsychological investigations of OCD provide some support for frontal lobe dysfunction, although this has not been unequivocal. Flor-Henry and co-workers (1979) studied 11 subjects with adult-onset OCD employing age- and sex-matched controls to find frontal—especially *dominant* frontal—deficits. They proposed that associated dominant temporal and parietal dysfunction stemmed from the failure of frontal inhibitory responses. Others (Insel et al., 1983) could not confirm frontal lobe findings. Behar and co-workers (1984) found signs of immaturity among 16 adolescent subjects on two measures reflecting frontal lobe function. The performance of 6 subjects on another test suggested "neurodevelopmental immaturity." Neurological soft signs, such as synkinesia, were seen in 5 of the 7 adolescents. Cox and co-workers (1989) suggested deficits in regulatory functions localized to the frontal lobe, although they did not confirm dominance of the frontal hemisphere. Few measures supported right-left hemispheric differences. The group underscored that findings were independent of impairment from OCD, implying a stable deficit that was unrelated to severity.

Psychoanalytic Theories

Psychoanalytic theories of OCD have not been subjected to rigorous, systematic scientific research. A rich anecdotal literature exists, but its reliability and validity remain untested.

Freud had observed obsessions and compulsions early in his investigations into the unconscious (1953a). What he termed obsessive-compulsive neurosis was an undifferentiated complex comprised of features from what we now call OCD and obsessive-compulsive personality disorder. He considered that obsessional symptoms, especially shame and overconscientiousness, resulted from a failure to defend oneself from unconscious aggressive drives that originate during the period of "anal" organization. During this period, he proposed, strong aggressive and sexual drives emerge when the ego is too weak to defend against powerful superego prohibitions. As a result, the ego responds with symptoms of "overconscientiousness, cleanliness, and piety," and libidinal impulses regress from genital to anal-sadistic organization.

Anna Freud proposed that the failure of two ego functions promoted obsessional neuroses: *fusion* of sexual and aggressive drives from the id, which ordinarily permits the infant to contain destructive, annihilating drives and maintain the attachment to the caretaker; and *synthesis*, which creates harmony out of "opposing strivings" before they reach consciousness (Freud, 1966). This hypothesis is of interest in light of studies suggesting that the frontal lobe, a region that is important in the inhibition or modification of sexual and aggressive impulses, may be impaired in OCD. As a consequence of these ego deficits, Anna Freud offered, patients with obsessional neuroses are unsuccessful in their mastery of ambivalence, including the resolution of sexual and aggressive urges or "intrasystemic contradictions" in the id, such as feelings of love-hate, masculinity-femininity, and so on (Freud, 1966).

Anna Freud (1966) also was impressed with the dysynchrony in the two mechanisms, which she believed lead to obsessional neurosis. Thus, the neurosis would be brought about in two ways: as a consequence of

the precocious maturation of ego and superego in comparison to the id, or when there is normal maturation of all three psychic structures followed by id regression. In the first case, the capacity to use defenses residing in thought develop during the anal stage. But, in either case the result is a punitive, intolerant response from the ego and superego occurring simultaneously with heightened anal-sadistic impulses (Freud, 1966). In both mechanisms, constitutional and environmental contributions are acknowledged. Defenses characterized by undoing, intellectualization, reaction formation, and isolation are prominent.

LABORATORY STUDIES

There are no pathognomonic laboratory findings in OCD. Appropriate laboratory evaluation follows from the findings of the history, physical, mental status, and psychological examination. An electrocardiogram, complete blood count with differential and baseline blood chemistries, including electrolytes, as well as liver function tests, blood urea nitrogen, and creatinine may be necessary before commencing somatic treatment. Copper measures for Wilson's disease are unnecessary in the absence of psychotic symptoms or physical findings of tics or chorea. Only when focal neurological findings are observed are CT or MRI scanning warranted. Karyotypes may be obtained for patients with abnormal appearance. Electroencephalography is indicated only when a seizure disorder is suspected.

Psychological tests provide a detailed picture of intellectual function, severity of acute stressors, and characteristic defensive structures in OCD patients. Standardized tests, such as the Wechsler Intelligence Scales for Children edition III (WISC-III) or the Kaufman Assessment Battery for Children (K-ABC) for younger children, are appropriate for determining intellectual level. Projective tests, including the Rorschach, Thematic Apperception Test, Draw-a-Person, and Adolescent Multiphasic Personality Inventory, can also be useful in identifying current sources of stress and characteristic defense patterns.

Severity measures of obsessions and compulsions are discussed below. In addition, the parents-on-child version of the Child Behavior Checklist (CBCL) (Achenbach and Edelbrock, 1983) can help discover other dysfunctional behaviors.

DIFFERENTIAL DIAGNOSIS

The differential diagnosis depends upon which system of classification is used to define OCD. Table 63.2 offers a partial list of disorders in which obsessions or compulsions may be seen. Though rare, there are specific brain disorders ("organic brain syndromes") that display OCD (Drummond and Gravestock, 1988; Frye and Arnold, 1981; McKeon et al., 1984).

The DSM-IV handles disorders comorbid with OCD by requiring that the content of the obsessions not be "restricted" to any coexistent disorder. Although this eliminates some difficulties, it creates others; the ability to discern the degree of "unrelatedness" can be a problem. Like DSM-III-R, DSM-IV combines a heterogeneous group of disorders and co-morbid features (Leonard et al., 1993; Swedo et al., 1989) under the term OCD on the basis of presence of a single symptom. Many different disorders and comorbid symptoms with different etiologies

Table 63.2. Disorders Manifesting Obsessions and/or Compulsions

Anorexia nervosa	Phobias
Body dysmorphic disorder	Posttraumatic stress disorder
Delusional disorder (all types)	Schizophrenia
Depression	Schizotypal personality
Hypochondriasis	Somatization disorder
Obsessive-compulsive personality disorder	Somatoform disorders
Organic mental disorder[a]	Trichotillomania
Panic disorder	Tourette's syndrome
Pervasive developmental disorder	"Fear of AIDS"

[a] Specifically arising from CNS trauma, tumors, toxins.

are subsumed under this one label. An important caveat emerges when working under this diagnostic scheme. If treatment decisions are to be relevant to the patient's needs, clinicians are obligated to conduct thorough diagnostic assessments in order to detect coexisting conditions that present in addition to OCD (Towbin et al., 1987). Failing to do so risks ignoring findings that are relevant to treatment. Similarly, if research is to be generalizable and valid, researchers are obligated to provide an equally complete evaluation of sample subjects (Towbin et al., 1987).

Care should be taken not to equate *subclinical* obsessions/compulsions and OCD, especially in adolescents. Subclinical phenomena appear to be stable features that do not interfere with development (Flament et al., 1988).

Inexperienced clinicians mistake obsessive-compulsive personality disorder (OCPD) for OCD. The majority of patients with OCD neither exhibit nor develop OCPD. Although persons with OCPD may have rigid routines, needs for orderliness, hoarding behaviors, and indecisiveness, they usually do not experience these as ego-dystonic. Their compulsive behaviors do not cause them anxiety and, ordinarily, do not result in impairment. Impairment in OCPD results from patterns of beliefs or behaviors, not from isolated symptoms. OCPD often undergoes phases of exacerbation and remission and particular characteristics may escalate when a patient is stressed. Conversely, patients with OCD generally are not emotionally cold, unexpressive, ungiving, or especially rigid about moral or ethical matters. Furthermore, hoarding, list making, and rigid scheduling behaviors are uncommon among compulsions reported by patients with OCD (Rasmussen and Tsuang, 1986).

Differentiating psychosis from the overvalued ideas of obsessional patients can be vexing. Like DSM-III-R, DSM-IV permits schizophrenia or delusional disorders to coexist with OCD. When such comorbid syndromes arise it can be very trying to apply definitions contending that OCD patients possess the insight to know that their obsessions originate in their minds and are not imposed by external sources. When insight is absent, treatment, prognosis, and etiology may be reconsidered. Clinicians should consider comorbid diagnoses when patients do not display insight.

"Fear of AIDS" consists of obsessional fears and preoccupations about contracting AIDS (Wagner and Sullivan, 1991; Fisman and Walsh, 1994). Although blood tests permit a positive diagnosis of AIDS, a clinician cannot give a diagnosis of hypochondriasis confidently to those with negative or equivocal serologic results. The long incubation period and high risks to adolescents who do not practice safe sex means that those with "fear of AIDS" constitute a group whose concerns can be neither completely refuted nor confirmed. Many cases straddle the boundary between subthreshold obsessions and OCD.

EVALUATION AND TREATMENT

Evaluation

The critical first step in the treatment of children with OCD is evaluation. Children often feel embarrassed about their symptoms and underreport impairment. Frequently, children fear that their symptoms are bizarre and "crazy." They are most likely to describe symptoms to a clinician who resists confrontation, conveys acceptance, and respects privacy; it takes time for the patient to reveal his or her fears fully. Consequently, assessment usually cannot be completed in one meeting.

An adequate evaluation of OCD must sample multiple sources. It is desirable to gather history from the patient alone, from his or her parents alone, and from the family together. Helpful information can be obtained from teachers on academic performance, peer relationships, areas of impairment, and tasks presenting special challenges. Siblings may provide valuable information on family responses to the patient.

The objectives of individual meetings are to estimate the extent of impairment, the developmental level attained by the patient, and the associated diagnoses and symptoms that are hampering progress. The clinician needs to learn about the patient's strengths and weaknesses, fears and aspirations, achievements and disappointments. Impairment

created by symptoms often permeates home, school, work, peer relations, and self-image. This dictates assessing the patient's adjustment in each of these domains. Although it may be tempting to use meetings with the patient to conquer denial, root out secrets, and unmask obsessions, fostering a relationship is critical.

Whatever modalities will be used, the clinician's relationship with the patient is crucial for several reasons. First, most children with OCD are apprehensive and secretive. They are anxious about treatment and their symptoms. The relationship with the clinician can reassure and absorb much of the anxiety in a way that promotes discussion and treatment. Second, many patients are uneasy discussing their thoughts or rituals because the content is scatological or sexual. Patients must feel that the clinician will understand the distress they experience and can be trusted with the unacceptable content of their symptoms. Third, when treatments require a lengthy trial period or cause increasing anxiety, the relationship with the clinician must be a sturdy one if treatment is to be sustained. Fourth, since treatment frequently is not completely effective, many patients have a chronic course. The relationship established with a clinician may be a long one and must be capable of sustaining both parties over years.

The family may provide information on the extent to which symptoms interfere with the patient's life, but the family also may unwittingly perpetuate them. Situationally, genetically, and psychologically OCD can be a familial disorder. The aims of the family evaluation are to characterize the prevailing family dynamics and identify the extent to which the patient's symptoms affect the family. This means learning the significance of the patient's symptoms to the parents, how the parents understand their child, and the family's responses to the patient's behaviors. These aims are most readily accomplished with direct observation and in interaction with the family. A critical question is whether concomitant family treatment may be needed to change patterns of communication, alter affiliations, and clarify sources of conflict. When parental psychopathology aggravates the patient's condition parental treatment may be necessary.

Meeting with parents alone provides time to both educate them and learn sensitive information from them. Information about the parents and their marriage, parental disappointment, concern, and frustration about their child or each other, and potentially confidential information about family history or about their own symptoms should be obtained without the patient. A second major aim of the meeting with parents alone is to teach and reassure them about their child's illness. They may fear that their child is psychotic or untreatable, feel guilty that they have caused their child's condition, or fear that the clinician is going to blame them for their child's difficulties or compete with them for their child's affection. Meetings are opportunities to reassure and solidify a collaborative relationship with parents.

Creating an arena where symptoms and stresses can be discussed and monitored may not be conducive to achieving a thorough overview of all the domains of strength and difficulty. Standardized instruments are more effective for general assessment and screening. Standardized instruments may not convey the quality of difficulties or the impact of symptoms on the patient and others, but they do review a number of behaviors or domains. They also permit the clinician to assess severity in comparison with clinical populations. Two instruments have been used with children and may assist a general clinician in this way: the Leyton Obsessional Inventory (LOI) (Berg et al., 1986; Cooper, 1970) and the Children's Yale-Brown Obsessive Compulsive Scale (Y-BOCS) (Goodman et al., 1989). Further investigation of the reliability, age range, and pragmatics of the Y-BOCS will likely be needed before it reaches general acceptance for children.

Treatment

A variety of treatments have been applied to children with OCD, although only behavioral approaches and medications have been systematically studied. Adjunctive family treatment and individual psychotherapy are usually necessary. There is a role for inpatient hospitalization under some circumstances.

BEHAVIORAL THERAPY

Behavioral treatments have been systematically investigated for adults (Foa et al., 1985; Marks et al., 1980) and children (March et al., 1994) with OCD. There are many reports of single case studies without control groups (Wolff & Wolff, 1991). Behavioral techniques such as self-observation, extinction, operant conditioning, and modeling have been used with adolescents (Wolff and Wolff, 1991). Interpreting these studies means considering the many design flaws also embedded in the early pharmacological research (Towbin et al., 1987). The combination of flooding and response prevention appeared to produce favorable results with adults and adolescents who suffer from compulsions (Steketee, et al., 1982). This method uses direct and imaginary exposure to the feared object or event followed by thwarting any opportunity to engage in symptom reactions. A patient with contamination fears about garbage would thrust his or her hand into a filled garbage can and be restricted from washing for a period of hours. Reported rates of improvement are near 90% in achieving moderate to complete improvement (Foa et al., 1985) and correlate with neuroanatomical changes (Baxter et al., 1992). A modification of this technique, which may be less threatening to children and adolescents, is *graduated* exposure with response prevention (Wolff and Wolff, 1991; March et al., 1994). March and co-workers (1994) employed a cognitive-behavioral method plus exposure and response prevention to treat 15 children of whom 9 (60%) achieved at least a 50% reduction in symptoms that was sustained for 18 months. Despite many design shortcomings, there is suggestive evidence that behavioral interventions can be useful in the treatment of OCD. The best results with these techniques are achieved by those who are trained and experienced in applying them.

PHARMACOLOGICAL TREATMENT

Much of the early systematic investigation of medication was plagued by problems in diagnosis and measurement, which made it difficult to generalize and interpret the findings (Towbin et al., 1987). Today, a variety of agents that share properties inhibiting serotonin reuptake, appear to be useful in the treatment of OCD. The choice of the most effective treatments will depend not only upon the presence of OCD, but also on what other psychopathology is present. The choice of pharmacological agents in OCD may depend on the presence of panic disorder, psychotic or schizotypal features, depression, or Tourette's disorder. It should also be remembered that there are reports of responses to a host of agents in virtually every class of psychotropic medication (Towbin et al., 1987).

In order to determine whether a patient will respond to medication, it is crucial that sufficient doses be given for a sufficient duration. A majority of studies suggest that an adequate trial has been offered when the patient receives the maximum allowable dose or the maximum dose tolerated for 12 weeks. Gradual reductions are strongly recommended when discontinuing these medications.

The most studied medications in the treatment of OCD are potent serotonin reuptake inhibitors (SRIs), which also affect other neurotransmitter systems. Examples of these agents are clomipramine (Flament et al., 1985; Insel et al., 1983), fluoxetine (Fontaine and Chouinard, 1986; Riddle et al., 1990), and fluvoxamine (Price et al., 1987), as well as the newer selective serotonin reuptake inhibitors sertraline (Chouinard et al., 1990) and paroxetine. Currently, none are approved for use in children.

In adolescent patients, clomipramine has been studied most (De-Veaugh-Geiss et al., 1992). Initial studies reported an average 46% symptom reduction in 74% of patients (Flament et al., 1985). These results correlated with the findings from adult trials, where an average 30% reduction occurred (Insel et al., 1983). The improvement occurred in a broad variety of patients in both studies and was independent of symptom type, age of onset, or response to previous medications. Flament and co-workers (1987) found that response correlated with platelet 5-HT concentration and MAO activity; lower 5-HT concentration was associated with greater symptom severity, and high 5-HT concentrations appeared to predict clinical response to clomipramine. The specificity of serotonergic effects of clomipramine in the treatment of OCD symptoms was suggested by two studies. In a double-blind, placebo-controlled investigation of desipramine versus clomipramine (Leonard et al., 1989), desipramine was no more effective than placebo in reducing OCD symptoms in adolescents. Later, a double-blind substitution study (Leonard et al., 1991) suggested substantially higher relapse rates on desipramine compared to clomipramine.

Side effects from clomipramine can be problematic. Anticholinergic side effects, including dizziness, xerostomia, blurred vision, postural hypotension, tachycardia, sedation, and constipation can occur and generate noncompliance. Side effects may be diminished by beginning with very low doses and gradually increasing until symptom reduction is achieved. The maximum recommended dose is 5 mg/kg/day or 250 mg/day. Electrocardiograms and liver function studies at 3-month intervals are advised during dosage adjustment and maintenance for the 1st year of treatment and then every 6 months thereafter.

Compared to clomipramine, fewer side effects are reported with the bicyclic agent fluoxetine (Pigott et al., 1990). Double-blind, placebo-controlled trials with children suggest that it is effective in controlling OCD symptoms (Riddle et al, 1992). Doses beginning with 5 mg/day and increasing gradually to a maximum of 60 mg/day are most commonly used. Of the reported side effects, the most frequent are agitation, insomnia, anorexia, dizziness, xerostomia, and increased anxiety. Fluoxetine also may cause a disturbing akathisia. Concerns about suicidal ideation and aggression have also been raised (King et al., 1991; Riddle et al., 1991).

Fluvoxamine has a single ring structure. Side effects are reputedly less common and include orthostatic hypotension and nausea. Doses beginning at 25 mg/day and increasing gradually up to a maximum of 5 mg/kg/day or 300 mg/day have been employed (Price et al., 1987). In an open-label study, Apter and co-workers (1994) employed doses of 100–300 mgs in 14 adolescents with OCD. Nine of 14 (62%) had a reduction in Y-BOCS scores of 8 or more.

Some patients with OCD without associated diagnoses fail adequate trials of these agents. Although the use of polypharmacy is generally to be avoided, when an adequate trial fails an augmentation strategy may be useful. As with refractory depression, the addition of lithium, triiodothyronine, or L-tryptophan may be useful. Of these, the use of both lithium and L-tryptophan has been reported to be effective (Rasmussen, 1984). Serious toxic reactions have been observed when fluoxetine is augmented with L-tryptophan; this combination is discouraged (Steiner and Fontaine, 1986). Buspirone may also increase serotonergic activity in conjunction with SRIs, but the evidence of success with buspirone augmentation is equivocal (Grady et al., 1993; Markovitz et al., 1990). Preliminary work (McDougle et al., 1994) suggests that patients with Tourette's syndrome, tics, or a family history of tics who are refractory to SRIs alone may benefit from the addition of dopaminergic blocking agents, such as haloperidol or pimozide. In addition, a small minority of SRI-refractory OCD patients who did not have tics or a family history of tics also improved with addition of dopaminergic blocking agents.

PSYCHODYNAMIC PSYCHOTHERAPY

Psychodynamic psychotherapy may be indicated when children have conflicts, associated with their obsessions or compulsions, that interfere with their optimal development. The use of psychodynamic psychotherapy for patients with OCD does not mean that a clinician has determined that the symptoms have a psychodynamic etiology. Psychodynamic treatment has a role in the treatment of reactions or conflicts that accompany OCD. Examples of these concerns might include insecurities related to family dysfunction or divorce, damage to self-esteem, inappropriate expectations, perfectionistic strivings, the regulation of sexual or aggressive impulses, and the impact of a potentially chronic illness during the developmental years. Also, patients may adopt defenses that obstruct their recovery. Psychotherapy geared to diminishing the impact of these impediments can reduce the stress experienced by patients and promote their treatment.

INPATIENT TREATMENT

In the majority of cases, it is not necessary to hospitalize patients in order to evaluate their symptoms thoroughly. However, patients and their families do encounter crises when symptoms spiral completely out of everyone's control, the family's capacity to support the patient is thoroughly depleted, symptoms are dangerous, or a course of adequate treatment fails. Although these circumstances can pressure clinicians to initiate additional interventions quickly, it should be remembered that, usually, crises emerge from chronic strains that accumulate over time. Initiating treatments without a sufficient understanding of these strains may undermine subsequent therapy.

In a crisis, the patient may benefit from hospitalization as an alternative to precipitous changes in outpatient treatment. Hospitalization can reduce the burden on parents to manage and contain uncontrollable symptoms and reduce the impossible demands on the patient to improve instantly. It reduces the risk of intervening improperly. The primary objectives of hospitalization are to provide rapid, objective assessment of the severity of the patient's impairment outside the home, to facilitate simultaneous initiation of psychological, family, and pharmacological treatments, and to diminish symptoms by reducing stresses and anxiety.

OUTCOME AND FOLLOW-UP DATA

Outcome from an episode of OCD ranges from complete, permanent remission to relentless decline. Points along this continuum include complete remission with discrete recurrent episodes, partial remission (chronic low to moderate symptoms), and partial remission punctuated by severe flareups (Goodwin et al., 1969). Studies sampling patients self-referred for treatment cannot point to a generalizable conclusion about outcome. Rasmussen and Tsuang (1986) suggest that, in adults, "continuous" illness with fluctuating severity is most common (84%) and a deteriorating course is next most common (15%). Others (Rachman and Hodgson, 1980) reported 2-year spontaneous remission rates of 65%. Mawson and co-workers (1982) followed their treatment cohort of 40 patients over 2 years and discovered greater than 80% improvement on all measures for the 37 subjects available. But when hospitalized patients are sampled, improvement reaching levels of "greatly improved" or more declines to 30% (Goodwin et al., 1969; Weiner et al., 1976).

There is one prospective study of a nonclinical adolescent cohort. Berg and co-workers (1989) resampled a public high school adolescent cohort selected for OCD and "subclinical" obsessions or compulsions 2 years later. Initially, 12 students had LOI scores >25; only one had sought treatment. Follow-up results suggested that those with "subclinical" obsessions and compulsions did not worsen. Two years following initial contact, the mean LOI interference scores of those diagnosed with OCD diminished by 7.6 points to a level beneath the cutoff for clinically significant impairment. The authors note this could reflect actual improvement or methodological unreliability. Five of 16 (31%) of those initially diagnosed with OCD had OCD 2 years later. The most likely

predictors of an OCD diagnosis after 2 years were previous diagnosis of OCD and presence of another psychiatric diagnosis with OC features. This supports the concept of OCD as a heterogeneous disorder with waxing and waning symptoms. The 69% recovery rate approaches the spontaneous adult remission rate proposed by Rachman and Hodgson (1980) and Goodwin and others (1969).

In a prospective study of an adolescent clinical cohort Swedo and co-workers (1989) evaluated 27 adolescents who participated in clinical trials of clomipramine at the NIMH. Twenty-five seen 2–5 years subsequent to successful clinical trials continued to have depression or anxiety, despite improvement in OCD. Bolton and co-workers (1983) reviewed the outcomes of 15 adolescent in- and outpatients 9–48 months following family and behavioral treatment. A "good" response to treatment occurred in 66%. Leonard and co-workers (1993) reviewed records of 54 adolescents at 3.5 (range 2–7) years after treatment. Although 94% had some symptoms, 57% did not meet criteria for OCD; only 19% were worse than on initial evaluation. Seventy percent remained on medication. Poor response to medication, presence of tics, and parental psychopathology predicted a poorer outcome (Leonard et al., 1992).

FUTURE RESEARCH

Future research in OCD offers exciting possibilities. It affords opportunities to discover answers to basic, far-reaching questions. The chance to learn the prevalence of childhood OCD is anticipated with the completion of an NIMH-sponsored, multi-site study of childhood disorders. Improved semi-structured interviewing methodology may produce the most accurate diagnoses and reliable estimates of impairment yet. A clearer idea of OCD prevalence in childhood may emerge. In addition, new pharmacological probes and imaging techniques will refine our understanding of the neurophysiology of serotonin and dopamine and their role in OCD. Purer agonists and antagonists that act at specific subtype sites may uncover more details of serotonin physiology, relationships between brain structures, and complex frontal, basal ganglia, and thalamic pathways. The lines of inquiry in genetics are already charted. Family study methodology has provided important clues to patterns of transmission. Genetic linkage will be investigated using recombinant DNA techniques in large family pedigrees displaying a high density of illness or in sibling pairs. With such techniques, research may identify specific genetic loci for OCD subgroups. Products of these genes can reveal the molecular biology of OCD and provide clues about the relationship between physiology and psyche. While learning about these genetic sites, risk and protective factors contributing to severity and outcome can be studied and understood.

Clinically there is also cause for optimism. Interest in OCD has produced well-informed clinicians with greater diagnostic and treatment skills. Self-help organizations, such as the OC Foundation (P.O. Box 9573, New Haven, CT 06535), open the possibility of informing the public and relieving the isolation of many persons with OCD. As organizations and clinicians educate the public, persons who fear treatment or have been disappointed in previous efforts may receive treatment. They can benefit from this new knowledge. The use of specific behavioral techniques, dynamically informed family treatments, psychotherapy, and medications can offer improvement for a majority of seriously ill patients now.

References

Achenbach TM, Edelbrock CS: *Manual for the Child Behavior Checklist and Revised Behavior Profile.* Burlington, VT, Thomas M. Achenbach, 1983.

Alexander GE, Crutcher MD, DeLong MR: Basal ganglia-thalamocortical circuits: Parallel substrates for motor, oculomotor, "prefrontal" and "limbic" functions. *Prog Brain Res* 85:119–146, 1990.

Anthony JC, Folstein M, Romanoski AJ, et al: Comparison of the Lay Diagnostic Interview Sched-

ule and a standardized psychiatric diagnosis. *Arch Gen Psychiatry* 45:667–677, 1985.

Apter A, Ratzoni G, King RA, et al: Fluvoxamine open-label treatment of adolescent inpatients with obsessive compulsive disorder or depression. *J Am Acad Child Adolesc Psychiatry* 33(3):342–348, 1994.

Austin LS, Lydiard RB, Ballenger JC, et al: Dopamine blocking activity of clorimipramine in patients with obsessive compulsive disorder. *Biol Psychiatry* 30:225–232, 1991.

Baldessarini RJ, Marsh E: Fluoxetine and side effects. *Arch Gen Psychiatry* 47:191–192, 1990.

Barr LC, Goodman WK, McDougle CJ, et al: Tryptophan depletion in patients with obsessive compulsive disorder who respond to serotonin reuptake inhibitors. *Arch Gen Psychiatry* 51(4):309–317, 1994.

Baxter LR, Phelps ME, Mazziotta JC, et al: Local cerebral glucose metabolic rates in obsessive-compulsive disorder. *Arch Gen Psychiatry* 44:211–219, 1987.

Baxter LR, Schwartz JM, Bergman KS, et al: Caudate Glucose Metabolic Rate Changes with both drug and Behavioral Therapy for Obsessive Compulsive Disorder. *Arch Gen Psychiatry* 49:681–689, 1992.

Baxter LR, Schwartz JM, Mazziotta JC, et al: Cerebral glucose metabolic rates in nondepressed patients with obsessive-compulsive disorder. *Am J Psychiatry* 145:1560–1564, 1988.

Behar D, Rapoport JL, Berg C, et al: Computerized tomography and neuropsychological test measures in adolescents with obsessive compulsive disorder. *Am J Psychiatry* 141:363–369, 1984.

Berg C, Rapoport JL, Flament M: The Leyton Obsessional Inventory-Child Version. *J Am Acad Child Adolesc Psychiatry* 25:84–91, 1986.

Berg CA, Rapoport JL, Whitaker A, et al: Childhood obsessive- compulsive disorder: Two year prospective follow-up of a community sample. *J Am Acad Child Adolesc Psychiatry* 28:528–533, 1989.

Berman L: Obsessive compulsive neurosis in children. *J Nerv Ment Disease* 95:26–39, 1942.

Black A: The natural history of obsessional neurosis. In: Beech HR (ed): *Obsessional States.* London, Methuen, 1974, pp. 19–55.

Black DW, Noyes R, Goldstein RB, et al: A family study of obsessive compulsive disorder. *Arch Gen Psychiatry* 49:362–368, 1992.

Bolton D, Collins S, Steinberg D: The treatment of obsessive compulsive disorder in adolescence: A report of fifteen cases. *Br J Psychiatry* 142:456–464, 1983.

Calabrese G, Colombo C, Bonfanti A, et al: Caudate nucleus abnormalities in obsessive-compulsive disorder: measurement of MRI signal intensity. *Psychiatry Res* 50(2):89–92, 1993.

Carey G, Gottesman II: Twin and family studies of anxiety, phobic and obsessive disorders. In: Klein DF, Rabkin J (eds): *Anxiety: New Research and Changing Concepts.* New York, Raven Press, 1981, pp. 117–136.

Charney DS, Goodman WK, Price LH, et al: Serotonergic function in obsessive-compulsive disorder. *Arch Gen Psychiatry* 45:177–189, 1988.

Chouinard G, Goodman WK, Greist, et al.: Results of a double-blind placebo controlled trial of a new serotonin uptake inhibitor, sertraline, in the treatment of obsessive compulsive disorder. *Psychopharmacol Bull* 26:279–284, 1990.

Cooper J: The Leyton Obsessional Inventory. *Psychol Med* 1:48–64, 1970.

Cox C, Fedio P, Rapoport IL: Neuropsychological testing of obsessive compulsive adolescents. In: Rapoport JL (ed): *Obsessive-Compulsive Disorder in Children and Adolescents.* Washington, DC, American Psychiatric Press, 1989, pp. 73–85.

DeVeaugh-Geiss J, Moroz G, Biederman J, et al: Clomipramine hydrochloride in childhood and adolescent obsessive-compulsive disorder—a multicenter trial. *J Am Acad Child Adolesc Psychiatry* 31(1):45–49, 1992.

Dowson, JH: The phenomenology of severe obsessive-compulsive disorders. *Br J Psychiatry* 131:75–78, 1977.

Drummond LM, Gravestock S: Delayed emergence of obsessive-compulsive disorder following head injury. *Br J Psychiatry* 153:839–842, 1988.

Esquirol JED: *Des Maladies Mentales* (Vol 2). Paris, Baillière, 1838.

Fisman SN, Walsh L: Obsessive compulsive disorder and fear of AIDS contamination in childhood. *J Am Acad Child Adolesc Psychiatry* 33(3)349–353, 1994.

Flament M, Rapoport IL, Berg CZ, et al: Clomipramine treatment of childhood obsessive compulsive disorder: A double blind controlled study. *Arch Gen Psychiatry* 42:977–983, 1985.

Flament MF, Rapoport JL, Murphy DL, et al: Biochemical changes during clomipramine treatment of childhood obsessive-compulsive disorder. *Arch Gen Psychiatry* 44:219–226, 1987.

Flament MF, Whitaker A, Rapoport JL, et al: Obsessive compulsive disorder in adolescence: An epidemiologic study. *J Am Acad Child Adolescent Psychiatry* 27:764–772, 1988.

Flor-Henry P, Yendall LT, Koles ZJ, et al: Neuropsychological and power spectral EEG investigations of the obsessive-compulsive syndrome. *Biol Psychiatry* 14:119–130, 1979.

Foa EB, Steketee GB, Ozarow BI: Behavior therapy with obsessive-compulsives. In: Mavissakalian M, Turner SM, Michelson L (eds): *Obsessive-Compulsive Disorder. Psychological and Pharmacological Treatment.* New York, Plenum, 1985, pp. 49–131.

Fontaine R, Chouinard G: An open clinical trial of fluoxetine in the treatment of obsessive-compulsive disorder. *J Clin Psychopharmacol* 6:98–101, 1986.

Freud, A: Obsessional neurosis: A summary of psychoanalytic views. *Int J Psycho-Anal* 47:116–122, 1966.

Freud S: Introductory lectures on psychoanalysis. In: Strachey J (ed): *The Standard Edition of the Complete Psychological Works of Sigmund Freud* (Vol 15). London, Hogarth Press, 1953a. (Originally published 1917).

Freud S: Notes upon a case of obsessional neurosis. In: Strachey J (ed): *The Standard Edition of the Complete Psychological Works of Sigmund Freud* (Vol 10). London, Hogarth Press, 1953b. (Originally published 1909).

Frye PE, Arnold E: Persistent amphetamine induced compulsive rituals: Response to pyridoxine (B6). *Biol Psychiatry* 16:583–587, 1981.

Garber HJ, Ananth JV, Chin LC, et al: Nuclear magnetic resonance study of obsessive-compulsive disorder. *Am J Psychiatry* 146: 1001–1005, 1989.

Goodman WK, Price LH, Rasmussen SA, et al: The Yale-Brown Obsessive Compulsive Scale. I: Development and reliability. *Arch Gen Psychiatry* 46:1006–1012, 1989.

Goodwin DW, Guze SB, Robins E: Follow-up studies in obsessional neurosis. *Arch Gen Psychiatry* 20:182–197, 1969.

Grady TA, Pigott TA, L'Heureux F, et al: Double blind study of adjuvant buspirone for fluoxetine treated patients with Obsessive Compulsive Disorder. *Am J Psychiatry* 150:819–821, 1993.

Green RC, Pittman RK: Tourette's syndrome and obsessive-compulsive disorder. In: Jenike MA, Baer L, Minichiello WE (eds): *Obsessive-Compulsive Disorders: Theory and Management.* Littleton, MA, PSG Publishing, 1986.

Helzer IE, Robins, LN, McEvoy LT, et al: A comparison of clinical and diagnostic interview schedule diagnoses. *Arch Gen Psychiatry* 42:657–667, 1985.

Hoehn-Saric R, Pearlson GD, Harris GJ, et al: Effects of fluoxetine on regional cerebral blood in obsessive-compulsive patients. *Am J Psychiatry* 148:1243–1245, 1991.

Hollander E, DeCaria C, Nitescu A, et al: Noradrenergic function in obsessive compulsive disorder: Behavioral and neuroendocrine responses to clonidine and comparison to healthy controls. *Psychiatry Res* 37:161–177, 1991.

Hollingsworth C, Tanguay P, Grossman L: Long-term outcome of obsessive-compulsive disorder in childhood. *J Am Acad Child Psychiatry* 19:134–144, 1980.

Hoover CF, Insel TR: Families of origin in obsessive compulsive disorder. *J Nerv Ment Dis* 172:207–215, 1984.

Hunter R, MacAlpine I: *Three Hundred Years of Psychiatry.* London, Oxford University Press, 1963.

Insel TR: Toward a neuroanatomy of Obsessive Compulsive Disorder. *Arch Gen Psychiatry* 49:739–745, 1992.

Insel TR, Akiskal H: Obsessive-compulsive disorder with psychotic features: Phenomenologic analysis. *Am J Psychiatry* 143:1527–1533, 1986.

Insel TR, Donnelly EF, Lalakea ML, et al: Neurological and neuropsychological studies of patients with obsessive-compulsive disorder. *Biol Psychiatry* 18:741–751, 1983.

Insel TR, Gillin JC, Moore A, et al: Sleep in obsessive compulsive disorder. *Arch Gen Psychiatry* 112:1372–1377, 1982.

Insel TR, Kalin NH, Guttmacher LB, et al: Dexamethasone suppression test in obsessive compulsive disorder. *Psychiatry Res* 6:153–160, 1982.

Insel TR, Mueller EA, Alterman, I, et al: Obsessive-compulsive disorder and serotonin: Is there a connection? *Biol Psychiatry* 20:1174–1188, 1985.

Insel TR, Murphy DL, Cohen RM, et al: obsessive-compulsive disorder: A double blind trial of clomipramine and clorgyline. *Arch Gen Psychiatry* 40:605–612, 1983.

Jaspers K, *General Psychopathology.* Chicago, University of Chicago Press, 1963, pp. 133–137.

Judd L. Obsessive compulsive neurosis in childhood. *Arch Gen Psychiatry* 12:136–143, 1965.

Karno M, Golding J, Sorenson SB, et al: The epidemiology of obsessive-compulsive disorder in five US communities. *Arch Gen Psychiatry* 45:1094–1099, 1988.

Kellner CH, Jolley RR, Holgate RC, et al. Brain MRI in obsessive compulsive disorder. *Psychiatry Res* 146:1001–1005, 1991.

King RA, Riddle MA, Chappell PB, et al: Emergence of self-destructive phenomena in children and adolescents during fluoxetine treatment. *J Am Acad Child Adolesc Psychiatry* 30:179–186, 1991.

Kramer H, Sprenger J: *Malleus Maleficarum* (M Summers trans.). London, Pushkin Press, 1928, pp. 175–179.

Laplane D, Levasseur M, Pillon B, et al: Obsessive compulsive and other behavioral changes with bilateral basal ganglia lesions: A neuropsychological, magnetic resonance imaging, and positron tomographic study. *Brain* 112:699–725, 1989.

Leckman JF, Goodman WK, North WG, et al: Elevated levels of CSF oxytocin in obsessive compulsive disorder: Comparison with Tourette's Syndrome and health controls. *Arch Gen Psychiatry* 51:782–792, 1994.

Lelliott PT, Noshirvani HF, Basoglu M, et al: Obsessive compulsive beliefs and treatment outcome. *Psychol Med* 18:697–702, 1988.

Lenane MC, Swedo SE, Leonard H, et al: Psychiatric disorders in first degree relatives of children and adolescents with obsessive-compulsive disorder. *J Am Acad Child Adolesc Psychiatry* 29:407–412, 1990.

Leonard HL, Lenane MC, Swedo SE, et al: Tics and Tourette's Syndrome: A two to seven year follow-up of 54 obsessive compulsive children. *Am J Psychiatry* 149:1244–1251, 1992.

Leonard HL, Swedo SE, Lenane MC, et al.: A double-blind desipramine substitution during long-term clomipramine treatment in children and adolescents with obsessive compulsive disorder. *Arch Gen Psychiatry* 48:922–927, 1991.

Leonard HL, Swedo SE, Lenane MC, et al: A 2–7 year follow-up of 54 obsessive-compulsive children and adolescents. *Arch Gen Psychiatry* 50:429–439, 1993.

Leonard HL, Swedo SE, Rapoport JL, et al.: Treatment of childhood obsessive compulsive disorder with clomipramine and desipramine: A double-blind crossover comparison. *Arch Gen Psychiatry* 46:1088–1092, 1989.

Luxenberg JS, Swedo SE, Flament MF, et al: Neuroanatomical abnormalities in obsessive-compulsive disorder detected with quantitative X-ray computed tomography. *Am J Psychiatry* 145: 1089–1094, 1988.

Machlin SR, Harris GJ, Pearlson GD, et al: Elevated medial-frontal cerebral blood flow in obsessive-compulsive patients: A SPECT study. *Am J Psychiatry* 148:1240–1242, 1991.

March JS, Mulle K, Herbel B: Behavioral psychotherapy for children and adolescents with obsessive compulsive disorder: An open trial of a new protocol driven treatment package. *J Am Acad Child Adolesc Psychiatry* 33(3):333–341, 1994.

Marks I, Stern R, Mawson D, et al: Clomipramine and exposure for obsessive compulsive rituals: I and II. *Br J Psychiatry* 136:1–25, 1980.

Markovitz PG, Stagno SJ, Calabrese JR. Buspirone augmentation of fluoxetine in obsessive-compulsive disorder. *Am J Psychiatry* 147(6):798–800, 1990

Maudsley H: *Pathology of the Mind.* London, Macmillan, 1895.

Mawson D, Marks IM, Ramm L: Clomipramine and exposure for chronic obsessive-compulsive rituals. III: Two year follow-up and further findings. *Br J Psychiatry* 140:11–18, 1982.

McDougle CJ, Goodman WK, Leckman JF, et al: Haloperidol addition in fluvoxamine-refractory obsessive compulsive disorder. *Arch Gen Psychiatry* 51:302–308, 1994.

McKeon I, McGuffin P, Robinson P: Obsessive-compulsive neurosis follow head injury: A report of four cases. *Br J Psychiatry* 144:190–192, 1984.

McKeon P, Murray R: Familial aspects of obsessive-compulsive neurosis. *Br J Psychiatry* 151: 528–534, 1987.

Nordahl TE, Benkelfat CC, Semple WE, et al: Cerebral glucose metabolic rates in obsessive-compulsive disorder. *Neuropsychopharmacology* 2: 23–28, 1989.

Noshirvani HF, Kasvikis Y, Marks IM, et al: Gender divergent aetiological Factors in Obsessive-Compulsive Disorder. *Br J Psychiatry* 158: 260–263, 1991.

Pauls DL, Leckman IF: The inheritance of Gilles de la Tourette syndrome and associated behaviors: Evidence for a genetic hypothesis. *N Engl J Med* 315:993–997, 1986.

Pauls DL, Towbin KE, Leckman JF, et al: Gilles de la Tourette syndrome and obsessive compulsive disorder: Evidence supporting a genetic relationship. *Arch Gen Psychiatry* 43:1180–1183, 1986.

Pigott TA, Pato M, Bernstein SE, et al: Controlled comparisons of clomipramine and fluoxetine in the treatment of obsessive-compulsive disorder: Behavioral an biological results. *Arch Gen Psychiatry* 47:926–932, 1990.

Pittman RK: Pierre Janet on obsessive compulsive disorder. *Arch Gen Psychiatry* 44:226–233, 1987.

Price LH, Goodman WK, Charney DS, et al:

Treatment of severe obsessive-compulsive disorder with fluvoxamine. *Am J Psychiatry* 144:1059–1061, 1987.

Rachman S, Hodgson R: *Obsessions and Compulsions.* Englewood Cliffs, NJ, Prentice-Hall, 1980.

Rapoport JL, Wise SP: Obsessive compulsive disorder: Evidence for a basal ganglia dysfunction. *Psychopharmacol Bull* 24:380–384, 1988.

Rasmussen SA: Lithium and tryptophan augmentation in clomipramine-resistant obsessive-compulsive disorder. *Am J Psychiatry* 141:1283–1285, 1984.

Rasmussen SA, Tsuang MT: Clinical characteristics and family history in DSM-III obsessive-compulsive disorder. *Am J Psychiatry* 143: 317–322, 1986.

Rettew DC, Swedo S, Leonard HL, et al: Obsessions and Compulsions across time in 79 Children and Adolescents with Obsessive Compulsive Disorder. *J Am Acad Child Adolesc Psychiatry* 31: 1050–1056, 1992.

Riddle MA, Hardin MT, King R, et al: Fluoxetine treatment of children and adolescents with Tourette's and obsessive compulsive disorders: Preliminary clinical experience. *J Am Acad Child Adolesc Psychiatry* 29:45–48, 1990.

Riddle MA, King RA, Hardin MT, et al: Behavioral side effects of fluoxetine in children and adolescents. *J Child Adolesc Psychopharmacol* 1:193–198, 1991.

Riddle MA, Scahill L, King R, et al: Obsessive compulsive disorder in children and adolescents: Phenomenology and family history. *J Am Acad Child Adolesc Psychiatry* 29:766–772, 1990.

Riddle MA, Scahill L, King R, et al: Double-blind, crossover trial of fluoxetine and placebo in children and adolescents with obsessive-compulsive disorder. *J Am Acad Child Adolesc Psychiatry* 31: 1062–1069, 1992.

Robins L, Helzer JE, Weissman MM, et al: Lifetime prevalence of specific psychiatric disorders in three sites. *Arch Gen Psychiatry* 41:949–958, 1984.

Rudin E: Ein Beitrag zur Frage der Zwangskrankheit, insobesondere ihrere hereditaren Beziehungen. *Arch Psychiat Nervenk* 191:14–54, 1953.

Sawle GV, Hymas NF, Lees AJ, et al: Obsessional slowness: Functional studies with positron emission tomography. *Brain* 114:2191–2202, 1991.

Steiner W, Fontaine R: Toxic reaction following the combined administration of fluoxetine and L-tryptophan: Five case reports. *Biol Psychiatry* 21: 1067–1071, 1986.

Steketee GS, Foa EB, Grayson JB: Recent advances in the behavioral treatment of obsessive compulsives. *Arch Gen Psychiatry* 39: 1365–1371, 1982.

Swedo SE, Leonard HL, Schapiro MB, et al. Sydenham's Chorea: Physical and psychological symptoms of St. Vitus Dance. *Pediatrics* 91(4):706–713, 1993.

Swedo SE, Pietrini P, Leonard HL, et al. Cerebral Glucose Metabolism in Childhood Onset Obsessive Compulsive Disorder: Revisualization during pharmacotherapy. *Arch Gen Psychiatry* 49:690–695, 1992.

Swedo SE, Rapoport IL, Leonard HL, et al: Obsessive-compulsive disorder in children and adolescents: Clinical phenomenology of 70 consecutive cases. *Arch Gen Psychiatry* 46:335–345, 1989.

Swedo SE, Schapiro MB, Grady CL, et al: Cerebral glucose metabolism in childhood onset obsessive-compulsive disorder. *Arch Gen Psychiatry* 46: 518–527, 1989.

Thoren P, Asberg M, Cronholm B, et al: Clomipramine treatment of obsessive-compulsive disorder. I: A Controlled clinical trial. *Arch Gen Psychiatry* 37:1281–1285, 1980.

Towbin KE: Obsessive-compulsive symptoms in Tourette's syndrome. In: Cohen DJ, Bruun RD, Leckman JF (eds): *Tourette's Syndrome and Tic Disorders.* New York, Wiley-Interscience, 1988, pp. 137–151.

Towbin KE, Leckman JF, Cohen DJ: Drug treatment of obsessive compulsive disorder: A review of findings in the light of the diagnostic and metric limitations. *Psychiatr Dev* 1:25–50, 1987.

Towey J, Bruder G, Hollander E, et al.: Endogenous event-related potentials in obsessive compulsive disorder. *Biol Psychiatry* 28:92–98, 1990.

Wagner KD, Sullivan MA: Fear of AIDS related to obsessive compulsive disorder. *J Am Acad Child Adolesc Psychiatry* 30:740–742, 1991.

Weizman A, Carmi M, Hermesh H, et al: High affinity imipramine binding and serotonin uptake in platelets of eight adolescent and ten adult obsessive compulsive patients. *Am J Psychiatry* 143:335–340, 1986.

Welner A, Reich T, Robins E, et al: Obsessive-compulsive neurosis: record follow-up and family studies. *Compr Psychiatry* 17:527–539, 1976.

Wolff PR, Wolff LS: Assessment and treatment of obsessive-compulsive disorder in children. *Behav Modif* 15(3):372–393, 1991.

Zohar J, Insel TR: Obsessive-compulsive disorder: Psychobiological approaches to diagnosis, treatment and pathophysiology. *Biol Psychiatry* 22: 667–687, 1987.

Zohar J, Insel TR, Berman KF, et al: Anxiety and cerebral blood flow during behavioral challenge. *Arch Gen Psychiatry* 46:505–510, 1989.

Zohar J, Insel TR, Zohar-Kadouch RC, et al: Serotonergic responsibility in obsessive compulsive disorder. *Arch Gen Psychiatry* 45:167–177, 1988.

Zohar A, Ratzoni G, Pauls DL, et al: An Epidemiologic Study of Obsessive Compulsive Disorder and Related Disorders in Israeli Adolescents. *J Am Acad Child Adolesc Psychiatry* 31(6):1057–1061, 1992.

64 SOMATOFORM DISORDERS

Elaine Davidson Nemzer, M.D.

DEFINITION

There are psychological aspects to all medical conditions and biological variables in all psychological disorders. The links between psyche (mind) and soma (body) are complex and incompletely understood. Mind-body interactions are most clearly apparent in the somatoform disorders.

The term *somatoform disorders* is used in DSM-IV (American Psychiatric Association, 1994) to name the group of disorders characterized by physical symptoms that cannot be explained by a neurological or general medical condition. "General medical" is the preferred term in DSM-IV for what were previously called "organic" conditions. Somatic symptoms, the primary manifestation of the somatoform disorders, are therefore presumed to be due to psychological factors.

In somatoform disorders the symptoms are not produced voluntarily. This differs from factitious disorder and malingering, in which the symptoms are intentionally produced. Somatoform disorders also differ from the DSM-IV diagnosis of psychological factors affecting medical condition in that the latter diagnosis requires the presence of a general medical illness.

The category of somatoform disorders includes seven diagnoses: conversion disorder, pain disorder, somatization disorder, hypochondriasis, body dysmorphic disorder, undifferentiated somatoform disorder, and somatoform disorder not otherwise specified. Of these, conversion disorder has been studied the most in children.

1. *Conversion disorder* is defined in DSM-IV as a symptom or deficit in sensory or motor function that suggests a neurological or general medical (organic) disorder, but apparently is due to psychological conflicts or stressors. The symptom is not produced intentionally and cannot be explained by known pathophysiological mechanisms. Most conversion symptoms resemble neurological disorders, such as paralysis, anesthesia, coordination disturbances, blindness, or seizures.

2. *Pain disorder* was called somatoform pain disorder in DSM-III-R, and psychogenic pain disorder in DSM-III. It is characterized by pain with no physical findings to account for the pain or its intensity. DSM-IV defines two types of pain disorder: one in which psychological factors are judged to be predominant, and another that is associated with both psychological factors and a general medical condition. Pain due exclusively to a medical condition is not a psychiatric disorder. In the past, children with unexplainable pain (e.g., recurrent headaches, abdominal pain, chest pain) were diagnosed as having conversion disorder. There is little in the literature to date that differentiates pain disorder from conversion disorder in children. In fact, unexplainable pain is often an associated symptom in children with other conversion symptoms (Kotsopoulos, 1986). Further research may clarify whether psychogenic pain alone signifies a different etiology, course, or prognosis in children.

3. *Somatization disorder* is characterized by a chronic pattern of recurrent and multiple somatic complaints for which no physical cause can be found despite repeated medical evaluations. Complaints are usually presented in a dramatic and exaggerated way and often include complaints of a sexual nature. Symptoms usually begin in adolescence or early adulthood. There is controversy over whether somatization disorder can be diagnosed in preadolescent children. At least one series of case reports supports the validity of prepubertal diagnosis (Livingston and Martin-Connici, 1985).

4. *Hypochondriasis* is defined as a preoccupation with the fear of having a serious illness despite medical reassurance to the contrary. The hypochondriac bases this fear on misinterpretation of normal body sensations such as heartbeats, peristalsis, or minor abnormalities such as mild cough. Barsky (1993) correlates the tendency to amplify bodily sensations to the development of hypochondriasis. Although this disorder can begin at any age, its primary age at onset is young adulthood. It is commonly associated with anxiety, depression, and compulsive or narcissistic traits (Williams, 1985). Hypochondriasis is obviously similar to somatization disorder and may share a common etiology and course.

5. *Body dysmorphic disorder* (dysmorphophobia) is defined as a preoccupation with some imagined defect in appearance in a normal-appearing person. Many adolescents show an increase in body awareness, are acutely self-conscious, and tend to question the normalcy of their body and appearance. Body dysmorphic disorder is, therefore, a difficult diagnosis to make in an adolescent. According to several case reports, this disorder is associated with schizoid, narcissistic, and obsessional personality traits (Braddock, 1982; Thomas, 1984). Phillips et al. (1993) suggest that body dysmorphic disorder is more closely related to mood and obsessive-compulsive disorder than to

the other somatoform disorders. Their series of 30 adults revealed an early age of onset (average of 15 years) and a chronic, waxing and waning course.

6. *Undifferentiated somatoform disorder* is defined as medically unexplainable, chronic symptoms that do not meet the criteria for somatization disorder.

7. *Somatoform disorder not otherwise specified*, is used for less chronic somatoform symptoms that do not meet criteria for a specific somatoform disorder.

This chapter focuses on conversion disorder and somatization disorder.

HISTORICAL NOTE

Semantic imprecision and changes in terminology have hampered the scientific study of somatoform disorders. A brief review of the history of these terms may provide some clarification.

Conversion symptoms were recognized as a clinical entity by the ancient Greeks. Their term *hysteria* referred to unexplained physical symptoms. It was originally thought to be a disorder in women due to abnormal movement of the uterus. Until recently, the term continued to be used for any unexplainable symptom (De Vaul, 1980).

In 1859, Paul Briquet published his extensive observations of patients with multiple chronic, unexplainable physical symptoms (Briquet, 1859). His was the first attempt to describe scientifically the syndrome of "hysteria."

Charcot, Bernheim, and Janet studied and treated hysterical symptoms with hypnosis. Janet proposed the concept of "dissociation," in which ideas can be split off or dissociated from conscious awareness, but can still affect functioning.

Building on these concepts, Freud hypothesized that the affect and painful memories of a traumatic event can be "dissociated" from conscious awareness and then "converted" into a somatic symptom that symbolizes some aspect of the traumatic episode. Dissociation and conversion were considered to be key mechanisms in the etiology of hysterical symptoms. The traumatic event was usually of a sexual nature. The influence of psychoanalytic theory led to the change in terminology from *hysteria* to *conversion hysteria*.

In 1952, DSM-I was published. It modified the term *conversion hysteria* to *conversion reaction*. *Dissociative reaction* was used to refer to the mental manifestations of hysteria: amnesias, fugue states, and multiple personality.

The DSM-II, published in 1968, refurbished the term *hysteria* in the form of "hysterical neurosis, conversion type" and "hysterical neurosis, dissociative type." Because *hysteria* had acquired so many meanings and connotations (including pejorative ones), it had lost much of its usefulness as a diagnostic label. The name *Briquet's syndrome* was adopted to refer to the chronic multisymptom somatoform disorder.

The DSM-III (1978), attempting to clarify the nomenclature, retained *hysterical neurosis* only parenthetically and put the preferred terms *conversion disorder* and *dissociative disorder* in separate categories. Similarly, *Briquet's syndrome* became *somatization disorder*, and *hysterical personality* became *histrionic personality*.

Some feel that dissociative and conversion disorders should again be categorized together (as in DSM-II) because both often occur in the same individuals and are considered to be linked by the same underlying psychological mechanism, namely, dissociation (Nemiah, 1985).

DSM-IV maintains the terms conversion disorder and somatization disorder, but makes significant changes in diagnostic criteria for these disorders. DSM-IV simplifies the criteria for somatization disorder to make it easier to use in clinical settings. However, the DSM-IV criteria for conversion disorder reflect conceptual differences as compared to its predecessors.

DSM-III and DSM-III-R broadened the category of conversion disorder to include autonomic symptoms, such as vomiting, and endocrine dysfunction, such as pseudocyesis (false pregnancy). DSM-IV returns to a narrower view of conversion disorder, restricting it to neurological symptoms involving the special sensory or voluntary nervous system. Thus, autonomic symptoms are excluded from the conversion disorder category and fall under the headings of "undifferentiated somatoform disorder" or "somatoform disorder not otherwise specified." A diagnostic category of "autonomic arousal disorder" was proposed, but current research data were deemed insufficient to support its inclusion in DSM-IV.

Separating autonomic from sensory-motor symptoms in the diagnosis of conversion disorders may at times seem arbitrary. Especially in children, conversion-like disorders may have a mixture of motor, sensory, and autonomic symptoms (Looff, 1970). Psychological factors are identified by a temporal relationship between an environmental stressor or conflict and the onset or exacerbation of the symptom.

PREVALENCE AND EPIDEMIOLOGY

There are few studies on the incidence of childhood conversion disorders, and the reports are conflicting. This is due to lack of agreement on definitions and diagnostic criteria, as well as differing populations, settings, and referral patterns. The fact that conversion symptoms generally present in a primary care setting, and often resolve without psychiatric evaluation or treatment, adds to the difficulty in determining true incidence. Children with conversion symptoms who are referred for psychiatric evaluation probably represent a more chronic form of the disorder. Given these factors, it is not surprising that estimates of the incidence of conversion disorder vary widely.

Among patients seen in outpatient child psychiatry clinics in developed countries, the incidence of conversion disorder has been reported in the range of 1.3–5% (Goodyer, 1981; Herman and Simonds, 1975; Proctor, 1958). The incidence of conversion disorder reported among pediatric inpatients receiving psychiatric consultation ranged from 4–22% (Herman and Simonds, 1975; Maloney, 1980; Siegel and Barthel, 1986). Cultural factors may contribute to a higher incidence of conversion disorder in less-developed countries. A recent study in India found that 30% of inpatients and 15% of outpatients were diagnosed with conversion disorder, mostly pseudoseizures (Srinath, 1993).

Psychological factors can cause alterations of bodily functions (such as stomachache and vomiting) even in preschoolers (Prugh, 1983). However, there is a general consensus that conversion disorder with sensorimotor symptoms rarely occurs in children younger than 5 years of age (Goodyer, 1981; Volkmar et al., 1984). Conversion disorder is much more common in adolescents than in younger children (Prazar, 1987; Rutter and Hersov, 1985).

Among adolescents and adults with conversion disorder, females usually predominate (Pomeroy and Stewart, 1981; Prazar, 1987; Volkmar et al., 1984). Most studies of prepubertal children have found equal numbers of boys and girls affected (Caplan, 1983; Stevens, 1986). However, some studies show a predominance of girls with conversion disorder, even in the preadolescent age group (Goodyer, 1981; Volkmar et al., 1984).

It is commonly thought that the incidence of conversion disorder is higher in less educated or less sophisticated populations, such as rural residents, immigrants, and lower socioeconomic groups. Prazar (1987) maintains that there is no correlation between conversion symptoms and socioeconomic status, although less sophisticated patients may present with more bizarre and less physiologically explainable symptoms. Proctor (1958) noted a higher incidence among African American children, but this has not been consistently seen (Herman, 1975).

CLINICAL DESCRIPTION

Conversion disorder and somatization disorder are two types of somatoform disorder. Conversion disorder occurs as an episode, usually time-limited, of one or a few symptoms. In contrast, somatization disorder represents a chronic, recurrent, multisymptom syndrome. Both conversion disorder and somatization disorder can occur in the same individual.

Conversion Disorder

The possible manifestations of conversion disorder are innumerable. It can mimic almost any physical disease. Alteration or loss of motor functions can present as weakness, paralysis of limbs (including monoplegia, paraplegia, and hemiplegia), ptosis, gait disturbances, aphonia, tics, or tremors. Astasia-abasia (the inability to stand or to walk) is an especially dramatic conversion symptom. Children with this symptom have wild staggering and jerky movements and appear to be unable to keep their balance. However, they rarely fall or injure themselves.

Loss or alteration of sensory functions is also possible. Common conversion symptoms include unilateral or bilateral blindness or deafness, restricted visual field (tunnel vision), and "stocking-glove" anesthesias and paresthesias. Both sensory and motor impairments conform to the child's idea of the functional unit and not to actual anatomical pathways. Some authors note that when one limb is affected by paralysis or anesthesia, it is usually the left (Ford and Folks, 1985; Mai and Merskey, 1980).

Pain (especially headache or abdominal pain) may occur alone or with other conversion symptoms. If pain presumed to be of psychological origin is the only symptom, it should technically be diagnosed as *pain disorder*. In clinical settings, unsubstantiated pain is often considered a conversion symptom. Unusual syndromes, such as intractable coughing, sneezing, or hiccuping, as well as recurrent vomiting have all been reported. Pseudoseizures (sometimes called hysterical seizures) are common conversion symptoms that can mimic petit mal, grand mal, or psychomotor seizures. Pelvic thrusting or other coitus-like movements during an apparent seizure have been associated with psychogenic origin in a number of reports (Goodwin et al., 1979; Gross, 1979; Looff, 1970).

In many cases there is not a "pure" somatoform symptom, but one that develops secondary to or together with a general medical condition. Often, a mild illness or injury precedes a conversion disorder. An example is a child with a shoulder sprain who later develops the inability to use that arm. In other cases, children with a known medical (organic) disorder develop similar conversion symptoms as well. A classic example is that of a child with a documented seizure disorder who also manifests pseudoseizures.

Although there is initially no demonstrable pathology in conversion disorder, prolonged conversion symptoms, such as paralysis, can cause disuse atrophy of muscles, demineralization of bones, and contractures. Other potential complications include iatrogenically induced problems from multiple diagnostic tests, therapeutic trials with potentially toxic medications, and unnecessary surgery.

Often, the conversion symptom presents acutely, with a rapid onset. At other times, onset can be vague and the progression of severity gradual or fluctuating. Sometimes there is one dramatic symptom (e.g., bilateral lower limb paralysis); in other cases there are multiple or changing symptoms.

Conversion symptoms in children usually occur after a significant psychosocial stressor, often of a sexual nature. Almost invariably, there are family conflicts and communication difficulties (Maloney, 1980). Often, there is an unresolved grief reaction. Many studies have noted the presence of a family model for the illness or disability. If a loved one has died, sometimes a symptom experienced by the deceased may be a model for the conversion symptom. A common example is chest pain suffered by a child whose father has died of a myocardial infarction. Inappropriate lack of concern ("la belle indifférence") sometimes occurs with conversion symptoms, but its presence is variable in children and should not be considered an essential characteristic of the syndrome.

Some studies suggest that conversion symptoms usually develop in a child with preexisting vulnerabilities within a troubled family milieu. These vulnerabilities can include learning disabilities (Silver, 1982);

academic problems; sexual abuse, especially incest (Goodwin et al., 1979; Gross, 1979); and previous physical and psychological problems (Volkmar et al., 1984). Others report that children with conversion disorder tend to be overly compliant, conscientious, and perfectionistic prior to the onset of their illness (Leslie, 1988).

Conversion symptoms have been seen in persons with all personality types, although individuals with histrionic personality traits are thought to be more predisposed to conversion symptoms. The concept of predisposing personality traits is not easily applied to children. Identifying premorbid personality characteristics is especially difficult in children. Furthermore, many of the characteristics considered histrionic (low tolerance for frustration, egocentricity, immaturity, dependency, emotional lability) can be normal qualities at certain developmental stages in children.

Many feel that conversion symptoms never occur as an isolated syndrome but only as part of a variety of psychiatric conditions, ranging from adjustment disorder, separation anxiety, and depression to psychosis and dementia (De Vaul, 1980). From this viewpoint, the primary usefulness of the conversion disorder label is to differentiate the symptom from a general medical (organic) condition.

Somatization Disorder

Somatization disorder is a chronic syndrome characterized by multiple unexplained somatic complaints. It is most commonly diagnosed in women and often associated with histrionic personality disorder, substance abuse, depression, and suicidal behaviors, as well as antisocial and interpersonal difficulties. Somatization disorder usually begins in adolescence. Briquet observed that 20% of the cases he studied began before puberty (Mai and Merskey, 1980). The phenomenon of somatization is recognized to be common in children and adolescents. However, the diagnosis of somatization disorder is rarely made before adulthood, because the diagnostic criteria are extensive and include chronicity of several years.

The criteria for somatization disorder include a history of many physical complaints, resulting in impaired functioning or the seeking of treatment, beginning before age 30 and persisting for several years. The DSM-IV requires a specified number of medically unexplained symptoms in four different categories: pain, gastrointestinal, sexual, and pseudoneurological (conversion). Since the symptom list includes complaints involving menstruation, pregnancy, and sexual intercourse, there is bias against making the diagnosis in children. A modification of the criteria to make it more applicable to children has been suggested (Livingston and Martin-Connici, 1985).

Although the diagnosis of somatization disorder in childhood is controversial, there is some support for the validity of prepubertal diagnosis. Livingston and Martin-Connici (1985) reported on five children aged 10–12 who met DSM-III criteria for somatization disorder. In addition to somatization disorder, these children, seen on a child psychiatry inpatient unit, had other significant behavioral problems: antisocial, histrionic, and seductive behaviors.

Adolescents who somatize (but who may not meet criteria for somatization disorder) have been noted by several observers to have a negative self-image (Garrick et al., 1988), as well as stressful life events (Robinson et al., 1988).

There is a high incidence of somatic concern even in nonclinical populations of adolescents. A longitudinal population-bound study of children and adolescents found that 40% worry about their health often, and 20% worry about it ''all the time'' (Orr, 1986). Females tend to worry more than males. Despite the prevalence of somatic concern and preoccupation with their bodies and appearance, this study suggests that *multiple* chronic complaints are uncommon in children and adolescents. The mean number of chronic complaints peaked in 13-year-olds, then decreased. Multiple somatic complaints were associated with anxiety, lowered self-esteem, family conflicts, health problems, and obesity. Overachieving females seem more prone than males to chronic somatic complaints.

Somatization disorder can cause significant impairment in academic and social functioning. Frequent absences from school affect both academic performance and involvement in extracurricular activities. Commonly, children with somatization disorder have difficulty maintaining peer relationships, do not accomplish age-appropriate developmental tasks, are excessively dependent on parents, and have low self-esteem. They are also subject to multiple unnecessary hospitalizations, diagnostic tests, medication trials, and surgical procedures.

Often, in both conversion disorder and somatization disorder, there are concurrent and associated physical and psychiatric disorders. The psychiatric disorders can include anxiety disorder, attention deficit/hyperactivity, conduct disorder, depression, separation anxiety with school refusal, schizophrenia, or mania. Cognitive disorders due to a general medical condition can also predispose children to conversion disorders and somatic complaints. These are discussed below in the section on differential diagnosis.

ETIOLOGY AND PATHOGENESIS

A number of theories have been proposed to explain the etiology and pathogenesis of somatoform disorders. Seven theoretical perspectives will be discussed: biological factors, psychodynamics, trauma and abuse, learning theory, emotions and communication, family systems theory, and environmental and social influences. These paradigms should not be seen as mutually exclusive. Rather, they are different factors that may interact in a given patient to produce a somatoform disorder.

Biological Factors

There is convincing evidence that genetic factors play a significant role in predisposing an individual to somatoform disorders, especially somatization disorder. Adoption studies have found somatization disorder to be 5–10 times more common in female first-degree relatives of probands with somatization than in the general population (Cloninger, 1986). There are also genetic links to antisocial personality and alcoholism. Cantwell (1972) suggested genetic associations between somatization disorder, antisocial behavior, and attention deficit disorder with hyperactivity.

Somatization disorder may be associated with a number of neuroprocessing dysfunctions. These deficits include low pain thresholds, impaired verbal communication, and a pattern of information processing characterized by distractibility, impulsiveness, and failure to habituate to repetitive stimuli (Cloninger, 1986). These deficits may explain the tendency of these individuals to somatize.

Psychodynamics

Traditionally, psychodynamic theories have been prominent in explaining the etiology of conversion symptoms. In this view, an unconscious intrapsychic conflict, wish, or need is ''converted'' into a somatic symptom. The symptom expresses symbolically some aspect of the conflict and, at the same time, protects the individual from conscious awareness of it. By keeping the wish or need unconscious, the symptom minimizes anxiety and thus provides primary gain. There is also secondary gain as the symptom provides an escape from unwanted consequences or responsibilities.

Engel (1962) describes several determinants in the choice of the symptom: (a) physical manifestation of an unacceptable wish and the defense against it, (b) revival of a ''memory trace'' of a previous physical sensation or state, (c) identification with an important figure who suffered from the symptom, and (d) punishment for an unacceptable wish or impulse directed against a loved one.

Some critics of the psychoanalytic approach hold that the symptom does not necessarily have symbolic meaning, but may be related to more general unconscious conflicts involving dependency needs or performance anxiety.

Trauma and Abuse

Trauma (especially physical and sexual abuse in early childhood) is an etiological factor in post-traumatic stress disorder and multiple personality disorder, and it may also be a significant factor in the somatoform disorders. Briquet (1859) believed that traumatic or adverse life experiences were a factor in most cases of "hysteria." He noted that 30% of 87 children under 12 with hysteria had experienced abuse. Freud (1896), in his early writings, recognized the strong links between "hysterical" or "neurotic" symptoms in his adult patients, and a history of childhood sexual abuse, especially incest. However, his "seduction theory" was unpopular and Freud's writings shifted to an emphasis on fantasy and unconscious conflict as causative factors. Therefore, the prominent role of childhood abuse in the etiology of somatoform and dissociative disorders was not well appreciated. Recent years have seen renewed interest in, and extensive documentation of, a significant association between childhood physical and/or sexual abuse and conversion, somatization and dissociative disorders (Green, 1993; Livingston, 1993; Loewenstein, 1990; Morrison, 1989; Rimsza et al., 1988). Pseudoseizures, in particular, have been shown to be highly correlated to a history of sexual abuse (Bowman, 1993).

Learning Theory

Learning theory can be valuable in explaining the etiology of somatoform disorders. A child with an injury or illness quickly learns the benefits of the sick role and may be reluctant to recover. The disabling symptom is more likely to recur if each episode of pain or disability is reinforced by increased parental solicitude and avoidance of unpleasant responsibilities, such as attending school.

Vicarious learning is also involved in the development of somatoform disorders. The child who sees a sick sibling receiving extra parental attention may well imitate the sibling's symptoms. Having a role model in the family for the illness has been highly correlated with the development of somatoform disorders (Kriechman, 1987; Maloney, 1980).

Emotions and Communication

Physical symptoms have been called a form of body language for people who, for various reasons, have difficulty expressing emotions verbally. Since children, by virtue of their developmental stage, have concrete thinking and limited vocabulary, physical symptoms may well be used to communicate distress. The child's dependent status may also predispose him or her to more covert forms of expression if open revelations—such as disclosures of sexual abuse or incest and expressing anger toward parents—would expose the child to rejection or retaliation from caregivers.

Conscientious, perfectionistic, or high-achieving children who try hard to live up to parents' demanding expectations may not be able to admit to themselves or to their parents that they feel they are under too much pressure. An inability to stand is a good metaphor for feeling overburdened—"I can't stand it!"

Similarly, families in which the expression of emotions is discouraged may inadvertently foster the development of physical symptoms. This is also the case in cultures where psychiatric illnesses, such as depression and anxiety, are stigmatized. An anxious or depressed child may have little choice but to develop a somatic complaint or disabling symptom to express his or her misery.

Family Systems Theory

Minuchin (Minuchin et al., 1975) first proposed the family systems model to explain the development of psychosomatic disorders. In this theoretical framework, the child and his illness are viewed within the context of a family network with reciprocal interactions. Specific patterns of family interaction can initiate or maintain somatization in the symptomatic child. Also, the child's symptoms play a role in maintaining family homeostasis.

Minuchin's ideas were originally developed from his work with the families of children with eating disorders and physical illnesses, such as asthma and diabetes mellitus. Many of his principles are also applicable to families of children with somatoform disorders.

In this model, families of somatizing children typically employ four specific transactional patterns: enmeshment, overprotection, rigidity, and lack of conflict resolution. In addition, the sick child enables the family to avoid conflict. Enmeshment is shown by excessive closeness, lack of privacy, and blurring of interpersonal boundaries. Overprotection is evident when family members worry excessively about each other's health and safety. This overprotection may mean that the child is prevented from engaging in age-appropriate endeavors (such as sports or social activities). Rigidity as a familial trait is manifested by a strong aversion to change and trouble with normal transition points (such as puberty). Rigid families find it very difficult to alter their patterns of interaction to allow for age-appropriate increases in autonomy and responsibility. Excessive aversion to conflict results in much effort being devoted to avoid points of disagreement. Consequently, conflict is rarely resolved.

Environmental and Social Influences

Cultural factors can play a significant role, both in the tendency to somatize and in the choice of symptoms. In cultures that are less sophisticated regarding psychological and emotional needs, somatic symptoms are often the presenting complaints for underlying anxiety and depression. In many rural areas mental health services are not available, but there is access to medical care for physical symptoms.

Authoritarian and religiously fundamental cultures may promote conversion symptoms and somatization by fostering sexual repression and by inhibiting the free expression of thoughts and feelings.

In some cultures it is common for people to believe that hexes, voodoo, or other mystical or magical powers can cause physical problems for those under the spell. Such believers will report physical symptoms if they are convinced a spell has been cast on them. In addition, faith healers, with their emphasis on dramatic cures, may encourage the development of physical symptoms in aspiring volunteers.

LABORATORY STUDIES

Patients with confusing somatic symptoms are often subjected to exhaustive batteries of tests. This is rarely necessary and may be counterproductive. Lengthy evaluations tend to reward the sick role. The diagnosis of conversion disorder or somatization disorder should not be a diagnosis of exclusion; it should be made based on positive findings. There should be clear evidence that normal function is possible and a positive history of psychosocial stress and/or intrapsychic conflict.

Careful and sensitive inquiry should be made to uncover stressors, especially trauma and sexual abuse. The presence of dissociative symptoms (e.g. trances, amnesias, alternate personalities) or post-traumatic symptoms (e.g., hypervigilance, startle reactions, flashbacks) are strong clues that presenting somatic complaints may be due to conversion disorder.

A thorough physical examination, with close attention to mental status as well as a complete psychosocial history, is basic to any diagnosis that attributes somatic symptoms to a psychological cause. There are biological and psychological tests that are helpful in the diagnostic process.

Biological Tests

In a patient with sensory and/or motor impairment, the following signs in a physical exam are highly suggestive of conversion disorder: normal deep tendon reflexes and an absent Babinski reflex, decreased vibratory sense on the affected side despite bone transmission, resistance to movement of the paralyzed extremity, and sharp lines of demarcation of anesthesia that do not conform to known nerve distribution.

A patient who is asleep (or unaware of the observer) may move the "paralyzed" limb. A person with conversion blindness will usually manage to avoid obstacles while walking. Such observations lend support to the diagnosis of conversion disorder.

The Amytal interview has been used extensively in adults and also can be effective in children (Weller et al., 1985). This procedure can be therapeutic as well as diagnostic. The conversion symptoms usually disappear transiently or even permanently after Amytal infusion. This can be helpful in convincing both doctors and parents that the symptoms are indeed a conversion reaction. Careful interpretation is necessary since, rarely, even true neurological impairments can improve partially with Amytal infusion.

Video-electroencephalographic monitoring is used in the diagnosis of conversion seizures (also called pseudoseizures or hysterical seizures). A clinical seizure is simultaneously videotaped and monitored by EEG. If there is no electrical evidence of a seizure, the event is very likely a conversion symptom. Because of this procedure, the diagnosis of pseudoseizures has increased in recent years (F.S. Wright, personal communication, 1989).

Psychological Tests

A wide range of psychological testing can be used in the assessment of children with somatoform disorders, including (a) screening instruments, (b) personality profiles, (c) projective tests, and (d) neuropsychological testing.

Screening instruments include scheduled interviews and rating scales. These identify children with somatic complaints and possible somatoform disorder. Other concurrent and possibly preempting diagnoses, such as depression, separation anxiety, attention deficit disorder, and schizophrenia, can be sought in a systematic way. The Child Behavior Checklist, devised by Achenbach, is a rating scale with both parent and teacher versions, as well as different formats for various age groups. It has a somatic concern scale. It is best used as a screening tool and should not be relied on alone to make the diagnosis. The Dissociative Experiences Scale (Bernstein and Putnam, 1985), devised for adults, is a self-report rating scale that may be helpful in encouraging the disclosure of dissociative symptoms. To date, this instrument has limited validity data in an adolescent population (Silberg). The Child Dissociative Checklist (Putnam) may also be of value in screening for dissociative symptoms. The identification of dissociative symptoms in a child or adolescent with suspected conversion disorder would provide strong support for a diagnosis of somatoform disorder.

Comprehensive structured interviews, such as the Diagnostic Interview for Children and Adolescents (DICA) and the Diagnostic Interview Schedule for Children (DISC), are useful. They include questions on somatization. As are rating scales, they should be part of a comprehensive work-up.

The Minnesota Multiphasic Personality Inventory (MMPI) is a much-used personality inventory for adults that has scales for both hysteria and hypochondriasis. The similar Personality Inventory for Children (PIC) has been used in the diagnosis of somatoform disorders in children. However, its value in differentiating general medical (organic) symptoms from conversion symptoms has been disputed (Prichard et al., 1988).

Projective testing includes the Thematic Apperception Test (TAT), the Children's Apperception Test (CAT), the Rorschach, and sentence completion. Projective material can also be obtained from drawings, such as Draw-a-Person and Kinetic Family Drawing. These may help clarify underlying psychological issues, such as dependency needs, repressed anger, and family conflicts. However, since children with emotional problems can also have physical illness, these tests alone cannot confirm a diagnosis; rather, they add to the evidence upon which a case for a somatoform diagnosis can be built.

Neuropsychological testing can be helpful when there is suspicion of cognitive deficits, learning disabilities, and/or a neurological syndrome. Learning disabilities may be a source of academic underachievement and psychological stress due to lowered self-esteem and parental conflict. Unrecognized learning disabilities were major etiological factors in at least two cases of conversion disorder (Silver, 1982).

DIFFERENTIAL DIAGNOSIS

Making the diagnosis of a conversion disorder or somatization disorder is often a challenge for even the most experienced clinician. All general medical causes for the symptom need to be considered as well as other psychiatric disorders that can present with physical symptoms, such as depression and anxiety.

Accurate diagnosis is made even more difficult by the fact that general medical, somatoform, and other psychiatric disorders can occur concurrently in the same patient. For example, a child with a mild ankle sprain can develop a conversion symptom of hemiparesis and have an underlying depression or separation anxiety with school refusal.

"True" Physical Illness

Some general medical conditions present with confusing and fluctuating signs and symptoms that can initially appear to be psychosomatic. Examples of these disorders include temporal lobe epilepsy, hemiplegic migraine, and multiple sclerosis. Factors weighing in favor of a nonpsychiatric medical diagnosis include positive findings on physical examination and laboratory studies, chronicity, and appropriate concern regarding the disability.

Conversely, factors favoring a psychological basis include recent psychosocial stressors, considerable secondary gain, previous conversion or dissociative symptoms, and family interaction that encourages somatization. Of course, true physical illness, especially in a child, also causes familial stress, engenders overprotection, and results in secondary gain. All these factors need to be carefully evaluated.

Affective Disorder

Affective disorder, especially depression, often presents with somatic symptoms (McCauley et al., 1991). These symptoms will be accompanied by dysphoria, disturbances in appetite and sleep, suicidal thoughts, and low self-esteem if major depression is the underlying cause.

Mania can also be associated with dramatic physical symptoms. The pressured speech; elevated, irritable, or expansive mood; and sleep and energy changes that are part of the syndrome of mania usually make the diagnosis obvious.

Anxiety Disorder

Children with anxiety disorders commonly have physical complaints. Headaches, stomachaches, and even nausea and vomiting are often triggered by separation fears in children with separation anxiety disorder. These symptoms may also be precipitated by fears of people in children with social phobias. Similar symptoms are common in overanxious children with performance anxieties. A temporal relationship between the symptoms and the anxiety-provoking circumstances usually clarifies the diagnosis.

Psychosis and Cognitive (Organic Brain) Disorder

Psychosis, especially psychotic depression, can present with physical symptoms or somatic delusions. Psychosis can be differentiated from somatoform disorder by evidence of thought disorder, social withdrawal, and impaired functioning.

Delirium and dementia of any etiology (e.g., toxic, metabolic, infectious) can also present with somatic symptoms and needs to be considered in the differential diagnosis. Impairment in cognitive functioning will be evident on mental status examination if such a disorder is present.

Malingering

Malingering is the intentional production of symptoms or signs of illness or disability in order to obtain a clearly recognizable goal. The goal can be to avoid school or military service or to acquire drugs or money. Malingering is not considered a mental disorder. In adults, malingering may be associated with antisocial personality.

In children, malingering may be difficult to distinguish from conversion disorder and somatization disorder, since the latter also enable a child to avoid school and other unwanted activities. School avoidance can be associated with a number of problems, including conduct problems, depression, separation anxiety, and overanxious or social phobic disorders. It is therefore unwise to diagnose a child as a "malingerer." Many cases of conversion disorder or somatization disorder may have both volitional and nonvolitional aspects. Academic stress, peer problems, family dysfunction, sexual abuse, and individual psychopathology may be involved. Because of the complexity of factors involved in somatoform disorders, the diagnosis of malingering should be avoided in dealing with adolescents and children.

Factitious Disorder

Factitious disorder is the intentional production of signs and symptoms of illness in order to maintain a patient role (Cassem, 1987). Examples of factitiously induced symptoms include heating a thermometer to simulate fever, injecting fecal material subcutaneously to produce an abscess, or ingesting toxic substances such as anticoagulants. This disorder has its onset primarily in young adulthood, but adolescent cases have been reported (Reich et al.,1977). It has been associated with borderline personality traits and substance abuse disorders (Livingston, 1992).

Factitious disorder by proxy (Munchausen by proxy) is a syndrome in which a caregiver induces signs of illness in a child. The child's "illness" or "disability" is utilized by the caregiver (often the mother) for her own psychological needs. A high index of suspicion and good detective work usually enable the clinician to differentiate the factitious disorders from both true physical disease and other somatoform disorders (see Chapter 101).

TREATMENT

Since the presenting symptoms in somatoform disorders are physical, the primary care physician is usually consulted first. Diagnosis and treatment begin at that level and may lead to psychiatric referral.

Primary Care

Extremely important to a successful outcome of somatoform disorders is the manner in which the initial work-up, diagnosis, preliminary treatment, and, if necessary, psychiatric referral are handled. The pediatrician or family practitioner will ideally take a complete medical and psychosocial history, especially noting any recent stressors. A thorough physical and mental status examination should also be performed. It is highly advisable to examine the child both with and without parents present. Physical findings may change and important information may more likely be divulged if the child's privacy and confidentiality are respected.

The physician should explain to both the child and parent that a comprehensive evaluation of the symptom will include exploring both physical and psychological factors. A discussion such as this assures the family that psychological factors are legitimate areas of concern. It also facilitates the disclosure of relevant history and decreases the stigma attached to psychogenic etiology. A balanced approach is also wise because often both psychological and biological factors are involved, and it is the relative contributions of each that need to be sorted out.

When evidence has been obtained that strongly suggests that the symptom or syndrome has significant psychological aspects, this should be presented to the patient and family in a supportive and nonjudgmental way. The physician can point out associations between the onset of the symptom and recent environmental stressors, such as moving to a new city, academic difficulties, parents' marital problems, or the death of a relative.

Once a somatoform diagnosis has been made, further diagnostic evaluation should be discouraged, despite pressure from parents to continue testing. Proceeding with a series of ever more sophisticated tests and consultations with specialists will entrench the patient role and reinforce the belief in an general medical etiology.

Merely making the diagnosis and linking it to psychosocial stressors can often be therapeutic. Parents may gain a better understanding of their child's level of distress and initiate environmental changes. This can include relatively simple interventions, such as change in class placement or increased parental attention.

Reassurance and suggestion from the physician that the symptom will improve are often helpful, as is the skillful use of placebos. Hypnosis or Amytal infusion can also be dramatically effective in alleviating conversion symptoms.

Physical therapy and prescribed exercises are often used to treat conversion disorders when motor symptoms are involved. This is often well accepted by the patient and encourages the symptomatic child to take an active role in the recovery process. It also provides a face-saving way to give up the symptom.

In cases of somatoform disorder involving a time-limited environmental stressor, where individual and family pathology are not prominent, interventions that focus on symptom removal may be sufficient. However, many cases require a more in-depth approach, and referral for psychiatric treatment is necessary.

Families of children with somatoform disorders are often initially resistant to psychological interpretation and treatment. The referral needs to be made in a way that will be accepted by both parents and child. They should be assured that close communication will be maintained between the primary care physician and the treating psychiatrist. A team approach is best and gives a message to the family that all aspects of their child's health are being addressed. This approach also avoids having the child and family feel that they are being "abandoned" out of frustration.

If somatic symptoms continue, it is often helpful to have scheduled appointments with the primary care physician at regular intervals. This allows opportunities to reassure the patient and family and avoids rewarding the sick role. In addition, regular examinations will identify any changes in physical findings that may call into question the somatoform diagnosis.

Psychiatric Treatment

In some cases, the referral for psychiatric treatment comes from a primary care physician. In other cases, the referral comes from school personnel, court officials, and/or children's welfare agencies because of excessive school absence that is often associated with somatoform disorders. Close liaison with these professionals is a valuable part of the therapeutic process. This is especially important when motivation for psychiatric treatment is low.

The treatment of somatoform disorders can encompass the full range of psychotherapeutic approaches. Modalities to be used include individual psychotherapy, family therapy, group therapy, and parent guidance.

Individual psychotherapy can utilize a number of theoretical frameworks. Psychodynamic principles (especially useful with conversion symptoms) can help a child gain insight into unconscious conflicts and understand how psychological factors have influenced the maintenance of the symptoms. Cognitive and behavioral approaches can also be valuable. It is crucial to identify and eliminate sources of secondary gain in order to avoid reinforcing the symptom. Behavior modification techniques, such as earning points for going to school despite feeling sick, provide incentives for recovery and reward the patient's mastery over the symptoms.

Psychosomatic children are often hypersensitive to physical sensations and misinterpret them. Educating them about physiological mechanisms can help them to sort out normal sensations and anxiety from symptoms of true illness. Relaxation training, biofeedback, and hypnotherapy can be useful modalities in teaching children to deal with their anxiety-related symptoms.

Many children with somatoform disorder are shy and unassertive and have difficulty expressing feelings. Additional goals of individual therapy include improving self-esteem, promoting assertiveness, and teaching nonsomatic ways to express distress. Family therapy and parent guidance are essential in the treatment of conversion disorder and somatization disorder. Parents and children need to be made aware of the patterns of family interaction that have fostered somatization. Goals of family therapy include development of healthier modes of interaction and improved communication. Any problems within the marital relationship need to be addressed as well.

Group therapy can be very helpful. These children often have poor peer relationships. Within the context of group therapy, somatizing children can find support to learn better coping strategies, decreased dependency on parents, and improved social skills.

It is important to recognize and treat underlying or coexisting psychiatric disorder, such as psychosis, affective disorder, anxiety, or attention deficit disorder. These disorders may require appropriate pharmacological interventions. Body dysmorphic disorder has been found to respond to serotonin re-uptake inhibitors such as clomipramine and fluoxetine (Phillips, 1993). If learning disabilities and school placement problems are a factor, educational interventions (e.g. special classes, tutoring) may be required.

If outpatient treatment is ineffective, psychiatric hospitalization may be necessary. Removal of the child from a pathological home environment to a group or foster home is necessary in some cases, especially if ongoing physical or sexual abuse is suspected.

OUTCOME

Transient conversion symptoms of the type seen by general practitioners and pediatricians generally have a good prognosis. Many symptoms remit spontaneously with minimal intervention after a few days or weeks (Prugh, 1983). Other children with conversion disorder who require inpatient treatment and/or psychiatric consultation have a less benign prognosis.

Some children (predominantly girls) with conversion disorder go on to develop somatization disorder. Others develop other psychiatric disorders, especially anxiety disorders and personality disorders. In one series of 20 children with conversion disorder, 40 % continued to have physical or psychiatric symptoms 1-3 years after initial assessment (Kotsopoulos and Snow 1986). In a long-term follow-up study of hospitalized children with somatoform disorders, more than two-thirds continued to have significant disability as adults (Robins and O'Neil, 1953).

The need for thorough evaluation is emphasized in several follow-up studies in which a significant percentage of the children, originally diagnosed with hysteria or conversion disorder, were later found to have a general medical (organic) condition that completely or partially explained their symptoms (Caplan, 1983; Robins and O'Neil, 1953; Woodbury et al., 1992). While some of these cases were misdiagnosed as conversion disorders, several authors (Rivinius et al., 1975) have hypothesized that early subclinical impairments in disorders such as multiple sclerosis or nervous system tumors may trigger a predisposed individual to develop a conversion disorder (Caplan and Nadelson, 1980).

Somatization disorder in children and adolescents usually has a fluctuating course and often develops into a chronic adult form that can be disabling. These children are vulnerable to unnecessary surgery and procedures and academic difficulties due to poor school attendance.

Group Conversion Disorder

Group conversion disorder, often termed *mass hysteria*, is an uncommon but dramatic phenomenon. It is of special interest to child psychia-

trists because it occurs most often among school-age children and adolescent girls.

The term refers to the occurrence of physical symptoms with no known general medical cause in a group of people in close proximity. The somatic symptoms appear to be contagious. Common symptoms include nausea, abdominal pain, headache, itching, dizziness, dyspnea, and fainting. These episodes usually occur in settings such as schools, factories, sports events, or rock concerts.

Historical reports of group conversion disorder date back to the early Middle Ages. "Tarantism," or outbreaks of dancing mania, in 13th-century Europe is now thought to represent a group conversion disorder. The dancers shared the belief that the nocturnal bite of a spider caused them to dance. Similar events occur in other human cultures. Hexes, spirits, witchcraft, insect bites, food poisoning, nerve gas, insecticides, and viruses have been alleged causal agents in conversion disorder epidemics.

Characteristics of the phenomenon of group conversion disorder were well described by Elkins (Elkins et al., 1988). Adolescent girls are especially vulnerable to this disorder. There are often preexisting physical and/or psychological stressors. Physical stressors can include heat, exertion, and fatigue. Psychological stressors can include low morale, political tension, and recent loss or separation. The apparent transmission is by visual and/or auditory contact. It is characterized by rapid spread and usually rapid remission. Relapses can occur if the patients are returned to the original setting and circumstances. Often the index case has high status within the group (Rutter and Hersov, 1985). There is usually a high degree of group cohesiveness among affected members. "Outsiders" are rarely affected.

The following responses are recommended:

1. Promptly recognize the phenomenon.
2. Avoid extensive searches for environmental agents, which reinforces the behavior and prolongs the outbreak.
3. Defuse the group's anxiety by authoritatively explaining the real causal factors (such as stress) and negating the alleged causes.
4. Isolate symptomatic individuals from one another and from the rest of the group.
5. Eliminate secondary gain.
6. Elicit cooperation from sources that may inadvertently encourage the maintenance of symptoms (such as news reporters).

These interventions usually lead to prompt recovery of all those affected. A child psychiatrist who is knowledgeable about group conversion disorder can serve as a valuable consultant in effectively treating this phenomenon.

RESEARCH DIRECTIONS

Many of the published works on childhood somatoform disorders are derived from small-series case reports and retrospective chart reviews. Few systematic empirical studies have been done. Many questions remain to be answered. Among them are the following:

1. What is the real incidence of conversion disorder?
2. Should a duration criterion be added to distinguish transient conversion symptoms (lasting hours or days) from more chronic conversion disorders?
3. What factors contribute to good outcome?
4. What interventions are most effective in the treatment of somatoform disorders?
5. Can somatization disorder be diagnosed accurately in children? Can early intervention prevent more serious adult psychopathology?
6. What is the relationship, if any, between personality variables and somatoform disorder?
7. How often is physical or sexual abuse a factor in conversion and somatization disorder?

CASE ILLUSTRATION

A.L., a 9-year-old girl, was brought to an emergency room following an episode of unresponsiveness and paralysis. A good student, with no history of behavioral problems, A.L. lived with her maternal grandmother and two older sisters in a public housing project.

Following a mild reprimand from a teacher over an argument with a peer, A.L. returned home from school complaining of dizziness and stomach pain. After falling off a sofa, she was found limp and unresponsive by her grandmother. After a few minutes, A.L. was able to open her eyes but could not move or speak. She was transported by emergency squad to the hospital. Within 2 hours of arrival she was able to move all of her limbs. The next day she regained the ability to speak but had no memory of the episode. There was no personal or family history of seizure disorder. She was hospitalized for 4 days for diagnostic testing. Physical examination, computed axial tomography (CAT) scan, toxicology screen, and EEG were all normal.

A psychiatric interview revealed that, 2 years before, A.L. had witnessed her mother's fatal stabbing by a female neighbor during an argument. The argument had escalated from a dispute between the other woman's child and A.L. At age 7, A.L. was a key witness in the murder trial, where she testified in the judge's chambers. The case was now up for appeal, and A.L. soon would be expected to testify in court.

A.L. recounted the details of her mother's death in a dramatic and emotionally detached manner. Aside from this inappropriate affect, the mental status exam was entirely normal. A.L. and the grandmother were given an explanation of the psychological origin of the episode of unresponsiveness. They were reassured that no general medical problem was found. Psychiatric treatment was recommended, and they were referred to a local children's guidance center. No appointments were kept, and the family was lost to follow-up.

Comment

A.L. was unable to openly express her fears about having to testify in court and confront her mother's murderer. In addition, the teacher's reprimand may have reactivated guilt feelings that she indirectly caused her mother's death by arguing with the murderer's child. The choice of symptoms—dizziness, abdominal pain, becoming limp and unresponsive—may have been a reenactment of the memory of her mother's injury and death. The inability to speak may have related to her ambivalence about testifying in court.

Without psychotherapy to help this child deal with her unresolved grief and guilt surrounding her mother's death, she is at high risk for a recurrence of conversion symptoms or the development of other psychiatric disorders.

CASE ILLUSTRATION

B.H., a 15-year-old girl, was admitted to a children's hospital neurology service because of severe intractable headaches. A complete work-up, including a CAT scan, spinal tap, magnetic resonance imaging, and EEG, found no general medical problems other than a mild scoliosis. A psychiatric consultation was requested.

Further history revealed that B. H. had frequent school absences due to illness every year since kindergarten. These illnesses included colds and ear infections, mild asthma, nausea and vomiting, as well as headaches and menstrual cramps. She often requested to leave school early because of "not feeling well." B.H. was a capable student, but her grades were barely passing because of her frequent absences. She had only one friend.

Her father was a large, domineering, and authoritarian man; he was disabled due to back problems. Her mother had frequent headaches, was chronically depressed, and looked to her daughter for emotional support. The marital relationship was poor.

In the initial consultation, B.H. appeared depressed and tearful. She complained of sleep and appetite problems of 2 months' duration. She expressed anger at her parents for being strict and overprotective and allowing her very little freedom or privacy. She was intimidated by her father's "violent temper." She felt helpless about the situation: "It's no use. They never listen to me."

The diagnoses of major depression and probable somatization disorder were made, and she was referred for further psychiatric treatment. After 3 weeks on antidepressant medication, B.H.'s mood improved and the headaches became less frequent, although other somatic problems continued. She still did not return to regular school attendance and received home tutoring at her parents' insistence. The parents abruptly withdrew B.H. from treatment after they were confronted about family issues.

B.H. made a suicide attempt several months later, and the family resumed treatment with another psychiatrist who was able to establish a therapeutic relationship with both B.H. and her parents. B.H.'s somatic symptoms decreased, and her school attendance improved.

Comment

This case illustrates a number of points regarding somatization disorder. At 15, B.H. did not meet DSM-IV criteria for somatization disorder. However, it is likely that she would, eventually, if this pattern continued for several years. Somatizing families such as this often have difficulty utilizing psychotherapy and are often resistant to therapeutic interventions. B.H. had difficulty communicating openly with her parents. Both parents had health problems that provided ample models for use of somatic symptoms. By being overly solicitous of her health and safety, they rewarded dependency and discouraged attempts toward normal adolescent strivings for autonomy.

References

American Psychiatric Association: *Diagnostic and Statistical Manual of Mental Disorders* (4th ed). Washington, American Psychiatric Press, 1994.

Barsky AJ, Cleary PD, Sarnie MK, et al: The course of transient hypochondriasis. *Am J Psychiatry* 150:484–488, 1993.

Bernstein E, Putnam FW: Development, reliability and validity of a dissociation scale. *J Nerv Ment Dis* 174:727–735, 1986.

Bowman ES: Etiology and clinical course of pseudoseizures: relationship to trauma, depression and dissociation. *Psychosomatics* 34:333–342, 1993.

Braddock L: Dysmorphophobia in adolescence: A case report. *Br J Psychiatry* 140:199–210, 1982.

Briquet P: *Traité de l'Hystérie*. Paris, J-B Ballioere and Fils, 1859.

Cantwell DP: Psychiatric illness in the families of hyperactive children. *Arch Gen Psychiatry* 27:414–417, 1972.

Caplan HL: Hysterical "conversion" symptoms in childhood. Dissertation, University of London. Cited in: Levine MD, Carey WB, Crocker AC, et al: *Developmental-Behavioral Pediatrics*. Philadelphia, Saunders, 1983.

Caplan LR, Nadelson T: Multiple sclerosis and hysteria: Lessons learned from their association. *JAMA* 243:2418–2421, 1980.

Cassem NH: Functional somatic symptoms and somatoform disorders. In: Hackett TP, Cassem NH (eds): *Massachusetts General Hospital Handbook of General Hospital Psychiatry* (2nd ed). Littleton, MA, PSG Publishing, 1987, pp. 126–153.

Cloninger CR: Somatoform and dissociative disorders. In: Winokur G, Clayton P (eds): *The Medical Basis of Psychiatry*. Philadelphia, Saunders, 1986, pp. 123–151.

De Vaul RA: Hysterical symptoms. In: Hall RCW (ed): *Psychiatric Presentations of Medical Illness*. New York, SP Medical and Scientific Books, 1980, pp. 105–116.

Elkins GR, Gamino LA, Rynearson RR: Mass psychogenic illness, trance states, and suggestion. *Am J Clin Hypn* 30:267–275, 1988.

Engel GL: *Psychological Development in Health and Disease*. Philadelphia, Saunders, 1962.

Freud S: The etiology of hysteria (1896). In: *Complete Psychological Works of Sigmund Freud*. London, Hogarth, 3:191–221, 1962.

Ford CV, Folks DG: Conversion disorders: An overview. *Psychosomatics* 26:371–383, 1985.

Garrick T, Ostrov E, Offer D: Physical symptoms and self-image in a group of normal adolescents. *Psychosomatics* 29:73–80, 1988.

Goodwin I, Simms M, Bergman R: Hysterical seizures: A sequel to incest. *Am J Orthopsychiatry* 49:698–703, 1979.

Goodyer I: Hysterical conversion reactions in

childhood. *J Child Psychol Psychiatry* 22:179–188, 1981.

Green A: Child sexual abuse: immediate and long term effects and intervention. *J Am Acad Child Adolesc Psychiatry* 32:890–902 (1993).

Gross M: Incestuous rape: A cause for hysterical seizures in four adolescent girls. *Am J Orthopsychiatry* 49:704–708, 1979.

Herman RM, Simonds IF: Incidence of conversion symptoms in children evaluated psychiatrically. *Mo Med* 72:597–604, 1975.

Kotsopoulos S, Snow B: Conversion disorders in children: a study of clinical outcome. *Psychiatr J Univ Ottawa* 11:134–139, 1986.

Kriechman A: Siblings with somatoform disorder in childhood and adolescence. *J Am Acad Child Adolesc Psychiatry* 26:226–231, 1987.

Leslie SA: Diagnosis and treatment of hysterical conversion reactions. *Arch Dis Child* 63:506–511, 1988.

Livingston R: Somatization in child, adolescent, and family psychiatry. *Psychiatr Med* 10:13–22, 1992.

Livingston R, Martin-Connici C: Multiple somatic complaints and possible somatization disorder in prepubertal children. *J Am Acad Child Psychiatry* 24:603–607, 1985.

Loewenstein, RJ: Somatoform disorders in victims of incest and child abuse. In: Kluft RP, ed. *Incest Related Syndromes of Adult Psychopathology*. Washington, DC: American Psychiatric Press, 1990, pp. 76–107.

Looff DH: Psychophysiological and conversion reactions in children. *J Am Acad Child Psychiatry* 9: 318–331, 1970.

Mai FM, Merskey H: Briquet's Treatise on Hysteria. *Arch Gen Psychiatry* 37:1401–1405, 1980.

Maloney MI: Diagnosing hysterical conversion reactions in children. *J Pediatr* 97:1016–1020, 1980.

McCauley E, Carlson GA, Calderon R: The role of somatic complaints in the diagnosis of depression in children and adolescents. *J Am Acad Child Adolesc Psychiatry* 30:631–635, 1991.

Minuchin S, Baker L, Rosman BL, et al: A conceptual model of psychosomatic illness in children. *Arch Gen Psychiatry* 32:1031–1038, 1975.

Morrison JR: Childhood sexual histories of women with somatization disorder. *Am J Psychiatry* 146:239–241, 1989.

Nemiah JC: Somatoform disorders. In: Kaplan HI, Sadock BI (eds): *Comprehensive Textbook of Psychiatry* (4th ed). Baltimore, Williams & Wilkins, 1985, pp. 924–942.

Orr D: Adolescence, stress and psychosomatic issues. *J Adolesc Health Care* 7 (suppl):975–1085, 1986.

Phillips KA, McElroy SL, Keck PE Jr, et al: Body dismorphic disorder: 30 cases of imagined ugliness. *Am J Psychiatry* 150:302–308, 1993.

Pomeroy IC, Stewart MA: Conversion symptoms. In: Gabel SM (ed): *Behavioral Problems in Childhood. A Primary Care Approach*. New York, Grune & Stratton, 1981, pp. 341–345.

Prazar G: Conversion reactions in adolescents. *Pediatr Rev* 8:279–286, 1987.

Prichard CT, Ball ID, Culbert I, et al: Using the personality inventory for children to identify children with somatoform disorders: MMPI findings revisited. *J Pediatr Psychol* 3:237–245, 1988.

Proctor JT: Hysteria in childhood. *Am J Orthopsychiatry* 28:394–406, 1958.

Prugh DG: *The Psychosocial Aspects of Pediatrics*. Philadelphia, Lea & Febiger, 1983. pp. 41–44.

Putnam FW, Helmers K, Trickett, PK: Development, reliability and validity of a child dissociative scale. *Child Abuse Negl*, in press.

Reich P, Lazarus IM, Kelly MI, et al: Factitious feculent urine in an adolescent boy. *JAMA* 238: 420–421, 1977.

Rimsza ME, Berg RA, Locke C: Sexual abuse: Somatic and emotional reactions. *Child Abuse Negl* 12:201–208, 1988.

Rivinus TM, Jamison DL, Graham PI: Childhood organic neurological disease presenting as psychiatric disorder. *Arch Dis Child* 50: 115–119. 1975.

Robins E, O'Neil P: Clinical features of hysteria in children. *Nerv Child* 10:246–271, 1953.

Robinson DP, Greene IW, Walker LS: Functional somatic complaints in adolescents: Relationship to negative life events, self-concept, and family characteristics. *J Pediatr* 113:588–593, 1988.

Rutter M, Hersov L: *Child and Adolescent Psychiatry: Modern Approaches* (2nd ed). Oxford, UK, Blackwell Scientific Publications, 1985, pp. 373–375.

Siegel M, Barthel RP: Conversion disorders on a child psychiatry consultation service. *Psychosomatics* 27:201–204, 1986.

Silberg JL, Stipic D, Taghizadeh F: Dissociative disorders in adolescents. In: Noshpitz J (ed): *Handbook of Child and Adolescent Psychiatry*, in press.

Silver LB: Conversion disorder with pseudoseizures in adolescence: A stress reaction to unrecognized and untreated learning disabilities. *J Am Acad Child Psychiatry* 21:508–512, 1982.

Srinath S, Bharat S, Girimaji S, et al: Characteristics of a child inpatient population with hysteria in India. *J Am Acad Child Adolesc Psychiatry* 32:4, 1993.

Stevens H: Is it organic or is it functional, is it hysteria or malingering? *Neuropsychiatry* 9: 241–254, 1986.

Thomas CS: Dysmorphophobia: A question of definition. *Br J Psychiatry* 144:513–516, 1984.

Volkmar FR, Poll J, Lewis M: Conversion reactions in childhood and adolescence. *J Am Acad Child Psychiatry* 23:424–430, 1984.

Weller EB, Weller RA, Fristad MA: Use of sodium amytal interviews in pre-pubertal children: Indications, procedure and clinical utility. *J Am Acad Child Psychiatry* 24:747–749, 1985.

Williams DT: Somatoform disorders. In: Shaffer D, Ehrhardt AA, Greenhill LL (eds): *The Clinical Guide to Child Psychiatry*. New York, Free Press, 1985, pp. 192–207.

Woodbury, MM, De Maso DR, Goldman SJ: An Integrated Medical and Psychiatric Approach to Conversion Symptoms in a four-year-old. *J Am Acad Child Adolesc Psychiatry* 31:1095–1097, 1992.

65 Dissociative Identity Disorder/Multiple Personality Disorder

Dorothy Otnow Lewis, M.D., and Catherine A. Yeager, M.A.

There is a certain historical irony in the fact that, as psychoanalysis waxed, the diagnosis of multiple personality disorder waned; for to observe the phenomenon of multiple personality disorder is to see the unconscious played out before one's very eyes. Multiple personality disorder is unbelievable to those who have never seen it. Perhaps it would be more accurate to say that multiple personality disorder is unbelievable to those who have not recognized it, since many, if not most, clinicians have seen it but have failed to recognize it. The signs, symptoms, and behaviors that together constitute the disorder are characteristics that we have been taught to associate with other syndromes; hence patients manifesting them are usually given other diagnoses. In the case of multiple personality disorder, it would be safe to say that, for the most part, seeing has been disbelieving.

How can a person have two, three, four, even more different personalities or states of conscious being, each relatively independent of the others and often unaware of their existence? Impossible? And yet, the gradually expanding clinical literature, which reports increasing numbers of cases, attests to the improved ability of clinicians to see and also recognize the syndrome, at least in adults.

In 1994, the American Psychiatric Association changed the name of the phenomenon to *dissociative identity disorder*, a more scientific and less metaphysical sounding designation than *multiple personality disorder*. Thus, for all intents and purposes, in the United States, multiple personality disorder (MPD) has disappeared. However, the definition of dissociative identity disorder (DID) is essentially the same as the previous DSM-III-R definition of MPD. As currently described in DSM-IV (1994), DID is manifested by the following:

A. The presence of two or more personality states (each with its own relatively enduring pattern of perceiving, relating to, and thinking about the environment and self).

B. At least two of these identities or personality states recurrently take control of the person's behavior.

C. Inability to recall important personal information that is too extensive to be explained by ordinary forgetfulness.

D. Not due to the direct effects of a substance or a general medical condition. Note: In children, the symptoms are not attributable to imaginary playmates or other fantasy play.

Clinicians may have misgivings about the existence of the disorder, but there is a consensus regarding etiology. DID/MPD is caused, in the overwhelming majority of cases, by early, ongoing, excruciating physical and/or sexual abuse. Until recently, this conclusion rested exclusively on retrospective material from adult patients. Even today, relatively few cases of DID/MPD have been reported in children and adolescents, although the past decade has witnessed a marked increase in the number of recorded cases.

History of Multiple Personality Disorder in Children

The first report of a case of what we would now designate childhood MPD or childhood DID was reported by Despine in 1840 (Ellenberger, 1970). Despine described Estelle, an 11-year-old girl who experienced visions, went into trance-like states, was comforted by the voices of angels, and found herself unable to walk. Through the use of hypnosis, or what then was called animal magnetism, Despine was able to bring to light the existence in Estelle of an alternate personality whose likes and dislikes differed from Estelle's; and this alternate was able to walk. Over time Despine observed in Estelle spontaneous fluctuations from one state of consciousness to the other. By means of hypnosis, and in a relatively brief time period, Despine was able to fuse the two personalities and thereby enable his patient to walk once more.

For almost a century and a half, Estelle remained the only reported case of the diagnosis and treatment of DID/MPD in a child. Then, in 1979, in a course given under the auspices of the American Psychiatric Association, Kluft described the diagnosis and treatment of an 8-year-old boy who suffered from DID/MPD. Since then, more and more clinicians have braved the skepticism, often the scorn, of their peers and have reported the recognition of the phenomenon of DID/MPD in children and adolescents (Bowman et al., 1985; Coons, 1985; Dell and Eisenhower, 1990; Fagan and McMahon, 1984; Hornstein and Putnam, 1992; Hornstein and Tyson, 1991; Kluft, 1984a, 1985, 1986; Lewis, 1991; Malinbaum and Russell, 1987; Riley and Mead, 1988; Vincent and Pickering, 1988; Weiss et al., 1985; Tyson, 1992). In a remarkable paper, published in 1988, Riley and Mead described the phenomenon of DID/MPD in a 3-year-old physically and sexually traumatized child. The child manifested two clearly distinct identities, each amnestic for the behaviors of the other. At the time that the chapter on DID/MPD for the first edition of this text was written, the youngest patient the author had evaluated was 7 years of age. Over the past 3 years, the authors of this chapter for the second edition have had the opportunity to evaluate over 20 children and adolescents with signs and symptoms meeting the criteria for a diagnosis of DID/MPD or dissociative disorder-not otherwise specified. Three of these children were between $3\frac{1}{2}$ and $4\frac{1}{2}$ years of age at the time of their referrals to the Bellevue Dissociative Disorders Clinic. Gradually, a diagnosis that 10 years ago was practically unknown to child psychiatrists has become a recognized entity, having specific, objectively identifiable characteristics.

EPIDEMIOLOGY

Until recently, DID/MPD was thought to be quite rare in adults and almost nonexistent in children. As recently as 1986, based on treatment figures for Orange County, California, Schafer (1986) estimated a prevalence rate of only 1 per 10,000. This very low estimate reflected, no doubt, the disfavor into which the diagnosis in adults had fallen during the first three-quarters of the 20th century. It was a time when the diagnosis of schizophrenia held sway, especially in the United States, an era when patients with other disorders such as bipolar mood disorder and DID/MPD, not to mention other dissociative states, tended to be considered schizophrenic. In the mid 1980s, however, as clinicians became less skeptical about the existence of DID/MPD and more skilled at its identification in adults, the number of cases reported in the literature began to increase. Ross (1989), a pioneer in the epidemiologic study of DID/MPD, used the Dissociative Disorders Interview Schedule (DDIS) to examine a sample of the adult population of Winnipeg, Canada. He reported finding that 11.2% of the individuals interviewed had some type of dissociative disorder, and that approximately 3% gave responses to the DDIS consistent with a diagnosis of DID/MPD. After reviewing his protocols individually, Ross concluded that only 6 individuals, or 1.3% of his sample, had symptoms similar to those of patients suffering from the full fledged disorder (Ross, 1991).

The prevalence of dissociative disorders in clinical populations, in contrast to the general population, is substantially higher. In a study of adult psychiatric inpatients, Ross and colleagues (Ross et al., 1990) found that 20.7% had a dissociative disorder, including 5.4% with signs and symptoms consistent with a diagnosis of DID/MPD. Kronson et al. (1990) reported that, in a sample of 100 substance abusing adults, 39% also met criteria for the diagnosis of a dissociative disorder; of these, he found that 14% had DID/MPD. Among 38 patients diagnosed with an eating disorder, McCallum and colleagues (1992) found that 29% were also severely dissociative, including 10% with DID/MPD.

The true prevalence of dissociative disorders in the general population of both children and adults is still unknown. Two recent studies have looked at the prevalence of dissociative symptomatology in child and adolescent psychiatric populations. Ross (1991) found that 35% of adolescents undergoing evaluations at a psychiatric facility had some type of dissociative disorder, including 17% with DID/MPD. Hornstein and Tyson (1991) reported that 5% of children admitted to a psychiatric inpatient unit over a year's time were diagnosed with a dissociative disorder, including 3% with DID/MPD. In our own study of 24 boys at a residential treatment center who were both emotionally disturbed and severely abused, one-third of the group had a dissociative disorder, including 6 with signs, symptoms, and behaviors consistent with a diagnosis of DID/MPD. Clearly, DID/MPD and other dissociative disorders are much more common among emotionally troubled children than has hitherto been appreciated. Therefore, assessment for the presence of dissociative symptoms should be a routine part of the psychiatric evaluation of all children and adolescents.

Estimates of the ratio of female-to-male DID/MPD cases have ranged from 2:1 to 14:1 (Bliss, 1980; Putnam et al., 1986; Stern, 1984). However, these figures are skewed. Violent behaviors are common manifestations of the disorder. Psychiatrically disturbed, aggressive males are more likely than their female counterparts to be channeled to the criminal justice system, and the nature of their psychopathology is less likely to be recognized. In our own experience, the ratio of males to females has depended on the sample of subjects or patients in question. In our clinic population, females predominate. However, in our male criminal samples, it was not uncommon to diagnose a previously unrecognized dissociative disorder.

Although DID/MPD is most commonly recognized in patients in their late 20s and early 30s (Bliss, 1980; Kluft, 1984b; Putnam et al., 1986), retrospective data suggest that the illness almost invariably begins in early childhood (Kluft, 1984a). However, when a child who experiences dissociative states does come to the attention of the mental health system, the disorder is usually misdiagnosed. Even in adult patients, the average period of time between initial psychiatric assessment and accurate diagnosis has been reported to be approximately 7 years (Coons et al., 1988; Putnam, 1989).

CAUSES

Physical and Sexual Abuse

When children are the victims of early, ongoing, extreme physical, sexual and/or psychological abuse they cannot endure it. If they are to survive, they must escape. Their immaturity, their small size, their limited strength preclude physical escape. However, the young human being is endowed with the innate capacity to escape mentally from that which is physically and emotionally intolerable. It would seem that children's intrinsic abilities to lose themselves in fantasy play to a far greater degree than can adults (Putnam, 1991) has special survival value. When they are repeatedly subjected to intolerable pain, children dissociate; that is, they spontaneously self-hypnotize and in so doing carry themselves to safety. They remove themselves mentally from the experience at hand. To them, the event is either not happening or it is happening to someone else. They are safe in some special sanctuary of the mind. At these times, the child's perceptions, thoughts, emotions and behaviors are somehow cut off, isolated from his or her usual consciousness or awareness and unavailable for normal recall.

Children as a group are far more suggestible or hypnotizable than adolescents or adults (Gardener, 1974; Place, 1984; Williams, 1981). It is as though nature had provided its most vulnerable human creatures with a special survival mechanism. Thus, dissociation can be conceptualized as an automatic, primitive, protective, psychological defense against extraordinary pain. And, at least in the authors' experience, the nature and degree of pain that engenders this psychological defense is almost unthinkable. The dissociative defense is not invoked lightly; it is not squandered, at least at first, on trivial events. In our clinical experience, children who repeatedly resort to dissociation, those who suffer from DID/MPD, are the ones who have been placed on heated burners, tied to hot radiators, bound hand and foot, brutally beaten, hanged in closets by their wrists, repeatedly raped and sodomized. They are children who have been prostituted, forced to star in pornographic films and, occasionally, children whose bodies and souls are tortured in bizarre rituals.

Whether or not all children who are subjected to ongoing torture of a particular intensity will dissociate is a question that remains to be answered. There is evidence that adult individuals vary in their capacities to be hypnotized. Since dissociation seems to be a self-hypnotic phenomenon, investigators have extrapolated from their findings regarding hypnosis and have inferred from them the existence of inborn differences in the susceptibility to dissociation (Frischolz, 1985; Hilgard, 1965; Spiegel and Spiegel, 1978). In a study of twins, Morgan (1973) reported greater similarities in hypnotizability between monozygotic than dizygotic twins. Others (Hilgard, 1970; Tellegen and Atkinson, 1974) have reported differences in people's abilities to become absorbed in imaginative materials. They have reported that an enhanced capacity to become entranced with movies and other kinds of fantasy material is associated with both hypnotizability and dissociation. Braun and Sachs (1985) have spoken of "a natural inborn capacity to dissociate." Braun (1985) has invoked evidence of DID/MPD in several generations of a given family to support the theory of a genetic predisposition to the disorder.

The above findings do not necessarily bespeak a genetic etiology for the differences in dissociative tendencies among people. It is possible that early, intensely painful experiences engender, within the young human organism, a special ability later on to flee into fantasies, trances, and dissociative states. Consistent with this hypothesis was Hilgard's (1970) finding that hypnotizability scores correlated significantly with the severity of the punishments that his subjects recalled. Others have reported that early childhood traumatic experiences are associated with increased tendencies to dissociate as adolescents and adults (Chu and Dill, 1990; Fink and Golinkoff, 1990; Nash et al., 1984; Putnam, 1991; Sanders and Giolas, 1991; Sanders et al., 1989). Thus, susceptibilities to dissociation that, in adults, may seem to be innate, may actually be the sequelae of early severe abuse.

The exact timing, quality, intensity and duration of abuse required to engender DID/MPD is not known and, perhaps, cannot be ascertained scientifically. Certainly, no civilized society would try to examine this question experimentally. Furthermore, the very function of dissociation is to erase painful experiences from consciousness. And, as any clinician who has worked with patients suffering from DID/MPD knows, even the memories of alternate personalities who experienced the pain can be unreliable. Recollections of early events are often confused and dis-

torted, and they are hard to verify with outside sources. Sometimes the abuse began so early in life that the capacity to think in terms of time or to verbalize were not yet developmentally established.

Retrospective reconstructions of the timing of abuse, based on the age at which adult DID/MPD patients recall the first emergence of alternate personalities, place the onset of the disorder prior to age 12 years and usually between the ages of 4–6 years (Bliss, 1986; Putnam, 1986). However, our own work at the Dissociative Disorders Clinic at Bellevue Hospital suggests that, in many cases, abusive treatment began much earlier—as did the dissociative symptomatology to which it gave rise. We have seen children aged $3\frac{1}{2}$–$4\frac{1}{2}$ years with all of the signs and symptoms of DID/MPD well established, and with histories suggesting that their disorders had been active for 2 years prior to clinic referral. We have also examined several adults suffering from DID/MPD with infantile preverbal alternate personalities. In one of these cases, abuse by the mother beginning in the second week of life could be verified. We have even evaluated a $4\frac{1}{2}$-year-old severely abused child who had a 2-year-old alternate personality that could neither control his bowel movements nor walk. Thus, our clinical data suggest that the phenomenon of DID/MPD is often the result of abuse that begins in the very first months and years of life.

A major impediment to the documentation of abuse in children with DID/MPD stems from the fact that, often, the very individuals upon whom we rely to obtain a history are themselves perpetrators or facilitators of the maltreatment. If they are aware of their own abusive treatment or that of other family members, they are unlikely to disclose it. In addition, many perpetrators suffer from severe dissociative symptoms and, consequently, are unaware of their own maltreatment of the child. In a remarkable paper on the parenting capacities of 75 women suffering from MPD, Kluft (1987a) reported that 16% of his sample "were grossly abusive to the extent of injuring, molesting, or placing their children at risk."

For all of these reasons, it is impossible to determine exactly the nature, degree, and timing of the kinds of abusive experiences that bring into being DID/MPD. What can be stated with a reasonable degree of medical certainty is that ongoing, repetitive abuse, usually of a sexual as well as a physical nature, starting sometimes during the first months of life and persisting well into childhood, engenders the disorder.

Because DID/MPD is such an unbelievable phenomenon, and because of its close association with hypnotic states, the question of whether or not it can be induced by therapists in an otherwise healthy person has arisen. According to Braun (1984), the idea that multiple personality could be created by means of hypnosis originated with Janet (1889). Janet ascribed the ability of his patient, Madame B, to recognize her children only while in a trance state to her having been hypnotized during her first delivery. Prince (1890), too, attributed this patient's symptoms of multiple personality to her having been hypnotized frequently.

Through hypnosis, Harriman (1942) was able to induce certain phenomena associated with MPD, such as automatic writing. Similarly, Leavitt (1947) claimed to induce alternate personalities through hypnotism. Kampman (1976) also reported the creation of secondary personalities in highly hypnotizable subjects. Indeed, in the 1970s clinicians (Bowers et al., 1971; Gruenwald, 1977) cautioned against the unintentional creation or reinforcement of alternate personalities.

More recently, clinicians experienced in treating patients with multiple personalities have questioned the ability of therapists to create entire personalities. They contrast the full-blown alternate personalities of true DID/MPD cases—personalities with wide ranges of affects and detailed life histories—with the kinds of stereotypic behavioral changes induced by hypnotic suggestion. However, it is not uncommon for new personalities to appear during therapy, personalities of which the therapist was initially unaware. Usually, in our own experience, these personalities preexisted therapy but chose to remain hidden. Often, a therapist encounters major players in the dissociative system months or even years after the onset of therapy. Furthermore, dissociation is a habit of mind, an automatic response to perceived danger. Hence, new alternate personalities can come into being in the course of therapy, but not necessarily as a result of therapy. After all, throughout the patient's life, different personalities or fragments of personalities have come into being to deal with different conflicts and stressors. That new personalities should be discovered or should come into being during the course of therapy is completely consistent with the rest of the phenomenology of the condition.

Initially, the capacity to enter into a trance or hypnotic state, experience oneself in another world or situation, and block out immediate pain are protective and, therefore, adaptive. The psychophysiologic mechanisms that enable these kinds of transformations to occur are not yet understood. They are the normal responses of a child to overwhelming threat. Over time, however, dissociation seems to become a habitual way of functioning. This initially adaptive mechanism becomes pathological when these kinds of episodes occur frequently, apparently spontaneously, usually in response to what the child experiences subjectively as impending danger or discomfort, and interfere with the child's memory, sense of self, and ability to function normally in the real world. Dissociation occurs along a continuum of severity, ranging from brief amnesias to "the appearance of alter identities that exchange control over the individual's behavior" (Putnam, 1993).

THE CLINICAL PICTURE

It is harder to diagnose DID/MPD in children than in adults. The switches from one personality to another may be brief, even fleeting, and may go unnoticed. The characteristics of alternates are often less fixed and their differences less pronounced, so that when changes from one personality to another occur, they may be attributed simply to mood swings. Symptoms and behaviors characteristic of the disorder also mimic numerous other, more commonly recognized, psychiatric disorders. Many of the signs, symptoms and behaviors of the illness (e.g., communicating with vivid imaginary companions, behaving like an animal, changing voice and demeanor, having peculiar beliefs or convictions) are easily dismissed as child's play, as the products of an overactive imagination. Further complicating the recognition of the disorder is the fact that the history of abuse, practically the *sine qua non* of the illness, is concealed by both children and caretakers. The major explanation for the failure to recognize the disorder, of course, is that most clinicians question its very existence; and, one cannot see what one does not believe exists.

Assuming a willingness to consider the diagnosis, what will the clinician encounter? The most common sign in children suffering from DID/MPD is a tendency to fall into trance-like states and become oblivious to the environment. Over time, in the course of an evaluation, the clinician will most likely observe this phenomenon. Even prior to witnessing the behavior in the office, the clinician will hear complaints from teachers or caretakers that the child seems to blank out and fails to respond to questions or instructions. Teacher reports will state that the child "spaces out" or daydreams and does not pay attention in class. This particular symptom is often so prominent that it leads clinicians to wonder whether the child suffers from a seizure disorder. At the Bellevue Dissociative Disorders Clinic we have evaluated a 10-year-old child whose lapses were so severe, beginning at age 7 years, that at another clinic she was treated with stimulant medication for narcolepsy. Usually, however, lapses or trances are less obviously pathological and are dismissed as manifestations of boredom or simply a refusal to pay attention and concentrate. It is from these lapses or altered states of awareness that the majority of other signs and symptoms associated with DID/MPD derive.

Although these trance-like states may appear to others to be random, they actually often occur in response to some negative stimulus that has a special, idiosyncratic meaning for the child. A teacher raises her voice and momentarily sounds like an abuser; a sentence or word in a workbook awakens a painful memory and the child is off to his or her own world. When this happens in class or at home, the child may simply stare into space and become unresponsive. The child flees psychologically to his or her secret, imaginary sanctuary.

Often, however, a word or a nudge on the playground acts as a sudden reminder of past horrors. At these times, the transition from ordinary consciousness to a dissociated state, the flight to psychological safety, may be marked externally by the flicker of an eye or a shudder or a shake of the head. In a blink, the child has whisked himself or herself away, and an alternate personality or identity has emerged to cope with the potentially threatening situation. It is at such times that ordinarily meek, docile children may curse out or even assault whoever was perceived, for the moment, as the enemy. Later on, the child is ignorant of what transpired while alternates were in command. Often, the attitudes and behaviors of alternates are anathema to the child, who later disavows them. Adults who witness these sudden behavioral changes tend to describe the child at such times as "not himself" or even as "possessed."

Thus, from the initial tendency to fall into trances in order to dissociate from the here and now, springs the other paramount symptom of DID/MPD: amnesia.

The amnesias of children with DID/MPD are often spotty. Sometimes children can recall certain happy events of very early childhood, such as visits to the park with a parent, but are confused about or totally amnestic about abusive experiences. It is also not uncommon for a sexually or physically abused child to recall an abusive event, but misidentify the perpetrator. Even more perplexing is the fact that some children are unaware of their amnesias and will consequently deny any loss of memory. Several of the children evaluated at the Bellevue clinic were so confused about their pasts that they spontaneously complained of being unable to determine what was real and what was a dream. Further compromising the tenuous hold on reality of traumatized children are the nightmares, flashbacks, and episodes of apparent sleepwalking that they suffer.

The trances, lapses, amnesias, and personality switches also wreak havoc with academic performance. When children are "spaced out" or in alternate states they are oblivious to what is being taught. When confronted with homework that they find impossible to do, they accuse teachers of never having taught them the material. Sometimes, one personality does the homework or studies for the test but the child (i.e., the "usual" personality) appears for the test and draws a blank. Scores on intelligence tests and achievement tests are often erratic, causing perfectly intelligent, capable children to be labeled learning disabled or even retarded. On the other hand, sometimes particular alternate personalities are especially talented academically and may produce a piece of work that the teacher finds hard to believe was produced by the child. Homework papers and other assignments vary from messy and indecipherable to neat and flawless. It is the flawless productions that cause teachers to reprimand the child with such statements as, "I know you can do better than this," in response to poorer performances. Yet, in contrast to the folklore that insists that individuals with DID/MPD are exceptionally bright, we have evaluated several children, adolescents, and adults at the Bellevue Dissociative Disorders Clinic who, in addition to suffering from DID/MPD, were of borderline intelligence or severely learning disabled.

Since, as will be discussed, almost all children hear their other personalities speak to them in their heads, some children are able to call upon their academically proficient other selves to coach them when they do homework or take tests. These beings are perceived by the children as helpful imaginary friends. Thus, occasionally, an alternate personality improves performance. But, for the most part, alternates cannot be relied upon, and their erratic, unpredictable appearances and different developmental levels, more often than not, produce disastrous academic consequences. The same lapses and switches that compromise academic performance give rise to severe behavioral problems in school settings. Several children whom we have evaluated have described imaginary friends who entertain them and tell them jokes at times of stress. Reviews of the school records of these children reveal comments such as, "laughs inappropriately in class." Sometimes, alternate personalities, again in the guise of imaginary friends, give unfortunate advice. For example, one 9-year-old girl, who was forever getting into trouble for "having a fresh mouth," would hear her alternate personality whisper, "Say 'dumb' to the teacher."

Sometimes, alternate personalities appear briefly to take objects, break things, or shout insults or curses. They may disappear as quickly as they arrived, leaving the bewildered child to deal with the consequences of their acts. In one instance, a 10-year-old girl suddenly grabbed a book from the hands of a classmate. When a teacher who witnessed the act confronted her, the 10-year-old flatly denied taking the book, although it was still in her hands. Sometimes, children suffering from DID/MPD, like their adult counterparts, will find objects in their rooms or in their pockets and have no idea how they got there. As a result of appropriating the property of others and then totally denying having done so, these dissociative children are labeled thieves and liars. When the evidence against them is strong and the denials are vociferous, such children are often called pathological liars. Reviews of school records reveal somewhat more tactful descriptions of these kinds of behaviors. One of the most frequent comments in the records of these children is, "This child refuses to take responsibility for his or her own behavior."

A major function of alternate personalities is to protect the child. Unfortunately, they are, as Vonnegut would say, "stuck in time." They misperceive relatively mild disagreement or reprimands in the same way as life threatening events of old, and, in response, lash out. In their zeal to help the child, alters can become dangerously aggressive, throwing desks, even seriously injuring other children. It is understandable that puzzled clinicians, called in to consult on these cases, diagnose the child as suffering from one or more of the disruptive disorders. We, like others who have worked with these kinds of children (Hornstein and Putnam, 1992) have found that previous clinicians almost invariably diagnosed attention deficit hyperactivity disorder and/or conduct disorder.

As is evident from the above description, children suffering from DID/MPD are changeable. One moment they may be sweet and agreeable, the next they are having a tantrum or assaulting a playmate. They may start the day being gregarious and end it as withdrawn and depressed, even self-mutilative or suicidal individuals. If their behavioral and academic problems have not already earned them a disruptive disorder diagnosis, then these fluctuations may cause them to receive the diagnosis of a mood disorder. Sometimes they do indeed suffer from such a disorder as well as DID/MPD. More often, however, the apparent mood changes reflect the characteristics of different personalities. Certain personalities function as entertainers or as competent guides through the social world; others keep the memories of pain and weep silently; still others took pain for the child and are contemptuous of the child for his or her weakness. These particular personalities berate the child, and encourage the child to burn or cut his or her arms or to run in front of a car. Thus, together, these different personalities manage to create the appearance of a severe unipolar or bipolar mood disorder.

One of the most common symptoms of children who suffer from DID/MPD is auditory hallucinations. They hear the voices of alternate personalities speak to them and to each other. They also receive instructions from them. Often, they talk aloud to their voices. Caretakers, listening to these conversations from the other side of a closed door, sometimes think that the child is playing with a friend, so different are the voices overheard. Several children and adolescents whom we have evaluated have also experienced vivid, grotesque, visual hallucinations of blood and body parts, apparent flashbacks to overwhelming experiences. Sometimes, children will report a hierarchy of imaginary companions that has the quality of a fixed delusion. As children report their experiences, they often become confused, contradictory, and momentarily inarticulate. They stutter; they pause and look upward, as if seeking help, before resuming speech. Sometimes, they stop altogether and completely lose their train of thought. The combination of command hallucinations,

voices speaking to each other, delusional beliefs, illogical thought patterns, and blocking sometimes leads clinicians to a diagnosis of schizophrenia. We have found, as have others (Kluft, 1987b; Putnam, 1989; Ross et al., 1990) that this cluster of signs and symptoms is far more commonly found in patients with DID/MPD than in schizophrenic patients.

Thus, children with DID/MPD, like their adult counterparts, have a plethora of signs, symptoms, and behaviors suggestive of many different kinds of medical and psychiatric disorders. If their clinic and emergency room or hospital records can be obtained, the clinician will often find that the child has visited numerous doctors and treatment centers and received a multiplicity of diagnostic procedures ranging from barium enemas to MRIs and EEGs. Depending on the personality state of the child at the time of evaluation, he or she may have been treated with stimulant medication, antidepressants, antipsychotics, antiepileptics, antacids, stool softeners, enemas, or all of the above. When none of these interventions has lasting benefit (although at first any one of them may seem to help), such children are dismissed either as having a disruptive disorder or as malingerers.

The Nature of Alternate Personalities in Children and Adolescents

The trances, the amnesias, and all the behaviors that follow from them are like the cloud cover, or better, the dust storm underneath which hide the child's alternate personalities. A principle to keep in mind is that each and every alternate has a function or reason for being. Without him, her, or "it," the child, on some level, feels he or she cannot survive. Therefore, all personalities or aspects are important, and their memories, thoughts, and feelings must be understood and respected.

The alternate personalities of children are remarkably similar to those of adults and they serve very similar functions. Their major functions are to protect the child from experiencing physical and emotional pain, and they do this in a variety of ways. By taking the child's place at the time abuse is occurring, they anesthetize the child. For this reason, the child is often unaware of the source of some scars on his or her body, and ignorant of the very existence of others. Sometimes, alternates function as violent protectors, attacking both real and imagined or misperceived abusers. Alternates who take the pain may also be violent protectors. Unfortunately, with children as with adults, these kinds of alternates tend to be contemptuous of the part of the child's being that could not endure the torture. Such alternates frequently retaliate against the weaker parts, deliberately hurting the child or telling the child to hurt or kill himself or herself. Other protector alternates may be in charge of helping the child run away and escape. Still others protect by keeping the memories that are too painful to be recalled. Among the ranks of the alternates who endured and remember atrocities will be found the most aggressive and dangerous personalities. Therapists are often amazed to discover within this group a personality who turns out to be the aggressor himself or herself. In a feat of mental gymnastics, the child creates within himself or herself the very figure who most severely and repeatedly inflicted punishment. It was the therapist, Lillian Gross, M.D. who, five years ago, first alerted the authors of this chapter to the existence of this almost unbelievable occurrence. Since then, in the cases of 5 adults and 3 children, we have made the acquaintance of 8 "parent" or "close relative" alternates (5 abusive mothers, an abusive father, an abusive male cousin and an abusive uncle); these personalities caused the children or adults to perform, on themselves or others, the very same punitive or sexual acts to which they were subjected.

Closely related to the aggressor personalities are the seductive, sexually precocious entities. They serve several functions. Often, they act as if they enjoy the sexual abuse to which the child has been or is being subjected. Sometimes, they perform explicit sexual acts that the child was forced to perform for the abuser or for the camera of the abuser. We have seen a 4½-year-old child who was used in pornographic films scuffle with a male anatomically correct doll, stamp on its genitals, fall on top of it, twist its arms while holding it between her legs and, in a voice strangely similar to the child's mother's voice, call it a bastard. Shortly thereafter, when the doll was placed out of reach, the child lay back with bent knees and beckoned toward the doll, purring, "I need him!" This sexy alternate explained to the therapist, "I was there and she (meaning the child) was supposed to run." In another case, the male alternate of a 7-year-old girl who was forced to perform oral sexual acts on her sister, explained in a deep voice, "I did things her (the 7-year-old's) sister didn't like." Note how the seductive alternates of both young children refer to the children in the third person (i.e., "*she* was supposed to run," "things *her* sister didn't like").

Within this alliance of protectors, there may also lurk deceiver personalities or identities whose function it is to fool the outsider. These may take on different apparent identities, causing the therapist to believe an agreement is being made with the child when that aspect of the child is, for all intents and purposes, asleep and unable to enter into any reliable contract.

Not all alternates are aggressive or sexually inappropriate. In fact, many demonstrate an extraordinary sweetness. It is as though all of the child's negative feelings and behaviors have been taken by the aggressor personalities, leaving other personalities consisting of pure goodness, gentleness, and compassion. These more benign entities also protect in important ways. In fact, sometimes they are the first to make an appearance, coming at a time when the child feels especially alone and vulnerable, and comforting the child. These benevolent beings keep the child company, amuse the child, and may even encourage the child to do well at school. Within this group of tender beings, the baby or babies can almost always be found. We have treated four children, a 3¾-year-old girl, a 4½-year-old boy and two 9-year-old girls, each of whom had a 1- or 2-year-old alternate. These entities tended to protect by virtue of their very vulnerability. Who would dare harm a tiny baby, sucking its thumb or unable to walk? Several of our adult patients have reported the existence of another sort of baby alternate, one that cries continually or is thought of as dead or near dead. These personalities seem to represent vestiges of the original tortured child.

The phenomenon of the dead or near-dead infant raises the question of exactly who the real person or so-called host-personality really is, and whether or not a host always exists. Therapists tend to think of the host as the child who first walked into the office. We tend to imagine the existence of a solid, core personality from which other personalities diverge. However, in the case of children who were maltreated from infancy and onward throughout the first years of childhood, the core may never have been established and all interactions thereafter may be with shadows or derivatives of the original traumatized being.

Children who suffer from DID/MPD, like their adult counterparts, usually have no idea of the nature of their disorder. They know only that they seem to have imaginary friends who are in their heads or in other parts of their bodies, or who come to them from afar and who both help and torment them. Figure 65.1 is a self-portrait by a 6-year-old boy, showing his alternate personality who, as he described him, "lives in my heart."

Figure 65.2A shows the drawing by an 8-year-old boy of his alternate personality, Joe, who, he explained, lived in a scalloped area of his brain (Fig. 65.2B). This boy drew other compartments in his brain, volunteering the information that others lived there but he didn't know who they were.

Individual experiences and cultural practices influence the nature of alternate personalities. Strong defenders are often identified as the latest superhero or TV character. Angry alternates who urge destructive acts are identified by some children as a devil. Benign personalities sometimes receive names such as Angelica. Many children who dissociate name their inner friends after cousins or schoolmates, making it hard for therapists to know whom the child is describing. Is it a real or an imaginary friend?

One type of alternate personality that, in our experience, has been especially characteristic of young children is the animal alternate. Figure

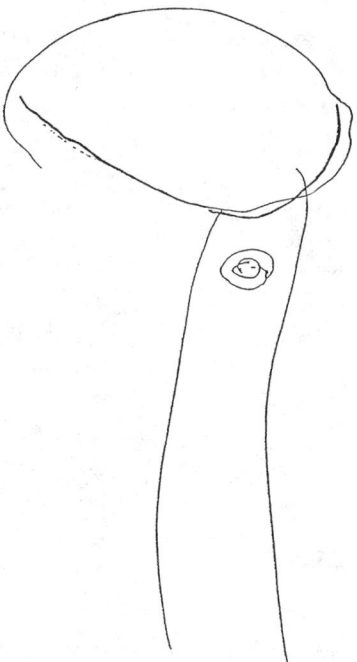

Figure 65.1. Self portrait of a 6-year-old boy with DID/MPD, depicting the place where his alternate personality lives—"in my heart."

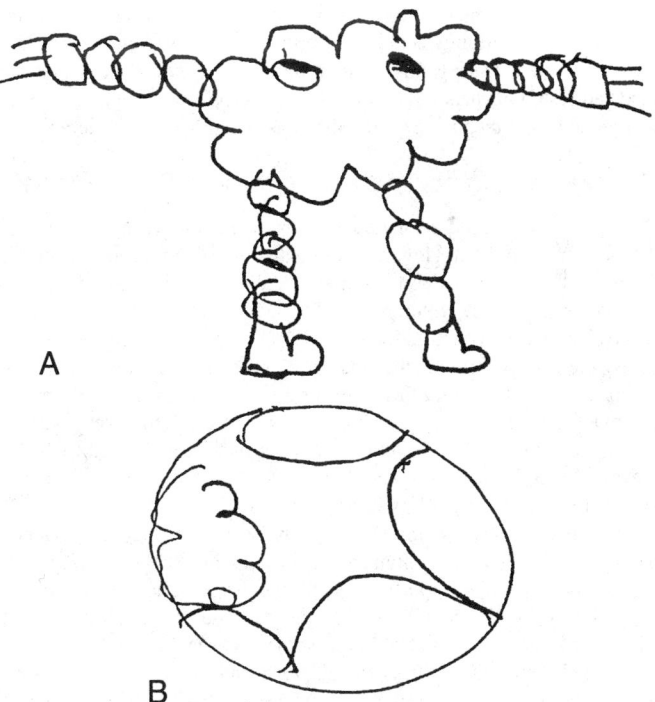

Figure 65.2. A, Picture drawn by an 8-year-old boy with DID/MPD of his alternate personality, "Joe." B, Picture drawn by the same boy, depicting the place in his brain where "Joe" lives.

65.3 was drawn by a 10-year-old child with DID/MPD. Listed are her numerous alternate personalities. Her most powerful alternate personality was a bull, depicted here as occupying half of her body.

In our experience, animal alternates have tended to be protectors. For example, one 4½-year-old severely abused boy, when threatened, became a tiger, growled, and bared his teeth. On one occasion, he actu-

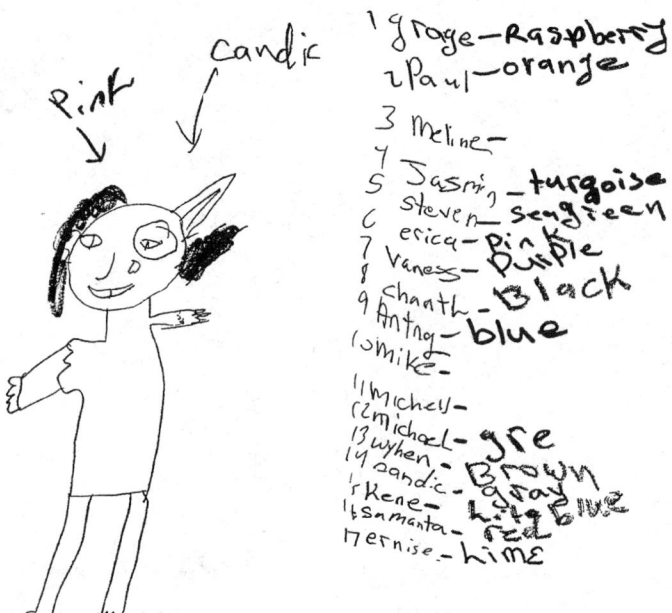

Figure 65.3. Picture, drawn by a 10-year-old girl, depicting a powerful alternate personality, a bull, as taking over half of her body. Also listed are her numerous other alternate personalities.

ally bit his foster mother. Another 8-year-old boy who was referred to the clinic with numerous dissociative symptoms, seemed to have a dog as an imaginary companion. We did not realize that the dog periodically took control of the boy's behavior until we reviewed the tapes of a therapy session. During this session, the boy periodically covered his face and rested his head on a table near a microphone. The microphone had picked up a menacing growl that was inaudible to the therapists.

Imaginary Companions vs. Alternate Personalities

Many normal children have imaginary companions or special toys that seem real to them. How might one distinguish between the normal fantasy life of children and the pathological dissociative experiences of severely traumatized children with DID/MPD? It is not always easy, especially in very young children.

By the time a child reaches the age of 6 or 7 years, most imaginary companions are long gone. Thus, the existence of an imaginary companion much beyond age 7 may be cause for concern. However, even 4- and 5-year-olds seem to have a good sense of what is real and what is make-believe. If they are asked directly whether their friend is "real" or "pretend," they usually will identify it as "pretend."

In a recent study we conducted on the nature of imaginary friends in abused, dissociative children and in normal school children, we found that, although similar proportions of children reported having had imaginary friends, by 10 years of age the normal children had all dispensed with their fictional playmates. Many of the dissociative children, on the other hand, reported that their imaginary friends were still active parts of their lives. The functions of the imaginary friends for the normal children were also of a very different quality. All of their imaginary friends, whether human or animal, were benign, played games with them and offered good advice. The imaginary friends of the dissociators were not always benevolent. Sometimes they frightened them or encouraged them to perform aggressive or self-injurious acts.

Sometimes it is possible to trace retrospectively the evolution of an imaginary friend as it turns into an alternate personality. In one case, a 38-year-old woman, Alice, had but one alternate personality, a vicious male named Frankie. As a child, Alice, an only child, had convinced friends and neighbors that she had a brother. During adolescence, this imaginary brother was experienced as an inner voice. Eventually, Alice's

hallucinated brother took over control and behaved in aggressive ways toward others. Alice was amnestic for long periods of time when Frankie was "out." In fact, prior to the recognition of Alice's dissociative disorder, a diagnosis of complex partial seizures had been made and Alice had been treated with antiepileptic medication. Thus, we know clinically that, in certain severely abused children, imaginary companions may evolve into alternate personalities. Exactly how this phenomenon comes about neurophysiologically remains to be understood.

Many of the indicators of possible DID/MPD in children are also characteristic of normal children (e.g., imaginary companions, spacing out, or day dreaming) and others are seen in a variety of different kinds of diagnoses (e.g., conduct disorder, attention deficit hyperactivity disorder). Several clinical researchers have created lists of its most prevalent signs, symptoms, and behaviors (Fagan and McMahon, 1984; Hornstein and Putnam, 1992; Kluft, 1985; Peterson, 1990; Putnam, 1993). These characteristics include: autohypnotic or trance-like states, amnesias, fluctuations in mood, fluctuations in abilities, disavowed behaviors (e.g., lying or stealing and denying having done so), marked behavioral changes (e.g., from aggressive to overly good), rapid regressions in behavior, evidence of active imaginary companions, auditory hallucinations, flashbacks, apparent sleepwalking, amnesia for abuse, hysterical symptoms, fluctuating physical complaints, and referring to the self in the third person. Refractoriness to various forms of psychotherapy and medication directed at treating other diagnoses is also frequently part of the history. Several investigator-clinicians have reported often finding other family members who suffer from the same type of disorder. We would add to this list: difficulty distinguishing fantasy from reality (e.g., believing certain experiences were dreamed), acting like an animal (e.g., growling or making other animal sounds; moving in animal-like ways), using different names at different times, and having different writing styles. The clinician must keep in mind that any one of the above characteristics is common to other disorders, and there is no fixed number of them that unequivocally indicates the existence of DID/MPD. However, the extraordinary number of diverse signs, symptoms, and behaviors should raise a strong suspicion of DID/MPD in the clinician's mind. Once the suspicion is raised, the clinician should be prepared to conduct the kind of evaluation most likely to bring to light DID/MPD if it exists in the child.

Psychosomatic Symptoms and Phenomena

Children who suffer from DID/MPD tend to complain of the very same kinds of physical symptoms as do their adult counterparts.

Headaches

A history of frequent, sometimes severe headaches is common. At least some of these headaches occur in response to conflicts among alternates regarding primacy. For example, a 9-year-old child with a history of early, ongoing, extreme sexual abuse by a male relative experienced severe headaches when alternates argued over whether or not to visit with the former abuser. When these headaches occurred during therapy sessions, they tended to subside when the therapist indicated that everyone's feelings were important and that alternates should quiet down and take turns expressing themselves.

Seizures and Narcolepsy

Seizure-like symptoms are also commonly part of the picture in children suffering from DID/MPD. The Dissociative Disorders Clinic at Bellevue has evaluated several children and adults with seizure-like symptoms who had undergone extensive neurological evaluations prior to referral to our clinic. In one case, that of a teenage girl, an ostensible seizure in our waiting room, manifested by apparent loss of consciousness and rapid jerking of the head back and forth, subsided in response to the therapist's instruction that "the voices stop arguing." The therapist learned later on in treatment that one alternate personality took pleasure in inflicting these ''seizures'' on another. We have evaluated 3 children with DID/MPD whose symptoms led previous doctors to suspect (and in one case treat) narcolepsy. In all of these cases, the children would suddenly seem to fall asleep for no reason discernible to observers. These apparent ''attacks'' occurred in response to perceived threats in the children's environments. Of note, in at least one case, the episodes occurred only at home or in the company of family members, never at school.

Anesthesias and Scarring

Children and adolescents with DID/MPD often report being anesthetic to certain kinds of physical maltreatment. They are often amnestic for events that resulted in severe scarring. One personality of a school-age girl completely denied physical abuse, whereas another recalled it graphically. This child was observed to ''space out'' and go into a trance when the therapist examined her back and discovered numerous scars that appeared to have resulted from whippings and burns. Children also often have scars from self-inflicted scratches, cuts, or burns. The alternate personalities of children, like those of adults, rarely appreciate that they and the child are one; there is often animosity among different personalities who enjoy inflicting harm on each other.

Paralyses

Conversion symptoms, including apparent paralyses, have also been observed in children with DID/MPD. One 4½-year-old, severely traumatized boy had episodes when he claimed to be unable to walk. During therapy it was learned that the boy had an infant personality who could not yet walk.

Visual, Auditory, and Speech Alterations

The kinds of differences in visual acuity and hearing reported to exist among the alternate personalities of adult patients may well exist in children, but they go unrecognized. At the Bellevue clinic, although we have not tested the visual acuity of different personalities, we have occasionally observed a slight strabismus in one personality not present in the others. The animal alternates of young children seem hyperalert to aspects of their surroundings; they are fleet of foot and quick to lash out at what they perceive to be threats. It is also common in children to have one or more personalities who cannot or will not speak. Sometimes the alternate is reported to be too young to speak. In one case, alternate personalities were mute but had written language and, notably, their penmanship differed markedly from each other's. In another case, a 12-year-old boy had one alternate personality who spoke so rapidly that it was hard to understand him. Yet another boy, an adolescent, had an alternate personality who spoke with an Irish brogue. It is not unusual to meet personalities who use inflections and figures of speech that the child, in his usual state, would not use.

Handedness and Writing

It is common in adult patients for alternate personalities to demonstrate changes in handedness (Putnam et al., 1986). At the Bellevue clinic, we have treated two children, a 7-year-old and a 13-year-old, who spontaneously changed writing hands when a particular alternate came forward. Figure 65.4, A and B, illustrates the right- and left-handed writings of the 13-year-old.

The handwriting of personalities changes not only with handedness, but also according to the developmental stage of the alternate personality. Although usually the writing of alternate personalities is either of the same maturity as the child or younger, we have seen one child whose adult personality had far better penmanship than did the child himself. (See section: Use of Schoolwork and Journals for examples of these phenomena.)

Gastrointestinal and Genitourinary Problems

Boys and girls with DID/MPD often suffer from and have histories of a variety of gastrointestinal and genitourinary complaints. Some of

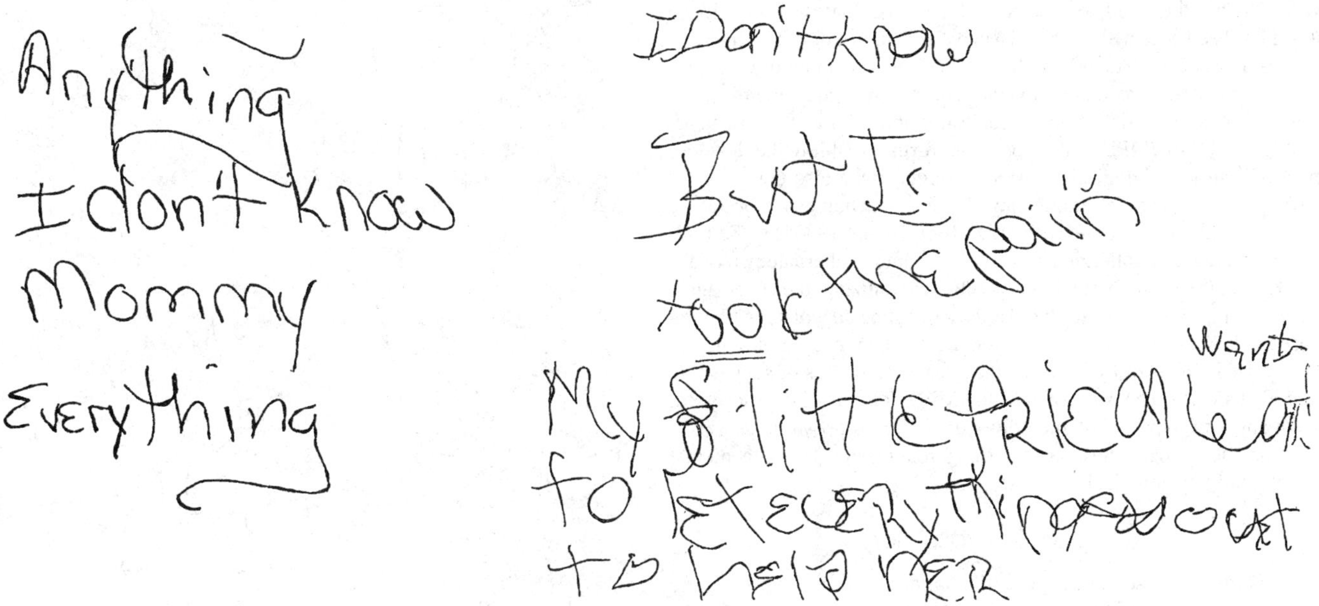

I don't know
But I took the pain.
My little friend wants to let everything out to help her.

Figure 65.4.   A, Writing sample of a 13-year-old, right-handed female patient with DID/MPD. B, Writing of left-handed alternate personality of the same 13-year-old girl.

these complaints (e.g., painful defecation) are the direct result of sexual abuse. We have found a history of constipation and encopresis to be especially common among sexually traumatized boys and girls. Unfortunately, the etiology of their disorders was rarely recognized prior to referral to the Bellevue Dissociative Disorders Clinic, and many of the examinations, tests, and treatments (e.g., digital rectal examinations, barium enemas, suppositories) further traumatized these already abused children. These children, like other sexually abused children, often have long histories of doctor visits for nausea and vague abdominal pains for which no medical cause can be found. In one case of a sexually abused adolescent boy, one of his female personalities experienced episodic gagging whenever "she" relived the experience of fellatio by an older male relative. An adolescent girl could not tolerate using toothpaste because it reminded her of the semen she had been forced to swallow.

In summary, our experiences at the Bellevue clinic suggest that most, if not all, of the psychosomatic and related phenomena described as characteristic of adults with DID/MPD can also be found in children with the disorder.

Neurophysiological Investigations

Studies of the neurophysiological differences among alternate personalities have focused on adults. They have included studies of galvanic skin response (Brende, 1984; Larmore et al., 1977; Ludwig, 1972; Putnam, et al., 1989), electromyography, (Larmore et al., 1977), electroencephalographic changes (Cocores et al., 1984; Coons et al., 1982; Larmore et al., 1977; Ludwig et al., 1972; Thigpen and Cleckley, 1954), differences in evoked potentials (Braun, 1983a; Denson-Gerber, 1986; Larmore et al., 1977; Ludwig et al., 1972; Putnam, 1984), differences in regional cerebral blood flow (de Vito et al., 1985; Lefkof et al., 1984; Mathew et al., 1985; Saxe et al., 1992), differences in autonomic functions, such as heart rate and respiration (Bahnson and Smith, 1975) and differences in cognitive functioning (Armstrong and Loewenstein, 1990; Erickson and Rappaport, 1980; Coons and Stern, 1986; Lovitt and Lefkof, 1985; Ludwig et al., 1972; Silberman et al., 1988; Wagner et al., 1983). These data, taken together, indicate that physiologic differences do exist among alternate personalities, and that some of these differences cannot be feigned by subjects pretending to suffer from DID/MPD. On the other hand, to date, none of the physiologic tests mentioned above has been accepted as a valid and reliable indicator of the disorder. Studies have tended to be small and findings contradictory (Coons, 1988). Nonetheless, as more clinicians come to recognize the disorder, larger, more systematic, controlled investigations of the phenomena associated with DID/MPD will be possible, further enabling the development of neurophysiological measures to identify the disorder.

One of the most intriguing physiological phenomena reported to occur in children and adults with DID/MPD (Braun, 1983b) is the finding of differences in allergic susceptibilities among alternate personalities. Kroger (1979) reported desensitizing, resensitizing, then once again desensitizing a boy to the urticarial effects of eating chocolate. Although these kinds of phenomena are poorly understood, they resemble some of the reported effects of hypnosis on the allergic responses of suggestible individuals who do not suffer from DID/MPD. Reports of the successful treatment with hypnosis of such diverse conditions as warts, psoriasis, acne, and ichthyosis attest to the strong relationship between mental activity and physiological response.

Diagnostic Evaluation

As is true of most other psychiatric diagnoses, there are no specific biological tests for DID/MPD. On the other hand, as mentioned in the section on clinical characteristics of the disorder, different personalities may demonstrate different electroencephalographic characteristics, particularly when visual or auditory evoked potentials are studied. A detailed neurological assessment may also demonstrate differences between personalities, particularly regarding touch and pain sensitivity. Differences have been reported in types of divergent eye movements

(i.e., strabismus) among several personalities, a phenomenon that the authors have also observed on several occasions. These are subtle changes that are hard to take note of during the course of an interview. However, videotaping allows one to recognize changes in expression and in eye movement that are missed during the clinical evaluation itself. Subtle changes in voice timbre that are not immediately recognizable during interviews may also be identified on audiotape. Differences in the galvanic skin responses of personalities may also be elicited. These kinds of tests, however, at present, are really more appropriate for research than for diagnostic purposes, and many of the phenomena that distinguish personalities from each other can be imitated by actors playing different roles.

We have found that the psychological test results of children with DID/MPD may be misleading. Fluctuations in developmental level, skills, and attention during testing sometimes lead to gross underestimates of intelligence. Differences among personalities are sometimes revealed most clearly on projective tests. In fact, depending on the personality being tested, a child's projective responses may range from perfectly normal to blatantly psychotic. Another helpful exercise is to have the child and the alternates draw a person or a self-portrait. These drawings of persons can range from age-appropriate to infantile and primitive, depending on the personality performing the task. Also, individuals with personalities of the opposite sex sometimes draw sexually ambiguous figures of the opposite sex.

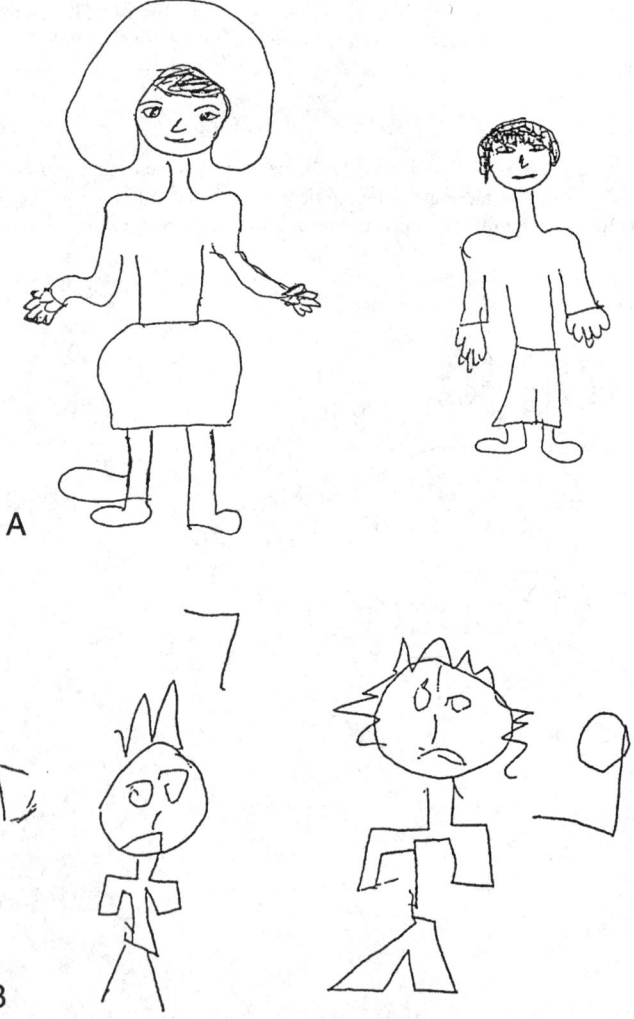

Figure 65.5. A, Drawings of a girl and boy made by a 13-year-old girl with DID/MPD. B, Drawings made by an infantile alternate personality of this same adolescent girl.

The drawings in Figure 65.5 were done by Karen, a young adolescent girl. The first set of drawings (Fig. 65.5A) was done by her usual personality in response to the requests: Draw a person . . . . Now draw the opposite sex. The second set (Fig. 65.5B) was done by a younger personality in response to the same requests. Note the immaturity of the drawing as well as the sexual confusion (i.e., the boy figure, on the left, is wearing a dress, and the girl figure, on the right, is wearing slacks).

We have also asked children to draw a picture of their brain. Figure 65.6A shows the picture of his brain, drawn by an 8-year-old boy. Figure 65.6B shows a picture of his brain drawn by the child approximately 30 minutes later in response to the very same request. At the time of the second drawing, this child was in an alternate personality state and had no memory of having drawn the first picture.

The simplest task of all is to ask each personality to write his or her name. Not only does handwriting vary, but the very ability to write at all may differ from personality to personality. Some personalities may simply make an "X" or a special sign because they are illiterate; others may have an immature way of lettering, characteristic of a small child; and others may be too young to write at all. The way in which the child grasps the writing instrument also tells a lot about the age of the personality in control at the time.

The Use of Schoolwork and Journals

Any written materials produced by the patient (child or adult) in the course of an evaluation may be influenced by the examiner and,

consequently, may be suspect. Therefore, it is especially helpful, diagnostically, to find graphic evidence of the phenomenon of DID/MPD that antedates the evaluation. All children from kindergarten on are required to produce written work at school. We have found these productions to be invaluable sources of documentation. A careful examination of all available written homework and classroom exercises can not only confirm the diagnosis of DID/MPD, but can also furnish information regarding the names, identities, and functions of alternate personalities. Sometimes the content of these extraordinary caches can even document the nature of the abuse endured by a child.

Figures 65.7–65.10 come from homework papers, classroom exercises, and journals of children with signs, symptoms, and behaviors meeting the DSM-IV criteria for a diagnosis of DID/MPD.

Figure 65.7 illustrates 4 different signatures found in the homework of a 12-year-old boy. They portray the different developmental levels of several of his personalities.

Figure 65.8 illustrates the age-appropriate signature found at the top of the work sheets of an 8-year-old boy with DID/MPD; below it, is the signature of an immature alternate; and below that, is the crossed out name of an alternate (Mikey), followed by the child's given name.

Figure 65.9 illustrates the markedly different handwritings found in the school journal of an 8-year-old boy with DID/MPD. This right-handed child had several alternate personalities, some who were his own age, some several years younger, and one who was a left-handed baby.

Figure 65.10 was found in the schoolwork of an 8-year-old boy who had been severely sexually abused by a stepfather.

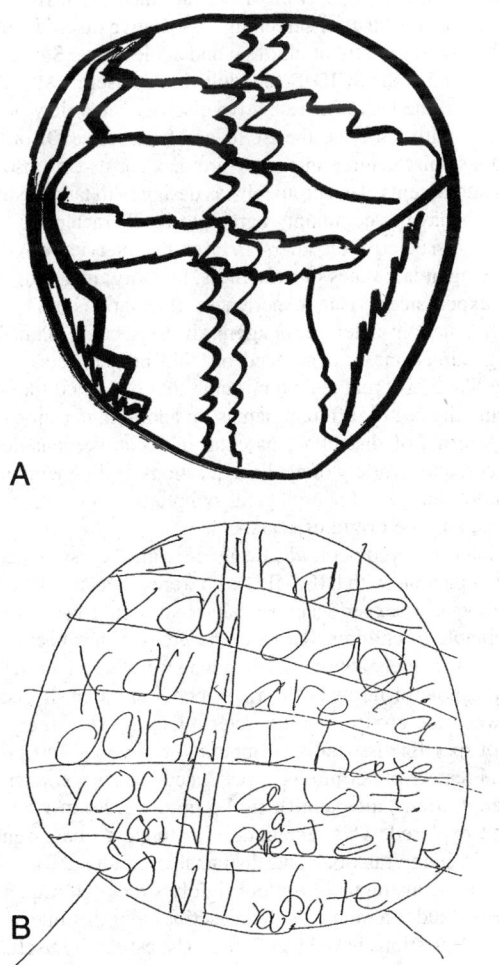

Figure 65.6. A, Picture drawn by an 8-year-old boy with DID/MPD, depicting his brain. B, Picture drawn minutes later by the alternate personality of the same 8-year-old boy, depicting his brain.

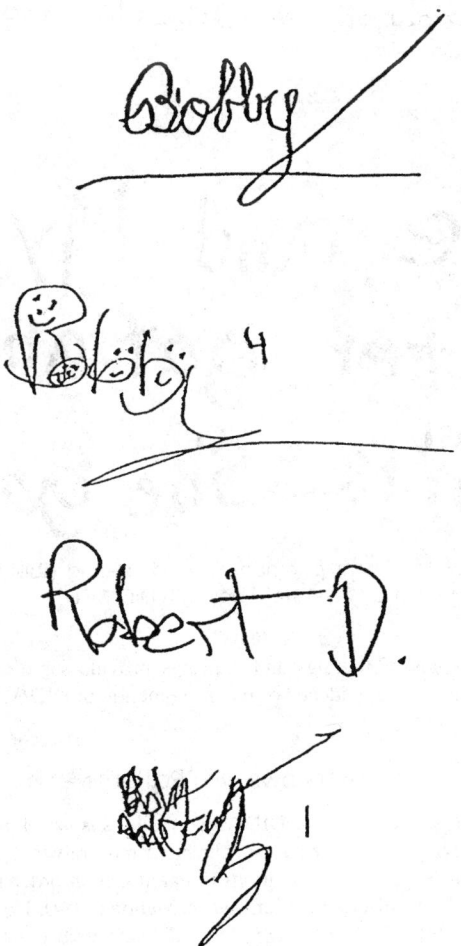

Figure 65.7. Four different signatures found in the schoolwork of a 12-year-old boy with DID/MPD.

dean

Do on

NAME [scribbled signature] Dean

Figure 65.8. Three different signatures found in the schoolwork of an 8-year-old boy with DID/MPD: the first, his usual signature; the second, the signature of a younger personality; the third, the signature of a personality named Mikey, hastily scribbled out and replaced.

he is coming home I missed
him he is bringing me some thing
I am geting him some thing too

Me and My Siter got a new Bike She got

Figure 65.9. Different penmanship and spelling ability from the school journal of an 8-year-old boy with DID/MPD.

These kinds of writings and drawings provide some of the most objective, untainted evidence of the phenomenon of DID/MPD in children.

Interviews with Patients

Whereas the diagnosis of DID/MPD in adults is based primarily on clinical interviews with the patient, clinicians must rely to a great extent on the knowledge and observations of caretakers in order to evaluate children with the disorder. Fagan and McMahon (1984), Hornstein and Putnam (1992), and Kluft (1985) have all created checklists of items commonly seen in children and adolescents with dissociative disorders. More recently, Peterson (1990) has reviewed these lists and identified the signs, symptoms, and behaviors most commonly cited. To the best

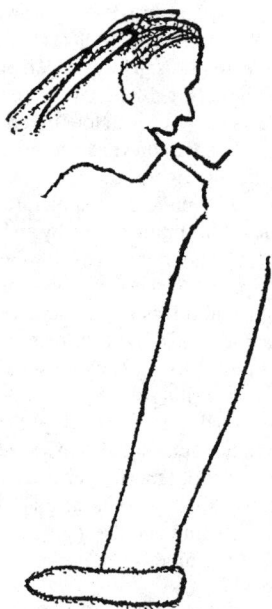

Figure 65.10. Drawing found in a notebook of a sexually abused 8-year-old boy with DID/MPD.

of our knowledge, Reagor et al. (1992) are the only investigators who have created a checklist for screening dissociative disorders using questions to be asked directly of children and adolescents. Steinberg (1995) has suggested that the SCID-D for adults is also useful with adolescents.

Because of the lack of dissociative disorders interview protocols for use directly with children, the Bellevue Dissociative Disorders Clinic designed a semistructured interview protocol for its own use with children and adolescents. This protocol was designed to tap the signs, symptoms, and behaviors commonly agreed to be characteristic of children with severe dissociative disorders. In brief, the interview covers in detail the following areas: states of awareness, memory, imagination, moods, auditory experiences, visual experiences, fluctuations in skills or handwriting, fluctuations in temper or aggressiveness, being blamed for doing or saying things one is convinced one did not do or say, feeling or sounding like a different person or being told one acted like a different person, and the use of different names. In addition, questions are posed regarding forms of discipline, parental dissociative behaviors, sexual experiences, and a variety of medical questions dealing with gastrointestinal, genitourinary, and neurological symptoms, accidents, loss of consciousness, and the origin of scars.

This interview protocol was designed with the assistance of some of our adult patients with DID/MPD who were especially gifted at asking about dissociative experiences in ways that would be understandable and acceptable to children. To date, the protocol has been pilot tested on a group of severely abused children who were in residential treatment and on a sample of normal 5th grade school children. It distinguished well between the groups and interrater reliability (i.e., the presence or absence of specific dissociative symptoms) was good. This protocol has the special feature of permitting experienced interviewers, familiar with all of the questions, a certain flexibility in the order in which they are asked and explored. This technique was found to be essential when interviewing highly anxious and distractable children, who are unable to tolerate the constraints of a more rigidly structured sequence.

Space precludes a more detailed description of this interview. However, certain questions have been found to be especially useful for diagnostic purposes and hence will be mentioned.

All of the children and adolescents whom we have evaluated and who were found to suffer from DID/MPD experienced auditory hallucinations. However, many, at first, were reluctant to report them. The following phraseology, suggested to us by an adult suffering from DID/MPD, seemed to enable children to confide their auditory experiences: "We know from what you (or your mother) have told us that you went through some pretty hard times. Many kids who have been through a lot or are feeling lonely can talk to someone in their heads and not feel so alone. Could (can) you ever do that?"

The following question regarding switching from one state or personality to another—and also suggested by an adult patient with DID/MPD—has also been useful: "You know the way someone can change channels on a TV? Well, some kids, if they need to be especially big and strong, or if they want to play around like a baby, can switch and become big and strong or get little. Can you do that?" Several children and adolescents have described switches into big, powerful, protector personalities in response to this question.

Finally, the following question seems to be especially useful in understanding the child's inner life when he or she appears to be "spaced out" or in a trance. We ask: "Many children who have been through a lot or who have been hurt are able to get away from it, to space out and go to a special place in their head and not feel it. Could (can) you do that?" Often one finds that children who suffer from DID/MPD have created a special place in their minds where they can escape physical and emotional pain. Most children have such a clear picture of the place (it can range from a closet to a paradise) that they can draw it in detail. The clinician who is let in on the existence of this secret retreat can make excellent use of it diagnostically and therapeutically. During the evaluation the therapist can ask the child to fade into or go to his or her special place and allow alternates to come forth and share their knowledge and feelings. Over the course of treatment, the special place can also be a safe haven from which the child can watch and listen to what alternates have to say; thus, they learn about experiences that previously were too painful to remember consciously. By making use of the special place (i.e., the child's ability voluntarily to self-hypnotize) the clinician need rarely make use of more formal hypnotic techniques.

The content of the diagnostic interviews with children resembles closely that of adults. The goal is to learn the identities of personalities, when they first appeared, their functions then and at the time of the evaluation, their attitudes toward each other, and the memories they hold of which the child is unaware.

A word of caution regarding the discovery of alternate personalities: Until the time that the child is evaluated, the very existence of these entities was a secret kept from the rest of the world, and usually from the child as well. Alternate personalities in children as well as adults perceive this secrecy as vital for survival. They may, therefore, consider the clinician's discovery of their existence to be a betrayal by the child. Thus, they may attempt to harm or kill the child in retaliation for exposing them. For this reason, after almost every session, and especially after the first session in which we learn of alternates, we end the session by expressing gratitude and admiration for all alternates, and we ask for a promise from all not to hurt themselves or to hurt each other. When there is a holdout (e.g., "Juan says 'no'") we reinforce our commitment to all and express confidence that the "holdout" will abide by the rules. When in doubt, we hospitalize.

Differential Diagnosis

The signs, symptoms, and behaviors of children and adolescents with DID/MPD mimic a multiplicity of other, more commonly made diagnoses. These include attention deficit hyperactivity disorder, complex partial seizures, mood disorders, schizophrenic disorders, borderline states, and conduct disorder. Tables 65.1–65.6 list many of the signs, symptoms, and behaviors common to DID/MPD and to the disorders for which DID/MPD is most frequently mistaken.

We found that among a group of severely abused, dissociative children in residential treatment, the most common diagnosis received prior to admission was attention deficit hyperactivity disorder. This diagnosis tended to be made because of their frantic, hyperactive behaviors and

Table 65.1. Signs and Symptoms of DID/MPD that Cause It to Be Confused with Schizophrenia

1. Hearing voices
2. Command hallucinations
3. Hearing voices talking to each other
4. Feeling controlled from outside
5. Having a hierarchy of "imaginary" companions
6. Apparent illogical thought processes

Table 65.2. Signs and Symptoms of DID/MPD that Cause It to Be Confused with Psychomotor Seizures

1. Dream-like states
2. Blackouts/loss of time
3. Impaired memory for acts, violent and otherwise
4. Appearing as though in a trance
5. Out-of-body experiences

Table 65.3. Signs and Symptoms of DID/MPD that Cause It to Be Confused with Hyperactivity, Attention Deficit Disorder

1. Restlessness and difficulty concentrating
2. Fluctuating academic abilities (e.g., math, spelling, language skills)
3. Tantrums
4. Problems following instructions
5. Impaired memory for learned material
6. Changes in maturity of handwriting

Table 65.4. Signs and Symptoms of DID/MPD that Cause It to Be Confused with Conduct Disorder/Antisocial Personality

1. Fights with peers and authority figures
2. Episodic violence
3. Apparent lying
4. Apparent stealing
5. Inappropriate sexual behaviors
6. Running away
7. Use of aliases
8. Apparent lack of feelings or guilt when describing violent acts

Table 65.5. Signs and Symptoms of DID/MPD that Cause It to Be Confused with Manic-Depressive Disorder

1. Mood swings
2. Episodic rages
3. Suicidal behaviors
4. Long periods without sleep
5. Inappropriate sexual behaviors/hypersexuality
6. Grandiosity
7. Self-mutilation

Table 65.6. Signs and Symptoms of DID/MPD that Cause It to Be Confused with Borderline Personality Disorder

1. Psychosomatic pain
2. Mood swings
3. Binge eating
4. Suicidal behaviors/self-mutilating behaviors
5. Episodic rages
6. Unstable interpersonal relationships/poor social adaptation/impulsivity
7. Episodic psychotic symptoms

their apparent distractibility. Unlike most other children with attention deficit hyperactivity disorder, however, these children periodically experienced auditory hallucinations, retreated into trance-like states, and were amnestic for discrete periods of time. Their responses to stimulant medication were also equivocal.

The trance-like states and memory lapses of dissociative children often cause them to be diagnosed as having seizure disorders. At our clinic at Bellevue, we have seen dissociative children who seem to have sleep attacks and who even fall to the ground. These episodes tend to occur in the presence of others, at times of stress, and usually are not accompanied by the loss of urine or feces. Unlike epileptic attacks, during these spells dissociative children can hear and respond to the therapist's suggestions (e.g., ''I want everyone to calm down. Everyone is safe. Now, when I count to 3 you will wake up and feel fine'').

Children with DID/MPD exhibit rapidly changing moods as they switch from one personality to the next. The changes are so striking that they sometimes appear to be evidence of a bipolar disorder. However, in bipolar illness moods are usually of greater duration, and switches from sad to happy are not instantaneous. In DID/MPD, sometimes one personality keeps the sad memories and weeps; often, that personality is identifiable by its voice, demeanor, or apparent developmental state. Again, in DID/MPD, in addition to mood changes, children have memory lapses, trance-like episodes and other signs and symptoms of dissociation.

Almost all children who suffer from DID/MPD experience auditory hallucinations and, when these are revealed, a misdiagnosis of schizophrenia is often made. Children with DID/MPD, like their adult counterparts (Kluft, 1987; Ross, 1989), have numerous first rank symptoms (e.g., command hallucinations, voices arguing in their heads, feeling controlled from outside). Periodically, as they switch from one personality state to another, their thought processes may become confused, vague, and illogical. However, children with DID/MPD usually relate to others with a normal range of affect when they are in their usual personality state. The amnesias, trances, and changes in voice and demeanor also distinguish them from children with the kinds of psychoses traditionally designated as schizophrenic.

Children who suffer from DID/MPD often behave in dangerous, aggressive ways. They run away, deny behaviors that they cannot recall, and are considered to be liars. In one personality state they may appropriate someone else's belongings and subsequently express bewilderment when they are accused of stealing. Sometimes they are cruel to peers and animals. Alternate personalities that have learned to become oblivious to pain may appear cold and unempathic. All of these attributes often result in the child's being diagnosed as having a conduct disorder. A thorough, unprejudiced evaluation, however, will bring to light the child's other symptoms that are indicative of dissociation. The discovery of a history of auditory hallucinations, amnesias, trances, fluctuating academic performance, and markedly differing penmanship should distinguish the child with DID/MPD from the child who simply has behavioral problems.

A word should be said regarding the diagnosis of borderline personality disorder. Whether or not this diagnosis is appropriate for children may be debatable, but the diagnosis tends to be made. The psychosomatic pain, the mood swings, the impulsivity, the unstable interpersonal relationships, the self mutilation, and the episodic psychotic symptoms characteristic of adult patients who are called ''borderline'' are also characteristic of children and adults with DID/MPD. It is likely that many, if not most, children and adults considered ''borderline'' suffer from dissociative disorders of varying intensities. Therefore, the very consideration of such a diagnosis in a child should alert the clinician to the strong likelihood that he or she is dealing with a severely dissociative child.

Because of its tendency to mimic other conditions, there is no single, easy way of making the diagnosis of DID/MPD in children. The multiplicity of symptoms, the fluctuating moods and behaviors, and the invariable history of amnestic states or well-documented behaviors for which the child denies responsibility, as well as a history of having received several different diagnoses in the past will alert the clinician to the possibility of DID/MPD. Another clue to the diagnosis is that children with DID/MPD have often received a variety of different medications (e.g., stimulants for attentional problems, antipsychotic medications for hallucinations, antiepileptic medication for trances). However, the attentional problems of DID/MPD do not respond to stimulants; the hallucinations are untouched by antipsychotics; and the trances continue in spite of antiepileptic medications. A history of abuse, practically the *sine qua non* of the disorder, cannot be relied upon to make the diagnosis because the child and caretaker are often amnestic of the abuse or protective of each other, and they are reluctant to tell what they know.

This confusing conglomeration of neuropsychiatric phenomena described above should in and of itself indicate to the clinician the need for the kind of diagnostic evaluation described.

Treatment

Clinicians who have treated adults and children suffering from DID/MPD have reported that progress toward integration is easier and more rapid with children than with adults (Hornstein and Tyson, 1991; Kluft, 1985, 1990; Putnam, 1989). In children, personalities tend to be less fixed in quality and less invested in separateness. However, we have found that this greater flexibility or malleability in children is often counterbalanced by the fact that children are often still in the care of extremely troubled families whose childrearing practices engendered the disorder to begin with. Often, parents themselves suffer from dissociative disorders and are unaware of their own abusive behaviors. In these cases, we have found that children are unable to make much, if any, progress until their parent's psychopathology is addressed. As Hornstein and Tyson (1991) suggest, when a child with DID/MPD fails to make progress or regresses to more seriously disturbed behaviors, it is likely that events in the home are reigniting feelings of endangerment. Often, siblings as well as parent figures must be assessed and even engaged in treatment if the child is to feel secure at home. It is not unusual to discover that older siblings have continued to intimidate a child after parental abuse has subsided.

We have found improvement to be most rapid in cases in which formerly severely abused children have been placed in excellent foster or adoptive homes. When a child is in a secure home we often include the surrogate parent in therapy sessions. In so doing, we teach parents to recognize the phenomena characteristic of DID/MPD and deal fairly and lovingly with all of the child's alternate personalities.

Once a diagnosis has been made, and a therapeutic alliance created, the tasks of learning about the experiences of each personality, working through trauma, and sharing knowledge are similar to those of working with adult patients. Care must be taken with children as well as adults to show empathy and respect for each personality, while encouraging all to work together. Usually, the child's most problematic behaviors result from the actions of one or more aggressive protector personalities. We have found it useful to recognize the power of these angry entities, to interpret their original need to be strong in order to protect the child, and to suggest that his or her power might better be used in new, helpful ways, such as in sports. One 10-year-old boy with whom we used this strategy became his baseball team's pitcher and the season's most valuable player.

The therapist must be able to use his or her imagination freely enough to identify the kinds of imagery that will permit the individual child to understand what he or she has experienced and to come to terms with what has been learned. We have found that, over time, as children feel increasingly safe, and as the needs, fears, and functions of different personalities are addressed, their distinct characteristics begin to blur and they become so similar to each other and to the child as to be almost indistinguishable from one another. Unfortunately, we have also found that months of progress can be undone when an apparently recovered child has been forced once again into the company of a former abuser.

Research Directions

Clearly, DID/MPD in children is fertile ground for psychodynamic and psychophysiologic exploration. The autonomic, electroencephalographic, and immunologic differences among alternate personalities make the disorder especially useful for the study of mind-body interactions. The fact that it is common for several individuals in the same family to suffer from the disorder makes it a promising research area for the study of the intergenerational transmission of symptoms and behaviors. The relationship of early trauma to the development of DID/MPD makes the illness especially relevant to studies of child abuse and of normal and pathological child development. The timing, nature, and duration of abusive experiences sufficient to engender the phenomenon remain to be understood. Above a certain age, are human beings invul-

nerable to the disorder? Will the disorder always respond to appropriate therapy or, after a certain period of time, is integration impossible? Will the disorder ever resolve over time on its own if a traumatized, dissociative child is given proper nurturing? What is the role of hypnosis in the diagnosis and treatment of children? When, if ever, are medications helpful?

From the point of view of child psychiatry and of the welfare of children, the most important questions must concern the early identification of the signs, symptoms, and behaviors associated with the development of DID/MPD. What does the disorder look like in infancy, childhood, and adolescence? The answers to these kinds of questions will lead to a better understanding of the incidence, prevalence, and early manifestations of the disorder and, hence, will have significance for prevention as well as treatment.

References

Armstrong JG, Loewenstein RJ: Characteristics of patients with multiple personality and dissociative disorders on psychological testing. *J Nerv Ment Dis* 7:448–454, 1990.

Bahnson CB, Smith K: Autonomic changes in a multiple personality patient. *Psychosom Med* 37:85–86, 1975.

Bliss E: Multiple personalities: A report of 14 cases with implications of schizophrenia and hysteria. *Arch Gen Psychiatry* 37:1388–1397, 1980.

Bliss E: Sociopathy and criminality. In: Bliss E (ed): *Multiple Personality, Allied Disorders, and Hypnosis*. New York, Oxford University Press, 1986, pp. 175–183.

Bowers MK, Brecher-Marer S, Newton BW, et al: Therapy of multiple personality. *Int J Clin Exp Hypn* 19:57–65, 1971.

Bowman ES, Blix S, Coons PM: Multiple personality in adolescence: Relationship to incestual experiences. *J Am Acad Child Adolesc Psychiatry* 24:109–114, 1985.

Braun BG: Neurophysiologic changes in multiple personality. *Am J Clin Hypn* 26:84–92, 1983a.

Braun BG: Psychophysiologic phenomena in multiple personality and hypnosis. *Am J Clin Hypn* 26:124–130, 1983b.

Braun BG: Hypnosis creates multiple personality: Myth or reality. *Int J Clin Exp Hypn* 32:191–197, 1984.

Braun BG: The transgenerational incidence of dissociation and multiple personality disorder: A preliminary report. In: Kluft, RP (ed): *Childhood Antecedents of Multiple Personality*. Washington, DC, American Psychiatric Press, 1985, pp. 127–150.

Braun BG, Sachs RG: The development of multiple personality disorder: predisposing, precipitating, and perpetuating factors. In: Kluft, RP (ed): *Childhood Antecedents of Multiple Personality*. Washington, DC, American Psychiatric Press, 1985, pp. 37–64.

Brende JO: The psychophysiological manifestations of dissociation. *Psychiatr Clin North Am* 7:41–50, 1984.

Chu JA, Dill DL: Dissociative symptoms in relation to childhood physical and sexual abuse. *Am J Psychiatry* 147:887–892, 1990.

Cocores JA, Bender AL, McBride E: Multiple personality, seizure disorder, and the electroencephalogram. *J Nerv Ment Dis* 172:436–438, 1984.

Coons PM: Children of parents with multiple personality disorder. In: Kluft RP (ed): *Childhood Antecedents of Multiple Personality*. Washington, DC, American Psychiatric Press, 1985.

Coons PM: Psychophysiologic aspects of multiple personality disorder: A review. *Dissociation* 1:47–53, 1988.

Coons PM, Bowman ES, Milstein V: Multiple

personality disorder: A clinical investigation of 50 cases. *J Nerv Ment Dis* 176:519–527, 1988.

Coons PM, Milstein V, Marley C: EEG studies of two multiple personalities and a control. *Arch Gen Psychiatry* 39:823–825, 1982.

Coons PM, Sterne AL: Initial and follow-up psychological testing on a group of patients with multiple personality disorder. *Psychol Rep* 58:43–49, 1986.

Dell PF, Eisenhower JW: Adolescent multiple personality disorder. *J Am Acad Child Adolesc Psychiatry* 29:359–366, 1990.

Densen-Gerber J: The occurrence of stigmata in multiple personality/dissociative states. In Braun, BG (ed): *Proceedings of the Third International Conference on Multiple Personality/Dissociative States, P74*. Chicago, Rush-Presbyterian-St. Luke's Medical Center, 1986.

Despine A: *De l'Emploi du Magnétisme Animal et des Eaux Minérales dans le Traitement des Maladies Nerveuses, Suivi d'une Observation Très Curieuse de Guérison de Nevropathie*. Paris: Bailière, 1840.

de Vito RA, Braun BG, Karesh S, et al: Regional cerebral blood flow studies in multiple personality disorder. In Braun, BG (ed): *Proceedings of the Second International Conference on Multiple Personality/Dissociative States*. Chicago, Rush University Press, 1985.

Diagnostic and Statistical Manual of Mental Disorders-IV. Washington, DC, American Psychiatric Press, 1994.

Ellenberger HF: *The Discovery of the Unconscious: The History and Evolution of Dynamic Psychiatry*. New York, Basic, 1970.

Erickson M, Rappaport D: Findings on the nature of the personality structures in two different dual personalities by means of projective and psychometric testing. In: Rossi EL (ed): (Vol 3) *The Collected Papers of Milton Erickson: Investigations of Psychodynamic Processes*. New York, Irvington, 1980.

Fagan J, McMahon PP: Incipient multiple personality in children: Four cases. *J Nerv Ment Dis* 172:26–36, 1984.

Fink D, Golinkoff M: Multiple personality disorder, borderline personality disorder and schizophrenia: A comparative study of clinical features. *Dissociation* 1:43–47, 1990.

Frischholz MA: The relationship among dissociation, hypnosis, and child abuse in the development of multiple personality disorder. In: Kluft, RP (ed): *Childhood Antecedents of Multiple Personality*. Washington, DC, American Psychiatric Press, 1985, pp. 99–126.

Gardener GG: Hypnosis with children and adolescents. *Int J Clin Exp Hypn* 22:20–38, 1974.

Gruenwald D: Multiple personality and splitting phenomena: A reconceptualization. *J Nerv Ment Dis* 164:385–393, 1977.

Harriman PL: The experimental production of some phenomena of multiple personality. *J Abnorm Soc Psychol* 37:244–255, 1942.

Hilgard ER: *Hypnotic Susceptibility*. New York, Harcourt, Brace and World, 1965.

Hilgard ER: *Personality and Hypnosis: A Study of Imaginative Involvement*. Chicago, University of Chicago Press, 1970.

Hornstein N, Putnam FW: Clinical phenomenology of childhood and adolescent dissociative disorders. *J Am Acad Child Adolesc Psychiatry* 31:1077–1085, 1991.

Hornstein N, Tyson S: Inpatient treatment of children with multiple personality/dissociative disorders and their families. *Psychiatr Clin North Am* 14:631–648, 1991.

Janet P: *L'automatisme Psychologique*. Paris, Felix Alcon, 1889.

Kampman R: Hypnotically induced multiple personality: An experimental study. *J Clin Exp Hypn* 24:215–227, 1976.

Kluft RP: Multiple personality in childhood. *Psychiatr Clin North Am* 7:121–134, 1984a.

Kluft RP: Treatment of multiple personality disorder. A study of 33 cases. *Psychiatr Clin North Am* 7:9–29, 1984b.

Kluft RP: Childhood multiple personality disorder: Predictors, clinical findings, and treatment results. In: Kluft RP (ed): *Childhood Antecedents of Multiple Personality*. Washington, DC, American Psychiatric Press, 1985, pp. 167–196.

Kluft RP: Treating children who have multiple personality disorder. In: Braun BG (ed): *Treatment of Multiple Personality Disorder*. Washington, DC, American Psychiatric Press, 1986.

Kluft RP: The parental fitness of mothers with multiple personality disorder: A preliminary study. *Child Abuse Negl* 11:273–280, 1987a.

Kluft RP: First-rank symptoms as a diagnostic clue to multiple personality disorder. *Am J Psychiatry* 144:293–298, 1987b.

Kluft RP: Multiple personality disorder in children: An update. In: van Dyck R, Spinhoven P, van der Does AJW, et al (eds): *Hypnosis: Current theory, research, and practice*. New York, Brunner/Mazel, 1990.

Kroger WS: *Clinical and Experimental Hypnosis in Medicine, Dentistry, and Psychology* (2nd ed). Philadelphia, Lippincott, 1979.

Kronson J, Ross CA, Koensgen S, et al: Dissociative disorders among chemically dependent individuals. In: Braun BG (ed): *Proceedings of the Seventh International Conference on Multiple Personality/Dissociative States*. Chicago, Rush-Presbyterian-St. Luke's Medical Center, 1990.

Larmore K, Ludwig AM, Cain RL: Multiple personality: An objective case study. *Br J Psychiatry* 131:35–40, 1977.

Leavitt MC: A case of hypnotically produced secondary and tertiary personalities. *Psychoanal Rev* 34:274–295, 1947.

Lefkof GD, Lovitt R, Bonte F, et al: Psychophysiciologial and personality aspects of multiple personality disorder. Paper presented at the First International Conference on Multiple Personality and Dissociative States, Chicago, 1984.

Lewis DO: Multiple Personality. In: Lewis M (ed): *Child and Adolescent Psychiatry: A Comprehensive Textbook*. Baltimore, Williams & Wilkins, 707–715, 1991.

Lovitt R, Lefkof G: Understanding multiple personality with the comprehensive Rorschach system. *J Pers Assess* 49:289–294, 1985.

Ludwig AM, Brandsma JM, Wilber CB, et al: The objective study of a multiple personality: Or are four heads better than one? *Arch Gen Psychiatry* 26:298–310, 1972.

Malinbaum R, Russell AJ: Multiple personality disorder in an 11-year-old boy and his mother. *J Am Acad Child Adolesc Psychiatry* 26:436–439, 1987.

Mathew RJ, Jack RA, West WS: Regional cerebral blood flow in a patient with multiple personality disorder. *Am J Psychiatry* 142:504–505, 1985.

McCallum KE, Lock J, Kulla M, et al: Dissociative symptoms and disorders in patients with eating disorders. *Dissociation* 4:227–235, 1992.

Morgan AH: The heritability of hypnotic susceptibility in twins. *J Abnorm Psychol* 82:55–61, 1973.

Nash MR, Lynn SJ, Givens DL: Adult hypnotic susceptibility, childhood punishment, and child abuse: A brief communication. *Int J Clin Exp Hypn* 32:6–11, 1984.

Peterson G: Diagnosis of childhood multiple personality. *Dissociation* 3:3–9, 1990.

Place M: Hypnosis and the child. *J Child Psychol Psychiatry* 25:339–347, 1984.

Prince M: Some of the revelations of hypnotism: Post-hypnotic suggestion, automatic writing and double personality. *Boston Med Surg J* 122:463–467, 1890.

Putnam FW: The psychophysiologic investigation of multiple personality disorder. *Psychiatr Clin North Am* 7:31–39, 1984.

Putnam FW: The scientific investigation of multiple personality disorder. In: Quen J (ed): *Split Minds Split Brains: Historical and Current Perspectives*. New York, New York University Press, 109–126, 1986.

Putnam FW: *Diagnosis and Treatment of Multiple Personality Disorder*. New York, Guilford, 1989.

Putnam FW: Dissociative disorders in children and adolescents: A developmental perspective. *Psychiatr Clin North Am* 14:519–531, 1991.

Putnam FW: Dissociative disorders in children: Behavioral profiles and problems. *Child Abuse Negl* 17:39–45, 1993.

Putnam FW, Guroff J, Silberman E, et al: The clinical phenomenology of multiple personality disorder: Review of 100 recent cases. *J Clin Psychiatry* 47:285–293, 1986.

Putnam FW, Zahn TP, Post RM: Differential autonomic nervous system activity in multiple personality disorder. *Psychiatry Res* 31:251–260, 1989.

Reagor PA, Kasten JD, Morelli N: A checklist for screening dissociative disorders in children and adolescents. *Dissociation* 5:4–19, 1992.

Riley RL, Mead J: The development of symptoms of multiple personality disorder in a child of three. *Dissociation* 1:41–46, 1988.

Ross CA: Epidemiology of multiple personality disorder and dissociation. *Psychiatr Clin North Am* 14:503–517, 1991.

Ross CA, Anderson G, Fleisher WP, et al: Scheiderian symptoms in multiple personality disorder and schizophrenia. *Compr Psychiatry* 31:111–118.

Ross CA, Huber S, Norton GR, et al: The Dissociative Disorders Interview Schedule: A structured interview. *Dissociation* 2:169–189, 1989.

Ross CA, Miller SD, Bjornson L, et al: Structured interview data on 102 cases of multiple personality disorder from four centers. *Am J Psychiatry* 147:596–601, 1990.

Sanders B, Giolas MH: Dissociation and childhood trauma in psychologically disturbed adolescents. *Am J Psychiatry* 148:50–54, 1991.

Sanders B, McRoberts G, Tollefson C: Childhood stress and dissociation in a college population. *Dissociation: Progress in the Dissociative Disorders* 2:17–23, 1989.

Saxe GN, Vasile RG, Hill TC, et al: SPECT imaging and multiple personality disorder. *J Nerv Ment Dis* 180:662–663, 1992.

Schafer DW: Recognizing multiple personality patients. *Am J Psychother* 40(4):500–511, 1986.

Silberman EK, Putnam FW, Weingartner H, et al: Dissociative states in multiple personality disorder: A quantitative study. *Psychiatry Res* 15:253–260, 1988.

Spiegel H, Spiegel D: *Trance and Treatment*. New York, Basic Books, 1978.

Steinberg M: Diagnosis and assessment of dissociation in children and adolescents. *Child Adolesc Psychiatr Clin North Am*, 1995.

Stern CR: The etiology of multiple personality. *Psychiatr Clin North Am* 7:149–160, 1984.

Tellegen A, Atkinson G: Openness to absorbing and self-altering experiences (''absorption''), a trait related to hypnotic susceptibility. *J Abnorm Psychol* 83:268–277, 1974.

Thigpen CH, Cleckley H: A case of multiple personality. *J Abnorm Soc Psychol* 49:135–151, 1954.

Tyson GM: Childhood multiple personality disorder/dissociation identity disorder: Applying and extending current diagnostic checklists. *Dissociation* 5, 1:20–27, 1992.

Vincent M, Pickering MR: Multiple personality disorder in childhood. *Can J Psychiatry* 33:524–529, 1988.

Wagner EE, Allison RB, Wagner CF: Diagnosing multiple personalities with the Rorschach: A confirmation. *J Pers Assess* 47:143–149, 1983.

Weiss M, Sutton PJ, Utecht AJ: Multiple personality in a 10-year-old girl. *J Am Acad Child Adolesc Psychiatry* 24:495–501, 1985.

Williams DT: Hypnosis as a psychotherapeutic adjunct with children and adolescents. *Psychiatr Ann* 11:47–54, 1981.

66 SLEEP DISTURBANCES AND DISORDERS

H. Allen Handford, M.D., Richard E. Mattison, M.D., and Anthony Kales, M.D.

From the day of a child's birth, his or her sleep patterns are a matter of primary concern to the parents, second only to feeding patterns. Because in the early weeks and months of life, feeding and sleeping frequently alternate with periods of crying, often interrupting parental sleep cycles, it is only natural for parents to be concerned if their child's sleep is irregular, frequently interrupted, or if the infant is slow to sleep throughout the night. Parental concern about sleeping habits is established very early in a child's life. Thus, it is logical that sleep disturbances and disorders will come to the attention of professionals working with children throughout the childhood years.

In the psychiatric assessment, diagnosis, and treatment of children and adolescents, a history of variations in the usual patterns of the sleep-wake cycle is often reported. Such alterations may be either transitory phenomena or manifestations of normal phases of development. However, they may also appear as signs or symptoms of specific sleep disorders or of a number of other mental and emotional disorders of childhood. It is, therefore, essential to have a full understanding of sleep, sleep patterns, and all of their various manifestations to diagnose and manage these disorders appropriately.

For our purposes, we will define childhood as the period extending from birth to the completion of adolescence, or approximately 18 years of age. Although sleep disturbances may be transitory and relatively benign, sleep disorders, in general, are characterized by greater severity and duration, and degree to which they significantly disrupt or interfere with the child's daily functioning. Thus, the disruptions of sleep that we will cover are those of more than occasional duration and more than minimal severity. They will include specific sleep disorders that often are related to emotional or physical alterations associated with specific phases of development. Using DSM-IV criteria (APA, 1994), sleep disorders may be divided into four major groups: the dyssomnias, which show disturbance in the duration, type, and pattern of sleep; the parasomnias, which consist of experiences a child may have during sleep that are directly related to the sleep process and sleep stages; sleep disturbances that frequently accompany the common major child psychiatric disorders seen in clinical practice; and sleep disorders due to general medical conditions or substance abuse.

SLEEP-WAKE PATTERNS IN CHILDREN

Development of Sleep/Wakefulness Cycle

The newborn infant alternates between sleep and wakefulness every 3 or 4 hours, with awakenings usually related to hunger. The periods of wakefulness during the day gradually lengthen, the number of naps dwindles, and nighttime sleep periods grow longer. A definite diurnal cycle is established at 5 weeks in the majority of infants (Kleitman, 1963). Sleeping through the night, or "settling," was found in 70% of infants by 3 months of age (Moore and Ucko, 1957). It takes about 5 years for the infant to develop the single night-day cycle that will be retained throughout the balance of childhood and adulthood.

Newborn children sleep about 16 hours a day and, by the 16th week of life, an extended, uninterrupted period of nocturnal sleep may reach 8.5 hours (Kleitman and Englemann, 1953; Parmelee et al., 1964). Sleep requirements diminish to 12 hours plus a 1-hour nap at 2–3 years of age; in studies of normal preschool children, duration of sleep at 2 years was about 10 hours (Kohler et al., 1968). Requirements for sleep further decrease to about 9 hours at 8–12 years of age (Ross et al., 1968). Nocturnal sleep time stabilizes at about 8 hours in young adulthood and remains there through midlife. With old age, nighttime sleep shortens, mostly because of frequent and prolonged awakenings (Feinberg and Carlson, 1968).

The development of the diurnal cycle is most likely related to maturation of the CNS, since the ability to sustain prolonged periods of sleep and wakefulness appears to depend on an increasingly higher level of organization of the CNS. Infants who have suffered some type of prenatal injury or trauma, such as anoxia, develop the ability to sustain sleep without interruption at a later age (Preston, 1945).

Learning and conditioning are also involved, in terms of the child's response to the family's patterns of sleep-wake behavior (Anders and Weinstein, 1972; Parmelee et al., 1964). From a practical standpoint, the sleep of the infant gradually becomes similar to that of the parents and is, therefore, less disturbing to parents; as this occurs, the infant is able to sleep for more prolonged periods and, predominantly, at night (Kleitman, 1963).

Sleep Stage Patterns

Early sleep laboratory studies by Aserinsky and Kleitman (1953) focused on the assessment of sleep in children, first with regard to slow eye movements and, later on, rapid eye movement (REM) sleep. Subsequently, Rechtschaffen and Kales (1968) published the first manual standardizing terminology, techniques, and scoring systems of adult stages of sleep. This was followed by a similar manual that standardized terminology, techniques, and criteria in newborn infants (Anders et al., 1971).

Three basic sleep states occur in infants: active-REM sleep and quiet-non-REM (NREM) sleep—which are considered precursors of REM and NREM sleep—and indeterminate sleep (Anders et al., 1971). At term, the approximate percentages of the sleep phases are as follows: active-REM sleep, 50%; quiet-NREM sleep, 35%; and indeterminate sleep, 15% (Parmelee et al., 1967). In the infant, frequent sucking movements are observed during REM sleep, as well as fine twitches, grimaces, tremors, and smiles. Indeterminate sleep, which is poorly organized, is derived from the concept of transitional sleep. It is considered an immature state that is characteristic of premature infants but is also present in full-term infants and infants with various abnormalities (Anders et al., 1971).

The proportion of the various sleep phases in the newborn also changes considerably within a short period of time. The percentage of REM sleep decreases progressively after birth to a level of 20–25% in childhood, which is maintained with slight variation throughout life

(Feinberg and Carlson, 1968; Roffwarg et al., 1966). Since premature and full-term infants spend approximately two-thirds of the day asleep, the total REM time for this group is considerably higher than the total REM time for any other age group, where the total sleep time is invariably less. By about 3 months of age, the EEG patterns of quiet sleep can be divided into various stages of NREM sleep. The combined percentage of stages 3 and 4 sleep (slow-wave sleep) is highest in childhood, about 20–30% of total sleep time. It decreases to 10–20% in young adults and diminishes even further after middle age. Stage 4 sleep is virtually absent in the elderly (Feinberg and Carlson, 1968; Roffwarg et al., 1966).

Whereas the adult REM-NREM cycle is 90 minutes, the cycle length in infants is approximately 50 minutes (Stern et al., 1969). Immature infants have even shorter cycles, and premature infants of less than 34 weeks gestational age do not show any sleep cycling (Dreyfus-Brisac, 1970). Between the ages of 3–8 months, the cycle length remains essentially the same, but the proportion of quiet sleep to active sleep within a cycle doubles (Stern et al., 1969). This age-related shift in the proportion of NREM to REM sleep is thought to indicate maturation of the CNS. REM sleep, which is characterized by irregular respiration and heart rate, is considered an archi-sleep or primitive sleep. NREM sleep, a more highly controlled state, with more regular respiration and heart rate, is regulated by higher cerebral centers, including the cortex.

The temporal sequences of REM and NREM sleep within a sleep cycle also change with age. Newborn infants frequently initiate sleep with a period of REM sleep and have relatively equal amounts of REM sleep in the first and second halves of a sleep period (Roffwarg et al., 1966). In contrast, adults begin sleep with about 70–100 minutes of NREM sleep and have a much larger proportion of REM sleep in the last third of the night's sleep (Feinberg and Carlson, 1968).

CLINICAL SLEEP EVALUATION

History

An adequate sleep/wakefulness history is essential for the accurate evaluation and proper management of any sleep disorder of infancy, childhood, or adolescence (A. Kales et al., 1980d). A description of the disorder, its frequency, severity, development, and associated circumstances should be obtained. It is important to procure a complete, 24-hour profile of active and quiescent periods. The history should include a description of the chronological development of sleep patterns and any reports of difficulties with sleep as well as difficulties with feeding and toilet training. The pattern and level of achievement of all developmental milestones should be noted. The history also should ascertain the presence or absence of prenatal infections or illnesses of the mother, trauma in relation to the birth process, or history of fetal distress. Also, the occurrence of infections or injuries during infancy and childhood must be determined.

The child's psychological adjustment is then thoroughly evaluated (A. Kales et al., 1980d). In addition, the maturity, competency, and emotional health of the parents is assessed, as well as the influence on the child of grandparents, baby sitters, and other significant individuals. Changes in residence or sleeping environment are noted; for example, sleep disturbance may appear among foster children who are moved frequently from one home to another.

Differential Diagnosis

In young children, it is important to differentiate between sleep difficulty that is secondary to immaturity of the CNS or other organic factors and that which is due to a disturbance in the mother-child relationship. If this distinction is not made, the mother may assume responsibility for the disturbance even when she is not at fault and, through her guilt and anxiety, superimpose psychological difficulties on the original problem.

It is also important to determine whether the sleep problem has been present since birth or early infancy, or whether it appeared after the normal development of sleep patterns and behavior. The infant or young child is more likely to present with a sleep disturbance that has existed since birth or early infancy. In these cases, the physician is primarily concerned with the possibility of physiological immaturity or organic conditions, such as birth trauma, infection, thyroid dysfunction, or other physical illness. After such developmental and organic factors have been ruled out, the mother-child relationship must be evaluated to determine whether it is the primary factor causing the disorder or whether it is contributing to another, underlying disorder. It is important to differentiate between sleep difficulty caused by separation anxiety and chronic resistance to going to sleep (Spock, 1957). Sleep disturbances associated with separation anxiety usually occur in the 2nd or 3rd year and are associated with the symptom of fear, while marked resistance to going to sleep usually occurs in the 1st year.

In children more than 3 years of age, it is more likely that the sleep problem has been acquired. Here, the physician assesses psychological, environmental, or organic causes, as well as developmental milestones that can account for the temporal development of the sleep disturbance. In children of this age and older, psychiatric disorders that may have a sleep problem as a symptom must be considered.

In the 3–5-year-old child with sleep difficulties, the factors mentioned above are evaluated, as well as the child's relationship with peers and his or her adjustment to nursery school or other preschool activities. In the child who is more than 5 years old, general daytime behavior and adjustment are thoroughly assessed, including evaluations of the child's adjustment at school, relationship with peers, and general social adaptation.

When an adolescent presents with a sleep difficulty, a thorough assessment of the patient's adjustment in school, peer relationships, and relationships with parents or parental figures is indicated—especially in terms of issues of dependence and independence, response to authority, and need to rebel. The physician also determines whether there is a history of delinquency or other types of acting-out behavior. Psychiatric disorders, such as depression, must also be ruled out.

DYSSOMNIAS

Primary Insomnia

Unlike adults or adolescents, younger children and, of course, infants are less likely to complain about their sleeplessness themselves than do their parents. Thus, insomnia in children may best be defined as observable prolonged or abnormal sleeplessness. The DSM-IV characterizes insomnia as a problem in initiating sleep, maintaining it, or not feeling rested after an apparently normal nocturnal sleep period (nonrestorative sleep). Insomnia may be related to other mental disorders in children, which we will discuss later in this chapter.

In one epidemiologocal study, 14% of 3-year-olds were found to have problems with persistent waking at night, and 12%, difficulty in falling asleep. In 8-year-olds, 12% had trouble falling asleep, and 3% were troubled by waking at night (Richman et al., 1982).

Sleep difficulty in children tends to have causes that are different from those in adults (Ferber, 1989; J. Kales et al., 1984). The problem, even in younger children who are less than 2 years of age, does not seem to be a neurodevelopmental one (Anders and Keener, 1985; Anders et al., 1980). Rather, it seems to be related more to interactional patterns between parents and their children and to parental reaction to short-term transitory behavior problems that have become more chronic. In a study of 23 infants 6 months of age, Keener et al. (1988) found that "variations in night waking were associated with differing patterns of infant signaling (crying for parents on awakening) and self-soothing (putting oneself back to sleep) and parental care giving at bedtime and during the night" (p. 770). Infants fed to sleep were more likely to signal on awakening. The more a parent becomes overinvolved in the child's sleep, the more likely it is that a sleep problem, including insomnia, will develop (Ferber,

1989). Often, the child is not able to return to a normal sleep pattern because of the degree of involvement of the parent. Anders et al. (1992), using all-night time-lapse video recordings of 21 infants at 3 weeks, 3 months, and 8 months of age, found that, by 3 months of age, infants who were awake when put in their cribs at bedtime were more likely to return to sleep on their own when they awoke later in the night than those who were put in their cribs asleep. At 8 months of age, "problem sleepers" were all males who were put to crib already asleep. No other sleep factors were predictors. In a similar study, Minde et al. (1993) found, in 12- to 36-month-old children, that good sleepers woke as frequently as poor sleepers, but the latter had more behavior problems, more difficult temperament, and adverse medical histories. Comparing the mothers of 20 sleep-disordered toddlers with 21 mothers of toddlers without sleep disorders, Benoit et al. (1992) found that 100% of the former mothers were insecure with respect to attachment, as compared to only 57% of the controls.

Changing patterns of feeding may frequently affect sleep patterns in infants (Ferber, 1989). In contrast, preschool and school-age children have few sleep difficulties, except as they relate to lack of limit setting or bedtime struggles—where the child wishes to remain up and active with the parents. It is recommended that excessive napping or sleeping during the day be restricted in children, particularly those of school age, to prevent interference with the normal length or onset of nocturnal sleep (Ferber, 1989).

Fears of nightmares may also occur, giving rise to insomnia problems (J. Kales et al., 1984). In a comprehensive review, King et al. (1992) addressed the issue of children's nighttime fears, their variation according to level of cognitive development, their causes, and successful treatment approaches without medication. Infants fear direct environmental stimuli; preschoolers, imaginary creatures; and school children, representations of real sources of anxiety in their environment—such as the possibility of health problems, physical injury, or school failure. With regard to treatment of night fears, "emotive imagery," where the children are trained to imagine a superhero who helps them to be brave in the face of the fears, was most successful. Parents have been successfully taught to help their own children with this method, strengthened by positive reinforcement. In a related study, Connell et al. (1987) reported on 6 children, 3 males and 3 females, between the ages of 10–12 years who developed severe phobic anxiety at bedtime subsequent to exposure to the death of a relative or close friend. Psychotherapy with them focused on their confused concepts of the relationship between sleep and death. Pollock (1994), in a 5-year prospective study, also reported that emotional distress, as well as chronic medical conditions, commonly caused night-waking at age 5, but less frequently by age 10.

Because insomnia in children seems to be more of a psychosocial problem based on the relationship between parent and child, treatment is addressed primarily through psychological or behavioral means. Richman et al. (1985) found that behavioral methods of treatment improved the bedtime disturbances and night waking (childhood equivalents of adult insomnia) of 35 children aged 1–5 years, whereas treatment with medication (trimeprazine) of 22 children with severe waking problems showed no permanent effect on sleep patterns (Richman, 1985).

Minde et al. (1994), reporting on a study of the effects on daytime mother-child interactions of a treatment program for severely sleep-disturbed children aged 12–36 months, found that relatively simple interventions, such as the father putting the child to bed instead of the mother, helped to improve the total mother-child relationship.

Adolescents seem to have an increased need to sleep during the daytime. In one study, (Price et al., 1978), 13% of adolescents were classified as having difficulty sleeping through the night on a regular basis. Similar findings have been reported for an adolescent psychiatric outpatient population (Monroe and Marks, 1977). Morrison et al. (1992), reporting on 943 adolescents from the general population, found that 10% reported difficulty falling asleep. Also, whether male or female, those who had sleep problems showed more DSM-III disorders, namely anxiety, depression, inattention, and conduct disorder. Carskadon (1990) reported accident proneness, daytime sleepiness, and behavior and mood problems in adolescents getting insufficient sleep. Based on a large survey of more than 1000 metropolitan households (Bixler et al., 1979), only 11% of adult chronic insomniacs reported the onset of their disorder in adolescence (between the ages of 11–20 years), suggesting that chronic insomnia is relatively uncommon in this age group. However, because insomnia in the adult population is frequently associated with depressive or dysthymic disorders, appropriate diagnosis and clinical treatment of those conditions in adolescents with antidepressant medication may serve to relieve symptoms of insomnia (see below). For adolescents who ruminate obsessively about their insomnia, long half-life benzodiazepine medications—with close monitoring for excessive daytime sleepiness and possible development of dependency—may be beneficial, not only to improve sleep induction and maintenance but also to reduce daytime anxiety (Kales et al., 1976).

In adolescents, insomnia unrelated to other primary psychiatric disorders may also appear as delayed sleep phase syndrome (DSPS) (Ferber and Boyle, 1983; Thorpy et al., 1988). DSPS consists of a chronic involuntary delay in falling asleep at night when desired and an inability to awaken at an appropriately scheduled time in the morning. Successful treatments of DSPS in adolescents with behavioral approaches (Cashman and McCann, 1988), sleep phase-advance techniques (Thorpy et al., 1988) or high doses of methylcobalamin (Vitamin B_{12}) (Ohta et al., 1991) have all been reported to foster the establishment of an appropriate 24-hour sleep pattern, resulting in improved school performance, mood, and behavior.

CASE ILLUSTRATION

A 14-year-old girl presented with the primary complaint of difficulty falling asleep at night. She would remain awake 1–2 hours after going to bed. Psychotherapy revealed an obsessional preoccupation with the need for a full night's sleep. This disturbance eventually resolved in the course of psychotherapy and she returned to her normal sleep pattern.

Primary Hypersomnia

Hypersomnia, or daytime somnolence, affects about 5 in 100 people in the general population, with a slight male predominance (Bixler et al., 1979). In children it tends to appear more often as they approach or enter adolescence.

Carskadon and Dement (1987) describe the evolution of daytime sleepiness in adolescents. In their study of 33 children, free of sleep complaints, who maintained a stable 10-hour sleep time, they assessed whether the need for sleep actually gradually decreased as youngsters entered adolescence. The study indicated that sleep needs did not change significantly during adolescence. Total sleep appeared to remain at a stable level when the opportunity existed to have a continuous 10 hours of sleep. There were some differences between males and females. The only changes noted during the adolescent years were that the combined duration of slow-wave sleep stages relative to other stages tended to decline.

In a case of hypersomnia, the relatively rare disorder Kleine-Levin syndrome should be considered (Billiard, 1989). This disorder is a periodic condition characterized by episodes of continuous daytime hypersomnolence associated with hyperphagia, irritability, aggression, sexual disinhibition, and mental disturbances, with a slight male predominance. The initial onset of this disorder is often related to an ill-defined flu-like condition. Diffuse paroxysmal slowing is found in the EEG. Treatment of this disorder has included amphetamines and lithium carbonate, but a definitive cure has not been achieved.

CASE ILLUSTRATION

A 16-year-old male experienced the onset of hypersomnolence during holiday home visits from a residential school. These visits would be characterized by excessive holiday food intake, followed by a 1- to 2-week period of hypersomnolence and a drunken-like condition in the daytime. Medical work-up confirmed the diagnosis of Kleine-Levin syndrome. Onset had been related to a flu-like illness approximately 1 year previously.

Narcolepsy

Narcolepsy is a disorder consisting of excessive somnolence in the nonsleep or daytime hours (Guilleminault et al., 1976; A. Kales et al., 1982; Roth, 1980). The general population prevalence among both adults and children is less than 1 in 1000 (Roth, 1980). Age of onset for narcolepsy tends to be late adolescence or young adulthood.

Children with narcolepsy have excessive daytime sleepiness, with irresistible sleep attacks usually occurring in conjunction with one or more of three auxiliary symptoms: cataplexy, sleep paralysis, and hypnagogic hallucinations (Guilleminault et al., 1974, 1976; A. Kales et al., 1982; Roth, 1980). The sleep attacks may last from a few seconds to 30 minutes and may be precipitated by sedentary, monotonous activity, such as watching television, reading, or sitting in class.

Cataplexy, present in about 60–80% of patients with narcolepsy (Hishikawa and Kaneko, 1965; Roth, 1980), is a brief (lasting a few seconds to about 2 minutes), sudden, complete or partial loss of muscle control that may cause the person to collapse while remaining conscious. This loss of muscle tone frequently occurs in relation to strong emotional experiences such as laughter, surprise, or anger. In patients who have cataplexy, REM periods usually occur at or shortly after sleep onset (Hishikawa and Kaneko, 1965; A. Kales et al., 1982; Roth, 1980), rather than preceded by the 70 to 90 minutes of non-REM sleep seen in normal persons.

With sleep paralysis, there is a temporary loss of muscle tone and a resulting inability to move, most often occurring on awakening. Hypnagogic hallucinations are vivid hallucinatory perceptions (usually visual or auditory) that occur even in normal children.

Sleep attacks and certain manifestations of the auxiliary symptoms of narcolepsy appear to be closely related to the neurophysiological mechanisms of REM sleep (Broughton, 1971; Hishikawa and Kaneko, 1965; Rechtschaffen and Dement, 1969). Two lower brainstem centers discharge together during REM sleep. The nucleus reticularis pontis caudalis stimulates an ascending activating system, producing EEG patterns of arousal, REM bursts, autonomic irregularity, myoclonic twitches, and pontogeniculooccipital spikes. Conversely, the locus ceruleus triggers a descending inhibitory system, causing areflexia and loss of muscle tone (Broughton, 1971).

Sleep attacks may involve a dysfunction of the activating part of the reticular formation in addition to a dysfunction of REM mechanisms (Broughton, 1971; Roth, 1980). The intense muscle atonia of cataplexy and sleep paralysis is probably more directly related to stimulation of the descending inhibitory pathway, whereas hypnagogic hallucinations can be viewed as dream-like experiences accompanying REM sleep.

Hereditary factors are clearly involved in the development of narcolepsy; 10%–50% of patients have an affected first-degree relative (Broughton, 1971; Hishikawa and Kaneko, 1965; Guilleminault et al., 1974; A. Kales et al., 1982; Kessler et al., 1974; Nevsimalova-Bruhova and Roth, 1972; Rechtschaffen and Dement, 1969). Genetic studies have revealed HLA antigen markers in the majority of narcoleptic patients (Langdon et al., 1984); In addition, both clinical and polygraphic characteristics of the disorder, such as disturbed nocturnal sleep and abnormal timing of REM sleep, suggest the presence of a chronobiological abnormality (Leckman and Gershon, 1976). Narcolepsy is unrelated to epilepsy; their respective symptoms are easily distinguishable (Guilleminault et al., 1976; A. Kales et al., 1982; Roth, 1980).

Treatment of narcolepsy has consisted primarily of therapeutic naps and the use of stimulant substances, such as methylphenidate or pemoline (A. Kales et al., 1987b). Tricyclic medications may also be considered when cataplexy is a problem, although they are used with caution in children because of their anticholinergic side effects and association with cardiac conduction defects.

CASE ILLUSTRATION

A 17-year-old boy evaluated in a sleep disorders clinic complained, ``I've been sleepy and tired since 7th grade.'' He reported feeling sleepy and fatigued during the day, falling asleep in classes, and taking a 3–4-hour nap at home after school. After getting a driver's license, he could drive no longer than an hour before stopping because of irresistible sleepiness. During the past 12 months he had also been experiencing sudden buckling of the knees, dropping of the jaw, slurred speech, and, on one occasion in the car with his father, sudden complete paralysis and inability to talk. In the sleep laboratory, he presented no evidence of sleep apnea but, on 3 successive nights, demonstrated decreased sleep latencies of 35 and 25 minutes and sleep onset REM. He was diagnosed as having narcolepsy with cataplexy. The treatment recommended included methylphenidate stimulant medication for the narcolepsy, imipramine for cataplexy, and appropriate driving precautions.

Breathing-Related Sleep Disorder (Sleep Apnea)

Breathing-related sleep disorder (sleep apnea) is a condition characterized by intermittent periods of cessation of breathing during sleep (Block, 1980: Guilleminault, 1987; Guilleminault and Dement, 1978; A. Kales et al., 1985; A. Kales et al., 1987b; Lugaresi et al., 1978; Sadoul and Lugaresi, 1972). These periods last more than 10 seconds and are often followed by loud and prolonged snoring sounds. Two general types of sleep apnea are described, obstructive and central. The former is characterized by mechanical obstruction of the airway, whereas the latter is secondary to CNS dysfunction. Some examples of sudden infant death syndrome (SIDS) have been thought to be due to central sleep apnea (Guilleminault, 1987; Steinschneider, 1975).

Significant sleep and breathing disorders (sleep apneas) have been reported in 0.7% of 4–5-year-olds (Ali et al., 1992). Habitual snoring (12.1%) has been associated with daytime sleepiness, restless sleep, and hyperactivity.

Obstructive apnea may frequently be seen secondary to enlarged tonsils in children (Guilleminault, 1987). Other less frequent anatomic causes include mandibular malformation, micrognathia, acromegaly, and glottal web (A. Kales et al., 1987b). A strong positive correlation exists between sleep apnea and obesity and between sleep apnea and certain endocrinopathies, such as hypothyroidism (Guilleminault, 1987).

Patients with obstructive sleep apnea typically have a history of excessive daytime sleepiness, sleep attacks, and repetitive nocturnal breathing cessation associated with loud snoring and gasping sounds (Block, 1980; Guilleminault, 1987; Guilleminault and Dement, 1978; A. Kales et al., 1985; A. Kales et al., 1987b; Lugaresi et al., 1978; Sadoul and Lugaresi, 1987). Although virtually every patient with apnea reports loud snoring as an associated symptom, not every snorer has or develops sleep apnea. Additional symptoms may include excessive body movements during sleep, sweating, secondary enuresis, cognitive impairment, and early morning headaches. Significant sleep and breathing disorders have been reported in 0.7% of 4- to 5-year-olds (Ali et al., 1993), and habitual snoring (12.1%) has been associated with daytime sleepiness, restless sleep, and hyperactivity.

When sleep apnea syndrome is suspected, parents should be questioned as to whether the child exhibits loud snoring or interrupted nocturnal breathing (Block, 1980; Guilleminault, 1987; Guilleminault and Dement, 1978; A. Kales et al., 1987b; Lugaresi et al., 1978; Sadoul and Lugaresi, 1972). A thorough physical examination must be undertaken, including the careful inspection of the upper airway, neck, and jaw. Whenever sleep apnea is suspected, a thorough sleep laboratory evaluation with recording of respiration and monitoring of hemoglobin oxygen saturation is necessary to confirm the diagnosis and to determine the type (central, obstructive, or mixed) and severity (number and duration of nightly episodes and lowest oxygen saturation) of the condition.

Severity, as determined by the sleep laboratory indices and level of daytime functioning, should be considered when deciding on the treatment for a child with sleep apnea (Block, 1980; Guilleminault and Dement, 1978; A. Kales et al., 1987b; Lugaresi et al., 1978, Sadoul and Lugaresi, 1972). When the etiology is secondary to tonsillar or adenoidal hypertrophy, a tonsillectomy and adenoidectomy is often curative. In other cases, the treatment options are not always as convenient or successful. Weight reduction can be helpful in some cases where the condition is secondary to obesity (Lugaresi et al., 1978; Sadoul and Lugaresi, 1972). Other nonsurgical options, not well tested in children, include a dental orthosis and continuous positive airway pressure (CPAP) (A. Kales et al., 1987b). In the past, in many cases, a tracheostomy was used to relieve the symptoms and possible long-term adverse effects of sleep apnea (Handford et al., 1984).

CASE ILLUSTRATION

An 8-year-old boy with classical hemophilia A (factor VIII deficiency ≤1%) was referred to a sleep research and treatment center after a period of stuporous hypersomnia. History revealed daytime sleep attacks and dull and uncoordinated behavior on arising in the morning. He was also reported to be falling asleep frequently in the classroom and experiencing declining academic ability. Physical examination revealed hypertrophy of the tonsils and cardiac enlargement with evidence of left-sided failure. Because of the potential seriousness of the condition, sleep laboratory studies were conducted. These revealed the presence of severe obstructive sleep apnea, with more than 500 events recorded in an 8-hour period, each lasting 20–40 seconds. During apneic periods, minimum O_2 saturation was 20% or less. Because the patient did not show improvement after tonsillectomy, a permanent tracheostomy was undertaken in order to place an open tracheostomy tube during sleeping periods (Handford et al., 1984). Five-year follow-up revealed that significant improvement resulted from all initial measures. At age 18, however, death occurred secondary to pulmonary complications of HIV infection.

PARASOMNIAS

Sleepwalking and Sleep Terror Disorders

Sleepwalking (somnambulism) and sleep terrors (formerly called night terrors) are much more common in children than in adults (Jacobson et al., 1969; A. Kales et al, 1980c; A. Kales et al., 1987a; J. Kales et al., 1980). About 15% of children are estimated to have had at least one sleepwalking episode (Jacobson et al., 1969), compared with 2.5% of the general adult population (Bixler et al., 1979). Sleep terrors are reported as a problem for 1–3% of all children and are considered to be disorders of impaired arousal (Broughton, 1968). These conditions usually begin in late childhood or early adolescence and generally cease by late adolescence (A. Kales et al., 1980b; A. Kales et al., 1987a; J. Kales et al., 1980). In a sample of 50 sleepwalkers, only 3 began sleepwalking after age 18 (A. Kales et al., 1980a).

A sleepwalking episode usually lasts less than 20 minutes. During this period, patients generally have blank expressions, behave as if they are indifferent to the environment, and show low levels of awareness and reactivity. After awakening, they usually do not remember the events that occurred during the episode (Broughton, 1968; Jacobson et al., 1969).

Table 66.1.   Clinical Characteristics of Sleepwalking and Night Terrors

Episodes occur early in night
Confusion on waking and minimal recall of event
High risk for injury
Family history of sleepwalking or night terrors usually present
Onset usually in childhood or early adolescence
Most often outgrown by late adolescence
Psychopathology suspected if onset is in adulthood

Adapted from Kales A, Soldatos CR, Kales JD. Sleep disorders: insomnia, sleepwalking, night terrors, nightmares, and enuresis. *Ann Intern Med* 1987;106:582–592.

The sleep terror episode has the additional and often dramatic characteristics of extreme vocalization and motility, excessive autonomic discharge, and intense terror or panic (Broughton, 1968; J. Kales et al., 1980). These episodes generally occur within a more restricted range than do sleepwalking episodes; for example, fewer patients with sleep terrors report leaving their homes during the event (J. Kales et al., 1980). Sleepwalking and sleep terrors are believed to share a common neurophysiological substrate and, thus, share many clinical and physiological similarities (A. Kales et al., 1987a), as summarized in Table 66.1.

Genetic (A. Kales et al., 1980a), developmental (A. Kales et al., 1980c), organic (J. Kales et al., 1979), and psychological factors (A. Kales et al., 1980b; A. Kales et al., 1987a; J. Kales et al., 1980) have been identified as causes of both sleepwalking and sleep terrors. In a study of a large sample of patients, a family history for either or both conditions was present in 80% of probands with sleepwalking episodes and in 96% of those with sleep terrors (J. Kales et al., 1979). Frequent onset of these disorders in childhood, with termination by late adolescence, strongly suggests the role of maturational factors (A. Kales et al., 1980c; A. Kales et al., 1987a; J. Kales et al., 1980). Also, in a group of children with somnambulism, an "immaturity factor" (sudden, rhythmic, high-voltage, slow activity) has been identified in the EEG pattern during sleep (Jacobson et al., 1969). In a few cases, febrile episodes have been noted to precede the onset of somnambulism (J. Kales et al., 1979).

Psychological factors are not usually prominent in children who develop these disorders early in childhood (A. Kales et al., 1980c; A. Kales et al., 1987a; J. Kales et al., 1980). However, sleep terrors as well as other sleep disturbances, such as inability to fall asleep and nightmares, have been described as symptoms of posttraumatic stress disorder in children (Benedek, 1985). Children who develop these disorders and continue to have them as adults, are much more likely to show significant psychopathology when evaluated as adults. Sleep terrors need to be differentiated from temporal lobe epilepsy, which rarely occurs only at night (J. Kales et al., 1980). EEG studies have confirmed that sleepwalking and sleep terrors are rarely manifestations of seizure activity (Soldatos et al., 1980; Tassinari et al., 1972).

The most important consideration in managing children and adolescents with sleepwalking or night terror episodes is protection from injury (A. Kales et al., 1980c; A. Kales et al., 1987a; J. Kales et al., 1980). Attempts to interrupt sleepwalking and night terror episodes should be avoided because intervention often confuses and frightens the child even more. Specific safety precautions may include special latches for outside doors and bedroom windows and sleeping accommodations on the ground floor. An important aspect of management is counseling and reassuring the parents that children with these disorders will usually outgrow the conditions by late adolescence, if not sooner.

In at least one reported case study (Garland and Smith, 1991), the simultaneous acute onset of sleep terrors, somnambulism, and spontaneous daytime panic attacks occurred in a 10-year-old boy from a family with a history of panic attacks. Under treatment with imipramine, the night terrors resolved within 10 days and the panic attacks within one month as the medication was increased. After 4 months, medication was discontinued without recurrence of either disorder. Lask (1988) reported

the successful elimination of sleep terrors and sleepwalking by behavioral alteration of the sleep pattern, i.e., charting the approximate time of the episodes each night and then waking the child 10–15 minutes before (when autonomic arousal was observed). Relief of the disorders occurred within a week, both initially and if there was recurrence. Psychotropic drugs (e.g., diazepam, imipramine) for controlling sleepwalking and night terrors should be used cautiously in children and only if the disorders are frequent, intense, and very disruptive (Lask, 1988).

CASE ILLUSTRATION

A 16-year-old boy reported, "They tell me I get up at night and walk around." His parents reported that, since the age of 5 years, he would abruptly awaken during the first third of the night frightened, disoriented, somewhat unresponsive and screaming. These episodes seemed to cluster around stressful events in his life and would occur every 3–4 months. In addition, in the past year he had a dramatic episode in which, while sleeping at a friend's house, he arose while asleep, exited from the house, walked through several backyards to his own home, retrieved the house key from the garage, entered the house, and returned to his own bed for the rest of the night without awakening. No such activity was recorded during 3 nights in the sleep laboratory but, based on history, the diagnoses of sleep terror disorder and sleepwalking disorder were made. Management with diazepam at bedtime and bedroom security measures were recommended.

Nightmare Disorder

The problem of chronic nightmares usually begins early in life; the condition's onset for about half of adult patients with nightmares is before age 10 (A. Kales et al., 1980b). In a sample of 900 schoolchildren aged 6–12 years, 22% reported nightmares (Vela-Bueno et al., 1985).

Nightmares are most often associated with fears of attack, falling, or death, and, in many patients, the nightly themes recur (A. Kales et al., 1980b; A. Kales et al., 1987a). Nightmares occur during periods of REM sleep and, thus, are most likely to occur late in the night, when REM sleep periods increase in duration (A. Kales et al., 1980b). The characteristics of nightmares easily differentiate them from the more dramatic sleep terrors (Broughton, 1968; A. Kales et al., 1980b; A. Kales et al., 1987) (Table 66.2), which occur during slow-wave sleep early in the night and, generally, are not well remembered, if at all.

When nightmares occur in childhood, they are most often related to specific developmental phases (A. Kales et al., 1980a; A. Kales et al., 1987a; Mack, 1965). They are especially frequent during the preschool and early school years because a child between the ages of 3–8 may at times be unable to distinguish between reality, fantasy, and dream content. Because the child has an active fantasy life during this developmental period, fears of imaginary figures and misperceptions of shadows and objects frequently trouble the child while he or she is preparing to go to sleep, thereby predisposing the child to fears during the night. Nightmares in children have also been associated with febrile illness (Karacan et al., 1968). When they occur frequently in late childhood

Table 66.2.   Differentiation of Night Terrors and Nightmares

Characteristic	Night Terrors	Nightmares
Vocalization	Intense	Limited
Autonomic activity	Marked increase	Slight increase
Arousal	Difficult	Easy
Motility	Marked	Limited
Recall	Minimal	Vivid
Sleep stage	NREM sleep	REM sleep

Adapted from Kales A, Soldatos CR, Kales JD. Sleep disorders: insomnia, sleepwalking, night terrors, nightmares, and enuresis. *Ann Intern Med* 1987;106:582–592.

and adolescence, nightmares are more suggestive of psychopathological causes (A. Kales et al., 1980b).

The family of a child who has nightmares needs to know and be reassured that the children frequently experience nightmares as part of normal development (A. Kales et al. 1980b; A. Kales et al., 1987a). Otherwise, they might treat the child as if he or she were psychologically disturbed. Also, minimizing the child's exposure to potentially traumatic experiences, such as terrifying movies and television programs or frightening bedtime stories, can also be helpful (A. Kales et al., 1987a). In general, pharmacotherapy is not indicated in this population.

CASE ILLUSTRATION

A 4-year-old girl complained of frequent nightmares of monsters. One especially vivid dream was of her two younger sisters being killed by a monster while she survived. This dream was particularly disturbing to her and resulted in her crying and going to her parents' bedroom. Historically, there was a detailed history of sibling rivalry problems, as well as parental discord and a tendency on the part of the parents to favor the two younger siblings over this child. She was also having serious behavior problems. A brief focused course of therapy for the child and for the parents proved helpful for relief of the nightmare symptom.

Enuresis

Enuresis is defined as bedwetting that occurs after bladder control should have been achieved, usually between the ages of 2–3 years (A. Kales et al., 1987a). This condition is among the most distressing of childhood sleep disorders for both child and parents, and its impact frequently persists long after the disorder has ceased. Between the ages of 3–12, about 10–15% of children still wet the bed at night (Essen and Peckham, 1976). The prevalence decreases with age, reaching about 3% at age 12 (A. Kales et al., 1987a.

This sleep disorder exists in two forms: primary (persistent) and secondary (acquired or regressed) enuresis (A. Kales et al., 1987a). In primary enuresis, children are never able to stop bedwetting for more than a month. Often, they have a family history positive for the disorder and usually have a small functional bladder capacity (A. Kales et al., 1987a; Starfield, 1967). Patients with secondary enuresis may be dry for months or years before bedwetting begins once again. Primary enuresis is, by far, the most prevalent of the two types, and both forms of the disorder are more prevalent in boys (Rutter et al., 1973).

Sleep laboratory studies have shown that enuresis is related more to time of night than to sleep stages (A. Kales et al., 1977; Mikkelsen et al., 1980). A common misconception is that enuresis occurs primarily during REM sleep. Two-thirds of all enuretic episodes occur during the first third of the night, predominantly during non-REM sleep (A. Kales et al., 1977). If the child is not awakened and given a change of clothes after an episode of bedwetting, the sensation of wetness may later be incorporated into a dream about bedwetting during the next REM period (Pierce et al., 1961).

Genetic and maturational factors underlie primary enuresis, with the major problem being a smaller than normal functional bladder capacity (Starfield, 1967). Anatomical abnormalities of the genitourinary system have been causative in only a small percentage of patients with enuresis (Starfield, 1972). Although general population surveys have shown an association between psychiatric disorders and enuresis (Rutter et al., 1973), most children with primary enuresis are actually free from any problems (other than bedwetting) affecting their behavior. Thus, in children with primary enuresis, psychopathological disorders, when they are present, are predominantly the effects rather than the causes of their enuresis.

In secondary enuresis, psychological factors are usually the etiologi-

cal agents (A. Kales et al., 1987a), for example, a significant event that disrupts the child's life, such as the birth of a new sibling or the parent's separation or divorce. However, bedwetting may also be a symptom of diabetes mellitus, diabetes insipidus, nocturnal epilepsy, severe mental retardation, or neurological disorders.

Determining whether a child has primary or secondary enuresis is critical to the effective management of the patient (A. Kales et al., 1987a). Therefore, evaluation of the patient with enuresis should include a thorough history, with specific attention to the development and clinical course of bedwetting, life events at the onset of bedwetting, and family history of this disorder (A. Kales et al., 1980d). General growth and development, as well as parental attitudes and expectations regarding toilet training, are evaluated.

Physical examination and urinalysis are also required for a complete assessment. Only 1–4% of children with enuresis are found to have genitourinary abnormalities (Starfield, 1972). To determine the baseline functional bladder capacity, the physician should have the child refrain from voiding as long as possible and then measure the volume of urine voided (Starfield, 1967).

The physiological, psychological, and behavioral principles (Doleys, 1977) in the management of primary enuresis are listed in Table 66.3. (See also Chapter 54). Given the psychological difficulties that typically underlie secondary enuresis, psychotherapeutic management is usually indicated (A. Kales et al., 1987a). Such an approach may range from parental education to psychodynamic treatment for the child and family. In taking this approach, it is important to explore the specific life-stress events usually found to have precipitated the onset of the enuresis. In young adults with enuresis unrelated to organic factors, psychotherapy is indicated.

In the pharmacological management of enuresis, imipramine has long been the drug of choice (A. Kales et al., 1977; A. Kales et al., 1987a; Werry et al., 1975). However, its use should usually be limited to older children and adolescents, and then only for relatively short time periods. The dosage approved by the Food and Drug Administration (FDA) is 1–2.5 mg/kg of body weight, or 25–75 mg daily in an average child. Fritz et al. (1994) confirm that imipramine is efficacious in 73% of reported cases at a dosage level of 2.5 mg/kg; side effects are rare. Responses improve with increased measured serum levels, but these levels varied at least 700% between subjects at equal dosage levels, indicating that there is limited usefulness overall in determining therapeutic serum levels. Because of the potential for cardiotoxicity, a baseline electrocardiogram should be obtained and higher doses should be avoided.

Table 66.3.   Principles in the Management of Primary Enuresis

1. Physiological
   Decreased functional bladder capacity is often present.
   Bladder training exercises are indicated to increase capacity and sphincter control: Child drinks increased amounts of water and withholds daytime urination for gradually increasing time periods; child is trained to stop and start urination.
   Most children eventually outgrow disorder as bladder capacity increases.
2. Psychological
   The case of a child with enuresis is frequently mishandled.
   Guilt, shame, and anxiety are often superimposed on problem.
   Parental counseling and reassurance are critical.
   Psychotherapy may be indicated.
3. Behavioral conditioning
   Bell and pad are placed in the bed at night.
   Bell or buzzer awakens child after first drops of urine.
   Complications include anxiety and skin irritation.
   Initial success rate is 75%, but there is a high relapse rate.
4. Pharmacological
   Imipramine markedly decreases frequency of urination.
   Difficulty with urination may be a side effect.
   A high relapse rate occurs after withdrawal of drug therapy.
   Recommended mainly for older children with persistent enuresis.

Adapted from Kales A, Soldatos CR, Kales JD. Sleep disorders: insomnia, sleepwalking, night terrors, nightmares, and enuresis. *Ann Intern Med* 1987;106:582–592.

The antidiuretic hormone desmopressin (DDAVP) has also been employed with success in enuretic children. It is described as being more expensive but clinically safer than imipramine and as having fewer side effects (Shaffer, 1994).

CASE ILLUSTRATION

A 9-year-old boy who was placed at age 6 in a residential school because his unmarried mother was unable to care for him, experienced nightly enuresis. Further evaluation revealed a history of grossly inadequate mothering before and continuing maternal rejection after placement. The boy responded to weekly play therapy and a course of 50 mg of imipramine at night with a marked decrease in enuretic episodes. However, there were periodic recurrences whenever his mother demonstrated unpredictability and open rejection with regard to holiday home visits.

SLEEP DISORDERS RELATED TO ANOTHER MENTAL DISORDER

Reporting on the comparison of a university psychiatric outpatient clinic population of 150 children and adolescents with a nonclinical sample of 309 subjects, Simonds and Parraga (1984) found that a significantly higher prevalence of restless sleep, limb movements, nightmares, night terrors, reluctance to go to sleep, needing to sleep with others, bedtime rituals, fears of dying, and daytime overactivity distinguished the clinical from the nonclinical population. Certain characteristic sleep problems were also associated with specific psychiatric disorders and will be described in this section.

Pervasive Developmental Disorder (Autistic Disorder)

Sleep disturbances are frequently observed in children with pervasive developmental disorder (PDD) or autistic disorder (Hosino et al., 1984; Segawa, 1982). However, because of their frequent perseverant motor activity, these children are very difficult to assess in the sleep laboratory. In general, children with PDD or autism tend to continue their restlessness or stereotyped activities into the usual hours of sleep, often having difficulty falling asleep and showing nocturnal or early-morning awakening patterns.

Sleep patterns of 75 autistic children showed that 65% had sleep disturbance beginning very early in life (Hosino et al., 1984). The form that the disturbance takes can be both difficulty falling asleep and remaining asleep. This study suggested that the sleep disturbance of these children was closely related to the severity of their disorder and their overall prognosis. Rutter (1968) reported that 43% of nonverbal autistic children showed problems with sleep, as compared with 30% of verbal autistic children. Environmental factors were also found to contribute to sleep disturbance, which was decreased by means of psychotherapy or play therapy (Segawa, 1982).

Rett's syndrome, an autistic-like neurological disorder appearing primarily in girls, also is characterized by changes in normal sleep patterns (Glaze et al., 1987). REM sleep is decreased in percentage. Respiratory patterns are abnormal during waking hours, characterized by disorganized breathing and compensatory hyperpnea, but nocturnal respirations are usually normal.

Attention-Deficit/Hyperactivity Disorder and Conduct Disorder

Data on children with attention-deficit/hyperactivity disorder (ADHD) indicate that certain alterations in sleep patterns are associated with this common childhood psychiatric disorder (Busby et al., 1981; Kaplan et al., 1987; Khan, 1982). One study reported a marked reduction of REM latency (Khan, 1982), while another found a lengthened REM latency (Busby et al., 1981). Ramos-Platon et al. (1990) reported a large number of nocturnal awakenings and a high increase of slow-wave sleep percentage in attention deficit disorder (ADD) and that ADD with hyperactivity and ADD without hyperactivity show distinct hypnographical correlates, indicating that they may be different clinical states. These findings support the hypothesis that ADHD is related to deficient control of the arousal level, either hypo or hyperarousal, perhaps at the level of the reticular formation. Hyperarousal may occur in situations with new stimuli and hypoarousal in situations that require sustained attention (Douglas, 1984).

Clinically, some of these children are reported by their parents to experience light sleeping and restlessness at night, while others report a very deep sleep once the child has attained the sleep state. Studies of these children at home also suggest a significant increase in body movements during sleep (Porrino et al., 1983). Comparing psychiatric clinical with nonclinical children, Simonds and Parraga (1984) found that ADHD children had significantly more snoring, head banging, restless sleep, and nighttime awakening problems. Palm et al. (1992) found 3 ADHD children in a series of 10 to have short daytime sleep latencies suggestive of daytime hypersomnolence.

Based on their review of the literature on sleep problems in ADHD children, Barkley et al., 1990; Busby and Pivik, 1985; Dahl et al., 1991; Dahl and Puig-Antich, 1990; Greenhill et al., 1983; Hunt et al., 1985, and Wilens et al., 1994, concluded that difficulty falling asleep and shorter sleep duration—often a stimulant-induced insomnia in these medicated children—constituted a problem calling for additional treatment. Based on their clinical experience, they advised the use of clonidine at bedtime in 4–7-year-old ADHD children, at a dosage of 0.05 mg, titrated upward to as high as 0.4 mg, to improve sleep. Although not FDA approved for use in children, clonidine has been demonstrated to be effective as an alternative to stimulant medication in ADHD where insomnia is a problem (Hunt et al., 1985).

Conduct disorder, which widely overlaps with ADHD due to the secondary behavioral effects of the chronic inability to focus attention and control behaviors, has shown a similarity to ADHD in terms of increased slow-wave sleep EEG activity (Coble et al., 1984). This finding further substantiates the close relationship between the two disorders that is observed clinically.

Developmental Reading Disorder

In a controlled study of sleep patterns of 24 8–10-year-old boys with developmental reading disorder (Mercier et al., 1992), findings included significantly more stage 4 sleep, less REM sleep, a longer REM onset latency, and an extended initial non-REM (NREM) cycle. Such factors could conceivably impair information processing and contribute to the cognitive deficits seen in these children.

Depressive Disorder

Because sleep disturbance is one of the primary vegetative symptoms reported in major depression, it could be assumed that depressed children may have abnormal sleep patterns. Hawkins et al (1985) reported extended sleep in depressed patients aged 17–25 years. Compared with age-matched normal control subjects, these depressed patients had almost double the length of extended sleep when allowed to sleep as long as they wanted.

A group of depressed children 9–14 years of age showed decreased REM latencies (Emslie et al., 1987), which is in agreement with some previous data by Lahmeyer et al., 1983. However, Puig-Antich (1987) found the opposite and concluded that depressed children seemed to differ from depressed adults due to developmental factors. This suggested that sleep disturbance might not be a reliable criterion for the diagnosis of depressive disorder in prepubertal children. However, further work by Emslie et al. (1990) with 25 hospitalized, depressed prepubertal children compared with 20 age-matched healthy controls, and by

Kutcher et al. (1992) with 23 matched teenagers with major depression, again showed reduced REM sleep latencies in both age groups. The depressed children and adolescents also had an increase in sleep latency and an increase in REM sleep, but without stage 4 differences.

As do 30–70% of depressed adults, experimentally sleep-deprived, depressed adolescents show a significant decrease in depression severity, with a persistence of one day after recovery sleep. These findings suggest a common pathophysiology in depressed adolescents and adults and a relationship between depression and sleep regulation (Naylor et al., 1993). Dahl et al. (1992) have shown a blunting of sleep growth hormone (GH) beginning with sleep onset in suicidal adolescents with major depressive disorder (MDD). This is in contrast to adolescents with MDD who were non-suicidal and to prepubertal MDD subjects who showed an increase in sleep GH. This finding, plus other sleep onset changes, may be a combined result of depression and developmental changes in adolescence and is comparable to the blunting of GH stimulated by sleep in recurrently depressed adults. The possible significance of this finding is that MDD occurring in adolescence may be related to sleep dysregulation and age-related hormonal changes, combined.

Generalized Anxiety Disorder and Posttraumatic Stress Disorder

The sleep findings in generalized anxiety (formerly overanxious) disorder and posttraumatic stress disorder may be fairly specific (van der Kolk, 1987). They are often characterized by nightmares relating to specific traumatic events or experiences, that is, traumatic, physically injuring episodes, such as falling off one's bicycle or being in an automobile accident. Depending upon their intensity, such traumatic events may result in recurrent nightmares depicting the episode. In addition, there may be difficulty getting to sleep as a result of these same psychological factors. Significant sleep disruption in children may also follow involvement in a major disaster (Benedek, 1985; Dollinger, 1986).

Some evidence has been reported in the stress literature that corticosteroid receptors are increased in the hippocampal area of the brain subsequent to traumatic stress in experimental animals (van der Kolk, 1987). The hippocampal area has often been associated with dream activity. However, there are no sleep laboratory studies confirming such findings in children.

Treatment considerations suggest that a combination of psychotherapy, behavior therapy, and anxiety-reducing medications, such as benzodiazepines, are useful in preventing or alleviating this condition. This approach appears more helpful if administered at the time of the traumatic event or shortly thereafter (Dollinger, 1986).

Tourette's Disorder

Tourette's patients have very disturbed sleep patterns (Glaze et al., 1983; Hashimoto et al., 1981; Mendelson et al., 1980). One study found an increased percentage of stages 3 and 4 sleep, a decreased percentage of REM sleep, and an increased number of awakenings during a nocturnal session (Glaze et al., 1983). Sudden, intense arousal was also seen in stage 4 sleep, including combativeness. In addition, Tourette's disorder is frequently associated with other sleep disorders, including enuresis and sleepwalking. Sverd and Montero (1993) have reported on the presence of obstructive sleep apnea and SIDS in the pedigrees of Tourette's disorder families. Dopaminergic mechanisms are cited in the pathogenesis of this illness (Glaze et al., 1983). Treatment with a dopamine-

blocking agent, such as haloperidol or pimozide, results in some improvement in the sleep patterns of these patients.

Brain Dysfunction and Mental Retardation

Sleep disturbances are commonly reported in brain-injured and mentally retarded children. Circadian rhythm sleep disorder (formerly sleep-wake schedule disorder), where an individual's circadian sleep-wake pattern varies significantly from the sleep-wake schedule for the person's environment, has been reported to have appeared after a closed head injury, suggesting that the insomnia that follows head injuries may represent such a disorder (Patten and Lauderdale, 1992). Irregular sleep-wake rhythms appear in patients with Down's syndrome and severe mental retardation, as well as in autistic behavior with retardation and Rett's syndrome (Okawa and Sasaki, 1987; Segawa, 1982). Prader-Willi syndrome, characterized by hypotonia, mental retardation, obesity, hypogonadism, and hyperphagia, also includes excessive daytime somnolence, with or without obstructive sleep apnea (Okawa and Sasaki, 1987; Vela-Bueno et al., 1984). Other disorders of retardation also show sleep changes, indicating that malfunctions in sleep patterns may be characteristic of brain dysfunction in general.

In a review paper on sleep studies in a variety of mentally handicapped children, Stores (1992) reports sleep spindle abnormalities in stage 2 NREM sleep and increases in stage 4 NREM sleep. In children with tuberous sclerosis and mental handicap, more than 90% had sleep disturbances, even more so when seizures were present. In epilepsy, severe sleep problems are also seen (Quine, 1991), with marked instability of sleep stages—apart from nocturnal seizures or medication effects. In their study of 200 children with severe mental handicap, 33% who had sleep problems were epileptic, while only 13% of those without these problems were epileptic. The authors believe that this is strongly suggestive of a neurological component in sleep disorders and indicative of the wide prevalence of sleep problems in epilepsy.

GENERAL RESEARCH DIRECTIONS

Sleep research in children should be expanded to include larger numbers of studies on more children with primary sleep disorders and on sleep problems accompanying specific psychiatric disorders and mental retardation syndromes. Only in this manner can sufficient data be collected to permit generalizations about specific distinguishing characteristics of sleep disorders of children. In addition, this data must be correlated with various stages of the metabolic development of children's brains, since changes in brain function, relative to the maturation of neurotransmitter systems occurring during childhood, may influence the nature of sleep dysfunction associated with psychiatric disorders (Puig-Antich, 1986).

Technical improvements in sleep laboratory polysomnographic assessment of children, including telemetry and computerized methods, will also enhance the ability of clinical investigators to gather the data necessary to better understand these disorders in children. As a result of these changes, clinicians will be able to determine more accurately what diagnostic methods are most appropriate for children with sleep disorders and what treatments will be most effective.

Finally, in the past decade there has been a dramatic increase in the use of multiple psychopharmacological agents in children (Campbell and Cueva, 1995a and b). As a result, controlled studies to measure their effects on child sleep patterns, and changes in those patterns that may affect daytime behavior, are a ripe area for new sleep research.

References

Ali NJ, Pitson DJ, Stradling JR: Snoring, sleep disturbance, and behaviour in 4–5 year olds. *Arch Dis Child* 68:360–366, 1993.

American Psychiatric Association: *DSM-IV.* Washington, DC, 1994.

Anders TF, Carskadon MA, Dement WC: Sleep and sleepiness in children and adolescents. *Pediatr Clin North Am* 27:29–43, 1980.

Anders TF, Emde R, Parmelee AH Jr (eds): *A Manual of Standardized Terminology, Techniques and Criteria for Scoring States of Sleep and Wakefulness in Newborn Infants.* Los Angeles, UCLA Brain

Information Service, NINDS Neurological Information Network, 1971.

Anders TF, Halpern LF, Hua J: Sleeping through the night: A developmental perspective. *Pediatrics* 90:554–560, 1992.

Anders TF, Keener M: Developmental course of nighttime sleep-wake patterns in full-term and premature infants during the first year of life. *Sleep* 8: 173–192, 1985.

Anders TF, Weinstein P: Sleep and its disorders in infants and children: A review. *Pediatrics* 50: 312–324, 1972.

Aserinsky E, Kleitman N: Regularly occurring periods of eye motility and concomitant phenomena during sleep. *Science* 118:273–274, 1953.

Barkley RA, McMurray MB, Edelbrock CS, et al: Side effects of methylphenidate in children with attention deficit hyperactivity disorder: a systemic, placebo-controlled evaluation. *Pediatrics* 86: 184–192, 1990.

Benedek EP: Children and psychic trauma: A brief review of contemporary thinking. In: Eth S, Pynoos RS (eds): *Post-Traumatic Stress Disorder*. Washington, DC, American Psychiatric Press, 1985, pp. 3–16.

Benoit D, Zeanah CH, Boucher C, et al: Sleep disorders in early childhood: Association with insecure maternal attachment. *J Am Acad Child Adolesc Psychiatry* 31:86–93, 1992.

Billiard M: The Kleine-Levin syndrome. In: Roth T, Dement WC (eds): *Principles and Practices of Sleep Medicine*. Philadelphia, Saunders, 1989, pp. 377–378.

Bixler EO, Kales A, Soldatos CR, et al: Prevalence of sleep disorders in the Los Angeles metropolitan area. *Am J Psychiatry* 136:1257–1262, 1979.

Block AJ: Respiratory disorders during sleep. Part I. *Heart Lung* 9:1011–1024, 1980.

Broughton RI: Sleep disorders: Disorders of arousal? *Science* 159:1070–1078, 1968.

Broughton R: Neurology and sleep research. *Can Psychiatr Assoc J* 16:283–293, 1971.

Busby K, Firestone P, Pivik RT: Sleep patterns in hyperkinetic and normal children. *Sleep* 4:366–383, 1981.

Busby K, Pivik RT: Auditory arousal thresholds during sleep in hyperkinetic children. *Sleep* 8: 322–341, 1985.

Campbell M, Cueva J: Part I. Psychopharmacology in child and adolescent psychiatry: a review of the past seven years. *J Am Acad Child Adolesc Psychiatry* 34:1262–1272, 1995a.

Campbell M, Cueva J: Part II. Psychopharmacology in child and adolescent psychiatry: a review of the past seven years. *J Am Acad Child Adolesc Psychiatry* 34:1262–1272, 1995b.

Carskadon MA: Patterns of sleep and sleepiness in adolescents. *Pediatrician* 17:5–12, 1990.

Carskadon MA, Dement WC: Sleepiness in the normal adolescent. In: Guilleminault C (ed): *Sleep and Its Disorders in Children*. New York, Raven Press, 1987, pp. 53–66.

Cashman MA, McCann BS: Behavioral approaches to sleep/wake disorders in children and adolescents. In: Hersen M, Eisler RM, Miller PM (eds): *Progress in Behavior Modification*. London, Sage Publications, 1988, pp. 215–283.

Coble P, Taska L, Kupfer D: EEG sleep "abnormalities" in preadolescent boys with a diagnosis of conduct disorder. *J Am Acad Child Psychiatry* 23: 438–447, 1984.

Connell HM, Persley GV, Sturgess JL: Sleep phobia in middle childhood—A review of six cases. *J Am Acad Child Adolesc Psychiatry* 26:449–452, 1987.

Dahl RE, Pelham WE, Wierson M: The role of sleep disturbances in attention deficit disorder symptoms: a case study. *Pediatr Psychol* 16(2):229–239, 1991.

Dahl RE, Puig-Antich J: Sleep disturbances in child and adolescent psychiatric disorders. *Pediatrician* 17:32–37, 1990.

Dahl RE, Ryan ND, Williamson DE, et al: Regulation of sleep and growth hormone in adolescent

depression. *J Am Acad Child Adolesc Psychiatry* 31: 615–621, 1992.

Doleys DM: Behavioral treatments for nocturnal enuresis in children: A review of the recent literature. *Psychol Bull* 84:30–54, 1977.

Dollinger SJ: The measurement of children's sleep disturbances and somatic complaints following a disaster. *Child Psychiatry Hum Dev* 16:148–153, 1986.

Douglas VI: The psychological processes implicated in ADD. In: Bloomingdale LM (ed): *Attention Deficit Disorder: Diagnostic, Cognitive, and Therapeutic Understanding*. New York, Spectrum, 1984, pp. 147–162.

Dreyfus-Brisac C: Ontogenesis of sleep in human prematures after 32 weeks of conceptional age. *Dev Psychobiol* 3:91-121, 1970.

Emslie G, Roffwarg H, Rush A: Sleep EEG findings in depressed children and adolescents. *Am J Psychiatry* 144:668–670, 1987.

Emslie GJ, Rush AJ, Weinberg WA, et al: Children with major depression show reduced rapid eye movement latencies. *Arch Gen Psychiatry* 47: 119–124, 1990.

Essen J, Peckham C: Nocturnal enuresis in childhood. *Dev Med Child Neurol* 18:577–589, 1976.

Feinberg I, Carlson V: Sleep variables as a function of age in man. *Arch Gen Psychiatry* 18:239–250, 1968.

Ferber R: Sleeplessness in the child. In: Kryger MH, Roth T, Dement WC (eds): *Principles and Practice of Sleep Medicine*. Philadelphia, Saunders, 1989, pp. 633–639.

Ferber R, Boyle MP: Delayed sleep phase syndrome versus motivated sleep phase delay in adolescents. *Sleep Res* 12:239, 1983.

Fritz GK, Rockney RM, Yeung AS: Plasma levels and efficacy of imipramine treatment for enuresis. *J Am Acad Child Adolesc Psychiatry* 33:60–64, 1994.

Garland EJ, Smith DH: Simultaneous prepubertal onset of panic disorder, night terrors, and somnambulism. *J Am Acad Child Adolesc Psychiatry* 30: 553–555, 1991.

Glaze DG, Frost JD Jr, Jankovic J: Sleep in Gilles de la Tourette's syndrome: Disorder of arousal. *Neurology* 33:586–592, 1983.

Glaze DG, Frost JD, Zoghbi HY, et al: Rett's syndrome: Characterization of respiratory patterns and sleep. *Ann Neurol* 21:377–382,1987.

Greenhill L, Puig-Antich J, Goertz R, et al: Sleep architecture and REM sleep measures in prepubertal children with attention deficit disorder with hyperactivity. *Sleep* 6:91–101, 1983.

Guilleminault C: *Sleep and Its Disorders in Children*. New York, Raven Press, 1987.

Guilleminault C, Carskadon M, Dement WC: On the treatment of rapid eye movement narcolepsy. *Arch Neurol* 30:90–93, 1974.

Guilleminault C, Dement WC (eds): *Sleep Apnea Syndromes*. New York, Liss, 1978.

Guilleminault C, Dement WC, Passouant P: Narcolepsy. In: Weitzman ED (ed): *Advances in Sleep Research* (Vol 3). New York, Spectrum, 1976.

Handford HA, Cadieux RJ, Kales A, et al: Tracheostomy for sleep apnea in a hemophilic child. *Am J Pediatr Hematol Oncol* 6:346–349, 1984.

Hashimoto T, Edno S, Fukuda K, et al: Increased body movement during sleep in Gilles de la Tourette syndrome. *Brain Dev* 3:31–35, 1981.

Hawkins DR, Taub JM, Von de Castle RL: Extended sleep (hypersomnia) in young depressed patients. *Am J Psychiatry* 142:905–910, 1985.

Hishikawa Y, Kaneko Z: Electroencephalographic study on narcolepsy. *Electroencephalogr Clin Neurophysiol* 18:249–259, 1965.

Hosino Y, Watanabe H, Yashima Y, et al: An

investigation of sleep disturbance of autistic children. *Folia Psychiatr Neurol Jap* 38:45–51, 1984.

Hunt RD, Minderaa RB, Cohen DJ: Clonidine benefits children with attention deficit disorder and hyperactivity: Report of a double-blind placebo-crossover therapeutic trial. *J Am Acad Child Psychiatry* 24:617–629, 1985.

Jacobson A, Kales JD, Kales A: Clinical and electrophysiological correlates of sleep disorders in children. In: Kales A (ed): *Sleep: Physiology and Pathology*. Philadelphia, JB Lippincott, 1969. pp. 109–118.

Kales A, Cadieux RJ, Bixler EO, et al: Severe obstructive sleep apnea. I: Onset, clinical course, and characteristics. *J Chron Dis* 38:419–425, 1985.

Kales A, Cadieux RJ, Soldatos CR, et al: Narcolepsy-cataplexy. I: Clinical and electrophysiologic characteristics. *Arch Neurol* 39:164–168, 1982.

Kales A, Caldwell AB, Preston TA, et al: Personality patterns in insomnia: Theoretical implications. *Arch Gen Psychiatry* 33:1128–1134, 1976.

Kales A, Kales JD, Jacobson A, et al: Effects of imipramine on enuretic frequency and sleep stages. *Pediatrics* 60:431–436, 1977.

Kales A, Soldatos CR, Bixler EO, et al: Hereditary factors in sleepwalking and night terrors. *Br J Psychiatry* 137:111–118, 1980a.

Kales A, Soldatos CR, Caldwell AB, et al: Nightmares: Clinical characteristics and personality patterns. *Am J Psychiatry* 137:1197–1201, 1980b.

Kales A, Soldatos CR, Caldwell, AB, et al: Somnambulism: Clinical characteristics and personality patterns. *Arch Gen Psychiatry* 37:1406–1410, 1980c.

Kales A, Soldatos CR, Kales JD: Taking a Sleep history. *Am Fam Physician* 22:101–108, 1980d.

Kales A, Soldatos CR, Kales JD: Sleep disorders: Insomnia, sleepwalking, night terrors, nightmares, and enuresis. *Ann Int Med* 106:582–592, 1987a.

Kales A, Vela-Bueno A, Kales JD: Sleep disorders: sleep apnea and narcolepsy. *Ann Int Med* 106: 434–443, 1987b.

Kales JD, Kales A, Bixler EO, et al: Biopsychobehavioral correlates of insomnia. V: Clinical characteristics and behavioral correlates. *Am J Psychiatry* 141:1371–1376, 1984.

Kales JD, Kales A, Soldatos CR, et al: Sleepwalking and night terrors related to febrile illness. *Am J Psychiatry* 136:1214–1215, 1979.

Kales JD, Kales A, Soldatos CR, et al: Night terrors: Clinical characteristics and personality patterns. *Arch Gen Psychiatry* 37:1413–1417, 1980.

Kaplan BJ, McNicol J, Conte RA, et al: Sleep disturbance in preschool-aged hyperactive and non-hyperactive children. *Pediatrics* 80:839–844, 1987.

Karacan I, Wolff SM, Williams RL, et al: The effects of fever on sleep and dream patterns. *Psychosomatics* 9:331–339, 1968.

Keener MA, Zeanah CH, Anders TF: Infant temperament, sleep organization, and nighttime parental interventions. *Pediatrics* 81:762–771, 1988.

Kessler S, Guilleminault C, Dement WC: A family study of 50 REM narcoleptics. *Acta Neurol Scand* 50:503–512, 1974.

Khan AU: Sleep REM latency in hyperkinetic boys. *Am J Psychiatry* 139:1358–1360, 1982.

King NJ, Tonge BJ, Ollendick TH: Night-time fears in children. *J Paediatr Child Health* 28: 347–350, 1992.

Kleitman N: *Sleep and Wakefulness* (rev ed). Chicago, University of Chicago Press, 1963.

Kleitman N, Englemann TG: Sleep characteristics of infants. *J Appl Physiol* 6:269–282, 1953.

Kohler WC, Coddington RD, Agnew HW: Sleep patterns in 2-year-old children. *Pediatrics* 72: 228–233, 1968.

Kutcher S, Williamson P, Marton P, et al: REM latency in endogenously depressed adolescents. *Br J Psychiatry* 161:399–402, 1992.

Lahmeyer HW, Poznanski EO, Bellur SN: Sleep in depressed adolescents. *Am J Psychiatry* 140:1150–1153, 1983.

Langdon N, van Dam M, Welsh KI, et al: Genetic markers in narcolepsy. *Lancet* 2:1178–1180, 1984.

Lask B: Novel and non-toxic treatment for night terrors. *Br Med J* 297:592, 1988.

Leckman JF, Gershon ES: A genetic model of narcolepsy. *Br J Psychiatry* 128:276–279, 1976.

Lugaresi E, Coccagna G, Mantovani M: Hypersomnia with periodic apneas. In: Weitzman ED (ed): *Advances in Sleep Research* (Vol 40). New York, Spectrum, 1978.

Mack JE: Nightmares, conflict, and ego development in childhood. *Int J Psychoanal* 46:403–428, 1965.

Mendelson WB, Caine ED, Goyer P, et al: Sleep in Gilles de la Tourette syndrome. *Biol Psychiatry* 15:339–343, 1980.

Mercier L, Pivik RT, Busby K: Sleep patterns in reading disabled children. *Sleep* 16:207–215, 1993.

Mikkelsen EJ, Rapoport IL, Nee L, et al: Childhood enuresis. I: Sleep patterns and psychopathology. *Arch Gen Psychiatry* 4:166–170, 1980.

Minde K, Faucon A, Falkner S: Sleep problems in toddlers: Effects of treatment on their daytime behavior. *J Am Acad Child Adolesc Psychiatry* 33:1114–1121, 1994.

Minde K, Popiel K, Leos N, et al: The evaluation and treatment of sleep disturbances in young children. *J Child Psychol Psychiatry* 34:521–533, 1993.

Monroe LJ, Marks PA: MMPI differences between adolescent poor and good sleepers. *J Consult Clin Psychol* 45:151–152, 1977.

Moore T, Ucko LE: Night waking in early infancy. Part I. *Arch Dis Child* 32:333–342, 1957.

Morrison DN, McGee R, Stanton WR: Sleep problems in adolescence. *J Am Acad Child Adolesc Psychiatry* 31:94–99, 1992.

Naylor MW, King CA, Lindsay KA, et al: Sleep deprivation in depressed adolescents and psychiatric controls. *J Am Acad Child Adolesc Psychiatry* 32:753–759, 1993.

Nevsimalova-Bruhova S, Roth B: Heredofamilial aspects of narcolepsy and hypersomnia. *Schweiz Arch Neurol Neurochir Psychiatr* 110:45–54, 1972.

Ohta T, Ando K, Iwata T, et al: Treatment of persistent sleep-wake schedule disorders in adolescents with methylcobalamin (Vitamin B$_{12}$). *Sleep* 14:414–418, 1991.

Okawa M, Sasaki H: Sleep disorders in mentally retarded and brain impaired children. In: Guilleminault C (ed): *Sleep and Its Disorders in Children*. New York, Raven Press, 1987, pp. 269–290.

Palm L, Persson E, Bjerre I, et al: Sleep and wakefulness in preadolescent children with deficits in attention, motor control and perception. *Acta Paediatr* 81:618–624, 1992.

Parmelee AH Jr, Wenner WH, Akiyama Y: Sleep states in premature infants. *Dev Med Child Neurol* 9:70–77, 1967.

Parmelee AH Jr, Wenner WH, Schulz HR: Infant sleep patterns: From birth to 16 weeks of age. *J Pediatr* 65:576–582, 1964.

Patten SB, Lauderdale WM: Delayed sleep phase disorder after traumatic brain injury. *J Am Acad Child Adolesc Psychiatry* 31:100–102, 1992.

Pierce CM, Whitman RM, Mass TW, et al: Enuresis and dreaming. *Arch Gen Psychiatry* 4:166–170, 1961.

Pollock JI: Night-waking at five years of age: Predictors and prognosis. *J Child Psychol* 35:699–708, 1994.

Porrino L, Rapoport J, Behar D, et al: A naturalistic assessment of the motor activity of hyperactive boys, I. Comparison with normal controls. *Arch Gen Psychiatry* 40:681–687, 1983.

Preston M: Late behavioral aspects found in cases of prenatal, natal and post-natal anoxia. *J Pediatr* 26:353–366 1945.

Price VA, Coates TJ, Thoresen CE: Prevalence and correlates of poor sleep among adolescents. *Am J Dis Child* 132:583–586, 1978.

Puig-Antich J: Psychobiologic markers: Effects of age and puberty. In: Izard CE, Read PB, Rutter M (eds): *Depression in Young People*. New York, Guilford Press, 1986, pp. 342–381.

Puig-Antich J: Psychobiologic markers of prepubertal major depression. *J Adolesc Health Care* 8:505–529, 1987.

Quine L: Sleep problems in children with mental handicap. *J Ment Defic Res* 35:269–290, 1991.

Ramos-Platon MJ, Vela-Bueno A, Espinar-Sierra J, et al: Hypnopolygraphic alterations in attention deficit disorder (ADD) children. *Intern J Neurosci* 53:87–101, 1990.

Rechtschaffen A, Dement WC: Narcolepsy and hypersomnia. In: Kales A (ed): *Sleep: Physiology and Pathology*. Philadelphia, Lippincott, 1969, pp. 119–130.

Rechtschaffen A, Kales A (eds): *A Manual of Standardized Terminology, Techniques, and Scoring Systems for Sleep Stages of Human Subjects* (Public Health Service NIH no. 204). Washington, DC, US Government Printing Office, 1968.

Richman N: A double-blind drug trial of treatment in young children with waking problems. *J Child Psychol Psychiatry* 26:591–598, 1985.

Richman N, Douglas J, Hunt H, et al: Behavioural methods in the treatment of sleep disorders—a pilot study. *J Child Psychol Psychiatry* 26:581–590, 1985.

Richman N, Stevenson I, Graham PJ: *Pre-School to School: A Behavioral Study*. New York; Academic Press, 1982.

Roffwarg H, Muzio I, Dement W: Ontogenetic development of the human sleep-dream cycle. *Science* 152:604–619, 1966.

Ross II, Agnew HW, Williams RL: Sleep patterns in pre-adolescent children: An EEG-EOG study. *Pediatrics* 42:324–335, 1968.

Roth B: *Narcolepsy and Hypersomnia*. Prague, Avicenum- Czechloslovak Medical Press, 1980. (Revised and edited by R. Broughton).

Rutter M: Concepts of autism—a review of research. *J Child Psychol Psychiatr* 9:1–25, 1968.

Rutter M, Yule W, Graham P: Enuresis and behavioral deviance: Some epidemiological considera-

tions. In: Kolvin L, MacKeith RC, Meadow SR (eds), *Bladder Control and Enuresis*. Philadelphia, Lippincott, 1973, pp. 137–147.

Sadoul P, Lugaresi E (eds): Hypersomnia with periodic breathing, symposium. *Bull Physiopathology Respir* 8:965–1288, 1972.

Segawa M: Child neurological approach to infantile autism. *Jpn J Dev Disabil* 4:184–197, 1982.

Shaffer D: Enuresis. In: Rutter M, Taylor E, Hersov L (ed) *Child and Adolescent Psychiatry* 3rd ed. London, Blackwell, 1994, pp 505–519.

Simonds JF, Parraga H: Sleep behaviors and disorders in children and adolescents evaluated at psychiatric clinics. *J Dev Behav Pediatr* 5:6–10, 1984.

Soldatos CR, Vela-Bueno A, Bixler EO, et al: Sleepwalking and night terrors in adulthood: Clinical EEG findings. *Clin Electroencephalogr* 11:136–139, 1980.

Spock B: Sleep problems in the early years. *Postgrad Med* 21:272–274, 1957.

Starfield B: Functional bladder capacity in enuretic and nonenuretic children. *J Pediatr* 70:777–781, 1967.

Starfield B: Enuresis: Its pathogenesis and management. *Clin Pediatr* 11:343–350, 1972.

Steinschneider A: Implications of the sudden infant death syndrome for the study of sleep in infancy. *Minn Symp Child Psychol* 9:106–134, 1975.

Stern E, Parmelee AH, Akiyama Y, et al: Sleep cycle characteristics in infants. *Pediatrics* 43:65, 1969.

Stores G: Sleep studies in children with a mental handicap. *J Child Psychol Psychiatr* 33:1303–1317, 1992.

Sverd J, Montero G: Is Tourette syndrome a cause of sudden infant death syndrome and childhood obstructive sleep apnea? *Am J Med Genet* 46:494–496, 1993.

Tassinari CA, Mancia D, Dalla Bernardina B, et al: Pavor nocturnus of non-epileptic nature in epileptic children. *Electroencephalogr Clin Neurophysiol* 33:603–607, 1972.

Thorpy MJ, Korman E, Spielman AJ, et al: Delayed sleep phase syndrome in adolescents. *J Adolescent Health Care* 9:22–27, 1988.

van der Kolk B: The trauma spectrum: The interaction of biological and social events in the genesis of the trauma response. *J Trauma Stress* 1:273–290, 1987.

Vela-Bueno A, Bixler EO, Dobladez-Blanco B, et al: Prevalence of night terrors and nightmares in elementary school children: A pilot study. *Res Commun Psychol Psychiatr Behav* 10:177–188, 1985.

Vela-Bueno A, Kales A, Soldatos CR, et al: Sleep in the Prader-Willi syndrome: Clinical and polygraphic findings. *Arch Neurol* 41:294–296, 1984.

Werry JS, Dowrick PW, Lampen EL, et al: Imipramine in enuresis—psychological and physiological effects. *J Child Psychol Psychiatry* 16:289:299, 1975.

Wilens TE, Biederman J, Spencer T: Clonidine for sleep disturbances associated with attention-deficit hyperactivity disorder. *J Am Acad Child Adolesc Psychiatry* 33:424–426, 1994.

67 ADJUSTMENT DISORDER

David A. Tomb, M.D.

It is a given in psychiatry that, in certain circumstances, stress can cause psychopathology (Rutter, 1983). Conditions that result from physical and psychosocial stressors have been part of practically every recent psychiatric nosology. There has been considerable uncertainty, however, about the proper way to classify that psychopathology. Do most stress-induced conditions disappear with decrease of the stress, or do they take on a life of their own? Do such conditions mimic exactly other psychiatric conditions, or do they have unique features? Stressors can worsen most major psychiatric illnesses, but can they cause them *de novo*? These and similar questions have received various answers over the years, but certainty necessitates future research.

Adjustment disorder is one current category that weds stress and psychopathology. Unfortunately, it is all too often a catch-all diagnosis for any collection of clinical symptoms associated with stress or trauma (Strain et al., 1993). It is a comfortable label to many professionals because it is perceived as minor, hopeful, and nonstigmatizing—all of which may be misleading (Newcorn and Strain, 1992). But when used in such a vague and adaptable way, it is frequently misapplied in place of a more specific and accurate diagnosis.

Although considered a common condition, adjustment disorder has received very little serious research attention. Most conclusions and recommendations about this condition are based primarily on clinical experience rather than on carefully controlled data collection or on experimental results. Nevertheless, considerable clinical wisdom has accumulated, so that we are able to recognize and treat successfully most such individuals.

DEFINITION

Adjustment disorder is a specific diagnosis, not a nebulous category. The current DSM-IV diagnosis is a refinement of a number of similar diagnoses developed over the years and variously called reactive, transient, situational, and adjustment disorders. The Group for the Advancement of Psychiatry Committee on Child Psychiatry (GAP) in 1966 used *reactive disorder* to describe a generally (but not exclusively) transient disorder caused by an emotionally traumatic event that reflected a conscious conflict between the child and his or her environment. The DSM-II (1968) described a set of "transient situational disturbances" that not only were transient and of any severity, but also were "acute reactions to overwhelming environmental stress" and tended to remit upon the disappearance of the stress. They were further categorized by the patient's developmental stage and included adjustment reactions of infancy, childhood, and adolescence. Although DSM-II specified that the symptoms were caused by an overwhelming stress, it accepted stressors as mild as the birth of a sibling. The DSM-III (1980) renamed this category *adjustment disorder* and required that specific objective criteria be met to make the diagnosis. The DSM-III also defined eight subtypes based upon symptom patterns, excluded very minor symptom pictures as well as psychotic reactions (reclassified as brief psychotic reactions), and removed the developmental stage (age) requirement. With minor variations, this classification was continued in DSM-III-R. Instead, DSM-IV (1994) has made several substantial changes, including deleting 3 of the previous 9 adjustment disorder subtypes and allowing for a chronic form of the disorder that may last longer than 6 months after the stressor has ceased, if the stressor has enduring consequences.

The DSM-IV has defined an adjustment disorder as a maladaptive reaction occurring within 3 months of one or more identifiable psychoso-

cial stressors. The stressor may be single or multiple, recurrent or continuous, minor or severe, common or unique—in short, the stressor need only be a psychosocial event that precedes the symptoms and that the patient and/or therapist view as stressful and responsible for the symptoms. The maladaptive reaction must be severe enough to impair school (or work) performance, hinder social activities or interpersonal relationships, and/or be in "excess of a normal and expectable reaction to the stressor(s)." Further, the reaction must remit within 6 months after the disappearance of the stressor (acute form), but may last for longer with a chronic stressor or a stressor with long-lasting consequences (chronic form).

The DSM-IV also recognizes that the patient's vulnerability is as important to symptom production as is the exact stressor, and specifies that the disturbance must be something other than "one instance of a pattern of overreaction to stress" or an exacerbation of another mental illness. Moreover, as is common with other diagnoses in DSM-IV, adjustment disorder is age independent, being defined primarily by its symptom picture rather than by the age at which symptoms occur.

Although clear in most respects, the definition of adjustment disorder presents some ambiguity. One of the most telling problems lies not with the severity of the stressor, but with its chronicity. If a stressor is continuously present or frequently recurrent, does the disturbance become something other than an adjustment disorder at some point? Patients with chronic symptoms due to ongoing stress, who also do not meet criteria for another diagnosis, fit the chronic form within this nosology, but for how long is this meant to last? In addition, sometimes it is exceptionally difficult, in the clinical situation, to differentiate between a parent-child problem or an uncomplicated bereavement and an adjustment disorder. This difficulty arises, in part, because the severity of both stressors and symptoms is continuous rather than discrete. Diagnostic reliability depends to an uncommonly large degree on clinical judgment.

One further requirement of the diagnosis that is particularly pertinent to adjustment disorders is that the type of psychosocial and/or environmental problems experienced during the previous year be categorized on Axis IV. A specific list is provided that includes items such as educational problems, problems with primary support group, and housing problems. In multiproblem families, several items may need to be listed. Of course, in any disorder that results from a stressor, that stressor is likely to be reflected in the past year's problems (Noshpitz and Coddington, 1990).

PREVALENCE AND EPIDEMIOLOGY

Although data are limited, clinical impression suggests that adjustment disorder may be the most common childhood psychiatric diagnosis (Thomsen, 1990) or may be second in frequency only to conduct disorders, and then only in selected populations. A few studies help with clarification in clinical settings, although no information is currently available about the prevalence of adjustment disorder in the general population. Even the most modern and complete community survey, the National Institute of Mental Health Epidemiologic Catchment Area (ECA) program, used as its basis a measure that did not screen for adjustment disorder and so provides little information (Regier et al., 1988).

Prevalence figures vary widely. Andreasen and Wasek (1980) report adjustment reaction in 5% of all new psychiatric adolescent and adult in- and outpatients seen during a 4-year period in an Iowa teaching hospital and clinic. In contrast, Jacobson et al. (1980) found that between 3.4%–10.1% of children seen in 4 separate general medical settings suffered from mental illness and that one-quarter to more than one-half of those children received the diagnosis of transient situational disturbance. It was the most common psychiatric diagnosis in 3 of the 4 settings. Among adolescents, females appear to outnumber males (Lewinsohn et al., 1993).

The occurrence of adjustment disorder among children experiencing significant stress is also uncertain, yet some indicators exist (Kaffman and Elizur, 1983; Van Eerdewegh et al., 1982). Older studies (Pless and Rohmann, 1971) suggest that approximately 30% of children suffering a chronic medical illness develop psychological symptoms. This agrees with more recent work (Kovacs et al., 1985), which found that 33% of children newly diagnosed with insulin-dependent diabetes mellitus (IDDM) developed an adjustment disorder within the 1st 3 months. Studies of community disasters as well have found that approximately one-third of children suffer symptoms of a severity approximating the adjustment disorders (e.g., Gleser et al., 1981).

The New York Longitudinal Study of Temperament (Chess and Thomas, 1984) sheds further light on prevalence by noting that adjustment disorder was the primary diagnosis in 40 of the 45 children in their study who developed a mental illness prior to 13 years of age. The majority of cases occurred in the 3–5 age group, and mild cases predominated. Although the number of afflicted children was small, the findings are particularly significant, since their sample flowed from a healthy population that during the course of the study developed illness, rather than from a self-selected population of psychiatric patients. Thus, their figure compares the relative frequency of children in the general population who develop an adjustment disorder to those who develop other mental illnesses.

Limited epidemiological information is currently available, although it is likely that adjustment disorder is more common among children from violent and disorganized households and from communities characterized by turmoil and change, such as those of the inner city.

CLINICAL DESCRIPTION

The DSM-IV permits an adjustment disorder to display a variety of symptoms as long as they are in excess of expected reactions or result in impaired functioning. It then subdivides the symptom patterns into 6 different adjustment disorder subtypes. However, although it is often possible to anticipate that a child experiencing significant stress will develop a reaction, it is as yet impossible to anticipate the specific form that reaction will take. (Occasionally, the specific presentation appears to represent an exaggeration of the child's baseline personality.) Moreover, the presentation may change with time; a child who experiences ongoing stress may demonstrate more than one clinical picture over the course of the illness. Finally, even though conceptualized as a less serious category, adjustment disorder may occasionally end in death (Runeson, 1992).

Although this scheme is logical and the subtypes are clinically recognizable, they currently possess little documented reliability or validity. In fact, the adjustment disorder category itself, when applied to children, is as yet highly unreliable (Werry et al., 1983; Rey et al., 1988). Further evidence will be required before the subtypes described below deserve a permanent place in psychiatric nosology.

Adjustment Disorder with Anxiety

This category is used when the predominant symptoms are nervousness, worry, and jitteriness. There are no studies that document its validity, although an anxious reaction to stress is well known to occur among children and adolescents. Subsyndromal levels of anxiety are common among children and certainly compose a major portion of the differential diagnosis. The remainder of the differential of this subtype includes generalized anxiety disorder, panic disorder, posttraumatic stress disorder, and organic anxiety disorder, all of which have symptoms of greater severity and, often, greater specificity.

Adjustment Disorder with Depressed Mood

Considered by some to be the most common subtype among adults (Andreasen and Wasek, 1980), adjustment disorder with depressed mood is also common among children and may be only slightly less common among adolescents as well. However, evidence for any position is scanty.

This diagnosis requires a predominance of such symptoms as depressed mood, tearfulness, and feelings of hopelessness. Thus, the clinical picture is that of a mild depression, without symptoms like guilt or psychomotor retardation. The differential diagnosis is broad in that it includes not only key mood disorders, such as major depression; dysthymia; and bipolar disorder, depressed, but also uncomplicated bereavement. The latter condition can be viewed as a normal variant of adjustment disorder—serious depressive symptoms in response to the loss of a loved one that, however, are an expected reaction to such a severe stress.

Other possible diagnoses are organic mood disorder, depressed, and several Axis II conditions that can present with depression. Both of these conditions can present diagnostic problems. Organic mood disorder, depressed, is sometimes difficult to differentiate from adjustment disorder with depressed mood because both share symptoms and both are found in children experiencing the stress of acute or chronic medical illnesses. Axis II disorders of the borderline and histrionic types, particularly in adolescents, are likely to present with depressive symptoms and develop in an individual from a turbulent environment.

Adjustment Disorder with Disturbance of Conduct

This subtype requires the violation of the rights of others (e.g., vandalism and fighting), as well as other conduct-disordered behavior, such as truancy, reckless driving, and defaulting on legal responsibilities. It is particularly common in adolescents (Andreasen and Wasek, 1980) but can also occur in children. It is presumably more common in children from violent, rejecting homes, in children who have given early evidence of antisocial behavior, and possibly in children with an attention deficit hyperactivity disorder diathesis. The primary differential, of course, is with conduct disorder and oppositional defiant disorder (Rey et al., 1988) but it also needs to include the lesser degree of misbehavior found in the V Code category of childhood or adolescent antisocial behavior. Limited evidence suggests a poor prognosis in children who react to stress with this behavior pattern.

Adjustment Disorder with Mixed Disturbance of Emotions and Conduct

As the name implies, this subtype includes emotional and conduct manifestations. It is presumably uncommon in adults but will be of occasional use with children and adolescents. The most common pattern seems to be disordered behavior with a depressed mood, often with suicide attempts (Schreiber and Johnson, 1986), although other combinations are possible. The most likely differential is with the combination of a conduct disorder and a full emotional disorder of some type. Few data are available about this condition.

Adjustment Disorder with Mixed Anxiety and Depressed Mood

This diagnosis requires emotional symptomatology of both depression and anxiety. Clinical lore suggests that such unstructured emotional responses are more likely in children and adolescents than in adults, although there are few data to substantiate this impression. Some clinicians argue that this may be one of the more common presentations of adjustment disorder in youth. The differential is with the two coincident but independent emotional disorders.

Adjustment Disorder Unspecified

This, of course, is the "wastebasket" diagnosis for those unusual or uncertain presentations that are too diffuse for the above categories to contain. It may include such features as massive denial of illness, markedly regressed behavior, or a preoccupation with fantasies. It also contains presentations that had previously been subtypes in DSM-III-R, such as physical complaints, social withdrawal, and work or academic inhibition. Some of these may be more common in children than adults, such as the child who responds to stress with stomach pain or headaches or who withdraws from most previously enjoyed events.

ETIOLOGY AND PATHOGENESIS

The particulars of the fit between a specific stressor or stressors and a specific child with unique vulnerabilities determine whether or not an adjustment disorder will develop. Our understanding of this process, however, is sketchy, so that we are unable to predict such a disorder except in the most obvious cases of extreme stress or striking vulnerability. Nor, as mentioned before, are we able to predict what type of adjustment disorder will appear.

The Nature of the Stressor

Debate continues about the importance of specific stressor characteristics on production of an adjustment disorder (Noshpitz and Coddington, 1990). Obviously, the stressor's intensity is vital, but little research is available to help identify other important features, and even the severity of the stressor is problematic. The stressor may be grossly traumatic, but it may also be apparently minor, like the loss of a boyfriend, a poor report card, or moving to a new neighborhood. Stressors thought to have particular significance include those that involve a loss (Hetherington et al., 1982), an interpersonal relationship failure, frequent moves (Wood et al., 1993), physical or sexual abuse, cognitive impairment, a lengthy duration or frequent recurrence, or cognitive uncertainty. However, most of these impressions come from clinical experience alone. It is generally acknowledged, for example, that problems that follow in the wake of a head injury are more likely to lead to an adjustment disorder than if the injury was to an arm or leg. Likewise, it is felt that the more chronic or recurrent a stressor, the more likely it is to produce a disorder—yet this is modified greatly by the support that the child receives from those around him or her. The child who suffers from a chronic illness is less likely to be impaired if there is consistent parental support and if the illness is viewed as understandable and something to be worked around or overcome. Thus, the nature of the stressor, in some cases, seems almost to be of secondary importance.

A question is often raised about whether specific stressors produce specific types of adjustment disorders. Again, research is limited. One comparison study of school-age children (Felner, 1975) found that those who had lost a parent were more likely to withdraw, while those from recently divorced families were more likely to react aggressively. On the other hand, Kovacs, in her study of children with newly diagnosed IDDM, found that of the 36% that received a psychiatric diagnosis, approximately one-third developed adjustment disorder with depressed mood, one-third an adjustment disorder with mixed emotional features, and one-third a variety of other presentations, including anxiety and phobias (Kovacs et al., 1985). Findings from numerous studies on sexually abused children suggest that they also develop a variety of emotional responses: The most common diagnosis associated with this form of stressor appears to be adjustment disorder with mixed emotional features (Sirles et al., 1989). Serious physical illness can produce one or more subtypes of adjustment disorders: Rait et al. found that 52% of chronic cancer patients suffer from an adjustment disorder (Rait et al., 1988). It may be, however, that all current studies of the relationship between stress and symptoms suffer from an insufficiently sophisticated concept of what is a stressor and, thus, are uniformly unreliable. In short, work that attempts to link stressors to specific reaction patterns is still in its infancy, but findings to date are not very convincing for a close, one-to-one stressor-response relationship.

Clearly, stressors are in the eye of the beholder: They have subjective as well as objective aspects. Although stressors come in all forms, crucial to their pathogenic potential is their *perception* by the patient as stressful. The most difficult of situations, when engaged with enthusiasm and viewed as a challenge rather than as a stress, is unlikely to result in an adjustment disorder. Thus, children who are well prepared for surgery often find that experience benign, but if they are unprepared and anticipate it with dread, they are much more likely to be psychologically symptomatic (Wolfer and Visintainer, 1979). Because of the insufficient explanatory power of stressors considered in isolation, recent attention has focused more on the specific sensitivities of the individual child.

The Vulnerabilities of the Child

The most important factor in the development of an adjustment disorder is the vulnerability of the child. That vulnerability depends upon characteristics of both the child and his or her environment (Woolston, 1988). Key factors intrinsic to the child include age, gender, intellectual and emotional maturation, ego development and coping skills, temperament, and past experiences. Extrinsic factors center around the parents and their support, expectations, understanding, skills, and maturity, but include the support of the child's larger environment as well.

INTRINSIC FACTORS

Age is a problematic variable. On one hand, younger children are at greater risk of developing an adjustment disorder because they have fewer coping resources. Yet, at the same time, they are less likely to perceive the full impact of a stressor or even to understand a stressor as stressful. On the other hand, periods of particular vulnerability exist for certain kinds of stressors. Separation from the parents and the birth of a sibling are naturally traumatic for the younger child but not for the adolescent. School performance and heterosexual relationships are of particular importance for adolescents but less so for the younger child. Adolescents as a group are particularly sensitive to stressors influencing their autonomy and self-esteem. Age, then, is important but in a multidimensional way.

Gender needs to be considered, but its influence on symptom development seems secondary. Men appear more vulnerable at all ages and across all types of stressors. The reasons for this are unknown, but its effect is to put boys at risk of developing adjustment disorders.

Intellectual and emotional immaturity is also a risk factor. An adjustment disorder can be thought of as the child's ineffective and counterproductive efforts to cope: Poorly developed ego and coping skills make such a disorder more likely since such skills are easily overwhelmed by stress. The vulnerability is increased whether that immaturity reflects youth, upbringing, or cerebral impairment. Thus, both the overprotected, dependent child and the brain-damaged child are at increased risk for an adjustment disorder in the face of unexpected demands.

Temperament has a major impact on the likelihood of a disorder's developing (Chess and Thomas, 1986). Both the "difficult" child and the "slow-to-warm-up" child may have difficulty adjusting to the demands of a rapidly changing, environment. On the other hand, some very adaptable children utilize counterproductive mechanisms in an effort to cope with unreasonable stressors, ultimately precipitating a disorder. There is no fixed rule governing the interaction of temperament and stress, yet that interaction plays a central role in symptom development.

Another central factor is past experience. A child who has been sensitized to a stressor through life experience is more likely to react poorly to it than is a child without such negative associations. Other children damaged by repeated traumas of many kinds, both physical and psychological, may react to any stressor poorly, even if those traumas are in the distant past. Past experience can increase vulnerability through several mechanisms, from changing a child's perception of what is stressful to effecting a physiological change in the nervous system, and must always be considered.

EXTRINSIC FACTORS

Presumably, an adjustment disorder sometimes may be prevented with proper support. Typically, this means support from and protection by the parents. Unfortunately, all too often the parents and the family have provided the stressor(s) that initiated the disorder in the first place. Moreover, even if they are not the source of the stress, they may have provided an atmosphere that has allowed a stressor to take its toll (Handford et al., 1986). Parent-child relations are woven into the fabric of each adjustment disorder, and no case can be appropriately managed without taking family issues into account.

Direct trauma brought by a parent upon a child is an obvious potential source for an adjustment disorder. Equally contributory, however, can be an environment of neglect that provides the child with no protection from external stressors and no sense of basic worth, both of which help ward off distress. Likewise, parents can be too protective and in so doing make the child vulnerable to external stressors by providing unrealistic expectations about the child's relationship to the world. Although hard to prove, flaws in the parent-child relationship probably contribute to the development of most cases of adjustment disorder.

The other extrinsic factor that modifies vulnerability is, of course, the larger environment itself. Surprisingly, this may play a secondary role. Most healthy children can tolerate markedly stressful settings if they have parental support and protection. Even if the environmental stressors are severe, such as those of children raised in a war zone, the reactions to this abnormal environment can be minimal if the child senses a fundamental safety. On the other hand, the vulnerable child is at risk anywhere: For example, a spoiled, dependent child can develop an adjustment disorder in response to the demands of a thoroughly normal environment.

DIFFERENTIAL DIAGNOSIS

The differential diagnoses of the specific subtypes of adjustment disorder were reviewed above as part of their clinical descriptions. However, several general points need to be made.

Symptomatically, adjustment disorders are on a continuum between normal (although distressed) reactions and specific psychiatric disorders. If symptoms are moderately severe or if daily functioning is disturbed, it is unlikely a normal reaction. If a clear-cut stressor is involved and/ or if the symptoms are not specific and severe, other psychiatric conditions are equally unlikely. However, even if caused by an obvious stressor, when the symptoms are extreme, specific diagnoses such as brief reactive psychosis or posttraumatic stress disorder (PTSD) may be required.

A diagnosis that occasionally may cause confusion is PTSD. Unlike the typical case of adjustment disorder, PTSD is more likely to be caused by a severe stressor and must produce a response of ''intense fear, helplessness, or horror.'' In addition, the symptom picture of PTSD includes some features not present in adjustment disorder, such as reexperiencing the traumatic event, avoiding stimuli associated with the trauma, emotional numbing, and psycho-physiological arousal. However, there is a gray zone between classic cases of these two disorders that can promote uncertainty.

Not all cases that are initially, and accurately, diagnosed as adjustment disorder remain so. Some children develop a condition that meets the criteria for adjustment disorder, then never recover. When 6 months have gone by following the disappearance of the stressor and the child has not improved, an alternative diagnosis is often required. The question is then raised as to whether this should have been the diagnosis all along. In most cases there is no answer to that question.

TREATMENT

Even though some cases remit without intervention, adjustment disorder is not a minor condition requiring no treatment (Cole et al., 1991). It is painful for the patient and the patient's family, likely to worsen if the illness and its underlying causes are not addressed, and often responsive to vigorous and appropriate treatment.

Treatment begins with a thorough evaluation, including a search for physical causes for any physical symptoms present. Because adjustment disorder can mimic so many different psychiatric disorders, such other conditions must be sought in the hope of finding a specific treatment for the child's difficulties.

The next step is to remove the stressor, if possible. Treatment is greatly facilitated if the stressor can be eliminated or ameliorated. However, often that cannot be done. Divorce, parental death, irreversible physical damage, and similar traumas require adjustment rather than removal.

The core of treatment typically centers around both working with the child individually to address his or her concerns and working with the family about many of the same issues. The conceptual approach and techniques used, of course, depend in part on the age of the child and the therapist's assessment of what the patient is likely to tolerate and at what pace. Treatment generally should be brief and focused, with an emphasis on the child's adjustments to the difficulties he or she has experienced. The stressor must not be ignored, particularly if chronic; rather, the child should be allowed (or encouraged) to express fear, dismay, resentment, and anger. Avoid, except temporarily and for very well-determined reasons, fostering regression or the hope of a magical recovery. A supportive, problem-solving approach often works well, but an insight-oriented focus may be required if dynamic issues are prominent. It is occasionally possible to change the *meaning* of the trauma for the child and thereby decrease its significance as a stressor and improve the course. Individual therapy becomes indispensable when the family is destructive or has few resources upon which to draw. Finally, some techniques, such as relaxation therapy, are useful symptomatically (Platania-Solazzo, 1992).

Because the family is bound up in so many of the stressors faced by these children, as well as in the solutions attempted, family therapy is an equally essential mode of intervention. This also should be supportive and should pay attention to the parent's distress, if present, over their child's plight, as well as to their need to grieve. The family should be involved in any efforts at behavioral management and environmental manipulation, if they can participate constructively.

There is limited research in this area; treatment relies heavily on clinical judgment. However, work in a number of different settings, and with adjustment disorder patients of several different types, strongly suggests that active treatment of these children is both useful (Galante and Foa, 1986) and necessary (Ravenscroft, 1982).

OUTCOME AND FOLLOW-UP DATA

Adjustment disorder is conceptualized as a transient disorder. Prior diagnostic schemes referred to it with terms such as transient situational disorder, while DSM-IV expects that it usually lasts no longer than 6 months. If it goes beyond this period of time, another diagnosis generally is found. Thus, adjustment disorder should be considered time-limited. Of the few studies that exist of adjustment disorder, some suggest that its symptoms may indeed last a short time, even if the stressor is chronic (Kovacs et al., 1985).

It is also conceptualized as reversible: Theoretically, if the stressor is removed, the disorder should improve. This, however, is not always the case. Time and treatment both play roles in its disappearance (Fabrega et al., 1987), yet, not uncommonly, what was initially viewed as an adjustment disorder (and therefore transient) goes on to become something else (Andreasen and Hoenk, 1982). Andreasen's study suggests that perhaps one-half of adolescents originally diagnosed with adjustment disorder ultimately require another diagnosis. Chess concurs in that she found a tendency for more severe cases to become chronic (Chess and Thomas, 1984).

It is unclear what promotes chronicity. Suggestions include severe stress (and, thus, potentially a blending of the diagnosis with PTSD), chronic stress, and the "vulnerable child." This issue has been rarely studied.

Unfortunately, this condition also is not without its residua. If a patient responds to a stressor with a counterproductive and unhealthy coping mechanism, he or she runs the risk of making that mechanism permanent. Thus, the child who temporarily adjusts to a stressful situation by developing physical symptoms may find the sick role comforting in other unpleasant circumstances and come to rely on it habitually, much to the child's detriment.

RESEARCH DIRECTIONS

Adjustment disorder has not been well studied. In part, this reflects the vagueness and unreliability of the diagnosis, in part, its presumed reversibility, and in part, the sense that it is a minor and unimportant condition. None of these assumptions are completely accurate.

Although far from perfect, DSM-IV is helping to increase the diagnostic reliability of adjustment disorder and has made it a condition that can be studied because it can be identified. Equally important is that it is no longer considered a completely benign disorder (Horowitz, 1986). It doesn't necessarily get better when the stressor is removed, it can induce a serious although temporary suicidal state, and it can progress to a chronic, incapacitating state. More positively, it also may respond to treatment—professional interest and activity can be vital. Taken together, these features of adjustment disorder make it a condition thoroughly worth studying, and a valuable candidate for future research attention.

References

American Psychiatric Association: *Diagnostic and Statistical Manual of Mental Disorders* (2nd ed). Washington, DC, American Psychiatric Press, 1968.

American Psychiatric Association: *Diagnostic and Statistical Manual of Mental Disorders* (3rd ed). Washington, DC, American Psychiatric Press, 1980.

American Psychiatric Association: *Diagnostic and Statistical Manual of Mental Disorders* (3rd ed, rev). Washington, DC, American Psychiatric Press, 1987.

American Psychiatric Association: *Diagnostic and Statistical Manual of Mental Disorders* (4th ed). Washington, DC, American Psychiatric Press, 1994.

Andreasen NC, Hoenk PR: The predictive value of adjustment disorders: A follow-up study. *Am J Psychiatry* 139:584, 1982.

Andreasen NC, Wasek P: Adjustment disorders in adolescents and adults. *Arch Gen Psychiatry* 37:1166, 1980.

Chess S, Thomas A: *Origins and Evolution of Behavior Disorders.* New York, Brunner/Mazel, 1984.

Chess S, Thomas A: *Temperament in Clinical Practice.* New York, Guilford, 1986, p. 200.

Cole W, Turgay A, Mouldey G: Repeated use of psychiatric emergency services by children. *Can J Psychiatry* 36:739, 1991.

Fabrega H, Mezzich JE, Mezzich AC: Adjustment disorder as a marginal or transitional illness category in DSM-III. *Arch Gen Psychiatry* 44:567, 1987.

Galante R, Foa D: An epidemiological study of psychic trauma and treatment effectiveness for children after a natural disaster. *J Am Acad Child Psychiatry* 25:357, 1986.

Gleser GC, Green BL, Winget C: *Prolonged Psychosocial Effects of Disaster: A Study of Buffalo Creek.* New York, Academic Press, 1981.

Handford HA, Mayes SD, Mattison RE, et al: Child and parent reaction to the Three Mile Island nuclear accident. *J Am Acad Child Psychiatry* 25:346, 1986.

Hetherington EM, Cox M, Cox R: Effects of divorce on parents and children. In: Lamb M (ed): *Nontraditional Families: Parenting and Child Development.* Hillsdale, NJ, Erlbaum, 1982.

Horowitz MJ: Stress-response syndromes: A review of posttraumatic and adjustment disorders. *Hosp Community Psychiatry* 37:241, 1986.

Jacobson AM, Goldberg ID, Burns BJ, et al: Diagnosed mental disorder in children and use of health services in four organized health care settings. *Am J Psychiatry* 137:559, 1980.

Kaffman M, Elizur E: Bereavement responses of kibbutz and non-kibbutz children following the death of the father. *J Child Psychol Psychiatry* 24:435, 1983.

Kovacs M, Feinberg TL, Paulauskas S, et al: Initial coping responses and psychosocial characteristics of children with insulin-dependent diabetes mellitus. *J Pediatr* 106:827, 1985.

Lewinsohn PM, Hops H, Roberts RE, et al: Adolescent psychopathology: I. Prevalence and incidence of depression and other DSM-III-R disorders in high school students. *J Abnorm Psychol* 102:133, 1993.

Newcorn JH, Strain J: Adjustment disorder in children and adolescents. *J Am Acad Child Adolesc Psychiatry* 31:318, 1992.

Noshpitz JD, Coddington RD: *Stressors and the Adjustment Disorders.* New York, Wiley, 1990.

Platania-Solazzo A, Field TM, Blank J, et al: Relaxation therapy reduces anxiety in child and adolescent psychiatric patients. *Acta Paedopsychiatr* 55:115, 1992.

Pless IB, Rohmann KI: Chronic illness and its consequences. *J Pediatr* 79:351, 1971.

Rait D, Jacobsen PB, Lederberg MS, et al: Characteristics of psychiatric consultations in a pediatric cancer center. *Am J Psychiatry* 145:363, 1988.

Ravenscroft K: Psychiatric consultation to the child with acute physical trauma. *Am J Orthopsychiatry* 52:448, 1982.

Regier DA, Boyd JH, Burke JD, et al: One-month prevalence of mental disorders in the U.S.: Based on five epidemiologic catchment area (ECA) sites. *Arch Gen Psychiatry* 45:977, 1988.

Rey JM, Bashir MR, Schwarz M, et al: Oppositional disorder: Fact or fiction? *J Am Acad Child Adolesc Psychiatry* 27:157, 1988.

Runeson BS: Youth suicides unknown to psychiatric case providers. *Suicide Life Threat Behav* 22:494, 1992.

Rutter M: Stress, coping, and development: Some issues and some questions. In: Garmezy N, Rutter M (eds): *Stress, Coping, and Development in Children.* New York, McGraw-Hill, 1983.

Schreiber TJ, Johnson RL: The evaluation and treatment of adolescent overdoses in an adolescent medical service. *J Natl Med Assoc* 78:101, 1986.

Sirles EA, Smith JA, Kusama H: Psychiatric status of intrafamilial child sexual abuse victims. *J Am Acad Child Adolesc Psychiatry* 28:225, 1989.

Strain JJ, Newcorn J, Wolf D, et al: Considering changes in adjustment disorder. *Hosp Community Psychiatry* 44:13, 1993.

Thomsen PH: Child and adolescent psychiatric inpatients in Denmark. *Nord Psykiatr-Tidsskr* 44:337, 1990.

Van Eerdewegh MM, Bieri M, Parrilla RH, et al: The bereaved child. *Br J Psychiatry* 140:23, 1982.

Werry JS, Methven RI, Fitzpatrick J, et al: The interrater reliability of DSM-III in children. *J Abnorm Child Psychol* 11:341, 1983.

Wolfer, JA, Visintainer MA: Prehospital psychological preparation for tonsillectomy patients. *Pediatrics* 64:646, 1979.

Wood D, Halfon N, Scarlata D, et al: Impact of family relocation on children's growth, development, school function, and behavior. *JAMA* 270:1334, 1993.

Woolston JL: Theoretical considerations of the adjustment disorders. *J Am Acad Child Adolesc Psychiatry* 27:280, 1988.

68 BORDERLINE DISORDERS

Kenneth S. Robson, M.D.

The human mind delights in finding pattern—so much so that we often mistake coincidence or forced analogy for profound meaning.
—Stephen Jay Gould

Borderline disorders in childhood, unlike their adult counterpart, are elusive phenomena when subjected to clinical scrutiny. Nevertheless, clinicians continue to find the borderline child concept a useful one despite legitimate concerns about its scientific validity (Greenman et al., 1986; Shapiro, 1982; Towbin et al., 1993). The diagnostic specificity of borderline personality disorder in the adult nomenclature appears to be relatively sound and involves a vast literature of its own (Stone, 1980). However, the continuity between the adult disorder and childhood borderline states remains unclear (Greenman et al., 1986; Kestenbaum, 1982). This chapter restricts its primary focus to the prepubertal age group.

It is difficult to disentangle the definition of borderline disorders in childhood from its historical origins. As Greenman and her colleagues (1986) point out, "Definitions of the syndrome remain a confusing mixture of the concepts and language of developmental psychology, descriptive psychopathology and psychoanalytic theory." Like many other nosologic concepts in child and adolescent psychiatry, the borderline disorders began as a "trickle down" from general psychiatry's growing awareness of patients whose presentation was neither psychotic nor neurotic but somewhere in between or on the border. Initial clinical descriptions by Mahler et al. (1949), Weil (1953), Ekstein and Wallerstein (1954), and Geleerd (1968) placed these children in the spectrum of childhood psychosis or schizophrenia. All of these authors noted the rapid fluctuations in ego states, proneness to primitive regressions, disturbed interpersonal relationships, and severe, diffuse anxiety of panic proportions characteristic in these children.

Anna Freud presented a paper in 1956, entitled "The Assessment of Borderline Cases." She highlighted clinical features of deep levels of regression, massive developmental arrests, withdrawal of libido from the object world and displacement onto the body or self, inability to receive comfort from others, and specific ego defects such as poor reality testing, poor synthetic functions, and inadequate development of age-appropriate defense mechanisms (Freud, 1969). Engel (1963), in describing the psychological test patterns of these children, and Rosenfeld and Sprince (1963), Frijling-Schreuder (1970), and Towbin et al. (1993), all emphasized, among other behaviors, anxiety related to fears of annihilation or disintegration and extreme forms of loneliness. The latter authors noted that borderline children "feel like toddlers whose mothers are permanently out of the room." Elegant and still highly relevant clinical subgroupings, detailed below, were subsequently developed by Pine (1982).

Thoughtful clinicians, while convinced that borderline phenomenology in prepubertal children was genuine, remained concerned that the net was so wide that issues of validity could not be tested. Hence Vela et al. (1982), using the major published studies described above, developed a set of "consensus criteria" yielding one proposed route toward diagnostic specificity. Bemporad et al. (1982) made a similar effort to establish diagnostic criteria. Petti and Law (1982) and Greenman et al. (1986) utilized the Diagnostic Interview for Borderlines to demonstrate that adult criteria could be used to classify prepubertal children (see below). Greenman's research raises questions about the validity and utility of the term *borderline* in these children. Despite such doubts, however, most clinicians continue to define and describe their child patients in this way. Noting that both "childhood schizophrenia" and

"borderline syndrome of childhood" suffer from lack of diagnostic specificity and discontinuity with adult disorder bearing the same name, Towbin and his colleagues (1993) suggest multiple complex developmental disorder as a more accurate, rigorous, and testable nosologic entity; these authors established "first-cut" validity of their criteria, which conform most closely to DSM-IV in format.

PREVALENCE AND EPIDEMIOLOGY

Epidemiologic studies of borderline children are few in number and of varying quality. All such studies suffer from the lack of syndromic and diagnostic specificity noted above. As a result, cross-study comparisons are relatively unreliable.

Chiland and Lebovici (1977) studied an "unselected" population of 66 school children, ages 7–9, from a district in Paris. Nine of these children were diagnosed borderline, and by 16–20 years of age, 5 of these 9 index patients remained subject to psychotic decompensation. These authors were impressed with the "silence" of the clinical presentation in this nonclinical population. Dahl (1976) followed up 322 admissions to a child psychiatric inpatient service 20 years later and reported that 6 were initially diagnosed as borderline psychotic. Three of these 6, at 20 years, had had no further psychiatric admissions, 2 were diagnosed borderline schizophrenic, and 1 as a schizoid character disorder. Aarkrog (1977) reviewed 100 admissions to an adolescent psychiatric unit; 50 were diagnosed psychotic and 50 borderline. Fifty-three patients suffered from some childhood psychiatric problem(s), of which 21 were identified as borderline; the adolescent diagnoses of these 21 patients are not described. Wergeland (1979) studied 29 cases diagnosed borderline between 2 and 13 years of age; follow-up from 5 to 20 years later revealed that 5 remained borderline psychotic, 4 were manifestly psychotic, 6 were severely neurotic, 3 were moderately neurotic, and 11 were symptom-free. Kestenbaum (1982) describes case histories of 7 children diagnosed borderline in childhood; 14- to 30-year follow-up diagnoses included anxiety neurosis, schizophrenia, bipolar disorder, schizotypal personality disorder, schizoid personality disorder, schizoaffective disorder, and borderline personality disorder. Lofgren and her colleagues (1991) followed up a group of children diagnosed "borderline" 10–20 years earlier. There were no Axis I diagnoses of affective disorders or schizophrenia, but Axis II diagnoses were prevalent; only three of 19 subjects were diagnosed borderline personality disorder, but overall outcome was poor.

Taken as a group, these reports hardly satisfy rigorous epidemiologic standards. The most compelling point they make is how *variable* is the clinical outcome of these children. Whether this validity more accurately reflects the diversity of the initial populations or the discontinuity of the development psychopathology of these conditions awaits more carefully designed prospective studies. But the *improvement* of some of these children with time seems most important to understand.

CLINICAL DESCRIPTION

The earliest clinical descriptions of borderline children emphasized broad, common features rather than discrete signs and symptoms. The umbrella for these features, as described by Pine (1982), involves "failures in the developmental lines associated with major ego functions or central aspects of object relationship." Pine emphasizes malfunctions in the sense of reality and/or reality testing, failure in the development of signal anxiety, shifting levels of object relations, and too great a dependence of the child's ego structure on the presence of a primary object. He notes that these children seem "peculiar" and suggests that this quality reflects violations of age-linked, normal developmental expectations. Pine correctly observes that the panic anxiety many of these children experience is a major source of interference in opportunities for mastery of new developmental demands.

From his substantial experience, Pine (1982) then proposes a series of clinical presentations that characterize subgroupings of borderline children. These subtypes include

1. *Shifting levels of ego organization:* This group is characterized by rapid regressions to disordered thinking and affective withdrawal that are ego-syntonic.
2. *Internal disorganization in response to external disorganizers:* Usually the product of disorganized social environments (abuse and neglect, addiction, criminality, violence, etc.), these children may present with suicide/homicide attempts, hallucinations, or thought disorder but rapidly integrate when hospitalized and appear normal; their fragile ego functions seem intact only in structured settings free of environmental assault.
3. *Chronic ego deviance:* In this group of children, the primitive regressions noted above are present on an ongoing basis rather than in the face of stress; their regressive symptomatology is more or less fixed and may become heightened in a close relationship with a diagnostician/therapist.
4. *Incomplete internalization of psychosis:* Certain children, usually those with a psychotic mother, reactively present major regressions when separated from that parent and integrate upon reunion; the regressed behavior reflects primitive incorporation to maintain fusion with the parent.
5. *Ego limitation:* This group of inhibited, dull, culturally deprived children exhibits severe impoverishment of language, cognition, affect, and relatedness and ever-growing damage to developmental progress.
6. *Schizoid personality:* The hallmarks of this population are a "sharply constricted and undeveloped affective life . . . emotional distance in human relationships and preoccupation with their own . . . fantasy life" (Pine, 1982).
7. *Splitting of good and bad images of self and others:* Often "sweet and good" on the surface, these children reveal an inner preoccupation with hate and violence and homicidal and world-destruction fantasies that become frightening to the child or therapist because of the child's precarious control.

Pine is cited here in detail because his broad cameos ring true to clinical experience with borderline children. His typology provides an aerial view of the terrain, particularly as it relates to process and the emergence of the condition's contours over time.

The discrete clinical "building blocks" of which Pine's descriptions are composed also merit attention and have been described by several authors (Andrulonis, 1990; Greenman et al., 1986; Vela et al., 1982). Andrulonis assessed specific clinical phenomena against a control population; his data are carefully derived. His inventory closely parallels earlier clinical descriptions as well. Those findings that appeared to discriminate 45 borderline children from controls, in order of significance, included the following:

1. Anger/rage/temper tantrums
2. Primitive/aggressive responses on projectives
3. Excessive/primitive fantasy life
4. Depressed mother
5. Impulsivity
6. Aggression toward others
7. Peer problems
8. Attention deficit hyperactivity disorder (ADHD)
9. Early separation
10. Borderline mother
11. Use of phenothiazines
12. Speech problems
13. Adopted status
14. Depression/chronic sadness
15. Repetitive wish to be killed by someone
16. Overanxious

The items in this inventory were all significant at or beyond the .05 level of significance (Andrulonis, 1990); the first nine were significant at the .001 level of significance. The wide-angle lens of Pine and the close-up lens of Andrulonis provide a focused view of the clinical presentations of these children.

Towbin et al. (1993) condense and simplify the above descriptions in elaborating criteria for multiple complex developmental disorder that include:

1. Regulation of affective state and anxiety that is impaired beyond that seen in children of comparable mental age;
2. Consistent impairments in social behavior and sensitivity (compared with children of similar mental age);
3. Impaired cognitive processing (thinking disorder);
4. No diagnosis of autism;
5. Duration of symptoms longer than 6 months. These authors do not specify posttraumatic symptoms in their classification scheme despite increasing clinical evidence supporting their importance.

ETIOLOGY AND PATHOGENESIS

It is difficult, of course, to describe stable, reliable etiologic influences and pathogenetic processes for a concept/syndrome as blurred as borderline disorder of childhood. The population of children that meet an agreed-upon definition with exclusion criteria does not exist. And while adult criteria for borderline personality disorder in DSM-III can be used successfully with children (Greenman et al., 1986; Petti and Law, 1982), that classification has limited validity. Furthermore, etiologic terms such as "poor self-object differentiation" or "impaired separation-individuation" are used to describe the clinical disorder.

Rutter's (1988) flagship paper on the perspective of developmental psychopathology should ultimately help in sorting out etiologic signal from noise. Rutter defines this perspective as "a set of research approaches that capitalize on developmental variations and psychopathologic variations to ask questions about mechanisms and processes." He emphasizes the crucial importance, within this framework, of *continuities* and *discontinuities* rather than rate of disorder per se. The aim is to "go beyond the identification of risk factors to the delineation of the *chain of operations* by which these factors lead to disorder." Age is the key variable in the developmental vector, both in research strategies and data analysis. Different definitions of normality/abnormality are critical psychopathological variables, and, relevant to borderline disorders in childhood, there is no interest in what constitutes a "case." There is no prior assumption about continuity between normality and illness, but rather a focus on continuities/discontinuities themselves. Rutter notes that caseness becomes a "crucial feature of the research" and is not a methodologic problem to be circumvented. Interest also focuses on how to subdivide abnormalities and situation-specific versus pervasive behaviors. Finally, to understand the mechanisms and processes that lead to disorder, he emphasizes the importance of causal chains "in which the end product is the result of many linkages over time." Delineation of the mechanisms involved in these chains of indirect connections is the primary route toward causal questions. And since such linkages can permit varied outcomes, there is equal interest in discontinuities and continuities in behaviors and/or syndromes (Rutter, 1988).

Utilization of the perspective of developmental psychopathology in studying childhood borderline disorders would be extremely valuable in establishing etiologic and pathogenetic mechanisms. In the absence of such studies, existing research can be loosely grouped into biological, psychological/developmental, and familial/social arenas.

The significant presence of ADHD, neurodevelopmental delays, and unusual central nervous system sensitivities in populations of borderline children has led a number of authors to suggest that nonspecific ''organic'' factors contribute to outcome (Bemporad et al., 1982; Bergman and Escalona, 1949; Marcus et al.,1982; Milman, 1979). Since such neurodevelopmental vulnerabilities are represented in all the major disorders of childhood, only when studied as part of causal chains (Rutter, 1988) will their contributions become apparent. Genetically, in family studies of both adult and childhood borderline disorders, schizophrenia does not exceed normal population rates (Andrulonis, 1990; Stone, 1980). Conversely, affective disorders and alcohol/substance abuse are overrepresented in the families of certain borderline children. Andrulonis (1990) has identified a subgroup of such children, primarily girls, in which he feels the affective disorder is the major psychopathologic mechanism. Once again, experimental models utilizing causal chains are essential to the delineation of the role of all biological and genetic variables in the shaping of childhood borderline disorders.

The influence of psychological and developmental mechanisms in these disorders is widely described in the literature (Pine, 1982). Disturbances in the mother-child relationship leading to incomplete separation/individuation, splitting, and faulty development of ego functions have been suggested (Kernberg, 1982; Shapiro, 1978). Perhaps related, some authors have noted the presence of early separations in the lives of some borderline children (Andrulonis, 1990; Bradley, 1979); the mechanism(s) for such influence remain obscure. Hence Pine's (1982) descriptions of the internal psychological structure and developmental lines of borderline children wisely avoid implicating *specific* etiologic and pathogenetic issues.

Family studies shedding light on childhood borderline disorders have just begun. Combrinck-Graham (1989) reviews this perspective and discusses the important concepts within family systems theory, noting that ''the interaction between the self and the object world is constantly being regulated in the family; that it is not just a property of the individual's ego structure, formed in early life . . . but it is a continuing process.'' She emphasizes that individual dysfunction is ''inseparable from its context, the family context being the most immediate.'' Within this view an individual borderline child cannot exist. Key etiologic variables relate to concepts of faulty family boundaries, unpredictable proximity between family members, and lack of appropriate hierarchical structure. The family systems perspective is powerful. Furthermore, this perspective, like that of developmental psychopathology, involves process over time and interactive mechanisms; these two models have a good fit with each other. Since ''family strife'' (Rutter, 1988) contributes variance to most forms of child psychopathology, a research design involving both developmental psychopathology and family systems theory should prove useful. Goldman et al. (1993) documented significantly higher rates of psychopathology in the families of children and adolescents with borderline personality disorder. Depressive, substance abuse and antisocial disorders were prominent. Bleiberg (1994) emphasizes family disruption and early loss of parent figures in his review of this topic. And it is not surprising that ''family stability'' was the only predictor of good follow-up outcomes in the work of Lofgren et al. (1991).

Childhood sexual abuse is being reported with increasing frequency in adolescent and adult borderline patients (Herman et al., 1989; Westen et al., 1990). Other studies are beginning to emphasize the role of sexual abuse and incest in children diagnosed borderline (Bleiberg, 1994). Famularo et al. (1991) describe a high incidence of sexual abuse in such children and suggest that the diagnosis of borderline personality disorder in childhood may *represent* posttraumatic stress disorder. In such studies, the isolation of sexual abuse as an independent variable is virtually impossible, complicating the exclusive focus upon this aspect of disturbed family process. How such experiences are mediated over time, whether they are important per se or as part of dysfunctional family process, and how the role of trauma may lead to altered biological

structure are some of the issues that suitably designed research could address. Only with studies of this kind will our understanding of etiologic and pathogenetic mechanisms in borderline children advance.

DIFFERENTIAL DIAGNOSIS

It should be apparent that differential diagnostic considerations are exceedingly complicated with borderline children. Earliest efforts relied upon intuition and the ''feeling'' of the clinical observer. Vela et al. (1982) developed six ''consensus criteria'' of common clinical features in major studies to date. These criteria include disturbed interpersonal relationships; disturbances in the sense of reality; excessive intense anxiety; excessive severely impulsive behavior; ''neurotic-like'' symptoms; and uneven/distorted development. Bemporad et al. (1982), on the basis of their experience with 24 latency-age children, proposed diagnostic criteria that involved fluctuation of functioning, nature and extent of anxiety, thought content and process, relationships to others, and lack of control. The overlaps between these two studies are evident. What is also evident is the breadth of the diagnostic net and the lack of both validity and specificity that such breadth carries with it. Of equal diagnostic concern are the variable outcomes of children diagnosed using these criteria (Kestenbaum, 1982). The importance of the developmental psychopathology model to this problem is strikingly clear.

Andrulonis (1990) has followed a population of 45 children initially studied at 5–12 years of age who met DSM-III and Gunderson criteria for borderline personality disorder. This group was matched with 45 control children. The primary behaviors differentiating the borderline children from control subjects are noted earlier in this chapter. Aggression and rage, ADHD, excessive use of fantasy, impulsivity, and poor relationships were especially significant. These behaviors do relate to the Vela et al. (1982) and Bemporad et al. (1982) criteria. Andrulonis followed this population and subdivided his sample into the following subgroups: (*a*) a developmental group characterized by early emotional trauma, abuse, neglect, and faulty separation/individuation; (*b*) an affective disorders group, and (*c*) a group where ADHD/learning disabilities and episodic dyscontrol were primary. Andrulonis believes that girls with borderline personality disorder are more likely to evolve toward affective disorders in later life, while boys evolve toward episodic dyscontrol syndromes and substance abuse.

Other reports, however, call the validity of the borderline diagnosis in childhood into question (Greenman et al., 1986; Gualtieri et al., 1983). Greenman and her colleagues completed a retrospective study of 86 hospitalized children, ages 6–12, and successfully differentiated a borderline and nonborderline group using a modified version of the Diagnostic Interview for Borderlines (DIB-R). However, these authors concluded that the ''relative paucity of significant differences between the children identified as borderline and . . . nonborderline raises questions about the validity and utility of the term.'' Petti and Vela (1990) suggest that classification of these children into at least two subgroups—borderline personality disorder/borderline spectrum and schizotypal personality disorder/autism/schizophrenia spectrum—is supportable. The diagnostic classification of Towbin et al. (1993) has already been described and appears to have merit as both a clinical and research tool.

A word should be said about other diagnostic tools used with these children. Psychological testing (Engel, 1963; Leichtman and Shapiro, 1982) reveals and highlights the clinical features described above. Such testing does not increase diagnostic specificity. No valid and reliable laboratory tests are at present available.

A major confounding problem in all considerations of differential diagnosis is that of developmental process and the passage of time, as discussed by Rutter (1988). As Shapiro (1982) has emphasized and Greenman and her colleagues demonstrated (1986), the diagnosis has to mean something to make a difference. At present there are too many pathways that children diagnosed as borderline may take into adult life to be certain about the scientific value of the nosologic use of that term.

TREATMENT

Despite diagnostic uncertainty, there is a seriously disturbed pool of highly dysfunctional children and families often labeled borderline whom clinicians must treat. Problems in the management of these children are similar in some respects to those encountered in treating children with learning dysfunctions (disabilities); the awesome armamentarium of diagnostic discussions and methodologies available contributes relatively little to altering the narrow but important range of existing therapeutic interventions.

Elsewhere (Robson, 1994) this author has proposed a model of therapeutic intervention based upon enhancing empathic capacities and reducing overstimulation and lack of modulation in the caretaking environment. The psychotherapies (especially family work), pharmacotherapies, and milieu/behavioral therapies converge around those dual goals. Of course, this approach needs linkage to specific symptom modification, so essential to managed care providers. But as child clinicians know, many aspects of effective treatment(s) require time. And in the absence of outcome studies, the choice of intensive, individual child psychotherapy requires careful scrutiny. It is this author's opinion that family-oriented interventions are superior in cost-effectiveness, benefit to the patient, and diminished risk of further undermining parental self-esteem; in this enterprise parents are viewed as colleagues. The therapeutic work focuses upon the issues discussed by Combrinck-Graham (1989).

Pharmacologic interventions specific to these children are reviewed by Petti (1982). Since publication of that report, little has appeared in the literature to suggest drug/symptom specificity. There are reliable data supporting antidepressants' lack of efficacy in managing affective disorders in children and adolescents (N. Ryan, personal communication, 1989). Controlled studies exploring the use of β-blockers and/or opium antagonists in modifying rage attacks and violent impulsiveness

would be helpful. Certainly, the judicious use of all pharmacologic agents approved for children may be useful when clinically indicated and safely administered.

The use of hospital settings for such children seems mainly justified in the management of crises such as suicide/homicide risk or acute psychotic regressions. In some instances, brief hospitalization may accelerate diagnostic assessment and integrated treatment planning. On the other hand, many if not most of these children require and appear to benefit from structured day programs, with behavior management a central part of the therapeutic milieu (Hanson et al., 1982). Newer studies underline the critical importance of early acquisition of self-control in predicting good developmental outcome (Mischel et al., 1989.) Given the impulsiveness of most borderline children, a focus on self-control in all areas of therapeutic effort seems especially important. Long-term work appears essential (Bleiberg, 1994; Towbin et al., 1993).

RESEARCH DIRECTIONS

Whether using the borderline concept in childhood moves the clinical knowledge base ahead is in question. However, that issue seems less significant than the children (and families) it so labels. In the author's opinion, priority should be given to (*a*) studies involving the developmental psychopathology model (Rutter, 1988) that focus upon individual symptoms (Zeitlin, 1986) and family context (Combrinck-Graham, 1989) in elucidating causal chains that lead to disorder and (*b*) rigorous and unbiased efforts to document therapeutic efficacy and outcome using the least resources to do the most, where and when that is possible. Convincing data that demonstrate significant improvement in the developmental course of these children over time should encourage both clinicians and researchers to bring hope and energy to bear on these children's lives.

References

Aarkrog T: Borderline and psychotic adolescents: Borderline symptomatology from childhood—Actual therapeutic approach. *J Youth Adolesc* 6:187–197, 1977.

Andrulonis PA: Borderline personality subcategories in children. Paper presented at the Annual Meeting of the American Psychiatric Association, New York, May 1990.

Bemporad JR, Smith HF, Hanson G, et al: Borderline syndromes in childhood: Criteria for diagnosis. *Am J Psychiatry* 139:596, 1982.

Bergman P, Escalona SK: Unusual sensitivities in very young children. *Psychoanal Study Child* 3–4: 333, 1949.

Bleiberg E: Borderline disorders in children and adolescents: The concept, the diagnosis, and the controversies. *Bull Menninger Clin* 58:169, 1994.

Bradley SJ: The relationship of early maternal separation to borderline personality in children and adolescents: A pilot study. *Am J Psychiatry* 134:424, 1979.

Chiland C, Lebovici S: Borderline or prepsychotic conditions in childhood—A French point of view. In: Hartocollis P (ed): *Borderline Personality Disorders.* New York, International Universities Press, 1977.

Combrinck-Graham L: The borderline syndrome in childhood: A family systems approach. *J Psychother Fam* 5:31–34, 1989.

Dahl V: A follow-up study of a child psychiatric clientele with special regard to the diagnosis of psychosis. *Acta Psychiatr Scand* 54:106, 1976.

Ekstein R, Wallerstein J: Observations on the psychology of borderline and psychotic children. *Psychoanal Study Child* 9:344, 1954.

Engel M: Psychological testing of borderline children. *Arch Gen Psychiatry* 8:426, 1963.

Famularo R, Kinscherff R, Fenton T: Posttraumatic stress disorder among children clinically diagnosed as borderline personality disorder. *J Nerv Ment Dis* 179:428, 1991.

Freud A: The assessment of borderline cases. In: *The Writings of Anna Freud* (Vol 5). New York, International Universities Press, 1969.

Frijling-Schreuder ECM: Borderline states in children. *Psychoanal Study Child* 24:307, 1970.

Geleerd E: Borderline states in childhood and adolescence. *Psychoanal Study Child* 13:279, 1968.

Goldman SJ, D'Angelo EJ, DeMaso DR: Psychopathology in the families of children and adolescents with borderline personality disorder. *Am J Psychiatry* 150:1832, 1993.

Greenman DA, Gunderson JG, Cane M, et al: An examination of the borderline diagnosis in children. *J Psychiatry* 143:998, 1986.

Gualtieri T, Koriath U, Van Bourgondien ME: Borderline children. *J Autism Dev Disord* 13:67, 1983.

Hanson G, Bemporad JR, Smith HF: The day and residential treatment of the borderline child. In: Robson KS (ed): *The Borderline Child.* New York, McGraw-Hill, 1982, p. 235.

Herman JL, Perry JC, van der Kolk BA: Childhood trauma in borderline personality disorder. *Am J Psychiatry* 146:490, 1989.

Kernberg PF: Borderline conditions: Childhood and adolescent aspects. In: Robson KS (ed): *The Borderline Child.* New York, McGraw-Hill, 1982, p. 101.

Kestenbaum CJ: The borderline child at risk for major psychiatric disorder in adult life. In: Robson KS (ed): *The Borderline Child.* New York, McGraw-Hill, 1982, p. 49.

Leichtman M, Shapiro S: A clinical approach to the psychological testing of borderline children. In:

Robson KS (ed): *The Borderline Child.* New York, McGraw-Hill, 1982, p. 121.

Lofgren DP, Bemporad J, King J, et al: A prospective follow-up study of so-called borderline children. *Am J Psychiatry* 148:1541, 1991.

Mahler M, Ross J, Defries Z: Clinical studies in benign and malignant cases of childhood psychosis. *Am J Orthopsychiatry* 19:295, 1949.

Marcus J, Ovsiew F, Hans S: Neurological dysfunction in borderline children. In: Robson KS (ed): *The Borderline Child.* New York, McGraw-Hill, 1982, p. 171.

Milman DH: Minimal brain dysfunction in childhood: Outcome in late adolescence and early adult years. *J Clin Psychiatry* 12:371, 1979.

Mischel W, Shoda Y, Rodrigues ML: Delay of gratification in children. *Science* 244:933, 1989.

Petti TA: Psychopharmacologic treatment of borderline children. In: Robson KS (ed): *The Borderline Child.* New York, McGraw-Hill, 1982, p. 235.

Petti TA, Law W: Borderline psychotic behavior in hospitalized children: Approaches to assessment and treatment. *J Am Acad Child Psychiatry* 21:197, 1982.

Petti TA, Vela RM: Borderline disorders of childhood: An overview. *J Am Acad Child Adolesc Psychiatry* 29:327, 1990.

Pine F: A working nosology of borderline syndromes in children. In: Robson KS (ed): *The Borderline Child.* New York, McGraw-Hill, 1982, p. 83.

Robson KS: *Manual of Clinical Child Psychiatry,* Revised Edition, Washington, DC, American Psychiatric Press, 1994.

Rosenfeld SK, Sprince MP: An attempt to formulate the concept "borderline." *Psychoanal Study Child* 18:603, 1963.

Rutter M: Epidemiological approaches to developmental psychopathology. *Arch Gen Psychiatry* 45: 486, 1988.

736 Section VI / Syndromesdefault

Shapiro ER: The psychodynamics and developmental psychology of the borderline patient: A review of the literature. *Am J Psychiatry* 135:1305, 1978.

Shapiro T: The borderline syndrome in children: A critique. In: Robson KS (ed): *The Borderline Child*. New York, McGraw-Hill, 1982, p. 11.

Stone MH: *The Borderline Syndromes*. New York, McGraw-Hill, 1980.

Towbin KE, Dykens EM, Pearson GS, et al: Conceptualizing "borderline syndrome of childhood" and "childhood schizophrenia" as a developmental disorder. *J Am Acad Child Adolesc Psychiatry* 32: 775, 1993.

Vela R, Gottlieb W, Gottlieb E: Borderline syndromes in childhood: A critical review. In: Robson KS (ed): *The Borderline Child*. New York, McGraw-Hill, 1982, p. 31.

Weil A: Certain severe disturbances of ego development in children. *Psychoanal Study Child* 8:271, 1953.

Wergeland H: A follow-up study of 29 borderline psychotic children 5 to 20 years after discharge. *Acta Psychiatr Scand* 60:465, 1979.

Westen D, Ludolph P, Misle B, et al: Physical and sexual abuse in adolescent girls with borderline personality disorder. *Am J Orthopsychiatry* 60:55, 1990.

Zeitlin H: *The Natural History of Psychiatric Disorders in Childhood*. New York, Oxford University Press, 1986.default

69 ALCOHOL AND DRUG ABUSE IN ADOLESCENTS

Roger L. Cambor, M.D., and Robert B. Millman, M.D.

The use of psychoactive drugs to alter perceptions, feeling states, or behavior is common among young people in Western society. Although the overall use of mind-altering substances among high school age adolescents has fluctuated over the past two decades, studies indicate that from 50% to 80% of school-age children use licit and illicit drugs for recreational (nonmedicinal) purposes. By the age of 18, in the United States, most young people have used drugs to "get high."

For many people experimentation with psychoactive substances may be short-lived and have no psychosocial or medical sequelae. In other cases the drug use may be acutely dangerous or likely to lead to more destructive drug-taking patterns. The clinician asked to evaluate or treat an adolescent with a substance abuse problem must attempt to distinguish normal patterns of experimentation from patterns of abuse that suggest serious abuse or dependency. In a substantial minority of cases, initial experimentation may lead to a pattern of repetitive use marked by phenomena such as tolerance, withdrawal (discussed more fully in the following section), and/or multiple substance use with resultant deterioration in functioning. Serious disability may result from the acute effects of the abused drug, as in the case of an overdose, or from medical conditions related to drug toxicity or the route of administration (such as toxic or viral hepatitis and HIV spectrum disorders). Rates of accidental deaths, homicides, and suicides are increased among drug users (Blum and Richards, 1979; Hein et al., 1979). Psychiatric disorders may be exacerbated or possibly precipitated by drug abuse. Tobacco and alcohol use patterns established in childhood and adolescence lead to the morbidity and premature death associated with lung cancer and alcohol-related diseases. Adolescents who become chemically dependent often experience disruption of relationships with family, teachers, and "straight" peers and deterioration of school and work performance. Alienation from the non-drug-abusing social world can progress to an extent wherein the adolescent lives to sustain his or her habit through drug sales or other criminal activities and is alone except for the company of fellow users.

The first section of this chapter covers terminology, epidemiology, predisposing factors, and patterns of drug abuse among children and adolescents. A second section describes issues relevant to diagnosis and some general principles regarding treatment. A third section offers a brief overview of the pharmacology, acute and chronic effects, and specific treatment considerations for the various categories of abused drugs. The final section of the chapter discusses general principles regarding recognition, referral, and treatment of adolescents with drug problems.

DEFINITIONS

Drug abuse refers to the taking of a psychoactive substance in a manner that violates current medical, legal, religious, or social practices. In DSM-III-R (American Psychiatric Association, 1987), psychoactive substance abuse is characterized as maladaptive and lasting for a period greater than 1 month and is distinguished from psychoactive substance dependence by lack of withdrawal symptoms (Table 69.1). The DSM-III-R comments that abuse patterns are most likely to be found in those recently commencing drug use and to involve substances such as cannabis, cocaine, and psychedelics. Abuse is a useful concept which describes behavior seen among addicts early in the history of their drug use and in nonaddicted individuals for brief periods often during adolescence, young adulthood, or in the context of stressful life events. Many individuals who abuse drugs do not progress to addiction or dependence. Social deviance related to drug use appears to be a useful criterion for diagnosing drug abuse as it appears to hold true for different cultures (Woody, 1993).

The clinical distinction between abuse and dependence in DSM-III-R was somewhat vague, since the criteria were taken from the dependence definition. The authors of DSM-IV have attempted to optimize the definition of abuse, by dropping the requirement for the continuous presence of symptoms for a 1-month period or longer, and by expanding the criteria for Psychoactive Substance Abuse to include legal problems stemming from the drug use, and problems fulfilling social role obligations. According to DSM-III-R and DSM-IV, one cannot resume "abusing" after becoming "dependent." Thus the same pattern of substance use might be classified as either abuse or dependence in a given individual at different time points. Although the DSM-IV criteria for drug dependence will be the dominant nosologic system for academic (and

Table 69.1. Criteria for Substance Abuse

A. A maladaptive pattern of substance use leading to clinically significant impairment or distress, as manifested by one (or more) of the following, occurring within a 12-month period:
  (1) recurrent substance use resulting in a failure to fulfill major role obligations at work, school, or home (e.g., repeated absences or poor work performance related to substance use; substance-related absences, suspensions, or expulsions from school; neglect of children or household)
  (2) recurrent substance use in situations in which it is physically hazardous (e.g., driving an automobile or operating a machine when impaired by substance use)
  (3) recurrent substance-related legal problems (e.g., arrests for substance-related disorderly conduct)
  (4) continued substance use despite having persistent or recurrent social or interpersonal problems caused or exacerbated by the effects of the substance (e.g., arguments with spouse about consequences of intoxication, physical fights)
B. The symptoms have never met the criteria for Substance Dependence for this class of substance.

Reprinted with permission for the *DSM-IV*. Copyright 1994, American Psychiatric Association.default insurance purposes), there have been no studies to validate the criteria among adolescents; other competing models of dependence may be more useful (Bukstein and Kaminer, 1994).

In general, addiction, or psychoactive substance dependence, denotes a pattern of substance use and related activities that is pervasive, destructive, or disabling to the user and beyond his or her control. In order to merit the DSM-III-R diagnosis of psychoactive substance dependence, an individual had to satisfy at least three of nine criteria presented. The authors of DSM-IV have proposed a more restrictive and probably more useful definition of Psychoactive Substance Dependence, which retains criteria from DSM-III-R relating to compulsive drug use and overwhelming involvement with the drug, while requiring evidence of physiologic dependence in the form of tolerance and withdrawal. In the physiologically dependent substance user, one sees upon cessation of drug use a predictable constellation of autonomic or other physical signs, accompanied by psychological and behavioral changes. This phenomenon is termed the withdrawal syndrome and is relatively specific for the various classes of abused drugs. Protracted withdrawal symptoms may be seen for several weeks to months, and may closely resemble other psychiatric conditions, particularly depressive disorders, anxiety states, and even psychotic disorders. Clinicians should be aware of the possibility of a protracted withdrawal syndrome in cases of recently detoxified addicts with psychiatric symptoms, yet must also be cognizant of the comorbidity of Psychoactive Substance Dependence with other Axis 1 disorders. Psychiatric symptoms in withdrawing addicts may require prompt intervention, but may respond differently to pharmacologic management, and may have different implications for treatment (Woody, 1993). Most protracted abstinence states resolve within 6 weeks, hence clinicians should wait before assigning other psychiatric diagnoses except in cases where another Axis 1 diagnosis was clearly established prior to the current substance use episode.

Tolerance to a particular substance refers to the diminution of psychoactive effects at a given dose over time. The user then requires an increase in dosage or frequency of administration to achieve a particular state of intoxication or to alleviate withdrawal symptoms. Substances producing tolerance to other substances, usually within a class (e.g., sedatives), are said to exhibit cross-tolerance (Millman, 1979).

Detoxification is the term applied to the procedures and medications involved in withdrawing patients from the drug they are dependent upon. Hospitals, outpatient clinics, sobering up stations, or other drug treatment facilities may be detoxification sites, as can be the home. Abrupt cessation of drug use can precipitate a withdrawal syndrome in the physiologically dependent individual. In the case of alcohol and the sedative drugs, delirium and life-threatening seizures can ensue. Detoxification from these substances is best managed in a controlled medical setting: An equivalent amount of cross-tolerant drug is substituted for the abused substance and then is gradually tapered. Opiate detoxification can be managed in a similar manner, and although the withdrawal syndrome is not life threatening, it may be sufficiently uncomfortable or anxiety producing to precipitate rash action, including suicide attempts. The guiding principle of drug detoxification involves gradual dosage decreases to prevent fulminant withdrawal symptoms and minimize discomfort (Table 69.2).

Psychoactive Substance Dependence tends to be chronic and relapsing in its course. The first 3–12 months are a critical period during which there are often relapses to substance use prior to sustained abstinence, which is termed recovery or remission. DSM-IV distinguishes between early and sustained remission. Sustained remission can be said to occur only after the addict has not met any of the dependence criteria for a full year.

EPIDEMIOLOGY

The epidemiology of adolescent drug abuse in America during the past 25 years resembles a large puzzle with most of the pieces missing. What we do know about the incidence and prevalence of drug abuse

Table 69.2. Criteria for Substance Dependence

A maladaptive pattern of substance use, leading to clinically significant impairment or distress, as manifested by three (or more) of the following, occuring at any time in the same 12-month period:

(1) tolerance, as defined by either of the following:
   (a) a need for markedly increased amounts of the substance to achieve intoxication or desired effect
   (b) markedly diminished effect with continued use of the same amount of the substance

(2) withdrawal, as manifested by either of the following:
   (a) the characteristic withdrawal syndrome for the substance (refer to Criteria A and B of the criteria sets for withdrawal from the specific substances)
   (b) the same (or a closely related) substance is taken to relieve or avoid withdrawal symptoms

(3) the substance is often taken in larger amounts or over a longer period than was intended

(4) there is a persistent desire or unsuccessful efforts to cut down or control substance use

(5) a great deal of time is spent in activities necessary to obtain the substance (e.g., visiting multiple doctors or driving long distances), use the substance (e.g., chain-smoking), or recover from its effects

(6) important social, occupational, or recreational activities are given up or reduced because of substance use

(7) the substance use is continued despite knowledge of having a persistent or recurrent physical or psychological problem that is likely to have been caused or exacerbated by the substance (e.g., current cocaine use despite recognition of cocaine-induced depression, or continued drinking despite recognition that an ulcer was made worse by alcohol consumption)

Specify if:
With Physiological Dependence: evidence of tolerance or withdrawal (i.e., either Item 1 or 2 is present)
Without Physiological Dependence: no evidence of tolerance or withdrawal (i.e., neither Item 1 nor 2 is present)

Course specifiers (see text for definitions):
Early Full Remission
Early Partial Remission
Sustained Full Remission
Sustained Partial Remission
On Agonist Therapy
In a Controlled Environment

Reprinted with permission from the *DSM-IV*. Copyright 1994, American Psychiatric Association.

among this cohort comes from probability surveys such as the National High School Senior Survey, a well-mounted survey of 135 high schools and approximately 17,000 young people (Johnston, O'Malley, and Bachman, 1990, 1993, 1994). Studies of treatment programs, emergency room reports (Drug Abuse Warning Network or DAWN), arrest rates and death rates, and the National Household Surveys are additional sources of epidemiologic data. A major problem is the use of retrospective self-report data, given that most drug use is illicit and/or deemed unacceptable by parents, teachers, and many peers. Surveys using self-report data may provide conservative estimates of use for all classes of drugs due to underreporting. Moreover, drug users as a group tend to have difficulties in school: Antisocial behavior, truancy, and school failure are increased in proportion to involvement with drugs. It is thus unlikely that heavy drug users of high school age, particularly those from the inner city, are proportionately represented in surveys such as the National High School Senior Survey.

Changes in patterns of drug use, such as the explosion of crack abuse in the inner cities, often happens rapidly, making surveys outdated by the time of publication. Moreover, the categorizing of data, such as grouping by age, often varies from study to study, precluding comparison of one study to another. Most epidemiologic studies do not provide data to distinguish compulsive from noncompulsive patterns of use and are therefore of limited relevance to the clinician. Emergency room visit data, arrest rates, and drug-related deaths (though they are the only way to get at rarer behaviors such as heroin abuse) pertain to the failures among drug abusers; it is difficult to know how many controlled users there are. With these limitations in mind, it is nonetheless possible to make some generalizations regarding drug use patterns among adolescents over the past 20–30 years.

During the past 30 years, illicit drug use in America has evolved from an infrequent phenomenon (seen primarily in members of inner city minority groups and among artists and entertainers) through a period of epidemic increase to the current situation: higher endemic levels of use in all socioeconomic groups and in all regions of the country. This trend began as an increase in marijuana use during the mid-1960s, primarily among urban males. Use then spread to more rural areas and to females. Following the initial increase in marijuana use, a rapid increase in drug use of all types, including psychedelics, opiates, sedatives, stimulants, and cocaine, occurred from 1967 to 1977. By 1979 illicit drug use had peaked, with a lifetime prevalence rate of 65% among high school seniors for use of any illicit drug; use has fallen since then (Johnston et al., 1988).

Marijuana is by far the most frequently abused illicit substance. The annual prevalence rate for marijuana use among seniors dropped from 51% in 1979 to 23.9% in 1991, only to rise to a level of 26% from 1991 to 1993. The proportion of daily users shows a similar pattern, having decreased from 10.7% in 1978 to 2% in 1991, then rising to a level of 2.4% among seniors in the class of 1993 (Johnston et al., 1993, 1994). Daily marijuana use statistics represent individuals involved in compulsive marijuana use; daily marijuana use increases the risk of further experimentation with harder drugs and is frequently elicited in the histories of those who develop other drug abuse problems. Between ages 10 to 12 young people often initiate drug use with beer and wine; they progress to marijuana somewhat later, then may experiment with other harder drugs. In later adolescence or young adulthood, there is often a return to the drugs that were used earlier, perhaps in response to the increased appreciation of danger associated with particular drug classes (Kandel and Logan, 1984). The recent increase in the prevalence of daily marijuana use among seniors is thus worrisome, and is consistent with several other indicators, suggesting that American youth is entering another phase of increasing drug use.

Increases in the use of stimulants, inhalants, and especially the use of LSD and other hallucinogens have occurred in parallel with the increase in marijuana use; this trend occurs in 8th, 10th, and 12th grade students. The perception of risk associated with illicit drug use has fallen correspondingly during the past 2 years, reflecting a softening of attitudes, associated with increasing patterns of drug use among high school students (Johnston et al., 1994).

Use of the licit substances alcohol and tobacco exceeds use of any of the other classes of drugs and has remained relatively stable over the past 10 years. The lifetime prevalence of alcohol use among seniors is currently 88%. Daily prevalence declined from 6.9% to 5% between 1979 and 1985 (Johnston et al., 1986) but has remained stable since then. More troubling is the reported frequency of heavy drinking (five or more drinks in a row in the preceding 2 weeks), which remains at the 1975 level of 37%. Daily cigarette use has remained at 20% since 1981, which is discouraging in view of the downward trends of other drug use as well as vigorous legislative and media efforts to reduce smoking rates (Johnston et al., 1990).

Changes in the epidemiology of cocaine and crack cocaine use require further comment. Cocaine use increased among high school seniors by twofold over the years 1976–1979 (annual prevalence increased from 6% to 12%), then remained stable until 1985, when significant increases in annual and monthly use were observed. In the period from 1986 to 1988, annual use dropped from 13% to 8% and has continued to decline. Cocaine use has not increased over the past two years, however, the overall increase in illicit drug use in combination with more permissive attitudes regarding drug taking may foreshadow a pending rise in the rate of cocaine use among adolescents, and should concern those involved with health issues among the young.

It is the authors' impression that the statistical decline is not reflective of the seriousness of cocaine and crack use in youthful populations. Crack cocaine probably became available in 1985 or the early part of

1986. During this time an increasing number of respondents in the National High School Senior Survey reported smoking cocaine (Johnston, 1993). Those reporting daily use of cocaine, or difficulty controlling use, doubled in number. The last survey reported a leveling off of crack use. According to the National Household Survey, annual prevalence rates of crack rose to 4% in 1985 and 1987, then declined to 3.1% in 1988. Crack use has become concentrated among inner city inhabitants, many of whom are dropouts or otherwise inaccessible to high school surveys. Yet the impact of cocaine and crack use on the inner city is increasing. Records of emergency room visits related to crack increased by 10-fold in Manhattan from 1985 to 1987; the number of neonates testing positive for cocaine in New York City increased 5-fold from 1986 to 1988; 60% of those arrested in Washington, D.C., tested positive for cocaine in 1988, an increase of 20% from 1986; and violent crimes in association with cocaine and crack are on the increase. Clinical research studies with cocaine users indicate that prices have decreased by as much as 50% to 75% over the past 5 years as the drug has become increasingly available; a gram of cocaine sold for $25 to $50 at the time of this writing. In certain inner city minority areas, cocaine and crack use have become remarkably prevalent. The spread of crack into the suburbs of major cities and more recently to rural areas has not been documented in a major study, though it is unquestionably occurring. The crack cocaine phenomenon illustrates the limitations of current epidemiological perspectives on substance abuse.

Although the use of cocaine and crack has declined among high school students since the late 1980s, overall drug use has increased. The rate of marijuana use rose sharply from 1991 to 1993, along with the increased rates of stimulant and psychedelic use. Cigarette smoking also increased during this time, while the perceived danger of drug use decreased among high school students (Johnston, Bachman, and O'Malley, 1994). An increasing concern in many urban areas is the renewed interest in heroin, which appears to be replacing crack as a drug of choice among adolescents and young adults.

FACTORS ASSOCIATED WITH DRUG USE IN ADOLESCENTS

The fact that some adolescents develop drug problems while most do not, despite phases of experimentation with drugs, is of clinical and theoretical interest. Many studies have identified variables distinguishing drug-using from non-drug-using populations. These factors comprise a wide spectrum, ranging from interpersonal factors such as attitudes, cognitive style, personality, and development, to family dynamics, peer group orientation, and larger trends in terms of societal values and media influences. Unfortunately, the available research is of limited usefulness due to methodological shortcomings. At present we do not understand how these many variables and risk factors interact within an individual. Nor is it possible to say which among several contributing factors is most important or necessary for the development of a drug problem. Similarly, it is impossible to predict who will develop a drug problem at some point in his or her life. Prospective longitudinal studies are needed to address such issues. Despite the limitations of our present knowledge, it is important that the clinician be aware of the determinants of drug use when evaluating patients presenting with drug problems.

Developmental Factors

In the course of normal development, the adolescent undergoes profound changes in self outlook and in views of those in the outside world. The adolescent's body matures, developing secondary sexual characteristics during puberty. The influence of peers increases, while parental influences tend to diminish or are actively rebelled against. The adolescent develops a capacity to reason and make decisions. Drug use may be associated with any of the dynamic factors seen in normal adolescent development.

Cognitively, the adolescent progresses from what Piaget termed a stage of concrete operations (ages 8–11) to the stage of formal operations (age 12 and over). As the adolescent's thinking becomes more abstract and hypothetical, the range of potential behaviors to explore expands. The adolescent perceives the inconsistencies and irrationalities of adults and can rationalize behaviors that adults consider deviant (teachers or parents are seen as ''out of touch'' or hypocritical). Parental influence in matters of life-style diminishes during this period, while concerns about the esteem of peers, particularly the need to conform within a peer group, become predominant. This has direct relevance to cigarette, alcohol, and other drug use. Although the adolescent knows that his or her parents don't approve of smoking cigarettes, cutting classes, listening to loud rock music, or taking drugs, it may be more important at this time to be popular and have a feeling of ''fitting in.'' The adolescent may use the parents' own behaviors as examples justifying his or her actions, or may refer to other adults with views similar to his or her own. Typically the need to conform within a peer group peaks at mid-adolescence, then diminishes. However, there is great variability among individuals. Within a given family certain members may be more susceptible to peer pressure than others.

Psychological Factors

Many studies have documented the presence of abnormal psychological characteristics in adolescent substance abusers. Drug abusers have been found to possess low self-esteem (Braucht et al., 1973), a high degree of dissatisfaction and pessimism (Coan, 1973), a greater need for social approval, and less social confidence. They tend to be more anxious, more impulsive, and less assertive than individuals without drug problems (Jarvik et al., 1977; Williams, 1973). Drug abusers have been described as having an external locus of control (they believe that life is controlled by external factors or forces such as chance or fate) (Williams, 1973). Drug users may tend to enter into adult roles earlier than nonusers. Despite these suggestive findings, no data from prospective studies have identified psychodynamic patterns or psychopathologic syndromes specific to drug users. Hence there is no evidence supporting the notion of an ''addictive personality'' (Millman, 1978; Zinberg, 1975). In evaluating the adolescent with a drug problem, it is necessary to identify underlying personality characteristics and areas of psychological conflict. The drug use is then explored in terms of its meaning to the patient.

Antisocial behaviors are often seen in drug using adolescents and young adults, and the psychiatric syndromes of conduct disorder and antisocial personality disorder have long been associated with drug and alcohol use. Substance abuse may necessitate antisocial behaviors (which are secondary in many cases), may influence or be influenced by the course of the conduct disorder, or may function as a risk factor for antisocial personality disorder (ASP) in conduct disordered patients (Bukstein, Brent, and Kaminer, 1989) Cloninger (1981) has described a particularly severe form of alcoholism in males who begin drinking heavily during adolescence; this form of alcoholism, termed Type II, is inheritable and associated with criminality in probands and their fathers; however, it may be argued that Type II alcoholics are in fact individuals with primary ASP and secondary alcoholism. ASP has been shown to affect the age of onset, course, and treatment response among alcoholic men, and appears to be an independent risk factor for the development of alcoholism (Hesselbrock et al., 1991). When evaluating the drug or alcohol using adolescent who exhibits antisocial behavior, a critical question involves the onset of antisocial behaviors; when they precede the drinking or drug use, a primary diagnosis of ASP is warranted.

Attention deficit hyperactivity disorder (ADHD) is often associated with alcohol or drug use, but does not appear to constitute a discrete risk factor for the development of addiction. Conduct disorder is often seen in patients with attention deficit disorder, and this appears to explain the association with drug or alcohol dependence, rather than the impulsivity, and hyperactivity of ADD (Alterman and Tarter, 1986). Treatment of ADD with stimulants does not appear to be a risk factor for later drug or alcohol dependence.

Drug abuse may represent a behavioral strategy for coping with stress-related affective states in some individuals. Marijuana, alcohol, sedatives, and opiates are often used in attempts to control unbearable affects such as rage, shame, depression, or anxiety. These painful emotional states may result from conflict at school due to poor performance, among peers as in the case of social anxiety, at home in a dysfunctional family system, or within the psychologically fragile individual. The use of substances in such cases could be viewed as a form of self-medication (Khantzian et al., 1974). Some authors postulate that a variety of behaviors often seen in drug using adolescents (restlessness, school apathy, and promiscuity, among others) may represent depressive states (Carlson and Cantwell, 1980; Gallemore and Wilson, 1972).

The incidence of severe psychopathology is increased among compulsive drug users (Khantzian et al., 1974). The choice of drug may provide an indication of the type and degree of underlying psychopathology: Opiates are effective antipsychotic agents and may be chosen by an individual who realizes that his or her thoughts are becoming disorganized or paranoid. Adolescents with borderline personality disorder may use sedatives, opiates, or alcohol to relieve dysphoric feelings of rage and emptiness. Alcohol is effective in suppressing panic attacks and social phobic symptoms and may be used to treat an underlying anxiety disorder. The prevalence of social phobic symptoms among alcoholics deserves further study, as it is undoubtedly high. It is important to inquire about negative experiences when interviewing adolescent drug users. Compulsive drug users with psychiatric problems will avoid drugs that intensify their anxiety, psychosis, or other symptoms. These individuals tend to avoid stimulants, hallucinogens, and marijuana and confine their use to the sedative and opiate drugs.

The pattern in which drugs are taken may be indicative of underlying psychopathology (Zinberg, 1975). Chaotic thought processes, as in the borderline or psychotic individual, may be mirrored by drug taking of a wide variety of drug classes, with frequent overdoses and other adverse sequelae. The so-called ''garbage head'' may take pride in his ability to ingest as many drugs of all types as often as desired. In such individuals primitive feelings of omnipotence and invulnerability are inextricably bound with the behavior of multiple drug taking and the state of overdose.

Withdrawal states or detoxification from compulsive drug use is often accompanied by dramatic changes in mental status. Delirium associated with sedative or alcohol use reflects disturbance of arousal processes. Psychosis or major affective episodes may be seen in those individuals with underlying psychiatric disorders during withdrawal from sedatives, alcohol, or opiates. Depressive states can also be induced by compulsive drug use and will often resolve during detoxification.

Conditioned learning appears to play a role in drug taking patterns among compulsive users. Various aspects of the drug-taking experience—social, sexual, relief of psychological distress, and other environmental attributes—eventually come to serve as stimuli for further drug craving and drug-taking behavior. Conditioned cues from the environment may be particularly important as a factor in relapse among recovering addicts (Childress et al., 1986). Treatment strategies involving extinction of conditioned cures through repeated exposure have been devised for cocaine abusers, but at this time no conclusions can be drawn about the efficacy of such treatments (O'Brien et al., 1988).

Social Factors

The social world of the adolescent often plays a contributing role in the development of a drug abuse problem. Family influences are among the earliest and most important. Adolescents raised in families where a parent or sibling has a drug or alcohol abuse problem are more likely to abuse drugs themselves (Bewley et al., 1974; Borland and Rudolph, 1975; Demone, 1973; Gergen et al., 1972; Kandel, 1973). In addition to modeling behaviors, parental attitudes or perceived parental attitudes can influence the adolescent's decision-making regarding drug, alcohol, or cigarette use (Hunt et al., 1971). Dysfunctional family dynamics involving parental rejection, instability, or divorce are associated with an increased incidence of drug use among children (Braucht et al., 1973; Gergen et al., 1972; Seldin, 1972; Wechsler and Thurn, 1973).

Children in lower socioeconomic groups are more likely to develop drug problems than those in higher socioeconomic groups (Borland and Rudolph, 1975; Gergen et al., 1972; US Public Health Service, 1976; Wechsler and Thurn, 1973). The impact of socioeconomic status on drug-taking patterns may relate to educational problems more so than to income. An adolescent in a college preparation curriculum or who has parents who went to college is less likely to develop a drug abuse problem. Peer influences may also be important as a socioeconomic factor associated with drug use. Smoking, drinking, and taking drugs are most often done in the company of peers, particularly in the early stages of use.

Peer influence on drug-taking practices is poorly understood; however, it may derive from perceived supportive attitudes of peers, or from adolescent notions about normal behavior (if everyone is doing it, then the behavior must be normal). Excessive reliance on one's peers is associated with a higher risk of developing a drug problem (Kandel, 1982). This condition may be more likely to arise in lower socioeconomic groups, where single-parent families are common and parental influence may be compromised by drug use. What is most impressive about crack-addicted mothers is their total neglect of parenting during periods of drug use.

The media play a facilitating role in drug abuse, largely through advertising of cigarettes and alcohol. People who drink alcohol or smoke are portrayed as being sexy, manly, sophisticated, or independent in commercials and other advertisements. This image is tailor-made for the adolescent consumer who seeks to define himself or herself within the adult social world but is not at all certain where he or she belongs. By adopting certain behaviors suggesting an image perceived to be desirable, the adolescent in effect mimics an adult personality. Other drugs such as marijuana and cocaine are not advertised commercially but rather are glamorized and sensationalized in movies, music, and television.

Sexual Factors

Adolescents are typically preoccupied with sex and sexual performance. Drugs such as sedatives, alcohol, opiates, or marijuana, when used in small quantities, may alleviate anxieties and inhibitions surrounding sexual behaviors and improve performance. Some young men are unable to perform unless intoxicated. Methaqualone has long enjoyed popularity among adolescents due to its reputation as a sex-enhancing drug. Cocaine use is frequently associated with sexual behaviors, though the connection may be more a matter of economics (prostituting) than direct drug effects. The ritualistic behaviors that one sees among cocaine users extend to sexual practices. A thorough history of sexual behaviors should be obtained from all compulsive cocaine users. Rituals involving masturbation, voyeurism, bondage, and other fetishes should be inquired about in addition to prostitution. Higher dosages of most drugs tend to impair erection and sexual performance and may exacerbate underlying anxiety rather than relieve it. Compulsive drug users who develop tolerance require increasing amounts of the particular drug of choice and tend to have decreased interest in sex and impaired sexual performance (Millman, 1978).

DRUG ABUSE AND ACQUIRED IMMUNE DEFICIENCY SYNDROME

Drug users, particularly those using via an intravenous route and/or involved in heavy crack cocaine use, are at high risk of contracting the human immunodeficiency virus (HIV-1). Intravenous drug use is the second most frequent risk behavior associated with HIV/AIDS exposure in the United States and Europe and accounts for the majority of cases involving heterosexual and perinatal transmission. Intravenous drug use, reported in 27% of AIDS cases in the United States in 1989 (Hahn et al., 1989), has remained at the same percentage during the early to mid 1990s (Centers for Disease Control, 1994b). Behaviors closely associated with HIV infection among drug users include sharing of needles among intravenous users, sexual contact with an infected person, and compulsive cocaine use, particularly by the smoking or intravenous routes (Turner and Miller, 1989).

Patterns of intravenous drug use vary widely. In the case of intravenous heroin users, injection may occur on a periodic basis ("weekend warriors"), sporadically ("chippies"), or as compulsive use three to four times daily to ameliorate withdrawal symptoms. Intravenous users may continue to use with those who initiated them to drug use, may change groups, or may use with a sexual partner. "Running buddies" often develop sexual relationships. Cocaine use is equally variable, often occurring in binges during which the user will administer the drug multiple times over the course of 1 to several days. During a binge the cocainist will neither sleep nor eat but will continue to sniff, inject, or smoke crack until he or she reaches a point of physical or financial exhaustion. Heroin and cocaine may be combined in a "speedball"; the heroin serves to smooth the dysphoria of the cocaine "crash."

Compulsive intravenous drug use requires a steady supply of drugs and injection materials. Users will often inject shortly after purchasing drugs to minimize the possibility of arrest, especially if they are experiencing withdrawal symptoms. Shooting galleries in large cities provide a facility for the purchase and use of injectable drugs. These are frequently located in abandoned buildings or dealers' apartments. "House works" are provided for a fee, resulting in the sharing of equipment.

Intravenous drug paraphernalia consists of five elements, each a potential source of contamination by HIV or other infectious agents. These are known as the "works" and include the syringe, the needle, the cooker, cotton, and rinse water. A description of the process of intravenous heroin injection best demonstrates the risk for infection. The heroin is put into the cooker (a bottle cap or spoon). A small amount of water is added to the cooker to dissolve the powder. The solution may be heated with a match to help sterilize the solution. (Cocaine and amphetamine are readily dissolved at room temperature; hence, they are not cooked.)

A piece of cotton is used to strain impurities in the process of drawing up the liquid into the syringe. Infected blood can be pushed out of the needle or syringe into the cotton in the process of drawing a new shot. A small amount of water is again added to the cotton to extract any remaining drug, enhancing the possibility of contamination. A likely source of contamination is through infected blood that remains in the syringe between uses. Intravenous users often "boot" the syringe during an injection: They will insert the needle, draw blood to ensure they are in the vein, then inject it, repeating the sequence several times before the needle is withdrawn from the vein. "Booting" ensures that the drug has been completely removed from the syringe. Contamination may occur if a droplet of infected blood remains inside or outside the needle (Turner and Miller, 1989).

Water is used to prevent clotting between injections. Bleach, alcohol, and hydrogen peroxide and liquid dish detergent may be used to disinfect the equipment. For this to be successful, the cleanser must be flushed to the highest level of the user's injection, and the needle must be flushed and dipped. Disinfectants may dissolve the silicon lubricant of the syringe plunger, rendering it stiff and difficult to operate. Intravenous drug users are often reluctant to use disinfectants for this reason.

Epidemiological data regarding intravenous drug users are fraught with methodological limitations and should be viewed as conservative in terms of numbers of users and illustrating broad trends. Studies of those in treatment are most accurate but represent a minority of the intravenous drug-using population. A recent review of the literature on HIV seroprevalence rates among drug users cites figures varying from 0–65% for different regions of the country. The Northeast and Puerto Rico have the highest rates, up to 65%. Urban centers such as Atlanta, Detroit, and San Francisco show seroprevalence rates of approximately 5–10%, though these are increasing. Seroprevalence rates are increased among blacks and Hispanics, probably due to needle-sharing practices.

The estimated number of seropositive intravenous drug users is thought to be between 61,000 and 398,000, or 5–30% of the population (Hahn et al., 1989). A recent study of alcoholics and drug users entering treatment through inpatient and outpatient community health centers in San Francisco revealed that minority subjects (blacks and Hispanics) were less likely to have been HIV tested, and were more likely to have misrepresented or misunderstood test results than nonminority subjects (Lindan et al., 1994). White subjects also misrepresented HIV test results in this study, though less frequently. This study suggests that epidemiological statistics regarding HIV seroprevalence among addicts and alcoholics, particularly in minority populations, should be viewed with caution. The findings also indicate the importance of clarifying whether clients understand the meaning of test results.

An estimated 250,000, or 25%, of the total population of intravenous drug users in this country live in New York State. The majority live within the five boroughs of New York City. A recent study of intravenous drug users in Manhattan indicates that the human immunodeficiency virus entered this group in the mid-1970s. The years 1979 through 1983 marked a period of rapid spread of the virus, following which seropositivity rates have stabilized in the range of 55% to 60%, which are below those for hepatitis B. The authors attribute the stabilization in seropositivity rates to a balance occurring between conversion of seronegative individuals to seropositive status, to individuals' leaving intravenous use, to risk reduction strategies, and to the rising death rate of intravenous drug users (Des Jarlais et al., 1989). A Swedish study recently estimated the mortality rate and causes of death of all diagnosed HIV positive intravenous drug users in the Stockholm area from 1986 to 1990. In Sweden 90% of all intravenous drug users are HIV tested, so the results of this study are representative of the intravenous drug using population in Stockholm as a whole. Of the 472 HIV positive subjects, 69 subjects died during the study observation period, 52 of these from violence or opiate overdose. Patients in methadone maintenance programs (MMTP) were less likely than non-methadone-maintained patients to die from these causes (relative risk of 25% for MMTP patients). The authors concluded that methadone maintenance programs contribute to a higher survival rate among HIV seropositive intravenous drugs users by providing psychosocial support, medical treatment, and control of opiate use (Fugelstad et al., 1995). Additional support for this hypothesis comes from a study of 156 HIV seropositive intravenous drug users in Scotland. The study suggest that continuing heroin use in itself may have an accelerating effect on the progression to AIDS, in comparison to methadone maintenance (Ronald, Robertson, and Elton, 1994).

The increased risk for HIV infection observed in black and Hispanic intravenous opiate users may also be related to concurrent cocaine use. A study of 633 intravenous opiate users in San Francisco demonstrated a significant increase in seropositivity rates among those who also used cocaine on a daily basis. Blacks had a higher rate of daily cocaine use. High-risk behaviors such as use in shooting galleries and sharing of equipment were increased among daily cocaine users (Chaisson et al., 1989). Cocaine use may be a marker indicating a constellation of high-risk behaviors among opiate users (Weiss, 1989).

Sexual activity varies considerably in the drug-using population. Some opiate users are relatively inactive, while others, particularly cocaine and crack abusers, engage in frequent unprotected sexual encounters with multiple partners. Despite efforts aimed at educating drug users in regard to safer sexual behaviors, particularly those who use needles, few seem to comply, even after reducing intravenous opiate use or adopting safer methods of injection. Many male intravenous drug users are sexually involved with females within the heterosexual non-drug-using population. Cocaine "binges" are frequently associated with promiscuous sexual behavior. In urban areas "crack houses" provide sites for heavy cocaine use over considerable periods of time, involving multiple persons. The exchanging of sexual favors for crack is common among females who inhabit "crack houses." Other cocaine and crack users support themselves by prostitution. Although prostitutes report an increase in the use of condoms in the work setting, they are less likely to use them in personal relationships. Of the 78,000 cases of AIDS reported in the United States as of 1988, 20% occurred in heterosexuals exposed to an infected intravenous user (Weiss, 1989). By 1993, this percentage had increased to 42% (Centers for Disease Control, 1994a). In a study of 222 adolescent crack cocaine users (Fullilove et al., 1990), 41% reported a past history of sexually transmitted disease, while 50% reported combining crack use with sexual relations. Statistics that can relate heavy crack use or frequenting of "crack houses" to AIDS are unavailable. Despite the increasing number of heterosexual AIDS cases, and the difficulties in treating drug addicts, several studies indicate that prevention programs can be effective in reducing the risk of transmission of HIV in high-risk populations (McCusker et al., 1993). A review of the literature on HIV prevention (Choi and Coates, 1994) states that there is unequivocal evidence for the effectiveness of AIDS prevention programs in producing lasting behavioral change among addicted populations. Successful programs tend to be sustained, intensive in terms of patient contact and provision of services, and emphasizing available alternative to high risk behaviors, such as in needle exchange programs. Community outreach programs among minority and homeless populations have also been shown to be effective (Choi and Coates, 1994).

DRUGS OF ABUSE

Alcohol

Alcohol is the psychoactive substance most frequently used by adolescents. The vast majority of high school age students will have experimented with alcohol by the time of graduation. Among seniors, 38% admitted to heavy use of alcohol (five or more drinks in a row during the preceding 2 weeks) (Johnston et al., 1988). It is therefore difficult in many cases to distinguish between normative social drinking patterns and those suggesting compulsive use. *Problem drinking* refers to a pattern of involvement with alcohol that produces clearly deleterious effects on functioning and/or health. Alcoholism is marked by behavior that centers on the acquisition and use of alcoholic beverages and is associated with physiologic dependence. In general, there has been a recent trend toward earlier onset of alcohol use among adolescents. This is especially true of inner city children, who may begin drinking by the age of 10 or 12. Increasing numbers of females now appear to initiate alcohol use during this childhood period (Blane and Hewitt, 1977). Research suggests that genetic and familial factors may increase the risk of developing alcoholism (Goodwin, 1984).

Most adolescents drink in a manner that is congruent with their sociocultural environment. Most have parents who use alcohol; drinking usually occurs during social functions. Early drinking in adolescence is often marked by infrequent episodes of heavy drinking; the children try to get as intoxicated as possible. The sedative effects of alcohol may be used to alleviate feelings of anxiety or depression. Anxiety in social settings is a common example of such use. Drinking may enable the adolescent to temporarily feel less awkward and more a part of the social milieu. It should be noted that drinking may actually exacerbate anxiety or depression, through the CNS depressant effects of alcohol or via the withdrawal syndrome. The dysphoria following a bout of heavy drinking can serve to reinforce the drinking behavior. In extreme cases a pattern of compulsive use may develop. When excessive drinking occurs in an otherwise functional adolescent, it is useful to inquire about recent stressful events in the areas of family, social, or sexual activity.

Alcohol is often used to counteract or heighten the effects of other psychoactive drugs. Marijuana or stimulant use frequently produces anxiety as a side effect. Alcohol is then used to take the edge off the high. Opiate and other CNS depressant drugs are potentiated by alcohol; the combination results in a more prolonged and profound period of intoxication. In some cases the individual may become a compulsive user of both substances. Some cocaine users require large amounts of alcohol in order to consume a maximal amount of cocaine during a binge; others find cocaine necessary during drinking episodes, for similar reasons. Abuse of multiple substances is often part of a cluster of dysfunctional behaviors that occurs in conjunction with other psychiatric symptoms among disturbed adolescents. In these cases it can be difficult to ascertain whether substance abuse is an etiological factor or a secondary symptom. Some young people who are chemically dependent on cocaine find that after a period of abstinence from the drug, the resumption of alcohol may lead to overwhelming desires for cocaine.

Alcohol is a CNS depressant, similar in effects to the minor tranquilizers such as benzodiazepines and the sedative depressants such as the barbiturates. For social drinkers, the degree of intoxication corresponds to the blood alcohol level and is influenced by the amount consumed, the rate of gastric emptying, and absorption by the small bowel. Ingestion of food interferes with intestinal absorption, as do congeners in alcoholic beverages. In nontolerant individuals a blood alcohol level of 100 mg/ml is associated with a state of mild sedation and intoxication. The anxious individual feels a lessening of anxiety, and social interaction may be enhanced. Sexual activity may become more enjoyable. At levels between 100 and 200 mg/ml, visuomotor skills, integration of sensory information, and sexual performance become impaired. Blood alcohol levels above 200 mg/ml are associated with severe intoxication and sedation. Chronic alcohol abuse often leads to development of tolerance, permitting the alcoholic to function despite relatively high blood concentrations (200–400 mg/ml). When the blood alcohol level exceeds 450 mg/ml, extreme lethargy, stupor, and comatose states occur in tolerant and nontolerant persons. Recent evidence demonstrates that women are less able to metabolize alcohol compared to men and that they are liable to increased intoxication at a given alcohol amount (Frezza et al., 1990).

Alcohol alters the metabolism of many drugs, including sedatives, cocaine, and opiates. The liver damage caused by chronic alcohol use can alter the metabolism of a second drug. A more direct effect occurs through the suppression of oxidative metabolism, as occurs when benzodiazepines such as diazepam and chlordiazepoxide are taken in combination with alcohol. This process may account for the prolonged sedative effects observed in combined alcohol-sedative use. Alcohol accelerates the metabolism of cocaine through the induction of hepatic microsomal enzymes. This results in the accumulation of cocaine metabolites, which compound the hepatotoxic effects of alcohol (Hoyumpa, 1984). Cross-tolerance occurs between alcohol and other sedatives but not with opiates. Alcohol potentiates opiate effects, due to the additive effects of these sedating drugs. The relatively narrow range of tolerance of alcohol may make the combination of alcohol and other sedatives or opiates lethal.

In young persons the acute effects of alcohol, rather than chronic sequelae, are an important cause of death and disability through overdose, accidents, violent behavior, homicide, and suicide.

ALCOHOL WITHDRAWAL

Persistent intake of large quantities of alcohol can lead to the development of physiological dependence. Sudden cessation of drinking will then result in a characteristic pattern of behavioral and physiological signs and symptoms. Acute alcohol withdrawal is characterized by autonomic hyperactivity, restlessness, agitation, tremulousness, and hyperreflexia. Symptoms become noticeable as early as 4–6 hours following the last drink and will persist with varying intensity over the next 48–72 hours before subsiding or remitting. Auditory or visual hallucinations may accompany the withdrawal state (alcoholic hallucinosis). Seizures are seen, though not frequently, 12–24 hours after cessation of drinking. Delirium tremens is unusual in the adolescent population. This syndrome peaks at 72–96 hours after drinking and consists of global confusion, disorientation, severe agitation, visual and tactile hallucinations, and marked autonomic hyperactivity. It is potentially life-threatening and should be considered a medical emergency requiring hospitalization.

A protracted abstinence syndrome has been observed in some alco-

holics following detoxification: Depression, anxiety, tremulousness, and insomnia may persist for several months. Though poorly understood, this syndrome has potential significance as a cause of relapse during the early phase of recovery.

Management of Alcohol Withdrawal

Prior to referral and treatment, adolescents with potential alcohol problems should be evaluated by a substance abuse expert. There is a real danger of overtreatment here; some young people are prematurely referred to treatment programs that are unduly restrictive or authoritarian when they might have been managed in less restrictive programs that would be less stigmatizing. Detoxification of the alcohol-dependent patient is best managed by trained personnel in a supervised setting. Patients should be hospitalized in a medical setting, or referred to alternative treatment centers specialized in the management of withdrawal. These include nonmedical detoxification centers (sobering up stations), therapeutic communities, or structured outpatient programs.

The presence of underlying medical illness increases the risk for delirium during alcohol detoxification. It is essential to establish whether conditions such as cerebral trauma, subdural hematoma, HIV infection, pneumonia, or liver disease are present upon initial examination of the patient. Treatment of conditions complicating the alcoholism should be prompt in order to minimize the patient's risk during detoxification. It is recommended that patients be given multivitamins. In cases of compulsive use, thiamine 50–100 mg should be administered intramuscularly on a daily basis.

Various agents have been used successfully to suppress withdrawal symptoms. Benzodiazepines are recommended as agents of choice due to their efficacy and relatively low toxicity. Chlordiazepoxide (Librium) and diazepam (Valium) are long-acting, with pharmacologically active metabolites, providing relatively stable blood levels between doses. Clinically, patients will be more comfortable than if they are treated with longer-acting benzodiazepines or sedatives. Chlordiazepoxide (25–100 mg) or diazepam (5–20 mg) every 6 hours is a useful initial dosage regimen. The dosage should then be tapered over the next 5–7 days. In the event that severe agitation occurs, higher and more frequent dosages may be needed (Sellers and Kalant, 1976), and the overall length of detoxification prolonged. More recently, carbamazepine (Tegretol) has been shown to be effective in the management of alcohol withdrawal. Dosages of 600–800 mg/day in divided doses are initiated upon hospitalization, then maintained over the next 5 days and decreased over 3 days. Carbamazepine appears to be similar to benzodiazepines in terms of efficacy and may be superior in reducing symptoms of anxiety and depression in the setting of detoxification (Bjorkqvist et al., 1976).

If a delirium (delirium tremens) occurs during alcohol detoxification, the following points should be kept in mind: First, benzodiazepines are not treating the delirium per se. The delirium will run its course despite the dosage of benzodiazepines administered. In some cases the delirium may increase in severity with excessive doses. To treat an alcoholic delirium, benzodiazepines should be used in amounts that will sedate the patient sufficiently for him or her to be manageable by hospital staff. If underlying medical problems are resolved, the delirium will resolve in 4–10 days. As the patient becomes less agitated, the dose of benzodiazepines should be reduced. Second, sensory deprivation may increase the severity of hallucinations and agitation during alcohol withdrawal. A nurse or counselor should be available to make regular contact with the patient, orienting him or her to reality. If possible, patients should be encouraged to be active and maintain a regular schedule.

A variety of long-term treatment settings are available to the adolescent with compulsive alcohol use. Following detoxification, severely dependent patients should be referred to a residential facility for a rehabilitation period of 2–6 weeks. Intensive outpatient care and day hospitals may also be an option. The indications for inpatient care vary with the individual but include (a) medical or psychiatric sequelae that are life-threatening; (b) a withdrawal syndrome that may be medically dangerous, such as that seen in high-dose alcohol or depressant use or with extensive polydrug abuse; (c) repeated failure in the outpatient setting; (d) a home or social situation that is a powerful reinforcement for the maintenance or resumption of drug-taking patterns; and (e) to enhance motivation in the face of persistent denial and resistance.

Inpatient options include psychiatric hospitals for those with coexisting psychiatric disorders, rehabilitation programs for those with uncomplicated chemical dependency, and therapeutic communities for young people with long-term problems and social deprivation who need a longer-term program. In such settings the compulsive drinker may be helped to come to terms with his or her alcoholism and its consequences. Denial is often quite profound and is a serious obstacle to successful treatment of these behaviors. Educational lectures, group and individual counseling, as well as family interventions within a highly structured and supervised environment designed to provide external control of the drinking behavior are helpful. Pharmacologic treatments include Antabuse, an aldehyde dehydrogenase inhibiting agent that inhibits the metabolism of alcohol, causing an accumulation of acetaldehyde after alcohol intake. The Antabuse reaction is marked by flushing, nausea, cramps, and vomiting. Treatment with Antabuse should be initiated after the patient has been abstinent from alcohol for a minimum of 12 hours, in order to avoid a toxic reaction. A loading dose of 500 mg is given on the first day, followed by a daily dose of 250 mg; this medication should be begun prior to discharge in those who have had previous relapses. Antidepressants such as desipramine and fluoxetine have been shown to reduce cravings for alcohol in compulsive drinkers (B. Mason, personal communication, 1989; Naranjo et al., 1986) in recent studies and may be useful additions to nonpharmacological treatment. Work by Volpicelli and others in a double-blind, placebo-controlled study of alcoholic veterans showed the efficacy of naltrexone (50 mg per day) in reducing drinking days, alcohol craving, somatic distress, and relapse rates when compared to placebo. The mechanism of naltrexone's actions in alcoholics is unclear, but preclinical work in animal models suggests that the reinforcing effects of alcohol are mediated through endogenous opiod systems, thus naltrexone may produce effects by blocking or attenuating the highfrom alcohol (Volpicelli et al., 1995).

Depressants

Abuse of sedative hypnotics is relatively common among adolescents seen in medical settings for drug-related problems. In adult populations sedative hypnotic drugs are prescribed for treatment of insomnia, anxiety states, depression (inappropriately), and muscle spasm; however, this is generally not the case with adolescents. The abuse of ''street'' (illicitly obtained) sedative drugs is more common among younger patients. Frequently abused drugs in this class include benzodiazepines such as diazepam (Valium), lorazepam (Ativan), alprazolam (Xanax), and triazolam (Halcion); short-acting barbiturates, particularly pentobarbital (Nembutal) and secobarbital (Seconal); various other hypnotics such as glutethimide (Doriden), methaqualone (Quaalude), ethchlorvynol (Placidyl), and amitriptyline (Elavil), an antidepressant with sedative properties. These drugs are often referred to as ''pills'' or ''downs.''

Patterns of recreational use are quite variable: Amounts of one or two hypnotic doses may be used intermittently in social settings. Compulsive sedative users may ingest 10–20 times the therapeutic dose on a daily basis for prolonged periods. Polydrug abuse is frequent in this population. Users describe the high from sedatives as a feeling similar to that preceding sleep in normal individuals. Anxiety is reduced, and a feeling of freedom or aggressiveness is often reported. Sexual anxiety is diminished, and sexual activity is felt to be more pleasurable when low doses are used. Violent behavior is sometimes seen in sedative abusers, perhaps from the disinhibiting effects of the drugs. Heavy users have a high incidence of premorbid psychiatric symptoms and may choose sedatives as a way of controlling anxiety, anger, paranoia, or other dysphoric affects (Kamali and Steer, 1976).

Sedative hypnotics produce a depressant effect on nervous tissue, skeletal and smooth muscle, and cardiac muscle. At low doses the CNS is most affected. Benzodiazepine drugs have been studied extensively and appear to exert their effects on the CNS through interactions with high-affinity receptors in the brain and spinal cord. Benzodiazepine receptors (BZRs) are associated with gamma-aminobutyric acid (GABA) receptors. Benzodiazepines appear to enhance the functions of GABA receptors by permitting the passage of chloride anions through a channel in the receptor complex. The resultant movement of chloride through the neuronal cell membrane causes changes in polarization and thereby alters excitability. GABA receptors serve to inhibit presynaptic and postsynaptic neuronal transmission throughout the CNS (Haefly, 1986). CNS effects range from mild sedation to coma, depending on the potency of the drug, the dosage used, the route of administration, and constitutional factors. Tolerance rapidly develops to all the depressants, though the range is more narrow than is the case with opiate drugs. Acute depressant poisoning may occur by accident, as a result of the combination with opiates or alcohol, or by intent in a suicidal attempt. Cross-tolerance develops between all depressants and alcohol.

Physical dependence results from chronic administration of sedatives. The withdrawal syndrome is similar to that produced by chronic alcohol use and varies in duration and severity depending on the primary drug of abuse, the dosage, and duration of use. Depressant withdrawal may be life-threatening, in contrast to opiate withdrawal. Symptoms of mild withdrawal include restlessness, anxiety, tremulousness, and insomnia. The more severe syndrome may involve seizures (usually within the first several days), delirium, and cardiovascular collapse due to hyperthermia and tachycardia. Barbiturate withdrawal usually resolves in 8–10 days, while longer-acting benzodiazepines can produce seizures at this time and a protracted delirium. Duration of use is an important risk factor in the development of withdrawal. In recent studies of benzodiazepine users taking the equivalent of 20–40 mg of diazepam per day, 43% experienced withdrawal symptoms after 8 months of use, while the incidence increased to 100% after 1 year's use (Salzman, 1989). High-potency benzodiazepines with short half-lives produce withdrawal symptoms that are abrupt in onset and severe in character. Alprazolam (Xanax) and triazolam (Halcion) are noteworthy for producing severe withdrawal syndromes.

MEDICAL MANAGEMENT

Acute depressant poisoning may require hospitalization and intensive care. A careful history regarding the specific drug of abuse, dosage, circumstances of the overdose, and the extent of chronic use (if any) should be obtained from the patient, family, or friends. A history of depression, past suicidal behavior, or recent traumatic life events should alert the examiner to a possible suicidal attempt. Psychiatric evaluation is indicated in such cases to establish the severity of suicidal behavior and the need for further psychiatric intervention. If the patient has a history of compulsive sedative use of several months' duration or more, hospitalization is indicated for the purpose of controlled detoxification. The daily dose of sedatives is estimated, then converted to an equivalent amount of a long-acting agent such as diazepam by means of a conversion table (see Table 69.3). The total daily dose is administered in divided doses every 6 hours to ensure that the patient is observed closely throughout the day for the emergence of withdrawal symptoms. Diazepam 5–10 mg can be administered on an as-needed basis between standing doses if the patient shows evidence of withdrawal. Sufficient drug should be administered to produce a mild intoxication, marked by inconstant, slow nystagmus on lateral gaze, slight dysarthria, and ataxia. The presence of elevated vital signs, agitation, or hyperreflexia indicates that the patient is receiving an inadequate dose of sedative. After 1 or 2 days the daily requirement of sedatives should be established. The daily dosage may then be tapered at a rate of 10% of the previous day's dose per day. The rate of taper should not be fixed, however, but adjusted as necessary to the patient's clinical status. Detoxification from sedatives is often quite a lengthy process, requiring several weeks of hospitaliza-

Table 69.3.   Sedative Hypnotics Equivalency Table Phenobarbital 30 mg is equivalent to:

Generic Name	Dose (mg)
Benzodiazepines	
alprazolam (Xanax)	0.5-1
chlordiazepoxide (Librium)	25
clonazepam (Klonopin)	1
clorazepate (Tranxene)	15
diazepam (Valium)	10
flurazepam (Dalmane)	15
lorazepam (Ativan)	2
oxazepam (Serax)	10
temazepam (Restoril)	15
Barbiturates	100
amobarbital (Tuinal)	
butabarbital	100
butalbital	100
pentobarbital	100
secobarbital (Seconal)	100
Glycerols	400
meprobamate (Miltown)	
Piperidinediones	250
glutethimide (Doriden)	
Methaqualone	300

From Smith D: Benzodiazepine dependence potential: Current studies and trends. *J Subst Abuse Treat* 1:163–167, 1984.

tion. Patients who are dependent on opiates in addition to sedatives should be withdrawn from sedatives first, while being maintained on suitable doses of methadone. Withdrawal from the opiates may then be accomplished.

It is not rare to encounter a sedative abuser claiming to use amounts in excess of 100 mg of diazepam (or its equivalent) per day. A study of such subjects indicated that detoxification can be safely managed using a starting dose of 40% of the reported daily intake (Harrison et al., 1984), followed by a 10% per day taper. Recent studies indicate that carbamazepine may be effective in the treatment of sedative withdrawal. Carbamazepine in doses of 400–800 mg/day appears to reduce withdrawal symptoms, through mechanisms that are unclear, permitting more rapid discontinuation of sedatives (Reis et al., 1989). Patients detoxified from sedatives often experience a protracted abstinence syndrome consisting of sleep disturbances, anxiety, depression, headaches, and muscle aches lasting for several months. The presence of such symptoms may increase the risk of relapse for an individual. The role of carbamazepine in the treatment of protracted abstinence states has not been defined. The danger of relapse is substantial; compulsive sedative users should be referred for long-term rehabilitation following discharge from the inpatient unit.

Stimulants

CNS stimulants are commonly referred to as "ups" and "speed." The most frequently abused stimulant drugs include cocaine, amphetamines (amphetamine, dextroamphetamine, and methamphetamine), ephedrine derivatives, methylphenidate (Ritalin), phenmetrazine (Preludin), and diethylpropion (Tepanil). Adult stimulant users are typically success-oriented individuals who attempt to enhance performance through drug effects. Others may work at jobs that require sustained concentration over long periods, such as truck drivers or those in military service. Tolerance to stimulants develops in many cases, resulting in the administration of large daily doses. Often the stimulant user will develop a secondary problem with sedatives, which are used to promote sleep and counteract unpleasant side effects.

Adolescent stimulant users are more interested in the mood-elevating properties of these drugs in contrast to adults. Methamphetamine ("crystal" or "meth") is preferred, due to its central effects. These drugs may be taken orally, as in the case of diet-pill abusers, but are more commonly insufflated or injected intravenously. The "rush" experienced by stimulant users is described as a feeling of well-being, vigor, physical power,

and intelligence. After 4–6 hours the rush subsides and is followed by feelings of dysphoria, anxiety, and depression. The "crash" following stimulant use can be quite profound; suicidal and other violent behaviors are not unusual at this time. As tolerance develops, the compulsive user will administer larger doses at more frequent intervals. Alcohol and other depressants are used to reduce symptoms of crashing and promote sleep. A binge of compulsive stimulant use may often last for days, during which time the user will administer the drug multiple times per day without sleeping or eating. Following this, a period of hypersomnolence often occurs, associated with lethargy and apathy. Stimulants may be used in combination with opiate drugs as a "speedball." Recently a smokeable form of methamphetamine known as ice appeared in the Hawaiian islands and areas of the East Coast. This preparation permits rapid delivery of high concentrations of drug to the brain and results in a profound rush and a prolonged period of intoxication (12–24 hours). Ice users frequently have psychotic symptoms associated with violent behaviors while intoxicated. The use of ice is increasing dramatically in California and Hawaii and may represent the early stages of an epidemic pattern of spread, similar to that seen with crack cocaine during the last 3 years.

Cocaine is an alkaloid derivative of the coca plant (*Erythroxylon coca*), a shrub that grows in the Andes region of South America. The active agent is contained in the plant leaves, which have been used for their stimulant properties for 1500 years. The Incas considered the coca plant to be divine in origin and administered the drug by the chewing route: wads of coca leaf were mixed with lime (from ash) and chewed throughout the day. Oral administration is still prevalent throughout large areas of South America. Taken in this manner, the stimulant and euphoriant effects of the drug are less intense and less reinforcing (Kleber, 1988).

Cocaine use became widespread in Europe and America in the late 19th century. Promoted by such prominent physicians of the time as Sigmund Freud, whose 1884 treatise on cocaine, *Uber Coca*, was considered the definitive reference on the subject until the 1970s, cocaine was used to treat conditions as diverse as hysteria, syphilis, and asthma. A coca wine, Vin Mariani, was endorsed by numerous celebrities for its invigorating properties; Coca Cola was marketed as a nonalcoholic alternative to Vin Mariani. The cocaine in Coca Cola was replaced by caffeine in 1903.

Cocainism became popular in Europe and America; injection of cocaine, as well as intranasal administration of the drug, was practiced during this time by "cocainists." By the early 1900s an epidemic of compulsive cocaine use associated with severe psychiatric sequelae led to the inclusion of the drug in the Harrison Narcotics Act of 1914. This legislation prohibited the use of cocaine (and heroin) in proprietary medicines and required the registration of manufacturers and distributors (Kleber, 1988).

From 1920 to 1960 cocaine use in America was restricted to a small number of individuals: artists, those in the entertainment industry, the very affluent, and some of the very poor. During the 1960s renewed interest in cocaine occurred as part of an epidemic increase in drug use of all types. In the 1970s cocaine use became widespread among entertainers, members of the cultural elite, professional athletes, and members of the business and banking community. Cocaine was viewed as a glamorous drug—exotic, expensive, glorified in the popular media, and proclaimed nonaddictive by the medical establishment.

Use among adolescents escalated dramatically from the mid-1970s through the 1980s. In 1984 16% of high school seniors had tried cocaine, while 5.8% reported current (within 30 days) usage (Johnston et al., 1988). According to a 1994 survey, cocaine use has fallen to 6.1%, and current use declined to 1.3% (Johnston et al., 1994). These figures do not, however, reflect the increase of use among inner city adolescents, due to the high truancy and drop-out rate in this population. The current epidemic of crack cocaine use is primarily confined to the underprivileged in the inner cities but has spread to suburban areas, small towns, and rural areas throughout the country. No accurate estimates of the number of crack users nationwide are available, though the high school regular senior survey reported a stable use pattern at 1.4%. Recent figures suggest that 250,000–600,000 people are regular or heavy users of crack in New York State; 25–40% of these are thought to be adolescents (*State of New York Anti-Drug Abuse Strategy Report*, 1989). Higher estimates of the extent of cocaine and crack use in urban areas may be assumed based upon (*a*) the increased number of arrests in major urban areas where the arrestee is positive for cocaine, (*b*) the increased amount of violent crime, (*c*) and the increased number of babies born with cocaine in their bodies. An estimated 50,000 babies born in the past year were positive for cocaine (Johanson and Fischman, 1989).

Cocaine is processed for consumption in several steps: Initially the leaves are soaked in vats of sulfuric acid for several days, producing a liquid. The liquid is mixed with lime, gasoline, ammonia, and other chemicals to make cocaine base. The base is further refined with the addition of acetone, ether, and hydrochloric acid to form a powder, cocaine hydrochloride. Cocaine hydrochloride is an acid salt that is administered by oral ingestion or, more commonly, by insufflation or injection. This form of cocaine is less bioavailable than the base or "free-base" form. The price of cocaine powder has dropped by 50–75% in recent years. A gram can be purchased on the street for as little as $25–50.

"Free-basing" cocaine involves chemical extraction of the cocaine base, which can then be vaporized at a lower temperature and inhaled. Free-basing began in the late 1970s among heavy cocaine users. The extraction process involves use of volatile substances, with a substantial risk of injury through combustion of the solvents. Crack cocaine first appeared in the Bahamas in 1983 and within 2 years had reached New York City. Crack is similar to free-base cocaine in that the base form is ignited and inhaled. The major difference is in the extraction process, which is quite simple. Powder cocaine (hydrochloride) is dissolved in water; baking soda is added to the mixture, which is then heated in an oven or over a flame. Impurities settle to the bottom of the solution, leaving brownish crystals of the cocaine base. These are allowed to harden into small chunks, or they may be pressed into various shapes for distribution. The name *crack* refers to the crackling or popping sound producing when the cocaine is ignited.

The attractiveness of free-basing and crack is due to the immediate, intense rush it gives, which results from greater bioavailability of the drug and rapid absorption through the pulmonary vascular bed. The pharmacokinetics of free-base cocaine are similar to those of intravenous injection. The effects of crack are felt immediately and subside within 5 minutes. The crash symptoms that follow are profound. This form of cocaine is highly reinforcing because of the rapid onset and rapid waning of effects. Crack sells for as little as $5–10 per rock on the street. Users will typically spend $50–200 or much more during a binge. Violent behavior and sexual promiscuity are frequent among crack users. In urban areas such as Manhattan, Detroit, and Los Angeles, crack is ubiquitous and may be purchased at any time. Crack houses are apartments occupied by dealers, which are made available to customers for prolonged periods of crack use. Children as young as 6 years of age are often recruited as lookouts in inner cities. There is a trend toward distribution by adolescents under the age of 14, who are not subject to existing criminal statutes. Many of these children are able to make considerable amounts of money and become the primary income source for the family. In distinction to some of the other illicit drugs, as many girls use the drug as boys. The economic attractiveness of the crack market in otherwise impoverished urban ghettos cannot be overemphasized.

PHARMACOLOGY

Stimulants produce an experience of increased alertness and enhanced physical and cognitive functioning when taken at low doses. Cocaine use is also associated with a sense of euphoria and well-being. All stimulants are monamine oxidase inhibitors, producing transient ele-

vations in brain concentrations of dopamine and catecholamines. In animal models the reinforcing properties of stimulant drugs appear to require the integrity of dopaminergic pathways in the forebrain and mesolimbic areas, though the picture in humans is more complex. Chronic cocaine use is thought to deplete brain stores of monoamines, particularly dopamine, producing compensatory alterations in monoamine receptor number and function (Dackis and Gold, 1987). Recent research also suggests that cocaine may exert some of its psychoactive properties through the serotonergic system (Reith et al., 1983) or by a process called "kindling," involving limbic structures (Post, 1987). No single theory regarding the effects of cocaine on brain function adequately explains the clinical phenomena seen in compulsive users. Tolerance develops to the stimulant properties of these drugs, and to a lesser degree to the euphorigenic properties of cocaine. Cross-tolerance to various amphetamines is seen, but the effect does not generalize to other stimulants. Abrupt cessation of stimulant use does not produce the autonomic hyperactivity, tremor, and delirium seen with alcohol and sedatives. Nor does the gooseflesh, bone pain, diarrhea, and sweating of opiate dependence occur. The crash period marked by depression and somnolence following compulsive cocaine or other stimulant use is thought by some to be the equivalent of acute withdrawal, suggesting physiological dependence. More chronic symptoms of lethargy, apathy, anxiety, and depression can persist for weeks following cessation of cocaine use and may be a powerful reinforcement for continued use. These states may reflect alterations in brain functioning, as previously mentioned.

ADVERSE EFFECTS

Adverse effects from stimulant cocaine use include those associated with intravenous administration: Hepatitis, HIV infection, endocarditis, and abscesses are common. Other medical complications of cocaine use include cardiac arrhythmias, rupture of the ascending aorta, cerebral infarction and infection, hyperpyrexia, seizures, myocardial infarction, and sudden death. Abruptio placentae, low birth weight and impaired interactive behaviors, and structural fetal abnormalities have been associated with cocaine use in pregnancy. Long-term cognitive and emotional deficits in the offspring of cocaine-abusing mothers have been postulated and are under investigation (Kaye et al., 1989). Crack cocaine use has additional effect on the pulmonary system and has been associated with acute respiratory failure and bronchospasm as well as pneumomediastinum and pneumopericardium (Cregler and Mark, 1986).

Psychological distress is associated with stimulant use and is almost invariably seen in compulsive users. Paranoid ideation and stereotyped behaviors, including sexual rituals, are not unusual. The degree of paranoia depends on the duration and extent of use, route of administration, use of multiple substances, and underlying psychological stability of the user. To combat the increasingly dysphoric effects of cocaine and crack use, most users take other drugs. Adolescents are likely to use alcohol or marijuana, though depressant pills and heroin are also used (Estroff et al., 1989). Multiple dependencies are not uncommon. Psychotic states can be induced in almost anyone given enough stimulants for sufficient time. These episodes closely resemble symptoms of acute decompensation in schizophrenics but are usually transient, lasting hours to days (Estroff et al., 1989). Violent and/or antisocial behavior may occur during periods of paranoia. Severe depression and suicidal behavior are also not infrequent, particularly during the early phases of abstinence. Panic attacks may occur during acute intoxication, and in some cases a stimulant-induced panic disorder may persist during periods of abstinence. Prolonged psychotic or depressive episodes should alert the clinician to the likelihood of an underlying psychiatric disorder.

Treatment of the adolescent stimulant abuser depends on the pattern of use and personal characteristics of the user and unfortunately may ultimately become a question of financial resources. Occasional users may respond to a combination of support, education, and help with life stresses if present. Hospitalization or residential treatment should be considered for compulsive users. There are few such programs for adolescents, particularly those in inner city areas. Antidepressant medications may be helpful for depressive symptoms associated with abstinence and appear to reduce the preoccupation with cocaine among compulsive users. Desipramine and the dopamine agonists bromocriptine and amantadine appear to be helpful in the initiation and maintenance of abstinence. Medication should be reserved for patients who are unable to remain abstinent without pharmacotherapy (Gawin, 1988). Twelve-step programs such as Alcoholics Anonymous or Cocaine Anonymous have often been of significant value in the maintenance of sobriety, though some young people are loathe to attend these meetings.

Opiates

Opiates have been used for centuries in religious, medical, and recreational settings. Heroin is the opiate abused most frequently by adolescents, though the annual prevalence is low (0.6% in 1989) (Johnston, 1990). Morphine, codeine, Dilaudid, and synthetic opioids such as Darvon, Percodan, and methadone are also subject to abuse. The history of heroin abuse typically begins with intranasal use (''snorting''), which may or may not progress to intradermal (''skin-popping'') or intravenous use as the user develops tolerance and dependence (a ''habit''). Intravenous injection is often the end result of opiate use due to the considerable addictive properties of this class of drugs and the cost of maintaining a habit, which can be as high as $100–150 per day. Intravenous use is more cost-effective as a route of administration. For the compulsive user, life revolves around the obtaining and use of heroin and the ever-present withdrawal syndrome. The adolescent heroin addict often withdraws from the culture, family, friends, and school, assuming a negative or ''junkie'' identity. Behavior becomes more deviant, often antisocial or criminal; the user's sole concern is the prevention of withdrawal. When heroin is not available, other opiates such as methadone or sedatives are substituted.

The likelihood of underlying psychiatric disturbance in opiate abusers is variable and appears to be related to the culture of their socioeconomic group. Opiate abuse is relatively common among inner city adolescents, few of whom are likely to exhibit other major psychiatric symptoms (e.g., schizophrenia). The drug is much more difficult to obtain and abuse is less common in middle-class populations; opiate abusers are therefore more deviant within that group. Middle-class opiate abusers are more likely to demonstrate additional psychopathology. Opiate abuse and dependence may also be a result of the attempt to self-medicate underlying psychiatric symptoms, including personality disorders and psychotic symptoms. The antipsychotic properties of opiate drugs are currently under investigation. Depression is frequently seen in adolescent and adult opiate abusers and is likely to be a result of the chronic neurochemical alterations induced by the drug.

PHARMACOLOGY

Tolerance to opiates develops rapidly with regular use. Abrupt cessation of opiate use in compulsive users results in an abstinence syndrome, which begins within hours of the last dose and persists for several days. Intense urges to use the drug are accompanied by nausea, diarrhea, rhinorrhea, gooseflesh, and bone pain. Profuse sweating, dilated pupils, lethargy, and yawning also occur. Opiate users experiencing withdrawal suffer from anxiety, restlessness, and depression and often experience the symptoms as life-threatening. In fact, this is rarely the case; however, the profound dysphoria that an opiate addict experiences during withdrawal may result in extreme behaviors such as criminal activity or suicide attempts. Cross-tolerance occurs among all opiate drugs.

A protracted abstinence syndrome consisting of depression, anxiety, and insomnia frequently occurs in chronic opiate users. Psychotic episodes may occur during and after detoxification from opiates. In such cases one should suspect the presentation of an underlying psychotic disorder, which the patient has medicated with opiates. Opiate drugs

exert their effects by acting on receptors located in the brain, spinal cord, and nervous tissue throughout the body. Endogenous opiates including endorphins, enkephalins, and dynorphins are morphine-like substances produced by the body and act at the same receptor sites as exogenously administered opiates. Endogenous opiates are capable of producing analgesia and tolerance. The function of these substances is not well understood but is thought to involve the regulation of affective states, appetite, and the experience of pain. Chronic heroin or other opiate abuse may lead to alterations in the production or action of endogenous opiates by a neural feedback mechanism and cause relative deficiency of the latter when the exogenous opiate use is discontinued.

ADVERSE REACTIONS

Adverse reactions from opiates include those associated with intravenous use (see previous discussion of cocaine use). A majority of acute deaths from opiate use are due to acute heroin reactions, characterized by cyanosis, pulmonary edema, respiratory depression, and coma.

TREATMENT

Acute opiate overdose is characterized by profound sedation (often to the extent of coma), respiratory depression, and pinpoint pupils. Treatment consists of general resuscitative measures and administration of naloxone, an opiate antagonist. Naloxone is given in a dose of 0.1 mg/kg intramuscularly or intravenously every 2–4 hours as needed. A positive response is indicated by increased alertness, increased respiratory rate and minute volume, and dilated pupils. Naloxone should be administered in all cases of suspected opiate overdose and may have to be repeated if a long-acting opiate such as methadone was used.

Opiate detoxification may be accomplished in specialized outpatient settings, during hospitalization, or within a residential facility such as a therapeutic community. The most effective agent for this purpose is methadone, a long-acting synthetic opiate with a half-life of 24 hours. Methadone can be administered in a single daily dose or in divided doses. Dosages of 20–40 mg/day will usually be sufficient to suppress abstinence symptoms; higher doses should be used with great caution. If opiates in pill form are the drug of abuse, a conversion table may be used to estimate the daily requirement of methadone (Table 69.4). The initial dose is tapered gradually over the next 2 weeks or longer. Patients who are simultaneously addicted to opiates and sedatives should be detoxified in an inpatient setting. Detoxification should begin with the sedative; the dose of methadone is kept constant at a level high enough to prevent withdrawal, but low enough to prevent undue sedation. Clonidine, an antihypertensive agent, has also proven useful to effect detoxification. It is particularly indicated in the outpatient setting and when the daily opiate dose has been relatively low.

When treating adolescent heroin addicts, particularly when the period of addiction has been short, an attempt should be made to refer them to

Table 69.4.   Opiate Equivalency Table

	Oral	Intramuscular
Methadone	1 mg	0.5 mg
Heroin	1–2 mg	0.4 mg
Morphine	3–4 mg	1 mg
Dilaudid	½ mg	0.15 mg
Codeine	30 mg	13 mg
Meperidine	20 mg	7.5 mg
Paregoric	7–8 mg	
Laudanum	3 mg	
Dromoran	1 mg	
Levo-dromoran	½ mg	0.2 mg
Pantopon	4 mg	
Percodan	3–4 mg	1.5 mg
Darvon	60 mg	24 mg
Talwin	9 mg	6 mg

Adapted from Lowinson JH, Ruiz P, eds. Clinical problems and perspectives. Baltimore: Williams & Wilkins, 1981.

a therapeutic community, or rehabilitation program that has a specialized adolescent track. A prolonged period in a highly structured environment is often necessary to combat the denial so prevalent in this population, to allow protracted abstinence symptoms and craving to wane, and to teach the relapse prevention techniques necessary for them to remain abstinent. Long-term outpatient programs are indicated after the period of institutionalization. Outpatient treatment alone is rarely successful for hardcore adolescent addicts.

The alternative to detoxification is stabilization on methadone, followed by referral to an outpatient program for prolonged methadone maintenance. For many heroin abusers methadone maintenance permits a return to normal functioning, without producing the symptoms of intoxication and withdrawal associated with short-acting opiate use. Relapse to opiate use is frequent in nonpharmacological treatment programs and is of particular concern in the case of intravenous users, who increase their risk for HIV exposure. This is a difficult decision in the case of youthful addicts since they may have to remain on methadone for long periods of time. Methadone maintenance is the treatment of choice in cases of compulsive opiate use in young people, where there has been relapse after a nonpharmacological course of treatment. A well-run methadone program will also provide nonpharmacological services to the patient in the form of group and individual counseling, and psychiatric or medical evaluation and treatment when needed.

Hallucinogens

Hallucinogens are among the oldest of psychoactive drugs; their use has been documented for centuries, mostly in religious and other community rituals of primitive peoples worldwide. In the context of primitive cultures, hallucinogen use facilitates the experience of a shared, collective consciousness (Millman and Beeder, 1994). In twentieth century America, the use of hallucinogens has primarily occurred among white, middle-class youth. Hallucinogen use became relatively widespread in the 1960s as part of the rejection of mainstream culture; during the late 1960s hallucinogen use affected as many as 1 million people. Hallucinogen use declined during the 1980s, at the time of the cocaine epidemic; however in the past 2–3 years, as the use of cocaine has declined among American teenagers, the use of hallucinogens appears to be increasing (Johnston et al., 1994).

Drugs of this class include lysergic acid diethylamide (LSD), psilocybin, mescaline, and the substituted amphetamines, such as MDA and MDMA. MDMA, 2, 5-di-methoxy-4-dimethaxy-4-methylamphetamine, formerly known on the street as DOM and STP, has recently been used more widely by middle-class young people under the street name "Ecstasy" (Climko et al., 1987; Dowling et al., 1987). Phencyclidine (PCP, "angel dust") is an anesthetic that has also been abused for its hallucinogenic properties. PCP use occurs in all socioeconomic groups, though it has been most widely used in inner city minority groups in certain geographical areas. LSD is available in liquid form, impregnated in sugar cubes or paper, or as a capsule or tablet for oral ingestion. Most hallucinogen use occurs on an intermittent basis; weekly, monthly, or less frequent "trips" are taken. "Acid heads" are individuals who use hallucinogens regularly, sometimes on a daily basis for prolonged periods. Severe psychopathologic disorders often accompany hallucinogen use in these instances. Chronic PCP use, in particular, is associated with severe social dysfunction and coexistent psychiatric illness.

The current state of hallucinogen use among American use is exemplified by two phenomena: "rave" parties and musical concerts featuring The Grateful Dead, a rock band whose original members have performed together since the heyday of the psychedelic era in the late 1960s. Rave parties are a major venue for psychedelic use among adolescents in urban areas on the east and west coast. "Raves" probably originated in Europe in the 1980s, then became popular in this country sometime over the past few years. Rave parties occur in large spaces, restaurants, halls, warehouses, or even abandoned buildings. Groups of young people, often minors, gather to ingest large quantities of hallucinogens, and

dance to loud "techno" music: instrumental synthesizer music with a driving beat, played by disc jockeys. Dealers of hallucinogens are ubiquitous, and usually have distinctive clothing: A backpack indicates that one is selling drugs (Millman and Beeder, 1994). Raves are unique in that the drugs of choice are hallucinogens, and within the psychedelic experience the music creates a context of anonymity shared by all. People can get out of themselves, yet be a part of something larger, which is tangible. Rave parties go on for long periods, during which the participants will dance themselves to the point of exhaustion.

Music concerts performed by the rock band The Grateful Dead were another venue for psychedelic drug use among young people. The band performed for 25 years, and had a large repertoire of songs which featured extended improvisational segments. "Dead Heads" are fans of the Grateful Dead who followed the recordings, touring schedule, and other movements of the band in an obsessive, almost religious manner. Grateful Dead concerts were tightly orchestrated and highly ritualized; Dead Heads were familiar with the entire ritual down to its smallest elements, which appeared to be important in the establishment of a structured collective experience. The group ritual involved thousands of Dead Heads, and progressed to a collective psychedelic experience as the evening passed, and the drugs (mostly LSD) took effect.

PHARMACOLOGY

The psychoactive effects of hallucinogens are usually preceded by a brief period of central sympathomimetic activity, with mydriasis, tachycardia, piloerection, and increased alertness as prominent features. The quality of the trip varies, depending on the drug, dose, surroundings, and individual characteristics of the user. Hallucinogens produce alterations in perception, thought, feeling, and behavior that may be bizarre in character. Perceptions are distorted: Visual after-images flow into ongoing visual perceptions; objects appear to melt. Thoughts assume unusual clarity, and the user may experience a merging with the environment. The sense of time is also distorted. True hallucinations with loss of insight are rare, although they may occur repeatedly in certain predisposed individuals. Moods may vary from euphoria to paranoia or panic states. Changes in mood are often abrupt. The duration of hallucinogen intoxication depends upon the drug; LSD intoxication persists for 12–24 hours and that from MDMA or PCP 4–8 hours, although visual distortions and fatigue may persist somewhat longer.

The psychoactive effects of hallucinogens appear to result from the activation of 5HT2 postsynaptic receptors located in the locus coeruleus and on interneurons in the cerebral cortex (Aghajanian, 1994). It is speculated that the actions on neurons in the locus coeruleus may account for certain of the perceptual changes, while the cognitive and associational alterations may be related to actions on cortical interneurons. The atypical antipsychotic drugs, clozapine and risperidone have been shown to block the effects of psychedelic drugs on 5HT2 receptors in animal models, and may find utility as agents for the treatment of psychedelic intoxications or "bad trips."

Tolerance to the effects of hallucinogens develops rapidly, so that repeated daily doses become ineffective after a few days. Cross-tolerance occurs between several of the hallucinogens, involving unknown mechanisms. Physical dependence on hallucinogens has not been reported.

ADVERSE EFFECTS

Hallucinogen use is rarely associated with physiologic toxicity; there are no reported deaths attributable to the direct effects of hallucinogens. Spontaneous abortion has been observed in women exposed to LSD during pregnancy. "Bad trips" are not infrequent among hallucinogen users and represent the most common adverse reaction to this class of drugs. This syndrome is characterized by an acute panic state, with associated symptoms of breathlessness, fear of bodily harm, or concerns that the user is losing his or her sanity. Symptoms usually remit within several hours. "Flashbacks" are transient episodes occurring weeks to months after a hallucinogenic experience, during which the adolescent will reexperience aspects of the hallucinogenic state without having taken drugs. These episodes are usually mild and very brief; however, severe flashbacks can occur with accompanying psychotic behavior. Prolonged psychotic episodes are infrequently seen; these typically occur in predisposed adolescents taking large doses of hallucinogens. It is possible though not proven that prolonged or permanent psychotic states that were precipitated by hallucinogen use might have occurred in the absence of the drug.

The acute effects of low doses of phencyclidine are similar to those produced by LSD. Violent behaviors and psychoses are relatively more common among PCP users, however. High doses of PCP have been associated with severe toxic reactions and death. The symptoms of PCP toxicity include nystagmus, incoordination, hypertension, and hyperreflexia. The syndrome may progress to extreme muscular rigidity, with arrhythmias, convulsions, and coma.

TREATMENT

Treatment of the adolescent experiencing a bad trip requires a warm, supportive environment with continual reassurance that the drug effects are temporary. Regular contact by hospital personnel is critical for the first 12–24 hours, after which the majority of patients will be substantially improved. Agitated patients may be given benzodiazepines via the oral or intramuscular route. Flashbacks are treated with reassurance and psychotherapy (in severe cases). Prolonged psychotic episodes following hallucinogen administration are treated with neuroleptics, as with functional disorders.

Toxic reactions due to high doses of PCP often require hospitalization and intensive supportive care. Excretion of phencyclidine is enhanced by acidification of the urine. This can be accomplished by the use of ammonium chloride, 75 mg/kg/day in divided doses, or ascorbic acid 500 mg every 4 hours. In milder cases, cranberry juice and 1 or 2 g of ascorbic acid are given four times daily.

Inhalants

Inhalant drugs comprise a wide variety of substances, such as organic solvents, glues, amyl nitrate, nitrous oxide, and others. These substances are volatile or gaseous and are inhaled for their psychoactive effects. Amyl nitrate ("poppers") is in widespread use among certain groups of adolescents. Use generally occurs in a social setting, particularly to enhance sexual experiences. The effects are immediate in onset and consist of a flushing sensation, rapid heart rate, dizziness, and a feeling of hilarity. Postural hypotension with loss of consciousness may occur, but other adverse effects are rare. The effects of amyl nitrate subside within a few minutes. Organic solvents (toluene in glue) are sometimes abused. Administration involves application of the solvent within a plastic bag that is wrapped around the head. The bag serves as a reservoir of vapors, which are then inhaled. The high is brief and resembles the initial effects of alcohol intoxication. Accidental suffocation from the plastic bag has been occasionally seen in solvent users. Aerosol sprays containing fluorocarbons are also inhaled for similar reasons.

Nitrous oxide ("laughing gas" or "whippets") is used in dental procedures and as an aerosol propellant in the restaurant industry for the delivery of whipped cream. Gas from the cartridges may be inhaled through the nozzle of a canister, producing a brief period of intoxication and hilarity. In rare cases compulsive use of massive quantities may occur. Such use may be associated with a delusional state, which resolves in a few days following cessation of use. Adverse effects in occasional users are rare, although respiratory depression is associated with forced inhalation of nitrous oxide.

TREATMENT

Intermittent users of inhalants may not require specific treatment. Chronic compulsive users, especially "glue sniffers," are likely to have underlying psychopathology and often require long-term treatment.

Cannabis

Marijuana is the most frequently used illicit substance among American adolescents. Current estimates indicate a lifetime prevalence for marijuana use of 44% among high school seniors (Johnston et al., 1990). Rates are likely to be higher among drop-outs. Experimentation with marijuana has become a part of normal development among some teenagers in this country. Marijuana and hashish are derived from *Cannabis sativa*, a hemp plant that grows throughout the world. The active ingredient in both forms of cannabis is delta-9-tetrahydrocannabinol. Marijuana refers to the combined mixture of dried stems, seeds, and leaves of the plant. Hashish contains compressed resins from the flowering tops of the cannabis plant and is several times more potent than marijuana.

Patterns of cannabis use vary from intermittent social use to compulsive day-long use. Daily use occurs in approximately 10% of those who have tried marijuana. Daily use is associated with an increased rate of school difficulties, deviant behaviors, and use of other drugs. Most compulsive users of hard drugs such as cocaine and heroin have a history of daily marijuana use at some earlier point in their drug use careers. Daily marijuana users have a higher rate of associated psychiatric disorders (Millman and Sbriglio, 1986).

Marijuana may be smoked from a pipe or, more commonly, rolled into cigarettes ("joints"). Hashish is usually smoked in a pipe. Both forms may be ingested orally, in combination with food or beverages. The effects of cannabis are felt within minutes after inhalation and persist for an hour or two before subsiding. Oral ingestion results in delayed effects that tend to persist for several hours. Metabolites of cannabis persist in the body for several days. There is some evidence to suggest that the psychoactive effects are also prolonged. Acute physiological effects are dose related and include an increase in heart rate, dry mouth, fine tremors of the fingers, and altered sleep patterns. Orthostatic hypotension and loss of consciousness occur infrequently.

The psychoactive effects of cannabis depend largely on the mood and expectations of the users, the circumstances of use, previous experiences with the drug, and the route of administration. The perception of visual and tactile stimuli is often enhanced. Drowsiness is common, as is an increase in appetite and sometimes binge eating ("munchies"). Time perception is altered. The effects on mood range from feelings of relaxation and well-being to depression and acute anxiety states. Short-term memory is impaired, as is the ability to perform complex motor tasks, such as driving. Some tolerance develops to the physiologic and psychoactive effects of the drug. A mild withdrawal syndrome consisting of irritability, restlessness, and sleep disturbances has been described under experimental conditions of heavy use. This does not appear to be a problem clinically though some young people find themselves unable to cease using the drug. In these individuals there is a profound craving for the altered state of consciousness induced by the drug.

ADVERSE EFFECTS

Considerable controversy exists as to the possible adverse effects of chronic cannabis use. No deaths have been reported due to cannabis overdose. Marijuana smoke contains 50–100 times more benzpyrene, hydrocarbons, and tar than cigarette smoke. However, an increased incidence of lung cancer among marijuana smokers has not been documented, so that the risk relative to cigarette smoking is unclear. Chronic marijuana users have an increased incidence of bronchitis, sinusitis, and nose and throat inflammations. Reproductive functioning may be affected by chronic marijuana use: Reduced testosterone levels, altered sperm morphology, abnormalities in menstruation, and an increased incidence of spontaneous abortion have been reported though not clinically confirmed. The meaning of the findings is unclear. Similarly, the findings of in vitro reduction of T lymphocytes and inhibition of DNA, RNA, and protein synthesis are of unknown significance.

The most common adverse effects associated with cannabis use are psychological and are similar to those produced by hallucinogens. Acute panic reactions, depersonalization paranoia, and depression are relatively common. These reactions usually resolve within several hours. Prolonged psychotic reactions are suggestive of an underlying psychiatric disturbance. Flashbacks do occur but are rare. An amotivational syndrome has been observed in some chronic users who become apathetic, are unable to pursue goals, and exhibit magical thinking. Whether this condition represents a drug-induced change in brain functioning is controversial (Millman and Sbriglio, 1986). An alternative explanation is that disturbed adolescents may be predisposed to heavy marijuana use as a means of coping with overwhelming anxiety and other psychiatric symptoms. In turn, the drug may render them less able to successfully negotiate the rites of adolescent passage.

Treatment of an acute cannabis reaction requires firm, supportive reassurance. The patient should be reminded that the feelings he or she is experiencing are drug-induced and will soon resolve ("talking down"). Sedatives may be used in cases of severe agitation or violent behavior. Chronic users should be thoroughly evaluated and treated for other psychiatric or social problems.

EVALUATION OF THE ADOLESCENT DRUG USER

Obtaining an accurate history is critical to the evaluation process. Determining whether there is a drug problem and the extent of it requires a careful drug and psychiatric history. Additional information from friends and family is often useful. Adolescents are peer oriented and often mistrustful of authority figures. There is often profound denial around drugs and drug-related sequelae. Adolescents abusing drugs on an intermittent or social basis who have an acute toxic reaction may honestly feel that they are no different from most of their friends. Adults who seem critical or judgmental are dismissed as "out of touch" or not understanding the world the adolescent lives in. The attitude of the physician must be one of interested and knowledgeable concern, if he or she hopes to get a reasonably truthful story. The inexperienced clinician will often fail to get useful information because he or she is unable to allay the patient's unspoken fear of criticism, punishment, or betrayal of confidence. The latter issue is best dealt with at the beginning of the interview by telling the patient, "What you say to me is between the two of us, but if I think that you have a problem that is life-threatening or really dangerous to you, I will have to tell your parents."

Adolescents experience profound developmental changes in physical and cognitive abilities; it is a time when they attempt to find out who they are. Experimentation with sex, substances, and behaviors that may appear deviant or risky is a way in which the adolescent finds out about himself or herself. Experimentation is not therefore bad or abnormal, but understandable. This understanding should be conveyed by the interviewer. A related adolescent tendency is to feel invulnerable, in the light of newfound physical, sexual, and cognitive powers. Denial of unpleasant feelings, thoughts, or experiences and externalizing one's problems onto the environment occur in normal teenagers. It is important to adolescents that they view themselves and are treated by others as independent and self-sufficient persons. Bad experiences due to intermittent drug use will be difficult for adolescents to acknowledge to themselves or to the clinician. Beneath a veneer of "machismo," sullenness, or indifference, the astute clinician sees a person who is frightened and demoralized. He or she may want to be helped, but without being made to feel guilty or ashamed.

The assessment of adolescents who are compulsive drug users is more complicated due to the multiple areas of dysfunctional behavior seen in this population. Presentation to a medical facility typically involves a crisis. Failure in school, motor vehicle accidents, violent fights involving knives or guns, suicide attempts, overdoses, and criminal behaviors are among the many modes of entry into the medical system. Drug abuse should be suspected in all adolescent cases who are brought to a doctor's office or emergency room or clinic for evaluation. The adolescent presenting in this manner may have compelling reasons for concealing information relating to his or her drug use. A useful strategy when interviewing such a patient is to calmly confront him or her with your suspicion: "I think that there are some important things that you may be afraid to tell me. I can understand why you would be afraid to trust me, but I can't help you if you won't be honest with me." The skillful handling of confidentiality issues is critical in such cases. If the patient is unwilling to cooperate with the interviewer, secondary sources of information, such as friends, family, or others, must be used. The interviewer must attempt to identify the drug or drugs of abuse, the route of administration, and the duration and frequency of use. A history of tolerance and withdrawal symptoms is obtained, and the presenting problem is characterized in terms of current drug intoxication or withdrawal. It is critical to determine whether a detoxification regimen should be instituted. In many instances withdrawal symptoms have not yet occurred due to relatively brief involvement, an intermittent or binge pattern of use, or choice of drug. Despite this, the drug use may still be out of control and the patient chemically dependent. Most adolescents with chemical dependence will have difficulties in one or many areas of functioning. Family relationships are almost always impaired; lying, stealing, fighting, and running away from home should be inquired about. If the patient presents a picture of normalcy, parents and siblings must be questioned to determine whether changes in behavior have occurred. If a drug problem exists, the patient may have exhibited particular drug-related behaviors, including lying, evasion, unexplained or sudden absence, or a change in daily routine. Theft of objects or cash from the home frequently occurs, creating intense mistrust. The patient often denies such problems and will blame the family for treating him or her unfairly. Nevertheless, a history of theft is highly suggestive of drug abuse or dependence.

Adolescent drug abusers tend to associate with other people like them. A recent change of friends should be inquired about. Social withdrawal in a previously outgoing teenager is another indicator of a possible drug problem. Academic and athletic performance tends to deteriorate as the adolescent becomes more involved in obtaining and using drugs. Functioning in these areas should be clarified in the interview of the patient, then corroborated by the family. It is also critical to learn from the patient which drugs he or she prefers, which drugs cause which effects, and how much time the adolescent spends getting, using, and thinking about them.

The diagnosis of chemical dependence may be resisted by the family. When the evidence is substantial, the physician must present the findings gently and firmly and perhaps attempt to explore the patient's or family's resistance to acknowledging the problem.

It may be difficult to determine whether adolescents have a drug problem, a psychiatric problem, or both. Many of these young people will present with symptoms and signs of a variety of psychiatric disorders. At the outset of treatment it may not be possible to delineate which came first, the psychopathology or the drug taking. Whereas drug use may be an attempt at self-medication of preexisting psychopathology in some people, chronic psychoactive drug taking almost invariably leads to psychiatric symptoms. In general, drug abuse should be considered primary, and treatments should be focused on this issue (Millman, 1986). At a later point in the patient's course, the psychiatric symptoms may become less evident as the drug effects wane.

Physical Examination

Physical examination of the drug-abusing patient should provide information regarding the presence of intoxication or withdrawal states, routes of drug administration, and the medical sequelae of drug use. The following are abnormalities that may be seen during examination of drug users:

APPEARANCE

Extreme states of anxiety or agitation suggest intoxication with stimulants, cocaine, and/or hallucinogens. Agitation may also be seen in cases of alcohol or sedative withdrawal and opiate withdrawal. Lethargy suggests recent alcohol, sedative, or opiate use.

VITAL SIGNS

Elevated vital signs are seen with stimulant intoxication and sedative or alcohol withdrawal.

SKIN

"Tracks" are scars or multiple injection marks following the course of a vein. They usually occur on the forearm, wrist, dorsum of the hand, antecubital area, or ankle and are the hallmark of intravenous drug use. Abscesses may also be seen in cases of intravenous or subcutaneous ("skin-popping") needle use. Jaundice is indicative of liver disease and may be associated with intravenous drug use or alcohol use. A rash occurring on the skin of a drug user may be a sign of secondary syphilis. Syphilis in an intravenous drug user or prostitute may be associated with HIV infection. Excoriations ("cocaine bugs") are suggestive of compulsive cocaine or crack cocaine use.

LYMPHATICS

Careful palpation for lymph node enlargement should be performed in any patient with compulsive drug use, a history of intravenous drug use, or a history of prostitution. Multiple enlarged lymph nodes are often observed in otherwise healthy intravenous drug users. HIV testing is indicated in any drug user with generalized lymphadenopathy.

HEENT

Pinpoint pupils occur in cases of acute opiate intoxication. Widely dilated pupils may be due to stimulant use or opiate withdrawal. Nystagmus is frequently seen with drug intoxication of various types, particularly sedatives and PCP. Marijuana intoxication is associated with conjunctival vascular congestion, though this is not a specific finding and may be seen with other drugs. Scleral icterus suggests jaundice secondary to liver disease. Chronic sinusitis ulcerations of the nasal mucosa and perforation of the nasal septum may be associated with cocaine insufflation. Oral thrush may result from poor nutrition or underlying immunosuppression due to HIV infection.

CHEST

Bronchospasm or asthmatic exacerbations are common in crack users. A chronic productive cough often occurs. Apical crackles suggest tuberculosis and, possibly, underlying HIV infection. The signs of pneumopericardium or pneumomediastinum may suggest crack use.

HEART

Tachycardia, irregular heartbeat, and ectopies are suggestive of cocaine intoxication. Murmurs at the lower left sternal border may indicate endocarditis with tricuspid valve involvement.

ABDOMEN

Hyperactive bowel sounds may occur during opiate withdrawal. Tenderness and enlargement in the right upper quadrant suggest hepatitis or liver disease, which may occur in intravenous drug users and alcoholics.

GENITALS

A thorough examination should be performed in all cases of intravenous use, prostitution, or crack cocaine use. Herpetic vesicles, syphilitic chancres, and discharge from the penis or vagina suggesting sexually transmitted disease should be sought. Anal warts are also quite common in sexually active drug abusers.

EXTREMITIES

Edema due to venous insufficiency occurs in chronic intravenous users. All drug abusers and particularly those engaged in prostitution should be examined for evidence of trauma, including fractures of the extremities.

NEUROLOGICAL

Mental status abnormalities such as lethargy, agitation, and impaired attention are consistent with drug intoxication or withdrawal. A history of fighting, accidents, or other forms of head trauma should be inquired about in such cases. Ataxia is suggestive of alcohol or sedative intoxication. Hyperreflexia occurs during alcohol or sedative withdrawal and frequently occurs in PCP intoxication.

Laboratory Evaluation

When drug or alcohol abuse is suggested, a urine toxicological screen may be indicated. If chronic drug abuse or dependence is suspected, the specimen should be obtained under observation to minimize the possibility of obfuscation. In cases of acute alcohol intoxication, blood alcohol levels may be ordered although the intoxication often resolves by the time the results are available. When ordering a urine drug screen, it is important to be sure to assay for the suspected drug of abuse. Certain assays, for example, PCP and diazepam, must often be requested in writing. In cases of compulsive use, more extensive laboratory evaluation is necessary. Patients who are chemically dependent are more likely to have underlying medical problems. The following tests are routinely ordered in the initial evaluation of adolescents: complete blood count with differential white blood cell count, electrolytes, blood urea nitrogen and creatinine, liver function tests, hepatitis serologies, VDRL, thyroid function tests. A chest X-ray and EKG are also part of routine evaluation in this population. A tetanus toxoid inoculation and PPD are administered during intake. Patients who are at risk for AIDS should be encouraged to submit to HIV testing. Informed consent must be obtained, and counseling is indicated both before the test is performed and when the results are available.

Emergency Treatment

Overdoses of sedatives, stimulants, opiates, or hallucinogens are frequently encountered in the emergency room setting. The adolescent brought to the emergency room because of bizarre behaviors, acute psychosis, coma, or respiratory or circulatory collapse is most likely to be suffering from a drug overdose. Drug overdoses can be fatal if misdiagnosed or improperly managed. Emergency room personnel should be familiar with common drugs of abuse and the management of drug poisoning involving these agents. Opiates and sedative hypnotics, often in combination with alcohol, are responsible for the vast majority of coma-inducing poisonings. Drug screens of urine, blood, and stomach contents should be obtained in all emergent situations; however, acute clinical management will be dictated by history and neurological examination. Blood gases and continuous cardiac monitoring may be necessary in cases of sedative or opiate overdose, which presents as profound CNS depression and pinpoint pupils. Naloxone (Narcan), an opiate antagonist, will reverse the symptoms of opiate intoxication and should be administered if there is even the possibility of an acute opiate reaction. Naloxone should be given in a dose of 0.1 mg/kg intramuscularly or intravenously every 2–4 hours as needed.

Overdose with a stimulant or hallucinogen usually presents as a toxic psychosis with agitation, confusion, paranoid delusions, perceptual distortions, and hallucinations.

MANAGEMENT OF ACUTE COCAINE TOXICITY

Acute cocaine poisoning represents a medical emergency requiring prompt intervention. The patient who presents with acute cocaine poisoning may be agitated, psychotic, hyperpyrexic, hypertensive, or acidotic, or may exhibit various combinations of these features. After establishing an airway, vital signs should be closely monitored. Supplemental oxygen and intravenous glucose should be administered to offset the hypermetabolic state. Naloxone may be considered, particularly in cases of intravenous cocaine use, since combined use of cocaine and heroin in a "speedball" is fairly common.

Evacuation of stomach contents by means of an Ewald tube is recommended in cases of oral ingestion. Cocaine is absorbed by activated charcoal. This may be administered with water in a slurry. Marked abdominal pain and leukocytosis may represent bowel gangrene, which warrants immediate surgical intervention. Cocaine is sometimes transported by sequestration in small packets, which are then swallowed. This "body packing" can be detected using an abdominal X-ray film. Intervention may or may not be required, depending on the condition of the packets within the gastrointestinal tract. Leakage can occur, causing acute poisoning; obstruction is another complication. Surgical intervention may be necessary in these instances.

Cardiovascular complications from acute cocaine poisoning may be quite severe. Hypertension is managed with β-blockers; however, cases of paradoxical hypertension have been reported with propranolol. More recently, labetalol has been recommended due to its combination of α- and β-adrenergic blocking effects. Ventricular tachycardia is best managed by use of phenytoin, while calcium channel blockers appear to be effective for supraventricular arrhythmias.

Seizures occurring in the setting of acute cocaine poisoning should be controlled by use of diazepam; if diazepam is not effective, phenytoin may be added. Metabolic acidosis increases the risk for seizures and arrhythmias and should be corrected with bicarbonate. Hyperthermia is controlled by cooling with ice packs. Agitation is managed with reassurance in a quiet environment. In cases of severe agitation, short or intermediate acting benzodiazepines are effective (Loper, 1989). Emergency management of such patients should take place in a calm and supportive atmosphere and consists of verbal reassurance ("talking down") and low-dose diazepam for severe agitation. Acute symptoms usually resolve within hours. The patient may then be admitted, or referred for further evaluation and treatment or follow-up.

Referral and Treatment

Various inpatient and outpatient substance abuse treatment programs are available to the adolescent with a drug abuse problem. The primary care physician should be sufficiently knowledgeable to refer the patient to an appropriate program or to a substance abuse professional for further evaluation (Millman and Botvin, 1983). The range of available programs is quite wide and includes psychiatric and nonpsychiatric inpatient detoxification units, inpatient rehabilitation programs based upon the disease model of chemical dependency and informed by Alcoholics Anonymous principles, therapeutic communities (Phoenix House, Daytop Village), and a variety of outpatient and day hospital programs. Self-help groups such as Alcoholics Anonymous, Cocaine Anonymous, Alanon, and Alateen are often a critical aspect of treatment, though some young people are not comfortable with the style and procedures of these fellowships. Some programs employ chemotherapeutic techniques such as methadone, while others emphasize an abstinent, drug-free approach. Most programs offer counseling or psychotherapy. Comprehensive programs designed specifically for adolescents appear to be the most effective means of providing care and preventive services (Semlitz and Gold, 1986). The following criteria may be used to guide treatment planning and referral:

1. Continued follow-up by primary clinical provider if:
   a. provider is knowledgeable in these areas;
   b. substance abuse is intermittent, experimental, and appropriate for age and sociocultural group;
   c. no significant psychopathology is present;
   d. function in educational, social, and vocational spheres is unimpaired;
   e. reasonable progress is taking place in developmental tasks; and
   f. no antisocial behavior is present.
2. Referral to specialized practitioner or treatment program if:
   a. uncertainty or lack of experience on the part of practitioner is present;
   b. frequent, regular, or compulsive drug abuse is found;
   c. psychopathology requiring evaluation and treatment is present;
   d. impaired function in educational, social, legal, or occupational spheres is found; and
   e. certain circumstances prevail (e.g., when a specialized unit is available); in such situations, evaluation on an inpatient basis is needed.
3. Referral to inpatient drug-treatment program or specialized hospital if:
   a. compulsive or addictive drug use is present (e.g., adolescent is brought for evaluation intoxicated or actively abusing drug);
   b. there is impaired function in educational, social, legal, or occupational spheres;
   c. imminent danger is posed to physical or mental health of the patient;
   d. persistent antisocial behavior is found (e.g., stealing or dealing);
   e. failure at prior outpatient treatment has occurred;
   f. psychopathology requiring behavioral and/or pharmacological management is present; and
   g. there is behavior presenting danger to self or others that requires containment or physical restraint.

References

Aghajanian GK: Serotonin and the action of LSD in the brain. *Psychiatr Ann* 24(3):137–144, 1994.

Alterman AI, Tarter RE: An examination of selected typologies: hyperactivity, familial and antisocial alcoholism. In: Galanter M (ed): *Recent Developments in Alcoholism* (Vol 4). New York, Plenum, 1986.

American Psychiatric Association: *Diagnostic and Statistical Manual of Mental Disorders* (3rd ed, rev). Washington, DC, American Psychiatric Press, 1987.

Bewley B, Bland J, Harris R: Factors associated with the starting of cigarette smoking by primary school children. *Br J Prevent Soc Med* 28:37–44, 1974.

Bjorkqvist SE, Isohanni M, Makela R, et al: Ambulant treatment of alcohol withdrawal symptoms with carbamazepine: A formal multicentre double-blinded comparison with placebo. *Acta Psychiatr Scand* 53:333–342, 1976.

Blane HT, Hewitt LE: *Alcohol and Youth: An Analysis of the Literature, 1960–1975* (Contract ADM 281-75-0026). Washington, DC, National Institute on Alcohol Abuse and Alcoholism, 1977.

Blum R, Richards L: Youthful drug use. In: Dupont RI, Goldstein A, O'Donnel J (eds): *Handbook on Drug Abuse*. Washington, DC, US Department of Health, Education and Welfare Office of the President, National Institute on Drug Abuse, 1979, pp. 257–267.

Borland BL, Rudolph JP: Relative effects of low socioeconomic status, parental smoking and poor scholastic performance on smoking among high school students. *Soc Sci Med* 9:27–30, 1975.

Braucht GN, Brakarsh D, Follingstad D, et al: Deviant drug use in adolescence: A review of psychosocial correlates. *Psychol Bull* 79:92–106, 1973.

Bukstein OG, Brent DA, Kaminer Y: Comorbidity of substance abuse and other psychiatric disorders in adolescents. *Am J Psychiatry* 146(9):1131–1141, 1989.

Bukstein O, Kaminer Y: The nosology of adolescent substance abuse. *Am J Addict* 3(1):1–13, 1994.

Carlson GA, Cantwell DP: Unmasking masked depression in children and adolescents. *Am J Psychiatry* 137:445–449, 1980.

Centers for Disease Control: Heterosexually acquired AIDS—United States, 1993. *MMWR* 43(9):155–159. March 11, 1994a.

Centers for Disease Control: Update: impact of the expanded AIDS surveillance case definition for adolescents and adults on case reporting—United States, 1993. *MMWR* 43(9):160–170. March 11, 1994b.

Centers for Disease Control: U.S. Public Health Service recommendations for human immunodeficiency virus counseling and voluntary testing for pregnant women. *MMWR* 44(RR-7):July 7, 1995.

Chaisson RE, Bacchetti P, Osmond D, et al: Cocaine use and HIV infection in intravenous drug users in San Francisco. *JAMA* 261:561–565, 1989.

Childress AR, McLellan, O'Brien CP: Role of

conditioning factors in the development of drug dependence. *Psychiatr Clin North Am* 9:413–426, 1986.

Choi HK, Coates TJ: Prevention of HIV infection. *AIDS* 8:1149–1155, 1994.

Climko RP, Roehrich H, Sweeney DR, et al: Ecstasy: A review of MDMA and MDA. *Int J Psychiatry Med* 16:359–370, 1987.

Cloninger CR, Bohman M, Sigvardsson S: Inheritance of alcohol abuse: cross-fostering analysis of adopted men. *Arch Gen Psychiatry* 36:861–868, 1981.

Coan RW: Personality variables associated with cigarette smoking. *J Pers Soc Psychol* 26:86–104, 1973.

Cregler LL, Mark H: Medical complications of cocaine abuse. *N Engl J Med* 315:1495–1500, 1986.

Dackis C, Gold AS: Neurotransmitter and neuroendocrine abnormalities associated with cocaine use. *Psychiatr Med* 3:461–483, 1987.

Demone HW: The nonuse and abuse of alcohol by the male adolescent. In: Chafetz M (ed): *Proceedings of the Second Annual Alcoholism Conference* (Publication no. [HSM]73-9083). Washington, DC, US Department of Health, Education and Welfare, 1973.

Des Jarlais DC, Friedman SR, Novick DM, et al: HIV-1 infection among intravenous drug users in Manhattan, New York City, from 1977 through 1987. *JAMA* 261:1008–1012, 1989.

Dowling GP, McDonough ET III, Bost RO: "Eve" and "Ecstasy": A report of five deaths associated with the use of MDEA and MDMA. *JAMA* 257:1615–1617, 1987.

Estroff TW, Schwartz RH, Hoffmann NG: Adolescent cocaine abuse: Addictive potential, behavioral and psychiatric effects. *Clin Pediatr* 28:550–555, 1989.

Frezza M, di Padova C, Pozzato G, et al: High blood alcohol levels in women: The role of decreased gastric alcohol dehydrogenase activity and first-pass metabolism. *N Engl J Med* 322:95–99, 1990.

Fugelstad A, et al: Mortality among HIV-infected intravenous drug addicts in Stockholm in relation to methadone treatment. *Addiction* 90:711–716, 1995.

Fullilove RE, Fullilove MT, Browser BP, et al: Risk of sexually transmitted disease among black adolescent crack users in Oakland and San Francisco, Calif. *JAMA* 263:851–855, 1990.

Gallemore JL, Wilson WP: Adolescent maladjustment or affective disorder? *Am J Psychiatry* 129:608–612, 1972.

Gawin FH: Chronic neuropharmacology of cocaine: Progress in pharmacotherapy. *J Clin Psychiatry* 49(suppl):11–16, 1988.

Gergen MK, Gergen KJ, Morse SM: Correlates of marijuana use among college students. *J Appl Soc Psychol* 2:1–16, 1972.

Goodwin DW: Studies of familial alcoholism: A review. *J Clin Psychiatry* 45:14–17, 1984.

Haefly W: Biological basis of drug induced intolerance, rebound, and dependence. Contribution of recent research on benzodiazepines. *Pharmacopsychiatry* 19:353–361, 1986.

Hahn RA, Onorato IM, Jones TS, et al: Prevalence of HIV infection among intravenous drug users in the United States. *JAMA* 261:2677–2683, 1989.

Harrison M, Busto U, Naranjo CA, et al: Diazepam tapering in detoxification for high dose benzodiazepine abuse. *Clin Pharmacol Ther* 36:527–533, 1984.

Hein K, Cohen MI, Litt JF: Illicit drug use among urban adolescents: A decade in retrospect. *Am J Dis Child* 133:38–40, 1979.

Hesselbrock MN: Gender comparison of antisocial personality disorder and depression in alcoholism. *J Subst Abuse* 3(2):205–219, 1991.

Hoyumpa A: Alcohol interactions with benzodi-azepines and cocaine. *Adv Alcohol Subst Abuse* 3:21–34, 1984.

Hunt WA, Barnett LW, Branch LG: Relapse rates in addiction programs. *J Clin Psychol* 27:455–456, 1971.

Jarvik ME, Cullen JW, Gritz ER, et al: Research on Smoking Behavior (National Institute on Drug Abuse Research Monograph 17, DHEW Publication no. [ADM] 78-581). Washington, DC, US Government Printing Office, 1977, p. 383.

Johanson CE, Fischman M: The pharmacology of cocaine related to its abuse. *Pharmacol Rev* 41:3–52, 1989.

Johnston LD, Bachman JG, O'Malley P: Reporting on their 1989 National Survey of American High School Seniors and their 10th National Survey of American College Students. University of Michigan, News and Information Services, Feb. 9, 1990.

Johnston LD, Bachman JG, O'Malley P: Reporting on the 1993 results of the 19th annual National Survey of American High School Seniors and their 3rd annual survey of eighth and tenth graders. University of Michigan, News and Information Services, January 31, 1994.

Johnston J, O'Malley P, Bachman J: *Drug Use among American High School Students, College Students and Other Young Adults* (National Institute on Drug Abuse, DHHS Publication no. [ADM] 86-1450). Washington, DC, US Government Printing Office, 1986.

Johnston J, O'Malley P, Bachman J: *Illicit Drug Use, Smoking and Drinking by America's High School Students, College Students, and Young Adults, 1975–1987* (DHHS Publication no. [ADM] 89-1602). Washington, DC, US Government Printing Office, 1988.

Johnston LD, O'Malley PM, Bachman JG: National surbey results on drug use from monitoring the future study, 1975–1992. Rockville, MD, U.S. Department of Health and Human Services, 1993.

Kamali K, Steer RA: Polydrug use by high school students: Involvement and correlates. *Int J Addict* 11:337–342, 1976.

Kandel D: Adolescent marijuana use: Role of parents and peers. *Science* 181:1067–1081, 1973.

Kandel D: Epidemiological and psychosocial perspectives on adolescent drug use. *J Am Acad Child Psychiatry* 21:328–347, 1982.

Kandel DB, Logan JA: Patterns of drug use from adolescence to young adulthood: Periods of risk for initiation, continued use and discontinuation. *Am J Public Health* 74:660–666, 1984.

Kaye K, Elkind L, Goldberg D, et al: Birth outcomes for infants of drug abusing mothers. *NY State J Med* May:256–261, 1989.

Khantzian EJ, Mack JE, Schatzberg AF: Heroin use as an attempt to cope: Clinical observations. *Am J Psychiatry* 131:160–164, 1974.

Kleber HD: Cocaine abuse: Historical, epidemiological and psychological perspectives. *J Clin Psychiatry* 49(suppl):3–6, 1988.

Lindan CP, et al: Levels of HIV testing and low validity of self-reported test results among alcoholics and drug users. *AIDS* 8:1149–1155, 1994.

Loper KA: Clinical toxicology of cocaine. *Med Toxicol Adverse Drug Exp* 4:174–185, 1989.

McCusker J, Stoddard AM, Zapka JG, Lewis BF: Behavioral outcomes of AIDS educational interventions for drug users in short term treatment. *Am J Pub Health* 83(10):1463–1465, 1993.

Millman RB: Drug and alcohol abuse. In: Wollman BB, Egan J, Ross AC (eds): *Handbook of Mental Disorders in Childhood and Adolescence.* Englewood Cliffs, NJ, Prentice-Hall, 1978, pp. 238–267.

Millman RB: Drug abuse, addiction, and intoxication. In: Beason P, McDermott W, Wynguarden JB (eds): *Cecil Textbook of Medicine* (15th ed). Philadelphia, Saunders, 1979, pp. 672–714.

Millman RB: Considerations on the psychotherapy of the substance abuser. *J Subst Abuse Treatment* 3:103–109, 1986.

Millman RB, Beeder AB: The new psychedelic culture: LSD, Ecstasy "rave" parties and The Grateful Dead. *Psychiatr Ann* 24(3):148–150, 1994.

Millman RB, Botvin GJ: Substance use, abuse and dependence. In: Levine MD, Carey WB, Crocker AC, et al (eds): *Developmental Behavioral Pediatrics.* Philadelphia, Saunders, 1983, pp. 683–708.

Millman RB, Sbriglio R: Patterns of use and psychopathology in chronic marijuana users. *Psychiatr Clin North Am* 9:533–545, 1986.

Naranjo CA, Sellers EM, Lawrin MO: Modulation of ethanol intake by serotonin uptake inhibitors. *J Clin Psychiatry* 47:16–22, 1986.

O'Brien CP, Childress AR, Arndt IO, et al: Pharmacological and behavioral treatments of cocaine dependence: Controlled studies. *J Clin Psychiatry* 49(suppl):17–22, 1988.

Post RW: Chronic cocaine administration: Sensitization and kindling effects. In: Fisher S, Raskin A, Uhlenhuth EH: *Cocaine: Clinical and Biobehavioral Aspects.* New York, Oxford University Press, 1987.

Reis R, Roy-Byrne PP, Ward NG, et al: Carbamazepine treatment for benzodiazepine withdrawal. *Am J Psychiatry* 146:536–537, 1989.

Reith MEA, Sershen H, Allen DL. et al: A portion of (3H) cocaine binding in brain is associated with serotonergic neurons. *Mol Pharmacol* 23:600–606, 1983.

Ronald PJM, Robertson JR, Elton RA: Continued drug use and other cofactors for progression to AIDS among injecting drug users. *AIDS* 8:339–343, 1994.

Salzman C: Grand rounds presentation. New York, Payne Whitney Clinic, February 27, 1989.

Seldin NE: The family of the addict: A review of the literature. *Int J Addict* 7:97–107, 1972.

Sellers EM, Kalant H: Alcohol intoxication and withdrawal. *N Engl J Med* 294:752–762, 1976.

Semlitz L, Gold M: Adolescent drug abuse. Diagnosis, treatment, and prevention. *Psychiatr Clin North Am* 9:455–473, 1986.

State of New York Anti-Drug Abuse Strategy Report. New York, The Governor's Statewide Anti-Drug Abuse Council, 1989.

Turner C, Miller H (eds): *AIDS, Sexual Behavior Intravenous Drug Use.* Washington, DC, National Academy Press, 1989, pp. 186–255.

US Public Health Service: *Teenage Smoking: National Patterns of Cigarette Smoking, Ages 12 through 18, in 1972 and 1974* (DHEW Publication no. [NIH] 76-931). Washington, DC, US Government Printing Office, 1976.

Volpicelli JR, Clay KL, Watson NT, O'Brien CP: Naltrexone inthe treatment of alcoholism; predicting response to naltrexone. *J Clin Psychiatry* 56(suppl7):39–44, 1995.

Wechsler H, Thurn D: Alcohol and drug use among teenagers: A questionnaire study. In: Chefiz M (ed): *Proceedings of the Second Annual Alcoholism Conference* (DHEW Publication no. [HSM] 73-9083). Washington, DC, US Government Printing Office, 1973.

Weiss SH: Links between cocaine and retroviral infection. *JAMA* 261:607–609, 1989.

Williams AF: Personality and other characteristics associated with cigarette smoking and young teenagers. *J Health Soc Behav* 14:374–380, 1973.

Woody G, Schuckit M, Weinreib R and Yu E: A review of the substance use disorders section of the DSM-IV. *Psychiatr Clin North Am* 16:1:21–32, 1993.

Zinberg NE: Addiction and ego function. In: Eissler RS, Freud A, Kris M, et al (eds): *The Psychoanalytic Study of the Child.* New Haven, CT, Yale University Press, 1975.

70 ACUTE RESPONSES TO EXTERNAL EVENTS AND POSTTRAUMATIC STRESS DISORDER

Lenore C. Terr, M.D.

Children respond to horrifying events with mental mechanisms that lead to acute and, at times, chronic psychological disorders. The events that cause these disturbances are usually ones that, through their intensity, their threats to the child or to someone else, their unusual nature, and their suddenness or quality of surprise, break past the child's ordinary coping and defensive mechanisms, rendering the child temporarily, utterly helpless. "Traumatic events" of childhood are almost always outside the range of what would have been expected in the course of an ordinary childhood. In other words, a divorce in the family would not, in and of itself, qualify as a traumatic event, but a parental knifing in the midst of that divorce, witnessed by the child or involving a direct threat to the child, most likely would. Current requirements under DSM-IV would include as qualifying events only those that threaten the child's life or physical integrity or those that the child witnesses, experiences, or is confronted with, having to do with someone else's threatened death or loss of physical integrity (American Psychiatric Association, 1994).

Traumatic events do not always create psychic trauma. In order for a "traumatic experience" to occur, mental adjustments to the traumatic event must take place. For the child's mind to take in and to adjust to a traumatic event, the child (*a*) must understand that he or she is in danger or is witnessing something terrible, (*b*) must sense his or her own extreme helplessness, and (*c*) must perceive (register) and store an implicit or explicit traumatic memory. Once the child appreciates the dangerousness, the threat, and the inability to do anything about it, and then processes this memory, the child will very likely experience either a single symptom or a number of psychological symptoms that comprise "posttraumatic stress disorder" or psychic trauma. Single findings of psychic trauma or a few minor findings may currently be considered an "adjustment disorder, with anxiety," although the specific posttraumatic symptoms may linger for years and may influence the child's later development. If there is considerable dissociation, along with a few single symptoms of trauma, the condition may also be called "acute stress disorder."

HISTORICAL NOTE

From the time of the Civil War on, it was recognized that some fighting men suffered from extreme stress on the battlefield and later experienced a number of physical and mental symptoms. Over the next 60 or 70 years, terms such as *battle fatigue* and *shell shock* were used to characterize some of these mental syndromes of war, most of which were probably posttraumatic. In 1920 Freud, in considering adults who had endured World War I, defined psychic trauma as a "breach" in the "stimulus barrier." In updated words, trauma was caused by a highly intense, unexpected event that penetrated past the ordinary coping and defensive operations. In 1926 Freud went on to define the key emotional response in psychic trauma as the sense of "utter helplessness." Freud's 1920 and 1926 definitions were quite modern and remain operational today (Freud, 1920/1955, 1926/1959).

Little was known about the psychic traumas of childhood, however, until two psychoanalytic trends—the direct study of children and the retrospective reconstruction of the childhoods of adults—began to stimulate valuable reports in the 1940s. David Levy published a landmark study in 1945 on the psychic traumas connected with childhood surger-

ies, analogizing children's responses to the responses of soldiers in World War II. Levy's work led to a new humanism on the pediatric ward. But it did not move child psychiatry toward intense study of childhood psychic trauma. Marie Bonaparte (1945) and Phyllis Greenacre (1949), both adult analysts, published interesting case reports in which the recovery of early traumatic memories assisted their older patients' recoveries. But this type of single case report did not set a trend toward reconstruction of childhood traumas in adults or direct psychoanalytic observations of traumatized children.

Anna Freud and her group at Hampstead studied a number of young children who had been evacuated from London during the blitz (Freud and Burlingham, 1943) and a small group of children who had been liberated from German concentration camps (Freud and Dann, 1951). Freud and her colleagues concerned themselves with child-parent relationships and parental loss. Although these Hampstead studies profoundly influenced child psychiatry as a field, they did not significantly clarify the mechanisms of psychic trauma. As a matter of fact, the most influential trend of the later 1940s and 1950s insofar as psychic trauma was concerned was the idea that "nervous" mothers created "nervous" children. It was believed that, if parents or guardians maintained complete calm under frightening circumstances, children would not be traumatized (Carey-Trefzger, 1949; Mercier and Despert, 1943; Solomon, 1942).

In the mid-1950s a significant field study of psychic trauma in school-age Mississippi children who had endured a tornado at a Saturday afternoon movie matinee was undertaken by Block et al. (1956). This team from the National Institute of Mental Health interviewed and surveyed the affected children's parents only. The conclusion that anxious parents created anxious children was almost an inevitable result of the study design itself. The study, however, did set an important trend because it looked at the results of a single traumatic event in a large group of children.

The stress and coping researches of the 1960s and 1970s defined many of the mechanisms that children use in dealing with ongoing stress. This research was particularly good in highlighting the protective functions that schools could fulfill for children who lived in stress-filled environments (Rutter et al., 1979). It also demonstrated that a child's innate capacities of intelligence, humor, and relatedness (Garmezy, 1987), as well as a child's basic character structure (Murphy and Moriarty, 1976), could be protective. Coping and stress research, however, did not specifically deal with the mental effects of the most extreme events, the traumatic ones.

In the late 1970s two important field projects began to shift the field's attention toward traumatized children. The first was Gaynor Lacey's (1972) follow-up of the October 21, 1966, Aberfan, Wales, mining disaster that destroyed an entire school. Lacey reported on 56 children who consulted him in his psychiatric practice in the 5 years that followed the event. He detailed a number of signs and symptoms that affected these children who had been away from their parents at the time they were traumatized. C. Janet Newman (1976), in reporting upon 11 children who had endured the February 1972, Buffalo Creek, West Virginia, flood, demonstrated how pessimistic and fantasy-ridden these traumatized children had become. Newman's paper also presented the drawings of very young children who had endured the disaster. Their artistic products carried the stamp of developmental immaturity, while at the same time conveying horror equal to anything an adult might experience.

In 1976 a school bus carrying 26 youngsters in Chowchilla, California, was captured by three kidnappers. The children were driven into a gully where they were transferred from the bus into blackened vans. They drove about for 11 hours in total darkness. They then were transferred into a buried truck trailer and covered with gravel and rocks. After 16 or 17 hours of confinement underground, the children were able to effect their own escape. This entire group was studied individually and prospectively from 1977 (Terr, 1979) through 1980–1981 (Terr, 1983a). Their parents or guardians were also interviewed. They were matched in 1980–1981 to a control group of school children more than 100 miles away (Terr, 1983b).

The Chowchilla study outlined the key manifestations of trauma observed in children and early adolescents. These symptoms and signs are summarized in the "Clinical Findings" section of this chapter.

INCIDENCE, PREVALENCE, AND EPIDEMIOLOGY

The incidence of psychic trauma in the Chowchilla school bus kidnapping was 100%. Regardless of the child's prior developmental, psychiatric, and medical history, his or her parental relationships, the relationships of his or her parents to the community, his or her past psychic trauma, and/or stressful events inside the family, the child would suffer from psychic trauma if the traumatic event was extreme enough and was directly experienced. The factors mentioned above, however, did appear to influence the severity of the individual's clinical condition at 4–5 years following the event (Terr, 1983a).

The control group against Chowchilla, the McFarland-Porterville group (Terr, 1983b), served as a small and very preliminary "prevalence" study of psychic trauma. Life attitudes, dreams, play patterns, fears, ideas about the future, and past frightening events were collected from interviews with 25 "normal" children (randomly selected and then age-, race-, and sex-matched to the Chowchilla group). The school principals and registrars had eliminated from this control group children already known to be trauma victims. Of this group of 25 "normal" children, 10 children appeared to be suffering from either extreme fright or psychic trauma. Although this study was small and quite preliminary, the prevalence of symptoms of psychic trauma in a normal population of school-age children appeared to be much higher than would have been expected.

In 1986, Galante and Foa published an epidemiological study of children following the devastating earthquakes that occurred in southern Italy. They concluded that the usual nonspecific screening instruments for childhood psychopathology were inadequate to determine the incidence and prevalence of childhood psychic trauma. In another study of children who survived a ferry disaster, Yule and Williams (1990) also demonstrated that commonly used screening instruments did not adequately pick up the extreme events that were occasionally experienced in childhood. Yule and Williams's study further demonstrated that children's self-reports were superior to parental reports or teacher reports, especially if any of these three was to be relied upon alone.

Pynoos et al. (1987) studied a sample of youngsters who attended a school that had been attacked by a sniper. Among those children under direct threat (in the playground), there was a 94.3% incidence of posttraumatic stress disorder. Psychic trauma was also found in 88.9% of those children who had been at the school during the attack. Among those children who had been at home or on school vacation when the sniper attacked, on the other hand, the incidence of psychic trauma was 45%. This study demonstrated that the full range of symptoms qualifying for a posttraumatic disorder was most likely to occur in those individual children for whom the dose of exposure to the traumatic event was the most extreme. Nader et al. (1990) conducted a 1-year follow-up study of this same sniper-exposed sample. At that time, bereavement for the child who had died in the sniper shooting was more commonly associated with posttraumatic stress disorder than were other factors. Those

children with the most direct exposure to the sniper attack continued to exhibit the most severe posttraumatic stress reactions.

In an incident in which there are varying doses of exposure to the threat, one does not expect a 100% incidence of psychic trauma. Also, when the threat is less obvious to a group of children, one may not see much posttraumatic disorder at all. Handford et al. (1986) studied 35 households for children's (ages 6–19) posttraumatic responses after the Three Mile Island Nuclear Power Plant accident. Although their anxiety scores were higher than normative levels for children, no child in this group received a diagnosis of posttraumatic stress disorder. Earls et al. (1988) used diagnostic interviews with 32 children (6–17 years old) from 20 households after a previously forecast flood forced family evacuations and damaged their property. A number of children in this group showed single findings of posttraumatic stress disorder, but none of them met the criteria for the full diagnosis.

It appears that children may suffer from bothersome symptoms of posttraumatic stress disorder without attaining the number or spread of symptoms necessary to achieve the diagnosis. Shannon et al. (1994) did a large study of 5,687 school children (ages 9–19) from Berkeley County, South Carolina, 3 months after Hurricane Hugo hit their rural area with unanticipated force (much of the county had not been evacuated). More than 5% of this sample reported sufficient symptoms to be classified as suffering from posttraumatic stress syndrome. But many more children had some symptoms. Girls reported more symptoms related to the emotional processing of the trauma than did boys. Boys reported more symptoms connected with behavioral and cognitive processing of the trauma than did girls. The presence of posttraumatic stress disorder (PTSD) symptoms after Hurricane Hugo were closely related to the severity of the storm, as experienced by the child, the amount of home damage, and the family displacement that had resulted (Lonigan et al., 1994). Children's level of trait anxiety (as measured by the Revised Children's Manifest Anxiety Scale (RCMAS)) and their reported emotional reactivity at the time of the hurricane also strongly influenced whether or not they experienced posttraumatic symptoms. In an earlier paper on the Hurricane Hugo effects by Lonigan et al. (1991), it was found that higher levels of impact (fierceness of the storm, homelessness, etc.) were accompanied by more PTSD symptoms or by a few symptoms endorsed at a high intensity level (on the Frederick's PTSD Reaction Index (1985)).

In a British study of 334 preadolescent and adolescent school children who had been aboard the sinking ship *Jupiter* on October 21, 1988 (one pupil, one teacher, and two seamen died), Joseph et al. (1993) found that half of the group met DSM-III-R criteria for PTSD. This, of course, was a far more intense and unanticipated situation than the South Carolina hurricane. Furthermore, it was a situation that children experienced apart from their families. But it was also a situation that caused bothersome symptoms in numbers of children who did not satisfy the full criteria for PTSD.

Although general psychiatric diagnostic structured interviews are not particularly sensitive or specific to the problems of psychic trauma, the Diagnostic Interview Schedule was used by Davidson et al. (1991) in an epidemiological catchment area (ECA) study to assess the prevalence of posttraumatic stress disorder in 2,985 adult subjects in a southeastern community. The lifetime prevalence of PTSD was 1.3%, and the 6-month prevalence was 0.44%. In another ECA study, interviewing only heads of Midwestern households regarding symptoms of PTSD in their families, Helzer et al. (1987) found a prevalence of 1% in the total group of 2,493 participants. Fifteen percent of participants, however, had experienced some, though not enough, of the symptoms of posttraumatic stress following a "frightening event" to have qualified for this diagnosis. Again, this study implies that physicians and mental health professionals may be called upon to treat bothersome symptoms in children who do not meet the full current criteria for PTSD.

It appears that a number of untreated children, who qualify for the diagnosis of posttraumatic stress disorder within a few months of a traumatic incident, lose their full qualifications for the diagnosis within a year or two. Of 808 children exposed to devastating brush fires in Australia, McFarlane et al. (1987) found that the frequency of the PTSD symptom complex was 94% 2 weeks after the fires, but 47% at the 9-month mark. Milgram et al. (1988) reported that 40% of children in a bus accident met the criteria for PTSD 1 month afterward, but by 9 months after the accident, the prevalence had diminished to 20%. These observed diminutions in prevalence rates may have to do, in part, with the original intensity of the exposure.

CLINICAL FINDINGS IN CHILDHOOD TRAUMA

Traumatized children present different clinical pictures if they are seen early in the course of the condition (within days), later following the event (weeks to months), or very late (years afterward). They also present somewhat different clinical pictures with their different developmental stages. Furthermore, they may appear different clinically when they were raised in cultures different from ours. For these reasons the diagnostic process in childhood psychic trauma is somewhat more complex than it is in adults.

Early Traumatic Responses (Within Minutes to Days)

At the moment a child is traumatized, the child usually retains full physical and emotional control. Bladder and bowel functions remain intact. Screaming rages or fits of misbehavior are highly unusual. One little boy, age 25 months, went ''limp'' but retained full consciousness during an airplane crash. From most children's behavior, it appears that children usually are silent during traumatic events, although they are capable of speech (Terr, 1979). Some children recall experiencing ''funny'' feelings in their stomachs, strange sensations on their skin, or dizziness. Children, however, do not ordinarily exhibit more massive evidences of physiological disturbances, such as blood pressure changes, heart malfunctions, difficulty breathing, or unconsciousness.

From the first, many children begin thinking retrospectively about why the horrifying event took place, why they were ''chosen,'' and what they could have done to avoid it. Turning points and retroactive reason for the event are sought. This tendency has been termed ''omen formation'' (Terr, 1979), ''cognitive reappraisal'' (Pynoos, 1989), and ''causal attribution'' (Joseph et al., 1991). It tends to last years in the course of the posttraumatic condition. In fact, Joseph's group found that causal attributions were significantly associated with other symptoms of PTSD in adults following the Herald Free Enterprise shipping disaster.

Children remember single, shocking events in extraordinary detail. It is highly unlikely that a child will have a fuzzy memory or an absent memory of such a one-time experience unless (a) the child was traumatized in a series of events or by a single event with long-lasting consequences such as the death of a family member or friend (Terr, 1991); (b) the child was below age 28–36 months at the time of the trauma and thus developmentally unable to lay down, store, and/or retrieve verbal memories (Terr, 1988); or (c) the child was unconscious, delirious, or suffered a concussion during the event(s) (Terr, 1990).

While memories of trauma—in those children paying attention and old enough to remember—stay remarkably clear, the details of these memories may become distorted through initial or ongoing misperceptions. Time, for instance, often becomes elongated or shortened, depending upon the original length of the event (Terr, 1984). Time placements may become ''skewed'' as events that came later are misplaced by the child into simultaneous or preceding positions. The child may misperceive the appearance of a person connected with the traumatic event, especially if that person was a stranger when the event took place (Terr, 1979, 1984). The child may also visually hallucinate (Terr, 1979, 1985). These tendencies often distort some of the ''facts'' children remember as part of their verbal narratives (Terr, 1994). The tendency to hallucinate or to suffer visual illusions may continue long into the course of the posttraumatic disorder. In fact, some children who do not misperceive early in the course of their traumas may begin to do so later (Terr, 1984,

1985). They may see ''ghosts,'' sense ''presences,'' or catch glimpses of perpetrators who are actually locked up in prison or are dead.

Pynoos and Nader found that some of the children who had been exposed to the Los Angeles sniper shooting of their elementary school tended to distort the amount of space between themselves and the sniper's gun (1989). Children, who were close, reported the shooting as further away than it had actually been. Children who were more removed ''saw'' it as closer. Although traumatized children may misjudge the relative danger of their own positions, they also tend to remember their own bodily orientations and placements with great detail (Terr, 1990). This placement memory may be sketched out in maps or drawings. For some children who initially cannot recapture much of a traumatic experience in words, such drawings may unlock a significant segment of their experience. A child's remembered placement in connection with a traumatic event may help to retrieve other parts of the memory that are less amenable to spontaneous recovery.

Traumatic imagery may come back to younger children upon reminders or while they are resting—at leisure or before sleep. Older adolescents may find their activities interrupted by more sudden flashbacks. In the first weeks after a traumatic event a young child may have trouble falling asleep and remaining asleep. He or she may have problems paying attention in school and in learning. If a child originally felt confused, detached, or numb, this sense may also continue for some time. Three months after Hurricane Hugo, Lonigan et al. (1994) described more numbing and detachment in those children who had experienced a sense of sadness initially connected with the storm.

Fears come up almost immediately in psychic traumas. They are of two types: (a) fear of a repetition of some literal, specific aspect of the traumatic experience and (b) fear of a ''mundane'' item, such as of the dark, being separated from parents, being alone, being outside, and strangers. Fears, though early to come in the course of the externally generated stresses of childhood, are late to go. As opposed to sleep difficulties and problems with attention, which are usually short-lived following a single, unrepeated traumatic event, fears continue for long periods of time. The American diagnostic manuals, while speaking of avoidances, do not use the word ''fears'' in their diagnostic lists. In children, however, fears are far more striking than are the associated avoidances.

In the first few weeks following a traumatic event, an affected child may develop dreams that literally repeat the experience. On the other hand, nonverbal children tend to dream unremembered terror dreams. Nonverbal children may also sleepwalk or sleeptalk (Terr, 1979). The ability to dream with remembered content is a developmental step (Mack, 1968). Traumatic dreaming, therefore, is not a consistent finding in traumatized children, especially in those who were very young when originally traumatized (Terr, 1987, 1988).

Children begin to play out, draw, dramatize, or tell their stories of trauma within days to a few weeks of the event. These repeated creative attempts to master overwhelming frights are characteristic of childhood. Posttraumatic play is grim, monotonous, and, at times, dangerous (Terr, 1981). Usually, the linkage between the play and the trauma is not evident to the child. This play often also escapes significance to the child's parents. Posttraumatic play, however, is transparent to a mental health professional because it is such a literal recreation of the original psychic dilemma. The traumatized child is very likely to play in the psychiatrist's office, even though he or she may also play secretly at home. To facilitate observing this play, the child might be asked to bring some favorite toys from home to the office, or the child psychiatrist might provide trauma-reminiscent toys among the other toys in the playroom (MacLean, 1977; Shapiro, 1973). In general, however, highly suggestive toys do not have to be introduced to the consulting room in order for the psychiatrist to observe posttraumatic play in traumatized children. The power of the childhood drive to play in the aftermath of terror impels the child to play, no matter what toys are offered. As a matter of fact, this kind of play demands so much repetition that even the traumatized adolescent, well beyond the age-range of the usual ''pretend'' player, may play posttraumatically when given sophisticated options such as tape recorders, air brushes, poetry recitations, or dramatic scenarios (Terr, 1990).

Responses to Psychic Trauma Within Months

In the course of a few months most of the full range of traumatic findings become evident in children, though some symptoms may begin to fade. Fears may extend. Repeated dreams, if they ever were a problem, are now fully evident. Memories remain intact. Sleeplessness, irritability, and school behavioral or learning problems may begin to resolve. Recollections of the event upon reminder, or when the mind is at rest, are active and can be quite bothersome.

Within months, however, one new type of repetitive behavior frequently emerges. This repetition, termed reenactment because it is not defined by children as ''fun,'' is often problematic (Terr, 1979). Reenactments of trauma may be single—one sudden unexplained action by the child reminiscent of some feeling engendered by the event or reminiscent of a defense that went into operation at the time. Reenactments may also be multiple, so frequently repeated that they lead to permanent personality changes. The child may victimize others because he once felt the victim himself. The child may retreat into passivity again and again because it was once ''dangerous'' to be outgoing. The most extreme character changes following psychic trauma come from the multiple, long-standing, violent, and, often, intrafamilial traumas (Kiser et al., 1991; Terr, 1990). But less-extensive character changes on the basis of reenactment may also follow from single traumas (Terr, 1983a).

Responses to Psychic Trauma Within Years

As the years go by, the traumatized child or adolescent and the family become more and more resistant to the idea of obtaining professional help. The child may not mention the traumatic events, even in a psychiatric interview, unless specifically requested to tell ''the worst thing that ever happened.'' He or she may refuse to enter treatment, although others suggest it and even offer to pay for it (Terr, 1980a).

Posttraumatic ''anniversary reactions'' sometimes become noticeable to others as the years go by. For the child, the connections may be lost as time obscures the old traumatic causality. However, resurgences of symptoms at times or in places reminiscent of the original traumatic event are quite common.

For children not at the center of a traumatic event, the full diagnostic criteria of posttraumatic stress disorder may not be met over the years. Some trauma-related fears fade. By progressively conditioning themselves to face feared objects, by moving away from a town where horrifying events happened, and by living ''safely'' for a period of time after a terrible event, children may eliminate some posttraumatic fears. It is rare, however, to find a traumatized child who is completely fear-free long after a traumatic event (Terr, 1983a). Fourteen months following the Los Angeles sniper attack, 78.9% of those children who had been on the playground during the shooting still felt afraid when they thought about the event, and 63.2% of them felt specifically fearful that a sniper attack would happen again (Nader et al., 1990). Fear appears to be a long-lasting finding.

Preoccupation with the traumatic event also remains a striking long-term finding. In his 26-month parent and teacher questionnaire follow-up of the Australian brush fires, McFarlane (1987) found that a third of the children were still dwelling on the event.

Over a long period of time traumatized children also limit their expectations for the future. The 4- to 5-year follow-up study of the Chowchilla kidnapping victims (Terr, 1983a) revealed that 23 of the 25 children had trouble envisioning a full, long life, a career, or a marriage. Several of these children envisioned world catastrophe. In the control group against Chowchilla (Terr, 1983b), it was found that problems in envisioning the future also accompanied the trauma that was discovered in this control sample. Future foreshortening is an important late finding of childhood trauma.

Comorbidity

Childhood posttraumatic stress disorder often coexists with attention deficit hyperactivity disorder. McLeer and her group showed (in clinic-referred groups of 31 and of 92 sexually abused children, 1988, 1992) that 48.4 and 43.9% of them, respectively, met the DSM-III-R criteria for PTSD. When a smaller group of these children was given the Schedule for Affective Disorders and Schizophrenia (K-SADS-E) interviews, 44% qualified for PTSD, while 33.3% qualified for a diagnosis of attention deficit disorder with hyperactivity (1992). There was also a high incidence of conduct disorders in this sexually abused group. When McLeer's team used KSADS-E to compare a group of 36 children referred to their clinic for sexual abuse with 23 children referred to the clinic for problems unrelated to sexual abuse, they found that attention deficit disorder was the most common diagnosis in both groups (1994). It, thus, appeared that children of various diagnoses may be referred to clinics when their attention and/or conduct problems become too much for the adults who provide them care. In a new study, McLeer et al. picked a group of children not referred to their clinic, but rather, untreated, sexually abused youngsters who were recruited directly from the Department of Human Services. They found comorbidity in these children with the other anxiety disorders and depressive spectrum disorders (S.V. McLeer, personal communication, 1993), rather than with the attention or conduct disorders.

There are a number of other disorders that also appear to be comorbid with PTSD of childhood. Simple phobias, separation anxiety disorders, and dissociative disorders, for example, may be diagnosed following traumatic occurrences. This may, however, represent an overlapping of symptoms, rather than a true comorbidity (McLeer et al., 1994). On the other hand, Kinzie et al. found major depressive disorder in Cambodian refugees who had emigrated to America after the terrifying Pol Pot regime. There was significant coexistence of PTSD with the depressive disorders in this group (1986, 1989). In older traumatized children and adolescents, substance abuse may also coexist or may originate secondarily to the PTSD.

Garbarino's Chicago-based group has shown that children who experience war or community violence are at greater risk for developmental impairment, physical damage, and race hatred (1991, 1992). A number of adult character disorders may also develop secondarily to childhood traumas; or they may coexist with these traumas (Terr, 1991).

Psychic Trauma at Various Phases of Development

Children traumatized below approximately age 28–36 months are incapable of putting their traumas to full narrative accounts or to full verbal memory (Terr, 1988). A spurt in hippocampal development around the age of 3, at about the time children begin to speak fluidly in phrases (Terr, 1994), probably enables a child above age 3 to begin verbally to remember a whole traumatic event. Despite failure to remember traumatic events fully and explicitly, infants and toddlers demonstrate fears, difficulties envisioning a future, posttraumatic play, reenactment, and some dreams and night terrors. This means that implicit memories of the traumas have been laid down and stored (Terr, 1988). Young traumatized children, in other words, tend not to remember with the clarity that children traumatized at older ages do, but they tend to fear specifically, to reenact, and to limit their projections for the future based upon entirely ''pictorial,'' ''feel,'' or ''habit'' memories. These memories are handled in other parts of the brain than the hippocampus.

Some adolescent responses to traumatic events may begin to resemble those of adults rather than those of younger children. Adolescents may, for instance, suffer quick, intrusive, unwelcome flashbacks similar to the flashbacks that adults experience (Horowitz, 1976; Terr, 1979). Adolescents play games of pretend less than they do in the latency years, and, therefore, they may not give a history of posttraumatic play. Adolescents may experience more sleeplessness, inattentiveness, and irritability than latency-age children. These developmental variations in the traumatic responses of adolescents are quite uneven. Traumatized adolescents experience posttraumatic symptoms, but their particular symptom clusters depend on their individual development.

Gender may influence the kind and extent of PTSD symptoms a child suffers (Lonigan et al., 1994). Girls and young children in the South Carolina hurricane cohort were more likely to have suffered PTSD symptoms. Similarly, Green et al. (1991, 1994) found in their studies 2 and 14 years after the Buffalo Creek flood that women had higher rates of PTSD than did men. Lest one consider the gender issue to be closed, however, Garbarino and Kostelny (1996) found that among 158 Palestinian children living with political violence on the West Bank in 1990, the boys were more susceptible to negative outcomes than were the girls.

Younger children (ages 6–9) were more vulnerable to political violence, Kostelny and Garbarino found, than were older children (ages 12–15). However, in reviewing the Buffalo Creek disaster data, Green et al. (1991) found that preschoolers, because they had fewer avoidant symptoms, qualified as having fewer PTSD symptoms than school-age and adolescent children. Green's group hypothesized that this finding might be artifactual because very young children would have been less able to put their avoidant symptoms into words and because young children's avoidant behaviors might have been more difficult to observe.

As time goes on in a child's development, a trauma may be rethought and reexperienced emotionally from the vantage point of the child's new developmental phase (Terr, 1990). As time goes on, trauma victims may also be retraumatized because they unconsciously reenact (Russell, 1986). Some of this reenactment is dangerous to the self or others. Trauma victims may also be retraumatized because some of them live in violent families or in violent communities where the risk for new trauma is high.

ETIOLOGY AND PATHOGENESIS

Psychic trauma is environmentally determined. If the traumatic event is intense enough, any child will be traumatized (Pynoos et al., 1987; Terr, 1979). This environmental origin does not mean, however, that once traumatized, a child will not be modified biologically. Organic-style visual hallucinations have been noted to occur while traumatic events are proceeding (Terr, 1979). This implies an almost immediate and massive release of neurotransmitters in the brain upon traumatic impact. There are three major systems in the brain that have thus far been implicated, though not proven, as contributing to the biology of posttraumatic stress: (a) the internal opiate system, (b) the noradrenergic system, and (c) the hypophysical pituitary-adrenal system.

Pitman et al. (1990) postulated that brain endorphins might cause the psychic numbing that is observed in trauma. The internal opiate system hypothetically causes the victim to fail to respond, to avoid, to shut off feelings. Pitman's group gave the morphine antagonist, naloxone, to 8 pain-resistant Vietnam veterans, and found that these veterans' pain and emotional responses became more normal. This preliminary experiment implied that active internal opiates operated in some trauma. When the pituitary releases adrenocorticotropic hormone (ACTH) in order to regulate the levels of cortisol in the body, β-endorphins are also simultaneously released in the brain (Dent et al., 1981). These β-endorphins may stimulate trauma-seeking behaviors and the tendencies to self-medication or self-mutilation that are observed in some adult trauma victims (Kosten and Krystal, 1988).

A second brain system that might be responsible for some of the changes observable in childhood trauma is the catecholaminergic system. Ornitz and Pynoos (1989) studied traumatized children's startle responses in order to understand related biological mechanisms (most likely in the catecholaminergic system). Startle responses ordinarily become more muted and controlled as development progresses. These investigators reported on a boy of 8 who underwent an apparent 4-year regression in the quality of his startle responses after he witnessed a murder.

In a study of rhesus monkeys, Kraemer et al. (1984) showed that monkeys, who were socially isolated during their 1st year of life, exhibited hypersensitive stereotypic responses to low doses of amphetamine administered 2–3 years after their isolation. These monkeys showed greater increases in cerebrospinal fluid norepinephrine than did normal monkeys. This implies a long-term change in central noradrenergic responses following extreme stress in early childhood (Rosen and Fields, 1988).

One preliminary study of children, done at the University of Minnesota (Jensen et al., 1991), offered some data on brain norepinephrine and dopamine responses in sexually abused and physically abused boys. These groups were compared to normal nonabused and psychiatrically referred, nonabused boys. The boys were compared regarding their growth hormone release, as stimulated by two central-acting catecholamine stimulants or agonists—clonidine, which acts to block α_2-adrenergic receptors, and L-dopa, which blocks dopaminergic activity. There were differences between the sexually abused and physically abused boys: the sexually abused boys exhibited an increased growth hormone response to clonidine and a decreased growth hormone response to L-dopa; the physically abused boys exhibited a decreased growth hormone response to clonidine and an increased response to L-dopa.

A third possible site of action of trauma on the brain is the hypothalamic-pituitary-adrenal axis. Corticosteroids are powerful agents around the body, and corticosteroid-releasing factors operate inside the brain as neurotransmitters. When cortisol was measured in the 24-hour urine specimens of traumatized veterans, the veterans' cortisol levels were found to be low (Mason et al., 1986). When these veterans' usually high serum norepinephrine was calculated as a ratio to their urinary cortisol, this norepinephrine/cortisol ratio began to define a difference between traumatized and schizophrenic or bipolar-disordered veterans. Although these ratios are not presently used for clinical purposes, and although they do not in any direct way apply to children, they may eventually point the way to a biological hypothesis of childhood stress. McEwen et al. (1987) suggested that stress-altered norepinephrine/cortisol ratios may produce brain changes through the actions of genomes. These are slow, relatively long-lasting changes; and they may stand in contrast to the relatively quick actions of the catecholamines.

Some investigators into the biology of trauma (Yehuda et al., 1990) believe that a changed, ongoing interrelationship between the noradrenergic system of the brain and the hypothalamic-pituitary-adrenal axis accounts for some of the symptom patterns that are noted in trauma. Excitatory responses (symptoms like posttraumatic repetitions and startle responses) might come from the stimulating effects of the corticosteroids on the noradrenergic functions of the brain cells. Inhibitory responses (symptoms like numbing and avoidances) might come from the effects of corticosteroids on the genetic activities of the brain.

A group at Emory University, working with young laboratory rats, has hypothesized that corticotropic substances released inside brain cells may be essential to the biological expressions of childhood trauma (C. Nemeroff, personal communication, 1994). This is a new area of investigation that may relate to some of the long-standing changes observed in traumatized children.

The interrelationships between the three major biological systems thus far implicated in PTSD are complex. Yet these are crucial to our understanding of externally generated disorders. Proofs are not available. We will need many more studies of children and of young animals before a full biological understanding of trauma emerges.

Psychological studies having the most bearing upon the mechanisms of psychic trauma are those dealing with (a) memory (Ceci et al., 1987; Johnson and Foley, 1984; Loftus and Davies, 1984), (b) visual perceptions (Chance and Goldstein, 1984), and (c) time sense (Fraisse, 1963). These studies are tailored only to the responses of normal children in nontraumatic circumstances. However, they are relevant because they deal with whether children can witness events reliably. Traumatized children exhibit perceptual and memory responses that are different from those of normal youngsters (Terr, 1994). A study of adults' memories for upsetting stories that they recently heard also implies that stressful memories are handled differently in the brain from bland memories (Cahill et al., 1994). This kind of memory response deeply concerns the legal system, where children must often serve as witnesses (Benedek and Schetky, 1985; Pynoos and Eth, 1984; Terr, 1980b). A child below the approximate age of 28–36 months is usually unable to form a complete, remembered narrative of his or her trauma (Terr, 1988). The child who cannot remember an ordeal in words is almost always able to show through his or her symptoms, however, that the trauma was perceived and implicitly remembered.

Once a child is traumatized, the child's family is also often found to be directly or indirectly traumatized (Terr, 1989). It is important to evaluate family members, including those who were removed from the traumatic events at the time it happened. Entire communities, including those who were elsewhere, have been shown to suffer psychic trauma when massive catastrophes strike (Erikson, 1976).

Traumatic symptoms tend to spread by rumors, folk tales, child "gossip," and play. Indirect victims may pick up isolated symptoms without any exposure to the event itself. This, of course, relates to the question of whether television or films can traumatize children. Laurel Kiser, of the University of Tennessee, Memphis, did an interesting study (1993) in this regard. Dan Rather of CBS News had predicted on national television in the fall of 1990 that a massive earthquake would be coming to the New Madrid Fault area in December 1990. Kiser's group studied randomly selected children both before and after this disaster failed to materialize. Children living near the fault were found to have experienced a significant upsurge of posttraumatic symptoms, not from any exposure to an earthquake, but from their exposures to the TV show and the surrounding talk in their communities.

Cultural influences may favor certain symptoms over others following traumatic events. A long-term study of Cambodian refugee children, conducted by researchers from the Oregon Health Sciences University, showed a high prevalence of depressive symptoms, along with posttraumatic symptoms, both 1 and 3 years after these children moved to America. Avoidant behaviors were very common in this group, even in those adolescents who did not have a diagnosis of PTSD (Kinzie et al., 1986, 1989; Sack et al., 1986). Different symptom patterns emerge in other cultures. Ziv and Israeli (1973) studied Israeli children who were under direct bombardment in the Golan Heights versus children who had been away from the war zone. These children were asked for self-reports regarding anxiety. There were no differences between the children of the two kibbutzim that were compared. Later, the Ziv team studied the same two groups for indirect physiological measures of anxiety. They found a significant difference between the two groups regarding the amount of nighttime teeth-grinding (bruxism). Apparently, Israeli cultural expectations for childhood stoicism in the face of adversity had influenced those youngsters who lived on the Golan Heights to minimize the anxiety in their self-reports.

DIFFERENTIAL DIAGNOSIS

The main problem in differentiating traumatized children from normal ones is the problem of determining: (a) Did an event actually happen? (b) Was the child actually exposed to this event? (c) Does the child have sufficient posttraumatic symptomatology to qualify under the current diagnostic requirements?

Questions about whether the traumatic event ever happened can often, but not always, be answered by checking third-party reports—pediatrician and hospital records, police documents, newspaper accounts, neighbors' testimony, and the testimony of eyewitnesses. Parental histories are important in this regard, but further documentation from other sources is often also necessary. Is it possible to speak to the siblings? To the neighbor children or peers from school? To the police? Occasionally the police are so suggestive in their questioning of children that "true" stories are suspect. Previous mental health treatments of the child or parental influences on the child may also be suggestive. It is

often necessary for the child/adolescent psychiatrist to review videotapes, transcripts, and therapeutic notes in order to help determine whether a certain child participated in the event in question. A child may develop a few, isolated posttraumatic signs and symptoms of low intensity simply from being told about a frightening event. However, the chances of developing a full-blown posttraumatic stress disorder in connection with suggestion from parents, police, or therapists are slim. Therefore, the best psychiatric proofs of a child's exposure to a traumatic event are the external corroborations from outside reports and the internal confirmations from the child's own symptom complex (Terr, 1994).

No child's memory per se ("story") can be assessed in a vacuum. Truisms in our field—that plenitude of details indicates veracity; that "seeing the memory" vouches for its reality; that the use of child language indicates truthfulness; that consistency of these stories over time confirms the child's reliability—all of these, though often right, have been proven wrong through a few, but notable, exceptions. Exceptions make it impossible to rely on memories alone. Children with proven traumas often retain false details as part of their memories about these real exposures (Terr, 1979, 1981). Thus, it is necessary to rely on both internal and external confirmations when assessing a child's trauma—and, in a sense, the professional must function at times as a medical detective.

Some childhood trauma is complicated by accompanying conditions. If a long-term horrifying series of events or one single event causes the death of an important figure in a child's life, the child will be bereaved as well as traumatized (Eth and Pynoos, 1985; Kinzie et al., 1986; Pynoos and Eth, 1984). If a long series of procedures, connected with a serious childhood illness, is administered to a child, the child may become traumatized, as well as physically ill and depressed (Nir, 1985; Stoddard et al., 1989; Stuber et al., 1991). If old psychic trauma becomes laden with characterological attempts to compensate for the trauma, the child may be diagnosed as having a "personality disorder" or a "conduct disorder." In a study of 27 physically abused versus 27 nonabused boys, Pelcowitz et al. (1994) found, in fact, that the physically abused boys were more at risk for behavioral and social disorders than for PTSD. Some PTSD symptoms may have been masked, perhaps, by the much more pressing characterological problems. One study of adolescents in residential treatment (Doyle and Bauer, 1989) suggested that rigorous use of the diagnostic criteria for PTSD be employed in assessing these cases. These authors suggested that PTSD be occasionally rediagnosed in order to identify what current traumatic reminders are precipitating otherwise unexplained adolescent behaviors.

LABORATORY STUDIES

At present, there are no clinically accepted laboratory studies that help to clinically differentiate PTSD from other conditions. A study by Perry (1992) of adolescents in a residential treatment setting showed that those traumatized in childhood had tachycardia, alterations in α_2 platelet receptors, and a marked reduction of symptoms in response to clonidine. These tests, however, were more useful to research than to the child's assessment.

At present, psychological testing does not include tests that are specific enough indicators of trauma to be particularly helpful. Draw-a-Person tests or Draw-a-Family tests occasionally pick up a posttraumatic drawing, but these tests were not designed for such purposes.

Susan McLeer and her Philadelphia-based research team has conducted a number of studies over the years that rely on standardized instruments to assess childhood symptoms of PTSD. She has suggested (1992) that three of these, which differentiate PTSD children from non-PTSD children, might be helpful in clinical practice—the Child Behavior Checklist (CBCL (Achenbach, Edelbrock, 1983)), the PTSD Reaction Index (Frederick, 1985a, 1985b), and the KSADS-E (Orvaschel et al., 1981, 1982). Wolfe et al. (1989) studied the psychometric properties of one of the subscales of the CBCL, which appears useful in assessing PTSD children. The PTSD Reaction Index may also be helpful in documenting a child's symptom severity, as well as in monitoring a child's treatment response over time. None of these instruments, however, currently serves as a standard assessment tool.

Clinical Interviews

The child interview and play session provide the most useful diagnostic instruments in finding posttraumatic disorder of childhood. One may ask the child to tell the story of "the worst thing that ever happened." Or, if the trauma is recent, one may ask for the story of what brings the child to the office. At some point during the diagnostic process, the story—if the child remembers—should be obtained in the child's own words. Care must be taken not to ask suggestive or leading questions, though cues are often needed before a young child even understands what the psychiatrist is inquiring about (Terr, 1994). One also asks the child for symptoms and assesses the child for the signs of trauma. Other psychiatric conditions are also assessed in the child, as are any developmental, health, or family problems. A free play session and a drawing period is also observed whenever possible. Two or three such observations will pick up repetitions of play themes and of modes of play. What the child says about the play or drawings is equally important to the play product itself.

TREATMENT

Prevention

Disastrous episodes at schools (such as the murder, accidental death, or suicide of a peer) and in communities (earthquakes, tornados, hurricanes, etc.) require early responses from child psychiatrists (Terr, 1989). School-related emergencies may be first managed through school assemblies and ceremonies that are aimed at education, clarification, and ventilation of the children's feelings (Terr, 1992a). At times, children can be handled in large groups with "minimarathon" sessions that emphasize the sharing of experiences, symptoms, and stories of heroism (Terr, 1992b). Smaller groups at schools that have felt the impact of a trauma are often organized by counselors and mental health professionals. Best friends and close classmates of a dead child, for instance, might participate in a regularly meeting small group, whereas distant acquaintances might meet only once or twice. Teachers also require considerable guidance during such postdisaster periods (Eth, 1992; Eth et al., 1985; Pynoos and Nader, 1988).

School-centered prevention groups may proceed up to 2 hours at a time. Drawing, poetry making, and story writing may be incorporated. The idea is to allow a group of children to tell their various stories and then to show that each individual has put his or her own emphasis to the very same happening. The group is encouraged to discuss certain common symptoms. Suggestions are made for desensitizing fears and nightmares, and for regaining a sense of personal control. (How do you call the police? How do you alert adults when you need help? etc.) Each child in a group is encouraged to speak at least once. Children who suffer intense symptoms or a number of symptoms may be identified during these group sessions and referred for individual psychotherapy.

Some child and adolescent psychiatrists have learned in recent years how to work with television, radio, and newspapers when mass disasters affect their communities (Terr, 1992a). Stemming the tide of mass hysteria is a worthwhile goal. Radio call-in shows have been found to serve good purposes (Blaufarb and Levine, 1972). Early ventilation of feelings has long been known to prevent some of the posttraumatic casualties that otherwise might occur (Grinker and Spiegel, 1945; Levy, 1939).

Medication

Early in the course of a posttraumatic or acute stress disorder, an occasional child (and/or the child's family) may require medication. Although medication has not thus far been shown to handle the entire posttraumatic problem, it may be a useful adjunct. Despite the need for

more data, however, the pharmacological treatment of childhood PTSD has barely been studied.

Clonidine, a centrally acting drug that is sometimes used for Tourette's syndrome, may help (in the same dose ranges as those for Tourette's) those children who have significant avoidant symptoms, startle responses, or trauma-related depressions (Kinzie and Leung, 1989). Propranolol, a β-blocking agent, was shown in an uncontrolled, unblinded study (Famularo et al., 1988) to relieve some of the symptoms of childhood posttraumatic stress disorder. The authors administered three divided doses of propranolol per day. A single dose of propranolol, calculated according to the child's weight, can also be used 30–40 minutes before the child must face a trauma-reminiscent situation (the dog-bite victim, for instance, who must walk home every day from school past the neighborhood dogs). Major drugs, such as the tricyclic antidepressants, may be used in traumatized children and adolescents, especially in those who exhibit strongly phobic or compulsive features as part of their disorder. But cautions regarding the cardiac side effects of these medications must be heeded. To mobilize those adult family members unable to help a child after a devastating event, quick-acting benzodiazepines, such as lorazepam or alprazolam, may be helpful to parents or guardians over short periods of time.

It is important to note, however, that in trauma, medication must be considered an adjunct to treatment, not the sole mode of therapy.

Group and Family Therapy

Group treatments for psychic trauma have been reported as quite effective, especially for groups in which everyone was exposed to the same event. It is important that all of the children in such groups be encouraged to speak out. It is also important that the group leader pick up and deal immediately with symptom contagion. Art work, poetry sharing, and dramatization are useful adjuncts to family and group therapy. In groups where there is considerable variance, from "severely traumatized" down to "untouched by the event," it is important for the group leader to eventually regroup the participants, releasing from that group those who have remained unaffected by posttraumatic symptomatology.

Individual Psychotherapy

Cognitive behavioral treatments have been used since the 1960s (see Silverman and Geer, 1968; Kipper, 1976) to desensitize posttraumatic dreams and fears in adults. More recently, Deblinger et al. (1990) reported an open clinical trial of cognitive behavioral therapy in 19 sexually abused and traumatized children. Each of the major categories of posttraumatic symptoms improved with this treatment. Although some children's individual symptoms persisted when the behavioral treatment ended, no one in this group of 19 met the full diagnostic criteria for PTSD any longer. One interesting behavioral modification technique that has appeared effective in managing posttraumatic nightmares and visualizations is to encourage the child to plan corrective endings before falling asleep and to will himself or herself to redream the repeated dream (Garfield, 1984). Since some childhood posttraumatic nightmares occur at not-quite-fully REM or stage 4 phases of sleep, these dreams come under partial conscious control. A reworked dream may serve to stop an entire dream series. But, although it is extremely useful, an entire trauma cannot be worked out behaviorally without more general interventions.

Play therapy is extremely useful in the individual treatment of the traumatized child (Gardner, 1971; Gil, 1991; Terr, 1983c; Webb, 1991). Drawing the scene of the event may help the child to speak fully about that event (Pynoos and Eth, 1986). Drawing also unlocks emotions, both in doing the art and in reviewing the art work. Speaking about the art helps both the patient and the therapist to unlock the personal meanings of the trauma. Children's drawings inspire the child to associate, and these associations should be jotted down, so that the psychiatrist can use them later in clarifying and interpreting the trauma. Winnicott's Squiggle Game is applicable to psychic trauma (Shapiro, 1983; Winnicott, 1971), as is David Levy's preset play (1939). It is important in presetting play that the psychiatrist give enough alternatives to the child in order to avoid oversuggestion, e.g., a lion, a tiger, and a bear, for instance, to a child mauled by a bear; three different commercial airplane toys to a child who crashed on a specific plane. Play therapy may be accomplished with indirect interpretations about "that puppet" or "that little girl." It can, however, be accompanied by direct interpretations aimed straight at the child.

Psychotherapy with traumatized children and adolescents may incorporate any or all of the techniques noted above. Psychotherapy can, however, be effective when only talk is involved. As long as there is some ventilation of feelings, exposure and discussion of symptoms, and clarification and interpretation of the child's defenses and coping strategies, psychotherapy will very likely help the victim. Talking therapies and play therapies should offer the child a "context" in which to view his or her trauma—a historical and a social perspective within the youngster's family, school, community, and the world. Perspective offers young traumatized people a tool with which to gain distance from their terrors. Given a fuller context, the traumatized child eventually realizes that the personal disaster occurred as a moment in life, not as a full life plan or a governing instant that controls all of life.

"Randomness" is also an important message of hope to a child, especially the child traumatized outside the bounds of the family. For children traumatized inside their own families, issues of betrayal, overexcitement, and personal responsibility must be considered. The messages "You are not alone" and "You are not the only one" are also very meaningful to traumatized children. The specific fears inspired by psychic trauma are different from the fears inspired in the course of an ordinary, internal development. These internal and external fears can eventually be separated by the child in psychotherapy. External fears can be overcome through behavioral modification. They also yield to playing games or discussing solutions with "corrective dénouements" (Gardner, 1971). Defensive elaborations following from the trauma must retreat before concluding therapy. In other words, a child should have found other ways to handle current situations beside dissociating, splitting, repressing, displacing, etc.

When trauma is compounded with grief and/or extreme anger, other measures must be taken. A London-based group (Black and Kaplan, 1988; Hendricks et al., 1993), for instance, has done interesting treatments with children whose fathers killed their mothers. They suggest therapeutic visits to the old neighborhood and to the mother's grave. They also suggest extreme care about child placements, and therapeutic awareness of when the father is getting out of prison. This group also urges that mourning takes place as part of the child's treatment.

OUTCOME

Childhood psychic trauma is amenable to treatment. The disorder is not, however, fully curable. Trauma leaves a "scar"—damaged attitudes about the future, pessimistic "one day at a time" philosophies, and unpredictable, intractable tendencies to repeat. As time goes on, we will develop better ideas about how to repair the more permanent damages wrought by outside events. But the better preventive programs we establish—for instance, well-regulated day care programs; better earthquake, tornado, hurricane, and volcano warnings; mechanisms for keeping drunk drivers off the highways; mechanisms for monitoring known pedophiles; gun control legislation—the fewer childhood trauma victims we will need to treat. And the better compliance from the public and the agencies to provide immediate treatment to young victims of known personal and general disasters, the better the eventual outcomes will be.

RESEARCH DIRECTIONS

There are a number of possible avenues of research in the still relatively wide open field of childhood trauma. Studies of the brains of knowingly killed children (as opposed to other childhood deaths) may eventually reveal what specific neurotransmitters were released during the trauma. Other physiological experiments on laboratory animals or living child subjects (within limits, of course) may also give us clues as to brain mechanisms in trauma.

Long-term follow-up studies of various kinds of traumas in various kinds of childhood groups may eventually reveal what happens when a traumatized child grows up. Epidemiological studies of large populations using more sophisticated surveys and structured interviews may also demonstrate how much childhood trauma goes undetected and how many traumatic symptoms—and with what intensity—affect children, whether or not they qualify for the PTSD diagnosis. Studies on how distant traumatic events impact the lives of normal children are also needed. Treatment outcome studies must eventually be done so that we will have more data-based information on preferable modes of practice.

CASE ILLUSTRATION

A 13-month-old child was removed by the authorities from her home because her 3-week-old baby sister was found murdered, shaken and bitten to death by one or more adults. Her father was put in prison for manslaughter. Her mother was not arrested. Upon coming into foster care, this little girl bit herself, bit others, shrieked in terror at the sight of overweight women (resembling her mother), and had difficulty using language with meaning. She clung to her foster mother, and often pinched her own genitals with no apparent provocation. She had great difficulty becoming socialized—completing her toilet training or playing with peers, for instance. She often stared incomprehensively into space. She attacked young babies and had to be watched almost every minute.

At age 3, this child came to the writer for evaluation because her mother had reestablished visitation, on the theory that eventually she would take the child back. This little girl trembled for hours before these visits occurred, and she returned quiet, with a blank face and eyes, and the tendency to talk about dead cats and babies. The writer of this chapter noted that the 3-year-old youngster feared the nutcracker doll on her shelf, the Zuni snake on her table, and the wooly sheep she kept on a child-sized table. The child stared at these items and trembled. The child would not touch the office baby doll, and when a tiny toy cat was presented to her for play, she enucleated the cat's eye, later pronouncing the small toy animal dead. When shown the photograph of a sleeping baby from a magazine ad, she screamed "Dead baby! Dead baby!" When asked to talk about what had happened when she was a little girl, this child said she did not know.

Here was a case in which a child had been gravely traumatized at the age of only 1 year, when she could not attain narrative memory. It is very likely that a cat had been blinded and killed by this biological family before or at the time the baby was bitten and shaken to death. It was also likely that this child herself had been treated similarly to the baby. It was also likely that this child had been sexually misused and injured. Upon receiving a letter from the child psychiatrist, the court temporarily put the idea of maternal visits or reunification aside.

The child, who lived at a great distance from the writer, came to her psychiatric office once a month. She developed a great love for tea parties, spending session after session deciding who could attend, which "bad" characters might be added without danger, and what requirements these characters must meet if they were to stay. She eventually revealed that she was afraid of an entire racial group (because they resembled her parents). She revealed that it "felt good" to mutilate her own leg with a pierced spoon (her foster parents stopped this behavior by immediately coming down hard about it). Each of this child's problems was discussed with her—her fears of bad events, of bad people, and of what could eventually happen to children. At age 3½ this child began drawing pictures of naked adults, with breasts, pubic hair, and blood on their mouths, dripping down the pages. She was told she might have seen something like this when she was too young to remember. (The decision to tell her this rested on the manslaughter conviction, the pathologist report about the dead baby, the report of a Stanford University pediatrician that had seen the adult bite marks on this 13-month-old child at the time she was brought into foster care, and on the child's current symptoms.)

When she was 4½ years old, this little girl was examined under anesthesia in a University of California San Francisco operating room (she had had a diffuse urinary stream). Her vagina was found to be stretched well-beyond the limits for a child of this age. Her urethra was scarred so extensively that a meatotomy had to be performed. This procedure cured her previous problems with urinating. It also created a convincing report that could be used in court.

The writer of this chapter informed the judge handling this child's custody of the injuries that now had been corrected by the surgical team. The writer made the point that a parent would have had to be—at the very least—exceedingly negligent to allow a 1-year-old to be injured in this way. The Court took this letter under advisement and required another letter explaining all past and current psychiatric symptomatology. A full hearing was then held regarding parental rights. The natural father signed off his paternal rights in prison, saying he did not care. The natural mother came to the hearing with an attorney, a social worker who believed in her, and her own protestations of innocence. The Court, acting on the psychiatric symptoms and the surgical findings in the little girl, terminated all parental rights.

At the time of this writing, this little girl, now 5 years old, has been adopted by her foster parents. The child rejoiced about the event, dressing up for the occasion and inviting some of her family to a real tea party in the psychiatrist's office. She has recently been told by this writer about the baby who died and about her own condition when she came to her foster parents. Her new mother took her to place flowers on the baby's grave. The writer gave this child a verbal story, and her new parents offered her a chance to visit her dead sister's grave in order to provide her a context for a previously inexplicable set of behaviors. With this new context, the little girl understands her life more fully and is ready to look forward, rather than acting blindly on her past. Her behavior is much improved, and she is adjusting to a regular kindergarten classroom in the public schools. Her behavior is no longer dangerous or self-harming. She is no longer fearful in most situations. It is anticipated that she will stop once-monthly therapy by the end of this year, perhaps moving to a once-seasonal series of brief evaluations to make sure that her development continues in a positive direction.

References

Achenbach TM, Edelbrock C: *Manual for the Child Behavior Checklist and Revised Child Behavior Profile.* Burlington, VT, University of Vermont Press, 1983.

American Psychiatric Association: *Diagnostic and Statistical Manual of Mental Disorders* (4th ed). Washington, DC, American Psychiatric Association, 1994.

Benedek E, Schetky D: False allegations of sexual abuse in child custody and visitation disputes. In: Schetky D, Benedek E (eds): *Emerging Issues in Child Psychiatry and the Law.* New York, Brunner/Mazel, 1985.

Black D, Kaplan T: Father kills mother: Issues and problems encountered by the child psychiatric team. *Br J Psychiatry* 153:624–630, 1988.

Blaufarb H, Levine J: Crisis intervention in an earthquake. *Soc Work* 17:16–19, 1972.

Block D, Silber E, Perry S: Some factors in the emotional reactions of children to disaster. *Am J Psychiatry* 113:416–422, 1956.

Bonaparte M: Notes on the analytic discovery of a primal scene. *Psychoanal Study Child* 1:119–125, 1945.

Cahill L, Prins B, Weber M, et al: β-Adrenergic activation and memory for emotional events. *Nature* 371:702–704, 1994.

Carey-Trefzger C: The results of a clinical study of war-damaged children who attended the Child Guidance Clinic, The Hospital for Sick Children, Great Ormond Street, London. *J Ment Sci* 95:535–559, 1949.

Ceci S, Ross D, Toglia M: Suggestibility of children's memory: Psychological implications. *J Exp Psychol* 116:38–49, 1987.

Chance J, Goldstein A: Face-recognition memory: Implications for children's eyewitness testimony. *J Soc Issues* 40:69–86, 1984.

Davidson JR, Hughes D, Blazer DG, et al: Posttraumatic stress disorder in the community: An epidemiological study. *Psychol Med* 21:713–721, 1991.

Deblinger E, McLeer SV, Henry D: Cognitive behavioral treatment for sexually abused children suffering posttraumatic stress: Preliminary findings. *J Am Acad Child Adolesc Psychiatry* 19:747–752, 1990.

Dent RRM, Guilleminault G, Albert LH, et al: Diurnal rhythm of plasma immunoreactive beta-endorphin and its relationship to sleep stage and plasma rhythms of cortisol and prolactin. *J Clin Endocrinol Metab* 52:942–947, 1981.

Doyle JS, Bower SK: Posttraumatic stress disorder in children: Its identification and treatment in a residential setting for emotionally disturbed youth. *J Traum Stress* 2:275–288, 1989.

Earls F, Smith E, Reich W, et al: Investigating psychopathological consequences of a disaster in children: A pilot study incorporating a structured diagnostic interview. *J Am Acad Child Adolesc Psychiatry* 27:90–95, 1988.

Erikson K: *Everything in Its Path.* New York, Simon & Schuster, 1976.

Eth S: Clinical response to traumatized children. In: Austin LS (ed): *Responding to Disaster: A Guide for Mental Health Professionals.* Washington, DC, American Psychiatric Press, 1992.

Eth S, Pynoos R: Interaction of trauma and grief in childhood. In: Eth S, Pynoos R (eds): *Post-Traumatic Stress Disorder in Children.* Washington, DC, American Psychiatric Press, 1985.

Eth S, Silverstein S, Pynoos RS: Mental health consultation to a preschool following the murder of a mother and child. *Hosp Community Psychiatry* 36:73–76, 1985.

Famularo R, Kinscherff R, Fenton T: Propranolol treatment of childhood posttraumatic stress disorder, acute type: A pilot study. *Am J Dis Child* 142:1244–1247, 1988.

Fraisse P: *The Psychology of Time.* New York, Harper & Row, 1963.

Frederick CJ: Children traumatized by catastrophic situations. In: Eth S, Pynoos R (eds): *Post-traumatic Stress Disorders in Children.* Washington, DC, American Psychiatric Press, 1985a.

Frederick CJ: Selected foci in the spectrum of posttraumatic stress disorders. In: Murphy LJ (ed): *Perspectives on Disaster Recovery.* East Norwalk, CT, Appleton-Century-Crofts, 1985b.

Freud A, Burlingham D: Infants without families. In: *The Writings of Anna Freud* (Vol 3). New York, International Universities Press, 1967. (Originally published 1943.)

Freud A, Dann S: An experiment in group upbringing. *Psychoanal Study Child* 6:127–168, 1951.

Freud S: Beyond the pleasure principle. In: Strachey J (ed): *The Standard Edition of the Complete Psychological Works of Sigmund Freud* (Vol 18). London, Hogarth Press, 1955. (Originally published 1920.)

Freud S: Inhibitions, symptoms, and anxiety. In: Strachey J (ed): *The Standard Edition of the Complete Psychological Works of Sigmund Freud* (Vol 20). London, Hogarth Press, 1959. (Originally published 1926.)

Galante R, Foa D: An epidemiological study of psychic trauma and treatment effectiveness after a natural disaster. *J Am Acad Child Adolesc Psychiatry* 25:357–363, 1986.

Garbarino J, Dubrow N, Kostelny K, et al: *Children in Danger: Coping with the Consequences of Community Violence.* San Francisco, Jossey-Bass, 1992.

Garbarino J, Kostelny K: The effects of political violence on Palestinian children's behavior problems: A risk accumulation model. *Child Development* 67:33–45, 1996.

Garbarino J, Kostelny K, Dubrow N: *No Place to Be a Child: Growing Up in a War Zone.* New York, Lexington Books, 1991.

Gardner R: *Therapeutic Communication with Children: The Mutual Storytelling Technique.* New York, Science House, 1971.

Garfield P: *Your Child's Dreams.* New York, Ballantine, 1984.

Garmezy N: Stress, competence, and development. *Am J Orthopsychiatry* 57:159–174, 1987.

Gil E: *The Healing Power of Play: Working with Abused Children.* New York, Guilford, 1991.

Green BL, Grace MC, Vary MG, et al: Children of disaster in the second decade: A 17 year follow-up of Buffalo Creek survivors. *J Am Acad Child Adolesc Psychiatry* 33:71–79, 1994.

Green BL, Korol M, Grace MC, et al: Children and disaster: Age, gender, and parental effects on PTSD symptoms. *J Am Acad Child Adolesc Psychiatry* 30:945–951, 1991.

Greenacre P: A contribution to the study of screen memories. *Psychoanal Study Child* 3/4:73–84, 1949.

Grinker R, Spiegel J: *Men under Stress.* Philadelphia, Blakiston, 1945.

Handford HA, Mayes SD, Mattison RE, et al: Child and parent reaction to the Three Mile Island nuclear accident. *J Am Acad Child Adolesc Psychiatry* 25:346–356, 1986.

Helzer JE, Robins LN, McEvoy L: Posttraumatic stress disorder in the general population: Findings of the Epidemiologic Catchment Area Survey. *N Engl J Med* 317:1630–1634, 1987.

Hendricks H, Black D, Kaplan T: *When Father*

Kills Mother: Guiding Children through Trauma and Grief. London, Routledge, 1993.

Horowitz M: *Stress Response Syndromes*. New York, Aronson, 1976.

Jensen JB, Pease JB, Bensel R, et al: Growth hormone response patterns in sexually or physically abused boys. *J Am Acad Child Adolesc Psychiatry* 30:784–790, 1991.

Johnson M, Foley M: Differentiating fact from fantasy: The reliability of children's memory. *J Soc Issues* 40:33–50, 1984.

Joseph SA, Brewin CR, Yule W, et al: Causal attribution and psychiatric symptoms in survivors of the Herald Free Enterprise disaster. *Br J Psychiatry* 159:542–546, 1991.

Joseph SA, Brewin CR, Yule W, et al: Causal attributions and post-traumatic stress in adolescents. *J Child Psychol Psychiatry* 34:1286–1302, 1993.

Kinzie JD, Leung P: Clonidine in Cambodian patients with posttraumatic stress disorder. *J Nerv Ment Dis* 177:546–550, 1989.

Kinzie JD, Sack WH, Angell RH, et al: The psychiatric effects of massive trauma on Cambodian children. *J Am Acad Child Adolesc Psychiatry* 25:370–376, 1986.

Kinzie JD, Sack WH, Angell RH, et al: A three-year follow-up of Cambodian young people traumatized as children. *J Am Acad Child Adolesc Psychiatry* 28:501–504, 1989.

Kipper D: The desensitization of war-induced fears. *Curr Psychiatr Ther* 16:41–47, 1976.

Kiser L, Heston J, Hickerson S, et al: Anticipatory stress in children and adolescents. *Am J Psychiatry* 150:87–92, 1993.

Kiser LJ, Heston J, Millsap PA, et al: Physical and sexual abuse in childhood: Relationship with posttraumatic stress disorder. *J Am Acad Child Adolesc Psychiatry* 30:776–783, 1991.

Kosten TR, Krystal J: Biological mechanisms in posttraumatic stress disorder: Relevance for substance abuse. In: Galanter M (ed): *Recent Developments in Alcoholism*. New York, Plenum, 1988.

Kraemer GW, Ebert MC, Lake CR, et al: Hypersensitivity to D-amphetamines several years after early social deprivation in rhesus monkeys. *Psychopharmacology* 82:266–271, 1984.

Lacey G: Observations on Aberfan. *J Psychosom Res* 16:257–260, 1972.

Levy D: Release therapy. *Am J Orthopsychiatry* 9:713–736, 1939.

Levy D: Psychic trauma of operations in children. *Am J Dis Child* 69:7–25, 1945.

Loftus E, Davies G: Distortions in the memory of children. *J Soc Issues* 40:51–68, 1984.

Lonigan CJ, Shannon MP, Finch AJ Jr, et al: Children's reactions to a natural disaster: Symptom severity and degree of exposure. *Adv Behav Res Ther* 13:135–154, 1991.

Lonigan CJ, Shannon MP, Taylor CM, et al: Children exposed to disaster. II: Risk factors for the development of posttraumatic symptomatology. *J Am Acad Child Adolesc Psychiatry* 33:94–105, 1994.

Mack J: Nightmares, conflict, and ego development in childhood. *Int J Psychoanal* 46:403–428, 1968.

MacLean G: Psychic trauma and traumatic neurosis. *Can Psychiatr Assoc J* 22:71–76, 1977.

Mason JW, Giller EL, Kosten TR, et al: Urinary free-cortisol levels in posttraumatic stress disorder patients. *J Nerv Ment Dis* 174:145–149, 1986.

McEwen BS, Brinton R, Harrelson A, et al: Modulatory interactions between steroid hormones, neurotransmitters, and neuropeptides in hippocampus. In: Nerozzi D, Goodwin F, Costa E (eds): *Hypothalamic Dysfunction in Neuropsychiatric Disorders*. New York, Raven Press, 1987.

McFarlane AC: Post-traumatic phenomena in a longitudinal study of children following a natural disaster. *J Am Acad Child Adolesc Psychiatry* 26:764–769, 1987.

McFarlane AC, Policansky SK, Irwin C: A longitudinal study of the psychological morbidity in children due to a natural disaster. *Psychol Med* 17:727–738, 1987.

McLeer SV: Post-traumatic stress disorder in children. In: Burrows G, Roth M, Noyes R Jr (eds): *Handbook of Anxiety 5: Contemporary Issues and Prospects for Research in Anxiety Disorders*. New York, Elsevier, 1992.

McLeer SV, Callaghan M, Henry D, et al: Psychiatric disorders in sexually abused children. *J Am Acad Child Adolesc Psychiatry* 33:313–319, 1994.

McLeer SV, Debliner E, Atkins MS, et al: Post-traumatic stress disorder in sexually abused children. *J Am Acad Child Adolesc Psychiatry* 27:650–654, 1988.

McLeer SV, Deblinger E, Henry D, et al: Sexually abused children of high risk for post-traumatic stress disorder. *J Am Acad Child Adolesc Psychiatry* 31:875–879, 1992.

Mercier M, Despert L: Effects of war on French children. *Psychosom Med* 5:226–272, 1943.

Milgram NA, Toubiana YH, Klingman A, et al: Situational exposure and personal loss in children's acute and chronic stress reactions to a school bus disaster. *J Traum Stress* 1:339–352, 1988.

Murphy L, Moriarty A: *Vulnerability, Coping and Growth*. New Haven, CT, Yale University Press, 1976.

Nader K, Pynoos R, Fairbanks L, et al: Children's PTSD reactions one year after a sniper attack at their school. *Am J Psychiatry* 147:1526–1530, 1990.

Nader K, Yasuda P, et al: Stress responses after pediatric bone marrow transplantation: Preliminary results of a prospective longitudinal study. *J Am Acad Child Adolesc Psychiatry* 30:16–21, 1991.

Newman CJ: Children of disaster: Clinical observations at Buffalo Creek. *Am J Psychiatry* 133:306–312, 1976.

Nir Y: Post-traumatic stress disorder in children with cancer. In: Eth S, Pynoos R (eds): *Posttraumatic Stress Disorders in Children*. Washington, DC, American Psychiatric Association, 1985.

Ornitz E, Pynoos R: Startle modulation in children with post-traumatic stress disorder. *Am J Psychiatry* 146:866–870, 1989.

Orvaschel H, Puig-Antich J, Chambers W, et al: Retrospective assessment of prepubertal major depression with the Kiddie-Sads-E. *J Am Acad Child Psychiatry* 21:392–397, 1982.

Orvaschel H, Weissman MM, Padier W, et al: Assessing psychopathology in children of psychiatrically disturbed parents: A pilot study. *J Am Acad Child Psychiatry* 20:112–122, 1981.

Pelcowitz D, Kaplan S, Goldenberg B, et al: Posttraumatic stress disorder in physically abused adolescents. *J Am Acad Child Adolesc Psychiatry* 33:305–312, 1994.

Perry BD: Neurobiological sequelae of childhood trauma: Posttraumatic stress disorder in children. In: Murberg M (ed): *Catecholamine Function in Posttraumatic Stress Disorder: Emerging Concepts*. Washington, DC, American Psychiatric Press, 1992.

Pitman RK, Van der Kolk BA, Orr SP, et al: Naloxone reversible stress induced analgesia in posttraumatic stress disorder. *Arch Gen Psychiatry* 47:541–547, 1990.

Pynoos R: Post-traumatic stress disorder in children and adolescents. In: Garfinkel B, Carlson G, Weller E (eds): *The Medical Basis of Child and Adolescent Psychiatry*. Philadelphia, Saunders, 1989.

Pynoos R, Eth S: The child as witness to homicide. *J Soc Issues* 40:87–108, 1984.

Pynoos R, Eth S: Witness to violence: The child

interview. *J Am Acad Child Adolesc Psychiatry* 25:306–319, 1986.

Pynoos RS, Nader K: Psychological first aid and treatment approach to children exposed to community violence: Research implications. *J Traum Stress* 1:445–473, 1988.

Pynoos RS, Nader K: Children's memory and proximity to violence. *J Am Acad Child Adolesc Psychiatry* 28:236–241, 1989.

Pynoos R, Frederick C, Nader K, et al: Life threat and post-traumatic stress in school age children. *Arch Gen Psychiatry* 44:1057–1063, 1987.

Rosen J, Fields R: The long-term effects of extraordinary trauma: A look beyond PTSD. *J Anxiety Disord* 2:179–191, 1988.

Russell D: *The Secret Trauma*. New York, Basic Books, 1986.

Rutter M, Maughan B, Mortimore P, et al: *Fifteen Thousand Hours: Secondary Schools and Their Effect on Children*. London, Open Books, 1979.

Sack W, Angell RH, Kinzie JD, et al: The psychiatric effects of massive trauma on Cambodian children. II: The family, the home, and the school. *J Am Acad Child Adolesc Psychiatry* 25:377–383, 1986.

Shannon MP, Lonigan CJ, Finch AJ Jr, et al: Children exposed to disaster. I: Epidemiology of post-traumatic symptoms and symptom profiles. *J Am Acad Child Adolesc Psychiatry* 33:80–93, 1994.

Shapiro S: Preventive analysis following a trauma. *Psychoanal Study Child* 28:249–285, 1973.

Shapiro T: The unconscious still occupies us. *Psychoanal Study Child* 39:547–568, 1983.

Silverman I, Geer J: The elimination of a recurrent nightmare by desensitization of a related phobia. *Behav Res Ther* 6:109–111, 1968.

Solomon J: Reactions of children to black-outs. *Am J Orthopsychiatry* 12:361–362, 1942.

Stoddard FJ, Norman DK, Murphy JM, et al: Psychiatric outcome of burned children and adolescents. *J Am Acad Child Adolesc Psychiatry* 28:589–595, 1989.

Stuber ML, Nader K, Yasuda P, et al: Stress responses after pediatric bone marrow transplantation: Preliminary results of a prospective longitudinal study. *J Am Acad Child Adolesc Psychiatry* 30:16–21, 1991.

Terr L: Children of Chowchilla. *Psychoanal Study Child* 34:547–623, 1979.

Terr L: Personal injury to children: The civil suit claiming psychic trauma. In: Schetky D, Benedek E (eds): *Child Psychiatry and the Law*. New York, Brunner/Mazel, 1980a.

Terr L: The child as a witness. In: Schetky D, Benedek E (eds): *Child Psychiatry and the Law*. New York, Brunner/Mazel, 1980b, pp. 207–221.

Terr L: ''Forbidden games'': Post-traumatic child's play. *J Am Acad Child Psychiatry* 20:740–759, 1981.

Terr L: Chowchilla revisited. *Am J Psychiatry* 140:1543–1550, 1983a.

Terr L: Life attitudes, dreams, and psychic trauma in a group of ''normal'' children. *J Am Acad Child Psychiatry* 22:221–230, 1983b.

Terr L: Play therapy and psychic trauma: A preliminary report. In: Schaefer C, O'Connor K (eds): *Handbook of Play Therapy*. New York, Wiley-Interscience, 1983c.

Terr L: Time and trauma. *Psychoanal Study Child* 39:633–666, 1984.

Terr L: Remembered images and trauma. *Psychoanal Study Child* 40:493–533, 1985.

Terr L: Children's nightmares. In: Guilleminault C (ed): *Sleep and Its Disorders in Children*. New York, Raven Press, 1987, pp. 231–242.

Terr L: What happens to the early memories of trauma? A study of twenty children under age five at the time of documented traumatic events. *Am J Child Adolesc Psychiatry* 27:96–104, 1988.

Terr L: Family anxiety after traumatic events. *J Clin Psychiatry* 50(suppl):15–19, 1989.

Terr L: *Too Scared to Cry*. New York, Harper & Row, 1990. (Paperback, New York, Basic Books, 1992.)

Terr L: Childhood traumas: An outline and overview. *Am J Psychiatry* 148:10–20, 1991.

Terr L: Large-group preventive treatment techniques for use after disaster. In: Austin LS (ed): *Responding to Disaster: A Guide for Mental Health Professionals*. Washington, DC, American Psychiatric Press, 1992a.

Terr L: Mini-marathon groups: Psychological "first aid" following disasters. *Bull Menninger Clin* 56:76–86, 1992b.

Terr L: *Unchained Memories: True Stories of Traumatic Memories, Lost and Found*. New York, Basic Books, 1994.

Webb NB: *Play Therapy with Children in Crisis: A Casebook for Practitioners*. New York, Guilford, 1991.

Winnicott DW: *Therapeutic Consultations in Child Psychiatry*. New York, Basic Books, 1971.

Wolfe VV, Gentile C, Wolfe DA: The impact of sex abuse on children: A PTSD formulation. *Behav Ther* 20:215–228, 1989.

Yehuda R, Southwick SM, Perry BD, et al: Interactions of the hypothalamic-pituitary-adrenal axis and the catecholaminergic system in posttraumatic stress disorder. In: Giller EL (ed): *Biological Assessment and Treatment of Post-Traumatic Stress Disorder*. Washington, DC, American Psychiatric Press, 1990.

Yule W, Williams R: Post-traumatic stress reactions in children. *J Traum Stress* 3:279–295, 1990.

Ziv A, Israeli R: Effects of bombardment on the manifest anxiety level of children living in kibbutzim. *J Consult Clin Psychol* 40:287–291, 1973.

71 PHARMACOKINETICS IN CHILDREN AND ADOLESCENTS

Paul D. Clein, M.D., and Mark A. Riddle, M.D.

Children and adolescents respond differently than adults to psychotropic medications. These differences are due to both pharmacokinetic and pharmacodynamic factors. *Pharmacokinetics* is concerned with biological processes that lead to changes over time in drug concentration in body tissues and fluids. This process is primarily responsible for determining how long a drug effect will last. Both the therapeutic and adverse effects of any medication are related to its concentration at the target tissue, the time required to achieve an effective concentration, and the duration of time that an effective concentration is maintained. Changes during development in drug absorption, distribution, metabolism, and excretion may affect the delivery of drug to the target tissue. *Pharmacodynamics* is concerned with the biochemical and physiological effects of drugs and their mechanisms of action. Pharmacodynamics relates a drug's concentration to its drug effect, which may be either desirable or undesirable. The effects of a medication may change during development as brain regions or neurotransmitter systems develop and mature at different rates.

The purpose of this chapter is to review pharmacokinetic factors that influence drug disposition during development. First, basic pharmacokinetic principles that are shared by children, adolescents, and adults are reviewed. Next, the broad pharmacokinetic differences that distinguish the pediatric population from adults are examined. This is followed by a review of specific factors affecting drug disposition, with an emphasis on developmental influences. Finally, clinically relevant drug-specific factors during development are discussed, concentrating on medications commonly used in child and adolescent psychiatry.

BASIC PHARMACOKINETIC PRINCIPLES

An understanding of pharmacokinetic principles is crucial for safe, effective patient care. Pharmacokinetic factors are often the critical variables in a variety of clinical decisions. These decisions include choosing between different medication forms within the same drug class, switching between these different forms, adjusting dosages, and correctly utilizing and interpreting therapeutic drug monitoring (i.e., plasma drug levels) (Preskorn, 1993b).

Pharmacokinetics can be functionally conceptualized as having four distinct phases: absorption, distribution, metabolism, and excretion. Absorption and distribution are primarily responsible for determining the speed of onset of drug effect, while the processes of metabolism and excretion terminate the action of the pharmacologic agent by removing the active form of the drug from the body. Taken together, these four phases determine the duration of drug activity (Paxton and Dragunow, 1993).

Once a drug gains entry to the bloodstream, it is diluted in the plasma, bound at varying degrees to plasma proteins, and then either excreted by the kidneys or carried to the liver and transformed to a more water-soluble (and usually inactive) metabolite, which can then be excreted in urine, bile, or feces. This complicated and interdependent series of events is designed to reduce the effect of the foreign molecule, with the ultimate goal of eliminating the drug from the body. If the dose of a drug is sufficiently large to withstand this pharmacokinetic assault, then a fraction of the drug molecules will endure to produce its pharmacodynamic effect (Paxton and Dragunow, 1993).

There are many definitions and equations that, when taken together, define the complex scientific discipline of pharmacokinetics. The knowledgeable clinician, however, needs only to comprehend several key concepts to have a competent, working understanding of the pharmacokinetic principles that underlie the fate of administered drugs. Practically all psychotropic medications follow *first-order kinetics*, meaning that the amount of drug eliminated is proportional to the amount of drug circulating in the bloodstream. This is fortunate because first-order kinetics provide a linear or roughly 1:1 relationship between dosage changes and plasma concentration changes. If metabolizing or eliminating mechanisms become saturated, however, *zero-order kinetics* prevails. This results in a fixed amount of drug being eliminated per unit of time, regardless of the plasma level. Some drugs, such as fluoxetine and alcohol, demonstrate zero-order kinetics at all clinically relevant doses rather than just at saturation doses, making the relationship between dose changes and subsequent plasma levels much less predictable (Janicak et al., 1993).

For drugs that follow first-order kinetics, the concepts of biologic *half-life* and *steady-state concentration* are most germane to the practicing clinician. The half-life is the time required for the concentration of drug to decrease by one-half. In clinical practice, this parameter is usually assessed by measuring the decay of plasma or serum drug concentration and is referred to as the plasma (or serum) half-life. The plasma half-life of a drug may not be the same as the half-life for the whole body. This is especially true for drugs that are taken up by tissues and then released from these tissues into blood, such as highly lipophilic (i.e., having an affinity for fat) drugs, which may be taken up and stored in fat and then released slowly. Nevertheless, plasma half-life values can be useful when determining dosing intervals. At consistent dosing intervals, it is the plasma half-life that determines the plasma steady-state concentration. This is defined as an equilibrium between the amount of drug ingested and the amount of drug eliminated, resulting in no net change in plasma concentration over time. Steady-state concentration is reached in a time equal to six half-lives, but it is clinically useful to recognize that greater than 90% of steady-state concentration is reached at four half-lives. Conversely, if drug intake is abruptly stopped, it takes a time equal to six half-lives for almost complete elimination.

PHARMACOKINETICS IN CHILDREN AND ADOLESCENTS

There are many pharmacokinetic similarities between the adult and pediatric populations. This is expected because many characteristics shared across age groups are genetically determined. The wide interindividual variability seen in adults is also present in children. Indeed, these genetic influences on protein binding, metabolism, and elimination can be much more salient than those influences attributed to age.

Nonetheless, children and adolescents do display unique pharmacokinetic properties. Unfortunately, data on children are scarce and fall considerably behind that available in adults (Gilman and Gal, 1992; Kauffman and Kearns, 1992). The result of this informational dearth is that dosage recommendations and therapeutic ranges utilized clinically in children and adolescents are, at least initially, extrapolated from adult studies, often hastily and arbitrarily (Gilman and Gal, 1992). The appropriate dose of a psychotropic medication in the pediatric age group should be empirically determined; a proportionately reduced adult dose based on body weight is frequently subtherapeutic or toxic. In addition, infants, children, and adolescents are not a homogenous group in terms of drug distribution patterns (Jatlow, 1987). These differences can be especially dramatic around the time of puberty, when the release of gonadal hormones can strongly influence plasma drug concentrations (Morselli and Pippenger, 1982).

Although pharmacokinetic data in children and adolescents are limited, one basic observation is suggested clinically: *Children and adolescents require larger, weight-adjusted doses of most medications than do adults to achieve comparable blood levels and therapeutic effects* (Jatlow, 1987). This appears to be mostly a function of shorter half-life due to an increased rate of metabolism and elimination, rather than different genetic manifestations at different ages (Geller, 1991).

FACTORS AFFECTING DRUG DISPOSITION

Absorption

Drugs gain entry into the body through a variety of portals. The bioavailability of a medication in the systemic circulation is determined by its absorption and, for orally administered medications, the *first pass* effect of liver metabolism. Absorption depends heavily on the route of entry, with intravenous administration being the equivalent of 100% absorption. Oral administration is by far the most common portal of entry and unfortunately is also the most unpredictable in terms of final bioavailability. Drugs given orally are absorbed in aqueous solutions through either the stomach or, as is the case with most psychotropic medications, the small intestine. The major factors influencing gastrointestinal absorption are pH-dependent diffusion and gastric emptying time. The drug then enters the portal circulation, where it is taken to the liver for first-pass metabolism.

Little information is available regarding the effect of age on the absorption of psychotropic medications, although there are several theoretic considerations regarding the influence of this process in children and adolescents. For instance, in children, stomach contents tend to be less acidic than in adults, causing weakly acidic drugs to be more ionized. Because it is the un-ionized fraction that is absorbed from the stomach, weakly acidic drugs may be absorbed more slowly in children. This process theoretically could affect anticonvulsants, amphetamines, and antidepressants (Taylor, 1994). Another theoretical concern is that children generally have fewer and less diverse intestinal microflora. Since drugs such as phenothiazines can be absorbed or metabolized in the gut wall, this may help explain why some children either are resistant to phenothiazine medication or require a surprisingly large oral dose (Taylor, 1994). Another factor that could reduce overall absorption is that intestinal transit time appears to be shorter in young children, which could result in incomplete uptake of slow-release preparations (Gilman, 1990).

It is important to remember that despite the theoretical considerations outlined previously, there are no data indicating a generally reduced absorption of orally administered drugs in children (Jatlow, 1987). Winsberg and colleagues (1974) reported that the absorption of imipramine is rapid and complete in prepubertal children. Anecdotal information and clinical experience suggest that absorption of certain psychotropic medications may be even more rapid in children than in adults. Rapid absorption, however, may not be desirable because it results in greater peak-to-valley fluctuations in blood levels. This does not affect the final average steady-state level but may be important because drug

toxicity can be a function of peak plasma concentration (Janicak et al., 1993). A high plasma level following rapid absorption theoretically could help explain the cardiac toxicity seen in children with certain psychotropic medications. Cardiac toxicity, owing to the artificial stabilization of necessarily excitable membranes, is as much a function of peak plasma concentration as it is of the steady-state tissue concentration (Janicak et al., 1993).

First-Pass Effect

An orally administered drug is absorbed from the gastrointestinal tract and must first enter the portal circulation, where it passes through the liver before reaching the systemic circulation. During this first pass, a considerable portion of the drug is hepatically metabolized (see later). Thus, a smaller portion of the drug enters the systemic circulation than was absorbed from the gastrointestinal tract. Note that intravenous administration completely avoids this first degradative step. Intramuscular and subcutaneous routes also avoid first-pass metabolism but depend heavily on blood supply for absorption, which can vary from 20 to 100%. Rectal administration results in both mesenteric and hemorrhoidal absorption, the latter of which bypasses the portal circulation, allowing for an overall decreased first-pass metabolism (McLeod and Evans, 1992).

Distribution

Following absorption, drugs are distributed into the intravascular and various extravascular spaces. Numerous physical factors can influence the distribution of a drug throughout the body: the size of body water compartments and adipose tissue depots, cardiac output, regional blood flow, organ perfusion pressure, permeability of cell membranes, acid-base balance, and binding to plasma and tissue proteins (Morselli, 1977). Each of these factors may change during development, resulting in changes in the distribution of a drug and, subsequently, in its pharmacological effect.

The two most important factors affecting distribution that change substantially during development are fat stores and the relative proportion of total body water to extracellular water. The relationship between the amount of drug absorbed (D), plasma concentration (Cp), and volume of distribution (Vd) can be summarized by the simple equation: $Cp = D/Vd$. Note that the larger the Vd, the smaller the Cp.

The volume of distribution (Vd) of highly lipophilic drugs, which includes most neuroleptics and antidepressants, is affected substantially by the proportion of body fat. The proportion of body fat is highest in the 1st year of life, followed by a steady decrease until an increase occurs prepubertally (Jatlow, 1987). Hence, children and adolescents at different ages have varying degrees of fat stores. Within the pediatric population, however, these differences appear to have only a minimal effect on age-related changes in drug disposition (Jatlow, 1987). In general, however, children tend to have a proportion of body fat less than that found in adults (Brown, 1991). Hence, in children, one would expect to find a larger plasma concentration (Cp) with lipophilic drugs when compared with adults after being given the same weight-adjusted dose. It has been demonstrated, however, that children actually exhibit a *lower* plasma concentration (Cp) than do adults under these conditions. Therefore, other mechanisms (such as increased metabolism) must explain the lower plasma concentration of lipophilic drugs in children (Jatlow, 1987).

The relative volume of extracellular water is high in children and tends to decrease with development. For example, total body water decreases gradually from about 85% of body weight in a small premature infant to about 70% in the full-term newborn to about 60% in the 1-year-old infant, a level that is generally maintained throughout adulthood. Similarly, extracellular water decreases gradually from about 40–50% of body weight in the newborn to about 15–20% by age 10–15 years (Edelman et al., 1952; Fetner and Geller, 1992; Friis-Hansen, 1961; Yaffe and Juchau, 1974). Thus, drugs that are primarily distributed in body water (e.g., lithium) would be expected to have a lower plasma concentration in the pediatric population compared with that in adults because the volume of distribution is higher in children.

Following absorption and first pass through the liver, drugs are transported in the general circulation in two forms, which are in dynamic equilibrium: bound to plasma protein or unbound (free). Only the unbound drug is usually available for passage across membranes, pharmacological effects, metabolism, and excretion. Although drug protein binding may be reduced in young children (Milsap and Szefler, 1986), it does not appear to be an important developmental factor in older children and adolescents. For example, in a study of 7- to 10-year-old children, plasma protein binding of imipramine ranged from 78 to 86%, levels comparable to those reported in adults of 77–95% (Winsberg et al., 1974). The clinician, however, must keep in mind that environmental influences can greatly affect the protein-binding equilibrium. For instance, febrile illness and antibiotic treatment, both very common in children, may significantly increase the amount of circulating protein and also affect the percent binding of various psychotropic medications (Geller, 1991). It is therefore prudent to monitor serum levels and medication side effects carefully during these times.

A final theoretic consideration in children and adolescents is the relative permeability of the blood-brain barrier when compared with that in adults. This increased permeability could result in an increased bioavailability of drugs in the CNS. This relative "porousness," however, would concomitantly permit greater amounts of protein to enter the cerebrospinal fluid. Any drug that crosses the blood-brain barrier but also substantially binds to proteins, such as the anticonvulsants, would in effect then have its bioavailability reduced (Taylor, 1994).

Metabolism

Most drugs are lipid soluble, which is usually a necessary requirement for absorption, distribution, and availability at receptor sites. To be effectively excreted, however, lipophilic drugs need to be metabolized to more polar or hydrophilic (e.g., having an affinity for water) forms. Enzymes that catalyze these metabolic reactions are found in greatest abundance in the liver, the main organ of drug metabolism, but also in the wall of the small intestine, skeletal muscles, kidneys, and lungs.

Although some drugs are excreted unmetabolized (e.g., lithium), most drugs undergo extensive biotransformation in the liver (Janicak et al., 1993). Phase 1 metabolic reactions, including hydroxylation, reduction, and hydrolysis, convert drugs to forms more suitable for elimination. The products of phase 1 reactions, referred to as metabolites, are usually less active and less toxic than the parent compound. A notable possible exception is desipramine, the demethylated active metabolite of imipramine. In phase 2 reactions, metabolites generated from phase 1 reactions are conjugated with glucuronic acid, sulfate, or glycine and excreted in the urine or other body fluids. It is clinically important to note that some drugs are never metabolized in a phase 1 reaction and instead simply undergo conjugation by glucuronic acid. This conjugative reaction may occur in almost any organ and therefore is not solely dependent on hepatic function. Hence, drugs such as the 3-hydroxybenzodiazepines (e.g., lorazepam, oxazepam, temazepam) are rapidly cleared at equal rates regardless of age as long as renal function is normal (Janicak et al., 1993).

Hepatic microsomal enzymes responsible for the metabolism of most psychotropic medications are subject to many environmental influences. These influences most commonly include various disease states and the concomitant administration of other drugs. Drugs such as phenobarbital, phenytoin, carbamazepine, alcohol, and nicotine classically *induce* microsomal enzymes, making them more active and resulting in a reduced plasma concentration for other drugs metabolized by these same enzymes. Conversely, commonly used drugs such as fluoxetine, paroxetine, cimetidine, β-blockers, phenothiazines, and valproic acid *inhibit* microsomal enzymes, resulting in a higher and potentially toxic plasma concentration for other drugs utilizing the same metabolic pathway (Callahan et al., 1993).

The relatively higher dosage requirement of most psychotropic drugs in children is most commonly explained by increased hepatic metabolic capacity. In general, metabolic pathways for many drugs function at a low level during the perinatal period, mature by about 6 months of age, peak between the ages of 1 and 5 years, and decline gradually to adult values by about 15 years of age (Morselli, 1977; Morselli and Pippenger, 1982). Liver weight is also proportionally greater in children than in adults. For example, the liver of a 2-year-old child weighs about 40–50% more, on a gram of liver to kilogram of body weight basis, than that of an adult; the liver weight of a 6-year-old child is about 30% more (Alvarez et al., 1975). Thus, in children, relatively larger milligram-per-kilogram doses of most drugs are needed to achieve comparable steady-state plasma levels.

In a classic study of drug metabolism rates in children, Alvarez and colleagues (1975) administered the model drugs antipyrine and phenylbutazone to 10 normal adults and 10 children ranging in age from 1 to 8 years. Both drugs are substrates for the cytochrome P-450-dependent liver microsomal enzyme systems. An oral dose of antipyrine is completely absorbed and completely metabolized by the liver and is not bound to plasma proteins (Brodie and Axelrod, 1950). Phenylbutazone is also completely absorbed and extensively metabolized by the liver but differs from antipyrine in being extensively bound to plasma proteins (Burns et al., 1953). The children metabolized both drugs at about twice the rate of adults: Mean half-lives were 6.6 hours in children and 13.6 hours in adults for antipyrine, and 1.7 hours in children and 3.2 hours in adults for phenylbutazone (Alvarez et al., 1975). The relatively larger hepatic mass in proportion to body weight in children was postulated by the authors as the explanation for these findings.

There are also some medications that, when administered to children, produce metabolites that are either not normally present in adults or are produced in higher concentrations. An example of this is the 4-en metabolite of valproic acid. This metabolite is associated with a rare fatal, idiosyncratic hepatotoxicity reaction, a phenomenon occurring almost exclusively in children receiving valproic acid (Gilman, 1990).

Excretion

The kidney is the most important organ for drug excretion. Three mechanisms are involved in the renal excretion of drugs: glomerular filtration, tubular secretion by active transport mechanisms, and reabsorption.

Water solubility is by far the most important factor in determining the kidney's ability to excrete a drug. Most unchanged drugs are hydrophobic and therefore must be metabolized before excretion, becoming more polar and hence more water soluble. Lithium is a notable exception to this generality because it is excreted unchanged by the kidney.

In contrast to hepatic function, renal functioning in infants approximates that of adults. Beyond early infancy, developmental changes in renal functions apparently do not contribute substantially to age-related differences in psychotropic drug disposition, with the probable exception of lithium (Jatlow, 1987).

DRUG-SPECIFIC FACTORS DURING DEVELOPMENT

Table 71.1 lists the psychotropic medications for which data on serum half-life ($t_{1/2}$) are available for children and adolescents. The half-lives of these same medications in adults are also listed for comparison. Compared to a more comprehensive table that lists all the psychotropic medications commonly used in child and adolescent psychiatry (Spencer et al., 1995), this list is relatively short and dramatically illustrates just how little data are available in the pediatric population for even commonly prescribed drugs. Because systematic pharmacokinetic studies in children have not been performed for most psychotropic medications, this leaves the clinician in the unenviable position of either extrapolating the adult data or relying on clinical experience and anecdotal reports. Unfortunately, this is frequently insufficient and can seriously hamper

Table 71.1. Serum Half-lives of Various Psychotropic Medications (in hours)

Medication	Half-life in Adults	Age Range in Children	Half-life in Children	Reference for Child Data
Psychostimulants				
Dextroamphetamine	10.25	5–12	6.8 ± 0.5	Brown et al., 1979
Methylphenidate	2–7	6–13	2.5–3.4	Gaultieri et al., 1982
Pemoline	12	8.0 ± 1.4	7.05 ± 1.99	Collier et al., 1985
		5–12	8.6	Sallee et al., 1985
Antidepressants				
Clomipramine	24	5–19	5–17	Dugas et al., 1980
Mianserin	32 ± 6	6–12	10 ± 2	Winsberg et al., 1987
Nortriptyline	24	5–12	20.8 ± 7.2	Geller et al., 1984
		13–16	31.1 ± 19.8	Geller et al., 1987
Neuroleptics				
Chlorpromazine	16–37	0.3–17	7.74 ± 0.65	Furlanut et al., 1990
Droperidol	103–127[a]	3.5–12	101.5 ± 26.4[a]	Grunwald et al., 1993
Haloperidol	24.1 ± 8.9	2–10	18.6 ± 12.2	Yhoshida et al., 1993
Anticonvulsants				
Carbamazepine	26[b]/5[c]	—[d]	32[b]/3[c]	Leppik, 1992[e]
Valproate	9[b]/15[c]	—[d]	5[b]/14[c]	Leppik, 1992[e]
Other				
Clonidine	12–16	—[d]	8–12	Hunt et al., 1990[e]
Diazepam	15–60	—[d]	15–21	Morselli, 1977[e]
				Morselli et al., 1978[e]
Diphenhydramine	9.2 ± 2.5	8.9 ± 1.7	5.4 ± 1.8	Simons et al., 1990
Lithium	24	9–12	17.9 ± 7.4	Vitiello et al., 1988

[a] Half-life in minutes.
[b] Half-life at initiation of treatment.
[c] Half-life after long-term administration.
[d] Half-life determined from composite of various sources.
[e] Reference citation is review article.

the delivery of effective clinical care to children who require medications for emotional and behavioral disorders.

Recommendations for dosages and therapeutic blood level monitoring for specific medications are beyond the scope of this chapter and can be found in other chapters within this textbook. The following discussion describes selected drug-specific factors that affect disposition during development.

Psychostimulants

In contrast to other psychotropic medications, the psychostimulants (methylphenidate, *d*-amphetamine, and pemoline) have been more widely studied in children than in adults.

Methylphenidate exhibits a very low rate of plasma protein binding (15%), making small doses pharmacodynamically active (Perel and Dayton, 1976). This factor, combined with the low lipophilic nature of methylphenidate, makes metabolism very rapid. Although there is not general agreement regarding the effect of food on the absorption of stimulants, this appears to have little influence when considering their overall pharmacokinetics (Patrick et al., 1987). The use of serum levels with the psychostimulants is not practical for a variety of reasons. Chief among these are wide fluctuations of blood levels, large interindividual variations, and no clear correlation of blood level with clinical response.

Methylphenidate has a plasma half-life of 2–3 hours in prepubertal children (Gaultieri et al., 1984, 1982; Hungund et al., 1979; Shaywitz et al., 1982), whereas the plasma half-life of *d*-amphetamine is 6–7 hours (Brown et al., 1979). Because these medications are commonly administered only two or three times a day in clinical practice, plasma concentrations decline substantially over each dosing interval. In fact, in most instances, plasma levels of methylphenidate and *d*-amphetamine are generally negligible prior to administration of the morning dose. The half-life is so short in proportion to dosing that a steady state is not achieved. Hence, plasma concentrations attained during the first few hours after a dose are determined more by such factors as absorption, first-pass effect, and volume of distribution than by plasma half-life (Jatlow, 1987). Although esterases may be more important than hepatic microsomal enzymes for the metabolism of methylphenidate, existing data support the contention that children metabolize methylphenidate

and *d*-amphetamine faster do than adults (Furlanut et al., 1990; Gualtieri et al., 1984; Rane and Wilson, 1976).

Pemoline has also been shown to have a shorter half-life in children (7–8 hours) compared with that in adults (11–13 hours) (Collier et al, 1985; Sallee et al., 1985). Sallee and colleagues (1985) demonstrated an increasing half-life with long-term use, leading to increased plasma levels and suggesting nonlinear kinetics. This finding has been used to support the clinical lore that pemoline has a delayed onset of action, typically 3–4 weeks (Dugas et al., 1980). It should be noted, however, that in a more recent study Sallee and colleagues (1992) demonstrated a positive effect of pemoline on neuroprocessing within 2 hours of administration and also found no clinical evidence of tolerance to the drug effect following 3 weeks of treatment. Pelham and colleagues (1990) also determined that pemoline exhibited beneficial clinical effects on the 2nd or 3rd day of the administration that were roughly equivalent to standard methylphenidate, sustained-release methylphenidate (Ritalin-SR), and sustained-release dextroamphetamine (Dexedrine Spansules). Collier et al. (1985) noted stable blood levels of pemoline over time, suggesting first-order kinetics. Further research is required to elucidate these issues.

From a pharmacokinetic standpoint, the sustained-release preparations (e.g., Ritalin-SR and Dexedrine Spansules) differ significantly from the regular formulations. The sustain-released preparations are slower to reach maximum serum concentrations and also attain lower peak plasma levels (Birmaher et al., 1989). Several research reports have drawn attention to the importance of pharmacokinetic considerations when using psychostimulant medications in children. Pelham and colleagues (1987) compared the standard methylphenidate formulation with the long-acting preparation (Ritalin-SR). Both formulations contained the same active ingredient and total daily dose. Although both forms were found to be effective and to demonstrate detectable effects 1 hour postingestion, the standard formulation exhibited superiority on several important measures of disruptive behavior, whereas the sustained-release preparation was found to have a slower onset of action on a cognitive measure of performance. This finding, along with anecdotal information, led to the belief that the sustained-release preparation was not as clinically effective as the standard methylphenidate formulation. It was theorized that this was due to a "ramp effect" in which the therapeutic efficacy of stimulants in attention deficit hyperactivity disorder correlated with the rate of absorption of the drug rather than with the final plasma concentration, rendering the slow release preparations less effective.

In a more recent, well-designed study, however, Pelham and colleagues (1990) compared the standard methylphenidate formulation with Ritalin-SR, Dexedrine Spansules, and pemoline. Interestingly, all four psychostimulants were found to have a generally equivalent, beneficial effect on the continuous performance task measure within 2 hours postingestion. Additionally, the continuous performance task improvement was as large at 9 hours as at 2 hours postingestion, suggesting that the major beneficial effect was not obtained during the absorption phase and was not related to the rate of absorption. In fact, pemoline and Dexedrine Spansules were found to be most consistently beneficial to the test group. Larger-scale studies in children and adolescents comparing the different psychostimulant medications are required to clarify their differences and to help guide clinical treatment further.

Neuroleptics

The elimination of most neuroleptics is affected by hepatic metabolism. Children receiving a constant dose of the phenothiazine chlorpromazine show declining plasma levels over time, suggesting autoinduction of hepatic enzymes (Rivera-Calimlim et al., 1979). Furlanut and colleagues (1990) demonstrated a shorter plasma half-life of chlorpromazine in children as compared with that previously found in adults. This replicated the earlier findings of Rivera-Calimlim (1979, 1982). Similar findings have been demonstrated with the butyrophenones, haloperidol (Morselli et al., 1982, 1983, 1979; Yoshida et al., 1993), and droperidol (Grunwald et al., 1993).

It has also been shown, however, that children actually require *smaller* weight-adjusted neuroleptic doses than do adults to achieve the same therapeutic effect (Morselli et al., 1982; Rivera-Calimlim et al., 1979). Hence, children, when compared with adults, require an increased milligram-to-kilogram dose to achieve the same plasma concentration but clinically require a lower milligram-to-kilogram dose to achieve the same therapeutic effect. This suggests that there may be a pharmacodynamic difference at the level of the developing brain, rather than only a pharmacokinetic difference. Indeed, this has been demonstrated by Seeman and colleagues (1987) who found that children have a greater density of dopamine D-1 and D-2 receptors than do adults. This suggests that children may be more sensitive to the effects of neuroleptics than are adults, and this phenomenon has been observed clinically (Verghese et al., 1991).

Tricyclic Antidepressants

Tricyclic antidepressants (TCAs) also undergo extensive hepatic metabolism. An increased metabolism of tricyclic antidepressants probably accounts for their shorter half-life in children and adolescents, which has been repeatedly demonstrated (Dulcan, 1990; Geller et al., 1984, 1987; Jatlow, 1987; Morselli et al., 1978; Potter et al., 1982). Thus, in children, higher doses (milligram-per-kilogram) of tricyclics (e.g., imipramine, desipramine, clomipramine, amitriptyline, and nortriptyline) are usually administered to attain comparable adult plasma or serum levels (Puig-Antich et al., 1987).

When considering TCAs, children and adolescents should not be viewed as a homogenous group. Prepubertal children metabolize tricyclics more rapidly than do adolescents, and preschool children (age 3–5 years) metabolize TCAs the most rapidly of all (Ryan, 1990; Wilens et al., 1993). Geller and colleagues (1984, 1987) demonstrated that the plasma half-life of nortriptyline in 5- to 12-year-olds ranged from 11 to 42 hours, whereas in 13- to 16-year-olds, it ranged from 14 to 77 hours. The clinician should also be cognizant that approximately 5–10% of children are likely to be *slow hydroxylators* of TCAs, resulting in dramatically prolonged tricyclic half-life and increased peak plasma

levels (Potter et al., 1982). This characteristic is genetically determined, and hence the rate that it occurs in children should approximate that found in adults.

The highly lipophilic TCAs are readily taken up and stored in body fat. Children, however, have relatively less body fat in proportion to weight than do adults. If a TCA is abruptly discontinued in a child, there is relatively less TCA available to leach back into the systemic circulation from the fat stores. This makes a rapid TCA-withdrawal syndrome much more likely to occur in children than in adults.

The lack of demonstrated efficacy of TCAs in double-blind, placebo-controlled studies in the treatment of childhood depression does not appear to be a pharmacokinetic phenomenon because frequent dosing has adequately addressed this issue (Geller, 1991).

Anticonvulsants

Children appear to eliminate antiepileptic drugs at a more rapid rate and to require relatively higher weight-adjusted doses than adults require to achieve therapeutic plasma concentrations (Gilman, 1991; Leppik, 1992; Taylor, 1994). Although a lower volume of distribution and increased protein binding in children may contribute to this finding, the shorter half-lives are generally attributed to an increased hepatic metabolism (Cloyd et al., 1993; Jatlow, 1987; Taylor, 1994).

Valproic acid has been shown to be an inhibitor of microsomal enzymes, which results in autoinhibition and the potential to cause very high serum levels of concomitantly administered medications that utilize the same metabolic pathway. Carbamazepine, on the other hand, is very well-known for its microsomal induction and autoinduction characteristics, resulting in lower plasma levels over the initial 4–6 weeks of administration despite constant dosing. This autoinduction phenomenon dissipates rapidly after the first 6 weeks of treatment.

Lithium

Although lithium obeys first-order kinetic principles, the factors governing its disposition are uniquely different from those of other psychotropic medications. It is rapidly absorbed into the gastrointestinal tract, there is no binding to plasma proteins, it is distributed almost exclusively in body water owing to its hydrophilic nature, and it is excreted unchanged in the urine without undergoing any metabolic degradation (Viesselman et al., 1993).

As previously discussed, elimination of lithium is almost entirely dependent on renal mechanisms, which tend to be more efficient in children (Rane and Wilson, 1976). There are several possible explanations for the increased rate of renal excretion of lithium in children. Children, when compared with adults, exhibit relatively greater total body water, a larger fluid intake, and an increased glomerular filtration rate, all resulting in a higher renal clearance of the drug (Geller, 1991; Janicak et al., 1993; Jatlow, 1987). Half-life in the pediatric population is approximately 10–12 hours and has been shown to be shorter in children than in adults (Vitiello et al., 1988).

There have been attempts to measure serum lithium levels indirectly by measuring the lithium level in saliva. Unfortunately, salivary lithium pharmacokinetic characteristics are individual-specific and require multiple blood draws to establish a saliva-to-serum ratio. This fact makes measurement of saliva lithium levels an impractical alternative to serum monitoring in children (Geller, 1991).

Benzodiazepines

Among the benzodiazepines, only diazepam has been studied from a developmental pharmacokinetic perspective. Morselli and colleagues (Morselli, 1977; Morselli et al., 1978) found that the plasma half-life of diazepam was longer in adults (mean 24 hours) than in children (mean 17 hours) or infants (10 hours). Kanto et al. (1978) also showed children to metabolize diazepam more rapidly than adults. Age-dependent changes in hepatic microsomal enzymes are the most likely explanation

Table 71.2. Selective Serotonin Reuptake Inhibitor Half-lives in Adults

Selective Serotonin Reuptake Inhibitor	Half-life after Single Dose	Half-life after Multiple Doses
Fluoxetine	1.9 days	5.7 days
Norfluoxetine	7 days	7–15 days
Sertraline	26 hr	Essentially unchanged
Paroxetine	10–16 hr	21 hr
Fluvoxamine	15 hr	19.5–22.5 hr (approx.)

Data from van Harten J: Clinical pharmacokinetics of selective serotonin reuptake inhibitors. *Clin Pharmacokinet* 24(3):203–220, 1993.

for these changes. As alluded to earlier, the 3-hydroxybenzodiazepines (e.g., lorazepam, oxazepam, temazepam) are not directly metabolized by hepatic microsomal enzymes prior to conjugation and hence do not demonstrate the same age-dependent changes in disposition that are observed for diazepam.

Selective Serotonin Reuptake Inhibitors

The most commonly used selective serotonin reuptake inhibitors (SSRIs) in clinical practice include fluoxetine, sertraline, paroxetine, and fluvoxamine. With the possible exception of the psychostimulants, in no other class of medications are pharmacokinetic considerations more important in choosing between the various drug forms available. There are few data regarding the pharmacokinetics of the SSRIs in children and adolescents, but the limited information available suggests that extrapolation from the adult data is probably appropriate. The critical pharmacokinetic differences between the various SSRIs encompass three main considerations: half-life, autoinhibition, and drug:drug interactions.

The half-life data for adults for the various SSRIs are listed in Table 71.2. Only fluoxetine has a pharmacologically active metabolite (norfluoxetine) that is thought to contribute to the overall clinical effect profile (van Harten, 1993). The longer half-lives of fluoxetine and its primary metabolite, norfluoxetine, clearly set them apart from the other SSRIs. This is clinically salient since it requires a time equal to six half-lives to achieve a steady state or, conversely, to eliminate the drug completely from the bloodstream. There are advantages to long half-life drugs: Missing one or two doses does not greatly affect the serum level, and abrupt discontinuation can result in a built-in autotaper, possibly avoiding a withdrawal syndrome. Long half-life drugs, however, also result in long periods of time that must pass before a steady state is achieved or before a drug is completely eliminated from the bloodstream. This can delay the assessment of dosage adjustments and clinical efficacy. Long half-life drugs may also be undesirable if untoward side effects occur, if drug:drug interactions become important, or if the clinician wishes to administer a different medication whose metabolism is affected by the continued presence of the long half-life drug.

Table 71.2 also illustrates that, after multiple dosing, the half-lives of most of the SSRIs increase. This is most likely due to autoinhibition (i.e., drugs inhibiting their own metabolism), which results in nonlinear

pharmacokinetics (van Harten, 1993). This nonlinearity has been demonstrated in fluoxetine (Bergstrom et al., 1988), norfluoxetine (Boyer and Feighner, 1991), paroxetine (Kaye et al., 1989), and fluvoxamine (van Harten, 1993). It should be noted that nonlinearity in paroxetine demonstrates extensive intersubject variability and that linear, first-order kinetics are often found in many subjects who take paroxetine regularly. Dose proportionality and linearity have been demonstrated for sertraline (Ronfeld et al., 1988), which appears to obey first-order kinetic principles across the clinically relevant dosage ranges (Murdoch and McTavish, 1992; Preskorn, 1993a, 1993b; Preskorn et al., 1993).

In vitro studies on human hepatic microsomes have shown that *all* of the SSRIs have the potential to inhibit the functional integrity of the cytochrome P-450 system in the liver (Crewe et al., 1992; Preskorn, 1993a; van Harten, 1993). This enzyme system is primarily responsible for the oxidative metabolism, biotransformation, and subsequent elimination of many drugs, including the tricyclic antidepressants (Preskorn, 1993a). There are significant differences, however, among the SSRIs in terms of the particular isoenzymes inhibited and the relative potency of inhibition (van Harten, 1993). A list of these specific drug:drug interactions is beyond the scope of this chapter, but the clinical implication is that, when using any of the SSRIs, great care should be exercised to identify and consider these potentially dangerous interactions.

Pharmacokinetic data for the SSRIs in children are badly needed to help guide clinical treatment. For example, although fluoxetine and norfluoxetine have long half-lives, children tend to metabolize drugs faster than do adults. This combination of factors could result in a once-daily dosing regimen for fluoxetine in children. This regimen may contrast sharply with the other SSRIs, which, owing to their shorter half-lives, would probably require a multiple-dosing schedule throughout the day. Pharmacokinetic research in children could help clarify these and other issues germane to half-life, autoinhibition, and drug:drug interactions.

Clonidine

Pharmacokinetic studies of clonidine in children and adolescents have not paralleled its rapidly escalating use in the clinical population. Clonidine has no active metabolites, and its excretion is evenly divided between hepatic and renal mechanisms. Half-life in children is shorter (8–12 hours) than that found in adults (12–16 hours) (Hunt et al., 1990).

CONCLUSIONS

A fundamental understanding of developmental pharmacokinetics is a necessary prerequisite to the safe, effective administration of psychotropic medications to children and adolescents. Unfortunately, despite the increasing use of psychotropic medications in the treatment of children with severe behavioral and emotional disorders, few pharmacokinetic studies of children are available to guide clinical practice. Although generalizations can be made and extrapolated from the adult literature, these are frequently insufficient and ineffective. As new medications become available to child and adolescent psychiatrists, more pharmacokinetic research will be needed.

References

Alvarez AP, Kapelner S, Sassa S, et al: Drug metabolism in normal children, lead poisoned children and normal adults. *Clin Pharmacol Ther* 17:179–183, 1975.

Bergstrom RF, Lemberger L, Faird NA, et al: Clinical pharmacology and pharmacokinetics of fluoxetine: A review. *Br J Psychiatry* 153(3, suppl):47–50, 1988.

Birmaher B, Greenhill LL, Cooper TB, et al: Sustained release methylphenidate: Pharmacokinetic studies in ADDH males. *J Am Acad Child Adolesc Psychiatry* 28:768–772, 1989.

Bourin M, Couetoux de Tertre A: Pharmacokinetics of psychotropic drugs in children. *Clin Neuropharmacol* 15(suppl 1):224A–225A, 1992.

Boyer WF, Feighner JP: Pharmacokinetics and drug interactions. In: Feighner JP, Boyer WF (eds): *Selective Serotonin Re-uptake Inhibitors*. Chichester, Wiley, 1991, pp. 81–88.

Brodie BB, Axelrod J: The fate of antipyrine in man. *J Pharmacol Exp Ther* 98:97–104, 1950.

Brown CS: Treatment of attention deficit hyperactivity disorder: A critical review. *Ann Pharmacother* 25:1207–1213, 1991.

Brown GL, Hunt RD, Ebert MH, et al: Plasma levels of *d*-amphetamine in hyperactive children. *Psychopharmacology* 62:133–140, 1979.

Burns JJ, Rose KR, Chenkin R, et al: The physiological disposition of phenylbutazone (Butazolidin) in man and a method for its estimation in biological material. *J Pharmacol Exp Ther* 109:346–357, 1953.

Callahan AM, Fava M, Rosenbaum JF: Drug interactions in psychopharmacology. *Psychiatr Clin North Am* 16(3):647–671, 1993.

Cloyd JC, Fischer JH, Kriel RL, et al: Valproic acid pharmacokinetics in children. IV: Effects of age and antiepileptic drugs on protein binding and intrinsic clearance. *Clin Pharmacol Ther* 53(1):22–29, 1993.

Coffey BJ: Anxiolytics for children and adolescents: Traditional and new drugs. *J Child Adolesc Psychopharmacol* 1:57–83, 1990.

Collier CP, Soldin SJ, Swanson JM, et al: Pemoline pharmacokinetics and long term therapy in children with attention deficit disorder and hyperactivity. *Clin Pharmacokinet* 10:269–278, 1985.

Crewe HK, Lennard MS, Tucker CT, et al: The effect of selective serotonin re-uptake inhibitors on cytochrome P4502D6 (CYP2D6) activity in human liver microsomes. *Br J Pharmacol* 34:262–265, 1992.

Dugas M, Zarifian E, Lehuezey MF, et al: Preliminary observations of the significance of monitoring tricyclic antidepressant plasma levels in the pediatric patient. *Ther Drug Monit* 2:307–314, 1980.

Dulcan MK: Using psychostimulants to treat behavior disorders of children and adolescents. *J Child Adolesc Psychopharmacol* 1:7–20, 1990.

Edelman IS, Haley HB, Schloerb PR, et al: Further observations on total body water. I: *Surg Gynecol Obstet* 95:1–12, 1952.

Fetner HH, Geller B: Lithium and tricyclic antidepressants. *Psychiatr Clin North Am* 15:223–241, 1992.

Friis-Hansen B: Changes in body water compartments during growth. *Acta Paediatr* 110:46, 1956.

Friis-Hansen B: Body water compartments in children: Changes during growth and related changes in body composition. *Pediatrics* 28:169–181, 1961.

Furlanut M, Benetello P, Baraldo M, et al: Chlorpromazine disposition in relation to age in children. *Clin Pharmacokinet* 18:329–331, 1990.

Geller B: Psychopharmacology of children and adolescents: Pharmacokinetics and relationships of plasma/serum levels to response. *Psychopharmacol Bull* 27(4):401–409, 1991.

Geller B, Cooper TB, Chestnut EC, et al: Nortriptyline pharmacokinetic parameters in depressed children and adolescents: Preliminary data. *J Clin Psychopharmacol* 4:265–269, 1984.

Geller B, Cooper TB, Schluchter MD, et al: Child and adolescent nortriptyline single dose pharmacokinetic parameters: Final report. *J Clin Psychopharmacol* 7:321–323, 1987.

Gilman JT: Therapeutic drug monitoring in the neonate and pediatric age group. *Clin Pharmacokinet* 19(1):1–10, 1990.

Gilman JT: Carbamazepine dosing for pediatric seizure disorders: The highs and lows. *Ann Pharmacother* 25:1109–1112, 1991.

Gilman JT, Gal P: Pharmacokinetic and pharmacodynamic data collection in children and neonates. *Clin Pharmacokinet* 23(1):1–9, 1992.

Greenblatt DJ: Basic pharmacokinetic principles and their application to psychotropic drugs. *J Clin Psychiatry* 54:9(suppl):8–13, 1993.

Greenhill LL: Pharmacologic treatment of attention deficit hyperactivity disorder. *Psychiatr Clin North Am* 15:1–27, 1992.

Grunwald Z, Torjman M, Schieren H, et al: The pharmacokinetics of droperidol in anesthetized children. *Anesth Analg* 76(6):1238–1242, 1993.

Gualtieri CT, Hicks RE, Patrick K, et al: Clinical correlates of methylphenidate blood levels. *Ther Drug Monit* 6:379–392, 1984.

Gualtieri CT, Wargin W, Kanoy R, et al: Clinical studies of methylphenidate serum levels in children and adults. *J Am Acad Child Psychiatry* 21:19–26, 1982.

Hungund BL, Perel JM, Hurwick MJ, et al: Pharmacokinetics of methylphenidate in hyperkinetic children. *Br J Clin Pharmacol* 8:571–576, 1979.

Hunt RD, Capper L, O'Connell P: Clonidine in child and adolescent psychiatry. *J Child Adolesc Psychopharmacol* 1:87–102, 1990.

Janicak PG: The relevance of clinical pharmacokinetics and therapeutic drug monitoring: Anticonvulsant mood stabilizers and antipsychotics. *J Clin Psychiatry* 54:9(suppl):35–41, 1993.

Janicak PG, Davis JM, Preskorn SH, et al (eds): Pharmacokinetics. In: *Principles and Practice of Psychopharmacotherapy*. Baltimore, Williams & Wilkins, 1993, pp. 59–79.

Jatlow PI: Psychotropic drug disposition during development. In: Popper C (ed): *Psychiatric Pharmacosciences of Children and Adolescents*. Washington, DC, American Psychiatric Press, 1987, pp. 29–44.

Jefferson JW: The use of lithium in childhood and adolescence: An overview. *J Clin Psychiatr* 43:174–177, 1982.

Kanto J, Sellman K, Haataja M, et al: Plasma and urine concentrations of diazepam and its metabolites in children, adults, and in diazepam intoxicated patients. *Int J Clin Pharmacol* 16:258–264, 1978.

Kauffman RE, Kearns GL: Pharmacokinetic studies in paediatric patients. *Clin Pharmacokinet* 23(1):10–29, 1992.

Kaye CM, Haddock RE, Langley PF, et al: A review of the metabolism and pharmacokinetics of paroxetine in man. *Acta Psychiatr Scand* 80(suppl 350):60–75, 1989.

Leppik IE: Metabolism of antiepileptic medication: Newborn to elderly. *Epilepsia* 33(suppl 4):S32–S40, 1992.

McLeod HL, Evans WE: Pediatric pharmacokinetics and therapeutic drug monitoring. *Pediatr Rev* 13(11):413–421, 1992.

Milsap RL, Szefler SJ: Special pharmacokinetic considerations in children. In: Evans WE, Schentag JJ, Jusko WJ (eds): *Applied Pharmacokinetics: Principles of Therapeutic Drug Monitoring*. Spokane, Applied Therapeutics, 1986, pp. 294–330.

Morselli PL: *Drug Disposition during Development*. New York, Spectrum, 1977.

Morselli PL, Pippenger CE: Drug disposition during development. In: *Applied Therapeutic Drug Monitoring*. Washington, DC, American Association of Clinical Chemistry, 1982, pp. 63–70.

Morselli PL, Bianchetti G, Dugas M: Haloperidol plasma level monitoring in neuropsychiatric patients. *Ther Drug Monit* 4:51–58, 1982.

Morselli PL, Bianchetti G, Dugas M: Therapeutic drug monitoring of psychotropic drugs in children. *Pediatr Pharmacol* 3:149–156, 1983.

Morselli PL, Bianchetti G, Durant G, et al: Haloperidol plasma level monitoring in pediatric patients. *Ther Drug Monit* 1:35–46, 1979.

Morselli PL, Cuche H, Zarifian E: Pharmacokinetics of psychotropic drugs in the pediatric patient. In: Mendlewicz J, van Praag HM, Karg S (eds): *Childhood Psychopharmacology: Current Concepts. Advances in Biological Psychiatry*. Basel, Karger, 1978, pp. 70–86.

Murdoch D, McTavish D: Sertraline: A review of its pharmacodynamic and pharmacokinetic properties, therapeutic potential in depressive illness, and prospective role in the treatment of obsessive-compulsive disorder. *Drugs* 44:604–624, 1992.

Patrick SK, Mueller RA, Gualtieri CT, et al: Pharmacokinetics and actions of methylphenidate. In: Meltzer HY (ed): *Psychopharmacology: The Third Generation of Progress*. New York, Raven Press, 1987, pp. 1387–1396.

Paxton JW, Dragunow M: Pharmacology. In: Werry JS (ed): *Practitioner's Guide to Psychoactive Drugs for Children and Adolescents*. New York, Plenum, 1993, pp. 23–55.

Pelham WE, Greenslade KE, Vodde-Hamilton M, et al: Relative efficacy of long-acting stimulants on children with attention deficit-hyperactivity disorder: A comparison of standard methylphenidate, sustained-release methylphenidate, sustained-release dextroamphetamine, and pemoline. *Pediatrics* 86(2):226–237, 1990.

Pelham WE, Sturges J, Hoza J, et al: The effects of sustained release 20 and 10 mg Ritalin b.i.d. on cognitive and social behavior in children with attention deficit disorder. *Pediatrics* 80:491–501, 1987.

Perel JW, Dayton PG: Methylphenidate. In: Usdin E, Forrest I (eds): *Psychotherapeutic Drugs. Part II*. New York, Marcel Dekker, 1976, pp. 1287–1316.

Potter WZ, Calil HM, Sultfin TA, et al: Active metabolites of imipramine and desipramine in man. *Clin Pharmacol Ther* 31:393–401, 1982.

Preskorn SH: Pharmacokinetics of antidepressants: Why and how they are relevant to treatment. *J Clin Psychiatry* 54:9(suppl):14–34, 1993a.

Preskorn SH: Pharmacokinetics of psychotropic agents: Why and how they are related to treatment. *J Clin Psychiatry* 54:9(suppl):3–7, 1993b.

Preskorn SH, Burke MJ, Fast GA: Therapeutic drug monitoring. *Psychiatr Clin North Am* 16(3):611–645, 1993.

Puig-Antich J, Perel JM, Lupatkin W, et al: Imipramine in prepubertal major depressive disorders. *Arch Gen Psychiatry* 44:81–89, 1987.

Rane A, Wilson JT: Clinical pharmacokinetics in infants and children. *Clin Pharmacokinet* 1:2–24, 1976.

Rivera-Calimlim L: Problems in therapeutic monitoring of chlorpromazine. *Ther Drug Monit* 4:41–49, 1982.

Rivera-Calimlim L, Griesbach PH, Perlmutter R: Plasma chlorpromazine concentrations in children with behavioral disorders and mental illness. *Clin Pharmacol Ther* 26:114–121, 1979.

Ronfeld RA, Shaw GL, Tremaine LM: Distribution and pharmacokinetics of the selective 5-HT uptake blocker sertraline in man, rat, and dog. *Psychopharmacology* 96(suppl):269, 1988.

Rudorfer MV: Pharmacokinetics of psychotropic drugs in special populations. *J Clin Psychiatry* 54:9(suppl):50–54, 1993.

Ryan ND: Heterocyclic antidepressants in children and adolescents. *J Child Adolesc Psychopharmacol* 1:21–31, 1990.

Ryan ND: The pharmacologic treatment of child and adolescent depression. *Psychiatr Clin North Am* 15:29–40, 1992.

Sallee FR, Pollock BG: Clinical pharmacokinetics of imipramine and desipramine. *Clin Pharmacokinet* 18(5):346–364, 1990.

Sallee F, Stiller R, Perel J, et al: Oral pemoline kinetics in hyperactive children. *Clin Pharmacol Ther* 37:606–609, 1985.

Sallee FR, Stiller RL, Perel JM: Pharmacodynamics of pemoline in attention deficit disorder with hyperactivity. *J Am Acad Child Adolesc Psychiatry* 31:244–251, 1992.

Seeman P, Bzowej NH, Guan HC, et al: Human brain dopamine receptors in children and aging adults. *Synapse* 1:399–404, 1987.

Shaywitz S, Hunt RD, Jatlow P, et al: Psychopharmacology of attention deficit disorders: Pharmacokinetic, neuroendocrine and behavioral measures following acute and chronic treatment with methylphenidate. *Pediatrics* 69:688–694, 1982.

Simons KJ, Watson WTA, Martin TJ, et al: Diphenhydramine: Pharmacokinetics and pharmacodynamics in elderly adults, young adults and children. *J Clin Pharmacol* 30:665–671, 1990.

Spencer T, Wilens T, Biederman J: Psychotropic medication for children and adolescents. *Child Adolesc Psychiatr Clin North Am* 4:97–121, 1995.

Tamayo M, Fernandez de Gatta MM, Garcia MJ, et al: Population pharmacokinetics of imipramine in children. *Eur J Clin Pharmacol* 43:89–92, 1992.

Taylor E: Physical treatments. In: Rutter M (ed): *Child and Adolescent Psychiatry*. Cambridge, Blackwell Scientific, 1994, pp. 880–899.

Teicher MH, Glod CA: Neuroleptic drugs: Indications and guidelines for their rational use in children and adolescents. *J Child Adolesc Psychopharmacol* 1:35–56, 1990.

Thomson AH, Brodie MJ: Pharmacokinetic optimisation of anticonvulsant therapy. *Clin Pharmacokinet* 18(5):346–364, 1990.

van Harten J: Clinical pharmacokinetics of selection serotonin reuptake inhibitors. *Clin Pharmacokinet* 24(3):203–220, 1993.

Verghese C, Kessel JB, Simpson GM: Pharmacokinetics of neuroleptics. *Psychopharmacol Bull* 27(4):551–563, 1991.

Viesselman JO, Yaylayan S, Weller EB, et al: Antidysthymic drugs. In: Werry JS, Aman MG (eds): *Practitioner's Guide to Psychoactive Drugs for Children and Adolescents*. New York, Plenum, 1993, pp. 239–268.

Vitiello B, Behar D, Malone R, et al: Pharmaco-

kinetics of lithium carbonate in children. *J Clin Psychopharmacol* 8:355–359, 1988.

Weller EB, Weller RA, Fristad MA: Lithium dosage guide for prepubertal children. Preliminary report. *J Am Acad Child Adolesc Psychiatry* 25:92–95, 1986.

Whitaker A, Rao U: Neuroleptics in pediatric psychiatry. *Psychiatr Clin North Am* 15:243–276, 1992.

Widdowson EM: Changes in body proportions and composition during growth. In: Davis JA, Dobbing J (eds): *Scientific Foundations of Pediatrics*. London, Heinemann, 1974, p. 153.

Wilens TE, Biederman J: The stimulants. *Psychiatr Clin North Am* 15:191–222, 1992.

Wilens TE, Biederman J, Spencer T, et al: A retrospective study of serum levels and electrocardio-

graphic effects of nortriptyline in children and adolescents. *J Am Acad Child Adolesc Psychiatry* 32:2, 270–277, 1993.

Winsberg BG, Camp-Bruno JA, Vink J, et al: Mianserin pharmacokinetics and behavior in hyperkinetic children. *J Clin Psychopharmacol* 7: 143–147, 1987.

Winsberg BG, Perel JM, Hurwic MJ, et al: Imipramine protein binding and pharmacokinetics in children. In: Forrest IS, Carr CJ, Usdin E (eds): *The Phenothiazines and Structurally Related Drugs*. New York, Raven Press, 1974, pp. 425–431.

Yaffe SJ, Juchau MR: Perinatal pharmacology. *Annu Rev Pharmacol* 14:219–238, 1974.

Yoshida I, Sakaguchi Y, Matsuishi T, et al: Acute accidental overdosage of haloperidol in children. *Acta Pediatr* 82(10):877–880, 1993.

72 PRINCIPLES OF PSYCHOPHARMACOTHERAPY AND SPECIFIC DRUG TREATMENTS

Wayne Hugo Green, M.D.

This chapter reviews selected topics and representative drugs used in child and adolescent psychopharmacology. The initial portion of the chapter discusses the relationships among psychopharmacology, symptoms and diagnoses, some aspects of psychopharmacologic research, and general principles of childhood and adolescent psychopharmacology. The remainder of the chapter focuses on the psychopharmacologic agents that are presently the most important in the clinical practice of child and adolescent psychiatry. The FDA-approved uses of the standard drugs are summarized. As the prescription of drugs for "off-label" indications is becoming increasingly important and frequent, the most pertinent literature concerning such uses is also reviewed.

PRINCIPLES OF PSYCHOPHARMACOLOGY

Psychiatric Diagnosis and Psychopharmacology

One major difficulty with the official American Psychiatric Association nomenclature found in DSM-IV (American Psychiatric Association, 1994) and with most current psychiatric nomenclatures is that usually etiology is not taken into account in formulating a diagnosis. This is because, at our present state of knowledge, we do not know the etiologies of many conditions. Hence, we are often treating specific constellations of behavioral symptoms without understanding adequately their biological and genetic underpinnings and how they interact with their psychosocial and physical environments. For example, autistic disorder is not etiologically homogeneous but has a multitude of causes.

Theoretically, drugs may be effective for a given psychiatric disorder by correcting the condition(s) leading to it or by influencing events somewhere along the usually complex pathways between the hypothesized abnormality(-ies) and its subsequent psychological and/or behavioral consequences. Thus, some psychoactive drugs may be effective in several dissimilar disorders because they influence or modify neurotransmitters and psychoneuroendocrine events in the brain along or near the end of these interacting, partially confluent, or final common pathways. Other psychoactive drugs appear to exert their therapeutic effects through entirely different mechanisms in different diagnostic entities (e.g., imipramine in treating depression, attention deficit hyperactivity disorder (ADHD), and enuresis).

Some patients with a specific diagnosis (e.g., ADHD, autistic disor-

der, or schizophrenia) will not have a satisfactory clinical response or will be refractory to a specific drug—even one known to be highly effective in statistically significant double-blind studies. For example, only about 75% of ADHD children treated with stimulants will show favorable responses, necessitating trial on nonstimulant drugs for the other 25% (Green, 1995b). Among those responding favorably to stimulants, however, there will be a spectrum; some children will respond extremely well, others will benefit but to a lesser degree. Also, some children with ADHD (or an earlier equivalent diagnosis) will respond unfavorably to one stimulant drug but favorably to another.

There are increasing numbers of reports in the literature that utilize combinations of medications in treating child and adolescent psychiatric disorders. These reports usually concern either treatment-resistant patients, most of whom have one or more comorbid diagnoses, who have had an unsatisfactory response to trials of single drugs, or patients who have experienced only mild or modest improvement or who cannot tolerate higher dosages because of untoward effects.

Polypharmacy also has a rational appeal. Sometimes it may permit two different target symptoms to be more adequately addressed, e.g., hyperactivity and tics. It may allow lower doses of each of two or more medications, resulting in fewer, less intense, or diminished risk of untoward effects, e.g., when the addition of another drug may result in satisfactory control of symptoms with a reduction in dosage of an antipsychotic drug.

Disadvantages of polypharmacy include unknown potential interactions of drugs, many of which are being used for off-label indications in children and younger adolescents, and the lack of double-blind placebo-controlled studies of their untoward effects and short- and long-term efficacy. Clinically, it always remains extremely important to continue to evaluate the impact of the family and psychosocial environment on the child or adolescent and to resist any temptation to attempt to solve any remaining problems only with the right combination of medications. Usually satisfactory resolution of psychiatric disorders in children and adolescents will require additional individual and/or family therapies.

Wilens et al. (1995) have provided a useful review of the current status of combined pharmacotherapy in child and adolescent psychiatry. Walkup (1995) has offered algorithms for the treatment of children and adolescents diagnosed with ADHD, mood disorder, and psychosis, which include systematic trials of various combined medications for patients who are treatment-resistant or who do not respond to standard pharmacotherapy with single agents. Green (1995b) reviewed the literature on polypharmacy in children and adolescents with ADHD alone and with comorbid disorders and noted that nonstimulant medications, e.g., tricyclics, selective serotonin reuptake inhibitors (SSRIs), and clonidine, have been used in combination with stimulants as adjunctive drugs for their synergistic effects or to augment partial but inadequate responses to stimulant medications.

Psychopharmacologic Research

The most scientifically rigorous proofs of drug efficacy are double-blind crossover studies in which the drug under investigation is compared with placebo or a standard treatment and is statistically found to be significantly better than placebo or equal to or better than the standard treatment.

Statistics, however, inform us about groups of patients, not individuals. Hence, if etiologically dissimilar groups are subsumed under the same diagnosis, a few patients may truly benefit, but their improvement could be so diluted by the larger majority who did not benefit that the drug may show no statistically significant benefit. Some researchers now note if there are strong individual responders in a drug study even when there is no statistical difference between experimental and control groups. Thus, individual case reports, studies of relatively small numbers, and open studies should not be summarily dismissed. The fact that a drug is statistically significantly better than another drug or placebo doesn't necessarily mean that the drug is a satisfactory treatment for a given condition or a specific child or adolescent. The drug may be effective only in certain environments (e.g., a laboratory) and not generalize to more ordinary circumstances, or it may improve only certain symptoms but not affect other major target symptoms to a clinically meaningful degree, or the overall improvement may be relatively modest, with significant symptoms or deficits remaining.

As psychiatric diagnosis becomes more refined and the etiology and pathogeneses of homogeneous subgroups are delineated, more specific and rational psychopharmacology will follow. Similarly, drugs are being developed with increasing neurotransmitter specificity and they are being used to modify certain symptoms or behaviors across diagnostic categories.

General Principles of Administering Psychoactive Medication to Children and Younger Adolescents

INDICATIONS FOR USE

Diagnosis and Treatment Plan

A complete psychiatric assessment, including appropriate psychological tests, resulting in a working diagnosis and comprehensive treatment plan; appropriate physical and laboratory examinations; and baseline behavioral measurements should be completed as minimum prerequisites prior to the initiation of psychopharmacotherapy. Treatment with psychoactive drugs should always be part of a more comprehensive treatment regimen and rarely, if ever, is appropriate as the sole treatment modality for a child or adolescent.

The legal guardian/caretaker and the child or adolescent patient, to the degree appropriate to the patient's age and psychopathology, should participate in formulating the treatment plan. The use of medication, including expected benefits and possible short- and long-term untoward effects, should be reviewed with them in understandable terminology. Their informed consents should be obtained and included in the clinical record.

It is essential to assess carefully the attitude and reliability of the persons who will be responsible for administering the medication. Unless there is a positive or at least honestly neutral attitude toward medication and some therapeutic alliance with the parents, it will be difficult

or unfeasible to make a reliable assessment of drug efficacy and compliance. One must also be confident that the parents will not withhold medication if their child appears to be doing well, increase the medication without the physician's approval if the patient's behavior worsens, or administer the drug to the child as a punishment. Likewise, to store and administer medication safely on an outpatient basis requires a responsible adult, especially if there are young children in the home or if the patient is at suicidal risk.

Diagnosis and Target Symptoms

It is essential to make an accurate diagnosis and to identify and quantify target symptoms in order to choose an efficacious drug and to assess the results of medication. The target symptoms must be of sufficient severity and must interfere so significantly with the child's or adolescent's current functioning and future development that the potential benefits of the drug will justify the risks accompanying its administration. Medication must be chosen with respect to both diagnosis and target symptoms. Thus, the symptom "hyperactivity" is present in numerous childhood psychiatric disorders. All hyperactivity, however, is not the same and one must be aware of the diagnosis. A hyperactive youngster with ADHD would be expected to respond favorably to the administration of a stimulant, while a schizophrenic youngster who exhibited marked hyperactivity would usually be treated with an antipsychotic to address the psychotic symptomatology. In fact, stimulant drugs, the drugs of choice in ADHD, are considered to be relatively contraindicated in schizophrenia and may cause worsening of psychotic symptoms.

BASELINE ASSESSMENTS PRIOR TO INITIATION OF MEDICATION

All patients should have a complete medical history and physical and neurological examinations. This is essential to identify any organic factors contributing to the psychiatric symptomatology and any coexisting medical abnormalities. In addition, since all drugs may cause untoward physical and psychological effects, baseline physical, laboratory, and behavioral assessments prior to initiation of psychopharmacotherapy are mandatory.

Because relatively little information is available concerning the long-term untoward effects of psychoactive drugs on the growth and development of children and adolescents, as well as the potential medicolegal ramifications, particularly when drugs are used for off-label indications (i.e., uses that have not been approved for advertising as efficacious and safe by the Food and Drug Administration (FDA)), the premedication workup should be comprehensive.

Physical Examination

This should include recording baseline temperature, pulse and respiration rates (TPR), and blood pressure. Height and weight should be entered on standardized growth charts, such as the National Center for Health Statistics Growth Charts, so that serial measurements and percentiles may be plotted over time (Hamill et al., 1976). A pregnancy test should be considered for any adolescent who might be pregnant, as drugs may have known or unknown adverse effects on the developing fetus.

Laboratory Tests and Diagnostic Procedures

The following are recommended: a complete blood count (CBC), differential, and hematocrit; urinalysis; blood urea nitrogen (BUN) level; blood chemistries, including serum electrolytes [sodium (Na^+), potassium (K^+), chloride (Cl^-), carbon dioxide (CO_2) content, calcium (Ca^{2+}), and phosphate (PO_4^{3-})]; and liver function tests, including aspartate aminotransferase (AST) or serum glutamic oxaloacetic transaminase (SGOT), alanine aminotransferase (ALT) or serum glutamic pyruvic transaminase (SGPT), alkaline phosphatase, lactic dehydrogenase

(LDH), and bilirubin (total and indirect). Serum lead level determination is recommended for children under 7 years of age and older children when indicated.

A baseline ECG should be performed prior to the administration of tricyclic antidepressants and lithium, as both can cause cardiac abnormalities. The ECG should be monitored with dose increases and periodically thereafter if tricyclics are used.

Blanz and Schmidt (1993) consider monitoring of EEG at baseline and during treatment with clozapine mandatory. An EEG may be considered if antipsychotics, tricyclics, and lithium will be administered, as all these drugs have been associated with either a lowered threshold to seizures or other EEG changes.

Thyroid function tests (triiodothyronine resin uptake (T_3RU), thyroxine (T_4), and thyroid-stimulating hormone (TSH)) are also recommended prior to the use of tricyclic antidepressants and lithium. Lithium has been reported to cause hypothyroidism, with lower T_3 and T_4 levels and elevated I^{131} uptake. Abnormal thyroid function can aggravate cardiac arrhythmias that may occur as an untoward effect of tricyclic antidepressants (*Physicians' Desk Reference* (PDR), 1995).

Because lithium has been reported to have adverse effects on renal function in adults, baseline studies are essential. In healthy children and adolescents, a baseline serum creatinine and urinalysis are usually adequate (Jefferson et al., 1987). If kidney disease is suspected or abnormalities found, complete urinalysis including specific gravity, BUN level, 24-hour urine volume, and 24-hour urine for creatinine clearance and protein should be performed, and a renal consultation should be obtained.

Baseline Behavioral Assessment

Baseline observations and careful characterizations of both behavior and target symptoms must be recorded in the clinical record. These should include direct observations by the clinician, as well as those reported to occur in other locations, such as the home and school, by other reliable observers. It is important to include usual eating and sleeping patterns, as these may be altered by many drugs. These observations should be described both qualitatively and quantitatively (amplitude and frequency), and the circumstances in which they occur noted. This is essential both to rate objectively the efficacy of the drug over time and to provide essential information for other clinicians who may later treat the patient. To be able to assess the efficacy of a specific medication, a baseline observation period, with reasonably stable or worsening target symptoms, is necessary. Other than in emergency situations (e.g., a violent, physically assaultive psychotic teenager), observation of the patient for a minimum of 7–10 days is recommended before initiating psychopharmacotherapy. For inpatients, this will permit assessment of the combined effects, upon the patient's psychopathology and symptoms, of (*a*) hospitalization and a therapeutic milieu and (*b*) the removal of the identified patient from his or her living situation. For outpatients, this observation period will give the clinician an opportunity to see the impact of the clinical contact and assessment on the symptom expression of the patient and the psychodynamic equilibrium of the family. During this observation period, many children and adolescents, both inpatients and outpatients for whom medication was being considered, will improve sufficiently so that psychopharmacotherapy will no longer be indicated.

Rating Scales.   Rating scales are an essential component of psychopharmacological research. They provide a means of recording serial qualitative and quantitative measurements of behaviors, and interrater reliability can be determined. Two of the most influential publications concerning rating scales and psychopharmacological research in children are special issues of the *Psychopharmacology Bulletin*, "Pharmacotherapy of Children" (1973) and "Rating Scales and Assessment Instruments for Use in Pediatric Psychopharmacology Research" (1985).

Although rating scales are also valuable in nonresearch settings, they tend to be used less in clinical practice. Perhaps the most frequently used are the various Conners rating instruments: Conners Teacher Questionnaire; Conners Parent-Teacher Questionnaire; and Conners Parent Questionnaire (*Psychopharmacology Bulletin*, 1973, pp. 219, 222, and 231–234). The Conners Parent-Teacher Questionnaire has only 11 items and can be completed in a short time. It is helpful in treating children and adolescents with ADHD, and serial ratings provide a good estimate of efficacy of response to medication in the classroom and home environments.

It is essential to record an accurate, baseline rating in the clinical record before beginning psychopharmacotherapy in children or adolescents who have or are at risk for developing abnormal involuntary movements (e.g., patients diagnosed with autistic disorder, tic disorders, severe mental retardation, or treated with antipsychotics). This is essential both to follow the patient's clinical course and to differentiate among recrudescence of preexisting involuntary movements, stereotypies, mannerisms, and any subsequent withdrawal dyskinesias or new stereotypies that may occur when medication, particularly an antipsychotic, is discontinued. Although the baseline data can be documented in the clinician's note, the use of a rating scale such as the Abnormal Involuntary Movement Scale (AIMS) ("Rating Scales and Assessment Instruments," 1985, pp. 1077–1080) that assesses abnormal movements is recommended. This will make it less likely that an area that should be assessed will be omitted and will also provide quantitative ratings for following the clinical course. This is helpful to the initial treating physician but especially useful if it becomes necessary for other physicians to use the clinical records at a later time in treating the patient.

CHOICE OF DRUG

In general, it is recommended that an FDA-approved, standard medication for the patient's age, diagnosis, and target symptoms be chosen initially. Factors such as selecting the drug with the least risk of serious untoward effects; known previous response(s) of the patient to psychotropic medication; the responses of siblings, parents, and other relatives with psychiatric illnesses to psychotropic medication; and the clinician's own previous experience in using the medication should also be weighed in choosing the initial and, if necessary, subsequent drugs.

In this chapter, standard treatments are considered those treatments that have been approved by the FDA for advertising and interstate commerce. This implies that the drug has demonstrated clinical efficacy and that its use is substantially safe. The FDA's legal authority over how marketed drugs are used, the dosages employed, and related matters is limited to regulating what the manufacturer may recommend and must disclose in the package insert or labeling. However, "The prescription of a drug for an unlabeled (off-label) indication is entirely proper if the proposed use is based on rational scientific theory, expert medical opinion, or controlled clinical studies" (American Medical Association, 1993, p. 14).

A substantial body of clinical and investigational experience in using FDA-approved drugs in children below the recommended age for use and in using approved drugs for non-FDA-approved (off-label) indications has accumulated over the past two decades. Lithium and tricyclic and SSRI antidepressants are, at present, the most clinically important of these. There appears to be a growing consensus among child psychiatrists that the risks of using lithium and some of the tricyclic and SSRI antidepressants for off-label indications are preferable to using antipsychotics, which increase the risks of impairing cognitive functioning and of developing tardive dyskinesia, or other drugs with less favorable profiles of untoward effects. This is elaborated further, as specific drugs are discussed.

DRUG INTERACTIONS

All psychoactive drugs may have significant interactions with other medications. It is essential to ascertain any medication, prescription or otherwise, that the patient may be taking concurrently and to evaluate the potential interaction. If substance abuse is known or suspected, screening of urine and/or blood for toxic substances may be indicated.

Drug interactions are not reviewed extensively in this chapter; the package insert, current PDR (1995), current *Drug Interactions and Side Effects Index* (1995), *Drug Interactions in Psychiatry* (Ciraulo et al., 1995), or other suitable reference should be consulted. When appropriate and with the patient's consent, any other physicians treating the patient should be contacted so that a comprehensive treatment regimen that addresses both the psychiatric and physical disorders can be developed safely.

REGULATION OF MEDICATION

Selecting Initial Dosage

It is recommended that the treating physician initially prescribe a low dose, which for most patients will be either ineffective or inadequate. Although this cautious approach may take longer to reach a therapeutic dose, it is worthwhile for several reasons. First, pharmacokinetics vary not only among various age groups but also among individuals of a specific age. For genetic and other reasons, some individuals may be highly sensitive and responsive to a given medication, while others are relatively resistant or nonresponsive. By beginning with a low dose, one will avoid starting at a dose that is already in excess of the optimal therapeutic dose for a few patients, and those children and adolescents who are good responders at low dosages of medication will not be missed. If the initial dose is too high, the therapeutic range for these individuals will not be explored, and only untoward effects, which may at times even be confused with worsening of target symptoms, will be seen. Hence, a potentially beneficial medication may be needlessly excluded. For example, with stimulants, a worsening of behavior may occur when optimal therapeutic levels for a specific patient have been exceeded. Second, with some drugs (e.g., methylphenidate), there is no significant relationship between serum level and clinical response. Third, an excessive initial dosage may also cause behavioral toxicity, particularly in younger children. Behavioral toxicity may occur before other side effects and includes such symptoms as worsening of target symptoms, hyperactivity or hypoactivity, aggressiveness, increased irritability, mood changes, apathy, and decreased verbal productions (Campbell et al., 1985). Fourth, some untoward effects of the drug may be eliminated or minimized; e.g., acute dystonic reactions appear to be related in most cases both to serum levels and to the rapidity of increase in serum level, and sedation may be less of a problem if dosage is increased gradually (Green et al., 1985).

Titration of Medication and Determining the Optimal Dose

The goal of the clinician is to achieve meaningful therapeutic benefits for the patient with the fewest possible untoward effects. Here again it is recommended that risks versus gains be assessed. To do so scientifically, however, it is necessary to explore the dose range of a patient's response. Therefore, unless there are extenuating circumstances, it is usually advisable to continue raising the dose level until one of the following events occurs: (*a*) an entirely satisfactory remission of symptoms is achieved; (*b*) the upper limit of the recommended dosage or a higher dose, if the clinician feels it is safe based on the literature and/or his or her experience, has been reached; (*c*) untoward effects that preclude a further increase in dose have occurred; or (*d*) after a measurable improvement in target symptoms, a plateau in improvement or a worsening of symptoms occurs with further increases in dose.

Unless this is done, an injustice may be done to the patient. This occurs most frequently when there is some behavioral improvement and the treating psychiatrist stabilizes the dosage at that point. Further significant improvement that might have occurred had a higher dose been given is missed. Hence, it is recommended that the next higher dose or two should be explored. If there is significant additional improvement, the therapist in conjunction with the patient and his or her parents can make a judgment as to whether the benefits from this outweigh the risks from the additional dosage.

Once the upper limit of the therapeutic dose range has been explored for a specific patient, the lowest possible dose that produces the desired effects should be determined. In clinical practice, this may be a compromise, and amelioration of target symptoms to an acceptable degree may occur only when some untoward effects are also present. This is considered the optimal dose for the specific patient.

In those cases where either no significant therapeutic benefit occurs or untoward effects prevent employment of a clinically meaningful therapeutic dose, a trial of a different medication must be considered. Clinicians should not continue to prescribe drugs in doses that do not have significant therapeutic effects.

Times chosen for administration of the drug and the number of times the drug is administered per day should be related to the pharmacokinetics of the drug (e.g., stimulants are most frequently given around breakfast and lunch, while antipsychotics may initially be given three or four times daily to reduce the risk of sedation and acute dystonic reactions). Once dosage is stabilized, it may be clinically useful to administer only once or twice daily those medications that have longer half-lives if that can be done safely (e.g., it may be possible to give the entire daily dose of an antipsychotic at bedtime). Tricyclic antidepressants, however, should not routinely be given in one daily dose, as the resulting higher serum levels would increase the likelihood of cardiac toxicity.

Dosage Increases

Changes in medication level should be made based on the clinical response of the patient, and the rationale for each change should be documented in the clinical record. Knowledge of the characteristic time frame of response for a particular drug and diagnosis should influence these decisions. Thus, the clinician may increase dosage once or twice weekly in some cases when using stimulants or neuroleptics. On the other hand, the clinical efficacy of tricyclic antidepressants may not be fully apparent for several weeks when they are used to treat major depressive disorder. Once daily dosage has reached a level that is usually associated with clinical response, increasing the dose because of a failure to respond during the first 2 or 3 weeks of treatment is not psychopharmacologically sound practice unless serum drug levels are being monitored and are felt to be in the subtherapeutic range.

UNTOWARD EFFECTS (SIDE EFFECTS)

All drugs, including placebos, have untoward effects or side effects. Actually, if one excludes allergic and idiosyncratic reactions, many untoward effects are as much a characteristic of the pharmacological makeup of a specific drug and as predictable as the drug's therapeutic effects. Individual patients may vary as much in their development of untoward effects to a drug as in their therapeutic responses to it.

It is sometimes useful to think of untoward effects as the "unwanted effects" of the drug for the specific patient and therapeutic indication. For a different patient and situation, an untoward or side effect will actually become the desired therapeutic action of the drug. For example, sedation, which may be an untoward effect when a benzodiazepine is prescribed for anxiety, is the desired result when a benzodiazepine is prescribed as a soporific.

Many untoward effects are related to dose or serum levels, but others are not. They may occur almost immediately (e.g., an acute dystonic reaction) or be delayed for years (e.g., tardive dyskinesia). They may be life threatening or fatal, or relatively innocuous. There is also evidence that the untoward effects of a specific drug may differ according to age and/or diagnosis of the subjects. For example, haloperidol produced excessive sedation in hospitalized school-age aggressive conduct-disordered children on doses of 0.04–0.21 mg/kg/day (Campbell et al., 1984b) but not in preschoolers with autistic disorder on doses of 0.019–0.217 mg/kg/day (Anderson et al., 1984)

A thorough knowledge of the most important and frequent side effects of the medications considered is essential and will often play a decisive role in which medication is selected and/or the dosage schedule. For example, if a schizophrenic youngster has insomnia, the clinician may select a low-potency antipsychotic and adjust the dosage schedule so that any sedation will aid the child in falling asleep. As an added benefit, the risk of an acute dystonic reaction is lower than if a high-potency antipsychotic were chosen.

Likewise, the management of unwanted effects is a vital component of pharmacotherapy. In clinical practice, careful attention to unwanted effects and flexibility may enable one to obtain a satisfactory clinical result with a minimal or acceptable level of side effects. Thus, one can adjust medication levels slowly and in small increments, or one can divide doses unequally over the day (e.g., giving more in the morning or more before bed, or the entire daily dose at bedtime).

It is essential that the clinician examine the patient frequently for the development of side effects during the period when the medication is being regulated, at regular intervals during maintenance therapy, and during scheduled periodic withdrawals of the medication. For example, with antipsychotics one should look particularly for sedation and extra-pyramidal side effects, the development of abnormal movements, and, during drug withdrawal periods, any evidence of a withdrawal dyskinesia. It has been reported that fine wormlike (vermicular) movements of the tongue may be an early sign of tardive dyskinesia and that discontinuation of the medication may prevent further development of the syndrome (PDR, 1995).

MONITORING OF SERUM LEVELS OF DRUGS AND/OR THEIR METABOLITES

Clinically, the monitoring of serum levels is useful to verify compliance and to be certain that adequate therapeutic serum levels are available (i.e., that values fall within the therapeutic window), and thus to avoid discontinuing a trial of medication before clinically effective serum levels have been reached or, conversely, to avoid inadvertently reaching toxic serum levels.

Regular determinations of serum levels of drug and/or metabolites should be considered mandatory for children and adolescents who are being administered lithium or a tricyclic antidepressant. The therapeutic ranges of antiepileptic drugs being used for psychiatric indications such as aggressive behavior are usually considered to be about the same as when used for controlling seizures. Serum levels are reviewed below under the specific drugs.

Serum level monitoring is potentially very important when there is minimal correlation between dose and serum level, and serum levels are correlated significantly with clinical response and/or potentially serious untoward effects. For example, Puig-Antich et al. (1987) have emphasized that they found no predictors of total maintenance plasma levels, including dosage, in their prepubertal subjects treated with imipramine for major depressive disorder. They also reported that positive therapeutic response to imipramine in prepubertal children was strongly correlated with serum levels over 150 ng/ml. Serum levels of tricyclic antidepressants may vary widely among individuals receiving the same dosage; hence, monitoring is especially helpful both in ascertaining that therapeutic levels have been achieved and in avoiding potentially cardiotoxic levels.

On the other hand, a detailed review of the pharmacokinetics and actions of methylphenidate concluded that "blood MPH [methylphenidate] levels are not statistically related to clinical response, nor are they likely to prove clinically helpful until this lack of correlation is understood" (Patrick et al., 1987, p. 1393).

LENGTH OF TIME TO CONTINUE MEDICATION

Children and adolescents are immature, developing organisms. Because of concerns about long-term untoward effects, such as tardive and withdrawal dyskinesias and growth retardation, and our inadequate knowledge of other long-term untoward effects of psychopharmacological agents on biological and psychological maturation, there is unanimous agreement that medication should be given for as short a period

as possible. It is to be hoped, especially when there is a significant psychosocial etiological factor, that medication will augment the child's response to other therapeutic interventions and enhance his or her social and academic functioning, maturation, and development. Once real gains are made and internalized, the cycle of failure broken, and maladaptive patterns replaced with more appropriate ones, it may be possible to discontinue the drug and maintain therapeutic gains. Even in chronic conditions with strong biological underpinnings, such as pervasive developmental disorder, schizophrenia, and depression, psychoactive medication may at times be reduced or even discontinued.

Hence, it is mandatory to discontinue psychotropic medications (or to attempt to do so) on a regular basis, certainly no less frequently than every 6 months to 1 year unless prior attempts have resulted in significant deterioration. Rapidly metabolized drugs such as methylphenidate and amphetamines may be discontinued abruptly; however, it is recommended that most medications, especially those with longer serum half-lives, be gradually reduced rather than stopped abruptly, to minimize the likelihood of developing withdrawal syndromes. For example, Gualtieri and his colleagues (1984) reported both physical withdrawal symptoms, such as decreased appetite, nausea and vomiting, diarrhea and sweating, and acute behavioral deterioration, in about 10% of children and adolescents following their withdrawal from long-term treatment with antipsychotics. Both types of withdrawal symptoms ceased spontaneously within 8 weeks.

If a withdrawal dyskinesia emerges upon discontinuing an antipsychotic, every effort should be made to keep the patient off antipsychotics.

In significant numbers of cases, medication may be no longer required or adequate symptom control can be maintained on a lower maintenance dose. On the other hand, with the passage of time, occasionally higher doses may be required to maintain gains. Although this may indicate tolerance or a worsening of the psychiatric disorder, in some cases it could be a consequence of normal weight gain or maturational/developmental changes.

For example, Sleator et al. (1974) administered a 1-month-long period of placebo to 28 of 42 hyperactive children who had been treated with methylphenidate for 1–2 years. Eleven of the 28 were able to continue performing adequately behaviorally and academically without medication. Seventeen of the 28 showed worsening during the placebo period; of the 17, 10 functioned well when their initial dose was resumed, while 7 needed an increase in dose to maintain their original gains.

"Drug holidays" may also be employed to minimize the amount of medication taken over time. The feasibility and type of drug holidays vary with diagnosis and the severity of the disorder. When medication is needed primarily for classroom functioning, as with some ADHD children, it is often not given on holidays and weekends and during school vacations.

SPECIFIC DRUG TREATMENTS

In this section, psychopharmacological agents are discussed by class. Each class of drugs is introduced with general comments, including indications for use and the most common untoward effects. Then specific drugs of each class are reviewed individually; standard, FDA-approved treatments are discussed first. Unless otherwise noted, all dosage recommendations are for oral administration. Some off-label treatments reported in the literature to be efficacious and that are used clinically by some practitioners are also discussed. It is recommended that these drugs be used conservatively, that is, only by experienced physicians, and primarily after standard treatment regimens have proven unsuccessful. Most of these studies illustrate a particular point or provide the reader with some of the evidence not readily accessible elsewhere. This evidence ranges from reasonably convincing to merely suggesting a possible alternative for a seriously disturbed patient who has not responded satisfactorily to any standard approved treatment. Excellent reviews of the older literature that support the standard psychopharmacological treatments of children and adolescents discussed below are easily accessible (for references see Green, 1995a).

Table 72.1. Diagnoses in Childhood and Adolescence for Which Psychopharmacotherapy May Be Therapeutically Indicated

DSM-IV Diagnoses	Medication	DSM-IV Diagnoses	Medication
Attention deficit/hyperactivity disorder	Stimulants Tricyclic antidepressants Antipsychotics Clonidine Guanfacine Fluoxetine Clomipramine MAOIs Bupropion	Overanxious disorder of childhood (subsumed under generalized anxiety disorder in DSM-IV)	Benzodiazepines Diphenhydramine Fluoxetine Buspirone Hydroxyzine
Conduct disorder (severe, aggressive)	Antipsychotics (thioridazine, haloperidol, and chlorpromazine) Lithium Propranolol Carbamazepine Trazodone Clonidine	Panic disorder	Tricyclic antidepressants Alprazolam Clonazepam
		Pervasive developmental disorders	Haloperidol Fluphenazine Naltrexone Fenfluramine Clomipramine Buspirone Clonidine
Encopresis	Lithium	Posttraumatic stress disorder (acute)	Propranolol
Enuresis	DDAVP Imipramine Benzodiazepines Carbamazepine Amphetamines Clomipramine Desipramine	Schizophrenia	Antipsychotics
		Selective mutism	Fluoxetine
		Separation anxiety disorder	Imipramine Chlordiazepoxide Fluoxetine Alprazolam Buspirone Clomipramine Clonazepam
Intermittent explosive disorder	Propranolol	Sleep disorders Primary insomnia	Benzodiazepines Diphenhydramine Hydroxyzine
Major depressive disorder	Antidepressants Lithium augmentation Lithium for prophylaxis	Circadian rhythm sleep disorder	Benzodiazepines Diphenhydramine Hydroxyzine
Manic episode (acute and maintenance)	Lithium Antipsychotics Valproic acid	Sleep terror disorder	Benzodiazepines Imipramine Carbamazipine
Mental retardation (with severe behavioral disorder and/or self-injurious behavior)	Thioridazine Chlorpromazine Haloperidol Lithium Propranolol Naltrexone	Sleepwalking disorder	Benzodiazepines Imipramine
Obsessive-compulsive disorder	Clomipramine Fluoxetine Fluvoxamine Clonazepam	Tourette's disorder	Haloperidol Pimozide Clonidine Desipramine Nortriptyline Fluoxetine

From Green WH: *Child and Adolescent Clinical Psychopharmacology* (2nd ed). Baltimore, Williams & Wilkins, 1995.

Although always important, informed consent, preferably written, is very important if FDA-approved drugs are used for nonapproved (off-label) indications. It should be documented that the parents or legal guardians and, when appropriate, the patient are cognizant of the situation. If standard approved treatments for a significantly disabling disorder have been tried with little or no success, a clinical trial of an off-label use of a drug is much more easily justified. The physician is advised to become thoroughly familiar with the official package circular provided by the manufacturer of the drug or the relevant entry in the latest edition and supplements of the PDR (1995) before prescribing any drug.

Table 72.1 lists the most common psychiatric diagnoses in children and younger adolescents for which psychopharmacotherapy may be therapeutically indicated. Where a specific drug or class of drugs is generally preferred for a particular condition, an attempt has been made to rank them in order of preference.

Sympathomimetic Amines and Central Nervous System Stimulants

These drugs, commonly referred to as stimulants, are the drugs of choice for treating ADHD. Bradley's 1937 report on the use of racemic amphetamine sulfate (Benzedrine) in behaviorally disordered children is usually cited as the beginning of child psychopharmacology as a discipline. Since this initial report, more research has been published on the stimulants and ADHD than on any other childhood disorder. Double-blind placebo-controlled studies have found consistently that stimulants are significantly superior to placebo in improving attention span and in decreasing hyperactivity and impulsivity.

Normal prepubertal boys and college-age men reacted similarly to patients diagnosed with ADHD when given single doses of dextroamphetamine; they exhibited decreased motor activity and generally improved attentional performance (Rapoport et al., 1978a, 1980a). Earlier teachings that stimulants have a paradoxical effect in hyperactive children are incorrect, and a positive response to stimulant medication cannot be used to validate the diagnosis of ADHD.

UNTOWARD EFFECTS

There is some evidence that, overall, the untoward effects of methylphenidate occur less frequently and with less severity than those from dextroamphetamine (Conners, 1971; Gross and Wilson, 1974). Gross and Wilson noted that side effects were infrequently severe enough to make immediate discontinuation of medication necessary—1.1% of 377 patients for methylphenidate, and 4.3% of 371 patients for dextroamphetamine.

The most frequent and troublesome immediate untoward effects include insomnia, anorexia, nausea, abdominal pain or cramps, headache, thirst, vomiting, lability of mood, irritability, sadness, weepiness, tachycardia, and blood pressure changes. Many of these symptoms diminish over a period of up to a few weeks, although the cardiovascular changes may persist.

Beginning in 1972, disturbances in growth, both height and weight, have been reported in conjunction with use of stimulant medication, and the long-term consequences of these untoward effects have been of particular concern (Safer et al., 1972). There has been controversy about how significant these changes are. Mattes and Gittelman (1983) reported significant decreases in height and weight percentiles in children treated with methylphenidate over a 4-year period. A controlled study found a significant reduction in growth velocity during the period of time that stimulants are actively administered (Klein et al., 1988). Despite this adverse effect on growth during the active treatment phase, it appears that an accelerated rate of growth or growth rebound occurs once a stimulant is discontinued, and that there is usually no significant compromise of ultimate height attained (Klein and Mannuzza, 1988). It seems likely, however, that some children are at greater risk for growth suppression than others, and careful serial heights and weights should be plotted on a growth chart (e.g., the National Center for Health Statistics Growth Chart) (Hamill et al., 1976) for any child receiving stimulants.

Stimulants can exacerbate existing tics and precipitate tics de novo and stereotypies. There is disagreement among experts as to whether stimulants should be given to persons with tics, Tourette's disorder, or a family history of either. At the present time, a conservative approach would consider the stimulants relatively or absolutely contraindicated in treating such children (Green, 1995a).

A few children treated with stimulants may develop a clinical picture resembling schizophrenia. This most frequently occurs when untoward effects such as disorganization are misinterpreted as a worsening of presenting symptoms, and the dosage is further increased until prominent psychotomimetic effects occur. This may also occur when stimulants are administered inadvertently to children with borderline personality disorders or schizophrenia, conditions in which stimulants are usually contraindicated. In most cases, the psychotic symptomatology improves rapidly following discontinuation of the drug (Green, 1989).

Some parents express concern that treatment with stimulants will predispose their child to later drug abuse or addiction. Most available evidence indicates that this is not the case. Although drug abuse itself is of major concern in our culture, children who have been treated for their ADHD with stimulants appear to be at no greater risk than control subjects for drug or alcohol abuse as teenagers and adults (Weiss and Hechtman, 1986).

The stimulants are the most frequently prescribed psychiatric drugs during childhood. In 1987 it was conservatively estimated that in the United States, 750,000 youth were being treated with medication for hyperactivity or inattentiveness (Safer and Krager, 1988). In Baltimore county, 6% of all public elementary school students were receiving such medication; methylphenidate accounted for 93% of the drugs prescribed, and other stimulants, another 6% (Safer and Krager, 1988). Because methylphenidate is the most commonly prescribed drug for ADHD, it will be used to illustrate the use of the stimulants, despite its having appeared on the scene considerably later than dextroamphetamine sulfate.

METHYLPHENIDATE (RITALIN)

Indications in Child and Adolescent Psychiatry

FDA approved for treating ADHD and narcolepsy.

Dosage Schedule for Treating ADHD

- Children under 6 years old: Not approved for use.
- Persons 6 years and over: Start with 5 mg once or twice daily and raise dose gradually 5–10 mg/week. Maximum daily dosage is 60 mg.

- Optimal dose usually is between 0.3 and 0.7 mg/kg/dose administered two or three times daily (total daily dose range from 0.6 to 2.1 mg/kg/day) (Duncan, 1990).

Dose Forms Available

- Tablets: 5 mg, 10 mg, 20 mg
- Sustained release tablets (Ritalin-SR): 20 mg

Administration of methylphenidate with meals does not appear to adversely affect the absorption, or the pharmacokinetics of methylphenidate and may diminish problems with appetite suppression (Patrick et al., 1987).

Methylphenidate and the Treatment of ADHD

An improvement of target symptoms can be seen within 20 minutes after a therapeutically effective dose is given. Peak blood levels occur 1–2½ hours after administration (Gualtieri et al., 1982), and serum half-life is about 2½ hours (Winsberg et al., 1982). Because of these pharmacokinetics, the most frequent times of dosage are before leaving for school and during lunch hour. This dosage schedule usually ensures adequate serum levels during school hours, which for most children is the foremost consideration. Sustained release tablets make once-daily dosage possible for some children.

Children who develop significant behavioral or attentional difficulties in the late afternoon or early evening may do so because of a return to baseline behavior as serum levels decline into subtherapeutic levels and/or because of a rebound effect as the drug wears off (Rapoport et al., 1978a). A third dose of medication given in the afternoon may be helpful for some such children. A recent study, however, suggests that psychostimulant rebound effects are not clinically significant for the large majority of children (Johnston et al., 1988).

Insomnia may also occur. It is clinically important to distinguish those children whose insomnia is an untoward effect of the drug from those children whose insomnia may be due to the recurrence of behavioral difficulties as the medication effect subsides. For the first group of children, a reduction in milligram dosage of the last dose of the day may be necessary. For the latter group, an evening dose or a dose about an hour before bedtime may be helpful.

There is some evidence that methylphenidate may lower the convulsive threshold; however, this may not be clinically significant at usual doses (for review see Green, 1995a). It is recommended that it be discontinued if seizures develop de novo or increase in frequency.

Reports of Interest

Methylphenidate has been investigated in the treatment of hyperactive children diagnosed with autistic disorder. Although most of the earlier literature states that stimulants are contraindicated for such children and cause a worsening in behavior and/or stereotypies, recent studies have reported that methylphenidate is effective in treating some children with autistic disorder who also exhibit such symptoms as hyperactivity, impulsivity, short attention spans, and aggression (Birmaher et al., 1988; Strayhorn et al., 1988). Until additional research corroborates these studies in larger samples, the efficacy of methylphenidate in treating autistic children or hyperactive subgroups of them must be regarded as unproven.

DEXTROAMPHETAMINE SULFATE (DEXEDRINE)

Indications in Child and Adolescent Psychiatry

FDA approved for treating ADDH (an earlier equivalent of ADHD) and narcolepsy.

Dosage Schedule for Treating ADHD

- Children under 3 years old: Not approved for use.
- Children 3–5 years: Begin with 2.5 mg daily; raise by 2.5-mg increments once or twice weekly; titrate for optimal dose.

- Persons 6 years and over: Begin with 5 mg daily; raise by 5-mg increments once or twice weekly; usual maximum dose is less than 40 mg/day.
- Optimal dose is usually between 0.15 and 0.5 mg/kg/dose administered two or three times daily (total daily dose range, 0.30–1.5 mg/kg/day) (Duncan, 1990).

Dose Forms Available

- Elixir: 5 mg/5 ml
- Tablets: 5 mg
- Sustained release capsules (Spansule): 5 mg, 10 mg, 15 mg

Dextroamphetamine and the Treatment of ADHD

Dextroamphetamine sulfate (Dexedrine) is the only amphetamine frequently used in treating ADHD and is the only stimulant approved by the FDA for administration to children as young as 3 years of age. Therefore, it is officially the drug of choice for children up to age 6 years, when most clinicians appear to prefer methylphenidate. In addition, if methylphenidate does not provide satisfactory benefit in controlling symptoms of ADHD, it is recommended that dextroamphetamine and/or pemoline be tried before moving on to another class of drugs.

Amphetamines may obtund the maximal electroshock seizure discharge and have been reported to prevent typical 3-per-second spike-and-dome petit mal seizures and to abolish the abnormal EEG pattern in some children (Weiner, 1980). Dextroamphetamine may thus be the stimulant of choice for individuals who have seizures or who are at risk for developing them.

Report of Interest

Geller et al. (1981) reported that dextroamphetamine administered to two children with pervasive developmental disorder and ADHD improved their attention spans with no significant worsening of behavior.

MAGNESIUM PEMOLINE (CYLERT)

Indications in Child and Adolescent Psychiatry

FDA approved for the treatment of ADHD.

Dosage Schedule for Treating ADHD

- Children under 6 years old: Not recommended for use.
- Persons 6 years and over: The initial recommended daily dose of pemoline is 37.5 mg. This may be increased weekly by 18.75 mg until satisfactory clinical benefit occurs, untoward effects prevent further increase, or the maximum daily dose of 112.5 mg is reached.

Dose Forms Available

- Tablets: 18.75 mg, 37.5 mg, 75 mg

Considerations in Use of Magnesium Pemoline

Magnesium pemoline elicits CNS changes that are similar to those of methylphenidate and amphetamines, but it is structurally dissimilar to those drugs and has minimal sympathomimetic effects. Its serum half-life is approximately 12 hours. About 50% of pemoline is excreted unchanged by the kidneys; the liver metabolizes the remainder.

The advantages of pemoline over the sympathomimetic amines include minimal untoward cardiovascular effects; a longer serum half-life, permitting a single morning dose daily (if sustained release forms of the other stimulants are not available to the patient); and (probably) a less intense rebound effect than methylphenidate and dextroamphetamine. The disadvantages of pemoline are that its clinical effect is not as great as that of dexedrine and methylphenidate, and improvement occurs gradually rather than promptly (Conners et al., 1972). If the manufacturer's recommended titration regimen is followed, significant clinical benefit from pemoline is often apparent only after 3–4 weeks. Another concern is hepatotoxicity. Elevated liver enzymes occur in a small percentage, perhaps 1–3%, of children treated with magnesium pemoline; these abnormalities appear to be reversible following drug withdrawal, but it is essential to monitor liver function regularly throughout the duration of therapy (PDR, 1995).

FENFLURAMINE (PONDIMIN)

Indications for Use in Child and Adolescent Psychiatry

Fenfluramine, a sympathomimetic amine with antiserotonergic properties, is approved by the FDA only as a short-term adjunct in the treatment of exogenous obesity in persons 12 years of age or older.

Reports of Interest

Fenfluramine has been investigated in the treatment of ADHD and autistic disorder. Clinically fenfluramine was not efficacious, and it had no beneficial effects on motor activity or behavioral ratings in the treatment of ADHD (Donnelly et al., 1989).

Fenfluramine is better known for the initial reports on its use in the treatment of autistic disorder, the rationale for which was that fenfluramine decreases serotonin levels, which have been found to be elevated in about 30% of mentally retarded and autistic children. Aman and Kern (1989) reviewed 25 published studies of fenfluramine used in treating subjects with autistic disorder. They concluded that fenfluramine may improve social relatedness and attention span and decrease stereotypies and excessive motor activity in some autistic children. However, broader areas of functioning as measured by IQ tests and assessment of communicative abilities did not appear to be affected. Untoward effects reported included lethargy, weight loss, irritability, restlessness, night awakenings, aggressiveness to self or others, diarrhea, and increased stereotypies.

Antipsychotic Drugs

Although in adults these drugs, also commonly referred to as neuroleptics or major tranquilizers, are used primarily to treat psychoses, in children they have additionally been used to treat other common nonpsychotic psychiatric disorders. One reason for this seems to be that the antipsychotics won by default; they were among the earliest psychoactive drugs used in child psychiatry, and the competition hadn't arrived yet. In addition, the risk of untoward effects such as cognitive dulling and irreversible tardive dyskinesia had not been fully appreciated. As clinical and research experience in child psychopharmacology progresses and other drugs become available, however, the use of these drugs in children is becoming more circumscribed, and indications for their use in children are more and more closely approaching those for which they are prescribed in older adolescents and adults.

At the present time, antipsychotics are the drugs of first choice in childhood for schizophrenia and autistic disorder. There is, however, some evidence that antipsychotics are not as effective clinically in schizophrenia with childhood onset as in schizophrenia occurring in later adolescence and adulthood (Green, 1989).

Shapiro and Shapiro (1989) concluded that antipsychotics were also the drugs of choice for treating chronic motor or vocal tic disorder and Tourette's disorder when psychosocial, educational, or occupational functioning was so impaired that medication was required. Although probably indicated in acute mania, paranoia, and schizoaffective disorder, these disorders are rarely diagnosed in childhood, and there is little information available on them.

Antipsychotics are also clinically effective in severely aggressive, conduct-disordered children, and some are approved for use in such children. The use of antipsychotics in the mentally retarded continues to be controversial, but they are frequently prescribed for institutionalized patients. In optimal doses, however, antipsychotics are effective in de-

Table 72.2.   Antipsychotic Drugs

Drug	Chemical Classification	Therapeutically Equivalent Oral Dose (mg)	Effects			Approved Age for Use	Usual Optimal Dose/Maintenance Dose Range
			Sedation	Autonomic[a]	Extrapyramidal Reaction[b]		
Chlorpromazine[c] Thorazine (SmithKline Beecham)	Phenothiazine: Aliphatic compound	100	+++	+++	++	Over 6 months	See text
Thioridazine[c] Mellaril (Sandoz)	Phenothiazine: Peridine compound	100	+++	+++	+	2 years	See text
Clozapine Clozaril (Sandoz)	Dibenzodiazepine	50	+++	+++	0?	16 years	See text
Mesoridazine Serentil (Boehringer Ingelheim)	Phenothiazine: Piperidine compound	50	+++	++	+	12 years	No specific doses for children
Chlorprothixene Taractan (Roche)	Thioxanthene	45	+++	+++	+/++	Over 6 years	10–25 mg 3 to 4 times daily
Loxapine Loxitane (Lederle)	Dibenzoxazepine	15	++	+/++	++/+++	16 years	As per adults
Molindone Moban (DuPont)	Dihydroindolone	10	++	+	+	12 years	No specific doses for children
Perphenazine[c] Trilafon (Schering)	Phenothiazine: Piperazine compound	10	++	+	++/+++	12 years	No specific doses for children
Trifluoperazine[c] Stelazine (SmithKline Beecham)	Phenothiazine: Piperazine compound	5	++	+	+++	6 years	See text
Thiothixene[c] Navane (Roerig)	Thioxanthene	5	+	+	+++	12 years	No specific doses for children
Fluphenazine[c] Permitil (Schering) Prolixin (Princeton)	Phenothiazine: Piperazine compound	2	+	+	+++	Not recommended for children	—
Haloperidol[c] Haldol (McNeil)	Butyrophenone	2	+	+	+++	3 years	See text
Pimozide[d] Orap (Gate)	Diphenylbutylpiperidine	10	+	+	+++	Over 12 years	0.2 mg/kg/day or maximum, 10 mg/day

Adapted from American Medical Association: *Drug Evaluations Annual 1994.* Chicago, American Medical Association, 1993.
[a] α-Antiadrenergic and anticholinergic effects.
[b] Excluding tardive dyskinesis, which appears to be produced to the same degree and frequency by all agents except clozapine with equieffective antipsychotic doses. Clozapine has produced agranulocytosis; therefore, recommendations for its use are limited (see text).
[c] Available genetically.
[d] Only indicated for Tourette's disorder that has not responded to other standard treatments.

creasing irritability, sleep disturbances, hostility, agitation, and combativeness and may improve concentration and social behavior in agitated, severely retarded individuals (American Medical Association, 1993). Aman and Singh (1988) cautioned that the influential studies of the mentally retarded by Breuning that showed significant detrimental effects resulting from antipsychotics appear to have been fabricated.

Table 72.2 summarizes representative antipsychotic drugs commonly used in child and adolescent psychiatry. It compares their relative potencies and expectable potential sedative, autonomic, and extrapyramidal untoward effects with chlorpromazine, the prototype of the antipsychotics. FDA age limitations and recommended dosages for approved use in children and adolescents are also given when available.

Although it is usually recommended that antipsychotics initially be administered in divided doses, most frequently three or four times daily, once the optimal dose is established, their relatively long serum half-lives usually permit either once daily dosage (e.g., before bedtime) or twice daily dosage, in the morning and before bedtime.

UNTOWARD EFFECTS

While antipsychotic drugs may have numerous serious untoward effects, those of greatest concern in children and adolescents are the effects of sedation on cognition and the extrapyramidal syndromes, in particular the concern over the possible development of irreversible tardive dyskinesia.

Both high-potency and low-potency neuroleptics are effective when given in equivalent doses, but they differ in the frequency and severity of their untoward effects. Usually, the higher-potency neuroleptics cause less sedation, fewer autonomic side effects, and more untoward extrapyramidal effects, and the lower-potency neuroleptics cause greater sedation, more autonomic side effects, and fewer extrapyramidal effects (Baldessarini, 1990). Because of the great importance of minimizing any cognitive dulling in school children and in the mentally retarded, whose cognition is already compromised, high-potency less-sedative antipsychotics are often preferred. Over a period of days to weeks, however, considerable tolerance often develops to the sedative effects of high-dose low-potency antipsychotics, and they are still useful when untoward effects are carefully monitored (Green et al., 1992).

Significant numbers of children and adolescents receiving antipsychotic medication develop extrapyramidal syndromes. The reported prevalence of neuroleptic-induced tardive dyskinesia and withdrawal tardive dyskinesia in children and adolescents has ranged from 0 to 51% (Wolf and Wagner, 1993). It is believed that the risk of developing tardive dyskinesia that will become irreversible increases with both total cumulative dose and duration of treatment. No cases of irreversible tardive dyskinesia developing in children or adolescents have been reported; the longest neuroleptic-free persistent tardive dyskinesia was reported to last was $4\frac{1}{2}$ years. Usually withdrawal dyskinesias resolve within a few weeks to a few months after discontinuation of the neuroleptic (Wolf and Wagner, 1993).

Baldessarini (1990) has identified six types of extrapyramidal syndromes associated with the use of antipsychotic drugs:

A. Effects usually appearing during drug administration
　1. Acute dystonic reactions: Period of maximum risk is 1–5 days after initiation of neuroleptic therapy. There is also increased

risk following increments in dose. Acute dystonic reactions respond rapidly to anticholinergic antiparkinsonian drugs (e.g., diphenhydramine (Benadryl) 25 mg orally or intramuscularly).

2. Parkinsonism: Period of maximum risk is 5–30 days after initiation of neuroleptic therapy. Symptoms respond to antiparkinsonian medication (e.g., benztropine (Cogentin) 1–2 mg given two or three times daily usually provides relief within a day or two).

3. Akathisia (motor restlessness): Period of maximum risk is 5–60 days after initiation of neuroleptic therapy. It may or may not respond to antiparkinsonian drugs. Propranolol may be helpful (Adler et al., 1986). Dosage reduction may be necessary.

4. Neuroleptic malignant syndrome: Can occur within weeks after initiation of neuroleptic therapy. Symptoms include severe muscular rigidity, stupor, catatonia, hyperpyrexia, labile pulse and blood pressure, and occasionally myoglobinemia. It can persist for up to 2 weeks or longer after medication is discontinued and can be fatal. Antiparkinsonian drugs are not useful. Immediate discontinuation of medication and hospitalization are mandatory.

B. Late-appearing syndromes (after months or years of treatment)

1. Tardive dyskinesia: Occurs while on medication. There is no adequate treatment; antiparkinsonian drugs may worsen the condition. However, there is some evidence that the atypical antipsychotic clozapine produces little or no tardive dyskinesia when it is the only neuroleptic ever used. Clozapine may significantly decrease or eliminate existing symptoms of tardive dyskinesia during the period it is prescribed (Mozes et al., 1994), but upon its discontinuation, some or all of the improvements in the symptoms of tardive dyskinesia usually recur (Small et al., 1987).

2. Rabbit syndrome (perioral tremor): May be a late variant of parkinsonism. It may respond to antiparkinsonian medication.

In addition, a withdrawal dyskinesia may emerge when neuroleptic medication is withdrawn or the dose reduced. Withdrawal dyskinesias can occur for two different reasons. First, antidopaminergic drugs, including antipsychotics, can suppress tardive dyskinesia; thus, decreasing their serum levels can "unmask" ongoing tardive dyskinesia. Second, Baldessarini (1990) points out that a "disuse supersensitivity" to dopamine agonists may also occur following withdrawal of antidopaminergic drugs and suggests that this phenomenon may explain withdrawal dyskinesias that resolve within a few weeks.

Because of such risks, antipsychotics should be given only to children and adolescents for whom no other potentially less harmful treatment is available; for example, while effective in some children diagnosed with ADHD, antipsychotics should not be used unless both stimulant and other nonstimulant medications have been treatment failures (Green, 1995b).

CHLORPROMAZINE (THORAZINE)

Indications in Child and Adolescent Psychiatry

In addition to being approved for uses similar to those for adults, including psychotic disorders, it is approved "for the treatment of severe behavioral problems in children marked by combativeness and/or explosive hyperexcitable behavior" (package insert). It is also noted that dosages over 500 mg/day are unlikely to further enhance behavioral improvement in severely disturbed mentally retarded patients.

Chlorpromazine may lower the threshold to seizures; another antipsychotic should be chosen for seizure-prone individuals.

Dosage Schedule for Children and Adolescents

- Infants under 6 months of age: Not recommended.
- Children over 6 months to 12 years of age with severe behavioral problems or psychotic conditions:

a. oral: 0.5 mg/kg every 4–6 hours as needed. Titrate upwards gradually. In severe cases, higher doses may be required.

b. rectal: 1 mg/kg every 6–8 hours as needed.

c. intramuscular: 0.5 mg/kg every 6–8 hours as needed. Maximum daily intramuscular dose for a child under 5 years or under 22 kg is 40 mg; for a child 5–12 years of age or 22–45 kg, maximum daily dose is 75 mg.

- Adolescents: Depending on severity of symptoms, begin with 10 mg three times daily to 25 mg four times daily, orally. Titrate upward with increases of 20–50 mg twice weekly. For severely agitated patients, 25 mg may be given intramuscularly and repeated if necessary in 1 hour. Any subsequent intramuscular medication should be at 4- to 6-hour intervals.

Dose Forms Available

- Tablets: 10 mg, 25 mg, 50 mg, 100 mg, 200 mg
- Syrup: 10 mg/5 ml
- Suppositories: 25 mg, 100 mg
- Concentrate: 30 mg/ml, 100 mg/ml
- Injectable: 25 mg/ml

THIORIDAZINE (MELLARIL)

Indications in Child and Adolescent Psychiatry

In addition to psychotic disorders, thioridazine has FDA approval for treating:

severe behavioral problems in children marked by combativeness and/or explosive hyperexcitable behavior (out of proportion to immediate provocations), and in the short-term treatment of hyperactive children who show excessive motor activity with accompanying conduct disorders consisting of some or all of the following symptoms: impulsivity, difficulty sustaining attention, aggressiveness, mood lability, and poor frustration tolerance. (package insert)

Dosage Schedule for Children and Adolescents

- Children under 2 years old: Not recommended.
- Children 2–12 years: Start with a low dose, such as 10 mg daily or 10 mg twice daily, and titrate upward for optimal therapeutic effect, to a maximum of 3 mg/kg/day. More severely disturbed children may initially require 25 mg once or twice daily.
- Older adolescents: As in adults, a maximum of 800 mg/day is permitted to minimize the likelihood that pigmentary retinopathy will develop. The initial dose depends on the severity of the disorder; frequently 25–50 mg twice or three times daily is an appropriate starting dosage.

Dose Forms Available

- Tablets: 10 mg, 15 mg, 25 mg, 50 mg, 100 mg, 150 mg, 200 mg
- Concentrate: 30 mg/ml, 100 mg/ml
- Suspension: 25 mg/5 ml, 100 mg/5 ml

TRIFLUOPERAZINE (STELAZINE)

Indications in Child and Adolescent Psychiatry

One manufacturer has a specific disclaimer that trifluoperazine has not been proven effective in the management of behavioral complications in patients with mental retardation and recommends it only for the treatment of psychotic individuals and the short-term treatment of nonpsychotic anxiety in individuals with generalized anxiety disorder who have not responded to other medications (PDR, 1995).

Dosage Schedule for Children and Adolescents

- Children under 6 years old: Not recommended.
- Children 6–12 years: A starting dose of 1 mg once or twice daily, with gradual upward titration, is recommended. Dosages in excess of

15 mg/day are usually required only by older children with severe symptoms.

- Adolescents: 1–5 mg twice daily. Usually the optimal dose will be 15–20 mg/day or less; occasionally up to 40 mg/day will be required. Titration to optimal dose may usually be accomplished within 2–3 weeks.

Dose Forms Available

- Tablets: 1 mg, 2 mg, 5 mg, 10 mg
- Concentrate: 10 mg/ml
- Injectable: 2 mg/ml. (One manufacturer notes there is little experience using intramuscular trifluoperazine with children and recommends 1 mg intramuscularly once, or maximally twice, daily if necessary for rapid control of severe symptoms (PDR, 1995, p. 2401).)

HALOPERIDOL (HALDOL)

Indications in Child and Adolescent Psychiatry

Haloperidol is approved for the treatment of psychotic disorders and Tourette's disorder. After treatment failures with psychotherapy and nonneuroleptic medication, haloperidol is approved for use for treating two groups of children:

[those with] severe behavioral problems . . . of combative, explosive hyperexcitability (which cannot be accounted for by immediate provocation) [and] in the short-term treatment of hyperactive children who show excessive motor activity with accompanying conduct disorders consisting of some or all of the following symptoms: impulsivity, difficulty sustaining attention, aggressivity, mood lability, and poor frustration tolerance. (package insert)

Shapiro and Shapiro (1989) concluded that the most effective neuroleptics in the treatment of tics and Tourette's disorder were haloperidol, pimozide (Orap), fluphenazine (Prolixin, Permitil), and penfluridol (Semap, an investigational drug).

Dosage Schedule for Children and Adolescents (Psychotic Disorders, Tourette's Disorder, and Severe Nonpsychotic Behavioral Disorders)

- Children under 3 years old: Not recommended.
- Children 3–12 years (weight, 15–40 kg): Begin with 0.5 mg daily; titrate upward by 0.5-mg increments at 5- to 7-day intervals. Therapeutic ranges are usually from 0.05 to 0.075 mg/kg/day for nonpsychotic behavioral disorders and Tourette's disorder; for psychotic children the upper range is usually 0.15 mg/kg/day. A few children may require lower doses, e.g., 0.25 mg/day. In severe cases higher doses may be required.
- Adolescents (over age 12): Depending on severity, 0.5–5 mg two to three times daily. Higher doses may be necessary for rapid control in some severe cases.

Dose Forms Available

- Tablets: 0.5 mg, 1 mg, 2 mg, 5 mg, 10 mg, 20 mg
- Concentrate: 2 mg/ml
- Injectable: (haloperidol lactate) 5 mg/ml: Safety not established for children. If necessary, in acutely agitated adolescents 2–5 mg may initially be given intramuscularly. Additional medication may be given every 1–8 hours, as determined by ongoing evaluation of the patient.

Haloperidol in the Treatment of Schizophrenia with Childhood Onset

Green et al. (1992) administered haloperidol on an open basis to 15 hospitalized children under 12 years of age diagnosed with schizophrenia. They reported the optimal dose to range between 1 and 6 mg/day. Acute dystonic reactions occurred in about 25% of the children despite low initial doses and gradual increments of the drug.

Spencer et al. (1992) administered haloperidol to 12 patients (9 males, 3 females; ages 5.5–11.75 years) in an ongoing double-blind placebo-controlled study of hospitalized children diagnosed with schizophrenia. Optimal haloperidol dose ranged from 0.5 to 3.5 mg/day (range, 0.02–0.12 mg/kg/day; mean, 2.02 mg/day). Haloperidol was significantly better than placebo on staff Global Clinical Judgments ($P = .003$) and on 4 of 8 Children's Psychiatric Rating Scale items selected for their pertinence to schizophrenic: ideas of reference ($P = .04$); persecutory ($P = .01$) and other thinking disorders ($P = .04$); and hallucinations ($P = .04$). Two children (16.7%) experienced acute dystonic reactions. All 12 improved on haloperidol and were discharged on that medication.

Haloperidol in the Treatment of Autistic Disorder

At the present time, haloperidol is the most well-studied drug used in the treatment of autistic disorder and is recommended as the drug of first choice. In a study of 40 autistic children, ages 2.33–6.92 years, haloperidol in optimal doses of 0.5–3 mg/day yielded global clinical improvement and decreased significantly symptoms of withdrawal, stereotypies, abnormal object relationships, hyperactivity, fidgetiness, negativism, and angry and labile affect (Anderson et al., 1984). A high rate of dyskinesias, however, remains a problem. Significant numbers of autistic children (22%; 8 of 36) developed tardive dyskinesia or withdrawal dyskinesias in a prospective study in which 0.5–3 mg/day of haloperidol were administered for from $3\frac{1}{2}$ to $42\frac{1}{2}$ months, so close monitoring is necessary (Perry et al., 1985).

In autistic disorder, stereotypies existing at baseline may be suppressed by administration of haloperidol. When the drug is withdrawn, there is potential for confusion between reappearance of stereotypies and a withdrawal dyskinesia; this is of especial concern if a physician unfamiliar with the child at baseline assumes treatment responsibilities for the child while he or she is on maintenance medication.

Haloperidol in the Treatment of Aggressive Conduct Disorders

In a double-blind placebo-controlled study of 61 treatment-resistant hospitalized children, ages 5.2–12.9 years, with undersocialized aggressive conduct disorder, both haloperidol and lithium were found to be superior to placebo in ameliorating behavioral symptoms (Campbell et al., 1984). Optimal doses of haloperidol ranged from 1 to 6 mg/day. The authors reported that at optimal doses the untoward effects of haloperidol appeared to interfere more significantly with the children's daily routines than did those of lithium.

Atypical Antipsychotic Drugs

CLOZAPINE (CLOZARIL)

Clozapine, an "atypical" antipsychotic drug, is a tricyclic dibenzodiazepine derivative whose CNS antidopaminergic activity is greater at limbic dopamine receptors than at striatal dopamine receptors. This may explain the remarkably low incidence of extrapyramidal symptoms. The manufacturer reports that no confirmed cases of tardive dyskinesia directly attributable to administration of only clozapine have been reported (PDR, 1995).

Because of the increased risk for serious and potentially life-threatening untoward effects, especially agranulocytosis and seizures, that has been reported in patients receiving clozapine, its administration is appropriate only for severely dysfunctional patients with schizophrenia who have not responded satisfactorily to adequate trials of at least two other standard antipsychotic drugs, or who cannot tolerate the untoward effects present at therapeutic dose levels.

The manufacturer noted that safety and efficacy of clozapine have not been established in persons under 16 years of age.

Dosage Schedule for Children and Adolescents

- Children and adolescents under 16 years of age: Not recommended.
- Adolescents at least 16 years of age: Initially a dose of 25 mg once or twice daily is recommended. The dose can be increased daily by 25–50 mg, if tolerated, to reach a target dose of 300–450 mg by 2 weeks' time. Subsequent dose increases of a maximum of 100 mg may be made once or twice weekly. Total daily dosage should not exceed 900 mg.

Dose Forms Available

- Tablets: 25 mg, 100 mg

UNTOWARD EFFECTS OF CLOZAPINE

Agranulocytosis is reported to occur in association with administration of clozapine in 1–2% of patients; however, with weekly monitoring and discontinuation of treatment if white blood cell counts dropped significantly, all but 11 cases of agranulocytosis reported in the United States following clozapine administration have been reversible. From its approval in late 1989 through January 1994, a total of 317 cases of agranulocytosis and 11 fatalities were reported among the more than 68,000 patients who had received clozapine (PDR, 1995). Administration of clozapine is also associated with an increased incidence of seizures that is apparently dose dependent. At doses below 300 mg/day, about 1–2% of patients develop seizures; at moderate doses of 300–599 mg/day, about 3–4% develop seizures; at high doses of 600–900 mg/day, about 5% of patients develop seizures.

Other untoward effects include adverse cardiovascular effects such as orthostatic hypertension, tachycardia, and ECG changes.

Because of the relatively high risk of patients developing agranulocytosis, at the present time in the United States clozapine is available only through distribution systems that monitor hematological functioning through weekly blood tests prior to dispensing medication for the following week to the patient.

Reports of Interest

Siefen and Remschmidt (1986) administered clozapine to 21 inpatients, 12 of whom were below 18 years of age (average age, 18.1 years). Their patients had an average of 2.4 inpatient hospitalizations and had been tried on an average of 2.8 different antipsychotics without adequate therapeutic response or with severe extrapyramidal effects.

Clozapine was administered over an average of 133 days. The average maximum dose was 415 mg/day (range, 225–800 mg/day), and the average maintenance dose was 363 mg/day (range, 150–800 mg/day). In addition, 11 of the 21 subjects were administered one or more other unidentified drugs during about half of the time they were receiving clozapine.

About 67% of symptoms that did not respond satisfactorily to prior treatment with antipsychotics disappeared or improved markedly in 11 (52%) of patients and showed at least slight improvement in an additional 6 (29%) patients. Four patients had no changes or worsening of over half of their psychopathologic symptoms during clozapine therapy. Positive symptoms of schizophrenia improved more than negative symptoms. Specifically, improvements in incoherent/dissociative thinking, aggressiveness, hallucinations, agitation, ideas of reference, anxiety, inability to make decisions, psychomotor agitation, motivation toward achievement, impoverished and restricted thinking, and ambivalent behavior were reported. Symptoms such as lack of self-confidence, fear of failure, psychomotor retardation, irritability, slowed thinking, blunted affect, and unhappiness showed no improvement or deteriorated during treatment with clozapine (Siefen and Remschmidt, 1986).

The most frequent untoward effects observed early in treatment with clozapine were daytime sedation, dizziness, tachycardia, orthostatic hypotension, sleepiness, and increased salivation. No patients developed agranulocytosis, and the hematological changes that occurred in about 25% of patients were clinically insignificant and normalized during continued maintenance on clozapine (Siefen and Remschmidt, 1986).

Schmidt et al. (1990) reported a total of 57 cases of children and adolescents (age range, 9.8–21.3 years; mean 16.8 years; 30 males and 27 females) who were treated with clozapine. Forty-eight patients were diagnosed with a schizophrenic disorder, 5 with schizoaffective disorder; 2 with monopolar manic disorder and 2 with pervasive developmental disorders. These patients had a mean duration of illness of 19.4 months (range, 0–74 months) prior to this hospitalization, which was the first for 16 patients, the second for 16 patients, and the third or more for the remaining 25 patients. Clozapine was begun on average about 3 months after hospitalization following treatment failures with other antipsychotics and concern about chronicity, intolerable untoward effects, or uncontrolled excitation. Average dose during the length of hospitalization was 318 mg/day (range, 50–800 mg/day); average dose at discharge was somewhat lower, 290 mg/day (range, 75–800 mg/day). Thirty-five patients received only clozapine. In 22 cases, one or more additional other neuroleptics, primarily phenothiazines, were administered simultaneously, but in about half of these cases the additional drugs were tapered off and discontinued so that eventually 80% of the patients were on clozapine only. Mean duration on clozapine during hospitalization was 78 days (range, 7–355 days) and 17 (31%) patients were discharged on clozapine.

Clozapine was discontinued in 15 (28%) of the patients between the 8th and 132nd day of treatment (average 50th day) when they were taking a mean dose of 143 mg/day (range, 25–350 mg/day) for the following reasons: insufficient antipsychotic effect in 7 cases; poor compliance and a change to depot medication in 5 cases; and severe untoward effects in 3 cases (cholinergic delirium, seizure, and questionably clinically significant decrease of erythrocytes to 2.3 million).

The authors reported that two-thirds of the patients significantly improved in the whole range of symptoms. Paranoid-hallucinatory symptoms and excitation responded best followed by a reduction in aggressivity. Clozapine was less effective in decreasing agitation and improving negative symptoms and these symptoms sometimes worsened. Untoward effects were noted in all subjects. These included increased heart rates of 94–109 beats/minute in 37 (65%) patients (during the first 8 weeks only); daytime sedation in 29 (51%) patients; hypersalivation in 20 (35%) patients; orthostatic hypotension in 20 (35%) patients; and 15 (26%) patients had an unspecified rise in temperature. Abnormal movements were observed in 9 patients including tremor (6 cases), akathisia (1 case) and unspecified extrapyramidal symptoms in 2 cases. During the first 16 weeks of clozapine, a significant decrease of various hemoglobin parameters including number of erythrocytes was observed but did not reach pathological values; a relative shift from lymphocytes to neutrophils was seen in the differential during the first 2 weeks. There was a reversible increase of liver enzymes, which peaked during the 3rd and 4th weeks. On EEGs, there was evidence that clozapine induced increased neuronal disinhibition, e.g., spike discharges, and a shift of background activity to lower frequencies. Pathological EEG changes were present in 30 (55%) of patients on clozapine compared to 17 (30%) of patients before clozapine (P < .01). One patient developed a seizure (Schmidt et al., 1990). The authors later noted that they considered EEG monitoring before and during treatment with clozapine to be mandatory (Blanz and Schmidt, 1993).

Mozes et al. (1994) treated with clozapine four children, 3 males and 1 female, 10–12 years of age, who were diagnosed with schizophrenia and had not responded satisfactorily to other neuroleptics. Clozapine was begun in doses of 25–100 mg/day and titrated upward. Three patients had significantly reduced symptomatology in less that 2 weeks. Further decreases in both positive and negative symptoms occurred during the next 10–15 weeks of treatment. All four children improved significantly on the Brief Psychiatric Rating Scale (BPRS) with a mean reduction of 41 within 15 weeks. At the time of the report, patients had been in treatment between 23 and 70 weeks and maintenance dosage ranged from 150 to 300 mg/day. The most frequent untoward effect was drooling, which spontaneously decreased over time; drowsiness, experienced by 3 patients, peaked during the first week and then gradually faded away. Excitatory EEG changes occurred in 3 patients, and dosage was not increased to decrease the likelihood of seizures. Of note, two cases of tardive dyskinesia caused by previous neuroleptic drugs disappeared on clozapine.

Clozapine appears to be an important addition to the therapeutic armamentarium in treating adolescents diagnosed with schizophrenia who do not respond satisfactorily to standard antipsychotics. There are few reports on its use in prepubertal children diagnosed with schizophrenia. As such children frequently respond less satisfactorily to treatment with standard antipsychotics, specific investigations of clozapine will be necessary to determine its efficacy in this age range (Green and Deutsch, 1990; Green et al., 1992).

RISPERIDONE (RISPERDAL)

Risperidone, recently approved by the FDA for use in treating psychotic disorders, is a benzisoxazole derivative. It improves both positive and negative symptoms of schizophrenia. Importantly, it has a low incidence of extrapyramidal untoward effects and it does not have the significantly increased risks of agranulocytosis and seizures of clozapine. Chronic patients diagnosed with schizophrenia who have had poor responses to conventional antipsychotic medications have shown significant improvement on risperidone. Although risperidone with its favorable therapeutic efficacy and untoward effect profile is a highly promising new drug, studies of its efficacy and safety in children and adolescents under 16 years of age are not yet available.

Antidepressants

At the present time the tricyclics are probably still the most important antidepressants used in the treatment of children and younger adolescents. However, even though not approved for treatment of depression in children and younger adolescents, SSRI antidepressants are being prescribed with increasing frequency because of their significantly safer untoward effect profile, in particular, reduced risks of cardiotoxicity and lethality of overdose. For these reasons, Ambrosini et al. (1993) recommend prescribing SSRIs and not tricyclics to patients with suicidal and/or impulsive tendencies.

TRICYCLIC ANTIDEPRESSANTS

The tricyclic antidepressants have FDA approval for the treatment of depression in persons with a minimum age of 12 years. Imipramine is additionally approved for the treatment of enuresis in persons at least 6 years of age. There is, however, a considerable body of literature suggesting that tricyclic antidepressants are effective in the treatment of ADHD, school phobia (separation anxiety disorder), and disorders of sleep (sleep terror disorder and sleepwalking disorder), and in some children with major depressive disorder who were treated on an open basis. Clomipramine, another tricyclic antidepressant, has been shown to be effective in the treatment of childhood obsessive compulsive disorder (Flament et al., 1985). A literature review of the use of tricyclic antidepressants in children and adolescents with major depression found them to be clinically effective in several open studies, but no double-blind placebo-controlled study has reported that tricyclics were superior to placebo (Ambrosini et al., 1993).

TRICYCLIC ANTIDEPRESSANTS AND CARDIOTOXICITY

At least five sudden deaths have been reported in children taking tricyclic antidepressants. Although these deaths have not been proven to be cardiac related, cardiac arrhythmias, particularly tachyarrhythmias, are suspected. Four of the sudden deaths occurred in children taking desipramine and two of these occurred after exercise. Four of the deaths occurred in children 9 years old or younger and the fifth in a 12 year old.

A 6-year-old girl taking imipramine for chronic school phobia and separation anxiety died 3 days after the dose had been raised to 300 mg (14.7 mg/kg) at bedtime (Saraf et al., 1974). Sudden deaths were reported in three boys treated with desipramine (''Sudden Death,'' June 1, 1990). These were two 8-year-old boys diagnosed with ADD (one received desipramine for 2 years at an unknown dose and one received the same drug for 6 months at 50 mg/day) and a 9-year-old boy whose diagnosis, dose, and duration of desipramine administration were not reported. All three of the boys had plasma levels in the therapeutic or subtherapeutic ranges (''Sudden Death,'' June 1, 1990). A fourth child, a 12-year-old girl who had been prescribed a single daily 125-mg dose of desipramine for the treatment of ADD, died a few days after the dose was increase to 50 mg three times daily; she was found unconscious after playing tennis and retiring for a nap and was not successfully revived (Riddle et al., 1993).

Several reports, editorials, and comments rapidly followed the report of these deaths. It became clear how little is known about the cardiac effects of tricyclics in prepubertal and even older subjects. Basically the response has been to be even more cautious when administering tricyclics to children but also to adolescents (Geller, 1991). In particular, it is recommended that a rhythm strip be obtained at baseline, during titration of medication, and at maintenance levels, emphasizing measurement of the QT_c to aid in identifying potentially vulnerable children (Riddle et al., 1991). Elliot and Popper (1990/1991) recommended obtaining ECGs at baseline, at a dose of about 3 mg/kg/day and at a final dose of not greater that 5 mg/kg/day and using the following parameters as guidelines for cardiovascular monitoring in children and adolescents receiving tricyclic antidepressants:

PR interval: less than or equal to 210 msec
QRS interval: widening to no more than 30% over baseline
QT_c interval: less than 450 msec
Heart rate: maximum of 130 beats/minute
Systolic blood pressure: maximum of 130 mm Hg
Diastolic blood pressure: maximum of 85 mm Hg

Although a more conservative viewpoint would be to obtain an ECG after each dose increase, Elliot and Popper (1990/1991) have pointed out that simply increasing the frequency of ECG monitoring does not necessarily reduce the risk of sudden death.

Cardiovascular toxicity of tricyclic antidepressants is of concern in all age groups but especially in children and younger adolescents. Of particular concern is the slowing of cardiac conduction as reflected on the ECG by increases in P-R, QRS, and QT_c intervals, cardiac arrhythmias, tachycardia, and heart block.

Schroeder et al. (1989) reported that the cardiovascular effects of desipramine in 20 children, ages 7–12 years, who were treated with an average dose of 4.25 mg/kg/day (maximum 5 mg/kg/day) were a 21% increase in cardiac rate and a 2.5% increase in the Q-T interval. Arrhythmias and clinically meaningful blood pressure changes did not occur. The authors concluded, concerning potential cardiotoxicity, that desipramine was safe in children without heart disease, although ECG monitoring was essential (Schroeder et al., 1989).

Baldessarini (1990) noted that children are more sensitive to cardiotoxic effects of tricyclic antidepressants than are adolescents and adults and suggested that this increased vulnerability may be related to the relative efficiency with which they convert tricyclic antidepressants to potentially cardiotoxic 2-OH metabolites. However, Wilens and colleagues (1992) studied steady-state serum concentrations of desipramine (DMI) and 2-OH-desipramine (OHDMI) in 40 child, 36 adolescent, and 27 adult psychiatric patients. Serum levels of desipramine per weight-corrected dose rose from 50 ng/ml:mg/kg in children (age range, 6–12 years) to 56 ng/ml:mg/kg in adolescents (age range, 13–18 years) to 91 ng/mg:mg/kg in adults (age range, 19–67 years). Contrary to expectations, OHDMI levels also increased with age from 17 ng/ml:mg/kg in children to 20 ng/ml:mg/kg in adolescents and to 26 ng/ml:mg/kg in adults. The results did not support the hypothesis that children would develop relatively higher levels of OHDMI than adolescents and adults because of more efficient hepatic oxidative metabolism of DMI. Children were either more efficient in clearing both DMI and OHDMI than adults or absorbed DMI relatively inefficiently. In fact, the data supported the clinical impression that children and adolescents usually require higher mg/kg doses of DMI than adults to reach similar serum DMI and OHDMI concentrations (Wilens et al., 1992).

In a subsequent study, Wilens et al. (1993) analyzed the effects of serum levels of DMI and OHDMI on ECGs in 50 child, 39 adolescent, and 30 adult psychiatric patients treated with DMI. With these expanded numbers of subjects, children and adolescents continued to have lower serum levels of DMI and OHDMI for weight-corrected doses than adults. Children and adolescents showed no significant associations between serum drug and metabolite levels and heart rate or conduction (PR and QRS) intervals, although there was a weak relationship between sinus tachycardia and higher total DMI plus OHDMI levels. When data from all 119 subjects were combined, there was a modest correlation among DMI, OHDMI, and DMI plus OHDMI serum levels and PR and QRS intervals; however, the authors concluded these were not likely to be clinically significant in any age group. About 10% of the subjects had combined DMI plus OHDMI serum levels of >250 ng/ml, which may increase risk of cardiovascular toxicity. The authors recommended monitoring serum levels, a baseline ECG, and ECGs with dosage increases when the total daily dose was over 3 mg/kg (Wilens et al., 1993).

Because routine ECGs may not record infrequent cardiac arrhythmias, Biederman et al. (1993) examined 24-hour ECG recordings and echocardiographic findings in 35 children and 36 adolescents receiving long-term (1.5 ± 1.2 years) desipramine therapy for psychiatric disorders. Compared with untreated healthy children, subjects' ECGs had significantly higher rates of single or paired premature atrial contractions and runs of supraventricular tachycardia and decreased rates of sinus pauses and junctional rhythm. DMI levels correlated significantly only with paired premature atrial contractions. All echocardiographic findings but one were normal; the abnormal one was felt to be caused by a pericardial effusion of viral origin and not to be drug related. Overall the data supported prior impressions that treatment with desipramine at usual therapeutic doses and serum levels is associated with minor and benign cardiac effects (Biederman et al., 1993).

Individuals have marked variations in their metabolism of tricyclic antidepressants that are of significant clinical importance. About 7% of the general population has a genetic variation that results in decreased activity of the cytochrome P-450 isoenzyme PA450IID6 (PDR, 1995, p. 943). Such individuals metabolize tricyclic antidepressants more slowly than usual and may develop toxic serum levels at therapeutic doses of less than 5 mg/kg. Individuals taking the same oral dose of desipramine have been reported to have up to a 36-fold variation in plasma levels (PDR, 1995, p. 1417). Dugas and his colleagues (1980) have recommended administering tricyclic antidepressants to children in two or three divided doses daily if over 1 mg/kg/day is given to avoid or minimize untoward effects related to peak serum levels. Long-acting preparations (e.g., imipramine pamoate capsules) are designed for once daily dosing; their use is not recommended in children and younger adolescents because of their high unit potency and greater sensitivity of the age group to cardiotoxic effects.

The above studies appear to conclude that tricyclic antidepressants in the usual clinical dose range (under 5 mg/kg/day) and at usual serum drug and metabolite levels (<250 ng/ml of DMI plus OHDMI) are usually associated with minor and clinically benign effects on cardiac function in all age ranges and that children and adolescents are not at significantly greater risk for developing such effects than are adults. As the number of sudden deaths is so small, the causal mechanism(s) are unknown, and no specific cardiac finding has any known predictive value, clinically it must be mandatory to monitor both ECG changes and serum drug and metabolite levels and to keep them within recommended parameters whenever tricyclic antidepressants are prescribed.

Discontinuing tricyclic antidepressants abruptly may result in a predictable withdrawal syndrome. Symptoms may include dizziness, nausea, vomiting, headache, malaise, sleep disturbances, hyperthermia, irritability, and worsening of psychiatric status. Hence, a gradual tapering of dose over a period of 10 days to 2 weeks is recommended.

IMIPRAMINE (TOFRANIL)

Because imipramine has been the most widely used clinically and has been more thoroughly studied in children than the other tricyclics, it will serve as the prototype. Discussions of other tricyclics follow that of imipramine.

Indications in Child and Adolescent Psychiatry

Imipramine is approved for use in treating depression in persons over 12 years old and for the treatment of enuresis in children at least 6 years old. Manufacturers state that a maximum dose of 2.5 mg/kg should not be exceeded in children (PDR, 1995).

Untoward Effects. Imipramine has many untoward effects, some of which are potentially life threatening. Cardiovascular effects, including arrhythmias, tachycardia, blood pressure changes, impaired conduction, and heart block and a decreased seizure threshold are particularly worrisome.

Imipramine and the Treatment of Enuresis

Although the pharmacological treatment of enuresis has been shown to be effective, imipramine should not be employed until possible organic etiologies have been ruled out by appropriate tests. It should be emphasized that behavioral therapies (e.g., conditioning with a bell and pad apparatus) are the treatments of choice for functional enuresis. There is a tendency for some children to become tolerant of imipramine's antienuretic effects, and many children relapse after medication withdrawal. Imipramine's antienuretic effect occurs rapidly and appears to be unrelated to its antidepressant effects; it may directly inhibit bladder musculature and increase outlet resistance (American Medical Association, 1986). Desmopressin acetate nasal spray (DDAVP), a synthetic analog of the natural hormone arginine vasopressin, may also be effective in some cases that do not respond satisfactorily to other treatments (package insert).

A trial of imipramine may occasionally be indicated when safer and more efficacious methods have failed and the symptom is psychologically handicapping or distressing to the patient or, perhaps, when rapid control is essential to permit a child to go to summer camp or travel.

Fritz et al. (1994) reviewed prior studies of plasma levels of imipramine (IMI) and DMI, its metabolite, in enuretic children treated with imipramine and reported on levels in 18 additional patients. Efficacy was moderately but significantly related to increasing levels of mg/kg dosage. Intersubject plasma combined IMI and DMI levels varied at least 7-fold at every dosage. The combined IMI and DMI levels at 2.5 mg/kg averaged 136.0 ng/ml (range, 35–170 ng/ml) for complete responders, 116 ng/ml (range, 37–236 ng/ml) for partial responders, and 96.0 ng/ml (range, 60–157 ng/ml) for nonresponders. The authors noted that despite the lack of a clear therapeutic window, serum level monitoring is useful in identifying subjects with low serum levels and suboptimal responses; in such cases, the dose of imipramine may be raised before concluding that the medication is ineffective. Knowledge of the serum level is essential, however, to avoid the danger of further dose increases, resulting in toxic serum levels in nonresponsive subjects who have relatively high serum levels.

The most frequent untoward effects reported in the treatment of enuretic children with imipramine are nervousness, sleep disorders, tiredness, and mild gastrointestinal disturbances (PDR, 1995). It is suggested that bed wetters who void soon after falling asleep benefit if imipramine is given earlier and in divided doses (e.g., 25 mg in midafternoon and 25 mg before bed) (PDR, 1995).

786 Section VII / Treatment

Recommended Dosage Schedule for Treating Enuresis

- A maximum dose of 2.5 mg/kg should not be exceeded because of the possibility of developing ECG abnormalities. Doses over 75 mg/day do not increase efficacy and do increase untoward effects (PDR, 1995).
- Children under 6 years old: Not approved for children this age.
- Children 6–11 years: Begin with 25 mg 1 hour before bedtime. If this dosage is not effective within 1 week, it may be increased to a maximum dose of 50 mg.
- Persons 12 years of age and up: Proceed as above, with the option to increase the dose to a maximum of 75 mg.

Reports of Interest

Imipramine and the Treatment of Childhood (Prepubertal) Major Depressive Disorder. Puig-Antich and his colleagues (1987) investigated the use of imipramine in prepubescent children diagnosed with major depressive disorder (MDD). In a double-blind placebo-controlled study of 38 subjects, there was no significant difference between response to imipramine (56%; 9 of 16 subjects) and response to placebo (68%; 15 of 22 subjects).

These authors also studied total maintenance plasma level (imipramine plus desipramine) in 30 prepubescent children and found a positive correlation between plasma level and clinical response. Responders had significantly higher ($P < .007$) mean maintenance total plasma levels (284 ± 225 ng/ml) than nonresponders (145 ± 80 ng/ml). The authors reported that a maintenance total plasma level of 150 ng/ml was the most important differentiating point between responders and nonresponders. Eighty-five percent of subjects (17 of 20) whose values were above 150 ng/ml had positive responses, but only 30% (3 of 10) of children with lower values responded positively. The authors also found nothing, including dosage, that predicted plasma levels (Puig-Antich et al., 1987). This is consonant with the finding that combined imipramine and desipramine steady-state plasma levels varied 6-fold (from 56 to 324 ng/ml) in 11 boys, all receiving 75 mg/day of imipramine (Weller et al., 1982).

Other important findings of Puig-Antich and his colleagues (1987) were (*a*) the more severe the pretreatment depressive symptoms, the less likely was a favorable response to imipramine ($P < .008$); (*b*) prepubescent children with the Research Diagnostic Criteria (RDC) psychotic subtype of MDD were much less likely to have a favorable response to imipramine than were nonpsychotic depressed children ($P < .05$); and (*c*) some children would require dosages over 5 mg/kg/day to reach plasma levels in the range associated with positive response.

These authors also reported that the following untoward effects were found in over 30% of the children treated with imipramine: excitement, irritability, nightmares, insomnia, headache, muscle pain, increased appetite, abdominal cramps, constipation, vomiting, hiccups, dry mouth, bad taste, sweating, flushed face, drowsiness, dizziness, tiredness, and restlessness. Similar untoward effects were present in the placebo group, although at lower frequencies. The untoward effects were severe enough in 17 of the 30 children to prevent upward titration to 5 mg/kg/day; cardiac side effects were responsible for 10 of these. Nine children had increases in the P-R interval to the maximum, and one child's resting heart rate reached 130 beats/minute. No child on placebo showed ECG changes from baseline, whereas nearly every child receiving imipramine had at least minor changes (Puig-Antich et al., 1987).

Imipramine and the Treatment of Adolescent MDD. Thirty-four adolescents with MDD treated with imipramine in an open study with monitoring of plasma imipramine levels showed some differences from prepubescent children (Ryan et al., 1986). Imipramine was titrated to a dose of 5 mg/kg/day, and the adolescents had an overall positive response rate of 44% (15 of 34), but there was no relationship between positive response and higher plasma imipramine levels. Another difference between the adolescents and prepubertal children with MDD was that, as a group, nonpsychotic subjects did not respond more favorably

than the psychotic subtype. The authors hypothesized that adolescents with MDD were less responsive to imipramine because of an antagonistic effect of sex hormones, levels of which increase during adolescence (Ryan et al., 1986).

Imipramine and the Treatment of ADHD. There is a considerable literature attesting to the clinical efficacy of imipramine in the treatment of ADHD, although most studies find stimulants superior. The development of tolerance to the therapeutic effects of imipramine by some children presents difficulties. Although imipramine does not have FDA approval for use in ADHD, some clinicians consider imipramine or another tricyclic the next drug of choice if a patient does not respond to stimulants.

The mechanism of action of imipramine in ADHD is different from that in depression; it is more rapidly effective, and often lower doses are required. Mean dosages reported in the literature have ranged from 20 to 173.7 mg/day.

While no official recommendations for age or dose exist, based on the literature and experimental protocols, the following dose schedule is suggested for treating children over 6 years of age who are diagnosed with ADHD. All monitoring prerequisites for tricyclic antidepressants should be followed rigorously. Begin with a low dose, either 25 mg or 0.5 mg/kg/day and slowly titrate upward with increases of 25 mg. Maximum dose should not exceed 2.5 mg/kg/day.

Imipramine and the Treatment of School Phobia (Separation Anxiety Disorder). Imipramine has been used with considerable success in treating school-phobic children (for review see Klein et al., 1980, pp. 712–718). Klein et al. (1980) emphasize that imipramine is effective in reducing separation anxiety but that anticipatory anxiety may continue to be problematic. Imipramine doses of between 75 and 200 mg/day were effective for school-phobic children between 6 and 14 years of age; however, children with severe separation anxiety without school phobia sometimes responded to doses as low as 25–50 mg/day (Klein et al., 1980).

School-phobic children who responded to imipramine were found to show at least some improvement when doses reached 125 mg/day; once improvement began, further dose increases usually produced additional benefit. Response was usually maximal within 6–8 weeks. It was suggested that maintenance be continued for a minimum of 8 weeks following remission of symptoms and then tapered and discontinued (Klein et al., 1980).

Ballenger and colleagues (1989) reported that three children with panic disorder who also had severe separation anxiety and agoraphobia responded well to a combination of imipramine and alprazolam, a benzodiazepine.

Imipramine and the Treatment of Somnambulism and Night Terrors. Four children with night terrors, two children with somnambulism, and one child with both disorders were treated with imipramine (10–50 mg at bedtime). The sleep disorders remitted completely in all children (Pesikoff and Davis, 1971).

NORTRIPTYLINE (PAMELOR)

Nortriptyline is approved by the FDA for the treatment of symptoms of depression in adolescents and adults. The drug is not recommended for use in the pediatric age group, as its safety and effectiveness have not been established in children.

Dosage Schedule for Children and Adolescents

- Children: Not recommended.
- Adolescents: Manufacturer recommends giving a total of 30–50 mg/day in either divided doses or a single dose. (See, however, recommendations of Geller and her colleagues, below.)

Dose Forms Available

- Capsules: 10 mg, 25 mg, 50 mg, 75 mg
- Oral solution: 10 mg/5 ml

Reports of Interest

Nortriptyline in the Treatment of MDD in Children and Adolescents. There are no double-blind placebo-controlled studies establishing nortriptyline's superiority over placebo in treating MDD in children and adolescents. In an open study of 22 children, 6–12 years old, who were diagnosed with MDD, Geller et al. (1986) found that therapeutic efficacy correlated with nortriptyline plasma levels. Responders in the fixed dosage part of the study had significantly higher mean mg/kg daily doses and mean nortriptyline steady-state plasma levels than nonresponders. All subjects with steady-state nortriptyline plasma levels of at least 60 ng/ml responded, as did 4 of 7 children with levels ranging from 40 to 59 ng/ml. Seven of the 8 nonresponders recovered when nortriptyline was increased to reach steady-state nortriptyline plasma levels between 60 and 100 ng/ml. Ultimately, 21 of the 22 subjects had good clinical response, with minimal and transient side effects, and all ECGs remained within recommended parameters for prepubertal children.

Geller and her colleagues (1989) enrolled 72 prepubescent children, ages 6–12 years, who were diagnosed with MDD nondelusional type by RDC (Spitzer et al., 1978) and DSM-III (1980) criteria, in a double-blind placebo-controlled study of the efficacy of nortriptyline. The study design was a 2-week single-blind placebo washout phase followed by an 8-week random assignment double-blind placebo-controlled phase. All subjects were outpatients and most had coexisting separation anxiety. The children were chronically depressed: 96% had been ill for at least 2 years, and 50% had had MDD for 5 or more years before entering the study. Of the 72 subjects entering the study, 12 (16.7%) responded during the placebo phase, 10 were discontinued for various reasons during the active treatment phase, and 50 (24 on placebo and 26 on nortriptyline) completed the study.

The initial dose necessary to achieve a steady-state nortriptyline level of 80 ± 20 ng/ml was estimated from 24-hour plasma levels. Any necessary adjustments to obtain mean steady-state plasma levels of nortriptyline and of total, *trans-*, and *cis*-10-hydroxynortriptyline (10-OH-NT) were made during the first 4 weeks of the double-blind phase.

Both the nortriptyline and the placebo groups had a low rate of positive response (30.8% on nortriptyline and 16.7% on placebo), and there was no significant difference between them. There was no significant correlation between mean nortriptyline plasma level and response, or between mean nortriptyline plus mean total, *cis-*, or *trans*-10-OH-NT plasma levels and response. Because of the poor response rate and the unlikelihood of finding a statistical difference between the placebo and active groups if the protocol were completed, Geller et al. (1989) stopped their study at this point.

Geller et al. (1990) enrolled 52 postpubertal adolescents, ages 12–17 years, diagnosed by RDC (Spitzer et al., 1978) and DSM-III (1980a) criteria with MDD in a random assignment double-blind placebo-controlled study of nortriptyline. Adolescents with delusional symptoms were not enrolled. Subjects had scores on the Children's Depression Rating Scale (CDRS) and the Kiddie Global Assessment Scale (KGAS), placing them in the severe range of pathology. Of the 31 subjects completing the study, 27 (87.1%) of subjects had a duration of symptoms for at least 2 years: 10 (32.3%) between 2 and 5 years and 17 (54.8%) more than 5 years.

The study was comprised of a 2-week single-blind placebo washout phase and an 8-week double-blind placebo-controlled phase. Initial dose necessary to achieve a steady-state nortriptyline level of 80 ± 20 ng/ml was estimated from 24-hour plasma levels. Mean nortriptyline plasma level was 91.1 ± 18.3 ng/ml.

Of the 52 subjects enrolled, 17 (32.7%) responded to placebo by the end of week 2, and 4 additional subjects dropped out for other reasons. Of the 31 completing the study, 12 were assigned to nortriptyline and 19 to placebo. The results of the study showed such a low rate of response to nortriptyline that the study was terminated early. Only 1 (8.3%) of 12 subjects receiving nortriptyline responded, while 4 (21.1%) of the

19 subjects on placebo responded. (The one responder to nortriptyline went on to have a bipolar course.) Subjects with higher nortriptyline levels achieved significantly worse scores on the CDRS ($P = .002$). There were, however, no significant differences between the two groups on final CDRS or KGAS scores.

It is most interesting that 17, or about one-third of enrolled patients, with chronic and severe depression responded to placebo within 2 weeks. However, 13 of the 17 placebo responders relapsed, 9 of them within 1–4 weeks (Geller et al., 1990).

Nortriptyline Dosage Schedule for Children and Adolescents. Geller et al. (1987) reported that 41 children 5–12 years old had a significantly shorter mean nortriptyline plasma half-life (20.8 ± 7.2 hours; range, 11.2–42.5 hours) than 32 adolescents 13–16 years old (31.1 ± 19.8 hours; range, 14.2–76.6 hours). Geller et al. (1985) also found that correlations between mg/kg dose of nortriptyline and steady-state plasma levels were not significant in 33 children and adolescents 5–16 years of age. The clinical significance of these data, including the interindividual variation of half-life by as much as 6- or 7-fold, prompted Geller et al. (1987) to advise that nortriptyline should be administered twice daily for all patients up through 16 years of age. Plasma level monitoring is essential to be sure of achieving therapeutic plasma nortriptyline levels and to avoid reaching toxic levels.

AMITRIPTYLINE (ELAVIL, ENDEP)

Study of Interest

Kashani et al. (1984) performed a double-blind crossover study comparing amitriptyline and placebo in nine prepubertal depressed children. Dosage ranged from 45 to 110 mg/day. Six (66.7%) of the subjects improved on amitriptyline, which was not significant ($P < .09$).

DESIPRAMINE (NORPRAMIN)

Study of Interest

Rapoport et al. (1980b) found that 75 mg of desipramine at bedtime had a short-term antienuretic effect that was not statistically different from that of imipramine.

CLOMIPRAMINE (ANAFRANIL)

Indications in Child and Adolescent Psychiatry

Clomipramine, a tricyclic antidepressant, is approved by the FDA for the treatment of obsessions and compulsions in patients at least 10 years of age who have been diagnosed with obsessive compulsive disorder.

Clomipramine itself has potent inhibitory effects on the neuronal reuptake of serotonin as compared to the neuronal reuptake of norepinephrine; however, its primary metabolite desmethylclomipramine effectively inhibits norepinephrine uptake. Flament and colleagues (1987) compared 29 children and adolescents (age range, 8–18 years; mean age, 13.9 ± 2.5 years) with obsessive compulsive disorder with control subjects on peripheral measures of serotonergic and noradrenergic function. The authors noted that a high pretreatment level of platelet serotonin was a strong predictor of a favorable clinical response and that clomipramine treatment produced a very marked decrease in platelet serotonin concentration for all patients ($P < .0001$). Clomipramine treatment also produced a trend toward reduction in platelet monoamine oxidase (MAO) activity ($P = .11$) and increased peripheral noradrenergic function. Plasma level of norepinephrine in standing subjects increased significantly ($P < .008$). These data suggest that clomipramine's inhibition of serotonin uptake may be essential to its antiobsessional effect (Flament et al., 1987).

Clomipramine has a long half-life. The mean half-life of a single 150-mg dose is 32 hours, and the mean half-life of its major metabolite, desmethylclomipramine, is 69 hours. Steady-state serum levels usually occur within to 1–2 weeks at a given daily dosage. Children and adolescents under 15 years of age had significantly lower plasma concentrations for a given dose than did adults (package insert). Bioavailability of clomipramine is not significantly altered by food, and administering it during initial titration in divided doses with meals helps to reduce gastrointestinal side effects. Clomipramine is metabolized in large part to its major bioactive metabolite desmethylclomipramine; both compounds are ultimately metabolized into their glucuronide conjugates by the liver. The metabolites are excreted through the bile duct and the kidneys.

Untoward Effects

The most significant risk of clomipramine appears to be the development of seizures. Risk for seizures is cumulative and increased from 0.64% at 90 days to 1.45% at 1 year. Other untoward effects that occur in children and adolescents include somnolence, tremor, dizziness, headache, sleep disorders, increased sweating, gastrointestinal effects (dry mouth, constipation, dyspepsia, anorexia), fatigue, cardiovascular effects (postural hypotension, palpitation, tachycardia, and syncope), abnormalities of vision, urinary retention, and dysmenorrhea in females and ejaculation failure in males (package insert). Because of reports of blood dyscrasias, a complete blood count should be determined in patients who develop fever and sore throat during the course of treatment.

Dosage Schedule for Children and Adolescents

- Children under 10 years old: Not recommended.
- Children at least 10 years old and adolescents: Initial dose of 25 mg/day titrated upward to a daily maximum of 100 mg or 3 mg/kg/day, whichever is less, over the first 2 weeks. Subsequently dosage may be increased gradually to a maximum of 200 mg/day or 3 mg/kg/day, whichever is less. After the optimal dose has been determined, clomipramine may be given in a single bedtime dose to minimize daytime sedation.

Dose Forms Available

- Capsules: 25 mg, 50 mg, 75 mg

Untoward Withdrawal Effects

Abrupt withdrawal of clomipramine may result in withdrawal symptoms similar to those of tricyclic antidepressants used to treat depression.

Reports of Interest

Flament et al. (1985) found clomipramine to be significantly superior to placebo in a placebo-controlled double-blind crossover study of 19 subjects whose ages ranged from 10 to 18 years (mean age, 14.5 ± 2.3) who were diagnosed with severe primary obsessive compulsive disorder. The dose range was 100–200 mg/day (mean, 141 ± 30 mg/day). The data suggested that clomipramine has a direct antiobsessional action that is independent of any antidepressant effect. In fact, 10 of the subjects had been previously treated with other tricyclics without significant benefit. Flament et al. (1987) increased the number of their subjects to 29 (age range, 8–18 years; mean age, 13.9 ± 2.5 years) and reported the continued efficacy of clomipramine; mean daily dose of clomipramine was 134 ± 33 mg/day.

Leonard et al. (1989) compared the efficacy of clomipramine and desipramine in the treatment of severe primary obsessive compulsive disorder in 49 child and adolescent subjects (31 males and 18 females; mean age, 13.86 ± 2.87 years; range, 7–19 years). In a 10-week crossover design, clomipramine was markedly superior to desipramine in decreasing obsessive-compulsive symptoms on several rating scales. In addition, when desipramine was administered following improvement on clomipramine, subjects experienced relapse rates similar to those for placebo in the Flament (1985) study.

Administration of clomipramine was begun at 25 mg/day for children weighing 25 kg or less and at 50 mg/day for subjects weighing over 25 kg (Leonard et al., 1989). Dosage was increased weekly by an amount equal to each subject's initial dose. Maximum dosage did not exceed 250 mg/day or 5 mg/kg/day. The mean dose of clomipramine at week 5 was 150 ± 53 mg/day, with a range of 50–250 mg/day. The most common side effects reported were dry mouth, tremor, tiredness, dizziness, difficulty sleeping, sweating, constipation, poor appetite, and weakness.

DeVeaugh-Geiss et al. (1992) reported a multicenter trial in which 60 children and adolescents, ages 10–17 years and diagnosed with obsessive compulsive disorder, were administered clomipramine in a 10-week, double-blind, fully randomized, parallel groups, placebo-controlled study. Thirty-one patients were assigned to the clomipramine group and 29 to the placebo group; except for an excess of males in the clomipramine group, the groups were comparable. Placebo was administered to all patients under single-blind conditions for the first 2 weeks. During the active drug stage, the initial daily dose was 25 mg of active drug or placebo; over the next 2 weeks, this was titrated to either 75 or 100 mg daily based on weight. Subsequent increases to a maximum of 3 mg/kg/day or 200 mg were permitted at the discretion of the investigator. Twenty-seven subjects in each group completed the study. Untoward effects were typical of the tricyclic antidepressants.

The patients receiving clomipramine improved significantly compared to those in the placebo group. On the Yale-Brown Obsessive Compulsive Scale (Y-BOCS) the clomipramine group had a mean reduction in score of 37% and the placebo group a reduction of 8% ($P <$ .05), and on the NIMH Global Scale the groups had reductions of 34 and 6%, respectively ($P <$ .05).

Selective Serotonin Reuptake Inhibitors

The SSRIs currently approved by the FDA for the treatment of depression in adults include fluoxetine hydrochloride (Prozac), sertraline hydrochloride (Zoloft), and paroxetine hydrochloride (Paxil); in addition, fluvoxamine maleate (Luvox) and fluoxetine hydrochloride have recently been approved for the treatment of obsessive compulsive disorder. The SSRIs are chemically unrelated to each other or to tricyclic, tetracyclic, and other antidepressants currently used in clinical practice (PDR, 1995). As SSRI suggests, at therapeutic levels, these drugs act primarily to inhibit serotonin reuptake; they also have relatively little effect on catecholaminergic (norepinephrine) reuptake mechanisms. At least five types and several subtypes of serotonin receptors with both distinct and overlapping functions have been identified in the CNS (Sussman, 1994a). These SSRIs have differing specificity for the serotonin receptors whose reuptake they inhibit, which explains their efficacy in treating disorders other than depression and the fact that they have somewhat different untoward effects. SSRI antidepressants also do not have clinically significant direct effects on the adrenergic, muscarinic, or histaminergic systems, resulting in fewer and less severe untoward effects than the tricyclic antidepressants. The most common untoward effects of the SSRIs parallel the symptoms caused by administration of exogenous serotonin and include headache, nausea, vomiting, diarrhea, nervousness, sleep disturbance, and sexual dysfunction (Sussman, 1994a).

SSRIs are of great interest to child and adolescent psychiatrists for several reasons: (a) the efficacy of tricyclic antidepressants in treating MDD in both children and adolescents has not been supported by double-blind, placebo-controlled studies; (b) there have been several reports of sudden death in children being treated with tricyclics, leading to particular concern about their cardiotoxicity in younger patients (SSRIs have a significantly safer untoward effect profile, including decreased cardiotoxicity and lethality in overdose.); (c) although significant, the untoward effects of SSRIs are more tolerable than those of tricyclic and monoamine oxidase inhibitor (MAOI) antidepressants; (d) SSRIs may be administered once daily; and (e) SSRIs appear to have potential in treating a spectrum of childhood psychiatric disorders in addition to depression, including obsessive compulsive disorder with and without comorbid Tourette's disorder, ADHD, and bulimia nervosa.

Because sertraline and paroxetine were approved more recently than fluoxetine, there is very little published data concerning their use in children and younger adolescents; therefore, these drugs will be noted only briefly. It is quite likely, however, that with additional clinical experience in this age group the SSRIs may become the agents of choice in treating depression and obsessive compulsive disorder in children and adolescents.

FLUOXETINE HYDROCHLORIDE (PROZAC)

Peak plasma levels of fluoxetine at usual clinical doses occur after 6–8 hours. Fluoxetine is metabolized by the liver; active and inactive metabolites are excreted by the kidneys. About 95% of fluoxetine is bound to plasma proteins. It may take up to several weeks for steady-state plasma levels to be achieved, but once obtained, they remain steady. Once stable serum levels are reached, the elimination half-life is 4–6 days for fluoxetine and 4–16 days for norfluoxetine, its active metabolite (PDR, 1995).

Indications in Child and Adolescent Psychiatry

Not approved by the FDA for use with children and younger adolescents. At the present time, the safety and efficacy of fluoxetine for children and younger adolescents remain to be elucidated.

Dosage Schedule for Older Adolescents and Adults

An initial morning dose of 20 mg/day of fluoxetine is recommended; there is evidence that this may frequently be the optimal dose (Altamura et al., 1988). Food does not seem to affect its bioavailability significantly. The full antidepressant action may take 4 weeks or longer to develop. If inadequate clinical response does not occur after several weeks, the dosage may be increased gradually to a maximum of 80 mg/day. It is recommended that, once 20 mg/day is exceeded, the medication be taken in divided portions twice daily, in the morning and at noon.

Dosage Schedule for Children and Younger Adolescents

Although not approved by the FDA for administration to children and younger adolescents for any indication, studies including patients is this age range are appearing in the literature with increasing frequency. Riddle et al. (1992) noted that 20 mg/day may be too high a dose for some children and suggested that an initial dose of 10 mg/day of fluoxetine is the most common starting dose given to children by most clinicians. Sandler (1993) suggests starting with only 5 mg/day in children and increasing dosage slowly.

Dose Forms Available

- Pulvules: 10 mg, 20 mg
- Liquid: 20 mg/5 ml

Untoward Effects

The most frequent troublesome untoward effects are anxiety, nervousness, insomnia, drowsiness, dizziness or lightheadedness, fatigue, nausea, diarrhea, weight loss, and excessive sweating. They are reported more frequently, and anticholinergic effects and sedation less frequently, than with the tricyclics (PDR, 1995).

Riddle et al. (1990/1991) reported the behavioral side effects of fluoxetine in 24 children and adolescents with various diagnoses, age range, 8–16 years. Mean dose was 25.8 ± 9.0 mg/day for the 12 subjects who developed fluoxetine-induced behavioral side effects such as restlessness, hyperactivity, insomnia, an internal feeling of excitation, subtle impulsive behavioral changes, and suicidal ideation (King et al., 1991;

Riddle et al., 1990/1991). Hypomania and mania have also been reported to occur in children and adolescents treated with fluoxetine (Jerome, 1991; Venkataraman et al., 1992)

Reports of Interest

Fluoxetine in the Treatment of Major Depressive Disorder in Children and Adolescents. Joshi and colleagues (1989) reported on their treatment with fluoxetine of 14 patients (8 males, 6 females) ranging in age from 9 to 15 years (average age, 11.25 years) who were diagnosed with major depression by DSM-III-R criteria and who had not responded adequately to tricyclic antidepressants, had serious untoward effects from tricyclics, or could not be treated with tricyclics for medical reasons. Ten (71.4%) of the subjects responded favorably within 6 weeks to fluoxetine 20 mg administered in the morning. Side effects were limited to transient nausea and hyperactivity in one patient each and did not require discontinuation of the drug.

Simeon and coworkers (1990) treated 40 adolescents (22 females, 18 males; ages 13–18 years, mean age 16 years) who were diagnosed with major depression unipolar type by DSM-III criteria, who also had baseline Hamilton Depression Scores of at least 20, with fluoxetine in a double-blind, placebo-controlled 8-week study. Fluoxetine was begun at a daily dose of 20 mg, increased to 40 mg after 4–7 days, and increased to a daily dose of 60 mg during the 2nd week. Thirty subjects completed the study divided equally between medication and control groups. About two-thirds of patients in each group showed moderate to marked clinical global improvement with significant improvement by week three. With the exception of disturbances of sleep, all symptoms showed slightly greater improvement in subjects treated with fluoxetine than in those receiving placebo, but differences were not significant. Patients taking fluoxetine, however, experienced a small but significantly greater weight loss than those receiving placebo. Untoward effects were usually mild and transient, and none necessitated discontinuation of medication. Those most frequently reported were headache, vomiting, insomnia, and tremor. There were no significant differences in the effects of fluoxetine and placebo on heart rate or blood pressure.

Thirty-two patients were successfully followed-up 8–46 months later (mean 24 months) at ages 15–22 years (mean, 18 years). No significant differences were found between the fluoxetine and placebo groups, or between responders and nonresponders to the initial clinical trial. Although both groups showed further overall improvement, psychosocial functioning was still poor in over one-third of the patients, and 50% of the subjects still required professional help (Simeon et al., 1990).

Fluoxetine in the Treatment of Children and Adolescents with Attention Deficit Hyperactivity Disorder

Barrickman et al. (1991) reported on 19 children and adolescents (age range, 7–15 years) diagnosed with ADHD and treated for 6 weeks in an open study with fluoxetine hydrochloride. Initial daily dose was 20 mg in the morning; subsequent doses were individually adjusted. Average daily dose was 27 mg (0.6 mg/kg); range, 20–60 mg. Nine subjects took 20 mg/day; 8 took 40 mg/day and 2 took 60 mg/day. Most subjects improved within a week after a therapeutic dose was reached. Ratings were made on a large number of standardized instruments. Eleven subjects (58%) were rated moderately or very much improved after 6 weeks; 8 had minimal improvement. Side effects were minimal and all remitted spontaneously or with dose reduction except mild sedation in one case. In particular, there were no reports of loss of appetite or significant changes in weight. Only one subject experienced nervousness, and none had insomnia or developed suicidal ideation.

Fluoxetine in the Treatment of Children and Adolescents Diagnosed with Obsessive Compulsive Disorder

In an open clinical study, Riddle et al. (1990) treated with fluoxetine 10 children (5 males, 5 females: age range, 8–15 years; mean age, 12.2 years) diagnosed with obsessive compulsive disorder only or with both obsessive compulsive disorder and Tourette's disorder. Dosage ranged from 10 to 40 mg/day, with 80% of the patients receiving 20 mg/day; duration of treatment ranged from 4 to 20 weeks. Four of the patients with Tourette's disorder concomitantly received additional medication for treatment of their tics. Fifty percent were considered responders to fluoxetine and were rated much improved; response rates were similar in patients with obsessive compulsive disorder alone and in those with both diagnoses. The most common untoward effect was behavioral agitation/activation characterized by increased motor activity and pressured speech. It occurred in 40% of the patients and usually started within the first few days: symptoms were most severe during the first 2–3 weeks but remained until medication was discontinued. No significant changes in blood pressure, pulse, weight, laboratory tests, or ECG were observed (Riddle et al., 1990).

Riddle and his colleagues (1992) reported a randomized, 20-week, double-blind, placebo-controlled, fixed-dose study with crossover after 8 weeks, of fluoxetine in treating 14 subjects (6 males and 8 females; age range, 8.6–15.6 years; mean age, $11.8 + 2.3$ years) diagnosed with obsessive compulsive disorder by DSM-III-R criteria. Subjects received 20 mg of fluoxetine or placebo. For various reasons, 13 subjects completed the first 4 weeks, 11 subjects completed the first 8 weeks, and only 6 subjects satisfactorily completed the entire 20 weeks. Comparison of between-group differences at 8 weeks was for 13 subjects, carrying the 4-week data forward to 8 weeks for the two subjects who dropped out during that time. The seven subjects receiving fluoxetine showed significant decrease on the Children's Yale-Brown Obsessive Compulsive Scale (CY-BOCS) total score (mean decrease = 44%, $P = .003$), obsessions score (mean decrease = 54%, $P = .009$), and compulsions score (mean decrease = 33%, $P = .005$) and on the Clinical Global Impression for Obsessive Compulsive Disorder (CGI-OCD) (mean decrease = 33%, $P = .0004$). The 6 subjects on placebo also showed reduction in their obsessive-compulsive symptomatology on the CY-BOCS of 27% and on the CGI-OCD of 12%, but they were not significant. When the two groups were compared, the improvement of subjects of fluoxetine was significantly greater than those on placebo on the CGI-OCD ($P = .01$) but not on the CY-BOCS ($P = .17$). The most frequently reported untoward effects were insomnia, fatigue, motoric activation, and nausea. Preexisting chronic motor tics worsened in two subjects; however, fluoxetine was continued and the tics subsided to negligible levels over the subsequent 2 years. A subject with comorbid diagnoses of MDD, separation anxiety, and oppositional disorder developed suicidal ideation, which resolved after fluoxetine was discontinued.

Of the 6 subjects initially on fluoxetine who crossed-over to placebo at 8 weeks, 3 dropped out at week 12 because of worsening of symptoms with a mean increase of 53% ± 37% in CY-BOCS scores; a fourth subject was worse at week 20 on the CY-BOCS; and the remaining two showed improvement (decrease) in their CY-BOCS scores. Although 3 of the 4 subjects who crossed-over from placebo to fluoxetine had shown substantial reductions in their CY-BOCS scores during the placebo period, further reduction in these scores were present at 20 weeks. Overall, these results complement findings in adults and suggest that fluoxetine is both safe and effective for 20 weeks in treating children and adolescents with obsessive compulsive disorder (Riddle et al., 1992).

SERTRALINE HYDROCHLORIDE (ZOLOFT)

Sertraline hydrochloride is approved by the FDA for the treatment of depression. Safety and efficacy have not been established for its use in children.

Dosage Schedule for Older Adolescents and Adults

An initial daily dose of 50 mg given either in the morning or at night is recommended. Full antidepressant response may be delayed for up to several weeks in some patients. Some patients may benefit from increases to a maximum of 200 mg/day. Dose changes should be at least a week apart because of sertraline's 24-hour elimination half-life.

Dosage Schedule for Children and Younger Adolescents

Not established.

Dose Forms Available

- Tablets (scored): 50 mg, 100 mg

PAROXETINE HYDROCHLORIDE (PAXIL)

Paroxetine hydrochloride is approved by the FDA for the treatment of depression. Safety and efficacy have not been established for its use in children.

Dosage Schedule for Older Adolescents and Adults

The recommended initial daily dose is 20 mg, usually administered in the morning. Full antidepressant response may be delayed for up to several weeks. Some patients may benefit from higher doses and paroxetine may be titrated upward with weekly increases of 10 mg recommended. (package insert)

Dosage Schedule for Children and Younger Adolescents

Not established.

Dose Forms Available

- Tablets (scored): 20 mg, 30 mg

TRAZODONE HYDROCHLORIDE (DESYREL)

Trazodone hydrochloride is chemically unrelated to tricyclic, tetracyclic, and other currently approved antidepressant agents. Although it is a serotonin reuptake inhibitor, it is unlike the SSRIs above in that its metabolites have significant effects on other neurotransmitter systems and their receptors (Cioli et al., 1984). It is approved for the treatment of patients diagnosed with major depressive episode, both with and without prominent symptoms of anxiety. Although trazodone's antidepressant activity is not fully understood, in animals it selectively inhibits serotonin reuptake in the brain and potentiates behavioral changes induced by 5-hydroxytryptophan.

Pharmacokinetics of Trazodone

It is recommended that trazodone be ingested soon after eating. When taken in this manner, up to 20% more drug may be absorbed than when taken on an empty stomach and maximum serum concentration is achieved more slowly (in about 2 hours rather than 1 hour) and with a lesser peak. This appears to diminish the likelihood of developing dizziness and/or lightheadedness. Trazodone is eliminated through the liver (about 20% biliary) and the kidneys (about 75%). Elimination is biphasic: the initial half-life is between 3 and 6 hours; this is followed by a second phase with a half-life between 5 and 9 hours.

Contraindications for Trazodone Administration

Known hypersensitivity to the drug is a contraindication.

Interactions of Trazodone with Other Drugs

Increased phenytoin levels have been reported when administered concomitantly with trazodone. Trazodone should not be administered with MAOIs, as the effects of their interaction are unknown.

Untoward Effects of Trazodone

The most common side effects include drowsiness, dizziness/lightheadedness, dry mouth, and nausea/vomiting. Priapism, which has necessitated surgical intervention and resulted in some cases of permanent impairment of sexual functioning, has been reported (incidence about 1:15,000). Male patients with a prolonged or inappropriate erection should be informed to immediately discontinue trazodone and contact their physician or, if it persists, go to an emergency room.

Indications for Use in Child and Adolescent Psychiatry

Trazodone is approved only for the treatment of major depressive disorder in individuals at least 18 years old. The drug is not recommended for use in the pediatric age group, as its safety and effectiveness have not been established for this age group.

Dosage Schedule for Children and Adolescents

USPDI (1992) reports the following pediatric doses guidelines when trazodone is used as an antidepressant:

- Children under 6 years old: Dosage not determined.
- Children 6–18 years old: Begin with 1.5–2 mg/kg/day in divided doses. Titrate dosage gradually at 3- to 4-day intervals to a maximum of 6 mg/kg/day.

Dose Forms Available

- Tablets: 50 mg scored, 100 mg scored
- Dividose tablets: 150 and 300 mg (both tablets scored to divide into 3 equal parts)

Reports of Interest

Trazodone in the Treatment of Children and Adolescents with Significant Aggression. Fras (1987) reported successfully treating with a daily dose of 200 mg of trazodone a 15-year-old male hospitalized for recurrent violence. Because of a misunderstanding, following discharge the dose was significantly decreased and at times omitted altogether. Repeated angry outbursts and threats of violence developed within a week and the patient became morose. Upon resumption of a daily dose of 200 mg, the patient returned to the previous stability and cooperativeness and remained so for 8 months of follow-up.

Ghaziuddin and Alessi (1992) noted the relationship of the expression of aggression and decreased levels of serotonin in the CNS and the successful use of trazodone to control aggressive behavior in adults with organic mental disorders. They administered trazodone to 3 boys, 7, 8, and 9 years old, with primary diagnoses of severe disruptive behavioral disorders; two of them were inpatients. Trazodone was initiated at doses of 25 mg once or twice daily and increased gradually. Improvement of symptoms was noted within 7–10 days at a mean dose of 0.35 mg/kg/day of trazodone (about 75 mg/day). In all 3 cases, marked deterioration of behavior occurred upon discontinuing the medication and aggressiveness decreased to former treatment levels once medication was resumed.

One boy had no reported untoward effects; one experienced mild sedation during the first week but this remitted with no dosage change. The third experienced spontaneous erections on 100 mg/day; because of concerns about reported priapism, dosage was reduced to 75 mg daily and behavioral control deteriorated. When 1000 mg daily of L-tryptophan (which has been subsequently withdrawn from the commercial market) was added, behavior markedly improved again. No ECG changes were noted in any of the boys. The authors note that further studies will be needed to determine the efficacy and safety of trazodone in treating aggressive children.

Zubieta and Alessi (1992) reported an open study of 22 inpatients (18 males and 4 females; age range, 5–12 years; mean age, 9 ± 2 years) with severe, treatment-refractory, behavioral disturbances. They were diagnosed with disruptive behavioral and mood disorders often with comorbidity. Six of the children continued to receive neuroleptics for psychotic symptoms during the trial of trazodone. An initial dose of 50 mg of trazodone at bedtime was begun an average of 23 ± 20 days after admission. It was titrated over a period of about 1 week to the maximum dose tolerated given in 3 divided doses. The 13 children designated as responders received a mean dose of 185 ± 117 mg/day (4.8 ± 1.7 mg/kg/day) of trazodone for a mean of 27 ± 13 days. The 7 nonresponders received a mean dose of 158 ± 70 mg/day (4.7 ± 2.0 mg/kg/day) for a mean of 24 ± 11 days. One patient was dropped from the study for severe orthostatic hypotension and a second for reported painful erections (not priapism). The other children tolerated any untoward effects that occurred. The most frequent was orthostatic hypotension (50%) but this diminished over a few days and did not require clinical intervention; 27% of children reported drowsiness, 9% nervousness, 9% anger. Dizziness, increased fatigue, and nocturnal enuresis each occurred in one child (4.5%).

Target symptoms that improved most frequently were impulsivity, hyperactivity, "involvement in dangerous activities," cruelty to people, frequency of physical fights, arguing with adults, and losing one's temper. Symptom improvement usually occurred within a few days of the initial administration of trazodone as contrasted to the several weeks of continuous administration typically required for its antidepressant effects to occur. At telephone follow-up 3–14 months later (mean 8.8 ± 4.2 months), 9 of the 13 responders were successfully contacted. Eight of the children continued to receive a mean trazodone dose of 241 ± 128 mg/day (range 100–800 mg/day); this was the only neuroleptic taken at follow-up, the neuroleptics 3 children were taking at discharge having been withdrawn within 2 months after discharge. The ninth child had an unsatisfactory response and his medication was changed to a combination of carbamazepine and pemoline. Overall, parents rated their children's improvements at 70 ± 20 (range 50–90) on a subjective overall rating of efficacy scale ranging from 0 to 100 (Zubieta and Alessi, 1992). Trazodone appears to be a potentially useful drug in treating acute and chronic behavioral disorders that have not responded to other treatments and merits further investigation.

Aminoketones

BUPROPION HYDROCHLORIDE (WELLBUTRIN)

Bupropion hydrochloride is an antidepressant of the aminoketone class. It is not related chemically to the tricyclics, tetracyclics, or other known antidepressants. It has been approved by the FDA for treating depression in individuals at least 18 years of age.

Indications in Child and Adolescent Psychiatry

- Children and adolescents under age 18: Not approved for any use.
- Adolescents at least 18 years of age: Used to treat depression, especially major depressive disorder.

Dosage Schedule for Children and Adolescents

- Children and adolescents under 18 years of age: Not recommended.
- Adolescents at least 18 years of age: An initial dosage of 100 mg twice daily is suggested. Based on clinical response, this may be increased to 100 mg three times daily, but not before day 4 of treatment. If no clinical improvement occurs within 4 weeks, dosage may gradually be increased. Because of increased risk of seizure, a dose of 150 mg should not be exceeded within a 4-hour time period. The maximum daily dosage should not exceed 450 mg.

Dose Forms Available

- Tablets: 75 mg, 100 mg

Contraindications for Bupropion Hydrochloride Administration

- Known hypersensitivity to bupropion hydrochloride and seizure disorders are contraindications.

- A current or prior diagnosis of bulimia or anorexia nervosa is also a contraindication, as a higher incidence of seizures is reported when bupropion is administered to such patients.
- Concurrent administration with any drug that reduces the seizure threshold is a relative contraindication.

Interactions of Bupropion Hydrochloride with Other Drugs

There are relatively few data available on this subject. Increased adverse experiences were reported when the drug was administered concomitantly with L-dopa. MAOIs may increase the acute toxicity of bupropion. Bupropion should not be administered concurrently with an MAOI. At least a 14-day period off MAOIs should precede initiation of treatment with bupropion hydrochloride.

Untoward Effects of Bupropion Hydrochloride

Of particular clinical concern is the finding that seizures have been associated with about 4 of 1000 (0.4%) patients treated with bupropion at doses of 450 mg/day or less. This is about 4-fold the incidence of seizures reported with other approved antidepressants, and the incidence of seizures increases with higher daily doses. On the other hand, Clay et al. (1988) note that bupropion's positive effects on memory performance may be unique among antidepressants and that other antidepressants either have no effect or a negative effect on memory performance.

The most common untoward effects were reported to be agitation, dry mouth, insomnia, headache, nausea, vomiting, constipation, and tremor.

Ferguson and Simeon (1984) reported no adverse (or positive) effects on cognition on a cognitive battery in 17 children with attention deficit disorder or conduct disorders who were treated in an open trial with bupropion.

Reports of Interest

Bupropion Hydrochloride in the Treatment of ADHD. Simeon et al. (1986) treated 17 male subjects (age range, 7–13.4 years; mean, 10.4 years) with bupropion in a 14-week single-blind uncontrolled study. Fourteen subjects were diagnosed with ADDH; of these, 8 were additionally diagnosed with conduct disorder, undersocialized aggressive type, and 2 with overanxious disorder. Eleven of the subjects had prior drug treatment; of these, 8 had shown no improvement. Four weeks of placebo were followed by 8-weeks of bupropion and then 2 weeks of placebo. The initial dose of bupropion was 50 mg/day; this was increased to 50 mg twice daily during the 2nd week and to a maximum of 50 mg three times daily during the 3rd week. No subjects responded to the baseline placebo. On drug, 5 patients showed marked improvement, 7 moderate improvement and 2 mild improvement on Clinical Global Improvement scale ratings. Significant improvements also occurred on the Children's Psychiatric Rating Scale (CPRS), Conners Parents and Teachers Scales, and self-ratings. Although not significant, group means for all 9 cognitive test variables showed improvement. Optimal dose was 150 mg/day in 15 cases and 100 mg/day and 50 mg/day in the other two subjects. Untoward effects were reported to be infrequent, mild, and transient.

Clay et al. (1988) reported that bupropion hydrochloride was safe and efficacious in treating prepubertal children diagnosed with ADHD. The authors' clinical impression was that children with additional prominent symptoms of conduct disorder responded particularly well to bupropion.

Thirty prepubertal children diagnosed with ADHD were enrolled in a double-blind placebo-controlled study and individually titrated to optimal doses of bupropion (Clay et al., 1988). Optimal doses ranged from 100 to 250 mg/day (3.1–7.1 mg/kg/day; mean, 5.3 ± 1 mg/kg/day). Subjects receiving bupropion showed statistically significant improvement on the Clinical Global Impressions Improvement and Severity Rating scales, the Self-Rating Scale, and on digit symbol and delayed recall on the Selective Reminding Test. Improvement that did not reach

significance was also reported on the Conners Parent Questionnaire and the Conners Teacher Questionnaire. The only serious side effect noted was an allergic rash in two children.

Clay et al. (1988) also noted that some children who had previously not responded satisfactorily to stimulants had a good response to bupropion. On the other hand, some subjects who had never received stimulants and who did not respond well to bupropion responded well when methylphenidate was openly prescribed at a later time.

Casat et al. (1989) administered bupropion to 20 children and placebo to 10 children in a parallel groups design, double-blind comparison study. All subjects were diagnosed with attention deficit disorder with hyperactivity. Decreases in symptom severity and overall clinical improvement were noted in physician ratings, and hyperactivity in the classroom settings was significantly decreased on the Conners Teachers Questionnaire.

Although confirmation of these findings is needed, bupropion may be an alternative treatment for ADHD that does not respond to standard therapies.

MONOAMINE OXIDASE INHIBITORS

Although effective antidepressants, monoamine oxidase inhibitors are usually not recommended for use in children and adolescents because of their potentially very serious drug interactions and untoward effects. Purposeful or accidental noncompliance with dietary prohibitions may result in ingestion of food containing tyramine and consequently a severe hypertensive crisis. Hence, the use of these agents should be reserved primarily for those children and adolescents who have not responded to other psychopharmacological agents, who have severe symptoms that significantly impair their functioning, and who are not at unacceptable risk (e.g., impulsive, suicidal) for following rigid dietary demands.

Lithium Carbonate

At the present time, lithium carbonate is approved by the FDA only for the treatment of manic episodes of bipolar disorders and for maintenance therapy of bipolar patients at least 12 years of age with a history of mania. Over the past two decades, however, lithium carbonate has been investigated in the treatment of many child and adolescent disorders, but especially in the treatment of children with severe aggression directed toward self or others, children with bipolar or similar disorders, and behaviorally disturbed children whose parents are known lithium responders. One major impetus for this research is that neuroleptics, which are frequently used to control severe behavioral disorders and sometimes mania, may cause cognitive dulling when used in sufficient dosage to control symptoms and carry a risk of causing tardive dyskinesia when used on a long-term basis (Platt et al., 1984).

LITHIUM TOXICITY AND UNTOWARD EFFECTS

One major difficulty associated with lithium carbonate is its low therapeutic index: Lithium toxicity is closely related to serum levels and may occur at doses close to therapeutic levels. Hence, it is essential that a laboratory capable of determining serum lithium levels rapidly and accurately be readily available to the clinician. For accuracy and serial comparisons, determinations of serum lithium levels should be made when lithium concentrations are relatively stable, and at the same time each day. Typically, blood is drawn immediately before the morning dose.

Although some patients who are unusually sensitive to lithium may exhibit toxic effects at serum levels below 1 mEq/liter, for most patients, mild to moderate untoward effects occur at serum levels between 1.5 and 2 mEq/liter, and moderate to severe reactions occur at levels of 2 mEq/liter and above. Younger subjects may be at greater risk than adults for developing untoward effects at lower serum lithium levels. Many untoward effects have been reported to occur in children at serum levels well below 1 mEq/liter (Campbell et al., 1984a). Patients and their caretakers should be alerted that clinically significant variations in lithium levels (both increases and decreases) have been reported following increased perspiration (e.g., during illness, hot weather, or vigorous exercise), dehydration, and dietary changes (see Green, 1995a, for review).

Fine tremor, polydipsia, and polyuria may be present throughout treatment. Nausea and malaise may occur initially but usually subside with ongoing treatment. Weight gain, headache, and gastrointestinal complaints may also occur. Lithium toxicity may be heralded by diarrhea, vomiting, muscular weakness, sedation, and impaired coordination. Increasingly severe and life-threatening toxic effects, including cardiac arrhythmias and severe CNS difficulties, occur with further elevations in serum lithium levels. Neuroleptic malignant syndrome has been reported in patients who were administered neuroleptics and lithium simultaneously.

As up to two-thirds of an acute dose of lithium is excreted in the urine within 6–12 hours (Baldessarini, 1990), lithium carbonate is usually administered three to four times daily (controlled release tablets are given twice daily) to avoid toxic serum levels.

LITHIUM CARBONATE (ESKALITH, LITHANE, LITHOBID), LITHIUM CITRATE SYRUP (CIBALITH-S)

Indications in Child and Adolescent Psychiatry

FDA approved for the treatment of manic episodes of manic-depressive illness and maintenance therapy of manic-depressive patients with a history of mania who are at least 12 years of age.

Dosage Schedule for Treating Acute Mania and Maintenance Therapy

- Children under 12 year old: Not approved for use.
- Persons 12 years of age and older: Dosage must be individually regulated according to clinical response and serum lithium levels.

Serum lithium levels should be monitored twice weekly during the acute manic phase and until both serum level and clinical condition have stabilized. During maintenance therapy during remission, serum lithium levels should be ascertained at least bimonthly, and cardiac, thyroid, and kidney functions periodically monitored.

Typically doses of approximately 1800 mg/day will achieve the serum lithium levels of between 1 and 1.5 mEq/liter necessary to control symptoms during acute mania. During long-term maintenance, serum lithium levels usually range between 0.6 and 1.2 mEq/liter; this usually requires a divided daily dose of between 900 mg and 1200 mg of lithium carbonate (PDR, 1995).

The therapeutic dosages of lithium carbonate used in treating children over 5 years of age with various disorders do not differ significantly from those used in treating older adolescents and adults, and the principles of administration are essentially the same (Campbell et al., 1984a).

Forms Available

- Lithium carbonate tablets: 300 mg
- Lithium carbonate capsules: 300 mg
- Lithium carbonate controlled release tablets: 300 mg, 450 mg
- Lithium citrate syrup: 8 mEq/5 ml (equivalent to 300-mg tablet)

Reports of Interest

Mood Disorders (Mania, Bipolar Disorder), Behavioral Disorders with Mood Swings, and/or Patients Whose Parent(s) Are Lithium Responders. DeLong and Aldershof (1987) reported that 66% of 59 children diagnosed with bipolar affective disorder, 82% of 11 children with emotionally unstable character disorder, and 71% of 7 offspring of lithium-responsive parents were treated successfully with lithium.

Disorders with Severe Aggression, Especially When Accompanied by Explosive Affect (e.g., Conduct Disorder), Including Self-Injurious Behavior (e.g., in Mental Retardation). In a double-blind placebo-controlled study of 61 treatment-resistant hospitalized children with undersocialized aggressive conduct disorder, both haloperidol and lithium were found to be superior to placebo in ameliorating behavioral symptoms (Campbell et al., 1984b). Optimal doses of lithium carbonate ranged from 500 to 2000 mg/day (mean, 1166 mg/day); corresponding serum levels ranged from 0.32 to 1.51 mEq/liter (mean, 0.993 mEq/liter). The authors noted that lithium caused fewer and milder untoward effects than haloperidol and that these did not appear to interfere significantly with the children's daily routines. There was also a suggestion that lithium was particularly effective in diminishing the explosive affect and that other improvements followed (Campbell et al., 1984b).

DeLong and Aldershof (1987) reported that rage, aggressive outbursts, and, interestingly, encopresis responded favorably to lithium pharmacotherapy in children with behavioral disorders associated with a variety of neurological and medical diseases, including mental retardation.

Anxiolytics

Benzodiazepines were the most frequently prescribed drugs in the United States for the 12 years prior to 1980; in 1978 alone, 68 million prescriptions for benzodiazepines were written for about 10 million individuals; over half of these were for diazepam (Ayd, 1980). Greenblatt et al. (1983) noted that by 1980 the trend toward increasing use of the benzodiazepines had reversed, perhaps subsequent to publicity about abuse of and addiction to the minor tranquilizers. There continues to be great concern regarding the abuse and addiction potential of the benzodiazepines, and in 1989 New York State began requiring all prescriptions for benzodiazepines to be written on triplicate forms, as for other controlled drugs.

Benzodiazepines appear to be prescribed to both older adolescents and adults for muscle relaxation and relief of anxiety and tension, sleep disorders, and seizures. In children, however, they are used primarily for treatment of sleep and seizure disorders and are used much less commonly for their anxiolytic and muscle relaxant qualities (Coffey et al., 1983).

Surprisingly little is known about the use of benzodiazepines in child and adolescent psychiatric disorders. In their important 1974 monograph, Greenblatt and Shader, after reviewing the use of benzodiazepines in children and adolescents, stated, "At present it is doubtful that the benzodiazepines have a role in the pharmacotherapy of psychoses or in the treatment of emotional disorders in children" (p. 88). More recently, the literature concerning their use in children has been reviewed by Campbell et al. (1985) and Simeon and Ferguson (1985). Most published reports have been open studies, and many were comprised of diagnostically heterogeneous subjects; results were discrepant. Diazepam and chlordiazepoxide were the drugs most frequently employed.

At the present time, the only psychiatric conditions occurring in childhood for which there is a convincing rationale for the use of a benzodiazepine as the drug of choice are sleep terror disorder and sleepwalking disorder; however, these conditions are not usually treated with pharmacotherapy unless they are unusually frequent or severe. Both sleep terror disorder (pavor nocturnus) and sleepwalking disorder (somnambulism) usually occur "during the first third of the major sleep period (the interval of nonrapid eye movement (NREM) sleep that typically contains EEG delta activity, sleep stages 3 and 4)" (American Psychiatric Association, 1987, pp. 310, 311). As benzodiazepines decrease stage 4 sleep, they theoretically might be of therapeutic value in these conditions. There is evidence of effectiveness in open studies; three children with somnambulism and pavor nocturnus and four children with insomnia were treated with 2–5 mg of diazepam near bedtime; all seven responded favorably (Glick et al., 1971). However, no controlled study of benzodiazepines in these disorders has yet been published.

On the other hand, benzodiazepines are theoretically contraindicated in treating sleep disturbance in psychosocial dwarfism (psychosocially determined short stature), as they would further compromise nocturnal secretion of growth hormone, which occurs maximally during sleep stages 3 and 4 (slow-wave sleep) (Green, 1986).

Werry concluded that, if pharmacotherapy is necessary for certain childhood sleep disturbances, including insomnia and night waking and night terrors and somnambulism, "probably" benzodiazepines are indicated, and that they are "possibly" indicated for some kinds of anxiety (Rapoport et al., 1978). Klein et al. (1980) suggested that benzodiazepines might be useful in treating residual anticipatory anxiety in school-phobic youngsters whose separation anxiety had been alleviated by treatment with imipramine. In a study of 50 enuretic children and adolescents, diazepam was significantly better than placebo (Kline, 1968).

Simeon and Ferguson (1985) reported that some overly inhibited children may show a lasting behavioral improvement following brief (not exceeding 4–6 weeks) treatment with a benzodiazepine. They attributed the improvement to an interaction between disinhibition facilitated by the medication and social learning. Consistent with this, they noted that children and adolescents with impulsivity and aggression who were under significant environmental stress should not be treated with benzodiazepines, as the disinhibition could result in worsening of behavior (Simeon and Ferguson, 1985).

Most of the literature suggests that benzodiazepines usually worsen symptoms in psychotic children. They also do not appear to be helpful in ADHD and mental retardation with behavior disorder (Campbell et al., 1985).

UNTOWARD EFFECTS

The most common untoward effects of benzodiazepines are manifestations of their being CNS depressants: Oversedation, fatigue, drowsiness, ataxia, and confusion progressing to coma may occur at high doses. When reduction of anxiety is the target symptom, benzodiazepines should be administered in divided doses to minimize sedation.

"Paradoxical reactions," episodes of marked dyscontrol and disinhibition, have been reported in children and adolescents. Symptoms have included acute excitation, increased anxiety, increased aggression and hostility, rage reactions, loss of all control and going wild, hallucinations, insomnia, and nightmares.

USE OF THE BENZODIAZEPINES IN CHILD AND ADOLESCENT PSYCHIATRY

At the present time, there are no specific clinical guidelines for treating any of the childhood psychiatric disorders with benzodiazepines, and if they are used, manufacturers' recommendations for children should not be exceeded. It is recommended that the need for benzodiazepines be reassessed frequently and that they be discontinued within a relatively short period of time, usually within a few weeks.

Table 72.3 gives usual daily dosages for the two benzodiazepines most commonly used in child and adolescent psychiatric disorders and for a benzodiazepine commonly used for nighttime sedation.

Table 72.3.   Some Representative Benzodiazepines

Benzodiazepine (Trade Name) (Estimated Serum Half-life)	Minimum Age Approved for Any Use	Usual Daily Dosage
Chlordiazepoxide (Librium) (half-life: 24–48 hr)	6 years	5 mg 2 to 4 times/day; max 30 mg/day
Diazepam (Valium) (half-life: 30–60 hr)	6 months	1–2½ mg 3 to 4 times per day; titrate as needed and tolerated
Flurazepam (Dalmane) (half-life: 47–100 hr)	15 years	15–30 mg at bedtime
Alprazolam (Xanax) (half-life: 12–15 hr)	18 years	See text

Reports of Interest

Alprazolam (Xanax).   Cameron and Thyer (1985) successfully treated with alprazolam a 10-year-old girl with severe nightly attacks of pavor nocturnus. Initially 0.5 mg of alprazolam was given at bedtime for 1 week; the dose was increased to 0.75 mg nightly for the next 4 weeks, and then the medication was tapered off. Attacks of night terrors ceased on the first night and there had not been a single recurrence at follow-up 9 months later.

Pfefferbaum et al. (1987) used alprazolam to treat anticipatory and acute situational anxiety and panic in 13 patients, ages 7–14 years, who were being treated for concomitant cancer. Treatment was begun 3 days prior to, and continued through the day of, the stressful procedures. This study was conducted under an Investigational New Drug permit, and maximum dosage allowed was 0.02 mg/kg/dose or 0.06 mg/kg/day; the higher dosage reported was on a single child for whom the FDA granted permission to increase doses incrementally by 0.25 mg to a maximum of 0.05 mg/kg/dose or 0.15 mg/kg/day. Initial doses were 0.005 mg/kg or lower and were titrated upward based on efficacy while monitoring untoward effects. Total daily dose ranged from 0.375 to 3 mg (0.003–0.075 mg/kg/day). Subjects were rated on four scales measuring anxiety, distress, and panic. The subjects' improvement was statistically significant ($P < .05$) on three scales and reached borderline significance on the fourth scale. Untoward effects were minimal, mild drowsiness being the most frequently reported.

Simeon and Ferguson (1987) administered alprazolam openly to 12 children and adolescents, ages 8.8–16.5 years (mean, 11.5 years), who were diagnosed with overanxious and/or avoidant disorder. After a 1-week placebo baseline period, to which none of the subjects responded, alprazolam was titrated individually over a 2-week period to maximum daily dosages from 0.50 to 1.5 mg. The total period of active treatment with alprazolam lasted 4 weeks. Seven of the 12 showed at least moderate improvement on several rating scales; no child worsened. Ratings by clinicians showed significant improvement of anxiety, depression, and psychomotor excitation; parents reported significant improvement of anxiety and hyperactivity on questionnaires; and teachers reported significant improvement on an anxious-passive factor. Improvement in the subjects' sleep problems was frequently reported by parents. The few untoward effects were mild and transient. Ferguson and Simeon (1984) reported no adverse effects of alprazolam on cognition or learning at therapeutically effective doses.

Simeon and Ferguson (1987) also noted that the subjects who responded best to alprazolam and who continued improved after the drug was stopped had good premorbid personalities and prominent symptoms of inhibitions, shyness, and nervousness. Patients with poor premorbid personalities and poor family backgrounds tended to develop negative symptoms of disinhibition such as increased aggressiveness and impulsivity, especially at higher doses, and relapsed following drug withdrawal.

Simeon et al. (1992) reported a double-blind, placebo-controlled study of alprazolam in 30 children and adolescents (23 males and 7 females; age range, 8.4–16.9 years; mean, 12.6 years) who had primary diagnoses of overanxious disorder (N = 21) or avoidant disorder (N = 9). Clinical impairment ranged from moderate to severe.

Placebo was administered for 1 week and followed by random assignment to a 4-week period of either placebo or alprazolam. Medication was tapered with placebo substitution during the 5th week. During the 6th week all subjects received only placebo. Patients who weighed under 40 kg received an initial dose of 0.25 mg alprazolam; heavier patients were given an initial dose of 0.5 mg alprazolam. The maximum daily dosage permitted was 0.04 mg/kg. Medication was increased at 2-day intervals until optimal dose was achieved. At completion of the active drug phase, the average daily maximum dose was 1.57 mg (range 0.5–3.5 mg). Untoward effects were few and minor, e.g., dry mouth and feeling tired, and at these doses did not appear to interfere with academic performance.

There was a strong treatment effect in both groups. At the time of completion of the double-blind period, alprazolam was superior to placebo based on clinical global ratings, but the differences were not significant. There were strong individual responders in both groups. After tapering off medication and the final week of placebo, there was a slight relapse with recurrence of original symptoms among the subjects on alprazolam while subjects on placebo showed no further change or continued to improve. The authors noted that doses employed were relatively low and were administered for only 4 weeks and suggested that higher doses and longer trials be investigated in the future. They also recommended that alprazolam be tapered more gradually over a period of several weeks.

Klein and Last (1989) reported Klein's unpublished data from a clinical trial of alprazolam in children and adolescents whose separation anxiety disorder did not respond to psychotherapy. Alprazolam was clinically effective when administered to 18 subjects, ages 6 years to 17 years, for 6 weeks in daily doses of 0.5–6 mg/day (mean, 1.9 mg/day). Parents and the psychiatrist judged that over 80% of the subjects improved significantly, while 65% of the subjects rated themselves as improved.

Azaspirodecanediones

BUSPIRONE HYDROCHLORIDE (BUSPAR)

Buspirone hydrochloride is a relatively new drug with anxiolytic properties that is not pharmacologically related to the benzodiazepines or barbiturates. Buspirone has a high affinity for $5-HT_{1A}$ serotonin receptors, which is associated with anticonflict activity in animals and predicts clinical anxiolytic activity (Sussman, 1994b). It does not appear to have significant affinity for benzodiazepine receptors or to affect γ-aminobutyric acid (GABA) binding (PDR, 1995). Buspirone does not have cross-tolerance with the benzodiazepines, does not suppress panic attacks, and lacks anticonvulsant activity; hence, it does not block the withdrawal syndrome that may occur when benzodiazepines and other common sedative hypnotic drugs are abruptly discontinued. At therapeutic doses it is less sedating than the benzodiazepines. In addition, no evidence of physical or psychological dependence or a withdrawal syndrome has been reported, and it appears to have low abuse potential even by individuals at increased risk for drug dependency. It is not classified as a controlled (Schedule II) substance.

Buspirone has been approved by the FDA for advertising as clinically effective for the management of anxiety disorders or the short-term relief of the symptoms of anxiety. It has been reported that, unlike benzodiazepines, which have an immediate anxiolytic effect, buspirone may take as long as 1–2 weeks for its antianxiety effect to develop. Symptom improvement may continue for at least 4 weeks, with psychic symptoms of anxiety improving sooner than somatic symptoms of anxiety (Feighner and Cohen, 1989).

Indications in Child and Adolescent Psychiatry

Buspirone is approved only for treatment of anxiety disorders and the short-term relief of anxiety in individuals at least 18 years old. Its safety and efficacy in children and adolescents remain to be determined.

Dosage Schedule for Treating Anxiety

- Children and adolescents: Not recommended.
- Persons 18 years old and older: Initiate treatment with 5 mg three times daily. Titrate to optimal therapeutic response by increases of 5 mg every 2–3 days to a maximum daily dose of 60 mg. Usual optimal doses in clinical trials were 20–30 mg/day in divided doses.

Dose Forms Available

- Tablets (scored): 5 mg, 10 mg

Pharmacokinetics of Buspirone Hydrochloride

Peak plasma levels occurred between 40 and 90 minutes after an acute oral dose of buspirone. Average elimination half-life after single doses of 10–40 mg of buspirone is usually between 2 and 3 hours.

Contraindications for Buspirone Hydrochloride Administration

Known hypersensitivity to buspirone is a contraindication. It is recommended that buspirone not be used concomitantly with monoamine oxidase inhibitors.

Interactions of Buspirone Hydrochloride with Other Drugs

The knowledge of the effects of concomitant administration of buspirone and other drugs is very limited; hence buspirone should be used cautiously with other drugs. There are reports that patients receiving MAOIs have developed elevated blood pressure when given buspirone.

Untoward Effects of Buspirone Hydrochloride

The untoward effects most frequently reported by adults taking buspirone include dizziness (12%), drowsiness (10%), nausea (8%), headache (6%), insomnia (3%), and lightheadedness (3%). Of note, however, drowsiness and insomnia were reported to occur with approximately equal frequency in subjects taking placebo; hence, these effects may not have been related to buspirone per se (PDR, 1995).

Reports of Interest

Buspirone Hydrochloride in the Treatment of Autistic Disorder. Because of buspirone's serotonin-inhibiting properties, Realmuto et al. (1989) treated four autistic children 9 or 10 years of age with buspirone 5 mg administered three times daily for 4 weeks, followed by a week-long washout period and 4 weeks of 10 mg twice daily of either fenfluramine or methylphenidate. Two of the four children showed decreased hyperactivity while on buspirone. None of the children experienced adverse untoward effects from buspirone.

Buspirone Hydrochloride in the Treatment of Overanxious Disorder with School Phobia. Kranzler (1988) reported a single case study in which a 13-year-old adolescent diagnosed with overanxious disorder, school refusal, and intermittent enuresis was administered buspirone. A previous trial of desipramine yielded some improvement but was discontinued at the patient's request because of untoward effects. Buspirone was begun at 2.5 mg three times daily. At 5 mg three times daily, some drowsiness occurred, particularly in the morning. Dosage was eventually stabilized at 5 mg twice daily. Scores on the Hamilton Anxiety Rating Scale dropped from 26 to 15 and stabilized, with improvement in phobic anxiety, insomnia, depressed mood, cardiovascular symptoms, and anxious behavior. The enuresis did not improve.

Buspirone Hydrochloride in the Treatment of Aggression. Quaison and her colleagues (1991) treated with buspirone hydrochloride a hospitalized 8-year-old boy diagnosed with conduct and attention-deficit hyperactivity disorders. Dosage was begun at 5 mg t.i.d. and titrated gradually to 15 mg t.i.d. By day 10 there was notable decrease in his aggressive and assaultive behavior, and the need for time outs or seclusion ceased altogether.

Ratey and coworkers (1989, 1991) reported that buspirone hydrochloride in doses of 15–45 mg/day was useful in treating 20 developmentally disabled and mentally retarded adults (age range, 18–63 years) for symptoms of anxiety, aggression, and self-injurious behaviors (SIBs). The decrease in aggressive behavior was independent of anxiety effects. The authors hypothesized that buspirone reduced aggression through its interaction with the serotonergic systems and that, at low dosage levels (although not necessarily at the higher doses of 30–60 mg/day used for its anxiolytic-antidepressant effects), buspirone may act as a serotonin agonist, especially in brains with low serotonin activity. However, it remains to be seen if buspirone hydrochloride will be efficacious and safe when its use is extended downward in age.

Antihistamines

DIPHENHYDRAMINE (BENADRYL)

Diphenhydramine has been used for over 40 years to treat psychiatrically disturbed children (Effron and Freedman, 1953). Although this is still not an FDA-approved use (PDR, 1995), it is reviewed here as child psychiatrists continue to find it clinically effective. In addition, if carefully titrated, it is among the safest drugs used in the psychopharmacotherapy of children.

Fish (1960) reported that diphenhydramine is most effective in behavioral disorders associated with anxiety and hyperactivity, but that it also could be useful in moderately (not severely) disturbed children with organic or schizophrenic (including autistic) disorders. A later study of 15 children, however, found no significant difference in behavioral improvement between diphenhydramine in doses of 200–800 mg/day and placebo (Korein et al., 1971).

Diphenhydramine may also be effective as an anxiolytic, reducing anxiety before producing drowsiness or lethargy, in children up to 10 years of age. However, it shows a marked decrease in efficacy when administered to older children; they respond like adults with untoward effects of malaise or drowsiness. Thus, for older children, diphenhydramine is useful primarily as a bedtime sedative to treat insomnia and/or nighttime anxiety (Fish, 1960).

The administration of diphenhydramine is contraindicated in newborn or premature infants. Its use is permitted only in children who weigh over 20 pounds (9.1 kg), and a maximum dose of 300 mg/day or 5 mg/kg/day is recommended. Maximum activity occurs in about 1 hour and lasts about 4–6 hours; thus, it is usually administered three to four times daily.

Young children appear to tolerate a higher dose per unit of weight than do adolescents and adults. Fish (1960) found that a dose range of from 2 to 10 mg/kg/day, with an average daily dose of 4 mg/kg, was most effective in treating her behaviorally disturbed youngsters.

The most frequent untoward effects are anticholinergic effects and sedation. Children do seem more tolerant than adolescents and adults to the sedative effects of diphenhydramine, but the clinician should still be alert to any cognitive dulling that may interfere with learning. Young children may sometimes be excited rather than sedated by diphenhydramine. It is cautioned that overdose may cause hallucinations, convulsions, or death, particularly in infants and young children.

Antiepileptic Drugs

The use of antiepileptic drugs for treatment of psychiatric disorders in children and adolescents was reviewed by Stores in 1978. He concluded that "while some of the antiepileptic drugs show possibilities as psychotropic agents, their use in children with nonepileptic conditions such as behavior or learning disorders of childhood cannot be justified except as a carefully controlled research exercise" (Stores, 1978, p. 314).

At the present time, most clinical interest in this area appears to be centered upon the use of carbamazepine and, to a lesser extent, valproic acid (valproate).

CARBAMAZEPINE (TEGRETOL)

Evans et al. (1987) attribute the increased interest in carbamazepine's use in child and adolescent psychiatry in part to both the increased awareness of the serious untoward long-term complications of neuroleptics and the finding that the untoward effects of carbamazepine are less formidable than initially thought. In particular, the serious blood

dyscrasias, agranulocytosis and aplastic anemia, are very rare. The risk of developing these disorders when treated with carbamazepine is 5 to 8 times that of the general population; agranulocytosis occurs in about 6 per million and aplastic anemia in about 2 per million of the untreated general population (PDR, 1995).

Although approved only for treating certain kinds of seizure disorders and neuralgias, carbamazepine has been used to treat many psychiatric disorders. In adults, perhaps the best known of these is the treatment of lithium-resistant bipolar disorder. There is evidence carbamazepine has acute antimanic and antidepressive effects as well as longer-term prophylactic action in treating bipolar disorder (Post, 1987). Post notes that more severe and dysphoric mania and a rapidly cycling course, variables associated with a poor response to lithium, appear to correspond to better responses to carbamazepine. It has been suggested that the efficacy of carbamazepine in psychiatric disorders may be secondary to its hypothesized ability to inhibit limbic system kindling. Kessler et al. (1989) reported that three psychotic adults improved markedly when carbamazepine was substituted for their neuroleptic medication and suggested criteria to identify affectively ill patients who may have a primary or superimposed organic mood disorder and who might benefit from carbamazepine.

Remschmidt (1976) reviewed data from 28 clinical trials, 7 double-blind and 21 open studies, with a total of over 800 nonepileptic child and adolescent subjects who were treated with carbamazepine. Positive clinical results were found for target symptoms of hyperactivity or hypoactivity, impaired concentration, aggressive behavioral disturbances, and dysphoric mood disorders. In addition to these behavioral effects, Remschmidt suggested these patients also experienced positive mood changes, increased initiative, and decreased anxiety.

Groh (1976) reported on 62 nonepileptic children treated for various abnormal behavioral patterns with carbamazepine. Of the 27 who showed improvement, most had a "dysphoric or dysthymic syndrome," the most important features of which were emotional lability and moodiness, which were felt to cause most of the other behavioral abnormalities.

Kuhn-Gebhart (1976) reported symptom improvement in a large number of nonepileptic children who were treated with carbamazepine for a wide variety of behavioral disorders. The author reported that 30 of the last 50 patients treated showed good or very good responses; 10 had discernible improvement, 9 had no change in behavior, and 1 deteriorated. The author noted that the more abnormal the EEGs of these nonepileptic patients, in general, the better the response, and that many of the good responders came from stable homes and poorer results were more frequent in subjects from unfavorable homes.

Puente (1976) reported an open study in which carbamazepine was administered to 72 children with various behavioral disorders who did not have evidence of neurological disease. Fifty-six children completed the study. The usual optimal dose was 300 mg/day (range, 100–600 mg/day). Carbamazepine was given for an average of 12 weeks (range, 9–23 weeks). Twenty symptoms were rated on a severity scale at the beginning and end of the treatment. Individual symptoms were present in as many as 55 and in as few as 2 of the 56 children. Over the course of treatment, a decrease in symptom expression of 70% or more occurred in 17 of 20 symptoms in at least 60% of the subjects. Interestingly, all 6 children (100%) with night terrors responded positively, as did 16 (94%) of the 17 children with other sleep disturbances. Anxiety present in 47 children improved in 34 (72%). Enuresis improved in 8 of 9 children (89%), and aggressiveness, present in 46 children, improved in 32 (70%). The most frequent untoward effects were transient drowsiness in about 20%, nausea and vomiting in about 4%, and urticaria in 4%.

Kafantaris et al. (1992) reported an open pilot study in which 10 children (9 male, 1 female; age range, 5.25–10.92 years, mean age, 8.27 years) diagnosed with conduct disorder and hospitalized for symptoms of explosive aggressiveness were treated with carbamazepine. Five of the subjects had previously failed to respond to a trial of lithium. After a 1-week baseline period, carbamazepine was administered in 3 divided doses beginning at a total of 200 mg/day and titrated to a maximum of 800 mg/day or a serum level of 12 μg/ml over a period of from 3 to 5 weeks. Optimal dose range was 600–800 mg/day (mean, 630 mg/day) with serum levels from 4.8 to 10.4 μg/ml (mean, 6.2 μg/ml). Target symptoms of aggressiveness and explosiveness declined significantly on all measures compared to baseline ratings. On the Global Clinical Consensus Ratings, 4 subjects were rated as markedly improved, 4 as moderately improved, 1 as slightly improved, and 1 as showing no improvement. Three of the lithium nonresponders showed marked improvement and one showed moderate improvement; the fifth did not respond to either drug. Untoward effects during regulation and at optimal dose included fatigue (2/10), blurred vision (2/10), and dizziness (1/10). Untoward effects above optimal dose included diplopia (2/10), mild ataxia (2/10), mild dysarthria (1/10), headache (2/10), and lethargy (1/10). One child experienced worsening of preexisting behavioral symptoms and loosening of associations, which were felt to be manifestations of behavioral toxicity. Overall the untoward effects were transient and were decreased to tolerable levels or eliminated by reduction in dose. White blood counts remained within normal limits although 4 children had reductions from baseline determinations.

Evans et al. (1987) have reviewed the use of carbamazepine in treating children and adolescents with psychiatric disorders including hyperkinesis, aggression, impulsivity, and emotional lability. They note the lack of systematic, well-controlled studies. These authors also address the important issue of the behavioral toxicity of carbamazepine and note that its untoward effects on mood and behavior may resemble the target symptoms for which it is being prescribed.

Carbamazepine's status in treating child and adolescent psychiatric disorders still remains to be elucidated. While there are indications that it is being used by clinicians with increasing frequency to treat many neuropsychiatric disorders that have failed to respond satisfactorily to more standard therapies, and positive results have been reported in open trials, further research is necessary to determine its efficacy for specific disorders, and which symptoms or patients are most likely to respond well.

Opiate Antagonists

Opiate antagonists have been investigated in the treatment of mentally retarded persons with SIB and in the treatment of autistic disorder. Deutsch (1986) has given a theoretical rationale for the use of opiate antagonists in the treatment of autistic disorder. Naltrexone (Trexan), a long-acting, potent opiate antagonist, is a potentially useful agent in a subgroup of autistic children who have elevated endorphin (opioid peptides) levels.

Reports of Interest in Children Diagnosed with Autistic Disorder

Although there are case studies and open studies with some encouraging data, Campbell et al.'s 1993, 8-week double-blind study in which 41 hospitalized children, 2.9–7.8 years of age (mean, 4.9 years) and diagnosed with autistic disorder, were treated with naltrexone or placebo did not support the efficacy of naltrexone in this population. All their subjects received placebo during the first 2 weeks while baseline data were obtained. Following this, subjects were randomly assigned to naltrexone or placebo for the next 3 weeks; the final week all subjects again received placebo. Twenty-three patients were assigned to the naltrexone group and 18 to the placebo group. The initial dose was 0.5 mg/kg/day of either placebo or active drug given in the morning; dose was increased to 1.0 mg/kg/day after 1 week and maintained at that level, as untoward effects were minimal and did not require a reduction in dose. Naltrexone did not improve the core symptoms of autism. The only significant finding was a modest decrease in hyperactivity on 3 different measures. It did not improve discriminate learning significantly more than placebo. Naltrexone was not better than placebo in reducing SIB, but 6 of 8

subjects with SIB who had severity rating of mild or above on the Aggression Rating Scale who received naltrexone experienced rebound (increase) in SIB during the final placebo period, whereas only one child in the placebo group exhibited worsening of SIB during that time. The authors concluded that it remains to be determined whether naltrexone is efficacious in treating moderate to severe SIB. Its use cannot be recommended as a first line treatment for patients diagnosed with either autistic disorder or SIB.

β-Adrenergic Blockers

PROPRANOLOL (INDERAL)

Although initially used primarily in controlling hypertension, angina pectoris, various cardiac arrhythmias, and other medical disorders, there has been considerable interest in propranolol's use in general psychiatry.

Propranolol is a nonselective β-adrenergic receptor blocking agent and is the most frequently used drug in this class. Propranolol and other β-adrenergic blocking agents reduce peripheral autonomic tone, thereby lessening somatic symptoms of anxiety such as palpitations, tremulousness, perspiration, and blushing. There is evidence that the β-adrenergic blocking agents significantly reduce these peripheral, autonomic, physical manifestations of anxiety but may not affect the psychological (emotional) symptoms of anxiety (Noyes, 1988). Noyes concludes from his review of the literature (1988) that β-blockers are relatively weak anxiolytics compared to benzodiazepines and should be used for generalized anxiety disorder, primarily in patients for whom the use of benzodiazepines is contraindicated.

In adults, propranolol has been investigated in treating anxiety disorders, including generalized anxiety, performance anxiety (stage fright), social phobia, and posttraumatic stress disorder; panic disorder and agoraphobia; and episodic dyscontrol and rage outbursts (Hayes and Schulz, 1987; Noyes, 1988). It has also been used in schizophrenia. Propranolol is effective in the treatment of some antipsychotic-induced akathisias (Adler et al., 1986).

There are few reports of the use of these drugs in psychiatrically disturbed children and adolescents. Williams et al. (1982) administered propranolol to 30 subjects (11 children, 15 adolescents, and 4 adults) with organic brain dysfunction and uncontrolled rage outbursts that had not responded to other treatments. The subjects had various psychiatric diagnoses, including 15 with the dual diagnoses of conduct disorder, unsocialized, aggressive type, and attention deficit disorder with hyperactivity; 7 with the dual diagnoses of conduct disorder, unsocialized, aggressive type, and attention deficit disorder without hyperactivity; 3 with conduct disorder only; 3 with intermittent explosive disorders; and 2 with pervasive developmental disorders. Thirteen had IQs in the retarded range, and 8 had borderline IQs. The authors reported that 80% of their subjects demonstrated moderate to marked improvement on follow-up between 2 and 30 months (mean, 8 months) later. Optimal dosages of propranolol ranged from 50 to 960 mg/day (mean, 160 mg/day). All untoward effects were transient and reversible with dosage reduction. Most of the patients were additionally treated with other medication: 13 subjects received anticonvulsants, 6 antipsychotics, and 3 stimulants; 21 had ongoing psychotherapy (Williams et al., 1982).

Two 12-year-old boys treated with propranolol for episodic dyscontrol and aggressive behavior showed marked improvement (Grizenko and Vida, 1988). Dosage was begun at 10 mg three times daily and gradually increased to 50 mg three times daily.

Famularo et al. (1988) reported that 11 children (mean age, 8½ years old) diagnosed with posttraumatic stress disorder (PTSD), acute type, had significantly lower scores on an inventory of PTSD symptoms during the period they were receiving propranolol, compared with scores before and after the drug. Dosage was begun at 0.8 mg/kg/day and administered in three divided doses; it was increased gradually over 2 weeks to approximately 2.5 mg/kg/day. Untoward effects prevented raising dosage to this level in only three cases. Propranolol was maintained at this level for 2 weeks and then tapered and discontinued over a 5th week. The authors emphasized that their subjects had presented in agitated, hyperaroused states and that propranolol might be useful during this particular stage of the disorder (Famularo et al., 1988).

At present, although there are some encouraging initial data, the use of propranolol and the β-blockers in children and adolescents must be regarded as preliminary. In particular, propranolol's use in anxiety disorders remains to be elucidated.

α-Adrenergic Agonists

CLONIDINE (CATAPRES)

Clonidine, a centrally acting antihypertensive agent, has been used for treating hypertension in older adolescents and adults; its safety and efficacy in children have not been established. It has, however, been investigated in treating children and adolescents diagnosed with ADHD and/or Tourette's disorder who have not responded to standard treatments.

Clonidine is an α-adrenergic stimulating agent that acts preferentially on presynaptic α-2 neurons to inhibit noradrenergic activity (Hunt et al., 1985). The authors note that the positive results suggest that the norepinephrine system may be important in causing behavioral and cognitive abnormalities in at least some children with ADHD.

Peak plasma levels of clonidine occur between 3 and 5 hours after ingestion, and plasma half-life is between 12 and 16 hours (PDR, 1995). Leckman et al. (1985), however, give somewhat different pharmacokinetic data, stating that clonidine's half-life is about 8–12 hours in adolescents and adults, while in prepubertal children it is considerably shorter, approximately 4–6 hours. Between 40 and 60% of the drug is excreted unchanged by the kidneys within 24 hours after oral ingestion, and about 50% is metabolized by the liver (PDR, 1995).

The Use of Clonidine in ADHD

Hunt et al. (1982) reported an open pilot study in which clonidine 3–4 μg/kg/day was administered orally to four children between 9 and 14 years of age diagnosed with ADHD for 2–5 months. Improvement was noted by parents and teachers. The authors noted that distractibility often persisted but the children were nevertheless more able to return to and complete tasks.

Hunt et al. (1985) conducted a double-blind placebo crossover study of 12 children (mean age, 11.6 $\pm$ 0.54 years). Ten children completed the study. Seven subjects had previously received stimulant medication; in four cases stimulants had been discontinued because of significant side effects. Parents, teachers, and clinicians all noted statistically significant improvements on clonidine for the group as a whole. The best responders were children who had been overactive and who were uninhibited and impulsive, which, in turn, had impaired their opportunities to use their basically intact capacities for social relatedness and purposeful activity.

The most frequent untoward effect was sedation occurring about 1 hour after ingestion and lasting 30–60 minutes. In all cases but one, tolerance to this effect developed within 3 weeks. Mean blood pressure decreased about 10% on clonidine (Hunt et al., 1985).

During the placebo period, parents, teachers, and clinicians noted significant deterioration in overall behavior for the group, with symptoms usually returning between 2 and 4 days after discontinuing the medication (Hunt et al., 1985).

Hunt (1987) compared the efficacies of clonidine (administered both orally and transdermally) and methylphenidate in an open study of 10 children diagnosed with ADHD, all of whom had ratings by both parents and teacher of more than 1.5 SDs above normal on the Conners behavioral rating scales. Eight subjects (7 males, 1 female; mean age, 11.4 (SD $\pm$ 0.6) years; age range, 6.7–14.4 years) completed the protocol. Subjects received placebo, low-dose (0.3 mg/kg) methylphenidate, or high-dose (0.6 mg/kg) methylphenidate. Each of these conditions was

randomized for a period of 1 week. All subjects then received an open trial of clonidine 5 μg/kg/day administered orally for 8 weeks. Eight subjects completed the open trial with positive results and were then switched from tablets to transdermal clonidine skin patch. Both clonidine and methylphenidate were significantly more effective than placebo, and clonidine in both dosage forms was equally effective to methylphenidate (Hunt, 1987). Children reported they felt more "normal" on clonidine than on methylphenidate. Transdermal administration was preferred to oral administration by 75% of the children and their families, partly because the embarrassment of taking pills at school was avoided but also because it was more convenient. Local irritation from patches, however, at times prevented their use.

Hunt (1987) noted that clonidine appears to increase frustration tolerance but does not decrease distractibility. He noted that an additional small dose of methylphenidate may be safely added to help focus attention and that this combination frequently necessitates a much lower dose of methylphenidate than would be required if it were the only drug used (Hunt, 1987).

Clonidine was begun at 0.05 mg and increased every other day until a dose of 4–5 μg/kg/day (about 0.05 mg four times daily) was attained (Hunt et al., 1985). When a transdermal patch was used, Hunt (1987) found that its efficacy wore off and had to be replaced in 50% of subjects after 5 days rather than the 7 days stated by the manufacturer. He also noted that in three of his eight subjects, an oral dose of 0.2 mg/day had to be increased to 0.3 mg/day when clonidine was administered transdermally, to maintain the same degree of symptom control.

Discontinuing Medication

Clonidine should be gradually reduced over a period of 2–4 days to avoid a possible hypertensive reaction and other withdrawal symptoms such as nervousness, agitation, and headache (PDR, 1995).

Dose Forms Available

- Tablets: 0.1 mg, 0.2 mg, and 0.3 mg (all single scored)
- Transdermal Therapeutic System (skin patch): programmed delivery in vivo of 0.1 mg, 0.2 mg, or 0.3 mg clonidine per day for 1 week.

At present, although clonidine is an unapproved treatment for ADHD, it may prove useful in treating a subgroup of ADHD children who do not respond well to stimulants. Clonidine may be considered also as an alternative treatment for some ADHD children who have chronic tics or who develop side effects of sufficient severity to preclude the use of stimulants (Hunt et al., 1985).

The Use of Clonidine in Tourette's Disorder

Cohen et al. (1980) reported that clonidine was clinically effective in at least 70% of 25 patients between 9 and 50 years of age diagnosed with Tourette's disorder who either did not benefit from haloperidol or could not tolerate untoward effects of that medication. Dosage was begun at 1–2 μg/kg/day (usually 0.05 mg/day) and gradually titrated up to a maximum of 0.60 mg/day. Most patients did best with small doses three to four times daily. Shapiro and Shapiro (1989), however, found clonidine to be only rarely effective in treating unselected patients with tics and Tourette's disorder.

Cohen et al. (1980) delineated five phases of treatment response to clonidine. Phase 1 occurred within hours or days; patients felt calmer, less angry, more in control. Phase 2 began about 3–4 weeks after initiation of clonidine and usually coincided with a therapeutic dose of 3–4 μg/kg/day (0.15 mg/day). The patient recognized progressive benefits, characterized by decreased compulsive behavior, further behavioral control, and decreased phonic and motor tics. In phase 3, a plateauing of improvement started at about the 3rd month. Phase 4 set in 5 or more months after beginning; an increase in dosage up to 4–6 μg/kg/day (0.30 mg/day) of clonidine was needed to maintain clinical improvement. Phase 5 may begin when further tolerance to clonidine occurs at a dose considered too high to increase further.

A review of the use of clonidine in Tourette's disorder (Leckman et al., 1982) noted discrepant results among studies. The reviewers estimated that about 50% of subjects improved meaningfully. Behavioral symptoms showed the most improvement, and maximum benefit could take from 4 to 6 months. A minority of patients didn't respond, and a few worsened.

Leckman et al. (1985) reported a 20-week, single-blind placebo-controlled trial of clonidine in 13 patients, ages 9–16 years, diagnosed with Tourette's disorder. This was followed by a 1-year open clinical trial. The mean dose of clonidine was 5.5 μg/kg/day (range, 3–8 μg/kg/day) (0.125–0.3 mg/day of clonidine). There was significant improvement in motor and phonic tics and associated behavioral problems. Forty-six percent of subjects were unequivocal responders and another 46% responded equivocally. Of interest is the fact that 9 of the 13 patients of Leckman et al. also had an additional diagnosis of ADHD. As noted above, some children with ADHD have symptoms that also respond to clonidine.

Dosage. Bruun (1983) has provided useful guidelines for prescribing clonidine for Tourette's disorder. She suggests initiating daily dosage at 0.025 mg twice daily for small children and at 0.05 mg twice daily for older children and adolescents. Medication is titrated upward gradually, with increases no greater than 0.05 mg/week; this slow pace often prevents untoward effects from interfering with the treatment. Usual optimal daily dose is between 0.25 and 0.45 mg. Doses above 0.5 mg/day may be required, but untoward effects (e.g. drowsiness, fatigue, dizziness, headache, insomnia, and increased irritability) become more troublesome. Bruun (1983) notes that drowsiness may occur at very low doses and suggests that no further increases in dosage be made until drowsiness subsides. Some patients note a decrease in beneficial effects 4–5 hours after their last dose, and treatment is usually more effective for all patients, with total daily dosage administered in three or four smaller doses (Bruun, 1983).

Although presently not an approved treatment, there is evidence some children and adolescents with Tourette's disorder respond favorably with significant symptom reduction when treated with clonidine.

Clonidine may be regarded as a possible treatment for those youngsters with Tourette's disorder who have not responded satisfactorily or who have intolerable untoward effects to standard treatments.

CONCLUSIONS

The advancement of child and adolescent psychopharmacology continues at a brisk pace, although considerably less than its adult counterpart. New drugs continue to be approved that have greater specificity of action and markedly more favorable untoward effect profiles than older medications, e.g., the new SSRIs and the atypical antipsychotics. Unfortunately, very few of the early studies of these drugs leading to their approval by the FDA included patients in the pediatric age range and this was often limited to a few older adolescents. Hence, although there are increasing numbers of open studies of these drugs in children and adolescents and some double-blind, placebo-controlled studies, there is still a paucity of reliable data concerning their efficacy and safety and most are not approved by the FDA for use in this age range and such use is presently off-label.

There is also an increasing proportion of reports in the literature that are concerned with polypharmacy. These reports most frequently concern patients who have not responded adequately to a drug, and a second medication is added to augment or enhance its effect. These are open studies of at most a few patients. Lithium, SSRI antidepressants, and antiepileptics, especially carbamazepine and valproate, are frequently used at the present time.

These rapid advances are exciting and most reports are encouraging; however, they are in relatively uncharted waters. Although major funded researchers certainly publish some statistically insignificant data and treatment failures, open studies, case reports, letters, and reports of polypsychopharmacy in single or small numbers of patients usually herald successes or report significant untoward effects. Reports of a single or a few cases saying drugs a and b were tried and had no therapeutically useful effect are rare in the published literature. As clinicians, we must be ever alert to this bias, proceed cautiously, and monitor appropriate parameters as we expand and improve our therapeutic repertoires and include our younger patients among those who benefit from the advances in psychopharmacology.

References

Adler L, Angrist B, Peselow E, et al: A controlled assessment of propranolol in the treatment of neuroleptic-induced akathisia. *Br J Psychiatry* 149:42–45, 1986.

Altamura AC, Montgomery SA, Wernicke JF: The evidence for 20 mg a day of fluoxetine as the optimal dose in the treatment of depression. *Br J Psychiatry* 153(suppl 3):109–112, 1988.

Aman MG, Kern RA: Review of fenfluramine in the treatment of the developmental disorders. *J Am Acad Child Adolesc Psychiatry* 28:549–565, 1989.

Aman MG, Singh NN (eds): *Psychopharmacology of the Developmental Disabilities.* New York, Springer-Verlag, 1988.

Ambrosini PJ: Pharmacotherapy in child and adolescent major depressive disorder. In: Meltzer HY (ed): *Psychopharmacology: The Third Generation of Progress.* New York, Raven Press, 1987, pp. 1247–1254.

Ambrosini PJ, Bianchi MD, Rabinovich H, et al: Antidepressant treatments in children and adolescents. I: Affective disorders. *J Am Acad Child Adolesc Psychiatry* 32:1–6, 1993.

American Medical Association: *Drug Evaluations Annual 1994.* Chicago, American Medical Association, 1993.

American Psychiatric Association: *Diagnostic and Statistical Manual of Mental Disorders* (3rd ed). Washington, DC, American Psychiatric Association, 1980.

American Psychiatric Association: *Diagnostic and Statistical Manual of Mental Disorders* (3rd ed, rev). Washington, DC, American Psychiatric Association, 1987.

American Psychiatric Association: *Diagnostic and Statistical Manual of Mental Disorders* (4th ed). Washington, DC, American Psychiatric Association, 1994.

Anderson LT, Campbell M, Grega DM, et al: Haloperidol in the treatment of infantile autism: Effects on learning and behavioral symptoms. *Am J Psychiatry* 141:1195–1202, 1984.

Ayd FJ Jr: Social issues: Misuse and abuse. *Psychosomatics* 21(suppl 10):21–25, 1980.

Baldessarini RJ: Drugs and the treatment of psychiatric disorders. In: Gilman AF, Rall TW, Nies AS, et al (eds): *Goodman and Gilman's the Pharmacological Basis of Therapeutics* (8th ed). New York, Pergamon, 1990, pp. 383–435.

Ballenger JC, Carek DJ, Steele JJ, et al: Three cases of panic disorder with agoraphobia in children. *Am J Psychiatry* 146:922–924, 1989.

Barrickman L, Noyes R, Kuperman S, et al: Treatment of ADHD with fluoxetine: A preliminary trial. *J Am Acad Child Adolesc Psychiatry* 30: 762–767, 1990.

Biederman J, Baldessarini RJ, Goldblatt A, et al: A naturalistic study of 24-hour electrocardiographic recordings and echocardiographic findings in children and adolescents treated with desipramine. *J Am Acad Child Adolesc Psychiatry* 32:805–813, 1993.

Birmaher B, Quintana H, Greenhill LL: Methyl-phenidate treatment of hyperactive autistic children. *J Am Acad Child Adolesc Psychiatry* 27:248–251, 1988.

Blanz B, Schmidt MH: Clozapine for schizophrenia (letter to the editor). *J Am Acad Child Adolesc Psychiatry* 32:223–224, 1993.

Bradley C: The behavior of children receiving benzedrine. *Am J Psychiatry* 94:577–585, 1937.

Bruun R: TSA medical update: Treatment with clonidine. *Tourette Syndrome Assoc Newslet,* Spring, 1983.

Campbell M, Anderson LT, Small AM, et al: Naltrexone in autistic children: Behavioral symptoms and attentional learning. *J Am Acad Child Adolesc Psychiatry* 32:1283–1291, 1993.

Campbell M, Green WH, Deutsch SI: *Child and Adolescent Psychopharmacology.* Beverly Hills, CA, Sage, 1985.

Campbell M, Perry R, Green WH: The use of lithium in children and adolescents. *Psychosomatics* 25:95–106, 1984a.

Campbell M, Small AM, Green WH, et al: Behavioral efficacy of haloperidol and lithium carbonate: A comparison in hospitalized aggressive children with conduct disorder. *Arch Gen Psychiatry* 41: 650–656, 1984b.

Cioli V, Corradino C, Piccinelli D, et al: A comparative pharmacological study of trazodone, etoperidone, and 1-(*m*-chlorophenyl)piperazine. *Pharmacol Res Commun* 16:85–100, 1984.

Ciraulo DA, Shader RI, Greenblatt DJ, et al (eds): *Drug Interactions in Psychiatry* (2nd ed). Baltimore, Williams & Wilkins, 1995.

Coffey B, Shader RI, Greenblatt DJ: Pharmacokinetics of benzodiazepines and psychostimulants in children. *J Clin Psychopharmacol* 3:217–225, 1983.

Cohen DJ, Detlor J, Young JG, et al: Clonidine ameliorates Gilles de la Tourette syndrome. *Arch Gen Psychiatry* 37:1350–1357, 1980.

Conners CK: Recent drug studies with hyperkinetic children. *J Learn Disabil* 4:476–483, 1971.

Conners CK, Taylor E, Meo G, et al: Magnesium pemoline and dextroamphetamine: A controlled study in children with minimal brain dysfunction. *Psychopharmacologia (Berlin)* 26:321–336, 1972.

DeLong GR, Aldershof AL: Long-term experience with lithium treatment in childhood: Correlation with clinical diagnosis. *J Am Acad Child Adolesc Psychiatry* 26:389–394, 1987.

Deutsch SI: Rationale for the administration of opiate antagonists in treating infantile autism. *Am J Ment Defic* 90:631–635, 1986.

DeVeaugh-Geiss MD, Moroz G, Biederman J, et al: Clomipramine hydrochloride in childhood and adolescent obsessive-compulsive disorder—A multicenter trial. *J Am Acad Child Adolesc Psychiatry* 31:45–49, 1992.

Donnelly M, Rapoport JL, Potter WZ, et al: Fenfluramine and dextroamphetamine treatment of childhood hyperactivity. *Arch Gen Psychiatry* 46:205–212, 1989.

Drug Interactions and Side Effects Index. Oradell, NJ, Medical Economics, 1995.

Duncan MK: Using psychostimulants to treat behavioral disorders of children and adolescents. *Child Adolesc Psychopharmacol* 1:7–20, 1990.

Effron AS, Freedman AM: The treatment of behavioral disorders in children with Benadryl. *J Pediatr* 42:261–266, 1953.

Evans RW, Clay TH, Gualtieri CT: Carbamazepine in pediatric psychiatry. *J Am Acad Child Adolesc Psychiatry* 26:2–8, 1987.

Famularo R, Kinscherff R, Fenton T: Propranolol treatment for childhood posttraumatic stress disorder, acute type. *Am J Dis Child* 142:1244–1247, 1988.

Feighner JP, Cohen JB: Analysis of individual symptoms in generalized anxiety—A pooled, multistudy double-blind evaluation of buspirone. 1. *Neuropsychobiology* 21:124–130, 1989.

Fish B: Drug therapy in child psychiatry: Pharmacological aspects. *Compr Psychiatry* 1:212–227, 1960.

Flament MF, Rapoport JL, Berg CJ, et al: Clomipramine treatment of childhood obsessive-compulsive disorder: A double-blind controlled study. *Arch Gen Psychiatry* 42:977–983, 1985.

Flament MF, Rapoport JL, Murphy DL, et al: Biochemical changes during clomipramine treatment of childhood obsessive-compulsive disorder. *Arch Gen Psychiatry* 44:219–225, 1987.

Fras I: Trazodone and violence (letter to the editor). *J Am Acad Child Adolesc Psychiatry* 26:453, 1987.

Fritz GK, Rockney RM, Yeung AS: Plasma levels and efficacy of imipramine treatment for enuresis. *J Am Acad Child Adolesc Psychiatry* 33:60–64, 1994.

Geller B, Cooper TB, Chestnut EC, et al: Child and adolescent nortriptyline single-dose kinetics predict steady-state plasma levels and suggested dose: Preliminary data. *J Clin Psychopharmacol* 5:154–158, 1985.

Geller B, Cooper TB, Chestnut EC, et al: Preliminary data on the relationship between nortriptyline plasma level and response in depressed children. *Am J Psychiatry* 143:1283–1286, 1986.

Geller B, Cooper TB, Graham DL, et al: Double-blind placebo-controlled study of nortriptyline in depressed adolescents using a "fixed plasma level" design. *Psychopharmacol Bull* 26:85–90, 1990.

Geller B, Cooper TB, McCombs HG, et al: Double-blind placebo-controlled study of nortriptyline in depressed children using a "fixed plasma level" design. *Psychopharmacol Bull* 25:101–108, 1989.

Geller B, Cooper TB, Schluchter MD, et al: Child and adolescent nortriptyline single dose pharmacokinetic parameters: Final report. *J Clin Psychopharmacol* 7:321–323, 1987.

Geller B, Guttmacher LB, Bleeg M: Coexistence of childhood onset pervasive developmental disorder and attention deficit disorder with hyperactivity. *Am J Psychiatry* 138:388–389, 1981.

Ghaziuddin N, Alessi NE: An open clinical trial of trazodone in aggressive children. *J Child Adolesc Psychopharmacol* 2:291–297, 1992.

Glick BS, Schulman D, Turecki S: Diazepam (Valium) treatment in childhood sleep disorder. *Dis Nerv Syst* 32:565–566, 1971.

Green WH: Psychosocial dwarfism: Psychological and etiological considerations. In: Lahey BB, Kazdin AE (eds): *Advances in Clinical Child Psychology* (Vol 9). New York, Plenum, 1986, pp. 245–278.

Green WH: Schizophrenia with childhood onset. In: Kaplan HI, Sadock BJ (eds): *Comprehensive Textbook of Psychiatry* (5th ed). Baltimore, Williams & Wilkins, 1989, pp. 1975–1981.

Green WH: *Child and Adolescent Clinical Psychopharmacology* (2nd ed). Baltimore, Williams & Wilkins, 1995a.

Green WH: The treatment of attention-deficit hyperactivity disorder with nonstimulant medications. *Child Adolesc Psychiatr Clin North Am* 4:169–195, 1995b.

Green WH, Deutsch SI, Campbell M, et al: Neuropsychopharmacology of the childhood psychoses: A critical review. In: Morgan DW (ed): *Psychopharmacology: Impact on Clinical Psychiatry.* St. Louis, Ishiyaku EuroAmerica, 1985, pp. 139–173.

Green WH, Padron-Gayol M, Hardesty A, et al: Schizophrenia with childhood onset: A phenomenological study of 38 cases. *J Am Acad Child Adolesc Psychiatry* 31:968–976, 1992.

Greenblatt DJ, Shader RI: *Benzodiazepines in Clinical Practice.* New York, Raven Press, 1974.

Greenblatt DJ, Shader RI, Abernethy DR: Current status of benzodiazepines (I). *N Engl J Med* 309:354–358, 1983.

Grizenko N, Vida S: Propranolol treatment of episodic dyscontrol and aggressive behavior in children (letter to the editor). *Can J Psychiatry* 33:776–778, 1988.

Groh C: The psychotropic effect of Tegretol in non-epileptic children, with particular reference to the drug's indications. In: Birkmayer W (ed): *Epileptic Seizures—Behaviour—Pain.* Bern, Hans Huber, 1976, pp. 259–263.

Gross MB, Wilson WC: *Minimal Brain Dysfunction.* New York, Brunner/Mazel, 1974.

Gualtieri CT, Quade D, Hicks RE, et al: Tardive dyskinesia and other clinical consequences of neuroleptic treatment in children and adolescents. *Am J Psychiatry* 141:20–23, 1984.

Gualtieri CT, Wafgin W, Kanoy R, et al: Clinical studies of methylphenidate serum levels in children and adults. *J Am Acad Child Psychiatry* 21:19–26, 1982.

Hamill PVV, Drizd TA, Johnson CL, et al: *N.C.H.S. Growth Charts, 1976* (Monthly Vital Statistics Reports, Health Examination Survey Data, National Center for Health Statistics Publication [HRA] 76-1120). 25(suppl 3):1–22, 1976.

Hayes PE, Schulz SC: Beta-blockers in anxiety disorders. *J Affect Disord* 13:119–130, 1987.

Hunt RD: Treatment effects of oral and transdermal clonidine in relation to methylphenidate: An open pilot study in ADD-H. *Psychopharmacol Bull* 23:111–114, 1987.

Hunt RD, Cohen DJ, Shaywitz SE, et al: Strategies for study of the neurochemistry of attention deficit disorder in children. *Schizophr Bull* 8:236–252, 1982.

Hunt RD, Minderaa RB, Cohen DJ: Clonidine benefits children with attention deficit disorder and hyperactivity: Report of a double-blind placebo-crossover therapeutic trial. *J Am Acad Child Psychiatry* 24:617–629, 1985.

Jerome L: Hypomania with fluoxetine (letter). *J Am Acad Child Adolesc Psychiatry* 30:850–851, 1991.

Johnston C, Pelham WE, Hoza J, et al: Psychostimulant rebound in attention deficit disordered boys. *J Am Acad Child Adolesc Psychiatry* 27:806–810, 1988.

Joshi PT, Walkup JT, Capozzoli JA, et al: The use of fluoxetine in the treatment of major depressive disorder in children and adolescents. Paper presented at the 36th Annual Meeting of the American Academy of Child and Adolescent Psychiatry, New York, October 11–15, 1989.

Kafantaris V, Campbell M, Padron-Gayol MV, et al: Carbamazepine in hospitalized aggressive conduct disorder children: An open pilot study. *Psychopharmacol Bull* 28:193–199, 1992.

Kashani JH, Shekim WO, Reid JC: Amitriptyline in children with major depressive disorder: A double-blind crossover pilot study. *J Am Acad Child Psychiatry* 23:348–351, 1984.

Kessler AJ, Barklaye NE, Jefferson JW: Mood disorders in the psychoneurologic borderland: Three cases of responsiveness to carbamazepine. *Am J Psychiatry* 146:81–83, 1989.

King RA, Riddle MA, Chappell PB, et al: Emergence of self-destructive phenomena in children and adolescents during fluoxetine treatment. *J Am Acad Child Adolesc Psychiatry* 30:179–186, 1991.

Klein DF, Gittelman R, Quitkin F, et al: *Diagnosis and Drug Treatment of Psychiatric Disorders: Adults and Children.* Baltimore, Williams & Wilkins, 1980.

Klein RG, Mannuzza S: Hyperactive boys almost grown up. III: Methylphenidate effects on ultimate height. *Arch Gen Psychiatry* 45:1131–1134, 1988.

Klein RG, Landa B, Mattes JA, et al: Methylphenidate and growth in hyperactive children: A controlled withdrawal study. *Arch Gen Psychiatry* 45:1127–1130, 1988.

Kline AH: Diazepam and the management of nocturnal enuresis. *Clin Med* 75:20–22, 1968.

Korein J, Fish B, Shapiro T, et al: EEG and behavioral effects of drug therapy in children: Chlorpromazine and diphenhydramine. *Arch Gen Psychiatry* 24:552–563, 1971.

Kranzler HR: Use of buspirone in an adolescent with overanxious disorder. *J Am Acad Child Adolesc Psychiatry* 27:789–790, 1988.

Kuhn-Gebhart V: Behavioural disorders in non-epileptic children and their treatment with carbamazepine. In: Birkmayer W (ed): *Epileptic Seizures—Behaviour—Pain.* Bern, Hans Hubert, 1976, pp. 264–267.

Leckman JF, Cohen DJ, Detlor J, et al: Clonidine in the treatment of Tourette syndrome: A review of data. In: Friedhoff AJ, Chase TN (eds): *Gilles de la Tourette Syndrome.* New York, Raven Press, 1982, pp. 391–401.

Leckman JF, Detlor J, Harcherik DF, et al: Short- and long-term treatment of Tourette's syndrome with clonidine: A clinical perspective. *Neurology* 35:343–351, 1985.

Leonard HL, Swedo SE, Rapoport JL, et al: Treatment of obsessive-compulsive disorder with clomipramine and desipramine in children and adolescents: A double-blind crossover comparison. Arch Gen Psychiatry 46:1088–1092, 1989.

Mattes JA, Gittleman R: Growth of hyperactive children on maintenance regimen of methylphenidate. Arch Gen Psychiatry 40:317–321, 1983.

Mozes T, Toren P, Chernauzan N, et al: Clozapine treatment in very early onset schizophrenia. J Am Acad Child Adolesc Psychiatry 33:65–70, 1994.

Noyes R: Beta-adrenergic blockers. In: Last CG, Hersen M (eds): Handbook of Anxiety Disorders. New York, Pergamon, 1988, pp. 445–459.

Patrick KS, Mueller RA, Gualtieri CT, et al: Pharmacokinetics and actions of methylphenidate. In: Meltzer HY (ed): Psychopharmacology: The Third Generation of Progress. New York, Raven Press, 1987, pp. 1387–1395.

Perry R, Campbell M, Green WH, et al: Neuroleptic-related dyskinesias in autistic children: A prospective study. Psychopharmacol Bull 21:140–143, 1985.

Pesikoff RB, David PC: Treatment of pavor nocturnus and somnambulism in children. Am J Psychiatry 128:778–781, 1971.

Physicians' Desk Reference (49th ed). Oradell, NJ, Medical Economics, 1995.

Platt JE, Campbell M, Green WH, et al: Cognitive effect of lithium carbonate and haloperidol in treatment resistant aggressive children. Arch Gen Psychiatry 41:657–662, 1984.

Post RM: Mechanisms of action of carbamazepine and related anticonvulsants in affective illness. In: Meltzer HY (ed): Psychopharmacology: The Third Generation of Progress. New York, Raven Press, 1987, pp. 567–576.

Psychopharmacology Bulletin. Special issue. US Department of Health, Education, and Welfare pub. no. (HSM) 73-9002, 1973.

Puente RM: The use of carbamazepine in the treatment of behavioural disorders in children. In: Birkmayer W (ed): Epileptic Seizures—Behaviour—Pain. Bern, Hans Huber, 1976, pp. 243–252.

Puig-Antich J, Perel JM, Lupatkin W, et al: Imipramine in prepubertal major depressive disorders. Arch Gen Psychiatry 44:81–89, 1987.

Quiason H, Ward D, Kitchen T: Buspirone for aggression (letter to the editor). J Am Acad Child Adolesc Psychiatry 30:1026, 1991.

Rapoport JL, Buchsbaum MS, Weingartner H, et al: Dextroamphetamine: Its cognitive and behavioral effects in normal and hyperactive boys and normal men. Arch Gen Psychiatry 37:933–943, 1980a.

Rapoport JL, Buchsbaum MS, Zahn TP, et al: Dextroamphetamine: Cognitive and behavioral effects in normal prepubertal boys. Science 199:560–563, 1978.

Rapoport JL, Mikkelsen EJ, Werry JS: Antimanic, antianxiety, hallucinogenic and miscellaneous drugs. In: Werry JS (ed): Pediatric Psychopharmacology: The Use of Behavior Modifying Drugs in Children. New York, Brunner/Mazel, 1978, pp. 316–355.

Rapoport JL, Mikkelsen EJ, Zavadil A, et al: Childhood enuresis: Psychopathology, plasma tricyclic concentration and antienuretic effect. Arch Gen Psychiatry 37:1146–1152, 1980b.

Rating scales and assessment instruments for use in pediatric psychopharmacology research. Psychopharmacol Bull 21:713–1124, 1985.

Ratey JJ, Sovner R, Mikkelsen E, et al: Buspirone therapy for maladaptive behavior and anxiety in developmentally disabled persons. J Clin Psychiatry 50:382–384, 1989.

Ratey J, Sovner R, Parks A, et al: Buspirone treatment of aggression and anxiety in mentally retarded patients: A multiple-baseline, placebo lead-in study. J Clin Psychiatry 52:159–162, 1991.

Realmuto GM, August GJ, Garfinkel BD: Clinical effect of buspirone in autistic children. J Clin Psychopharmacol 99:122–125, 1989.

Remschmidt H: The psychotropic effect of carbamazepine in non-epileptic patient, with particular reference to problems posed by clinical studies in children with behavioural disorders. In: Birkmayer W (ed): Epileptic Seizures—Behaviour—Pain. Bern, Hans Huber, 1976, pp. 253–258.

Riddle MA, Geller B, Ryan N: Another sudden death in a child treated with desipramine. J Am Acad Child Adolesc Psychiatry 32:792–797, 1993.

Riddle MA, Hardin MT, King R, et al: Fluoxetine treatment of children and adolescents with Tourette's and obsessive-compulsive disorders: Preliminary clinical experience. J Am Acad Child Adolesc Psychiatry 29:45–48, 1990.

Riddle MA, King RA, Hardin MT, et al: Behavioral side effects of fluoxetine in children and adolescents. J Child Adolesc Psychopharmacol 1:193–198, 1990/1991.

Riddle MA, Scahill L, King RA, et al: Double-blind, crossover trial of fluoxetine and placebo in children and adolescents with obsessive-compulsive disorder. J Am Acad Child Adolesc Psychiatry 31:1062–1069, 1992.

Ryan ND, Puig-Antich J, Cooper T, et al: Imipramine in adolescent major depression: Plasma level and clinical response. Acta Psychiatr Scand 73:275–288, 1986.

Safer DJ, Krager M: A survey of medication treatment for hyperactive/inattentive students. JAMA 260:2256–2258, 1988.

Safer D, Allen RP, Barr E: Depression of growth in hyperactive children on stimulant drugs. N Engl J Med 287:217–220, 1972.

Sandler SB: What psychotropic drugs can—and can't—do for your patients. Contemp Pediatr 120–122; 127–130; 132, 134–136, March 1993.

Schmidt MH, Trott G-E, Blanz B, et al: Clozapine medication in adolescents. In: Stefania CN, Rabavilas AD, Soldatos CR (eds): Psychiatry: A World Perspective (Vol 1). Proceedings of the VIII World Congress of Psychiatry. Amsterdam, Excerpta Medica, 1990, pp. 1100–1104.

Shapiro AK, Shapiro E: Tic disorders. In: Kaplan HI, Sadock BJ (eds): Comprehensive Textbook of Psychiatry (5th ed). Baltimore, Williams & Wilkins, 1989, pp. 1865–1878.

Siefen G, Remschmidt H: Behandlungsergebnisse mit Clozapin bei schizophrenen Jugendlichen [Clozapine in the treatment of adolescents with schizophrenia: Treatment outcome]. Z Kinder Jugendpsychiatr 14:245–257, 1986. (English translation by the Ralph McElroy Co., provided by the manufacturer.)

Simeon JG, Ferguson HB: Recent developments in the use of antidepressant and anxiolytic medications. Psychiatr Clin North Am 8:893–907, 1985.

Simeon JG, Dinicola VF, Ferguson HB, et al: Adolescent depression: A placebo-controlled fluoxetine treatment study and follow-up. Prog Neuropsychopharmacol Biol Psychiatry 14:791–795, 1990.

Sleator ED, von Neumann A, Sprague RL: Hyperactive children: A continuous long-term placebo-controlled follow-up. JAMA 229:316–317, 1974.

Small JG, Milstein V, Marhenke JD, et al: Treatment outcome with clozapine in tardive dyskinesia, neuroleptic sensitivity, and treatment resistant psychosis. J Clin Psychiatry 48:263–267, 1987.

Spencer EK, Kafantaris V, Padron-Gayol MV, et al: Haloperidol in schizophrenic children: Early findings from a study in progress. Psychopharmacol Bull 28:183–186, 1992.

Spitzer RL, Endicott J, Robins E: Research diagnostic criteria. Arch Gen Psychiatry 335:773–782, 1978.

Stores G: Antiepileptics (anticonvulsants). In: Werry JS (ed): Pediatric Psychopharmacology: The Use of Behavior Modifying Drugs in Children. New York, Brunner/Mazel, 1978, pp. 274–315.

Strayhorn JM, Rapp N, Donina W, et al: Randomized trial of methylphenidate for an autistic child. J Am Acad Child Adolesc Psychiatry 27:244–247, 1988.

Sudden death in children treated with a tricyclic antidepressant. Med Lett 32(June 1):53, 1990.

Sussman N: The potential benefits of serotonin receptor-specific agents. J Clin Psychiatry 55(1, suppl):45–51, 1994a.

Sussman N: The uses of buspirone in psychiatry: J Clin Psychiatry Monograph 12(1):3–19, 1994b.

USPDI (United States Pharmacopeial Dispensing Information): Drug Information for the Health Care Professional. Rockville, MD, United States Pharmacopeial Convention, 1992.

Venkataraman S, Naylor MW, King CA: Mania associated with fluoxetine treatment in adolescents. J Am Acad Child Adolesc Psychiatry 31:276–281, 1992.

Walkup JT: Clinical decision making in child and adolescent psychopharmacology. Child Adolesc Psychiatr Clin North Am 4:23–40, 1995.

Weiner N: Norepinephrine, epinephrine, and the sympathomimetic amines. In: Gilman AG, Goodman LS, Gilman A (eds): Goodman and Gilman's The Pharmacological Basis of Therapeutics (6th ed). New York, Macmillan, 1980, pp. 138–175.

Weiss G, Hechtman LT: Hyperactive Children Grown Up: Empirical Findings and Theoretical Considerations. New York, Guilford, 1986.

Weller EB, Weller RA, Preskorn SH, et al: Steady-state plasma imipramine levels in prepubertal depressed children. Am J Psychiatry 139:506–508, 1982.

Wilens TE, Biederman J, Baldessarini RJ, et al: Developmental changes in serum concentrations of desipramine and 2-hydroxydesipramine during treatment with desipramine. J Am Acad Child Adolesc Psychiatry 31:691–698, 1992.

Wilens TE, Biederman J, Baldessarini RJ, et al: Electrocardiographic effects of desipramine and 2-hydroxydesipramine in children, adolescents, and adults treated with desipramine. J Am Acad Child Adolesc Psychiatry 32:798–804, 1993.

Wilens TE, Spencer T, Biederman J, et al: Combined pharmacotherapy: An emerging trend in pediatric psychopharmacology. J Am Acad Child Adolesc Psychiatry 34:110–112, 1995.

Williams DT, Mehl R, Yudofsky S, et al: The effect of propranolol on uncontrolled rage outbursts in children and adolescents with organic brain dysfunction. J Am Acad Child Psychiatry 21:129–135, 1982.

Winsberg BG, Kupietz SS, Sverd J, et al: Methylphenidate oral dose plasma concentrations and behavioral response in children. Psychopharmacology 76:329–332, 1982.

Wolf DW, Wagner KD: Tardive dyskinesia, tardive dystonia, and tardive Tourette's syndrome in children and adolescents. J Child Adolesc Psychopharmacol 3:175–198, 1993.

Zubieta JK, Alessi NE: Acute and chronic administration of trazodone in the treatment of disruptive behavioral disorders of children. J Clin Psychopharmacol 12:346–351, 1992.

73 Intensive Individual Psychodynamic Psychotherapy: The Therapeutic Relationship and the Technique of Interpretation

Melvin Lewis, M.B., B.S., F.R.C.Psych., D.C.H.

GOALS

The goals of intensive individual psychodynamic psychotherapy may include reduction of anxiety, improvement in self-esteem, increased frustration tolerance, disappearance of symptoms, better coping strategies, disappearance of symptoms, better coping strategies, appropriate independence, good relationships with peers and adults, satisfactory and satisfying schoolwork, feelings of pleasure and joy, and a sense of resumption of development.

HISTORICAL NOTE

Hermine Hug-Hellmuth, in Vienna in 1920, was the first child analyst to describe a *technique* of play in child analysis, especially in the preparatory phase, although she did not develop a concept of play in therapy. Melanie Klein, in Berlin, was the first to develop the *concept* of play in therapy and made extensive use of play with interpretation, using a wide range of small toys and wooden human figure representations. Melanie Klein read her first paper in Budapest in 1919 (Klein, 1920). David Levey presented the first American report on play therapy in 1925 (Harrison, 1980). Later, in 1927, Anna Freud repeated Hug-Hellmuth's earliest account of the elements of child analysis (McLean and Rapper, 1991). Meanwhile Freud, in 1923, had stated the essential goals for treatment: "to make the best of him [or her] that his [or her] inherent capacities will allow and so to make him [or her] as efficient and as capable of enjoyment as is possible" (Freud, 1923/1955).

GENERAL METHOD

The general method essentially involves a trusting, confidential, real relationship between a trained, motivated, caring, and accepting person who offers help to a person who needs that help. Usually there is agreement between therapist and parent about the type of theory used. Generally, opportunities are provided for the verbal expression of feelings, increasing self-knowledge, and improving self-mastery (Karasu, 1977; Langs, 1982; Paolino, 1981). The therapy is usually divided into periods of 30–50 minutes given from one to four times a week in a suitable office setting. Although numerous methods, techniques, and theories have been categorized (London, 1982) and described (Kazdin, 1988; Varma, 1974), unequivocal superiority of any one method has not been established (Luborsky et al., 1975; McDermott, 1977; Schaefer 1977; Wolman et al., 1978).

BECOMING A CHILD THERAPIST

How does one become a child therapist? First, it has to be said that neither the amount nor the kind of training are very reliable guides to the eventual effectiveness of a therapist: Highly trained psychotherapists often achieve no more with their patients than do those with much less experience (Strupp, 1979). Victor Raimy once observed that "psychotherapy is an undefined technique applied to unspecified cases with unpredictable results. For this technique, rigorous training is required" (quoted in London, 1964). Supervision and continuous case conferences with acknowledged experts are the generally accepted methods of acquiring psychotherapy skills. The amount required varies with the en-

dowment and needs of the individual psychotherapist. In a brief (8-month) longitudinal study of 12 beginning psychiatric residents, Buckley et al. (1982) found that appropriate use of clarification, confrontation, management of resistance, and the ability to deal with negative transference could be learned with supervision and experience, while the capacity for empathy and awareness of countertransference did not change during the period of the study (Buckley et al., 1982) There is some evidence that ordinary communication skills and empathic understanding can be taught very quickly (Bird, 1980; Ivey, 1980; MacGuire, 1980; Matarazzo, 1978) and that the rest is experience. There is no evidence that a personal analysis must be a part of psychotherapeutic training (Marks, 1982).

INDICATIONS

The question of when intensive individual psychodynamic psychotherapy in childhood is the treatment of choice nowadays often resolves into the question of to what degree multiple other forms of therapy are indicated and available for a particular child with a particular diagnosis. Diagnosis is thus an essential prerequisite and for this purpose must go beyond the categories of DSM-IV (American Psychiatric Association, 1994) or ICD-10 to a comprehensive developmental formulation that will provide a useful basis for treatment planning (Shapiro, 1989).

Rarely does a single form of psychiatric treatment suffice for the child. In most instances, various combinations of treatment modalities are necessary, including individual psychotherapy, pharmacotherapy, behavior therapy, family therapy, educational remedies, counseling, environmental changes, group therapy, and concomitant work with the parents. For example, multimodal treatment has been found to bring about significant improvement in children with attention deficit hyperactivity disorder (Satterfield et al., 1980). (An account of the steps in planning multimodal treatment for children and adolescents is given by Looney (1984).) Nevertheless, the same principles of psychodynamic psychotherapy are operative no matter what other treatments are required.

Pure, solitary, intensive, individual psychodynamic psychotherapy for the child alone is indicated with confidence only when the child's problem is primarily intrapsychic and there is no other known factor amenable to treatment of any other kind. Such is rarely the case. Conversely, when the child's problems are more external than internal or internalized, and other etiologic factors are recognized, one becomes less confident in the solitary use of intensive individual psychotherapy. Thus, there may also be present various current conflicts and frustrations, losses, physical illness, and other stresses, as well as other psychiatric diagnoses, that may require the addition of one or more of the previously mentioned interventions.

INTERPRETATION AS AN ESSENTIAL ELEMENT

No matter what accompanying treatments are necessary, when individual intensive or psychodynamic psychotherapy is used, the same essential elements of the process unfold, albeit modified by the age, diagnosis, and presence of these other factors, with or without the other forms of treatment. The basic requirements for psychodynamic psychotherapy for children, together with a broad description of the stages and various components of the ongoing clinical work, have been described by McDermott and Chan (1984). Brief psychotherapy with children, adolescents, and their families has been described by Dulcan (1984). This chapter focuses on the particular essential elements of interpretation in intensive individual psychodynamic psychotherapy.

Intensive individual psychodynamic psychotherapy is based largely on psychoanalysis, which specifically places great importance on interpretation (making the unconscious or preconscious conscious), particularly interpretation of the transference, as the principal therapeutic agent (Lewis, 1974). This holds true whether one is treating a preschool child (Neubauer, 1972), a school-age child (A. Freud, 1946/1950, 1968), or an adolescent (Bion, 1962) and across a wide range of diagnoses (Witmer, 1946).

Cognitive perspectives also inform psychotherapy, and some mention of cognitive-developmental and information-processing considerations are made in the sections below. (For a more comprehensive account of cognitive development and clinical applications, see Chapter 11.)

For purposes of discussion, intensive individual psychodynamic psychotherapy can be approached as a process with three major phases: initial phase, middle phase, and termination phase.

Initial Phase

THERAPEUTIC ALLIANCE

The major goal of the initial phase is to foster a therapeutic alliance between therapist and child. This goal is usually achieved by enabling the child to experience a nonjudgmental, understanding response to his or her behavior. The actual relationship is an important therapeutic agent in its own right, as well as the soil in which the seed of an interpretation may flourish. A positive actual relationship, therefore, is encouraged.

To foster a therapeutic alliance, the child must first be given some understanding by the parents of why he or she is being brought to a therapist and what therapy is like. Essentially, the child can be told that, in addition to himself or herself, others such as parents or teachers are concerned about how the child is feeling and/or behaving and that the child's parents believe the child may be troubled or upset, possibly by something he or she is not aware of.

Next, the parents may tell the child that talking with someone who understands children may help them and the child understand what may be troubling the child. The child can be told that the parents know of such a person, and the parents can describe the person, the setting, and the arrangements to the child. The child should then be encouraged to ask any questions, and the parents should be prepared to answer truthfully and accurately.

The therapist can set the scene by first seeing the child in a suitable playroom and by making sure that he or she knows by what name the child likes to be called (and that the child knows the therapist's name). The child will begin to feel understood and will also ally more with the therapy if the therapist can offer an early interpretative statement that provides the child with some insight yet does not arouse undue anxiety. In order to do this, a series of preparatory statements, including setting statements, attention statements, reductive statements, and situational statements, is useful (Lewis, 1974).

Setting Statements

A child may first be told in language appropriate to the child's developmental level that this is a time set aside for the child so that he or she can allow himself or herself to think freely and begin to understand why he or she sometimes feels troubled. The child should also be told that sometimes the therapist will intervene, but with the understanding that it will always be in the interest of helping the child understand himself or herself better.

Attention Statements

Next, the child's attention can be directed to the content of his or her actions or verbalizations. Sometimes attention is drawn to a coincidence that the child has perceived but has not, or professes not to have, registered; more frequently, attention is drawn to certain paradoxes. The immediate aim is to free the child to produce new material and to consolidate existing gains (Devereux, 1951). In the course of the child's play, the therapist may, for example, provide a verbal counterpart to the action being portrayed, to an affect that might be present, or to the conspicuous absence of certain persons, actions, or affects.

CASE ILLUSTRATION

An 8-year-old boy with a severe school phobia repeatedly enacted a war scene in which the general was attacked and almost killed. Many fantasies were contained in this play, but one prominent feature was the absence of any female, not only in this play item but in any other play. After attention was drawn to this "fact," the child recognized his fear of attack from his mother, his wish to attack her, his resentment that his father was often attacked and offered him no protection, the displacement of his aggression toward his mother to his father, and his anxiety about even mentioning his mother.

This is different from a direct translation of possible symbolic representation in the play. The play characteristic to which attention is here drawn is in bold relief and capable of being understood by the child. This point is made to draw the distinction from more subtle paradoxes, which are not readily perceived, at least not by the younger child who is in the preoperational stage of cognitive development. In fact, attention statements can be easily understood by a preoperational child since they relate to more or less concrete perceptions within the play and require only short-term memory and limited "chunking" (defined as "aggregates of related, facts, concepts, or percepts"; see Chapter 11).

Reductive Statements

Certain statements reduce apparently disparate behavioral patterns to a common form that has hitherto not been noticed by the child. Thus, a child may manifest certain kinds of behavior whenever he or she is, say, angry. The child may not have been aware of this anger.

CASE ILLUSTRATION

In the course of the treatment of a 10-year-old boy, it was noticed that there were recurring episodes of mocking, insulting, or denigrating behavior toward the therapist. Each of these episodes was related in time to one of the frequent trips away from home that the boy's mother would take. His resentment at being left behind, together with his anxiety at being left alone with his father, led to the behavior just described. This type of behavior could be reduced to a single behavioral reaction to underlying rage and anxiety precipitated by the temporary loss of his mother. When the child was told of this relationship, he reacted first of all by an intensification of the behavior pattern but subsequently was able to recognize for the first time his underlying feelings, when he stated, "My parents are always nice to me when we do fun things, but they don't help me with the serious things when I'm unhappy."

The child here was manifesting a more or less fixed defense, which, in the example given, was brought into sharper relief. A certain level (concrete operations) of cognitive development, including some capacity to take distance from and observe affects, must be available to the child for this to occur.

Situational Statements

Situational statements naturally follow from those previously described. For example, the child now aware of his or her anger can be shown the situations that give rise to this anger and how in certain instances he or she has repeatedly brought about such situations, either in current relationships or in the transference. However, the degree of directness with which such situational statements may be made varies with the emotional and cognitive levels of the child. Children who are in the oedipal or preoedipal phases and are at the preoperational stage of cognitive development probably need to have these statements made to them in the context of the play, either through dolls and puppets, or indirectly through some other hypothetical child or children. Children who are postoedipal and at the stage of concrete operations can usually be approached directly.

In the very young child, feelings seem to be almost exclusively experienced in response to an external event and seem to be viewed by the child as controlled by that external event (e.g., receiving a present produces a happy feeling, mother leaving gives rise to sad or angry feelings). Subsequently, feelings are more or less contained within the body but still not under the control of the child. Next, feelings come to be felt as part of one's self; that is, the child can conceptualize a feeling, first as a somewhat diffuse internal experience and then as multiple, different emotions that are more or less controlled as the self becomes more differentiated. During the preoperational stage, children find it difficult to experience two emotions simultaneously, perhaps because the child is still tied to the immediate perception (e.g., a drawing of a face has either a smile or a downturned mouth (Nannis, 1988)). Very shortly, children can experience opposite feelings, but at first only sequentially (e.g., happy first, sad later (Harter, 1983)). Once the child is at the concrete operational stage, achieves the operation of conservation, decenters, and is more or less freed from being tied to immediate perception, the child can then experience two opposite feelings simultaneously; that is, the child can begin to experience, understand, and tolerate ambivalence (i.e., being angry at someone one loves).

Middle Phase

The essence of the middle phase of psychotherapy is the interpretation of the transference and "working through." Notwithstanding the difficulties of the initial phase, a child soon understands one of the goals of psychotherapy: the attempt to gain an understanding of the way he or she feels and behaves. After the initial phase of treatment, the child realizes that everything he or she says and does is subject to use by the therapist. Consequently, the child's play that follows is part of the associative process in the context of therapy. In certain respects, however, the developmental difference between the child and the adult influences the form of these associations. The child is much more susceptible to current reality, which exerts a powerful influence on his or her play. The play is often goal directed and not freely associative. Again, the child has a tendency to act rather than think, giving at least the impression of an overemphasized aggressive transference (A. Freud, 1965). Further, in school-age children especially, the play is often characterized by organization, reflecting a developmental shift. Lastly, the child may become totally absorbed in his or her play and may then be unable to exercise an observing function.

At the same time, in addition to play, a child also communicates through most of the other elements that constitute "free association." That is, the child talks, pauses, shows affects, exhibits mannerisms, portrays attitudes, and moves about in space. It is this total picture, viewed as a whole over the course of several hours, that enables the therapist to discern, or infer, an associative thread. And it is this overall connection that can often be grasped by the child.

TRANSFERENCE

In the course of discerning this total picture, a true transference—that is, those previously fixed conflicts and compromise symptoms of the child that are now being experienced currently by the child in relation to the therapist (Harley, 1967) can usually be observed. Again, the developmental differences between child and adult modify, but do not eradicate, this emerging transference in three ways: First, to the extent that the child is normally dependent, the parents with whom the original conflict was concerned are still with the child and continue to exert their influence on the child. Second, the child is not an equal of the therapist; he or she is still a child relating to an adult as well as a patient relating to a therapist. Thus, besides the mutual respect that should exist between patient and therapist, the child also has certain expectations of the adult, such as appropriate birthday and holiday greetings and gifts (Temeles, 1967). Third, the continuing development of the child continues to modify the transference, especially during shifts from the oedipal to postoedipal and eventually adolescent stages. In addition, fixations that occurred earlier may be modified with the increased range, flexibility, and shifts of defenses that occur with the development of the child.

For all these reasons, the transference in child psychotherapy is incomplete and more unstable than the transference in the therapy of an adult. Nevertheless, to the extent that there is a transference, however modified, it is available for interpretation. The more common situation in work with children is one in which a relatively simple current displacement from parent to therapist is recognized and interpreted. Even within such apparently simple displacements, however, elements of a transference can be found, and when they are interpreted, they throw light on the child's current behavior.

RECONSTRUCTION

Linking the complexities of the child's current behavior with his or her earlier fantasies may be helpful to the child. This earlier material may be derived from the personal myth of the child or may be hypothesized from reconstruction. The striking aspect of a reconstruction is that it helps the child "make sense' out of what was previously discomforting and/or perplexing. Further, it occasionally helps a child by confirming what was probably an essentially correct perception by the child at the time, but which has since undergone distortion. The conceptual abilities of the child are such that the child often attributes affects the child thinks he or she perceives in the parents as resulting from thoughts or wishes of his or her own. Further, the child frequently projects his or her own fantasies and affects onto the parents and subsequently acts against the parents, whom the child now regards as, say, dangerous or angry. At the same time, reconstructions are sometimes barely tolerated by the child when the child is still close to the reconstructed period. The preoperational child too may have particular difficulty in distinguishing fantasies from reality (Piaget, 1929). On the other hand, the child who is at the stage of concrete operations may have particularly strong defenses—specifically, various reaction formations, such as guilt against aggressive impulses, shame about exhibitionistic urges, and disgust when regressive impulses become threatening—and may accordingly develop a resistance to any exploration of anxiety-arousing impulses.

PROCESS OF INTERPRETATION

Some further general points on the process of making an interpretation may now be considered. Loewenstein (1951), whose account would have been more complete had he placed greater emphasis on the interpretation of unconscious, or at least preconscious, material, described the following steps:

1. Show the patient that certain common elements exist in a series of events.
2. Point out the similar behavior of the patient in each of these situations.
3. Demonstrate that such behavior was manifested in circumstances that all involved, for example, competitive elements, and where rivalry might have been expected.
4. Point out that (say) rivalry does exist unconsciously but is replaced by another kind of behavior, such as (say) avoiding competition.

5. Show that this behavior originates in certain critical events of the patient's life and encompasses reactions and tendencies that can be grouped together.

In the stages just outlined, the interpretation of mechanism, as opposed to that of content or affect, is significant. Further, it can also be seen that there is a gradual transition from preparatory intervention, through confrontation, to an interpretation containing a genetic component. Ferenczi once described his own experiences as he proceeded in the steps just outlined: "One allows oneself to be influenced by the free associations of the patient; simultaneously one permits one's own imagination to play on these associations; intermittently one compares new connections that appear with previous products . . .without, for a moment, losing sight of, regard for, and criticism of one's own biases" (quoted in Kris, 1951).

Essentially, one might speak of an interactive process in the therapist involving empathy, self-observation, and clinical judgment.

The description given by Erikson (1940) is remarkably similar. Speculations are first derived from the observer's impressions, associations, and recollections, for example, "It was as if . . . ." The observer also associates past impressions in the same child, from other children, or from data derived from the parents. The therapist reflects on the latent possibilities that the associations may possibly correspond to a genetic or associative connection in the child's mind and pictures what the child is doing under the observer's eyes and what the child is said to have done in other situations. This all leads up to the interpretation. Erikson then describes three steps in making the interpretation. First, there are observations, feelings, and reflections that lead to interpretational hints. For example, a symbolic equation or metaphor may make it possible to recognize a play act as alluding to and standing for an otherwise manifestly avoided item (a person, an object, an idea), or a play arrangement may prove to represent a special effort on the part of the child to rearrange in effigy his or her psychological position in an experienced or expected danger situation. Such an arrangement usually corresponds to the child's defense mechanisms. Second, these hints are then subject to further observations and reflections and emerge as a conviction in the observer's mind in the form of the reconstruction of a genetic sequence or of a dynamic configuration pertaining to the patient's inner or outer history. Finally, the therapist may proceed to convey part of these reconstructions to the child whenever the therapist feels the time has come to do so. Erikson considers the last step to be the therapeutic interpretation.

The significant point here is the step-by-step progression in working with children implied in Erikson's statement that "the observer may proceed to convey parts of these reconstructions to the child whenever he feels the time has come to do so" (Erikson, 1940). However, it is important to keep in mind here the developmental level of the child, since massive interpretations given to a young child are more likely to be heard as interfering noises than helpful statements, with a consequent heightening of resistance and play disruption or, worse, a play inhibition.

In short, the therapist, while still engaging with the child, takes mental distance from the immediate transaction and tries to place the immediate observations into the context of what has previously taken place. The therapist can do this by a kind of mental "playback." Material from previous sessions is not only "played back" mentally, but is also translated to a higher level of abstraction, which enables the therapist to formulate to himself or herself "what is going on" as a basis for formulating an interpretation. The therapist then mentally translates this back to the level of the child and the immediate situation and makes his or her interpretation at that level.

GENERAL GUIDELINES FOR INTERPRETATION

Multiple Appeal

As a general rule, interpretations are probably more effective when they have "multiple appeal" (Hartman, 1951). The therapist also decides clinically when to interpret the past, current reality, the transference, or all three.

Sequence

A number of other guidelines for the order of interpretation have been suggested. Resistances or defenses should be interpreted before the instinctual derivatives (Loewenstein, 1951). One should defer interpreting a symptom representing an important unconscious conflict until a strong therapeutic alliance has been established. One should also start with interpretation of still-mobile defense traits in preference to rigid, characterologic defenses. In spite of these guidelines, individual situations may be handled in several different ways, depending on the developmental level of the child and the stage of therapy. Take, for example, the following situation: An 8-year-old boy wanted to take along some tracing paper belonging to his therapist on the eve of his going on a car trip with his mother and father, the anticipation of which had already aroused considerable anxiety.

What were the possibilities here for interpretation?

1. The therapist could simply have confronted the child with his wish to take something along. At the particular stage in the therapy of this child, however, this would have been redundant, although it might have been useful as a building block, or an "attention statement" for future use.
2. The therapist could have shown the child how anxious he was about the trip with his parents, but doing so might have forced the child to face his anxiety too abruptly, with insufficient time for "working through" (see below), and without the therapist's ongoing support.
3. The therapist might conceivably have tried to link this wish with the boy's reactions in other similar situations in which he had become anxious, but this could not be done without the previous steps.
4. The therapist might also have interpreted the patient's wishes toward the therapist for protection, but in this patient such a move might have left the patient feeling exposed and defenseless.
5. The therapist might have made the connection for the child between this coming event and earlier events in his life, but this intervention might have had little use for this particular patient, since he did not yet have a clear idea of his feelings about the coming event.
6. It might then be asked whether anything should be said at all. Something should be said, but something that will temporarily buttress the child and offer support, at the same time that both the defense and the fear are being interpreted. For example, the therapist could say to the child, "How nice it will be to have something to take along, especially if you are worried about the trip." There would be no need to interpret the positive transference aspect at this point, since the movement is in a forward direction. The therapist might also decide to include an aspect of the transference, but in a supportive way. The therapist might say, for example, "I think you would like to have something of mine with you on this trip." He might then allow the child to keep the paper and reserve for a later date any further exploration of the act: "Why don't you take the paper with you? When you come back we can talk again about how you feel when you have to take a trip with your mother and father."

These examples are not meant to be recommendations of specific things to say but rather illustrations of underlying principles. The choice of level and wording depends on such factors as the diagnosis, the stage of the therapy, and the developmental level of the child. A 6-year-old child at the beginning of psychotherapy might experience his or her anxiety on the eve of such a trip as ego-syntonic and fail to understand an interpretation of the anxiety. On the other hand, a 10-year-old who was more advanced in therapy might well experience such anxiety as inappropriate and ego-alien and might find such an interpretation useful.

Timing

An interpretation is probably well timed when the therapist thinks that the statement at that moment will help to consolidate existing gains and elicit new material (Devereux, 1951). Devereux described an interpretation as being "timely" when it is capable of being utilized by the patient, and this in turn can occur only if the patient understands it.

Focus of Interpretation

When should an interpretation be made in the play, and when should it be taken out of the play? When attention statements are made, the interpretations are clearly made "in the play." Reductive statements imply that the child is receptive to statements about himself or herself, that is, "out of the play," while transference interpretations in their most effective form are made quite distinctly "out of the play," given the earlier steps of preparation. (The use of play in psychotherapy with children has been extensively described in Chapter 74 and elsewhere (Beiser, 1979; Buxbaum, 1954; Haworth, 1964; McDermott and Harrison, 1977; Winnicott, 1971)).

Tact

Tact is required when significant developmental differences are considered. A young child may have great difficulty in tolerating ambivalence and may find it especially difficult to accept a hostile or aggressive wish or fantasy. This reluctance may be overcome by placing within a fuller context the anger, say, that is to be interpreted. For example, one might more tactfully say to a child, "It is very hard to be angry at someone you love."

Glover (1930) tried to be more specific with regard to tact, stating that the interpretation should be delivered as a plain statement in terms devoid of active emotional stress, to prevent an immediate, overwhelming conscious conviction on the patient's part that his or her therapist was in a state of countertransference. Glover also cautioned about the use of wit, the exploitation of the comic, and the shelter provided by technical expressions. It is usually preferable to refer to the child's parents as "mother" or "father." Only with a very young child would one use such terms as "mommy" and "daddy," and then only because they are developmentally appropriate.

Wording

Wording should be specific and concrete; the interpretation should also be worded to fit the individual situation. Again, the therapist is cautioned to avoid using the same defense mechanism as the patient uses, for example, laughing things off and minimizing them. Interpretations appear to gain when they contain an element of time, for example, "now," "before," "at the age of" "after this happened."

Wording is particularly critical with young children, not only from the point of view of the level of cognitive development but also from the point of view of what the child can accept in his or her dependent position with respect to the parents and of the child's own struggle against regressive pulls or progressive pushes. The child attaches greater meaning to certain words than does the adult, and it becomes necessary for the therapist to understand these special meanings.

Inexact and Incomplete Interpretation

Glover (1930) distinguished between inexact and incomplete interpretations in psychoanalysis. An incomplete interpretation was termed by Glover a "preliminary interpretation." For example, one would interpret a so-called genital fantasy before an anal fantasy. He contrasted this with an inexact interpretation, when one might never interpret the anal fantasy at all. That is to say, if the interpretation of the genital fantasy was regarded as the complete interpretation, then the interpretation was ipso facto inexact.

An interpretation is never complete until the immediate defensive reactions following on the interpretations are subjected to investigation. The complete interpretation is really the complete treatment: "Every construction is an incomplete one. . . . As a rule he (the patient) will not give his assent until he has learnt the whole truth—which often covers a very great deal of ground" (Freud, 1937/1964).

COUNTERTRANSFERENCE

In work with children, the therapist is particularly prone to countertransference phenomena. For example, there is a much greater "regressive pull" (Bornstein, 1948). The therapist must learn to recognize the feelings aroused in himself or herself so that he or she can deal with the child in a way that is helpful. One's own feelings are a vital instrument for understanding the child. At the same time, if the therapist is not aware of, or not clear about, the nature of his or her aroused feelings and their sources (both external and internal), he or she may be hampered in working effectively with the child. Indications that countertransference feelings may be at work include the following:

1. The therapist may fail to recognize where a child is in his or her development. Expectations will then not be commensurate with the child's maturational and developmental capacities. Unrealistic goals, alternating with despair, may then be experienced by the therapist.

2. The regressive pull experienced by the therapist playing and working with a child may give rise to the temptation to identify, compete, and/or act out with the child, or infantilization of the child may occur.

3. A misreading of the child's relationship to the therapist may occur, in which the relationship is seen as realistic when in fact it may be a transference from the child's feelings toward his or her parents. Therapists are usually well aware of a child's aggressive feelings but may be less aware of a child's seductiveness toward an adult (parent).

4. Remnants of the therapist's own childhood relations with his or her brothers and sisters may be an important source of the therapist's ambivalence to the child. For example, excessive concern—or lack of concern—for a child's climbing on a chair or approaching a tall column of heavy building blocks may mask an underlying wish that the child will hurt himself or herself and may be associated with guilt feelings when the child does stumble or fall. Such a feeling of guilt may come about because of the partial unsuspected fulfillment of an unacceptable wish.

5. The stirring up of old conflicts within the therapist, when exposed to certain behavior in the child, may cause anxiety in the therapist. For example, uncontrolled aggression, sex play, or masturbation may be upsetting to the therapist.

6. Sometimes the therapist may transfer old feelings from his or her own childhood onto the parents of the child. The therapist may then overidentify with the child in his or her struggle with his or her parents. Rescue fantasies may then occur. Conversely, the therapist may erroneously identify with the parents (perhaps through an identification with the aggressor mechanism) and consequently exercise unnecessary, even punitive, controls against the child who is acting too aggressively or sexually for the therapist's comfort.

7. Sometimes the therapist simply cannot understand the meaning of certain behavior in a child. Of course, there are times when all of us find some item or other of behavior inexplicable. However, the persistent drawing of a blank in understanding a repeated item of behavior should lead to the suspicion of an interference by one's own conflicts—an emotional blind spot, so to speak.

8. A therapist may find himself or herself feeling depressed or uneasy during his or her work with children. Assuming the therapist is not suffering from a true depression, the possibility exists that emotions from old conflicts have been aroused and are interfering with the therapist's functioning. Occasionally, a therapist may find himself or herself aroused and experiencing great affection for a child. This too may interfere with his or her work with the child.

9. Countertransference may be at work when the therapist permits, or even encourages, acting out in the child; for example, a therapist may suggest to a child that he or she must stand up for himself or herself and hit back. On occasion a therapist may even feel the impulse to act out with a child.

10. A therapist may need and solicit the admiration obtained by having the child like him or her. This too may represent a deeper, unconscious need of the therapist and may not be in the best interest of the child.
11. Conversely, repeated arguing with a child may suggest that the therapist has not only become involved but has become enmeshed with the child.
12. Recurring countertransference problems commonly arise in relation to specific characteristics of a child. For example, a retarded child may evoke guilt and defenses against such guilt within the therapist, or omnipotent rescue fantasies, both of which may then be acted out. Passive, hostile children may arouse anger in a therapist. Aggressive children may evoke counteraggression. Sexually attractive children and adolescents of the same or opposite sex as the therapist may threaten the therapist, leading to either vicarious and "excessive" exploitation of sexual issues or denial and avoidance.

WORKING THROUGH

It is clear that working through is necessary to sustain any therapeutic effect (Greenacre, 1956). The defensive conflicts remain somewhat structured unless they are dealt with repetitively in relation to various behaviors, events, and feelings. Historically, working through was first emphasized from the point of view of being of educative value and compared with mourning and the progressive detachment of the individual libido from the organized tensions and aims that permeated the later life. This view is insufficient.

Another concept, that of the corrective emotional experience, is really an aspect of working through, at least in its more modern construction. Originally, the idea involved replenishment of earlier deficiencies through the current relationship. This appealing idea unfortunately proved to be too simplistic. Among other things, it failed to take into account the power of the unconscious repetition compulsion. The concept has some merit, however, if it is modified to provide the child in the here-and-now with a reaction different from his or her previous experiences, a reaction that is now more appropriate and does not perpetuate the malignant interactions to which he or she has become accustomed. This update of the concept is of course consonant with the concept of working through. Finally, with the rise of ego psychology, the recognition of the need for consistent work with the patterns of defense and the affects related to them once more becomes paramount (Bornstein, 1948).

From a developmental point of view, working through with children poses a special problem. The chief difficulty lies in the fact that the live parents are usually present and may continue to exert a reinforcing influence upon the child's original conflicts. Sometimes this interference can be alleviated by concomitant work with the parents, through some form of psychotherapy or through regular meetings between the parents and the child's therapist. Occasionally, it becomes clear that the child cannot work through a conflict while in the home, and an alternative plan may become necessary, such as boarding school in the case of an older child. Sometimes the difficulty is insuperable at the time, and the therapy must be interrupted until the child is in a more advantageous situation for therapy. Occasionally, it is possible to hold the child in therapy until such a situation occurs. In some instances the child can be helped to understand the repetitive and reinforcing behavior of the parents and his or her involvement in precipitating or responding to their behavior. If the influence of the parents is not too strong, the child can be helped to modify his or her own behavior in this regard, to interrupt the vicious cycle.

Termination Phase

The criteria for termination ideally include some actual achievement (as opposed to a "flight into health" (Train, 1953)) of the goals of therapy: reduced anxiety, improved self-esteem, increased frustration tolerance, disappearance of symptoms, better coping strategies, relative independence, good relationships with peers and adults, satisfying schoolwork, feelings of pleasure and joy, and a sense of resumed developmental progress.

In almost every instance, these achievements are judged clinically rather than measured scientifically. Clinically, there is no such thing as a perfect therapy (or for that matter, a perfect patient or therapist). Every therapy eventually stops, and when it does the child should be more or less along the road toward these laudable goals. A child may even have gained a better understanding of himself or herself and may no longer need to act out so much of his or her infantile longings, frustrations, and feelings, and may have learned instead more adaptive ways, say, to love and be loved. But in some cases, the therapy simply stops because there is a sense of diminishing returns, the resistances are too great, the treatment is inappropriate, or for various other reasons the treatment is a failure. In one survey of terminated analytic cases (N = 49), only 14% terminated by mutual agreement among parent, therapist, and child (A. Freud, 1971).

The actual phase of termination is a useful period to explore issues of separation, reactions to loss, dependency versus independence, and anxiety about progressive developmental movements. Some children undergo a temporary regression, manifested by a reappearance of their presenting symptoms, in the face of leaving the therapist and returning, as it were, to the family. Others are able to "reconstruct" and recall the beginning of their treatment rather than reenact it through regressive behavior. Depending on the frequency, duration, and intensity of the psychotherapy, a reasonable period of time is required to deal with these issues. Thus, when the question of whether to terminate has been decided, preferably by mutual agreement, a termination date is set that will allow a suitable amount of time for the termination phase. This period may vary from 6 weeks to 3 months or so.

Follow-up communication is often helpful in consolidating the work of the termination phase.

THERAPEUTIC ACTION AND THEORY

Many attempts have been made to describe the therapeutic effects of interpretation in terms of the insight achieved (Rothstein, 1989). However, children (and adults) may achieve insight yet fail to improve emotionally or behaviorally. Further, some children (and adults) may show remarkable improvement without any evidence of insight at all. This latter phenomenon suggests other therapeutic modes may be at work, including the beneficial effects of a loving, compassionate, respectful, and dedicated relationship, the child's feeling of being understood, and the enlightening feeling that may result from new, positive life experiences.

The particular type of interpretation that will produce a so-called therapeutic insight, that is, a structural change, has been given different names, as has the actual therapeutic insight. For example, "transference" (Fenichel, 1945) or "mutative" (Strachey, 1934) interpretations may produce "emotional," "psychological," "ostensive" (Richfield, 1954), or "dynamic" insights as opposed to "intellectual," "descriptive," or "neutral" (Reid, 1952) insights. The significant point presumably is that shifts from unconscious to conscious awareness are thought to occur only after derivatives of the original feeling are recognized with an experiential sense of conviction and worked through. Bergler (1945) considered that the whole process of working through is centered chiefly in the correct handling and mobilization of the feeling of guilt. Devereux (1951) felt that an interpretation (which consists of supplying an unconscious closure element) is effective when practically all conscious and preconscious material pertaining to the neurotic gestalt has been produced. Loewenstein (1951) believed that the therapeutic effect is due to a psychic process in which each of the following parts has its respective place: (*a*) the overcoming of resistances, (*b*) the working through, (*c*) the remembering and reliving of repressed material, and (*d*) the effect of the reconstruction.

Anticipated changes resulting from psychotherapy are also to some extent a function of normal development. Therefore, all of the factors that facilitate normal development will also facilitate the desired changes in psychotherapy.

The experience with the psychotherapist not only is a corrective one but also represents an oasis phenomenon for the child, who now finds himself or herself, at least temporarily, in a relatively protected, facilitating environment that enables development to proceed by reducing the impact of trauma and the acting-out tendencies in the child. Another way of putting this is to say that the child in psychotherapy finds himself or herself, at least momentarily, at a distance from the acute upset of the current developmental turmoil, whether it be a too exciting, sexualized relationship with a parent, a sadomasochistic relationship with a parent, a grief reaction at the birth of a sibling, or frightening fantasies of bodily harm.

The child is also afforded an opportunity for confirmation of his or her essentially correct perception of his or her parents, leading to a strengthening of reality testing and an increase in self-esteem. The play of the child, as well as the use of words, inasmuch as they represent an intermediate stage between action and thought, provides a handle by which the child grasps affects and is enabled to delay. Most important, the play itself undergoes a development that carries with it a significant shift from primary process to secondary process.

The dyadic therapeutic relationship provides an introspective opportunity for the child and also serves to foster an identification with an appropriate adult model. Indeed, the child may "borrow" strength, clarity, and organization from the psychotherapist as the child struggles to deal with an acute development crisis. Further, the loving relationship in itself and the feeling of being understood have important therapeutic effects, perhaps regardless of any insight that may have been achieved (Rothstein, 1989). Another significant therapeutic force is the change from despair to hope, leading to a therapeutic optimism. Concomitant work with other family members also leads to shifts in the dynamic equilibrium within the family; releases the child and parents from their locked-in, fixed positions; and allows development to proceed. Lastly, the extended moment of time, the opportunity to examine in detail, itself contributes to clearer, more direct communications for all concerned.

EVALUATION OF OUTCOME OF PSYCHOTHERAPY

Evaluation of the effectiveness of psychotherapy is in general a complex undertaking (Heinecke and Ramsey-Klee, 1986; Kazdin, 1988; Strupp, 1977), and such research is plagued by methodological problems (Hine, 1982). Parloff (1982) reviewed nearly 500 rigorous, controlled studies providing research evidence on outcome. Parloff concluded that all forms of psychological treatment are comparably effective in producing therapeutic benefits and that such benefits are reliably superior to those found in controls. More recent outcome studies (Casey and Berman, 1985; Weisz et al., 1987) have not contradicted this global conclusion, although Weiss and Weisz (1990) reported that (a) behavioral treatments are associated with significantly larger effect sizes than nonbehavioral treatments, (b) most studies of child psychiatry in actual clinical practice show very small effects (Weisz et al., 1992), and (c) psychodynamic treatments have an effect size that is even smaller than client-centered treatments (0.01 versus 0.56, respectively). Shirk and Russell (1995), however, have expressed concern about major methodological flaws in many of the studies used in the Weiss et al. meta-analytic approach and have suggested that all such flawed studies should be excluded from meta-analytic comparisons. Improved methodology in studies of child psychotherapy remains an important goal for future studies. (For a critical review of the psychotherapies, see Chapter 81.)

Ultimately, outcome in psychotherapy is a value judgment, requiring that the therapist recognize the multiple values, criteria, and factors that go into such judgments. Research on psychotherapy with children in particular is especially sparse (Barrett et al., 1978; Levitt, 1971; Shaffer, 1984). More focused research is needed. Marans (1989) has suggested specific questions concerning which aspects of the therapeutic process are especially useful for a particular child.

In one controlled, albeit limited, study, longer and more intensive treatment was independently associated with a greater likelihood of reliable improvement, particularly among children with severe overanxious or generalized anxiety disorders, although the majority of older (>11 years), severely disordered children remained diagnosable at termination. Moreover, if severely disordered children were treated nonintensively (once- or twice-weekly psychotherapy), more than half (56.5%) got worse or showed no improvement. Less severely disordered children were as likely to benefit from nonintensive treatment as from intensive treatment (Target and Fonagy, 1994).

Acknowledgments. *This chapter is modified from an earlier publication (Lewis, 1974).*

References

American Psychiatric Association: *Diagnostic and Statistical Manual of Mental Disorders* (4th ed, rev). Washington, DC, American Psychiatric Association, 1994.

Barrett CL, Hampe IE, Miller K: Research on child psychotherapy. In: Garfield SL, Bergin AE (eds): *Handbook of Psychotherapy and Behavior Change* (2nd ed). New York, Wiley, 1978, pp. 411–435.

Beiser HR: Formal games in diagnosis and therapy. *J Am Acad Child Psychiatry* 18:480–491, 1979.

Bergler E: "Working through," in psychoanalysis. *Psychoanal Rev* 32:449–480, 1945.

Bird J: Teaching medical interviewing skills: A comparison of medical and non-medical tutors. In: *Research in Medical Education: Proceedings of the Association of American Medical Colleges*. Washington, DC, Association of American Medical Colleges, 1980.

Blos P: *On Adolescence: A Psychoanalytic Interpretation*. New York, Free Press, 1962.

Bornstein B: Emotional barriers in the understanding and treatment of young children. *Am J Orthopsychiatry* 18:691–697, 1948.

Buckley P, Conte HR, Plutchik R, et al: Learning dynamic psychotherapy: A longitudinal study. *Am J Psychiatry* 139:1607–1610,1982.

Buxbaum E: Technique of child therapy. *Psychoanal Study Child* 9:297–333, 1954.

Casey RJ, Berman JS: The outcome of psychotherapy with children. *Psychol Bull* 98:388–400, 1985.

Devereux G: Some criteria for the timing of confrontations and interpretations. *Int J Psychoanal* 32:19–24, 1951.

Dulcan MK: Brief psychotherapy with children and their families: The state of the art. *J Am Acad Child Psychiatry* 23:544–551, 1984.

Erikson EH: Studies in the interpretation of play. *Genet Psychol Monogr* 22:557–671, 1940.

Fenichel O: *The Psychoanalytic Theory of Neurosis.* New York, Norton, 1945.

Freud A: *The Psycho-Analytic Treatment of Children.* New York, International Universities Press, 1950. (Originally published 1946.)

Freud A: *Normality and Pathology in Childhood.* New York, International Universities Press, 1965.

Freud A: Indications and contraindications of child analysis. *Psychoanal Study Child* 23:37–46, 1968.

Freud A: Problems of termination in child analysis. In: *The Writings of Anna Freud* (Vol 7). New York, International Universities Press, 1971, pp. 3–21.

Freud S: Two encyclopedia articles. (a) Psychoanalysis. In: Strachey J (ed and trans): *The Standard Edition of the Complete Psychological Works of Sigmund Freud* (Vol 18). London, Hogarth Press, 1955, pp. 235–263. (Originally published 1923.)

Freud S: Constructions in analysis. In: Strachey J (ed and trans): *The Standard Edition of the Complete Psychological Works of Sigmund Freud* (Vol 23). London, Hogarth Press, 1964, pp. 257–269. (Originally published 1937.)

Glover E: The "vehicle" of interpretations. *Int J Psychoanal* 11:340–344, 1930.

Greenacre P: Re-evaluation of the process of working through. *Int J Psychoanal* 37:439–444, 1956.

Harley M: Transference developments in a five-year-old child. In: Geleerd ER (ed): *The Child Analyst at Work.* New York, International Universities Press, 1967, pp. 115–141.

Harrison SI: Individual psychotherapy. In: Kaplan HI, Sadock BJ (eds): *Comprehensive Textbook of Psychiatry* (3rd ed). Baltimore, Williams & Wilkins, 1980, pp. 2647–2667.

Harter S: Children's understanding of multiple emotions: A cognitive developmental approach. In: Overton W (ed): *The Relationship between Social and Cognitive Development.* Hillsdale, NJ, Erlbaum, 1983, pp. 147–194.

Hartmann H: Technical implications of ego psychology. *Psychoanal Q* 20:31–43, 1951.

Haworth MR (ed): *Child Psychotherapy*. New York, Basic Books, 1964.

Heinecke C, Ramsey-Klee: Outcome of child psychotherapy and a factor affecting outcome. *J Abnorm Psychol* 74:553–560, 1986.

Heine FR, Werman DS, Simpson DM: Effectiveness of psychotherapy: Problems of research on complex phenomena. *Am J Psychiatry* 139:204–208, 1982.

Ivey AE: *Counselling and Psychotherapy: Skills, Theories and Practice*. Englewood Cliffs, NJ, Prentice-Hall, 1980.

Karasu TB: Psychotherapies: An overview. *Am J Psychiatry* 134:851–863, 1977.

Kazdin AE: *Child Psychotherapy: Developing and Identifying Effective Treatments*. New York, Pergamon, 1988.

Klein M: Der Familien roman in Statu Nascendi. *Int Z für Psychoanalyse* 6: 1920.

Kris E: Ego psychology and interpretation in psychoanalytic therapy. *Psychoanal Q* 20:15–30, 1951.

Langs R: *Psychotherapy*. New York, Aronson, 1982.

Levitt EE: Research on psychotherapy with children. In: Bergin AE, Garfield SL (eds): *Handbook of Psychotherapy and Behavior Change*. New York, Wiley-Interscience, 1971, pp. 474–494.

Lewis M: Interpretation in child analysis. *J Am Acad Child Psychiatry* 13:32–53, 1974.

Loewenstein RM: The problem of interpretation. *Psychoanal Q* 20:1–14, 1951.

London P: *The Modes and Morals of Psychotherapy*. New York, Holt, Rinehart & Winston, 1964.

London P, Klerman EL: Evaluating psychotherapy. *Am J Psychiatry* 139:709–717, 1982.

Looney JG: Treatment planning in child psychiatry. *J Am Acad Child Psychiatry* 23:529–536, 1984.

Luborsky L, Singer B, Luborsky L: Comparative studies of psychotherapies: Is it true that "Everyone has won and all must have prizes?" *Arch Gen Psychiatry* 32:995–1008, 1975.

MacGuire P: Teaching medical students to interview psychiatric patients. *Bull R Coll Psychiatry* 4: 188–190, 1980.

MacLean G, Rappen U: *Hermine Hug-Hellmuth*. New York, Routledge, 1991.

Marans S: Psychoanalytic psychotherapy with children: Current research trends and challenges. *J Am Acad Child Adolesc Psychiatry* 28:669–674, 1989.

Marks I: Personal psychotherapy in the training of a psychiatrist? *Bull R Coll Psychiatry* 6:39–40, 1982.

Matarazzo R: Research on the teaching and learning of psychotherapeutic skills. In: Garfield S, Bergin AR (eds): *Handbook of Psychotherapy and Behavior Modification* (2nd ed). New York, Wiley, 1978, pp. 941–966.

McDermott JF, Chan WF: Stage-related models of psychotherapy with children. *J Am Acad Child Psychiatry* 23:537–543, 1984.

McDermott JF, Harrison SI (eds): *Psychiatric Treatment of Children*. New York, Aronson, 1977.

Nannis E: Emotional understanding and child psychotherapy. In: Shirk S (ed): *Cognitive Development and Child Psychotherapy*. New York, Plenum, 1988, pp. 91–115.

Neubauer PB: Psychoanalysis of the preschool child. In: Wolman BB (ed): *Handbook of Child Psychoanalysis*. New York, Van Nostrand Reinhold, 1972, pp. 221–252.

Paolino TJ: *Psychoanalytic Psychotherapy*. New York, Brunner/Mazel, 1981.

Parloff MB: Psychotherapy research evidence and reimbursement decisions: Bambi meets Godzilla. *Am J Psychiatry* 139:718–727, 1982.

Piaget J: *The Child's Conception of the World*. New York, Harcourt Brace, 1929.

Reid JR, Finesinger JE: The role of insight in psychotherapy. *Am J Psychiatry* 108:726–734, 1952.

Richfield J: An analysis of the concept of insight. *Psychoanal Q* 23:390–408, 1954.

Rothstein A (ed): *How Does Treatment Help? On the Modes of Therapeutic Action of Psychoanalytic Psychotherapy*. Madison, WI, International Universities Press, 1989.

Satterfield J, Satterfield B, Cantwell D: Multimodal treatment: A two year evaluation of 61 hyperactive boys. *Arch Gen Psychiatry* 37:915–919, 1980.

Schaefer CE, Millman HL: *Therapies for Children*. San Francisco, Jossey-Bass, 1977.

Shaffer D: Notes on psychotherapy research among children and adolescents. *J Am Acad Child Psychiatry* 23:552–561, 1984.

Shapiro T: The psychodynamic formulation in child and adolescent psychiatry. *J Am Acad Child Adolesc Psychiatry* 28:675–680, 1989.

Shirk SR, Russell RL: Effectiveness of psychotherapy. *J Am Acad Child Adolesc Psychiatry* 34: 972, 1995.

Strachey J: The nature of the therapeutic action of psychoanalysis. *Int J Psychoanal* 15:127–159, 1934.

Strupp H, Hadley S: Specific vs. nonspecific factors in psychotherapy. *Arch Gen Psychiatry* 36: 1125–1136, 1979.

Strupp HH, Hadley SW: A tripartite model of mental health and therapeutic outcomes. *Am Psychol* 32:187–196, 1977.

Target M, Fonagy P: Efficacy of psychoanalysis for children with emotional disorders. *J Am Acad Child Adolesc Psychiatry* 33:361–371, 1994.

Temeles MS: Gift-giving. *Bull Philadelphia Assoc Psychoanal* 17:31–32, 1967.

Train GF: Flight into health. *Am J Psychother* 7: 463–486, 1953.

Varma V (ed): *Psychotherapy Today*. London, Constable, 1974.

Weiss B, Weisz JR: The impact of methodological factors on child therapy effectiveness. *J Am Acad Child Adolesc Psychiatry* 31:703–709, 1990.

Weisz J, Weiss B, Alicke M, et al: Effectiveness of psychotherapy with children. *J Consult Clin Psychol* 55:542–549, 1987.

Weisz JR, Weiss B, Donnenberg GR: The lab versus the clinic: Effects of child and adolescent psychotherapy. *Am Psychol* 47:1578–1588, 1992.

Winnicott DW: *Therapeutic Consultations in Child Psychiatry*. New York, Basic Books, 1971.

Witmer HL (ed): *Psychiatric Interviews with Children*. Cambridge, MA, Harvard University Press, 1946.

Wolman BB, Egan J, Ross AO (eds): *Handbook of Treatment of Mental Disorders in Childhood and Adolescence*. Englewood Cliffs, NJ, Prentice-Hall, 1978.

74 Use of Play in Psychodynamic Psychotherapy

Henry P. Coppolillo, M.D.

The essence of psychodynamically oriented psychotherapy is the communication and exploration of the patient's subjective states and convictions even when these are dimly perceived by the patient or are unconscious. This is an arduous task when it is undertaken with an adult, who usually comes to the psychotherapeutic situation with a well-developed repertoire of signals, signs, and symbols as communicative vehicles. With the child, the task becomes more difficult since his or her complement of culturally validated signals and symbols is as yet incomplete. The play of the child can often more than compensate for this immaturity. In this chapter the use of play as a vehicle for therapeutic effectiveness and the conditions that facilitate that use are explored. A word of caution: Many of the concepts regarding psychotherapy are deceptively easy to understand. It is their application in the living situation that is difficult. For this reason, beginning psychotherapists to become competent must avail themselves of competent supervision as a necessary companion piece to texts and to reading and hearing case presentations.

HISTORICAL NOTES ON THE PSYCHOLOGY OF PLAY

It is beyond the purpose of this chapter to explore the ideas of all who have been interested in play. Suffice it to say that play has been scrutinized by members of disciplines as widely disparate as military theory (war games) and philosophy of religion (Berger, 1969). Closer to our interest, one of the first psychodynamic considerations of play is found in Freud's (1955) development of the concept of the repetition compulsion. The repeated tossing and retrieving of a spool of thread by a small boy whose parents were away was used by him as an example of the wish to master a trauma. Waelder (1933) extended the understanding of the broad and varied psychological functions that play serves.

Hug-Hellmuth (1913, 1921) wrote the formal articles on the use of play in the therapeutic situation when she described the psychoanalysis of children. By the time that Kline (1932) and Anna Freud (1946) published their texts on the use of play in the treatment of children, the modality had become broadly accepted and utilized by therapists.

By 1940, child therapists had begun to utilize play in therapeutic efforts that conceived of specific, more restricted goals than did psychoanalysis. Levy (1939) aimed at achieving a therapeutic effect with a cathartic resolution of conflict or need tension through the child's play. Allen (1942) described the use of the play situation to develop and sustain the relationship that he felt had central therapeutic significance in the child's life. A variation in the technique of using play was suggested by Solomon (1955) as he guided the child's play in an effort to help the child achieve psychological integration.

A relatively more subtle conceptual variation is to be found in Virginia Axline's work (1947). Basing her ideas on the Rogerian concepts of ''client centered therapy,'' she used play to reflect back to the child his states, wishes, or convictions without attempting interpretations of unconscious motives or conflicts. The articulation of that which the child conveyed was considered therapeutically effective.

A moving and profoundly significant explanation of the meaning of play is offered by Peter Berger (1969) in his book *A Rumor of Angels*. Berger follows the historian Huizinga, C.S. Lewis, and Freud in ascribing to the very nature of human beings the wish to be joyful, playful, and to seek pleasure. He then proposes that it is in play that this joy and exuberance can emerge most easily, because, in play, portions of reality can be suspended. The portions of reality that he believes are most important to suspend are pain and death. At the same time he describes the preservation and extension of parts of reality through the principle of transcendence. By transcendence he means ''phenomena that are to be found within the domain of our 'natural' reality but that appear to point beyond that reality'' (pp. 65–66). Berger then proposes that human beings tend to order or organize their realities and possess an ''intrinsic impulse to give cosmic scope to this order'' (p. 70). In play then human beings can suspend certain painful aspects of their reality, even as they preserve other components of that reality and live out the wish to maintain order and pleasurable predictability in their universe. In a beautiful passage he summarizes his views by describing the play of children (p. 74).

> Some little girls are playing hopscotch in the park. They are completely intent on their game, closed to the world outside it, happy in the concentration. Time has stood still for them or more accurately, has been collapsed into the movements of the game. The outside world has for the duration of the game, ceased to exist. And, by implication (since the little girls may not be very conscious of this), pain and death, which are the law of the world, have also ceased to exist. Even the adult observer of this scene, who is perhaps all too conscious of pain and death, is momentarily drawn into beatific immunity.

Although Berger is not a clinician and his philosophical exploration may not have direct bearing on the technical uses of play in therapy, below we see how closely his thoughts parallel the thinking of a clinician who used play with great therapeutic effectiveness.

D. W. Winnicott (1953), in his timeless paper on transitional objects, articulated concepts that are useful for understanding the developmental and therapeutic functions of play. He proposed that, in addition to the capacity of a child to experience external reality and the internal world, an intermediate area of experience is available to the child to which internal and external experiences both contribute. He called this the intermediate area of experience, and the objects that were experienced in this way he called ''transitional objects.'' Concrete objects as well as songs, rhymes, or even the babbling of an infant can be experienced in the intermediate area. According to Winnicott, having the intermediate area of experience available to him, the child can begin to relieve the strain of relating internally generated wishes with the rigidity of external reality; once acquired, this mode of attaining self-soothing continues throughout life. Winnicott further states that ''This intermediate area is in direct continuity with the play area of the small child who is 'lost in play''' (p. 96). For example, a bored or sad child may pick up a teddy bear to play with. The child can easily appreciate the external reality of its button eyes, soft fur, and the inviting demeanor its manufac-

turer provided. But as he brings it into the intermediate area of experience, it becomes a transitional object and, as such, is also appreciated as a soothing companion, the reciprocator of a loving hug or even the worthy opponent in a wrestling match for the championship of the child's preschool class. The teddy bear has been transformed from a toy into a character in a drama that reveals the wishes and impulses, the convictions and visions of the little author who provided him his script. Bringing a physical entity into the intermediate area of experience allows the entity to be imbued with qualities currently significant to the child. Those elements of the subjects inner world that are brought into the intermediate area and are thus attached to an object can be played with and mastered with just the right intensity. If a child becomes disturbed by the intensity of his own aggression when playing with his teddy bear he can readily turn his attention to the real qualities of the toy and thus escape the threat of his own impulses until he is ready once more to face them in play. It is this capacity's persistence that allows adults to transform a combination of sound waves into the *Eroica* or the *Appassionata* and allow great visions or tender images to sweep away the tedium of daily living without losing the ability to address the reality of daily living when necessary.

Rapaport (1951, 1958) envisioned how the ego would be handicapped by the extremes of being totally engrossed by events of the external world or responsive only to the impulses and images of the inner world. In the former condition the person would be oppressed by stimulus slavery, while in the latter state we would have to say he was handicapped by madness. Transitional objects become excellent vehicles for maintaining a balance between the tides of stimuli from the external and internal worlds. When a child takes an object or a story or song into the intermediate area of experience, he takes with it a quantity of reality that is reliably there but is unobtrusive when he imbues the object with qualities that serve to play out a wish or impulse from his inner world. If his wishes or impulses become too threatening to him, he can attend to the realistic qualities of the object more fully. If the reality of the toy is insufficient to provide him relief from tedium, he can suspend some of that reality (Coppolillo, 1976). These are the conditions of this kind of play that render it invaluable as a vehicle for the modulated, manageable expressions of the inner states of the child. The thinking of Berger, Winnicott, and Rapaport had many points of overlap and concordance even though they developed their ideas quite independently and were addressing different aspects of life and theory. The work of Peller (1954) on the function of play in development seems also to coincide with their thinking as she states ''Small quantities of anxiety are mastered in play'' and further asserts that unconscious impulses can be acted out in play without reaching awareness (p. 181). In this chapter the work of these authors is the theory that supports the suggestions for using play as a psychodynamically therapeutic tool. (For a more extensive review of the literature on this topic, see Gardner, 1979.)

Play in this chapter is considered as both an adjunct to communication and as a vehicle of communication between child and therapist that reveal to the therapist states of the child's inner world. These states may include (but are not limited to) misconceptions and misinformation about himself or herself or misconceptions about the child's world. These states may contain unrealistic wishes, anxiety laden impulses, conflicts, and frightening expectations of retaliations. Of course this is not to say that even as the child is struggling with these conflicts other phenomena are not occurring simultaneously. For example, it would be surprising if the child were not enjoying the growing relationship with a caring and warm therapist even as they are struggling to understand the origins of an irrational fear. Or for some children the time playing in the presence of the therapist may be one of the few moments in their lives when they feel soothed. Deconditioning or relearning may be occurring, or perhaps the narcissistic gratification of being the only object of the therapist's attention may be helpful to the child. Conflict resolution often combines with these other bonuses of human relatedness to produce therapeutic benefits.

PRECONDITIONS NECESSARY FOR THERAPEUTIC PLAY

There are times in the course of a treatment process that play loses its usefulness as a communicative or therapeutic tool. This may happen even when the therapist seems to be conducting the sessions in a technically correct manner and has his or her own internal world in order in terms of fatigue, personal gratifications, and countertransferences (Coppolillo, 1987). Often the causes for the derailment of the process may be found in the preparation of the child and the therapist to conduct therapy. For this reason some attention must be paid to conditions that will make the play an activity that is considered therapeutic by both the clinician and child, rather than one in which something will hopefully happen that will somehow benefit the child. A brief review of these conditions may be helpful.

Conditions Regarding the Therapeutic Environment

PHYSICAL ENVIRONMENT

The physical conditions that are necessary to conduct safe and dignified psychotherapy are more fully discussed elsewhere (Coppolillo, 1987). Here it is sufficient to say that the physical environment needs to be safe, sufficiently well contained to convey the notion of confidentiality to the child, and provided with considerations that will allow the adults waiting for the child to be comfortable, especially if they must sit with a younger child while the patient is in the consulting room.

There is some question as to whether a separate "play area" is desirable or not. There are advantages and disadvantages on both sides of the question. A separate play area sometimes invites the child to make an artificial distinction between "talking time" and "playing time" and to therefore resent or resist inferences made by the therapist from the play. On the other hand, a single office may have rugs, furniture, and paintings that, to the therapist's horror, the child may damage. If the child senses this concern, it may inhibit his or her play or spontaneity. Giving some thought to the problem will allow the therapist to compensate for one or the other disadvantage.

Another specific issue that arises is that of how to equip the play area. Some therapist's play areas look like a toy store with the variety of games and equipment that are on display. Others prefer to have only a small number of toys and drawing materials immediately available. Anna Freud (Sandler et al., 1980) is quoted as saying, "The special role of the toy as a therapeutic agent has been greatly overvalued" (p. 39). By this she meant that the use the child makes of the toy is by far more revealing than the choice of the toy itself. Children can use checkers to build a wall between themselves and some imagined threat and may use blocks to play a competitive game with the therapist. In addition, an important issue is what toys the therapist feels allow him or her to most comfortably assume an attitude of inquiry. If the therapist is vulnerable to compulsive reactions of neatness when his or her child patient is ruining a model by smearing glue all over it, it would be a good idea not to have models to build on his or her shelf. If the therapist finds himself or herself sliding into unproductive competitive feelings with a youngster, board games may not be the toys he or she would choose to have on display. One suggestion might be to have a few basic items of play in the office like some drawing and coloring material, a doll family and simple doll house, some toy vehicles and perhaps some toy soldiers. If the child then appears to want or need other things to play with, he can be asked as the treatment progresses if or how other toys will help both therapist and child to understand his or her worries or problems. This keeps the ultimate purpose of the play in the child's mind. What the therapist should keep in mind is that, in the optimal situation, it is the benign interest and attentive inquiry of the therapist that is helpful to the child and engages him or her and not the allure of the toys. If the child cannot use this interest and attention (and where else in life can a child get 45 minutes to an hour of undivided attention from an adult), this inability needs to be addressed and worked through and not bypassed with the seductive appeal of toys.

PRECONDITIONS IN THE THERAPIST

We must hope that the therapist will come into the therapeutic sessions well rested, with few worries of his or her own, sufficiently confident that his or her own skills and techniques are adequate to help most children (so that the child does not *have to* get well for the sake of the therapist), and with enough play in his own personal life to ensure that the child is playing for the child's own reasons and not the therapist's. These are conditions to strive for, of course, and not ones that must be attained every minute of every day. If they were constant essentials, few of us could ever treat anyone. But if the therapist does detect a persistent disturbance in any of the conditions mentioned, it is essential that remediation through environmental or psychological change take place in the therapist for the therapist's own and the patient's sake.

In addition to this unending self-scrutiny that the therapist must undergo, there is of course the intellectual preparation that is required to make play meaningful in terms of what it can reveal about the child's developmental achievements and arrests, as well as about the current state of his or her psychological organization. This requires a vivid, living picture of stages and processes in development as well as mental images of how children function in health and illness. Training in the recognition of these states as well as education in theories of human development make it possible for the clinician to utilize the rich, profound revelations that play provides.

PRIOR TO PLAY

Before all else, a history of the child's development as well as that of the difficulties that bring him to the clinical situation must be gathered (Coppolillo, 1987; Simmons, 1981). Usually this history is gathered from the parents. The therapist must recall that we are all vulnerable to retrospective falsification, and especially when the historian is as emotionally involved as most parents are with their children. Remember too that the clinician is not just interested in whether a phase of development was deemed to be "normal." More often than not, normal is judged by whether or not the child was troublesome to the adults around him. It is most useful to learn of the style in which the child faced the stress of a new developmental phase; the defenses used in adapting to it, and whether or not there was pride in leaving behind old modes of adaptation and enthusiasm in adopting new talents. In short, conjuring an image of the living child as he or she developed is far more productive than pasting a label of "normal" or "abnormal" across a developmental phase.

The same considerations may be applied to the history of the difficulties that brought the child to the clinical situation. In this segment of the preparation, however, the clinician must anticipate and deal with two conditions that may become obstacles to the treatment later. The first of these is that the people who referred the child or who are paying the bill may expect that the therapist will act as their agent. The situation can become critical if a school or court has referred the child and awaits guidance from the therapist. If there is any question of about who the therapist is representing, every effort must be made to clarify expectations at this stage of the treatment process. If they are not clarified, later in the treatment the child may sense divided responsibility in the therapist and may feel that the therapist has betrayed him or her.

A second related issue occurs when, without meaning to do so, people bring a child to the clinical situation to be made *good*, and not necessarily *well*. If the therapist inadvertently participates in trying to make the patient good, he or she joins the multitude of people who must seem to the child to wish only that he or she behave in a certain manner and to care but little about the anguish or the forces that the child feels so powerless to resist. If the child reaches this conclusion, acquiescence may be possible, but revelation of his inner world is unlikely.

CASE ILLUSTRATION

A 16-year-old girl was treated, with parental approval, after the juvenile court had adjudicated her "an unruly child." She had run away from home twice in 6 months and was returned both times by the police. It was only after she became convinced that her therapist was *her* agent and not insistent on her behaving in any predetermined manner that she could reveal that she was running away from an incestuous situation at home. She had turned to a number of adults in her environment for help and had encountered blank stares or deaf ears. Running away from home, the very action that was labeled "bad" and for which she had been sent to therapy, had been the most adaptive action she felt she could have taken under the circumstances. Had the therapist been intent on making her *good* by convincing her of the evils of running away she would have probably not revealed her secret.

After the history is gathered, the more formal aspects of treatment begin, and it is in this phase that we come to see what an important asset the initiative of the child can be to the treatment. Yet let us review for a moment the manner in which many children are brought to our offices. One day the mother or the father says "you are having trouble with such and so, and we are going to see a doctor about this." Often without further explanation the child is taken to the family car, where he or she sits *passively*, until he or she is escorted to a strange waiting room, where once more the child *passively* waits until initiative is further taken from the child by his being led into the consulting room. Then the child is invited to become *active*. How strange this must seem to the child! One way to avoid this dilemma is to come to an agreement with the parents about the time that the child can be seen. If it is possible, make more than 1 hour available in order to allow the child a choice in case there is some activity that is especially important to *the child* that might compete with the agreed-upon hour. Then ask the parents to have the child call to make the appointment. Some parents say that the child would not call, but few children actually refused to do so. When they do call from the safe environment of their home, the therapist can demonstrate awareness and respect for the fact that the child has activities that are important to him or her, and also demonstrate that language or concepts that will leave the child hopelessly perplexed will not be used. An added advantage of this is that it demonstrates to the child that what he or she has to say or show will be heeded (Coppolillo, 1987).

The therapeutic alliance, as essential for any child therapy as it is for adult work, has already begun with the phone call. In the succeeding hours it must be continued, developed, and fortified. It must be stated as well as demonstrated to the child that no conclusions will be reached without the child's awareness and, whenever possible, participation. The child must come to realize that the clinician will not "spring something" on him or her through a gimmick or a ploy, and that the work that will be done will be accomplished with cooperative respect. The child will produce the data that the clinician and child will examine together to reach conclusions. Phrases like "We'll put our heads together to see if we can figure out what things mean" are helpful in forging and reforging the therapeutic alliance. As part of this alliance and of the therapeutic contract, the therapist must convey to the child the message that play will be primarily for the purpose of helping them both to understand what causes some of the child's troublesome feelings and behavior to occur. To fail to mention this and then, when the child is lost in play, to interpret the play tends to make the child feel what we feel when in a social situation we make a painfully revealing slip of the tongue and that is then "interpreted" by a "parlor analyst" who feels impelled to interpret the slip for all to hear. The child is far less troubled when he knows that his play will be used for revelation and the interpretation begins with a phrase something like, "I wonder if your play means that . . .".

While the suggestions in the preceding paragraphs apply to the whole phase of the beginning of treatment, it should be remembered that the foundations for the therapeutic alliance are laid during the first contacts with the family. To ignore this may mean that, if treatment is recommended after the diagnostic workup, the therapist may have to undo some distasteful or even frightening convictions that the parents or child may have drawn about the child's treatment during the early contacts with the therapist.

Another necessary element in treatment planning that influences the therapeutic alliance is setting the number of times per week and the hours that the patient will be seen. While it may not be possible to accommodate the child's wishes as to the time that he or she can be seen, thoughtful consideration to the child's schedule will be a powerful support to the alliance.

Setting the frequency of the sessions requires consideration of a number of variables. The finances of the parents and the therapist's fees are one variable. The nature of the pathology and what its treatment will require should, of course, be the central consideration. But there is another issue that is more frequently not considered. The child's improvement in the therapeutic sessions counts for little if there is not concomitant improvement in his or her feelings and behavior in the everyday world. This requires working through of the conflicts uncovered in the treatment. Often this working through cannot be accomplished in the home environment because, in the adaptation that the family group has made to the child's behaviors, the parents inadvertently keep the conflict alive. In addition to consultations with the parents, the child needs a milieu in which he or she is free to try out the different behaviors that result from the resolution of conflicts. If the child is scheduled so tightly that he or she has little or no time for spontaneous play with peers or for the relaxation that supports spontaneity, scheduling more sessions may be counterproductive, especially if the scheduled treatment hours are at the expense of his "free time." Setting times should therefore be done with an eye to how the therapeutic hours will influence and be influenced by the rest of the child's daily life.

CASE ILLUSTRATION

A 9-year-old girl was being seen for a delayed and inhibited grief reaction occasioned by the loss of her father when she was 4. She had been given hours before school largely because her after school hours were filled with all manner of activities (which were also used as defenses against the recognition of her unremitting loneliness). A phase of her therapy that was shallow and unproductive had lasted for several months. During this phase she had taken to drawing a number of "wilderness scenes" in which the woods and mountains she drew contained various animals that were depicted and described as busily going about their customary activities without interacting in any way. When the therapist commented on the absence of interaction and that the animals must be lonely, she first associated to the idea that if they stayed busy they would not fight, and then to the more general notion that if they stayed busy they would not feel any disturbing affects. After the therapist likened this to her staying busy in general and in her treatment hours in specific, she could acknowledge that she was afraid that if she cried during her treatment hour she would go to school with red eyes and everyone would wonder why. It was only after a conference with her mother, a reduction of the after school activities that she had scheduled, and the setting of her appointments after the school day that she could begin to see that the reluctance to experience and show sad affects was based on her fear that her grief would upset her mother (and in the transference, her therapist). It was only when the real concern that she would be embarrassed by her red eyes in school could be addressed that she could address the *neurotic* conviction that her negative affects would disintegrate her mother. Few defenses are as effective as a bit of reality that is used as a defense.

Having attended to the notion that events prior to formal therapy may influence the therapy itself, we can turn to those technical considerations that will render the process of play useful for therapy.

PLAY IN THE SERVICE OF PSYCHOTHERAPY

A paradox to be reckoned with in the use of play is that play is so revealing that we sometimes fail to see what it conceals. If in watching a child play we come to a conclusion prematurely and misunderstand the significance of the play or understand only one part of the play, the misunderstanding or partial understanding can be used as a defense against revealing more important significances. The therapist must be ready to wait for the cues and learn to avoid taking for granted assumptions made from his or her own past experiences.

CASE ILLUSTRATION

Joey, a bright boy of 6, was being treated for his tendency to isolate himself from his parents and his passive disobedience at home and at school. He had been in treatment before, which his parents had deemed ineffective and had terminated. His former therapist stated that all Joey had wanted to do was to play board games. In one of the early sessions of his second treatment Joey picked up some checkers and went to the table where children usually played. The therapist, sure that the child again wanted to play a board game picked up the checker board on his way to the table, and as he picked it up he remembered the comments of Joey's former therapist. He replaced the board and sat down to see what Joey would do. Joey said nothing but began to use the checkers as blocks. He built a wall between himself and the therapist, commenting on how difficult it was to build a good wall with checkers. The therapist answered that if Joey really wanted to show him how important a wall was, he would get some blocks with which he could more easily build a wall. The blocks became unnecessary. The discussions about walls between people were necessary and revealing.

Even the therapist's very natural presupposition that Joey wanted to play a board game with him would have lead to a compliant and counterproductive defense on Joey's part in this instance. Thus the adage: "Wait until the cues are clear to make an inference or an interpretation."

Generally there are four ways that children play during their treatment hours. They can become lost in play and play alone in the presence of their therapist. They can play alone but with a demand, either explicitly stated or conveyed implicitly through body language, that the therapist watch their play attentively. They may play with the therapist in unstructured play with no rules other than that the game evolve. They may express a wish to play a structured game such as a board game, guessing game, or a hiding game. The meaning of each of these modes will eventually become clear if the therapist keeps a number of principles in mind.

The first of these principles is that while minding the content of the play the therapist must also notice the process by which the play is chosen and how it progresses.

CASE ILLUSTRATION

Tommy was a boy of 10 with little self-esteem despite a remarkable talent for drawing and better than average intelligence. In the course of his treatment he would suddenly break off discourse or some form of play and would ask to draw. He would then engross himself so deeply in his drawing that he would not attend to questions about the content of his picture or the techniques he had used to produce it. When finished with what was usually a remarkably good drawing he would present it to the therapist and give bland, nonrevealing answers to anything that he was asked about the picture. One day he came to the office ahead of his mother and announced that he wanted to draw a picture. Before the therapist and Tommy could move to the inner office the mother arrived and announced that she had to tell the therapist that Tommy had gotten grades that were far below his competence in a number of his classes. The therapist waited until they were in the inner office then recalled that Tommy felt his compelling desire to draw on a number of occasions when they had discussed or gotten close to discussing issues that Tommy felt would cast him in a bad light. When the therapist mentioned that he had just begun to notice when Tommy wanted to draw, Tommy himself said "Yeah. When I get in trouble." By noticing the process rather than being stuck on the content of the drawings, the therapist and Tommy found great amounts of material to explore together.

Another issue to contemplate is that of body language that serves communication during play. Recall the pinched, tight control of the perfectionistic youngster who is attempting to draw the perfect picture to win approbation. Think of the increasingly less purposive movements of the impulsive child who gets "carried away" by aggressive impulses while playing with toy soldiers. And who can ignore the apathy and anhedonia conveyed by the lack of tone and movement of the depressed child?

CASE ILLUSTRATION

Annie, a 4-year-old who had lost her mother, displayed both the longing for close contact as well as the rejection of substitute relationships in her play. On a number of occasions she demanded that the therapist sit on the floor near a doll house as she played with the dolls. Several times she stumbled "accidentally" or had another accident which would land her in the therapist's lap. On other occasions she would clearly avoid any physical contact with the therapist. In one instance she asked the therapist to fix the clothes on the doll with which she was playing. As the therapist reached for the doll she was handing him she shrank away. The therapist, by asking her to notice her movement, made it possible to discuss her ambivalence about feeling close to anyone else while mourning her mother.

The third issue that requires attention as play progresses is the above-mentioned countertransference that can occur at any point. These are subtle and can be insidiously destructive to the therapeutic process. Countertransference may take any number of forms. They are facilitated by the regressive pull of the child's immaturity and his or her play and generated by a variety of states and conflicts in the therapist. Lewis offers a list of examples of countertransference in the preceding chapter on intensive, individual psychotherapy of children (see Chapter 73). The only comment to add here is that when countertransferences occur in a positive form, as in the wish to rescue the child, or to defend the child, or to be protective of the child or when he or she is already being protected, they are much more difficult to detect. Negative feelings toward the child become a foreign body in the awareness of the therapist more readily than those that are compatible with our self-image of loving, caring adults. But positive countertransferences can be as destructive to the process as negative ones (Coppolillo, 1969). Rather than think of these as sins that must be abolished, it is useful to view them as additional cues to consider regarding the nature of the transaction.

The therapist who understands that he or she is vulnerable to rejection may, for example, come to understand that a feeling of irritation or boredom is being occasioned by a withdrawn child's need or wish to become ''lost'' in solitary play in order to avoid the burden of relating. Again, the therapist who depends on the affection of the child may find that the child seeks play that he or she thinks will please the therapist in order to charm or seduce the therapist away from recognizing conflicted, negative feelings in more spontaneous play.

Finally, an eye must be kept on the content of the play. Here the help of the child is needed in order to ascertain in what way the play is significant *to the child*. Questions about what is happening in the play can be asked both when the child is playing alone and when the play is interactive. When the child has assigned the therapist a role in the play and demands that he or she act out the role, asides or stage whispers can be used as parentheses in which the questions may be posed.

CASE ILLUSTRATION

A 4-year-old child, whose mother had suffered a serious accident after the child had been sent to bed for her afternoon nap, was playing out her fear and chagrin about being coerced to go to sleep. She made the dolls with which she was playing be sent to bed by the therapist and then had them hop out of bed to ask for drinks, food, and other favors.

Child, holding the doll in the therapist's face: ''I want some milk.''

Therapist, in a stage whisper behind his hand: ''What does he say?''

Child, in a stage whisper: ''He says 'go to bed.'''

Therapist, gruffly: ''Go to bed!''

Child puts the doll in the doll bed while she pretends to be crying.

Therapist, again in a stage whisper: ''What do you wish he had said?''

Child: ''Why can't you sleep, little girl?''

His inquiry allowed the therapist to then meet her plea for understanding instead of coercion.

In addition to inquiry about the content of the play, the therapist must continually look for the associations that may explain the shift from one play activity to another.

CASE ILLUSTRATION

An 8-year-old boy, son of a physician, had played ''going to doctor school'' in the therapist's office by looking through an anatomy text. When it became clear to the therapist that the child was demonstrating more than a passing interest in the genitalia and breasts in the female illustrations, he asked him if the medical school play was to hide his embarrassment at his curiosity about women's bodies. The boy was able to acknowledge this. Later in treatment the therapist noticed that on several occasions the boy returned to the medical school play after having talked about his sister. With some gentle questioning the therapist discovered that the boy was chronically anxious and stimulated due to the fondling and exploration to which he had been subjected by an older sister.

On occasion, a seemingly disconnected or spontaneous comment during play offers a revealing association.

CASE ILLUSTRATION

A 4-year-old boy, brought to treatment for voluntary retention of feces and fear of using the potty, became obsessed with flat tires in play. The toy cars he played with always developed flat tires. He drew cars with flat tires and requested repeatedly that the therapist draw cars with flat tires for him. On one occasion when the therapist was drawing one of these cars for him, the boy commented that the therapist had a big belly. When the therapist asked him what he meant and how it was connected to the cars, the boy answered ''your belly is round and not flat.'' Having made the connection of flatness between car tires and bellies, the boy could tell of when he was riding with his father in the car when they had a blowout that sent the car out of control and frightened him. He could then say that he was afraid of getting flat (out of control) if he went to the bathroom.

Finally, the therapist must allow some disciplined play to his own creativity and imagination in making abstractions about the content and process of the play that he is observing. For example, if a child is playing with cars and labels one a fire truck, another a police car, and still another an ambulance, the abstraction that would occur to the therapist that would tie them together would be responses to an emergency. Then, depending on the age of the child, and with his history in mind, the therapist might be able to determine if the child was in the process of mastering a trauma that he had experienced, like a home fire, or was symbolically conveying anxiety about something unpredictable or uncontrollable occurring such as an impulse getting out of hand.

And so, by having the patience and interest to wait for the cues, the serenity to keep an eye on his or her own countertransference, the imagination and creativity to envision patterns of significance in the content and process of the child's play, the therapist can, with tact and kindness, return to the child, in a manageable form that which the child has anxiously revealed symbolically in his or her play.

CONCLUSIONS

Theoretical considerations often provide frames of reference that permit the user of a technique disciplined creativity in the use of that technique. Instituting rules for the use of a technique often does just the opposite, by simply constricting rather than enabling. For this reason, a brief review of how the above-mentioned concepts of Winnicott and Rapaport, as they specifically apply to the therapeutic use of play, is indicated.

Winnicott (1953) demonstrated how bringing an object into the ''intermediate area of experience'' alleviated the strain of relating external reality to the inner world of wishes and subjective convictions.

Rapaport (1951, 1958) described how attending to the inner world of drives and impulses, as well as to one's own values and self system, presents a stimulus barrier to the world of external reality and shelters one from slavery to external circumstances. He continued his exploration by noting that, conversely, human beings were not simply expressions of sublimated drive activities. Both the autonomous functions of the ego and attentions to external reality provide the human being with a measure of autonomy from the inner world.

Integrating the work of these two authors (Coppolillo, 1976) permits us to appreciate the powerful effects of play in the adaptation of the human being to his or her environment. In the therapeutic use of play, we may join Winnicott (1965) in considering the immersion into play as providing a ''holding environment'' (pp. 50–51). The privacy, and the nonthreatening and nonintrusive qualities of the ambience then act as a shield against any coercive qualities the child may ascribe to the external world, and thus increase the child's sensitivity to his or her inner world. At the same time, ''the reality'' of the therapist's presence, his or her absence of fear or anxiety about the child's impulses, the regularity of the hours, and the therapist's commitment to understanding rather than judging, reassure the child that his or her own impulses will not be overwhelming. Into this setting a toy, game, or an idea can be taken into the intermediate area by the child and there further regulate and titrate the amount of anxiety the child can tolerate as either fear of his or her impulses or dangers ascribed to the external world. For example, if the child is playing out destructive fantasies with the use of soldiers and an impulse to destroy becomes too transparent or intense, the child may turn his or her attention to the realistic quality of the soldiers and decide that they are too small, too few, or just toys. If aspects of reality become too coercive or boring, the child may allow himself or herself to be a bit more lost in the unrealistic quality of the play and imbue the toy with more aggression or more creative ways to bring down the opposing general. With each new awareness achieved through these adventurous explorations, the child becomes more secure, expansive, and above all, more confident that the revelations his or her play brings will be useful and not threatening or destructive. In this way, more profound and subtle issues can be addressed in the process of play until one day, with that bit of sadness that accompanies all developmental steps, child and therapist recognize that the healing brought by play no longer needs the catalytic action of the therapist. Even without being aware of it, the child has developed another function for play, another way to find healing and soothing.

References

Allen FH: *Psychotherapy with Children.* New York, Norton, 1942.

Axline V: *Play Therapy.* Boston, Houghton Mifflin, 1947.

Berger P: *A Rumor of Angels.* New York, Doubleday, 1969.

Coppolillo HP: A technical consideration in child analysis and child therapy. *J Am Acad Child Psychiatry* 8:411–435, 1969.

Coppolillo HP: The transitional phenomenon revisited. *J Am Acad Child Psychiatry* 15:36–48, 1976.

Coppolillo HP: *Psychodynamic Psychotherapy of Children.* Madison, CT, International Universities Press, 1987, pp. 9–10.

Freud A: *The Psycho-analytical Treatment of Children.* London, Imago, 1946.

Freud S: *Beyond the Pleasure Principal.* London, Hogarth Press, 1955.

Gardner RA: Helping children cooperate in therapy. In: Harrison SI (ed): *Basic Handbook of Child Psychiatry* (Vol 3). New York, Basic Books, 1979, pp. 414–433.

Hug-Hellmuth H von: *Aus dem Seelenleben des Kindes.* Leipzig, Deuticke, 1913.

Hug-Hellmuth H von: On the technique of child analysis. *Int J Psychoanal* 2(3/4):287–305, 1921.

Klein M: *The Psychoanalysis of Children.* London, Hogarth Press, 1932.

Levy D: Release therapy. *Am J Orthopsychiatry* 9(4):713–736, 1939.

Peller L: Libidinal phases, ego development and play. *Psychoanal Study Child* 9:178–198, 1954.

Rapaport D: The autonomy of the ego. *Bull Menninger Clin* 15:113–123, 1951.

Rapaport D: The theory of ego autonomy. *Bull Menninger Clin* 22:13–35, 1958.

Sandler J, Kennedy H, Tyson R: *The Technique of Child Psychoanalysis.* Cambridge, MA, Harvard University Press, 1980, p. 39.

Simmons JE: *Psychiatric Examination of Children* (3rd ed). Philadelphia, Lea & Febiger, 1981.

Solomon JC: Play technique and the integrative process. *Am J Orthopsychiatry* 25(3):591–600, 1955.

Waelder R: The psychoanalytic theory of play. *Psychoanal Q* 2(2):220–224, 1933.

Winnicott DW: Transitional objects and transitional phenomena. *Int J Psychoanal* 30:89–97, 1949.

Winnicott DW: *The Maturational Process and the Facilitating Environment.* New York, International Universities Press, 1965:50–51.

75 CHILD AND ADOLESCENT BEHAVIOR THERAPY

Lawrence A. Vitulano, Ph.D., and Jacob Kraemer Tebes, Ph.D.

HISTORY

Behavior therapy refers to a set of related assumptions, principles, and techniques that are rooted in learning theory and used to change human behavior. Although the intellectual foundations of behavior therapy date back to the 17th-century empiricism of Locke and the 19th-century utilitarianism of Bentham, behavior therapy's more recent past can be divided into two relatively distinct periods: an early history dating from approximately the turn of the 20th century to the early 1950s, and a more recent period dating from the 1950s to the present.

The early history of behavior therapy is characterized by seminal contributions from key figures that frequently were not recognized for their relevance to human problems until the mid-20th century. Examples of this are the work of Ivan Pavlov (1927) on the conditioned reflex, Edward Thorndike (1911) on connectionism and the law of effect, and John B. Watson (1913) on behaviorism. Watson and his colleagues, Rosalie Raynor (Watson and Raynor, 1920) and Mary Cover Jones (Jones, 1924a, 1924b), were particularly influential in drawing popular attention to the importance of behavioral principles of conditioning in shaping human behavior. In addition, they were the first to show that these principles could be used to ameliorate infant and childhood problems. Despite these and other efforts, behavioral approaches were overshadowed during this period by the prevailing *zeitgeist*, then dominated by psychoanalysis and the emerging child guidance movement. Even a 1938 appeal by Arnold Gesell, a leader in that movement, for professionals to pay greater attention to behavioral principles had little impact on the use of behavioral approaches (Ross, 1971). The subsequent influence in the 1940s of Carl Rogers and his client-centered therapy further delayed the acceptance of behavioral approaches (Meyers and Craighead, 1983).

It was not until the 1950s that mental health professionals began to adopt behavioral approaches more widely for the treatment of mental disorders. This period was marked by a critical evaluation of the limitations of traditional therapeutic approaches to human problems and an eagerness to consider more scientifically based approaches. Works by Skinner (1953), Wolpe (1958), Eysenck (1960), and Bandura (1963) were particularly influential in demonstrating how learning theory principles could be used to ameliorate human problems. Patients with psychoses, severe anxiety neuroses, and autism became candidates for the application of the behavioral strategies and techniques identified in these works because few of the traditional approaches offered much hope for symptom improvement (Ferster and DeMyer, 1962; Ross, 1981). The success of these approaches in the 1950s and early 1960s with the most seriously disturbed adults and children enhanced the credibility of behavior therapy and increased its acceptance among professionals (Kazdin, 1978). This heralded the appearance of a host of behavioral journals during the 1960s, which began to provide a scientific basis for the field. Success with more disturbed patients also prompted professionals to begin to apply behavioral approaches to a wider range of problems, particularly to those presenting in outpatient settings. This prompted behavior therapists to reconceptualize the role of cognitions in changing behavior, such that they came to be viewed not only as a potential *target* of treatment but also as a possible *mechanism* for behavior change (Myers and Craighead, 1983a). The integration of cognitions into behavior therapy, coupled with developments in the emerging field of information processing, sparked the development of social learning theory and cognitive behavioral approaches in the late 1960s and early 1970s (Myers and Craighead, 1983a). These latter approaches dramatically increased behavior therapy's scope, the settings in which it could be practiced, and its potential for human betterment. Today, behavior therapy includes such a diverse array of therapeutic principles, practices, targets, and settings that it may be more accurate to use the term behavioral *interventions* to describe the additional preventive, promotive, and consultative efforts within the field.

BASIC ASSUMPTIONS

Behavior therapy rests on a common set of assumptions that distinguish it from other forms of therapy. The primary assumption is that most behavior develops and is maintained according to the principles of learning (Herbert, 1988; Johnson et al., 1986; O'Leary and Wilson, 1987; Rimm and Masters, 1979). Learning may be defined as a process in which behavior is initiated or is changed in reaction to internal or external stimuli that are not the result of "native response tendencies, maturation, or temporary states of the organism" (Hilgard and Bower, 1966, p. 2). Specific behavior therapy techniques are derived from each of the four types of learning: respondent conditioning, operant conditioning, cognitive-behavior modification, and social learning.

The principles of respondent conditioning are perhaps the most widely known among these. Respondent conditioning is based on the observation that certain behaviors, known as *respondents* (e.g., salivation, increased heart rate), are elicited involuntarily in response to certain stimuli (e.g., having food in one's mouth or being startled by a loud noise). Such behaviors are known as *unconditioned reflexes* or *unconditioned responses* because they occur "automatically" in response to a particular stimulus. Stimuli that are able to elicit such responses are known as *unconditioned stimuli*. When unconditioned stimuli are paired repeatedly with a previously neutral stimulus, eventually the neutral stimulus is able to elicit a conditioned response that usually resembles the unconditioned reflex. This was first demonstrated by Pavlov (1927) in a now-classic experiment with dogs, in which he paired a previously neutral stimulus—a bell—with the presentation of food, such that eventually his dogs began to salivate merely at the sound of the bell. Respondent conditioning in humans was first demonstrated by Watson and Raynor (1920) in their experiment with Albert, an 11-month-old infant. After allowing Albert to play comfortably with a furry white rat, the experimenters began to startle Albert with a loud noise (an unconditioned stimulus) whenever he began to play with the rat. After only seven pairings, Albert's pronounced startle to the noise was capable of being elicited exclusively by the sight of the rat, thus revealing a conditioned fear response. Importantly, Albert's fear also was elicited to a lesser degree when he was in the presence of other furry animals and objects, illustrating the related principle of *stimulus generalization*. Seligman (1971) has argued that humans are more "prepared" to be conditioned to certain objects, thus accounting for the observation that persons are more likely to be conditioned to some objects rather than others.

Another form of learning is *operant conditioning*. Based on Thorndike's observation that behavior is strengthened or weakened by its consequences, operant conditioning was first identified by Skinner (1938, 1953) as involving behaviors that could be modified or maintained by their consequences. Skinner termed such behaviors *operants* because they operate on the surrounding environment to generate consequences. Thus, behavior that is followed by pleasant consequences is likely to increase in frequency, while behavior followed by unpleasant consequences is likely to decrease in frequency. Operants differ from respondents in two primary ways: (*a*) They involve voluntary behavior that is "emitted" (i.e., as thoughts or actions) rather than "elicited" (i.e., as involuntary reflex responses), and (*b*) in the stimulus-response science of behavior, they are linked to properties of the response (e.g., its strength, frequency, duration) rather than to those of the stimulus (Hilgard and Bower, 1966). Since Skinner (1953) argued that most human behavior is operant in character, he advocated that the principles of operant conditioning be used to solve many types of behavior problems, an approach known today as applied behavioral analysis.

A third type of learning is *cognitive behavior modification* (Beck, 1976; Ellis, 1962; Mahoney, 1974; Meichenbaum, 1977). This has been described as an attempt to integrate internalism with behaviorism because of the primacy of cognitive and symbolic processes in mediating behavior (Meichenbaum, 1977). A basic assumption of cognitive behavioral approaches is that cognitive processes (e.g., attributions, cognitions, expectations, beliefs) influence one's behavior and affect. Irrational and faulty cognitive processes foster the development of maladaptive behavior patterns that are best reversed directly through the modification of maladaptive cognitions. Techniques such as cognitive restructuring and problem solving are common tools used by cognitive behavioral therapists to correct maladaptive cognitive processes that are believed to cause behavioral problems. Cognitive behavioral approaches do not concern themselves with intrapsychic, biological, neurological, or genetic factors in the development of child behavior problems (Kendall, 1985). Rather, a major focus of cognitive behavioral approaches is determining how cognition and behavior influence the development of child behavior problems. Although cognitive behavioral approaches place less emphasis on the influence of affective, familial, and social processes on human behavior, they seek to integrate understanding of these processes with cognitive and behavioral factors in order to produce change (Kendall, 1993).

Social learning theory, also known as *social cognitive theory*, describes the final category of learning (Bandura, 1963, 1969, 1977, 1986). Social learning theory is an attempt to integrate the two types of conditioning theories with our understanding of cognitive processes. According to Bandura (1977), learned behavior is governed by three types of regulatory processes: paired stimulus-response events (as in respondent conditioning), environmental consequences (as in operant conditioning), and symbolic cognitive processes (described partially in cognitive behavior modification). The most important among these are cognitive processes, and particularly those that involve observational learning, a process in which behavior change occurs by observing a model. For example, a child who views another child being rewarded for a particular behavior is more likely to perform similar behaviors. The centrality of observational learning in social learning theory is one of its distinguishing features. Another important feature is the view that behavior is characterized by "triadic reciprocality"; that is, behavior is determined by the reciprocal interplay among three forces: behavior, cognitive and other personal factors, and environmental influences (Bandura, 1986). A final distinguishing characteristic of social learning theory is that it emphasizes one's capacity for self-directed change. These latter two characteristics are clear departures from the more deterministic view of human nature and causality offered by respondent and operant conditioning theories, and to a lesser extent by cognitive behavior modification (Bandura, 1986). (For a more complete discussion of theories of learning, see Chapter 9 by Kazdin in this volume.)

A second major assumption of behavior therapy is that observable behavior should be the primary focus of therapy (Kazdin, 1985a; Rimm and Masters, 1979). Subjective experiences such as feelings and cognitions, as well as psychophysiological processes such as electrodermal activity, are viewed as integral and essential elements of the therapeutic enterprise as long as observable behavioral referents for their occurrence are identified. In general, behavior therapists eschew treatment formulations that hypothesize a distal underlying cause for an observed behavior, preferring instead to focus on environmental contingencies proximal to the behavior in question. In this connection, although behavior therapists acknowledge the importance of biological and genetic factors that may contribute to the emergence of a problem behavior, they seek to identify and modify environmental contingencies that are presumed to maintain it in the here and now.

A third major assumption of behavior therapy is that treatment techniques should be empirically based (Johnson et al., 1986; O'Leary and Wilson, 1987; Rimm and Masters, 1979). Many of the techniques behavior therapists employ were derived from laboratory experiments and have their roots in experimental psychology. As a result, behavior therapists view their work as an "applied science" (O'Leary and Wilson, 1987), because it involves the application of these techniques to clinical problems. A related by-product of this development is that behavior therapists emphasize the setting of clear and precise goals in treatment, which enables them to validate treatment goals and outcomes empirically.

A fourth major assumption of behavior therapy, related to the above, is that treatment should be action oriented and directive (London, 1986; Rimm and Masters, 1979). This assumption is based on the belief that action, rather than insight, is the primary mechanism for change, and that symptom change is the appropriate focus of treatment rather than some ill-defined and unspecifiable "underlying cause." The primacy of action means that behavior therapists take an active, directive role in treatment ("homework" is assigned for patients to complete between sessions, specific treatment goals and strategies are discussed directly with patients, behavioral contracts between therapist and patient or between parents and child are negotiated in the session, etc.). Practice is encouraged, interpretation is rarely used, and empathic listening is employed as long as it promotes the accomplishment of behaviorally based treatment objectives.

A fifth and final major assumption of behavior therapy is that behavior change is best maintained through enlisting the help of key persons in the client's environment (Herbert, 1988; Kazdin, 1985a). In the case of children, this usually means teaching behavioral principles to parents, teacher, and other family members and establishing a treatment plan that provides for the generalization or "transfer" of treatment from the clinic to the child's natural environment, such as the home or school. Underlying this assumption is the belief that much behavior is situation specific and that proximal environmental contingencies can best be addressed by training key persons in the child's environment who can help maintain therapeutic gains.

BEHAVIOR THERAPY TECHNIQUES

The techniques of child and adolescent behavior therapy can be categorized as attempting to produce either of two kinds of behavior change: (*a*) to strengthen, develop, or maintain behavior, or (*b*) to reduce or eliminate behavior. Although these techniques can be employed for a wide range of problem behaviors, only the most common applications are summarized below.

Techniques to Strengthen, Develop, or Maintain Behavior

In operant conditioning, *reinforcement* is the process by which behavior is strengthened by its consequences. In the case of *positive reinforcement*, a reward (or reinforcer) is presented after the occurrence of the desired behavior; in *negative reinforcement*, the reward involves removal of an aversive stimulus after the desired behavior occurs. Both positive and negative reinforcement differ from punishment because their purpose is to *increase* the likelihood that a particular behavior will occur. Punishment, on the other hand, is aimed at *reducing* the incidence of a particular behavior. Reinforcers can be either tangible (i.e., involving concrete, material items, such as food, money, privileges, opportunities to engage in specific activities or behaviors, and removal of sanctions) or intangible (i.e., involving social or related items, such as encouragement, praise, and smiles) (Herbert, 1988). In addition, reinforcers can be external (i.e., obtained from others) or internal (i.e., provided to oneself). An important property of reinforcement is that behavior is strengthened differentially by the schedule of reinforcement one uses. Reinforcement that is administered immediately after each time a desired response occurs is known as *continuous reinforcement*. Other types of reinforcement schedules involve some form of *intermittent reinforcement*. In a *fixed interval* schedule, the child is reinforced after a specific time period, regardless of what response is emitted, while in a *variable interval* schedule the rate varies randomly around a specific average at which reinforcement is administered. A *fixed ratio* schedule administers reinforcement after a specified number of the child's desirable responses,

while a *variable ratio* schedule administers a reinforcer randomly around a specific average of desirable responses on the part of the child. In general, learning that results from intermittent schedules of reinforcement—and in particular, variable interval or ratio schedules—is more stable and difficult to change than that acquired through continuous reinforcement. Compulsive gambling is an example of how an intermittent reinforcement schedule can lead to behavioral persistence and high rates of responding.

Positive and negative reinforcement are techniques frequently used to teach children skills to compensate for behavioral, learning, and other skill deficits. In addition, reinforcement is often employed in combination with other techniques used to strengthen or eliminate behaviors.

A second important behavioral change technique is *stimulus discrimination training*. This involves reinforcing a particular response in the presence of one stimulus while not reinforcing that response in the presence of another stimulus. Stimulus discrimination training enables the child to learn how to discriminate when and under what conditions it is most appropriate to emit a particular response, and when it is not. Three techniques are used in stimulus discrimination training: shaping, fading, and chaining (Martin and Pear, 1983). *Shaping* involves reinforcing closer and closer approximations of behavior in order to produce the final desired behavior. Thus, a teacher of a severely mentally retarded child might initially reward the child for standing near a desk, then sitting in the desk, then engaging in playful behavior while sitting in the desk, then for on-task classroom behavior while sitting in the desk. This is accomplished by varying when and under what conditions reinforcement is provided. *Fading* involves gradually changing a stimulus that controls a response so that eventually a new, alternative stimulus produces the same response. Thus, an autistic child who only mimics the word *shoe* might be provided with a reinforcer (e.g., praise, hugs, tokens) every time he or she repeats shoe in the presence of an additional prompt, such as "What's on your foot? Shoe." Gradually the prompt shoe is faded until the child is able to respond directly to the question "What's on your foot?" *Chaining* involves reinforcing more and more of the stimulus-response links that comprise a complex chain of behavior, such as using a fork to eat. This procedure usually involves the use of shaping or fading techniques to achieve stimulus control of the desired behavior. Thus, in chaining one might demonstrate an entire behavior to be learned and then reinforce a child in his or her attempts to complete the entire behavior, as well as for specific successive approximations of the behavior as is done in shaping. Shaping, fading, and chaining are commonly used in conjunction with other behavioral techniques, such as reinforcement, to teach children skills to compensate for behavioral, social, or other skill deficits.

Conditioned reinforcement is also used to strengthen, develop, or maintain behavior. In conditioned reinforcement, a particular stimulus—the conditioned reinforcer—signals the likelihood that reinforcement is forthcoming. Over time, the stimulus itself becomes reinforcing (i.e., it becomes conditioned) because of its association with the receipt of reinforcement. Thus, parental praise is a conditioned reinforcer because it signals the likelihood that other reinforcers, such as food, privileges, affection, and so on, are forthcoming. Tangible conditioned reinforcers that can be earned and exchanged for other reinforcers are typically referred to as *tokens*. A behavioral program that uses tokens systematically to produce behavior change is known as a *token economy*. Token economies have been used with considerable success in a wide variety of settings, such as schools, inpatient units, and group homes, as well as in the home by parents (Kazdin, 1977).

Contingency contracting is another behavioral technique, which is primarily used to increase specific behaviors, but may also be used to reduce inappropriate or unwanted behaviors (Herbert, 1987; Kazdin, 1989; Spiegler and Guevremont, 1993). Contracts may be verbal or written and may be used in conjunction with conditioned reinforcers, such as tokens, to reinforce target behaviors. Written contingency contracts should specify the following in unambiguous terms: (*a*) the responsible parties involved (e.g., the parent(s) and the child); (*b*) the

What (child _____) agrees to do:	What (parents _____) agree to do:
1. *Get ready for school.* Wake up on his own, get dressed for school, pack all homework and school materials, and get out to the school bus on time every day.	1. *Make breakfast, buy supplies, and reward each day and week.* Make breakfast by 7:00 AM every day. Buy all school supplies. Give (child _____) $1/day for being ready and a $5/week bonus if he or she makes all days of the week.
2. *Complete homework.* Complete daily homework, complete at least 20% of work on longer homework projects each day, and study at least 30 extra minutes each day.	2. *Give (child _____) the car.* Allow (child _____) to use the car for one outing on the weekend if 75% or more of all three homework tasks are completed. If 100% of all homework tasks are completed, (child _____) may use the car two or more times on the weekend when it's available.
3. *Complete chores.* Take out trash on Tuesday nights, clear dinner table on Mondays and Thursdays, and throw dirty clothes in his or her bedroom hamper by Friday morning.	3. *Pay weekly allowance.* Pay (child _____) weekly allowance of $10 on Friday at 6:00 PM.
4. *Engage in "fair fighting."* When arguing with (parents _____), (child _____) will not: • call them names • intimidate them physically • hit them	4. *Engage in "fair fighting."* When arguing with (child _____), (parents _____) will not: • bring up sore points from the past • impose a punishment without further listening to (child's _____) version of what happened

Note: Each week, if more than one area above is not met, (child _____) will be grounded for 1 week (must stay in the house with no TV or use of telephone after 6 PM).

I agree to abide by the above contract to the best of my ability.

_____   _____
(child)   (mother)

                                                          _____
                                                          (father)

Figure 75.1. Sample contract between (child _____) and (parents _____) from the week beginning Sunday, _____.

target behavior(s) to be increased (e.g., studying, school attendance) or eliminated (e.g., smoking, physical aggression toward a sibling); (*c*) the consequences for completing or failing to complete the target behavior (i.e., the behavioral contingencies); and (*d*) the time interval during which the contract is in effect (e.g., weekly, monthly). For some contracts, it may also be necessary to specify *who* will monitor some target behaviors (e.g., a teacher) or *how* those behaviors will be monitored (e.g., daily school report). An example of a written behavioral contract that parents might use to increase several specific target behaviors of an adolescent is found in Figure 75.1.

Modeling represents a behavioral change technique that involves having a child observe a model engage in a particular sequence of behavior for the purpose of producing behavior change. Three types of modeling have been identified: live, symbolic, and participant (Bandura, 1969). In *live modeling*, a child observes a model engaging in the target behavior in vivo; in *symbolic modeling*, a child views the model on film or videotape or imagines himself or herself engaging in the behavior; and in *participant modeling*, a child observes a model engaging in the target behavior in vivo and then attempts that same behavior. Modeling can have a number of different effects: acquisition of a new behavior, social facilitation of observed behavior, enhancement of environmental influences, arousal of specific emotions, disinhibition of behaviors that were previously avoided, and extinction of behaviors associated with persons or objects that were observed (Bandura, 1986). (The latter two involve effects that reduce or eliminate problem behaviors.)

A final set of behavioral change techniques that can be used to strengthen, develop, or maintain behavior, as well as to reduce or eliminate behavior, is skills training approaches. Two types of skills training

approaches are most commonly described: *social skills training* and *cognitive skills training.* The aim of social skills training approaches is to teach children skills necessary to interact in socially appropriate ways with peers and adults. Typically, skills are taught in an analogue or laboratory setting through a combination of behavioral techniques, such as positive reinforcement, modeling, coaching, instruction, role playing, and behavioral rehearsal (Hops et al., 1985). For example, an extremely shy boy may be taught how to interact more assertively with peers by first viewing a model perform the target behavior and then being praised for each successive approximation of that behavior during a role play. Therapist and child then rehearse this procedure until the child is ready to interact assertively with peers. Such techniques have been used extensively to teach appropriate social skills to socially isolated and withdrawn children, to mentally retarded and autistic children, and to children who are overly aggressive and antisocial (Dumas, 1989; Hansen et al., 1989; O'Leary and Wilson, 1987).

Cognitive skills training approaches are a related type of technique that emphasizes teaching children cognitive skills that are presumed to mediate successful task performance. Also known as *self-instructional training, problem-solving training,* or *self-control training* (depending on the goals of the treatment), cognitive approaches are based on the cognitive behavioral assumption discussed earlier, in which faulty cognitions mediate maladaptive behavior. As opposed to social skills training approaches, which emphasize teaching behavioral skills, these approaches focus on teaching children covert cognitive mediational techniques, such as corrective self-statements and covert verbalizations to help regulate their behavior in various situations. In most training programs, the children use self-statements to identify the problem, generate alternative solutions, decide on one solution, evaluate the outcome of their choice, and provide covert positive self-reinforcement (Dumas, 1989). This approach has been employed successfully to promote adjustment to a wide variety of behavior problems in very young children, as well as in older children and adolescents. Although summarized here as a technique to strengthen, develop, or maintain behavior, cognitive skills training approaches are often used to reduce or eliminate childhood impulsivity, aggression, or fears (Dumas, 1989; Christoff and Myatt, 1987; Kendall and Braswell, 1985; Meyers and Craighead, 1983).

Techniques to Reduce or Eliminate Behavior

In operant conditioning, *extinction* refers to the process in which reinforcement is withheld after an operant response so as to reduce the frequency of its occurrence. Ironically, undesirable behaviors usually *increase* in frequency for a brief period immediately following the introduction of an extinction procedure, although gradually they disappear in the absence of reinforcement. A common example of extinction is when parents attempt to help their young infant sleep for longer periods through the night. If a parent responds immediately to the infant's cries after it is put to bed by holding it, the infant learns to associate crying at bedtime and being held. To unlearn or extinguish this operant response, a parent allows the infant to cry a few minutes before responding. If this practice is followed on successive nights by gradually increasing the parent's response delay intervals by 5 minutes on each occasion, the infant's crying will slowly be extinguished, so that it learns to fall asleep alone. Although useful as a procedure to reduce or eliminate some undesirable behaviors, extinction is usually not appropriate for the elimination of destructive or disruptive behaviors, which may require more direct intervention (Johnson et al., 1986).

A technique for the reduction of problem behaviors that combines some of the properties of extinction with those of reinforcement is *differential reinforcement*. In this technique, reinforcement is given for the nonoccurrence or low rate of occurrence of the problem behavior. Three types of differential reinforcement have been identified: *differential reinforcement of other behavior* (DRO), *differential reinforcement of incompatible behavior* (DRI), and *differential reinforcement of low rates of behavior* (DRL). In a DRO procedure, a child is reinforced for not emitting the problem behavior during a specified time or response interval. In effect, what is being reinforced is every behavior *other* than the problem behavior. In a DRI procedure, a child is reinforced for emitting an appropriate behavior that is topographically incompatible with the problem behavior during a specified time or response interval. For example, a child who has trouble remaining on-task during class is reinforced for completing a specified number of assignments or for working on an assignment for a specified length of time. In a DRL procedure, a child is reinforced for emitting low rates of the problem behavior during a specified time or response interval. Thus, a child who frequently leaves his or her seat during class is reinforced for leaving the seat only twice during a specified time interval. DRO and DRL procedures provide the least amount of stimulus control in that alternative problem behaviors may be reinforced during a specified interval, along with appropriate behaviors. This is not the case with a DRI procedure since the emission of appropriate or prosocial behaviors is required for reinforcement to occur. Differential reinforcement procedures are readily incorporated into school or institutional settings and are particularly effective in the reduction of disruptive, aggressive, and self-injurious behaviors (O'Leary and Wilson, 1987; Martin and Pear, 1983; Repp and Dietz, 1979).

Punishment is a technique used to reduce or eliminate undesirable behavior through the introduction of an aversive stimulus or removal of a positive stimulus after an operant response. Scolding, spanking, or removal of privileges (e.g., watching television, going outside to play) are examples of punishment, if these are presented contingent on a child's behavior and reduce the frequency of that behavior. Punishment procedures differ from extinction procedures because they usually bring about a rapid decrease in the frequency of problem behaviors, thus making them particularly effective techniques for the reduction of self-injurious and aggressive behaviors and certain kinds of disruptive behaviors. Nevertheless, punishment also has many disadvantages that recommend against its regular use. It tends to suppress behavior temporarily rather than actually change it and may produce serious and unwanted side effects (Johnson et al., 1986; Johnston, 1972; Kazdin, 1984), such as (*a*) the elicitation of fear responses that may become conditioned to the punisher or punishing situation; (*b*) the promotion of escape responses, such as physical or emotional withdrawal, after punishment is terminated; (*c*) the strengthening of behaviors that motivate the child to avoid the aversive situation and thus reduce the chance that more desirable behaviors can be learned; (*d*) reinforcement (and thus strengthening) of the undesirable behavior through negative attention the child receives during punishment; and (*e*) observational learning of other undesirable behaviors that may be modeled by the punisher for the child, such as aggressive physical or verbal behavior and disrespect for the rights of others.

Three common punishment procedures are time out, response cost, and overcorrection. In a *time out* procedure, the child is removed from the setting in which the misbehavior occurs and is placed in a restrictive environment for a brief period. The lack of opportunity to obtain reinforcers by having to remain in such an environment usually results in a rapid suppression of misbehavior. In the typical application of this procedure, the child is warned that a time out will follow if the misbehavior continues. If the child does not heed the warning, he or she is sent to the time out room (or area) and asked to remain there for 10 minutes (3–5 minutes for very young children). At the end of the designated time, the child is allowed to return to the previous setting. Time out has been widely used with success in classroom and institutional settings, as well as in the home. It has been found to be a particularly effective punishment technique for the reduction of disruptive or aggressive behavior, which is easily reinforced by peers (Foxx and Shapiro, 1978; Hobbs and Forehand, 1977).

Response cost is another common punishment procedure in which a reinforcer is removed contingent upon misbehavior so as to reduce the future probability of its occurrence. Typically, response cost procedures are used in conjunction with a token economy program, but they may also be used in the home by parents who have established "contingency contracts" with their child, usually an adolescent. In such contracts, the parents agree to provide the child with rewards or privileges (e.g., use of the family car, extended use of the telephone) in return for completion of specific behaviors on the part of the child (e.g., coming home before curfew, cleaning one's bedroom). If the child does not keep the contract, payment is made by removal of agreed-upon rewards or privileges. In the appropriate use of this procedure, the child is informed in advance that he or she will be penalized a specified amount of rewards, privileges, or tokens for a particular misbehavior. When a misbehavior occurs, rewards, privileges, or tokens are removed. This procedure has been used to reduce the incidence of a wide range of problem behaviors, such as disruptions in the classroom, crying, perseverative speech, aggressiveness, and hyperactivity (Rimm and Masters, 1979). Response cost differs from time out because the child is not removed from the opportunity to gain reinforcers, making it particularly effective in promoting self-control and self-management.

A final, frequently used punishment procedure is *overcorrection*. Overcorrection involves having the misbehaving child correct the consequences of the misbehavior. In *restitutional overcorrection*, the child is required not only to restore the environment to its original state prior to the misbehavior but also to improve it (e.g., a child who defaces a roommate's poster may be required to save enough money to replace the poster, as well as to do the roommate a particular favor). In *positive practice overcorrection*, the child is required to practice positive behaviors that are incompatible with the misbehavior (e.g., a messy eater may be required to practice eating correctly). Although these two procedures are usually not used in combination, for some problem behaviors, such as bed-wetting, their combined use has met with success (e.g., a bed wetter is required to remove wet linen, remake the bed, and then repeatedly practice leaving the bed, walking to the toilet, and returning to the bed) (Azrin et al., 1974). Major characteristics of overcorrection procedures are (a) they relate directly to the misbehavior by requiring the child to complete a chain of behavioral responses that are topographically similar to a correct response; (b) they are intended to have the child experience the effort required by others to correct the consequences of the misbehavior; (c) they are instituted immediately after the misbehavior so as to reduce the likelihood that positive reinforcement from the behavior can occur; and (d) "graduated guidance" is used to enforce completion of the overcorrection requirement, whereby the enforcing adult manually assists the child through completion of the overcorrection response (Foxx and Bechtel, 1982). Although overcorrection has been shown to be effective in reducing the incidence of a wide range of aggressive, self-injurious, and self-stimulatory behaviors, as well as inappropriate toileting and oral behaviors (e.g., vomiting, drooling), it is an aversive procedure that holds considerable potential for abuse if not used with caution and discretion.

Desensitization refers to a broad class of related "exposure training" behavioral techniques that are based on classical conditioning principles and used to reduce children's fears. In desensitization, a child is gradually exposed to a conditioned stimulus (e.g., a dog, taking a test, being separated from one's mother) until the fear is extinguished. *Participant modeling* and *symbolic modeling* have each been used to desensitize a child from a conditioned stimulus. In participant modeling, the child observes another person (usually a child) in the presence of the feared stimulus and then is reinforced for gradually approaching the stimulus until the fear disappears. In symbolic modeling, the conditioned fear is extinguished by having a fearful child view a film in which an initially fearful child gradually overcomes the fear.

The most common form of exposure training to reduce fears is *systematic desensitization*. In this technique, the child first works with the therapist to establish a hierarchy of fears about the anxiety-provoking stimulus. In order for desensitization to have the potential for success, this hierarchy must be as detailed as possible. A sample hierarchy is presented in Table 75.1 for a child with test anxiety.

Once the fear hierarchy is established, the child is helped to feel relaxed by talking to the therapist or a parent, playing quietly with peers, or eating a favorite food. An alternative approach used regularly in systematic desensitization with adults is to have the child engage in deep muscle relaxation prior to exposure training (Cautela and Groden, 1978). Relaxation is intended to function as an incompatible response to anxiety. Once the child is relaxed, the therapist asks the child to imagine the least distressing scene in the fear hierarchy and to indicate if the scene remains distressing (e.g., if the child is seated in an armchair, he or she may be instructed to lift an index finger to indicate distress). If the scene continues to elicit anxiety, the child is instructed to relax

for a few seconds, and then the procedure is repeated with the same scene until it no longer elicits anxiety on three successive presentations. The therapist repeats this procedure with each successive distressing scene in the hierarchy until the child no longer reports being distressed by the feared stimulus. Typically, no more than three to five scenes can be presented per session.

A variation of this technique called *in vivo desensitization* has been developed, in which the child undergoes exposure training to the hierarchy in vivo rather than through imaginal responses (Morris and Kratochwill, 1983). The effectiveness of both systematic and in vivo desensitization is enhanced when the therapist has the child practice between sessions those items that no longer elicit anxiety and when practice is accompanied by positive reinforcement (Johnson et al., 1986).

A related exposure training technique that may be used as an alternative to desensitization is *flooding* (also known as *implosion therapy* when applied in vivo). Widely used with adults, flooding involves having the child come in contact with the most feared item in the hierarchy, either in vivo or in imagination, until the fear is extinguished. Although flooding has been effective with children when graded desensitization procedures have not met with success (Yule et al., 1974), its use with children raises ethical concerns about children's informed consent and voluntariness of participation in such a potentially upsetting procedure.

In addition to the behavioral reduction techniques discussed above, a number of the techniques described earlier have met with considerable success in reducing or eliminating problem behaviors in children. Techniques such as modeling, self-instructional training, problem solving, and contingency contracting have been used extensively to treat problems such as aggressiveness, impulsivity, antisocial behavior, fears, and substance abuse.

BEHAVIORAL ASSESSMENT

Behavioral assessment is the process of identifying target behaviors and their controlling conditions by several different methods, in order to assist the clinician in developing an appropriate treatment plan. Traditional assessment approaches hypothesize the operation of traits or personality constructs from *within* the individual. Behavioral assessment approaches hypothesize the operation of specific behavior patterns or states *outside* of the individual. Although the distinction between these two approaches may be extremely subtle in practice (e.g., in the assessment of a child's cognitions and affects), conceptually it is an important one, since it focuses the assessment on current circumstances in the client's environment rather than on enduring underlying traits or states.

Traditional assessment approaches attempt to uncover the individual's personality structure, arrive at a diagnosis, and finally, offer a prognosis. In contrast, behavioral assessment methods gather data that are directly, rather than inferentially, related to a treatment program and its evaluation. Behavioral assessment can be viewed as a dynamic process that involves (a) problem identification and target behavior selection, (b) choice and design of a treatment program, (c) periodic measurement of results during treatment, and (d) evaluation of the final treatment outcome (Bornstein et al., 1984). Since all treatments are not equally effective and vary in their efficacy according to several client-therapist factors, such as the client's age and potential for compliance, family support, and the therapist's expertise in behavioral assessment, the choice and design of a treatment program is based, as much as possible, on the relevant therapy outcome literature. Once a treatment program has been selected, periodic reassessment of its efficacy and suitability throughout the treatment phase is essential.

Models of Assessment

There are several widely used models of behavioral assessment. Kanfer and Saslow's S-O-R-K-C model (Kanfer et al., 1969) is a comprehensive method that assesses the stimulus (S), the organism's biological conditions (O) and behavioral response (R), the contingencies and

Table 75.1.   Sample Items of a Desensitization Hierarchy for Test Anxiety for a 14-Year-Old Student[a]

10	Attending class
20	Hearing the teacher announce that there will be a test at the end of the week
30	Attending class the day after the test has been announced
40	Doing homework in that same subject the day after the test has been announced
50	Attending class 3 days before the test
60	Studying for the test at home 3 nights before the test
70	Attending class 2 days before the test
80	Studying for the test at home 2 nights before the test
85	Attending class the day before the test
90	Talking to classmates about the test 2 days before the test
100	Sitting in class just before the exam is passed out

[a] Items are ranked according to the amount of subjective anxiety they elicit, from 10 (lowest) to 100 (highest).

schedules of reinforcement (*K*), and relevant consequences (*C*). The BASIC ID model of Lazarus (1973) is a multimodal assessment of behaviors (*B*), affects (*A*), sensations (*S*), imagery (*I*), cognitions (*C*), interpersonal relationships (*I*), and drugs and general physical state (*D*). Peterson (1968) has proposed a functional analysis of behavior model that involves systematic observations of the problem behavior and the stimulus conditions (antecedents and consequences) that give rise to it, followed by experimental manipulation of a functionally related condition that causes the behavior.

One particularly useful and comprehensive model for behavioral assessment is the Behavioral Assessment Grid (BAG) developed by Cone (1978). This model divides assessment into a tripartite conceptual scheme of behavioral contents, methods of assessment, and types of generalizability. The behavioral *contents* area of the BAG refers to the three domains that behavior therapists typically assess for behavioral responses: cognitive (subjective), motor, and physiological. For example, a child's fear may be assessed as a worry in the cognitive domain, as behavioral avoidance in the motor domain, or as a biochemical response to a stimulus in the physiological domain. These are believed to be distinct yet potentially overlapping areas of behavioral functioning. The *methods* component of the BAG refers to the many types of indirect and direct measurement techniques that can be used to make a behavioral assessment. Indirect methods include behavioral interviews, self-reports, and ratings by others. Direct methods include self-observations or observations by others in analogue or naturalistic situations under free play conditions or role play instructions. Lastly, the *universes of generalizations* component of the BAG refers to the extent to which measurements obtained are generalizable across multiple contexts. Specifically, six "universes" of generalizability have been identified as particularly relevant to consider when making a behavioral assessment: dimension (of behavior that is assessed), method (used to make the assessment), setting (in which the assessment is made), time (when the assessment is made), item (which aspect of a dimension is assessed), and scorer (who makes the assessment). Thus, the BAG model allows for three domains of behavioral contents by eight methods of data collection by six universes of generalization, resulting in a theoretically possible matrix of 144 different combinations of behavioral assessments. Although existing assessment measures do not fit into each of these 144 categories, the BAG model provides a useful framework within which one can conceptualize and classify behavioral assessment instruments and measures.

Assessment Strategies

There are a variety of behavioral assessment strategies, which range from the least to the most direct in terms of the method of data collection (Cone, 1978).

INTERVIEWS

Behavioral interviews are an integral element of the assessment process (Morganstern, 1988). The objective during the initial phase of the behavioral interview is to establish rapport with the child, regarded as a necessary but not sufficient ingredient for successful treatment. During this phase, the child is assured of the confidential nature of the relationship and informed of under what conditions of danger to self or others that confidentiality will be broken. After the child presents the problem, the therapist probes for additional information regarding the initiation, frequency, and controlling conditions surrounding the problem behaviors. In the case of very young children, it is common to conduct a verbal interview with the parents and a play interview with the child in order to obtain a sample of the child's behavior.

Structured interviews are another type of indirect assessment strategy and a relatively recent addition to the classic behavioral assessment protocol for children (Morrison, 1988). There are currently three major structured interview measures in use with children: the Diagnostic Interview for Children and Adolescents (DICA) (Herjanic et al., 1975), the

Diagnostic Interview Schedule for Children (DISC) (Costello et al., 1984), and the Schedule for Affective Disorder and Schizophrenia for School-Age Children, Present Episode Version (K-SADS-P) (Chambers et al., 1985). The DICA is a 60- to 90-minute interview of both the child and parent in three parts, conducted by trained interviewers. The DISC involves two 45- to 60-minute separate interviews with both the child and parent by trained interviewers and provides a DSM diagnosis. Lastly, the K-SADS-P is a semistructured interview of both the parent and child that assesses four areas (affect, anxiety, conduct, and psychosis) in two time periods (the past week and when the current episode was at its worst). It takes about 60 minutes to complete each interview.

SELF-REPORTS AND RATINGS BY OTHERS

Self-reports and ratings by others can be obtained through the use of various rating scales, which vary in terms of their validity and reliability (Morrison, 1988). Such self-report scales increasingly are being used by behavior therapists to assess symptom severity and also to monitor treatment effects. Some of the most widely used self-report instruments are discussed below.

The Children's Depression Inventory (CDI) is a 27-item scale adapted from the Beck Depression Inventory that provides information on a child's cognitive, affective, and behavioral signs of depression (Kovacs and Beck, 1977). It can be self-administered or read to children, as well as completed by parents. The Child Behavior Checklist (CBCL) is an empirically derived questionnaire that asks respondents to rate the occurrence of 118 problem behaviors of childhood or adolescence on a three-point scale (Achenbach, 1978; Achenbach and Edelbrock, 1979). Although the version that is the most widely used is the parent form, teacher and youth self-report forms have also been developed. The CBCL is one of the most carefully designed, empirically sound, and comprehensive instruments available for the assessment of children's problems. It also includes additional items that provide a gross assessment of a child's social competencies. The Conners Teacher Rating Scale (Conners, 1973) is a 39-item self-report measure whose items are rated on a four-point scale. It is most commonly used in the assessment and treatment of hyperactivity since it is sensitive to changes from both behavioral interventions and psychopharmacological treatment. The Conners Parent Rating Scale (Conners, 1970) is also available for parent reports, and both scales come in short-form versions. The Fear Survey Schedule for Children-Revised (Ollendick, 1983) is an 80-item self-report measure that is rated on a three-point scale. It differentiates phobic from nonphobic children and also identifies etiological factors such as separation anxiety, school phobia, and recent physical illness.

SELF-OBSERVATION

Self-observation, one of the oldest methods of direct behavioral assessment, includes the simple tabulation of behaviors by check marks or counters as well as behavioral monitoring by more sophisticated electronic devices that measure physiological responses such as heart rate and blood pressure. These measures are employed in several self-control procedures, such as weight reduction, tic control, and nail-biting cessation. Self-observation is less expensive and intrusive than the use of outside observers, allows monitoring to occur for longer periods of time and across a greater number of settings, and is particularly appropriate when monitoring infrequently occurring behaviors. It is important to note that self-monitoring can be a highly reactive process for clients, one that can precipitate dramatic behavior change in a favorable direction.

DIRECT OBSERVATION

Direct observation can be conducted in the natural environment as well as in analogue situations. An example of the use of direct observation in an analogue situation is the use of the Behavioral Avoidance Test (BAT) to measure phobic behavior in children. The BAT is the most commonly employed direct observational procedure to assess specific fears (Wells and Vitulano, 1984). During the BAT, the clinician records the distance from and time a client will spend with a feared object. Although this procedure is very useful in providing concrete evidence of the nature and extent of a specific fear under controlled conditions, it can be quite reactive to demand characteristics, such as telling a child to try harder.

Direct observation of role plays is also used in behavioral assessment, in either naturalistic or analogue situations. During a role play, clients are asked to imagine themselves in various situations and then to respond in their typical manner. Role plays in naturalistic and analogue situations are frequently used in the assessment of social skills deficits in children.

TREATMENT APPLICATIONS

Anxiety Disorders

Anxiety disorders include that group of disorders whose symptoms are primarily characterized by anxiety and avoidance behavior. This category of disturbances includes phobic disorders, panic disorders, generalized anxiety disorders, and obsessive compulsive disorders. Although fears and anxieties are common and transitory throughout childhood (Lapouse and Monk, 1959), more severe and persistent phobic reactions in childhood that are not considered to be age- or stage-specific require the attention and treatment of professionals. Thorough assessment of children's fears should include an evaluation of the three-channel response system of subjective feelings and thoughts, behavioral avoidance, and physiological activity (Graziano et al., 1979).

Assessment in all three channels facilitates treatment planning and enhances treatment efficacy. For example, for a child who exhibits avoidance behavior (i.e., the motor system or channel), reinforced practice would be an essential component of the treatment; for a child who reports considerable subjective anxiety (i.e., the cognitive channel), self-control strategies would be recommended; and finally, for a child who experiences somatic symptoms when confronted with the feared stimulus (i.e., the physiological channel), relaxation training would be indicated. Typically, however, treatment plans for anxiety disturbances usually are more complex because they involve two or three different channels of behavioral disruption. For example, a treatment plan for a child who experiences fear in all three channels might begin with relaxation training (physiological), move to self-instructional training (cognitive), and then advance to the use of participant modeling (motor) in combination with self-instructional training. Thorough reviews of the use of various behavioral techniques, such as relaxation training, systematic desensitization, flooding, implosion, modeling, self-control training, and operant procedures to treat childhood anxiety disorders are available (Siegel and Ridley-Johnson, 1985; Straus, 1987; Wells and Vitulano, 1984).

Despite the controversy over the etiology and definition of school phobia, behavior therapy has generally been successful in its remediation. Techniques such as systematic desensitization, participant modeling, and contingency contracting have been particularly efficacious (Ollendick and Mayer, 1984). Obsessive compulsive disorders, on the other hand, have been shown to be responsive to in vivo exposure procedures when combined with response prevention techniques (Baer and Minichiello, 1990; Grayson et al., 1982). For example, compulsive handwashers are encouraged to touch contaminated objects and then refrain from washing in order to break the negative reinforcement chain. Although there has been less success in the treatment of obsessional behaviors, the most promising strategy appears to be imaginal exposure to obsessional thinking for a prolonged period of time of 30 minutes or more (i.e., avoidance response prevention) in order to extinguish the anxiety response (Rachman and Hodgson, 1980). The treatment of obsessive-compulsive disorder symptoms in children and adolescents with Tourette's syndrome is best approached as part of a comprehensive, multimodal therapeutic plan (King et al., 1993). Finally, it should be noted that much of childhood anxiety may in fact be secondary to social skill deficits in anxious children. Such children initially may lack the necessary skills to interact in a feared situation and fail to acquire those skills because of successful avoidance behaviors, while their peers continue to learn interaction skills (Wells, 1981). The obvious treatment program for these children is to augment fear reduction techniques with social skills training (Christoff and Myatt, 1987).

Depression

Behavioral researchers and clinicians maintain that childhood depression represents a complex amalgam of symptoms that vary in degree and kind according to a child's developmental level. Thus, children who are depressed in early childhood may show evidence of excessive crying, loss of appetite, and temper tantrums, while those of middle childhood (ages 6–8) may exhibit dysphoria, somatization, and impulsive behaviors, and those of late childhood (ages 8–12) may display poor self-esteem, social isolation, self-depreciating behaviors, and hopelessness (Kaslow and Rehm, 1985; Kovacs and Beck, 1977). The complexity of this symptom picture, coupled with the considerable overlap between these and other symptoms of disorder in childhood and adolescence (Kendall et al., 1989), has led behavioral investigators to argue that the most effective intervention for childhood depression is to treat specific symptoms of the disorder, such as self-depreciating behaviors, social withdrawal, and low activity level (Kaslow and Rehm, 1983; Puig-Antich, 1982).

There is growing evidence that this strategy is effective (Reynolds and Coats, 1986; Stark, 1990; Stark et al., 1987, 1991). Among the various behavioral techniques, self-control training has demonstrated the greatest efficacy in the treatment of depression for children (ages 9–12) and adolescents. Self-control training in the treatment of depression involves teaching the child to monitor negative self-attributions, evaluate the validity of those attributions, and reinforce positive alternative attributions. Children are also taught to set realistic goals and standards for performance, refrain from punitive self-statements, and utilize positive self-statements as reinforcers. Finally, in order to compensate for the tendency of depressed children to attribute success to luck or chance, children are taught to view success as resulting from their own stable and internal competencies and to view failure as emanating from external factors outside of their control (Hughes, 1988; Rehm, 1977). Controlled outcome studies using these techniques in either 10- or 12-session interventions delivered over a 5-week period have resulted in significant reductions of depressive symptomatology immediately after treatment as well as at 5–8 weeks follow-up, in comparison to waiting list control groups (Reynolds and Coats, 1986; Stark et al., 1987).

Two other behavioral approaches have also been successful in the treatment of depression: problem-solving training and relaxation training. Problem-solving training has emphasized teaching children problem-solving skills for use in social and interpersonal situations, such as identifying and expressing feelings appropriately, generating alternative courses of action and considering their consequences, and implementing the solution that best fits the situation (Stark et al., 1987). Relaxation training, on the other hand, has been found to be successful in reducing depressive symptoms in adolescents (Reynolds and Coats, 1986). Adolescents are taught to identify the link among stressors, muscle tension, and depressive symptomatology and then are trained in relaxation techniques.

The success of self-control and problem-solving training with children and of relaxation and self-control training with adolescents attests to the considerable promise of behavioral treatments for childhood and adolescent depression. At the present time, however, the key ingredients of behavior change remain unknown. Among the cognitive-behavioral treatments (i.e., self-control training and problem-solving training), there is a common emphasis on having the child engage in more pleasant activities and use self-monitoring to track depressive symptoms (Hughes, 1988). Among all three treatments, there is a common emphasis on providing the child with an enhanced sense of control over symptoms.

Conduct Disorder and Antisocial Behavior

Conduct disorder and antisocial behavior in children are characterized by externalizing behaviors such as aggression, truancy, firesetting, stealing, and other social rule violations. The level of dysfunction it entails is extensive, involving significant disruption in the home, at school, in peer relations, and in cognitive processes. Its prevalence in community samples is relatively high, and its demand on clinical services is great, accounting for up to one-third to one-half of clinic referrals (Kazdin et al., 1989). In addition to its significant social and personal costs in the short run, the effects of conduct disorder and antisocial behavior frequently extend well into adulthood, manifested in such problems as criminal behavior, alcoholism, problems at work or school, significant disruptions in interpersonal relations, and other psychosocial difficulties (Kazdin, 1987; Robins, 1981; Rutter and Giller, 1983).

Two types of behavioral interventions have demonstrated success in the treatment of conduct disorder and antisocial behavior: problem-solving skills training and parent training. Problem-solving skills training (PSST) utilizes behavioral rehearsal, role playing, modeling, corrective feedback, and social reinforcement to teach children interpersonal cognitive problem-solving skills, such as generating solutions, means-ends and consequential thinking, and perspective taking (Kazdin et al., 1987). The intervention is delivered in 20–25 sessions once or twice per week. Recent controlled studies have demonstrated that problem-solving skills training, as opposed to relationship therapy or an attention placebo control intervention, is effective in reducing antisocial behavior in severely disturbed clinic-referred children ages 7–13 at posttreatment as well as after a 1-year follow-up (Kazdin et al., 1987, 1989). Despite these reductions in antisocial behavior, the incidence of problem behaviors of PSST children remained significantly higher than that found in community samples (Kazdin et al., 1989).

A second approach to the treatment of conduct disorder and antisocial behavior in children and adolescents is behavioral parent training. A variety of such treatment programs have been developed and have demonstrated considerable success in reducing antisocial behavior when compared with no treatment or alternative interventions (Wells and Forehand, 1985). The most widely evaluated parent-training approach is the program developed by Patterson and his colleagues (Patterson, 1975, 1982; Patterson and Guillion, 1968; Patterson and Reid, 1973; Patterson et al., 1982, 1992; Wiltz and Patterson, 1974). In this program, parents are taught basic behavioral principles and techniques (e.g., reinforcement, time out, response cost, conditioned reinforcement, contingency contracting) and how to apply these to specific interactions with their child. Next, parents are trained extensively through program manuals and weekly training sessions to observe, identify, track, and record deviant and prosocial behaviors on the part of their child. As part of this training, parents are asked to identify two prosocial and two problem behaviors to track and monitor over a 3-day period. In order to facilitate monitoring, it is not uncommon for the therapist to call parents daily to assist in the completion of this task. Finally, the therapist works directly with parents to help them design and implement a token reinforcement system for use in the home. Children are praised for appropriate behavior as well as provided with points that can be exchanged daily for reinforcers. Noncompliance or misbehavior is managed through the use of a time out (from reinforcement) or response cost (loss of points) procedure. The therapist uses a variety of behavioral procedures to teach parents necessary skills, such as modeling, behavioral rehearsal, and role playing.

Related behavioral parent training programs have also been developed for use with younger clinic-referred children, ages 2–8 (Forehand and McMahon, 1981; Webster-Stratton et al., 1988). Such programs usually teach parents how to (a) observe, identify, and monitor their child's behavior; (b) reinforce prosocial and appropriate behavior; (c) extinguish minor aggressive or destructive behavior through ignoring; (d) give clear and concise one-time commands upon the appearance of misbehavior; (e) provide a single warning of impending consequences for failure to comply with a command; and (f) use a 3- to 5-minute time out to punish noncompliance (Wells and Forehand, 1985). In general, since positive reinforcement for prosocial behavior is often quite successful in reducing aggressive and destructive behavior in younger children, it is recommended that these techniques be implemented first before more punitive techniques are applied.

Overall, behavioral parent training programs for children and adolescents with conduct disorder or antisocial behavior have been very effective in reducing the problem behaviors of referred children to levels observed in nonreferred peers. These effects are maintained up to 1 year posttreatment (Fleischman and Szykula, 1981), with some benefits persisting for over 10 years (Baum and Forehand, 1981; Forehand and Long, 1988). Such programs also appear to have some impact on reducing maternal depression and enhancing the prosocial behavior of other children in the family (Kazdin, 1985b). Importantly, these programs have been found to be least effective when implemented in brief, time-limited treatment (10 hours or less rather than 50–60 hours) or by an inexperienced therapist, or with families who have significant marital, psychological, or social adjustment difficulties (Kazdin, 1988; Wells and Forehand, 1985). When such difficulties are observed during the course of treatment, the therapist is advised to deal with marital conflicts and other potential barriers to effective treatment implementation directly, as part of a more comprehensive intervention strategy (Griest and Wells, 1983). Recent studies have shown that a combined approach of PSST and parent training is most effective in the treatment of antisocial behavior in children (Kazdin et al., 1992).

Attention Deficit Hyperactivity Disorder

Evidence is compelling that behavior therapy in combination with psychostimulant medication currently is the treatment of choice for attention deficit hyperactivity disorder (ADHD) (Rapport, 1987). In studies comparing these two treatments, neither alone has been found to demonstrate efficacy consistently across relevant outcomes, such as reduced impulsivity and motor activity and improved attention, concentration, academic performance, and social relations (Barkley, 1985; O'Leary and Wilson, 1987; Rapport, 1987). While this may be due in part to the complexity inherent in diagnosing this disorder accurately (Barkley, 1981, 1991; Rapoport and Ismond, 1984), a picture is beginning to emerge which suggests that these two treatments may each have a differential impact and thus be most effective when used in combination.

The psychostimulant medications most frequently prescribed for the treatment of children with ADHD are methylphenidate, dextroamphetamine, and pemoline, with methylphenidate by far the most commonly used and investigated of these in the United States (Safer and Krager, 1983). Controlled outcome studies have shown methylphenidate to be effective in reducing impulsivity (Ayllon et al., 1975; Brown and Sleator, 1979; Rapport et al., 1985) and motor activity level (Porrino et al., 1983), improving attention, concentration, and on-task behavior (Rapport et al., 1986, 1987), and enhancing social relations with adults and peers (Barkley, 1977; Barkley et al., 1984; Whalen et al., 1981, 1989). Despite widespread positive effects in these domains, psychostimulant medication generally has faired poorly in demonstrating short- or long-term effectiveness on learning and performance on academic tasks (Barkley and Cunningham, 1978; Hechtman, 1985; O'Leary, 1980), although there is evidence that some kinds of learning may be responsive to methylphenidate at higher dosage levels than are commonly employed (Rapport, 1987; Rapport et al., 1982; Vyse and Rapport, 1989).

Behavioral treatments for children with ADHD, on the other hand, consistently have demonstrated efficacy in enhancing learning and improving academic performance (Ayllon et al., 1975; Barkley, 1985; O'Leary, 1980; Pelham et al., 1980), in some cases by as much as 1.6 years of growth over the course of 1 year of treatment (Satterfield et al., 1979). Behavioral treatments have also been shown to be effective in reducing impulsivity and motor activity and enhancing attention and concentration, although findings from these studies are less clear and at times contradictory (Barkley, 1985; Gittelman-Klein et al., 1976; O'Leary and Wilson, 1987).

Behavioral interventions are most effective when implemented in three arenas: the home, the classroom, and with the individual child. Home interventions usually involve teaching parents observational and behavior management skills for use in rewarding appropriate behavior and extinguishing inappropriate behavior. Typically, parents are taught to use positive as well as conditioned (token) reinforcement to strengthen their child's ability to play independently and to engage in prosocial interactions with others. In addition, parents are trained in the use of time out and response cost procedures so that they can provide mild punishment for misbehavior and noncompliance with house rules. Successful school interventions have emphasized similar techniques, although a token economy system used in combination with response cost is usually an essential component of such programs. Finally, self-control techniques, such as self-monitoring, self-evaluation, and goal setting have also been used with ADHD children. Although these techniques have demonstrated only limited effectiveness, when used alone or in combination with psychostimulant medication they hold promise when combined with the parent or teacher components of a comprehensive behavioral treatment program (O'Leary and Wilson, 1987; Whalen et al., 1985).

Pervasive Developmental Disorders and Autism

Pervasive developmental disorders (PDDs) consist of infantile autism and pervasive developmental disorders (not otherwise specified). The essential features of effective treatment of PDD include a thorough assessment of functional behaviors and their controlling variables. Since PDD involves impairment in social interaction and communication skills, the selection of target behaviors for modification should focus upon key deficits that have a generalizing effect on several areas of functioning. Attentional and social skills training are two such areas that appear to have far-reaching educational and interpersonal ramifications.

Behavioral treatment techniques for these disorders generally fall into two categories: suppressing unwanted behaviors and teaching new skills. Early attempts at perceptual and sensory processing and integration training (Ornitz and Ritvo, 1968) based on a neurological theory of deficits have shown inconsistent results. Several different techniques have since been used with success to reduce unwanted behaviors, such as time out (Foxx and Shapiro, 1978), overcorrection (Foxx and Azrin, 1973), and punishment (Rincover et al., 1979). New skills are taught by using reinforcement, stimulus discrimination training, and social skills training, and by providing clear instructions (Harris and Handleman, 1987). For example, a child who has difficulty responding to social cues might respond to shaping and prompting techniques that can be used to teach such basic skills as making eye contact and sitting still. Once these latter skills are acquired, they can be used to teach the more complex and related skills of attention and observation (Koegal and Schreibman, 1977). Parent training and sibling involvement in behavioral interventions have also been used to enhance the effectiveness of such training programs (Harris, 1973, 1984; Lovaas et al., 1973; Schreibman et al., 1983).

Historically, the long-term prognosis for a return to normal functioning in children with PDD or autism has been very poor. However, a recent controlled outcome study by Lovaas and his colleagues (1987; Lovaas et al., 1989; McEachin et al., 1993) on the intensive treatment of autistic children under 4 years old is very encouraging. The treatment involved a minimum of 40 hours per week of one-to-one adult contact with the child for a period of over 2 years. Student therapists as well as the child's parents were trained to provide the intensive home-based treatment, which consisted of operant procedures aimed at promoting cognitive, verbal, and social skills. At the conclusion of the controlled trial, 47% (9 of 19) of the children who participated in the treatment were enrolled in regular 1st-grade classrooms and were reported as "indistinguishable" from their classroom peers by school personnel. None of the children in a nonintervention group were enrolled in regular 1st-grade classes. In addition, the nine children attending 1st-grade classes exhibited dramatic gains in IQ from pretreatment to posttreatment. This pattern of differences between experimental and control groups was maintained at a subsequent follow-up of these children when they reached a mean age of 11.5 years (McEachin et al., 1993).

Mental Retardation

The dramatic expansion of behavior therapy techniques has revolutionized the field of mental retardation therapy over the past 3 decades (Reber, 1992; Whitman and Johnston, 1987). The most effective behavioral interventions have been developed for the mildly and moderately retarded, a group that comprises about 98% of the total population of retarded persons (Grossman, 1983). In general, the goals of behavior therapy with the mentally retarded do not involve treatment for psychiatric disorders but rather focus on promoting adaptation in three major areas of skill deficits: self-control, social skills, and academic performance.

Self-control problems have been treated with a wide variety of techniques, such as overcorrection for self-stimulatory behavior (Foxx and Azrin, 1973), differential reinforcement of other behaviors for the reduction of stereotypies (Eason et al., 1982), and a variety of other operant techniques (Berkson, 1983). As a last resort, punishment has been used effectively to reduce unwanted behaviors (Barrett et al., 1981). Remarkable success has also been demonstrated in the acquisition of social skills among the mentally retarded, especially in the areas of communication skills and daily living skills. In general, reinforcement techniques have been applied in programs designed to improve expressive language skills (Handleman, 1984), to foster understanding and ability to follow directions (Lancioni et al., 1984), and to acquire basic personal and home living skills (Schadlock et al., 1984). Finally, academic performance has been enhanced through the implementation of behavioral interventions. Basic classroom learning skills have been taught with the help of interventions that promote eye contact and increase on-task behavior (Bornstein and Quevillon, 1976; Zigler and Hodapp, 1985).

Enuresis and Encopresis

Behavior therapy has been found to be particularly effective in the treatment of enuresis and encopresis. Of the two kinds of enuresis, diurnal (daytime) and nocturnal (nighttime), the latter is usually more persistent and troublesome to parents and child. Two types of behavioral treatment have been used with success in the treatment of nocturnal enuresis: the urine alarm and dry bed training. The urine alarm was first popularized as the bell and pad treatment for enuresis in 1938 by Mowrer and Mowrer (1938). Although a number of modifications of the original bell and pad procedure have been developed over the years, the essential procedure remains the same. The child sleeps with a pad under a sheet that has been wired with an electrical current and serves as a urine sensor. When urine wets the pad, an alarm goes off and wakes parents and child. After using the toilet, the child makes the bed and resets the alarm before returning to sleep. Conditioning is believed to occur through either one or both of the following mechanisms: (*a*) the repeated pairing of the alarm and voiding (i.e., classically conditioned reinforcement), such that the child comes to inhibit voiding and sleep through the night, or (*b*) stimulus discrimination training, whereby the child is wakened when bladder distension cues are near their peak (i.e., when there is a full bladder) and, as a result, learns to wake and void when these cues are present.

Recent reviews have found this technique to be effective in 75–80% of cases, with relapse rates of 30–41% (Doleys, 1977, 1985; O'Leary and Wilson, 1987). Of those children who relapse, just over two-thirds remain continent after reinitiation of the procedure. Typically, training is completed within 5–12 weeks.

Two modifications of the standard urine alarm treatment have been found to reduce relapse considerably (Doleys, 1985). The first involves use of an intermittent reinforcement schedule in which the child is awakened on only 50–70% of wetting episodes. The second involves use of an overlearning procedure in which the child is asked to consume liquid 1 hour before bedtime, usually beginning with 10 ounces and building up to 32 ounces over a few weeks. Overlearning is believed to promote generalization of learning to an increased range of bladder capacity and distension (Young and Morgan, 1972).

A second behavioral treatment found to be effective in eliminating nocturnal enuresis is dry bed training (DBT) (Azrin et al., 1974; Said et al., 1991). This treatment incorporates a number of behavioral techniques: positive practice, positive reinforcement, punishment, and the urine alarm. In DBT the child is wakened during the night, asked to go to the toilet if any urge to void is present (positive practice), and then allowed to return to bed with praise for completing this onerous task (positive reinforcement). The urine alarm is also used as part of the treatment, and in the usual manner, the child is required to clean and change wet sheets in the event of an accident (punishment). Usually the child is also verbally reprimanded for a wet bed (punishment) and praised for staying dry (positive reinforcement). This procedure is followed on successive nights (and, in some applications, repeatedly throughout a single night) until the child remains dry for 2 weeks. Parent training manuals have been written to make this treatment accessible to the public (Azrin and Besalel, 1979; Azrin and Foxx, 1974).

There is some evidence that DBT is slightly more effective than the urine alarm, particularly in reducing relapse and achieving faster results, although evidence from various studies is inconclusive (O'Leary and Wilson, 1987; Ronen et al., 1992; Young and Morgan, 1972). Since this procedure requires considerable effort on the part of parents and child, clinicians must determine whether the additional benefits of DBT over and above those of the urine alarm outweigh the very real possibility of treatment noncompliance.

Behavior therapy has also been shown to be effective in the treatment of functional encopresis, which is defined in DSM-IV as the repeated passage of feces in inappropriate places more than once per month after the age of 4 and occurring for a period of 6 consecutive months (American Psychiatric Association, 1994). Recommended effective behavioral treatments for encopresis involve the use of (a) positive and conditioned reinforcement, sometimes in combination with mild punishment, or (b) regular pants checks in combination with positive and conditioned reinforcement plus full cleanliness training (FCT). Laxatives or suppositories are also often employed as an adjunct to treatment, so as to promote the passage of fecal material. Treatments based on reinforcement (with or without mild punishment) involve training the parent to praise the child or deliver a conditioned reinforcer contingent upon the child's passage of feces on the commode (Ashkenazi, 1975; Wright and Walker, 1976; Young and Goldsmith, 1972). In the initial stages of this treatment, sometimes it is necessary to provide reinforcement for successive approximations of the appropriate behavior, for example, rewarding the child for passing feces in the pants while in the bathroom. This treatment usually eliminates encopresis within 15–20 weeks in the majority of cases.

A second, slightly more efficient treatment for encopresis, which is also carried out by parents and supplemented by laxatives or suppositories as necessary, is comprised of three components: (a) periodic pants checks (usually 1–2 hours apart), (b) FCT after soiling, and (c) positive reinforcement for clean pants checks (Young and Morgan, 1972). FCT is implemented when soiling is discovered during a pants check. After a show of displeasure by the parent, the child is required to wash the soiled underpants for 20 minutes and then must take a 20-minute bath in cool water. Successful pants checks result in praise as well as the awarding of conditioned reinforcers, such as tokens or points, which

can be accumulated and exchanged for privileges, treats, or special activity time with one or both parents. This technique usually results in the elimination of functional encopresis in 10–15 weeks and is effective with the majority of cases (Young and Morgan, 1972).

Applications of Behavior Therapy in Diverse Settings

One of the major advantages of behavior therapy is its applicability to a wide range of settings. Behavior therapy has been used with success in family interventions, school and community interventions, residential settings, and in the delivery of pediatric services. These diverse applications of behavioral approaches have promoted the delivery of services and treatments to previously underserved populations.

FAMILY INTERVENTIONS

Two types of behavioral interventions have been widely used with families: behavioral parent training and behavioral family therapy. Parent behavioral training programs differ according to the behavioral skills emphasized (e.g., contingency management, conflict resolution, problem solving, positive parent-child interactions, contingency contracting) and the problem behavior being addressed (e.g., fostering independence for a mentally retarded child, reducing a child's fears, decreasing a parent's likelihood to engage in physically abusive behavior, promoting effective parent-child communication, and reducing parent-adolescent power struggles) (Graziano, 1977; Twardosz and Nordquist, 1987). Despite this wide-ranging focus, behavioral parent training programs have shown a promising record of efficacy relative to other forms of treatment.

Behavioral family therapy, on the other hand, is an emerging area of family intervention that combines family systems theory with learning theory. Family systems theory is used to formulate the presenting problem in the context of key parameters of family functioning, such as family communication, boundaries, power, affectivity, and family life cycle status. Learning theory is used to formulate the presenting problem in terms of behavioral contingencies that maintain or exacerbate the problem or that function to block effective problem solving. These perspectives are then combined in a treatment plan that may include teaching family members to identify feelings and thoughts during family interactions; reinforcing effective communication within the session; pointing out behavioral contingencies that inadvertently strengthen problem behaviors within the family; using modeling, role plays, and behavioral rehearsal in the session to teach contingency contracting or behavioral management skills (e.g., time out); and assigning homework for family members to practice skills taught in the session.

SCHOOL AND COMMUNITY INTERVENTIONS

School and community interventions are another rapidly growing arena for behavioral interventions. Behavioral treatments are well suited for implementation in school settings because they often can be delivered effectively in a group context. The school, in particular, provides an excellent opportunity for implementing behavioral interventions at multiple levels. Children referred for treatment often can be seen individually or in groups in the school setting by a school psychologist, social worker, or counselor (Hughes, 1988). In addition, high-risk or normal children can participate in behaviorally based classroom interventions that seek to promote competencies or prevent problem behaviors, such as substance abuse (Snow et al., 1987). These programs frequently are compatible with other types of behavioral interventions, such as parent training programs delivered in the same setting (Tebes et al., 1989). Community interventions provide further opportunities for behavioral interventions implemented at multiple levels. Such programs can augment school-based or parent training programs, can involve a variety of community organizations in their implementation, and can utilize the popular media to enhance the impact of the intervention (Pentz et al., 1989).

RESIDENTIAL SETTINGS

Behavioral interventions are also common in residential treatment programs for children and youth. The most common form of behavioral intervention in these settings is the use of a token economy system as part of the treatment milieu. Such interventions typically provide steps in which children can gain more and greater privileges as they progress through the program. Token economies have been implemented with success in a variety of settings, such as those used to treat delinquent youths and mentally retarded children and adolescents (Kazdin, 1977).

PEDIATRIC BEHAVIORAL MEDICINE

Finally, over the past 2 decades, behavior therapy has begun to expand its applications to pediatric settings in hospitals. Pediatric behavioral medicine is the new, rapidly expanding, interdisciplinary field involved with the prevention and treatment of emotional and behavioral problems related to child and adolescent health and illness. While there is no specific theoretical orientation to the field of pediatric behavioral medicine, in practice it is the application of behavior modification principles in the medical arena. Pediatric behavioral medicine and its parent field of behavioral medicine usually are characterized by three types of interventions: (a) direct treatment of medical problems such as pain (Varney et al., 1982) and hypertension (Lutzker and Martin, 1981); (b) the development of programs to enhance compliance to medical procedures and regimens, such as fear reduction programs before surgery (Lutzker and Martin, 1981) and compliance programs for juvenile diabetics (Lowe and Lutzker, 1979); and (c) health education, in which knowledge and skills training are provided in such areas of health behavior as accident prevention, nutritional compliance, and medical advice (Finney and Christopherson, 1984). The emergence of the relatively new field of behavioral medicine has expanded traditional medicine beliefs to include a more important role for the emotional factors that influence the development and course of many physical disorders and their most efficacious treatment.

RELATED APPROACHES
Hypnosis

HISTORY

A field related to child and adolescent behavior therapy is *hypnotherapy*. Although hypnosis has been practiced for thousands of years, much skepticism remains regarding the legitimacy of its therapeutic use (Kroger, 1977; Olness and Gardner, 1988). The history of modern hypnosis begins with Franz Anton Mesmer (1734–1815), who in the late 18th century claimed that magnetic fluid imbalances in the human body were the cause of many somatic and psychological diseases. His dramatic "cures" involved staring into his patients' eyes while they held onto iron rods attached to a large tub of iron filings and allegedly were demagnetized of their illnesses (Tinterow, 1970). Mesmer was discredited by the distinguished Franklin Commission, which had been established by King Louis XVI to investigate mesmerism. Several of Mesmer's followers tried to defend mesmerism, but not until the late 19th century did Jean-Martin Charcot (1835–1893), the French neurologist, give hypnosis a new measure of scientific credibility by describing it in neurological terms. James Braid (1795–1869) coined the term hypnosis from the Greek word for sleep, *hypnos*, and he is now remembered as "the father of hypnosis." Finally, Freud was initially interested in Charcot's work with hysteria through hypnosis but abandoned this interest in favor of free association in psychoanalysis.

DEFINITION

The definition of hypnotherapy is complicated because it encompasses a wide variety of theories and techniques. Basically, hypnotherapy is a treatment modality that utilizes an altered state of consciousness (i.e., hypnosis) in its overall treatment plan. Much of the work in hypnotherapy is viewed as instilling "an attitude of hope in the context of mastery" (Olness and Gardner, 1988, p. 89). Most popular theories define hypnosis as an altered state of consciousness involving some combination of heightened awareness, increased suggestibility, intense interpersonal relationship, or direct unconscious access. These theories are primarily physiological, psychological, or some combination of the two. The physiological theories suggest selective inhibition of brain centers, while the psychological theories emphasize the subject's hypersuggestibility. It is clear, however, that the process of undergoing hypnotic trance can affect physiology through altering autonomic nervous system responses, such as lowering blood pressure or reducing muscle tone. However, the studies of physiological responsivity are unreliable because one's exact physiological response is also related to the level of arousal developed by the imagery of the specific hypnotic trance. Not all hypnosis induces the same response.

TECHNIQUE

Formal hypnotic trance induction can be achieved in a variety of ways. In general, the child is first offered an explanation of the process that includes a methodology for relaxing and imagining, while therapeutic rapport is established. During the induction phase, the child is often asked to concentrate and focus on a visual fixation point on the ceiling until his or her eyelids became heavy and he or she closes them. Then, a deepening technique would enhance relaxation by means of any simple counting or breathing procedure, for example. Obviously, there are a limitless number of hypnotic induction techniques utilizing visual imagery, auditory imagery, movement imagery, storytelling, ideomotor techniques, progressive relaxation, eye fixation, distraction, and other individual and group variations (Olness and Gardner, 1988). Although children below the age of 7 have a limited responsiveness to standard techniques, children between 7 and 14 years of age reach their peak in hypnotic susceptibility (Place, 1984). Often there is a temporary decline during adolescence, when trust in adults is typically diminished, until the pattern is stabilized again during adulthood. Olness and Gardner report the use of tactile and kinesthetic stimulation techniques with very young preverbal children. There appear to be no significant sex differences during childhood regarding susceptibility (Cooper, 1966). However, the data are confounded when we consider informal hypnosis in the style of Milton Erickson and his followers (Erickson and Rossi, 1981). These methods involve indirect unconscious suggestion without the use of a bona fide trance induction. The child may or may not even know that a hypnotic technique was employed, since the doctor appears to be simply talking in some strange metaphor or asking the child to imagine something silly and absurd. These techniques can become quite sophisticated and appear subtle to the untrained eye. Some of the best professional training programs in hypnotherapy are organized by the American Society of Clinical Hypnosis in Des Plaines, Illinois, and the Society for Clinical and Experimental Hypnosis in Liverpool, New York.

APPLICATIONS

The clinical uses of hypnotherapy are limited only by the creativity of the therapist. In general, hypnotherapy is underutilized in the treatment of children, but it is often considered valuable in the areas of pain and habit control, pediatric medical problems, and stress reduction. As long as hypnosis is not used as an exclusive technique outside of a professional therapeutic context, there is little danger involved in its use. The major contraindications are situations where its use aggravates existing problems (ignoring acute pain, which is a warning signal) or avoids more effective treatment of the problem (medication or surgery). Hypnotherapy can be helpful in the treatment of headache (Olness and MacDonald, 1981, 1987; Olness et al., 1987), chronic and acute pain (Crasilneck and Hall, 1973; Hilgard and Hilgard, 1975; Russo and Varni,

1982), severe burns (Wakeman and Kaplan, 1978), obesity (Haber et al., 1979), compliance and pain control during medical procedures (Olness and Gardner, 1988), asthma (Kohen, 1986), dermatological problems (Mirvish, 1978; Olness, 1977), enuresis (Mirvish, 1978; Stanton, 1979), nausea associated with chemotherapy (Cotanch et al., 1985; Hockenberry and Cotanch, 1985; Kohen et al., 1984; Zeltzer et al., 1984), stress reduction, and other problems of childhood and adolescence. There have been several dramatic claims of clinical cures of terminal disease through the use of hypnosis and positive imagery, but there are no properly controlled studies to support these claims (Lucas, 1985). In the broader context of good treatment, hypnosis can be a useful adjunct to behavioral treatment. The reader is referred to *Hypnosis and Hypnotherapy with Children* (Olness and Gardner, 1988) for a further review and excellent discussion of this topic.

Biofeedback

Biofeedback is a treatment method that utilizes physiological feedback instrumentation to train individuals in the regulation of their body responses, such as muscle tone, heart rate, blood pressure, and cortical brain activity (Blumenthal, 1985). Originally, biofeedback technology developed out of experimental attempts to operantly condition autonomic nervous system responses (Miller, 1969). Several models over the past two decades have attempted to explain the process of biofeedback: learning theory, body awareness, cybernetics, hypnosis, and others. Some of the major applications of biofeedback are (*a*) electromyography (EMG) feedback for muscle relaxation in the treatment of tension headaches (Budzynski, 1978), hypertension (Patel, 1977), cardiovascular disease (Cheatle and Weiss, 1982), muscular rehabilitation (Basmajian, 1981), and temporomandibular joint (TMJ) pain (Scott and Gregg, 1980); (*b*) thermal feedback of skin temperature in the treatment of migraine headaches (Blanchard and Andrasik, 1982) and Raynaud's disease (Surwit et al., 1978); (*c*) feedback of electrodermal (EDR) activity for treatment of hyperhydrosis; and (*d*) electroencephalographic feedback of cortical brain arousal in the treatment of neurological disorders. Due to the cost and inconvenience of the equipment, biofeedback has lost some relative popularity among the vast array of relaxation therapies, yet it still remains helpful for some clients.

ISSUES IN CHILD AND ADOLESCENT BEHAVIOR THERAPY

Common Criticisms

Two of the most common criticisms of behavior therapy is that it results in symptom substitution as opposed to lasting therapeutic change and that it fails adequately to take into account clinical process issues that arise during the course of treatment.

SYMPTOM SUBSTITUTION

Perhaps the most well-known criticism of behavior therapy is that it results in symptom substitution. This criticism is based on the belief, grounded in psychoanalytic theory, that the goal of behavior therapy is to provide symptomatic relief as opposed to treatment for a symptom's underlying cause. According to this view, the alleviation of a particular symptom will result in the appearance of a new symptom until the underlying cause is addressed.

A number of behavior therapists have questioned the logical basis for this view (Bandura, 1969; Kazdin, 1982; Sloane et al., 1975; Wolpe, 1978). For example, since critics who argue for the inevitability of symptom substitution following behavioral treatment do not specify which symptom will appear, when, and under what conditions, how can a valid test ever be made of the charge? Furthermore, how would one know whether a symptom arising following behavior therapy was a consequence of the treatment and not merely a new symptom? And finally, since all types of intervention—behavioral or otherwise—inevitably result in both intended and unintended positive and negative effects, why should behavior therapy be singled out for criticism when such effects are endemic to therapy per se? Logical considerations aside, evidence is lacking for symptom substitution following behavioral interventions (Kazdin, 1982), although there is considerable evidence that behavioral interventions have wide-ranging beneficial effects beyond specific target symptoms (Casey and Berman, 1985; Durlak et al., 1991; Herbert, 1988; Hersen and Bellack, 1985; Weisz et al., 1987).

CLINICAL PROCESS

Another frequent criticism of behavioral interventions is that clinical process factors that emerge over the course of treatment are not taken into account. Factors such as the therapist-client relationship and the nature of the therapeutic interaction are focal examples of such processes. Critics have asserted that this is because behavior therapists do not adequately attend to these issues in treatment or even eschew the clinical value of doing so.

To some extent, these criticisms are accurate. For many years, behavior therapists spent much of their time emphasizing the need to attend more to the *tasks* of treatment than to process issues. An example of this can be found in the early behavior therapy literature in which the therapist was described essentially as a "social reinforcement machine" (Krasner, 1962). Someone with only a cursory knowledge of actual behavior therapy practice could easily be led to believe that behavior therapists regard themselves merely as technicians who find little merit in fostering the therapeutic alliance and responding genuinely and with empathy to their clients. Although the reasons for this early emphasis are not entirely clear, a prevailing experience among behavior therapists in the 1950s and 1960s was excitement over the emerging technologies being used in treatment and a belief that this represented significant strides away from previous approaches. The cost of embracing this "techno-therapist" vision, however, was that much of the writing about behavior therapy excluded some of the *essentials* of successful treatment, behavioral or otherwise: the need to build a strong working alliance with one's client and to use that alliance to weather disruptions (i.e., resistances) in the treatment so as to facilitate therapeutic gains.

In recent years, behavior therapists have begun to focus on the merits of the clinical process in promoting the therapist-client relationship and in facilitating effective clinical interactions (Fishman and Lubetkin, 1983; Herbert, 1988; Hersen and Bellack, 1985; Kazdin, 1988; Sloane et al., 1975). Ironically, some behavior therapists have argued that such factors are even more important to the success of behavioral interventions since the therapist is usually more actively engaged with the client over the course of treatment in setting goals collaboratively and in implementing them through the use of a variety of interactive techniques (Fishman and Lubetkin, 1983).

Ethical Issues

The ethical concerns of child and adolescent behavior therapy are no different, in principle, from those found in any other area of psychotherapeutic practice (Keith-Spiegel and Koocher, 1985). The 1970s saw a growing legal and public demand for increased accountability on the part of all therapists for their clinical practices. This led to a published report on the ethical practice of behavior therapy by the Association for the Advancement of Behavior Therapy (Azrin et al., 1977). The report sought to protect clients' rights in such areas as therapeutic goal setting, quality and appropriateness of treatment, voluntary participation, confidentiality, and the competency of the therapist.

Ideally, behavior therapists encourage young clients together with their parents to set their own goals for treatment in consultation with their therapist. This minimizes the chance for the treatment to be unduly influenced by the therapist's personal biases. Behavior therapy practice insists that therapists make clear their biases to their clients, establish an explicit treatment contract, and monitor progress periodically in order to determine whether continued treatment is warranted. Alternative methods of treatment should always be considered, and clients must remain aware of their treatment options as well as their voluntary and confidential participation in any treatment program.

Since so much of behavior therapy occurs in the context of research to evaluate treatment efficacy, these standards apply to clinical as well as research protocols. Special guidelines have also been developed for use whenever more aversive techniques of punishment are implemented as part of the treatment (American Psychological Association, 1981). Although interventions based on such techniques can affect incidental behavior not targeted for change, they are justifiable as a final treatment of choice for self-injurious and otherwise unmanageable children exhibiting dangerous behaviors. Finally, behavior therapists believe that the ethical practice of therapy involves selecting an intervention strategy well suited to the presenting problem. Such a choice should be based upon empirical evidence of the treatment's long-term effectiveness, relative efficiency, likely side effects and response covariation, overall safety, the potential for compliance, and the potential consequences of not offering treatment.

New Directions

Over the past 2 decades, behavior therapy has clearly established itself as a major force in mental health treatment, prompting a reconsideration of previous approaches to practice. Two examples of this changing view are the current value placed on the use of integrative approaches to practice and the considerable interest in more and better treatment outcome studies. Currently, the trend in mental health care is toward a greater integration of therapeutic approaches. Therapists of all persuasions are moving toward a pragmatic eclecticism rooted in empirical evidence (Bornstein et al., 1985), rather than defending their own turf. This open-mindedness is prompted by the reality that most clinical data are equivocal and that therapeutic behavior change is difficult to achieve. Such a perspective will permit clinical researchers to begin to specify which treatments work with which persons and under what conditions (Kazdin, 1988).

The emphasis on treatment specificity is currently a major issue in the field of child and adolescent behavior therapy and is one that underlies the current interest in more and better treatment outcome studies. Such studies need to utilize more adequate controls, employ larger sample sizes to be able to detect true differences among sample groups (not only between treatment versus placebo or waiting list control groups but also among groups that receive differing treatments), and examine more comparable treatments to determine relative differences in their effectiveness on similar disorders. At the present time, clinical research-

ers generally have failed to utilize samples that are large enough to detect the small differences that presumably exist between two or more treatments (Kazdin and Bass, 1989) and have generally compared a heterogeneous mix of treatments for widely varying clinical populations (Kazdin, 1993). In addition, treatment outcome studies need to include three-channel assessments of children's functioning as well as assessment of other relevant domains in the child's life, such as family functioning, school performance and adjustment, and peer relations.

Another promising direction for behavior therapy is the increased design and implementation of self-control and self-management interventions. Not only are these approaches efficacious (Durlak et al., 1991; Dush et al., 1989), but they also foster the development of such basic competencies as independence and self-control, are relatively easy to use, and are readily accessible through self-help books and tapes that can serve as an adjunct to treatment and, in some cases, produce equivalent results (Webster-Stratton et al., 1989).

Pediatric behavioral medicine is another exciting and growing field in child and adolescent behavior therapy that holds future promise (Lewis and Vitulano, 1988). As one of the fastest growing interdisciplinary fields, its potential to improve the care and treatment of children with health-related problems is great, particularly in such areas as stress management, pain reduction, treatment compliance, and the care of chronically ill children.

Finally, the development of preventive and promotive interventions is also likely to be a major arena for behavioral approaches. Such interventions often include common behavioral techniques (e.g., skills training, role playing, behavioral rehearsal, self-monitoring) that can easily be incorporated into natural settings for children, such as schools (Weissberg et al., 1991). The recent implementation of life skills training programs in schools in which children are taught social skills, self-control, and other behaviorally based skills in order to reduce high risk behavior that may lead to AIDS and other problems faced by children and youth is one recent example of a preventive behavioral intervention (Barth, 1993). Behavioral approaches also figure prominently in recent interventions aimed at promoting resilience among children at risk, such as those surviving a natural disaster, being regularly exposed to community or family violence, growing up in extreme poverty, or being reared by a severely mentally ill parent (Rolf and Johnson, 1994; Tebes, 1994).

Behavior therapy's emphasis on an empirically based science of behavior, coupled with its applicability to a wide range of settings, has enabled it to grow into a field that addresses many of the problems of childhood and adolescence and offers efficacious interventions for their prevention and treatment.

References

Achenbach TM: The Child Behavior Profile. I: Boys aged 6 through 11. *J Consult Clin Psychol* 46: 478–488, 1978.

Achenbach TM, Edelbrock CS: The Child Behavior Profile. II: Boys aged 12–16 and girls aged 6–11 and 12–16. *J Consult Clin Psychol* 47: 223–233, 1979.

American Psychiatric Association: *Diagnostic and Statistical Manual of Mental Disorders* (4th ed). Washington, DC, American Psychiatric Association, 1994.

American Psychological Association: Ethical principles and guidelines. *Am Psychol* 36:633–686, 1981.

Ashkenazi A: The treatment of encopresis using a discriminative stimulus and positive reinforcement. *J Behav Ther Exp Psychiatry* 6:155–157, 1975.

Ayllon T, Layman D, Kandel NJ: A behavioral-educational alternative to control of hyperactive children. *J Appl Behav Anal* 8:137–146, 1975.

Azrin NH, Besalel VA: *Parent's Guide to Bedwetting Control: A Step-by-Step Method*. New York, Simon & Schuster, 1979.

Azrin NH, Fox RM: *Toilet Training in Less Than a Day*. New York, Simon & Schuster, 1974.

Azrin NH, Sneed TJ, Foxx RM: Dry-bed training: Rapid elimination of childhood enuresis. *Behav Res Ther* 12:147–156, 1974.

Azrin NH, Stuart RB, Risley TR, et al: Ethical issues for human services. *Behav Ther* 8:V–VI, 1977.

Baer L, Miniciello WE: Behavior therapy for obsessive compulsive disorder. In: Jenike MA, Baer L, Minichiello WE (eds): *Obsessive Compulsive Disorders: Theory and Management*. Chicago, Year Book, 1990, pp. 203–232.

Bandura A: *Principles of Behavior Modification*. New York, Holt, 1969.

Bandura A: *Social Learning Theory*. Englewood Cliffs, NJ, Prentice-Hall, 1977.

Bandura A: *Social Foundations of Thought and Action: A Social Cognitive Theory*. Englewood Cliffs, NJ, Prentice-Hall, 1986.

Bandura A, Walters RH: *Social Learning Theory and Personality Development*. New York, Holt, Rinehart & Winston, 1963.

Barkley RA: A review of stimulant drug research with hyperactive children. *J Child Psychol Psychiatry* 18:137–165, 1977.

Barkley RA: *Hyperactive Children: A Handbook for Diagnosis and Treatment*. New York, Guilford, 1981.

Barkley RA: Attention deficit disorders. In: Bornstein PH, Kazdin AE (eds): *Handbook of Clinical Behavior Therapy with Children*. Homewood, IL, Dorsey Press, 1985, pp. 158–217.

Barkley RA: Diagnosis and assessment of attention deficit-hyperactivity disorder. *Comp Ment Health Care* 1:27–43, 1991.

Barkley RA, Cunningham CE: Do stimulant drugs improve the academic performance of hyperkinetic children? *Clin Pediatr* 17:85–92, 1978.

Barkley RA, Karlsson J, Strzelecki E, et al: Effects of age and Ritalin dosage on the mother-child interactions of hyperactive children. *J Consult Clin Psychol* 52:750–758, 1984.

Barrett RP, Matson JL, Shapiro ES, et al: A comparison of punishment and DRO procedures for treating stereotypic behavior of mentally retarded children. *Appl Res Ment Retard* 2:247–256, 1981.

Barth RP: Promoting self-protection and self-control through life skill training. *Children and Youth Serv Rev* 15:281–293, 1993.

Basmajian JV: Biofeedback in rehabilitation: A

review of principles and practices. *Arch Phys Med Rehabil* 62:469, 1981.

Baum CC, Forehand R: Long-term follow-up assessment of parent training by use of multiple outcome measures. *Behav Ther* 12:643–652, 1981.

Beck AT: *Cognitive Therapy and the Emotional Disorders*. New York, International Universities Press, 1976.

Berkson G: Repetitive stereotyped behaviors. *Am J Ment Defic* 8:239–246, 1983.

Blanchard EB, Andrasik F: Psychological assessment and treatment of headache: Recent developments and emerging issues. *J Consult Clin Psychol* 50:859, 1982.

Blumenthal JA: Relaxation therapies and biofeedback: Applications in medical practice. In: Cavenar JO (ed): *Psychiatry* (Vol 2). Philadelphia, Lippincott, 1985.

Bornstein PM, Quevillon RP: The effects of a self-instructional package on overactive preschool boys. *J Appl Behav Anal* 9:179–188, 1976.

Bornstein PH, Bornstein MT, Dawson B: Integrated assessment and treatment. In: Ollendick TE, Hersen M (eds): *Child Behavioral Assessment: Principles and Procedures*. New York, Pergamon, 1984.

Bornstein PH, Kazdin AE, McIntyre TJ: Characteristics, trends, and future directions in child behavior therapy. In: Bornstein PH, Kazdin AE (eds): *Handbook of Clinical Behavior Therapy with Children*. Homewood, IL, Dorsey Press, 1985.

Brown RT, Sleator EK: Methylphenidate in hyperkinetic children: Differences in dose effects on impulsive behavior. *Pediatrics* 64:408–411, 1979.

Budzynski T: Biofeedback in the treatment of muscle-contraction (tension) headache. *Biofeedback Self Regul* 3:409, 1978.

Casey RI, Berman IS: The outcome of psychotherapy with children. *Psychol Bull* 98:388–400, 1985.

Cautela JR, Groden I: *Relaxation: A Comprehensive Manual for Adults, Children, and Children with Special Needs*. Champaign, IL, Research Press, 1978.

Chambers WI, Puig-Antich J, Hirsch M, et al: The assessment of affective disorders in children and adolescents by semistructured interview: Test-retest reliability of the Schedule for Affective Disorders and Schizophrenia for School-Aged Children, Present Episode Version. *Arch Gen Psychiatry* 42:696–702, 1985.

Christoff KA, Myatt RI: Social isolation. In: Hersen M, Van Hasselt VB (eds): *Behavior Therapy with Children and Adolescents*. New York, Wiley, 1987, pp. 512–535.

Cheatle MD, Weiss T: Biofeedback in heart rate control and in the treatment of cardiac arrhythmias. In: White L, Tursley B (eds): *Clinical Biofeedback: Efficacy and Mechanisms*. New York, Guilford, 1982.

Cone ID: The behavioral assessment grid (BAG): A conceptual framework and taxonomy. *Behav Ther* 9:882–888, 1978.

Conners CK: Symptom patterns in hyperkinetic, neurotic, and normal children. *Child Dev* 41:667–682, 1970.

Conners CK: Rating scales for use in drug studies of children. *Psychopharmacol Bull* 23:24–84, 1973.

Cooper LM, London P: Sex and hypnotic susceptibility in children. *Int J Clin Exp Hypn* 14:55–60, 1966.

Costello EI, Edelbrock CS, Dulcan MK, et al: *Testing of the NIMH Diagnostic Interview Schedule for Children (DISC) in a Clinical Population*. Final Report to the Center for Epidemiological Studies, National Institute for Mental Health. Pittsburgh, University of Pittsburgh, 1984.

Cotanch P, Hockenberry M, Herman S: Self-hypnosis as antiemetic therapy in children receiving chemotherapy. *Oncol Nurs Forum* 12:41–46, 1985.

Crasilneck MB, Hall JA: Clinical hypnosis in problems of pain. *Am J Clin Hypn* 15:153–161, 1973.

Doleys DM: Behavioral treatments for nocturnal enuresis in children: A review of the recent literature. *Psychol Bull* 84:30–54, 1977.

Doleys DM: Enuresis and encopresis. In: Bornstein PM, Kazdin AE (eds): *Handbook of Clinical Behavior Therapy with Children*. Homewood, IL, Dorsey Press, 1985, pp. 412–440.

Dumas IE: Treating antisocial behavior in children: Child and family approaches. *Clin Psychol Rev* 9:197–222, 1989.

Durlak JA, Fuhrman T, Lampman C: Effectiveness of cognitive-behavioral therapy for maladapting children: A meta-analysis. *Psychol Bull* 110:204–214, 1991.

Dush DM, Mirt ML, Schroeder ME: Self-statement modification in the treatment of child behavior disorders: A meta-analysis. *Psychol Bull* 106:97–106, 1989.

Eason LJ, White MJ, Newsom C: Generalized reduction of self-stimulatory behavior: An effect of teaching appropriate play to autistic children. *Anal Intervention Dev Disabil* 2:157–169, 1982.

Ellis A: *Reason and Emotion in Psychotherapy*. New York, Lyle Stuart, 1962.

Erickson MN, Rossi EL: *Experiencing Hypnosis: Therapeutic Approaches to Altered States*. New York, Irvington, 1981.

Eysenck, HI: *Behavior Therapy and the Neuroses*. New York, Pergamon, 1960.

Ferster CB, DeMyer MK: A method for the experimental analysis of behavior of autistic children. *Am J Orthopsychiatry* 32:89–98, 1962.

Finney IW, Christopherson ER: Behavioral pediatrics: Health education in pediatric primary care. In: Mersen M, Eisler RM, Miller PM (eds): *Progress in Behavior Modification*. New York, Academic Press, 1984.

Fishman ST, Lubetkin BS: Office practice of behavior therapy. In: Hersen M (ed): *Outpatient Behavior Therapy: A Clinical Guide*. New York, Grune & Stratton, 1983.

Fleischman NJ, Szykula SA: A community setting replication of a social learning treatment for aggressive children. *Behav Ther* 12:115–222, 1981.

Forehand R, Long N: Outpatient treatment of the acting-out child: Procedures, long-term follow-up data, and clinical problems. *Adv Behav Res Ther* 10:129–177, 1988.

Forehand R, McMahon RI: *Helping the Noncompliant Child: A Clinician's Guide to Parent Training*. New York, Guilford, 1981.

Foxx RM, Azrin N: The elimination of autistic self-stimulatory behavior by overcorrection. *J Appl Behav Anal* 6:1–14, 1973.

Foxx RM, Bechtel DR: Overcorrection. *Prog Behav Modif* 13:227–281, 1982.

Foxx RM, Shapiro ST: The timeout ribbon: A nonexclusionary timeout procedure. *J Appl Behav Anal* 11:125–136, 1978.

Gittelman-Klein R, Klein DF, Abikoff H, et al: Relative efficacy of methylphenidate and behavior modification in hyperkinetic children: An interim report. *J Abnorm Child Psychol* 4:361–379, 1976.

Grayson I, Foa EB, Steketee G: Habituation during exposure treatment: Distraction vs. attention-focusing. *Behav Res Ther* 20:323–328, 1982.

Graziano AM: Parents as behavior therapists. In: Hersen M, Eisler RM, Miller PM (eds): *Progress in Behavior Modification*. New York, Academic Press, 1977, pp. 251–298.

Graziano AM, DeGiovanni IS, Garcia KA: Behavioral treatment of children's fears: A review. *Psychol Bull* 86:804–830, 1979.

Griest DL, Wells KC: Behavioral family therapy with conduct disorders in children. *Behav Ther* 14:37–53, 1983.

Grossman IN (ed): *Classification in Mental Retardation*. Washington, DC, American Association of Mental Deficiency, 1983.

Haber CM, Nitkin R, Shenker LR: Adverse reactions to hypnotherapy in obese adolescents: A developmental viewpoint. *Psychiatr Q* 51:55–63, 1979.

Handleman IS, Powers, MD, Harris SL: Teaching of levels: An analysis of concrete and pictorial representations. *Am J Ment Defic* 8:625–629, 1984.

Hansen DI, Watson-Perczel M, Smith IM: Clinical issues in social-skills training with adolescents. *Clin Psychol Rev* 9:365–392, 1989.

Harris SL: *Families of the Developmentally Disabled: A Guide to Behavioral Intervention*. Elmsford, NY, Pergamon, 1983.

Harris SL: The family of the autistic child: A behavioral-systems view. *Clin Psychol Rev* 4:227–239, 1984.

Harris SL, Mandlertian IS: Autism. In: Hersen M, Van Masselt VB, (eds): *Behavior Therapy with Children and Adolescents: A Clinical Approach*. New York, Wiley, 1987, pp. 224–240.

Hechtman L: Adolescent outcome of hyperactive children treated with stimulants in childhood: A review. *Psychopharmacol Bull* 21:178–191, 1985.

Herbert M: *Behavioral Treatment of Children with Problems: A Practice Manual* (2nd ed). London, Academic Press, 1988.

Herjanic B, Herjanic M, Brown F, et al: Are children reliable reporters? *J Abnorm Child Psychol* 3:41–48, 1975.

Hersen M, Bellack AS: General considerations. In: Hersen M, Bellack AE (eds): *Handbook of Clinical Behavior Therapy with Adults*. New York, Plenum, 1985, pp. 3–22.

Hilgard ER, Bower GM: *Theories of Learning* (3rd ed). New York, Appleton-Century-Crofts, 1966.

Hilgard ER, Milgard IR: *Hypnosis in the Relief of Pain*. Los Altos, CA, William Kaufman, 1975.

Hobbs NA, Forehand R: Important parameters in the use of timeout with children: A re-examination. *J Behav Ther Exp Psychiatry* 8:365–370, 1977.

Hockenberry MI, Cotanch PM: Hypnosis as adjuvant antiemetic therapy in childhood cancer. *Nurs Clin North Am* 20:105–107, 1985.

Hops M, Finch W, McConnell S: Social skills deficits. In: Bornstein PM, Kazdin AE (eds): *Handbook of Clinical Behavior Therapy with Children*. Homewood, IL, Dorsey Press, 1985, pp. 543–598.

Hughes IT: *Cognitive Behavior Therapy with Children in Schools*. New York, Pergamon, 1988.

Johnson JM, Rasbury WC, Siegel LI: *Approaches to Child Treatment*. New York, Pergamon, 1986.

Johnston JM: Punishment of human behavior. *Am Psychol* 27:1033–1054, 1972.

Jones MC: A laboratory study of fear: The case of Peter. *Pedag Sem* 31:308–315, 1924a.

Jones MC: The elimination of children's fears. *J Exp Psychol* 7:883–390, 1924b.

Kanfer FH, Saslow G: Behavioral diagnosis. In: Franks CM (ed): *Behavior Therapy: Appraisal and Status*. New York, McGraw-Hill, 1969.

Kaslow NJ, Rehm LP: Childhood depression. In: Morris RI, Kratochwill TR (eds): *The Practice of Child Therapy: A Textbook of Methods*. New York, Pergamon, 1983.

Kaslow NJ, Rehm LP: Conceptualization, assessment, and treatment of depression in children. In: Bornstein PH, Kazdin AE (eds): *Handbook of Clinical Behavior Therapy with Children*. Homewood, IL, Dorsey Press, 1985, pp. 599–657.

Kazdin AE: *The Token Economy: A Review and Evaluation*. New York, Plenum, 1977.

Kazdin AE: *History of Behavior Modification: Experimental Foundations of Contemporary Research*. Baltimore, University Park Press, 1978.

Kazdin AE: Symptom substitution, generalization, and response covariation: Implications for psychotherapy outcome. *Psychol Bull* 91:349–365, 1982.

Kazdin AE: Behavior therapy. In: Cavenar JO (eds): *Psychiatry* (Vol 2). Philadelphia, Lippincott, 1985a, pp. 1–10.

Kazdin AE: *Treatment of Antisocial Behavior in Childhood and Adolescence*. Newbury Park, CA, Sage, 1985b.

Kazdin AE: *Conduct Disorder in Childhood and Adolescence*. Newbury Park, CA, Sage, 1987.

Kazdin AE: *Child Psychotherapy*. New York, Pergamon, 1988.

Kazdin AE: *Behavior Modification in Applied Settings* (4th ed). Homewood, IL, Dorsey Press, 1989.

Kazdin AE, Bass D: Power to detect differences between alternative treatments in comparative psychotherapy outcome research. *J Consult Clin Psychol* 57:138–147, 1989.

Kazdin AE, Bass B, Siegel T, et al: Cognitive-behavioral therapy and relationship therapy in the treatment of children referred for antisocial behavior. *J Consult Clin Psychol* 57:522–535, 1989.

Kazdin AE, Esveldt-Dawson K, French NH, et al: Problem-solving skills training and relationship therapy in the treatment of antisocial child behavior. *J Consult Clin Psychol* 55:76–85, 1987.

Kazdin AE, Siegel T, Bass D: Cognitive problem-solving skills training and parent management training in the treatment of antisocial behavior in children. *J Consult Clin Psychol* 60:733–747, 1992.

Keith-Spiegel P, Koocher GP: *Ethics in Psychology*. New York, Random House, 1985.

Kendall PC: Toward a cognitive-behavioral model of child psychopathology and a critique of related interventions. *J Abnorm Child Psychol* 13:357–372, 1985.

Kendall PC, Braswell L: *Cognitive-Behavioral Therapy for Impulsive Children*. New York, Guilford, 1985.

Kendall PC, Cantwell DP, Kazdin AE: Depression in children and adolescents: Assessment issues and recommendations. *Cognit Ther Res* 13:109–146, 1989.

King RA, Vitulano LA, Riddle MA: The treatment of obsessive-compulsive disorder in Tourette's syndrome. In: Kurlan R (ed): *Handbook of Tourette's Syndrome and Related Tic and Behavioral Disorders*. New York, Marcel Dekker, 1993, pp. 401–422.

Koegel RL, Schreibman L: Teaching autistic children to respond to simultaneous multiple cues. *J Exp Child Psychol* 24:299–311, 1977.

Kohen DP: Applications of relaxation/mental imagery (self-hypnosis) to the management of asthma: Report of behavioral outcomes of a two-year, prospective controlled study (Abstract). *Am J Clin Hypn* 28:196, 1986.

Kohen O, Olness K, Colwell S, et al: The use of relaxation-mental imagery (self-hypnosis) in the management of 505 pediatric behavioral encounters. *Dev Behav Pediatr* 5:21–25, 1984.

Kovacs M, Beck AT: An empirical-clinical approach towards a definition of childhood depression. In: Schulterbrandt IG, Raskin A (eds): *Depression in Children: Diagnosis, Treatment, and Conceptual Models*. New York, Raven Press, 1977, pp. 1–25.

Krasner L: The therapist as a social reinforcement machine. In: Strupp NH, Luborsky L (eds): *Research in Psychotherapy* (Vol 2). Washington, DC, American Psychological Association, 1962.

Kroger WS: *Clinical and Experimental Hypnosis in Medicine, Dentistry and Psychology*. Philadelphia, Lippincott, 1977.

Lancioni GE, Smeets PH, Oliva DS: Teaching severely handicapped adolescents to follow instructions conveyed by means of three-dimensional stimulus configurations. *Appl Res Ment Retard* 5:107–123, 1984.

Lapouse R, Monk MA: Fears and worries in a representative sample of children. *Am J Orthopsychiatry* 29:803–813, 1959.

Lazarus AA: Multimodal behavior therapy: Treating the "BASIC ID." *J Nerv Ment Dis* 156:404–411, 1973.

Lewis M, Vitulano LA: Child and adolescent psychiatry consultation-liaison services in pediatrics: What messages are being conveyed? *Dev Behav Pediatr* 9:388–390, 1988.

London P: *The Modes and Morals of Psychotherapy* (2nd ed). Cambridge, MA, Hemisphere, 1986.

Lovaas OI: Behavioral treatment and normal educational and intellectual functioning in young autistic children. *J Consult Clin Psychol* 55:3–9, 1987.

Lovaas OI, Koegel RL, Simmons IW, et al: Some generalization and follow-up measures on autistic children in behavior therapy. *J Appl Behav Anal* 6:131–166, 1973.

Lovaas OI, Smith T, McEachin II: Clarifying comments on the young autism study: Reply to Schopler, Short, and Mesibov. *J Consult Clin Psychol* 57:165–167, 1989.

Lowe K, Lutzker JR: Increasing compliance to a medical regimen with a juvenile diabetic. *Behav Ther* 10:57–64, 1979.

Lucas RA: Hypnosis. In: Cavenar JO (ed): *Psychiatry* (Vol 2). Philadelphia, Lippincott, 1985.

Lutzker JR, Martin JA: *Behavior Change*. Monterey, CA, Brooks/Cole, 1981.

Mahoney MI: *Cognition and Behavior Modification*. Cambridge, MA, Ballinger, 1974.

Martin G, Pear J: *Behavior Modification: What It Is and How to Do It* (2nd ed). Englewood Cliffs, NJ, Prentice-Hall, 1983.

Meichenbaum DH: *Cognitive Behavior Modification*. New York, Plenum, 1977.

Meyers AW, Craighead WE: Cognitive behavior therapy with children: A historical, conceptual, and organizational overview. In: Meyers AW, Craighead WE (eds): *Cognitive Behavior Therapy with Children*. New York, Plenum, 1983, pp. 1–18.

Miller NE: Learning of visceral and glandular responses. *Science* 163:434–445, 1969.

Mirvish I: Hypnotherapy for the child with chronic eczema: A case report. *S Afr Med J* 54:410–412, 1978.

Morganstern KP: Behavioral interviewing. In: Bellack AS, Hersen M (eds): *Behavioral Assessment: A Practical Handbook* (3rd ed). New York, Pergamon, 1988.

Morris RI, Kratochwill TR: *Treating Children's Fears and Phobias: A Behavioral Approach*. New York, Pergamon, 1983.

Morrison RL: Structured interviews and rating scales. In: Bellack AS, Hersen M (eds): *Behavioral Assessment: A Practical Handbook* (3rd ed). New York, Pergamon, 1988.

Mowrer OH, Mowrer WM: Enuresis: A method for its study and treatment. *Am J Orthopsychiatry* 8:436—459, 1938.

O'Leary KD: Pills or skills for hyperactive children. *J Appl Behav Anal* 13:191–204, 1980.

O'Leary KD, Wilson GT: *Behavior Therapy: Application and Outcome* (2nd ed). Englewood Cliffs, NJ, Prentice-Hall, 1987.

Ollendick TN: Reliability and validity of the Revised Fear Survey Schedule for Children (FSSC-R). *Behav Res Ther* 21:685–692, 1983.

Ollendick TN, Mayer JA: School phobia. In: Turner SM (ed): *Behavioral Theories and Treatment of Anxiety*. New York, Plenum, 1984.

Olness K: In-service hypnosis education in a children's hospital. *Am J Clin Hypn* 20:80–83, 1977.

Olness K, Gardner G: *Hypnosis and Hypnotherapy with Children* (2nd ed). Philadelphia, Grune & Stratton, 1988.

Olness K, MacDonald I: Self-hypnosis and biofeedback in the management of juvenile migraine. *J Dev Behav Pediatr* 2:168–170, 1981.

Olness K, MacDonald I: Headaches in children. *Pediatr Rev* 8:307–311, 1987.

Olness K, MacDonald J, Uden D: A prospective study comparing self-hypnosis, propranolol, and placebo in management of juvenile migraine. *Pediatrics* 79:593–597, 1987.

Ornitz EM, Ritvo ER: Perceptual inconsistency in early infantile autism. *Arch Gen Psychiatry* 18:76–98, 1968.

Patel CH: Biofeedback-aided relaxation and meditation in the management of hypertension. *Biofeedback Self Regul* 2:1, 1977.

Patterson GB, Guillion ME: *Living with Children*. Champaign, IL, Research Press, 1968.

Patterson GB, Reid JB: Intervention for families of aggressive boys: A replication study. *Behav Res Ther* 11:383–394, 1973.

Patterson GR: *Families: Applications of Social Learning to Family Life*. Champaign, IL, Research Press, 1975.

Patterson GR: *Coercive Family Process*. Eugene, OR, Castalia, 1982.

Patterson GR, Chamberlain P, Reid JB: A comparative evaluation of a parent-training program. *Behav Ther* 13:638–650, 1982.

Pavlov IP: *Conditioned Reflexes: An Investigation of the Physiological Activity of the Cerebral Cortex*. London, Oxford University Press, 1927.

Pelham WE, Schnedler RW, Bologna NC, et al: Behavioral and stimulant treatment of hyperactive children: A therapy study with methylphenidate probes in a within-subject design. *J Appl Behav Anal* 13:221–236, 1980.

Pentz MA, Dwyer IN, MacKinnon DP, et al: A multicommunity trial for the primary prevention of adolescent substance abuse. *JAMA* 261:3259–3266, 1989.

Peterson DR: *The Clinical Study of Social Behavior*. New York, Appleton-Century-Crofts, 1968.

Place M: Annotation hypnosis and the child. *J Child Psychol Psychiatry* 25:339–347, 1984.

Porrino LI, Rapoport IL, Behar D, et al: A naturalistic assessment of the motor activity of hyperactive boys. *Arch Gen Psychiatry* 40:681–687, 1983.

Puig-Antich J: Major depression and conduct disorder in prepuberty. *J Am Acad Child Psychiatry* 21:118–128, 1982.

Rachman S, Hodgson R: *Obsessions and Compulsions*. Englewood Cliffs, NJ, Prentice-Hall, 1980.

Rapoport IL, Ismond DR: *DSM-III Training Guide for Diagnosis of Childhood Disorders*. New York, Brunner/Mazel, 1984.

Rapport MD: Attention deficit disorder with hyperactivity. In: Hersen M, Van Hasselt VB (eds): *Behavior Therapy with Children and Adolescents: A Clinical Approach*. New York, Wiley, 1987, pp. 325–361.

Rapport MD, DuPaul GI, Stoner G, et al: Attention deficit disorder with hyperactivity: Differential effects of methylphenidate on impulsivity. *Pediatrics* 76:938–943, 1985.

Rapport MD, DuPaul GJ, Stoner G, et al: Comparing classroom and clinic measures of attention deficit disorder: Differential, idiosyncratic, and dose-response effects of methylphenidate. *J Consult Clin Psychol* 54:334–341, 1986.

Rapport MD, Jones IT, DuPaul GJ, et al: Attention deficit disorder and methylphenidate: Group and single-subject analyses of dose effects on attention in clinic and classroom settings. *J Clin Child Psychol* 16:329–338, 1987.

Rapport MD, Murphy A, Bailey JS: Ritalin vs. response cost in the control of hyperactive children: A within-subject comparison. *J Appl Behav Anal* 15:205–216, 1982.

Reber M: Mental retardation. *Psychiatr Clin North Am* 15:511–522, 1992.

Rehm LP: A self-control model of depression. *Behav Ther* 8:787–804, 1977.

Repp AC, Deitz DE: Reinforcement-based reductive procedures: Training and monitoring performance of institutional staff. *Ment Retard* 5:221–226, 1979.

Reynolds WM, Coats KI: A comparison of cognitive-behavioral therapy and relaxation training for the treatment of depression in adolescents. *J Consult Clin Psychol* 54:654–660, 1986.

Rimm DC, Masters IC: *Behavior Therapy: Techniques and Empirical Findings*. Orlando, FL, Academic Press, 1979.

Rincover A, Cook R, Peoples A, et al: Using sensory extinction and sensory reinforcement principles for programming multiple adaptive behavior change. *J Appl Behav Anal* 12:221–233, 1979.

Robins LN: Epidemiological approaches to natural history research: Antisocial disorders in children. *J Am Acad Child Psychiatry* 20:566–580, 1981.

Rolf J, Johnson J: *Intervention*. Invited address to the Conference on the Role of Resilience in Drug Abuse, Alcohol Abuse, and Mental Illness. Washington, DC, National Institute on Drug Abuse, 1994.

Ronen T, Wozner Y, Rahav G: Cognitive intervention in enuresis. *Child Fam Behav Ther* 14:1–14, 1992.

Ross AO: *Child Behavior Therapy*. New York, Wiley, 1981.

Russo D, Varni IW (eds): *Behavioral Pediatrics: Research and Practice*. New York, Plenum, 1982.

Rutter M, Giller H: *Juvenile Delinquency: Trends and Perspectives*. New York, Penguin, 1983.

Safer DI, Kroger JM: Trends in medication treatment of hyperactive school children. *Clin Pediatr* 22:500–504, 1983.

Said JA, Wilson PH, Hensley VR: Primary versus secondary enuresis: Differential response to urine-alarm treatment. *Child Fam Behav Ther* 13:1–13, 1991.

Satterfield IN, Cantwell DP, Satterfield BY: Multimodality treatment. *Arch Gen Psychiatry* 36:965–974, 1979.

Schadlock RL, Gaswood LS, Perry PB: Effects of different training environments on the acquisition of community living skills. *Appl Res Ment Retard* 5:425–438, 1984.

Schreibman L, O'Neill RE, Koegel RL: Behavioral training for siblings of autistic children. *J Appl Behav Anal* 16:129–138, 1983.

Scott DS, Gregg IM: Myofacial pain of temporomandibular joint: A review of the behavioral-relaxation therapies. *Pain* 49:231, 1980.

Seligman MEP: Phobias and preparedness. *Behav Ther* 2:307–320, 1971.

Siegel LI, Ridley-Johnson R: Anxiety of childhood and adolescence. In: Bornstein PH, Kazdin AE (eds): *Handbook of Clinical Behavior Therapy with Children*. Homewood, IL, Dorsey Press, 1985, pp. 266–308.

Skinner BF: *The Behavior of Organisms: An Experimental Analysis*. New York, Appleton-Century-Crofts, 1938.

Skinner BF: *Science and Human Behavior*. New York, Free Press, 1953.

Sloane RB, Staples FR, Cristol AN, et al: *Psychotherapy versus Behavior Therapy*. Cambridge, MA, Harvard University Press, 1975.

Snow DL, Grady K, Tebes JK: Adolescent decision-making program: Report of a longitudinal school-based preventive intervention. *Community Psychol* 20:13–14, 1987.

Spiegler MD, Guevremont DC: *Contemporary Behavior Therapy* (2nd ed). Pacific Grove, CA, Brooks/Cole Publishing, 1993.

Stanton HE: Short-term treatment of enuresis. *Am J Clin Hypn* 22:103–107, 1979.

Stark KD, Reynolds WM, Kaslow NJ: A comparison of the relative efficacy of self-control therapy and a behavioral problem-solving therapy for depression in children. *J Abnorm Child Psychol* 5:91–113, 1987.

Straus CD: Anxiety. In: Hersen M, Van Hasselt VB (eds): *Behavior Therapy with Children and Adolescents: A Clinical Approach*. New York, Wiley, 1987, pp. 109–136.

Surwit R, Pilon R, Fenton C: Behavioral treatment of Raynaud's disease. *J Behav Med* 1:323, 1978.

Tebes JK: *Resilience: Some Basic Assumptions*. Invited comments to the Conference on the Role of Resilience in Drug Abuse, Alcohol Abuse, and Mental Illness. Washington, DC, National Institute on Drug Abuse, 1994.

Tebes JK, Grady K, Snow DL: Parent training in decision-making facilitation: Skill acquisition and relationship to gender. *Fam Rel* 38:243–247, 1989.

Tinterow M: *Foundations of Hypnosis: From Mesmer to Freud*. Springfield, IL, Charles C Thomas, 1970.

Thorndike EL: *Animal Intelligence*. New York, Macmillan, 1911.

Twardosz S, Nordquist VM: Parent training. In: Herson M, Van Hasselt VB (eds): *Behavior Therapy with Children and Adolescents: A Clinical Approach*. New York, Wiley, 1987, pp. 75–105.

Vamey JW, Katz ER, Dash I: Behavioral and neurochemical aspects of pediatric pain. In: Russ DC, Varn JW (eds): *Behavioral Pediatrics: Research and Practice*. New York, Plenum, 1982.

Vyse SA, Rapport MD: The effects of methylphenidate on learning in children with ADDH: The stimulus equivalence paradigm. *J Consult Clin Psychol* 57:425–435, 1989.

Wakeman RI, Kaplan IZ: An experimental study of hypnosis in painful burns. *Am J Clin Hypn* 21:3–12, 1978.

Watson JB: Psychology as the behaviorist views it. *Psychol Rev* 20:89–116, 1913.

Watson JB, Raynor R: Conditioned emotional reactions. *J Exp Psychol* 3:1–14, 1920.

Webster-Stratton C, Kolpacoff M, Hollinsworth T: Self-administered videotape therapy for families with conduct problem children: Comparison with two cost-effective treatments and a control group. *J Consult Clin Psychol* 56:558–566, 1988.

Webster-Stratton T, Hollinsworth T, Kolpacoff M: The long-term effectiveness and clinical significance of three cost-effective training programs for families with conduct-problem children. *J Consult Clin Psychol* 57:550–553, 1989.

Weissberg RP, Caplan M, Harwood RL: Promoting competent young people in competence-enhancing environments: A systems-based perspective on primary prevention. *J Consult Clin Psychol* 59:830–841, 1991.

Weisz JR, Weiss B, Alicke MD, et al: Effectiveness of psychotherapy with children and adolescents: Meta-analytic findings for clinicians. *J Consult Clin Psychol* 55:542–549, 1987.

Wells KC: Assessment of children in outpatient settings. In: Hersen M, Bellack AS (eds): *Behavioral Assessment: A Practical Handbook* (2nd ed). New York, Pergamon, 1981.

Wells KC, Forehand R: Conduct and oppositional disorders. In: Bornstein PH, Kazdin AE (eds): *Handbook of Clinical Behavior Therapy with Children*. Homewood, IL, Dorsey Press, 1985, pp. 218–265.

Wells KC, Vitulano LA: Anxiety disorders in childhood. In: Turner SM (ed): *Behavioral Theories and Treatment of Anxiety*. New York, Plenum, 1984.

Whalen CK, Henker B, Buhrmester D, et al: Does stimulant medication improve the peer status of hyperactive children? *J Consult Clin Psychol* 57:545–549, 1989.

Whalen CK, Henker B, Dotemoto S: Teacher response to the methylphenidate (Ritalin) versus placebo status of hyperactive boys in the classroom. *Child Dev* 52:1005–1014, 1981.

Whalen CK, Henker B, Hinshaw S: Cognitive therapy for hyperactive children: Premises, problems, and prospects. *J Abnorm Child Psychol* 13:391–410, 1985.

Whitman TL, Johnston MB: Mental retardation. In: Hersen M, Van Hasselt VB (eds): *Behavior Therapy with Children and Adolescents*. New York, Wiley, 1987, pp. 184–223.

Wiltz NA, Patterson GR: An evaluation of parent training procedures designed to alter inappropriate aggressive behavior of boys. *Behav Ther* 5:215–221, 1974.

Wolpe J: Cognition and causation in human behavior and its therapy. *Am Psychol* 33:437–446, 1978.

Wolpe J: *Psychotherapy by Reciprocal Inhibition*. Stanford, CA, Stanford University Press, 1958.

Wright L, Walker CE: Behavioral treatment of encopresis. *Pediatr Psychol* 4:35–37, 1976.

Young GC, Morgan RT: Overlearning in the conditioning treatment of enuresis: A long-term follow-up study. *Behav Res Ther* 10:419–420, 1972.

Young IL, Goldsmith AD: Treatment of encopresis in a day treatment program. *Psychother Theory Res Pract* 10:231–235, 1972.

Yule W, Sacks B, Hersov L: Successful treatment of a noise phobia in an 11-year old. *J Behav Ther Exp Psychiatry* 5:209–211, 1974.

Zeltzer L, LeBaron S, Zeltzer PM: The effectiveness of behavioral intervention for reducing nausea and vomiting in children and adolescents receiving chemotherapy. *J Clin Oncol* 2:683–690, 1984.

Zigler E, Hodapp RM: Mental retardation. In: Cavenar JO (ed): *Psychiatry* (Vol 2). Philadelphia, Lippincott, 1985.

76 Cognitive Therapies

Theodore A. Petti, M.D., M.P.H.

Cognitive therapy (CT), rational emotive therapy (RET), and cognitive-behavioral therapy (CBT) have become exciting and innovative approaches to the therapy of disturbed and disturbing children and adolescents (the labels are often used interchangeably). With roots in a number of conceptual and theoretical schools, these approaches provide an impressive array of conceptual, assessment, therapeutic, and evaluative tools for treatment and prevention (Kendall, 1991, 1993; Petti, 1989). Clinicians who learn the basic theory and strategic techniques of CT, RET, and CBT will significantly increase their assessment and treatment skills.

This chapter attempts to illustrate the potential and practical value of all three models in the present and future development of child and adolescent psychiatry. RET and CT are similar in their focus on the role of cognitive distortions in the development and maintenance of psychopathologies. Differences include CT's emphasis on modifying underlying dysfunctional beliefs, while RET aims to change specific and dysfunctional self-statements (Meyers and Craighead, 1984b). CBT is a hybrid of cognitive, behavioral, affective, and social strategies (Kendall, 1993) in which behavior and feelings are altered through changes in thinking patterns (Werry and Wollersheim, 1989). The focus is on behavior and the cognitions needed for controlling and guiding feelings and behavior (Ellis and Bernard, 1983).

COGNITIVE THERAPY

Background and Conceptual Framework

The contributions of such diverse theorists as A. Adler, F. Alexander, K. Horney, S. Freud, G. Kelly, M. Arnold, R. Lazarus, A. Ellis, C. Rogers, and J. Piaget have been acknowledged in the development of CT (Weishaar and Beck, 1987). The empirical nature of the approach is ascribed to developments in behavior modification, especially those related to collaboratively developing an agenda for each session, operationalizing problems, testing hypotheses, eliciting feedback, assigning homework, and employing problem-solving techniques. In the cognitive therapy model, feelings and behavior are largely determined by how people structure situations or events in their own minds. Thoughts or images of an event are *cognitions*, which are shaped by classifying, interpreting, evaluating, and assigning meaning to the event based on underlying attitudes or assumptions (schemata) derived from earlier experiences. When, for example, danger is perceived, egocentric (i.e., Piagetian preoperational stage) mechanisms are activated, and primitive thinking is employed. Objective reality cannot be clearly distinguished from subjective thoughts and feelings. Cognitions have also been described as stream-of-consciousness awareness for verbal or pictorial events (Beck, 1967; Beck et al., 1979). Personal schemata generally develop early in life and can be either adaptive or maladaptive, universal or idiosyncratic, positive or negative (Harter, 1977; Wright, 1988).

The schemata are influenced by the child's developmental history prior to the onset of psychological distress. In stressful situations, latent negative schemata can be activated by circumstances similar to the original event or by an overwhelming of the child's coping abilities. *Automatic thoughts*, cognitions that tend to be repetitious and to occur without deliberation, are then invoked. The normal corrective process—refinement of the perception through testing against reality and prior experience, and then modification to reflect reality—fails to func-

tion in these instances. The result is the person's responding with exaggerated affect and deviant behavior. The automatic thoughts, only partially available to consciousness, are accepted as plausible without question. Closer scrutiny of these thoughts can reveal distortions and errors in logic. Psychiatric disorders result when the patient is sensitized to situations that evoke such *cognitive distortions* (systematic errors in reasoning). The consequent dysfunctional beliefs, attitudes, and assumptions become "silent" regulators of behavior. They override common sense and realistic responses, resulting instead in pathologic and disturbing emotional reactions (Beck, 1967; Beck et al., 1979; Weishaar and Beck, 1987). The negative cognitive triad of a negative view of the self, world, and future illustrates this principle (Beck, 1967; Beck et al., 1979).

The related depressogenic schemata (e.g., "I am really dumb. Nothing is ever going to go right for me") are latent and may be activated by a situation.

CASE ILLUSTRATION

Don, an 8-year-old boy with dysthymic and developmental reading disorders, felt overloaded with homework due to procrastination in completing assignments and not understanding a key concept needed to complete an English paper. As his depression deepened, Don lost the ability to objectively assess his negative thoughts and to adaptively process incoming information. His automatic thoughts precluded his seeking clarification in his textbook or from class notes. Cognitive distortions then followed.

Several types of cognitive distortions or systematic errors in reasoning are associated with depression and require attention in therapy (Beck, 1967; Beck et al., 1979; Weishaar and Beck, 1987).

1. *Arbitrary inference:* Specific conclusions are made contrary to or without confirming evidence (e.g., even though Don had always submitted papers in a timely fashion, he began to tell himself, "This material is so complicated that I will never get it and may as well give up now").
2. *Selective abstraction:* Details are taken out of context, and relevant data are ignored in conceptualizing an entire experience (e.g., Don thought, "The teacher doesn't like me at all. So I'll probably get a bad grade anyway." This was based on the teacher's not calling on Don when he had the answer to a question).
3. *Personalization:* Responsibility for external events is attributed to the self, with no basis for a connection (e.g., "I'm to blame for my parents' fighting." This caused Don to daydream considerably, to not concentrate, and to miss class material or assignments).
4. *Absolutistic, dichotomous thinking:* All experiences are placed in extreme categories, and the patient selects the most negative one (e.g., "I'll never learn to do that").

Anxiety disorders, agoraphobia, and other phobias are likewise conceptualized as responses to incorrect processing of situations (Weishaar and Beck, 1987). Cognitive therapy has been employed in treating a number of childhood disorders and is usually combined with other cognitive and behavioral methods (Robins and Hayes, 1993).

Strategies and Techniques

The goal of CT is to relieve symptoms and prevent future disorder. The therapist is active and directive. Questioning opens the belief system to scrutiny, with behavioral "experiments" serving as means to determine the validity of the underlying dysfunctional assumptions or beliefs. The behavioral experiments are generally developed and agreed upon in the session. This process has been labeled a collaborative empiricism, with the patient's active involvement being a critical feature. The patient must understand the rationale and objectives of each assignment or experiment and agree to its implementation. The collaborative relationship is enhanced through active elicitation of feedback from the patient regarding his or her perceptions of therapy-related issues, and it aids in handling transference and resistance issues.

Initial treatment strategies are directed at clarifying the model and its theory, defining the problem, and relieving symptoms. Training patients to identify their automatic thoughts and to treat them as testable hypotheses is key. Also central is a listing of problems and priorities for treatment, which is incorporated into an overall treatment plan and used to set agendas for each session. *Guided discovery* is a term denoting the process by which Socratic dialogue is employed in helping the patient learn to identify maladaptive conditions and underlying assumptions and to test them through consideration of alternatives. Behavioral change is expected to occur through the testing of these hypotheses, the subsequent development of more realistic, adaptive assumptions, and the increased use of congruent behaviors (Weishaar and Beck, 1987).

"Cognitive" techniques allow for identifying, testing, and correcting specific distortions in thinking through monitoring negative automatic thoughts; recognizing the interrelatedness of cognitions, affect, and behavior; examining evidence supporting the distorted cognitions; substituting reality-based interpretations for the distorted ones; and changing the dysfunctional, distorting beliefs (Beck, 1967). They explore the basis of faulty assumptions by operationally defining the assumptions, refining terms, developing measures of probability, and reassigning attribution. Other useful techniques include charting the occurrence of automatic thoughts and disturbed affects, exploring worst-case scenarios, and using imaging to convey self-concepts and fantasies. (A listing of additional cognitive or verbal techniques is available elsewhere (Beck, 1967).) Once an assumption is identified, the patient and therapist engage in a process of validity testing: determining its universal application, listing supporting evidence, and considering the pros and cons of modifying the assumption or implementing an experiment contrary to the expected result.

"Behavioral" techniques help patients bring forth and test their dysfunctional cognitions and change their behavior. Homework assignments are used in practicing social skills, increasing activity, time structuring, and carrying out exercises targeted to specific situations. Monitoring activity through mastery and pleasure ratings, behavioral rehearsals and role-playing, cognitive rehearsals, self-reliance training, graded task assignments, use of "diversion techniques," exposure to dreaded situations, and relaxation training are additional behavioral techniques of value in conducting CT (Beck, 1967; Petti et al., 1982; Robins and Hayes, 1993).

Application to Children and Adolescents

Several strategies to facilitate the successful use of CT in adolescents have been described (Bedrosian, 1981; Leahy, 1988; Petti et al., 1982; Wilkes and Rush, 1988). The need to interview the whole family in order to learn the context within which the symptoms occur and to get the family involved in treatment distinctly differs in all three models from standard work with adults. Bedrosian (1981) outlines a series of questions useful in addressing this issue. Often the parents, who have brought the youth for treatment, have their own distorted perceptions related to developmental issues of adolescence, which require modification. Similar distortions exist in teenagers (e.g., regarding physical appearance, sexuality, autonomy and control, competency, and peer status).

SPECIAL ISSUES

As in all psychotherapies, the nature of the therapeutic alliance with children and adolescents differs from that with adults. It is difficult to evaluate and test automatic thoughts in children, even after they have been acknowledged. The alliance can be jeopardized by premature confrontation of the dysfunctional cognitions. The youngsters may not perceive a need for treatment, believing that it is the parents' problem. Modifications to address these issues include examining everyone's view of the problem and acknowledging and accepting the teen's negative view of treatment. A more symptom-focused plan can be developed once the relationship jells. Wilkes and Rush suggest that offering to teach teens alternative ways of perceiving events is preferable to identifying and correcting logical errors. Use of a triple-column technique, with the headings "fear," "automatic thought," and "rational response" placed at the top of the columns, to deal with specific areas (e.g., noncompliance in keeping appointments), is recommended as well (Wilkes and Rush, 1988).

The techniques and principles of establishing rapport differ little from those applied in adult practice; conflict and threats to the relationship are minimized by modeling a style of information processing that contrasts significantly with that experienced in relation to the parents. However, the therapist must clarify that he or she cannot control the adolescent's behavior, that the therapist's evaluation of the teen is quite separate from his or her reaction to the adolescent's behaviors, and that the adolescent must feel in control of the flow of information considered and be involved at least in helping to set the agenda for the session (Bedrosian, 1981). Juveniles frequently have difficulty with lengthy, hour-long sessions; durations of 30 minutes supplemented by meetings with family members are usually better tolerated. Accepting teens' wish to end therapy upon cessation of symptoms is often necessary unless a risk of danger is evident (Bedrosian, 1981). Likewise, expectations for homework assignments are less than those for adults. Flexibly set standards and concrete assignments are necessary. Recordings of activities and behavioral experiments should be expected to be completed more often than cognitive tasks, which can provoke performance anxiety. Some children have difficulty learning to use the techniques. Determining their cognitive capacity to complete the assignments is critical (Forehand and Wierson, 1993).

DEVELOPMENTAL PERSPECTIVE

Leahy (1988) highlights the importance of taking a developmental perspective in the utilization of cognitive approaches with children and describes levels of depression related to development. One type, helplessness depression, frequently presents with the maladaptive assumption that a failure represents part of a long pattern, not succeeding calls for giving up. The primary attributional distortion is overgeneralization: Any failing means continued failing. Treatment is geared to assisting the child to cope with failure rather than to learn to master any individual task. The basic strategy is to help children view any targeted task as a learning opportunity and a challenge instead of as a situation in which they will be judged or evaluated. An adaptive cognition might be "It's good to learn from mistakes." Using such a strategy of self-vocalization in stressful, anxiety-provoking, performance situations helped Don from the preceding case illustration "feel better"—"I was able to go to the front of the class without acting weird."

Treatment of the second type, self-criticism depression, is based on developmental cognitive studies indicating that self-reflection, the capacity to develop internal standards, commonly reveals disparities between reality and idealized high demands expected of the self. This capacity for self-reflection occurs in late childhood or early adolescence and creates the conditions for guilt. It allows the teen to employ diverse cognitive distortions to support the negative cognitive triad. Self-punitive assumptions abound, which can also be displaced to others and result in depreciation of their value, distancing, and withdrawal from social interactions.

Leahy (1988) suggests use of a blackboard to illustrate concepts such as the "Bad Thought Monster" and the "Smart Thought Man (or Woman)" and to depict examples of types of thoughts for each, have them fight, and so forth, to illustrate conflict, maladaptive and adaptive cognitions, and the relationship between thoughts, feelings, and actions. He also suggests creating an exciting persona such as a "Zen warrior" with the "force" for correct thinking and gaining competence. Thus, the same treatment principles used with adults are creatively implemented in socializing youngsters to treatment (e.g., accepting behavioral assignments), identifying and changing underlying assumptions, and setting up experiments to challenge dysfunctional cognitions, commensurate with the cognitive-developmental level of the child. Facilitative modeling is a modification of treatment in which a parent is invited to some sessions to demonstrate interrelationships between thoughts and feelings and to serve as a role model for such behaviors as the sharing of negative self-statements and their correction.

Challenging assumptions is difficult with children, and the therapist may need to draw inferences from limited verbalizations. The Bad Thought Monster and Smart Thought Man (Woman) are particularly useful in providing examples. Puppets that easily look the part of such representations can also be useful. For children under 12 or those lacking formal operational thinking and the ability to abstract, Leahy (1988) recommends having the child commit adaptive thoughts to rote memory, with the therapist modeling such during the sessions. Less emphasis is placed on Socratic dialogue and more on role playing and reverse role playing in rational responding. Rational thoughts can be carried on flashcards and practiced as self-verbalizations during the day, with the parents being involved with this type of homework. In the initial socialization of the youngster to principles of the cognitive approach, the therapist may be usefully portrayed as "like a teacher" (Leahy, 1988). Drawing the analogy of therapist as coach may also assist in this process.

The following case represents an attempt to demonstrate the direct application of Beck's CT principles to the treatment of a disturbed child (Petti et al., 1982).

CASE ILLUSTRATION

John, age 12 years, was referred for suicidal ideation, recurrent depression, and refusal to eat or to go to school. We agreed that these problems, particularly his fear of eating outside his home, had contributed markedly to his dysphoria and would be the focus of our work. He developed an understanding of the interrelatedness of thoughts, feelings, and behaviors through the use of diagrams depicting his own feelings in positive and negative situations. We exposed several major cognitive distortions through role playing, assessing probabilities, monitoring predicted outcomes, homework ("experiments"), and other techniques. Our handling of an invitation he received for holiday dinner at a favorite relative's home illustrates some of these techniques. John's first response was to adamantly refuse to go or even to discuss the possibility. Exploration of this during the session revealed the underlying dysfunctional belief: "I'll get sick and puke all over. I'll be very embarrassed, and everyone will be upset with me." Thus the resulting automatic thought, "No! I am not going," and the block to further discussion became more understandable. John then estimated the probability or likelihood that any of the feared events expressed in his dysfunctional thoughts might actually occur (i.e., someone getting sick, getting scared of becoming ill, getting a nauseated feeling, being extremely embarrassed) on a scale from 0 to 100%. The estimated probabilities ranged from 80 to 100%. These were substantially reduced as we discussed his actual past related experiences. Proba-

bilities for pleasant experiences on the visit were likewise analyzed and modified. We then role played the visit and ultimately devised a set of thoughts that could be used when the automatic thought occurred. He practiced them during the session and agreed to do further practice at home and to record the actual outcome as part of our "experiment." John carried out his homework and reported that no one, including himself, had gotten sick, and he compared this outcome to his early and modified predictions. This became another part of our developing a more complete picture of his distorted cognitions and the means to address situations causing his fears and dysphoria. The parents were also involved in supporting his positive cognitions, adaptive responses, and overall program. Systematically collected data revealed progress in all areas.

Schrodt and Fitzgerald (1987) argue that in adolescents changes due to CT differ from those seen in adults and are better characterized as a generalized maturation of thinking style. The "curative" aspect of the therapeutic work is expected to result from modeling and identification with the cognitive processes or thinking of the therapist.

RATIONAL-EMOTIVE THERAPY

Background and Conceptual Framework

RET represents a natural link between CT and CBT. RET has been employed with children since the 1950s and was among the first cognitive approaches in the psychotherapy of disturbed youth (Bernard and Joyce, 1984; Ellis and Bernard, 1983; Waters, 1982). As with CT, RET focuses on cognitions and on the identification, then elimination, of sources causing symptoms. Unlike CT, it seeks profound and lasting personality change, emphasizes active disputation with the patient concerning fundamental dysfunctional thoughts, and teaches evaluation of actions. It focuses on the core of the underlying dysfunctional belief system within the structure of an interactional theory of personality and personality disorder and may be used with developmentally advanced teens, but requires levels of cognitive functioning generally beyond those of younger youth. For these younger children, general RET, "virtually synonymous with CBT," is used (Ellis and Bernard, 1983).

RET applies a panoply of action-oriented activities. In RET, *beliefs* express values and consist of one's appraisal and evaluation of the interpretation of reality and not the interpretation itself. *Assumptions* comprise both interpretations made about reality that can be assessed as true or false and the actual appraisal and evaluation of the interpretations, which can also be evaluated regarding extent of validity. *Irrational beliefs* within the RET framework are antiempirical assumptions held about the self or surrounding world that are formed early in life and are often fixed. In the RET model, emotional disorders are considered to occur following cognitive errors, either from (*a*) the interpretation of one's perceptions of a situation through empirical distortions of reality, or (*b*) the faulty *appraisal of the interpretation* through a negative evaluation of the inference with respect to one's life (DiGiuseppe and Bernard, 1983; Ellis and Bernard, 1983; Waters, 1982). The faulty appraisal of interpretations is considered the key to most emotional disturbance and to treatment. Distortions of reality can be corrected by adequate appraisal. A distorted perception will not result in significant levels of extreme arousal and pathology if it is appropriately appraised (Bernard, 1988).

RET, like CT, aims to modify or replace dysfunctional cognitive-emotive links and thus ameliorate specific emotional and behavioral problems, and to provide broad-based skills and strategies for solving diverse problems during and after treatment (Ellis and Bernard, 1983). Labeled "ABC(DE)," the therapeutic process is as follows: An activating event (A) is interpreted and analyzed in view of the person's belief (B) about what happened, which creates the emotional or behavioral consequence (C). In and after treatment, disputation (D) employs systematic challenge and question of the untenable hypotheses or irrational beliefs of absolutistic and imperative assumptions held about self, the world, and others in the environment. The new trust in the resulting cognitive-emotive and behavioral changes (E) occurs when the unrealistic assumptions and beliefs are reformatted into more sound and empirically valid statements.

Targeting distortions of inferences drawn during interpretation is a limited, less elegant, and short-lived solution (nonpreferential RET), while challenging the appraisal or evaluation of the interpretation (preferential RET) is the approach of choice if the child is capable and willing to engage in such an effort. RET assumes that children and adolescents are especially influenced by affective and behavioral interventions and susceptible to cognitive appeals through didactic teaching, persuasion, and information giving (Ellis and Bernard, 1983; Waters, 1982). The basic goal for both preferential and nonpreferential RET is the internalizing of a "philosophy of life/cognitive strategy that is more rational and realistic than the one [patients] commonly abide by when they get into difficulties" (Ellis and Bernard, 1983).

Adolescents and older children may in addition have the following as goals of treatment (Young, 1983): learning self-acceptance; learning to dispute personal imperatives (e.g., "musts," "shoulds," and "oughts" and "awfulizing"); and correcting misperceptions of reality. Young also suggests that adolescents can most easily grasp the irrationality of "I can't stand it" thinking and learn to challenge their conviction of being unable to handle inconvenience or discomfort.

Waters (1982) has listed seven goals of RET for younger children: identifying emotions correctly, establishing a vocabulary of terms to accurately describe emotions, distinguishing harmful from constructive feelings, distinguishing thoughts from feelings, being alert to self-talk, connecting self-talk and feelings, and developing rational coping statements.

Strategies and Techniques

The stages of RET consist of relationship building, assessment, skill building, and application of skills. A high level of rapport may not be required for successful treatment with children and adolescents (Bernard, 1988). The factors for developing a working relationship are similar to those for CT.

ASSESSMENT

Problem identification is the first phase of assessment. In this stage, determination is made of the actual existence of a problem and whether it belongs to the child or to individuals in the environment (e.g., parents, teachers) (DiGiuseppe and Bernard, 1983). The problem analysis phase follows and continues as an ongoing part of therapy. The dysfunctional cognitions, emotions, and behavior contributing to the disorder are determined and the subsequent insights integrated into the evolving treatment plan. Central concerns are expected to be revealed after higher levels of rapport are achieved in the therapeutic relationship. The assessment also addresses the child's cognitive strengths and weaknesses, the extent to which language may control the child's behavior, and the child's capacity to gain distance from the problem. The assessment should identify the antecedent and consequent conditions of the target behavior and the type and severity of maladaptive emotions, prior to the analysis of such dysfunctional cognitions, as (a) irrational self-statements and beliefs—self-defeating and irrational appraisal ("awfulizing," self-downing); and (b) causal attributions—appropriateness of beliefs regarding negative and positive events (e.g., negative outcomes are caused by factors related to the self; positive events are attributed to external factors). Additional components of the analysis are areas of strengths and skills, including coping self-statements and practical problem-solving skills—for example, generating several solutions to an interpersonal problem (alternative solution thinking) and predicting consequences of specific behavior (consequential thinking) (DiGiuseppe and Bernard, 1983).

Direct assessment measures, elaborated by DiGiuseppe and Bernard (1983) to access the self-talk of children and teens, are of great practical use in helping youngsters access their own thoughts and feelings, as well as in providing a mechanism for reporting self-talk. For the RET practitioner, they provide a window into the child's perceptions and verbal-language range and a basis for cognitive restructuring efforts. The following techniques may be of value for conducting most types of psychotherapy with children and some teens (DiGiuseppe and Bernard, 1983):

1. *Subjective Units of Discomfort Scale* (Wolpe, 1982): The child is asked to think of the worst feeling he or she has had or can imagine. This feeling is given a 100 rating and then compared to absolute calm, rating 0. The child is then asked, "From this scale, for (situation) how do you rate yourself at this moment, or when you are exposed to—?"

2. *Emotional (feeling) scales:* Children are asked to rate the impact of a particular emotion experienced in a given situation on a 10-point scale. This enhances the child's ability to quantify the strengths of feeling states and to perceive the experience of several emotions from weak to strong.

3. *Emotional flashcards:* The therapist and child take turns play acting the emotion named on the card, while the other guesses at it or tells stories about the emotion. This increases emotional awareness.

4. *Emotional detective:* The child is asked to work on a "case" by investigating how the child or others handle feelings, with the report due at the next session.

5. *Peeling the onion:* The therapist keeps offering verbal prompts until the level of thought activating the dysfunctional thinking is exposed.

6. *Feeling charts:* Descriptors (e.g., pleasant-unpleasant, weak-strong, short-long) are used by the child to depict feelings.

7. *Emotional vocabulary building:* Children list the names of all the feelings they know, then are asked to consider a situation in which a particular feeling was experienced and, if possible, the preceding thoughts. This allows labeling each feeling with a definition and sensitizes children to a wider range of emotions. It also demonstrates the level of emotional understanding and provides an introduction to RET (Waters, 1982).

8. *Thought bubbles:* The aim here is to convey the notion of thoughts creating feelings and to assist children in making the connections. This can be done with a series of cartoons depicting temporally related scenes of a problem. The cartoons contain characters with dramatic expressions, and the child is asked to fill the accompanying bubble with thoughts of the character.

9. *Sentence completion:* Incomplete sentences concerning problem areas are presented, which the child is requested to complete. These elicit the presence or absence of coping self-statements, beliefs, practical and emotional problem-solving skills (e.g., "When the girl gets teased before class, she thinks . . .").

10. *Think-aloud:* Children are asked to think aloud as they attempt to complete a task. This provides a picture of the affective quality of their self-talk (e.g., fear of visiting the dentist for an examination).

11. *TAT-like approach:* Pictures of ambiguous situations are shown, and the child is asked to create a story about the thoughts and feelings of the characters and explore alternative options in that situation.

12. *Expansion:* Verbal prompts expand abbreviated self-talk, for example, as the child expresses thoughts experienced in a problematic situation, the therapist asks questions and gives verbal instruction to expand the content ("What thoughts came after . . .?" "Tell me more about . . .").

13. *Words "and," "but," and "because":* These are used to facilitate tuning in to and reporting automatic self-talk when the child ends an incomplete sentence about a thought.

14. *Instant replay:* Developed for parents and children to use to keep track of unpleasant emotions arising from specific situations and

events occurring during the prior week, the "rerun" asks them to play back their related thoughts and feelings.

15. *Guided imagery:* The child is asked to relax, to vividly imagine a problem situation, and to describe feelings and related self-talk.

SKILL BUILDING

The third stage, skill acquisition and skill building, consists of training to use problem-solving skills and to help the child or adult take responsibility for their emotions by controlling their feelings through rational thinking and use of such skills. Teaching youngsters to change inappropriate to appropriate feelings frequently involves changing irrational, extreme responses to moderate and more realistically appropriate feelings and actions (e.g., changing self-defeating responses from rageful ones, or feeling panicky to feeling annoyed or apprehensive) in order to allow more goal-oriented actions (Waters, 1982).

DiGiuseppe (1981) suggests that initial efforts with children should be directed to helping them build a schema with a vocabulary of feelings and responses and a framework for their application. To illustrate how changes in feelings and behavior are possible, the contrasting differences in results between a child's usual negative behavior and what can be expected from more appropriate, less disturbing behavior, achieved by use of alternate strategies, should be discussed. The need to get out of an "emotional fog" and to calm down before taking action is another principle to discuss early on in the process of problem solving.

Teaching the specifics of "ABC," the next step, focuses on awareness of self-talk and the connections between beliefs, feelings, and antecedent events. Older children are taught the difference between rational and irrational beliefs and other critical thinking skills (e.g., absolute versus conditional thinking; consequential thinking; discriminating fact from opinion, inference, and assumption; learning to take a perspective on a situation; and disputing irrational thinking). Younger children practice coping self-statements in learning how cognitive change can occur and influence B and C in the ABC paradigm (DiGiuseppe and Bernard, 1983; Waters, 1982).

Since younger children may have difficulty with the terms *rational* and *irrational*, Waters (1982) suggests substituting *helpful* and *harmful*, respectively. Helpful beliefs are based in reality and result in more acceptable feelings and actions and in getting what you want. Harmful beliefs result in self-defeating thoughts, destructive and nonacceptable feelings, and failure to attain one's desires. A set of questions based on the question, "Is there enough evidence to conclude that this thought is true?" allows the child to reasonably challenge beliefs.

CASE ILLUSTRATION

Fred, a verbal young teen with borderline and schizotypal features, is overly attached and dependent on his grandmother. He asked her to help monitor his homework. Learning disabled but very bright, he frequently makes errors. When she suggests that a word may be misspelled or a sentence incomplete, an argument ensues since he inevitably challenges her point. Fred was finally able to share his underlying belief that being wrong was a sign of weakness and defeat. To accept her correction meant "submitting" and defeat. He learned to challenge the rationality or helpfulness of the belief by questioning the correctness of the appraisal and seeking evidence to try to support it. He decided that it was not so awful to have her point out errors, that he was really strong enough to accept such assistance, and that it could be much worse if she corrected in a belittling fashion or not at all. He learned that the harmful belief ran counter to his own needs and desires. Most critically, he came to understand that making errors did not make him any less worthwhile and that accepting corrective feedback could improve rather than diminish his stature as a person of worth.

Fred's case also illustrates a more sophisticated intervention. He had just received a poor grade from a recent exam. Beyond learning to dispute the concepts of "ain't it awful" or "I'm just stupid" with regard to that particular episode, he was able to look at the more general issue of what needs to be done when you have a learning handicap, and that it is different from being stupid or not having any control over the situation. He discussed what might be done differently in the future. The next step was to apply empirical analysis, a strategy to modify dysfunctional interpretations. As in CT, therapist and child agreed to design an experiment to evaluate his belief of being stupid. Fred agreed to pay closer attention to the teacher and write assignments and tests down in a notebook that would be kept up and brought home daily. We then compared the results of the next exam to his earlier experience. He tested whether he (a) would do poorly again or not, to see if he did have some control over the situation and (b) could do well, contrary to his belief that he was always doomed to fail. His belief was that he had done everything possible and that he had no control over his grades. Fortunately, the behavioral structure he imposed on his schoolwork demonstrated that organizational skills and not stupidity accounted for his poor performance.

Rational-emotive imagery (REI) (Ellis and Bernard, 1983; Waters, 1982) is another strategy that asks the child to imagine a mental picture depicting a situation that generates an extreme emotion. The child is asked to change the feeling to a milder form (e.g., from hating and greatly fearing a bully to a strong dislike and worry about the bully). Once this is done, the link between thought and emotional change is highlighted for present and future use.

APPLICATION OF SKILLS

Implementation of the newly learned rational thinking skills outside the therapy session is the final stage of RET. Homework assignments are the major vehicle in effecting this task. This involves, for example, practicing the skills; monitoring their effect and associated feelings; listing personal demands; listing thoughts, feelings, and behaviors related to specific events; completing a self-concept inventory; and using positive self-talk as a reinforcer (Bernard, 1988). This phase requires considerable effort by both therapist and child, as major changes in thinking, feeling, and acting are being attempted. The relationship must be sufficiently established to weather the expectations placed on the child. Bernard suggests that youngsters with a problematic history of completing homework are at greatest risk for similar problems with RET. Development of a system of reinforcers in cooperation and collaboration with the parents can be useful in overcoming resistance to completing the homework or in overcoming a well-entrenched set of bad habits. The therapist can also focus on irrational beliefs within the session to deal with this difficult issue (Bernard, 1988). In children with cognitive deficits rather than distortions, training in such CBT models as interpersonal cognitive problem solving (ICPS) (Spivack and Shure, 1974) is most appropriate.

ROLE OF PARENTS

Involvement of the parents in all stages of assessment and treatment facilitates a successful outcome. Assessment provides a guide of the extent to which parental behaviors and beliefs influence the child's problems. Goals and principles to use in work with the parents have been developed (Bernard, 1988), and the same four stages are applicable, from the development of rapport to practice of skills outside the sessions. Likewise, problem identification and problem analysis of difficulties that exist within the family are analogous to those for the children. The focus is to assist the parents in overcoming their own and the child's difficulties by developing an understanding of their basic dysfunctional beliefs and an awareness of more constructive alternatives. Participation in homework for themselves is also expected, including better control of emotions, distinguishing rational from irrational ideas, implementing behavioral changes, and use of child-related literature (Bernard, 1988).

COGNITIVE-BEHAVIORAL THERAPY

Background and Conceptual Framework

CBT, a major force in the treatment of children, is based on developments from the behavior therapy movement of the late 1960s and the thrust of psychology in a "cognitive" direction. A number of workers have been credited for their major contributions to this growth (Kendall, 1993; Mahoney, 1993; Petti, 1989). The evolution occurred along three paths: (a) advances in cognitive and developmental psychology (Bandura, 1977; Meichenbaum, 1977; Petti, 1989; Shirk, 1988); (b) evolution of self-control procedures from the operant model, including Bandura's (1977) concept of reciprocal interaction between individuals and their environment; and (c) the contributions of CT and RET as noted above.

Primary CBT goals are concordant development of efficient and adaptive modes of responding to problematic situations and the elimination or reduction of maladaptive and inappropriate behaviors. This is accomplished by developing and internalizing self-controls skills and reflective problem-solving strategies. CBT integrates the concept from behavior therapy that antecedent and consequent environmental factors contribute to overt behaviors with concepts from cognitive and rational-emotive therapies that emphasize the role cognitions play in dealing with environmental stimulation and changing overt behavior (Craighead et al., 1985). Cognitive distortions and cognitive deficiencies associated with deviant or dysfunctional behavior are the focus of concern (Kendall, 1993). A multimodal approach to treatment is considered necessary in order to address the multidimensional factors that contribute to and maintain the psychopathology. Underlying assumptions have been summarized by Cohen and Schleser (1984): (a) active problem-solving is expected in childhood; (b) discrimination, extraction, and analysis of data and subsequent planning are characteristic of problem-solving; and (c) styles of problem-solving change with developmental progression. The child is assumed to be an active participant in and interpreter and recorder of experiences. The developmental implications and skill levels of the child are considered essential to planning treatment strategies. Cognitive therapies with adults can successfully focus on their distorted processing of information and world views. In most children and many adolescents, however, the issue of distorted cognitions is considered of less importance than the lack of effective strategies for controlling behavior (Braswell and Kendall, 1988) and the prominence of impulsive cognitive styles over more reflective styles (Cohen and Schleser, 1984). The need to differentiate between the presence of cognitive deficiencies, distortions, or both is critical in helping the child build a new "cognitive template" to identify and solve problems (Kendall, 1993).

With age, children become more reflective (Leahy, 1988; Roberts and Nelson, 1984). Strategies for implementing CBT interventions must also consider the developmental levels of the child's cognitive skills (Durlak et al., 1991) and attentional, memory, and related skills. Achieving a level of formal operations allows the teen to attend selectively to tasks, to employ deductive reasoning and problem solving, and to learn strategies that can be applied in a flexible manner. Those who have attained the concrete level of operations can appreciate the usefulness of a strategic approach to problem solving but may not be able to focus their attention or may get excessively involved in the problematic situation and thus may lose details in the process. They need to be made aware of the value of employing a mnemonic strategy. Preoperational and preschool children function on a here-and-now basis. They are incapable of planning for a problem-solving situation (Cohen and Schleser, 1984).

Generalization of change to other situations, settings, or environments is a major consideration in conceptualizing strategy. Problem identification, goals of treatment, and sequence of planned intervention strategies are dependent on the child's level of development (Roberts and Nelson, 1984). Increasing a child's ability to accurately report experiences to evaluate his or her own performance situation and to self-monitor mood is considered a major objective of cognitive behavioral interventions.

Strategies and Techniques

Many types of CBT models exist; the titles of these approaches include cognitive-developmental (Harter, 1977), cognitive training, cognitive behavior modification (Meichenbaum, 1977), cognitive-behavioral-psychosituational (Grieger and Boyd, 1983), and others (Dobson, 1988; Dryden and Golden, 1987; Meyers and Craighead, 1984a). The basic strategies are generally similar. Most of the variants emphasize one facet of CT, RET, or CBT over another, depending on the developmental level of the child, the targeted behavior, and the techniques to be employed. For example, Trautman and Rotheram-Borus (1988) suggest that an effective cognitive-behavioral program for depressed youth should begin with an assessment focusing on "idealistic positivism": concentrating on positive aspects of the child and family, giving compliments and providing prompts for more information, emphasizing loving bonds and family strengths, reframing negative perceptions into a positive context, building a positive therapeutic relationship, and modeling positive behaviors. The problem list is also accompanied by a list of strengths.

ASSESSMENT AND TREATMENT

Assessment issues for general use with CBT are nicely reviewed by Roberts and Nelson (1984). These include the role of developmental processes, identification of target behaviors, evaluating outcome, and relationships between measures for verbal and motor behavior. Also outlined by these workers are cognitive and behavioral assessment strategies related to academic and social problem solving. Rating scales, checklists, measuring academic performance, and behavioral observations are also considered.

Several standardized scales and approaches have been devised to assess the family structure in CBT with conduct-disordered children and teens (DiGiuseppe, 1988). Understanding the extent to which children have the cognitive repertoire needed to understand therapeutic interpretations and their causal/attributional/locus of control style is considered a critical aspect of assessment (Shirk, 1988). Braswell and Kendall (1988) list a number of other behavior rating scales, performance measures, and self-report instruments used to assess children's self-talk, expectancies, and attributional style.

Differentiation between internalizing and externalizing disorders may be a means of selecting treatment strategies. Internalizing disorders (e.g., depression and anxiety disorders in older children and teens) might best be treated through recognizing and testing "mistaken misperceptions, expectations, and/or attributional preferences," while externalizing conduct-disordered children with deficiencies in effectively mediating their behavior might be approached through training in verbal mediation techniques (e.g., self-control and more reflective problem-solving approaches) (Braswell and Kendall, 1988). Even within the same diagnostic category, several different CBT methods and strategies might be considered. Multiple approaches to particular types of disorders are available. These include depression and suicidality (Clarke et al., 1992; Leahy, 1988; Matson, 1989; Petti et al., 1980, 1982; Reynolds and Coats, 1986; Rotheram-Borus et al., 1994; Stark et al., 1987, 1991; Trautman and Rotheram-Borus, 1988); hyperactivity and impulsivity (Finch et al., 1993b; Hinshaw and Erhardt, 1991; Meichenbaum and Goodman, 1971; Ronan and Kendall, 1990; Whalen et al., 1985; Williamson et al., 1981); anxieties, fears, and phobias (Braswell and Kendall, 1988; Grace et al., 1993; Grieger and Boyd, 1983; Kendall, 1993); aggression (Camp and Ray, 1984; Finch et al., 1993a; Lochman, 1992; Polyson and Kimball, 1993); delinquency (Kennedy, 1984); mental retardation (Whitman et al., 1984); learning disorders (Braswell and Kendall, 1988); posttraumatic stress (Deblinger et al., 1990); and conduct disorders (DiGiuseppe, 1983; Kazdin et al., 1992). Individual case descriptions in many of these works provide examples of how specific techniques are employed in assessment and treatment. Kendall (1993) lists general treatment strategies of CBT as modeling, building a coping template, rewards, enactive procedures, affective education, and training tasks and provides specific methods for each. The following describes representative cognitive behavioral models.

MODELS

Verbal Self-Instruction Training

Among the most widely used of CBT procedures, verbal self-instruction training (SIT) has been demonstrated to be effective in assisting impulsive and disruptive children who have deficits in controlling their own behavior. It has been demonstrated to be differentially effective in hyperactive children as compared with the effect of stimulant medication (Braswell and Kendall, 1988; Bugental et al., 1977) and enhances overt problem-solving ability. The procedures have also been demonstrated to be effective with learning-disabled children (Braswell and Kendall, 1988) and depressed adolescents (Reynolds and Coats, 1986; Stark et al., 1987). Meichenbaum's (1977) model provides a structure of procedures that includes an orientation to problem solving and training to (a) identify and define problems, (b) generate alternative solutions, and (c) select and then implement the most appropriate solution. The following vignette nicely describes this approach (Petti, 1989).

CASE ILLUSTRATION

Nine-year-old Joe was referred for severe hyperactivity and oppositional behavior present from the time of his adoption at age 6 years. His dysthymia was successfully treated with imipramine, but his impulsive and negative behavior persisted. His adoptive parents were most concerned about his ravenous "stealing, wolfing, and secreting" of sweets. He and his parents agreed to targeting this behavior for treatment. After collecting baselines for missing goodies, a self-control program was initiated. First Joe's thoughts, feelings, and actions were explored using the thought, "I want/need a cookie." A written sequence was developed, which was practiced out loud in the sessions for Joe to learn to use at home:

I want cookies!
What AM I supposed to do? (Think of available choices.)
I need to look at all my alternatives!
Grab it and take a chance on being punished, feeling guilty, etc.
Ask my mom or dad and expect . . .
Wait till later to ask and expect . . .
Which is my best choice?
How should I do it? and, later to discuss in therapy . . .
How well did I do? (Petti, 1989).

Joe refused to keep a log monitoring his thoughts, feelings, and success in maintaining control when faced with the urge. He did report verbally what occurred, and this compared well to parents' reports. His probability estimate for how successful he would be in controlling his behavior around sweets was less than 50%. Both he and his parents were therefore delighted at his close to 100% success rate. A similar approach was taken with other impulsive behaviors.

Interpersonal Cognitive Problem Solving

The components of this model are frequently incorporated into other types of CBT. The approach for children developed by Spivack and Shure (1974) has been shown to be an effective preventive intervention with poor urban preschools (Shure and Spivack, 1988), though the relationship between interpersonal cognitive problem solving skills and later social behavior has been questioned (Braswell and Kendall, 1988). ICPS assumes that people often become fixated on an ultimate goal and fail to think through strategies to solve typical interpersonal difficulties, consequences of their actions, and other options to achieve the same objectives. This in turn leads to frustration, aggressive behavior, or withdrawal. Interpersonal adjustment and avoidance of psychopathology is expected when the alternative-solution thinking and means-end thinking of ICPS are employed. The training in the Spivack and Shure (1974) model is conducted in 20-minute segments by a teacher who devotes the first 10 to 12 sessions to teaching language concepts of "not," "some," "all," "if . . ., then . . .," "same," and "different." The next 20 sessions concentrate on identifying and becoming sensitized to feelings of self and others. Concepts of "maybe and might," "because and why," "later, not now," and "after and before" are also taught. The final 15 or so sessions are devoted to problem solving. To the games and dialogues employed as means of mastering the concepts are added stories and role-playing games. The major skills of this section are (a) developing alternative solutions (i.e., "There is more than one way to solve everyday problems"); (b) consequential thinking (i.e., what might happen after a given action); and (c) solution-consequence pairing, in which the children suggest solutions to a problem, consider the consequences, and continue the process of pairing solutions to consequences. They ultimately learn to pair solutions with goals (Shure and Spivack, 1988).

Other problem-solving approaches have been described for both children and teens. The "turtle technique" involves withdrawing from a provoking situation and then using relaxation skills (Kendall and Braswell, 1985). Conflict resolution skills training can be effectively combined with a comprehensive treatment plan.

CASE ILLUSTRATION

In the treatment of a depressed, impulsive 12-year-old (Petti and Wells, 1980), situations provoking anxiety or anger were hierarchically arranged from least to most arousing. Scenes evoking the lowest level of arousal were addressed first through role playing of appropriate cognitive, behavioral, and verbal responses. The responses were first modeled by the therapist, then the youngster was coached in their use and was provided positive feedback as he role played each situation. The emotion-arousing situations were practiced until the patient's responses were satisfactory to both patient and therapist. Follow-up indicated better than adequate functioning.

CASE ILLUSTRATION

Jean is a 14-year-old girl with low-average intelligence and a long history of being sexually abused within a chaotic "family" setting. Her episodic dyscontrol became prominent after placement in a supportive preadoptive home. During an inpatient stay, her lack of interpersonal skills was evident. She had developed a knowledge of the basic language concepts required for this approach and had some appreciation for the feelings of herself and others. However, she was wedded to "satisficing"—taking the first available option that came to mind, which was usually based on long-standing distrust of others and was predominantly hostile, aggressive, and negative in nature. Several episodes on the unit were used to develop the concept of seeking to think of alternative explanations and responses, then to tie the options to possible consequences, and finally to anticipate the consequences of her actions when confronted with conflict. She then practiced this evolving skill around her desire to do what she wanted on an outing, in conflict with the desires of her caretaker. She was able to negotiate a compromise acceptable to all. This allowed her to then trust and to learn to discuss conflicting views and desires without assuming the worst before she even began the process. She ultimately felt more confident in relating to peers, staff, and family members. Initial preparation of significant others in the environment to be receptive to these changes can be the critical factor predicting the degree of successful outcome.

Self-Management Skills

These comprise several types of CBT interventions, including problem solving. Other categories include self-regulation, correspondence, and self-instructional training (Whitman et al., 1984). These approaches can prove useful with the mentally retarded, children with concrete thinking, and those with learning problems or low-average intelligence. Self-regulation involves (a) learning self-monitoring skills by accurately identifying and recording a specific type of behavior, (b) setting acceptable objectives, (c) evaluating the response, and (d) reinforcing oneself if the standard is met. Williamson and associates (1981) describe a modification of this approach with an extremely hyperactive, distractible young boy and the subsequent dramatic decrease in his need for stimulant medication. Correspondence training operates by rewarding children either for doing what they say they will, for accurately describing what they did, or for showing an appropriate response to a targeted situation described by the therapist and then actually performing it in a real situation. Once again, the focus of self-management-type interventions depends upon the individual child's skills. Autistic children have also benefited from these approaches (Whitman et al., 1984).

CONCLUSIONS

The cognitive therapies are varied and comprise amalgams of diverse contributions. It has been argued that they are simply extensions of the behavior therapies (Wolpe, 1982). However, collectively they do address in a systematic manner virtually all nine of the skills axes and methods to promote these skills considered by Strayhorn (1983) to be relevant to psychotherapy and preventive mental health. Combinations of treatment components are generally employed in most studies (Durlak et al., 1991).

The work of Stark and associates (1987) demonstrates the use of several of the techniques with school-age children to effect statistically significant decreases in depression in two treatment groups employing cognitive and behavioral principles, compared to another group on a waiting list. The self-control group learned to set realistic standards and subgoals for themselves, to positively reinforce themselves more, to punish themselves less, and to attribute the cause of good and bad outcomes in a more realistic fashion. They also learned to monitor themselves, especially in regard to pleasant activities. The other group, based on Lewinsohn's behavioral model, was taught the rationale for the model. They learned to monitor themselves, to schedule pleasant events, and to develop an awareness of the interdependency of depressed feelings, thoughts, and social behavior. Of equal importance, this study and others (D.A. Brent, unpublished manuscript, 1989; March et al., 1994; Rotheram-Borus et al., 1994) employed manuals for the consistent application of the intervention.

Overall, the cognitive therapies provide variable efficacy and long-term benefits (Abikoff, 1985; Durlak et al., 1991; Kendall, 1991, 1993; Lochman, 1992). The cognitive therapies provide opportunities for briefer therapies and for developing the mechanisms to evaluate our work in the cost-conscious environment of today. They allow multimodal assessment and intervention to meet the needs and developmental stages of individual children.

References

Abikoff H: Efficacy of cognitive training interventions in hyperactive children: A critical review. *Clin Psychol Rev* 5:479–512, 1985.

Bandura A: *Social Learning Theory*. Englewood Cliffs, NJ, Prentice-Hall, 1977.

Beck AT: *Depression: Clinical, Experimental, and Theoretical Aspects*. New York, Harper & Row, 1967.

Beck AT, Rush AJ, Shaw BF, et al: *Cognitive Therapy of Depression*. New York, Guilford Press, 1979.

Bedrosian RC: The application of cognitive therapy techniques with adolescents. In: Emery G, Hollon SD, Bedrosian RC (eds): *New Directions in Cognitive Therapy: A Casebook*. New York, Guilford Press, 1981, pp. 68–83.

Bernard ME: Enhancing the psychological adjustment of school-age children: A rational-emotive perspective. In: Dryden W, Trower P (eds): *Developments in Rational-Emotive Therapy*. Philadelphia, Open University Press, 1988, pp. 173–196.

Bernard ME, Joyce MR: *Rational-Emotive Therapy with Children and Adolescents: Theory, Treatment Strategies, Preventative Methods*. New York, Wiley, 1984.

Braswell L, Kendall PC: Cognitive-behavioral methods with children. In: Dobson KS (ed): *Handbook of Cognitive-Behavioral Therapies*. New York, Guilford Press, 1988, pp. 167–213.

Bugental DB, Whalen CK, Henker B: Causal attributions of hyperactive children and motivational assumptions of two behavior-change approaches: Evidence for an interactionist position. *Child Dev* 48:874–884, 1977.

Camp BW, Ray RS: Aggression. In: Meyers AW, Craighead WE (eds): *Cognitive Behavior Therapy with Children*. New York, Plenum, 1984, pp. 315–350.

Clarke G, Hops H, Lewinsohn PM, et al: Cognitive-behavioral group treatment of adolescent depression: Prediction of outcome. *Behav Ther* 23:341–354, 1992.

Cohen R, Schleser R: Cognitive development and clinical interventions. In: Meyers AW, Craighead WE (eds): *Cognitive Behavior Therapy with Children*. New York, Plenum, 1984, pp. 45–68.

Craighead WE, Meyers AW, Craighead LW: A conceptual model for cognitive-behavior therapy with children. *J Abnorm Child Psychol* 13:331–342, 1985.

Deblinger E, McLeer SV, Henry D: Cognitive-behavioral treatment for sexually abused children suffering post-traumatic stress: Preliminary findings. *J Am Acad Child Adolesc Psychiatry* 29:747–752, 1990.

DiGiuseppe RA: Cognitive therapy with children. In: Emery G, Hollon SD, Bedrosian RC (eds): *New Directions in Cognitive Therapy: A Casebook*. New York, Guilford Press, 1981, pp. 50–67.

DiGiuseppe R: Rational-emotive therapy and conduct disorders. In: Ellis A, Bernard ME (eds): *Rational-Emotive Approaches to the Problems of Childhood*. New York, Plenum, 1983, pp. 111–137.

DiGiuseppe R: A cognitive-behavioral approach to the treatment of conduct disorder children and adolescents. In: Epstein N, Schlesinger S, Dryden W (eds): *Cognitive-Behavioral Therapy with Families*. New York, Brunner/Mazel, 1988, pp. 183–214.

DiGiuseppe R, Bernard ME: Principles of assessment and methods of treatment with children. In: Ellis A, Bernard ME (eds): *Rational-Emotive Approaches to the Problems of Childhood*. New York, Plenum, 1983, pp. 45–88.

Dobson KS (ed): *Handbook of Cognitive-Behavioral Therapies*. New York, Guilford Press, 1988.

Douglas V, Parry P, Marton P, et al: Assessment of a cognitive training program for hyperactive children. *J Abnorm Child Psychol* 4:389–410, 1976.

Durlak JA, Fuhrman R, Lampman C: Effectiveness of cognitive-behavior therapy for maladapting children: A meta-analysis. *Psychol Bull* 110:204–214, 1991.

Dryden W, Golden WL (eds): *Cognitive-Behavioural Approaches to Psychotherapy*. Cambridge, Hemisphere Publishing Corp., 1987.

Ellis A, Bernard ME: An overview of rational-emotive approaches to the problems of childhood. In: Ellis A, Bernard ME (eds): *Rational-Emotive Approaches to the Problems of Childhood*. New York, Plenum, 1983, pp. 3–37.

Finch AJ Jr, Nelson WM III, Moss JN: Childhood aggression: Cognitive-behavioral therapy strategies and interventions. In: Finch AJ Jr, Nelson WM III, Ott ES (eds): *Cognitive-Behavioral Procedures with Children and Adolescents: A Practical Guide*. Boston, Allyn and Bacon, 1993a, pp. 148–205.

Finch AJ Jr, Spirito A, Imm PS, et al: Cognitive self-instruction for impulse control in children. In: Finch AJ Jr, Nelson WM III, Ott ES (eds): *Cognitive-Behavioral Procedures with Children and Adolescents: A Practical Guide*. Boston, Allyn and Bacon, 1993b, pp. 233–256.

Forehand R, Wierson M: The role of developmental factors in planning behavioral interventions for children: Disruptive behavior as an example. *Behav Ther* 24:117–141, 1993.

Grace N, Spirito A, Finch AJ Jr, et al: Coping skills for anxiety control in children. In: Finch AJ Jr, Nelson WM III, Ott ES (eds): *Cognitive-Behavioral Procedures with Children and Adolescents: A Practical Guide*. Boston, Allyn and Bacon, 1993, pp. 257–288.

Grieger RM, Boyd JD: Childhood anxieties, fears, and phobias: A cognitive-behavioral-psycho-situational approach. In: Ellis A, Bernard ME (eds): *Rational-Emotive Approaches to the Problems of Childhood*. New York, Plenum, 1983, pp. 211–239.

Harter S: A cognitive-developmental approach to children's expression of conflicting feelings and a technique to facilitate such expression in play therapy. *J Consult Clin Psychol* 45:417–432, 1977.

Hinshaw SP, Erhardt D: Attention-deficit hyperactivity disorder. In: PC Kendall (ed): *Child and Adolescent Therapy: Cognitive-Behavioral Procedures*. New York, Guilford Press, 1991, pp. 98–128.

Kazdin AE, Siegel TC, Bass, D: Cognitive problem-solving skills training and parent management training in the treatment of antisocial behavior in children. *J Consult Clin Psychol* 60:733–747, 1992.

Kendall PC: *Child and Adolescent Therapy: Cognitive-Behavioral Procedures*. New York, Guilford Press, 1991.

Kendall PC: Cognitive-behavioral therapies with

youth: Guiding theory, current status, and emerging developments. *J Consult Clin Psychol* 61:235–247, 1993.

Kendall PC, Braswell L: *Cognitive-Behavioral Therapy for Impulsive Children*. New York, Guilford Press, 1985.

Kennedy RE: Cognitive behavioral interventions with delinquents. In: Meyers AW, Craighead WE (eds): *Cognitive Behavior Therapy with Children*. New York, Plenum, 1984, pp. 351–376.

Leahy RL: Cognitive therapy of childhood depression: Developmental considerations. In: Shirk SR (ed): *Cognitive Development and Child Psychotherapy*. New York, Plenum, 1988, pp. 187–204.

Lochman JE: Cognitive-behavioral intervention with aggressive boys: Three-year follow-up and preventive effects. *J Consult Clin Psychol* 60:426–432, 1992.

Mahoney MJ: Theoretical developments in the cognitive psychotherapies. *J Consult Clin Psychol* 61:178–193, 1993.

March JS, Mulle K, Herbel B: Behavioral psychotherapy for children and adolescents with obsessive-compulsive disorder: An open trial of a new protocol-driven treatment package. *J Am Acad Child Adolesc Psychiatry* 33:333–341, 1994.

Matson IL: *Treating Depression in Children and Adolescents*. New York, Pergamon, 1989.

Meichenbaum D: *Cognitive-Behavior Modification: An Integrative Approach*. New York, Plenum, 1977.

Meichenbaum D, Goodman J: Training impulsive children to talk to themselves: A means of developing self-control. *J Abnorm Psychol* 77:115–126, 1971.

Meyers AW, Craighead WE (eds): *Cognitive Behavior Therapy with Children*. New York, Plenum, 1984a.

Meyers AW, Craighead WE: Cognitive behavior therapy with children: A historical, conceptual, and organizational overview. In: Meyers AW, Craighead WE (eds): *Cognitive Behavior Therapy with Children*. New York, Plenum, 1984b, pp. 1–18.

Petti TA: Individual psychotherapy in children. In: Kaplan HI, Sadock BJ (eds): *Comprehensive Textbook of Psychiatry* (Vol 2, 5th ed). Baltimore, Williams & Wilkins, 1989.

Petti TA, Wells K: Crisis treatment of a preadolescent who accidentally killed his twin. *Am J Psychother* 34:434–443, 1980.

Petti TA, Bornstein M, Delamater A, et al: Evaluation and multimodality treatment of a depressed prepubertal girl. *J Am Acad Child Psychiatry* 19: 690–702, 1980.

Petti TA, Kovacs M, Feinberg T, et al: Cognitive therapy of a 12-year-old boy with atypical depression: A pilot study. Paper presented at the Annual Meeting of the American Academy of Child Psychiatry, Washington, DC, October 1982.

Polyson J, Kimball W: Social skills training with physically aggressive children. In: Finch AJ Jr, Nelson WM III, Ott ES (eds): *Cognitive-Behavioral Procedures with Children and Adolescents: A Practical Guide*. Boston, Allyn and Bacon, 1993, pp. 206–232.

Reynolds WM, Coats KI: A comparison of cognitive-behavioral therapy and relaxation training for the treatment of depression in adolescents. *J Consult Clin Psychol* 54:653–660, 1986.

Roberts RN, Nelson RO: Assessment issues and strategies in cognitive behavior therapy with children. In: Meyers AW, Craighead WE (eds): *Cognitive Behavior Therapy with Children*. New York, Plenum, 1984, pp. 99–128.

Robins CJ, Hayes AM: An appraisal of cognitive therapy. *J Consult Clin Psychol* 61:205–214, 1993.

Ronan KR, Kendall PC: Non-self-controlled adolescents: Applications of cognitive-behavioral therapy. *Adolesc Psychiatry* 17:479–505, 1990.

Rotheram-Borus MJ, Piacentini J, Miller S, et al: Brief cognitive-behavioral treatment for adolescent suicide attempters and their families. *J Am Acad Child Adolesc Psychiatry* 33:508–517, 1994.

Schrodt GR, Fitzgerald BA: Cognitive therapy with adolescents. *Am J Psychother* 41:402–408, 1987.

Shirk SR: Causal reasoning and children's comprehension of therapeutic interpretations. In: Shirk SR (ed): *Cognitive Development and Child Psychotherapy*. New York, Plenum, 1988, pp. 53–89.

Shure MB, Spivack G: Interpersonal cognitive problem solving. In: Price RH, Cowen EL, Lorion RP, et al (eds): *14 Ounces of Prevention: A Casebook for Practitioners*. Washington, DC, American Psychological Association, 1988, pp. 69–82.

Spivack G, Shure MB: *Social Adjustment of Young Children: A Cognitive Approach to Solving Real-life Problems*. San Francisco, Jossey-Bass, 1974.

Stark K, Reynolds WM, Kaslow NJ: A comparison of the relative efficacy of self-control and behavior therapy for the reduction of depression in children. *J Consult Clin Psychol* 15:91–113, 1987.

Stark KD, Rouse LW, Livingston R: Treatment of depression during childhood and adolescence: Cognitive-behavioral procedures for the individual and family. In: Kendall PC (ed): *Child and Adolescent Therapy: Cognitive-Behavioral Procedures*. New York, Guilford Press, 1991, pp. 165–206.

Strayhorn JM: A diagnostic axis relevant to psychotherapy and preventive mental health. *Am J Orthopsychiatry* 53:677–696, 1983.

Trautman PD, Rotheram-Borus MJ: Cognitive behavior therapy with children and adolescents. In: Frances AJ, Hales RE (eds): *Review of Psychiatry* (Vol 7). Washington, DC, American Psychiatric Press, 1988, pp. 584–607.

Waters V: Rational emotive therapy. In: Reynolds CR, Gutkin TB (eds): *The Handbook of School Psychology*. New York, Wiley, 1982, pp. 570–579.

Weishaar ME, Beck AT: Cognitive therapy. In: Dryden W, Golden WL (eds): *Cognitive-Behavioral Approaches to Psychotherapy*. Cambridge, Hemisphere Publishing Corp., 1987, pp. 61–91.

Werry JS, Wollersheim JP: Behavior therapy with children and adolescents: A twenty-year overview. *J Am Acad Child Adolesc Psychiatry* 28:1–18, 1989.

Whalen CK, Henker B, Hinshaw SP: Cognitive-behavioral therapies for hyperactive children: Premises, problems, and prospects. *J Abnorm Child Psychol* 13:391–410, 1985.

Whitman T, Burgio L, Johnson MB: Cognitive behavioral interventions with mentally retarded children. In: Meyers AW, Craighead WE (eds): *Cognitive Behavior Therapy with Children*. New York, Plenum, 1984, pp. 193–228.

Wilkes TCR, Rush AJ: Adaptations of cognitive therapy for depressed adolescents. *J Am Acad Child Adolesc Psychiatry* 27:381–386, 1988.

Williamson D, Calpin I, DiLorenzo T, et al: Combining Dexadrine and feedback for the treatment of hyperactivity. *Behav Modif* 5:399–416, 1981.

Wolpe J: *The Practice of Behavior Therapy* (3rd ed). New York, Pergamon, 1982.

Wright IH: Cognitive therapy of depression. In: Frances AJ, Hales RE (eds): *Review of Psychiatry* (Vol 7). Washington, DC, American Psychiatric Press, 1988, pp. 554–570.

Young H: Principles of assessment and methods of treatment with adolescents: Special considerations. In: Ellis A, Bernard ME (eds): *Rational-Emotive Approaches to the Problems of Childhood*. New York, Plenum, 1983, pp. 89–110.

77 GROUP PSYCHOTHERAPY FOR CHILDREN AND ADOLESCENTS

Fern J. Cramer-Azima, Ph.D.

Group psychotherapy for children and adolescents has long been advocated as a treatment of choice. Young, active children can communicate with one another, often without words or symbolic reasoning, as if they have a private language. Therapists have the opportunity to observe the actual behavior of the children, to clarify the diagnosis, and to gradually interpret the meaning of their play and interactions. Psychotherapeutic and educational goals are provided in a safe, supportive, empathic setting where boundaries and rules are established by the thera-

pists. As for adolescents, group settings are particularly advantageous because of their specific need for relationships with their peers. Reciprocal exchange of thoughts and feelings permits self-disclosure in the group often not possible in individual therapy, where rebellious silences pervade the transference to parental authority figures. In the group the adolescents have a very high regard for what is acceptable and proper for others of their age group. Learning that problems are not unique and that they are shared by peers can promote faster sharing of information.

APPROACHES

Present group psychotherapeutic approaches for children stem from modifications of traditional activity therapy (Schiffer, 1977; Slavson, 1952) and group analytic models (Anthony, 1965). For young children these approaches are blended with psychoanalytically oriented play therapy (Ginnott, 1961; Phillips, 1985; Winnicott, 1971).

Activity Group Therapy

This approach, introduced by Slavson (1952), focuses on observation of the children's behavioral and motoric communications and is carried out in a permissive, empathic, supportive setting. The focus is on seeing how the child relates and copes with other children and physical objects within the group context. Transference interpretation is minimized. The therapist provides little structured activity and intervenes only when a child is in danger, is hurt, or threatens another child. Toward the end of the session, refreshments are provided.

Activity-Interview Therapy

This modification was formulated by Schiffer (1977) to provide additional structure to the original technique. The first part of the session allows group play with peers, followed by a structured discussion period. The fantasy produced in the play period is explored, with the therapist imparting meaning, insight, and transference interpretation. Additionally, the group dynamics and bonding with peers and the therapist solidify over time and provide the vehicle for the therapeutic change.

Group-Analytic Psychotherapy

This model was adapted by Anthony (1965) for nursery, latency, and adolescent groups. The therapist intervenes rarely with the nursery children, keeps to the background, and fits interpretation into the play themes. A specified "small table" technique was evolved, which concertized the space or territory of the table and room for each child and therapist and permitted observation of changes over time. For the latency group, a "small room" technique was used, in which a discussion group was followed by an activity phase. Repeated themes identify the children's conflicts, whether they are expressed in symbolic play, free associations, or in fantasies and dreams. The older latency children begin to demonstrate more of the specific group analytic factors introduced by Foulkes, such as socialization, mirroring, the condenser, and chain phenomena. The condenser is a sudden reaction to the group that is discharged by a particular event. The chain phenomenon is likened to the group's free-floating discussions, in which the topic is carried forward by each individual's response, followed by a condenser outburst. The specific roles of the scapegoat, stranger, and historian in the latency-age group are still highly relevant today. While the technical aspects of the approach may be modified, the therapist's psychodynamic understanding remains central.

Some 50 years later, present-day group approaches include pure or blended psychoanalytic, psychodynamic, behavioral, and cognitive models, combined with family and network interventions. The precise applications appear to be the result of the group therapist's theoretical training, the particular setting's philosophy, and the type of population that is in need of treatment.

Most therapists working in the field today utilize a developmental framework involving parents in parallel treatment for the younger children. The two major theoretical trends are psychoanalytically oriented and behavioral/cognitive approaches, both emphasizing here and now interactions. Unfortunately, in this age range there has been insufficient attention paid to the actual interactions within the matrix, the reciprocity patterns, and the changes over time of leader dominance and submissive followers within the group (Azima, 1982).

The group therapy area has suffered from an undue borrowing from individual therapy theory. For group theorists the historical premise is that the infant is embedded in a symbiotic group fusion and, developmentally, only gradually becomes individuated. Within the last 10 years there has been a revival of interest in interpersonal (Sullivan, 1953) and peer theories. Grunebaum and Solomon (1987) have concluded that the ability to master peer relationships and define friendship patterns involves a separate line of development from that of the mother-child dyad. These authors do not negate the importance of the parent-child relationship but emphasize the independence of peer competency. These authors have postulated that self-esteem and peer relationships are such interconnected phenomena that self-evaluation may be viewed in large measure as the inner experience of the esteem in which one is held by one's peers. Nowhere is the study of peer relationships more important than in child and adolescent group therapy.

As in all therapies, the essential ingredient is the analysis of content and process, which over time allows the unfolding and recapitulation of the past in the present context. The group affords an increased expression of thoughts and feelings, including projective biases that allow each member to be understood from many more points of view than a single therapist can hypothesize. Further, the projections open a window into the speaker's own pathology. The allies and dissidents actively demonstrate the variation in projective identifications, as if it were a system of revolving mirrors, reflecting intrapsychic and interpersonal coordinates for each and every member. The differing responses to the individual speakers promote the working through process and constitute a corrective monitoring system for the group therapist. Among other important features of multiperson therapy is the provision of a social context and the rebuilding of more accurate interpersonal relationships; the development of bonding, an esprit de corps or group climate that motivates and energizes the loyalty, intimacy, disclosure, and cohesion of the membership; the development of a group composition that permits stronger, better-functioning members to interact therapeutically with ego-weak, more pathological children; and the working through of dominant/submissive, independent/dependent roles, (Garland, 1992; Pfeifer, 1992; Spinner, 1992).

APPLICATIONS AND TECHNIQUES FOR CHILDREN'S GROUPS

Increasingly, community demands have led to the introduction of short-term models (Epstein, 1976; Scheidlinger, 1984) and the introduction of structure and innovative techniques to focus the attention of the emotionally disturbed child to allow self-disclosure. Frank (1983) introduced the concept of dramatic play for greater structure and therapeutic support for ego-weak children. Central to the controversy was the dilemma of whether the children's verbalizations were necessary for an interpretive approach (Charach, 1983; Sugar, 1974). Not only were many of the children nonverbal, but they also lacked the symbolic ability to communicate their thoughts and feelings.

Significant sociocultural changes have altered the concepts of latency and adolescence and have led to a modification in group composition, the roles of the members, and the functions and countertransferences facing the therapist (Azima, 1977). The bulk of referrals for clinic and day hospitals are for defiant, acting-out children from single-parent families in which the father is absent or plays a minor role. These children are often both witnesses and victims of psychological and physical abuse. Simultaneously, they are encouraged by television, music, and dance to act out more of their sexual and aggressive fantasies. These youngsters in the group are boisterous, outspoken, and use sexualized language and behavior.

COMPOSITION AND STRUCTURE

A major task facing the therapist is the selection and balancing of the composition of the group, orchestrating the number of acting-out children with the quieter, less demanding, more compliant ones and deciding upon the play, activities, or toys used to engage and interest the children. The reality is that there is no such thing as an ideal composition, and a group is formed with the available referred candidates. The stronger the group, the more very disturbed children can be included.

As a rule, the children are seen and evaluated with their parents. Often observing the children over time helps clarify the diagnosis (Anthony, 1965; Liebowitz and Kernberg, 1986).

AGE GROUPINGS, HETEROGENEITY, HOMOGENEITY, AND FREQUENCY

Preschool children, boys and girls ages 3–5, are seen in small groups of three, four, or five and usually by two therapists in a play or activity group. The more active or pathological the children, the greater the need for auxiliary personnel.

The latency therapy group is usually separated into early (ages 5–7), middle (ages 8–10), and late (ages 10–12) groups. Frequently these age groups are intertwined, and more attention is placed on the composition of the range of intelligence, physical size, and diagnoses of the children. In treatment groups, latency boys outnumber girls, at a ratio of 4:1 to 8:1, depending on the population being serviced. Presently there is some indication that there is a rise in girl referrals. The preponderance of boys in the groups necessitates that one of the therapists or special care counselors be male to provide a role model and to diminish acting-out behavior. It should be noted that some of the children from single-parent families are threatened by the presence of both male and female therapists.

At times the late latency group is combined with the preadolescent group. The older boys and girls usually do better in homogeneous groups with the same-gender therapist (Kennedy, 1989).

Frequency of sessions varies from once or twice a week to every day in a day hospital. A beginning group may tolerate only 15 minutes and gradually work up to 45 minutes or an hour.

PLAY, TOYS, AND SETTING

Play is the natural vehicle for the therapy, and in general, the less complicated and fewer the toys, the better fantasy play is encouraged. The fundamentals are a portable table and chairs, paper, pencil, crayons, playhouse, dolls, and play telephones. The toys should not be unduly stimulating but rather should focus on the projective nature of the action and production. Among the techniques useful in getting the children focused and "grouped" are the following: creating large murals or collages and playing the game of "Guess What I Have Made." Psychodramatic techniques are useful procedures, both when the children invent the characters and when the therapists provide a fishbowl from which a variety of themes outlined on paper slips may be drawn. This technique is especially helpful when a theme is being avoided, for example, dealing with the group bully, the sexually provocative child, a child who feels responsible for a divorce, or a child in the group who faces residential placement.

Through the play, the therapist and children begin to understand the meaning of the disclosures. Preparing the children to express themselves is antecedent to further working through of their problems.

SPECIALIZED GROUP APPROACHES

A "clown club" (Smith et al., 1985) has been introduced to provide a structured fantasy approach. The therapists dress up and play clowns, to the delight of the children. The psychodrama can be expanded to include the playing of good and bad witches, angry teachers or parents, and the like.

A variety of video techniques (Mallery and Novas, 1982) have been used with school-age children. Children can produce and watch their own videos. Replaying and redoing scenes allow the children actually to see their behavior and attempt to correct it by activities that strengthen organizational skills and memory. The video camera is an invaluable tool for diagnosis, research, and follow-up.

Kinetic group psychotherapy (Schachter, 1984) is a technique involving an activity period of exercises or games, followed by a verbal discussion period. The technique has been used with a wide range of children's problems, including childhood autism and depression.

The use of genograms (Davis et al., 1988) is a technique borrowed from family therapy with latency-age children. The children, aided by the therapist, map out the family constellation, which helps the children to focus on and question the events of the parents' marriage or separation, new alliances, and catastrophic events. The genograms are shared in the group and encourage each member to divulge hidden fears and learn to distinguish between reality and fantasy.

Other innovative techniques include storytelling, constructing and using masks, puppet plays, and group emblems. All such projective activities allow the children to reveal their problems in a nonthreatening manner. A sign of a maturing group process is when the children need less prepared structure from the therapists and suggest and create their own object world. Older, more verbal, intelligent, and stable children are capable of using a talking group as compared to a holding group for the ego-weak children.

For impulse-ridden children (Crawford-Brobyn and White, 1986), changes in the traditional models may be necessary. Some children can progress from working with another child in a dyad for a period of time to joining the group. The acting-out child may be able to tolerate only one of four group sessions, until tolerance is slowly built up. Schamess (1986) has reviewed a wide variety of differential diagnoses and corresponding group structures operating in outpatient treatment of latency-age children.

INTERACTIONAL PSYCHODYNAMIC GROUP PSYCHOTHERAPY

The model described in this chapter is applicable to all age groups. The specificities of the approach for children and adolescents include the provision of activity, play, and fantasy according to developmental level, temperament, diagnostic pathology, and goals of the treatment. The interactive context in the here and now, among the peers and the therapists, amplifies the precise nature of the communication difficulties and conveys over time the dysfunctional intrapsychic conflicts within the group paradigm. The degree of permissiveness, structure, and limit setting depends upon the activity level and explosiveness of the group and the degree to which regressive acting out is desired or can be tolerated. Greater vigilance is necessary with children who are overly aggressive than with shy children. The thrust of the model is to define the emerging object relations, symbolized by the choice of play objects, and the actual interactions with other group members. The psychodynamics of the group activities are partially translated into meaningful dialogues and understanding by the children. As the therapy progresses, modifications in the explanations and interpretations are appropriately made.

CASE ILLUSTRATION

David was a husky, attractive 7-year-old bully when he first came to the day hospital. He kicked the therapist and refused to have anything to do with the other children. His bravado covered his horrifying nightmares, his daily nausea in the car, and his inability to function in the classroom. When he started in the group, the members were working on a large mural. One youngster was drawing the clinic, another the roadway, and another the school car. At this point David became very agitated and wanted to scribble over the drawing. The group members became somewhat intimidated, and the therapists attempted to calm him down but to no avail. He was then told that, unfortunately, he could not manage the group that day and was asked to leave, with the comment "When you feel you are able to return and join the activity, please tell Sally (the Special Care Counselor who escorted the child from the room), knock at the door, and let us know when you are ready.'' It took several weeks before David was able to return to the group; when he did, he announced, ''I'll try it out.'' The other children greeted him with understanding. The group members were drawing different emotions on faces. David first drew an angry face with teeth; when he noticed that others were drawing happy or sad faces, he remarked that he often had such feelings himself. In a subsequent session two or three of the members played with hand puppets and through the play told David that they did not like to be hit. Two years later David was present when a new child joined the group. By chance he and this child again chose the puppets. When the younger child kept smashing the head of the puppet on the table, David said in a soothing voice, ''I know what it is like when you are so mad that your head feels like thunder.'' David worked through a considerable amount of rage. His somatic symptoms, including car sickness, largely disappeared, as did his repetitive drawing of cars. Such a child needed a gradual progression from dyadic to group therapy. His mother profited from parenting management. She was not a psychologically minded individual but was motivated to help her child and cooperated well with the program.

SPECIAL POPULATIONS

Child group therapy has been expanded widely into such problem areas as poor peer relations, low academic achievement, delinquency, and somatic and terminal illnesses.

Social skills groups emphasizing behavioral and cognitive models are used to improve peer relations for the shy, aggressive, impulsive, or narcissistic child. Immigrant children are helped by these short-term groups in learning how to make friends with a stranger or start or change schools.

Underachieving groups are helpful with retardation and attention deficit disorders, where token rewards and contingency models are used. The use of computer games and videotaping in these and other groups has proven to be helpful and enjoyable. Other behavioral techniques include contracting, targeting strategies, modeling, shaping, and imagery (Gaines, 1986).

School groups for problem children are possible when the parents give their consent and when the disorder is not unduly severe. In the latter case, referral is made to a clinic or day hospital. Berkowitz (1989) has described a consultation/supervisory model with teachers that allows them to run such groups.

Children of divorce groups utilize a variety of techniques to deal with the burgeoning effects of divorce on children. Some models include warm-up procedures, defined reading material, and homework preparation. Other models emphasize having children tell stories of their difficulties. Some children prefer to draw or write their stories.

Epstein and Bordiun (1985) have introduced a ''Could This Happen'' game. The children are faced with a number of stories, such as ''A father tells the child that the child's mother is a bad person. Could this happen?'' The group is structured into two teams who have to decide among four choices: (*a*) Yes, I'm sure it could happen; (*b*) Yes, I'm not sure, but I think this could possibly happen; (*c*) No, I'm not sure this could happen; and (*d*) I'm not sure, but I don't think this could happen. Team leaders are chosen, and the children become involved in the cognitive organization, learning to express themselves and share their experiences with the other children.

In heterogeneous groups, when there is some balance between children from intact families and those who live with one parent, there is the possibility of less negative circular feedback.

Groups for abused children face many complex issues (Schacht et al., 1990). These children have great difficulty in divulging secrets about their abusive parents. The fears of final separation or placement in a treatment facility are often sufficient for children to minimize their pain. Whether these children are treated in homogeneous or heterogeneous groups depends both on the setting and the numbers to be treated. Homo-

geneous groups are usually found in residential treatment facilities. Increasingly, in school settings counselors report a much more open divulgence by younger children of psychological, physical, and sexual abuse.

Follow-up studies of the effects of abuse have shown impairment in ego development and cognition, low self-esteem, and self-mutilating behavior (Green, 1978). Most therapists favor short-term structured groups, while a few advocate longer psychodynamic models. Dealing in the group context with the details of separation, visits to the delegated residential treatment center, visitation rights with parents, and so forth, allows the child to share feelings of shame, anxiety, fear, and rage. Parents of an abused child (Mara and Winston, 1990) are often very resistant to any treatment program. When, however, they recognize the danger of losing the child, and that there are other parents with whom they can share their shame, some accept the proposition (Cunningham and Matthews, 1982). Unless the parents become involved in the therapy, their children feel solely responsible and deserving of the abuse.

Unfortunately, abused children often perpetrate the same behavior upon other children, as, for example, an 8-year-old boy who had repeatedly witnessed the sexual acting out of his mother and was quite possibly involved in these behaviors. Now separated from his mother, his unsatisfied libidinal drives became more manifest in the group with the boys, whom he seduced into sexual play. The dilemma was how to feel empathic for this abused child while also preventing him from continuing this pattern in the treatment program.

It is likely that future groups will be necessary for the children born to surrogate mothers and those born with drug addiction or AIDS.

Crisis groups have been formed in emergencies to deal with the tragedies of earthquake, fire, suicide, and so forth. Joint student/staff groups allow swift abreaction of feelings and shared support.

Educational and preventive groups inform children about the dangers of smoking, drugs, going with a stranger, entering a car, or letting anyone, including a sibling, friend, or parent, violate their bodies and genitals.

Parent and family groups allow parents and families to become involved in the treatment of their children. The approaches vary among separate parent meetings and combined family and multiple family approaches (Epstein, 1976; Hoffman et al., 1981; Parmenter et al., 1987; Pasnau et al., 1976). In the day hospital or intensive treatment program of the latency-age child, parent involvement has become a mandatory part of the program. Parents and multiple family therapy groups are also included in treatment of a wide range of children's disorders, such as those resulting from the effects of divorce or abuse, autism, and chronic illness.

Peled and Edelson (1992) have reported on a 10 session group format for children of battered women. Children who are witnesses to violence and abuse of their mothers suffer significant trauma. Ability to speak about these events with their peers and therapists provide significant support in short-term, manually guided psychoeducational groups. Recently, Vardi and Bucholz (1994) have described groups for grandmothers who are raising their inner city children and who are overcome with depression and fears of incompetence. The groups last approximately a year, deal actively with issues of school, home maintenance, and daily problem solving.

Among newer applications are the treatment of mothers exhibiting postpartum depression, and their newborns (Clark et al., 1993). Mothers and infants are seen separately for 12 weekly group session. Part of each session includes a dyadic group for mothers and infants together. Two of the 12 group sessions include spouses or partners. The goals of the three-tier model include (*a*) alleviating the depression of the mother, to clarify her parenting needs with special emphasis on empathy, and providing for the infant's physical and social-emotional needs; (*b*) for the infants, stimulating and broadening of affective responses to others, providing comfort, encouraging self-worth, and fostering developmental skills; (*c*) for the mother-child dyad, focusing on the here and now interactions with the aim of fostering reciprocal enjoyable interactions and promoting the mother's parenting skills; and (*d*) for the family relationships, providing group therapy to help to define the nature of the depression, promote support, empathy, and joint problem solving. The authors' report is based on 5 years of time-limited groups, and the results are highly encouraging. The model presents an important preventive group model for infants at risk.

Trad (1994) has also elaborated an integrative sequential model of mother-infant psychotherapy, integrating the mother's individual therapy with mother observation of their infant's behavior with therapist, participation in mothers' group, and family therapy. This multimodal perspective allows therapists a broad intrapsychic interpersonal framework. The technique provides, in addition to a preventive approach for the rearing of infants, a prospective, longitudinal research methodology.

ADOLESCENT GROUP PSYCHOTHERAPY

Young Adolescent Group

The techniques used with the pubertal group (ages 12–14) approximate those used with latency-age children, namely, a combination of activities, play, drawing, psychodrama, and discussion periods. Most therapists tend to treat pubertal children in homogeneous groups with a same-sex therapist. These adolescents are often gauche and active and have difficulty in verbalization, especially the more pathological who are hospitalized or live in residential care. This age group works best on structured themes related to dependency, attachment, separation, and competition among others. Sessions in general are a maximum of 45–50 minutes in length. Both short-term and long-term models are used. In the latter category, Gordon (1989) has reported a 2-year group with aggressive boys that used the model of working through symbiotic attachment and gradually working toward individuation. Interpretations were made to the group as a whole, dealing with ongoing interpersonal themes, rather than on the intrapsychic material of any one member. Videotaping, music, projective art techniques, and board games (Kraft, 1986) are often stimulating for children of this age, who often are too timid to talk openly about their sexual abuse, drug use, inferiority fears, and marked ambivalence to parents.

Middle and Late Adolescent Groups

The age group of 15–19 years is most amenable to verbal psychotherapy. Outpatient models usually group the 15- to 18-year-olds. Increasingly, the adolescents referred for group psychotherapy suffer from depressive reactions, suicidal attempts, and borderline symptomatology, in addition to the usual range of behavior disorders linked to delinquency, rebellion against parents, school dropout, and drug and alcohol use. The more severely disturbed adolescents are hospitalized and placed in residential and treatment centers. School groups focus on learning disorders, low motivation, disruptive behavior, and the like. Outpatient clinic groups treat the largest number of adolescents, while private practice groups tend to cluster in the more affluent areas.

The average psychotherapy group size ranges from six to eight and includes both sexes (with the exception of the pubertal group); where possible, heterogeneous composition is preferable. Acutely psychotic, autistic, or very handicapped borderline youngsters are suitable for outpatient groups but may be placed in modified group forms in hospital and residential settings (Speers and Lansing, 1965; Stengel, 1987). The inclusion of borderline and very fragile adolescents depends upon the strength of the total membership, which acts as a type of absorption filter and control mechanism. Group sessions vary from 1 to 1½ hours, at the rate of once or twice a week, and may be either short- or long-term.

THEORETICAL CONSTRUCTS

Theories and techniques range among psychoanalytic, psychodynamic, psychodramatic, gestalt, transactional analysis, behavioral, cognitive, and system approaches. The choice of methods appears to be made by a combination of the therapist's theoretical orientation and the specificities of the adolescents being treated.

Within the psychoanalytically oriented framework, the approaches of Freud, Bion, and Kohut have been adapted to the group protocol. By and large, the developmental, interactive, and cohesive processes dictate whether individual or group address is used.

Identity Group Psychotherapy

Rachman (1989) has focused the theoretical model on the resolution of the adolescent's identity crisis within the group context and utilizes a blend of creative introspection, free thought, verbal and fantasy experimentation, and active techniques. The latter include role play, psychodrama, and dream interpretation, as well as specially devised scenarios to permit adequate self-disclosure and working through of problems.

Interactional Psychodynamic Group Psychotherapy

It is proposed that confrontation, empathy, and interpretation are the therapeutic triad underlying this approach and that all three stem from a common source (Azima, 1989). Confrontation accentuates the verbal enunciation of thoughts and feelings, while empathy involves the experiential process incorporating the other person's feelings and thoughts. It is postulated that the peers in the group are representative of varying confrontative and empathic styles. Some personalities are in need of a more confrontative approach, while others need longer nurturance and silent understanding. Interpretation occurs at the point in the therapeutic process when there has been sufficient empathic confrontation and clarification to uncover and give meaning to the underlying unconscious conflicts, and it should occur in synchrony with the individual and the group process.

CASE ILLUSTRATION

John was a 15½-year-old with marked narcissistic and grandiose features. For many sessions he boasted that he could live on his own, that he did not want to be in school, and that he had many friends. The other five group members could hardly get a word in, as he pontificated and analyzed everyone. Gradually certain members began to confront and question him and to express their annoyance. He soon revealed that his mother had divorced his alcoholic, abusive father and later married an older, quiet man. This man could not tolerate the patient, and he was moved into a small apartment with one of his brothers, who soon left, and he continued there alone. As these facts and feelings came out, he was amazed to regain the empathy of many group members. The therapist in the early stages had assumed an empathic, understanding approach with John and only gradually began to confront the narcissistic defenses. Although the patient was willing to interpret everybody else's problems, he could not accept other people's intruding into his inner life. Many sessions later, a pretty adolescent to whom John was clearly attracted told him in a direct, confronting manner that he would have a hard time making friends, especially with girls, because he was not truly interested in them, and that he was sure to make others very angry by his know-it-all manner. John was stunned, averted his gaze, bent over, and remained silent. He slowly lifted his head, and holding back his tears, he said, "I think you are right, and that's what I am afraid of."

Comment

It may be necessary to confront the silence of adolescent members very early, in an understanding way. The psychodynamic significances of the intrapsychic and interpersonal communications and interactions remain the cornerstone of interactional psychodynamic group psychotherapy (IPGP) approach. As in all psychotherapies, the goal is for the adolescent to develop self-understanding, independence, self-esteem, and interpersonal competence.

The preceding clinical example was taken from an outpatient, open-ended, heterogeneous group whose average patient attendance is 2 years. In this model, the goal is the development of autonomy and independence. Parents are seen only at intake and at the end of each year's group, with the adolescents' consent. Confidentiality is highly protected in this model, and this in turn promotes faster divulgence of material. This approach is made more possible in a country (such as Canada) that provides funds so that parents do not have to pay the bills. Additionally, in the Canadian system of health care, any adolescent over the age of 14 can request treatment without the parents' knowledge. Outpatient clinics and private practice group psychotherapy often involve a combination of psychopharmacology, combined individual and group therapy, and parallel or conjoint parent or family therapy. In long-term treatment necessitated by regressions or traumatic events, a combined network approach has been used effectively (Richmond, 1989).

Inpatient and residential treatment groups form an integral part of most adolescent units and residential treatment centers (Chase, 1991; Stein and Kymisses, 1989). The group format varies indefinitely according to the degree of pathology, intellectual level, longevity of the group, and number of absences of group members. Inpatient psychotherapy groups are advantageous in that they can focus on ongoing resistances and acting out in the group and the hospital network. Conformity and compliance as to weekend passes, attendance at meetings, and taking of medication are strengthened in the group context. The handling of confidentiality in inpatient groups is a delicate issue, and it seems wise to explain at the outset the team's sharing of information. In ward situations where adolescents are assigned to certain staff members, there is often conflict between the patients and different staff teams.

APPLICATIONS FOR SPECIAL POPULATIONS

The focus of this review is limited to those groups in which the emotional disorder is a primary focus for the psychotherapy group.

High school and college groups are often labeled counseling groups; more severely disturbed students are referred to other treatment facilities.

University mental health clinic groups play a very valuable role for young students dealing with problems of separation from family, difficulty in interpersonal and sexual identity relationships, reactive depressions, suicidal ideation, and psychotic reactions. Increasingly, eating disorders are being treated in adolescent groups. Azima (1992) discussed the limitations for homogenous versus heterogenous composition and the counterindication for the therapist of the psychodynamic group to combine both therapeutic and active control of the eating patterns.

Preventive and educational groups for AIDS, abortion, alcoholism, drugs, and the effects of divorce and the Holocaust are among the themes that increasingly are being offered by short-term groups (Bogdaniak and Piercy, 1987; Bratter, 1989; Gaines, 1986; Grant, 1988).

Groups for *learning-disabled adolescents* in residential treatment were described by Coché and Fisher (1989) as a way to develop cognitive and affective communication skills, learn how to deal with authority figures, develop problem-solving skills, and learn to accept one's learning disability and assume responsibility for improving and coping with it. An eclectic approach was used to foster self-esteem and to target various ego deficits. Often parents seeking schools for the learning disabled reject psychiatric treatment, blaming the child's or adolescent's problems on an inborn or organic etiology. An integrative approach combining academic skill building and psychotherapy is considered the most effective way of handling the two parts of this problem. Video (Cox and Lothstein, 1989) and group computer learning has been very advantageous for children and adolescents with reading, writing, and mathematics deficits. Each member can encourage, share, and suggest alternatives. Team competitions increase motivation and foster learning.

Therapy groups for delinquents have a long history (Raubolt, 1983). These difficult, conduct-disordered, acting-out, defiant adolescents often rebel against the authority model of individual psychotherapy, retreating into hostile silences and frequent absences. The inclusion of delinquents into group therapy depends on the degree of their motivation, their conscientiousness, and their degree of resistance. Among the theoretical constructs utilized with delinquents are the following: permissive, para-analytic, psychoanalytic, and directive. More recent techniques have rejected the traditional permissive models and have emphasized increased activity, limit setting, and early confrontation on the therapist's part, at times including individual behavioral contracts. The therapist dealing with delinquents must be a strong, fair authority figure who can be a logical advocate for both the adolescent and the laws of society. Significant countertransferential rage and fear are likely to be aroused in the therapist who is threatened by obscene dialogue, personal attack, and victimization.

Groups for adolescents addicted to alcohol and drugs (Bratter, 1989; Friedman and Glickman, 1986) (as well as groups for delinquents) are among the most difficult. Routinely such children are referred from individual and family therapists as nonworkable. Most of the time it is the law that coerces these addicted and delinquent youth into treatment. Drug and alcohol dependency reinforces their obsessive-compulsive personality characteristics. Prohibiting or limiting the use of drugs and alcohol must be part of the therapeutic contract. The group therapist must be a rational authority who confronts the group members with their self-abusive, at times suicidal, behavior. Unlike traditional approaches, group members are asked to keep in contact with one another and to try to monitor and control one another's "habit," and often the group therapist is committed to being available outside of the group therapy proper. The goal for these adolescents is the building of control and independence to replace impulsive obedience to their addicted cravings. Freedom of choice must replace the repetitive use of the behavior. Bratter (1989) proposes the following four therapeutic factors: (*a*) The group serves as a rational restraining force; (*b*) the group collectively learns how to confront one another's malignant addiction; (*c*) the group becomes a corrective emotional experience, identifying caring responsibility and suggesting viable alternatives; and (*d*) the group becomes a caring community within and outside of the therapy group proper.

Preventive and educational therapy groups are used increasingly, including, for example, goal-oriented groups for sexually abused adolescents (Corder et al., 1990; Furniss et al., 1988) and groups for adult children of abused, alcoholic, addicted, or divorced parents. Both younger and older adolescents who are grandchildren of Holocaust survivors have been seen with or without parents, and as a group they have made pilgrimages to rediscover family roots and the sites of the disaster. Inpatient groups for mothers who have lost a child through abortion, miscarriage, or death allow abreaction, grieving, and sharing of the traumatic loss. Groups for young victims of cancer, diabetes, and thalassemia add to the ever-growing list. In cases where drug regimens or use of needles, a respirator, or other procedures are necessary, conformity with the treatment plan is heightened by the group.

THE GROUP PSYCHOTHERAPIST: FUNCTIONS, REALITY ISSUES, AND COUNTERTRANSFERENCE

Aside from the obvious managerial duties of selecting, composing, and deciding upon time and place, the major focus of the group therapist is to forge a *therapeutic alliance* appropriate to the age level of the patient. It must be made clear to the group that the common goal is the understanding and solving of painful thoughts and behavior. Increasingly patients are being prepared, prior to and in the initial group sessions, to understand the functioning of the mind and the ability to analyze the self and to be responsible to uncover and talk about conflicts hidden in their inner worlds. A parallel task for the therapist is to orient the group members to be aware of their behavior with each other, to share thoughts and feelings, and to offer suggestions about how to deal with these problems.

Functioning in the group context puts greater stress on the therapist, especially with children who act out physically and regress rapidly (Azima, 1986). With adolescents there is the accompanying disrespect and rebellion against authority figures (Azima, 1973). The reports of homogeneous groups for young patients suffering from bulimia, anorexia, diabetes, migraine, thalassemia, and cancer indicate improvement in motivation and compliance with prescribed diets, exercise, and the use of medication.

A leader must solve the quandary of how to be a competent therapist and a respected authority figure, and not an admonishing disciplinarian. The reality is that therapists working with adolescents may suddenly experience eruptions of anger at and fear of some members, as well as showing undue sympathy and overprotectiveness to others. Consider the following examples: A sudden brawl breaks out; a member swears at and insults the therapist; an adolescent produces a gun or a knife; one of the group members breaks into the therapist's car. Should the therapist's disturbed reactions to any of these episodes be classified as countertransferential, or realistic? It is clear that more punitive rage can be activated in the group therapist working with children and adolescents than with adults. Furthermore, the scoffing, belittling attitudes of adolescents often cause narcissistic injury to the doctor's status.

There is general agreement that present-day child and adolescent group therapists have become more actively involved, less permissive, more spontaneous in their play, more confronting, and in general less distant in their relationship with group members. With adolescents, the therapist tries to assume an emotional/cognitive role model midway between the adolescent and the parent. Therapists with overclose identification with adolescents are put at risk of collusion, passivity, or acting out, while therapists with too distant an identification are rendered vulnerable to possible rebellion against parental figures. A good practice with adolescents is to assume an attitude of controlled curiosity and sophisticated ignorance, especially in the early stages of the group. An overintellectual approach on the part of the therapist is likely to produce silence, fear, withdrawal, and withholding in the group members.

Adding to the therapist's countertransference is the pressure from parents for the therapist to see the child from the parents' point of view. The therapist must be realistically empathic and not overjudgmental. Within the clinic or day hospital setting, the therapist is often caught in a tug of war between team members who side with or against the parent, teacher, or judge.

In many cases the therapist's reaction should not be classified as countertransferential unless there is evidence of ongoing behavior patterns that block or are destructive to the group process. Therapists who do not do well with this age group are usually unable to deal with the acting out, overplayfulness, and disregard for the status of authority figures. But it is precisely these defensive resistances that provide the first insight into the group members' problems. Therapists who have been raised in a strict, obedient fashion, with strong moral and ethical standards, may be more vulnerable to the adolescent age group. Fearing loss of control of their own anger, they become overly silent and permissive in their leadership.

Group psychotherapists who do not overcentralize their position are more likely to be perceptive of the interactive psychodynamics and to reflect on the variety of positive and negative feelings and thoughts that corroborate or differ from their own. The interactive interpersonal variations become a therapeutic tool for the therapist and in many instances dilute or eliminate countertransferential responses by clarifying and comparing the responses of other group members.

Some helpful qualities of the group therapist working with children and adolescents include comfort in a group, spontaneity, flexibility, playful creativity, and the ability to set adequate limits as a rational, empathic role model. Continuing clinical research in the area of child and adolescent group psychotherapy will, it is hoped, clarify and identify which therapeutic models are most effective with specified age groups, intelligence levels, and diagnoses.

CONTRAINDICATIONS

The question of contraindications of group psychotherapy for children depends not so much on the diagnoses, symptoms, or deviant behavior, but on the total composition of the group, the competence of the staff, the availability of support staff, and whether the treatment is carried out in residential or outpatient settings.

Special problems and hazards are presented by children who are explosive, cruel and vindictive, sexually acting out, overly autistic, seclusive, and depressed. Children with physical stigmata are often scapegoated. When children are enuretic or encopretic, entry into the group is usually postponed until adequate controls are developed. Children of very low intelligence do poorly in verbal psychotherapeutic groups but profit from socialization, compliance, and support groups. Homogeneous groups in residential treatments report better outcome with retarded and delinquent populations.

Some children entering day hospital programs may initially not be ready or capable of entering a psychotherapy group until they have adequate controls, are capable of listening to others, and are capable of expressing themselves. Younger children must usually be involved in multimodal therapeutic school programs with gradual transition to triadic therapies with another child or parent before group psychotherapy is possible. Short preparatory groups are necessary for children with poor frustration tolerance.

For adolescents, the basic contraindications outlined above also apply. For outpatient treatment of adolescents ages 15–18, contraindications include acute psychosis, heavy medication, drug addiction, and delinquent acting out. Again, it appears that motivation, psychological mindedness, and attraction to the norms of the adolescent peer group are the more critical variables. Additionally, an alliance must be articulated that sets the therapeutic goals for the group.

The selection of the specific therapeutic modality for children and adolescents should be made in a more sequential fashion, considering the developmental stage, the type of problem, and the degree of intrapsychic or interpersonal deficit. It may be that one child may need individual play therapy first, while another requires integration into a group. Additionally, the combination of individual, family, or group becomes realistic only if time and expense are not factors. It is likely that some patients are held in one fixed therapeutic modality too long before another is tried.

RESEARCH

Dies and Riester (1986) and Azima and Dies (1989) have summarized the pitfalls of research in the area of children and adolescents and have underlined the difficulties in instrumentation, statistical methodology, and lack of longitudinal follow-up of outcome studies. The majority of past studies report positive outcome with group psychotherapy from a qualitative, impressionistic point of view. Increasingly, studies are more rigorously planned. Present emphasis is less on the use of control groups and more on the use of contrast groups (i.e., comparing one therapeutic modality with another). Untreated controls are very difficult to find, and keeping children or adolescents on waiting lists is ethically untenable.

Toseland and Siporin (1986) in a thorough review of the literature identified 74 studies comparing individual and group treatment from 1969 to 1985 and concluded that group treatment was more effective than individual treatment in 25% of the cases. Narrowing this sample to 32 well-controlled experimental studies, the authors concluded that group therapy was more effective than individual therapy by 31%. Of this latter group, analysis of their data revealed six child and adolescent studies, four college studies, and two family studies. The findings revealed no statistically significant differences between individual and group treatments. There were indications that schoolchildren with self-control problems did better in group therapy when they were 12 and 13 years old; children with home problems such as noncompliance, tantrums, and fighting did better in family group therapy; adolescents with psychoses showed a trend for greater improvement in group therapy. The overall findings revealed no superiority for individual therapy in any of these studies and that there was an edge for group therapies.

Review of the adolescent research group literature (Azima, in press) indicates that homogeneous groups are specifically advantageous for the difficult patient, drug-addicted or psychosomatic patient, and for patients with eating disorders. Cognitive group therapies have proven particularly useful with depressed patients, and long-term therapies are indicated for the more dysfunctional children and adolescents.

Mitchell et al. (1990) studied eating disorders in 171 females (age range 18–40) and compared the efficacy of antidepressant drug therapy with structural manual-guided group therapy for a total of 12 weeks. The overall finding was that the addition of the antidepressant treatment to the intensive group psychotherapy component did not significantly improve outcome over intensive group psychotherapy combined with placebo treatment in relation to the eating disorder, but did result in greater improvement in the features of depression and anxiety. At 6-month follow-up (Pyle et al., 1990) of the participating 68 subjects of the initial study, 30% had relapsed. Initial treatment with group psychotherapy plus placebo or imipramine was associated with a lower relapse rate than initial treatment with the medication alone. The investigators also noted that neither attendance at the maintenance group sessions nor imipramine maintenance were associated with better outcome.

Fine et al. (1991) reported on the comparison of two forms of short-term group therapy for 66 outpatient adolescents clinically diagnosed as depressed. Subjects were randomly assigned to either a therapeutic support group or a social skills group. Post treatment, adolescents in the therapeutic support group showed greater decrease in depressive symptoms and significant increases in self-concept. At the 9-month follow-up, the adolescents in the therapeutic support groups maintained their improvements, but the adolescents in the social skills group had now caught up in their improvement between the post group and the follow-up assessments. The authors postulated that the original gains made in the therapeutic support group were necessary to alleviate the depression before members were able to profit from the problem-solving strategies taught in the social skills groups.

Increasingly, AIDS patients are being seen in group interpersonal formats. Levine et al. (1991) reported a pilot study of a single group of 6 patients (5 men, 1 woman) between ages 18 and 55 identified as HIV seropositive with major depression, who were being treated with fluoxetine. The group format consisted of 20 sessions combining psychoeducational, supportive, and cognitive orientations. A battery of tests, including scales for depression and anxiety, a symptom checklist, and a modified semistructured evaluation interview, was repeated at outcome for 4 of the patients and showed a decrease in depression, anxiety, and symptoms. The sample of the study is overly small to permit generalization but suggests a good methodology worthy of repetition.

The clinical research study of Furniss et al. (1988) was a case-by-case descriptive, nonstatistical follow-up of 10 sexually abused girls between the ages of 12 and 15 years who attended psychoanalytic-oriented group psychotherapy for 2 years and a follow-up of the progress of 9 girls. Seven of the 9 girls showed improvements in level of self-esteem, overall social adjustment, more positive relationships with peers, and a diminishment in display of sexualized and victim behavior. The girls were more open in their expression of trust, self-assertiveness, and anger and were able to discuss their trauma with parents. The therapy groups with both adolescents and parents were part of a multipronged treatment including individual and family therapy.

Present and future outcome research will likely be easier to carry out with the introduction of more efficient instrumentation, more sophisticated statistical methodology, and a concentration on short-term group modalities. The efficacy of outcome is now considered not only in terms of self-esteem, pleasure, and improvement in functioning in the home, school, and work, but also in terms of cost of the delivery of mental health care. Here group therapy has the advantage in that more children can be treated at less cost. It is clear that the research results support group therapy effectiveness, and children and adolescents are decidedly excellent candidates for this interpersonal treatment modality.

References

Anthony EJ: Group-analytic psychotherapy with children and adolescents. In: Foulkes SH, Anthony EJ (eds): *Group Psychotherapy*. Baltimore, Penguin Books, 1965, pp. 186–232.

Azima FJC: Transference-countertransference in adolescent group psychotherapy. In: Brandes NS, Gardner ML (eds): *Group Therapy for the Adolescent*. New York, Jason Aronson, 1973, pp. 101–126.

Azima FJC: Group therapy for latency children. *Can Psychiatry Assoc J* 21:210–212, 1977.

Azima FJC: Communication in adolescent group psychotherapy. In: Pines M, Rafelson L (eds): *The Individual and the Group*. New York, Plenum, 1982, pp. 133–145.

Azima FJC: Countertransference: In and beyond child group psychotherapy. In: Riester AE, Kratt IA (eds): *Child Group Psychotherapy, Future Tense*. Madison, CT, International Universities Press, 1986, pp. 139–155.

Azima FJC: Confrontation, empathy and interpretation issues in adolescent group psychotherapy. In: Azima FJC, Richmond LH (eds): *Adolescent Group Psychotherapy*. Madison, CT, International Universities Press, 1989, pp. 3–19.

Azima FJC: Adolescent group treatment. In: Harper-Guiffre H, MacKenzie KR (eds): *Group Psychotherapy for Eating Disorders*. Washington, DC, American Psychiatric Press, 1992, pp. 233–247.

Azima FJC: The status of adolescent group psychotherapy research. In: Kymissis P, Halperin D (eds): *Group Therapy with Children and Adolescents*. Washington, DC, American Psychiatric Press, in press.

Azima FJC, Dies KR: Clinical research in adolescent group psychotherapy: Status, guidelines and directions. In: Azima FJC, Richmond LH (eds): *Adolescent Group Psychotherapy*. Madison, CT, International Universities Press, 1989, pp. 193–223.

Berkowitz IH: Application of group therapy in secondary schools. In: Azima FJC, Richmond LH (eds): *Adolescent Group Psychotherapy*. Madison, CT, International Universities Press, 1989, pp. 99–123.

Bogdaniak RC, Piercy FP: Therapeutic issues of adolescent children of alcoholics (ADCA) groups. *Int J Group Psychother* 37:569, 1987.

Bratter TE: Group psychotherapy with alcoholically and drug addicted adolescents. In: Azima FJC, Richmond LH (eds): *Adolescent Group Psychotherapy*. Madison, CT, International Universities Press, 1989.

Charach R: Brief interpretive group psychotherapy with early latency age children. *Int J Group Psychother* 33:349–364, 1983.

Chase JL: Inpatient adolescent and latency age children's perspectives on the curative factors in group psychotherapy. *Group* 15:95–99, 1991.

Clark R, Keller A, Fedderly S, et al: Treating the relationships affected by postpartum depression: A group therapy model. *Two to Three, National Center for Clinical Infant Programs* 13:16–23, 1993.

Coché JM, Fisher JM: Group psychotherapy with learning disabled adolescents. In: Azima FJC, Richmond LH (eds): *Adolescent Group Psychotherapy*. Madison, CT, International Universities Press, 1989, pp. 125–135.

Corder BF, Haizlip T, DeBaer P: A pilot study for a structured time-limited therapy group for sexually abused pre-adolescent children. *Child Abuse Neglect* 14:243–257, 1990.

Cox E, Lothstein LM: Video self portraits: A novel approach to group psychotherapy with young adults. *Int J Group Psychother* 39:237–253, 1989.

Crawford-Brobyn J, White A: A two-stage model for group therapy with impulse ridden latency age children. In: Riester AE, Krait IA (eds): *Child Group Psychotherapy, Future Tense*. Madison, CT, International Universities Press, 1986, pp. 123–135.

Cunningham JM, Matthews KL: Impact of multiple-family therapy approach on a parallel latency age/parent group. *Int J Group Psychother* 32:91, 1982.

Davis L, Geikie F, Schamess G: The use of genograms in a group for latency age children. *Int J Group Psychother* 38:189, 1988.

Dies RR, Riester AE: Research in child group therapy: Present status and future directions. In: Riester AE, Kraft IA (eds): *Child Group Psychotherapy, Future Tense*. Madison, CT, International Universities Press, 1986, pp. 173–220.

Epstein N: Techniques of brief group therapy with children and parents. *Soc Casework* 56: 317–323, 1976.

Epstein YM, Bordiun CM: Could this happen? A game for children of divorce. *Psychother Theory Res Pract* 22:770–773, 1985.

Fine S, Forth A, Gilbert M, et al: Group therapy for adolescent depressive disorder. A comparison of social skills and therapeutic support. *J Am Acad Child Adolesc Psychiatry* 30:79–85, 1991.

Frank M: Modified activity group therapy with ego impoverished children. In: Buchholz ES, Mishne JM (eds): *Ego and Self Psychology*. New York, Jason Aronson, 1983, pp. 145–156.

Friedman AS, Glickman NW: Program characteristics for successful treatment of adolescent drug abuse. *J Nerv Ment Dis* 174:669–679, 1986.

Furniss T, Bingley-Mitler L, Van Elburg A: Goal oriented group treatment for sexually abused adolescent girls. *Br J Psychiatry* 152:97–106, 1988.

Gaines T: Applications of child group psychotherapy. In: Riester AE, Kraft IA (eds): *Child Group Psychotherapy, Future Tense*. Madison, CT, International Universities Press, 1986, pp. 103–121.

Garland JA: The establishment of individual and collective competency in children's groups as a prelude to entry into intimacy, disclosure, and bonding. *Int J Group Psychother* 42:395–405, 1992.

Ginnott H: *Group Psychotherapy with Children: The Theory and Practice of Play Therapy*. New York, McGraw-Hill, 1961.

Gordon R: Symbioses in the group: Group therapy for younger adolescents. In: Azima FJC, Richmond LH (eds): *Adolescent Group Psychotherapy*. Madison, CT, International Universities Press, 1986, pp. 43–51.

Grant W: Support groups for youth with the AIDS virus. *Int J Group Psychother* 38:237–251, 1988.

Green A: Psychiatric treatment of abused children. *J Am Acad Child Psychiatry* 17:356–371, 1978.

Grunebaum H, Solomon L: Peer relationships, self esteem and the self. *Int J Group Psychother* 37:475–573, 1987.

Hoffman TE, Byrne KM, Belnap KL, et al: Simultaneous semipermeable groups for mothers and their early latency-aged boys. *Int J Group Psychother* 31:83–98, 1981.

Kennedy JK: Therapist gender and the same-sex puberty age psychotherapy group. *Int J Group Psychother* 39:255–263, 1989.

Kraft IA: Innovative and creative approaches in child group psychotherapy. In: Riester AE, Kralt IA (eds): *Child Group Psychotherapy, Future Tense*. Madison, CT, International Universities Press, 1986, pp. 263–272.

Levine SH, Bystristky A, Baron D, et al: Group psychotherapy for HIV seropositive patients with major depression. *Am J Psychother* XLV:413–424, 1991.

Liebowitz JH, Kernberg PF: Diagnostic play groups for children: Their role in assessment and treatment planning. In: Riester AE, Kraft IA (eds): *Child Group Psychotherapy, Future Tense*. Madison, CT, International Universities Press, 1986, pp. 71–79.

Mallery B, Novas M: Engagement of preadolescent boys in group therapy: Videotape as a tool. *Int J Group Psychother* 32:453–467, 1982.

Mara B, Winton M: Sexual abuse intervention: A support group for parents who have a sexually abused child. *Int J Group Psychother* 40:63–78, 1990.

Mitchell JE, Pyle RL, Eckert ED, et al: Anti depressants vs group therapy in the treatment of bulimia. *Arch Gen Psychiatry* 47:149–157, 1990.

Parmenter F, Smith JC, Cecic BA: Parallel and conjoint short-term group therapy for school-age children and their parents: A model. *Int J Group Psychother* 37:239–254, 1987.

Pasnau RO, Meyer M, Davis LJ, et al: Coordinated group psychotherapy of children and parents. *Int J Group Psychother* 26:89–103, 1976.

Peled E, Edelson JL: Multiple perspectives in group work with children of battered women. *Violence Vict* 7:327–346, 1992.

Pfeifer G: Complementary cultures in children's psychotherapy groups: Conflict, coexistence, and convergence in group development. *Int J Group Psychother* 42:357–367, 1992.

Phillips RG: Whistling in the dark? A review of play therapy research. *Psychother Theory Res Pract* 22:752–760, 1985.

Pyle RL, Mitchell JE, Eckert ED, et al: Maintenance treatment and 6 month outcome for bulimia patients who respond to initial treatment. *Am J Psychiatry* 147:871–875, 1990.

Rachman AW: Identity group psychotherapy with adolescents: A reformulation. In: Azima FJC, Richmond LH (eds): *Adolescent Group Psychotherapy*. Madison, CT, International Universities Press, 1989, pp. 21–41.

Raubolt RR: The clinical practice of group psychotherapy with delinquents. In: Azima FJC, Richmond LH (eds): *Adolescent Group Psychotherapy*. Madison, CT, International Universities Press, 1989, pp. 143–162.

Richmond LH: A case presentation of a borderline adolescent in long-term psychotherapy. In: Azima FJC, Richmond LH (eds): *Adolescent Group Psychotherapy*. Madison, CT, International Universities Press, 1989, pp. 85–96.

Schacht A, Kerlinsky D, Carlson C: Group therapy with sexually abused boys: Leadership, projective identification and countertransference issues. *Int J Group Psychother* 40:401–418, 1990.

Schachter RS: Kinetic psychotherapy in the treatment of depression in latency age children. *Int J Group Psychother* 34:83–91, 1984.

Schamess F: Differential diagnosis and group structure in the outpatient treatment of latency age children. In: Riester AE, Kraft IA (eds): *Child Group Psychotherapy, Future Tense*. Madison, CT, International Universities Press, 1986, pp. 29–68.

Scheidlinger S: Short-term group psychotherapy for children: An overview. *Int J Group Psychother* 34:573–585, 1984.

Schiffer M: Activity-interview group psychotherapy: Theory, principles and practice. *Int J Group Psychother* 3:377–388, 1977.

Slavson SR: *Child Psychotherapy*. New York, Columbia University Press, 1952.

Smith JD, Walsh RT, Gavin MA: The clown club, a structured fantasy approach to group therapy with latency age children. *Int J Group Psychother* 35:27–33, 1985.

Speers RW, Lansing C: *Group Therapy in Childhood Psychosis*. Chapel Hill, NC, University of North Carolina Press, 1965.

Spinner D: The evolution of culture and cohesion in the group treatment of ego impaired children. *Int J Group Psychother* 42:369–381, 1992.

Stein MD, Kymisses P: Adolescent in-patient group psychotherapy. In: Azima FJC, Richmond LH (eds): *Adolescent Group Psychotherapy*. Madison, CT, International Universities Press, 1989, pp. 69–84.

Stengel BE: Developmental group therapy with autistic and other severely psychosocially handicapped adolescents. *Int J Group Psychother* 37:417–431, 1987.

Sugar M: Interpretive group psychotherapy with latency children. *J Am Acad Child Psychiatry* 13:648–666, 1974.

Sullivan HS: *The Interpersonal Theory of Psychiatry*. New York, Norton, 1953.

Toseland RW, Siporin M: When to recommend group treatment: A review of the clinical and the research literature. *Int J Group Psychother* 36:171–201, 1986.

Trad PV: Mother-infant psychotherapy: Integrating techniques of group, family and individual therapy. *Int J Group Psychother* 44:53–78, 1994.

Vardi DJ, Bucholz ES: Group psychotherapy with inner-city grandmothers raising their grandchildren. *Int J Group Psychother* 44:101–122, 1994.

Winnicott DW: *Playing and Reality*. London, Tavistock Publications, 1971.

78 FAMILY THERAPY

Kent Ravenscroft, M.D.

Evolving separately from psychiatry for several decades, family therapy has begun to reconverge because of new research and clinical trends in both areas. Child and adolescent psychiatry has recently rejoined this process after early forays.

The family therapy movement itself, though characterized by a wide diversity of theories, techniques, and partisan politics, collectively took a radically environmentalist point of view for several decades, emphasizing an interpersonal holistic "systems approach" to dysfunction and treatment. In essence, most family therapists embarked on the attempt to change the person exclusively through changing the family system, rather than changing the person and secondarily the family—avoiding for "systemic" reasons what they felt were diverting issues of individual biological differences, diagnostic classification, and differential therapeutics.

Though some leaders are currently moving further along these lines (a "new epistemology," theories of "system coevolution" and "ecosystemic approaches"), others are rediscovering the individuality of both family members and therapists, their private feelings and internal worlds, personal and family developmental history, and genetic biological contributions, weaving these deeply relevant areas into the mainstream of the "new systems thinking." This tentative new openness among family therapy schools is also facilitating cross-fertilization with other fields, especially medicine.

Until recently, however, most child and adolescent psychiatrists have felt disinclined to explore and integrate family therapy into their overall clinical approach because of these tensions and antipathies—given the positions taken historically by family therapy. This reaction has been heightened by the perception that family therapy is still of questionable value.

All this is changing, however, because of the establishment of clear and convincing evidence of the efficacy of family treatment and the emergence of the promising new biopsychosocial climate within the family therapy movement. Let us review these developments.

HISTORY OF FAMILY THERAPY

Psychoanalytic Roots: Evolution

The roots of family therapy in America go back to the early 1900s, nourished in practice by the emergence of the Child Guidance Movement (1909), orthopsychiatry, and marriage counseling. Psychoanalysis captured the imagination of psychiatry during this period, creating the ideal of separate confidential individual treatment. Yet Freud, with his brilliant discovery of the unconscious and depth psychology, pointed out the interplay of dyadic and triadic family influences on intrapsychic development. Johnson and Szurek observed the relationship between parental dysfunction and a delinquent's defective conscience (superego lacunae). Frieda Fromm-Reichman was exploring unidirectional dyadic maternal effects on schizophrenic offspring (the schizophrenogenic mother), following a linear causality model. At the same time in England, psychoanalytic object relations theory was being developed by Klein, Fairbairn, Guntrip, Bowlby, and Winnicott.

Radical Environmentalism: Revolution

While these evolutionary bridges between the human internal and external worlds were being built, a new radical environmentalist revolution was gathering momentum, predominantly during the post-World War II era. Social and interpersonal processes were being emphasized, including systems theory, circular causality, and teleological mechanisms, concepts that were to revolutionize family therapy theory and technique.

Pioneers of Family Therapy

Nathan Ackerman, a child psychiatrist and analyst trained at Menninger's Foundation in Topeka, was perhaps the first pioneer. Integrating analytic principles and a sense that individual dynamics and symptoms arose from similar parallel processes in parents, he worked actively with the whole family, often "tickling their defenses" as a diagnostic technique. Because of his influential position in established psychiatric circles, he did much to win acceptance for family therapy, and in 1960 he founded what is now called the Ackerman Family Institute in New York.

In other ways *Carl Whitaker* most typified such pioneers. In 1946 his early interest in families, spouses, and children shifted to schizophrenia, though he also initiated research on conjoint marital therapy. Whitaker, known for his freewheeling style and creative leadership, has encouraged use of countertransference and inclusion of all family members from grandparents to children. He is the founder of the *experiential family therapy school*. Ahistorical and antitheoretical, experiential family therapy emphasizes feeling-expression and promotes self-actualization. Though still vital in the hands of Whitaker and others, such as Virginia Satir, Walter Kempler, and Fred and Bunny Duhl, it has proven too amorphous and eclectic to teach easily in institutional settings.

During the early 1950s, the biological revolution in psychiatry had not begun, leaving the field desperate for effective new treatments for schizophrenia and other major mental illness. In Palo Alto, *Gregory Bateson* in 1952 arranged for *Jay Haley's* momentous work with Milton Erickson, the famous hypnotherapist who pioneered clinical work with special communications and paradoxical techniques. These ideas and approaches contributed substantially to the Palo Alto group's Schizophrenia Project and the development of *communications therapy*, which later became the basis for Haley's *strategic therapy*.

In 1953 Bateson recruited Don Jackson to Palo Alto. Jackson was already writing about schizophrenic family homeostatic mechanisms and completed Bateson's research team, which soon produced the world-famous paper "Toward a Theory of Schizophrenia" (Bateson et al., 1956). They hypothesized that a special form of communication deviance seen in schizophrenic families called the *double bind* was causing schizophrenia in offspring. Jackson, a strong proponent of conjoint family therapy and fresh from intense immersion with schizophrenics and their families at Chestnut Lodge, provided the actual clinical experience for what was primarily a theoretical research hypothesis. Only later did the group attempt to research it.

Based on the revolutionary communications family therapy model, Jackson established the Mental Research Institute in 1958, with Jules Riskin, Virginia Satir, and later Jay Haley, John Weakland, and Paul Watzlawick as staff. Satir was an important charismatic member of this group before moving on to develop her own family approaches. Later, Haley left to join Salvador Minuchin, founder of structural family therapy.

Structural family therapy was developed by *Salvador Minuchin* based on his innovative work with poor, multiproblem families during the early 1960s (Minuchin, 1974; Broderick and Schrader, 1991). Although he was not among the first wave of family theorists, who mainly saw middle-class patients, his brilliant and effective approach to this difficult population soon captured the attention of the field. As Director of the Philadelphia Child Guidance Clinic in 1965, he developed his world-famous training program with colleagues such as Montalvo, Haley, Rosman, Aponte, Walters, and Greenstein. Structural family therapy is now perhaps the most practiced and influential form of family therapy.

In 1951, *John Bell*, another family pioneer working at Clark University, was visiting John Sutherland, then Director of the Tavistock Clinic, who mentioned in passing that John Bowlby was beginning to see the families of his child cases (Broderick and Schrader, 1981). Intrigued by this idea, Bell began seeing families in an ongoing fashion. His method was predominantly *family group analytic therapy*, which is described in his book *Family Group Therapy* (Bell, 1961). Other significant family therapists using group analytic approaches, at least in part, were Rudolf Dreikurs, Christian Midlefort, John Foulkes, Wilfred Bion, Pierre Tourquet, and Robin Skynner. Group theory had a more dominant influence outside the United States. Only with the recent emergence of the Object Relations Family Therapy school have modern advances in group analytic thinking been reintroduced into the mainstream of the family therapy movement in England and the United States.

Theodore Lidz, trained at Hopkins in the 1940s, went to Yale in 1951 to continue his research interest in hospitalized schizophrenics. With Stephen Fleck, he developed the concepts of marital schism (overt marital distance and hostility) and skew (covert accommodation to a dysfunctional partner), and was particularly interested in intergenerational boundaries.

In 1952, *Lyman Wynne* went to the National Institute of Mental Health (NIMH) and began to develop the ideas of Talcott Parson and Lindemann through work with schizophrenics and their families (Broderick and Schrader, 1991). He was particularly interested in communication deviance in these families as a possible cause of schizophrenia. In collaboration with Margaret Singer and others, his famous Schizophrenia Project at NIMH yielded many creative family concepts such as the rubber fence, pseudomutuality, and pseudohostility. He attracted and facilitated many prominent family researchers, such as David Reiss (now Director, Family Research Center, George Washington University), Irving Ryckoff, Roger Shapiro, and John Zinner (Object Relations Family Therapy, Washington School of Psychiatry), and Helm Stierlin (Director, Family Therapy Research, Heidelberg).

Murray Bowen, trained in child psychiatry and psychoanalysis at the Menninger Clinic like Ackerman, became interested in 1951 in hospitalizing parents, especially mothers, with their schizophrenic children, much as Christian Midlefort had done in the late 1940s (Broderick and

Schrader, 1991). In 1954 Bowen came to NIMH, joining Wynne, to continue his conjoint parent hospitalization project, where he developed many of his seminal concepts, including parental triangulation of schizophrenic offspring as a transactional means of binding dyadic interpersonal tension. He hypothesized that multigenerational transmission of such tendencies might cause schizophrenia in a powerfully scapegoated child. Moving to Georgetown Medical School in 1959, he continued an immensely productive and influential career, developing a school of family treatment called *family systems therapy*.

In 1957, *Ivan Boszormenyi-Nagy*, an analyst with an interest in schizophrenia, families, and intergenerational loyalties, founded the Eastern Pennsylvania Psychiatric Institute, a major center for research and training in family therapy, and also the school of *contextual family therapy* (Broderick and Schrader, 1991).

DISILLUSIONMENT AND DIVERSIFICATION

As the schizophrenia research results gradually proved inconclusive or dubious, the initial excitement over the possibility of family approaches leading to a cure for schizophrenia diminished. At the same time, the explosion of family theories and techniques proved to be immensely rich and promising for families suffering from less biologically based dysfunction, leading to a crescendo of multidisciplinary interest and a proliferation of schools and training centers.

During the 1960s, as the biological revolution in psychiatry was well under way, family therapy continued to develop out of the mainstream of psychiatry and child psychiatry. Within this separatist climate, various positions were taken by the leading family proponents, based partly on systems theory and partly on old or new biases, including attitudes "anti-" the following: medical model, designated patient, individual symptoms; differential diagnosis and differential therapeutics; and individual therapy, especially psychoanalysis.

The ideal was pure family therapy on an outpatient basis without medication, adjunctive therapy, or other associated treatment programs—thought to maximize therapeutic leverage through a systems approach. Ignoring both individual interior mind-body subsystems and wider extended family and social ecosystems, this bordered on a remarkably narrow, even unsystemic, view surprisingly similar to that criticized in psychoanalysis at the other extreme.

In the late 1970s, 1980s, and early 1990s, along with major advances in psychiatry in general—and biological psychiatry in particular—family therapy research and practice has matured, with increasing signs of consolidation, integration, and rapprochement—both among schools of family therapy and between family therapy, psychiatry, and medicine in general. Major indicators of this are the development of differentially indicated specialized family therapy approaches for specific individual psychiatric and psychophysiologic illnesses, particular child and adolescent disorders, and specific family dysfunctions. Examples of this are family treatments for schizophrenia, manic-depressive illness, panic disorder, alcoholism, anorexia nervosa, bulimia, asthma, diabetes, delinquency, drug abuse, and conduct disorder.

While these approaches admittedly are not curative, they promote recovery from specific episodes and reduce recidivism, and even result in improvement among siblings in delinquency and conduct disorder. These represent more modest but specifiable outcomes as family therapy comes of age. The growing interest in family aspects of physical health (Wynne et al., 1992) and collaboration with the medical field are illustrated by the California Family Health Project (Fisher et al., 1993) and the relatively new journal, *Family Systems Medicine*.

Currently, in what is now called the "postmodern era" of family therapy (Anderson and Goolishian, 1990; Derrida, 1978; Foucault, 1988; Goldner, 1991) there are strong trends away from the cybernetic-biologic (Maturana and Varela, 1980) and strategic-instrumental approaches, towards a more gender-sensitive, feminist, second-order, social constructivist approach (Goolishian and Anderson, 1992)—one more collaborative and less concealed. This approach, more self-reflective and responsive to individual differences, follows a narrative paradigm using "therapeutic conversations" to understand every family member's and the therapist's relative perspective in a shared, not hierarchical, process of "transforming" the family's "story"—"recontextualizing" their way of perceiving and functioning.

Systemic schools of family therapy, though not discussing the "unconscious" per se, are in the process of a creative rediscovery of "internal maps," "internalized living history," the impact of development on current functioning, and the way family history may be embedded in the living relationship structures of the extended family, broadening their domains of interest in ways that converge on object relations family and couples therapy.

SELECTED SCHOOLS OF FAMILY THERAPY

Behavioral Approaches to Family Therapy

THE PARENT-TRAINING MODEL

Based on the assumption that child behavior is primarily a function of naturally occurring environmental contingencies (positive and negative reinforcement and punishment), behavioral approaches to family therapy developed initially within a *parent-training model* since the mid-1960s. Parents were thought to have parenting-skill deficits affecting the child's acquisition of prosocial skills in an adverse linear unidirectional fashion leading to escalation and maintenance of oppositional aggressive child behavior (Griest and Wells, 1983; Ollendick and Cerney, 1981; Patterson, 1982). According to Wells (1988), parent-training focused almost exclusively on teaching new skills for managing positive and negative child behavior by altering empirically identified inappropriate positive and negative parent behavior (Wells and Forehand, 1981). First providing a rationale to the parent for the use of each skill, the therapist defines the skill using examples and then models the skill. With the therapist acting the part of the child, the parent then practices each skill. Finally, under direct therapist supervision, the parent practices with the child, with specific homework assignments given between sessions (Wells and Forehand, 1985).

BEHAVIORAL FAMILY THERAPY

Even with overall positive outcome results for parent-training, several observations (treatment relapses, need for "booster sessions," or adjunctive interventions to retain gains) suggested the unidirectional parent-training model alone may not represent a complete enough approach for certain families with aggressive and oppositional children. Griest and Wells (1983) proposed an expanded behavioral family therapy model. Parental maladjustment is assessed before parent-training techniques are begun. When significant evidence of parental depression, anxiety, marital maladjustment, and social insularity are found, behavioral and cognitive-behavioral interventions are added to address these specific problem areas within the context of family or parent meetings.

FUNCTIONAL FAMILY THERAPY

An extension and integration of behavioral psychology and systems theory, *functional family therapy* was developed by *Alexander, Barton*, and colleagues at the University of Utah (Barton and Alexander, 1981). Assuming that the meaning of all behavior derives from the family context (systemic view) and that it is ultimately adaptive as an interpersonal outcome (behavioral view), functional family therapists see presenting symptoms as partially maladaptive yet legitimate and adaptive in their overall functional significance. Problem behaviors arise when they are the most currently available means to attain interpersonal functions or outcomes. When a subsystem and/or the family as a whole do not recognize and adapt well to the changing interpersonal outcomes sought by members over the course of the family life cycle, then problems and sometimes symptoms arise (Wells, 1988).

The functional family therapist first must assess the interpersonal outcomes of particular problematic behavioral sequences and then select and implement treatment strategies that maintain that interpersonal outcome in a more efficient less disruptive way. The therapist intervenes in two phases: a therapeutic and an educational phase.

During the "therapy" phase, the therapist helps the family relabel maladaptive person-specific definitions of problems into more functional relational terms by making relationship-oriented comments ("so you each have ways of walking out on each other rather then sticking with the problem") rather than content-oriented observations ("so you disagree on whether to have an allowance at all"). To reduce anger and defensiveness and create a new value or affect toward the behavior, the therapist provides new developmentally oriented and relationship-oriented optimistic labels that "relevance" behavior (redefining a 7-year-old's naughty lying as his immature way of getting things when feeling unheard by anxious conflicted parents), decreasing resistance and increasing interpersonal motivation for change (Barton and Alexander, 1981; Wells, 1988).

> During the "educational" phase, the therapist chooses systemically consistent behavioral strategies that provide the desired interpersonal goals for everyone in the family system but through more adaptive means, rebalancing interpersonal distance and closeness, for instance, arranging for the overburdened exasperated parents of the lonely, ignored, lying 7-year-old to provide him with short periods of dedicated quality time and one reasonable "wish" in exchange for more truthful cooperation and supervised independent activity at other times. Behavioral techniques such as contracting and modeling may be coupled with paradoxical reframing interventions.

Deriving from the behavioral-systems family therapy model, functional family therapy has received impressive empirical research support for its use with conduct-disordered delinquent adolescents, improving behavior and recidivism for both delinquent patients and their siblings. Since this population is notoriously difficult to treat, Wells (1988) feels that the results obtained by Alexander and his colleagues lend strong support to the use of this approach with other populations.

Systemic Approaches to Family Therapy

Representing a radical departure from linear theories of causation, systemic approaches to family therapy are based on cybernetics and general systems theory, introducing the concept of circular or reciprocal causality. Cybernetics theory holds that systems, including families, tend to maintain their equilibrium. According to general systems theory, living systems are characterized by a dynamic tension between homeostasis and change—balancing stability and self-preservation with change and adaptation. In families, symptoms are seen as often preserving family homeostasis. Disturbances in families result from overly rigid, homeostatic mechanisms taking precedence over flexible adaptive ones. During the family life cycle (Carter and McGoldrick, 1988; Ravenscroft, 1974), physical, emotional, and social development on any level within the family, as well as situational events, may disturb the family equilibrium, resulting in healthy growth and adjustment or maladaptive group reactions, individual symptoms, and dysfunction. Children and parents in dysfunctional families become caught up in a reciprocal spiral of interactions, mutually distorting each other's respective interlocking developmental life cycle phases (Combrinck-Graham, 1985; Stierlin and Ravenscroft, 1972).

STRATEGIC AND STRUCTURAL FAMILY THERAPY

Two of the major schools of family therapy—strategic and structural family therapy—are elegantly representative of the systemic approach and are conveniently described together, for both historical and technical reasons. Strategic family therapy is associated with several prominent practitioners, including Haley and Cloe Madanes of the Family Therapy Institute of Washington, D.C.; Selvini-Palazzoli and her associates at the Milan Family Studies Center; John Weakland and Paul Watzlawick

of the Mental Research Institute of Palo Alto; and Peggy Papp, Lynn Hoffman, and their associates at the Ackerman Institute of Family Therapy in New York. Structural family therapy is associated with Minuchin and his Philadelphia Child Guidance Center group. Because of the time Haley spent with Minuchin, his creative and constantly evolving approach to strategic family therapy converges most with the structural approach.

Strategic and structural family therapy share a common focus on observable as well as reported family behavior sequences as the underlying basis for analysis of symptoms and dysfunction in children, parents, and families. At the same time, these approaches differ in several distinctive ways.

Derived from communications therapy with its roots in Ericksonian therapy, cybernetics, and systems theory, strategic therapy takes a systemic (circular causality) view of problem-maintenance and a planned or strategic orientation to change. Interventions are based on deciphering family communication "rules" (metacommunication) underlying the behavior sequences that support the problems. Interventions are implemented through directives ("straight" or "paradoxical"), which interdict these rules, interrupting these repetitive interpersonal patterns. With no interest in insight, this approach circumvents resistance through these directives, which often seem illogical to the family (i.e., actually "prescribing" the symptom or the resistance) because they run counter to the family's usual self-defeating (homeostatic) attempts at problem solving (Nichols, 1984).

Structural family therapy takes the position that problems are the result of dysfunctional family structures that become evident only when the whole family is seen in action by the therapist. Family structure, its assessment, and interventions are based on an analysis of family subsystems, boundaries, alignments, and power. Subsystems are units of the family based on function, including the grandparental, marital-parental, and sibling subsystems. If a chronic rigid misalignment or cross-generational power coalition occurs between grandmother and son against daughter-in-law, this becomes a dysfunctional subsystem and results in problems for the marriage and often the children. In normal families, boundaries are firm enough to protect the autonomy and separateness of subsystems and individuals but permeable enough to insure mutual rapport, affection, and support. Enmeshed families have diffuse boundaries; disengaged families have very rigid boundaries. The goal of structural family therapy is to distinguish dysfunctional from functional family structures and then intervene by specific techniques to mend these dysfunctional subsystems, boundaries, and alignments—reestablishing a healthy family hierarchical structure.

Comparing strategic and structural therapy, then, strategic family therapy has a primary emphasis on the presenting problem and on the in-session family descriptions of behavior sequences maintaining it. A careful history of the presenting problem and how the family dealt with it then complete the assessment picture. Rather than intervening within sessions, strategic therapists use change-inducing directives and tasks assigned to be carried out at home between sessions that are carefully designed to alter these dysfunctional behavior sequences (Goldner, 1987).

Structural family therapy, on the other hand, focuses more on the structural problems underlying both the repetitive behavior sequences and the presenting problem and emphasizes in-session intervention techniques aimed at directly creating indicated structural changes in family relationships. With less historical interest in what goes on at home or descriptions of the presenting problem, the structural therapist encourages family enactments of the problem within the session in order to directly observe, assess, and intervene.

Four stages characterize the initial interview and highlight similarities and differences of techniques (Goldner, 1987): a *social stage*, a *problem stage*, an *interaction stage*, and a *goal-setting or intervention stage*. After the initial informal introductory *social phase* in which each adult and child is greeted on his or her level and put at ease (with seating choice and interaction noted), the therapist then moves into a more formally conducted *problem stage*. Talking first with the parents to acknowledge and support their hierarchical leadership position, the therapist explores the problem with each member, often leaving the problem child until last to convey impartiality and help put him or her at ease. Strategic therapists use an accepting circular process of inquiry, perfected by Selvini-Palazzoli's Milan Associates (Penn, 1982), to win confidence and obtain an intimate multiperspective history of the problem and its management. Structural therapists use specific joining techniques (systems maintenance, tracking, and mimesis) (Minuchin and Fishman, 1981) to win entry and acceptance.

During the interaction phase of the interview, various family patterns of coalition, boundary violation, facilitation, interruption, and disagreement are observed as the presenting problem is explored. Moving from social director to observer at this point, the strategic therapist encourages discussion while the structural therapist promotes an observable enactment or spontaneous behavior sequence demonstrating the problem.

> In the case of the lying 7-year-old, as the parents describe the problem with frustration and irritation, the therapist explores how the family has coped with it, while noting: that maternal grandmother cuts father off and sides with mother as they attempt to discuss what to do. Unnoticed in a corner, the 7-year-old and his little sister begin to squabble over a toy—suddenly drawing everyone's attention from the adult argument. When asked what happened, the boy says his sister took his toy; she protests she had it first. The women are noted to side with the daughter, the father with the son, though he soon backs away when confronted by wife and grandmother.
> Bringing this sequence to the family's attention, the structural therapist would move in directly during the session to shore up boundaries (mending cross-generational coalitions), helping grandmother to support her daughter's parenting and marriage by asking her not to interfere with their discussion, and helping the parents to remain united by not becoming split and aligned with different children—thus reestablishing the trigenerational structural hierarchy. Homework might be given such as observing any boundary violations and practicing boundary maintenance. The strategic therapist would wonder with grandmother and parents if this is what happens at home and then move into the goal-setting and prescription phase, perhaps giving the family paradoxical directives (prescribing the resistance) such as telling the grandmother to interfere sooner and more effectively to protect her daughter from a marital dispute, and the parents to side with the kids right away for the same reason. The children would be asked to practice lying and fighting at the first sign of parental disagreement over discipline to keep the parents from fighting directly.

Prescribing the covert function of these boundary and subsystem violations renders them explicit and voluntary. If the family complies with the therapist, they are brought under conscious control. If they resist and refrain, the dysfunctional structure changes and the problem resolves. The Haley group, and especially Selvini-Palazzoli's Milan Associates, make use of one-way mirror and team observation, advising or meeting with the therapist during the session to formulate verbal or written interventions. The Milan Associates have been particularly noted for disarming family resistance through the use of positive connotation (Selvini-Palazzoli et al., 1980)—a deeply empathic and respectful approach to each family member's personal (though reciprocally interlocked) point of view as part of their family formulations. The Milan group has, more recently, deemphasized positive connotation, emotional detachment from clients, neutrality, paradoxes, and the notion of "brief" therapy (Selvini, 1991), while stressing the importance of observer-family teamwork and mutual hypothesizing involving the whole family in order to understand and change symptomatic behavior.

EXTENDED FAMILY THERAPY

Because of their systemic emphasis on extended family and social networks, the family approaches of Bowen (family systems therapy), Laqueur (multiple family therapy), and Speck (network therapy) are considered together here (Nichols, 1984). A family presenting with an identified patient or child-centered problem is refocused onto adult, multigenerational family, and social support systems. Intergenerational processes within the wider kinship and social network are the theoretical and technical focus rather than exclusively within the immediate nuclear family.

A dominant influence in family therapy since the 1950s, Murray Bowen's continuing influence stems from his innovative and comprehensive system of family theory and technique, first developed at NIMH (1954–1959) and later at Georgetown Medical School (1959–present), in conjunction with Guerin, Fogarty, Kerr, Beal, Lorio, and Paddock. Except for Laqueur and Speck, Bowen has trained most extended family therapists.

Bowen's central idea is that, before one can differentiate one's self into a mature healthy personality, unresolved emotional attachments to one's family must be worked out rather than reactively rejected or passively accepted. Six interrelated concepts make up the core of Bowen's theory (Bowen, 1976; Nichols, 1984): emotional triangles, differentiation of self, nuclear family emotional system, family projection process, multigenerational projection system, and influence of sibling position.

When conflict exists between two people, often a third person is brought in ("triangled in") to defuse the tension. Since triangles are stabilizing and yet often insufficiently stabilizing, these old triangles are discarded in favor of new people being triangled in. In a family with a great deal of tension and a significant tendency toward emotional rejection or cutoffs, the available family members for triangulation will eventually be exhausted and the family will triangle-in outsiders—children, teenagers, a friend or colleague, a minister, or, hopefully at some point, a therapist.

Originally, fusion or lack of separation and independence, coming from past generations to the grandparents (multigenerational projection system), is transmitted to parents and then projected into the children (family projection process). In successive generations of a family, Bowen feels that the child least involved in a family process of fusion (undifferentiation) moves toward a higher level of self-differentiation, while the child most involved in the family's fusion moves to a lower level of differentiation, sometimes becoming mentally ill. Parents are not to blame for this, nor is the child, since the problem is the result of a multigenerational transmission process in which everyone is reciprocally involved (Nichols, 1984). Children also develop certain personality characteristics based on sibling position in their families (Bowen, 1976; Toman, 1969).

Bowen's family systems therapy prescribes family and individual differentiation, reversing the effects of this fusion process in overlapping stages by opening up closed relationships and resolving triangles in the extended family. The therapist, through the use of genograms (extended family maps of the patient's family), through education about family structure and functioning, and through supportive coaching, prepares the patient for the ultimate prescription of actual visits to parents, grandparents, and relevant extended family members to accomplish the actual reopening and reworking of excessive emotional dependency or emotional cutoffs. Although Bowen's theory is wide in scope, his choice of only individuals or couples for family treatment is among the narrowest (Nichols, 1984). Adult children are treated directly—actual children and families only indirectly. Yet Bowen feels that through triangulation with a neutral knowledgeable therapist and extended family visits, dyadic or personal tension can be reduced individually while family change occurs through resulting detriangulation and reciprocal readjustments throughout the family system.

In a social network extension of the family approach, Peter Laqueur developed *multiple family therapy*, bringing a number of inpatient families together with several therapists to promote curative group process, communication, and sharing as families rotated on and off an inpatient unit. Research and clinical work in this area have been carried out by Reiss and Costell (1977). Ross Speck and Carolyn Attneave, around family crisis situations where conventional approaches had failed, expanded therapy beyond the family to include social networks of 40–50 friends, relatives, and community members, promoting "retribalization" through multiple therapist marathon meetings, recreating a healing sense of family in community.

In the case of the lying 7-year-old, a family systems therapist would see the parental couple, refocusing their attention on their extended family. Through use of a family genogram, mother and father become aware that they are repeating familiar patterns from their families of origin (grandparents distant with female-dominated households and mother-daughter coalitions going back another generation). Currently maternal grandmother and grandfather are separated, with neither mother or father in touch with their opposite sex parent. The therapist would review these various cutoffs along sex lines, note the overly close exclusive relationship among the women, and coach the couple (and perhaps the grandmother if invited in) to explore each of these estranged relationships. As these impasses are explored and resolved, reciprocal realignments occur, with mother and maternal grandfather getting closer, rekindling grandmother's jealous interest and stirring some separateness from mother. Father's involvement with his mother stirs his wife's interest as well as paternal grandparental reinvolvement. As the parents get closer and maternal grandmother less dependently intrusive, the 7-year-old and his sister are noted to stop fighting—a result of increased parental teamwork, discipline, and support.

OBJECT RELATIONS FAMILY THERAPY

Many of the pioneers in family therapy, whether systems oriented or not, had psychoanalytic backgrounds and were variably influenced by Freud's predominantly intrapsychic theory. While several of these leaders felt family therapy required a revolutionary "systemic" departure from psychoanalytic concepts, others embarked on a more complex evolutionary approach to family work. Rather than concentrating on just what goes on *between* family members (i.e., interpersonal processes), they chose to study what goes on *within* family members *in relation to* what goes on *between* them (i.e., both intrapsychic and interpersonal processes). Convinced of the importance of the unconscious, the enduring impact of personal and family developmental history, and the integration of internal and external worlds, these pioneers found that the bridge between the intrapsychic and the interpersonal was provided by object relations theory.

Recently, a major new school of family therapy—*object relations family therapy*—has developed in Washington, D.C. (Scharff and Scharff, 1987), within the psychoanalytic family movement, integrating a more comprehensive group analytic approach to families with significant new developments in object relations theory. Emerging during the 1950s and 1960s from the family research group at NIMH under Lyman Wynne, early founders of this school were Roger Shapiro and John Zinner with contributions by Helm Stierlin (before going to Heidelberg), joined later by David and Jill Scharff, Bob Winer, Justin Frank, and Kent Ravenscroft. Their work has been heavily influenced by Klein, Bion, Fairbairn, Guntrip, and Winnicott, as well as other British object relations theorists associated with London's Tavistock Clinic (John Sutherland, John Bowlby, Sally Box, Hyatt Williams, and Pierre Turquet).

While early object relations theorists differed in their emphasis on the infant's or mother's relative contributions to individual intrapsychic development, they all stressed that internal psychological development occurred *in relation to* significant caretakers and not primarily between parts of the mind as stressed by Freud. Providing a major conceptual bridge between internal object relations and their manifestations in marital and family interpersonal relationships, Melanie Klein in 1946 introduced the concept of projective identification (Segal, 1973). Projective identification results from projection of parts of the self into another person followed by identification with and reaction to these perceived attributes. For instance, marital couples, who tend to select each other because of the mutuality of fit of their conscious and unconscious internal object needs, each project anxiety-provoking aspects of themselves into their spouses. Then, through unconscious collusion and mutuality of need, each spouse often tends to behave in a way that fulfills the other spouse's manifest fears and hidden wishes (Dicks, 1967; Frank, 1989). Thus, a couple's conscious reasons for marrying may be sabotaged to varying degrees by their unconscious needs through this reciprocal projective process.

If the couple is unable to contain their frustrations and tensions—and if they also have children—they often engage one or all of them in this same process of projective identification. When parents with individual or shared phase-specific conflicts enter certain vulnerable phases of the family child-rearing life cycle, their core conflicts become stimulated—like "ghosts in the nursery" (Fraiberg et al., 1975). Zinner and Shapiro (1972) developed the concept of delineation to describe the parental acts and statements communicating their internal images to their children based on a range of healthy to pathological projections.

Individuals, couples, and families often share a mutual developmental level based on their projective processes, reflecting a developmental hierarchy of projective identification (Ravenscroft, 1991; Zinner, 1989). "When a particular area is conflictual for all the members of the family, the projective identifications of the family members tend to interlock and condense in what are called 'shared unconscious family group assumptions'" (Winer, 1989), such as shared unspoken family positions like 'open conflict over, or expression of, sexual feelings will destroy this family.' Shapiro and Zinner (1976) developed the concept of unconscious family group assumptions, based, in part, on the small group theory of Wilfred Bion (1961). Winer goes on to point out that these shared unconscious assumptions tend to support and stabilize pathological internal object relations in the family, undermining the overall family task of promoting its members' development.

Introjective and projective identification are mutual processes going on between mother and baby, between spouses, parent and child, siblings, and also between the family group and the therapist (Scharff, 1992; Scharff and Scharff, 1987). The configuration of object relations that evolve between individual family members over the course of family development is initially largely determined by the nature of the marital relationship, with their own parental child-rearing life cycle (Ravenscroft, 1992) echoing the earlier dyads and triads of their own upbringing. During this reciprocal process, their children internalize not just each parent separately, but the parental couple as a pair, as well as the siblings, the sibship group, and the family as a whole. In family therapy, since experience with past generations is internalized and reenacted through present relationships, the family therapist can rediscover these interlocking sets of object relations, as they are reenacted among family members and with the therapist personally. In order to discover all these interrelationships, object relations family therapy emphasizes the inclusion of all family members, including grandparents, small children, and infants, with a particular emphasis on integrating the use of age-appropriate play and communication techniques (Scharff and Scharff, 1987; Zilbach, 1986) within the family therapy sessions.

To achieve full understanding, object relations family therapy employs active but nondirective listening, deeply personal communication, and carefully timed interpretations to promote insight. This is often achieved through the use of the therapist's own countertransference, which provides a major empathic guide to what is most troubling for the family at the moment. Use of countertransference is a major therapeutic technique—a hallmark of object relations family therapy. While this includes the well-known process of attending to personal reactions to individual transference and projection, it now also includes the therapist's own internal reaction to the interrelationships among the marital/parental couple, the sibship groupings, and the family as a whole. This represents a central new therapeutic position for the therapist to maintain in doing object relations individual, couples, and family therapy—one reflecting the cutting edge of the new integration of group analytic and object relations theory.

The stance of the therapist, whether seeing an individual family member, the parents, other indicated pairings, or the family as a whole, is what provides a special opportunity for deeper exploration and more intimate accurate therapeutic work. Compared to family systems approaches, family insight and understanding through such empathic exploration and interpretation are considered essential in bringing about family change in object relations family therapy. Scharff (1989, 1992) emphasizes that early in treatment the family's resistance to being helped is analyzed as well as the therapist's own countertransference resistances to becoming involved in painful family experiences. At the same time, object relations family therapists have paid particular attention to the indications for, and integration of, conjoint or sequential use of individual, couples, and family therapy for different ages, developmental issues, psychopathology, and family difficulties, as well as the indications for the use of either a single or collaborating therapist(s).

In object relations family therapy (Scharff and Scharff, 1987, 1991), there are three important concepts derived from an object relations understanding of development leading directly to special modifications in therapeutic technique: centered relating, centered holding, and contextual holding. Derived from Winnicott (1972), these concepts are relevant to the treatment situation precisely because the family's internal object relations are reenacted within the therapeutic setting itself, as if it were a facilitating parental container for the family and its members. By engaging the family through providing centered and contextual holding, the object relations family therapist assesses any developmental accomplishments, failures, and impasses at each level—individual, couple, and family. When seeing an individual family member, the therapist pays particular attention to the centered and contextual transferences to absent family members as they manifest with the therapist. With the couple the task is more complicated, requiring attention to both the transferences of the individual partners to each other and to the therapist, as well as their shared couples transference to the therapist. With the family, although all the intrafamilial and therapist transferences are of interest, the family therapist focuses primarily on the various group transference configurations, and in particular, any shared central and contextual transferences to the therapist and his or her therapeutic holding environment (Ravenscroft, 1993; Scharff, 1992). When working on each level, the therapist is particularly curious about why family members cannot hold each other in a developmentally appropriate way, given their respective stages in their individual and family life cycle (Ravenscroft, 1988).

Therapeutic interventions through clarification and interpretation are aimed at expanding the family's capacity to perform developmental holding functions for each other. Repairing self-holding and group-holding capacities on all levels within the family are essential goals for the object relations family therapist. Analysis and working through of the shifting contextual transference in couples and family work provides a major therapeutic basis for fundamental family change. Through the discovery and resolution of current pathological projective identification fueled by unhealthy internalized object relations, the family therapist helps the family to free itself from developmental, life-cycle impasses in order to achieve mutual growth and more healthy functioning in the present.

During the assessment and early treatment of the lying 7-year-old, an object relations family therapist would probably see the entire family, the couple, and the adults (parents and maternal grandmother). If indicated by history and the family sessions (or strongly desired by the parents), the 7-year-old might be seen, with and without his sister. Through an active, open inquiring stance, the therapist would support spontaneous family interaction and history telling, allowing their world view, the children's play, their themes, anxieties, and shared defenses to emerge naturally. The therapist (or cotherapists), depending on gender, might both hear about, see, and experience the distancing and collusion along sexual and generational lines—feeling the conflicted sexual anxiety and hostility at the core of the parental relationship and family—tension that drives them to a multigenerational repetition compulsion now manifesting in the sibling pair. Through the family's specific projective distortions and shared distrust of the therapist(s)' provision of a therapeutic holding environment and the parental couple's attempt to split a male-female cotherapist pair and/or attempts to ally along gender lines, the therapist(s) come to know the intimate issues separating the couple, pairing the women, inhibiting the men, interfering with their parenting, and now disturbing the son and daughter. The couple's shared projective identifications (including the grandmother in the adult triad and the children in the next generation) lead to reenactment of their internalized experience with their own parents and family groupings. Mother, for instance, has selected a shy inhibited more distant man to insure safety around her sexual and aggressive conflicts and

fear of intimacy. She also projects on to him her fear he will get too sexually and aggressively close to her and her daughter. Faulting him for his distance, she turns around and attacks him when he attempts more intimate involvement and discipline. His own issues and anxieties around aggressive dominating women and retiring fathers, stemming from his parental experience, mesh with her behavior, leading to the family's familiar repetitive pattern—leaving room for grandmother's involvement, given her related dynamics. Carefully timed interpretation of these issues, especially their appearance in the unguarded transparent play of the children, often permit warring colluding grown-ups to gain insight and contain destructive urges in the service of providing a less pathological more developmental atmosphere—for the children's sake. Empathic intimate understanding connecting feelings, shared behavior patterns, and personal family experience frees everyone to function on age-appropriate levels rather than being repetitively taken over by compelling old perceptions and patterns. Based on such awareness, the parental communication, disciplinary teamwork, and intimacy improve; grandmother is helped both to assume her proper place and to reach out to her estranged husband (or a new male friend or peers); and the children cease enacting parent-like male-female fights. As the son and father feel less anxious about their assertiveness and nurturing, lying and retiring disappear as issues. Resolution based on such insight is felt to heal on a deeper, more enduring level.

RESEARCH IN FAMILY THERAPY

Reviewing all research on the process and outcome in marital and family therapy, Gurman et al. (1986) conclude that it is "now established convincingly that, in general, the practice of family and marital therapy leads to positive outcomes. Family therapy no longer needs to justify itself on empirical grounds."

Family Therapy Outcome Research

Gurman et al. succinctly summarize major conclusions from this research as follows:

1. Nonbehavioral marital and family therapies produce beneficial outcomes in about two-thirds of cases, and their effects are superior to no treatment.
2. When both spouses are involved in therapy conjointly in the face of marital problems, there is a greater chance of positive outcome than when only one spouse is treated.
3. The developmental level of the identified patient (e.g., child/adolescent/adult) does not affect treatment outcomes significantly.
4. Positive results of both nonbehavioral and behavioral marital and family therapies typically occur in treatment of short duration, that is, 1–20 sessions.
5. Marital and family therapies at times may be associated with both individual (identified patient) and relationship deterioration.
6. A therapist "style" of providing little structuring of early treatment sessions and confrontation of highly affective material may be reliably associated with observed deterioration effects and is clearly more deterioration-promoting, in general, than a style of stimulating interaction and giving support.
7. Family therapy is probably as effective as, and possibly more effective than, many commonly offered (usually individual) treatments for problems attributed to family conflict.
8. There is no empirical support for the superiority of cotherapy compared with marital or family therapy conducted by a single therapist.
9. A reasonable mastery of technical skills may be sufficient for preventing worsening or for maintaining pretreatment family functioning, but more refined therapist relationship skills seem necessary to yield genuinely positive outcomes.
10. Certain family variables, for example, identified patient diagnosis, quality of family interaction, and family constellation, exert unreliable effects on clinical outcome. (Gurman et al., 1986, p. 572).

Since their monumental 1986 review, no subsequent large-scale review of outcome studies has been carried out (A.S. Gurman, personal communication, July, 1989). Asen et al. (1991) have reviewed more recent outcome studies, coming to the same conclusions.

Efficacy Research on Particular Family Treatment Methods

No method or school of family therapy has established incontrovertible evidence of overall effectiveness. Though some methods of family therapy are somewhat more specific about what they actually do in sessions, published descriptive reports are notoriously difficult to assess because of the absence of process data, making it problematic to evaluate what is effectively causing outcome treatment effects. Using all well-documented clinical and research reports in the literature, Gurman et al. (1986) have attempted to give "efficacy estimates" for 15 types of marital and family therapy, including all of the treatment methods not yet tested empirically:

> (1) . . . six have shown at least moderately positive evidence of efficacy with at least one clinical disorder or problem; (2) with the arguable exception (Gurman, 1981) of Psychodynamic Therapy, all the methods with at least moderately positive evidence of efficacy for some problems are highly directive in nature; (3) there are 4 disorders (schizophrenia, substance abuse, juvenile delinquency, marital discord) for which we now have at least moderately positive evidence of the efficacy of more than one method of family treatment; (4) there are 7 disorders for which at least moderately positive evidence exists that at least one method is effective.

They are quick to point out that the absence of evidence for efficacy does not mean a method is not efficacious. They note that, in fact, when most family therapy techniques are tested rigorously, significantly positive, and at times extremely impressive, outcomes are reported.

Just as the systems perspective has challenged the linear causality model of traditional psychotherapy with individuals and families, the shift to a systemic or circular view has challenged individual and family research. This approach stresses that ecologically valid holistic research must take into account both the system being researched and the research-researcher system within which it is occurring (Colapinto, 1979; Gurman, 1983; Tomm, 1983). To date, however, no family outcome research has been carried out using such ecosystemic ideas (Gurman et al., 1986), with the possible exception of Reiss (1984) and Asen et al. (1991). Though in systemic family research the diagnosis of the identified patient should be secondary to the diagnosis of the systemic dysfunction (family-level diagnosis), as yet no accepted system for family diagnosis exists. It is also questionable whether controlled studies of family efficacy should ever be based solely on family diagnosis without reference to individual diagnosis or illness (Goldstein, 1984).

Outcome Research with Specific Populations

Lange et al. (1993) reviewed the impact of the different family approaches in understanding and treating psychopathology for the following disorders: schizophrenia, mood disorders, anxiety disorders, psychoactive substance use disorders, eating disorders, and conduct disorders in children. They conclude that eclectic family-oriented interventions are useful in treating these disorders when applied flexibly and multidimensionally and when used in conjunction with psychopharmacological or other valid individual treatment approaches. Their results are in agreement with the growing emphasis on integration of family therapy schools advocated by Wynne (1988).

DISORDERS OF CHILDREN AND ADOLESCENTS

Major family therapy approaches are used to treat a wide variety of child and adolescent difficulties. Research results fall into three categories: psychosomatic disorders, juvenile delinquency and conduct disorders, and mixed emotional/behavioral disorders (Gurman et al., 1986).

PSYCHOSOMATIC DISORDERS

Minuchin and Fishman (1979) contrast the individual and contextual approaches to the psychiatric treatment of psychosomatic diseases in children, emphasizing the power of family-oriented techniques for these difficult conditions. A brief review of work in this area follows.

ANOREXIA NERVOSA AND BULIMIA

Researchers and clinicians have recommended family therapy for the treatment of eating disorders (Bruch, 1973; Crisp et al., 1974; Garner et al., 1982; Selvini-Palazzoli, 1978; Swift, 1982). Lange et al. (1993) point out that structural family therapy generates the most successful outcomes in treating psychosomatic and eating problems, exemplified by the well-known study by Minuchin et al. (1978) in which they successfully treated 53 anorexics and 4 diabetics and their families, concluding that a "psychosomatic family" does exist and is characterized by: enmeshment, overprotection, rigidity, and a lack of problem-solving skills. However, reanalysis of their data by Coyne and Anderson (1988) shows that there is no basis in their data for the concept of "a psychosomatic family" and that the patients did not protect the family through their symptoms, with the observed enmeshment, rigidity, and other "dysfunctions" being understandable responses to the medical crises and treatment approach. Coyne and Anderson (1989) warn against the use of the term "psychosomatic family" because it may keep the therapist from helping the families in a practical way with the medical crises. An attempt at replication of the Minuchin work by Kog and Vandereycken (1989) supports this judgment. Lange et al. (1993) note that studies by Grigg and Friesen (1989) and by Marcus and Wiener (1989), which focused entirely on eating disorders, gave additional support for the conclusions of Coyne and Anderson (1988, 1989) that there is no demonstrable "anorexogenic family structure." However, there is evidence showing that family factors do influence the emergence and maintenance of somatic and eating disorders and that a flexible family approach, including Minuchin's techniques, is clearly indicated and effective.

Compared with that on anorexia, there is only scant literature on bulimic families (Madanes, 1981; Schwartz, 1982). In a combined family and individual treatment study, using structural-strategic techniques with 30 consecutive adolescent and young adult bulimics and their families, Schwartz et al. (1983), reporting on 29 cases, found that 66% improved almost entirely and at follow-up maintained their improvement. These researchers added three additional characteristics to Minuchin's (now questionable) five anorexic features that are specific to bulimics: isolation, consciousness of appearance, and a special meaning attached to food and eating. Root et al. (1986) describe three different types of bulimic families, the perfect family, the overprotective family, and the chaotic family. Russell (1987), using control subjects for a group of 80 hospitalized anorexics and bulimics, comparing family therapy with individual supportive therapy, found that, for more acute patients hospitalized before age 19, family therapy was more effective than individual therapy, with a tentative trend for older patients to benefit more from individual therapy. A detailed single case study based on an object relations family therapy approach has been reported by Ravenscroft (1988). Families with members with eating disorders and that are characterized by high negative expressed emotion are currently being studied to see if specific interventions will make a difference in outcome (Szmukler, 1983).

CHRONIC ASTHMA AND DIABETES MELLITUS

Using psychosocial and physiological (blood sugar, respiratory functioning) measures, Minuchin et al. (1975), treating adolescents with chronic asthma and diabetes mellitus, obtained a 90% combined-sample improvement rate. Mrazek et al. (1991) have recently conducted studies on early-onset asthma, bringing parental factors more clearly into view.

JUVENILE DELINQUENCY AND CHILDHOOD CONDUCT DISORDERS

Already described in the behavioral family therapy section above, functional family therapy, developed by Alexander and his group at Utah, seems to be among the most effective treatments for "soft" delinquents (status offenses such as runaway, shoplifting, curfew violation), though their studies are unreplicated by other research groups and were conducted on predominantly Mormon families with unusually strong family ties. Delinquents were randomly assigned to functional family therapy, family and individual therapy, individual therapy alone, and no treatment. On the central measure of supportiveness/defensiveness, all families receiving family therapy improved. The control group deteriorated while those receiving only individual treatment remained the same. Taken with later studies, these data point to preventive effects of functional family therapy with "soft" delinquents, their families, and their siblings, as well as generally better adaptation to adolescent crises (Gurman et al., 1986, p. 574).

Also with demonstrated effectiveness are parent-training and behavioral family therapy (Wells, 1988). Patterson (1982) at the Oregon Social Learning Center developed with his colleagues what is generically known as "parent management training" for treatment of children with persistent conduct disorder of both the aggressive and nonaggressive types, now extensively researched over two decades (Forehand and Atkeson, 1977). resulting in several major trends: (*a*) superiority to no treatment; (*b*) treatment effects persisting to 18-month follow-up; (*c*) changes in classroom behavior subsequent to home intervention; (*d*) sibling improvement; and (*e*) reduction in maternal psychopathology, especially depression (Gurman et al., 1986). Reviewing controlled parent-training outcome studies, Wells (1988) concludes that parent-training (parent-management) is significantly more effective than no treatment for child oppositional and aggressive behavior disorders. Compared to other forms of therapy, parent-training is demonstrated to be equally efficacious or superior to other treatments for oppositional and aggressive behavior disorders, with no other therapy found to be superior (Wells, 1988).

One excellent study indicates that behavioral family therapy (Wells and Forehand, 1985), described earlier, is superior to parent-training alone for children with conduct disorder (Griest et al., 1982), improving short- and long-term parent-training results. An extensive review of "parent behavioral training" by Graziano and Diament (1992) shows that it is not only a very effective method for treating conduct disorders, but also for treating children with fears, enuresis, obesity, and stuttering.

MIXED CHILDHOOD AND ADOLESCENT DISORDERS

Reviews of family research studies involving child and adolescent identified patients (Gurman and Kniskern, 1978; Gurman et al., 1986; Masten, 1979) reveal that there are several dozen outcome studies focusing on different diagnoses and developmental levels. Unfortunately, in almost every instance, heterogeneous patient samples were selected (mixed, unclear, or inadequate diagnosis; inadequate severity measures; mixed developmental levels) precluding any significant specific meaningful theoretical or clinical conclusions. *In general, though, taken together these studies reliably indicate that, when any of the several well-known eclectic or well-defined family therapy methods is used, approximately two-thirds to three-quarters of cases can be expected to improve* (Gurman et al., 1986). Simpson (1991), in a controlled study comparing Milan Family Therapy with a combined behavioral, cognitive, and psychoanalytic individual therapy method, found that both approaches reduced a variety of symptoms in a population of 3- to 16-year-olds, with the Milan method changing family relationships in addition to the identified patient by using fewer sessions (but more therapists).

SCHIZOPHRENIA, ADDICTIVE, AFFECTIVE, AND ANXIETY DISORDERS

Moving beyond the psychosocial and biological revolutions, research and clinical work in psychiatry and family therapy are now embarking on a new "third revolution," based on a *biopsychosocial interactional model*. The interactional model embraces a more holistic open-systems ecosystemic perspective integrating body and brain, mind and person, family and community, medical science and art, and research subject

and researcher. While retaining the powerful family systems perspective, modern family approaches for major psychiatric disorders neither overlook individual constitutional vulnerability nor consider individual dysfunction secondary to family dysfunction. They recognize that it is legitimate at times to keep the focus on the identified patient while keeping the reciprocal family interactions in mind simultaneously.

As part of this approach, the psychiatrist/family therapist is not just a communications expert but also a medical management expert. The family is not just the object of intervention but the "real treatment team" for their sick member (Beels, 1988). As gatekeeper and crucial therapeutic ally, the family decides if the psychiatrist and his or her approach are taken in and whether they will work with him or her to carry out the treatment—empowering the physician instead of the other way around (Reiss, 1985).

SCHIZOPHRENIA

Pioneering leads by British investigators Brown et al. (1972) suggested that a core biological deficit in schizophrenics renders them particularly vulnerable to stressful interaction with critical intrusive family members. Following this lead, Vaughn and Leff (1976a, 1976b) focused on this family affective interactional style, called "expressed emotion" (EE). They found that patients living 35 hours or more per week with a high EE family (increased criticalness, overinvolvement, and hostility toward each other) had a high probability of relapse even on neuroleptics, compared with those exposed to decreased EE or spending less time (less than 35 hours) exposed to high EE. Those not on neuroleptics fared poorest.

American research by Goldstein et al. (1978) showed that family stress reduction and patient improvement followed psychoeducational family intervention around stress management. Stimulated by these findings, Goldstein and colleagues (Doane et al., 1981) followed a sample of 65 adolescents that they felt were at risk for developing schizophrenia based on the critical and intrusive nature of their family interaction when entering treatment. In fact, 5 years later, these parent behaviors had predicted the development of schizophrenia and schizophrenic-like disorders. The Goldstein and the Vaughn and Leff studies stimulated interest in methods aimed at reducing parental overinvolvement and intrusiveness.

Treating schizophrenics on optimal levels of neuroleptics but at high risk for relapse because of high EE families and other stressors, Falloon et al. (1982, 1985, 1993) utilized a home visit intervention called "behavioral family therapy" (interpersonal problem-solving, contingency management procedures, and family education) compared with outpatient individual supportive psychotherapy. This approach resulted in improvement in relapse (6 versus 44%), level of symptomatology, and social functioning at 9-month follow-up.

In summary, "these approaches forestall relapse but in no way provide 'prevention' per se" (Anderson et al., 1986); at the same time, it is clear that they result in specific areas of improvement in the patient's illness, clinical state, and quality of life (Gurman et al., 1986). It is also clear that, along with this improvement of the schizophrenic adolescent or adult, family morale and family life improve immeasurably as a result of these specific collaborative approaches with the family. Konstantareas (1990) has shown that for families with *autistic children* a combination of psychoeducation, behavior therapy, and family therapy yields the probability of improvement while conventional family therapy has failed to help these families.

SYSTEMS THEORY: REFRAMING RESEARCH

Reiss (1985) feels that family research, so elegantly typified by the above studies, nevertheless, still exclusively incorporates the idea that mental disorder represents a significant individual deficiency in interpersonal, cognitive, or affective function. Such research follows two lines of inquiry: "toxic" family interaction either is seen as distorting normal development, producing serious psychopathology, or tends to retard recovery from psychopathology whatever its etiology. There is another important group of scientific family studies, however, fundamentally reframing the perspective on pathogenesis. These studies investigate how the integrity and continuity of the family are supported, even strengthened, by psychopathology. Taking this seemingly paradoxical systems-level point of view, "psychopathology is viewed as a source of power and protection for the patient in the social world and a medium of communication, integration, and continuity for the family" (Reiss, 1985, p. 174). Fully integrated into complex, subtle, enduring patterns of family interaction, symptoms function as central integrating regulators of family life, not as maladaptive defects.

Two well-designed research studies in this new area are: (*a*) the research study of Straker and Jacobson (1979) on childhood encopresis both as the central regulator of autonomy and control in a family avoiding loss and growth and as part of a recurrent 2-week cyclic regulator of central family interaction; and (*b*) those of Wolin et al. (1980) on drinking behavior both as a central family ritual linking the couple pivotally with their alcoholic families of origin and as a major determinant of their children's alcoholic mate selection and drinking behavior. While the 2-week cycle documented by Straker and Jacobson expands our usual time perspective, Wolin et al. extend our clinical time frame to include psychopathology maintaining family patterns over time across two generations. Family research on inheritance and wills carries this supraordinate time perspective even further into past and future generations through financial and legal instruments.

ADDICTIVE DISORDERS

With regard to drug addiction, Stanton et al. (1982) found strong family structural ties, even when the drug user was not living at home; they also found poor generational boundaries, an inverted family hierarchy involving family decision-making by the younger generation and cross-generational coalitions involving the user. Their structural-strategic approach, and a comparable approach used by Romijn (1989), reduced drug abuse. Romijn (1992) also found this approach most effective for younger users living at home, improving their relations with their parents. Lange et al. (1993) stress that a strictly paradigmatic approach is counterproductive, compared to their effective combination of a structural/strategic approach with interventions in the sphere of communication and social skills. Family alcohol research has been growing steadily (Schaap et al., 1991). A well-recognized pattern of responsibility avoidance has also been found in alcohol-related wife-battering (Christensen, 1989). Studying alcoholic families, Steinglass et al. (1987) observed that alcoholic families have at least two distinct typologies, one when dry (not drinking) and one when wet, as well as a phasic drinking pattern indicating covert positive sustaining aspects to the wet phase. They concluded that alcohol served a short-term adaptive problem-solving function in the marriage. Wolin and Bennet (1984) observed that children of alcoholic families were protected against alcoholism through the preservation of family rituals. The style of drinking and where the alcohol is consumed are important (Jacob and Krahn, 1988; Jacob and Leonard, 1989). In treating (male) alcoholics, it is important to integrate alcohol-focused and marriage/family-focused approaches (O'Farrell and Cowles, 1989; O'Farrell et al., 1985; Sission and Azrin, 1986). Wife-battering, child-battering, and sexual abuse occur with increased frequency in alcoholic families, underscoring the importance of child psychiatric issues in recognizing and treating these families.

AFFECTIVE AND ANXIETY DISORDERS[a]

Children and spouses of adults with affective and anxiety disorders suffer significantly from these prevalent and incapacitating conditions.

---

[a] Parenthesis added by the author because a similar approach has been found to be useful with couples and families dealing with anxiety and panic disorders, often in conjunction with medication.

Outcome studies of affective, anxiety, and phobic disorders have indicated that behavioral treatments using the spouse as a collaborator in therapy are usually better than comparison treatments such as individual or group alone, though there is some controversy about this (Badenoch et al., 1984; Cobb et al., 1984; Gurman et al., 1986; Hafner et al., 1983). Using a collaborative family psychoeducational approach, the spouse and family are educated about the illness, its course, and its management, including expectable family group and individual reactions. Through this collaborative approach, "the therapist saves time and effort and gives the home atmosphere a sense of purpose, which contrasts markedly with the despair that usually hangs over a household of a depressed (or anxious[a]) person" (Beels, 1988). Such an approach pays significant dividends for the children involved.

In perhaps the best study of major affective disorder to date, Glick and Clarkin (*Inpatient Family Intervention for Affective Disorders*, Cornell University Medical Center, unpublished manuscript, 1985) used a modification of Anderson et al.'s (1981) psychoeducational family therapy with 54 consecutive inpatients. Family treatment goals were:

> helping family members accept and understand their depressed family member's current condition; identification of possible precipitating stressors and of potential future stressors; identification of stress-producing aspects of the family's interaction; planning to minimize and/or manage future stressors; and acceptance of the identified patient's need for post-discharge outpatient treatment (Gurman et al., 1986).

The study compared either the standard use of multimodal inpatient treatment (somatic, milieu, group, and individual therapy) or a multimodal approach with the addition of psychoeducational family therapy. At the 6-month mark, preliminary results indicated that, with the addition of family therapy, patients functioned better globally at discharge; females showed better symptomatic improvement, role functioning, and treatment compliance at follow-up while males did not; and families were in better alliance. Clarkin et al. (1990) underscored these findings when presenting the final results of their project. The studies of bipolar and major depression lead to the conclusion that psychoeducation alone is insufficient treatment for families with depressed patients. More active involvement of family members in treatment approaches is supported by a number of studies (Coyne, 1986; Lange and Ijzerman, 1989).

With regard to adult anxiety disorders, marital conflict appears, in part, to cause and sustain such disorders as agoraphobia and obsessive-compulsive disorder, even in the face of powerful, often shared, genetic contributions. Children are reciprocally involved in this process also. Some studies indicate that individual treatment has been associated with deterioration in a spouse or the marriage (Hafner, 1977, 1986), while these negative effects do not occur if the marital partner is included in spouse-aided treatment approaches (Bland and Hallam, 1981; Emmelkamp, 1980). Leaving out children, especially adolescent children, can also reduce effective family treatment and outcome. Gurman et al. (1986) conclude

> every study to date of the effectiveness of conjoint husband-wife therapy for adult affective and anxiety disorders has involved some variant of behavioral therapy, that is, behavioral marital therapy, exposure therapy, or problem-solving therapy (p. 582).

In panic disorders, it is important to distinguish between 'simple' and 'complex' agoraphobia (Chambless and Goldstein, 1980), the former explained entirely by intrapsychic (panic and fear of panic) stressors, and thus amenable to more individual behavioral approaches, while the latter is characterized by multiple interpersonal (family, marital) stressors as well as intrapsychic stressors requiring additional marital and family approaches (Stronkman et al., 1987).

FAMILY RESEARCH ON DIVORCE AND REMARRIAGE TREATMENTS

Among the few studied divorce treatment approaches, divorce mediation (Coogler, 1978) is indicated as most effective. To date, there has been no rigorous study of the effects of conjoint divorce treatment on the children of divorce, either as treatment participants or as beneficiaries (Gurman et al., 1986). The same is true for family treatment of remarried families. This having been said, it is important to stress that the work of Hetherington et al. (1979a, 1979b) and Wallerstein (Wallerstein and Blakeslee, 1989; Wallerstein and Kelly, 1980) clearly point out the short- and long-term child and family effects of divorce and single parenthood. Relatively new work takes into account an extended life cycle perspective including divorce, single-parent families, and remarriage as part of a normative process for families. This perspective is integrated with expectable stages of the divorce process, the family's stage of development (newly married, young children, adolescents, etc.), and family type (relationship or coping style). Treatment approaches specifically taking into account all these variables are now available (Ahrons and Rodgers, 1987; Isaacs et al., 1986; Kaslow and Schwartz, 1987; Whiteside, 1989).

Family Models and Typologies

There are no universally accepted models or typologies of family functioning, despite much clinical and research work in this area. Several of the more promising research and clinical approaches are mentioned here briefly for reference, including efforts by Beavers, Olson, and Reiss, the McMaster group, and family life cycle approaches.

BEAVERS SYSTEMS MODEL

Designed to utilize data from direct observation of family interaction rather than from self-reports, the Beavers systems model is based on a two-dimensional grid using ratings of (*a*) whole family competence and adaptability around task performance and (*b*) family interaction style. Using this grid, a clinically useful and empirically supported family typology is constructed. Applied now to a diversity of families with and without mental and physical disorders, the Beavers model can be used as an assessment instrument and starting point for therapy as well as an outcome measure (Beavers, 1982; Beavers and Voeller, 1983).

OLSON CIRCUMPLEX MODEL

Based on self-report and the analysis of a clustering of over 50 concepts developed to describe family and marital dynamics, the circumplex model of marital and family systems identifies and diagrams three dimensions of family behavior (cohesion, adaptability, and communication), leading to 16 types of marital and family systems. The diagram reveals the various combinations of marital and family cohesive forces leading to distance and closeness and capacity and willingness to adapt, as mediated through the facilitating function of communication. Based on this model, useful scales have been developed, called the Clinical Rating Scale (CRS) and the Family Adaptability and Cohesion Evaluation Scale (FACES), which have now gone through several modifications. These scales, and the constructs from the circumplex model, have proven useful clinical and research tools for assessing marital and family dynamics (Olson et al., 1983), stimulating considerable research and a certain amount of controversy about their validity and reliability (Green et al., 1991; Olson, 1991; Thomas and Olson, 1993).

REISS FAMILY PARADIGMS

Using a laboratory card sorting task, Reiss's group (Reiss, 1981) explored how families form a shared construct that reflects ''how the family may react to a variety of novel, challenging problems in its everyday life'' (Reiss, 1981, p. 68). They identified three parameters, which they called configuration, coordination, and closure. Where a family falls on all these parameters determines any given family's ''paradigm.'' Rather than implying pathology, specific family paradigms reflect the way a given family constructs reality when faced with challenges, describing how that family frames assumptions about the properties of the world. This laboratory approach has yielded interesting results with regard to a comparison among delinquent, normal, and schizophrenic families (Reiss, 1971), family perception of psychiatric wards, multiple family therapy groups (Costell et al., 1981; Reiss, 1981), and drug effects (Reiss and Salzman, 1973). This research converges with the clinical concept of family basic assumptions offered by the object relations family therapy school.

McMASTER MODEL OF FAMILY FUNCTIONING

Developed by a group led by Nathan Epstein at McMaster, this is a problem-oriented systems model of family functioning in health and illness that evolved from investigation of both normal and clinical populations. Taking a multidimensional approach to understanding family patterns of problem-solving, communication, roles, affective responsiveness, affective involvement, and behavior control, the McMaster model assumes that ''a primary function of today's family unit is to provide a setting for the development and maintenance of family members on the social, psychological, and biological levels'' (Epstein et al., 1982). In addition to clinical applications for assessment and treatment, this model has led to the McMaster Family Assessment Device (FAD) and Clinical Rating Scale (CRS).

FAMILY LIFE CYCLE

In recent years, a more complex family life cycle has been developed, including reciprocally related subcycles involving the marital-parental couple, the sibship, and the extended family (Carter and McGoldrick, 1988; Falicov, 1988). During the family life cycle, transitional phases and crises are inevitable as family members enter, develop, and exit from the family. A frequently used version of the family life cycle includes five main stages: the newly married couple, the family with young children, the family with adolescents, launching children out of the family, and the family in later life. The range of normal family process throughout the life cycle has come under more careful investigation (Walsh, 1982). Recently, Scharff and Scharff (1987), Joan Zilbach (1988), and Lee Combrinck-Graham (1988) have made contributions specific to children and adolescents in the family life cycle, and Ravenscroft (1993) has discussed developmental aspects of the unconscious life cycle for children, parents, and families. Given the prevalence of divorce and remarriage in our society, Carter and McGoldrick (1988) have modified the family life-cycle schema to deal with this continuum from divorce, through the single parent family to remarriage and stepfamily formation (Visher and Visher, 1979, 1988). Further modifications are emerging around adoption, foster parenting, primary grandparenting, and the impact of all the new forms of conception and reproductive technology (artificial insemination, in vitro, in vivo, surrogacy), as well as ethnicity, cultural and religious differences (Falicov, 1983; McGoldrick et al., 1982), socioeconomic factors, feminist issues, power, violence, and abuse (Goodrich et al., 1988; Luepnitz, 1988; McGoldrick et al., 1989; Miller, 1988), and sibling issues (Bank and Kahn, 1982). There is also major new work on adoption by Brodzinsky and Schechter (1990) and Benson et al. (1994) clarifying family issues and dynamics.

CLINICAL APPLICATION

Assessment

With regard to conducting family assessment and the initial family interview (Framo, 1980; Franklin and Prosky, 1973; Haley, 1973; Scharff and Scharff, 1987; Stierlin et al., 1980; Weber et al., 1985), there is still much theoretical and technical debate. Although each school approaches assessment in a different way, most would be interested in elucidating through various means the family's: structure, interaction patterns, extended family structure, stage in the life cycle, sociocultural context, developmental level, proneness to reenactments, resistance to treatment, strengths and resources, motivation and alliance, and capacity to solve problems.

A basic assessment and intervention approach (adapted from Grunebaum and Glick, 1985) might include the following:

> For *assessment*, bringing all relevant members of the family household unit together, including babies and grandparents; forming a therapeutic alliance with each member; learning what each person thinks the problem is and what they think the strengths of the family are (circular questioning, perfected by the Milan School (1980s); observing interaction; becoming aware of sources of difficulties beyond those in the immediate problem interactions (from biological to extended social systems problems); and evaluating to what extent the symptoms are the result of or maintained by the reciprocal interaction among people. They direct initial *interventions*, as well as further assessment, toward problem behaviors, preventing physical harm if present, strengthening parental-marital coalition if the problem is in a child, and fostering boundaries between overinvolved pairs. They recommend observing and exploring the reactions of the other family members to changes in the behavior of a member, intervening on issues interfering with family development, fostering clear and open communication, observing and listening carefully for the distorting attributions and expectations of the family members; exploring how mistaken attributions are rooted in past or present conflict; evaluating the balance of fairness and justice in the family; fostering changes in identification, aiding family role assumption, education, and demythologization, and making use of behavioral techniques adapted to the family problems.

The influence of specific schools or models of family therapy can be seen in many aspects of this integrated eclectic approach. Again, the stance and sequence the interviewer takes in the initial interview and throughout the assessment process (such as active physical and psychological interventions, semiformal interviewing techniques, homework prescriptions, directives and paradoxical directives, completion of genograms) can sometimes dramatically affect the nature of the relationship thereafter, altering alliance, resistance, and depth. Clearly, there are important clinical "tradeoffs" involved, which must be weighed by each family therapist depending on the clinical problem, treatment setting, expertise of the therapist, and time and funding available, among other things.

Essential to the process, however, is assessment of the family on all levels, from the biological and individual, up through various family subgroups and especially the marital-parental couple, to the whole family, and on into the extended family and familial-community social ecosystem. This assessment should attend to personal meaning and social significance, past history and future prospects, covert structure and overt patterns, and unconscious meaning and conscious significance. Through assessing the family on all levels, a therapist can best determine where the rate-limiting problems and impasses are interfering with change and development, where alliance and motivation are strongest, and how to prioritize and sequence interventions. Indications for individual, couples, or family therapy, as well as medication and other adjunctive therapies and settings, will follow naturally and surely from this systematic conceptual and clinical framework. On the other hand, if one doesn't have systematic information and experience with the family on all these levels, it is easy to miss crucial aspects of the case. Research and clinical experience point toward the importance of utilizing a flexible, integrated, multimodality approach to treatment.

Selection of Approach

Ideally, if a therapist were well-trained and comfortable with all therapies, including individual, couples, family, group, and biological, the selection of therapeutic approach would be determined by indications specific to a given case. In reality, many therapist and institutional variables understandably enter into this choice, such as: therapist personality style and background, clinical training and professional discipline, institutional and clinical policies and attitudes, insurance and reimbursement issues, proficiency and comfort with different modalities, experience with integration and sequencing of these modalities, familiarity with outcome research, personal biases, and countertransference issues (specific to the modality, type of case, or a particular case).

These considerations are true for any modality, and certainly true for family therapy, given its novelty, lingering controversies, and therapeutic complexity. In addition to the technical question of how to integrate and sequence family sessions with other modalities, a family therapist—especially a child and adolescent psychiatrist—must also consider how to include within family sessions both play and age-appropriate activities and communication for children of different ages. As with other modalities, the essential thing is sufficient training, adequate supervised experience, and personal comfort with child and family work. Though some gifted clinicians not previously trained in family therapy can learn one of the family approaches or develop "eclectically" by reading and occasional workshops, systematic training and resolution of subtle but repetitive countertransference issues can be accomplished only through fairly structured programs and longer term supervision.

The family approach is, first and foremost, an internal clinical stance, rendering the therapist open to all levels within the family-therapist system—a stance informed by a systematic holistic theoretical orientation. In order to achieve this degree of multilevel self and family integration, it is certainly best to know one approach thoroughly as a foundation for incorporation of new techniques than to simply collect scattered technical bits into either an unintegrated patchwork or a traditional individual therapy stance and orientation. Through learning any one family approach, a therapist internalizes the systemic interpersonal perspective. In effect, this new orientation reorganizes and reintegrates individual and biological perspectives into a more holistic, reciprocally interactional framework, doing away with the individual-family dichotomy just as the field has moved beyond the intrapsychic-interpersonal/mind-body problem in individual therapy. This represents for the developing therapist a successful bridging of the last frontier, moving clinical work and personal orientation in the direction of an open-systems perspective and approach. Any review or chapter on family therapy can only provide intellectual stimulation for such a perspective and a beginning guide or resource for further reading and development—and, hopefully, a possible selection of a personally congenial type of family training.

A review of research was placed before discussing clinical applications of family therapy because selection of family approaches should be guided by both research and clinical experience—and dominated by neither. The approach of this chapter is to select several of the more prominent schools of family therapy and present them more coherently. In practice, clinicians often use one approach they know well to treat a range of problems, referring cases that don't fit or respond—certainly a reasonable starting point. When a clinician happens to be well-versed in several schools, deciding which one to use for a given family becomes an issue. While being loosely "eclectic" has its utility and its risks, following a semistructured sequence (Beels, 1988) using techniques from different schools seems more promising, moving from the more practical and direct techniques to the more complex and indirect.

Following this strategy, a family therapist would first try techniques based on behavioral approaches, then structural, next strategic, then extended, and finally psychoanalytic object relations. More time, intensity, frequency, and technical expertise are assumed to be involved with progression along this continuum. In fact, with easier cases less time is needed for any approach, though the latter approaches often have more ambitious objectives of deeper structural change and family growth, if the family wants this in addition to symptomatic relief. While this sequence seems to be reasonable in terms of ease of learning and application, and can be quite useful up to a point, a major problem of incompatibility can arise for the family and therapist when moving from an initial active directive stance to a later more indirectly active, uncovering exploratory stance. This may be possible for some families in experienced hands. But often problems around trust and alliance emerge when attempting such technical transitions, resulting in mounting resistance that interferes with the shift into extended or object relations approaches.

In general, if a training center, institutional setting, or individual therapist is dynamically and developmentally oriented, and already works with parents and children on an intrapsychic as well as interpersonal basis, then dynamically oriented object relations family therapy would naturally be the most congruent and congenial family therapy approach. Behaviorally oriented programs and practitioners would normally opt for behavioral family therapy. Structural, strategic, and extended family approaches might fit with other settings or be indicated for specific conditions. Within any one of these major frameworks, an open-minded and progressive family-oriented child and adolescent psychiatrist would systematically attempt to integrate the relevant aspects of these other powerful theories and techniques. Despite their conceptual and political differences, family therapists of all schools increasingly reveal in their actual clinical work a convergence of techniques as they struggle with similar challenging family problems.

Family Therapy and Child and Adolescent Psychiatry

Child psychiatrists are ideally trained to work with children and parents throughout their individual and shared family life cycle, including competence in the therapeutic modalities of individual, parental-marital, and family work. As such, they are the only true generalists, capable of working with anyone and everyone at all stages of development on all levels of the biopsychosocial continuum. With this comprehensive approach, the overall objective is to determine to what extent pathology lies in the family as a whole, in one or more individual members, in the suprasystem (the outer environment with which the entire family system and its individuals interact), or in a combination of these, and then to plan appropriate treatment interventions (Grunebaum and Glick, 1985). Such is the ideal.

Child and adolescent psychiatrists are ideally positioned by training and speciality, with their sophisticated commitment to a developmental biopsychosocial perspective (Grunebaum and Belfer, 1986; Malone, 1974, 1979, 1985), to carry out such comprehensive clinical work and at the same time to contribute substantially to the new bridging research work in family therapy, while enriching their clinical competence and effectiveness with their child and adolescent patients and their families.

References

Ahrons CR, Rodgers RH: *Divorced Families: A Multidisciplinary Developmental View.* New York, Norton, 1987.

Anderson CM, Hogarty G, Reiss DJ: The psychoeducational family treatment of schizophrenia. In: Goldstein MJ (ed): *New Developments in Intervention with Families of Schizophrenics.* San Francisco, Jossey-Bass, 1981.

Anderson CM, Reiss DJ, Hogarty GE: *Schizophrenia and the Family.* New York, Guilford, 1986.

Anderson H, Goolishian HA: Beyond cybernetics. *Fam Process* 29:157–163, 1990.

Asen K, Berkowitz R, Cooklin A, et al: Family therapy outcome research: A trial for families, therapists, and researchers. *Fam Process* 30:3–20, 1991.

Badenoch A, Fisher J, Hafner RJ, et al: Predicting the outcome of spouse-aided psychotherapy for persisting psychiatric disorders. *Am J Fam Ther* 12:59–71, 1984.

Bank SPB, Kahn MD: *The Sibling Bond.* New York, Basic Books, 1982.

Barton CV, Alexander JF: Functional family therapy. In: Gurman AS, Kniskern DP (eds): *Handbook of Family Therapy.* New York, Brunner/Mazel, 1981, pp. 403–443.

Bateson G, Jackson DD, Haley J, et al: Toward a theory of schizophrenia. *Behav Sci* 1:251–264, 1956.

Beavers WR: Healthy, midrange, and severely dysfunctional families. In: Walsh F (ed): *Normal Family Processes.* New York, Guilford Press, 1982.

Beavers WR, Voeller MN: Family models: Comparing and contrasting the Olson circumplex model with the Beavers systems model. *Fam Process* 22:85–98, 1983.

Beels CC: Family therapy. In: Talbot JA, Hales RE, Yudofsky S (eds): *Textbook of Psychiatry.* Washington, DC, American Psychiatric Press, 1988, pp. 936, 946.

Bell JE: *Family Group Therapy* (Public Health Monograph 64, HEW). Washington, DC, US Government Printing Office, 1961.

Benson PL, Sharma AR, Roehlkepartain EC, et al: *Growing Up Adopted: A Portrait of Adolescents and Their Families.* Minneapolis, Search Institute, 1994.

Bion WR: *Experiences in Groups and Other Papers.* London, Tavistock, 1961.

Bland K, Hallam RS: Relationship between response to graded exposure and marital satisfaction in agoraphobics. *Behav Res Ther* 19:335–338, 1981.

Bowen M: Theory in the practice of psychotherapy. In: Guerin PJ (ed): *Family Therapy: Theory and Practice.* New York, Gardner Press, 1976.

Broderick CB, Schrader SS: The history of professional marriage and family therapy. In: Gurman AS, Kniskern DP (eds): *Handbook of Family Therapy.* New York, Bruner/Mazel, 1991.

Brodzinsky DM, Schechter MD: *The Psychology of Adoption.* New York, Oxford University Press, 1990.

Brown GW, Birley JLT, Wing JK: Influence of family life on the course of schizophrenic disorders: A replication. *Br J Psychiatry* 121:241–258, 1972.

Bruch H: *Eating Disorders: Obesity, Anorexia Nervosa, and the Person Within.* New York, Basic Books, 1973.

Carter B, McGoldrick M: *The Changing Family Life Cycle.* New York, Gardner Press, 1988.

Chambless DL, Goldstein A: The treatment of agoraphobia. In: Goldstein AJ, Foa EB (eds): *Handbook of Behavioral Interventions.* New York, Wiley, 1980.

Clarkin JF, Glick ID, Haas GL, et al: Inpatient family intervention for affective disorders. In: Keitner GI (ed): *Depression and Families: Impact and Treatment.* Washington, DC, American Psychiatric Press, 1990.

Cobb JP, Mathews AA, Childs-Clarke A, et al: The spouse as co-therapist in the treatment of agoraphobia. *Br J Psychiatry* 144:282–287, 1984.

Colapinto J: The relative value of empirical evidence. *Fam Process* 18:427–441, 1979.

Combrinck-Graham L: A model of family development. *Fam Process* 24:139–150, 1985.

Combrinck-Graham L: *Children in Family Contexts.* New York, Guilford Press, 1988.

Coogler OJ: *Structured Mediation in Divorce Settlement.* Lexington, MA, Lexington Books, 1978.

Costell R, Reiss DJ, Berkman H, et al: The family meets the hospital: Predicting the family's perception of the treatment program from its problem-solving style. *Arch Gen Psychiatry* 38:569–577, 1981.

Crisp AH, Harding B, McGuiness B: The starving hoarder and voracious spender: Stealing in anorexia nervosa. *J Psychosom Res* 245:225–231, 1974.

Christensen E: Alcohol as a component of wife-battering. In: Haario-Mannila W (ed): *Women, Alcohol and Drugs in Nordic Countries.* Helsinki, Nordic Council for Alcohol and Drugs, 1989.

Coyne JC: Strategic marital therapy for depression. In: Jacobson NS, Gurman AS (eds): *Clinical Handbook of Marital Therapy.* New York, Guilford, 1986.

Coyne JC, Anderson BJ: The 'psychosomatic family' reconsidered: Diabetes in context. *J Mar Fam Ther* 14:113–123, 1988.

Coyne JC, Anderson BJ: The 'psychosomatic family' reconsidered. II: Recalling a defective model and looking ahead. *J Mar Fam Ther* 15:139–148, 1989.

Derrida J: *Writing and Differences.* London, Routledge & Kegan Paul, 1978.

Dicks HV: *Marital Tensions.* London, Routledge & Kegan Paul, 1967.

Doane JA, West KL, Goldstein MH, et al: Parental communication deviance and affective style. *Arch Gen Psychiatry* 38:679–685, 1981.

Emmelkamp PMG: Agoraphobics' interpersonal problems: Their role in the effects of exposure in vivo therapy. *Arch Gen Psychiatry* 37:1303–1306, 1980.

Epstein NB, Bishop DS, Baldwin LM: McMaster model of family functioning: A view of the normal family. In: Walsh F (ed): *Normal Family Processes.* New York, Guilford Press, 1982, pp. 115–141.

Fairbairn WRD: Theoretical and experimental aspects of psycho-analysis. *Br J Med Psychol* 25:122–127, 1952.

Falicov CJ (ed): *Cultural Perspectives in Family Therapy.* Rockville, MD, Aspen Systems, 1983.

Falicov CJ: *Family Transitions: Continuity and Change over the Life Cycle.* New York, Guilford Press, 1988.

Falloon IRH, Boyd JL, McGill CW, et al: Family management in the prevention of exacerbations of schizophrenia. *N Engl J Med* 306:1437–1440, 1982.

Falloon I, Boyd JL, McGill CW: *Family Care of Schizophrenia.* New York, Guilford, 1985.

Falloon IR, Haoutyan K, Shanahan WJ, et al: A family-based approach to adult mental disorders. *Fam Process* 15:147–161, 1993.

Fisher L, Ransom DC, Terry HE, et al: The California Family Health Project. VII: Summary and integration of findings. *Fam Process* 32:69–86, 1993.

Forehand R, Atkeson B: Generality of treatment effects with parents as therapists. *Behav Ther* 8:575–593, 1977.

Foucault J: Technologies of the self (pp. 16–49) and The political technology of individuals (pp. 145–162). In: Martin LH, Gutman H, Hulton PH (eds): *Technologies of the Self: A Seminar with Michel Foucault.* London, Tavistock, 1988.

Fraiberg S, Adelson E, Shapiro V: Ghosts in the nursery: A psychoanalytic approach to the problems of impaired mother-infant relationships. *J Am Acad Child Psychiatry* 14(3):387–421, 1975.

Frank JA: Who are you and what have you done with my wife. In: Scharff JS (ed): *Foundations of Object Relations Family Therapy.* Northvale, NJ, Jason Aronson, 1989.

Framo JL: Marriage and marital therapy: Issues and initial interview techniques. In: Andolfi M, Zwerling I (ed): *Dimensions of Family Therapy.* New York, Guilford Press, 1980, pp. 49–71.

Franklin P, Prosky P: A standard initial interview. In: Bloch DA (ed): *Techniques of Family Psycho-*

therapy: A Primer. New York, Grune & Stratton, 1973, pp. 29–37.

Garner DM, Garfinkel PE, Bemis KM: A multidimensional psychotherapy for anorexia nervosa. *Int J Eat Disord* 1:3–46, 1982.

Goolishian HA, Anderson H: Strategy and intervention versus nonintervention: A matter of theory? *J Mar Fam Ther* 18(1):5–15, 1992.

Goodrich TJ, Rampage C, Ellman B, et al: *Feminist Family Therapy.* New York, Norton, 1988.

Goldner V: Family therapy. In: Shaffer D (ed): *The Clinical Guide to Child Psychiatry.* New York, Free Press, 1987, pp. 539–553.

Goldner V: Feminism and systemic practice: Two critical traditions in transition. *J Fam Ther* 13: 95–104, 1991.

Goldstein MJ, Rodnick EH, Evans JR, et al: Drug and family therapy in the aftercare of acute schizophrenia. *Arch Gen Psychiatry* 35:1169–1177, 1978.

Goldstein MJ: *Family Composition and Other Structural/Contextual Co-variates.* Paper presented at the NIMH State of the Art Conference on Family Therapy Research, Rockville, MD, 1984.

Graziano AM, Diament DM: Parent behavioral training. An examination of the paradigm. *Behav Mod* 16:3–38, 1992.

Green RG, Harris RN Jr, Forte JA, et al: Evaluating FACES III and the circumplex model: 2,440 families. *Fam Process* 30:55–73, 1991.

Green RG, Kolevzon MS, Vosler NR: The Beavers-Timberlawn model of family competence and the circumplex model of family adaptability and cohesion: Separate! But equal? (and commentaries). *Fam Process* 24(3):385–408, 1985.

Griest DL, Forehand R, Rogers T, et al: Effects of parent enhancement therapy on the treatment outcome and generalization of a parent training program. *Behav Res Ther* 20:429–436, 1982.

Griest DL, Wells KC: Behavioral family therapy for conduct disorders in children. *Behav Ther* 14: 37–53, 1983.

Grigg DN, Friesen JD: Family patterns associated with anorexia nervosa. *J Mar Fam Ther* 15: 29–42, 1989.

Grunebaum H, Glick ID: The basics of family treatment. In: Grunebaum H, Grinspoon L (eds): *Psychiatry Update* (Vol 2). Washington, DC, American Psychiatric Press, 1985.

Grunebaum H, Belfer ML: What family therapists might learn from child psychiatry. *J Mar Fam Ther* 12:415–423, 1986.

Gurman AS: Integrative marital therapy: Toward the development of an interpersonal approach. In: Budman S (ed): *Forms of Brief Therapy.* New York, Guilford, 1981.

Gurman AS: Family therapy research and the 'new epistemology.' *J Mar Fam Ther* 9:227–234, 1983.

Gurman AS, Kniskern DP: Deterioration in marital and family therapy. *Fam Process* 17:3–20, 1978.

Gurman ASS, Kniskern DP: *Handbook of Family Therapy* (Vols 1 and 2). New York, Brunner/Mazel, 1986, 1991.

Gurman AS, Kniskern DP, Pinsof WM: Research on the process and outcome of marital and family therapy. In: Garfield SL, Bergin AE (ed): *Handbook of Psychotherapy and Behavior Change.* New York, Wiley, 1986, pp. 565–624.

Hafner RJ: The husbands of agoraphobic women and their influence on treatment outcome. *Br J Psychother* 131:289–294, 1977.

Hafner RJ: Marital therapy for agoraphobia. In: Jacobson NS, Gurman AS (ed): *Clinical Handbook of Marital Therapy.* New York, Guilford, 1986.

Hafner RJ, Badenoch A, Fisher J, et al: Spouse-aided versus individual therapy in persisting psychiatric disorders: A systematic comparison. *Fam Process* 22:385–399, 1983.

Haley J: Strategic therapy when a child is presented as the problem. *J Am Acad Child Psychiatry* 12:641–659, 1973.

Hetherington EM, Cox M, Cox R: The aftermath of divorce. In: Stevens JH, Mathews M (ed): *Mother-Child, Father-Child Relations.* Washington, DC, National Association for Education of Young Children, 1979a, pp. 149–176.

Hetherington EM, Cox M, Cox R: The development of children in mother headed households. In: Hoffman H, Reis D (eds): *The American Family: Dying or Developing.* New York, Plenum, 1979b.

Hsu LKG: Outcome of anorexia nervosa: A review of the literature. *Arch Gen Psychiatry* 31: 609–618, 1980.

Isaacs MB, Montalvo B, Abelson D: *The Difficult Divorce.* New York, Basic Books, 1986.

Jacob T, Krahn GL: Marital interactions of alcoholic couples: Comparison with depressed and nondistressed couples. *J Consult Clin Psychol* 56:73–79, 1988.

Jacob T, Leonard KE: Alcohol-spouse interaction as a function of alcoholism subtype and alcohol consumption interaction. *J Abnorm Psychol* 97: 231–237, 1989.

Kaslow FW, Schwartz LL: *The Dynamics of Divorce: A Life Cycle Perspective.* New York, Brunner/Mazel, 1987.

Kog E, Vandereycken W: The facts: A review of research data on eating disorder families. In: Vandereycken W, Kog E, Vanderlinden J (eds): *The Family Approach to Eating Disorders.* New York, PMA, 1989.

Konstantareas MM: A psychoeducational model for working with families of autistic children. *J Mar Fam Ther* 16:59–70, 1990.

Lange A, Ijzerman L: The treatment of depression in an interactional context. In: Albersnagel F, Emmelkamp PM, van den Hoofdakker R (eds): *Depressien Theorie, Diagnostiek en Behandeling.* Lisse, Swets & Zeitlinger, 1989.

Lange A, Schaap C, van Widenfelt B: Family therapy and psychopathology: Developments in research and approaches to treatment. *J Fam Ther* 15: 113–146, 1993.

Lee C: Theories of family adaptability: Toward a synthesis of Olson's circumplex and the Beavers systems models (and commentaries). *Fam Process* 27(1):73–96, 1988.

Leff J, Kuipers L, Berkowitz R, et al: A controlled trial of social intervention in the families of schizophrenic patients. *Br J Psychiatry* 141: 113–134, 1982.

Luepnitz DA: *The Family Interpreted: Feminist Theory in Clinical Practice.* New York, Basic Books, 1988.

Madanes C: *Strategic Family Therapy.* San Francisco, Jossey-Bass, 1981.

Malone CA: Observations on the role of family therapy in child psychiatry training. *J Am Acad Child Psychiatry* 13:437–458, 1974.

Malone CA: Child psychiatry and family therapy: An overview. *J Am Acad Child Psychiatry* 18:4–21, 1979.

Malone CA: Family therapy and childhood disorder. In: Grunebaum H, Grinspoon L (eds): *Psychiatry Update* (Vol 2). Washington, DC, American Psychiatric Press, 1985.

Marcus MA, Wiener M: Anorexia nervosa reconceptualized from a psychosocial transcultural perspective. *Am J Orthopsychiatry* 59:346–354, 1989.

Masten AS: Family therapy as a treatment for children: A critical review of outcome research. *Fam Process* 14:323–335, 1975.

Maturana HR, Varela FJ: *Autopoiesis and Cognition: The Realization of Living.* Boston, D Reidel, 1980.

McDermott JF: Family therapy in child psychiatry: Introduction. *J Am Acad Child Psychiatry* 18: 1–3, 1979.

McGoldrick M, Pearce JK, Giordano J: *Ethnicity and Family Therapy.* New York, Guilford Press, 1982.

McGoldrick M, Anderson CM, Walsh M: *Women in Families: A Framework for Family Therapy.* New York, Norton, 1989.

Miller D: Family violence and the helping system. In: Combrinck-Graham L (ed): *Children in Family Contexts.* New York, Guilford, 1988.

Minuchin S: *Families and Family Therapy.* Cambridge, MA, Harvard University Press, 1974.

Minuchin S, Baker L, Rosman BO, et al: A conceptual model of psychosomatic illness in children. *Arch Gen Psychiatry* 32:1031–1038, 1975.

Minuchin S, Rosman BL, Baker L: *Psychosomatic Families.* Cambridge, MA, Harvard University Press, 1978.

Minuchin S, Fishman HC: The psychosomatic family in child psychiatry. *J Am Acad Child Psychiatry* 18:67–75, 1979.

Minuchin S, Fishman C: *Family Therapy Techniques.* Cambridge, MA, Harvard University Press, 1981.

Mrazek DA, Klinnert MD, Mrazek P, et al: Early asthma onset: Consideration of parenting issues. *J Am Acad Child Adolesc Psychiatry* 3(2):277–282, 1991.

Nichols MP: *Family Therapy: Concepts and Methods.* New York, Gardner Press, 1984.

O'Farrell TJ, Cowles KS: Marital and family therapy. In: Hester RK, Miller WR (eds): *Handbook of Alcoholism Treatment Approaches: Effective Alternatives.* New York, Pergamon, 1989.

O'Farrell, Cutter HS, Floyd FJ: Evaluating behavior in marital therapy for male alcoholics: Effects on marital adjustment and communication from before to after treatment. *Behav Ther* 16:147–167, 1985.

Ollendick TH, Cerney JA: *Clinical Behavior Therapy with Children.* New York, Plenum, 1981.

Olson DH: Commentary. *Fam Process* 30: 74–79, 1991.

Olson DH, Russell CR, Sprenkle DH: Circumplex model of marital and family systems. VI: Theoretical update. *Fam Process* 22:69–83, 1983.

Patterson GR: *Coercive Family Process.* Eugene, OR, Castalia, 1982.

Penn P: Circular questioning. *Family Process* 21: 267–280, 1982.

Ravenscroft K: Normal family regression at adolescence. *Am J Psychiatry* 131(1):3–35, 1974.

Ravenscroft K: Psychoanalytic family therapy approaches to the adolescent bulimic. In: Schwartz HJ (ed): *Bulimia: Psychoanalytic Treatment and Theory.* Madison, CT, International Universities Press, 1988, pp. 433–488.

Ravenscroft K: Changes in projective identification during couples therapy. Paper presented at the Twelfth Object Relations Family and Couples Therapy Conference, Washington School of Psychiatry, Washington, DC, March, 1991.

Ravenscroft K: The unconscious life cycle in families and couples. Paper presented at the Thirteenth Object Relations Family and Couples Therapy Conference, Washington School of Psychiatry, Washington, DC, March, 1992.

Ravenscroft K: Mourning and the contextual transference in family therapy. Paper presented at the Fourteenth Object Relations Family and Couples Therapy Conference, Washington School of Psychiatry, Washington, DC, March, 1993.

Reiss DJ: Varieties of consensual experience. III: Contrasts between families of normals, delinquents, and schizophrenics. *J Nerv Ment Dis* 152:73–95, 1971.

Reiss DJ: *The Family's Construction of Reality.* Cambridge, MA, Harvard University Press, 1981.

Reiss D: Theoretic versus tactical inferences, or, how to do family psychotherapy research without dying of boredom. Paper presented at the NIMH Conference on the State of the Art in Family Therapy Research, Rockville, MD, January 1984.

Reiss DJ: Family studies: Reframing the illness, the patient, and the doctor. In: Grunebaun H, Grinspoon L (eds): *Psychiatry Update* (Vol 2). Washington, DC, American Psychiatric Press, 1985, pp. 172–184.

Reiss D, Costell R: The multiple family group as a small society: Family regulation of interaction with non-members. *Am J Psychiatry* 134:21–24, 1977.

Reiss DJ, Salzman C: Resilience of family process: Effect of secobarbital. *Arch Gen Psychiatry* 28: 425–433, 1973.

Romijn C: *Family Therapy for Adolescent and Young Adult Drug Abusers.* Mijmegen, Institute for Applied Sociology, 1989.

Romijn C, Platt J, Schippers G, et al: Family therapy for Dutch drug abusers: The relationship between family functioning and success. *Int J Addict* 27:1–14, 1992.

Root MPP, Fallon P, Friedrich WN: *Bulimia: A Systems Approach to Treatment.* New York, Norton, 1986.

Russell GFM, Szmukler GI, Dare C, et al: An evaluation of family therapy in anorexia nervosa and bulimia nervosa. *Arch Gen Psychiatry* 44: 1047–1056, 1987.

Schaap CP, Schellekens I, Schippers GM: Alcohol and marital interaction: The relationship between male alcoholism, interaction characteristics and marital therapy. In: Schippers GM, Lammers SM (eds): *Contributions to the Psychology of Addiction.* Lisse, Swets and Zeitlinger, 1991.

Scharff DE, Scharff JS: *Object Relations Family Therapy.* Northvale, NJ, Jason Aronson, 1987.

Scharff DE, Scharff JS: *Object Relations Couple Therapy* (2nd ed). Northvale, NJ, Jason Aronson, 1991.

Scharff JS: Object relations theory and its application to family therapy. In: Scharff JS (ed): *Foundations of Object Relations Family Therapy.* Northvale, NJ, Jason Aronson, 1989, pp. 11–24.

Scharff JS: *Projective and Introjective Identification and the Use of the Therapist's Self.* Northvale, NJ, Jason Aronson, 1992.

Schwartz R: Bulimia and family therapy: A case study. *Int J Eat Disord* 2:75–82, 1982.

Schwartz DM, Barrett MJ, Saba G: Family therapy for bulimia. In: Garner D, Garfinkel P (eds): *Handbook of Psychotherapy for Anorexia and Bulimia.* New York, Guilford Press, 1983.

Segal H: *Introduction to the Work of Melanie Klein.* London, Hogarth Press, 1973.

Selvini M: Commentary on: Milan systemic family therapy: A review of ten empirical investigations. *J Fam Ther* 13:265–266, 1991.

Selvini-Palazzoli M: *Self-starvation.* New York, Jason Aronson, 1978.

Selvini-Palazzoli M, Boscolo L, Cecchin G, et al: Hypothesizing-circularity-neutrality: Three guidelines for the conductor of the session. *Fam Process* 19:3–12, 1980.

Shapiro RL, Zinner J: Family organization and adolescent development. In: Mileer E (ed): *Task and Organization.* London, Wiley, 1976, pp. 289–308.

Simpson L: The comparative efficacy of Milan family therapy for disturbed children and their families. *J Fam Ther* 13:267–284, 1991.

Simon FB, Steirlin H, Wynne LC: *The Language of Family Therapy: A Systemic Vocabulary and Sourcebook.* New York, Family Process Press, 1985.

Sission RW, Azrin NH: Family-member involvement to initiate and promote treatment of problem drinkers. *J Behav Ther Exp Psychiatry* 17:15–21, 1986.

Stanton MD, Todd TC, et al: *The Family Therapy of Drug Abuse and Addiction.* New York, Guilford Press, 1982.

Steinglass P, Bennett LA, Wolin SJ, et al: *The Alcoholic Family.* New York, Basic Books, 1987.

Stierlin H, Ravenscroft K: Varieties of adolescent 'separation conflicts.' *Br J Med Psychol* 45: 299–313, 1972.

Stierlin H, Rucker-Embden I, Wetzel N, et al: *The First Interview with the Family.* New York, Brunner/Mazel, 1980.

Straker G, Jacobson R: A study of the relationship between family interaction and individual symptomatology over time. *Fam Process* 18:443–450. 1979.

Stronkman G, Kromhout J, Van der Werff C: Methodical rigidity and the patient. *Directieve Therapie* 3:211–217, 1987.

Swift WJ: The long-term outcome of early onset anorexia nervosa: A critical review. *J Am Acad Child Psychiatry* 21:38–46, 1982.

Szmukler GI: A study of family therapy in anorexia. In: Darby PL, Garfinkel PE, Garner DM, et al (eds): *Recent Developments in Research.* New York, Alan R Liss, 1983.

Thomas V, Olson D: Problem families and the circumplex model: Observational assessment using the clinical rating scale (CRS). *J Mar Fam Ther* 19(2):137–148, 1993.

Toman W: *Family Constellation.* New York, Springer, 1969.

Tomm K: The hat doesn't fit. *Fam Ther Networker* 7:39–41, 1983.

Vaughn CE, Leff JP: The influence of family and social factors on the course of psychiatric illness: A comparison of schizophrenic and depressed neurotic patients. *Br J Psychiatry* 129:125–137, 1976a.

Vaughn CE, Leff JP: The measurement of expressed emotion in the families of psychiatric patients. *Br J Psychol* 15:157–165, 1976b.

Visher EB, Visher J: *Stepfamilies: A Guide to Working with Stepparents and Stepchildren.* New York, Brunner/Mazel, 1979.

Visher EB, Visher J: *Old Loyalties, New Ties: Therapeutic Strategies with Step Families.* New York, Brunner/Mazel, 1988.

Wallerstein JS, Blakeslee S: *Second Chances: Men, Women and Children a Decade after Divorce.* New York, Bantam Press, 1989.

Wallerstein JS, Kelly JB: *Surviving the Breakup.* New York, Basic Books, 1980.

Walsh F: Conceptualizations of normal family functioning. In: Walsh F (ed): *Normal Family Processes.* New York, Guilford Press, 1982, pp. 3–42.

Weber TT, McKeever JE, McDaniel SH: A beginner's guide to the problem-oriented first family interview. *Fam Process* 24:356–364, 1985.

Wells KC: Family therapy. In: Matson JL (ed): *Handbook of Treatment Approaches in Childhood Psychopathology.* Applied Clinical Psychology Series. 1988, pp. 45–61.

Wells KC, Forehand R: Childhood behavior problems in the home. In: Turner SM, Calhoun KS, Adams HE (eds): *Handbook of Clinical Behavior Therapy.* New York, Wiley, 1981.

Wells KC, Forehand R: Conduct and oppositional disorders. In: Bornstein PH, Kazdin AS (eds): *Handbook of Clinical Behavior Therapy with Children.* New York, Dorsey, 1985.

Whiteside MF: The role of the family therapist in divorce: Benevolent healer or agent of social change? *Fam Process* 28:357–367, 1989.

Winer R: *Introduction to Object Relations Theory.* Paper presented at the Washington School of Psychiatry Family Therapy Conference, Washington, DC, March, 1989.

Winnicott DW: The maturational process and the facilitating environment. London, Hogarth Press, 1972, pp. 37–55.

Wolin SJ, Bennet LA: Family rituals. *Fam Process* 23:401–420, 1984.

Wolin SJ, Bennet LA, Noonan DL, et al: Disrupted family rituals: A factor in the intergenerational transmission of alcoholism. *J Stud Alcohol* 41: 199–214, 1980.

Wynne LC: *The State of the Art in Family Therapy Research.* New York, Family Process Press, 1988.

Wynne LC, Shields CG, Sirkin MI: Illness, family theory, and family therapy. 1: Conceptual issues. *Fam Process* 31:3–18, 1992.

Zilbach JJ: *Young Children in Family Therapy.* New York, Brunner/Mazel, 1986.

Zilbach JJ: The family life cycle: A framework for understanding children in family therapy. In: Combrinck-Graham L (ed): *Children in Family Contexts.* New York, Guilford, 1988.

Zinner J: The family group as a single psychic entity: Implications for acting out in adolescence. *Int Rev Psychoanal* 1(1):179–186, 1974.

Zinner J: *A Developmental Spectrum of Projective Identification.* Paper presented at the Washington School of Psychiatry Family Therapy Conference, Washington, DC, March, 1989.

Zinner J, Shapiro RL: Projective identification as a mode of perception and behavior in families of adolescents. *Int J Psychoanal* 53:523–530, 1972.

79 PARENT WORK

Paula Armbruster, M.A., M.S.W., Susan Dobuler, M.S.W., Victor Fischer, M.S.W., and R. Kevin Grigsby, D.S.W.

The purpose of this chapter is to describe psychotherapeutic work with parents as a means of helping the child in child and adolescent psychiatric outpatient settings. This work begins with the evaluation and continues through the spectrum of therapeutic interventions.

Child behavior and parents' relationships with their children are rooted in part in the affective life and in the parents' unconscious issues and conflicts (Freud, 1969). Because of the proclivity of human beings to unconsciously replicate behavior patterns over time, the parent-child relationship often becomes the arena in which parents reenact with their children aspects of relationships with their own parents (Fraiberg, 1954, 1975). In theory, once the parents' intrapsychic issues and conflicts are identified, worked through, and resolved at some higher level of integration, the child should be less burdened with the parents' emotional legacies.

Hence, parent work relies primarily on principles that encourage parents to explore, uncover, and understand the ways in which they have repeated their own childhood experiences in patterns of behavior as adults, and especially where they have consciously or unconsciously reenacted these experiences with their child. In practice, parent work rests on the assumption of the validity of the theories of behavioral, cognitive, and psychodynamic treatments. Thus, prerequisites for doing parent work are skills in individual, marital, family, and group interventions based on these theories, as well as knowledge of child and adult development. Awareness of indications for psychoanalysis, psychological testing, and psychopharmacological therapy is also required for purposes of referral. Additionally, clinicians need to be familiar with services provided by schools, pediatricians, day care centers, and other community agencies that touch the lives of the child and his or her family.

ASSESSMENT OF PARENT

Before determining what type of intervention is needed, an assessment of the parent should be carried out. This assessment should include: (*a*) the nature of the parents' difficulty with the child, (*b*) individual attributes of the parent, and (*c*) motivation for treatment.

Nature of the Parents' Difficulty with Child. As a basis for treatment planning, the evaluator needs to consider the nature of the problem that has led parents to request assistance for their child. For instance, if one assesses the child's difficulty to be of a developmental nature, it may suffice to educate the parents about normal child development and parenting tasks at specific developmental phases.

If the problem involves the child's constitutional or organic vulnerabilities, the parents may need to be assisted in mourning the loss of their idealized child, in dealing with their feelings in having a less than perfect child, as well as how to best support the child and themselves (Solnit and Stark, 1961). If it is a child's mood or behavior for which the parents seek help, it is essential to involve them in a deeper exploration of the patterns and dynamics of their interrelationships with each other, the child, and other significant persons in the child's environment.

Individual Attributes of the Parent(s). Psychological awareness (psychological mindedness), an observing ego, and an ability to form and utilize a therapeutic relationship often are key in predicting good outcome in parent work. The presence of these attributes implies that the parent(s) will take some responsibility for the child's problem and that the child will not be blamed and brought to a mental health professional to be "fixed." If parent(s) are open to change and can modify rigid defenses, this augurs well for positive outcome.

Vaillant's (1977) hierarchy of primitive, neurotic, and healthy defenses is useful in assessing parental attributes. For example, parents exhibiting primitive defenses such as projection may have a guarded prognosis. Continuing with Vaillant's typology, a sense of humor (as opposed to sarcasm) about one's self in relation to one's child implies the ability to separate oneself from the parent/child conflict and can bode well for effective parent work. Parental level of anger (or rage) and how the individual deals with this emotion is also critical to assess.

Motivation for Treatment. Parents present themselves and/or their child for evaluation or treatment for both conscious and unconscious reasons. Conscious motivations may include a wish for relief from the parent/child conflict, for help in coping with the child's mood or behavior, or for an understanding of how the environmental or dynamic situation may be influencing the child. Parents may request education in parenting skills or in problem solving. As mentioned earlier, parents may also come with an implied attitude that the clinician should "fix" the child or find a magic cure. This attitude may reflect the parents' need to distance themselves from the child's behavior, perhaps in an effort to avoid guilt, blame, or responsibility. Some parents may find the child's behavior acceptable and congruent with the family style, and may have only brought the child for evaluation at the suggestion or request of the school, pediatrician, public welfare department, or some other referral agent. Such parents may have little motivation. Sometimes bringing the child as the identified patient may be a "ticket of admission" for the parent, who may have difficulty acknowledging initially his or her own problems. Whatever the conscious or expressed reasons for seeking help, the clinician seeks to identify underlying dynamics and to understand their nature.

A systematic guideline for the assessment of the parent(s) is shown in Table 79.1. The family history is indispensable for understanding the complexities of the child and his or her family. When taking a family history, it is important to know the family constellation: Who are the people in the life of the child? Age, cultural and religious affiliations, employment, education (SES), and living conditions are also relevant.

The marital history and individual history of each parent are other key components of the parent assessment. In taking a history, one often learns that an adult's relationship with his or her child mirrors the one he or she had with a father or mother. One may find that the child and his or her siblings are replicating the marital conflict. During history taking, dynamics such as repetition compulsion and primitive defenses (e.g., projective identification), which are having a deleterious effect on the child, may be revealed. The parents' own histories will influence how each of them cope with a child who is handicapped with pervasive developmental disorder, autism, Tourette's disorder, retardation, and other serious impairments (Lefley, 1987; McLoughlin, 1992). The family style, including the degree of affection and support available to family members, the degree of conflict/anger in the family, and how conflict/anger is handled, is crucial to assess. Whether the child is reacting to parental/family dynamics or bears his or her own serious mental illness, the individual history of each parent, the marital history, and the family style are all critical elements in understanding the child in the context of the family.

Table 79.1. Parent Evaluation Outline

Reason for referral
  By whom and for what reason
  Parents' concerns, their ''diagnosis'' and their prediction of the outcome.
Family history
  Family constellation: Identifying and *relevant* descriptive data regarding members of household, i.e., age, employment, cultural and religious affiliations; living conditions.
  Parent presentation: Impressions, including *relevant* physical presentation, degree of comfort or anxiety in interview situation, affective presentation, relative contribution of each parent, agreement or disagreement in describing the child.
  Individual history of each parent: Summary of significant personal, social, environmental, academic, psychiatric, and medical history. Relevant peer and family relationships. Strengths and weaknesses.
  Marital history: Describe adjustment in current marriage/previous marriages as significant.
  Family style: Discipline style of parents; how from parents'/caretakers' perspective does child compare with siblings (if any) and with parents when they were child's age.
Developmental history
  Include significant history of pregnancy, labor and delivery, infancy, sleeping, eating, toileting, motor development, language, play, sexuality, anxieties and fears, aggression, relationships.
School history/psychological testing
Medical/psychiatric history of child (as relevant)
Diagnostic formulation of family
Recommendations/disposition (indicate if recommendation accepted or not)

As alluded to earlier, possibly the most important issue to explore when evaluating the parents is whether or not they appear to be projecting their own conscious or unconscious conflicts onto the child or are in some other way using the child as a vehicle through which they may reenact an aspect of their own emotional histories or current life problems. If so, it must be further determined whether this conflict is limited to a relatively small area of the relationship or whether it tends to be all-inclusive. ''Good enough'' parents can identify and maintain parental, marital, and generational boundaries. Sometimes the parents' difficulties in maintaining such boundaries are part of a characterological problem.

TREATMENT

If the assessment determines that the parent is ready to continue and if the situation is a suitable one for outpatient clinic treatment, regular, usually weekly or semiweekly, appointments with both parent and child are scheduled. Optimally, but not always possible, the child usually sees his or her own therapist while, at the same time, the parents work with their therapist. The process that takes place is referred to as ''parent work'' rather than ''parent guidance,'' ''counseling,'' or some other denominator because these other terms are restrictive and are usually subsets of the larger domain of the interventions used with parents.

The services offered in the course of parent work following the evaluation are selected from a spectrum of potential interventions. It is not unusual to use a psychodynamic approach with one set of parents, and to use a cognitive/behavioral (''parent guidance'') approach with another, or both during the course of a given treatment. Even among that group of parents with whom the psychodynamic model is appropriate, the clinician might determine that marital therapy (Scarf, 1987) is the best way of treating one couple, while in the case of another family, she or he might make the assessment that intensive psychodynamic psychotherapy with only one member of the marital dyad is the intervention that is most likely to be effective (Chethik, 1976, 1989; Fromm-Reichmann, 1950). The goal is to free the child from the conflict that has been displaced from the marital to the parent-child relationship. If, in the course of this work, an issue arises that requires and is suitable for a more educative or informational approach, the work can shift from psychotherapy to parent guidance. In Hollis and Woods' (1981) topology, a pattern-dynamic intervention shifts to one of direct influence. When the emergent issue is resolved, the work may return to the more insight-oriented intervention. The clinician may also need to interact with others in the child's environment, such as noncustodial parents, stepparents, relatives, teachers, and other school personnel. In different cases, and at different times within a given case, although the *kind* of intervention may vary, the *goal* of change remains constant: to promote and maintain the healthy development of the child.

SPECTRUM OF INTERVENTIONS IN PARENT WORK

The flexible, selective use of clinically indicated different treatment modalities characterizes the framework proposed for parent work. These modalities can vary in depth, intensity, and duration, depending on the internal and external situation of the parent at a particular point in time. This spectrum of interventions includes but is not limited to: parent guidance, supportive therapy, brief insight psychotherapy, intensive psychodynamic psychotherapy, and psychoanalysis. Marital, group, and family therapy may also be utilized depending on the clinical issues.

Parent Guidance

Educative in essence, parent guidance is a cognitive/behavioral intervention directed at the parents' conscious level of understanding, motivation, and behavior. Parent guidance incorporates a variety of techniques, including providing parent education and information in child development and child management, environmental manipulation, and the use of community resources; behavior guidance (problem solving); and direct recommendations for behavior change (McDermott, 1975).

Providing information or education is the teaching of normal child development—what it means to be a child and what it means to be the parent of that child. Parents learn, for example, that all behavior is meaningful, that children respond to their parents' moods and behavior, and that parents need to provide consistent structure and limits in order to foster a sense of security for their child. In addition, specific skills can be taught didactically—such as how to negotiate the institutional environment to which the child must relate, and how to locate and utilize services and social supports. Thus, an overburdened single mother might be informed about how to access day care services or respite care available in the community in order to enable her to reduce the stressors that led to her family's referral to a child protective unit for evaluation. A parent may be advised to enlist the school's help in identifying whether a child has a learning disability or some other cognitive impairment. If the child does have such a disability, then the appropriate interventions need to be implemented.

Behavior guidance or problem solving (Perlman, 1957) is frequently used in parent work. It involves working through a parent-child impasse or conflict in an effort to learn alternative responses to problem behaviors. Guiding parents to an understanding of what may have precipitated or elicited the problem behavior can help them to recognize the chain of events that may have led to the parent-child impasse. Equally as important is that parents become aware of the impact of a positive response to the desired behavior. For example, if a parent always raises her or his voice in response to a child's oppositional behavior, resulting in another oppositional response on the part of the child, the parent might be helped to understand that this encourages the child to focus on the parent's raised voice rather than on the problem behavior. The use of ''time out'' (a behavioral approach) helps the parent to stop the negative behavior and gives the child an opportunity to correct his or her own behavior by thinking of alternatives. Time out also helps the parent to develop an effective strategy that is not merely an angry response to the child's misbehavior. Helping parents to understand the dynamics of these situations is critical in assisting them to develop constructive alternatives with which to respond to their child's undesirable behavior and simultaneously to learn to support the child's positive behavior.

CASE VIGNETTE

A parent complained that her 9-year-old-daughter would not stop whining. Any time that she tried to have her child complete assigned chores, they both would eventually become involved in a shouting match. Usually both mother and daughter would end up in tears and hours would sometimes pass before they spoke to one another. The chore remained uncompleted as well. When the mother was asked to describe the events that led up to one of these fiery exchanges, she described how her daughter would persist in whining if she was required to do something that she did not want to do, which was usually a simple chore. The mother would ask the child repeatedly to stop whining, with little or no response on the part of the daughter. This would lead to the mother becoming angry at the lack of response, as she saw this as her daughter not respecting her authority as a parent. The therapist suggested that the daughter's whining was an effort to "wear down" the mother so that the child would not have to complete her chores or to elicit attention from the mother, albeit negative. The next time that the child was requested to complete a chore and started whining, the mother was "coached" to:

1. Request that the chore be completed in very concrete language with a time limit. ("Pick up the toys in your room by 5:15 PM, please.")
2. Identify the problem behavior. ("You are whining.")
3. Instead of responding angrily to the whining, point out that the chore still needed to be done. ("Your toys need to be picked up by 5:15.")
4. Separate herself from the child by telling the child to take "time out" (in her room or other location away from the parent) for 9 minutes (1 minute for each year of age) to think about how she can change her behavior.
5. Develop alternative responses that the parent can use (restricting the child's access to toys if they are not picked up by the time limit).
6. Praise the child if and when she picks up the toys without whining.
7. Repeat the procedure again each time that the child starts to whine, until the desired chore is completed.

Upon utilizing this method, the parent explained that it felt awkward at first and that it was time consuming, but that eventually the child learned what to expect as a consequence of whining and that the whining ended.

CASE VIGNETTE

Direct recommendations or advice may be used when the clinician wishes to impart to the parent specific information or tactics to be used with a particular child, typically revolving around a particular point of conflict in the parent-child relationship.

The mother of an 8-year-old boy complained that he habitually had strewn his dirty play clothes on the floor of his room and refused to pick them up, this becoming the source of enormous friction between them. Once she had seen the connection between this behavior and the numerous difficulties she reported in the father-son relationship, it became possible for her to accept the advice that, because the child liked fancy sweatshirts and would often ask for them when accompanying his mother to the store, a strategy more effective than the punishment involved in her yelling would be to set up a token economy in which the child could earn points toward the sweatshirt of his choice by keeping his clothes off the floor of his room for a given period of time. Although the dynamics in the father-son relationship remained unresolved, this intervention proved moderately successful.

Occasionally, sharing written articles is helpful in working with parents. Discussion of such readings may be limited to the potential achieve-

ment of a specific child management task or extended to other relevant aspects of the parent/child relationship.

It must be emphasized that the giving of advice assumes the parents' ability to modify their behavior through a conscious decision (Hoffman, 1984). If a parent is unable to make use of such advice, the unconscious roots of this inability must be assessed and addressed. As in the case of the vignette presented immediately above, in order to ensure that the parent is accessible to a particular recommendation, it may be necessary to provide some insight-oriented work. This work would focus on the dynamics of the behavior that is the vehicle for the child's expression of his or her distress and that the parent perceives as "the problem."

The predominantly educative, or didactic, approaches described are most useful when parents feel reasonably adequate in their role and are relatively free of emotional conflicts, which directly interfere with their learning new ways of relating to their child (Langford and Olson, 1951).

Supportive Therapy

Often people can understand the pain of the other with whom they are in conflict only if they feel their own pain is understood. Thus, the use of empathy, reassurance, validation, and reflection constitutes a supportive intervention with parents. If the therapist acknowledges and supports the parents' feelings of grief, anger, or disappointment, the parents may be able to allow themselves, in turn, to be more supportive of their children. For example, the clinician might support the parents for their previous efforts to deal with the problem constructively on their own, and support their decision to seek professional help in dealing with the difficulty, as well as support their efforts to fill the parental role more effectively.

CASE VIGNETTE

A 9-year-old girl had been referred to a clinic because of her attacks on other children in her classroom when denied the exclusive attention of her female teacher. In discussing the problem, which had gone on for almost 2 years, the mother revealed that the child's behavior was problematic for her because "every time she does it and gets sent home, I have to leave my job and go get her." The mother was initially unaware of the child's displacement from her (the mother) to the teacher, how her own behavior was gratifying the child's wishes for her undivided attention, and other dynamic aspects of the situation. By adopting a supportive therapy approach at the outset of treatment, her feelings of anger and frustration were validated. Her efforts to deal responsibly with the child were then praised. As she began to experience some reassurance and was able to begin to regard the therapist as an ally, not a critic, she became open to the therapist's suggestions that she not gratify the child's wishes for her exclusive attention when they were expressed by behavior at school, and that within the child's home life, she make available the periods of exclusive attention that the child was demanding. This supportive work was combined with the therapist's intervention with the school's staff to help them find more effective ways of modifying the child's behavior than the repeated suspensions that had been employed to that point.

Brief Insight Psychotherapy

Brief insight psychotherapy on the parent-child relationship requires an exploration of the parents' own histories for the purpose of elucidating their relationship with the child and/or of understanding the nature of an obstacle in treatment (Chethik, 1976). For example, often a parent's own conflict around discipline, perhaps rooted in his or her own history of having been disciplined too harshly, inhibits or exaggerates the optimum balance necessary to effectively discipline the child. A clinician will then find that maladaptive patterns are repeated even after they are explored at a cognitive level. Going back to the parent's cache of past experience in order to understand the current conflict with the child may free the parent so that he or she will not have to displace past feelings onto the child (Cooper, 1961, 1974).

CASE VIGNETTE

The single, custodial father of an adolescent girl complained of her defiant attitude when he erratically attempted to enforce a weekend curfew. Initially, the therapist worked with the father in a supportive way around his efforts to provide appropriate limits for his daughter and attempted to help him see the relationship between his own inconsistency and his daughter's defiance. After several months of sporadic efforts to arrive at a contract with his daughter, interspersed with more frequent periods during which the father found reasons not to negotiate with her, the therapist felt it necessary to encourage the father to talk about his own experiences as a teenager with discipline and curfews. What emerged over some weeks was the father's feeling of having been unfairly prevented from having a more active social life by his father during his own adolescence, and importantly, his vow that when he became a parent he would show more tolerance for his children's desires for active social lives outside of the family circle. As these identifications with his daughter were explored, he was helped to see the difference between his past needs in coping with an overly restrictive parent, and his daughter's different need (especially given the circumstances of the divorce and the inaccessibility of the mother to the child) for sensitive, consistent, firm, limit-setting. While, as a result of this work, it seemed that the father had other issues that might profitably be explored in his own individual psychotherapy, the therapist, respectful of the reasons this man had originally come to the clinic, limited the insight-oriented work to those historical determinants revealed by the client that seemed clearly linked to current issues in the parent-child relationship.

Intensive Psychodynamic Psychotherapy

Intensive psychodynamic psychotherapy for parents is advised when it is assessed that more profound changes in a parent are necessary in order to allow a child to develop normally. For instance, a parent may be unable to benefit from other forms of parent work because of his or her rigid identifications and projections and/or a conflict may be so entrenched in the parent's characterological structure that it renders the parent unresponsive to the above-mentioned interventions. Suggesting individual psychotherapy to a parent may be interpreted, however, as a statement that the problem lies within the parent alone. For this reason, it is premature to suggest individual treatment if the parent has not adequately understood the connection, or the lack thereof, between his or her own conflicts and the dynamics of his or her relationship to the child. Also, as mentioned earlier, sometimes parents bring a child for mental health intervention when consciously or unconsciously they are looking for therapy for themselves, but are uncomfortable requesting help directly. In such cases, intensive psychotherapy may be what a parent is actually seeking.

CASE VIGNETTE

A 43-year-old mother, who lived in the house in which she had been born with her 78-year-old mother, presented her 4-year-old child for evaluation because of the child's daytime enuresis at nursery school, which the child had attended since 12 months of age. Though a practicing Catholic and outwardly conventional, the mother had sought out an unreliable man with whom she established a brief liaison. He terminated the relationship following the

birth of his daughter, ''just as I knew he would,'' in the mother's words. As the evaluation unfolded, it became clear that this mother had serious ego deficits, which often prevented her from acting in ways that promoted the child's security and independence. For example, although the child had an elaborately decorated room of her own, she still slept in a crib in her mother's bedroom, or, in her mother's bed. Out of doors, the child's range of activity was often constrained by a leash, and she was constantly reminded that ''little girls get lost, just like Pépé,'' a much-loved, and now lost, pet terrier. After a 5-month period of parent work, during which the majority of the sessions were utilized to help the mother begin to understand the degree of her enmeshment with her daughter, in a tearful session this woman cried, ''I'm so miserable . . . all I wanted was a perfect little girl to love, and I've messed that up, too. My problems are the reason she's got so many (problems).'' Out of this transaction grew a receptiveness and then a tentative commitment to accept twice per week treatment with the parent therapist in conjunction with her daughter's own psychotherapy.

Psychoanalysis

The recommendation that a parent enter psychoanalysis implies not only a certain rigidity of character in the parent, which itself might be the object of the analysis, but a high degree of motivation for improvement of self and of the relationship with the child. When a parent(s) is referred for analysis, the parent therapist may still need to be involved to help with issues that are specifically child focused.

CASE VIGNETTE

A 15-year-old girl was brought to the clinic because of suicidal ideation and other symptoms. Upon evaluation, it was learned that her mother was also depressed, in large part because her daughter's developmentally appropriate moves toward separation had rekindled long-buried conflicts regarding the mother's inability to successfully negotiate this phase of her own development. Because of the strong mutual identifications between mother and daughter, it seemed as if to some degree the daughter was expressing her mother's disorder. Because the mother was aware of her need for treatment, saw the connection between her own neurotic difficulties and her daughter's presenting symptoms, was intelligent, and had the appropriate economic resources, psychoanalysis was recommended for her. Her daughter's treatment was brief (6 months) and successful. The mother's analysis seemed to help her, suggesting a favorable prognosis.

KEY ISSUES TO BE CONSIDERED IN PARENT WORK: RELATIONSHIP, TRANSFERENCE/ COUNTERTRANSFERENCE, FLEXIBILITY, COLLABORATION

Relationship

The establishment of a relationship between the patient and the therapist is critical to the outcome of any intervention (Perlman, 1979; Taft, 1933). The results of outcome research suggest that often the determinants of therapeutic success lie in the personal qualities of the patient and the therapist and in their interactions, rather than in the particular therapeutic method employed (Frank, 1978). The case is no different in parent work, where a good match between parent and therapist is essential to treatment effectiveness. The therapist offers concern for the patient's welfare and encouragement for forming a trusting, confiding, nonjudgmental, emotional relationship (Parloff, 1986). This relationship becomes the basis for parent work as in any other therapeutic work.

Transference/Countertransference

Transference phenomena are present regardless of the level of intensity of the relationship between patient and therapist, or for that matter, regardless of the type of therapy that the therapist believes him or herself to be conducting. Understanding these phenomena is part of the foundation for any intervention that seeks to alter intrapsychic structure and functioning. The therapist is often perceived as the parent the patient wished for, as well as the parent he or she actually had. Also important is the countertransference, the role that the patient begins to take on for the therapist. In parent work especially, it is easy to judge a parent who, in the clinician's eyes, is mistreating a child. The temptation to "rescue" a child may be great. The clinician must always be especially sensitive to and aware of his or her own feelings and limitations.

While traversing the spectrum of treatment modalities, the clinician's role toward the parent changes somewhat. It is at times directive and at other times nondirective; it is both consultative and therapeutic; the clinician is at times a "real person," even when at other times he or she is the object in the transference. With these shifts in the therapeutic interaction, the transference/countertransference issues can change. The clinician needs to be alert to these subtle and not so subtle variations in the relationship.

Flexibility

In parent work it is important to recognize the need for flexibility in the relationships between the clinician and the parent. However, any discussion of flexibility is overridden by what is considered clinically useful and appropriate. Three modalities along the spectrum—parent guidance, supportive therapy, and brief insight psychotherapy—can be traversed fairly naturally without harm to the relationship. For example, in the case of a child who has a constitutional or organic impairment, supportive and insight-oriented therapy may be employed to help the parents mourn the loss of a normal child and to explore the implications of this loss, as well as parental guidance in enlisting community supports such as respite care and appropriate school placement. However, relationships formed in intensive psychodynamic psychotherapy, as well as in psychoanalysis, must be protected and structured as they develop; therefore, less flexibility is possible when working in these modalities. As noted earlier, in parent work, where the clinician exercises flexibility in drawing from a spectrum of interventions, awareness of the nature of the transference and the possible effects of these various interventions on the treatment relationship must be kept at the forefront of the clinician's attention.

Collaboration

Probably in no other therapeutic work is collaboration as essential as it is in a children's mental health setting. In order to ensure optimal therapeutic work with the child, communication between child and parent therapists is critical. The concept of a team approach for the child and parent treatment should drive the collaboration. For example, a team might comprise one therapist providing parent guidance or marital therapy, one engaging a parent in analysis, one treating one or two parents psychopharmacologically, in addition to the therapist(s) treating the child(ren), not to mention one or two group therapists. Although this is a bit extreme, the risks in lack of collaboration are obvious. Furthermore, patients are often able to sense, "tacitly; perhaps unconsciously" (Hartman and Hurn, 1960), lack of collaboration between therapists. Not only does this lack hinder the attainment of treatment goals, but with more impaired patients it risks "splitting" the clinicians, who may find themselves replicating the family dynamics. Experienced therapists have observed that the parallel and yet unified process occurring when child and parent therapists collaborate is comparable to the dynamics in dance when the music and movement come together.

Before leaving the subject of collaboration, a related issue needs discussion: referral for additional or complementary intervention. As mentioned earlier, in some cases a single clinician may be able to provide parent treatment initially and psychopharmacological invention subsequently; however, if the therapist does not have these skills, he or she must have the knowledge that such a referral is appropriate. The same is true for other modalities in which the parent therapist may not be versed (e.g., family, group, marital). Implicit in the referral is ongoing collaboration between the clinicians.

The concept of team collaboration also applies to nonclinicians who are involved with the child and family, such as pediatricians, school personnel, or other agencies with whom a child and his or her family has contact. This is particularly true in recent years when the so-called "dysfunctional family" has mustered a veritable army of resources. Current standards for intervention, such as wrap around services, integration of services, and case management, imply and often mandate close collaboration. Lack of collaboration among therapists and others involved in the family will prove confusing to the family, fertile ground for "splitting" as mentioned earlier and a barrier to positive outcome.

RESEARCH FINDINGS: PARENT WORK AND TREATMENT OUTCOME

Researchers have agreed that parent motivation and positive attitude toward treatment appear to be a "crucial factor" and the "only reliable finding" in predicting continuance in a child guidance clinic (Armbruster and Kazdin, 1994; Cole and Magnussen, 1967; Gould et al., 1985; McAdoo and Roeske, 1973; Novick et al., 1981; Pekarik and Stephenson, 1988). Agreement on the problem and mutual goals between therapist and parent appear to augur well for treatment (DeChillo, 1993; Lake and Levinger, 1960). Improving communication between therapist and parents and understanding parental expectations, perceptions, and attitudes have also been identified as key to treatment continuance (Singh et al., 1982). Madger and Werry (1966) have noted that "improvement generates resistance [in clinicians] as often as resistance is responsible for parents stating that their child is improved." In children's mental health this resistance to the "parents' point of view" (Madger and Werry, 1966) may be described as "clinic centrism" (Armbruster and Kazdin, 1994), "observer bias" (Madger and Werry, 1966), "staff bias" (Mirin and Namerow, 1991), and "blame" (Early and Poertner, 1993). Patients "vote with their feet" (Mirin and Namerow, 1991) when the match with the clinician is not comfortable and the offered service does not meet their needs. Chess and Thomas' (1986) concept of "goodness of fit" is useful to consider in this context. Examining the match between the proffered service and the child and family, as well as the tension between patients' goals and expectations and that of clinicians (Armbruster and Kazdin, 1994), is particularly important in parent work, as well as in other psychotherapeutic interventions.

A recent study (Armbruster and Fallon, 1994) found that the Family Environment Scale (FES) (Moos and Moos, 1986) was the only standardized measure (Children's Global Assessment Scale (C-GAS), Child Behavior Checklist (CBCL), Vineland, and Diagnostic and Statistical Manual of Mental Disorders, 4th edition (DSM-III-R) diagnoses were also administered) that distinguished between dropouts and continuers at a children's outpatient psychiatric clinic. Families who scored high on family cohesion on the FES were more likely to continue at the clinic. Studies support the associations between high marital conflict and poor adjustment in toddlers (Reid and Crisafulli, 1992) and distressed families predicting child behavior problems (Abidin et al., 1992). A "disturbed family system" will "likely take an early toll on the child"; conversely, problematic children often increase stress within families (Donenberg and Baker, 1993). Costello and Janiszewski (1990) note that referral for children's mental health service "has more to do with the impact of the child's behavior on parents and teachers" than with the intrinsic nature of the child's problem. Kazdin and colleagues have reported that when child treatment includes the parents, gains result in both child and parent functioning (Kazdin, 1985; Kazdin et al., 1992). Hence, findings underscore the importance of families and of working with them to support effective child treatment (Campbell et al., 1993; Hibb et al., 1993; Yama et al., 1993). Future models of the child psychiatric services are urged to pay "close attention to variables other than children's psychiatric symptom levels," such as parent characteristics (Jensen et al., 1990).

CONCLUSION

Successful parenting requires a delicate balance between being consistent and firm (setting limits, providing structure) and being nurturing and supportive. Clinicians must recognize the needs of the child, of the parent, of their own abilities, and of the limitations of any one modality at any particular time. With these limitations in mind, the therapist must constantly reassess the parent's abilities, motivations, and the nature of the problem with the child in order to choose the locus of intervention. Child and parent behavior is an "interactive process" (Donenberg and

Baker, 1993), exquisitely complex and deserving of thoughtful evaluation and sensitivity to the interaction of many variables. Parent work requires *creativity*, *flexibility*, and *fluidity*. In addition to these attributes on the part of the therapist, the possession of skills in many areas of the psychotherapeutic work ranging from cognitive/behavioral to psychodynamic are important. In order to make the right choice in terms of an appropriate treatment modality, the goal of parent work must always be kept in mind: to help the child by helping the parents. The challenge of parent work is to facilitate parents' understanding of their relationship with their child and to help them achieve some resolution of their own conflicts manifested in their behavior, especially when these behaviors are specific to the interactions with the child. If parent work is effective, the child's progress in treatment is enhanced and her or his growth is supported; secondarily, but no less important, parenthood as a developmental phase (Benedek, 1959) may be attained; and finally, the mental health of the family unit may be achieved.

References

Abidin RR, Jenkins CL, McGaughey MC: The relationship of early family variables to children's subsequent behavioral adjustment. *J Clin Child Psychol* 21:60–69, 1992.

Achenbach TM, Edelbrock C: *Manual for the Child Behavior Checklist and Revised Child Behavior Profile.* Burlington, VT, University of Vermont, Department of Psychiatry, 1981.

American Psychiatric Association: *Diagnostic and Statistical Manual of Mental Health Disorders* (4th ed). Washington, DC, American Psychiatric Press, 1987.

Armbruster P, Fallon T: Clinical, sociodemographic and systems risk factors for attrition in a children's mental health clinic. *Am J Orthopsychiatry,* 1994.

Armbruster P, Kazdin A: *Attrition in Child Psychology. Advances in Clinical Child Psychology* (Vol 16). New York, Plenum, 1994.

Benedek T: Parenthood as a developmental phase. *J Am Psychol Assoc* 7:389–417, 1959.

Campbell N, Milling L, Laughlin A, et al: The psychosocial climate of families with suicidal preadolescent children. *J Orthopsychiatry* 63(1): 142–145, 1993.

Chess S, Thomas A: *Temperament in Clinical Practice.* New York, Guilford Press, 1986.

Chethik M: Work with parents: Treatment of the parent-child relationship. *J Am Acad Child Psychiatry* 15:453–463, 1976.

Chethik M: *Techniques of Child Therapy Psychodynamic Strategies.* New York, Guilford Press, 1989.

Cole JK, Magnussen MG: Family situation factors related to remainders and terminators of treatment. *Psychother Theory Res Pract* 4:107–109, 1967.

Cooper S: New trends in work with parents: Progress or change? *Social Casework* 42:342–347, 1961.

Cooper S: *Treatment of Parents. American Handbook of Psychiatry* (Vol 2). New York, Basic Books, 1974.

Costello EJ, Janiszewski, S: *Who Gets Treated? Factors Associated with Referral in Children with Psychiatric Disorders.* 1990.

DeChillo N: Collaboration between social workers and families of patients with mental illness. *Fam Soc J Contemp Hum Serv* 104–112, 1993.

Donenberg G, Baker B: The impact of young children with externalizing behaviors on their families. *J Abnorm Psychol* 21(2):179–198, 1993.

Early T, Poertner J: Families with children with

emotional disorders: A review of literature. *J Natl Assoc Social Workers* 38(6):743–751, 1993.

Fraiberg S: Psychopathology of childhood. *Social Casework* 35:47–57, 1954.

Fraiberg S, Adelson E, Shapiro V: Ghosts in the nursery: A psychoanalytic journal of the problem of impaired infant-mother relationships. *J Am Acad Psychiatry* 387–422, 1975.

Freud A: The child guidance clinic as a center of prophylaxis and enlightenment. In: Weinreb J (ed): Recent Developments in Psychoanalytic Child Therapy. New York, International Universities Press, 1960.

Fromm-Reichmann F: *Principles of Intensive Psychotherapy.* Chicago, University of Chicago Press, 1950.

Gould MS, Shaffer D, Kaplan D: The characteristics of dropouts from a child psychiatry clinic. *J Am Acad Child Psychiatry* 24:316–328, 1985.

Hartman NM, Hurn P: Collaboration as a therapeutic tool. *Social Casework* 459–463, 1960.

Hibbs E, Hamburger S, Kruesi M, et al: Factors affecting expressed emotion in parents of ill and normal children. *Am Orthopsychiatr Assoc* 63(1): 103–112, 1993.

Hoffman MB: The parents' experience with the child's therapist. In: Cohen RS, Cohler BJ, Weissman SH (eds): *Parenthood: A Psychodynamic Perspective.* New York, Guilford Press, 1984.

Hollis F, Woods ME: *Casework: A Psychosocial Therapy* (3rd ed). New York, Random House, 1981.

Jensen PS, Bloedau L, Davis H: Children at risk: II. Risk factors and clinic utilization. *J Am Acad Child Adolesc Psychiatry* 5(29):804–811, 1990.

Kazdin A: *Treatment of Antisocial Behavior in Children and Adolescents.* Chicago, Dorsey Press, 1985.

Kazdin A, Siegal T, Bass D: Cognitive problem-solving skills training and parent management training in the treatment of antisocial behavior in children. *J Consult Clin Psychol* 60(5):733–747, 1992.

Lake M, Levinger G: Continuance beyond appreciation interviews at a child guidance clinic. *Social Casework* 91:303–309, 1960.

Langford WS, Olson E: Clinical work with parents of child patients. *Q J Child Behav* 3:240, 1951.

Lefley H: The family's response to mental illness in a relative. In: Lamb HR (ed): *Families of the Mentally Ill: Meeting the Challenges.* San Francisco, Jossey-Bass, 34:3–22, 1987.

Madger D, Werry JS: Defection from a treatment waiting list in a child psychiatric clinic. *J Am Acad Child Psychiatry* 5:706–720, 1966.

McAdoo WG, Roeske NA: A comparison of de-

fectors and continuers in a child guidance clinic. *J Consult Clin Psychol* 40:328–334, 1973.

McDermott FE: *Self-Determination in Social Work.* London, Routledge & Kegan Paul, 1975.

McLoughlin K: Professional supportive caring for children and adolescents with chronic neurobiological disorders. In: Peschel E, Peschel R, Howe C, Howe J (eds): *New Directions for Mental Health Services.* San Francisco, Jossey-Bass, 54:123–127, 1992.

Mirin SM, Namerow MJ: Why study treatment outcome? *Hosp Community Psychiatry* 42: 1007–1013, 1991.

Moos RH, Moos BS: *Family Environment Scale Manual* (2nd ed). Palo Alto, CA, Consulting Psychologists Press, 1986.

—Novick J, Benson R, Rembar J: Patterns of termination in an outpatient clinic for children and adolescents. *J Am Acad Child Psychiatry* 20: 834–844, 1981.

Parloff MB: Frank's common elements in psychotherapy: Non-specific factors and placebos. *Am J Orthopsychiatry* 56:521–530, 1986.

Pekarik G, Stephenson LA: Adult and child client differences in therapy dropout research. *J Clin Child Psychol* 17:316–321, 1988.

Perlman HH: *Social Casework: A Problem-Solving Approach.* Chicago, University of Chicago Press, 1957.

Reid WJ, Crisafulli A: Marital discord and child behavior problems: A meta-analysis. *J Abnorm Child Psychol* 18:105–117, 1990.

Scarf M: *Intimate Partners.* New York, Random House, 1987.

Shaffer D, Gould MS, Brasio J, et al: A children's global assessment scale (C-GAS). *Arch Gen Psychiatry* 40:1228–1231, 1983.

Singh H, Janes CL, Schechtman JM: Problem children's treatment attrition and parents' perception of the diagnostic evaluation. *J Psychiatr Treat Eval* 4:257–263, 1982.

Sparrow S, Balla D, Cicchetti D: *Vineland Adaptive Behavior Scales Survey Form Manual.* Circle Pines, MN, American Guidance Service, 1985.

Solnit A, Stark M: Mourning the birth of a defective child. *Psychoanal Study Child* 16:523–537, 1961.

Taft J: *The Dynamics of Therapy in a Controlled Relationship.* New York, Macmillan, 1933.

Vaillant G: *Adaptation to Life* (1st ed). Boston, Little, Brown, 1977.

Yama M, Tovey S, Fogas B: Childhood family environment and sexual abuse as predictors of anxiety and depression in adult women. *Am J Orthopsychiatry* 63(1):136–141, 1993.

80 PSYCHODYNAMIC PARENT PSYCHOTHERAPY: TREATING THE PARENT-CHILD RELATIONSHIP

Julian B. Ferholt, M.D.

Most parents who hurt their children are sincere in their commitment to treat their children well. They feel unreasonable anger and disappointment toward their children, but they are in love with those very same children. In addition, hurtful parents—while victims of their external situation and mental forces out of their control—almost always are still, to some extent, responsible for their hurtful behavior. These paradoxes remind us of the complexity of the inner lives of parents; they are the hallmark of an inner struggle to manage unwanted thoughts and feelings without acknowledging them.

Many characteristics of the parent, the child, and the surrounding context are important in creating and sustaining parenting problems, including parental personality disorders, psychiatric illnesses, drug dependence, physical illnesses, ignorance about child development, immaturity, unemployment, social isolation, personal losses, difficult children, marital disorders, family disorders, poverty, sexism, racism, and social violence. Yet, within the mind of the parent, a collection of unconscious thoughts and feelings about the child almost always lies at the heart of every significant parenting problem, and these unconscious forces have usually become relatively self-sustaining by the time parenting disorders are evaluated by clinicians.

Psychodynamic parent psychotherapy is an intervention designed to best promote relatively profound and permanent improvements in the content and regulation of those enduring, self-sustaining patterns of unconscious thoughts and feelings that drive a parent to hurt a child he or she loves. In practice, it turns out that parenting problems are often overlooked, and psychodynamic parent psychotherapy is not recommended as often as it should be. More importantly, treatment failures are common even when there are adequate conditions, including qualified therapists and suitable patients. Countertransference is by far the most prevalent cause of therapists' problems in treating defects in the parent-child relationship. In addition to countertransference, two other treatment problems are notable. First, it is difficult for therapists to keep the therapeutic focus on one area of the unconscious life of the parent, while adequately attending to other aspects of clinical situations that involve many different people with a variety of important problems. Second, it is difficult to manage the moral dilemmas that arise when a commitment to a parent's interests conflict with a parent therapist's commitment to help the child who is being hurt.

This chapter suggests that therapists can manage countertransference and other treatment obstacles better by embracing an approach that includes five practical cognitive schemes: (*a*) a formulation of the parenting disorder that is built around the concept of a defective parental mental portrait of the child; (*b*) an explicit attribution of moral responsibility to a parent who is hurting his or her child; (*c*) an outline of a nonreductionistic view of science; (*d*) a model of the mental stance of the parent therapist; and (*e*) an explicit advocacy for the optimal inner life of the child as the primary goal of the parent treatment. The chapter begins with a presentation of the defective mental portrait model of parenting disorders, followed by a description of countertransference in parent therapy. Then, the five cognitive schemes are outlined, two illustrative cases are presented, and the chapter ends with several practical suggestions.

DEFECTIVE PARENTAL MENTAL PORTRAIT OF THE CHILD

The concept of the defective parental mental portrait of the child is at the center of the clinical scheme that is being recommended to parent therapists as a framework to help them understand the nature of parenting problems, their development, underlying psychological mechanisms, and impact on the child. The scheme is a collection of useful clinical notions and it draws heavily from the interpersonal (Gill, 1983) and object relations (Kernberg, 1982) schools of psychoanalytic theory. It depends on classical intrapsychic psychoanalytic principles, and it is designed to embrace the biomedical, cognitive, family, and socioeconomic spheres as well.

The mental portrait of the child refers to a parent's enduring, global synthesis of all the remembered thoughts and feelings that are closely associated in that parent's mind with the subjective experience of a particular child (Ferholt, 1976; Ferholt et al., 1985). These remembered thoughts and feelings are more or less well organized, often hierarchically, to form a global mental synthesis that serves to represent a particular child in the mind of the parent. The global synthesis is best thought of as an enduring dynamic mental system, not simply a static composite or "average" memory. The mental portrait includes what is commonly called—in folk psychology (Bruner, 1990)—the meaning of the child to the parent and is informed by what others have written about as the mental representation (Kernberg, 1980; Sutherland, 1980), narrative story line (Schafer, 1992), working model (Greenson, 1960; Stern, 1985; Zeanah, 1989), or schema (in classical psychology). Since the mental portrait guides the perception, selection, and interpretation of new information and remembered thoughts and feelings about the child, it has a major impact on all the parent's behavior in relation to that child.

AN UNHEALTHY PARENTAL MENTAL PORTRAIT OF A CHILD

Since all parents lose empathy and hurt their children at times, disorders are distinguished from "good enough" situations primarily because they are pervasive, extreme, and long-lasting. A parenting disorder may also be designated in relation to the unique vulnerabilities of a particular child. Disorders of parental experience of the child are characterized by insufficient empathy, denigration or idealization, overinvolvement or remoteness, and a poor match with the actual characteristics of the child. The discrepancy between the parent's view of the child and reality stems from distorted perceptions, misinterpretations, confusions, overly simplistic interpretations, and even (unconscious) fabrications about the child.

When there is a very severe defect in regulation within the portrait, parents unconsciously experience the child predominantly in a prejudiced way. They may attribute mythical qualities to the child—most often with evil designs, but sometimes with godlike perfection (Miller, 1981). Also, a parent may experience a child as if he or she were someone or even something else (e.g., father, mother, sister, demon, monster, genius, angel, or god). In some of the most severe disturbances, the parental prejudices render the child in terms of conventional undesirable caricatures such as: the coldly calculating, self-aggrandizing villain; the wild, unsocialized primitive; the irresponsible, lazy, manipulative tramp; the tragic, fragile, suffering invalid; or the generous, powerful, brilliantly intelligent, creative, invulnerable leader. The case of Jason M., presented later in this chapter, illustrates a defect in a parental portrait so severe that it could not be sufficiently repaired. The second case, of Douglas T., illustrates a less severe case in which similar prejudices occur but are less predominant and more responsive to treatment.

DEVELOPMENT OF THE UNHEALTHY MENTAL PORTRAIT

The mental portrait begins with the parent's fantasies even before meeting the child. In the course of an adult's healthy development as a parent, the mental portrait of a child is repeatedly reworked to achieve higher levels of organization and complexity. Such ongoing development of the mental portrait is best viewed by parent therapists in terms of two interactive processes: (a) the components of the mental portrait are repeatedly reconciled with perceptions of the real child who is changing, and (b) the parent's mental representations of the child—initially tightly entangled with the parent's self-representations—are gradually separated in the parent's mind from those representations of the parent's self.

These two developmental processes in the portrait are best understood as dependent on a sequence of parental experiences formulated in terms borrowed from the study of psychological processes associated with grief and mourning after a loved one has died (Engel, 1962). If the mourning processes associated with the development of the mental portrait are significantly obstructed or distorted, the mental portrait will become defective. Significantly, the same etiological factors are common to pathological deviations in grieving and defective development of the mental portrait.

Viewed from the perspective of the grieving that the parent must achieve in the development of the healthy mental portrait, the causes of deviant, defective development include the following: ambivalence toward the loved one (e.g., a child that comes at a very bad time; a painful, physically damaging pregnancy and birth; or a child who is very difficult to care for), overwhelming intensity of the psychological loss itself (e.g., the child is deformed, handicapped severely, or almost dies—during gestation, at birth, in an accident, or from a potentially fatal illness), parental psychiatric disorder (e.g., depression), personality problems in the parent (e.g., pathological narcissism), lack of preparation for the loss (e.g., ignorance and misinformation about pregnancy, labor, delivery, and child care), lack of emotional support from loved ones after the loss (e.g., marital problems, or social isolation), and compounding losses from additional environmental stressors. The interaction of various factors at any one time may trigger disturbances in the development of the mental portrait of one child even in a parent who sustains healthy portraits of other children.

PSYCHOLOGICAL PROCESSES ASSOCIATED WITH DEFECTIVE REGULATION

Almost all the mental processes central to a defective mental portrait transiently distort the mental life of every parent. Again, problems are distinguished from good enough situations by degree, pervasiveness, and balance. In the intrapsychic sphere, problems in regulation of the mental portrait can be conceived in terms of problems of content and regulation in the mental portrait. Most commonly, there is a failure to manage adequately the boundary between the mental representation of the child, that of the parent's self, and that of each of the parent's own parents, although representations of other loved ones may sometimes play a role too. Many psychodynamic notions can help the therapist generate a useful intrapsychic understanding of the nature of particular aspects of the psychological processes that underlie the defective regulation. The ego mechanisms of defense are indispensable to such psychodynamic formulations, but more comprehensive notions are helpful in some cases (e.g., the child in the parent's mind as: "self-object," "symbiotic object," "unacceptable self," and even "sexual fetish" (Schreier, 1992)).

Two clinical concepts—identification and reactivation— are especially useful to describe dynamics in the intrapsychic sphere. When the child is very young, a healthy parent uses a variety of processes of internalization to "identify" strongly with that child. Such intense and irrational identifications help sustain sufficient commitment and interest in the child. But a strong, irrational kind of identification, inappropriately used, leads to defective regulation in which the mental representation of the parent's self and that of the child tend to become stuck in the fused state, stuck in a detached state, or alternate erratically from extreme detachment to extreme fusion. In a state of extreme fusion, characteristics of the child that are significantly different from the parent are overlooked; in a state of extreme detachment, the identifications needed to sustain an essential intuitive empathic knowledge of the child are impossible.

A healthy parent also experiences the eruption of repressed memories of childhood in the context of his or her identifications with a child, because that child is at the same age, in the same stage of development, or having experiences similar to those the parent had when the memory was created. This process—referred to as reactivation—is often a constructive impetus for continuing personality development in the parent. However, if the reactivated memories are very disturbing, then reactivation may contribute to defective regulation by causing tumultuous emotional responses or eliciting primitive defensive operations, especially denial and distortion of those aspects of the child that stimulated the intolerable reactivation (Coleman et al., 1953).

A set of interrelated concepts—including projective identification, extractive identification (Bollas, 1987, 1992), and introjective identification—are also useful in understanding some aspects of the defective mental portrait. Although historically connected to terms describing intrapsychic processes (e.g., projective identification (Klein, 1946)), these concepts have been expanded in current psychoanalytic theoretical writing so that they can be used as psychodynamic concepts to bridge the intrapsychic and interpersonal spheres (Tansey and Burke, 1989). In this discussion of the parent-child relationship, these bridging concepts refer to an interactive psychological process by which the parent places an attribute from his or her unconscious mental portrait directly into the mental life of the child—specifically into the child's unconscious self-representation.

These interactive processes—like the intrapsychic processes referred to earlier in this section—are ubiquitous in the relationship of a child to a parent, and they are usually compatible with healthy personality development. However, projective or extractive identifications can interfere with healthy development and are important aspects of defective regulation in an unhealthy mental portrait associated with parenting disorders. They may contribute to the development of the child's experience of a false self, when too many important aspects of the child are removed from his or her authentic self-portrait, and/or too many incompatible traits are placed into the child by the parent. In addition, particular unhealthy personality traits (e.g., defects in conscience—superego lacunae) may be unconsciously put into the child by a parent.

It is sometimes useful for the parent therapist to view the psychological processes of a defective portrait from the perspective of the family unit as a whole. At such times, concepts of group dynamics that apply only within the interpersonal sphere, such as delineations, designations, and scapegoating (Ackerman, 1958; Stierlin, 1977; Vogal, 1960; Zinner and Shapiro, 1972), are most useful. When group dynamics are in focus, the individual intrapsychic mechanisms and bridging psychological mechanisms mentioned above are subsumed within the interpersonal group concepts that the therapist is using at that time.

CONSCIOUS ASPECTS, GUILT, AND MORAL RESPONSIBILITY

Parents who consistently hurt a child they know and love are repeatedly aware, if peripherally and transiently, that something is wrong with what they are doing to the child and the way they are thinking about the child. These parents almost always deny this awareness at first, but in describing many specific interactions in detail, they usually indicate that they realize that they do things to make a bad situation worse, forget to do things that they know could make it better, feel some inappropriate emotions, and perhaps notice that people outside the web of the colluding family suspect a parenting problem. Very disturbed parents often have elaborate rationalizations for their abusive behavior and may even experience a dissociative state when they are doing something awful to their child. But even such parents are aware, to some degree, at some times, that something is very wrong; for example, they notice that they are lying to family and friends in a way that they were not before.

Therefore, most parents with a defective mental portrait of a child decide many times to deceive themselves and not to ask for help. These are decisions, made with more or less freedom, to continue to hurt their children in order to indulge their own desire to avoid both the guilt and shame, and also the embarrassment and other consequences that would result from others knowing. Such decisions are value choices for which parents are to some extent morally responsible. When parents think they are vulnerable to such self-accusation, they often try to escape from guilt, more or less consciously, by adopting a simplistic image of themselves (e.g., innocent victim, martyr, or handicapped person). To embrace such a simplistic caricature of themselves in relation to their children, parents must also adopt reciprocally extreme conscious positions about their children (e.g., abusing villain or cross to bear)—thus, increasing the child's mistreatment.

HARMFUL PARENTING BEHAVIORS FROM THE DEFECTIVE MENTAL PORTRAIT

A parent's conscious attitudes and feelings are communicated to the child in good part through planned, easily observable actions that include child-rearing practices. But, unconscious thoughts and feelings (e.g., loss of empathy, rejection, idealization, sexualization, and other disturbing aspects of the parent's inner life) influence the child primarily through nonverbal communication and the emotional tone surrounding words and overt actions—that is, unintentional, "microscopic" aspects of the parent's behavior, including: (a) the subtext of the parent's verbal communications, (b) the timing of intended actions, and (c) body language. The subtext, or latent content, of verbal communication is expressed through tone of voice (pitch, rhythm, and stress), sound patterns of selected words, slips, jokes, evoked images, connotations of words, and associative sequences. The timing of actions communicates meaning in relationship to the context of the action and state of reception in the child as a biological organism and psychological being. Body language is expressed through facial expressions, patterns of direct eye gaze, posture, gesture, proximity modulation, style of movement in the presence of the child, and ways of touching, avoiding touching, or even being touched.

IMPACT OF A DEFECTIVE PORTRAIT ON THE CHILD

Even the more transient and mild disorders in the mental portrait may cause profound mental anguish, but when there is an enduring and pervasive disorder, even a very resilient child will suffer pervasive and enduring personality disturbances. A defective portrait may also induce the onset and alter the course of many psychiatric disorders and physical illnesses—including those in which biological factors are usually preeminent. The deleterious impact of the defective parental mental portrait on a child's personality development can be formulated in many ways; three are very useful: (a) traumatic experiences have profound and enduring impact, (b) dysphoric experiences within parent-child interactions[a] have an incremental impact, and (c) the unique learning

experiences associated with internalization in love relationships—including projective identification and extractive identification—impose specific unconscious parental expectations on the personality of the child.

It is tempting to speculate that, in some cases involving very bad parenting of a vulnerable infant, global disturbances of brain function may be associated with deviations in postnatal structural development of the brain as well—deviations that could have long-term psychiatric and educational implications. Such a speculation is supported by the evidence that disturbances in the parental mental portrait can interfere with a child's central nervous system functioning enough to stop growth, precipitate asthma, diabetes, projectile vomiting, or dehydrating diarrhea. Further support comes from a variety of data derived from pediatrics and animal investigations, which document deviations in postnatal brain development associated with permanent significant abnormalities of perceptual and synthetic psychological functioning as a result of early and prolonged sensory deprivation or perceptual challenges. In addition, data associating child abuse, psychiatric disturbance, and neurobehavioral deviations in violent criminals are also suggestive, although it must not be forgotten that biologically damaged children are more likely to behave in ways that precipitate mistreatment by their caregivers.

Case illustration 1, describing Jason M., illustrates the devastating impact of a severe disorder of a parental mental portrait on a child in a family where child-rearing practices were by conventional standards "good enough."

CASE ILLUSTRATION 1: Jason M.

This case demonstrates the devastating psychiatric disorders, personality deviations, and physical problems that resulted when a vulnerable child was living with serious ongoing disorders in the emotional tone of the interactions with his parents, even while child-rearing practices were, for the most part, appropriate. Countertransference problems were responsible for the delay in diagnosing the parenting defect. The treatment reflects child advocacy and dual empathy. The father's defective mental portrait resolved, and the boy's situation was improved, but the mother's situation was so disturbed that she could not tolerate the psychodynamic parent psychotherapy, and the defective mental portrait of her son could not be repaired.

Case

Jason, age 7, was admitted to a combined medical and psychiatric research hospital ward for psychiatric evaluation and studies of his growth hormone regulation. He weighed 22 pounds and was 3 feet tall. (National averages for second graders are 50 pounds and 4 feet.) Prior to his admission to the hospital, Jason was spending long periods alone in his room, doing nothing but sitting on his bed—motionless and mute. He also had inconsolable screaming spells for no apparent reason, ate garbage, drank from toilet bowls, and ate his own vomitus. He almost never spoke at home and he usually acted unfriendly, angry, and demanding with his family.

As an infant, Jason had cried incessantly, rejected comfort, recoiled when held, ate so much that he vomited, and slept only during the day. In his 2nd year he clung to his mother and displayed frequent strong tempers with head banging and breath holding. During his 3rd year he became indifferent and listless, stopped growing, and developed the behavior problems that still were prominent 4 years later when he was hospitalized at age 7.

Jason's parents were middle class, educated, intelligent adults without any formally diagnosed, psychiatric disorder. They were "good enough" parents to their other children who were growing adequately and were well adjusted at home and at school. Before treatment, both mother and father accepted this bizarre situation almost without complaint. Supported by their pediatrician, they believed—without any supporting medical evidence—that Jason was brain damaged from birth and that, as a result, he could not help

---

[a] After Freud's rejection of the seduction theory, much psychoanalytic literature underestimated the role of the real parent on the child's experience; on the other hand, some recent literature underestimates the role of the child's distortions of memories of his or her parents (e.g., Masson (1984) and Miller (1991)). Psychoanalytic literature that appreciates the significant impact of the real parent without underestimating the influence of the child's fantasy and imagination on the child's mental experience of a parent includes the work of Bollas (1987, 1992), Miller (1981), Sperling (1974), and Sutherland (1980).

being self-centered, demanding, and unaffectionate. They did not physically abuse, sexually molest, or neglect Jason. After consulting their pediatrician, they had used child-rearing practices that were reasonable, considering their son's extreme behavior problems. In fact, they spent a lot of time trying to teach him self-help skills and appropriate social behavior.

Treatment Course

Once in the hospital, Jason was seen in individual psychotherapy, and his parents were seen in parent psychotherapy. He lived in a pediatric hospital environment with very intensive nursing, a school program and a ``child life'' program. Jason's abnormal growth hormone metabolism corrected itself (without medication) in days, and he began to grow at the rate of 1 cm per month. His social adjustment was excellent from the outset, his school work improved, and he was free of all his previous bizarre behavioral symptoms. There was no evidence of psychosis or brain damage of any kind. However, Jason's play therapy continued to reveal extensive abnormalities of his inner life, indicating deviant personality development.

Jason's father at first was perplexed when his son improved so rapidly in hospital, but he gradually recognized the family problems and accepted a psychosomatic formulation of the growth failure. He began to like Jason and to notice the boy's feelings. Jason's mother, on the other hand, became depressed, angry, and anxious as he improved—insisting that he was not really changing—even denying his measurable growth. As her anxiety escalated, she accused her husband and the medical staff of turning against her and lying about Jason's progress. She threatened to end the marriage. When she was not very angry, she was depressed with suicidal thoughts.

It became evident that the parents' detached, dehumanized view of their son as a brain-damaged retarded child had caused them to ignore Jason's loneliness and despair and their own sadness and anger. Jason no longer behaved like a brain-damaged child, Jason's father changed his impression of his son, but Jason's mother revealed a fixed ``negative portrait'' of Jason in her mind that she could neither change nor erase. She could see only his hidden anger and selfishness, completely mistrusting his sincere expressions of affection, sadness, and fear. She visited less and less often and was always angry when she did. Gradually, as treatment progressed, she relinquished her conscious conviction that Jason was possessed with evil; her overt anger diminished and she complained of feeling that there was a ``transparent wall'' between herself and her son. Yet, the discomfort they experienced with each other remained intolerable.

Mrs. M. confided that when he was still an infant she had developed a completely negative view of Jason and had been desperately frightened that he would ``destroy'' all she had obtained in life. She was self-critical and deeply depressed at the time, because she thought he was ``angry'' and ``disappointed'' with her. In our conversations she began to express her rage and to talk about fantasies in which she violently assaulted her son, attributing supernatural powers to him and using terms appropriate for a demon or an animal. As it turned out, Mrs. M.'s portrait of her son was modeled on similar sketches from her childhood, where she worked constantly but unsuccessfully for the approval and affection of her own depressed and bitter mother.

Comment

The outcomes of extremely serious cases, like this one, are variable. In some instances, it is possible to help parents as disturbed as Mrs. M. to alter significantly the character of the mental portrait of the child. In this case, however, Jason's mother was not able to tolerate the disorganizing impact of the treatment. Jason's mother and father decided, for reasons too complex to describe here, that Jason should live with supervised foster parents. The decision was experienced with great sadness by everyone, but it was accomplished in an atmosphere of honesty. While living in a foster home

where he came to be loved, and working in his own psychotherapy, Jason gradually began to understand that his mother's rejection was real and not imaginary, and that it was primarily the result of her own psychological problems and not because he was a bad or inadequate person.

PERSONAL RESPONSES OF THE CLINICIAN: COUNTERTRANSFERENCE

The enormous problems that clinicians have helping parents very often are the result of the strong emotional responses clinicians have to parenting problems. Surprisingly, even empathic, mature, experienced therapists working under favorable conditions experience emotional disturbances that are unusually frequent, severe, and tenacious, in response to parents who are hurting their children. These emotional disturbances impede the therapist's work in many ways; for example they lead therapists to overlook parenting problems in their evaluations, to recommend insufficient interventions, to lose empathy for parents in treatment, to assume a rigid prescriptive treatment style, or to allow the psychotherapy to drift away from the focus on parenting problems.

The countertransference reactions in parent therapy stem from many sources. It is painful to identify with a parent who is suffering in various ways. It is, also, painful to identify with the despair, rage, humiliation, and confusion of a child who is being hurt, because it reactivates early memories of being a hurt child, which are, in turn, associated with the superstitions, magical thinking, and unbearable global emotional states that are similar to fragmenting terror, homicidal rage, and hopeless despair. In addition, parents with character problems subject therapists to intense projective identifications that encourage empathic failures. All of these factors are difficult for qualified psychodynamic therapists, but not extraordinarily so. The most powerful factor creating countertransference errors in psychodynamic parent therapy is the intense psychic pain that is ubiquitously associated with the unusual demand placed on parent therapists to sustain dual empathy—simultaneous empathy for both a hurt child and a hurtful parent. The problem with this dual empathy is 2-fold—guilt associated with personal memories and existential anxiety. Dual empathy requires identifications that force a person to contemplate memories associated with guilt for hurting others in love relationships. While there are important differences among individuals, no one can avoid hurting others in love relationships, and no therapist, however empathic, kind, and mature, could ever become invulnerable to the guilt associated with memories of having hurt loved ones. Again, the most uncomfortable memories are those from early childhood, which are associated with primitive experiences of overwhelming, unforgiving, self-hating guilt and shame.

Dual empathy in the parent-child relationship creates an existential anxiety as well, because it forces a therapist to confront an aspect of our social reality that is universally ignored. Everyone denies, more or less, that the average, good enough person, in the course of his or her daily life, is responsible for regularly hurting even those people he or she loves, and for turning away from those who are being hurt by others. Thus, empathy for a parent who is hurting a child is very difficult to achieve, in part, because it demands that we embrace the partial responsibility we all bear for the ways we perpetrate or fail to oppose instances of mistreatment in the world.

Thus, simplistic and rigid moralism is central to most countertransference manifestations in this kind of therapy. Simplistic moralism leads therapists either to totally blame parents who are hurting their children or to totally exonerate them. In this way, therapists can avoid the pain associated with dual empathy. Simplistic moralism cannot be sustained without simplistic psychological thinking about the parent, the child, and the relationship.

A therapist who is blaming a parent may decide, inappropriately, that the parent has a severe character disorder. However, regardless of whether the character diagnosis is correct or not, a therapist committed to a simplistic moral position loses track of the psychological complexity of the parent's inner life in order to think of the parent, in a caricatured fashion, as a villain. Only a villain deserves unqualified blame, because he or she does not love a child and does not even try to honor conventional commitments to protect and nurture the child. Viewing the parent as a villain prohibits all empathy. In instances of blaming, therapists are not able to reliably overcome their anger, contempt, and frustration with the parents who persist in hurting their children.

Likewise, in the service of simplistic moral exoneration, therapists may minimize the parenting problem, especially by losing empathy for the child. Minimizing the parenting problem to exonerate a parent compromises any psychotherapy intended to address that parenting problem in a way that is self-evident. When therapists do remember the parenting problem accurately, they may still incorrectly exonerate parents without qualification by concluding that those parents have only the best intentions to love and treat their children well and are completely powerless to be less hurtful to those same children. In such instances, a parent may be caricatured psychologically as a helpless victim who is subject to the overwhelming power of unusual hardship—including a difficult child, as a martyr to the burdens of caring for a child that no parent could manage successfully, or as too incompetent, physically or mentally, to care for a child that most parents would enjoy.

Empathic failure associated with unqualified exoneration of the parent is less easy to comprehend than empathic failure associated with blaming; an appreciation of the various types of empathy and the components of the empathic process is needed. In contrast to instances of blaming, a therapist who simplistically exonerates a parent may retain a very full kind of empathy for many aspects of the parent's life experience outside the hurtful interactions with their child. In addition, an exonerating therapist may even maintain a capacity for some components of empathy for a parent's experience within the parent-child relationship. For example, the therapist may be able to intuitively share a parent's conscious experience of rage toward a crying child that can't be comforted.

However, the therapist who has completely exonerated a parent in the context of a countertransference disturbance will not be able to achieve a conceptual or imaginative empathy that encompasses the complexities and paradoxes that make up the unique conscious and unconscious subjective experiences of a hurtful parent who both loves and hates, and who is both victim of powerful forces and responsible perpetrator of mistreatment. For example, a therapist who simplistically exonerates a parent will not be able to share important aspects of guilt, shame, helplessness, or love that almost always accompany the rage that a hurtful parent consciously experiences for a crying child that cannot be comforted.

The impetus for a parent therapist to avoid the personal pain associated with dual empathy and to embrace simplistic moralism instead is so strong that the usual approaches to prevent and manage countertransference disturbances often turn out to be insufficient. A successful personal psychotherapy, although essential, cannot sufficiently eliminate the unconscious factors in therapists that stimulate such disturbances. Reducing the therapist's activity and increasing vigilance about following the ground rules limit some of the detrimental consequences, but do not adequately protect the therapy. Case consultations reduce the intensity of a particular disturbance transiently by clarifying or reinterpreting familiar unconscious factors that were already examined in a personal therapy, but the disturbances recur. Thus, additional approaches are needed.

It is suggested in this chapter that particular cognitive schemes can be used by a parent therapist to reduce countertransference and enhance empathy. Current psychoanalytic formulations clarify the role of conscious thought in the empathic process. Adequate empathy for a difficult psychotherapy is conceived to include much more than a therapist experiencing the affect of a parent without losing track of his or her separateness. Such empathy includes various kinds of conscious self-scrutiny, which is used primarily to detect and rectify various countertransference distortions and impediments. In addition, self-scrutiny is used to prepare

the way for a more complete kind of empathy that is sometimes referred to as imaginative imitation empathy (Buie, 1981). In this phase of empathy, a therapist actively and consciously projects his or her consciousness into the inner world of the parent, as an experiment in thinking and feeling, in order to intuitively grasp a more complete sense of the conscious and unconscious experience of that parent. The phase of self-scrutiny in empathy involves conscious cognitive processes. Thus, consciously held clinical schemes can be used by the parent therapist to support the empathic process and oppose countertransference. Four schemes that are particularly useful for this kind of therapy are briefly described below.

ATTRIBUTING MORAL RESPONSIBILITY TO A HURTFUL PARENT

An articulated, carefully reasoned attribution of moral responsibility to a parent for perpetrating harmful behavior toward the child is needed to help the therapist resist the simplistic moralism that is central to countertransference disturbances. In addition, therapists must be able to assess moral responsibility in order to guide parents to understand better their own conscious freedom of choice, responsibility, morality, and search for meaning, in the context of a treatment that primarily addresses unconscious mental phenomena.

The attribution of moral responsibility is very difficult to do accurately and constructively. Such an assessment requires systematic consideration of many different factors, including (*a*) intimate and extensive psychological data about powerful unconscious mental processes in the parent; (*b*) interpersonal, familial and other external forces impinging on the parent; (*c*) the degree of conscious awareness of the parenting problem; and (*d*) the relative freedom of choice that the parent had to act differently and to seek help in various contexts and at different times.

Even with such a full profile of data, it is very difficult to know how courageous and hard-working a parent has been at various times and in various contexts. Parents are often more desperate than they know and than anyone around them can tell at the time; also, acknowledging moral responsibility by relinquishing their own caricatured self-image of victim, martyr, or incompetent person can be extremely dangerous for some parents at some times in their lives. In view of these complexities, moral responsibility should be estimated initially, but then reevaluated often during the course of a treatment. The assessment should be done by the therapist, often with consultation, in a spirit of empathy and generosity.

A SCHEME OF VALID SCIENCE FOR PARENT THERAPY

It is suggested in this chapter that to help prevent the confused and simplistic psychological thinking that sustains the simplistic moralism of countertransference, a practical schematic summary of the nonreductionist paradigm of science that has emerged during this century should be kept in mind by the therapist. Epistemology is the area of philosophy concerned with the methods by which we know things and the grounds upon which we judge the limits and validity of what we know. A paradigm of scientific knowledge can be considered as one aspect of epistemological philosophy. The scientific paradigm of Newton and Descartes—dominant for the past 300 years of Western Civilization—tends to support the overly simplistic moralism involved in countertransference. In a fashion too complex to discuss in this chapter, the backbone of this scientific paradigm—experimentalism, reductionism, linear causation, objective neutrality, universalism, and radical materialism—are all factors that sustain countertransference and impede dual empathy in parent therapy (Ferholt et al., 1986; Hunter et al., 1991).

A new paradigm of science has been developed over the past century to correct logical and empirically demonstrated problems with the Newtonian-Cartesian approach. The contemporary approach is derived from work done in many disciplines (especially molecular physics, linguistics, cultural anthropology, psychology, literary criticism, and philosophy) and is now embraced by most philosophers and by many psychological theoreticians. The new paradigm of science is supportive of empathy and can be used to prevent and rectify countertransference reactions.

The modern paradigm is grounded in two fundamental assumptions about the limitations of our ability to know about the world. The first limitation stems from the knowledge that values, theories, and observations are always interacting, as are the observer and that which is being observed; the second, from the realization that while the world of external reality is infinite, the capacity of the human mind to apprehend is limited. Thus, every theory, mental model, or group of schematic statements, no matter how radical or extensive it attempts to be, must exclude most of the world. Since elements in the excluded realm affect elements in the sector of the world that is encompassed by the theory, every theory about some aspect of the world is inherently incomplete and to some extent incorrect (Harré, 1972; Koch, 1959–1963; Manicus and Secord, 1983). This contemporary paradigm is nonreductionist, systemic, value-based, and pragmatic; it is especially important to applications of the scientific method to psychological matters.

The reductionist paradigm of Newton dominated all science productively throughout the 17th, 18th, and 19th centuries of Western civilization almost without challenge, and it is still deeply ingrained in the traditions of scientific medicine and psychiatry. Unfortunately, the reductionist paradigm sustains countertransference at times of stress. Thus, without adopting a clinical scheme that outlines a contrasting paradigm of scientific thought, even the most intellectually and psychologically sophisticated parent therapists remain prone to engage in confused and simplistic thinking about a parent when there is strong internal pressure to avoid intense psychological pain.

The following six statements are recommended as a clinical scheme to insure valid scientific thinking in order to help psychodynamic parent therapists resist countertransference errors when their thinking is stressed by internal or external forces: (a) The conception of the whole cannot be reduced to the sum of its component parts, and summary statements about the parts of a whole cannot be subsumed by the conception of the whole (von Bertalanffy, 1968). For example, the parent-child relationship cannot be fully understood as a subunit of the family system; conversely, the family system cannot be fully understood by describing the marriage, the parent-child relationships, the sibling relationships, or each of the individual members. (b) The two domains of reality that are inherent in our thinking—mental reality (thoughts and feelings) and material reality (including behavioral and neurobiological phenomena)—are conceptually independent and equally valid. (c) Limited freedom of choice and moral responsibility are well-established "facts" within the domain of subjective experience (Searle, 1993). (d) The belief that sensory-based "empirical" research using the experimental design can be absolutely objective, value-free, or atheoretical is not valid. Thus, the experimental method is no longer thought to be the primary or superior building block of all valid and reliable knowledge of the world (i.e., science), but only one among many valuable kinds of systematic valid and reliable (scientific) approaches to observing and understanding the world, including mental and behavioral phenomena. (e) For most questions, especially those that are clinically important, causation in both material and psychological realms and at all levels of complexity is understood best within a model of dynamically interacting systems and subsystems. Thus, the relationship between "nature" and "nurture" in psychological development is interactive and complex, and the etiology of psychological disorders is multidetermined. (f) A theory is more or less true only in comparison to alternative theories and only in relation to a specific question (Ferholt et al., 1986). Therefore, well-accepted theories of psychological or behavioral causation developed around particular clinical or experimental questions should not be applied uncritically to very different clinical questions.

CHILD ADVOCACY: AN EXPLICIT TREATMENT GOAL

The primary treatment goal of psychodynamic parent psychotherapy suggested in this chapter is an explicit advocacy for the child's well-being, including a basic commitment to healthy qualities in the child's inner life. Child advocacy is suggested to buttress dual empathy for parent and child and to prevent the treatment from losing its focus on the parenting problem. Child advocacy also helps therapists to make the best treatment decisions when there is a moral dilemma created by a conflict of interest between parent and child. When therapists embrace child advocacy, they are making a moral commitment to work toward an optimal or "healthy" inner life for that child (O'Rourke et al., 1992), as defined by accepted norms of secular Western culture. Such norms are implicit in the aspects of child psychiatry, pediatrics, and child development, that are focused on achieving enduring changes in the mental life of children. Similarly, an implicit understanding of a "healthy" parental mental portrait is one that supports best the development of a healthy inner life for a child.

Many very useful clinical interventions for children or for parents are not primarily committed to enduring improvements in the child's inner life; they focus, instead, on ameliorating the child's overt behavioral and psychological symptoms and signs and restoring social adjustment. The ethical position implicit in such symptomatic treatments is legitimate, but different from that implicit in life-changing psychotherapies. Although the two ethical positions are usually complementary, they are sometimes incompatible. For example, in circumstances in which there is a parenting disorder, there may be a conflict between the two ethical positions, because the therapeutic goal for the child to achieve a good social adjustment to family life may be inconsistent with a primary commitment to relieve the child's inner pain or to support the development of healthy enduring patterns of inner life, usually referred to as personality. Similarly, as a practical matter, successful interventions to relieve symptoms and maladjustment often are associated with improvements in the child's inner life; however, sometimes they are not. For example, in some cases the child's inner life remains unhealthy although that child has become relatively asymptomatic. Thus, the child's personality development remains unprotected, although there may be acceptable social adjustment.

In practice, the evaluator uses the value-based child advocacy position to guide the decision to recommend psychodynamic parent psychotherapy in the first place. Similarly, during the course of a treatment in progress, it is used to decide when to encourage parents to engender personal risk and expense on behalf of their child. To make such treatment choices in an ethical fashion, the therapist must systematically balance costs and benefits considering the following factors (Hundert, 1987): (a) various accounts of the clinical situation as viewed from diverse perspectives, including many levels of organizational complexity (e.g., biological, psychological, behavioral, interpersonal, family, and social); (b) a wide variety of alternative actions including those from a diversity of theoretical and professional orientations (e.g., descriptive, psychoanalytic, cognitive-learning, existential, interpersonal and family systems); (c) the likely outcomes of such actions in the particular situation; (d) the likely risks and costs of such actions; and (e) at least six sources of relevant values—namely, the values of the parent in treatment, the psychiatrist's own values, and professional secular values of mental health (Sider, 1984), the values of any other parent, those of other important members of the family, and in some cases the values of the child as well.

The explicit advocacy position suggested in this scheme is the professional value position that allows a parent therapist to consciously and systematically do such a review of costs and benefits. Without an explicit scheme, the therapeutic goals remain implicit in parent therapy, and treatment decisions cannot be made fairly and intelligently. In addition, therapists are forced to make unavoidable ethical choices unilaterally and without sufficient disclosure to and consent from the parent(s) and sometimes the child as well. Thus, the essential trust in the therapeutic relationship is betrayed.

MODEL OF THE PSYCHOTHERAPEUTIC MENTAL STANCE

A model representing the frame of mind of the working therapist—the psychotherapeutic mental stance—is used in this approach to oppose the simplistic, rigid, and inappropriate application of various aspects of theory to the particular clinical problem at hand, because this mode of thinking is inadvertently used by parent therapists to mask and sustain countertransference. The tenets that are inappropriately applied by parent therapists to mask countertransference include all encompassing theories of personality development and the etiology of mental illness, doctrine associated with established schools of psychotherapy, specific therapeutic techniques and ground rules, and the results of selected systematic research.

The psychotherapeutic clinical stance is used in this scheme to refer to the general frame of mind that a therapist regularly assumes when performing this therapy. The stance draws upon many aspects of a therapist's personality. It is a version of that personality—a second self (Schafer, 1983)—that is shaped especially for a particular psychotherapeutic role. The therapeutic stance is quite consistent in any single therapist whenever he or she is at work, and it is relatively consistent in its main features among similar therapists doing the same kind of psychotherapy.

The stance is conceived to be the entire collection of enduring mental qualities, conscious and unconscious, that define the therapist's frame of mind at work. The stance includes, but is not limited to, those areas usually addressed in conventional psychodynamic theory in discussions of the therapeutic attitude. Thus, it is conceived to include consciously held scientific theories and knowledge, but much more as well. Three interacting aspects, in addition to theory and knowledge, are most often cited as especially important: (a) the real relationship or alliance with the parent, (b) the quality of the therapist's attention, and (c) the background emotional tone in the therapist's mind.

The quality of the stance in a particular therapist is dependent on many personality characteristics, including: maturity, wisdom, self-acceptance, self-knowledge, decency, personal ethics, personal views on scientific knowledge, self-discipline, and accrued personal experience. It is also dependent on many qualities of the therapist as a trained clinician, including general and specifically relevant scientific knowledge, favorite explanatory theories, unconscious assumptions acquired through professional experiences, and a repertoire of accrued clinical experience. However, all these personal and professional qualities are organized into a working stance around a cognitive framework built from a small group of theoretical schemes that the therapist has adopted to understand the clinical problem and the method selected to address that problem.

The various theories that are central to the organization of a therapist's stance are referred to as clinical theory in this discussion. A parent therapist regularly brings such clinical theory to mind in order to generate the best therapeutic stance and then strives to keep such theory near the front of his or her mind while engaging in a psychodynamic parent treatment in order to sustain that therapeutic stance even when under pressure. The clinical theory used in the stance is different from explanatory theory, findings in basic research, and psychoanalytic meta-theory in several ways. It is designed and evaluated in reference only to how well it helps to generate and sustain the best stance to accomplish selected goals for a particular group of patients with certain problems within a circumscribed range of clinical circumstances. In addition, it is designed pragmatically and particularly to serve a specific group of therapists using a particular set of available ideas and material resources.

The best clinical theory to support a stance for any psychotherapy needs to be practical, guiding the therapist's thinking by addressing three areas especially: (a) the nature of the particular clinical problem, which is, in this case, the defect in parenting; (b) the primary method selected to solve that clinical problem, which is, in this case, psychodynamic parent psychotherapy; and (c) the problems known to commonly impede the particular psychotherapy, which are, in this case, primarily manifestations of countertransference and moral dilemmas.

Even more specifically, the best clinical theory for psychodynamic parent psychotherapy is that theory that helps to create and sustain a frame of mind that will help a therapist to interact with a parent in a way that will repeatedly produce corrective transient states in that par-

ent's mind that will ultimately promote the growth of more enduring constructive characteristics. Such characteristics will, in turn, help the parent to interact with his or her child in ways that will repeatedly produce corrective transient states and then more enduring healthy personality qualities in that child—the ultimate goal of that particular parent therapy.

In most complicated psychotherapies, clinical theory is constructed best using ideas from many sources that are combined pluralistically (Havens, 1987)—not eclectically or syncretically. The best set of clinical theories for this kind of parent therapy relies especially on psychoanalysis, but it is not the simple application of psychoanalytic meta-theory. The general principles of therapeutic action developed for conventional insight-oriented psychodynamic individual psychotherapy of adult patients are still the main elements of the method of psychodynamic parent therapy; however, these principles are not sufficient. They must be modified and supplemented by the clinical schemes outlined in this chapter. Psychological formulations from outside analysis, clinical approaches from other established schools of psychiatry, and philosophical and ethical notions from outside of psychiatry are important ingredients.

Psychodynamic technical guidelines, the results of various kinds of systematic research, and many psychological theories of causation are indispensable to the work. These ideas are not applied directly. Instead, they are applied from within the therapeutic frame of mind organized around the central clinical theory outlined in this chapter. In this way, all general psychological theory and knowledge is subordinated to idiosyncratic pragmatic realities and the value-based goals of the particular treatment. The scheme of a therapeutic stance organized around clinical theory is used to help the parent therapist to avoid errors in practice that result from the inappropriate use of concepts to avoid the pain associated with dual empathy for the child and the parent.

PRACTICAL SUGGESTIONS FOR THE INITIAL PHASES OF TREATMENT

Severe disturbances in the parent-child relationship without overt abuse are often overlooked when the clinical evaluation of a child fails to include data revealing the thoughts and feelings of the parents and child about the relationship, along with direct observations of the emotional tone of their interactions. There are situations in which the evaluator should consider recommending psychodynamic parent psychotherapy although a parenting disorder is not the reason the evaluation was initiated; for example, in some cases when a psychiatric disorder is found in the child, parent therapy may be recommended initially, or after another kind of effective psychiatric treatment has ameliorated the child's symptoms, but not sufficiently improved a parenting problem. Psychodynamic parent therapy may be the best recommendation for some adults that complain of marital problems, or psychiatric symptoms, especially during pregnancy, the postpartum period, or during their child's adolescence.

Although a variety of possible arrangements can work for psychodynamic parent psychotherapy, in general, both parents should be involved in the treatment (conjointly, individually, or both). Too often, fathers still are neglected in or excluded from treatment (Ferholt and Gurwitt, 1982). Occasional sessions including the children and their parents, and sessions of the whole family are useful, but the children should most often be seen in concurrent individual therapies of their own, even if they are participating in family sessions, are not obviously disturbed, or are very young.

When it is clear that a parent has serious psychopathology, it is helpful for the parent therapist to insist at the outset on an individual therapy for the vulnerable parent, in addition to and concurrently with the parent therapy. Serious family crises do occur regularly in these treatments, and some are serious enough to cause concern about murder, suicide, divorce, a major psychiatric episode in a family member, or extrusion of the child (or one of the parents) from the family. In such cases, it is best if therapists arrange ongoing consultation to help them persevere as an advocate for the child's inner life.

PRACTICAL SUGGESTIONS FOR ONGOING TREATMENT

The therapist should deliberately strive to enhance a parent's self-respect in this kind of psychodynamic treatment by expressing appreciation for the parent's courage and discipline in the therapy and by identifying the stressors impinging on the parent and the pain associated with them. There are a growing number of psychotherapists who emphasize the interactive nature of the therapeutic relationship and who use carefully selected countertransference disclosures in their psychotherapy work (Bollas, 1987; Little, 1981; Searles, 1979; Tansey, 1989). Such disclosures can be especially helpful in psychodynamic parent psychotherapy by utilizing the ubiquitous intense countertransference disturbances to model a very important way that a parent can act to ameliorate the damage done to a child in the parent-child interactions and to enhance a parent's self-respect by seeing an esteemed therapist admit error without excessive shame or guilt.

Therapists should educate some parents to help them develop a parenting stance guided by the same ethical and psychological tenets underlying the parent psychotherapy. Such a parenting stance can be applied constructively to family decision-making and to a parent's conduct in interactions with a child. For example, when a child feels hurt and acts sullen or angry in response to a parent's behavior, it is not useful for the parent to view the event simply as a matter of the parent behaving inappropriately, nor simply as a matter of a child being overly sensitive. Rather, it is most useful to think of the interaction in terms of shared responsibility.

Often in such instances, a parent should learn ways to acknowledge responsibility for behaving in a way that hurt his or her child, even if the parent's behavior is conventionally appropriate, would not have hurt most children, or even this child at other times. Acknowledging responsibility for hurting the child may even be the best course for a parent who has acted only in response to angry, rude or destructive behavior from the child. Parents are advised to extend themselves to their children in this way to accommodate the vulnerability of children who feel insecure about themselves and/or unsafe in the relationship and the world. Many children are too vulnerable to think or talk about their part in an interaction until after their parents first concede some regret for hurting them. While these are simple truths, applying them over and over again in the context of the trials and tribulations of every day family life is extremely difficult.

In some cases, the therapist must also teach parents to avoid circumstances that elicit destructive states of mind, to recognize destructive mental states early when they inadvertently recur, and to manage them with discipline. (Ironically, this often requires that the parent recruit the help of others including at times the child who may have provoked the very state that the parent is trying to manage.)

CASE ILLUSTRATION 2: Douglas T.

This case illustrates the course of a parent treatment relatively free of countertransference disturbance. Dual empathy is sustained in good part because the therapist has adopted the clinical schemes purposed in this chapter. The actual implementation of a scheme to resist countertransference or to solve a moral dilemma is not as well illustrated in a successful treatment as it might be in a case illustrating a treatment failure. This case also demonstrates the characteristics of a more subtle disorder in the emotional tone of the parent-child relationship than that in Jason M.

Case

Douglas, age 7 years, in the 2nd grade, lived with a 3-year-old sister, an infant brother, and his parents who were both college edu-

cated, professionally trained, and financially secure. Over the past year, he had gradually developed an oppositional defiant disorder with anxiety symptoms. Douglas had early indications of poor neurobehavioral self-regulation, and as he grew older, he was unusually intolerant of frustrations and transitions, and prone to brief periods of exaggerated developmental anxieties, unusual fears, and withdrawal associated with sadness and self-criticism. On the other hand, Douglas also showed evidence of intrinsic resilience and acquired competence.

Douglas's psychiatric disorder developed in association with parenting problems and marital discord at the time his parents were forced to cope with severe environmental stressors. Both parents were competent and well-motivated; they wanted to address the family problems before they asked Douglas to be in a treatment. Thus, the initial child psychiatry intervention selected in this case was a parent psychotherapy, performed during weekly, 50-minute sessions, almost always attended by both parents.

Therapy

A trusting therapeutic relationship was built with both parents during the first months in the course of gathering data, discussing formulation and diagnosis, seeking solutions to pressing management problems, and providing a cognitive framework for sustaining empathy and understanding for Douglas. This was a kind of psychoanalytically informed psychoeducation offering a clinical theory of parenting to help create a better mental stance in the parents when they were interacting with their son. The parent counseling also focused on the organization of family life, the collaboration of the parents, and the practical management of difficult situations involving Douglas.

The parents came to feel less frightened, confused, and self-critical about their parenting, improved the schedule and behavioral rules within the household, criticized each other less, and arranged for the father to spend more time with his son and to take more leadership in discipline. They learned to anticipate difficult periods for their son, to avoid some, to prepare him better for others, and to respond more constructively when he did get very upset.

They also learned an unconventionally generous way to respond to their son's oppositional defiant behavior, based on an interactive interpretation that his symptomatic behavior depended on one-sided interpretations of their actions. They did this while sustaining a clear-cut although attenuated set of limits and expectations associated with unnegotiable, enforceable, reasonable consequences for transgressions. Over time, Douglas began to seem more comfortable and to behave better.

The nature and procedure of psychodynamic psychotherapy were explained, and gradually the conversations in the therapeutic sessions shifted focus to feelings the parents had for each other, those they each had when Douglas behaved in ways that hurt them, and those associated with their early memories about Douglas. The father's negative feelings, once exposed, were easily modified. Douglas's mother, on the other hand, discovered intense feelings of frustration, deprivation, guilt, shame, and anxiety in association with a tendency to slip into a frame of mind dominated by an ego-alien prejudice that reflected a negative mental portrait of her son. In this primarily unconscious frame of mind, Douglas was a self-centered, ungrateful, manipulative, dishonest, immoral person who was dominating, exploiting, and abusing her because she was not good enough for him no matter how hard she tried to make him happy. He dominated her by provoking her guilt, threatening to hurt her, and threatening to abandon her.

A crisis in the mother developed as she experienced an onslaught of very uncomfortable thoughts and feelings about interactions with her parents, now and in her difficult childhood. With a great deal of support from her husband at home and in the sessions, a strong relationship with the therapist, the help of several dear old friends, and a brief course of antidepressant medication, she managed to sustain herself during a period of intense grieving associated with uncovering very painful repressed memories of early experiences and a reconsideration of her current experiences with her parents. As the conversations about her past were elaborated, the therapist guided them to retain a focus on Douglas, and the connections between the feelings and thoughts she had about her mother and her son emerged without interpretation.

Over the time this work was being done in therapy, dramatic improvements occurred in the tone of the interactions between Douglas and both parents, his oppositional defiant disorder was resolved, his dysphoria was reduced significantly, and he became more expansive in his life outside the family. After 18 months (approximately 70 sessions) the parents were ready to stop the conjoint parent psychotherapy, and Douglas's mother decided to seek her own individual psychotherapy.

Comment

The psychiatric disorder in this child may well have been ameliorated by any one of a variety of interventions, or it may have even dissipated spontaneously when the stress on the parents decreased. Thus, the parent-child relationship would have improved as well; however, it is argued in this chapter that without a psychodynamic parent psychotherapy the improvements in the parent-child relationships would have, most likely, been more narrow, superficial, and transient, and the child's personality development would have been compromised.

CONCLUSIONS

In conclusion, a disorder of a parent's mental portrait of a child is always painful and destructive. If it is severe and persistent, it can create a tormented inner life for the child, destroy the qualities of personality we value in this culture, and contribute to the creation of an adult prone to crush the inner lives of others. Child psychiatrists and other mental health professionals responsible for children should (*a*) be proficient at discerning the presence of parenting disorders even in the absence of deviant child-rearing practices, (*b*) be competent at performing psychodynamic parent psychotherapy, and (*c*) engage parents in this kind of treatment more often. As advocates for the inner life of children, they should insist on such treatment when it is appropriate—even if health care managers try to promote only less expensive interventions focused on symptom reduction and social adjustment.

Acknowledgments. *The author wishes to acknowledge his appreciation to Robert J. Hoffnung and David E.K. Hunter who contributed to the preparation of this manuscript and extensively to the development of the ideas contained in it.*

References

Ackerman NW: *The Psychodynamics of Family Life.* New York, Basic Books, 1958.

Bollas C: *The Shadow of the Object: Psychoanalysis of the Unthought Known.* New York, Columbia University Press, 1987.

Bollas C: *Being a Character.* New York, Hill & Wang, 1992.

Bruner J: *Approaches to the Mind.* New York, Basic Books, 1990.

Bugental JFT: *The Search for Existential Identity.* San Francisco, Jossey-Bass, 1976.

Buie DH: Empathy: Its nature and limitations. *J Am Psychoanal Assoc* 29:281–307, 1981.

Coleman RW, Kris E, Provence S: The study of variations of early parental attitudes: A preliminary report. *Psychoanal Study Child* 7:20–47, 1953.

Eagle NE: *Recent Developments in Psychoanalysis: A Critical Evaluation.* New York, McGraw-Hill, 1984.

Engel GL: *Psychological Development in Health and Disease.* Philadelphia, Saunders, 1962.

Ferholt JB: A type of infant crisis. Presented November 22, 1976 at the fifth meeting of the National Advisory Council for Clinical Infant Programs at Mental Health Study Center, National Institute of Mental Health, Adelphi, MD.

Ferholt JB, Gurwitt AR: Involving fathers in treatment. In: Cath SH, Gurwitt AR, Ross JM (eds): *Father and Child: Developmental and Clinical Perspectives.* Boston, Little, Brown, 1982, pp. 557–568.

Ferholt JB, Hoffnung RJ, Hunter DEK, et al: Clinical investigators under severe stress: A critique of Garmezy's commentary. *J Am Acad Child Adolesc Psychiatry* 25:724–727, 1986.

Ferholt JB, Rotnem DL, Genel M, et al: A psychodynamic study of psychosomatic dwarfism: A syndrome of depression, personality disorder, and impaired growth. *J Am Acad Child Psychiatry* 24:49–57, 1985.

Flax J: Treating psychoanalysis: Feminist and postmodernist impulses within psychoanalytic theories and practices. Presented April 9, 1994 at annual scientific symposium of the Western New England Psychoanalytic Society at New Haven, CN.

Gill MM: The interpersonal paradigm and the degree of the therapist's involvement. *Contemp Psychoanal* 19:200–237, 1983.

Greenson RR: Empathy and its vicissitudes. *Int J Psychoanal* 4:418–424, 1960.

Harré R: *Philosophies of Science.* Oxford, England, Cambridge University Press, 1972.

Havens L: *Approaches to the Mind.* Cambridge, MA, Harvard University Press, 1987.

Hundert EM: A model for ethical problem solving in medicine, with practical applications. *Am J Psychiatry* 144:839–846, 1987.

Hunter DEK, Ferholt JB, Hoffnung RJ: Back to the future: In search of a psychodynamic family therapy in the treatment of families of individuals with prolonged mental illness. *J Fam Psychother* 2:81–96, 1991.

Kernberg OF: *Internal World and External Reality.* New York, Jason Aronson, 1982.

Klein M: Notes on some schizoid mechanisms. *Int J Psychoanal* 33:433–438, 1946.

Koch S: *Psychology: A Study of a Science* (Vol 1–6). New York, McGraw-Hill, 1959–1963.

Langs R: *Psychotherapy: A Basic Text.* New York, Jason Aronson, 1982.

Little MI: *Transference Neurosis and Transference Psychosis.* New York, Jason Aronson, 1981.

Manicus PT, Secord PF: Implications for psychology for the new philosophy of science. *Am Psychol* 38:399–413, 1983.

Margoles A: *The Empathic Imagination.* New York, Norton, 1989.

Masson JM: *The Assault on Truth: Freud's Suppression of the Seduction Theory.* New York, Macmillan, 1984.

Miller A: *Prisoners of Childhood: How Narcissistic Parents Form and Deform the Emotional Lives of Their Gifted Children.* New York, Basic Books, 1981.

Miller A: *Breaking Down the Wall of Silence: The Liberating Experience of Facing Painful Truth.* New York, Penguin Books, 1991.

O'Rourke K, Snider BW, Thomas JM, et al: Knowing and practicing ethics. *J Am Acad Child Adolesc Psychiatry* 31:393–396, 1992.

Schafer R: *The Analytic Attitude.* New York, Basic Books, 1983.

Schafer R: *Retelling a Life.* New York, Basic Books, 1992.

Scheirer HA: The perversion of mothering: Munchausen syndrome by proxy. *Bull Menninger Clin* 56:421–437, 1992.

Searle J: *The Rediscovery of the Mind.* Boston, MIT Press, 1993.

Searles HF: The patient as therapist to his analyst. In: Searles HF (ed): *Countertransference and Related Subjects.* New York, International Universities Press, 1979.

Sperling M: *The Major Neuroses and Behavior Disorders in Children.* New York, Jason Aronson, 1974.

Sider RC: The ethics of therapeutic modality choice. *Am J Psychiatry* 141:390–394, 1984.

Spence DP: *Narrative Truth and Historical Truth.* New York, Norton, 1982.

Stern D: *The Interpersonal World of the Infant: A View from Psychoanalysis and Development Psychology.* New York, Basic Books, 1985.

Stierlin H: *Psychoanalysis and Family Therapy.* New York, Jason Aronson, 1977.

Sutherland JD: The British object relations theorists: Balint, Winnicott, Fairbain, and Guntrip. *Am J Psychoanal* 28:829–860, 1980.

Tansey MJ, Burke WP: *Understanding Countertransference.* Hillsdale, NJ, McGraw-Hill, 1989.

Vogel EF, Bell NW: The emotionally disturbed child as the family scapegoat. In: Bell NW, Vogel EF (eds): *A Modern Introduction to the Family.* Glencoe, NY, Free Press, 1960, pp. 389–397.

von Bertalanffy L: *General Systems Theory.* New York, Braziller, 1968.

Zeanah CH, Benoit D, Hirshberg L, et al: A structured interview to assess mother's representations of their infants. Presented September 22, 1989 at the 4th World Congress of the World Association of Infant Psychiatry and Development at Lugano, Switzerland.

Zinner J, Shapiro RL: Projective identification as a mode of perception and behavior in families of adolescents. *J Psychoanalysis* 53:523–530, 1972.

81 THE PSYCHOTHERAPIES: A CRITICAL OVERVIEW

John Scott Werry, M.D., and Leah K. Andrews, M.B., Ch.B., F.R.A.N.Z.C.P.

The power of one person to comfort, to teach, or to influence others is a universal part of human experience, or in short has incontrovertible face validity. Psychotherapy is merely an attempt to capture this power within a healing context, to systematize it so that it becomes transmissible (and researchable) and to regulate it in a helping professional relationship for the protection of the consumer and therapist alike. In this section on treatment, there are a number of chapters addressing the various kinds of psychotherapy used with children and adolescents. In general, these chapters focus on the theory, practice, and clinical indications of particular methods. Beneficence of outcome, and an established place in the therapeutic armamentarium and in teaching programs in child and adolescent psychiatry, is largely assumed.

In this review, the field of psychotherapy is examined as a whole and subjected to critical scrutiny using the assumptions and value systems accepted in medicine and other helping professions—that is, the best way to establish efficacy and safety and to advance theory is through the scientific method, based on the null hypothesis, or as Bertrand Russell put it, not doubt, but dogmatic doubt.

However, the scientific basis of medicine is rather recent and made possible only by enormous growth first in the physical and then biological sciences during the last two centuries. Yet medicine is as old as the first civilizations, all of which have defined certain individuals as healers and expected them to care for—and cure—the sick and the dying whether they had the knowledge to do so or not. Given the lack of effectiveness and down right noxiousness of most medical remedies until the 20th century, the wonder is that medicine survived at all as a profession. Cynics might say that this is due mostly to the patient's fear of death and need to believe in a saviour and to the skill of the medical profession in disguising its impotence and chicanery, as portrayed by Racine, George Elliott, and Mark Twain among others. But also important in the continued survival of the medical profession is what is portrayed in the famous, if sentimental, 19th century painting "The Doctor" in the Tate Gallery in London in which late at night, a doctor sits, thoughtful and troubled, at the bedside of a sick child. It is said that the painter, Sir Luke Fildes, executed this work in gratitude for the most attentive care given to his child. (The fact that the child died, does not seem to have diminished this gratitude!) The physician was perceived as trying all remedies, but more importantly, as being there when needed and showing care and concern.

Medicine is thus equally a humanistic and a scientific profession, and the spectacular growth in technological knowledge has been matched, it seems, by increasing public concern about the diminution in personalized, humanistic care. In addition to its own value system, medicine is influenced by the political, economic, and cultural ecosystem that shapes its form and dictates its execution. It is thus necessary to temper any critique of what doctors do, with due consideration for all these factors beside the scientific.

Psychotherapy has some distinctive features that differentiate it from many other medical treatments. First, its practice is not limited by statute to licensed physicians, and there are those who will argue that the rules of medicine thus do not apply. However, it can be said equally that physicians who practice psychotherapy are still so obligated, and that should be one of the discernible differences between psychiatrists and nonmedical professionals. Second, while medicine did originally depend on charisma and caste to establish validity of treatment, this has gradually faded considerably in favor of hard data from well-designed clinical trials. For a variety of reasons, some of which reflect the sheer complexity of the subject though others are less worthy, traditional child psychotherapy was and is still largely dependent on charismatic leaders and innovators rather than on data (Werry, 1989).

ABOUT THIS REVIEW

Some terms need defining. *Psychotherapy* further unspecified encompasses all kinds of such treatment that are united by the common goal of healing within a professional relationship using psychological means alone, independent of the technique or underpinning theory, whether psychodynamic, client-centered, behavioral, individual, play, group, family, brief and long term, and so on. While the use of this generic term may appear simplistic or even demeaning, there is both utility and good reason for doing so. First, research has demonstrated that much of the therapeutic power stems from a set of variables common to all kinds of psychotherapy however different they may seem. Second, many kinds of child psychotherapy are insufficiently explicated to examine their putative differences from each other. Third, there are insufficient data to examine all kinds of child psychotherapy individually, and aggregating studies is necessary to get sufficient statistical power. Finally, those who think that their kind of psychotherapy is superior, despite insufficient data to support their contention, may be motivated to do the studies necessary to prove the point.

Unless otherwise stated, psychotherapy is described as applied to children. *Child* is taken to include infants, children, and adolescents.

This is not an exhaustive review of psychotherapy. Detailed analysis of individual studies is not undertaken since these already exist (e.g., Barrnett et al., 1991; Casey and Berman, 1985; Fauber and Long, 1991; Hazelrigg et al., 1987; Hengeller et al., 1993; Kazdin, 1991, 1993; Kovacs and Paulauskas, 1986; Ollendick, 1986; Tramontana, 1980; Shirk and Russell, 1992; Weisz and Weiss, 1993; Weisz et al., 1987, 1992). Rather, some basic questions are posed and some of these reviews used in response. The answers are cast in terms of their implications for research, training, and practice in child psychiatry. The most recent reviews (Weisz et al., 1995; Weisz, Donenberg, et al., in press; Weisz, Weiss, et al., in press) appeared too late to include details here but their content only underlines the questions posed and strengthens the answers.

SOME FUNDAMENTAL QUESTIONS ABOUT PSYCHOTHERAPY

1. Can psychotherapy be validly researched?
2. Does psychotherapy work?
3. If it works, just how good is it?
4. Is psychotherapy better than placebo?
5. Is one kind of psychotherapy better than another?
6. Can psychotherapy be taught?
7. Is more psychotherapy better than less?
8. Is psychotherapy better for some children than for others?
9. Is psychotherapy safer than biological therapies?
10. Is psychotherapy acceptable to consumers?
11. Is psychotherapy cost-effective?
12. Should psychotherapy be taught, and if so, in child psychiatry training?

1. Can Psychotherapy Be Validly Researched?

As all the cited reviews show, one of the more persistent problems in evaluating psychotherapy is the lack of sufficient good research to answer the questions under discussion. There are those who believe that psychotherapy is unmeasurable since it concerns the elemental nature of human beings not only within the individual, but also as interacting with others such as parents or therapists. Indeed, this argument was used to dismiss the findings of some of the first attempts to evaluate psychotherapy such as the American Institute of Psychoanalysis study of the 1960s. Most of the good research on traditional individual psychotherapy with children (excluding behavior therapy) was done in a flurry of optimism between 1963 and 1973 (Barrnett et al., 1991), with only a few since (see Weisz, Weiss, et al., in press). This suggests disillusionment with the results and the enormity of the task. The rise in popularity of competing methods like behavior therapy and family therapy may also be partly responsible for the siphoning off of both interest and serious researchers.

No one doubts that the task of researching psychotherapy is extremely complex and, as with applied research in humans, very difficult to pursue, but that should be a challenge not a deterrent. Science operates by removing only one skin of the infinitely layered onion of Nature at a time, and though the task will never be complete, the success of science in our everyday lives is there for all to see. Is any research about psychotherapy better than nothing? Clearly, if the result is meaningless nonsense, or worse, misleading sense, the answer must be no. But the rules for good psychotherapy research were set out many years ago (Heinecke and Strassman, 1975), and methodology by which to enact these rules, especially that derived from adult psychotherapy, have advanced considerably since then (Barrnett et al., 1991; Kazdin, 1991; Shirk and Russell, 1992). Add to this advances in the technology of measurement in psychiatry as a whole and in adult psychotherapy (Bergin and Garfield, 1994; Kazdin, 1991) and in other areas of child psychiatry (e.g., psychopharmacology), and there is now a formidable body of knowledge to facilitate this process.

However, there is a more compelling argument, which is being given increasing momentum by underwriters of health services (Krupnick and Pincus, 1992). The difference between an informal or even paid transaction between two persons in which one tries to share and relieve the burdens of another, and that between a psychiatrist and a patient, is that the psychiatrist is a physician bound by the rules of the profession and incurs certain privileges (most conspicuously status and higher fees) as a result. It would be hard to argue that a physician is not now bound by the following requirements: (*a*) The first treatments offered should be any that are known to be effective and safe. (*b*) If these are not available or have been tried and found ineffective, before pursuing other treatments, the degree of suffering or disability must be unsupportable and likely to continue to be so without treatment. (*c*) The consumer must be fully apprised of the uncertain nature of the treatment. These principles are illustrated to some degree in the case of *Oshoroff v. Chestnut Lodge* (Klerman, 1990), in which it was argued that Oshoroff was wrongly given psychotherapy instead of electroconvulsive therapy (ECT).

In any case, a reviewer does not get the sense from serious writers on psychotherapy (apart from gurus) that the dearth of good research in most forms of psychotherapy, except behavior therapy, is due to lack of tools to do the job (e.g., Barrnett et al., 1991; Shirk and Russell, 1992, 1995). What appears to be lacking is the will. While those who would defend child psychotherapy, especially the traditional forms, on the grounds that it has not been adequately studied (e.g., Shirk and Russell, 1992), such research as there is with children suggests that the findings do not differ qualitatively from the much vaster, more robust, and more active field of psychotherapy research in adults (Kazdin, 1991, 1993). Thus, it is possible to draw on this fund of knowledge (e.g., Andrews, 1993) to make tentative statements for child psychotherapy where child data are inadequate. Further, the issues of methodological

complexity and shortcomings in studies have been overstated. It has been shown (Weiss and Weisz, 1990; Weisz et al., 1995b) that even when the effect of methodological flaws are partialled out in meta-analyses, substantial effects of psychotherapy are still discernible.

There is one serious criticism that clinicians may legitimately level at research in psychotherapy—in order to meet the requirements of rigor (and publication within the time span imperative to success in promotion, reputation, and grantsmanship!): There is little resemblance between what researchers study and what practitioners do (Kazdin, 1991, Weisz et al., 1992). For example, Kazdin (1991) listed seven major differences such as subject recruitment, locus, duration and theoretical orientation of treatment, and involvement of parents. There is also the issue of adequate follow-up since delayed (sleeper) effects have been demonstrated (Kazdin, 1993). The answer to this problem seems to be clear—there is a need for practitioners to research themselves or actively promote and assist in the process, rather than have unfriendly and ununderstanding researchers speaking for what they do. If psychotherapists fail to do this, then they have no right to complain that research rarely reflects the real world of clinical practice. How to bridge this gap has been discussed in detail by Weisz, Donenberg, et al. (in press).

2. Does Psychotherapy Work?

There is enough research in over 200 studies to be able to give a tentatively affirmative answer to this question (Kazdin, 1991). With the exception of one reviewer (Levitt, 1957, 1963), all others, especially the meta-analyses (Barrnett et al., 1991; Weisz et al., 1987, 1992; Weisz, Weiss, et al., in press) involving over 250 studies, conclude that, *independent of the kind of psychotherapy, treatment is better than no treatment*. Some have been concerned that this comforting convergence of results conceals serious problems of methodology, which either inflate the efficacy (Shirk and Russell, 1992, 1995) or raise doubts about the validity of conclusions (Barrnett et al., 1991; Heinecke and Strassman, 1975). While these concerns do have some legitimacy, as already noted they have been overstated, especially when there are sufficient studies for a meta-analysis (Weiss and Weisz, 1990; Weisz et al., 1995). Thus, it seems quite in order to say that the evidence *does* favor efficacy and thus that the practitioner can claim that psychotherapy is a *legitimate treatment*, though, as will be seen below, this statement is subject to caveats regarding for whom, for how long, and for which kinds of psychotherapy.

3. If It Works, Just How Good Is It?

If, as just concluded, psychotherapy is better than no psychotherapy, just how often is it so and to what degree? In their meta-analysis of over 100 studies, Weisz et al. (1987) found the effect size was 0.79, that is, that 79% of children were better off treated than not, a very substantial proportion. Only 6% of children were made worse. In clinical practice then, this means that the odds of psychotherapy helping are very high—provided, of course, that approximately the same criteria for selecting patients used in most studies are applied—which they are not (Kazdin, 1991), though the algebraic summation of these differences is probably zero, since some would favor and others disadvantage practice. This may explain why Weisz et al. (1987) did not find much difference between genuine clinic and "analog" studies (e.g., recruited subjects).

However, the actual *amount* of benefit produced is less impressive, accounting for less than 20% of the outcome variance (Weiss and Weisz, 1990). This suggests that the *average effect* of psychotherapy is rather small, though most practitioners would probably consider a 20% improvement as realistic and valuable. It should be noted too, as discussed in more detail below under cost/benefit, that the measures used may not do justice to the flow on effects of psychotherapy beyond mere clinical improvement.

4. Is Psychotherapy Better Than Placebo?

In his review of adult psychotherapy, Andrews (1993) points out that, while psychotherapy has been demonstrated to be better than no treatment, there are few studies that try to find out if psychotherapy is better than "placebo" or, in short, has effects not solely dependent on expectancy, ordinary human caring, status of the therapist, and what Andrews calls "good clinical care." Even in adult psychotherapy, this question remains unanswerable (Andrews, 1993). Of all the psychotherapies, behavior therapy has by far the greatest amount of evidence to suggest that its effect extends beyond mere placebo (Andrews, 1993), though there are those who would query the clinical relevance of some of its effects.

Nearly all the studies of child psychotherapy compare its effects against no treatment or alternative forms of psychotherapy, making estimate of the placebo effect impossible. Kazdin (1991) points out that it is extremely difficult to design effective placebo-type procedures. For example, how does the researcher ensure that therapists have the same commitment and enthusiasm to the placebo as practicing therapists have to their treatment? What are the ethical and legal implications of common placebo conditions such as random assignment to treatment/no treatment? These issues may be complex but cannot be avoided. If differences between placebo and psychotherapy emerge, then second stage research to tease out the variables responsible for the superiority becomes economically and ethically justifiable.

There are other possible indicators of more than just nonspecific effect beyond placebo-controlled studies, such as if one treatment were to be clearly better than another (as behavior therapy so seems, at least in some circumstances [Weisz et al., 1987; Weisz, Weiss, et al., in press]) or there were differential effects on symptom areas consistent with the objectives of differing treatments. Though not definitive, these kind of effects could indicate that, despite expense and difficulty, a properly controlled study was worth pursuing. Only behavior therapy seems to have given these indirect indicators much attention, though its favored paradigm of baseline/treatment/baseline/reversal/baseline still does not totally eliminate the possibility of placebo effects (and other errors).

5. Is One Kind of Psychotherapy Better Than Another?

In their review, Casey and Berman (1985) concluded that there was no difference among therapies, though protagonists for traditional psychotherapy seem to have been unaware of the fact that there were sufficient data to compare only behavior and client-centered therapy. Weisz et al. (1987) criticized the way that Casey and Berman's evaluative methods had disadvantaged behavioral studies, added more studies, and concluded in their meta-analysis that behavior therapy was clearly superior to other therapy in children. Similar conclusions were reached by Andrews (1993) for adult psychotherapy, for which he estimated the size of the superiority to average at least half a standard deviation. In rebuttal, Shirk and Russell (1992, 1995) concluded that it is not possible to say that behavior therapy is superior to psychodynamic psychotherapy in children because the studies of the latter have been so flawed as to make them invalid. Kazdin (1991) also felt that the issue was undecided because of lack of data in most methods other than behavioral. However, Weiss and Weisz (1995) found little support for this hypothesis using meta-analysis.

Thus, while the answer is still not clear, there is some indication that behavior therapy may be superior to other forms of psychotherapy (though only by half a standard deviation, which may not be a great deal in terms of clinical effect). This is particularly true if the symptom focus of behavior therapy is accepted as a legitimate focus of all psychotherapy. Other forms of psychotherapy do themselves a disservice in their persistent reluctance to conduct research, since most of the apparent superiority of behavior therapy resides not only in a lot more data but also in the rather narrower and therefore more measurable targets (Kazdin, 1991; Weisz, Weiss, et al., in press).

6. Can Psychotherapy Be Taught?

Training is taken as essential for the practice of any kind of psychotherapy, and some modes, notably psychoanalysis, go to extraordinary lengths in training. However, is there any evidence that these training programs improve efficacy and efficiency of therapy? Hengeller et al. (1993) point out that there are some 2000 or so training programs in family therapy in the United States, yet none seems to have been evaluated. It may be noted in passing, however, that psychotherapy is not alone in ignoring this problem since medical education itself operates largely from implied rather than demonstrated efficacy—which may explain why medical curricula undergo radical reforms with such regularity.

Research on training in child psychotherapy has suggested that it has little discernible effect on therapist efficacy (Shirk and Phillips, 1991), and in fact, the evidence suggests that training may have negative effects (Weisz et al., 1987). Again, in the carefully controlled Newcastle study (Kolvin et al., 1988), it was found that untrained teacher aides were more effective than psychologists. A similar result was found by Weisz, Weiss, et al. (in press). However, most of the studies examining this issue are seriously flawed in that training was often confounded with other critical variables (such as method of psychotherapy). Also against the value of training, graduates of training programs often view their training as seriously defective, though this may be not so much a problem with training per se but with the way it is done. Finally, there is lack of apparent difference in efficacy of therapists from differently oriented training programs (Shirk and Phillips, 1991). There are, however, persistent indications that some *persons* make better therapists than others (Bergin and Garfield, 1994; Shirk and Phillips, 1991). Also, the type of problem treated may interact with training in a complex way (Weisz, Weiss, et al., in press).

Collectively, these uncomfortable facts suggest that whatever is needed to do psychotherapy may well be acquired by the trainee before and/or after training is undertaken—because the critical ingredient in psychotherapy may not be so much theoretical framework or technique, but some nonspecific personal capacity to relate to other human beings, melded into the combination of other humane or common sense things that go to make up Andrews' "good clinical care." If this be so, it is hardly surprising that a training program has little impact on a trainee who has been learning human relationships for most of the life span and will continue to do so. Shirk and Phillips (1991) point out that because of the lack of any real effort to relate research findings to the practice of psychotherapy, training lacks the kind of explicit goals that might just improve its efficacy.

7. Is More Psychotherapy Better Than Less?

The average duration of treatment varies greatly across psychotherapies, practitioners, and researchers. It is therefore reasonable to ask is more better than less? While analogies are hazardous, pharmacotherapy accepts that there is an optimum dose—too low and it is ineffective, too high and it becomes poisonous. Research on dose effects of psychotherapy in adults (see Andrews, 1993; Koss and Butcher, 1986; Orlinsky and Howard, 1986) is limited, most of it is flawed to some degree, and there are almost no comparative data on really long-term treatment (2 years or more); but the general conclusion is that the dose-response relationship is logarithmic. Most of the gain occurs within the first 10–20 sessions, the size of the effect is enhanced by therapist and patient knowing that therapy is time limited, and effect may even diminish in some patients with longer periods (Koss and Butcher, 1986).

There are little data in child psychotherapy on dose effects (Kazdin, 1993), but what there is does not support the idea that more is better (Casey and Berman, 1985). There is also the disconcerting fact that dosage is dictated largely by patients rather than by therapists and by what underwriters will pay rather than by clinical considerations (Andrews, 1993). If psychotherapists want to convince underwriters that more is better, they will have to do some urgent research in these days when the push is to reduce health care costs (Krupnick and Pincus, 1992). The adult literature (Orlinsky and Howard, 1986) and a recent study in children (Fonagy and Target, 1994) suggests that such research is worth pursuing.

8. Is Psychotherapy Better for Some Children Than for Others?

One of the more dramatic changes in child psychiatry since 1980 has been the rise of disorder-based classification. Pharmacotherapy has now disorder-specific indications and it seems plausible that diagnosis would affect psychotherapy too, and indeed this seems to be the case in adults (Andrews, 1993). Child psychotherapy seems to have been slow to catch up with these advances, and there is little or no study of diagnosis-specific indications, though there are minimal data on broad problem clusters such as externalizing versus internalizing problems. Generally, these have failed to showed any differences (Weisz et al., 1987; Weisz, Weiss, et al., in press). However, recent work (Fonagy and Target, 1994; Kazdin, 1993) suggests that this question is still worth investigating and that the failure to find differences thus far is probably tied to the powerful ''placebo'' effect, the lack of specific problem-oriented objectives, and ways to address these in most psychotherapies except behavioral ones.

Other variables that ought to affect the efficiency and the type of psychotherapy needed (and are common clinical issues), but that are only just beginning to be addressed, are comorbidity, concurrent pharmacotherapy, age, socioeconomic class, family variables, and culture (Armbruster and Kazdin, 1994; Fauber and Long, 1991; Fonagy and Target, 1994; Kazdin, 1991, 1993; Tharp, 1991; Tramontana, 1980; Weisz et al., 1987). For example, Weisz, Weiss, et al. (in press) found that adolescent females may do better, suggesting that more attention to these variables is required.

9. Is Psychotherapy Safer Than Biological Therapies?

It is also often assumed that psychotherapies are preferable to pharmacotherapy because they are less ''invasive'' (and can therefore present no risk to life or limb). This may be true at a physiological level, but psychotherapy is clearly not free from ''side effects'' of stress and emotional upheaval during treatment and may make an unknown percentage of patients worse (Andrews, 1993) though this number appears quite small in children (Weisz et al., 1987). Also, up to 50% of child patients never complete treatment to the satisfaction of the therapist (Armbruster and Kazdin, 1994). The causes of this are complex (and could include rapid response) but may help to conceal adverse outcomes. Pharmacotherapy recognizes the need to monitor closely side and adverse effects. The lack of data on side and adverse effects of child psychotherapy clearly needs addressing, since it reflects practice based on unproven assumptions of safety and efficacy.

10. Is Psychotherapy Acceptable to Consumers?

The fact that many children are considered unsuitable for psychotherapy, that up to 50% of those selected may drop out of treatment (Armbruster and Kazdin, 1994), and that some patients/families report negative experiences (Andrews, 1993; Weisz et al., 1987) suggests that there is a gap of unknown size between consumers and therapists. The causes of this are complex but deserve careful study since acceptability to young people and families is likely to be an important variable in efficacy.

11. Is Psychotherapy Cost-Effective?

This issue was reviewed in detail for adult psychotherapy by Krupnick and Pincus (1992) who concluded that, despite an impressive body of research attesting to the power of psychotherapy to alleviate destructive and painful illness, data needed to assess cost-effectiveness were lacking. Though underwriters and administrators seem to think otherwise, this is a most complex issue, too much so to discuss here. (Interested readers are referred to the cited article and its reference list.) However, by way of example, one of the bigger problems was the failure of a substantial body of outcome research to use measures critical to the cost/benefit equation on the impact of treatment on functions such as education, creativity, work, social obligations, health, and social costs, rather than the usual estimates of improvements in illness-related variables (such as depressive or anxiety symptoms). Again, because of even greater paucity of data, the view with children is even more opaque. Though it seems agreed that psychotherapy is effective with children to some, if rather modest, degree (Weiss and Weisz, 1990), no answer can be given as to whether it is cost/effective. On the other hand, the long-term costs of *not* treating children are equally unknown but are probably enormous (see Kazdin, 1993). This suggests that good studies utilizing the principles outlined by Krupnick and Pincus (1992) are likely to show the worth of psychotherapy in terms acceptable to the business persons who increasingly control both public and private resources for health care. It is worth noting too that it is not just a question of psychotherapy showing its worth—it will need to be shown that other methods such as social reforms or government policies will not do much better for considerably more children.

While the cost/benefit of child psychotherapy is unknown, there are some indicators that cost/efficiency could be improved a great deal.

First, it does not make economic sense to use highly trained expensive staff such as psychiatrists to do what the research suggests can be done as well by less trained staff (e.g., Kolvin et al., 1988; Weisz, Weiss, et al., in press). However, there are a few signs that, in some areas, better trained staff may do better. It should also be noted that supposedly ''untrained'' staff in most studies had very experienced supervisors (Weisz et al., 1987). It may be more a matter of moving to the executive role in a team than discontinuing involvement with psychotherapy altogether. It is likely that Andrews' (1993) concept of good clinical care can be delegated but that management plans, treatment manuals, and some kinds of specific or complex treatments will, rather like complex surgery, still have to done by experienced therapists.

Second, it seems likely that most of the benefit from psychotherapy comes in under 10–20 sessions and is facilitated by knowledge in both parties that treatment will be time-limited (Koss and Butcher, 1986). Therefore, any longer term therapy should be for the exceptional case only. For example, the fact that there is a crude logarithmic relationship between duration of therapy and effect (Orlinsky and Howard, 1986) means that the law of initial values applies. That is, where the disability or suffering is very large, longer treatment, though ever-diminishing in effect, may still produce sizeable changes simply because there is so far to go. However, the decision to extend treatment should be based on demonstration that psychotherapy is effective and, if so, for which particular disorders.

Third, behavior therapy seems more efficient than other psychotherapies and it seems reasonable to make this the treatment of first choice (after good clinical caring). In addition, behavior therapy is remarkable for its emphasis on delegation of therapy by explication of targets, process, and outcome, reducing costs further. Until research can show what are the advantages of pursuing other forms of treatment and for which patients (as indeed seems most likely it could, if it did the research), it is hard to justify them, in the first instance.

Fourth, it is customary in some forms of therapy (e.g., family therapy, group therapy) to use cotherapists and there may be further discussions among cotherapists and supervisors after each session. While this is laudable in terms of peer quality assurance, it doubles or trebles the cost of the treatment. Of course, this is offset if the alternative would be multiple, individual treatments. Research to see if cotherapists and supervisors improve efficiency to the degree that they increase costs is sorely needed.

Fifth, in some disorders, other treatments such as biological ones are likely to be far more cost-effective. For example, methylphenidate produces much larger effects in the core symptoms of attention deficit hyperactivity disorder than do psychotherapies of any kind (Barkley et al., 1993) though there remain many problems that medication does not touch.

12. Should Psychotherapy Be Taught and, if so, in Child Psychiatry?

This question brings together all the issues raised in its 11 predecessors and serves as a suitable summary and conclusion to this review.

(a) The most signal finding is the lack of good data by which to make critical decisions about the teaching and practice of psychotherapies, especially those that dominate in child psychiatry. Paradoxically, in view of their popularity, the traditional psychotherapies have been little studied in the last 15 years (Barrnett et al., 1991). Family therapy fares a little better (Hengeller et al., 1993) in that there seems to be more research activity, though not nearly enough has been addressed to outcome. No other method comes close to behavior therapy in amount and quality of research (Kazdin, 1993; Weisz et al., 1987; Weisz, Weiss, et al., in press).

(b) Such data as there are reveal some disquieting findings that are at odds with the certainty with which psychotherapy is taught, practiced, and marketed, making it seem, at times, more like a religion than a professional activity (Werry, 1989). For example, there are serious doubts about the specificity of different treatments (except behavior therapy), the value of training, the high costs of psychotherapy, and socioeconomic and cultural limitations in application. Inexplicably, despite this, traditional and family therapies continue to flourish and form a centerpiece of most training programs in child psychiatry.

(c) In child psychiatry as a whole, there is currently a sense of excitement, an intellectual renaissance. Though fueled largely by biological psychiatry including taxonomy, epidemiology, molecular biology, and psychopharmacology, behavioral scientists are increasingly lending their specialized research and theoretical knowledge to round out this medical subspecialty, as any issue of the *Journal of the American Academy of Child and Adolescent Psychiatry* makes clear. Amid this intellectual ferment, psychotherapy still depends too much on tradition, charisma, extended preceptorship, assertion, and presumption of beneficence.

Hopefully, the sleeping giant is beginning to awake as the generally impressive papers and reviews cited here show, though these are almost exclusively by nonmedical behavioral scientists. Three papers, one of child analysis comparing disruptive behavior-disordered with emotionally disturbed children (Fonagy and Target, 1994), one of family therapy with serious juvenile offenders (Hengeller et al., 1993), and one on treatment dropout from psychotherapy (Armbruster and Kazdin, 1994), are but the most recent examples. However, child therapy still lags behind the intellectual activity in adult psychotherapy.

(d) There is good reason to teach and practice behavior therapy since it has a clear advantage in efficacy and in volume of supporting data, and its approach is generally more transmissible and heuristic. But child psychiatrists need to overcome their idea that this is something that only psychologists do, and move on to master, teach, practice, and supervise it.

(e) Teaching and practice of forms of psychotherapy other than behavioral are less defensible unless they are perceived for the moment as simply part of good clinical caring, in which case, it is unlikely that prolonged training, high fees, long-term, or intensive treatment can be justified. The fact that many practitioners currently earn their living from long-term or traditional psychotherapies does not mean that child psychiatry training and practice can be exempt from the painful radical restructuring that is a feature of the 1990s economic world. As long as child psychiatry belongs to and wishes to avail itself of the privileges of being part of medicine, it must adhere to the fundamental ethical values that no treatment can be assumed to be effective and safe—it must be demonstrated to be so.

(f) The strongest justification for continuation of nonbehavioral psychotherapies is in research and in care of the severely ill, where proven treatments have failed. Even then, these treatments should ordinarily be delegated to less highly paid personnel to reduce cost—until such time, if ever, it is clearly demonstrated that child psychiatrists can do it better.

(g) This review has not touched on the issue of whether or not personal psychotherapy may have a place in the training of child psychiatrists. However, since training has not yet been clearly demonstrated to improve efficiency as a therapist, it seems premature to assume that personal psychotherapy could either. While personal experience with psychotherapy may be helpful to individual child psychiatrists, it also risks promoting pseudo-understanding and quelling enquiry if a similar model is used in the individual's working life. Furthermore, most personal psychotherapy takes considerable time and incurs financial costs, both of which diminish the amount of time available for other just as important learning experiences.

(h) As discussed in the introduction, psychotherapy may be justified as an essential part of medicine's other arm—humanistic concern and care for the sick and their relatives (Pardes, 1990). Psychiatry must maintain its current prerogative among medical specialties of being able to take time to listen to children and their families and thus to exercise the traditional medical activity of humane clinical caring (Pardes, 1990). In view of the lack of distinctive effects in different kinds of psychotherapy, it seems likely that many practitioners of psychotherapy, when faced with a distressed patient, abandon most of the theoretical orthodoxy they were taught in favor of what seems sensible, caring, and ethical.

Those practitioners who conceptualize children's suffering, handicaps, and maladaptations within traditional frameworks have no need to change if it enables them to deliver this most important element of medical care. But there is a substantial difference between such a position and promulgating, teaching, or practicing most psychotherapies as proven treatments for child psychopathology, especially within child psychiatry, which is supposed to show medicine's scepticism toward treatment and proper regard for the cost of health care.

(i) Looking at the dramatic remedicalization of psychiatry in the last two decades (Wilson, 1993) and the main thrust of current research, it seems clear that the role of the child psychiatrist in the 21st century increasingly will resemble that of other physicians (that is, performing diagnostic assessments encompassing medical, psychological, social, and cultural issues; participating in multidisciplinary case conferences; delegating administration of all except especially skilled treatments) and thus will differ substantially from that of many teachers in the past who spent much of their time on psychotherapy. Unless it can be shown that psychotherapy greatly enhances effectiveness in diagnosis and delivery of good clinical caring, there seems little justification for the predominance of nonbehavioral psychotherapy in child psychiatry training. Since skill in psychotherapy and clinical caring seems more related to personal qualities than to training, it may make more sense to concentrate on better selection of medical students and psychiatric trainees.

(j) The time has come for psychotherapy to undergo a painful personal analysis and confront the nagging perennial questions about psychotherapy, using the tools of science: What do we know about psychotherapy that is derived from research, not assertion or tradition? How can this knowledge be used to determine what sort of psychotherapy should be given, to which patients, for how long, at what cost, and by whom? How should psychotherapy be taught, if at all? What is needed is more research, more intellectual curiosity, and more excitement and less complacency, less dogma, less training, and less unexamined clinical practice.

References

Andrews G: The essential psychotherapies. *Br J Psychiatry* 162:447–451, 1993.

Armbruster P, Kazdin AE: Attrition in child psychotherapy. In: Ollendick TH, Prinz RJ (eds): *Advances in Clinical Child Psychology* (Vol 16). New York, Plenum, 1994.

Barkley RA, DuPaul GJ, Costello A: Stimulants. In: Werry JS, Aman MG (eds): *Practitioner's Guide to Psychoactive Drugs for Children and Adolescents*. New York, Plenum, 1993.

Barrnett RJ, Docherty JP, Frommelt GM: A review of child psychotherapy research since 1963. *J Am Acad Child Adolesc Psychiatry* 30:1–14, 1991.

Bergin AE, Garfield SL: *Handbook of Psychotherapy and Behavioral Change* (4th ed). New York, Wiley, 1994.

Casey RJ, Berman JS: The outcome of psychotherapy with children. *Psychol Bull* 98:388–400, 1985.

Conners CK: Teachers' questionnaires. *Psychopharmacol Bull* 21:823–827, 1985.

Fauber RL, Long N: Children in context: The role of the family in child psychotherapy. *J Consult Clin Psychol* 59:813–820, 1991.

Fonagy P, Target M: The efficacy of psychoanalysis for children with disruptive disorders. *J Am Acad Child Adolesc Psychiatry* 33:45–55, 1994.

Hazelrigg MD, Cooper HM, Borduin CM: Evaluating the effectiveness of family therapies: An integrative review and analysis. *Psychol Bull* 101: 428–442, 1987.

Heinecke CM, Strassman LH: Towards more effective research in child psychotherapy. *J Am Acad Child Psychiatry* 14:561–568, 1975.

Henggeler SW, Borduin CM, Mann BJ: Advances in family therapy: Empirical foundations. In: Ollendick TH, Prinz RM (eds): *Advances in Clinical Child Psychology* (Vol 15). New York, Plenum, 1993.

Kazdin AE: Effectiveness of psychotherapy with children and adolescents. *J Consult Clin Psychol* 59: 785–798, 1991.

Kazdin AE: Psychotherapy for children and adolescents: Current progress and future research directions. *Am Psychol* 48:644–657, 1993.

Klerman GL: The psychiatric patient's right to effective treatment: Implications of Osheroff v Chestnut Lodge. *Am J Psychiatry* 147:409–418, 1990.

Kolvin I, MacMillan A, Nicol AR, et al: Psychotherapy is effective. *J R Soc Med* 81:261–266, 1988.

Koss MP, Butcher JN: Research on brief psychotherapy. In: Garfield SL, Bergin AE (eds): *Handbook of Psychotherapy and Behavioral Change* (3rd ed). New York, Wiley, 1986.

Kovacs M, Paulauskas S: The traditional psychotherapies. In: Quay HC, Werry JS (eds): *Psychopathological Disorders of Childhood* (3rd ed). New York, Wiley, 1986.

Krupnick JL, Pincus HA: Cost effectiveness of psychotherapy: A plan for research. *Am J Psychiatry* 149:1295–1305, 1992.

Levitt EE: The results of psychotherapy with children: An evaluation. *J Consult Psychol* 21: 189–196, 1957.

Levitt EE: Psychotherapy with children: A further evaluation. *Behav Res Ther* 1:45–51, 1963.

Morrow-Bradley C, Elliot R: Utilization of psychotherapy research by practising psychotherapists. *Am Psychol* 41:188–197, 1986.

Ollendick TH: Behavior therapy with children and adolescents. In: Garfield SL, Bergin AE (eds): *Handbook of Psychotherapy and Behavioral Change* (3rd ed). New York, Wiley, 1986.

Orlinsky DE, Howard KI: Process and outcome in psychotherapy. In: Garfield SL, Bergin AE: *Handbook of Psychotherapy and Behavioral Change* (3rd ed). New York, Wiley, 1986.

Pardes H: Defending humanistic values. *Am J Psychiatry* 147:1113–1119, 1990.

Quay HC: Classification. In: Quay HC, Werry JS (eds): *Psychopathological Disorders of Childhood* (3rd ed). New York, Wiley, 1986.

Shirk SR, Philips JS: Child therapy training: Closing the gaps with research and practice. *J Consult Clin Psychol* 59:766–776, 1991.

Shirk SR, Russell RL: A re-evaluation of estimates of child therapy effectiveness. *J Am Acad Child Adolesc Psychiatry* 31:703–710, 1992.

Shirk SR, Russell RL: Effectiveness of psychotherapy (letter). *J Am Acad Child Adolesc Psychiatry* 34:973–974, 1995.

Tharp RG: Cultural diversity and the treatment of children. *J Consult Clin Psychol* 59:799–812, 1991.

Tramontana MG: Critical review of research on psychotherapy with adolescents: 1967–1977. *Psychol Bull* 88:109–143, 1980.

Weiss B, Weisz JR: The impact of methodological factors on child psychotherapy outcome research: A meta-analysis for researchers. *J Abnorm Child Psychol* 18:639–670, 1990.

Weiss B, Weisz JR: Relative effectiveness of behavioral versus nonbehavioral child psychotherapy. *J Consult Clin Psychol* 63:317–320, 1995.

Weisz JR, Donenberg GR, Han SS, et al: Bridging the gap between lab and clinic in child and adolescent psychotherapy. *J Consult Clin Psychol*, in press.

Weisz JR, Weiss B: *Effects of Psychotherapy with Children and Adolescents*. Newbury Park, CA, Sage Publications, 1993.

Weisz JR, Weiss B, Alicke MD, et al: Effectiveness of psychotherapy with children and adolescents: A meta-analysis for clinicians. *J Consult Clin Psychol* 55:542–549, 1987.

Weisz JR, Weiss B, Donenberg GR: The lab versus the clinic. Effects of child and adolescent psychotherapy. *Am Psychol* 47:1578–1585, 1992.

Weisz JR, Weiss B, Han SS, et al: Effects of psychotherapy with children and adolescents revisited. A meta-analysis of treatment outcome studies. *Psych Bull*, in press.

Werry JS: Family therapy: Professional endeavour or successful religion? *J Fam Ther* 11:377–382, 1986.

Wilson M: DSM-III and the transformation of American psychiatry: History. *Am J Psychiatry* 150: 399–410, 1993.

82 CHILD AND ADOLESCENT PARTIAL HOSPITALIZATION

Jerry D. Heston, M.D., Laurel J. Kiser, Ph.D., and David B. Pruitt, M.D.

BACKGROUND AND DEFINITION

Partial hospitalization has been used historically as an umbrella term describing many varieties of alternative care. With the advent of managed care and health care reform, less costly and less restrictive treatment modalities are in increasing demand. In order to provide definition for these alternatives, which stretch along the continuum of psychiatric care between inpatient and outpatient office visits, three levels of ambulatory mental health services have been outlined (Kiser et al., 1993). The most intense level of services functions as an alternative to or prevention of inpatient hospitalization. The other levels of care function as intermediate, maintenance care or step-up programs from outpatient. Partial hospitalization (PH), as traditionally defined, is the prototype of a hospital diversion program.

In the mental health care delivery system, partial hospital and intensive outpatient services are analogous to outpatient surgery. These services represent a specific modality along the continuum of care, offering more intensity than outpatient services without the iatrogenic effects of hospitalization. Like inpatient services, partial hospital programs (PHPs) strive to provide intense, highly structured treatment. They do so by utilizing a variety of therapeutic modalities: individual, group, and family therapy; educational or vocational therapy; recreation and activity therapy; and medical and nursing services. This multimodal treatment requires an interdisciplinary staff typically drawn from psychiatry, psychology, social work, educational or vocational therapy, occupational or recreational therapy, and nursing. The American Association for Partial Hospitalization (AAPH) in 1991 published this definition: Partial hospitalization is a time-limited, ambulatory, active treatment program that offers therapeutically intensive, coordinated, structured clinical services within a stable therapeutic milieu (Block et al., 1991, p. 1).

HISTORY

The history of partial hospitalization for children and adolescents is brief. The first programs were for adults in Russia (late 1930s), Canada (late 1940s), and England (early 1950s). The Menninger Clinic introduced the concept to the United States when it opened its unit in the mid-1950s. In 1963, the Community Mental Health Center Act mandated comprehensive services including partial hospitalization for children and adolescents. This movement had three main origins: deinstitutionalization, interest in the role of family and community, and movement to cost-effective treatment alternatives.

Throughout the 1970s and 1980s and into the present, the modality has been severely underutilized (Novello, 1979; Prevost, 1981). With only 2% of those in need of treatment receiving services in partial hospital programs (Krizay, 1989) and the majority of programs operating below 75% capacity (AAPH, 1994a), underutilization is a major problem for the survival of many programs.

Three clinical issues contribute to underutilization of partial hospitalization. First, for providers, it is difficult to serve moderately to severely disturbed children and adolescents in an open system with less restrictiveness and a less structured environment. Second, for families, it requires major commitments to family therapy, to transportation, and to keeping a difficult child at home. Third, for referral sources who are more accustomed to and better trained to treat severely dysfunctional patients in inpatient programs, it necessitates a shift in conceptualization and behavior.

Historically, other factors related to low utilization of partial programs include a lack of definition, criteria, and outcome data, with consequent funding limitations. In fact, reimbursement policies serve as a major impediment to wider use of partial hospital services. Traditionally, the vast majority of policies with mental health care benefits had better coverage for inpatient than for outpatient services and no coverage for partial hospitalization services. Therefore, instead of treating the child in the least restrictive, least expensive environment, the clinician and family were forced to utilize more restrictive, more expensive programs (Leibenluft and Leibenluft, 1988; Novello, 1979; Weithorn, 1988). Finally, the nature of the health care industry during the 1980s favored creation of new hospital beds, rather than partial hospitalization programs. Current industry trends, however, promise major changes in the service delivery system.

Now, in the 1990s, the emphasis of health care delivery returns to cost-containment with increased interest in community, family-based alternatives, managed care, and accountability. Managed care focuses on eliminating unnecessary inpatient services with efforts directed toward development of systems favoring outpatient practices (Hoge, 1992). Although early indications from managed care pointed to their desire to assure both quality and efficiency, fiscal management frequently translates to either rationing care or providing the cheapest services for the shortest length of time possible regardless of clinical decision-making and effectiveness data (VandenBos, 1990).

These trends are creating major shifts in the delivery and funding of mental health care, including substantial growth in the number of partial hospitalization programs, development of freestanding partial hospitalization chains, increased utilization of acute partial hospitalization for patient stabilization using inpatient admission criteria, and rapid development of a variety of intensive outpatient treatment options. New funding opportunities for ambulatory mental health services include passage of federal regulations offering partial hospital services to Civilian Health and Medical Program Uniformed Services (CHAMPUS) enrollees and the development of more inclusive and flexible benefit plans. In fact, a liberal benefit for partial hospitalization and other intensive nonresidential treatment alternatives is included in most health care reform packages.

THEORETICAL ISSUES

Two basic philosophies of care provide the basis for child and adolescent partial hospital programs. First, partial hospital programs strive to treat patients requiring intensive therapeutic intervention with the least amount of disruption to their normal daily functioning. This requires partial programs to define the limits between when patients can be treated safely in an outpatient setting and when they require the restrictiveness of hospitalization. Thus, partial hospital programs are designed to maintain a balance between treatment in the least restrictive environment and risk management.

Second, partial hospitalization encourages programs to take advantage of the "open system" inherent in the concept. This philosophy emphasizes the use of family supports and strengths and community agencies and programs. Two major sequelae result from this philosophy of care. Partial programs invite the patient and the patient's family to maintain a higher level of functioning than do treatment settings that remove the patient from the home. Philosophically, this translates into a program of therapeutic interventions designed to maintain power within the parental/familial subsystem and to view that subsystem as competent in providing care for the child. Interventions are structured to alter dysfunctional interactional patterns rather than remove the child from these interactions. Translated into program policy, partial programs use only techniques and treatment strategies that a family can also use at home.

Additionally, partial programs promote reliance on community support systems and programs whenever possible. Benefits of this approach include limiting the development of dependence on the treatment team, expansion of and appropriate use of resources, decreased lengths of stay, and improved adjustment following discharge (Herz, 1982). This unique combination of providing "security and structure while simultaneously promoting patient responsibility and autonomy" (Hoge et al., 1988, p. 208) may be the particular advantage of this modality.

The philosophies underlying partial hospitalization can be accomplished in programs with a variety of theoretical orientations. Behaviorally oriented programs utilize principles of learning theory. The goals of a behavioral program are, consequently, to teach desirable behaviors and to extinguish undesirable ones. The majority of partial hospital programs, although not operating exclusively from this orientation, use some form of behavioral system to reinforce appropriate patient behavior (Kiser et al., 1986). Psychoanalytic programs focus on structuring a therapeutic environment in which behaviors and other symptoms are analyzed and interpreted. Another approach uses a psychoeducational orientation with the classroom as the basic structure for program design. "Students" rather than "patients" usually receive psychotherapy in conjunction with classroom instruction. Programs using systems theory emphasize the theoretical proposition that many different areas of a child's life influence the child's functioning: biologic, intrapsychic, family, peers, school, work, neighbors, religious affiliation, and others. Within a systems orientation, programs are challenged to assess problems and intervene on a multilevel basis (Kiser and Pruitt, 1991). Some programs are based on a medical model in which all patients receive psychiatric diagnoses and treatment is prescribed by a child and adolescent psychiatrist (Novello, 1979).

These orientations differ in the manner in which they view the child, his or her problem(s), and the treatment program. Although many theoretical orientations are possible within an organization, the model used should be consistent across the continuum of care. Conflicting models established between components of care may cause confusion for the staff as well as for the patient and family.

GOALS OF TREATMENT

The functions of partial hospital and intensive outpatient treatment differ according to the level of care offered (Glasscote et al., 1977; Kiser et al., 1993). Partial hospitalization and other intensive nonresidential treatment options function to provide short-term, crisis intervention as an alternative treatment to hospitalization or an intensive transition setting in order to shorten a hospital stay. Less intensive ambulatory modalities provide support and maintenance for patients in order to avoid long-term hospitalization or residential care. Finally, intensive outpatient services provide a step up in care for patients for whom one or two office visits per week is insufficient. Another goal or function of ambulatory mental health services can be extensive evaluation involving observation, identification of problem areas, diagnosis, and formulation of treatment plans (Casarino et al., 1982).

CLINICAL ISSUES

Indications

The need for partial hospital programs to define target populations is essential for continued viability of the modality (Leibenluft and Leibenluft, 1988). In many ways, the intensity, yet openness, of partial hospitalization, suggests the types of patients appropriate for this mode. Individual programs define their target population by establishing admission criteria. From a programmatic standpoint, evaluation to determine appropriateness for partial hospitalization includes (Novello, 1979; Zimet and Farley, 1985):

1. Level of impulse control—ability to control suicidal, homicidal, and runaway ideation, and abuse of drugs or alcohol.
2. Level of functional impairment—difficulty functioning in a variety of areas including school, social activities, community, home; level of intellectual and academic functioning appropriate to educational structure of the program.
3. Parental support—able to provide adequate control and support at home during evenings and weekends; able to engage in treatment process; able to provide transportation.
4. Physical health—no requirement for 24-hour medical care.
5. Ability to pay.

A decision matrix, assessing both level of impulse control and parental support and structure, is another valuable tool for assessing appropriateness for admission (Kiser et al., 1991) (Fig. 82.1). Level of impulse control can be viewed along a continuum with some patients demonstrating no problems and other patients requiring a more structured, locked treatment environment due to problems with behavior control. On the other axis the continuum of family functioning (support and commitment

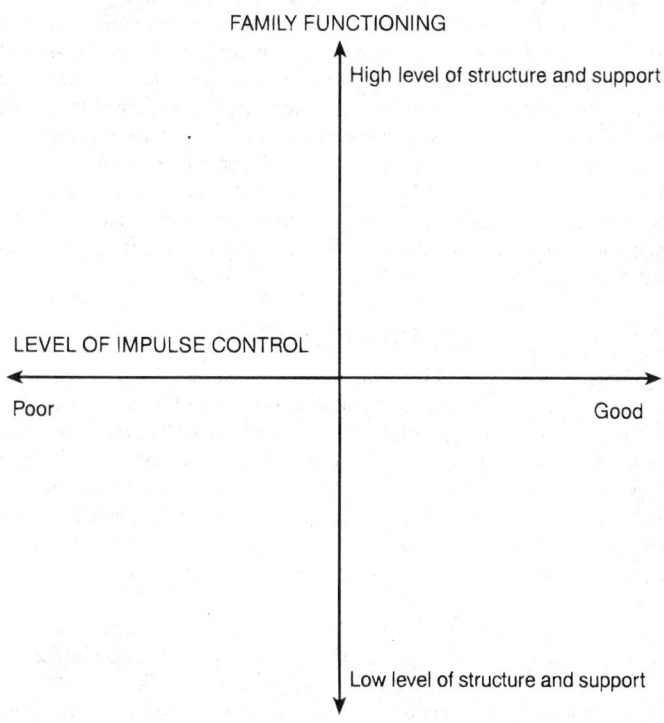

Figure 82.1. Decision matrix: risk management assessment. (From Kiser LJ, Heston JD, Millsap PA, et al: Testing the limits: Special treatment procedures for child and adolescent partial hospitalization. *Int J Partial Hospitalization* 7(1):39, 1991.)

to treatment) is evaluated. It is expected that families will work with the partial hospital program to encourage their child to comply with program limits. Families who are unable or unwilling to participate in this manner are less likely to provide the daily support and structure needed by the patient, who is therefore unlikely to derive significant benefit from partial hospital treatment.

PROGRAM OF THERAPEUTIC ACTIVITIES

The clinical components, that is, each patient's daily activities, are based upon an individual treatment plan developed by the treatment team (Block et al., 1991; Kiser et al., 1986). Continuous monitoring of the patient's response to treatment dictates any alterations in this plan. Therapeutic progress is monitored weekly by the entire multidisciplinary staff, and periodically a treatment update is prepared and the patient's case is reviewed by the entire treatment team. Progress to date on problems is reviewed, new problems are discussed, and progress toward discharge is monitored.

A distinguishing characteristic of a partial hospital program is the intensity of diverse clinical components. These components most often include individual, group, family, medical management, activities, and education. The Standards and Guidelines published by AAPH stipulate that 50% of the time spent in the program is active treatment (Block et al., 1991).

Individual

Individual therapy is offered by most partial hospital programs in the United States (AAPH, 1994a; Kiser et al., 1986), usually on a weekly or semiweekly basis with a mean of 1.60 hours per week (Kiser et al., unpublished manuscript). Like individual therapy in other settings, it provides the patient with an opportunity to develop a close, interpersonal relationship with an adult other than a parent and an opportunity to work on intrapsychic problems.

The wealth of information available to the individual therapist through contacts with the patient in other parts of the program makes individual therapy in partial hospitalization different from outpatient individual psychotherapy. An example of this occurs when a depressed child denies withdrawal from peers, but is frequently observed sitting alone during milieu periods. For this reason individual therapy frequently progresses at a faster rate during a partial hospitalization than in outpatient therapy. Differences between individual psychotherapy in partial hospital and inpatient settings are also significant and mainly due to the openness of the partial hospital system. Individual therapy in partial hospitalization can utilize material from daily encounters with parents, siblings, and peers to address dysfunction in these areas.

Group

Group psychotherapy plays an important role in partial hospital programming by allowing peers to develop the ability to deal with problems through the expression of feelings and experiences in a safe environment. This therapy also provides an opportunity for work on group dynamics, including cohesion, roles, and norms. As with all group work, it is important that the structure and content of the group be appropriate for the developmental levels of the patients involved. As with individual therapy, therapists in a partial hospital program have direct knowledge about patient functioning in multiple areas, thus allowing immediate and specific feedback to the group members.

Family

The use of family therapies by many programs is consistent with the research, which demonstrates that family structure is predictive of successful completion of treatment and follow-up (Prentice-Dunn et al., 1981). Family involvement in treatment may take a variety of forms including traditional family therapy, multifamily groups, parent education classes, and parent support groups.

Family therapy provides an opportunity to focus on family dynamics in order to facilitate change in the home environment. Within a partial hospital program, this therapy allows intensive work on family conflict and family structure on a day-to-day basis. Because the patients return home to the family each evening, new skills can be practiced and evaluated in a continuous manner.

Another important benefit to family therapy in a partial hospital system is the ability to establish consistent rules and limits for the child both at home and at the program. One powerful difference between family treatment in this environment and that of an inpatient unit is the emphasis in partial hospitalization on maintaining parental authority. In partial hospitalization, parents are involved in every level of decision-making and problem-solving. Parents are, in effect, viewed as co-therapists.

Medical Management

The extent of medical involvement in the management of patients in partial hospital programs varies depending upon the theoretical background of the program. Trends recently, however, are toward emphasizing aspects of the medical model in partial hospital programs regardless of their basic theoretical approaches. As various forces work toward decreasing rates of hospitalization in children and adolescents, more severely disturbed patients and those with combined medical and psychiatric disorders will be referred to partial hospital programs. Management of somatic complaints, eating disorders, elimination disorders, as well as other physical problems demands strong medical involvement. This underscores the importance of the medical and nursing aspects of care within these programs.

Medical management includes an initial assessment of the patient's physical as well as psychological health status. Both medical and psychiatric diagnoses are assigned. This may involve direct physical examinations done by a physician associated with the program or, in those programs that are more community based, consultation and liaison with the patient's pediatrician. It is the responsibility of nurses and physicians to identify specific health problems that may be important factors in the overall functioning of the patient. These problems may be treated directly or referred to a community physician. Referrals often serve to educate and guide families in accessing needed health care services and to use these resources effectively.

Pharmacotherapy, another aspect of medical management, may be practiced within the structure of a partial hospital program with advantages over other therapeutic settings. As on an inpatient unit, observations from multiple viewpoints are available to determine specific indications for medications. The ability to monitor new medications or changes in regimens is augmented by daily contact with the patient and information about the patient's status in many different activities. This use of medication within a structured environment is frequently seen as an advantage to pharmacotherapy developed on an outpatient basis. Also, in distinction to an inpatient hospitalization, the family is able to provide ongoing feedback about medication response, side effects, or other concerns about medication.

Therapeutic Activities

Recreation, movement, art, occupational, and milieu therapies, as well as community field trips, provide staff and peer support for appropriate behavior in social settings. Patients learn constructive ways to use leisure time in activities that foster team work, cooperation, and task commitment. Milieu therapy is a constant in partial hospital scheduling to create an environment that allows children and adolescents successful social interaction. Community morning meetings are a part of the milieu creating an opportunity for patients to assume an active role in structuring their day, to discuss problems occurring on and off the unit, and to make the transition from the outside to the more structured partial hospital environment. Frequent field trips and involvement in community events are consistent with the partial hospitalization belief that children and adolescents should remain active members of the community.

Behavior Modification Programs

The behavioral system is based upon the principles of learning theory and behavior modification. The most common systems delineate desired behaviors and their reinforcements and undesirable behaviors and their consequences. The developmental level of the patient population must be considered in designing a viable behavioral system. Consistency and feedback to patients about their performance are significant to the success of any reinforcement system.

Within a partial hospital program, behavior modification plans can be adapted and tailored to the needs of a specific patient and his or her family. Plans are developed with active and ongoing involvement from the family. These behavioral programs may be designed in a therapy session and used immediately when the patient returns home in the evening. Problems may be identified quickly and adaptations made daily with input from the therapist, other staff members, and the family. This is in marked contrast to behavioral plans developed on an inpatient unit that are not used by the family until after discharge when they are removed from the support of the hospital.

Education

Just as much of a child's life revolves around school and related activities, much of the programming in partial hospitalization revolves around school issues and educational therapy. Different programs meet the needs for educational services in very different ways; however, intensive programs offering a school component provide a minimum of 3 hours of education daily (Block et al., 1991). On the other hand, acute programs with lengths of stays under 2 weeks might provide educational experiences based upon a "homebound" model. Obtaining fiscal support for the educational portion of treatment is an area of concern, with piecemeal funding often requiring that programs meet several sets of standards and answer to several local and state agencies.

The steps of educational therapy include (a) an assessment of current levels of functioning and a diagnosis of specific learning problems; (b) development of an individualized educational plan; (c) a therapeutic classroom designed to provide structured learning activities that meet individual needs, stress adaptive learning skills, remediate learning deficits, and foster success; and (d) liaison with community schools. Partial hospital programs also utilize the educational environment to aid children in dealing appropriately with the frustrations encountered in the school setting, including dealing with authority and assuming responsibility for work.

Special Populations

Proponents of partial hospitalization suggest that it is a viable treatment mode for many special populations (juvenile offenders, those with eating disorders, and alcohol and drug abusers), as well as for nonpsychiatric populations (patients with head trauma, epilepsy, etc.). Several reports of programs designed for adolescent offenders have appeared in the literature (Comer, 1985; Gaylor, 1979). Treatment emphasis for offenders that results in generally positive outcomes appears to be intensive group therapy and social, recreational, and special educational services.

Another special population described in the literature is preschoolers. Special emphasis in partial hospital programs for young children is placed upon play, communication and language, socialization, skill development, and parent-child interaction. Young children benefiting from treatment in a therapeutic preschool include those with developmental delays, victims of physical and sexual abuse, and those with other severe emotional/behavioral disturbances (Rogers and Lewis, 1989).

Health care reform and the interest in development of cost-effective treatments have resulted in programs that address the psychosocial as well as physical needs of chronically ill pediatric patients. Patients with eating disorders, sickle cell disease, asthma, diabetes, and other disorders may benefit from specialized partial hospital treatment provided by health care professionals from appropriate pediatric specialties.

LIMITATIONS AND COMPLICATIONS

As various theoretical, ethical, economic, and other factors discussed earlier continue to discourage the use of hospitalization, PHPs will be challenged to manage patients whose behavioral symptoms and impulsivity have escalated to the point that special treatment procedures are indicated. Policies and procedures for dealing with patients displaying aggressive, acting out behaviors, noncompliance with program rules, and suicidal or runaway ideation are a necessary part of partial hospital programming (Kiser et al., 1991). Special treatment procedures designed for use in child and adolescent partial hospitalization programs must adequately address the issue of safety, involve the family and the community, and yet maintain the patient in the least-restrictive environment.

Management of patients' behavior on the unit necessitates policies that address seclusion, physical holding, and restraints. Often partial hospitalization programs simply do not offer these services because the belief is that they are appropriately utilized only on inpatient units. Other partial hospital programs use quiet room and physical holding policies, which do not violate the mandate of the program, in other words, procedures that can also be used by parents and guardians in the home environment. The quiet room and physical holding are used sparingly with adolescents; immediate transfer to a secure facility may be indicated for an aggressive or acutely psychotic, disruptive adolescent. Manual and chemical restraints are typically not used in PHPs.

Just as programs must develop policies to help patients control their behavior that are compatible with the program's theoretical basis and intensity of treatment, they must address similar issues with other problems both on the unit and at home. For example, PHPs may be able to treat patients with significant suicidal ideation if they are able to maintain appropriate levels of observation and plan for continued supervision after program hours using family therapy, telephone contact, beeper services, or other interventions. Runaway patients may similarly be placed in PHPs, given policies for structure after hours and ability to liaison with community resources such as runaway homes or other community emergency shelters. Thus, intensive programs that are designed to serve as alternatives to inpatient treatment are able to treat severely disturbed patients using policies that address program structure, family resources, and community involvement.

Due to the intensity of programming, the developmental level and the severity of illness of patients treated, and the lack of restrictiveness, most programs operate with very small staff-to-patient ratios. A typical ratio is one staff person to fewer than four patients (Kiser et al., 1995), with a recommended range from 1:3 through 1:6 (Block et al., 1991). Even with small staff-to-patient ratios, the high intensity of the programs results in staff stress and burnout (Kiser et al., 1986; Novello, 1979). A fuller explanation no doubt lies in the philosophy of the approach: maintaining severely affected patients in the least restrictive environment.

Crisis Management and Hospital Liaison

Partial hospital programs that attempt to shorten or eliminate hospitalization must have adequate policies and procedures to handle the emergencies that prompt immediate admission to the program and the inevitable crises that develop during treatment. While general principles are described above in the discussion of some of the limitations and challenges of PHPs, specific details of crisis management should be identified. These organizations should have an emergency system integrated into their program. The following recommendations meet these crisis management needs (Kiser et al., 1986): (a) An on-call child and

adolescent psychiatrist available 24 hours per day, 365 days per year; (b) additional on-call services to help families resolve conflicts that do not require hospitalization or major changes in treatment plans, staffed primarily by partial hospital professionals; and (c) an established affiliation with both pediatric and psychiatric inpatient units. In the case of hospital-based programs, this should be addressed in policies regarding transfer between PH and inpatient units. In freestanding PHPs, formal affiliations with hospitals must be made so that admissions can occur quickly and safely for patients with acute emergencies.

Less intense ambulatory programs must also develop emergency plans. These might include policies to admit patients to the PHP within a number of days and consultation with a psychiatrist to assist with decisions regarding emergency management and possible hospitalization.

DISCHARGE AND AFTERCARE SERVICES

Discharge planning is an integral part of treatment planning in partial hospitalization, beginning during the initial intake and continuing throughout the treatment process as discharge goals are formulated and clarified. During the course of treatment, progress toward discharge is continually monitored by the treatment team with input from the patient's family.

The following principles govern the discharge planning process: (a) patients receive treatment in the least restrictive environment that provides the structure and intensity necessary; (b) patients receive treatment for the shortest time possible in order to reach maximum treatment benefit; and (c) discharge planning is done in a fashion that maximizes a successful transition to the patient's new setting (either more or less structured). Thus, discharge planning involves attention to issues of termination, liaison with community resources (inpatient settings, school settings, etc.), development of aftercare plans, and follow-up to encourage compliance with aftercare recommendations.

ROLE OF THE CHILD AND ADOLESCENT PSYCHIATRIST

Physician involvement in partial hospitalization varies according to the theoretical model of the program and the level of treatment intensity offered. In those programs that de-emphasize the medical model and function mainly as intensive outpatient programs, psychiatrists may function as consultants. Other programs that are designed as intense psychiatric treatment settings and serve as alternatives to hospitalization are usually more medically oriented and follow a traditional attending psychiatrist model.

In those programs that are designed as intensive outpatient services, psychiatrists may be contracted to function as consultants to provide specific, limited services. These services include initial psychiatric evaluation and diagnosis as well as monitoring pharmacotherapy. The psychiatrist is not a part of the treatment team and is usually not involved in the day-to-day care of the patients or administration of the program. While the advantages of this model are financial and logistical, saving the program the cost of a full-time specialist in a profession that is relatively undersupplied, the main disadvantage is the lack of physician input into the overall treatment of patients.

In other partial hospital programs, psychiatrists function as attending physicians and members of the treatment team. This model of psychiatric involvement is usually seen in programs that are designed as intensive, acute treatment programs serving as alternatives to hospitalization. Under this model the physician can be seen as the team leader, orchestrating the treatment provided. The use of Engel's (1980) biopsychosocial model of medical practice is particularly congruent with the philosophy of partial hospital. Physician involvement is not limited to the specifics of medical management, but includes substantial input into program administration and direction. The cost disadvantage may be counteracted by the preference of insurance companies and Medicaid to reimburse for medically directed services.

Table 82.1.   Advantages and Disadvantages of Partial Hospitalization for Children and Adolescents

Advantages

1. Partial hospitalization allows the patient to remain with his/her family.
2. Partial hospitalization encourages the family to be responsible for the patient while providing opportunities to learn new patterns of interaction.
3. Partial hospitalization provides partial care for the patient, thus removing that burden from the parents for a portion of each day.
4. Partial hospitalization may provide the patient with a break from a dysfunctional family system and a chaotic environment.
5. Partial hospitalization avoids the iatrogenic effects of inpatient treatment, such as dependency and dehumanization.
6. Partial hospitalization provides the freedom for patients to continue involvement in extracurricular activities, such as part-time work, social affairs, etc.
7. Less social stigma is attached to partial hospitalization than inpatient services.
8. Transitions from either less intensive or more intensive treatment are facilitated by partial hospitalization.
9. Partial hospitalization allows for more flexibility in scheduling the frequency and intensity of treatment than inpatient hospitalization.
10. Comprehensive psychiatric evaluations can be accomplished without totally disrupting the child's or adolescent's environment.
11. Typically, partial hospitalization is able to offer a greater variety of therapeutic experiences than do most hospital units.

Disadvantages

1. Sometimes it is necessary to temporarily remove a child or adolescent from his/her home environment.
2. The openness of partial hospitalization results in a higher level of risk involved in treating some patients with disorders of impulse control.
3. Partial hospitalization is more stressful for staff because of the increased risks and the necessity of dealing with everyday, life problems.
4. Partial hospitalization makes it easier for children and families to drop out of treatment than do inpatient programs.
5. Problems of transportation and living arrangements are frequently encountered in partial hospitalization.
6. Partial hospitalization interferes with normal daily activities, such as school, athletics, etc.
7. The cost to parents for partial hospitalization may be substantially higher than for more expensive inpatient services.

As managed care grows and continues to influence psychiatric care, physicians may be expected to help programs, patients, and their families negotiate appropriate financial coverage for treatment. This assistance may come in clarifying diagnoses and outlining treatment options. Frequently physicians in partial hospital programs are called upon to participate in physician-to-physician reviews of cases that have been tagged as questionable by the managed care company. The effective psychiatrist will be called upon to document rationale for treatment in a partial hospital program and should be familiar with advantages that this treatment setting has over others. As this aspect of psychiatry evolves with health care reform, physician involvement is also expected to change and adapt.

In order to provide a summary of partial hospital's indications and limitations, the advantages and disadvantages of the modality are presented in Table 82.1.

CASE ILLUSTRATION

The case of Tammy, a 16-year-old, black girl admitted to a PHP following a suicide attempt, is presented to illustrate the use of partial hospitalization in emergency care. Tammy was first seen in a pediatric emergency room on a Saturday morning by a psychiatry resident who determined that, although she had continued suicide ideation, she did not have a specific plan, and could be treated without hospitalization. Over the weekend the resident contacted Tammy and her family twice by phone and arranged for her to be admitted to a partial hospital program on Monday morning. During her first few days in the program, she was monitored closely by the staff, and her suicide potential was evaluated at the end of each day by the medical director. During the 1st week her suicide ideation resolved in response to the support and structure of the program. At the end of her 2nd week in the partial hospital program she was stabilized, started on antidepressant medication, and moved to outpatient family and group therapy following stated commitments to follow-up by the patient and her parents. The use of partial hospitalization prevented a psychiatric inpatient admission for this acutely symptomatic adolescent.

CASE ILLUSTRATION

Other aspects of day treatment are highlighted in the case of Jamie, a 15-year-old white boy who was admitted to a medium intensity partial hospital program. During a hospitalization for a life-threatening suicide attempt, his family's managed care company decertified his admission, saying he was no longer at acute risk for suicide. Due to Jamie's continued serious depressive symptoms and chronic family dysfunction, his case was determined to be inappropriate for routine outpatient management. He was admitted to a PHP with a strong family systems orientation. Over the course of his 8-week treatment he was able to develop a therapeutic alliance with his individual therapist, and significant family restructuring was accomplished. The consulting child and adolescent psychiatrist was able to manage Jamie's medication and monitor his suicide potential regularly. After discharge he continued in outpatient therapy and was able to attend school successfully. This partial hospital enrollment allowed for prompt discharge from the hospital and consolidation of progress in a highly structured system.

RESEARCH AND EVALUATION

As partial hospital and intensive outpatient services take a more central role in mental health care delivery, it is critical to establish quality standards and to differentiate these services offered from other services currently on the market. Evaluating quality of care and treatment outcome are integral components of this process.

Quality of Care

Partial hospital and other nonresidential hospital alternatives share many common treatment goals and techniques and differ in important ways from both inpatient treatment and outpatient office visits. Accordingly, the measurement of quality in this modality presents some unique challenges. Using the underlying philosophies, the unique therapeutic aspects, the distinctive treatment procedures, as well as the historical problems and promises of the field, specific quality indicators can be formulated.

Several specific quality indicators of effectiveness for partial hospital and intensive outpatient services include valid and accurate admission criteria, standards of care, and low negative, critical treatment incidents. As an alternative treatment modality, it is incumbent upon partial hospital and other ambulatory mental health services to establish admission criteria that reliably and validly discriminate between patients who need intervention at a more intensive level than outpatient visits, yet at a less restrictive level than 24-hour care. Having targeted an appropriate patient population, the standardization of services rendered as well as special treatment procedures needs to assure that the care offered provides the safety and security necessary for intensive treatment in a nonresidential setting.

Additional unique quality indicators include specific aspects of cost efficiency and patient satisfaction. Providing intensive treatment within a nonresidential environment mandates the use of outside resources and the reliance on strengths within the family and community for augmenting treatment, both of which translate into cost-efficient care. For partial hospitalization, two specific areas of patient satisfaction become applicable, the patient's feelings regarding receiving treatment as an outpatient and the family's sense of contentment with their role in the treatment process.

Finally, for partial hospitalization, viability is a critical factor, both at the level of the individual program and industrywide. Increased utilization, cost-containment, and internalization of quality are integral to survival of the modality. It is incumbent upon leaders in the field as well as policy-makers in managed care to improve patterns of utilization if alternative, intermediate forms of mental health care are to fulfill a role in the overall continuum of mental health services.

Treatment Outcome

Research on treatment effectiveness and outcome in psychiatry involves a complex constellation of factors, and major problems are encountered, including providing an objective, standardized definition of effectiveness and solving methodological constraints such as difficulties of selection procedures and randomization (Moskowitz, 1980). The scope of the research literature on the effectiveness of child and adolescent partial hospitalization is not yet broad enough to provide definitive information.

Limited research has been done on treatment effectiveness or outcome with child and adolescent samples. A summary of the studies conducted to date on adolescents in partial hospital programs indicates generally positive outcomes with improvement in interpersonal relationships and school performance (Corky and Zimet, 1987; Kettlewell et al., 1985). Review of studies on treatment outcome with children suggests 66–90% of patients demonstrated improvement and successful return to community-based schools. Studies suggest that family functioning (structure and stability) is a major factor in improvement (Prentice-Dunn et al., 1981; Sack et al., 1987) while others conclude that the younger children showed greater benefits from treatment in partial hospital settings than did older patients (Blom et al., 1973; Prentice-Dunn et al., 1981). Baenen et al. (1986), following a review of outcome studies, generally reported improvements in behavioral, academic, and family role functioning following partial hospitalization with a variety of aftercare services needed.

Movement to partial hospitalization away from traditional treatment modes would be alarming and irresponsible without treatment comparisons. It is essential to look at treatment effectiveness of partial hospital settings in comparison to effectiveness of other modalities. Again, published research has not been as extensive as desired. The literature on child and adolescent populations contains three studies that compare treatment outcomes in partial hospitalization and residential settings (Goldfarb and Goldfarb, 1966; Leone et al., 1986; Valesquez and Lyle, 1985). Overall, the findings suggest that partial hospitalization is equally effective with some patients on some variables, is more effective with some patients on some variables, and is less effective with some patients on some variables. Clearly, partial hospital advocates must continue to compare outcomes from different treatment modalities, from various partial program models, as well as compare treatment outcomes of specific populations.

One of the major difficulties encountered in the area of outcome measurement is the lack of standardization of outcome variables and instruments. Five areas of outcome measurement are recommended for partial hospitalization including cost of services, utilization of services postdischarge, severity of symptoms, level of functioning, and satisfaction (AAPH, 1994b). Standardized assessment of these variables is a goal with the objective of providing industrywide information regarding expected outcomes.

CONCLUSION

Partial hospitalization represents an important part of the continuum of psychiatric care available to children and adolescents with a wide array of disorders and allows these patients treatment in less restrictive settings than hospitals. In the current era of health care reform, this and other ambulatory mental health services will likely be in increased demand. As policies encourage such options, it is necessary to be aware of differences between partial hospital programs so that patient needs can be matched with program variables such as theoretical orientation, targeted populations, types of treatments offered within the program, staffing patterns, and the degree of structure provided. Issues related to quality of care, therapeutic outcome, and cost-effectiveness must also be considered. With careful review it is possible to identify intensive PHPs that serve as alternatives to inpatient hospitalization, those that function as transitions between highly restrictive treatments and outpatient services, and programs that serve as intensive outpatient programs.

It should be noted that, although partial hospitalization is an established concept and has a significant history, the field is in transition, as is health care in general. In the years to come, several questions will require answers. What position will partial hospitalization play as intensive outpatient services are expanded? What policies and procedures should be developed regarding intensive, freestanding programs versus step-down programs? Where does partial hospital treatment end and intensive outpatient begin?

PHPs will also face broader challenges as overall concepts of health care develop. How will partial hospital programs integrate with other children's services such as special education systems, juvenile courts, and state departments of child protection and human services? How will they fit into large health care organizations to provide prevention and related services? How will the concept of partial hospitalization evolve as health care reform progresses? We hope the closing decade of the 20th century brings answers to these important questions and the further development of this exciting mode of treatment.

References

American Association for Partial Hospitalization: *Outcomes Measurement Protocol.* American Association for Partial Hospitalization, Alexandria, VA, 1994.

Baenen RS, Stephens-Parris MA, Glenwich DS: Outcome in psycho-educational day programs: A review. *Am J Orthopsychiatry* 56:263–270, 1988.

Block BM, Arney K, Campbell DJ, et al: *Standards and Guidelines for Child and Adolescent Partial Hospitalization.* American Association for Partial Hospitalization, Alexandria, VA, 1991.

Blom GE, Farley GK, Ekanger C: *A Psychoeducational Treatment Program: Its Characteristics and Results.* Denver, University of Colorado Medical Center Press, 1973.

Casarino JP, Wilner M, Maxey JT: American Association for Partial Hospitalization (AAPH) standards and guidelines for partial hospitalization. *Int J Partial Hospitalization* 1(1):5–21, 1982.

Comer R: Day treatment of adolescents: An alternative to institutionalization. *J Counseling Dev* 64(1):74–76, 1985.

Corky CL, Zimet SG: Relationships with family and friends in young adulthood. *Int J Partial Hospitalization* 4:97–115, 1987.

Engel GL: The clinical applications of the biopsychosocial model. *Am J Psychiatry* 137:533–544, 1980.

Gaylor ML: Treating the adolescent offender in a rural partial hospitalization program. In: *Proceedings Annual Conference on Partial Hospitalization.* Boston, Federation of Partial Hospitalization Study Group, 1979.

Glasscote R, Kraft AM, Glassman S, et al: *Partial Hospitalization for the Mentally Ill.* Washington, DC, Joint Information Service 28:448–450, 1977.

Goldfarb W, Goldfarb N, Pollack RC: Treatment of childhood schizophrenics. *Arch Gen Psychiatry* 14:119–128, 1966.

Herz MI: Research overview in day treatment. *Int J Partial Hospitalization* 1:33–34, 1982.

Hoge MA, Davidson L, Hill WL, et al: The promise of partial hospitalization: A reassessment. *Hosp Community Psychiatry* 43:345–354, 1992.

Hoge MA, Farrell SP, Munchel ME, et al: Therapeutic factors in partial hospitalization. *Psychiatry* 51:199–210, 1988.

Kettlewell PW, Jones JK, Jones RH: Adolescent partial hospitalization: Some preliminary outcome data. *J Clin Child Psychol* 14:130–144, 1985.

Kiser LJ, Culhane DP, Hadley TR: The current practice of child and adolescent partial hospitalization: Results of a national survey. *J Am Acad Child Adolesc Psychiatry* 34:1336–1342, 1995.

Kiser LJ, Pruitt DB: A systems approach for day treatment. In: Farley GK, Zimet SG (eds): *Day Treatment for Emotionally Disturbed Children.* Vol 2: *Models and Their Efficacy.* New York, Plenum, 1991.

Kiser LJ, Heston JD, Millsap PA, et al: Testing the limits: Special treatment procedures for child and adolescent partial hospitalization. *Int J Partial Hospitalization* 7(1):37–53, 1991.

Kiser LJ, Lefkowitz PM, Kennedy LL, et al: Visions: The continuum of ambulatory mental health services. *Behav Healthcare Tomorrow* 2(4):14–16, 1993.

Kiser LJ, Prudden K: *Overview of the partial hospitalization industry.* American Association for Partial Hospitalization. Alexandria, VA, 1994.

Kiser LJ, Pruitt DB, McColgan EB, et al: A survey of child and adolescent day treatment programs: Establishing definitions and standards. *Int J Partial Hospitalization* 3(4):247–259, 1986.

Krizay J: *Partial Hospitalization. Facilities, Cost, and Utilization.* Washington, DC, American Psychiatric Association, Office of Economic Affairs, 1989.

Leibenluft E, Leibenluft RF: Reimbursement for partial hospitalization: A survey and policy implications. *Am J Psychiatry* 145:1514–1520, 1988.

Leone P, Fitzmartin R, Stetson F, et al: A retrospective follow-up of behaviorally disordered ado-

lescents: Identifying predictors of treatment outcome. *Behav Disord* 11(2):87–97, 1986.

Moskowitz JS: The effectiveness of day hospital treatment: A review. *Community Psychol* 8: 155–165, 1980.

Novello JR: Day hospital treatment of adolescents. In: Novello JR (ed): *The Short Course in Adolescent Psychiatry.* New York, Brunner/Mazel, 1979.

Prentice-Dunn S, Wilson DR, Lyman RD: Client factors related to outcome in a residential and day treatment program for children. *J Clin Psychol* 21: 189–196, 1981.

Prevost J: Partial hospitalization—Dynamics of under-utilization. Proceedings of the Annual Conference on Partial Hospitalization, San Diego. Boston, American Association for Partial Hospitalization, 1981.

Rogers SJ, Lewis H: An effective day treatment model for young children with pervasive develop-

mental disorders. *J Am Acad Child Adolesc Psychiatry* 28(2):207–214, 1989.

Sack WH, Mason R, Collins R: A long-term follow-up study of a children's psychiatric day treatment center. *Child and Human Dev* 18(1):58–68, 1987.

VandenBos GR: U.S. mental health policy, proactive evolution in the midst of health care reform. *Am Psychol* 48:283–290, 1990.

Velasquez JS, Lyle CG: Day versus residential treatment for juvenile offenders: The impact of program evaluation. *Child Welfare* 64(2):145–156, 1985.

Weithorn LA: Mental hospitalization of troublesome youth: An analysis of skyrocketing admission rates. *Stanford Law Rev* 40(40):773–838, 1988.

Zimet SG, Farley GK: Day treatment for children in the United States. *J Am Acad Child Psychiatry* 24: 732–738, 1985.

83 PSYCHIATRIC INPATIENT SERVICES

Joseph L. Woolston, M.D.

HISTORY

Just as child psychiatry as a specialty is only 35 years old, inpatient child psychiatry is virtually a fledgling treatment modality. Although the first few inpatient units were started in the 1920s and 1930s (American Psychiatric Association, 1957; Barker, 1974), their treatment remained narrowly focused on children with postencephalic brain disorders, and their numbers remained small for nearly four decades. In the 1970s a confluence of scientific, political, and fiscal factors produced a rapid rise in child psychiatric inpatient services.

This reached its apogee in the mid-1980s with a proliferation of child and adolescent units in both general and specialty psychiatric hospitals. The best of these services provided comprehensive, multimodal evaluation and treatment for several months duration (Harper and Geraty, 1985). However, by the early 1990s, enormous fiscal and political pressures (Woolston, 1993) have resulted in a halt to the expansion in the total number of inpatient beds as well as a dramatic reduction in the average length of stay (National Association of Private Psychiatric Hospitals, 1992).

Current child psychiatric inpatient units are deeply embedded in the milieu of the hospital environment and therefore are quite distinct from other institutionally based treatments of emotionally and behaviorally disturbed children and adolescents. However, children and adolescents have been, and continue to be, treated in a variety of other nonpsychiatric, institutional settings, including juvenile detention, social welfare, and educational systems. To date, the choice of treatment settings has been determined more by politics and custom than by diagnostic need. Until the middle of the 20th century, serious mental illness in children was thought to be rare, and therefore psychiatric hospitalization was rare. On the other hand, at the beginning of the century, child welfare facilities such as orphanages and shelters for the homeless housed the largest group of institutionalized children. In 1935 Congress authorized Aid to Families with Dependent Children (AFDC), which provided federal welfare funds for home care. Concurrently, professionals and politicians came to believe that "normal" children did not require the expensive course of institutional programs, so that many children in welfare facilities were deinstitutionalized.

Unfortunately, the juvenile detention system experienced a concurrent increase in children, completely offsetting the trend of deinstitution-

alization in the child welfare system. Specifically, admissions to all types of juvenile correctional facilities increased 9-fold from 1923 until 1979. This burgeoning use of the juvenile detention system was reversed by the passage of the Juvenile Justice and Delinquency Prevention Act in 1976 by the U.S. Congress. Between 1975 and 1979, the rate of detention for juvenile offenders decreased by 68% (Weithorn, 1988).

Two sets of legal decisions by the United States Supreme Court, one that supported the requirement for mental health coverage in insurance plans (*Massachusetts v. Metropolitan*) and the other that broadened the rights of parents to hospitalize their children voluntarily (*Parham v. J.R.*), served to accelerate this trend. As a result of these various influences, in the mid-1970s, the rate of admission to psychiatric hospitals began to increase as the rate of institutionalization in the juvenile detention system began to decline. The more recent trend in the mid-1990s toward greatly reduced lengths of stay in psychiatric hospitals has apparently been offset by a corresponding increase in placements in residential treatment programs, juvenile detention, and group homes. This phenomenon of shifting children and adolescents from one institutional setting to another as a result of nontherapeutic or nonclinical forces has been described as transinstitutionalization (Weithorn, 1988).

In the 1970s the transinstitutional shifts not only resulted in a higher rate of psychiatric admissions for minors but also changed the specific type of psychiatric facility to which they were admitted. In 1970 the rate of children's admissions to private for-profit psychiatric hospitals was 9.3 per 100,000 children or one-fourth of the rate of admissions to federal, state, and county public hospitals (37.8 per 100,000). During the 1970s, admissions of minors to public hospitals declined by 30% and admissions to private for-profit hospitals increased almost 100% so that in 1980 the rate of admissions of minors was about the same for both types of institutions. The rate of admissions of minors to private nonprofit general hospitals with inpatient services increased slightly from 63.3 per 100,000 in 1970 to 68.5 per 1000,000 in 1980 (U.S. Department of Health and Human Services, 1986). In addition to reduced admission rates to public hospitals, the average length of stay dropped from 74 days in 1970 to 54 days in 1980. Lengths of stay remained constant in private for-profit psychiatric hospitals at 36 days and increased slightly in general hospitals from 9 to 14 days (U.S. Department of Health and Human Services, 1986).

In the late 1980s and early 1990s, three separate forces combined to reverse this trend of increased inpatient utilization, especially in the private psychiatric hospitals. First, the proportion of money spent on mental health services had become unacceptably distorted toward inpatient services. For example, in 1986 residential and inpatient mental treatment for minors used up 78% of the $3.5 billion spent on all of mental health services in the United States. Partial hospitalization and various outpatient services accounted for 22% or $0.77 billion. For one specific insurance program, CHAMPUS, in 1989, the total mental health costs were $613 billion, of which $500 million was for inpatient psychiatric care in general, and $305 million for child and adolescent inpatient care in particular. Thus, nearly one-half (49.75%) of the entire CHAMPUS mental health costs for 1989 were accounted for by the hospital and residential treatment of children and adolescents (United States House of Representatives Select Committee on Children, Youth and Families, 1992). This rapid escalation of hospital costs combined with the national recession of the late 1980s to stimulate the development of cost saving strategies like managed care review and institutionally negotiated contracts with capitated reimbursements.

A second major brake on the rapid growth of hospitalization for minors was a nationally publicized series of criminal and unethical scandals, which rocked private psychiatric hospitals (United States House of Representatives Select Committee on Children, Youth and Families, 1992). A third, and apparently much more positive force has been the trend toward intensive, noninstitutional psychiatric treatments. Examples of this trend include federal legislation such as the Children and Adolescent System Services Program (CASSP); innovative state programs in Alaska, Vermont, and California; parent advocacy groups such as National Alliance of the Mentally Ill (NAMI); and support from foundations from organizations like the Robert Wood Johnson Foundation. All of these various programs emphasize the need for multiple services (e.g., mental health, welfare, education, recreation, and housing) to be available in a seamless fashion to children and family. Rather than requiring the child and family to accommodate to the demands of various institutions, the programs seek to develop individualized integrated services customized to the needs of the child. These various reform-oriented groups have attempted to reconceptualized inpatient units as the most restrictive and rarely used component of an integrated system of care rather than as the most accessible but disconnected fragment in a mental health nonsystem.

DIMENSIONS OF PSYCHIATRIC SERVICES FOR CHILDREN

These extraordinarily rapid and constant changes in inpatient psychiatric treatment have been accompanied by numerous growing pains. The model (and perhaps modal) child and adolescent inpatient service of the mid-1980s was a 10- to 20-bed unit dedicated to comprehensive evaluation and treatment with a length of stay of several months (Harper and Geraty, 1985; Woolston, 1989). More recently, in the early 1990s, the average length of stay has dropped to several weeks. This change has resulted in a focus on crisis intervention and evaluation rather than on longer term treatment. Such facilities are specialty units in general or larger psychiatric hospitals and are staffed with a multidisciplinary treatment team including child psychiatrists, pediatricians, psychologists, social workers, nurses, and teachers. High technology diagnostic testing, including brain imaging, electroencephalography, and chromosomal analysis is frequently employed (Woolston and Riddle, 1990). Treatment is characterized by an orchestrated blend of milieu, family, pharmacological, and individual therapies. For these and other reasons, children and adolescents may receive intensive evaluation and short-term treatment in hospital programs but then be unable to progress to less restrictive and less expensive but longer term treatments. This increasing intensity of treatment provided in inpatient units has tended to cut off such services from their historically related programs provided by educational, juvenile detention, and social welfare agencies. The very same medical, financial, and political forces that have promoted the growth

of these inpatient units have created artificially rigid boundaries with these other related treatments. Typically, children may receive public or private insurance funding for a relatively short hospital treatment but are without benefits to cover intensive outpatient or residential treatment. Ironically, the shortening of hospital lengths of stay to several weeks frequently results in a more disruptive hospital experience since welfare agencies, schools, and outpatient treatment programs cannot respond to the newly identified needs of the child before discharge.

Although the psychiatric treatment of children and adolescents is sometimes conceived of as a relatively homogeneous treatment modality, considerable heterogeneity actually exists in inpatient facilities. While inpatient units can be characterized by a large variety of factors, the following six dimensions account for most of the variance: level of restrictiveness of treatment, length of stay, type of psychiatric disorder, developmental level of patient, hospital organization or affiliation, and philosophy of treatment. Although each of these dimensions is distinct, they are obviously interdependent. For example, children with severe, chronic disorders, such as mental retardation and autism, frequently need very long-term treatment. Their families usually do not have the financial resources to pay for such treatment, so that the treatment facilities must rely on some form of public funding. A completely different constellation of factors is represented by adolescents with adjustment disorders. They are frequently treated in emergency or acute services funded by private insurance. Despite such clustering, these six dimensions provide a useful guide to understanding the current heterogeneity of services.

Level of Restrictiveness of Treatment

Perhaps the fundamental dimensions of inpatient child psychiatry is level of restrictiveness of treatment. By definition, inpatient treatment is the most restrictive modality, by virtue of its being an out-of-home, institutional setting. However, level of restrictiveness can vary considerably among psychiatric hospitals by such variables as whether admissions are voluntary or involuntary, the unit is locked or unlocked, participation by parents is encouraged or discouraged, and visits to the home community are facilitated or prevented.

This dimension of restrictiveness indicates part of the explanation for the rapid shifts among the population of mental hospital, welfare institutions, and juvenile detention facilities. All three sets of institutions, while supposedly treating children with quite different diagnostic descriptions, have in common the most restrictive treatment setting. Thus, from the point of view of funding or licensing agencies, hospitals, juvenile detention centers, and state institution shelters have virtually nothing in common. From the point of view of level of restrictiveness, all three facilities are nearly identical: They are highly restrictive, out-of-home, institutional placements.

LENGTH OF STAY

Length of hospital stay is both reflective of other dimensions of a hospital program and a determinant of constraints on these very same dimensions. Attempts to apply rational prospective payment systems (e.g., diagnostic related group system) to inpatient child psychiatry have shown that the major determinant of length of stay is funding availability or explicit program limitations, rather than patient diagnosis (Christ et al., 1989). Traditional groupings of lengths of stay include emergency (up to 3 days), acute (less than 4 weeks), short-term (1–3 months), intermediate (3–5 months), and long-term (greater than 9 months). Although these divisions are somewhat arbitrary, they both reflect and organize treatment philosophy, psychiatric diagnosis, type of patient served, and institutional organization. For example, very short-term lengths of stay preclude comprehensive interventions since the necessary relationships cannot be formed and evaluations cannot be completed. In addition, therapies that require a definite time period, such as some medication trials or educational programming, are not feasible. However, such short-term lengths of stay may be minimally disruptive to the child's important social relationships. In contrast, hospital programs with very long lengths of stay can reasonably attempt such goals as character change and academic disability remediation but run the risk of deleterious institutionalization effects.

Psychiatric Disorder

The typical psychiatric disorders of a specific inpatient population are determined by such factors as length of stay and institutional organization, and in turn determine other variables, such as philosophy of treatment. The broad groupings of psychiatric disorders include adjustment disorders, mixed behavior/affective disorders, eating disorders, adolescent/adult onset psychosis, substance abuse, pervasive developmental disorders, childhood onset psychosis, and mental retardation. Although the basic rudiments of diagnostic grouping exist, surprisingly little is known about the most basic aspects of the phenomenology of serious childhood-onset psychiatric disorders, including such aspects as natural history, epidemiology, etiology, and associated comorbidity (Woolston et al., 1989). The current state of ignorance about these fundamental issues places major constraints on specificity of treatment design as well as on intervention outcome evaluation.

Developmental Stage

Hospital programs designed for the treatment of children and adolescents usually stratify their units according to the developmental age of their patients. Not surprisingly, hospital facilities follow the same developmental groups as do education programs. These include programs for children up to 3 years (infant/toddler/preschool), 4–14 years (elementary/middle school), and 16–19 (high school/college). A program that is relatively homogeneous in developmental age automatically defines some of the constraints of psychiatric diagnosis, philosophy of treatment, and level of restrictiveness. For example, programs for adolescents will typically treat patients with eating disorders, affective/behavior disorders, substance abuse, and adolescent-onset psychotic disorders, whereas programs for young children will focus on pervasive developmental disorders, disruptive behavior disorders and, less frequently, childhood-onset eating disorders. Organization of elements of the treatment programming, such as the type of milieu and family therapy employed, will be greatly influenced by the developmental stage of the patient.

Institutional Organization/Affiliation

Another dimension defining hospital treatment is related to institutional organization or affiliation. One fundamental dichotomy is between publicly funded/affiliated hospitals and private hospitals. The publicly funded hospitals may be local, state, or federal, or some mixture of all three. Until recently, publicly funded hospitals have tended to be large psychiatric hospitals for severely and chronically disturbed children who frequently come from socially disadvantaged families. Because of the long-term, chronic nature of the psychiatric disturbance and relatively poor funding, these public hospitals tend to focus on benign environmental amelioration as a treatment philosophy. In these ways, some programs may more closely resemble residential treatment centers than inpatient services. The recent trends of deinstitutionalization and diminishing public funded hospitals have combined to result in shortened lengths of stay and decreased admission rates. Unfortunately, because few alternative mental health services for poor, chronically disturbed children have been implemented, the juvenile detention, social service, and education systems may well be forced to resume their previous roles in providing services. The other fundamental type of institutional organization group, nonpublicly funded hospitals, occurs as either nonprofit or for-profit hospitals. Typically, inpatient units in nonprofit private institutions are part of a general medical hospital that provides a full array of medical, surgical, and psychiatric services. These hospitals may be primary (local), secondary (state based), or tertiary (regional) facilities; each

level has an attendant structure of resources and typical patient population. Psychiatric inpatient treatment in general hospitals is quite heterogeneous. Some general hospitals do not have discrete children's psychiatric units. Instead, patients are admitted to general medical or pediatric units in so-called "scattered beds." Typically, children treated in these settings receive crisis intervention and then are discharged within 1–7 days. On the other hand, discrete, dedicated child psychiatric inpatient units in general hospitals offer comprehensive evaluation and treatment services by a multidisciplinary treatment team. Lengths of stay in these units range between 10 and 60 days. Although the median length of stay reported for psychiatric inpatients in general hospitals is 14 days, this number is probably a meaningless average between these two disparate groups in a bimodal distribution. Even within this special group of dedicated child inpatient units in general hospitals, there is considerable variation in philosophy of treatment, length of stay and developmental/diagnostic characteristics of the patients.

For-profit private proprietary psychiatric hospitals have experienced tremendous growth in the past decade. In 1971, about 6,500 children and adolescents were admitted to proprietary psychiatric hospitals, whereas by 1980 about 17,000 children under 18 were admitted. By 1984, 23,000 adolescents (ages 13–17) alone were admitted to these hospitals, and by 1986, 38,000 teenagers were hospitalized (Weithorn, 1988). The explanation for this explosive growth of proprietary psychiatric hospital admissions is multifaceted but probably devolves on four main factors: diminished availability of juvenile detention and child welfare systems; increased funding provided by private insurance and Medicaid; increased social instability due to divorce, moves, and social disruption; and the relaxation of the statutory rights of minors by the Parham decision of the U.S. Supreme Court in 1979 (Weithorn, 1988). This rapid growth of proprietary psychiatric hospital admissions have been accompanied by a storm of controversy and criticism that focused on excessive and inappropriate hospitalization of adolescents as a result of unprofessional and unethical admission policies (United States House of Representatives Select Committee on Children, Youth and Families, 1992; Weithorn, 1988; Woolston, 1993). This rapid proprietary hospital growth and its attendant abuses has had a number of consequences. Closer scrutiny by third-party payers and licensing agencies has occurred. This has resulted in numerous hospital closures and consolidations.

Philosophy and Goals of Treatment

The philosophy and goals of treatment espoused by various psychiatric inpatient services occur in a continuum ranging from custodial care to comprehensive evaluation and treatment of the child, family, and the important social environment. Although less ambitious treatment philosophies may reflect a callous or unethical approach to disturbed children, they may equally likely emerge from a realistic appraisal of fiscal, social, and clinical realities. Frequently, the level of intensity of the philosophy of treatment is highly correlated with the severity/chronicity of the psychiatric disturbance and the adequacy of funding. As the severity/chronicity of a disturbance increases and/or the level of funding decreases, the intensity of treatment diminishes.

CUSTODIAL CARE

Custodial care is geared toward preventing harm from befalling the patient, whether from inability to provide self-care or from injury. Custodial care is usually the dominant treatment philosophy only for the most severely disturbed psychotic and retarded children. Ironically, the only other setting in which custodial care is the prominent treatment philosophy is for acute, "social" admissions of relatively high-functioning children who need protection from their parents.

ENVIRONMENTAL AMELIORATION

The next level of treatment philosophy is nonspecific, benign, environmental amelioration. Specifically, the institution provides good nutrition, safe and pleasant surroundings, medical care, appropriate recreational activities, and an adequate education. While this level of treatment is rarely the officially stated philosophy of a hospital program, it may be the de facto treatment goal because of inadequate staffing and treatment planning. For institutions like child welfare agencies that provide services for children who are considered "normal," environmental amelioration may actually be an appropriate and desirable level of treatment.

SELECTED EVALUATION AND TREATMENT

The next level of treatment is selected evaluation and treatment of some aspect of the child and his or her important social environment. For example, many traditional psychiatric hospitals and residential treatment centers focus on evaluating and treating the child's psychiatric and behavioral problems. These programs emphasize milieu and individual as well as special education programs and parental counseling therapies (Harper and Geraty, 1985).

Of all the specific treatment modalities currently employed, milieu therapy encompasses the broadest range and is most specific to this form of treatment philosophy. Milieu therapy has its roots in the writings of Aichorn (1935), Bettelheim (1950), Redl and Wineman (1952), and Trieschman et al. (1969). These authors emphasized the use of the child's "Life-Space Model," the notion that every aspect of the child's physical and social environment is important in therapeutic understanding and treatment. Although milieu therapy at first focused upon an individual psychoanalytic understanding of the child, it has successively incorporated concepts of group, occupational, recreational, and behavioral therapies to create a multimodal therapeutic life experience. Although the specifics of each milieu program are different depending upon the psychiatric diagnoses and the developmental levels of the patient, the overall principles are similar (Cotton, 1993).

Individual therapies are considered to be all those interventions directed specifically toward the individual patient. They include individual psychodynamics psychotherapy, cognitive psychotherapy, individual behavior therapy, and pharmacotherapy. While these therapies are employed in a similar manner and for the same indications as they are for nonhospitalized patients, modifications are necessary to account for greater frequency and intensity of treatment and greater severity of psychiatric disturbance in the patient.

Regardless of the specific array of the treatment, inpatient psychiatry requires active coordination of the program. This issue of creating a coherent, well-synthesized treatment program fashioned out of many different treatment elements and employing many different clinicians is a major challenge for hospital treatment. Staton and Schwartz (1954) highlighted the frequently described phenomenon of significant clinical deterioration of patients when the coherence and consistency of the hospital program is destroyed by poor communication, divergent clinical opinions, and strongly held, emotionally charged differences among staff members.

Special education programs are an important, albeit much neglected, component of hospital programs. Perhaps the majority of children hospitalized on psychiatric inpatient units have a significant cognitive (e.g., mental retardation or borderline intellectual functioning) and/or academic (e.g., specific developmental learning disability) disorder (Woolston et al., 1989). The identification of these disorders and the subsequent development of remedial teaching strategies can play an important part in a child's treatment. Unfortunately, wide regional variation occurs in the level of funding available for these educational services. Services may vary from 2 hours of tutoring in the child's bedroom to 8 hours of special education in a comprehensive school setting. As lengths of stay diminish below 4 weeks, linkages with the child's original school becomes more difficult and providing a bona fide school curriculum becomes increasingly difficult.

In the service of maximizing the impact of these therapies on the child, those programs that use this level of treatment philosophy tend to disconnect the child from the important social environment, the family, and local school. While family therapy or parent counseling may be offered, it occurs in parallel and quite separate from the active hospital treatment of the child. This level of treatment philosophy is heavily influenced by the traditional medical model of hospitalization: The child is sick; the hospital treatment is to cure the child's illness; when cured, the child can return home. While this model works well for some acute illnesses, it is not appropriate for many chronic conditions, whether they are medical or psychiatric. Because such definite "fixing" of the child is not possible, changing the child's important social environment to be more suitable to the child's developmental needs may be as important as changing the child.

COMPREHENSIVE EVALUATION AND TREATMENT

The highest level of treatment philosophy aims at comprehensive evaluation and treatment of the child, the child's important environment, and the interaction of the two. An appreciation of the complex and powerful effect of the evolving interaction between the child and his or her important social environment follows from understanding the concept of a transactional risk model (Woolston, 1989). The transactional risk model rests on the concept of "goodness of fit" proposed by Chess and Thomas (1984), as well as concepts of resilience proposed by such authors as Garmezy (1983), Rutter (1979), and Werner and Smith (1982).

Articulation of this transactional model is a relatively recent development in inpatient treatment of children and awaits testing and development to determine its applications and problems. This model may provide a guide for both the orchestration of specific treatment modalities in an inpatient unit and the development of a network of services linking inpatient and outpatient programs to provide the most comprehensive and least restrictive treatment. Perhaps of greatest importance, this treatment philosophy attempts to address a major problem for hospital treatment: How can the gains achieved during the hospitalization be generalized and continued in less restrictive, more normative settings? In addition to "fixing" the child or, less frequently, "fixing" the family, this treatment philosophy attempts to ameliorate the interaction between the child and his or her environment so that the child's developmental potential will be maximized.

In the current climate of several-week hospitalizations, a major focus is on developing a more comprehensive, more appropriate outpatient system of care. This development entails bringing the new information learned about the child and family to the professionals who provide social services, education, and mental health services. In order to accomplish this development of a new system of individualized care, the inpatient facility must have preestablished linkages with an array of services such as school systems, day treatment, in-home services, therapeutic foster care, protective services, medical providers, traditional outpatient services, housing resources, and recreational programs.

FUTURE DIRECTIONS OF INPATIENT SERVICES FOR CHILDREN

The current status of inpatient child psychiatry is characterized by an exciting ferment of rapid development with a huge perceived need for treatment, but with a nearly total absence of data about the mechanisms to meet this need (Manderscheid et al., 1993). The further development of inpatient psychiatry will occur in response to the acquisition of more refined knowledge. Specifically, research is needed to increase understanding in several areas, including basic phenomenology about childhood-onset psychiatric disorders and their association with psychosocial stressors, the development and refinement of specific treatment strategies, the utilization of biomedical diagnostic and treatment techniques, and the implementation of an integrated network of mental health services with an appropriate, nondiscriminating funding basis.

References

Aichorn A: *Wayward Youth.* New York, Viking Press, 1935.

American Psychiatric Association: *Psychiatric Inpatient Treatment of Children.* Baltimore, Lord Baltimore Press, 1957.

Barker P: History. In: Barker P (ed): *The Residential Psychiatric Treatment of Children.* New York, Wiley, 1974.

Bettelheim B: *Love Is Not Enough.* New York, Free Press, 1950.

Chess S, Thomas A: *Origins and Evolutions of Behavior Disorders from Infancy to Early Adult Life.* New York, Brunner/Mazel, 1984.

Christ AE, Andrews H, Tsemberis S: Fiscal implications of a childhood disorder DRG. *J Am Acad Child Adolesc Psychiatry* 28:279–733, 1989.

Cotton N: *Lessons from the Lion's Den. Therapeutic Management of Children in Psychiatric Hospitals and Treatment Centers.* San Francisco, Jossey-Bass, 1993.

Garmezy N: Stressors of childhood. In: Garmezy N, Rutter M (eds): *Stress, Coping and Development in Children.* New York, McGraw-Hill, 1983, pp. 43–102.

Harper G, Geraty R: Hospital and residential treatment. In: Michels R (ed): *Psychiatry.* New York, Basic Books, 1985.

Manderscheid R, Rae DS, Narrow WE, et al: Congruence of service utilization estimates from the epidemiologic catchment area project and other sources. *Arch Gen Psychiatry* 50:108–114, 1993.

National Association of Private Psychiatric Hospitals 1987–1991: *Annual Report.* Washington, DC, National Association of Private Psychiatric Hospitals, 1992.

Redl F, Wineman D: *Control from Within.* New York, Free Press, 1952.

Rutter M: Protective factors in children's responses to stress and disadvantage. In: Rutter M (ed): *Primary Prevention of Psychopathology: Social Competence in Children* (Vol 3). Hanover, NH, University Press of New England, 1979.

Stanton AH, Schwartz MS: Pathological excitement and hidden staff disagreements. In: Stanton AH, Schwartz MS: *The Mental Hospital.* New York, Basic Books, 1954, pp. 342–365.

Trieschman AE, Whittaker JK, Bendtro LK: *The Other 23 Hours.* Chicago, Aldine Publishing, 1969.

United States House of Representatives Select Committee on Children, Youth and Families: *Special Hearing, The Profits of Misery: How Inpatient Psychiatric Treatment Bilks the System and Betrays Our Trust.* Washington, DC, U.S. Government Printing Office, 1992.

U.S. Department of Health and Human Services: *Children's Mental Health: Problems and Services,* Background Paper. Washington, DC, U.S. Government Printing Office, 1986, pp. 24–26.

Weithorn LA: Mental hospitalization of troublesome youth: An analysis of skyrocketing admission rates. *Stanford Law Rev* 40:773–838, 1988.

Werner EE, Smith RS: *Vulnerable but Invincible: A Study of Resilient Children.* New York, McGraw-Hill, 1982.

Woolston JL: Transactional risk model for short and intermediate term psychiatric inpatient treatment of children. *J Am Acad Child Adolesc Psychiatry* 28: 38–41, 1989.

Woolston JL: Crisis in psychiatric hospital care of children and adolescents: The paradox of simultaneous overuse, misuse, and abuse and underuse. Presented at the Annual Meeting of the American Psychiatric Association, San Francisco, CA, 1993.

Woolston JL, Riddle MA: The role of advanced technology in inpatient child psychiatry: Leading edge or useful aid? *J Am Acad Child Adolesc Psychiatry* 29:905–908, 1990.

Woolston JL, Rosenthal S, Riddle MA, et al: Childhood comorbidity of affective/anxiety and behavior disorders. *J Am Acad Child Adolesc Psychiatry* 28:707–713, 1989.

84 RESIDENTIAL TREATMENT

Melvin Lewis, M.B., B.S., F.R.C.Psych., D.C.H., Jeffrey W. Summerville, M.S.W., C.I.S.W., M.H.S.A., and Paul N. Graffagnino, M.D.

DEFINITION

Residential treatment centers (RTCs) are defined by the National Institute of Mental Health (Stroup et al., 1988) as psychiatric organizations serving children and meeting the following criteria:

1. It is an organization, not licensed as a psychiatric hospital, whose primary purpose is the provision of individually planned programs of mental health treatment services in conjunction with residential care for its residents.
2. It has a clinical program within the organization that is directed by either a psychiatrist, psychologist, social worker, or psychiatric nurse who has a master's and/or a doctoral degree.
3. It serves children and youth primarily under age 18.
4. The primary reason for the admission of 50% or more of the children and youth is mental illness, which can be classified by DSM-II/ICDA-8 or DSM-III/ICD-9-CM codes, other than those codes for mental retardation, substance (drug)-related disorders, and alcoholism. (We would now add DSM-IV/ICD-10 CM codes.)

HISTORY AND ORIGINS

In 1729 the first U.S. orphanage was founded by Ursuline nuns in New Orleans to provide care for a group of children whose parents had died in a smallpox epidemic. This is the origin of the custodial, or residential, component of residential treatment in the United States. Religious institutions remained prominent in offering custodial care for many years. Recognition of the developmental differences characteristic of children gradually led to the formation of the specialties of pediatrics and child psychiatry and, in the 1880s, to the emergence of numerous special agencies for children. In the 1900s mental health professionals—particularly psychoanalysts, child psychiatrists, psychologists, and social workers—began discovering and applying psychodynamic theories in the care and treatment of children. The main needs of the developing child were increasingly recognized, and comprehensive programs designed to meet those needs were planned. This program development constituted the first treatment component of residential treatment. Group living experiences; educational, physical health, and creative opportunities; and psychotherapy for children and their families, individually and in groups, began to replace rigid custodial care, with its strong moral and discipline-oriented attitudes.

The field of residential treatment for children subsequently developed on an empirical basis to provide multiple models of treatment to suit different needs. The different models also reflected different theories of child development. Thus, psychoanalysis and learning theory initially provided significant foundations for two polar treatment approaches, between which various admixtures of the two could be found. Subsequently, other theoretical models were introduced, including a goodness-of-fit model and various cognitive and behavioral approaches.

A view that has gained ground conceptualized the residential experience as a whole—group living, on-grounds schools, and psychotherapy—as constituting each child's therapy. Working under this view, all staff members are in full communication as they deal therapeutically with the children, their parents, and, in some cases, the whole family. Combined treatment modalities are used, including milieu therapy, family therapy, parent work, psychodynamic psychotherapy (individual, group), behavior therapy, pharmacotherapy, recreational therapy, art therapy, music therapy, and special education.

Table 84.1 Trends in Residential Treatment Bed Occupancy

	1972	1978	1984	1986	1988	1990[a]
Number of children	19,384	20,384	16,745	24,547	25,547	27,785
Number of facilities	340	375	322	437	440	501

[a] Statistics drawn from unpublished data, NIMH, 1994.

STATISTICS, TRENDS, AND FUNDING

In 1990 approximately 68,729 emotionally disturbed children in the United States received residential treatment in 501 facilities representing a total bed capacity of 29,756, with a year-end census of 27,785. The figures show a general increase in growth over the past two decades in the number of treatment beds available. There was a period of temporary decline in the early 1980s and a period of slight growth between 1986 and 1988 (Table 84.1).

Statistics published by the National Institute of Mental Health in 1991 note the following trends in residential treatment. In 1988 California and Massachusetts had the highest number of RTCs, 48 and 38, respectively. Other states with 15 or more RTCs were Colorado, Illinois, Minnesota, Ohio, Pennsylvania, and Wisconsin. Approximately 70% of RTCs had 50 or fewer beds. Twenty percent had 50–75 beds. Ten percent had over 100 beds. Over 33% of children were in residential treatment facilities having more than 100 beds.

In 1988 28% of RTC patients were black and 10% were Hispanic. Mental illness was considered the major disability of 94% of RTC admissions. Only 1–2% were diagnosed as alcohol or drug abusers. Occupancy rates increased from 87% in 1977 to over 95% in 1983 and remained over 95% throughout the 1980s.

Indicators of higher turnover rates and shorter lengths of stay began to appear, and from 1986 to 1988 there was a dramatic increase in the number of RTCs that offered partial care and outpatient treatment services. In 1988 RTCs provided services to 6.5% of the total population under 18 receiving psychiatric services.

An estimated $359.1 million was spent to maintain RTCs in 1977. By 1983 the figure had risen to $573 million, an increase of 60%. In 1988 the figure rose to $1.3 billion. However, in constant dollars this represents an increase of less that 5%. In 1988, of funds available for RTCs, 70% came from state and local government sources, 5% came from federal funds, 10% from client fees, and 12% from all other sources.

CONTINUUM OF RESIDENTIAL GROUP CARE OF CHILDREN

Historically, children are placed in the continuum of group care through the channels of the social welfare, juvenile justice, and mental health service delivery systems. According to the National Survey of Residential Group Care–1981, conducted by the University of Chicago, 3914 facilities in the United States operated with a total daily census of 125,323 (Young and Dore, 1989). Children classified as being in facilities for emotionally disturbed children accounted for 16% of the total in the year 1981 (Table 84.3). RTCs account for only a portion of the reporting facilities. Placement of children in different categories of facilities does not represent an accurate differentiation of children by diagnosis. The type of placement a child receives is also influenced by factors such as economic status, race, and geographical location.

STAFF AND SETTING

The professional staff of a residential treatment center includes child care workers, teachers, social workers, psychiatrists, pediatricians, nurses, and psychologists.

There were dramatic increases in the number of staff working in RTCs between 1984 and 1988. This increase followed a time of decline from 1978 to 1984. In 1978 RTCs employed 22,443 full-time equivalent (FTE) staff. The number dropped 5% in 1984 to 21,211. Between 1984 and 1988 the number of FTEs working in RTCs nearly doubled, reaching 39,186. In 1988 there were only 103 full-time psychiatrists working in RTCs with an additional 808 psychiatrists working part-time in RTCs. There were 370 full-time doctoral level psychologists and 472 part-time psychologists. Social workers with MSWs comprise the largest number of professionally degreed staff, reaching 2,753 full-time and 328 part-time staff in 1988. Registered nurses with Master's degrees numbered 163 full-time and 36 part-time in 1988. The percent distribution of FTE staff has remained relatively stable over the past decade (Table 84.2).

The Joint Commission on Mental Health of Children made the following structural or setting recommendations in 1979:

> In addition to space for therapy programs there should be facilities for a first-rate school and a rich evening and weekend activity program and there should be ample space for play, both indoors and out. Facilities should be small, seldom exceeding 60 in capacity with 100 a maximum limit, and should make provision for children to live in small groups. The centers should be located near the families they serve and be readily accessible by public transportation. They should be located for ready access to special medical and educational services and to various community resources, including consultants. They should be open institutions wherever possible; locked buildings, wards, or rooms should only rarely be required. In designing residential programs, the

Table 84.2 Number, Percent Change in Number, and Percent Distribution of Full-time Equivalent (FTE) Staff in Residential Treatment Centers (RTCs), by Staff Discipline, United States, January 1978 and 1984 and December 1988

Staff Discipline	Number of FTE Staff/Percent Change in Number (1978–1984)/(1984–1988)			Percent Distribution		
	1978	1984	1988	1978	1984	1988
Psychiatrists	140	240 (+71%)	449 (+187%)	0.6	1.1	1.1
Psychologists	497	820 (+65%)	1274 (+155%)	2.2	3.9	3.3
Social workers	2196	2283 (+4%)	4211 (+184%)	9.8	10.8	10.7
Registered nurses	324	485 (+50%)	821 (+169%)	1.4	2.2	2.1
Other (BA+)	7667	6723 (−12%)	12934 (+192%)	36.1	31.7	33.0
Other (BA−)	5640	4746 (−16%)	10451 (+220%)	25.9	22.4	26.6
Administration/maintenance	5979	5914 (−1%)	9046 (+153%)	26.6	27.9	23.1

Note: Table amended from NIMH published statistics, 1988 and 1991. Listings for psychologists, social workers, and nurses include both BA, MA, and Doctoral level staff functioning in those designated roles.

Table 84.3   Number of Children and Youth, 1966 and 1981, by Type of Facility

Type of Facility	Number of Children and Youth			
	1966		1981	
	N	%	N	%
Dependent and neglected	60,459	(39)	24,533	(20)
Pregnant	5,835	(4)	1,676	(1)
Temporary shelter	1,832	(1)	3,893	(3)
Delinquent	55,000	(35)	40,335	(32)
Status offenders	0[a]	—	4,754	(4)
Detention	10,875	(7)	15,423	(12)
Substance abuse	0[a]	—	1,629	(1)
Emotionally disturbed	13,876	(9)	20,397	(16)
Psychiatric	8,028	(5)	12,683	(10)
Total	155,905	(100)	125,323	(99)[b]

© 1989. Child Welfare League of America. Used with permission. This table was originally published in Young T, Dore M, Pappenfort D: Trends in residential group care: 1966–1981. In: Balcerzak EA (ed): *Group Care of Children Trends Toward the Year 2000.* Washington, DC, Child Welfare League of America, 1989.
[a] Not recognized as a type of facility in 1966.
[b] Figures do not equal 100% due to rounding.

guiding principle should be this: Children should be removed the least possible distance—in space, in time, and in the psychological texture of the experience—from their normal life setting. (p. 43)

The actual design of the building should take into account the physical, cognitive, and emotional needs of children between 6 and 15 years of age. Private or shared bedrooms, separate showers and bath facilities for boys and girls, communal living rooms and dining rooms, safe and easy access to recreational facilities and classrooms, and therapists' offices close to the group living area are some of the requirements. Units serving specific age groups are preferred.

Most residential treatment centers gradually increase in size; as they do so, the number of children in each residential unit tends to increase. At the same time, Marsden et al. (1970) found that the duration of treatment seems to shorten as this growth occurs. Older children tend to remain in residence for shorter periods of time than do younger children.

INDICATIONS

The child's lack of age-appropriate internal controls and need for more consistent external controls, as well as the child's need for intensive specialized treatment, constitute basic indications for residential treatment. Such children may present with moderately severe symptoms of antisocial and aggressive behaviors; they may have psychotic symptoms, including loose associations and hallucinations; or they may exhibit precipitous, severe regressions. Bed-wetting is a common symptom. Most, if not all, children referred for residential treatment have severe learning problems.

Genetic factors, organic brain damage, neurochemical dysfunctions, and adverse psychological experiences in the child, together with psychosis and other psychiatric disorders in the parents and an impoverished socioeconomic climate, are major causative factors. A history of parental deprivation, loss, seduction, incest, sexual and physical abuse, and physical injury is common, as is a history of multiple foster home placements.

Using the DSM-IV classification (American Psychiatric Association, 1994) the clinical diagnoses most often attached to the child include pervasive developmental disorders (not otherwise specified), attention deficit hyperactivity disorder, specific developmental disorders, conduct disorder, dysthymia, major depressive disorder and anxiety disorders.

Referral, Intake, and Admission

Most children who are referred for residential treatment have been seen previously by one or more professional persons, such as a school psychologist, pediatrician, or members of a child guidance clinic, juve-

nile court, or state welfare agency. Unsuccessful previous attempts at outpatient treatment and foster home or other custodial placement often precede residential treatment. Consequently, considerable data are usually available to and are usually required by the intake staff of the residential treatment center; however, residential centers differ in the evaluation and decision-making process used for selecting children for admission. Satisfactory studies comparing admission criteria and outcome correlations have not been done. The type of child referred to a particular institution is often idiosyncratic to that institution. The age range of the children varies from institution to institution, but most children are between 5 and 15 years of age. Boys are referred more frequently than girls.

An initial review of the data enables the intake staff to determine whether a particular child is likely to benefit from their particular treatment program. The next step usually involves interviews with the children and their parents by various staff members, such as a therapist, a group living worker, and a teacher. Psychological testing and neurological examinations are performed when indicated, if these have not already been done. Children and their parents should be prepared for these interviews. A useful practice is to have the child spend a day at the center, both in class and on a residential unit.

During this admission and diagnostic process, a comprehensive profile of each child is established. There is at present no standard profile in use. Structured interview schedules are useful. A mental status examination of the child is essential.

The needs of each child, the skills of the staff, the balance of the patient population, and estimates of the prognosis are some of the variables weighed when children are accepted for admission. The parents may or may not be available for treatment. This entire evaluation and assessment process forms the basis on which the total staff reaches a decision and makes a tentative treatment plan. A preplacement visit by the children and their families is usually arranged to help prepare each child for admission.

TOTAL STAFF COLLABORATION

Group cohesiveness among the staff improves performance. Johnson (1982) described the measures that promote such cohesiveness: meetings to discuss team process issues, acquisition of leadership skills, clear lines of authority and role expectations, training programs, total team participation in decisions, and prompt expressions of support, concern, and empathy by the leadership. The cooperative attitude of administrative leaders sets the tone for residential treatment staff. Haley (1980) suggested that success in therapy might be determined in part by what happens among the professional staff. Resolving communication problems, sharing perceptions and experiences, clarifying transference and countertransference issues, and providing a means by which staff can receive feedback on how well they are doing are matters that are as important for the staff as they are for the children.

ADMINISTRATION

Administration of an RTC requires sound business practices in regard to defining the organization's purpose and mission, securing adequate financial and personal resources, clarifying lines of authority and accountability, and developing responsive programming. RTC administrators must be involved in statewide and national professional and political organizations, as changes in health care and social service policies require rapid adaptive changes in RTC programming and funding. In the past decade, strong state and national consortiums of residential treatment facilities have been developed to play a vital role in assessing the changing needs of children, advocating for children's services, and sharing resources.

In addition to employing sound business practices, administrators of RTCs must understand the impact of severely disturbed children on the individual and group functioning of the staff. This has become more important in recent years as psychiatric hospital stays and other factors have led to RTCs' admitting even more seriously disturbed children, many on psychotropic medication, than they had in years past. Administrative commitment to a supervisory process that acknowledges the impact of severely emotionally and behaviorally disturbed children on all agency staff is essential. R. Howenstine (unpublished manuscript, 1984) suggests that a key administrative role in achieving staff collaboration is to conceptualize interdepartmental collaboration and conflict management as a vehicle for identifying, containing, and dealing with the aspects of the children's pathology that are internalized by the staff. Brown (1983) provides a theoretical and systematic approach to managing conflict at departmental interfaces from a management perspective, focusing on six major opportunities for change: (*a*) alter perception, (*b*) alter communication, (*c*) alter behavior, (*d*) alter the interface, (*e*) alter one or both departments, and (*f*) alter organizational context.

CHILD CARE WORK

By far the largest amount of time in the child's life in a residential treatment setting is spent in group living. Northrup (1982) maintains that it is the child care worker in group living who is usually responsible for the improvement in deeply disturbed children in residential treatment. These workers' use of ''good enough parenting'' allows them to serve as role models for the children. Child care workers also offer a structured environment that constitutes a therapeutic milieu. Tasks are defined within the limits of the child's abilities; incentives, such as increased privileges, encourage the child to progress rather than regress. Every member of the staff is important; for example, the dietary staff may have a special role and meaning for some children for whom food and its associations have special significance, including feelings of security, deprivation, love, and aggression.

Children often select one or more staff members with whom to form a relationship through which they express, consciously and unconsciously, many of their feelings toward their parents. The child care staff should be able to recognize such transference reactions and to respond to them in a way that is different from the children's expectations based on previous or even current relationships with their parents. Sometimes, the child care workers know enough about a child to make an interpretation to the child when it seems appropriate—the so-called life-space interview (Redl, 1959). However, the child care worker must also be aware of the countertransference problems stimulated by the child's behavior and, indeed, by other staff members in what is essentially a large, close, familylike community.

To maintain consistency and balance, the group living staff must communicate freely and regularly with one another and with the other professional and administrative staff members of the residential setting, particularly the child's teacher and therapist. The group living worker has perhaps the most potential among the staff members to produce therapeutic gains.

The child care staff members must recognize any tendency toward being the good, or bad, parent in response to the child's splitting behavior. This tendency in a staff member may become manifest as a pattern of blaming other staff members for the child's disruptive behavior. Similarly, the child care staff must recognize and avoid such individual and group countertransference reactions as sadomasochistic and punitive behavior toward a child.

A common milieu dilemma occurs when the child care worker has to differentiate the approaches needed for, say, the conduct disordered or psychotically disturbed children in their care from an understandable tendency to want to apply a consistent approach to all children. Therapists and consultants need to be called upon to educate child care staff regarding the developmental and psychodynamic needs of each child and how different techniques might be applied while maintaining unit cohesiveness and avoiding countertransference problems.

The structured setting should offer growth-promoting experiences and opportunities for facilitating and improving the adaptive behavior of the children. Particular deficiencies such as speech and language deficits, intellectual retardation, inadequate peer relationships, bed-wetting, poor feeding habits, or attention deficits may be at the base of the children's poor academic performance in school and their unsocialized behavior, including temper tantrums, fighting, and withdrawal, and require particular attention.

Behavior therapy principles are also applied, particularly in group work with children. In the course of group therapy, behavior that is socially adaptive and appropriate may be awarded points. At the end of the session, all the children receive a prize of, say, candy, but the child who has the most points gets first choice. Behavior therapy is a component of the total therapeutic effort of the residential center.

Unfortunately, many child care workers feel frustrated and confused, and they experience job dissatisfaction. Rick and Charlesworth (1982) suggested that this is partly because they do not have sanction to cross certain professional boundaries. Child care workers and other professionals—psychiatrists, psychologists, social workers, teachers—need to recognize the problem as a systems issue and should participate in education and accommodation aimed at realignment of professional roles. There is a corresponding need for a career development ladder for child care workers.

PHYSICAL HEALTH

Many children referred to RTCs have physical health problems, including poor nutrition, dental problems, and frequent infections. Attention must therefore be paid to health care. Particular attention must be given to adequate hygiene, and standard universal safety precaution procedures should be followed. On-staff registered nurses are indispensable, along with a panel of physician consultants.

SCHOOL PROBLEMS

Children in residential treatment frequently have severe learning disabilities, as well as disruptive behavior, and usually they cannot function in a regular community school. A thorough diagnostic assessment of a child's specific learning difficulties is required as a basis for a rational approach to the application of specific remedial measures (Table 84.4).

A special on-grounds school setting is usually required. Some of the characteristics of this on-grounds school include staff who are skilled in special educational assessments; a low teacher-to-student ratio; specialized learning equipment including computers and word processors; and a curriculum designed to captivate the children's interest and motivate them to begin learning again.

The teacher is also often in the same relationship to the children as the group living worker and can offer them a structured environment, a model for identification, and a clarifying interpretation of their behavior, when appropriate. The teacher must be in free and regular communication with the other professional staff members, including the group living

Table 84.4 Evaluation Process for Assessment of School Difficulties in the Child

1. Pediatric history: birth, development, personal, social, family, school, previous illnesses, life events
2. Specific strengths: sports, creative arts
3. Specific symptoms or skill delays, or both: reading, writing, arithmetic, directionality, visual and auditory sequencing, memory, coordination, attention
4. Associated behavior, personality trait or difficulties: adaptations, defenses, self-esteem, anxiety, depression
5. Comprehensive pediatric physical examination and diagnostic consultations: visual, auditory, speech, and language evaluations
6. Neurodevelopmental examination
7. Psychiatric and psychological assessment
8. Educational assessment

Table 84.5. The Educational Process in Residential Treatment

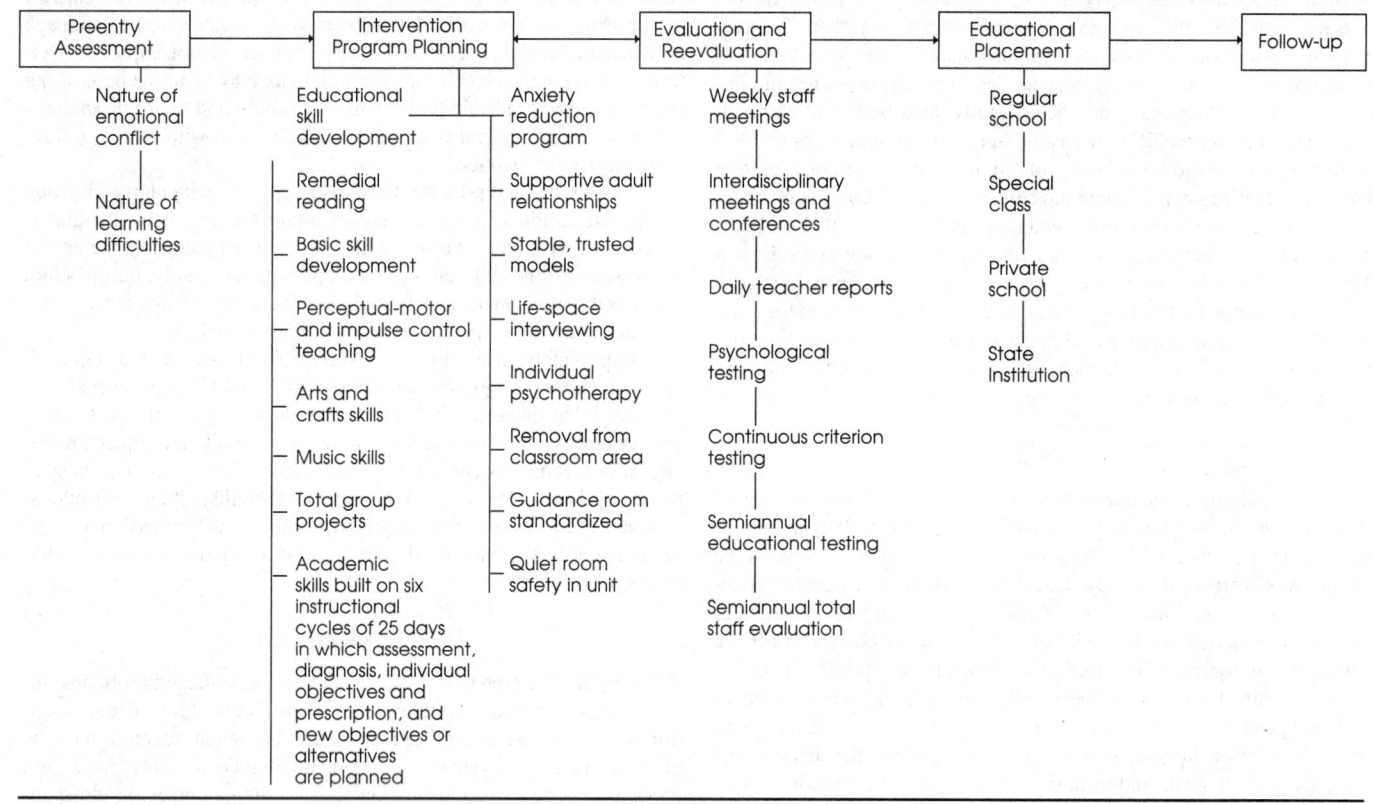

Preentry Assessment	Intervention Program Planning		Evaluation and Reevaluation	Educational Placement	Follow-up
Nature of emotional conflict	Educational skill development	Anxiety reduction program	Weekly staff meetings	Regular school	
Nature of learning difficulties	Remedial reading	Supportive adult relationships	Interdisciplinary meetings and conferences	Special class	
	Basic skill development	Stable, trusted models	Daily teacher reports	Private school	
	Perceptual-motor and impulse control teaching	Life-space interviewing	Psychological testing	State Institution	
	Arts and crafts skills	Individual psychotherapy	Continuous criterion testing		
	Music skills	Removal from classroom area	Semiannual educational testing		
	Total group projects	Guidance room standardized	Semiannual total staff evaluation		
	Academic skills built on six instructional cycles of 25 days in which assessment, diagnosis, individual objectives and prescription, and new objectives or alternatives are planned	Quiet room safety in unit			

From Lewis M: Residential treatment. In: Kaplan HI, Sadock BJ (eds): *Comprehensive Textbook of Psychiatry* (Vol. 4). Baltimore, Williams & Wilkins, 1985, p.1800.

staff and the children's therapists. Table 84.5 shows some of the components of the educational process.

A major goal of the on-grounds school is to motivate the children to learn. This is done, in part, by providing multiple success experiences at whatever level the child is capable. While the children are in school, the school should have full responsibility for dealing with them. School staff should take advantage of what is known about the child as they attempt to improve the children's self-esteem, motivate them to learn, and provide opportunities for them to acquire adaptive skills. Comer (1980) notes that the child and adolescent psychiatrist can offer useful consultations to school staff members in this regard, and the child care workers and therapists can offer support to the teachers in understanding and managing a particular child.

If the location of the RTC permits, the occasional child may attend a nearby public school, if indicated, while remaining in the residential program.

THERAPY

Traditional modes of psychotherapy have a definite place in residential treatment. These modes include intensive individual psychotherapy with the child; group therapy with selected children; individual or group therapy or both for parents; and in some cases, family therapy. However, several modifications need to be kept in mind.

The child relates also to the total staff of the setting and therefore needs to know that what transpires in the therapist's office is shared with all professional staff members. The therapist informs the child that what they discuss and do in individual therapy will not be revealed to other family members or to other children in the residential center but will in most instances be shared with professional staff members within the setting itself. Indeed, psychotherapeutic encounters often continue outside the setting of the therapist's office. Psychotherapy within a residential setting can hardly proceed without a full knowledge of the daily life of the child with peers and staff members in the group living situation and in the school. In addition, group living and school experiences can be made more meaningful if the therapist communicates freely and frequently with the child care worker and the teacher.

THE PARENTS

Concomitant work with the parents is essential. The child usually has a strong tie with the parent, no matter how disturbed that parent may be. Sometimes the parent is idealized by the child but repeatedly fails the child. Sometimes the parent has an ambivalent or unrealistic expectation that the child will return home. In some instances, the parent must be helped to enable the child to live in another setting when that is in the best interest of the child. Most residential treatment centers offer individual or group therapy with the parents, couples therapy, and, in some cases, conjoint family therapy.

The therapist who works with the child should also be the person who works closely with the family to help them deal with their feelings of guilt regarding placing the child and with their tendencies to overcompensate for this placement by trying to indulge the child. Wild swings of ambivalence and reaction formation toward children before admission are sometimes replaced by hostility after they enter residential treatment.

Similarly, the parents need help when the children go home for a visit. The children's behavior often represents a demand for reparations in the form of constant demands for attention, sometimes virtually compelling their families to rearrange their schedules around the children's wishes. Children almost become tyrants during these visits, leading the parents to resent them since they are unable, without instructional help from the staff, to set limits. Children may also present a distorted picture of their parents to the staff as part of an unconscious attempt to ward off anxiety through splitting and projection.

CASE MANAGEMENT

All components of residential treatment must be effectively coordinated with regard to each specific child. The program should be carefully tailored to meet the needs of each specific child. Individualized treatment goals and objectives should be written with input from the therapist, teacher, child care worker, psychiatrist, psychologist, child, parent, referral source, and accountable funding source. Clinical social workers are specifically trained in the coordination of child and family services, as well as in individual psychodynamics and group dynamics. Clinical social workers increasingly play a case management role in residential treatment facilities, in addition to providing specific modes of therapy. In most RTCs the clinician assigned to the child is also designated the case manager and is responsible for coordinating and integrating the work of the school, child care department, and clinical department, as well as that of the parent/guardian and accountable funding source. The case manager must have the responsibility and authority to ensure coordination and consistency of programming for designated children. In most RTCs the clinician must also, of necessity, play a broader role in overall program management and the coordination of treatment teams. A particularly challenging problem must be faced by the clinician who serves as the case manager and therapist for the same child at the same time. The child and adolescent psychiatrist can serve a useful role as consultant to the case manager.

THE ROLE OF THE CHILD AND ADOLESCENT PSYCHIATRIST

The presence of a fully qualified child and adolescent psychiatrist is essential for the staff of any residential treatment center serving children and adolescents and their families. The exact administrative position may vary from that of chief administrator to medical director to psychiatric consultant, and must be clearly understood by administrator and psychiatrist. Whatever the position and title, there are certain clinical, consultative, and educational services the psychiatrist should be asked to provide.

The need for the psychiatrist in RTCs has continued to increase in recent years because of a number of changes that have occurred in the mental health delivery system and the resultant changes in the needs of the children and adolescents who are being admitted and treated. For example, relatively long-term inpatient psychiatric hospitalization has nearly disappeared in the United States. Many of the young patients who must be discharged under current criteria are not ready or able to be returned to their families even with the provision of the most extensive and sophisticated types of "wrap-around" services.

Thus RTCs are receiving young patients with more serious, and less well-stabilized, psychiatric illnesses than in the past. To meet the challenge of this situation, the psychiatrist must be available to have significant input and responsibility in the intake process, in the communication with the referral source, in the initial evaluation and treatment planning, and in particular, in the increasingly complex psychopharmacological regimens the referring hospital may have initiated for many of the incoming young people.

As a corollary to the above changes, there is an increasing need to be able to use referral to the short-term inpatient psychiatric hospital for emergency situations affecting the patient's safety or for severe regressive episodes that the RTC is not able to handle. Here again the psychiatrist's role is crucial in helping the staff of the RTC make decisions in a given case, and in communication with the receiving hospital during the referral stage, after the patient has been admitted and during the planning for the return to the RTC.

The well-functioning RTC calls for a carefully orchestrated and multifaceted effort by all staff members, who come from many disciplines and from all departments (including "nonclinical" areas such as housekeeping, dietary, maintenance, and business office) whose goal is to help the individual child and his or her family. The psychiatrist must become integrated into the organization in such a way as to be able to help provide the unique understanding of the complexities of the individual child and to help in the ongoing and often changing need for balance in the many approaches concurrently being used to help that child.

It is important that the specific duties and functions of the psychiatrist be carefully spelled out, understood, and clarified when necessary. Among these it is recommended that the following should be included:

1. *Direct case consultation with the clinicians:* The psychiatrist consults once a week for 30–45 minutes individually with each clinician, discussing the issues of that person's caseload as indicated. Both client-centered and consultee-centered case consultation should be offered (Caplan, 1970). Especially important is a discussion of any psychopharmacological treatment of a given child for whom the psychiatrist and the nonpsychiatric clinician may be collaborating.

2. *Participation in case conferences with team members:* At least 1–2 hours per week of the psychiatrist's time should be available as needed for participation in conferences dealing with any and all issues regarding a given child, ranging from crises to milieu dilemmas to longer range treatment problems.

3. *Direct psychiatric evaluation of children:* Whenever needed, the psychiatrist will be available to evaluate a given child for various purposes, including intake evaluations, evaluations upon admission, evaluations for psychopharmacological treatment, evaluations for psychiatric emergencies, and direct consultative evaluations to explore clinical issues as requested by staff clinicians.

4. *Continuous case conference with clinicians:* A weekly 1-hour conference is suggested, led by the psychiatrist, at which one of the clinicians presents, for a series of weeks, an informative treatment process. Should there be clinical trainees in the agency, their supervisors may want them to be present at such a conference.

5. *In-service educational conferences:* The psychiatrist provides talks and seminars and participates in panel presentations on topics of interest to all staff of the agency.

6. *Informal visits to classrooms, living units, and other residential activities:* As the consultant becomes more familiar to staff and clients, communication is enhanced and the consultant's contributions in more formal meetings is enhanced.

7. *Participation in agency committees and working groups:* On an as needed basis the psychiatrist should be available to make contributions to agency groups.

8. *Administrative consultation:* In many agencies the administrators and the psychiatrist will have developed a relationship such that the psychiatrist may be asked to provide consultation on the development of new programs, revision of existing programs, or other related problems (Caplan, 1970).

9. *Direct monitoring of patients on psychotropic medications:* The psychiatrist must take responsibility not only for prescribing the medications, but must on a regular basis follow the patients directly. A useful way to do this might be to conduct a weekly "medication clinic" wherein the psychiatrist spends approximately $\frac{1}{2}$ hour evaluating each child, reviewing the chart, and writing a progress note. In an agency of 40 residents, 20 of whom are on medication, for example, the "medication clinic" would last for about $2\frac{1}{2}$ hours each week in order that each patient be seen once a month.

10. *Medication rounds with agency nursing staff:* Once a week a systematic review of charts should be done with appropriate documentation of findings and recommendations. The psychiatrist and nurse conduct the review, but input by other staff members is welcome.

In most residential treatment centers the psychiatrist does not have complete responsibility for the treatment of a given child or adolescent, but must in some aspects act as a consultant, in some as collaborator, and in the matter of medication, as the responsible physician. It is important that the psychiatrist and agency staff members understand and remain aware of these interrelationships at all times.

ADMINISTRATION OF MEDICATION

Medication is most helpful when there is a clear indication or target symptom for a particular drug; it may help the child engage in a therapeutic relationship and may facilitate attention and learning. Sometimes a drug is a useful additional measure during the stress of the initial period of residential treatment, or later at times of crisis. Many children with thought disorders or hallucinatory experiences can be maintained in the RTC only with appropriate antipsychotic medications. As noted above, many children admitted are already receiving medications.

Inasmuch as the total staff, the child, and the family are all involved, it is important to develop a well-understood medication procedure. The initial request for medication may arise from the child, a parent, or any staff member and is then processed by the child's therapist. A full discussion by the entire staff is necessary to clarify the goals for medication use and its anticipated effects on the child. Impulsive proposals for the use of medication are sometimes made by staff members who feel frustrated and desperate in their efforts to manage especially difficult behavior. Countertransference problems are sometimes an unrecognized motivation.

The child should have as thorough an understanding as possible of the medication's effect and the reasons for taking it. Children may have special fears about taking psychotropic medication. Often, these fears and unrealistic expectations are elaborations of statements or attitudes of peers, staff members, parents, or other family members.

It is important to talk with the child's parents or guardians about the proposal for medication. In addition to obtaining informed consent, the staff can correct misunderstandings and can encourage the parents to develop a reasonable, supportive attitude toward the child's use of medication. To achieve this end, the following procedure is useful:

1. The therapist, in consultation with the staff, the child, and the parents, defines the target symptoms, the expected goals, and the anticipated effects of the medication. The therapist explains the procedures to the parents.
2. A careful history is taken of significant previous illnesses or allergies in the child or family members and of any history of previous drug experience.
3. The child's physical state is reviewed.
4. A baseline mental status examination is performed, and various behavior ratings may be made.
5. Informed consent is obtained in writing from the parents or legal guardians.
6. All this information is made available to the entire staff for discussion. For this purpose, a brief synopsis of the drugs commonly used should be available to the staff, and the therapist should prepare a summary that follows a standard outline for all to read. A key decision-making conference should then be held.
7. After the decision is made, appropriate laboratory tests are performed, and the medication is prescribed and administered.

Over the past decade the numbers of children admitted to residential treatment centers with severe psychiatric disorders and those taking psychotropic medications have increased steadily. It is not uncommon now that 30–50% of residents are on such medications. Appropriate medical records and written procedures and protocols for psychopharmacological therapy must be in place. These should include the following:

1. *Medical records:* The child's medical records relevant to psychotropic medications should include doctor's orders, prescriptions, laboratory reports, reports from other hospitals or facilities, progress notes, documentation of medication reviews with the nursing staff, copies of informed consent and authorizations by parents or guardians.
2. *Written protocols for psychopharmacotherapy:* These should include procedures for initiating therapy (including the issues as described above) and for maintaining and discontinuing therapy. Staff are sometimes reluctant to discontinue medication because they fear a return of difficult behavior in the child. The reluctance may take the form of rationalizations such as upcoming vacations, schedule changes, room changes, staff changes, parent visits or other possible stresses. The clinical reasons for discontinuing medication should therefore be carefully documented.
3. *Protocols for laboratory and other studies:* For a given medication, or for a given category of medications, the specific schedules of studies including vital signs, laboratory studies, abnormal involuntary movement scale (AIMS) testing, rating scales, checklists of side effects, ECGs, and other tests should be documented for the premedication phase, for the times of changes of dosage, and for the ongoing maintenance phase. Behavior changes in relation to itemized target symptoms and initial behavior ratings should be regularly documented.
4. *Procedures for discharging clients on medications:* Before discharge it is important to have established which outside practitioner will take responsibility for continuing the treatment and to document that the parent or guardian accepts the responsibility to carry this out.

COMMUNICATION

To maintain the necessary communication in the residential staff, the staff members must meet as a total group, without an agenda, at least once a week. These meetings allow feelings to come to light that may otherwise remain hidden and silently ferment. Role conflicts; countertransference problems; treatment blind spots; and residential center policies with regard to such issues as limit setting, outside visits, treatment approaches, and work with such agencies as an outside school and a welfare agency are some of the subjects that are discussed. Greater staff cohesion, collaboration, and commitment occur when all staff members are involved in every aspect of the child's treatment. Recent contributions from social system theory have enabled residential treatment center staff members to view their interaction as part of a complex social system, constituting a further aid to communication.

To monitor the course of treatment, the staff must also attend regular comprehensive case review conferences, at which reports from group living, school, and therapy staff members are presented and discussed, along with additional data derived from neurological examinations and psychological tests. Diagnoses and treatment goals often need to be revised as the child becomes better known to the staff. The revision may go in either direction; that is, a psychotic process may gradually be revealed or a child may show strong restitutive capacities once he or she is in a stable environment. Colligan et al. (1981) developed an organizational grid to provide a visual representation of the factors involved in residential treatment. The grid evaluates diagnostic information from four developmental dimensions: physiological, emotional, sociobehavioral, and cognitive-academic. The effects of these dimensions on family, school, and group living can then be monitored.

COURSE OF TREATMENT

Children who enter a residential center may experience anxiety and feelings of loss, as well as some relief. They may temporarily deal with this anxiety or relief by exhibiting good behavior and a strong apparent wish to please. This so-called honeymoon period, which may last from a few days to a few months, soon gives way to the reemergence of the children's characteristic behavior patterns, albeit in modified form. The children seem to attempt to reestablish many of the characteristics of their relationships with adults and peers. The slow and difficult task of working through unconscious attitudes and fantasies that perpetuate their now maladaptive behavior constitutes a major part of the total therapeutic effort, which may last for 2 or more years. There is no single course of treatment because the variables are many, including the strengths and weaknesses of the particular child, the strengths and weaknesses of the parents, the skills of the staff, and the degree to which a suitable discharge plan can be put into effect.

TERMINATION

As termination and discharge approach, earlier feelings of loss are often reevoked, and temporary regression may occur, with heightened acting-out behavior, sometimes of an aggressive kind. Intense anxiety about abandonment may also reappear. The borderline child especially needs a great deal of support at this time. It is necessary to arrange preplacement visits to avoid precipitous changes in the child's life.

DISCHARGE PLANS AND FOLLOW-UP CARE

Children, parents, and staff all anticipate with ambivalence the time of leaving. Expectations—some realistic, others unrealistic—tinged with apprehension and anxiety about real or imagined problems abound. In a sense, preparation for departure begins at admission. Actual preparation for leaving should be a planned process, with the child's best interests being of paramount importance. It is important that the children at all times participate in planning their future lives.

Cure, whatever that may mean, is rarely an attainable goal for children in residential treatment. Improved object relations and social adaptation, ability to function in an outside school and later at work, and the working through of certain kinds of trauma are more realistic goals for the child. Similar goals obtain for the parents. The degree to which these goals are achieved is sometimes difficult to determine. The outcomes that may occur range from no change at all to improvement in the whole family.

The range of disposition plans varies according to the outcome. Return to the family with or without further outpatient treatment, day treatment, placement in a group or foster home, boarding school, further residential treatment, or custodial care are some common options. Many residential treatment centers have developed some of these options as part of their own programs, so that a child may be admitted, say, into a day treatment program or into a day treatment and on-grounds school program, with full residential treatment reserved as a possible option, or vice versa.

Intensive residential treatment should be seen as a phase of treatment rather than as the one definitive treatment. Both the children and their families are usually vulnerable people. Some may always show a tendency to paranoid behavior when under stress. The residential treatment home may well need to continue to represent the core of stability for these children as they progress through adolescence and young adulthood.

RESULTS

Many attempts at follow-up studies have been made, but unfortunately, numerous serious methodological problems plague research in this area. Most studies of outcome are subjective and difficult to evaluate. Criteria for diagnosis, treatment, and outcome are not sufficiently well defined for research purposes, and the intervening variables make controlled studies virtually impossible. Clinical impressions suggest that good residential treatment programs do provide a beneficial experience for the child during the period of residential treatment and may lead to more satisfactory development and functioning in the child than would otherwise have occurred had the child not been admitted.

Taylor and Alpert (1973) found, however, that the degree of change that children achieved in residential treatment was not significantly related to postdischarge adaptation. Lewis et al. (1980) similarly found that the majority of children who had received about 2 years of residential treatment in one particular setting fared poorly at follow-up according to the objective measures they used to assess outcome. Thus, improvement made in residential treatment did not determine the degree of adjustment experienced on return to the home and community. Instead, Lewis et al. found that ecological factors and postdischarge factors were important in determining outcome. Successfully adjusted children showed a greater increase in family and community support during enrollment and also received more help from community agencies and special school programs.

Lewis et al. also noted that, during the course of residential treatment, crucial attachments are formed between the children and the staff members and recommended that these attachments be protected. Thus, the same residential facility staff should be prepared in many instances to continue their commitment and attachment to the children and their families through and beyond adolescence. In effect, the residential treatment center in many instances should serve as a secure base until adulthood. Without that security, the hard-won gains achieved during residential treatment for the vulnerable child and adolescent are essentially undone.

Wenning (1988) reported a high recidivism rate and a high rate of affective conditions in a follow-up study of children diagnosed as borderline while in residential treatment.

FUTURE TRENDS IN RESIDENTIAL TREATMENT

The place of residential treatment in the continuum of childrens' services and the vitality of residential treatment programs face serious social, political, and economic challenges in the years ahead. The dearth of follow-up studies demonstrating the efficacy of residential treatment continues to plague its advocates in the face of increased demands for results and cost-effectiveness. Many state and federal policymakers emphasize family preservation or alternative family placement for children currently utilizing residential treatment. Residential treatment is increasingly seen as a treatment of last resort, and therefore, child and family pathology is increasingly serious at the point of admission. Staff recruitment and staff retention are serious problems for many residential treatment organizations as budgetary constraints limit resources in many areas for childrens' services. The statistical trend toward an aging society not only increases the demand for resources for the elderly but also potentially pits the elderly against the very young in the increasing competition for mental health, medical, and social services. The resources needed to combat the AIDS epidemic and the rapid rise of drug abuse and drug-related violence increase the strain on all social service resources. Emotionally disturbed children are not a voting constituency, and historically their families have not been an effective political force in advocating for their specific needs. Residential treatment organizations often act as advocates for disenfranchised children but are often discredited as being biased or self-serving in their advocacy.

Davis et al. (1989) report that traditional long-term residential treatment facilities are adapting their programs and treatment foci to attempt to meet the changing needs of children and adolescents. Children are presenting with more intensive treatment needs, while family and community resources have diminished for a large population of children. Consumer demands for results and accountability have increased, and agencies must offer a larger range of specialized clinical services to children who are in residential treatment.

Residential treatment facilities have responded by developing subacute intensive treatment services within existing facilities. These include 90-day intensive assessment units, 30- to 90-day alcohol/drug treatment units, physical/sexual abuse and trauma response teams, specialized foster care and adoption services, aftercare and independent living programs, outreach family support services, and family preservation services such as Home Builders.

In response to consumer demand for results and accountability, many residential treatment facilities have adapted their programs to be in compliance with the standards of the Joint Commission on Accreditation of

Healthcare Organizations (JCAHO). JCAHO provides comprehensive standards for residential treatment in the areas of administrative and clinical management, patient management, special treatment services, patient services, and environmental management. JCAHO standards emphasize professional staff organization and development, program evaluation, patient safety, patient rights, and all aspects of quality assurance (Joint Commission on Accreditation of Healthcare Organization, 1989).

The Civilian Health and Medical Plan for the Uniformed Services (CHAMPUS) and the American Psychiatric Association have also played a major role in developing comprehensive quality assurance standards and in implementing a peer review system for residential treatment. As of July 1989, 108 JCAHO-approved residential facilities also met CHAMPUS quality assurance requirements and were being monitored through a peer review process.

References

American Psychiatric Association: *Diagnostic and Statistical Manual of Mental Disorders* (4th ed, rev). Washington, DC, American Psychiatric Association, 1994.

Brown D: *Managing Conflict at Organizational Interfaces*. Reading, PA, Addison-Wesley, 1983, pp. 81–116.

Caplan G: *The Theory and Practice of Mental Health Consultations*. New York, Basic Books, 1970, pp. 32–34.

Colligan RC, Roberts MD, Miner RA: An organizational grid for residential staff conferences. *Milieu Ther* 1:41, 1981.

Comer JP: *School Power*. New York, Free Press, 1980.

Davis R, Myers B, Sorbo P: Managing through change. In: *Contributions to Residential Treatment 1989*. Washington, DC, American Association of Residential Centers, 1989, pp. 51–56.

Haley J: *Leaving Home*. New York, McGraw-Hill, 1980.

Johnson S: Staff cohesion in residential treatment. *Child Care Q* 2:204, 1982.

Joint Commission on Accreditation of Healthcare Organizations: *Consolidated Standards Manual 1989*. Chicago, Joint Commission on Accreditation of Healthcare Organization, 1989.

Joint Commission on the Mental Health of Children: *Crisis in Child Mental Health: Challenge for the 1970s*. New York, Harper & Row, 1970.

Lewis M, Lewis DO, Shanok SS, et al: The undoing of residential treatment. *J Am Acad Child Psychiatry* 19:160–171, 1980.

Marsden G, McDermott J, Miner D: Residential treatment of children: A survey of institutional characteristics. *J Am Acad Child Psychiatry* 9:332, 1970.

Northrup G: The direct care worker in residential treatment. *Milieu Ther* 2:32, 1982.

Redl F: A strategy and technique of the life space interview. *Am J Orthopsychiatry* 29:1, 1959.

Rick F, Charlesworth J: Role and function of child care working. *J Child Care* 1:35, 1982.

Stroup A, Witkin M, Atay J, et al: *Residential Treatment Centers for Emotionally Disturbed Children 1983* (Mental Health Statistical Note no. 188). Rockville, MD, National Institute for Mental Health, 1988.

Taylor DA, Alpert SW: *Continuity and Support Following Residential Treatment*. New York, Child Welfare League of America, 1973.

Wenning K: *Borderline Children Two to Eight Years Later: A Follow-Up Study*. Unpublished doctoral dissertation, Northampton, MA, Smith College School of Social Work, 1988.

Young T, Dore M, Pappenfort D: Trends in residential group care: 1966–1981. In: *Group Care of Children Trends Toward the Year 2000*. Washington, DC, Child Welfare League of America, 1989.

85 SOCIAL SKILLS TRAINING FOR CHILDREN

Roger D. Cox, Ph.D., and Eric Schopler, Ph.D.

In recent years, there has been an increase in interest in the development of social competence and social skills in children (Asher and Coie, 1989; Dunn and McGuire, 1992). This interest has been widespread, as physicians, child psychologists, and educators have all focused on the implications of poor social skills development in children. In DSM-IV (American Psychiatric Association, 1994), newly included disorders of childhood disintegrative disorder, Asperger's syndrome, and Rett's disorder all involve primary difficulties involving social relatedness. These newly included diagnostic categories continue to expand the childhood disorder listing of psychopathology involving core deficits of social problems (e.g., autism) and others that include as associated features problems in social skills (e.g., learning disorders). With the growing interest has come a burgeoning number of published papers focusing on interventions that attempt to correct social deficits. These assorted intervention efforts have come to be loosely categorized under the global heading "social skills training programs." This chapter addresses the issues related to program development in social skills training.

RATIONALE FOR SOCIAL SKILLS TRAINING

The current interest in social skills development in children is the result of the contributions of several researchers/theorists. One particularly important early influence was H.S. Sullivan (1953), who first emphasized the importance of early childhood friendships in his writings on personality development and the interpersonal theory of psychiatry. Among other things, Sullivan suggested that the development of same-sex friends during middle childhood is important in the development of intimacy. These same-sex friendships provide an important context for the later development of heterosexual relationships during adolescence. In addition to his widely recognized contribution to individual psychotherapy and the interpersonal aspects of therapist-patient relationships, Sullivan provided an early focus on the importance of early social com-

petence in children, complete with warnings about the implications of failed social skill development for functioning during both childhood and later adult life.

Another major milestone occurred 20 years later as researchers began consistently to report that children who had demonstrated problems in peer relationships during the early elementary school years had a higher incidence of later emotional disturbance than did children with satisfactory peer relationships (Cowen et al., 1973; Roff et al., 1972). Following these early reports, there is now a consistent body of research that supports the notion that the adequacy of childhood peer relations is one of the best predictors of mental health status in adulthood (Hartup, 1967; Hartup and Sancillio, 1986).

Finally, researchers have reported that peer relationships are stable over time, suggesting that over periods of weeks or even years both positive and negative relationships remain consistent (Bryan, 1967; Cole and Dodge, 1983; Dodge et al., 1986).

Taken together, it is not surprising that clinicians and educators have become interested in developing interventions that can assist children with social deficiencies. Consequently, increasing numbers of reports of social skills training programs continue to be published. It should be noted, however, that the development of social skills training programs is based on several assumptions that are seldom specified and even less often the direct focus of investigation.

ASSUMPTIONS ABOUT SOCIAL SKILLS TRAINING FOR CHILDREN

Number 1: A Causal Link Connects Social Skillfullness and Peer Acceptance/Popularity

A body of literature exists describing the characteristics of children who are popular or who have good friendship patterns (Dodge et al.,

1986; Gottman, 1983). It is certainly true, and not surprising, that children who are selected by other children as those they would like to sit by or play with generally display behaviors described by researchers as socially skillful. However, it is still an unproven assumption that training a child with poor social skills to show more of the behaviors of the socially skillful will automatically result in a change in popularity. This is an important assumption to verify because it is not the social skillfulness per se that is the final goal of social skills training programs. Rather, peer acceptance and increased pleasure in social interactions on the part of trainees are the main goals.

Number 2: Social Skills Can Be Trained in Controlled Settings and Generalized to Informal, Uncontrolled, Real-World Situations

Social skills training is typically conducted under the supervision of adult teachers/therapists. The differences between the training sessions and the social opportunities that occur in the world are numerous and significant. Social skills training usually involves some combination of role play, coaching, feedback in the form of social praise, and repetition of preselected social exchanges. In addition, many training programs are increasingly using videotaping as a means of allowing a more detailed review of social responses by trainees. Real-world social settings typically are spontaneous, fluid, and unstructured. None of the structured aspects of social skills training activities occur outside of the training session.

This is an important assumption because of the futility of training in social skills if generalization cannot or does not naturally occur.

Number 3: It Is Possible to Identify and Teach Required Social Skills for Children of Differing Developmental Levels and with Differing Handicapping Conditions

The assumption that it is possible to identify the requisite social skills needed underlies all attempts to provide social skills training. And yet, one could suggest that our current knowledge about social skills is meager and poorly conceptualized. The behaviors labeled as social skills cross numerous boundaries of social, cognitive, emotional, and communicative functioning.

No comprehensive listing of identified components of social skillfulness in children has been developed. Yet it is possible to list a few components that have been the target of social skills training:

1. Conflict resolution;
2. Social initiation;
3. Group entering skills;
4. Assertiveness skill development;
5. Conversational skills;
6. Joint attention skills;
7. Sensitivity training skills;
8. Compliance to authority training;
9. Communication request skill training.

This listing makes clear some of the problems of attempting to summarize or describe social skill training efforts. The range of skills being taught under the general heading "social skills training" may not be closely related. Even as researchers continue to develop intervention programs aimed at specific skills, it remains impossible to describe the interrelationships among the components of social skillfulness.

Number 4: Social Competence Deficits in Children Result from a Lack of Knowledge of Appropriate Behaviors or a Lack of Behavior Skill in Producing Those Behaviors

This is an important assumption because it supports the notion of *training social skills*. There could be a number of other reasons why a child does not display appropriate social behaviors. It is possible that the child knows what is expected and knows how to show the appropriate behavior, but is not motivated enough to make the effort to show appropriate skill. It is also possible that the child has feelings of inadequacy and fears that an attempt to show the correct behavior will fail, leading to increasing anxiety when he or she tries to implement the behavior. A final example is the child who is angry and hostile with authority figures. This child might not show appropriate social skills, in part, as an attempt to show rejection of adult/authority values.

These alternative explanations for poor social skills are meant as examples, not as a comprehensive list of possible reasons for the skill deficits. However, the interventions recommended for children should be matched to therapist's assumptions about why social skills levels are deficient in a child. Social skills training would not necessarily be the treatment approach of choice for children whose deficits are not due to a lack of knowledge.

DEFINITION OF SOCIAL SKILLS TRAINING

Almost all attempts to define social skills refer back to the general concept of social competence. Many definitions of social competence have been presented (Hops, 1983; McFall, 1982). The definitions of two authors seem to best capture the important aspects of social competence: Howlin (1986) suggested that "the essence of social behavior consists of the ability to relate to others in a mutually reinforcing and reciprocal fashion and to adapt social skills to the varying demand of interpersonal contexts" (p. 103). Putallaz and Gottman (1982) suggest that social competence is composed of "those aspects of social behavior that are important with respect to preventing physical illness or psychopathology in children and adults" (p. 7).

Taken together, these two definitions present the basis for social skills training. Howlin (1986) emphasizes the importance of mutually reinforcing reciprocal interactions. Putallaz and Gottman (1982) emphasize the importance of selecting social competencies that are somehow related to adaptive functioning, both physically and emotionally.

SOCIAL SKILLS TRAINING: WHO SHOULD RECEIVE IT?

One interesting aspect of social skills training is that it is apparently considered a viable treatment option for children with almost all types of mental or emotional handicaps. From one perspective, such a conclusion is reasonable. The development of appropriate social behaviors for all children born into a society is one of the primary responsibilities of the family, specifically the parents. Nonhandicapped children learn social skills as a result of the informal training that occurs within families and neighborhoods. So, in a sense, all social skills are taught to children, with some children learning the skills better than others.

The literature on social skills training seems to reflect the assumption that social skills can indeed be taught, even when the normal socialization of the child has resulted in deficits in social skills attainment. Regardless of type or degree of handicap, social skills training has been attempted for most of the problem areas of childhood. Numerous references to social skills training are found in the literature on three areas of childhood psychopathology: children with learning disabilities, autistic children, and mentally retarded children (mild to severe). In addition, there are increasing reports of social skills training efforts focused on delinquent offenders involved with the courts. Programs for this population are naturally targeted for older children and young adolescents. The following listing presents additional conditions for which social skills training has been reported as a treatment modality in recent professional publications:

1. Severely emotionally and behaviorally disturbed children;
2. Neglected and rejected children;
3. Blind, socially withdrawn, multihandicapped children;
4. Fragile X males with mental retardation;
5. Isolated preschool-age children;
6. Retarded children with severe productive language disabilities.

This tendency to attempt social skills intervention across disability groups is paralleled by the proliferation of interventions across the full age range of childhood, from preschool to adolescence and young adulthood.

SOCIAL SKILLS TRAINING: WHAT SHOULD BE TRAINED?

One of the major problems of social skills training programs is the wide range of skills and abilities trained. If fact, almost all interventions aimed at children have some social quality that can, if the researcher/ clinician chooses, be called social skills. For example, communication is often considered a social skill (Ross et al., 1982) because it serves to establish and maintain interpersonal contact. However, communication can occur at both nonverbal and verbal levels, and the general label of communication can be subdivided into numerous categories, including conversational discourse skills, conflict negotiation, and assertiveness skills.

The result of this overlap between social skills and communication is that the literature on social skills and communication abilities is difficult to separate and subsequently difficult to categorize. Depending on the background and training of the clinician/researcher, intervention programs examining many of the same skills are often conceptualized somewhat differently. It is relatively easy to remedy this problem by conceptualizing communication skills as a subheading of social skills. What is more difficult is to decide what aspects of human social interactions should not be categorized as social skills. This chapter focuses on only the most widely taught social and communication skills.

The goals of social skills training are usually determined by the nature and extent of the handicapping conditions of the children served. Social skills training efforts vary from targeting advanced skills to programs that focus on the basic, lower-level abilities common to all human interactions. In the section that follows, the basic, lower-level skills are discussed.

SOCIAL SKILLS FOR PRESCHOOL AND LOW-FUNCTIONING CHILDREN

When children are young preschoolers, low functioning, or have autism or related pervasive developmental disorders, the goals of social skills training are simple and uncomplicated.

Olley (1986) describes the assessment of social skills using the Treatment and Education of Autistic and Related Communication Handicapped Children (TEACCH) social skills curriculum with autistic children. Olley includes primitive skills: proximity, social initiation, and social response. These basic skills are mastered in the normal population during the preschool years (Hartup, 1967; Mueller, 1972; Savitsky and Watson, 1975). For the young, severely handicapped autistic child, all three of them are often lacking. When there are deficits in social initiation (including reaching out for something, pointing at an object out of reach, or other nonverbal actions), this becomes an obvious starting point for social skills training. Likewise, when a child is oblivious to the initiations of others or is intentionally nonresponsive to overtures by others, social skills training typically begins there.

Three main approaches to social skills training are usually employed (Lord, 1994). Although these overlap, they can be described separately. First is the behavioral approach involving contingency and contiguity. More recently these have been broadened to involve the natural teaching situations (Koegel and Koegel, in press; Koegel et al., 1994). The second is a developmental approach, assuming that learning will be easier and generalized better when developmental readiness is taken into account (Lord et al., 1993). The third is the ecological approach with emphasis on participating in normal community functions, on age-appropriate tasks, in the least restrictive environment (Dyer and Peck, 1987).

Other low-level social skills targeted with autistic and severely/profoundly retarded children include eye contact, simple social cause and effect (e.g., touch person and he or she will laugh), and reciprocal turn taking (e.g., child takes a block, then adult takes a block). Thus, assessment and intervention programs for this population focus on all these basic factors that actually set the context for social interactions (Olley, 1986).

A number of general social skills have been reported for children during the early preschool years. These skills are usually labeled positive social behaviors and include the following specific skills: laughing and/ or smiling (giving positive attention), sharing and/or compromising, giving objects spontaneously to peers, and showing affection and/or acceptance (Charlesworth and Hartup, 1967; Stone and LaGreca, 1986).

Early skills training efforts directed at developmentally handicapped preschoolers attempted to increase the frequency of their interactions with peers (Allen et al., 1964), but this strategy was not successful on its own. In fact, some efforts to increase the frequency led to an increase in aggressive responses by trainees (Kirby and Toler, 1970). The frequency approach to training was replaced by efforts to teach positive social behaviors (Sisson et al., 1985; Strain, 1977). Various targeted behaviors for preschoolers have included general social skills and specific social abilities. Some examples of targeted training skills for preschoolers are as follows: entering ongoing peer activities (Evers and Schwartz, 1973; O'Conner, 1969), sharing (Barton and Bevirt, 1981), giving affection and praise (Rogers-Warren and Baer, 1976), smiling and laughing with peers (Keller and Carlson, 1974), and even training socially effective play behaviors (Hendrickson et al., 1986).

SOCIAL SKILLS FOR ELEMENTARY SCHOOL CHILDREN

Children at the developmental level of the average elementary school child have rapidly developing social skills. As mentioned earlier, however, the sophistication and subtlety of the skills developed during this time render a simple categorization of the skills learned, such as "positive social behaviors," relatively meaningless. It is known that children in this age range spend increasing amounts of time with peers, and that most of their interactions with peers are positive. Though many of the specifics of positive peer interaction are poorly understood at present, it appears that the elementary school child generally becomes increasingly facile at modifying his or her behavior in response to the needs of friends and acquaintances (Hartup, 1967). Beyond that general statement, our knowledge is somewhat limited. It has been suggested that sharing and cooperative actions increase and play an increasingly important role in peer relationships in middle childhood (Radke-Yarrow et al., 1983). But is has also been suggested that young children are capable of showing sensitivity and understanding of the feelings and intentions of others even as toddlers. The increase in the powers of understanding, sensitivity, and intimacy in young elementary school-age children has only recently begun to be researched and studied (Dunn, 1993).

In part, and perhaps because of the relatively low number of studies on normal social development during middle childhood, intervention studies have focused on general, globally defined goals. Because of the obvious importance of being able to enter a social group and be accepted, several studies have looked at the skills needed to join groups or be accepted by others (Gresham and Nagle, 1980). The complexity of the skills required for children to make successful entries emphasizes how subtle and sophisticated the required skills are. School-age children who are successful at making an entry into a group of peers use subtlety and tact. Initially, the successful child waits and hovers around the edge of the group. Next, the child begins to mimic the activities enjoyed by the group. Then, the child will begin to comment on the activities of the group, slowly moving closer to the participants before attempting to enter. Any activities or actions that draw attention away from the group tend to be responded to negatively by group members. Actions such as attention seeking, self-comments, or disruptions in group activities tend to have negative consequences for the newcomer (Dodge et al., 1983; Putallaz and Gottman, 1981). Sharing and playing cooperatively have been the focus of interventions (Oden and Asher, 1977). Ladd (1981) attempted to train the skills of giving support, giving attention, and giving help to peers. Making positive praise statements and giving compliments were the training goals of a study by LaGreca and Santogrossi (1980).

Studies of social skills training in the middle childhood years have also focused on communication skills training. To a degree, this has resulted from the increasing understanding that children resolve conflict through the use of conversation (Putallaz and Gottman, 1981). The verbal strategies used by these older children are different from the more physical or aggressive methods younger children use to resolve conflicts. The goals of social skills training programs with a communication focus have generally been based on the clinical intuition and judgment of the researchers. School-age children have been taught to ask open-ended questions of others (Minkin et al., 1976). Other researchers have taught the children to share information about themselves (LaGrecca and Mesibov, 1981) or to give suggestions and advice to other children in a socially appropriate way (Ladd, 1981). LaGreca and Santogrossi (1980) taught children to use good eye contact and give positive feedback in order to communicate an active interest in conversation with a peer, and a peer tutor program for autistic children has been implemented (Lord, in press). One study attempted to teach learning-disabled middle childhood subjects to stay on a subject of conversation and to generate new topics of conversation when old ones failed (LaGrecca and Mesibov, 1981). Recently, Koegel and Koegel (in press) have written about the successes that can be obtained with autistic students when the correct motivational components are included within a communication skills training program that shares many of the goals of the described social skills interventions.

SOCIAL SKILLS FOR ADOLESCENTS

As with the younger children, a wide range of social skills have been selected to be taught to the adolescent. Depending on the level of handicap of the adolescent involved in the training, the sophistication of the training program may range from basic to advanced. Many of the training goals and objectives relating to basic skills remain relevant for lower-functioning adolescents. However, mildly handicapped adolescents may be capable of handling an advanced level of skill training; in some cases, programs for advanced adolescents may not be noticeably different from programs developed for adult clients (e.g., sensitivity training, assertiveness training, conversational skill training).

One recent approach to social skills training with adults has focused on higher-level autistic adolescents (Mesibov, 1986). The goals for these high-functioning autistic clients were an interesting mix of basic and higher-level skills. Areas for training fell into the following categories: (a) lack of interaction, especially the reciprocal interactions of normal social exchanges; (b) difficulties in comprehending rules; (c) difficulties with attention; (d) problems with communication; and (e) lack of positive social experiences.

Client goals typically reported for programs dealing with adolescents with less pervasive and less socially handicapping conditions are higher than those of Mesibov's program. For example, the following were the goals in a program for adolescents with behavior problems: (a) to develop listening abilities, (b) to develop respect for the opinions of others, (c) to become aware of both one's own and others' emotions, and (d) to recognize and diminish derogatory remarks made about others (Mills, 1987).

The goals of some social skills training programs for adolescents who have been involved with the court system are even more ambitious (Henderson and Hollin, 1983). In studies with this group of adolescent clients, the focus is often on recognizing and appropriately managing conflict, decreasing disruptive behavior, and advancing problem-solving skills (Hazel, 1982; Larson and Gerber, 1987).

In summary, it seems that current efforts in social skills training are based on the belief that any and all measured deficits in social abilities can and should be ameliorated through training. The specific list of what is trained in the various studies depends on the disability group being trained, the degree of mental and social handicap of the group, and the social and communicative competence of the subjects. Not surprisingly, higher-level social skills are targeted at higher functioning groups, while lower-level skills are taught to the more pervasively developmentally disordered children.

SOCIAL SKILLS TRAINING: HOW SHOULD TRAINING BE CONDUCTED?

Most social skills training programs are conducted with groups of targeted low social skill children. Group training has the advantage of providing a social context for participants. Individual training is done when an isolated case of poor social skills is found, and grouping with other similarly handicapped children is not possible.

Training Techniques in Social Skills Interventions

Perhaps because there are so many gaps in our current understanding of social skills development and remediation, many studies use multiple approaches in attempting to train social behaviors. This shotgun approach is not necessarily unwarranted, but it does reflect our current limited knowledge about human social behaviors.

In almost all reported studies of social skills training, a number of techniques are involved. Often the training involves a basic core of teaching techniques, which often includes *modeling* (watching a skilled trainer/peer demonstrate the desired behavior with a peer (Lord, in press), *instructions* (verbal or nonverbal directions to the participant to try the modeled behaviors), and *performance feedback* (verbal or tangible rewards for participating in the lesson). In some studies, *role play* (play-acting various parts of a social interaction) and *rehearsal* (opportunities to practice the social activity several times) are included in the training package. One example of a study using all of these techniques was an attempt to train two autistic children (a 10-year-old girl and a 9-year-old boy) in interpersonal skills (Taras et al., 1988). In this study the two children were taught to refrain from perseveration, to make eye contact, and to show appropriate affect among other targeted social behaviors. The techniques used included the five mentioned above plus tangible and social reinforcers. Though positive outcomes were reported and the training package was considered useful, no determination can be made about the contribution of any particular training technique.

Elaborations of these training techniques in different studies are often innovative and interesting to children. For example, in one study of multiply handicapped children (ages 8–13), the trainers used hand puppets to model skills taught and used brief role play sessions. Tokens were also used to shape and reinforce the desired behaviors (Wallander and Hubert, 1984).

One might expect that a group leader would be necessary for social skills training to effectively provide participants with all the content to be taught. In early training trials, the teaching of social skills was directly managed by a group leader or social skills teacher who controlled sessions, often running discrete trials of the social situations for which training was needed (Donnollan et al., 1984). Generally, most social skills activity programs do have group leaders, but the role of the group leader seems to be becoming less noticeable as training models evolve. At present, social skills groups are relying more on the use of peer tutors. Though this has been a recent development, studies of social skills training involving peers with learning-disabled, socially disadvantaged youth and autistic children have been in the literature for a number of years (Cloward, 1972; Gartner et al., 1972; McHale, 1983; Strain et al., 1979). In some programs peer tutors are called coaches or trainers, but the role seems to be much the same. Generally, these are same-age children who are recruited in a variety of ways to be paired with the handicapped children during the targeted social settings. Interestingly, the inclusion of the peer tutors has resulted in a number of changes in social skills groups for children of all ages.

One study of preschool male children comparing the effectiveness of teacher-antecedent interventions (teacher directs the activities) with peer-antecedent interventions (peer prompts the responses by the participant) found different effects for the two conditions. Peer initiation procedures reliably increased the social responses of the autistic children. However, the teacher-antecedent condition led to increases in both initiations and responses of the autistic preschool male children (Odom and Strain, 1986). Though it may be tempting to conclude that teacher-initiated interventions provide a wider range of responses, it is also true that teacher-initiated interventions are always farther away from the natural social interactions of children in unstructured, natural environments. Therefore, it is highly possible that the short-term gain of having teacher-directed interventions may not sustain itself in studies of the generalization of treatment effects over time. It should also be noted that preschool children generally need more supervision and guidance in developing cooperative play and prosocial activities than do school-age children.

For programs involving children of all ages, the inclusion of peer tutors has had one consistently positive effect. When one includes non-handicapped peers in a planned series of social activities, it becomes apparent that considerable attention needs to be given to making sure that each participant, handicapped or nonhandicapped, has a good time at the activity. Attendance by targeted children can often be made mandatory, as participation in the social skills activity is assumed to be beneficial. But participating peer tutors are usually in attendance in a voluntary role, and if activities become rigid, forced, or repetitive, it will probably be difficult to keep them in the program. Mesibov (1986) has responded to this challenge with several creative ideas. First, he has as a major goal that participants in the program have fun with activities. This is accomplished by providing a snack time at the beginning of activities with his autistic adolescents and their peer coaches/trainers. While the food is a motivator for many participants, the informal atmosphere of eating and talking together often allows for many of the program goals to be addressed as well. In addition, with these verbal, high-functioning autistic clients, each meeting is used to allow participants and peer coaches/trainers to tell jokes. Though the jokes may be no more sophisticated than the "knock-knock" variety, the important fact is that participants enjoy the time and share the experience of humor and laughter.

SUMMARY AND FUTURE DIRECTIONS IN SOCIAL SKILLS TRAINING

The proliferation of social skills training activities for children in the past 10–15 years reflects a growing awareness of the social deficits of children with a wide range of childhood psychopathologies. Without a doubt, direct intervention is needed to assist these children with their marked social problems. Social skills training models are still in the earliest stage of development, and the following issues continue to interfere with the development of more effective training models.

Long-term Effectiveness of Social Skills Training

The long-term effectiveness of social skills training for children has not been demonstrated consistently to generalize beyond the training settings, nor have the gains been found to persist after the termination of training sessions. Initially, social skill researchers were satisfied demonstrating that social skills could be taught to low-skill children in training sessions. And recently, as described earlier in this chapter, considerable effort has been given to extending social skills training to different disability groups and children of differing ages.

These minor advances in extending the model of training social skills to a broader population of children leave unanswered the difficult question of why it is so difficult for children to show robust and persistent skill improvement outside the training environment.

Part of the problem can be found in the limitations of the social skills training model most widely used in published research. For the most part, researchers in this area espouse some variant of a cognitive-behavioral theory of social skills development. From this perspective, it is the perceptions of social obligation that must first be taught, followed by the social rules for a given situation. The child must have the communicative and behavioral skills necessary to carry out a complex series of actions, and his or her success in this is complicated by the fact that another person (or persons) is an active, dynamic participant in the social exchange.

Perhaps social skills training should move away from the cognitive-behavioral model based on learning theory and toward the richer, vastly more complex model of human relationships. Recently Greenberg and Speltz (1988) have suggested that the intervention approaches with conduct-disordered children have failed to understand the emotional or social-cognitive delays or deficits in either parent or child (or both) that lead to children's conduct disorders. In other words, these authors suggest that conduct disorders in children are really better conceptualized as problems in parent-child relationships. It is also possible that social skills training would be better conceptualized as "peer relationship training," with a focus on the dyadic relationships often found in programs involving peer tutors. The focus on the peer relationships would replace the preoccupation with cognitive-behavioral deficits that is now in vogue.

From this perspective, social skills training programs are supervised locations for developing, nourishing, and expanding on close personal relationships. Our ability to develop the comprehensive set of social perceptions and social rules seems limited at present, suggesting that social skills training will soon reach an impasse, if it hasn't already done so. It would appear that there is much to be gained and little to be lost by exploring new and unexplored relationship issues when thinking about the future of social skills training. Recently, there has been some encouraging work that has begun to develop social skills programming through relationship issues (Duck, 1993; Dunn, 1993).

DETERMINATION OF ANTICIPATED OUTCOME OF SOCIAL SKILLS TRAINING

Though clinicians and educators have become invested in developing training packages and programs to remediate social skills deficits in children, there is a lack of understanding about the relationship between social skills and outcome variables of importance. The acceptance of the unproven assumption that popular children must somehow be children with good social skills contributes little toward the development of realistic social skills training programs for handicapped children. Even with a successful outcome in a social skills program, one would not expect an autistic child to be selected as one of the most popular children in a class (Olley, 1986).

Recently, Gresham (1985) has suggested that a social validity approach to social skills deficits may be helpful. According to Gresham's notion, social skills that lead to or predict important outcomes in the child's present or future life should be selected as goals for training. This would mean that acceptance by peers; social skills valued by parents, siblings, and teachers; and skills that would lead to socially valued adult status (e.g., independence, employment, and responsibility) would be the guiding principles behind the selection of specific social skills goals. Popularity with peers as measured by sociometric peer nomination techniques would be relatively less important when following this approach.

Effects of Social Skills Training on Peer Tutors

It is possible that one of the major benefits of social skills training programs that use peer tutors will prove to be the change wrought in the cognitions and behaviors of the peer tutors. When observing programs that use peer tutors over time, one quickly develops an appreciation for the change in peer tutors' sensitivity to, acceptance of, and openness with their paired handicapped participant. It is always possible to train the peer tutors to be miniature versions of the adult trainer, which will not necessarily lead to the positive changes mentioned. But if social skills activities are arranged so that all participants have fun and share pleasant experiences, with help provided by the adult trainer when necessary, much of the change in the social skills of the trained participants can be traced to changes in the attitudes and behaviors of the peer tutors. And in fact, this is a highly desirable goal for social skills groups. The ability of a nonhandicapped child to accommodate to the social deficits of a handicapped child will always be greater than that possible in the other direction. For no matter how good social skills training can become, it is not likely to cure any of the psychopathologies of the participants. But when the peer tutor can learn to accept and enjoy social activities involving leisure activities with handicapped children, a worthwhile goal will have been achieved. Perhaps social skills training programs in the future will be considered supervised, supportive places for the social abilities of handicapped and nonhandicapped children to intertwine and reach a comfortable level of social interaction.

References

Allen KE, Hart B, Buell JS, et al: Effects of social reinforcement of isolate behavior of a nursery school child. *Child Dev* 35:511, 1964.

American Psychiatric Association: *Diagnostic and Statistical Manual of Mental Disorders* (4th ed). Washington, DC, American Psychiatric Association, 1994.

Asher SR, Coie JD: *Peer Rejection in Childhood.* New York, Cambridge University Press, 1989.

Barton EJ, Bevirt J: Generalization of sharing across groups: Assessment of group composition with preschool children. *Behav Modif* 5:503, 1981.

Bryan TH: Peer popularity of learning disabled children: A replication. *J Learn Disabil* 9:307, 1976.

Charlesworth R, Hartup WW: Positive social reinforcement in the nursery school peer group. *Child Dev* 38:993, 1967.

Cole JD, Dodge KA: Continuities and changes in children's social status: A five-year longitudinal study. *Merrill-Palmer Q* 29:261, 1983.

Cloward R: Studies in tutoring. *J Exp Educ* 36:14, 1972.

Cowen EL, Pederson A, Babigian J, et al: Long-term follow-up of early detected vulnerable children. *J Consult Clin Psychiatry* 41:438, 1973.

Dodge KA, Pettit GS, McClaskey CL, et al: Social competence in children. *Monogr Soc Res Child Dev* 51 (Serial no 213), 1986.

Dodge KA, Schlundt DC, Schocken I, et al: Social competence and children's sociometric status: The role of peer group entry strategies. *Merrill-Palmer Q* 29:309, 1983.

Donnellan AM, Mosaros RA, Anderson JL: Teaching students with autism in natural environments: What educators need from researchers. *J Special Educ* 18:505, 1984.

Duck S (ed): *Learning about Relationships.* Newberry Park, CA, Sage, 1993.

Dunn J: *Young Children's Close Relationships: Beyond Attachment.* Vol 4: *Individual Differences and Development Series.* Newberry Park, CA, Sage, 1993.

Dunn J, Mcquire S: Sibling and peer relationships in childhood. *J Child Psychol Psychiatry* 33:67–105, 1992.

Dyer K, Peck CA: Current perspectives on social/communication curricula for students with autism and severe handicaps. *Educ Treatment Child* 10:338–351, 1987.

Evers W, Schwartz JC: Modifying social withdrawal in preschoolers. The effects of filmed modeling and teacher praise. *J Abnorm Child Psychol* 1:248, 1973.

Gartner A, Kohler M, Riesman F: *Children Teach Children.* New York, Harper & Row, 1972.

Gottman JM: How children become friends. *Monogr Soc Res Child Dev* 48 (Serial no. 210), 1983.

Greenberg MT, Speltz ML: Attachment and the ontogeny of conduct problems. In: Belsky J, Nezworksi T (eds): *Clinical Implications of Attachment.* Hillsdale, NJ, Erlbaum, 1988, p. 177.

Gresham FM: Strategies for enhancing the social outcomes of mainstreaming: A necessary ingredient for success. In: Meisel CJ (eds): *Mainstreaming Handicapped Children.* Hillsdale, NJ, Erlbaum, 1985, p. 117.

Gresham FM, Nagle RJ: Social skills training with children: Responsiveness to modeling and coaching as a function of peer orientation. *J Consult Clin Psychol* 48:718, 1980.

Hartup WW: Peer relationships. In: Mussen PM (ed): *Handbook of Child Psychology* (Vol 4). New York, Wiley, 1967, p. 103.

Hartup WW, Sancillo M: Children's friendships. In: Schopler E, Mesibov GB (eds): *Social Behavior in Autism.* New York, Plenum, 1986, p. 61.

Hazel JS: Social skills training with court adjudicated youth. *Child Youth Serv* 5:117, 1982.

Henderson M, Hollin C: A critical review of social skills training with young offenders. *Criminal Justice Behav* 10:316, 1983.

Hendrickson JM, Strain PS, Tremblay A, et al: Functional effects of peer social initiations on withdrawn preschool children. *Behav Mod* 13:502, 1986.

Hops H: Children's social competence and skill: Current research practices and future directions. *Behav Ther* 14:3, 1983.

Howlin P: An overview of social behavior in autism. In: Schopler E, Mesibov GB (eds): *Social Behavior in Autism.* New York, Plenum, 1986, p. 103.

Keller MG, Carlson PM: The use of symbolic modeling to promote social skills in children with low levels of social responsiveness. *Child Dev* 45:912, 1974.

Kirby FD, Toler HC: Modification of preschool isolate behavior: A case study. *J Appl Behav Anal* 3:309, 1970.

Koegel LK, Koegel RL: Motivating communication in children with autism. In: Schopler E, Mesibov GB (eds): *Learning and Cognition in Autism.* New York, Plenum, in press.

Koegel RL, Frea WD, Surratt AV: Self management of problematic social behavior. In: Schopler E, Mesibov GB (eds): *Behavioral Issues in Autism.* New York, Plenum, 1994, pp. 81–94.

Ladd GW: Effectiveness of a social learning method for enhancing children's social interaction and peer acceptance. *Child Dev* 52:171, 1981.

LaGreca AM, Mesibov G: Facilitating interpersonal functioning with peers in learning disabled children. *J Learn Disabil* 14:197, 1981.

LaGreca AM, Santogrossi DA: Social skills training with elementary school students: A behavioral group approach. *J Consult Clin Psychol* 48:220, 1980.

Larson KA, Gerber MM: Effects of social metacognitive training for enhancing overt behavior in learning disabled and low achieving delinquents. *Except Child* 54:201, 1987.

Lord C: Early social development in autism. In: Schopler E, Mesibov GB (eds): *Preschool Issues in Autism.* New York, Plenum, 1994, pp. 61–88.

Lord C: Facilitating social inclusion: Examples from peer intervention programs. In: Schopler E, Mesibov GB (eds): *Learning and Cognition in Autism.* New York, Plenum, in press.

Lord C, Bristol M, Schopler E: Early intervention for children with autism and related developmental disorders. In: Schopler E, Mesibov GB (eds): *Preschool Issues in Autism.* New York, Plenum, 1993, pp. 199–219.

McFall RM: A review and reformulation of the concept of social skills. *Behav Assess* 4:1, 1982.

McHale S: Changes in autistic children's social behavior as a function of interaction with nonhandicapped children. *Am J Orthopsychiatry* 53:81, 1983.

Mesibov GB: A cognitive program for teaching social behaviors to verbal autistic adolescents and adults. In: Schopler E, Mesibov GB (eds): *Social Behavior in Autism.* New York, Plenum, 1986, p. 265.

Mills MC: An intervention program for adolescents with behavior problems. *Adolescence* 22:91, 1987.

Minkin N, Braukman CJ, Minkin BL, et al: The social validation and training of conversational skills. *J Appl Behav Anal* 9:127, 1976.

Mueller E: The maintenance of verbal exchanges between young children. *Child Dev* 43:930, 1972.

O'Conner RD: Modification of social withdrawal through symbolic modeling. *J Appl Behav Anal* 2:15, 1969.

Oden S, Asher SR: Coaching children in social skills for friendship making. *Child Dev* 48:495, 1977.

Odom SL, Strain PS: A comparison of peer-initiation and teacher-antecedent interventions for promoting reciprocal social interaction of autistic preschoolers. *J Appl Behav Anal* 19:59, 1986.

Olly JG: The TEACCH Curriculum for teaching social behavior to children with autism. In: Schopler E, Mesibov GB (eds): *Social Behavior in Autism.* New York, Plenum, 1986, p.351.

Putallaz M, Gottman JM: An interactional model of children's entry into peer groups. *Child Dev* 52:986, 1981.

Putallaz M, Gottman JM: Conceptualizing social competence in children. In: Karolay P, Steffen JJ (eds): *Advances in Child Behavior Analysis and Therapy.* New York, Gardner, 1982, p. 1.

Radke-Yarrow M, Zahn-Waxler C, Chapman M: Children's prosocial dispositions and behavior. In: Mussen PH (ed): *Handbook of Child Psychology.* New York, Wiley, 1983, p. 469.

Roff M, Sells SB, Golden MM: *Social Adjustment and Personality Development in Children.* Minneapolis, University of Minnesota Press, 1972.

Rogers-Warren A, Baer DM: Correspondence between saying and doing: Teaching children to share and praise. *J Appl Behav Anal* 9:335, 1976.

Ross HS, Lollis SP, Elliot C: Toddler-peer communication. In: Rubin KH, Ross HS (eds): *Peer Relationships and Social Skills in Childhood.* New York, Springer-Verlag, 1982, p. 173.

Sacks O: A neurologist's notebook: An anthropologist on mars. *The New Yorker* 70:106–125, 1994.

Savitzky JC, Watson MJ: Patterns of proxemic behavior among preschool children. *Represent Res Soc Psychol* 6:109, 1975.

Sisson LA, Van Hasselt VB, Hersen M, et al: Peer interventions: Increasing social behaviors in multihandicapped children. *Behav Mod* 9:293, 1985.

Stone WL, LaGreca AM: Development of social skills in children. In: Schopler E, Mesibov GB (eds): *Social Behavior in Autism.* New York, Plenum, 1986, p. 35.

Strain PS: An experimental analysis of peer social initiations on the behavior of withdrawn preschool children: Some training and generalization effects. *J Abnorm Child Psychol* 5:445, 1977.

Strain PS, Kerr M, Ragland E: Effects of peer-mediated social imitation and prompting/reinforcement on the social behavior of autistic children. *J Autism Dev Discord* 9:41, 1979.

Strain PS, Shores RE, Timm MA: Effects of peer social behavior on the behavior of withdrawn preschool children. *J Appl Behav Anal* 10:289, 1977.

Sullivan HS: *The Interpersonal Theory of Psychiatry*. New York, Norton, 1953.

Taras ME, Matson JL, Leary C: Training of social interpersonal skills in two autistic children. *J Behav Ther Exp Psychiatry* 19:275, 1988.

Wallander JL, Hubert NC: Training and generalization methods to improve social skills deficits in children. *Scand J Behav Ther* 13:274, 1984.

86 CONSULTATION WITH YOUTH SHELTERS, GROUP HOMES, FOSTER CARE HOMES, AND BIG BROTHERS/BIG SISTERS PROGRAMS

R. Kevin Grigsby, D.S.W., L.C.S.W.

The continuum of services offered by child welfare programs presents a challenge to mental health professionals. These services have been developed to serve children and adolescents, who are a diverse group with multiple and varied needs. The system that is designed to serve and protect children is at times overwhelmed by the sheer numbers of children needing assistance and the needs of those children (Foster care system, 1990). Child-serving agencies are often ill-equipped to deal with children who present with problems that require more than minimal services. When faced with children who are not easily served, child-serving agencies will often turn to child mental health professionals for consultations or technical assistance. This chapter offers practical advice to the mental health clinician who is called upon to provide a consultation to child-serving agencies such as emergency youth shelters, residential group homes, foster care homes, Big Brothers/Big Sisters programs, and others.

THE CONTINUUM OF SERVICES IN CHILD WELFARE

Since the early part of the 20th century, the child welfare field has evolved into a complex, multidimensional matrix of services and programs. Although these programs and services may vary from community to community and from state to state, it appears that a continuum of services, which vary in level of intensity, has developed. In the least intense mode, child advocates lobby for and support policy initiatives that seek to improve or maintain children's rights. Services include community-based emotionally supportive programs offered to children, such as those of Big Brothers/Big Sisters of America. In a moderately intense mode, home-based intensive family preservation services are offered to families where children are at risk for out-of-home placement (Adnopoz et al., 1991; Frankel, 1988; Morton and Grigsby, 1993). More intensive services may utilize out-of-home placement of children to provide for the care of children whose parents cannot or have not provided those children with an adequate level of care. Out-of-home placement varies in intensity in that children may be placed into a foster care setting with relatives, with licensed foster parents, in an emergency youth shelter, in a group home, or in a more institutional setting such as a residential treatment center.

Youth shelters, group homes, and foster homes are representative of a portion of the child welfare service continuum. Various providers of these services may call upon mental health professionals for assistance because these programs are not typically staffed by mental health professionals. Even so, many of the children and youth that they serve present with a wide range of problems that include behaviors commonly dealt with by mental health providers in more intensive programs, such as community mental health centers and hospitals.

WHAT IS CONSULTATION?

Kadushin (1977) offers a list of representative definitions of *consultation* from the human services literature. For the purpose of this discussion, Boehm's (1956) definition appears to be the most useful:

> Consultation is an educational process whereby expertness in knowledge or skill is made available for the purposes of help with the solution of a problem by the provider of the consultation to the recipient of consultation, the latter assuming the responsibility for seeking the consultation and the use, nonuse or partial use of the fruits of the consultation. (p. 241)

This chapter concerns itself with the "expertness in knowledge and skill" that relates specifically to the area of child and adolescent psychiatry. This is an important distinction, as many times consultation is requested related to agency functions or problems that are not specifically related to the area of knowledge and skill in child psychiatry. For example, the consultant may be asked to offer help regarding dealing with employee absenteeism. While the consultant may wish to explore the area further in order to clarify clinical issues (are employees not coming to work because they are feeling too frustrated with the clients?), it is important to remember that employee absenteeism may be a problem that requires "expertness in knowledge and skill" that is outside the realm of child psychiatry. Consequently, the consultant may find himself or herself acting to refer agency personnel to other "experts" (such as employee assistance programs) for help. The consultant may spend a great deal of time helping agency personnel refine questions so that the real problems or issues can be addressed.

TYPES OF CONSULTATION

It is unlikely that the consultant will meet with a specific problem that can be easily identified. If this were the case, the consultant's help probably would not have been requested in the first place. Rather, the consultant may be met by a situation that is unclear and by a group of workers who are very frustrated because their attempts to intervene may have failed. In fact, unsuccessful intervention may have worsened the situation. The first task of the consultant is to ascertain the type of help that is needed; it can be categorized into one of two types: (*a*) *clinical* consultation and (*b*) *programmatic* consultation.

Clinical consultation is usually related to an individual person, family, or group. By and large, the consultant is asked to "reveal" information about the person, family, or group that will somehow improve the agency's ability to serve that particular "unit of intervention." Quite often, clinical consultation takes place on the "turf" of the consultant. For example, a foster mother may be having a difficult time dealing with the behavior of a child and request that the child welfare worker arrange for her to meet with the consultant to discuss methods of dealing with the child. The foster mother then meets with the psychiatric consultant at the local child guidance clinic for several sessions in order to make use of the clinician's insight related to the foster child's behavior.

Programmatic consultation usually relates to groups or classes of persons who are served by the provider. This type of consultation may be offered on the consultant's "turf," but it is usually offered on-site through actual observation or participation by the consultant. Both types of consultation are directed toward improving services, but the goals may differ significantly in that clinical consultation is directed toward smaller, specifically identified units of intervention, while programmatic consultation is directed toward broader organizational change.

Types of consultation closely related to programmatic consultation are training, education, and supervision of agency volunteers and employees. These types of consultation are covered in more depth elsewhere in the literature but are discussed briefly, as they pertain to the programs in the child welfare continuum.

COMMON THEMES IN CONSULTATION

There are five closely related themes that the mental health consultant to programs of this type should be able to address. These are the themes of separation, loss, identity, continuity, and crisis (Siu and Hogan, 1989). All children who are placed in youth shelters, foster homes, and group homes have to deal with these themes. Children involved in Big Brothers/Big Sisters programs have also had to deal with some of these issues, although the degree of intensity may be less, as they have not necessarily had an out-of-home placement. The consultant may not be directly asked about any of these themes by the agency or persons asking for help. It is imperative, however, that the consultant be cognizant of the importance of these issues to the children involved in the programs. Further, the consultant should utilize his or her status as an expert to raise the consciousness of the agency or program staff to the need for consideration of these factors in the day-to-day operation of the program.

Another common area of consultation is related to the understanding of and management of "acting-out behavior." The consultant should recognize that agency and program staff may often use this term incorrectly; however, that is usually of little consequence. Rather, it is important to recognize that when program personnel describe behavior as "acting out," they may be indicating that they do not have an understanding of this child, or of the child's behavior. This is a cue that the program personnel may be asking the consultant to make use of his or her "expertness" in order to help them understand and deal with the problem child or behavior on both the individual and programmatic level. Helping the program personnel know which behaviors are beyond their scope of intervention is also important. For example, a youth shelter program may not be able to offer shelter to a child who is actively setting fires. Most shelters do not offer the type of close behavioral monitoring that is necessary in order to appropriately serve these children. A referral to a more intensive program may be necessary, and the shelter personnel may need to be supported in their refusal to admit the child who sets fires.

In general, the common themes addressed in dealing with children who are being served by these programs are no different from those themes that are dealt with in evaluating or treating children and youth in the child guidance clinic. The difference is that the consultant is one step removed from the child as the agency or program personnel are assisted through consultation.

CONSULTATION WITH YOUTH SHELTERS

Youth shelters have traditionally been called upon to provide safe haven for runaway and homeless youth. As the population of homeless youth has increased, and as the problems of this population group have become complex (Shane, 1989), the pressures on both the shelters themselves and the state child welfare agencies have increased. Data suggest that the complexity and urgency of the problems of runaway and homeless youth may overwhelm programs that are not prepared to serve children and youth with serious problems including depression (General Accounting Office, 1989, p. 27; Kurtz et al., 1991) and histories of maltreatment (Kufeldt and Nimmo, 1987; Powers et al., 1990). Forty-nine percent of all children placed into shelter care by the Connecticut Department of Children and Youth Services (DCYS) during a 12-month period had a history of psychiatric hospitalization and/or residential treatment (Connecticut Department of Children and Youth Services, 1986).

Another indicator of the intensity of the problems faced by shelters is seen in a national survey of 139 shelter facilities that found "depression" to be the most frequently listed presenting health problem (78%). Suicidal tendencies were reported as a "common presenting health problem" by 56% of the shelters. A survey completed by the National Association of Social Workers (Survey reveals, 1992) found that 20% of the children and youth surveyed had attempted suicide. "Severe psychological or psychiatric problems" were reported by 37% (National Network of Runaway and Youth Services, 1984). Substance abuse is also a chronic problem of many homeless and runaway youth (Southeastern Network of Youth and Family Services, 1990).

Although many of the youth entering shelters have lived with a parent or relative within the past year (General Accounting Office, 1989, p. 20), many have experienced a history of multiple placements in foster or group care. Seventy-two percent of the youth placed into shelters by the Connecticut Department of Children and Youth Services during a 12-month period had a history of three or more out-of-home placements, with a mean number of placements of 6.44 (Connecticut Department of Children and Youth Services, 1986). A Canadian study found that a significant portion of youth living "on the street" (46%) had left a foster home or other form of government-sponsored care (Kufeldt et al., 1992).

In spite of the high level of need, service delivery to this population has historically been difficult, and services that are available have often been fragmented or distant. Although some shelters provided basic mental health services as long ago as a decade (Gordon, 1978), a survey of all the runaway and youth shelters in Connecticut revealed that none of the 10 shelters had on-site mental health evaluations or treatment available in 1986 (Douglas House Shelter and Yale Child Study Center, 1986). A model for mental health consultation at shelters for homeless and runaway youth has been developed (Grigsby, 1993) that makes use of naturalistic methods to provide mental health consultation that is both clinical and programmatic in nature. This model assumes that there is not only a need to understand the individuals who are placed in the shelter, but also a need to understand the "culture" of the shelter environment, if the consultant is to be successful in both the clinical and programmatic senses. In this model, the consultant assumes the role of "credentialed expert," as described by Snow et al. (1986), a role that was also employed and found to be useful in a study of homelessness. This allows the consultant to enter the "culture" of the shelter in a way similar to that of the field researcher or ethnographer entering a foreign culture and attempting to study that culture as a participant observer. Schein (1987) explicates the "clinical perspective" as being different from that of ethnography in that "clinicians enter an organization . . .if they are requested to do so by someone in the organization or someone acting on the organization's behalf seeking some kind of help" (p. 24). An understanding of the shelter is necessary before any meaningful programmatic consultation can take place. As the consultant begins to understand the shelter, the behaviors of both residents and staff may be better understood. The shelter staff also begin to accept the consultant as someone who "has been there" and who has an understanding of the day-to-day operations of the shelter. On-site involvement also leads to the formation of relationships between the consultant and the residents, and between the consultant and the shelter staff. As the consultant is accepted as a person who has an understanding of the situation, the staff and residents will begin to approach the consultant for help. In order to get to this point, however, many weeks of on-site participant observation may be necessary. Eventually, the consultant will be able to gain enough trust that he or she will be able to offer consultation about residents without waiting to be solicited for advice. As clinical consultation regarding individual residents becomes routine, programmatic consultation can then begin to take place. In one consultation effort at a shelter in New Haven, Connecticut, the rate of unplanned discharge was reduced from 43.5 to 18% within a 6-month period through the use of this model (Grigsby, 1993). By taking the clinician out of the clinic and placing him or her in the community, the work of both the mental health professional and the community staff can be enhanced as trust is built. The gulf between the mental health professional and the community staff is reduced, and a statement of the value of the shelter program and its staff is made.

This consultation is not treatment. Rather, it is the use of clinical skills, insight, and knowledge to support those who work on the front line with homeless youth. The consultation helps them to understand the strengths as well as the pathology of the individual clients and helps them to gain insight into the group dynamics within the shelter facility itself.

In providing programmatic consultation to emergency youth shelters, the limitations of the facilities and programs may require that the consultant advocate for major change in programming so that the facilities are better able to meet the needs of the children that are referred. In a less sophisticated sense, a consultant may become aware that modifying or altering the present program may still fall far short of what is needed. In these cases, the consultant may need to work toward developing a model or prototype program that will better serve the needs of clients. Grigsby and Miller (1989) argue for the creation of a shelter care program for homeless, at-risk youth that is designed to accommodate youth who have a history of psychiatric problems and who are in need of mental health evaluation and intervention. In order to insure that shelter programs serve the best interests of children, this model promotes a nonjudgmental philosophy that encourages the admission of children in need while considering the limitations of the emergency youth shelter. For this reason, the model makes specific recommendations about the types of clients who *cannot* be appropriately served in a shelter care setting.

CONSULTATION WITH GROUP HOMES

Community-based living facilities for youth have come into wide use over the past several years. Although these facilities have been used for various types of persons (the mentally ill, the physically handicapped, recovering substance abusers), this discussion is limited to group homes for clients who are dependent youths, emotionally disturbed youths, and/or socially maladjusted youths (Shostak, 1987). Group homes for these types of youth usually serve children who have reached adolescence. These facilities can be distinguished from other residential facilities by their small size, their reliance on other community resources such as public schools, and the lack of restraints on the movement of the residents within the community (Shostak, 1987, p. 14). As traditional foster care homes have been less and less available (Foster care system, 1990), group care facilities have come into greater demand. In order to meet this demand, there was a sizable increase in the number of residential group care facilities of this type between 1965 and 1981. Even so, there was a "decrease in the relative proportion of residential group care for dependent, neglected, or abused children and youth" (Dore et al., 1984, p. 493). This was accompanied by a reduction in facility size (Dore et al., 1984, p. 494), which suggests that a change in the orientation of services may have taken place during the period of 1966–1981. Dore and Kennedy (1981) argue that three major principles have affected the delivery of services over the past 20 years. The movement toward deinstitutionalization, normalization, and the right to treatment has caused changes to take place within the child welfare system that have greatly affected the clientele and programs at group homes. In a sense,

there has been an impetus to improve the services offered in order to meet more effectively the needs of the population served at these facilities. It appears, however, that there is a paucity of published literature regarding the effectiveness of these programs. Studies of children who have been terminated from foster care have "generally combined group homes with larger facilities and foster families, disregarding potential differences in the clients and the outcomes of these programs" (Shostak and Quane, 1988, p. 30). One study that examined youths who had left group homes found that group homes were only short-term placements for many children and that many left prematurely (Shostak and Quane, 1988, p. 33). Group home directors who were interviewed reported that they felt that "the high percentage of premature terminations was due largely to a recent trend toward assigning more seriously disturbed or maladjusted youths to group homes" (Shostak and Quane, 1988, p. 30). A study of the quality of care in group homes in the Los Angeles County area found that all of the group homes studied provided "good basic care; that is, food, clothing, education, recreational activities, and interventive medical care" but that there was "a particularly troubling problem for group homes" in obtaining and retaining qualified, caring, and competent staff (Cohen, 1986). Generally, these research questions are reflective of the problems and issues that are presented to the mental health consultant. Group home administrators often request consultation to help them (a) obtain, retain, and train child care personnel; (b) prevent premature discharge or termination; (c) evaluate and briefly intervene with problem residents; and (d) develop treatment plans and strategies for dealing with seriously disturbed or maladjusted youth who are placed in the group homes.

The mental health consultant can be most helpful to these programs by focusing on the unique situation of each facility while promoting the generic knowledge offered by the theory base of child psychiatry. In other words, the application of clinical knowledge acts as a guide to help the group home personnel understand the needs and behavior of residents and, to some degree, of staff themselves. The consultant can then guide the program personnel to better serve the group home residents.

CONSULTATION WITH FOSTER HOMES

Children who are placed in out-of-home care are placed into a variety of settings including youth shelters, group homes, or foster homes. Generally, foster homes are the "placement of choice" whenever possible, because it is felt that they offer the most homelike environment for children who have often experienced significant turmoil in their lives and have required protective service intervention. Foster homes offer latency-age and younger children an environment that is temporary in nature and that offers the child the care and nurturance that is needed at the time of placement. Persons who become foster parents must go through a procedure of licensing, but they usually do not have any special training in dealing with children, except for their own life experiences. In recent years, therapeutic foster homes and "special" foster homes (such as homes specifically designed for HIV-infected children) have been developed, which make use of foster parents who have a high degree of training. Foster parents are often in need of help in order to understand and manage the behavior of children who are placed into care within the foster home. For example, foster parents may approach the mental health consultant for help with a specific problem they are experiencing with a child, such as nocturnal enuresis. Usually the foster family has attempted to deal with the problem by making use of their own resources and understanding. If this has failed, they may then approach the consultant for help. It is important, however, that the consultant recognize that the foster parents may also need help with feelings of frustration or failure that they may have because they were unable to deal with the problem on their own. The consultant must consider this as he or she helps the foster family to understand the problem through the use of the knowledge base of child psychiatry. In a sense, the consultant must move through a series of roles as educator, clinician, and "coach" as he or she helps the foster family to deal with the problem at hand.

In some cases, child welfare workers will need assistance in understanding the nature of parent-child, sibling-sibling, and grandparent-child attachment relationships. Too often, workers underestimate the need for visitation and are not "cognizant of the importance of encouraging and maintaining attachments between children in foster care and persons to whom they are attached" (Grigsby, 1994). The mental health consultant must remember to advocate for the child's best interest, even if visitation requires a great deal of effort on the part of the child welfare worker.

In some cases, programmatic consultation is requested with regard to the operation of foster homes. The mental health consultant may be asked to train a group of foster parents around some issue or issues pertinent to caring for foster children. For example, a group of foster parents who are providing foster care for adolescents may ask for help with trying to deal with the behavior of these foster children. A time-limited, group-oriented training module for these foster parents on understanding adolescents is one possible option. Information should be presented in such a way that it can be specifically related to the children that these foster parents have in their homes. Child psychiatric knowledge should be applied to both the generic and unique situations encountered by these parents. Additionally, the consultant should be prepared to offer consultation to foster parents that is child specific. This may need to be done outside of the group situation, however.

CONSULTATION WITH BIG BROTHERS/BIG SISTERS PROGRAMS

Big Brothers/Big Sisters programs offer children from single-parent families the opportunity to engage in a relationship "with an adult friend who can provide regular assistance, understanding, and acceptance" (Big Brothers/Big Sisters, 1988, p. 978). Usually the adult friend and the child are of the same gender. Big Brothers/Big Sisters of America is an organization of federated local agencies that are administered by local, volunteer boards of directors (Big Brothers/Big Sisters, 1987, 1988). The programs make use of adult volunteers who have limited training in working with children but who receive supervision and support from professionally trained social workers employed by the local Big Brothers/Big Sisters programs. These programs will often request consultation that is related to helping volunteers have a better understanding of the needs and behavior of the children that they serve. At times, these programs may request training workshops that are intended to help volunteers have a better understanding of the children who are involved. Training that is requested is often related to the five common themes of separation, loss, identity, continuity, and crisis (Siu and Hogan, 1989). Consultation may also be requested on a specific child or a specific problem area, such as thumb-sucking or fighting with siblings. It is important to remember that the consultant is asked to bring "expertness" on the subject and that a better understanding of the subject area can be reached if the consultant is able to present the material in a manner that is relevant. In the case of Big Brothers/Big Sisters programs, the presentation should be case specific, if possible, as volunteers appear to be most accepting if they feel that the issues are personally relevant. While a discussion of theory may be fruitful when working with group home or youth shelter personnel, it may not be as useful when consulting with volunteer foster parents or Big Brothers/Big Sisters.

THE LIMITS OF CONSULTATION

As Boehm (1956) relates in his definition of consultation, the recipient of the consultation is responsible for the "use, nonuse or partial use of the fruits of the consultation" (p. 241). It is the nature of the consultant's role to have little control over the operation of the consultee's program. In the hospital or clinic setting, the mental health professional has a great deal of responsibility and, to a degree, the concomitant control. The lack of control that is inherent in the consultant's role is at times frustrating to mental health professionals. Even though the consultant may offer concrete advice relating to a situation in a program, the program personnel may choose to disregard the consultant's advice or to make only partial use of the consultant's advice. By not utilizing the consultant's advice, a situation may get worse. The consultant may be sought out for further help at that point, and it may be difficult for the consultant to refrain from expressing his or her displeasure that the initial advice was disregarded or modified. This is the nature of consultation. The consultant may experience a great deal of frustration and at times may be tempted to "take over" as the agency director, supervisor, or foster parent. It is obvious that this is not helpful. Therefore, the consultant must be cognizant of and agree to the limitations of the consultant role from the outset of the consultant-consultee relationship.

CONCLUSIONS

Child-serving agencies must deal with many children whose needs are varied and broad. Although these agencies are charged with meeting the needs of children, they are at times ill-equipped to do this. When these agencies are overwhelmed or faced with situations of crisis, they may call upon mental health professionals for help. Quite often, these agencies have difficulty in articulating the type or degree of problem that they are having. First, the mental health consultant must help the requesting person or persons to define the problem and refine the questions that they wish to have addressed. Second, the consultant must be clear about his or her role as a helper in the problem-solving process. The consultant must recognize the limits of his or her knowledge and power and must be ready to assist in locating an appropriate source of help if the problem or problems encountered fall outside of the scope of the consultant's knowledge base in child psychiatry. Third, the consultant must recognize that, even though issues related to insight, unconscious motivation, and acting out may be encountered and dealt with in the consultation process, that "the consultant's function is essentially educational, that learning develops out of a relationship, but that this relationship need not be therapeutic" (Stein, 1956, p. 249). Finally, by taking the time to understand the culture of the consultation site through a naturalistic or ethnographic intervention, the consultant is better able to understand the point of view of the client. This allows the mental health consultant's knowledge of child psychiatry to be most useful to agency personnel, to volunteers, and to the children who are served by these programs.

References

Adnopoz DJ, Grigsby RK, Nagler SF: Multiproblem families and high-risk children and adolescents: Causes and management. In: Lewis M (ed): *Child and Adolescent Psychiatry: A Comprehensive Textbook*. Baltimore, Williams & Wilkins, 1991, pp. 1059–1066.

Big Brothers/Big Sisters of America: In: *The Encyclopedia Americana* (international ed). Danbury, CT, Grolier, 1987, pp. 733–734.

Big Brothers/Big Sisters of America: In: Daniels PK, Schwartz CA (eds): *Encyclopedia of Associa-*tions (28th ed). Detroit, Gale Research Co., 1994, p. 1232.

Boehm W: The professional relationship between consultant and consultee. *Am J Orthopsychiatry* 26: 241–248, 1956.

Cohen NA: Quality of care for youth in group homes. *Child Welfare* 65:481–493, 1986.

Connecticut Department of Children and Youth Services (DCYS): *Runaway and Homeless Youth Shelter Record Survey*. Hartford, CT, Connecticut Department of Children and Youth Services, 1986.

Dore MM, Kennedy KG: Two decades of turmoil: Child welfare services, 1960–1980. *Child Welfare* 60:371–382, 1981.

Dore MM, Young TM, Pappenfort DM: Comparison of basic data for the National Survey of Residential Group Care Facilities: 1966–1982. *Child Welfare* 63:485–495, 1984.

Douglas House Shelter and Yale Child Study Center: *Mental Health Services to Shelters Survey* (mimeograph). New Haven, CT, Douglas House Shelter and Yale Child Study Center, 1986.

Foster care system reeling, despite law meant to help. *New York Times* September 21:A1, A18, 1990.

Frankel H: Family-centered, home-based services in child protection: A review of the research. *Soc Serv Rev* 62:137–157, 1988.

General Accounting Office: *Homelessness: Homeless and runaway youth receiving services at federally funded shelters.* Washington, DC, Department of Health and Human Services, United States Government Printing Office, 1989.

Gordon JS: The runaway center as community mental health center. *Am J Psychiatry* 135:932–935, 1978.

Grigsby RK: Mental health consultation at a youth shelter: An ethnographic approach. *Child Youth Care Forum* 21:247–261, 1993.

Grigsby RK: Maintaining attachment relationships among children in foster care. *Families in Society* 75:269–276, 1994.

Grigsby RK, Miller MH: A prototype shelter program for homeless, at-risk youth. Paper presented to the Connecticut Shelter Directors Association, Middletown, CT, September 1989.

Jarvis SV: *Drug use among runaway and homeless youth: A southeastern perspective.* Athens, Georgia, The Southeastern Network of Youth and Family Services, Inc., 1990.

Kadushin A: *Consultation in Social Work.* New York, Columbia University Press, 1977.

Kufeldt PD, Nimmo M: Youth on the street: Child abuse and neglect in the eighties. *Child Abuse Negl* 11:531–543, 1987.

Kufeldt PD, Durieux M, Nimmo M, et al: Providing shelter for street youth: Are we reaching those in need? *Child Abuse Negl* 16:187–199, 1992.

Kurtz PD, Jarvis SV, Kurtz GL: Problems of homeless youths: Empirical findings and human services issues. *Soc Work* 36:309–314, 1991.

Morton ES, Grigsby RK (eds): *Advancing Family Preservation Practice.* Newbury Park, CA, Sage, 1993.

National Network of Runaway and Youth Services: *Health and Educational Survey.* Washington, DC, National Network of Runaway and Youth Services, Inc., March 1984.

Powers JL, Eckenrode J, Jaklitsch B: Maltreatment among homeless and runaway youth. *Child Abuse Negl* 14:87–98, 1990.

Schein EH: *The Clinical Perspective in Fieldwork.* Beverly Hills, CA, Sage, 1987.

Shane PG: Changing patterns among homeless and runaway youth. *Am J Orthopsychiatry* 59: 208–213, 1989.

Shostak AL: *Group Homes for Teenagers.* New York, Human Sciences Press, 1987.

Shostak AL, Quane RM: Youths who leave group homes. *Public Welfare* 46:29–36, 1988.

Siu S-F, Hogan PT: Common clinical themes in child welfare. *Soc Work* 34:339–345, 1989.

Snow DA, Benford RD, Anderson L: Fieldwork roles and informational yield. *Urban Life* 14: 377–408, 1986.

Stein HD: The use of the consultant: Discussion. *Am J Orthopsychiatry* 26:249–251, 1956.

Survey reveals plight of young runaways. *NASW News* February 37:8, 1992.

87 OTHER ORGANIC TREATMENTS
David A. Tomb, M.D.

The landscape of psychiatry is littered with speculative and ineffective organic therapies. Treatments such as allergen extracts for behavior problems and optometric training (Metzger and Werner, 1984) or vestibular dysfunction correction (Polatajko, 1985) for learning disabilities have no justification at this time. Other treatments may have had a place once but are currently outmoded, for example, insulin coma therapy and Metrazol convulsion therapy. Still other therapies are showing promise in adult psychiatry, but as yet have no basis of experience or research in child psychiatry, for example, light therapy for seasonal affective disorder and sleep schedule alteration for depression.

Psychotherapy and psychopharmacology remain the primary credible treatments in child psychiatry. Electroconvulsive therapy (ECT) should be considered in a few, very select cases. Psychosurgery is experimental and has no current clinical role. Finally, a host of nutritional therapies dot the landscape, which, although they frequently do no harm, possess uncertain and unlikely clinical value.

ELECTROCONVULSIVE THERAPY

ECT with adults, although controversial in some circles, has become routine. Standard, safe, and acceptable methods of administering ECT are available (Glenn and Weiner, 1985). Patients for whom ECT is the appropriate treatment can be readily identified and agreed upon by most experts (Small et al., 1986). Moreover, when administered correctly and for proper indications, ECT is undeniably safe and effective (Crow and Johnstone, 1986).

Professional opinion is much more divided about the usefulness of ECT with children and adolescents. Although ECT has been administered to children for many years by a small number of practitioners, it is not commonplace. In fact, discussion of its appropriateness with this population often adopts the overtones of polemics rather than science. This may partly be due to a scarcity of scientific studies: There are no controlled studies of ECT applied to children and adolescents. Clinical practice is based exclusively on clinical experience, a few open and poorly conducted studies on small populations of patients, a handful of case studies, and extrapolation from the science and clinical use of ECT with adults. Thus, current treatment must by necessity be based on an unstable foundation.

ECT was first administered to significant numbers of children in the early 1940s. Bender (1947) reported using ECT on 98 "schizophrenic" children under the age of 12, with some as young as 3 years of age. The patient population was mixed; although her clinical descriptions are vague, it is likely that many would not be considered schizophrenic by today's standards. She felt that almost all the children improved in their social functioning, even though their "schizophrenic" symptoms remained (e.g., disturbances in thought, language symbol formation, and stereotyped movements). Moreover, she found the complications associated with this large series of ECT treatments (most patients received approximately 20 treatments, but some children as many as 40) to be minimal: one fractured vertebra, one "recurring grand-mal convulsions," and four children with "organic-type mental disturbances with excitement and confusion" that lasted about 2 weeks.

Clardy and Rumpf (1954) later restudied a subpopulation of Bender's original sample and took issue with her optimistic findings. They believed both that the original diagnosis of childhood schizophrenia was in error and that the outcome was less positive than presented by Bender. In fact, they found only 9 of a study population of 32 children to still deserve their original diagnosis; they believed that most displayed primary behavior disorders, while some warranted a research diagnosis of "psychopathic personality." They found the majority of children with schizophrenia to be unimproved, while when viewed retrospectively most of the others showed few effects, either positive or negative, from their ECT treatment.

An additional early positive report was that of Heuyer et al. (1947), who found that 11 of 12 children suffering from depression, mania, or delirium improved with ECT, while none of 17 other children who suffered from a mixture of other conditions, including schizophrenia, recovered. Unfortunately, due to the lack of diagnostic clarity, this early research has little to teach us. This literature does suggest, however, that children can receive ECT without obvious harm, if also without obvious benefit.

The issue of effectiveness has been addressed in more recent times by a series of case studies (Bertagnoli and Borchardt, 1990). Early on, Gillis (1955) reported the dramatic recovery of a "schizophrenic" 12-year-old boy treated with ECT. By today's nosology, this case would likely be considered a form of a major depression. Other single-case studies have followed in a similarly positive vein: a 14-year-old boy with mania (Warneke, 1975), a 16-year-old girl with catatonic schizophrenia (Perkins and Tanaka, 1979), a 12-year-old girl with mania (Carr et al., 1983), a 17-year-old boy with depression and organic brain damage (Mansheim, 1983), an 11-year-old boy with major depression (Black et al., 1985), an 18-year-old girl with rapidly cycling bipolar disorder (Berman and Wolpert, 1987), and a 13-year-old prepubescent boy with repeated stuporous depression (Powell, 1988). Although it is in the nature of single-case studies to report successes, these papers do indicate the presence of a small population of seriously disturbed children who appear to respond to ECT. All of these patients had failed to improve with appropriate medications, and all ultimately received ECT because they presented serious clinical management problems and were, in several cases, *in extremis*. Moreover, none of these youths experienced difficulty with side effects from the ECT. More recently there has been a report in the French literature on the successful treatment of 9 teenagers, ages 15–19, with ECT (Paillere-Martinot et al., 1990). This report has been confounded, however, by the diverse conditions suffered by these teens, conditions that ranged from acute schizophrenia to delusional mania. Finally, Schneekloth and colleagues (Schneekloth et al., 1993) report successful outcomes in 20 youth receiving ECT for serious affective and schizophreniform disorders, while Fink (Fink, 1993) argues for careful studies to place the use of ECT in young people on a firm scientific footing.

Less favorable is the report by Guttmacher (1988), who studied four children, ages 12–15, retrospectively and found only one to have improved to any extent with ECT. The diagnoses of these young adolescents included major depression, psychotic depression, catatonic schizophrenia, and pervasive developmental disorder. Only the child with psychotic depression seemed to respond to ECT. Of equal importance, three of the patients had seizures lasting longer than 4 minutes, and two required pharmacological intervention to terminate those seizures. Until further research clarifies the issue, prolonged seizures should be considered a risk of ECT in children and adolescents, and preparations should be made to intervene if necessary. On challenge by McGough et al. (1989), Guttmacher reported an additional negative case, a prepubescent early teenager with severe depression who failed to respond to a series of 11 ECT treatments. Idupuganti and Mujica (1988) also reported very modest improvement in a 16-year-old girl with symptoms of catatonia.

There is a long, if unreported, history of giving ECT to adolescents in the United States (Asnis et al., 1978). ECT has been administered to children less frequently. As the above cases indicate, there are psychiatrically impaired children for whom ECT is useful, necessary, and even lifesaving; it should remain in our clinical armamentarium. Although some experienced clinicians feel that, on average, ECT is somewhat less effective in children than in adults, the risk:benefit ratio is favorable in carefully selected cases. However, conservative treatment still requires that electroshock be administered to children and adolescents "as a last resort," after vigorous psychotherapy and psychopharmacology have proven ineffective. In addition, it should be given carefully, only with indicated patients, and only with proper safeguards.

The technique of ECT administration to children and adolescents is similar to that with adults. ECT requires a thorough medical evaluation, a proper setting such as an operating room and recovery area in a hospital, and the presence of appropriate equipment and medical personnel trained to administer anesthesia to young people. The ECT protocol involves preanesthesia and procedure anesthesia, unilateral nondominant electrode placement, and the induction of a cerebral seizure with an ample electrical stimulus. Some practitioners feel that children require stimulus levels lower than those required to produce a seizure in adults (McGough et al., 1988), but require approximately the same number and spacing of treatments as do adults. Six to 12 treatments should be sufficient for most patients; more than a dozen treatments probably should be avoided unless the condition is undeniably life-threatening.

The only youths for whom ECT should be considered are those with profound melancholic or psychotic depression or those with uncontrolled mania. It might be considered for lesser degrees of depression if the illness is incapacitating and if the child proves supremely sensitive or unresponsive to medication. Occasionally a stuporous, catatonic state might require ECT, although those that respond are more likely related to the affective disorders than to schizophrenia. The temptation to use ECT in other conditions should be resisted.

Before giving ECT, legal and ethical safeguards should be firmly in place. The American Psychiatric Association currently recommends that ECT in a child 12 or under should require the evaluation and concurrence of two psychiatrists, not otherwise involved with the case, who are experienced with ECT and with the treatment of children. For youths 13 and older, one external reviewer should be involved. These are sensible recommendations. Moreover, informed consent should always be sought. The child should be helped to understand the procedure in accord with his or her developmental level. The parents must be fully informed about the reasons for, and the process and the risks of, ECT. Before the procedure, they must be told about temporary amnesia, confusion, and headache. ECT should never be described as a panacea or as a desperation procedure but rather as a safe, appropriate treatment in very select cases.

PSYCHOSURGERY

Psychosurgery currently has little place in child psychiatry. Although CNS surgery that alters pathology is an essential part of medicine, surgery on normal tissue to alter behavior is not. A case can be made that occasionally severely ill and hopelessly refractory adults benefit from psychosurgery (Baer et al., 1995; Smith et al., 1976; Tippin and Henn, 1982), and in fact, small positive series have been obtained with severe depressions, chronic anxiety states, obsessive-compulsive disorder, or a combination of these problems. There is little reason to doubt that a few patients do improve markedly with psychosurgery and without unfortunate sequelae. It is also likely that the number of potential patients for such procedures will shrink with time since the very patients most responsive to psychosurgery—those with depression, anxiety, and compulsions—are also those to whom recent psychopharmacological advances apply.

On the other hand, the child is a developing organism whose outcome is unpredictable until adulthood (if then). Those children who are psychiatrically impaired need to "prove" that their impairment is so severe and intractable as to require psychosurgery. Such proof takes time, and typically decisions about surgery should wait until the child matures.

Pediatric psychosurgery has a long, but spotty, history. It has never been used routinely for any single condition nor in great numbers of conditions. It has, however, been performed occasionally, experimentally, in the most difficult of cases, and with variable and unpredictable success in a number of different conditions (Holland et al., 1958). Incapacitating anxiety and obsessive-compulsive states may respond, as does depression, but the original opinion that psychosurgery was an effective treatment for schizophrenia seems unwarranted.

There are better and more treatments available today than were available in the heyday of psychosurgery several decades ago. As our options and their effectiveness have improved, the place of psychosurgery as a viable treatment for children has receded to the point of disappearance.

NUTRITIONAL THERAPIES

The value, or lack of value, of nutritional therapy for childhood psychiatric disorders seems to be a controversy that will not die. Even the boundaries of this debate are hard to define; it involves not only individuals from numerous professional and nonprofessional disciplines but also a seemingly endless list of possible substances in the diet, which either should be present and aren't, or are present and shouldn't be. It is also not clear what disorders are diet related, if any; the list of contenders certainly includes attention deficit hyperactivity disorder (ADHD) and learning disabilities, but may also include nonspecific aggressiveness, autism, childhood schizophrenia, and others. Moreover, much of the debate has been conducted in the public arena, and typically the issues have not been subjected to careful scientific scrutiny. (It reflects the state of the field that the most broad-based recent review of this area by a careful scientist was published as a popular, rather than scientific, book (Conners, 1989)). As a result, the value of nutritional therapy, in part or in whole, has neither been proved nor disproved.

Many of the speculations surrounding the effects of nutrients and nutritional therapy on behavior rest on shaky ground. In spite of decades of enthusiastic but undisciplined publishing, for example, support for the basic tenets of orthomolecular psychiatry and megavitamin therapy remains elusive. Likewise, structuring a diet around esoteric tests such as hair analysis for mineral content is suspect, not only because the tests are exceptionally sophisticated and potentially unreliable (Bailey, 1989), but also because correction of any putative abnormalities has not been shown to affect behavior. However, a few nutritional interventions are worth attention. Most of these focus on the role of diet in generating hyperactivity, aggression, and learning disabilities.

It is hard to determine what should be excluded from the diet. Feingold (1975) postulated that hyperactive behavior in children was due to food allergy and eschewed artificial food flavors and colors. He prescribed an almost unobtainably complex elimination diet as the cure, a regimen that has not been supported by several double-blind efforts to test his hypothesis (e.g., Goyette et al., 1978). On the other hand, other efforts to identify contributory substances in the diet have been more positive. An example is Egger's effort (Egger et al., 1985) to test the hypothesis of food allergy by administering an oligoantigenic diet (few varieties of food) to which were then sequentially added excluded foods. Sixty-two of 76 previously overactive children were believed to be improved. The other type of evidence typically presented to validate the food allergy hypothesis has been the occasional child who "unequivocally" is made worse by a specific food or substance. This is proof of a sort, according to Conners (1989), who relates a compelling example of a 4-year-old boy who became aggressive upon consuming aspartame. Unfortunately, this clinical evidence finds limited support in careful large-scale studies. It may be that food additives influence a limited and unpredictable subpopulation of the ADHD group of children.

Other dietary substances run into similar problems in efforts to prove culpability. Refined sugar, like food additives, has been thought to cause hyperactivity and aggression, yet many attempts to prove this hypothesis by challenging normal (Rosen et al., 1988) and "sugar sensitive" hyperactive children (Kruesi et al., 1987; Milich and Pelham, 1986) with sugar have been negative. This may be, as Connors suggests (1989, p. 99), a more complex process that involves the interaction of several other crucial variables, such as patient age, as well as the protein and carbohydrate intake at the time of sugar consumption. Past research designs may just not have been sophisticated enough to capture the legitimate effects of diet. In any case, the issue of sugar's influence on behavior remains unsettled, although its effect is likely to be somewhat subtle.

A final class of compounds for which confusing evidence of a dietary effect exists is the minerals. Problems have been attributed to too little iron, too much lead, too little zinc, and too much cadmium. All of these elements can be neurotoxic, yet the best evidence for a behavioral effect at normally encountered levels occurs with lead. Needleman was able to correlate lowered IQ and nonadaptive classroom behavior to elevation of dentine lead levels in 1st- and 2nd-grade schoolchildren (Needleman et al., 1979). Other studies have also emphasized the disruptive effects of elevated lead on behavior and intelligence. However, effective treatment for this condition remains speculative, although chelation has been suggested (David et al., 1976).

CONCLUSIONS

Organic treatments, except for psychopharmacology, have little to offer child psychiatry. Each possible modality has its detractors, and only ECT has a broad enough base of clinical support to be considered useful, and then only in select cases. Psychosurgery has no place in current treatments. Nutritional therapies lack power and precise applications, yet are worthy of further study.

References

Asnis GM, Fink M, Saferstein S: ECT in metropolitan New York hospitals: A survey of practice, 1975–1976. Am J Psychiatry 135:479, 1978.

Baer L, Rauch SL, Ballantine HT, et al: Cingulotomy for intractable obsessive compulsive disorder. Arch Gen Psychiatry 52:384, 1995.

Bailey DN: Drug screening in an unconventional matrix: Hair analysis. JAMA 262:3331, 1989.

Bender L: One hundred cases of childhood schizophrenia treated with electric shock. Trans Am Neurol Soc 72:165, 1947.

Berman E, Wolpert EA: Intractable manic-depressive psychosis with rapid cycling in an 18-year-old woman successfully treated with electroconvulsive therapy. J Nerv Ment Dis 175:236, 1987.

Bertagnoli MW, Borchardt LM: A review of ECT for children and adolescents. J Am Acad Child Adolesc Psychiatry 29:302, 1990.

Black DW, Wilcox JA, Stewart M: The use of ECT in children: Case report. J Clin Psychiatry 46:98, 1985.

Carr V, Dorrington C, Schrader G, et al: The use of ECT for mania in childhood bipolar disorder. Br J Psychiatry 143:411, 1983.

Clardy ER, Rumpf EM: The effect of electric shock treatment on children having schizophrenic manifestations. Psychiatr Q 28:616, 1954.

Conners CK: Feeding the Brain. New York, Plenum, 1989.

Crow RJ, Johnstone EC: Controlled trials of electroconvulsive therapy. Ann NY Acad Sci 462:12, 1986.

David OJ, Hoffman SP, Severd D, et al: Lead and hyperactivity, behavioral response to chelation: A pilot study. Am J Psychiatry 133:1155,1976.

Egger J; Graham PI, Carter CM, et al: Controlled trial of oligoantigenic treatment in the hyperkinetic syndrome. Lancet 1:541, 1985.

Feingold BF: Why Your Child Is Hyperactive. New York, Random House, 1975.

Fink M: Electroconvulsive therapy in children and adolescents. Convuls Ther 9:155, 1993.

Gillis A: A case of schizophrenia in childhood. J Nerv Ment Dis 121:471, 1955.

Glenn MD, Weiner RD: Electroconvulsive Therapy: A Programmed Text. Washington, DC, American Psychiatric Press, 1985.

Goyette CH, Conners CK, Petti TA, et al: Effects of artificial colors on hyperkinetic children: A double blind challenge study. Psychopharmacol Bull 14:39, 1978.

Guttmacher LB, Cretella H: Electroconvulsive therapy in one child and three adolescents. J Clin Psychiatry 49:20, 1988.

Heuyer G, Dauphin M, Lebovici S: La practique de l'electrochoc chez l'enfant. Z Kinder Jugenpsychiatr 14:60, 1947.

Holland NC, Newman EG, Hohman LB: Effects of lobotomy in childhood diseases of the nervous system. Dis Nerv Sys 19:201, 1958.

Idupuganti S, Mujica R: Hemifacial flushing during unilateral ECT (letter). Am J Psychiatry 145:1037, 1988.

Kruesi MJP, Rapoport JL, Cummings EM, et al: Effects of sugar and aspartame on aggression and activity in children. Am J Psychiatry 14:1487, 1987.

Mansheim P: ECT in the treatment of a depressed adolescent with meningomyelocele, hydrocephalus, and seizures. J Clin Psychiatry 44:385, 1983.

McGough JJ, McCall WV, Shelp FE: ECT in children and adolescents (letter). J Clin Psychiatry 50:106, 1989.

Metzger RL, Werner DD: Use of visual training for reading disabilities: A review. Pediatrics 7:824, 1984.

Milich R, Pelham WE: Effects of sugar ingestion on the classroom and playgroup behavior of attention deficit disordered boys. J Consult Clin Psychol 154:714, 1986.

Needleman HL, Gunnoe C, Leviton A, et al: Deficits in psychologic and classroom performance of children with elevated dentine lead levels. N Engl J Med 300:689, 1979.

Paillere-Martinot ML, Zivi A, Basquin M: Use of electroconvulsive therapy in adolescence. Encephale 16:399, 1990.

Perkins IH, Tanaka R: The controversy that will not die is the treatment that can and does save lives: Electroconvulsive therapy. Adolescence 14:607, 1979.

Polatajko HI: A critical look at vestibular dysfunction in learning-disabled children. Dev Med Child Neur 27:283, 1985.

Powell JC: Pre-pubertal depressive stupor: A case report. Br J Psychiatry 153:689, 1988.

Rosen LA, Bender ME, Booth SR: Effects of sugar (sucrose) on children's behavior. J Consult Clin Psychol 56:583, 1988.

Schneekloth TD, Rummans TA, Logan KM: Electroconvulsive therapy in adolescents. Convuls Ther 9:158, 1993.

Small IF, Milstein V, Miller MI, et al: Electroconvulsive treatment—Indications, benefits, and limitations. Am J Psychother 40:343, 1986.

Smith JS, Kiloh LG, Cochrane N, et al: A prospective evaluation of open prefrontal leucotomy. Med J Aust 10:731, 1976.

Tippin J, Henn FA: Modified leukotomy in the treatment of intractable obsessional neurosis. Am J Psychiatry 139:1601, 1982.

Warneke L: A case of manic-depressive illness in childhood. Can Psychiatr Assoc J 20:195, 1975.

88 PRIMARY PREVENTION

Naomi I. Rae Grant, M.B., B.S., F.R.C.P.(C.), F.R.C.Psych.

The prevalence rate of emotional and behavioral disorders among children and adolescents is high, almost one in five; furthermore, evidence suggests that the rate of disorders has increased with each generation over the past 20 years. There is evidence of the earlier onset of depression (Cross National Collaborative study, 1992), higher suicide rates in the 15- to 24-year-old group (Klerman et al., 1985), and increased scores both on externalizing and internalizing disorders among children and adolescents in a recent community survey (Achenbach and Howell, 1993).

The one in five prevalence figure is not unique or limited to only one particularly deprived geographic area. In a review of five community surveys (Costello, 1989), the prevalence rate in four different jurisdictions was found to vary over a narrow range between 17.6 and 22.2%. Not only are such disorders common, but comorbidity is present in over two-thirds of children and adolescents who have an emotional or behavioral disorder (Offord et al., 1987).

It has been suggested that community surveys tend to overestimate the rate of disorder among a target population, and certainly more information is still needed on the severity of the disorders identified in community surveys and on the extent of associated problems. It is now clear, however, that the disorder can be remarkably tenacious. Recent longitudinal studies have emphasized the high rates of persistence of conduct disorder (Offord et al., 1992) and attention deficit hyperactivity disorder among children followed up into adolescence and adulthood (Weiss and Hechtman, 1993).

It is not known to what degree children and their families detected as disordered in community surveys would accept diagnostic and treatment services even if such services could be offered. In the province of Ontario, where health care, including child mental health services, is fully funded, the biggest barrier to treatment is lack of availability of resources. In the Ontario Child Health Study, a community survey of over 3000 children between the ages of 4 and 14 years, fewer than one in six children had been seen by any mental health or social service in the previous 6 months (Offord, 1987). Finally, those children who do receive treatment have been found to be not necessarily those most in need, in terms of degree of impairment (Offord, 1982).

Even if all of the children and adolescents with disorders who require and would accept treatment could be offered treatment, therapeutic methods for those conditions for which they are effective are very expensive, time consuming, and require highly trained personnel. There will never, in the foreseeable future, be adequate treatment resources, and the implications are clear that other means of reducing the risk for disorder in the childhood population must be found (Offord et al., 1989).

If the prevalence rates of psychiatric disorder in these surveys were reduced to 10%, there is wide acceptance that this 10% of the child population would have clinically important conditions with serious associated impairments, including learning problems, physical health problems, and substance abuse (Institute of Medicine, 1989). The findings in these surveys merit urgent consideration and have implications for the delivery of child psychiatric services, for training, and for research (Rae Grant et al., 1989a).

The evidence for the enormous discrepancy between needs and resources is not a new phenomenon and has been repeatedly decried over the past 40 years. Numerous conferences, commission reports, and papers have recommended that some of our resources be put into prevention. There have been many influential people in the field of child mental health who have cited such evidence to argue for a preventive stance over the past three decades (Berlin, 1972; Caplan, 1964, 1976; Eisenberg, 1961). Prevention programming, research in the preventive intervention area, and prevention training have, however, been slow to develop.

BARRIERS TO PREVENTION

Barriers to prevention efforts have been not only operational but also paradigmatic, ethical, and ideological. Operational impediments have included the difficulty with the definition of prevention, the difficulty in proving that the reduction of risk by preventive intervention during childhood does indeed result in the reduction of mental disorders in adulthood, the lack of research tools in the area, the lack of funding opportunities, the lack of a cadre of trained researchers, and the lack of a body of well-researched intervention studies that would conclusively prove the effectiveness of primary prevention.

PARADIGMATIC BARRIERS

For many clinicians, changing the emphasis from treating "psychopathology" to promoting mental health or preventing disorder requires a paradigm shift and necessitates a recognition that the target is the population of children at risk, not just those identified and referred to hospitals or clinics and from focusing on the disordered individual to intervening in the risk environment. Garmezy (1983) emphasized that for decades mental health researchers devoted their energies to the study of patterns of maladaptation and incompetence. As Rutter (1985) pointed out, it is only comparatively recently that it has become fashionable to study the development of individuals who overcome childhood circumstances of disadvantage and stress and to study the factors that are supportive or protective to children under stressful circumstances.

ETHICAL BARRIERS

There has been an understandable fear of "promising too much" and of actually doing harm by intervening in high risk populations where disorder does not yet exist. The McCord studies about the negative effects of treatment with juvenile delinquents in comparison with a control, untreated group, have emphasized the dangers of labeling and intervening without clear knowledge of the possible effects (McCord, 1992).

IDEOLOGICAL BARRIERS

Children in North American culture are still regarded as belonging primarily to their parents. No special knowledge or skill is considered requisite for becoming a parent. Children are not generally regarded as a resource for the future, and therefore there has been little concerted societal effort to safeguard their development. Insufficient resources are devoted to ensuring that they receive the basic necessities of attention in order to develop cognitively, socially, and emotionally.

PREVENTION: THE STATE OF THE ART

There is finally some indication that things are changing. As recently as 1988 the American Psychological Association reviewed 300 primary prevention projects and found only 14 that met their scientific criteria. Since that time, the legitimacy of the field has gradually been established

Figure 88.1. (From Institute of Medicine: *Reducing Risks for Mental Disorders: Frontiers for Preventive Intervention Research.* Mrazek PJ, Haggerty RJ (eds): Washington, DC, National Academy Press, 1994.)

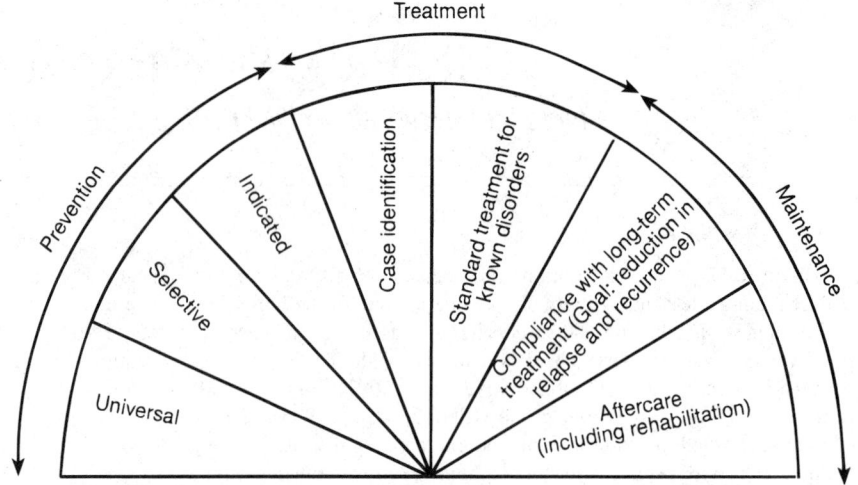

The Mental Health Intervention Spectrum for Mental Disorders

and, as Lorion et al. (1994) have described, individually and together, mental health scientists, policymakers, and service providers have argued for the inclusion of prevention in public health policies. More importantly, they have successfully lobbied for the allocation of federal funds to support the consolidation of existing knowledge, the establishment of research priorities, and the development of a national network of prevention research centers. As a result, the number of projects using randomized controlled trials has not only increased dramatically, but several projects have been funded for replication trials in multiple sites (Institute of Medicine, 1994). In Canada the Federal Health and Welfare Project Brighter Futures and the Ontario Consortium of Ministries project ''Better Beginnings, Better Futures'' (1990), which supports 11 intervention projects for disadvantaged families and children from prebirth to age 8, suggests that the federal and provincial governments are beginning to support primary prevention albeit still at the demonstration project level. The thrust of Project Prevention by the American Academy of Child and Adolescent Psychiatry (1990) and the inclusion of primary prevention as one of the topics in the guidelines for training in child and adolescent psychiatry by the Canadian Academy of Child Psychiatry suggest that perhaps, at last, primary prevention is also beginning to be taken seriously by the subspecialty.

WHAT IS PRIMARY PREVENTION?

If we agree that primary prevention is at least one of the ways in which to begin to tackle the discrepancy between needs and resources, the next problem is one of definition.

Interventions were first categorized according to the classic public health distinctions among primary, secondary, and tertiary interventions (Caplan, 1964), the term *primary prevention* refers to efforts to decrease the prevalence of disorder through reducing its incidence, i.e., prevention in its literary sense. *Secondary prevention* refers to interventions designed to reduce the prevalence of disorder, i.e., treatment. *Tertiary prevention* refers to efforts designed to minimize the sequelae of established disorders, i.e., rehabilitation.

Bloom (1968) used the term primary prevention to cover two separate and distinct areas: (*a*) those activities that come under the heading of specific protection or disease prevention, and (*b*) those geared to the promotion of health. He pointed out that specific protection interventions usually require more traditionally trained health professionals to implement them, whereas health promotion activities necessitate a more educational paradigm. For the purpose of this chapter, the term *primary prevention* includes both specific protection and mental health promotion.

Gordon (1983) proposed an alternate classification scheme for the

prevention of physical diseases: *a universal preventive measure* is one which is desirable for everyone in the eligible population. In this category are included measures that can be confidently advocated (those in which the benefits outweigh the costs) for the general population. Examples include prenatal care, immunization, and the use of seat belts.

Selective preventive measure is indicated when a subgroup of the population is at risk for a particular condition and when the balance of benefits against risk and cost can be justified. Risk groups for mental disorders may be identified on the basis of biological, psychological, or social risk factors known to be associated with the onset of mental disorders. Examples of selected interventions include home visitation and infant day care for high risk mothers and preschool programs for all children from disadvantaged neighborhoods.

Indicated preventive interventions are targeted to high risk individuals with detectable symptoms or signs foreshadowing mental conditions or markers indicating predisposition for mental disorders but who do not meet DSM-IV criteria, for example, the provision of a parent/child training program for parents of preschool children with aggressive behavior.

This classification is the one used by the Committee on the prevention of mental disorders in a recently published report (Institute of Medicine, 1994). The range of intervention activities is perhaps best understood as existing on a continuum with health promotion at one end and rehabilitation at the other end of the spectrum (Fig. 88.1).

PREVENTION AND TREATMENT

Whereas treatment focuses on the individual, deals with referred patients, and has a remedial aim, in prevention the focus is on a target group or a population at risk but not identified individually, and the aim is protection or competence enhancement (Fig. 88.2).

CONCEPTS IN PRIMARY PREVENTION

The same risk factors or correlates may produce many different emotional and behavioral outcomes. A review of community surveys and longitudinal epidemiological studies emphasizes that the markers for disorder are multifactorial (Offord et al., 1987, 1989; Rutter, 1989). It has become evident that most risk factors other than genetic factors are not specific to a single disorder. It is the aggregation of risk factors with appropriate weighting of the relative importance of each factor that will yield the targets with the most potential for prevention of later onset of mental disorders (Institute of Medicine, 1994). In order to look at possible opportunities for intervention, we need to be concerned not only with child factors but also with family environments, with stressful life events, with the communities in

Treatment	Prevention
Focuses on individual	Focuses on group or population
Referred patients or clients	Unreferred persons or groups
Identified "problem"	At risk
Aim is remedial	Aim is protective
Restores status quo	Enhances competence

Figure 88.2. Prevention is not treatment.

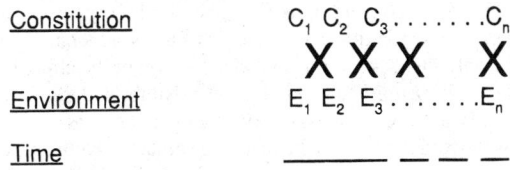

Figure 88.3. The transactional model of organism-environment reciprocity. (Adapted from Sameroff AJ, Chandler MJ: Reproductive risk and the continuum of caretaking casualty. In: Horowitz FD, Hetherington M, Scarr-Salopatek S (eds): *Review of Child Development Research* (Vol 4). Chicago, University of Chicago Press, 1975, pp. 187–244.)

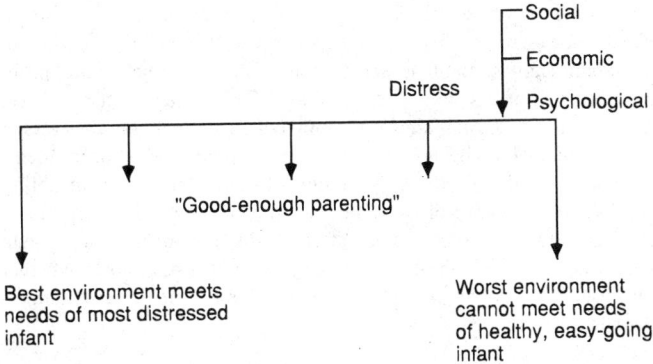

Figure 88.4. Continuum of child-caring causality. (Adapted from Sameroff AJ, Chandler MJ: Reproductive risk and the continuum of caretaking causality. In: Horowitz FD, Hetherington M, Scarr-Salopatek S (eds): *Review of Child Development Research* (Vol 4). Chicago, University of Chicago Press, 1975.)

which families live, with the institutions that influence children, and with the interaction of all these domains.

Lee Robins (1970) first described the concept of causal chains, by which one situation or event leads to another, which leads to an outcome. Robins suggested that one could intervene at any point along the causal chain; for example, take the chain

unresponsive parenting → lack of language stimulation → language delay → learning difficulties → behavior disorder

Intervention could be aimed at improving parental responsiveness or at providing another responsive adult in the nurturing environment; these would be preventive interventions for the child, whereas attempting to provide speech therapy or remediate a learning disability or attend to the behavior disorder later on would be treatment interventions.

Sameroff (1987) modified Robin's concept of causal chains to include a bidirectional framework; in other words, how things turn out is a complex result of the interaction between the child and the environment at different points in time, as parent and child each in turn affect the other and change the outcome (Fig. 88.3).

Things go wrong when the family environment is just not able to meet the needs of the child, either because the child is too impaired or temperamentally difficult or because the parents lack responsiveness due to their own lack of nurturing, psychiatric illness, or overwhelming environmental distress. Sameroff and Chandler (1975) have described this as the continuum of caretaking casualty; at one end of this continuum is an adaptive family environment that can meet the needs of the most distressed infant, and at the other end is the disordered family environment that cannot meet the needs of the least distressed, most healthy, normal, temperamentally easy newborn. In between are the majority of average environments that provide "good enough" parenting (Fig. 88.4).

It is evident that adverse conditions in the growing child's environment do not necessarily produce adverse outcomes. However, it is becoming increasingly clear that the combination of risk factors in the child and risk factors in the family environment, particularly if these are multiple, is likely to predispose children to negative outcomes. For example, Lewis et al. (1989), in developing a theory of the genesis of violence, followed 95 formerly incarcerated delinquents. She found that there was an interactive effect between intrinsic vulnerability and abusive, violent families and that it was the combination of severe impairment and severe abuse that was most closely associated with extreme aggression in adulthood. She suggested, first, that children who are

neuropsychiatrically and cognitively intact are better equipped than are multiply handicapped children to resist models of family violence and are able to choose among alternative styles and make rational judgments. Second, severe abuse engenders rage, which psychiatrically and cognitively impaired individuals find particularly difficult to control. Third, where child abuse involves shaking, battering, or other injury to the central nervous system, it may create the very psychiatric, neurological, and cognitive vulnerabilities described. Finally, impaired children, because they are hyperactive and impulsive, often invite abuse.

Outcomes, in summary, depend on the interaction of a number of factors:

1. The number of risk factors in the wider environment;
2. The number of stressors/risk factors in the family environment;
3. The vulnerability of the child;
4. The timing and nature of particular stressful and life experiences;
5. The resilience of the child (protective factors);
6. Protective factors in the family environment;
7. Protective factors in the wider environment.

George Albee (1979) has developed an equation that attempts to capture all these different factors:

$$Incidence = \frac{organic\ factors\ and\ stress}{competence,\ coping\ skills,\ and\ available\ supports}$$

Risk Factors

Garmezy (1983) has defined risk factors as "those factors which, if present increase the likelihood of a child developing an emotional disorder in comparison with a randomly selected child from the general population." To qualify as a risk factor a variable must be associated with an increased probability of disorder and must antedate the onset of disorder. Variables that may constitute risk factors at one life stage may or may not put an individual at risk at a later stage of development. These factors can include biological and genetic attributes of the child, family factors, and community factors that impinge on the child and family environment.

RISK FACTORS IN THE CHILD

Risk factors in the child can lead to a state of vulnerability in which other risk factors may then impact; for example, a prematurely born infant is more vulnerable than a full-term, healthy sibling in a suboptimal family environment. Other innate risk factors that render the child vulnerable include adverse prenatal conditions such as drug or alcohol ingestion in pregnancy, developmental delay (late walking and talking) (Werner and Smith, 1982), and below average intelligence. Links have been shown between early language disabilities and later development of behavior disorders (Dattilo and Camarata, 1991). Children who are temperamentally difficult are more likely to show later behavioral problems than children who are less difficult (Earls, 1981; Reitsma-Street et al., 1985). It is the combination of infant difficulty with family stress or dysfunction that has been found to contribute to later behavior problems (Maziade et al., 1989). Similarly, chronic illness and functional disability (Cadman et al., 1986) place a child at increased risk for externalizing disorder, and chronic conditions affecting the central nervous system place a child at the highest risk (Rutter, 1977). It is not known whether this is due to the cognitive damage itself or the resulting difficult temperament of the child.

RISK FACTORS IN THE FAMILY ENVIRONMENT

Family dysfunction (Quinton et al., 1984) involves a number of different aspects: factors that have to do with family adversity, disruption, and stress; factors that interfere with the parent/child interaction, and factors that interfere with optimal parenting practices. Marital discord in families has been persistently found to predict disruptive behavior problems in boys, especially in combination with maternal depression (Rutter and Giller, 1983). It is the extent of discord and conflict between the parents, whether or not they are separated, that is associated with risk for antisocial behavior (Hetherington et al., 1985). The effects of witnessing parental violence have recently been shown to predispose boys to use violence as a means of conflict resolution (Jaffe et al., 1990).

Factors that interfere with the development of parent/child relationships include parental alcoholism (Quinton et al., 1984); maternal alcohol problems, found to have the greatest effect on the behaviors of younger boys (Avison, 1992); parental psychiatric illness (Rutter and Quinton, 1984), especially maternal depression (Avison, 1992); and criminality in parents (West and Farrington, 1982). Poor maternal education has been found to correlate with poor school achievement but not with emotional disorder in children (Offord et al., 1985). Dysfunctional parenting practices, especially harsh, erratic, and abusive forms of discipline, have been found to predispose to conduct disorder. Patterson et al. (1992) have systematically documented how coercive behavior on the part of both child and parent, combined with parental inconsistency, creates negative reinforcement patterns in which child aggression and coercion are reinforced. The combination of inadequate supervision, parental criticism, harsh and inconsistent discipline, and rejecting attitudes toward a child have been described by Patterson et al. to have a specific effect in producing antisocial behavior in children.

COMMUNITY FACTORS

Community factors that impinge on children and their families include the impact of poverty (Offord et al., 1989). Having a parent on social assistance has been found to have a particularly detrimental effect on children, especially girls (Offord, 1987). Overcrowding (Rutter and Quinton, 1977) and living in subsidized housing (Rutter, 1981) have also been found to be risk factors for conduct problems (Hawkins et al., 1992b). Poverty appears to have its effect due to the aggregation of risk factors, that is, the number of life stresses and daily hassles that inevitably have an impact on family interactions and relationships in a way that changes what Rutter has described as the "under the roof culture of the family." Low income has been found to be one of the most powerful risk factors for conduct disorder in young children (Kolvin et al., 1988; Offord et al., 1986).

Schools have been found to have the power to either enhance or detract from intellectual and social growth and can thus function as community risk or protective environments for children and adolescents.

Urban areas typically have higher rates of delinquency. Even within cities there is marked variation in crime rates by neighborhood. In early childhood it is evident that a positive family environment is able to protect children from the effects of the wider community environment

but, as the child grows older, the peer, school, and community effects become more powerful.

MULTIPLE RISK FACTORS

Adverse conditions in the environment do not always necessarily produce adverse outcomes. It is becoming clear that it is the combination and number of risk factors in the child and risk factors in the family environment that is likely to predispose children to negative outcomes. For example, Greenberg et al. (1993) have suggested that there are four domains of risk that are interrelated to produce early onset conduct disorder. These are contributions from the child's organic or temperamental difficulties; family factors such as family adversity, disruption and stress; ineffective parenting and socialization of the child; and problems in the early parent/child relationships. Rutter and Quinton (1977) suggested that a 4-fold increase in the amount of stress in childhood produced a 24-fold increase in the incidence of later psychiatric disorder. Not all subsequent studies have replicated this exponential effect, but it is quite clear that multiple risk factors markedly increase the preponderance of adverse outcomes.

Sameroff (1987) found that families with seven or more risk factors had children who scored 30 IQ points below families with no risk factors.

Resilience

Resilience has been described as the capacity for successful adaptation, positive functioning, or competence despite high-risk status, chronic stress, or following prolonged or severe trauma (Egeland et al., 1993). These authors view resilience in terms of a transactional process within an organizational framework. Developmental outcomes are determined by the interaction of genetic, biological, psychological, and sociological factors in the context of environmental support (Cicchetti and Schneider-Rosen, 1986).

Protective Factors

Rutter (1985) defined protective factors as "those factors that modify, ameliorate or alter a person's response to some environmental hazard that predisposes to a maladaptive outcome." Because they modify risk factors, however, they do not necessarily foster normal development in the absence of risk factors. Research into protective factors is less well developed than risk factor research, and several conceptual and methodological issues remain to be resolved (Luthar, 1993), but there is evidence that a core set of individual characteristics and sources of support can buffer the effects of both biological and psychosocial risks during childhood (Institute of Medicine, 1994). Protective factors can be considered under the headings of factors within the child, the family, and the community.

CHILD FACTORS

Child factors include positive temperament (Rutter, 1985), above-average intelligence (Rutter et al., 1970), and measures of social competence, which include academic achievement, participation and competence in outside school activities, and the ability to relate easily to others. Rae Grant et al. (1989b) found that the ability to get along with teachers, parents, and peers, and having friendships, were strongly protective for adolescents. Children who are easygoing and responsive call forth the best from not only their parents but later from teachers, peers, and other adults in their environment. Above average intelligence may allow a child not only to succeed academically but also develop problem-solving skills. In adolescence having a sense of coherence and internal locus of control has been cited as a protective factor (O'Grady and Metz, 1987).

FAMILY FACTORS

Favorable family factors include supportive parents, family closeness, and adequate rule setting (Werner and Smith, 1982). A supportive relationship with even one parent was found to provide a substantial protective effect for children living in severely discordant, unhappy homes (Rutter, 1975). There is consistent evidence that the nature and quality of children's interaction with their parents affects their interpersonal behaviors, social competence, and school performance (Amato, 1989; Dornbusch, 1989). Smaller family structure with spacing of more than 2 years between siblings has been found to be protective (Werner and Smith, 1992).

COMMUNITY FACTORS

Community factors include the relationships that children develop outside the family with peers, significant other adults, and the institutions with which they come in contact. These have been found to have the potential to exert significant positive or negative effects. Good schools were found not only to positively affect academic achievement but also to reduce the rate of truancy and school drop-out and juvenile court appearances for children in disadvantaged areas in inner London (Rutter et al., 1979).

Three clusters of protective factors were found to differentiate the resilient group from other high risk children who developed serious and persistent problems in childhood and adolescence in the Kauai Longitudinal Study (Werner and Smith, 1992). These were:

1. At least average intelligence and temperamental attributes that elicited positive responses from family members and other adults;
2. Good relationships with parents or parent substitutes;
3. An external support system that rewarded competence and provided a sense of coherence.

Interactions of Risk and Protective Factors

Garmezy et al. (1984) have proposed three possible models for the ways in which risk factors and protective factors interact to produce competence in children:

1. The compensatory model, in which stresses, risk, and vulnerability factors combine additively. It is the aggregation of risk factors rather than the presence of any specific single factor that impairs development. Infancy risk factors appear to be magnified synergistically when family environments in childhood are negative or when children are subjected to stressful life events (O'Grady and Metz, 1987).
2. The challenge model, which describes a curvilinear relationship in which stress enhances competence as long as it is not excessive. This model has been described as one of ''inoculation'' (Werner and Smith, 1982) or ''steeling'' (Anthony, 1974). Successive, moderately challenging experiences strengthen coping capacities (Murphy and Moriarty, 1976).
3. The protective model, which suggests that protective factors modulate or buffer the impact of stressors as variables by, for instance, improving coping adaptation and competence building.

Anthony (1974), quoting Jacques May, makes an analogy that is useful in depicting this relationship. He suggests that we imagine three dolls, one of glass, one of plastic, and one of steel, each of which is exposed to a blow from a hammer. The first doll breaks down completely, the second carries a permanent scar, and the third merely gives out a fine metallic sound. The glass doll is obviously at risk from external forces because of its ''constitution.'' It could also have been mishandled after leaving the factory or might have been neglected by its owner and thus have been exposed to being chipped or cracked. The cumulation of risk experiences may leave the doll in a heightened state of susceptibility. To carry the analogy further, Anthony suggests that one might imagine a protective coating of some sort being applied to the glass doll to reduce its vulnerability and protect it from further trauma.

PATHWAYS FROM CHILDHOOD TO ADULTHOOD

In discussing the ways in which early events might be linked to later outcomes, Rutter (1989) emphasized that not only continuities but also discontinuities are found between events in childhood and subsequent adult outcomes; for example, some risk pathways turned into more adap-

tive routes because of adventitious happenings (e.g., more positive environments or events such as positive school experiences). Children at risk early in life who subsequently had good school experiences and completed their secondary education were three times more likely to show planning in their choice of life career or marital partner. Similarly, the presence of marital support in mothers who had been earlier at risk because of institutional experiences was found to lead to good social functioning and good parenting, in contrast with those who did not receive good marital support.

Werner and Smith (1982) suggest that the interaction of risk and protective factors is a balance between the power of the person and the power of the social and physical environment. A balance is necessary throughout life, although different factors assume different degrees of importance at different developmental stages. These authors suggest that constitutional factors are most important during infancy and childhood and interpersonal factors are more important during adolescence.

How Do Preventive Interventions Work?

The aim, in summary, is to reduce the number of risk factors either in the child, in the parent-child environment, or in situations in the wider environment with which the child comes into contact. Not all risk factors need to be reduced. Even reducing some in a multirisk situation is likely to result in more advantageous outcomes for children. Conversely, if the number of protective factors can be increased either in the individual child or in the parenting environment or by increasing support systems available to the child, then resilience is likely to be increased (Fig. 88.5).

Levels of Preventive Intervention

Kessler and Albee (1977) have suggested that anything that improves the quality of children's lives can be considered within the realm of primary prevention. Within this broad range, there are a large number of avenues of approach (Fig. 88.6). It is possible to target the individual child, his or her parents, the interaction between the parents and child, or, at the community level, the institutions with which children come into contact, including schools, hospitals, and social agencies. At the wider, sociopolitical level, it is possible to try to influence government policies and legislation, which may have an impact on the environment in which children grow.

Catalano and Dooley (1980) have described interventions directed

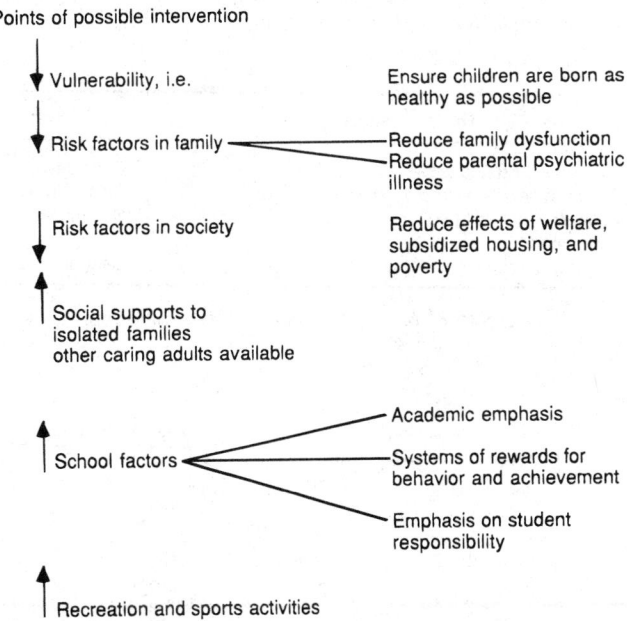

Points of possible intervention

Vulnerability, i.e. — Ensure children are born as healthy as possible

Risk factors in family — Reduce family dysfunction / Reduce parental psychiatric illness

Risk factors in society — Reduce effects of welfare, subsidized housing, and poverty

Social supports to isolated families other caring adults available

School factors — Academic emphasis / Systems of rewards for behavior and achievement / Emphasis on student responsibility

Recreation and sports activities

Figure 88.5. Points of possible intervention.

at the wider environment as proactive and those directed at individual levels as reactive and point out that mental health professionals usually prefer to work in the reactive arena and are reluctant to tackle the more daunting tasks of attempting to influence government policies that might effect a reduction in stress in the wider environment that impinges on the child and family.

At the child and family levels, preventive intervention may attempt to reduce the number of risk factors impinging on the child or to improve the competence of children to deal with stress. Moving from the case level to target interventions aimed at children at the community level recognizes the large number of children who are at risk; working with a target group of children at risk reduces the danger of labeling individual children and utilizes interventions that can reach a larger population more efficiently. This is not a new idea; Eisenberg (1961), over 25 years ago, coined the term *the multiplier effect* to describe the benefits of the child psychiatrists working with people who work directly with children. Providing seminars on behavioral management for the staff of a day care center, for example, rather than working directly with children referred from that center to a therapeutic day treatment program indirectly reaches many more children and provides the day care staff with skills they can use with subsequent groups of children (E. Shaver, personal communication, 1987). An example of a communitywide program is furnished by moving from interventions with individuals at risk to interventions aimed at changing a risk situation (Fig. 88.7). There is evidence now that targeting the risk situation posed by high school entry, a stressful transition for many teenagers, by changing the environment of the high school for entering 9th grade students is a more powerful and simpler intervention than working with groups of students to prepare them for moving from junior high to high school (Felner and Adan, 1988).

An outstanding example of moving from intervening at the level of the child at risk to intervening with the risk environment was described by Olweus in 1987; instead of teaching individual children to cope with bullying by aggressive peers, a national program was developed and successfully carried out in Norway to reduce bullying throughout the entire school system (Olweus, 1991). The primary emphasis of the multicomponent prevention program was to educate the community, families, and school personnel on the scope of the bully-victim problem and potential solutions.

Prevention Research

Price (1987) points out that there are four stages in carrying out a successful intervention research program:

Focus on Intervention	Level
Individual child and/or family	Case Level
Group (type) of children or families	Class Level
Local environment (e.g., institutions, agencies, neighborhoods)	Community Level
Wider environment areas	Central Level

Figure 88.6.   Intervention at different levels.

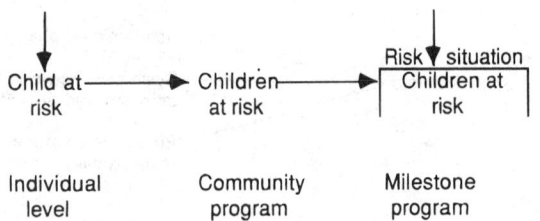

Figure 88.7.   Paradigm shift, or moving from interventions with the child at risk to interventions in the risk situation.

1. Assessment of the degree of risk in a target population;
2. Formulation of the plan of intervention;
3. Assessment of the effects of the intervention;
4. Wide dissemination of the knowledge gained.

Prevention intervention research requires evidence of risk in a population or target group, outcome specifications, the development of a hypothesis about the genesis of the risk factors, and a rationale for the connection between the planned intervention and such risk factors. There are particular problems in this field since, as Price has pointed out, new conceptual and methodological tools are needed to assess the degree of risk and to measure the effectiveness of various interventions.

Because prevention research always involves the community in some way, a partnership between the researcher and the community is highly desirable. The issue to be studied must be a problem or disorder that is a matter of concern to the community to be involved in the research, for example, the school, community, or neighborhood. A method of designing, conducting, and analyzing programs within the preventive intervention research cycle has recently been described (Institute of Medicine, 1994) (Fig. 88.8).

Promising Preventive Interventions

There are now a sizable number of well-planned, well-evaluated prevention projects in the child and adolescent area. Such programs include unique program components, strong research designs, a longitudinal follow-up of children and families, and use of multiple relevant outcome measures that measure short-term (proximal) as well as long-term (distal) results.

PRENATAL/INFANT DEVELOPMENT PROGRAMS

The age of children served by these programs has ranged from pre-birth to 4 years. Most programs consist of home visiting by a nurse or nonprofessional home visitor who calls on at-risk families. Programs during pregnancy often focus on such risk factors as inadequate diet, smoking, and alcohol and drug abuse. Family planning as well as interventions geared toward improving mother-child interaction and providing education regarding the child's normal physical and psychological development are the major emphases during the infant and toddler stages. Reducing social isolation and employment training for the mother are also important program components. Examples of two such programs follow.

One of the most frequently cited of the prenatal and early infancy projects (Olds et al., 1986) was selected as a model primary prevention project by the American Psychological Association. The project was carried out in a small semirural county in the Appalachian region of New York. The project emphasized a strong outreach component, including biweekly visiting by a nurse at home. Prenatal care, pediatric care, and a variety of social services were made available. The program recruited 384 poor single mothers who were all below 25 weeks of gestation. The emphasis was on building the nurse-parent relationship and providing parent education. During the last trimester of pregnancy, education was aimed at improving the diet; monitoring weight gain; eliminating cigarettes, alcohol, and drugs; identifying signs of pregnancy complications; encouraging regular rest; and preparing for labor and delivery and for care of the newborn infant. Infancy education emphasized improving the parents' understanding of temperament, promoting the infant's social, emotional, and cognitive development, and promoting the physical health of the child. Mothers were encouraged to make appropriate use of the health care system to make plans regarding subsequent pregnancies, returning to school, and finding employment. Efforts were made to enhance informal support and to link with formal services. Free transportation was provided if necessary.

The program found multiple positive outcomes. At the end of 3 years there were reduced rates of child abuse and neglect, fewer emergency room visits and accidents, better home environments, and more use of formal services and informal social supports. The program is now being

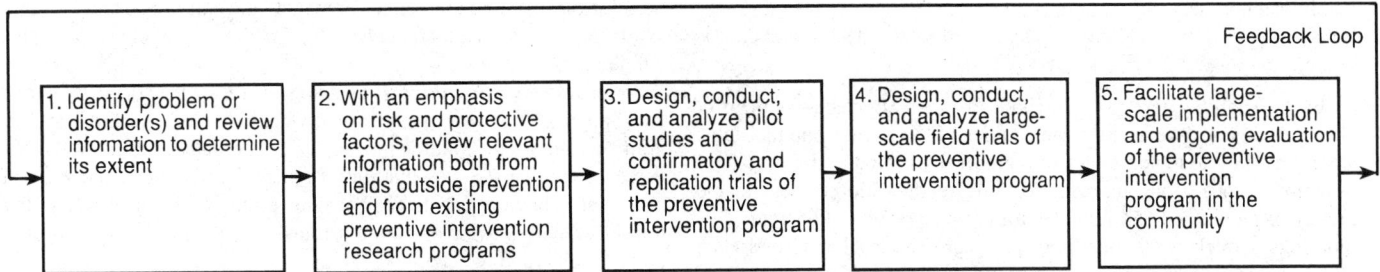

Figure 88.8. The preventive intervention research cycle. Preventive intervention research is represented in *boxes 3* and *4*. Note that although information from many different fields in health research, represented in *boxes 1* and *2*, is necessary to the cycle depicted here, it is the review of this information, rather than the original studies, that is considered to be part of the preventive intervention research cycle. Likewise, for *box 5*, it is the facilitation by the investigator of the shift from research project to community service program with ongoing evaluation, rather than the service program itself, that is part of the preventive intervention research cycle. Although only one feedback loop is represented here, the exchange of knowledge among researchers and between researchers and community practitioners occurs throughout the cycle. (From Institute of Medicine: Designing, conducting and analyzing programs within the preventive intervention research cycle. In: Mrazek P, Haggerty RJ (eds): *Reducing Risks for Mental Disorders. Frontiers for Preventive Intervention Research.* Washington, DC, Institute of Medicine, National Academy of Sciences, 1994, p. 362.)

Table 88.1 Short-Term Effects of Prenatal/ Infancy Programs

Children
  Better physical health
  Better nutrition provided by parents
  Fewer low birth weight babies
  Fewer feeding problems
  Fewer accidents and emergency room visits
  Reduced incidence of child abuse
Parents
  Better social support networks
  Greater confidence
  Improved parenting skills
  Better parent-child interactions
  More stable marital relationships
  Less abuse of children
  Longer time periods between pregnancies
  More frequent, appropriate use of other services

Table 88.2. Long-Term Effects of Prenatal/ Infancy Programs

Children
  Less aggressiveness and distractibility in school
  Less delinquency
  Better attitudes toward school
  Better social functioning
  Higher rates of prosocial attitudes
Parents
  More registration in school by mothers
  More high school completion by mothers
  Higher rates of family employment

replicated by Olds in an urban area with a different high risk group in order to test out the generalizability of the intervention.

The Yale Child Research Project (Seitz et al., 1983) was a comprehensive family support project for economically disadvantaged adolescent first-time mothers with their infants from birth to 30 months, with long-term follow-up. The program emphasized family support, social work, pediatric care, day care, and psychological services to meet the needs of each family. At 30 months the program children showed better language development and adaptive functioning than did the control group children. Five years later, the program children had higher IQ scores and better school achievement and school attendance than did randomly chosen children from the same neighborhood. More program mothers were employed, had attained additional education, and had smaller families than did the mothers in the comparison families. At a 10-year follow-up, the program children continued to have better school attendance, and boys were found to be less likely to require special education.

A review of 30 publications describing prenatal/infancy prevention programs in North America, England, and Australia (Ministry of Community and Social Services, 1990) found that the programs with greatest impact had multiple components, were of long duration (2–5 years), began prenatally, and had home visits as a major component. It was concluded that there was evidence of both short-term and long-term positive effects (Tables 88.1 and 88.2).

A more recent review of prenatal/infant preventive intervention research programs (Institute of Medicine, 1994) that have been used during infancy to target babies and their parents include high-quality prenatal and perinatal care, childhood immunization, regular home visitation, parenting education, promotion of healthy parent/infant interaction, appropriate cognitive and language stimulation, well baby care, family support, and center-based infant day care. This review demonstrates that it is possible to adhere to a rigorous protocol for a complex, comprehensive human development study across several sites that show diversity in their characteristics.

PRESCHOOL PROGRAMS

Research in primary prevention programming for preschool age children has been both intensive and extensive. This is due, in large part, to the Headstart Compensatory Preschool Program begun in 1960 for disadvantaged children. The effectiveness of such programs to produce positive changes is well documented (Consortium for Longitudinal Studies, 1983; Woodhead, 1988; Zigler and Valentine, 1979). Higher-quality preschools are associated with positive educational outcomes in terms of lower rates of retention in grade, fewer referrals to special education, and lower rates of school drop-out in high school. Social and emotional development is enhanced, as evidenced by increased social competence and more positive attitudes and motivation in school. Long-term positive outcomes include lower rates of juvenile crime and arrest, higher rates of employment and earnings, self-sufficiency in early adulthood, and fewer teen pregnancies.

Recent preschool interventions (Institute of Medicine, 1994) have addressed several risk factors that are related to the major developmental tasks of the preschool period, including the acquisition of language skills to prepare the child to read and write and the development of impulse control (Hawkins and Catalano, 1992). Prevention efforts that address these issues have adopted a number of approaches including:

Center-based early education;
Home visiting to provide a variety of support and educational services;
Parent training and education to teach skills in caregiving and effective
  behavior management;

Family support services;
Policy initiatives that address issues of child safety, health, and education.

In the High/Scope Perry Preschool Program (Berrueta-Clement et al., 1984), 3- and 4-year-olds from families of low socioeconomic status were randomly assigned either to a group that attended the preschool program or to a group that did not. Fifty-eight children were in the preschool group, and 65 in the control group. The school operated five mornings a week for 7 months of the year. The teacher visited each child's home on a weekly basis. This program was unique because of the long-term follow-up and the analysis of the children's later social, correctional, and vocational outcomes, which revealed the following:

1. The children who had attended the preschool showed improved school achievement in the elementary and middle school grades.
2. In high school they made better grades and had fewer failing grades.
3. They spent fewer years in special education.
4. At age 15 the preschool group were found to place a higher value on education.
5. At age 19 the preschool group had higher scores on a literacy and a competence test. They had better jobs and higher earnings and were more likely to be self-supporting. There was reduced use of welfare assistance, fewer arrests, and less self-reported antisocial behavior. The girls had fewer pregnancies and births.

A recent review of effective preventive intervention programs at the preschool level (Institute of Medicine, 1994) has demonstrated that multicomponent interventions that address multiple risk factors have proved effective in improving the family management practices and in facilitating the cognitive and social development of children in high risk family situations. There is also some evidence that such interventions have shown effects in promoting prosocial behavior and preventing behavior problems.

Early childhood interventions can also have positive long-term effects on academic performance and social adjustment and in reducing risks of later disorders in children from at-risk families.

PRIMARY SCHOOL INTERVENTIONS

Middle to late childhood is a period of rapid cognitive and social development. Children who cannot perform academic tasks expected by grade 4 and who show social incompetence, impulsivity, and aggressive behavior during this period are at high risk for developing such disorders as conduct disorder, depressive disorder, and substance abuse. Poor parenting practices, high levels of conflict in the family, and low degree of bonding between children and parents appear to increase the risk for disorder (Institute of Medicine, 1994).

Interventions in this age group have been focussed on the enhancement of social and academic competence.

Two types of primary prevention programs have been geared for primary school children: child centered and system centered or "ecological."

Child-Centered Programs

Most programs for school-age children are child centered and focus on the development of specific skills or competencies: affective education, social problem solving, coping with stress, and extracurricular skills development.

Affective Education. The programs strive to enhance children's social and emotional development by increasing the child's awareness of how feelings, attitudes, and values influence interpersonal and intrapersonal functioning. Such programs assume that improvement in emotional and social development will improve behavior (Durlack, 1985).

The results have been disappointing and flawed by methodological weaknesses, including lack of controls, nonspecific program effects, and inadequate follow-up. However, affective education remains popular

because there are commercially prepared curriculum packages readily available and because it coincides with the philosophy of educating the whole child.

Interpersonal Cognitive Problem Solving. Developed by Shure and Spivak (1982), the Interpersonal Cognitive Problem Solving Program teaches young children how to derive alternative solutions to interpersonal problems. Shure and Spivak report significant enhancement of prosocial behaviors and fewer behavior problems 1 and 2 years after training. The behavior of children trained by their mothers improved both at home and at school.

Social Skills/Assertiveness Skills Approaches. Rotheram et al. (1982) implemented a program for children in grades 4 through 6 in classes identified by teachers and school administrators as lacking in social skills. The children were randomly assigned to one of three programs. Better behavior, achievement, and popularity were reported by teachers among the classes who received the training 2 months and 1 year later.

Other social skills training programs include those of Lochman et al. (in press), which followed up a group of 31 aggressive boys 3 years post intervention. The experimental group had lower rates of drug and alcohol use and higher levels of problem-solving skills but not lower rates of delinquency or classroom problem behaviors.

Programs Aimed at Enhancing Academic Achievement. Reciprocal relationships between achievement and early depression (Kellam and Rebok, 1992) and the evidence that poor academic achievement predicts both later drug abuse and delinquency (Hawkins et al., 1992a) has led to the investigation of enhancement of academic skills as a component of preventive intervention.

The Community Epidemiological Preventive Intervention: Mastery Learning and Good Behavior Game (Kellam and Rebok, 1992) found positive effects on reading achievement in the first graders in 19 ethnically and sociodemographically mixed public schools in Baltimore, Maryland. The gains were found among those students with initially low reading scores and showing depressive symptoms. In addition the Good Behavior Game program had positive effects on aggressive and shy behavior (Kellam et al., 1994).

Individual tutoring has been shown to produce significant improvements in reading and math achievement in reading and math among low achieving socially rejected fourth graders, and the effects on reading scores were maintained 1 year later (Coie and Krehbiel, 1984).

The Seattle Social Development Project (Hawkins et al., 1992b) targeted first graders in eight Seattle schools. The initial universal preventive intervention program lasted 4 years. It was a multicomponent intervention project and sought to reduce risks in family, school, and peer environments. The students in the remaining six schools were randomly assigned to experimental and control classrooms. The intervention included teacher training and supervision, also the use of Spivak and Shure's Interpersonal Cognitive Problem Solving Curriculum and parent training in grades 1, 2, and 3.

Results were reported soon after children entered the fifth grade (Hawkins et al., 1992b). Fewer children in the experimental group reported having initiated alcohol use and delinquent behavior and also reported more positive results than control children for parent management, family communication, family involvement, and attachment to school.

A major criticism of the early child-centered school-based primary school prevention programs was their narrow focus and brief duration. The newer programs, described briefly above, have integrated the programs into the regular classroom curriculum activities and thus build in generalizability.

School Ecology Programs

These programs were aimed at altering the organization of a school.

The Yale New Haven Primary Prevention Project was first implemented in 1968 (Comer, 1976, 1980). This is a well-researched, ecologically based program that not only has been run successfully for over 20 years but also has been replicated in 14 primary schools. The program model consists of a school planning and management team, a parent participation program, a mental health team, and attention to the specific educational needs of the children. Comer emphasizes that the program is a process, not a product, which results in the creation of a sense of community and direction for parents, school staff, and students. The program's results include improved academic achievement, improved attendance, reduced incidence of behavior problems, improved staff attendance, reduced staff turnover, and markedly improved parent involvement in school activities.

At follow-up 3 years later, 24 8th-grade students who had attended the school showed significant differences in academic scores and measures of self-confidence, in comparison with 24 matched students (Cauce et al., 1987). After further testing with increasingly more rigorous design, the School Development Program is now being used in more than 100 schools throughout the United States, and the Rockerfeller Foundation has awarded funding for national dissemination of the intervention. A randomized controlled study of the intervention is currently underway in Maryland (Jessor, 1993).

INTERVENTIONS AT THE JUNIOR HIGH SCHOOL LEVEL

The developmental risk factors associated with early adolescence have been described by Hamburg (1992). Children appear to be at greatest risk for the initiation of substance abuse and antisocial behaviors between the ages of 12 and 15 years. Efforts at reducing antisocial behavior among this age group have focused largely on preventing, or at least delaying, the onset of substance abuse.

DRUG ABUSE PREVENTION PROGRAMS

Many approaches to drug abuse prevention in the schools have been tried. Consistently effective interventions have included at least two components (a) classroom-based training in skills to identify and resist influences to use drugs and (b) encouragement to adopt norms against drug use during adolescence. Social influence training (Ellickson and Bell, 1990) provides instruction, modeling, and role play. Hansen and Graham (1991) have examined the relative contribution of the two components in a universal four condition experimental study, the Adolescent Alcohol Prevention Trial, of 3011 seventh graders at 12 junior high schools. Overall, the students of those classrooms that received the normative education program had significantly reduced rates of alcohol and marijuana consumption.

The strategy of establishing a clear consensus regarding norms have apparently some limitations and risks. Ellickson and Bell (1990), for example, found that, although their curriculum was effective in preventing tobacco use in grade 7 for nonusers, it was counterproductive for those students who were already smoking!

MULTICOMPONENT INTERVENTIONS

Some drug abuse prevention programs have combined school-based curriculum interventions with interventions focused on parents, community leaders, and the media to promote greater consistency of clear normative standards regarding alcohol and other drug use.

Pentz et al.'s (1989) results so far are encouraging but have not yet been reported in full (Institute of Medicine, 1994).

ECOLOGICAL INTERVENTION AT THE HIGH SCHOOL LEVEL

Felner and Adan (1988) describe an ecological intervention designed to reduce the stressful effects of transition to high school in vulnerable students, including disadvantaged and minority students as well as those who had a history of frequent school moves. Academic scores for such students showed significant declines in school performance following transition to high school (Felner et al., 1981). The School Transition Environment Program (STEP) was designed to reduce the difficulty of the transitional tasks for students. It has two basic elements: reorganization of the social system and a changed role for the teachers.

All academic classes are taken with other STEP students, and all STEP classrooms are located in close proximity to one another. Thus, the students no longer need to adapt to continually shifting peer groups in each of the classes or to navigate around a large, unfamiliar institution. All incoming students are assigned to a home room in which the teacher's role has been redefined to serve as the primary link between the students, their parents, and the rest of the school. The teachers provide counseling for the students and help them choose courses. Home room counseling periods last longer than is usual, and each student has an individual counseling session every 4–5 weeks. STEP teacher training includes basic listening skills, identification of educational and emotional problems, and knowledge of referral mechanisms. The results of the program include no decrease in academic performance in grade 9, no increase in absenteeism, and stable scores on self-concept.

On follow-up it was found that there was a 43% drop-out rate for control subjects, compared with a 21% rate for STEP students; no STEP students required special programming because they were in danger of failing; there were fewer increases in measures of behavioral dysfunction; there was less substance abuse; and there was less delinquency.

Felner (Institute of Medicine, 1994) has now combined the school restructuring components of STEP with curriculum changes suggested by the Carnegie Council and applied the program in 50 schools with 22,000 children.

PROGRAMS IN INSTITUTIONS AND AGENCIES FOR CHILDREN

Pediatric hospital practice has changed dramatically over the past two decades with the introduction of the shorter hospital stay and day surgery and attention being devoted to the importance of the psychosocial aspects of pediatric care, including the introduction of child life programs (predominantly in children's hospitals). Hospitalization still remains, however, a traumatic event, particularly for children under the age of 6. Attempts at preventing the adverse effects of hospitalization have recently been reviewed (Byrne and Cadman, 1987). These include preparation for hospitalization, increasing the amount of contact with parents during the hospitalization, and decreasing the length of the hospital stay.

Children who are admitted to the care of a local authority have long been known to constitute a high risk group (Rutter, 1984). Issues of attachment and separation in foster care and adoption and ways of minimizing potentially deleterious effects have been discussed in detail by Steinhauer (1988). Successful attempts to reduce the replacement rate of children from one foster home to another by working individually with the children are described by Schaeffer et al. (1981). Whether improved recruitment, training, and support to foster parents would be equally effective remains to be researched.

A review of the literature on preventive interventions designed to reduce the harmful sequelae of adoption (Jerome et al., 1987) identified two major types of interventions: improved screening techniques for adoptive parents and the provision of support for adoptive parents. Adequate research in these areas still remains to be carried out.

PREVENTION AT THE COMMUNITY LEVEL

Attempts to increase the protective qualities of the environment and to reduce the opportunities for antisocial behavior can have beneficial effects (Rutter, 1980). Jones and Offord (1989) have clearly demonstrated that a recreation program (nonschool skill development), offered to a population of poor children living in an Ontario housing project, resulted in a reduced rate of vandalism as compared to that seen for children at a control housing complex.

PREVENTION AT THE CENTRAL/NATIONAL LEVEL

It has been known for over 20 years and it is well documented that the incidence of premature births and birth complications in at-risk populations can be reduced by nutritional advice, dietary supplements, and good prenatal care for all (Ryan, 1972). Early identification of complications of pregnancy, such as multiple pregnancy, toxemia, and placenta previa, combined with arrangements for specialized care of such high-risk pregnancies, were found to reduce the incidence of birth problems and resultant damage and disability in children (Wynn and Wynn, 1976). This was achieved through a good primary care service available to all pregnant mothers, along with the ensured provision of regional specialized perinatal units. Nations providing outreach health programs have been able to reach as much as 98% of the population (Fox, 1978).

A national program for the prevention of preterm births was proposed and applied throughout France as part of a program to reduce perinatal deaths and morbidity of perinatal origin (Papiernik et al., 1985). During the 12-year period of the program, the proportion of women visiting the antenatal clinic during the first trimester of pregnancy almost doubled and the percentage never seen before delivery decreased 6-fold. In the early years of the project, women with a higher educational level showed the greatest response rates. Within 4 years the middle school group attendance equalled that of those of higher educational level, and within 8 years the lower school group norms came close to the initial value of the group with the highest education.

The same time-lag pattern showed in terms of the decline in the preterm birth rate across the different socioeconomic status groups.

The low birth weight rates and the rates of preterm birth were significantly reduced following the institution of the prevention program (Papiernik et al., 1985).

A study conducted in Martinique also showed a lack of difference in pregnancy outcomes between socioeconomic classes after a prevention program had been implemented (Gougon et al., 1984).

In the United States, in recent years, there have been increases in infants at risk for developmental problems and in infants and children already showing such problems (Rikel and Allen, 1987). Deteriorating neighborhoods, unemployment, family violence, and lack of access to medical care have all contributed to this problem (The Center for the Study of Social Policy, 1992). Societal and macroeconomic solutions to these problems are urgently needed.

Interventions with Families in Transition and Situation Stress

INTERVENTION WITH CHILDREN OF SEPARATION AND DIVORCE

Children of divorce are recognized as being at an increased risk for emotional and behavioral problems. The immediate and longer-term effects of parental separation and divorce on children and adolescents and the effects under different family circumstances and for children of different ages have become clearer (Hetherington et al., 1979, 1985). Opportunities for preventive intervention in situational groups, both for children and for parents, are many and suggest that the stress of these events could he mitigated.

Pedro-Carroll and Cowen (1985) in their Children of Divorce Intervention Program sought to reduce the risk and enhance adaptation among children of divorce. A subsequent modification of the study suggests the promise of selective preventive intervention focusing on the enhancement of social competence during elementary grades for children who have recently experienced parental separation. Unfortunately, the subject still needs to be researched. Studies of intervention with children of separation and divorce have suffered from methodological weaknesses, including small sample sizes and selection of subjects mostly from clinic populations or possessing a limited range of demographic characteristics (Rae Grant and Robson, 1988).

A more recent review of these interventions has been carried out by Grych and Fincham (1992). However, adequately evaluated, randomized, controlled trials of primary prevention programs with these groups, though promising, remain to be carried out.

INTERVENTIONS WITH CHILDREN WITH CHRONIC MEDICAL ILLNESS

Children with chronic medical illness and functional limitations have been found to be at increased risk for emotional and behavioral disorders. Cadman et al. (1986) reviewed three randomized, controlled trials of interventions aimed at reducing the risk. All three showed positive results; however, one had serious methodological flaws, the results of the second did not reach significance, and the data from the third were preliminary.

CHILDREN OF PSYCHIATRICALLY ILL PARENTS

The degree of disturbance in children of psychiatrically ill parents can be seen as a function of the intensity, frequency, duration, and severity of parental dysfunction; the degree of genetic loading for a particular disorder; the availability of an alternate, caring adult; the intensity and duration of exposure to the parental dysfunctional behavior; and the degree of psychosocial distress experienced by the child (Garmezy and Rutter, 1983).

Recent research suggests that interactions between genetically determined traits and selected environmental factors affect the expression of the disease. Silverman (1989) suggests that some of the risk factors in the family environment, such as poor communication patterns, ineffective parenting, and lack of structure, may be modifiable. Infant vulnerability could be reduced by special attention to prenatal nutrition, decreasing birth complications, and facilitating mother-child bonding. In middle childhood the goal of intervention should be to increase the child's ability to process information and to attend to appropriate internal and external cues. Recent research has identified the need to decrease communication deviation and to change patterns of inappropriately expressed emotion in families at risk (Doane et al., 1985).

Goodman and Isaacs (1984) suggested three goals for preventive intervention:

1. To improve the stability of the family system by decreasing marital discord and separation, developing more consistent parenting techniques, and increasing the availability of family supports;
2. To foster the ability of the mother to meet the children's needs by improving parenting skills and parent-child communication;
3. To minimize the pathology to which the children are exposed by improving the child's reality testing, coping skills, and problem-solving skills, and by providing social support networks.

Cohler (Cohler and Musick, 1984) recommended continued support for children at risk throughout childhood and adolescence, and Silverman (1989) suggested that risk assessments should be carried out yearly up to the age of 21 in children of psychiatrically ill parents through pediatric/medical checkups and, later on, at times of life transitions.

Current preventive intervention research designs, such as those for children of divorce, could be applied to other groups of high-risk children. For example, work has begun in designing and field testing interventions for children of alcoholics (Springer et al., 1992), but these have not yet been well evaluated. Work has also begun with children of depressed parents. Clinical and educational interventions for family members based on studies of resilient adolescents exposed to parental depression have been developed and are being tested (Beardslee et al., 1993).

Preventing Psychiatric Problems in Children Following Natural Disasters

Pynoos and Nader (1989) point out that a disaster is one of the very few life stresses for which early access to children is authorized as a public health measure. The authors confirmed that the degree of exposure to life threat in children of school age determined the severity of posttraumatic stress disorder, a pattern that continued to be present at follow-up 14 months later. Parental and family function was a major mediating factor.

Pynoos and Nader suggest that the following risk factors should be taken into consideration in devising a prevention program: age of the child (very young children may be somewhat protected, as they do not perceive the full extent of the threat); perception of the cause of the disaster as being natural rather than human-made; separation of the child from parents or siblings; and situations of multiple adversity. The major goals of preventive interventions suggested by Pynoos include ameliorating traumatic stress reactions and facilitating grief work following the event.

Possible intervention strategies include the following:

1. Predisaster training in schools where there is a high risk of natural disaster;
2. Disaster evacuation plans that, as far as possible, preclude separation of young children from parents;
3. The protection of children from unnecessary exposure to the injured, mutilated, and dead;
4. The provision of psychological first aid for preschool to grade 1 children, which should include repeated concrete clarifications, consistent care, and help in verbalizing fears, feelings, and complaints;
5. Cautioning older children about an increased posttraumatic tendency toward impulsive behavior and risk taking (Systematic research is needed in the development of age-appropriate techniques for use in early intervention.);
6. Goals for good family work should include giving children a sense of being supported, establishing a sense of physical security, validating children's affective responses, and providing assistance in dealing with traumatic reminders by accepting the children's renewed anxiety and by offering reassurance;
7. School-based mental health intervention program elements should include consultation with school administration, the training of teachers, and education of children and parents;
8. Special procedures are needed to help reintegrate injured children into school and to help bereaved children.

At the classroom level, the staff should identify and address misconceptions, rumors, and fears and engage children in drawing and symbolic representation of the events. Pynoos suggests that children should be screened according to levels of risk and that early case finding should be followed by therapeutic consultation, the goal being to assist the child in exploring subjective experiences and understanding the meaning of his or her responses.

Galante and Foa (1986) describe the reaction to a devastating earthquake in which 4000 were killed and tens of thousands were rendered homeless in 116 villages damaged by the earthquake. Six months later, all the children were tested to identify the numbers and locations of those at risk. A treatment program was implemented in the village with the largest number of children at risk. The intervention consisted of a week-long series of group sessions lasting 1 hour for children in grades 1 through 4. The intervention objectives included giving the children permission to communicate openly, to discuss their fears, to demonstrate that being afraid was common, and to discuss myths and erroneous beliefs about earthquakes. There was a significant difference between the pretest and posttest scores at 1-year follow-up. The authors conclude that the most important factors are the availability of family support systems, reestablishment of the daily routine as quickly as possible, rapid resumption of school services, and the provision of structured opportunities for children to discuss and work through their fears and experiences.

Summary

A review of the literature in primary prevention and health promotion with children and adolescents suggests that interventions that influence the child's environment in the most effective way for the longest period of time are the most powerful. The target environment varies, depending on the age and stage of development of the child. Thus, for the infant the intervention of most importance involves the parent-child interaction. At the preschool level, both the family and the preschool environment are important. With the primary-school-age child, environmental intervention will affect not only families but also primary school and nonschool activities. It is evident that interventions that attempt to change the ecological situation surrounding the child are more effective than those directed only at the child. Again, interventions that attack risk situations may be simpler and more effective than those that are developed at the level of the individual at risk.

POSSIBLE ROLES FOR THE PSYCHIATRIST IN PRIMARY PREVENTION

As Consultant: Community Education and the Use of the Multiplier Effect

For the practicing clinician, there are many opportunities to use consultation and community education skills by utilizing knowledge gained in training, research, and clinical practice to move from the case level to the class level of intervention. For example, at an outpatient child psychiatric clinic, a careful review of children on the waiting list showed an increase in the number of school-age boys referred by school personnel because of disruptive behavior, poor peer relationships, and inattentiveness in class. From the assessment material, it became readily apparent that the behavior complained of in about 50% of the cases had appeared subsequent to parental separation. The clinic improved their waiting-list time by triaging the children whose behavior was reactive into age-matched groups in which discussion of the problems of parent separation could be addressed.

The problem could equally well be posed at the systems level rather than the individual case level, by intervening at the school level. The average teacher knows little about the research findings on the effects of separation on boys of this age. One possible solution might be to suggest that a professional development day be set aside in that school area to discuss this topic and suggest ways in which teachers could better understand and cope with the children's behavior in the classroom. Working with school personnel to help them to allow children to discuss such issues or setting up groups for children and parents within the school situation to address the topic are other possibilities for preventive intervention.

As Psychiatric Consultant to the Agencies with Which Children Come into Contact

The aim here would be to work with agencies, programs, and staff members in order to attempt to avoid the sequelae of stressful situations; for example, the psychiatrist could work with staff in family agencies to devise interventions that would reduce the number of foster home placements or that would support children of at-risk parents more successfully in their own homes. Target groups might include children of parents with psychiatric problems or those with developmental disability, who are clearly at high risk for emotional, behavioral, and learning problems. Family preservation services such as the Homebuilders program in Tacoma, Washington, pioneered this type of intensive, multicomponent service for families at high risk for out-of-home placement of the children. The most rigorous evaluation was a New Jersey study that compared 214 eligible families randomly assigned to a Homebuilders program or a control group. The results suggested that intensive family preservation services are effective in avoiding some out-of-home placements in the short term, but long-term results are less impressive (Feldman, 1991a, 1991b). New models of service for these at-risk families are desperately needed.

Another much needed selected intervention would be with agencies who work with children known to have been abused. Family court clinics and child welfare department staff need assistance in providing early intervention services for such children in order to offset some of the proximal and distal effects of child maltreatment, which are now becoming better recognized. A preventive intervention research program to reduce the further traumatization of abused children in the court system has been successful and has been described by the Child Witness Project (1991).

As Liaison Psychiatrist

The aim here is to work with colleagues in obstetrics, pediatrics (particularly neonatal and pediatric intensive care units), burn units, and oncology units in order to assist in providing an environment for child patients and support for their families that will reduce the emotional and behavioral complications of medical conditions.

As Educator

The academic child psychiatrist may have an opportunity to give input to the undergraduate medical program and in so doing may attempt to redress the overemphasis during training on individual deviance, disease, and psychopathology with an equal emphasis on health and competence promotion, methods of reducing individual and group vulnerability to stress, and thinking in terms of the needs of target populations as well as the needs of individuals (Rae Grant, 1982). Medical students who go on to become family physicians have many opportunities for supporting good parent-child interaction, facilitating normal social growth and development, and identifying remediable problems. However, normal child development and parent-child interaction are inadequately emphasized in the medical school curriculum. Consultation to family practice units offers the opportunity to work with residents in family medicine. Experience in seven family medicine units in southwestern Ontario suggests that topics such as parent/child relationships, parenting practices, child maltreatment, the disruptive behavior disorders, eating disorders, and affective disorders in childhood and adolescence are popular topics with the residents. Evaluation of the effectiveness of such consultation work is urgently needed.

As Facilitator of Community Prevention Projects

Child psychiatrists who are interested in the social ecology of the area in which they practice and in whether this is a good place for children to grow up may be interested in being involved in an interagency coordinating group and leading or taking part in the planning of community intervention projects. Psychiatric support to the public health unit in their outreach to families at risk is readily accepted and urgently needed.

Psychiatric support to recreation services may allow for the development of training programs for recreation counsellors to reach out to children in disadvantaged areas and to attract children to recreation activities and to maintain them in such programs.

As Researcher

The field of epidemiology has developed rapidly over the past decade and has provided a much clearer picture of the prevalence and demographic markers for emotional, behavioral, and learning problems. With this backdrop, the opportunity for hypothesis generation, development of primary intervention programs to test hypotheses, and for evaluation studies is much clearer than it has been in the past. To this end it will be important to foster opportunities for support for young career investigators in primary prevention.

As Advocate

The child psychiatrist who is in a position to review the effect of various legislative actions on children and their families and how they may enhance or detract from their ability to cope with their environment has an opportunity to act as a participant on committees and planning commissions at various levels of government, either as an individual or as part of a psychiatric association group.

Child psychiatrists are in a good position to advocate for better programs to assist the children of economically deprived populations (Tanguay et al., 1984). Childhood poverty is common in North America. Fourteen million children under 16 years old live in economically deprived circumstances (Institute of Medicine, 1989; Shah et al., 1987). The incidence of poverty is highest among children of single mothers, unemployed parents, Native Americans, and recent immigrants.

BASIC CONDITIONS NECESSARY FOR NORMAL CHILD MENTAL HEALTH

In medicine in general and in psychiatry in particular, we attempt to deal with child, adolescent, and adult problems in a doctor-patient relationship when the social infrastructure requisite for normal physical, emotional, and psychological development of all children is not yet being met for a large percentage of the population. Psychiatry can adapt McDermott's (1966) model, which suggests that there are five stages in the growth of medical care in underdeveloped countries, ranging from primitive to modern, to understand the changes that will be needed to ensure that all children's physical and emotional needs will be met. The first stage in change away from the most primitive sort of society is the introduction of measures that are not customarily regarded as being related to disease at all, such as eating off the table instead of eating off the floor. Second come the more complex aspects of development: roads, dams, bridges, communications; the provision of a safe water supply; the draining of swamps; and the use of insecticides to combat malaria. The third stage includes intermittent professional care (e.g., immunization every 2–3 years). The fourth stage is the introduction of the classic patient-physician relationship. The fifth stage is that of modern metropolitan medicine.

The mental health analogy to eating off the table instead of the floor may perhaps be regarded as having been achieved with the introduction of child labor and child protection acts. However, the analogous second and subsequent stages in the paradigm have not been met. A large proportion of the population lacks adequate housing, transportation, facilities for recreation and education, adequate nutrition and antenatal care during pregnancy, and adequate cognitive and language stimulation, as well as affectional care, during the first 2 years of life. The physical, social, learning, and emotional deficits caused by social disadvantage have been clearly identified by cohort studies such as the one carried out by the National Children's Bureau in the United Kingdom (Davie et al., 1972). By the age of school entry, the child's potential learning capacity has already been promoted or retarded by the preschool environment.

Even where service is provided, it is evident that the system of delivery is so fragmented that it may do more to promote than relieve family disintegration, conflict, or personal anxiety. Reliance on therapist-patient methods to reach the children most at risk fails in situations of social disintegration.

The rate of change in society is such that the gap between needs and resources is increasing rather than decreasing. A sizable proportion of the childhood population is not being provided with the basic minimum requirements for normal social, emotional, and intellectual growth needed to reduce the predisposition of children to such disorders. There is evidence that not only is the situation not improving for high-risk children and their families but, in recent years, there have been notable increases in the number of infants and children at risk for developmental impairments and in infants and children already showing such problems (Rickel and Allen, 1987).

While more research into specific interventions with groups at risk for particular conditions and in situations of particular risk remains to be carried out, a review of the literature suggests that there are a sufficient number of well-designed studies to indicate that certain risk factors can be reduced and to suggest ways of increasing the number of protective factors in order to balance the coping/disorder equation. Rutter (1990) suggests that we need to focus especially on the protective processes that bring about changes in life trajectories. He included among them those that reduce the risk impact, those that reduce the likelihood of negative chain reactions, those that promote self-esteem and self-efficacy, and those that open up opportunities. Such a change in the balance of the equation would allow a larger percentage of the child population to move into the normal developmental trajectory.

References

Achenbach TM, Howell CT: Are American children's problems getting worse? A 13 year comparison. *J Am Acad Child Adolesc Psychiatry* 32(6): 1145–1154, 1993.

Albee GW: Primary prevention. *Can Ment Health* 27:5–9, 1979.

Amato PR: Family process and the competence of adolescents and primary school children. *J Youth Adolesc* 18:39–53, 1989.

American Academy of Child and Adolescent Psychiatry: *Prevention in Child and Adolescent Psychiatry: The Reduction of Risk for Mental Disorders.* Office for Substance Abuse Prevention and the American Academy of Child and Adolescent Psychiatry, Washington, DC, 1990.

Anthony EJ: The syndrome of the psychologically invulnerable child. In: Anthony EJ, Koupernik C (eds): *The Child and His Family: Children at Psychiatric Risk* (Vol 3). New York, Wiley, 1974, pp. 99–121.

Avison WR: Risk factors for children's conduct problems and delinquency; The significance of family milieu. Paper presented at the American Society of Criminology Annual Meeting, New Orleans, 1992.

Beardslee WR, Salt P, Porterfield K, et al: Comparison of preventive interventions for families with parental affective disorder. *J Am Acad Child Adolesc Psychiatry* 32(2):254–263, 1993.

Berlin I: Prevention of mental and emotional disorders in childhood. In: Wolman BJ (ed): *Manual of Child Psychopathology.* Vol 1: *The Issues.* New York, McGraw-Hill, 1972, pp. 1088–1109.

Berrueta-Clement JR, Schweinhart LJ, Barnett WS, et al: *Changed Lives: The Effects of the Perry Preschool Program on Youth Through Age 19.* Michigan, High/Scope Press, 1984.

Bloom BL: The evaluation of primary prevention programs. In: Roberts LM, Greenfield NS, Miller NH (eds): *Comprehensive Mental Health.* Madison, WI, University of Wisconsin Press, 1968, p. 117.

Byrne CM, Cadman D: Prevention of the adverse effects of hospitalization in children. *J Prev Psychiatry* 3:167–190, 1987.

Cadman D, Boyle MH, Offord DR, et al: Chronic illness and functional limitation in Ontario children: Findings of the Ontario child health study. *Can Med Assoc J* 135:761–767, 1986.

Caplan G: *The Principles of Preventive Psychiatry.* New York, Basic Books, 1964.

Caplan G: The family and the support system. In: Caplan G, Killilea M (eds): *Support Systems and Mutual Help.* New York, Grune & Stratton, 1976.

Catalano R, Dooley D: Economic change in primary prevention. In: Price RH, Ketterer RF, Bader BC, et al (eds): *Prevention in Mental Health: Research, Policy and Practice* (Vol 1). Beverly Hills, CA, Sage, 1980.

Cauce AM, Comer JP, Schwartz D: Long term effects of a systems-oriented school prevention program. *Am J Orthopsychiatry* 57:127–131, 1987.

Center for the Study of Social Policy with the Annie E. Casey Foundation: *Kids Count Data Book.* Washington, DC, Center for the Study of Social Policy, 1992.

Child Witness Project: *Reducing the System-induced Trauma for Child Sexual Abuse Victims through Court, Preparation, Assessment and Follow-up.* London, London Family Court Clinic, 1991.

Cicchetti D, Schneider-Rosen K: An organizational approach to childhood depression. In: Rutter M, Izard C, Read PR (eds): *Depression in Young People: Developmental and Clinical Perspectives.* New York, Guilford Press, 1986, pp. 71–134.

Cohler B, Musick JS (eds): *Risk and Intervention among Psychiatrically Impaired Parents and Their Young Children.* (New Directions for Mental Health Series). San Francisco, Jossey-Bass, 1984.

Coie J, Krehbiel G: Effects of academic tutoring on the social status of low-achieving, socially rejected children. *Child Dev* 55:1465–1478, 1984.

Comer JP: Improving the quality and continuity of relationships in two inner-city schools. *J Am Acad Child Psychiatry* 15:535–545, 1976.

Comer JP: *School Power: Implications of an Intervention Project.* New York, Free Press, 1980.

Consortium for Longitudinal Studies: *As the Twig is Bent . . . .* Hillsdale, NJ, Erlbaum, 1983.

Costello EJ: Developments in child psychiatric epidemiology. *J Am Acad Child Adolesc Psychiatry* 28:836–841, 1989.

Cross National Collaborative Group: The changing rate of major depression. *JAMA* 268(21): 3098–3105, 1992.

Dattilo J, Camarata SM: Facilitating conversation through self-initiated augmentative communication treatment. *J Appl Behav Anal* 24:369–378, 1991.

Davie R, Butler N, Goldstein H: *From Birth to Seven: A Report of the National Child Development Study.* London, Longman, 1972.

Doane JA, Falloon IRH, Goldstein MJ, et al: Parental affective style and treatment of schizophrenia: Predicting course of illness and social functioning. *Arch Gen Psychiatry* 42:34–42, 1985.

Dornbusch SM: The sociology of adolescence. In: Scott WR, Blake J (eds): *Annual Review of Sociology* (Vol 15). Palo Alto, CA, Annual Reviews Inc, 1989, pp. 233–259.

Durlack JA: Primary prevention of school maladjustment. *J Consult Clin Psychol* 53:623–630, 1985.

Earls F: Temperament characteristics and behavior problems in three-year-old children. *J Nerv Ment Dis* 169:367–373, 1981.

Egeland B, Carlson C, Sroufe LA: Resilience as process. *Dev Psychopathol* 5:517–528, 1993.

Eisenberg L: The strategic deployment of the child psychiatrist in preventive psychiatry. *J Child Psychol Psychiatry* 2:229–241, 1961.

Ellickson PL, Bell RM: Drug prevention in junior high: A multisite longitudinal test. *Science* 247: 1299–1305, 1990.

Feldman LH: *Assessing the Effectiveness of Family Preservation Services in New Jersey within an Ecological Context.* Trenton, New Jersey Division of Youth and Family Services; Bureau of Research, Evaluation and Quality Assurance, 1991a.

Feldman LH: Evaluating the impact of intensive family preservation services in New Jersey. In: Biegel DE, Wells K (eds): *Family Preservation Services: Research and Evaluation.* Newbury Park, CA, Sage, 1991b, pp. 47–71.

Felner RD, Primavera J, Cauce AM: The impact of school transitions: A focus for preventive efforts. *Am J Community Psychol* 9:449–459, 1981.

Felner RD, Adan AA: The school transitional environmental project: An ecological intervention and evaluation. In: Price RH, Cowen EL, Lorion RP, et al (eds): *14 Ounces of Prevention.* Washington, DC, American Psychological Association, 1988, pp. 111–122.

Fox M: Predictive neurology or clinical mythology. Paper presented at the Canadian Psychiatric Research Institute Symposium on Early Diagnosis, London, Ontario, May 31, 1978.

Galante R, Foa D: An epidemiological study of psychic trauma and treatment effectiveness for children after a natural disaster. *J Am Acad Child Adolesc Psychiatry* 25:357–363, 1986.

Garmezy N: Stressors of childhood. In: Garmezy N, Rutter M (eds): *Stress, Coping and Development in Children.* New York, McGraw-Hill, 1983, pp. 43–84.

Garmezy N, Rutter M: *Stress, Coping and Development in Children.* New York, McGraw-Hill, 1983.

Garmezy N, Masten A, Tellegen A: The study of stress and competence in children. *Child Dev* 55: 97–111, 1984.

Goodman SH, Isaacs ID: Primary prevention with children of severely disturbed mothers. *J Prev Psychiatry* 2:387–402, 1984.

Gordon R: An operational classification of disease prevention. *Public Health Rep* 98:107–109, 1983.

Goujon H, Papiernik E, Maine D: The prevention of preterm delivery through prenatal care: An intervention study in Martinique. *Int J Gynaecol Obstet* 23:423–433, 1985.

Greenberg MT, Speltz ML, DeKlyn M: The role of attachment in the early development of disruptive behavior problems. *Dev Psychopathol* 5:191–214, 1993.

Grych JH, Fincham FD: Interventions for children of divorce: Toward greater integration of research and action. *Psychol Bull* 111:434–454, 1992.

Hamburg DA: *Today's Children; Creating a Future for a Generation in Crisis.* New York, Basic Books, 1992.

Hansen WB, Graham JW: Preventing alcohol, marijuana, and cigarette use among adolescents: Peer pressure resistance training versus establishing conservative norms. *Prev Med* 20:414–430, 1991.

Hawkins JD, Catalano RF: *Communities That Care. Action for Drug Abuse Prevention.* San Francisco, Jossey-Bass, 1992.

Hawkins JD, Catalano RF, Miller JY: Risk and protective factors for alcohol and other drug problems in adolescence and early adulthood: Implications for substance abuse prevention. *Psychol Bull* 112(1):64–105, 1992a.

Hawkins JD, Catalano RF, Morrison DM, et al: The Seattle Social Development Project. Effects of the first four years in protective factors and problem behaviors. In: McCord J, Tremblay R (eds): *The Prevention of Antisocial Behavior in Children.* New York, Guilford Press, 1992b.

Hetherington EM, Cox M, Cox R: Family interactions and the social, emotional and cognitive development of children following divorce. In: Vaughan JC, Brazelton JB (eds): *The Family: Setting Priorities.* New York, Science and Medicine Publishers, 1979.

Hetherington EM, Cox M, Cox R: Long-term effects of divorce and remarriage on the adjustment of children. *J Am Acad Child Psychiatry* 24:518–530, 1985.

Institute of Medicine: *Children and Adolescents with Mental, Behavioral and Developmental Disorders: Mobilizing a National Research Initiative.* Washington DC, Institute of Medicine, National Academy of Sciences, 1989.

Institute of Medicine: Designing, conducting and analyzing programs within the preventive intervention research cycle. In: Mrazek P, Haggerty RJ (eds): *Reducing Risks for Mental Disorders. Frontiers for Preventive Intervention Research.* Washington, DC, Institute of Medicine, National Academy of Sciences, 1994, p. 362.

Jaffe PG, Hurley DJ, Wolfe D: Children's observations of violence. 1: Critical issues in child development and intervention planning. *Can J Psychiatry* 35(6):466–470, 1990.

Jerome L, Cohen J, Westhues A: A review of the literature on the prevention of harmful sequelae of adoption. *J Prev Psychiatry* 3:261–277, 1987.

Jessor R: Successful adolescent development among youth in high-risk settings. *Am Psychol* 48(2): 117–126, 1993.

Jones MB, Offord DR: Reduction of anti social behavior in poor children by nonschool skill-development. *J Child Psychol Psychiatry* 30:737–750, 1989.

Kellam SG, Rebok GW: Building developmental and etiological theory through epidemiologically based preventive intervention trials. In: McCord J, Tremblay RE (eds): *Preventing Antisocial Behavior: Interventions from Birth through Adolescence.* New York, Guilford Press, 1992, pp. 162–195.

Kessler M, Albee GW: An overview of the literature of primary prevention. In: Albee GW, Joffe JM (eds): *Primary Prevention of Psychopathology. The Issues* (Vol I). Hanover, NH, University Press of New England, 1977, pp. 351–399.

Klerman GL, Lavori PW, Rice J, et al: Birth cohort trends in rates of major depressive disorder among relatives of patients with affective disorder. *Arch Gen Psychiatry* 42:689–693, 1985.

Kolvin FJ, Miller JW, Fleeting M, et al: Social and parenting factors affecting criminal-offence rates: Findings from the Newcastle thousand family study (1947–1980). *Br J Psychiatry* 152:80–90, 1988.

Lewis DO, Lovely R, Yeager C, et al: Toward a theory of the genesis of violence: A follow-up study of delinquents. *J Am Acad Child Adolesc Psychiatry* 28:431–436, 1989.

Lochman JE, Coie JD, Underwood MK, et al: Effectiveness of a social relations intervention program for aggressive and nonaggressive rejected children. *J Consult Counsel Psychol* 61(6):1053–1058, 1993.

Lorion RP, Myers TG, Bartels DA: Preventive intervention research. In: Ollendick TH, Prinz RJ (eds): *Pathways for Extending Knowledge of Child/ Adolescent Health and Pathology.* New York, Plenum, 1994.

Maziade M, Cote R, Bernier H, et al: Significance of extreme temperament in infancy for clinical status in pre-school years: 1. *Br J Psychiatry* 14:535–543, 1989.

McCord J: The Cambridge-Somerville study: A pioneering longitudinal-experimental study of delinquency prevention. In: McCord J, Trembley RIE (eds): *Preventing Antisocial Behavior. Interventions from Birth through Adolescence.* New York, Guilford Press, 1992.

McDermott W: Medical institutions and the modification of disease patterns. *Am J Psychiatry* 122:1398–1406, 1966.

Ministry of Community and Social Services: *Better Beginnings Better Futures: An Integrated Model of Primary Prevention of Emotional and Behavioral Problems.* Toronto, Queen's Printer for Ontario, 1990.

Offord DR: Primary prevention: Aspects of program design and evaluation. *J Am Acad Child Psychiatry* 211:225–230, 1982.

Offord DR: Prevention of behavioral and emotional disorders in children. *J Child Psychol Psychiatry* 28:919, 1987.

Offord DR, Alder RJ, Boyle MH: Prevalence and sociodemographic correlates of conduct disorder. *Am J Soc Psychiatry* 6:272–278, 1986.

Offord DR, Boyle MH, Fleming JE, et al: Ontario Child Health Study: Summary of selected results. *Can J Psychiatry* 34:483–491, 1989.

Offord DR, Boyle MH, Racine Y, et al: Outcome, prognosis and risk in a longitudinal follow up study. *J Am Acad Child Adolesc Psychiatry* 31(5):916–923, 1992.

Offord DR, Boyle MH, Szatmari P, et al: The Ontario Child Health Study. II: Six month prevalence of disorder and rates of service utilization. *Arch Gen Psychiatry* 44:832–836, 1987.

Offord DR, Last JM, Barrette PA: A comparison of the school performance, emotional adjustment and skill development of poor and middle class children. *Can J Public Health* 76:174–178, 1985.

O'Grady D, Metz JE: Resilience in children at high risk for psychological disorder. *J Pediatr Psychol* 12:3–23, 1987.

Olds D, Henderson C, Chamberlin R, et al: Improving the delivery of prenatal care and outcomes of pregnancy: A randomized trial of nurse home visitation. *Pediatrics* 77:16–28, 1986.

Olweus D: Bully/victim problems among school children: Basic facts and effects of an intervention program. In: Rubin K, Pepler D (eds): *The Development and Treatment of Childhood Aggression.* Hillsdale, NJ, Erlbaum, 1991.

Papiernik E, Bouyer J, Dreyfus J, et al: Prevention of Preterm Births; A perinatal study in Hagunau, France. *Pediatrics* 76(2):154–158, 1985.

Patterson GR, Chamberlain P, Reid JB: A comparative evaluation of a parent training program. *Behav Ther* 13:638–650, 1982.

Patterson GR, Reid JB, Dishion TJ: *Antisocial Boys. Oregon Social Learning Center.* Eugene, OR, Castalia, 1992.

Pedro-Carroll JL, Cowen EL: The children of divorce intervention program: An investigation of the efficacy of a school-based prevention program. *J Counsel Clin Psychol* 53:603–611, 1985.

Pentz MA, Dwyer JH, Mackinnon DP, et al: A multicommunity trial for the primary prevention of adolescent drug abuse. *JAMA* 261:3259–3266, 1989.

Price RH: Linking intervention, research and risk factors. In: Steinbert JA, Silverman MM (eds): *Preventing Mental Disorders: A Research Perspective.* Rockville, MD, US Department of Health and Human Services, 1987, pp. 48–56.

Pynoos RS, Nader K: *Prevention of Mental Disorders, Alcohol and Other Drug Use in Children.* Washington, DC, US Department of Health and Human Services, 1989, pp. 225–271.

Quinton D, Rutter M, Liddle C: Institutional rearing, parenting difficulties and marital support. *Psychol Med* 14:107–124, 1984.

Rae Grant NI: Implications of primary prevention for the training of the child psychiatrist. *J Am Acad Child Psychiatry* 21:219–224, 1982.

Rae Grant NI, Offord DR, Munroe Blum H: Implications for clinical service, research and training. *Can J Psychiatry* 34:492–499, 1989.

Rae Grant NI, Thomas H, Offord DR, et al: Risk, protective factors, and the prevalence of behavioral and emotional disorders in children and adolescents. *J Am Acad Child Adolesc Psychiatry* 28:262–268, 1989.

Rae-Grant Q, Robson BE: Moderating the morbidity of divorce. *Can J Psychiatry* 33:443–452, 1988.

Reitsma-Street M, Offord DR, Finch T: Pairs of same-sexed siblings discordant for antisocial behavior. *Br J Psychiatry* 146:415–423, 1985.

Rickel AU, Allen L: *Preventing Maladjustment from Infancy through Adolescence.* Newbury Park, CA, Sage, 1987.

Robins LN: Follow-up studies investigating childhood disorders. In: Hare EH, Wing JK (eds): *Psychiatric Epidemiology.* London, Oxford University Press, 1970.

Rotheram MJ, Armstrong M, Booraem C: Assertiveness training in fourth and fifth grade children. *Am J Community Psychol* 10:567–582, 1982.

Rutter M: Protective factors in children's responses to stress and disadvantage. In: Kent MW, Rolf SEJ (eds): *Primary Prevention of Psychopathology: Social Competence in Children* (Vol 3). Hanover, NH, University Press of New England, 1975.

Rutter M: *Changing Youth in a Changing Society.* Cambridge, MA, Harvard University Press, 1980.

Rutter M: Stress, coping and development: Some issues and some questions. *J Child Psychol Psychiatry* 22:323–356, 1981.

Rutter M: Resilience in the face of adversity: Protective factors and resistance to psychiatric disorder. *Br J Psychiatry* 147:598–611, 1985.

Rutter M: Pathways from childhood to adult life. *J Child Psychol Psychiatry* 30:23–51, 1989.

Rutter M: Psychosocial resilience and protective mechanisms. In: Rolf J, Master AS, Cicchetti D, et al. (eds): *Risk and Protective Factors in the Development of Psychopathology.* Cambridge, Cambridge University Press, 1990.

Rutter M, Giller H: *Juvenile Delinquency: Trends and Perspectives.* New York, Penguin Books, 1983.

Rutter M, Quinton D: Psychiatric disorder: Ecological factors and concepts of causation. In: McCurck H (ed): *Ecological Factors in Human Development.* Amsterdam, North Holland Publishing, 1977.

Rutter M, Quinton D: Parental psychiatric disorder: Effects on children. *Psychol Med* 14:853–880, 1984.

Rutter M, Maughan B, Mortimore P, et al: *Fifteen Thousand Hours: Secondary Schools and Their Effects on Children.* Cambridge, Harvard University Press, 1979.

Rutter M, Tizard J, Whitmore K: *Education, Health and Behavior.* London, Longman, 1970.

Ryan TJ: *Poverty and the Child: A Canadian Study.* Toronto, McGraw-Hill, Ryerson, 1972.

Sameroff AJ: Transactional risk factors and prevention. In: Steinberg JA, Silverman MM (eds): *Preventing Mental Disorders: A Research Perspective.* Rockville, MD, US Department of Health and Human Services, 1987, p. 76.

Sameroff AJ, Chandler MJ: Reproductive risk and the continuum of caretaking casualty. In: Horowitz FD, Hetherington M, Scarr-Salopatek S (eds): *Review of Child Development Research* (Vol 4). Chicago, University of Chicago Press, 1975, pp. 187–244.

Schaeffer MH, Kiliman G, Friedman MJ, et al: Children in foster care: A preventive service and research program for a high risk population. *J Prev Psychiatry* 1:47–56, 1981.

Seitz V, Apfel N, Rosenbaum L, et al: Long-term effects of projects Head Start and follow through: The New Haven Project. In: *Consortium for Longitudinal Studies: Lasting Effects of Preschool Programs.* Hillsdale, NJ, Erlbaum, 1983, p. 7.

Shah CP, Kahan M, Krauser J: The health of children of low-income families. *Can Med Assoc J* 137: 485–490, 1987.

Shure M, Spivak G: Interpersonal cognitive problem solving. *J Community Psychol* 10:344–357, 1982.

Silverman MM: Children of psychiatrically ill

parents: A prevention perspective. *Hosp Community Psychiatry* 40:1257–1265, 1989.

Springer F, Phillips J, Cannady LP, et al: CODA: A creative therapy program for children in families affected by alcohol or other drugs. *J Community Psychol; OSAP Special Issue*, 1992, pp. 55–74.

Steinhauer PD: The preventive utilization of foster care. *Can J Psychiatry* 33:459–467, 1988.

Tanguay P, Shaffer D, Hamburg BA, et al: Child psychiatric aspects of preventive psychiatry. *J Prev Psychiatry* 2:211–233, 1984.

Thomas A, Chess S: *Temperament and Development.* New York, Brunner/Mazel, 1977.

Weiss G, Hechtman LT: *Hyperactive Children Grown Up* (2nd ed). New York, Guilford Press, 1993.

Werner EE, Smith RS: *Vulnerable but Invincible: A Longitudinal Study of Resilient Children and Youth.* New York, McGraw-Hill, 1982.

Werner EE, Smith RS: *Overcoming the Odds: High Risk Children from Birth to Adulthood.* New York, Cornell University Press, 1992.

West D, Farrington D: *Delinquency: Its Roots, Careers and Prospects.* London, Heinemann, 1982.

Woodhead M: When psychology informs public policy: The case of early childhood intervention. *Am Psychol* 43:443–454, 1988.

Wynn A, Wynn M: *Prevention of Handicap and Perinatal Origin: An Introduction to French Policy and Legislation.* London, Foundation for Education Research in Childbearing, 1976.

Zigler EF, Valentine J (eds): *Project Head Start: A Legacy of the War on Poverty.* New York, Free Press, 1979.

89 CHILD PSYCHIATRIC EMERGENCIES

David A. Tomb, M.D.

Child psychiatry has few life-threatening emergencies. However, many clinical situations demand emergency attention because they are perceived as emergent by those involved. Most frequently this occurs when the family system is fragmented, the parents overwhelmed or absent, the child distressed, and the child's environment (school, clinic, physicians) concerned but without ready answers. The general principles of recognition, evaluation, and treatment that apply to all emergencies are described below. In addition, several well-defined, specific emergencies are also discussed.

GENERAL PRINCIPLES

Definition and Presentation

Most children are fundamentally dependent upon their parents or other key adults in their environment. Because of this, it is those adults, not the child, who typically define a situation as an emergency. Thus, if the parents (or other referring sources) feel too anxious, angry, or inadequate to help a child manage or master his or her problems, they are likely to declare the situation beyond control and seek immediate help. Even those few conditions that appear to be emergencies in their own right, such as an acute psychosis or a depression associated with a serious suicide attempt, often require adult participation to reach general attention.

Occasionally, however, older children or adolescents will seek emergency help on their own. It is unusual for school-age children to ask for help independently when in crisis, but when they do, they often have come from homes in which the parents are abusive. These children may turn in desperation to relatives, school authorities, or other adults, who then initiate treatment. Adolescents, on the other hand, are more likely to seek emergency care by themselves. Such youths frequently come from homes in which the parents are nonsupportive, unapproachable, abusive, or absent. In reacting against their environment, the teenagers may have frightened themselves with their own self-destructive impulses and thus may be asking for someone to directly intervene in their behalf. On the other hand, an occasional adolescent, frightened by the developmental need to separate from his or her parents and develop autonomy, may react with acute anxiety, depression, or misbehavior, which can lead to an emergency presentation (Kalogerakis, 1992).

Rarely does an emergency present without warning. Almost invariably the acute event has been preceded by a long period of marginal adjustment on the part of the child and impaired relationships within the family. Likewise, the primary cause of the acute presentation is as likely to be a recent impairment of the parents' functioning as it is to be a worsening of any prior psychopathology in the child. A child in crisis typically reflects a family system in crisis.

Although many emergency patients are brought for treatment by their parents, some present at the request of other referral sources. Most common among these sources are the school, the juvenile court, the police, health and mental health agencies, other community agencies, the family physician or pediatrician, and neighbors. Each of these sees a different spectrum of children and childhood pathology, has a different set of expectations of normal behavior, and has a different crisis point for insisting that the child get immediate help, but any of them may occasionally make a referral.

Likewise, although many child and adolescent emergencies come to attention through a hospital emergency room, even more appear directly on the doorstep of the child or adult psychiatrist, community agency, or general physician. What little is known about clinical differences among these populations, based upon either referring source or the setting in which they seek help, is described below.

Demographics

Adolescents make up the bulk of child psychiatric emergencies. Approximately 75–80% of those patients referred or self-referred for immediate help are 13 years old or older (Morrison, 1975). What few studies are available have consistently found more girls than boys seeking emergency treatment, particularly among middle and older teenagers, in spite of a predominance of boys in most psychiatric outpatient clinic populations. In part this reflects a tendency for girls in crisis to be self-destructive and to be viewed as having a psychiatric problem, while boys are more likely to act out and be handled by the police and courts.

The socioeconomic group and setting from which a child comes seem to be equally important factors in determining the likelihood that the child in crisis will present to the psychiatric system. For example, the acutely acting-out, aggressive delinquent from a lower class, inner city setting is likely to be handled by the courts, while a similar child from an upper class suburb is more likely to find his or her way to an emergency room and a psychiatrist. In part this reflects a realistic appraisal by experienced workers in the area about what resources are available: There is no point in seeking emergency psychiatric help for a lower-class child when none exists in the community or when no reimbursement is available to pay for such care.

Although it varies with the setting, in most communities almost one-half of psychiatric emergencies are for suicidal threats or behavior. This is particularly true if an exclusively adolescent population is examined. Almost a quarter of other adolescent presentations, mostly among males, are for assaultive, destructive, and violent behavior. Moreover, both the suicidal and the violent behavior are as frequently related to a diagnosis of adjustment disorder as to diagnoses of depression and conduct disorder, respectively. Additional common presenting psychiatric conditions found among child psychiatric patients include anxiety states (often with medical complaints), school refusal, somatoform disorders, psychoses, and a mixture of personality disorders.

The most common factor precipitating a crisis for the child is a crisis in the family, particularly one that threatens family stability or involves object loss through divorce, abandonment, illness, or death. Usually something perceived as being of great significance will have happened within the family shortly prior to the onset of the emergency. It is essential to identify that event. Other frequent precipitants include peer and school problems, a move to a new neighborhood, legal difficulties for the child (or parent), and medical illness with or without hospitalization.

EVALUATION

The elements of the child and adolescent psychiatric evaluation are elaborated elsewhere in this volume and won't be repeated here. Although the emergency situation brings its own special requirements to the evaluation, it also demands attention to the normal information and procedures of child psychiatry. Thus, even within the context of an emergency, interview style must vary with the child's age and developmental level, as must the sophistication of the information shared. The assessment must contain a review not only of the child's intellectual and emotional functioning but also of his or her social, interpersonal, educational, and physical functioning as well. It is necessary to obtain a history of recent events, trauma, drug use, and maladaptive behavior. Equally important is a review of the family structure and relationships, including strengths and weaknesses, and an assessment of the child and family's place within the community. Although some of this type of information may seem incidental or unduly "academic" in the flush of an emergency setting, long-lasting solutions are unlikely without appreciation of the personal, family, and community features in which the child's immediate problem is embedded.

However, an emergency brings with it some additional requirements. First, there is the need for an immediate evaluation. This typically reflects the distress and expectations of the parents and, in addition, may be required by the severity of the child's illness. On the other hand, the need to intervene quickly may also be caused by the fact that a crisis situation is often highly charged with negative emotion. Child and parent may be highly polarized, often viewing the other as culpable, and any delay in generating a dialogue may result in a further hardening of the parent's position, with a concomitant deterioration of the child's behavior. This destructive spiral can sometimes be prevented by immediate and vigorous intervention.

An additional and related reason for an immediate response is that many crises carry with them a brief window of opportunity during which entrenched and rigid ways of relating within a family temporarily become more flexible. There is a passing moment when those caught up in the crisis are more willing to listen, learn, and change. Parents and children both may be more forthcoming, and information long concealed may be revealed. Unfortunately, unless hooked into the process of change at that crisis-provoked moment, the system typically settles back into the status quo, denial of problems reasserts itself, and the family disappears from treatment.

The actual interview of the child may be unusually easy or unusually difficult. The child may have precipitated a crisis and be "ready to talk" or feel coerced into treatment and be resistant to initial approaches. Even though presenting symptoms such as a theft or a physical attack on the parents may show the child in a bad light, do not become confrontational or accusatory. Little will be gained, and as additional information is gathered and the picture changes, a critical opportunity may be lost. Of course, always search for signs of serious psychiatric disturbance such as psychosis or major depression. Also, the specifics of the child's history may be suspect. Children who have participated in generating a crisis may be so taken aback by the emotions they have created in others that they will minimize feelings and behavior ("I didn't really try to kill myself; I just took a couple of pills").

The symptoms that appear when the family is under stress often reflect long-standing problems of disturbed and chaotic family communications and bitter child and parent interactions. It is essential to look for and identify these maladaptive patterns. The symptom itself may be the tip of the iceberg. In fact, the current crisis may actually be only one in a series of crises, and the current symptom only one in a series of symptoms. Frequently families become adept at focusing on the child's presenting symptoms while denying underlying family pathology, a defense mechanism that must be recognized when it occurs. Parents who are anxious, disorganized, or actively destructive all too frequently fail to appreciate the direct results of their behavior on their children, effects that may be readily apparent to concerned outside observers. Such family dysfunction and scapegoating demand intervention, when possible.

It is equally important to note the degree of family intactness. Even if not disorganized and chaotic, a family without strong emotional bonds among its members is dysfunctional. On the other hand, if those bonds exist among key members, and if there are a sufficient number of competent and supportive adults present, the family can weather most acute emotional storms. As the relationship among family members becomes better defined, it becomes important to know who really initiated the request for emergency care, since that will often identify both the most imperiled part of the system and what factors led to the crisis.

DIAGNOSIS

Although accurate diagnosis is essential, frequently the presenting symptom has little diagnostic significance and represents merely a measure of the child's distress. However, the standard diagnoses must be looked for, both in the child and in the involved adults. Occasionally the most effective intervention that can be made in a child psychiatric emergency is to identify and treat psychopathology in the parent.

Because adjustment disorder is the most common diagnosis in most studies of child crises, often the diagnosis is less useful than the identification of precipitants to the crisis, such as physical abuse or object loss. Other specific diagnoses that occasionally present as emergencies in their own right and that are considered in greater depth below include dysthymia and major depression, psychotic disorders (particularly those that have their onset in adolescence, such as schizophrenia), anxiety disorders, dissociative and somatoform disorders, anorexia nervosa, conduct disorder, substance abuse, separation anxiety disorder, and medical problems with concomitant psychiatric symptoms. However, almost any other psychiatric diagnosis can accompany a child in crisis if external conditions warrant.

TREATMENT

The principles of treatment of the child psychiatric emergency are the principles of crisis intervention (Khan, 1979; Sargent et al., 1984). As we have seen, a crisis is an opportunity for change, and every effort should be made to maximize the child's and family's cooperative efforts to resolve the crisis. However, therapy is also directed by the diagnosis. If the child (or parent) suffers from a major psychiatric disorder such as depression or schizophrenia, its presence requires specific treatments.

The first order of business is to ensure the safety of the child. This usually means safety from self-harm or from an abusive environment. In most states the physician is responsible for determining if a child is safe and for acting on that determination. Hospitalization is the usual way of ensuring safety when little is provided by the environment. If the child is suicidal, very depressed, labile and impulsive, very distressed, psychotic, or has failed at intensive outpatient treatment, it may initially be necessary to concentrate on gaining control of the child rather than on investigating any underlying psychotherapeutic issues, so hospitalization is probably indicated. If a child's home environment appears unsafe and unpredictable, and if the child is sufficiently distressed to receive a psychiatric diagnosis, hospitalization may again be appropriate. Such inpatient stays are usually brief. In some communities, less restrictive but safe environments like foster and group homes are available, yet placement in them often takes several days to arrange.

Another form of ensuring the child's safety occurs when the child is panicky or traumatized. The child who has been raped, physically abused, or acutely damaged in some other way requires psychological protection in the form of support, reassurance that the worst is past, and sensitive attention to critical or affect-laden issues. Frequently, however, efforts to reach out to such children may be rebuffed by the child in his or her distress; gentle persistence may be required. Just as often, particularly in cases of rape or some other damage by a third party, the parents may demand more immediate attention than the child. If the parents are so upset that they interfere with care of the child, it is often necessary to assign a staff member to deal solely with them.

The other responsibility during a crisis is to ensure that those around the youth are safe. This issue is considered below in the discussion of aggressive and violent behavior.

Following the initial diagnostic assessment and after guaranteeing safety, it is essential to establish communication with the child and between the child and family. Both must be encouraged to recognize the problem and commit to finding solutions. Ideally the therapist should meet with the entire family and should be forthright in modeling accurate communication about central issues that led to the crisis. Everyone involved needs to understand that the current problem is probably not "just a temporary crisis" but rather must be viewed within the context of past personal and family history. Finally, whether or not hospitalization is necessary, every effort should be made to avoid allowing the child's role as patient to further scapegoat him or her in the eyes of the family.

SPECIFIC CHILD PSYCHIATRIC EMERGENCIES

Abuse

Both physical and sexual abuse can present with either acute or delayed emergency symptoms, in both males and females (Bergman and Brismar, 1992).

Acutely, the abuse may be obvious (rape, serious physical injury) or disguised (incest, moderate physical abuse by a parent). Typically, sexual abuse is more frequently overlooked in preadolescent and adolescent children due to their reluctance to make any leading comments (Campis et al., 1993). If obvious, it is essential to treat the child with sensitivity and support and to immediately intercede to prevent further damage if necessary. If disguised, maintain a high index of suspicion: expect denial, resistance, and hostility from the abusing party (e.g., a physically abusive mother or a sexually abusive father).

Chronic abuse can produce a range of psychopathology such as depression and anxiety that may eventually lead to a crisis presentation (see Chapters 99 and 100). Most prominent are features such as severe depression with suicidal and psychotic characteristics, poor impulse control and interpersonal aggression, substance abuse, significant anxiety and panic, and hysterical and dissociative symptoms. Many of these children can present acutely, yet the underlying cause of their distress may also be disguised.

Aggression and Violence

Although much is known about the pathogenesis, clinical presentation, and treatment of violent behavior (Reid and Patterson, 1989; Tardiff 1989), its evaluation and clinical management in the acute setting remains as much art as science. This is particularly true of children and adolescents for whom aggressive behavior is a final common pathway expressing a multitude of etiologies. In all youths it is multidetermined, but it may reflect predominantly biological factors in some cases (e.g., psychosis, delirium, low serotonin levels) and predominantly psychosocial factors in others (e.g., past history of abuse).

With younger children, the importance of psychosocial variables is undeniable in most individuals. Most aggressive younger children seem to be reacting against interpersonal forces in their environment: inconsistent or abusive parenting, lack of appropriate limit setting, unreasonable demands. Even the rare child who becomes violent under the influence of psychosis, severe attention deficit hyperactivity disorder, or a seizure shows the modifying effect of psychosocial factors. Adolescents perhaps exhibit more primarily biological conditions that are associated with aggression, such as bipolar disorder, schizophrenia, and major depression, yet psychological factors greatly influence even these disorders.

Violent children and adolescents are seen in crisis when the adults in their environment feel unable to control them. The younger child is more likely to be seen within the mental health system, while the adolescent may initially come to the attention of the courts.

Wherever these youths surface, the first duty of the therapist is to ensure both the safety of the child and the safety of those around him or her. This is less of a problem with the younger child, but the adolescent presents many of the same problems as the violent adult. In the emergency setting the violent adolescent may need to be approached in force and restraints and medication used to control behavior, although it certainly is preferable to employ a gentler approach and "talk him down." If thoroughly out of control, both the older child and the adolescent may need to be hospitalized.

In the process of controlling the assaultive youth, it is necessary to draw some diagnostic conclusions. Diagnosis dictates both psychosocial and pharmacologic therapy to some extent. For example, a conduct-disordered teenager or one high on drugs will be treated differently from a psychotic youth, regardless of the modalities employed.

Psychopharmacologic approaches to the violent youth emphasize the need to tailor medication to diagnosis (Stewart et al., 1990). Although almost anyone who is extremely agitated can be controlled with antipsychotic medication (droperidol or haloperidol are both effective in adults), there is limited literature on their use or safety as an acute "chemical straightjacket" in children or adolescents. Benzodiazepines may also be effective in the agitated, aggressive youth who needs to "settle down." A better practice, but one not always effective in or suitable for the emergency situation, is to use a medication that has been found to be effective in treating the underlying condition: Antipsychotics for schizophrenia, autism, and other psychoses; lithium for bipolar disorder; stimulants for attention deficit disorder; anticonvulsants for epilepsy.

Whatever interventions are chosen for the aggressive or violent youth, it is necessary to utilize the crisis as merely a setting in which to initiate longer term follow-up treatment. Without such continuity, this potentially dangerous behavior is likely to recur.

AIDS

The incidence of AIDS, though small, is rising among children. Most cases (85%) develop in very young children and have been acquired in utero or perinatally (Falloon et al., 1988), typically from mothers who use intravenous street drugs or have been sexually involved with infected men. Older children with AIDS may have survived from infancy, been inoculated via blood product transfusion, or been the victim of sexual abuse by an infected individual. Adolescents, particularly those from lower socioeconomic groups and those who are runaways, are at markedly increased risk for developing AIDS via heterosexual or homosexual transmission or from infected needles. However, these infected youths rarely are diagnosed until their 20s, due to the long latency of the virus.

The initial diagnosis of AIDS in a child is surrounded by a sense of emergency. Typically this distress comes from the mother or the health professionals involved. Although the mother is often known to be infected and thus the child known to be at risk, the diagnosis of AIDS promotes a sense of despair, anger, and hopelessness that must be addressed in the service of providing the best care for the child. Occasionally, however, the child's illness is the first indication to the mother that she herself has AIDS. In such a case the child's mother and family require immediate attention. Frequently the child will outlive the parent.

More commonly the real concern is on the part of the health professionals, since the need to care for a child with AIDS may be a new experience for many. Irrational fear of infection and a resultant reluctance to be involved with the child may predominate in otherwise devoted professionals and require education about the infinitesimally small likelihood of infection for careful staff.

The other crisis associated with AIDS occurs when the older infected child attempts to integrate into the community. Although the American Academy of Pediatrics recommends that a child with AIDS attend school unless he or she has oozing skin lesions, lacks control of body secretions, or bites others (American Academy of Pediatrics Committee on Infectious Diseases, 1986), schools and the parents of other children frequently resist. The atmosphere can become heated and the child be further stigmatized, so such situations must be handled with sensitivity. In addition, occasionally these immunodeficient children are best served by avoiding school, particularly during episodes of infectious illness.

Anorexia and Bulimia

The diagnosis of anorexia nervosa requires a body weight at least 15% below the minimum expected. Not uncommonly, however, patients will come to attention rather suddenly, with weights dangerously lower than that minimum standard; weights as low as 50% of expected are occasionally compatible with life. Significant weight loss may often go unnoticed, even by pediatricians and therapists, because of these patients' well-documented skills at deception: wearing loose-fitting clothing, drinking water just before weighing, attaching weights to the hems of a nightgown, and so forth. An emergency occurs when the family or treating professional suddenly discovers how physically compromised the patient is; serious complications of starvation (Bhanji and Mattingly, 1988) include life-threatening cardiac arrhythmias, apparently reversible cerebral atrophy with dilated lateral ventricles, vomiting and abdominal pain, severe constipation, abnormal liver function tests, reduced resistance to infection, hypoglycemia, hypothalamic-pituitary disturbances, and the superior mesenteric artery syndrome. The mortality rate for severe anorexia nervosa, particularly for cases discovered late, probably exceeds 15–20%.

Bulimia nervosa may be equally life threatening in severe cases, although the overall mortality rate and therapeutic intractability seems to be somewhat less than with anorexia nervosa. Because of the patient's need to hide induced vomiting, the illness may not be recognized by professionals until vomiting patterns are well established and the patient is medically unstable. Of particular concern are hypokalemia (Bonne et al., 1993) and other electrolyte disturbances, which can lead to altered cardiac function and kidney damage. Aspiration pneumonia is infrequent but potentially serious.

Aggressive intervention is usually required with the eating-disordered patient who presents as an emergency. Because patients with severe forms of either anorexia or bulimia are highly resistant to treatment, hospitalization is usually required (Yates, 1990). Often this is contrary to the patient's wishes and must be an involuntary admission. However, it can be life saving. An intensive medical evaluation must be completed on admission, including ECG and blood work, to identify the presence of any serious cardiac or other medical problems.

Anxiety Disorders

Although a disorder of excessive anxiety (generalized anxiety disorder) does occur in children and adolescents, it seldom escalates to create an emergency. On the other hand, severe or repeated stress, such as that found with a serious or painful medical illness, a periodically chaotic household, or a strange and frightening environment like a hospital, occasionally can produce an acute anxiety state in a child who then requires emergency intervention to help him or her regain control. Moreover, the occasional anxieties, fears, and phobias that are common phenomena among children can cause a new or nervous mother to declare an emergency in her child and seek immediate help. There are, however,

several other anxiety disorders that can reach crisis proportions: separation anxiety disorder, panic disorder, and posttraumatic stress disorder.

Separation anxiety disorder or school phobia may develop suddenly when a child is faced with leaving home or going to school for the first time. It also may develop slowly when the child gradually becomes more reluctant to leave home or more symptomatic (headaches, stomachaches, terrifying fears) when he or she does (Last and Strauss, 1990). In either case, symptoms can reach emergency proportions when the issue of leaving is forced. What is more, because treatment requires in part the rapid return to the school setting, it probably is appropriate at times for a crisis atmosphere to prevail in the service of returning the child to school quickly.

Panic disorder, although uncommon, does occur in adolescence and childhood (Black and Robbins, 1990; Hayward et al., 1989; Moreau and Weissman, 1992). It often goes unrecognized as a psychiatric disturbance. Until understood by both child and parent and effectively treated, attacks generally are dealt with as emergencies.

Although posttraumatic stress disorder is a well-recognized psychological response to overwhelming trauma (Schwartz and Perry, 1994; Terr, 1990), few patients suffering from this disorder present with a psychiatric emergency. A few teenagers may have frightening flashbacks, and occasionally younger children may be troubled by fears (see Chapter 70) that cause the parents to seek help for them. Otherwise, the greatest help that can be provided in a crisis setting is at the time of the incident that produces the syndrome. At that time the children need support, acceptance, explanation and clarification, and a chance to describe and ventilate if they are able. Most important, they need to be encouraged to begin ongoing therapy that will be aimed at allowing them to work through their experience.

Conduct Disorder

Conduct disorder is common and multidetermined. Also, as Lewis (Chapter 51) points out, it is frequently associated with other significant psychiatric pathology. Because much of the symptomatology associated with conduct disorder can present in an acute fashion (runaway, physical aggression, firesetting), children and adolescents bearing such a diagnosis often are seen in emergency settings, and often with juvenile court involvement. When presenting as an emergency, it is essential that such a child receive a careful diagnostic review to look for psychiatric and neurologic diagnoses other than conduct disorder, since failure to recognize alternative causes for symptomatology leads to inappropriate and ineffective interventions.

Encouragement for such a determined diagnostic approach is particularly necessary for these children since their brash, rejecting, unpleasant, and frequently hostile interpersonal style often leads to a rapid negative countertransference on the part of the examiner, followed by premature diagnostic closure. This can be a mistake for all involved, but particularly for the child.

A clinical presentation that can mimic conduct disorder but that must be distinguished from it is that which occurs in the youth displaying acute delinquent behavior. A diagnosis of conduct disorder requires symptoms with a duration of at least 6 months. On the other hand, many children will react to difficult life circumstances or to serious internal psychopathology such as major depression or psychosis with transitory delinquent behavior. Moreover, because the behavior is new and frequently upsetting for those adults responsible for the youths, these children are perhaps more likely to present as emergencies than are those with true conduct disorders. For these reasons it is especially important that any youth with such new symptoms be carefully evaluated for personal or interpersonal pathology and treated accordingly.

Depression and Suicide

Threatened suicide or an unsuccessful suicide attempt is the most common emergency in child psychiatry. Although attempted suicide is described in detail in Chapter 61 of this volume, such a crisis demands that the therapist possess a core of knowledge that allows a rapid assessment of potential risk, followed by safe management of the emergent situation.

Most patients who threaten or attempt suicide kill themselves neither at that time nor at any time in the future: Many suicide threats are transparent attempts to achieve some other goal and reflect impaired interpersonal communications and relations. However, some children *do* commit suicide; it is therefore essential to recognize those characteristics of the child and his or her environment that increase potential lethality. The difficulty, of course, with a mere detailing of risk factors is that such statistical measures have only indirect predictive value for the individual child. More important, perhaps, is the gestalt that surrounds the suicidal episode, that is, the sense and degree of hopelessness and desperation encountered and whether or not any long-lasting changes can be made to improve the situation.

There is a small group of crucial risk factors that must be reviewed in each case: age, sex, presence of depression, presence of conduct disorder, drug abuse, prior suicide attempt, family history of suicide, access to weapons, and possibly "general psychopathology and general family upset." The risk to those below 14 years of age is minor; it increases dramatically during middle and older adolescence. Males, particularly white males, are at greatest risk, even though teenage girls make three times as many attempts. Major depression with accompanying symptoms of poor self-esteem, hopelessness and helplessness, loneliness, and a sense of guilt may be the most important risk factor (Robbins and Alessi, 1985), although it is not necessary to be depressed to commit suicide. Almost as important as depression, for reasons that are not clear but that may relate to decreased impulse control and low self-esteem, is the presence of a conduct disorder and its associated chronic difficulty with authority. Antisocial males are almost as likely to harm themselves as to harm others, a fact made more likely if they also abuse drugs and alcohol, since the impaired judgment and impulse control that accompany the intoxicated state can be deadly (Rich et al., 1986). Moreover, all of the above are made worse if there is ready access to a gun, the most common method of successful suicide among teenage males. Traditional risk factors of prior suicide attempts and family history of suicide apply to adolescents as well. Finally, there is a high level of nonspecific individual and family distress and psychopathology in the majority of successful suicides: most successful suicides occur at home (Saccomani et al., 1992).

In evaluating the individual patient, it is essential to determine the patient's intention:

1. Why does he or she want to die? Peculiar and flawed rationales and fantasies for considering suicide are common and often responsive to intervention.
2. Was there a suicide plan and a lethal method? (Note, however, that an ineffective method may be employed in the presence of real distress and a serious attempt, while a lethal method may be used inadvertently in a suicide gesture, particularly in the younger child.)
3. Are there any organic factors (including intoxication) that might decrease impulse control?
4. What was the degree of premeditation? (Is the child "preoccupied with dying"?)
5. How much turmoil, abuse, violence (Deykin et al., 1985), neglect, and lack of support is present within the family?
6. Does the child believe, rightly or wrongly, that he or she is not wanted or cared for?

Intervention begins with an attempt to develop rapport with the child and the family. Even if significant risk factors are present, hospitalization can frequently be prevented if there is a support system in place that can respond to the child's needs and provide a safe environment so that outpatient psychotherapy can be undertaken. In the emergency setting, it is the task of the therapist not only to identify risk factors, assess the child's motivations toward suicide, and establish the family's level of commitment but also to work with the child and family during the crisis to try to develop a new (although possibly transient), higher level of support and stability, which will see the child through the following several days until therapeutic interventions begin to have their effects. However, often stable family support can't be developed, and the child must be hospitalized for his or her own protection, or alternative community support services (see Chapter 105) must be identified before the youth can be released. Also, occasionally the child may be too disturbed (panicked, psychotic) to be safe in any setting except a hospital.

Whatever the resolution of the immediate crisis, treatment of a suicide attempt remains incomplete unless plans for follow-up care, however brief, are made. Even the most inspired intervention in the emergency room may come undone when the child and family return to their "natural environment," so a follow-up visit typically is a necessity.

Dissociative Disorders

These disorders will occasionally appear during the teenage years, and even in children. Although the presentations are not always emergent, frequently the symptoms are so startling to the child (e.g., depersonalization disorder) or to the parents (e.g., amnesia) that a sense of crisis prevails. Only multiple personality disorder (see Chapter 65) generates symptoms, such as aggressive or self-destructive acts, that produce an emergency in their own right (Kluft, 1984). Even though the spectrum of dissociative disorders is known to exist in children and adolescents, research into their clinical presentations and treatment in this group is limited.

Drug Abuse

Drug and alcohol abuse is increasingly common among youths, particularly the use of crack cocaine among inner city youth and alcohol abuse among teenagers of all groups. Acute intoxications and drug reactions frequently present as psychiatric emergencies, and the details of their identification and management are thoroughly described in Chapter 69. It is worth emphasizing, however, that acute drug presentations may actually be embedded in, and disguise, a more primary psychiatric emergency. Thus, a major depression, psychosis, or environment of abuse may be overlooked in the turmoil that surrounds a drug-related emergency; yet if the relationship between the drug problem and the broader psychiatric pathology goes unrecognized, little long-lasting improvement will occur. Final evaluation and disposition of a drug-related presentation should include the family and should wait until intoxication or any other acute reactions are resolved; otherwise, crucial underlying processes may be missed.

Firesetting

Few events in psychiatry are more likely to generate a sense of emergency than the discovery that a child has set a significant fire, particularly a fire that has resulted in major property loss or the loss of life. The parents may be frantic, social service agencies may demand immediate help, and the police are frequently involved. Acute upset in the child is likely caused by the magnitude of what he or she has done and by the concern of those around him. Usually such situations are emergencies primarily by virtue of the distress of the adults involved, although rarely the child is suffering from an acute psychiatric disorder such as psychosis or an organic mental disorder.

Typically, if the child suffers from a disorder at all, it is a chronic one, such as attention deficit hyperactivity disorder in younger children and conduct disorder in adolescents (Gaynor and Hatcher, 1987). There is often a history of previous firesetting episodes or other misbehavior on the child's part. Family malfunction is also common: Younger children may be left unsupervised frequently and allowed to play with matches; older children may be acting out in response to family psychopathology or expressing their own character pathology. Although the current event is likely to be the most serious in a series of past difficulties, there is often little relationship between the amount of damage caused by the fire and the degree of child or family psychopathology (see Chapter 55).

Assessment and treatment should begin immediately. No treatment of firesetting is complete without vigorously looking for and addressing those dysfunctional family interactions that seem often to underlie such behavior. Although careful outcome studies are lacking, seemingly effective treatments exist for firesetters. Typically, they directly get the child to recognize the impulse to set fires and then help him or her identify its underlying motivations. Although much of this can be done on an outpatient basis, in select cases the emergency presentation will resolve into an inpatient stay. Occasionally this is to ensure community safety. It is useful for the child, family, and social/legal system to understand that therapy is available and that long-lasting change can occur.

Psychosis

Psychotic disorders in youths are brought to emergency attention more frequently than one would expect, given the length of time they take to develop. Generally the psychotic presentation of acute schizophrenia or bipolar illness develops over weeks or months, and when viewed retrospectively, the symptoms often are felt by family members probably to have been present for some time. Unfortunately, the symptoms are often denied or ignored by those around the patient until the situation becomes emergent, at which time the physician is confronted with the need to force both hospitalization and antipsychotic medication.

Most acute psychotic presentations occur in adolescents who are developing or have developed schizophrenia or bipolar disorder, particularly those who abuse drugs or alcohol (Kutcher et al., 1992), although brief psychotic reactions in response to substance abuse (hallucinogens, crack cocaine, phencyclidine (PCP), inhalants, etc.) must always be considered. Occasionally medical illness produces a delirium that mimics a typical functional psychosis, although the medical history and presence of confusion help distinguish the two.

Runaway

Runaway youths are common and represent a major child mental health problem in the United States (see Chapter 106). Many such youths never come to professional attention, either through their own or their family's reluctance. More commonly, however, a distraught parent will seek emergency help for a recalcitrant teenager who has just returned

from running away, or a community agency will request immediate intervention with a runaway youth who has just been "dropped in its lap."

In either case, the typical rules of crisis intervention in child psychiatry should be followed. It can be difficult initially to develop rapport with these adolescents (relatively few children are runaways), who may be wary around adults, but it is well worth the effort since the keys to resolving their acute as well as their long-term problems often lie with improved communication between them and the adults in their family and their environment. Every effort should be made to engage these youth in treatment and to provide initial, even if temporary, solutions to their concerns, since the likelihood of losing contact with them is high and the damage done by chronic runaway behavior is profound.

Somatoform Disorders

The only somatoform disorder likely to present as an emergency is conversion disorder. Conversion symptoms typically appear as complex and dramatic medical symptoms that develop rapidly and demand immediate attention. They occur most frequently in teenage girls but can develop at almost any age and in either sex.

Because medical symptoms predominate, pediatricians usually are the physicians first involved. Psychiatrists typically enter the picture only after a careful physical evaluation and laboratory testing finds no medical disorder. Not infrequently, however, conversion symptoms complement and embellish real biological pathology, so organic disease must not be ruled out too quickly.

In spite of the drama of the symptom, the patient may be surprisingly calm ("la belle indifference"). Often, however, the parents make up for this calm with their own desperate efforts to get help for their child, thus adding to the emergency atmosphere. In addition, a recent stress frequently has helped precipitate the symptom in the first place, making the situation even more turbulent.

It is important that treatment begin as quickly as possible after the diagnosis is made, that is, after physical illness and malingering have been eliminated. Allowed to remain untreated psychologically, the symptom may become persistent. Thus, at the same time that the patient is presenting as a medical emergency, the child and parents are being encouraged to see the connection between the physical symptoms and psychological mechanisms. Hypnosis or an Amytal interview to remove symptoms during the acute presentation may dramatically improve the symptoms on occasion.

References

American Academy of Pediatrics Committee on Infectious Diseases: School attendance of children and adolescents. *Pediatrics* 77:430, 1986.

Bergman BK, Brismar BG: Do not forget the battered male! *Scand J Soc Med* 20:179, 1992.

Bhanji S, Mattingly D: *Medical Aspects of Anorexia Nervosa*. London, Butterworth, 1988.

Black B, Robbins DR: Panic disorder in children and adolescents. *J Am Acad Child Adolesc Psychiatry* 29:36, 1990.

Bonne OB, Block M, Berry EM: Adaptation to severe chronic hypokalemia in anorexia nervosa: A plea for conservative management. *Int J Eat Disord* 13:125, 1993.

Campis LB, Hebden-Curtis J, DeMaso DR: Developmental differences in detection and disclosure of sexual abuse. *J Am Acad Child Adolesc Psychiatry* 32:920, 1993.

Deykin EY, Alpert JJ, McNamarra JJ: A pilot study of the effect of exposure to child abuse or neglect on adolescent suicidal behavior. *Am J Psychiatry* 142:1299, 1985.

Falloon J, Eddy J, Roper M, et al: AIDS in the pediatric population. In: DeVita V, Hellman S, Rosenberg S (eds): *AIDS: Etiology, Diagnosis, Treatment, and Prevention*. Philadelphia, Lippincott, 1988.

Gaynor J, Hatcher C: *The Psychology of Child Firesetting*. New York, Brunner/Mazel, 1987.

Hayward C, Killen JD, Taylor CB: Panic attacks in young adolescents. *Am J Psychiatry* 146:1061, 1989.

Kalogerakis MG: Emergency evaluation of adolescents. *Hosp Community Psychiatry* 43:617, 1992.

Khan AU: *Psychiatric Emergencies in Pediatrics*. Chicago, Year Book, 1979.

Kluft RP: Multiple personality in childhood. *Psychiatr Clin North Am* 7:121, 1984.

Kutcher S, Kachur E, Marton P, et al: Substance abuse among adolescents with chronic mental illnesses. *Can J Psychiatry* 37:428, 1992.

Last CG, Strauss CC: School refusal in anxiety-disordered children and adolescents. *J Am Acad Child Adolesc Psychiatry* 29:31, 1990.

Moreau D, Weissman MM: Panic disorder in children and adolescents: A review. *Am J Psychiatry* 149:1306, 1992.

Morrison GC: *Emergencies in Child Psychiatry*. Springfield, IL, Charles C Thomas, 1975.

Reid JB, Patterson GR: The development of antisocial behaviour patterns in childhood and adolescence. *Eur J Personality* 3:107, 1989.

Rich CL, Young D, Fowler RC: San Diego Suicide Study: Young versus old subjects. *Arch Gen Psychiatry* 43:577, 1986.

Robbins DR, Alessi NE: Depressive symptoms and suicidal behavior in adolescents. *Am J Psychiatry* 142:588, 1985.

Sargent J, Silver M, Hodas G, et al: Crisis intervention in children and adolescents. *Clin Emerg Med* 4:245, 1984.

Stewart JT, Myers WC, Burket RC, et al: A review of the pharmacotherapy of aggression in children and adolescents. *J Am Acad Child Adolesc Psychiatry* 29:269, 1990.

Tardiff K: *Assessment and Management of Violent Patients*. Washington, DC, American Psychiatric Press, 1989.

Terr L: *Too Scared to Cry*. New York, Harper & Row, 1990.

Yates A: Current perspectives on the eating disorders. II: Treatment, outcome, and research directions. *J Am Acad Child Adolesc Psychiatry* 29:1, 1990.

90 THE CONSULTATION PROCESS IN CHILD AND ADOLESCENT PSYCHIATRIC CONSULTATION-LIAISON IN PEDIATRICS[a]

Melvin Lewis, M.B., B.S., F.R.C.Psych., D.C.H., and Patricia K. Leebens, M.D.

Recent studies have demonstrated the clear association between physical disorders and psychiatric disturbances in children and adolescents (Shugart, 1991; Steiner et al., 1993). Psychiatric assessments of randomly selected hospitalized pediatric patients suggest that as many as two-thirds of children admitted to pediatric wards would benefit from a child or adolescent psychiatry consultation (Shugart, 1991). Coexistent medical and psychiatric problems in pediatric patients appear to contribute to more complex diagnostic assessments, increased health care costs, and less satisfactory outcomes compared to those in patients without comorbidity (Steiner et al., 1993). The child psychiatric consultation, then, is an important intervention to help improve the care of hospitalized pediatric patients and their families.

This chapter summarizes common psychological responses in hospitalized children and adolescents and outlines the child and adolescent psychiatric consultation process.

PSYCHIATRIC CONSULTATION IN PEDIATRICS

The process of child and adolescent psychiatry consultation-liaison in hospital pediatrics rests on a broad foundation that includes a knowledge of normal development (Knobloch et al., 1980; Lewis and Volkmar, 1990), psychopathology, diagnosis and treatment (Lewis, 1991a), and a familiarity with pediatrics and pediatric hospital practices. The purpose of the consultation, the characteristics of the patient and the patient's family and their reactions to the hospitalization, the nature of the patient's illness or injury, and the nature of the relationship between pediatrics and child and adolescent psychiatry all influence the consultation-liaison process. An understanding of the child's concept of his or her body, of how these concepts change with development, and of children's (and family) reactions to illness is particularly useful (Lewis and Schonfeld, 1994) as well.

CHILDREN'S CONCEPT OF THE BODY AND ILLNESS

The child's developing concept of the body is reflected in the child's behavior, verbalizations, and drawings of the body (DeLeo, 1977). Initially, the infant seems to experience the body as an external object that either gratifies or causes discomfort. Thus, the infant appears to be either content and oblivious of the body or appears enraged and cries vigorously when the threshold for bodily discomfort is exceeded. There

appears to be very little ability in the infant to comprehend or tolerate discomfort or to delay gratification.

By the time children enter preschool, there is clear evidence they possess some knowledge about the body, as well as an increasing capacity to take care of the body. For example, 3-year-old children are curious about the body, can name body parts, including eyes, nose, and mouth, and are concerned about cuts and "booboos." Very young children seem to view the body as a kind of fluid-filled sac that, if punctured, will ooze precious fluids. Maintaining body integrity is paramount at this developmental stage, and even minor injuries may seem catastrophic to the child. Band-Aids are very reassuring at this time. At this age, also, a simple knowledge of internal organs is beginning, usually with those organs related to direct experience, e.g., stomach and stomachache.

In kindergarten, children 4 or 5 years of age can draw a simple representation of the body. Frequently they will draw a single circle within which simple features are drawn, e.g., dots for eyes and nose, a single line for the mouth, and a scribble for hair (the child frequently identifies the sex of the person "by the hair"). Limbs are represented by simple "stick" lines with an indeterminate number of digits emanating from the end of the stick limbs. Simple knowledge of internal organs (e.g., a heart in the shape of a valentine) begins to develop.

As children develop, more details appear in their pictures of the body. By 5 or 6 years children can identify the jaw, temples, forearms, and shins. From ages 5 or 6, also, children will draw a circle for the head and an ellipse for the torso and will add more detail, e.g., eyebrows and ears. Articles of clothing also become more detailed between 7 and 10 years.

When the child approaches the cognitive stage of formal operations (usually ages 12 and older), the proportions of the body are more realistically represented, and such advances as profile views and representation of movement appear. Knowledge of physiological functions of certain bodily organs begins to develop; however, adolescents, who might be expected to have a good working knowledge of major anatomical organs and functions, may still be surprisingly ignorant of certain body parts and functions.

Children's concepts of illness follow a similar developmental sequence (Lewis, 1994a). In infants there appears to be no concept of illness other than an external agent (the body) that is attacking the infant and causing discomfort. Very young children who are in the early stages of concrete operations seem to conceive of illness as a result of "immanent justice," i.e., the illness is a punishment for misdeeds committed or imagined and for which the child feels guilty.

The preschool child develops a "contagion" theory of illness—that is, illness is caused by a germ, or "bug." Usually the germ or bug is large and imaginary and "infects" in ways imagined by the child. By school age the child develops a more sophisticated knowledge of the

[a] An earlier version of this chapter by Melvin Lewis was published in Lewis M, King RA (eds): Consultation-Liaison in Pediatrics (Child and Adolescent Psychiatry Clinics of North America). Philadelphia, WB Saunders, 1994, pp. 439–448.

causes of illnesses and the relationship between symptoms and medical treatments. At this developmental age, children may ask many more questions as they attempt to sort out their understanding of the symptoms, illnesses, and treatments that affect their bodies.

Again, adolescents, while cognitively more capable of understanding illness, are often psychologically immature and sometimes behave as though they believe they are invincible and immortal. In any event, earlier concepts may persist or reappear as part of the regression that often occurs with illness. Thus, feelings of guilt may accompany the onset of certain illness, and children and adolescents may have an inaccurate or incomplete understanding of how they became ill.

TYPES OF REQUESTS FOR CONSULTATION

Requests from pediatricians for child psychiatry consultation in the hospital may fall into the following categories.

Emergencies

The most common emergency that stimulates a psychiatric consultation is attempted suicide, usually by overdose or physical self-injury, in an adolescent. Other emergencies, also usually seen in the emergency room, include physical abuse (sometimes presenting as Munchausen syndrome by proxy), sexual abuse, drug abuse, acute agitation, acute psychotic reactions, and family crises. In addition, such conditions as anorexia nervosa with critical weight loss may require urgent hospital care.

Emergency consultation on the pediatric ward may be requested for the diagnosis and management of major disruptive behaviors in a child or parent. The consultation may merge into concomitant psychiatric treatment during the hospitalization or may entail making arrangements for psychiatric care following the pediatric hospitalization. Other emergent consultations on the pediatric wards may be requested for the diagnosis and management of delirium caused by a wide range of medical conditions (e.g., brain infections and trauma, drug intoxications or interactions, adrenal, hepatic, pancreatic, or renal failure, burns and electrolyte imbalance, and space-occupying lesions) that severely affect the metabolism and function of the brain.

Differential Diagnosis of Somatoform Symptoms

Anxiety and depression may be the underlying cause of such pediatric symptoms as recurrent abdominal pain, headache, and failure to thrive. Somatoform disorders, including somatization disorder, body dysmorphic disorder, conversion disorder, and pain disorder characteristically present with symptoms that at first glance suggest a physical disorder, but for which psychological factors are of major etiological importance. The request for consultation and diagnosis may come late in the hospitalization, often after an exhaustive, and often expensive, somatic workup has taken place.

Collaborative Care of Children with Stress-Sensitive Illnesses

Acute episodes of certain illnesses, including asthma, diabetic acidosis, and ulcerative colitis, are often precipitated by psychological stress in children who are particularly vulnerable and in whom the psychological component of the illness is especially prominent. Psychological assessment and care may be essential for the comprehensive treatment of such a child.

Diagnosis and Care of Children with Psychiatric Symptoms following a Somatic Illness

Some illness seems to linger long after the acute phase in the form of a prolonged postillness depression that may last for a long time. For example, acute infectious mononucleosis and other viral infections are often followed by symptoms of depression that may last for weeks or months.

Chronic Illness

Chronic pediatric illness of almost any kind, with recurrent hospitalization, is a psychological risk factor for children (Lewis, 1994a). The rate of psychiatric illness in children with both chronic medical conditions and disability is three times greater than in noncompromised children for conditions such as attention deficit hyperactivity disorder, overanxious disorder, depression, and conduct disorder (Cadman et al., 1987).

Reactions to Major Pediatric Treatment Techniques

Certain kinds of pediatric treatment evoke serious psychological symptoms. Bone marrow transplantation, in particular, gives rise to considerable anxiety and depression (see Chapter 95). Extensive surgical repair for injury and burns (see Chapter 98), especially in young children, may give rise to acute behavioral problems. Psychiatric assessment and care may be essential to the child's successful participation in the medical treatment.

Reactions to Pediatric Illness or Trauma

Lastly, every child with a pediatric illness or trauma requiring hospitalization experiences a psychological reaction (Lewandowski and Baranoski, 1994). The degree of the reaction varies with the developmental level and premorbid state of the child, the state and reaction of the family, and the seriousness of the illness. The more serious the illness (e.g., leukemia) or injury (especially head injury), the more likely it is that behavioral reactions will arise.

PSYCHOLOGICAL RISK FACTORS

In general, psychological disturbances are more likely to occur when any of the specific risk factors listed in Table 90.1 are present.

Other psychological risk factors include impaired function, immobilization, disfigurement, and loss of autonomy in the child. Additional parental reactions that may increase the risk of psychological disturbance in the child include parental feelings of loss and grief, guilt, depression and anxiety, exhaustion, and isolation, as well as the effects of marital strain, financial drain, and disruption of routine family functioning.

Characteristics of the treatment team or the treatment process may also increase the risk of psychological disturbances in pediatric inpatients. In general, psychological distress is more likely to occur in the presence of any of the following risk factors:

1. Use of multiple medical consultants (sometimes with conflicting opinions) without adequate, available, and/or clearly designated leadership;

Table 90.1. Risk Factors for Psychological Disturbances in Hospitalized Pediatric Patients

1. Premorbid psychopathology in the patient
2. Poor parent-child relationships
3. Psychiatric disturbance in either parent
4. Infancy age group
5. More severe or ambiguous medical diagnoses
6. Chronic illness and multiple hospitalizations
7. Inadequate psychological preparation for hospital and invasive procedures
8. Parents' inadequate understanding of the illness, including unrealistic expectations, and debilitating parental reactions, including feelings of extreme helplessness and pessimism
9. Involvement of other nonmedical agencies (department of child services, police, law) interested in the patient's welfare

Table 90.2.   Signs of Psychological Distress in Pediatric Patients

1. Biopsychological symptoms
    Malaise, pain, irritability, disturbances in appetite and sleep
2. Increased attachment behavior
    Clinging, demanding, heightened separation anxiety
3. Regression
    Thumb-sucking, regression in developmental milestones (i.e., speech,
        bladder and bowel control, self care)
4. Passivity and withdrawal
    Feelings of helplessness and powerlessness
5. Aggressiveness and acting out
    Tantrums, combativeness, and oppositional behavior
6. Frightening fantasies about illness and procedures
    Ideas of punishment, fear of mutilation and bodily harm
7. Anxiety and mobilization of defenses
    Denial, projection, phobic symptoms, conversion symptoms
8. Precipitation or aggravation of premorbid psychiatric symptoms

2. The hospital staff's inadequate response to or understanding of the psychological meaning of the illness, injury, and/or hospitalization to the child and other family members;
3. The hospital staff's inadequate awareness of their transference and countertransference feelings about the child, the family, and the illness or injury.

SIGNS OF PSYCHOLOGICAL DISTRESS

Some of the common signs of psychological distress associated with pediatric illness are shown in Table 90.2.

MODELS OF CONSULTATION

Several models of consultation-liaison have been developed in response to the kinds of consultations requested by pediatricians and to the kinds of psychological reactions prominent in hospitalized pediatric patients and their families (Lewis, 1994b).

Anticipatory Model

This model derives in part from an earlier concept of "anticipatory pediatrics" (Senn, 1947) and is especially useful when serious psychological reactions to an anticipated procedure are to be expected. For example, children undergoing bone marrow transplantation, and their families, can benefit from a pretreatment psychiatric consultation to assess the strengths and vulnerabilities of the family and to prepare the child and family accordingly (Atkins and Patenaude, 1987). When the expected psychological reaction does occur, the psychiatric consultation team is then already in place and informed, and in a much better position to offer further help. Sometimes the prior assessment process may be used to help avert serious psychological reactions.

Case Finding Model

A modified form of the anticipatory model derives from the liaison work that can be offered to the pediatric staff on the ward. Thus, through the use of regular weekly ward meetings with pediatric and nursing staff (Lewis, 1962), early detection or anticipation of psychological problems can help alleviate stress and possibly prevent severe psychological reactions. Unfortunately, the preventive and therapeutic uses of such liaison meetings are not directly reimbursable by most third party payers, and the cost has to be absorbed into the general cost of the hospital care (Fritz, 1990; Lewis, 1994b). This liaison function is invaluable, but rarely receives adequate financial support. In some instances, the liaison work may lead to a formal consultation request (which is usually then reimbursable).

Education and Training Model

The consultant can make a useful contribution to the pediatric hospital care of infants, children, and adolescents through regular case confer-

ences and discussions. Often this is most appreciated in the context of acute care units, such as a pediatric intensive care unit. Training for pediatricians can also be enhanced by the use of a study group (Lewis and Colletti, 1973). Training of child psychiatrists and child psychologists in consultation and liaison in pediatrics can be facilitated by direct, on-the-case supervision as well as by indirect supervision, case conferences, and regular seminars.

Emergency Response Model

This model uses a 24-hour emergency on-call roster and is mostly used for emergency room calls, but may also apply in the case of urgent consultation requests on the wards. Attempted suicide in an adolescent is a frequent reason for an emergency child psychiatry consultation in an emergency room, while the need for containment, restraint, or structure for a behaviorally out-of-control child on the wards (King and Lewis, 1994) is a common reason for an urgent response by the consultant.

Continuing and Collaborative Care Model

In many pediatric illnesses there is a need for consistent, collaborative, and concurrent pediatric and psychiatric treatment. Typical illnesses that require such care include anorexia nervosa, bulimia, and obesity. Children with recurring or chronic pain may also benefit from ongoing collaborative approaches for pain management, including behavioral approaches (Cardona, 1994) and psychopharmacological approaches (Green, 1994).

None of these models is mutually exclusive. Indeed, a good child and adolescent psychiatric consultation-liaison service in pediatrics should incorporate all of the above models for comprehensive consultative care.

BASIC CONSULTATION PROCESS

The psychiatric consultation is generally facilitated when the consultant is part of a team consisting of a child psychiatrist, child psychologist, social worker, developmental pediatrician, and child psychiatry clinical nurse specialist. The team approach allows for comprehensive understanding of the medical, psychiatric, and social issues that may be involved in a referral, as well as for greater coordination of services within the hospital and at the time of outpatient referral. Attention to the following factors will enhance every form or model of consultation.

AVAILABILITY

Prompt, practical, and understandable recommendations (Leslie, 1992) from an easily available psychiatric consultant are the foundation of effective consultation and liaison work. The presence on the ward of the child psychiatrist at ward rounds, conferences, or other meetings is useful. Liaison work in particular facilitates accessibility, provides opportunities for informal suggestions, and may prepare the way for more formal consultation requests.

RELATIONSHIPS

Collaboration is much more likely to occur when there are good relationships based on mutual respect and friendship between pediatrician and child psychiatrist. As pediatricians and child psychiatrists work in different ways (Burket and Hodgin, 1993; Fritz, 1990), misunderstandings may occur regarding the urgency of a referral or the speed of response needed (Black et al., 1990). Understanding how each other functions in practice can encourage smoother collaboration between pediatricians and child psychiatrists (Lewis, 1994b). Good relationships between pediatric and psychiatric colleagues make communication easier and more straightforward, reduce the tendency for acting out of ambivalent feelings, and ultimately improve the care of patients and families.

LEVELS OF CONSULTATION

Five levels of consultation should always be kept in mind:

1. The inner life of the child;
2. The dynamics of the relationship between the child and his or her family;
3. The relationship between the child and family and the various ward staff;
4. Interdisciplinary dynamics operating among attending pediatricians, housestaff, nurses, social worker, child psychiatrist, child psychologist, and other consulting specialists;
5. In some instances, the relationship of the hospital staff to an outside agency, including state departments of children's services, police, or law.

PREPARATION FOR THE CONSULTATION

In preparing to respond to a request for psychiatric consultation, the following questions provide a useful checklist to review before going ahead with the clinical interviews:

1. *Who* is requesting the consultation? A consultation request must come ultimately from the physician responsible for the care of the hospitalized child and should include a brief written request by the responsible physician.
2. *What* is (are) the consultation question(s)? The question or questions must be clear and should be of a kind that can reasonably be answered in the often brief period of time that the child is on the ward and in the context of the particular ward environment.
3. *When* was the request made, and what is the time frame? In some instances, there simply may not be sufficient time before discharge in which to perform a reasonable consultation.
4. *Why* is the request being made at this time? Sometimes the ostensible reason for the request covers a hidden agenda, e.g., a pending court appearance, a possible custody conflict, or, in some instances, a conflict among hospital staff.
5. *How* much workup has been done or should be done (and by whom) before proceeding with the consultation? Since the available time is often brief, prior information about the child and family may enable the child psychiatrist to focus on specific areas.
6. Have the child and parents been informed and suitably prepared? Occasionally parents may refuse to have a psychiatrist see their child. The cooperation of the parents is needed for a satisfactory consultation.

PROCEDURE

A flexible interview approach is often required for completing consultations on a pediatric ward. One may have to improvise through the use of a few portable materials (e.g., paper, pencil, crayons, deck of cards, and small rubber doll figures) and by adapting to frequent interruptions and lack of privacy on a pediatric ward.

The psychiatric evaluation is of necessity detailed and complex and should not be rushed, if possible (Leslie, 1992). If the time available for the consultation is not adequate to complete the necessary evaluation, the focus of the consultation should be adjusted or the evaluation should be deferred to a time or setting (i.e., the inpatient psychiatric unit or the outpatient psychiatric clinic) when a more appropriate assessment can be made.

Ideally one would first interview the patient's parents, but this may not be feasible. Suitable preparation of the child and parents by the requesting pediatrician usually reduces the child's and parents' reluctance, if any, to speak with a psychiatric consultant; however, the complete assessment of the child may still require multiple interviews with the child and parents. The basic items of a mental status examination (Lewis, 1991b) will need to be performed and additional inquiries or tests ordered as needed. A thorough knowledge of the patient's treatment and medication regimen is particularly necessary when evaluating a

patient for delirium or other possible medication-induced conditions (e.g., depression, anxiety, psychosis, agitation).

Very useful information about the child and family can often be gathered from the observations of such ward staff as nurses, child life specialists, and social workers. Also, conversations with a variety of the patient's health care providers (inpatient and outpatient) may be necessary to sort out treatment issues that may be in conflict and contributing to the psychological stress of the patient and/or the patient's family. Clarification of any pending legal or social service issues may also be necessary to comprehend the patient's current stressors.

REPORT

The findings of the consultation should first be reported to and discussed with the requesting pediatrician. Subsequently, and with the agreement of the pediatrician, one communicates as necessary and as appropriate with the parents and their child and key ward staff. The written consultation note should be relatively brief and should be organized in such a manner as to be easily read and understood. Useful headings might include (*a*) a brief statement of the question and the purpose of the consultation; (*b*) a concise summary of pertinent historical data; (*c*) the important findings, both positive and negative, from the mental status examination (MSE) and comprehensive psychiatric evaluation; (*d*) diagnosis, using a standard multiaxial classification (e.g., DSM-IV or ICD-10); (*e*) a brief diagnostic formulation and summary; and (*f*) a recommended treatment/management plan or suggestions for further workup.

CONFIDENTIALITY

A hospital chart is not a particularly private or confidential record; it may be seen by the parents or child as well as other people. For this reason the words used must be carefully chosen to avoid offense, slander, or potential dissemination of possibly damaging information. The written record is at the same time a legal document carrying the consultant's signature and should be written with that in mind.

FOLLOW-UP

Follow-up after a consultation by inquiring of the requesting pediatrician about the subsequent course of the child is helpful. The consultant obtains general information about the accuracy of the psychiatric assessment and the effectiveness of the intervention, and the pediatrician often appreciates the psychiatrist's continuing interest. Follow-up studies of matched pediatric patients who received psychiatric consultations and those who did not can help assess the efficacy of psychiatric interventions in hospitalized pediatric patients (Shugart, 1991).

IMPEDIMENTS TO CONSULTATION-LIAISON IN PEDIATRICS

Difficulties that may interfere with a well-functioning consultation-liaison service (Anders, 1977, 1982; Burket and Hodgin, 1993; Eisenberg, 1967; Fritz, 1990; Jellinek, 1982; Kanner, 1937; Lawrence and Adler, 1992; Leslie, 1992; Lewis, 1973, 1994; Lewis and Vitulano, 1988; Lourie, 1962; Oke and Mayer, 1991; Rothenberg, 1979; Senn, 1946; Shugart, 1991; Wright et al., 1987) include the following:

1. The failure of some child psychiatrists to understand how pediatricians function in practice, and vice versa;
2. A perceived, or real, lack of availability of child psychiatrists;
3. Professional identity problems in both disciplines;
4. Different perceptions of patients (health versus disorder);
5. Different interviewing techniques (''anamnesis'' versus ''listening'');
6. Anxiety among pediatricians in dealing with the emotional problems of children and their families;
7. Transference and countertransference issues;

8. Time constraints in both pediatric rotation training schedules and inpatient load;
9. Financial considerations, including inadequate funding for child psychiatry consultation-liaison services in pediatrics (many, if not most, services are simply reimbursed on a fee-for-service basis);
10. Ambivalent support for the concept of coordinated multidisciplinary care for the whole child and his or her family;
11. Limited opportunities for continuity of care in pediatric training;
12. Compartmentalized, disease-oriented research rather than collaborative biopsychosocial research;
13. Inadequate outcome studies.

None of these impediments is irremediable. With positive motivation and cooperation among all the disciplines involved, one should expect to have a thriving child and adolescent psychiatric consultation-liaison service in pediatrics (Lewis and Vitulano, 1988).

RESEARCH DIRECTIONS

Future national health policies and plans may result in an increased role for child psychiatry consultation in pediatrics. Furthermore, advances in pediatric medical knowledge and technology may lead to growth in child psychiatric consultation and liaison in the near future. Bone marrow and solid organ transplantation, neonatal and pediatric intensive care, and prolonged survival from cancer, cystic fibrosis, chronic renal disease, and other once fatal pediatric conditions not only illustrate the effects of technology on pediatrics but also identify new regions of pediatrics in which the expertise of the consultation-liaison child psychiatrist is relevant.

Increased awareness about the coexistence of psychiatric and medical problems in pediatric patients has contributed to the development of pediatric medical-psychiatric units (Fritz, 1990; Sexson and Kahan, 1991; Steiner et al., 1993) and triple-board programs, which prepare physicians to be board eligible in pediatrics, general psychiatry, and child and adolescent psychiatry. However, the role of the consultation-liaison child psychiatrist in this setting, as well as in the general pediatric setting, continues to need clarification (Fritz, 1990).

Problems of training, funding, and organization continuously need to be addressed, particularly in the changing health care environment. New ethical and legal issues continue to arise and need to be considered as well. And perhaps most importantly, the design of research projects with clear short-term and long-term outcome measures (e.g., hospital length of stay, improved compliance with medical care, decreased utilization of medical services, improved functioning, or improved quality of life) are needed to assess the efficacy and cost-effectiveness of particular psychiatric consultation-liaison interventions (Shugart, 1991).

References

Anders TF: Child psychiatry and pediatrics: The state of the relationship. *Pediatrics* 60:616–620, 1977.

Anders TF, Niehans M: Promoting the alliance between pediatrics and child psychiatry. In: Sherman M (ed): *Pediatric Consultation-Liaison (Psychiatric Clinics of North America)*. Philadelphia, Saunders, 1982, pp. 241–258.

Atkins DM, Patenaude AF: Psychosocial preparation and follow-up for pediatric bone marrow transplant patients. *Am J Orthopsychiatry* 57:246–252, 1987.

Black D, McFadyen A, Broster G: Development of a psychiatric liaison service. *Arch Dis Child* 65:1373–1375, 1990.

Burket RC, Hodgin JD: Pediatricians' perceptions of child psychiatry consultations. *Psychosomatics* 34(5):402–408, 1993.

Cadman D, Boyle M, Szatmari P, et al: Chronic illness, disability, and mental and social well-being: Findings of the Ontario Child Health Study. *Pediatrics* 79:805–813, 1987.

Cardona L: Behavioral approaches in the pediatric patient to pain and anxiety. In: Lewis M, King R (eds): *Consultation-Liaison in Pediatrics (Child and Adolescent Psychiatric Clinics of North America)*. Philadelphia, Saunders, 1994, pp. 449–464.

DeLeo JH: *Child Development Analysis*. New York, Brunner/Mazel, 1977.

Eisenberg L: The relationship between psychiatry and pediatrics: A disputatious view. *Pediatrics* 39:645–647, 1967.

Fritz GK: Consultation-liaison in child psychiatry and the evolution of pediatric psychiatry. *Psychosomatics* 31(1):85–90, 1990.

Fritz GK, Bergman AS: Child psychiatrists seen through the pediatricians' eyes: Results of a national survey. *J Am Acad Child Psychiatry* 24:81–86, 1985.

Green W: Pharmacological approaches in the pediatric patient to pain and anxiety. In: Lewis M, King R (eds): *Consultation-Liaison in Pediatrics (Child and Adolescent Psychiatric Clinics of North America)*. Philadelphia, Saunders, 1994, pp. 465–483.

Jellinek MS: The present status of child psychiatry in pediatrics. *N Engl J Med* 306:1227–1230, 1982.

Kanner L: The development and present status of psychiatry in pediatrics. *J Pediatr* 11:418–435, 1937.

King RA, Lewis M: The difficult child. In: Lewis M, King RA (eds): *Consultation-Liaison in Pediatrics (Child and Adolescent Psychiatric Clinics of North America)*. Philadelphia, Saunders, 1994, pp. 531–541.

Knobloch H, Stevens F, Malone AF: *Manual of Developmental Diagnosis*. New York, Harper & Row, 1980.

Lawrence J, Adler R: Childhood through the eyes of child psychiatrists and pediatricians. *Aust NZ J Psychiatry* 26:82–90, 1992.

Leslie SA: Paediatric liaison. *Arch Dis Child* 67:1046–1049, 1992.

Lewandowski LA, Baranoski MV: Psychologic aspects of trauma. In: Lewis M, King RA (eds): *Consultation-Liaison in Pediatrics (Child and Adolescent Psychiatric Clinics of North America)*. Philadelphia, Saunders, 1994, pp. 513–529.

Lewis M: The management of parents of acutely ill children in the hospital. *Am J Orthopsychiatry* 32:60, 1962. (Abstracted in *Psychosomatics* 3:491, 1962.)

Lewis M (ed): *Child and Adolescent Psychiatry. A Comprehensive Textbook*. Baltimore, Williams & Wilkins, 1991.

Lewis M (ed): Psychiatric assessment of infants, children and adolescents. In: *Child and Adolescent Psychiatry. A Comprehensive Textbook*. Baltimore, Williams & Wilkins, 1991, pp. 447–463.

Lewis M: Chronic illness as a psychological risk factor in children. In: Carey W, McDevitt S (eds): *Individual Differences as Risk Factors for the Mental Health of Children*. New York, Brunner/Mazel, 1994a, pp. 103–112.

Lewis M: Consultation process in child and adolescent psychiatric consultation-liaison in pediatrics. In: Lewis M, King R (eds): *Consultation-Liaison in Pediatrics (Child and Adolescent Psychiatric Clinics of North America)*. Philadelphia, Saunders, 1994b, pp. 1–10.

Lewis M, Colletti RB: Child psychiatry teaching in pediatric training. The use of a study group. *Pediatrics* 52:743–745, 1973.

Lewis M, Schonfeld D: The role of child and adolescent psychiatric consultation and liaison in assisting children and their families in dealing with death. In: Lewis M, King R (eds): *Consultation-Liaison in Pediatrics (Child and Adolescent Psychiatric Clinics of North America)*. Philadelphia, Saunders, 1994, pp. 613–627.

Lewis M, Vitulano LA: Child and adolescent psychiatry consultation-liaison services in pediatrics: What messages are being conveyed? *J Dev Behav Pediatr* 9:388–390, 1988.

Lewis M, Volkmar F: *Clinical Aspects of Child and Adolescent Development* (3rd ed). Philadelphia, Lea & Febiger, 1990.

Lourie RR: The teaching of child psychiatry in pediatrics. *J Am Acad Child Psychiatry* 1:477–489, 1962.

Oke S, Mayer R: Referrals to child psychiatry—A survey of staff attitudes. *Arch Dis Child* 66:862–865, 1991.

Rothenberg MB: Child psychiatry-pediatric consultation liaison services in the hospital setting: A review. *Gen Hosp Psychiatry* 1:281–286, 1979.

Senn MJE: Relationship of pediatrics and psychiatry. *Am J Dis Child* 711:537–549, 1946.

Senn MJE: Anticipatory guidance of the pregnant woman and her husband for their roles as parents. In: *Problems of Early Infancy (Transactions of the First Conference)*. New York, Josiah Macy, Jr. Foundation, 1947, pp. 11–16.

Sexson SB, Kahan BB: Organization and development of pediatric medical-psychiatric units. *Gen Hosp Psychiatry* 13:296–304, 1991.

Shugart MA: Child psychiatry consultations to pediatric inpatients: A literature review. *Gen Hosp Psychiatry* 13:325–336, 1991.

Steiner H, Fritz GK, Mrazek D, et al: Pediatric and psychiatric comorbidity. Part I: The future of consultation-liaison psychiatry. *Psychosomatics* 34(2):107–111, 1993.

Wright HH, Eaton JS, Butterfield PT, et al: Financing of child psychiatry pediatric consultation-liaison programs. *J Dev Behav Pediatr* 8:221–226, 1987.

91 COLLABORATION BETWEEN CHILD PSYCHIATRISTS AND PEDIATRICIANS IN PRACTICE

Richard H. Granger, M.D., and Elsa L. Stone, M.D.

Nowhere in the life span is the bond between psyche and soma closer than it is in infancy and childhood. Because of this, adequate and responsible health care for children demands close collaboration between pediatrics and child psychiatry. However, the two fields have developed from different roots and along different paths, and the relationship between them has been stormy and ambivalent from the outset. Interestingly, the ambivalence has slowly swung from pediatricians' fears that the child psychiatrists were invading their territory (Brenneman, 1931) to the more recent fears of child psychiatrists that behavioral pediatricians are threatening their turf (Work, 1989). The truth, as usual, is somewhere in between.

The long-term discomfort and arms-length interaction between the two fields has been most unfortunate in its adverse effect on the care of children. The straight physical-organic health care of children (both ambulatory and inpatient) has been inadequately informed by knowledge and skills from the mental health fields, although it has been repeatedly demonstrated that such knowledge and skills can decrease pain, suffering, and time of recovery from injury and illness and can therefore improve outcomes (Granger, 1990). At the same time, the care of children with all kinds of psychological or developmental problems is often begun too late or not at all because of difficulties in the referral process. Even a relatively neutral area like the development of first-rate child care facilities for young children has suffered because pediatricians and child mental health workers have all too seldom worked together to develop facilities that would address all aspects of care—accident and illness protection as well as cognitive, social, and psychological development.

Those who write about these issues suggest that (in addition to time constraints and financial considerations) differences in personality and temperament, in training, in theoretical framework, and in therapeutic approach between the practitioners of the two fields mark and perpetuate the tensions between them (Greene, 1984; Lewis and Vitulano, 1988; Work, 1989). There is, as always, some ground for these beliefs, but the arguments as presented are often self-serving and usually ignore the fact that there are, in both fields, individuals with a wide spectrum of personalities, training, understanding, and approach to children and families. Whatever the truth, there has been little attempt to go beyond the perceived differences to find the common ground that might serve the attempts of both groups to improve the welfare of children. It is the purpose of this chapter to suggest to both professions areas in which their joint work is crucial to the well-being of children and ways in which that joint work may be achieved.

BACKGROUND

Collaboration is most commonly thought of as occurring around the needs of individual children and families in psychological distress. This is not a small group. Although earlier surveys suggested much smaller numbers, in the last 20 years increasing numbers of studies have indicated that 12–15% of children are in need of direct, intensive mental health services, and that 20–40% could benefit from services that were at least informed by knowledge and skills from the mental health fields (Garralda and Bailey, 1989; Starfield et al., 1980, 1984; Sturner et al., 1980). In the socioeconomically high-risk populations commonly seen in inner city hospitals and clinics and in other areas where poverty, broken families, and drug use are common, it is likely that developmentally based mental health services are needed by 100% of the children. The increase is due partly to demographic changes, such as the increasing percentage of single-parent, poor, minority families; the huge increase in drug abuse; and the increased mobility of the population. The increase is also due to increased sophistication on the part of those performing the surveys in the recognition of such problems in children. It is of note that surveys by pediatric professionals have begun to match those of mental health professionals in this respect (Garralda and Bailey, 1989; Starfield et al., 1980, 1984; Sturner et al., 1980).

Emotionally disturbed or developmentally aberrant children are not the only group around whom collaboration is needed. Chronically ill children, children with life-threatening injuries and illnesses, and children with psychosomatic illness also benefit from care that is offered collaboratively by health and mental health resources. And, as suggested above, there are many child care environments—both health care and general care environments—that would be better for children if they were planned collaboratively by the same groups. While this is already happening in some areas and in some institutions, it is still far from the norm.

PROBLEMS

A major issue seems to be a failure of communication. Both the willingness and the vocabulary to facilitate mutual understanding are often missing on both sides of the interface. Potential interchanges bog down in stereotypes and expectations on both sides that are neither reasonable nor based on any understanding of the other side's problems and capabilities. Pediatricians and psychiatrists seem, rather, to expect criticism from each other, and communications seem more aimed at deflecting that criticism than at reaching common ground. The most commonly cited stereotypes suggest that pediatricians are more concrete, more goal oriented, and more comfortable with quick fixes and short interventions, and less interested in family dynamics issues. They also suggest that psychiatrists are more contemplative, theoretical, and comfortable with uncertain and slower progress and more in touch with their own feelings and reactions to patients. These stereotypes, presented in this way, present antithetical portraits and almost guarantee that personnel on each side will not be able to work together. While there are good reasons to believe that these stereotypes are not all smoke, it is important to remember that stereotypes are essentially descriptions of a mean and that they do not, in fact, describe any individual satisfactorily. There is a great variety in both professions, and each side needs to understand the individual(s) with whom he or she is working, rather than trying to respond to the stereotype.

The psychiatrist needs to understand that an increasing number of pediatricians are interested in and have had some training in the psychological and developmental aspects of pediatric care (Zebal and Friedman, 1984). More and more pediatric departments now include in their training programs personnel who are trained in mental health disciplines. Although *behavioral pediatrics* is now a term in general use and suggests the application of behavioral modification techniques as the treatment of choice, it is not true that most or all pediatricians interested in families and development teach or practice this sort of work. In fact, the majority of programs still emphasize the existence of the unconscious and an understanding of its workings based on all the great theoretical frameworks of the last century, Freud as well as Piaget. It is certainly true, given the nature of pediatricians and primary care practice, that pediatricians intervening in psychosocial areas will probably do so in a more action-oriented mode. But this does not mean that they do not understand the rationale of and the need for the slower, deeper pace of dynamically informed psychotherapy.

It may well be true that the majority of pediatric practitioners are not yet very sophisticated in developmental/psychological work, but more and more of them are now learning to incorporate these areas into their practices. The child psychiatrist will have to interact with pediatricians who are at all levels of understanding and interest, and he or she needs to be able to differentiate among them in order to have any chance for collaborative work. Obviously, if the referring pediatrician is neither interested nor knowledgeable about these issues, he or she may not want to participate in any active collaboration. There may be times when this fact is both frustrating and irritating to the child psychiatrist, and when it truly interferes with the ability to do the best possible work. But there is an increasing number of pediatricians who can do so and who want to do so, and they will make collaborative efforts richly rewarding for the child psychiatrist. One finding of many studies is that both child psychiatrists and pediatricians are better able to collaborate with one another when they have been trained in a place where they worked with trainees and professionals in the other discipline (Bergman and Fritz, 1985).

The pediatrician has often known the child and family for many years—not infrequently from birth—and has both background information and a long-term overview that can illuminate family dynamics, motivations to treatment, likelihood of continuation, and treatment success. The relationship is complicated in that the pediatrician may have a closer alliance with the parents than with the child, and the child psychiatrist may need to understand the available information in that context.

THE NATURE OF COLLABORATION

There are several ways in which pediatricians and child psychiatrists may become involved in a working relationship around a case. First, the most classic mode is the referral by a pediatrician directly to a child psychiatrist of a child and family that he or she feels to be in trouble. Second, child psychiatrists may have cases referred to them by other sources—parents or relatives, schools, community agencies, lawyers—with (or sometimes without) the knowledge of the pediatrician. Third, many pediatricians maintain some ongoing contact with one or more child psychiatrists around cases in their practices that manifest emotional or developmental problems in the context of acute or chronic serious disease. Each of these referral modes is likely to bring about a different type of collaboration.

Referral by Pediatricians

In the first mode the pediatrician essentially indicates his or her confidence in the child psychiatrist by asking him or her to take the case on for evaluation and treatment. Sometimes the family will be well prepared for the referral, and at other times they will not be. Sometimes the referral will be both thoughtful and appropriate, and at other times it will seem more like an impulsive rejection of the child and family by the pediatrician. This will depend both on the sophistication of the pediatrician and on the anxiety level of the parents. The pediatrician may have made more effort to prepare the family than is evident on their first visit, and the psychiatrist should withhold judgment on this issue. It is important for the child psychiatrist to remember that the pediatrician is usually asking him or her to share the burden of managing what has become, for the pediatrician, a difficult and problematic family and/or child. At the very least, collegiality suggests that the psychiatrist try to sort these factors out on behalf of both the patients and the pediatrician, rather than just abandoning them in turn.

For many pediatricians the process of assessing the mental health needs of a child and family is a difficult one, and the act of suggesting and making a referral often puts a strain on the pediatrician-family relationship. Although some parents initiate this process themselves, the great majority of them are still strongly ensconced in some level of denial and are resentful of the pediatrician's intervention. The child psychiatrist can help strengthen the pediatrician-family relationship by the way in which he or she supports the actions of the pediatrician and encourages and facilitates the family's maintenance of close ties with the pediatrician. Child guidance agencies often do this quite poorly. By the agency's refusal to communicate with the pediatrician, they give the family a message about the pediatrician that is, at the very least, ambiguous and ambivalent. Sometimes this results in the family's leaving the pediatrician, but at other times the ongoing tie to the pediatrician is stronger than the developing tie to the mental health agency, and the result is the shortening or interruption of treatment. The private child psychiatrist should be aware of all the possibilities and dangers in these dynamics and should act accordingly. The child will certainly continue to need access to ongoing health supervision and illness treatment, and it is not likely to be desirable that such access be blocked or changed in the middle of psychiatric treatment. One way the psychiatrist can help in this process is by providing regular and periodic feedback to the pediatrician about the status and progress of treatment. He or she is likely to get useful feedback from the pediatrician in turn about new or ongoing illnesses or complaints. Especially if the family has more than one child, the pediatrician is likely to have continuing contact with the family in a way that can provide important information for the therapist.

There is no suggestion in this that confidentiality should be breached. However, over the years a dangerous mystique has arisen about this issue. It certainly is no longer true that most patients wish to hide all evidence of their being in treatment or that they want no communication to occur between the therapist and other important caretakers in the child's life. In the authors' experience most families, if asked, encourage ongoing contact between the child psychiatrist and the pediatrician. There is no need for the therapist to provide the pediatrician with details of dynamics or treatment process. He or she should merely make a brief phone call or provide a short note about the continuing nature of the treatment.

In regard to this mode of referral, it is important to note that many pediatricians choose to refer many kinds of cases to mental health professionals other than psychiatrists—social workers, psychologists, even other psychologically oriented pediatricians. A major reason for this is the pediatricians' belief that child psychiatrists are less available, less responsive, and less communicative than these other professionals. But there is also evidence that pediatricians often do not understand what types of problems child psychiatrists are trained to deal with (Fritz and Bergman, 1985).

Referral by Other Sources

When the referral comes to the child psychiatrist from a source other than the pediatrician, the child psychiatrist may assume that the pediatrician does not know about the problem or is not interested in it. This may sometimes be true, but it is not a safe or useful conclusion. In these cases, just as in those above, the therapist should ask for permission to communicate directly with the pediatrician. If the family really does not want such communication they will not hesitate to say so. However, even in these cases it is likely that the pediatrician may have a great deal of information that will be both useful and germane to the evaluation and treatment process. Occasionally the family may want to exclude the pediatrician specifically because he or she does know a great deal about the family, and the family wants an unbiased, "blind" opinion about the problem from the psychiatrist. This dynamic is seldom useful to the child, and the psychiatrist may want to examine his or her options in these cases. Finally, inasmuch as the pediatrician has ongoing supervision of the health of the child, he or she may be able to provide some insights into other areas in the child's life about which neither the child nor the parents may be forthcoming.

Ongoing Consultation with Pediatricians

In the course of busy ambulatory practice, pediatricians assume the management of many children with difficult and complicated illnesses and difficult and complicated families and psychosocial situations. Studies of pediatric primary care practices (Goldberg et al., 1984; Starfield et al., 1980, 1984; Sturner et al., 1980) reveal that between a fourth and a half of all well-child visits to pediatricians revolve primarily around psychosocial issues. The pediatrician may choose to ignore all the signs and symptoms involved in this, but he or she will almost certainly need and want to manage some of them more directly. In doing this, pediatricians often want consultation from a mental health colleague, and many of them have developed some ongoing pattern of presenting such issues to a child psychiatrist in their area—if they are lucky enough to have one. This consultation may take the form of telephone calls or of more formalized meetings. It may be seen as an intrusion by the psychiatrist, but this type of contact is useful in helping the pediatrician assess the kind of help available from the mental health field, and from individual colleagues in particular. It is an important and valuable service that the child psychiatrist would do well to foster in his or her community. Such initial calls often lead to referrals for more extensive evaluation and treatment, but even if they do not, they create a goodwill that cannot be overestimated. The need for such consultation is especially clear and acute around emergency situations such as suicide attempts, but it is equally important for less dangerous and acute problems as well.

There is now, in some communities, a specialized form of this type of collaboration that has been in place for varying periods of time (Granger, 1985; Solnit, 1968a, 1968b). In this model a group of pediatricians meets regularly with one or two child psychiatrists to discuss difficult cases from the pediatricians' practices. The pediatricians present the cases to the group, and the group discusses them under the leadership of the psychiatrist and, perhaps, a senior pediatric colleague as well. The ongoing nature of the group provides more benefit for its members than just the case discussions themselves. The members, pediatricians and psychiatrists alike, come to see the group as a support in the continuing struggle against the vicissitudes of practice. Pediatric members of the group unquestionably develop both knowledge and skills in the management of psychological and developmental problems in their practices. Psychiatrists often use the process to keep up with the changing biological factors in pediatric practice, many of which impinge on the etiology and treatment of psychological disease. In fact, studies in the educational field suggest that the only mode of continuing education that actually results in changed behavior among practitioners is the one in which they interact around cases from their own practices in a continuing manner.

One common ground for collaborative work between pediatricians and child psychiatrists is the use of the concept of temperament in pediatric practice (Carey, 1986, 1994; Chess and Thomas, 1986). Temperament measurements can be useful, for example, in educational discussions with parents as well as in formulating first-time intervention measures when an interference with the "goodness of fit" has given rise to behavioral problems in the child (Cameron et al., 1994; see also Chapter 13). The concept of temperament has also proven useful in the collaborative care of certain children with chronic illness (Lewis, 1994) and with the uninfected child in an HIV-affected family (Lewis, 1995).

The collaborative relationship also opens the door for the possibilities of joint research between child psychiatrists and pediatricians. Some of the most interesting aspects of clinical case management come out of such collaborations. And there is ample room in the process—especially in the group process outlined above—for more definitive intervention research in pediatric practice settings. Such research can be set up to conform with good psychological practice and can be carried out in multiple practice settings in such a way as to offer truly useful information on the possibilities of what might be called preventive mental health.

CASE ILLUSTRATION

Mr. and Mrs. George, a couple in their late 30s, have two children, John, age 9 years, and David, age 6 years. From birth David had numerous illnesses, and when sick he was always loud, irritable, and inconsolable. Despite his robust appearance and normal development, Mrs. George was convinced there was something seriously wrong with him. The pediatrician, Dr. Jones, performed an immune evaluation, which was normal, and resisted pressure to be more aggressive. When David was 2 years old the frequency of his illnesses subsided, but the complaints about him did not. Mrs. George wanted tight control of her children, and David resisted. When David was 3½ Mrs. George described him as "fresh" and felt her household was ruled by his temper.

Shortly after this he fell from his bicycle and sustained a facial injury with temporary paralysis of his lower facial nerve. At age 4½ he developed colitis secondary to antibiotic therapy for otitis. From this point on, crampy abdominal pain became the focus and currency of communication between mother and child. Organic disease was present: Toxin from *Clostridium difficile* was found on several occasions. But the pain often occurred without signs of active disease and even despite findings of a normal colon on examination. Three months following the onset of the abdominal pain, the mother became willing to discuss the emotional component with the pediatrician. She was distressed because David had said he hated her and "when I grow up I am going to get a knife and kill you." She did not believe her husband would be willing to get help for David, but he proved very willing to talk to the pediatrician about David.

Mr. George was mostly concerned with the physical nature of David's illness, but Mrs. George felt that David had ruined her life. Although originally wanting many children, she had begun to refuse to have sexual relations with her husband when David was young because David was "so tough." When David was 2, she had her tubes tied. She felt she should be able to produce perfect children; she believed her first child was perfect, and David was her failure. She also believed that David was just like her—testing, challenging, being difficult.

The parents agreed to a psychiatrically oriented developmental assessment of David. He was found to be a bright, competent boy who desperately felt the need to be in control of all things and who had no ability to get help from others when things were out of control, as when he was sick. He had very little ability to express his feelings other than by outbursts of anger, and the recommendation was that he undergo psychotherapy.

The feedback session for the parents was held jointly by the developmentalist and the pediatrician. Throughout the discussion of the results, the mother fumed and said very little. The father remained calm but inscrutable. The pediatrician was certain they would be looking for a new pediatrician. Surprisingly, the next day the mother phoned the pediatrician to apologize for her behavior and to request the name of a therapist for David. Her husband had told her that the description he had heard of David was exactly like his image of her, and he did not want his son to have the same difficulties as an adult that she had.

Thus, David began to work with Dr. Morgan, a child psychiatrist. During the treatment the mother has been helped by Dr. Morgan to confront the pediatrician, Dr. Jones, with the mother's anger about the diagnosis and management of David's illness. She has also been helped to enter psychotherapy for herself. David's behavior has improved significantly, and he is finally venting his rage about all that was done to him.

As David became less of a problem, Mrs. George brought John to Dr. Jones with complaints of headache that Mrs. George believed to be the result of an osteoma of the skull. She said that she had had an osteoid osteoma of the skull during adolescence that had caused her to have headaches, especially with activity, and that had to be removed. She claimed to have had a similar tumor 3 years previously in another area of the skull, which was also removed. She believed this to have been a large growth, which if unremoved was about to cause her to have seizures. She was terrified of hospitals and had a hard time coping with this. John was convinced she was going to die and spent several sessions with Dr. Jones discussing his feelings. Dr. Jones was unable to support Mrs. George's suspicion on clinical examination of John or on skull film. Discussion with the neurosurgeon who removed the second lesion from Mrs. George revealed that the lesion had actually been very small, and he believed that it was asymptomatic, nonfamilial, and at no time likely to have caused seizures.

Dr. Jones and Dr. Morgan are in close contact. It is apparent that physical illness is somehow important for Mrs. George and that she is under considerable stress at this point. David has begun with some abdominal pain again, but John's headaches, if they ever existed, seem no longer to be a concern. Knowledge that Mrs. George is apparently more upset provides a cogent explanation for David's abdominal pain and allows Dr. Jones to be more conservative in its management. Conversely, knowledge of Mrs. George's problem with headaches and osteomas—real and imagined—opens new areas of exploration for Dr. Morgan and for Mrs. George's therapist as well.

Comment

Physical illness is often accompanied by emotional stress; emotional stress increases the propensity for physical illness. In susceptible families these facts can create a spiraling problem of increasing magnitude. In such families, focusing on only one side of the equation—either side—rarely produces a satisfactory solution to a family's needs. Nowhere is there a greater need for the professionals to understand the multidetermined interactions of the whole family constellation and to adhere to the concept of treating the whole child. Managing both the physical and the psychological needs of the child and family most often requires collaboration between and among professionals, and this in turn necessitates close communication between child psychiatrist and pediatrician.

SUMMARY

Given the differences between their disciplines, pediatricians and child psychiatrists have not up to now found it easy to collaborate. However, more and more of them are managing to do it and, as they get more experienced at the process, are finding it a rewarding way to manage their professional lives. The process results in improvement in the management of health care for children that neither discipline can achieve alone. It can only be hoped that more and more pediatricians and child psychiatrists will discover the satisfactions and rewards of true collaboration.

References

Bergman AS, Fritz GK: Pediatricians and mental health professionals: Patterns of collaboration and utilization. *Am J Dis Child* 139:155, 1985.

Brenneman J: The menace of psychiatry. *Am J Dis Child* 42:376, 1931.

Cameron JR, Rice D, Hansen R, et al: Developing temperament guidance programs within pediatric practice. In: Carey WB, McDevitt SC (eds): *Prevention and Early Intervention*. New York, Brunner/Mazel, 1994, pp. 226–336.

Carey WB: Temperament in pediatric practice. In: Chess S, Thomas A (eds): *Temperament in Clinical Practice*. New York, Guilford, 1986, pp. 218–239.

Carey WB: Specific uses of temperament data in pediatric behavioral interactions. In: Carey WB, McDevitt SC (eds): *Prevention and Early Intervention. Individual Differences as Risk Factors for the Mental Health of Children*. New York, Brunner/Mazel, 1994, pp. 215–225.

Chess S, Thomas S: *Temperament in Clinical Practice*. New York, Guilford, 1986.

Fritz GK, Bergman AS: Child psychiatrists seen through pediatricians' eyes: Results of a national survey. *J Am Acad Child Psychiatry* 24:81, 1985.

Garralda ME, Bailey D: Psychiatric disorders in general paediatric referrals. *Arch Dis Child* 64:1727, 1989.

Goldberg ID, Roghmann KJ, McInerny TK, et al: Medical health problems among children seen in pediatric practice: Prevalence and management. *Pediatrics* 73:278, 1984.

Granger RH: One to six: The pediatrician's role in mastery and individuation. In: Green M (ed): *The Psychosocial Aspects of the Family: The New Pediatrics*. Lexington, MA, DC Heath, 1985, p. 65.

Granger RH: The psychological aspects of physical trauma. In: Touloukian R (ed): *Pediatric Trauma* (2nd ed). St. Louis, Mosby, 1990, p. 90.

Greene CM: Mutual collaboration between child psychiatry and pediatrics: Resistances and facilitation. *J Dev Behav Pediatr* 5:315, 1984.

Lewis M: The special case of the uninfected child in the HIV-affected family. In: Geballe S, Gruendel J, Andiman W (eds): *Forgotten Children of the AIDS Epidemic*. New Haven, Yale University Press, 1985, pp. 50–63.

Lewis ML, Vitulano LA: Child and adolescent psychiatry consultation-liaison services in pediatrics: What messages are being conveyed? *J Dev Behav Pediatr* 9:388, 1988.

Solnit AJ: Child analysis and paediatrics: Collaborative interests. *Int J Psychoanal* 49:280, 1968a.

Solnit AJ: Eight pediatricians and a child psychiatrist. In: Bibring GL (ed): *The Teaching of Dynamic Psychiatry*. New York, International Universities Press, 1968b, p. 158.

Starfield B, Gross E, Wood M, et al: Psychosocial and psychosomatic diagnoses in primary care of children. *Pediatrics* 66:159, 1980.

Starfield B, Katz H, Gabriel A, et al: Morbidity in childhood: A longitudinal view. *N Engl J Med* 310:824, 1984.

Sturner RS, Granger RH, Ferholt JB, et al: The routine "well child" examination. *Clin Pediatr* 19:251, 1980.

Work NH: The "menace of psychiatry" revisited: The evolving relationship between pediatrics and child psychiatry. *Psychosomatics* 30:86, 1989.

Zebal BH, Friedman SB: A nationwide survey of behavioral pediatric residency training. *J Dev Behav Pediatr* 5:331, 1984.

92 THE CHILD'S COGNITIVE UNDERSTANDING OF ILLNESS

David J. Schonfeld, M.D.

Physicians realize how difficult it is to provide adequate and effective explanations of illness and proposed treatment to their adult patients. Medical education has left the physician with a qualitatively different way of understanding illness, both physical and mental, that is beyond the grasp of the lay public. Explanations must be translated by the physician so that the patient can understand. This is not a simple process of merely replacing unfamiliar medical terminology with words from the patient's own vocabulary, but often involves the much more difficult task of restructuring the explanation to comply with a conceptual framework that is comprehensible to the patient. When the patient is a child, the clinician is confronted with a broad range of conceptual frameworks, some of which may initially seem idiosyncratic. The challenge of ensuring effective communication therefore becomes far greater, but is of no less importance.

The prospect of determining each child's unique conceptual framework for understanding illness may at first seem difficult. Fortunately, systematic research has been conducted that provides important insights into the developmental process by which children obtain an understanding of the fundamental concepts of physical illness, such as causality, prevention, and treatment. These cognitive-developmental studies (Burbach and Peterson, 1986) demonstrate that there is a systematic and predictable sequence by which children acquire these concepts to explain both general physical illness, as well as specific conditions such as AIDS (Schonfeld et al., 1993). This developmental process is comparable to that of the acquisition of causal understanding as described by Piaget (Piaget, 1929). According to Piaget's model (Brewster, 1982; Ginsburg and Opper, 1969; Perrin and Gerrity, 1981; Piaget and Innhelder, 1969), as the result of biologic maturation and the accumulation of experience, the child progresses through four sequential stages of cognitive development: the sensorimotor period (infancy), the preoperational period (early childhood, roughly 2–7 years), the concrete operational period (middle to late childhood, roughly 7–11 years), and the formal operational period (adolescence to adulthood). Although experience has shown that children often progress through these stages at a faster rate than was initially predicted by Piaget, the nature and sequence of these stages, described by Piaget as invariate, have been confirmed by extensive research. Children in the preoperational period rely on direct personal experiences and have little ability to generalize to related situations or to appreciate multiple aspects of one situation; their thought processes tend to be empirical rather than logical. Later stages involve an increasing ability to utilize logical thought processes, with abstract thought attained only during the formal operational period. Later stages also are characterized by the child's increasing ability to differentiate self from others and to distinguish internal wishes, needs, and thoughts from the realities of the external world.

Efforts to promote the child's adjustment to physical illness and its treatment require an appreciation of this developmental process. Effective support and assistance is predicated on an understanding of not only the child's feelings but also the child's beliefs about being ill (Bibace and Walsh, 1980). For example, it is often assumed that children fear blood drawing because of the pain associated with the procedure, and reassurances thereby take the form of "It will only hurt a little." In reality, the child's feeling of fear may be related to a belief that the phlebotomist will remove too much blood and the child will die (Licamele, 1987). In this situation the reassurances offered will be ineffective, and the child will be left to deal, alone, with a terrifying misconception about the treatment process. Efforts to facilitate the child's adjustment to physical illness and its treatment must therefore be based on an appreciation of the child's knowledge of the relevant concepts of illness. Otherwise the ill child will be left, as depicted by Anna Freud, "to submit uncomprehendingly, helplessly and passively" to both the illness and the treatment process (Freud, 1977, p. 2).

The child's knowledge and understanding of the concepts of illness can thereby be viewed as vital determinants of the child's adjustment to illness. The focus of this chapter is to review what is known of the developmental process by which children acquire an understanding of the concepts related to illness and the implications of this knowledge for clinicians.

PRIOR RESEARCH

On the basis of a review of the cognitive-developmental literature on children's concepts of physical illness, Burbach and Peterson (1986) concluded that there exists a positive relationship between the level of understanding of the concepts of illness and the child's chronologic age/cognitive maturity that is consistent with Piaget's theories of cognitive development. Wide variability in children's understanding as a function of age was noted across studies; similar but somewhat lesser variation persisted when analysis was conducted as a function of cognitive-developmental level (frequently measured in terms of Piagetian tasks). Global estimates of a child's cognitive abilities are thereby often inaccurate predictors of the level of understanding of concepts about illness; on

average, the understanding of the causality of illness typically lags behind that of general causality (Perrin and Gerrity, 1981). Children bring their own personal experiences to bear on their understanding of illness; some of these experiences may promote understanding of the concepts for a particular child, whereas others may have been negative experiences that only serve to heighten anxiety and interfere with the acquisition of knowledge. It is not surprising, then, that it is still unclear what role personal experience with illness plays in the process by which children develop an understanding of the concepts of illness (Burbach and Peterson, 1986; Perrin et al., 1991). For this reason, in the sections to follow, the focus is not on what "a typical child" knows or thinks at a particular age. When possible, generalizations about representative age ranges are provided, but the emphasis is on an overview of the process and not a time line. Clinicians are advised not to rely on age-based normative data but to develop instead an appreciation of the process of cognitive development in this area. Simple inquiry into the child's views and understanding will then identify the child's level of comprehension and lead to an appreciation of the child's unique misconceptions and concerns.

Immanent Justice, Guilt, and Shame

With increasing cognitive maturity (and age), children's understanding of the causality of illness increases in a predictable manner. Younger children, lacking an adequate explanation for the cause of illness, are apt to resort to explanations that attribute the cause of illness to immanent justice, "the belief that a form of natural justice can emanate from inanimate objects," wherein misdeeds will be automatically punished. Such a belief leads to the acceptance of personal guilt and shame for the etiology of illness. It is hypothesized that magical thinking and immanent justice concepts are employed by the young child in preference to the concept of chance, thereby allowing the child to retain the illusion of order and personal control in what would otherwise appear to be a random and often unfair world (Wilkinson, 1988, p. 60). Freud also appreciated the child's tendency to assume guilt for personal illness: "[Illness] appears to the child as a confirmation of the belief that wrongdoing, however secretly performed, is open to punishment, and that other, still undetected misdeeds, whether actually carried out or merely contemplated in fantasy, will likewise be followed by retribution of some kind" (Bergmann and Freud, 1965, p. 138). As one 11-year-old boy related about his diagnosis of polio 2 years prior: "I was charged with having polio. I had to plead guilty, and my sentence was life imprisonment in a wheel chair" (Bergmann and Freud, 1965, p. 96).

Research has shown that explanations based on immanent justice are more persistently utilized for ailments for which the child has limited personal experience and for which another explanation is not readily available (Siegal, 1988). With increasing cognitive maturity and with the accumulation of experience with illness, the child will more likely reject the notion that illness and misbehavior are linked, and instead acquire more accurate perceptions of personal control over illness and recovery (Burbach and Peterson, 1986). It is hoped that, by providing the child with more appropriate explanations for the cause of illness, the child will be able to abandon immanent justice explanations at an earlier age (Kister and Patterson, 1980). Such immanent justice explanations can be expected to result in guilt and/or shame, impede competent understanding of the etiology of disease and thereby hinder attempts to promote compliance with preventive health measures and treatment regimens, and impair adjustment and coping to illness of self and significant others. Recently, it has been demonstrated that even preschoolers will dismiss immanent justice as an explanation for familiar ailments with which they have had personal experience (e.g., colds) while retaining this concept in their explanations of causality for ailments with which they are less familiar (e.g., toothaches) (Siegal, 1988). Such findings lend support for the role of personal experience, and indirectly education, in advancing the child's understanding of the causality of illness.

Further Understanding of Illness Causality

As children begin to develop an understanding of the true causes of physical illness, the concept of contagion appears in their explanations for the causality of disease. Younger children (preoperational stage) initially tend to overextend the concept of contagion to include noncontagious illness; the concept is applied most appropriately by children reaching the later stages of cognitive development (concrete and formal operational stages) (Kister and Patterson, 1980; Potter and Roberts, 1984). Yet in appropriate circumstances, proper discriminant application of the concept of contagion is within the grasp of children as young as the preschool level. Siegal (1988) demonstrated that most preschool children in his study (the mean age for study participants was $4^{11}/_{12}$ years) were able to accurately attribute contagion to the common cold and to differentiate this from certain noncontagious ailments (e.g., a scraped knee). As such, it was concluded that knowledge of the causes of illness is within the cognitive grasp of very young children, offering support for the incorporation of causal knowledge into health education efforts for children even at the preschool level.

Subsequent to the acquisition of the knowledge that illness can be contagious, an understanding of the physical process by which this can occur must be developed by the child. Such an understanding typically takes the form of a germ theory. In a study of Scottish nursery children (3–5 years in age), Wilkinson (1987) describes the early stages of children's understanding of the role of germs in the spread of disease. Initially, the child is unfamiliar with the word and will often confuse *germ* with *bug* (and thereby *insect*) in addition to other terms—''I don't know what a germ is but I have heard of a German person.'' They view germs within their own magical and egocentric context: ''Germs are not there all the time. They come when mummies go away.'' And they attempt to draw on concrete experiences to explain what they look like. Many children in Wilkinson's study stated that germs were blue and 1–9 inches in diameter, and although they had not seen one, they claimed ''I think I will see one one day.'' Discussion with parents disclosed that the children were drawing these images from a television commercial for a cleaner wherein hidden imaginary blue germs were destroyed by the application of the product. Little understanding is seen at this age as to how germs are transmitted or cause illness. One mother, attempting to have her son describe the nature of germs, inquired, ''Why are you made to wash your hands before eating?'' His reply illustrated his lack of comprehension: ''So my plate doesn't get dirty.''

Perrin and Gerrity (1981) found that by about 9 or 10 years of age, children generally believe that illness is caused by germs but still have little understanding of how this is accomplished once the germ is internalized. By about 12 or 13 years of age, illness is seen as the result of multiple causes; with this comes an appreciation of the role of host factors and the beginning of an understanding of the subtle interactions between host and agent in the causality of disease and the recovery from illness. It is therefore not until at least adolescence that the child can associate apparently unrelated symptoms (e.g., headache and rash) and view them as belonging to one illness, and can identify and relate the various phases of an illness into a coherent progression of one disease process. During the formal operational period, children also develop an increased understanding of their bodies, which allows an appreciation of internal physiologic structures and functions that is demonstrated in the emergence of physiologic explanations for the causality of illness in early adolescence (Bibace and Walsh, 1980). Only at this stage, with this improved understanding of internal physiology and the causality of illness, can the child be expected to comprehend many of the simplest treatment regimens that adults take for granted, such as the use of oral antibiotics to treat an ear infection or the use of injections of insulin in diabetes.

IMPLICATIONS

Knowledge of what children understand about illness and its treatment at various stages of cognitive development has practical implica-tions for child psychiatry consultations to clinicians. It provides a framework for offering guidance on how to approach discussions about illness and its treatment with children, both to advance their understanding and coping skills and to promote their attainment of an active role in the decision-making process for their health care. As children acquire increasing knowledge about the concepts related to illness and the cognitive skills to process this information, they become more able to accurately report symptoms of illness, comply with the treatment regimens prescribed, adjust to the illness and its treatment, and make informed decisions regarding preventive health measures.

The Child's Ability to Report Symptoms

Young children, with their immature understanding of disease processes, may fail to report important symptoms of serious illness. This may be due, in part, to a lack of sensitivity to the relevant internal cues and objective signs of even serious illness (Pidgeon, 1985). But even when aware of their symptoms, egocentrism and magical thinking may lead them to withhold this information from caregivers, preferring instead to rely on internal mechanisms of dealing with the illness. They may assume that if they do not wish to be ill, then they will not be ill; they may worry that the mere vocalization of their concerns may be sufficient to bring their fears to reality. Children who persist with immanent justice explanations for the causality of illness may also be disinclined to voice their symptoms out of shame or fear of retribution. These issues are particularly relevant for children with chronic illnesses that require prompt recognition and management of often subtle internal symptoms, such as hypoglycemia in the child with diabetes.

The Child's Compliance with Treatment

Attempts to communicate effectively with children about illness and its treatment will also maximize efforts to enlist the child's cooperation in the treatment process. Such efforts should maintain as a long-term goal the child's attainment of an active role in the decision-making process in the child's own health care. In times of frustration it is easy to lose sight of this goal, such as when a child with asthma is noncompliant with treatment and is warned, ''If you don't take your medicine, you'll have to go to the emergency room and get a needle,'' but is not provided with a developmentally appropriate explanation of the treatment process. Parents will need help in appreciating that such threats may yield temporary compliance, but at the expense of reinforcing maladaptive concepts of illness, that may, in the long run, lead to decreased compliance. This approach might be justifiable if it were shown that the concepts of illness were beyond the grasp of children and that illness in the child could be effectively prevented through compliance with recommendations. Both assumptions are incorrect. First, the preceding discussions illustrate that an understanding of the concepts of illness is possible even in very young children, if given appropriate explanations and provided with constructive learning experiences. Second, even if children were able to fully comply with all the numerous restrictions and requirements placed on them by their parents in the hopes of preventing illness (e.g., to get enough sleep, to eat the right food, to dress correctly), many will still get ill. If the only explanations provided about the causality of illness reinforce immanent justice, then the child is left with no other recourse but to accept self-blame for personal illness. Hospitalization and increasingly invasive medical management, when required, is then not perceived as a result of the natural process of the disease but instead as a personal failure on the part of the child. The child feels he or she has failed and is being punished; in addition to feeling ill and frightened, the child is now apt to feel angry and rejected. As one child remarked about his failure to be discharged from the hospital: ''I did everything the doctors told me to do, and now they won't let me go home.'' He had been told in simple terms what he needed to do to get better, but had not been given explanations that he could understand of how these procedures would influence his illness. After complying fully with the requirements placed on him and failing to become well and be discharged, he was understandably hurt and angry.

The Child's Adjustment to Illness and the Treatment Process

Explanations for children about their illness and treatment should seek not only to achieve compliance but also to promote the child's understanding. The explanations should be presented in a manner that is consistent with the current level of understanding of the child, or perhaps slightly advanced (Bibace and Walsh, 1980; Brewster, 1982). These explanations should aim to replace frightening misconceptions and supply constructive information in a manner that will promote coping and adjustment. This is, of course, an ongoing process. Children need to be questioned about their understanding of the explanations provided, thereby allowing the discussion to become a true dialogue. Vocabulary used should be simple and direct. Indeed, even adult patients misinterpret terminology at a rate that exceeds the expectations of most physicians. In one study of women attending a public health clinic, 80% of patients confused ''anemia'' with ''enema,'' and over 50% defined ''well-nourished'' as ''nervous body'' (Collins, 1955).

When under stress, such as during an acute illness, children often regress in their developmental abilities and are least amenable to techniques to advance their developmental progress. Even in this setting, recognition of children's current level of functioning will still have practical implications for efforts to restructure their thinking and provide support during the illness. For example, when constructing a plan to help control pain for a child in the preoperational period, the connection between the medication taken orally and the relief of the pain can be emphasized, but more concrete measures that will be reassuring to the child (e.g., application of a heating pad for abdominal pain) should also be employed. As much as possible, the use of intramuscular pain medication should be avoided, realizing the child's tendency to associate treatment with punishment and to fail to comprehend the logic of giving a painful intramuscular injection to treat abdominal pain. And in selecting the oral medication to be given, knowledge of the child's cognitive abilities regarding comprehension of quantity and number may have further practical implications; it may be preferable when the dose of pain medication is to be adjusted to give two 15-mg pills instead of one 30-mg pill, or to use elixir instead, because of the even clearer concrete representation of increasing dose with increasing amount (Clark, 1985). Appreciation of children's understanding of their illness and its treatment and knowledge of their cognitive abilities can thereby provide guidance not only in the selection of explanations but also in the selection of the most appropriate techniques for the delivery of health care.

Research also has shown that, parallel to the process of conceptual development wherein children acquire an understanding of the causes of illness, children also develop increasing appreciation for the intent of medical procedures. Brewster (1982) describes three stages in this process: The child initially views the procedures as punishment, is subsequently able to understand the intent of the procedures but feels that the staff will be empathetic only if the child outwardly expresses pain, and, finally, is able to infer both empathy and intention. In order to enlist their cooperation and to decrease their anxiety and fear surrounding the procedures, it is important that children be prepared for procedures with information and explanations that are consistent with their level of understanding of the relevant concepts. Preoperative teaching for the child in the preoperational period, for example, might focus on acquainting the child with what the concrete experiences will be (e.g., what the room will look like, who will be there), whereas preparation for the child in the formal operational period might also include a more detailed discussion of the procedure, including mention of anatomical and physiologic principles within the cognitive grasp of the more mature child (Perrin and Gerrity, 1981).

Programs to prepare children psychologically for procedures have been shown to be effective in helping them cope with the associated anxiety. A recent study (Edwinson, 1988) demonstrated that such programs are effective in reducing anxiety, even in the setting of emergency surgical procedures (e.g., acute appendectomy), when compared with standard, unstructured preoperative preparation. Recent research is also just beginning to empirically demonstrate that preparation programs for hospitalization and medical procedures that are consonant with the child's cognitive-developmental level are more effective in decreasing distress and anxiety in response to procedures when compared to preparations that are not designed with these concepts in mind (Rasnake and Linscheid, 1989).

Preventive Health Education for Children

Health education only at the time of illness or hospitalization may not be the most effective means of advancing the child's understanding of illness. During times of illness, as in other stressful periods, children will often regress in their developmental abilities. At these times they will be least prepared to understand the situation confronting them, least able to benefit from educational efforts to promote this understanding, but most in need of this information to facilitate adjustment and successful coping. This observation provides a strong argument for the need to promote the acquisition of these concepts prior to the time they are needed to deal with acute crisis in the form of illness. Health education efforts, then, should begin when the child is well, with the aim of promoting increased understanding, knowledge, and skills in this area. Recent research has demonstrated that developmentally appropriate health education in elementary school can advance young children's conceptual understanding and factual knowledge of illness (Schonfeld et al., 1995). Children should be taught to do more than ''just say no'' to bad health decisions; they should be helped to understand the rationale behind these choices and to acquire the skills to make informed and responsible health decisions that affect them in the future. For health education to be effective, it must be developmentally based so that discussions coincide with the child's level of understanding.

Physicians should utilize preventive health visits during the pediatric years to educate not only the parents but also the child. Unfortunately, research has shown that little time is spent by the pediatrician during pediatric visits talking directly to the child. In one study of children 4–7 years of age attending private pediatric practices for routine health maintenance visits or visits for minor illness, only about 5% of the discussion during these visits was directed by the physician toward the child. Interviews of the children after the visits illustrated that most of them desired more information about their medical problems; their concerns were well formed and relevant to the reason for the current visit, yet these concerns were not addressed by either the parent or physician. In fact, explanations about treatment and symptoms were not provided to the children in this setting, and the children were treated instead as passive recipients of health care (Perlman and Abramovitch, 1987).

Other studies have shown similarly low rates of communication between physicians and child patients. This is unfortunate, as children are interested in clinical information even at a young age and are capable of comprehending the information if it is presented in an appropriate manner. Pediatricians should take advantage of this opportunity to advance the child's understanding of the concepts of physical illness in a salient and relevant context—that of the child's own medical visit. One reason for this oversight may relate to the observation that pediatricians, and other health care professionals who work with children, are unfamiliar with the developmental stages of children's understanding of illness: ''Professionals do not operate with an intuitive sense about cognitive development. . . .They lack an understanding of the important qualitative differences in the very basic ways in which children at different stages of development see, interpret, and understand the world around them'' (Perrin and Perrin, 1983). A recent study (Lewis et al., 1991) demonstrated that a brief educational intervention targeted to (5- to 15-year-old) children, parents, and physicians can enhance physician-child communication and rapport during pediatric office visits and allow children to take a more active and effective role in their health care.

CONCLUDING REMARKS

The focus of this chapter has been on the cognitive process by which children develop an understanding of their illness and treatment, and on the implications of this for health care professionals. It should be emphasized that such a cognitive-developmental approach to viewing the child's understanding of illness is not in conflict with other theories that aim to explain the child's psychological reaction and behavioral response to the illness experience. Conscious understanding (cognitive factors) is only one component of the child's response to illness. Unconscious developmental fantasies, too, may alter the child's perceptions of the illness and treatment process, despite the presence of mature cognitive abilities. For example, a fear of surgery may be heightened by underlying castration anxiety (Lewis, 1982). Even adolescents who have reached the formal operational stage of cognitive development may still be overwhelmed by anxiety from unconscious developmental conflicts. These conflicts may distort their perceptions and result in misconceptions and fears out of proportion to what would be predicted by a purely cognitive-developmental approach. An integrated approach to viewing the ill child that incorporates both the child's cognitive abilities and an appreciation of the psychological factors pertinent to his or her personality development is therefore likely to yield the most insight into the complex process by which the child comes to understand, accept, and respond to both the illness and treatment process.

Subsequent chapters highlight the child's unique response to specific illnesses and components of the treatment process (such as hospitalization and surgery). An increased appreciation of the stages of children's understanding of illness will allow the physician to communicate more effectively with children, in order to improve their medical care, minimize their anxiety and fear, and promote their adjustment to illness and its treatment. Health care professionals will thus be able to assist the children to acquire the requisite skills to become increasingly active and effective partners in their health care management.

References

Bergmann T, Freud A: *Children in the Hospital.* New York, International Universities Press, 1965.

Bibace R, Walsh M: Development of children's concepts of illness. *Pediatrics* 66:912–917, 1980.

Brewster A: Chronically ill hospitalized children's concepts of their illness. *Pediatrics* 69: 355–362, 1982.

Burbach D, Peterson L: Children's concepts of physical illness: A review and critique of the cognitive-developmental literature. *Health Psychol* 5: 307–325, 1986.

Clark E: Pain assessment, intervention and evaluation. In: Milch R, Freeman A, Clark E (eds): *Palliative Pain and Symptom Management for Children and Adolescents.* Alexandria, VA, Children's Hospice International and Division of Maternal and Child Health, 1985.

Collins G: Do we really advise the patient? *J Fla Med Assoc* 42:111, 1955.

Edwinson M: Psychologic preparation program for children undergoing acute appendectomy. *Pediatrics* 82:30–36, 1988.

Freud A: The role of bodily illness in the mental life of children. In: Eissler R, Freud A, Kris M, et al (eds): *Physical Illness and Handicap in Childhood.* New Haven, CT, Yale University Press, 1977, pp. 1–12.

Ginsburg H, Opper S: *Piaget's Theory of Intellectual Development.* Englewood Cliffs, NJ, Prentice-Hall, 1969.

Kister M, Patterson C: Children's conceptions of the causes of illness: Understanding of contagion and use of immanent justice. *Child Dev* 51:839–846, 1980.

Lewis C, Pantell R, Sharp L: Increasing patient knowledge, satisfaction, and involvement: Randomized trial of a communication intervention. *Pediatrics* 88:351–358, 1991.

Lewis M: *Clinical Aspects of Child Development: An Introductory Synthesis of Developmental Concepts and Clinical Experience* (2nd ed). Philadelphia, Lea & Febiger, 1982.

Licamele W, Goldberg R: Childhood reactions to illness and hospitalization. *Am Fam Physician* 36: 227–232, 1987.

Perlman N, Abramovitch R: Visit to the pediatrician: Children's concerns. *J Pediatr* 110:988–990, 1987.

Perrin E, Gerrity S: There's a demon in your belly: Children's understanding of illness. *Pediatrics* 67:841–849, 1981.

Perrin E, Perrin J: Clinicians' assessments of children's understanding of illness. *Am J Dis Child* 137:874–878, 1983.

Perrin E, Sayer A, Willett J: Sticks and stones may break my bones . . . Reasoning about illness causality and body functioning in children who have a chronic illness. *Pediatrics* 88:608–619, 1991.

Piaget J: *The Child's Conception of the World.* New York, Harcourt Brace Jovanovich, 1929.

Piaget J, Innhelder B: *The Psychology of the Child.* New York, Basic Books, 1969.

Pidgeon V: Children's concepts of illness: Implications for health teaching. *Matern Child Nurs J* 14: 23–35, 1985.

Potter P, Roberts M: Children's perceptions of chronic illness: The roles of disease symptoms, cognitive development, and information. *J Pediatr Psychol* 9:13–27, 1984.

Rasnake L, Linscheid T: Anxiety reduction in children receiving medical care: Developmental considerations. *J Dev Behav Pediatr* 10: 169–175, 1989.

Schonfeld D, Johnson S, Perrin E, et al: Understanding of AIDS by elementary school children—A developmental survey. *Pediatrics* 92:389–395, 1993.

Schonfeld D, O'Hare L, Perrin E, et al: A randomized, controlled trial of a school-based, multifaceted AIDS education program in the elementary grades: The impact on comprehension, knowledge and fears. *Pediatrics* 95:480–486, 1995.

Siegal M: Children's knowledge of contagion and contamination as causes of illness. *Child Dev* 59:1353–1359, 1988.

Wilkinson S: Germs: Nursery school children's views on the causality of illness. *Clin Pediatr* 26: 465–469, 1987.

Wilkinson S: *The Child's World of Illness: The Development of Health and Illness Behavior.* Cambridge, Cambridge University Press, 1988.

93 PREMATURITY, BIRTH DEFECTS, AND EARLY DEATH: IMPACT ON THE FAMILY

Richard Oberfield, M.D., and H. Paul Gabriel, M.D.

HISTORICAL NOTE

While the topics discussed in this chapter represent forms of family crises experienced since the dawn of humanity, the child and adolescent psychiatric literature was relatively sparse in these areas until approximately 25 years ago. Prior relevant literature appeared in the early 20th century, when the topic of loss and its psychological implications was discussed by Freud (1957a) in the classic paper "Mourning and Melancholia." While normative mourning was utilized by Freud in order to understand the more pathological state of melancholia, his interest appears to have legitimized the normative experience as an area for further study. It was not until the 1940s, however, that a formal descriptive study appeared in the literature. In 1944 Erich Lindemann and his colleagues reported on studies of acute traumatic loss in families who had lost a close relative in the catastrophic "Coconut Grove" fire in Boston. In one case vignette unrelated to the fire, they alluded to mothers of infants who had died being especially vulnerable to severe grief reactions. Many of the victims in this study were very young servicemen and their escorts and might therefore be considered to be late adolescents.

In the 1950s child and adolescent psychiatrists began more specific inquiries into the stresses of prematurity as a family crisis. Dane Prugh, one of the first consultation-liaison child psychiatrists, published in 1953 an anecdotal and theoretical article on parents and premature infants. Slightly later, Gerald Caplan, the founder of community psychiatry and his associates studied families with premature infants as a paradigm for acute stress in normative families (Caplan et al., 1965).

The term sudden infant death syndrome was not present in the medical nomenclature until the 1970s. Furthermore, although the term crib death had been used in the pediatric literature, no family studies were conducted, most likely because these families were inaccessible at the time. Instead, efforts were directed toward parents with children dying in the hospital (Solnit and Green, 1959). In 1961 Solnit and Stark directed their attention to parents of children with birth defects, particularly the retarded. All of these early papers were primarily descriptive and anecdotal in nature, with theoretical postulates and management approaches being suggested. It was not until the mid-1960s that formal studies of significant numbers of parents began to appear in the literature.

In 1963 Friedman and his associates studied prospectively the parents of 27 children admitted to the National Cancer Institute and followed the parents' adaptation to their child's illness irrespective of the course of illness (Freidman et al., 1963a). Special emphasis was placed on families whose children had died, and for the first time, measurement of corticosteroids in the parents' urine was used during the study to document the biological effects of chronic stress (Friedman et al., 1963b). These studies can be said to have ushered in the modern era of family studies of a more specific nature, which have produced management techniques in dealing with parents in the premature intensive care unit, the general hospital unit, and at home.

THE FAMILY AND PREMATURE BIRTH

Early Studies and Crisis Theory

The premature birth of a baby has been viewed historically in psychiatry as a crisis for the family as a whole. The crisis has been described as a period of normative emotional disequilibrium, during which individuals demonstrate symptoms resembling psychopathology, (Caplan, 1960; Caplan et al., 1965; Friedman et al., 1963b; Kaplan and Mason, 1960). Early authors, such as Prugh (1953), highlighted the mother's emotional responses to the baby, staff care givers, and family members. He pointed out that the complex psychological reactions on the part of the mother included anxiety, particularly related to lack of confidence as a caretaker, guilt about the prematurity, resentment and disgust toward the baby, and competition and jealousy toward nursing staff. Furthermore, Prugh described an "emotional lag" or period of alienation on the part of the mother during the first few days, as well as an occasional tendency to overprotection. Suggested interventions included early contact with the baby, provision of information, encouragement of emotional expression, involvement of the father and other family members, and discussion groups of mothers on the ward.

Caplan, in another early description in the literature, studied 30 cases of prematurity (Caplan, 1960). He depicted "healthy" and "unhealthy" outcomes based upon the mother's sensitivity to the infant's needs, her respect for and satisfaction of these needs, and the maintenance of other family relationships. Caplan related the patterns of parental response to their cognitive grasp of the situation, their handling of associated feelings, and their seeking help.

Kaplan and Mason (1960) presents the hypothesis that maternal reactions to the stress of the premature birth are usefully described as acute emotional disorders. Unique psychological tasks related to the prematurity were enumerated sequentially. The first task included preparation for the possible loss of the child ("anticipatory grief"). The second task

related to the mother's failure to deliver a normal full-term baby. (They noted that the first two tasks were often associated with grief and depression). The third task was the resumption of the process of relating to the baby, which had been interrupted by the premature birth. The fourth task related to the mother's understanding and attention to the baby's special needs and growth patterns. These authors further described pathological deviations from the normative accomplishment of the tasks. These included maladaptive denial and failure to respond positively to the progress of the baby.

In a pivotal integrative paper, Caplan et al. (1965) described patterns of parental response to the crisis of prematurity. They defined the crisis state as analogous to Lindemann's (1944) classical description of bereavement. Caplan et al. more fully elaborated "healthy" and "unhealthy" adaptations to the premature birth. For instance, they questioned whether the parents continuously attempted to gather information about the baby with little subsequent distortion of facts. Did they acknowledge ambivalent feelings about the premature baby, with accompanying verbal and nonverbal expression? Was there an active seeking of help for the family, related to the child's special needs and the need of the parents for emotional expression?

Development and Bonding

Somewhat later, there appeared many articles in the literature relating to the association between premature birth, neonatal complications, developmental difficulties, and subsequent problems with bonding between the mother and baby. Several authors postulated a link between dysfunction in bonding and later potential for abuse and or neglect (Elmer and Gregg, 1967; Hunter et al., 1978; Klein and Stern, 1971). This association has remained controversial and was not confirmed by other investigators (Minde, 1980; Steele and Pollock, 1974). Several researchers describe the behavioral and interactional difficulties that preterm babies have during the first years of life (Als, 1981; Als and Brazelton, 1981). They and others also presented the difficulties parents have in engaging the attention of the babies (Als, 1981; Als and Brazelton, 1981; Brown and Bakeman, 1980; Field, 1979).

Minde et al. (1983) in a well-controlled study of 184 low birth weight infants in a neonatal intensive care unit demonstrated that parents of "sick infants" interacted far less with them than parents of well babies. Furthermore, they found that this pattern continued at home after discharge from the hospital. Bidder et al. (1974), comparing mothers' attitudes to their preterm and term babies, found that the mothers perceived the preterm baby to be "weaker" than the term babies. They highlighted two specific periods of particular anxiety for the mother: immediately after the birth and when the baby goes home.

Jeffcoate et al. (1979) compared attitudes of parents of preterm infants to those of parents of full-term infants. They found that there was evidence of some disturbance in parent-child relationships in the preterm group. This consisted of delays in maternal attachment, negative maternal perception, and continuing parental anxiety about caretakers. Two of their sample of preterm infants had been abused or neglected. Jeffcoate and colleagues emphasized the need for ongoing psychological support for these parents.

Silcock (1984) utilized the previously mentioned four-task framework of Caplan et al. to investigate the intensity of maternal experience of these tasks, mothers' success in dealing with them, and the relationship between successful task completion and later mother-infant interaction. The author studied 24 mothers of preterm infants and found that the ability to cope with the crisis was correlated with better mother-infant relationship at 1 month and 4 months of age. She also ascertained that the degree of intensity of emotion accompanying each task varied widely among the mothers and related to individual prior life experience.

In a recent study, Macey et al. (1987) reported that mothers of preterm infants felt overprotection toward them, were apprehensive about surrogate caretakers, and believed the baby's birth had had an initially negative effect on the family. These authors also noted that preterm infants demonstrated less exploratory play and stayed closed to their mothers while at play.

Specific Family and Network Issues

In the past 2 decades, rapid advances in technological care of the preterm neonate have resulted in the need for adaptation of corresponding psychosocial care. Liberalized contact between family members and the baby has become routine in the vast majority of special care nurseries. As a result of such increased access, several authors have maintained that the emphasis of concern on the part of the mother has shifted from her own feeling of psychological loss to the outcome for the baby (Klaus and Kennell, 1983; Pederson et al., 1987).

Many writers have alluded to the significance of networks of social and emotional support to aid parents who are dealing with a preterm birth crisis (Bidder et al., 1974; Blackburn and Lowen, 1986; Fox and Feiring, 1985; Pasco and Earp, 1984; Prugh, 1953). Pederson et al. (1987), utilizing an interview format, confirmed the continuing need for such a supportive network to aid the mother in particular with the ongoing stress of caring for the infant. They reported that husbands, parents, and members of church were viewed as the major sources of ongoing support.

The stresses a premature infant places on the marital unit have been investigated by several authors (Leifer et al., 1972; Trause and Kramer, 1983). Leifer et al. (1972) showed that parents of such an infant are at increased risk for divorce. However, this finding was not confirmed by another clinical investigation (Boyle et al., 1977). Trause and Kramer (1983) evaluated a middle-income group of parents of premature infants in comparison with a group of parents of healthy full-term infants. They found that the premature birth caused a crisis in the immediate postpartum period, but the stress decreased significantly after discharge home. With passage of time, parents of preterm infants reported themselves to be ''more attuned to each other'' than parents of full-term infants. They also found that mothers in both groups consistently rated themselves as more distressed than the fathers.

Blackburn and Lowen examined the impact of premature birth on grandparents (1986). Referring to the grandparents as the ''forgotten grievers.'' In a retrospective exploratory study they ascertained that intense stress was experienced by grandparents as well as parents. The stress was exacerbated by the fact that the grandparents, lacking direct access to physicians, were forced to rely on the distressed parents as their sources of information about the infant.

In a study of mothers of preterm versus full-term infants, Crinc et al. (1983) confirmed the positive effects of social network support on lowering overall stress and increasing positive parenting interactive behaviors. Beckman and Pokorni (1988) recently reported that stresses related to preterm birth are specific but also change over time. They found that lowered levels of stress were associated with the continuity of informal, intimate environmental support.

Although of significant clinical interest, the majority of these studies of network support suffer from small sample size and lack of adequate control groups.

Management

In the literature there is overwhelming agreement among authors about the type and frequency of psychosocial intervention that are most constructive for the families of premature infants. Liberal access to the babies by family members is desirable, particularly in light of technological advances in neonatal intensive care units that otherwise tend to isolate babies for extended period of time. Harper et al. (1976), in a retrospective questionnaire format study of 58 families, determined that perceived parental anxiety correlated with the degree of the infants's illness. However, despite the associated anxiety the parents felt at the time, parents did maintain much contact with the infants and would have been opposed to more restricted contact. They noted that even parents of babies who died expressed no regrets about the time spent with the infant in the intensive care unit.

The other area of uniform agreement among authors in the field pertains to the need for continuity of psychosocial contact and support of the family. Members of the extended family network may provide informal continuing support over time. Just as significant to long-term adaptation appears to be continuity of medically based psychosocial follow-up. Child psychiatrists may play an integral liaison role within this framework of continuing psychosocial attention.

CASE ILLUSTRATION

A middle-class primiparous mother has given birth to a 1500-g 30-week infant. It has been 3 days since the birth, and the mother has recently been discharged from the outlying community hospital from which the baby was transferred on day 1. The pediatrician states that the mother became quite distraught after viewing the baby for the first time. She appeared to be overwhelmed by the technological equipment, became quite tearful, and stated, ''He doesn't look human.'' The head nurse called the neonatology fellow, who attempted to be reassuring. However, the mother remained tearful and was unable to interact with the baby. The neonatology fellow is requesting advice about further management at this point.

Comment

This is a typical child psychiatry liaison problem in a major teaching hospital setting. The primary role for the psychiatrist is first to review with the neonatologist and senior nursing personnel about the psychosocial issues and tasks confronted by their families. These include feelings of failure and disappointment in relation to the ''expected'' baby, the challenges of physical care, and anxiety about other caretakers. The importance of early psychological bonding to the infant should be emphasized as well.

The next step is for the psychiatrist to provide support and supervision while the psychosocial intervention is performed by the pediatric staff. The neonatologist should be encouraged to arrange meetings with both parents, which is often difficult since fathers of premature infants often distance themselves from the stressful situation. In addition, nursing staff need to be strongly encouraged, despite frequent subtle opposition, to assist the mother in overcoming her ambivalence and anxiety by involving her in the infant's physical care. The mothers often feel inept in dealing with the premature baby, and these reactions are usually modified with a modest amount of educated staff effort.

BIRTH DEFECTS AND THE FAMILY

History and Special Considerations

The birth of a child with congenital abnormalities presents the family with a severe crisis that shares some features of a premature birth but has specific characteristics of its own. Although there is usually less uncertainty about the survival of the child compared to the situation of premature birth, the defective baby's birth is generally associated with mourning over the loss of the expected child (Solnit and Stark, 1961). In addition, continuing conflicts surrounding the appearance of the baby, and the difficulties of physical care of the deformed child complicate the family crisis as well. The societal stigma often associated with physically defective children is a continuing issue for the parents and siblings and must be considered in planning psychosocial intervention strategies.

Descriptions of family adaptation to the birth of an infant with congenital abnormalities began appearing in the literature in the 1950s and 1960s. Schonell and Watts (1957) wrote about the effects of a ''subnormal child'' on the family unit. This early report from Australia, focusing on a heterogeneous group of retarded children, documented the frustration experienced by, and lack of information and of psychosocial supports provided to, parents who were attempting to rear their children at home.

In their paper on the crisis of the birth of a child with congenital abnormalities, Solnit and Stark (1961) referred to the acute grief reaction originally described by Lindemann (1944). They referred to the initial shock, denial, and sense of disequilibrium observed in these families. In addition, they utilized a "theoretical approach founded on the psychoanalytic explanation of the process of mourning as applied to the mother's reactions to the birth of a defective child" (Solnit and Stark, 1961). Referring to the original descriptions by Freud (1957a, 1957b, 1961), and later by Engel (1961), Solnit and Stark explained the mother's psychological reaction as relating to the loss of the image of the expected baby. During the pregnancy, the mother's normative anticipatory process of expecting a healthy baby is acutely interrupted by the birth of a child with congenital abnormalities and possibly disabilities. Furthermore, her reaction is influenced by her own past experiences with family members and significant life events. Solnit and Stark suggested that because of the acute crisis, there is no time for the mother to work through the loss of the expected child before there is a demand to bond to the ambivalently viewed new baby. Although the emphasis of these authors was focused upon the mother's emotional reactions, their advice was to clarify continuously to both parents the situation and needs of the new infant. They also strongly suggested that the mother view the new child as soon as possible, a step that had often been omitted based on a well-intentioned attempt to spare the mother pain.

Family Stress in Relation to Specific Birth Defects

Another early description of the psychosocial sequelae of the birth of a child with birth defects was by Tisza and Gumpertz (1962), writing about infants with cleft palate. They described parents who, after experiencing the initial shock and disbelief components of acute grief, became obsessed with etiology (e.g., genetic linkages, which are associated with guilt). They emphasized the need for early imparting of information about the baby to the parents, preferably by the physicians, who should be available to answer the variety of questions posed. They described occasionally pathological overcloseness between mother and child, based on the mother's viewing the child as an extension of herself.

Family stress in relation to an infant born with spina bifida was studied in Wales by Hare et al. (1966) via the use of a prospective interview format. Many of the parents reported that the medical staff did not seem to appreciate their initial worries and concerns. The study pointed to the fact that many mothers were unable to comprehend much of what was explained to them soon after the delivery. The parents also expressed a keen interest in meeting with other parents of spina bifida children.

Walker et al. (1971), in a prospective questionnaire study of 107 British families of infants with spina bifida, reported the parents' dissatisfaction with the manner in which they were informed about the abnormality. The parents complained of chronic tension in the home, difficulties with siblings, and a sense of isolation due to the arrival of the baby. Walker et al. suggested to physicians that a psychosocial team closely monitor these at-risk families.

Very few investigators have applied a psychoanalytic point of view to the issue of birth defects and parental reaction. Lax (1972), in an anecdotal report of only a few patients, described the mother's "narcissistic trauma" in relation to the arrival of the impaired child. Interestingly, she noted that the severity of the mother's depressive reaction was often unrelated to the magnitude of the birth defect (Lax, 1972). Lax emphasized preexisting personality features in the mother as clinical clues to her adaptation and acceptance of an impaired child. She presented a dramatic illustration of the rejection by the mother of a newborn with a large nevus of the cheek: "Upon seeing the child for the first time, the mother turned away and said: 'She's ugly—it can't be a two-faced monster' (referring to the normal side of the child's face and the deformed one)" (Lax, 1972, p. 341).

Studies of Heterogeneous Defects

Johns (1971), in an Australian study, performed a prospective 6-month investigation of 12 consecutive infants born with a congenital abnormality. Initially and subsequent reactions of the mothers and family were observed. Johns found that parents of children with more visible or more severe defects were the most anxious and most accessible to offers of psychological help. Facially disfiguring lesions were of particular concern to the parents. The author suggested an early but brief announcement to the parents of the abnormal finding, an early statement of the plan to correct the deformity, ready access to genetic counseling, and continuing emotional monitoring and support.

A large sample of parents of 20 children with a wide range of malformations was reported by Drotar et al. (1975). The malformations included Down's syndrome, cleft palate, and congenital heart disease. They arranged structured interviews after the birth of the child (elapsed time ranged from 7 days to 5 years). They emphasized the more adaptive elements in the coping of these parents, which had previously been largely overlooked. Successive stages of parental reactions were outlined by this group as components of a normative pattern; shock; denial (feelings of unreality); a mixture of sadness, anger, and anxiety; eventual adaptation; and reorganization. According to Drotar and colleagues, often seen in the middle phases of coping were mixtures of sadness, rejection, hatred, and fears of becoming attached to babies who might die. The last stage, reorganization, included positive long-term acceptance of the child with mutual support between parents. These investigators emphasized the importance of early physical contact (bonding) with the child, referring to earlier work by Klaus and Kennell (1970). They maintained that the early initiation of a relationship, specifically through physical care, served as a major means of anxiety reduction in the parents.

The descriptive studies noted above, although clinically rich in detail, generally lack relevant control groups and large sample size of subjects.

Effect on the Marital Relationship and Siblings

The significant effects of the arrival of a child with a birth defect on the marital relationship have been studied by several clinical investigators. Tew and associates (1974), utilizing a prospective interview format, were the first researchers to note significant deterioration in the couple bond after the birth of an atypical child. The divorce rate of the index parents (of offspring with spina bifida) was twice that of the control group and the national average (in Wales). Only one-fourth of the index families appeared to be free of marital difficulties; mothers pregnant at the time of the marriage appeared to be at the greatest risk for divorce or separation subsequent to the birth. Martin (1975), in a slightly later study, also documented a high rate of marital breakdown in families of babies with spina bifida.

Drotar et al. (1975) underlined the importance of synchrony between the parents and their reactions. Parents who were viewed to be "out of synch" with each other were more prone to emotional separation coinciding with the stresses on the family of such a child.

Gath (1977) reported on a prospective controlled study of 30 families of Down's syndrome infants. This author found few differences in the mental or physical health of the two groups of parents, but marital rupture or severe disharmony was found in nine of the families with a child with Down's syndrome and in none of the controls.

Very little work has been presented in the literature regarding the specific reactions of siblings to the arrival and presence of a child with birth defects and/or physical handicaps. In a clinically descriptive case study, Poznanski (1969) pointed to the resolution of stress and conflict in the family through displacement onto a "well" sibling. The author pointed to the frequent overinvolvement on the part of the mother with the handicapped child, and her lack of sensitivity to the more subtle needs of the other siblings. According to Poznanski, this constellation of dynamics often led to "behavioral reactions as a consequence of emotional neglect."

Intervention and Counseling Techniques

Intervention strategies for counseling families of defective infants have been discussed in the literature since the 1960s. Focusing on 140 families of infants with Down's syndrome, Giannini and Goodman (1963) emphasized the point that, through immediate crisis intervention counseling, families were better able to participate in decision-making relating to institutional placement outside the home. Goodman (1964), in reference to the same population with Down's syndrome, recommended group counseling for the parents to provide peer support, as well as counseling in the home if possible.

The British Working Party (1971) suggested to clinicians guidelines of communication with the parents of an abnormal child. They recommended that a familiar staff person tell the parents as soon as possible to prevent unfortunate discovery of the problem by the parents. They warned of psychological reactions to be expected, such as anger, projection of blame and guilt onto staff, and, at times, temporary rejection of the infant. A multidisciplinary team approach including the pediatrician and medical social worker was suggested for communications with the family during the crisis.

In a description of work with families with children with Down's syndrome, Golden and Davis (1974) emphasized that clinicians should carefully evaluate their own feelings about the child in order to better counsel the family. They found that a surprising number of parents are able to accept raising these children at home if their questions are answered and psychosocial needs met.

Drotar et al. (1975), as a result of their study of parents of children with congenital malformations, suggested pediatric management guidelines. Familiarity on the part of the physician with the predictable psychological stages of adaptation to the birth crisis is critical. Furthermore, they stated, "Since the parents' initial shock and disbelief limit the amount of information that they can absorb in regarding their child's condition, information regarding the child's handicap may have to be communicated very clearly and repeated many times" (Drotar et al., 1975, p. 716). Again, early physical contact with the baby was highly urged in order to minimize the parents; feelings of estrangement.

Drotar and associates recommended that young housestaff officers be assisted by more senior staff physicians in intervening with these parents. Family counseling by the physician during the infant's 1st year of life was strongly urged to maximize the development of the child within the family. Van Riper and associates, in a recent study of 90 parents of children with Down's syndrome, found that pediatric house officers often avoided interacting with parents of the affected child. They suggested that all involved clinicians need to adopt a more interactional and positive approach to the family (Van Riper et al., 1992).

The physician's role in management is critical and requires both an understanding of the psychological reactions of the parents and a willingness to deal with personal responses to these infants.

CASE ILLUSTRATION

Mrs. C., a 32-year-old mother, gave birth to a baby boy with Down's syndrome. This was the first child for the mother, a college professor, and her husband, a 36-year-old attorney. The mother had carefully arranged her work schedule around the planned birth and expected to resume teaching soon afterward. The father was present for the delivery, which was by natural childbirth. Amniocentesis had not been performed during the pregnancy.

When the baby was born, Mrs. C. noticed the concerned expressions of doctors, nurses, and her husband. Mr. C.'s first instinct was to protect his wife, but he was encouraged by the medical staff to show her the infant. There was medical evidence of an endocardial cushion defect for which surgery would most likely be indicated by age 5.

Mrs. C.'s response was to reject the baby due to his physical appearance, future retardation, and cardiac status. She refused to breast-feed the infant and directed much of her anger toward the nursing staff, whom she felt were forcing her to deal with the child. Although the father expressed concern about the future, he was certain that he preferred to keep the baby at home. Mrs. C. continued to be obsessed with the stigma of having such a child and expressed the desire to place him in an institution since he'd "never be perfect."

A pediatric social worker was enlisted to discuss disposition options with the parents. The child psychiatrist was regularly consulted by the social worker regarding the counseling.

This case underlines several important features and implications of psychosocial support in relation to modern pediatric practice. Since there are too many children born with congenital defects for all to be seen by child psychiatrists, the management of these families is best undertaken by social workers or child life specialists, with psychiatric consultation and intervention as needed.

The families generally experience such psychological reactions as shock, a sense of unreality, denial, sadness, anger, rejection of the baby, and eventually adaptation. It is crucial that the family members work through the mourning process of the loss of the "expected" intact child and be encouraged to involve themselves rapidly in the physical care of the infant. In our society, nonvisible remediable physical defects and nonmentally handicapping conditions are more readily accepted by the family. On the other hand, facial deformities and retardation syndrome elicit more severe emotional reactions in family members.

Although some families do eventually place defective, particularly retarded, infants in institutional settings, it is generally agreed that the outcome for children with special handicapping conditions is better if they are raised in the home environment.

THE FAMILY AND EARLY INFANT DEATH

History and Medical Considerations

Sudden death in infancy has been familiar to clinicians for centuries. Over the past three decades, it has been described more specifically, and its etiology has been aggressively studied. Known prior to 1970 as crib death or cot death, it has been referred to as sudden infant death syndrome (SIDS) since that time. SIDS is responsible for the death of approximately 7000 infants per year in the United States and is the most frequent cause of death of babies between 1 week and 1 year of age (Swoiskin, 1986). A recent study demonstrated a SIDS mortality of 1.40 per thousand live births and this represented 14.1% of all infant deaths (Goldberg, 1992). Peak incidence of SIDS is between 2 and 4 months of age. An increased incidence is associated with premature and low birth weight infants, lower socioeconomic status, nonwhite ethnicity, younger age of mother, smoking during pregnancy, and male sex of baby (Hoffman, 1987; Valdes-Dapena, 1980).

Over the years, the hypothesized causes of sudden infant death have been numerous. In the remote past, it was thought to be associated with "overlying" or smothering by the parents (Templeman, 1892). In the 1930s, spasm of the glottis and cardiac failure were suggested (Goldbloom and Wigglesworth, 1938). Other theories of causation have included enlarged thymus gland, allergy to cow's milk, suffocation from bedding, infection, and cardiac immaturities (Weinstein, 1978). More recent research has been focused on sleep apnea, enzyme irregularities, and chronic oxygen deficiency (Naeye, 1974; Steinschneider, 1975). Newer theories have pertained to brainstem function and metabolism, cardiac predisposition, and possible genetic linkages (Giulian et al., 1987; Kinney, 1987; Sadeh et al., 1987). Beal (1992), in a recent study, found a slightly increased incidence of SIDS in siblings, which may be attributable to biological or environmental factors. The definitive etiology remains obscure at present, and researchers may ultimately conclude that the syndrome is related to multiple factors.

Psychological Reactions

It has often been noted in the literature that the acute psychological reaction of the family to SIDS death is extremely intense and severe in quality. Most authors refer to Lindemann's (1944) description of normative acute grief reactions as a reference point. These descriptions included various somatic symptoms, guilt secondary to perceived negligence, and anger and hostility directed toward health professionals. Pathological or "morbid" grief reactions presented by Lindemann and observed among SIDS parents include delayed mourning, overactivity without a sense of loss, alteration in relationship to friends and relatives, furious hostility directed against specific persons, schizophrenia-like symptoms, and agitated depression.

According to Friedman (1974), the intensity of reaction to the loss of the infant is related to the absence of "anticipatory mourning." The parents lack the time to prepare themselves psychologically for the overwhelming event. In addition, the death occurs in otherwise healthy infants, the etiology is unclear, and parents often feel blamed or responsible for the child's death (Friedman, 1974).

Descriptive Studies

Bluglass (1981), in a review of psychosocial aspects of SIDS, stated that few well-controlled prospective studies have been done relating to bereavement, and none at all in relation to SIDS. However, some descriptive studies of family reaction to SIDS have been reported. Bergman et al. (1969) delineated the acute phase of family reactions to the sudden death of the baby. They mentioned feelings of disbelief, anger, helplessness, severe guilt, and loss of meaning to life. Parents felt they were "losing their minds," and there was associated disruption of usual routines. Following the death, they described some of the parents demonstrating denial of the event and experiencing persistent dreams of the child. Hostility to friends and relatives was common as well.

DeFrain and Ernst (1978), in a clinical study of 32 parents of infants who died of SIDS, found through mailed questionnaire responses, that SIDS was the most severe crisis the parents had ever encountered. In addition, they found that the majority of parents suffered feelings of personal guilt and other psychological difficulties and that relatives were also affected. An interesting finding of their study was that 60% of the parents who had experienced SIDS had moved from their hometowns within 2 ½ years of the death. They also reported that behavioral difficulties were found in siblings and that better psychological recovery of the family was associated with higher income.

Cornwell et al. (1977) reported on a small Australian prospective questionnaire study. They stated that three families sought formal psychiatric attention for severe difficulties (e.g., delusional hypochondriasis, severe depression, extreme anxiety). In addition, marital difficulties were common (one-third of the group), siblings were noted to be overanxious, and "anniversary reactions" were usual. Physical health was reported to have deteriorated, with the emergence of psychosomatic symptoms. They also noted parents' overprotective tendencies toward surviving siblings. There was a preoccupation with subsequent fertility, and thoughts of a "replacement child" were common. The questionnaire studies may be critiqued on the basis of sample bias; specifically, it is possible that the families who replied to the questionnaire were more disturbed and dysfunctional than were the nonrespondents. The prominent role of guilt in the reaction of SIDS parents, which is exacerbated by the mysterious etiology, was discussed by Salk (1971). In an anecdotal summary, he argued that parents who are prone to self-blame are more likely to do so after SIDS death due to the ambiguity of cause. He underemphasized the role of the physician in helping families to cope with the crisis of SIDS.

Smialek (1978) conducted a 2-year follow-up study involving 351 families, most of which (75%) had lost a baby to SIDS. (The remaining 25% lost infants suddenly due to other causes.) In addition to the common psychological reactions noted by other clinicians, the author found that certain parents expressed "relief" at the death due to extreme ambivalence about the child. She noted that the stages originally described by Kauubler-Ross (1969) in relation to dying patients were useful in understanding the adaptation of parents to sudden infant death.

Zebal and Woolsey (1984) recently reviewed parent's reactions to sudden infant death and emphasized the relative youth of the parents, for whom this may have been the first death experience. Consequently, the parent may misinterpret normative grief reactions and fear they are becoming mentally ill. The authors noted that individuals in the surrounding social network tend to underestimate the intensity and duration of the grief reaction and are therefore less supportive than they might be. Furthermore, police investigations and legal proceedings are usually involved, which heightens the initial stress. Parents are not infrequently accused of child abuse and or neglect pertaining to the death of the infant.

Family Adaptation

A "long-term adaptation" model with key transitional points was presented by Zebal and Woolsey (1984) in their review. After several days or weeks, the initial shock or denial reactions give way to the acute grief reactions described previously. Six or 8 weeks later, the reality of death is more clear, coinciding with the gradual withdrawal of external supports. Four to 6 months after the death, there is a shift to future-oriented concerns. Significant dates (birthdays, holidays) are associated with anniversary reactions. After 1–2 years, consideration of a new pregnancy usually occurs; if a pregnancy occurs, there is heightened anxiety about the vulnerability of the baby to SIDS and other dangers.

Several authors have noted that there are sex differences among the parents regarding their psychological adaptation to SIDS (Benfield et al., 1978; Cornwell et al., 1977). Benfield and coworkers reported on 50 parent pairs whose children had died suddenly (Benfield et al., 1978). They noted that fathers appeared to experience less intense and more accelerated "grief work" due to involvement in practical matters (funeral arrangements, etc.). They postulated differences in societal expectations for men and women regarding expression of grief and mourning. Mandell, in a clinical study of paternal response, described fathers of SIDS infants as driven to "keep busy" through increasing involvement with work; they also demonstrated stoicism and a limited ability to verbalize feelings or ask for support (Mandel et al., 1980).

Marital Issues

Regarding the effect on the marital bond, Benfield et al. noted that, in couples where communication was poor, it appeared that critical emotional issues were avoided for extended periods of time (Benfield et al., 1978). Zebal and Woolsey (1984) noted that the differing styles of adaptation of men and women can lead to difficult interactional cycles in the marriage. There is often misunderstanding of the respective styles of grieving, which often leads to conflict. Mandell (1980) observed that, of his study sample of 28 parent pairs who had lost babies, six marriages had dissolved after the death.

Several authors have referred to the desire of some parents to replace the dead infant with another child. Cornwell found that most parents he studied seemed to be aware of the psychological risks of replacing a lost child (Cornwell et al., 1977). Rowe et al. (1978), in a follow-up study of 26 families who had experienced perinatal death, found that a prolonged grief reaction in the parents was associated with early subsequent pregnancy. The implication of this work is that the necessary grief work had been interrupted by the new pregnancy and birth.

Effect on Siblings

The effects of SIDS on surviving siblings has been presented often in the literature, although there have been no published long-term longitudinal studies. Most authors highlight the particular difficulties older siblings have in dealing with the infant's death, due to preexisting rivalrous feelings. Cain et al. (1964) described the sense of responsibility and guilt reactions the older children suffer. They noted distorted views about the concept of death, death phobias, and a subsequent feeling of deprivation experienced by the surviving sibling. Halpern (1972) mentioned the tendency of some mothers to project blame and guilt onto the older sibling, which may lead to behavioral problems. He also described painful anniversary reactions experienced by the family, which affect surviving siblings.

Several authors have presented the frequent occurrence of behavioral difficulties in siblings of SIDS infants, as well as the tendency on the part of the parents to overprotection of the remaining siblings (Cornwell et al., 1977; Mandell et al., 1988). Williams (1981) studied a group of surviving siblings and noted developmental age-specific differences in response. He found that the children between 6 and 9 years of age showed the least direct expression of their distress. The younger children (preschool age) were confused and angry, and the older children (over 10 years) demonstrated an adult-like pattern of grief. Gaffney (1992) has recently described that well-intentioned attempts to spare the feelings of the siblings often result in increasing isolation and tendencies to fantasize in a maladaptive manner.

Swoiskin (1986) also noted age-specific developmental reactions and cautioned that misleading euphemisms about the baby's death often exacerbated the emotional reactions of the surviving siblings. She also described occasional parental distancing from a sibling, related to idealization of the lost child.

Burns et al. (1986), in a questionnaire study of 50 siblings of 43 families, noted that 54% of them experienced extended grief reactions, lasting over 1 year. In a recent prospective interview study of 45 surviving sibs of 36 families, Mandell and colleagues (1988) described changes in sleep patterns, social interaction, and parent-child interaction. They noted that these behavioral changes reflected both patterns of adjustment by the child and persistence of parental concerns.

Effect on Grandparents

In a recent questionnaire study, DeFrain et al. (1992) examined the psychological and social impact of SIDS on surviving grandparents. The loss of the baby was found to be devastating for them as well, with mixed emotional reactions of disbelief, anger, guilt, anxiety, and depression identified. They described difficulties inherent in grieving for the baby, while at the same time attempting to console and comfort their own grown children. Bereavement support groups were found to be quite helpful for the grandparents involved.

Interventions and Counseling Techniques

In the two decades of active recognition of SIDS, much has been written about intervention and management techniques. Most authors have pointed to the tendency of medical staff to avoid dealing actively with the psychosocial issues confronting these families. Referring to the work by Kennell et al. (1970), correlating more adaptive mourning with prior physical contact with the infant, the majority of clinical investigators have urged increased visual and physical contact between the parents and the dead infant. Many authors suggest that autopsies be routinely performed, in order to decrease the atmosphere of confusion, ambiguity, and mystery surrounding the death of the infant (Bergman, 1974, 1979; Weinstein, 1978). Any available information should be rapidly transmitted to the family by the medical and nursing staff to minimize tendencies of self-blame or blame of others. Powell (1991) has suggested that providing medical information to the family within the first 3 months after the death leads to more normative grief reactions and acceptance. The vast majority of investigators suggest that the medical team, including active involvement by the physician, participate in ongoing psychosocial follow-up of the affected families.

More specific counseling interventions have been suggested in the literature. To foster mutual support, Salk (1971) recommended regular group meetings of parents of infants who have died of SIDS. Goldberg (1992) has suggested that group parental sessions comprised of recently affected parents and "veterans" are quite effective and should contain a significant educational component regarding recent medical research findings in SIDS. Smialek (1978) outlined a multiple-step counseling model based on a large prospective study of 351 families of sudden death infants. These steps include accepting parents' grief reactions, encouraging ventilation of feelings, clarifying misconceptions about the death, allowing private access to the dead infant, and assisting with autopsy and funeral arrangements. Smialek advised that siblings be permitted to attend the funeral of the infant to encourage their grieving process.

Zebal and Woolsey (1984), and later Woolsey (1988) writing independently, made the point that many families experience a withdrawal of social support several months after the death of the infant. Buschbacker et al. recently reported that relatives in the extended family network are often unable to provide necessary support due to their own grieving (Buschbacker and Delcampo, 1987). Most authors agree that a network of aid should be arranged to be available to the family over an extended period of time, considering that the grieving process for the lost child often takes place over years. The network might include other parents, whose infants have died of SIDS, family members, friends, and members of the psychosocial/medical team. Many states provide services through SIDS Information and Counseling Projects and the National SIDS Foundation.

In a recent critical review of adaptation following perinatal loss, Zeanah (1989) makes several important points. He maintains that hospital management of these families, including encouragement to view the deceased baby, has not been based on adequately tested assumptions. He also states that other specific areas need to be more systematically tested as well, including differing mourning patterns of mothers and fathers, differentiation of grief and mourning during the course of bereavement, and advice-giving about subsequent pregnancies.

Davis et al. (1989), in a recent investigation about subsequent pregnancy, interviewed mothers about the advice they had received from physicians about postponing pregnancy. Significantly, they found that, regardless of the specific advice given, most mothers felt that their individual psychosocial situations had not been considered enough at the time. They note that physicians and other caregivers may be most effective and helpful by educating parents about the advantages and disadvantages of postponing pregnancy, in order to help them make a more informed decision.

CASE ILLUSTRATION

A 19-year-old mother gave birth to a 4 ½-pound baby girl after a 36-week gestation. This was the mother's second pregnancy; there was a 2½-year-old brother at home at the time of the birth. The baby had been delivered by cesarean section due to premature onset of labor and fetal distress. There had been a possible history of alcohol or drug abuse; the mother tested negative for HIV infection. She had also been a cigarette smoker throughout the pregnancy. Apgar scores were 7 and 6, and the baby was observed for 3 days in the neonatal intensive care unit for labored breathing.

The infant was doing well until age 2 months, when she had several episodes of apnea at home, none requiring resuscitation. After a careful evaluation, it was decided not to place the child on a cardiorespiratory monitor.

At age 5 months, the older brother, now almost 3 years of age, discovered the baby not moving in her crib. He reported this to the mother, who impulsively yelled out "What did you do to her?" The boy had previously demonstrated some behavioral difficulties indicative of sibling rivalry. The baby was rushed to the pediatric emergency room, where she was pronounced dead. Counseling was recommended to the family at the time, but they did not seek help,and little outreach by hospital staff took place.

Several weeks later, the parents brought their son to the pediatric emergency room one evening, complaining that he had a cough and chest congestion that worried them. In the course of the evaluation, mother herself presented vague somatic complaints, stated she felt she was "going crazy" because she saw visions of her daughter choking, and feared she was losing control of her temper with the son. The child psychiatrist was consulted.

It was ascertained that the father was attempting to support his wife, but he indicated that he was in danger of losing his job if he kept attending to the problems at home. Extended family members were unavailable, and the parents felt rather isolated and helpless, particularly in relation to their son's behavioral problems. The child was also demonstrating nightmares and new animal phobias. Counseling was arranged for the child and family by the pediatric social worker, and the primary pediatrician made himself available for continuing support. One year after the death of the infant, all family members were functioning more adaptively, the brother was enrolled in nursery school, and the parents were considering another pregnancy.

Comment

This case presents a rather classic paradigm of the problems SIDS families encounter. The families demonstrate the following general characteristics: the mothers tend to be young, multiparous, of low socioeconomic level, and cigarette smokers. The pregnancies are relatively complicated and are more prone to premature birth. The infants often present with difficulties at birth, which may resolve acutely, are discharged home, and later experience episodes of apnea that presage the sudden death.

The acute psychological reaction to such an event often involves displacement of blame onto a family member, such as an older sibling, or medical staff. Fathers frequently present as somewhat distant, stoic, and relatively unsupportive of the mother's emotional state.

Ideally speaking, follow-up visits should be planned at the time the infant arrives at the emergency room. However, these families are too often inadequately followed, and those without network support often experience delayed emotional sequelae. Typically, well-intentioned friends, family members, and physicians suggest premature replacement of the infant, which may lead to exacerbation of symptoms on the part of the parents. A sibling who feels guilt about the death may present with symptoms. The mothers frequently develop psychosomatic or depressive features.

Immediate psychological intervention is usually necessary; involvement of the father and surviving siblings is critically important. Continuous monitoring by the pediatrician and pediatric social worker is indicated, with psychiatric consultation as needed. Outcome and prognosis depend on premorbid adjustment as well as on management by the interdisciplinary team.

CONCLUSIONS

The immediate effect of potential and acute loss of an infant on the nuclear family is the major theme of this chapter. Each condition presents young and relatively inexperienced parents with a crisis for which they have usually had little preparation and no prior education. Furthermore, in our technologically and medically advanced culture, with its overinvestment in physical beauty, high intelligence, and medical expertise, the negative impact of prematurity, disability, and death tends to be exaggerated. It is almost impossible for the average American to comprehend that there are parts of the world where infant morbidity and mortality are daily experiences. Actually, this was, and in a few places still is, true of the United States well into the 20th century. Universally, the potential or actual loss of an infant is a severe stressor for the family.

Prematurity represents a state of suspended animation for most parents. Even large premature infants with good prognoses induce anxiety and symbolize potential death and disability. Furthermore, the specter of mental retardation, an anathema in our society, presents parents with a long period of ambiguity and chronic anxiety. During this period, they must be helpless observers rather than active participants. Recent research has indicated that the active involvement of parents in the care of their premature infants can be helpful in alleviating both the guilt and the anxiety related to loss and impairment. Even if the ultimate complexities of bonding have yet to be fully delineated, this is a practice and useful approach in the prematurity nursery. Clearly, child psychiatrists have important roles to fulfill both in helping staff members to deal with increased parental participation and in the direct management of family members with intense distress related to their infants' fragility.

Parents whose infants are born with congenital anomalies may face a lifetime of adjustment to a child who places special demands upon them. While some congenital anomalies are not obvious to the culture at large or are surgically remediable, those presenting visible deformities to the world or resulting in mental retardation place special emotional burdens on the parents. This situation usually requires the health care professional to deal with both chronic guilt and often significant ambivalence on the part of one or both parents. In addition, considering the social and economic burdens that must be endured, major realistic stressors must be recognized and attended to if the family is to remain a viable unit.

Lastly, the literature on sudden infant death has been reviewed. While infant mortality has been a reality throughout human history, the psychological study of families experiencing the death of an infant or child is a very recent endeavor. Mourning, in a secular society, has evolved from being a primary purview of the religious counselor to the legitimate scientific pursuit of the psychological investigator. Counseling efforts are now being introduced and implemented in hospitals and clinics to provide support for families with children who die suddenly at home or in the hospital. Child psychiatrists have important roles to fill at all levels of liaison activity regarding SIDS, be it in direct consultation and service or in training and supervision of other health care professionals.

It is clear that there will never be enough child and adolescent psychiatrists to treat all families of premature, disabled, and deceased infants. Knowledge of normative responses has advanced to the point where basic skills can be utilized by and transmitted to others who can provide basic services. However, there is much to be learned about the short- and long-term sequelae of such stressful situations upon individuals and family systems with preexisting psychopathology. For such families, child and adolescent psychiatrists are uniquely suited to play a further role in research and treatment.

References

Als H: *Infant Individuality: Assessing Patterns of Very Early Development.* New York, Basic Books, 1981.

Als H, Brazelton TB: A new model of assessing the behavioral organization in preterm and fullterm infants—Two case studies. *Child Psychiatry* 20: 239–263, 1981.

Beal S: Siblings of sudden infant death syndrome victims. *Clin Perinatol* 19(4):839–848, 1992.

Beckman P, Pokorni J: A longitudinal study of families of preterm infants: Changes in stress and support over the first two years. *J Special Educ* 22: 55–65, 1988.

Benfield DG, Leib S, Vollman JH: Grief responses of parents to neonatal death and parent participation in deciding care. *Pediatrics* 62:171–177, 1978.

Bergman AB: Psychological aspects of sudden unexpected death in infants and children. *Pediatr Clin North Am* 21(1):115–121, 1974.

Bergman AB: The sudden infant death syndrome—What can you do? *Med Times* 107:32–36, 1979.

Bergman AB, Pomeroy M, Beckwith B: the psychiatric toll of the sudden infant death syndrome. *Gen Pract* 40:(6):99–105, 1969.

Bidder R, Crowe E, Gray O: Mothers' attitudes to preterm infants. *Arch Dis Child* 49:766–770, 1974.

Blackburn S, Lowen L: Impact of an infant's premature birth on the grandparents and parents. *J Obstet Gynecol Neonatal Nurs* 14:173–178, 1986.

Bluglass K: Psychosocial aspects of the sudden infant death syndrome (''cot death''). *J Child Psychol Psychiatry* 22(4):411–421, 1981.

Boyle M, Griffen A, Fitzhardinge P: The very low birthweight infant: Impact on parents during the preschool years. *Early Hum Dev* 1:191–201, 1977.

British Working Party: The birth of an abnormal child: Telling the parents. *Lancet* 2:1075–1077, 1971.

Brown J, Bakeman R: Relationships of human mothers with their infants during the first year of life. Effects of prematurity. In: Bell R, Smotherman W (eds): *Maternal Influences on Early Behavior.* Holliswood, NY, Spectrum, 1980.

Burns E, House ID, Ankenbauer M: Sibling grief in reaction to sudden infant death syndrome. *Pediatrics* 78:485–487, 1986.

Buschbacher V, Delcampo R: Parents' response to sudden infant death syndrome. *J Pediatr Health Care* 1:85–90, 1987.

Cain AC, Fast I, Erickson M: Childrens' disturbed reactions to the death of a sibling. *Am J Orthopsychiatry* 34:741–745, 1964.

Caplan G: patterns of parental response to the crisis of premature birth. *Psychiatry* 23:365–374, 1960.

Caplan G, Mason E, Kaplan D: Four studies of crisis in parents of prematures. *Community Ment Health J* 1:149–161, 1965.

Cornwell J, Nurcombe B, Stevens L: Family response to loss of a child by sudden infant death syndrome. *Med J Aust* 1:656–658, 1977.

Crinc KA, Greenberg MT, Ragozin A, et al: Effects of stress and social support on mothers of premature and full-term infants. *Child Dev* 54:209–217, 1983.

Davis D, Stewart M, Harmon R: Postponing pregnancy after perinatal death: Perspectives on doctor advice. *J Am Acad Child Adolesc Psychiatry* 28:481–487, 1989.

DeFrain JD, Ernst L: The psychological effects of sudden infant death syndrome on surviving family members. *J Fam Pract* 6(5):985–989, 1978.

DeFrain J, Jakub D: The psychological effects of sudden infant death on grandmothers and grandfathers. *Omega J Death Dying* 24(3):165–182, 1992.

Drotar D, Baskiewicz A, Irvin N, et al: The adaptation of parents to the birth of an infant with a congenital malformation: A hypothetical model. *Pediatrics* 56(5):710–717, 1975.

Elmer E, Gregg G: Developmental characteristics of abused children. *Pediatrics* 40(596):602, 1967.

Engel GI: Is grief a disease? A challenge for medical research. *Psychosom Med* 23:18–22, 1961.

Field TM: Interaction patterns of preterm and term infants. In: Field TM (ed): *Infants Born at Risk: Behavior and Development.* Jamaica, NY, SP Medical and Scientific Books, 1979, pp. 333–356.

Fox N, Feiring C: High-risk birth. In: Harel S, Anastasiow N (eds): *The At-Risk Infant: Psycho/Socio/Medical Aspects.* Baltimore, Paul H Brookes, 1985.

Freud S: Mourning and melancholia. In: Strachey J (ed): *The Standard Edition of the Complete Psychological Works of Sigmund Freud* (Vol 14). London, Hogarth Press, 1957a.

Freud S: On narcissism: An introduction. In: Strachey J (ed): *The Standard Edition of the Complete Psychological Works of Sigmund Freud* (Vol 14). London, Hogarth Press, 1957b.

Freud S: The ego and the id and other works. In: Strachev J (ed): *The Standard Edition of the Complete Pyschological Works of Sigmund Freud* (Vol 19). London, Horgarth Press, 1961.

Friedman SB: Psychological aspects of sudden unexpected death in infants and children. *Pediatr Clin North Am* 21(1):103–111, 1974.

Friedman S, Chodoff P, Mason J, et al: Behavioral observations on parents anticipating the death of a child. *Pediatrics* 32:610–625, 1963a.

Friedman S, Mason J, Hamburg D: Urinary 17-hydroxycorticosteroid levels in parents of children with neoplastic disease. *Psychosom Med* 25(4):364–367, 1963b.

Gaffney D: Sudden infant death syndrome: Loss and bereavement. *N Jersey Med* 89(9):680–682, 1992.

Gath A: The impact of an abnormal child upon the parents. *Br J Psychiatry* 130:405–410, 1977.

Giannini MJ, Goodman L: Counseling families during the crisis reaction to mongolism. *Am J Ment Defic* 67:740–747, 1963.

Giulian G, Gilbert E, Moss R: Elevated fetal hemoglobin levels in sudden infant death syndrome. *N Engl J Med* 316:1122–1126, 1987.

Goldberg J: The counseling of SIDS parents. *Clin Perinatol* 19(4):927–938, 1992.

Goldbloom A, Wigglesworth FW: Sudden infant death in infancy. *Can Med Assoc J* 38:119–129, 1938.

Golden DA, Davis JG: Counseling parents after the birth of an infant with Down syndrome. *Child Today* 2:7–37, 1974.

Goodman L: Continuing treatment of parents with congenitally defective infants. *Soc Work* 9:92–97, 1964.

Halpern W: Some psychiatric sequelae to crib death. *Am J Psychiatry* 129:398–401, 1972.

Hare EH, Laurence KM, Payne H, et al: Spina bifida and family stress. *Br Med J* 2:757–760, 1966.

Harper RG, Sia C, Sokal S, et al: Observations on unrestricted parental contact with infants in the neonatal intensive care unit. *J Pediatr* 69:441–445, 1976.

Hoffman HJ: Diptheria tetanus-pertussis immunization and SIDS: Results of NICHHD cooperative epidemiological study of SIDS risk factors. *Pediatrics* 79:598–611, 1987.

Hunter R, Kilstrom N, Kraybill E, et al. Antecedents of child abuse and neglect in premature infants: A prospective study in a newborn intensive care unit. *Pediatrics* 61:629–635, 1978.

Jeffcoate IA, Humphrey ME, Lloyd IK: Disturbance in parent-child relationship following preterm delivery. *Dev Med Child Neurol* 21:344–352, 1979.

Johns N: Family reactions to the birth of a child with a congenital abnormality. *Med J Aust* 7:277–282, 1971.

Kaplan D, Mason E: Maternal reactions to premature birth viewed as an acute emotional disorder. *Am J Orthopsychiatry* 30:539–552, 1960.

Kennell I, Slyter H, Klaus M: The mourning response of parents to the death of a newborn infant. *N Engl J Med* 283:344–349, 1970.

Kinney H: *Brainstem Maturation in the Sudden Infant Death Syndrome.* Abstract (National Institute of Child Health and Human Development, Projects Concerned with SIDS Primary FY, 1987: Project No. R012099102). Boston, Children's Hospital Corporation, 1987.

Klaus M, Kennell I: *Parent-Infant Bonding.* St. Louis, CV Mosby, 1982.

Klaus M, Kennell I, Plumb N, et al: Human maternal behavior at the first contact with her young. *Pediatrics* 46:182, 1970.

Klein M, Stern L: Low birthweight and the battered child syndrome. *Am J Dis Child* 122:15–18, 1971.

Kauubler-Ross E: *On Death and Dying.* New York. Macmillan, 1969.

Lax RF: Some aspects of the interction between mother and impaired child: Mother's narcissistic trauma. *Int J Psychoanal* 53:340–341, 1972.

Leifer AD, Leiderman CR, Barnell CR, et al: Effects of mother-infant separation on maternal attachment behavior. *Child Dev* 43:1203–1205, 1972.

Lindemann E: Symptomatology and management of acute grief. *Am J Psychiatry* 101:141–149, 1944.

Macey TJ, Harmon RJ, Easterbrooks MA; Impact of premature birth on the development of the infant in the family. *J Consult Clin Psychol* 55(6):846–852, 1987.

Mandell F, McAnulty E, Reece R: Observations of paternal response to sudden unanticipated infant death. *Pediatrics* 65:221–225, 1980.

Mandell F, McClain M, Reece R: The sudden infant death syndrome: Siblings and their place in the family. *Ann NY Acad Sci* 533:129–131, 1988.

Martin P: Martial breakdown in families of patients with spina bifida cystica. *Dev Med Child Neurol* 17:557–564, 1975.

Minde K: *Bonding of Parents to Premature Infants: Theory and Practice* (Monographs in Neonatology Series). New York, Grune & Stratton, 1980, pp. 291–313.

Minde K, Whitelaw A, Brown J, et al. Effect of neonatal complications in premature infants on early parent-infant interactions. *Dev Med Child Neurol* 25:763–777, 1983.

Naeye RL: Hypoxemia and the sudden infant death syndrome. *Science* 186:837–838, 1974.

Pasco J, Earp J: The effect of mothers' social support and life changes on the stimulation of their children in the home. *Am J Public Health* 74:358–360, 1984.

Pederson D, Bento S, Graham C, et al: Maternal emotional responses to preterm birth. *Am J Orthopsychiatry* 57(1):15–21, 1987.

Powell M: The psychological impact of Sudden Infant Death Syndrome on siblings. *Ir J Psychol* 12(2):235–247, 1991.

Poznanski E: psychiatric difficulties in siblings of handicapped children. *Clin Pediatr* 8:232–234, 1969.

Prugh D: Emotional problems of the premature infant's parents. *Nurs Outlook* 1(8):461–464, 1953.

Rowe J, Clyman R, Green C, et al: Follow-up of families who experience a perinatal death. *Pediatrics* 62:166–170, 1978.

Sadeh D, Shannon D, Abbaud S, et al: Altered cardiac repolarization in some victims of sudden infant death syndrome. *N Engl J med* 317:1501–1505, 1987.

Salk L: Sudden infant death: Impact on family and physician. *Clin Pediatr* 10(5):248–250, 1971.

Schonell F, Watts BH: A first survey of the effects of a subnormal child on the family unit. *Am J Ment Defic* 61:210–219, 1957.

Silcock A: Crises in parents or prematures: An Australian study. *Br J Dev Psychol* 2:257–268, 1984.

Smialek Z: Observations on immediate reactions of families to sudden infant death. *Pediatrics* 62:160–165, 1978.

Solnit A, Green M: Psychological considerations in the management of deaths on pediatric hospital services (part I). *Pediatrics* 24:106–112, 1959.

Solnit A, Stark M: Mourning and the birth of a defective child. *Psychoanal Study Child* 16:523–537, 1961.

Steele B, Pollock C: A Psychiatric Study of Parents Who Abuse Infants and Small Children (2nd ed). Chicago, University of Chicago Press, 1974.

Steinschneider A: Implication of the sudden infant death syndrome for the study of sleep in infancy. *Minn Symp Child Psychol* 9:106–134, 1975.

Swoiskin S: Sudden infant death: Nursing care for the survivors. *J Pediatr Nur* 1(1):33–39, 1986.

Tew BJ, Payne H, Laurence KM: Must a family with a handicapped child be a handicapped family? *Dev Med Child Neurol* 16(suppl 32):95–98, 1974.

Templeman C: Two hundred and fifty eight cases of suffocation of infants. *Edinb Med J* 38:322–329, 1892.

Tisza VB, Gumpertz E: Parents' reaction to the birth of a child with cleft palate. *Pediatrics* 30:86–90, 1962.

Trause MA, Kramer LI: The effects of premature birth on parents and their relationship. *Dev Med Child Neurol* 24:459–465, 1983.

Valdes-Dapena M: Sudden infant death syndrome: A review of the medical literature (1974–1979). *Pediatrics* 66(4):597–610, 1980.

Van Riper M, Pridham K, Ryff C: Symbolic interactionism: A perspective for understanding parent-nurse interactions following the birth of a child with Down's syndrome. *Matern Child Nurs J* 20(1):21–39, 1992.

Walker JH, Thomas M, Russell IT: Spina bifida and the parents. *Dev Med Child Neurol* 13:462–476, 1971.

Weinstein S: Sudden infant death syndrome: Im-

pact on families and a direction for change. *Am J Psychiatry* 135:831–834, 1978.

Williams M: Sibling reaction to cot death. *Med J Aust* 2:227–231, 1981.

Woolsey S: Support after sudden infant death. *Am J Nurs* 10:1348–1351, 1988.

Zeanah C: Adaptation following perinatal loss: A critical review. *J Am Acad Child Adolesc Psychiatry* 28:467–480, 1989.

Zebal BH, Woolsey BF: SIDS and the family: The pediatrician's role. *Pediatr Ann* 13:237–261, 1984.

94 PSYCHIATRIC ASPECTS OF CANCER IN CHILDHOOD AND ADOLESCENCE

John P. Glazer, M.D., and Todd M. Ivan, M.D.

Cancer is the leading cause of death due to illness in childhood and adolescence, except in infancy (Vaughan, 1987). At the same time, dramatic improvements in survival have occurred over the past 30 years, in large part because of the development of a complex array of treatments, including chemotherapy, radiotherapy, surgery, and bone marrow transplantation. It is these fundamental characteristics—the continued importance of childhood cancer as a contributor to terminal childhood illness, the technological complexity and adverse neuropsychiatric effects of treatments for cancer, and the psychological issues faced by long-term survivors of childhood cancer—that define the tasks for child and adolescent psychiatrists working in pediatric oncology.

Following a discussion of methodological issues, this chapter reviews psychological aspects of cancer in childhood and adolescence, taking a longitudinal perspective. First, psychological issues for children and adolescents with cancer at the time of diagnosis, during treatment, and during long-term survival or terminal illness is presented. Next, psychological aspects of specific settings in pediatric oncology, such as bone marrow transplantation, medical procedure pain, and cranial radiation, are considered. Finally, psychotherapeutic, psychopharmacological, and other psychosocial interventions for the child and adolescent with cancer are discussed.

METHODOLOGICAL AND CONCEPTUAL ISSUES

Chronic physical illness in childhood and adolescence is an established risk factor for psychological disturbance (Pless and Nolan, 1989), and involvement of the CNS enhances this risk (Rutter et al., 1970).

Thus, all pediatric patients with cancer would be expected to be at increased risk of psychiatric disorder, and important subpopulations may be especially vulnerable: The two most prevalent pediatric malignancies are acute lymphoblastic leukemia (ALL) and tumors of the brain and CNS (Miller, 1989). Children with ALL commonly receive 1800–2400 rad of cranial radiation (CRT) for the purpose of presymptomatic treatment of presumed leukemic foci within the CNS (Poplack, 1989); CRT is associated with neurocognitive toxicity (Rowland et al., 1984). Together, ALL and brain tumors account for about 40% of all cancer in childhood and adolescence (Miller, 1989); thus, because of either neurotoxic treatment or direct CNS involvement by the malignancy itself, a major fraction of young people with cancer may be at major psychiatric risk.

Controlled studies on the efficacy of psychosocial interventions in the prevention and treatment of psychological disturbance in chronically ill youth are scarce (Gortmaker, 1990; Pless and Nolan, 1989; Rutter,

1982). Particularly striking is the lack of studies of individual psychotherapy for children and adolescents with cancer (Pless and Nolan, 1989). Given the demonstrated efficacy of individual and group psychotherapy for adults with cancer (Massie et al., 1989), the need for such studies in pediatric oncology is compelling.

There is no established theory of the way chronic illness predisposes to psychological disturbance in childhood. A common formulation is that illness serves as a "stress" and that the psychological task for the ill child is "adaptation" to or "coping" with this stress. In this model, provision of additional social supports, typically through parent- or patient-based support groups, is thought to be therapeutic (Pless and Nolan, 1989). However, systematic studies of the role of stress are limited (Rutter, 1982). For example, in a controlled study to examine the role of environmental stress in producing emotional disturbance in a large group of children with myelodysplasia and cerebral palsy, a causal link could not be demonstrated (Breslau, 1990).

On the other hand, this model is attractive in that it conceives of psychological dysfunction in chronically ill children as a crisis occurring in the course of normal development rather than as psychopathology (Futterman and Hoffman, 1970; Silberfarb, 1982; Spinetta, 1982). In a prospective study of children undergoing bone marrow transplantation that speaks directly to the role of environmental stress as a mediator of psychological disturbance, for example, Stuber et al. (1989) reported a high incidence of posttraumatic stress disorder.

Improved survival from cancer in childhood and adolescence has come at the expense of increased treatment toxicity, which may include second malignant neoplasms, gonadal dysfunction, growth failure, and neuropsychiatric sequelae, among other effects (Meadows and Hobbie, 1986; Rowland et al., 1984). Pediatric oncologists are increasingly turning their attention to providing formal, long-term medical and psychosocial follow-up for their patients, even after cure of the initial malignancy, and are beginning to consider psychosocial factors as legitimate outcome variables in the design of cancer treatment protocols (Meadows and Hobbie, 1986; Mulhern et al., 1989).

Assessment instruments used in populations of healthy children to determine the prevalence of psychiatric disorders may not be suitable for children and adolescents with cancer. Heiligenstein and Jacobson (1988) have recently reported, for example, that the Children's Depression Rating Scale (CDRS) fails to discriminate depressed from nondepressed 7- to 15-year-old pediatric patients with cancer. The problem resides in the overlap between symptoms of physical impairment and those of depression.

Also, categorical psychiatric diagnosis may not be the best approach, in the sense that behavior that would reflect symptom formation in a physically well child may be adaptive for the child with cancer (Futterman and Hoffman, 1970). Denial, considered a primitive psychological defense in psychoanalytic terms, for example, is often adaptive in pediatric patients with cancer (Koocher and O'Malley, 1981, p. 161).

One alternative to categorical psychiatric diagnosis is the construct designated *quality of life* (Mulhern et al., 1989a; Schipper and Levitt, 1985). This term seems to represent an attempt to place value on some feature or features of human experience (Jonsen et al., 1982). Several authors (Hinds, 1990; Rosenbaum, 1990) emphasize the subjective sense of *well-being* as central to the determination of quality of life. What has become clear is that any assessment of quality of life must be multidimensional (Ivan and Glazer, 1994). The traditional definition of therapeutic success in oncology as the duration of absolute or cancer-free survival makes it difficult to compare psychosocial and functional outcome across treatment protocols and inhibits the evaluation of psychosocial interventions. It also misses the essential point: that one's experience of life transcends simple measures of its duration.

Schipper and Levitt's Functional Living Index for Cancer (1985) assesses physical, occupational, social, and psychological functioning in adults in a single self-report measure. Lansky's Play Performance Scale for Children (PPSC) (Lansky et al., 1985) and the Vineland Adaptive Behavior Scales (Sparrow et al., 1984) have been suggested as candidate quality of life instruments for use in pediatrics (Mulhern et al., 1989a). Mulhern et al. (1989a) have proposed the following characteristics for a pediatric quality of life measure:

1. It should allow assessment of "physical function, occupational or school performance, social adjustment, and 'self-satisfaction.'"
2. It should allow an estimation of psychosocial functioning prior to the diagnosis of cancer.
3. It should be suitable for prospective longitudinal studies of psychosocial functioning in children and adolescents with cancer, as well as allowing for child and parental ratings and supranormal premorbid performance.

Civin (1989) suggests that the central issue in pediatric cancer treatment at the present state of knowledge is that of weighing the relative importance of additional improvements in survival on the one hand and the quality of that survival on the other. Adults with cancer, for example, sometimes choose treatments associated with a lower chance of cure but greater preservation of physical function (Schipper and Levitt, 1985). Resolution of these difficult issues in clinical care and investigation requires scientifically sound methods for measuring the quality of survival. As stated by Schipper and Levitt (1985), "Clinical trials analysts measure tumor size, disappearance, reappearance, and survival. Patients measure quality of life" (p. 1116).

PSYCHIATRIC DISORDER IN CHILDREN AND ADOLESCENTS WITH CANCER

At Diagnosis

Several watershed events in the longitudinal course of cancer in childhood are particularly stressful; these include the diagnostic period, cancer relapse, and the point at which successful survivors come to the end of treatment.

The period surrounding the diagnosis of cancer is typically described as a time of emotional crisis for the child (Lansky et al., 1983; Pfefferbaum, 1989). Kupst and Schulman (1980), for example, assessed 43 children 16 years old or younger within 48 hours of being informed of a diagnosis of leukemia, using direct clinical observation and videotaped interviews. Anxiety was judged to be present in 54–70% (depending on observer) of subjects; however, as a group, subjects were judged to be "coping" adequately, and depression was rarely observed. Powazek et al. (1980), however, using a variety of self-report measures in a similar population, found anxiety present in only 8% of study subjects, compared to 45% of mothers. Finally, in their retrospective study of 114 long-term survivors of childhood cancer, Koocher and O'Malley (1981) found that loss of social relationships during the diagnostic period and a reaction of "shock and distress" on learning the diagnosis were associated with poor psychological adjustment.

FAMILY FACTORS

Weisman and Worden's (1976) work established the importance of social supports to the psychological well-being of adults with cancer. The family is often viewed as the chief source of social support for children (Blotcky et al., 1985). Fife et al. (1987) divided 10 subject families of children with cancer into "functional" or "dysfunctional" categories, based in part on their effectiveness in managing stressful events prior to the onset of their child's leukemia. The only episode of noncompliance—refusal to take prescribed chemotherapy—occurred in a child of one of the "dysfunctional" families, suggesting that prior family functioning is an important predictive factor. Similarly, Blotcky et al. (1985) reported that high levels of subjective parental distress were predictive of hopelessness in a group of school-age children with cancer 3 months after diagnosis. Also, parental coping behaviors best suited to reducing distress in parents themselves were different from those that reduced feelings of hopelessness in their children.

Psychosocial assessment at the time of diagnosis in pediatric oncology should include obtaining a psychiatric history of the patient, parents, and siblings and should focus on the identification of families with a history of poor coping with previous stressful life events and those in which parental distress is high. The poor fit between coping strategies that diminish psychological distress in parents and those that benefit their children with cancer strongly suggests a role for family-centered psychotherapy, particularly for families selected on the basis of these risk factors. Koocher and O'Malley's findings (1981) of a relationship between long-term adjustment and both the manner of response to learning the cancer diagnosis and the resilience of social relationships during the diagnostic period suggest that important individual premorbid psychological variables also mediate outcome.

Psychiatric Disorder during Treatment: Depression

Clinical studies of psychiatric disorder during cancer treatment have largely focused on depression. Kashani and Hakami's study was probably the first to address categorical psychiatric diagnosis in a pediatric oncology population (1982). In this study, a child psychiatrist interviewed each of 35 children and adolescents with cancer and their parents during outpatient clinic visits. Study subjects were between 6 and 17 years old and between 1 month and 10 years since their cancer diagnosis. Major depressive disorder was diagnosed in 17% of the study population, compared to 1.9% and 4% in child and adolescent control subjects, respectively.

Kaplan et al. (1987), using the Beck Depression Inventory (BDI) and the Child Depression Inventory (CDI) to longitudinally assess a heterogeneous group of 17 adolescents and 21 children with cancer, found that depression scores for the adolescent subjects were comparable to, and those for children were lower than, those in the control groups. Finally, in a retrospective chart review study, Rait et al. (1988) reported an incidence of major depressive disorder of 12% in a sample of 58 pediatric and young adult cancer inpatients referred for psychiatric consultation.

The spectrum of results of these studies reflects the heterogeneity of study subjects and methods of assessment—inpatients and outpatients at varying stages of illness were assessed using clinical interviews or self-report measures—and the limitations of existing assessment methodology. The CDI, for example, has been shown to detect less depression in a pediatric oncology sample than in control groups of healthy children or child psychiatric inpatients (Worchel et al., 1988), and, as mentioned above, the CDRS, a clinician-rated instrument, overestimates the severity of depression in children with cancer (Heiligenstein and Jacobson,

1988). Deletion of the "somatic" subscale from the CDRS yields an instrument, the CDRS-Revised, that correlates more closely with clinician judgments of depression severity in a subject population. This work exemplifies the refinements needed in the assessment of affective disturbances in children and adolescents with cancer, in whom "depression" may account for as much as 20% of psychiatric referrals (Rait et al., 1988).

Long-term Survival

Long-term survival, the sine qua non of success in pediatric oncology, is most visible for ALL because of its frequency and the dramatic improvements in outcome achieved since the 1950s. As depicted in Table 94.1, equally optimistic results have been achieved for Hodgkin's disease and Wilms' tumor (and some bone sarcomas not shown in the table), but it is important to remember that, for many other children with cancer, the outlook is less optimistic. Numerically, the most important example of the latter category is brain tumors, which are almost as frequent as ALL but have 5-year survival rates of only 10–40%.

Long-term survival, moreover, has come at the expense of adverse late effects, both medical and psychological (Lansky et al., 1986; Meadows and Hobbie, 1986). Late medical effects include short stature, sterility, major organ system failure, and, most tragically, second malignant neoplasms (Meadows and Hobbie, 1986). An early example of a direct relationship between improved survival and enhanced neuropsychiatric toxicity was the introduction of cranial radiation during remission induction in ALL. Historically, after prolonged bone marrow remissions in ALL became possible with multidrug chemotherapy, the CNS became the most frequent site of relapse, and this complication is often the harbinger of bone marrow relapse and a fatal outcome. Prophylactic cranial radiation was found to markedly reduce the frequency of CNS relapse and became a standard feature of treatment (Poplack, 1989) but is associated with neuropsychological toxicity, as discussed below.

Another example is the treatment of the roughly one-third of children with ALL who present at diagnosis with unfavorable prognostic indicators; until recently, prolonged, disease-free survival in this group was achievable in only 30–40% of cases; newer treatment protocols have achieved levels closer to 70% (Civin, 1989). However, one recent study has reported severe gonadal toxicity in a group of children with ALL treated with an aggressive regimen that includes 10 chemotherapeutic agents plus cranial radiation (Quigley et al., 1989). The question of the balance between treatment efficacy and toxicity in pediatric oncology is the subject of active debate (Civin, 1989; Meadows et al., 1989). Studies of *psychological* outcome in long-term survivors of childhood cancer are a crucial part of this issue. Selected major features of eight studies of psychological outcome in long-term survivors are summarized in Table 94.2 (Fritz et al., 1988; Greenberg et al., 1989; Holmes and Holmes, 1975; Koocher and O'Malley, 1981; Lansky et al., 1986; Mulh-

ern et al., 1989b; Teta et al., 1986; Wasserman et al., 1987); two of these are described in more detail (Fritz et al., 1988; Koocher and O'Malley, 1981).

Koocher and O'Malley (1981) comprehensively assessed 114 long-term childhood cancer survivors retrospectively, using self-report measures of anxiety, depression, and self-esteem, and assignment of a "combined adjustment rating" from independent interview data of a psychiatrist and psychologist. In this study, 53 of the 114 subjects (47%) were judged to exhibit at least "mild" psychological symptoms. Of the total, 26% had "mild" symptoms without functional impairment, 10% were moderately symptomatic and unimpaired, and 11.2% had moderate or severe symptoms and functional impairment. Psychiatric interviews revealed more anxiety and depression and lower self-esteem in the 47% judged "poorly adjusted" than in the 53% judged "well adjusted." Paralleling the interview findings, among several psychological and demographic variables assessed using standardized measures, levels of depression and anxiety and low self-esteem accounted for the greatest proportion of the variance in overall adjustment. Compared to a control group of children with chronic, non-life-threatening illnesses, the group of cancer survivors exhibited significantly poorer overall adjustment and lower self-satisfaction. Finally, well-adjusted survivors in this study used denial adaptively and were more likely to have been informed promptly of their diagnosis of cancer.

Fritz et al. (1988) reported on a cohort of 52 children and adolescents at least 2 years after successful completion of treatment for cancer. Mean age was 9.7 years at diagnosis and 15.9 years when studied. Antecedent variables most closely associated with outcome in this study were those in the *psychosocial* category: Direct communication during treatment between the child patient and his or her peers, schoolmates, and family was predictive of successful academic, social, and physical functioning and high "global adjustment" scores (based on videotaped interviews); peer support during treatment was associated with high global adjustment. Of the illness-related variables, only physical impairment was significantly associated with any outcome variable: Greater physical impairment was predictive of depression and lower global adjustment scores. Interestingly, the severity of the medical aspects of the cancer experience, as measured by the nature of the diagnostic process and prognosis, and the difficulty of the treatment protocol was not related to psychological outcome. Depression, using the CDRS, was definitely absent in 80% of the subjects, definitely present in three subjects (6%), and questionably present in seven (14%).

Among the eight studies depicted in Table 94.2, several variables emerge as apparent mediators of psychological outcome. Illness-related communication was addressed by two of the studies. Koocher and O'Malley (1981) assessed timeliness in communication of the diagnosis of cancer as a predictor of psychological outcome, and Fritz et al. (1988) studied the degree to which the child patient communicated with others about his or her illness as an antecedent variable. Both studies found greater communication predictive of favorable psychological outcome. In a related study of 16 6- to 10-year-old children with leukemia, Spinetta and Maloney (1978) found that openness of family communication about the child's illness, as judged by their mothers, was associated with the ill child feeling close to family members, satisfied with self, and nondefensive. The presence of support from peers was also found to be correlated with favorable adjustment (Fritz et al., 1988; Koocher and O'Malley, 1981).

Physical disability was predictive of psychological maladjustment in three of four studies (Fritz et al., 1988; Greenberg et al., 1989; Mulhern et al., 1989b; but not in Koocher and O'Malley, 1981). Studies of chronically ill children in general have confirmed this association, especially in boys (Pless and Nolan, 1989).

Several of the studies found that children younger at the time of diagnosis were better adjusted (Fritz et al., 1988; Greenberg et al., 1989; Koocher and O'Malley, 1981).

Finally, two studies suggest a link between cancer treatment toxicity and psychological outcome. Mulhern et al. (1989b), using the Child Behavior Checklist, reported that administration of prophylactic cranial radiation, known to produce cognitive impairment (Fletcher and Cope-

Table 94.1.   Incidence and Approximate 5-Year Survival for Selected Childhood Malignancies

Cancer Type	Annual Incidence[a]	5-Year Survival (%)
ALL	29.4	75
ANLL[b]	10.6	20–35
Hodgkin's disease	7.3	90
Wilms' tumor	7.7	90
Brain tumors	24.5	
Medulloblastoma	5.5	40
Astrocytoma	NA	20
Glioma	15.9	10

Adapted from Rowland J: Developmental stage and adaptation: Child and adolescent model. In: Holland J, Rowland J (eds): *Handbook of Psychooncology.* New York, Oxford, 1989, p. 520. Miller R: Frequency and environmental epidemiology of childhood cancer. In: Pizzo P, Poplack O (eds): *Principles and Practice of Pediatric Oncology.* Philadelphia, Lippincott, 1985.
[a] Per million population.
[b] ANLL, acute nonlymphoblastic leukemias; NA, not available.

Table 94.2. Studies of Psychological Outcome in Long-term Survivors of Childhood Cancer

Reference	Study Subjects	Controls	Design	Outcome Measures	Selected Results
Holmes and Holmes (1975)	124 ≥ 10-yr survivors. Cancer dx 1–15 yr.	None	Retrospective mailed questionnaire	Self-report via questionnaire	7.3% with "serious impairment" (mental or physical)
Koocher and O'Malley (1981)	114 5- to 32-yr survivors. Cancer dx < age 18 yr.	22 with nonfatal chronic illness treated ≥ 5 yr ago	Retrospective	Rutter/Graham interview; self-report measures of anxiety, depression, self-esteem; "Combined Adjustment Rating"	(1) 53% well-adjusted; 35% psychological symptoms, no functional impairment; 11.2% symptomatic and impaired. (2) Poorer adjustment in cancer survivors than in controls.
Lansky et al. (1986)	39 5- to 10-yr survivors. Cancer dx age 10–18 yr.	Nearest age sibs	Retrospective	Semistructured interview	15% with history of treated depression, alcoholism, or suicide attempts. Results for controls not given.
Teta et al. (1986)	450 5- to 34-yr survivors. Cancer dx ≤ 19 yr.	587 sibs	Retrospective	SADS-L	*Lifetime major depression* 　 Subjects　Controls M　15%　　12% F　22%　　24% *Suicide attempts and psychiatric hospitalizations:* Subjects and controls not significantly different.
Wasserman et al. (1987)	40 ≥ 5-yr Hodgkin's survivors. Mean age cancer dx 12.8 yr.	None	Retrospective	DSM-III diagnosis by semistructured interview	15% with psychiatric disorder
Fritz et al. (1988)	52 survivors 2–7 yr off treatment. Mean age cancer dx 9.7 yr.	None	Retrospective	Children's Depression Rating Scale; observer ratings of school, social, physical functioning; "Global Adjustment Rating"	6% definitely depressed; 14% questionably depressed; 80% not depressed. *Global adjustment:* 61% good or excellent; 26% average; 14% marginal or poor.
Mulhern et al. (1989)	183 ≥ 2-yr survivors. Mean age cancer dx 2.7 yr.	None	Retrospective	Child Behavior Checklist	3- to 4-fold higher incidence of abnormalities in behavior and social competence compared to instrument norms
Greenberg et al. (1989)	138 ≥ 2-yr survivors. Mean age cancer dx 3.6 yr.	92 well-child clinic patients	Retrospective	Child Depression Inventory; Piers-Harris Self-Concept Scale; Norwicki-Strickland Locus of Control Scale for Children; Family Environment Scale	*Depression:* no difference between subjects and controls. *Self-concept:* Subjects significantly poorer than controls. *Locus of control:* Subjects significantly more external than controls.

land, 1988), was predictive of psychological disturbance in long-term survivors, and Greenberg et al. (1989) found that the severity of several adverse medical late effects, including cognitive impairment, predicted depression and poor self-concept in survivors.

To summarize, several points regarding outcome studies in long-term childhood cancer survivors should be emphasized.

First, the data on long-term psychological outcome in child and adolescent cancer survivors are conflicting; several authors speak with prognostic optimism (Fritz et al., 1988; Greenberg et al., 1989; Teta et al., 1986), yet caution seems warranted. The finding that 15% of the cohort reported by Lansky et al. (1986) had histories of psychiatric intervention for depression, suicidal behavior, or alcoholism, and the finding by Mulhern et al. (1989b) of a 3- to 4-fold higher incidence of disturbances in social competence and behavior on the Child Behavior Checklist compared to instrument norms, cannot be ignored.

Second, of the three long-term survivor studies that used controls, Koocher and O'Malley (1981) found significantly more maladjustment among cancer survivors than in survivors of non-life-threatening chronic illness; Greenberg et al. (1989) found significantly lower self-concept in cancer survivors than in control well-child outpatients; and Teta et al. (1986) found no difference in the lifetime prevalence of major depressive disorder in survivors compared to sibling controls.

Third, antecedent variables that may predict psychological disturbance in survivors, based upon their identification in one or more studies, include inadequate social and peer support; limited illness-related communication between the child and his or her family, physician, and peers; concealment of the diagnosis; physical impairment as a result of cancer or its treatment; and the severity of late medical sequelae, such as gonadal failure, cognitive impairment, or major cosmetic effects.

Fourth, the availability of mental health services for children and

Table 94.3. Depression and Long-term Survivors of Childhood Cancer

Reference	Results
Fritz et al., 1988	*Measure:* Children's Depression Rating Scale (clinician rated) *Depression* Definite　　　6% Questionable　14% Absent　　　　80%
Greenberg et al., 1989	*Measure:* Children's Depression Inventory (self-report) *Depression:* Same in subjects and controls and less than for instrument norms
Teta et al., 1986	*Measure:* SADS-L *Depression:*　Subjects　Controls M　　　15%　　12% F　　　22%　　24%
Lansky et al., 1986	*Measure:* Interview 15% with history of depression, suicide attempt, or alcoholism requiring treatment

adolescents with cancer and their families is widely recommended (Koocher and O'Malley, 1981). Since openness of communication and preservation of family and social ties are predictive of favorable psychological outcome, psychotherapeutic intervention may be crucial when communication and socialization are compromised.

Fifth, methodological limitations must be kept in mind. Studies to date have been retrospective, and a variety of observer-rated, self-report, and interview-based outcome measures were used. This diversity is illustrated in Table 94.3, which lists the four long-term survivor studies in which depression was measured.

Sixth and last, it is probable that no single style of coping is associated with a favorable adjustment to cancer; individual differences are the rule and must be kept in mind when interventions are contemplated. Fritz et al. (1988) state:

> Individuals . . . who were . . . well adjusted, free of depression, successful at school, and popular with friends used different coping styles. Some well-adjusted survivors had embraced their cancer and had become experts and advocates; others had encapsulated the illness and acknowledged it as little as possible. Assertiveness and argumentativeness toward caregivers were associated with good outcome, as were compliance and passivity. A concrete, nonphilosophical approach served some survivors well, while others ascribed a larger purpose of meaning to the illness. . . . The present findings underscore the need for understanding and acceptance of individual response styles in the planning of psychosocial interventions. (p. 560)

The Terminally Ill Child with Cancer

Current figures indicate that there are about 2200 annual cancer deaths in children under 15 years of age in the United States (Miller, 1989). Thus, although the current psychological literature in pediatric oncology reflects a shift in emphasis from the psychological tasks of "adapting to the imminence of death to one of coping with uncertain survival" (Eisenberg, 1981), the extensive older literature devoted to terminal illness in childhood is as relevant today as it was in the past (Glazer, 1990).

Spinetta et al. (1973), Waechter (1971), Bluebond-Langner (1977), and others have extended earlier studies of the acquisition of a concept of death by healthy children (Anthony, 1940; Nagy, 1948) to those who have a life-threatening illness. This work has shown that terminally ill children are capable of acquiring a mature understanding of the realities of death and dying as early as age 4–6 years (Solnit and Green, 1963; Spinetta et al., 1973). In the early work of Richmond and Waisman (1955), the authors noted that children dying of cancer infrequently verbalized fears of dying; the results of two controlled studies, however, indicate that terminally ill children with cancer are significantly more anxious than their chronically but not fatally ill counterparts (Spinetta et al., 1973; Waechter, 1971), even though they may not verbalize their distress.

Psychological care of the terminally ill child and his or her family requires the utmost in sensitivity by caregivers who are themselves uniquely vulnerable in this clinical setting (Solnit, 1983; Solnit and Green, 1963; Spinetta, 1974). A flexible approach that respects each child's and family's unique psychological needs and the creation of an atmosphere of open communication that avoids a "conspiracy of silence" (Karon and Vernick, 1968), which leaves the child feeling isolated and alone, are essential (Bluebond-Langner, 1977; Spinetta, 1974; Waechter, 1971).

At no time in a child's life are the basic human discomforts of physical pain, loneliness, and anxiety more appropriate concerns of the caregiver than at the end of life (Solnit, 1983). Thus, aggressive management of cancer pain, reassurance to the dying child that he or she will not be left alone, and relief of the psychological discomforts of anxiety and depression are essential. Psychotherapeutic intervention may be particularly helpful when the needs of the child cannot be fully met by parents who themselves face the psychological task of disengaging from a child they are about to lose. Finally, home care for the dying child, the preference of some families, should be made an available option (Fortunato and Komp, 1979; Mulhern et al., 1983).

SPECIFIC CLINICAL PROBLEMS

School Phobia and Regressive Symbiosis

Futterman and Hoffman (1970) reported a single case of school phobia in a 7½-year-old girl with leukemia, in a series of 25 children with leukemia. Their patient's two school-avoidant episodes occurred in conjunction with leukemic relapse on the first occasion and during an intercurrent respiratory infection on the second; both episodes resolved with

resolution of the intercurrent medical problem. The authors suggest that psychodynamic factors operative in the child's family prior to the diagnosis of leukemia at age 2½, in combination with exaggerated parental sensitivity to separation from their daughter following diagnosis, set the stage for school phobia at those times when leukemic relapse or other medical problems brought parental anxiety over the impending permanent separation from the child, through death, out in the open.

Lansky et al. (1975) reported school phobia in over 10% of a series of children with leukemia, compared to a prevalence of about 1% in the general population and roughly 5% in studies of children who were psychiatrically referred (Hersov, 1985).

Whether because of school avoidance or for legitimate medical reasons, children with cancer experience frequent school absences (Cairns et al., 1982; Wasserman et al., 1987), and, as discussed below in the section on intervention, medical caregivers have a crucial role to play in facilitating the reentry of youthful cancer patients into their peer culture and the educational settings they left behind at the time of diagnosis. Both are essential ingredients in favorable psychological adjustment.

Finally, Lansky and Gendel (1978) described a clinical syndrome they termed "symbiotic regressive behavior" in 12 children and adolescents with cancer among 300 such patients reviewed by the authors. As a group, these patients exhibited a spectrum of profoundly regressed behaviors, which included resumption of bottle-feeding, loss of speech milestones, and assumption of a fetal position. Severe separation anxiety on the part of the children and their mothers and withdrawal of the mother-child dyad from family and social contacts were seen in all cases; psychosis occurred in 2 children and school phobia in 5. Pathological mourning was common in the parents following the deaths of these children. The authors suggest that early psychosocial intervention for all families with a child with cancer is the best preventive measure, treatment often being unsuccessful once the symbiotic regressive pattern is established. It should be noted that this report appeared in an era of uniformly fatal outcome for most childhood cancers; whether such severe psychological reactions have diminished in frequency with improved prospects for survival is unknown.

Noncompliance

In those pediatric cancer patients with curable malignant neoplasms, provision of anticancer treatment is literally life-saving; thus, compliance with recommended treatments is crucial. Using the assay for urinary 17-ketosteroids of Smith et al. (1979), Lansky et al. (1983) reported that in a series of 31 2- to 14-year-old children with leukemia, fully 42% of the sample were noncompliant with treatment, and none of the patients were compliant 100% of the time. Although the frequency of noncompliance was unrelated to patient gender, important gender differences were detected in the psychological correlates of compliance and noncompliance: Parent personality variables were related to compliance behavior in boys, while patient variables were decisive in girls. The most important predictors of compliance in this study were anxiety in the parents of male patients and anxiety in the female patients themselves.

Age also appears to be an important determinant of noncompliance. Tebbi et al. (1986) studied compliance with chemotherapy in a series of 46 patients with cancer ranging in age from 2.5 to 23 years (mean age, 6.9 years) and detected important age effects: The mean age of patients was 9.5 years for those who never missed a dose of prescribed chemotherapy, 10.5 years for those who missed occasional doses, and 17.4 years for those who frequently missed doses. Finally, noncompliance in adolescents with cancer may be associated with aversive medical procedures and side effects of chemotherapy.

CASE ILLUSTRATION

R., a 15-year-old girl with newly diagnosed Hodgkin's disease, was referred to a pediatric oncology program after refusing her second cycle of chemotherapy at another center because it upset her stomach. Family and psychiatric history revealed that the patient had made three suicide attempts during the 2 years prior to the diagnosis of cancer and that her mother had failed to obtain medical or psychiatric care for her daughter after each of these episodes. The patient's mother, a single parent, felt overwhelmed by the needs of her daughter and unable to set limits upon her increasingly provocative behaviors. Mental status examination of the adolescent revealed psychomotor slowing, depressed mood, withdrawal, and tearfulness. She expressed indifference to the knowledge that, without treatment, which she continued to refuse, she would die. Psychiatric hospitalization was arranged initially without the patient's consent. After a week on a psychiatric unit for adolescents, and after her oncologist showed her her chest radiograph, which demonstrated tumor regression following her first course of chemotherapy, the patient's affect brightened, and she granted permission for administration of her next cycle of chemotherapy.

Compliance with treatment in pediatric oncology may be related to several factors, including age, normative psychological variables in patients and in parents, aversive treatments, and as a correlate of serious psychopathology and self-destructiveness. In the latter instance, timely psychiatric intervention is essential. In the more common situation in which compliance issues are less overt, management guidelines are less clear; however, data from studies performed to date suggest that adolescents should be regarded as being at particularly high risk.

Distress Related to Medical Procedures and Chemotherapy

The performance of multiple invasive medical procedures such as diagnostic bone marrow aspiration and diagnostic as well as therapeutic lumbar puncture are facts of life for a majority of pediatric patients with cancer, especially during the early intensive phase of treatment. Several studies have found that, both for the patient (Wasserman et al., 1987) and for parents (Kupst and Schulman, 1980), treatment-associated distress may cause more acute suffering than the psychological reaction to the illness itself. As noted, these treatment side effects have been linked to noncompliance with anticancer treatment. For some diagnostic categories, adolescents with cancer have a poorer prognosis than younger children (Simone et al., 1975); poor compliance may be a contributing factor (Dolgin et al., 1989).

In perhaps the only naturalistic study of treatment-related distress in children and adolescents with cancer to date, Dolgin et al. (1989) surveyed psychological and behavioral symptoms in a prospective, longitudinal study of 94 consecutively diagnosed 3- to 19-year-old pediatric oncology patients. A key finding was that adolescents exhibited a higher rate of symptom formation, particularly anxiety and nausea and vomiting, than younger patients, and the prevalence of symptoms in adolescents increased over the 6-month course of the study, while it decreased in the younger patients. For example, 7 months postdiagnosis, 71% of the adolescents exhibited anticipatory anxiety, and 36% exhibited anticipatory nausea or vomiting in the 24-hour period prior to scheduled administration of chemotherapy. Although this study did not specifically address the response to invasive medical procedures, it suggests that the day-to-day experience of pediatric patients in active treatment for cancer involves significant psychological distress and that adolescents are at particular risk.

A variety of psychological and pharmacological interventions have been evaluated in the management of medical procedure-associated distress in the pediatric oncology setting (Zeltzer et al., 1989). Psychological approaches include preparatory information giving, hypnosis, and emotive imagery and distraction. Among these techniques, the demonstration of efficacy in controlled clinical trials appears to be most convincing for hypnosis (Olness, 1989), and Kuttner et al. (1988) have

recently shown that hypnosis may be effective in children with cancer undergoing medical procedures as young as 3 years of age.

Using standardized outcome measures, Jay et al. (1987) reported the results of a clinical trial comparing a nonhypnotic psychological intervention, pharmacological intervention, and a control condition in which no specific intervention was provided in a series of 56 3- to 13-year-old children with cancer scheduled to undergo three or more bone marrow aspirations. The psychological intervention consisted of a "package" of nonhypnotic modalities including breathing exercises, imagery/distraction, and behavioral rehearsal. The pharmacological intervention was diazepam 0.3 mg/kg by mouth 30 minutes before the procedure. Results indicated that children in the psychological intervention group exhibited significantly less behavioral distress, reported significantly less pain, and had significantly lower pulse rates than control subjects. The diazepam group did not exhibit significant differences on any of these measures compared to controls; however, the possibility that a higher dosage would have been efficacious was not addressed in this study.

Among pharmacological approaches to painful medical procedures, a variety of agents have been used, including benzodiazepines, chloral hydrate, narcotics, nitrous oxide, and combinations of agents from more than one class. One study found that chlorpromazine served as an effective anxiolytic and antiemetic in chemotherapy patients (Relling et al., 1993). Midazolam has been advocated as an effective anxiolytic and amnestic agent in lumbar puncture and bone marrow aspiration (Friedman et al., 1991). In general, controlled clinical trials of pharmacological intervention for painful pediatric procedures have not been reported, and practices vary widely across centers (Zeltzer et al., 1989). General anesthesia, widely used in Europe for this indication, is infrequently used in the United States; however, in one United States pediatric oncology center, favorable results have been reported for children undergoing bone marrow aspiration of lumbar puncture (Fisher et al., 1985). Appropriate attention to drug toxicity is crucial when pharmacological intervention is used, and the presence of a pediatric anesthesiologist is also essential when certain agents are used (Zeltzer et al., 1989). A rational approach to the use of sedative, anesthetic, and analgesic medications to lessen the trauma of medical procedures in pediatric cancer patients has been proposed (Table 94.4). Selected local anesthetic agents and their uses are summarized in Table 94.5.

Children undergoing the same medical procedure vary in the magnitude of distress they exhibit (McGrath and Craig, 1989). Zeltzer et al. (1989) suggest that different approaches to procedure pain management should be used with children to the extent that a given child benefits from a sense of personal control over the procedure situation. These authors propose that *psychological* techniques enhance a sense of mastery in children benefiting from a sense of control of medical procedures, while *pharmacological* intervention with such children may be contraindicated since agents such as narcotics and sedatives impair personal control. Children who present with severe anxiety, on the other hand, are more appropriate candidates for pharmacological intervention, especially when anxiety is so great that a procedure simply cannot be performed without prompt and significant anxiety reduction. The data of Zeltzer et al. (1989), using a laboratory paradigm involving cold water arm immersion, suggest that psychobiologically "pain tolerant" and "pain sensitive" children can be distinguished, and that these two groups will benefit from distinct interventions for reducing the distress of medical procedures.

Finally, two additional factors that must be considered in the approach to procedure pain are the effect of the presence of parents during procedures and the importance of conditioned aversive responses. An essential concept is that the absence of protest from a child undergoing a procedure is not synonymous with lack of distress. Studies have shown that children are more likely to inhibit expressions of distress when unaccompanied by a parent during medical procedures (Shawn and Routh, 1982). Ross and Ross (1984) found that 99% of a group of over

Table 94.4. Possible Approaches to Specific Procedures

Painless Procedures (CT and MRI scans)	Mildly Painful Procedures (finger sticks, intravenous cannulation, venipunctures)	Lumbar Punctures	Bone Marrow Aspirations
1. Preparation 2. Age of child may require use of agent: chloral hydrate (when agent is necessary), midazolam, rembutal	1. Preparation 2. Parental presence	1. Preparation 2. Parental presence	1. Preparation 2. Parental presence

	3. EMLA[a] or local anesthetic
	4. Clustering of procedures so that minimal sticks are necessary
		3. EMLA and/or buffered lidocaine
		4. Benzodiazepines for selected children
			3. EMLA or local anesthetic
			4. Analgesics
			  a. If intravenous access: intravenous fentanyl and intravenous midazolam 5 min before the procedure or general anesthetic
			  b. If no intravenous access: oral morphine and oral midazolam 1 h before the procedure or oral diazepam and ketamine or general anesthesia

	5. Behavioral approaches (bubble blowing, use of party blowers, other distractions or imaginative techniques)	5. Distraction and/or hypnotic techniques	5. Behavioral cognitive approaches

From Pomietto M, Schechter N: Cancer, AIDS, and Sickle-Cell Related Pain. Proceedings of the Third International Symposium on Pediatric Pain, Philadelphia, June 6–9, 1994.
[a] EMLA, eutectic mixture of lidocaine 2.5% and prilocaine 2.5% for topical use.

Table 94.5. Selected Local Anesthetics and Their Uses for Painful Procedures

EMLA
  Local anesthetic cream consisting of prilocaine and lidocaine, which goes through intact skin.
  Requires 60 min under an occlusive dressing; not studied for newborns or children under 1 month.
  Appropriate for reservoir access, lumbar punctures, venous cannulations, blood drawing, and for local anesthesia associated with bone marrow aspirations.
Lidocaine
  Injectable local anesthetic
  Works typically within 2–5 min
  Injected through small-gauge needle, burns upon infiltration
  Can be buffered with sodium bicarbonate to reduce associated burning (lidocaine to bicarbonate, 9:1)
TAC
  Combination of tetracaine, adrenalin, and cocaine
  Can be placed in a gauze pad and placed over open wounds
  Provides adequate anesthesia for suturing
  Should not be used on digits, eyes, or mucous membranes
Bupivicaine
  Long-acting, local anesthetic
  Typically used during epidural anesthesia, may be used in surgical incisions to give prolonged anesthesia postoperatively

From Pomietto M, Schechter N: Cancer, AIDS, and Sickle-Cell Related Pain. Proceedings of the Third International Symposium on Pediatric Pain, Philadelphia, June 6–9, 1994.

700 children reported that the "thing that helped most" in coping with a pain experience was the presence of a parent.

The issue of the conditioning effects of painful medical procedures is also essential, since for most children with cancer, frequent repetition of procedures is the rule. Thus, maximal intervention with the very first invasive procedure, often a bone marrow aspiration performed when the child first presents for diagnostic evaluation, has been recommended.

Chemotherapy-associated nausea and vomiting is mediated via dopaminergic neural pathways; thus, dopamine antagonists such as prochlorperazine, droperidol, and metoclopramide have been widely used in the treatment of these conditions. The serotonergic neural pathways are also involved, and the serotonin-blocking agent ondansetron has been found effective (Grunberg, 1990). Nausea and vomiting in pediatric patients with cancer have been reported to respond to a variety of pharmacological (van Hoff and Olszewski, 1988) and psychological (Redd et al., 1987) interventions. Conditioned anticipatory nausea and vomiting triggered by stimuli associated with previous chemotherapy experience can be a particularly difficult management problem (Redd, 1989).

Effects of Cranial Radiation

The importance of the CNS as a sanctuary site for leukemic cells inaccessible to systemically administered antileukemic drugs was recognized in the late 1950s and early 1960s as a direct result of the early successes of chemotherapy in producing prolonged remissions. As children began to live longer, the CNS became the most common site of relapse; when this occurs, bone marrow relapse generally follows, and prognosis for long-term survival diminishes substantially. These developments led in the 1970s to the routine inclusion of CNS preventive therapy in treatment protocols for all children with ALL during induction, using a combination of CRT and intrathecal methotrexate. The incidence of CNS leukemia was reduced from roughly 80 to 10% with this approach (Poplack, 1989).

Subsequent to the routine inclusion of CNS preventive therapy for children with ALL, more than 40 studies have addressed the issue of the adverse neurobehavioral effects of this procedure, which may be associated with learning impairment severe enough to require special education in 8–30% of patients (Blatt and Bleyer, 1989). In their comprehensive review of these studies, Fletcher and Copeland (1988) conclude that CNS preventive therapy is associated with cognitive impairment, that children under 5 years of age are at higher risk for these effects, and that a causal role is more clearly established for CRT than for intrathecal chemotherapy.

Neuropsychological assessments of recipients of CNS preventive therapy have found that nonverbal cognitive functions are preferentially impaired. Rourke (1987) has suggested that these specific neuropsychological abnormalities may be etiologically related to lesions of white matter found on neural imaging and autopsy studies of these children (Fletcher and Copeland, 1985). Finally, from a pilot study of cerebrospinal fluid (CSF) monoamine metabolites in children with ALL, Glazer et al. have data to suggest that metabolic degradation products of dopamine and serotonin are elevated in the CSF of children receiving CRT, compared to nonradiated control subjects (J. Glazer et al., unpublished data, 1990), suggesting an additional means by which the effects of neurotoxic treatments for cancer can be investigated and monitored.

Mulhern et al. (1992) conducted a review of the literature on the neuropsychological outcomes of children treated for primary CNS tumors. Twenty-two studies summarizing the experience of 544 patients were analyzed to assess the relationship between known risk factors for neuropsychological impairment following treatment. Cranial radiation, volume, and age at time of treatment were of primary importance in the development of neuropsychological sequelae. Interestingly, tumor location was not found to be a factor. Riva et al. (1989) found that medulloblastoma patients (who were treated with resection and chemo-radiotherapy) had poorer cognitive performance than did those treated for astrocytoma (by resection alone).

Because of the adverse effects of CNS irradiation, alternative regimens are being sought that are equally effective in preventing CNS leukemia but less toxic to the CNS. To date, these approaches have included reducing the dose of CRT and eliminating CRT altogether from the regimens of patients with favorable prognostic features (Poplack, 1989). The occurrence of adverse CNS effects as a direct result of a treatment that dramatically improves medical outcome, and the modification of treatment to reduce these adverse effects while maintaining treatment efficacy, typifies the challenge currently facing pediatric oncology to preserve the quality of life associated with therapies that enhance absolute survival.

Bone Marrow Transplantation

Transplantation of histocompatible bone marrow, usually obtained from a sibling, may be lifesaving for some children and adolescents with leukemia, lymphoma, or neuroblastoma who would otherwise die (Ramsay, 1989). Bone marrow transplantation (BMT) is a unique therapeutic modality, in that the child must endure a hospital stay of several weeks in a single isolation room and is prepared for the transplant with doses of total body irradiation and chemotherapy that, without the transplant, would be lethal (Atkins and Patenaude, 1989). BMT is curative in up to 50% of cases when performed for a pediatric malignancy (Trigg, 1988); the other 50% of children succumb, most often due to relapse or infection.

Psychological issues commonly encountered in children undergoing transplantation include struggles over control and medical treatment compliance (Atkins and Patenaude, 1987; Gardner et al., 1977; Patenaude et al., 1979), dependency (Gardner et al., 1977; Patenaude et al., 1979), and reluctance to leave the protected environment, to which magical qualities may be attributed, as discharge approaches (Atkins and Patenaude, 1987; Freund and Siegal, 1986; Gardner et al., 1977; Patenaude et al., 1979). Strong attachments often develop between transplant patients in adjacent beds, and survivor guilt has been described in successfully transplanted patients when "the patient in the other bed" dies (Patenaude and Rappeport, 1982). Psychological issues for bone marrow donors, often children, have also been described, particularly feelings of guilt arising if the recipient dies (Freund and Siegel, 1986; Gardner et al., 1977).

For the child's family, the disruption of relocation of part or all of the family to a distant transplant center is a major stress (Atkins and Patenaude, 1987; Patenaude et al., 1979). Patenaude et al. (1979) describe the difficult psychological task faced by the families of gravely ill children for whom transplantation is contemplated: "When a family chooses a still experimental treatment that may be fatal over palliative treatments or no treatment and certain death, their decision raises questions that have no answers" (p. 412).

Stuber et al. (1989, 1991) reported findings of a prospective, longitudinal study of children undergoing BMT. Seven of the eight children studied exhibited "mild" symptoms of posttraumatic stress disorder (PTSD) before their transplants, with worsening of PTSD symptoms after transplantation. Preliminary data from existing descriptive studies suggest that intensive psychosocial support for parents, psychotherapy with the child bone marrow recipient, and provision of liaison support to bone marrow transplant staff are useful interventions (Atkins and Patenaude, 1987; Freund and Siegel, 1986; Patenaude et al., 1979). Please refer to Chapter 95 for a more detailed discussion of bone marrow transplantation.

PSYCHOSOCIAL INTERVENTION IN CHILDHOOD CANCER

The Chronically Ill Child

Several studies have addressed psychological and functional outcome in children with a variety of chronic physical illnesses as a function of psychosocial intervention. Pless and Satterwhite (1975) studied the effect of a nonprofessional family counseling intervention on the psychological functioning of a group of 98 chronically ill children; there were 56 treated families and 42 untreated control families. Children in the treated families functioned significantly better on several outcome measures. Stein and Jessop's (1984) randomized study of a team-based home care program for families of chronically ill children also demonstrated a beneficial effect.

In contrast, in a randomized, controlled trial of intervention by a social worker with families of chronically ill children at Montreal Children's Hospital, no significant difference in outcome, using the Child Behavior Checklist, could be demonstrated between children in treated families compared to children in untreated families (Nolan et al., 1987).

Psychosocial Intervention for the Child and Adolescent with Cancer

The outcome studies discussed in the previous section suggest that many young people with cancer cope remarkably well with the stress of their illness. These studies also indicate, however, that a spectrum of psychological disturbances may be exhibited, which includes subjective symptoms such as anxiety, depression, and lowered self-esteem, and dysfunctional behaviors such as school refusal, academic failure, and noncompliance with medical treatment. Antecedent psychosocial variables that appear to be associated with these symptoms and behaviors include poor illness-related communication, dysfunctional social and family relationships, lack of peer support, and poor family coping with previous life stresses.

A central task in any psychosocial intervention strategy should be the facilitation of normal psychological development. The model described in Section I, in which chronic illness is conceived as a developmental crisis rather than as a cause of psychopathology, is therefore useful in considering psychosocial interventions. In this context, the age of the cancer experience is related to psychological outcome, as found in some of the long-term survivor studies (Fritz et al., 1988; Koocher and O'Malley, 1981). Onset during the preschool years seems to be protective (Koocher and O'Malley, 1981). On the other hand, the experience of illness during adolescence presents the unique developmental challenge inherent in the occurrence of increased dependency on parents and health care providers at precisely that point in development at which the emergence of autonomous functioning is a crucial task (Fritz et al., 1988; Koocher and O'Malley, 1981, p. 8).

Psychoneuroimmunology

The interrelationship of the brain and immune system has been well documented (Yudofsky, 1994); examples include innervation of immune end organs, and the presence on lymphocytes of receptors for numerous neurohumors, including gonadal steroids, endorphins, enkephalins, adrenocorticotropic hormone (ACTH), vasointestinal peptide, cholecystokinin, neurotensin, acetylcholine, and serotonin (Gorman and Kertzner, 1990). These neuroanatomic and neuorohumoral relationships are paralleled by clinical studies suggesting that psychotherapeutic interventions in patients with cancer are beneficial not only with respect to psychological outcome but biological outcome and survival as well. In the pioneering study of Spiegel et al. (1989), mean survival in a cohort of women with metastatic carcinoma of the breast randomly assigned to receive group psychotherapy was double that of the control group (36 versus 18 months), a statistically significant difference. Fawzy et al. (1990a, 1990b) randomly assigned adults with stage I malignant melanoma to group psychotherapy or control groups, finding significantly reduced psychological distress, enhanced long-term coping, and significantly more robust cellular immune function (as determined by increased numbers of natural killer cells and other immune measures) in those randomized to receive group psychotherapy. A subsequent report of the same study population (Fawzy et al., 1994) indicated that the cohort receiving group psychotherapy also exhibited significantly prolonged melanoma-free survival.

Studies of this kind, while not yet reported in pediatric oncology populations, illustrate the limitations of reductionistic categorization of human disease into "organic" and "functional" and have reinvigorated the field of psychosomatic medicine.

Psychotherapy

Several studies have established the therapeutic efficacy of individual and group psychotherapy for adults with cancer in relation to several outcome measures, including improved mood and self-esteem (Massie et al., 1989).

In one of the few such intervention studies in pediatric oncology, Kupst et al. (1984) studied roughly 50 families of children with leukemia using a prospective, longitudinal design beginning at the time of diagnosis, with formal assessments at 6 months and 1 and 2 years, using several outcome measures of family functioning and coping. Outcome was assessed as a function of three levels ("no," "moderate," or "total") of psychosocial, family-based intervention by master's-level social workers or counselors. Psychosocial intervention in this study was predictive of adequate coping by families at 6 months but not at 1 or 2 years after diagnosis; however, even families in the "no" intervention group had some contact with the research team, for which a beneficial effect cannot be excluded.

CASE ILLUSTRATION

R., a 6-year-old boy with neuroblastoma refractory to conventional oncologic treatment, underwent bone marrow transplantation with the aim of cure of the malignancy. Initially cooperative and cheerful, noncompliance with isolation requirements and refusal to take prescribed medication developed several weeks later. A consulting child psychiatrist found the child to be sad and withdrawn; in the second evaluation session, the child depicted in play a sadistic "doctor" who kept stuffed animal "patients" trapped alone in a room. After these initial contacts, the child began verbalizing to his primary nurse his anger at being left alone when she went to care for her other patient, an infant. Compliance with isolation and medication soon improved and the child's affect brightened. Twice weekly psychotherapy continued during the remaining hospital course.

The frequency with which fundamental psychodynamic themes, such as separation anxiety in preschool children, fantasies of illness as retribution for wrongdoing in school-age children, and conflicts over dependency and autonomy in adolescents, appear among seriously ill children and adolescents (Schowalter, 1970) argues strongly for a role for psychotherapy in this setting. Equally important is the need in this group of patients for a psychotherapeutic approach that respects each patient's unique configuration of defenses, particularly the vicissitudes of denial about life threat and prognosis (Koocher and O'Malley, 1981; Solnit, 1983). The current challenge is to define as carefully as possible in prospective longitudinal studies the specific indications for intervention with psychotherapy, the relative benefits of individual, group, and family modalities, and outcome.

Psychopharmacotherapy

Pfefferbaum-Levine et al. (1983) treated eight pediatric cancer patients, ranging in age from 4 to 16 years, with imipramine or amitriptyline for a spectrum of symptoms including sadness, anxiety, sleep disturbance, cancer pain, and anorexia. Categorical DSM-III diagnoses were not reported. Medication dosages ranged from 0.7 to 1.9 mg/kg/24 hours, and plasma tricyclic levels ranged from 24 to 295 ng/ml. The

authors report generally favorable responses to drug treatment, anxiety and sleep disturbance being especially responsive. The authors caution, however, that the multiplicity of medications administered to patients in this study, including analgesics for cancer pain, and the limited period of follow-up, limit the conclusions that can be drawn. While no studies of the selective serotonin reuptake inhibitors in the pediatric cancer patient exist, judicious use in select patients may prove beneficial, and the favorable side effect profile of these agents is appealing.

Maisami et al. (1985) reported that a constellation of symptoms, including depressed mood, withdrawal, separation anxiety, and an escalating requirement for analgesics in three children terminally ill with cancer, ages 7, 9, and 14 years, responded to a combination of amitriptyline and haloperidol, at dosages of 1–2 mg/kg/24 hours and 0.05–0.10 mg/kg/24 hours, respectively. Improved mood, reduction in separation anxiety, reduced narcotic analgesic dosage requirement, and improved accessibility to psychotherapy were features of response among these three patients. Two patients exhibited recurrent symptoms when medication was discontinued. This report is also limited by its small sample size and lack of a control group.

Cancer pain, moreover, may be a confounding variable; since some tricyclic antidepressants exert a narcotic analgesic-sparing effect (Massie and Lesko, 1989), it is possible that the findings of Maisami et al. (1985) could be an artifact of enhanced analgesia. In another important study, Steif and Heiligenstein (1989) reported that, of a group of 43 pediatric cancer patients consecutively referred for psychiatric consultation and evaluated using a semistructured interview based on the children's version of the Schedule of Affective Disorders and Schizophrenia (K-SADS), 20% of the sample were judged as having inadequately treated cancer pain as the etiology of presenting psychiatric symptoms. In all but one case, psychiatric symptomatology markedly improved or resolved with adequate pain control. The authors conclude that a formal pain assessment should be routinely included in psychiatric evaluations of children and adolescents with cancer.

Psychoactive Drugs and Cancer Pain

Clinical studies have demonstrated conclusively that physical pain due to illness in hospitalized children and adolescents is underrecognized and undertreated (Schechter, 1989; Schechter et al., 1990). Controlled clinical trials in adults have established the efficacy of certain tricyclic antidepressants in a variety of chronic pain states (Watson et al., 1982), and these agents are in wide use as adjuvants to narcotic analgesics and in the treatment of insomnia in adult cancer patients with pain (Portenoy and Foley, 1989).

Tricyclic agents may also be effective in treating deafferentation pain (due to nerve injury) (Miser and Miser, 1989b). No controlled trials of these agents have been reported for children and adolescents with cancer, but their use has been cautiously recommended (Miser and Miser, 1989a). In one recent case, imipramine was reported to be effective in treating a child with peripheral neuropathic pain due to the chemotherapeutic agent vincristine, a common cause of this condition (Heiligenstein, 1989). Amitriptyline is the tricyclic most often recommended, because of its sedative effects and its activity as a serotonin reuptake inhibitor, since serotonin appears to play a role in pain modulation (Miser and Miser, 1989b).

Finally, anecdotal reports suggest that the psychostimulants methylphenidate and dextroamphetamine may be useful for pediatric patients with cancer pain who require doses of narcotic analgesics that produce excessive sedation (Miser and Miser, 1989b). Like the tricyclics, these agents also enhance narcotic analgesia. One possible setting for an intervention with psychostimulants might be that of a terminally ill child requiring high doses of opioids for adequate pain relief, but who wishes to be sufficiently alert to be interactive with his or her family as long as possible. Finally, it should be noted that one neuroleptic, methotrimeprazine, has been shown to have analgesic activity.

DELIRIUM

Delirium is characterized by reduced ability to maintain attention to external stimuli, disorganized thinking, disturbances of the sleep-wake cycle and level of psychomotor activity, perceptual disturbances, and disorientation (American Psychiatric Association, 1987). Delirium is common in hospitalized adults with cancer (Fleishman and Lesko, 1989) and also occurs in children (Glazer, 1990), although systematic surveys have not appeared. Etiologies include drug toxicity, infection, hypoxia, and metabolic imbalances, among others (Cassem and Hackett, 1987).

The occurrence of delirium in a critically ill child or adolescent requires a thorough medical and psychiatric differential diagnostic assessment and should not be ascribed to "ICU psychosis," since treatable medical causes may be discovered (Cassem and Hackett, 1987). Delirium that is frightening to a patient or accompanied by behavioral dyscontrol that interferes with care may require psychopharmacological intervention with an antipsychotic agent. This may be difficult in a child too ill to tolerate orally administered medication, while the intramuscular route is painful and often contraindicated because of thrombocytopenia. Several authors discuss the use of intravenous haloperidol in the treatment of delirium in medically ill adults, including those with cancer (Adams, 1988; Cassem and Hackett, 1987; Fleishman and Lesko, 1989), and this approach has also been used successfully in pediatric oncology (E. Heiligenstein, personal communication, 1990). Regardless of route, haloperidol is probably the antipsychotic of choice because of its relative lack of effect on blood pressure or respiration and its low anticholinergic potency. Acute dystonic reactions, possible reversal of the pressor effects of dopaminergic agents, and neuroleptic malignant syndrome must be kept in mind when neuroleptics are used in a medical setting.

Thus, uncontrolled reports suggest that psychoactive agents including tricyclic antidepressants, neuroleptics, and the psychostimulants may have a role in the amelioration of a spectrum of symptoms in children and adolescents with cancer, including depression, anxiety, vegetative disturbances, delirium, and vincristine neuropathy. Novel uses as adjuvants in the treatment of cancer pain—to enhance the analgesic efficacy of narcotic agents, to promote sleep in the pediatric cancer patient with pain, and to counteract narcotic-induced somnolence—should be evaluated. The relationship between presenting psychiatric symptoms in pediatric patients with cancer and cancer pain appears to be an important one requiring further study. Controlled clinical trials will help specify indications and dosage guidelines for these agents. In the meantime, psychopharmacological agents are likely to be employed in pediatric oncology; their use requires exquisite attention to drug toxicity in this uniquely vulnerable group of patients who are already receiving highly toxic chemotherapeutic agents. Child and adolescent psychiatrists skilled in pediatric psychopharmacology have a unique role to play in the evaluation and treatment of these patients.

Other Interventions

THE SCHOOL

School attendance is an important predictor of long-term psychosocial functioning (Perrin and Maclean, 1988); pediatric patients with cancer routinely experience school absences, which in one study ranged from 8 weeks to more than a year, averaging 6 months (Wasserman et al., 1987). In this study, 40% of a cohort of long-term survivors of Hodgkin's disease reported difficulty with peers upon their return to school; teasing about hair loss and other physical attributes and fear of contagion were the major issues. Cognitive limitation related to neurotoxic cranial radiation is also an educational issue for some pediatric patients with cancer (Fletcher and Copeland, 1988). Educators must be equipped with both factual knowledge of cancer, needed to avoid prejudices based on misinformation, and programmatic flexibility, needed to take multiple absences and cognitive limitations into account. Medical professionals are in an excellent position to provide classroom teachers and other school personnel with needed information (Koocher and O'Malley, 1981; Spinetta and Deasy-Spinetta, 1986).

THE HOSPITAL

Repeated hospitalization per se is associated with adverse psychosocial sequelae (Rutter, 1982); controlled studies have demonstrated the beneficial effects of preparative programs for children facing hospitalization (Ferguson, 1979). Also, Kash and Holland (1989) have shown that provision of psychiatric liaison services to professional staff of an adult oncology unit was associated with a perception by their patients of more empathic care. Such a study would be very useful in a pediatric oncology setting.

SOCIETY

Lansky has reviewed the financial burdens imposed on the family of the child with cancer; these include many nonmedical, and therefore nonreimbursable, costs (Lansky et al., 1989). Socioeconomic disadvantage, moreover, is related to adverse psychological outcome in childhood cancer (Fritz et al., 1988). Survivors of childhood cancer also commonly encounter employment and insurance discrimination, which have been associated with psychological distress (Koocher and O'Malley, 1981). It is of interest in this context that, in one follow-up study (Mulhern et al., 1989b), socioeconomic background was not predictive of outcome; the institution at which this study was conducted provided transportation, meals, and lodging for patients and parents. Thus, whether by educating insurance companies about the lack of excessive absenteeism in survivors of cancer (Koocher and O'Malley, 1981) or by direct economic assistance, influences on psychological outcome may involve concrete interventions directed at societal problems.

MISCELLANEOUS INTERVENTIONS

A summer camp experience for children and adolescents with cancer has been shown to facilitate information sharing, which as discussed above, is associated with beneficial psychological effects (Bluebond-Langner et al., 1990).

CONCLUSIONS AND FUTURE DIRECTIONS

Jellinek (1987) has noted the "increasing complexity, range, and stress associated with pediatric illness" (p. 453), a description that applies well to pediatric oncology. The child and adolescent psychiatrist consultant in pediatric oncology must be a skillful psychotherapist and psychopharmacologist and ideally should also possess a comfortable working knowledge of pediatrics (Herzog and Jellinek, 1987). Pfefferbaum (1989) and Lansky (1974) and others have suggested that child psychiatrists should serve as members of the pediatric oncology treatment team, participating in hospital rounds and related activities on a regular basis. The quality of the lives of young people with cancer will be enhanced by the participation of child and adolescent psychiatrists in their care, whose knowledge of individual, family, and group psychodynamics, pharmacological approaches to the relief of physical pain and psychological distress, and behavioral medicine can serve the goals of facilitating normal development in those who survive cancer and of relieving suffering in those who do not.

As we look to the future, four priorities for thoughtful clinical investigation can be identified. First, characterization of psychological morbidity in long-term survivors in prospective longitudinal studies using outcome measures properly suited to the unique characteristics of this group of patients are needed, and these should be linked to controlled assessments of psychosocial interventions. Second, individualized responses to medical procedure pain and nausea and vomiting due to chemotherapy must be further characterized so that the high levels of distress, especially in adolescents, can be reduced through individually tailored management programs. Third, in collaboration with our colleagues in oncology, methods should be developed that allow the quality as well as the quantity of survival to be incorporated as outcome measures in cancer treatment protocols. Finally, efforts should be made to elucidate the basic mechanisms responsible for the adverse neurobehavioral effects of treatments for cancer, particularly cranial radiation, using current neurochemical and neuroimaging technology, in the hope that a more favorable balance between treatment efficacy and toxicity can be achieved.

References

Adams F: Emergency intravenous sedation of the delirious medically ill patient. *J Clin Psychiatry* 49(suppl 12):22–26, 1988.

Adams M: Helping the parents of children with malignancy. *J Pediatr* 93:734–738, 1978.

American Psychiatric Association: *Diagnostic and Statistical Manual of Mental Disorders* (3rd ed, rev). Washington, DC, American Psychiatric Association, 1987, p. 100.

Anthony S: *The Child's Discovery of Death*. New York, Harcourt Brace, 1940.

Atkins DM, Patenaude AF: Psychosocial preparation and follow-up for pediatric bone marrow transplant patients. *Am J Orthopsychiatry* 57:246, 1987.

Blatt J, Bleyer WA: Late effects of childhood cancer and its treatment. In: Pizzo PA, Poplack DG (eds): *Principles and Practice of Pediatric Oncology*. Philadelphia, Lippincott, 1989, pp. 1003–1025.

Blotcky AD, Raczynski JM, Gurwitch R, et al: Family influences on hopelessness among children early in the cancer experience. *J Pediatr Psychol* 10:479, 1985.

Bluebond-Langner M: Meanings of death to children. In: Feifel A (ed): *New Meanings of Death*. New York, McGraw-Hill, 1977, pp. 48–66.

Bluebond-Langner M, Perkel D, Goertzel T, et al: Children's knowledge of cancer and its treatment: Impact of an oncology camp experience. *J Pediatr* 116:207, 1990.

Breslau N: Does brain dysfunction increase children's vulnerability to environmental stress? *Arch Gen Psychiatry* 47:15–20, 1990.

Cairns NU, Klopovich P, Heame E: School attendance of children with cancer. *J Sch Health* 52:152, 1982.

Cassem NH, Hackett TP: The setting of intensive care. In: Hackett TP, Cassem NH (eds): *Massachusetts General Hospital Handbook of General Hospital Psychiatry* (2nd ed). Littleton, MA, PSG Publishing, 1987, pp. 353–379.

Chang PN, Nesbit ME, Youngren N, et al: Personality characteristics and psychosocial adjustment of long-term survivors of childhood cancer. *J Psychosoc Oncol* 5:43–58, 1987.

Civin CI: Reducing the cost of the cure in childhood leukemia (Editorial). *N Engl J Med* 321:185, 1989.

Dolgin MJ, Katz ER, Ziltzer LK, et al: Behavioral distress in pediatric patients with cancer receiving chemotherapy. *Pediatrics* 84:103, 1989.

Eisenberg L: Foreword. In: Koocher G, O'Malley J (eds): *The Damocles Syndrome*. New York, McGraw-Hill, 1981, pp. xi–xv.

Fawzy FI, Cousins N, Fawzy NW, et al: A structured psychiatric intervention for cancer patients. I: Changes over time in methods of coping and affective disturbance. *Arch Gen Psychiatry* 47:720–725, 1990a.

Fawzy FI, Kemeny ME, Fawzy NW, et al: A structured psychiatric intervention for cancer patients. II: Changes over time in immunological measures. *Arch Gen Psychiatry* 47:729–735, 1990b.

Fawzy FI, Fawzy NW, Hyun CS, et al: Malignant melanoma. Effects of an early structured psychiatric intervention, coping, and affective state on recurrence and survival 6 years later. *Arch Gen Psychiatry* 50(9):681–689, 1993.

Ferguson BF: Preparing young children for hospitalization: A comparison of two methods. *Pediatrics* 64:656, 1979.

Fife B, Norton J, Groom G: The family's adaptation to childhood leukemia. *Soc Sci Med* 24:159, 1987.

Fisher DM, Robinson S, Brett CM, et al: Comparison of enflurane, halothane and isoflurane for outpatient pediatric anesthesia. *Anesthesiology* 63:647, 1985.

Fleishman S, Lesko LM: Delirium and dementia. In: Holland JC, Rowland JH (eds): *Handbook of Psychooncology: Psychological Care of the Patient with Cancer*. New York, Oxford University Press, 1989, pp. 342–355.

Fletcher JM, Copeland DR: Neurobehavioral effects of central nervous system prophylactic treatment of cancer in children. *J Clin Exp Neuropsychol* 10:495–537, 1988.

Fortunato RP, Komp PM: Death at home for children with acute lymphoblastic leukemia. *Virginia Med Monthly* 106:124, 1979.

Freund BL, Siegel K: Problem in transition following bone marrow transplantation: Psychological aspects. *Am J Orthopsychiatry* 56:244, 1986.

Friedman AG, Mulhern RK, Fairclough D, et al: Midazolam premedication for pediatric bone marrow aspiration and lumbar puncture. *Med Pediatr Oncol* 19(6):499–504, 1991.

Fritz G, William J, Amylan M: After treatment ends: Psychosocial sequelae in pediatric cancer survivors. *Am J Orthopsychiatry* 58:552, 1988.

Futterman EN, Hoffman I: Transient school phobia in a leukemia child. *J Am Acad Child Psychiatry* 9:477, 1970.

Gardner GG, August CS, Githens J: Psychological issues in bone marrow transplantation. *Pediatrics* 60:624, 1977.

Glazer JP: Life-threatening pediatric illness in a high technology age: The paradigm of childhood cancer. In: Michels R et al (eds): *Psychiatry* (Vol 2). Philadelphia, Lippincott, Chapter 74, 1990.

Glazer JP, Riddle MA, Anderson GM, et al: CSF 5-HIAA increases with whole brain radiation in childhood leukemia. 38th Annual Meeting, American Academy of Child and Adolescent Psychiatry, San Francisco, October, 1991 (Abstract).

Gortmaker S, Walker D, Weitzman M, et al: Chronic conditions, socioeconomic risks, and behavioral problems in children and adolescents. *Pediatrics* 85:267–276, 1990.

Greenberg HS, Kazak AE, Meadows AT: Psychologic functioning in 8- to 16-year-old cancer survivors and their parents. *J Pediatr* 114:488, 1989.

Grunberg SM: Making chemotherapy easier. *N Engl J Med* 332:846, 1990.

Heiligenstein E: Tricyclics for pain (Letter). *J Am Acad Child Adolesc Psychiatry* 28:804, 1989.

Heiligenstein E, Jacobson PB: Differentiating depression in medically ill children and adolescents. *J Am Acad Child Adolesc Psychiatry* 27:716, 1988.

Hersov L: School refusal. In: Rutter M, Hersov L (eds): *Child and Adolescent Psychiatry* (2nd ed). Oxford, Blackwell, 1985, pp. 382–399.

Herzog DB, Jellinek MS: Child psychiatric consultation. In: Hackett TP, Cassem NH (eds): *Massachusetts General Hospital Handbook of General Hospital Psychiatry* (2nd ed). Littleton, MA, PSG Publishing, 1987, pp. 477–495.

Hinds P: Quality of life in children and adolescents with cancer. *Semin Oncol Nurs* 6:285–291, 1990.

Holmes HA, Holmes FF: After ten years, what are the handicaps and life styles of children treated for cancer? *Clin Pediatr* 14:819, 1975.

Ivan TM, Glazer JP: Quality of life in pediatric psychiatry: A new outcome measure. *Child Adolesc Psychiatr Clin North Am* 3(3):599–611, 1994.

Jay SM, Elliott CH, Katz ER, et al: Cognitive behavioral and pharmacologic interventions for children undergoing painful medical procedures. *J Consult Clin Psychol* 55:860, 1987.

Jellinek MS: The hospitalized child: General considerations. In: Hackett TP, Cassem NH (eds): *Massachusetts General Hospital Handbook of General Hospital Psychiatry* (2nd ed). Littleton, MA, PSG Publishing, 1987, pp. 462–476.

Kaplan SL, Busner J, Weinhold C, et al: Depressive symptoms in children and adolescents with cancer: A longitudinal study. *J Am Acad Child Adolesc Psychiatry* 26:782, 1987.

Karon M, Vernick J: An approach to the emotional support of fatally ill children. *Clin Pediatr* 7:274, 1968.

Kash KM, Holland JC: Special problems of physicians and house staff in oncology. In: Holland JC, Rowland JH (eds): *Handbook of Psychooncology: Psychological Care of the Patient with Cancer*. New York, Oxford University Press, 1989, p. 654.

Kashani J, Hakami N: Depression in children and adolescents with malignancy. *Can J Psychiatry* 27:474, 1982.

Koocher G, O'Malley J: *The Damocles Syndrome*. New York, McGraw-Hill, 1981.

Kupst MJ, Schulman JL: Family coping with leukemia in a child: Initial reactions. In: Schulman JL, Kupst MJ (eds): *The Child with Cancer: Clinical Approaches to Psychosocial Care Research in Psychosocial Aspects*. Springfield, IL, Charles C Thomas, 1980, pp. 111–128.

Kupst MJ, Schulman JL, Maurer H, et al: Coping with pediatric leukemia: A two-year followup. *J Pediatr Psychol* 9:149, 1984.

Kuttner L, Bowerman M, Teasdale M: Psychological treatment of distress, pain, and anxiety for young children with cancer. *J Dev Behav Pediatr* 9:374, 1988.

Lansky LL, List MA, Lansky SB, et al: Toward the development of a play performance scale for children (PPSC). *Cancer* 56:1837, 1985.

Lansky S: Childhood leukemia: The child psychiatrist as a member of the oncology team. *J Am Acad Child Psychiatry* 13:499, 1974.

Lansky S, Gendel M: Symbiotic regressive behavior patterns in childhood malignancy. *Clin Pediatr* 17:133, 1978.

Lansky S, List M, Ritter-Sterr C: Psychological consequences of cure. *Cancer* 58:529, 1986.

Lansky S, List MA, Ritter-Sterr C: Psychiatric and psychological support of the child and adolescent with cancer. In: Pizzo PA, Poplack DG (eds): *Principles and Practice of Pediatric Oncology*. Philadelphia, Lippincott, 1989, pp. 885–896.

Lansky S, Lowman JJ, Vats T, et al: School phobia in children with malignant neoplasms. *Am J Dis Child* 129:42, 1975.

Lansky S, Smith ST, Cairns MU, et al: Psychological correlates of compliance. *Am J Pediatr Hematol Oncol* 5:87–92, 1983.

Maisami M, Schmer BH, Coyle JT: Combined use of tricyclic antidepressants and neuroleptics in the management of terminally ill children: A report on three cases. *J Am Acad Child Psychiatry* 24:487, 1985.

Massie MJ, Lesko LM: Psychopharmacological management. In: Holland JC, Rowland JH (eds):

Handbook of Psychooncology: Psychological Care of the Patient with Cancer. New York, Oxford University Press, 1989, p. 475.

Massie MJ, Holland JC, Straker N: Psychotherapeutic interventions. In: Holland JC, Rowland JH (eds): *Handbook of Psychooncology: Psychological Care of the Patient with Cancer.* New York, Oxford University Press, 1989, pp. 455–469.

McGrath PJ, Craig KD: Developmental and psychological factors in children's pain. *Pediatr Clin North Am* 36:823, 1989.

Meadows A, Hobbie W: The medical consequences of cure. *Cancer* 58:524, 1986.

Meadows AT, Robison LL, Sather H: Potential long-term toxic effects in children treated for acute lymphoblastic leukemia (Letter). *N Engl J Med* 321:1830, 1989.

Miller RW: Frequency and environmental epidemiology of childhood cancer. In: Pizzo PA, Poplack DG (eds): *Principles and Practice of Pediatric Oncology.* Philadelphia, Lippincott, 1989, p. 5.

Miser AW, Miser JS: Management of childhood cancer pain. In: Pizzo PA, Poplack DG (eds): *Principles and Practice of Pediatric Oncology.* Philadelphia, Lippincott, 1989a, pp. 923–932.

Miser AW, Miser JS: The treatment of cancer pain in children. *Pediatr Clin North Am* 36:979, 1989b.

Mulhern RK, Fairclough DL, Smith B, et al: Maternal depression, assessment methods, and physical symptoms affect estimates of depressive symptomatology among children with cancer. *J Pediatr Psychol* 17(3):313–326, 1992a.

Mulhern RK, Hancock J, Fairclough D, et al: Neuropsychological status of children treated for brain tumors: A critical review and integrative analysis. *Med Pediatr Oncol* 20:181–191, 1992b.

Mulhern RK, Horowitz ME, Ochs J, et al: Assessment of quality of life among pediatric patients with cancer: Psychological assessment. *J Consult Clin Psychol* 1:130, 1989a.

Mulhern RK, Lauer ME, Hoffman RG: Death of a child at home or in the hospital: Subsequent psychological adjustment of the family. *Pediatrics* 71:743, 1983.

Mulhern RK, Wasserman AL, Friedman AG, et al: Social competence and behavioral adjustment of children who are long-term survivors of cancer. *Pediatrics* 83:18, 1989b.

Nagy M: The child's theories concerning death. *J Genet Psychol* 73:3, 1948.

Nolan T, Zvagulia I, Pless IB: Controlled trial of social work in childhood chronic illness. *Lancet* 2:411–415, 1987.

Olness K: Hypnotherapy: A cyberphysiologic strategy in pain management. *Pediatr Clin North Am* 36:873, 1989.

Patenaude AF, Rappeport JM: Surviving bone marrow transplantation: The patient in the other bed. *Ann Intern Med* 97:915, 1982.

Patenaude AF, Szymanski L, Rappeport J: Psychological costs of bone marrow transplantation in children. *Am J Orthopsychiatry* 49:409, 1979.

Perrin JM, Maclean WE Jr: Children with chronic illness: The prevention of dysfunction. *Pediatr Clin North Am* 35:1325, 1988.

Pfefferbaum B: Common psychiatric disorders in childhood cancer and their management. In: Holland JC, Rowland JH (eds): *Handbook of Psychooncology Psychological Care of the Patient with Cancer.* New York, Oxford University Press, 1989, pp. 544–561.

Pfefferbaum-Levine B, Kumor K, Cangir A: Tricyclic antidepressants for children with cancer. *Am J Psychiatry* 140:1074, 1983.

Pless I, Nolan T: Risks for maladjustment associated with chronic illness in childhood. In: Shaffer D, Philips I, Enzer N (eds): *Prevention of Mental Disorders, Alcohol and Other Drug Use in Children and Adolescents.* Washington, DC, US Department of Health and Human Services, 1989, pp. 191–244.

Pless IB, Satterwhite B: Chronic illness. In: Haggerty JR, Roghmann KJ, Pless IB (eds): *Child Health and the Community.* New York, Wiley, 1975, pp. 78–94.

Pomietto M, Schechter N: Cancer, AIDS, and Sickle-Cell Related Pain. Proceedings of the Third International Symposium on Pediatric Pain, Philadelphia, June 6–9 1994.

Poplack DG: Acute lymphoblastic leukemia. In: Pizzo PA, Poplack DG (eds): *Principles and Practice of Pediatric Oncology.* Philadelphia, Lippincott, 1989, pp. 323–366.

Portenoy RK, Foley KM: Management of cancer pain. In: Holland JC, Rowland JH (eds): *Handbook of Psychooncology: Psychological Care of the Patient with Cancer.* New York, Oxford University Press, 1989, pp. 369–382.

Powazek M, Payne JS, Goff JR, et al: Psychosocial ramifications of childhood leukemia: One year post-diagnosis. In: Schulman JL, Kupst MJ (eds): *The Child with Cancer: Clinical Approaches to Psychosocial Care Research in Psychosocial Aspects.* Springfield, IL, Charles C Thomas, 1980, pp. 143–155.

Quigley C, Cowell C, Jimenez M, et al: Normal or early development of puberty despite gonadal damage in children treated for acute lymphoblastic leukemia. *N Engl J Med* 321:143, 1989.

Rait DS, Jacobsen PB, Lederberg MS, et al: Characteristics of psychiatric consultations in a pediatric cancer center. *Am J Psychiatry* 145:363, 1988.

Ramsay NKC: Bone marrow transplantation in pediatric oncology. In: Pizzo PA, Poplack DC (eds): *Principles and Practice of Pediatric Oncology.* Philadelphia, Lippincott, 1989, pp. 971–990.

Redd WH: Management of anticipatory nausea and vomiting. In: Holland JC, Rowland JH (eds): *Handbook of Psychooncology: Psychological Care of the Patient with Cancer.* New York, Oxford University Press, 1989, pp. 423–433.

Redd WH, Jacobsen PB, Die-Trill M, et al: Cognitive/attentional distraction in the control of conditional nausea in pediatric cancer patients receiving chemotherapy. *J Consult Clin Psychol* 55:391, 1987.

Relling MV, Mulhern RK, Fairclough D, et al: Chlorpromazine with and without lorazepam as antiemetic therapy in children receiving uniform chemotherapy. *J Pediatr* 123(5):811–816, 1993.

Richmond JB, Waisman HA: Psychologic aspects of management of children with malignant diseases. *Am J Dis Child* 89:42, 1955.

Riva D, Pantaleoni C, Milani N, et al: Impairment of neuropsychological functions in children with medulloblastomas and astrocytomas in the posterior fossa. *Child's Nerv Sys* 5(2):107–110, 1989.

Rosenbaum P, Cadman D, Kirpalani H: Pediatrics: Assessing quality of life. In: Spilker B (ed): *Quality of Life Assessment in Clinical Trials.* New York, Raven Press, 1990, pp. 205–215.

Ross D, Ross S: The importance of type of question, psychological climate, and subject set in interviewing children about pain. *Pain* 19:71, 1984.

Rourke BP: Syndrome of nonverbal learning disabilities: The final common pathway of white-matter disease/dysfunction? *Clin Neuropsychol* 1:209, 1987.

Rowland J, Glidwell O, Sibley R, et al: Effects of different forms of central nervous system prophylaxis on neuropsychologic function in childhood leukemia. *J Clin Oncol* 2:1327, 1984.

Rutter M: Prevention of children's psychosocial disorders: Myth and substance. *Pediatrics* 70:883, 1982.

Rutter M, Tizard J, Whitmore K: *Education, Health and Behavior.* London, Longman Group Ltd, 1970.

Schechter NL: The undertreatment of pain in children: An overview. *Pediatr Clin North Am* 36:781, 1989.

Schechter NL, Altman A, Weisman S (eds): Report of the consensus conference on the management of pain in childhood cancer. *Pediatrics* 86(suppl):813–834, 1990.

Schipper H, Levitt M: Measuring quality of life: Risks and benefits. *Cancer Treat Rep* 69:1115, 1985.

Schowalter JE: The child's reaction to his own terminal illness. In: Schoenberg AC, Carr D, Peretz D, et al (eds): *Loss and Grief.* New York, Columbia University Press, 1970, pp. 51–69.

Shawn E, Routh D: Effect of mother presence on children's reaction to aversive procedures. *J Pediatr Psychol* 7:33–44, 1982.

Silberfarb PM: Research in adaptation to illness and psychosocial intervention: An overview. *Cancer* 50(suppl):1921, 1982.

Simone J, Versoza M, Rudy J: Initial features and prognosis in 363 children with acute lymphocytic leukemia. *Cancer* 36:2099, 1975.

Smith SD, Rosen D, Trueworthy RC, et al: A reliable method for evaluating drug compliance in children with cancer. *Cancer* 43:169, 1979.

Solnit AJ: Changing perspectives: Preparing for life or death. In: Schowalter IE, Patterson PR, Tallmer M, et al (eds): *The Child and Death.* New York, Columbia University Press, 1983, pp. 3–18.

Solnit AJ, Green M: The pediatric management of the dying child. Part II: The child's reaction to the fear of dying. In: Solnit AJ, Provence SA (eds): *Modern Perspectives in Child Development.* New York, International Universities Press, 1963, pp. 217–228.

Sparrow SS, Balla DA, Cicchetti DV: *Vineland Adaptive Behavior Scales.* Circle Press, MN, American Guidance Service, 1984.

Spiegel D, Bloom JR, Kraemer HC, et al: Effect of psychosocial support on survival in patients with metastatic breast cancer. *Lancet* 2:888–891, 1989.

Spinetta JJ: The dying child's awareness of death: A review. *Psychol Bull* 81:256,1974.

Spinetta J: Behavioral and psychological research in childhood cancer: An overview. *Cancer* 50(suppl):1939, 1982.

Spinetta JJ, Deasy-Spinetta P: The patient's socialization in the community and school during therapy. *Cancer* 58:512, 1986.

Spinetta JJ, Maloney LJ: The child with cancer: Patterns of communication and denial. *J Consult Clin Psychol* 46:1540, 1978.

Spinetta JJ, Rigler D, Karon M: Anxiety in the dying child. *Pediatrics* 52:841, 1973.

Steif BL, Heiligenstein EL: Psychiatric symptoms of pediatric cancer pain. *J Pain Symptom Manage* 4:191, 1989.

Stein REK, Jessop DJ: Does pediatric home care make a difference for children with chronic illness? Findings from the pediatric ambulatory care treatment study. *Pediatrics* 73:845, 1984.

Stuber M, Nader K, Yasuda P, et al: PTSD after pediatric bone marrow transplantation. Paper presented at annual meeting of the American Academy of Child and Adolescent Psychiatry, New York, 1989. (Abstract NR-54)

Tebbi CK, Cummings M, Zevon MA, et al: Compliance of pediatric and adolescent cancer patients. *Cancer* 58:1179, 1986.

Teta MI, Delpo MC, Kasl SV, et al: Psychosocial consequences of childhood and adolescent cancer survival. *J Chronic Dis* 39:751, 1986.

Trigg M: Bone marrow transplantation for treatment of leukemia in children. *Pediatr Clin North Am* 35:933, 1988.

Van Hoff I, Olszewski D: Lorazepam for the control of chemotherapy-related nausea and vomiting in children. *J Pediatr* 113:146–149, 1988.

Vaughan VC: The field of pediatrics. In: Behrman R, Vaughan VC (eds): *Nelson Textbook of Pediatrics* (13th ed). Philadelphia, Saunders, 1987, pp. 2–3.

Waechter EH: Children's awareness of fatal illness. *Am J Nurs* 71:1168, 1971.

Wasserman AL, Thompson EI, Wilimas IA, et al:

The psychological status of survivors of childhood/adolescent Hodgkin's disease. *Am J Dis Child* 141: 626, 1987.

Watson CP, Evans RI, Reed K, et al: Amitriptyline vs. placebo in post herpetic neuralgia. *Neurology* 32:671, 1982.

Weisman AD, Worden JW: The existential plight in cancer: Significance of the first 100 days. *Int J Psychiatr Med* 7:1, 1976.

Worchel FF, Nolan BF, Willson VL, et al: Assessment of depression in children with cancer. *J Pediatr Psychol* 3:101, 1988.

Yudofsky S (ed): *The American Psychiatric Press Textbook of Psychiatry*. Washington, DC, American Psychiatric Press, pp. 569–571, 1994.

Zeltzer LK, Jay SM, Fisher DM: The management of pain associated with pediatric procedures. *Pediatr Clin North Am* 36:941, 1989.

95 PSYCHIATRIC ISSUES IN PEDIATRIC BONE MARROW AND SOLID ORGAN TRANSPLANTATION

Jonathan A. Slater, M.D.

Both bone marrow transplantation (BMT) and solid organ transplantation (SOT) have undergone a revolution in the past 20–30 years, evolving from primarily experimental procedures to accepted treatment for a variety of diseases and varieties of end-stage organ failure (House and Thompson, 1988; Surman, 1989). The history of pediatric cardiac transplantation was reviewed by Addonizio (1990). Dr. Christiaan Barnard performed the first adult cardiac transplant in 1967, though the patient lived only 17 days. In 1967, Kantrowitz transplanted a heart into a 2-week-old infant who survived for several hours, and in 1968, Denton Cooley transplanted a new heart and lungs into a 2-month-old, who also survived for several hours. Though government-sponsored treatment of end-stage renal disease was instituted in 1972, almost 20 years following the first successful renal transplant in 1954 (using an identical twin as donor), poor success rates during the 1970s, due primarily to infection, rejection, and donor shortages, caused a relative moratorium on transplantation of other organs during this time period (Surman, 1989).

In the late 1970s, however, positive results at Stanford University, which had persisted with its heart transplant program, led to a resurgence of interest in heart transplantation. The experience with children and adolescents, however, remained quite limited. With the introduction of a new immunosuppressant, cyclosporine, in 1980, success rates began to improve, due to both a decreased rate of infection and improved management of rejection episodes. Following this, the number of centers performing heart transplantation soared, and the experiences with greater numbers of patients led to efforts at heart transplantation in infants and children. The progression from the laboratory into mainstream medicine was thus facilitated by the development of immunosuppressant medications, improvements in operative technique, more careful immunological subtyping and matching, greater refinement in the candidate selection process, and growing experience in the medical management of transplant patients (Parkman, 1986; Surman, 1989).

The historic "Baby Fae" xenograft (nonhuman donor) received much media attention in 1984. In 1985, Dr. Leonard Bailey successfully performed a neonatal cardiac allotransplantation (human heart as donor), and during the mid-1980s, the number of transplants in children increased exponentially. Between 1984 and 1988, the International Heart Transplantation Registry recorded 583 cardiac transplantations in patients under the age of 20; prior to 1980, there were fewer than five transplants a year performed on patients in this age group (Addonizio, 1990).

The first allogeneic BMT was reported in 1969, in a 5-year-old with severe combined immunodeficiency syndrome (Meuwissen et al., 1969). For BMTs in particular, statistics have been cited that indicate that about half of all BMTs have taken place in the pediatric population (Wiley and House, 1988). The number of BMTs rose as chemotherapy and immunological techniques improved, and the types of illnesses treated

extended to soft tissue tumors, immunological and metabolic diseases, and leukemia (Stuber, 1993). BMT is a mainstay of treatment for early acute lymphoblastic leukemia (ALL) or acute myelogenous leukemia (AML), chronic myelogenous leukemia (CML), and some solid tumors in children (Parkman, 1986; Trigg, 1988). The application of transplant technology to the pediatric population has thus often been center stage in this process for both SOT and BMT, with an exponential rise in the number of transplants performed (see Tables 95.1 and 95.2).

Research into the quality of posttransplantation life, which was reviewed by Surman (1989), helped push SOT transplantation into the forefront of accepted medical technology for end-stage or incurable conditions. The role of psychiatric involvement developed in the setting of: the implicit ethical issues surrounding allocation of a resource (the donated organ) in which the demand far exceeds the supply; as psychosocial factors in candidate selection (such as the potential for noncompliance) became identified as important in affecting outcome; and as neuropsychiatric complications such as delirium, anxiety, depression, and the psychological impact of the transplantation process on the patient and family became recognizable.

The United Network for Organ Sharing (UNOS), an outgrowth of the National Transplant Act of 1984, is under the directorship of the Health Resources and Service Administration, which sets standards about transplant success rates, criteria for review, and application to function as a transplant center (Surman, 1989). UNOS directs the national Organ Procurement and Transplantation Network (OPTN) and United States Scientific Registry on Organ Transplantation. All transplant centers, organ procurement agencies, and tissue typing laboratory in the country participate. UNOS administers the allocation and distribution of organs utilizing a computerized list that is managed by strict scientific criteria, including organ type, tissue match, blood type, length of time on the waiting list, geographical distance if applicable (heart, heart-lung, lung, liver, pancreas), and immune status.

Research into the psychiatric aspects of transplantation in children has been limited, though child psychiatric involvement in a consultation-liaison role represents a standard component of the transplant team. It has become increasingly evident, however, that the psychiatric ramifications in the world of SOT and BMT represent paradigms of modern, high-technology medicine today that are generalizable to many pediatric medical conditions and treatments (Stuber et al., 1991). Issues involving informed consent/assent, ethical and quality of life concerns, developmental considerations, pain and anxiety management, noncompliance, and the effects of acute and chronic illness on the patient and family transcend this particular field, though perhaps no where else are they all found in such a compelling, poignant manner.

The child psychiatrist's task in consulting to a transplant team in a similar way, perhaps, requires the use of all of one's professional skills

Table 95.1. Number of Transplants in the United States, 1988–1993, by Recipient Age and Type of Transplant

Year	Age	Kidney[a]	Liver	Pancreas	Heart	Heart-Lung	Lung	Total
1988	0–5	126	257	1	60	2	0	446
	6–17	531	151	0	64	9	1	756
1989	0–5	122	321	0	95	2	1	541
	6–17	510	132	0	58	5	3	708
1990	0–5	124	335	0	138	3	2	602
	6–17	517	178	4	84	3	7	793
1991	0–5	129	342	2	178	2	7	660
	6–17	507	158	0	83	8	26	782
1992	0–5	126	325	1	153	4	6	615
	6–17	465	168	1	82	6	31	753
1993	0–5	151	338	4	162	7	7	669
	6–17	496	186	2	109	7	29	829

Source: UNOS OPTN and Scientific Registry data.
Modified from Stuber ML: Psychiatric aspects of organ transplantation in children. *Psychosomatics* 34:379–387, 1993, with permission.
From Slater JA: Psychiatric aspects of transplantation in children and adolescents. *Child Adolesc Psychiatr Clin North Am* 3(3):557–598, 1994, with permission.
[a] Cadaveric and liver donor data pooled.

Table 95.2. Five-Year Survival Probability (±95% Confidence Interval) after Bone Marrow Transplantation for Children Less Than 19 Years of Age with Acute Lymphoblastic Leukemia, Acute Myelogenous Leukemia, and Severe Aplastic Anemia by Disease, Disease State, and Donor Type[a]

Disease State	5 Year Probability			
	N	HLA-Identical Sibling	N	Alternative Donor[a]
Acute lymphoblastic leukemia				
1st remission	270	64 ± 6%	54	46 ± 14%
≥2nd remission	651	41 ± 4%	219	36 ± 8%
Relapse	180	22 ± 7%	82	11 ± 8%
Acute myelogenous leukemia				
1st remission	473	62 ± 5%	61	42 ± 15%
≥2nd remission	87	47 ± 11%	36	31 ± 16%
Relapse	134	24 ± 8%	57	13 ± 9%
Severe aplastic anemia ±10%	458	(Andrykowski, 1994) ± 4%	114	43

[a] Includes other related and unrelated donors.
[a] The raw data presented here were obtained from the Statistical Center of the International Bone Marrow Transplant Registry. The analysis has not been reviewed or approved by the Advisory Committee of the IBMTR. The IBMTR database contains reports for 2876 children less than 19 years of age receiving bone marrow transplants for ALL, AML, and SAA, transplanted in the 10-year period 1984–1993.

Table 95.3. Possible Etiologies for End-stage Organ Disease in Children

Heart	Liver (Stewart et al., 1989, 1991a, 1991b, 1992)	Kidney (Grimm and Ettenger, 1992)	Lung (Quitell, personal communication, 1993)
Congenital malformations	Extrahepatic biliary atresia	Urologic abnormalities	Cystic fibrosis
Cardiomyopathies	α_1-Antitrypsin deficiency	Focal segmental glomerulonephritis	Pulmonary hypertension
	Intrahepatic biliary hypoplasia	IgA nephropathy	Interstitial lung disease
	Idiopathic cirrhosis	Henoch-Schönlein purpura	Congenital heart disease
	Hepatoma	Hemolytic-uremic syndrome	
	Chronic active hepatitis	Membranoproliferative glomerulonephritis	
	Tyrosinemia	Metabolic disease	
	Sclerosing cholangitis	Wilms' tumor	
	Hamartoma		

Above three tables from Slater JA: Psychiatric aspects of transplantation in children and adolescents. *Child Adolesc Psychiatr Clin North Am* 3(3):557–598, 1994, with permission.

in a setting where individual and family psychotherapy, psychopharmacological intervention, behavior therapy, liaison to other staff, and the understanding of medical illness and procedures are all required.

This chapter reviews the psychiatric issues involved in pediatric SOT and BMT, with the overall focus being the role of the consultation-liaison child and adolescent psychiatrist.

GENERAL ISSUES IN THE PEDIATRIC TRANSPLANT POPULATION

The literature on the psychiatric aspects of transplantation in the pediatric population has recently been reviewed (Sexson and Rubenow, 1992; Slater, 1994; Stuber, 1993). Stuber (1993) notes many of the salient aspects specific to transplantation in the pediatric population,

which include effects on donor supply secondary to size, longer waiting periods, and the ethical implications of using living-related donors or organs from anencephalic infants. The effects of transplantation on identity and self-concept formation are just beginning to be studied, and pediatric transplant recipients differ from many of their adult counterparts in that they are not regarded as having "caused" the conditions that necessitate transplantation (Stuber, 1993).

SOT has become recognized as a legitimate treatment for many types of end-stage organ failure (Table 95.3). The number of children on waiting lists at the time of writing, the number of transplants performed annually by organ, and survival rates are detailed in Tables 95.4, 95.1, and 95.5, respectively. Analogous data on BMT patients are presented in Table 95.2. The dilemma in allocation of solid organ donations is presented in Table 95.6, which indicates how many children die on the waiting list.

Table 95.4.   Number of Child/Adolescent (<18 Years Old) Registrations on the National Transplant Waiting List 3/31/94

Age (years)	Kidney	Liver	Heart	Heart-Lung	Lung	Total
0–5	74	267	83	5	7	476
6–10	104	105	20	7	13	259
11–17	462	108	44	13	65	704

Source: UNOS OPTN and Scientific Registry data.

Table 95.5.   Three-Month, 1-Year, and 2-Year Graft/Patient Survival Rates: October 1, 1987–December 31, 1991

Type	Age at Time of Transplant	N	3-Month Survival (%)	1 Year Survival (%)	2 Year Survival (%)
Graft survival					
Cadaveric donor	0–5	227	72.7	65.7	64.5
Kidney transplants	6–18	1350	82.5	75.2	67.8
Living donor	0–5	262	88.1	85.3	82.5
Kidney transplants	6–18	1042	93.4	90.1	84.9
Patient survival					
Liver transplants	0–5	1299	78.3	73.0	68.7
	6–18	707	84.4	79.3	76.9
Heart transplants	6–5	364	81.5	69.3	64.0
	6–18	260	88.2	80.8	73.3
Lung transplants	6–5	8	100.0	60.0	60.0
	6–18	33	80.5	53.5	32.1

Source: UNOS OPTN and Scientific Registry data.
Modified from Stuber ML: Psychiatric aspects of organ transplantation in children. *Psychosomatics* 34:379–387, 1993, with permission.
From Slater JA: Psychiatric aspects of transplantation in children and adolescents. *Child Adolesc Psychiatr Clin North Am* 3(3):557–598, 1994, with permission.

Table 95.6.   Percentage of Possible Recipients Who Died While on Waiting List, 1988–1992, by Age (Number of Deaths Divided by Number of Patients)

Transplant Type	0–5 Years	6–18 Years	18+ Years	Overall
Heart	23.3	17.2	13.2	13.8
Liver	7.9	6.4	7.0	8.6
Kidney	2.4	1.5	3.6	3.5
Lung	19.7	15.0	11.3	11.7

Data from UNOS, 1988–1992.
Modified from Stuber ML: Psychiatric aspects of organ transplantation in children. *Psychosomatics* 34:379–387, 1993, with permission.
From Slater JA: Psychiatric aspects of transplantation in children and adolescents. *Child Adolesc Psychiatr Clin North Am* 3(3):557–598, 1994, with permission.

Stages of the Transplant Experience

The transplantation experience may be viewed as a series of stages with common elements for different patients and families (Table 95.7). Patients and families develop an integrative narrative about this experience, which is continuously revised as events occur and time passes, putting their individualized stamp on the experience.

THE PRETRANSPLANT EVALUATION

Much of the literature on psychosocial assessment of transplant candidates has been in the adult literature (Freeman et al., 1992; Levenson and Olbrisch, 1993), though recently this has been described in the pediatric population (Sexson and Rubenow, 1992; Slater, 1994). In the pediatric population, the decision to transplant is one probably less mediated by psychiatric factors. A multidisciplinary transplant team represented by pediatrics, surgery, psychiatry/psychology, nursing, and social work is oriented more toward identifying risk factors for psychopathology and noncompliance, and ensuring that there are adequate social supports. The child and adolescent psychiatrist performs a dual function. As a consultant, he or she conducts a thorough psychiatric evaluation

of the patient and family, with an emphasis on identifying psychopathology or potential risk factors for adjustment reactions or noncompliance. The consultant role also includes periodic neuropsychiatric assessment and the brief treatment of patients and families with a variety of modalities that may extend into the posttransplant period and perhaps arguably should in many circumstances (Stuber et al., 1991).

As the psychiatric liaison, the child and adolescent psychiatrist performs an equally important function as someone who can function as an intermediary, communicating a level of understanding about the patient and family's experience to the rest of the medical staff. In addition to this, however, the psychiatrist may serve a supportive or directive function for the other members of the transplant team, who may struggle with feelings triggered by particular patients, clinical situations, or ethical dilemmas. He or she is very much a part of the "family" composed of the transplant team, patient, and patient's family.

Transplant teams are comprised of individuals who may conceptualize the psychiatrist's role in different ways, and expectations and/or priorities should be specified prior to evaluation or suggested interventions. For instance, lung transplantation in an adolescent cystic fibrosis patient with a history of noncompliance will carry a particular focus. The evaluation of the family consisting of a 2-year-old and 5-month-old twins, where one of the twins has a serious cardiomyopathy requiring transplantation, will be different. The pediatrician's focus in the first case may be trying to develop a formulation of the causes of noncompliance and the likelihood of successful intervention to address this problem. In the latter case, the availability of family supports and the psychological state of the mother may be of more concern. Little data are available on parental factors that may correlate with postoperative morbidity, and more are needed (Stuber, 1993).

Transplantation is all the more compelling because, with the exception of kidney transplantation, SOT and BMT are treatments of last resort, without which the patient would likely die. Urgency is less on the pediatric nephrology service, since these children can survive on dialysis without transplantation, which may thus be considered more electively.

CASE ILLUSTRATION

Psychiatric consultation was requested when the father of a child who received a cardiac transplant punched a hole in the wall and repeatedly threatened nursing staff in the aftermath of his son's cardiac arrest. Psychotherapy with this man was not possible due to what appeared to be his limited ability to have insight into the underlying causes for his anger, which was believed to be a sense of helplessness and tremendous desperation, as well as the wish to fix blame to somebody or some thing for what had happened to his son. While it was important to help the staff understand what this man was going through, it was perhaps more important to ensure they felt protected. Security was called, and definitive limits were set for this man with regard to verbal and nonverbal threats.

The pretransplant evaluation should be part of the multidisciplinary assessment of the transplant candidate, the purpose of which should be explained to the family by the primary physician. Psychiatric consultants may best be conceptualized as experts in child development, pain and anxiety management, and the psychological responses to transplantation. He or she is an important member of the transplant team who can provide emotional support to the patient and family during an unusual crisis that anyone would find extremely distressing and help prepare them emotionally for transplantation. The child and adolescent psychiatrist can also serve a vital function in helping to communicate the child's needs to his or her family and the rest of the transplant team. If framed in this manner by the primary physician, the evaluation will rarely be met with resistance by the family. It is important that there be continuity of care with respect to psychiatric services, since the pretransplant evalu-

Table 95.7. Psychosocial Issues Facing Parents

Preoperative	Perioperative	Long-term Postoperative
Initial hospital experience	First 24 hours	Return home
Loss of control	Anxiety	Adaptation of new parenting role
Denial of medical reality	Numbness/shock	Fear of rejection/death
Building trust in staff	First 2 weeks	Readjustment in family structure
Waiting at home	Exhilaration/new beginning	Long-term issues
Concrete tasks	Cease fire period	Continued public involvement in transplant issues
Financial burdens	Realignment in parent/child interaction	Uncertainties about the future
Public involvement	Emotional integration of organ	
Guilt	Remainder of hospitalization	
Death of donor	Roller coaster period	
Competition for limited organs	Fear of rejection/infection	
Burden of informed consent	Lack of control/powerlessness	
Anger	Continued guilt/fear of death	
Loss of control	Isolation/marital stress	
Feeling forgotten/abandoned	Preparation for discharge	
Depression	Realization of hospital dependency	
Endless wait	Building confidence	
Child's deteriorating condition		

From Gold LM, Kirkpatrick BS, Fricker FJ, et al: Psychosocial issues in pediatric organ transplantation: The parents' perspective. *Pediatrics* 77:738–749, 1986. Reproduced by permission of *Pediatrics* © 1986.

ation can form the basis for a trusting relationship that will affect the receptivity of future interventions and allow a greater depth of understanding in the patient's and family's experience.

The pretransplant evaluation must encompass the standard elements of child psychiatric evaluation. In addition, however, the consultant must be familiar with the medical problems for which transplantation is being considered, as well as have a working understanding of transplantation itself from a medical and surgical perspective. In so doing, he or she will be more likely seen as an integral part of the transplant team. The consultant should ascertain whether other members of the transplant team have specific concerns about a patient or family.

The child or adolescent patient and his or her family have reactions simply to the fact that they are being evaluated for transplantation (see "Diagnosis" below). Such reactions may cover the range from denial to panic, with different family members often reacting differently. In some cases, extended family members or siblings are not told about the evaluation. In others, grandparents and siblings are present at the evaluation and clearly impact upon the process itself. Evaluation is often complicated by the fact that it is occurring in an urgent setting with a critically ill child, and parents are required to digest relatively quickly a great deal of complicated information about a subject about which they know nothing, in the setting of acute anxiety and fear, leaving them overwhelmed, which often makes true informed consent impossible.

In other cases, small children with cardiomyopathies may not visibly appear that ill, taxing the capabilities of parents to overcome the understandable inclination to use denial. These children may nevertheless have borderline cardiac function and be subject to fairly rapid decompensation. They may therefore be listed for transplantation because the relatively long waiting periods for small children could make organ procurement difficult. Parents may later look back on videotaped footage of their child prior to transplantation and wonder how they did not realize the child was sick. Listing the child early may also give the transplant team more time to familiarize themselves with the family and vice versa. Prior to meeting with the family, the psychiatric consultant can benefit from information concerning the reactions of the family to the evaluation procedure.

Parents and patients may ask the psychiatric consultant questions about medical or surgical aspects of transplantation, such as survival rates, that are best referred back to the pediatrician or surgeon. With prepubertal children, it is often helpful to meet with the parents first, as in a standard child psychiatric evaluation. Adolescents may wish to meet with the psychiatric consultant first, or with his or her parents; at some point, adolescents and children should be interviewed alone, since they often will reveal feelings not expressed in the presence of their parents. The child and adolescent psychiatrist should begin the consulta-

tion by asking the parent and/or patient about conceptions and expectations about the psychiatric evaluation, to allow appropriate clarifications to be made.

The psychiatric pretransplant evaluation can be diagnostic as well as educational and potentially therapeutic. Elements of this evaluation should include:

1. Getting to know the patient and family and vice versa: Will they be able to function as part of a "team?"
2. How is the patient/family experiencing the pretransplant evaluation and the prospect of transplantation? Significant "psychoeducation" may take place by helping to "normalize" the patient/family's reactions to the transplant experience.
3. Obtaining a history of the medical/surgical problem, prior illness experience, and the "parallel" emotional or psychiatric history. This includes:
   a. an assessment of the patient's and family's coping styles. Certain coping styles may be predictive of fewer adjustment problems in the setting of a chronic illness and include "positive self-talk, attention diversion, relaxation, thought stopping, task orientation, talk(ing) with someone, and good problem solving activity," as opposed to "catastrophizing" strategies such as the "focus on negative affect or fear, anxious anticipation, escape or avoidance, worry/rumination, self-denigration and self-blame, (and) fear of unlikely consequence" (Olson et al., 1993).
   b. obtaining a description of the temperament of the child/adolescent
   c. past and present psychopathology in patient, parents, siblings
   d. nature of past procedures, hospitalizations, surgeries, and reactions to same, including "secondary" psychopathology, giving consideration to affective (depression, anxiety), cognitive (confusion, distortion), and behavioral (tantrums, oppositional behavior, noncompliance, posttraumatic phenomena) parameters
   e. risk factors for noncompliance
   f. history of drug or alcohol abuse in the adolescent
4. Assessing the quality of the child/adolescent-caregiver(s) relationship and family dynamics
5. Detailed developmental, neuropsychiatric, social and school history
6. Mental status examination and neurocognitive assessment of the child/adolescent
7. Assessment of how socioeconomic factors may have impacted upon the management or course of the child/adolescent's illness, and concerns over how these factors may be of concern regarding life after transplantation. Are psychosocial supports adequate?
8. What the patient/family understand about the process of transplantation, from being listed, to the surgery itself, postoperative course,

and immunosuppressant medication. Much of this information may not routinely be given to the patient until there is consideration for formal listing, but the family often has many misconceptions about this process, perhaps from what they have read or heard from other families. Are parents able to give informed consent, and is the child/adolescent able to give informed assent/consent? Is the family and adolescent accepting of long-term medication administration and care? (Modified from Slater JA: Psychiatric aspects of transplantation in children and adolescents. *Child Adolesc Psychiatr Clin North Am* 3(3):557–598, 1994, with permission.)

Other factors will influence the response to hospitalization at the time of transplantation:

1. The age of the child and developmental level. Younger children are more prone to cognitive distortions common to the Piagetian preoperative stage, regression, fantasies of intended harm, mutilation, and separation fears. They will be less likely to understand the rationale of procedures, nature of pathophysiology and course of an illness.
2. The number of prior hospitalizations early in life. Repeated hospitalizations between the ages of 6 months and 4 years may increase the risk of later psychiatric disorder (Mrazek, 1984; Quinton and Rutter, 1976).
3. Hospital characteristics, such as visitation policies and quality of the Child Life Department. (From Slater JA: Psychiatric aspects of transplantation in children and adolescents. *Child Adolesc Psychiatr Clin North Am* 3(3):557–598, 1994, with permission.)

At the conclusion of the evaluation, which may take several interviews, a concise formulation should integrate data, which have been gathered into a form easily "digestible" by nonpsychiatric colleagues. This formulation should identify psychopathology, describe coping styles, and address possible predictors of resilience or noncompliance and the adequacy of social supports. The psychiatric consultant should indicate areas where misconceptions exist regarding information presented to the family by other members of the transplant team and relay this back to his or her colleagues.

The diagnostic impressions and therapeutic recommendations should be communicated to both the referring physician as well as to the patient and family. This should be done both verbally, and in the form of a written note, a copy of which may be given to the parents as well, if appropriate, which may help "demystify" the psychiatrist's role, as well as educate. Recommendations should correlate with problem areas identified in the formulation and may include, for example, preparation for transplantation with play or videotapes, the teaching of relaxation techniques for anxiety reduction, social service intervention to clarify medical insurance, or contact with other transplant families.

Families commonly look forward to hearing suggestions from the psychiatrist for helping them through the arduous process of transplantation. If immediate follow-up is not felt to be necessary by the consultant and family, the family should be told how the consultant can be reached. If the patient is in the hospital, continued follow-up is advised. When the psychiatric consultant communicates with colleagues, judgment should be exercised with respect to patient confidentiality about issues not relevant to the transplantation process; this should be discussed with the patient and family. Care should be exercised about what is written in the hospital record, since in many ways this is a public document.

DIAGNOSIS

The reactions of the patient and family to the diagnosis of a medical problem serious enough to warrant transplantation occur within the context of the prior medical history. A chronically ill child who has already had several surgeries for congenital heart disease presents a different scenario from a previously well child who noticed a lump in his cheek initially assumed to be an abscess that turns out to be a Burkitt's lymphoma (see Case Illustration below). These differences may seem obvious, but what all patients and families come to share is an extreme

fear of uncertainty associated with the unknown, fears of pain—emotional and physical—and on some level the fear of death.

Parents may react differently (Gold et al., 1986), some in more of an assertive, information-seeking mode, acting proactively for their children, and others with more passivity and increased reliance on medical staff for direction. The psychiatric consultant can be of great assistance in helping parents to act in their own (and the child's) best interests and become more aware of how their individual coping styles affect them.

CASE ILLUSTRATION

Adolescents themselves may have a powerful sense of denial. An adolescent, on being told that he needed a heart transplant, said: "Really how to figure how I felt back then, basically a thirteen year old kid is invincible in his own mind. I remember I was playing football and my dad pulled me over. He didn't want to tell me, but then he finally told me, and I'm like, 'All right dad, can I go back in the game?' And he was like, 'Yeah, go ahead.' Because at thirteen you don't think of what a transplant means. You don't know the dangers, the risks, or anything." (From Slater JA: Psychiatric aspects of transplantation in children and adolescents. *Child Adolesc Psychiatry Clin North Am* 3(3):557–598, 1994, with permission.) "One adolescent with severe heart disease confided that when she was around her parents, she used to bite her lips to make them turn red, so they would not realize she was cyanotic" (Slater, 1994).

CASE ILLUSTRATION

The consultation-liaison child and adolescent psychiatrist was called by a senior colleague to see his relative, an 8-year-old boy with newly diagnosed Burkitt's lymphoma. The patient's father was in a state of shock, unable to believe that what he thought was a simple abscess was in actuality a malignancy for which his son would receive emergent bone marrow transplantation. The fact that, like many chemotherapy protocols, the one his son would receive was experimental further overwhelmed this man. In desperation, he began frantically calling different centers that do BMTs to compare protocols, and in fact he began to wonder if a mistake had been made when the pathology slides were read or that they had somehow been switched. He became irritable and sleep-deprived, and to further complicate matters, he did not want his son told that he had a malignancy, fearing it would overwhelm and terrify him. The staff reacted powerfully to this scenario, and many meetings with the family and staff in various combinations were needed.

Many stresses impacted upon the psychiatrist, including the feelings associated with referral from a senior colleague, the need to accurately assess the father's mental status and intervene appropriately, the need to consider the best interests of the boy, and the need to liaison with other staff. All of this happened rapidly in the setting of diagnosis leading to BMT within several days.

Diagnosis itself may thus represent a trauma that may manifest post-traumatic symptoms, requiring intervention. Parental misconceptions about or lack of exposure to the process of transplantation, such as donor allocation and wait listing, further complicates matters. In this setting, parents are asked to organize themselves cognitively and make terribly difficult decisions in a short time frame that will impact on the survival of their child; it is often an impossible quandary. They may find it difficult to communicate with one another openly about fears, due to concerns over destabilizing the spouse, and may suffer in solitude. Parents may focus on concrete details like survival statistics to attempt to center themselves in the face of a feeling of overwhelming helplessness and anxiety over entrusting their child's life to people whom they barely know, who are recommending procedures about which parents may be completely ignorant. Illusions of control over the events of one's life seem to be obliterated.

Alternative treatments may be sought that may potentially delay medical intervention, such as the case of a family who made phone calls around the world: ''Maybe somebody will tell us that there's a doctor in the Philippines who has found a Papaya serum that can cure cardiomyopathy'' (Slater, 1994).

BEING LISTED

If recommended, informed consent for transplantation is obtained following evaluation, when families are educated about the indications, risks and benefits, and process of transplantation. Being listed represents a ''point of no return'' (Slater, 1994), and families typically experience great anxiety about the future that may include confusion over how UNOS manages the wait list for organs. Parents are in a sense formally committing their child's future to events and personnel over which they have little control, often with a feeling of blind faith that things will work out positively, knowing full well they might not. The ''roller coaster'' metaphor has been used by many families in describing the process of a building up of tension, followed by a fearful though perhaps exhilarating but out of control descent (Slater, 1994).

Parents of young children wonder how they should explain to their children what will be happening to them, and how to prepare them. Here, the child and adolescent psychiatrist can be of great assistance.

CASE ILLUSTRATION

A 3½-year-old boy named Steven who had a cardiomyopathy was listed for heart transplantation. The consulting psychiatrist, using dolls and stuffed animals, engaged Steven in a story about a little boy named ''Chris'' who had become ill. Using some elementary drawings and a heart cut from red construction paper, he explained what the heart did, and how it had become sick in this little boy. In the play, he told how the boy's heart was too sick even for medicine to help, but that he had to somehow be helped.

''What could we do?'' asked the psychiatrist.

''I don't know,'' responded Steven.

''Well, we could get him a new one,'' said the psychiatrist.

Following that, Steven and the psychiatrist acted out the heart operation many, many times over a period of days, using an actual anesthesia mask and as many ''real'' props as possible, including miniature intravenous poles, operating room tables, tape, bags of intravenous solution, masks, gloves, etc. Each time Steven would become more involved, insisting on the operation, and emphasizing specific aspects of it, such as the use of the mask or saying good-bye to the mommy or daddy in the operating room.

At one point, the psychiatrist said, ''You know, Steven, you are like the little boy in our story in some ways.''

''How?''

''Well, you are in the hospital because your heart is sick too. And we have tried to give you medicine to make you better, but it isn't working, so, like Chris, we are going to have to give you a new heart.''

Steven's reactions to the preceding play intervention were carefully discussed with his mother prior to the sessions with him, and at an appropriate pace, more details about the story were layered on in successive versions, incorporating aspects of Steven's experience, all within the play. Chris, for example, was so tired of waiting in the hospital for so long, but this was explained to be due to the fact that he was too sick to go home. His new heart could come at any moment! He had an especially hard time saying good-bye to his mommy when she went home for Saturday night and his father stayed over with him, because he feared his mommy might never come back—but this was not true, for she always did.

Additional observations were made about Steven's negative reaction toward his father on these occasions, and his father's anger at this treatment, which his father took personally. Counseling with the father was directed at explaining how beneath Steven's rejecting behavior was anxiety over his mother's absence and his failing

to understand and accept her need for a night's sleep. Specific suggestions were given to facilitate the ''transfer'' between parents, which included the father bringing something special with him on visits, phone contact with his mother on the nights when she was absent, coaching his mother to address Steven's underlying fears that she would not return, and helping his father adopt more of a ''holding environment'' for the boy's anger and frustration.

In the play, much of Steven's underlying anxieties were fleshed out in the character of Chris, and all of the details of surgery and postoperative care, including pain management and medication administration, were added. Steven would react excitedly to the psychiatrist's entrance, eagerly gathering his stuffed animals and recreating the stories over and over. In another version, it was ''ET, the ''Extraterrestrial'' who had the heart problem and was far from home, in the clutches of doctors who were trying to do him harm. Even ET was eventually successfully transplanted and returned home.

He would often ask the psychiatrist to supply voices:

''Have him (Chris) say 'good-bye' to his parents again,'' or ''have his mommy tell him she will be coming back.''

When the actual time of Steven's transplantation approached, after some initial reluctance, and to his mother's surprise, he said ''Okay, let's go!'' In the operating room, he calmly held the mask to his face himself, said good-bye to his parents, and was successfully transplanted.

Children and adolescents may react with mixtures of fear, anxiety, depression, confusion, and existential angst, which is mediated by cognitive level and the tendency to regress. This may take the form of oppositional behavior and irritability. They often wonder ''Why is this happening to me? What did I do wrong?'' (Slater, 1994).

CASE ILLUSTRATION

''One twelve year old girl who was constantly in tears whenever the subject of transplantation came up: ''I had never had surgery before, any kind. And just the thought of having your heart taken out. There were just so many questions: 'Am I going to live?' 'Is it going to hurt?' 'How long is it going to take?' 'How am I going to recover?' 'Am I going to be normal?'''

CASE ILLUSTRATION

An 8-year-old boy who came from a religious family and was refusing transplantation, put his parents in an extremely difficult position. His mother felt tormented that if she signed the consent against his will and he did not survive, that she would never be able to forgive herself. After considerable work with a child psychiatrist, the underlying fear was revealed. The boy said that under no circumstances would he allow someone else to be killed so that he could have a new heart. With the help of a hospital chaplain, this boy's misconceptions were corrected, and he was successfully transplanted'' (Slater, 1994). (Both above illustrations from Slater JA: Psychiatric aspects of transplantation in children and adolescents. *Child Adolesc Psychiatr Clin North Am* 3(3):557–598, 1994, with permission.)

Older children and families may benefit from viewing a videotape about children and adolescents who have had transplants. One such film about cardiac transplantation in children includes interviews with donor families, as well as a family who lost a child following transplantation (Slater, 1992). Seven families have watched the film prior to cardiac transplantation. All have had positive reactions. Samples have included:

''The first reaction was relief that these kids existed, that they were apparently healthy. Our son could survive. It really worked. When we actually saw the donor families talking, it was enormously sad and moving, but in a positive way that somehow helped me.''

''I felt reassured that I had no choice and that it was the only decision possible, as I listened to the parents of the child who died wrestle with their guilt over having put her through the surgery, knowing she would die without it.''

''It made me feel better even though I cried during certain parts. It helps but it hurts at the same time.''

''It was a helpful film which confirmed the emotions we went through . . . it also provided firsthand knowledge of what we would go through . . . you realize that no matter who you are or what walk of life you come from, you all have the same concerns, fears, anxieties and questions.''

''It was hard to see the donor parents' sadness, talking about their son. It is so hard to think about the donor family, yet it's something I always find myself thinking of.''

WAITING

The waiting period, between the time a child is listed for a transplant and the arrival of the donor organ, can last from days to months. This can be tantamount to psychological torture, since the transplant can happen at any moment or not at all. Either alternative can be devastating. Intervening complications such as infection can temporarily remove the child from the waiting list. Median waiting times to transplant by organ are depicted in Table 95.8.

CASE ILLUSTRATION

One parent commented that ''waiting for the heart is like sitting in a tunnel with no light in either direction, there's no where to go.''

Another described this period: ''Waiting for the heart is a very helpless and scary feeling. You can't do anything. As a mother and as a parent, you're used to being able to take care of your children. If they have a fever you take them to the doctor, you put cold soaks, you give them Tylenol. If they have colds you give them fluids. You can do a lot of things to cure little illnesses that they have. You can't do anything when you're waiting for a heart.'' (From Slater JA: Psychiatric aspects of transplantation in children and adolescents. *Child Adolesc Clin North Am* 3(3):557–598, 1994, with permission.)

Parents may consider interfacing with the community, either to request assistance in meeting the extraordinary costs of transplantation or in an effort to publicize the need for a donor organ with the hope that this will make a difference. Such exposure can have costs for the family in terms of loss of privacy, but may be seen as necessary.

Parents often regard the issue of organ procurement with ambivalence, as they wrestle with conflicting feelings that arise from survivor guilt or identification with the family who lost their child. On an emotional level, many parents fear they are ''wishing'' for another child to

die, though they ''rationally'' know they have no control over this event. On occasion, two children in the same hospital might need an organ of the same size and blood type, with one listed higher than the other because he or she is more critically ill, for example. Such a situation can cause tremendously conflicting feelings for parents who might feel they are in a sense ''competing'' for the same organ; guilty feelings often ensue.

As time goes by, the waiting period often seems to wear patients and families down. If the child is hospitalized, mothers will often literally move into the hospital for weeks or months at a time, such that marital relationships are entirely disrupted. Emotional and physical reserves of parents often become so depleted during a turbulent medical course, such that their own basis needs are neglected. As day-to-day events are responded to, often in turbulent cycles, the parents have little time to reflect upon what has happened or to replenish their emotional and physical reserves. The psychiatrist can often detect this trend and advise accordingly with simple suggestions that may act as ''permission'' for a guilt-ridden parent to leave the hospital temporarily, for example, to get a night's sleep or a decent meal. Parents may experience a sense of support and validation of their experience from speaking with the psychiatrist.

Parents commonly feel torn between the responsibilities of other children, work, and the child in the hospital, and may feel guilty about ''failing'' to meet all these demands, though the task may be impossible to carry out completely. If the family does not live in proximity to the hospital, these feelings can be exacerbated, as siblings are shunted off to other family members, often leading to resentment toward the parents and sometimes toward the sibling in the hospital. Siblings may have a variety of adjustment reactions, and the psychiatric consultant's duties may extend to counseling parents about issues with their other children, and on occasion, the psychiatric evaluation of siblings.

Parents may become resentful at what has happened to their lives and describe being short-tempered with one another. The parent in the hospital with the child may become resentful toward the working parent, who is not with the child day-to-day, dealing with events in the hospital. Marital problems that were present prior to transplantation are obviously worsened, and parents may become clinically depressed or develop anxiety disorders, such as one parent who developed panic attacks that required treatment.

''False alarms'' may add to the feeling of unpredictability and helplessness, when a parent(s) receives word about a possible donor organ that does not come to fruition. Such instances can be even more anticlimactic and potentially traumatizing if the parent has already said goodbye to the child, who is moved to the operating room. In one instance, a mother became seriously depressed, returned home, and could not leave her bed for a number of days.

The patients themselves may become progressively more irritable and obstinate, stressing their relationships with parents, who are often the objects of angry outbursts, which tests their abilities to both empathize and set limits with their children. In some cases, the parent(s) cannot take extended leave from work, and the child may spend much of his time in the hospital without visitors.

Table 95.8.   Median Waiting Time (in Days) to Transplant by Organ, 1988–1991

Year	Age	Kidney Median (days)[a]	Liver Median (days)	Heart Median (days)	Lung Median (days)
1988	0–5	269	75	29	NC[b]
	6–18	296	26	28	577
1989	0–5	238	63	33	NC
	6–18	317	55	36	653
1990	0–5	179	66	26	664
	6–18	346	40	30	446
1991	0–5	258	67	35	171
	6–18	423	77	60	235

Source: UNOS OPTN and Scientific Registry data.
Modified from Stuber ML: Psychiatric aspects of organ transplantation in children. *Psychosomatics* 34:379–387, 1993; with permission.
Modified from Slater JA: Psychiatric aspects of transplantation in children and adolescents. *Child Adolesc Psychiatr Clin North Am* 3(3):557–598, 1994, with permission.
[a] Living-related donor data excluded.
[b] NC, not calculated due to small N.

CASE ILLUSTRATION

In one such case, a 12-year-old boy developed strong, somewhat flirtatious attachments to some of the intensive care unit nurses, which became problematic when he began to engage in inappropriate behaviors, such as suddenly cutting one of the nurse's hair with a scissors when she turned around. He later bit off the end of a glass thermometer, saying he was just ''kidding around'' (Slater, 1994). The consulting psychiatrist felt that fueling these behaviors was the boy's sense of frustration and helplessness at the long waiting period, exacerbated by his parents being unable to visit him during the daytime, and his being semiconscious during a witnessed cardiac arrest and resuscitation several days prior to these behaviors. Psychotherapy with the boy allowed him to discuss his lack of feeling safe in the ICU, even in the presence of all the high-tech monitoring equipment. As a developing adolescent young man, he felt his body becoming weaker and weaker, which severely affected his self-image and emerging sexual identity. The psychiatrist also assisted the intensive care unit staff in setting limits with this young man, which led to an abatement in these behaviors.

SURGERY

When parents are notified that a suitable organ donor has been found, many report ambivalent feelings. One parent thought "Oh my God, it's here. Well, I don't want to go. I just felt like saying, 'Give it to the next person, we're not ready'" (Slater, 1994). On the way into the hospital, she and her husband felt the impulse to turn off the exit and return home with their daughter, who was listed for a heart transplant. Parents struggle with the responsibility they bear for committing their child to transplantation, knowing that there are operative and postoperative risks, and are sometimes tormented by the thought that somehow the child could almost magically survive without the transplant. The ambivalence is generally worse if the child is waiting for a transplant as an outpatient and is not critically ill at the time of transplantation. In either case, parents experience guilt over making decisions that expose the child to the potential trauma of hospitalization and surgery, despite knowing it is the only way to save their child. If the child does not fare well, parents need maximal support to help them cope with their sense of responsibility for the outcome, however "irrational" that might be.

The moment of separation just prior to surgery is a moment many parents recall as an indelible mark in their minds. As one parent described:

"I kissed her good-bye, turned toward the door to the operating room, and never turned around. It was because you make that separation, even though you still hear sound . . . . You just have to do it. If you turned around, I think the impulse would be so strong they'd probably have to restrain you and drag you out" (Slater, 1992).

Another recalled: "We certainly felt that we were leaving her in very capable hands, but there's all of the unknown questions, you know: 'Are you going to see this child again? Is everything going to go through okay?' And just simply walking away from it was a hard thing to do. Somehow I felt if I could just stay there it would be okay" (Slater, 1992).

During surgery, time is often telescoped for these parents who sit waiting to hear word on their child's progress. A visit from the psychiatrist at this time can be quite supportive.

Parents should be prepared both visually and descriptively for what they will see in the intensive care unit postoperatively. A preoperative visit and detailed description can often help defuse parents' acute shock of witnessing their child with an endotracheal tube, intravenous lines, indwelling chest tubes and other high-tech monitoring devices. Despite explanations prior to surgery, they are often overwhelmed and confused by the complicated medical management in the immediate postoperative setting, and this anxiety may be exacerbated by the presence of other critically ill children (Bradford, 1990).

The conduct and sensitivity of the intensive care unit staff can greatly affect parents' emotional state during this period, when postoperative sedation, analgesia, and the presence of an endotracheal tube make communication with their child difficult. As the child's level of awareness returns, he or she may be irritable, combative, or withdrawn, and the psychiatrist may assist in recommending pharmacological intervention or other behavioral techniques to help the child. The psychiatrist can be invaluable in helping to explain the nature of the child's experience to parents, as well as to staff (Bradford, 1990), and should conduct serial neuropsychiatric assessments. Strokes, metabolic derangement, medication effects, delirium, and hypoxia are among the many events that may compromise mental status in the perioperative period.

A common tendency among families is to compare their postoperative course with that of other families whom they have met. Unfortunately, though kidney transplant recipients can often be discharged within a week (Stuber, 1993), other SOT recipients may remain in the intensive care unit for that long and spend weeks or even months in the hospital, subject to unpredictable complications. In the often elated atmosphere of a successful transplant, it is easy for parents to think ahead to discharge, setting themselves up for inevitable disappointment at the first postoperative complication. Such events, like mild rejection episodes and postoperative fevers, are common, and can "burst the bubble" of the "honeymoon" phase described by some families immediately following transplantation. This deflation may herald the "roller coaster" ride that may continue, with cycles of high hopes and expectations alternating with periods of intense fear and worry. As the sense of reality sets in that the transplant is really not a "cure," patients and families may feel quite disillusioned. The psychiatrist can both help prepare them for this process, as well as allow expression of these feelings in a supportive setting.

Thus, speaking with other transplant recipients can have both positive and negative aspects. In one respect, feelings can be validated by others who have gone through the same experience. On the other hand, since these experiences are inevitably individualized and subject to so many variables, patients may experience a sense of frustration, failure, or disappointment if their expectations, which are modeled by the experiences of others, are not met.

As tubes and lines are withdrawn, and analgesia reduced, children can benefit from more contact with visitors and the child life department. Parents can read to their children, and videotapes can be viewed. Behavioral interventions such as guided imagery, story-telling, self-relaxation, and games such as "Game-boy" can continue to play a role during this period and be used to help children tolerate postoperative procedures. Such practices may decrease the need for sedation (Bradford, 1990; Bullock and Shaddy, 1993).

Developmental Considerations

As Stuber describes (Stuber, 1993a, 1993b), developmental issues impact on the child's and adolescent's experience of and response to transplantation in a manner different from that in adults. Parents must be involved in the decision-making process, and adolescent assent or consent is also essential. Developmental regressions compete with the demands for autonomy common to all phases of childhood. The impact of developmental factors on illness has been approached from many different models, including ego psychology, self-psychology, and cognitive psychology, and delineated by many including Anna Freud (1952) and others (Bauman, 1981; Nagera, 1976; Schowalter, 1971). Other writers have applied theories of affective development within the infant-caregiver dyad (Emde, 1989) to help understand how illness can impact on relationship formation (Parmelee, 1989). The application of Piagetian theory to the progression of the cognitive understanding of illness has been reviewed by Schonfeld (1991). Thompson and Vernon (1993) and Vernon and Thompson (1993) have recently reviewed the literature on the effects of hospitalization and directed interventions on children. Developmental theory has been applied specifically to transplantation as well (Sexson and Rubenow, 1992; Slater, 1994) (Table 95.9).

The patient-family system is exposed to the multiple stresses of acute and chronic illness, intrusive high-tech procedures, surgery, and hospitalization, often in an unrelenting fashion. Ethical issues, involving solid organ or bone marrow donations by family members, and quality of life issues may further complicate this picture. A fundamental purpose of the child and adolescent psychiatrist is to translate childhood experience into terms adults can understand and therefore respond to empathically.

When transplantation occurs in the infancy or early childhood, children are more likely to incorporate physical sequelae such as the scar and medical management (chronic medication and medical follow-up) into their developing identity and self-image. The subject of transplantation may be dealt with in a similar manner to adoption, explaining to

Table 95.9. Developmental Aspects of Transplantation

Age	Developmental Tasks	Potential Effects of Chronic Illness/Transplantation
0–18 months	Attachment/bonding (Bowlby) Basic trust (Erikson) Sensorimotor stage (Piaget) Physiological and affective regulation and sharing (intersubjectivity) Learning "Biobehavioral shifts" at 2–3, 6–9, 12, and 18–21 months with dramatic changes in social relationships, motor skills, affect, language (Emde, 1989)	Separation from caregivers is major stressor Difficulty transferring care (stranger anxiety 7–9 months) Disruption of biological rhythms Decreased confidence in infant vitality can affect the developing social relationship with the infant (Parmelee, 1989) Developmental regressions and disruption of "biobehavioral shifts" Potential disruption in developing social relationships Empathic responsiveness may be more difficult
18 months to 3 years	"Toddlerhood" Autonomy vs. shame/doubt (Erikson) Approaching preoperational stage (Piaget) Separation-individuation (Mahler) Language development	Pride in newly developing skills may be threatened Tendency to tantrum, ambivalence exacerbated problems accepting medication Symbolic thinking allows speech, but preoperational thinking may lead to "immanent justice" explanations, and heightened fears, e.g., about the aggressive intent of medical staff re: procedures (e.g., catheterization), may lead to heightened perception of pain Interference with play and its developmental and reparative function Coping mechanisms unstable, tendency to regress Prone to withdrawal, irritability, sleep/appetite disturbance Separation still a major stressor
3–6 years	"Initiative vs. guilt" (Erikson) Cognitive and motor development: writing, forming letters, self-care (hygiene), drawing Emergence into concrete operational stage at 6–7 years and evolution of understanding of illness along Piagetian lines	Development of initiative interfered with Phobias (e.g., pills, needles); pain modulated by fear Susceptibility to fears of bodily mutilation esp. in face of procedures Continuation of "immanent justice" theorizing, magical thinking, or later, fears of "contagion" Difficulty understanding the rationale for procedures Prone to regression (bedwetting, "baby talk"); cognitive distortions Problems accepting medication Possible neurodevelopmental delays
6–10 years	"Latency" (Freud) "Industry vs. inferiority" (Erikson) "Concrete operational" thinking (Piaget) Social involvement; groups Learning "3 R's"; hobbies Development of sense of "pride and mastery" through "affirming responses" of others Rapid physical development Moral development	School tasks/learning interfered with due to absences, possibly neuropsychiatric co-morbidity of illness Involvement with peer group affected Possible impairment of self-esteem Motor tasks (running, jumping, playing games) interfered with though transplantation generally increases endurance Decreased opportunities for mastery Regressive pulls toward dependency "Germ" or "contamination" theories of illness in early school-age
11–18 years	"Adolescence" Puberty: sexual maturation Formal operational thinking (Piaget) 80% function normally (Offer, 1991) Importance of attractiveness: body image as self-image, peer acceptance, and being part of the "group" Sexual identity consolidation "Second phase" of separation/individuation (Blos, 1962)) Females: importance of relationships Males: sense of masculinity may derive more from physical/sexual prowess Understanding of death and ability to conceptualize the future	Etiology of late rejection is often adolescent noncompliance Sexual maturation may be interfered with; normal discomfort with secondary sexual characteristics exacerbated Steroids may exacerbate moodiness, cause cushinoid changes, acne; cyclosporine and hirsutism Scar on chest (esp. with women) Problems with romantic relationships, heightened anxiety over sexuality Females may experience social isolation, men a sense of inferiority Chronic illness may threaten identity formation and the ability to formulate future roles and relationships Uncertainty of existence as a transplant recipient, chronic fears of rejection/infection may interfere with conceptualization of the future "Annuals" and other hospitalizations interfere with social functions Denial, sense of "invincibility," wanting to be "normal," defiant behavior may affect compliance

Adapted from Sexson S, Rubenow J: Transplants in children and adolescents. In: Craven J, Rodin GM (eds): *Psychiatric Aspects of Organ Transplantation.* Oxford, Oxford University Press, 1992, pp. 35–36, with permission. From Slater JA: Psychiatric aspects of transplantation in children and adolescents. *Child Adolesc Clin North Am* 3(3):557–598, 1994, with permission.

the child from an early age what has happened to him or her and helping the child develop a narrative and more complex understanding about who he or she is as time goes by. This openness and acceptance on the part of the parents that the transplant is not a "secret," but an integral part of the child's identity, may help facilitate adjustment and the child's acceptance of the requirements of life as a transplant recipient. Such issues apply to BMT as well, which is covered later in the chapter.

Though children may experience cognitive distortions, such as using "immanent justice" theorizing to explain that their illness may represent a punishment for misdeeds (Schonfeld, 1991), it is continually surprising to physicians and parents alike how much children do understand. For example, the parents of a 4-year-old who had undergone cardiac transplantation at age 2 felt that she had little recollection of the events and were amazed when she played out features of the hospitalization in exact detail when given miniature hospital props.

In communicating with a child or adolescent about his or her illness, transplantation, procedures, or other aspect of medical care, the accepted

approach is to be honest within a developmental orientation. In the pediatric transplant population, these distortions often occur alongside normal childhood curiosity. In the setting of heart transplantation, cultural symbols and metaphors invest this organ with tremendous meaning:

"We tend, in the medical world, to think of a heart as a pump. We've got to be reminded, sometimes by the patient, that the heart is an organ with a lot of mystery to it, if you will, a lot of history to it. The heart loves, the heart represents not simply that organ which sends the blood around, but that organ which we associate with some of our most wonderful human attributes. I mean love, heart as courage. We'll talk about an athlete who has heart; identifying the heart with valiant, courageous impulses. The heart with sentiment, with affection. Do we really think that one can take out a heart, and replace it with another heart, and not set off an extraordinary chain of associations on the part of the recipient? Will my new heart be valiant? Will my new heart be loving? Am I the same person now that I have a new heart? Am I that other person?" (From Slater JA: Psychiatric aspects of transplantation in children and adolescents. *Child Adolesc Psychiatr Clin North Am* 3(3):557–598, 1994, with permission.)

Children may wonder, for example, if it matters whether the donated organ comes from a male or female, black or white. Others queries have included children asking "how they will know whom to love, for example, when they receive their new heart: Should they still love their parents, or the family from which the donor heart came? They think of the sayings, 'I love you from the bottom of my heart,' or that someone's heart can 'break' because they miss someone, and apply this to the transplant experience and become understandably confused" (Slater, 1994).

Under the influence of tremendous anxiety, cognitive distortions can be exacerbated. This interface became apparent when a child began refusing her endocardial biopsies, because she believed that each time, more "pieces" of her heart were being removed, such that eventually it would fall into her stomach. In her play, she repeatedly tied her stuffed animals down to perform "biopsies" on them and soothed them by saying "it's going to be all right." This posttraumatic repetition could be perhaps understood as helping the child master her helpless feelings during catheterization. In ego psychological terms, one might characterize her as "identifying with the aggressor" or "turning passive into active."

Another child told his mother he was worried that other children in the playground would start coughing, as he did, if they overexerted themselves. This projection of one's own experience upon that of others is typical of the egocentrism in the preoperational Piagetian phase.

Latency or school-age children also respond to transplantation within a developmental frame. Interference with physical prowess in boys, and relationship development with peers in girls, can result from repeated hospitalization and illness. Academic performance can be affected by school absence or the neurocognitive sequelae of treatment, such as cranial irradiation in BMT. The development of self-esteem can be affected by the decreased opportunities for mastery that are normally associated with important affirming responses from role models.

Adolescent transplant recipients present unique challenges to the physicians working with them due to the seriousness of noncompliance, which is more prevalent in this age group. Adolescents react to contingencies of their illness, which undermine developmental needs for independence and control. The enforced dependency, though in line with regressive forces brought about by serious illness, may result in more demanding and boisterous behavior.

The psychological issues in this population have been reviewed by Stuber (1993b) who addresses several important points, including ethical concerns about the adolescent's right to refuse treatment, the need for systematic research to identify psychosocial predictors for outcome, specific developmental considerations such as the parents' involvement in the adolescent's "personal body functions and decisions," and the psychological reactions to implantation of a foreign organ. As Stuber notes, hearts may be imbued with more philosophical meaning. An adolescent who was approaching his birthday, for example, said that he felt strange that he would be turning 16, but his heart, who came from a donor 2 years younger, would be only 14. Over time he came to experience his new heart as an integral part of his identity and body.

Illness and medication side effects can dramatically affect appearance, and physical and sexual development, significantly impacting on the adolescent's identity and relationships, and making him or her more self-conscious. Prednisone can cause weight gain, acne, and a cushingoid appearance. Cyclosporine causes hirsutism. BMT is associated with hair loss and cachexia. Adolescents may desperately struggle with the need to be "normal" like their peers, while at the same time accepting that he or she is different. Their sense of a possible foreshortened future may interfere with plans for college, a career, and intimate relationships.

Adolescents may struggle with decisions about who to tell about the transplant. This question may have antecedents in failure to confide in friends about the illness leading to transplantation, such as an adolescent with cystic fibrosis who is listed for lung transplantation and has told her friends over the years that she has asthma. The issue of who to tell generally revolves around concerns over peer acceptance and may have painful aspects, such as one adolescent whose boyfriend's mother told her son not to get involved with the patient because she was a transplant recipient and might not live a long life.

Making it "public knowledge" that one is a transplant recipient can lead to celebrity status in school initially for an adolescent, but can also lead to intrusive questions about sexual functioning and other naive questions that must be fielded about life as a transplant recipient. An adolescent reported that he was initially treated like an invalid, and one classmate asked whether he had to carry oxygen with him on a date. These questions interestingly reflect the transplant candidates concerns early on as well, but will often not be addressed unless the consultant raises them in a sensitive way.

Adolescents often describe feeling out of step with their contemporaries, in terms of both concrete issues like missed social events, but also in terms of a sense that many of them describe that they have grown up too quickly and have lost a carefree quality they see in their friends:

"I guess at that point I just felt they weren't taking life serious, as seriously as they should. But I think in reality I was just taking it too seriously, like I felt like every minute was my last minute. And I was trying to be the best I could be because I thought maybe it was because I was bad that it happened to me. And I found that I was given this second life and I was making a mess of it because I was so tight and wound up about everything" (Slater, 1992).

Transplant recipients often talk about entering a health-related profession or other field where they can feel useful to others. One adolescent joined the volunteer fire department and relished in the idea of carrying a beeper with him; in fact, he used his fire fighting "on-call" schedule as a rationale for missing clinic appointments at times. Several have confided in me that they would rather be nurses, since they cannot see themselves as the one actually "causing" the pain, but understand what it is like to be the patient, and feel they could more sensitively soothe children in pain and fear. Many of their aspirations and specific commendations reflect on the importance of supportive care in the hospital and the important role of hospital staff at crucial junctures in their recovery.

Pain and Anxiety Management

The topic of pain and anxiety management in the pediatric transplant population has not been well studied or described (Green, 1994). There is a literature on this subject in the pediatric population, especially in the psychology and pediatrics journals (Abu-Saad, 1984; Bush, 1987; Kuttner et al., 1988; Manne et al., 1988, 1990; McGrath and Hillier, 1989; Siegel and Smith, 1989; Varni et al., 1987). Bush (1987) reviewed the literature on analgesic use in children, which suggests that children are undermedicated for pain as compared with adults undergoing similar procedures. Undermedication can exacerbate pain behaviors and disrupt the trust between the child and physician.

In addition, there is good reason to expect that this population can benefit greatly from cognitive-behavioral techniques designed to diminish pain and anxiety associated with biopsies, catheterizations, venipunctures and central line placement, surgery, bone marrow aspirations, lumbar punctures, and many other procedures that may potentially occur in these patients. These techniques have been used for such procedures in different populations (Bush, 1987), especially in pediatric cancer patients (Kuttner et al., 1988; Manne et al., 1990; McGrath and Hillier, 1989). Manne et al. (1990) described a behavioral approach designed to decrease anxiety in children with cancer who undergo repeated venipunctures (see also Cardona, 1994). A combination of parent coaching, distraction, and positive reinforcement was associated with a decrease in parental anxiety and report of the child's pain, and less distress for both child and parent.

One relevant study utilized such techniques during right ventricular endocardial biopsies in pediatric patients (Bullock and Shaddy, 1993), which are used to monitor for episodes of rejection in the cardiac transplant population. The techniques described included preparation, reassurance, deep breathing, imagery, distraction, and muscle relaxation. By the sixth biopsies, all patients discontinued the use of benzodiazepines, felt more in control, and reported less pain (which was associated with decreased autonomic measures). In addition, the length of time required to do the biopsies was diminished.

Bush (1987) and McGrath and Hillier (1989) have reviewed this literature from a developmental point of view, recommending an interdisciplinary approach. Early impressions that infants do not experience pain have been refuted, and it is clear that from several weeks of age, infants react to pain in gradually more differentiated patterns of response. Specific responses to painful stimuli, as well as anticipatory anxiety and avoidance behavior follow a typical developmental sequence along Piagetian lines. Cognitive factors impact on pain intervention in multiple areas that include the subjective pain experience, how to describe pain intervention measures, how to evaluate pain, how to implement the pain-reduction techniques, and how much children will retain after being taught techniques to help them manage pain (Bush, 1987). Prior experiences with pain are also modulators of later pain response (McGrath and Hillier, 1989).

Pain behaviors may serve communicative functions in families. Parental responses, including anxiety prior to a procedure and expectation of the child's fear or uncooperativeness, can significantly affect the child's experience of a painful stimulus and subsequent behavior. Heightened parental anxiety can thus exacerbate distress for a child undergoing a procedure (Bush, 1987; Manne et al., 1988). Family patterns of pain response are learned through modeling and reinforcement, and operant conditioning models have also been used to describe responses that reinforce pain behaviors as predominant coping strategies. In line with a learning model, instruments or even people that are associated with pain induction can later independently elicit anxiety, fear, avoidance, and complaints of pain. Nevertheless, most clinicians working in this area oppose a differentiation of pain between "psychogenic" versus "organic." Such a distinction can disrupt therapeutic alliances and is generally not relevant or able to be substantiated diagnostically or therapeutically.

In assessing pediatric pain, Bush (1987) suggests focusing on diminishing anticipatory anxiety, the prior history of pain experiences, and the environmental responses to pain behaviors. Varni (1987) underscores the importance of combining cognitive, behavioral, and physiological data in evaluating pain. In children, self-reported distress during a procedure may not habituate following repeated exposure though it may appear to lessen to an observer. Developmental and psychological factors, such as age and fearfulness, may be more operative (Manne et al., 1988). Adaptive coping mechanisms may include distraction, desensitization, information seeking, and parental presence. Visual analog scales (Bush, 1987; Varni et al., 1987) or "word descriptors" (Abu-Saad, 1984) have been used successfully in pain assessment in children to help quantify the fear or pain experience.

Psychological techniques in pain management have included hypnosis, distraction, and relaxation with the help of breathing exercises. Other interventions may address family factors that are operative in the child's pain experience. The preparation aspect of intervention may use a modeling principle in exposing children to educational videotapes or other children who are utilizing adaptive coping mechanisms. Younger children may benefit more from "imaginative involvement," a technique that takes advantage of their active fantasy life in creating stories and using hypnotic suggestions, than distraction (Kuttner, 1988).

In summary, the BMT and SOT pediatric population can undoubtedly benefit from psychological techniques to assist with anxiety, fear, and pain associated with the myriad of procedures that these patients experience. There may be long-term benefits as well, such as improved compliance and the possible decrease in potential posttraumatic symptomatology.

Posttransplant Life and Noncompliance

THE 1ST YEAR

Lifestyle is irrevocably changed following transplantation and evolves in parallel with the medical course and nature of follow-up. There seems to be a differentiation with respect to issues involved in early follow-up and late follow-up, and the end of the 1st year following transplantation may be an important marker.

Initially, there are frequent clinic visits and a necessary immersion in becoming versed with the requirements of transplant life. Complications may occur during the 1st year, as the immunosuppressant regimen is adjusted. One parent summed up this period by saying: "Life then was centered around the hospital. We lived transplant, we ate, we slept transplant. We were totally removed from the rest of our lives" (Slater, 1994).

Patients and families are more closely followed and monitored during the 1st year and exist in the aftermath of having survived a extraordinary ordeal and often describe having more powerful family bonds and pride in having weathered the ordeal. Being closer in time to the pretransplant and transplant experience, they may be more likely to treat their bodies and the new organ inside with respect. They are much more task-focused as they learn about administering medication and recognizing signs and symptoms of illness. Many of the social sequelae may not yet be apparent, because children and adolescents are just beginning to reenter their social milieu and might still be treated as quite special by peers, a time-limited but perhaps supportive influence on self-esteem. In addition, many of the physical side effects may not become fully in evidence. For all these reasons, adolescents may be less likely to be noncompliant during the 1st year.

Biopsies and catheterizations are more frequent in the early period following heart transplantation and tax the skills of most parents, who are used to having more latitude with respect to setting limits with their children. In the world of transplantation, there is often little room for negotiation: medication must be given, doctor's appointments must be kept, biopsies and catheterizations must be done.

LATE FOLLOW-UP POST TRANSPLANTATION

The end of the 1st year is often marked by an anniversary celebration by patient and families, and as routine follow-up diminishes in frequency, many families describe a discomfort with being more on their own, "waiting for the other shoe to drop" (Slater, 1994).

The uncertainty of posttransplant life is a background anxiety that some patients and families are more able to suppress than others, and unexpected complications, which can include rejection, seizures, alterations in renal function, infection, and posttransplant lymphoproliferative disorder, for example, can be powerful reinforcers for a constant background dread that may seriously affect patients and families. Other potential chronic effects of immunosuppressive therapy include hypertension, coronary artery disease (cardiac transplant patients), bone disease, cataracts, and growth reduction (Moskop, 1989).

Stuber (1993b) underscores salient clinical considerations in the adolescent population, such as anxiety, impaired self-esteem, noncompliance, depression, and posttraumatic stress disorder. One adolescent told me that he was troubled by the discontinuity in his conscious experience of the transplant, since he did not "see" the actual operation, but simply awoke with a scar on his chest and a new heart inside. He developed intrusive images of what he felt the actual operation looked like, seeing his heart repeatedly lifted out of his chest and replaced by another. Eventually, the treating psychiatrist obtained some videotaped footage of an actual heart transplant, which the adolescent eagerly watched, and later reported his intrusive thoughts had abated. He later brought this tape to school to show his classmates in health class.

Major depression can be differentiated from organic mental syndromes or constitutional symptoms secondary to depleting medical illness. Useful criteria in making this differentiation include the presence of cognitive correlates of depression, including hopelessness, guilt, low self-worth, and suicidal ideation, and the absence of signs and symptoms of delirium or encephalopathy on formal mental status examination (Stuber, 1993b).

Parents may also exhibit posttraumatic phenomena, such as a mother of a transplant recipient who nearly died waiting for an organ, who was tormented for months by intrusive images of her daughter's funeral.

Over time, parents struggle with normal developmental issues in relinquishing control and responsibility to their adolescent children, but this is exacerbated by heightened anxiety over whether the adolescent will be able to be compliant and recognize physical signs and symptoms. Events such as the adolescent leaving for college can have profound impact on a parent. As one mother described: "I think that this whole transplant life, is a life, and you can get lost in it. When my daughter went to college, she said, 'Mom, you know, like 'get a life.'"

"I said, 'But you are my life. I've been taking you back and forth, doing things with you, and watching you all this time—you have been my life.'

"She said, 'Yeah but mom, now you have to get a life'" (Slater, 1992).

There may continue to be residual issues among siblings and between healthy siblings and parents that originated in the need for the parents to be so preoccupied with the ill child. These feelings may have distorted relationship development within the family to such a degree that psychiatric treatment is warranted.

Outpatient individual or family psychotherapy can be of great assistance, especially during the 1st year following transplantation, when most of the acute adjustment to transplant life takes place, and psychiatric follow-up may be made easier by patients' frequent visits to the transplant clinic. During rehospitalizations for complications or routine biopsies or catheterizations, the psychiatric consultant should reevaluate, looking for the presence of any intercurrent psychopathology in the patient or family members or risk factors for noncompliance. The consultant should assess social adaptation, compliance behaviors, and the overall level of family and patient functioning, including school attendance and presence of any cognitive impairment. Appropriate referrals for neuropsychological testing or Committee on Special Education evaluation can be made.

NONCOMPLIANCE IN TRANSPLANT RECIPIENTS

Most of the literature on noncompliance in the transplant population involves adult renal transplant recipients or pool data from adults and children (DeLone et al., 1989; Dunn et al., 1990; Kiley et al., 1993; Rovelli et al., 1989a, 1989b; Schweizer, 1990), though some studies have looked specifically at the pediatric population (Beck, 1980; Foulkes et al., 1993; Korsch et al., 1973, 1978; Phipps and DeCuir-Whalley, 1989). There is literature on general noncompliance issues in medically adolescents that has been recently reviewed (Cromer and Tarnowski, 1989).

Shapiro and Fingeroth (unpublished data) reviewed the literature on noncompliance in the adult cardiac transplant population, and in their own study found a robust association between noncompliance and both global psychiatric risk and personality disorders. Global psychiatric risk was estimated clinically as low, moderate, or high by the psychiatrist after reviewing the prior psychiatric history. Included among the items scrutinized were any history of substance abuse, cognitive impairment, personality disorder, social stressors, prior level of functioning, previous history of noncompliance, social supports, interpersonal problems with treating physicians, and knowledge/expectations about transplantation. For those patients with high global psychiatric risk, 50% were noncompliant. Personality disorders were diagnosed clinically as being nonexistent, mild, moderate, and severe, with patients having severe personality disorders found to be noncompliant 100% of the time.

Korsch et al. (1973) examined the psychosocial outcome of 35 pediatric renal transplant recipients and found that, within a year, most normal family patterns had returned if the child was healthy, with most of the disruption in family functioning occurring during this year. Ten of the 35 patients had scores indicating maladjustment on personality measures, most apparent in the anxiety and self-esteem scales. Eight patients had psychopathology, with depression the "most specific test finding." Transplant patients with personality disturbances were more likely to be noncompliant. Seventeen of 19 of the older adolescents were in college or working. Eleven of 16 of the younger patients were in school. Leisure activities were age appropriate. Anxiety over rejection and side effects of steroids emerged as significant clinical issues.

Korsch (1978) found that risk factors for noncompliance with immunosuppressive medication included sex (female greater than male), adolescence, premorbid deviance on personality scores, absence of the father, and lack of community support and other resources.

Beck (1980) reported a 43% prevalence of noncompliance in a sample of pediatric renal transplant recipients and found that all of the noncompliant patients were adolescent. The noncompliant patients seemed to have less parental involvement in supervising their medication and attending clinic visits. An intervention program including counseling and instruction resulted in 5 of the noncompliant patients becoming compliant. None of this latter group of patients lost their grafts, as was the case with 6 other noncompliant patients. Notebooks in which medication administration and laboratory results were recorded have facilitated compliance.

Rovelli et al. (1989a) found noncompliance in renal, heart, and liver transplant recipients to be higher in the under 20 age group. After the initial 3-month period following transplantation, it was reported that noncompliance caused graft loss more frequently than unmanageable rejection episodes in compliant patients. Schweizer (1990) reported that clinic visit noncompliance was associated with medication noncompliance.

Factors that predict compliance in the outpatient setting have also not been well studied in the pediatric BMT population. One study in outpatient adolescents with cancer (not specific for BMT recipients) showed that nearly 50% were noncompliant with oral medication regimens (McConville et al., 1990). Risk factors for noncompliance included less developed concepts of illness, less perceived vulnerability, greater denial, and relatively decreased orientation toward the future (Tamaroff et al., 1992). A study that looked specifically at compliance in inpatient pediatric BMT recipients reported greater than 50% noncompliance rates as inpatients, most commonly found with oral antibiotics, and most prevalent in the preschool or school-age population (Phipps and DeCuir-Whalley, 1990). More research in this area is needed.

Hesse et al. (1990) suggested that noncompliance with corticosteroids may be more prevalent in the pediatric and adolescent population. Foulkes et al. (1993) found that compliance with different medications may vary within an individual's regimen and underscored the importance of assessing compliance to each medication.

Bradford (1990) reviewed other risk factors for noncompliance in chronic renal failure patients, which included "side effects, duration, and complexity (of medication); the doctor-patient relationship; family factors: instability or discord, poor communication, lack of support from family members, maternal mood, poor maternal understanding of treatment, and lack of supervision; poor understanding, perceived vulnerability and doubts about the effectiveness of the treatment" (Bradford, 1990). Periodic psychosocial assessment of transplant recipients as outpatients was recommended.

Preliminary results from a study of noncompliance in pediatric heart transplant recipients found noncompliance in 13/64 (20%) of patients and was significantly associated with adolescent age and "late" rejection occurring greater than 1 year following cardiac transplantation. In noncompliant patients, graft survival dropped off precipitously in stepwise fashion from 1 year posttransplant, such that only 30% graft survival was present at 5 years in these patients (Douglas et al., 1993). This is alarming because 8 of these patients lost their grafts (2 retransplantations and 6 deaths).

One of these patients maintained a powerful sense of denial and invincibility throughout the entire transplant experience. He later became secretly noncompliant with his medication, rejected the first heart, and almost died before being retransplanted. He eventually died several years later.

CASE ILLUSTRATION

This adolescent young man who was secretly noncompliant as a 13-year-old later confided: "I guess when you're that age you think you're invincible, especially after going through a transplant. I mean hey, you were close to death and you made it. You're even more invincible now. I mean you were just a normal invincible thirteen year old before, now you kind of feel I guess, for lack of a better word, *immortal*. Yeah you laughed in the face of death, big deal. But in the end, if you don't take your medicine, he's going to laugh back really hard. Probably why I needed a second transplant is one very big reason, stupidity: I was too proud to take my medicine in front of other kids. I had that, you know, the peer pressure, the look of someone turning around while I'm taking it. And it really got to me, it did. The reason I spoke up about not taking my medicine is that I realized I was hurting myself. I realized whether consciously or not I was committing suicide. Whether I actually thought of it that way or not, I was killing myself. So, while the doctors were going crazy trying to research every angle on this of why I could be getting sick, I just said, "Look, I wasn't taking my medicine, that's why I've been getting sick." I paid the price, losing a transplanted heart and having to go through it again was painful, not to mention I lost the trust of a lot of doctors." (From Slater JA: Psychiatric aspects of transplantation in children and adolescents. *Child Adolesc Psychiatr Clin North Am* 3(3):557–598, 1994, with permission.)

Based on available data, it would appear that risk factors for noncompliance in the pediatric transplant population include:

1. Adolescence;
2. Conduct disorder, sociopathy, or other significant personality disorder;
3. Affective disorder including major depression and perhaps other more chronic, indolent depression with impaired self-esteem such as dysthymia; possibly, the presence of another psychiatric disorder such as PTSD;
4. Family psychopathology, possibly an absent father, and poor supervision by parents;
5. Prior history of noncompliance;
6. Cognitive limitations and problems understanding the medication regimen by adolescents or parents;
7. Low perceived vulnerability and expectation of benefit from treatment, including a sense of a foreshortened future the patient feels powerless to affect;
8. Poor physician-patient relationship or continuity of care;
9. Inadequate resources to meet treatment requirements (including transportation, financial, etc.);
10. Poor understanding or acceptance of the need for commitment to treatment and follow-up.

Warning signs for noncompliance in this population may include (Douglas et al., 1993):

1. Late rejection;
2. Variations in cyclosporine levels or reluctance to have them drawn;
3. Casual reporting of missed doses of immunosuppressants;
4. Missed or delayed clinic appointments;
5. Not reporting illness.

Management issues should include treating noncompliance as a phenomenon with a differential diagnosis (Cromer and Tarnowski, 1989):

1. Direct physical assays should be used when possible to monitor compliance;
2. Interventions should be directed at presumed underlying causes and risk factors;
3. Treat noncompliance as an issue "shared" by the patient, family, and physicians and approach it from a task-oriented, problem-solving point of view;
4. Combine interventions that use closer monitoring (more frequent clinic visits), and help the patient with organization strategies (use of alarm watch, pill boxes, carrying extra doses of medication at all times);
5. Use psychiatric involvement and individual and/or family psychotherapy and pharmacotherapy if appropriate;
6. Manage pain adequately;
7. Consider increased involvement of parents or parental surrogates.

Adolescent issues impacted upon by transplantation should be anticipated even prior to surgery and discussed with the patient in an appropriate fashion to help identify potential problem areas. Noncompliance should be addressed early on with the patient and family, as a major side effect of treatment and serious cause of graft loss and death. This discussion should continue following transplantation. Specific areas that might be addressed include concrete help with side effects (helping to establish diet and exercise regimens, advice on removing excess hair, etc.) or peer issues. Adolescents as young as 10 years old, depending on their level of maturity, can often be taught to manage their own medication from the time they are in the hospital and should be put in touch with other transplant patients who can provide opportunities for modeling coping behaviors.

For adolescent patients in particular, outpatient follow-up should be considered as a routine measure. An early alliance between an adolescent and mental health specialist may be of great value in facilitating work later when the adolescent is at higher risk for noncompliance (see below) and allow early identification of risk factors and intervention.

In a study that looked at brittle diabetics (Moran et al., 1991), many of whom are presumed to have psychosocial factors that exacerbate their medical course, intensive inpatient psychotherapy 3 to 4 times weekly, for an average duration of 15 weeks, was associated with improved diabetic control, which was maintained at 1-year follow-up. One might extrapolate from such a preliminary study and suggest that severely noncompliant adolescent transplant patients should be hospitalized for a period of weeks to months in a medical facility that can provide a multidisciplinary approach to treatment that includes a strong psychiatric component. Hopefully, insurance companies will reimburse such services, which may have a strong impact on patient survival.

SPECIFIC ORGAN SYSTEMS

Bone Marrow Transplantation

OVERVIEW

The psychiatric aspects of BMT were reviewed in two recent articles by Andrykowski (1994) and Wolcott and Stuber (1992). The usage of BMTs has undergone a rapid increase since the late 1970s, due to better survival rates, its being used to treat a greater variety of illnesses, and the growth of alternative donor pools besides an identical twin sibling.

The procedure itself is offered only as a final option in diseases where conventional treatments will not or have not sufficed and that include leukemias, lymphomas, breast cancer, neuroblastoma, ovarian cancer, germ cell tumors, melanoma, multiple myeloma, and malignant gliomas (Abramowicz, 1992; Andrykowski, 1994; Trigg, 1988; Wolcott and Stuber, 1992). In the pediatric population, BMTs have also been used to treat aplastic anemia and congenital metabolic and immunological disorders. Cytotoxic drugs, often in combination with total body irradiation, are used to wipe out the patient's own bone marrow over a 4- to 10-day period, while the patient remains in relative isolation, often in specialized laminar air flow rooms, with visitors generally required to wear gowns, gloves, and masks. Healthy marrow is then delivered via intravenous infusion. BMTs are categorized by the source of the marrow to be transplanted, which is either autologous, allogeneic, or syngeneic.

Autologous BMTs utilize the patient's own marrow, harvested prior to BMT, and is utilized in lymphomas, sarcomas, and advanced breast cancer (Andrykowski, 1994). Immunosuppressant medication is not necessary, and there is less risk of "graft versus host disease" (GVHD), where the infused white blood cells react to the host as being foreign and mount an immune reaction.

Allogeneic transplants are used to treat hematologic malignancies and immune disorders (Andrykowski, 1994) and use human lymphocyte antigen (HLA)-matched marrow from a family member or other donor, with the benefit that tumor cells are not part of the infused marrow (Abramowicz, 1992). GVHD is more common than with autologous BMTs. Syngeneic transplants utilize marrow from an identical sibling donor.

Bone marrow transplantation typically involves a hospitalization of at least 5–6 weeks and can require a much more lengthy hospitalization of several months due to the high rate of complications, with a mortality rate of 5–20% with autologous transplants and 10–30% with allogeneic transplants (Abramowicz, 1992; Andrykowski, 1994). Patients with leukemia generally fare better, with disease-free survival at 2 years approaching 60% with early leukemia, than those with solid tumors (Table 95.2). Many factors have been associated with survival rates, including the type of tumor, stage of tumor prior treatment, age and physical state of the recipient, origin of the marrow, type of chemotherapy used prior to transplantation, the actual transplant protocol used, and the experience of the transplant center itself (Abramowicz, 1992).

Following discharge, patients are often in a compromised state, with normal immune function not recurring for up to 1–2 years post transplant, thus placing the patient at moderate risk for dangerous infections and requiring a strict care regimen on the part of the patient and family. Acute GVHD occurs and runs its course within 30–100 days post transplant and commonly affects the liver, gastrointestinal tract, and skin. GVHD is differentiated from rejection in solid organ transplantation where the host is mounting the immune response. Chronic GVHD occurs later and does not resolve, though it can be managed medically (Andrykowski, 1994).

Thus, even though the patient may survive the initial malignancy, postoperative morbidity may include infections, GVHD, graft failure, primary malignancy relapse, secondary malignancies, and a multitude of treatment-associated side effects that may affect a variety of organ systems, including cognitive function (Andrykowski, 1994; Wolcott and Stuber, 1992). Recovery can thus be broken down into the acute phase in the hospital, a slower subacute phase that may last months following discharge, and a significantly prolonged stage "of adjustment and rehabilitation" (Wolcott and Stuber, 1992). Conceptualization of the process in phases, as in solid organ transplantation, can lend itself to a better understanding of the psychological sequelae.

Psychosocial or psychiatric evaluation of BMT candidates may play a less crucial role in the selection process, since bone marrow is a "renewable resource" whose supply is not limited as in solid organ transplantation. Nevertheless, due to the expense of the procedure, its significant medical and psychological morbidity, and debate over the allocation of health care resources, there may be an increasing pressure to establish priorities along guidelines that take into account survival rates and quality of life (Andrykowski, 1994). Research has been extremely limited, especially in the pediatric population, to look at psychosocial variables that may predict compliance and medical/psychological outcome in patients and families.

PSYCHIATRIC SEQUELAE AND INTERVENTION

The neuropsychiatric sequelae and psychological adjustment in pediatric bone marrow transplant recipients and their families is amassing some literature (Andrykowski, 1994; Dermatis and Lesko, 1990; Gardner et al., 1986; Kramer et al., 1992; McConville et al., 1990; Parkman, 1986; Patenaude et al., 1979; Pfefferbaum et al., 1977, 1978; Pot-Mees, 1987; Smedler et al., 1990; Stuber, 1993b; Stuber et al., 1991; Trigg, 1988; Wiley and House, 1988; Wolcott and Stuber, 1992; Wolcott et al., 1987).

The experience of pediatric BMT can be conceptualized in terms of emotional stages (Patenaude et al., 1979; Pfefferbaum et al., 1978). Pfefferbaum (1978) describes a 10-stage process, with implications for the need for psychological management. Many of these stages have correlates in solid organ transplantation previously discussed. Chronological hallmarks include:

1. The exigencies of the informed consent/assent process and living-donor considerations such as putting a healthy sibling at risk. Many authors note the unrealistic expectations on the part of the patient and family that often accompany this stage (Patenaude et al., 1979; Pfefferbaum et al., 1978). Psychological distress in parents during this stage has been studied (Dermatis and Lesko, 1990) and suggests that parents experience a variety of psychiatric symptoms that may inversely correlate with the quality of the communication between parents and the physician. Parents may not fully grasp all aspects of the informed consent process, and single parents may be more at risk for psychiatric symptoms. Psychological intervention may be especially important during this stage to facilitate communication and the use of coping strategies.
2. Pretransplant evaluation (similar to that in solid organ transplantation).
3. Effects of separation from school, home, and friends.
4. The intense feelings of "separation and helplessness" during the child's being isolated for several hours for total body irradiation and the inevitable chills, nausea/vomiting, and diarrhea that follow.
5. "Transplant day" with the specific risks of general anesthesia and bleeding for the donor. The bone marrow infusion itself may be a somewhat "anticlimactic event, greater in symbolic than immediate medical significance" (1979). The isolation of the sterile room may pose a significant stressor.
6. The "waiting period," during which time the family "settles in" to the hospital, and parents may attempt to counter feelings of helplessness by carefully following blood counts with attendant anxieties.
7. Watching for the donated marrow to "take," approximately 2 weeks following the infusion, with children sometimes feeling a sense of "responsibility for the outcome, . . . assuming "blame for infiltrated intravenous lines, unsuccessful venipunctures, nausea, diarrhea, and even results of blood counts." Patenaude et al. (1979) describe the "vacillation between . . . fear and hope."
8. Medical complications and psychological reactions to "waiting again" for marrow activity to stabilize, with children perhaps most prone to withdrawal, depression, and irritability; parents feeling "rejected and embarrassed"; and the possible decrease in support from family members who may become less available, as well as from the staff itself.
9. Anxiety over reentering the social milieu as discharge approaches, due to the change in physical appearance (hair loss, weight loss, cushingoid changes), and the inevitable disappointment that the child is not "well."
10. The "relative isolation," dietary restrictions, chronic medication administration, and uncertainty that characterizes life following discharge (Pfefferbaum, et al., 1978). BMT survivors may be even more physically compromised than solid organ transplant recipients. The enforced dependency and reliance of the child upon a single figure, often the mother, poses a significant stressor for the entire family (Patenaude et al., 1979).

The child and adolescent psychiatrist is perhaps best utilized as an integral member of the BMT team who makes contact with the family during their initial evaluation and serves as a liaison to the rest of the hematology-oncology team. Pretransplant evaluation of the patient, family, and living-related donor, as well as neuropsychiatric assessment and family support during the procedure are also important avenues for both treatment and prevention of psychiatric morbidity. Attention should be paid to the relationship between the referring physician or institution and the hospital administering the BMT, since the patient may likely return to the original hospital at some point, and families may experience complicated feelings about the two institutions, with potential feelings of abandonment, issues over transferring care, or possible splitting mechanisms (Atkins and Patenaude, 1987).

A waiting period between the decision to transplant and BMT itself may occur due to the availability of hospital beds, financial factors, or identification of suitable nonrelated or related donors. Like the waiting period in solid organ transplantation, this can be associated with ambivalence about the procedure, significant anxiety over intercurrent survival or progression of illness, and the psychological consequences of possibly not living near the transplant center (Andrykowski, 1994). In the case of a living-related donor, donor feelings may be less ambivalent since an organ is not being "sacrificed" (Gardner et al., 1977), as compared with kidney donation, for example, where recipient guilt is common. In BMTs, the donors may nevertheless experience guilt and perhaps added pressure, since the request for marrow donation does not involve the irretrievable loss of an organ. Solid organ donation may represent a sacrifice that makes absolution from further responsibility, or ambivalence about donating, more "justifiable" (Gardner et al., 1977). Other siblings may feel "relief" as well as feeling "left out" (Patenaude et al., 1979). All these factors may impact on parents, siblings, and patients alike (Pot-Mees, 1987), and mothers of BMT recipients may be particularly prone to these sequelae since they may spend an extraordinary amount of time in the hospital with their child.

Simply identifying and assisting the family in coping with the extensive array of individual stressors can represent tremendously supportive interventions. These stressors may alter family roles and finances and include long geographical distance from home, the tremendous fear of death, and the tendency for attention to center around the BMT recipient to the exclusion of other family members. The latter can evoke feelings of both guilt and resentment over individual needs not being met (Andrykowski, 1994). Addressing these problems is paramount, because psychiatric sequelae can affect the relationships between the members of the team working with the child and his or her family network, which can have deleterious affects on the BMT recipient (Andrykowski, 1994). The psychiatric consultant can be of great help in assisting the rest of the medical staff in their understanding and management of the patient and family. He or she may also be of great assistance to parents in helping them to manage both their own feelings and the reactions of their children.

Behavioral and affective responses in pediatric BMT recipients may include depression, sleep difficulties, anxiety, apathy, withdrawal, irritability, and regression, as well as organic mental syndromes from neurotoxic CNS irradiation, chemotherapy, and infectious and metabolic effects (Andrykowski, 1994). Often children experience a gradually decreasing tolerance and increasing opposition to procedures, along with increasing fearfulness and separation anxiety, which may all cause havoc for parents (Gardner et al., 1977; McConville et al., 1990). For the child, the need for intravenous hyperalimentation due to decreased oral intake, the denial of symptoms due to the (legitimate) fear of further intervention, and pronounced helplessness and dependency may further complicate the medical aspects of the procedure (McConville et al., 1990).

Mental status assessment may often be complicated by the presence of a dynamic interplay of these factors. BMT recipients are acutely affected by the medical course of other similar patients in the hospital and, in the setting of another patient's death, may undergo a complex series of reactions that include denial and distancing, a heightened fear of death due to identification, and survivor guilt (Patenaude and Rappeport, 1982); psychological intervention is indicated in such circumstances.

Decompensation and death provide unique challenges to all involved in the care of the child and adolescent. Concerns over quality of life and minimizing the suffering of a child compete with the wish to save the child and may present conflicts among staff and family members.

There are also psychological effects on the patient and family, which relate to the source of the marrow and the subsequent success or failure of the graft, which may not be unlike analogous issues in living-related organ donation in kidney or liver transplantation (Wolcott and Stuber, 1992). Death of the BMT recipient presents unique psychological sequelae for a family member who has donated marrow and may feel guilty that somehow his or her marrow was faulty (Freund and Siegel, 1986) or that he or she failed to save the recipient.

In the author's experience, BMT may be more stressful for the transplant team, with guilty feelings perhaps more easily aroused, since the children are necessarily made so visibly sick by this extended procedure. Many solid organ transplant recipients, in contrast, may look significantly better soon following transplantation. Heart transplant recipients, for example, no longer appear cyanotic and may be out of the intensive care unit in several days, soon enjoying relatively greater physical activity in comparison with what may have been a fairly compromised pretransplant state. The physical changes secondary to immunosuppressant medication, so distressing to the adolescent patient, appear later.

Psychopharmacologic and psychotherapeutic intervention in the pediatric cancer population was reviewed by McConville et al. (1990). Medications have included anxiolytics, antidepressants, and low-dose neuroleptics to manage anxiety and depressive symptomatology during both the acute and terminal phases of illness. Psychotherapeutic techniques range from work with the family, to teaching hypnosis and behavioral relaxation exercises to help patients tolerate painful procedures and decrease overall anxiety levels. Especially with respect to the latter, supportive collaboration with other medical staff is an essential aspect of the psychiatrist's role.

Hospital staff can play a significant role in helping the patient and family prepare for discharge realistically and assist the family in concrete planning about resuming activities, helping parents understand the likely reactions of siblings, and helping parents anticipate the effects of changes in marital roles (Freund and Siegel, 1986). Discharge from the hospital is also accompanied by stressors that are associated with the return home and reentry into the social milieu. These issues are similar to those confronted by solid organ transplant recipients, but complicated by the fact that recovery may be slower in the BMT population. Patients are not physically well and often exhibit the continuation of adjustment reactions, with consequent effects on siblings. There is a required preoccupation with cleanliness and minimizing exposure to potential pathogens that represents a constant reminder of the precarious line that is being traversed. These concerns often take on a compulsive quality.

Disruption of the marital relationship is common, due to the enforced separation during hospitalization, the reformulation of roles, and potentially conflicting coping styles, and preexisting difficulties are magnified tremendously (Freund and Siegel, 1986). A sense of "anger and betrayal" may be evoked in the patient and family when the transplant has not provided a cure (Atkins and Patenaude, 1987). This feeling may be exacerbated in the setting of post-BMT complications. Depression and impaired self-esteem may result when expectations meet with disappointment (Freund and Siegel, 1986). Individual psychotherapy, including play therapy with younger children, may facilitate psychological adjustment and the expression of feelings associated with the illness and procedure (Atkins and Patenaude, 1987). "Open communication, maintenance of hope, and the positive use of denial" may predict a more positive outcome, though clinical course may be a powerful predictor of psychopathology (McConville et al., 1990).

Though denial may be adaptive in children and adolescents in helping to maintain self-esteem, caregivers can play a significant role in addressing issues that would not voluntarily be raised and provide guidance as to the timing of education concerning these issues for the child/adolescent and family (Wolcott and Stuber, 1992).

Denial, however, may not necessarily be adaptive. Stuber (1991) noted persistent symptoms of posttraumatic stress in 3- to 7-year-olds for more than 1 year post BMT. Symptomatology appeared most pronounced around the time immediately following discharge from the hospital when anxiety over survival is high. Denial and avoidance were the most prominent PTSD symptom. Stuber theorizes that the more "chronic, nonimminent" nature of a threat that is internal and not external may be more likely to lead to denial and avoidance. This reaction "may seem the only possible response when the traumatic event is perpetrated by adults who are said to be acting in the child's interest, with the permission and assistance of parents." She also suggests that the simple fact of asking children about symptoms may be therapeutic. Intrusive, repetitive preoccupation may be evident only in the child's play. If one does not ask about symptoms or observe the play of these children, necessary treatment may be delayed because of the nature of this phenomenon, where symptoms are less dramatic and more insidious, and early intervention will thus be compromised.

These data should guide future early psychiatric treatment in this patient population and probably others who experience life-threatening illness with high-tech, dramatic, invasive interventions. It also has implications for follow-up care, due to the probability that denial will affect how and when medical help is accessed. The occurrence of late psychological effects of BMT questions the view expressed by some to put "the BMT experience behind them" and suggests a more direct approach to dealing with issues surrounding the illness and its sequelae.

Specific sequelae for pediatric BMT recipients may include learning disabilities, growth retardation, and infertility. Significant motor delays and subtle impairments of performance in perceptual and fine motor tasks have been reported in children between 3 and 11 years of age treated with BMT accompanied by total body irradiation (Smedler et al., 1990). Children in this age group were more significantly subject to these effects than were older children and adolescents, and cranial irradiation may be the significant factor in predisposing to neurocognitive deficits (Kramer et al., 1992). Cognitive deficits seem to be related to the dose of cranial irradiation or intrathecal methotrexate, and such sequelae can have significant effects on the developing child's school performance and self-esteem. Low-dose cranial irradiation may be associated with less cognitive sequelae (Kramer et al., 1992).

Other long-term sequelae include sterility in most patients following BMT, with consequent effects on sexual identity and romantic relationships, as well as self-esteem. Sexual dysfunction is also common, such as problems in vaginal lubrication in women and impotence and/or retarded ejaculation in men (Andrykowski, 1994). Psychological intervention may address these effects and provide appropriate counseling, which may mitigate and help differentiate between effects that are secondary to treatment/illness and social and/or psychological factors such as affective illness (Andrykowski, 1994).

Kidney Transplantation

Adjustment following kidney transplantation seems to be influenced by developmental factors. Preschool children exhibit the most rapid rates of growth increase and improved social functioning, with adolescents experiencing the greatest degree of social and emotional problems. Bernstein (1977) reported risk-taking behavior, school phobia, and depression in 4 adolescents of the 32 renal transplant patients he studied. Korsch (1973) examined outcome in pediatric renal transplant recipients and found that most negative effects on family functioning occurred during the 1st year. A subset of patients (10/35) had maladjustment on personality measures that consisted of problems with anxiety and self-esteem; these patients were at higher risk for noncompliance. Depression was the "most specific test finding." Seventeen of 19 adolescents were working or in college, and 11 of 16 younger patients were in school. Important concerns in this population included steroid-induced side effects and apprehension about rejection.

Several studies have indicated that quality of life improves following

renal transplantation in the pediatric population (Almond et al., 1991; Brownbridge and Fielding, 1991; Cole, 1991; Khan et al., 1971; Poznanski et al., 1978; Reynolds et al., 1991). Denial seems operative as a defense against fears of rejection and may lessen as patients enter their twenties. Disturbances in autonomous functioning associated with enforced dependency on adults may lead to social isolation, impaired self-esteem, and depression. In particular, impaired social functioning in particular may put children at risk and may be exacerbated by prolonged school absence (Khan et al., 1971). The continuation of peer relationships is especially important in adolescents, and specific interventions might focus on the maintenance of "social networks" (Melzer et al., 1989).

There may be a role for preemptive transplantation prior to the progression to end-stage renal disease requiring dialysis to attempt to avoid the metabolic and psychological impact of chronic renal disease (Cole, 1991), and transplantation has been advocated as the preferred treatment in end-stage organ failure (Almond et al., 1991; Brownbridge and Fielding, 1991). Improved physical health following transplantation has been postulated to have a positive effect on psychosocial outcome in the patient and family (Reynolds et al., 1991). Brownbridge and Fielding (1991) found psychosocial adjustment in transplant recipients to be superior to that in hemodialysis or peritoneal dialysis.

However, despite reports of improved physical, emotional, and cognitive functioning, renal transplant recipients continue to experience the problems associated with chronic immunosuppression, impaired growth, anxiety over rejection, and delayed sexual maturation (Reinhart and Kemph, 1988). Cognitive deficits may persist, especially if the onset of disease was at an earlier age, and there was a longer period of time with end-stage organ failure prior to transplantation (Sexson and Rubenow, 1992), as is the case with liver failure (see below). Child psychiatry has been described as having a significant role in addressing these issues and in helping to facilitate adjustment.

Liver Transplantation

The role of the consultation-liaison psychiatrist in liver transplantation cases has been described by Pinard and Minde (1991) and Krener (1987). Psychosocial effects have been discussed by Bradford (1991), who noted that competition for organs, maternal overprotectiveness, and enhanced dependency by the child on parents may impact significantly on the family. Cognitive deficits may persist, although posttransplant life is generally marked by fewer hospitalizations, shorter lengths of stay, and fewer medications.

Windsorova et al. (1991) have studied the emotional adaptation of pediatric liver transplant recipients and found that, as a group, they did not display any more behavioral disturbance, anxiety, depression, or effects on self-concept than did a control group of diabetic children. Compared with normative data, however, the liver transplant recipients showed indications of greater anxiety and depression on projective testing. Multidimensional assessments of psychosocial functioning were deemed more sensitive for identifying such phenomena than was parental or patient report.

Others have assessed quality of life in liver transplant recipients (Chin et al., 1991; Windsorova et al., 1991). In Chin's sample (1991), all but one school-age child had returned to school, with quality of life described as good or excellent in all. However, in 7 of 12 children older than 5 years of age, maladaptive behavior was reported, which may have been related to the degree of hepatic encephalopathy that persisted following transplantation. Zamberlan (1992) identified problems in socialization and peer relations, which were associated with feelings of loneliness and vulnerability, in the 20 school-age liver transplant recipients she studied. Psychiatric intervention, especially during the 1st year following transplantation has been recommended (Sexson and Rubenow, 1992; Zamberlan, 1992).

The most comprehensive data on neuropsychological outcome in pediatric liver transplant recipients have been published by Stewart

(1989, 1991a, 1991b). In one series (1989), 15 of 29 children had delays in cognitive or motor function prior to transplantation, which were associated with earlier onset of liver disease. Following transplantation, 4 of 11 patients with cognitive delays, and 5 of 10 with motor delays had improvements great enough to place them within the normal range at 1-year follow-up. As a group, improvement in cognitive function did not reach significance. Improvement on the Social Scale of the Child Behavior Checklist (Achenbach and Edelbrock, 1983) was found at 1-year follow-up in children who were transplanted at 4 years of age or older. Enhanced functioning was reported with peers, in sports, and in the ability to take on greater home responsibilities. Prednisone exerted robust effects on linear growth, and gains in head circumference were most notable in children younger in chronological age.

Neuropsychological deficits were found in these patients (Stewart et al., 1991a, 1991b), in a variety of parameters including learning and memory, abstraction and concept formation, visual-spatial function, and motor function. When matched against a control group of cystic fibrosis patients (1991b), the liver transplant patients had greater impairments in intellectual/academic function, learning and memory, abstraction and concept formation, visual-spatial function, and motor skills. Significantly more liver transplant recipients were receiving special services in school, though less than a third were receiving the services they needed.

The greater impairment in functioning in the liver transplant patients was postulated to be related to the effects of hepatotoxins on the developing brain, though other factors, such as acute illness requiring invasive surgery, were not controlled for.

Ethical factors involving living-related liver donation, often from a parent to the child, was reviewed by Singer et al. (1989). UNOS Scientific Registry Data indicate that the number of living liver donors has been increasing since 1989, when 2 were reported, to 1993, when 35 such donors were recorded.

Heart Transplantation

Neuropsychological function in cardiac transplantation recipients has been reviewed in the adult population (Nussbaum and Goldstein, 1992), but few studies exist in the pediatric population. In one series of 54 infants with congenital heart disease who were transplanted at 4 months of age or less, 80% of these infants survived the 1st year, and 89% were neurologically normal at 14 months posttransplantation (Trimm, 1991). Normal language functioning was found in the 77% old enough to be assessed, and normal audiologic function was found in 90%. The Bayley Scale of Infant Development was administered sequentially, and when their scores were averaged, all but 2 infants fell within 2 standard deviations of the mean on the Mental Developmental Index, and all but 2 infants fell within 2 standard deviations of the mean on the Psychomotor Developmental Index.

Adolescents with congenital heart disease that was surgically corrected earlier in childhood, like other chronically ill children, may be at higher risk for later behavior and adjustment problems (Utens et al., 1993). Studies examining the psychosocial outcome of pediatric cardiac transplantation are limited, but in a multicenter study, Uzark et al. (1992) reported that these children's level of function approaches that of their peers, with 93% attending school and able to participate in athletics. Nevertheless, this sample of 49 children, who averaged 21 months posttransplant and whose mean age was 10.4 years, showed less social competence and more frequent behavior problems relative to the norm on the Child Behavior Checklist (Achenbach and Edelbrock, 1983). Such problems were associated with impaired self-concept and higher anxiety levels, as well as the inclination not to discuss feelings. The authors hypothesized that depression and behavior problems were related to personality and interpersonal factors, such as the adolescent's not feeling accepted by or communicating well with peers. Families experienced relatively high stress levels without a concomitant increase in resources to assist in coping with the stress. Psychosocial assessments, enhancing

communication between family members, and cognitive work with adolescents were suggested.

Other authors have looked at psychosocial adaptation in this population (Gold et al., 1986; Lawrence and Fricker, 1987; Lawrence et al., 1987; Suszycki, 1988; Uzark and Crowley, 1989) or addressed clinical issues more descriptively (Slater, 1994). Lawrence and Fricker (1987) found that quality of life in 7 children who had received heart transplants was characterized by a return to normalcy. Uzark and Crowley (1989) note that pretransplant stress levels secondary to chronic and sometimes life-threatening illness are superimposed on the transplantation scenario, resulting in powerful effects on family function that relate to doubts about the child's vitality, financial pressure, marital tension, and potential distance from the social milieu. Multidisciplinary intervention from social work, nursing, and mental health workers can be of enormous help.

Heart-Lung and Lung Transplantation

Warner (1991) published data from a series of pediatric patients in end-stage respiratory failure referred for heart-lung transplantation and found that two-thirds died at some point during the referral, evaluation, or surgery process. He underscored the necessity for careful screening of these patients to avoid putting them through additional trauma that would be associated only with a poor outcome, though for some children heart-lung transplantation represents a desperate but viable final option. Five children of 10 transplanted had returned to school and other age-appropriate activities.

Research on psychosocial or neuropsychiatric outcome in lung or double-lung transplantation is quite sparse. In one series, four of the seven pediatric patients who underwent heart-lung or lung transplantation are currently alive, with all school-age children back at school and doing well emotionally (Quitell, personal communication, 1993). Indications for transplantation included decompensation in the context of pseudotruncus type 6, pulmonary hypertension, pulmonary fibrosis, and pulmonary atresia.

CASE ILLUSTRATION

One of the children who received a single lung transplant at 16 months of age is currently approximately 1½ years post surgery. He was reportedly delayed neurodevelopmentally prior to transplantation, but has made significant gains since his surgery. Following his birth, he had spent only 2 months at home before being admitted to the hospital, where he spent the next 14 months until he was transferred to another medical center and transplanted.

At that time, the medical staff was concerned about the lack of time that his parents spent with him. It almost seemed as if they had "dropped him off" to have a transplant, and there were large stretches of time that the baby was alone in his hospital room, unlike many of the other children whose parents literally hover by the child's bedside and never leave. The staff became concerned about whether this constituted neglect, but following transplantation, it became apparent that the parents had been completely misjudged, as they became model parents, "never skipping a beat" according to their pediatrician.

In retrospect, upon further evaluation, it became apparent that these parents had never had the opportunity to bond with their child, since he had been admitted to the hospital in an extremely compromised state so soon after birth. His mother had been completely overwhelmed and had never had the opportunity to "feel like a mother." With the multitude of nurses who were necessarily caring for her baby, she felt without a role. A follow-up conversation with this family was reflective of a beaming father, proud and loving toward his son who was reported as "just like any other three-year old" except for some speech and language problems (From Slater JA: Psychiatric aspects of transplantation in children and adolescents. *Child Adolesc Psychiatr Clin North Am* 3(3):557–598, 1994, with permission.)

Comment

This case illustrates the importance of consideration of impaired maternal-/paternal-infant bonding in the case of some severely impaired infant transplant candidates, and the need to both help the parents develop some role in their care, and to use this knowledge in assessing the relationship between caregivers and their baby.

In summary, available neuropsychiatric and psychosocial follow-up studies in this population indicate that the quality of life is generally improved following transplantation; many of these children, in fact, would not be alive without transplantation. Following surgery, many have increased levels of physical activity and school attendance, and cognitive function may be improved in some. Nevertheless, many have persistent cognitive deficits due to the effects of chronic illness and circulating neurotoxins during brain development. Transplantation is another stressor superimposed on a stressed family system, with sequelae for siblings and marital relationships. For the transplant recipient, studies suggest that they are at risk for depression, behavioral problems, and impaired self-esteem, which probably relates to the social problems for which these patients are also at risk. Anxiety symptomatology, including school refusal and posttraumatic symptomatology, may also be more common in this population. For these reasons, neuropsychological testing and early psychiatric evaluation and intervention are recommended.

PSYCHOPHARMACOLOGICAL ASPECTS OF TRANSPLANTATION

Neuropsychiatric side effects of immunosuppressant and antiinfectious agents used in transplantation and aspects of psychopharmacological intervention in this population were reviewed by Trzepacz (1993a, 1993b, and see Tables 95.10 and 95.11). Important considerations of drug use in this population include altered pharmacokinetics due to drug interactions and impaired hepatic, renal, or cardiac function. Children have both altered pharmacodynamics, due to developmental factors in neural pathways and neurotransmitter systems, and altered pharmacoki-

netics due to differences in distribution, absorption, and metabolic rates (Teicher and Baldessarini, 1987).

Hepatic metabolic rate is relatively high in infancy compared with that in adults, decreases around the time of puberty, and reaches adult levels during adolescence; in infancy, kidney function approximates adult levels (Jatlow, 1987). Neuroleptic drugs and tricyclics are generally metabolized more rapidly in children, though dosing must be considered in the context of dose-response curves, which show that children may respond to lower serum levels of neuroleptics and tricyclics (Jatlow, 1987). Diazepam seems to be more rapidly metabolized in children, but this may not be true of some other benzodiazepines, in which case hepatic transformation is not a predominant mode of metabolism. Higher glomerular filtration rates in childhood compared with those in adults may be responsible for the need for higher lithium dosing (mg/kg) in children. Children also metabolize antiepileptic drugs more rapidly than do adults, resulting in increased dosing requirements. Though no published data exist for psychopharmacologic intervention for child or adolescent transplant recipients, stimulants, tricyclics, and selective serotonin reuptake inhibitors (SSRIs) have all been used anecdotally.

ETHICAL ISSUES IN TRANSPLANTATION

Significant ethical dilemmas exist in every aspect of the transplantation process, from informed consent, recipient selection, and organ procurement and allocation, to issues involved in extended medical care (Lewis, 1974, 1993; Lowy and Martin, 1992; Moskop, 1989; Sexson and Rubenow, 1992). A relative shortage of donor organs in comparison to need, and the relative high cost of transplantation, which can run into the hundreds of thousand of dollars, means that many patients who need transplants cannot get them. Significant controversy has surrounded the establishment of criteria to make such decisions (Lowy and Martin, 1992). Using psychosocial factors to help decide who shall receive organs has been controversial, especially in children and adolescents.

Measures directed at increasing the donor pool, issues surrounding informed consent in nonrelated donors, and the use of artificial devices, anencephalic infants, or xenografts (nonhuman donors) are also relevant issues (Lowy and Martin, 1992; Sexson and Rubenow, 1992). Some areas have enacted legislation requiring that families be asked to donate organs of a deceased relative, which has ethical implications in terms of the emotional effects of such a request and the deliberation that must follow, including what the deceased would have "wanted."

Controversy has surrounded the management of the wait list itself, as Moskop (1989) notes, such as whether adolescents should receive priority over adults. In addition, patients with certain blood types, such as "O," and adult males, tend to wait longer for organs (UNOS Scientific Registry Data). There may be an underutilization of parents who would potentially donate organs of a child (Morris et al., 1992).

The concept of "beneficence" implies that physicians must act in the best interests of the patient, though application of this concept becomes complicated by the medical and psychological sequelae of the intervention itself, such as in the case of transplantation (Moskop, 1989; Sexson and Rubenow, 1992). Consideration of whether transplantation is in the best interests of an adolescent who is expected to be noncompliant is further clouded.

Informed consent involves a three-step process that includes mental competency, understanding, and freedom from coercion (Moskop, 1989). An explanation of expected medical, psychosocial, and neuropsychiatric outcome is an essential part of this process. Lewis (1974) points out that true informed consent is often a "myth." With respect to parents, the ability to make decisions about the welfare of their child in the context of serious medical illness or impending death is seriously affected by information overload, the overwhelming pressure to save the child, and an implicit or explicit recommendation by the physician.

The concept of autonomy has been interpreted to allow "mature minor" or "emancipated minor" statutes, such that adolescents as young as 14 or 15 years of age have the right to consent to or refuse

Table 95.10. Possible Central Nervous System Side Effects of Immunosuppressants and Antiinfectious Agents

	Potential Neuropsychiatric Side Effects
Immunosuppressants	
Cyclosporine	Tremor, anxiety, delirium, ataxia, seizures, visual hallucinations, disorientation
	Less common: cerebral blindness, paresthesias, dysarthria, paresis
Corticosteroids	Depression, delirium, mania
Azathioprine	None
OKT3	Tremor, aseptic meningitis, seizures, delirium, ?encephalopathy
FK 506	Headache, anxiety, tremor, restlessness, insomnia, paresthesias, vivid dreams, nightmares, delirium (esp. with levels > 3 ng/ml)
Antiinfective agents	
Antivirals	
Acyclovir	Tremor, confusion, lethargy, major depression with psychotic features, seizures, agitation, confusion, abnormal EEG patterns
DHPG	Headache, confusion, seizures, and hallucinations
Alpha Interferon	Irritability, depression, anxiety, delirium
Antibiotics	
Ciprofloxacin	Restlessness, dizziness, tremor, headache, insomnia, hallucinations, delirium
Cephalosporins	Disorientation, restlessness, anxiety, hallucinations
Sulfonamides	Depression, ataxia, visual and auditory hallucinations
Antifungals	
Amphotericin B	Restlessness, confusion, delirium
Metronidazole	Depression, hallucinations, agitation

Adapted from Trzepacz PT, DiMartini A, Tringali R: Psychopharmacological issues in organ transplantation. Part I: Pharmacokinetics in organ failure and psychiatric aspects of immunosuppressants and anti-infectious agents. *Psychosomatics* 34(3):199–207, with permission. From Slater JA: Psychiatric aspects of transplantation in children and adolescents. *Child Adolesc Clin North Am* 3(3):557–598, 1994, with permission.

Table 95.11.   Aspects of Psychopharmacologic Treatment in Transplant Recipients

Psychopharmacologic Agent	Metabolism/Elimination	Increases Levels of Psychopharmacologic	Potential Side Effects/Comments
Antidepressants			
Tricyclics	Hepatic Metabolites renally excreted	Hepatic failure Renal failure Acidemia Hypoalbuminemia Fluoxetine increases tricyclic levels	Orthostatic hypotension Type IA antiarrhythmics May increase digoxin levels Dry mouth, constipation Blurred vision, mydriasis Urinary retention Sinus tachycardia
Fluoxetine Norfluoxetine	Hepatic	Hepatic failure	Nausea, insomnia Nervousness, headache Fluoxetine $T_{1/2}$ = 4 days Norfluoxetine $T_{1/2}$ = 7 days Can cause elevated plasma levels of cyclosporine, some benzodiazepines, some antiarrhythmics, β blockers, lithium, neuroleptics, and some anticonvulsants
Trazodone	Excreted mainly in urine		Orthostasis Ventricular ectopy (rare) Useful in low doses for sleep
Sertraline	Hepatic		Favorable side effect profile Less potent P-450 inhibitor than fluoxetine w/shorter $T_{1/2}$ (26 hours)
MAOIs	?Hepatic	?Hepatic failure	Should not be used in transplant recipients
Psychostimulants	Hepatic metabolism. Pemoline and d-amphetamine are also partially excreted unchanged in urine	Hepatic failure Renal insufficiency	May be useful in treating depression in medically ill Useful in ADHD in pediatric transplant recipients
Buproprion	Hepatic metabolism Renal elimination	Hepatic failure Renal insufficiency	Low incidence of cardiac arrhythmias
Lithium	Renal elimination	Cyclosporine ?Methylprednisolone Renal failure	Hepatic disease will not affect levels, though fluctuating renal function, electrolyte changes, and fluid status can. Can be used in cardiac disease
Neuroleptics	Hepatic metabolism Renal elimination	Hepatic failure Renal insufficiency	Useful for acute sedation and in steroid-induced mania Haldol is neuroleptic of choice in transplant patients
Anxiolytics			
Benzodiazepines	Hepatic	Hepatic failure Renal insufficiency in some	Respiratory depression Cognitive dysfunction Sedation, esp. in cirrhosis and can precipitate hepatic encephalopathy
Oxazepam Lorazepam Temazopam	Oxazepam and lorazepam are glucuronidated in the liver, which is less affected by liver disease		Short $T_{1/2}$ No active metabolites Not as affected by cirrhosis as long $T_{1/2}$ benzodiazepines
Alprazolam	Hepatic metabolism Renal elimination	Hepatic failure Renal insufficiency	Rapid tapering can precipitate withdrawal reactions with restlessness, agitation, irritability, insomnia, seizures, delirium
Buspirone	Liver	Liver disease	No tolerance, respiratory depression, sedation, or cognitive deficits

Adapted from Trzepacz PT, DiMartini A, Tringali R: Psychopharmacological issues in organ transplantation. Part II: Psychopharmacologic medications. *Psychosomatics* 34(4):290-298, with permission. From Slater JA: Psychiatric aspects of transplantation in children and adolescents. *Child Adolesc Clin North Am* 3(3):557-598, 1994, with permission.

treatment. Nevertheless, developmental issues such as the relative emphasis on physical factors in adolescence may cause a disparity in what is considered in one's best interest in adolescence compared with that in adulthood and complicate the consideration of cosmetic side effects as a reason for refusing treatment. In addition, parents generally play a vital role in supporting their adolescents and have rights to help determine what is in their adolescent's best interest (Moskop, 1989).

Cognitive factors obviously play a powerful role with respect to informed consent earlier in childhood. However, as children mature, an "absence of dissent" can be determined, and the level of "assent," or "emotional consent," the nature of the child's emotional response to what is being asked, can be ascertained (Slater, 1994).

Ethical issues surround solid organ or bone marrow donation from a multitude of angles. Psychologically, all transplant recipients have reactions to the donation process, and specific feelings about the donor have been studied in the adult population (Bunzel et al., 1992). From the point of view of the recipient, feelings include guilt, a sense of responsibility, and identification with the donor family.

The wish for contact between donor and recipient is a phenomenon that occurs in both directions. Psychologically, the donor-recipient connection is imbued with tremendous meaning. One adolescent organ recipient felt that "they (the donor's family) are my family inside. I have their blood running through my veins" (Slater, 1994).

The parent of a child who had received a cardiac transplant reflected: "It's really impossible to put into words the way you feel about what they went through. I mean it's a true, deep empathy, except you know you didn't quite cross that line. And you're grateful you didn't, but you feel badly enough getting as close to that line as you did. I can't imagine what it would be like to lose a child, or maybe the problem is that I can, and that's what's so frightening, and that's what's so hard." (From Slater JA: Psychiatric aspects of transplantation in children and adolescents. *Child Adolesc Psychiatr Clin North Am* 3(3):557-598, 1994, with permission.)

While the right to privacy is protected, anonymous contact is possible under certain circumstances. Sympathy cards, thank you notes, and photographs have been sent. Many donor families simply desire the knowledge that the recipient is doing well, and often the recipient has curiosity about from where the organ came. Nevertheless, the two parties may not share the same wishes for giving or receiving information. For the donor's family, it may be too painful to be exposed to the child that has lived while theirs has died. For the recipient, it might be too difficult to have contact with the family who donated their child's organs to allow him to live and is mourning their own child's death.

As Rothman (1992) notes, one stands in awe of donor families, who in the midst of such tragedy and traumatic loss are able to think of the welfare of another child and family. A mother who donated the organs of her deceased son recounted her feelings:

"At first there was a little apprehension, but the apprehension is more than compensated with compassion, and that any of your fears that you do have, which are right to feel, would really be smoothed over tremendously by making your child available in a sense to being a donor; and that it is such a wonderful gift. There is no greater gift of giving life to someone else. And its rewards are not just—in a sense, they will never be monetary—but it's more precious than gold. And it's the wisdom to be able to . . . you're not really giving up anything. That's what love really is about, it's being able to give." (From Slater JA: Psychiatric aspects of transplantation in children and adolescents. In: Lewis M (ed): *Child Adolesc Psychiatr Clin North Am* 3(3):557–598, 1994, with permission.)

With respect to living-related organ or bone marrow donation, can the decision to donate ever be "voluntary" (Lewis, 1974; Lowy, 1992; Singer et al., 1989)? What about situations where two children in the same family require donor kidneys but only one parent is immunologically compatible? Other considerations include the morbidity and risk associated with making the donation, and the effect on family relationships for both the sibling who donates and the siblings who do not (Lewis, 1974; Sexson and Rubenow, 1992). The feelings surrounding the death of a child reached dramatic proportions when a parent once pleaded with me to allow her to donate her own heart to her dying daughter.

Lewis (1974) wrote extensively on the case of an identical twin confronting the decision to donate a kidney to her sister, where it appeared that overt refusal was an impossibility. In this situation, the child psychiatrist had to consider the impact of this decision on the relationship between the sisters, the donor's current state and later development, and the emotional state of the family. All of this was felt difficult to predict (Lewis, 1974):

"She might have a nagging sense of loss, emptiness, and resentment at losing her kidney; but she might feel a greater sense of loss if she were to lose her sister. She might develop a fantasy of being anatomically united with her sister; on the other hand, she might experience a precipitous increase in individuation if her sister were to become more and more different and eventually die. She might feel a sense of increased self-esteem from giving her kidney, and might feel guilty later if she had not given her kidney."

Both girls initially did well, though the donor developed persistent somatic anxiety, and somatization symptomatology developed in other family members as well. When Lewis (1993) reported anecdotally on follow-up 14 years later, the twins had drifted apart both geographically and emotionally. The donor twin continued to have a fantasy that since she and her sister were twins, each having one functioning kidney, that the donor symbolically still had two kidneys.

Bereavement work is an inevitable consequence for the child and adolescent consultation-liaison psychiatrist in this setting and represents perhaps the most difficult task one could face. Feelings of tremendous loss, sadness, and impotence are often engendered in the psychiatrist, who nevertheless can play an enormously supportive role simply by his presence. One family later thanked the child psychiatrist for being at the bedside so their child did not die alone. Involvement with these families is different from the typical work in child psychiatry. I have personally attended funerals and received cards from such families years later.

Lastly, consideration given to transplanting a child while he or she is still relatively stable and not in dire need of the organ has ethical implications as well. Transplanting a child earlier in the course of what appears to be a disease that will result in end-stage organ failure may also decrease persistent cognitive deficits presumably caused by circulating neurotoxins, by shortening the time that the child is exposed to them. It will also lessen the chances that the child will die waiting for an organ.

CONCLUDING COMMENT

Transplantation inexorably alters life for the patient and family who endure it. A change in perspective or philosophy inevitably accompany adjustment to posttransplant life. Many adolescents describe a change in priorities, such that they are not as troubled by trivial matters and are better able to appreciate life. At the same time, however, these patients and their families often live life day-by-day, with an omnipresent uncertainty lurking in the background. As one adolescent described, "I was worried about what to wear, and now, you know, I'm worried about whether I'm going to live" (Slater, 1994).

The role of the child and adolescent psychiatrist in this drama may be as deep as he or she is willing to allow. There exists the opportunity for much collaboration with physician colleagues and a flexibility of roles in the physician-patient relationship that may be unique to this type of work, in which the psychiatrist can truly function as a member of a "family" composed of the transplant team, patient, and patient's family. Being around this "family" can be awe-inspiring at times and quite painful at others. In a sense, it is a privilege to be involved with these children and adolescents. More systematic research is obviously needed to help identify risk factors for noncompliance and other secondary psychiatric morbidity, to develop a clearer understanding of psychosocial and neuropsychiatric sequelae, and to help formulate intervention strategies.

"There is a strange heroism and poignancy to their stories, some sense that a miracle has taken place, but also the lament of two childhood's lost in the act of one being saved. Perhaps this is the ultimate paradox of organ transplantation in children" (Slater, 1994).

References

Abramowicz M (ed): Bone marrow transplants for malignant diseases. *Med Lett* 34(877): August 21, 1992.

Abu-Saad H: Assessing children's responses to pain. *Pain* 19:163–171, 1984.

Achenbach TM, Edelbrock C: *Manual for the Child Behavior Checklist and Revised Child Behavior Profile*. Burlington, University of Vermont, 1983.

Addonizio LJ: Cardiac transplantation in the pediatric patient. *Prog Cardiovasc Dis* 23(1):19–34, 1990.

Addonizio LJ: In: Second Chance: Heroes of Heart Transplantation in Children (documentary film). Slater JS (writer/producer). New York, Steve Shane Productions, 1992.

Addonizio LJ, Hsu DT, Smith CR, et al: Late complications in pediatric cardiac transplantation recipients. *Circulation* (suppl IV) 82(5):295–301, 1990.

Almond PS, Morell PH, Matas AJ, et al: Trans-planted children with long-term graft function have an excellent quality of life. *Transplant Proc* 23(1): 1380–1381, 1991.

Andrykowski MA: Psychiatric and psychosocial aspects of bone marrow transplantation. *Psychosomatics* 35(1):13–24, 1994.

Atkins DM, Patenaude AF: Psychosocial preparation and follow-up for pediatric bone marrow transplant patients. *Am J Orthopsychiatry* 57(2):246–252, 1987.

Bauman S: Physical aspects of the self. A review of some aspects of body image development in childhood. *Psychiatr Clin North Am* 4:455–470, 1981.

Beck DE, Fennell RS, Yost RI, et al: Evaluation of an educational program on compliance with medication regimens in pediatric patients with renal transplants. *J Pediatr* 96:1094, 1980.

Bernstein DM: After transplantation—The child's emotional reaction. *Am J Psychiatry* 127:9, 1971.

Bernstein DM: Psychiatric assessment of the adjustment of transplanted children. In: Simmons R, Klein S, Simmons R (eds): *Gift of Life: The Social and Psychological Impact of Organ Transplantation*. New York, Wiley, 1977, pp. 199–247.

Bibace R, Walsh M: Development of children's concepts of illness. *Pediatrics* 66:912–917, 1980.

Blohme I, Gabel H, Brynger H: The living donor in renal transplantation. *Scand J Urol Nephrol* 64(suppl):143–151, 1981.

Blos P: *On Adolescence: A Psychoanalytic Interpretation*. New York, The Free Press of Glencoe, 1962.

Bradford R: Psychological guidelines in the management of paediatric organ transplantation. *Arch Dis Child* 65:1000–1003, 1990.

Bradford R: Children's psychological health status—The impact of liver transplantation: A review. *J R Soc Med* 84:549–553, 1991.

Brownbridge G, Fielding DM: Psychosocial adjustment to end-stage renal failure: Comparing hemodialysis, continuous ambulatory peritoneal dialysis and transplantation. *Pediatr Nephrol* 5: 612–616, 1991.

Bullock E, Shaddy R: Relaxation and imagery techniques without sedation during right ventricular endomyocardial biopsy in pediatric heart transplant patients. *J Heart Lung Transplant* 12:59–62, 1993.

Bunzel B, Wollenek G, Grundbock A: Living with a donor heart: Feelings and attitudes of patients toward the donor and the donor organ. *J Heart Lung Transplant* 11(6):1151–1155, 1992.

Bush JP: Pain in children: A review of the literature from a developmental perspective. *Psychol Health* 1:215–230, 1987.

Cardona L: Behavioral approaches to pain and anxiety in the pediatric patient. *Child Adolesc Psychiatr Clin North Am* 3(3):446–465, 1994.

Chadwick O, Rutter M, Thompson J, et al: Intellectual performance and reading skills after localized head injury in childhood. *J Child Psychol Psychiatry* 22:117–137, 1981.

Chin S, Shepherd RW, Cleghorn GJ, et al: Survival, growth and quality of life in children after orthotopic liver transplantation: A 5 year experience. *J Paediatr Child Health* 27:380–385, 1991.

Cole BR: The psychosocial implications of preemptive transplantation. *Pediatr Nephrol* 5: 158–161, 1991.

Cromer BA, Tarnowski KJ: Noncompliance in adolescents: A review. *Dev Behav Pediatr* 10(4): 207–215, 1989.

DeLone P, Trollinger JH, Fox N, et al: Noncompliance in renal transplant recipients: Methods for recognition and intervention. *Transplant Proc* 21(6): 3982–3984, 1989.

Dermatis H, Lesko LM: Psychological distress in parents consenting to child's bone marrow transplantation. *Bone Marrow Transplant* 6:411–417, 1990.

Dixon D: Religious and spiritual perspectives on organ transplantation. In: Craven J, Rodin GM (eds): *Psychiatric Aspects of Organ Transplantation*. Oxford, Oxford University Press, 1992, pp. 131–144.

Douglas J, Hsu D, Addonizio L: Late rejection as a major indicator of noncompliance in pediatric heart transplant patients. Abstract presented at the Annual Meeting of the American Heart Association, Dallas, 1993.

Dunn J, Golden D, Van Buren CT, et al: Causes of graft loss beyond two years in the cyclosporine ear. *Transplantation* 49(2):349–353, 1990.

Emde R: The infant's relationship experience: Developmental and affective aspects. In: Sameroff AH, Emde RN (eds): *Relationship Disturbances in Early Childhood: A Developmental Approach*. New York, Basic Books, 1989, pp. 33–51.

Ettinger RB, Rosenthal JT, Marik JL, et al: Improved cadaveric renal transplant outcome in children. *Pediatr Nephrol* 5:137–142, 1991.

Festa RS, Tamaroff MH, Chasalow F, et al: Therapeutic adherence to oral medication regimens by adolescents with cancer. I: Laboratory assessment. *J Pediatr* 120(5):807–811, 1991.

Foulkes L, Boggs SR, Fennell RS, et al: Social support, family variables, and compliance in renal transplant children. *Pediatr Nephrol* 7:185–193, 1993.

Freeman A, Davis L, Libb JW, et al: Assessment of transplant candidates and prediction of outcome. In: Craven J, Rodin GM (eds): *Psychiatric Aspects of Organ Transplantation*. Oxford, Oxford University Press, 1992, pp. 9–21.

Freud A: The role of bodily illness in the mental life of the child. In: Eissler RS, et al (eds): *The Psychoanalytic Study of the Child*. New York, International Universities Press, 1952, pp. 69–81.

Freund BL, Siegel K: Problems in transition following bone marrow transplantation: Psychosocial aspects. *Am J Orthopsychiatry* 56(2):244–252, 1986.

Gardner GG, August CS, Githens J: Psychological issues in bone marrow transplantation. *Pediatrics* 60:4(Part 2):625–631, 1977.

Gold LM, Kirkpatrick BS, Fricker FJ, et al: Psychosocial issues in pediatric organ transplantation: The parents' perspective. *Pediatrics* 77:738–749, 1986.

Green W: Psychopharmacologic treatment of pain and anxiety in the pediatric patient. *Child Adolesc Psychiatr Clin North Am* 3(3):465–483, 1994.

Grimm P, Ettenger R: Pediatric renal transplantation. *Adv Pediatr* 39:441–493, 1992.

Hesse UJ, Roth B, Knuppertz G, et al: Control of patient compliance in outpatient steroid treatment of nephrologic disease and renal transplant recipients. *Transplant Proc* 22(4):1405–1406, 1990.

House RM, Thompson TL: Psychiatric aspects of organ transplantation. *JAMA* 260:535–539, 1988.

Jatlow PI: Psychotropic drug disposition during development. In: Popper C (ed): *Psychiatric Pharmacosciences of Children and Adolescents*. Washington, DC, American Psychiatric Press, 1987, pp. 27–44.

Khan A, Herndon C, Ahmadian S: Social and emotional adaptations of children with transplanted kidneys and chronic hemodialysis. *Am J Psychiatry* 127:1194–1198, 1971.

Kiley DJ, Lam CS, Pollak R: A study of treatment compliance following kidney transplantation. *Transplantation* 55(1):51–56, 1993.

Koocher GP, O'Malley JE: *The Damocles Syndrome*. New York, McGraw-Hill, 1981.

Korsch BM, Fine RN, Negrete VF: Noncompliance in children with renal transplants. *Pediatrics* 61: 872–876, 1978.

Korsch BM, Gardner JE, Fine RN, et al: Kidney transplantation in children: Psychosocial follow-up study on child and family. *J Pediatr* 83:399–408, 1973.

Kramer JH, Crittendon MR, Halberg FE, et al: A prospective study of cognitive functioning following low-dose radiation for bone marrow transplantation. *Pediatrics* 90:447–450, 1992.

Krener P: Psychiatric liaison to liver transplant recipients. *Clin Pediatr* 26:93–97, 1987.

Kuttner L, Bowman M, Teasdale M: Psychological treatment of distress, pain, and anxiety for young children with cancer. *Dev Behav Pediatr* 9:374–381, 1988.

Lawrence KS, Fricker FJ: Pediatric heart transplantation: Quality of life. *J Heart Lung Transplant* 6:329–333, 1987.

Levenson J, Olbrisch M: Psychosocial evaluation of organ transplant candidates. *Psychosomatics* 34(4):314–323, 1993.

Lewis K: Kidney donation by a 7-year-old identical twin child: Psychological, legal, and ethical considerations. *J Am Acad Child Psychiatry* 13: 221–245, 1974.

Lewis M: Letter to the editor. *J Am Acad Child Adolesc Psychiatry* 32:876, 1993.

LoBiondo-Wood G, Bernier-Henn M, Williams L: Impact of the child's liver transplant on the family: Maternal perspective. *Pediatr Nurs* 18(5):461–466, 1992.

Lowy F, Martin D: Ethical considerations in transplantation. In: Craven J, Rodin GM (eds): *Psychiatric Aspects of Organ Transplantation*. Oxford, Oxford University Press, 1992, pp. 108–120.

Manne S, Jacobsen P, Redd WH, et al: Correlates of self-reported pain during venipuncture in pediatric oncology outpatients. Paper presented at the Ninth Annual Meeting of the Society of Behavioral Medicine, Boston, April 1988.

Manne SL, Redd WH, Jacobsen PB, et al: Behavioral intervention to reduce child and parent distress during venipuncture. *J Consult Clin Psychol* 58: 565–571, 1990.

McConville BJ, Steichen-Asch P, Harris R, et al: Pediatric bone marrow transplants: Psychological aspects. *Can J Psychiatry* 35:769–775, 1990.

McGrath PA, Hillier LM: The enigma of pain in children: An overview. *Pediatrician* 16:6–15, 1989.

Melzer SM, Leadbeater B, Reisman L, et al: Characteristics of social networks in adolescents with end-stage renal disease treated with renal transplantation. *J Adolesc Health Care* 10:308–312, 1989.

Meuwissen H, Gatti R, Terasaki P, et al: Treatment of lymphopenic hypogammaglobulinemia and bone marrow aplasia by transplantation of allogeneic marrow. *N Engl J Med* 2811:691–696, 1969.

Moran G, Fonagy P, Kurtz A, et al: A controlled study of the psychoanalytic treatment of brittle diabetes. *J Am Acad Child Adolesc Psychiatry* 30(6): 926–935, 1991.

Morris J, Wilcox T, Frist W: Pediatric organ donation: The paradox of organ shortage despite the remarkable willingness of families to donate. *Pediatrics* 89(3):411–425, 1992.

Moskop JC: Organ transplantation in adolescence: Moral issues. *Pediatr Ann* 18(4):246–253, 1989.

Mrazek DA: Effects of hospitalization on early child development. In: Emde RN, Harmon RJ (eds): *Continuities and Discontinuities in Development*. New York, Plenum, 1984, pp. 211–225.

Nagera H: Children's reaction to hospitalization and illness. *Child Psychiatry Hum Dev* 9:3–19, 1978.

Nussbaum PD, Goldstein G: Neuropsychological sequelae of heart transplantation: A preliminary review. *Clin Psychol Rev* 12:475–483, 1992.

Offer D, Boxer AM: Normal adolescent development: Empirical research findings. In: Lewis M (ed): *Child and Adolescent Psychiatry: A Comprehensive Textbook*. Baltimore, Williams & Wilkins, 1991, pp. 266–278.

Olson AD, Hohansen SG, Powers LE, et al: Cognitive coping strategies of children with chronic illness. *Dev Behav Pediatr* 14:4, 1993.

Parkman R: Current status of bone marrow transplantation in pediatric oncology. *Cancer* 58: 569–572, 1986.

Parmelee AH: The child's physical health and the development of relationships. In: Sameroff AH, Emde RN (eds): *Relationship Disturbances in Early Childhood: A Developmental Approach*. New York, Basic Books, 1989, pp. 145–161.

Patenaude AF, Rappeport JM: Surviving bone marrow transplantation: The patient in the other bed. *Ann Intern Med* 97:915–918, 1982.

Patenaude AF, Szymanski L, Rappeport J: Psychological costs of bone marrow transplantation. *Am J Orthopsychiatry* 49:409–422, 1979.

Pfefferbaum B, Lindamood M, Wiley F: Pediatric bone marrow transplantation: Psychosocial aspects. *Am J Psychiatry* 134:1299–1301, 1977.

Pfefferbaum B, Lindamood M, Wiley F: Stages in pediatric bone marrow transplantation. *Pediatrics* 61:625–628, 1978.

Phipps S, DeCuir-Whalley S: Adherence issues in pediatric bone marrow transplantation. *J Pediatr Psychol* 15:459–476, 1990.

Pinard L, Minde K: The infant psychiatrist and the transplant team. *Can J Psychiatry* 36(6): 442–446, 1991.

Pot-Mees CC: Psychosocial consequences of bone marrow transplantation in children: A preliminary communication. *J Psychosoc Oncol* 5:73–81, 1987.

Poznanski EO, Miller E, Salguero C, et al: Quality of life for long-term survivors of end-stage renal disease. *JAMA* 239:2343–2347, 1978.

Quinton D, Rutter M: Early hospital admissions and later disturbances of behavior: An attempted replication of Douglas' findings. *Dev Med Child Neurol* 18:447–459, 1976.

Rasbury WC, Fennell RS, Morris MK: Cognitive functioning of children with end-stage renal disease before and after successful transplantation. *J Pediatr* 102(4):589–592, 1983.

Reinhart JB, Kemph JP: Renal transplantation for children: Another view. *JAMA* 260(22):3327–3328, 1988.

Reynolds JM, Garralda ME, Postlethwaite DG: Changes in psychosocial adjustment after renal transplantation. *Arch Dis Child* 66:508–513, 1991.

Rothman D: In: Second Chance: Heroes of Heart Transplantation in Children (documentary film). Slater JS (writer/producer). New York, Steve Shane Productions, 1992.

Rovelli M, Palmeri D, Vossler E, et al: Noncompliance in organ transplant recipients. *Transplant Proc* 21(1):833–834, 1989a.

Rovelli M, Palmeri D, Vossler E, et al: Noncompliance in renal transplant recipients: Evaluation by socioeconomic groups. *Transplant Proc* 21(6): 3979–3981, 1989b.

Schonfeld DJ: The child's cognitive understanding of illness. In: Lewis M (ed): *Child and Adolescent Psychiatry: A Comprehensive Textbook*. Baltimore, Williams & Wilkins, 1991.

Schowalter JE: Psychological reactions to physical illness and hospitalization in adolescence. *J Am Acad Child Psychiatry* 10:684–699, 1971.

Schweizer RT: Noncompliance in organ transplant recipients. *Transplantation* 49:374–377, 1990.

Sexson S, Rubenow J: Transplants in children and adolescents. In: Craven J, Rodin GM (eds): *Psychiatric Aspects of Organ Transplantation*. Oxford, Oxford University Press, 1992, pp. 33–49.

Shapiro PA, Williams DL, Foray AT, et al: Psychosocial variables and outcome of heart transplantation. *Transplantation*, in press.

Siegel LJ, Smith KE: Children's strategies for coping with pain. *Pediatrician* 16:110–118, 1989.

Singer PA, Siegler M, Whitington PF, et al: Ethics of liver transplantation with living donors. *N Engl J Med* 321:620–622, 1989.

Slater JA: In: Second Chance: Heroes of Heart Transplantation in Children (documentary film). Slater JS (writer/producer). New York, Steve Shane Productions, 1992.

Slater JA: Psychiatric aspects of transplantation in children and adolescents. *Child Adolesc Psychiatry Clin North Am* 3(3):557–598, 1994.

Slater JA: Child development. In: Cutler J, Marcus E (eds): *Essentials of Psychiatry*. Philadelphia, Saunders, 1996, in press.

Smedler AC, Ringden K, Bergmen H, et al: Sensory-motor and cognitive functioning in children who have undergone bone marrow transplantation. *Acta Paediatr Scand* 79:613–621, 1990.

Stewart S, Campbell RA, McCallon D, et al: Cognitive patterns in school-age children with end-stage liver disease. *Dev Behav Pediatr* 13(5):331–338, 1992.

Stewart SM, Hiltebeitel C, Nici J, et al: Neuropsychological outcome of pediatric liver transplantation. *Pediatrics* 87:367–376, 1991a.

Stewart SM, Silver CH, Nici J, et al: Neuropsychological function in young children who have undergone liver transplantation. *J Pediatr Psychol* 16(5):569–583, 1991b.

Stewart SM, Uauy R, Waller D, et al: Mental and motor development, social competence, and growth one year after successful pediatric liver transplantation. *J Pediatr* 114:4, Part 1, 1989.

Stuber ML: Psychiatric aspects of organ transplantation in children. *Psychosomatics* 34:379–387, 1993a.

Stuber ML: Psychological care of adolescents undergoing transplantation. In: McNarney ER, Kreipe RE, Orr DP, et al: *Textbook of Adolescent Medicine*. Philadelphia, Saunders, 1993b.

Stuber ML, Nader K, Yasuda P, et al: Stress responses after pediatric bone marrow transplantation: Preliminary results of a prospective longitudinal study. *J Am Acad Child Adolesc Psychiatry* 30: 952–957, 1991.

Surman OS: Psychiatric aspects of organ transplantation. *Am J Psychiatry* 146:972–982, 1989.

Suszycki LH: Psychosocial aspects of heart transplantation. *Soc Work* May-June:206–209, 1988.

Tamaroff MH, Festa RS, Adesman AR, et al: Therapeutic adherence to oral medication regimens by adolescents with cancer. II: Clinical and psychologic correlates. *J Pediatr* 120(5):812–817, 1992.

Teicher MH, Baldessarini RJ: Developmental pharmacodynamics. In: Popper C (ed): *Psychiatric Pharmacosciences of Children and Adolescents*. Washington, DC, American Psychiatric Press, 1987, pp. 45–80.

Thompson RH, Vernon DT: Research on children's behavior after hospitalization: A review and synthesis. *J Dev Behav Pediatr* 14:28–35, 1993.

Trigg ME: Bone marrow transplantation for treat-

ment of leukemia in children. *Pediatr Clin North Am* 35:933–938, 1988.

Trimm F: Session VII: Physiologic and psychological growth and development in pediatric heart transplant recipients. *J Heart Lung Transplant* 10:5, Part 2, 1991.

Trzepacz PT, DiMartini A, Tringali R: Psychopharmacological issues in organ transplantation. Part I: Pharmacokinetics in organ failure and psychiatric aspects in immunosuppressants and anti-infectious agents. *Psychosomatics* 34(3):199–207, 1993.

Utens EM, Verhulst FC, Meijboom FJ, et al: Behavioral and emotional problems in children and adolescents with congenital heart disease. *Psychol Med* 23:415–424, 1993.

Uzark K, Crowley D: Family stresses after pediatric heart transplantation. *Prog Cardiovasc Nurs* 4: 23–27, 1989.

Uzark KC, Sauer SN, Lawrence KS, et al: The psychosocial impact of pediatric heart transplantation. *J Heart Lung Transplant* 11:1160–1167, 1992.

Varni JW, Thompson KL, Hanson V: The Varni/Thompson Pediatric pain questionnaire. I: Chronic musculoskeletal pain in juvenile rheumatoid arthritis. *Pain* 28:27–38, 1987.

Vernon TA, Thompson RH: Research on the effect of experimental interventions on children's behavior after hospitalization: A review and synthesis. *J Dev Behav Pediatr* 14:36–44, 1993.

Warner JO: Heart-lung transplantation: All the facts. *Arch Dis Child* 66:1013–1017, 1991.

Wiley FM, House KU: Bone marrow transplant in children. *Semin Oncol Nurs* 4:31–40, 1988.

Windsorova D, Stewart SM, Lovitt R, et al: Emotional adaptation in children after liver transplantation. *J Pediatr* 119:880–887, 1991.

Wolcott D, Stuber M: Bone marrow transplantation In: Craven J, Rodin G (eds): *Psychiatric Aspects of Liver Transplantation*. Oxford, Oxford University Press, 1992, pp. 189–204.

Wolcott DL, Fawzy FI, Wellisch DK: Psychiatric aspects of bone marrow transplantation: A review and current issues. *Psychiatr Med* 4:299–317, 1987.

Younger S: Organ donation and procurement. In: Craven J, Rodin GM (eds): *Psychiatric Aspects of Organ Transplantation*. Oxford, Oxford University Press, 1992, pp. 121–130.

Zamberlan K: Quality of life in school-age children following liver transplantation. *Matern Child Nurs J* 20:167–229, 1992.

96 Psychiatric Aspects of Pediatric Disorders

Philip J. Graham, F.R.C.P., F.R.C.Psych., and Jeremy Turk, M.D., M.R.C.Psych.

Handicapping chronic illness in childhood is a common occurrence, even in the developed world. Approximately one in six children suffer in this way, some from apparently minor conditions, such as a patch of eczema in a conspicuous site, others from far more serious, potentially fatal diseases.

Psychosocial factors may be relevant in the understanding and management of such children in a variety of ways. They may be significant in etiology, and in this connection it should be noted that they may vary considerably in etiological importance in children with the same physical condition. For example, in one child with bronchial asthma, psychosocial factors may be the paramount influence, while in another, of no significance. In contrast, handicapping childhood illness must by defini-

tion always be seen to have at least some impact on psychosocial aspects of the life of the child and his or her family.

Issues of impact, coping, and adaption to pediatric illness have been widely researched and discussed (Breslau, 1985; Cadman et al., 1987; Eiser, 1993; Maddison and Raphael, 1965; Mattson, 1972). It is clear that although there are certainly some common themes, the interrelationships between psychosocial factors and illness vary considerably according to the specific condition or conditions from which the child is suffering (Graham, 1991), a concept that has governed the format of this chapter.

Related issues concerning other aspects of pediatric illness will be found in other sections of this book, namely, psychosocial aspects of brain dysfunction (Chapter 59), psychogenic pain (Chapter 102), sensory disorders (Chapter 49), the impact of hospitalization (Chapters 90 and 103), and consultation/liaison and the role of the child and adolescent psychiatrist in the pediatric setting (Chapter 90).

CLASSIFICATION

The classification of psychological conditions associated with chronic physical disorders presents some problems and these have been addressed in a new fashion in DSM-IV (American Psychiatric Association, 1994). The DSM-IV classification has abolished the category of "organic mental disorder" on the reasonable grounds that this phrase inappropriately implies that most mental disorders are non-organic. The procedure is therefore as follows. Any general medical condition from which the child or adolescent suffers should be coded on Axis 3. If it is judged there are Psychological Factors affecting the Medical Condition, this should be coded as 316 on Axis 1. This code (316) may be appropriate for a variety of reasons, because mental disorders may adversely affect the medical condition in a number of ways. For example, such factors can influence the *course* of the general medical condition (and this might be inferred by a close temporal association), or they may interfere with *treatment* of the general medical condition. "Psychological or behavioral factors that influence general medical conditions include Axis 1 disorders, Axis 2 disorders, psychological symptoms or personality traits that do not meet the full criteria for a specific mental disorder, maladaptive health behaviors, or physiological responses to environmental or social stressors" (American Psychiatric Association, 1994). When coding 316, one of these preceding factors should be specified, and if more than one type of factor is present, the most prominent should be named. The mental disorder, psychological symptoms, and other relevant symptoms should also be separately coded on the appropriate axis.

If there is evidence from the history, physical examination, or laboratory findings that a general medical condition is responsible for a psychiatric disorder, then the appropriate coding should be used. Thus, the code 293.83 is used for a mood disorder which is due to a specific medical condition. The medical condition is then separately specified. Similar codes exist for other mental disorders, e.g., 293.89 for anxiety disorder due to a general medical condition.

Mental disorders occurring in parents as a result of the impact of a chronic disorder in a child will, of course, require separate classification.

The International Classification of Diseases (ICD-10) retains a main section (F00–F09) for organic, including symptomatic, mental disorders (World Health Organization, 1992). ICD-10 also has an additional code (F54) for classifying psychological and behavioral factors associated with disorders or diseases classified elsewhere.

CHROMOSOMAL ABNORMALITIES

Down Syndrome (Trisomy 21)

BACKGROUND INFORMATION

This condition, which if present is now almost always recognized at birth, is revealed by a characteristic facial and bodily appearance. Affected children have slanting eyes with epicanthic folds, a short nose with a flat nasal bridge, and white (Brushfield) spots in the iris; there is an increased incidence of cataracts and strabismus. The fingers are short, the little finger is in-curved, and there may be a single (rather than the normal double) palmar crease. The children are short in stature and may show muscular hypotonia, sometimes with associated atlantoaxial instability. Associated gut and cardiac abnormalities are relatively common, respiratory infections and serous otitis media occur frequently, and there is an increased incidence of leukemia.

The condition occurs in about 1 in 660 children and is responsible for about one-third of all cases of severe mental handicap (IQ less than 50). Most (about 95%) cases are due to the presence of an additional chromosome at position 21, but in about 5% there is a translocation

defect with displacement of part of a chromosome from elsewhere to position 21. Mosaicism may occur, the degree of learning disability being proportional to the number of cells demonstrating the trisomy. There is a definite tendency for the condition to occur with increased frequency with increasing maternal age.

COGNITIVE DEVELOPMENT

By about the age of 5 years the mean IQ level of children with Down syndrome is around 45, with the great majority falling within the range of 25–70. However, the early development of such children is often very little retarded (Carr, 1970), and this may mean that in the early years parents are unrealistically optimistic. Rates of intellectual development become increasingly slower as children get older (Hodapp and Zigler, 1990). Much of this decline appears to occur in the earliest years, although IQ declines also may occur later in development. Further, professional exaggeration of the benefits of early intervention may also be misleading. Certainly early stimulation programs do promote development, and home-reared children achieve higher educational attainments (though not higher IQ) in reading and arithmetic than do non-home-reared children (Carr, 1988), but there is no evidence that achievement of intelligence within the normal range is other than a most unusual outcome. With policies directed towards mainstreaming, many children with Down syndrome are educable within ordinary schools, but all will need programs tailored to their special educational needs. Children with Down syndrome continue to develop well into their late teens, and there is now evidence of a slight but consistent rise in intelligence up to the age of 21 years (Carr, 1988). In later adulthood, however, individuals with Down syndrome are likely to develop neuropathological changes in the brain similar to those occurring in dementia of the Alzheimer type (Blackwood et al., 1988).

IMPACT ON THE FAMILY

The birth of a handicapped child will, of course, have a significant impact on family life, and the presence of a child growing into adulthood but only achieving partial independence will alter the lives of both parents and siblings in a most significant way. Depression in mothers of affected children is more common than it is in the general population, and this is often related to the experience of loss of the normal child the mother expected to have (Bicknell, 1983). Guilt feelings are not usually a prominent feature. Rates of divorce are not higher in these parents (Carr, 1988; Gath and Gumley, 1984), and a significant number of parents speak positively of the experience of bringing up a child with this condition. The life of siblings is certainly affected. Behavioral problems in siblings are more often found if the child with Down syndrome has very disturbed behavior (Gath and Gumley, 1987). In addition, there is a higher rate of emotional and behavioral problems in the older sisters in these families, possibly due to their carrying an undue burden of care (Gath, 1974). Academically and socially, siblings do as well as their peers (Gath and Gumley, 1987).

PSYCHIATRIC ASPECTS

Children with Down syndrome do not show increased rates of behavioral and emotional disturbance compared to children in the general population and show lower rates than other children with comparable levels of learning disability. In particular, they only rarely develop autism and the hyperkinetic syndrome, although both these conditions have been described in affected children. Early reports that children with Down syndrome are particularly placid and compliant are accurate only insofar as they reflect comparisons with other children with mental handicap. Efforts at empirical evaluation of the proposed personality stereotype in Down syndrome have produced mixed and contradictory results. While recent research does support the association of certain descriptive adjectives with a diagnosis of Down syndrome (e.g., clownish, sociable, affectionate) it may be that children are being rated by observers on the known stereotype rather than on their actual personality (Gibbs and Thorpe, 1983). Also, the issue of variability within the syndrome itself is being reappraised. Green and colleagues (1989) found a small but important subgroup of the children with Down syndrome to have notably impaired attentional abilities, both quantitatively and qualitatively. There was some association between poor attention and lower cognitive functioning but these were not synonymous. A minority of children affected with Down syndrome show extremely eccentric and bizarre behavior, with ritualistic habits and mannerisms unrelated to autism. In general, however, of the autosomal disorders, Down syndrome stands out by virtue of the relatively low rates of serious psychiatric disturbance such as autism and hyperactivity (Turk, 1994a). However these do occur in some individuals with Down syndrome and can be severe (Pueschel et al., 1991). Psychiatric management of behavioral problems in affected children will not differ from that undertaken with other children with learning difficulties.

Gonadal Dysgenesis (Turner's Syndrome)

This sex chromosome abnormality is usually characterized by a single X chromosome, one sex chromosome being absent. Some children show a mosaic chromosomal pattern, with a variety of sex chromosomal arrangements in some cells (especially XX) and an absent sex chromosome in others. Ten to twenty percent have duplication of one arm of the X chromosome with loss of the other arm ("isochromosome X"). In rare instances there may be an X chromosome/autosome translocation or ring formation of the X chromosome with loss of variable amounts of chromatin.

Features of the condition include short stature, failure of gonadal development with primary amenorrhea, and, less commonly, webbed neck and a wide carrying angle at the elbow. Approximately one-third also have coarctation of the aorta. The condition usually presents with growth delay in childhood or with absent periods in puberty. It has been noted that chromosomal short arm loss is associated with short stature and other visible clinical signs while long arm loss produces streak gonads (Ferguson-Smith, 1965).

Cognitive development is characterized by a normal or near-normal verbal intelligence but defective visuospatial skills. Difficulties with arithmetic and spatial orientation are relatively common (Silbert et al., 1977). These specific learning difficulties correlate with magnetic resonance imaging findings—in particular, diminished right parieto-occipital lobe volumes (Murphy et al., 1993). Social relationships are often impaired, and there may be other behavioral problems. A national study of over 200 girls with Turner syndrome demonstrated difficulties in other areas including social anxiety, shyness, communication difficulties, and attentional problems (Skuse et al., 1994). This does not appear to be due to the short stature itself; comparisons with children with other types of short stature suggest that girls with Turner's syndrome are specifically at risk for these types of difficulty (McCauley et al., 1986). Girls with Turner's syndrome, however, show a stronger feminine sex role identity than do girls with constitutional short stature (Downey et al., 1989).

Counseling for children with Turner's syndrome and, where appropriate, their parents is likely to focus on difficulties arising from short stature and learning problems in school. Later, in the immediate prepubertal stages, girls should be counseled about their sexual anomaly and the implications for normal childbearing frankly discussed. Recent treatments with estrogens, androgens, and growth hormone hold promise for improving growth and sexual development and are currently being evaluated.

Fragile X Syndrome

This condition was first discovered when it was shown that, if cells of affected individuals are cultured in a folate-deficient medium, a proportion will, on careful examination, be seen to show a hypochromic site at q27.3 on the long arm of the X chromosome in males, and on one of the two X chromosomes in females. This condition is now known to be associated with an abnormal expansion of CGG base triplet repeats at position Xq27.3 which can grow transgenerationally and causes local hypermethylation and consequent interference with protein transcription (Fu et al., 1991; Verkerk et al., 1991). Expansion size may be related to degree of intellectual impairment. Laboratory examination of chromosomes is problematic, as even in fragile site-positive individuals, only a relatively small proportion of cells, between 1% and 50%, show the characteristic chromosomal defect. It is therefore necessary to examine at least 50 cells in any at-risk individual, and even this number might not be adequate. Variations in methods of cell culture and observer variation are currently another potential cause of unreliability in laboratory diagnosis and a reason why some laboratories identify higher rates of affected individuals than do others. A fragile site in over 2% of cells analyzed is now generally reckoned to confirm the diagnosis (Hagerman and Sobesky, 1989), but this threshold may change as knowledge advances. It is important to note that the number of cells demonstrating the fragile site bears *no* relationship to the nature and degree of intellectual impairment. Newer techniques involving DNA analysis by means of Southern blot and polymerase chain reaction technology should preferably be used to make the diagnosis.

PATTERN OF INHERITANCE

Although the condition is a sex-linked cause of mental retardation and more common in males, the pattern of inheritance is not that of a simple sex-linked Mendelian disorder. Only four-fifths of affected males show cognitive defects, and about one-third of carrier females are themselves mentally retarded (Davies, 1989). The condition may be transmitted from unaffected carrier males to their progeny, who may themselves suffer mental retardation. Fragile X accounts for approximately 10% of all boys with severe mental retardation of no obvious cause (Webb et al., 1986) and for 6–10% of unexplained mild mental retardation (Thake et al., 1987). It is therefore at least the second commonest form of mental retardation known.

CLINICAL FEATURES

Given the problems with laboratory diagnosis and the pattern of inheritance, it is not surprising that there is also uncertainty as to what exactly constitutes the physical and behavioral phenotype. A proportion of affected individuals, probably the majority, show characteristic physical stigmata, particularly a high forehead, prominent supraorbital ridges, "simple" protruding ears, a prominent jaw, and postpubertal macroorchidism. (Simko et al., 1989; Thake et al., 1985). There may also be a high arched plate, joint hypermobility, and soft velvety skin. Possible cardiovascular complications include aortic root dilatation and mitral valve prolapse (Turk et al., 1994). Additionally, the trajectory of intellectual development shows a characteristic profile whereby the rate of development remains parallel to that of nondisabled peers up until puberty when the discrepancy widens (Hagerman et al., 1989). Intellectual development certainly continues but at a slower rate. This has been found to be due to specific difficulties in the sequential processing of information (taking a string of information a bit at a time) which becomes more marked over time (Hodapp et al., 1991). This contrasts with the earlier developing simultaneous information processing skills and is required increasingly throughout development. All the above intellectual anomalies are witnessed in female carriers, most of whom have average intellectual functioning (Miezejeski et al., 1986). Female carriers also often display difficulties with "executive function" skills: planning ahead, attending, sustaining effort, generating problem-solving strategies, using feedback, self-monitoring, and shifting responses (Mazzocco et al., 1992). These abilities are thought to be subsumed by the frontal lobes.

The mental retardation that occurs in this condition may be associated with autism or autistic features, and strong suggestions have been made that fragile X individuals are particularly prone to autism. It now seems likely (Peyton et al., 1989) that autism does not occur to a greater extent in fragile X-associated mental retardation than in other forms of mental retardation, although the majority of males with fragile X may have some autistic-like features (Hagerman, 1989), most notably hand flapping, hand biting, and poor eye contact due to gaze aversion (Wolff et al., 1989).

It seems that fragile X syndrome accounts for no more than 2–3% of cases of typical autism (Bailey et al., 1993). The presence of typical autism in fragile X syndrome is probably no higher than in learning disabled populations generally. However, it is the *profile* of disturbances rather than the presence or absence of a discrete diagnosis which often typifies the condition (see Turk et al., 1994, for review). The poor eye contact is usually attributed to *gaze aversion* (Wolff et al., 1989). Hyperactivity has been reported as the presenting feature in nonretarded boys with fragile X syndrome (Hagerman et al., 1989). Recent research suggests that while boys with fragile X are not more overactive than other learning disabled children, they do display poorer concentration spans with more restlessness and fidgetiness. These impairments tend not to improve developmentally as they do in non-fragile X learning disabled individuals. Here then is another example of the *trajectory* of development being as important as the exact nature of the impairments (Turk, 1994b). The hyperactivity and attentional deficits will often respond partially to stimulant medication such as methylphenidate (Hagerman et al., 1988).

Most prepubertal males with fragile X syndrome are mildly retarded. Reading and spelling skills are relatively advanced in contrast with poor arithmetic performance (Kemper et al.,1988). Speech is frequently "cluttered" with frequent dysfluent, rapid, tangential remarks and poor topic maintenance (Hanson et al., 1986). The simultaneous presence of visuospatial difficulties, impaired constructional ability, and shortened digit span may be indicative of nondominant hemisphere dysfunction (Crowe and Hay, 1990). However, neuroimaging studies suggest midline abnormality in the form of hypoplasia of the cerebellar vermis (Reiss et al., 1991).

Genetic counseling is problematic. Bearing in mind that about 6–10% of children with unexplained mild mental retardation (IQ 50–70) show fragile sites (Thake et al., 1987), it is advisable to request laboratory investigation of chromosomes of all individuals with IQs below 70, specifically requesting DNA examination for fragile X syndrome. A positive result from an experienced laboratory requires explanation to the parents, who should be advised that further male children have about a one in two chance of mental retardation and female children a roughly one in six chance of being affected. These figures are based on knowledge that about 10% of males and 70% of females with a fragile site are of normal ability (Bundey, 1987).

Klinefelter's Syndrome

This condition is usually associated with an XXY chromosome karyotype, though this is not invariable. The phenotype is characterized physically by long legs and male appearance, but a small penis and testes and, at puberty, gynecomastia and absent secondary sexual characteristics.

The psychological significance of the condition lies in the fact that children often show delayed onset of language with impairment in expressive language plus visual-motor and sensory integration problems (Mandoki et al., 1991). There is a slightly reduced average IQ, but the condition is compatible with high intelligence (Ratcliffe et al., 1990). Although emotional problems do occur, there is no significant increase in child psychiatric disorder. However, there have also been reports of XXY boys being introverted, quiet, unassertive, and passive, with low levels of activity and tending to withdraw from group activities. Ratcliffe et al. (1982) also found Klinefelter boys to be more tender minded, apprehensive, and insecure with peer group relationship problems and little sexual interest in girls.

Chromosome investigation should be requested in children with the characteristic appearance, as a positive result implies later infertility for which counseling will be needed. There is no reason why a positive result should influence decisions on psychiatric intervention.

XYY Syndrome

Children with this karyotype are often unusually tall but show no other clearly characteristic physical features. The condition was once thought to be associated with criminal behavior, but the evidence for this is weak. However, children in the general population with the karyotype are definitely more likely to have early language delay and later reading (but not arithmetical) retardation (Ratcliffe et al., 1990). In childhood they do show high rates of emotional but not conduct disorder, and psychiatric referral occurs more frequently than in the general population. Psychological intervention should not, however, be influenced by the presence of the karyotype, which will in any case usually be unsuspected (Ratcliffe and Field, 1982).

Prader-Willi and Angelman Syndromes

Angelman's syndrome and Prader-Willi syndrome have created interest due to their strikingly different behavioral phenotypes despite relatively similar deletions on the long arm of chromosome 15. Individuals with Prader-Willi syndrome display marked obesity due to hyperphagia. Absence of satiety is important. There may also be a lack of the normal need to vary the nature of food eaten in order to ensure continuing appetite. Unpredictable tantrums, violent outbursts, and stubbornness are common (Hall and Smith, 1972) as well as skin picking. Developmental changes in the behavioral phenotype have been clearly documented (Donaldson et al., 1994). Decreased fetal movements herald hypotonia, poor feeding, and an abnormal, weak, or absent cry. In infancy these tendencies predispose to failure to thrive. Expressive language and articulation problems are also noted around this time. Hyperphagia develops throughout childhood with consequent obesity. Behavior problems including skin picking and temper outbursts in response to frustration evolve combined with an apparent decreased sensitivity to pain. Intellectual abilities are uneven. Visuospatial skills seem good yet arithmetic and short-term memory processing present particular difficulties. By adolescence, obsessional tendencies often manifest as tantrums in response to trivial changes in routine.

PSYCHOSOCIAL ASPECTS

Associated psychiatric problems in Prader-Willi syndrome are relatively common. Anxiety reactions and obsessive-compulsive symptoms are often prominent, but aggressive behavior is most unusual (Whitman and Accardo, 1987). Such symptoms may be a response to the stress of experiencing food restriction in the presence of excessive appetite.

The most challenging aspect of management is the prevention and treatment of the severe obesity (Laurance, 1985). Strict food restrictions should be undertaken from an early age. Behavior modification has been used and has produced weight reduction, though this is difficult to sustain. Appetite suppressants are of little value.

Parents need a great deal of support to cope with the special problems in management of children with this condition and benefit particularly from membership in the Prader-Willi Syndrome Association.

In contrast Angelman's syndrome individuals lack these features and tend to display a happy disposition with paroxysmal laughter, jerky ataxic gait, and a tendency towards an open mouth with tongue protrusion (Clayton-Smith, 1993). Mental retardation is usually extreme (Robb et al., 1989). Behavior may lead observers to attribute to these individuals a highly sociable tendency with an intense desire to communicate. This may be so for some, but the evidence suggests that autistic tendencies are common with substantially delayed social and communication skills even when their often severe mental retardation is taken into account (Sales and Turk, 1991). Studies of communication development in Angelman's syndrome suggest that these children develop very few words and have difficulty in using gestural or sign systems (Jolleff and Ryan, 1993). The research also suggests that this typical lack of speech is not due to mental retardation alone (Penner et al., 1993). Neonatal observations in Angelman's syndrome include feeding problems and an abnormal high-pitched cry (Clayton-Smith, 1993). Sleep requirements are also reported as being reduced. The need for sleep does increase with age and some adolescents may even sleep longer than usual (Clayton-Smith, 1993).

CONGENITAL MALFORMATIONS

Cleft Lip and Palate

This is a relatively common condition, occurring in about 1.4 in 1000 births. It is largely genetically determined, with a concordance rate of 40% in monozygotic twins and 5% in dizygotic twins and siblings. Maternal exposure in early pregnancy to certain drugs such as lithium and hydantoin increases the risk. Surgical repair of the lip is now carried out at 1–2 months of age, and repair of the palate between 12 and 18 months, so that in the 1st year or so the baby requires a dental plate and/or a special teat for feeding. Cosmetic results are now excellent; however, even successfully operated children are liable to develop serous otitis media, with subsequent recurrent hearing problems. The presence of other congenital defects, especially congenital heart disease, may also complicate the outcome.

PSYCHOSOCIAL ASPECTS
Early Management

The appearance of the baby after birth is naturally very shocking to parents. It is now normal practice for both parents to be prepared for the appearance of the child before they first see it together. An early explanation of the surgical treatment is given with before-and-after photographs of successfully treated children. It is important that parents are also prepared for the immediate postoperative appearance of the child, as this is also unsightly.

In the first few weeks of the baby's life, parents require a great deal of both emotional support and practical help. Feeding difficulties are common, partly because of the anatomical problem and partly because of the anxiety and guilt parents naturally feel and sometimes transmit to their babies in these circumstances. Psychological intervention may be indicated at this point.

Later in childhood, although there is no evidence of raised rates of emotional and behavioral disorders in affected children (Richman, 1983), an imperfect repair is likely to elicit teasing from other children. Deformities of the mouth and teeth are particularly likely to elicit peer rejection (Lansdown and Polak, 1975). Teachers tend to underestimate the intelligence of bright children with unsatisfactorily repaired clefts (Richman, 1978). The presence of undetected hearing problems may also lead to a misdiagnosis of mental retardation, and children benefit from follow-up programs offering the combined advice of an audiologist and a speech therapist.

Psychiatric problems may center around feelings of inferiority and an exaggerated sense of feeling rejected, with low self-esteem. Counseling that provides behavioral advice on improving social skills will often be effective, but a minority of affected children. usually those who have experienced additional family problems, may require more formal psychotherapy.

Hypospadias

In about one in 350 male infants, the external meatus of the penis is on the undersurface rather than at the tip. In severe cases (chordee) the penis may be bowed ventrally. Surgical treatment is undertaken at variable points in time, but rather than carry out two-stage or three-stage operations between the ages of 2 and 5, there is now a tendency to operate in single-stage operations within the first 2 years of life, often before a year. Postoperative complications requiring reoperation are relatively common.

PSYCHOSOCIAL ASPECTS

The site of the malformation makes it unsurprising that parents often have particular anxieties about it. They are often too embarrassed to talk openly about it to friends and family and may be concerned about the later sexual potency and fertility of their son. If operation is delayed beyond 2 or 3 years, the boys themselves may feel different from others because they have to urinate sitting down and cannot join in those important male competitions involving demonstrating prowess in producing a powerful stream.

Follow-up studies of variable quality, summarized by Schultz (1983), have suggested that in later life adults who have been operated on for hypospadias in childhood are less likely to marry and have children than controls. They may suffer from feelings of inadequacy and avoid competitive activities. Sexual intercourse is experienced later and less frequently than is the case with controls.

It is uncertain whether these unsatisfactory outcomes are the result of hormonal changes related to the malformation, parental anxieties transmitted to their offspring, or internalized psychological difficulties perhaps related to the timing of the operation. There are no studies relating outcome to early or late hormonal status or comparing psychological outcome in relation to timing of the operation. However, it is obviously desirable for parents to have the opportunity to share their anxieties as early as possible, not least because they may well be misinformed about the nature of the condition. Parents and children (where age appropriate) need preparation for the operative procedures. Follow-up should include opportunities for the boy to express any fears of permanent mutilation he may have. It is probable that sexual counseling in adolescence of boys who have experienced hypospadias operative procedures would have a preventive effect in relation to later sexual dysfunction, though there do not appear to be studies investigating this issue. Certainly those counseling adolescents and young men for sexual dysfunction should be aware that feelings of inferiority may be related to the presence of an earlier anatomical abnormality.

Undescended Testes (Cryptorchidism)

This condition occurs in about 1% of males over the age of 3 months. Management first involves ensuring the testes are not merely unusually retractile. True cryptorchidism is now initially treated hormonally; if this is unsuccessful, orchidopexy is performed. The operation used to be performed around age 5–7, when many boys found it a frightening and unpleasant experience, even given adequate preparation and explanation. There was, however, no evidence of long-term adverse psychosocial consequences (Cytryn et al., 1967). Modern approaches involve surgical treatment before the age of 2 years. This makes adequate preparation for the child more difficult, but parents can be reassured that discomfort will be relatively short-lived. There is also no evidence of long-lasting adverse effects if the operation is carried out at this earlier age.

Congenital Heart Disease

Congenital defects of the heart occur in about 1 in 150 children and represent the commonest congenital malformation. About 10% of children with such defects have an additional associated congenital abnormality. The etiology may be genetic or may arise as a result of exposure to toxic or infective agents (e.g., rubella virus) in the early stages of pregnancy. Investigations of defects by noninvasive techniques such as echocardiography or invasive tests such as cardiac catheterization will, in themselves, prove threatening to some parents and children. Subsequent surgery has become increasingly successful in the short-term, although the results in adolescence and adult life for more recently developed operations remain uncertain. Cardiac transplantation is now used as early as the 1st year of life for previously inoperable multiple cardiac lesions.

PARENTAL REACTIONS

Most congenital heart disease presents in the first few weeks or months of life and, in considering psychological reactions to diagnosis of the condition, it is obviously parental reactions that are of most immediate importance. Studies of parental responses to the realization that their child has a heart defect suggest that high levels of anxiety are prominent (Garson et al., 1978). This is not surprising, for, at least in popular mythology, the heart is seen (along with the brain) as *the* vital organ necessary for life, and indeed medical judgment also defines death partly in terms of cessation of heart function. Anxiety may be compounded by guilt, parents not infrequently worrying whether they themselves caused the defect in some way during the pregnancy. If the lesion is asymptomatic and detected only by routine examination, then there may be active denial.

In contrast, the presence of such symptoms as cyanosis, dyspnea, feeding difficulties, and slow weight gain may elicit mild or more serious levels of overprotection. Parents may find themselves getting up frequently during the night to check on their infant's welfare. Anxiety may cause feeding times to become a battleground, with parents knowing that a successful operation may only be possible if sufficient weight is gained and infants and toddlers resenting pressure to eat more than they want.

Consequently, explanations to parents and, where appropriate, to children need to be very carefully and systematically undertaken. These should cover the nature of the defect, the various investigative procedures, and the nature of the surgery to be performed. Drawings and models can be helpful. The use of puppets has been found helpful with older children (Cassell and Paul, 1967). Explanations need to be repeated at each stage of investigation and as surgery is approached.

Teams of physicians, surgeons, nurses, play specialists, and social workers in cardiac surgery centers have found different solutions to the issues of explanation and preparation. In general, it is helpful if there is a systematic approach and set of procedures so that parental anxieties are routinely considered. On the other hand, it is also important for specialist staff to recognize that the personalities, patterns of relationships, and fantasies of each parent are unique and require individual concern (Glaser and Bentovim, 1987). Blanket explanations or the use of videos without the opportunity for discussion are therefore unlikely to be very effective.

When older children require operative procedures or reoperation and during the period of follow-up after successful operation, communication with the child becomes increasingly relevant. Again, models and drawings are useful aids to communication, and the child should have the opportunity to express his or her own unique fears and fantasies.

BEHAVIORAL AND EMOTIONAL PROBLEMS

The rates of behavioral and emotional problems in operated children depend to some degree on operative success (Kramer et al., 1989), but not on diagnostic group (Utens et al., 1993). Asymptomatic children are unlikely to have higher rates of problems than are healthy control subjects. On the other hand, children with physical impairment following surgery do appear to have higher levels of anxiety and impulsiveness as well as a greater sense of inferiority when compared to physically fit children and healthy control subjects (Kramer et al., 1989). Parents may not be aware of the underlying concerns that children experience. Yet their perception of the severity of the lesion contributes greatly to the psychosocial adjustment of the child (DeMaso et al., 1991).

COGNITIVE DEVELOPMENT

The fact that operative procedures may need to be accompanied by hypothermia and disturbances of cerebral circulation has stimulated a number of studies of the cognitive development of operated children.

Obviously a small number will suffer serious brain damage. Once these have been excluded, the intelligence of children operated on for serious defects is about 10 points lower than that of normal controls, that is, significantly reduced but well within the average range (Haka-Ikse et al., 1978). The fact that the intelligence level is not associated with the severity of surgical complications suggests that other factors, such as inherited potential, minor episodes of cerebral circulatory disturbance before or after operation, or parental anxiety, may be responsible.

Finally, newer techniques of heart and heart-lung transplantation require consideration. Psychological aspects of these procedures when carried out in childhood have so far been little researched, but parental anxieties are naturally intense. Specific fears concerning the nature of the donor, the viability of the transplant, and its capacity to develop in a way that continues to meet the needs of the growing child may or may not be expressed, but parents should always be given the opportunity to discuss them. The greatest anxieties of the surgical team will probably center around the immunological status of the child postoperatively, rather than around the operation itself and parents will benefit from discussion of this issue as early as possible. There is preliminary evidence (E. Serrano, personal communication, September, 1995) that the quality of family functioning before transplantation is associated with compliance with medical treatment after surgery, and noncompliance is linked to a poor outcome.

RESPIRATORY DISEASE

Asthma

BACKGROUND INFORMATION

Episodic recurrent resistance to air flow in the lungs producing wheezing or coughing may be precipitated by infection, exercise, exposure to allergens, or psychological stress. In many children attacks are precipitated by all of these, individually or in combination, at different times. The prognosis is extremely variable, with some children having only one or two attacks and others (a minority) experiencing chronic disability that persists into adulthood. Severe chronic forms of the condition may require treatment with steroids, with their attendant complications. Such children, and others with disabling recurrent attacks, will also require preventive treatment between episodes with cromolyn sodium.

In its mild form the condition is chronic, occurring in 5–10% of the child population. Although there is an inherited component, it is likely that environmental factors, including poor social conditions, atmospheric pollution, exposure to infective agents and allergens, and psychological stress, play a more important part.

PSYCHOSOCIAL ASPECTS
Etiological Factors

Whereas the role of genetic and immunological factors in the primary etiology of this condition remains well established, the role of psychological factors remains controversial. Specific patterns of family interaction, to be described below, are present in children shortly after they develop asthma, but these patterns could be secondary to the frightening nature of the condition. There is no evidence that the onset of asthma is produced by significant life changes (Horwood et al., 1985). Longitudinal studies of psychological development in children at risk for asthma because of their family history have, however, illuminated this issue further. It seems that early problems in parental coping do predict later development of asthmatic attacks (Mrazek et al., 1991).

On the other hand, there is no doubt that once asthma is established, in some children—perhaps as many as a quarter to a third—attacks may be precipitated by emotion, usually excitement, fear, anger, or frustration. The mechanisms whereby stress produces wheezing are not fully understood, but it is clear that intense emotion can reduce pulmonary flow rate (Tal and Micklich, 1976). Immune systems can be influenced by activation of hypothalamic-limbic-midbrain circuits, and such activation can occur following interpretation of a psychologically meaningful stimulus at the cerebral level. Release of chemical mediators triggering an asthma attack probably occurs either as a result of the influence of these neuroregulatory pathways or following a hypersensitivity reaction to allergens. Various forms of respiratory behavior associated with emotional expression, such as laughing or crying, may also act as direct, specific triggers of attacks, possibly as a result of a conditioning mechanism.

Family Factors

A severe, acute attack of asthma is one of the most frightening problems for junior pediatric staff so it is not surprising that parents are often panic-stricken; parental attitudes are often affected for a not insignificant period of time. Mrazek et al. (1987) have shown that insecure attachment is more common in severely asthmatic preschool children in comparison with healthy control subjects; Williams (1975) and Kashani et al. (1988) have found that parents of asthmatic children are indeed unusually anxious. Family studies of children with asthma, in comparison with healthy and diabetic children, have demonstrated that the families of asthmatic children tend to rigidity and overinvolvement or enmeshment in their relationships (Gustafsson et al., 1987). In this study, extreme overinvolvement in non-steroid-dependent children was specifically linked to low immunoglobulin E concentrations, suggesting that in these families immunological mechanisms were less important.

The importance of parent-child relationships in the precipitation of asthma attacks was demonstrated in a classic study described by Purcell and Weiss (1970). Parents of selected non-steroid-dependent asthmatic children were encouraged to live for 2 weeks away from their home in which their children continued to reside, looked after by substitute parents. The children thus continued to be exposed to the same allergens in the domestic environment. In a significant number of children there was a considerable reduction in the number of attacks, followed by an increase when their parents returned. The anxiety of the parents in this study, produced by their separation from their children, was often intense. In contrast to these parents, a small minority deny that attacks worry them and behave as if the attacks have not occurred. Such an attitude of denial can be dangerous if, as sometimes happens, the child is consequently not given essential medical treatment.

PSYCHOLOGICAL DEVELOPMENT

Although there is no evidence that asthmatic children have a specific type of personality (Herbert, 1965), it is clear that children with asthma do show a somewhat higher rate of emotional disturbance than do healthy children. Disturbance rates are not markedly elevated, and most children with asthma do not show such problems. However, raised levels of disturbance have been shown in asthmatic preschool children (Mrazek et al., 1987), in the middle years of childhood (Graham et al., 1967), and throughout the whole childhood age range (Kashani et al., 1988; McNichol et al., 1973). Although the evidence is not consistent, most studies (e.g., McNichol et al., 1973) show that the more severely physically disabled the child, the greater the likelihood of disturbance. Children with low allergic potential, as assessed by skin tests and immunological investigations, tend to show a higher rate of disturbance, but again the evidence is not conclusive (Block, 1968). There are no specific types of behavioral or emotional disturbance, and severely asthmatic children may be either more aggressive and demanding or more anxious than other children (McNichol et al., 1973). There is some evidence, however (Mrazek et al., 1987; Williams, 1975), that asthmatic children do have specific conflicts in their feelings of dependency and need for independence. Again, it is difficult to know whether such conflicts arise from the frightening experience of the asthma or are responsible for it, at least to some degree, in the first place.

The impact of asthma on different aspects of a child's life has been reviewed by Nocon (1991). The educational progress of children with asthma may be somewhat retarded (Mitchell and Dawson, 1973), and the frequent absences from school such children suffer may be, to some degree, responsible. For example, Hill et al. (1989) found 9% of a total population of asthmatic children ages 5–11 had lost time from school

in the previous year, and in 1.7%, many of whom were inadequately treated, more than 10 days had been lost in that time. Educational problems may be related directly to medication prescribed for the asthma, and it is significant that Rachelefsky et al. (1986) found in a double-blind study that school performance and behavior were affected adversely by the use of the bronchodilator theophylline. Steroid medication does not appear to have directly adverse effects of this type (Bender et al., 1987).

PSYCHOLOGICAL ASPECTS OF MANAGEMENT

The role of the health professional in the management of asthma has been discussed by Matus (1981), who places special emphasis on the important issue of noncompliance in treatment. Certainly an understanding of family dynamics and of the child's perception and understanding of the illness will contribute to clarification of noncompliance issues. Children who seem to precipitate attacks deliberately need careful mental health evaluation. Discussion of means of avoiding the stresses that trigger attacks may be helpful. There is evidence that family therapy as an adjunct to pediatric management can result in improvement not just in psychological adjustment but also in measures of lung function (Lask and Matthew, 1979). Similarly, a behavioral self-management program for children with asthma has demonstrable effectiveness (Colland, 1993). Although most children with asthma do improve significantly and indeed may be permanently symptom-free before adulthood, in a minority this does not occur. It is particularly in these more severe and chronic cases that mental health professionals may play a valuable role in evaluating the need for residential schooling. Lask (1993) has discussed indications for referral of children with asthma to a psychologist or psychiatrist.

Cystic Fibrosis

BACKGROUND INFORMATION

In this condition the function of the exocrine glands is affected, so that their secretions are abnormally viscid. The most common presentations are intestinal obstruction (due to meconium ileus) at birth, and chronic lung and pancreatic disease. Significant clinical features from a psychological point of view are the chronicity of the condition, with repeated relapses requiring hospitalization during childhood; the need for heavy involvement of the parents in home care, especially postural treatment to drain the lungs; and the poor, though improving, prognosis. About 85% of children who survive the very early years live at least into early adulthood, and much longer survival does occur. Nevertheless the quality of life is often seriously impaired.

The condition is inherited as an autosomal-recessive and occurs in about 1 in 2000 births. There is a roughly equal sex ratio. The locus of the gene responsible for a majority of sufferers from the condition is now more clearly known, and antenatal counseling can now be given with a greater degree of accuracy of risk.

PSYCHOSOCIAL ASPECTS

The impact of the condition of the child and the rest of the family will, at least to some degree, depend on the age at which the diagnosis is made and the severity of the disorder. Diagnosis may be made at or before birth. At birth the child may present with meconium ileus. Much later in childhood or adolescence the diagnosis may be made as a result of investigation for recurrent chest infections or failure to thrive. In many children the need for repeated hospitalizations interrupts schooling, places extra financial burdens on the family, and adds to the stress on families. The final course of the condition is very variable, with death sometimes supervening in a sudden, unexpected manner because of a particularly fulminant infection; much more commonly, serious invalidism is delayed until adulthood. The development of heart-lung transplantation may now further improve the prognosis, although early experience is not particularly encouraging.

Parental involvement in treatment might be expected to result in the development of overprotective attitudes, and Burton's (1975) extensive study confirms this expectation. However, more recently Walker et al. (1987) have found that parents of affected children did not perceive themselves as less strict with their children than other parents. They are, however, more likely to become depressed, and such depression is linked more to the parents' subjective feelings about the severity of the condition than to objective ratings of severity.

Although most children with cystic fibrosis are reasonably well adjusted psychologically to their predicament (Bywater, 1981; Drotar et al., 1981; Gayton et al., 1977), there is some evidence that they do show significantly higher rates of behavioral disturbance. Cowen et al. (1986), in an uncontrolled study using behavioral methods with established norms, found higher than expected rates of behavioral problems, especially delinquency in younger children, cruelty in girls, and immature behavior in boys. Depression and anxiety are more common in older adolescents and adults, whereas younger sufferers more commonly show eating problems (Pearson et al., 1991). But disturbed children are in a minority, and the level of disturbance is related to some degree to the amount of social support the family receives (Frydman, 1981). In fact, psychosocial family variables such as emphasis on personal growth and a balanced family coping style are fairly strongly predictive of longitudinal trends in respiratory function (Patterson et al., 1993). Although schooling is often interrupted, there is no evidence to show that educational attainment is significantly affected.

The adjustment of siblings of children with cystic fibrosis has also been a matter of concern. Parental involvement with a sick child may result in a good deal of jealousy, although parents are often well aware of this danger and do their best to minimize it. Siblings also show somewhat higher rates of behavioral disturbance than do children in the general population (Cowen et al., 1986). There is some evidence that younger siblings are more likely to be disturbed than those older than the affected child, perhaps because older children are often better able intellectually to understand the problem and indeed to take some part in caring for the sick child (Burton, 1975).

PSYCHOSOCIAL ASPECTS OF MANAGEMENT

Ensuring that both parents, seen together, often on several occasions, have a real understanding of the genetic nature of the condition and its implications for further pregnancies is an important component of management. Parents should be encouraged to have the same level of expectations for self-help and behavior as they do for their unaffected children.

Good communication between parents and unaffected as well as affected children is associated with better family functioning (Burton, 1975), and mental health professionals may be helpful in promoting such communication. Groups of parents (Bywater, 1984) of children with this condition have been found helpful in providing mutual support. Parents should be encouraged at an early stage to acknowledge to their children that the condition is long lasting and cannot be expected to go away, though periods of good health can certainly be anticipated. Children should know they will always have symptoms from time to time and that these may become more severe as time goes on. There are particular difficulties in communication, as is not infrequently the case when there is more than one affected child in the family. It is, however, surprising to what degree it remains possible for good communication to occur, especially when pediatricians and mental health professionals do not collude with natural tendencies toward denial.

METABOLIC DISORDERS

Diabetes

BACKGROUND INFORMATION

Diabetes mellitus occurs in two main forms, insulin dependent (juvenile type) and non-insulin dependent; the latter is usually, though not always, adult in onset. Seriously obese children and adolescents may suffer from non-insulin-dependent diabetes, but discussion in this section will be limited to insulin-dependent diabetes mellitus (IDDM). The condition is not uncommon, and the prevalence is 1–2 per 1000 in school-age children. Treatment of IDDM involves insulin replacement and dietary control. Most children require two daily injections of insulin, although some can be managed on a once-daily basis. A small number of well-motivated older children can manage the use of a permanently established infusion pump. Dietary control requires more regular meals and snacks than most children find easy to accept, and there is a need to modify diet if variable levels of exercise are undertaken. Many children suffer from brief hypoglycemic attacks and need to be taught how to recognize these as well as prevent or abort them. The condition is lifelong, and vascular complications frequently ensue, though not usually during childhood.

STRESS AND PHYSIOLOGICAL MECHANISMS

The fact that glucose homeostasis is maintained partly by the catabolic actions of the catecholamines epinephrine and norepinephrine makes it reasonable to consider whether psychological stress might have a direct physiological effect on the progress of the condition and, in particular, on insulin requirements to prevent hyperglycemia. Baker et al. (1969) showed that a stressful interview produced an increase in urinary epinephrine and that this effect could be inhibited by the prior administration of a β-adrenergic blocking substance. However, in a carefully controlled experimental study, Kemmer et al. (1986) have shown that although exposure to stressful situations does result in moderate elevation of catecholamines and cortisol, there is no change in circulating levels of glucose, ketones, or free fatty acids. It therefore seems unlikely that stress has a direct physiological effect producing hyperglycemia.

PSYCHOLOGICAL EFFECTS OF HYPO- AND HYPERGLYCEMIA

Significant decrements in cognitive performance occur with short-term variations of both the hypoglycemic and hyperglycemic types. Thus Holmes (1986; Holmes et al., 1983) found performance on a complex reaction time task to be impaired both with high (more than 16.7 mmol/liter) and low (less than 3.3 mmol/liter) levels of blood glucose. Interestingly, in this study the subjects were unaware of their poor performance even though this was obvious to the outside observer.

INTELLECTUAL DEVELOPMENT

Children with IDDM show somewhat higher rates of learning problems than do children in the general population (Gath et al., 1980). Cognitive impairment is related in childhood, though not in adulthood, to the length of time since the onset of the condition. Ryan et al. (1985) found no differences between later-onset adolescents with IDDM and matched sibling controls on a range of cognitive tasks. However, children diagnosed before 5 years of age showed significant deficits on predominantly visuospatial and memory tasks, as well as on tests of educational attainment, such as reading. Very early-onset diabetes (before 5 years) was found to have the most marked effects on right hemisphere functioning (e.g., visuoconstructional problem solving and recall of visual information), with later-onset IDDM having more specific effects on left hemisphere function, as assessed, for example, by verbal concept information and reading and spelling skills. There is also a suggestion (Rovet et al., 1987) that affected girls show these cognitive problems more consistently than do boys.

BEHAVIORAL AND EMOTIONAL DISTURBANCES

The rates of disturbance in children with diabetes have been extensively studied (Johnson, 1988), and most, though not all (Gath et al.,

1980), find increased rates of problems in this group. Most (e.g., Lavigne et al., 1982) find that diabetic boys show higher rates of disturbance than do girls. There is also evidence concerning the effect of length of illness and age on rates of disturbance. Rovet et al. (1987), for example, found higher rates in boys who were late onset as compared to those who were early onset (before 5 years), and Cassileth et al. (1984), studying adults, found that improved mental health ratings are associated with length of time since diagnosis, suggesting that after a period of adjustment to the illness, rates of disturbance fall. A wide range of behavioral problems is described, and there is no particular behavioral profile found in children with diabetes. High rates of anxiety, depression, low self-esteem, aggression, anger, obsessive-compulsive symptoms, hyperactivity, and schizoid symptoms have all been reported by different workers.

Attempts to relate rates of disturbance to quality of control have led to some rather surprising findings. In particular, it seems that children who are particularly well or rigidly controlled, as indicated by low glycosylated hemoglobin (a physiological means of assessing good long-term control), have higher rates of behavioral problems (Close et al., 1986; Fonagy et al., 1987). In contrast, Rovet et al. (1987) found diabetic children classified as having a significant level of disturbance to have more episodes of ketoacidosis, though the differences in rates were small. It seems there is some possibility, perhaps because they are at increased risk of hypoglycemic episodes, that rigidly controlled children show higher rates of disturbance then less rigidly controlled children.

A significantly sized group of diabetic youngsters in early and middle adolescence present with particular difficulties in biochemical control (Kovacs et al., 1992). These patients with brittle diabetes may require repeated hospitalizations, and there are often major associated psychiatric problems, including attempted suicide (Kaminer and Robbins, 1988). There is a tendency to assume that poor biochemical control necessarily implies poor compliance with treatment, but this may well not be the case. There is indeed a weak and inconsistent relationship between treatment compliance and biochemical control (Glasgow et al., 1987), but even when youngsters with the problem are admitted to a hospital under well-controlled conditions, achieving a satisfactory biochemical result may not be easy. Uncontrolled studies (e.g., White et al., 1984) suggest that children with poor biochemical control usually come from families with multiple social problems, but in a controlled study of a total population of diabetic children, Marteau et al. (1987) found no relationship between control and social class, family income, or employment status of the parents. On the other hand, these workers did find that poor control was strongly linked to relationship problems within the family. It does seem reasonably well established that families of children with poor diabetic control show disturbed relationships. In this connection, the investigation carried out by Minuchin (1974), though uncontrolled, suggests that overprotection of the children, lack of flexibility, and poor conflict resolution are frequently found. It is much less clear (Johnson, 1988) whether such disturbance is primary or secondary to the very considerable stress that uncontrolled diabetes in a child puts on family life. The management of diabetes within the home provides numerous ready-made foci for conflict. Normal difficulties in separation may be heightened if the child refuses to cooperate with urine testing, regular insulin injections, or dietary requirements. An overdose of insulin can be threatened by a teenager who is depressed and/or manipulative.

IMPLICATIONS FOR MANAGEMENT

Coping behavior in children with this chronic illness can be enhanced by pediatric management involving early and repeated full explanations of the condition and its implications. As the child gets older, advice on insulin management should include discussion of ways in which children should, at a pace with which they feel comfortable, take responsibility for their own injections, urine testing, exercise, and diet. Metabolic control is improved when youngsters with this condition are encouraged to take responsibility for what is indeed within their control, but are not

blamed for factors over which they have little or no power (Brown et al., 1991).

Cognitive and learning problems in children with diabetes require careful appraisal by psychologists aware of the possibility that hypoglycemic episodes may be impairing concentration and affecting attention in the school setting.

The psychiatric appraisal of the child with poor biochemical control, requiring repeated hospital admissions for recurrent ketoacidosis, is a crucial part of the assessment of such a problem and should be routine in these circumstances. An interview with the whole family to assess communication about the diabetes and other aspects of family function will usually be clarifying, and seeing the teenager alone will often reveal significant depressive and angry feelings. Mental health professionals should retain an open mind on the issue of whether disturbed family relationships are primary or secondary to the biochemical problems and will need to work closely with pediatricians and endocrinologists in devising management programs tailored to the individual needs of the child and family. Family therapy sessions supplementing pediatric management may enable autonomy issues to be successfully surmounted and communication improved. Behavioral methods, with rewards for the achievement of short-term goals in treatment compliance, may break a vicious cycle of treatment failure and depression, anger, and low self-esteem. Boardway and colleagues (1993) showed that stress management training for the older diabetic adolescent can reduce the impact of specific diabetes-related problems, though it did not benefit metabolic control. Incidentally, there is currently a lack of follow-up studies into adulthood of poorly complying adolescents with diabetes: the results of such studies could clarify important management issues.

Phenylketonuria

BACKGROUND INFORMATION

This condition is due to an inborn error of metabolism in which the lack of the enzyme phenylalanine hydroxylase blocks conversion of phenylalanine to tyrosine, with the resultant accumulation of phenylpyruvic acid, phenylacetic acid, and phenylacetylamine. Competitive inhibition of transport of tyrosine and tryptophan across the blood-brain barrier results in defective myelin production and maturation of gray matter.

The condition occurs in about 1 in 15,000 live births and is inherited as an autosomal-recessive. Neonatal screening on the 4th or 5th day after birth is now undertaken in most economically developed countries and is virtually 100% effective in identifying cases. Dietary treatment is immediately instituted in affected children. This consists of a highly restricted diet, low in phenylalanine, in which most essential substances are provided in a special milk-substitute preparation. The diet used to be relaxed before puberty but is now usually maintained at least in modified form well into adolescence. Uncontrolled relaxation of the diet results in decrements in intelligence in younger children and may precipitate the development of brain syndromes in older patients (Smith et al., 1991). In the childbearing years affected women are at great risk for bearing mentally retarded children because of transfer of brain-toxic substances across the placenta. Such fetal brain damage can be prevented if these women go on a low phenylalanine diet during pregnancy, beginning before conception when planning a child (Drogari et al., 1987).

INTELLECTUAL DEVELOPMENT

Before dietary treatment, affected children were usually, although not always, severely mentally retarded and often had associated psychiatric problems, especially hyperkinesis and autism (Hackney et al., 1968). Epilepsy was common. With current forms of treatment a normal level of intelligence is obtained, and comparisons with control subjects in the general population and with siblings suggest that well-treated children do reach their full intellectual potential. However, even relatively small deviations in biochemical control in early life result in some lowering of IQ. Both the American collaborative study (Holtzman et al., 1986) and the United Kingdom study (Smith et al., 1990) show small but definite decrements in IQ if diet is relaxed in the middle years of childhood.

BEHAVIORAL AND EMOTIONAL DEVELOPMENT

Rates of behavioral deviance are definitely higher in treated children with phenylketonuria than in the general population (Smith et al., 1988). Affected children show more mannerisms, fidgetiness, restlessness, and poor attention, and are more solitary, anxious, and miserable. Behavioral deviance is inversely related both to IQ and to the quality of biochemical control in the early years, but these are, of course, closely related.

The restrictiveness of the diet inevitably places very heavy demands on parents in the early years, and as the child reaches school age, social life is inevitably affected to some degree. Conflicts over diet may become a focus of family tensions (Kazak et al., 1988), and counseling can be helpful here. The high rates of behavioral and emotional disturbance are probably produced both by the direct effects of brain dysfunction and by the increased strain on families produced by the condition and, more especially, its treatment.

Lesch Nyhan Syndrome

This very rare X-linked recessive condition arises as a result of a defective enzyme hypoxanthine-guanidine phosphoribosyl transferase. As well as moderately severe mental retardation, it is accompanied by choreoathetosis, spasticity, and, of particular psychiatric significance, intractable self-injurious behavior. Self-mutilation is often a major problem, with biting of the lips, cheeks, and knuckles, and head-banging as prominent features (Nyhan, 1972).

The behavior of affected boys can sometimes only be contained by the use of restraints such as helmets and mouth guards, but some success has been reported with the use of operant conditioning techniques (McGreevy and Arthur, 1987).

Hypopituitarism

Failure of secretion of the pituitary gland is most commonly manifest by growth failure due to growth hormone (GH) deficiency, though deficiency of other secretions of the anterior pituitary, especially thyroid stimulating hormone (TSH) and adrenocorticotropic hormone (ACTH) may also occur.

GH deficiency may arise from idiopathic hypopituitarism, hypopituitarism of known cause, hypothalamic dysfunction, or target cell unresponsiveness to GH. It occurs in about 1 in 10,000 live births and is four times as common in males as in females. The condition is treatable by the use of GH. Recently the occurrence of Jacob-Kreutzfeld disease in patients treated with human pituitary extract has led to a switch to commercially manufactured GH. Growth delay caused by hypopituitarism and other forms of clear-cut organic etiology must be distinguished for management purposes from those cases in which no sign of a disease process can be identified (normal short stature), as well as those produced by environmental deprivation (Skuse, 1987).

Unless hypopituitarism is produced by a disease process such as a tumor affecting other aspects of brain function, there is usually little evidence of cognitive delay, though visuomotor abilities may be mildly affected. Specific learning difficulties are, however, common, and in the absence of cognitive deficits, these are most likely to be due to anxiety about school attendance in children who are very much smaller than their peers.

In contrast, the social behavior of very small children may be markedly affected. They are not only small in stature, but their facial appearance is also immature, so that, in contrast, for example, to very short children with achondroplasia, there is really no way of telling from their appearance that they are much older than they seem. They may show social withdrawal, especially as adolescence approaches, or may adopt an inappropriate social role, consistently behaving like much younger children. Clowning, often irritating to parents and teachers, has also been described as a means of gaining social acceptance. Disturbed parent-child relationships may occur as a result of anxieties parents naturally feel about the amount the child is eating, and indeed there may be severe feeding difficulties in the first few years of life.

If instituted in the prepubertal period, treatment of short stature due to GH deficiency by GH injection on a regular basis has a marked positive effect on growth. However, follow-up studies to adulthood suggest that social adjustment in later life may be affected in the long-term, as rates of employment and marriage are significantly lower than in normal-height siblings and the general population (Dean et al., 1986). This unsatisfactory outcome might be prevented if as Drotar et al. (1980) suggest, parents and children are counseled using anticipatory guidance. For example, children may be encouraged to role play in situations where they are being mistaken for a much younger child.

Intersex Disorders

These are conditions in which sexual appearance is ambiguous or in which there is inconsistency in the features of sexual differentiation. The criteria for sexual differentiation include chromosomal structure, internal morphology, external morphology (the appearance of the external genitalia), the pattern of sex hormone secretion, gender identity (the degree to which individuals perceive themselves as male or female), gender role (pattern of sex-typed behavior), and choice of sex object. Although chromosomal or gonadal sex are sometimes suggested to be the indicators of true sex, there is no logical justification for this, and indeed gender identity and role might just as reasonably be regarded as the best indicators.

In so-called true hermaphroditism, the gonads contain both ovarian and testicular tissue. Conditions of this type are extremely rare. More common is male and female pseudo-hermaphroditism, in which chromosomes and gonads are clearly differentiated, but the external genitalia are ambiguous. Thus in male pseudohermaphroditism, the chromosome structure is XY, and testes are present although there is cryptorchidism and the external genitalia have a female appearance.

Congenital adrenal cortical hyperplasia (CAH) when it occurs in chromosomal females causes female pseudohermaphroditism and is by far the most common intersex condition. It results from an inherited (autosomal recessive) enzyme defect, usually of 21-hydroxylase. This affects steroid production, and there is excessive androgen excretion in utero and subsequently. In boys this produces precocious puberty. Girls present at birth with ambiguous genitalia. A salt-losing syndrome is often associated. The condition is diagnosable after birth and treatable with steroids.

The decision as to which sex the child should be reared as should be made as soon as possible after birth, when the condition has been investigated and the diagnosis made. Decision making should involve parents, pediatricians, and the pediatric surgeon, and psychological or psychiatric input is often helpful. At this stage, the most relevant consideration is the likely external appearance after plastic surgery.

Issues of reassignment of sex after a period in which the child has been brought up in one sex role require very careful consideration, with much psychological or psychiatric input. In general, reassignment of sex after age 2 or 3 presents very considerable problems and involves a major family crisis, as gender identity and parental perceptions are relatively fixed by this time (Money and Erhardt, 1972). Reassignment has been described at puberty with 5-reductase deficiency in males brought up pubertally as females, but this has occurred in a closed community where the condition is relatively common and accepted by members of the community (Imperato-McGinley et al., 1979).

Although the physical outcome of CAH is usually satisfactory given early diagnosis, psychosocial outcome may be much less so (Hochberg et al., 1987). Chromosomal girls raised as females tend to be tomboyish in manner and, postpubertally, have a higher than expected rate of homosexuality (Money et al., 1984). Chromosomal girls raised as males usually have a small penis even after surgical reconstruction and show poor peer relationships and later low sexual potency. If early reassignment of CAH chromosomal females raised as boys is possible, this should be discussed with parents.

Children with intersex conditions and their parents are likely to benefit from continued psychological and psychiatric counseling (Money, 1975). Practical advice concerning how to deal with situations in which, for example, the child's genitalia may be seen by other children will be helpful. Information about the future can be presented in a positive manner. For example, parents and, as they get older, children, can be told that marriage will be possible, as well as child rearing, though this may need to be by adoption. Self-esteem is often closely linked to a clearly defined sexual identity, and children with intersex conditions may need special encouragement for their performance in school or in recreational activities so that they can maintain a good self-image. Counseling for children and families should not be discontinued after the prepubertal years, but should continue well into adolescence, when new difficulties may need to be faced.

Hypothyroidism

BACKGROUND INFORMATION

Although acquired forms of hypothyroidism do occur, by far the most common form of hypothyroidism is congenital and is due either to a developmental abnormality of the thyroid gland or to an inborn error of metabolism. Congenital hypothyroidism occurs in about 1 in 4000 live infants and is much less common in black infants. Neonatal screening programs to detect the condition have now been introduced in most economically developed countries. Treatment with daily replacement therapy is relatively simple and should not impose a significant burden on families with an affected child.

The success of infant screening programs means that it is now becoming increasingly rare to identify hypothyroidism as a cause of slow intellectual development. Nearly all studies report early treated cases have IQs within the normal range, with small deficits of 5–10 points compared to control subjects (e.g., Murphy et al., 1986). Some studies report specific deficits in neuromotor and language function (Rovet et al., 1992). The earlier the treatment and the less severe the form of disease, as measured by physiological parameters, the better the outcome. Nevertheless, thyroid function should be checked in any child with slow psychological development when no other physical or environmental cause is evident.

BEHAVIORAL AND EMOTIONAL DEVELOPMENT

Children with late-treated hypothyroidism show high rates of behavioral deviance, especially high levels of activity and attentional difficulties. However, early-treated children detected by screening have no excess of behavioral disturbance at follow-up into the early school years, though a higher than expected number of affected 6-month-olds may show "difficult temperament" (Rovet et al., 1984). Emotional and behavioral problems in early-treated children with this condition are therefore likely to be related to factors unconnected to their thyroid dysfunction, though a small minority of those treated with thyroxine do seem to be adversely affected by the medication (Rovet et al., 1993).

THYROTOXICOSIS

This condition is extremely rare in infants and young children; it occurs slightly more frequently in older children and adolescents. Although they are not commonly the presenting features, anxiety, emotional lability, overactivity, and restless sleep may accompany the classic clinical picture of increased appetite, loss of weight, tachycardia, fine tremor, and enlargement of the thyroid gland. The condition should be borne in mind when a child presents with recent onset of hyperactivity. As with adults, stress may be of possible importance in the precipitation of the condition (see e.g., Morillo and Gardner, 1979), but no systematic studies have been carried out to verify this suggestion.

BLOOD DISORDERS

Hemophilia

BACKGROUND INFORMATION

In this condition, one of the factors necessary for blood clotting (factor VIII or IX) is absent and excessive bleeding occurs, in severe cases spontaneously and in milder cases after minor trauma. In severe conditions, less than 1% of the missing factor is present. In these circumstances the condition is likely to be chronically handicapping, with most physical damage occurring as a result of bleeding into the joints and bruising of soft tissues, producing pressure on vital structures. Treatment of the severe condition after the first 3 or 4 years can now largely be carried out on an outpatient or home care basis, with first parents and then the child taking responsibility for venipuncture and infusion of the factor in a plasma concentrate. Moderate or mild forms mainly require special precautions to be taken after trauma or before such minor operations as tonsillectomy and dental extractions.

The condition is present in about 1 in 15,000 boys and is inherited as an X-linked recessive. Consequently, 50% of the sons of carrier women are affected.

PSYCHOSOCIAL ASPECTS

Mild and moderate forms of the condition do not usually have any significant effects on the child or the family. There may be some degree of parental overprotection, but if this persists after counseling, there are probably other factors present to explain this parental attitude.

A minority of parents of severely affected children become seriously overprotective, and among these, resentment and bitterness over the child's condition is common (Mattson and Gross, 1966). A few parents function by using denial and show inappropriately little anxiety about the condition. The situation can be complicated by the fact that, in some children, spontaneous bleeding may sometimes occur after emotional stress, perhaps as a result of autonomic effects on capillary walls (Mattson and Gross, 1966).

Severely affected children are often outgoing in personality, and their enjoyment of sports and play-fighting may be particularly exasperating to parents and teachers. Younger children may be unusually clumsy with knives and scissors, perhaps because they have been deprived of appropriate experience with them.

The great majority of even severely affected children can and do now attend normal schools and achieve well educationally (Markova et al., 1980).

In management of the condition it is particularly important that there be good communication between family and pediatrician and that the parents and child know precisely what to do if unusual bleeding occurs. Parents also need reassurance that their children can use knives and scissors if supervised. Parents who continue to be overprotective or whose children show emotional or behavioral disturbance require skilled counseling. Teachers in the ordinary schools such children attend also need information and counseling about the condition.

In the early 1980s a number of hemophiliac children were given HIV-infected plasma concentrate and a high proportion of these have developed AIDS. Affected boys and their families have needed a great deal of counseling and support to cope with this massive additional stress, not only because of the actual risks to the boys' own future but also because of the understandable but misguided concerns of the parents of normal children attending the same schools.

Sickle Cell Disease

BACKGROUND INFORMATION

This is a group of conditions in which there has been a mutation of the β-globin gene. As a result of the abnormality of the red blood cells, both chronic anemia and blockage of small blood vessels occurs. When such blockages arise, they can give rise to acutely painful episodes, so-called vaso-occlusive crises. The condition occurs primarily in black children. Treatment involves preventive health maintenance with the use of prophylactic penicillin, as well as exchange transfusions during crises.

PSYCHOSOCIAL ASPECTS

Not surprisingly, patients with this painful condition have been found to differ both by showing more internalizing (depressive) symptoms, and more externalizing behavior difficulties than their siblings (Brown et al., 1993a). Painful episodes are often intractable even to skilled and experienced management. However, there is some evidence that certain pain-coping strategies, especially those in which the sufferer takes an active, positive approach rather than adopts passive adherence to suggested regimes with negative thinking, require less support from health services (Gil et al., 1993).

Leukemia

BACKGROUND INFORMATION

Cancer of the white blood cells (leukemia) is the most common form of malignancy in childhood, and there is an annual incidence of about 1 in 25,000 children. Acute lymphoblastic leukemia is the most common form. The condition usually presents with a period of nonspecific malaise, perhaps with unusual susceptibility to infection. After a few weeks, episodes of bleeding or the presence of unusual pallor lead to blood testing, and the diagnosis is rapidly made. The etiology is unknown, but there is no good evidence that psychological stress is of importance. Treatment is likely to involve chemotherapy over 2 to 3 years, with intrathecal injections in the first few weeks. Cranial radiotherapy is also now routinely used to prevent secondary CNS deposits. With this form of treatment the outlook has improved, so that 5-year survival (usually indicating a permanent cure) can be expected in 50–60% of affected children.

PSYCHOSOCIAL ASPECTS
Cognitive Development

There is now good and generally consistent evidence from over 20 studies that the cranial irradiation involved in treatment results in about a 10-point full-scale IQ decrement (Cousens et al., 1988). This is probably largely due to the effect of brain dysfunction rather than to psychological trauma. The size of the decrement has been found in follow-up studies to be greater in younger children irradiated below the age of 4 years, but this may be related to the length of follow-up rather than specifically to the age of the child. The size of the IQ decrement may be misleading in relation to the learning ability of the child in that although the IQ may be well within the normal range, the child may have serious problems in learning new material. Radiotherapy following relapse may be associated with further IQ decrements (Christie et al., 1994).

Child and Family Reactions

At the time of diagnosis there is characteristically a period when parents are shocked and question the diagnosis. Repeated explanations of the complicated regimen of treatment with reiteration of the uncertainty of the prognosis are necessary. Parents often find it hard to believe that the physician cannot be more precise in predicting outcome. As the picture unfolds, with or without relapses, and the outlook becomes clearer, family functioning usually improves markedly over time, but Brown and colleagues (1993b) found that about one-third of mothers of children with leukemia showed a DSM III-R psychiatric diagnosis. Kupst and Schulman (1988) have found that good coping is particularly related to the level of family support, the quality of the marital relationship, the lack of other stresses, and the presence of open family communication.

Specific stresses that may be particularly painful to the child and the family include medical failure to make the diagnosis in the disease's very early stages. In the early stages of treatment repeated injections often come to be feared by the child. Short-term side effects of treatment may include nausea and vomiting, as well as hair loss. The child may be embarrassed in school by his or her appearance. The need to protect the child against infection may result in serious anxiety, especially in the school setting, and school refusal may occur for this and other reasons.

IMPLICATIONS FOR MANAGEMENT

Pediatricians and oncologists will need to spend a considerable amount of time in explanations to parents and in preparing children for unpleasant investigations or forms of treatment. The involvement of mental health professionals is invaluable for a variety of reasons. Parents may require counseling to maintain positive communication with each other and with the child. If treatment fails, there needs to be discussion concerning terminal aspects of care, especially the relief of pain and discomfort; with older children the parents may need help in continuing to communicate. For most older children, an open approach to communication will seem desirable to parents, the child, and physicians and nurses, but this may not always be the case. Professional staff support will be necessary, especially for relatively inexperienced nursing staff who may be severely stressed in their interactions with parents and child. A sensitive discussion of these issues, especially from the point of view of nursing staff, is available in Gyulay (1978).

RENAL DISEASE

Disorders of the urinary tract of particular psychiatric significance include urinary infections, which may occasionally raise suspicion of sexual abuse (see Chapter 100), enuresis (see Chapter 54), and the various congenital and inflammatory conditions leading to chronic renal failure.

Failure of kidney function may occur at any stage during childhood, from infancy to adolescence. Children with this debilitating condition will, if it is progressive, require peritoneal dialysis and eventually kidney transplantation. Psychological problems are in excess of healthy control subjects, but most do not show psychiatric disorders (Garralda et al., 1988). In general, the more severe the physical problems, the more likely is the child to show emotional difficulties, particularly anxiety, loneliness, and overdependency on parents.

Posttransplantation psychological difficulties are more likely to occur in children with antecedent personality problems (Korsch et al., 1978), although family distress has usually declined considerably by 1 year posttransplantation. Children with chronic renal failure are at risk of psychological disturbance, and mental health professionals may have a useful part to play in this aspect of management (Drotar and Ganofsky, 1977). When they reach adulthood, survivors of pediatric dialysis and transplant programs may be less socially mature than other people, but their quality of life is not substantially impaired (Reynolds et al., 1993).

GASTROINTESTINAL DISORDERS

Crohn's Disease

Background Information

This chronic inflammatory condition mainly affects the ileum, but other parts of the alimentary tract may be affected also. It presents with abdominal pain, weight loss, and diarrhea. Malabsorption often produces growth failure. Treatment with medication is often only variably successful, and resection of the gut is frequently undertaken in adolescence.

PSYCHOSOCIAL FACTORS

Psychological factors are no longer thought to be of primary significance in the etiology, but stress may be one of a number of factors producing relapses. Children suffering from this condition are often chronically miserable and unhappy, and this probably occurs partly because of the debilitating, unpleasant nature of the disease. The rate of emotional disturbance in sufferers is about four times that of control subjects (Steinhausen and Kies, 1982), and sufferers are more likely to feel their fate is no longer in their own hands and to have a predominantly external locus of control (Engstrom, 1991a). Patients with this condition have low self-esteem (Raymer et al., 1984). The presence of psychopathology is related to growth failure but not to other clinical measures. Mothers of children with inflammatory bowel disease, both Crohn's and ulcerative colitis (discussed below), have very high rates of distress (Engstrom, 1991b). Management of the condition should include psychological support. Interpretive psychotherapy is unlikely to be helpful, although it may reveal significant psychopathology. McDermott and Finch (1967), for example, found long-standing compulsive personality traits in girls and passive-aggressive or dependent features in boys. If stoma surgery is undertaken, careful psychological as well as physical preparation will improve results (Lask, 1988).

Ulcerative Colitis

BACKGROUND INFORMATION

Acute episodes of noninfective inflammation of the colon and rectum characterize this chronic condition. Bloody diarrhea is often associated with abdominal pain and, less frequently, anorexia, nausea, and vomiting. Both intestinal and nonintestinal complications are common and long-term; the risk of intestinal cancer is one of the reasons for undertaking gut resection in chronic cases.

PSYCHOSOCIAL FACTORS

A considerable psychiatric literature, mainly written in the 1950s and early 1960s, ascribed primary etiology to psychological factors, especially the presence of unconscious hostility and severe personality disturbances mainly of obsessional type. Subsequent studies, especially those of Feldman et al. (1967), failed to confirm these suggestions, although emotional stress can certainly precipitate relapse and play a significant part in the maintenance of this condition.

Children suffering from the condition have high rates of emotional disturbance (Raymer et al., 1984; Steinhausen and Kies, 1982), but this is likely to be largely secondary to the distressing nature of the condition. Stoma surgery, if it results in symptom relief, is often associated with considerable psychological improvement.

Supportive psychotherapy, delivered either by the pediatrician responsible for physical management or by a mental health professional working as part of the team, is often helpful (McDermott and Finch, 1967), but psychiatric referral will be more clearly indicated where there is a significant associated psychiatric disorder, a not infrequent occurrence. As with Crohn's disease, preparations for stoma surgery should include discussion of the psychological as well as the physical aspects of this form of surgical treatment.

JUVENILE RHEUMATOID ARTHRITIS

Background Information

This is a group of conditions in which one or a number of joints are affected by an inflammatory process. Classification of this group is not fully satisfactory, but subdivisions include systemic, polyarticular, and pauciarticular forms of the disease. About 25% of children, particularly those who are rheumatoid factor-positive, develop a chronic form of the condition characterized by limitation of movement, deformity, and pain. The prevalence of chronic arthritis in children is about 1 in 1500. The etiology of these conditions is poorly understood, but there is probably an interaction of genetic, infective, and immunological factors. There is no good evidence that psychological stress is of primary importance

in etiology, although Heisel (1972) provides some inconclusive evidence for life changes and consequent stress playing some part.

Psychosocial Features

Psychosocial factors are relevant to many aspects of the management of the chronic form of this disease. There is conflicting evidence as to whether children with arthritis have a higher than expected rate of behavioral and emotional problems. McAnarney et al. (1974) found an association, but with the paradoxical finding that it was the least physically handicapped children who showed the most disturbance. More recently, Billings et al. (1987), Wallander et al. (1988), and Daltroy et al. (1992) have found little or no excess of psychiatric problems in this condition; and these studies appear better controlled, and their findings seem to have great validity.

Nevertheless, children with chronic arthritis certainly have many psychosocial problems related to their condition. In young, severely affected children, a poor self-concept may be experienced (Ungerer et al., 1988). Older children, especially those with a poor self-concept, spend less time with friends and relatives than do normal children. Sexual anxieties are common in both sexes, and girls in particular are prone to depression (Wilkinson, 1981).

Pain is perhaps the most unpleasant feature of the condition. Beales et al. (1983) found that younger children appear to experience less pain than older children and adults, possibly because the young child does not attach such unpleasant meaning to the pain every time it is experienced. Mothers are generally less positive than their children about the impact of the condition on family life (Ennett et al., 1991). The psychosocial functioning of both parents is closely rated to fluctuations in the child's symptomatology (Timko et al., 1992).

The management of arthritis requires that children and parents consider ways in which disability can be lessened. There is a danger of social isolation, particularly as the youngster moves into the teenage years. The affected adolescent may need counseling concerning sexual anxieties, and a positive attitude toward careers will prevent adolescents from developing depressive ideas that there is no place for them in the adult world.

INFECTIOUS DISEASES

Intrauterine Infections

Infection contracted in utero may cause brain damage and have a marked effect on postnatal psychological and psychosocial functioning.

Congenital rubella is now, as a result of successful immunization programs, relatively rare in the United States but still occurs with some frequency in the United Kingdom and other countries where immunization coverage is less comprehensive. The fetus is particularly at risk of infection in the first 4 months of gestation. Sequelae identifiable at, or soon after birth, include a wide range of neurological disorders, cataracts, and sensorineural deafness.

Mental retardation occurs in about half of affected cases, and in those children in whom mental retardation occurs, it is commonly associated with characteristic childhood autism. Visual impairment also increases the risk of autism and autistic features (Chess and Fernandez, 1980), though of markedly atypical type and better prognosis. The autism is usually of early-onset but may also occur after a period of normal development. Management of autism should be similar to that for children when the etiology is unknown, but, of course, the genetic implications will be different.

Cytomegalovirus (CMV), a form of herpesvirus, occurs widely among pregnant women (50–60% in the United States), but only about 1% of infants are infected with CMV at birth. About 10% of these have disseminated infections, which may produce brain damage leading to hearing loss and mental retardation. Interpretation of the results of survey evidence is complicated by the fact that the condition is more common among socioeconomically deprived groups.

Other intrauterine infections that may produce cerebral damage or dysfunction include other viral conditions (e.g., herpes simplex), syphilis, and protozoal infections such as toxoplasmosis. Congenital HIV infection is discussed in Chapter 97.

Postnatal Infectious Disease

Infectious diseases, especially upper and lower respiratory tract and gastrointestinal infections, are the most common conditions affecting young children and are responsible for most absences from school and health professional consultations during this age period. Psychosocial factors are relevant in understanding the etiology and outcome, and mental changes are occasionally prominent in symptomatology.

ETIOLOGY

Although the extent of exposure to the infective agent and the child's immunological state will be the main determinants, psychosocial factors may nevertheless be relevant in causation. Children living in poor social conditions are more prone to infection than are those from privileged groups. There is a relationship between the frequency of infection and social class (Colley, 1976). More specific adverse social factors, such as overcrowding and damp housing, have also been identified as significant (Martin et al., 1987).

Stressful circumstances may also predispose to infection. Many years ago Meyer and Haggerty (1962) showed, for example, a link between the occurrence of β-hemolytic streptococcal infection and a period of family stress.

MANIFESTATION

Acute infections are often accompanied by irritability and/or tiredness. When the physical manifestations are nonspecific, as is sometimes the case with urinary infections and meningitis, infections may, especially in the young child, be mistaken for behavioral or emotional disorders. Infections that involve invasion of brain tissue or the meninges or that produce an acute toxic state may result in an acute or subacute delirious state. Episodes of drowsiness will alternate with states of agitation in which the child may be confused and disoriented and may visually hallucinate. Differential diagnosis involves exclusion of poisoning, either accidental or non-accidental, and epilepsia partialis continuans.

POSTINFECTIVE STATES

Encephalitis and meningitis may result in permanent brain damage, producing long-term motor abnormalities. This is an unusual outcome, occurring, for example, in about 3–7% of children suffering bacterial meningitis. Hearing defects following meningitis are relatively more common (10%), and these may lead to learning difficulties (Sell, 1983). Learning problems may also occur as a result of specific visuospatial or visuomotor deficits following *Hemophilus influenzae* meningitis (Taylor et al., 1984). These sequelae are more likely to arise if the meningitis has been contracted before the age of 1 year (Chamberlain et al., 1983). It should be remembered that follow-up studies are usually only carried out on the most seriously affected children admitted to specialist centers, and long-term morbidity rates may, overall, be lower than those described here.

It has been suggested that following encephalitis, specific behavioral and personality changes such as irritability, aggression, and withdrawal may occur in children in the absence of overt brain damage (Sabatino and Cramblett, 1968). It is difficult to know whether such effects arise as a result of brain dysfunction or as a consequence of the frightening experiences (e.g., hospitalization, separation from parents, physical investigations such as lumbar punctures and brain scans) that children experience while suffering from encephalopathic illnesses.

Progressive dementia leading to a fatal outcome is fortunately rare in postinfective states but occurs in subacute sclerosing panencephalitis

(SSPE), a complication of infection with measles virus, occurring months or years after the initial infection. The early signs of this condition often include irritability, moodiness, and a deterioration in schoolwork, so that a psychiatric disorder is frequently suspected. Later an obvious organic deterioration supervenes, and myoclonic jerking may be observed. A pathognomonic EEG pattern with regularly occurring bursts of high-voltage spike wave activity occurring on a background of slow activity confirms the presence of the condition.

Postviral fatigue syndromes are also described in children. In this condition (known as myalgic encephalomyelitis or ME syndrome in the United Kingdom) children suffer from weakness and exhaustion following even small amounts of exercise. There may also be more nonspecific symptomatology such as inattention, irritability, withdrawal, muscle aches and pains, and depression. There is controversy over the nature of this condition. When it occurs, as it sometimes does, in epidemic form, sufferers have been shown to have a preexisting tendency to anxiety and somatic symptoms. Further, although viral etiology is claimed and indeed raised coxsackievirus B titers have been identified more commonly in groups of sufferers than in control subjects, viral studies in individuals are often negative. Untreated, this condition may last months or even years (David et al., 1988). Gradual physical rehabilitation with a positive approach to an increase in physical activity usually results in speedier recovery. Depressive disorders may also occur in classic form following viral infections (see Chapter 60).

ECZEMA

Dryness and scaling of the skin may be limited to the limb flexures but may also be widespread and disfiguring. The condition nearly always begins in the first 5 years, and usually in the first few months of life. It usually has a benign prognosis for full recovery before school age, but in a small minority of cases it continues at least until the middle school years. The condition is probably caused by an inherited immunological dysfunction, and most patients have elevated immunoglobulin E levels and T cell abnormalities. Onset may be associated with the introduction of artificial milks or mixed feeding; occasionally attacks may be precipitated by ingestion of particular food substances.

Psychosocial Aspects

There is no convincing evidence that psychosocial factors are important in the primary etiology of eczema, but they may be of significance in its maintenance, and psychological distress with disturbed family relationships is relatively common in severe forms of the condition. Further, exacerbations of the condition are accompanied by significant increases in the rate of behavior problems (Daud et al., 1993).

The intractable itching and scratching that may occur can result in parents' developing anxiety, depression, and anger toward their children, who, they may believe, should be able to resist the temptation to scratch and exacerbate the condition. Children may themselves become depressed for similar reasons. The involvement of parents, especially the mother, in the application of bandages and in frequent bathing may result in the development of an overprotective, enmeshed relationship. Alternatively, one or both parents may feel repelled by the condition and have problems in cuddling or even holding the child. Thus difficulties in the development of attachment may occur (Rauch and Jellinek, 1988).

The relatively benign prognosis and coping capacities of most families mean that specific psychological interventions are not usually indicated, but such intervention may be helpful in intractable cases. In these circumstances an educational approach to parental counseling directed toward more effective limit setting and self-understanding of ambivalent feelings may be helpful (Koblenzer and Koblenzer, 1988). Family sessions in which parents and children are encouraged to communicate both positive and negative feelings may improve symptomatology. Behavior modification, with reinforcement of behaviors alternative to scratching, has occasionally been successful, and a controlled trial of hypnosis in children has been concluded with small but definite benefit to the treated group.

CONCLUSIONS

Psychological and physical interactions do indeed vary considerably between different pediatric diseases, depending on their nature, treatment, and outcome. Further, although the significance of psychosocial factors will vary between children suffering from the same condition, within the practice of every primary care pediatrician, specialist pediatrician, and pediatric surgeon there will be a significant proportion of children who require special attention from this point of view. This has implications for the training of both pediatricians (Graham and Jenkins, 1985) and child psychiatrists. It also brings with it the implication that psychiatric and psychological expertise should be readily available in every setting where chronically ill children are assessed and treated.

References

American Psychiatric Association: *Diagnostic and Statistical Manual of Mental Disorders* (4th ed). Washington, DC, American Psychiatric Press, 1994.

Bailey A, Bolton P, Butler L, et al: Prevalence of the fragile X anomaly amongst autistic twins and singletons. *J Child Psychol Psychiatry* 34:673, 1993.

Baker L, Barcai A, Kay R, et al: Beta adrenergic blockade in juvenile diabetes: Acute studies and long-term therapeutic trial. *J Pediatr* 75:19, 1969.

Beales JG, Keen JH, Holt PJ: The child's perception of the disease and the experience of pain in juvenile chronic arthritis. *J Rheumatol* 10:61, 1983.

Bender BG, Belleau L, Fukuhara JT, et al: Psychomotor adaptation in children with chronic severe asthma. *Pediatrics* 79:723, 1987.

Bicknell J: The psychopathology of handicap. *Br J Med Psychol* 56:167, 1983.

Billings AG, Moos RH, Miller JJ, et al: Psychosocial adaptation in juvenile rheumatic disease: A controlled evaluation. *Health Psychol* 6:343, 1987.

Blackwood DHR, St Clair DM, Muir WJ, et al: The development of Alzheimer's disease in Down's syndrome assessed by auditory event-related potentials. *J Ment Defic Res* 32:439, 1988.

Block J: Further consideration of psychosomatic predisposing factors in allergy. *Psychosom Med* 30: 202, 1968.

Boardway RH, Delamater AM, Tomakowsky J, et al: Stress management training for adolescents with diabetes. *J Pediatr Psychol* 18:29, 1993.

Breslau N: Psychiatric disorder in children with physical disabilities. *J Am Acad Child Psychiatry* 24: 87, 1985.

Brown RT, Kaslow NJ, Doepke K, et al: Psychosocial and family functioning in children with sickle cell syndrome and their mothers. *J Am Acad Child Adolesc Psychiatry* 32:545, 1993a.

Brown RT, Kaslow NJ, Madan-Swain A, et al: Parental psychopathology and children's adjustment to leukemia. *J Am Acad Child Adolesc Psychiatry* 32:554, 1993b.

Brown RT, Kaslow NJ, Sansbury L, et al: Internalising and externalising symptoms and attributional style in youths with diabetes. *J Am Acad Child Adolesc Psychiatry* 30:921, 1991.

Bundey S: The fragile X syndrome. *Practitioner* 23:910, 1987.

Burton L: *The Family Life of Sick Children*. London, Routledge & Kegan Paul, 1975.

Bywater M: Adolescents with cystic fibrosis: Psychosocial adjustment. *Arch Dis Child* 56:538, 1981.

Bywater M: Coping with a life-threatening illness: An experiment in parents' groups. *Br J Soc Work* 14:117, 1984.

Cadman D, Boyle M, Szatmari P, et al: Chronic illness, disability, and mental and social well-being: Findings of the Ontario Child Health Study. *Pediatrics* 79:805, 1987.

Carr J: Mental and motor development in young Mongol children. *J Ment Defic Res* 14:205, 1970.

Carr J: Six weeks to twenty-one years old: A longitudinal study of children with Down syndrome and their families. *J Child Psychol Psychiatry* 29: 407, 1988.

Cassell S, Paul M: The role of puppet therapy on the emotional responses of children hospitalized for cardiac catheterization. *J Pediatr* 71:233, 1967.

Cassileth BR, Lusk EJ, Strouse TB, et al: Psychosocial status in chronic illness. A comparative analysis of six diagnostic groups. *N Engl J Med* 311:506, 1984.

Chamberlain RM. Christie PM, Holt K. et al: A study of schoolchildren who had identified virus infection during infancy. *Child Health Care Dev* 9:29, 1983.

Chess S, Fernandez P: Neurologic damage and behavior disorder in rubella children. *Am Ann Deaf* 125:998, 1980.

Christie D, Battin M, Leiper AD, et al: Neuropsychological and neurological outcome after relapse of lymphoblastic leukaemia. *Arch Dis Child* 70:275, 1994.

Clayton-Smith, J: Clinical research on Angelman syndrome in the United Kingdom: Observations on 82 affected individuals. *Am J Med Genet* 46:12, 1993.

Close H, Davies AG, Price DA, et al: Emotional difficulties in diabetes mellitus. *Arch Dis Child* 61: 337, 1986.

Colland VT: Learning to cope with asthma: a behavioural self-management programme for children. *Patient Educ & Counselling* 22:141, 1993.

Colley JRT: Epidemiology of respiratory disease in childhood. In: Hull D (ed): *Recent Advances in Paediatrics* (no. 5). London, Churchill Livingstone. 1976.

Cousens P, Waters B, Said J, et al: Cognitive effects of cranial irradiation in leukaemia: A survey and meta-analysis. *J Child Psychol Psychiatry* 29: 839, 1988.

Cowen L, Mok J, Corey M, et al: Psychologic adjustment of the family with a member who has cystic fibrosis. *Pediatrics* 77:745, 1986.

Crowe SF, Hay DA: Neuropsychological dimensions of the fragile X syndrome. Support for a nondominant hemisphere dysfunction hypothesis. *Neuropsychologica* 28:9, 1990.

Cytryn L, Cytryn E, Rieger E: Psychological implications of cryptorchidism. *J Am Acad Child Psychiatry* 6:131, 1967.

Daltroy LH, Larson MG, Eaton MH, et al: Psychosocial adjustment in juvenile arthritis. *J Pediatr Psychol* 17:277, 1992.

Daud LR, Garralda ME, David TJ: Psychosocial adjustment in preschool children with atopic eczema. *Arch Dis Child* 69:670, 1993.

David AS, Wessely S, Pelosi AJ: Post-viral fatigue syndrome: Time for a new approach. *Br Med J* 296:696, 1988.

Davies K: *The Fragile X Syndrome*. Oxford, Oxford University Press, 1989.

Dean HJ, McTaggart TL, Fish TL, et al: Long-term social follow-up of growth hormone deficient adults treated with growth hormone during childhood. In: Stabler B, Underwood LE (eds): *Slow Grows the Child. Psychosocial Aspects of Growth Delay*. Hillsdale, NJ, Erlbaum, 1986, p. 73.

DeMaso DR, Campis LK, Wypij D, et al: The impact of maternal perception and medical severity on the adjustment of children with congenital heart disease. *J Pediatr Psychol* 16:137, 1991.

Donaldson MDC, Chu CE, Cooke A, et al: The Prader-Willi syndrome. *Arch Dis Child* 70:58, 1994.

Downey J, Erhardt AA, Morishima A, et al: Gender role development in two clinical syndromes: Turner's syndrome versus constitutional short stature. *J Am Acad Child Adolesc Psychiatry* 26:566, 1989.

Drogari E, Smith I, Beasley M, et al: Timing of strict diet in relation to fetal damage in maternal phenylketonuria. *Lancet* 2:927, 1987.

Drotar D, Doershuk C, Stern R, et al: Psychological functioning of children with cystic fibrosis. *Pediatrics* 67:338, 1981.

Drotar D, Ganofsky MA: Mental health intervention with children and adolescents with end-stage renal disease. *Int J Psychiatry Med* 7:179, 1977.

Drotar D, Owens R, Gotthold J: Personality adjustment of children and adolescents with hypopituitarism. *Child Psychiatry Hum Dev* 11:59, 1980.

Eiser C: *Growing Up with a Chronic Disease*. Philadelphia and London, 1993.

Engstrom I: Family interaction and locus of control in children and adolescents with inflammatory bowel disease. *J Am Acad Child Adolesc Psychiatry* 30:913, 1991a.

Engstrom I: Parental distress and social interaction in families with children with inflammatory bowel disease. *J Am Acad Child Adolesc Psychiatry* 30:904, 1991b.

Ennett S, Devellis BM, Earp JA, et al: Disease experience and psychosocial adjustment in children with juvenile rheumatoid arthritis: Children's versus mother's reports. *J Pediatr Psychol* 16:557, 1991.

Feldman F, Cantor D, Soll S, et al: Psychiatric study of a consecutive series of 34 patients with ulcerative colitis. *Br Med J* 3:14, 1967.

Ferguson-Smith MA: Karyotype-phenotype correlations in gonadal dysgenesis and their bearing on the pathogenesis of malformations. *J Med Genet* 2: 142, 1965.

Fonagy P, Moran GS, Lindsay MKM, et al: Psychological adjustment and diabetic control. *Arch Dis Child* 62:1009. 1987.

Frydman MI: Social support, life events, and psychiatric symptoms: A study of direct, conditioned and interaction effects. *Soc Psychiatry* 16:69, 1981.

Fu Y-H, Kuhl DPA, Pizzuti A, et al: Variation of the CGG repeat at the Fragile X site results in genetic instability: Resolution of the Sherman Paradox. *Cell* 67:1047, 1991.

Garralda ME, Jameson RA, Reynolds JM, et al: Psychiatric adjustment in children with chronic renal failure. *J Child Psychol Psychiatry* 29:79, 1988.

Garson A, Benson RS, Ivler L, et al: Parental reactions to children with congenital heart disease. *Child Psychol Hum Dev* 9:86, 1978.

Gath A: Siblings' reactions to mental handicap; a comparison of brothers and sisters of Mongol children. *J Child Psychol Psychiatry* 15:187, 1974.

Gath A, Alison-Smith M, Baum D: Emotional, behavioural and educational disorders in diabetic children. *Arch Dis Child* 55:371, 1980.

Gath A, Gumley D: Down syndrome and the family: Follow-up of children first seen in infancy. *Dev Med Child Neurol* 26:500, 1984.

Gath A, Gumley D: Retarded children and their siblings. *J Child Psychol Psychiatry* 28:715, 1987.

Gayton WF, Friedman SB, Tavormina JF, et al: Children with cystic fibrosis: Psychological test findings of patients. siblings and parents. *Pediatrics* 59:888, 1977.

Gibbs MV, Thorpe JG: Personality stereotype of non-institutionalised Down syndrome children. *Am J Ment Defic* 87:601, 1983.

Gil KM, Thompson RJ, Keith BR, et al: Sickle cell disease pain in children and adolescents: change in pain frequency and coping strategies over time. *J Paediatr Psychol* 18:621, 1993.

Glaser D, Bentovim A: Psychological aspects of congenital heart disease. In: Anderson RH, Macartney FJ, Shinebourne EA, et al (eds): *Paediatric Cardiology* (Vol 2). Edinburgh, Churchill Livingstone, 1987.

Glasgow RE, McCaul KD, Schafer LC: Self care behaviors and glycemic control in type 1 diabetes. *J Chronic Dis* 40:399, 1987.

Graham P: *Child Psychiatry: A Developmental Approach.* Oxford, Oxford University Press, 1991.

Graham P, Jenkins S: Training of paediatricians for psychosocial aspects of their work. *Arch Dis Child* 60:777, 1985.

Graham P, Rutter M, Yule W, et al: Childhood asthma: A psychosomatic disorder? Some epidemiological considerations. *Br J Prev Soc Med* 21:78, 1967.

Green JM, Dennis J, Bennets LA: Attention disorder in a group of young Down's syndrome children. *J Ment Defic Res* 33:105, 1989.

Gustafsson PA, Kjellman N-IM, Ludvigsson J, et al: Asthma and family interaction. *Arch Dis Child* 62:258, 1987.

Gyulay JE: *The Dying Child.* New York, McGraw-Hill, 1978.

Hackney IM, Hanley WB, Davidson W, et al: Phenylketonuria: Mental development, behaviour and termination of the low phenylalanine diet. *J Pediatr* 72:646, 1968.

Hagerman R: Behaviour and treatment of the fragile X syndrome. In: Davies KE (ed): *The Fragile X Syndrome.* Oxford, Oxford University Press, 1989.

Hagerman RJ, Murphy MA, Wittenberger MD: A controlled trial of stimulant medication in children with the Fragile X Syndrome. *Am J Med Genet* 30:377, 1988.

Hagerman RJ, Schreiner RA, Kemper MB, et al: Longitudinal IQ changes in Fragile X males. *Am J Med Genet* 33:513, 1989.

Hagerman RJ, Sobesky WE: Psychopathology in fragile X syndrome. *Am J Orthopsychiatry* 59:142, 1989.

Haka-Ikse K, Blackwood MJA, Steward DJ: Psychomotor development of infants and children after profound hypothermia during surgery for congenital heart disease. *Dev Med Child Neurol* 20:62, 1978.

Hall BD, Smith DW: Prader-Willi Syndrome: a resume of 32 cases including an instance of affected first cousins, one of whom is of normal stature and intelligence. *Pediatrics* 81: 286, 1972.

Hanson DM. Jackson AW, Hagerman RJ: Speech disturbances (cluttering) in mildly impaired males with the Martin-Bell/Fragile X syndrome. *Am J Med Genet* 23:195, 1986.

Heisel JS: Life changes as etiological factors in juvenile rheumatoid arthritis. *J Psychosom Res* 16:411, 1972.

Herbert M: Personality factors and bronchial asthma: A study of South African Indian children. *J Psychosom Res* 8:353, 1965.

Hill RA, Standen PJ, Tattersfield AE: Asthma, wheezing and school absence in primary schools. *Arch Dis Child* 64:246, 1989.

Hochberg Z, Gardos M, Benderly A: Psychosexual outcome of assigned females and males with 46XX virilising congenital adrenal hyperplasia. *Eur J Pediatr* 146:497, 1987.

Hodapp RM, Dykens EM, Ort SI, et al: Changing patterns of intellectual strengths and weaknesses in males with Fragile X syndrome. *J Autism Dev Disord* 21:503, 1991.

Hodapp RM, Zigler E: Applying the developmental perspective to individuals with Down syndrome. In: Cicchetti B, Beeghly M (eds): *Children with Down Syndrome: A Developmental Perspective.* New York, Cambridge University Press, 1990, pp. 1–28.

Holmes CS, Hayford JT, Gonzalez JL, et al: A survey of cognitive functioning at different glucose levels in diabetic persons. *Diabetes Care* 6:180, 1983.

Holmes DM: The person and diabetes in psychosocial context. *Diabetes Care* 9:194,1986.

Holtzman MA, Kronmal RA, Doorninck W, et al: Effect of age at loss of dietary control on intellectual performance and behavior of children with phenylketonuria. *N Engl J Med* 314:593, 1986.

Horwood L, Fergusson D, Shannon F, et al: Social and familial factors in the development of early childhood asthma. *Pediatrics* 75:859, 1985.

Imperato-McGinley J, Peterson RE, Gautier T, et al: Androgens and the evolution of male gender identity among male pseudohermaphrodites with 5-reductase deficiency. *N Engl J Med* 300:1233, 1979.

Johnson SB: Psychosocial aspects of juvenile diabetes. *J Child Psychol Psychiatry* 29:729, 1988.

Jolleff N, Ryan MM: Communication development in Angelman's syndrome. *Arch Dis Child* 69:148, 1993.

Kaminer Y, Robbins D: Attempted suicide by insulin overdosage in insulin-dependent diabetic adolescents. *Pediatrics* 81:526. 1988.

Kashani JH, Konig P, Shepperd JA, et al: Psychopathology and self-concept in asthmatic children. *J Pediatr Psychol* 13:509, 1988.

Kazak AE, Reber M, Snitzer L: Childhood chronic disease and family functioning: A study of phenylketonuria. *Pediatrics* 81:224, 1988.

Kemmer FW, Bisping R, Steingruber HJ, et al: Psychological stress and metabolic control in patients with type 1 diabetes mellitus. *N Engl J Med* 314:1078, 1986.

Kemper MB, Hagerman RJ, Altshul-Stark D: Cognitive profiles of boys with the fragile X syndrome. *Am J Med Genet* 30:191, 1988.

Koblenzer CS. Koblenzer PJ: Chronic intractable atopic eczema. Its occurrence as a sign of impaired parent-child relationship and psychologic development arrest: Improvement through parent insight and evaluation. *Arch Dermatol* 124:1673, 1988.

Korsch BM, Fine RM. Megrete VP: Non-compliance in children with renal transplants. *Pediatrics* 61:872, 1978.

Kovacs M, Goldston D, Scott Obrosky D: Prevalence and predictors of pervasive non-compliance with medical treatment among youths with insulin-dependent diabetes mellitus. *J Am Acad Child Adolesc Psychiatry* 31:1112, 1992.

Kramer HH, Awiszos D, Sterzel U, et al: Development of personality and intelligence in children with congenital heart disease. *J Child Psychol Psychiatry* 30:299, 1989.

Kupst M-J, Schulman JL: Long-term coping with pediatric leukemia: A 6 year follow-up study. *J Pediatr Psychol* 13:7, 1988.

Lansdown R. Polak L: A study of the psychosocial effects of facial deformity in children. *Child Care Health Dev* 1:85, 1975.

Lask B: Psychological aspects of gastro-intestinal disorder. In: Milla P, Muller D (eds): *Paediatric*

Gastroenterology (2nd ed). London, Churchill Livingstone, 1988.

Lask B: Psychological treatments for childhood asthma. *Arch Dis Child* 67:891, 1993.

Lask B, Matthew D: Childhood asthma-a controlled trial of family psychotherapy. *Arch Dis Child* 54:116, 1979.

Laurance BM: The Prader Willi syndrome. *Mat Child Health* 10:106, 1985.

Lavigne JV, Traisman HS, Marr TJ, et al: Parental perceptions of the psychological adjustment of children with diabetes and their siblings. *Diabetes Care* 5:420, 1982.

Maddison D, Raphael B: Social and psychological consequences of chronic disease in childhood. *Med J Aust* 2:1265, 1965.

Mandoki MW, Sumner GS, Hoffman RP, et al: A review of Klinefelter's syndrome in children and adolescents. *J Am Acad Child Adolesc Psychiatry* 30:167, 1991.

Markova I, Macdonald K, Forbes C: Integration of haemophiliac boys into normal schools. *Child Care Health Dev* 6:101, 1980.

Marteau TM, Bloch S, Baum D: Family life and diabetic control. *J Child Psychol Psychiatry* 28:823, 1987.

Martin CJ, Platts SD, Hunt SM: Housing conditions and ill-health. *Br Med J* 294:1125, 1987.

Mattson A: Long-term physical illness in childhood: A challenge to psychosocial adaptation. *Pediatrics* 50:801, 1972.

Mattson A, Gross S: Social and behavioral studies on hemophiliac children and their families. *J Pediatr* 68:952, 1966.

Matus I: Assessing the nature and clinical significance of psychological contributions to childhood asthma. *Am J Orthopsychiatry* 51:327, 1981.

Mazzocco MM, Hagerman RJ, Cronister-Silverman A, et al: Specific frontal lobe deficits among women with Fragile X gene. *J Am Acad Child Adolesc Psychiatry* 31:1141, 1992.

McAnarney ER, Pless IB, Satterwhite B, et al: Psychological problems in children with chronic juvenile arthritis. *Pediatrics* 53:523, 1974.

McCauley E, Ito J, Kay T: Psychosocial functioning in girls with Turner's syndrome and short stature: Social skills, behavior problems and self-concept. *J Am Acad Child Psychiatry* 25:105, 1986.

McDermott J, Finch S: Ulcerative colitis in children: Reassessment of a dilemma. *J Am Acad Child Psychiatry* 6:512, 1967.

McGreevy P, Arthur M: Effective behavioural treatment of self-biting by child with Lesch-Myhan syndrome. *Dev Med Child Neurol* 29: 536, 1987.

McNichol KM, Williams HE, Allen J, et al: Spectrum of asthma in children. III: Psychological and social components. *Br Med J* 4:16, 1973.

Meyer RJ, Haggerty RJ: Streptococcal infections in families. *Pediatrics* 29:539, 1962.

Miezejeski CM, Jenkins EC, Hill AL. et al: A profile of cognitive deficit in females from Fragile X families. *Neuropsychologia* 24:405, 1986.

Minuchin S: *Families and Family Therapy.* London, Tavistock, 1974.

Mitchell RG, Dawson B: Educational and social characteristics of children with asthma. *Arch Dis Child* 48:467, 1973.

Money J: Sex education and infertility counseling. In: Gardner LI (ed): *Endocrine and Genetic Disease of Infancy and Childhood.* Philadelphia, Saunders, 1975, p. 1228.

Money J, Ehrhardt AA: *Man and Woman, Boy and Girl: The Differentiation and Dimorphism of Gender Identity from Conception to Maturity.* Baltimore, Johns Hopkins University Press, 1972.

Money J, Schwartz M, Lewis VG: Adult emotional status and fetal hormonal masculinisation: 46

XX congenital virilising adrenal hyperplasia and 46 XY androgen insensitivity syndrome compared. *Psychoneuroendocrinology* 9:405, 1984.

Morillo E, Gardner LI: Bereavement as an antecedent factor in thyrotoxicosis of childhood. Four case studies with survey of possible metabolic pathways. *Psychosom Med* 41:545. 1979.

Mrazek DA, Casey B, Anderson I: Increasing attachment in severely asthmatic pre-school children: Is it a risk factor? *J Am Acad Child Psychiatry* 26:516, 1987.

Mrazek DA, Klinnert MD, Mrazek P. et al: Early asthma onset: consideration of parenting issues. *J Am Acad Child Adolesc Psychiatry* 30:277, 1991.

Murphy DGM, Decarli C, Daly E, et al: X-chromosome effects on female brain: a magnetic resonance imaging study of Turner's syndrome. *Lancet* 342:1197, 1993.

Murphy G, Hulse JA, Jackson D, et al: Early treated hypothyroidism: Development at 3 years. *Arch Dis Child* 61:761, 1986.

Nocon A: Social and emotional impact of childhood asthma. *Arch Dis Child* 66:458, 1991.

Nyhan WL: Behavioral phenotypes in organic genetic disease. *Pediatr Res* 6:1, 1972.

Patterson JM, Budd J, Goetz D, et al: Family correlates of a ten year pulmonary health trend in cystic fibrosis. *Pediatrics* 91:383, 1993.

Pearson DA, Pumariega AJ, Seilheimer DK: The development of psychiatric symptomatology in patients with cystic fibrosis. *J Am Acad Child Adolesc Psychiatry* 30:290, 1991.

Penner KA, Johnston J, Faircloth BH, et al: Communication, cognition and social interaction in the Angelman syndrome. *Am J Med Genet* 46:34, 1993.

Peyton JB, Steele MW, Wenger SL, et al: The fragile X marker and autism in perspective. *J Am Acad Child Adolesc Psychiatry* 28:417, 1989.

Pueschel SM, Bernier JC, Pezzullo JC: Behavioural observations in children with Down's syndrome. *J Ment Defic Res* 35:502, 1991.

Purcell K, Weiss J: Asthma. In: Costello C (ed): *Symptoms of Psychopathology*. New York, Wiley, 1970, p. 597.

Rachelefsky GS, Wo J, Adelson J, et al: Behavior abnormalities and poor school performance due to oral theophylline use. *Pediatrics* 78:1133, 1986.

Ratcliffe SG, Bancroft J, Axworthy D, et al: Klinefelter's syndrome in adolescence. *Arch Dis Child* 57:13, 1982.

Ratcliffe SG, Butler GE, Jones M: Edinburgh study of growth and development of children with sex chromosome abnormalities. In: Hamerton J, Robinson A (eds): *Birth Defects*, Original Article Series. New York, Alan R Liss, 1990.

Ratcliffe SG, Field MA: Emotional disorders in XYY children: Four case reports. *J Child Psychol Psychiatry* 23:410, 1982.

Rauch P, Jellinek MS: Psychosocial development in children with cutaneous disease. In: Schachnar LA, Hansen RC (eds): *Psychiatric Dermatology*. New York, Churchill Livingstone, 1988.

Raymer D, Weininger O, Hamilton JR: Psychological problems in children with abdominal pain. *Lancet* 8374(i):439, 1984.

Reiss AL, Aylward E, Freund LS, et al: Neuroanatomy of Fragile X syndrome: The posterior fossa. *Ann Neurol* 29:26, 1991.

Reynolds JM, Morton MJS, Garralda ME, et al: Psychosocial adjustment of adult survivors of a paediatric dialysis and transplant programme. *Arch Dis Child* 68:104, 1993.

Richman LC: The effect of facial disfigurement on teachers' perceptions of ability in cleft palate children. *Cleft Palate J* 15:115, 1978.

Richman LC: Self-reported social, speech and facial concerns and personality adjustment of adolescents with cleft lip and palate. *Cleft Palate J* 20:108, 1983.

Robb SA, Pohl KRE, Baraitser M, et al: The "Happy Puppet" syndrome of Angelman: review of the clinical features. *Arch Dis Child* 64:83, 1989.

Rovet J, Daneman D, Bailey JD: Psychologic and psychoeducational consequences of thyroxine therapy for juvenile acquired hypothyroidism. *J Pediatr* 122:543, 1993.

Rovet J, Ehrlich R, Hoppe M: Behaviour problems in children with diabetes as a function of sex and age of onset of disease. *J Child Psychol Psychiatry* 28:477, 1987.

Rovet J, Ehrlich R, Sorbara DL: Neurodevelopment in infants and pre-school children with congenital hypothyroidism: Etiological and treatment factors affecting outcome. *J Pediatr Psychol* 17:187, 1992.

Rovet J, Westbrook D-L, Ehrlich RM: Neonatal thyroid deficiency: Early temperamental and cognitive characteristics. *J Am Acad Child Psychiatry* 23:10, 1984.

Ryan C, Vega A, Drash A: Cognitive deficits in adolescents who developed diabetes early in life. *Pediatrics* 75:921, 1985.

Sabatino D, Cramblett H: Behavioral sequelae of California encephalitis virus infection in children. *Dev Med Child Neurol* 10:331, 1968.

Sales S, Turk J: Angelman's syndrome: Is there a behavioural phenotype? Paper presented at the annual workshop of the Society for the Study of Behavioural Phenotypes, London, 1991.

Schultz JA: Timing of elective hypospadias repair in children. *Pediatrics* 71:342, 1983.

Sell SR: Long-term sequelae of bacterial meningitis in children. *Pediatr Infect Dis* 2:90, 1983.

Silbert A, Wolff PH, Lilienthal J: Spatial and temporal processing in patients with Turner's syndrome. *Behav Genet* 7:11, 1977.

Simko A, Hornstein L, Soukup S, et al: Fragile X syndrome: Recognition in young children. *Pediatrics* 83:547, 1989.

Skuse D: The psychological consequences of being small. *J Child Psychol Psychiatry* 28:641, 1987.

Skuse D, Percy E, Stevenson J: Psychosocial functioning in the Turner syndrome: A national survey. Paper presented at the annual meeting of the British Paediatric Association, University of Warwick, 1994.

Smith I, Beasley MG, Ades AE: Intelligence and quality of dietary treatment in phenylketonuria. *Arch Dis Child* 65:472, 1990.

Smith I, Beasley MG, Ades AE: Effect on intelligence of relaxing the low phenylalanine diet in phenylketonuria. *Arch Dis Child* 66:311, 1991.

Smith I, Beasley MG, Wolff OH, et al: Behavior disturbance in 8 year old children with early treated phenylketonuria. *J Pediatr* 112:403, 1988.

Steinhausen H-C, Kies H: Comparative studies of ulcerative colitis and Crohn's disease in children and adolescents. *J Child Psychol Psychiatry* 23:33, 1982.

Tal A, Micklich DR: Emotionally induced decreased pulmonary flow rates in asthmatic children. *Psychosom Med* 38:190, 1976.

Taylor HG, Michaels RH, Mazur PM, et al: Intellectual neuropsychological and achievement outcomes in children 6–8 years after recovery from *Haemophilus influenzae* meningitis. *Pediatrics* 74:198, 1984.

Thake A, Todd J, Bundey S, et al: Is it possible to make a clinical diagnosis of the Fragile X Syndrome in a boy? *Arch Dis Child* 60:1001, 1985.

Thake A, Todd J, Webb T, et al: Children with the fragile X chromosome at schools for the mildly mentally retarded. *Dev Med Child Neurol* 29:711, 1987.

Timko C, Stovel KW, Moos RH: Functioning among mothers and fathers of children with chronic rheumatic disease: A longitudinal study. *J Pediatr Psychol* 17:705, 1992.

Turk J: Profile of autistic disturbances in children with genetically determine learning difficulties. Paper presented at the winter meeting of the Royal College of Psychiatrists, London, 1994a.

Turk J: Attentional deficits in boys with Fragile X syndrome: Evidence for a characteristic development profile. Paper presented at the annual meeting of the British Paediatric Association, University of Warwick, 1994b.

Turk J, Hagerman RJ, Barnicoat A, et al: The Fragile X syndrome. In Bouras N (ed): *Mental Health and Mental Retardation—Recent Advances and Practices*. Cambridge, Cambridge University Press, 1994, pp. 135–153.

Ungerer JA, Horgan B, Chaiton J, et al: Psychosocial functioning in children and young adults with juvenile arthritis. *Pediatrics* 81:195, 1988.

Utens EM, Verhulst FC, Meijboom FJ, et al: Behavioural and emotional problems in children and adolescents with congenital heart disease. *Psychol Med* 23:415, 1993.

Verkerk AJMH, Pieretti M, Sutcliffe JS, et al: Identification of a gene (FMR-1) containing a CGG repeat coincident with a breakpoint cluster region exhibiting length variation in Fragile X syndrome. *Cell* 65:905, 1991.

Walker LS, Ford MB, Donald WD: Cystic fibrosis and family stress: Effects of age and severity of illness. *Pediatrics* 79:239. 1987.

Wallander JL, Varni JW, Babani L, et al: Children with chronic physical disorders. Maternal reports of their psychological adjustment. *J Pediatr Psychol* 13:197, 1988.

Webb TP, Bundey S, Thake A, et al: The frequency of the fragile X chromosome among schoolchildren in Coventry. *J Med Genet* 23:396, 1986.

White K, Kolman M-L, Wexler P, et al: Unstable diabetes and unstable families: A psychological evaluation of diabetic children with recurrent ketoacidosis. *Pediatrics* 73:749, 1984.

Whitman BY, Accardo PJ: Behavioral symptomatology in Prader-Willi syndrome adolescents. *Am J Med Genet* 28:897, 1987.

Wilkinson VA: Juvenile chronic arthritis in adolescence: Facing the reality. *Int Rehabil Med* 3:11, 1981.

Williams JS: Aspects of dependence-independence conflict in children with asthma. *J Child Psychol Psychiatry* 16:199, 1975.

Wolff PH, Gardner J, Paccia J, et al: The greeting behaviour of Fragile X males. *Am J Ment Retard* 93:406, 1989.

World Health Organization: *International Classification of Diseases* (10th ed). Geneva, World Health Organization, 1992.

97 NEUROBIOLOGICAL AND PSYCHOSOCIAL ASPECTS OF HIV INFECTION IN CHILDREN AND ADOLESCENTS

Penelope Krener, M.D.

DESCRIPTION OF THE EPIDEMIC

Human immunodeficiency virus type I (HIV-I) brings about slow destruction of the immune system and the central nervous system after an asymptomatic, infective latency period of about 10 years (Haseltine, 1989). Acquired immunodeficiency syndrome (AIDS) was initially an epidemic identified in gay men and recipients of blood products contaminated with the virus (Jones et al., 1992). The epidemic is now spreading most rapidly among intravenous drug users and their sexual partners. Children at risk for HIV infection are infants of intravenous drug users, sexually abused youngsters whose molesters may be bisexual or IV drug users, those who have received blood products between 1982 and 1985, adolescents who use needles, gay adolescents, and those who are sexually active with multiple partners or intravenous drug users. Over one-fifth of all people with AIDS in the United States are between 20 and 29 years (Centers for Disease Control and Prevention (CDC), 1992). Cases in adolescents ages 13–19 are increasing rapidly (American Academy of Pediatrics (AAP) Task Force on Pediatric AIDS, 1993), and the long latency of the virus (Rees, 1987) implies that many adults were infected when they were teenagers. The CDC definitions used for national surveillance are periodically updated to incorporate new findings among women and children. The 1993 version includes a diagnosis of AIDS based on a CD4 cell count of $<200/\mu l$ of blood. This replaces older definitions based on a changeable list of opportunistic infections and malignancies (DesJarlais, 1994).

Seroprevalence varies from low-risk groups such as military recruits, who have a prevalence rate of 0.03% (Braverman and Strasberger, 1992b), to homeless youth in New York City shelters, who have a seroprevalence rate of 0.8% (Miller et al., 1990). A sample of adolescents attending sexually transmitted disease (STD) clinics have a rate of 2.2% (Braverman and Strasberger, 1992b). The progression of the epidemic in children and adolescents shows the same greater prevalence in poor and minority groups as that described in current patterns of increasing spread in adults (Report of Presidential Commission, 1988). AIDS is expected to move into the top five causes of childhood death in the next few years. HIV infection is spreading most rapidly among young populations, especially those who are in the midst of the epidemic of IV drug abuse. Poor and minority children and families are differentially infected with HIV because risk factors for the infection overlap with poverty and substance abuse (Rogers and Williams, 1994). Eighty-five percent of the children who have acquired AIDS perinatally, 71% of women with AIDS, and more than 50% of adolescents with AIDS are black or Hispanic (Coye, 1989).

Heterosexual spread of HIV-I accounts for significant risk for teenage boys. The male-to-female ratio of AIDS is higher in adolescents (4:1) than in adults (9:1). Twelve percent of adolescents with AIDS are partners of high-risk males; this is a much higher proportion of heterosexually transmitted cases than that (2.5%) in adults (AAP Task Force on Pediatric AIDS, 1993).

The HIV-I virus eludes the immune response induced by traditional vaccine procedures because its surface coating closely resembles the surface of normal cells, it mutates rapidly, it may enter a latent intracellular stage, and it may be transferred from cell to cell directly without being visible to the immune system (Haseltine, 1989). Even if a vaccine or cure for AIDS were at hand, psychiatrists would be called on to respond to psychosocial sequelae of the epidemic for the next generation.

INFANTS AND CHILDREN

Vertical Transmission

Perinatal transmission accounts for approximately 80% of pediatric HIV infections and is the most rapidly increasing route of infection with HIV in children (Hutto et al., 1991). Over 20,000 women in the United States have been diagnosed with AIDS; most are of childbearing age and are poor or women of color (Cotton et al., 1994). Rates of transmission of HIV to her fetus from an infected mother range from 20 to 50%, depending upon factors such as maternal T-cell count. In 1984 about 100 cases of pediatric AIDS had been reported to CDC. In 1988 almost 600 cases were reported. In 1992 almost 700 new cases were reported to CDC of children who had acquired the infection perinatally (Oxtoby, 1994), while new cases of transfusion-acquired AIDS cases have dropped to almost zero (Rogers, 1994). Detecting HIV infection in the newborn nursery is compromised by local legal constraints on informed consent for testing and by the fact that antibody measured at birth may be maternal antibody. This requires postponing certainty diagnosis for the infant, as more than half of newborns testing seropositive may not go on to develop HIV because seropositivity reflects maternal infection. Infected infants not identified in the nursery may be diagnosed later either by monitoring their serostatus or when they develop failure to thrive and frequent infections. The asymptomatic mother may learn that she harbors HIV when her infant is diagnosed with AIDS; this is a double catastrophe for the family, and one that necessitates intense psychosocial support. Although some infants with congenital HIV infection deteriorate and die within months, many youngsters infected perinatally with HIV do not manifest illness until early childhood and live into their school years slowly developing chronic illness. Management of HIV-positive infants requires consistent follow-up to evaluate developmental plateauing, nutrition, and interaction with caregivers. Parental dysfunction due to multiple risk factors, including substance abuse or chaotic life situations, must be assessed, which can be a difficult task in busy pediatric settings. Infants have special needs for immunization, for protection against usual childhood illnesses, for nutritional support, and for repeated careful developmental reassessment. When neurologic involvement develops, it is particularly important to try to provide a stable environment with consistent caregivers (Krener, 1987).

Youth with Hemophilia

By June 1982, when the first case of AIDS-related pneumonia in a hemophiliac without other risk factors was reported to CDC, HIV-I had permeated the hemophilia population, efficiently disseminated by the method of extracting factor VIII from pooled blood. Ninety percent of patients with less than 1% factor VIII have become seropositive in some areas. Effective blood bank monitoring and heat-treated factor VIII concentrates have been used since 1985, so currently children infected by blood and blood products are a small and declining proportion of those infected. Hemophilia organizations have responded early and effectively to the need for psychological and organizational resources for children with HIV. As a risk group, children with hemophilia do not suffer from the sociological disadvantages of those perinatally infected through substance abuse in impoverished urban areas. They do, however, have other risk factors that may complicate early assessment of neuropsychological damage resulting from HIV-I infection. These may result from the illness itself. For example, a high incidence of subtle neuropsychological deficits was found in neuropsychological batteries administered by psychologists blind to serostatus in hemophiliac children both seropositive and seronegative for HIV (Whitt et al., 1993).

Hemophilia is a condition that requires major modification of life patterns to minimize its complications; this fact, together with its genetic transmission, make it a central feature of the experience of the hemophiliac child within his family. The intrusion of a lethal virus into the very vehicle for treatment of the condition has placed a simultaneous sentence of death upon several members of hemophiliac families and has done so through the same medical means around which they had organized their hope of living in health. Moreover, the prevalence of the infection in the hemophiliac community means that the group with whom the hemophilia patient may identify, and from whom he may derive support, are also infected, ill, or dying.

The psychological consequences are therefore profound, despite anecdotal information that infected hemophiliac youth appear to have curiously better survival times. Child psychiatrists consulting to hemophilia services must prepare to work with a multidisciplinary team, as is customary, to help youngsters live optimally with a chronic medical condition, and must now employ their particular training to evaluate insidious neurodegenerative processes brought about by the virus and to help treat the rage and grief resulting from the succession of losses it will create in the hemophiliac community.

Children Infected by Sexual Molestation

HIV infection resulting directly from child sexual abuse has been described. Perpetrators may derive from any social background but there is significant overlap of child sexual molestation with substance abuse disorders, with disturbed function or disorganization in families, and with other sexual difficulties. Sexual assault, one of the most underreported crimes, more commonly has adolescent victims rather than adult women. Female adolescents are at highest risk for completed rape and all other forms of sexual assaults (Protherow-Smith, 1989). Stratified random sampling of youths seen in public health clinics shows that a history of physical abuse, sexual abuse, or rape is related to practicing HIV risk behaviors (Cunningham et al., 1994).

The painful documentation of details of molestation or rape by examining and interviewing young victims is familiar to pediatricians and child psychiatrists. Evaluation of risk for HIV exposure complicates an already delicate and difficult process, as it may pose procedural challenges of assessing serostatus of accused molesters. Legalities of obtaining informed consent for testing and bioethical dilemmas about disclosure of results are not well worked out for children and adolescents. Child psychiatrists may need to become involved in developing individualized case solutions.

ADOLESCENT PATTERNS OF RISK AND TRANSMISSION: SEX, DRUGS, AND RUNNING AWAY

Sex

Adolescents in the United States are sexually active. The median age of first intercourse is now under 17 years (D'Angelo, 1994); by age 20, 75% of females and 80% of males have had intercourse (Braverman and Strasberger, 1992a). Their sexual practices include oral sex and anal intercourse, during which 70% do not use condoms. One in six of sexually active teenagers has had a STD (Braverman and Strasberger, 1992b). One in 10 teenage women become pregnant each year (Braverman and Strasberger, 1992a), with cumulative risk of pregnancy up to age 20 being almost 40%, and 125,000 to 200,000 adolescents become involved in prostitution each year (DiClemente, 1989).

National data on adolescents with AIDS show that 73% were infected by intravenous drug use or sexual activity, and 22% through exposure to infected blood products (Braverman and Strasberger, 1992b). Regional differences account for some local differences in proportions. A recent (Moscicki et al., 1993) study of high-risk behaviors in adolescents compared responses of youths attending a university-based clinic, a planned parenthood neighborhood clinic, and an inner city public health clinic. All groups had high rates of anal intercourse (21%), unprotected vaginal sex (95%), and oral sex (73%), but there were higher rates of homosexual experiences and multiple partners in the public health clinic, and higher rates of substance abuse associated with sexual activity in the other two clinics. Hence, the authors caution against ascribing particular risk behaviors to particular populations. Adolescents with psychiatric symptomatology are at higher risk for HIV infection for several reasons. They have a high prevalence of sexual activity, with ensuing STDs, and are likelier to have intercourse with multiple partners and to have experienced sexual abuse or forced sex. They are more likely to have associated substance abuse, and dual diagnoses are frequent in adolescents admitted to both privately and publicly funded inpatient units. Not uncommonly they practice self-injurious behaviors alone, or in groups, with shared cutting implements (DiClemente et al., 1989), a newly identified risk behavior.

One adolescent in 10 struggles with the problem of same-sex orientation (Braverman and Strasberger, 1992a). Teenagers attracted to their own sex are also sexually active and may have special vulnerabilities because they preferentially seek older partners and because the urgent connection between their sexuality and their emerging identity may propel them into risky sexual behavior. Sex between males accounts for about half of the non-transfusion-associated cases of AIDS among boys between 13 and 19 (AAP Committee on Adolescents, 1993). Gay youth are likelier to become runaways if conflict within the family revolving around sexuality issues is intolerable. There are few studies of adolescent homosexuality beyond individual case reports of therapy. Remafedi (1987) anonymously interviewed 29 gay and bisexual male teenagers. The majority had school problems related to sexuality, substance abuse, and or emotional difficulties warranting mental health intervention. Half had had sexually transmitted diseases, had been runaways, or had had trouble with the law. A minority had been victims of sexual assault or had been involved in prostitution. In a sample of patients in a private university-maintained inpatient unit in San Francisco, 25% of the males reported having sexual intercourse with other males, and half were youngsters who reported sexual abuse and forced sex (DiClemente et al., 1989). Gay youngsters are likelier to have emotional disorders, in part stemming from reactions to homophobic responses to their emerging identity, and these may interfere with their caring for their own health and maintaining protective assertiveness when pressured to engage in unsafe sexual practices.

Drugs

The rapid spread of the epidemic of drug use demands that all psychiatrists be familiar with substance abuse disorders. Adolescents do not always say "no" to intravenous or other drugs. Findings of a 1986 national study by the National Institute for Drug Abuse were that 1% of high school seniors reported having used heroin through needle injections. In some inner city areas, where drug use and addiction is a socially contagious environmental hazard, this figure may be much higher. The proportions of IV drug use related AIDS cases vary widely; 93% of cases have been reported from 13 states. Importantly, it has been found that drug users can learn about retroviral transmission, and, if given the means, will choose to protect themselves against infection using clean needles (DesJarlais and Friedman, 1994).

Runaways

Runaways are subject to many sources of risk for HIV infection (Stircof et al., 1991). The Department of Health and Human Services

(DHHS) estimates a million youngsters run away from home each year, and one quarter remain homeless and on the streets (DHHS, 1986a). Runaways range from 12 to 17 years (mean 15.3 years). Eighty-five percent are sexually active. A similar percent use illegal drugs, and 5% use IV drugs (DHHS, 1986b). Problems with the law are reported in 78% of boys and 47% of girls. Thirty-four percent of runaway girls become pregnant. Of runaways found to have dropped out of or to have been expelled from school 71% were boys, and 44% were girls. Thirty-four percent report having been physically abused or neglected at home, and 63% are "throwaways" or are homeless by mutual agreement of parents and teens. This group has a wide variety of medical problems and health-endangering behaviors including prostitution and drug abuse. Many cite their same-sex orientation as the reason for leaving home. Whitaker et al. (1990), studying teenage shelter users, found them to have a psychiatric profile largely indistinguishable from adolescents attending a psychiatric clinic, with 30% being found to be depressed, 18% antisocial, and 41% depressed and antisocial. Fifty percent had considered suicide and half of these had attempted suicide. Runaway teens are at greater risk for infection and are unarmed with the psychological resources needed to translate health care information into personal patterns of protection. Although they are a difficult population to track, evidence indicates that they are becoming infected with HIV at higher rates than their age mates. Limited street surveys in Newark, New Jersey, and a more comprehensive survey at Covenant House in New York City found HIV infection rates among teenagers living on the street from 7–18% (Coye, 1989).

NEUROPSYCHIATRIC MANIFESTATIONS OF HIV IN PEDIATRIC PATIENTS

HIV-I Invasion of the Brain

The brain is a primary site of HIV infection in infants and children, leading to calcification of basal ganglia (Epstein et al., 1988) and impaired brain growth (Epstein et al., 1987). The prevalence of HIV-I-related CNS disease in infants and children is unknown, but a recent estimate at the National Cancer Institute was 30–40% in symptomatic children referred for antiretroviral therapy (Brouwers et al., 1994). Central manifestations are the result of direct viral infection of the brain. The virus can be recovered in CSF before it can be detected in blood (Haseltine, 1989; Jacobson and Siegelman, 1985; Pumerola-Sune, 1987) and has been estimated to cause CNS dysfunction in 50–90% of children (Scott, 1988). In children as well as infants, CNS involvement may complicate developmental delay caused by nutritional and situational factors related to chronic illness (Epstein et al., 1987; de la Monte et al., 1987). Central nervous system events include acute encephalitis in the early stage of infection before the host immune response has mobilized. Infection may be asymptomatic, or aseptic meningitis may occur at any point. Clinical severity of AIDS dementia complex (ADC) is correlated well with the neuropathology that afflicts white rather than gray matter. Motor symptoms involve legs before arms, and clumsiness precedes weakness of gait. The magnetic resonance imaging (MRI) may show discrete areas of increased signal in white matter. The computerized tomography (CT) and MRI both may show cortical atrophy and ventricular dilation, but also may be normal. CT scans show variable degrees of cerebral atrophy and decreased attenuation in white matter. Recent findings implicate altered astrocyte function as part of HIV-I neuropathogenesis. Interventions should be directed at reducing the viral load in the CNS and blocking viral or cellular products that mediate neuronal damage (Brouwers et al., 1994).

Clinical Features

ADC may occur at any point in the disease, with increasing likelihood as the illness progresses (Report of the Presidential Commission, 1988). Unanswered questions are how early after infection does the virus affect the brain, and what is the course of ADC? The finding of Grant et al. (1987), that asymptomatic HIV-positive persons had neuropsychological abnormalities, received lively attention. The balance of evidence indicates that a mild degree of impairment can be detected in 20–33% of medically asymptomatic HIV-positive adults (Martin, 1994).

Cognitive slowing may be evidenced by simple reaction times and decision-making speed on a detection and decision task, more so if the HIV-positive person is symptomatic. Abnormalities of spatial attention and of controlled processing have been found (Martin et al., 1992a, 1992b). Such impairments exhibit a pattern consistent with subcortical dysfunction (Marsh and McCall, 1994). Early symptoms are impaired attention and concentration, memory loss, slowed information processing, mild frontal lobe dysfunction, and difficulty with performance of complex sequential mental activities. ADC is chronically progressive with subcortical dementia and a variable constellation of cognitive, motor, and behavioral disturbances. ADC becomes progressively likelier later in the course of the disease, and opportunistic CNS infections may supervene toward the end (Price et al., 1990).

CDC defines the dementia as "clinical findings of a disabling cognitive or motor dysfunction interfering with occupational activity or loss of behavioral milestones affecting a child." It is a diagnosis of exclusion after CSF examination and CT or MRI. Most symptomatic HIV-I-infected children have some degree of neurological and neuropsychological impairment (Brouwers et al., 1994). This is influenced by the disease stage and age of the child. Static encephalopathy has been described in about 25% of symptomatic children. Progressive encephalopathy has a higher incidence in infants and young children and has been reported as a first manifestation in perinatally infected children. The course for perinatally infected children may be better than previously thought (Tovo et al., 1992).

Diagnostic Assessment

Neuropsychological testing will establish a baseline and allow distinguishing between static encephalopathy, with cognitive development occurring below the expected curve and with a flatter slope, and progressive encephalopathy, which leads to a more rapid decline in function. Brouwers et al. (1994) set forth a test schedule and a recommended test battery for core assessment and for periodic monitoring. It is important to test general intelligence, but also attention, expressive behavior, language skills, memory, concept formation, and motor development. Behavior and personality should also be assessed, as psychosocial factors may influence cognitive performance to some degree. For example, deficits in physical growth affect social adaptation, and depression may influence attention and cognitive effort on testing. Because the goal of testing is to estimate the child's optimal level of functioning, it is important to avoid testing the child near the time of painful or disturbing procedures.

It is possible that other factors may influence abnormal performance on neuropsychological test batteries (Maj et al., 1994). Global neuropsychiatric impairment was significantly increased in asymptomatic seropositive subjects in two of five research centers in an international WHO Neuropsychiatric AIDS study. Subjects in Zaire and Kenya with higher education were less likely to have an impaired performance than those in Brazil, Germany, or Thailand. The authors discuss these findings in the context of a "cerebral reserve" theory, namely, that redundancy of cerebral networks may be reduced by organic or psychosocial factors such as malnutrition, presence of other diseases affecting the CNS, or lack of social and educational stimulation.

In children this is a crucial issue for studies parallel to those underway with adults (Van Gorp et al., 1989). The child's developing brain with incomplete education might be one lacking in "cerebral reserve," particularly if that child resides in an impoverished environment and has complications of his or her chronic illness that have caused the child to miss school and other educational opportunities. The normal test variation in IQ measurement may be up to 10 points, but declines in IQ secondary to HIV infection may be faster and steeper in very young children. It is not known if this is due to increased vulnerability or to the timing of infection at a cognitively more critical stage (Weiner et al., 1992). Note that cognitive functioning may not decline as fast as other regulatory functions; also behavioral deterioration with bizarre features, in the presence of relatively intact cognitive function, has been described. Observed attention disorder symptoms with or without hyperactivity, may be due to AIDS encephalopathy or to a different base rate for attention disorders in the vulnerable population or to emotional symptoms secondary to stresses of a chronic and incurable illness.

Diagnostic characterization should be done by neuropsychological testing rather than by clinical screening, with a careful cognitive history probing for slowed thinking; poor attention, memory and concentration, or derailment; speech problems; and word-finding problems. Pediatric patients should be followed with annual WISC-R examinations and semiannual tests of memory and psychomotor speed. Diagnostic assessment should distinguish between direct and indirect effects of seropositivity upon cognition. Direct effects of HIV-related CNS disease would likely lead to steady decline in cognitive abilities, flat affect, loss of expressive language, loss of initiative, and possibly agitation. Indirect effects, mediated by HIV-related stress, social alienation, family disorganization, chronic tension, and physical debilitation, might include distractibility, irregular school performance, and behavioral and emotional symptoms such as depression, hyperactivity, regression, and sleep disturbance. The course of the direct effects of ADC is ameliorated by the antiviral azidothymidine (AZT) (Brouwers et al., 1990; Yarchoan et al., 1988). The indirect effects upon cognition and functioning require a psychosocial intervention.

TREATMENT

Newer Treatment Approaches

Discussion of medical treatment for HIV infection is not the focus of this chapter except insofar as it affects the child's experience of illness. For an excellent review of the protean physical manifestations of the disease, the reader is referred to the Guidelines for the Care of Children and Adolescents with HIV Infection Report of the New York State Department of Health AIDS Institute Criteria Committee for the Care of HIV-Infected Children (Nicholas et al., 1991). An established treatment is passive intervention with immunoglobulins rich in HIV-specific antibodies, monoclonal antibodies, and CD4 receptor analogs. Newer treatments include biologic and immunoregulatory interventions to resist the progression of the infection. An example is the use of interleukin-2, with the goal of supporting the growth of T cells, which has been used in children with primary immunodeficiency disease and malignancy and after bone marrow transplantation. Trials of combining this with antiretroviral therapy are planned by the National Cancer Institute Pediatric Branch.

Such treatments are difficult to explain to a small child. Also their access is limited to few patients. There are obstacles to carrying out trials in small children because pharmaceutical companies may be reluctant to perform clinical studies in infants and children, fearing greater liability or calculating that there may not be a significant financial advantage after approval of drugs for infants and children. It has been argued (Amman and Duliege, 1994) that, given that the causative agent, HIV-I, is the same in infants and children as it is in adults, and given that AIDS is a life-threatening illness, a separate demonstration of efficacy of antiviral agents in clinical trials in children is not required, but rather, research focus should be on unique pharmacokinetics and safety of the drugs in pediatric patients.

Psychosocial Treatment of HIV Spectrum Disease: The Contribution of the Psychiatrist

HIV infection is a chronic illness necessitating multiple clinic visits, many hospitalizations, successions of medications, nutritional and growth compromise (McKinney et al., 1993), missed school, and often, developmental delay (Christ, 1985). Care should be comprehensive and aimed at secondary prevention. The crucial figure in the child's care is the pediatrician who will optimize the child's health and manage the complications of the disease when they occur.

Psychosocial assessment must be comprehensive, to allow the pediatric team to maximize medical compliance, and to tailor the treatment insofar as possible to the child's needs. The Pediatric Branch of the National Cancer Institute has developed a psychosocial program that is comprehensive, child-centered, and family-focused. It commences with a full psychosocial assessment including the family (or adoptive, foster, or extended family) constellation, the child's preillness and current personality profile and level of functioning, the family history, beliefs, attitudes and relationships, and estimation of their community support (Weiner and Septimus, 1994; Weiner et al., 1992). Most children should be cared for in their own home, or in a foster home if parents are ill or deceased. Regular clinic care, ideally in a clinic staffed by a multidisciplinary team and geared to treating children with AIDS, should minimize the need for hospitalizations. Treatment includes monitoring nutrition, administering gamma globulin and/or AZT, and treating intercurrent adventitious infections.

Placement in group homes and institutional settings is often resorted to for AIDS orphans, but diluted parenting and exposure to a larger number of children in their living setting may compromise secondary prevention of complications of HIV positivity for small children. Children with AIDS should attend school (American Academy of Pediatrics, 1986; Black, 1986; CDC, 1988a; Rubenstein, 1986) unless they have problems handling secretions, exhibit biting behavior, or have open skin sores. The immunodeficient child should be protected as much as possible from contagious illnesses in the school population. As with all chronic childhood illnesses, losses and missed childhood experiences result from the HIV disease; however, family losses compound this and bereavement is a complicating concomitant. Discrimination may be an added obstacle to implementing recommendations for the child, and the intervention of the physician may be called for in ways not expected in the care of children with other chronic illnesses.

Orchestration of care between medical and psychiatric care providers and coordination with schools is indicated in managing this phase of the illness. Psychiatric advocacy can specifically address the clinical need for coordinated care in order to optimize the child's development and minimize erosion of skills and morale. More importantly, the child psychiatrist has special skill in diagnostic discernment between neurological, psychiatric, and environmental causes of developmental failure.

The psychiatrist caring for patients caught in the AIDS epidemic must use flexible skills. Clinical skills are needed for assessment of developmental, neuropsychiatric, and affective impacts upon the patient. Because AIDS is a life-threatening STD, all physicians must be able to take competent and thorough sexual histories. Families require both extensive evaluation and supportive intervention. Patients with HIV spectrum disease present most difficult problems in all diagnostic areas; DSM-IV Axis I diagnoses may include developmental, organic, affective, and severe adjustment disorders. Axis II diagnoses are common, in part produced by the same family dysfunction and social impoverishment that leads to drug abuse and makes poor and minority young patients differentially become victims of HIV infection. Axis III diagnoses are frequent as the illness progresses. Axis IV levels of psychosocial stress are typically high, and Axis V global assessment of functioning may fluctuate rapidly. Knowledge of pediatric liaison, community drug treatment, psychotherapy, family therapy, child development, neuropsychiatric assessment, and pharmacotherapy are demanded of clinicians who encounter AIDS in pediatric populations.

Bioethical judgment is challenged by the particular difficulties involving rights of minor patients. Decisions about testing for and disclosure of seropositivity must incorporate knowledge of risk factors, balancing the risk of continued exposure and risky behavior against the possible incidence of false-positive test results. Ingenious approaches must be individually devised for helping adolescents who may be in crisis but who do not have families that can emotionally support them. Effective and collegial interdisciplinary clinical functioning is necessary because few psychiatric interventions are possible without taking into account the management of medical, social, and educational professionals who also serve the patient. Accurate clinical assessment of the young patient is the foundation for all other intervention choices, and children with AIDS may not maintain clinical plateaus. Decisions about what information to give children and who should give it, must be made with reference to the child's level of cognitive development, the family's stage of disclosure in their community, and the relationship between the child and the medical caregiver.

Consultation-liaison skills are essential for operating in a multidisciplinary field. Psychiatric consultants must be prepared to help caregivers of children with AIDS deal with four feeling patterns not usually encountered in pediatrics: fear, contempt, grief, and burnout.

1. Fear.   External reassurances that buoy our ordinary healthy denial of death are lacking in the case of AIDS, an illness that is epidemic, largely invisible, and fatal to young patients. Fear of contagion is inevitable, regardless of the cognitive understanding that the means of spread is not through casual contact. Most medical services dealing with AIDS patients undergo progressive mastery of such fear (Krener, 1987), but each psychiatric consultant must be prepared to sensitively assess the stage of mastery within the service to which he or she consults and to devise responses at its current level of need.

2. Contempt.   The sociological pattern of pediatric exposure to HIV infection in the poor and minority residents of inner cities and in those whose use of sex and drugs may be stigmatized often means there is a general sociological gap between AIDS patients and their caregivers. Countertransference feelings of contempt for families whose behavior they blame for the child's illness may be difficult for medical and mental health personnel to acknowledge. Skilled psychiatric consultation may detoxify negative feelings interfering with care by bringing them into words, and by helping to show that the infected parent is also a victim.

3. Grief.   Pediatricians and obstetricians frequently state that they have selected their specialty because they enjoy fostering life rather than dealing with illness and death. They may be more vulnerable to personal grief when their young patients die; they require the support of their colleagues to deal with that grief.

4. Burnout.   Burnout, the well-described constellation of exhaustion, depersonalization, and feeling of failure, is described increasingly among those who care for patients with AIDS. This is contributed to by professional exhaustion as the epidemic accelerates and also by the fact that individual clinicians may not be able to experience a recovery period between the losses of their patients. Support from psychiatric colleagues can help physicians and nurses who undertake the care of AIDS patients to also take care of themselves.

Care of the Individual and Family

The family's attitudes and knowledge about illness in general and AIDS in particular will influence how they help the child to understand it. The physician has an important role in transmitting accurate information and alleviating unnecessary fears (Krener and Miller, 1989; Lusher et al., 1991). Professionals must first, therefore, assess the family's knowledge level and their explanatory model of illness. Information should be presented to children at their cognitive developmental level (O'Brien and Pfeifer, 1993). Extensive resources are available for children explaining HIV prevention and the nature of the infection (Burr and Emery, 1994). Techniques such as incomplete stories and the creation of drawings can assist children in communicating to a trusted adult or a therapist, even if what they are trying to say contains feelings that they may have learned to mute or disguise (Weiner et al., 1994). Mothers have been assisted to make videotapes that after their death their children can keep and watch. Such tapes are created in a supportive setting, with help to organize the powerful affects within them, and are considered ''work in progress,'' which may be completed over many months.

Adaptation to Specific Clinical Settings

Inpatient psychiatric units will see increasing numbers of youth with HIV infection (AAPAC 1989 Policy Statement, Binder, 1987). The patient's fear of dying and dread of stigmatization may be met with fear of infection and avoidance of a person with a terminal illness by staff unless special training and support is offered to health care providers. Dementia and depression late in the course may prolong psychiatric hospitalizations, but third party carriers may deny reimbursement, placing inpatient units in a familiar conflict between program needs and patient needs.

Outpatient treatment of dual diagnosis and substance-abusing youth must incorporate outreach and interpersonally direct approaches, a departure from the more familiar and traditional techniques of office-based psychotherapy based upon a therapeutic alliance. The therapist must keep up-to-date, as different patterns of street drug use and new illegal products increase even more rapidly than pharmaceutical research and published knowledge in medical pharmacology. Inquiry about drug use may yield scant information if it is indirect or brief. Clinical reevaluation of substance-abusing youth is necessary with each encounter. Difficult instructions, which include communicating antibody test results, should not be discussed with patients who are intoxicated, as they may be unable to incorporate important information or to control their emotional reactions to it. Even if the youngster with a substance abuse disorder understands risk factors in the physician's office, he or she may disregard use of clean needles and practice of safe sexual behaviors when under the influence of drugs and immersed in the intensity of sexual and drug exchange.

NEEDS OF FAMILIES WITH INFECTED MEMBERS

Medical Care and Psychiatric Care

Since 45% of white and 88% of nonwhite children with AIDS acquired the disease from a parent who is an IV drug user, their medical and mental health providers must be conversant with subculture and minority values and customs in order to work with their families as is routinely necessary in the care of a chronically ill child. Allowance must also be made for the fact that the parenting person may herself be ill; the mother of an infant with AIDS may be caring for that infant while becoming progressively weaker. Many infants outlive their parents, and displacement to public or foster care follows a long siege of having illness nursed by an ill parent (AAP Committee on Infectious Disease, 1987). Local prejudice and fear of AIDS may require parents to chose between living with secrecy or with stigma. They may struggle with the child's frequent complications and downhill course without the usual community supports that may be available to families with chronically ill children. The lack of practical neighborhood supports, such as help with transportation to clinic appointments or baby-sitting for siblings, may be added to the difficulties of obtaining medical care. The child with HIV disease requires the care of several specialists—pediatrician, neurologist, infectious disease specialist, and child psychiatrist (Belfer et al., 1988). It is likely that even using current patterns of pediatric care with subspecialty consultation, such specialized pediatric management might result in fragmented care. The active process of reorganization of health care delivery patterns has the effect of further restructuring access to specialty consultation. Moreover, the adult family member with HIV disease may require the care of a parallel group of specialists, as well as requiring management of psychosocial problems resulting from drug use or poverty. This challenges the family to a double round of medical evaluations and follow-up visits. The present health-care delivery system, already strained by incompatibility between its middle-class social values and economic models and the inner city utilization patterns, is unable to accommodate the disproportionate numbers of HIV infections in poor areas (Report of Presidential Commission, 1988). Minority risk populations must be targeted for medical, obstetrical, nutritional, and mental health services, and for drug abuse treatment, education, and counseling. In practice, low socioeconomic (SES) families with multiple problems must travel to different sites for care, to methadone maintenance clinics, Medicaid agencies, prenatal clinics, pediatric clinics, and welfare offices. Referrals may be difficult to implement and follow-up may be limited.

However, children with better outpatient care need fewer hospitalizations. Models for the sort of program needed for children with HIV are culturally sensitive, federally sponsored, comprehensive care systems, such as the National Cancer Institute's Pediatric Oncology Program and the Developmental Disabilities Program supported by the Offices of Human Development Services and of Maternal and Child Health. Child psychiatrists need to become part of such model programs and need to advocate their replications in local communities. Public Law 99-457 established a program in 1990 to provide early intervention services to handicapped or developmentally delayed infants and toddlers (0–24 months). Children whose developmental delay is caused by AIDS are eligible for such services but require advocacy and referral in order to access them.

Extended Families and Extensions of Families

IV drug abuse in families of children with AIDS brings with it family dysfunction, poverty, and poor compliance with medical recommendations. Grandmothers may take on the care of ill grandchildren after burying their own children. New programs for caring for infants *in loco parentis* are demanded, particularly in areas with high prevalence of AIDS infection in children. These include more integrated health care models, programs to place boarder babies, and increase in subsidized medical foster homes. More than half of newborns testing seropositive may not go on to develop HIV because their measured seropositivity reflects maternal infection. If they are placed in out-of-home placements, they need a normal family environment to avoid developmental problems resulting from early isolation, abandonment, and stigmatization.

Statutes for protection of the rights and safety of children, although variable from state to state, have all required reexamination in the face of the AIDS epidemic. If the parents are deceased and other relatives are uninvolved, the State has full responsibility, but if a parent has voluntarily placed the child in foster care, then the parent retains the right of approval. If the State has legal responsibility for the child, it may seek parental approval before making any decision involving the child. Children who are wards of state may have no one to sign for their participation in experimental or innovative investigational treatment programs so that they cannot receive state-of-the-art care, which might reduce symptoms and complicating illnesses and improve quality of life.

CDC recommends against group settings for HIV-infected children under 3 years of age because they are highly susceptible to opportunistic infections. The cost of group home care is often higher than cost of family care plus associated support services, and parenting is spread thinner. In advocating for and supporting children who have lost their birth families, the child psychiatrist must join in the task of recruiting and maintaining foster families. Evaluations that encourage certification of relatives as foster parents, entitled to the same payments and support as other foster parents, will enlarge the pool. Foster parents may experience rejection or disapproval by friends and relatives for bringing a child with AIDS into their home to raise along with their own family. They will need particular guidance to know how to explain to their own children and to their children's friends the illness and death of the foster child. Potent opportunities for secondary prevention of the psychological toll of AIDS in children exist through psychological support for extended families and foster families. Such support must be extended on an outpatient or outreach basis, in collaboration with clinics, social services, and volunteers. The currently inadequate reimbursement modes for such powerful augmentors of psychiatric skill should be challenged by psychiatrists interested in carrying out this work.

THE MISSION OF EDUCATION

The greatest potential cultural influence of AIDS may be on psychological and psychosexual development of young people. A culture that properly prepares its youth to survive and thrive must therefore educate them about coexisting with HIV-I. This education must begin in early childhood and must take forms that children can understand at each developmental level. Thus, children ages 2–7, whose thought is prelogical, require quite specific information, but it should be presented in ways that do not excite irrational fears in small people whose thinking is still magical. Thus, one might explain "AIDS is a very bad illness, but it is hard to catch, so it is OK to shake hands with a friend who has AIDS" (Burr and Emery, 1994). Children ages 7–10 years, whose thought is at the concrete logical stage, have a better understanding of cause and effect and absorb much information through the media, but still need very specific information about concrete ways in which AIDS is and is not transmitted. Children over 11 years begin to develop formal logical thinking and can think about multiple factors influencing events. They have the cognitive potential for appreciating how they could avoid AIDS through their actions as adolescents. However, in adolescents other, noncognitive factors may jeopardize their putting this information to use.

The challenge of changing teens' behavior through education is central to questions of mastery, perceived self-effectiveness, and learning, which are integral therapeutic issues for practicing psychotherapists (Sandberg et al., 1988). Educators have responded to the epidemic by providing information to youth. Large-scale surveys show this has been successful (DiClemente et al., 1986).

But does knowledge about HIV infection cause youths to change their behavior? The AIDS epidemic demonstrates how rudimentary our skills are to solve the problem of helping young people connect knowledge with action and to affect adolescent behavior (Price, 1985, 1986; Quackenbush, 1989). Only 15% of adolescents in a Massachusetts survey indicated that they had changed their sexual behavior because of concern abut AIDS (Strunin and Hingson, 1987), and among respondents who had changed their behavior only 20% used methods that were effective against AIDS. Sexually active middle school adolescents were less knowledgeable than their abstinent peers about HIV and less fearful of HIV while expressing less tolerance for people with AIDS (Brown et al., 1992). The same inverse relationship between prejudice and safe behaviors has been observed by others (Westerman and Davidson, 1993).

The urgent public health challenge is to reduce transmission of HIV by reducing the private behaviors involving drugs and sex which are known to spread the virus. This requires connecting knowledge about the illness to behavior change. It should be recognized that abstinence, while a good goal, is not a realistic goal for the half of teenagers of high school age who have experienced sexual intercourse or for the 20% who have had more than one partner (CDC, 1992). As only 20% of youths in some samples use condoms, it is important to persuade the other 80% to change their behavior. Therefore, the issue for education goes beyond mere transmission of knowledge. Education is a continuum that can be conceptualized as having four stages:

1. *Knowledge:* the communication of information accurately in a culturally meaningful and cognitively appropriate way. This is a challenge to be met by designing media bits, pamphlets, and educational materials. These should be developmentally appropriate (Schonfeld et al., 1993).

2. *Belief:* the affective arousal within the learner, which activates attention to the information, empathy for those who are affected by it, and the like. The enhancement of high school programs about AIDS by presentations from persons with AIDS has been well recognized and is an example of mobilizing affect of the audience to belief that AIDS is a disease that can afflict them or people like themselves.

3. *Conviction:* At this stage the learner connects the information directly with himself or herself and determines upon behavior change. This requires the perception of vulnerability and self-efficacy.

4. *Mastery:* The learner practices and masters the skills needed to effectively change behavior.

Much attention has been given to the issue of education as prevention, and published reports suggest that most adolescents surveyed have been educated at stage 1 of the above four stages. Adolescents in schools have been found to have absorbed information about the epidemic. A CDC survey using a questionnaire for anonymous self-administration was developed collaboratively by representatives of 24 state and local departments of education and carried out in 6 cities and 9 states. Sample sizes at sites ranged from 778 to 7013 students. Findings showed that 89–96% of respondents believed students their age should be taught about AIDS in school, 83.3–98.4% knew that AIDS is transmitted by sharing needles, and 88.3%–98.1% knew AIDS is transmitted through sexual intercourse. However, there was no evidence of progression of education toward stage 4, leading to reduction of behaviors that would put youngsters at risk for infection with HIV. Simultaneously with indicating their knowledge, respondents reported ongoing risk-taking behavior. In each site, older students reported more sexual activity and injecting more illegal drugs, with boys reporting both more often than girls (CDC, 1988a).

Modification of sexual behavior to avoid unwanted pregnancy has not occurred in spite of consistent educational attempts. Overall, about one-third of sexually active adolescents nationwide use no contraception, and only a small percentage report the consistent use of condoms (Hein, 1989). Because AIDS is a sexually transmitted disease, education about AIDS must surmount the same obstacles that have thwarted other sex education efforts.

Gay boys pose particular problems for education (Remafedi, 1987). They are potentially alienated because their sexual needs are counter to mainstream social mores. Prejudice and fear may interfere with absorbing information and changing behavior. They preferentially select older partners and thus expose themselves to a group with higher prevalence of HIV seropositivity. Rejection by family and peers may propel them into a reckless search for intimacy and acceptance and into urgent and unfamiliar situations where they cannot assert themselves easily or control whether they have protected sexual experiences. Hence every encounter between a health care provider and an adolescent may be an opportunity for education. Simple, specific questions, asked in a nonjudgmental fashion, are the best approach to discovering what the teen believes and what he or she practices. If the questions do not assume the gender of the partner (e.g., ''Are you sexually active with boys, girls, or both?''), then the youngster who is fearful of a negative judgment about his or her developing same-sex preference may be able to give and receive information. Listening for the teen's level of information will enable the physician to connect their comments to his educational level. For example abstinence is a ''health choice'' for an adolescent who is not sexually active, while a teen who is sexually active may need help with assertiveness skills or demonstration of the use of a condom.

Adolescents who exist in cultural streams not identified as the mainstream may bring responses from their own experiences to educational programs developed for their age mates. Rotheram-Borus et al. (1991) have shown that adolescents experience different sequences of sexual milestones depending upon their experience. Runaways, youth who have been sexually abused or had forced sex, and black youth may progress through the expected sequence of psychosexual milestones, dating, kissing, breast petting, genital petting, and intercourse, in different order. Ethnic differences may be present in frequency of such behaviors as oral sex. Minority adolescents, in comparison to their white counterparts, are less knowledgeable about AIDS overall, and particularly ill-informed about the effectiveness of condoms as a protective barrier to prevent infection (DiClemente et al., 1987a, 1987b). Minority teens, runaways, and substance-abusing adolescents are at special risk because of higher prevalence of sexually transmitted diseases in these groups, combined with the multiple risks associated with poverty. School-based AIDS education programs will fail to reach these high-risk groups: dropouts who are intravenous drug users, minorities, runaways and homeless youth, and pregnant teenagers.

High-risk adolescents are currently least well able to access systems of care and support. The findings of Whitaker (1990) and others about the patterns of psychiatric stress in street youth suggest that cognitive impairment may interfere even with acquisition of the first (knowledge) stage of education, and affective symptomatology may interfere with being able to connect information to the learner's belief. Chaotic lifestyle and present-oriented survival mode interferes with translating a clear belief that AIDS might kill one into a conviction that one should avoid exposure to it; if a cold hungry teenager living on the street is offered $50 for sex by a john, it is unlikely that he or she will bargain about whether a condom will be acceptable.

A small number of important studies probe the progression from stage 1, transmission of knowledge, toward stages 3, conviction that one's behavior must change, and 4, training in skills needed to change. An early large-scale survey conducted with 1,326 high school-age adolescents in San Francisco reported that 92% could identify the route of HIV transmission as sexual intercourse, but only 60% realized that condoms would reduce risk of infection (DiClemente et al., 1986). Strunin and Hingson (1987) showed that adolescents in a low-prevalence area had not changed their sexual practices or methods of contraception as a result of the AIDS epidemic. Brown et al. (1988) have found that translation of knowledge into behaviors is affected by attitude and coping style. These studies point to the root of the problem of public health education—exposure to health information does not predictably lead to change in behaviors directly affecting health. Rotheram-Borus et al. (1991) have shown that high-risk behavior declines and use of condoms increases in New York City runaways who participate in group sessions focused on personal attitudes and skill acquisition. These changes persisted for 6 months. Inner city black teenage boys participating in a 5-hour intervention showed persistent decline in risk behaviors after 3 months. Most effective are programs that prepare youths for decision-making, resisting peer pressure, and negotiating risk reduction (Brown and Lourie, 1994).

LEGAL AND ETHICAL ISSUES

Primary Prevention and Limiting the Spread of the Epidemic

The AIDS epidemic has presented bioethical and legal challenges at every turn and for each subpopulation of people with AIDS. Classical theoretical concepts in medical ethics are spotlighted; these are patient interests versus patient rights, communal interests versus societal investment, and individualism versus community good (Twomey and Fletcher, 1994).

HIV-infected infants and children find themselves in situations for which the precedents are unclear, beginning with prenatal diagnosis. The diagnosis of HIV-I infection in asymptomatic infants is established by positive virus culture, polymerase chain reaction, or p24 antigen. However, these tests may have false-negative results in half of the infants who are subsequently found to be infected. If a method were available for prenatal diagnosis of HIV-I infection, then counseling regarding the risk of vertical transmission would be possible. It is important for such a diagnostic technique to be without risk of infecting an otherwise healthy fetus. At present there is still the risk of missing the diagnosis in an infected fetus and also of making the diagnosis wrongly because of maternal contamination of fetal specimen (Viscarello and Landers, 1994). Still at issue is the question of whether prenatal screening should be routine. The National Pediatric HIV Resource Center Workshop has recommended prenatal HIV counseling and routine availability of HIV testing as the standard of prenatal care (Cotton et al., 1994). Physicians do not have established guidelines for counseling parents and expectant parents on options; this requires each physician to make their own determination, and might create concern, for example, if the physician disagrees with the parent's decision to carry through the pregnancy.

The disproportionate dissemination of the virus among women of color and their children is due to its association with substance abuse. This spotlights the already unequal distribution of human services and health care between the rich and the poor in U.S. society. It has been observed that the AIDS epidemic has brought about a questioning of the social value of people with AIDS (Twomey and Fletcher, 1994) so that the existing rights-based ethics of medical care must be supplemented by an ethics of caring. These social issues magnify concerns about access to involvement in research trials on clinical care, and protection of subjects' privacy. The increasing number of AIDS orphans, a poorly represented constituency, raises questions about how to obtain rights for children who do not have secure legal status in a family. For example, it is difficult in many states to legally include children in foster care in clinical research.

Consent and confidentiality are not easily separated issues. The AIDS epidemic is catalyzing the process of defining these issues for young patients (Schoenberg, 1989). Informed consent for medications for children is inherently complex because both the child and the legal caregiver must be engaged in the consent process (Krener and Mancina, 1994), and both the competence of that caregiver and their honest advocacy for the child's best interests are assumed traditionally, but may not be optimal. The issue of informed consent has never been entirely clear in the case of adolescents who fail to understand or who do not fully desire the recommended treatments for which their parents sign. Informed consent takes on new meaning when the context is testing for the presence of HIV. How can a clinician or researcher be satisfied that an adolescent fully comprehends the implications of a positive HIV test result upon future education, employment, insurability, and social acceptance? Is it preferable to insist upon parental consent for testing when this may result in either an obstacle to care for the adolescent or an abuse of the adolescent's confidentiality about his or her sexual behavior? Confidentiality and disclosure issues, which may be clear in concept, are more difficult to ensure in practice, when many people have access to the identities of the subjects, even if those people are well-meaning. The promise to maintain confidentiality may be an empty one when medical records are accessible to so many. Is it preferable to protect the patient's confidentiality by withholding information from his or her medical record?

Because vertically transmitted HIV is an infectious disease that is likely to affect two persons, there are ethical dilemmas about how to proceed if only one (the mother) may need treatment, and if the treatment may harm the other (the infant). Should pregnancy be regarded as an exclusionary factor for participation in drug trials for HIV? If the fetus is uninfected, is the risk of its exposure to antiviral drugs justified?

At the present time the law is far behind the surge of the AIDS epidemic and is tossing heavily in its wake. Change in the legal net will be woven slowly from the threads of many bioethical dilemmas. Tactical decisions about bioethical issues require tailoring a solution to each clinical situation after detailed study. Psychiatrists will be called upon to provide special skills to explore individual factors in clinical decision-making, which might lead to policy or law.

Secondary Prevention: How to Live with the Fox in the Hen House?

Being infected with HIV engages each seropositive person in a long, losing war. Life, however, goes on even in wartime. Psychiatrists are practiced in staying the course with patients who have chronic illnesses; a substantial proportion of DSM-IV Axis I diagnoses are, in fact, chronic or relapsing conditions. In a multidisciplinary team, consultation-liaison psychiatrists have an important role in helping patients accommodate to and sustain themselves during their illness.

Acculturation to chronic illness is gradual. Cooperation with the physician is necessary for optimal management, and an inner process of hope or endurance is necessary for extending survival. Clinicians may subsume several obstacles to cooperation under the label "medical noncompliance." These include unfamiliarity with the medical system, lack of comprehension of the treatment, denial, and active resistance to or sabotage of the treatment. For adolescents, additional obstacles are

their developmental need to disengage themselves from their families and their self-experience as immortal. The succession and interplay of these factors requires further investigation.

Sociologically, pediatric patients whose infection has come about through IV drug use in the family are members of a group whose previous poor socialization to health care delivery may have resulted from adaptation to those health care systems available to them that delivered services only in an impersonal or emergency fashion. Even if the parents of the child with AIDS were entirely motivated to cooperate with comprehensive multidisciplinary services, practical obstacles to their doing so include illness in care providers and difficulties with mechanics such as transportation to clinic appointments, which might be posed by poverty or the need for secrecy about the child's illness. Research is needed to delineate patterns of utilization and extra needs for support of high-risk mother-infant pairs. Outcome of treatment for the infections and neurological manifestations of AIDS in childhood must include evaluation of the child's physical development and also his or her cognitive and emotional development. However, research tools are lacking to sensitively describe the cognitive development of children against the background noise of chaotic families, parental substance abuse, low SES, and loss.

Clinical research with AIDS patients is inextricable from clinical contacts; communication must be coordinated among caregivers in several subspecialties and with a range of training from volunteers to National Institutes of Mental Health grant principal investigators. Extreme physical, emotional, and social pressures exist for all members of the research treatment care team. They must deal not only with the sadness of childhood pain and weakness that is directly illness related, but also with poverty, parental drug abuse, and homelessness, which disproportionately beset these children. Interaction with housing authorities, local school districts, public assistance programs, drug abuse treatment authorities, and community health clinics is unavoidable. Countless "research" hours are consumed by telephone calls, conferences, and numerous other interactions required to support HIV children and their families.

What Are the Rights of Juveniles in AIDS Research?

Established guidelines exist for carrying out clinical research in which minors are subjects (National Commission for the Protection of Human Subjects of Biomedical and Behavioral Research, 1978). However, the application of these to research into a lethal illness in minors who may not have parents, and who may not be in traditional medical settings, is difficult. Medicolegal problems may arise where there are major ethical issues. In the case of children and adolescents with HIV spectrum disease, the issues are confidentiality and consent: consent to participate in research or to receive investigational treatments. One of the first ethical questions to arise with adults is that of the duty to warn sexual contacts, if the infected partner cannot be persuaded to do so (Gostin and Curran, 1987). This problem is present for adolescents as well. Rosnow RL, Rotheram-Borus MJ et al. (1993) have explored certain of these issues and identified painful questions that result from the psychosocial vulnerability of the pediatric populations in whom AIDS is spreading most rapidly. They give examples of consent dilemmas in determining when is it necessary to obtain parental consent when conducting research with children. In the case of teen runaways living on their own, are they mature minors? Confidentiality is a core issue in adolescent psychiatry and is a specially charged one in the case of AIDS. The authors query what criteria determine when clinical concerns override concerns for confidentiality and give the example of gay youth who wish to participate in a research program but do not want their parents to know of their sexual preference.

CONCLUSION

Psychiatrists working with children and adolescents will become involved in caring for victims of AIDS unless their practice excludes sexually active adolescents, inpatient psychiatry, consultation-liaison activities, victims of sexual abuse, gay men, and patients with dual diagnoses. The field of psychiatry encompasses several areas of specialized knowledge about management of chronic illness, dealing with death and bereavement, adolescent psychiatry, and cognitive development, areas in which support is vitally needed by clinicians who deal with AIDS patients on a day-to-day basis. Psychosocial research questions, which have become compelling as a result of the epidemic, include questions about neuropsychiatric functioning, cognitive change through education, patient resilience, and bioethical rights of juveniles, and are currently among the most vital questions in the field.

References

American Academy of Child and Adolescent Psychiatry: *Policy Statement. AIDS and Psychiatric Hospitalization of Children and Adolescents.* Washington, DC, AACAP, 1989.

American Academy of Pediatrics Committee on Adolescents: Homosexuality and adolescence. *Pediatrics* 92:631–633, 1993.

American Academy of Pediatrics Committee on Infectious Diseases: School attendance of children and adolescents with human T lymphotrophic virus III/lymphadenopathy-associated virus infection. *Pediatrics* 77:430–432, 1986.

American Academy of Pediatrics Committee on Infectious Diseases: Health guidelines for the attendance in daycare and foster care settings of children infected with human immunodeficiency virus. *Pediatrics* 79:466–469, 1987.

American Academy of Pediatrics Task Force on Pediatric AIDS: Adolescents and human immunodeficiency virus infection: The role of the pediatrician in prevention and intervention. *Pediatrics* 92:626–630, 1993.

Amman AJ, Duliege AS: Biologic and immunomodulating factors in treatment of pediatric AIDS. In: Pizzo PA, Wilfert CM (eds): *Pediatric AIDS: The Challenge of HIV Infection in Infants, Children, and Adolescents* (2nd ed). Baltimore, Williams & Wilkins, 1994, pp. 689–712.

Belfer ML, Krener PKG, Miller FB: AIDS in children and adolescents. *J Am Acad Child Adolesc Psychiatry* 27:147–151, 1988.

Binder R: AIDS antibody tests on inpatient psychiatric units. *Am J Psychiatry* 144:176–181, 1987.

Black JL: AIDS: Preschool and school issues. *J Sch Health* 56(3):93–95, 1986.

Braverman PK, Strasburger VC: Adolescent sexuality. Part 1: Adolescent sexual activity. *Clin Pediatr* 658–666, November 1993.

Braverman PK, Strasburger VC: Adolescent sexuality. Part 3: Sexually transmitted diseases. *Clin Pediatr* 26–37, January 1994.

Brouwers P, Balman AL, Epstein L: Central nervous system involvement: Manifestations evaluation, and pathogenesis. In: Pizzo PA, Wilfert CM (eds): *Pediatric AIDS: The Challenge of HIV Infection in Infants, Children, and Adolescents* (2nd ed). Baltimore, Williams & Wilkins, 1994, pp. 433–456.

Brouwers P, Moss H, Wolters P, et al: Effect of continuous-infusion zidovudine therapy on neuropsychologic functioning in children with symptomatic human immunodeficiency virus infection. *J Pediatr* 117:980–985, 1990.

Brown LK, Fritz GK: Children's knowledge and attitudes about AIDS. *J Am Acad Child Adolesc Psychiatry* 27:505–508, 1988.

Brown LK, Lourie K: Changing adolescents' HIV-related attitudes and behaviors: The challenge and the opportunity. *Curr Opin Pediatr* 6(4):428–433, 1994.

Brown LK, DiClemente RJ, Beusoleil NI: Comparison of human immunodeficiency virus related knowledge, attitudes, intentions and behaviors among sexually active and abstinent young adolescents. *J Adolesc Health* 13:140–143, 1992.

Burr CK, Emery LJ: Speaking with children and families about HIV infections. In: Pizzo PA, Wilfert CM (eds): *Pediatric AIDS: The Challenge of HIV Infection in Infants, Children, and Adolescents* (2nd ed). Baltimore, Williams & Wilkins, 1994, pp. 923–936.

Centers for Disease Control: Guidelines for effective school health education to prevent the spread of AIDS. *MMWR* 37(47):717–721, 1988a.

Centers for Disease Control: HIV-related beliefs, knowledge, and behaviors among high school students. *MMWR* 37(S-2):1–13, 1988b.

Centers for Disease Control and Prevention: National Center for Infectious Diseases, Division of HIV/AIDS. *HIV/AIDS Surveillance, Year End Edition, Cases Reported through December 1992.* Bethesda, MD, US Department of Health and Human Services, US Public Health Service, 1992a.

Centers for Disease Control and Prevention: Sexual behavior among high school students. *MMWR* 40:885–888, 1992b. Christ AE: Reactions of children to illness, hospitalization, surgery and physical disabilities. In: Simons RC (ed): *Understanding Human Behavior in Health and Illness.* Baltimore, Williams & Wilkins, 1985, pp. 281–286.

Cotton D, Currier JS, Wofsy C: Information for caretakers of children about women infected with HIV. In: Pizzo PA, Wilfert CM (eds): *Pediatric AIDS: The Challenge of HIV Infection in Infants, Children, and Adolescents* (2nd ed). Baltimore, Williams & Wilkins, 1994, pp. 83–93.

Coye MJ: Families living with AIDS. Presentation at 5th International Pediatric AIDS Conference, Los Angeles, September 6–8, 1989.

Cunningham RM, Stiffman AR, Doré P, et al: The association of physical and sexual abuse with HIV risk behaviors in adolescence and young adulthood: Implications for public health. *Child Abuse Negl* 198(3):233–248, 1994.

D'Angelo L: HIV infection and AIDS in adolescents. In: Pizzo PA, Wilfert CM (eds): *Pediatric AIDS: The Challenge of HIV Infection in Infants, Children, and Adolescents* (2nd ed). Baltimore, Williams & Wilkins, 1994, pp. 71–82.

de la Monte SM, Schooley RT, Hirsch MS, et al: Subacute encephalomyelitis of AIDS and its relation to HTLV-III infection. *Neurology* 37:562–569, 1987.

Department of Health and Human Services: *An Occasional Report on Runaway and Homeless Youth Data.* Summary data on youth identified as "possibly" suicidal. Washington, DC, Office of Human Development Services, 1986, pp. 1–7.

Department of Health and Human Services: *An Occasional Report on Runaway and Homeless Youth Data.* Summary data on alcohol and drug abuse among youth. Washington, DC, Office of Human Development Services, 1986.

DesJarlais DC, Friedman SR: AIDS and the use of injected drugs. *Sci Am* 270(2):82–89, 1994.

DiClemente RJ: Prevention of human immunodeficiency virus infection among adolescents: The interplay of health education and public policy in the development and implementation of school-based, AIDS education programs. *AIDS Educ Prev* 1(1):70–78, 1989.

DiClemente RJ, Boyer CB: Ethnic and racial misconceptions about AIDS. *Focus: A Review of AIDS Research* 2(3):287–291, 1987.

DiClemente RJ, Boyer CB, Morales ES: Prevention of AIDS among adolescents: Strategies for the development of comprehensive risk-reduction health education programs. *Health Educ Res* 2:287–291, 1988.

DiClemente RJ, Pies CA, Stoller EJ, et al: Evaluation of school-based AIDS education curricula in San Francisco. *J Sex Res* 26:188–198, 1989.

DiClemente RJ, Ponton LE, Hartley D, et al: Prevalence of HIV-related high-risk sexual and drug-related behaviors among adolescents with severe emotional disturbances: Preliminary results. In: Woodruff JO, Doherty D, Garrison-Athey J (eds): *Troubled Adolescents and HIV Infection: Issues in Prevention and Treatment.* Washington, DC, CASSP Technical Assistance Center, Georgetown University, 1989.

DiClemente RJ, Zorn J, Temoshok L: Adolescents and AIDS: A survey of knowledge, attitudes and beliefs about AIDS in San Francisco. *Am J Public Health* 76:1443–1445, 1986.

DiClemente RJ, Zorn J, Temoshok L: The association of gender, ethnicity, and length of residence in the Bay Area to adolescents' knowledge and attitudes about acquired immune deficiency syndrome. *J Appl Soc Psychol* 17:216–230, 1987.

Epstein LG, Goudsmit L, Paul DA, et al: Expression of human immunodeficiency virus in cerebrospinal fluid of children with progressive encephalopathy. *Ann Neurol* 21:397–340, 1987.

Epstein LG, Shearer LR, Goudsmit L: Neurological and neuropathological features of human immunodeficiency virus in children. *Ann Neurol* 23:19–23, 1988.

Gostin L, Curran WJ: AIDS screening, confidentiality and the duty to warn. *Am J Public Health* 77:361–365, 1987.

Grant I, Atkinson JH, Hesselink JR, et al: Evidence for early central nervous system involvement in the acquired immunodeficiency syndrome (AIDS) and other human immunodeficiency (HIV) infections. *Ann Intern Med* 107:828–836, 1987.

Haseltine WA: Prospects for the medical control of the AIDS epidemic. *Daedalus* 118(3):1–21, 1989.

Hein K: AIDS in adolescents: Exploring the challenge. *J Adolesc Health Care* 10:10S–35S, 1989.

Hutto C, Parks WP, Lai S, et al: A hospital based prospective study of perinatal infection with human immunodeficiency virus type 1. *J Pediatr* 118:347–363, 1991.

Jacobson HG, Seigelman SS: Intracranial lesions in the acquired immunodeficiency syndrome. *JAMA* 253:393–396, 1985.

Jemmott JB, Jemmott LS, Fong GT: Reduction in HIV risk-associated sexual behaviors among black male adolescents: Effects of an AIDS prevention intervention. *Am J Public Health* 82:372–377, 1992.

Jones DS, Byers RH, Bush TJ, et al: Epidemiology of transfusion-associated acquired immunodeficiency syndrome in children in the United States, 1981–1989. *Pediatrics* 89:123–127, 1992.

Krener PKG: Impact of the diagnosis of AIDS on hospital care of an infant. *Clin Pediatr* 26:30–34, 1987.

Krener P, Mancina R: Informed consent or informed coercion? Decision making in pediatric psychopharmacology. *J Pediatr Psychopharmacol* 4(3):183–200, 1994.

Krener PKG, Miller FB: Psychiatric response to HIV spectrum disease in children and adolescents. *J Am Acad Child Adolesc Psychiatry* 28:596–605, 1989.

Lusher JH, Operskalski EA, Aledort LH, et al: Risk of human immunodeficiency virus type 1 infection among sexual and nonsexual household contacts of persons with congenital clotting disorders. *Pediatrics* 88:242–249, 1991.

Maj M, Statz P, Janssen R, et al: WHO Neuropsychiatric AIDS Study, Cross-sectional Phase II. Neuropsychological and Neurological Findings. *Arch Gen Psychiatry* 51:51–61, January 1994.

Marsh NV, McCall DW: Early neuropsychological change in HIV infection. *Neuropsychology* 8(1):44–48, 1994.

Martin A: Clinically significant cognitive dysfunction in medically asymptomatic human immunodeficiency virus-infected (HIV+) individuals? *Psychosom Med* 56:18–19, 1994.

Martin EM, Sorensen DJ, Edelstein HE, et al: Decision-making speed in HIV-1 infection: A preliminary report. *AIDS* 6:109–113, 1992a.

Martin EM, Sorensen DJ, Robertson LC, et al: Spatial attention in HIV-1 infection: A preliminary report. *J Neuropsychiatry* 4:288–293, 1992b.

McKinney RE, Robertson WR, Duke Pediatrics AIDS Clinical Trials Unit: Effect of human immunodeficiency virus infection on the growth of young children. *J Pediatr* 123:579–582, 1993.

McKirnan DJ, Johnson T: Alcohol and drug use among "street" adolescents. *Addict Behav* 11:201–205, 1986.

Miller HG, Turner CF, Moses LE (eds): *AIDS: The Second Decade*. Washington, DC, National Academy Press, 1990, pp. 152–159. Moscicki A, Millstein SG, Broering J, et al: Risks of human immunodeficiency virus infection among adolescents attending three diverse clinics. *J Pediatr* 122:813–820, 1993.

Moscicki A, Millstein SG, Broering J, et al: Risks of human immunodeficiency virus infection among adolescents attending three diverse clinics. *J Pediatr* 122:813–820, 1993.

National Commission for the Protection of Human Subjects of Biomedical and Behavioral Research: *Research involving children: Report and recommendations*. DHEW (OS)77-004 Appendix, DHEW (OS)77-005. Washington, DC, US Government Printing Office, 1977.

National Commission for the Protection of Human Subjects of Biomedical and Behavioral Research: *Belmont Report: Ethical principles and guidelines for the protection of human subjects of research*. DHEW (OS)78-0012 Appendix I, DHEW (OS)78-0013 Appendix II, DHEW (OS)78-0014. Washington, DC, US Government Printing Office, 1978.

Nicholas SW, Leung J, Fennoy I: Guidelines for nutritional support of HIV-infected children. J Pediatr 119(1, part 2):S59–62, 1991.

O'Brien ME, Pheifer WG: Physical and psychosocial nursing care for patients with HIV infection. *Nurs Clin North Am* 28:303–316, 1993.

Oleske JM, Minnefor AB: Acquired immune deficiency syndrome (AIDS) in children. In: Ma P, Armstrong D (eds): *Acquired Immune Deficiency Syndrome and Infections of Homosexual Men*. Stoneham, MA, Yorke Medical Books, 1984.

Oxtoby MJ: Vertically acquired HIV infection in the United States. In: Pizzo PA, Wilfert CM: *Pediatric AIDS: The Challenge of HIV Infection in Infants, Children, and Adolescents* (2nd ed). Baltimore, Williams & Wilkins, 1994, pp. 3–20.

Parks WP, Scott GB: An overview of pediatric AIDS: Approaches to diagnosis and outcome assessment. In: Broder S (ed): *AIDS: Modern Concepts and Therapeutic Challenges*. New York, Marcel Dekker, 1987.

Price JH: AIDS, the schools, and policy issues. *J Sch Health* 56(4):137–140, 1986.

Price JH, Desmond S, Kukulka G: High school students' perceptions and misperceptions of AIDS. *J Sch Health* 55(3):107–109, 1985.

Price RW, Sidtis J, Rosenblum M: The AIDS dementia complex and HIV 1 brain infection: a pathogenetic model of virus-immune interaction (Research publication no. 68). New York: Association of Research in Nervous and Mental Disease, 1990, p. 269–290.

Protherow-Smith D: Drug treatment planning, sexuality and privacy, management of fertility. *J Adolesc Health Care* 10:5–8, 1989.

Pumarola-Sune T, Navia BA, Cordon-Cardo C, et al: HIV antigen in the brains of patients with the AIDS dementia complex. *Ann Neurol* 21:490–496, 1987.

Quackenbush M: Educating youth about AIDS. *Focus: A Review of AIDS Research* 2(3):1–10, 1987.

Rees M: The sombre view of AIDS. *Nature* 326:343–345, 1987.

Remafedi G: Adolescent homosexuality: Psychosocial and medical implications. *Pediatrics* 79:331–337, 1987.

Report of the Presidential Commission on the Human Immunodeficiency Virus Epidemic. Washington, DC, Government Printing Office, June 1988.

Rogers M: Families living with AIDS. 5th International Pediatric AIDS Conference, Los Angeles, September 6–8, 1989.

Rogers M, Williams W: AIDS among racial/ethnic minorities—United States 1993. MMWR 43(35):644–647, 653–655, 1994.

Rosnow RL, Rotheram-Borus MJ, Ceci SJ, et al: The institutional review board as a mirror of scientific and ethical standards. *American Psychologist* 48(7):821–826, 1993.

Rotheram-Borus MJ, Koopman C, Bradley JS: Barriers to successful AIDS prevention programs with runaway youth. Paper prepared for Knowledge Development Workshop: "Issues in Prevention and Treatment of AIDS among Adolescents with Serious Emotional Disturbance." Sponsored by Georgetown University Child Development Center, NIMH Child and Family Support Branch and Health and Behavior Research Branch, National Institute on Drug Abuse, June 1988. Washington DC, personal communication, 1988.

Rotheram-Borus MJ, Koopman C: Sexual risk behaviors, AIDS knowledge, and beliefs about AIDS among runaways. *Am J Public Health* 81(2):208–210, 1991.

Rotheram-Borus MJ, Koopman C, Haignere C, et al: Reducing HIV sexual risk behaviors among runaway adolescents. *JAMA* 266(9):1237–1241, 1991.

Rubenstein A: Schooling for children with acquired immune deficiency syndrome. *J Pediatr* 109:301, 1986.

Sandberg DE, Rotheram-Borus MJ, Bradley J, et al: Methodological issues in assessing AIDS prevention programs. *J Adolesc Res* 3(3–4):413–418, 1988.

Schoenberg SK: Adolescents and AIDS. *J Adolesc Health Care* 10:45, 1989.

Schonfeld KJ, Johnson SR, Perrin EC, et al: Understanding of acquired immunodeficiency syndrome by elementary school children: A developmental survey. *Pediatrics* 92:389–395, 1993.

Scott GB: Clinical manifestations of HIV infection in children. *Pediatr Ann* 17:365–370, 1988.

Stircof RL, Kennedy JT, Nattell TC, et al: HIV seroprevalence in a facility for runaway and homeless adolescents. *Am J Public Health* 81(suppl):50–53, 1991.

Strunin L, Hingson R: Acquired immunodeficiency syndrome and adolescents: Knowledge, beliefs, attitudes and behaviors. *Pediatrics* 79:825–828, 1987.

Tovo PA, deMartino M, Gabiano C, et al: Prognostic factors and survival in children with perinatal HIV-1 infection. *Lancet* 339:1249–1253, 1992.

Twomey JG, Fletcher JC: Ethical issues surrounding care of HIV-infected children. In: Pizzo PA, Wilfert CM (eds): *Pediatric AIDS: The Challenge of HIV Infection in Infants, Children, and Adolescents* (2nd ed). Baltimore, Williams & Wilkins, 1994, pp. 713–724.

US Department of Health and Human Services: *Coping with AIDS*. DHHS Publication no. (ADM) 85-1432. Washington, DC, US Department of Health and Human Services, 1986.

Van Gorp WG, Satz, P, Hinkin C, et al: The neuropsychological aspects of HIV-1 spectrum disease. *Psychiatr Med* 7:59–78, 1989.

Viscarello RR, Landers DV: Advances in prenatal diagnosis of HIV-1 infection. In: Pizzo PA, Wilfert CM (eds): *Pediatric AIDS: The Challenge of HIV Infection in Infants, Children, and Adolescents* (2nd ed). Baltimore, Williams & Wilkins, 1994, pp. 207–218.

Weiner L, Septimus A: Psychosocial support for child and family. In: Pizzo PA, Wilfert CM (eds): *Pediatric AIDS: The Challenge of HIV Infection in Infants, Children, and Adolescents* (2nd ed). Baltimore, Williams & Wilkins, 1994, pp. 809–828.

Weiner L, Best A, Halpern A: Children speaking with children and families about HIV infection. In: Pizzo PA, Wilfert CM (eds): *Pediatric AIDS: The Challenge of HIV Infection in Infants, Children, and Adolescents* (2nd ed). Baltimore, Williams & Wilkins, 1994, pp. 937–963.

Weiner L, Moss H, Davidson R, et al: Pediatrics: The emerging psychosocial challenges of the AIDS epidemic. *Child Adolesc Social Work J* 9:381–407, 1992.

Weiner LS, Spencer ED, Davidson R, et al: National telephone support groups: A new avenue toward psychosocial support for HIV-infected children and their families. *Soc Work Groups* 16(3):55–71, 1993.

Westerman PL, Davidson PM: Homophobic attitudes and AIDS risk behavior of adolescents. *J Adolesc Health* 14:208–213, 1993.

Whitaker A, Johnson J, Shaffer D, et al: Uncommon troubles in young people: Prevalence estimates of selected psychiatric disorders in a non-referred adolescent population. *Arch Gen Psychiatry* 47:487–496, 1990.

Whitt JK, Hooper SR, Tennison MB, et al: Neuropsychological functioning of human immunodeficiency virus-infected children with hemophilia. *J Pediatr* 122:52–59, 1993.

Yarchoan R, Mitsuya H, Broder S: AIDS therapies. *Sci Am* 259:110–119, 1988.

98 CARE OF INFANTS, CHILDREN, AND ADOLESCENTS WITH BURN INJURIES

Frederick J. Stoddard, M.D.

Fire over the ages has inspired awe, wonder, fear, allegory, and myth from Hephaestus, the Greek god of fire, peaceful but ugly and deformed and wed to the beautiful Aphrodite, to Daedalus, flying too near to the sun, losing his wings, and plunging to his death. The Jews escaped Egypt through a miracle: "the Lord went before them by day in a pillar of a cloud, to lead them the way; and by night in a pillar of fire, to give them light" (Exodus 13:21). A Mother Goose nursery rhyme catches the child's wish for a mother's rescue with "Ladybug, ladybug, fly away home. Your house is on fire, and your children will burn." For authors and poets, fire can be an image of mental awakening, as in "A World Lit Only by Fire" (Manchester, 1992) and "The Poets light but lamps . . ." (Dickinson, No. 883), and feelings, "Some say the world will end in fire, some say in ice. From what I've tasted of desire, I hold with those who favor fire . . ." (Frost, 1923). Also pertinent is Tennyson as he catches the power of language to assuage with "But for the unquiet heart and brain/A use in measured language lies; The sad mechanic exercise, Like dull narcotics numbing pain." (In Memoriam, 5, st 2). We feel these evocative images, e.g., fear and rescue, ugliness and beauty, death and miracle, each day in the care of burned children.

HISTORY

The era of intensive research and treatment of burns began over 50 years ago during World War II at the Massachusetts General Hospital after the Cocoanut Grove Fire in Boston on November 28, 1942. Cobb and Lindemann chronicled the posttraumatic reactions of the survivors of that fire (Cobb and Lindemann, 1943). Lindemann, in a classic paper about them, also described the symptomatology and management of their acute grief (Lindemann, 1944). Since then, images of war have made plain for all to see the catastrophe wrought by fire. Drawings by child and adult survivors of Hiroshima, photographs from Korea, televised images from Vietnam, films depicting a nuclear holocaust, and the tragedy of Bosnia have riveted the world's attention. Such images evoke terror but also compassion, and a positive benefit of such compassion is the near miraculous care now available for children with burns.

The Shriners Hospitals joined with the Massachusetts General Hospital and Harvard Medical School in 1968 to build the Shriners Burns Institute, recently rebuilt, where free care is provided to burned children. The Shriners also built pediatric burn hospitals in Cincinnati, Galveston, and now at UC-Davis. Awareness in the 1960s and 1970s of the high rate of burns to children led to the founding of pediatric burn units in children's hospitals and general hospitals throughout the United States and Canada. There are now designated burn centers for children in most major cities of the United States, Canada, Europe, and many other countries. In the last 20 years new research has led to improved methods of resuscitation and transport, excision and grafting (Sheridan et al., 1994b), cardiovascular and infection control, artificial skin and skin substitutes (Sheridan et al., 1994a), plastic surgical techniques (Salisbury, 1992), and other advances. Together, these have improved outcomes.

Child psychiatrists such as Norman Bernstein (Bernstein, 1976) and Richard Galdston (Galdston, 1972), a child psychoanalyst, were pioneers in the psychiatric care of burned children, their families, and in work with the "burn team." Stoddard (1982a) initially highlighted a develop-

mental approach to pain of burned children, and an adult psychiatrist, Samuel Perry, and colleagues spearheaded the focus on undertreatment of pain in children and adults through a national survey of burn units (Perry and Heidrich, 1982). Trauma surgeons and plastic surgeons, nurses, anesthesiologists, pediatricians, psychologists, social workers, physical therapists, cosmetologists, burn survivors, and many others have contributed to major advances in prevention, education, research, and treatment. Although acute care of serious burns is specialized, most mental health professionals, at some time in their careers, provide or supervise treatment for patients who have been burned, as well as care of their siblings and families.

ORGANIZATIONAL AND RESEARCH ISSUES

The organization of care differs from some other pediatric areas: in large centers burns tend to be a subspecialty in many of the fields mentioned above. As managed care forces increased generalization of services, that trend toward specialization may reverse somewhat. The American Burn Association and the International Society for Burn Injuries are the principal scientific organizations sponsoring meetings to educate physicians, nurses, other professionals, and the public. The Phoenix Society is the international self-help group for children and adults with burns and their families, which has been instrumental in advancing the care and understanding of burned individuals.

Psychological aspects of burns are an active research area, especially pain and outcome studies. As surgical research and improved treatment have increased survival rates, there is new focus on pain as a crucial variable increasing stress and probably adversely affecting psychological outcome (Patterson, 1993). Improving pain relief (Kavanaugh et al., 1991; Ptacek et al., 1994) and increasing focus on psychological interventions is providing increased hope to children and their families and may be improving outcomes, but pain remains undertreated (Marvin et al., 1991). As comprehensive care improves, burn care personnel and the families are helping disfigured children and adolescents resume normal lives, enabling them to adapt to handicaps. *Research with burned children* can pose ethical and human studies dilemmas because the research benefits to them and others are balanced against risks of their age, critical condition, and exposure to many procedures; Levine (1991) wisely presents an ethical overview pertinent to such research with children.

EPIDEMIOLOGY

There are more than 2.5 million burn injuries in the United States and Canada each year and thousands of deaths (Collins, 1990; Stats Canada, 1989), of which about 35% are children. The United States has one of the highest rates of burn injury in the world. Of 625,000 people who visit emergency rooms with burns, about 100,000 are hospitalized, many of them children (American Burn Association: Annual Burn Facility Survey Data 1991, unpublished; National Center for Health Statistics, 1989). Fire and burn injuries are the second leading cause of accidental deaths in children for ages 1–4, and the third leading cause of injury and death for ages 1–18 (National Center for Health Statistics, 1989). Most burns are preventable. Preventive public health laws for fire retardant sleepwear and lowered hot water heater temperatures in public housing have reduced burns to children. However, further laws are needed, e.g., for self-extinguishing cigarettes, which is pending in Congress, since cigarettes cause many burn deaths. Many infants and young children are burned due to scalds. Other common types of burns are flame, electrical, ingestion, and chemical (McLaughlin and Crawford, 1985). These may be the result of poor housing, overcrowding, child abuse or neglect, parental substance abuse or depression, risk-taking behavior, match play or firesetting (see also Chapter 55), suicide attempt (Table 98.1), or war.

Child abuse or neglect (see Chapter 99) is a frequent cause of burns. The child psychiatrist collaborates with the surgeon, nurse, and social worker in suspected cases, and psychiatric assessment skills may confirm child abuse where other methods fail to do so. This type of burn is common, with abuse accounting for 6–20% of pediatric burns in different units, including some fatalities. Hight et al. (Renz and Sherman, 1993) found 13–24 months to be the period of maximum risk of abuse. The most common type of inflicted burn is a scald, with other types (cigarette, hot iron, or radiator) much less common. Renz and Sherman (1993) prospectively studied abusive scald burns and found that all 30 children, a mean age of 22.5 months, had buttocks burns, 80% had complications, and four died of sepsis. Indicators suggesting abuse include a changing history of what occurred, a past history of "accidents," an inattentive parent, a consistently passive, withdrawn child who is "numb" to pain, and physical findings suggestive of abuse, e.g., a burn distribution not consistent with the history, other physical signs of abuse,

and fractures. When abuse is suspected, reporting to the appropriate state social agency is mandated and an investigation follows, with subsequent interventions as indicated. When support and explanation are provided to the parents or caretakers as to why filing a report is required, they will often accept counseling as part of burn care, although in some cases they withdraw from unit staff. Recognition of abuse or neglect is very important since these children are at increased risk for subsequent injury and death.

UNDERMEDICATION FOR PAIN

Pain is very severe during acute treatment, especially during debridement of the burn wound (dressing changes, "tubbing" or "tanking"), but pain management has been inadequate and may be a source of staff conflict. While the reasons are not fully understood, some of the reasons for undermedication by doctors and nurses seem to be: (a) lack of education about pain management, (b) fear of respiratory depression and other side effects, (c) reluctance to systematically obtain self-ratings of pain, (d) false confidence: "I know what pain in children looks like," and (e) lack of attention to adequate doses of opiates required with curariform drugs. Perry (1984), in a reflective article about this issue with adult burn unit staff, found (a) that preservation of the patient's pain unconsciously preserved the boundary of the patient as a definable being, separate from staff, and (b) that pain responses helped to confirm for the staff that the patient was alive; it was not a sadistic wish to cause pain but, rather, a reluctance to eliminate it. He suggested that

Table 98.1. Adolescent Survivors of Self-inflicted Burns

Age/Sex	DSM-III Diagnosis	% Burn	Risk-Rescue Ratios	Previous Suicide Attempt	Previous Psychiatric Treatment	History of Mental Illness	Family Abuse of Patient	Adult Intact Family	Religion
14/F	Depression[a]	60–70	50	Yes	Unknown	Yes	Yes	Yes	Muslim
14/F	MDD; conduct aggressive[b]	93	56	Yes	Yes (1–2 times per week psychotherapy with psychiatrist stopped by guardian)	Unknown	Yes	Yes	Fundamental Christian
15/F	MDD; alcohol and cannabis abuse, aggressive conduct disorder	80	71	Yes	Yes; chose to discontinue treatment 1 previous 1 month hospitalization	Yes	Yes	Yes	Fundamental Christian
15/M	MDD; mixed mental disorder (learning disability)	90	63	No	No (but did see school counselor)	No	No	No	
15/M	MDD; ? mental retardation[c]	96	56	Yes	Yes	Unknown	No	No	Unknown
16/M	Schizophrenia or depression[d]	73	56	No	Yes (parents discontinued psychiatric treatment)	Unknown	Unknown	Yes	Catholic
17/M	Atypical depression atypical PDD, enuresis, phobia	90	71	No	Educational psychological evaluation only	Yes	No	No	Fundamental Christian
18/F	Schizophrenia	80	71	Yes	Yes (3 times per week by psychologist)	Unknown	Unknown	Yes	Jewish
16/M	MDD with psychosis	15	63	No (but recently caused and escaped a severe accident)	Yes (weekly with school psychiatrist and 4 psychiatric visits)	Yes	Yes	Yes	Mormon
18/F	MDD with hypomania; narcissistic character disorder	80 Propane	71	Yes	Yes (4 interviews by child psychiatrists; parents refused to follow hospitalization advice)	Yes	Yes	Yes	Catholic
16/M	Schizophrenic disorder, paranoid type[e]	27 Electrical	56	Yes	Yes. Psychiatric hospitalization 1 year preburn EEG inconsistent with psychomotor seizures on 1 occasion; another normal.	Yes. Paternal grandfather suicide; paternal uncle epileptic	No	Yes	Catholic

[a] There is diagnostic uncertainty in this case.
[b] MDM, major depressive disorder; PDD, pervasive developmental disorder.
[c] This patient died of his burns and related complications.
[d] There is diagnostic uncertainty in this case.
[e] There is diagnostic uncertainty in this case. Different psychiatrists at different hospitals at different times diagnosed him as major affective disorder, manic type with psychosis and schizophrenic disorder. Patient responded to lithium carbonate, and later in a second episode to haloperidol.

Table 98.2. Pain Management Guidelines from Shriners Burns Institute, Boston

I. Pharmacological managment of ventilated acute patients
  A. Background
    1. Pain
      a. Morphine sulfate intermittent i.v. bolus 0.05–0.1 mg/kg every 2 hours may need to be increased gradually
      b. Morphine sulfate continuous infusion
         Dose: Start at 0.05 mg/kg/hour
      c. Naloxone (Narcan) for reversal if needed for airway crises
    2. Anxiety
      a. Midazolam (Versed) intermittent i.v. bolus for patients without adequate comfort with analgesics
         Dose: 0.04 mg/kg slow push every 4–6 hours
      b. Midazolam (Versed) continuous infusion for patients with ongoing need for anxiety management not alleviated by other intervention
         NOTE: *Reversible neurologic abnormalities have been reported in critically ill children following long-term midazolam use.*
         Dose: starting at 0.04 mg/kg/hour
      c. Flumazinil (Mazicon) for reversal if need for airway crisis
         Dose: 0.2–1.0 mg given at rate of 0.2 mg/min; may take 6–10 minutes for peak effect. Wait >1 minute between doses. Too rapid administration may cause seizures
  B. Procedural, similar to above
  C. Transitional issues for weaning mechanical ventilation (omitted here but available)
II. Pharmacological management of nonventilated acute patients
  A. Background
    1. Pain
      a. Morphine sulfate immediate release (MSIR) on a consistent schedule
         Dose: 0.3–0.6 mg/kg enterally every 4–8 hours
      b. Morphine sulfate, intermittent i.v. bolus to supplement enteral morphine
         Dose: 0.05 mg/kg i.v. every 2–4 hours
      c. Morphine sulfate continuous infusion when enteral administration is not effective or patient NPO
         Dose: starting at 0.05–0.1 mg/kg/hour
    2. Anxiety
      a. Enteral or i.v. lorazepam on consistent schedule for patients unable to achieve adequate level of comfort from analgesic or other measures
  B. Procedural
    1. Pain
      a. MSIR 1 hour prior to procedure
         Dose: 0.05 mg/kg i.v.
         NOTE: use pulse oximetry monitoring for patients receiving multiple bolus doses; morphine effects may exceed the duration of the procedure.
      b. Morphine sulfate i.v. bolus ½ hour prior to procedure
         Dose: 0.05 mg/kg i.v.
         NOTE: use pulse oximetry as above
    2. Anxiety
      a. Enteral or i.v. lorazepam ½ hour prior to procedure for patients unable to achieve adequate level of comfort from analgesics or other measures
         Dose: 0.04 mg/kg i.v. or p.o.
  C. Transitional issue: pharmacologic management during changeover from parenteral to enteral route; opiate weaning
    1. Pain
      a, b, c opiates tapered 10–20% every 24–48 hours; MSIR, 10–25% every 24–72 hours
      d. Acetaminophen may be appropriate when tapering MSIR dose
    2. Anxiety. Lorazepam taper 25% per day over 4–7 days. Psychiatric consultation if needed
III. Pharmacologic management of acute rehabilitative patient
  A. Background
    1. Pain
      a. MSIR, similar to above
      b. MS Contin (morphine sulfate sustained release) for patients able to swallow tablet
         Dose: Based on 24-hour dose requirement of MSIR. Administer one-half daily dose every 12 hours.
    2. Anxiety
      a. Lorazepam
      b. Consider different longer acting medication: psychiatric consultation
  B. Procedural
    1. Pain.
      a. MSIR
    2. Anxiety
      a. Lorazepam 0.04 mg/kg p.o. ½ hour prior to procedures
IV. Reconstructive or routine postoperative, similar to III above.

Modified from Daly W, Sheridan R, Stoddard R, et al: Taking the conflict out of pain management: An institutional approach. Proceedings of the 26th Annual Meeting of the American Burn Association, Orlando, FL, April 20–24, 1994, p. 206.

consultants be aware of possible unconscious factors, identify and differentiate them from pain management, and encourage appropriate levels of analgesic use. Hospital pain guidelines (e.g., Table 98.2), collaboratively developed and monitored, may reduce this problem.

PAIN MANAGEMENT

The pain problems for burn patients are mainly acute rather than chronic. Prior to treatment of pain, physicians and nurses identify the location and source of pain, its usual intensity, course, and duration, and its response to treatment. Pain does correlate with endorphin levels (Fig. 98.1) and with the extent and depth of burn in children (Carr et al., 1993). Several years ago analgesics were withheld from a hateful adolescent girl with massive self-inflicted burns and a history of drug abuse, since her constant complaining about pain was viewed as manipulative; a research study later revealed that her endorphin levels had been negligible and that she should have been receiving high doses of morphine. Unfortunately endorphin levels are not rapidly available, but self ratings are usually sufficient. For infants (Porter, 1993) behavioral measures (facial expression, body movement, behavioral state, and cry), as well as physiologic parameters (heart rate, blood pressure, respiratory rate, and O_2 saturation, if available, and epinephrine, norepinephrine, growth hormone, and cortisol), are used to monitor pain response. Pain relief in infants improves surgical outcomes (not yet studied in burns), and there is need for a reliable and valid infant pain index.

For any child who cannot communicate, e.g., due to use of curariform drugs or intubation, estimates of maximum analgesic requirement for body weight are made. The only easily used assessment for pain and pain relief for conscious patients is self-rated pain ratings, preferably recorded on each shift and at each dressing change. When such ratings, performed consistently and reliably, are not present, there is little basis for evaluation of pain treatment, although clinical judgment and nurses' ratings are still used. Matthews et al. (1993) point to limitations of each but indicate particular strengths of self-report measures such as the Faces Scale, Visual Analogue Scale, and Oucher Scale. Of observational scales

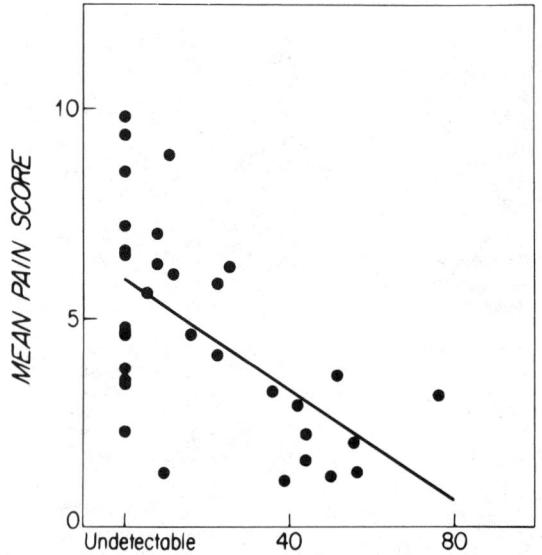

Figure 98.1. Mean pain score versus initial β-endorphin level during burn dressing change. The relationship of the initial (before analgesic and burn dressing change) β-endorphin plasma immunoactivity and mean pain score for the time of burn dressing change. (Szyfelbein SK, Osgood PF, Carr DB: The assessment of pain and plasma B-endorphin immunoactivity in burned children. *Pain* 22:173, 1985.)

Table 98.3. Developmentally Targeted Approaches to Pain Treatment

General principles
1. Assess extent and depth of burn, temperament, developmental stage, family relationshps, past pain response, complications, and cultural background.
2. Specify staff member, e.g., primary nurse, to develop consistent relationship outside the pain-producing situations.
3. Individualize treatment with multiple biological and psychological modalities for pain from burn (''background''), surgery, dressing changes, physical therapy, etc.
4. Prepare the parent or guardian well to also assist to decrease fear and increase security including use of favorite objects, especially for infants and toddlers.
5. Prepare child emotionally in his/her native language with developmentally appropriate modes of communication (using verbal protocol, picture book, play).
6. *Encourage child's participation (Kavanaugh et al., 1991), which may lessen medication.*
7. *Adequate dosages of medication (usually morphine) are essential in the acute, intermediate, and rehabilitative phases (Table 98.2).*
8. Record self-ratings of pain or, for infants, behavioral ratings.
9. Evaluate adequacy of pain regimen, including side effects, e.g., during ''pain rounds.''
10. Change treatment when pain does not lessen, usually by increasing dosages.

I. Pharmacological
  A. Antiinflammatory, e.g., acetaminophen, NSAID
  B. Antianxiety and antineuropathic
    1. Benzodiazepines
    2. Antidepressants
  C. Opioid
    1. Morphine i.v.
    2. Morphine p.o.
    3. Fentanyl i.v.
    4. Other opiates
    5. Patient-controlled analgesia (PCA)
II. Additional psychological and other therapies: to supplement pharmacologic therapy or for procedures of mild-to-moderate pain intensity
  A. Hypnosis and self-hypnosis
  B. Focused visual imagery
  C. Relaxation
  D. Distraction
  E. Transcutaneous electrical nerve stimulation (TENS)
  F. Biofeedback

---

these authors favor the Childrens Hospital of Eastern Ontario Pain Scale (CHEOPS). The most easily used self-rating scale is a simple 1–10 visual analogue scale rating or asking the child to rate the pain from 0–10, with 0 as none and 10 as the most severe pain (Szyfelbein, Osgood, Carr, et al., 1985). A variety of scales are in use for young children, e.g., the Faces Pain Scale, which pictures faces rated from 0, a happy face that ''doesn't hurt at all,'' through 5, a sad crying face ''hurting as much as you can imagine.'' The range of developmentally targeted approaches for use in managing pain is shown in Table 98.3.

Of the psychological methods, the behavioral method involving the child's participation developed by Kavanaugh, Lasoff, McEttrick, and others was designed to increase the ''locus of control'' in burned children themselves (Kavanaugh et al., 1991). The method involves preparation for each step of the burn dressing change and increases the children's control over that aversive experience by encouraging their help in removing bandages and in other steps. It leads to fewer maladaptive behaviors, improved outcomes, and lower dosages of narcotics. Tarnowski et al. (1987) described a similar behavioral method, ''self-mediated debridement,'' with similar results in one patient in a ''within-subjects repeated reversal design.''

Kuttner (1993), following Olness and Gardner, highlights the effectiveness and practicality of *hypnosis* for burn pain in children and notes that education of parents and encouraging their presence is desirable. She describes practical hypnotic methods in 3- to 6-year-olds and in older children, stating that maximum hypnotizability is in children, and advocates its rapid use, short-term, and indicates that capacity for self-hypnosis is the ideal end point, giving maximal control. It is probable that this method is underused, given its relative ease with children.

PHARMACOLOGICAL TREATMENT

Opiates and Benzodiazepines

Pharmacological treatment is the primary intervention to relieve pain in children. Pain treatment is important for biological as well as psychological reasons: the stress it causes disrupts metabolic, autonomic, and thermoregulatory as well as immune functions; it also can ''adversely affect morbidity and mortality'' (Carr et al., 1993). Recent studies have clarified the effectiveness of morphine in relieving pain, using either intravenous or oral administration of the drug (Carr et al., 1993). The doses used are much higher than doses used for most other purposes as demonstrated in Table 98.2 (Daly et al., 1994), which is a protocol incorporating current research on pharmacological pain and anxiety management. Self-reported pain ratings are to be documented.

Gaukroger (1993) carefully reviewed all aspects of *patient-controlled analgesia* (PCA) and noted its unsuitability for preschool and mentally retarded children. Berde et al. (1991) evaluated PCA in a randomized, prospective comparison with intramuscular administration of morphine for postoperative analgesia and found excellent results for PCA with children 6–18 years old. Doyle et al. (1994) studied children after surgery (not burns) with the finding that those treated with higher dose morphine had less pain and the lower dose group had more hypoxemic episodes. Carr et al. (1993) state that ''although PCA has been successfully used in acutely burned children, it lends itself more easily to the more manageable postoperative pain of patients returning for reconstructive surgery.''

Adjuvants, which enhance the effect of opiates can make the difference between presence and absence of pain relief. Most common in current use are low dose benzodiazepines, acetaminophen, and nonsteroidal antiinflammatory drugs (NSAIDs) and less common are low dose methylphenidate, amphetamine, tricyclic antidepressants, and haloperidol. Except for benzodiazepines, these have had no formal study in burned children.

The benzodiazepines in common use, depending on pain severity and duration of action desired include: *short-acting*, midazolam (Sheridan et al., 1994), lorazepam, oxazepam, and triazolam; and *long-acting*, chlordiazepoxide, diazepam, clonazepam, and flurazepam. In a study of three acutely burned children at our center (F.J. Stoddard, L. Baer, L. Rizzone, unpublished, 1992), clonazepam caused excessive sedation and anorexia in combination with morphine in two subjects but was effective in the third, a child with a family history of panic disorder.

There are few indications for use of psychotropic drugs with acutely burned children other than management of pain, anxiety (Tables 98.2 and 98.3), or delirium. Major tranquilizers are rarely necessary to control severe burn delirium, agitation, or severe insomnia. In the rare instances when benzodiazepines are unsuccessful, or paradoxically cause disinhibition or agitation, the drug of choice for children over 12 is short-term use of intravenous haloperidol in low doses (0.5–2.0 mg slow i.v. push) for only 24–48 hours, while the cause (e.g., sepsis, metabolic change, etc.) is being identified and treated. It has few cardiovascular effects and is rapidly effective; in the author's experience in two of approximately 75 cases, rapid infusion of haloperidol appeared to cause brief reversible hypotension in children, and these two children were under 10 years old. Continuous ECG and blood pressure monitoring at the time of administration is indicated if used with young children. Although dystonia can occur with continued use, requiring an anti-Parkinsonian agent, that has not occurred with short periods of intravenous use, while the therapeutic benefits are marked. A recent study of haloperidol use in children with burns also found it useful (Brown et al., 1996).

Despite wide use in acutely burned children, the only studies to date of symptom response to psychotropic agents have been with analgesics, and the small study of clonazepam for anxiety. Occasional children with attention deficit hyperactivity disorder (ADHD) who were previously taking a stimulant may require it in the course of burn treatment; a side benefit is that it can enhance analgesics as well. The reasons for generally not using other psychotropic agents are possible interactions or toxic effects, e.g., from lithium, further compromising acute burn treatment. A severe psychotic disorder, not due to the burn or burn treatment, would usually be managed with haloperidol due to its relative lack of cardiovascular risk. Also, a few children with minor (<10%) burns may require psychotropic agents for preexisting conditions, usually with little risk of complications.

Drug side effects and, rarely, toxicity occur, especially with opiates, benzodiazepines, and haloperidol. Neuroleptic malignant syndrome may occur, and symptoms can be almost the same as malignant hyperthermia from anesthetics. Opiate or benzodiazepine tolerance, dependence, and withdrawal do occur. The withdrawal syndrome from opiates includes abdominal cramps, vomiting, diarrhea, tachycardia, hypertension, diaphoresis, restlessness, and insomnia; it is reversed by opiate agonists. Abrupt withdrawal from benzodiazepines may cause anxiety, dysphoria, or insomnia but also full-scale withdrawal with abdominal cramps, vomiting, sweating, tremors, and convulsions. Some symptoms occur even several days later after gradual withdrawal. Resuming and then slowly tapering the benzodiazepine usually reverses the withdrawal symptoms. Although some patients become dependent on opiates and benzodiazepines, *addiction (i.e., severe drug abuse) is almost never caused by analgesia for burn pain*, despite the concerns of many staff about this, especially with adolescents. Dependence is effectively managed, once the patient no longer needs the medication, by gradual tapering, including with occasional adolescent substance abusers who may have required higher doses of opiates at first than others. The use of a clonidine patch has been effective in eliminating moderate opiate withdrawal symptoms. In children the combination of opiates and benzodiazepines may contribute to respiratory depression, delirium, anorexia, and excess sedation (American Psychiatric Association, 1990). Severe opiate side effects can be reversed by naloxone, and benzodiazepine toxicity by flumazenil, but this may cause seizures. Taking these risks into account, the judicious use of medications and careful monitoring normally results in predictable and reliable reductions in pain and anxiety.

PHASES OF BURN RECOVERY: ACUTE PHASE

Three postburn phases occur after a burn, which have both neurobiological and psychological features. These are *acute*, *intermediate*, and *rehabilitative*. Psychiatric assessment and treatment are adapted to each phase. The full range of psychiatric knowledge and skills are used in work with burned infants, children, adolescents, and their families.

Diagnostic Assessment

From the time of admission, assessment and treatment proceed together. Orientation, explanation, and preparation for what has occurred and is to come are linked with assessment of the child's and parent's responses to these interventions. Communication is best when it is at the child's stage of development (Gaffney, 1993; Stoddard, 1982) and in the child's and parents' language. Since the child is often confused in the strange burn unit setting, afraid of dying regardless of wound severity, and anxious about pain, the initial history may be obtained from others, but it is important to elicit it from the child when possible. The child responds positively to reassurance about his or her condition and efforts to create familiarity and comfort. Relief of pain lessens fear and confusion. When parents understand, feel support and reassurance, then they can assist and be successful in calming their child. Once an initial secure and trusting staff-parent alliance is established, additional history emerges that may clarify preburn risk factors such as a toddler's new motor skills, homelessness or poverty, firesetting, child neglect or abuse, and parental substance abuse, mental disorder, or criminality. Similarly, postburn emotional reactions such as fear, guilt, denial, grief, or withdrawal become evident.

An important early diagnosis to be alert for is *delirium (293.0)* since the confused, agitated, or aggressive patient can cause self-injury by abrupt events such as unplanned pulmonary extubation or pulling out intravenous lines. EEG abnormalities associated with burn delirium have been demonstrated in adults (Andreasen et al., 1977), and Antoon et al. (1977) described seizures in 10 of 20 subjects. Delirium in burned children is common and "alerts staff to the patient's unstable medical condition and can be the first indicator of opiate side effects, sepsis, metabolic disturbance, CNS injury or a combination of these. Prompt diagnostic evaluation of the delirious child, treatment of the causative factors, symptomatic relief, environmental change, and increased personal contact with staff and family are indicated" (Stoddard, 1990). Antoon et al. (1972) studied the etiology of burn encephalopathy in 20 children and found the etiology to be hypoxia due to smoke inhalation in 6 cases, sepsis in 4, a combination of the two in 2, and hyponatremia in 4 cases; of the survivors, only one had residual neurological impairment; 10 patients died and 5 had complete neuropathological examinations, 1 with *Pseudomonas* meningitis, 1 with sepsis, and 3 with minimal findings. While delirium remains a sign of complications, modern treatment has reduced the mortality rate to a fraction of what it was.

The stress of an acute moderate or severe burn is extraordinary, a shock that may involve loss of possessions and of loved ones, as well as injury to the child's own body. Many children with burns manifest *acute stress disorder (308.3)* . The burn unit offers an opportunity for case identification, assessment, and intervention including referrals for developmental, neurological, and educational evaluation of at risk children who would otherwise not receive them. For this reason, it is important to complete or initiate assessment even during brief hospitalizations when indicated.

Developmental Neurobiology

The child's body is able to respond remarkably to trauma such as a massive burn, but it is less certain how resilient the child is emotionally. "A massive catecholamine release occurs immediately after burn injury both from the adrenal medulla and the autonomic nervous system" (Demling, 1990). The body goes through three phases. First, an acute shock or resuscitation phase occurs, with decreased metabolism, dulling of severe pain, and many other acute changes requiring intensive treatment, especially fluid replacement. Second, after a few days there occurs a hypermetabolic or recovery phase with an increase in the metabolic rate of about two times normal during which the hypothalamus seems to select a higher temperature set point and which is associated with increases in plasma catecholamines, cortisol, glucagon, and growth hormone (Demling, 1990; Wilmore, 1974). In the presence of pain and anxiety, the brain can increase the hypermetabolic response (Demling, 1990). In infants and children today, unless complications occur, the excision of burn-damaged tissue and coverage of the burn wounds with skin grafts results in healing often in 1–3 months, even with large wounds. The acute and intermediate treatments are often accompanied by severe chronobiological changes, including for some a reversal of the day-night sleep-wake cycle due to round-the-clock treatments; as healing progresses, the sleep-wake cycle gradually returns to its preburn pattern although sleep disorders, day napping, and enuresis are common posttraumatic symptoms (Kravitz et al., 1993; Murphy et al., 1989). Third, during the rehabilitative phase, wound healing is completed and metabolism gradually returns to normal a few months after discharge.

Neurobiological Phases Postburn

ACUTE STRESS DISORDER (DSM-IV)

The physiological changes briefly outlined above appear to be mirrored by changes in brain function and mental status in those patients who are not so sedated that they cannot be evaluated. Some of the mental states commonly seen during acute treatment, which may reflect or relate to the systemic phases described above, include acute stress disorder, delirium, pain syndromes, sleep disorders, depression, and eventually recovery. The hypermetabolic response may appear as a pseudomanic delirious state with confusion, anxiety, and agitation; later, associated with catecholamine depletion, a state of depression usually develops, with depressive mood, interpersonal withdrawal, and decreased appetite (Gold et al., 1988). This is not true in all cases, and there are children, whose pain and anxiety are controlled, who are mentally clear and conversant as deep fascial excisions or amputations of burned areas are about to be or have just been done; in all cases, psychiatric assessment, surgical preparation, and psychotherapeutic support are essential.

In the child, adequate relief of pain and anxiety, together with rapid healing, may lessen the probability of acute stress disorder, posttraumatic stress disorder (PTSD), or major depression. Charney et al. (1993) describe a model that shows a central role for the locus ceruleus, ventral tegmental area, and especially the amygdala in facilitating the "encoding of traumatic memories" through "fear conditioning, extinction, and sensitization." Interestingly, the postulated neurotransmitter systems involve norepinephrine, dopamine, opioids, and corticotropin-releasing factor. These are some of the same systems activated in severe burns, and drugs affecting these systems are frequently required for complications arising during burn treatment: cardiovascular, renal, pain, and metabolic disturbances. However, studies reflecting central neurobiological effects in burned children have included mainly endorphins and cortisol.

Some of the common phenomena in acute burn treatment affecting and being affected by neurobiological systems include: neurotoxins (anoxia, CO), delirium, catecholamine depletion and depression, opiate dependence/side effects/withdrawal, and benzodiazepine dependence/side effects/withdrawal. Endorphins, and probably endogenous benzodiazepines (Rothstein et al., 1992), and the receptor systems involved affect the response to trauma and to medications. It is not known whether residual neurodevelopmental abnormalities follow burn trauma treated by modern methods.

NEUROBIOLOGY OF THE INTERMEDIATE PHASE

This phase, after the patient has survived and is healing, is somewhat less stressful. Physiological responses such as a conservation-with-drawal reaction or post acute stress depression seem to be normal after burn trauma. Hospitalization is not free of stress, and it is this period for which Gilboa et al.'s (1994) term "continuous traumatic stress" may be most fitting. Stress occurs throughout burn treatment, not only acutely and then after it is all over (PTSD), but continuously to varying degrees. Vulnerable children with prior comorbid conditions, e.g., anxiety, affective, or disruptive behavior disorders, may have special difficulty adapting to the frequent stresses of burn care and benefit from resumption of psychotropic medications if they were temporarily stopped. Other neurobiological changes occur commonly in burn care secondary to acute surgical use of potent agents such as dopamine, curare, analgesics, or ketamine. Complications may emerge including infection, organ failure, or metabolic disturbance, any of which can contribute to the occurrence of delirium.

A special, but increasing problem in burn care is HIV infection and AIDS (Blumenfield and Schoeps, 1993). Children are less commonly infected than adult burn patients, but it is important for staff to adhere strictly to universal precautions. Generally the acute issues of burn treatment take precedence over HIV interventions unless AIDS is in the late stages. For children it can be especially tragic if they survive burns only to learn that they are infected due to any cause, including transfusions, a rarity now, as transfusions are much less used and the blood supply is carefully screened. Adverse events such as needle sticks do occur; such events and staff fears are addressed using standard hospital policies and procedures.

POSTTRAUMATIC STRESS DISORDER

In the assessment of neurobiological sequelae of burns, the child psychiatrist's medical expertise and skills in diagnosis and treatment become important. As the child becomes more active, stress disorders such as PTSD may become chronic. For children, DSM-IV PTSD criteria have now been modified to include "disorganized or agitated behavior" in the response to trauma, and posttraumatic play, "frightening dreams without recognizable content," and "trauma specific reenactment" as evidence of reexperiencing. Alternative criteria for diagnosis are being developed for children ages 0–4 (Scheeringa et al., 1995). Formal study of PTSD has rarely been done with burned children, the largest being a follow-up study (F.J. Stoddard, J.M. Murphy, L. Rizzone, unpublished, 1994) of 60 children ages 7–19 with mean burn size of 38% body surface. The findings are consistent with their earlier study of 30 children (Stoddard et al. 1989a), that is, that at least $\frac{1}{4}$ to $\frac{1}{3}$ of burned children manifest PTSD, but over 50% have posttraumatic symptoms. Large burns and facial burns increased risk of PTSD. They concluded that PTSD symptoms are widespread among burned children and that treatment to prevent and alleviate PTSD is indicated. Kravitz et al. (1993) had consistent findings, with a similar incidence of sleep disorders. They studied sleep disorders in 82 children, mean duration postburn 7.3 years, 41 boys and 41 girls with a mean burn size of 44% (range 2–91% total body surface). They found that a subgroup of 30 children reported nightmares. Of the 55 reporting dreams, 45 reported normal childhood topics, 6 burn injury-related topics, and 5 burn treatment-related topics. Some of the "normal" topics may be burn-related also, e.g. monsters, kidnapping, being killed, scary movies, dying, being locked up, parents dying, or a sibling harmed. Topics clearly related to the burn were reliving of the event, smelling smoke, and dreaming of others who died in the fire, and screaming, "Fire." Topics related to treatment included pain from dressing changes, anesthesia induction, fear of dying in the operating room, dreaming scars are gone, and fearing a burned hand will be amputated. In that study, nightmares involved clear disorders of arousal with screaming, thrashing, sweating, yelling, etc. They found sleep walking in 7% of subjects. Similar to Stoddard et al. (1989a, 1989b), they found a history of enuresis in 24% of subjects.

The outcome of PTSD after burns is not known, although studies suggest some attenuation of symptoms after the first few months. Research studies are confirming the clinical finding that cognitive interventions for children with PTSD may assist their coping. PTSD is not the only disorder afflicting these children, and an intervention may benefit them in other areas also, e.g., phobia, depression, enuresis, and ADHD. Ongoing psychotherapeutic intervention is indicated, and adding a psychopharmacological intervention, e.g., clonazepam, sertraline, or fluoxetine, is done if anxiety or depressive symptoms associated with PTSD require it. Reports of cognitive-behavioral therapy for PTSD in other traumatized children are relevant (Deblinger et al., 1990), and Solomon et al. (1992) reviewed the literature on all aspects of PTSD treatment, highlighting the potential value of behavioral, cognitive, and pharmacological therapies, but mainly in adult studies.

INTERMEDIATE PHASE: EFFECTS ON PSYCHOLOGICAL DEVELOPMENT

Psychological Interventions

INDIVIDUAL

There is a shift from the acute into the intermediate phase once survival is assured and most burn wounds are grafted, although the patient may not be ambulatory. During this period it is possible to more fully assess mental status and to begin differentiating issues of mourning the prior body image, grief over loss of loved ones, depression, and posttraumatic stress disorder. In addition, assessment and diagnosis of neurological or preexisting psychiatric impairment becomes feasible. The child's or adolescent's emerging awareness of their functional losses and cosmetic disfigurement are eased by responsive staff and supportive, informed family members. "Healing well" or "looking good" surgically does not mean that the child or parent see the raw wounds or new grafts in the same way, especially if they expected a return to previous appearance. When a child requests a mirror, the curiosity and emerging self-awareness about facial burns and appearance can unsettle a nurse or parent, leading to the question of whether or not the child is ready or may react with too much anxiety or depression. While each situation must be individually assessed, in most cases children benefit when such requests are honored, but with exploration of their expectation and adequate support nearby when they first view themselves. Modes of intervention usually include brief consultative checks, and for those in most distress, several sessions of 15–30 minutes per week focussed on the issues mentioned above as well as preparation for forthcoming surgery, return to home and school, and rehabilitation.

FAMILY

Adaptation of the parents and family usually follows the course of the child's recovery. Remarkably similar feelings and defensive responses are observed in the child and family. Psychotherapeutic support, especially regarding guilt feelings, and grief work with parents, often in several sessions per week, during this phase assists the parents and enables them to support the child's coping through this phase.

GROUP THERAPY

Some hospitals with many burned children provide groups varying from brief psychotherapy to education to rehabilitation. At the Shriners Burns Institute in Boston, three types of group interventions have been used for over 15 years. The author has conducted a weekly inpatient *children's group* with a resident, nurse, or teacher, for children 2–12 years old, which varies from preschoolers to school age to preadolescents, depending on which children are in the hospital. This is a semistructured play group in which children introduce themselves, say why they are in the hospital and how they were burned, play with puppets and toys, draw, and then clean up the toys and prepare to say good-bye. The children readily express their feelings and fantasies in displacement to the consistent "Curious George" puppet who, while a troublemaker, is very curious about the children's puppets' understanding of their burns, pain, surgery, dreams, scars, peer ridicule, etc. While at first hesitant to participate, they become attached to the group. When they are again readmitted, they ask for the "children's group"; once they become adolescents, they remember it with a smile since they usually enjoy it despite occasional painful topics. An *adolescent group* for hospitalized adolescents, and a *parent group* for parents of acute patients are also provided, focusing on education about treatment, grief, response to hospitalization, surgery, stigmatization, and discharge and reentry issues. In England, Rivlin et al. (1986) conducted similar groups, which the parents rated as helpful, using a multidisciplinary approach.

REHABILITATIVE PHASE: BODY IMAGE AND PLASTIC AND RECONSTRUCTIVE SURGERY

After surviving and healing from the burn, the child's surgical follow-up care is transferred to the plastic and reconstructive surgeon if not previously involved. The acute surgical service and plastic and reconstructive surgical services are often linked, which assists transition from one to the other. The child psychiatrist and mental health team learn through their patients and the plastic surgeons about the various surgical and nonsurgical options available for scars, disfigurement, functional impairment or loss, and amputations. Plastic surgeons of necessity develop psychological skills in evaluating burned patients and may seek psychiatric consultation for some cases (Goin and Goin, 1981). Since much of acute treatment, even with recent changes, is outside of the control of the child and family, a central psychological goal at this point in care is to increase the child's and parents' roles in the choice of treatment, its timing, and the long-term plan (Cahners and Kartiganer, 1990; J. Remensnyder, unpublished, 1979). While staff responses assist the patient in seeing himself or herself anew (Solnit and Priel, 1975), the consultant in turn, through the eyes of the child, becomes aware of the experience of being burned.

Seeing Through the Eyes of a Burned Child: The Developing Body Image

Interviewing a burned child and observing the child's play provide a window on the child's body image development, the interference in that development caused by the burn and painful treatments, and, usually, the psychological adaptation and recovery that follow. The early concept was summarized by Fenichel as "the sum of the mental representations of the body and its organs, the so-called body image, [which] constitutes the idea of I and is of basic importance for the future formation of the ego" (Stoddard, 1982b). A more contemporary definition derives from the functions of body image and the developmental levels at which it operates (Shontz, 1974). The functions it serves are sensory register; instrument for actions; source of drives; a stimulus to the self (as in arousal, pain, and proprioceptive experiences); a stimulus to others (appearance identifies attractiveness or can be a stigma); an expressive instrument; and a private world. Disorders may occur at any cognitive level of body image experience including body schemata, body self, body fantasy, or body concept, and there are associated defense patterns and symptoms. Parental attitudes toward the child's physical defects help to shape body image development (Stoddard, 1982b). Some scarred individuals have no disorder of body image, while others with little or no scar may have significant body image disorder (body dysmorphic disorder (300.7), i.e., there is no necessary relationship between external appearance and internalized body image.

The issue of "how first was the body imaged?" is of practical relevance in the care of burned children. Recent research on infancy (see Chapter 20) pertains to the impact of burns on children 0–3 years old and on older children. Intricate attachment processes begin prenatally and continue seamlessly in the mother-child relationship following birth. Observations reveal that a burned infant is emotionally traumatized in the following ways: pain is felt and localized; the sense of safety and security in attachment to the mother is threatened or even shattered; the recovery from that experience or those experiences depends on the reestablishment of the attachment and the signs of responsivity present before the burn. What does this imply for body image development? A disturbance results from disruption of the protective mother-infant dyad for development of body image with its attendant affects and relational interactions. That appears in behavior as increased helplessness, sleep and feeding disturbances, and affective withdrawal in infants; social restriction and loss of acquired skills in the toddler; and problems in development of control over new fears and other feelings in 2- to 3-year-olds, e.g., aggression, problems with excretory functions, nightmares, play constriction, and play reenactment of the burn trauma or burn treatments (Scheeringa et al., 1995).

Hospitalization for a burn is often an early separation experience, which reveals the child's capacity to form and be consoled bodily by transitional objects, including a father or nurse who may represent a transitional relationship or surrogate. The capacity to create such relationships bodes well for the prognosis of the child and resembles hypnosis in its intensity and capacity to soothe. Body image is a relatively stable part of the self-concept by age 2–3 and is modified by growth, puberty, trauma, and aging. Burns in childhood and adolescence may leave an emotional "scar" as well as the physical one and may profoundly alter the subsequent body image, self-esteem, and interpersonal relations as well as ego functioning (Stoddard, 1982b). However, body image disturbance may not be inevitable, as suggested by a study of children ages 5–15 with matched controls using human figure drawings, which did not find significant differences in body image, except for increasing body image disturbance in both burned and unburned adolescents (Jessee et al., 1992).

This change in the child's body image and associated feelings such as sadness, shame, or pride may be seen in self-portraits (Figs. 98.2–98.4). Also, body image revision occurs through plastic surgery, often allowing another stage of reintegration of body image and optimally a degree of healing of the prior damage to appearance and self-

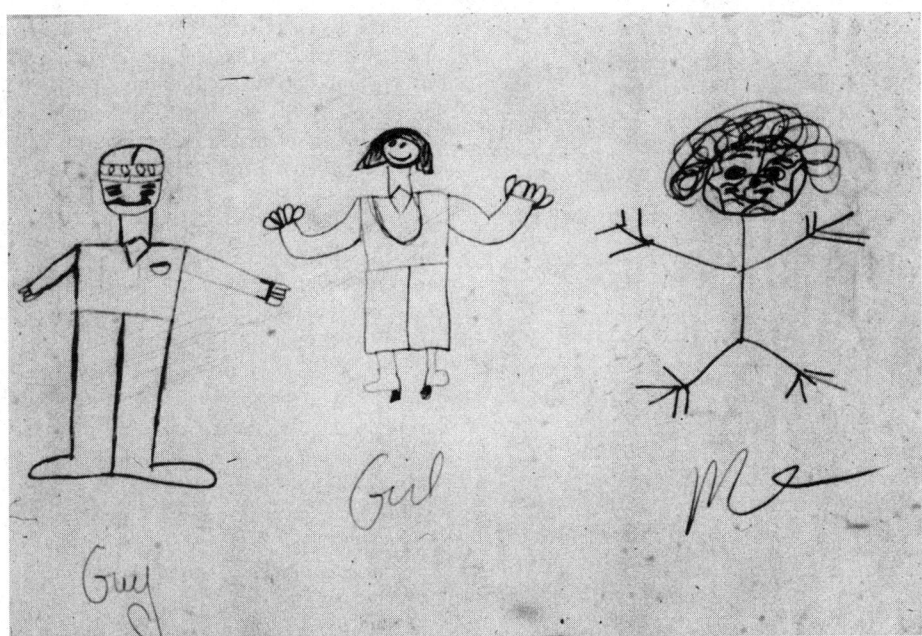

Figure 98.2. Portraits, including self, by a facially burned girl.

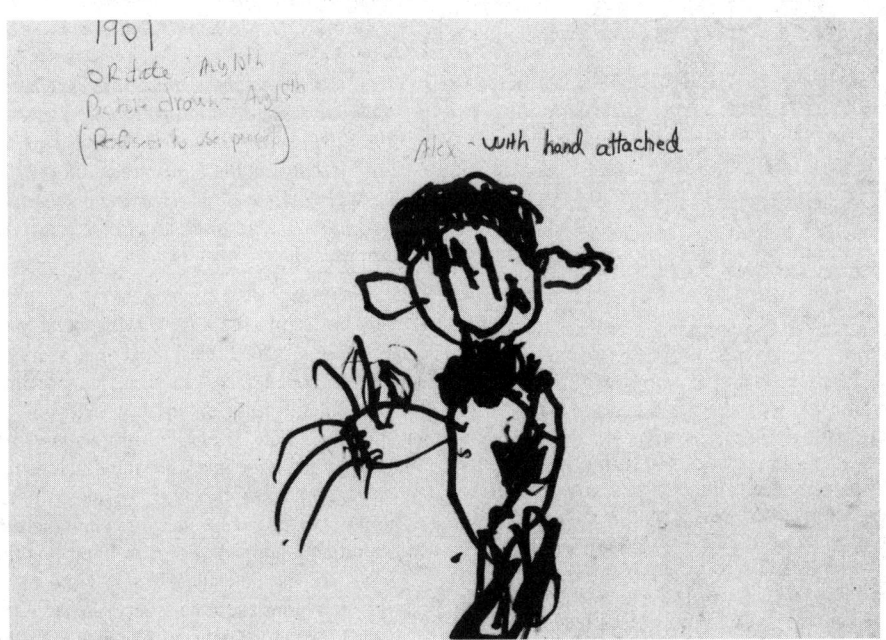

Figure 98.3. Accurate self-portrait by boy with severe burns with his hand surgically attached to his groin during a phase of a reconstructive procedure.

image. Focussed short-term supportive and educational psychotherapy is helpful, and a protocol for short-term therapy addressing body image issues is being developed (Pruzinsky and Doctor, 1994).

Psychological Trauma: Burns, Body Image, and Reintegration

In the last 20 years facially burned individuals have become commonplace on TV, in movies (*Nightmare on Elm Street*), and even in plays (*Phantom of the Opera*), but only occasionally with compassion or explanation, and most commonly in horror films. An exception was an award-winning pediatric film by Andrew Maguire, ''Here's Looking at You, Kid,'' a documentary about a boy with facial burns and his and his mother's experiences afterward. Television and film have familiar-

ized the public with scarring from burns. Notwithstanding, or sometimes because of, publicity, children are subjected to ridicule with epithets such as ''monster,'' ''french fry,'' and ''Freddie Krueger.'' Clear explanation by children with burns to peers about their injuries, and unequivocal leadership and support by teachers and parents directly addressing such problems, may reduce their frequency.

CASE ILLUSTRATION: SIBLING STIGMATIZATION REDUCED BY OUTREACH TO THE SCHOOL

Paul is a white boy who sustained deep full-thickness burns over 90% of his body, an inhalation injury, and renal failure at age 19 months in a house fire, surviving only because of heroic measures

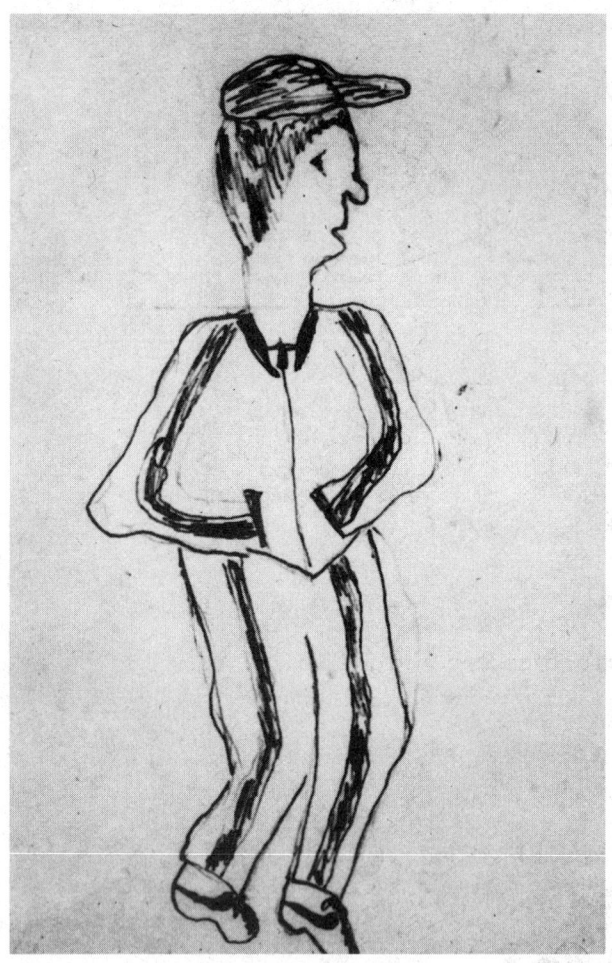

Figure 98.4. Self-portrait by boy with facial and hand burns.

MacGregor and Bernstein reported that social isolation or "social death" was common among the severely disfigured (Bernstein, 1976). Recent studies do not confirm this, at least in the United States, which may mean that they and others succeeded in helping to lessen the stigma of burns by stimulating improved surgical and psychological techniques and by advocating vigorously for equal social, educational, and occupational opportunity. However, social stigmatization is prevalent in cultures where disability is seen "as a form of punishment. The individual with a disability, his or her family, or an ancestor, according to the particular belief system, has been either cursed by God or the Gods, sinned or violated a taboo. . . . Others may seek to distance themselves from those who have incurred such 'evil'" (Groce and Zola, 1993).

Note to the Reader: Figures 98.5 through 98.9 are included not to offend but to inform and usefully prepare the consultant for feelings associated with seeing and talking with burned children. Most burns are much less severe. While such images are seen in surgical texts or on rounds, they are rare in psychiatric writing. The reader may progress through feelings of shock, revulsion, disgust, sadness, and even despair on viewing them—all normal reactions of new staff on ward rounds, and which scarred children and adolescents also experience from others at home, school, and at times in intimate relationships. Consultants may feel at first unable to comprehend or discuss these kinds of injuries or disfigurement, which many children and families survive and effectively cope with. Nevertheless, these cases all demonstrate positive emotional recoveries that are common today after severe burns. Such pictures are "dehumanized," standing alone, and therefore more upsetting than talking with the child. A child psychiatry fellow, completing his 3-month rotation, observed thoughtfully that he no longer "sees," i.e., reacts to, the scarring since he relates to the children as people. This gradual adaptation is a common experience among burn unit staff.

and 6 months of hospitalization at the Shriners Burns Institute. Three years later, his older brother, Bobby, was brought to a local clinic by his mother because Bobby was being isolated by his peers and had been beaten up severely by neighborhood boys who ridiculed him because his disfigured little brother "was a monster." Bobby was fighting with his peers about this and at the same time deeply resenting Paul and all of the special attention he had received. Their mother felt helpless and sought child psychiatric assistance after Bobby slammed the door on Paul to prevent children who were passing by from seeing him. In addition to caring for Paul, this single mother on welfare was caring for younger twins requiring frequent trips to downtown specialty clinics at Childrens' Hospital because of respiratory distress syndrome. They lived in a tough, low income suburban neighborhood.

The clinic child psychiatrist, together with the special education outreach team from the Shriners Hospital and Bobby's school, arranged a school outreach presentation about burns, disfigurement, and burn prevention. The teacher who conducted the presentation told a special assembly of 300 first and second graders and teachers how Paul had survived almost miraculously through use of skin grafts. She also explained about "same and different" using a book *We're Different We're the Same* and illustrated that M & M's are different colors but taste the same. She emphasized how different each child's feelings may be and "what it feels like to be teased." She reported that the faculty and students were very receptive to her presentation and that Bobby's class looked forward to helping Paul feel welcome when entering school next year. The boys' mother soon reported that children were now coming to their house to visit the boys, and that they looked forward to coming to Bobby's birthday party, whereas before none of the children had socialized with them at all.

One need only see a child with facial burns (Fig. 98.5), amputated fingers (Fig. 98.6), breast or genital scars to appreciate some of the damage to appearance and sometimes to internalized body image, as well as the suffering endured, and to realize how irrational thinking and prejudice can be elicited in response. And yet, burn treatment is remarkably effective in preserving life, reducing suffering, and in restoring appearance and function. Burns do not inevitably cause psychopathology but can, especially in vulnerable children whose burn care and familial support do not meet their emotional needs.

What are the key questions in child psychiatric evaluation before plastic and reconstructive surgery? What issues are involved perioperatively? Of primary importance are *secure relationships* with the family and with the doctor and treatment team. Another factor is the *capacity to tolerate fear and anxiety* associated with rehospitalization. Other factors involve the *results of preparation and consent for surgery*: (*a*) realistic awareness of scars and functional impairments, i.e., the indications for surgery; (*b*) the child's wish or willingness to have the surgery at this time; (*c*) the parents' wish for the child to have surgery at this time; and (*d*) understanding of the procedure and the capacity to communicate it. Anxiety often blocks understanding, and multiple explanations may be necessary. If there is significant psychopathology (Table 98.1), review of records and preoperative assessment are indicated to reduce complications. Suicide is very rare in patients who were not suicidal preburn (Stoddard, 1993), and the rate appears to be the same or less than in the general population. However, screening for suicide risk is important in all cases of depression, and also for those enduring long, stressful, or potentially disfiguring procedures or complications. On occasion, a child will refuse surgery at the operating room door due to acute anticipatory anxiety. Emotional support and benzodiazepines given early

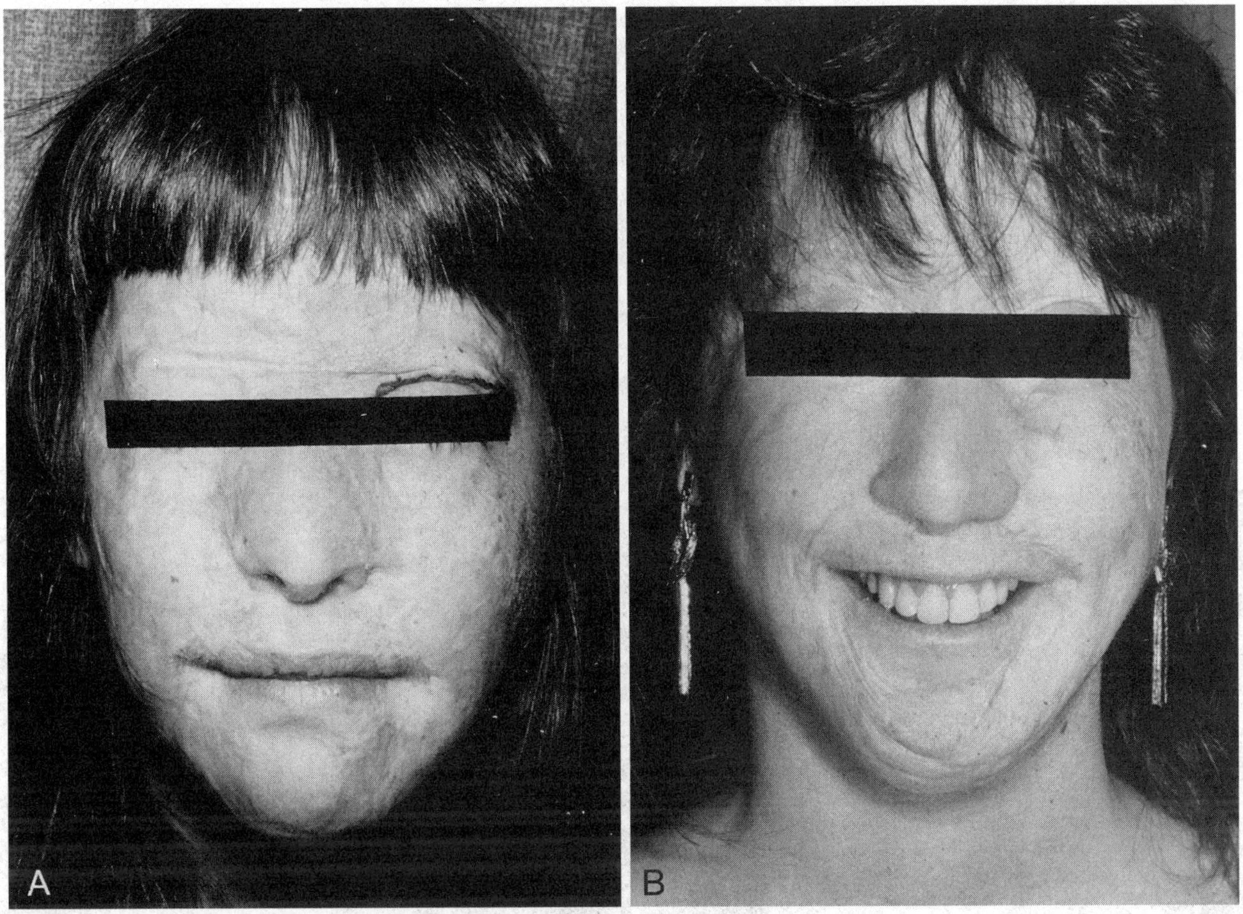

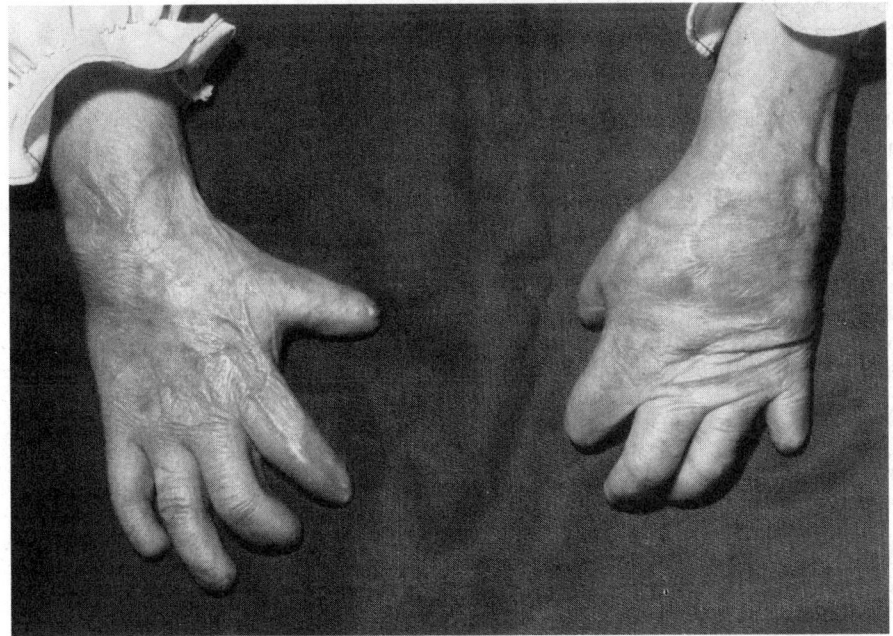

Figure 98.5.   Facial burns before and after reconstructive surgery in a girl at ages 6 and 16.

Figure 98.6.   An 8-year-old girl, who became a pianist, with healed hand burns, amputated digits, but no reconstruction.

often relieve it, while being certain that the child participates in choosing "if, when, and what" surgery is effective if the child's wishes were not a part of the decision. Other preoperative problems include: unrealistic expectations of "perfect" surgical results, embarrassment or shame related to severe disfigurement, and resurgence of PTSD symptoms such as flashbacks or nightmares. Supportive, reality-oriented psychothera-

peutic interventions usually allow the patient to cope and progress with a reasonable and hopeful attitude toward surgery.

In order to perform a psychiatric consultation to the patient, surgeon, and staff, some understanding of the surgery (Feldman, 1984; May and Moses, 1992; Salisbury, 1992)—standard and newly developed—is essential. This includes split thickness skin grafts and releases of con-

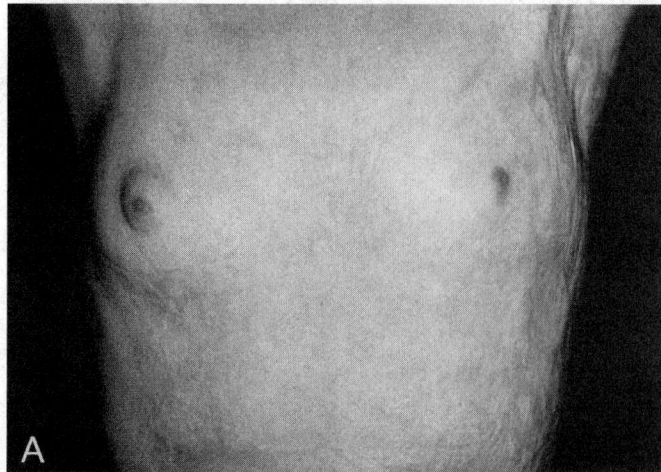

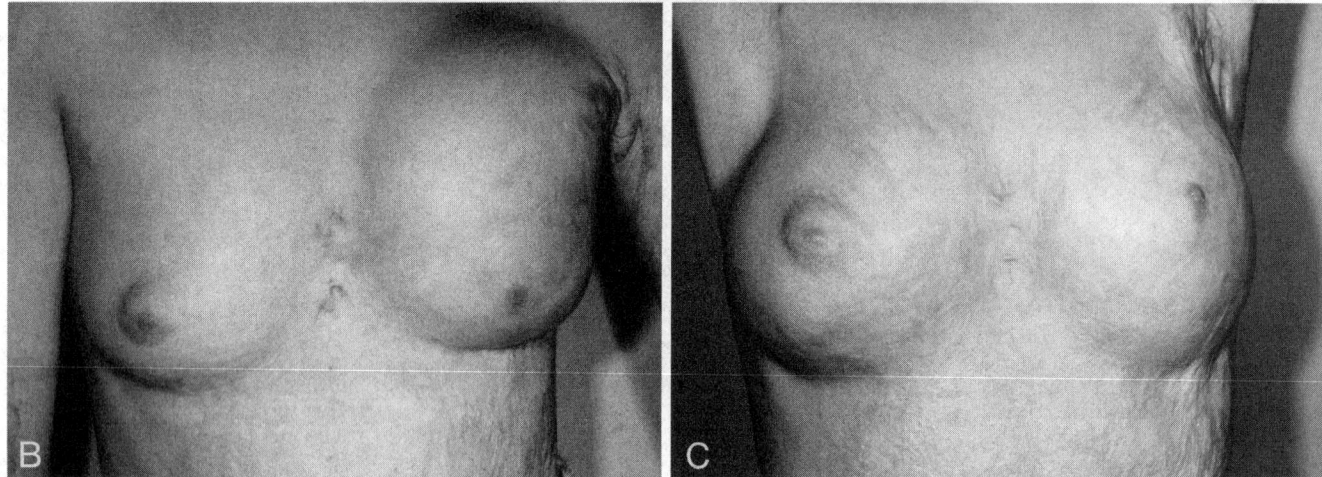

Figure 98.7.   **A**, Healed breast burns in a 14-year-old. **B**, Breasts being reconstructed through use of tissue expanders (balloons inflated with saline). **C**, Postoperative result at age 15 after reconstruction.

tractures, and such dramatic advances as facial resurfacing, restoration of scalp and hair with scalp expanders and flaps, microsurgery to the hand with reconstruction of usable opposition and other digits, breast reconstruction with or without expanders or implants, amputations and prosthetic placement, and even penile/scrotal or vaginal repair or reconstruction. The reason for a consultation, while seemingly broad, often narrowly concerns the patient's reactions to a recent surgical procedure and its success or failure in the child's, parent's, and doctor's eyes. Children undergoing such procedures benefit from psychiatric collaboration, reassessment, support, and, at times, treatment.

SEXUAL DEVELOPMENT

As children with burns approach and pass puberty, they, like others their age, become more concerned with attractiveness, loving and being loved, and sexuality. Their sense of self is revised and some become very self-conscious, covering their scars and avoiding being seen in public such as in locker rooms and beaches. Others become counterphobic and may be promiscuous or abuse substances in an effort to cope with conflict over self-image and self-esteem. Their requests for surgery involve wishes to appear normal, e.g., to repair scalp scars and have normal hair, to have asymmetrical breasts repaired and made symmetrical (Fig. 98.7), or to repair a facial scar that may cause peer ridicule. Most adolescents, including those with genital burns, which usually heal well (Figs. 98.8 and 98.9), become sexually active and many become parents. Finding a supportive partner, accepting of their burn injuries, aids sexual adjustment. Some studies indicate that women with burns

have a lower level of sexual satisfaction than men, but this has not been studied in adolescents. Continued individual, family, and group psychotherapy assists with difficult personal, sexual, social, educational, and occupational transitions. Those who have not had such services or who live far from the centers where they are available may benefit from burn camps in their region (Doctor, 1992). Although some of these adolescents are followed in medical centers for plastic and reconstructive surgery, many do not receive counseling to assist them emotionally or with education about drugs, contraception, HIV, childbirth education, or parenting skills.

For over 20 years several centers have provided ''reentry programs'' after discharge (Cahners and Kartiganer, 1990) through the hospital social service, special education, and other departments to assist with prompt return to school of burned children after discharge, rather than home tutoring, which was formerly common and increased morbidity and social isolation. This often involves school outreach educational programs to reduce peers', parents', and teachers' fear of disfigured children and to support reentry.

LONG-TERM TREATMENT

Psychological Interventions

INDIVIDUAL

Many children are not seen for psychological follow-up after their acute burn. This group may be most likely to have unexpressed feelings that may shape development, influencing avoidance behavior and, in

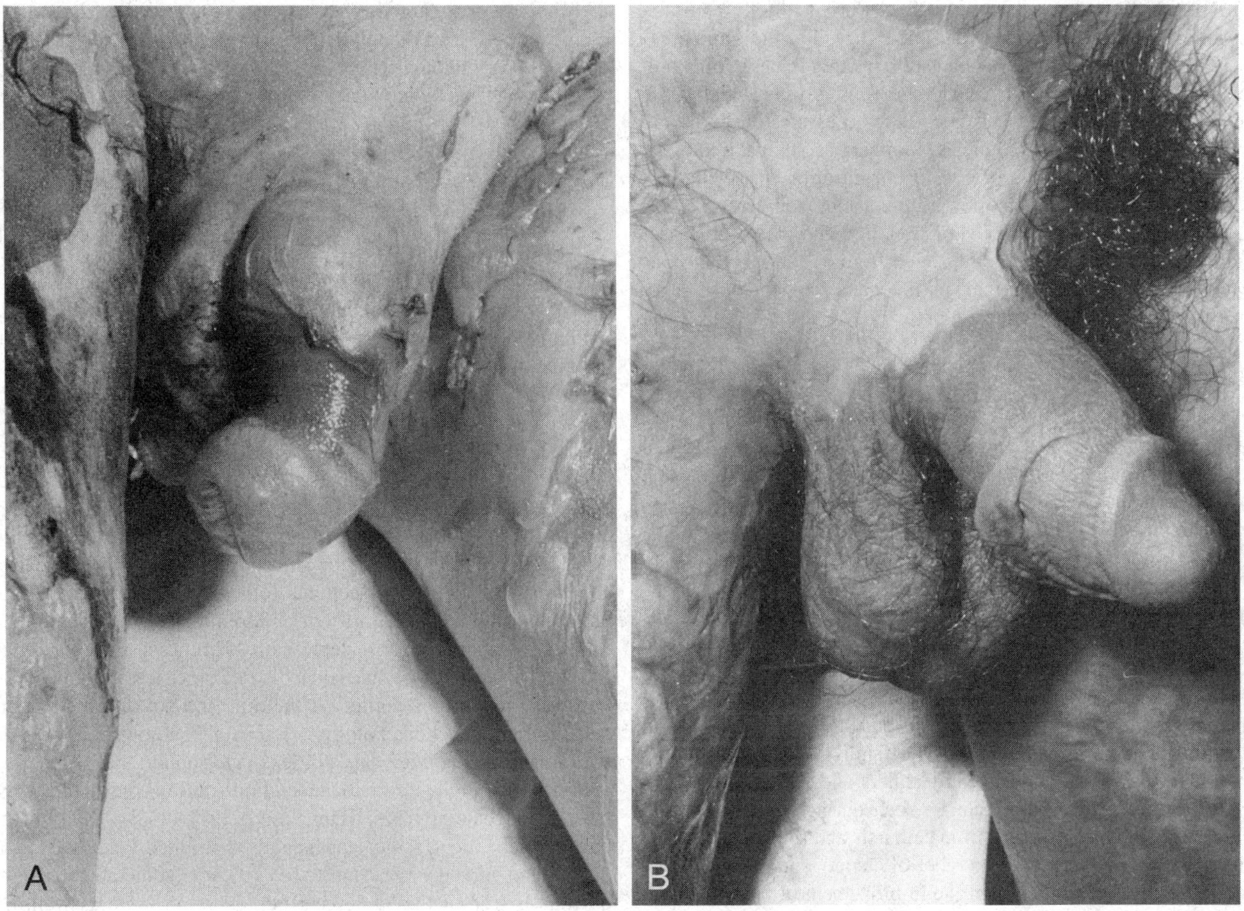

Figure 98.8.   **A**, Burn to penis in a 3-year-old. **B**, His healed perineal scar at 15 years with full recovery of function.

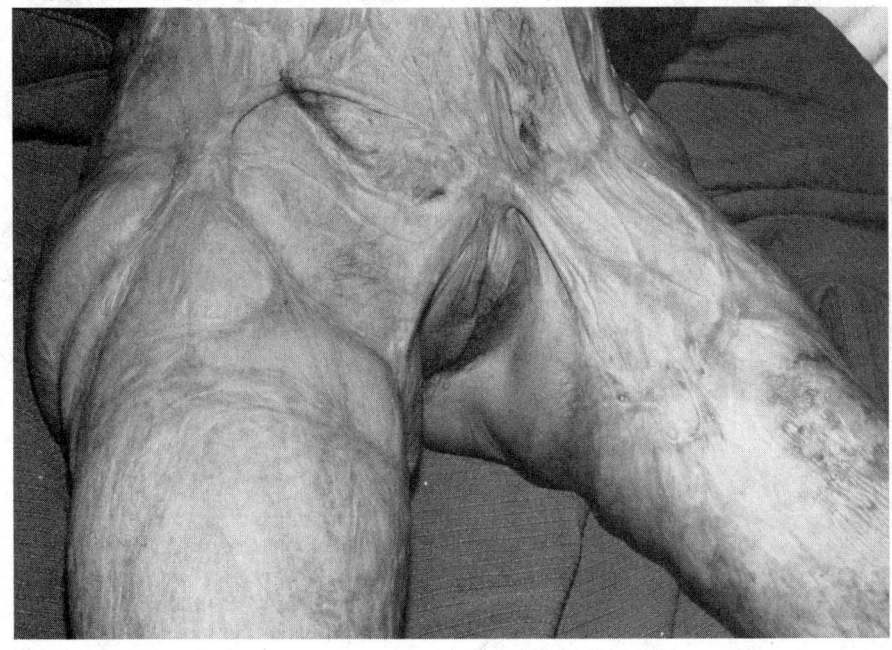

Figure 98.9.   Burn causing severe genital and leg scarring in an 8-year-old girl who had no reconstruction, accepted her scars with the help of supportive parents, and later married and gave birth to a child.

some cases, learning problems, phobia, or depression. The most common psychotherapeutic approaches are through plastic surgical clinics, during rehospitalization, or in groups. These medically oriented follow-ups address specific burn-related concerns and encourage the child's and family's mastery over new, often developmentally related issues. Collaborative long-term monitoring with plastic surgeons is indicated for "at risk" children. Referral to outside agencies is necessary for those with emotional difficulties or who require psychopharmacological treatment. A few patients receive long-term weekly insight-oriented psychotherapy. Those therapies are directed toward enhancing self-esteem, body image, interpersonal relatedness, and autonomy, and in several cases the children and adolescents were separated from or had lost their parents. Mental health teams at regional burn centers provide consultative guidance to therapists in distant locations.

FAMILY

Parents and families may be at greater risk for impairment than the children themselves. Cahners and Kartiganer (1990) observe parental guilt for the injury as the most painful, persistent emotion. They state that "Parents often blame themselves rather than attributing an occurrence to fate or the improbable. This creates a diminished sense of worth as a parent and many self-doubts as a person. Guilt impedes coping mechanisms and emotional recovery." Cella et al. (1988) found a high rate of depression in mothers years after the burn injury. Rizzone et al. (1994) found an incidence of PTSD of 52% in mothers of burned children, which is higher than that found in any study of children or adults with burns. Meyer et al. (1994) found increased stress in mothers correlating with increased stress in their children who had survived burns, and in earlier studies that family support and the family value of autonomy was critical to the child's adjustment. Cahners and Kartiganer (1990) observed over many years that parents, seen during follow-up clinic visits in group, are able to benefit from catharsis and mutual support in outpatient parent groups focused on relief of anxiety and guilt feelings, grief work, feelings about the scars, and improvement of family coping skills.

GROUP

In some clinics and camps, groups are led by social workers, psychologists, or child psychiatrists. At the author's hospital, a social worker and psychologist lead a weekly *adolescent group* for 13- to 21-year-olds, primarily for outpatients returning to clinic. This group provides support for teenagers as they return and focuses on their family lives, adolescent body image issues, peer relations, school, drugs, sexuality, and choices for surgical reconstruction and/or the specialized cosmetics available. Social workers conduct a weekly *group for parents* of children returning to clinic for plastic surgical follow-up visits (Cahners and Kartiganer, 1990). As with most of these groups, the membership varies weekly but most parents are well known from their child's acute admission, and many have returned to clinic from other states or countries. The groups address topics such as how to parent a burned child, grief, assistance with feelings about plastic surgery, rehabilitation issues, resolution of unrealistic expectations from surgery, and help with referrals to social, educational, or occupational resources in their areas. Salient information from the groups is shared in the weekly psychosocial rounds. Recently, social workers and volunteers have started self-help groups by mail (Cahners, 1992) and by telephone.

Psychopharmacological Treatment

During readmission, other frequent diagnostic indicators for psychopharmacological treatment include anxiety disorders, anticipatory phobic reactions before surgery or procedures, PTSD, depression, ADHD, and enuresis. Treatment of the anxiety disorders with benzodiazepines has been effective, as has PTSD with psychotherapy together with benzodiazepines and selective serotonin receptor inhibitors (SSRIs), and

depression with SSRIs or tricyclic antidepressants. Skin rashes, which can be caused by any drug, have the potential of complicating burn care and should be monitored. The association of cardiac toxicity and possible death with tricyclic antidepressants (Biederman, 1991; Biederman, et al., 1995), although very rare, has led us to obtain Holter monitors and repeat ECGs on any burned child receiving them (see Chapter 72). Since enuresis is common among burned children, behavioral interventions and the bell and pad are the initial interventions, but intranasal aqueous vasopressin and imipramine are also treatment options.

OUTCOME FOLLOWING CHILDHOOD BURN INJURIES

This is a challenging subject for review. There are many small studies varying in quality, a few larger ones, and several doctoral theses, most available only as abstracts. In addition, the quality of burn and reconstructive treatment has improved over the last 25 years, which probably makes earlier studies invalid in predicting outcomes for recently treated children and young adults. Of recent authors, there are two viewpoints on the outcome data: Tarnowski et al. (1991) in their review assert that "collectively, findings indicate that there exists little empirical data to support the contention that the majority of pediatric burn victims exhibit severe poor post-burn adjustment," and Blakeney et al. (1993) essentially agree. While the author (Murphy et al., 1989; Stoddard et al. 1989a, 1989b) in a cross-sectional follow-up study of severely burned children found that a majority of children manifested mental disorders (anxiety including PTSD, depression, disruptive behavior, enuresis), 20% had no disorders; while some disorders existed preburn, the study's aim was to identify disorders at the time and not differentiate preburn and postburn psychopathology. Even using Tarnowski et al.'s review, their assertion that there exists little data to support that severe postburn adjustment is premature may depend on what is considered "severe," but may have some basis. Many studies (Table 98.4) have found postburn anxiety, depression, and behavior problems. Several, including ours, found burned adolescents to be especially vulnerable to depression, but this is true of the adolescent population at large as well. Several studies, including ours, have found positive correlations between psychopathological symptoms and visible disfigurement (especially facial) and the size of burn injury. However, other studies, such as those by Blakeney et al. (1993), did not. While several studies are satisfactory, none are excellent. In this author's view, there is need for more research with structured diagnostic interviews, not only surveys, and large sample sizes including large and small burns, matched controls, longitudinal design, and especially inclusion of surgical, psychological, and other treatment variables.

What are the likely explanations for the conflicting findings regarding outcomes? First, *preburn psychopathology* does not disappear postburn, but it is difficult to measure reliably retrospectively: It is rarely reported. Second, *selection bias* is present in nearly all studies, especially those not specifying sampling methods, and is difficult to eliminate in tertiary referral centers. Third, *time since burn varies widely*. Fourth, *other pediatric handicaps and chronic illnesses* have been shown to be associated with increased psychopathology (Perrin and MacLean, 1988) and this could be true for burns, as our outcome study suggests. Fifth, *treatment interventions of all kinds are not described and their effects analyzed.*

The Death of a Child

A child's death (see Chapter 104) from burns is a most tragic loss of life due to a usually preventable injury. Parents and family may have little preparation if the death occurs quickly, as it can from massive burns, respiratory burns, or sepsis. Their grief can be almost unbearable and the presence of empathic staff especially consoling. When there is more time for parental participation and preparation, such as in cases of brain death, the grieving process can proceed in stages. Sensitive emotional and ethical (see Chapter 126) issues arise with consent for

Table 98.4. Outcome Studies of Burned Children

Author	No. Patients	BSA[a]	Age at Burn	Duration after Burn	Summary	Control	Quality E/S/U
Long and Cope, 1961	19	"Small" to "severe"	1–16	Inpatients	4 categories: anxiety, regression/depression, aggression, guilt; severe preburn family pathology.	No	S
Woodward, 1959, 1961	198				81% "emotionally disturbed" compared with only 17% preburn; had comparison group and concluded it is not true burned children specially selected and already disturbed.	Yes	S+
Vigiliano et al., 1964	10 (26)	15%	4–17		*Method:* Interview and testing. *Results:* 9 disturbed children suspicious, aloof, immature, anxious, body image disturbances. Also: 8/10 mothers especially disturbed and guilty.	No	S−
Galdston, 1972	100	Severe	0–16½	Inpatients	⅔ under age 5 when burned; withdrawal; sleep disorders; regressed speech; hallucinoses; loss of self; ⅓ of parents had preburn marital discord.	No	S
Goldberg, 1974	22 facial burns; 26 congenital heart disease	Severe	Under 11–15	2–11 years	"The group with the invisible disability were higher on all 10 measures including vocational aspirations, self-image and work values."	Yes	S+
Wright, 1974	12 12 Controls	5–50%	8–13	1–5 years	*Method:* CMAS, Peabody, Rorschach, DAP. *Results:* Few differences between experimental and control children; mothers of burned children significantly more depressed than controls.	Yes	S+
Goldberg et al., 1975	34	? Facial burns	12–18	1 year	Semistructural interview and Goldberg scale *Results:* Adolescents with a burn injury may be affected by degree of facial disfigurement.	No	S
Chang and Herzog, 1976	14	Severe	6–18	? 1 year	*Method:* Interview or questionnaire. *Results:* 75% continued school (of 20); 2/14 delinquents.	No	S−
Cain et al., 1988	68/98	Severe	1–18	2 years	*Method:* 30 interviewed; 35 by questionnaire *Results:* chronic stress and grief in families; need more social supports; 1 sibling suicide.	No	S+
Kuehnle, 1980	21	3–81%	9–15	5–7 years	*Method:* Interview, WAIS, Soares Self-Perception, etc. *Results:* "Burn injury generally does not become a handicap. Personal adjustment is affected by severity and visibility. Social and academic adjustment by caretaker attitudes. Vocational adjustment by visibility. Increased emotional problems with facial disfigurement."	No	S+
Herndon et al., 1986	12	89% (82% 3rd degree)	9 months to 12 years	1.4–3 years	*Method:* Child mental status; developmental history; Louisville Behavior Checklist for Children >4. *Results:* Moderate to severe problems with body image, self-esteem, anxiety, fears, relationships and active mastery. Louisville checklist: 11% with lack of sense of self, excess anxiety, soiling, major depression, hypersensitivity, antisocial behavior, 17% hyperactive. 17% no scale elevations. 25% immature and inhibited. 33% with excessive fear, aggression and neurotic somatic complaints.	No	S+
Knudson-Cooper, 1981	165	2–85%	8 months to 16 years		*Method:* Interview and tests *Results:* Most adjusted well; 30% of sample married and in their 20's.	No	S
Byrne et al., 1986	145/337	"Minor" and "major"	1–12 years		*Method:* Achenbach Behavior Profile. PAIS, Family Environment Scale. *Results:* 69% of children were doing well. The more socially competent children had more severe burns. More middle class socially competent families, with mothers who viewed their children's adjustment positively, had more socially competent children.	No	S
Rivlin, 1983	106/1510	?	1–16	Early postburn	Hospitalized referred sample over 5 years, not random. Main problems were anxiety (61%), depression (21%), behavior (18%)	No	S+
Campbell and La Clave	286 (all admissions)	10–50%	1 month to 18 years mean = 4.9 years	6 months to 5 years	*Method:* Psychiatric interview; Piers Harris; Spielberger; Alpern-Boll Self-Help. *Results:* DSM-III major depression in 11.9%, Buttocks 51.5% and genitals 49% depressed. Race and child abuse correlated with depression.	No	S+
Blakeney et al., 1988	38	5–91%	5 months to 17 years	2–15 years	Sampling not specified. Older adolescents and adults burned as children. Used MMPI, Suicide Probability Scale, and FES. Found them "within normal limits."	No	S
Tarnowski et al., 1989	68	>10%; mean = 18.7%	1–5 years	2–17 years	Ratings by mother. Assessed with CBCL. All scores WNLs.	No	S

(continued)

Table 98.4. *continued*

Author	No. Patients	BSA[a]	Age at Burn	Duration after Burn	Summary	Control	Quality E/S/U
Stoddard et al. (initial 30 reported in 1989a, 1989b)	90 (random sample)	1–98%	1–17 years	1–17 years	*Method:* Children 7–19 parent interviewed. Diagnostic Interview for Children and Adolescents; Spielberger; CGAS; Social Concept Scale; Pediatric Sympt. Checklist. *Results:* Phobia in 47%; PTSD in 23%; OA 33%; Depressive disorder 43% (present 17%); enuresis 30% (present 10%). Disorder correlated with size and facial.	Yes	
Blakeney et al., 1993	25	80–99	11 months to 15 years	1–19	Sampling not specified. Assessed with CBCL, Teacher Report, Piers-Harris Children's Self-Concept Sale, Parenting Stress Index. As a group within normal limits. Signif. family stress and impact.	No	S
Maron, 1991	90	<29 to >60 mean = 28%	1 month to 17 years	2–18 years	CBCL by mother: 9% behavior problem T scores in ''clinical range.'' Degree of disfigurement and social support predictive.	No	S+
Jessee et al., 1992	32	1–100 50% ''entire body burns''	5–15 years	~5 years	Nonrandom sample. Human figure drawing test to assess body image. No significant difference from matched nonburned controls.	Yes	S
Blakeney et al., 1993	25	80–99	11 months to 15 years	1–19 years	Sampling not specified. Assessed with CBCL, Teacher Report, Piers-Harris Children's Self-Concept Scale, Parenting Stress Index. As a group within normal limits. Significant family stress and impact.	No	S
Kravitz et al., 1993	82	,2–91 (mean = 43.8%)	30 months to 20 years	>1 year mean = 7.3 years	Consecutive acute admissions 1989–1990. RN assessment form. Parent/child sleep history questionnaire. Nightmares 37%, bedwetting 24%, sleepwalking 18%, daytime naps in 63%.	No	E–
Meyer et al., 1994	38	15–100	6.6 ± 4.6 years	4.6–20 years	Stratified random sample. Mothers completed CBCL, Parenting Stress Index, and 8 State Questionnaire. Mothers reporting children as troubled are stressed. Children WNL on CBCL. No correlation with burn size.	No	S+
Abdullah et al., 1994	49	15–99	5–18 years	1–6 years	Nonrandom. Piers-Harris Children's Concept Scale. Increased visible scars associated with lower self-ratings of physical appearance and ''happiness and satisfaction.''	No	S+

[a] BSA, body surface area burned; CMAS, Children's Manifest Anxiety Scale; DAP, Draw-A-Person test; WAIS, Wechsler Adult Intelligence Scale; PAIS, Psychosocial Adjustment to Idleness Scale; E/S/U, excellent/satisfactory/unsatisfactory; MMPI, Minnesota Multiphasic Personality Inventory; FES, Family Environment Scale; CBCL, Children's Behavior Checklist; WNL, within normal limits; CGAS, Children's Global Assessment Scale; Ped. Sympt. Checklist: Pediatric Symptom Checklist; OA, other anxiety disorder.

DNR orders and organ donation, as reuse of body tissues for transplants increases (Fratianne et al., 1992; Hammond and Ward, 1989; Petro and Salzberg, 1992). Such decisions are made with the burn team, led by the surgeon, together with the family. The burn team, supported by the mental health team, provide much needed support after the death to the grieving family and assist with their transition to gaining support from friends and community. Follow-up, usually by the social worker, is sustaining to the family both soon after the death and on subsequent anniversaries. Other children (and their parents) present on the burn unit may react with alarm, sadness, somatization, posttraumatic play, and fear of their own death. Sensitivity and developmentally appropriate responses to the child aid their coping with yet another unexpected trauma (Rizzone, L., D. S. Chedekel, unpublished, 1995).

STAFF SUPPORT

The burn unit is a most challenging place to work and psychiatric consultative skills are highly valued. An understanding of consultative principles, models, impediments, and process is useful prior to initiating consultation (Lewis, 1994). Witnessing horribly injured children, seeing, smelling, and touching their burned flesh, and causing pain as part of treatment for an infant or child may evoke anxiety, sadness, and guilt, but also satisfaction and pride in providing needed treatment to an injured child. Turnover can be frequent on stressed units, but it is reduced by appropriate administrative leadership and staff support and loyalty develops. While some units may appear focused on technology to the exclusion of feelings, women physicians in all specialties as well as in allied professions have moderated ''macho'' attitudes and contributed to a greater focus on emotional sustenance of both children and staff. The burn unit offers unparalleled opportunities to learn, provide treatment, and teach in areas such as pain, stress, grief, healing, consultation, and diagnosis and treatment in the acute care setting.

The aura of the burn unit is special and, for many, intimidating at first. Strong staff cohesion may make the burn team like the elite ''Marine Corps'' or battlefield station of the medical center, with a staff ''tough enough'' to treat such severe, frightening injuries. The image of the patient on the burn unit is of a ''monster,'' frightening to see and whose handicaps can be crippling—an image at great variance from the real child who speaks, feels, creates, and has relationships, whether with minimal or extensive scarring. Other scary images associated with the burn unit are of death and burning in hell, but also more hopeful ones of rebirth, as in the phoenix rising up from the ashes. The surgeon and others on the team may be both pitied (''how can you stand to work there?'') and idealized as a superhero, savior, or god invested with the magical powers of healing science.

Entry by New Staff

Arrival at the burn unit may be a ''culture shock'' for doctor, nurse, patient, and family alike. New staff, trainees, medical students, and graduate students alternately tend naturally to withdraw emotionally or to identify with the child's suffering, at times overly so. For example, a new researcher said of a boy with massive healed burns, ''He must be in so much pain.'' On my asking the boy about it later, he told me he had no pain and was only concerned with his computer game! There is a usual sequence of emotional adaptation following arrival on a burn unit: shock and dismay, curiosity and fear, frustration and helplessness, and sadness with often persistent feelings and images on return home, appearing as anxiety dreams, and even for some, a questioning of professional identity and goals (Jellinek, 1993). Bernstein (1976) pointed out how the feelings of shock often mobilize staff to use their skills on behalf of the patients and thereby to master their fear, frustration, and sadness.

When new staff arrive, I explain that they can expect feelings such as those above. One resident said how it had helped to have heard from me that I too, even after many years there, feel the stress of the burn unit. It is also helpful to them to know that the feelings of horror wane as they come to know the children and their families and join the burn team, enhancing feelings of competence. Knowing about the usual course of the three phases postburn is a hopeful approach in the face of such stress. They learn too that preparation of patients for these phases assists their transitions and hopefulness. Further, it is helpful to provide assurance that mentors are available to listen and provide validation or advice when needed.

Teaching Empathy

The psychiatrist and other mental health professionals demonstrate listening skills, communication, compassion, reflection, and constructive therapeutic action. Sensitivity to shame and embarrassment (Lazare, 1987) during rounds when the children's or adolescents' bodies are exposed to groups of staff, or where discussions may be overheard, is crucial to prevent humiliation or involuntary exposure to unwelcome information. It is important to encourage empathy in those "steeled" against feelings and also to convey understanding of inevitable overidentifications with children or their relatives, who evoke feelings reminiscent of their own children, families, or of their own life experience. Such transference and countertransference experiences are frequent, and supervision and experience can assist with these intimate feelings. For instance, a primary nurse transiently wept with grief over the suffering of a child to whom she had to cause pain. This child reminded her of her own, and she was grateful to share her feelings off the unit and then return to her work. In another instance, a doctor became the target of much fear, blame, and rage over a child's disruptive behavior and had to voice his feelings of frustration, despair, and inadequacy before resuming his work. Others can be less aware of their feelings, acting them out within the clinical situation. Such feelings are easily aroused when parents' rage is evoked, when disruptive boys resist helpful nurses and insult them, or when staff are in conflict over what course of action to take, e.g., with critically ill or dying children. In such situations, group consultation is most effective (Jellinek, 1993).

Staff Consultation

The presence of the psychiatrist validates attention to emotional and diagnostic and treatment issues that might otherwise be avoided, often with adverse effects on patient and family care and staff morale. An overall goal is to support staff cohesion and prevent "burnout." Scrubbing and gowning and entering isolation areas or the operating room conveys a willingness to talk with the patient or surgical staff "where they are." The consultative approach is ideally informed, consistent, flexible, and responsive to the situation. Admitting ignorance, reviewing the cases, and helping implement constructive recommendations is an effective way to join the team. The consultant models developmental and family assessment skills, and respect and advocacy for children, since others on the unit may have limited experience with infants and children.

In the situations of staff conflict, various interventions are possible. The psychiatrist reflects upon his or her own feelings, realizing that another team member reacts similarly, sometimes also carrying home feelings of fear, helplessness, or dread at returning the next day. While ultimate responsibility for treatment is the surgeon's, the spoken or unspoken burdens are shared with nurses, who are often "in the middle" (Jameton, 1992), and with all other staff. The nurse is more likely to know the child's situation, but may feel conflict between duty and irritation when decisions are made or not made that do not agree with her or his sense of what is good care. Routine teaching rounds, psychosocial rounds, or informal or formal acute or plastic surgical rounds, separately or in combination, may be effective for "venting" feelings and working through the issues. Support groups for nurses or other staff are held to discuss and process stress and morale issues together. The primary nursing management system seeks to achieve that aim within the nursing care team.

Communication is enhanced in many ways. Since consultation is not continuously available, staff is sustained by knowing when the consultant is available and the times of next meetings. Crises call for special meetings, including surgeon, nurse, and consultant, the other involved team members, and at times the family and patient. Respect for defenses, which can interfere with empathy, but which are necessary for staff to cope, is important. Defenses include denial, transient regressions, distancing from the situation, and overinvolvement and are often bridged by more senior members of the burn team who help master the situation. Having the psychiatrist on the team "puts behavior into a positive developmental and group-process perspective. Through emphasis on the normal and expectable phases of burn trauma recovery, the usual course of burn hospitalization for different age groups, and the impact of various burn treatments on children and families with different backgrounds and styles" the psychiatrist increases levels of mental health expertise among burn team members (Ravenscroft, 1982).

Departure from the Burn Team

When staff leave the burn unit, their leavings demonstrate their attachment and sense of involvement. The collected staff often tells residents and trainees in rounds how they will be missed. When seasoned senior staff leave, the departure can be so painful that those on the unit may react wondering "how will we manage without them?." The farewells and testimonials are proof of their dedication and the appreciation for their work and convey to those who continue that their efforts are worth the hardships. Sensitivity to administrative changes, team cohesion, losses, and the staff's adaptation is useful in maintaining the consultative alliance.

CONCLUSIONS

Burn injuries are prevalent worldwide among infants, children, and adolescents. Treatment of burns has progressed over the last 50 years to a point where most children treated in burn units survive even massive burn injuries. The priorities in psychiatric care are pain management; diagnosis and treatment of delirium, stress disorders and depression; psychotherapeutic support of the child and family throughout the postburn phases; and support for the dying child and consolation for the family, including follow-up. A reflective attitude assists the consultant's gradual adaptation to the stresses of being on the burn unit. Critical psychological interventions are infant-parent support, encouraging participation by the child in care, aiding school reentry, aiding adaptation to body image change, and aiding social mastery during stress developmental periods such as adolescence. Rehospitalization for plastic and reconstructive surgery, while stressful, is also an opportunity for emotional processing and reintegration. The child psychiatrist and mental health team experience—and support surgical, nursing, and other staff who endure—significant emotional stress together with satisfaction from care of children and their families on the burn unit.

References

American Psychiatric Association: *Benzodiazepine Dependence, Toxicity, and Abuse*. A Task Force Report of the American Psychiatric Association. Washington, DC, American Psychiatric Association, 1990.

American Psychiatric Association: *Diagnostic and Statistical Manual of Mental Disorders* (4th ed). Washington, DC, American Psychiatric Press, 1994.

Andreasen NJ, Hartford CE, Knott JR, et al: EEG changes associated with burn delirium. *Dis Nerv Syst* 38:27–31, 1977.

Antoon A, Volpe JJ, Crawford JD: Burn enceph- alopathy in children. *Pediatrics* 50(4):609–616, 1972.

Berde CB, Lehn BM, Yee JD, et al: Patient-controlled analgesia in children and adolescents: A randomized, prospective comparison with intramuscular administration of morphine for postoperative analgesia. *J Pediatr* 118:460, 1991.

Bernstein N: *Emotional Care of the Facially Burned and Disfigured*. Boston, Little, Brown, 1976.

Biederman J: Sudden death in children treated with a tricyclic antidepressant. *J Am Acad Child Adolesc Psychiatry* 30(3):495–498, 1991.

Biederman J, Thisted R, Greenhill L, et al: Debate forum: Negative. Resolved: Cardiac arrhythmias make desipramine an unacceptable choice in children. *J Am Acad Child Adolesc Psychiatry* 34(9):1241–1248, 1995.

Blakeney P, Herndon D, Desai M, et al: Long-term psychosocial adjustment following burn injury. *J Burn Care Rehabil* 9:661, 1988.

Blakeney P, Meyer W, Moore P, et al: Psychosocial sequelae of pediatric burns involving 80% or greater total body surface area. *J Burn Care Rehabil* 14:684, 1993.

Blumenfield M, Schoeps MM: *Psychological Care of the Burn and Trauma Patient*. Baltimore, Williams & Wilkins, 1993.

Brown RL, Henke A, Greenhalgh, et al: The use of haloperidol in the agitated, critically ill pediatric patient with burns. *J Burn Care Rehabil* 17:34–38, 1996.

Byrne C, Love B, Browne G, et al: The social competency of children following burn injury: A study of resilience. *J Burn Care Rehabil* 7:247–252, 1986.

Cahners SS: Young women with breast burns: A self-help "group by mail." *J Burn Care Rehabil* 13:44, 1992.

Cahners SS, Kartiganer PP: The social worker and the family: A long term relationship in burn care. In: Martyn JAJ (ed): *Acute Management of the Burned Patient*. Philadelphia, Saunders, 1990.

Campbell JL, LaClave LJ: Clinical depression in paediatric burn patients. *Burns* 13(3):213–217, 1987.

Carr DB, Osgood PF, Szfelbein SK: Treatment of pain in acutely burned children. In: Schechter N, Berde CB, Yaster M (eds): *Pain in Infants, Children and Adolescents*. Baltimore, Williams & Wilkins, 1993.

Cella DF, Perry SW, Poag ME, et al: Depression and stress response in parents of burned children. *J Pediatr Psychol* 13:87–99, 1988.

Chang FC, Herzog B: Burn morbidity: A follow-up study of physical and psychological disability. Ann Surg 183:34–37, 1976.

Charney DS, Deutsch AY, Krystal JH, et al: Psychobiologic mechanisms of posttraumatic stress disorder. *Arch Gen Psychiatry* 50:301, 1993.

Cobb S, Lindemann E: Neuropsychiatric observations after the Cocoanut Grove fire. *Ann Surg* 117(6):814–824, 1943.

Collins JC: *Types of Injuries by Selected Characteristics, 1985–87*, Data from the National Health Survey, Series 10, No. 175, DHHS Publication No (PHS) 91-1503, Hyattsville, MD, National Center for Health Statistics, December 1990.

Daly W, Sheridan R, Stoddard F, et al: Taking the conflict out of pain management: An institutional approach. Proceedings of the 26th Annual Meeting of the American Burn Association, Orlando, FL, April 20–24, 1994, p. 206.

Deblinger E, McLeer SV, Henry D: Cognitive behavioral treatment for sexually abused children suffering from post traumatic stress. Preliminary findings. *J Am Acad Child Adolesc Psychiatry* 29(5):747–752, 1990.

Demling RH: Pathophysiological changes after cutaneous burns and approach to initial resuscitation. In: Martyn JAJ (ed): *Acute Management of the Burn Patient*. Philadelphia, Saunders, 1990, pp. 18, 93.

Doctor ME: Burn Camps and Community Aspects of Burn Care. *J Burn Care Rehabil* 13:68–76, 1992.

Doyle E, Mottart KJ, Marshall C, et al: Comparison of different bolus doses of morphine for patient-controlled analgesia in children. *Br J Anaesth* 72:160, 1994.

Feldman JJ: Reconstruction of the burned face in children. In: Serafin D, Georgiade N (eds): *Pediatric Plastic Surgery*. St. Louis, Mosby, 1984, pp. 594–596.

Fratianne RB, Brandt C, Yurko L, et al: When is enough enough? Ethical dilemmas on the burn unit. *J Burn Care Rehabil* 13:600, 1992.

Gaffney A: Cognitive developmental aspects of pain in school-age children. In: Schechter N, Berde CB, Yaster M (eds): *Pain in Infants, Children and Adolescents*. Baltimore, Williams & Wilkins, 1993, pp. 75–85.

Galdston R: The burning and healing of children. *Psychiatry* 35:57, 1972.

Gaukroger PB: Patient-controlled analgesia in children. In: Schechter N, Berde CB, Yaster M (eds): *Pain in Infants, Children and Adolescents*. Baltimore, Williams & Wilkins, 1993.

Gilboa G, Friedman M, Tsur H: The burn as a continuous traumatic stress: Implications for emotional treatment during hospitalization. *J Burn Care Rehabil* 15:86, 1994.

Goin JM, Goin MK: *Changing the Body: Psychological Effects of Plastic Surgery*. Baltimore, Williams & Wilkins, 1981.

Gold PW, Goodwin FK, Chrousos GP: Clinical and biochemical manifestations of depression. Relation to the neurobiology of stress. *N Engl J Med* 319(6):348–353, and 319(7):413–420, 1988.

Goldberg RT: Adjustment of children with invisible and visible handicaps: Congenital heart disease and facial burns. *J Counsel Psychol* 21:428–432, 1974.

Goldberg RT, Bernstein NR, Crosby R: Vocational development of adolescents with burn injury. *Rehabil Counsel Bull* 18:140–146, 1975.

Groce NE, Zola IK: Multiculturalism, chronic illness, and disability. *Pediatrics* 91(5):1048–1055, 1993.

Hammond J, Ward CG: Decision not to treat: "Do not resuscitate" order for the burn patient in the acute setting. *Crit Care Med* 17:136, 1989.

Herndon DN, LeMaster J, Beard S, et al: The quality of life after major thermal injury in children: An analysis of 12 survivors with ≥80% total body, 70% third degree burns. *J Trauma* 26:609–619, 1986.

Jameton A: Nursing ethics and the moral situation of the nurse. In: Friedman E (ed): *Choices and Conflict*. Chicago, American Hospital Publishing, 1992, pp. 101–109.

Jellinek MS, Todres ID, Catlin EA, et al: Pediatric intensive care training: Confronting the dark side. *Crit Care Med* 21(5):775–779, 1993.

Jessee PO, Strickland MP, Leeper JD, et al: Perception of body image in children with burns, five years after burn injury. *J Burn Care Rehabil* 13:33–38, 1992.

Kane JM, Lieberman JA (eds): *Adverse Effects of Psychotropic Drugs*. New York, Guilford, 1992.

Kavanaugh CK, Lasoff E, Eide Y, et al: Learned helplessness and the pediatric burn patient: Dressing change behavior and serum cortisol and beta endorphin. *J Pain Symptom Manage* 6:106–177, 1991.

King B, Moss L, Tuohig G, et al: Compliance with DNR policy in a regional burn center. Proceedings of the American Burn Association, Cincinnati, March 24–27, 1993, p. 109.

Knudson-Cooper MS: Adjustment to visible stigma: The case of the severely burned child. *Soc Sci Med* 15:31–44, 1981.

Kolko DJ, Kazdin AE: The emergence and recurrence of child firesetting: A one-year prospective study. *J Abnorm Child Psychol* 20(1):17–37, 1992.

Kravitz M, McCoy BJ, Tompkins DM, et al: Sleep disorders in children after burn injury. *J Burn Care Rehabil* 14:83–90, 1993.

Kuehnle KJ: The burn injury: A study of the factors leading to a handicap. (EdD dissertation, Harvard University). *Dissertation Abstracts International*, Vol 40–11, Section B, p. 5391, 1979.

Kuttner L: Hypnotic interventions for children in pain. In: Schechter N, Berde CB, Yaster M (eds): *Pain in Infants, Children and Adolescents*. Baltimore, Williams & Wilkins, 1993.

Lasoff EM, McEttrick MA: Participation versus diversion during dressing changes: Can nurses' attitudes change? *Issues Comp Pediatr Nurs* 9:391–398, 1986.

Lazare A: Shame and humiliation in the medical encounter. *Arch Intern Med* 147:1653–1658, 1987.

Lewis M: The consultation process in child and adolescent consultation and liaison psychiatry. In: Lewis M, King RA (guest eds): *Child and Adolescent Psychiatric Clinics of North America*. Philadelphia, Saunders, 1994, pp. 439–448.

Levine RJ: Respect for children as research subjects. In: Lewis M (ed): *Child and Adolescent Psychiatry: A Comprehensive Textbook* (1st ed). Baltimore, Williams & Wilkins, 1991.

Lindemann E: Symptomatology and management of acute grief. *Am J Psychiatry* 101:141–148, 1944.

Long RT, Cope O: Emotional problems of burned children. *N Engl J Med* 264:1121–1127, 1961.

Manchester W: *A World Lit Only by Fire: The Medieval Mind and the Renaissance, Portrait of An Age*. Boston, Little, Brown, 1992.

Maron MT: Psychological adjustment of children and adolscents following burn injuries. (PhD dissertation, Virginia Commonwealth University). *Dissertation Abstracts International*, Vol. 52–03, Section B, p. 1728, 1991.

Marvin JA, Carrougher G, Bayley B, et al: Burn nursing delphi study: Setting research priorities. *J Burn Care Rehabil* 12:190–197, 1991.

Matthews JR, McGrath PJ, Pigeon H: Assessment and measurement of pain in children. In: Schechter N, Berde CB, Yaster M (eds): *Pain in Infants, Children and Adolescents*. Baltimore, Williams & Wilkins, 1993.

May JW, Moses MH: Soft tissue injuries of the hand. In: Burke JF, Boyd RJ, McCabe CJ (eds): *Trauma Management*. Chicago, Year Book, 1988, pp. 352–357.

McLaughlin E, Crawford JD: Types of burn injury. *Pediatr Clin North Am* 23:41, 1985.

Meyer WJ, Blakeney P, Moore P, et al: Parental well-being and behavioral adjustment of pediatric survivors of burns. *J Burn Care Rehabil* 15:62–68, 1994.

Murphy JM, Stoddard FJ, Norman DK, et al: *Final Report of the Psychiatric Interview Study of Burned Children and Adolescents*. April 25, 1989, Boston, Shriners Hospitals for Crippled Children.

National Center for Health Statistics: *Hospital Discharge Abstract Survey*, 1989.

National Fire Protection Association: *Fire Incident Reporting System Data*, 1990.

Patterson DR, Everett JJ, Bombardier CH, et al: Psychological effects of severe burn injuries. *Psychol Bull* 113(2):362–378, 1993, p. 369.

Perrin JM, MacLean WE: Biomedical and psychosocial dimensions of chronic illness in childhood. In: Karoly P (ed): *Handbook of Child Health Assessment: Biosocial Perspectives*. New York, Wiley, 1988.

Perry SW: Undermedication for pain on a burn unit. *Gen Hosp Psychiatry* 6:308–316, 1984.

Perry S, Heidrich G: Management of pain during debridement: A survey of US burn units. *Pain* 13:267, 1982.

Petro JA, Salzberg CA: Ethical issues of burn management. *Clin Plast Surg* 19(3):615, 1992.

Porter F: Pain assessment in children: Infants.

In: Schechter N, Berde CB, Yaster M (eds): *Pain in Infants, Children and Adolescents*. Baltimore, Williams & Wilkins, 1993.

Pruzinsky T, Doctor M: Body images and pediatric burn injury. In: Tarnowski KJ (ed): *Behavioral Aspects of Pediatric Burn Injuries*. New York, Plenum, 1994, pp. 169–192.

Ptacek JT, Patterson DR, Montgomery BM, et al: The relationship between pain during hospitalization and disability at one month post-burn. Proceedings of the American Burn Association Meeting, Orlando, FL, 1994, p. 46.

Ravenscroft K: The burn unit. *Psychiatr Clin North Am* 5:419–432, 1982.

Renz BM, Sherman R: Abusive scald burns in infants and children: A prospective study. *Am Surg* 59:329–334, 1993.

Rizzone L, Stoddard FJ, Murphy JM: Posttraumatic stress disorder in mothers of burned children and adolescents. *J Burn Care Rehabil* 15:158–163, 1994.

Rivlin E: The psychological trauma and management of severe burns in children and adolescents. *Br J Hosp Med* 40:210–215, 1988.

Rivlin E, Forshaw A, Polowyi G, et al: A multidisciplinary group approach to counselling the parents of burned children. *Burns* 12(7):479, 1986.

Rothstein JD, Garland W, Puia G, et al: Purification and characterization of naturally occurring benzodiazepine receptor ligands in rat and human brain. *J Neurochem* 58:2102–2115, 1992.

Salisbury RE (guest ed): Burn rehabilitation and reconstruction. *Clin Plast Surg* 19(3):551–756, 1992.

Scheeringa MS, Zeanah CH, Drell MJ, et al: Two approaches to the diagnosis of posttraumatic stress disorder in infancy and early childhood. *J Am Acad Child Adolesc Psychiatry* 34(2):191–200, 1995.

Sheridan R, McEttrick M, Bacha G, et al: Midazolam infusion in pediatric patients with burns who are undergoing mechanical ventilation. *J Burn Care Rehabil* 15:515–518, 1994.

Sheridan RL, Hegarty M, Tompkins RG, et al: Artificial skin in massive burns—Results to ten years. *Eur J Plast Surg* 17:91–93, 1994a.

Sheridan RL, Tompkins RG, Burke JF: Management of burn wounds with prompt excision and immediate closure. *J Intensive Care Med* 9:6–19, 1994b.

Shontz FC: Body image and its disorders. *Int J Psychiatr Med* 5:461–472, 1974.

Solnit AJ, Priel B: Psychological reactions to facial and hand burns in young men. *Psychoanal Study Child* 30:549–566, 1975.

Solomon SD, Gerity ET, Muff AM: Efficacy of treatments for posttraumatic stress disorder. *JAMA* 268:633–638, 1992.

Stoddard FJ: Coping with pain: A developmental approach to treatment of burned children. *Am J Psychiatry* 139(6):736, 1982a.

Stoddard FJ: Body image development in the burned child. *J Am Acad Child Psychiatry* 21:502–507, 1982b.

Stoddard FJ: Psychiatric management of the acute burn patient. In: Maartyn JAJ (ed): *Acute Care of the Burn Patient*. Philadelphia, Saunders, 1990.

Stoddard FJ: A psychiatric perspective on self-inflicted burns. *J Burn Care Rehabil* 14:340, 1993.

Stoddard FJ, Wilens TE: Delirium. In: Jellinek MS, Herzog DB (eds): *Psychiatric Aspects of General Hospital Pediatrics*. Chicago, Year Book, 1990, p. 254.

Stoddard FJ, Chedekel D, Shakun L: Dreams and nightmares of burned children. In: Barrett D (ed): *Trauma & Dreams*, in press, 1995.

Stoddard FJ, Norman DK, Murphy JM: Diagnostic outcome study of children and adolescents with severe burns. *J Trauma* 29(4):471–477, 1989a.

Stoddard FJ, Norman DK, Murphy JM, et al: Psychiatric outcome of burned children. *J Am Acad Child Adolesc Psychiatry* 28(4):589–595, 1989b.

Stoddard FJ, Stroud L, Murphy JM: Depression in children after recovery from severe burns. *J Burn Care Rehabil* 13:340, 1992.

Szyfelbein SK, Osgood PF, Carr DB: The assessment of pain and plasma B-endorphin immunoactivity in burned children. *Pain* 22:173, 1985.

Tarnowski KJ, McGrath ML, Calhoun MB, et al: Pediatric burn injury: Self- versus therapist-mediated debridement. *J Pediatr Psychol* 12(4):567–579, 1987.

Tarnowski KJ, Rasnake LK, Gavaghan-Jones MP, et al: Psychosocial sequelae of pediatric burn injuries: A review. *Clin Psychol Rev* 11:371–398, 1991.

Tarnowski KJ, Rasnake LK, Linscheid TR, et al: Behavioral adjustment of pediatric burn victims. *J Pediatr Psychol* 14(4):607, 1989.

Vigliano A, Hart LW, Singer F: Psychiatric sequelae of old burns in children and their parents. *Am J Orthopsychiatry* 34:753–761, 1964.

Watkins PN, Cook EL, May SR, et al: Psychological stages in adaptation following burn injury: A method for facilitating psychological recovery of burn victims. *J Burn Care Rehabil* 9:376, 1988.

Wilmore DW, Long CL, Mason AD, et al: Catecholamines: Mediator of the hypermetabolic response to thermal injury. *Ann Surg* 180:653–669, 1974.

Woodward J: Emotional disturbances of burned children. *Br Med J* 1:1009–1013, 1959.

Woodward J, Jackson DM: Emotional reactions of burned children and their mothers. *Br J Plast Surg* 13:316–324, 1961.

Wright L, Fulwiler R: Long range emotional sequelae of burns: Effects on children and their mothers. *Pediatr Res* 8:931–934, 1975.

99 PHYSICAL ABUSE AND NEGLECT

Sandra J. Kaplan, M.D.

Physical abuse and neglect of children and adolescents are major public health problems. The Revised 1988 Study of the National Incidence and Prevalence of Child Abuse and Neglect of the National Center on Child Abuse and Neglect of the United States Department of Health and Human Services (Sedlak, 1991) estimated that more than 1,400,000 million children in the United States experience abuse or neglect, and that 1,200 to 5,000 children died that year as a result of maltreatment (Sedlak, 1991). The abuse and neglect of children has been associated with the development of aggressive behaviors in victims that are directed toward society (Alfaro, 1978; Kashani et al., 1992; Lewis, 1985; Lewis et al., 1979; Widom, 1989), toward other family members (Kaufman and Zigler, 1987; Oliver, 1993; Straus and Gelles, 1986; Straus et al., 1980), and toward themselves (Deykin et al., 1985; Green, 1978b; Livingston et al., 1993; Pfeffer, 1986; Rotheram and Bradley, 1987).

Cruelty toward children has been described throughout history, with children being viewed as parental property (Wolfe, 1987). However, in the United States, medicine has focused on child maltreatment only since 1946, when Caffey described fractures of the long bones in multiple stages of healing in children with subdural hematomas (Caffey, 1946). Early efforts on behalf of maltreated children focused on the development of legislation to protect children. Child maltreatment reporting laws were instituted in all 50 states.

Psychiatric studies of maltreating families and psychiatric treatment programs are still in the early stages of development. The pediatrician Kempe and his child psychiatric colleague Steele at the University of Colorado were largely responsible for the current focus on child maltreatment on the part of American medicine, including psychiatry (Steele and Pollack, 1968). They and their colleagues Silverman, Droegenmueller, and Silver described the battered child syndrome in 1962 (Kempe et al., 1962).

PHYSICAL ABUSE

Definitions

Definitions of physical abuse vary with (*a*) cultural practices regarding corporal punishment; (*b*) cultural values (i.e., privacy versus interdependence); and (*c*) biological predispositions, such as the higher activity levels of Anglo neonates versus Chinese neonates (Gabarino and Etaba, 1983). According to Straus and Gelles (1988), 6.9 million children are physically abused each year. This is when abuse is defined as whether the child was hit with an object, kicked, bitten, punched, beaten up, burned, scalded, or threatened or attacked with a knife or gun. The same authors, however, report that 97% of children from 0 to 3 years old were physically punished.

Physical abuse has been defined by the Child Abuse Prevention, Adoption, and Family Services Act of 1988 (Public Law 100-294) as "the physical injury of a child under 18 years of age by a person who is responsible for the child's welfare, under circumstances which indicate that the child's health or welfare is harmed or threatened thereby, as determined in accordance with regulations prescribed by the Secretary of Health and Human Services."

Persons responsible for a child's welfare include employees of a residential facility, any staff of a facility, or any staff providing out-of-home care. The New York State Family Court Act (1976) defines physical abuse as "the situation which results when a parent or other person legally responsible for a child less than 18 inflicts or allows to be inflicted upon such child physical injury by other than accidental means" (Family Court Act, 1971).

Straus and Gelles, the principal investigators of the National Incidence Studies of Violence in America, define child abuse as the use by a parent of any of the acts of the Severe Violence Index of the Conflict Tactics Scale. Severe violence is defined by this scale as kicking, biting, hitting with a fist, hitting or trying to hit with something, beating up, threatening with a gun or a knife, or using a gun or a knife (Straus and Gelles, 1980).

Incidence

In their 1985 study of violence in America, Straus and Gelles (1986) found that the rate of physical abuse toward children and adolescents was 19 per 1000 children ages 3–17 years.

Straus and Gelles's earlier 1975 study of violence in America involved in-person interviewing utilizing the Conflict Tactics Measure (Straus and Gelles, 1986). That study indicated that 36 per 1000 children 3–17 years of age were abused. Their 1985 study indicated that 19 per 1000 children 3–17 were abused, but that study involved telephone rather than in-person interviews. This methodological difference, as well as increased public awareness and legislation regarding child abuse, may have accounted for the decrease in rates reported by the second study.

The 1986 National Incidence and Prevalence Study of the National Center on Child Abuse and Neglect estimated that 22.6 per 1000 or 1,424,400 children in the United States were maltreated that year (Sedlak, 1991). The majority of these cases (64%) involved neglect. The rate of physical abuse reported by this study was 4.9 per 1000 children, or 311,500 children. Females experienced more overall abuse than did males (Sedlak, 1991).

The exact incidence of child abuse in the United States is unknown due to reporting biases and investigatory procedural constraints. The probability that an abuse report will be filed is increased for ethnic minorities, the poor, urban residents, and those who utilize public rather than private sources of health care. The ability of a child protective service to document or substantiate abuse varies with the source of the report. Physicians' reports have been found to be most likely to be substantiated by investigatory agencies (Eckenrode et al., 1988).

Age of Onset of Abuse

Severity of abuse found by the 1986 Child Abuse and Neglect Incidence and Prevalence Study varied inversely with the age of the child victim. Most fatalities occurred in younger children (U.S. Department of Health and Human Services, 1988). Daro and Mitchel (1990) reported that more than 50% of fatalities involved children less than 1 year old. Child abuse involving prepubertal children is most often reported in single-parent, ethnic minority, low-income families, while the majority of adolescents reported as abused in the United States during 1977 were white and from intact two-parent families who earned at that time more than $11,000 per year (U.S. Department of Health and Human Services, 1981). Fathers are more often indicated as the perpetrators of physical abuse of adolescents, while mothers are more often indicated as perpetra-

tors of physical abuse of prepubertal children (Straus et al., 1980). Most studies of abuse involving adolescents report that, although such abuse sometimes began in early childhood and was continued into adolescence, in the majority of cases the onset of abuse began during adolescence (Libbey and Bybee, 1979; Lourie, 1979; Straus et al., 1976).

The onset of abuse during adolescence has been explained by Lourie (1979), Libbey and Bybee (1979), Garbarino et al. (1984), and Pelcovitz et al. (1984) to relate most often to interpersonal conflicts around adolescent developmental tasks and parental midlife crises, rather than as a result of socioeconomic stress, as is often the case with the abuse of younger children. Parental psychopathology as hypothesized in the Pelcovitz et al. study was an additional risk factor for abuse in families of abused adolescents.

Physical Examination Findings

Every child suspected of being physically abused or neglected should be given a physical examination (American Medical Association, 1992; Kessler and Hayden, 1991). The American Medical Association (AMA) Diagnostic and Treatment Guidelines Concerning Child Abuse and Neglect (Council on Scientific Affairs, AMA, 1985) state the following in terms of diagnostic physical findings: "Characteristically, the injuries are more severe than those that could reasonably be attributed to the claimed cause" (Council on Scientific Affairs, AMA, 1985).

Physical signs of abuse include bruises and welts on the face, lips, mouth, ears, eyes, neck, head, trunk, back, buttocks, thighs, and/or extremities, forming regular patterns that often resemble the shape of the article used to inflict the injury (e.g., hand, teeth, belt buckle, or electrical cord); burns inflicted with cigars or cigarettes, especially on the soles, palms, back, or buttocks; immersion burns (stocking or glove-like on extremities, doughnut-shaped on buttocks or genitals) or patterned burns resembling an electrical appliance (e.g., iron, burner, or grill); fractures of the skull, ribs, nose, facial structures, or long bones, frequently with multiple or spiral fractures in various stages of healing; lacerations or abrasions; rope burns on wrists, ankles, neck, torso, palate, mouth, gums, lips, eyes, ears, or external genitalia; bruises of the abdominal wall; intramural hematoma of the duodenum or proximal jejunum; intestinal perforation; ruptured liver, pancreas, or spleen; ruptured blood vessels, kidney, or bladder; and central nervous system injuries, including subdural hematoma (often a product of blunt trauma or violent shaking), retinal hemorrhage, or subarachnoid hemorrhage (often a product of shaking) (Council on Scientific Affairs, AMA, 1985).

Etiology of Abuse

The prevailing model of the etiology of abuse is the ecological one (Belsky, 1980), which views child abuse as the consequence of the interactions of parental vulnerabilities (mental illness, substance abuse), child vulnerabilities (low birth weight, difficult temperament), a particular developmental stage (adolescence, toddler), and social stressors (lack of social supports, poverty, single parenthood, minority ethnicity, lack of acculturation, four or more children in a family, young parental age, stressful events, exposure to family violence) (Belsky, 1980; U.S. Department of Health and Human Services, 1988).

Psychopathology of Abused Children and Adolescents

Studies of psychiatric disturbance in referred-for-treatment child abuse victims have found the children to be impulsive, hyperactive (Martin and Beezley, 1977), depressed (Green, 1978a; Kaplan et al., 1986), conduct disordered (Kaplan et al., 1986; Kinard, 1980), learning impaired (Kline and Christiansen, 1975; Salzinger et al., 1984), and, frequently, substance abusers (Kaplan et al., 1986). Studies of child and adolescent psychiatric populations have often found these children to have histories of physical child abuse (Kashani et al., 1987a, 1987b). Lewis (1985; Lewis et al., 1979) and Alfaro (1978) found that delinquent and violent adolescents also frequently had histories of physical abuse. More specifically, children with a depressive symptomology were found to have more likely been physically abused than nondepressive children (Allen and Tarnowski, 1989; Kazdin et al., 1985). Kaufman (1991) found that 18% of her sample of maltreated children (abused and/or neglected) met criterion of major depression and 25% met criteria for dysthymia.

Salzinger et al. (1984) found that maltreatment victims who had been referred for treatment, and to a lesser extent their siblings, showed significantly more conduct disturbance, hyperactivity, tension, and anxiety than did a nonmaltreated comparison group. In an analysis of data utilizing the Diagnostic Interview for Children and Adolescents (DICA) (Herjanic and Reich, 1982; Reich et al., 1982) on a referred sample, they found that abused children and adolescents were significantly more often diagnosed as having depression, alcohol abuse, conduct disorders, and attention deficit disorders than were a comparison group of nonmaltreated children and adolescents (Kaplan et al., 1986).

Kaufman (1991) found a prevalence of 18% of 56 maltreated children being diagnosed as having major depressive disorder and 25% as having dysthymic disorder. Pelcovitz et al. (1993) reported in a comparison study of physically abused adolescents and nonabused adolescents, who were not referred for treatment, that the abused adolescents were more often diagnosed as having depressive disorders and conduct disorders than were the nonabused adolescents.

None of the above-mentioned studies of behavioral dysfunction included any analyses of commonly suggested risk factors for child psychopathology, such as parental psychopathology (Weissman et al., 1984; Wolkind and Rutter, 1985), lack of family cohesion and adaptability (Wolkind and Rutter, 1985), lack of perceived parental supportiveness (Keller et al., 1986), marital discord (Illfeld, 1977), prolonged separation of a child from a parent (Rutter, 1971; Wolkind and Rutter, 1973), or head trauma (Rutteret al., 1983). The Kaplan et al. study (1986) was the only one that did any analysis of psychiatric illness in parents of abused children. In that study, abused children of psychiatrically disturbed parents were more often diagnosed as having a psychiatric disorder than were nonabused children with a psychiatrically disturbed parent. Since these risk factors are frequently present in child abuse, future research on the association of child mental illness and abuse will be improved by adjusting for the presence of these risk factors.

Suicide and Abuse

An association between abuse and suicide has been found in studies of abused children and adolescents, of adolescent suicide attempters, and of mothers who attempt suicide. Self-mutilation was reported in abused and neglected children by Green (1978b). Deykin has reported that adolescents who attempted suicide had more often been reported as abuse victims than had nonattempters (Deykin et al., 1985). Pfeffer (1986) reported frequent child abuse in families of children who attempted suicide, and Farber et al. (1984), Kaplan (1986), and Rotheram and Bradley (1987) reported high rates of suicide attempts in adolescent runaways. Garbarino and Farber have reported high rates of adolescent abuse in runaway youth (Farber et al., 1984; Garbarino et al., 1984).

In a recent preliminary report on adolescent suicide of New York City metropolitan area adolescents, Shaffer (1987) reported that conduct disorders, substance abuse, and, less frequently, depression, as well as family discord and family histories of suicide and other exposure to suicide appeared to be risk factors for adolescent suicide. These same psychiatric disorders have been reported in child and adolescent abuse victims (Kaplan et al., 1986). Child-abusive behaviors were also found more often in mothers who attempted suicide than in a comparison group of nonsuicidal mothers (Hawton et al., 1985). Parental suicide attempts are known to be major risk factors for adolescent suicide (Shaffer, 1989).

The etiology of the association between suicidal behavior and physical abuse remains to be studied. It may be secondary to modeling of aggressive behavior within the family or to exposure to the suicidal behavior of family members. It may also be secondary to increased biological risk in these families for disorders highly associated with suicide: affective disorders, substance abuse, and impulsive conduct disorders (Kaplan et al., 1983, 1986; Shaffer, 1987). Finally, the adolescent as well as his or her parents and family may be socially isolated and therefore at increased risk for suicide (Salzinger et al., 1983; Shaffer and Fisher, 1974; Spinetta and Rigler, 1972).

Psychopathology of Parents of Maltreated Children

Comparative studies, although reporting an increased incidence of psychopathology in abusive parents, have been limited by the failure to use structured diagnostic interviews (Estroff et al., 1985; Paulson et al., 1976; Smith et al., 1973), by study populations inadequately defined as abusive (Bland and Orn, 1986), by the fact that they relied on cases referred for treatment, and because they indiscriminately combined parents of child and adolescent abuse victims. These studies have reported maltreating parents as depressed (Bland and Orn, 1986; Kaplan et al., 1983; Wolfe, 1985), aggressive (Kaplan et al., 1983; Wolfe, 1985), having increased somatic concerns, exhibiting an imbalance in the proportion of negative to positive and aversive control behaviors when interacting with the target child, having more physical and verbal aggressive behaviors when interacting with the child, and having increased arousal and reactivity to any aversive child stimuli when compared to nonmaltreating parents (Wolfe, 1985).

In a study of a referred sample that used diagnostic structured interviews and distinguished between parents of abused children and adolescents, it was found that there was significantly more diagnosed psychopathology in maltreating than in nonmaltreating parents. Mothers in abusive families were more frequently diagnosed as having a depressive disorder, while fathers, usually the perpetrating parent, were more often diagnosed as having alcoholism, antisocial personality disorders, or labile personalities. Mothers of maltreated children were more often diagnosed as having drug abuse than were mothers of maltreated adolescents (Kaplan et al., 1983).

Intergenerational Transmission of Abuse

Abuse during childhood has been associated with increased risk that its victims will abuse their own offspring (Kaufman and Zigler, 1987; Oliver, 1993; Straus and Gelles, 1980). In a critical review of this area, Kaufman and Zigler (1987) suggested that approximately one-third of those who were physically abused, sexually abused, or severely neglected will maltreat their offspring. They reported that the presence of one supportive parent during childhood, a supportive spousal relationship, and fewer stressful events during adulthood may buffer against the intergenerational transmission of abuse.

Social Isolation of Abusive Families

Social competence has been found to be impaired both in child abuse victims and in their parents (Salzinger et al., 1983, 1984). It has been found that mothers of abused children and adolescents were less often employed outside their homes and were more socially isolated, particularly with respect to peers. As a result, outsiders were found to have less access to the family interactions of abusive families than to those of comparison families (Salzinger et al., 1983). This type of social isolation may be hypothesized to lead to a lack of child-rearing acculturation of the abusive parent (Salzinger et al., 1983).

CASE ILLUSTRATION

Four-year-old Carol was referred for an evaluation when her teacher made a child abuse complaint to the State Central Register for Child Abuse Reports. A family evaluation by a social worker revealed the following:

Carol is the older of two children, both of whom live with their parents in a two-bedroom apartment. Her problems began with the birth of her sister 3 months ago. Her teacher noticed a change in her behavior at school. She began pushing other children and hit a classmate with a wooden block, causing a laceration of the classmate's lip. When Carol's teacher took her aside to talk about her behavior, she noticed what seemed to be belt marks on Carol's abdomen and forehead. Carol's sister was "colicky" and slept only for short periods of time throughout the day and night. She stopped crying only when her mother held her. Her mother therefore had little time for Carol, and Carol's father took over her care on evenings after day care and on weekends. He began to drink more than usual, a half a bottle of wine each evening, and became increasingly irritable. He and his wife argued over her attention to the infant and the requirement that he take care of Carol. Carol, who was a bright, curious, talkative 4-year-old, constantly asked questions and often asked to carry the baby. When refused, she would lie on the floor and have a tantrum. Since her sister's birth, she also began to have difficulty falling asleep and awoke repeatedly during the night.

Carol's father was unable to cope with her demands for attention and often told her to shut up and slapped her when she continued her demands. On many occasions he responded to her tantrums or repeated questions by hitting her with his belt.

When interviewed, Carol presented as a lively and attractive little blue-eyed blond girl dressed in jeans, tee shirt, and sneakers. She related appropriately and warmly to the interviewer and easily separated from her parents in the waiting room. Her intelligence appeared to be above average, as indicated by fund of knowledge, vocabulary, and drawings of a person and of geometric forms. About her sister, Carol said, "She's a bad girl. She cries all the time. I get hit when I cry, but no one hits the baby." When asked about fights at the day care center, she said, "I hit Robert (her playmate) because he pulls my hair." She said she is afraid to go to sleep because she has bad dreams of an old man killing her.

Carol's changed behavior included temper tantrums at home, fighting with other children at school, and having trouble falling asleep. These few symptoms are not indicative of a syndrome that would justify the diagnosis of a disorder. Therefore, Carol at that time was given the residual diagnosis of adjustment disorder with mixed disturbance of emotions and conduct.

Carol, along with her mother and father, began a family therapy program that included parenting training and behavioral therapy for Carol, coordinated with the day care center. Her father was persuaded to join Alcoholics Anonymous, has stopped drinking, and has been able to control his anger at his daughter. Six months later, Carol's aggressive behavior had ceased. She was doing well with peers and in her academic work, was sleeping throughout the night, and had stopped having temper tantrums (Kaplan, 1989a).

EMOTIONAL ABUSE

Emotional abuse has been defined in the Study of the National Incidence and Prevalence of Child Abuse and Neglect (U.S. Department of Health and Human Services, 1988) as follows:

Close Confinement (Tying or Binding and Other Forms)
Tortuous restriction of movement, as by tying a child's arms or legs together or binding a child to a chair, bed, or other object or confining a child to an enclosed area (such as a closet) as a means of punishment.
Verbal or Emotional Assault
Habitual patterns of belittling, denigrating, scapegoating, or other nonphysical forms of overtly hostile or rejecting treatment, as well as threats of other forms of maltreatment (such as threats of beating, sexual assault, abandonment, etc.).
Other or Unknown Abuse
Overtly punitive, exploitative, or abusive treatment other than [that] specified under other forms of abuse, or unspecified abusive treatment. This form includes attempted or potential physical or sexual assault, deliberate withholding of food, shelter, sleep, or other necessities as a form of punishment, economic exploitation, and unspecified abusive actions.

Garbarino has further defined emotional abuse and has applied a developmental approach as clarification. He views emotional abuse as

a pattern of psychically destructive behavior inflicted by an adult upon a child. This pattern may take five forms: rejecting, isolating, terrorizing, ignoring, or corrupting (Garbarino et al., 1986). Garbarino illustrated these patterns according to stages of child development, as follows:

1. Rejecting
   a. *Infant:* Parent refuses to accept an infant's primary attachment.
   b. *Preschooler:* Parent excludes child from family activities.
   c. *School-age child:* Parent conveys negative definitions of self to the child.
   d. *Adolescent:* Parent refuses to acknowledge the changing social roles expected of the child.
2. Terrorizing
   a. *Infant:* Parent intentionally violates child's tolerance for change and intense stimuli.
   b. *Preschooler:* Parent uses extreme gestures to threaten or intimidate child.
   c. *School-age child:* Parent places child in a double-bind ("Damned if you do, damned if you don't") (Garbarino et al., 1986).
   d. *Adolescent:* Parent threatens to expose and humiliate the child.
3. Ignoring
   a. *Infant:* Parent fails to respond contingently to infant's spontaneous behavior.
   b. *Preschooler:* Parent displays lack of affect toward and does not engage child in activities of socialization.
   c. *School-age child:* Parent does not protect child or intervene on child's behalf when made aware of the need for help.
   d. *Adolescent:* Parent abdicates the parental role and does not have an interest in the child.
4. Isolating
   a. *Infant:* Parent withholds from the child interactions with parents or other parenting persons.
   b. *Preschooler:* Parent teaches child to avoid contact other than with the parent.
   c. *School-age child:* Parent discourages peer relationships.
   d. *Adolescent:* Parent attempts to prevent socialization by prohibiting organized and other activities outside the home.
5. Corrupting
   a. *Infant:* Parent reinforces the development of inappropriate behavior (such as sexual) or creates an addiction (exposure to drugs, alcohol).
   b. *Preschooler:* Parent reinforces aggressive and/or sexualized behaviors.
   c. *School-age child:* Parent reinforces aggressive, sexualized criminal behaviors, or the abuse of substances.
   d. *Adolescent:* Parent promotes in child socially prohibited forms of sexual, aggressive, criminal, or substance-abusing behaviors.

Incidence

The National Incidence of Child Abuse and Neglect Study (U.S. Department of Health and Human Services, 1988) estimated the incidence of emotional abuse as stated in Table 99.1.

NEGLECT

Definitions

Giovannoni (1988) generally defined child neglect as follows:

While abuse is considered an act of "commission," neglect is considered an act of "omission." Neglect is perpetrated by caretakers of children who: fail to fulfill their caretaker obligations to children. Neglect occurs in the following three situations: 1. Neglect is due to a parenting problem present; 2. Neglect is due to social deviance of the caretaker secondary to caretaker problems such as substance abuse, mental retardation, mental illness, criminality, or secondary to other problems; 3. Neglect is associated with the physical abuse or sexual abuse of the child.

This definition may be further broken down into the following three categories, discussed at length below: physical neglect, educational ne-

Table 99.1. Incidence of Specific Forms of Emotional Abuse during 1986 in the United States

Form	1986 (Rates)[a]	1986 (Totals)[b]
Close confinement	0.18	11,100
Verbal or emotional assault	2.1	129,900
Other or unknown abuse	0.9	54,600
Total	3.0	188,100

Adapted from US Department of Health and Human Services. Study of the national incidence and prevalence of child abuse and neglect. Washington, DC, US Department of Health and Human Services, 1988, Revised Report, Sedlak, A., 1991.
[a] Per 1000 children in the population.
[b] Total number of children rounded to the nearest 100; not adjusted by population totals.

glect, and emotional neglect (U.S. Department of Health and Human Services, 1988).

PHYSICAL NEGLECT

Refusal of Health Care
Failure to provide or allow needed care in accordance with recommendations of a competent health care professional for a physical injury, illness, medical condition, or impairment.

Delay in Health Care
Failure to seek timely and appropriate medical care for a serious health problem that any reasonable lay person would have recognized as needing professional medical attention.

Abandonment
Desertion of a child without arranging for reasonable care and supervision. This category included cases where children were not claimed within 2 days and where children were left by parents/substitutes who gave no (or false) information about their whereabouts.

Expulsion
Other blatant refusals of custody, such as permanent or indefinite expulsion of a child from the home without adequate arrangement for care by others, or refusal to accept custody of a returned runaway.

Other Custody Issues
Custody-related forms of inattention to the child's needs other than those covered by abandonment or expulsion. For example, repeated shuttling of a child from one household to another due to apparent unwillingness to maintain custody, or chronically and repeatedly leaving a child with others for days/ weeks at a time.

Inadequate Supervision
Child left unsupervised or inadequately supervised for extended periods of time or allowed to remain away from home overnight without the parent/ substitute knowing (or attempting to determine) the child's whereabouts.

Other Physical Neglect
Conspicuous inattention to avoidable hazards in the home; inadequate nutrition, clothing, or hygiene; and other forms of reckless disregard of the child's safety and welfare, such as driving with the child while intoxicated, leaving a young child unattended in a motor vehicle, and so forth.

EDUCATIONAL NEGLECT

Permitted Chronic Truancy
Habitual truancy averaging at least 5 days a month was classifiable under this form of maltreatment if the parent/guardian had been informed of the problem and had not attempted to intervene.

Failure to Enroll/Other Truancy
Failure to register or enroll a child of mandatory school age, causing the child to miss at least 1 month of school; or a pattern of keeping a school-age child home for nonlegitimate reasons (e.g., to work, to care for siblings, etc.) an average of at least 3 days a month.

Inattention to Special Educational Need
Refusal to allow or failure to obtain recommended remedial educational services, or neglect in obtaining or following through with treatment for a child's diagnosed learning disorder or other special education need without reasonable cause.

EMOTIONAL NEGLECT

Emotional neglect is defined by the 1988 National Center on Child Abuse study as "a parent providing inadequate nurturance/affection, exposing a child to chronic or extreme spouse abuse, permitting a child to abuse drugs or alcohol, permitting other maladaptive behavior, or refusing a child psychological care."

Incidence

The 1986 National Incidence and Prevalence of Child Abuse and Neglect Study indicated that the incidence of neglect was as follows: physical neglect, 8.1 per 1000 children; educational neglect, 4.5 per 1000 children; and emotional neglect, 3.2 per 1000 children (Sedlak, 1991).

Physical Examination Findings

Typical findings are as follows:

1. *Physical neglect:* Malnutrition, repeated pica, constant fatigue, poor hygiene, clothing inappropriate for weather or setting (Council on Scientific Affairs, AMA, 1985).
2. *Medical neglect:* Lack of appropriate medical care for chronic illness, absence of appropriate immunizations or medications, absence of dental care, absence of necessary prostheses such as eyeglasses or hearing aid, discharge from treatment against medical advice.
3. *Emotional neglect:* Delays in physical development and failure to thrive (Council on Scientific Affairs, AMA, 1985).

Psychopathology of the Neglected Child

The effects of neglect have been studied even less frequently than those of abuse. In one of the very few studies on neglect, Egeland (1985) reported that physically neglected children at 12 months were more likely than nonneglected children to have insecure attachments. At 24 months, neglected children were more likely to be noncompliant and easily frustrated, as compared with controls. At 42 months they were rated as more likely to have low self-esteem and self-assertion, less flexibility, and less self-control, and to have a difficult time dealing with frustration. They lacked persistence and enthusiasm on educational tasks. They were more dependent and lacked enthusiasm and interest in the preschool environment. In elementary school they had attentional problems, low self-assertion, low self-esteem, and greater internalizing behaviors. They were also reported as socially isolated by teachers. Egeland found emotionally neglected children more likely than control children to show declines on cognitive testing, insecure attachment, avoidance of emotional contact, depression, and aggressive behavior.

In the United States during 1985, 58 per 1000 couples experienced severe assault (spouse abuse), which included kicking, biting, punching, hitting with an object, beatings, and threats or harm with guns or knives (Straus and Gelles, 1986). Children often witness the spouse abuse incidents of their parents. These children are, according to child treatment reporting laws, considered to be emotional neglect victims by virtue of this exposure. Child witnesses of spouse abuse have been described as having separation anxiety, sleep disturbances, psychosomatic symptoms (Wolfe, 1987), generalized fearfulness and withdrawal from conflict, impaired social competence, and conduct disorders (Jaffee et al., 1990; Wolfe et al., 1986). Witnessing spouse abuse during childhood has been associated with increased risk for becoming either a spouse abuse perpetrator or a spouse abuse victim (Straus et al., 1980).

Psychopathology of Neglectful Parents

Neglectful mothers were found to be less verbally responsive to their children than nonneglectful mothers (Aragona and Eyberg, 1981). Neglectful mothers were also found by Aragona to use more direct commands, less verbal praise or acknowledgment, and more critical statements when interacting with their children than were nonneglectful mothers (Aragona and Eyberg, 1981).

Zuravin (1988) reported that maternal depression was more often associated with physical neglect than with physical abuse of children.

Gaudin et al. (1993) found neglectful parents to be more depressed and more socially isolated than were nonneglectful parents.

Parents who perpetuate spouse abuse have been frequently found to have substance abuse disorders (Kaplan, 1989b), while their nonviolent spouses frequently had been diagnosed as having depressive disorders (Kaplan et al., 1988).

EXPOSURE TO SUBSTANCES IN UTERO

Currently there is a United States epidemic of children being born to substance abusive mothers. The U.S. General Accounting Office (1990) reported that 325,000 prenatally drug exposed infants are born annually in the United States, and that approximately 100,000 of these are exposed to cocaine as well as to other illicit drugs and alcohol used with cocaine.

There have been reports of infants exposed to substances in utero having smaller head circumferences than non-drug-exposed infants (Griffith et al., 1993) and having problems with hyperarousability with prolonged crying, sleeping and feeding difficulties, tonicity and attentional problems, low birth weight, and seizures (Chasnoff, 1989). Rodning et al. (1989) reported that preschoolers exposed to illicit substances in utero when compared with non-substance-exposed preschoolers had lower developmental quotient results on the Bayley Developmental Assessment Test, deficits in spontaneous play and representational play, less secure attachment behaviors, attentional problems with a disorganization of intentionality, and an absence of the impression of delight and pleasure.

Treatment and assessment needs of the in utero substance-exposed infant and preschooler include comprehensive programs for parents and children with the following available services: cognitive, language, and mental health assessments of infants and children; dyadic assessment of infant/child-parent attachment; parenting and extended family functioning enhancement strategies; and special education, speech and language, and mental health services for children; and substance abuse, mental health, and vocational assessments and programs for parents.

CASE ILLUSTRATION

Charles, a 3-year-old, was referred by his day care center for psychiatric evaluation because of withdrawn behavior and sad affect, which alternated with aggressive behavior toward peers. Day care staff also reported that Charles was frequently absent from the center. Family history revealed that both parents used cocaine and had frequent physical arguments. Charles had often witnessed his father beating his mother. During psychiatric evaluation of Charles, his affect was depressed. Intelligence was above average, as indicated by fund of knowledge. There were no motor abnormalities. Charles spoke of concerns about his mother's safety and of his father getting ''mad and hurting mommy.'' He said, ''Mommy sleeps a lot when I'm home'' and said that he spent most of his time alone at home ''watching TV.'' Both of his parents were diagnosed as having cocaine abuse. Treatment recommendations included (a) play therapy for Charles; (b) cocaine abuse treatment for both parents; (c) marital therapy, with the primary goal being the cessation of spouse abuse; and (d) parent counseling to enhance parental child-rearing capacities and understanding of child development.

TREATMENT OF CHILD ABUSE AND NEGLECT

Since parental psychopathology is a high-risk factor for child or adolescent psychopathology in violent families, treatment programs for these families must include treatment for parental mental illness, including substance abuse, as well as treatment for the abused child or adolescent.

Specific treatment and prevention strategies for both family violence and adolescent psychopathology and suicidal behavior will be better informed based on further understanding of their association. In fact,

the low rate of compliance with treatment in cases of adolescent suicide attempts suggests that adolescent suicide attempters may come from families that are very similar to adolescent abuse families and that they may therefore require treatment strategies similar to those designed for child abuse. Despite a considerable literature on the diagnosis of child abuse and initial phases of management, there is a dearth of information regarding long-term psychotherapeutic management. There are virtually no empirical studies evaluating effectiveness of therapeutic modalities or techniques with this population.

The majority of child abuse treatment programs have, as their major focus, treatment of the abusing parent, with little treatment of the maltreated child. This model views abuse and neglect as a consequence only of parental psychopathology. In contrast, a multidimensional or ''ecological'' view of child abuse (Belsky, 1980) defines treatment needs more broadly than the parental psychopathology model. Main and Goldwyn (1988) and Wolfe (1987) have emphasized the importance of focusing on the interactive aspect of the cycle of maltreatment and the importance of changing the negative mode of parent-child interactions. In addition to possible emotional disturbances in parents, other variables are seen as contributors to abuse and neglect. These include vulnerability of the child, family dysfunction, and environmental stress factors such as parental unemployment and the degree to which social support systems exist and operate for parents. In this view, child abuse occurs as a function of the degree to which the parents' environment tends to enhance or to undermine good parenting. When support is adequate, parental propensities toward violence are controlled. When there is little social support, violent propensities manifest themselves.

Effective treatment programs recognize the multidimensional nature of the etiology of family violence. The multidisciplinary treatment team needs to aim its interventions at variables operating at all levels of the problem: individual psychopathology, family dysfunction, stress, and lack of social supports. In a study done from 1979 to 1981 of 19 child maltreatment clinical demonstration programs funded by the National Center on Child Abuse and Neglect, serving 1000 families, Daro (1988) found that clinicians rated families who received family therapy and group therapy for between 13 and 18 months of treatment as having made the most progress and being the least likely to have a relapse of child maltreatment necessitating rereporting. Parental substance abuse was associated inversely with treatment progress, as were greater numbers of types of maltreatment exhibited by a family prior to referral.

In a study of physically abusive families who had a child in out-of-home placement because of abuse, low socioeconomic status, older age of child, greater severity of abuse, and/or victim's school behavioral problem predicted poor outcome of social service agency rehabilitative effort and the need for permanent out-of-home care for victims (Barth et al., 1985–1986).

Parent Treatment

There is an unusually high dropout rate when abusive parents are referred to traditional community mental health clinics. Given the probability that the parents came from a family environment where needs for nurturance and dependency were often met with rejection and violence, it is not surprising that these parents often view authority figures with suspicion and mistrust. Initial resistance and missed appointments should be viewed as almost inevitable components of early phases of therapy. In order to get beyond the parents' lack of basic trust, outreach to these families must be made in a manner not usually needed with nonabusive parents. This includes staff being available to them on a 24-hour basis and the availability of evening treatment time in order to involve all parents. The psychotherapy of the parents is viewed as having two primary components. The first is the provision of intense emotional support and positive models of parenting. The tendency of these parents to make unrealistic demands on their children is dealt with directly by teaching them appropriate developmental expectations and effective, nonpunitive child-rearing techniques. The second component is traditional psychotherapy aimed at insight and conflict resolution. Until a solid, trusting therapeutic relationship is established, this is often done in the context of individual psychotherapy. In later stages, conjoint family sessions deal with the interactional issues, such as the scapegoating of the abused child and marital conflict (Kaplan et al., 1981).

Child Treatment

Abused children are at risk for serious behavioral and emotional disorders, developmental disorders, and learning problems. To screen for these problems, complete medical, developmental, and psychiatric evaluations should be performed on all abused and neglected children. School records should be reviewed. Referral for more appropriate educational placement is frequently indicated, as is referral for individual psychotherapy. The goal in psychotherapy is not only to overcome the emotional problems of abuse but also to facilitate emotional development in a manner that will overcome the intergenerational cycle of abuse.

LEGAL ASPECTS OF ABUSE AND NEGLECT

All states have reporting laws mandating that professionals in the areas of health care, social service, law enforcement, and education report suspected cases of child abuse or neglect. In approximately 20% of reported cases, children alleged to be abused or neglected become involved in court proceedings (Besharov, 1971). The purposes of these proceedings are to determine whether abuse or neglect occurred, the services required for family rehabilitation, and the need for custodial disposition.

In most states, abused and neglected children involved in court proceedings receive court-appointed attorneys called law guardians or guardians ad litem. The Federal Child Abuse Prevention and Treatment Act of 1974 mandated that states must provide children with representation independent of that of their parents for those children involved in judicial proceedings. The role of these attorneys is to act as advocates for the rights of the child client and the desires of that child. The duty of the law guardian is to permit inclusion of all relevant evidence and argument in behalf of the child client.

HOSPITAL MANAGEMENT

Child abuse and neglect are frequently diagnosed and reported by hospitals, with children being routinely hospitalized following these reports. Many hospitals have developed child protection teams to assess cases of child abuse and neglect. These teams, which often include mental health professionals, cooperate with the state agencies responsible for receiving and investigating child abuse reports and formulating treatment recommendations.

PREVENTION

Three types of child maltreatment primary prevention strategies are currently being utilized. The first is competency enhancement, such as parent education programs. The second is preventing the onset of maltreating behaviors through, for instance, media campaigns, crisis hotlines, and community socialization programs for parents. The third is the targeting of high-risk groups, such as single, adolescent, low-socioeconomic status parents and those with complicated pregnancies and deliveries, to attend programs that increase parent-child contact and provide family support, such as visiting nurses or home visiting parent aides (Rosenberg and Repucci, 1985). The effectiveness of these programs still remains to be studied since there has been little prevention outcome research done utilizing comparison groups.

One methodologically sophisticated study of high-risk mothers did indicate that providing visiting nurses reduced rates of maltreatment, enhanced parents' positive perceptions of their infants, improved the health of high-risk mothers, and reduced prematurity rates for their children, as compared with those who did not receive these services (Rosenberg and Repucci, 1985).

ROLE OF THE PSYCHIATRIST

Psychiatrists can make important contributions to child abuse and neglect case management by consulting to social service agencies, hospitals, and courts, as well as by establishing and participating in treatment programs designed for these families.

Children and parents in child maltreatment cases are often not routinely screened for psychopathology and substance abuse, so that the prevalence of psychopathology and substance abuse has probably been underestimated and untreated. In a survey of hospitals with pediatric beds and of child protective services in the New York City metropolitan area, Kaplan and Zitrin (1983a, 1983b) found that the majority of abused and neglected children and their parents were not being assessed by psychiatrists or psychologists, nor were psychiatrists or psychologists members of child protection committees in most hospitals surveyed (Kaplan and Zitrin, 1983b). In a study of abused children and their parents in cases reaching the Manhattan Family Court, more than half of these children and more than half of their parents had not had psychiatric evaluations prior to court proceedings, despite having been known to multiple social agencies prior to court referral. When psychiatric consultation was available to law guardians in family court proceedings, their initial legal custody plans for the children were modified following psychiatric consultation in 21 of 40 cases (Kaplan, 1981). It is therefore recommended that psychiatrists become involved as members of hospital child protection committees and that routine psychiatric evaluations of parents and children, as well as frequent psychological testing to screen for developmental and learning disabilities and regular review of school records, should be done by agencies involved in planning for these families.

Child maltreatment poses a particular challenge to psychiatry. Child and adolescent mental health treatment compliance depends on parental as well as child and adolescent motivation. Medical neglect reports should be considered by psychiatry when treatment compliance problems exist. This route to overcome resistance to essential mental health treatments for children and adolescents is often overlooked by psychiatrists.

CONCLUSIONS

Child maltreatment efforts directed at understanding, preventing, and intervening in this area are in the pioneering stages. Maltreated children, their parents, and their relatives are at risk for the development of mental disorders, substance abuse, and aggressive behaviors. In addition to the need to advocate for the improvement of environmental stressors, the cessation of exposure of children to family violence, improved parenting, and child development education for parents and children, psychiatry must advocate an increase in child maltreatment mental health services.

References

Alfaro J: *Summary Report on the Relationship between Child Abuse and Neglect and Later Socially Deviant Behavior.* New York, Select Committee on Child Abuse, 1978.

Allen DM, Tarnowski KJ: Depressive characteristics of physically abused children. *J Abnorm Child Psychol* 17(1): 1–11, 1989.

American Medical Association: *Diagnostic and Treatment Guidelines on Child Physical Abuse and Neglect,* AA22: 92–407, 20 M, 6/91.

Aragona J, Eyberg S: Neglected children: Mothers' report of child behavior problems and observed verbal behavior. *Child Dev* 52:596–602, 1981.

Barth R, Snowden L, Broeck E, et al: Contributors to reunification or permanent out of home care for physically abused children. *J Soc Serv Res* 9: 31–45, 1985–1986.

Belsky J: Child maltreatment: An ecological integration. *Am Psychol* 35:320–335, 1980.

Besharov DJ: *McKinney's Consolidated Laws of Book 29A. Part I Family Court Act.* St. Paul, MN, West Publishing, 1971.

Bland R, Orn H: Psychiatric disorders, spouse abuse and child abuse. *Acta Psychiatr Belg* 86: 444–449, 1986.

Caffey J: Multiple fractures in the long bones of infants suffering from chronic subdural hematoma. *AJR* 56:163–173, 1946.

Chasnoff I, Schnoll S, Burns W, et al: Disorganized/disoriented attachment relationships in maltreated infants. *Dev Psychol* 25:525–531, 1989.

Council on Scientific Affairs, American Medical Association: AMA diagnostic and treatment guidelines concerning child abuse and neglect. *JAMA* 254: 796–800, 1985.

Daro D: *Confronting Child Abuse: Research for Effective Program Design.* New York, Free Press, 1988.

Daro D, Michel L: *Current Trends in Child Abuse Reporting and Fatalities: The Results of the 1989 Annual Fifty State Survey.* Chicago, National Center on Child Abuse Prevention Research, 1990.

Deykin E, Alpert J, McNamarra J: A pilot study of the effect of exposure to child abuse or neglect on suicidal behavior. *Am J Psychiatry* 142:1299–1303, 1985.

Eckenrode J, Powers J, Doris J, et al: Substantiation of child abuse and neglect reports. *J Consult Clin Psychol* 56:9–16, 1988.

Egeland B: The consequences of physical and emotional neglect on the development of young children. Paper presented at symposium of the National Center on Child Abuse and Neglect, Chicago, November 10, 1985.

Estroff T, Herrera C, Gaines R, et al: Maternal psychopathology and perception of child behavior in psychiatrically referred and child maltreatment families. *J Am Acad Child Psychiatry* 23:649–652, 1985.

Family Court Act: *McKinney's Consolidated Laws* (Book 29A, Part I). St. Paul, MN, West Publishing, 1971.

Farber E, Kinast C, McCord W, et al: Violence in families of adolescent runaways. *Child Abuse Negl* 8:295–299, 1984.

Garbarino J, Ebata A: The significance of ethnic and cultural differences in child maltreatment. *J Marriage Fam* Nov:733–783, 1983.

Garbarino J, Guttmann E, Seeley J: *The Psychologically Battered Child* (1st ed). San Francisco, Jossey-Bass, 1986, pp. 25–29.

Garbarino J, Sebes J, Schellenbach D: Families at risk for destructive parent-child relations in adolescence. *Child Dev* 55:174–183, 1984.

Gaudin JM, Polansky NA, Kilpatrick AC, et al: Loneliness, depression, stress, and social supports in neglectful families. *Am J Orthopsychiatry* 63(5): 597–605.

Giovannoni J: Overview of issues on child neglect. In: *Child Neglect Monograph: Proceedings from a Symposium.* Washington, DC, Clearinghouse on Child Abuse and Neglect Information, 1988, pp. 1–6.

Green A: Psychopathology of abused children. *J Am Acad Child Psychiatry* 17:92–97, 1978a.

Griffith DR, Azuma SD, Chasnoff IJ: Three-year Outcome of Children Exposed Prenatally to Drugs. *J Am Acad Child Adolesc Psychiatry* 33(1):20–27, 1993.

Green A: Self-destructive behavior in battered children. *Am J Psychiatry* 135:579–582, 1978b.

Hawton K, Roberts J, Goodwin G: The risk of child abuse among mothers who attempt suicide. *Br J Psychiatry* 146:486–489, 1985.

Herjanic B, Reich W: Development of a structured psychiatric interview of children: Agreement between child and parent on individual symptoms. *J Abnorm Psychol* 10:307–324, 1982.

Illfeld F: Current social stressors and symptoms of depression. *Am J Psychiatry* 134:161–166, 1977.

Jaffee PG, Hurley DJ, Wolfe D: Children's observations of violence. I: Critical issues in child development and intervention planning. *Can J Psychiatry* 35:466–470, 1990.

Kaplan S: Child psychiatric consultation to attorneys representing abused and neglected children. *Bull Am Acad Psychiatry Law* 9:140–148, 1981.

Kaplan S: No one hits the baby. In: Spitzer R, Gibbon M, Skodol A, et al (eds): *DSM-III-R Casebook Diagnostic and Statistical Manual of Mental Disorders* (3rd ed, rev). Washington, DC, American Psychiatric Press, 1989a, pp. 346–348.

Kaplan S: Parental psychopathology according to type in maltreatment presentations. Paper presented at annual meeting of the American Psychiatric Association, San Francisco, 1989b.

Kaplan S, Zitrin A: Psychiatrists and child abuse. I: Case assessment by child protective services. *J Am Acad Child Psychiatry* 22:253–256, 1983a.

Kaplan S, Zitrin A: Psychiatrists and child abuse. II: Case assessment by hospitals. *J Am Acad Child Psychiatry* 22:257–261, 1983b.

Kaplan S, Ganeles D, Samit C, et al: The family crisis program: An overview. *North Shore Univ Hosp Clin J* 4:19–24, 1981.

Kaplan S, Montero G, Pelcovitz D, et al: Psychopathology of abused and neglected children. Paper presented at the International Congress of Child Psychiatry and Allied Professions, Paris, France, July 1986.

Kaplan S, Pelcovitz D, Salzinger S: Psychopathology in nonviolent women in violent families. In: Anthony EJ, Chiland C (eds): *The Child in His Family.* New York, Wiley, 1988.

Kaplan S, Pelcovitz D, Salzinger S, et al: Psychopathology of parents of abused and neglected children. *J Am Acad Child Psychiatry* 22:238–244, 1983.

Kaplan W: Runaway youth: Psychiatric aspects. Paper presented at Child Psychiatry Grand Rounds Presentation, North Shore University Hospital, Manhasset, NY, February 10, 1986.

Kashani J, Beck N, Hoeper E, et al: Psychiatric disorders in a community sample of adolescents. *Am J Psychiatry* 144(3):584–588, 1987a.

Kashani JH, Daniel AE, Dandoy AC, et al: Family violence: Impact on children. *J Am Acad Child Adolesc Psychiatry* 31(2):181–189, 1992.

Kashani JH, Hoeper EW, Beck N, et al: Personality, psychiatric disorders, and parental attitude among a community sample of adolescents. *J Am Acad Child Adolesc Psychiatry* 26:879–885, 1987b.

Kaufman J: Depressive disorders in maltreated children. *J Am Acad Child Adolesc Psychiatry* 302: 251–265, 1991.

Kaufman J, Zigler E: Do abused children become abusive parents? *Am J Orthopsychiatry* 57:186–192, 1987.

Keller M, Beardslee W, Dorer D, et al: Impact of severity and chronicity of parental affective illness on adaptive functioning and psychopathology in the children. *Arch Gen Psychiatry* 43:930–937, 1986.

Kempe CH, Silverman FN, Steele BF, et al: The battered child syndrome. *JAMA* 181:17–24, 1962.

Kessler DB, Hayden P: Physical, sexual, and emotional abuse of children. *Clin Symp* 43(1): 1991 (Physical Assessment).

Kinard E: Emotional development in physically abused children. *Am J Orthopsychiatry* 50:689–696, 1980.

Kline D, Christiansen J: *Educational and Psychological Problems of Abused Children, Final Report 1975.* (ERIC Document Reproduction Service no. ED 121041).

Lewis D: Biopsychosocial characteristics of children who later murder: A prospective study. *Am J Psychiatry* 142:1161–1167, 1985.

Lewis D, Shanok S, Pincus J, et al: Violent juvenile delinquents: Psychiatric, neurological, psychological, and abuse factors. *J Am Acad Child Psychiatry* 18:307–319, 1979.

Libbey R, Bybee R: The physical abuse of adolescents. *J Soc Issues* 35:101–126, 1979.

Livingston R, Lawson L, Jones J: Predictors of self-reported psychopathology in children abused repeatedly by a parent. *J Am Acad Child Adolesc Psychiatry* 32(5):948–953, 1993.

Lourie I: Family dynamics and the abuse of adolescents: A case from a developmental phase specific model of child abuse. *Child Abuse Negl* 3:967–974, 1979.

Main M, Goldwyn R: *Predicting Rejection of Her Infant Son from Mother's Representation of Her Own Experience: Implications for the Psychopathology.* Newbury Park, CA, Sage, 1988.

Martin H, Beesley P: Behavioral observations of abused children. *Dev Med Child Neurol* 13:373–387, 1977.

Oliver JE: Intergenerational transmission of child abuse: Rattles, research, and clinical implications. *Am J Psychiatry* 150:1315–1324, 1993.

Paulson MJ, Schwemer FT, Bendel RB: Clinical application of the P, Ma, and (PH) experimental MMPI scales for further understanding of abusive parents. *J Clin Psychol* 32:558–564, 1976.

Pelcovitz D, Kaplan S, Goldenberg B, et al: Post traumatic stress disorder in physically abused adolescents. *J Am Acad Child Adolesc Psychiatry* 33:3, 1994.

Pelcovitz D, Kaplan S, Samit C, et al: Adolescent abuse: Family structure and implications for treatment. *J Am Acad Child Psychiatry* 23:85–90, 1984.

Pfeffer CR: *The Suicidal Child.* New York, Guilford Press, 1986.

Reich W, Herjanic B, Weiner Z, et al: Development of a structured psychiatric interview for children: Agreement on diagnosis comparing child and parent interviews. *J Abnorm Child Psychol* 10: 302–306, 1982.

Rodning C, Beckwith L, Howard J: Prenatal exposure to drugs: Behavioral distortions reflecting CNS impairment. In: Cramer J, Wiggins R (eds): *Drug Abuse and Brain Development.* Arkansas, Intox Press, 1989.

Rosenberg M, Repucci ND: Primary prevention of child abuse. *J Consult Clin Psychol* 53:576–585, 1985.

Rotheram MJ, Bradley R: Evaluation of imminent danger for suicide among youth. *Am J Orthopsychiatry* 57:1, 102–110, 1987.

Rutter M: Parent-child separation: Psychological effects on the children. *J Child Psychol Psychiatry* 12:233–260, 1971.

Rutter M, Chadwick O, Shaffer D: Head injury. In: Rutter M (ed): *Developmental Neuropsychiatry.* New York, Guilford Press, 1983.

Salzinger S, Kaplan S, Artemyeff C: Mother's personal social network and child maltreatment. *J Abnorm Psychol* 22:253–256, 1983.

Salzinger S, Kaplan S, Pelcovitz D, et al: Parent and teacher assessment of children's behavior in child maltreating families. *J Am Acad Child Psychiatry* 23:58–64, 1984.

Sedlak A: *National Incidence and Prevalence of Child Abuse and Neglect: 1988, Revised Report.* Rockville, MD, Westat, 1988.

Shaffer D: A critical look at suicide prevention in adolescence. Paper presented to the Society for Adolescent Psychiatry, New York, April 29, 1987.

Shaffer D: Youth suicide, epidemiology, risk factors, prevention and biology. Paper presented at North Shore University Hospital/Cornell University Medical College, Manhasset, NY, December 1, 1989.

Shaffer D, Fisher P: The epidemiology of suicide in children and adolescents. *J Child Psychol Psychiatry* 15:275–291, 1974.

Smith S, Hanson R, Nobel S: Parents of battered babies: A controlled study. *Br Med J* 4:388–391, 1973.

Spinetta J, Rigler D: The child-abusing parent: A psychological review. *Psychol Bull* 77:296–304, 1972.

Steele BF, Pollack C: A psychiatric study of parents who abuse infants and small children. In: Heifer RE, Kempe CH (eds): *The Battered Child*. Chicago, University of Chicago Press, 1968.

Straus M, Gelles R: Societal change and change in family violence from 1975 to 1985 as revealed by two national surveys. *J Marriage Fam* 48:465–479, 1986.

Straus M, Gelles R, Steinmets S: *Behind Closed Doors: Violence in the American Family*. New York, Anchor Press, 1980.

US Department of Health and Human Services: *National Study of the Incidence and Severity of Child Abuse and Neglect*. no. OHDS 81-30325. Washington, DC, US Department of Health and Human Services, 1981.

US Department of Health and Human Services: *Study Findings: Study of the National Incidence and Prevalence of Child Abuse and Neglect*. Washington, DC, US Department of Health and Human Services, 1988, pp. 5–8.

Weissman M, Prusoff B, Gammon G, et al: Psychopathology of the children (ages 6–18) of depressed and normal parents. *J Am Acad Child Psychiatry* 23:78–84, 1984.

Widom CS: Child abuse, neglect, and adult behavior: Research design and findings on criminality, violence, and child abuse. *Am J Orthopsychiatry* 59:355–367, 1989.

Wolfe D: Child abusive parents: An empirical review and analysis. *Psychol Bull* 97:462–482, 1985.

Wolfe D: *Implications for Child Development and Psychopathology*. Newbury Park, CA, Sage, 1987, p. 12.

Wolfe DA, Zak L, Wilson S, et al: Child witness to violence between parents: Critical issue in behavioral and social adjustment. *J Abnorm Child Psychol* 14:95–104, 1986.

Wolkind S, Rutter M: Children who have been "in care": An epidemiological study. *J Child Psychol Psychiatry* 14:97–105, 1973.

Wolkind S, Rutter M: Separation, loss and family relationships. In: Rutter M, Hersov L (eds): *Child and Adolescent Psychiatry: Modern Approaches* (2nd ed). Oxford, Blackwell Scientific, 1985.

Zuravin S: Child abuse, child neglect and maternal depression: Is there a connection? In: *Child Neglect Monograph: Proceedings from a Symposium*. Washington, DC, Clearinghouse on Child Abuse and Neglect Information, 1988, pp. 20–45.

100 CHILD SEXUAL ABUSE AND INCEST

Arthur H. Green, M.D.

DEFINITION AND PREVALENCE OF CHILD SEXUAL ABUSE

Child sexual abuse may be defined as the use of a child as an object of gratification for adult sexual needs or desires. Incest refers to the sexual exploitation of a child by another family member. The legal definition of incest is cohabitation between persons related to a degree where marriage would be prohibited by law. Sexual abuse ranges in severity from gentle fondling to forcible rape resulting in physical injury. Sexually abused children can range in age from infants to young adults. Girls are reported as victims of sexual abuse five times more often than boys (American Humane Association, 1981). The most common forms of sexual abuse encountered by girls are exhibitionism, fondling, genital contact, masturbation, and vagina, oral, or anal intercourse by a male perpetrator. Boys are usually subjected to fondling, mutual masturbation, fellatio, and anal intercourse. About half of child victims are involved in repeated incidents of sexual abuse; in many cases the molestation may take place over a period of years.

Prevalence

There has been a dramatic increase in the incidence of sexual abuse in this country in the past 15 years. The National Incidence Study carried out in 1979–1980 by the National Center for Child Abuse and Neglect (1981) estimated that 44,700 cases of sexual abuse occurred in the United States during a 12-month period. By 1993, that number had risen to an estimated 300,000 (National Center on Child Abuse Prevention Research, 1994). While most sexual offenders against children are male, the National Incidence Study (1981) reported the percentage of female abusers to be 13% in the case of female victims and 24% for male victims.

Retrospective surveys of women estimate a higher prevalence of sexual abuse during their childhood. Russell (1983) reported that 38% of a community population of randomly selected women who were interviewed in San Francisco had experienced sexual contact with an adult during childhood. Wyatt (1985) discovered that 45% of a community sample of Afro-American women in Los Angeles had had unwanted sexual contact during childhood. Bagley and Ramsay (1986) found that 22% of women surveyed in Calgary, Canada, had been molested during childhood. The higher estimates of victimization obtained from these retrospective surveys suggest that most cases of child sexual abuse are never reported. In Russell's (1983) study only 2% of intrafamilial and 6% of the extrafamilial sexual abuse cases were reported to the police or child protective services.

Surveys of college students report a somewhat lower incidence of sexual abuse. Finkelhor's (1979) survey of 530 female college students documented a 19% incidence of sexual abuse during childhood and adolescence. Nine percent of a population of 266 male students had also been victimized. Fromuth (1983) reported that 22% of 482 female college students had had unwanted sexual contact with adults. Seidner and Calhoun (1984) indicated that 11% of 595 female students and 5% of 490 male students had been molested during childhood and adolescence. The lower incidence of sexual abuse among these college students might be due to a sampling bias reflected by predominantly white, middle-class populations. Both the community and college surveys indicate that one-fifth to two-fifths of adult women and almost one-tenth of adult men were sexually abused during childhood. According to Finkelhor (1986), the mean ratio of eight random sample community surveys that interviewed both men and women is 2.5 women for every man sexually victimized. This corresponds to a breakdown of total victims into 71% females and 29% males.

DESCRIPTION OF THE FAMILY DYNAMICS OF INCEST

Parental Patterns of Dominance and Submission

The incestuous family has been universally described as disturbed and dysfunctional. Although some typical characteristics of incestuous families have been widely observed, there is considerable variation in the family psychopathology.

The most frequently described pattern is the rigid, patriarchal family structure, with the father maintaining his dominant position through force and coercion. The marital relationship is unable to satisfy the strong dependency needs of the mother and father, who were often deprived during their own childhoods. The family system is closed, and outsiders are viewed with suspicion. Some domineering incestuous fathers may use violence as a means of securing power and control over the family (Weinberg, 1955). However, not all incestuous fathers are violent; some initiate sexual activity through subtle coercion and escalating sexual contacts rather than through physical force.

On the other hand, an opposite pattern has been reported, where the mother is domineering and the father passive. These fathers feel powerful only in the incestuous relationship with the child (Cavallin, 1966). There is a significant imbalance of power in each type of parental configuration in most incestuous families.

Sexual Problems

Sexual problems are common in the marital relationship of incestuous families. The husband's sexual frustration due to the wife's sexual unavailability may precipitate some cases of incest. Some incestuous fathers have a strong pedophilic component to their sexuality; these men are more sexually aroused by children than by their spouses. These individuals are also likely to experience additional paraphilias (i.e., exhibitionism, voyeurism, sexual masochism, etc.) and are sexually aroused by young children other than their daughters or stepdaughters. Groth (1982) made a distinction between "fixated" and "regressed" sexual offenders. The fixated offenders demonstrate an arrest in their psychosexual development and are sexually aroused by prepubertal young children, especially boys. They rarely engage in sexual relationships with peers and seldom marry. The regressed offenders, on the other hand, demonstrate a primary sexual arousal to peers. They frequently marry and appear to have adequate relationships with their wives and children. They become sexually aroused by children when their adult relationships become conflictual. According to Groth, regressed offenders are usually aroused by young girls.

Social Isolation

Social isolation is frequently observed in incestuous families. Weinberg (1955) described an "endogamic" type of incestuous father who is unable to establish gratifying social relationships outside of the family. These fathers turn toward their children when sexually frustrated, rather than pursuing extramarital contacts. Summit and Kryso (1978) described incest occurring in a "rustic environment" where families accept sibling and intragenerational incest as routine practices.

Role Confusion

Role confusion is common in incestuous families. The mother frequently delegates marital and homemaking roles to the daughter (Meiselman, 1978). The father often assumes the nurturing, caretaking role, but he provides this in a sexual context (Mrazek et al., 1981). Unfortunately, the incestuous relationship might be the only source of intimacy and affection for the child. The father often uses his daughter as a surrogate wife, expecting the child to supply him with sexual gratification and emotional support and depending on her to perform housekeeping chores. The daughter's fixation on her father as a sexual object usually precludes her achieving normal adolescent heterosexual peer relationships.

Alcohol Abuse

Alcohol abuse has been frequently implicated as a precipitating factor in incest. Kaufman et al. (1954), Cavallin (1966), and Gebhard et al. (1965) described a high incidence of alcoholism in incestuous fathers. Aarens et al. (1978) maintained that incest offenders were more likely to be involved in alcohol than were nonincestuous child molesters. These investigators also reviewed the literature and discovered that alcohol was involved in 30–40% of all cases of child molestation. It is likely that alcohol has an inhibition releasing influence on the sexual abuser.

Blurring of Physical and Psychological Boundaries

Incestuous families exhibit patterns of enmeshment within the family system (Brooks, 1982) and disengagement from the outside world. There is confusion regarding intergenerational boundaries and there is little respect for members' physical space, privacy, and belongings. There is often a lack of modesty concerning nudity and toileting and poor limit setting. The rigid boundaries between the incestuous family and the outside world are in sharp contrast to the blurred intergenerational boundaries.

Denial

Denial is the most prominent defense mechanism used by the family members. The father may use denial by regarding the incest as "sex education" for his daughter. The mother is unable to recognize and process the obvious signs of incest because this would jeopardize the relationship with her husband. The child uses denial and constriction of affect for several purposes: It serves as a protection against shame and guilt, it blots out awareness of the father's deviancy, and it preserves the intactness of the family.

SIBLING INCEST

Sexual contact between siblings is the most common form of incest, even though incestuous activity between daughters and their fathers or stepfathers is more frequently reported.

Finkelhor's (1979) survey of New England college students revealed that while only 1% of the girls had been molested by their fathers or stepfathers, 15% had had sexual relations with a sibling. Ten percent of the male students had participated in sibling incest. Ninety percent of the girls and 80% of the boys had been 12 or under at the time.

Sibling incest, however, is reported much less frequently than parental incest. For example, an analysis of sexual abuse hotline reports by Pierce and Pierce (1985) revealed that fathers and stepfathers were the perpetrators in 62% of the sexual abuse cases, while only 6% of the cases involved sibling incest. The discrepancy between the survey and reporting data might have occurred because sibling incest is less likely to be disclosed, as it is less disruptive to family functioning and might be less damaging to the child than parent incest.

PSYCHOLOGICAL SEQUELAE OF CHILD SEXUAL ABUSE

Until the mid-1980s, the literature dealing with the impact of child sexual abuse had been limited to anecdotal clinical observations and uncontrolled studies. A critical review of the sexual abuse literature reveals the following methodological deficiencies: (a) failure to employ comparison or control groups, (b) small sample size, (c) failure to control for psychological impairment antedating sexual abuse, (d) confounding independent variables (e.g., physical abuse in addition to sexual abuse), (e) failure to use standardized assessment instruments, and (f) lack of discrimination between short- and long-term psychological sequelae. Despite these methodological weaknesses, there appears to be some consensus among the clinical observations concerning immediate and long-term sequelae of sexual abuse.

The sequelae will be divided into general psychopathology and specific disorders in sexual behavior and gender identity.

General Psychopathology

Recent studies of sexually abused children using standardized instruments reveal the presence of significant psychiatric impairment. Merry and Andrews (1994) reported that 63.5% of 66 sexually abused children evaluated with the Diagnostic Interview Schedule for Children warranted an Axis I diagnosis on DSM-III-R. The most common diagnoses were oppositional defiant disorder, anxiety disorders, depressive disorders, posttraumatic stress disorder, and attention deficit hyperactivity disorder. Earlier research carried out by Gomes-Schwartz et al. (1985) assessed levels of emotional distress in 156 sexually abused children using the Louisville Behavior Checklist. Seventeen percent of preschoolers, 40% of school-age children, and 24% of adolescents demonstrated significant impairment consisting of anxiety, depression, destructive behavior, phobic reactions, and deficits in intellectual, physical, and social development. Each group of sexually abused children displayed more behavioral problems than their normal peers but fewer problems than children attending a child psychiatry clinic. The major areas of psychopathology can be categorized as follows: anxiety disorders and dissociation, depression, and aggressive behaviors.

ANXIETY DISORDERS

Fearfulness and anxiety-related disorders have been frequently described as immediate or short-term sequelae in sexually abused children. Anxiety-generated symptoms such as sleep disturbances, insomnia, nightmares, phobic avoidance, and somatic complaints were recognized by early investigators (Adams-Tucker, 1982; Browning and Boatman, 1977; Kempe and Kempe, 1978; Lewis and Sarrel, 1969). Sgroi (1982) described fear reactions of sexual abuse victims, extending to all males. Anderson et al. (1981) reported "internalized psychosocial sequelae" (sleep and eating disturbances, fears, phobias, depression, guilt, shame, and anger) in 67% of adolescent female victims of intrafamilial sexual abuse. Severe cases of child sexual abuse have recently been placed in the context of posttraumatic stress disorder (PTSD). Goodwin (1985) described posttraumatic symptoms in child victims of incest (i.e., fear, startle reactions, reenactment of the trauma, flashbacks, sleep disturbance, and depressive symptoms) by adapting Kardiner's descriptions (1941) of "shell-shocked" combat veterans to victims of child sexual abuse. Subsequent research was designed to identify symptoms of PTSD in sexually abused children according to DSM-III-R criteria.

Kiser et al. (1988) observed that 9 of 10 children from 2 to 6 years old who were sexually abused in a day care setting manifested symptoms of PTSD. The most frequently observed symptoms were acting as if the traumatic event was reoccurring because of environmental stimuli, avoiding activities reminiscent of the traumatic event, and intensification of symptoms after exposure to events resembling the molestation.

McLeer et al. (1988) reported that 48% of sexually abused girls from 3 to 16 years of age evaluated at a child psychiatry outpatient clinic met DSM-III-R criteria for PTSD. The symptoms included reexperiencing phenomena, avoidance behavior, and autonomic hyperarousal. Seventy-five percent of children abused by natural fathers and 25% abused by trusted adults exhibited symptoms of PTSD as opposed to none of the children abused by an older child.

DISSOCIATION

Dissociation, an alteration in consciousness resulting in an impairment of memory or identity, may be regarded as a primitive defense against potentially disorganizing types of psychological trauma. Kluft (1985) and Putnam (1984) observed dissociation in sexually abused children that led to multiple personality disorder (see Chapter 65). Signs of early dissociation in children are forgetfulness with periods of amnesia, excessive fantasizing and daydreaming, trancelike states, somnambulism, the presence of an imaginary companion, sleepwalking, and blackouts. According to Braun and Sachs (1985), the two major predisposing factors for multiple personality disorder are a natural inborn capacity to dissociate and exposure to severe overwhelming trauma.

Hysterical symptoms appear to be closely related to dissociation. Freud (1896) regarded hysterical symptoms as symbols of repressed memories of childhood seduction emerging from the unconscious that are provoked by situations that may be linked to the original trauma. Gross (1979) and Goodwin et al. (1989) reported hysterical seizures in adolescents who experienced incest. The hysterical symptoms were interpreted as the child's attempt to "wall off" traumatic impressions of the incest through primitive defenses of denial, isolation of affect, and splitting.

DEPRESSION AND LOW SELF-ESTEEM

Sgroi (1982) described depression, guilt, and low self-esteem along with a sensation of permanent damage or "damaged-goods syndrome"

as pivotal issues in sexually abused children. More recent research has confirmed the negative impact of sexual trauma on the child victim's affect and self-esteem. Livingston (1987) documented major depressive disorder with psychotic features in 10 of 13 sexually abused child psychiatric inpatients using the Diagnostic Interview for Children and Adolescents (Herjanic, 1977) as a standardized psychiatric interview. Sansonnet-Hayden et al. (1987) reported a 71% incidence of major depression in sexually abused adolescent inpatients, based on the Diagnostic Interview Schedule for Children. These sexually abused adolescents had a much higher incidence of suicide attempts than nonabused inpatients. Cavaiola and Shiff (1988) also reported a greater severity of depressive symptoms and more suicide attempts in sexually abused adolescent inpatients than in nonabused inpatients. Friedrich et al. (1986) observed that 46% of a sample of 61 sexually abused girls had significantly elevated scores on the internalizing scale of the Child Behavior Checklist, which includes behaviors described as fearful, inhibited, depressed, and overcontrolled.

INCREASED AGGRESSION

Angry reactions and poor impulse control have been noted by several authors (Adams-Tucker, 1982; Browning and Boatman, 1977; Simari and Baskin, 1982; Steele and Alexander, 1981). The aggression is usually directed toward both parents. The previously mentioned study by Friedrich et al. of 61 sexually abused girls revealed that 39% had elevated scores on the externalizing scale of the Child Behavior Checklist, indicating aggressive, antisocial, and undercontrolled behavior. In a recent study by Merry and Andrews (1994), oppositional defiant disorder was diagnosed in 20% of 66 sexually abused children.

OTHER SYMPTOMS

Impaired peer relationships have been frequently reported in sexually abused children. Tsai and Wagner (1981), Adams-Tucker (1982), and Knittle and Tuana (1980) described inadequate social skills, difficulties in personal relationships, and social withdrawal in child victims of sexual abuse. Sgroi (1982) described how incestuous families discourage the incest victim from separation-individuation and peer relationships. Herman (1981) described runaway behavior in sexually abused adolescents.

Poor school performance has been reported by DeFrancis (1969), Goodwin et al. (1989), and Sgroi (1982).

DISTURBANCES IN SEXUAL BEHAVIOR AND GENDER ROLE

One might expect that premature exposure to coercive and frightening sexual activity cloaked in secrecy would have an adverse impact on the child's psychosexual development, gender identity, and future capacity for sexual intimacy. Sexual hyperarousal and sexual acting out, with a tendency to repeat and reenact the incest experience, have been frequently described in victims of sexual abuse. Brant and Tisza (1977) postulated that these children provoke additional sexual contact as a means of obtaining pleasure and need satisfaction and as a technique for mastering the original trauma. James and Meyerding's (1977) retrospective study of adult female prostitutes revealed that 36% reported incest in childhood. Yates (1982) described the eroticization of preschool children by incest, with the degree of eroticization being proportional to the duration and intensity of the sexual contact. The victimized preschoolers were orgastic and/or maintained a high level of sexual arousal. Many of these children were unable to differentiate affectionate from sexual relationships and were aroused by routine physical or psychological closeness. Friedrich (1988) also documented disturbances in sexual behavior in two controlled studies. One study demonstrated a higher incidence of sexual behavior problems in 20 sexually abused boys between 4 and 7 years old than in a comparison group of 23 nonabused boys with a history of conduct disorder. Another study reported frequent sexual behavior problems in sexually abused children of both sexes compared with nonabused children who were psychiatric outpatients and nonabused normal children.

On the other hand, many studies cite phobic reactions and sexual inhibition in sexually abused children (Goodwin, 1985; Sgroi, 1982) and in adult incest survivors (Bess and Janssen, 1982; Brooks, 1982; Herman, 1981). In essence, there seems to be two contrasting adaptive styles in sexual abuse victims, one seeking mastery through active repetition of the trauma and the other coping by avoiding sexual stimuli.

In addition to abnormal sexual behavior, disturbances in sexual identity and sexual object choice have been documented in sexually abused girls and boys. Aoisa-Karpas et al. (1991) reported gender identity problems in adolescent girls, ages 12–19, who had been victims of sexual abuse. These girls demonstrated significantly greater gender identity conflict than nonabused psychiatric and nontreated controls. The abuse victims reported greater male identification for gender role behavior with regard to their choice of male fantasy roles in early childhood play. The authors suggest that the adolescent victims of sexual abuse experience difficulties in the formation and consolidation of a stable female identity due to an identification with the more dominant abusive father rather than with the disengaged mother.

In a similar study, Cosentino (1991) reported that sexually abused female children and adolescents manifested significantly more masculine gender role behavior and gender identity conflict than comparison groups of nonabused girls attending a child psychiatry outpatient clinic and a pediatric clinic. The sexually abused girls experienced extreme unhappiness about being female and a strong preference to become a boy. Many of these girls rejected their female genitalia. They more actively participated in rough and tumble play, had a greater interest in traditionally masculine clothing, and manifested a greater tendency to associate with male peers than the nonabused girls.

Similar gender identity problems have been documented in sexually abused boys. Meyer and Dupkin (1985) and Zucker and Kuksis (1990) described case histories of sexually abused boys who displayed effeminate behavior with cross-dressing, and played with girls. Meyers (1989) and Dimock (1988) reported male identity confusion in adult males who were sexually abused as boys. Many of these men engaged in sexually compulsive behavior and engaged in homosexuality. Homophobia, conflicted sexual orientation, and sexual dysfunction were also described in these men. Finkelhor (1984) found that male college students who had been molested by an older man were four times as likely to be involved in homosexual activity than a nonabused control group.

ADULT SURVIVORS OF SEXUAL ABUSE AND INCEST

The study of adult survivors of sexual abuse and incest offers a longitudinal perspective to the long-range defensive adaptation of sexual abuse victims. Many of the symptoms and psychiatric disorders exhibited by these survivors are similar to those seen in recently molested children, but there are also some significant differences in the way a sexual abuse victim adapts to the trauma one generation later.

Anxiety symptoms such as chronic tension, sleep disturbances, nightmares, and somatic complaints have been reported to be more frequent in former sexual abuse victims than in nonabused comparison groups (Briere, 1984; Briere and Runtz, 1985; Sedney and Brooks, 1984). Linderg and Distad (1985) described sleep disturbance, guilt, intrusive imagery of the incest, feeling of detachment, and sexual dysfunction in women who had been molested in childhood. These authors regarded these symptoms as manifestations of delayed or chronic posttraumatic stress disorder.

Depressive symptoms in formerly molested adults have been described by Bagley and Ramsay (1986), Peters (1985), and Sedney and Brooks (1984). Low self-esteem has been documented in adult survivors of child sexual abuse by Bagley and Ramsay (1985), Courtois (1979), and Herman (1981), while suicidal behavior has also been observed in this population (Briere, 1984; Sedney and Brooks, 1984).

Borderline personality disorder has been frequently observed in adult female survivors of sexual abuse and incest (Herman et al., 1989; Stone et al., 1988). Herman and van der Kolk (1987) attribute the higher incidence of borderline personality disorder in women to the more widespread sexual victimization of girls. Herman et al. (1989) regard borderline personality disorder as a complicated posttraumatic syndrome in which the subjects fail to perceive the connection between their current symptoms and their abusive childhood experiences. These authors maintain that the memories of victimization become integrated in the total personality organization and become ego syntonic.

Substance abuse has been reported as a common problem in adult survivors of sexual victimization in childhood (Briere, 1984; Goodwin et al., 1990). Considerable numbers of incest victims and survivors of child sexual abuse become dependent on drugs and alcohol during adolescence and early adulthood. Clinical experience with adolescent and adult survivors of sexual abuse reveals that these substances help blot out painful memories and affects associated with the victimization. Multiple personality disorder and dissociation have been frequently documented in adult incest survivors (Briere and Runtz, 1988; Putnam et al., 1986). Severe sexual and/or physical abuse inflicted during childhood has been considered to be the primary etiological factor in multiple personality disorder (Coons and Milstein, 1986; Putnam et al., 1986).

Several researchers have documented a higher incidence of sexual dysfunction in adult incest survivors than in nonabused controls (Briere, 1984; Herman, 1981; Meiselman, 1978). Commonly described symptoms of sexual dysfunction include promiscuity, decreased sex drive, an inability to enjoy sexual activity, and sexual avoidance.

Women survivors of childhood sexual abuse appear to be vulnerable to revictimization later in life. They are more prone to rape (Russell, 1986) and spouse abuse (Briere, 1984). Miller et al. (1978) reported a higher incidence of child sexual abuse in the histories of women victimized by multiple rape than in first-time rape victims.

There is considerable evidence linking childhood sexual victimization with subsequent child molesting in men (Groth and Freeman-Longo, 1979; Seghorn et al., 1987). Although females are less likely to molest children, there is a very high incidence of prior sexual abuse in these female sexual offenders (Green and Kaplan, 1994; McCarty, 1986). It is likely that the sexual offenses represent a reenactment of the original childhood molestation and an identification with the perpetrator. The sexually arousing component of the childhood victimization appears to be an important factor in the reenactment.

NATURE OF THE TRAUMA IN CHILD SEXUAL ABUSE

Both the child victims and adult survivors of sexual abuse exhibit pathological anxiety, affective dysregulation, impulsivity, and dissociative defenses that contribute to considerable psychological distress. They differ in that the adult survivors are less consciously preoccupied with their victimization because of the substantial passage of time and the absence of the perpetrator. The adults have a wider variety of defenses at their disposal so that the original traumatic memories and affects become absorbed into personality traits and identifications that may become ego syntonic and appear to be unrelated to the original trauma. Because the adults are more removed from the original trauma, they are more likely to experience delayed posttraumatic stress reactions elicited by events evoking memories of the sexual victimization than acute PTSD symptoms.

MODELS OF SEXUAL ABUSE

Finkelhor and Browne (1986) proposed a model to explain the traumatic effects of sexual abuse. They identified four trauma-causing or "traumagenic" factors:

1. Traumatic sexualization occurs through the sexual stimulation and reinforcement of the child's sexual responses, so that the child learns to use sexual behavior to gratify numerous nonsexual need. This leads to inappropriate and premature sexual activity, a confused sexual identity, and deviant patterns of sexual arousal.

2. Powerlessness refers to helplessness during the sexual assault, leading to fear and anxiety.
3. Stigmatization describes the child's senses of being damaged and blamed for the molestation, which might be reinforced by peers and family members. This leads to shame, guilt, and low self-esteem.
4. Betrayal refers to the child's sharp disillusionment when he or she is cruelly sexually exploited by a trusted parent or caretaker from whom love and protection are expected. Betrayal may lead to a generalized distrust of others, hostility, and anger.

This traumagenic model is a useful guide in understanding the impact of sexual abuse and might be applied in designing research and intervention strategies. However, this model fails to differentiate acute and chronic traumatic events and the interaction between them. Terr (1991) conceptualized sexual abuse as a long-standing multiple trauma, or ''Type II'' trauma, which produces profound character changes such as denial, repression, dissociation, self-hypnosis, and identification with the aggressor, etc. This is in contrast to a discrete catastrophic event producing PTSD, which she labeled a ''Type I'' trauma. However, this model fails to explain the frequent occurrence of PTSD in sexually abused children due to the traumatic nature of certain types of sexual abuse. Green (1988) added a temporal and developmental perspective to account for the development of immediate and long-term sequelae. He describes sexual abuse as the repeated infliction of sexual and aggressive stimulation superimposed upon a chronic background of pathological family interaction, including stigmatization, betrayal, role reversal, sexualization, and a breaching of the child's physical and psychological boundaries. The acute sexual assault includes traumatic sexualization and powerlessness and produces fearfulness and anxiety-related symptoms such as nightmares, sleep disorders, hypervigilance, psychosomatic symptoms, and dissociative reactions that may satisfy criteria for PTSD in some cases. The underlying chronic family dysfunction results in stigmatization, betrayal, guilt, shame, low self-esteem, mistrust, depression, and pathological defenses. The interaction between these acute and long-term variables is likely to potentiate their pathological impact.

The severity of both the acute and long-term symptoms would depend on the following variables: (a) age and developmental level of the child; (b) the child's preexisting personality; (c) onset, duration, and frequency of the abuse; (d) degree of coercion and physical trauma; (e) the nature of the relationship between the child and the perpetrator; (f) the family's response to the disclosure; (g) the institutional response; and (h) the availability and quality of therapeutic intervention.

CLINICAL EVALUATION OF INTRAFAMILIAL CHILD SEXUAL ABUSE

The assessment of a potential case of child sexual abuse should be carried out by a trained mental health professional—psychiatrist, psychologist, psychiatric nurse, or social worker who has special expertise with children and families involved in child sexual abuse. The evaluator should have a knowledge of child development, child psychopathology, family dynamics, and the signs, symptoms, and sequelae of child sexual abuse. He or she should also be familiar with the phenomenon of false allegations and its manifestations and should understand the typical psychopathology of incestuous families and sexual offenders. The clinician should be aware of his or her own feelings and reactions regarding sexual behavior and sexual victimization of children, to avoid countertransference reactions.

Assessment of the Child

Prior to interviewing the child, a detailed history should be obtained, including a developmental survey, a medical history (including the presence of genital and anal symptoms), information about the development of sexual behavior and sexual interests, family attitudes regarding sex and modesty, and some information about the child's usual behavior and coping to provide a contrast between pretraumatic and posttraumatic

functioning. The history should be designed to elicit the presence of typical sequelae of child sexual abuse as previously described.

The child will often require a longer period of evaluation than the usual child psychiatric patient, as incest victims are often very defensive and resistant to direct questioning. In some cases, several interviews might be required to establish rapport and trust before focusing on the sexual abuse allegations. If the child is able to talk about the sexual abuse, detailed descriptions of the events should be obtained where possible (e.g., type of molestation, frequency, duration, location, nature of threats by offender, etc.). If the child is unable to verbalize memories and feelings regarding the molestation, his or her perceptions of the event may be elicited indirectly through play, fantasy, and dreams. Drawings are often a valuable tool in providing information about the sexual abuse. The drawing of genitalia, precocious sexualized representations, and the exaggeration or avoidance of sexual features are often indicators of sexual molestation.

Anatomically correct dolls may be used as an aid in the assessment of preschool children who may have difficulty verbalizing their experience. The dolls are, however, frequently misused by unskilled or biased evaluators, who may use them in a leading manner. The dolls are controversial, and the following criticisms have been made about their use in sexual abuse evaluations: (a) there is no commonly accepted, standard protocol for their use; (b) there is an absence of available norms on how sexually abused and nonabused children interact with the dolls; (c) the dolls may be sexually overstimulating and induce nonabused children to engage in sex play; and (d) use of the dolls promotes interviewer error and misuse. Although Everson and Boat (1994) argue that these criticisms of the anatomical dolls are not supported by recent research, the use of the dolls as a diagnostic test has not been recommended by any of the major guidelines for sexual abuse evaluations formulated by major mental health organizations (Everson and Boat, 1994).

Leading questions should be avoided during the interview. The credibility of the child is weakened if he or she is unable to remember details of the alleged molestation and if the stories are varying and inconsistent, if the child uses adult sexual terminology, if the molestation is described matter of factly with little or no affect, and if the child is unduly suggestible. Assessment of the child can usually be completed in four to six visits.

Evaluation of the Parents

A separate psychiatric examination of each parent should complement the assessment of the child. This should include a family history with information concerning a background of physical or sexual abuse and family violence, a sexual history, information regarding impulse control, substance abuse, cognitive and psychiatric impairment, and a history of the marital relationship. The alleged perpetrator should be questioned about sexual dysfunction and the presence of other paraphilias (i.e., exhibitionism, voyeurism, sexual sadomasochism, etc.) that may be associated with pedophilia. Fathers or father surrogates should be asked about their degree of participation in routine child care activities such as bathing, diapering, and toileting of the child.

Observation of the Child with Each Parent

MOTHER-CHILD INTERACTION

The mother-child interaction provides a baseline for the assessment of the relationship between the child and the alleged perpetrator. One should document the degree of spontaneity, warmth, and closeness in their contact, and the amount of maternal control of the child's behavior. Most mothers who discover that their child may have been sexually abused by their partner are shocked and distraught and initially find the allegations incredible. But they are protective of the child and encourage him or her to describe what happened. Mothers making false allegations of sexual abuse often control the child by monitoring his or her responses through eye contact or subtle facial expressions. The child may respond by "checking" with the mother before proceeding. These mothers often pressure the child to discuss the alleged molestation and encourage the child to disparage the father.

FATHER-CHILD INTERACTION

A child who has been molested by a father or stepfather is likely to exhibit some form of fearfulness, anger, or discomfort during their encounters. However, a benign, "normal" appearing father-child interaction might occur in cases of "gentle" fondling of a preschooler or young child who is unable to appreciate the inappropriate and deviant nature of this experience. In cases of false allegations, there is often a striking discrepancy between the child's negative attitudes toward the father in the (accusing) mother's presence and his or her spontaneous and affectionate behavior when observed alone with the father and free from the mother's influence. The child's wishes should be heeded if he or she is firmly opposed to meeting with the alleged perpetrator.

INTERVENTION

The immediate goal of intervention in cases of child sexual abuse is to modify the abusive environment so that the child is no longer at risk for molestation; that is, the perpetrator should no longer have access to the child. Treatment of the child begins with crisis intervention to deal with his or her acute anxiety-related symptoms pertaining to the molestation and the ensuing family crisis. Intervention is also designed to prevent the development of the long-term sequelae of sexual abuse. Since the incestuous family is severely dysfunctional, treatment of the child is supplemented by intervention with the family members. Incestuous fathers are usually removed from the home, but they may benefit from individual or group psychotherapy, or a behavioral intervention if there is a pedophilic component to their incestuous behavior. Intervention with the mother is geared to promoting a more supportive and protective maternal response to the child victim. Additional treatment issues that must be addressed with the mother are guilt, anger toward the spouse, loss and depression associated with the breakup of the marriage, and anger toward the child for usurping her role as a sexual partner. Under certain conditions, family therapy and dyadic treatment can be helpful.

Group therapy for the child victim might be useful as a primary treatment modality or as an adjunct to individual psychotherapy. It may be particularly effective in adolescent and preadolescent victims of sexual abuse because it offers peer support, facilitates discussion of sensitive issues, and helps the members overcome their sense of isolation and stigmatization.

Individual psychotherapy or play therapy helps the victim to resolve conflicts and symptoms that interfere with relationships with peers and family, academic functioning, and self-esteem.

The literature on intervention is flawed by a paucity of treatment outcome studies. However, two recent studies have demonstrated the efficacy of cognitive behavioral intervention with sexually abused children. Deblinger (1995) compared the effectiveness of a variety of cognitive behavioral interventions with sexually abused children 7 to 13 years old (child only, child plus mother, mother only) with the treatment received by abused children who were referred to community agencies. The children assigned to the child only or parent-child intervention exhibited fewer depressive and PTSD symptoms than the children referred to the community. The children assigned to interventions including direct work with a parent exhibited fewer externalizing symptoms at posttreatment compared with the community sample. Cohen and Mannarino (1995) demonstrated a greater reduction in behavior problems, including abnormal sexual behavior, in sexually abused preschool children receiving short-term cognitive behavioral treatment compared with an abused cohort receiving nondirective supportive therapy. Several group therapy outcome studies have been reported using standardized instruments to measure posttreatment improvement. James (1977) and Verleur et al.

(1986) found that sexually abused girls demonstrated more improvement in self-esteem after treatment than did untreated control groups. Nelki and Watters (1989) documented a significant decline in problematic behaviors exhibited by sexually abused children at the end of group therapy, according to parent rating scales.

There is an obvious need for more treatment outcome studies using standardized instruments to determine the efficacy of intervention with sexually abused children and their families, and whether a diminution or reversal of symptoms persists over time.

MAJOR TREATMENT ISSUES IN INDIVIDUAL PSYCHOTHERAPY

Betrayal and the Establishment of Trust

Much of the beginning phase of therapy is designed to overcome the child's fear of betrayal and to establish a supportive, trusting relationship. The experience of sexual exploitation and coercion by a parent from whom love and nurturance is expected generates a feeling of betrayal that is easily generalized and displaced onto other parental and authority figures and is inevitably encountered in the therapeutic relationship. The child is often afraid of being seduced by a male therapist and is concerned about the ability of a female therapist to act in a protective manner. The therapist can eventually interpret these transference reactions by tracing them back to the original feelings of betrayal and disillusionment with the parents. After a period of "testing" behavior, the child gradually views the therapist as reliable, predictable, and trustworthy. This newly acquired sense of trust may then be applied to extratherapeutic relationships.

Acute Traumatization and Anxiety-Related Symptoms

Even in the absence of further victimization, the child might still exhibit anxiety-related symptoms, sometimes in the form of posttraumatic stress disorder. Some victims appear to be fixated on the trauma; they reenact the traumatic elements of their molestation in play, dreams, fantasies, and artistic productions. The main therapeutic goal is to identify and interpret the unconscious link between the repetitive play activity and the original traumatic experiences. Once this connection is made, the child will be able to verbalize the traumatic memories and express the painful affects in words rather than in action.

Some sexually abused children will utilize phobic and avoidant defenses instead of reenacting their molestation. They will avoid peer contact and intimacy and situations associated with sexuality, i.e., dancing, dating, undressing in front of others, etc. The therapist might explain to the child that the phobic, avoidant coping style that was adaptive in the incestuous environment is burdensome and unnecessary in normal settings. The child must be taught to differentiate benign individuals from sexual predators.

Stigmatization

The stigmatization of the child by the incestuous relationship results in shame, guilt, low self-esteem, and depression and may lead to suicidal behavior. These feelings of shame and guilt are intensified if the child is blamed for participating in the sexual activity. The therapist must challenge the victim's perception that he or she is responsible for the sexual acts. It must be emphasized that the child who is coerced into a sexual activity by a parent or other adult cannot be regarded as culpable in any way. The offender's behavior should be labeled as "sick" and inappropriate.

Role Confusion

The incest victim is prematurely burdened with parental roles, serving the father as a sexual partner and confidant and assuming the mother's household and caretaking responsibilities. These role reversals are in direct conflict with the child's needs for protection and nurturance. The child victim of incest maintains an infantile attachment to the father in spite of the pseudoadult facade and is discouraged from establishing normal peer relationships, which are prerequisite for independent functioning. In the treatment setting, the child's need to please and ingratiate the therapist at the expense of his or her own needs may be interpreted and linked to the child's previous need to please the parents. The therapist should encourage the child to engage in age-appropriate childhood activities and foster peer relationships.

Premature Sexualization

Child incest victims exhibit two contrasting coping styles in response to their experiences of premature sexual stimulation. One seeks mastery through repetition and reenactment of the molestation and the other through avoiding sexual stimuli. Each of these responses is based on a weakening of normal repression. The aim of psychotherapy is to control the acting out and avoidance patterns while encouraging the use of higher level defenses such as repression, sublimation, and intellectualization. This may be carried out by a variety of therapeutic maneuvers, such as limit setting, educational techniques, interpretation, and desensitization. The child is encouraged to verbalize memories of the incest experience instead of acting them out or avoiding them. The therapist must set limits on the child's hypersexual seductive behavior when it surfaces during therapy sessions. The child is gradually able to internalize these prohibitions. The child's use of ''identification with the aggressor'' as a component of the seductive behavior may be interpreted. The child also must be taught to differentiate routine physically affectionate behavior from behavior with a sexual intent and is encouraged to respect his or her own bodily privacy and that of others.

Countertransference Reactions

The major countertransference problem confronting therapists who work with sexually abused children is the tendency to overidentify with the victim, become enraged with the abuser, and develop exaggerated rescue fantasies. This situation may lead to an intolerance for the child's positive feelings toward the perpetrator or encourage the child to vent his or her own anger prematurely. These therapists easily become impatient with the progress of therapy and cannot tolerate the child's resistance and hostility, which threaten the rescue mission.

Working with sexually abused children may elicit the therapist's own unconscious childhood sexual feelings about child sexual abuse and sexuality. If a therapist is uncomfortable about sexual matters, this might be communicated to the child, who would then be reluctant to discuss his or her victimization.

References

Aarens M, Cameron T, Roizen J, et al: *Alcohol, Casualties and Crime.* Berkeley, CA, Social Research Group, 1978.

Adams-Tucker C: Proximate effects of sexual abuse in childhood: A report on 28 children. *Am J Psychiatry* 139:1252–1256, 1982.

Aiosa-Karpas C, Karpas R, Pelcovitz D, et al: Gender identification and sex role attribution in sexually abused adolescent females. *J Am Acad Child Adolesc Psychiatry* 30:266–271, 1991.

American Humane Association: *National Study on Child Neglect and Abuse Reporting.* Denver, American Humane Association, 1981.

Anderson SC, Bach CM, Griffith S: Psychosocial sequelae in intrafamilial victims of sexual assault and abuse. Paper presented at the Third International Conference on Child Abuse and Neglect, Amsterdam, The Netherlands, April 1981.

Bagley C, Ramsay R: Sexual abuse in childhood: Psychosocial outcomes and implications for social work practice. *J Soc Work Hum Sexuality* 4:33–47, 1986.

Bess BE, Janssen Y: Incest: A pilot study. *Hillside J Clin Psychiatry* 4:39–52, 1982.

Brant R, Tisza V: The sexually misused child. *Am J Orthopsychiatry* 47:80–90, 1977.

Briere J: The long-term effects of childhood sexual abuse: Defining a post-sexual abuse syndrome. Paper presented at the Third National Conference on Sexual Victimization of Children, Washington, DC, April 1984.

Briere J, Runtz M: Symptomatology associated with prior sexual abuse in a non-clinical sample. Paper presented at the Annual Meeting of the American Psychological Association, Los Angeles, 1985.

Briere J, Runtz M: Post sexual abuse trauma. In: Wyatt GE, Powell GJ (eds): *Lasting Effects of Child Sexual Abuse.* Newbury Park, CA, Sage, 1988.

Brooks B: Familial influence on father-daughter incest. *J Psychiatr Treat Eval* 4:117–124, 1982.

Browning DH, Boatman B: Incest: Children at risk. *Am J Psychiatry* 134:69–72, 1977.

Cavaiola A, Schiff M: Behavioral sequelae of physical and/or sexual abuse in adolescents. *Child Abuse Negl* 12:181–188, 1988.

Cavallin H: Incestuous fathers: A clinical report. *Am J Psychiatry* 122:1132–1138, 1966.

Cohen JA, Mannarino AP: Treatment for sexually abused preschoolers. *J Am Acad Child Adolesc Psychiatry*, in press, 1995.

Cosentino CE: Cross-gender behavior and gender conflict in sexually abused girls. *J Am Acad Child Adolesc Psychiatry* 32:940–947, 1993.

Courtois C: The incest experience and its aftermath. *Victimology Int J* 4:337–347, 1979.

Deblinger E: Cognitive behavioral intervention for treating post-traumatic stress disorder in sexually abused children: A treatment outcome study. Paper presented at the San Diego Conference on Responding to Child Maltreatment, San Diego, CA, January, 1995.

DeFrancis V: *Protecting the Child Victim of Sex Crimes Committed by Adults.* Denver, American Humane Association, 1969.

Dimock P: Adult males sexually abused as children. *J Interpersonal Violence* 3:203–221, 1988.

Everson MD, Boat BW: Putting the anatomical doll controversy in perspective; an examination of the major uses and criticisms of the dolls in child sexual abuse evaluations. *Child Abuse Negl* 18:113–129, 1994.

Finkelhor D: *Sexually Victimized Children.* New York, Free Press, 1979.

Finkelhor D: *A Sourcebook on Child Sexual Abuse.* Beverly Hills, Sage, 1986.

Finkelhor D, Brown A: Initial and long-term effects: A conceptual framework. In: Finkelhor D (ed): *Sourcebook on Child Sexual Abuse.* Beverly Hills, Sage, 1986.

Freud S: The etiology of hysteria. *The Standard Edition of the Complete Psychological Works of Sigmund Freud* (Vol 3). London, Hogarth Press, 1962 (1896), pp. 191–221.

Friedrich WN: Behavior problems in sexually abused children; an adaptational perspective. In: Wyatt GE, Powell GJ (eds): *Lasting Effects of Child Sexual Abuse.* Beverly Hills, Sage, 1988.

Friedrich WN, Urquiza AJ, Beilke R: Behavioral problems in sexually abused young children. *J Pediatr Psychol* 11:47–57, 1986.

Fromuth ME, Burkhart BR: Long-term psychological correlates of childhood sexual abuse in two samples of college men. *Child Abuse Negl* 13:533–542, 1989.

Gebhard P, Gagnon J, Pomeroy W, et al: *Sex Offenders: An Analysis of Types.* New York, Harper & Row, 1965.

Gomes-Schwartz B, Horowitz J, Sauzier M: Severity of emotional distress among sexually abused preschool, school age and adolescent children. *Hosp Community Psychiatry* 36:503–508, 1985.

Goodwin JM: Post-traumatic symptoms in incest victims. In: Eth S, Pynoos R (eds): *Post-Traumatic Stress Disorder in Children.* Washington, DC, American Psychiatric Press, 1985.

Goodwin JM, Cheeves K, Connell V: Borderline and other severe symptoms in adult survivors of incestuous abuse. *Psychiatr Ann* 20:22–32, 1990.

Goodwin JM, Zouhar MS, Bergman R: Hysterical seizures in adolescent incest victims. In: Goodwin J (ed): *Sexual Abuse: Incest Victims and Their Families.* Chicago, Year Book, 1989.

Green AH: Child maltreatment and its victims. *Psychiatr Clin North Am* 11:591–610, 1988.

Green AH, Kaplan MS: Psychiatric impairment and childhood victimization experiences in female child molesters. *J Am Acad Child Adolesc Psychiatry* 33:954–961, 1994.

Gross M: Incestuous rape: A cause for hysterical seizures in four adolescent girls. *Am J Orthopsychiatry* 49:704–708, 1979.

Groth AN: The incest offender. In: Sgroi S (ed): *Handbook of Clinical Intervention in Child Sexual Abuse.* Lexington, MA, Lexington Books, 1982.

Groth AN, Freeman-Longo R: *Men Who Rape: The Psychology of the Offender.* New York, Plenum, 1979.

Herjanic B: *Diagnostic Interview for Children and Adolescents.* St. Louis, MO, Washington University 1977.

Herman JL: *Father-Daughter Incest.* Cambridge, MA, Harvard University Press, 1981.

Herman JL, van der Kolk BA: Traumatic antecedents of borderline personality disorder. In: van der Kolk BA (ed): *Psychological Trauma.* Washington, DC, American Psychiatric Press, 1987.

Herman JL, Perry JC, van der Kolk BA: Childhood trauma in borderline personality disorder. *Am J Psychiatry* 146:490–495, 1989.

Horowitz M: *Stress-Response Syndromes.* New York, Jason Aronson, 1976.

James J, Meyerding J: Early sexual experiences as a factor in prostitution. *Am J Psychiatry* 134:1381–1385, 1977.

Kardiner A: The traumatic neuroses of war. In:

Arieti S (ed): *American Handbook of Psychiatry* (Vol 1). New York, Basic Books, 1941.

Kaufman I, Peck A, Tagiuri L: The family constellation and overt incestuous relations between father and daughter. *Am J Orthopsychiatry* 24: 266–279, 1954.

Kiser LJ, Ackerman BJ, Brown E, et al: Posttraumatic stress disorder in young children: A reaction to purported sexual abuse. *J Am Acad Child Adolesc Psychiatry* 27:645–649, 1988.

Kluft R: *Childhood Antecedents of Multiple Personality*. Washington DC, American Psychiatric Press, 1985.

Knittle B, Tuana S: Group therapy as primary treatment for adolescent victims of intrafamilial sexual abuse. *Clin Soc Work J* 8:236–242, 1980.

Lewis M, Sarrell P: Some psychological aspects of seduction, incest and rape in childhood. *J Am Acad Child Psychiatry* 8:606–619, 1969.

Linberg F, Distad L: Post-traumatic stress disorders in women who experienced childhood incest. *Child Abuse Negl* 9:329–334, 1985.

Livingston R: Sexually and physically abused children. *J Am Acad Child Adolesc Psychiatry* 26: 413–415, 1987.

McCarty L: Mother-child incest: Characteristics of the offender. *Child Welfare* 65:447–458, 1986.

McLeer SV, Deblinger E, Atkins MS, et al: Posttraumatic stress disorder in sexually abused children. *J Am Acad Child Adolesc Psychiatry* 27:342–353, 1988.

Meiselman K: *Incest: A Psychological Study of Causes and Effects with Treatment Recommendations*. San Francisco, Jossey-Bass, 1978.

Merry SN, Andrews LK: Psychiatric status of sexually abused children 12 months after disclosure of abuse. *J Am Acad Child Adolesc Psychiatry* 33: 939–944, 1994.

Meyer JK, Dupkin C: Gender disturbance in children; an interim clinical report. *Bull Menninger Clin* 49:236–239, 1985.

Miller J, Moeller R, Kaufman A, et al: Recidivism among sex assault victims. *Am J Psychiatry* 135:1103–1104, 1978.

Mrazek P, Lynch M, Bentovim A: Recognition of child sexual abuse in the United Kingdom. In: Mrazek P, Kempe H (eds): *Sexually Abused Children and Their Families*. New York, Pergamon, 1981.

Myers MF: Men sexually assaulted as adults and sexually abused as boys. *Arch Sex Behav* 18: 203–215, 1989.

National Center on Child Abuse and Neglect: *Study Findings: National Study of Incidence and Severity of Child Abuse and Neglect*. Washington, DC, Department of Health, Education, and Welfare, 1981.

National Center on Child Abuse Prevention Research: *Current trends in child abuse reporting and fatalities: The results of the 1993 annual fifty state survey*. Chicago, The National Committee for Prevention of Child Abuse, 1994.

Nelki J, Watters J: A group for sexually abused young children. *Child Abuse Negl* 13:369–377, 1989.

Peters SD: Child sexual abuse and later psychological problems. Paper presented at the American Psychological Association, Los Angeles, 1985.

Pierce R, Pierce L: The sexually abused child: A comparison of male and female victims. *Child Abuse Negl* 9:191–199, 1985.

Putnam FW: The psychophysiologic investigation of multiple personality disorder. *Psychiatr Clin North Am* 7:31–40, 1984.

Putnam FW, Guroff JJ, Silberman EK, et al: The clinical phenomenology of multiple personality disorder; review of 100 recent cases. *J Clin Psychiatry* 47:285–293, 1986.

Russell DE: The incidence and prevalence of intrafamilial and extrafamilial sexual abuse of female children. *Child Abuse Negl* 7:133–146, 1983.

Russell DE: *The Secret Trauma: Incest in the Lives of Girls and Women*. New York, Basic Books, 1986.

Sansonnet-Hayden H, Haley G, Marriage K, et al: Sexual abuse and psychopathology in hospitalized adolescents. *J Am Acad Child Adolesc Psychiatry* 26: 753–757, 1987.

Sedney MA, Brooks B: Factors associated with a history of childhood sexual experience in a nonclinical female population. *J Am Acad Child Psychiatry* 23:215–218, 1984.

Seghorn T, Prentky R, Boucher R: Childhood sexual abuse in the lives of sexually aggressive offenders. *J Am Acad Child Adolesc Psychiatry* 26: 262–267, 1987.

Seidner AL, Calhoun KS: Childhood sexual abuse: Factors related to differential adult adjustment. Paper presented at the Second National Conference for Family Violence Researchers, Durham, NH, 1984.

Sgroi S: *Handbook of Clinical Intervention in Child Sexual Abuse*. Lexington, MA, Lexington Books, 1982.

Simari CG, Baskin D: Incestuous experiences within homosexual populations: A preliminary study. *Arch Sex Behav* 11:329–344, 1982.

Steele B, Alexander H: Long-term effects of sexual abuse in childhood. In: Mrazek PB, Kempe CH (eds): *Sexually Abused Children and Their Families*. Oxford, Pergamon, 1981.

Stone M, Unwin A, Beacham B, et al: Incest in female borderlines: Its frequency and impact. *Int J Fam Psychiatry* 9:277–293, 1988.

Summit R, Kryso J: Sexual abuse of children: A clinical spectrum. *Am J Orthopsychiatry* 48: 237–251, 1978.

Terr LC: Childhood traumas: An outline and overview. *Am J Psychiatry* 148:10–20, 1991.

Tsai M, Wagner N: Incest and molestation: Problems of childhood sexuality. *Med Times* 16–22, 1981.

Verleur D, Hughes RE, Bobkin de Rios M: Enhancement of self-esteem among female adolescent incest victims: A controlled comparison. *Adolescence* 21:843–854.

Weinberg K: *Incest Behavior*. New York, Citadel Press, 1955.

Wyatt GE: The sexual abuse of Afro-American and white American women in childhood. *Child Abuse Negl* 9:507–519, 1985.

Yates A: Children eroticized by incest. *Am J Psychiatry* 139:482–485, 1982.

Zucker KJ, Kuksis M: Gender dysphoria and sexual abuse: A case report. *Child Abuse Negl* 14: 281–283, 1990.

101 MUNCHAUSEN SYNDROME BY PROXY

Brian W.C. Forsyth, M.B. CH.B. F.R.C.P.(C.)

DEFINITION AND HISTORICAL NOTE

Definition

Munchausen syndrome by proxy is a disorder in which a person persistently fabricates symptoms of illness on behalf of another, so causing that person to be regarded as ill (Meadow, 1977). In instances involving children, it is almost exclusively their mothers who are fabricating the illness. The severity of the disorder and the extent of the fabrication are variable: In the least severe cases mothers only report false symptoms, and the physical harm to the children is only that resulting from the medical investigations carried out in attempting to diagnose the illnesses; at the other end of the spectrum are instances in which mothers have caused severe physical harm to their children or have even caused the death of their children in the continued pursuit of making their children appear ill. Although a form of child abuse, there are characteristics of this syndrome that set it apart from other types of abuse.

Historical Note

In 1951 Asher first used the eponym Munchausen syndrome to describe adults who consistently fabricate symptoms of illness for themselves, leading to numerous medical investigations and frequently to surgical operations. The syndrome was named after Baron von Munchausen of Hanover, who lived in the 18th century and was renowned for telling greatly embellished stories about his adventures in the wars against the Turks. His tales became even more fantastic when written by a friend, Rudolf Eric Raspe, who published a pamphlet (1948) retelling some of the stories. In 1976 Sneed and Bell used the term "the dauphin of Munchausen" to describe a case in which a 10-year-old boy presented with factitious recurrent urinary calculi and in which the mother was suspected of colluding with the child in fabricating the symptoms. The following year, Meadow (1977) coined the term *Munchausen syndrome by proxy* in his report of observations of two cases in which mothers repeatedly caused their children to be ill. Prior to this time, there had been reports in the literature of cases referred to as "non-accidental poisoning" in which children repeatedly presented as diagnostic dilemmas and were found to have been poisoned by a parent (Lansky and Erickson, 1974; Rogers et al., 1976). Such cases are now considered to be variants of Munchausen syndrome by proxy. Subsequent to Meadow's initial report, there have been other suggestions for a title for the syndrome; these have included the names Meadow's syndrome or Polle syndrome, but these have now given way to the more commonly used Munchausen syndrome by proxy (Lazoritz, 1987; Meadow and Lennert, 1984; Verity et al., 1979).

PREVALENCE AND EPIDEMIOLOGY

Although the true prevalence remains unknown, Munchausen syndrome by proxy is almost certainly a rare disorder. It is likely, however, that like other forms of child abuse, more cases will be diagnosed as physicians become increasingly aware of the syndrome.

In 1987 Rosenberg conducted an extensive review of the literature and summarized all the published reports. These included 117 children in 97 families. In nearly all instances the perpetrator was the mother; in one case, it was an adoptive mother. In another report, a babysitter who herself had Munchausen syndrome had caused the death of two children and suffocated a third. It is uncertain, however, whether this latter case shares all the characteristics of Munchausen syndrome by proxy. Only very rarely have there been cases reported in which the father was the perpetrator or appeared to be complicit in the fabrication of illness (Meadow, 1984; Makar and Squier, 1990).

The diagnosis has been made in children of all ages between 1 month and 21 years. Rosenberg reports the mean age at time of diagnosis is 40 months, with the mean time interval between the onset of symptoms and time of diagnosis being 15 months. There is a report of one instance in which the condition started prior to the child's birth with the mother inducing preterm delivery (Goss and McDougall, 1992). There is an approximately equal prevalence among male and female children.

CLINICAL DESCRIPTION

The variety of medical symptoms in children who present with Munchausen syndrome by proxy is extensive and includes practically all organ systems. Generally the illness appears to be multisystem, and the children may appear to have different types of illness at different times. Bleeding is the most common presentation and accounted for 44% of the 117 cases included in Rosenberg's review of the literature. The apparent bleeding may be from many different sites, including the gastrointestinal, genitourinary, and respiratory systems. Seizures accounted for 42% of the cases, central nervous system depression for 19% of the cases, and apnea was present in 15% of the cases. Diarrhea was a presenting symptom for 11%, vomiting for 10%, and fever for 10%. Altogether Rosenberg listed 68 different presentations or pathologic findings. The means by which the perpetrators caused the symptoms or abnormal findings are just as diverse and illustrate the severity and horrifying nature of the syndrome: One mother had put bleach in her child's eye, causing the appearance of a periorbital infection; others had repeatedly suffocated their children so as to simulate recurrent apnea or seizures. Other mothers caused sepsis by putting fecal material into their children's intravenous lines.

In approximately one-quarter of cases in Rosenberg's review, the mother had simulated an illness but had not actually done anything directly to the child to cause harm. These were instances where the mother had done something such as putting drops of her own blood in her child's urine or contaminating the specimen. In these instances, although the mother does not herself physically harm the child, she does continue to collaborate with the physicians as distressing and often painful investigations and procedures are carried out.

Bools et al. (1992) have pointed out that there is a significant amount of comorbidity among cases of Munchausen syndrome by proxy: In a review of 56 cases, 29% had a history of failure to thrive and 25% had a history of either non-accidental injury or neglect. Siblings also might have a history of such findings or might themselves have been the subjects of fabricated illnesses. This appears to be particularly true among cases that have presented as apnea and which, in fact, are due to suffocation (Light and Sheridan, 1990; Meadow, 1990; Alexander et al., 1990). When children present with apnea, Munchausen syndrome by proxy should always be considered if there is a history of death of a sibling or if serious episodes of apnea have occurred only in the presence of one person.

Description of the Mother

These mothers often have had prior extensive exposure to the health care system. This, in some instances, has been from past training and work experience as either a nurse, medical receptionist, or other health care professional. In Meadow's (1982) description of 17 families, 9 of the mothers had such a background, and Rosenberg (1987) reported that 27% of 97 mothers had a nursing background and another 3% had worked in medical offices. In other cases, the mother herself has had Munchausen syndrome and therefore has brought to her experience as a mother both her own psychopathology and often a vast knowledge of medicine, hospitals, and medical practice acquired from her experiences prior to her child's birth.

A striking characteristic of the mothers is that they are nearly always considered exemplary in all their interactions with medical staff. This is in contrast to adults with Munchausen syndrome and also to parents who provoke sickness behavior in their children and refuse to accept psychological mechanisms (Kaplan and Sadock, 1988; McKinlay, 1986). Both of these groups are often described as demanding and difficult. In Munchausen syndrome by proxy, the mothers often develop close relationships with the nurses and doctors with whom they come in frequent and continued contact. These relationships sometimes traverse the more usual boundaries between parent and medical staff and may include such things as helping the nurses in their duties, eating meals with the doctors, or maintaining social contact with the medical personnel outside of the hospital. However, these mothers tend to be unavailable for genuine interpersonal interactions, and hospital staff often report subjective feelings of uneasiness or of feeling intrusive in the mother's presence (Zitelli et al., 1987).

The quality of the mother's care for her child is also notable. These mothers are often considered model parents who are extremely attentive to their children. They take over the care of their children to a greater degree than is usual in hospitals. They often live in the hospital and remain with the child constantly. It has been noted, however, that the care given to the child can be of an excessive nature; for example, the child may be dressed in inappropriately lavish clothing, or the hospital room may be stocked with an outrageous number of toys (Zitelli et al., 1987).

One striking quality of the mother that may be important in recognizing the syndrome is her inappropriate affect when given information about the severity of her child's illness or when discussing invasive medical investigations. There is a bland acceptance, rather than obvious distress, and she appears to be relatively at ease with medical uncertainties (Zitelli et al., 1987). In one report, the mother was even described as appearing euphoric as her child became sicker (McGuire and Feldman, 1989).

Besides fabrication of symptoms of illness, these mothers often fabricate extensively about other parts of their lives. An example of this is a mother who reported that she had just completed a law degree and was working toward a masters degree in Russian history, both of which were false (Guandolo, 1985). Certainly an important element of the syndrome is the mother's ability to converse with the medical staff about her child's illness in a very knowledgeable and medically sophisticated manner. The other fabrications often serve to add to the mother's appearance as an intelligent person or as someone who has achieved despite adversity.

Description of the Father

In contrast to the mother's constant presence, the father may have very little involvement in his child's care and sometimes does not even visit the hospital. This is particularly noteworthy considering the severity of the child's illness. Often, these fathers have jobs that keep them away from the family for prolonged periods of time (Meadow, 1982). The marital relationship between the parents is often poor, although in some instances the child's apparent illness serves to bring the parents closer together.

ETIOLOGY AND PATHOGENESIS

The substantial number of reports of Munchausen syndrome by proxy are largely to be found in pediatric journals; only a few cases have been reported in the psychological or psychiatric literature (Chan et al., 1986; Lansky and Erickson, 1974; Nicol and Eccles, 1985; Palmer and Yoshimura, 1984; Waller, 1983). Among the cases reported, there are only a few in which there has been an extensive psychiatric evaluation, and even fewer that have undergone psychotherapy. Despite the paucity of cases, these reports do provide some understanding of the underlying psychopathology and knowledge of features that are common to most cases. However, the full extent to which some of the descriptions are generalizable and an understanding of the limits of the spectrum of the disorder remain undefined.

Three major etiological factors appear to be important in the pathogenesis of the disorder. These include the mother's experience of abuse or rejection in her own childhood, her pathological relationship with her child, and the rewarding effect of the medical care system on the mother. In addition, in some cases there have been other associated psychopathological symptoms.

Abuse or Rejection of the Mother

These mothers often have experienced abuse in their own childhoods or have felt rejected by one or both parents (Krener and Adelman, 1988; McGuire and Feldman, 1989; Palmer and Yoshimura, 1984). The experience of rejection continues into adult life, and there is often a poor marital relationship (Meadow, 1982). The mothers often feel isolated and have a decreased sense of self-worth.

Pathological Relationship with Child

These mothers have an extremely close, symbiotic relationship with their children. The child is viewed as very precious but also as somehow damaged and susceptible to illness or harm. Meadow (1977), in his first description of the syndrome, described a child who had been a "long-awaited baby" and who was born after the mother had taken a fertility medication. The child described by Nicol and Eccles (1985) was born after a pregnancy in which there had been a threatened miscarriage at 12 weeks' gestation, an antepartum hemorrhage at 36 weeks, and termination of breastfeeding because of cracked nipples when the child was 5 weeks old. In this regard, cases of Munchausen syndrome by proxy are similar to those seen in the vulnerable child syndrome in which the mother develops an abnormally overprotective relationship with the child following a severe illness early in the child's life (Green and Solnit, 1964). Obviously, there is the important difference that in the vulnerable child syndrome, although the mother views her child as abnormally susceptible to illness, she does not cause her child to be ill. In Munchausen syndrome by proxy there is the complicated and contradictory situation of a mother being excessively concerned about what may be minor complaints and actually causing illness herself.

The contradictory relationship between mother and child is extremely complex and not fully understood. In the case reported by Nicol and Eccles (1985), they describe the mother as experiencing the failure of breastfeeding as "a personal deprivation and attack on herself by the baby." This distorted perception is explained as a protective identifica-

tion in a stressed person with an abnormal coping mechanism. In the case described by Palmer and Yoshimura (1984), the mother herself had Munchausen syndrome and incorporated her daughter as an integral part of herself. In this way the child experienced both the love and self-hate of the mother.

Effect of the Medical Care System

Important components in the development of the syndrome are the behavior of the doctors, the hospital environment, and the effect that both have on the mother. In the report by Nicol and Eccles (1985), the mother reported that "she found, in her general practitioner, a source of support and kindness and this reinforced the pattern of very regular attendance at the surgery." Guandolo (1985) has commented that "illness is the ticket of admission to a place where understanding and caring relieved the feelings of hopelessness and isolation." The interaction, however, is more complex than just the mothers' feelings of being supported. With the increasing severity of illness of their children, these mothers feel a sense of self-worth and importance that is otherwise lacking in their lives. One mother, after confessing to repeatedly suffocating her child, reported that whenever she did it, she experienced a similar feeling to that which she had felt on her graduation day. This mother, during one of the times her child was being resuscitated in the hospital, was overheard by a nurse calmly telling other mothers on the ward that she had already had a child die from a similar episode. This, in fact, was a fabrication but serves to illustrate the mother's need to make the situation even more dire so as to gain greater sympathy and appear the more heroic. The hospital environment contributes to these feelings of importance. Chan et al. (1986) described a mother who would visit the intensive care unit just to talk to other mothers, and Meadow (1984) has described another mother who had some nursing training and who would help teach nursing students. There obviously becomes an increasing need for the mother to gain admission to the hospital through her child's illness.

Another factor is the pleasure gained from the contact with the doctors. In the case discussed by Nicol and Eccles (1985), the mother reported that she liked to feel that she "was being considered by intelligent people." There appears to be an additional element in which the mother gains pleasure from outwitting the doctors. It becomes a bizarre game in which the mother matches herself against the specialists, and as one problem is resolved, another one is created.

Associated Psychopathology

As Meadow (1985) has stated, "Many mothers who have perpetrated Munchausen syndrome by proxy have been referred to psychiatrists, and many have had detailed psychological testing. Usually the tests are normal and no disorder is apparent to the psychiatrist." This likely speaks to the misdirected focus of these evaluations rather than to a true lack of psychopathology. It is true, however, considering the severity of the nature of the disorder, that for the majority of cases, there is a surprising lack of associated psychiatric symptoms. There are, however, reported cases that have an extensive history of prior psychiatric illness, and there is likely a spectrum of symptoms.

Of the 97 mothers reported by Rosenberg (1987), 12 were described as suicidal, 7 before the disclosure of the Munchausen syndrome by proxy and 5 after the disclosure. Of the psychiatric disorders described, depression was noted most commonly, hysterical personality disorder was noted several times, and borderline personality, narcissistic personality disorder, and unspecified personality disorder were noted only occasionally. Ten percent of the mothers were noted to have Munchausen syndrome themselves, and another 14% had some features of Munchausen syndrome.

Because only a few cases have been examined and reported in detail, it is perhaps more helpful to look at these. They serve to demonstrate a spectrum of illness rather than a universal picture. Chan et al. (1986)

describe a mother who demonstrated several features consistent with both narcissistic and borderline personality disorders. She was explosive, was constantly seeking attention, displayed sadomasochistic tendencies, showed marked shifts in attitude and affect, and presented a sense of entitlement. Her primary defenses seemed to be denial and splitting. In the report by Nicol and Eccles (1985) of a mother's progress in psychotherapy, they describe an important part of the pathogenesis of the abuse as being the mother's affect, which included infantile rage as a central component together with crushingly low self-esteem. In the report by Palmer and Yoshimura (1984) of a mother who herself had Munchausen syndrome, psychological testing "revealed a profoundly needy individual whose reality testing was impaired. She perceived the world as a malevolent place and people as attacking. Thought processes were distorted and interpersonal boundaries were blurred. Coping strategies included extreme forms of denial, projection and paranoid vigilance."

The fabrication of illness and the often continued denial does not have the fixed quality of a delusion, although the mother does not appear to be consciously lying (Waller, 1983). It has been described as "quasi-delusional" and Waller has commented that "the disturbance in thought content and behavior may be a dissociative phenomenon or a form of pseudologia phantastica or pathological lying in which the parent comes to believe, at least intermittently, the fantasy that the child has a primary rather than a factitious illness." Mothers who have confessed to the perpetration of injury on their children have been able to describe the incident but have little recollection for the details and describe themselves as committing the act in a disassociated-like state.

PSYCHIATRIC DESCRIPTION OF THE CHILD

There is very little in the literature describing the children in this disorder. The one striking comment, however, is that the children, particularly older children, collude with their mothers in the ongoing deception. In the original report of Sneed and Bell (1976), it was the 10-year-old boy who was presenting the pebbles as renal calculi. A 2½-year-old girl at our institution did not cry out when her mother, in what must have been a painful process, produced signs of gastrointestinal bleeding by excoriating her anal canal. Furthermore, these children, like children who have been repeatedly physically abused, quickly learn to passively tolerate medical procedures. Other symptoms that have been described include feeding disorders among infants and toddlers and withdrawn, hyperactive, or oppositional behavior among preschoolers (McGuire and Feldman, 1989).

SPECTRUM OF THE DISORDER

Meadow (1985), in reporting on what he terms mild cases, raises questions regarding the limits of the definition of the disorder. He points out that, at times, parents often exaggerate their children's symptoms or may perceive that a problem is present when it is not apparent to the doctor. This is particularly true for some parents who consider their children allergic and limit their exposure to various foods and things in the environment. Certainly some of these parents share a number of the same characteristics as those more severe cases of parents who actually cause their children to be ill (Warner and Hathaway, 1984).

It is also important to ask the question of when, in an individual case, does Munchausen syndrome by proxy begin, recognizing that some cases start with parental concerns surrounding a real illness and that these concerns, at some stage, overflow into fabricated illness. Also, is it only the lack of the medical knowledge that prevents others from developing Munchausen syndrome by proxy? In fact, the syndrome has been described as only one end of a spectrum of parental behaviors surrounding chronic and factitious illnesses of children (Libow and Schreier, 1986; Krener and Adelman, 1988; Eminson and Postlethwaite, 1992). It is important, however, that we recognize the significant differences in the psychopathology of the parent who injures her child or

causes her child to appear ill and the parent who repeatedly presents as overconcerned about her child's illness. What appears to set Munchausen syndrome by proxy apart is the synergistic effect of the mother's prior experience of abuse or rejection, her pathological symbiotic relationship with her child, and the powerful rewarding effects of her interaction with the medical environment. McKinlay (1986) describes the parent "who provokes sickness behavior in the child, refuses to accept psychological mechanism, seeks multiple opinions and insists on repeated investigations" and points out that this type of parent is often combative or has a contemptuous style, which is very different from the exemplary, ingratiating parental style seen in Munchausen syndrome by proxy. The former does not appear to experience the elevation of self-worth and feeling of importance that seem so much a part of Munchausen syndrome by proxy. There is, however, a striking similarity between these cases and Munchausen syndrome by proxy in the symbiotic relationship between mother and child and the way in which the child colludes with the mother in continuing the illness (Woollcott et al., 1982).

TREATMENT

The management of Munchausen syndrome by proxy often proves to be extremely difficult. There are a number of reasons why this is true: First, there is the difficulty of making the diagnosis—it often goes unsuspected for a long time, and then, even when suspected, it is often difficult to be sure that one's suspicions are in fact correct; second, the disbelief that the diagnosis engenders often serves to sabotage overall management; and last, psychotherapy is extremely difficult when the therapist is reliant on the patient's telling the truth, something that rarely happens in these cases, at least initially.

Medical Management

The warning signals that should alert a physician to the possibility of a factitious illness have previously been identified by Meadow (1982) and are shown in Table 101.1. Once it is suspected that an illness may be fabricated, the physician needs to establish the diagnosis with certainty. This is often an arduous and time-consuming task. Obviously the safety of the child and protection from further harm are of utmost importance during this time.

The physician should review the medical history in detail and distinguish those complaints that may have been fabricated from those that were definitely real; complaints that occurred when only the mother was present need to be separated from those witnessed by others; details of the medical, psychiatric, personal, and social history, as presented by the mother, need to be verified. This may require careful and detailed histories from other family members.

Detailed descriptions of the mother's behavior and incidents that occurred while in the hospital may provide a profile consistent with

Table 101.1. Warning Signals of Munchausen Syndrome by Proxy

1. Persistent or recurrent illness that cannot be explained.
2. Discrepancies between the history, clinical findings, and general health of the child.
3. Working diagnosis is a rare disorder, or experienced clinicians have "never seen a case like it before."
4. Symptoms and signs occur only in the mother's presence.
5. A mother who is extremely attentive and always in the hospital.
6. A child who is frequently intolerant to treatments.
7. A mother who appears less worried about her child's illness than is the medical staff.
8. Seizures that do not respond to appropriate therapy.
9. Families in which sudden unexplained infant death has occurred.
10. A mother with previous medical or nursing experience or who has an extensive history of illness.

Adapted from Meadow R. Munchausen syndrome by proxy. *Arch Dis Child* 67:92–98, 1982.

Munchausen syndrome by proxy. A number of laboratory methods have been used to confirm fabricated symptoms. These include biochemical analyses of blood and urine samples, typing of blood to determine if it is the child's or the mother's, and analyzing recordings from apnea monitors. Continuous observation of the mother by nursing staff is extremely difficult and usually not possible. Also, it is often not possible to exclude the parents from the hospital for a long enough time to establish a temporal association between the symptoms and the presence of the mother. Video surveillance of the mother and child in the hospital has also been carried out. This, like searching a mother's personal belongings, creates ethical and legal problems. However, these need to be weighed against the risks to the child, and if there is no recourse, video surveillance may need to be carried out (Meadow, 1987; Williams and Bevan, 1988).

Once the diagnosis has been established, the mother needs to be confronted and informed of the doctor's knowledge about what is going on and the course of action that needs to be taken to ensure the safety of the child. Other family members also need to be notified and the diagnosis explained to them. Because the child in most instances has been abused and because continued protection is needed for the child, the protective services agency needs to be notified, and legal services need to be involved.

The Role of the Psychiatrist

From a review of the literature it would appear that in the past psychiatrists have seldom played a significant role in the management of Munchausen syndrome by proxy. This is most likely because psychiatrists have had little experience and a poor understanding of this relatively recently described syndrome. However, reports of cases being successfully managed in psychotherapy suggest that child psychiatrists have a very important role to play in ensuring an optimal outcome for these children and parents.

One difficulty is that although it is a psychiatric disorder, the clinical presentation is medical, and often the apparent lack of psychiatric symptoms precludes a reason for the psychiatrist's involvement. Once the diagnosis is suspected, however, the child psychiatrist's contribution can be very important in a number of different ways.

HELPING TO ESTABLISH THE DIAGNOSIS

Even though the mother may not herself request psychiatric help, once the diagnosis is suspected, a reason should be sought for the child psychiatrist to meet with the mother. Because care needs to be taken not to sabotage the overall management plan by giving the mother warning that she is under suspicion, the reason might be that the psychiatrist can often be helpful to families with children with chronic illnesses. The history taken at this time should include family, social, and psychiatric information, but the most important focus, and that likely to be most acceptable to the mother, is around the child's illness. In reviewing the details of the child's life and illness, the child psychiatrist may be able to obtain an understanding of the special meaning of this child to the mother and of the symbiotic relationship between mother and child. An example of this is a mother's description of how much more worried she had been about her daughter (the child now presenting with illness) than she had been about her older child, a son, although both had been on home monitoring because of concern about apnea (see case illustration below). When the daughter, who was named after the mother, was 8 weeks old, the mother heard of another child who had died of sudden infant death syndrome (SIDS). Since that time, she had feared that her daughter would die and was compulsively careful about the apnea monitor in a way that she described as being very different from when her son was on the monitor. With her son, she had often turned the monitor around so that she could not see all the flashing digital lights and alarms; with her daughter it was intolerable for her not to see these. It is the ability to elicit this quality of the relationship between the mother and child that might be most helpful in the interview. The child psychiatrist, with his or her training and experience in understanding the relationship

between mother and child, is likely to be more helpful in assessing this quality of the relationship than would someone without training in child psychiatry (Meadow, 1985; Eminson and Postlethwaite, 1992). During the assessment, the child psychiatrist may also be able to elicit other information that provides evidence of fabrication or is indicative of other psychiatric symptoms associated with Munchausen syndrome by proxy. The child psychiatrist should also be able to provide an assessment of the degree of psychological disturbance experienced by the child and should be key in planning how this should be addressed.

DEVELOPING A THERAPEUTIC RELATIONSHIP

A potentially important part of the early assessment is to provide an opportunity for the mother to start to develop a therapeutic relationship with the psychiatrist. Because in most of the cases reported in the literature the psychiatrist has only been involved once the mother has been confronted, it is unclear whether an earlier meeting, prior to the confrontation, might be beneficial, or whether the mother's later realization that the psychiatrist was complicit in the suspicion of her might be detrimental to ongoing treatment. It seems likely, however, that the mother could accept reassurance that the psychiatrist is intent on helping her and that she could therefore maintain the trust necessary for ongoing therapy. It may therefore be an important opportunity if the psychiatrist doing the early assessment could continue to provide ongoing treatment, though in some centers this is not always possible.

CONFRONTATION

The aim of the confrontation is to explain to the mother that the clinicians know that she is harming her child and the effects this could have. She should be informed of the steps that will be taken to protect her child and to provide help for her and her family. Meadow (1985) has suggested that confrontation of the mother is best done by the pediatrician alone, without other professionals or family members being present. Although this may be true for someone like Meadow, who has such a vast experience with this syndrome, it may not necessarily be true in instances where the pediatrician has had no prior experience of Munchausen syndrome by proxy. In these cases, it may be helpful to have a child psychiatrist present to help in the process. It is important, however, that the pediatrician be the one who confidently affirms what has been going on. The child psychiatrist then is able to speak of it as a psychiatric problem and can outline what is likely to happen, while at the same time being supportive.

At this stage, only a few mothers will confess to what they have been doing, although at times there are remarks that serve as tacit admission of the activity. The majority of mothers continue to deny their activity, often in a very convincing way, although sometimes in a remarkably calm, affectless manner. It is not helpful to try to prove to the mother that you are right and she is wrong, nor is it helpful to counter every explanation she provides.

Following the confrontation, some mothers have become extremely agitated, acutely psychotic, or depressed and suicidal (Palmer and Yoshimura, 1984). An assessment may need to be made regarding the need for psychiatric hospitalization. Needless to say, it is critically important that the child be protected from the mother at this time, because she may have a heightened need for the child to be truly sick.

ASSISTING STAFF IN UNDERSTANDING THE DYNAMICS OF THE CASE

For medical and social services staff this may be an extremely difficult problem to deal with, particularly if they have had no prior experience with or knowledge of the syndrome. The emotional responses of the staff are made more complicated by the fact that some might have known the family for a long time and developed close relationships with the mother and child. For some people, there is complete disbelief; for others, there is anger at the mother and feelings of guilt that they have participated in harming the child or have not been more astute in correctly identifying the problem at an earlier time. Group discussions are helpful in both informing staff about the syndrome and providing them an opportunity to express their feelings. It is also helpful to provide written material about the syndrome for staff to read.

The psychiatrist may also play an important role in providing protective services workers and lawyers with an understanding of the syndrome and may even appear as an expert witness in the courts. In this way, the psychiatrist can help to facilitate an appropriate legal course of action. The psychiatrist's role in this may have important ramifications in later treatment: The assertion of the severity of the disorder and the danger to the child, together with a noncritical view of this as a psychiatric disorder, may have therapeutic implications for the mother.

PSYCHOTHERAPY

As noted previously, there is at present very little information available in the literature concerning psychotherapy of mothers and children with Munchausen syndrome by proxy. Palmer and Yoshimura (1984) have emphasized that the following are important determinants of how a case should be managed: "the degree and duration of abuse; the parent's psychological state; whether the reaction to the confrontation is denial or acknowledgment of behavior; resistance or willingness to engage in treatment; and whether the child is perceived as part of herself or as a separate entity." Obviously, each of these factors might be an important indicator of the accessibility of the individual to psychotherapeutic intervention, but an adverse factor should not necessarily be considered a contraindication to therapy.

Nicol and Eccles have provided details of their case in which the mother initially denied the allegations but later confessed when faced with the possibility that her children might be placed in foster care. The mother, in this case, continued in therapy on a weekly basis for 6 months and then biweekly for a further 6 months. From early on it was "clear that the mother had a strong wish to understand herself, that she was intelligent, and that she had a capacity to bring active and painful feelings to therapy sessions." General themes of therapy included the complex reasons for the abuse, where a full realization of the danger she had put her child in gradually emerged. Other important themes were her relationship with her parents and fears about her child's health that first originated during her pregnancy.

OUTCOME

The final outcome for children with Munchausen syndrome by proxy is very variable and likely dependent both on the severity of the disorder and the treatment provided. The mother who in addition to Munchausen syndrome by proxy has other psychiatric disorders and the child who has been involved in the fabrication of symptoms for many years are likely more difficult to treat than those with a simpler presentation. This is likely true for those mothers who themselves have Munchausen syndrome, which is often very difficult to treat successfully (Mayo and Haggerty, 1984). The child whose symptom of illness has been caused by a more dangerous activity (for example, suffocation) is obviously more at risk of dying than the child whose symptom was due to less dangerous methods (for example, a mother's putting blood in her child's urine).

Of the 19 children reported by Meadow (1982), 2 died. Of the 17 survivors, 8 were removed from their families, and 7 continued to live with their families and were free of all symptoms 1 to 4 years later. The remaining 2 children who lived with their families continued to be taken to the doctor with minor complaints only. In Rosenberg's (1987) review of the 117 cases reported in the literature, 9% died. The leading causes of death were suffocation and poisoning. It needs to be noted that children have died after the diagnosis has been made and the mother confronted. Also, the abuse of a second child might continue even after a first child in a family has died. Eight percent of the survivors had permanent disfigurement or permanent impairment of function.

The psychiatric sequelae, both for the mother and child, have been less well described. Certainly, some of these children have continued to fabricate illness for themselves, and the child with Munchausen syndrome by proxy has grown up to be the adolescent or adult with Munchausen syndrome (Meadow, 1985). Of the 12 children described by McGuire and Feldman (1989), 11 were described as having adverse effects that included immaturity, abnormal relationships with their mothers, separation problems, and aggressive behavior. Some children have expressed fears of poisoning and death, and at least 2 children have required psychiatric hospitalization (Rogers et al., 1976).

In some cases, once the family has been confronted with the diagnosis, the fabrication of illness has stopped, and the condition appears resolved. However, the psychological sequelae for these children remain unknown, and in the vast majority of cases it is unrealistic to expect that the mother's focus on medical concerns will completely disappear.

CONCLUSION

In this condition, perhaps more so than any other, there needs to be extensive collaboration between the child psychiatrist and pediatrician, as well as with the other services involved (Meadow, 1985; Bentovim, 1985; Eminson and Postlethwaite, 1992). The role of the psychiatrist may be very different from that with other psychiatric diagnoses, particularly when a case is first diagnosed. It is hoped that with our increased understanding of this syndrome and an appropriate psychiatric approach to management, there will be an improvement in outcome for both the children and their mothers.

CASE ILLUSTRATION

A 10-month-old girl was admitted to hospital for the fourth time over a 3-month period. Each admission was for treatment of unilateral periorbital swelling and inflammation. The presumed diagnosis was recurrent periorbital cellulitis, and on each admission she was treated with intravenous antibiotics. While on treatment, her eye would sometimes improve, then inexplicably become worse. Numerous consultations and diagnostic studies were carried out. On the final admission, corneal ulcers were noted. Suspicions had already been aroused, and at this time the pH of the conjunctival fluid was tested and found to be more alkaline than that of the other eye. A diagnosis of Munchausen syndrome by proxy was made.

This child was the younger sibling of a 3-year-old boy who had had bacterial meningitis in the neonatal period and had developed apnea when 8 weeks old. He was started on apnea monitoring at home and then, at the age of 11 months, started having seizures. The index child was also reported to have apnea starting at 8 weeks of age. She was monitored at home and had a number of significant apneic episodes. Three of these episodes occurred in the hospital: At the start of each occasion the mother was alone with the child, and when called, the medical staff found the child cyanosed and with gasping respirations. Later, once the correct diagnosis was realized, a recording stored in memory in the apnea monitor was reviewed and showed that prior to the last episode of apnea, the monitor had been switched off for 2 minutes and that when it was switched on again, the child was apneic. The mother had been the only one present during this interval, and there was no reasonable explanation for why the monitor had been switched off.

A child psychiatrist experienced in Munchausen syndrome by proxy was consulted, and the mother was confronted with both the pediatrician and psychiatrist present. She appeared extremely upset and denied all allegations. Her husband and other family members were disbelieving but agreed to the plan of management "in case it were true." The management included referral for ongoing psychotherapy and initiation of plans with the protective service agency to ensure continued protection of the children. Because placement of the children with members of the extended family was a consideration, a family meeting was called to ensure that everyone believed what had happened and understood the seriousness of the disorder. Prior to this meeting taking place, the mother confessed to what she had done. She sought help from her psychiatrist and, at the meeting, was able to talk about her problem and ask for help from her family. At the court hearing it was decided that the children should be placed in the custody of their father and paternal grandparents, with the mother to have supervised visitation and to continue in psychotherapy.

Comment

In this instance, the mother shared many characteristics described in cases of Munchausen syndrome by proxy. She had been abused as a child, her parents were divorced, and she had little contact with her father. Her relationship with her husband was described as good, but he had three jobs and was seldom at home. She herself had not had frequent illnesses, nor did she have nursing training, but she had become acquainted with medical care and technology with her first child. She considered her second child to be very special and was very concerned that she might die. She was extremely attentive to her child, stayed in the hospital constantly, and was very friendly with the medical staff.

In this case, the mother developed a trusting relationship with the child psychiatrist right from the time when she was most distressed, following the confrontation. The family meeting was extremely helpful in ensuring the family's continued attention to the safety of the children and support for the mother. It should be noted, however, that in some respects this case was less complex than many and less difficult to manage.

References

Alexander R, Smith W, Stevenson R: Serial Munchausen syndrome by proxy. *Pediatrics* 86:581–585, 1990.

Asher R: Munchausen syndrome. *Lancet* 1:339–341, 1951.

Bentovim A: Munchausen's syndrome and child psychiatrists (Letter). *Arch Dis Child* 60:688, 1985.

Bools CN, Neale BA, Meadow SR: Co-morbidity associated with fabricated illness (Munchausen syndrome by proxy). *Arch Dis Child* 67:11–19, 1992.

Chan DA, Salcedo JR, Atkins DM, et al: Munchausen syndrome by proxy: A review and case study. *J Pediatr Psychol* 11(7):1–80, 1986.

Eminson DM, Postlethwaite RJ: Factitious illness: recognition and management. *Arch Dis Child* 67:1510–1516, 1992.

Goss PW, McDougall PN: Munchausen syndrome by proxy—a cause of preterm delivery. *Med J Aust* 157:814–817, 1992.

Green M, Solnit AJ: Reactions to the threatened loss of a child: A vulnerable child syndrome. *Pediatrics* 34:58–66, 1964.

Guandolo VL: Munchausen syndrome by proxy: An outpatient challenge. *Pediatrics* 75:526–530, 1985.

Kaplan HI, Sadock BJ: *Synopsis of Psychiatry, Behavioral Sciences, Clinical Psychiatry* (5th ed). Baltimore, Williams & Wilkins, 1988, pp. 396–399.

Krener P, Adelman R: Parent salvage and parent sabotage in the care of chronically ill children. *Am J Dis Child* 142:945–951, 1988.

Lansky SB, Erickson HM: Prevention of child murder. *J Am Acad Child Psychiatry* 13:691–698, 1974.

Lazoritz S: Munchausen by proxy or Meadow's syndrome? *Lancet* 2:631, 1987.

Libow JA, Schreier HA: Three forms of factitious illness in children: When is it Munchausen syndrome by proxy? *Am J Orthopsychiatry* 56:602–611, 1986.

Light MJ, Sheridan MS: Munchausen syndrome by proxy and apnea (MPBA)—a survey of apnea programs. *Clin Pediatr* 29:162–168, 1990.

Makar AF, Squier PJ: Munchausen syndrome by proxy: Father as a perpetrator. *Pediatrics* 85:370–373, 1990.

Mayo JP, Haggerty JJ: Long-term psychotherapy of Munchausen syndrome. *Am J Psychother* 38:571–579, 1984.

Meadow R: Munchausen syndrome by proxy: The hinterland of child abuse. *Lancet* 2:343–345, 1977.

Meadow R: Munchausen syndrome by proxy. *Arch Dis Child* 57:92–98, 1982.

Meadow R: Fictitious epilepsy. *Lancet* 2:25–28, 1984.

Meadow R: Management of Munchausen syndrome by proxy. *Arch Dis Child* 60:385–393, 1985.

Meadow R: Video recording and child abuse. *Br Med J* 294:1629–1630, 1987.

Meadow R: Suffocation, recurrent apnea, and sudden infant death. *J Pediatr* 117:351–357, 1990.

Meadow R, Lennert T: Munchausen by proxy or Polle syndrome: Which term is correct? *Pediatrics* 74:554–556, 1984.

McGuire TL, Feldman KW: Psychologic morbidity of children subjected to Munchausen syndrome by proxy. *Pediatrics* 83:289–292, 1989.

McKinlay I: Munchausen's syndrome by proxy (Letter). *Br Med J* 293: 1308, 1986.

Nicol AR, Eccles M: Psychotherapy for Munchausen syndrome by proxy. *Arch Dis Child* 60:344–348, 1985.

Palmer AJ, Yoshimura GJ: Munchausen syndrome by proxy. *J Am Acad Child Psychiatry* 234:503–508, 1984.

Raspe RE: *Singular Campaigns and Adventures of Baron Munchausen* (Carswell J, ed). London, Cresset Press, 1948.

Rogers D, Tripp J, Bentovim A, et al: Non-accidental poisoning: An extended syndrome of child abuse. *Br Med J* 1:793–720, 1976.

Rosenberg D: Web of deceit: A literature review of Munchausen syndrome by proxy. *Child Abuse Negl* 11:547–563, 1987.

Sneed RC, Bell RF: The dauphin of Munchausen: Factitious passage of renal stones in a child. *Pediatrics* 58:127–130, 1976.

Verity GM, Winckworth C, Burman D, et al: Polle syndrome: Children of Munchausen. *Br Med J* 2:422–423, 1979.

Waller DA: Case report: Obstacles to the treatment of Munchausen by proxy syndrome. *J Am Acad Child Psychiatry* 22:80–85, 1983.

Warner O, Hathaway MJ: Allergic form of Meadow's syndrome (Munchausen by proxy). *Arch Dis Child* 59:151–156, 1984.

Williams C, Bevan VT: The secret observation of children in hospital. *Lancet* 1:780–781, 1988.

Woollcott P, Aceto T, Rutt C, et al: Doctor shopping with the child as proxy patient: A variant of child abuse. *J Pediatr* 101:297–301, 1982.

Zitelli BJ, Seltman MF, Shannon RM: Munchausen's syndrome by proxy and its professional participants. *Am J Dis Child* 141: 1099–1102, 1987.

102 RECURRENT NONORGANIC ABDOMINAL PAIN: CURRENT CONCEPTS

Ian S. Goldberg, M.D., and H. Paul Gabriel, M.D.

DEFINITION

Recurrent abdominal pain (RAP) is defined by Apley and Nalsh (1958) as "at least three episodes of incapacitating pain over not less than three months." The syndrome is generally found in tense children of school age who may be experiencing stress at school or at home. There may be associated nonorganic headaches or limb pains, although physical examination is normal.

Subvarieties have been called periodic syndrome (pain, vomiting, headache, and low-grade fever) (Apley and MacKeith, 1968) or cyclical vomiting (recurrent abdominal pain and vomiting). RAP may be viewed as part of a spectrum of disorders from transient normal variants to persistent conversion disorders.

CLASSIFICATION

In the DSM-IV (American Psychiatric Association, 1994) RAP is coded within the Somatoform Disorders as "Pain Disorder with Psychological Factors, DSM-IV: 307.80." Two subtypes are recorded: acute, where the pain is less than 6 months in duration and chronic, where the pain is at least 6 months in its duration.

HISTORICAL NOTE

Serious inquiry into the nature of RAP in childhood, predominantly of nonorganic etiology, began after the end of World War II. The British seemed to have led the way with Trotter's (1941) term ''disharmonious mental states'' in childhood, laying down a conceptual groundwork for research thinking. Most notable were the studies of Apley and Nalsh (1958), who ultimately studied 1000 children over an extended period.

PREVALENCE AND EPIDEMIOLOGY

RAP is more common in girls and unusual before 5 years of age (Green, 1967); 12.3% of girls compared to 9.5% of boys are affected, with more than 25% of all girls at 9 years of age affected (Apley and Nalsh, 1958). Apley found no somatic complaints in the small number of children below 5 years of age, but between 5 and 10 years of age a 10% to 12% incidence in boys was noted. A late peak at age 14 was seen within the male population, followed by a steady decline. The incidence in girls paralleled that of boys up to 8 years of age, rose markedly at 9, and then declined in a fashion similar to that of boys.

In a study of 5- and 6-year-olds, in a newly established town in northern England, Faull and Nicol (1986) found that 34% were suffering from RAP, although school worriers (20%), overeaters (24%), and users of pain for secondary gain (20%) were overrepresented in their high figures.

Stone and Barbero (1970) likened the chronic and recurrent symptoms of childhood RAP to the functional gastrointestinal illness in adults known as irritable bowel syndrome. They reviewed 102 hospitalized children with RAP, paying particular attention to medical and family history. The significance of early problems for the later emergence of chronic symptoms remains unclear, but the following were found: 41% of the pregnancies had nausea and vomiting of more than 5 months's duration, resulting in ''excessive tiredness necessitating protracted bed rest or even in hysterical paralysis''; 31% had complicated labors and delivery, with 12% requiring a cesarean section. Infancy was marked in 19% by respiratory distress and bowel obstruction, with 30% developing colic lasting more than 3 months. Most significant was the evidence for medical illness in the parents (56% mothers and 44% fathers), with about 50% of the illness in both parents being focused on the gastrointestinal tract.

Stone and Barbero (1970) also noted that ''25% of all parents had lost a parent by death or divorce before they were 20 years of age; 33% of such losses occurred before the child (with RAP) was 10 years of age.'' This event is a particularly traumatic one for any child and may, as Wasserman et al. (1988) postulate, relate to the pain symptom at a stage of development when death is not well understood (Lewis, 1982) or understood but still frightening and anxiety provoking (Sarafino, 1986), especially in children who still depend on their parents and who fear abandonment (Poznanski, 1973). Lapouse and Monk (1959) report that children with RAP were found to have twice the prevalence found in the general population with regard to worries about their parents and themselves. Apley (1967) records a six times higher frequency rate of abdominal complaints in the parents and siblings of the RAP group as compared to matched controls.

Although MacKeith and O'Neill (1951) described anxiety, anger, or grief as determinants of attacks, a temporal relationship was not always evident. Parents in 67% of Stone and Barbero's (1970) study related onset of symptoms to events such as ''excitement, punishment or familial disturbance,'' often (23%) in association with a school activity. Bain (1974) noted that ''a great deal of abdominal pain and other vague somatic symptoms begin in September after school starts!'' Psychogenic complaints may be an integral component of school phobia (Schmitt, 1971).

A recent epidemiological study in Sweden (Alfven, 1993c) further elaborated that an increased frequency of RAP was noted in schools which drew children from a lower socioeconomic status. Significant urban stress was noted in the histories of these patients: recent immigration, poverty, and unstable family circumstances. While reflecting a Swedish focus, this study may have relevance to the incidence of RAP in other countries.

CLINICAL DESCRIPTION

Although RAP is defined by Apley in criteria that may appear somewhat broad, the morbidity is extensive. Green (1967) found that 50% had symptoms for less than 1 year, with the remaining 50% symptomatic for up to 5 years. Furthermore, the afflicted may have had up to seven attacks per day, lasting minutes to hours. Attacks may be separated by weeks or months in the less symptomatic patient. Onset tends to be gradual, and the quality of the pain mild and moderate rather than severe or colicky (Green, 1967). Green observed that nausea, pallor, vomiting, dizziness, headache, and faintness may precede or accompany the pain. The site of the pain is variable. It is often poorly localized to the epigastrium or perineum region. Not surprisingly, these symptoms are rapidly taken for serious medical problems, and such patients usually find themselves in their pediatrician's office.

There is no pathognomonic personality profile of a child or adolescent presenting with psychogenic pain symptoms. However, most are described as anxious and sensitive, with a tendency toward being fearful, inhibited, and overcontrolled (Apley, 1975; Friedman, 1972; Hodges et al., 1985; Hughes and Zimin, 1978; Lambert, 1941; Wasserman et al., 1988). Christensen and Mortenson (1975) stated that psychogenic abdominal pain occurred in ''sensitive'' children who have a family history of abdominal pain. They defined sensitivity as a ''combination of genetic predisposition, an environment conducive to modeling, plus a tendency to internalize.''

These authors also speculated that the determining factor for symptom formation may not be the level of emotional tension in the RAP children but their manner of coping. Gordon (1983) reported that children with RAP are sadder and tend to be socially isolated compared to ''externalizers.'' Such affects, combined with peer and adult isolation, mean that there are fewer people in these children's lives with whom they can discuss their worries, resulting in symptoms of anxiety. Sharrer and Ryan-Wenger's (1991) study indicates that RAP children have a more limited repertoire of coping mechanisms compared to a matched control group and feel their skills are equivalently less effective in reducing stress. Kanner (1957) noted that stomachache is a common complaint of the emotionally upset child, a finding corroborated by other authors (Apley, 1967; Friedman, 1972; Hodges et al., 1986). Other forms of the expression of emotional disturbance include undue fears, nocturnal enuresis, sleeping difficulties, and, most commonly, appetite problems, food fussiness, and difficulties at school (Apley, 1967).

ETIOLOGY AND PATHOGENESIS

Neuropsychobiological mechanisms for pain have been postulated. Noxious stimuli are transmitted via myelinated A-delta fibers or unmyelinated C-fibers, depending on whether the pain is sharp and well localized or dull and poorly localized. These peripheral fibers transmit the impulses afferently to cell bodies in the dorsal root ganglia. Through synapses in the dorsal horn of the spinal cord, via the spinothalamic and other tracts, impulses are conveyed to synapses in the thalamus and brainstem. From these secondary neurons, fibers terminate in the subcortical areas, limbic system, and postcentral gyrus of the cortex (Avery and First, 1989).

The mechanism of peripheral or spinal triggering is complex (Wall, 1984). Chemical mediators (including bradykinins, prostaglandins, potassium, and others in the peripheral unmyelinated sensory afferents) and neuropeptides (such as the undecapeptide substance P) have been implicated at the dorsal horn level of the sensory afferents.

Avery and First (1989) and First et al. (1993) indicate that there is modulation of afferent impulses. The transmission is gated at the dorsal horn level by large A-fibers, by descending tracts within the brainstem and other rostral sites, and by neurochemical transmitters. Neurotransmitters involved in this downward modulation are endorphins, norepinephrine, serotonin, and enkephalins.

Perceptual inputs from the higher brain functions may actively influence the site and experience of pain (Busbaum and Fields, 1984), although the exact pathways of such higher inputs are not understood. There may be some genetic loading in some families where the symptom is reproduced from one generation to the next, with conditioned reflexes possibly playing a part in the triggering mechanisms referred to above (Zeltzer et al., 1992).

Alfven, in a more recent series of controlled studies, postulates that RAP children have chronically tender and tense muscles when compared to a control group (Alfven, 1993a). He further elaborated that the RAP group showed greater sensitivity in the striated muscles of the abdomen, linking his preliminary clinical findings to a biological basis, specific to RAP children (Alfven, 1993b).

PSYCHOLOGICAL THEORIES

Family

Recurrent abdominal pain is usually part of the child's pattern of reaction to emotional stress, often reflecting a family pattern (Apley, 1975). Friedman (1972) noted that children with RAP commonly experience such stresses as psychological illness in one or both parents; marital discord; parental preoccupation with illness; parental absence; school problems; difficulty in handling aggressive, hostile, or sexual feelings; and unsatisfying parent-child relationships.

Zeltzer et al. (1992) postulated that inconsistent parental responses over whether the pain is a fabrication or not can lead to exaggerated symptom expression "to get their parents to notice their distress." Allowing the children to stay home encourages "secondary gains" by inadvertently discouraging their participation in stressful situations, e.g., sports competitiveness or social interactions.

There may also be a tendency for these children to internalize (Wasserman et al., 1988) and/or identify, consciously or unconsciously, with family somatization (Kriechman, 1987; Maloney, 1980) through learning experiences (Leybourne, 1972), the result of which seems to indicate the influence of a conscious component to the child's symptoms.

Another suggestion is that family secrets and myths may play a role (Karpel, 1980; Richtsmeier and Waters, 1984). Somatization may enable family members to reveal such secrets symbolically and covertly, while consciously denying their existence (Avery, 1982; Kriechman, 1987). Themes of secrets are often highly charged, involving sexual conflicts and threatened object loss. The family myth may refer to a shared belief held by family members resulting in patterns of interactions that provide a way of avoiding unpleasant psychological issues. The child's symptoms become pivotal to this avoidance.

Psychoanalytic Theory

Psychoanalytic theory proposes that pain is an organizer of body image, contributes to self-object differentiation, and may become linked with phase-specific unconscious fantasies (Frances and Gale, 1975). There is no single, encompassing psychoanalytic theory of RAP in children. Major contributors include Freud (1905/1964), Weiss (1934), Gloyne (1954), Engel (1959), and Basch (1976). Wasserman et al. (1988), as noted earlier, suggested that internalization is a major factor in the anxiety experienced by the child.

LABORATORY STUDIES

Because the early symptoms of RAP can mimic many potentially serious disorders, and because families of RAP children tend to be some-

what insistent on an organic etiology, most pediatricians first perform a basic group of laboratory tests, including a complete blood count, sedimentation rate, urinalysis, and stool guaiac. When there is serious doubt, amylase, total protein, and albumen levels, liver function tests, and stool cultures for bacteria and parasites may be obtained. Some pediatricians recommend a lactose hydrogen breath test, although the evidence for a lactose intolerance malabsorption etiology for RAP is conflicting (Barr et al., 1979; Lebenthal, 1980). If these tests are normal and the history is strongly suggestive of RAP, no further testing should be done.

DIFFERENTIAL DIAGNOSIS

The potential etiologies for most psychogenic pains, in adults or children, may be vast and certainly pose problems (Herzog and Harper, 1981). Dunger et al. (1986) note that it is sometimes difficult to reassure ourselves and the parents that significant disease has indeed been ruled out. An organic lesion is present in 5% to 10% of the pediatric population with recurrent pain symptoms (Apley, 1975; Faull and Nicol, 1986; Green, 1967; Hodges et al., 1985).

Organic RAP is usually consistent and localized, related to daily events, apt to interrupt sleep, and may penetrate to the back (Avery and First, 1989). There are also usually fewer of the nonintestinal symptoms (such as fatigue, dizziness, and headache) associated with organic disorders.

The most common organic cause of RAP is colonic distention secondary to constipation. Certain foods may precipitate this disorder in a child who has some degree of malabsorption, perhaps secondary to lactose or sucrose intolerance, pancreatic insufficiency, or celiac disease. Food allergies or excessive use of some ingredients, such as caffeine or carbonated beverages, may cause intermittent pain. More than 100 organic causes have been recorded as causing RAP (Bain, 1974).

Among the patients whose symptoms appear more psychogenic in nature, 74% have definitive anxiety classified under an adjustment disorder with anxious or mixed moods or an anxiety syndrome of childhood (Wasserman et al., 1988). The figure for anxiety rises to 87% when attention deficit hyperactivity disorder is included.

Anxiety and depression are often found in both RAP patients and their parents. Hodges et al. (1985) emphasized that both parents of a child with RAP demonstrated significant anxiety levels, mothers outweighing fathers 40% to 25%. Both these figures represent a standard deviation above the mean for men and women with respect to manifestations of anxiety. Children with RAP were confirmed to have higher levels of anxiety than healthy children in the study focusing on anxiety. Twenty-five percent of the mothers of children with RAP had a mild level of depression, but the children did not demonstrate significant levels of depression.

TREATMENT

Once the family is reassured that an organic problem is not evident, explanations that the child is experiencing tension and perhaps other upsetting emotions should be offered. The family should be given every opportunity to express their worries and concerns. Explorations of psychological stress and conflicts in the child and in the family are important. External environmental stresses at home and in the school should be explored and relieved as appropriate.

Individual psychotherapy, family therapy, and behavioral modification may all be indicated. Liebman et al. (1976) note that an integrated psychiatric-pediatric, family-oriented treatment program is an efficient and successful approach to RAP. The pediatrician's relationship to the child-family psychiatrist is pivotal in de-emphasizing repeated medical reevaluations in order to diminish the parents' dependency on an organic focus, guide them to cope more confidently, and appropriately assist the child in his or her ability to master symptoms. This becomes especially important for improved school attendance and functioning. Thus a treatment plan must include an ongoing relationship with relevant school personnel.

In summary, the pediatrician and psychiatrist must demonstrate a consistent approach to the patient, the parents, and the school.

OUTCOME AND FOLLOW-UP DATA

The prognosis for RAP appears to be poor (Wasserman et al., 1988). Some authors (Apley, 1975; Apley and Hale, 1973) reported symptoms persisting into adulthood in a third of the children. Others (Christensen and Mortenson, 1975) report a 50% figure. Friedman (1972) followed up 74 children he had reviewed 1 to 3 years earlier who had complained of a variety of psychogenic pains (predominantly abdominal pain and headache) and found that 69% were much improved or symptom-free, 9% were worse, and in 14% there was a small improvement.

Outcome studies are often methodologically flawed. Reports of symptom experience may not be adequately validated or adequately related to the time at which follow-up occurred, varying in some intra-studies as well as interstudies from months to years. Rigorous studies on the influence of puberty or treatment modalities are equally lacking, although Friedman (1972) states the rate of improvement in his study was unchanged in the untreated or treated group with psychogenic pain.

Avery and First (1989) state that the prognosis is worse when symptoms are of more than 6 months' duration, the onset is prior to 5 years of age, the child is a male, and other family members have a functional disorder. Prognosis is improved if there is an emotionally available pediatrician who recommends psychiatric intervention.

King (1991) in his review states that outcomes are varied: "informal psychotherapy by the pediatrician did not cure the pain," referring here to a long-term follow-up series done by Apley and Hale (1973), nor did it affect those with persisting pain, in comparison to a controlled, untreated group. He reports more optimistic studies but adds they were uncontrolled.

Rutter (1994) continues to cite the literature over the last two decades as reflecting a guarded outcome for these children, viewing RAP, as most psychiatric authors do, as a significant disruption in childhood. Like most, he urges stronger focus on controlled outcome studies.

CASE ILLUSTRATION

A 9-year-old girl in a regular 4th grade class is referred by her pediatrician after two negative evaluations for vague abdominal pains over the past 6 months. She has in addition begun to show occasional school reluctance with this complaint, with "whiny" complaints of pain but usually compliant attendance with urging.

Relevant history from her mother, a rather depressed woman who suffers from dysmenorrhea herself, reveals the following. The family is intact with a 12-year-old sister who is well and a father who is a tense "workaholic" businessman. He spends long hours away from home and travels a good deal. Mother is a housewife and feels overburdened since losing her mother about 1 year ago. She describes the marriage as "all right" but is clearly concerned that her husband might leave her and openly wonders if he might be having an affair as their sexual life has been poor since her mother's last illness 18 months ago. She strongly denies any disagreements or arguments in the household and is certain that her daughter knows nothing about the tensions in the marriage. She describes her child as very "good" both at home and at school, getting excellent grades, and always helping her mother. The child and her father get along well but spend little time together. Sleeping, eating, and

peer-group activities have been limited since the onset of her stomach pains but have not stopped.

Evaluation of the patient revealed a hesitant, shy girl who claimed not to understand why she was seeing a psychiatrist for her stomachaches. She played appropriately and related quite well to the examiner after a warm-up period. All aspects of her mental status were within normal limits, but she demonstrated strong elements of denial throughout the interview. This was most blatant in areas related to family issues and problems, sources of anxiety such as school, and tension contributing to her pain syndrome. She was not very accepting of the idea that talking to someone might help her recurrent abdominal pain.

Comment

While not universal, these families often present with a number of common thematic issues. There are usually "secret" instabilities within the marriage. One or another of the parents has or has had a pain problem. This is usually the mother, and she often presents with depressive phenomenology. In addition, loss and threatened loss play a part. Fathers tend to be absent or distant in these families. The children who suffer from recurrent abdominal pain appear to have some traits in common with children who have eating disorders. They often have histories of being compliant overachievers with poor insight and strong themes of denial.

The initial phase of psychotherapy in such cases involves creating a nonjudgmental, therapeutic environment, open to dialogue and play; encouraging functional integrity with respect to school attendance, peer relationships, and family interactions; and avoiding confrontation or premature interpretation.

Long-term psychotherapeutic goals include relieving somatic preoccupation through linking experience with its affective component, as well as improving family communication around dependency-independency issues in particular and resolution of family conflicts in general.

RESEARCH DIRECTIONS

Over the past decade, research into RAP/psychogenic pain syndromes has attempted to focus on biopsychosocial influences. Asnes et al. (1981) emphasize that such a diagnosis is made not by exclusion of an organic etiology but rather by the presence of positive symptoms and psychosocially deviant influences.

Research in the psychologically complex field of RAP continues to require more rigorous methodology. Development perspectives on etiology and the continuity or discontinuity of symptomatology over time (Rutter, 1987) need to be delineated more clearly, as do RAP-specific psychopharmacological trials, for example, using anxiolytics and antidepressants.

Woodbury's review (1993) urges further exploration into RAP children with attention deficit hyperactivity disorder, learning disorders, and those with histories of sexual abuse. She suggests researching the parents of the RAP group, those who have similar diagnoses and those who abuse substances and/or have a borderline personality disorder.

Outcomes of those treated in therapy (individual, family, behavioral, group, etc.) equally require a more thorough review.

Children with RAP feel pain; it has a reality for them. Those seen by a child psychiatrist usually are functionally impaired. Such children often present with far more psychosocial pathology than the single symptom of pain and thus may present a special subgroup in which pain represents only a part of the total picture.

References

Alfven G: Preliminary findings on increased muscle tension and tenderness and recurrent abdominal pain in children. A clinical study. *Acta Paediatr* 82:400–403, 1993a.

Alfven G: The pressure pain threshold (PPT) of certain muscles in children suffering from recurrent abdominal pain of non-organic origin. An algometric study. *Acta Paediatr* 82:481–483, 1993b.

Alfven G: The covariation of common psychosomatic symptoms among children from socio-eco-

nomically differing residential areas. An epidemiological study. *Acta Paediatr* 82:484–487, 1993c.

American Psychiatric Association: *Diagnostic and Statistical Manual of Disorders* (4th ed). Washington, DC, American Psychiatric Association, 1994.

Apley J: The child with recurrent abdominal pain. *Pediatr Clin North Am* 14:63, 1967.

Apley J: *The Child with Abdominal Pains* (2nd ed). Oxford, Blackwell Scientific Publications, 1975.

Apley J, Hale B: Children with recurrent abdominal pain: How do they grow up? *Clin Res Br Med J* 3:7, 1973.

Apley J, MacKeith RC: *The Child and His Symptoms*. Oxford, Blackwell Scientific Publications, 1968.

Apley J, Nalsh N: Recurrent abdominal pains: A field survey of 1,000 school children. *Arch Dis Child* 33:165, 1958.

Asnes RS, Santulli R, Bemporad JR: Psychogenic chest pain in children. *Clin Pediatr* 20:788–791, 1981.

Avery ME, First LR (eds): *Pediatric Medicine* (1st ed). Baltimore, Williams & Wilkins, 1989, pp. 414–415, 551–556.

Avery NC: Family secrets. *Psychoanal Rev* 69:471, 1982.

Bain HW: Chronic vague abdominal pain in children. *Pediatr Clin North Am* 21:991, 1974.

Barr RG, Levine MD, Watkins JB: Recurrent abdominal pain of childhood due to lactose intolerance: A prospective study. *N Engl J Med* 300:1449, 1979.

Basch MF: The concept of affect: A reexamination. *J Am Psychoanal Assn* 26:759, 1976.

Busbaum AI, Fields HL: Endogenous pain control systems: Brainstem spinal pathways and endorphin circuitry. *Annu Rev Neurosci* 7:309–338, 1984.

Christensen MF, Mortenson O: Long-term prognosis in children with recurrent abdominal pain. *Arch Dis Child* 50:110, 1975.

Dunger, DB, Pritchard J, Hesman S, et al: The investigation of atypical psychosomatic illness. *Clin Pediatr* 25:341, 1986.

Engel G: "Psychogenic" pain and the pain-prone patient. *Am J Med* 26:899, 1959.

Faull C, Nicol AR: Abdominal pain in six year olds: An epidemiological study in a new town. *J Child Psychol Psychiatry* 27:251, 1986.

First LR, Masland R, Berde C, et al: Approach to pain in general pediatrics. In: Avery ME, First LR (eds): *Pediatric Medicine* (2nd ed). Baltimore, Williams & Wilkins, 1993, pp. 63–69.

Frances A, Gale L: Proprioceptive body image in self-object differentiation. *Psychoanal Q* 44:107, 1975.

Freud S: Three essays on the theory of sexuality. In: Strachey J (ed): *The Standard Edition of the Complete Psychological Works of Sigmund Freud*, Vol 7. London, Hogarth Press, 1964. (Originally published 1905)

Friedman R: Some characteristics of children with "psychogenic" pain. *Clin Pediatr* 11:331, 1972.

Gloyne HF: Psychosomatic aspects of pain. *Psychoanal Rev* 41:135, 1954.

Gordon M: Responses of internalizing and externalizing children to clinical interview questions. *J Am Acad Child Adolesc Psychiatry* 22:444–446, 1983.

Green M: Diagnosis and treatment: Psychogenic abdominal pain. *Pediatrics* 40:84, 1967.

Herzog D, Harper G: Unexplained disability—Diagnostic dilemmas and principles of management. *Clin Pediatr* 20:761, 1981.

Hodges K, Kline J, Barbero G, et al: Anxiety in children with recurrent abdominal pain and their parents. *Psychosom Med* 26:859, 1985.

Hodges K, Kline JJ, Barbero G, et al: Depressive symptoms in children with recurrent abdominal pain in their families. *J Pediatr* 107:622, 1986.

Hughes MC, Zimin R: Children with psychogenic abdominal pain and their families. *Clin Pediatr* 17:569, 1978.

Kanner L: *Child Psychiatry*. Springfield, IL, Charles C Thomas, 1957.

Karpel MA: Family secrets. *Fam Process* 19:295, 1980.

King R: King R & Noshpitz J (eds): *Pathways of Growth, Vol.2, Psychopathology*. New York, Wiley, 1991, pp. 536–544.

Kirsner JB, Palmer WC: The irritable colon. *Gastroenterology* 34:491, 1958.

Kriechman AM: Siblings with somatoform disorders in childhood and adolescence. *J Am Acad Child Adolesc Psychiatry* 2:226, 1987.

Lambert J: Psychiatric observations in children with abdominal pain. *Am J Psychiatry* 98:451, 1941.

Lapouse R, Monk MA: Fears and worries in a representational sample of children. *Am J Orthopsychiatry* 29:803, 1959.

Lebenthal E: Recurrent abdominal pain in childhood. *Am J Dis Child* 134:347, 1980.

Lewis M: *Clinical Aspects of Child Development*. Philadelphia, Lea & Febiger, 1982.

Leybourne P, Churchill S: Symptom discouragement in treating hysterical reactions of childhood. *Int J Child Psychol* 1:111, 1972.

Liebman R, Honig P, Berger H: An integrated treatment program for psychogenic pain. *Fam Process* 15:397, 1976.

MacKeith R, O'Neill D: Recurrent abdominal pain in children. *Lancet* 2:278, 1951.

Maloney MJ: Diagnosing hysterical conversion reactions in children. *J Pediatr* 97:1016, 1980.

Poznanski EO: Children with excessive fears. *Am J Orthopsychiatry* 43:428, 1973.

Richtsmeier AM, Waters DB: Somatic symptoms as family myth. *Am J Dis Child* 138:855, 1984.

Rutter M: Psychopathology and development: Links between childhood and adult life. In: Rutter M, Hersov L (eds): *Child and Adolescent Psychiatry* (2nd ed). Oxford, UK, Blackwell, 1987, pp. 720–739.

Rutter M, Hersov L (eds): *Child and Adolescent Psychiatry* (3rd ed). Oxford, UK, Blackwell, 1994, pp. 706–707.

Sarafino EP: *The Fears of Childhood: A Guide to Recognizing and Reducing Fearful Status in Children*. New York, Human Sciences Press, 1986.

Schmitt BD: School phobia—the great imitator: A pediatrician's viewpoint. *Pediatrics* 48:433, 1971.

Sharrer VW, Ryan-Wenger N: Measurements of stress and coping among school-aged children with and without recurrent abdominal pain. *J School Health* 61(2):86, 1991.

Stone RT, Barbero GJ: Recurrent abdominal pain in childhood. *Pediatrics* 45:732, 1970.

Trotter W: *Collected Papers of Wilfred Trotter*. London, F.R.S., 1941.

Wall PD: The painful consequences of peripheral injury. *J Hand Surg* 9:37, 1984.

Wasserman AL, Whitington PF, Rivara FP: Psychogenic basis for abdominal pain in children and adolescents. *J Am Acad Child Adolesc Psychiatry* 27:179, 1988.

Weiss E: Bodily pain and mental pain. *Int J Psychoanal* 15:1, 1934.

Woodbury MM: Recurrent abdominal pain in child patients seen at a pediatric gastroenterology clinic. *Psychosomatics* 34:6, 485–493, 1993.

Zeltzer LK, Barr RG, McGrath PA, et al: Pediatric pain: interacting behavioral and physical factors. *Pediatrics* 90(5, pt 2):816, 1992.

103 CHRONIC PEDIATRIC ILLNESS AND MULTIPLE HOSPITALIZATIONS

David A. Mrazek, M.D., F.R.C.Psych.

CONCEPTUAL OVERVIEW

It is estimated that more than 3 million American children suffer from some type of chronic illness (Schoenborn and Marano, 1988). Given the scope and pervasiveness of pediatric problems, serious physical illness should be conceptualized as one of the most important early risk factors for emotional disturbance and given a high priority in national efforts to prevent negative sequelae. One factor that has complicated efforts to develop an intervention strategy is the wide variability that exists in the results of studies designed to demonstrate the association between the occurrence of early illnesses and subsequent problems in emotional development. The range of adaptation to physical illness is broad. Some children seem to thrive heroically despite enduring long periods of unquestionable adversity, while others succumb to despair as they struggle to meet the demands created by the symptoms and treatment of their illnesses. In many ways, this variability is completely parallel to children's responses to other major risk factors, which include divorce (Heatherington, 1989) and child abuse (Mrazek and Mrazek, 1987).

There are two quite different approaches to building a framework from which to understand the emotional impact of medical illnesses on children. The first strategy is to look for commonalities across the different types of medical diseases. Using this approach, investigators have described a set of characteristics typical of ill children that includes a high prevalence of problems with self-esteem and peer relationships. These difficulties are similar to those that characterize physically healthy children who grow up in highly stressful environments and can probably be considered to be generic sequelae of early adversity. While this is a useful approach for arriving at an overview of the scope of the national problem created by pediatric illness, it provides less guidance for the clinician faced with how to help a particular child with a specific chronic disease.

An alternative approach is to try to focus on the unique characteristics of a given illness, with the goal of defining factors that place an individual child suffering from a specific set of physical symptoms at risk for problems in adaptation. Such a perspective is best organized by considering children within their family and social contexts, thereby allowing for a more complete developmental understanding of their current adjustment. This leads to an analysis of the interactions of illness-specific risk factors, familial risk factors, and social/environmental risk factors. More important, this approach is compatible with considering the role of protective factors in the child, family, and community that can be therapeutically supported to mediate the potential pathogenic impact of negative influences. Risk factor analysis has been used in studies designed to clarify interactional processes that result in the development of psychopathology in physically well children (Rutter and Garmezy, 1983). Further identification and definition of the protective mechanisms should be a high priority, as they provide the promise of yielding new knowledge that can be used to create interventions designed to facilitate adaptation. This chapter will focus primarily on chronic illness-specific risk and chronic illness-specific protective factors within the broader context of the child's support system. A complete therapeutic response to children with chronic physical illnesses, and their families, requires considering chronic illness-specific factors within a more extensive analysis of all major risk and protective factors.

ILLNESS-SPECIFIC RISK FACTORS

Illness-specific risk factors are the characteristics of specific chronic diseases that place children at increased risk for emotional disturbance. Physically ill children are not immune to the negative effects of poverty, parental dysfunction, divorce, and abuse. Additionally, they must cope with hardships imposed on them by their physical symptoms, limitations of function, and disruptive and unpleasant treatments. On a more positive note, they benefit from illness-specific protective factors, such as the support provided by sensitive physicians and nursing staff. These beneficial influences can be further potentiated by protective influences that are not illness-specific, such as secure parental attachments and family cohesiveness. Many of the innovations in pediatric care and hospitalization, such as systematic preparation for procedures and liberal rooming-in policies, should be conceptualized as illness-specific protective factors.

Of most central importance in analyzing the coping of an ill child's family is the simple realization that being diagnosed as having a serious chronic illness does not mean that a child is doomed to depression, rejection, or isolation. Chronic illness should be viewed as a condition characterized by a set of serious challenges that can either be overcome or result in an emotional defeat. Every pediatrician can provide anecdotes of particularly competent children who have faced the adversity of dreadful illnesses with great courage and have achieved a sense of accomplishment in managing their symptoms effectively. These stories of victories are retold in part because the success of these patients to some degree reflects the skill and support of their doctor in their shared battle against disease. It is more difficult to focus on the family and child who do not succeed. Helping children who cannot overcome the emotional traumas associated with a serious medical illness often becomes the central role of the child psychiatrist in a pediatric setting. The need for psychiatric involvement becomes even more evident at

the point that illness-specific risk factors begin to contribute to the development of overt psychopathology in either the child or the parents.

Impact of Time of Onset

Few specific studies have focused on the differential impact of the time of onset of chronic illnesses. However, a guiding therapeutic principle has been that the painful and frightening symptoms of chronic illnesses are most difficult for young children to manage, in part because of their inability to fully understand the nature of either the medical problem or the treatment. The exception to this may be very young infants, who may be spared the association that links physical traumas with the as yet incompletely differentiated significant caregiver. During infancy, primitive defense mechanisms may contribute to amnesia for the trauma itself. A review of children's cognitive appraisal of illness highlights this point and demonstrates the link between cognitive development and the capacity to cope with medical procedures (Brewster, 1982). In contrast, the onset of a serious illness during adolescence can be particularly stressful for quite a different set of developmental reasons. Body image, personal identity formation, and peer acceptance are major issues for the young adolescent, and the onset of a chronic illness during the teenage years can completely disrupt the normal process of self-development. In some cases the adaptations that children have made to the early onset of disease can be effective throughout the elementary school years, but with puberty they can begin to fail in the face of the stressors associated with establishing a sexual relationship or beginning to assume greater independence from family support systems. Depressive symptoms clearly increase during adolescence, with a concomitant increase in suicidal ideation and risk.

Nature of the Etiology of the Illness

The understanding that the child and family have concerning the reason that the child developed the illness can have a major impact on their capacity to adapt to it. Here, rational and irrational elements always to some degree coexist. Genetic illnesses have perhaps the most problematic implications in that there is frequently a powerful tendency on the part of even well-adjusted parents to blame themselves and each other for a "familial taint" that has been passed on to one of their children. However, other etiologies that include infections and trauma can also result in similar self-recrimination on the part of both the child and the parents.

In contrast, diseases that seem to be "an act of God" may provide less direct interpersonal stress for the patient and family, as there is a less evident target for the designation of blame. Instead, a classic phase of denial and grief, characterized by a vain search for an answer to the inevitable "why me" question, is a part of the process.

In both cases, the therapeutic task is to shift away from a preoccupation with *why* and move toward focusing on the challenges of *what* treatment should be instituted and *how* the family can adapt. The exception to this rule is when the etiology of the illness is clearly genetic and a quantifiable risk for future children in the family must be addressed. After the pediatrician or genetic counselor explains what the risk for future children actually is, the child psychiatrist can play an important role in the process of helping families to realistically integrate and act on this new information.

Certainty of Diagnosis

If the diagnosis can be determined with certainty, the child and family can begin the process of coming to grips with whatever life changes are required to manage the illness. In those cases where a long period of uncertainty follows the onset of physical symptoms, a variety of negative processes emerge that can disrupt the doctor-family relationship. This is particularly compounded in the case in which the diagnosis is unnecessarily delayed as a result of error or confusion, and it is eventually determined that a specific treatment could have been provided earlier in the course of the illness that would have had a positive impact on the patient's long-term prognosis.

As a general rule, dealing with a defined stressor is less difficult than coping with the unknown. This principle often provides guidance to the medical team, who may be overtly uncomfortable with the painful news of the diagnosis of a chronic illness and be tempted to delay the actual naming of the disease for months. This avoidance is most common in the case of a terminal illness, when both family and physicians may find it unbearable to explain to a young child that he or she will not recover. In some cases, a suggestion is made that the child psychiatrist break the news to the child, based on the rationale that he or she is particularly skillful in speaking directly with children and dealing with their emotional responses. While this is an acceptable plan and far superior to a prolonged pretense, it is usually more productive for the child psychiatrist to play the role of the facilitator in a process that includes the family and pediatrician. The goal of this effort is to establish an openness about the child's life expectancy in a manner that the child can understand, which will allow the family and physician to make informed decisions that include the child's input and wishes.

Degree of Deformity and Disability

Deformity and disability clearly increase the impact of chronic illness on the capacity of the child and family to cope with the disease. Chronic illness is usually associated with some degree of limitation, but to the degree that the child can compensate for these losses, these limitations provide much less of a potential risk for impairment of growth and emotional development. Studies that have focused on the degree of impairment have often found an association with increased psychopathology.

A somewhat different set of considerations is raised when a major deformity in body image results from the disease or its treatment. While the negative impact of the deformity is obviously present throughout development, the most specific period of vulnerability occurs during early and middle adolescence. One of the most central issues is the support of significant others who provide the critical emotional reassurance that, despite disfigurement, the child is still a valued part of the family and community. A particularly effective strategy to normalize the child's experience is to encourage a peer group experience with children with similar deformities who have made an adequate adjustment.

Prognosis and Course of the Illness

While by definition chronic illnesses tend to be persistent, the ultimate prognosis of the illness is a major factor in adaptation. When a reasonable hope exists that the illness will either remit completely or eventually provide little disability, an optimistic stance by the medical team and family is highly adaptive. A similar approach is indicated when the illness falls in the category described as the "Damocles syndrome" (Koocher and O'Malley, 1981). In these cases, a dreadful outcome is possible, but the best strategy is still to assume an optimistic stance, as remission is a realistic possibility. In contrast, terminal illnesses provide a set of specific challenges to both the family and caretakers. After achieving the first step, open acknowledgment of the impending death of the child, a long process of adapting to the reality of the loss of the child begins. Denial is a common defense and must be dealt with sensitively, as few stressors for a family are as disruptive as the death of a child, and parents often need time to find ways to mobilize family supports and reorganize future hopes and expectations.

THE CHRONIC ILLNESSES

While many chronic illnesses exist, the most common serious diseases and their estimated prevalence are listed in Table 103.1. Less serious illnesses occur frequently during childhood, but these are for the most part self-limiting problems that are rarely associated with severe

Table 103.1.   Prevalance of Serious Chronic Conditions in Children in the United States in 1987

Disease	Number per 1000
Asthma	52.5
Migraine	8.4
Anemia	7.5
Epilepsy	4.1
Arthritis	2.8
Diabetes	2.0
Leukemia	0.42

Results, except for the prevalence of leukemia, derived from Schoenborn CA, Marano M: *Current Estimates from the National Health Interview Survey: United States, 1987* (Vital and Health Statistics, Series 10, No. 166. DHHS Pub. No. (PHS) 88-1594). Washington, DC, US Government Printing Office, 1988.

emotional sequelae that require child psychiatric intervention. Five quite distinct chronic illnesses are reviewed in this chapter to serve as models of the clinical issues presented by this wide range of pediatric disease. (Further information on the illnesses selected [asthma, epilepsy, cystic fibrosis, diabetes, and malignancies] may be found in Chapters 59, 94, and 96.)

Asthma

Asthma affects more than 1 in 20 American children and is the most prevalent chronic illness of childhood. Incidence estimates in other countries vary widely, reaching a maximum rate of 1 in 10 in New Zealand. In many ways, asthma is the prototypic psychosomatic illness. While there is no question that there is a demonstrable physical component to asthma, both acute and chronic stressors directly affect the management of the illness (Mrazek, 1988).

Asthma is defined as a reversible reactive airway disease triggered by a variety of immunological and nonimmunological factors. It is familial in nature, with a significantly increased risk of the disease occurring in other family members. While serum immunoglobulin E may play a role in the expression of symptoms in many patients with asthma (Burrows et al., 1989), the disease is heterogeneous in presentation, suggesting that different mechanisms may be prominent in different patients.

The onset of asthma usually occurs quite early in life, with approximately 75% of children developing the illness within their first 3 years (Falliers, 1970). However, asthma can begin for the first time at any age. This presents an interesting clinical issue in that dealing with the alarming and often rapid onset of intense chest tightness and respiratory distress can be a particularly frightening problem for children younger than 3 years of age. Thus early onset can have a significantly greater impact on subsequent emotional development. Later onset, during adolescence, is relatively unusual and in many ways less difficult to adapt to than other illnesses arising during the teenage years, in large part because of the availability of increasingly effective pharmacological control of symptoms and the absence of visible physical symptoms.

The etiology of asthma is complex and still not well understood. Despite clear evidence of increased familial risk of developing the illness, twin studies unequivocally demonstrate that environmental factors are necessary for the expression of the disease. Environmental factors that have been considered to be salient include early respiratory infection, difficulties in parenting (Mrazek et al., 1991), and excessive exposure to a highly antigenic environment in infants with elevated levels of immunoglobulin E (Mrazek et al., 1990). Exposure to cigarette smoke is a nonspecific irritant that may affect onset. The wide range of potential factors involved in the expression of the disease complicates the process of attributing causality to specific experiences that have been hypothesized to be associated with the onset of the child's illness. Like all illnesses with a genetic basis, the alleles that a child has at specific gene sites determine the likelihood of disease expression. However, potential therapeutic strategies targeted at familial behavior may well delay or prevent the onset of the symptoms (Mrazek, 1993).

The establishment of the diagnosis can be difficult in the first months of life. It has been a common practice among some pediatricians to consciously avoid making the diagnosis in the first years of life for fear of "stigmatizing" the child. The rationale for this strategy was that if the disease was not viewed as chronic, it would have a less detrimental impact on the child's development. One strategy is to diagnose wheezing in infancy as "bronchiolitis," despite the fact that the attacks may be occurring without a clear concurrent infection. While it is true that this practice avoids an early confrontation with the potential long-standing nature of the problem, it also may postpone early intensive management of the illness. In summary, overly optimistic reassurance that a child may well "grow out of asthma" may inadvertently lead to inadequate treatment of the illness.

Asthma rarely has any visible stigmata. However, in the 5% to 10% of asthmatic children who become steroid-dependent, striking changes in appearance can occur. These children often suffer from chronic respiratory insufficiency, which may result in the development of a "barrel chest." Furthermore, steroid treatment can cause cushingoid stigmata and delay growth, resulting in permanent short stature.

The issue of limitation of activity is important. A natural parental tendency is to shelter asthmatic children from the rigors of intense exercise. This is clearly inadvisable. Strunk et al. (1989) demonstrated the beneficial impact of improved fitness on the adaptation of asthmatic children. For the majority of children with asthma, an active program of normalization of their activities is the appropriate clinical approach.

The prognosis of asthma is complex. For the majority of children with mild asthma, there is little risk of a fatal attack and good reason to expect that with proper management there will be a high probability of remission of symptoms. Consequently, appropriate treatment which includes pharmacological, environmental, and psychological interventions usually results in the control of symptoms. A permanent "cure" or remission is less likely.

The prognosis is less clear for children with steroid-dependent asthma. In these children, the risk for a fatal episode may approach 5%. These severely asthmatic children must learn to pay close attention to their physiological state because responding to early warning signs of respiratory distress is often critical in order to reach help in time to reverse bronchoconstriction and to avert a respiratory arrest. Prescription of steroids is a complicated issue. While steroid control is essential in these children, the side effects of prednisone can be disturbing. Negative reactions to steroid treatment are particularly common in young adolescents, who are most self-conscious, but this is the precise developmental period when children seem to be at most risk for a fatal episode (Strunk et al., 1985). A set of risk factors associated with fatal episodes has been established and essentially creates a profile of children at increased risk. The three most prominent features of this profile are a history of seizures, documented affective disturbance, and demonstrated conflict between the child's family and the medical caregivers.

CASE ILLUSTRATION

Sybil was a 12-year-old chronically asthmatic girl with a life-long history of unremitting asthma, complicated by serious steroid side effects. She was admitted to a tertiary treatment center to comprehensively review the management of her symptoms. She had been treated at a well-known children's hospital with little improvement despite her more than 40 admissions. She had received chronic steroid treatment to control her airway reactivity, which had resulted in severe cushingoid stigmata and retardation of growth, to the extent that she appeared to be the size of a 7-year-old. Her steroid treatment had resulted in the development of scoliosis, which further complicated her ability to breathe.

Sybil was an extremely intelligent child, with an IQ of 152. Despite her multiple hospitalizations and many school absences, she was able to score above grade level in basic academic skills. While her nuclear family was intact, her father had developed chronic pancreatitis secondary to heavy use of alcohol and had become increasingly depressed.

During a 4-month intensive hospitalization, Sybil's steroid dose was dramatically reduced. She received intensive psychotherapy, which provided her a more realistic perspective on her range of abilities, and she made a readjustment in personal goals that included a shift away from a desire to be a competitive ice skater to a focus instead on ambitious but obtainable academic objectives. During this 4-month period, her depressive affect improved dramatically, and she was able to communicate openly with her family about her feelings in a way that had never occurred previously.

Sybil's asthma was acutely sensitive to emotional factors. This was well illustrated early during her hospitalization when she developed an episode of acute respiratory distress that was not relieved by oral medication or injections of epinephrine. A plan for an immediate transfer to the intensive care unit (ICU) for an intravenous aminophylline infusion and the possibility of mechanical ventilation was instituted. While waiting for transfer to the ICU, she requested that her therapist hypnotize her to relieve her intense anxiety. She proved to be a good subject, and hypnosis resulted in a complete remission of her acute respiratory distress within minutes. This remission was persistent, and no ICU admission was required.

On returning to her home, Sybil's course deteriorated dramatically. She became resistant to medical treatment and became acutely depressed. Her father's emotional problems became more severe, and intense family conflict was a daily experience. Despite antidepressant medication, she developed intense suicidal ideation. She announced to the psychiatrist whom she had begun to see regularly that she would not see him again because she was going to die before their next session. Three days later she had an acute episode of asthma and expired in the family car on the way to the emergency room.

Epilepsy

Many quite heterogeneous central nervous system disorders can be broadly classified as chronic epilepsy. Epilepsy defined as persistent major motor seizures affects approximately 4 children per 1000. Onset of seizures occurs throughout childhood and onset in the first years of life is particularly common. Genetic etiologies are unusual, which influences the focus of parental attribution of blame. The level of anxiety associated with the diagnosis of epilepsy is clearly linked to the family's beliefs regarding prognosis and etiology. While a single febrile seizure is rarely a cause of persistent concern, focal seizures that suggest central nervous system pathology have a major impact on both the child and family. Harrison and Taylor (1976) examined the long-term outcome of a sample of children with seizures and found a mortality rate of 10.1%. In this sample, 24.2% of the children developed chronic epilepsy. As with many physical illnesses, chronicity and severity of symptoms are among the key factors influencing subsequent deviations in emotional development. Similarly a wide range of psychosocial stressors have been reported to be associated with the onset or recurrence of seizures, including quite discrete events such as the occurrence of sexual abuse (Greig and Betts, 1992).

Onset in adolescence can be particularly disturbing, as key expectations for greater independence can be dramatically altered by the uncertainty created by episodic seizures. It has long been demonstrated that children with seizures are at increased risk for emotional disturbance. In the Isle of Wight study, 28.6% of children with uncomplicated epilepsy and 58.3% of children with documented lesions above the brainstem suffered from emotional disturbance (Rutter et al., 1970). More recent studies report similar rates of psychopathology (Hoare and Kerley, 1991). These rates have been consistently found to be considerably higher than rates of psychopathology in children with other chronic physical illnesses, suggesting that pathological features of the central nervous system increased the likelihood of behavioral disturbance (Howe et al., 1993).

The differential diagnosis of epilepsy can be complex. An initial seizure can be clinically difficult to differentiate from an episode of loss of consciousness that may be due to cardiac or functional factors. Confusion in establishing the nature of the episodes can result in both loss of confidence in the medical team and considerable fear about the nature of the underlying pathology.

While epilepsy does not result in persistent physical deformity, the emotional stigmata of an epileptic attack have been well documented. Taylor (1987) suggested that prejudice against epileptics is in part the result of a publicly perceived association between epilepsy and madness, mental deterioration, and death. This notion is reinforced by the unsettling similarity between a sudden epileptic attack and an imagined fatal collapse. There are often real limitations in the epileptic child's ability to function, particularly as related to participating in sports. The subsequent impact on self-esteem, coupled with the repeated experience of episodic loss of control is a substantial challenge for a developing child and requires pragmatic planning on the part of both the family and medical team to construct an appropriate strategy to maximize the opportunities for the child to develop an appropriate degree of autonomy and independence.

In a recent review, Hermann et al. (1990) adopted a risk factor strategy for predicting the occurrence of psychopathology in epileptics. One hundred and two adults were studied. For the majority, their disease began during childhood and adolescence, and the mean duration of their illness was more than 16 years. A set of predictive risk factors was identified. Illness-specific risk factors included early onset of symptoms and a perception of being stigmatized. Additionally, their adjustment to seizures, as defined by the experience of embarrassment, disturbance of self-esteem, and sense of personal rejection, were features associated with development of psychiatric symptoms. Non-illness-specific factors associated with disturbance included more frequent adverse life events, financial stress, and vocational difficulties. A major positive impact on emotional symptoms in epileptic patients has been reported to be associated with successful surgical intervention (Seidman-Ripley et al., 1993).

Cystic Fibrosis

Cystic fibrosis is an autosomal recessive genetic illness affecting only about 0.05% of white children and fewer black or Asian children. In Caucasian populations, about 5% of adults are carriers of the gene. The expression of the symptoms of cystic fibrosis occurs almost universally during infancy and involves multiple organ systems. Physical problems include chronic bronchial airway obstruction, often leading to infection, and maldigestion subsequent to pancreatic defects. An alternative name for this illness is mucoviscidosis, which describes the increased viscosity of secretions that is the common origin of many of the symptoms, including those of the lung, pancreas, liver, intestine, and genitals. Because the initial presentation of the illness can involve either pulmonary or gastrointestinal symptoms, the initial onset is often difficult to recognize. There has been a dramatic increase in the lifespan of children with cystic fibrosis. While previously it had been unusual for children to live to adulthood, the median survival rate has increased beyond 20 years. Sexual development is usually delayed, and 98% of the males are sterile (Taussig et al., 1976). Pregnancy in females with cystic fibrosis is associated with increased risk of deterioration in respiratory functions, but has been successfully managed with intensive medical support.

Since the diagnosis of cystic fibrosis usually occurs in infancy or early childhood, the child and family must quickly learn to cope with medical problems. Caring for a child with cystic fibrosis requires considerable effort and a major time commitment because of the need for frequent physical therapy to decrease the occurrence of pulmonary com-

plications. Burke et al. (1989) examined the occurrence of obsessive-compulsive symptoms in children with cystic fibrosis and found modestly elevated scores but no overt obsessive-compulsive disorder. Given the demands of cystic fibrosis, obsessive attention to self-care may well be a good coping strategy and serve a protective function in minimizing disease sequelae.

Despite its early onset, adolescents with cystic fibrosis often experience the management of their physical symptoms in a way that allows academic and peer activities to be particularly stressful. Problems that typically become more acute during the teenage years include maldigestion, associated unpleasant flatus, concerns about self-esteem related to sexual potency, and an increasing awareness of the reality of a compromised lifespan. Despite these difficulties, some patients do marry and have reported that their sexual relationships are satisfactory (Levine and Stern, 1982).

Given that the disease is clearly hereditary in etiology, genetic counseling is an important component to include in a comprehensive plan for supporting these families. Because of the high level of phenotypic expression of the disease in infants with the homozygous recessive genotype, one in four subsequent children born to parents of a child with cystic fibrosis will also develop the illness. With the development of methods to determine the genotype of the fetus in utero, much of the uncertainty about future pregnancies can be resolved. Somewhat ironically, since both parents must be carriers of the illness for their children to develop the disease, there is less possibility of attributing blame to one parent. Given the need for early intensive treatment, the establishment of the initial diagnosis is an important factor involved in establishing a strong and supportive doctor-family relationship.

Studies have suggested variable frequencies of co-occurrence of emotional disturbance in children with cystic fibrosis. Some studies have reported that children with cystic fibrosis have no increased incidence of psychiatric disturbance (Blair et al., 1994) and that they have normal intellectual and academic abilities (Thompson et al., 1992). However, a recent comparison of four chronic pediatric illnesses suggested that methodological issues of ascertainment of psychopathology in physically ill children may result in lower estimates of psychopathology. Twenty-five percent of the school aged children with cystic fibrosis within this sample were diagnosed with a psychiatric disorder (Canning, 1994).

Illness-specific risk factors have been hypothesized to be mediated by protective factors such as positive familial involvement and high-quality medical support. Steinhausen et al. (1983) examined a set of hypothesized risk factors thought to be associated with psychological disturbance. Only one of these, severity of illness, was illness-specific. The other risk factors included parental pathology, disturbed parenting, and socioeconomic difficulties. The entire set of risk factors, including severity of illness, was responsible for nearly 37% of the variance in the occurrence of psychiatric disturbance in this sample. Approximately one-third of the children were diagnosed as having severe emotional disturbance, and another 22% had less severe problems.

The occurrence of maternal depression has been examined in the mothers of children with cystic fibrosis based on both their guarded prognosis and the large burden of care that is required as part of their treatment. Mothers of children with cystic fibrosis report higher levels of depression and greater levels of emotional strain than do the fathers of these children (Quittner et al., 1992). Other studies have linked maternal distress with higher levels of adjustment problems in these children (Thompson et al., 1994).

Venters (1981) showed an association between competent family functioning and the child's adjustment. Two characteristics, seeking out social support during stressful periods and the ability of the family to understand the illness within a broader religious or philosophical frame of reference, were shown to be associated with better outcome. While a broad range of problems has been reported to occur in families with a child with cystic fibrosis, Petzel et al. (1984) identified concerns about treatment and premature death as being the most salient issues for children with cystic fibrosis and their families.

Insulin-Dependent Diabetes Mellitus

Juvenile onset insulin-dependent diabetes mellitus (IDDM) is a disease of the islet cells of the pancreas characterized by a deficiency in the production of insulin. It is not a common illness of very young children but does occur in about 0.2% of school-age and adolescent children. Because of its delay in onset, it presents an interesting contrast to the problems associated with lifelong chronic physical illness. It has been suggested that less evidence of psychopathology has been demonstrated in diabetic children when compared to children with other serious physical illnesses that begin in infancy. Possible factors that contribute to a better outcome would include (a) later onset, with less negative impact on early emotional development; (b) a more effective mode of treatment; and (c) minimal early central nervous system involvement.

Questions have arisen related to the role of stress in the initial onset of diabetes. Barglow et al. (1986) reported no significant association between psychopathology in diabetic mothers and the subsequent development of "developmental deficits" in their offspring when obstetrical and perinatal factors other than diabetes were well controlled. Chase and Jackson (1981) reported an association between stressor scores and serum glucose and triglyceride concentrations in an adolescent sample. Gustafsson et al. (1987) documented an association between disturbed family interaction and diabetic control in adolescents, as measured by elevated glycosylated hemoglobin (HbA_1) 5 years after the initial assessment.

While associations between poor emotional adjustment and difficulty in control of diabetic symptoms have been repeatedly observed, the nature of the relationship is not clear. It is often suggested that poor emotional regulation subsequently interferes with medical compliance. However, the alternative view that poor chemical control causes emotional disturbance remains a viable, although unproven, hypothesis.

While there is a strong familial propensity for the development of diabetes, the genetic risk is less clear than for illnesses with an established pattern of inheritance, such as cystic fibrosis. Diagnostic issues are for the most part less of an issue than the therapeutic issues associated with management of the illness. Wilkinson (1987) suggested that two of the characteristics of IDDM that result in later disturbance are its impact on so many aspects of everyday living and the high degree of personal responsibility required to manage the illness. In his study of adult diabetics, as many as 18% of the sample were diagnosed with psychiatric disorder. Depression and anxiety were the most frequently reported symptoms.

Little physical deformity initially results from IDDM. However, children experience considerable anxiety related to fears of hypoglycemic or hyperglycemic coma and later vascular complications (Moran, 1984). Some interference with normal function is a key problem in adolescence, when restrictions in activity and dietary compliance can be particularly problematic. White et al. (1984) studied the association between potential stressors and poor diabetic control in children with very labile IDDM. Ketoacidosis was sometimes associated with "intercurrent illness" (15–30%) and dieting indiscretions and insulin mismanagement (5–10%). However, most of these children came from families with multiple problems that were believed to be highly associated with their poor control. All but 4 of the 30 children that they studied became labile after psychosocial intervention.

IDDM shares some of the features of other illnesses with uncertain outcome. While most children survive well into adulthood, the fear of diabetic sequelae and the occurrence of severe ketoacidotic episodes can be upsetting for children. Gath et al. (1980) demonstrated a number of cognitive difficulties in diabetic children between the ages of 9 and 10 whose duration of diabetes was 3.5 years. A correlation was shown between poor diabetic control and (a) the presence of a psychiatric disorder, (b) problems in reading, and (c) adverse psychosocial factors in the family background. More recent neuropsychological studies of children with onset of disease prior to 5 years of age have found impairment in abstract/visual reasoning subscales of the Stanford-Binet Intelli-

gence Scale, even in children with only mild hypoglycemia (Golden et al., 1989).

Kovacs et al. (1985) studied a group of school-age diabetic children and found no evidence of increased life stress or psychiatric disturbance preceding diagnosis. She described two patterns of coping in these children. One was characterized by some social withdrawal and sadness in 64% of the children. The remaining 36% met criteria for psychiatric disorder, with depressive syndromes being most prominent. Ninety-three percent of the children recovered from these reactions to the diagnosis within the first year of their illness. In a study of the rehospitalization of diabetic children, externalizing symptoms were shown to be correlated with readmission prompting recommendation of appropriate intervention of these problems as a preventive measure (Kovacs et al., 1994)

Fonagy et al. (1987) conducted a well-controlled study to examine psychological factors that affected management of children with IDDM. Psychological disturbance in both the children and the parents predicted low glycosylated hemoglobin concentration in the children and accounted for 44% of the variance in blood glucose control. Their findings suggested that as many as one-third of the children with IDDM have appreciable emotional and behavioral problems. However, children perceived as having problems were less often responsible for the care of the illness. The authors conclude that children under 12 are often unable to manage the self-care regimens prescribed to treat their illness. The importance of parental involvement in maintaining optimal diabetes management has been clearly demonstrated and well accepted (Weist et al., 1993).

Pediatric Malignancies

Pediatric malignancies are rare and can begin at any time in childhood. The leukemias are the most common, occurring in 4.2 children per 100,000 and are commonly diagnosed between the ages of 2 and 4. A generation ago, childhood malignancies were considered fatal illnesses, but due to the dramatic improvements in chemotherapy and radiation treatment, leukemia is now more appropriately considered a chronic illness, given that the current 5-year survival rate is in excess of 50%. Clearly, this places malignancies in an intermediate position between terminal and stable conditions. For this reason, Koocher and O'Malley (1981) have aptly referred to these illnesses as "the Damocles syndrome."

The etiologies of most malignancies remain quite unclear. While some evidence of increased genetic risk for some subtypes of leukemia has been determined, many cases appear to occur sporadically. While various hypotheses related to infectious or immunological mechanisms leading to leukemia have been put forward, the diagnosis usually comes as a shock with little sense of parental responsibility.

Malignancies vary in their difficulty of diagnosis. Leukemias can be asymptomatic for months. However, once the suspicion of leukemia is raised, the definitive diagnosis can be reliably confirmed through laboratory examination. Given the importance of aggressive early treatment, any delay in establishing the diagnosis presents an important psychological issue in the care of the family.

For the most part, leukemias result in only minimal physical deformity, although bruising and wasting can be a problem in the later stages of the illness. In contrast, solid tumors that require surgical intervention result in radical and abrupt changes in the child's body image. In many ways, adolescence is a particularly difficult time for the onset of these illnesses and the often quite extensive treatment that is required.

Considerable controversy currently exists regarding the frequency of emotional disturbance occurring in children with malignancies. Clearly, some studies (Eiser, 1979; Greenberg et al., 1989; Kupst et al., 1984) suggest relatively low levels of either emotional or behavioral disturbance. Sawyer et al. (1986) reported significant differences in behavioral and emotional problems between affected children with leukemia and siblings in the 2-year period following onset of diagnosis. A longer term follow-up some 4 years after the initial evaluation (Sawyer et al., 1989) showed considerable normalization of the functioning of leukemic patients, with the only remaining difference between the patients and siblings being problems in school performance as noted by both teachers and parents. Three possible explanations for these persistent findings are (a) the direct effect of central nervous system irradiation on neuropsychological functioning, (b) the documented large number of school days missed, and (c) the lasting impact of documented earlier emotional and behavioral problems that had occurred primarily in school-related areas. The treatment of the illness should be considered an illness-specific risk factor to the degree that repeated, painful bone marrow biopsies and other invasive procedures are required. This can be particularly difficult for children with early onset.

The cranial irradiation literature suggests that aggressive treatment can result in neuropsychological damage (Stehbens and Kisker, 1984), particularly if administered before 8 years of age (Moehle and Berg, 1985). Pavlovsky et al. (1983) reported that children with cranial irradiation plus intrathecal methotrexate treatment had the greatest number of psychological sequelae and associated abnormal computed tomography (CT) scans. Brouwers et al. (1984) again noted associations with CT scans. Specifically, greater neuropsychological deficits and attention deficit problems were noted in patients with evidence of atrophy. In the relatively few patients who showed calcification, the greatest deficits were noted. Long-term follow-up of survivors of acute lymphoblastic leukemia has revealed a greater likelihood of being placed in special education programs, but they generally have good outcomes. Dosage of cranioradiotherapy and earlier age at diagnosis were found to be important education-related risk factors (Haupt et al., 1994).

The effect of chronic illness should not be considered in isolation to other concurrent stresses. This is illustrated by Kalins et al. (1980), who documented the non-illness-specific stressors occurring in the families of physically ill children. A higher frequency of other serious life events was noted to have occurred in families with sick children than had been expected. However, independent studies have noted an association between "family cohesion and adaptation" and better psychological outcome in adolescent cancer survivors across a range of stressful experiences (Rait et al., 1992).

Mulhern et al. (1981) described the differences in the relative perception of the nature of the prognosis for recovery by physicians, parents, and children. Physicians had the most negative view of prognosis, parents an intermediate view, and children the most optimistic perspective. While this is probably an appropriate therapeutic posture to maintain, the authors point out that it does provide an explanation for studies that find few affective and emotional symptoms in children with serious disease, suggesting that denial may be an adaptive form of coping with the seriousness of their medical prognosis.

CASE ILLUSTRATION

An example of an adaptive response to an overwhelming disability was demonstrated by George. George was 16 and was the second of four children in a middle-class, upwardly mobile family. George was not chronically ill as a young child but rather was an outstanding athlete, playing three sports in high school and competing in the state finals in track and field. During his senior year in high school, he suddenly developed intense pain in his right leg, and the diagnosis of osteosarcoma in his right tibia was quickly made. The necessity of an immediate amputation and the serious nature of his prognosis were openly discussed with George and his family in a sensitive and thorough manner. Surgery was performed without delay.

For George, the impact of the loss of his leg was enormous. Given that at this point in his development, his appearance and athletic ability were central components of his identity, one might have predicted a negative outcome. Instead George responded in an extremely positive and forward-looking manner. His adaptive and spir-

ited recovery was strongly supported by his family, who could both acknowledge the severity of the illness and at the same time were emotionally available to him. A very aggressive postoperative rehabilitation program was planned that included visits by teenage amputees to the hospital before George's discharge. By the time he was ready to return home, he had heard from an enormous number of his classmates, and the family had the unshakable conviction that he would persevere. On follow-up, no depressive symptoms had developed, and George continued to be an outstanding student at his high school and went on to a prestigious university.

EFFECTS OF MULTIPLE HOSPITALIZATION

A pediatric hospitalization, like a chronic illness, should be considered an experience during which a child will be exposed to a set of illness-specific risk factors that could have a negative impact on subsequent adaptation (Mrazek, 1986). Substantial evidence exists to suggest that a single hospitalization, particularly if sensitively handled, has relatively minimal impact on long-term development (Quinton and Rutter, 1976). However, as is true with many stress factors, multiple exposure can greatly increase the potential negative impact of the experience. A complex multivariate model designed to analyze the impact of hospitalization should include five sets of variables: (a) the nature of the disease, (b) the nature of the hospital experience, (c) the sociocultural context of the hospitalization, (d) the adaptive abilities of the parents, and (e) the child's capacity to cope with the illness. Developmental considerations are particularly important. While little evidence exists that very early hospitalization occurring within the first 6 months of life is associated with later difficulty, a number of studies over the years have suggested that a child between 1 and 4 years of age may be particularly sensitive (Illingworth and Holt, 1955; Mrazek et al., 1985; Prugh et al., 1953). Many developmental features contribute to this being a more vulnerable period, including (a) the reality that the parent is perceived as the primary attachment figure but is often unable to modulate the experience of hospitalization, resulting in a stress on the primary caregiving relationship; (b) the child's wish to establish a sense of independence and autonomy at this time, which is often undermined by the passive, dependent position required during the hospitalization; and (c) the child's preoperational cognitive abilities. This last factor results in the inability to rely on therapeutic strategies based on concrete cognitive operations that include the effective use of anticipatory preparation.

The response of the parents to hospitalization remains one of the critical clinical considerations. The basic objective during acute hospitalizations is to provide a sense of emotional security for the child. To the degree that the parents are unable to cope with their own anxieties about the child's illness, they will have limitations on their ability to modulate the experience for the child. It is critical for parents to take an active role in providing emotional support. This includes the realization that their physical presence is important, as well as is their providing some "emotional translation" of the sometimes bewildering experiences that can be particularly frightening to a preschool child. This is best accomplished by assuming a proactive stance. Even in a maximally sensitive hospital, the emotional needs of a child in a medical crisis will necessarily take a back seat to what is perceived as the primary mission of the pediatric team, providing state-of-the-art intensive medical treatment. In this climate, the parent is often the critical link between the system and the child. It is often advisable for the medical team to encourage parents to assume this role and become a partner in the provision of their child's care. If they can successfully achieve this goal, it is often an effective method of coping with their own anxiety.

Much attention has been focused on the protective factors that mediate the frightening and painful aspects of hospitalization. The evolution of Child Life programs is a good example of the development of protective strategies. The alliance between the medical team and the family is of central importance. A trusting and communicative relationship with the pediatrician will decrease the anxiety level of both parents and child. This trust can be potentiated by nurses, who have become increasingly sophisticated in being able to identify parents who are having difficulties with coping and are able to organize nursing plans that include emotional support for the family. An example of this approach is consciously organizing the management of painful procedures to maximize the support of the parents while minimizing the association between the pain and presence of the parents.

The child psychiatrist providing pediatric liaison is a critical part of the treatment team. In addition to the classic role of diagnostician and therapist able to intervene at moments of family crisis, child psychiatrists have increasingly taken a proactive role in the development of systems designed to help families deal with the experience of hospitalization. One very specific aspect of this role is the responsibility of ensuring both cognitive and emotional understanding of the implications of medical procedures and the prognosis of the illness. All too often, misunderstandings about medical care can arise that lead to major disruptions in the emotional equilibrium of the child. Ensuring that both the family and the child have a good understanding of the need for medical procedures and the implications of proceeding in a particular clinical direction is a cornerstone of appropriate care for ill children.

In analyzing the impact of hospitalization on an individual child, two variables are basic. These are the severity of illness and the duration of the discomfort of necessary therapeutic procedures. Minde et al. (1982, 1983) developed a morbidity scale to monitor these variables in infants. This approach highlights the specific needs of some families, who may cope well during early phases of an illness but become worn down in the face of what eventually becomes a prolonged and overwhelming experience.

Several specific aspects of hospital organization of pediatric services facilitate this process. Ensuring that attachment figures can be available to younger children throughout the hospitalization is of central importance. Other factors that minimize the negative impact of long hospital stays include (a) the opportunity to have educational and tutorial experiences that ensure minimal delays or problems in learning; (b) maintenance of close contact between support figures, particularly friends and classmates; and (c) development of a supportive peer network with other children who also require prolonged hospitalization.

SUMMARY

In conceptualizing the impact of chronic medical conditions on child development, it is helpful to integrate the stressful aspects of illness into

Table 103.2. Illness-Specific Risk Factors

1. Onset	Particularly difficult developmental periods include early childhood (6 months to 5 years) and early adolescence.	
2. Etiology	Illnesses that are the result of some environmental exposure (trauma or infection) or inherited genes provide specific stressors on the family.	
3. Diagnosis	Prolonged delay in diagnosis or misdiagnosis have a negative impact on the family-doctor relationship.	
4. Deformity	Physical deformity and disability negatively influence both the development of self-image and availability of support.	
5. Prognosis	The more negative the prognosis, the greater the risk posed to adaptive emotional development.	

a broader systems perspective on early childhood adaptation. Similarly, both illness-specific and nonspecific protective factors must be considered. This approach is somewhat of a compromise between the general position that all chronic illnesses have a similar impact on development and the most specific view that a particular set of emotional conflicts are related to each individual disease. There actually seems to be some truth in both views. Illnesses that have a long, unremitting course share characteristics, as do illnesses with uncertain prognoses, with early onset, and with parallel etiologies. To the degree that the illness-specific characteristics of various diseases are similar, their emotional sequelae should be similar (Table 103.2).

RESEARCH DIRECTIONS

The need to have ongoing prospective longitudinal studies is overwhelmingly apparent in a review of the multiple cross-sectional studies of physically ill children. When considering problems with a genetic etiology, the optimal plan would be to recruit a sample of children prior to the onset of illness and follow them longitudinally. Where illnesses have more spontaneous onsets, the best approach is a study that is designed to follow children after initial diagnosis. Any prospective longitudinal study should include the documentation of not only the key characteristics of the illness itself but also of the familial risk and protective factors that simultaneously influence development. Through the judicious examination of how these factors interact, it is probable that primary prevention strategies can be developed to minimize the emotional sequelae of physical illness. Given the prevalent nature of these problems, the implications of early intervention for physically ill children are of substantial public health importance.

References

Barglow P, Berndt DJ, Burns WI, et al: Neuroendocrine and psychological factors in childhood diabetes mellitus. *J Am Acad Child Psychiatry* 25:785–793, 1986.

Blair C, Cull A, Freeman CP: Psychosocial functioning of young adults with cystic fibrosis and their families. *Thorax* 49:798–802, 1994.

Brewster AB: Chronically ill hospitalized children's concepts of their illness. *Pediatrics* 69:355–362, 1982.

Brouwers P, Riccardi R, Poplack D, et al: Attentional deficits in long-term survivors of childhood acute lymphoblastic leukemia (ALL). *J Clin Neuropsychol* 6:325–336, 1984.

Burke P, Meyer V, Kocoshis S, et al: Obsessive-compulsive symptoms in childhood inflammatory bowel disease and cystic fibrosis. *J Am Acad Child Adolesc Psychiatry* 28:525–527, 1989.

Burrows J, Jennings PH, Harvey E, et al: Association of asthma with serum IgE levels and skin-test reactivity to allergens. *N Engl J Med* 26:307–320, 1989.

Canning EH: Mental disorders in chronically ill children: Case identification and parent-child discrepancy. *Psychosom Med* 56:104–108, 1994.

Chase HP, Jackson GG: Stress and sugar control in children with insulin-dependent diabetes mellitus. *J Pediatr* 98:1011–1013, 1981.

Eiser C: Psychological development of the child with leukemia: A review. *J Behav Med* 2:141–157, 1979.

Falliers C: Treatment of asthma in a residential center. *J Allergy Clin Immunol* 28:513–521, 1970.

Fonagy P, Moran GS, Lindsay, MKM, et al: Psychological adjustment and diabetic control. *Arch Dis Child* 62:1009–1013, 1987.

Gath A, Smith MA, Baum DJ: Emotional, behavioural, and educational disorders in diabetic children. *Arch Dis Child* 55:371–375, 1980.

Golden MP, Ingersoll GM, Brack CI, et al: Longitudinal relationship of asymptomatic hypoglycemia to cognitive function in IDDM. *Diabetes Care* 12:89–93, 1989.

Greenberg HS, Kazak AE, Meadows AT: Psychologic functioning in 8- to 16-year old cancer survivors and their parents. *J Pediatr* 114:488–493, 1989.

Greig E, Betts T: Epileptic seizures induced by sexual abuse. Pathogenic and pathoplastic factors. *Seizure* 1(4):269–274, 1992.

Gustafsson PA, Cederblad M, Ludvigsson I, et al:

Family interaction and metabolic balance in juvenile diabetes mellitus. A prospective study. *Diabetes Res Clin Pract* 4:7–14, 1987.

Harrison RM, Taylor DC: Childhood seizures: A 25-year follow-up. *Lancet* 1:948–951, 1976.

Haupt R, Fears TR, Robison LL, et al: Educational attainment in long-term survivors of childhood acute lymphoblastic leukemia. *JAMA* 272:1427–1432, 1994.

Heatherington EM: Coping with family transitions: Winners, losers, and survivors. *Child Dev* 60:1–14, 1989.

Hermann BP, Whitman S, Wyler AR, et al: Psychosocial predictors of psychopathology in epilepsy. *Br J Psychiatry* 156:98–105, 1990.

Hoare P, Kerley S: Psychosocial adjustment of children with chronic epilepsy and their families. *Dev Med Child Neurol* 33:201–215, 1991.

Howe G, Feinstein C, Reiss D, et al: Adolescent adjustment to chronic physical disorders—I. Comparing neurological and non-neurological conditions. *J Child Psychol Psychiat* 34:1153–1171, 1993.

Illingworth RS, Holt KS: Children in hospital: Some observations or, their reactions with special reference to daily visiting. *Lancet* 271(2):1257–1262, 1955.

Kalins IV, Churchill MP, Terry GE: Concurrent stresses in families with a leukemic child. *J Pediatr Psychol* 5:81–92, 1980.

Koocher GP, O'Malley JE (eds): *The Damocles Syndrome.* New York, McGraw-Hill, 1981.

Kovacs M, Feinberg TL, Paulauskas S, et al: Initial coping responses and psychosocial characteristics of children with insulin-dependent diabetes mellitus. *J Pediatr* 106:827–834, 1985.

Kovacs M, Obrosky DS, Stiffler L: Biomedical and psychosocial predictors of early rehospitalization among children with insulin-dependent diabetes mellitus: A longitudinal study. *Pediatr Ann* 23:(6):300–305, 1994.

Kupst MJ, Schulman JL, Maurer H, et al: Coping with pediatric leukemia: A two-year follow-up. *J Pediatr Psychol* 9:149–163, 1984.

Levine S, Stern R: Sexual function in cystic fibrosis. Relationship to overall health status and pulmonary disease severity in 30 married patients. *Chest* 81:422–428, 1982.

Minde K, Perrotta M, Orter C: The effect of neonatal complications in same-sexed premature twins on their mother's preference. *J Am Acad Child Adolesc Psychiatry* 21:445–452, 1982.

Minde K, Whitelaw A, Brown J, et al: The effects of neonatal complications in premature infants on early parent-infant interactions. *Dev Med Child Neurol* 25:763–777, 1983.

Moehle KA, Berg RA: Academic achievement and intelligence test performance in children with cancer at diagnosis and one year later. *Dev Behav Pediatr* 6:62–64, 1985.

Moran GS: Psychoanalytic treatment of diabetic children. In: Solnit AJ, Eissler RS, Neubauer PB (eds): *The Psychoanalytic Study of the Child.* New Haven, CT, Yale University Press, 1984, pp. 407–447.

Mrazek DA: Pediatric hospitalization: Understanding the stress on families from a developmental perspective. In: Christie M (ed): *The Psychosomatic Approach: Contemporary Practice of Whole-Person Care.* Cichester: Wiley, 1986, pp. 91–111.

Mrazek DA: Asthma: Psychiatric considerations, evaluation, and management. In: Middleton E, Reed CE, Ellis EF (eds): *Allergy: Principles and Practice* (3rd ed). St. Louis, Mosby, 1988, pp. 1176–1196.

Mrazek DA: Psychosomatic processes and physical illnesses. In: Zeanah C (ed): *Handbook of Infant Mental Health.* New York: Guilford, 1993, pp. 350–358.

Mrazek DA, Anderson IS, Strunk RC: Disturbed emotional development of severely asthmatic preschool children. *J Child Psychol Psychiatry* 26(suppl 4):81–94, 1985.

Mrazek DA, Klinnert M, Brower A, et al: Predictive capacity of elevated serum IgE for early asthma onset. *J Clin Immunol* 85:194, 1990.

Mrazek DA, Klinnert M, Mrazek P, et al: Early asthma onset: Consideration of parenting issues. *J Am Acad Child Adolesc Psychiatry* 30:277–282, 1991.

Mrazek PI, Mrazek DA: Resilience in child maltreatment victims: A conceptual exploration. *Child Abuse Negl* 11:357–366, 1987.

Mulhern RK, Crisco II, Camitta BM: Patterns of communication among pediatric patients with leukemia, parents, and physicians: Prognostic disagreements and misunderstandings. *J Pediatr* 99:480–483, 1981.

Pavlovsky S, Castano J, Leiguarda R, et al: Neuropsychological study in patients with ALL. *Am J Pediatr Hematol Oncol* 5:79–86, 1983.

Petzel SV, Bugge I, Warwick WJ, et al: Long term adaptation of children and adolescents with cystic fibrosis: Identification of common problems and risk factors. In: Blum RW (ed): *Chronic Illness and Disabilities in Childhood and Adolescence.* Orlando, FL, Grune & Stratton, 1984, pp. 413–427.

Prugh DG, Straub EM, Sands HH, et al: A study of the emotional reactions of children and families to hospitalization and illness. *Am J Ortho Psychiatry* 23:70–106, 1953.

Quinton D, Rutter M: Early hospital admissions and later disturbances of behaviour: An attempted replication of Douglas' findings. *Dev Med Child Neurol* 18:447–459, 1976.

Quittner AL, DiGirolamo AM, Michel M, et al: Parental response to cystic fibrosis: A contextual analysis of the diagnosis phase. *J Pediatr Psychol* 17:683–704, 1992.

Rait DS, Ostroff JS, Smith K, et al: Lives in a balance: Perceived family functioning and the psychosocial adjustment of adolescent cancer survivors. *Fam Proc* 31:383–397, 1992.

Rutter M, Garmezy N: Developmental Psychopathology. In: Mussen PH (ed): *Handbook of Child Psychology: Vol. 4. Socialization, Personality and Social Development* (4th ed). New York, John Wiley & Sons, 1983, pp. 775–911.

Rutter M, Graham P, Yule W: *A Neuropsychiatric Study in Childhood* (Clinics in Developmental Medicine Nos. 35/36). London, Heinemann/Spastics International Medical Publications, 1970.

Sawyer M, Crettenden A, Toogood I: Psychological adjustment of families of children and adolescents treated for leukemia. *Am J Pediatr Hematol Oncol* 8:200–207, 1986.

Sawyer MG, Toogood I, Rise M, et al: School performance and psychological adjustment of children treated for leukemia. *Am J Pediatr Hematol Oncol* 11:146–152, 1989.

Schoenborn CA, Marano M: *Current Estimates from the National Health Interview Survey: United States, 1987* (Vital and Health Statistics, Series 10, No. 166. DHHS Pub. No. (PHS) 88-1594). Washington, DC, US Government Printing Office, 1988.

Seidman-Ripley J, Bound V, Andermann F, et al: Psychosocial consequences of postoperative seizure relief. *Epilepsia* 34:248–254, 1993.

Stehbens JA, Kisker CT: Intelligence and achievement testing in childhood cancer: Three years postdiagnosis. *Dev Behav Pediatr* 5:184–188, 1984.

Steinhausen H, Schindler H, Stephan H: Correlates of psychopathology in sick children. An empirical model. *J Am Acad Child Psychiatry* 22:552, 1983.

Strunk RC, Mrazek DA, Fukuhara JT, et al: Physiologic and psychological characteristics associated with deaths due to asthma in childhood. *JAMA* 254:1193–1198, 1985.

Strunk RC, Mrazek DA, Fukuhara JT, et al: Cardiovascular fitness in children with asthma correlates with psychologic functioning of the child. *Pediatrics* 84:460–464, 1989.

Taussig L, Cohen M, Sieber O Jr: Psychosexual and psychosocial aspects of cystic fibrosis. *Med Aspects Hum Sex* 10:101–102, 1976.

Taylor DC: Epilepsy and prejudice. *Arch Dis Child* 62:209–211, 1987.

Thompson RJ, Gustafson KE, George LK, et al: Change over a 12-month period in the psychological adjustment of children and adolescents with cystic fibrosis. *J Pediatr Psychol* 19:189–203, 1994.

Thompson RJ, Gustafson KE, Meghdadpour S, et al: The role of biomedical and psychosocial processes in the intellectual and academic functioning of children and adolescents with cystic fibrosis. *J Clin Psychol* 48:3–10, 1992.

Venters M: Familial coping with chronic and severe childhood illness. The case of cystic fibrosis. *Soc Sci Med* 15A:289–297, 1981.

Weist MD, Finney JW, Barnard MU, et al: Empirical selection of psychosocial treatment targets for children and adolescents with diabetes. *J Pediatr Psychol* 18(1):11–28, 1993.

White K, Kolman ML, Wexler P, et al: Unstable diabetes and unstable families: A psychosocial evaluation of diabetic children with recurrent ketoacidosis. *Pediatrics* 73:749–755, 1984.

Wilkinson G: The influence of psychiatric, psychological and social factors on the control of insulin-dependent diabetes mellitus. *J Psychosom Res* 31:277–286, 1987.

104 DYING AND DEATH IN CHILDHOOD AND ADOLESCENCE

Melvin Lewis, M.B., B.S., F.R.C.Psych., D.C.H., Dorothy Otnow Lewis, M.D., and David J. Schonfeld, M.D.

Dying is a transitional state during which the child and the family may look to the physician for understanding, support, and direction. However, a physician may experience anxiety in the presence of a dying child because of (*a*) the feelings of impotence, failure, and anxiety that are aroused in a physician when confronted with his or her own limitations and mortality, (*b*) the regressive pull the child's loneliness, abandonment, neediness, and insecurity evoke in the physician, and (*c*) the difficulty of dealing with the parents' anxiety, depression, anger, resentment, and denial.

Yet there is probably almost nothing that the child or parent fears, imagines, feels, or experiences that cannot be discussed with the child in an honest way. The basis for the discussion is a trusting relationship.

Children in particular soon learn whom they can trust and hence to whom they can open up. Indeed, the child often senses more accurately what the adult can tolerate than the adult senses how much the child can assimilate, and the child acts accordingly.

CHILDREN'S CONCEPTS OF DEATH

The child's reaction to his or her own dying or the death of others is related in part to his or her concept of death (Schonfeld, 1993), which in turn is related to the child's developmental stage (Table 104.1).

The stages in the child's understanding of the concepts of death have been well studied (Hostler, 1978; Kastenbaum, 1967; Smilansky, 1987; Speece and Brent, 1984; Wass, 1984). Four major concepts related to death have been noted consistently: irreversibility, finality (also termed nonfunctionality), causality, and inevitability (also termed universality). Failure to comprehend each of these concepts impairs the child's ability to mourn successfully (Table 104.2). Speece and Brent (1984), in a recent review of the literature, concluded that most studies found the age of acquisition of the three concepts they reviewed (irreversibility, nonfunctionality, and universality) to occur between 5 and 7 years; earlier studies citing an older age of acquisition were typically noted to have significant procedural flaws.

During the first few years, the child ordinarily has virtually no con- cept of death other than that of a disappearance. However, when faced with traumatic events, such as the death of a parent, children under the age of 5 may develop what seems to be a precocious understanding of death. In general, the role of personal exposure to death of others has been controversial; although several studies have shown that such personal experience may promote the acquisition of the concepts of death (Kane, 1979; Reilly et al., 1983), other studies have failed to support this conclusion (Jenkins and Cavanaugh, 1986; Townley and Thornburg, 1980). Cross-cultural comparisons (Florian and Kravetz, 1985; Schonfeld and Smilansky, 1989; Wass et al., 1979) have also illustrated significant cultural variations and important cross-cultural consistencies, suggesting that although the underlying developmental framework is likely to be robust across cultures, various sociocultural variables may have a significant and profound impact on the rate of acquisition of important individual concepts.

Children between 5 and 10 years of age (approximately) continue to clarify their concepts of death but are still at times confused. For example, a child may say, "When I die, my heart stops, I can't see, and I can't hear. But if I'm buried, how will I breathe?" Some of the child's difficulty in thinking clearly about death is developmental, but some of the difficulty is emotional. If the child of this age has a heightened concern about a part of his or her body and its functioning, the child may tend to think of death in terms of the harm to that part of his

Table 104.1. Death and Childhood

	Before		During			After		
			Sudden	Acute	Chronic			
Child	Ideas on death	Death and stage anxieties						
0–5	Abandonment Punishment	Fear of loss of love	Avoidance of pain Need for love	Withdrawal Separation anxiety				
5–10	Concept of inevitability Confusion	Castration anxiety	Guilt (bad) Regression Denial	Guilt (religious) Regression, Denial				
10–15	Reality	Control of body and other developmental tasks	Depression Despair for future	Depression Despair, anxiety, anger				
	Sudden	Acute	Chronic			Sudden	Acute	Chronic
Parents		Anxiety Concern Hopefulness	Premature mourning, anticipatory grief, guilt, reaction formation and displacements, need for information	Disbelief Displaced rage Accelerated grief Prolonged numbness	Desperate concern Denial Guilt	Denial Remorse Resurgence of love	Guilt Mourning	Anger at M.D., need for follow-up, overidealizing, fantasy loss	Remorse Relief and guilt
Siblings 0–5	Reactions to changes in parent (sense of loss of love and withdrawal)					1. Respond to reaction of parents		
5–10	Concern re: their implication Fearful for themselves					2. Survivor guilt		
10–15	Generally supportive							
Staff	Anxiety Conspiracy of silence		Reaction: Withdraw Tasks 1. Correct distortions, e.g., "Am I safe?"; Will someone be with me?''; ''Will I be helped to feel better?'' 2. Comfort parents. 3. Allow hope and promote feelings of actively coping. 4. Protect dignity of patient.			Need for after-care of survivors Autopsy request tact Accurate information regarding disposal of body Delay billing		

From Lewis M, Clinical aspects of child development. Philadelphia: Lea & Febiger, 1982, pp. 326–327.

Table 104.2. Concepts of Death and Implications of Incomplete Understanding for Adjustment to Loss

1. *Irreversibility*
   Death is seen as a permanent phenomenon from which there is no recovery or return.
   Example of incomplete understanding:
   The child expects the deceased to return, as if from a trip.
   Implication:
   Failure to comprehend this concept prevents the child from engaging in the process of detachment from the deceased, a necessary first step in successful mourning.
2. *Finality (Nonfunctionality):*
   Death is seen as a state in which *all* life functions cease *completely.*
   Example of incomplete understanding:
   The child worries about a buried relative being cold or in pain; the child wishes to bury food with the deceased.
   Implication:
   May lead to preoccupation with physical suffering of the deceased and may impair readjustment.
3. *Inevitability (Universality):*
   Death is seen as a natural phenomenon that no living being can escape indefinitely.
   Example of incomplete understanding:
   The child views significant individuals (i.e., self, parents) as immortal.
   Implication:
   If the child does not view death as inevitable, he or she is likely to view death as a punishment (either for actions or thoughts of the child or the deceased), leading to excessive guilt and shame.
4. *Causality:*
   The child develops a realistic understanding of the causes of death.
   Example of incomplete understanding:
   The child who relies on magical thinking is apt to assume responsibility for death of a loved one by assuming bad thoughts or unrelated actions were causative.
   Implication:
   Tends to lead to excessive guilt that is difficult for the child to resolve.

Adapted from Schonfeld D. Crisis intervention for bereavement support: A model of intervention in the children's school. *Clin Pediatr* 1989;28:29.

or her body and its functioning, especially since the child also tends to think in concrete terms at this stage. Children in this age group with a terminal illness have been shown to have a marked awareness of the seriousness of their illness, even if never told that their illness is fatal, and a precocious understanding of personal mortality (Clunies-Ross and Lansdown, 1988; Spinetta, 1974).

Somewhere between 10 and 15 years of age, the average child acquires a grasp of the meaning of mortality (Kastenbaum, 1959). The child's reaction to death at this time is influenced more by his or her emotional struggles than by the child's intellectual capacities. Thus a young adolescent who is concerned with, among other things, sexual performance, control of impulses, physical intactness, and separation from parents may react with anxiety if any one of these sensitive conflict areas is involved in the fatal illness.

THE CHILD'S REACTION TO HIS OR HER OWN DYING

The very young child is mostly preoccupied with the discomfort of the illness, whether acute or chronic, and the separation and withdrawal that occur when hospitalization is necessary. A somewhat older child, although also troubled by pain and separation, interprets his or her illness according to his or her level of cognitive development and emotional conflicts. Thus he or she may interpret the illness as an act of "immanent justice" for the guilt he or she feels about some real or imagined misdeed. Usually the child shows regressive behavior in the face of the illness, hospitalization, and its treatment, and a fear of mutilation. Occasionally the child shows a denial of discomfort or dread (Solnit, 1965; Solnit and Green, 1959). An older child who is aware of the irreversibility of death may deny his or her own anxiety but may exhibit a depression, occasionally mixed with outbursts of anger and anxiety. This reaction is especially common in adolescents. On the other hand, some children are astoundingly courageous and steadfast in the face of death.

The range of reactions is great. In a sense, all that has gone before contributes to the child's understanding of death and his or her reaction

to it. Each child is an individual, and a myriad of variables influence the behavior of the child, the family, and the helping persons around the child.

REACTIONS OF OTHERS TO THE DEATH OF A CHILD

An important determinant of children's reaction to death is the reaction of those around them to death. Those others may be parents, siblings, or hospital staff members.

Reaction of Parents

GENERAL REACTIONS

The general reactions of parents have a chronological sequence, starting before and continuing during and after the moment of death. Initial shock and denial of the diagnosis may last from a few seconds to a few months. This stage may be followed by anger ("Why my child?") or guilt ("If only I had. . . ."). Sooner or later, the parent starts to bargain ("If he could only live to. . . ."). This stage is followed by normal grieving and mourning over the impending loss and by the beginning of separation. Finally, a stage of resignation or acceptance can be reached.

SPECIFIC REACTIONS

Reactions to a Rapid Death

When the death has occurred relatively rapidly (e.g., perhaps as a consequence of a brief illness), the period prior to death is filled with anxiety and concern. (For a discussion of sudden infant death syndrome [SIDS], see Chapter 93.) The parents may be desperately hopeful, but they may also have feelings of guilt and a need to deny the possibility of death as an eventual outcome. After a rapid death of their child, the parents may again feel some diffuse anger, which may be displaced onto the physician. This reaction may occur whether or not the physician has been diligent, but it is more likely to fester and be prolonged if the physician fails (out of his or her own discomfort) to show consideration at the time and to provide the opportunity for a follow-up interview. Over a period of time the parents will then go through their own characteristic mourning process. Their mourning may include some identification with the lost person and, occasionally, an overidealizing of the lost person (particularly in cases in which the parent also experiences the loss of what they had expected for the lost child). Further possible normal reactions (within limits) may include (a) a displacement of attitudes toward the dead child onto one or more of the surviving children, (b) attempts to fill the loss by another pregnancy, or (c) withdrawal for a time. These and other normal reactions, in general, should be respected and left alone. Extreme forms of defenses may be dysfunctional and are an indication for therapy (Krell and Rabkin, 1979).

Reactions to Prolonged Dying

Occasionally, premature mourning may occur, with anticipatory grief and withdrawal of interest in the dying child, perhaps accompanied by the displacement of warm feelings onto an infant child in the family. Often, unacceptable thoughts arise. For example, a parent may find himself or herself wishing that the child would finally die and relieve everyone of the emotional and financial burden and suffering. Such a wish may horrify a parent and lead to the immediate mobilization of certain defense mechanisms. A common defense mechanism is that of reaction formation: The parent becomes extraprotective in caring for the dying child. The parent may also feel guilty and express his or her guilt (and anxiety) by asking repetitive questions that require tactful answers.

As a chronically ill child nears death, the parents may be filled with remorse and may experience a resurgence of love. Rarely, a denial that death is imminent may remain in force. After the death of a chronically ill child, parents may feel a mixture of relief and guilt, perhaps with feelings of remorse being uppermost.

Reactions of Siblings

Siblings who are very young, especially those under the age of 5, feel the withdrawal of the parent intensely and consequently feel a loss of love. Young siblings may view the death as an abandonment, as punishment, as the realization of unacceptable wishes, or as all three. Children between about 5 and 10 years of age generally are somewhat more concerned for the dying child and may also be fearful for themselves. Although it is expected that older children usually can muster a supportive attitude and temporarily assume parental roles for the younger siblings at home, even teenagers feel and react to parental withdrawal and may ''act up'' during such a trying time. They too require special attention (Adams and Deveau, 1987). Children as well as adults may experience survivor guilt after the death of a child (Lifton, 1967). Some surviving children suffer serious symptoms and subsequent distortions of character structure (Cain et al., 1964). Through identification with the deceased, felt to be more common and dramatic in children than in adults, surviving children may also manifest conversion symptoms. In one series of conversion disorders in children, 58% were associated with unresolved grief reactions (Maloney, 1980).

Reactions of the Hospital Staff

Hospital staff members also experience anxiety in the presence of a dying child or a grieving parent (Solnit and Green, 1959), and they tend sometimes to deal with that anxiety by withdrawal and a conspiracy of silence. These reactions may hamper them from giving the dying child and his or her family the best care possible and may prevent the staff members from carrying out certain essential psychological tasks. Besides comforting the parents, such tasks include helping the child feel as active as possible in his or her attempts to cope with anxiety and allowing the child some hope. Furthermore, the privacy and dignity of the child require protection. Last, certain distortions require correction. The child, for example, may show his or her concern by asking such questions as ''Am I safe?'' ''Will someone be with me when I need them?'' ''Will I be helped to feel better?'' The need for tact carries through into the period of care for the survivors.

Survivors outside of the family will also need assistance in dealing with their grief. Psychiatrists are not infrequently consulted to provide crisis intervention for bereavement support in settings outside of the hospital, such as in the schools. Different techniques are often required to provide this type of intervention service and are described elsewhere (Schonfeld, 1989; Schonfeld and Kline, 1994).

CLINICAL CARE OF THE DYING CHILD

Talking with the Parents about Fatal Illness

The hardest task for the physician is to tell the parents that their child is fatally ill. The physician should take the parents into a private office and allow at the very least half an hour, uninterrupted by telephone calls or other tasks. He or she can begin by telling the parents the diagnosis and the nature of the illness. He or she might then go on to describe the treatment that is available to offer some relief for the child's symptoms. At some point, the physician will have to tell the parents that there is no treatment that can cure the child of the illness. Throughout this interview the physician should pause and give the parents every opportunity to express their feelings and ask questions. The physician must resist an understandable impulse to ''shut off'' the parents' grief. If the parents ask whether the child will die from the illness, the physician will have to say that the child will. If they do not ask, the physician should at some point attempt to clarify that the illness is progressive and that the child will die. At the same time, the physician must remember that the parents will not necessarily understand or accept what they have been told.

The physician should not end the interview then but should stay with the parents as they experience their shock (and perhaps anger) and grief.

The physician might then tell the parents how he or she plans to treat the child and help the parents feel some measure of participation in and control of the treatment.

The physician is obliged to tell the parents what to expect as the illness progresses. This information need not be given in full in the first interview; rather, it should be given in stages over an extended period. The goal is to give the parents information that will enable them to anticipate the child's needs at each stage. The parents usually will indicate by their questions what they need to know.

Regular contact with the parents should then be planned. The contact should take the form not of comments made in passing but of time set aside to talk, review, and listen in the privacy of an office. The physician should resist the natural impulse to avoid the parents or avoid the subject. In order to do this, the physician must recognize any impotence and anger he or she may feel in the face of death. The parents will come to trust the physician and feel safe expressing, if they so wish, some of their less acceptable feelings if they are sure that the physician is available and ready to listen. During these planned interviews, the physician can discuss with the parents their child's behavior, their management of the child, what to tell the child's siblings, and whether and in what way the parents would like their minister, priest, or rabbi involved. The parents should be reassured about their own handling of the situation, and the physician should feel free to share admiration for how well they are meeting the child's needs.

The physician may be asked for advice about religious rites for the sick. The practice of offering prayer with the child or administering the Sacrament of the Sick, although intended to comfort, may be anxiety arousing. Although it sometimes happens that the Sacrament of the Sick is given without the parents' consent, or even knowledge, most priests prefer to involve the parents and family first, and to have the family present in the room. However, administering the Sacrament of the Sick may cause as much upset in the family as in the child. The 1972 modification of the Sacrament of the Sick (''Ordo Unctionis,'' 1972) does not alter very much the way in which the child might experience the ritual. Indeed, there are no specific modifications for children other than those based on the judgment of the particular priest. The physician should discuss with the parents and the priest the child's needs and how the child might experience the praying or the Sacrament before any step is undertaken.

Talking with the Child

In regard to talking about death with the sick child, especially the young sick child, the parents' feelings and wishes must be respected. Some parents, for example, do not wish the child to be told that he or she is going to die, whereas others do. Some families need to use denial as a protective device.

There is no simple answer to the question of whether or not the particular child should be told. One useful approach is to discuss with the parents how they think they would respond if their dying child asked them whether he or she was going to die. There are several stages of response to such a question that might be suggested.

First, the child's reason for asking the question must be clarified. The child may be responding to the parents' or the hospital staff's anxious behavior, or the child may be concerned about such things as pain, mutilation, loneliness, and the needs of others. The child then can be given repeated opportunities to talk about what he or she is worried about.

Second, if the parents decide that they want the child to know that his or her illness is fatal, the process of telling the child about the illness and impending death should have the characteristics of a dialogue rather than of an announcement. Some children simply cannot understand and do not want to hear the truth; they should not be told. Others have to arrive slowly at the realization of the significance of their illness; it is too much for them to understand and grasp at one time.

Third, the child must be given hope. Even when the child is told that the illness is one that causes death, the child can and should be told that the physicians will do everything they can to fight the illness.

The adults must agree not only on how the child should be told but also on *who* should be the first to tell him or her. Sometimes the physician is not the right person to disclose this information. A parent or a member of the clergy who is close to the child may have a more sensitive understanding of the child's needs.

A discussion of this kind with parents often helps them to express some of their own concerns. It also promotes in them a feeling of trust and of being understood, as well as a feeling that they have some control over the care of their child. Nothing is so painful to the parents as their feeling of helplessness as their child's life ebbs.

Most important, the physician who has had a dialogue with the parents is prepared to have a dialogue with the child, always keeping in close touch with the parents. The physician, for example, can convey assurance while imparting to the child as much of the truth as the parents want and the child seems ready to know. There is no blueprint answer.

The ward staff members should be clear about who has the primary responsibility for talking with the parents and child about the seriousness of the illness. If it has been agreed on by the parents that the physician should talk with the child, the physician should first establish a relationship of trust with the child. Before the physician talks with the child, he or she should make sure that someone is available to be with the child after the physician has left the room, if the child so desires. The involved staff members should be informed about how much the child knows about the illness so that the child does not receive conflicting and therefore puzzling information. Ward staff members also experience anxiety when in the presence of a dying child or such a child's family. Their natural inclination to avoid these feelings may cause them to stay away from both the child and the grieving family. Such inclinations may be better controlled if the ward staff members have the opportunity to explore and share their feelings in meetings (Berman and Villarreal, 1983; Lewis, 1962).

Specific Management of the Child Who Is Dying

Kübler-Ross (1972) gives a beautiful description of a dying boy's expression of his thoughts and feelings:

[The dying] boy tried to paint what he felt like. He drew a huge tank and in front of the barrel was a tiny little figure with a stop sign in his hand. This to me represents the fear of death, the fear of the catastrophic, destructive force that comes upon you and you cannot do anything about it. If you can respond to him by saying it must be terrible to feel so tiny and this thing is so big, he may be able to verbally express a sense of smallness or impotence or rage. The next picture he drew was a beautiful bird flying up in the sky. A little bit of its upper wing was painted gold. When he was asked what this was, the boy said it was the peace bird flying up into the sky with a little bit of sunshine on its wing. It was the last picture he painted before he died. I think these are picture expressions of a stage of anger and the final stage of acceptance.

This description underscores the importance of one aspect of the care of the dying child: With the parents' permission and in the privacy of his or her own room, the young child should be given the opportunity on different occasions to express his or her concerns through drawings or through play with toys and dolls (Figs. 104.1 and 104.2).

If needed, and if the parents agree, the collaboration of a child psychiatrist here can be very helpful. The opportunity for expressive play may enable the child to exercise some control over his or her anxiety. If the child expresses concern about such problems as pain, loneliness, and fear through this play this fact should be noted mentally by the pediatrician or child psychiatrist. At another time, the child could be reassured, without reference to the play session, that the physicians will make sure that he or she does not have pain, that there will always be someone available to help him or her, and that everything will be done to help him or her feel better.

Patients—adults and children alike—feel threatened by the passivity imposed on them by illness. Every effort must be made to give the child a feeling of active participation in treatment. The child should be

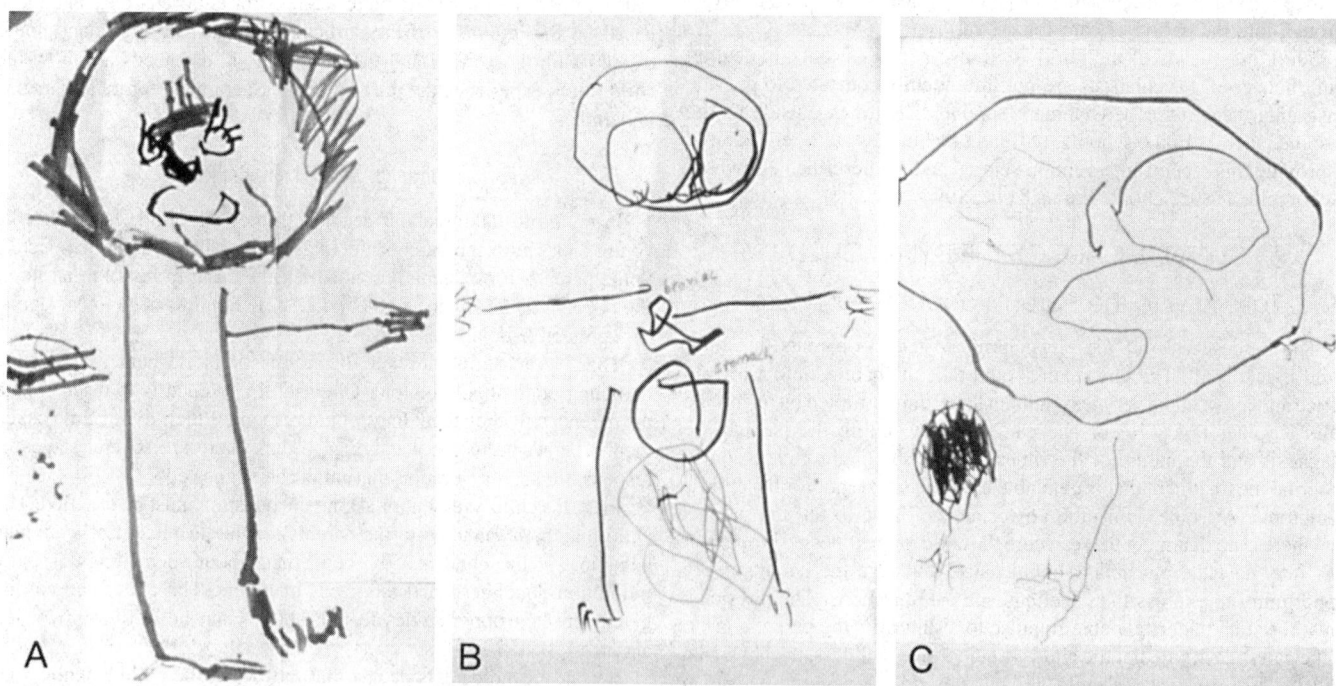

Figure 104.1. Self-portraits done by a 4-year-old female hospitalized with osteosarcoma. **A,** Self-portrait drawn within the 1st week of diagnosis. The body is intact; it is a very positive body image (i.e., profuse facial and body details, including eyelashes and hair). **B,** This portrait was drawn about a month after diagnosis. The patient was still hospitalized. Note the disintegration: The body is no longer intact, and the Broviac is highlighted, as is her stomach (she was experiencing nausea, and her Broviac became a prominent part of her experience of her body). **C,** This last drawing was done a week before death. Note the tumor looming largely in the picture. She died 3 months after diagnosis.

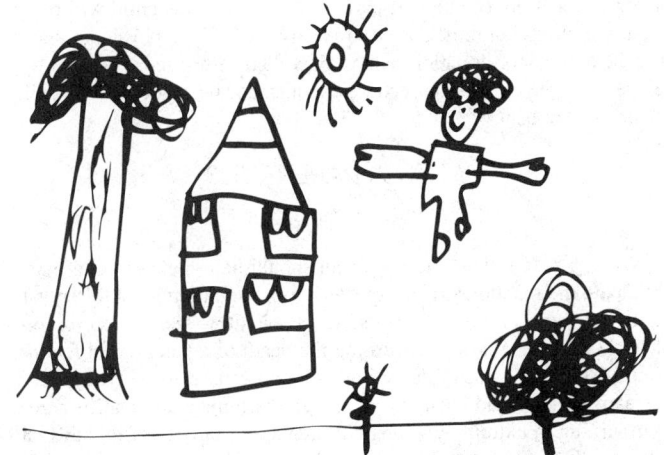

Figure 104.2. Self-portrait drawn by a school-age hospitalized patient dying of AIDS. The drawing expresses the child's sadness, isolation, and fears of death associated with this illness. The picture was drawn in black, and noteworthy are the major objects that appear to be floating in space with no roots, no foundation, and no sense of security. The house without a door offers no entrance or exit, implying perhaps little family support and isolation. The child is flying to heaven. He stated, ''This is me flying to home in heaven in the sky.''

informed at each stage what is being done, why it is being done, and what he or she can expect. Some feeling of hope needs to be provided. Last, the dignity of the child requires protection, and the child's privacy should be ensured.

Denial of death in a child, as in an adult, is a defense against anxiety, and it should be respected. Each person must be allowed his or her own way of dealing with the dread of death. At the same time, certain distortions should be corrected. For example, the child may require reassurance that the illness was not brought about by anything the child did (or thinks he or she did). Reactions that generate further anxiety, such as regression, should be gently but firmly controlled by the parents as well as by the hospital staff; excessive regressive behavior is uncomfortable for a child as well as for those caring for him or her.

Children vary in their capacity to deal with the inevitability of their impending death or with the diagnosis that implies impending death (Greenham and Lohmann, 1982). Some children, particularly older children, want to know, whereas others do not want to know or cannot comprehend. In some cases, older children and adolescents will possess the cognitive and emotional maturity to render them competent to take part in even the most difficult decisions in their medical care, including the decision to forego life-sustaining treatment for terminal illness (Leikin, 1989).

The Moribund Child

In a situation in which a child has no brain activity and is being kept ''alive'' by artificial methods, and there is no hope of spontaneous respiration or recovery of brain function, the physician must proceed with tact. First, before any decision is made to stop artificial life supports, the parents must be fully informed and prepared. The physician first might tell them that the child is being sustained by machines but that there is no possibility that the child will breathe on his or her own or will recover brain function; that is, the child in essence is dead. The physician should explain why this is so. In some instances, the parents have already considered the issue and will have decided to discontinue artificial life supports. Such parents may also have decided whether they want to be in the room at the time of death. Other parents may experience great anguish at the burden of deciding when to discontinue artificial respiration and may also prefer not to know exactly when it will be

stopped. In a tactful way, the physician can say to such parents that there is nothing more that can be done. Then when the parents do decide to discontinue artificial respiration, the physician should ask the parents where they want to be when it is discontinued.

The parents' wishes must be respected at all times; the child is theirs. The parents should not be rushed. It is usually their decision to make, and they need all the help they can get.

It is essential also that the parents feel a sense of unanimity with and security in the entire ward staff. Therefore, before the plan is carried out, the staff physician should discuss with all the ward staff members the steps just outlined and encourage them to express their thoughts and feelings. Patients tend to seek different answers from different staff members, and it is essential that all the staff members be aware of the way in which an individual case is being handled so that their responses do not conflict.

If the child dies suddenly without the parents being present, the parents should be informed of the death immediately, no matter what the time of day. The parents' sense of guilt at not being present when their child dies is an enormous one.

Management of Parents During Prolonged Illness in the Child

The many different reactions that parents may have when the period of dying is one of prolonged suffering necessitate sensitive management. Some parents may request other opinions regarding prognosis or treatment. Often they should be given this opportunity. Sometimes, however, a futile search for a magical cure may devastate a family emotionally and financially. The physician then should gently attempt to steer the parents toward a more realistic and helpful way of coping with their feelings of impotence. The physician can help parents by giving them opportunities to talk about their feelings in an accepting, nonjudgmental way. For example, parents often feel relieved when the physician reassures them that they are doing everything they can and that the physician knows how hard it is for them. The physician can also say, ''Many parents have told me how at times they had wished it would all finally end, and then felt bad about thinking that. But it's a natural thought to occur. We all have many kinds of thoughts. What is important is that you have done everything that could possibly be done.''

Questions may arise about child-rearing during the long period of time during which remissions occur and treatment is administered. While the child's condition is far from normal, there is often a wish on the part of the child to feel normal. Perhaps this represents in part the child's wish that he or she no longer had the disease, that there was no longer a need for painful treatments, and that he or she could talk freely with others about feelings of frustration, anger, and resentment.

At the same time, parents may be in a quandary about how to rear the child, siblings about how to relate to the child and deal with their guilt, and teachers about how to educate and deal with the child and the other children in the classroom. Once again, there is no blueprint answer; indeed, blanket recommendations (e.g., ''Treat the child normally'') may only burden the parents with more conflicts and guilt. Each situation must be thought out and managed individually, taking into account the many needs of the child, the parents, and the siblings.

Management of Siblings

Good medical management takes into account how the child's dying and death affect the child's siblings. Siblings of all ages need support and explanations, and the physician can help the parents provide them. The physician may suggest that the parents gather the family together and then give a simple explanation to all the children. The explanation should include the facts that Johnny is very ill, that everyone is doing his or her best to make the child as comfortable as possible, that the illness Johnny has could not be prevented, that it is no one's fault, and that it is necessary to figure out together how everyone can help. Later, individual children in the family may be given more information as they give evidence that they require it. If the siblings are told that death is near, they will also need help on how to conduct themselves in the presence of the dying child. The dying child needs their support, and they can give it by doing such things as making drawings for the child, bringing messages from others, and getting things he or she may need. If the dying child asks them whether he or she is going to die, they can say, "I don't know. I know it's a serious illness. Would you like me to ask Mommy and Daddy, or do you want to ask them yourself?"

When the child dies, in order to avoid hurt feelings, all the siblings should be told of the death at the same time if possible. A simple account of the death can be given if the children ask about it. It is better to avoid such statements as "He died in his sleep," especially when young children are present, because of the danger of engendering in them a fear of sleep.

A visit to the home by the physician is nearly always deeply appreciated by the parents and siblings of the dead child. If the physician has had a long-standing relationship with the family, he or she should ask about the funeral or memorial service and should attend the service. A physician who has provided extended care for a dying child may be remembered only for failing to attend the funeral service or convey his or her condolences.

Sometimes parents will ask whether a young sibling should attend the funeral. The physician first should decide whether the parents will probably be in control of themselves and who else will be present at the funeral who could support the child. For children under the age of 5, the funeral can be a puzzling experience unless it is explained and unless a great deal of support is given by a familiar and caring adult. Attendance also depends on cultural practices. Children above the age of 5 often can utilize the funeral rite in the same way adults do, especially if they have adults in attendance who can also explain to them their feelings and describe what is taking place. A child who does not wish to attend the funeral should not be made to feel guilty. Rather, arrangements should be made for the child to be in the company of an understanding adult during the time of the funeral. Older children should be encouraged to attend the rites and observe the rituals the adults are attending and observing, since, again, these practices usually help one to deal with the reality of death. If the older child chooses not to attend the funeral, the reason for the choice should be explored, but if the child continues to feel that he or she does not want to attend, this wish should be respected. Each person mourns in his or her own way. In no circumstance should the subject of the dead person be closed off. A wall of silence hampers the child as he or she struggles with the reality of the death and his or her feelings about death. Some of the specific ways of helping children understand the many facets of death have been described by Wolf (1958).

Other questions involving siblings may arise later. A younger sibling may ask to have some of the dead child's toys. The transfer can be done in a helpful way by suggesting that the dead child would have wanted his or her younger brother or sister to have his or her toys. Other decisions, such as rearranging the dead child's room or giving a sibling the dead child's room, might be deferred until most of the work of mourning has been done. Such decisions can probably be made on a rational basis then, when the mourners are less affected by their emotions.

Requesting Autopsy Permission or Organ Donation

A difficult task for the physician is requesting autopsy permission or organ donation. Because of the difficulties, the request is frequently made in a hasty, tactless manner. The physician must be aware that many families have strong feelings against such procedures. For example, Orthodox Judaism prohibits the permanent removal of organs. Despite the physician's medical curiosity and zeal to learn, he or she must resist pressuring a family into agreeing to a procedure to which it objects. On the other hand, the physician may legitimately describe an autopsy to the parents as a postmortem internal examination that determines the cause of death and the effects of the treatment given. He or she can honestly present to them the possible potential benefits of an autopsy

or organ donation to others. If parents ask whether the child will be cut open, the physician must answer honestly, even if the physician knows that the autopsy or donation request may then be refused. Families who refuse to agree to such procedures should not be made to feel guilty about their refusal.

WHEN A PARENT DIES
The Children

When a parent dies, the physician should help the surviving parent anticipate the reactions to be expected from the children. Children, particularly young children, are unable to tolerate—and therefore complete—the painful task of mourning the death of a parent. Sad feelings often are curtailed, and often the child quickly returns to everyday activities as if nothing had changed. Although the immediate manifestations of mourning in extremely young children are usually brief it is difficult to assess the impact of a parent's death on the child's future personality development. Occasionally, a child may express hostile feelings toward the surviving parent. The child may actually be angry at and feel abandoned by the parent who died. Since such feelings usually are experienced as unacceptable, the child displaces them onto the surviving parent. The expression of hostile feelings toward the surviving parent unfortunately invites punishment when it is misunderstood. Frequently, a child, by virtue of his or her still somewhat primitive way of viewing the world, is convinced that he or she caused the parent's death, either by not being a good child or by having at one time or another wished the parent dead. When the child provokes the surviving parent, he or she may in part be seeking punishment to assuage feelings of guilt. Therefore, it is necessary to prepare a parent for these reactions as well as to attempt to correct the child's fantasies.

The child who has lost a parent is a child at psychiatric risk. After a review of the literature on bereavement in childhood, the Institute of Medicine (Osterweis et al., 1984), recently summarized the factors that are associated with an increased risk of psychological morbidity for children following the death of a parent or sibling:

1. Loss in a child less than 5 years of age or during early adolescence.
2. Loss of a mother for girls less than 11 years of age and loss of a father for adolescent boys.
3. Premorbid psychological difficulties in the child or lack of prior knowledge about death.
4. When the relationship with the deceased had been conflictual or when the parent remarries and there is a poor relationship between the child and the stepparent.
5. When the surviving parent is psychologically vulnerable and excessively dependent on the child, or the environment is unstable and inconsistent.
6. When there is a lack of adequate family or community supports, or when the surviving parent is unable to access available supports.
7. When the death was unanticipated or the result of suicide or homicide.

Impairments in the child's capacity to form new, lasting relationships may show up later. Shame at being different may be experienced. Impaired sexual identity and conscience formation also may occur (Bonnard, 1962; Neubauer, 1960). In addition, the loss of a parent during childhood may predispose a child to attempt suicide during adolescence.

The family disruption and the reactions of the surviving parent may lead to a depression in the child. The presenting symptom may be a school learning problem or a behavior difficulty. Another hazard that sometimes occurs is a morbid attachment of the surviving parent to a child of either sex, particularly an adolescent. The adolescent in question may have great difficulty in separating from the parent or may develop along homosexual lines.

On the other hand, as development proceeds, the child may be able to continue the work of mourning on a piecemeal basis. As his or her cognitive capacity matures and reality testing is strengthened, the child may at some later date be able to express some of the feelings that he or she had earlier repressed. These feelings may include yearning and sadness, which may occur at times of special significance in the form of anniversary reactions (Fox, 1985), as well as anger and resentment.

The physician can help most if he or she can enable the parent, who is also in a state of mourning and withdrawal, to recognize the needs of the child. The child needs to know that there is someone he or she can depend on to meet his or her needs, and to whom feelings can be expressed. In some instances, the physician may appropriately support the parent in this role by making himself or herself available to the child, if the parent agrees. The pediatrician should suggest a consultation with a child psychiatrist if there is concern about the child's behavior.

The Surviving Parent

The death of a parent almost always disrupts a family. As much as possible, the physician should help the family to maintain its stability and to avoid making hasty decisions while the family is in a state of acute grief. The services of a relative or a homemaker may be helpful during this acute period. Some tact is required as the physician tries to steer a course that will not be experienced by the parent either as intrusive or as an abandonment.

The disruption in the family caused by the death of a parent is not confined to the period of mourning. Loss of income, reduction in the amount of time that can be spent with the children, changed roles for the surviving spouse, caretaking responsibilities for the older children in the family, and altered social relationships are some of the repercussions that continue to affect the family. The physician should remain accessible to members of the family. Sleep difficulties, psychosomatic disturbances, and school learning difficulties are some of the common signs of continuing distress that may require further psychiatric evaluation.

References

Adams D, Deveau E: When a brother or sister is dying of cancer: The vulnerability of the adolescent sibling. *Death Stud* 11:279–295, 1987.

Berman S, Villarreal S: Use of a seminar as an aid in helping interns care for dying children and their families. *Clin Pediatr* 22:175–179, 1983.

Bonnard A: Truancy and pilfering associated with bereavement. In: Lorand S, Schneer HL (eds): *Adolescence*. New York, Harper & Row, 1962.

Cain AC, Fast I, Erickson ME: Children's disturbed reactions to the death of a sibling. *Am J Orthopsychiatry* 34:741–752, 1964.

Clunies-Ross C, Lansdown R: Concepts of death, illness, and isolation found in children with leukaemia. *Child Care Health Dev* 14:373–386, 1988.

Florian V, Kravetz S: Children's concepts of death: A cross-cultural comparison among Muslims, Druze, Christians, and Jews in Israel. *J Cross-Cult Psychol* 16:174–189, 1985.

Fox S: Children's anniversary reactions to the death of a family member. *Omega* 15:291–305, 1985.

Greenham D, Lohmann R: Children facing death: Recurring patterns of adaptation. *Health Soc Work* 7:89–94, 1982.

Hostler S: The development of the child's concept of death. In: Sahler OJ (ed): *The Child and Death*. Saint Louis, Mosby, 1978, pp. 1–25.

Jenkins R, Cavanaugh J: Examining the relationship between the development of the concept of death and overall cognitive development. *Omega* 16:193–199, 1986.

Kane B: Children's concepts of death. *J Gen Psychol* 134:141–153, 1979.

Kastenbaum R: Time and death in adolescence. In: Feifel H (ed): *The Meaning of Death*. New York, McGraw-Hill, 1959.

Kastenbaum R: The child's understanding of death: How does it develop? In: Grollman E (ed): *Explaining Death to Children*. Boston, Beacon, 1967, pp. 89–108.

Krell R, Rabkin L: The effects of sibling death on the surviving child: A family perspective. *Fam Process* 18:471–477, 1979.

Kübler-Ross E: On death and dying. *JAMA* 221:174–179, 1972.

Leikin S: A proposal concerning decisions to forgo life-sustaining treatment for young people. *J Pediatr* 115:17–22, 1989.

Lewis M: The management of parents of acutely ill children in the hospital. *Am J Orthopsychiatry* 32:60–66, 1962.

Lifton RJ: *Death in Life*. New York, Random House, 1967.

Maloney M: Diagnosing hysterical conversion reactions in children. *J Pediatr* 97:1016–1020, 1980.

Neubauer PB: The one-parent child and his oedipal development. *Psychoanal Study Child* 15:286–309, 1960.

Ordo Unctionis Infirmorum Eorumque Pastoralis Curae. In: *Rituale Romanum*. Rome, Typis Polyglottis Vaticanis, 1972, pp. 10, 15.

Osterweis M, Solomon F, Green M (eds): *Bereavement: Reactions, Consequences, and Care*. Washington, DC, National Academy Press, 1984.

Reilly T, Hasazi J, Bond L: Children's conceptions of death and personal mortality. *J Pediatr Psychol* 8:21–31, 1983.

Schonfeld D: Crisis intervention for bereavement support: A model of intervention in the children's school. *Clin Pediatr* 28:27–33, 1989.

Schonfeld D: Talking with children about death. *Journal of Pediatric Health Care* 7:269–274, 1993.

Schonfeld D, Kline M: Members of the Crisis Intervention Committee: School-based crisis intervention: an organizational model. *Crisis Intervention* 1:155–166, 1994.

Schonfeld D, Smilansky S: A cross-cultural comparison of Israeli and American children's death concepts. *Death Stud* 13:593–604, 1989.

Smilansky S: *On Death: Helping Children Understand and Cope*. New York, Peter Lang, 1987.

Solnit AJ: The dying child. *Dev Med Child Neurol* 7:693–695, 1965.

Solnit AJ, Green M: Psychologic considerations in the management of deaths on pediatric hospital services. I: The doctor and the child's family. *Pediatrics* 24:106–112, 1959.

Speece M, Brent S: Children's understanding of death: A review of three components of a death concept. *Child Dev* 55:1671–1686, 1984.

Spinetta J: The dying child's awareness of death: A review. *Psychol Bull* 81:256–260, 1974.

Townley K, Thornburg K: Maturation of the concept of death in elementary school children. *Educ Res Q* 5:17–24, 1980.

Wass H: Concepts of death: A developmental perspective. In: Wass H, Corr C (eds): *Childhood and Death*. Washington, DC, Hemisphere, 1984, pp. 3–24.

Wass H, Guenther Z, Towry B: United States and Brazilian children's concepts of death. *Death Educ* 3:41–55, 1979.

Wolf AWM: *Helping Your Child to Understand Death*. New York, Child Study Association of America, 1958, pp. 7–44.

105 Multiproblem Families and High-Risk Children and Adolescents: Causes and Management

Jean Adnopoz, M.P.H., R. Kevin Grigsby, D.S.W., and Steven F. Nagler, A.C.S.W.

This chapter describes some of the environmental and intrafamilial factors common to multiproblem families, which place children at high risk for poor developmental, psychological, and educational outcomes, including out-of-home placement. The authors describe an intervention that focuses on the developmental needs of children within the context of addressing the family's complex needs.

MULTIPROBLEM FAMILIES: DESCRIPTIONS AND CAUSAL FACTORS

Most authors acknowledge that the multiproblem family arises from a multifactorial etiology and is not the result of a unitary condition (Bowlby, 1953). Disease, poverty, alcoholism, chemical dependency, mental deficiency, constitutional inadequacy, parental discord, social isolation, and lack of familial and community support are all thought to contribute to the making of families in which parents are unable to meet the psychological and physical needs of their children.

Parental conditions such as psychiatric disorders (Rutter and Quinton, 1984), substance abuse (Deutsch, 1983), chronic illness, impaired intellectual functioning, and disturbed emotional development alone are often predictive of poor developmental outcomes for children. When these conditions are joined with environmental stressors such as poverty, isolation, homelessness, and discrimination, the risk of family disintegration increases. Families who share these combined characteristics are commonly identified as multiproblem families (Kaplan, 1986; Spencer, 1963). Kilpatrick (1995) argues that "these families lack a leadership and control structure that is needed in order to meet basic nurturing and protection needs of members" (p. 4).

In recent decades the ability of families to provide for the needs of their children adequately has been compromised by the convergence of adverse environmental, psychosocial, psychological, physical, educational, and economic factors (Ford Foundation Executive Panel, 1989). The prevalence of these stressors on families appears to be increasing in the United States. For example, at present more than 12 million American children live in poverty (one in five). Each year, half a million children are born to mothers under the age of 17. Approximately 3.3 million children live in single-parent, female-headed households. Growing numbers of preschool children and their families are homeless (American Public Welfare Association, 1987; Ford Foundation Executive Panel, 1989; National Commission on Child Welfare and Family Preservation, 1991).

The effects on children of growing up within multiproblem families have been documented by Taylor and Newberger (1979), among others. Children in these families are more likely to present with symptoms of neglect and nonorganic failure to thrive. The health care provided for them is more likely to be episodic and illness oriented. Developmental delays, language difficulties, behavioral problems, and school failures are common. For some children, attendance at school may be further fragmented and episodic because of frequent family moves or homelessness.

The National Center for Children in Poverty (Klerman, 1991) reported that poor children experience more of many types of health problems than children in families with more adequate incomes. Rates of infant mortality, sudden infant death syndrome, unintended injuries, child abuse and infectious diseases, including AIDS and HIV infection, are higher among poor children. Poor and near poor children also suffer disproportionately high rates of problems related to nutrition, asthma, otitis media and other infectious diseases, as well as increased incidence of dental decay and lead poisoning.

The existence of multiple stressors often increases the impact of any particular stressor. The National Center for Children in Poverty stated that poor children on inadequate diets are likely to experience more frequent infectious disease than the non-poor, and to be sicker longer and more severely. Inadequate nutrition may also impact upon cognitive development and social behavior, particularly as undernourished children may be more apathetic and less responsive in social situations (Adnopoz, 1994b).

Numerous authors report that in addition to sharing etiological pathways, multiproblem families demonstrate certain similar characteristics (Geismar and Lasorte, 1964; Kaplan, 1986). Kaplan (1986) states that these families have "a number of problems that cut across many dimensions of family life" (p. 16). Multiproblem families have been found to evidence poor coping skills in intrapersonal, interpersonal, and environmental areas and have demonstrated difficulty negotiating the interrelationships between these spheres of functioning. In the social ecology of their environment, problems transcend a single level and often appear as a "web" or cluster of issues that eventually threatens to overwhelm the family.

Geismar and Lasorte (1964) describe this type of family as having difficulties in the following functional areas: developing relationships inside the family; developing relationships outside the family group, particularly in the neighborhood and in the community; and performing tasks concerned with the maintenance of health care and with the range of everyday economic and household practices that are designed to maintain the family as a physical unit.

Spencer (1963) states that the term *multiproblem family* describes

those families which are of public concern because of their social and economic cost to the community and are characterized by:
1. A "pathological" family type as shown by (*a*) inadequate or destructive parent-child relationships by both parents, (*b*) inadequate social functioning on the part of parents and/or children, and (*c*) extreme emotional immaturity of either or both parents.
2. Dependent and/or exploitative behavior toward the community and community agencies.
3. Persistent failure to respond to help or treatment offered.
4. A state of chronic dependency on the social services. (p. 12)

These families contribute to burgeoning social services costs through their inappropriate use of the caregiving system. Spencer places the responsibility upon the family for its frequent reliance on crisis care, remedial services, and public support. He concludes that chronic dependency upon public resources is not only costly but also represents an inefficient use of available resources.

Selig (1976) suggests that effective intervention can be designed for these families. He suggests that the term *multi-problem family* is a misnomer that places blame undeservedly. He believes that the problem lies within a "multi-problem delivery system" (p. 526) that offers fragmented social services. Selig identifies issues of accessibility, ownership, caregiver attitudes toward dysfunctional families, lack of coordination between providers, gaps in the service continuum, insensitivity to social and cultural distinctions, and lack of continuity of caregiving as central contributors to a troubled service system.

MULTIPROBLEM FAMILIES: PROBLEMS IN INTERVENTION

The association of such major societal problems as poverty, racial and ethnic discrimination, inadequate and substandard housing, and underclass status with multiproblem families discourages caregivers from working intensively with them. The behaviors of service providers suggest a lack of confidence in both the family's ability to institute change and in the service system's capacity to intervene positively. The providers' cynical attitudes toward these families are unwittingly supported by the families themselves, who because of their past futile experiences may be unable or unwilling to give expression to their need for help. As a result, they may appear uninterested in the interventions offered to them. Because issues of distrust, noncompliance, and failure to keep appointments frequently arise in working with multiproblem families, negative caregiver attitudes are further perpetuated. Families are blamed by providers for behaviors that when better understood are not symptomatic of the family's inability to accept responsibility and respond to the needs of its children but are rudimentary attempts by families to defend against the attitudes and behaviors of the service providers themselves. For example, a mother who fails to regularly visit her child in the hospital may be made to feel demeaned and inadequate by hospital staff when she does visit. Her failure to appear may represent an attempt to protect her self-esteem rather than an uncaring, neglectful attitude toward her child.

There are numerous barriers to successful intervention; some families may be resistant to interventions provided by "outsiders" who come from cultures, races, or socioeconomic groups from whom they feel alienated. Services may be inaccessible, especially for parents who have no alternative source of child care and must travel unassisted, with several small children. Language barriers may make communication between families and caregivers difficult. Caregivers may have little if any knowledge of the cultural differences, customs, and strongly held beliefs of the families they treat. Significantly, the service system may focus upon the family's failure, without assessing the family's strengths and attempting to build upon them. Although families do share responsibility for their situations, blaming the family for being in trouble is not useful.

The traditional social service delivery system has proven itself inadequate to meet the complex needs of multiproblem families. Unidimensional interventions designed to address specific problems in single spheres of functioning have not been an effective means of confronting the multidimensional problems that categorize these families. Recently service providers have been challenged to find innovative ways to reach these difficult-to-serve families. A variety of legislative, child welfare, and mental health initiatives have addressed the multidimensional needs of troubled families. The Adoption Assistance and Child Welfare Act of 1980 (Public Law 96- 272) required states to make "reasonable efforts" to keep children from out-of-home-placement; the Education for All Handicapped Children Act of 1975 (Public Law 94-142), rewritten in 1990 as the Individuals with Disabilities Education Act, requires that placement decisions be made on the basis of the least restrictive setting; the Child and Adolescent Service System Program (CASSP) of the National Institute of Mental Health, created in 1983; and the Mental Health Services Program for Youth (MHSPY), initiated in 1989 by the Robert Wood Johnson Foundation in 1989, all support the development of integrated, comprehensive service systems. The failures of the foster care system, combined with a rise in the number of children referred for placement (Knitzer and Cole, 1989), have put increased pressures upon policy makers and professionals to find new models of service that are responsive to the needs of children and families.

Most recently, in August of 1993, the United States Congress enacted a new Subpart 2 of Title IV-B of the Social Security Act entitled Family Preservation and Support Services. The new legislation strengthens the Adoption Assistance and Child Welfare Act of 1980, and authorizes funding that is expected to serve as an added stimulus for states to engage in broad-gauged consensus building, collaboration, and systems reform by providing family support and family preservation services (Adnopoz, 1994a).

As a result, new programs have emerged that attempt to make significant changes in the ways in which services are delivered by reducing the barriers to effective utilization. These programs tend to be family oriented, child centered, community and home based, and treatment focused. Crisis intervention, case management, skill building, and the provision of concrete services are often part of the available core service. These programs recognize that the most appropriate placement for a child is an adequately functioning family. Assisting isolated, disaffected, alienated families to function well enough to care adequately for their children requires a flexible, enlightened, and integrated service system whose purpose is clear and unambivalent.

In one program, developed by the authors, the doctrine of the best interests of the child constitutes the first of two organizing principles guiding intervention for multiproblem families in which a child is at risk of placement. The second principle recognizes the strengths of the ego support lent to the parent by the therapeutic team, whose role is to build a relationship through which the path to behavior change can be negotiated (Lewis and Stark, 1966; Soule et al., 1993).

TWO ORGANIZING PRINCIPLES FOR WORKING WITH MULTIPROBLEM FAMILIES

Anna Freud (1965) has stated that the best interests of the child are satisfied when the child's needs for affection, stimulation, and object constancy are met. The family unit is the institution society considers best suited to respond to these needs and to guide the child from dependence to independence (Caplan, 1978; Provence, 1979). Some families are unable to assume these responsibilities and to provide an environment supportive of healthy child development. In all cases children need adults (generally parents) to attend to their physical needs, to nurture them, to demonstrate that they are wanted and cared for, and to protect and guide them. They need to feel that they are important, that they matter.

Parents also have needs. Solnit (1968) has described these as needs for evidence of their competence as parents and for effective, esteem-enhancing assistance from their community in times of crisis. In the best of cases, children's needs are met in relatively strong, relatively self-sufficient families by parents or other adults who are capable of nurturing and committing themselves to these children. In the best of cases, parents' needs are in turn met by the extended family, loyal friends, and other support systems of the larger society. When parents meet children's needs, children are more likely to feel secure and valued. They are more likely to be equipped for the challenges of school and prepared for the challenges of life. They are more likely to grow into adulthood with the ability to nurture others.

However, when there is a confluence of parental inadequacies and environmental stressors, families are at greater risk of being dislodged from the mainstream of familial and societal supports. social isolation may lead to a pervasive sense of futility, and desperation. Erikson (1964) has noted that

defenseless as babies are, they have mothers at their command to protect the mothers, societies to support the structure of families, and to give a cultural continuity to systems of child care and training. this is necessary for the human infant to evolve humanly, for his development must provide that outer wholeness and continuity which, like a second womb, permits the child to develop his capacities in distinct steps, and to unify them.

If a child's environment does not provide that "outer continuity," the child's chances of growing and developing in a healthy way are diminished.

When families lack the intrapersonal and interpersonal means to satisfy the needs of individual family members, they cannot perform their crucial function as socializing agents for children. If they cannot perform that function, the individual family and society as a whole suffer losses (Lower East Side Family Union, 1976; Schorr and Schorr, 1988). The situation is particularly egregious for the children of poor families (Kaplan, 1986).

The motivation for behavioral change on the part of the parent is brought out by providing an *auxiliary ego* (Lewis and Stark, 1966), most frequently in the person of a family support worker, whose role is defined more fully later in this chapter. It is important to note here that the empathy, support, and acceptance the parent(s) receives, perhaps for the first time, can be sufficient to move the parent toward a higher and more appropriate level of functioning (Soule et al., 1993).

The argument for interventions that support the structure of the family is made even more compelling by the human and economic costs involved. As stated, the inability of families to meet the basic needs of children within the family constellation often leads to foster care placement and a consequent break in the child's relationship with the primary object. For some children, out-of-home placement may be clinically indicated. For the majority, however, the first separation will simply provide an easy pathway to additional placements and to the loss of important affective and nurturing ties. The current shortage of foster homes and the inability of states to ensure continuity of placement once a child is removed makes any removal of a child a significant risk, to be balanced carefully against maintenance of the child within the family. In addition, multiproblem families use public services such as crisis health care, police, special education, and mental health programs more frequently than other families. Therefore, efforts to stabilize these families and to improve their capacity to manage have important social and economic implications as well. Tracy and Whittaker (1987) and Tracy (1990, 1991) have demonstrated that identifying families appropriate for intervention and developing social support resources with those families has helped to stabilize and improve their capacity to manage with potential social and economic benefits.

INTERVENTION MODELS FOR WORKING WITH MULTIPROBLEM FAMILIES

As previously noted, pressures to reduce out-of-home placements and other expensive services have increased. There has been an explosion in the number of programs designed to help the multiproblem family function more effectively. These programs have recognized that an integrated, comprehensive approach can be a powerful strategy for helping families cope more effectively within a stressful environment (Kaplan, 1986).

Programs designed to serve multiproblem families recognize that families evidence difficulty across spheres of functioning. Because a negative synergism often exists within the complex, dynamic interrelationships among the family, its members, and the environment, interventions that are focused on only one problem area may be futile. In most instances, strategies for effective intervention address the interrelation of the intrapersonal, interpersonal, and environmental domains. The range of intrapersonal problems may include parental substance abuse (alcohol or drug), major mental or physical illness, mental retardation, chronic unemployment, and lack of job skills. Interpersonal problems include marital or partner conflict, child abuse or neglect, incidence of accidental or intentional injuries within the family, isolation or alienation from the extended family, absence of an extended family or other supportive personal relationships, and a history of foster

care placements. Environmental problems include a history of involvement with multiple social service agencies, persistent failure of social service interventions, homelessness, poverty, isolation, lack of transportation, as well as broader issues of service availability, institutional racism, and institutional sexism.

Several of the programs designed to serve multiproblem families make use of a generic model of family-centered, home based services that seek to accomplish the goal of preserving the family while addressing its interlocking problems (Edna McConnell Clark Foundation, 1985). Kaplan (1986) offers descriptions of several exemplary home based, family centered programs that have proven to be successful with multiproblem families. These programs have several common elements:

1. The family system is seen as the primary unit of treatment (Kaplan, 1986).
2. Services are provided to the family in their own home.
3. It is assumed, according to a growth model, that change within the family is possible; family strengths, not weaknesses, are pursued (Kaplan, 1986).
4. Services are provided on a time-limited basis.
5. Services focus on keeping families together and preventing unnecessary foster placement of children (Edna McConnell Clark Foundation, 1985).
6. Services are intensive; caseloads are low.
7. Concrete services and advocacy are provided.

While clinicians may draw upon a number of theories to guide the intervention with families, Grigsby (1993, 1994, 1995) argues that social attachment theory (Bowlby, 1969, 1973, 1980, 1988) is most useful as a guide for working with families of this type.

Some of these principles have been incorporated into the home based family preservation programs which began in the early 1970s, when the Homebuilder Program was developed in Tacoma, Washington. The program, then operated by a nonprofit agency, attempted to avert out-of-home child placement by offering intensive, short-term, home based therapy and casework to families in crisis, using a single, master's-level therapist as the in-home worker. This program model has spread across the country and has recently been implemented on both coasts. Other models of intervention have been developed as well, with similar strategies but with somewhat different elements. Length of intervention varies from 4 weeks to 6 months, services are provided by paraprofessionals or therapeutic teams, and time in the home varies from 5 to 18 hours weekly. Nelson (1990a, 1990b) and Nelson et al. (1990) offer descriptions of various service models and discuss their effectiveness.

Common to all programs is the provision of therapy in the home and its availability to all family members. Although the modality may differ, the move of the clinician from the traditional office or institutional setting to the family's setting has lessened resistance to treatment for parents and children. In addition, it has enabled the clinician to observe the family within its own environment and to identify more clearly and more quickly the range of the family's needs. Given the particular characteristics of multiproblem families and their historic rate of treatment failures, the ability to intervene clinically within the home environment appears to offer significant promise for improved outcomes.

As a result, most have viewed these programs optimistically. The popular press ("Why leave children with bad parents?" 1994, April 25) and some researchers (Frankel, 1988; Wald, 1988), however, have raised questions as to whether these programs are actually helping the children and families they are designed to serve. Wald (1988) argues that "family preservation cannot be an end in and of itself" and that "family preservation is appropriate only when it serves to protect and promote" the goal of the child's well-being. This is consistent with the point of view that the focus of family preservation programs should be the best interests of the child (Goldstein et al., 1973). One model program with such a focus is the Family Support Service (FSS) developed by the authors.

FAMILY SUPPORT SERVICE

FSS is a time-limited, 24-hour, in-home, voluntary program for families in which a child is at imminent risk of placement outside the home. It was developed in 1985 by the Yale Child Study Center in collaboration with the Connecticut Department of Children and Youth Services (DCYS) and with the support of the Edna McConnell Clark Foundation, which has played a significant role in the family preservation movement. The program is staffed by trained, crisis-oriented lay "family support workers," who join with master's level social work clinicians from the Yale Child Study Center to form a therapeutic team around each family in the program.

Six operating assumptions inform the work of the FSS. First, there are existing strengths in families that, once identified, can be utilized effectively by the therapeutic team. This assumption is significant because it represents a reversal of the traditional position of state child protection agencies, which by virtue of their legal mandate seek to identify family weakness, parenting failure, and degree of risk.

Second, utilization of a therapeutic team is a particularly effective means of serving multiproblem families, as it addresses the environmental and intrapsychic needs of the family simultaneously, while also providing mutual support for the team itself.

Third, the work of the lay family support worker is central to the program's ability to effect change within the family. Families who are often socially isolated members of society's underclass, with previous histories of health, mental health, and other problems and a historic inability to use the service system effectively, have significant difficulties in accepting and relating to traditional service providers. The FSS worker, a role model with whom they can identify, works with the families in their own homes, uses their own language, and understands their lifestyle. He or she is a critical and essential resource in breaking the cycle of isolation and reducing the distrust and distance that have frequently characterized the family's past relationships with other helpers.

Fourth, the social work clinician plays a flexible role. The clinician may function as psychotherapist, diagnostician, evaluator, case manager, service broker, or consultant to the FSS worker; the specific clinical role is determined by the needs of each individual case. The clinician works most frequently within the home and in the community and less frequently in the office.

Fifth, collaboration with other agencies is essential to the success of the intervention. FSS intervention is brief (8–12 weeks); it does not replace existing services and programs. Work with community agencies from the time of referral to the time of discharge is expected and necessary if the goals for the family are to be attained during this brief period and maintained over time.

Sixth and last, planning for discharge must begin at time of intake. Well-planned, intensive, and brief involvement is a potent vehicle for change. This final operating assumption is embodied in the first question asked when a case is accepted into the program: What are the criteria for discharge? The brevity of the intervention is intended to minimize the intrusion into the family; it also capitalizes on the crisis that commonly exists at the time of referral by bringing the problem areas into sharp focus and stabilizing the family so that it can go on to utilize other less intrusive and more familiar means of support.

The FSS program categorizes a family's risk for having a child removed in the following ways:

1. The referring child protection agency has decided that a child will be placed outside of the home within 5 days unless the family's resources can be rallied immediately.
2. A child already has been removed as a crisis response, but immediate return home may be indicated if additional internal and/or external support can be put into place quickly.
3. A referring worker's persistent discomfort about a child's health or safety propels a move toward placement, even though there may be

significant clinical uncertainty about the benefit to the child of removal from the biological family. These are often cases in which significant parental dysfunction coexists with evidence of a positive child-parent attachment.

The FSS process begins with an intake assessment in the family home. At this time, the parent(s), the FSS worker, the clinician, and the referring worker jointly establish the goals for the intervention. Initial visiting schedules are established, task assignments are made, and roles are clarified.

Family support workers visit with their family clients twice weekly at a minimum, often more. The worker attempts to establish a nonjudgmental, empathic relationship with the parent (or parents) and to arrange for concrete services for the family. It is not uncommon for the work to take place in the FSS worker's car, as she takes her clients to the welfare office, the supermarket, the Housing Authority, or medical appointments.

The social work clinicians screen and assess children and families for their service needs, keeping in mind the multiple environmental and intrafamily issues with which these families present. Their clinical formulations of individual and family dynamics and their ability to assign a priority to the order of addressing these problems are integral parts of case management and treatment. Clinicians and FSS workers are in frequent (often daily) contact, exchanging information and clinical impressions, which are used continually to monitor and evaluate case progress and refine intervention strategies.

FSS also has available a contingency fund for items such as security deposits, refrigerators, furniture, diapers, and food. The therapeutic team requests funding for its clients when such expenditures are thought to be important to maintaining a child in a family. For some families, this fund is used as a non-interest-bearing loan; for others it is given as a grant.

The task of the lay family support worker is to relate empathically to the parent/client as a nonjudgmental, caring role model and to assist the parent to obtain concrete services and negotiate appropriate service systems. Frequently, the sociocultural and personal background of the FSS worker resembles that of the client. This similarity can enhance the client's acceptance of the FSS worker as a trusted and knowledgeable person.

The role of the clinician is to apply clinical knowledge to the tasks of understanding underlying family dynamics and identifying both the parental behaviors and the environmental stressors upon which the efforts of the FSS worker can be focused. Less frequently, the clinician will be involved directly with the parent in brief psychotherapy.

The pairing of the family support worker with the clinician focuses the work in a specific and goal-directed way that is based in the family's reality. Attention is first directed toward identifying and meeting the immediate basic needs of the family. After issues of food, clothing, and shelter are addressed, other issues can be seen more clearly and the intrafamilial work begun. In the process of assisting the family to obtain the necessary concrete services, the worker and parent begin to establish the relationship out of which real change can come. This approach assists families to cope with the immediate crisis, avoid further deterioration, work to gain some insight into the family situation, and achieve reorganization at a higher level.

In addition to assessing the immediate needs of the family, the team also assesses its needs beyond the time of intensive intervention. Together the family support worker, the clinician, and the family identify other voluntary community resources that are appropriate, accessible, and available to address the family's longer-term needs. The professional status of the clinician facilitates access to certain services and makes possible more efficient case planning and transition. The FSS worker, with a working knowledge of grass-roots resources, often is able to cut through bureaucratic red tape to obtain services by utilizing contacts with line staff. The ability of the therapeutic team to relate to systems and services at two levels simultaneously makes possible more effective negotiation of the boundaries between agencies and systems than could be accomplished by either individual working alone. The use of the clinician-lay family worker team thus seems to address both the concrete and psychodynamic needs of families in a way that mobilizes difficult-to-reach multiproblem families.

Because threatened placement is a primary consideration for referral to programs such as FSS, it can be assumed that there is an existing concern for a child's safety. The active and continuous involvement of the FSS team with the state child protection agency is designed to encourage careful consideration and decision making focused on maintaining the child in the home when appropriate and possible, taking enlightened risks in the interests of continuity and consistency and unraveling and ameliorating the complex web of environmental and intrafamilial problems that beset these families. The FSS clinician provides a level of support and knowledge that enables the child protection worker to weigh alternatives carefully and to feel less anxious about leaving the child in the home. All those involved with the family thus can attend better to the real needs of the child and family. At the same time, the active involvement of the lay family worker ensures a watchful presence in the home and provides an assurance that concrete efforts will be made to improve the environment.

In summary, the team-structured FSS model holds promise for being an effective intervention with multiproblem families at high risk for poor child outcomes. The utilization of a therapeutic team to assess and address the concrete and psychodynamic needs of the child and family appears to be particularly effective.

CASE ILLUSTRATION

This case illustration offers an example of a team-structured intervention with a multiproblem family. This example has relevance for the child psychiatrist and/or other mental health clinician who is asked to evaluate, assess, and/or treat a child where the locus of the actual problem may be within the immediate family or family environment.

Mrs. M., a 32-year-old Hispanic mother of six children who ranged in age from 2 to 10 years, was referred for service 2 weeks after the sudden death of her husband. Mr. M. had negotiated all of the systems for her and for her family during his lifetime. Mrs. M. spoke only Spanish, was illiterate, and was reported by the Association of Retarded Citizens as being mentally retarded and probably unable to manage the affairs of her family. At the time of the initial home visit, Mrs. M. was in a deep state of mourning. Her children were reported to be delayed developmentally, to lack age-appropriate social skills, and to have little expressive language. In addition, the 7-year-old daughter, Maria, had difficulty controlling her impulsivity and aggression, and 2-year-old Juan appeared developmentally delayed, although further evaluation was needed to confirm the diagnosis.

At the time of referral the primary supports for the family were Mrs. M.'s minister and some paternal family members. However, the minister, who was a key influence in this family, strongly doubted that Mrs. M. could provide for the children adequately enough for them to remain at home.

By identifying family and personal strengths, the clinician and the family support worker made an initial assessment that Mrs. M. might possess the ability to function adequately as a parent if she had assistance in negotiating the various provider systems that would be essential to her family's health, welfare, and well-being. She would need help in such basic areas as managing money, making the home safe for her children, making and keeping appointments, and advocating for the special educational needs of her children. This initial impression was derived from Mrs. M.'s clear devotion to her children and their apparent attachment to her, her ability to protect them in a dangerous neighborhood, and the clinician's awareness of the fear and isolation Mrs. M. suffered because of her illegal alien status.

Because Mrs. M. already was in psychotherapy at a community clinic, the FSS clinician assumed the role of case manager and not of therapist. The family support worker began a twice-weekly visiting schedule. Both the clinician and the family support worker became involved in obtaining concrete services for Mrs. M. The family support worker transported her to the appropriate state agencies to help her qualify for survivor's benefits. She was accompanied to the housing project office to report a problem toilet and sink, as well as to clarify her rent situation. She was given a ride to the Department of Income Maintenance for the monthly budget verification she needed to settle the rent problem. The clinician visited Maria's school to discuss the appropriateness of her school placement with the principal. With the school's support, the clinician gained Mrs. M.'s permission to refer Maria to a child guidance clinic for a full psychiatric evaluation.

During the first month of FSS involvement with this family, Mrs. M. felt increasingly overwhelmed by the problems stressing her family. Mrs. M. believed that she was approaching a "nervous breakdown." Shortly afterward, while Mrs. M. and the family support worker waited together for the children at the bus stop, Mrs. M. confided that she would like to place all her children in foster care and arrange to see them only on the weekends. Although the aide was surprised and discouraged, she told Mrs. M. that she would bring her information that would help her to begin the placement process. At the next visit, the family support worker suggested the alternative possibility of a day care program for the children and a homemaker for Mrs. M. Mrs. M. was interested in exploring these possibilities because she had realized that she didn't want her children to be placed away from her. She just felt overwhelmed by caring for them alone. She wanted them at home. She also wanted help. Both the clinician and the family worker began to negotiate with other systems to find a homemaker and the day care program and to keep food on the family's table by maintaining the family's food stamps, which were suspended temporarily because of the family's illegal immigrant status.

At this time, the family support worker supplied clothes she had obtained from her own community contacts and helped the family to obtain food from emergency food banks. During the time of its involvement with Mrs. M., the FSS team also contacted the neighborhood health clinic to coordinate the family's health care and simplify the family's access to the health care system. At a case coordination meeting of all of the case-specific agencies involved with the M. family, which took place after a homemaker was found and the day care program was in place, the therapist from the child guidance clinic agreed to act as ongoing case manager. With these supports in place, the intervention was terminated.

Comment

There should be no illusion that this 12-week intervention provided a "cure." Mrs. M.'s limited intellectual functioning, her depression, and her continued mourning do suggest that her functioning over time will be impaired. However, she had taken responsibility when in the past she had taken none, and she had begun to play a more active role in caring for the multiple needs of her children and herself. A support system had been developed and activated for Mrs. M. and her children that required her to relate to only two primary caregivers: the pediatrician and the child guidance clinic. Six children were then enabled to remain together with their biological parent. The mother's potential dependency and inability to function were modified, and multiple problem areas were addressed with positive results. The alternatives for the M. family might have more than doubled the sense of loss and abandonment that the death of their father already had occasioned and might have left them at greater risk for disintegration and despair.

CONCLUSIONS

Many families experience more than one problem at a time; some are able to utilize services and mobilize their inherent strengths on their own behalf. Others are unable to recognize and draw upon their own strengths or make use of other resources that might be helpful to them. The combination of factors that leads to either effective capability or chronic dysfunction remains unclear. Models such as FSS potentially offer to both family and service systems significant hope of breaking chronic patterns of maladaptive family interactions and coping.

Multiproblem families present a challenge to service providers because of their difficulties across multiple spheres of functioning. The families are often in a state of chronic dependency upon community social services, which contributes to the burgeoning costs of mental health and social welfare. These families may also exhibit a persistent failure to respond to help that is offered, which adds to the frustration of the service providers, who may already have a lack of confidence in the family's ability to institute change and in the service system's capacity to intervene in a positive manner.

Because of the complex web of problems with which these families present, traditional social service approaches appear to be inadequate. Unidimensional interventions designed to address specific problems in isolation have not been effective in ameliorating the multidimensional problems of these families; however, confronting these multiple problems can be overwhelming to the service provider.

Two organizing principles are necessary in order to focus work with the multiproblem family. The first is the doctrine of "in the best interest of the child." Focusing upon the needs of the children creates a frame of reference by which the intervention can be measured. Without such focus, the work can be diffused, less purposive, overgeneralized, and difficult to assess. The second principle recognizes the centrality of the psychoanalytic concept of the auxiliary ego, which lends support to the parent as he or she moves toward a higher level of functioning (Lewis and Stark, 1966). The therapeutic team, often the family support worker, is critical in this regard. When this principle is utilized within the context of forming a personal relationship with the family, the family's and the helper's feelings of being overwhelmed can be managed. In addition to these two principles, moving the site of clinical treatment from the traditional setting to the home has been found to significantly reduce resistance to involvement and treatment disruptions.

Working with multiproblem families appears to require new approaches to treatment and redevelopment of clinical resources. This may have important implications for training and practice of psychiatrists and other mental health professionals. The FSS program at the Yale Child Study Center has intervened successfully with these families since 1985. This success is reflected in the program's ability to prevent out-of-home placement of children in over 85% of the families served. Other program models appear to be equally effective (Pecora et al., 1990); however, Dore (1993) argues that extremely poor families may need more and continuing service. Berry (1992, 1993) has shown that these types of programs may not be as successful with chronic, long-term neglecting families. It is the authors' belief that although there is still much to be learned about these programs, investment in families previously believed to be unavailable for treatment offers our best hope of preserving and assisting families in crisis.

References

Adnopoz J: Preserving families for children: An assessment of risks, benefits and options. Clinical Conference Presentation, Yale University School of Medicine Child Study Center, New Haven, CT, 1994a.

Adnopoz J: Effects of poverty on children. Paper presented at Social Advocacy Program, Temple Mishkan Israel, Hamden, CT, 1994b.

American Public Welfare Association and the Nationies for children: An assessment of risks, benefits and options. Clinical Conference Presentation, Yale University School of Medicine Child Study Center, New Haven, CT, 1994a.

Adnopoz J: Effects of poverty on children. Paper presented at Social Advocacy Program, Temple Mishkan Israel, Hamden, CT, 1994b.

American Public Welfare Association and the National Council of State Human Service Administrators: One Child in Four. Investing in Poor Families and Their Children: A Matter of Commitment. Washington, DC, American Public Welfare Association, 1987.

Berry M: An evaluation of family preservation services: Fitting agency services to family needs. Social Work 37:314–321, 1992.

Berry M: The relative effectiveness of family preservation services with neglectful families. In: Morton ES, Grigsby RK(eds): Advancing Family Preservation Practice. Newbury Park, CA, Sage, 1993, pp. 70–98.

Bowlby J: Special problems: Problem families, neglectful parents, the broken home, illegitimacy. In: British National Conference on Social Welfare: The Family: Report of the British National Conference On Social Work. London, National Council of Social Service, 1953.

Bowlby J: Attachment (2nd ed). New York: Basic Books, 1969.

Bowlby J: Separation. New York: Basic Books, 1973.

Bowlby J: Loss. New York: Basic Books, 1980.

Bowlby J: A Secure Base. New York: Basic Books, 1988.

Caplan G: Family support systems in a changing world. In: Anthony EJ, Chiland C (eds): The Child in His Family: Children and Their Parents in a Changing World. New York, Wiley, 1978.

Deutsch C: Children of Alcoholics: Understanding and Helping. Hollywood, FL, Health Communications, 1983.

Dore MM: Family preservation and poor families: When "Homebuilding" is not enough. Families in Society 74:545–556, 1993.

Edna McConnell Clark Foundation: Keeping Families Together: The Case for Family Preservation. New York, Edna McConnell Clark Foundation, 1985, p. 13.

Erikson E: Human strength and the cycle of generations. In: Insight and Responsibility. New York, Norton, 1964, p. 184.

Ford Foundation Executive Panel: The Common Good, Social Welfare, and the American Future. New York, Ford Foundation, 1989.

Frankel H: Family centered, home-based services in child protection: A review of the research. Soc Serv Rev 62:136–137, 1988.

Freud A: Safeguarding the emotional health of children. In: Goldstein J, Katz J (eds): The Family and the Law. New York, Free Press, p. 1059, 1965.

Geismar LL, Lasorte MA: Understanding the Multi-Problem Family. New York, Association Press, 1964.

Goldstein J, Freud A, Solnit A: Beyond the Best Interest of the Child. New York, Free Press, 1973.

Grigsby RK: Theories that guide intensive family preservation services: A second look. In: Morton ES, Grigsby RK (eds): Advancing Family Preservation Practice. Newbury Park, CA, Sage, 1993, pp. 16–27.

Grigsby RK: Maintaining attachment relationships among children in foster care. Families in Society 75(4):269–276, 1994.

Grigsby RK: Interventions to meet basic needs in high-risk families with children. In: Kilpatrick AC, Holland TP (eds): Assessing and Working with Families: An Integrative Model by Level of Functioning. Needham Heights, MA, Allyn & Bacon, 1995, pp. 69–84.

Kaplan L: Working with Multi-Problem Families. Lexington, MA, Lexington Books, 1986, pp. 6, 7.

Kilpatrick AC, Holland TP: Levels of family functioning. In: Kilpatrick AC, Holland TP (eds): Assessing and Working with Families: An Integrative Model by Level of Functioning. Needham Heights, MA, Allyn & Bacon, 1995, pp. 69–84.

Klerman LV: Alive and Well? A Research and Policy Review of Health Programs for Poor Young Children. National Center for Children in Poverty, Columbia University School of Public Health, New York, 1991.

Knitzer J, Cole ES: Family Preservation Services: The Program Challenge for Child Welfare and Child Mental Health Agencies. New York, Bank Street College of Education, 1989.

Lewis M, Stark MH: Family centered diagnosis and treatment in a pediatric clinic. Soc Casework 47:13–18, 1966.

Lower East Side Family Union: Annual Report. New York, Lower East Side Family Union, 1976.

National Commission on Child Welfare and Family Preservation: A Commitment to Change. Washington, DC: American Public Welfare Foundation, 1991.

Nelson K: Populations and outcomes in eleven family-based child welfare programs. In: Wells K, Biegel D (eds): Family Preservation Services: Research and Evaluation. Newbury Park, CA, Sage, 1990a.

Nelson K: How do we know that family-based services are effective? The Prevention Report. Oakdale, IA, National Resource Center On Family Based Services, 1990b, pp. 1–3.

Nelson KE, Landsman MJ, Deutelbaum W: Three models of family-centered placement prevention services. Child Welfare 69(1):3–21, 1990.

Pecora P, Fraser MW, Haapala D: Intensive home-based family treatment: Client outcomes and issues for program design. In: Wells K, Biegel D (eds): Family Preservation Services: Research and Evaluation. Newbury Park, CA, Sage, 1990, pp. 3–32.

Provence S: Changing families and child rearing. Paper presented at the Children's Advocacy Conference of the New England Children's Mental Health Task Force, Durham, NH, 1979.

Rutter M, Quinton D: Parental psychiatric disorder: Effects on children. *Psychol Med* 14:853–880, 1984.

Schorr L, Schorr D: *Within Our Reach: Breaking the Cycle of Disadvantage.* New York, Anchor Press, 1988.

Selig AL: The myth of the multi-problem family. *Am J Orthopsychiatry* 46:526–532, 1976.

Solnit A: In the best interests of the child and his parents. In: Levitt M, Rubenstein B (eds): *Orthopsychiatry and the Law.* Detroit, Wayne State University Press, 1968.

Soule CR, Massarene K, Abate K: Clinician-support worker teams in family preservation: Are two heads better than one? In: Morton ES, Grigsby RK (eds): *Advancing Family Preservation Practice.* Newbury Park, CA, Sage, 1993, pp. 39–55.

Spencer J: The multi-problem family. In: Schlesinger B (ed): *The Multi-Problem Family: A Review and Annotated Bibliography* (3rd ed). Toronto, University of Toronto Press, 1963, pp. 1–12.

Taylor L, Newberger EN: Child abuse and the International Year of the Child. *N Engl J Med* 301: 1205–1212, 1979.

Tracy EM: Identifying social support resources of at-risk families. *Social Work* 35:252–258, 1990.

Tracy EM: Defining the target population for family preservation services. In: Wells K, Beidel DE (eds): *Family Preservation Services: Research and Evaluation.* Newbury Park, CA, Sage, 1991.

Tracy EM, Whittaker JK: The evidence base for social support interventions in child and family practice: Emerging issues for research and practice. *Children and Youth Services Rev* 9:249–270, 1987.

Wald MS: Family preservation: Are we moving too fast? *Public Welfare* 46:33–38, 1988.

"Why leave children with bad parents?" *Newsweek* (1994, April 25):52–56,58.

106 THE RUNAWAY ADOLESCENT
David A. Tomb, M.D.

Approximately 1 million adolescents in the United States run away from home and live on the streets for at least part of each year. Perhaps 10% of all teenagers run sometime (Edelback, 1980). Many of these youths suffer significant and long-lasting physical and psychological damage, yet receive little or no care from any public or private agency (Robertson, 1988).

Our ability to anticipate and prevent running, and to remedy the effects of this experience, has been limited. In part this reflects a scarcity of careful empirical studies. However, it also reflects the impact of the runaway experience: Life on the street is so traumatic that when we study runaways it becomes difficult to distinguish which clinical features were antecedent and which were consequent to the runaway (Justice and Duncan, 1976). In spite of this, there is a growing appreciation of who these children are, what motivates them, what interventions will help, and, to a lesser degree, what the outcome of running away during adolescence is likely to be.

PREVALENCE

Runaway teenagers come from all social groups and geographical regions but most are urban youths from lower socioeconomic status (SES) levels. Fewer than half live with both parents, and those who do are likely to come from very large homes (Johnson and Peck, 1978). More than a quarter come from single-parent homes, while another quarter come from foster or group homes. Although the statistics are in dispute, girls predominate by a slim margin in most categories of runaways (Garbarino et al., 1985). Ninety percent of youths run fewer than 50 miles from home. Seventy percent of runaway episodes are brief (lasting 1–6 days), and follow a triggering incident (usually an argument with the parents); the child's focus remains on the home. However, as many as 15% of runaway adolescents are absent from home for many weeks or months: they develop an alternative identity that is streetwise and independent of their families. These youths may never return home. An additional group of runaway adolescents come and go from home numerous times over their teenage years; a dozen or more runaway episodes are not unusual. This group is more likely to come from an abusive environment and to have their instability complicated by drug and alcohol abuse.

Such a variable pattern of running away causes the figure of 1 million runaway adolescents in the United States each year to be very approximate. Definition is crucial. Fewer than 400,000 youths are absent from home for months or years. On the other hand, many adolescents who leave home briefly (usually to the house of a friend or relative) are never reported. To include them might swell the number of runaways into the millions. Also, those children who run numerous times further confuse the statistics. Perhaps the key point is that running away is a substantial problem badly in need of interventions, particularly considering the negative consequences of even a brief period of time spent on the streets.

RUNAWAY TYPOLOGY

Several detailed taxonomies are available that, with mixed success, attempt to categorize the complex phenomena of adolescent runaway (Adams et al., 1985; Dunford and Brennan, 1976; Homer, 1973; Jones, 1988; Miller, et al., 1990; Roberts, 1982a). Each incorporates one or more of the following organizing principles: the putative cause of running away, the family dynamics, the individual dynamics and/or psychopathology, sociocultural variables, the age of the adolescent, and the length of the runaway period.

The recent use of "runaway" as a diagnosis has been confused. Although DSM-II included the category of runaway reaction of childhood or adolescence, this was subsumed within conduct disorder, undersocialized nonaggressive type, in DSM-III. This latter diagnosis then disappeared completely in DSM-III-R and remains absent from DSM-IV, except as one of many possible criteria for conduct disorder. Runaway adolescents currently are to receive diagnoses for any specific conditions from which they suffer but not for their runaway behavior itself. At the very least, in most cases, this requires the "V" code of Parent-Child Relational Problem.

Although no single classification scheme has emerged as ideal for all purposes (Hartman et al., 1987), a typology based on the youth's reasons for running may be the most clinically useful, particularly when enriched by correlations with other important variables. Such a scheme must have at least two major categories: adolescents who "run from" home (runaway) and adolescents who are "pushed from" home (throwaway). It is essential, for clinical purposes, to know whether a child has chosen to leave home voluntarily or has been forced to leave by abusing or rejecting parents, even though this distinction frequently blurs in individual cases.

Runaway Youth

Most adolescents on the street have run from home rather than been driven out (Sharlin and Mor-Barak, 1992). Moreover, the majority of these youths have come from turbulent homes with fractured family relations and are actively escaping a situation perceived as intolerable (Council on Scientific Affairs, 1993). A smaller percentage are adventure-seeking teenagers who are actually "running to" the exciting life on the streets. In some cases there is intergenerational transmision of running away, as sequential generations of children from one family "hit the streets" (Plass and Hotaling, 1995). Although both groups deserve clinical attention, the former may be more in need of, and responsive to, intervention.

"RUNNING FROM" YOUTH

Many different situational and personal characteristics can predispose to runaway. Moreover, what a youth judges to be an acceptable reason for running differs with the culture and with the expectations of the youth's immediate peer group.

The most common reason for running away is a difficult home situation. A few adolescents are in homes that are truly intolerable by any standard; to escape from them may be both rational and healthy. These youths may be fleeing chronic physical or sexual abuse (Famularo et al., 1990; Farber et al., 1984), often at the hands of antisocial, alcoholic, or drug-abusing parents. They may suffer equally severe psychological abuse by rejecting, punitive, or chronically neglectful parents. A few homes are so disorganized that the children are essentially without a history; they watch a parade of adults pass through their lives and don't know in some cases even who their natural parents are. Such families are frequently well known to community agencies and the children are often removed before they have a chance to run. Occasionally, however, the children must escape by their own means and thus end on the streets as runaways. They may find more warmth and caring on the street than they ever encountered at home, and if they become part of a "substitute family," their run may become permanent. In recent years, the substitute family willing and eager to adopt such disaffiliated youth has been one of the antisocial gangs that grace the midsized and major cities in the United States. In fact, the majority of gang members seem to have come from such dysfunctional families.

More commonly, the homes of runaways are characterized by a lesser degree of turmoil and by verbal abuse and poor communication. Typically the children and parents battle over one or more issues that neither seems able or willing to resolve. Parents identify problems with the teenager's behavior that range from the mundane (dinner table deportment, jewelry selection, hair style) through the expected (school performance, dating habits, curfew) to the profound (drug and alcohol abuse, illegal activities). The adolescents, on the other hand, feel themselves unheard, controlled and powerless, and without respect. Common to all these settings, however, is a reliance by both parties on the child's leaving home to resolve interpersonal conflicts. Girls predominate, perhaps because parents are more controlling and demanding of them. Family ties are usually intact, although loose, and reconciliation typically remains possible.

Alternatively, a crisis in the home can precipitate a runaway. Divorce, infidelity, financial disaster, or tension among other family members can cause an adolescent to flee. This may occur if the youth senses a loss of support when most family resources are directed elsewhere, but it also may represent the adolescent's need to call attention to the family's distress in an effort to get help. With otherwise stable parent-child relations, such running away is usually brief but may recur if the crisis persists or returns. However, if the child personally experiences the crisis (pregnancy, sudden trouble with the law, homosexuality revealed), the likelihood that he or she will run depends primarily upon the reaction of the parents or on the expectation of an unacceptable reaction—and this depends in large part on the quality of the communications between parents and child.

Finally, some teenagers run from home as a manipulation. They may be seeking attention, trying to avoid punishment for a minor infraction, or trying to "let their parents know who is boss" (and have some fun while they are at it). This may occur with the adolescent whose parents have finally decided to crack down on increasingly unacceptable behavior. Such an episode is usually brief and done safely (e.g., run to a friend's house); it may be repeated if felt to be successful.

"RUNNING TO" YOUTH

A significant minority of youths run away from home initially to exercise their independence, to escape boredom and seek excitement, and because of the allure of being "on the street." Home life for most of these adolescents is not supportive and as likely to be characterized by minimal control and parental indifference as by overcontrol and abuse, although some of these youths appear to have normal relationships with their parents and to come from homes that seem relatively stable. Moreover, some report adequate (and even exceptional) school performance and uneventful peer relations. This diverse group of teenagers range from naive youngsters who have been inordinately influenced by pressure from their peers (and who often quickly return home after a brief adventure) to frankly antisocial adolescents for whom life on the streets differs little from the life they led before leaving home.

Throwaway Youth

Approximately one-quarter of runaway children are actually throwaways (abandoned, castaways, homeless, pushouts) (Gullotta, 1978). These difficult, traumatized adolescents have either been encouraged to leave or been forcibly ejected from their homes. They are slightly more likely to be girls, to be older than more typical runaways, and to display high levels of conduct disorder, school failure, and drug and alcohol use. Typically their homes are very disturbed and marked by abuse, violence, and neglect. However, infrequently the homes are relatively stable, but the child has been scapegoated: identified as the "bad seed," whose removal from the home will solve the family's problems. In either case, relations between parents and child are chronically impaired, and neither party sees hope. Efforts to repair the family are usually unsuccessful.

CLINICAL DESCRIPTION

Although several efforts to develop a psychological profile of adolescent runaways have been made (Adams and Munro, 1979; Jenkins, 1971; Pietropinto, 1985; Roberts, 1982a), no single description can encompass the diversity of runaway youths. However, that large group of runaway/throwaway youths who come from abusive and emotionally impoverished homes share some common psychological features.

Most studies find the majority of them to be demoralized and to have a poor sense of self. In spite of a spirit of bravado and defiance, they are insecure and frightened. They frequently see themselves as inadequate not only academically and occupationally but also socially and interpersonally. This often reflects reality since many of these youngsters have a long history of failures: Almost all have been poor students or had significant school difficulties, while many have received limited occupational training. They typically are uneasy around and avoid adults. They are likely to be ostracized as "losers" by their more successful peers and are most comfortable with an equally impaired peer group. Compared to their peers, they typically choose maladaptive ways of coping with stress, including running away (Roberts, 1982b). Finally, in spite of the apparent independence required to run away, many such youth are passive and dependent when given the chance (Benalcazar, 1982).

Coincident with this self-image of incompetence is a sense that they have little impact on their environment. They frequently feel powerless to influence their parents, and since many of their parents are controlling and abusive or, alternatively, neglectful and disinterested, this may also have a basis in reality. Nor do they feel that other adults in their environment, such as school teachers, respect them. As a result, leaving home becomes in part an effort to establish a sphere of self-esteem.

As might be expected, dysthymia and depression occur with increased frequency (Feitel et al, 1992). Estimates of depression among this population range from 20% to 80% (Hersch, 1988). Suicide attempts may occur in over one-third of this population (Rotheram-Borus, 1993). A key contributing factor to this pattern may well be the high incidence of previous and concurrent sexual abuse among runaways of both sexes (McCormack et al., 1986). As many as two-thirds or more of runaway females and one-third or more of runaway males (Janus et al., 1987) have been abused. Such experience is known to bring in its wake significant depression but also is associated with symptoms such as anxiety, dissociative episodes, sexual dysfunction and sexual acting out (Seng, 1989), substance abuse, conduct disorder, fear of adult men (by both males and females), and difficulty with close interpersonal relationships. These symptoms are frequently observed among runaways; past sexual exploitation may have contributed to the current clinical presentation of such a youngster.

Not only do they experience broad-based failure, but they actively adopt, or are forced to adopt, self-destructive behaviors likely to worsen that course (Greenblatt and Robertson, 1993). They frequently abuse alcohol and a variety of drugs even before they run from home, further compounding their problems. In fact, substance abuse may occasionally dominate the clinical picture, leading to daily disruptions and generalized failures and resulting in expulsion from the home. Chronic truancy and status offenses are also common; the typical runaway is more likely to be the petty rather than the serious offender. The increase in conduct disorder among runaways, although real, may partly reflect the runaway experience itself. Adolescents for whom the fundamental problem is conduct disorder are more likely to have run at an earlier age, to stay away longer, and to get into more serious trouble.

Although by far the most common psychiatric conditions to be found among runaways are depression, substance abuse, and conduct disorders, other psychopathology also occurs with increased frequency. Some youths are markedly anxious and deserve an anxiety disorder diagnosis. These adolescents also seem to be more likely to suffer from attention deficit hyperactivity disorder and learning disabilities, yet good evidence is currently not available. Certainly, though, studies have found the runaway adolescent to be restless, demanding, and impulsive (Goldberg, 1972). Deeply disturbed or psychotic children living on their own in the community are present with a modestly increased frequency. That they are not even more common probably reflects both their likelihood of being institutionalized once recognized and the difficulty such youngsters with significant psychological disorganization have surviving on the street.

Although the majority of runaways can be contained within the preceding description, a sizable subpopulation of adolescents fits better another general description entirely. These are the youths who envision running as an adventure (the "running to" group) and who have a value system consonant with life on the streets. They frequently are excitement-seeking, moderately antisocial adolescents who are likely to come and go from home as the mood suits them or to stay on the street for months or years if they find a niche of their own there. These are the teenagers most likely to exploit those around them and to slip into a more permanent antisocial life-style.

Finally, some runaway adolescents are indistinguishable from normal. They have a generally good relationship with their parents and maintain close ties throughout one or more runaway episodes. They have strong ties to their peers (who may be confused by, or participants in, the running behavior) and perform well in school. Psychopathology is not evident, and since the running episodes are brief, infrequent, and safely performed, the behavior produces few psychological repercussions.

Parental Patterns

To understand the runaway teenager, it is necessary to recognize that the parents' role in generating disturbed family interpersonal relations is usually at least as important as their child's. A poor parent-child relationship is the most consistent finding in the home of a runaway. Although some homes and parents are psychologically unremarkable, often the parents of the more persistent runaway adolescents have features in common.

Most of these parents are exceptionally critical of and dissatisfied with their children. Parent-child communications are typically negative; the parents provide little in the way of compliments or support (and the child reciprocates in kind). They establish a standard for behavior (often poorly defined) that the teenager often finds unattainable but then provides little help or counseling when the child fails. Their frustration and demands typically take the form of verbal abuse as well as occasional shoves or blows.

The communication of perpetual dissatisfaction with their child is usually accompanied by inconstant discipline. They are quite capable of being restrictive at times, particularly around specific issues such as dating and curfew, and lax at other times. The teenager interprets the restriction as parental rigidity and control and then rebels (or runs away). However, these efforts by the parents to make demands on their children typically are overlaid on a more fundamental pattern of disinterest and lack of supervision. Runaway adolescents are as likely to report that their parents have no time for or interest in them as they are to report that the parents are too demanding. Many of these parents are absorbed in their own problems and desires and give little time or energy to their children (latch key children). They are not there to help with schoolwork, intercede with teachers, or discuss problems. The children rightfully see themselves as incidental to the parents and are less willing to adapt themselves to their parents' wishes. There is little real comfort to be had in these families, and so the child looks elsewhere.

A significant minority of these parents displays real psychopathology as well. Antisocial personality disorder and drug and alcohol abuse are common. Parental disorganization and instability may also result from depression, psychosis, or low intelligence. In any case, the parents may need intervention separate from work with the family.

THE CONSEQUENCES OF RUNNING AWAY

Most teenagers leave home with a plan in mind. Unless their departure is precipitous, they usually are running to a friend's house, to a distant relative, or to a known location or town. Alternatively, they may be "hitting the road," but usually with one or more friends with whom they have planned their runaway. Girls frequently run to or with their boyfriends, who often provide them with money and a place to stay. Episodes of running often end when the money runs out. Many teens are quickly returned home by acquaintances or by the police, or they end up in shelters as a way station to home or alternative residential placements. These well-contained runaway episodes generally do little long-lasting damage, occasionally provide the teenager with enhanced self-esteem, and may be beneficial by mobilizing the family to get help. (Unfortunately, many first-time runaway youngsters return to angry parents who decide to "crack down," producing a worsening spiral.)

Prolonged runaway attempts are less benign (Young et al., 1987). Few adolescents survive on the street for lengthy periods without trauma; the street is a great leveler. Unless a youth is provided for by friends or family, the dominant issue of living on the street quickly becomes survival. One estimate suggests that within one month a youth on the street without resources will have to turn to crime to survive (Hersch, 1988). This means turning to theft and street hustles, prostitution, pornography, drug selling, and the exploitation of others. Among chronic street adolescents, three-quarters have been involved in prostitution, three-quarters with selling drugs, and three-quarters have been incarcerated. The longer adolescents are on the street, the more likely they are to find their way into trouble and into the courts.

More important, however, is the sheer physical danger of being on the streets. Violence (assault, battery, rape) and its associated injuries are the most serious problems a youth faces. Most street youths will be beaten or raped at some point. Some will become pregnant; some will receive permanent injury; some will be killed. In addition, their physical health will deteriorate. Skin infections, parasitic infections, respiratory and gastrointestinal diseases, dental problems, nutritional deficiencies, and medical conditions associated with drug abuse are common (Council on Scientific Affairs, 1989). Because of their hand-to-mouth existence, they risk exposure to the elements, exhaustion, and musculoskeletal problems. To make matters worse, hunger, fatigue, and drug-related cognitive impairments all compromise the teenager's ability to cope with routine stresses, let alone with the major challenges they face on the street.

All of these physical disabilities occur during a time when they have limited access to health care and limited ability to pay for it. Although some care can be provided to minors without parental consent in some states for certain conditions (e.g., pregnancy, venereal disease), most nonemergent care is unavailable unless the individual is an emancipated minor. But even if emancipated, they have the same difficulty in obtaining health care as does anyone who is indigent.

Besides violence and drug abuse, the other major risk to the physical health of the runaway is sexually transmitted disease (Rotheram-Borus et al., 1992a). Runaway youths are perhaps the most sexually active of all teenagers, and their rates of syphilis and gonorrhea are the highest of any group (Rotheram-Borus et al., 1992b; Zylke, 1989). This sexual activity, coupled with high rates of drug abuse, places runaways at high risk of exposure to AIDS. Although an epidemic of AIDS among runaway teenagers is unlikely due to the long latency of the disease, there is an epidemic of exposure to AIDS in progress (Hersch, 1988). In some inner city populations of runaway adolescents, the HIV seropositive rate may approach 10% with much of the exposure occurring through heterosexual contacts (Hein, 1987, 1989).

Prostitution (male and female) and pregnancy present other risks to runaways (Brown, 1979). As many as 900,000 adolescents are involved in prostitution each year; many, but not all of them, are runaways. Adolescent male prostitution is common, but female activity predominates. The average age of first intercourse for these girls is approximately 12 to 13, while the average age of beginning prostitution is 14 to 15. Prior traumatic sexual experiences are the norm: Many of these adolescent girls have been molested; half have been raped. Although some hardcore runaways prostitute for the money and glamour, most are trying to survive. With this group of runaways in particular, street drug use is extensive and other physical risks excessive (Yates et al., 1991a).

Teenagers pay a severe psychological price for life on the street; those who successfully adapt are usually the worse for it. Many of these youths are intensely lonely, fearful, and unhappy (Kufeldt and Nimmo, 1987). The longer they are on the street, the greater the number of demoralizing experiences they will have had. In fact, life on the streets itself can produce all of the symptoms usually associated with runaway adolescents. Running away often has forced them into a life they did not expect and do not want. However, they frequently have few options. Only 50% of chronic runaway teenagers have any possibility of returning home. As time goes by the consequences of running become long-lasting; they have effectively excluded themselves from an education and a career. Determination to succeed flags, and many of these youths become permanent members of the underclass.

TREATMENT

Runaway adolescents can be both difficult to treat as well as desperately in need of treatment. Perhaps the most formidable obstacle to treating them is that they rarely seek help (Brennan, 1978). Even those in medical need will frequently suffer rather than look for aid from adults, agencies, or shelters. In addition, they are frightened, defensive, hypersensitive, embittered, rebellious, and mobile—they don't stay in treatment long, they run away. Keeping them engaged requires tact, a nonjudgmental attitude, the development of a personal relationship (with someone), and, most frequently, patience. They are present oriented; because of the intensity of their feelings, they tolerate review of their past poorly. However, it is possible to have considerable impact if the child (and his or her family) is engaged skillfully at the right moment.

Most commonly runaways are reported missing by their parents and are brought to clinics or inpatient facilities by the parents, police, a relative, or a mental health worker. Occasionally their absence from the home goes unreported, and their status only comes to attention when they appear at a shelter or on the street. These "forgotten" adolescents are typically the most impaired. The Juvenile Justice and Delinquency Prevention Act of 1974 prevents the long-term incarceration of these youths, yet their treatment in the eyes of the law reflects state statute: Some states consider runaways to be juvenile delinquents and send them through the courts, while other states consider them status offenders and send them home or to treatment facilities.

Once identified, the first order of business is to provide a safe environment. This usually involves a rapid assessment of the home and perhaps a return there, but may mean finding a shelter, group home, or other social service facility as an alternate placement until an appropriate long-term setting can be found. It helps to have an assessment unit as part of the clinic or shelter and to have ready access to medical care, since these youths may be in poor health and need prompt attention. Although their skittishness and lack of cooperation may interrupt treatment, immediate provision of welcome medical care can entice them into a treatment-receptive stance. Although some professionals worry about it, providing medical and psychotherapeutic aid to runaway adolescents in need without parental consent is generally acceptable in the eyes of the law (Croxton, 1988; English, 1991).

Appropriate treatment usually depends upon the type of runaway and the length of time the teenager has been gone. Usually, however, the earlier the intervention, the better, although simply returning the child home rarely works. An effort at family therapy is essential for the "running from" youth (Ostensen, 1981). Such therapy is often effective, particularly if the running episode has been brief and if the family is basically stable but in acute crisis. More severely disabled families may respond to intervention; the focus needs to be on family stress rather than on the child's problems, on education in parenting skills, and on interpersonal skills training for all members. The parents need to learn to listen, to show affection, to develop consistency and parenting effectiveness, and to care. They need to be alerted to and to correct interpersonal distortions when they occur, and to avoid scapegoating the child in service of their own marital disputes. They often need to develop more realistic expectations for their child, and this typically requires a careful assessment of the child's capabilities.

Like the teenagers, the parents are also often resistant to treatment. They may consider their problems so serious that a bad result is inevitable or too confidential to talk about. They may be defensive or demoralized and without confidence. It is essential to engage them in therapy before they become hardened to their youngster's problems or disenchanted by any treatment efforts. In spite of the best efforts, some families will not follow through.

In general, the more chronic and complex the family's problems, the more broad-based the interventions needed. If the child has been out of the home for a long period, however, the family ties may be so weakened that returning home is unrealistic and formal family therapy of little value. Family therapy is generally not useful for chronic street kids.

"Running to" adolescents, particularly if they are moderately antisocial and enjoying their time away from home, are resistant to treatment. Often the most that can be accomplished is to help them find acceptable, legal, and even constructive outlets for their energies and enthusiasms. Throwaway adolescents typically are the most traumatized of all and need support and stable placement, if they will accept such help. They also occasionally respond to intensive individual psychotherapy, but due to their sensitivity and lack of trust, group therapy with peers is often a necessary and acceptable alternative.

Runaway adolescents are often difficult to engage in individual therapy, but when a therapeutic alliance develops, such treatment can be very effective. Many of these youngsters want to feel better and do better. Many want to return to school and be reintegrated into their community, only the hurdles seem overwhelming to them. The therapist must recognize their heightened defensiveness, anxiety, and impulsivity—it is impossible to be too gentle and supportive to many of these youths. If they are abusing drugs, every effort must be made to detoxify them. Issues around sexual abuse need to be addressed, yet the patient may respond with withdrawal, denial, cockiness, anger, or verbal abuse if the pace is too rapid. At least initially, the child needs to feel in control of the interviews. Many (most) of these youths can benefit from training in specific coping skills, well received often through role playing exercises with peers. Of course, identifying and treating specific psychiatric disorders such as depression, substance abuse, and psychosis is essential, as is the recognition of specific deficiencies such as learning disabilities. Perhaps even more than in most psychotherapies, however, success depends upon developing a personal relationship with the youngster that will weather the inevitable storms to follow.

Public and private resources of all types are inadequate for runaway adolescents. Some agencies avoid dealing with these teenagers in part because they can be difficult (Kufeldt, 1991). Comprehensive services with a continuum of care are needed but unavailable in most communities. This continuum should include not only medical care and individual psychotherapy but also runaway shelters for brief but safe stays, small group homes for longer stays, hostels and supervised but independent living apartments for selected older adolescents, carefully chosen foster homes, and secure facilities for very disturbed youths. However, some youths have trouble in any structured setting and may need to be treated for a while on the street (Kufeldt et al., 1992; Smart, 1991; Yates et al., 1991b). Emergency hotlines are available and advertised in some locations, and there are at least three runaway hotlines that serve a national or regional audience: National Runaway Switchboard (1-800-621-4000 [HIT-HOME]), Covenant House (New York) hotline (1-800-999-9999 [''nine-line'']), and National Center for Missing and Exploited Children (1-800-843-5678).

OUTCOME

Careful outcome studies are rare (Olson, 1980; Robins, 1958), based on few patients, and dated. Only limited conclusions can be drawn. Runaways, as a group, are failures in later life. They never make up for lost schooling or missed occupational opportunities. They tend to slip to the lowest SES group and frequently become dependent upon others (ironically, often their families) for support. Adult interpersonal relations are typically poor, and their sense of self remains low. The more significant their runaway activities as an adolescent (i.e., chronics or repeaters versus brief nonrepeaters), the more likely they are to fail as an adult. On the other hand, teenagers with brief, one-time runaway episodes may be indistinguishable from a normal group later in life.

There is insufficient information at this time to either go beyond these tentative conclusions or to explain them. It is not clear, for example, how much of runaway behavior or outcome is due to innate temperament and abilities and how much to parent-child conflicts and experience. It is clear, however, that the runaway adolescent is an individual deserving clinical and research attention.

RESEARCH DIRECTIONS

The research base with this population is inadequate. Even fundamental clinical questions go unanswered: How diversified or uniform are the personality characteristics of these children? Is drug use etiologic or secondary? What are the features that determine a priori whether a child will engage in a brief or a sustained runaway? What personal characteristics allow a child to succeed as a runaway? Which interventions are effective, if any, and with which populations (Podschun, 1993)? Numerous interwoven factors have made this a difficult group to study; they need to be specifically identified and teased apart.

Any research must be broad-based, or at least must recognize its limitations. Results differ depending upon the cultural and socioeconomic group studied, upon the location of the study, and upon the time of the study. Inner city runaways differ from suburban runaways; summer runaways may differ from those gone year-round. Outcome may vary with family structure, with drug use, with degree of criminality, and with interventions available. All results may vary with the generation studied; studies during the restless 1960s don't necessarily apply today. Serious hope of influencing the runaway problem awaits clarification of may of these basic issues and questions.

References

Adams GR, Gullota T, Clancy MA: Homeless adolescents: A descriptive study of similarities and differences between runaways and throwaways. *Adolescence* 20:715, 1985.

Adams GR, Munro G: Portrait of the North American runaway: A critical review. *J Youth Adolesc* 8:359, 1979.

Benalcazar B: Study of fifteen runaway patients. *Adolescence* 17:553, 1982.

Brennan T, Huizinga D, Elliott DS: *The Social Psychology of Runaways*. Lexington, MA, Lexington Books, 1978.

Brown ME: Teenage prostitution. *Adolescence* 14:665, 1979.

Council on Scientific Affairs, American Medical Association: Adolescents as victims of family violence. *JAMA* 270:1850–1856, 1993.

Council on Scientific Affairs: Health care needs of homeless and runaway youths. *JAMA* 262:1358, 1989.

Croxton TA, Churchill SR, Fellin P: Counseling minors without parental consent. *Child Welfare* 67:3, 1988.

Dunford FW, Brennan T: A taxonomy of runaway youth. *Soc Serv Rev* 50:457, 1976.

Edelback C: Running away from home. *J Fam Issues* 1:210, 1980.

English A: Runaway and street youth at risk for HIV infection: Legal and ethical issues in access to care. *J Adolesc Health* 12:504–510, 1991.

Famularo R, Kinscherff R, Fenton T, et al: Child maltreatment histories among runaway and delinquent children. *Clin Pediatr Phila* 29:713–718, 1990.

Farber ED, Kinast C, McCoard WD, et al: Violence in families of adolescent runaways. *Child Abuse Negl* 8:295, 1984.

Feitel B, Margetson N, Chamas J, et al: Psychosocial background and behavioral and emotional disorders of homeless and runaway youth. *Hosp Community Psychiatry* 43:155–159, 1992.

Garbarino J, Wilson J, Carbarino A: The adolescent runaway. In: Garbarino J et al (eds): *Troubled Youth, Troubled Families*. New York, Aldine Publishing, 1985.

Goldberg M: Runaway American. *Ment Hygiene* 56:13, 1972.

Greenblatt M, Robertson MJ: Life-styles, adaptive strategies, and sexual behaviors of homeless adolescents. *Hosp Community Psychiatry* 44:1177–1180, 1993.

Gullotta TP: Runaway: Reality or myth. *Adolescence* 13:543, 1978.

Hartman CR, Burgess AW, McCormack A: Pathways and cycles of runaways: A model for understanding repetitive runaway behavior. *Hosp Community Psychiatry* 38:292, 1987.

Hein K: AIDS in adolescence. *J Adolesc Health Care* 10:10C, 1989.

Hein K: AIDS in adolescents: A rationale for concern. *NY State J Med* 87:290, 1987.

Hersch P: Coming of age on city streets. *Psychol Today*, January:28, 1988.

Homer LE: Community-based resource for runaway girls. *J Soc Casework* 54:473, 1973.

Janus M, Burgess AW, McCormack A: Histories of sexual abuse in adolescent male runaways. *Adolescence* 22:405, 1987.

Jenkins RL: The runaway reaction. *Am J Psychiatry* 128:168, 1971.

Johnson NS, Peck R: Sibship composition and the adolescent runaway phenomenon. *J Youth Adolesc* 7:301, 1978.

Jones LP: A typology of adolescent runaways. *Child Adolesc Soc Work* 5:16, 1988.

Justice B, Duncan DF: Running away: An epidemic problem of adolescence. *Adolescence* 11:365, 1976.

Kufeldt K: Social policy and runaways. *J Health Social Policy* 2:37–49, 1991.

Kufeldt K, Durieux M, Nimmo M, et al: Providing shelter for street youth: Are we reaching those in need? *Child Abuse Negl* 16:187–199, 1992.

Kufeldt K, Nimmo M: Youth on the street: Abuse and neglect in the eighties. *Child Abuse Negl* 11:531, 1987.

McCormack A, Janus M, Burgess AW: Runaway youths and sexual victimization: Gender differences in an adolescent runaway population. *Child Abuse Negl* 10:387, 1986.

Miller AT, Eggertson-Tacon C, Quigg B: Patterns of runaway behavior within a larger systems context: the road to empowerment. *Adolescence* 25:271–289, 1990.

Olson L, Liebow E, Mannino FV, et al: Runaway children twelve years later. *J Fam Issues* 1:165, 1980.

Ostensen KW: The runaway crisis: Is family therapy the answer? *Am J Fam Ther* 9:3, 1981.

Pietropinto A: Runaway children. *Med Aspects Hum Sex* 19:175, 1985.

Plass PS, Hotaling GT: The intergenerational transmission of running away: childhood experiences of the parents of runaways. *J Youth Adolesc* 24: 335–348, 1995.

Podschun GD: Teen Peer Outreach-Street Work Project: HIV prevention education for runaway and homeless youth. *Public Health Rep* 108:150–155, 1993.

Roberts AR: Adolescent runaways in suburbia: A new typology. *Adolescence* 17:387, 1982a.

Roberts AR: Stress and coping patterns among adolescent runaways. *J Soc Serv Res* 5:15, 1982b.

Robertson JM: Homeless adolescents: A hidden crisis. *Hosp Community Psychiatry* 39:475, 1988.

Robins LN: Mental illness of the runaway: A 30-year follow-up study. *Hum Organization* 16:1, 1958.

Rotheram-Borus MJ: Suicidal behavior and risk factors among runaway youths. *Am J Psychiatry* 150: 103–107, 1993.

Rotheram-Borus MJ, Meyer-Bahlburg HF, Rosario M, et al: Lifetime sexual behaviors among predominantly minority male runaways and gay/bisexual adolescents in New York City. *AIDS Education Prevention*, Fall Suppl, 34–42, 1992a.

Rotheram-Borus MJ, Meyer-Bahlburg HF, Koopman C, et al: Lifetime sexual behaviors among runaway males and females. *J Sex Res* 29:15–29, 1992b.

Seng MJ: Child sexual abuse and adolescent prostitution: A comparative analysis. *Adolescence* 24:665–675, 1989.

Sharlin SA, Mor-Barak: Runaway girls in distress: motivation, background, and personality. *Adolescence* 27:387–405, 1992.

Smart DH: Homeless youth in Seattle. *J Adolesc Health* 12:519–527, 1991.

Yates GL, Mackenzie RG, Pennbridge J, et al: A risk profile comparison of homeless youth involved in prostitution and homeless youth not involved. *J Adolesc Health* 12:545–548, 1991a.

Yates GL, Pennbridge J, Swofford A, et al: The Los Angeles system of care for runaway/homeless youth. *J Adolesc Health* 12:555–560, 1991b.

Young RL, Godfrey W, Matthews B, et al: Runaways: A review of negative consequences. *Fam Relations* 32:275, 1987.

Zylke JW: Interest heightens in defining, preventing AIDS in high-risk adolescent population. *JAMA* 262:2197, 1989.

B/ Child Psychiatry and Education

107 SCHOOL CONSULTATION

Mary E. Schwab-Stone, M.D., and Christopher Henrich, B.A.

Mental health problems in our citizens have become of increasing concern in the last several decades. In schools, too, ever larger numbers of emotionally disturbed children with increasingly difficult learning and behavior problems concern more and more educators. Mental health professionals . . .are being asked to help educators with these problems . . ..It is clear that in the foreseeable future there will not be enough treatment time and trained personnel available to help disturbed youngsters and their parents. The collaboration of mental health personnel and educators in developing both preventive and therapeutic educational measures, therefore, becomes vital. (Berlin and Szurek, 1965)

There are many compelling reasons why child psychiatrists should engage actively in school consultation and in related school-based activities that support the mental health of children. The most pressing is that mental health services delivered in traditional clinic, hospital, and private office settings do not reach the majority of young people who suffer from psychiatric disturbance. School consultation provides a unique avenue for helping many children who would not otherwise come to psychiatric attention. It also extends knowledge to educators and other school-based professionals to help them work more effectively with psychiatrically disturbed and psychosocially stressed children. And, school consultation can serve as an entry point for the child psychiatrist who is curious about the functioning of schools, the social institution that, second only to the family, bears responsibility for promoting socialization, as well as for other key aspects of development. Finally, through such engagement with schools, the child psychiatrist may have the opportunity to promote ways of thinking and teaching that will promote the physical and mental health of young people.

Despite the compelling argument of need and the potential for mutually interesting interchange, the relationship between educators and mental health professionals has been described in terms such as tenuous (Mattison, 1993a) or ambivalent and uncertain (Comer, 1992). The paucity of collaborative research between educators and child psychiatrists and the lack of cross-fertilization by way of publication in each others' journals attests to a relationship that traditionally has been more distant than collaborative (Mattison, 1993a). This may be due to differences in theoretical orientation, as educators have generally been trained to utilize behavioral paradigms, and psychiatrists, psychodynamic ones (Mattison, 1993a). Also, some residual ill or ambivalent feeling may have been

sustained from the period in the 1960s and 1970s when community mental health centers were mandated to provide consultation to public agencies, an arrangement that led to the sense of psychiatristic consultants as uninvited "strangers bearing gifts" to other community agencies (Borus, 1984). Whatever the reason or combination thereof, many school systems are now actively seeking local child psychiatric consultants to advise on classroom management and on appropriate educational programming for psychiatrically disturbed children. Concurrently, child psychiatrists have achieved prominence through careful studies of school characteristics as they affect psychological health and development and through innovative proposals for school reform (e.g., Comer, 1993; Rutter et al., 1979).

In what is hopefully an improving climate for working relationships between educators and mental health consultants, it is timely for this chapter to: (*a*) review models that apply to school consultation, (*b*) consider some unique features of schools that child psychiatrists can learn about in order to be maximally effective as consultants, and (*c*) discuss the tasks of the child psychiatric consultant in some detail with reference to a frequently requested type of consultation—evaluation for special education services.

HISTORICAL PERSPECTIVE

In the two decades following World War II, awareness of the expanding population base and the numbers of untreated mentally ill stimulated a sense of urgency about providing community-based psychiatric services. In Caplan's words: "An outstanding challenge which today faces mental health specialists is connected with our realization that the number of actual or potential mentally disordered persons in the population exceeds our current capacity for remedial action" (Caplan, 1970, p. 3). With President Kennedy's message to Congress on mental health and mental retardation and the subsequent passage of Public Law (PL) 88-164, the Community Mental Health Centers Act of 1963, community mental health consultation became, for a time, an obligatory basic service (Caplan, 1970). Changes in the organization of the mental health care delivery system further stimulated the opening up of mental hospitals and the expansion of psychiatrists into a variety of community settings. The Community Mental Health Centers Act spawned the rapid growth of community mental health consultation and of thinking about a range of consultation models.

The discovery of the prevalence of mental illness in the United States did not initially advance the practice of school consultation because the few mental health workers who interacted with schools were pressured to work in places of greater need, such as Veteran Administration Hospitals (Alpert, 1976). Over time it became clear that, to address the problem of mental illness in the community, intervention in schools would be essential. Through the leadership of Caplan, Sarason, Berlin, and others, a literature on school consultation emerged, documenting the theoretical basis for and common clinical issues encountered in the growing field of school consultation.

MODELS OF CONSULTATION

After conducting a multidisciplinary literature search, West and Idol (1987) reported finding 10 different models of consultation. In most of these, consultation was conceptualized as an indirect method of problem-solving that provides remedial services for a current problem and increases the consultee's ability to handle such problems in the future (Gutkin and Curtis, 1982; West and Idol, 1987). The indirect nature of consultation is an important feature and one that, in psychiatry, distinguishes it from more traditional psychiatric processes of evaluation and treatment. It is also considered by many to be critical to the success of this type of consultation process. In schools, because it is indirect, the consultation process also allows the mental health consultant to reach many more children than would be possible through direct service. Indeed, if as Bergan estimated, 20% or more of children entering elementary school had at least moderate behavior problems (Bergan and Kratochwill, 1990), then the sense of urgency and level of need that Caplan articulated in 1970 are as relevant today as then.

Of the 10 models of consultation described by West and Idol (1987), three—the mental health model, the behavioral model, and the organizational model—are probably most widely known, and in child psychiatric consultation to schools, the mental health model in various forms is most commonly applied.

Mental Health Consultation

Caplan defines consultation as "the process of interaction between two professional persons—the consultant, who is a specialist, and the consultee, who invokes his help in regard to a current work problem with which the latter is having some difficulty . . .. The problem involves the management or treatment of one or more clients of the consultee, or the planning or implementation of a program . . . (for) such clients" (Caplan, 1963, p. 470). An essential feature in this conceptualization of consultation is that the consultee retains professional responsibility for the client and, in this capacity, is free to follow—or not—the recommendations of the consultant. Inherent in this is the collaborative, nonhierarchical nature of the relationship between the consultee and consultant. In the usual arrangement, this is facilitated by the consultant's being of a different profession from the consultee and by the consultant's "visiting" rather than membership status in the consultee's institution (Caplan, 1970). Caplan also stresses that the consultant's goals are both to be helpful with the problem that led to the consultation request and also to impart new knowledge and skills so that the consultee will become more capable of handling such problems in the future.

Caplan delineates four basic forms of consultation (Caplan, 1963; 1970): client-centered case consultation, program-centered administrative consultation, consultee-centered case consultation, and consultee-centered administrative consultation. In client-centered consultation, the consultant brings expertise to bear on problems the consultee is having in working with a client (or group of clients); in school consultation this is usually a student. While the consultant may deal primarily with the consultee, the focus nevertheless is on the client. In the program-centered administrative form of consultation, the consultant typically meets with a group of consultees to help reform troubled administrative programs or to advise in the development of a new program or policy. The last two forms of mental health consultation, consultee-centered case and consultee-centered administrative, are parallel in content (case versus program) to the first two forms. They differ in that the consultant focuses on the problems that the *consultee* has with either the client (student) or program rather than on the client or program per se. In consultation work in schools, an example of the consultee-centered case approach would be the consultation to a teacher about how he or she may be contributing to problems in working with a student (Alpert, 1976). Caplan (1963) proposes four types of consultee problem that can be addressed in this type of consultation: (*a*) lack of understanding, (*b*) lack of skill, (*c*) lack of objectivity, and (*d*) lack of confidence. As Caplan (1970) and Alpert (1976) point out, in real life the clean distinctions of the four-part typology often break down, with shifts in focus occurring in the course of the consultation process. Fritz (1993) further notes that, in the current climate for consultation work, consultee-centered consultation is hard to fund, rarely requested as such, and problematic for the maintenance of the egalitarian, collaborative relationship between consultant and consultee.

Applying principles of dynamic psychiatry to a broad range of consultation situations, Caplan's writings are filled with rich descriptions of case material and of mechanisms (e.g., simple identification, transference, characterological distortion) by which the consultee's work with a client becomes problematic or stymied (Caplan, 1963, 1970). Consultation skill lies in the accurate recognition of these processes and in the ability to work constructively with them toward the goal of "increased effectiveness in the work setting," that is, more effective work on the part of the consultee in the service of the client. Caplan is careful to delineate the major distinctions between consultation work and psychotherapy, which are quite fundamental and involve, for example, the nature of the contract and relationship between the consultee and the consultant, as well as the very different goals of these two activities (improving the consultee's work with his or her clients versus personal cure).

Berlin, another leader in school mental health consultation, notes the potentially unique opportunity that the mental health consultant has "to communicate and sometimes to demonstrate mental health principles to teachers" (Berlin, 1962, p. 671). Applying principles of ego psychology to the consultation process, Berlin focuses on teachers, with the goal of reducing anxieties and tensions that hinder effective classroom work with disturbed students. He notes that in sensitive areas it may be particularly useful to find strategies for externalizing the situation, such as through the use of examples from other contexts. Through the detailed joint exploration of difficulties in work with a particular student, the teacher is helped to identify critical choice points and to consider new, more adaptive solutions.

Sarason et al. (1966), recognizing the potential of schools for preventive mental health work, applies a social ecological approach to mental health consultation. Extrapersonal features of the institution, along with intrapsychic phenomena, are taken into account in examining problems between consultees and clients (students) (Alpert and Myers, 1983). Like the approaches of Caplan and Berlin, this approach commonly focuses on changing the teacher's perception of a problem with a student. Particular emphasis, however, is placed on the role of teachers in schools and on difficulties in relationships within the school as an institution (Alpert, 1976).

Behavioral Consultation

Bergan broadly defines behavioral consultation as "the application of behavioral theory and research in consultation services" (Bergan and Kratochwill, 1990, p. 3). Like behavioral therapists, behavioral consultants focus on changing the behavior of their clients through a problem-solving process designed to attain behaviorally defined goals (Bergan and Kratochwill, 1990). Different behavioral consultants subscribe to slightly different problem-solving processes, but most processes are fundamentally similar to that described by Bergan, which involves the following four stages: (*a*) problem identification, (*b*) problem analysis, (*c*) plan implementation, and (*d*) problem evaluation (Bergan and Kratochwill, 1990; Osterweil, 1987; West and Idol, 1987).

During the problem identification stage, the consultant and consultee determine if there is a problem and, if there is, how to define it. A problem occurs when an individual's (i.e., the client's) observed behavior is not what is desired and expected (i.e., by the consultee) (Bergan and Kratochwill, 1990). When the consultant and the consultee have defined a problem by establishing that a discrepancy exists between current and desired behavior, they establish goals for the resolution of the problem (Bergan and Kratochwill, 1990). It is important to note that the consultant is mainly responsible for defining the problem and formulating it in behavioral terms.

During the stage of problem analysis, the consultant and the consultee generate hypotheses about factors that influence the behavior and design a plan to solve the problem (Bergan and Kratochwill, 1990). Again, the consultee plays an integral role in problem analysis and plan development. Next, the plan is put into action. During the plan implementation stage, the consultant and consultee also collect data to assist in the final stage, problem evaluation. During evaluation, the consultant and the consultee determine whether their goals have been attained, whether new problems have arisen, and whether plan implementation should continue, be changed, or be terminated (Bergan and Kratochwill, 1990).

Behavioral consultation is popular, especially among educators, and it is the model of choice for many school psychologists. There are several distinctive features of the behavioral model: The consultee is viewed as a problem solver who contributes to all stages of the problem-solving process; the client is encouraged to develop problem-solving skills; the goals of consultation involve observable and measurable incidents of behavior; and the model defines the problems of individuals as related to the environment (Bergan and Kratochwill, 1990).

Organizational Consultation

Organizational consultation focuses on schools as systems and seeks to facilitate improvement in their functioning through the application of behavioral science concepts and the involvement of system members in the process of organizational change. According to this model, mental health and learning difficulties are symptomatic of an unhealthy educational system (Christ, 1991). Achieving optimal organizational functioning by introducing systemwide changes is seen as essential to improving the quality of life and facilitating the healthy productivity of its individual members. Overall, the goal of organizational development is to build ''self-renewing schools, schools that are able to adapt to current changes within the student body, community, and world while continuing to maintain an effective educational program'' (Schmuck, 1976, p. 627). Self-renewing schools are viewed as adaptive and changing and thus are not bound to particular structures and procedures.

An important feature of the organizational consultation process is the involvement of system members in the assessment, diagnosis, and transformation of the organization (Schmuck, 1976). Consultants work with and advise teachers and administrators to help them change their interpersonal and group methods of interaction. Thus, this model of consultation focuses on the organizational context, including the mode of communication and quality of relationships within the school. School ''culture'' is viewed as a powerful influence that must be understood and worked with to ensure the success of educational innovation and reform efforts (Schmuck, 1976).

SCHOOL CONSULTATION EFFICACY

Assessing the efficacy of school consultation is difficult because the practice of consultation tends to be naturalistic, has varying goals, and

because consultations are not performed in a standardized manner (Brent and Howell, 1983). As a result, consultants often assess efficacy anecdotally, and empirical attempts often suffer methodological problems. Nevertheless, some research reviews and results of two meta-analyses have shown school consultation to be an effective means of intervention (Medway, 1979; Sibley, 1986; see also Medway and Updyke, 1985, a meta-analysis of psychological outcome studies that utilized 54 controlled studies, predominantly, but not entirely limited to school consultation.) The two meta-analyses compared effectiveness across different models of consultation and concurred in the finding that there was no evidence for the superiority of any particular model (Medway and Updyke, 1985; Sibley, 1986; West and Idol, 1987).

Studies investigating relative preference for different models of school consultation have found that teachers prefer behavioral consultation to mental health consultation (Jason and Ferone, 1978; Medway and Forman, 1980), although school psychologists view mental health consultation as more effective (Medway and Forman, 1980). Teachers may prefer behavioral consultation because it provides them with a specific and directed plan of action that seems more readily applicable to the classroom setting. West and Idol note that preference for a particular model may depend on the stage of the consultation process, lending support ''to the concept of consultation as a complex, multi-dimensional process'' (West and Idol, 1987, p. 400), which warrants continued and more sophisticated efforts at evaluation.

PRACTICAL ASPECTS OF SCHOOL CONSULTATION

From the above review it is apparent that the novice consultant, preparing to embark upon school consultation work, has at hand a diverse set of theoretical approaches on which to draw and relatively little evidence from the research literature to constrain his or her work. In many ways it is up to the consultant to fashion a strategy for this undertaking and to begin what all agree is the evolving process of the consultation relationship. The remainder of this chapter is intended to have a pragmatic focus. It presents a series of issues that the consultant should consider in embarking on a consultative relationship with a school or school system and a framework that can be applied in conducting client or student-centered mental health consultations. The chapter closes with the brief presentation of a specific model developed for consultations in special education.

SCHOOLS AS SOCIAL INSTITUTIONS

In engaging with a school or school system to provide consultative services, the consultant is entering a social system that has well-specified and unique functions. These functions have developed historically to address society's needs for socializing and educating its young. Comer says, ''The school, like the family, is charged with preparing the young to become successful adult workers, members of families, and citizens'' (Comer, 1992, p. 2). This is a large mission, and accordingly children spend a considerable amount of time in schools each year through the span of the childhood and adolescent years.

Not surprisingly, to accommodate the goals that have been set for them, schools have developed into complex social institutions. They bring together people of different disciplines, levels of preparation, age, and experience (Comer, 1992) to function together to address the developmental needs of children. Viewed this way, an important aspect of the consultant's preparation is to become knowledgeable about and comfortable moving in this system. For example, schools have traditionally been hierarchical and fairly authoritarian in structure. Although innovative models of school reform are challenging the necessity and efficacy of that type of structure (e.g., Comer, 1993), it is nevertheless not uncommon for the consultant to encounter a fairly fixed structure with explicit lines of authority and relatively low tolerance for transgression. It may be very useful for the consultant to consider why schools may have developed in this manner, e.g., to institute externally a degree of structure that may be necessary in order to learn at a time when the child's internal capacities for self structure and regulation are still developing. At a practical level, this makes it easier to understand what may superficially appear to be unnecessary constraints on times available for meetings with staff or students or the necessity of communicating a seemingly straightforward request through a specific chain of authority. Also, an understanding of the structure and rules of school life can facilitate the consultant's ability to work effectively and without unproductive conflict and to appreciate the culture of school life as perceived through the eyes of the child.

SCHOOL CLIMATE

While it is useful for the consultant to become familiar with the structural and organizational aspects of school life, it is also important in getting to know a school to evaluate the process aspects of its functioning. School process refers to the nature and style of relationships and flow of information within the school (Purkey and Smith, 1983). The resulting "climate" of the school involves a number of components that have been variously conceptualized, but include, for example, dimensions such as orientation toward learning, level of conflict, promotion of independence, student involvement in school decision-making, etc. (Kasen et al., 1990). Research suggests that school climate influences both the academic achievement of students (Purkey and Smith, 1983; Rutter et al., 1979) and their emotional development (Kasen et al., 1990). But while there is general agreement that the climate of a school has an important impact on its students, it is less clear which specific factors are most influential. In a 1983 review of the literature, Purkey and Smith argue that many of the studies of effective schools focus on much too simple factors that have little effect on the development of students (e.g., class size) while the important factors are deeply rooted in the school's 'culture' and are therefore slow to change even when sweeping changes in policy are made.

From the perspective of the school consultant, evaluating school climate provides essential diagnostic information that will enhance the consultant's understanding of the experiences of both students and teachers (consultees) who study and work in the school. Over time and with the development of trust, the consultant may have the opportunity to influence decisions and attitudes that will sustain a positive and supportive context for student learning and development.

SCHOOL STAFF

The school system staff that the school consultant typically encounters includes teachers, guidance counselors, school psychologists, school social workers, and administrators (principals and assistant principals). Teachers spend the most time with and know the students best and as a result are an extremely valuable resource for the consultant (Mattison, 1993a). Teachers' roles differ depending on the age of the student. In elementary school, students spend most of their day with one teacher, while in middle and high school, students usually spend an hour or less with each of their teachers per day.

Guidance counselors, usually former teachers who have degrees in guidance counseling, are often the first school staff contacted by either student or teacher when a student has a problem (Mattison, 1993a). Guidance counselors frequently have access to mental health resources, but their roles and training vary. Although familiar with psychological principles, the impact of psychosocial stress, and fairly normative adjustment issues, they may not actually have much experience with psychiatric diagnostic thinking and nomenclature.

School psychologists have degrees in psychology and have probably been trained in the diagnosis and treatment of behavioral problems (Mattison, 1993a). School psychologists often perform much psychoeducational testing and may be involved in behavioral management or counsel-

ing. In working with children with learning disabilities and complex profiles of cognitive deficiencies and strengths, the consultant will often need to rely on the school psychologist's expertise in describing the impact of such conditions on the child's school functioning.

School social workers work with the families of students but may also share with the school psychologist the function of providing psychological interventions, usually in the form of group or individual treatments. The school social worker may be the key link to the family. The likelihood of achieving success with a classroom intervention may be considerably heightened by engaging the social worker to gain the parents' understanding and support for it. School social workers vary widely in their training and experience with psychiatric diagnostic and treatment principles.

Lastly, administrators are often alerted to problems with a student, and they may serve as a liaison between the school and the family. A principal's opinion concerning a student and/or capacity for involvement in the consultation process can determine the course of action taken by a school (Mattison, 1993a).

THE STUDENTS

In beginning consultation work at a school, it is extremely useful for the consultant to spend some time learning about the students in the school. This can be done by walking the halls, observing classes across the school's grade range, watching children play on the school grounds during recess, visiting the cafeteria, and attending art, music, or other enrichment activities. In particular, the consultant should get to know the special education classes, both the teachers and students. This background work is essential for developing a sense of the normative experience of growing up and going to school for the population from which consultation referrals will be generated. It provides an opportunity to begin assessing the school climate, as well as educating the consultant about the range of intervention options that exist within that school setting.

The consultant brings to the consultation process his or her expertise in the diagnostic assessment of psychopathology in children and adolescents and experience in identifying and working with dynamic issues. While the range and specific types of problems that lead to consultation requests will not be reviewed here, it is useful to have a framework for thinking about clinical presentations in the school context.

Briefly, a framework that we have found useful focuses on the developmental tasks of childhood, how schools support a normative progression along developmental lines, and why students who cannot meet the challenges posed at certain stages come to attention for special psychiatric help and/or educational services. Although a full discussion of this model is beyond the scope of the current chapter, a few examples will illustrate the general approach.

In the United States, most children are in school by at least age 6 years. Although today kindergarten is a fairly universal experience, and increasingly now children are attending day care and preschool, entry into first grade has generally been considered the beginning of formal schooling, with a more academic curriculum and, in many places, the start of full day programming. The child entering school faces a fairly extensive set of demands on his or her capacities across developmental lines. These include, for example, the requirement to separate from primary caregivers and to maintain a sense of sustenance and comfort that is sufficient to get through the day relatively emotionally intact. The child must tolerate and comply with what is probably a greater level of structure than has been previously imposed on his or her day. Activities requiring sustained attention are required. While the average 6-year-old is ready cognitively, emotionally, and socially for these challenges, it is also apparent that a certain number of children will not be so neatly on schedule. Some may be compromised in specific areas, for example, by difficulties with attention and/or activity regulation and impulsivity. The challenge of separation may overwhelm others with anxiety, or the stress of coping with peer interactions may send the socially immature child into behavioral outbursts. And some, albeit fewer, such as those with pervasive developmental disorder, will be unable to function across all or nearly all domains. It is common then for the consultant to become involved with cases characterized by a lack of developmental readiness for the challenges at hand. For some this will be constitutionally based; for others it may be rooted in stress from home and family issues. While the pervasively affected child will require a special classroom and supportive services, those for whom the "fit" problem is of a more limited nature may improve with therapy, medication, or merely clarification and reassurance for the teacher and some adjustment of classroom practices. Often sharing a developmental formulation with the teacher or other school staff is immensely useful and leads to constructive and creative ideas about the classroom management of the student's problem.

Generally speaking, school transitions are points of particular vulnerability since the new setting usually poses a new set of developmental challenges. Again, these challenges are ones that the child who is developing in a roughly normal manner will be able to negotiate with reasonable success. Those who are not ready may come to the consultant's attention over the course of the year following the transition. This can be seen in the transition to middle school, which occurs for most children at age 10 or 11 years. With the transition to middle school there is the expectation that the student will function with more autonomy. Children change teachers and classrooms; more homework is required; and expectations are heightened for the student to take a serious and independent interest in learning and schoolwork. Not surprisingly, at this stage the consultant hears of children who are suffering the cumulative effects of learning failure because they have been referred too late or because successful interventions were not found in their elementary school years. For other children, the family and home have not provided the degree of structure and support needed to develop the internal motivation to apply themselves in the more challenging and less personal middle school setting. For such youth the lure of street culture may become irresistible for its excitement and promise of easy access to material rewards. The sooner that such transition casualties are caught, the more likely they can be helped back onto the track. In addition to the obvious clinical role that the consultant can play in helping school staff work with and refer such youth, the consultant can, over time, educate consultees to adopt a developmental mode for conceptualizing student problems and for initiating timely consultation requests and referrals for treatment.

THE CONSULTANT

From their extensive literature review, West and Idol (1987) note that certain features of the successful school consultant consistently emerge. Not surprisingly, such characteristics include attributes such as cooperativeness, empathy, flexibility, emotional stability, warmth, and understanding (see West and Idol, 1987 for reference list). In terms of the process of the consultation, efficiency in responding to referrals, flexibility in applying psychological principles, and skill in eliciting information contributed to successful problem identification (Bergan and Tombari, 1976, cited in West and Idol, 1987). Collaborative skills are also noted to be critical to the perceived success of the consultation. Taken together this means school staff wish to be treated as professionals collaborating for the benefit of the students in their charge. Consultants who present as being available, concerned, and empathic gain trust and conduct consultations that are deemed successful.

SPECIAL EDUCATION CONSULTATION

An important and common type of school consultation for the child psychiatrist is the consultation to determine eligibility for special education. The Education for All Handicapped Children Act, PL 94-142, was enacted in 1975 and established the right of children with any number

of handicaps to an appropriate education and to related services needed for the child to benefit from that education. (See Appendix for discussion of legal background and issues relating to special education.) When a student's emotional and/or behavioral difficulties appear to be seriously interfering with his or her educational progress, a referral is made for an evaluation for special education. The labels applied in these situations vary; Mattison (1993b) uses perhaps the most common terminology, seriously emotionally disturbed (SED).

On referral for special education, the student enters the special education administrative structure, which prescribes a set of procedures for evaluating eligibility and determining the services to be provided to the student. In brief, a multidisciplinary team is convened to conduct the appropriate educational, psychological, medical, social work, and other evaluations. When the evaluations are complete, the team meets together with the parent(s) to review the results. The team determines whether the child meets the criteria for handicap on the basis of serious emotional disturbance (and also for other categories of handicap if relevant), and if so, an appropriate individual educational plan is developed. This plan includes goals to be met, the time expected to meet them, the educational setting that is appropriate, the amount of time to be spent in a separate classroom and in regular classrooms, the related services that are recommended and other considerations that the team may wish to note formally. In accordance with PL 94-142, SED students must be placed in the "least restrictive," most mainstreamed setting possible.

Mattison (1993b) notes the need for greater standardization in school consultation, citing particularly the need for a formalized approach to the consultation for determining special education eligibility. He emphasizes that these evaluations usually involve children with complicated, serious symptomatology who also often have families suffering from major concurrent stressors. Following is an outline of the consultation procedure we have used for these evaluations over the past 8 years. It is very similar to the excellent model described by Mattison (1993b). The reader is referred to this reference for a detailed description of the model and for very useful examples of forms, interview outlines, and a sample final consultation report.

A SPECIAL EDUCATION CASE EVALUATION

1. Review of Referral Packet

In the usual case, the consultation will be initiated with a referral summary from the school, a copy of the parent's signed consent for psychiatric evaluation (obtained by the school), and results of previous evaluations. Of particular use are the recent and past reports from the school psychological evaluation. The consultant should develop some ability to understand test scores, particularly for basic tests of intelligence and achievement. Of particular importance is the presence of a learning disability(ies), which should be described in the psychologist's report. A social work assessment may be present and may in some instances include an extensive developmental history. Various teacher reports and documentation of special education programming may also be provided. What is missing at times, however, despite the presence of a wealth of information, is documentation of the chronology of events leading to the current clinical state and referral for consultation.

2. Meeting with the Multidisciplinary Evaluation Team

This meeting allows team members to review their knowledge of the case with the consultant prior to his or her interviews with the student and parents. For the consultant it provides an opportunity to lace together the history if, as noted above, the chronology was not apparent from the materials in the referral packet. In this meeting the consultant can also learn about the concerns or worries that are too "soft" or unsubstantiated for staff to write about in their formal evaluation reports. The meeting also provides an important opportunity for the consultant to gauge staff feeling about the student and to assess whether there are programming outcomes that are desired by various members of the team.

3. Interview with the Parent(s)

The goals of this interview generally resemble those of parent interviews in other types of evaluation. The consultant seeks to gather history about the difficulties that have led to the consultation and to obtain history about other emotional and behavioral problems and treatments (past and present). Also to be covered are a review of psychiatric symptomatology, medical conditions, developmental history, family history (including psychiatric conditions of extended family members), assessment of the student's current social adjustment, and parental assessment of the student's strengths and positive aspects of coping. Additionally, the consultant should evaluate the parent(s)' understanding of the special education evaluation process and hopes or expectations about the outcome. The level of trust that the parent feels toward school staff may be critical to the ultimate success of an intervention and/or referral and should be assessed at this time.

4. Classroom Observation

When evaluating an elementary school age child, it is often very useful to schedule a classroom observation and it is usually best to do this prior to the individual interview with the child. Such an observation can yield considerable information about the student's capacity to function in the current classroom setting, about his or her peer relationships, and about the teacher's current strategies for dealing with the student's difficulties. It is usually not helpful to observe an older student in his or her classroom (and it can be unduly embarrassing for the student to be observed.)

5. Interview with the Student

This student interview is similar to the general psychiatric interview in covering an explanation of the nature of the interview and the "kind of doctor" the consultant is, a discussion of current and past difficulties, a review of relevant areas of symptomatology, inquiry about physical health and health concerns, and a discussion of home, friends, favorite activities and feelings about school. A mental status exam should be conducted and Mattison (1993b) notes the value of a systematic mini neuroeducational exam covering coordination and basic educational skills (e.g., reading, math, spelling). It is also useful to assess the student's hopes and expectations about the outcome of the current evaluation. An important feature of this type of consultation is that, beyond the conclusion of the evaluation, there is no expectation of a continued relationship with the consultant. As in any psychiatric evaluation, it is important to ask about anything that might shed light on the nature of the student's problems or be of potential use in disposition planning; however, uncovering techniques and extensive probing in affectively sensitive areas should be curtailed if their yield is not of direct relevance to the purpose of the consultation. There will not be an ongoing therapeutic relationship with the student, and he or she must return to school and cope with multiple academic and social demands for the rest of the day.

6. Team Meeting for Presentation of Consultant's Report and Collaborative Planning

After completing data gathering through the stages outlined above, the multidisciplinary team reconvenes to hear the results of the consultant's evaluation. At this meeting the consultant should present an overview of the history (with the level of detail determined by the group's general knowledge of this). It is extremely useful for the consultant to synthesize and summarize information contained in the initial packet along with the perspectives of the various team members; however, this should be done in a succinct manner that generates a sense of accord about the definition of the problem. Then, results of the parent interview, student interview, and classroom observation are presented, followed by the consultant's formulation. If the team agrees on the formulation, the consultant's program recommendations can often serve as a springboard for the discussion of an educational plan for the student. This phase should be viewed as a collaborative process among professionals with different areas of expertise. The consultant's unique contribution will be in conceptualizing and communicating about potential strategies for dealing with emotional and behavioral issues in the school setting. Together the team will agree on a specific plan and on how it will be implemented.

7. Feedback to the Parent(s) and Student

It should be noted that, in some places, the parent is present at this team meeting. Agreeing with Mattison (1993b) that it is far preferable for feedback to be given by the consultant accompanied by the educator who will have continued involvement with the student and family rather than in a larger group context, it is nevertheless the case that in some systems there is a strong precedent for having parents at the team planning meeting. When the parent(s) is present, the consultant must present findings in a style that is comprehensible, devoid of jargon, and recognizable to the parents as the story they have told the consultant. When the parent is not present, a separate feedback session should be scheduled relatively promptly, i.e., before the team members begin talking about and implementing aspects of the plan. In some instances, depending on the age of the student and the nature of the problem and plans, it will be important to include the student in the feedback session.

8. The Consultation Report

Often schools prefer to see a draft copy of the report at the time of the team meeting but allow some further work afterwards so that it can reflect planning decisions that were made collaboratively at the meeting. An excellent model for such a report is provided by Mattison (1993b, pp. 125–129).

SCHOOL CONSULTATION: THE FUTURE

In a 1990 article, Jellinek identifies four evolving trends affecting schools in the United States which, in various ways, concern child psychiatrists practicing school consultation. The first is the increasing demand for special services in the face of limited resources to pay for expensive, albeit often needed, services. The second issue is that of rising parental expectations for academic achievement and the expanding role of the school as an institution bearing increased responsibility for nurturing children and for preventing harmful behavior (e.g., substance use, suicide, high risk sexual behavior). The third issue involves the aging of the faculty of school teachers whose personal pressures and needs are new to school administrations accustomed to a younger faculty and higher rate of turnover. The fourth issue is the burden created by the interaction of the above as well as other complex stresses of modern life. Jellinek notes that it is critical for the child psychiatrist to understand the evolving economics, values, and pressures on local school systems, as these will affect the lives of the children and families with whom he or she works. Further, although the trends that Jellinek identifies are worrisome and speak to the enormous pressures on an essential social institution, they may also signal a unique opportunity for the school consultant to contribute in new and creative ways to the mental health of many children and to the viability of many schools in our communities.

Acknowledgment. *The authors gratefully acknowledge the valuable contributions of Margaret Briggs-Gowan, Ph.D., in the preparation of this chapter.*

References

Alpert JL: Conceptual bases of mental health consultation in the schools. *Prof Psychol* 7:619–626, 1976.

Alpert JL, Meyers J: *Training in Consultation.* Springfield, IL, Charles C Thomas, 1983.

Bergan JR, Kratochwill TR: *Behavioral Consultation and Therapy.* New York, Plenum, 1990.

Bergan JR, Tombari ML: Consultant skill and efficiency and the implementation of outcomes of consultation. *J Sch Psychol* 14:3–14, 1976.

Berlin IN: Mental health consultation in schools as a means of communicating mental health principles. *J Am Acad Child Psychiatry* 1:671–679, 1962.

Berlin IN, Szurek SA (eds): *Learning and Its Disorders.* Palo Alto, CA, Science and Behavior Books, 1965.

Borus J: Strangers bearing gifts: A retrospective look at the early years of community mental health center consultation. *Am J Psychiatry* 141:868–871, 1984.

Brent DA, Howell M: Data based program evaluation in a project involving mental health consultation to schools. *J Am Acad Child Psychiatry* 22:447–453, 1983.

Caplan G (ed): *Prevention of Mental Disorders in Children.* New York, Basic Books, 1961.

Caplan G: Types of mental health consultation. *Am J Orthopsychiatry* 33:470–481, 1963.

Caplan G: *The Theory and Practice of Mental Health Consultation.* New York, Basic Books, 1970.

Christ AE: School consultation. In: Lewis M (ed): *Child and Adolescent Psychiatry: A Comprehensive Textbook* (1st ed). Baltimore, Williams & Wilkins, 1991.

Comer JP: School consultation. In: Michels R, Cooper AM, Guze SB, et al (eds): *Psychiatry* (Vol 2). Philadelphia, Lippincott, 1992.

Comer JP: *School Power: Implications of an Intervention Project.* New York, Free Press, 1993.

Fritz GK: Introduction: What is consultation? In: Fritz GK, Mattison RE, Nurcombe B, et al: *Child and Adolescent Mental Health Consultation in Hospitals, Schools, and Courts.* Washington, DC, American Psychiatric Press, 1993.

Gutkin TB, Kurtis MJ: School-based consultation. In: Reynolds CR, Gutkin TB (eds): *The Handbook of School Psychology.* New York, Wiley, 1982, pp. 796–826.

Jason LA, Ferone L: Behavioral versus process consultation interventions in school settings. *Am J Community Psychol* 6:531–543, 1978.

Jellinek MS: School consultation: Evolving issues. *J Am Acad Child Adolesc Psychiatry* 29: 311–314, 1990.

Kasen S, Johnson J, Cohen P: The impact of school emotional climate on student psychopathology. *J Abnorm Child Psychol* 18:165–177, 1990.

Mattison RE: Consultation in the school environment. In: Fritz GK, Mattison RE, Nurcombe B, et al: *Child and Adolescent Mental Health Consultation in Hospitals, Schools, and Courts.* Washington, DC, American Psychiatric Press, 1993a.

Mattison RE: A model for SED case evaluation. In: Fritz GK, Mattison RE, Nurcombe B, et al: *Child and Adolescent Mental Health Consultation in Hospitals, Schools, and Courts.* Washington, DC, American Psychiatric Press, 1993b.

Medway FJ: How effective is school consultation? A review of recent research. *J Sch Psychol* 17(3):275–282, 1979.

Medway FJ, Forman SG: Psychologists' and teachers' reactions to mental health and behavioral school consultation. *J Sch Psychol* 18(4):338–348, 1980.

Medway FJ, Updyke JF: Meta-analysis of consultation outcome studies. *Am J Community Psychol* 13(5):489–505, 1985.

Osterweil Z: A structural process of problem definition in school consultation. *The School Counselor* 34:345–352, 1987.

Purkey SC, Smith MS: Effective schools: A review. *Elementary Sch J* 83:427–452, 1983.

Rutter M, Maughan B, Mortimore P, et al: *Fifteen Thousand Hours: Secondary Schools and Their Effects on Children.* Cambridge, MA, Harvard University Press, 1979.

Sarason SB, Levine M, Goldenberg II, et al: *Psychology in Community Settings.* New York, Wiley, 1966.

Schmuck RA: Process consultation and organization development. *Prof Psychol* 7:626–631, 1976.

Sibley SL: A meta-analysis of school consultation research. *Dissertation Abstr Int* 47(5-B):2145, 1986.

West JF, Idol L: School consultation (part 1): An interdisciplinary perspective on theory, models, and research. *J Learn Disabil* 20:388–408, 1987.

Appendix/ The Law As It Pertains to Special Education and School Consultation

Melissa D. Shannon, B.A., and Mary E. Schwab-Stone, M.D.

The Individuals with Disabilities Education Act (IDEA), also known as PL 102-119, passed by Congress in 1991, provides all children with disabilities the right to a free public education that includes special education and related services and that is designed to meet their unique needs. The underlying premise of the act is that all children with disabilities can learn and that their education should be appropriate to their individual needs (1). This law was first established in 1975, under the name of the Education for All Handicapped Children Act (EAHCA or Public Law 94-142), in response to congressional findings that 1 million children with disabilities were excluded entirely from the public school system and that nearly half of the nation's 8 million disabled children were not receiving appropriate education services to enable them to have full equality of opportunity (2). Children with emotional disabilities were among the most poorly served of disabled students, with studies revealing that the educational needs of 82% of children with emotional disabilities were not being met (3). The law was also enacted in response to federal lawsuits that challenged the denial of an appropriate education to children with disabilities on the grounds that this denial violated the precedent set by the *Brown vs. Board of Education* decision (4). The EAHCA was amended in 1986, through Public Law 99-457, to apply to children ages 3–5 years, inclusive. The law was revised again in 1991 (as IDEA) largely in response to a congressional finding that children with serious emotional disturbance (SED) remained severely underserved. Fewer than half the nation's children with SED were being identified and provided with appropriate services (5). Among other changes, IDEA ensured a smooth transition for children moving from early intervention programs (covered in another statute for at risk children, ages birth to 3 years) to preschool special education programs (6). IDEA stressed the importance of family support and involvement in a child's early intervention and preschool programs. This has been considered a critical provision of the bill as research indicates that one of the most consistent factors in successful preschool programs is family support and involvement (7).

IDEA defines "children with disabilities" to mean children with mental retardation, hearing impairments including deafness, speech or language impairments, visual impairments including blindness, orthopedic impairments, autism, traumatic brain injury, other health impairments (8), specific learning impairments, or serious emotional disturbance; and who by reason thereof need special education and related services. As of 1991, states may also expand eligibility to children ages 3–5 years who are experiencing developmental delays in one or more areas including social and emotional development (9).

IDEA defines "seriously emotionally disturbed" as a condition having one or more of the following over a long period of time, to a marked degree, and which adversely affects educational performance: an inability to learn that cannot be explained by intellectual, sensory, or health factors; an inability to build or maintain satisfactory interpersonal relationships with peers and teachers; inappropriate types of mood or behavior under normal circumstances; a general mood of unhappiness or depression; a tendency to develop physical symptoms or fears associated with personal or school problems. The term "related services" is defined in the statute to mean transportation as well as developmental, corrective, and other support services that may be required for the child with a disability to benefit from special education and includes the early identification and assessment of disabling conditions in children. These services may include speech pathology and audiology, psychological services, physical and occupational therapy, recreation, social work services, and counseling services. Medical services are covered for diagnostic and evaluative purposes only (10). IDEA defines "free appropriate public education" to mean special education and related services that have been provided at public expense, under public supervision, and in conformity with the individualized education program that is required under section 1414 (a) (5) of the act (11).

In order to create an appropriate education for an eligible child, IDEA places responsibility on the state to see that an individualized education program (IEP) is devised for each eligible child by a multidisciplinary team that must involve the child's parents. The IEP should describe the child's current educational ability and detail annual goals and short-term objectives for improvement in that child's performance. It should describe the special instruction and related services that will enable the child to meet those objectives (12). The evaluations must be conducted in the language used by the child and may not be racially or culturally discriminatory. The IEP must be reviewed and, where necessary, revised annually in order to ensure that a free and appropriate public education is tailored to the child's unique needs. The IEP must see that each child with disabilities be educated in the least restrictive context possible (13). This means that a child with disabilities is to be educated with nondisabled peers unless education in the classroom, with supplementary aids and services, cannot be achieved. Further, a child with disabilities is to be educated in the same public school he or she would attend if not disabled, and as close to home as possible; however, if the child's particular needs preclude this, another placement may be selected (14). This provision is particularly relevant to children with SED who have been removed from their educational settings for behavior problems that are related to their disabilities.

There are a number of potential roles in this process for child mental health consultants. At times, child psychiatrists and behavioral pediatricians are called upon to provide diagnostic assessments and medically based recommendations about a child's educational needs. The mental health consultant may also serve an integral role in pulling together recommendations of other medical or psychiatric evaluations. Also, the consultant may suggest certain specific strategies that can be imple-

mented in the child's classroom to address the objectives of the IEP. And, the mental health consultant can often play an important role in helping parents understand more fully the nature of a child's disturbance and its implications for the child's functioning at school.

The promise set forth in IDEA for all children with disabilities to receive free and appropriate public education to meet their unique needs is at times unfulfilled due to ambiguities in the law. Noticeably absent from the law is any substantive standard prescribing the level of education that each child should receive. The law requires only that a "free appropriate public education" meet the unique needs of a child with a disability so that the child may *benefit* from the instruction, but not necessarily reach his or her fullest potential (15). This ambiguity has caused much conflict between parents and schools with many parents initiating court cases. The lower courts have ruled that states must maximize the potential of handicapped children commensurate with the opportunities provided other children. However, in the case of *Board of Education v. Rowley*, the Supreme Court ruled that Congress did not impose any substantive standard to insure that states provide children who have disabilities with an education that helps them achieve their greatest potential, and that therefore a special education program must be provided that would allow a child to benefit from instruction (16).

Familiarity with basic aspects of the laws pertaining to special education and their application strongly enhances the child psychiatrist's effectiveness in the consultation process. A comprehensive and thoughtful discussion of these issues can be found in the chapter entitled "The Legal Rights of Children with Disabilities to Education and Developmental Services" by Miriam Berkman (17). In most states, the Department (Board) of Education can serve as a good source of information, and the National Information Center for Children and Youth with Disabilities is also a very useful resource (P.O. Box 1492, Washington, DC 20013-1492, phone (800) 695-0285).

Acknowledgment. *The authors gratefully acknowledge Miriam Berkman, J.D., M.S.W., who provided an extremely valuable review of this appendix and helpful suggestions and clarifications.*

References

1. Glennon T: "Disabling ambiguities: Confronting Barriers to the Education of Students with Emotional Disabilities," *Tennessee Law Review* 60:295–364, 1993.
2. 20 U.S.C. Chapter 33 1400 (b) 1995.
3. U.S.C.C.A.N 1975 1425, 1432.
4. Donohue DC: Clovis Unified School District v. California Office of Administrative Hearings (903 F.2nd 635): Restricting Related Services Under the Individuals with Disabilities Educa-

tion Act. *Journal of Contemporary Health Law and Policy* 8:407–428, 1992.
5. H.R. Rep No. 544, supra note 1. at 39 as cited in Glennon, p. 303.
6. Individuals With Disabilities Education Act Amendments of 1991 (PL 102-119) Legislative History, 316.
7. Ibid.
8. The Americans with Disabilities Act of 1990 defined disability in such a way as to include AIDS sufferers.
9. 20 U.S.C. Chapter 33, Sec 1401.

10. Ibid.
11. Ibid.
12. Ibid., Sec 1412.
13. Ibid., Sec 1401.
14. Glennon T. op. cit.
15. *Bd. of Ed. of Hendrick Hudson Central School Dist. v. Rowley*, 458 U.S. 176 (1982).
16. Ibid.
17. Berkman M: The legal rights of children with disabilities to education and developmental services. In: Cohen DJ, Volkmar FR (eds): *Autism and Pervasive Developmental Disorders: A Handbook* (2nd ed). New York, Wiley, in press.

108 EARLY CHILDHOOD EDUCATION
David Elkind, Ph.D.

The theory and practice of early childhood education, like that of so many other disciplines, has a long past and a short history. When education is taken in its broad sense, including everything a child is taught and learns during the first years of life, then early childhood education has existed for as long as humankind has been rearing children. However, in the narrow sense of education, nonparental instruction in knowledge, values, and skills, the education of young children is a relatively modern innovation.

In this chapter we will be concerned only with early childhood education in the narrow sense. In the first section we will look at some of the factors that have contributed to the rapid growth of early childhood

education in modern times. In the second section we will briefly review the contributions of some of the major figures in early childhood education as we know it today. Then in the third section we will highlight the basic parameters of early childhood education. In the closing section, we look at some of the major mental health issues raised by early childhood education in the United States today.

THE GROWTH OF EARLY CHILDHOOD EDUCATION

The growth of early childhood education in the modern era has many different roots. Darwin's theory of evolution, for example, transformed our ideas about the insane, the retarded, and children. Just as insanity and retardation came to be seen as natural phenomena, rather than as the work of the devil, children's behavior came to be viewed as reflecting their immaturity rather than their original sin. For each of these groups, humanitarian practices progressively replaced restriction and punishment.

Another factor that contributed to the growth of early childhood education was the establishment of socialist societies in countries such as China, Russia, and Israel. In these countries, the society, rather than the family, was to be the prime identity and allegiance of the individual. Accordingly, massive early childhood care programs were instituted, in part to enable women to join the work force, in part to weaken the strength of family bonds. In many ways, these state-supported programs were large-scale experiments in early childhood education. Unfortunately these were uncontrolled experiments, and we have no good way of assessing their effects.

In this country, a different type of social change eventually contributed to the growth of early childhood education, namely, the movement of farm families to the cities and factory work, as well as the waves of immigration around the turn of the century. Initially, in the United States, early childhood programs were introduced for the children of poor, two-parent working and often immigrant families. Many day schools, such as the "Home for Little Wanderers" in Boston, were founded in major cities in the first two decades of this century.

Although programs for young children began as a service for working mothers, after World War I many of these programs were institutionalized and redirected to serve the children of single mothers or those of troubled families. Day care programs were thus associated with social pathology. As a consequence, day care centers acquired a social stigma. Children who were in out-of-home programs for a full day were looked upon as unfortunate and underprivileged. The social stigma associated with day care is gradually being overcome, but some traces of that stigma may account, at least in part, for the continued resistance to early childhood education in some quarters.

Another contribution to the growth of early childhood education in this country was the nursery school movement. In contrast to the evolution of day care, the nursery school movement in America was directed toward children of middle-income parents. Between the two world wars, the nursery school movement flourished, and training schools for nursery school teachers, such as the Bank Street College of Education in New York, the Merrill Palmer School in Detroit, and the Nursery Training School in Boston, prepared young people to work with young children in nursery school settings.

In contrast to the day care programs, the nursery school program was a half-day affair and often involved the parents in one or another form of "guided observation." The contemporary growth of early childhood education has its roots in the nursery school movement, not day care programs. In fact, however, there is now so much overlapping that it would be hard to tell the difference between a good day care program and a good traditional nursery school program.

MAJOR CONTRIBUTORS TO CONTEMPORARY EARLY CHILDHOOD EDUCATION

Many writers, both within and outside the discipline of education, have contributed to the theory and practice of early childhood education. Among the most prominent of these are the contributors described below.

Heinrich Pestalozzi (1746–1826)

Pestalozzi was a Swiss educator who extended some of the ideas of the Enlightenment to early childhood education (Green, 1914). The spirit of the Enlightenment was to look to experience, rather than to authority, for true knowledge. Pestalozzi began several schools for children whom today we would call disadvantaged. None of these schools was very successful or lasted very long. This was probably more a result of Pestalozzi's limitations as an administrator than of the programs he initiated.

Pestalozzi was nonetheless a prolific writer and in his many books gave what is perhaps the first systematic approach to the education of infants and young children. In his most famous book, *Gertrude Teaches Her Children*, which takes the form of a series of letters to mothers, Pestalozzi described many exercises the mother could engage in with her child. These exercises were aimed at helping children develop their intellectual and physical abilities. These exercises were revolutionary in the sense that they took account of child development and catered to it. Up until that time young children were taught what adults thought they ought to know, namely, the catechism.

Although he was personally not successful in maintaining a school run accordingly to his own principles, Pestalozzi did influence many parents and other educators, who also began to look at what children needed to learn rather than at what adults wanted them to know.

Frederich Wilhelm Froebel (1782–1852)

Froebel is generally regarded as the originator of early childhood education as a distinct field of pedagogy (Froebel, 1893). Froebel believed that children could and should be taught outside the home as well as within it and that such education should be provided by trained teachers. He developed not only a curriculum for young children but also a training school to prepare teachers to work with young children.

Froebel is perhaps best known for his introduction of the kindergarten ("children's garden"), where children could learn through play. Froebel recognized the educational value of certain toys and advocated toys and play as the appropriate way of instructing young children. His kindergarten included blocks, pets, and simple games. The toys Froebel introduced for educational purposes, such as a ball, he termed "gifts." He believed that children could not only learn simple ideas such as "roundness" from playing with the ball but also begin to comprehend the shape of the earth and the concept of unity also implicit in the sphere.

Maria Montessori (1870–1952)

The first woman in Italy to gain admittance to and graduate from medical school, Maria Montessori (1964) laid the foundations for early childhood education as we know it today. After graduating from medical school, Montessori worked with retarded children, for whom she designed some innovative learning materials. She was then invited to set up an educational program for young children in a low-income housing project. Using untrained teachers and modifications of the materials she had devised for retarded children, she created what is known today as Montessori education.

Like Pestalozzi and Froebel, Montessori began with observations of how children engage in learning on their own. From these observations she not only was able to choose materials that were uniquely suited to the intellectual needs of young children, but she was also able to describe some general principles of early childhood education. For example, Montessori believed that young children should always be exposed to the object, property, or quality before they are given the name for that object, property, or quality. Put differently, she believed that sensory learning should precede symbolic learning.

Many of Montessori's innovations have become part of accepted early childhood teaching practice. For example, like Froebel, she believed that early childhood teachers had to be specially trained, and she worked out an elaborate training program of teacher preparation. Today, Montessori-oriented teacher training is one of the more rigorous early childhood teacher training programs in this country and abroad. Montessori teachers are particularly well schooled in the use of manipulative materials with young children.

In addition to rigorous teacher training, Montessori also introduced what are now staples of most early childhood classrooms—child-sized tables and chairs, dishes, and utensils. Other curriculum innovations were form boards, sandpaper letters, button and shoe lacing boards, and much more. Montessori believed that if the environment were properly prepared with the right learning materials, then children would spontaneously move to these materials and extract the most educational benefit from them. Since the 1960s Montessori programs have multiplied rapidly and are now in all of the states and in many public schools.

John Dewey (1858–1952)

Although trained as a philosopher, John Dewey became America's first original educator. Like Pestalozzi, Froebel, and Montessori, Dewey believed that childhood was a unique stage of life that should not be rushed. In addition, he believed that education should be practical—his brand of educational philosophy has been called *functionalism*—and should prepare children for the life they will experience outside of school. While Dewey was not opposed to classical education at some levels, he believed that children should also learn more practical skills (Dewey, 1916).

In addition to his contributions to educational philosophy, Dewey also introduced instructional innovations. Perhaps the most well known is what has come to be called the *project method*. Rather than teach subjects as separate and apart from one another, Dewey believed they could be taught in an integrated way if children were engaged in particular projects. In putting on a play, children would have to learn the lines (reading, vocabulary), build the sets (measurement and carpentry), and design and sew the costumes (history, measurement, sewing), as well as follow instructions and work cooperatively (social skills).

Dewey's ideas and methods became a major movement in the United States that lasted until the mid-1950s and was called *Progressive Education*. It disappeared from the scene for many different reasons, not the least of which is because, in distorted form, it had become associated with "permissiveness" (Cremin, 1961).

Sigmund Freud (1856–1939)

Freud's (1938) discoveries of infant sexuality, the stages of psychosexual development, and the Oedipus complex have had a significant impact upon early education. Although most of what Freud had to say about early childhood dealt with parent-child relationships, there were some implications for out-of-home care as well. This is particularly true with respect to children's play.

Whereas writers such as Froebel and Montessori saw play as an all-important mode of learning for young children, Freud saw play as comparable to a dream. Like a dream, play has both a *manifest* and a *latent* content. Children's play can reflect inner complexes and conflicts and also be a way of working them out. A child who has just returned from the doctor, for example, may play at being doctor as a way of relieving some of the anxiety aroused by that visit. The technique of play therapy has grown out of this recognition that children's play can have symbolic meaning. It is now generally recognized that the play of young children has both cognitive *and affective* value.

Erik Erikson (1902–1994)

Erik H. Erikson was trained as a child analyst but later departed significantly from analytic theory (Erikson, 1950). In his writings, Erikson focused upon the social dimensions of development and the evolution of such social orientations as trust and identity. Four of Erikson's eight stages of development occur in early childhood.

In Erikson's theory, we are born with a number of social potentials. How these potentials are realized depends very much upon the sort of experiences to which we are exposed, as well as upon our own unique characteristics. Each potential exists as a kind of polarity and has a particular time when the balance between the two opposing tendencies will be determined (although changes can occur at later ages as well).

To illustrate the relevance of the Eriksonian stages for early childhood education, we can look at the stage of initiative versus guilt, which

has its critical time around the ages of 4 and 5. If the child is given the opportunity to explore the world and undertake projects on his or her own, the child will develop a sense of initiative that is stronger than the sense of guilt. In contrast, if the child is constantly told what to do and corrected if he or she makes mistakes, then the child will acquire a sense of guilt that is greater than his or her sense of initiative.

Erikson's theory, then, has rather direct implications for the practice of early education, as well as for child rearing.

Jean Piaget (1896–1980)

Although he was trained as a philosopher and biologist, Jean Piaget's greatest contributions were to developmental psychology. Piaget elaborated a theory of intellectual development that has influenced many different disciplines, including early childhood education. While Piaget (1970) himself wrote about education in general terms, his work has had a major impact upon the pedagogy of young children.

From a theoretical point of view, Piaget's work has emphasized the importance of development and the fact that learning cannot accelerate growth. Piaget's theoretical work has been a major factor in the current effort by early childhood educators to get schools to provide "developmentally appropriate" practice for young children (Bredenkamp, 1987). In addition, Piaget's work on the development of children's understanding conceptions, such as number, has led to major curriculum innovations (Kamii, 1982).

Lev Vygotsky (1896–1934)

Although Vygotsky (Kozulin, 1990) was a contemporary of Jean Piaget, his work is only today becoming generally known in America. Thanks to changes in Russian policy, his works are being made available and translated at an increasing pace. Although he worked in many different areas of psychology, he is perhaps best known for his contributions to our understanding of the relationships between language and thought.

Vygotsky argued that there were two levels of development, that which was biological and which we share with animals and that which is sociological and unique to humans. Both animals and humans, to illustrate, employ tools or implements to attain desired goals—a process Vygotsky described as mediation. But only humans use language as a mediator and language is acquired socially and not as a biological given. Vygotsky believed that thought and language were initially a single undifferentiated activity and that they became separate only later in development. Initially language is entirely social, derived from hearing adults speak. As they develop, language becomes increasingly internalized (whispering is a step along the way) and individual rather than social.

Vygotsky, like Piaget, believed that children construct and reconstruct their ideas until they approximate those of the adult world. Nonetheless, he also contended that when adults mediate the child's learning, the child will arrive at the socialized concept earlier than if he or she has no adult model. Observing a parent use a spoon, for example, enables the child to use a spoon earlier than if he or she had never been witness to a model. The difference in time between the child's spontaneous attainment of a concept, and the time when the concept is attained with adult mediation is the "zone of proximal development." Vygotsky, like Montessori, believed that children could progress more effectively with a prepared environment and with adult modeling than if left to their own spontaneous devices.

It is important to emphasize that Vygotsky was not arguing that development could be quickened with adult intervention. Perhaps his position is best understood in contrast to that of Piaget. In general, Piaget believed that children spontaneously maximize their abilities given an average family environment. Vygotsky, in contrast, argued that children without adult mediation do not maximize their abilities but can quicken their development with the aid of adult mediation. There is a zone of undeveloped capacity that can be achieved with adult intervention, but this zone is limited by the child's native capacity.

MAJOR PARAMETERS OF EARLY CHILDHOOD EDUCATION

Every system of education presupposes a set of assumptions regarding the learner, the learning process, the knowledge to be required, and the aims of education. Contemporary early childhood education in America can be described within these parameters. It must be said that this description represents the views of mainstream early childhood education and does not purport to convey all the many varieties of early childhood education currently available.

The discussion of the parameters of early childhood education has implications for dynamic theories and for therapy with young children. For example, any theory or therapy applied to young children must take the child's developing mental powers into account. The therapist must understand the child's level of mental ability, what the child can and cannot do cognitively. A case in point is the writings of Melanie Klein. Although her books have raised important issues and concepts, she nonetheless seems to attribute too much to the young infant in the way of cognitive processes. For example, Klein (1957) suggests that young infants have aggressive fantasies. Yet Piaget's (1951) work demonstrates that children do not really have images before the 2nd year of life. Inasmuch as fantasy is comprised of images, the child could hardly engage in fantasy activity before he or she was capable of constructing images. From a developmental point of view, Klein is attributing too much mental ability to the young infant.

The Learner

Young children are first and foremost growing individuals. From this point of view, all children are seen as having the same basic learning abilities, which they may nonetheless attain at different ages. For example, we expect that all children (with the exception perhaps of the extremely retarded) will eventually attain the mental abilities that Piaget (1950) calls *concrete operations*, which enable young children to reason in a syllogistic way and to follow rules. While most children acquire these operations at about the age of 6 or 7, bright children may acquire them at the age of 4, whereas the slow child may attain them at the age of 8 or 9.

The view of children as endowed with developing abilities has many educational implications. What is important is to match the child's developing mental abilities with a curriculum that is nicely suited to those potentials. Curricula have to be studied to determine their "developmental difficulty," the level of mental ability required for their comprehension. For example, instruction in phonics requires children to have attained the concrete operations described earlier. This is true because children require these abilities to grasp that one and the same letter can represent different sounds and that the same sound can be represented by different letters. Teaching a child phonics before he or she can grasp that one and the same thing can be two things can be frustrating and demoralizing.

The Learning Process

From a developmental point of view, learning is always a creative activity. The child never simply copies information from the external world but always transforms it in significant ways. The Connecticut youngster who heard the Lord's Prayer as "Our Father who art in New Haven, Harold be thy Name" is not the exception but the rule. In effect this means that we cannot really separate the learning process from the content to be learned. Every different content engages us in a unique way. There are no disembodied learning principles that operate entirely apart from the content to be learned. Learning is always content oriented.

Here again this view of the learning process differs from the view of learning held by those who educate at the primary and secondary levels. At those levels there is a strong belief in the separation of learning and content. Currently, for example, there is a great deal of interest in teaching "thinking skills" (Baron and Sternberg, 1987) and "learning strategies" (Weinstein and Mayer, 1986). Such efforts reflect the belief that the learning or thinking process can be taught and learned apart from specific contents.

The issue here is what has been called transfer of training. To be sure, the developmental approach recognizes that such transfer occurs. But those who wish to teach thinking or learning skills assume that transfer is automatic and hence unconscious. A developmental approach, which argues for the necessity of content for the operation of learning and thinking, insists that transfer can only occur when the learner is consciously aware of content and is making the effort to generalize.

On the other hand, there is a growing recognition of the importance of individual learning styles, e.g., some children learn best through the visual modality, others through the auditory (Elkind, 1994). Learning styles, in contrast to thinking skills, are individual differences that do transfer from one type of learning task to another. Here again, however, the identification of learning styles means that we have to adapt our materials to the child's learning mode, not decide on our own what skills they should learn.

From a therapeutic point of view, this conception of the creative nature of learning means, for example, that the child's language always contains individual symbolic significance. In this respect, the developmental approach to learning would be in keeping with the creative role attributed to language by Jacques Lacan (1968).

The Nature of Knowledge

From an early childhood education perspective, knowledge is always a construction. That is to say, reality as we know it is never simply a copy of the external world but rather is a construction or creation that bears something of ourselves and something of the external world and that cannot be reduced to either one. To be sure, we all have the same sensory apparatus, and there are constants in the external world, so our individual realities are never entirely egocentric. But we never see the world exactly the same way as everyone else does.

To this individual difference dimension we must add the developmental one. As the child matures, so too do his or her mental abilities. As a consequence, the child must construct and reconstruct reality in the process of growing up. The same holds true for our memory of past reality. Each time the child attains a new, higher level of mental ability, he or she reconstructs the past. Memory is thus never a simple recall of previously stored images but rather an active, constructive process that transforms the information derived from earlier experience.

This way of viewing knowledge and memory implies an approach to curriculum different from that which is currently taken in our schools. The idea that knowledge is tied up with thought and action and should not be separated was first put forward by John Dewey (1916) and reiterated by Vygotsky. As mentioned earlier, in the project method, children engage in putting on a play, building a house, and so on. In the process they learn language, math, science, social cooperation, and much more. The project method speaks to the conviction that content is an integral part of the learning and knowing process and should not be separated from it.

From a therapeutic point of view, the idea of reality as a construction again has important implications. It suggests that realities can be different and not just right or wrong. The young child who believes that adults are all-powerful and all-knowing has a different reality from the adult, but it is not wrong from a developmental point of view. Indeed, that conception is as developmentally appropriate as the more negative perception of adults held by adolescents.

The rule that there can be different realities without these being necessarily right or wrong is as important in therapy as it is in education. A child's fear of a particular animal is very real for him or her, even though it appears baseless to us. Rather than try and disabuse the child of this fear, we need to accept it as a reality for the child and reassure the child that we will not allow the animal to do the child any harm. On the other hand, there are certainly some beliefs that are right or wrong (the Bastille was stormed in 1789 and not in 1960), and there are some evil realities. The difficult thing is always to make the right discriminations as to when we should bring in the value judgements of right or wrong, good and evil.

THE AIMS OF EDUCATION

The aims of early childhood education have been clearly enunciated by Jean Piaget. "The principle goal of education is to create men who are capable of doing new things . . . men who are creative, inventive and discoverers. The second goal of education is to form minds which can be critical, can verify, and not accept everything that is offered" (Ripple and Rockcastle, 1964).

According to Piaget, the legitimate aim of early childhood education is to produce self-motivated learners and critical thinkers. From a therapeutic point of view, this aim suggests that therapy be directed not solely at removing this or that problem but also at helping the child acquire an orientation and strategies that will enable him or her to deal with the later stresses of life more effectively and productively.

ISSUES IN EARLY CHILDHOOD EDUCATION

There are many different issues currently being debated regarding the education of young children. Only a few of these can be dealt with here.

The Effect of Early Childhood Education on the Infant

Today 57% of mothers with children under the age of 6 have jobs. In addition, more than half of the mothers with infants of less than 1 year of age are employed. This means that a large percentage of infants and young children is being cared for by relatives within the home or by paid caregivers outside the home. What effect is being cared for by nonparental figures going to have upon these children? There has been a long-standing debate on this issue. For example, in 1950 John Bowlby wrote: "The absolute need of infants and toddlers for the continuous care of their mothers will be borne on all those who read this book. . . . We must recognize that leaving any child under three years of age is a major operation to be undertaken with good and sufficient reasons" (p. 16).

Yet many contemporary researchers do not agree. They find that the critical issue is not the parent as caregiver but rather the *quality* of the care the child receives. When a child is cared for by an experienced, warm adult, with one adult caring for not more than three infants, and the environment is a safe, pleasant, and interesting one, there is no evidence of lasting untoward effects. According to one investigator, with quality child care of the sort described above "the major effect of day care seems to be a speeding up some of the child's social and intellectual skills during the preschool period" (Clarke-Stewart, 1982, p. 75). Likewise, the authors of a leading child development textbook conclude their review of the literature with the following statement: "There is little clear evidence that day-care is likely to cause disruption of the infant-parent attachment relationship. In fact, day-care may have positive effects for some infants, particularly when it is of high quality." (Hetherington and Park, 1993).

The real issue for contemporary working parents is to find quality, affordable child care. With such care, there is no evidence of any immediate or lasting harm to young children. There is, however, one important caveat. It does appear that children in child care settings, particular large day care settings, are more subject to communicable diseases than children cared for at home or the home of the caregiver.

Will Early Childhood Education Increase a Child's Intelligence or Give Him or Her an Academic Head Start?

One of the questions usually raised in relation to early childhood education is whether it will raise the child's IQ. This question is interest-ing because it is rarely, if ever, raised with respect to elementary or secondary education. If neither elementary nor secondary education is expected to raise a child's IQ, why should it be expected of early childhood education? And indeed, there is no evidence that early education will raise a child's IQ on any permanent basis.

It is still possible, however, that early education can give children who have it an edge over those who haven't. Does this in fact occur? Certainly some high-quality age-appropriate programs for disadvantaged children seem to have demonstrated long-term positive benefits (Schweinhart et al., 1985).

But these results cannot be generalized to all programs and to all children. A simple analogy may help to make the dangers of such generalizations concrete. Assume a group of children who are badly undernourished and who are well below their age norms for height and weight. If these children are now placed on a full calorie, nutritionally well-balanced diet, they will make quite noticeable progress in height and weight in a reasonably short period of time. If, however, you take a group of children who are already well nourished and at or above the norms for height and weight for their age group, a comparable regimen will have little or no effect.

Does this mean that advantaged children receive no benefits from early childhood education because it merely duplicates what they have at home? Not at all. The issue here is comparable to the one raised about home schooling. Yes, parents can and do successfully school their children at home, even through high school. This does not signify that early childhood programs are unimportant. It does mean that parents who have the time, energy, and commitment to home school can do so successfully. But parents who do not have the time, energy, and commitment to home school do need the public education to fill that role.

Exactly the same holds true for early childhood education. If parents have the time, energy, and commitment to provide an intellectually challenging environment at home, to have regular periods of time to spend with the child reading, talking, and engaging in other activities, and to have other children in the neighborhood over on occasion, there is really no need for the child to attend a preschool. But if the parent is not ready or able to devote the time and energy to providing that kind of experience, then a good preschool experience would be enriching and rewarding for the child.

Is Earlier Better?

The idea that earlier is better when it comes to early childhood education is widespread. It stems from the 1960s when many writers hoped that early childhood education might be the way to break the cycle of poverty. It was hoped that if disadvantaged children could be given a head start at the preschool level, that they would be on a level playing field with advantaged children when they entered school.

At that time the promise of early childhood education seemed unlimited. Jerome Bruner wrote that "we begin with the hypothesis that any subject can be taught effectively in some intellectually honest way to any child at any stage of development" (Bruner, 1962, p. 22.). It was hoped that if children were taught the basics of reading, writing, and arithmetic during the early years, then this would not only ensure them a head start but also insure them against failure later.

The idea that earlier is better was reinforced by the writing of Benjamin Bloom (1964), who contended that "general intelligence appears to develop as much from conception to age four as it does during the fourteen years from age four to eighteen" (pp. 207–208). Bloom went on to argue that because intelligence grows so rapidly in early childhood, it is the time to engage in serious instruction rather than play. The idea that little children are sponges ready and eager to soak up all the information we pour over them became a widespread and accepted conviction. It encouraged many parents to try to teach their infants and young children everything from reading to violin to karate.

But is early childhood a critical period for learning basic skills? It is certainly true that infants and young children are eager and avid learners. Yet what young children need to learn is not academic subjects and skills but rather the basics of the world in which they live. Young children need to learn sights, colors, sounds, shapes, textures, and tastes. They need to discover *up* and *down*, *behind* and *on top of*. They need to discover what floats and what sinks, to encounter the many forms, sounds, and smells of different animals and encounts.

Yes, infants and young children are avid learners, but they are eager to learn from their own explorations and discoveries and not from formal instruction. That is what all of the workers in early childhood education, from Pestalozzi to Piaget, have emphasized. The child needs to acquire a conception of the immediate fundamental world before he or she begins to learn the derived, symbolic world of formal instruction.

SUMMARY AND CONCLUSIONS

Early childhood education is a relatively modern innovation. It had its origins in the industrial revolution, the humanitarian thrust of the theory of evolution, and the emergence of socialist societies and communal child rearing. In the contemporary United States early childhood education has grown to accommodate the needs of two- and single-parent working families, as well as to provide a head start for disadvantaged children.

There are four basic principles of developmental early childhood education. The first is that the learner is an individual with growing mental abilities. A second principle is that learning is a creative process and necessarily involves both the subject and the object or material to be learned. The third principle is that knowledge is always a construction and always contains something of the subject as well as of the material to be known. Finally, the aim of developmental early childhood education is to produce active, self-motivated learners and critical thinkers.

There are many unresolved issues surrounding early childhood education. Among these are the questions of whether early childhood education can harm the child, whether it can improve the child's IQ, and whether it can give the child a head start.

In the United States early childhood education is coming into its own as a part of the educational system. It is increasingly recognized that early childhood education is not a ''size smaller'' 1st grade, that young children learn differently from older children and adults, and that they require their own curriculum, their own teaching modes, and their own method of evaluation. Early childhood education is coming to be accepted on its own terms.

References

Baron JB, Sternberg RJ: *Teaching Thinking Skills: Theory and Practice*. New York, Freeman, 1987.

Bloom B: *Stability and Change in Human Behavior*. New York, Wiley, 1964.

Bowlby J: *Child Care and the Growth of Love*. London, Penguin Books, 1950.

Bredenkamp S: *Developmentally Appropriate Practice*. Washington, DC, National Association for the Education of Young Children, 1987.

Bruner J: *The Process of Education*. Cambridge, Harvard University Press, 1962.

Clarke-Stewart A: The day care child. *Parents* September:72–75, 1982.

Cremin L: *The Transformation of the Schools*. New York, Vintage, 1961.

Dewey J: *Democracy in Education*. New York, Macmillan, 1916.

Elkind D: *A Sympathetic Understanding of the Child* (3rd ed.) Boston: Allyn & Bacon 1994.

Erikson E: *Childhood and Society*. New York, Norton, 1950.

Froebel F: *The Education of Man*. New York, D Appleton & Co., 1893.

Freud S: Infantile Sexuality. *The Basic Writings of Sigmund Freud*. New York, Random House, 1938, pp. 580–603.

Green JA: *The Educational Ideas of Pestalozzi*. New York, Greenwood, 1914.

Hetherington EM, Park RD: *Child Psychology: A Contemporary Viewpoint*. New York: McGraw-Hill, 1993.

Kamii C: *Number in Preschool and Kindergarten*. Washington, DC, National Association for the Education of Young Children, 1982.

Klein M: *Envy and Gratitude*. London, Tavistock Publications, 1957.

Kozulin A: *Vygotsky's Psychology*. Cambridge, MA: Harvard University Press, 1990.

Lacan J: *The Language of the Self*. New York, Delta, 1968.

Montessori M: *The Montessori Method*. New York, Schocken, 1964. (Originally published 1912)

Piaget J: *Play, Dreams and Imitation in Childhood*. New York, Norton, 1951.

Piaget J: *The Psychology of Intelligence*. London, Routledge & Kegan Paul, 1950.

Piaget J: *Science of Education and the Psychology of the Child*. New York, Orion, 1970.

Ripple RE, Rockcastle VO (eds): *Piaget Rediscovered: A Report of the Conference on Cognitive Studies and Curriculum Development*. Ithaca, NY, School of Education, Cornell University, 1964.

Schweinhart LJ, Weikart DP, Larner MB: Consequences of three preschool curriculum models through age 15. *Early Childhood Research Q* 1: 15–45, 1985.

Weinstein CE, Mayer RE: The Teaching of Learning Strategies. In: Witrock MC (ed): *Handbook of Research on Teaching* (3rd ed). New York, Macmillan, 1986.

109 Improving Psychoeducational Outcomes for African-American Children

James P. Comer, M.D., and Norris M. Haynes, Ph.D.

There has been a dramatic increase in problems facing families and children in the inner cities of urban America during recent years. These social difficulties are having significant negative impact on the school readiness and school success of African-American children in disproportionate numbers, resulting in an urgent need for us to improve psychoeducational outcomes for African-American children in our schools. Therefore, providing low-income African-American children with a successful school experience is one of the most important tasks facing the United States today. If these children remain undereducated in disproportionate numbers in this age of science and technology, all of our most troublesome social problems will be exacerbated—low productivity, dependency, substance abuse, crime, children having children, and others. Across the country in areas where such children are located in disproportionate numbers, they are often up to 2 years behind children from better-educated families. And in large urban centers, school dropout rates are as high as 50% (Children's Defense Fund, 1989). There is evidence that these youngsters can achieve at a much higher academic level (Comer, 1980, 1988).

While it is more difficult to document, some social and behavioral scientists and educators believe that many African-American young people from better-educated, middle-income families may not be achieving at the levels of their ability due to negative peer pressure, as well as insensitive schooling practices (Ogbu, 1986). If this is the case, the leadership group needed to improve opportunities for all African-Americans, which in turn would benefit all Americans, will not grow sufficiently rapidly or large enough.

There are several commonly suggested causes for the educational underachievement of low-income black children: school segregation, inadequate schools, low teacher expectations and bias, too few educational role models such as teachers, continuing insensitive schooling practices, as well as unemployment and its detrimental effects on families (Boykin, 1983; Clark, 1983; Haynes, 1993).

Some African-American children achieve despite these obstacles. In 1939 the first author entered an elementary school in East Chicago, Indiana, with three other black youngsters from a low-income community. The school was racially integrated, served the highest socioeconomic group in town, and was considered one of the best. All four students were from two-parent families. All four fathers made a living wage as laborers in the local steel mills. Despite similar intellectual potential, all three of the first author's friends had difficult educational and life outcomes—one died prematurely from alcoholism, a second spent a significant part of his life in jail, a third has been in and out of mental institutions. The more favorable outcome for the first author was due largely to the fact that his parents provided him with a preschool experience that gave him the confidence and kinds of skills necessary to elicit support in school. His parents interacted with school people in a way that encouraged support for him. And beyond home and school, a constructive social network of friends and kin, religious and other institutions, helped to make academic success possible for him. Although the second author was raised in another culture, Trinidad, where racism and segregation were not part of his educational experience, but class distinctions were, he also found that his mother's understanding of the importance of positive social relationships and the existence of a supportive network of caring adults and good friends were critical in his educational and social experiences. The notion that "it takes a village to raise a child" was very much true.

A similar experience is usually found among African Americans who have had academic success. Many, perhaps most, of today's educated, middle- and upper-income African Americans are from low-income backgrounds (Jaynes and Williams, 1989). Most educated blacks over 45 years of age, and a large percentage of the leadership group, attended racially segregated primary and secondary schools, even postsecondary schools (Jaynes and Williams, 1989). Also, many black children have not done well in racially integrated schools, even schools considered very good and serving middle- and upper-income families (Ogbu, 1986). And while unemployment is a serious problem and has probably served to increase the number of single-parent families, some black children of unemployed parents and low-income families do reasonably well in school (Clark, 1983). And how are we to explain the underachievement of black youngsters from middle- and upper-income families (Fordham, 1988)? In short, our usual explanations for school underachievement among African-American youngsters are simplistic, adynamic, and not very useful.

In the 1960s, in part because of his own experience, the first author began to speculate that the relationship experiences of students before school and in school and relationships between parents and school staff affect their development, and, in turn, their ability to achieve in school. Further, that if this is the case, the almost exclusive focus of schools on instruction and curriculum, without attention to issues of relationships and development, is probably at the root of the academic underachievement of many students. These relationship issues and their impact on academic learning have been given far too little attention.

Also, because of his own experience and his psychotherapeutic work with middle- and upper-income black children, the first author became aware of the troublesome racial identity problem that such young people face. (This is also a relationship issue.) Often without conscious intent, but because of historical situations and conditions, the society attributes characteristics to African Americans or blacks such as bad, unsuccessful, limited interest in academic learning, and the like. Being white or a member of the majority and more powerful group in the society—even when not in a majority in a particular situation, such as school—is characterized by opposite traits. Identification as a black person, then, can be problematic (Comer, 1972).

Recent events in New York, North Carolina, and Boston (in which African-American men have been falsely accused of brutal crimes by the perpetrators of these crimes to give credibility to their stories and to garnish national sympathy) reinforce pervasively accepted negative stereotypes of African Americans generally and African-American males in particular. African-American children are aware of these stereotypes and adversely affected by them, especially in terms of their self-evaluations and educational aspirations. Young African-American male students appear to be especially at risk. Relationships based on mutual acceptance and respect promote success, no matter the age, sex, race, or class of those involved. It is by the quality of these relationships that we determine the effectiveness of our social institutions, including our schools.

Why, then, has society largely ignored relationship issues in its efforts to improve education, particularly that of minority children? In part, because educational theory is influenced more by industrialization than by child development and the social and behavioral sciences. Society tends to understand teaching and learning as a mechanical process. Thus academic learning is thought of as an entirely cognitive (mechanical) process, willfully engaged in or rejected by the individual and facilitated or limited only by the individual's ability level.

In addition, social scientists usually analyze the behavior of societies, groups, and individuals in the here and now, as if it were unrelated to their histories. The impact of powerful structural forces created by political, economic, social, geographical, and other conditions is often ignored. The effects of these forces, positive and negative, are transmitted from generation to generation—parents to child—greatly influencing child development, subsequent social and academic performance in school and opportunities in life (Clark, 1983).

And finally, society's neglect of these known effects is due in part to societal guilt relative to the experience of Native Americans, Hispanics, and African Americans in particular. But even the European and Asian immigrant experience and the experience of groups isolated from the positive effects of scientific and technological changes (and not all were positive) have not been adequately explored to help us understand individual, group, and societal functioning, teaching, and learning in school. It is necessary to consider the effects of the black experience on the functioning of the community and individuals in order to understand the obstacles and opportunities involved in the education of African-American children.

What is needed is a theory of teaching and learning that looks beyond the child in school, that considers the complex interactions of children developing in families and family interactions in social networks within a larger society. The perspective must also include an understanding of the force of past social and economic conditions on the present. Thus in this chapter we will: (a) discuss the relationship dynamics of children developing in families, social networks, and the school; (b) explore the relative economic and social history of America, comparing the difference between European and Asian immigrants and African-Americans and the different and similar psychosocial consequences; (c) present a discussion of a child development program work in schools as a model of the complex problems involved, but also as a model for addressing them; and finally, (d) consider the role child and adolescent psychiatrists can play in influencing practices and policies relevant to the education of African-American young people.

The theory presented below grew out of our Yale Child Study Center-New Haven school system experience in schools over the past 25 years.

A THEORETICAL FRAMEWORK

Children are born totally dependent, with biological potentials that must be developed and aggressive drives that must be channeled and sublimated into the energy of learning, work, and play. They are also born with a capacity to form relationships. When competent caretakers (usually parents) provide for them, a strong emotional attachment and bond develops between the child and the caretakers. This enables parents and other caretakers to help them grow along many developmental pathways (Bowlby, 1952; Stern, 1977). At least five pathways are critical for future academic learning: social-interactive, psychoemotional, moral, speech-language, and intellectual-cognitive.

Families are enmeshed in a social network of friends, kin, and religious and social institutions (Erikson, 1963). Social networks or groups have a history that influences their attitudes, values, and ways, but also they live under contemporary conditions that establish and maintain a mainstream set of attitudes, values, and ways. And, generation after generation, mainstream parents transmit the ways of their group to their children as they interact with them from birth forward.

The school is a mainstream institution. When a child's growth is adequate along critical developmental pathways in his or her family and social network, and the culture and expectations of the network are similar to those of the school, most are adequately prepared to achieve in school at the level of their ability.

Development along critical pathways takes place through incidental experiences that children have with their caretakers, as well as through systematic teaching efforts on the part of the adults around them. For example, a 2-year-old who wants to play with the ball of another child does not know that he or she can't just take the ball. He or she may attempt to do so, and a struggle or fight may ensue. A caretaker intervenes and mediates. In the process the caretaker spells out several options for the aggressor—do something else until Johnny is through playing with the ball, play with Johnny if there is an interest on his part, or just go away. In the process the caretaker is helping the child grow along all the critical developmental pathways.

In this single incident the child learns appropriate social interaction. The impulse to hit or take is controlled, and sometimes the caretaker must help the child handle emotions or feelings related to being denied. What is right and wrong is learned. Language is involved, and thinking is involved. Thus development takes place along all the critical pathways.

More closely related to academic learning is reading. Parents who are part of the mainstream of the society usually read to their very young children. They often do so at the end of a busy day, and the child has the parent's total attention. Reading, then, is a special time and becomes a positively charged emotional experience. Children's stories often deal with the fears and anxieties they experience attempting to cope, with few skills, in a threatening world. Thus children want to hear the stories repeatedly. Eventually they memorize the words and associate them with the pictures on a page. Delighted parents, and other important adults in the lives of the children, often excitedly express their approval.

Children are programmed to seek the approval of adults. With approval, they want to read more and master other aspects of their environment in order to win the recognition of important adults around them. The motivation for learning and mastery, then, grows out of early relationships with important adults. The attitude about learning and positive learning experiences with parents and other primary caretakers at a very early age becomes the basis for a transference reaction with other adults, particularly school people, later in the development of the child.

Children who have been living in average expected mainstream environments approach the school experience, and the adults involved, with attitudes, values, and ways similar to those expected in school, and with development at a level necessary for the child to meet school tasks. Such children are able to interact appropriately with other students. They are able to sit still and listen or attend to a task when it's appropriate to do so. They are able to be spontaneous and curious when it's appropriate to do so.

Such behavior elicits a positive response from adults in the school environment and promotes positive transference between the child and school people. This permits a positive attachment and bond to take place between the child and school people, similar to, but not as strong as, the attachment and bond that took place at home between the child and the primary caretaker. The child then has the same need to please school people as to please parents at home. This enables school people to help students continue to grow along the critical developmental pathways.

Growth along these pathways—social-interactive, psychoemotional, moral, linguistic, and intellectual-cognitive—facilitates academic learning.

The desire and capacity to become a good academic learner grows steadily from birth. And the utility or benefits of academic learning accrue. Eventually the child develops an inner motivation to learn and achieve, and it is as powerful, if not more so, than the outside approval of teachers, other adults, and other external rewards such as money or gifts.

The preschool and school developmental experience is often different for children growing up in families that are marginal to and outside of the mainstream of the society and often under economic, racial, or other stresses. The relationship processes in such families less often lead to school success.

Income that is not adequate to enable heads of households to meet basic family needs is a source of excessive stress. Negative societal attitudes about minorities and poor people are stressors. They contribute to the increased frequency of divorce and to never-married single-parent families, in turn a major source of poverty. Children from poor families more often grow up in neighborhoods with a disproportionate number of social problems— delinquency and crime, violence, teenage pregnancy, welfare dependency, undesirable housing, and inadequate health care (Children's Defense Fund, 1989). And while successful families and social networks exist within such neighborhoods, there are extraordinary pressures interfering with the development of children at all times. Thus all such families are under stress.

Parents often lack education themselves or bear social and psychological scars related to their social status and conditions. They often sense exclusion and feel alienated from the mainstream of the society. They often carry some attitudes, values, and ways that are different from those of the mainstream. They often simply don't know mainstream expectations and ways (Lightfoot, 1978). Thus even when they want to prepare their children to succeed in school—a mainstream institution—they are not able adequately to do so.

For example, learning to negotiate and work things out rather than fight is expected in school. But in many nonmainstream communities children are expected to fight rather than negotiate. Many such families do not read to their children, take them on recreational-learning excursions, or otherwise give them the informal preschool learning and social skills needed to grow along the critical developmental pathways discussed above. By school age such children are underdeveloped, or differently developed, along the developmental pathways most related to academic learning. They often have skills that enable them to function adequately on the playground, the halls of the housing project, and a variety of other customary places, but such skills will elicit a negative staff response in school.

The preparation of most school people does not help them understand the behavior and apparent ability level of such children as underdevelopment, or different development. It is viewed as "bad" and "dumb," or evidence of inadequate learning potential. Most school staff attempt to change the behavior of the children through punishment. This often leads to even more troublesome behavior and accompanying low expectations on the part of students, and, in turn, to increased control efforts and continued low expectations by school staff. Some students eventually respond with severe acting out behavior, or withdrawal and apathy. This leads to hopelessness and despair among all in school settings (Edmonds, 1979).

Parents who had ambivalent feelings about the school in the first place—hoped that it would give their children a chance for greater success than they experienced, but feared that it wouldn't—are often brought into conflict with school people, or withdraw and avoid the school. The attachment and bonding that should occur between school staff and students does not occur, and the staff is not able to help the students invest strongly in the academic learning task. In the situation where parent-child bonding was not strong because of difficult social circumstances, inadequate bonding in school is doubly troublesome.

Prior to 8 or 9 years of age, most students are able to establish the level of attachment and bonding that enables adults to influence their behavior (Bowlby, 1952). But around this period the academic performance demands of the school (more abstract learning) begin to outstrip their performance preparation. Second, a child's cognitive capacity now enables him or her to understand his or her social status—at home and in the community, and in the classroom. And third, the thrust for independence is greater at this age (Flavell, 1985). These developments limit or facilitate mainstream aspirations and reduce the ability of adults to positively influence the behavior of young people. If constructive attitudes toward learning have not been internalized by this point, it can be difficult for adults to introduce them.

Students with a weak attachment and bond to the people and the program of the school, or with extraordinary pressures to belong to troublesome social networks outside of school, begin to pull away. It is at this point, around 3rd grade, that one sees the academic performance gain of children from families and communities under stress begin to level off.

As they confront the developmental issues of pre- and early adolescence, they "place" themselves in the social scheme of things. They learn to develop an understanding—correct or not—of their exclusion from, or their limited opportunities in, the mainstream of the society. Their source of self-affirmation is from their own families and social networks. In fact, when schools ask young people to achieve at a high level, they are often asking them to be different from their own parents—the people with whom they have the most important and powerful social ties.

Around 12 to 13 years of age they develop the cognitive capacity to consider hypothetical situations-not only what is, but what could be (Piaget, 1970). This ability not only widens their world but also makes it more complex. Simultaneously, numerous confusing physiological and body changes are taking place. Succeeding and belonging in groups—with attendant group pressures—become very important tasks at this point. In addition, in 7th grade, in many places, young people are required to change schools and make numerous social adjustments associated with doing so.

Most young people who are developing well and who are from the societal mainstream are able to manage these challenges with the average expected difficulty. But many capable young people go on a sharp psychosocial downhill course at this point, leading to school dropouts, teenage pregnancy, delinquency and crime, and other social problems. A disproportionate number of such youngsters—for reasons we will discuss—are African American (Children's Defense Fund, 1989).

By mid-adolescence—around 9th grade for most—social class and race-related expectations and occupational and career possibilities begin to greatly influence student performance. Many high-ability students from low-income backgrounds begin to do less well in school, often less well than the low-ability students from middle- and upper-class backgrounds (Fordham, 1988). Also, by this point, many students have serious academic deficiencies and negative attitudes and beliefs about themselves that make it difficult for them to perform adequately even when they desire to do so.

The situation for middle-class African-American youngsters is different, but still problematic. With adequate income, such families are under less stress and better able to prepare their children to meet the expectations of the school. Many such parents believe that their economic well-being will protect their children from negative societal attitudes and behaviors related to race. In fact, many avoid any discussion of race. At the other extreme, parents express angry and hostile feelings about racial injustice in a way that conveys powerlessness. They often encourage their children to be individuals, as if raceless, and as if they will not be forced to confront and manage racial issues in their lives (Fordham, 1988). These youngsters often receive the same message in school. A well-meaning professor once told the first author that he, the first author, had ability in spite of his race (*sic!*) (and encouraged him to go on for postgraduate work).

The developing young person has no way to understand the disproportionate number of problems he or she observes among African Americans. Such persons are not prepared to manage racial antagonisms, deliberate and unintentional, in ways that minimize the negative effects on their self-esteem. With little understanding of the experience, strength, and successes of their racial group, they cannot experience the level of positive identification with the group that is needed to better manage the racial antagonism in the larger society. In adolescence some young people from better-educated, middle-income black families, struggling to establish their identity, are drawn into behaviors defined by the society as black and internalized by some as "true" black behavior—low academic achievement, troublesome social performance, and the like (Fordham and Ogbu, 1986).

In order to appreciate fully these dynamics—and to develop effective education intervention programs—it is important to consider the historical and contemporary political, economic, and social structures and forces that created the economic, social, and psychological vulnerability of black families.

THE AFRICAN-AMERICAN EXPERIENCE

Over the past 150 years the United States has moved through four economic stages: agricultural, before 1860; late agricultural-early industrial, 1860–1900; mid- or heavy industrial, 1900–1945; late industrial-early scientific-technological, 1945–1980; postindustrial, high scientific-technological, after 1980. European and Asian immigrants arrived in the United States in large numbers prior to 1915. Most were able to maintain a reasonable degree of cultural continuity—religion, language, and other aspects of their culture—because they lived in ethnic enclaves, resulting in a reasonable degree of social cohesion (Lieberson, 1980).

Some had ties to financial resources in the old country. They obtained the vote in one generation. Cultural cohesion, the vote, and economic resources, together, permitted most groups to gain political, economic, and social power in one generation at a level that permitted their families to undergo four generations of change and development that paralleled economic change and development in the country (Lieberson, 1980).

Prior to 1900 heads of households could be uneducated and unskilled and earn a living in the economy, provide for themselves and their families, and give their children the kinds of experiences that enabled them to gain the moderate level of education and skill needed to succeed in the mid-industrial period between 1900 and 1945 (Wilson, 1987). Successful heads of households in this economy were able to give their children the kinds of experiences that enabled them to gain high levels of education and skill needed for the last stage of the industrial era, 1945 to 1980, and of course a similar process permitted most heads of households to prepare their children for the postindustrial era.

While such groups experienced numerous hardships, and as a consequence unsuccessful families living under stressful conditions are found in various areas of the country today, most did not experience significant group and family deterioration. The experience and outcome for a significant number of African Americans, Hispanics, and Native Americans was different. We will discuss only African-Americans here.

The African-American experience was characterized by cultural discontinuity (Franklin, 1947; Frazier, 1957). The sense of adequacy, worth, and direction given by culture was lost in the separation from Africa. Because the central organizing force of West African culture was tight-knit kinship and lineage groups with communal traditions, a slave culture—and ultimately, release into a society that highly valued independence and competition—was extremely traumatic. Slavery was a system of forced dependency, inherent inferiority, and no opportunity for a better future. These are three of the most problematic conditions that can be imposed on people who are then expected to function in a competitive economic and social system (Berry and Blassingame, 1982).

These conditions created negative psychosocial consequences among many. And they were transmitted from generation to generation, parents to children, among some, even down to the present day (Elkins, 1963). But many African Americans were protected to some degree by the ''Black Church,'' fashioned from aspects of African culture and Protestant religions in the South, and by living under better conditions of slavery. Also, southern rural culture tended to reinforce the church culture and facilitate effective family functioning (Comer, 1972; Frazier, 1962).

After slavery, blacks in large numbers were denied the vote and, in fact, denied in significant numbers right up until the 1960s, the middle of the last stage of the industrial era. Also, blacks had no ties to capital (Jaynes and Williams, 1989). Without the vote and capital, it was not possible for the black population to limit the level of racial antagonism, or racism. As a result, blacks were closed out of the political, economic, and social mainstream. Most black heads of households worked at the lowest levels of the economy—sharecroppers and tenant farmers, domestics and industrial laborers.

Without political and economic power, blacks were closed out of educational opportunities. In the eight states that had 80% of the black population, four to eight times as much money was spent on the education of a white child as on the education of a black one (Bose and Caliber, 1936). Where the black population was disproportionate in numbers, the disparity was as great as 25 times and more (Bose and Caliber, 1936). This situation continued into the 1940s, perhaps beyond. As late as 1964–1965, the combined endowment of two prestigious white women's colleges was half the endowment of Harvard. One-half of Harvard's endowment was greater than that of all black colleges put together (totalling more than 100) (Council for Financial Aid to Education, 1967).

Blacks were closed out of mainstream business and government participation. Educated blacks were limited to professional areas—teachers, physicians, nurses, and the like. As a result, the kind of information, contacts, and connections needed to make the social system work for its members was not available. Even the growing political power of the last two decades is in the absence of economic power; thus it is less useful in making the social system work for the entire black community. Despite these difficult conditions, the black population did reasonably well right into the 1950s (Wilson, 1987).

As late as 1950 only 22% of all black families were headed by single parents; now it's over 50% (Wilson, 1987). And black communities were reasonably safe. Today's serious conditions among a disproportionate segment of the black population began with (a) the mass migration of undereducated people from rural to urban areas in the 1940s and (b) with education increasingly becoming the ticket of admission to living wage jobs after 1945 (Wilson, 1987). Blacks were disproportionately undereducated, compared to other groups, and lacked the power to gain well-paying low-skill jobs. In addition, previous organizing cultural ties were lost with mass migration. Many families that once functioned well in the traditional church-based, extended family, rural culture of the South began to function less well under urban conditions.

Also, families functioning well in urban areas began to reduce family size, except for religious reasons. Families not functioning well did so less often. As a result, the growth in population over the last 40 years—among all groups—has been among low-income families operating under the greatest stress (US Bureau of the Census, 1985). And for the reasons cited, African-Americans have a disproportionate number of families operating under excessive stress.

Most industrial countries developed social and educational policies that facilitated family functioning in the 1940s and 1950s. This country did not do so to the same extent (Kamerman and Kahn, 1981). As a result, a number of minority group families—more than among groups able to undergo several generations of development and stabilization—are not able to give their children the kind of preschool experiences that will enable them to meet the expectations of the school. And for the reasons described above, some mainstream middle-class minority youngsters are affected. Thus too many minority group children are undereducated.

SCHOOL DEVELOPMENT PROGRAM AS A MODEL

In 1968 a Yale Child Study team (directed by the first author and made up of a social worker, a psychologist, and a special education teacher) began a collaborative project with the New Haven school system. This team worked in two schools in the inner city of New Haven as a subsystem of the school system. The plan was to develop a successful change process within these two schools, in collaboration with the parents and school staff, in a way that could be transmitted to all New Haven schools and beyond, eventually influencing national school policies and practices (Comer, 1980).

Work began in the Martin Luther King Elementary School, kindergarten to fourth grade, with approximately 300 students, and the Simeon Baldwin school, kindergarten to sixth grade, with approximately 350 students. After 5 years the team left Baldwin, already vastly improved but resistant to additional changes, and began to work in the Katharine Brennan school, a kindergarten to 5th grade school with a profile similar to that of the original schools. These schools were 99% black, and almost all the students were from poor families. The students ranked 32nd and 33rd of 33 city schools on standardized achievement tests. They were 19 and 18 months behind in achievement in language arts and mathematics by the 4th grade. Their attendance was among the lowest in the city, and there were serious behavior problems in both schools. Teacher turnover was common, and parent dissatisfaction with the schools was widespread.

By 1979, without a change in the socioeconomic make-up of the school communities, the children were at grade level on standardized achievement tests. The improvement process was institutionalized, allowing the team to leave these two schools in 1980. In 1984 the two schools, again with no change in the socioeconomic make-up, tied for the third and fourth highest levels of achievement in the city on standardized achievement tests, a year above grade level at King School and 7 months above grade level at Brennan School. King School's attendance had been first or second in the city for 5 of the previous 6 years, and Brennan School's attendance was improved and ranked first at least once during that period. Behavior problems were greatly decreased in both schools; teacher turnover was extremely rare, and there were no serious behavior problems (Comer, 1976, 1980).

What the team found initially in these school communities served to provide insight for the theoretical formulation described above. The parents and the students were largely the descendants of rural, southern African Americans, undereducated and working at the bottom of the job market, or not working and on public assistance. Many were experiencing significant economic and social stress. The underdevelopment and different development of their children made it difficult for them to meet the expectations of the school.

The school staff was not prepared to successfully adjust. The resultant difficult interactions between home and school, among school staff and between staff and students led to alienation, distrust, disrespect, inadequate student-staff attachment and bonding, difficult teaching conditions, and limited academic learning.

The Yale Child Study Center team took an ecological and child development perspective in identifying the problems and opportunities. The team realized that it would need to (a) change the difficult interactions among the adults into cooperative and collaborative interactions so that they would be able to support the level of child development that would make successful academic learning possible and (b) make teaching a gratifying experience. But the team could not mandate a change in the culture of the school—its beliefs, attitudes, values, and ways. Efforts to teach school people about child development and behavior, in the hope that they would apply their knowledge in the classroom, were unsuccessful. The team instead had to gradually develop mechanisms that permitted the staff and parents to carry out a process that allowed them to function in a way that changed the culture and/or climate of the school and promoted child development, teaching, and learning as needed.

The Child Study Center team used their clinical skills to help the staff work more effectively with children displaying behavior problems. With each success the team gained staff interest and appreciation for clinical methods. Eventually the team was able to share child development and child-rearing knowledge, skills, and sensitivity with the staff and help them appreciate how school attitudes, beliefs, values, and practices either facilitate or limit student growth and development, teaching and learning.

With school staff and parents, the team eventually developed a change process called the School Development Program, which has three mechanisms, three operations, and three guidelines designed to address the problems and opportunities found in all schools, but especially the more problematic ones in schools serving low-income minority students. The three mechanisms are the governance and management team, the mental health team, and the parents program. The governance and management team is representative of all of the adult stakeholders in the schools—parents, teachers, administrators, mental health team or support staff, the nonprofessional support staff, and so forth. This is the most important program element. It carries out the three critical operations—development of a comprehensive school plan, staff development based on the plan, and systematic assessment and modification of the program. This mechanism and these operations bring the key adults together in a way that enables them to establish agreement and to coordinate and carry out a program that reduces duplication and conflict, facilitates communication, and establishes mutual trust and respect. The comprehensive school plan focuses on carrying out activities that systematically serve to improve the climate of relationships and the academic program.

The mental health team brings together personnel usually found working separately in schools—social worker, psychologist, special education teacher, nurse, and the like. This team works with individual children, but the focus is on prevention. They often gain clues from individual student problems about the kind of building level changes that can be made that will reduce them. For example, difficult adjustments to transferring into the schools led to serious behavior problems among some students. Transfer problems were reduced by orientation sessions for new students at the classroom and building level, preventing immediate, sustained, and more serious problems. Problems of discontinuity in the lives of children, interfering with their ability to establish the kinds of attachments needed to trust and take chances, led to a program of keeping children with the same teacher for 2 years, with great success. A program for helping children in crisis greatly reduced disruptive acting-out behaviors. A "Discovery Room" enabled many withdrawn children, doubtful of their ability to manage in the school setting, to function adequately.

The mental health team person serving on the governance and management team helped that group to establish policies and practices that prevented student behavioral problems or reduced their adverse consequences. In the process he or she provided all adults in the school with knowledge about how children grow and develop, and how that is related to teaching and learning. The mental health team also helped staff members to interact well together and to develop a school climate that facilitated the work of all involved. Adults functioning well in a good climate, who are knowledgeable about child growth and development, can facilitate attachment and bonding, child growth and development, leading to adequate teaching and learning.

The third mechanism was the parents' program. Parents were involved at three levels—as members of the governance and management team, selected by other parents; as members of the parents group that put on activities with school staff in support of the school program; and as visitors and participants in school activities. A school social worker or teacher served as a liaison between the staff and the parent group and facilitated their work in the school. This reduced the likelihood of the development of an adversarial relationship.

During one period parents worked as assistants in the classroom, receiving a minimum wage for 10 hours and often volunteering 20 to 30 more. The presence of parents in the school working closely with school staff reduced the alienation and distrust between home and school. It facilitated the attachment and bonding between students and school staff and the program of the school. Many parents working in this way were motivated to go back to school themselves; at least seven went on to college and became professional people. The presence of a core of parents in school increased the social comfort of all parents in the school setting. Because of this and other things done to improve school operations and climate, parent turnout for school activities went from 15 in a school serving a little over 300 students to 400 in the same building 3 years later. Similar increases in parent participation were seen in almost every school district in which the team worked.

But school restructuring alone was not responsible for these outcomes. It was necessary to change the culture of the school from being punitive with low expectations to having a focus on supporting growth and development, cooperation, collaboration, and high expectations for all. The team's three working guidelines were designed to change the culture. The mechanisms and operations of the program generated and carried the new beliefs, attitudes, values, and ways, or culture.

The three guidelines were (a) a "no-fault" policy, (b) consensus decision making, and (c) an agreement that the members of the governance and management team could not paralyze the principal, but also that the principal could not ignore the input of team members. In this way, time was not wasted placing blame but was used to solve problems; decision making through consensus rather than voting kept groups focused on child development principles and avoided winner-loser behavior; and leadership was effective without being oppressive and was based on multiple perspectives. While the governance and management team generated the desired culture, its style permeated the school as all involved carried out the work set forth in the comprehensive school plan.

When the three mechanisms, the three operations, and the three guidelines were all working appropriately, everyone experienced ownership and responsibility for the school program, and a kind of synergism developed that gave the school hope and forward momentum. It enabled student growth and development to take place; adequate teaching and learning were then possible.

The team eventually developed a program that very systematically taught low-income minority group children the same skills that mainstream children from better educated families gain simply by growing up with their parents. The team developed units in politics and government, business and economics, health and nutrition, and spiritual and leisure time in which there was an integrated teaching of basic academic skills, social skills, and appreciation of the arts. The artistic programs enabled children to channel aggressive energy that would otherwise be harmful to themselves and others, or at least disruptive, into the energy of recreation and learning. The social skills students gained through these activities enabled them to elicit a positive response from teachers and other people in the mainstream of the society. This facilitated the needed attachment and bonding to mainstream people and programs and motivated young people to achieve. Because of the beneficial outcomes of this approach, the New Haven School System has established a social development program from elementary school through high school in which students are taught appropriate problem solving and decision making skills.

Because the team members are not educators, the team is not greatly involved in shaping the content of the curriculum. The team's process makes students available for and capable of learning curriculum content, who otherwise would not have been available or able. Also, the team supported the use of age-appropriate academic programs and activities. The team also supported a curriculum that recognized cultural diversity and urged that the curriculum contain material that would provide students with accurate information about the nature of the African-American experience.

The program has expanded nationally to approximately 500 schools in about 63 school districts. Although the majority of students in schools serviced by the program are of African American or other minority ethnic backgrounds, an increasing number of schools with majority white populations are opting to implement the program due to its demonstrated effects in improving the psychoeducational outcomes for large numbers of African-American and culturally diverse groups of students. Our own research (Haynes and Comer, 1993) and that of others (Becker and Hedges, 1992) have documented the program's effectiveness in improving the educational and psychosocial climate of schools resulting in enhanced student self-esteem, motivation, learning and achievement. The work of the mental health team in focusing attention on child development principles, proactive and preventive interventions, and child and family issues from a systems perspective has served to increase parents' involvement, their sense of efficacy in helping to raise and educate their children, and in turn resulted in significant reductions in school absenteeism and behavior problems.

THE CHILD AND ADOLESCENT PSYCHIATRIST

General psychiatrists focus more on the individual than on his or her environment. But because children are in a state of significant dynamic development and are dependent, the people and institutions around them (their critical environment) greatly affect their behavior. With greater appreciation of the power of people and institutions, child and adolescent psychiatrists can help promote policies and practices in organizations and institutions that promote growth and development. Child and adolescent psychiatrists have this opportunity in their work with families, the juvenile justice system, social welfare agencies, schools, and others. Schools probably offer the best opportunity to affect the most people under the best conditions.

Going to school is a normative function with no stigma attached to it. It is the final common pathway for almost all children today. It is strategically placed in the development pathway, early enough to compensate for potentially troublesome preschool experiences. School is the work of young people and is of long enough duration on a daily basis and over the years to significantly influence their development. Thus the child and adolescent psychiatrist should be involved in helping people engaged in every aspect of schooling, providing preventive and direct service, policy making, and research.

While most child and adolescent psychiatrists will not have full-time involvement in the way the Child Study Center team did, many are engaged in regular consultation, accept school referrals, and interact with school people regarding patients otherwise referred. Given the needs and training of most school people, child and adolescent psychiatrists are usually encouraged to work only with individuals or small groups and to address problem behaviors that appear child and family centered. But as child and adolescent psychiatrists enable teachers and administrators to help students, the child psychiatrist develops the trust and respect that allows him or her also to begin to look at school practices and policies that often interfere with student growth and development or that aggravates existing psychological problems. Sharing such insights often leads to the child psychiatrist's involvement in building-level staff development sessions. Such involvement provides even greater opportunities.

Through such sessions the child psychiatrist can help school staff understand how the fears and anxieties of students, the threat that school presents to many (and the related behaviors that arise), and the staff's own tendency toward control and punishment, make matters worse. Child psychiatrists can help staff understand that academic learning is more than a mechanical process in which students wilfully participate or refuse—that the affective component is important and that the motivation for learning grows out of relationships at home and school and between home and school. Child psychiatrists can help staff learn how their own behaviors promote either desirable or undesirable student responses. As the child psychiatrist and his or her team work with individual children, they can share their knowledge of child development and ways to promote growth and development with teachers, administrators, and parents.

Many schools lack orientation programs for new students, conflict resolution approaches, activities designed to promote cooperation and collaboration, and a focus on helping students develop inner discipline, self-motivation, and personal responsibility. Social problem solving and social skills are not taught systematically in most schools. Social activities are thought of as frills rather than as opportunities to help young people who are underdeveloped or differently developed grow and develop in ways that enable them to meet the expectations of the school. Child and adolescent psychiatrists are in a position to help school people understand how these skills and the resultant successes, confidence, and growth in self-esteem facilitate (a) bonding and attachment to school people and the program of the school and (b) teaching and learning.

Few school people understand the real or potential conflict that exists because of the income, education, racial, and other differences between home and school. And even fewer understand how, when, and why these differences influence academic learning. Child psychiatrists can help teachers understand the kinds of experiences that children from poor families need to be prepared for the level of abstract learning that is more required after 8 or 9 years of age, as well as the need to appreciate the effects of the thrust for independence among young people at this age and the later effects of social and racial status "placement" and/or identification with their respective groups. With such understanding, practices and programs can be devised at the building level to facilitate an appreciation for learning while enabling students to make a positive identification with their own group. And in some cases there will be opportunities to influence preservice programs and schools training future teachers and others, so that they will be better prepared to support the development of children in school once they are in practice.

Knowledge of how and why children learn and behave is also needed among policy makers. Decisions about the employment and use of social workers, psychologists, special education teachers, and the like depend on their understanding of child development and behavior, or lack of understanding. Likewise, school size and architecture, compensatory education programs, busing, school desegregation, the management of trauma, racial identification issues, class and race relations in general, gender issues, and a variety of other issues require knowledge of the behavioral and social sciences, held by child and adolescent psychiatrists. When child and adolescent psychiatrists are helpful with social issues at the building level, central office level school people are more likely to use them to help school board members, legislators, and the media better understand school district needs, opportunities, and limitations.

The surge in violence in recent years has resulted in significant demand for child psychiatric services in schools to address the devastating impact of this violence on children's lives. Children now, more than ever before, attend schools with such serious psychological problems as post-traumatic stress disorders, severe depression, behavior disorders and attention deficit problems, many of which result from exposure to the chronic violence in these children's lives. Our school-involved clinical consultants and crisis teams at the Yale Child Study Center provide significant and valuable interventions in New Haven schools to prevent and treat violence-related psychological problems among children. The result of these vital services is a very special collaborative relationship between the New Haven schools and our Yale Child Study Center in which our child psychiatrists, social workers, and psychologists participate in strategic planning and program development sessions with school officials. Very notable also is the police fellowship program directed by Dr. Steven Marans in which New Haven police officers are trained in child and adolescent development and psychology in order to improve their skills and increase their sensitivity (Marans, 1994).

Child and adolescent psychiatrists, because of their clinical focus, are probably better prepared than are other researchers to do the kind of research that is helpful in schools. The experimental research designs favored by nonclinicians take behavior out of context in a way that limits the value of their findings. The clinician looks at dynamic interactions in context, just as school people must do. In fact, school change leaders are suggesting that teachers be trained in a way that they can engage in the clinical practice of education. The participant-observer, ethnographer, case study approach child psychiatrists are more inclined to use is much more helpful. Child psychiatrists are in a good position to understand the insights and limitations of experimental design research findings and to use them appropriately and help school people do so.

Finally, training programs for child psychiatrists are probably least strong in preparing future psychiatrists to appreciate the impact of sociocultural, organization, and management effects and of history. However, a knowledge and understanding of the impact of family and social net-

work experiences on children, and an appreciation of historical, sociocultural, and organization and management effects, are easily gained. Future child and adolescent psychiatrists would be much better prepared to be helpful in every aspect of education if they had more systematic training in the effects of culture on institutions and individuals in homogeneous, heterogeneous, and complex societies (Coleman, 1966). The education of black students, and all other students, can be improved when we understand how societal, institutional, family, and/or group networks and individual development all interact to promote or limit student readiness for academic learning and teaching.

References

Becker J, Hedges LV: *A review of the literature on the effectiveness of Comer's School Development Program.* Unpublished paper prepared for the Rockefeller Foundation, 1992.

Berry MF, Blassingame J: *Long Memory: The Black Experience in America.* New York, Oxford University Press, 1982.

Bose D, Caliber A: *Statistics of the Education of Negroes*, 1929-30; 1931-32 (Bull. 133). Washington, DC, US Department of the Interior, Office of Education, 1936.

Bowlby J: The purpose of the family. In: *Maternal Care and Mental Health.* Geneva, World Health Organization, 1952.

Boykin AW: The academic performance of Afro-American children. In: Spence J (ed): *Achievement and Achievement Motives.* San Francisco, Freeman, 1983, pp. 321–371.

Children's Defense Fund: *A Vision for Americas Future.* Washington, DC, Children's Defense Fund, 1989.

Clark RM: *Family Life and School Achievement: Why Poor Black Children Succeed or Fail.* Chicago, University of Chicago Press, 1983.

Coleman JS: *Equality of Educational Opportunity.* Washington, DC, US Government Printing Office. 1966.

Comer JP: *Beyond Black and White.* New York, Quadrangle/New York Times Books, 1972.

Comer JP: Educating poor minority children. *Sci Am* 259:5, 1988.

Comer JP: Improving the quality and continuity of relationships in two inner-city schools. *Child Psychiatry* 15:2, 1976.

Comer JP: *School Power.* New York, Free Press, 1980.

Council for Financial Aid to Education: *1964-1965 Voluntary Support of America's Colleges and Universities.* New York, Council for Financial Aid to Education, 1967.

Edmonds R: Some schools work and more can. *Soc Policy* 9:28–32, 1979.

Elkins SM: *Slavery: A Problem in American Institutional and Intellectual Life.* New York, Grossett & Dunlap, 1963.

Erikson E: *Childhood and Society.* New York, Norton, 1963.

Flavell JH: *Cognitive Development.* Englewood Cliffs, NJ, Prentice-Hall, 1985.

Fordham S: Racelessness as a factor in black students' school success: Pragmatic strategy or pyrrhic victory? *Harvard Educ Rev* 58:1, 1988.

Fordham S, Ogbu JU: Black students' school success: Coping with the burden of "acting white." *Urban Rev* 18:3, 1986.

Franklin JH: *From Slavery to Freedom.* New York, Knopf, 1947.

Frazier EF: *The Negro in the United States* (rev ed). New York, Macmillan, 1957.

Frazier EF: *The Negro Church in America.* New York, Schocken Books, 1962.

Haynes NM: *Critical Issues in Educating African-American Children.* Langley Park, MD, IAAS Publishers, 1993.

Haynes NM, Comer JP: The Yale School Development Program: Process outcomes and policy implications. *Urban Educ* 28:166–199, 1993.

Jaynes GD, Williams RM Jr: *A Common Destiny.* Washington, DC, National Academy Press, 1989.

Kamerman S, Kahn AJ: Europe's innovative family policies. *Transatlantic Perspect* 2:9, 1981.

Lieberson S: *A Piece of the Pie: Black and White Immigrants Since 1880.* Berkeley, CA, University of California Press, 1980.

Lightfoot S: *Worlds Apart: Relationships between Families and Schools.* New York, Basic Books, 1978.

Marans S: Community violence and children's development: Collaborative interventions. *Children and Violence* 11:109–124, 1994.

Ogbu JU: Class stratification, racial stratification and schooling. In: Weis L (ed): *Race, Class and Schooling (Special Studies in Comparative Education, no. 17).* Buffalo, NY, Comparative Education Center, State University of New York at Buffalo, 1986.

Piaget J: Piaget's theory. In: Mussen PH (ed): *Carmichael's Manual of Child Psychology* (Vol 1). New York, Wiley, 1970.

Stern DN: *The First Relationship: Infant and Mother.* New York, Basic Books, 1977.

US Bureau of the Census: *Current Population Reports.* Washington, DC, US Government Printing Office, 1985.

Wilson WJ: *The Truly Disadvantaged.* Chicago, IL, University of Chicago Press, 1987.

110 SCHOOL AVOIDANCE, SCHOOL PHOBIA, AND TRUANCY

Ian Berg, M.D., F.R.C.P., F.R.C.Psych.

SCHOOL AVOIDANCE

In developed countries, education is provided for all children, and there is an expectation that they should attend school regularly to take advantage of the opportunities for learning that are offered. Penalties may be imposed if children fail to attend school without an adequate excuse (Berg and Nursten, 1996).

In the United States, attendance laws were passed early in the 19th century requiring 12 weeks at school in a year, but enforcement came only much later (Hersov, 1990). In Britain, the present system of compulsory schooling, backed by legal procedures that can be used if attendance is unsatisfactory, was introduced nearly 100 years ago. Throughout most of the 19th century, children were affected to a considerable extent by extreme poverty, crippling diseases, early death, and employment in

mines, agriculture, and factories, all of which made it difficult for any sort of national system of education to be organized. There were then few schools, and those that did exist often had poor facilities and inadequate teaching. However, there were some schools that attempted to encourage regular attendance. Inducements were sometimes offered in the form of a distribution of welfare benefits. Occasionally, lists of enrolled pupils who failed to attend regularly were displayed publicly as a means of deterring absence. A century ago, laws began to be enacted that enabled schools to be set up throughout the country, that compelled all children of specified ages to attend, and that also stated how regular attendance should be enforced. Courts were empowered to act when there was lack of compliance (Berg et al., 1988).

Despite this legal framework of mandatory education, many children have always had some time off school without adequate excuse. On average, at any one time in the United Kingdom, 10% of all children are out of school. Most are away with an acceptable reason, namely, a physical illness or a family holiday, but possibly as many as a third of them are off without adequate explanation. Community surveys have indicated what social, educational, and individual factors are associated with failure to go to school (Farrington, 1980; Fogelman and Richardson, 1974). Epidemiological studies have also shown that there is a small proportion of children who remain away from school for more than half the time they should be there (Berg et al., 1993; Galloway, 1980).

Generally, there is no strong relationship between the sex of the child and absence from school. In this respect there is a big difference between this problem and delinquency, which is so much more common in boys. However, there is a clear connection between absence from school and poor social circumstances, as well as lack of parental interest in the child's education (Fogelman et al., 1980). Factors within the school have also been found to be related to children's staying off (Reynolds et al., 1980; Rutter et al., 1979). It has also been found that a sizable proportion of children at school show considerable dislike of it and show some reluctance to attend (Mitchell and Shepherd, 1980; Moore, 1966). The simple fact of failure to attend school has also been considered to be an important indicator of antisocial conduct occurring in later life (Robins, 1978). It is important to view the problems of school phobia and truancy against the general background of school attendance.

SCHOOL PHOBIA (SCHOOL REFUSAL)

Difficulties in going to school may be due to emotional upset. This was probably first described by Jung in 1913 (Jung, 1961). Soon afterwards, Melanie Klein and Anna Freud also reported the psychotherapeutic treatment of children who had fear of going to school (Sayers, 1992). Broadwin (1932) reported several children who appeared afraid to go to school and stayed at home. Partridge (1939) also provided descriptions of children who did not go to school and who preferred to remain close to their mothers. They were generally well behaved. The term *school phobia* was later introduced (Johnson et al., 1941) essentially for neurotic difficulties in leaving mother that were manifested as fear of going to school. In Britain, an alternative term, *school refusal* was more generally employed for similar problems (Hersov, 1960b). In this chapter, to avoid confusion, the descriptive label school phobia will be used throughout, since the view is taken that school phobia and school refusal can be used interchangeably. There have been many papers and review articles on school phobia, and some of the best accounts of childhood anxiety and depression have appeared in them. It would seem that school phobia is often the presenting problem that brings disabling emotional disturbances to professional attention (Hersov and Berg, 1980).

Definition

School phobia is easier to describe than to define. Many children are referred to clinics for treatment who stay home, apparently unable to face the prospect of having to attend school, despite normal parental efforts to help bring about their attendance and despite the absence of any evidence that the child is antisocially inclined and is deliberately attempting to avoid going there. Such children tend to show emotional upset in various ways.

Although any clear set of defining criteria would appear to exclude some children who in all other respects would be considered to be suffering from school phobia, it is probably helpful to have in mind the following features and also to be aware of the pitfalls of applying them too rigidly (Berg et al., 1969):

1. *The child remains at home with the knowledge of the parents.* This is in marked contrast with truancy, which is often considered to be characterized by staying away from home as well as from school and attempts to conceal the absence from parents (Hersov, 1960a).
2. *There is an absence of severe antisocial behavior.* This is also in

marked contrast to truancy, which is often found to be associated with antisocial conduct (Hersov, 1960a).

3. *Parents make reasonable attempts to secure their child's attendance at school.* This distinguishes the problem from condoned absence (Kahn and Nursten, 1962), in which irresponsible parents allow the child to stay away from school.
4. *There is emotional upset at the prospect of having to go to school.* This may be confined to the situation of leaving home and/or going to school or may be part of a more general disorder characterized by anxiety and depression (Atkinson, et al., 1985; DeAldaz et al., 1987).

Problems associated with use of these criteria will be mentioned (Bools et al., 1990). Staying home during school hours, with parents knowing about it, often occurs when other features of school phobia are not evident (Belsen, 1975). Parents who are at work when the child should be at school are obviously less able to influence the situation. Sometimes parents, concerned about their child's getting into trouble wandering about, reluctantly accept that they are better off staying home. Mothers weighed down with family commitments in poor social circumstances may appear too easily prepared to accept the child's complaints of illness, and this can lead to unwarranted absence, with the child remaining at home. Occasionally, there is the situation of a child who is manifestly afraid to go to school, who hides in the vicinity of home or takes refuge with a friend or relative. However, in general, staying home in the knowledge of parents is a necessary, if not a sufficient, criterion for considering that school phobia exists. To this extent the term *home-bound school absence* (Waller and Eisenberg, 1980) is appropriate. Considering the second criterion of antisocial behavior, confusion may arise because some apparently school phobic children manifest aggressiveness and resistiveness at home toward members of the family. However, they do not show other antisocial tendencies, such as lying, stealing, destructiveness, or wandering from home, and characteristically appear rather timid with other children away from home. Regarding the third criterion, concerning parental attitudes, it can be difficult to distinguish the irresponsible permissiveness of the parent who encourages or condones absence from school and the oversolicitous attitudes of the typical school phobic child's parents who give way to their offspring's demands to avoid having to go to school because of fears of putting too much pressure on the child or because of their own difficulties in separation engendered by overclose emotional attachments (Eisenberg, 1958). The fourth criterion of emotional upset in the child also presents some difficulties when the reaction is almost entirely confined to the situation of having to attend school, is expressed as refusal and determined resistance without obvious fearfulness, or is mainly in the form of vague physical symptoms without any discoverable cause. This last situation has been referred to as the masquerade syndrome (Waller and Eisenberg, 1980).

It is possible that the syndrome of school phobia is an artifact created by the obvious need to treat children who are not fulfilling their legal obligations to go to school and at the same time have an emotional or affective psychiatric disorder. Severe separation anxiety can occur without refusal to go to school (Last et al., 1987), and school phobia can occur without separation anxiety or indeed much evidence of anxiety and/or depression other than in the immediate situation of school attendance (Bools et al., 1990; Smith, 1970). It will require further epidemiological surveys to clarify this issue.

Clinical Features

Many cases of school phobia manifest the interplay of two tendencies: avoidance behavior in relation to school and active seeking of situations providing comfort and security (Perugi et al., 1988). Unlike children displaying the common fears of childhood, such as those of insects, loud noises, or the dark, whose apprehension increases when the phobic stimulus is present, once in school, children with school phobia quite often appear to behave normally. The fear in their case appears to dissipate very rapidly, only to recur the next day at the prospect of having to go to school. So many reviews of school phobia are available (Berg, 1992; Hersov, 1990) that it is unnecessary to give yet another account of the protean manifestations of this condition; just some of the main features are outlined.

BACKGROUND CHARACTERISTICS

Boys and girls are approximately equally affected. The condition is most frequent in the early teenage years, although it can occur anytime a child is enrolled in school. No social class bias is apparent. Intelligence and educational achievement are in no way different from what would otherwise be expected. Children without brothers and sisters do not suffer from school phobia more than children with siblings, but there may be a tendency for younger children in the family to be affected (Berg et al., 1972). Correspondingly, parents tend to be older than would otherwise be the case.

ONSET AND COURSE

There is usually a gradual onset, with increasing upset on school mornings, although a sudden occurrence of the problem is by no means infrequent. Absence from school because of illness or holidays may precipitate school phobia, and there would seem to be a relationship with change of school, particularly to the more demanding educational settings a child moves to with increasing age. Stressful events at home, at school, or in the peer group outside school may be related to onset. Often, however, the problem comes on out of the blue (Gittelman-Klein and Klein, 1980). Some school days may be particularly avoided because of lessons or activities the child finds stressful, but in general it is most difficult for a child to get to school after the weekend at home. The distinction between problems of leaving home and of getting to school is not an easy one to make. So often both tendencies appear to be of equal importance and inextricably intermingled. Nevertheless, some workers in the field do make this distinction (Last, 1993). Efforts on the part of the child to overcome the problem vary enormously. At one extreme, the child gets ready for school and may even leave home, but cannot progress any further. At the other, there is total unwillingness to even contemplate return to school, refusal to get ready, staying in bed, and threats of self-harm or of running away. Emotional upset is manifested by obvious fearfulness, as well as by physical complaints that appear to be due to anxiety, such as anorexia, pallor, headaches, abdominal pain, diarrhea, and frequency of micturition. Depressive features, such as misery, tearfulness, and lack of enjoyment of things, are often found but are less persistent than anxiety (Berney et al., 1981). Manifestations of anxiety and depression overlap in many instances (Bernstein and Garfinkel, 1986). Although some school phobic children who show a very circumscribed difficulty in getting to school behave normally at home and with their friends, most affected youngsters are severely socially impaired by the condition. They appear concerned about being seen to be off school and often go out little or not at all; they cut themselves off from social contacts and become increasingly anxious and depressed. The problem can continue indefinitely if little or nothing is done about it. However, if efforts are made to restore regular school attendance by a combined effort of family, school, and professional workers involved with the problem, this is often successful, particularly in children under age 11 (Rodriguez et al., 1959) and in the more circumscribed school attendance difficulties (Kennedy, 1965). Otherwise, return to school and improvement in more general neurotic and affective disturbances are less likely to be satisfactorily achieved (Berg, 1970; Berg and Fielding, 1978).

ASSOCIATED PSYCHIATRIC DISORDERS

Although it has been known for a long time that symptoms indicating anxiety and depression are usual in children with school phobia (Berg

et al., 1969), it is only recently that efforts have been made to relate diagnostic classifications such as DSM-IV to the condition. In a study of children who met the DSM-III criteria for separation anxiety disorder (Last et al., 1987), about three-quarters were having difficulty going to school. Additional diagnoses were made in 90% of the entire sample: Half of them had overanxious disorder, and a third, major depressive disorder. An investigation of about 50 school phobic children ages 9–14 showed that approximately one-half had depression as assessed on well-defined criteria (Kolvin et al., 1984). Separation anxiety, more or less corresponding to DSM-III separation anxiety disorder, was found in only about a seventh of a group of Japanese school phobic children (Hoshino et al., 1987), a third of a sample of British school phobic students (Smith, 1970), and four-fifths of cases studied in New York (Gittelman-Klein and Klein, 1980). It is difficult to imagine that cultural factors are entirely responsible for discrepancies of these magnitudes. Referral practices determining the characteristics of samples of cases studied, differences in diagnostic criteria, and possibly unusually severe educational pressures, in the case of Japan, may have played a part (Chiland and Young, 1990).

In discussing the impact of the introduction of DSM-III on our understanding of school phobia, Werry (personal communication) suggested that, from what was known before this system of classification was introduced, there were indications that at least five different groups of disorders might be involved: separation anxiety disorder, phobic disorder, overanxious or avoidant disorder, mood disorder, some major psychiatric disorders, and an adjustment type of disorder. He went on to say that since the publication of several studies in which DSM-III diagnoses were made in relation to school phobia, the fact that several disorders were often present at the same time reduced the value of employing the classification. The frequent coexistence of separation anxiety, overanxiousness, and depressive disorders made the separation of different kinds of disorders in school phobia more difficult to sustain. Nevertheless, it seemed that phobic disorder remained somewhat distinct. Werry (1996) discusses the possible impact of the recent revisions of the International Classification of Disease (ICD-10) and DSM (DSM-IV) on categories that will be useful in cases of school phobia. In ICD-10, separation anxiety disorder of childhood (F93.0) will often be used. Phobic anxiety disorder of childhood (F93.1) is another category that will be employed. Social anxiety disorder of childhood (F93.2) will also be appropriate sometimes. Categories not limited to children will be useful in some instances: agoraphobia without panic disorder (F40.00), some other anxiety disorders (F41), reactions to severe stress and adjustment disorders (F43), somatoform disorders (F45), and mild depressive episodes (F32.0) are likely to be found in some school phobic children. In DSM-IV, all the categories that will be kept in the section of anxiety disorders of childhood or adolescence will be used in school phobia, particularly separation anxiety disorder (F93.0), which will be relevant when there are problems leaving parents not always connected with school. Of the DSM-IV disorders not confined to young people, specific phobia (F40.2), social phobia (F40.1), agoraphobia without history of panic disorder (F40.9), generalized anxiety disorder (F41.1), avoidant personality disorder (F60.6), posttraumatic stress disorder (F43.1), somatoform disorder (F45.0), and major depressive disorder single episode (F32) will all have a place.

Occurrence

The incidence of school phobia among referrals to child and adolescent psychiatric clinics has been reported as 11% (Chazan, 1962), 8% (Kahn and Nursten, 1962), and 4% (Smith, 1970). It thus forms a small, but not inconsiderable, part of the work of these services. In the cross-sectional Isle of Wight epidemiological survey of children ages 10–11 in the general population, the prevalence of school phobia was less than 3% of all psychiatric disorders (Rutter et al., 1970). A follow-up study at age 14 produced substantially more cases of school phobia in the Isle of Wight, but no precise prevalence figures were given (Rutter et al.,

1976). The severity of the manifestations of anxiety and depression that characterize school phobia, coupled with the severe social impairment that is also typical of the condition and the urgent need to do something about it that the legal requirement to attend school engenders would provide obvious reasons for most cases coming to professional attention. However, there is some evidence that a considerable number of school phobic children are not identified as such and are dealt with more generally as school attendance problems (Galloway, 1985). A nonclinical sample of 100 severe school attendance problems (Bools et al., 1990) contained a considerable proportion of children with school phobia, but only some of them had a classifiable ICD-9 emotional disorder. A study of 80 13- to 15-year-old children who failed to attend school for more than 40% of the time over several months (Berg et al., 1993) identified school phobia without an identifiable psychiatric disorder as well as school phobia accompanied by a DSM-IIIR anxiety/mood disorder; 15 children in the sample had one of the latter disturbances. Few had any contact with psychiatric services.

Dependency

A child's attachment to and reliance on parental figures is referred to as dependency (Bandura and Walters, 1963). School phobic children have often been described as overdependent on their parents and as being overprotected by them (Kahn and Nursten, 1962). A self-administered questionnaire, completed by mothers, was developed to measure dependency: the Self-Administered Dependency Questionnaire (SADQ) (Berg, 1974). Compared with children in the general population, young adolescents with school phobia were found to be more likely to require assistance in washing, dressing, and carrying out other domestic tasks. There was therefore some evidence for undue reliance on parents. In the case of school phobic girls, they were less willing than control subjects to travel around unaccompanied. The SADQ includes a preference rating, and it appeared that mothers of school phobic children were more likely to encourage dependency in their children than would be expected (Berg and McGuire, 1974). However, an investigation of family life variables failed to show that families containing a school phobic child are deviant in the way they live their lives, looking at contact with relatives and friends, leisure and work activities, and how household tasks are apportioned (Berg et al., 1981). Some deficiency in self-reliance in the child's makeup would therefore appear to be a feature of children who get school phobia.

Agoraphobia

The essentially adult disorder of agoraphobia is characterized by difficulties going out, traveling, and entering places from which escape is difficult, such as trains, buses, elevators, and crowded shops. There is a tendency to rely on the company of friends and relatives in going around, since their presence seems to reduce anxiety. Agoraphobia has been thought of as a complication of panic disorder, which consists of severe and regular anxiety attacks. However, since agoraphobia often occurs without panic disorder, the suggestion has been made that some predisposition exists as shown by previous school phobia or a dependent personality (Gelder, 1989). A small proportion of adults who suffer from agoraphobia have had the condition from before the end of the period of compulsory education (Marks, 1969). Transposing the features of adult agoraphobia to childhood and imagining how it would affect children, the result is very much what is observed with some children with school phobia who will not travel alone, who cannot go into school assembly, who are fearful of crowded playgrounds, and who rely excessively on their parents for comfort and security. Follow-up studies, in which adult psychiatric patients were asked if they had suffered from school phobia when they were young, showed an increased incidence compared with what would be expected in the case of affective and anxiety disorders generally, not just agoraphobia (Berg et al., 1974; Tyrer and Tyrer, 1974). It was also found that children of agoraphobic women were more likely to suffer from school phobia (Berg, 1976).

Outcome

A number of follow-up studies of school phobic children have been carried out (Gittelman-Klein and Klein, 1980). In one of them (Berg and Jackson, 1985), 160 young adolescents with school phobia were reviewed on average 10 years after treatment in an inpatient psychiatric unit, when they were of mean age 24. It was found that a third of them had required further treatment for psychiatric illness, mostly anxiety and depression. Five percent of the group had been readmitted to hospital because of severe affective disorders. Half were well on discharge after their treatment for school phobia, and they remained essentially free from further problems. The remainder had persistent but fluctuating symptoms and social impairment. More psychiatric illness had occurred than would have been expected. Similar findings were reported from a 15- to 20-year follow-up of 35 younger Swedish school phobic children. Outpatient psychiatric treatment had been given to about a third, compared with only a tenth of control subjects, and a tenth of ex-school phobic children were still living with their parents, compared with none of the control children (Flakierska et al., 1988).

Management

So much has been written about the treatment of school phobia (Berg, 1980, 1985b; Hersov, 1990) that it is necessary to include only a brief outline here. The principal aim is to bring about an early return to school (Hersov, 1980), since many of the symptoms of anxiety and depression that continue while the child is at home rapidly resolve once regular school attendance is restored. Management of associated psychiatric disorders is dealt with elsewhere in the book so is not given much attention in this chapter.

PARENTAL COUNSELING

Regular contact with parents is important, on their own or with the affected child and other members of the family, when appropriate. It may be difficult to persuade parents of the need to bring about an early return to school. The usual reasons are either that they have been told by teachers, doctors, or others that the child is too ill to go and must be treated first, or they believe there is some physical illness as yet undiagnosed that should be identified and dealt with before the child can be expected to return. Less commonly, parents have a fixed view that something is wrong at school and that the child should not go back until that is put right. The process of counseling is to help disabuse parents and secure their cooperation. When there is the question of undiagnosed physical illness, the condition called the masquerade syndrome (Waller and Eisenberg, 1980), persuading parents to accept that the problem is school phobia can take a little time. By rearranging hours of work, it may be that both parents can be there when it is time to go to school, so as to provide the child with more firm support. It may be necessary to accompany the child to school. It is sometimes only when the child realizes that the parents are at last determined to restore normal school attendance that resistance begins to crumble and progress is made. Counseling techniques along behavior modification lines can be used with parents to reduce their overprotectiveness and bolster their resolve, so that the child gets consistent cues and parent responses that help restore normal attendance (Yule et al., 1980).

ASSISTING THE CHILD

It is important to try to get the child's cooperation in going back to school. Regular individual counseling sessions may be helpful in achieving this. Initially there may be frank hostility, with the child refusing to cooperate in any way, but the situation usually improves with time, and it may help for the child to have some say in when and how return to school is brought about. Systematic desensitization can sometimes restore school attendance within 1–2 weeks (Chiland and Young, 1990; Yule et al., 1980) when simple counseling of parents and child proves inadequate to the task. Although there is some evidence that medication in the form of high doses of imipramine can supplement the methods of management described (Gittelman-Klein and Klein, 1980), this was subsequently not confirmed (Klein, personal communication), and a controlled trial of the related drug clomipramine (Berney et al., 1981) failed to show any beneficial effect. Some anxiolytic medication may be helpful in the initial stages of reintroducing the child to school.

PLACEMENTS

Change of school is often suggested as a means of overcoming school phobia. It is rarely successful, since the same problems arise at the new school and neither teachers nor other children have known the affected child under more normal circumstances. Sometimes special educational centers are available with transport provided, which can admit the child for a few weeks or months on a daily basis. The use of such units is recommended only when all attempts to get the child to normal school have failed. Special units normally have few children and a high staff: student ratio. Children with school phobia often find such centers acceptable and attend regularly without too much difficulty. From time to time, outpatient treatment, either alone or combined with a day placement, has no success, and admission to a residential center is required. Such centers are often part of psychiatric services and may be run on a weekly basis so that the child can be at home on weekends. There are often difficulties in getting the child to accept admission, but once this is accomplished, symptoms of emotional upset soon improve, and a planned return to school from home is arranged. Unit staff can be helpful in bringing this about. One or 2 days a week at the child's own school while he or she is still in the unit can be a useful stepping stone. The hospital admission has the added advantage of enabling associated psychiatric difficulties to be treated (Berg and Fielding, 1978) by such methods as family therapy, social skills training, psychotherapy, and behavior modification, as appropriate. Bringing about separation from the family by admission does appear to have a beneficial effect in itself and starts the process of rehabilitation, since the child usually attends the unit school and mixes with other children. Only rarely is admission to a boarding school, as a definitive solution to the problem, necessary. However, this may be the only answer when home circumstances warrant it (e.g., when there is mental or physical illness affecting a parent).

TRUANCY

Definition

Staying away from school without good reason with attempts to conceal the absence from parents is probably the most satisfactory definition of truancy (Fogelman et al., 1980), although the term is often used more loosely to cover any unwarranted failure to go to school (Robins, 1978).

Prevalence and Etiology

Teachers' estimates of truancy are often preferred to those of parents or children, for obvious reasons. In one survey carried out in Glasgow, teachers judged that 3% of boys and girls were truanting at any one time (ISTD, 1974). In the British National Child Development Study, teachers estimated that 8% of children had truanted in the previous year (Fogelman et al., 1980). There are probably more boys than girls among truants (Fogelman et al., 1980). Truancy predominantly affects poorer homes, where adverse social factors are evident, including large families, overcrowding, and multiple family problems (Farrington, 1980; Hersov, 1960). Some schools seem to foster truancy more than others (Reynolds et al., 1980; Rutter et al., 1979), possibly because of their more authoritarian regimes. There is a well-established relationship between truancy and poor educational achievement (Douglas and Ross, 1965; Fogelman and Richardson, 1974; Gittelman-Klein and Klein, 1980). There is a definite association between truancy and delinquency, even in girls

(Berg et al., 1985). The British Cambridge Study of Delinquent Development found truancy and delinquency to have similar backgrounds characterized by social adversity (Farrington, 1980).

Conduct Disorder

Psychiatric disorders characterized by antisocial behavior are common (Quay, 1986) but tend to be confused with hyperactivity and attention deficit disorders, which frequently coexist (Taylor et al., 1986; Trites and LaPrade, 1983). In ICD-10 (1988), truancy is given as one of the antisocial behaviors that occur in conduct disorders, but a recommendation is made that it should have persisted for 6 months before a child is considered as suffering from a conduct disorder on the strength of it. Two main varieties are described: unsocialized conduct disorder, in which there is a pervasive impairment of relationships with other children, and socialized conduct disorder, in which there is not. Conduct disorders have long been thought of as the basis of truancy (Hersov, 1960a). Suggestions that children who truant from school often fail to show the features of conduct disorders emerged from a general population survey of persistent absentees from school in Sheffield, England (Galloway, 1985), and in a clinical study of 100 children who persistently failed to attend school without adequate reason (Bools et al., 1990) who had been dealt with as disciplinary problems. It was found that about one-half of the group were typical truants, with a sex ratio of 3 boys to 1 girl. A cluster analysis indicated a group of 11 children, nearly all of whom had both truancy and a severe conduct disorder, but there was also another group of 68, 44 of whom were categorized as truants but who usually had no conduct disorder.

Clinical Features

Severity and persistence of truancy varies enormously. On the one hand, a child may take odd days off school because of some transient problem, and on the other, there may be persistent absence extending over weeks or months. Absence from school may be a solitary activity, or it may be in the company of others. The day may be spent wandering around, or the child may come home while the parents are at work (Belsen, 1975). Efforts are made to pretend that normal school attendance is continuing, and accusations of staying off school are frequently met with denials. From what has already been said in this chapter, educational backwardness is usually found to be associated with truancy, and when there is an associated conduct disorder, the situation is complicated by aggressiveness, destructiveness, poor personal relationships, wandering from home, dishonesty, and other antisocial activities, with or without delinquency. The family situation is, likewise, generally unsatisfactory in various ways, with severe social adversity creating stress in many instances. The child and adolescent psychiatrist is likely to encounter young teenagers who truant and who come into hospital having taken an overdose (Hawton, 1982).

Outcome

Severe and persistent truancy is an important forerunner of antisocial conduct occurring in adult life (Robins, 1978). This may take the form of criminal behavior with convictions in the courts (Farrington et al., 1989; Huissy and Howell, 1985; Loeber and Dishion, 1983). The importance of truancy as a predictor of antisocial tendencies in adult life is well established, but it should not be forgotten that many truants will develop normally without manifestations of deviant behaviour in later life.

Management

Truancy is normally dealt with as a social, legal, or educational problem by social work, law enforcement, and school agencies. The severity and duration of the problem and its associated difficulties, particularly the occurrence of delinquent acts, often determine the ways in which it is handled (Turner, 1974). Similar types of problems may go to juvenile court or be referred for psychiatric treatment (Gath et al., 1972), so there appears to be an element of chance about which agency is left to manage the problem.

Some schools are more assiduous than others about checking up on and finding ways of preventing school attendance problems, by keeping in close touch with parents, providing education in keeping with the needs of their pupils, and motivating children to keep coming to school (Boyson, 1974; Jones, 1980). Special day units are sometimes available, which have a high teacher:pupil ratio and offer a limited education, which truants sometimes find more acceptable than normal school (Galloway, 1980; Sproule, 1974).

In Britain, there are education welfare officers, employed by local education authorities, who have the task of enforcing school attendance (Clark, 1976). They keep an eye on school registers and visit homes where they suspect a child may be away from school without good reason. Parents and/or children may be taken to court if unwarranted absence from school continues. A series of randomly controlled trials carried out by juvenile court magistrates showed the value of courts supervising children who were persistently out of school without a satisfactory excuse in reducing unwarranted absence (Berg et al., 1988). Occasionally, children who continue to truant are taken into care or sent to residential schools when efforts to provide a solution to truancy have failed.

Confronted with the problem of truancy, the clinician will often be busy dealing with associated conduct problems, educational backwardness, and family disadvantage. Close liaison between home, school, and the professional agencies involved is essential in restoring and maintaining normal school attendance. Particular difficulties may be helped by clinical procedures. Thus, poor peer-group relationships may respond to social skills training. Social work counseling along behavioral lines may be helpful in motivating parents to keep in regular touch with school and take the child to school when appropriate. Very little has been written about the efficacy of routine clinical methods in truancy (Berg, 1985a). If the analogous problem of absconding from residential institutions is anything to judge by (Clarke, 1980), then close supervision, surveillance, and preventative activity by home and school will be the most useful approaches. Occasionally, children who come to clinics with problems of truancy have satisfactory homes, no educational backwardness, and few associated conduct problems. Clinical techniques such as counseling and behavior modification procedures, including the use of reinforcement, may be worth trying. Further work on the evaluation of different treatment approaches in truancy is urgently needed.

References

Atkinson L, Quarrington B, Cyr JJ: School refusal: The heterogeneity of the concept. *Am J Orthopsychiatry* 55:83–101, 1985.

Belsen WA: *Juvenile Theft: The Causal Factors.* London, Harper & Row, 1975.

Berg I: A follow-up study of school phobic adolescents admitted to an inpatient unit. *J Child Psychol Psychiatry* 11:37–47, 1970.

Berg I: A self-administered dependency questionnaire (SADQ) for use with the mothers of school children. *Br J Psychiatry* 124:1–9, 1974.

Berg I: School phobia in the children of agoraphobic women. *Br J Psychiatry* 128:86–89, 1976.

Berg I: School refusal in early adolescence. In: Hersov L, Berg L (eds): *Out of School.* Chichester, Wiley, 1980, pp. 231–249.

Berg I: Annotation: The management of truancy. *J Child Psychol Psychiatry* 26:325–331, 1985a.

Berg I: Management of school refusal. *Arch Dis Child* 60:486–488, 1985b.

Berg I, Fielding D: An evaluation of hospital inpatient treatment in adolescent school phobia. *Br J Psychiatry* 131:500–505, 1978.

Berg I, Jackson A: Teenage school refusers grow up. *Br J Psychiatry* 147:366–370, 1985.

Berg I, McGuire R: Are mothers of school phobic adolescents overprotective? *Br J Psychiatry* 124:10–13, 1974.

Berg I, Nursten J (eds): *Unwillingly to School* (4th ed). London, Gaskell, 1996.

Berg I, Brown I, Hullin R (eds): *Off School, in Court.* New York, Springer-Verlag, 1988.

Berg I, Butler A, Fairburn I, et al: The parents of school phobic adolescents—A preliminary investigation of family life variables. *Psychol Med* 11:79–84, 1981.

Berg I, Butler A, Franklin J, et al: DSM-IIIR disorders, social factors and management of school attendance problems in the normal school population. *J Child Psychol Psychiatry* 34:1187–1203, 1993.

Berg I, Butler A, McGuire R: Birth order and family size of school phobic adolescents. *Br J Psychiatry* 121:509–514, 1972.

Berg I, Goodwin A, Hullin R, et al: Juvenile delinquency and failure to attend school. *Educ Res* 27:226–229, 1985.

Berg I, Marks I, McGuire R, et al: School phobia and agoraphobia. *Psychol Med* 4:428–434, 1974.

Berg I, Nichols K, Pritchard C: School phobia, its classification and relationship to dependency. *J Child Psychol Psychiatry* 10:123–141, 1969.

Berney T, Kolvin I, Bhate SR, et al: School phobia: A therapeutic trial with clomipramine and short-term outcome. *Br J Psychiatry* 138:110–118, 1981.

Bemstein GA, Garfinkel BD: School phobia: The overlap of affective and anxiety disorders. *J Am Acad Child Psychiatry* 25:235–241, 1986.

Bools C, Foster J, Brown I, et al: The identification of psychiatric disorders in children who fail to attend school: A cluster analysis of a non-clinical population. *Psychol Med* 20:171–181, 1990.

Boyson R: The need for realism. In: Turner B (ed): *Truancy.* London, Ward Lock, 1974, pp. 52–61.

Broadwin IT: A contribution to the study of truancy. *Am J Orthopsychiatry* 2:253–259, 1932.

Chazan M: School phobia. *Br J Educ Psychol* 32:200–217, 1962.

Chiland C, Young JG (eds): *Why Children Reject School, Views from Seven Countries.* New Haven, Yale University Press, 1990.

Clark J: *Educational Welfare Officers.* Master's thesis, London, University of London, 1976.

Clarke R: Absconding from residential institutions for young offenders. In: Hersov L, Berg I (eds): *Out of School.* Chichester, Wiley, 1980, pp. 111–136.

de Aldaz EG, Feldman L, Vivas E, et al: Characteristics of Venezuelan school refusers, towards the development of a high-risk profile. *J Nerv Ment Dis* 175:402–407, 1987.

Douglas JWB, Ross J: The effects of absence on primary school performance. *Br J Educ Psychol* 35:28–40, 1965.

Eisenberg L: School phobia: A study in the communication of anxiety. *Am J Psychiatry* 114:712–718, 1958.

Farrington D: Truancy, delinquency, the home and the school. In: Hersov L, Berg I (eds): *Out of School.* Chichester, Wiley, 1980, pp. 49–64.

Farrington DP, Loeber R, Van Kammon WB: Long-term criminal outcomes of hyperactivity-impulsivity, attention deficit and conduct problems in childhood. In: Robins LN, Rutter M (eds): *Straight and Devious Pathways from Childhood to Adulthood.* Cambridge, Cambridge University Press, 1989.

Flakierska N, Lindstrom M, Gillberg C: School refusal: A 15–20 year follow-up of 35 Swedish urban children. *Br J Psychiatry* 152:834–837, 1988.

Fogelman K, Richardson K: School attendance: Some results from the National Child Development Study. In: Turner B (ed): *Truancy* London, Ward Lock, 1974, pp. 29–51.

Fogelman K, Tibbenham A, Lambert L: Absence from school: Findings from the National Child Development Study. In: Hersov L, Berg I (eds): *Out of School.* Chichester, Wiley, 1980, pp. 25–48.

Galloway D: Problems of assessment and management of persistent absenteeism from school. In: Hersov L, Berg I (eds): *Out of School.* Chichester, Wiley, 1980, pp. 149–170.

Galloway D: *Schools and Persistent Absentees.* Oxford, Pergamon, 1985.

Gath D, Cooper B, Gattom F: Child guidance and delinquency in a London borough. *Psychol Med* 2:185–191, 1972.

Gelder MG: Panic disorder: Fact or fiction. *Psychol Med* 19:277–283, 1989.

Gittleman-Klein R, Klein D: Separation anxiety in school refusal and its treatment with drugs. In: Hersov L, Berg I (eds): *Out of School.* Chichester, Wiley, 1980, pp. 303–320.

Hawton K: Attempted suicide in children and adolescents. *J Child Psychol Psychiatry* 23:497–503, 1982.

Hersov LA: Persistent non-attendance at school. *J Child Psychol Psychiatry* 1:130–136, 1960a.

Hersov LA: Refusal to go to school. *J Child Psychol Psychiatry* 1:137–145, 1960b.

Hersov LA: Hospital inpatient and daypatient treatment of school refusal. In: Hersov L, Berg I (eds): *Out of School.* Wiley, 1980, pp. 303–320.

Hersov LA: School refusal: An overview. In: Chiland C, Young JG (eds): *Why Children Reject School, Views from Seven Countries.* New Haven, Yale University Press, 1990, pp. 16–41.

Hersov L, Berg L (eds): *Out of School.* Chichester, Wiley, 1980.

Hoshino Y, Nikkuni S, Kaneko M, et al: The application of DSM-III diagnostic criteria to school refusal. *Jpn J Psychiatry Neurol* 41:1–7, 1987.

Huissy HR, Howell DC: Relationships between adult and childhood behaviour disorders. *Psychiatr J Univ Ottawa* 10:114–119, 1985.

ICD-10: *Draft of Chapter V.* Geneva, World Health Organization, 1988.

ISTD: Truancy in Glasgow. *Br J Criminol* 14:248–255, 1974.

Johnson AM, Falstein EI, Szureck SA, et al: School phobia. *Am J Orthopsychiatry* 11:702–711, 1941.

Jones A: The school's view of persistent non-attendance. In: Hersov L, Berg I (eds): *Out of School.* Chichester, Wiley, 1980, pp. 171–188.

Jung CG: 1913: A case of neurosis in a child. In: *Collected Works of CG Jung* (Vol 4). New York, Basic Books, 1961.

Kahm JH, Nursten JP: School refusal: A comprehensive view of school phobia and other failures of school attendance. *Am J Orthopsychiatry* 32:707–718, 1962.

Kennedy W: School phobia: Rapid treatment of 50 cases. *J Abnorm Psychol* 70:285–289, 1965.

Kolvin I, Berney TP, Bhate SR: Classification and diagnosis of depression in school phobia. *Br J Psychiatry* 145:347–357, 1984.

Last CG (ed): *Anxiety across the Lifespan, a Developmental Perspective*. New York, Springer, 1993.

Last CG, Francis G, Hersen M, et al: Separation anxiety and school phobia: A comparison using DSM-III criteria. *Am J Psychiatry* 144:653–657, 1987.

Loeber R, Dishion T: Early predictors of male delinquency: A review. *Psychol Bull* 94:68–99, 1983.

Marks I: *Fears and Phobias*. London, Heinemann, 1969.

Mitchell S, Shepherd M: Reluctance to go to school. In: Hersov L, Berg I (eds): *Out of School*. Chichester, Wiley, 1980, pp. 7–24.

Moore T: Difficulties of the ordinary child in adjusting to primary school. *J Child Psychol Psychiatry* 7:17–38, 1966.

Partridge JM: Truancy. *J Ment Sci* 85:45–81, 1939.

Perugi G, Delits J, Soriam A, et al: Relationships between panic disorder and separation anxiety with school phobia. *Compr Psychiatry* 29:98–107, 1988.

Quay NC: Classification. In: Quay NC, Werry JS (eds): *Psychopathological Disorders of Childhood* (3rd ed). Chichester, Wiley, 1986, pp. 1–33.

Reynolds D, Jones D, St Leger S, et al: School factors and truancy. In: Hersov L, Berg I (eds): *Out of School*. Chichester, Wiley, 1980, pp. 85–110.

Robins L: Sturdy childhood predictors of adult antisocial behaviour: Replications from longitudinal studies. *Psychol Med* 8:611–622, 1978.

Rodriguez A, Rodriguez M, Eisenberg L: The outcome of school phobia. *Am J Psychiatry* 116:540–544, 1959.

Rutter M, Graham P, Chadwick OFD, et al: Adolescent turmoil: Fact or fiction. *J Child Psychol Psychiatry* 17:35–56, 1976.

Rutter M, Maughan B, Mortimore P, et al: *Fifteen Thousand Hours*. London, Open Books, 1979.

Rutter M, Tizard J, Whitmore K: *Education, Health and Behavior*. London, Longman, 1970.

Sayers J: *Mothering Psychoanalysis. Helen Deutsch, Karen Horney, Anna Freud, Melanie Klein*. London, Penguin Books, 1991.

Smith SL: School refusal with anxiety: A review of 63 cases. *Can Psychiatry Assoc J* 15:257–264, 1970.

Sproule A: Local authority experiment. In: Turner B (ed): *Truancy*. London, Ward Lock, 1974, pp. 103–112.

Taylor E, Schachar R, Thorley G, et al: Conduct disorder and hyperactivity. I: Separation of hyperactivity and antisocial conduct in British child psychiatric patients. *Br J Psychiatry* 149:760–767, 1986.

Trites RL, LaPrade K: Evidence for an independent syndrome of hyperactivity. *J Child Psychol Psychiatry* 24:573–586, 1983.

Turner B: *Truancy*. London, Ward Lock, 1974.

Tyrer P, Tyrer S: School refusal, truancy and adult neurotic illness. *Psychol Med* 4:416–421, 1974.

Waller D, Eisenberg L: School refusal in childhood, a psychiatric paediatric perspective. In: Hersov L, Berg I (eds): *Out of School*. Chichester, Wiley, 1980, pp. 209–230.

Werry JS: *Psychiatric Diagnosis*. In: Berg I, Nursten J (eds): *Unwillingly to School*. London, Gaskell, 1996, pp. 211–227.

Yule W, Hersov L, Treseder J: Behaviour treatment in school refusal. In: Hersov L, Berg I (eds): *Out of School*. Chichester, Wiley, 1980, pp. 267–302.

C/ Child Psychiatry and Law

111 ADOPTION

Andre P. Derdeyn, M.D.

Adoption involves the child psychiatrist primarily in terms of clinical consultation and treatment of the child-adoptive parent family unit. This chapter focuses upon extrafamilial adoption, which currently comprises close to one half of adoptions. The other half of adoptions, intrafamilial adoption, is comprised of adoption by step-parents after divorce, adoption by fathers of their out-of-wedlock children, and adoption of family members by uncles, aunts, and grandparents. The major psychodynamic issues affecting children who experience intrafamilial adoption are quite different from those affecting children who are adopted extrafamilially and will not be discussed in this chapter.

ADOPTION AND SOCIAL CHANGE

Spanish immigrants brought to this country adoption modeled upon the Roman tradition, in which adoption primarily benefitted the adopter (Huard, 1956; Presser, 1971). The purpose of adoption soon changed to that of providing homes for children in need of parents. Adoption, like divorce, was an occasional event until well into the 1800s. If one wished to adopt or divorce, a petition was made to one's state legislature (Witmer et al., 1963). In 1851, Massachusetts was the first of the states to provide a general adoption law (Whitmore, 1876).

Until the middle of the 20th century, adoption by deed without involvement of public agencies or the courts was the rule. In Texas until 1931, a child could be adopted by filing with the county clerk a written statement of adoption (Jacobs and Goebel, 1952; *Texas Revised Civil Statutes*, 1925). If the natural parents were living, the statement of adoption was accompanied by a written transfer of parental authority. After World War II, as adoption became part of the child welfare system, the system of agency adoption with screening and preparation of parents and counseling with birth parents was established (Kadushin, 1976).

The number of children that young single women have given up for adoption has diminished due to increased use of contraception and wider availability of abortion, but probably most of all because of these mothers' choosing to raise their children. Adoption of healthy infants appears to be increasingly the domain of independent adoption arranged by individuals and their attorneys (Wells and Reshotko, 1986). Over the last decade, children from foreign countries have been adopted in great numbers (Hostetter and Johnson, 1989). Children who come from the foster care system and those with special physical or emotional needs are generally placed by public or private agencies. Because of the importance of the child welfare system to adoption and because consultation is often requested of child psychiatrists by public agencies, recent developments regarding termination of parental rights and the rights of foster parents will be presented in some detail.

The Child Welfare System and Adoption

The biggest problem in making adoption possible for children who are in need of it is concern for the rights of their parents (Derdeyn and Wadlington, 1977), or as Solnit (1987) has termed it, "witting or unwitting efforts of most adults to place fairness for the contending adults before the best interests of the child" (p. 455). A 1982 Supreme Court case further impeded the path to terminating the rights of parents of children in foster care so as to free them for adoption. The U.S. Supreme Court, in *Santosky v. Kramer*, found the New York State child neglect statute permitting termination of parental rights on the standard of proof by "fair preponderance" of the evidence that a child is permanently neglected was not adequate in terms of the parents' rights (*San-*

tosky v. Kramer, 1982). At the time, many other states were also using the "fair preponderance" standard. Due process regarding the parents' rights was found by the Supreme Court to require that allegations supporting termination of parental rights be proved by at least "clear and convincing evidence," making termination more difficult to accomplish. The rights of putative fathers to influence the fate of their offspring have also increased in a series of cases (*Caban v. Mohammed*, 1979; *Lehr v. Robertson*, 1983; *Quilloin v. Walcott*, 1978; *Stanley v. Illinois*, 1972), providing yet another potential hurdle to the legal process of adoption.

Some changes have taken place regarding the stability of foster placements and regarding foster parents' being allowed to adopt children in their care. The changes have resulted in large part because of increased public awareness of the problems facing children in care. Maas and Engler (1959) published their study of over 4000 children in foster care in 1959. Their data indicated that more than half of the children would remain in foster care for most of their childhood. A 1973 study of children in foster care in Massachusetts indicated that 60% had been in foster care between 4 and 8 years, with the average being over 5 years (Gruber, 1973). The Columbia University longitudinal study of children in foster care in New York City showed that two thirds of the 36% of children who remained in foster care at the end of 4 years had lost contact with their biological parents (Fanshell, 1976). In 1983 a class action suit was brought against the entire foster care system of Jackson County, Missouri, which encompasses Kansas City. Twenty-nine percent of the children had been placed in four or more homes within a span of less than 5 years. The longer a child remained in care, the more likely he or she was to experience movement from home to home (Mushlin et al., 1986). A federal court ordered specific improvements in foster care policies and practices (*G. L. v. Zumwalt*, 1983). That decision relied upon a doctrine that children in public care have a "right to freedom from harm" (*New York State Association for Retarded Children v. Rockefeller*, 1973).

Various schemes have been devised for stimulating permanency planning and activity in order either to return the foster child to the parental home or to make the child available for adoption (Bush and Goldman, 1982; Festinger, 1975; Seltzer and Bloksberg, 1987; Ten Broeck and Barth, 1986; Wiltse, 1985). The 1980 Adoption Assistance and Child Welfare Act (PL 96-272) stipulated federal requirements for a reporting and tracking system for children in foster care (Hartley, 1984).

The Foster Parent: More Rights and the Ability to Adopt

Traditionally foster parents have not been considered to have a legally recognizable interest in their foster child. When foster parents have attempted to contest removal of the child by the welfare agency or have attempted to adopt the child against agency wishes, courts have almost uniformly upheld the sanctity of the placement contract between foster parents and the agency and the rights of the biological parents (Katz, 1971). In the 1977 case of *Smith v. Organization of Foster Families*, the Supreme Court recognized that for a child

> who has been placed in foster care as an infant, has never known his natural parents, and has remained continuously for several years in the care of the same foster parents, it is natural that the foster family should hold the same place in the emotional life of a foster child, and fulfill the same socializing functions as a natural family. For this reason, we cannot dismiss the foster family as a mere collection of unrelated individuals. (pp. 844–845)

The Court, however, judged the procedures utilized by the State of New York to be constitutionally adequate for the protection of the foster care parent-foster child relationship. Any rights that foster parents accrue can benefit the foster children in their care because of the enhanced stability of the foster placement (Derdeyn, 1986).

Studies of children's experience in foster care and adverse publicity regarding various aspects of the public child care system have led to some significant changes with regard to foster parents' becoming adoptive parents (Coyne and Brown, 1986). In the past child welfare agencies selected adoptive and foster parents according to quite different standards. Now the requirements for foster and for adoptive parents vary little (Proch, 1981), and adoption by foster parents has recently become commonplace (Derdeyn, 1990; Meezan and Shireman, 1985). In 1974 the foster care agreements of 27 states specified that the child was not being placed for adoption and that the foster parents agreed not to attempt to adopt (Festinger, 1974). A 1981 survey found that foster parents were given a preference to adopt a child currently in their care in 43 states (Proch, 1981). Another development regarding foster parents is foster care/adoption or "risk adoption" (Lee and Hull, 1983).

In risk adoption, agencies place children who are not free for adoption but for whom adoption appears to be a likely outcome. The commitment of the foster family is for provision of foster care for as long as the child requires it and adoption if that is possible (Gill and Amadio, 1983; Lee and Hull, 1983). Risk adoption, similar to the development of the rights of foster parents to maintain the intactness of the foster home and the rights of foster parents to adopt, can contribute to enhancing continuity of care for foster children, either in stabilizing foster care placement or in permitting adoption.

Openness Versus Privacy in Adoption

Adoption policy of the last several decades has required that the biological parents voluntarily or by legal force terminate any right to the child, who is then, in a separate legal procedure, adopted by another family. In recent years, due to pressure from some adopted persons and advocacy on the part of some professionals, there is a lot of interest in and more adoptions taking place under conditions of "open" adoption (Belbas, 1987; Chapman et al., 1987; Demick and Wapner, 1988; Watson, 1988). This means that the birth parent meets the adoptive family and has some arrangement regarding sharing information or visiting after adoption. Probably an influence upon this practice is the fact that so many current adoptions are intrafamilial, where contact is made with the biological parent in the case of step-parent adoptions following divorce, and with grandparents and other relatives (Derdeyn, 1985). In addition, in extrafamilial adoption increasing numbers of older children are being adopted (Borgman, 1982). While some courts will not terminate a parent's rights to free a child for adoption because of vague interest on the part of the biological parent, or if the parent is not culpable, other courts will allow adoption with some continuing contact of the parent with older children (Derdeyn et al., 1978). Advocates of open adoption point out that a mother may not be able to accept the finality of relinquishment without knowledge or possibly contact in years to come, making her more likely to fight termination of her parental rights (Baran et al., 1976). While there is little controversy but some judicial resistance to adoption that includes a stipulation for visitation by biological parents for older children, there is no agreement in the adoption field that open adoption for infants is desirable (Triseliotis, 1987).

Some states have passed laws to open the sealed adoption record for adoptees wishing to make contact with birth parents. The birth parent is notified and is given the option to consent or to refuse the adoptee's request. If one birth parent has died or a birth parent does not consent, the adopted person may petition the court to open the birth record. The court then acts on the basis of weighing the interest of all the parties (Auth and Zaret, 1986; Weidell, 1984).

In the areas of joint custody and grandparent visitation, the courts and society are increasingly accepting of diminished family boundaries. In these instances, however, it is adults and not the children of divorce who have been motivated for change and have effected that change by political means (Derdeyn, 1985; Derdeyn and Scott, 1984). The desire for change in adoption is different from that in divorce, in that it is the adoptees themselves who are feeling the need to make changes in the structure of adoption to diminish the secrecy and mystery, and to provide knowledge of and contact with biological parents. Some years ago, Triseliotis (1973) suggested that people searching for biological parents might have unsatisfactory relationships with adoptive parents and poor self-images, while Sorosky et al. (1975) determined that their interview study established that was not the case. Today the desire to make some sort of contact with biological parents is widely accepted as a normal phenomenon devoid of implications of psychopathology or maladjustment (Anderson, 1988; Aumend and Barrett, 1984; Campbell et al., 1991). Clinical experience as well as some reports in the literature (Moran, 1994; Sorosky et al., 1974) indicate that making contact with birth parents is generally found to be arduous but ultimately relieving emotionally. It is becoming apparent that many women who relinquished a child have a desire to establish contact and gain some emotional relief from doing so (Field, 1992). In pointing out problems with the sealed record, Sorosky et al. (1976) mention that information given to adoptive couples at the time of adoption is limited, and often describes immature, confused, adolescent behavior characteristic of many biological parents at that stressful time in their lives. No one is provided with follow-up information as to what kind of people the biological parents might have become later in life.

The trend to open adoption continues, albeit slowly (Baran and Pannor, 1990; Sachdev, 1991). A survey regarding 1396 newly adopted children in California indicated that most of the adoptions were open. Two thirds of adoptive parents had met one or both of the birth parents. Agencies, typically protective of confidentiality, had 40% of their adoptions open while 80% of the independent adoptions were open (Berry, 1991). These adoptive families will be followed regarding the incidence and frequency of post-placement contact, and regarding the effect of openness upon the adoptive family unit (Berry, 1993).

ADOPTION OUTCOME

Reports of the incidence of adoption in children referred for outpatient treatment have established that adopted children are over-represented compared to their proportion in the population, which is usually estimated to be 3.5% (Schwam and Tuskan, 1979), and that they tend to be referred for externalizing, acting-out behaviors (Goodman et al., 1963; Humphrey and Ounsted, 1963, 1964; Menlove, 1965; Offord et al., 1969; Schechter, 1960; Schechter et al., 1964; Simon and Senturia, 1966). A study of 2148 international adoptees found that early neglect, abuse, and the number of changes of caretaking environment increased the risk of later maladjustment (Verhulst et al., 1992). Recent studies have continued to find an over-representation of adopted children and adolescents in outpatient clinics (Kotsopoulos et al., 1988) and on inpatient wards. A study of 3698 adolescents, 145 of whom were adopted, corroborates the over-representation of young adoptees in clinical settings. The adoptees did have more problems than the controls, but were also found to be referred more readily for lesser problems (Warren, 1992).

A 1985 study of inpatient adolescents found a great over-representation (over 21%) of adopted children, but no difference in diagnosis from the control group (Senior and Himadi, 1985). Senior and Himadi cite a number of studies of adopted inpatients. While one of the studies found a slight under-representation (Humphrey and Ounsted, 1963), the rest showed a significant over-representation: 9.4% of girls and 9.3% of boys (Work and Anderson, 1971), 7% of boys and 11% of girls (Kellman-Pringle, 1961), and 4.3% of both boys and girls (Kirk et al., 1966). A review of over 5000 patients registering for their first psychiatric hospitalization found a moderate over-representation of adoptees on the children's service and an under-representation on the adult service (Brinich and Brinich, 1982). Rogeness and colleagues (1988) found 8.7% of 763 consecutive admissions to a children's psychiatric hospital to be adopted. Dickson et al. (1990) found 11.7% of their inpatient population to be adopted.

Kim and associates (1988) found an over-representation of adoptees in their hospitalized children and an under-representation of adopted children referred to the regional juvenile court. These authors postulated that the relatively high socioeconomic status of adoptive parents was instrumental in their adoptive children's entering the psychiatric rather than the criminal justice network. A 1975 study of adopted children before the juvenile court found the children's parents to be extremely rejecting of them and the courts to be particularly harsh with them,

compared to a group of neglected children also referred by the court to the psychiatric clinic. The authors ascribed the difference in the court's dispositions in the two groups to the parents of neglected children defending their children and the parents of the adopted children failing to defend them or even requesting placement in correctional facilities (Lewis et al., 1975). A more recent study of 3280 juvenile delinquents did not find significant differences between adopted and non-adopted children in terms of their dispositions (Kim et al., 1992).

Studies carried out with school populations find some differences for the adopted group. Brodzinsky et al. (1984) studied 260 adopted and non-adopted children by means of maternal and teacher ratings. Adopted children were found to be higher in psychological and school-related problems and lower in social competence and school achievement than were non-adopted children. Lindholm and Touliatos (1980) compared 41 adopted and 2991 non-adopted children of a suburban school district by means of teacher ratings on a behavior problem checklist. Adopted children evidenced more conduct and personality problems. The Ontario Child Health Study, a community survey of 3294 children, 104 of whom were adopted, found that adopted boys had a significantly increased risk of psychiatric disorder versus non-adopted boys (Lipman et al., 1992, 1993).

Although adopted children and the adoptive family receive a disproportionate share of clinicians' attention, it is also evident from the literature that most adoptions go very well indeed. Kadushin (1967) reviewed a number of follow-up studies regarding children adopted in infancy (Brenner, 1951; Davis and Douck, 1955; Edwards, 1954; Fairweather, 1952, Fradkin and Krugman, 1956; Morrison, 1950; Nieden, 1951; Theis, 1924; Witmer et al., 1963) and found "success" rates of 78–86%. The younger the age of adoptive placement, the better the outcome (Humphrey and Ounsted, 1963; Kotsopoulos et al. 1993; Offord et al., 1969). Kadushin (1967) also carried out a follow-up interview study of children adopted over the age of 5 and found the adoptions to be successful in 73–82% of cases and unsuccessful in 13–18%.

With regard to the outcome of cross-cultural and interracial adoptions, which have become increasingly common in recent years, some data are available. The literature indicates that the adjustment of these children is indistinguishable from that of white children (Feigelman and Silverman, 1984; McRoy et al., 1982; Shireman and Johnson, 1986; Silverman and Feigleman, 1981; Tizard, 1991). However, the adoption of nonwhite children by white parents has been increasingly decried because of the loss to the child of a cultural heritage and related issues (Green, 1983; Shore, 1978). The scientific literature has as yet not adequately addressed these issues, although work in this area is beginning (Kim et al., 1979).

BENEFITS OF ADOPTION

Adoption is very desirable and constructive for those children who are in need of it. Although the fact and the mystery of being relinquished by parents is an important issue for every adopted person, it is the early life experiences that are surely the most problematic for children who are later adopted. Studies of children who moved from foster to adoptive families have found that immediate and long-term problems were greater when the move was made between 6 and 12 months than when it was made before 6 months (Yarrow and Goodwin, 1973; Yarrow and Klein, 1980). It was found that the deleterious effect was mitigated by high quality of care in the adoptive home.

The value of adoption to children is made particularly evident by studies that include children who have fates other than adoption. A group of children who spent their first 2–7 years in an institution was followed for a number of years. The children who were adopted were noted to be overly friendly with strangers and to be attention seeking, and to cause moderate to severe problems in the school situation. The children who were in foster care or who returned to their families, however, fared much worse (Tizard and Rees, 1975). Bohman and Sigvardsson (1980) identified 624 Swedish children who were candidates for adoption as infants. At 11 years of age they evidenced greater maladjustment than classmates, whether they had been adopted, had been placed in foster care, or had remained with their biological mother. At age 15, adjustment of the adopted children differed only slightly from that of their classmates, while children living in foster homes or with their biological mothers had a high degree of social maladjustment and/or scholastic underachievement. The military enlistment process at age 18 confirmed the findings at age 15. The adopted boys were indistinguishable from age-matched controls. Boys who remained with their mothers or were raised in foster homes scored lower in intelligence and psychological tests and were more frequently exempted from military service for social or psychiatric reasons than the adoptees (Bohman and Sigvardsson, 1990). Dumaret (1985) followed the progeny of 28 French mothers: 35 children were abandoned and adopted early in life by well-to-do families, 46 were raised by their biological mothers and/or her relatives, and 21 were raised in institutions or foster homes. In primary and secondary schools the percentage of school failure for the adopted group was 17%; for the biological family-raised group, 67%; and for the institutional or foster care group, 100% (all the institutional or fostered children had been excluded from the normal secondary school curriculum). Teachers' ratings of behavior showed both the adopted and family-raised groups of children to be more problematic than their classmates.

ADOPTION AND HEREDITY

Adoption affords a unique situation for study of the relative effects of heredity and environment regarding a variety of conditions. Some findings from this area of study follow.

Intelligence

An early study by Skodak and Skeels (1949) suggested a substantial influence of early environment in raising the average IQ of a group of adoptive children. The brighter children had brighter biological mothers, however, indicating that heredity was playing a role in individual differences, even while the environment was raising the IQs of the group of adopted children as a whole.

Subsequent studies have indicated that individual differences in IQ are substantially influenced by genetic differences among individuals, but that family environment also has a significant impact. The family environment may be more influential early in development and less influential later. A Texas study involved 300 adoptive families who adopted immediately after birth from a home for unwed mothers (Horn, 1983). Psychometric testing was carried out with the biological mother, the child, and both adoptive parents. As in the prior studies discussed, the adopted children were more influenced by their biological mothers than by the intellectual milieu of the adoptive family. A Minnesota study involved 176 adopted children, most of whom were black, and 143 biological children of the adoptive parents. The black and interracially adopted children were found to score above the average of the white population. Black children adopted in the first 12 months of life scored an average 20 points above comparable children being reared in the black community. The authors concluded that genetic differences did not account for a major portion of the IQ performance between racial groups, because black and interracial children reared in the culture of the tests and the schools performed as well as other adopted children in similar families. The adopted children scored below the natural children of the same families, however, a quite consistent finding in these types of studies (Scarr and Weinberg, 1983). In a French study (Duyme, 1988), school failures of 87 adopted children were related to the social class of their adoptive parents. The higher the parental social class, the fewer grades repeated by their adopted children.

Behavior Disorders

Studies in this area are notable for findings of significant hereditary predisposition and significant environmental effects of the adoptive home. Cadoret and Crowe (1983) found a marked increase in antisocial behaviors in adolescence when the adoptee had both a genetic factor and an adverse environmental factor such as psychiatric problems, antisocial

behaviors, or drinking problems in the adoptive home. Biological parents who were alcoholic or antisocial tended to have adopted-away offspring who met criteria for antisocial personality in adulthood. Two environmental factors significantly increased adoptee antisocial personality: placement in a home where there was an alcohol problem or antisocial behavior, and placement in a lower socioeconomic home for a child whose biological parents had exhibited criminality or delinquency (Cadoret et al., 1990). Duyme (1990) studied a series of 77 children relinquished at birth and adopted before age 3 whose biological mothers were of low socioeconomic status. The study found that the higher the social class of the adoptive parents, the lower the antisocial behavior rates in the adolescent adoptees.

ADOPTIVE CHILDHOOD: CHALLENGES AND DIFFERENCES

It is a testament to the complexities of the human mind that the fact of adoption makes the difference that it does. One could surmise that on the face of it, adoption should not make much difference to a child adopted early in life, for the child can have no perspective on the identity of the caretaking adults. Later, however, when the child is told of adoption, he or she must deal with the incomprehensible questions of who the other parents are and why they left him or her. Although the practice of telling children early of their adoption is almost universal, the benefits and liabilities remain unclear (MacIntyre and Donovan, 1990). Brodzinsky et al. (1981, 1984) have established that "being told" about adoption leads to a process of understanding on the basis of outside information provided and inside cognitive development. As in most areas of significant communications between parent and child, the parent's comfort regarding adoption is of utmost importance. The parent who can talk easily of adoption is likely to be able to observe the child's response and to gauge what is communicated to the child's response at a given time. The psychological separation process of adolescence does appear to be complicated by the fact of adoption, an issue that will be taken up later in a discussion of identity.

Adoptee's Images of Biological Parents and of Self

Many children "solve" the narcissistic injury and unfathomable mystery of having been given up for adoption by assuming that they were unlovable, dirty, too angry, or otherwise bad or unrewarding to their biological parents. Almost all such assumptions reflect diminished self- esteem (Nickman, 1985). A boy may think he was placed for adoption because he is a boy, and a girl may think it was because she is a girl.

> One adopted boy talked about how at the orphanage the children were not cared for and were fed slop. When his parents brought him home at 3 months, he vomited white stuff that he had been fed at the orphanage. At the orphanage they only cared for themselves and were just trying to get rid of all the little kids, which is what his real mother wanted to do also.

Some children deal with the injury and mystery by attributing the cause or blame to the biological parents. They assume their parents were bad, alcoholic, or mentally ill, their fathers criminal and their mothers prostitutes. This process of blaming their parents still does not leave the child unscathed, as the identification with "bad" parents can be quite strong.

Anxious Attachment

Many adopted children readily assume that abandonment or other loss could well happen again. This is probably enhanced by unconscious rage at having been abandoned previously, in that the parents may retaliate against the anger by "again" abandoning the child. For example, an adopted 13-year-old boy reported that his parents had gone for a few days to Israel. He immediately commented in what appeared to be a casual fashion that if something happened to them, he would have to be adopted again, and he sure would hate that.

Identity Issues at Adolescence

Knowledge about and experiences with one's parents and extended family contribute greatly to the establishment of a sense of identity. Erikson's (1959) definition of the sense of ego identity as "the accrued confidence that one's ability to maintain inner sameness and continuity is matched by the sameness and continuity of one's meaning for others" (p. 89) suggests the liabilities adoption might bring with it. Sants (1964) has written of the adolescent's experiencing "genealogical bewilderment."

Adolescents are curious about their own and their family's history. Adoptive children have a double handicap in this regard, in that they find it difficult to locate their own personal history within that of their family, and they are likely to experience their curiosity about their origins and early life as conflictual within themselves and difficult for their adoptive parents.

Many adult adoptees continually search faces for resemblances and wonder if a person talked with or observed might be a relative. Sants (1964) described adoptees' developing a fear of committing incest, and this has also been an issue in the author's clinical experience with adoptees.

The Family Romance of Freud

One of the central dynamic theories explaining the identity problems of adolescent adopted children is based upon concepts initially postulated by Freud. In normal development a fantasy of having a second set of parents who will only love and cherish the child commonly emerges to help the child deal with ambivalent feelings, frustration, and disappointment. Freud (1909/1959) describes the dynamics of the family romance fantasy as follows: "The child's sense that his own affection is not being fully reciprocated then finds a vent in the idea which is often consciously recollected from early childhood of being a stepchild or an adopted child" (p. 75). For non-adopted children, their purportedly adoptive parents are typically devalued and the imagined biological parents are idealized. The family romance for these children is adaptive because it displaces disappointment and anger at parents while maintaining the relationship with them (Rosenberg and Horner, 1991); it is then abandoned as the child moves into adolescence.

For the adopted child, the family romance is typically constructed of incomplete pieces of knowledge and of attitudes of adoptive parents regarding birth parents. The family romance does not ease the developmental path and then go away as it does for non-adopted children, but tends to be a continuing conflict-imbued focus for identity formation (Rosenberg and Horner, 1991).

ADOPTIVE PARENTHOOD: CHALLENGES AND DIFFERENCES

A Reciprocal Relationship between Parent and Child

Under the best of circumstances, there are challenges to the development of a reciprocal relationship between parent and child. There are differences of "fit" between parent and child in terms of responsiveness, activity level, and other characteristics, as well as problems such as parental depression and preoccupation with other issues in life. Because of genetic differences, the fit of parent and child may be especially problematic in adoption. At the least, the child is days old upon arrival at the adoptive home, or the child may be years old. The child's relationships may have been disrupted several times before, so that the child brings ambivalent attitudes to the relationship with the new parents. Differences in intelligence between the adoptive parents and the adopted child may create problems. The legal course of adoption, where the adoption is not finalized for many months, with the parents' being essentially on probation for that period of time, also can impede the relationship's development. Other issues of importance that can contribute to the parents' attenuated attachment are societal ambivalence regarding adoption and grandparents' disapproval of the adoption (Blum, 1983).

Infertility and Situations Where Pregnancy Is Medically or Genetically Contraindicated

Infertility has not usually been suspected by either of the adults, requiring of the prospective adoptive parent a painful alteration of self-concept. Medical problems of the woman and genetic liabilities of either spouse may lead to a choice not to conceive. Recognized and unrecognized anger toward the partner held responsible for the inability or the choice not to conceive may continue to contaminate family relationships.

The Fate of the Biological Child

Adoptive parents must acknowledge emotionally that the adopted child is a replacement of the child that they cannot have (Solnit and Stark, 1961). The danger here is that if the parents are not able to adequately grieve the wished-for biological child, the extent of their attachment to the adopted child may be affected. In addition, there may be a parental analogy to the child's confusion about having two sets of parents: the parent may maintain a fantasy about a dual identity of the child—the natural and the adopted child. Insufficient emotional acceptance for the adoption alternative may be accompanied by an idealized image of the natural child who might have been. In addition, the adopted child may be the target of some anger because of the child's not affirming the parental biological role and reminding the parent of what is not possible.

The Effect of Pregnancy

Most couples experience many months of preparation for parenthood throughout the pregnancy. The myriad manifestations of pregnancy serve as a focus to stimulate both parents to work through some of the changes occurring in the marital relationship. The birth of the new child is increasingly anticipated, and the pending loss of freedom and of being able to attend to one's own and each other's needs will unavoidably be faced due to various aspects of the pregnancy process. In adoption, these processes tend to be attenuated because there is no pregnancy, and often because it cannot be predicted when a child will become available for adoption.

The Adoptive Parents as Rescuer

There is a particular danger to the parent-child relationship if the parent views adoption as a rescue. When in the course of the conflict inherent in child-raising there is frustration of rescue fantasies, a very angry response from the adoptive parents too often results. Problems in this area may be closely connected to the issue of failure to work through the loss of the child one cannot have. When the child has had significant deprivation in the past and exhibits the characteristic sequelae of emotional withdrawal, indiscriminate friendliness, or provocative behavior, however, even the most capable adoptive parent is likely to feel rejected.

Entitlement or Ownership of the Child

Adoptive parents sometimes feel that their right to be the parents of the child is tenuous. This attitude may, in major part, be the result of insufficient resolution of the losses and issues inherent in the developmental process of adoptive parenthood. As a result, the adoptive parents may fail to take on the full role of parenthood in terms of confidently providing the guidance and control that seem to enhance feelings of security and self-confidence in younger children.

The Adoptee as Alien Child

For the biological mother, her child is, or was, part of her. For the adoptive mother, the child was part of someone else. This may relate at the mildest level to difficulties of attachment and of the parents' feeling entitled to the child. But there may also be implications for strongly negative parental attitudes. When there are difficulties in adoption, one can quite often observe that the parent has trouble accepting the adoptive child's expressions of instinctuality in a variety of areas—soiling, sexual curiosity, aggression, and, very frequently, eating (Brinich, 1980). The child's instinctual side is the target of strong and quick prohibitions and expressions of negative expectations. There may be a rather disconnected pair of internal representations, one acceptable and one not. Referral tends to revolve about behaviors in the instinctual sphere.

CLINICAL ISSUES

Parents who bring their adopted children to psychiatric facilities often have a high degree of concern regarding the child's behavior, typically sexual behavior in girls and aggressive behavior in boys. Particularly in the case of young children, the degree of parental concern is often far out of proportion to the actual behavior the child is exhibiting. An example of such overconcern is a 2-year-old referred for "stealing." A source of this concern relates to the parents' fantasies of the behavior and personalities of the people whose union produced the child and whose imagined weakness, immorality, or instability also led to the child's adoption. And again, in the adoptive parents' minds there may be a too readily available transition from "our good child" to "their bad child" (Brinich, 1980, p. 126). Another aspect of importance is guilt for having someone else's child. The adoptive parents' fantasies regarding the biological parents plus their guilt and fear that they might not deserve the child may predispose them to be overly concerned about the child's behavior. They may tend to look to the child for excessive reassurance to assuage their own anxiety about the child's becoming antisocial and their guilt about having someone else's child.

Johnson and Szurek (1952) described how parental concerns may lead to their acting in ways that may influence the child to engage in the behavior that the parents consciously least desire. Due to the parents' oversensitivity, there is a tendency to express unnecessary prohibitions about sexual and aggressive behavior. Parents may express unfounded but vocal allegations of drug use, may ask their adolescent daughter whether she kissed her date or "went further," or may otherwise express what the child eventually views as an expectation that he or she is going to do some of these things. As Johnson and Szurek state it, "Such constant checking, or such warning, means to the child that there is an alternate image of him in the parent's mind." The transmission to the child of an alternate, antisocial image on the part of the adoptive parents may have a peculiarly powerful effect upon the adopted child. The child's having two sets of parents makes it more difficult to fuse the intrapsychic good and bad parents' images of infantile object relations into a workable, realistic identification. On the parents' part, an analogous situation pertains. To use Erikson's (1968) terminology, the child may be particularly vulnerable to the development of a negative identity due to the unhappy combination of the child's fantasy that he or she could be living in another home and the adoptive parents' unfortunate expression of their negative expectations to the child.

Sources of the adoptive child's hostility to the adoptive parents have the usual developmental determinants as well as one unique to the adoptive situation: rage at having been abandoned. This can readily be displaced from the biological parents to the adoptive parents. The child's rejection of the adoptive parents may serve as an illusory reversal of the painful actuality of history, by way of identifying with the rejecting biological parents. Often all that is immediately evident is provocative behavior. Generally this antagonistic, aggressive behavior serves as a defense against feeling vulnerable and is one of the major reasons that adopted and foster children are referred for therapy in the first place. In the treatment situation, the therapist and any treating institution may become the objects of the adolescent's rejection. At breaks occasioned by the therapist's vacation or other activities, children often play out compensatory displays of strength (Sherrick, 1983), and adolescents tend to leave therapy or run away from the institution.

Another illusory reversal related to repair of narcissistic injury that is often exhibited by adopted children is the telling of incredible stories. Sherrick (1983) suggests this is a form of "fantasy lying" as described by Fenichel (1945, p. 529). Such stories relate to such things as possessing superior wealth and expensive automobiles and having great mental or physical attributes. These types of fantasies are surprisingly powerful and persistent. The children can be of normal physical and intellectual ability, may manifest minimal signs of emotional disturbance, and may be the object of considerable teasing by peers because of what is perceived as bragging. Yet the behavior continues unabated. This phenomenon is also quite resistant to psychotherapy, where interpretations of the meaning are often drowned out by a continuation or elaboration of the theme. Responses on the part of the therapist that are restricted to reflecting the wish to be wealthy, powerful, or famous are much more likely to be heard than are interpretations of what these stories are geared to accomplish in terms of repair of self-esteem. It is the impression of the writer that in many instances these fantasies are most responsive to improvements of self-esteem related to the development of an attachment to the therapist and to improvement in other relationships that result from the therapist's work with parents or residential school staff.

In order to counter the narcissistic injury and deny the meanings attributed to adoption, the child may develop a family romance in which the biological parents are assigned the greater wealth or finer personal qualities. This is often associated with inadequate resolution of hostility to the adoptive parents.

Brinich (1980) suggests that the core problem for some adopted children is to create a self-representation as a "wanted" child. He also points out some practical limitations of therapy: "All the psychoanalytic investigation and assistance in the world cannot undo the fact that the adopted child has been rejected or abandoned. This is one reason why adopted children present a particularly difficult therapeutic challenge" (p. 126).

When things do not go well in adoption, there is often a combination of some of the issues discussed above. Parents may have insufficiently worked through giving up the biological child and accepting adoption and the adopted child, and feel insufficient entitlement to and ownership of the child. Their overconcern about problematic behavior has had a paradoxical effect whereby the child has started to identify with the parents' apparent expectations and has started to act accordingly. The parents' lack of feelings of entitlement undermines their confidence, so that their efforts to direct and set limits are ineffective. Parental frustration leads to increasing hostility on their part, which triggers the child's separation anxiety. The child typically deals with the separation anxiety in a counterphobic manner in terms of provocative behavior (Stein and Derdeyn, 1980). For example, a 12-year-old behavior-disordered girl in a hostile impasse with her adoptive parents felt she would be treated much better by her biological mother, whose abuse of her had led to the child's removal from the home at age 5. The girl bitterly complained that her friends whose parents are divorced get to see both parents, but she would never to get to see her mother again. This girl, as do some adopted and foster children, idealized the lost biological parent and was aware of only hateful feelings for the adoptive parents. Increasingly, therapists are finding it helpful to involve the biological parents, when available, in the treatment of such disturbed adolescent adoptees (Blotcky et al., 1982).

In one study of a hospital population, it was found that adopted adolescents had significantly more runaway episodes and terminated hospitalization via a runaway more often than did the non-adopted adolescent population (Fullerton et al., 1986). Termination runaways were more likely to occur after a year of hospitalization among the adopted adolescents than among the non-adopted adolescents. The authors postulated that increasing anxiety about attachment might play a role, as well as "taking charge" of leaving the hospital in lieu of being discharged. Again, one can expect hypersensitivity to both attachment and loss in the disturbed adopted adolescent. These authors suggested that particular attention should be paid to the adolescent's dependency conflicts and defensive needs for inappropriate pseudo-autonomous actions. In other studies of inpatient adolescents, a trend was noted for these children to be discharged to placements out of the parental home (Senior and Himadi, 1985), and it was concluded that the parent-child relationship of hospitalized adopted adolescents were more problematic than those of hospitalized non-adopted adolescents (Weiss, 1984). Probably the trend favoring adoption to foster care is related to the apparently increasing frequency of adoption disruption (Barth et al., 1988; Elbow and Knight, 1987; Schmidt et al., 1988), which may occur most of all to children with special needs (Groze, 1986; Rosenthal et al., 1988). It is the author's impression that adolescents (and some younger children) whose adoptions are in the process of disrupting are appearing in disproportionate numbers on inpatient wards, particularly in public facilities.

COMMENT

Problems related to adoption commonly engage the child psychiatrist in areas of activity that this chapter has not entered. An adolescent's wish to learn more of his or her origins may prompt a referral. Typically, the adolescent, as well as being determined to learn more about biological parents if not also to make contact with them, also feels guilty and disloyal to the adoptive parents. Invariably such an adolescent can benefit from exploration of relationships with adoptive parents, of fantasies about biological parents, and of developmental issues which may be fueling the increasing curiosity about her origins. The adoptive parents usually feel threatened if not severely rejected by the adolescent's interest. The child psychiatrist involved in such a situation can help the child

and adoptive family to understand one another and to resolve further their unfinished business regarding adoption. Sometimes, as mentioned previously in the text, actually involving a biological parent may be helpful clinically.

The author's experience with adults in psychotherapy who contacted lost parents, whether the break in the relationship was due to adoption or hateful divorce, is that all of them achieved some relief from the questions answered and closure obtained regarding their earlier lives. All seemed better prepared to get on with their lives.

Consultation is often sought by courts and welfare departments regarding children in the child protection and foster care systems. Disputes regarding private adoption may also involve the child psychiatrist (Drotar and Stege, 1988). In addition to work with adopted children and their adoptive parents, the biological or adopted sibling of an adopted child may be the focus of treatment (Jacobs, 1988; Ward and Lewko, 1988). The relinquishing birth parent may seek treatment (Deykin et al., 1984; Geber and Resnick, 1988; Millen and Roll, 1985; Rynearson, 1982). When adoption fails, the child and adoptive parents tend to have great distress, which leads them to seek therapeutic help.

Adoption is constantly changing. The current trends include increasing numbers of international and of open private adoptions, and of agency adoptions of children from foster care. Adoption, however, continues to offer children who need homes the opportunity to be raised by people who desire to have a child and who have generally made difficult conscious decisions and gone to efforts that most biological parents do not even approach on their route to parenthood. This chapter of necessity focuses on differences and difficulties pertaining to adoption; the great majority of adoptions go well.

References

Anderson RS: Why adoptees search: Motives and more. *Child Welfare* 67:15–19, 1988.

Aumend SA, Barrett MC: Self-concept and attitudes toward adoption: A comparison of searching and nonsearching adult adoptees. *Child Welfare* 63:251–259, 1984.

Auth PJ, Zeret S: The search in adoption: A service and a process. *Soc Casework* 67:560–568, 1986.

Baran A, Pannor R: Open adoption. In: Brodzinski DM, Schechter MD (eds): *The Psychology of Adoption.* New York, Oxford University Press, 1990.

Baran A, Pannor R, Sorosky AD: The open adoption. *Soc Work* 21:97–100, 1976.

Barth RP, Berry M, Yoshikami R, et al: Predicting adoption disruption. *Soc Work* 33:227–233, 1988.

Belbas NF: Staying in touch: Empathy in open adoptions. *Smith College Stud Soc Work* 57:184–198, 1987.

Berry, M: The practice of open adoption: Findings from a study of 1396 adoptive families. *Child Youth Serv Rev* 13:379–395, 1991.

Berry M: Adoptive parents' perceptions of, and comfort with, open adoption. *Child Welfare* 72:231–253, 1993.

Blotcky MJ, Looney JG, Grace KD: Treatment of the adopted adolescent: Involvement of the biologic mother. *J Am Acad Child Psychiatry* 21:281–285, 1982.

Blum HP: Adoptive parents: Generative conflict and generational continuity. *Psychoanal Study Child* 38:141–163, 1983.

Bohman M, Sigvardsson S: A prospective, longitudinal study of children registered for adoption. *Acta Psychiatr Scand* 61:339–355, 1980.

Bohman M, Sigvardsson S: Outcome in adoption: Lessons from longitudinal studies. In: Brodzinski DM, Schechter MD (eds): *The Psychology of Adoption.* New York, Oxford University Press, 1990.

Borgman R: The consequences of open and closed adoption for older children. *Child Welfare* 61:217–226, 1982.

Brenner R: *A Follow-up Study of Adoptive Families.* New York, Child Adoption Research Committee, 1951.

Brinich PM: Some potential effects of adoption on self and object representations. *Psychoanal Study Child* 35:107–133, 1980.

Brinich PM, Brinich EB: Adoption and adaptation. *J Nerv Ment Dis* 170:489–493, 1982.

Brodzinsky DM, Pappas C, Singer LM, et al: Children's conception of adoption: A preliminary investigation. *J Pediatr Psychol* 6:177–189, 1981.

Brodzinsky DM, Singer LM, Braff AM: Children's understanding of adoption. *Child Dev* 55:869–878, 1984.

Bush M, Goldman H: The psychological parenting and permanency principles in child welfare: A reappraisal and critique. *Am J Orthopsychiatry* 52:223–235, 1982.

Caban v. Mohammed, 441 U.S. 380, 1979.

Cadoret RJ, Crowe RR: Evidence for gene-environment interaction in the development of adolescent antisocial behavior. *Behav Genet* 13:301–310, 1983.

Cadoret RJ, Troughton E, Bagford J, et al: Genetic and environmental factors in adoptee antisocial personality. *Eur Arch Psychiatr Neurol Sci* 239:231–240, 1990.

Campbell LH, Silverman PR, Patti PB: Reunions between adoptees and birth parents: The adoptees' experience. *Soc Work* 36:329–335, 1991.

Chapman CT, Dorner P, Silber K, et al: Meeting the needs of the adoption triangle through open adoption: The adoptive parent. *Child Adolesc Soc Work* 4:3–12, 1987.

Coyne A, Brown ME: Relationship between foster care and adoption units serving developmentally disabled children. *Child Welfare* 65:189–198, 1986.

Davis R, Douck P: Crucial importance of adoption homes study. *Child Welfare* 34:20–21, 1955.

Demick J, Wapner S: Open and closed adoption: A developmental conceptualization. *Fam Process* 27:229–249, 1988.

Derdeyn AP: Grandparent visitation rights: Rendering family dissension more pronounced? *Am J Orthopsychiatry* 55:277–287, 1985.

Derdeyn AP: Foster children: Continuity of relationships and the law. *Int J Fam Psychiatry* 7:303–317, 1986.

Derdeyn AP: Foster parent adoption: The legal framework. In: Brodzinski DM, Schechter MD (eds): *The Psychology of Adoption.* New York, Oxford University Press, 1990.

Derdeyn AP, Rogoff AR, Williams SW: Alternatives to absolute termination of parental rights after long-term foster care. *Vanderbilt Law Rev* 31:1165–1192, 1978.

Derdeyn AP, Scott E: Joint custody: A critical analysis and appraisal. *Am J Orthopsychiatry* 54:199–209, 1984.

Derdeyn AP, Wadlington WJ: Adoption: The rights of parents versus the best interests of their children. *J Am Acad Child Psychiatry* 16:238–255, 1977.

Deykin EY, Campbell L, Patti P: The postadoption experience of surrendering parents. *Am J Orthopsychiatry* 54:271–280, 1984.

Dickson LR, Heffron WM, Parker C: Children from disrupted and adoptive homes on an inpatient unit. *Am J Orthopsychiatry* 60:594–602, 1990.

Drotar D, Stege ER: Psychological testimony in foster parent adoption: A case report. *J Clin Child Psychol* 17:164–168, 1988.

Dumaret A: IQ, scholastic performance and behaviour of sibs raised in contrasting environments. *J Child Psychol Psychiatry* 26:553–580, 1985.

Duyme M: School success and social class: An adoption study. *Dev Psychol* 24:203–209, 1988.

Duyme M: Antisocial behaviour and postnatal environment: A French adoption study. *J Child Psychol Psychiatry* 31:699–710, 1990.

Edwards ME: Failure and success in the adoption of toddlers. *Case Conference* 1:3–8, 1954.

Elbow M, Knight M: Adoption disruption: Losses, transitions, and tasks. *Soc Casework* 68:546–552, 1987.

Erikson E: Identity and the life cycle. *Psychol Issues* 1:89, 1959.

Erikson EH: *Identity: Youth and Crisis.* New York, Norton, 1968.

Fairweather OE: Early placement in adoption. *Child Welfare* 31:3–8, 1952.

Fanshell D: Status changes of children in foster care: Final results of the Columbia University longitudinal study. *Child Welfare* 55:143–171, 1976.

Feigelman W, Silverman AR: The long-term effects of transracial adoption. *Soc Serv Rev* 58:558–602, 1984.

Fenichel O: Character disorders. In: *The Psychoanalytic Theory of Neurosis*. New York, Norton, 1945.

Festinger T: Placement agreements with boarding homes. *Child Welfare* 53:643–652, 1974.

Festinger T: The New York review of children in foster care. *Child Welfare* 54:211–245, 1975.

Field J: Psychological adjustment of relinquishing mothers before and after reunion with their children. *Aust NZ J Psychiatry* 26:232–241, 1992.

Fradkin H, Krugman D: A program of adoptive placement for infants under 3 months. *Am J Orthopsychiatry* 26:577–590, 1956.

Freud S: Family romances. In: Strachey J (ed): *Collected Papers* (Vol 5). New York, Basic Books, 1959, pp. 74–78. (originally published 1909)

Fullerton CS, Goodrich W, Bernian LB: Adoption predicts psychiatric treatment resistances in hospitalized adolescents. *J Am Acad Child Psychiatry* 25:542–551, 1986.

Geber G, Resnick MD: Family functioning of adolescents who parent and place for adoption. *Adolescence* 23:417–428, 1988.

Gill MM, Amadio CM: Social work and law in a foster care/adoption program. *Child Welfare* 62:455–467, 1983.

G. L. v. Zumwalt, 564 F. Supp. 1030, 1983.

Goodman JD, Silberstein RM, Mandell W: Adopted children brought to child psychiatric clinic. *Arch Gen Psychiatry* 9:451–456, 1963.

Green HJ: Risks and attitudes associated with extracultural placement of American Indian children: A critical review. *J Am Acad Child Psychiatry* 22:63–67, 1983.

Groze V: Special-needs adoption. *Child Youth Serv Rev* 8:363–373, 1986.

Gruber A: *Foster Home Care in Massachusetts*. Boston, Commonwealth of Massachusetts Governor's Commission on Adoption and Foster Care, 1973.

Hartley EK: Government leadership to protect children from foster care "drift." *Child Abuse Negl* 8:337–342, 1984.

Horn JM: The Texas adoption project: Adopted children and their intellectual resemblance to biological and adoptive parents. *Child Dev* 54:268–275, 1983.

Hostetter M, Johnson DE: International adoption. *Am J Dis Child* 143:325–332, 1989.

Huard LA: The law of adoption: Ancient and modern. *Vanderbilt Law Rev* 9:743–763, 1956.

Humphrey M, Ounsted C: Adoptive families referred for psychiatric advice. I: The children. *Br J Psychiatry* 109:599–608, 1963.

Humphrey M, Ounsted C: Adoptive families referred for psychiatric advice. II: The parents. *Br J Psychiatry* 110:549–555, 1964.

Jacobs AC, Goebel J: *Cases and Other Materials on Domestic Relations* (3rd ed). Brooklyn, Foundation Press, 1952.

Jacobs TJ: On having an adopted sibling: Some psychoanalytic observations. *Int Rev Psychoanal* 15:25–35, 1988.

Johnson AM, Szurek SA: The genesis of antisocial acting out in children and adults. *Psychoanal Q* 21:323–343, 1952.

Kadushin A: A follow-up study of children adopted when older: Criteria of success. *Soc Work* 12:22–23, 1967.

Kadushin A: Child welfare services—past and present. *Child Today* 5:16–23, 1976.

Katz S: Legal aspects of foster care. *Fam Law Q* 5:283–302, 1971.

Kellman-Pringle ML: The incidents of some supposedly adverse family conditions and of lefthandedness in schools for maladjusted children. *Br J Educ Psychol* 31:183–193, 1961.

Kim SP, Hong S, Kim BS: Adoption of Korean children by New York area couples: A preliminary study. *Child Welfare* 58:419–427, 1979.

Kim WJ, Davenport C, Joseph J, et al: Psychiatric disorder and juvenile delinquency in adopted children and adolescents. *J Am Acad Child Adolesc Psychiatry* 27:111–115, 1988.

Kim WJ, Zrull JP, Davenport CW, et al: Characteristics of adopted juvenile delinquents. *J Am Acad Child Adolesc Psychiatry* 31:525–532, 1992.

Kirk ND, Johassohn K, Fish AD: Are adopted children especially vulnerable to stress? *Arch Gen Psychiatry* 14:291–298, 1966.

Kotsopoulos S, Coté A, Joseph L, et al: Psychiatric disorders in adopted children: A controlled study. *Am J Orthopsychiatry* 58:608–612, 1988.

Kotsopoulos S, Walker S, Copping W, et al: A psychiatric follow-up study of adoptees. *Can J Psychiatry* 38(6):391–396, 1993.

Lee RE, Hull RK: Legal, casework, and ethical issues in "risk adoption." *Child Welfare* 62:450–454, 1983.

Lehr v. Robertson 103 S.Ct. 2985, 1983.

Lewis DO, Balla D, Lewis M, et al: The treatment of adopted versus neglected delinquent children in the court: A problem of reciprocal attachment? *Am J Psychiatry* 132:142–145, 1975.

Lindholm BW, Touliatos J: Psychological adjustment of adopted and nonadopted children. *Psychol Rep* 46:307–310, 1980.

Lipman EL, Offord DR, Racine YA, et al: Psychiatric disorders in adopted children: A profile from the Ontario child health study. *Can J Psychiatry* 37:627–633, 1992.

Lipman EL, Offord DR, Boyle MH, et al: Follow-up of psychiatric and educational morbidity among adopted children. *J Am Acad Child Adolesc Psychiatry* 32:1007–1012, 1993.

Maas N, Engler R: *Children in Need of Parents*. New York, Columbia University Press, 1959.

MacIntyre JC, Donovan DM: Resolved: Children should be told of their adoption before they ask. Debate Forum, Terr LC (ed). *J Am Acad Child Adolesc Psychiatry* 29:828–832, 1990.

McRoy RC, Zurcher LA, Lauderdale MC, et al: Self-esteem and racial identity in transracial and interracial adoptees. *Soc Work* 27:522–526, 1982.

Meezan W, Shireman JF: Antecedents to foster parent adoption decisions. *Child Youth Serv Rev* 7:207–224, 1985.

Menlove FL: Aggressive symptoms in emotionally disturbed adopted children. *Child Dev* 36:519–532, 1965.

Millen L, Roll S: Solomon's mothers: A special case of pathological bereavement. *Am J Orthopsychiatry* 55:411–418, 1985.

Moran RA: Stages of emotion: An adult adoptee's postreunion perspective. Child Welfare 73(3):249–260, 1994.

Morrison H: Research study in adoption. Child Welfare 29:7–9, 1950.

Mushlin MB, Levitt L, Anderson L: Court-ordered foster family care reform: A case study. *Child Welfare* 65:141–154, 1986.

New York State Association for Retarded Children v. Rockefeller, 357 F. Supp. 752, 1973.

Nickman S: Losses in adoption: The need for dialogue. *Psychoanal Study Child* 40:365–398, 1985.

Nieden MZ: The influence of constitution and environment upon the development of adopted children. *J Psychiatry* 31:91–95, 1951.

Offord DR, Aponte MA, Cross LA: Presenting symptomatology of adopted children. *Arch Gen Psychiatry* 20:110–116, 1969.

Presser SB: The historical background of the American law of adoption. *J Fam Law* 11:443–516, 1971.

Proch K: Foster parents as preferred adoptive parents: Practice implications. *Child Welfare* 60:617–625, 1981.

Quilloin v. Walcott, 434 U.S. 246, 1978.

Rogeness GA, Hoppe SK, Macedo CA, et al: Psychopathology in hospitalized, adopted children. *J Am Acad Child Adolesc Psychiatry* 27:628–631, 1988.

Rosenberg EB, Horner TM: Birthparent romances and identity formation in adopted children. *Am J Orthopsychiatry* 61:70–77, 1991.

Rosenthal JA, Schmidt D, Conner J: Predictors of special needs adoption disruption: An exploratory study. *Child Youth Serv Rev* 10:101–117, 1988.

Rynearson EK: Relinquishment and its maternal complications: A preliminary study. *Am J Psychiatry* 139:338–340, 1982.

Sachdev P: Achieving openness in adoption: Some critical issues in policy formation. *Am J Orthopsychiatry* 61:241–249, 1991.

Santosky v. Kramer, 455 U.S. 745, 1982.

Sants NJ: Genealogical bewilderment in children with substitute parents. *Br J Med Psychol* 37:133–141, 1964.

Scarr S, Weinberg RA: The Minnesota adoption studies: Genetic differences and malleability. *Child Dev* 54:260–267, 1983.

Schechter MD: Observations on adopted children. *Arch Gen Psychiatry* 3:21–32, 1960.

Schechter MD, Carlson PV, Simmons JQ, et al: Emotional problems in the adoptee. *Arch Gen Psychiatry* 10:109–118, 1964.

Schmidt DM, Rosenthal JA, Bombeck B: Parents' views of adoption disruption. *Child Youth Serv Rev* 10:119–130, 1988.

Schwam JS, Tuskan MK: Varieties of family structure. In: Noshpitz JD (ed): *Basic Handbook of Child Psychiatry* (Vol 1). New York, Basic Books, 1979, pp. 342–348.

Seltzer M, Bloksberg LM: Permanency planning and its effects on foster children: A review of the literature. *Soc Work* 32:65–68, 1987.

Senior N, Himadi E: Emotionally disturbed, adopted, inpatient adolescents. *Child Psychiatry Hum Dev* 15:189–197, 1985.

Sherrick I: Adoption and disturbed narcissism: A case illustration of a latency boy. *J Am Psychoanal Assoc* 31:487–513, 1983.

Shireman JF, Johnson PR: A longitudinal study of black adoptions: Single parent, transracial, and traditional. *Soc Work* 31:172–176, 1986.

Shore JN: Destruction of Indian families—beyond the best interests of Indian children. *White Cloud J* 1:13–16, 1978.

Silverman AR, Feigelman W: The adjustment of black children adopted by white families. *Soc Casework* 62:529–536, 1981.

Simon NM, Senturia AG: Adoption and psychiatric illness. *Am J Psychiatry* 122:858–868, 1966.

Skodak M, Skeels N: A final follow-up of one hundred adopted children. *J Cent Psychol* 75:85–125, 1949.

Smith v. Organization of Foster Families, 431 U.S. 816, 1977.

Solnit AJ: Child placement conflicts: New approaches. *Child Abuse Negl* 11:455–460, 1987.

Solnit A, Stark M: Mourning and the birth of a defective child. *Psychoanal Study Child* 16:523–537, 1961.

Sorosky A, Baran A, Pannor R: The reunion of adoptees and birth relatives. *J Youth Adolesc* 3(3):195–206, 1974.

Sorosky, AD, Baran A, Pannor R: Identity conflicts in adoptees. *Orthopsychiatry* 45:18–27, 1975.

Sorosky AD, Baran A, Pannor R: The effects of the sealed record in adoption. *Am J Psychiatry* 133:900–904, 1976.

Stanley v. Illinois, 405 U.S. 645, 1972.

Stein JM, Derdeyn AP: The child in group foster care. *J Am Acad Child Psychiatry* 19:90–100, 1980.

Ten Broeck E, Barth RP: Learning the hard way: A pilot permanency planning program. *Child Welfare* 65:281–294, 1986.

Texas Revised Civil Statutes, Articles 42, 44, 1925.

Theis SV: *How Foster Children Turn Out*. New York State Charities Aid Association, 1924.

Tizard B: Intercountry adoption: A review of the evidence. *J Child Psychol Psychiatry* 32:743–756, 1991.

Tizard B, Rees J: The effect of early institutional rearing on the behavior problems and affectional relationships of four-year-old children. *J Child Psychol Psychiatry* 16:61–73, 1975.

Triseliotis J: *In Search of Origins: The Experiences of Adopted Persons*. Boston, Beacon Press, 1973.

Triseliotis J: Adoption with contact. *Adoption Fostering* 11:35–39, 1987.

Verhulst FC, Althaus M, Bieman HJMV: Damaging backgrounds: Later adjustment of international adoptees. *J Am Acad Child Adolesc Psychiatry* 3:518–524, 1992.

Ward M, Lewko JH: Problems experienced by adolescents already in families that adopt older children. *Adolescence* 23:221–228, 1988.

Warren SB: Lower threshold for referral for psychiatric treatment of adopted adolescents. *J Am Acad Child Adolesc Psychiatry* 31:512–527, 1992.

Watson KW: The case for open adoption: ''I am convinced that openness truly serves those involved in adoption in the best way.'' *Public Welfare* 46:24–28, 1988.

Weidell RC: Unsealing sealed birth certificates in Minnesota. *Child Welfare* 63:113–124, 1984.

Weiss A: Parent-child relationships of adopted adolescents in a psychiatric hospital. *Adolescence* 19:77–88, 1984.

Wells K, Reshotko P: Cooperative adoption: An alternative to independent adoption. *Child Welfare* 65:177–188, 1986.

Whitmore WH: *The Law of Adoption in the United States, and Especially in Massachusetts*. Albany, NY, Munsell, 1876.

Wiltse KT: Ethical issues in permanency planning. *Child Youth Serv Rev* 7:259–266, 1985.

Witmer HL, Herzog E, Weinstein EA, et al: *Independent Adoptions: A Follow Up Study*. New York, Russell Sage Foundation, 1963.

Work HH, Anderson N: Studies in adoption: Requests for psychiatric treatment. *Am J Psychiatry* 127:948–950, 1971.

Yarrow LJ, Goodwin MS: The immediate impact of separation: Reactions of infants to a change in mother-figures. In: Stone LJ, Smith HT, Murphy LB (eds): *The Competent Infant*. New York, Basic Books, 1973.

Yarrow LJ, Klein RP: Environmental discontinuity associated with transition from foster to adoptive homes. *Int J Behav Dev* 3:311–322, 1980.

112 THE CHILD AND THE VICISSITUDES OF DIVORCE[a]

Judith S. Wallerstein, Ph.D., and Shauna B. Corbin, Ph.D.

Changes within the contemporary family are reshaping the experience of growing up in America. The steep rise in recent decades of the incidence of divorce is foremost among the changes that are profoundly influencing the lives of children and their parents. The number of children from divorced families more than doubled between 1960 and 1980 (Spanier and Glick, 1981). Demographers have estimated that 38% of all children born in the mid-1980s will experience the divorce of their parents (A.J. Norton, U.S. Bureau of the Census, personal communication). This phenomenon continues to newly affect no fewer than 1 million children each year.

Although many children weather the stress of marital discord and family rupture without psychopathological sequelae, a considerable number falter along the way. As a result, the high divorce rate has also had a notable effect on the makeup of clinical populations. Children of divorce are greatly overrepresented in outpatient psychiatric, family agency, and private practice populations relative to their presence within the general population (Furstenberg et al., 1983; Gardner, 1976; Kalter, 1977). Parental divorce and parental loss significantly predict mental health referrals for school-age children (Felner et al., 1975). A national survey of adolescents whose parents had separated and divorced by the time the children were 7 years old found that 30% of these children had received psychotherapy by the time they reached adolescence, compared with 10% of adolescents in intact families (Zill, 1983); by young adulthood, 40% had received psychological help. The representation of children from divorced families is even higher among inpatient populations. Although national figures are unavailable, many inpatient psychiatric facilities for adolescents report informally that 75–100% of their patients are from nonintact families. Overall, recent national data have shown that young people from single-parent or stepfamilies have a 2–3 times greater likelihood of experiencing emotional or behavioral problems,

and a higher incidence of learning problems, than those living with both biological parents (Zill and Schoenborn, 1990).

The divorce literature, which scarcely existed prior to the 1970s, has proliferated as a growing number of investigators in psychiatry, psychology, and sociology have examined the processes involved in family separation and marital dissolution. As a result, we have begun to acquire knowledge in many critical areas: the nature of the divorce process, the responses of children and adolescents by age and gender, the impact of divorce and parental conflict on parent-child relationships, factors in good and poor outcome in the short- and long-term perspectives, patterns of custody and visitation, the role of the father, the roots and dimensions of interparental conflict, and some of the issues that children and adults confront in remarriage. More recently, as findings from longitudinal studies have become available, we have been able to shed light on divorce-specific anxieties that emerge belatedly in the lives of children of divorce, when they enter young adulthood (Wallerstein and Blakeslee, 1989).

By and large, however, professional interest has not been directed toward issues of treatment. With the exception of mediation programs and school-based groups that have been developed in scattered areas of the country, and a few pilot and demonstration projects (some clinical, others primarily educational), there has been a paucity of preventive or clinical services specifically designed to respond to the new stress points of change in divorcing families or to the special needs of children and adolescents whose family structure has been temporarily or more lastingly weakened by marital distress and breakdown. The majority of families struggling with divorce have relied perforce on the traditional mental health services available in the community.

Additionally, much of the interest in exploring the theoretical issues inherent in the relatively new family forms that are being created (e.g., joint custody families; single-parent families in which one parent, usually the father, continues to visit; remarried and/or redivorced families) has centered around reassessing the role of the father in child development (Cath et al., 1982; Hanson and Bozett, 1985). And although it is widely acknowledged that the psychological theory that underlies established clinical interventions with children (whether in psychoanaly-

---

[a] Copyright Judith S. Wallerstein, Ph.D. This chapter is part of a book, in preparation, entitled *Helping the Family in Separation and Divorce: Advances in Theory and Practice*, by Judith S. Wallerstein and the clinical staff at the Center for the Family in Transition, Corte Madera, CA.

sis, family systems theory, or child development) was developed primarily within the paradigm of the intact two-parent family, there has been little theoretical exploration of how changes in family structure can or should modify the goals or approach of the clinician, either in work with parents, who find themselves cast in unfamiliar roles, or with the child, whose primary identification figures are often shifting and unclear.

THE NATURE OF DIVORCE

Divorce as a Process

Divorce is a process of social and psychological change in the individual and in family relationships that can extend over many years. It has no true counterpart in other crises of adult life. Although it was initially considered analogous to bereavement in the central significance of loss as the critical component of the adult experience, we have come to recognize that, in divorce, grief is only one of many powerful affects; rage, sexual jealousy, and unrequited love share equal power and significance (Wallerstein and Kelly, 1980). Divorce is not a time-limited event for the adults or the children involved, in part because a complex undulation of changes (many of them unanticipated and unforeseeable) leads up to and, in turn, is set into motion by the marital rupture. These changes often occupy a significant portion of the adult's postdivorce life. They typically occupy a significant portion of the youngster's childhood and adolescence and, as we are learning, of his or her own young adulthood.

Divorce can be broadly conceptualized as progressing through three successive phases (Wallerstein and Blakeslee, 1989). The ambience of the first, acute phase of dramatic and highly emotional responses is established by the fact that divorce in a family with children is rarely a mutual decision. Separation often occurs amid escalating spousal conflict, which can include physical violence between the parents. During this acute phase, in extreme cases, one or both parents may experience depression with suicidal ideation and may regress considerably in behavior. Similarly, one or both parents may experience ego-syntonic rage, which can reach paranoid dimensions. There is, in many of these people, a temporary weakening of ego control over aggressive and sexual impulses, accompanied by lapses in customary judgment. This acute phase may be relatively brief or it may extend over several years. Sometimes, the divorcing couple remains fixated in this acute phase for years, reenacting the separation drama again and again, in the vain hope of modifying the events or the ending but never obtaining relief from the narcissistic injury that was initially sustained. These reenactments may take place in the courts, or they may be played out in the many other arenas available when there are children from the broken marriage. In most instances, the acute phase is followed by a transitional phase in which the parents begin to disengage from each other's lives and move into new relationships and new work and home settings. The physical, social, and emotional environments of the family during this time may be in continual flux. This intermediate period may be relatively brief or it too may last for several years. Finally, with the onset of the third phase, comes the establishment of the relatively stable postdivorce single- or remarried-parent household, each of which has its own associated strains and gratifications.

Ongoing stresses confront many postdivorce families. Some of these stresses are rooted in convergent economic and social issues that communities have been reluctant to address, particularly those that affect the serious economic disadvantaging of women and children following divorce (Weitzman, 1985). Other reports describe the many complex psychological issues that adults face in reconstructing their postdivorce lives and how their tasks are affected by the number of years invested in the marriage, the age of the adult at the divorce, and the discrepant opportunities that are available to divorced men and women in the sexual, social, and economic marketplaces (Wallerstein and Blakeslee, 1989). Moreover, recent observations on remarriage have called attention to the many psychological differences between first and subsequent marriages and the complex challenges that a second marriage, with children, poses to all of the participants (Pasley and Ihinger-Tallman, 1987; Wallerstein and Blakeslee, 1989). These concerns have been reinforced by reports from demographers that the incidence of divorce in remarried families with children from a previous marriage is even higher than the divorce rate in first marriages (Pasley and Ihinger-Tallman, 1987).

EFFECTS OF DIVORCE ON THE PARENT-CHILD RELATIONSHIP

Diminished Parenting

Hess and Camara (1979) have pointed out that "for children, the threat of divorce lies in the disruption of relationships with the parents." This applies both to the availability of the parent and to the quality of the postdivorce relationship itself. Hetherington and her associates (1978, 1982) observed disorganization, deterioration of discipline, rising angers, and lowered expectations for appropriate social behavior by their children on the part of custodial mothers. Others (Santrock et al., 1982) have noted the more conflicted postdivorce relationship of children with an opposite-sex custodial parent. The impairment of relationships between parent and child may appear early in the separation and divorce process, or may remain latent, emerging only in young adulthood. Mother-child relationships that had previously weathered the storms of adolescence have been noted to deteriorate in young adulthood. This parallels Wallerstein's observed "sleeper effect" in young women from divorced families (Wallerstein, 1991).

Wallerstein (1985a) has suggested that a diminished capacity to parent is an expectable short-term consequence of divorce, which has the dangerous potential of becoming chronic when the custodial parent fails to reconstitute or becomes involved in new relationships that overshadow or replace the relationship with the child. This diminished capacity is most evident in the parent's decreased ability to separate the child's needs and reactions from those of the adult. She has proposed that the fantasy underlying the sometimes astonishing changes in the parent's relationship with the child is a conscious or unconscious wish to abandon the child coincident with the breakup of the marriage. As a fantasy, this impulse to leave the child behind may remain unacted upon, or it may unconsciously spur sudden flight or unexpected rejection by a parent of a child who had previously been well-cared for. Whatever the conscious or unconscious roots of the disrupted parent-child relationship may be, the consequence is that the child's fears of abandonment at the time of the breakup are powerfully reinforced by a parent's changed attitudes and behavior. Often these fears lead to a hypervigilant tracking of the parent's responses and an intense anxiety that can dominate the child's inner life and intrude upon his or her capacity to accomplish normative developmental tasks.

Wallerstein (1985a) has also proposed that a contrapuntal theme to the temporary rejection of the child at the time of the breakup is an intensified need of the parent for the child. This dependence on the child by one or both parents is often at the core of parental conflict and prolonged litigation over custody and visitation. In extreme cases, the dismantling of customary supports within the marriage, combined with the humiliation of the narcissistic injury inflicted by the divorce and the painful persistence of attachment to the divorcing partner, may result in severe ego regressions in parents whose previous functioning, separately or together, may have been at least adequate. Feeling suddenly bereft and in need of help, such parents turn to their children for help in warding off the threatened depression.

In many divorcing families the temporary dependence of the adult on the child is a transient phenomenon that has no lasting deleterious effects and may indeed be of benefit to a child suddenly elevated to unaccustomed importance. However, as Wallerstein (1985b) has pointed out, turning to a young son or daughter as a peer, or worse, as to a parent, may overwhelm the child with responsibility, placing the child at

serious risk if the intense dependence continues. For these overburdened children—out of worry, guilt, compassion, or, indeed, out of their conviction that it is their assigned task to keep the parent alive—may devote themselves entirely to maintaining the psychic functioning and physical needs of the ailing parent and relinquish their responsiveness to their own needs over many years.

CHILDREN IN HIGH-CONFLICT DIVORCE

The struggle for and through the children embodies the intense conflicts that often accompany the failing marriage. Although competition for a child's affection may occur in an intact, even well-functioning family, disruption of the family system and its resulting angers bring the parents' competitiveness into sharpened focus. It is not uncommon for angry, sometimes distraught parents to cast their children in a great many roles during postmarital battles, ranging from that of audience, whose presence appears to be a necessary backdrop for the parental fighting, to that of fully positioned battle allies. The children often range in their participation from astonished, frightened observers to denunciatory Greek chorus or, in some instances, ardent champions of one parent against the other.

Many of the anger-driven parent-child relationships that emerge at the time of the marital breakup are new alliances that diverge from the pattern that existed within the intact marriage. The child's conscious behavior may be powered by loyalty to the disrupted marriage or by the quixotic impulse to defend or rescue the parent who has been identified by the child (sometimes erroneously) as the victim. Not atypically, a child may take up the cause of the absent parent, representing his or her interests in the events of the custodial household. A child's active involvement in the marital battle is additionally fueled by the rise in physical violence between the parents that often erupts at the separation, even though it had never been a feature of the marriage (Wallerstein and Kelly, 1980).

Such alignments occur most often between a late latency or early adolescent child and the parent who has vehemently opposed the divorce. The adult's participation is almost always rooted in an entrenched sense of moral outrage at having been betrayed and cruelly exploited during the marriage. The avowed agenda of these alignments is likely to be the restoration of the failed marriage; the unspoken agenda is almost always revenge.

These anger-driven alliances serve a range of psychological purposes for both parent and child. The loneliness of the divorce period is reduced significantly by the new partnership. The child's own gnawing fear of being abandoned is alleviated by becoming the needy parent's trusted companion. Directing their anger outward against the absent parent serves as a powerful antidote to the intolerable pain of rejection and helplessness that the allied child and parent experience. Nor is it accidental that many children join cause with a parent with whom their relationship during the marriage had been tenuous or emotionally impoverished and take up an angry campaign against the parent they once had cherished. Additionally, for the child, the new alignment provides an opportunity to resolve any existing ambivalence of feeling toward the parents by creating a clear repository of virtue in one and villainy in the other.

There is evidence that such active alignments generally do not survive the adolescence of the young ally. Nevertheless, many young people come to adulthood complaining that their responses to the "villainous" parent had been governed by perceptions that they did not truly share. They regret deeply that they were not given the opportunity to form their own judgments, and their anger at having been cheated out of a true relationship with both parents is often intense. Some also express profound and pervasive guilt at having participated in lying or even more serious misbehavior directed at hurting their parent (Wallerstein and Blakeslee, 1989). These issues may underlie the negative shift seen in the maternal relationship once adolescence has been traversed (Zill et al., 1993).

One of the most significant findings in family research concerns the

serious hazard posed to the psychological health and development of children by continued exposure to high conflict between the parents, whether in the context of an intact marriage or as part of ongoing postdivorce antagonism (Emery, 1982). In one recent California study of 1,124 divorcing families, one-quarter were characterized by high levels of conflict at an average of $3\frac{1}{2}$ years postseparation (Maccoby and Mnookin, 1992). There is increasing interest in the plight and fate of children in such families and the impact of witnessing abuse and violence between the parents, especially if it is prolonged. The psychological effects and disturbances in parent-child attachments observed are not unlike those reported in families where the child has been the target of abuse directly. As yet, it is not clear whether this detrimental impact is mediated by the influence of the conflict on critical aspects of the parent-child relationship or whether it largely represents the intense reactions of the children who directly witness or overhear the fighting. Nor is it known whether children's reactions are primarily governed by the stimulation of seeing the parents fight, by the anxiety engendered from parents who appear to be out of control, by the fear that one or both parents—and perhaps the children as well—may be severely harmed, by complex issues of identification, or by some combination of all of these factors. The persistence of high conflict for many years, even after the parental divorce, may be particularly psychonoxious to children in that it appears to lack any remedy.

The link between parental conflict and the subsequent psychological adjustment of children represents one of the most fertile areas for increased theoretical understanding and new models of psychotherapeutic intervention. Johnston and Campbell (1988) have addressed the serious effects these lasting impasses create in some families after divorce, reporting severe reactions among the children, including impairment in reality testing. Adding to this concern is the report from a longitudinal study that, at 10 and 15 years postdivorce, many young people remembered with great clarity incidents of physical conflict between their parents and described having been continually haunted by those memories during their waking and dream lives throughout the postdivorce decade and well into their young adulthood. A significant number of these children from homes where there was physical and verbal abuse between parents during the intact marriage became involved, at entry into young adulthood, in abusive relationships of their own, although they had been separated by at least a decade from the trauma of witnessing their parents' quarrels (Wallerstein and Blakeslee, 1989).

At the cutting edge of research in this area is the work of Johnston and Roseby on the developmental impact of high-conflict divorce and of separations in the context of violent relationships. Children caught in such circumstances show problems in psychological separation and individuation and disturbances of gender and sexual identity (Johnston, in press; Roseby, 1993; Roseby and Wallerstein, in press).

EFFECTS OF DIVORCE ON CHILDREN

Initial Reactions

Children and adolescents experience parental separation and its immediate aftermath as an immensely stressful period in their lives. Indeed, for middle-class children in America, their parents' divorce is likely to be the central stress of their growing-up years. The family rupture evokes an acute sense of shock, intense anxiety, and profound sorrow. Many children can feel relatively content and even well parented within families in which one or both parents are unhappy. A surprising number (one-third in one study) did not know that their parents' marriage was troubled (Wallerstein and Kelly, 1980). Few youngsters experience relief with the divorce decision; those who do are usually older and have witnessed open conflict between their parents. Children's initial responses are typically governed neither by an understanding of the issues leading to the divorce nor by the fact that divorce has a high incidence in their community. To children, their own parents' divorce signifies the collapse of the structure that was responsible for providing them basic nurturance and protection, even when the family was performing poorly in this role.

The initial pain experienced by children and adolescents in response to a marital separation is compounded by their fantasies of the catastrophes they fear the divorce will bring in its wake. Children suffer with a pervasive sense of vulnerability as they experience the family breaking apart. They grieve over the loss of the intact family, including the hopes and dreams attached to it, and over the absence of the noncustodial parent. Often they must also confront the additional losses of familiar friends, neighborhood, and school. Children worry about their distressed parents. They are concerned about who will take care of the parent who has left and whether the custodial parent will be able to manage alone. They experience intense anger toward one or both parents for disrupting the family. Some of their anger is reactive and defends them against their own feelings of powerlessness, their concern about being lost in the shuffle, and the fear that their needs will be disregarded as the parents give priority to their own wishes and needs. They often feel a painfully divided loyalty, as if they were being forced to choose between their parents, even when this question has not been put before them. They may suffer with imagined guilt over having caused the divorce. This is especially likely among young children, or where the parents have fought over child-related issues. Young children sometimes decide heroically that it is up to them to mend the broken marriage.

The responses of children, particularly their sense of loneliness and social isolation, are also strongly influenced by the social context of the divorce. Children all too often must face the tensions and sorrows of divorce with little outside help. Fewer than 10% of children in one widely reported study (Wallerstein and Kelly, 1980) had any support at the time of the crisis from adults, other than relatives, who might have helped them, such as teachers, pediatricians, clergy, or family friends. Only 25% felt that grandparents came to their aid emotionally. Many children are poorly prepared by their parents for the impending upheaval, some not at all. Thus, it is a striking feature of divorce that when it occurs—unlike in bereavement or other stressful events that can occur in childhood—customary support systems, either through adult ignorance or diffidence, fall away.

Developmental Factors

Developmental factors are critical in the responses of children and adolescents at the time of the marital rupture. Despite significant individual differences in children, in their families, and in parent-child relationships, it appears that children's dominant concerns, their capacity to perceive and understand family events, their central psychological preoccupations and conflicts, their available repertoire of defenses and coping strategies, and the dominant patterning of their relationships and expectations, all primarily reflect their age and developmental stage at the time of the parental separation.

A major finding in divorce research has been these common patterns of response within age-related groups (Wallerstein and Kelly, 1980). The groups reported to share significant perceptions, responses, underlying fantasies, and behaviors are (a) the preschool ages 3—5, (b) young school or early latency ages 6½–8, (c) later latency ages 8–11, and (d) adolescent ages 12–18. The responses of young adolescents have also been differentiated from those in mid- and late adolescence (Springer and Wallerstein, 1983). It may be that the similarities observed within children's age groups represent their commonly shared responses to acute stress generally, not simply to marital rupture. Until recently, there has been no systematic research addressing the short- or long-term effects of divorce on infants and toddlers under 3 years of age. The newest work in this area is a longitudinal study in progress by Solomon and Wallerstein (1992), examining the effects of overnight visitation on the parent-child attachments of 100 children ages 12–18 months at the time of the family rupture. This is an important subgroup to understand, as many divorces occur within the first 2 years of marriage.

Observations about preschool children derived from longitudinal studies in two widely divergent regions, northern California and Virginia, are remarkably similar (Hetherington et al., 1982; Wallerstein and Kelly, 1980). Preschool children are likely to regress following one parent's departure from the home. The regression usually occurs in the most recent developmental achievement of the child. Intensified fears are frequent and are evoked by routine separations from the custodial parent during the day and at bedtime. Sleep disturbances are common. The preoccupying fantasy of many of these youngsters is fear of abandonment by both parents. Yearning for the departed parent is intense. Preschool children are likely to become irritable and demanding and to behave aggressively with parents, younger siblings, and peers.

Children ages 5–8 grieve openly for the departed parent. Many share the terrifying fantasy of replacement: "Will my daddy get a new dog, a new mommy, a new little boy?" Little girls weave elaborate Madame Butterfly fantasies, asserting that the departed father will someday return to them, that he loves them "the best." Many very young children cannot believe that the divorce is permanent. In their preoccupation with their fantasies, there is often a precipitous decline in their schoolwork (Wallerstein and Kelly, 1980).

For those 8½–12 years old, the central response often seems to be fierce anger at one or both parents. These children grieve over the loss of their intact world and suffer anxiety, loneliness, and a humiliating sense of their own powerlessness. They often see one parent as "good" and the other as "bad," and in this latency-age period, they appear especially vulnerable to the blandishments of a parent to participate in the marital battles. They also have a high potential for assuming an empathic and engrossing role in the care of a needy parent. School performance and peer relationships may consequently suffer (Wallerstein and Kelly, 1980).

Adolescents are also vulnerable to the impact of their parents' divorce. The incidence of acute depression, accompanied by suicidal preoccupation and acting out, is frequent enough to be alarming. Anger can be intense. Several instances have been reported of direct violent attacks on custodial parents by young adolescents who had not previously shown such behaviors (Springer and Wallerstein, 1983). Preoccupied with issues of morality, adolescents may sit in judgment on their parents' conduct around the divorce, and they may identify with one parent and do battle against the other. They are often anxious about their own future entry into adulthood, fearful that they may experience marital failure like their parents. Nevertheless, as researchers have pointed out, many adolescents show an impressive capacity to grow in maturity and independence as they respond to the family crisis and their parents' need for help (Weiss, 1979). The presence or absence of perceived fairness and integrity in their parents' postdivorce dealings with each other is not lost on them; yet, they are capable of considerable compassion for their parents' weaknesses and struggles, even as they continue to grapple with their own.

Gender Differences

Although it had been widely accepted by researchers that boys are more vulnerable than girls in both initial and long-term responses to divorce, this finding has been called into question by a critical analysis of the methodology employed in a range of studies (Zaslow, 1988, 1989). The picture is confusing, in part because the comparative developmental course of boys and girls in intact families, from infancy to young adulthood, is far from being clearly understood. The current state of our knowledge of divorce populations links gender differences to the different developmental stages. Thus, major differences between preschool boys and girls at approximately 4 years postseparation have been observed on a wide range of cognitive, social, and developmental measures (Hetherington et al., 1982). Although traditional sex-role typing in girls did not appear to be disrupted by divorce, boys scored lower on male preference and higher on female preference on the sex-role preference tests at this same time. The boys were also spending more time playing with girls and with younger children. They showed affective narrowness and a constriction in fantasy and play and were more socially isolated than their female peers.

Gender differences were observed as well in the California Children of Divorce Study (Wallerstein and Kelly, 1980). Although boys and girls did not differ in their overall psychological adjustment at the time of the marital breakup, 18 months later the boys' psychological adjustment had deteriorated, whereas that of the girls had improved, making for a significant gap between the two groups (Springer and Wallerstein, 1983). Guidubaldi (1985), in a national survey of elementary-school-age children 6 years postdivorce, found that boys, but not girls, tested significantly below a matched control group from intact families in academic achievement and social relationships. Other evidence suggests that, in general, marital turmoil has a greater impact on boys than on girls, both in divorced families and in intact, discordant families (Block et al., 1981; Emery, 1982; Rutter, 1970). In fact, a report of two national, longitudinal studies of divorce effects on children in Great Britain and the United States suggests that, at least for boys, negative symptoms that are usually considered divorce sequelae are actually apparent before the marital split (Cherlin et al., 1991).

A critical question is how much of the reported differential response between the sexes, if it does exist, is mediated by mother custody. One small study from the late 1970s found that latency-age children in the custody of the same-sex parent showed greater sociability and independence than did those boys and girls in the custody of the opposite-sex parent (Santrock and Warshak, 1979).

Finally, there is increasing evidence that adolescent girls in divorced and remarried families confront particular difficulties. Kalter has described special problems that girls from divorced families face in their relationships with their mothers, especially the difficulties of separating at adolescence (Kalter et al., 1985). Wallerstein's 10-year study (Wallerstein and Blakeslee, 1989) also reported that young women from divorced families often have a turbulent adolescence and a conflict-ridden entry into young adulthood. A significant number of young women at the 10-year mark were caught up in a web of short-lived sexual relationships, some with much older men. They described themselves as fearful of commitment, anticipating infidelity and betrayal. Many of the young women who encountered difficulties in late adolescence had done well during the early years after the divorce, when they were preschool and latency children. It may be that boys, especially oedipal and latency-age boys in mother-custody homes, have a more difficult time immediately following the divorce, whereas girls in mother custody find adolescence and entry into young adulthood particularly hazardous. Clearly, gender differences need to be explored further for the various age groups and within different family structures.

Long-Term Outcomes in Children

There is mounting evidence that the effects of divorce in a general population extend well beyond the previous expectation of a several-year, but limited, aftermath to the marital rupture. Wallerstein's research over a 10- and 15-year period (Wallerstein and Blakeslee, 1989) represents the most extended longitudinal study of children and adults following divorce. Her findings show ongoing as well as delayed effects that come to the fore during the years from midadolescence to young adulthood, as relationships with the opposite sex move to center stage. The ongoing effects associated with good or poor adjustment are likely to reflect the quality of life and the parent-child relationships within the postdivorce or remarried family. The delayed (often long-delayed) effects are more likely to reflect concerns associated with the possibility of repeating the failure of relationship between a man and a woman that the child observed during the marriage, as well as with the parents' subsequent failures in coparenting or new love relationships that the child may have observed. Where the postdivorce relationship that the parents develop with each other is more satisfactory, and where the parent individually is able to successfully reconstruct his or her life, the child's memories of the first poor parental relationship are less likely to be a disturbing influence.

Observations over the 10-year postdivorce period have led Wallerstein to propose that the inner developmental course of children of divorce is significantly altered by the parents' failed marriage and its frequently troubled, long-lasting aftermath (Wallerstein and Blakeslee, 1989; Wallerstein and Corbin, 1989). This is true whether or not the child falls into a more resilient group with better outcomes or into a more vulnerable group with poorer outcomes. The reports from the children over the many years of the follow-up suggest that the internal developmental tasks of establishing intimacy and trust in their own relationships with the opposite sex are felt to be persistently burdened to a greater or a lesser degree by the template of a failed man-woman relationship that these children carry within them. Additionally, the fears of disappointment, betrayal, and abandonment that are legacies of the failed parental marriage are often reinforced by extended periods of diminished parenting during the postdivorce period. When many find as well that the bond with the father does not survive transplantation into the alien, rocky soil of arranged visitation, this too adds to their sense of the unreliability of relationships.

There are other delayed effects of divorce that may not emerge until many years later. There is evidence that at adolescence the need for the father increases in both boys and girls, and that feeling rejected by the father at this critical development time may pose special hazards. For the young adult, relationships with both parents appear burdened by divorce—specific issues surrounding the normative events of separation from home and family, which are emotionally much more complicated if the custodial parent will be left alone. In brief, children of divorce face many tasks in addition to the usual ones of growing up. These tasks are formidable and may require more help than children in intact families in our society typically receive (Wallerstein, 1983). What seems very clear is that, over the years of their growing up, children of divorce find it necessary to work hard and consciously on the mastery of their experiences. It may be for this as well as other reasons that they continue to think of themselves as "children of divorce," as if that were their fixed identity (Wallerstein and Blakeslee, 1989).

Factors in Outcome

The initial responses of children do not predict long-term consequences for psychosocial adjustment, either for those who did well at the time of the divorce or for those who fared poorly. Nor do preliminary findings at the 15-year mark of the California Children of Divorce Study indicate that even 10-year outcomes have remained stable (Wallerstein and Blakeslee, 1989). There appears to be considerable shifting in individual adjustment as the young people now in their third decade of life either seek psychotherapy for themselves after several relationship failures or succeed in building gratifying heterosexual relationships and marriages. No single theme appeared among the children in this study who were well functioning immediately following the separation and divorce, or over the years that followed. Nor was there a single thread associated with poor outcome. Many of the children who looked good at the 10-year mark were well parented or had had considerable help along the way from a parent or grandparent. Only a few were helped by both parents. Visiting frequency or patterns of visiting were unrelated to outcome, but whether or not the child felt rejected by the father remained a critical factor. Some were fortunate enough to find adult mentors, and those who did showed particular promise in scholarship or athletics. Many had taken a great deal of responsibility for bringing themselves up.

Although in remarried families the stepparent can, on occasion, play a critical role in the child's development, the extent to which this occurs is unclear. In the cited 10-year study, few stepparents took on a central role in the child's life. Also, in a significant number of remarried families, the children felt excluded from the orbit of the remarriage. The latest national figures provide no clear support for the protective or mitigating influence of remarriage for children of divorce, although when divorce had occurred early in the child's life, parental remarriage seemed to offer some benefit to the child (Zill et al., 1993).

In the Wallerstein study, the amount of stress noted in the postdivorce family was considerable. One of two children experienced a second parental divorce. One of two continued to live with intense anger between their parents that did not subside over the years. Three of five felt rejected by one or both parents. There were additional economic stresses, and a quarter of the youngsters experienced a significant drop in their standard of living, which they did not recoup during the postdivorce decade.

In effect, in investigating the long-term adjustment of the child of divorce, we have confronted a rich mix of individual issues in the resiliency and vulnerability of child and parent, the individual talents and staying power of the child, the nature of the relationship between the child and each parent (especially the custodial parent), the extent to which the postdivorce coparenting relationship is relatively free from continued conflict that involves the child, and the encouragement and support available to the child from whatever other sources are available within or outside the family.

DISPUTED CUSTODY AND VISITATION

The most tragic children of divorce are those aptly described as "the children of Armageddon" (Watson, 1969), who are caught in the entrenched legal battles of their parents. There are no national figures available on the numbers of families involved in full-scale legal battles over custody and visitation, but based on an early estimate, it is likely that 10–15% of families with children struggle in the courts over many years, and that one-third of divorcing families return to court for modification of the initial orders (Freed and Foster, 1974). In the Maccoby and Mnookin study, researchers estimated that 10% of families encountered "substantial" legal conflict over custody and visitation, while 15% experienced "intense" legal conflict (Maccoby and Mnookin, 1992). Thus, although most families make custody and visitation arrangements without recourse to the courts, many relying on the advice of their attorneys, even private arrangements are very much influenced by court decisions, which cast a long shadow over all postdivorce arrangements, including those that were never in dispute (Mnookin and Kornhauser, 1979).

The causes of continued legal contest between divorcing spouses are complex and multidetermined. Fortunately, recent studies have begun to shed light on the interlocking issues that maintain the conflict at high intensity over many years. Johnston and Campbell (1988) have suggested a triad of factors that contribute to the impasse in the family: those that reflect psychopathology in the individual, those that derive from the marital relationship and the changed interaction between the partners, and those factors in the social surround that support the continued litigation and contribute to the increasing stress of the parties involved. In the individual, a history of repeated unmourned losses is not uncommon and may go hand in hand with a pathological dependence on the constant presence of the child. The severe narcissistic injury of the divorce may trigger a rage against the divorcing spouse that continues to bind the partners to each other via conflict over the children. The same psychodynamics may underlie child stealing.

There is growing recognition among mental health professionals that the adversarial system of the courts is not only poorly suited to resolving family conflict but also may intensify it by further dividing the hapless parents and adding to the stress on the family. As Gardner (1982) has noted, "the adversarial system is ill suited to deal optimally with custody conflicts, is psychically detrimental to children, and is therefore antithetical to good psychiatric practice." The Group for the Advancement of Psychiatry (1980) has recognized the impact of the entire family's interrelationships during the postdivorce years and strongly advocates that all family members should be examined before a court decision on custody or visitation is made. Practitioners have increasingly refused to appear as an expert witness for one side in a custody or visitation dispute and have insisted on meeting with both parents before rendering a recommendation to the court.

Mediation

Mediation has attracted considerable interest in recent years as the intervention of choice for disputing families (Coogler, 1978; Haynes, 1981). Reports from a study of mediation in four court systems (Hartford, Denver, Minneapolis, and Los Angeles) indicate that families who agree to make use of the mediation services in the courts are generally pleased with the process and outcome. A significant number of families, however, reject mediation even when it is made available without charge. There are many issues that continue to hinder the full realization of mediation's early promise. Recent research shows that severely conflicted parents are unable to make use of the mediation process successfully (Kressal et al., 1989). Still unresolved is the issue of whether mediation falls within the domain of the attorney or the mental health professional or whether they should work in concert with the disputing family. A critical issue is that the mediator's role may leave the child's interests without adequate protection, because mediators, by and large, lack training in child development or psychopathology and are unable, except from a common sense vantage point, to assess how the mediated agreement will influence the child. Furthermore, the mediation process makes the assumption that the child's interests will be protected by the parents, an assumption often unwarranted at divorce, especially in the case of intensely conflicted parents. Finally, whereas the judge is charged with protecting the best interests of the child, the mediator in most settings does not share this responsibility.

In 1981 California enacted mandatory mediation for divorcing families who are disputing custody or visitation. Reports from different jurisdictions within that state show a high settlement rate, ranging from 55 to 85% of the disputing families in the different counties, who then refrain from taking their case to court. There is still much to be learned about the nature of these agreements and their impact on the psychological adjustment of the children or their parents. Overall, however, the courts have considered mediation services to be of great benefit, and the availability of mediation services has increased rapidly within courts throughout the country.

Custody

The changing roles of men and women are mirrored in the courts and in legislation regarding custody and visitation. Early in the 1980s, the courts relied extensively on the concept of "the psychological parent," assuming that, except in unusual circumstances or for older children, the mother would fulfill this role. Our society has now moved away from the expectation that single-parent custody, combined with reasonable visitation with the noncustodial parent, is the legacy of divorce. Attention has increasingly focused on the contribution of the father as parent and as potential primary parent (Cath et al., 1982; Jacobs, 1982). Custodial arrangements have changed over the past 15 years (Maccoby and Mnookin, 1992). We still lack sufficient information about the extent of this change in the direction of joint custody. It is important, however, that during the 1980s over one-half of the states enacted legislation that permits joint custody. In several instances the public policy has leaned toward a presumptive preference for joint custody. In California, in 1988, legislation went against the presumption of joint custody; while acknowledging the importance of both parents for the child, it emphasized the necessity of matching the custody arrangement to the needs of the individual family. Clearly, community attitudes and social policy are in flux.

Joint custody remains a variously defined arrangement, differing not only among states but also even between local jurisdictions. Joint *legal* custody typically refers to an equally shared responsibility between parents for major decisions regarding their children's lives and well-being. Joint physical custody indicates that the child actually resides for substantial periods of time in each parent's home, although the proportion of time spent and the schedule of transitions between households may vary widely.

Joint physical custody can be properly regarded as a new family form. The motivation for its choice varies widely. Some parents select joint custody out of commitment to the child's continuing relationship with both parents; others, however, select this custody form out of the demands of the workplace; still others select joint custody because neither parent truly wishes to take responsibility for their child. Obviously the experience of the child will vary with the parents' motivation and emotional investment.

Researchers have raised the question as to how important the custody arrangement by itself is to the psychological adjustment of the child. Kline, in a sample of 93 white middle- and upper-class divorcing families, compared the psychological adjustment of those 38% of the children who were living in joint custody with that of the remaining group who were in sole custody (Kline et al., 1989). She and her colleagues found that neither the custody arrangement itself nor the frequency of access and visitation with the father influenced the child's psychological adjustment. The factors affecting the child's psychological and social adjustment, regardless of custody arrangement, were the prior psychological functioning of the parents and the degree of postdivorce hostility and conflict between the parents.

One study of intensely conflicted families, where the court had ordered joint custody over the considerable reluctance of one or even both parents, showed that children in involuntary custody situations looked seriously deteriorated in their psychological and social adjustment, school performance, and peer involvement, as observed over a several-year period. Both boys and girls seemed to suffer when frequent access to both parents was imposed on families locked in ongoing disputes (Johnston et al., 1989). This work addressed the very serious issue that has been raised in many jurisdictions as to whether the courts should award joint custody in the face of one parent's strong opposition. Findings from this study are very much in accord with the clinical opinions that practitioners have held over many years.

There is evidence from a number of studies that many children prefer joint custody to sole custody and that many children benefit from this arrangement (McKinnon and Wallerstein, 1986; Steinmann, 1981). Our knowledge at present indicates that, when it is entered into voluntarily by both parents with dedication and conviction, joint physical custody can be regarded as a viable family form. Under appropriate circumstances, it serves well, especially in the transition from divorce to remarriage. Joint custody does demand special effort and commitment from the parents, the ability of the formerly married partners to remain in close touch with each other's lives, and considerable flexibility from both child and parents (Wallerstein and Blakeslee, 1989). There is an insufficiency of research in this entire domain, especially on the long-term effects of joint custody. We especially await findings from the study of infants and young children to shed light on how the frequency of going back and forth from one home to another affects bonding and development.

PUBLIC POLICY AND DIVORCE RESEARCH

Although policy makers, legislators, and judges have increasingly sought support from the findings of behavioral science and guidance from the mental health professions, the accumulation of psychological knowledge has not kept up with the rapid evolution of family law. Knowledge about children and parent-child relationships in the postdivorce family is still fragmentary and insufficient to support many of the legislative changes in family policy that have found powerful adherents. The subtleties of psychological thinking and shadings of individual difference that are so critical to the perspective of the behavioral scientist translate poorly into the arenas of court and legislature. The several years of follow-up required to assess the impact of changed circumstances on altered family structure are ill-suited to the pressured agendas of the political and judicial process. Despite the widespread acknowledgment given to the important interface between family law and mental health, the major task of building cooperation and mutual understanding on a firm basis of empirical knowledge and shared values still lies ahead.

INTERVENTIONS

It is evident that many families need professional advice and guidance in negotiating their way through the complex and tangled pathway of divorce and the postdivorce years. Moreover, it is important not only to provide the services that they need but also to find ways to reach both adults and children at the appropriate times, namely, at the marital rupture and at critical turning points along the arduous road that lies ahead. Essentially, divorcing families confront two sets of divorce-related issues that fall within the domain of the clinician: those associated with the acute crisis engendered by the marital breakup and those associated with rebuilding the family, and subsequent families, that will provide a "holding environment" for children and adults during the postdivorce years. These two sets of issues translate into a series of immediate and long-term psychological and social tasks for adults and children (Wallerstein, 1983; Wallerstein and Blakeslee, 1989). They translate as well into two separate preventive and clinical agendas: one addressed primarily to the amelioration of the psychological disequilibria of the separation crisis and its immediate aftermath and a second addressed to building or restoring family structure and parent-child relationships within the postdivorce or remarried family (Wallerstein, 1990).

A third, clinical agenda is addressed to children who show relatively consolidated psychological disturbance. Although children in this group present clinical issues that are relatively familiar, the therapist's relationships with the parents and other significant adults will differ sharply from those with most intact families. Thus, for example, in the divorced family the issue of who bears primary financial responsibility for the child's therapy is often in dispute. The treatment itself, whatever its course, has a high potential for being caught within the continuing angers between the parents, and the therapist is likely to be identified by one or both as allied with "the other side." Furthermore, there is the thorny issue, which needs to be resolved on a case-by-case basis, as to which adults should be included in the therapist's relationship with the family. When and under what circumstances should a biological father who has had little contact with the child be seen? When should a stepparent be dealt with as the primary parent? When and how should live-in lovers be included? These multiple relationships need to be carefully assessed by the clinician not only for their bearing on the child but also because of their importance in constructing a network that will support the child's treatment.

Another critical issue that will influence treatment process and goals is that the development of a significant number of children is hindered by the continuing failure of their families to provide sufficient nurturance and protection to sustain the youngsters' developmental progress. As a consequence, in addition to addressing issues of neurotic conflict, the clinician may need to take a more supportive role. These supportive parameters, which so many of the children need, have implications not only for process but also for the duration of treatment.

Tasks of Divorce

The reorganization and readjustments required of the child of divorce, namely, the psychological tasks that need to be addressed, represent a major addition to the expectable tasks of childhood and adolescence in our society. In effect, the child of divorce faces a special set of challenges and carries an added burden, which may indeed require professional help at different points along the developmental course. The individual child's resolution of these tasks is profoundly influenced by the family ambience and by the extent to which the parents have made progress in resolving the many issues to which divorce gives rise. Nevertheless, it is the child who must carry the burden of mastery and resolution on the way to successfully achieved adulthood; there is no necessarily determining relationship between the resolution and adjustment achieved by either of the parents and the outcome for any particular child in the family. There is in fact a widening difference in outcome among siblings as they approach young adulthood (Corbin, 1988).

These readjustments are likely to stretch over the growing-up years and through adolescence. They are the coping tasks that are shaped by psychological threats to the child's psychic integrity and development. These tasks have been conceptualized as a hierarchical series, which follows a particular time sequence beginning with the critical events of parental separation and culminating at late adolescence and young adulthood. They represent the agenda for the child as well as for the therapy.

The psychological tasks, as formulated by Wallerstein (1983) are six in number. They fall into an unfolding sequence with varying time spans attached for the accomplishment of each. Task 1, *acknowledging the reality of the marital rupture*, and Task 2, *disengaging from parental conflict and distress and resuming customary pursuits*, need to be addressed immediately at the time of the decisive separation, and they are optimally resolved within the 1st year. The child's successful mastery of these two immediate tasks is tied to the maintenance of his or her appropriate academic pace and overall developmental agenda, after the initial dip at the time of crisis. But the child's successful mastery of divorce-engendered stress is only partially related to the early period following the marital rupture. Task 3, *the resolution of losses* (including the loss of the presence of one parent in the home), Task 4, *resolving anger and self-blame*, and Task 5, *accepting the permanence of the divorce*, will be worked and reworked by the child over many years. They, along with the final Task 6, *achieving realistic hope regarding relationships*, will become salient at adolescence and entry into adulthood.

Some Treatment Considerations

Various treatment modalities have been employed with this population to facilitate adjustment, including family therapy, individual psychoanalytically oriented therapy for the child, parent guidance, supportive group therapy for parents, and supportive group therapy for children. Cognitive behavioral approaches have been used, primarily in groups for children within school settings. In working with all of these modalities, it is important to keep in mind that treatment of the adult *qua* adult does not necessarily trickle down to help the child. Our own work of many years shows that parent-child relationships need to be addressed directly within the treatment and cannot be counted on to extend from the treatment of the parent as the primary patient to the child (Wallerstein and Blakeslee, 1989). The conjoint treatment of divorced parents and their children may place children in jeopardy. It is not uncommon for the child in a divorced family to be punished severely by disputing parents for statements that might have been acceptable within the framework of an intact family. The child's greater vulnerability in these families needs to be understood by the clinician.

The psychological assessment of both child and parent takes on special importance in work with a divorce population. A significant measure of responsibility for the selection of the treatment goals falls on the clinician. In the ordinary course of child psychotherapy, parents present their concerns, which provide the starting point for the therapeutic alliance. By contrast, divorcing families, especially those who come to a preventive program, bring multiple and conflicting overt and covert agendas, each of which may cancel out the other. These agendas range from the wish to reconcile the marriage to fantasies of Medea-like revenge, from the need to hear that the children are untroubled to well-founded serious concerns about their welfare. Nowhere is the difference between an intact family, however conflict ridden, and a disrupted family more evident than in the difficulty in arriving at a common treatment agenda.

An additional consideration in the clinician's greater responsibility for the agenda of the intervention is that often parents are unaware of what may be the grave psychological condition of the children. Time and again we have observed children in serious trouble, even in dire emergencies, whose normally attentive parents seem oblivious to the danger, caught up as they are in their own concerns. This is true not only of threats to psychological health of the child but also of a decline in the physical health of the child as well. Both need to come under the special scrutiny of the psychiatrist.

Finally, it should be noted that there is a considerable likelihood that children in these families will have witnessed severe verbal abuse or physical violence between the parents. Often the effects of such experiences will not show up initially in the symptomatology of the child. They may well be associated, however, with serious superego lacunae, deficits in object relations and identity, and skewed expectations regarding relationships between men and women, which, although they may not become manifest during childhood, may, if left untreated, come to the fore at subsequent developmental stages. The therapist is well advised to make appropriate inquiries about parental conflict in the child's history that may not be readily forthcoming and to attempt to engage the child in an exploration of his or her reactions to what may have been searing incidents.

Finally, it should be noted that treatment of children and parents in the separating and divorced family often depletes the therapist's emotional resources. The final scenes of the failed marriage are played out in the consulting room not only in the painful context of the verbal interactions but also, just as importantly, in the transference reactions of the client caught up in the crisis and in the subsequent countertransference responses of the clinician. There is an extraordinary lack of psychological distance between therapist and client as identifications move back and forth across the therapeutic interface. The most common countertransference is for the clinician to experience anxiety about the stability of his or her own intimate relationships (Wallerstein, 1990).

Future Directions in Interventions

There are indications of mounting community concern about the recent changes in the family in our society and their impact on children, particularly the initial and long-term effects of divorce. Whether this concern will translate into adequately funded preventive and clinical programs, we cannot predict. Thus far, mediation and court-based programs have traditionally excluded children, while school-based programs have typically excluded parents. Nevertheless, the possibility is greater that the decade of the future will see a proliferation of new and integrated educational and preventive programs that will address families at the time of the separation crisis. Such programs should ideally reach out to parents within a general divorcing population and provide them with guidance in regard to the many decisions that they face and with specific advice about how to restore parenting and how to help their children during the crisis and its often extended aftermath.

One such demonstration project has been developed in northern California at the Center for the Family in Transition, funded by private foundations. The outreach includes a letter sent to every family within the county that files for divorce. Children and adolescents are assessed individually and receive intensive counseling over an initial 3-month period, returning for brief follow-ups at the 1- and 2-year marks (Wallerstein, 1990). This model has been copied in several clinics within the United States and Canada. There has also been some recent interest in modifying the model to meet the demands of the private sector. The work of Johnston and her associates offers another important template for working with families in high-conflict situations.

Precisely because divorce draws a large segment of the general population, it provides an unprecedented opportunity for developing and testing models of prevention in mental health. And because the subgroups at greater risk can often be identified at the time of the separation, among both parents and children, the clinician is provided with the opportunity to offer a range of intervention programs early on. One such subgroup that may well receive increased attention are those high-conflict families who fall through the net of the mediation services provided by the court. It is possible that the courts will recognize the grave psychopathology among these children and their parents and develop referral networks within the private sector. The high incidence of allegations of physical and sexual abuse in divorcing families may also encourage the development of clinical services via a referral network attached to the courts.

Among the hopeful signs on this landscape is the new willingness of public, private, and parochial schools to recognize the link between the learning and behavioral problems of many children and the weakening in the family structure. School systems are increasingly willing to permit or even welcome groups for children within the school setting, especially in the elementary schools.

Finally, there is burgeoning recognition of the needs of children of divorce that emerge with new intensity at young adulthood. Group programs are being developed that primarily attract adults in their twen-

ties and thirties who find their shared experience a useful supplement to individual psychotherapy.

Overall, however, our society has been reluctant to undertake measures related to helping families deal with change. The mental health professions have not taken a leadership role, and children continue to lack a powerful voice raised on their behalf. Still critically needed are research that will address the large lacunae in our knowledge and programs in prevention and intensive clinical interventions that can push our knowledge far beyond its current compass. Both the research agenda and the intervention agenda appear to lengthen and to unfold before us as we come closer to understanding the psychodynamics of these new family forms.

References

Block JH, Block J, Morrison A: Parental agreement-disagreement on child rearing orientations and gender-related personality correlates in children. *Child Dev* 52:965–974, 1981.

Cath SH, Gurwitt AR, Ross JM: *Father and Child: Developmental and Clinical Perspectives.* Boston, Little, Brown, 1982.

Cherlin AJ, Furstenberg FF, Chase-Lansdale PL, et al: Longitudinal studies of effects of divorce on children in Great Britain and the United States. *Science* 252:1386–1389, 1991.

Coogler OJ: *Structural Mediation in Divorce Settlement.* Lexington, MA, Lexington Books, 1978.

Corbin SB: *Factors Affecting Long-Term Similarities and Differences Among Siblings following Parental Divorce.* Unpublished doctoral dissertation, Menlo Park, CA, Pacific Graduate School of Psychology, 1988.

Emery RE: Interparental conflict and the children of discord and divorce. *Psychol Bull* 92:310–330, 1982.

Felner RD, Stolberg AL, Cowen EL: Crisis events and school mental health referral patterns of young children. *J Consult Clin Psychol* 43:305–310, 1975.

Freed DJ, Foster HH: The shuffled child and divorce court. *Trial* 10:26–41, 1974.

Furstenberg FF, Nord CW, Peterson JL, et al: The life course of children of divorce: Marital disruption and parental contact. *Am Sociol Rev* 48:656–668, 1983.

Gardner RA: *Family Evaluation in Child Custody Litigation.* Cresskill, NJ, Creative Therapeutics, 1982.

Gardner RA: *Psychotherapy and Children of Divorce.* New York, Aronson, 1976.

Group for the Advancement of Psychiatry: *Divorce, Child Custody and the Family.* New York, Mental Health Materials Center, 1980.

Guidubaldi J, Perry JD: Divorce and mental health sequelae for children: A two-year follow-up of a nationwide sample. *J Am Acad Child Psychiatry* 24:531–537, 1985.

Hanson SMH, Bozett FW: *Dimensions of Fatherhood.* Beverly Hills, CA, Sage, 1985.

Haynes J: *Divorce Mediation.* New York, Springer, 1981.

Hess RD, Camara KA: Post-divorce family relationships as mediating factors in the consequences of divorce for children. *J Soc Issues* 35:79–96, 1979.

Hetherington EM, Cox M, Cox R: The aftermath of divorce. In: Stevens JH, Mathews M (eds): *Mother/Child, Father/Child Relationships.* Washington, DC, National Association for the Education of Young Children, 1978.

Hetherington EM, Cox M, Cox R: Effects of divorce on parents and children. In: Lamb ME (ed): *Nontraditional Families: Parenting and Child Development.* Hillsdale, NJ, Erlbaum, 1982.

Jacobs J: The effect of divorce on father: An overview of the literature. *Am J Psychiatry* 139:62–66, 1982.

Johnston JR: High conflict divorce. *Future Child* 4:1994.

Johnston JR: Problems in separation and individuation in children of high-conflict divorce. In: Cohen T et al (eds): *The Vulnerable Child* (Vol 2). Madison, CT, International Universities Press, in press.

Johnston JR, Campbell LEG: *Impasses of Divorce: The Dynamics and Resolution of Family Conflict.* New York, Free Press, 1988.

Johnston JR, Kline M, Tschann JM: Ongoing postdivorce conflict: Effects on children of joint custody and frequent access. *Am J Orthopsychiatry* 59:1–17, 1989.

Kalter N: Children of divorce in an outpatient psychiatric population. *Am J Orthopsychiatry* 47:40–51, 1977.

Kalter N, Reimer B, Brickman A, et al: Implications of divorce for female development. *J Am Acad Child Psychiatry* 24:538–544, 1985.

Kline M, Tschann JM, Johnston JR, et al: Children's adjustment in joint and sole physical custody families. *Dev Psychol* 25:430–438, 1989.

Kressal K, Pruitt DG, et al: *Mediation Research: The Process and Effectiveness of Third-Party Intervention.* San Francisco, Jossey-Bass, 1989.

Maccoby EE, Mnookin RH: *Dividing the Child: Social and Legal Dilemmas of Custody.* Cambridge, MA, Harvard University Press, 1992.

McKinnon R, Wallerstein JS: Joint custody and the preschool child. *Behav Sci Law* 4:169–183, 1986.

Mnookin RH, Kornhauser L: Bargaining in the shadow of the law: The case of divorce. *Yale Law J* 88:950–977, 1979.

Pasley K, Ihinger-Tallman M: *Remarriage & Stepparenting: Current Research & Theory.* New York, Guilford, 1987.

Roseby V: *Conflicts in Gender and Sexual Identity in Children of High-Conflict Divorce.* Paper presented at The Vulnerable Child Discussion Group, Meeting of the American Psychoanalytic Association, San Francisco, 1993.

Roseby V, Johnston JR: Clinical interventions with children of high conflict and violence. *Am J Orthopsychiatry* 65:48–59, 1995.

Roseby V, Wallerstein JS: Impact of divorce on latency-age children: Assessment and intervention strategies. In: Noshpitz J (ed): *Handbook of Child Psychiatry* (rev ed). New York, Basic Books, in press.

Rutter M: Sex differences in children's responses to family stress. In: Anthony EJ, Koupernik C (eds): *The Child in His Family.* New York, Wiley, 1970.

Santrock JW, Warshak RA: Father custody and social development in boys and girls. *J Soc Issues* 35:112–125, 1979.

Santrock JW, Warshak R, Lindbergh C, et al: Children's and parents observed social behavior in step-father families. *Child Dev* 53:472–480, 1982.

Solomon J, Wallerstein JS: *Infants after Divorce: Overnight Visitation and Family Relationships.* Washington, DC, Department of Health and Human Resources, Maternal and Child Health Grant MCJ-060616, in progress.

Spanier GB, Glick PC: Marital instability in the United States: Some correlates and recent changes. *Fam Relations* 31:329–338, 1981.

Springer C, Wallerstein JS: Young adolescents' responses to their parents' divorces. In: Kurdek LA (ed): *Children and Divorce.* San Francisco, Jossey-Bass, 1983.

Steinman S: The experience of children in a joint custody arrangement: A report of a study. *Am J Orthopsychiatry* 51:403–414, 1981.

Wallerstein JS: Children of divorce: The psychological tasks of the child. *Am J Orthopsychiatry* 53:230–243, 1983.

Wallerstein JS: Changes in parent-child relationships during and after divorce. In: Anthony EJ, Pollock GH (eds): *Parental Influences in Health and Disease.* Boston, Little, Brown, 1985a.

Wallerstein JS: The overburdened child: Some long-term consequences of divorce. *Soc Work* 30:116–123, 1985b.

Wallerstein JS: Preventive interventions with divorcing families: A reconceptualization. In: Goldston SE, Heinicke CM, Pynoos RS, et al (eds): *Preventing Mental Health Disturbances in Childhood.* Washington, DC, American Psychiatric Press, 1990a, pp. 167–185.

Wallerstein JS: Transferences and countertransferences in clinical interventions with divorcing families. *Am J Orthopsychiatry* 60:337–345, 1990b.

Wallerstein JS: The long-term effects of divorce on children: A review. *J Am Acad Child Adolesc Psychiatry* 30:349–360, 1991.

Wallerstein JS, Blakeslee S: *Second Chances: Men, Women and Children a Decade after Divorce.* New York, Ticknor and Fields, 1989.

Wallerstein JS, Corbin SB: Daughters of divorce: Report from a ten-year study. *Am J Orthopsychiatry* 59:593–604, 1989.

Wallerstein JS, Kelly JB: *Surviving the Breakup: How Children and Their Parents Cope with Divorce.* New York, Basic Books, 1980.

Watson A: The children of Armageddon: Problems of children following divorce. *Syracuse Law Rev* 21:231–239, 1969.

Weiss RS: Growing up a little faster. *J Soc Issues* 35:97–111, 1979.

Weitzman LJ: *The Divorce Revolution: The Unexpected Social and Economic Consequences for Women and Children in America.* New York, Free Press, 1985.

Zaslow MJ: Sex differences in children's response to parental divorce. I: Research methodology and postdivorce family forms. *Am J Orthopsychiatry* 58:355–378, 1988.

Zaslow MJ: Sex differences in children's response to parental divorce. II: Samples, variables, ages, and sources. *Am J Orthopsychiatry* 59: 118–141, 1989.

Zill N: *Divorce, Marital Conflict, and Children's Mental Health: Research Findings and Policy Recommendations.* Testimony before the Subcommittee on Family and Human Services, US Senate Committee on Labor and Human Resources, Senate Hearing 98-195. Washington, DC, US Government Printing Office, 1983, pp.90–106.

Zill N, Schoenborn CA: Developmental, learning and emotional problems: Health of our nation's children, United States, 1988. *Advance Data, Vital and Health Statistics of the National Center for Health Statistics.* Washington, DC, National Center for Health Statistics, no. 190, November 16, 1990.

Zill N, Morrison DR, Coiro MJ: Long-term effects of parental divorce on parent-child relationships, adjustment and achievement in young adulthood. *J Fam Psychol* 7(1):91–103, 1993.

113 LEGAL CONSIDERATIONS IN THE PSYCHIATRIC HOSPITALIZATION OF CHILDREN AND ADOLESCENTS

Stephen Wizner, J.D.

The mode and procedure of medical diagnostic procedures is not the business of judges. What is best for a child is an individual medical decision that must be left to the judgment of physicians in each case (1).

No area of medical practice affords a physician as broad and far-reaching discretion in the exercise of professional judgment as does psychiatric hospitalization of children and adolescents. Unlike the circumstances under which adults are admitted to psychiatric hospitals or wards—as voluntary patients, under short-term emergency procedures, or after a judicial hearing replete with due process protections and specific commitment criteria—children and adolescents, as a rule, may be confined at the request of a parent or guardian. In most states, only the admitting physician stands between a parent's desire to hospitalize a child, for whatever reason, and the child's interest in not being improperly or unnecessarily institutionalized. Even in those states that afford objecting minors some judicial review of their involuntary confinement, review procedures and substantive commitment standards tend to be less formal and precise than those applicable to adults.

In addition to the lack of procedural formality and precise commitment criteria, the "mental illness" that brings most minors to psychiatric hospitals in the United States is manifested by behavioral problems rather than by cognitive or affective disorders. The typical minor whose psychiatric hospitalization is sought by parent or guardian will be given a diagnosis of conduct disorder, personality disorder, adjustment reaction, or transient or situational disturbance. Only a relatively small proportion of hospitalized youngsters, less than one-third, are hospitalized for severe or acute mental illness, such as psychotic, organic, or serious affective disorders (2).

The reasons that some seriously disturbed minors who are hospitalized are diagnosed as having conduct disorders or a situational disturbance may reflect a reluctance to label a child as having a serious mental illness prematurely and the difficulty in diagnosing a child or adolescent without a significant history of psychiatric disturbance. Nevertheless, the fact is that most minors who are hospitalized are hospitalized because of conduct or personality disorders and do not suffer from serious mental illness.

In her 1988 study of psychiatric hospital admission rates of juveniles, psychologist Lois Weithorn reported that in 1980 there were 81,532 psychiatric hospital admissions of persons under the age of 18, of which 49,910, or 61%, were to private hospitals (3). The fact that large numbers of minors without serious psychiatric disorders are confined in mental hospitals is attributable to several factors, not the least of which is the absence of clear procedural protections and precise commitment standards.

During the 1970s the practice of parental volunteering of minors into psychiatric hospitals was the subject of scholarly criticism (4) and judicial disapproval (5) as a violation of the constitutional right of juveniles not to be confined in institutions without due process of law. These academic critics and lower court judges concluded that parental discretion, subject only to psychiatric ratification or acquiescence, was insufficient to protect the liberty interests of minors.

THE *PARHAM* DECISION

In 1979, in the case of *Parham v. J.R. and J.L.,* the United States Supreme Court upheld the practice of parental volunteering of minors into mental institutions, stipulating only that a physician at the admitting facility be "free to evaluate independently the child's mental and emotional condition and need for treatment" and that this physician "has the authority to refuse to admit any child who does not satisfy the medical standards for admission" (6).

The Court used the opportunity presented by the *Parham* case to constitutionalize a presumption that parents act in their children's best interests and therefore ought to be able to decide, free of state interference, that their children require psychiatric hospitalization. The Court sought to justify the state's failure to institute procedural safeguards by hypothesizing benign, and even beneficent, reasons the state might have for refusing to provide procedural protections for institutionalized children. The Justices speculated that a cumbersome or intrusive procedure might dissuade parents from taking advantage of state-provided health opportunities, to the detriment of their children and the public. Also, the Court inferred that the state could have an interest in assuring that psychiatrists and other staff spend their time treating patients, rather than preparing for and appearing in court. Nevertheless, balancing the interests of the parents and the state against the "risk of error" from the child's perspective, the Court concluded that "some kind of inquiry should be made by a 'neutral factfinder' to determine whether the statutory requirements for admission are satisfied." That "neutral factfinder" is the physician who approves the parent's decision to hospitalize the child.

The Justices were unwilling to accept the notion that children's rights might be violated by apparently well-meaning parents and predicted that the focus of an evidentiary hearing was likely to be an examination of the parents' motives rather than evaluation of the child's need for hospitalization.

The Court expressed concern about the possible antitherapeutic consequences of such a hearing, theorizing that it would exacerbate tension between parents and children and make the child's subsequent return home more difficult. Finally, the Court observed that the adversary system is not the best mechanism for discovering truth when psychiatric decisions are at stake.

Under the Supreme Court's ruling, the kind of inquiry that must occur is to be conducted by a staff physician at the admitting facility. The review of the admission decision should focus on "what is best for the child." "Informal, traditional medical investigative techniques" are satisfactory. There must be an interview with the child; mere review of records is not sufficient. Finally, periodic review is required, although the Court did not specify how frequently review must occur, nor whether it may be less formal than the preadmission screening.

On only one remedial point did the Supreme Court agree with the trial court. The danger to children who are state wards of becoming "lost in the shuffle" after being admitted to the hospital might necessitate some formal postcommitment review procedures.

The facts of the *Parham* case, which the lower court had found to be "representative" of the class of children volunteered into state mental hospitals, would appear to cast doubt on the presumption that parents (and guardians) always act in the best interests of their children. At the request of his mother, J.L. had been admitted to a state mental hospital in 1970 at the age of 6. His diagnosis was "hyperkinetic reaction of childhood." He was still there 5 years later when the case was filed because his parents would not take him home and, in fact, had voluntarily terminated their parental rights the year before. Hospital staff had recommended that J.L. be placed in a foster home, but that recommendation had not been carried out.

J.R., the other named plaintiff, had been declared a neglected child and removed from his parents' custody at the age of 3 months. He had been placed by state authorities in a succession of seven different foster homes and was eventually volunteered by social workers into a state mental hospital at the age of 7. His diagnosis was "unsocialized, aggressive reaction of childhood." More than 5 years later, when the lawsuit was filed, he remained in the hospital, solely because state authorities had failed to implement a hospital recommendation that he be placed in a foster home.

In the words of Justice Brennan in a dissenting opinion, "In these circumstances, I respectfully suggest, it ignores reality to assume blindly that parents act in their children's best interests when making commitment decisions and when waiving their children's due process rights" (7).

STATE LEGISLATION

Although the Supreme Court in *Parham* expressly rejected the views of academic critics, civil rights lawyers, and lower court judges, it left the door open for states to provide additional protections for minors beyond the minimum that it found to be constitutionally sufficient.

Virtually every state currently has legislation that applies to the admission (and discharge) of minors to psychiatric facilities. Because of the significant variance in standards and procedures contained in the various state statutes, it is essential for the physician contemplating psychiatric hospitalization of a child or adolescent to be familiar with the law in his or her own state (8).

Some state statutes merely enact into law the vague admonition of the Supreme Court that "some kind of inquiry" be made at the time of admission, and periodically thereafter, by a hospital physician to assure that hospitalization is appropriate. For example, the Arizona statute permits hospitalization of a minor upon application of a parent, guardian, or custodian, following a determination by the medical director of the admitting facility that the "child needs an inpatient evaluation or will benefit from care and treatment of a mental disorder or other personality disorder or emotional condition in the agency" and that "the evaluation or treatment goals can[not] be accomplished in a less restrictive setting" (9).

Other states, like Virginia (10), have extended to minors substantive and procedural protections similar or even identical to those afforded adults facing involuntary civil commitment. These may include the right of a minor, on his or her own, to be a voluntary patient and to enjoy the substantive and procedural protections afforded by the state's emergency and civil commitment statutes if he or she refuses to enter the hospital voluntarily. Typically, such statutes require that, in order to be involuntarily hospitalized, an individual must be found, by clear and convincing evidence, in a judicial proceeding where he or she is afforded the right to an attorney and other procedural protections, to be suffering from a mental illness that seriously disrupts functioning and causes the individual to be "dangerous" to himself or herself or others, or "gravely disabled," and that there is no less restrictive environment in which the individual can receive necessary treatment, care, and custody.

State laws differ in a variety of specific respects. For example, some states, like Idaho (11), do not require any type of review prior to the admission of a minor, beyond that conducted by the admitting physician. Other states, like Virginia (12), require a judicial commitment hearing for any person, including a minor, who is unwilling to accept voluntary admission or is incapable of making a voluntary admission decision.

Even those states that require judicial review of the involuntary admission of minors differ on the *timing* of such reviews. For example, Virginia (13) requires that the judicial commitment hearing *precede* admission and further requires a judicial order for a 48-hour emergency detention. In contrast, North Carolina (14) requires that a judicial hearing be held within 10 days *after* a minor is hospitalized.

Some states make such hearings mandatory. North Carolina (15) and Florida (16), for example, require a postadmission judicial hearing in *every* case. Other states, like Louisiana (17), provide for a postadmission judicial hearing only upon request by the minor or the parent or guardian.

State laws also differ in the form of judicial review provided and the procedural protections afforded to minors. For example, Connecticut (18) provides for an evidentiary hearing, with representation by court-appointed counsel, an independent psychiatric evaluation, and the right to present evidence and cross-examine witnesses. Virginia (19) goes beyond this, providing in addition a right to appeal a commitment decision to a higher court for a jury trial.

States that provide judicial hearings to minors differ with respect to the substantive criteria to be applied at such hearings. Connecticut (20), for example, requires a judicial finding that "the child suffers from a mental disorder, is in need of hospitalization for treatment, and such treatment is available, and such hospitalization is the least restrictive available alternative." New Mexico (21) requires a judicial finding "(1) that as a result of mental disorder or developmental disability the minor needs and is likely to benefit from the treatment or habilitation services proposed; and (2) that the proposed commitment is consistent with the treatment needs of the minor and with the least drastic means principle." Iowa (22) requires only that the court determine that hospitalization is "in the best interests of the minor and is consistent with the minor's rights," without further definition or specificity. In contrast, Virginia (23) requires that in order for a minor to be involuntarily committed the court must find that the minor "(i) presents an imminent danger to himself or others as a result of mental illness, or (ii) has been proven to be so seriously mentally ill as to be substantially unable to care for himself and (iii) that alternatives to involuntary confinement and treatment have been investigated and deemed unsuitable and there is no less restrictive alternative to institutional confinement and treatment."

Another important respect in which state laws differ is the age at which minors are entitled to invoke such legal protections as may exist. These age distinctions are of two basic types. First is the age at which a minor is deemed to be a "child" or "adult" for purposes of psychiatric commitment. For example, in Connecticut (24) a minor 16 years of age or older is covered by the *adult* voluntary and commitment statutes. Second, some state laws distinguish between minors of varying ages within statutes that apply specifically to children and adolescents. For example, Illinois (25) permits minors 12 years of age or older to request postadmission judicial review, while Virginia (26) grants the right to all minors, regardless of age, to request a preadmission judicial hearing.

Finally, in a small number of states, such as Oregon (27), the mental hospital admission statute applies only to *state* facilities.

THE RESPONSIBILITY OF THE PSYCHIATRIST

It is unlikely that either the Supreme Court decision in *Parham* or the wide variety of state legislation governing the admission of children and adolescents to psychiatric institutions will make a difference in the majority of cases of parental hospitalization of children for psychiatric treatment. In many, if not most, cases the decision to hospitalize a child is made by responsible parents and competent psychiatrists and only when there is no other way to provide necessary treatment. In such cases, whether a minor has a right to a hearing or exercises his or her right to a hearing, and regardless of the standards for commitment, the decision to hospitalize is likely to be the same.

However, there will remain a significant number of cases in which children and adolescents face unnecessary, or unnecessarily prolonged, confinement in mental institutions. State statutes will protect some of them. But there will continue to be young people, particularly in those states that have chosen not to enact detailed child commitment statutes, whose right to liberty must be protected, if at all, not by lawyers or courts but by the medical profession.

The psychiatrist called upon to make the decision to institutionalize or not must not allow himself or herself to be party to using the process of commitment to remove unruly or unwanted children from unpleasant situations. Particularly in light of the long stays of some children for lack of a home to which to return or a more appropriate placement, the admitting psychiatrist should see that discharge planning begins at the time of admission rather than at the time the child is ready for release.

Finally, the psychiatrist should realistically view the dangers inherent in forced hospitalization by taking the long view of treating a child's problems. More than determining whether the child can benefit from a stay in a hospital, the psychiatrist should ask how this period of institutionalization will likely affect the child's life over a period of years. What kind and quality of treatment will the child actually get? Will the family or state agency use this as a way to abdicate responsibility for the child? Will hospitalization improve the child's lot, taking into account the entire living situation, including the home to which the child may return? If a seemingly therapeutic short stay in a hospital stretches into an unnecessarily long period of time, will the benefits of the originally prescribed treatment be undone?

While it may be true, as Chief Justice Burger asserted in *Parham*, that "in the typical case" the decision to hospitalize a child is made cautiously, by competent, caring parents in consultation with well-trained and qualified psychiatrists, even the Chief Justice would have to concede that there are instances, such as those presented in the *Parham* case, involving uninformed and expedient decision-making by parents and other caretakers; conflicts of interest between children and their parents; abandonment of troublesome or intellectually limited children; use of mental institutions as asylums or as a form of incarceration; confinement of children and adolescents in understaffed, overly restrictive, depressing state institutions; and hospitalization of youngsters who could receive appropriate treatment in nonhospital, community-based programs.

In 1969 the Joint Commission on the Mental Health of Children reported that most state mental hospitals for children and adolescents provided little or inappropriate treatment because of shortages of professional staff, untrained aides, lack of educational and recreational programs, and outmoded facilities, and it concluded that, for these thousands of hospitalized youngsters, "instead of being helped, the vast majority are the worse for the experience" (28). More than a decade later, the Children's Defense Fund surveyed mental health facilities for children and adolescents and reported disturbingly similar findings (29).

Shortly after the Supreme Court's decision in the *Parham* case, Edward Futterman, a child psychiatrist, drafted a partial "dissenting opinion":

> While children do need protection from their own rebelliousness, they also need protection from arbitrary and capricious decision-making by parents and caretakers. While children do need protection from decision-making beyond their developmental capabilities, they also need protection from abandonment and from the use of the hospital as a form of incarceration. While parental responsibility, family autonomy and cooperation by families in the care of their children need to be respected, children need protection when

their own interests are in conflict with parental wishes. While children need to be protected in their access to necessary treatment, they need protection from the imposition of overly restrictive treatment approaches when less restrictive alternatives are available (30).

Parents' decisions to hospitalize their children may bear little relation to the severity of the child's mental condition or to the optimal therapeutic approach. Parents may simply not want to or not be able to continue living with a difficult child. Parental unwillingness to live with a difficult child may result in placement in a mental hospital because parents know of no other alternative, either because of a failure to devote sufficient effort to looking for appropriate services or inability to afford whatever appears to be available, or a combination of both (31).

Even if less restrictive alternatives exist, a youngster may be accepted for inpatient treatment by a psychiatric hospital because hospital staff are not required to investigate the availability of alternatives, may lack the time or competence to assist parents in identifying and making arrangements for nonhospital treatment, or may have a financial interest in accepting a child into their program.

Parents who have volunteered their child into a mental hospital may undercut the child's treatment by failing to cooperate in family therapy. Parents may be inconsistent or hostile in their attitudes toward their child's treatment and improvement and reluctant or unwilling to have their child return home, even when hospital staff conclude that the child should be discharged (32).

In addition to parent-child conflicts of interest and parental ignorance of less restrictive treatment alternatives, there are other causes of inappropriate hospitalization of children and adolescents. Admission is generally based on a short interview with the child, together with additional information supplied by the parent, guardian, or referring agency. Diagnosis is difficult, and diagnostic labels are vague. "Adjustment reaction" and "transient situational disturbance" are ambiguous and encompass a broad range of "normal" as well as "sick" behavior. Youngsters can spend extended periods of time in mental hospitals despite early findings of "no mental illness."

Often there is third-party pressure on the child, the parents, and the hospital. Judges, police, probation officers, social workers, and school personnel may recommend or insist upon psychiatric hospitalization, either for evaluation or treatment. All of these individuals may be acting from motives that, however well-intentioned, do not provide adequate protection against erroneous and unnecessary hospitalization.

Children and young adolescents may experience painful and traumatic psychological effects from being "locked up" in mental hospitals. Disruption in the continuity of relationships with adults is harmful for both young children and older adolescents. The committed child lives in a restrictive environment characterized by frequent staff turnovers and three different "shifts" of staff each day, making it difficult if not impossible to develop new, stable relationships. The committed child is denied the opportunity to explore the world. Instead he or she confronts an environment that places a premium on institutional efficiency and encourages compliant and passive behavior (33).

Because of the adverse effects of institutionalization on a child's cognitive, emotional, and social development, mental health professionals caution against hospitalization of a child, even in a superior facility, except when clearly necessary: "[N]o matter how good a treatment program for children in the state hospital is, hospitalization of an emotionally disturbed child is not the best answer . . . [The] basic experiences which a child needs in order to grow into an emotionally healthy, happy and productive adult . . . cannot be found in a hospital" (34).

Confinement in a mental hospital creates a special stigma not present in the placement of children in general hospitals or residential schools. The personal and social consequences of being labeled "mentally ill" are well documented in the professional literature (35). The label becomes "a double-edged blade . . . caus[ing] [the individual] to demean himself and to magnify social ostracism" (36).

The problem of stigmatization is magnified for children, who are more impressionable than adults, who are more likely to accept as true society's judgment that they are "crazy," and whose peer group is less tolerant of those who are "different."

For the child who requires psychiatric hospitalization, stigmatization is an unfortunate "side effect." But when a child is confined unnecessarily, the profound and long-term harm that results cannot be justified. A system that provides few procedural protections at the time of admission and no assurance that discharge will occur when therapeutically appropriate cannot protect children from the severe deprivation of liberty and other suffering caused by unnecessary, or unnecessarily prolonged, confinement in mental hospitals.

THE MEDICAL DECISION TO HOSPITALIZE A CHILD OR ADOLESCENT

There exist differing professional standards, and differences in professional practice, regarding the conditions and circumstances that warrant psychiatric hospitalization of children and adolescents. Other than in the *relatively* uncommon, clear cases involving suicidally depressed or dangerously psychotic juveniles, most minors whose hospitalization is sought by parents or other legal guardians manifest symptoms of conduct or personality disorders, adjustment reactions, or situational disturbances. Adults carrying such diagnoses would not be considered appropriate for involuntary commitment, since, as a rule, such persons do not pose an imminent risk of physical harm to themselves or others and are not wholly incapable of caring for themselves as a result of mental illness.

The National Association of Private Psychiatric Hospitals, the American Psychiatric Association, and the American Academy of Child and Adolescent Psychiatry have each issued standards for psychiatric hospitalization of children and adolescents (37). Notwithstanding their clinical language, the National Association guidelines are sufficiently general and behaviorally based that they could be used to justify the involuntary hospitalization of a wide range of acting out and nonconforming, as well as mentally ill and emotionally disturbed, youths. These guidelines include "self-defeating" or "self-destructive" behavior, inability "to attend to age-appropriate responsibilities," and "pronounced affective and/or behavioral disturbance" as reasons for psychiatric hospitalizations. An example of self-defeating or self-destructive behavior that might require "immediate acute-care hospitalization [as] the only reasonable intervention" is "sexual promiscuity," although the standards provide no definition of the type of sexual behavior to which that term ought objectively to apply. Behavior demonstrating "inability to function" that might justify hospitalization under these guidelines could be refusal to communicate with parents, angry outbursts, or participation in disapproved social activities, rather than doing homework, having

a job, participating in socially approved extracurricular activities, and spending time with one's family. Not only do the National Association guidelines emphasize behavioral disturbances, they lack a clear definition of the "mental disorders" that justify hospitalization.

The American Psychiatric Association (APA) standards provide a more "medical" definition of the type and severity of "mental disorder" that would justify the emergency or long-term psychiatric hospitalization of a minor: "'Mental disorder' means a substantial disorder of the child's cognitive, volitional, or emotional processes that grossly impairs judgment or capacity to recognize reality or to control behavior" (39). Under the APA guidelines, involuntary civil commitment of a minor would require a judicial finding "by clear and convincing evidence, that (a) the child has a mental disorder and that (b) the child is in need of treatment or care available at the institution for which certification is sought and that no less structured means are likely to be as effective in providing such treatment or care" (40).

The American Academy of Child and Adolescent Psychiatry standards are even more precise and medically based and assume that inpatient treatment should be employed only in situations where outpatient psychotherapy or other community-based treatment programs have been shown to be inadequate (41), and the youth is suffering from a severe problem that is primarily attributable to a "psychiatric disease" (42). Specific criteria justifying hospitalization under the American Academy standards include (a) "acute disabling symptoms of mental illness such as impaired reality testing, disordered or bizarre behavior, psychotic organic brain symptoms;" (b) "acute danger to property or self or others . . . attributable to primary psychiatric disease;" and (c) "severely impaired social or family or educational or vocational or developmental functioning" (43).

Whatever standards or guidelines are followed, the admitting physician who is called upon to make the decision whether or not to hospitalize a child or adolescent must exercise clinical judgment. He or she must determine whether the youngster suffers from a severe or acute disabling mental disorder that requires psychiatric treatment, whether he or she requires hospitalization in order to receive the treatment, whether such treatment is actually available in the hospital, whether he or she could obtain the treatment in a less restrictive setting or on an outpatient basis, and whether the potential benefits of involuntary psychiatric hospitalization outweigh the restriction of liberty, separation from family and friends, stigmatization, and other harms associated with institutionalization. In addition, the physician must carefully monitor the course of the treatment to ensure that the hospitalized juvenile does not spend any more time in confinement than is necessary to carry out the treatment plan, which should, in any event, be designed to help him or her return and adjust to life in the community as quickly as possible.

References

1. *Parham v. J.R.*, 442 U.S. 584,607–8(1979).
2. L.A. Weithorn, "Mental Hospitalization of Troublesome Youth: An Analysis of Skyrocketing Admission Rates," 40 *Stanford Law Review* 773, 788–89 (1988).
3. *Id.* at 783, n. 67.
4. *See* J. Ellis, "Volunteering Children: Parental Commitment of Minors to Mental Institutions," 62 *California Law Review* 840 (1974).
5. *See, e.g., J.L. v. Parham*, 412 F. Supp. 112 (M.D. Ga. 1976), *rev'd sub nom. Parham v. J.R.*, 442 U.S. 584 (1979); *Institutionalized Juveniles v. Secretary of Pub. Welfare*, 459 F. Supp. 30 (E.D. Pa. 1978), *rev'd*, 442 U.S. 640 (1979); *In re Rogers*, 19 Cal. 3d 921, 569 P.2d 1286, 141 Cal. Rptr. 298 (1977).
6. 442 U.S. at 607.
7. 442 U.S. at 632.
8. The review of state legislation that follows draws heavily on a state-by-state statutory analysis

contained in J. Knitzer, *Unclaimed Children: The Failure of Public Responsibility to Children and Adolescents in Need of Mental Health Services*, Washington, D.C.: Children's Defense Fund (1982), and L.A. Weithorn, "Mental Hospitalization of Troublesome Youth: An Analysis of Skyrocketing Admission Rates," 40 *Stanford Law Review* 773 (1988).
9. Arizona Revised Statutes, § 36-518 (Supp. 1986).
10. Virginia Code Annotated, § 37.1-67.3 (Supp. 1987), § 16.1-241(B) (1982), and Virginia Department of Mental Health and Mental Retardation, Departmental Instruction No. 60 (January 22, 1979).
11. Idaho Code, § 66-318 (Supp. 1987).
12. Loc. cit.
13. Loc. cit.
14. North Carolina General Statutes, § 122C-223(a) (1986). *See Protocol for the Admission of Children to Psychiatric Facilities* (North Carolina Council for Children, 1993), for a detailed de-

scription of the rights, roles, and responsibilities of children, lawyers, judges, and others in the psychiatric hospitalization of children pursuant to the North Carolina statute.
15. Loc. cit.
16. Florida Statutes Annotated § 394.467(2(a) (1987)).
17. Louisiana Revised Statutes, §§ 28:,54 and 57(F)-(G) (West Supp. 1987).
18. Connecticut General Statutes, § 17-205c, et seq., (1987).
19. Loc. cit.
20. Loc. cit.
21. New Mexico Statutes Annotated § 43-1-16.1(G)(1978).
22. Iowa Code Annotated. § 229.2 (West 1985).
23. Loc. cit.
24. Connecticut General Statutes, § 17a-75 (1991).
25. Illinois Annotated Statutes, chapter 91 1/2, paragraphs 3-505, 3-507 (Smith-Hurd Supp. 1986).
26. Loc. cit.
27. Oregon Revised Statutes, § 426.220(1) (1987).

28. *Crisis in Child Mental Health,* Joint Commission on the Mental Health of Children (New York: Harper & Row, 1969), p. 6.

29. Knitzer, J., op. cit.

30. Memorandum from Edward H. Futterman, M.D., Chairperson, American Psychiatric Association Council on Children, Adolescents and Their Families, to APA Commission on Judicial Action, et al., dated June 29, 1979.

31. *See* Ellis, op. cit., 851-52.

32. In general, children are more likely to stay longer in mental hospitals than are adults. *Crisis in Child Mental Health,* supra, p. 271. See also I. Rieger-Norbert, "Changing Concepts in Treating Children in a State Mental Hospital," *I Int. J. Child Psychotherapy* 89, 104 (1972): "[M]ost mentally ill children who are treated in a state hospital overstay, by months and even years, the optimum period required for their partial or total social restoration." A nationwide study reported that 40–50% of children and adolescents confined in mental hospitals are admitted inappropriately or remain hospitalized longer than necessary; Knitzer, op. cit. A recent national survey found that the average length of stay of children and adolescents in private psychiatric hospitals had decreased between 1990 and 1992, children from 36.4 days to 27.6 days, and adolescents from 33 days to 23.6 days. For adults during this same 2-year period, the average length of stay in private psychiatric hospitals declined from 19.6 days to 15.8 days. *National Association of Psychiatric Health Systems 1992*, Annual Survey: Final Report, summarized in *Hospital and Community Psychiatry*, v. 44, n.9 (Sept. 1993) at pp. 898–899. The survey did not include public psychiatric hospitals where nearly half of all hospitalized children and adolescents are confined and where the lack of private insurance constraints often results in longer periods of confinement than typically occur in private hospitals.

33. "[H]ospitalization in a mental institution is a serious and possibly injurious event in the life of an individual, particularly a child or adolescent. Institutionalized individuals are cut off from significant interpersonal relationships with family and friends, and from their usual life activities. Institutionalization creates a major discontinuity in a person's life. It also places him or her within an artificial, regimented, and restrictive environment that can seriously harm those not in need of such placement." Affidavit of Eli C. Messinger, M.D., filed on August 28, 1975, in the case of *Poe v. Weinberger,* Civ. No. 74-1800, U.S. District Court, District of Columbia.

34. I. Riegel-Norbert, op. cit., 104, 197. One study found no advantage in therapeutic results for adolescent inpatients when compared with a comparable group that had been treated as outpatients; K. Flomenhalt, "Outcome of Treatment for Adolescents," 9 *Adolescence* 57 (1974).

35. *See* J. Rabkin, "Public Attitudes Toward Mental Illness: A Review of the Literature," *Schizophrenia Bulletin 9,* 10 (Issue 10, Fall 1974).

36. *In re Ballay,* 482 F.2d 648, 669 (D.C. Cir. 1973).

37. National Association of Private Psychiatric Hospitals, Guidelines for Psychiatric Hospital Programs: Children and Adolescents (1989); American Psychiatric Association Council on Children, Adolescents, and their Families, Task Force on the Commitment of Minors: Guidelines for the Psychiatric Hospitalization of Minors (1981), *Am J Psychiatry* 139:7 (July 1982); American Academy of Child and Adolescent Psychiatry, Child and Adolescent Psychiatric Illness: Guidelines for Treatment Resources, Quality Assurance, Peer Review and Reimbursement (1987).

38. National Association Guidelines, 3–4.

39. APA Guidelines, § 1(g).

40. APA Guidelines, § 4(e)(iii).

41. American Academy Guidelines, 30, Core Guideline A.1.

42. American Academy Guidelines, 34–35, Specific Guideline I.A.

43. *Id.,* Specific Guidelines I.A. 1, 2,8 (emphasis added).

114 The Mental Health Professional in the Juvenile Justice System

Stephen Wizner, J.D.

Mental health professionals occupy a special place in the juvenile justice system. Because of the rehabilitative and therapeutic goals of the juvenile court and its expressed commitment to individualized, nonpunitive dispositions for children and adolescents who are brought before it, mental health professionals are frequently called upon to evaluate juveniles, to recommend treatment or other rehabilitative programs, and to provide consultation and expert testimony.

Juvenile court judges, probation officers, and attorneys defer to and rely upon the opinions and recommendations of mental health professionals. It is therefore important for the clinician who would provide services in the juvenile court to be familiar with its history, jurisdiction, and procedure, as well as with its limitations.

HISTORY OF THE JUVENILE COURT

Jane Addams and other turn-of-the-century social reformers brought the juvenile court into being in order to rescue misbehaving children from the harshness and rigidity of the adult criminal justice system (1). In contrast to the criminal justice system, designed to apprehend, prosecute, and punish offenders for the protection of society, the goals of the child-saving movement were the identification, evaluation, and treatment of maladjusted youths for their own benefit, and ultimately society's.

Beginning in Chicago in 1899 and eventually spreading throughout the country, the juvenile court (in some states called the family court) was envisioned as a humane, informal, treatment-oriented social agency that would "save" delinquent children from what the reformers saw as the failure of many immigrant and other impoverished parents to cope with the adverse effects on their children of an increasingly urban and industrial environment.

Initially, the jurisdiction of the juvenile court was broad, encompassing both criminal and noncriminal misbehavior. Children who had committed no crimes but who were alleged to be truant, disobedient, engaging in undesirable behavior, associating with unacceptable companions, or otherwise beyond the control of their parents ("ungovernable") were brought before the juvenile court, together with those who were charged with criminal offenses, in order that they might receive the treatment, discipline, and care they required. These so-called "status offenders" were treated the same as youths who were charged with criminal offenses, though in many jurisdictions they were given a different label, such as "persons in need of supervision" (PINS).

The juvenile justice reformers believed that juvenile misbehavior, criminal or otherwise, was not a law enforcement problem but a social-psychological problem of children and their families, requiring state interference with and assumption of the parental function of child rearing. It was possible, they believed, and therefore proper, to discipline, educate, and reform the errant and neglected children of the urban poor through the intervention of kindly judges, supportive probation officers, and well-meaning social workers and volunteers. If necessary, children were to be removed from their families and placed in rural reform or "training" schools where they would be subject to long hours of physical labor and strict discipline.

There were theoretical flaws and practical problems in the child-saver's program for curing juvenile delinquency. The coercive nature of involuntary court-imposed "therapy," however benevolently intended, must have seemed punitive from the child's perspective, since it was imposed as a consequence of the child's having engaged in disapproved conduct. The "treatment" provided—judicial admonition, probation supervision, counseling, and confinement in reform schools—was frequently both excessively intrusive and ineffective. Moreover, the theory was based on a simplistic and sentimental view of the nature of children and their psychological development and a naive and romantic faith in the extent to which youthful rebelliousness and antisocial behavior were amenable to treatment of the type offered by the juvenile court.

From the outset, juvenile courts lacked the resources even to attempt to carry out their program. Insufficient funds were appropriated by legislatures to enable juvenile courts to provide individualized justice or to implement costly treatment plans for the majority of juveniles who appeared before them. There were not enough qualified mental health professionals available to the court to perform the evaluation, referral, and treatment services that were required. As with many social reform movements, rhetoric outpaced reality.

In addition, the court's treatment-oriented approach was thought to provide insufficient protection for the community from certain juveniles who committed serious crimes or were repeat offenders. Thus, as early as 1903, only 4 years after the first juvenile court was established in Chicago, that court transferred 14 children to the adult criminal system (2). By the 1970s every state, the District of Columbia, and the federal government had laws authorizing or requiring the criminal prosecution in adult courts of certain minors found to be "not amenable to treatment" (3).

Critics have pointed to the unbridled discretion, rehabilitative pretensions, and punitive realities of the juvenile court. They have called for restriction of juvenile court jurisdiction, limitation of the discretion of juvenile court judges, diversion of petty (or first) offenders to nonjudicial alternatives, procedural safeguards, and improved facilities, resources, and treatment (4).

The rising tide of criticism of the juvenile court culminated in the 1960s and thereafter in legislative reforms and judicial decisions that mandated procedural protection for juveniles and narrowed the court's jurisdiction. The New York Family Court Act of 1962 introduced due process into that state's family courts. A major innovation of the act was its provision for "law guardians," independent lawyers who were appointed to represent juveniles who came before the court. In 1966 the United States Supreme Court decided the landmark case of *Kent v. United States,* holding that the transfer, or "waiver," of a juvenile to an adult criminal court was "an invitation to procedural arbitrariness," and a decision "of such tremendous consequences" that it ought not be made without a hearing that provided "the essentials of due process and fair treatment" (5).

In 1967, in *In re Gault,* the Supreme Court expanded on its decision in Kent and ordered the provision of due process protection to all juveniles in delinquency proceedings, characterizing the existing informal juvenile court procedure as "a kangaroo court" (6).

Finally, in 1977 the United States Congress enacted legislation requiring states seeking federal financial assistance for juvenile delinquency programs to cease confining status offenders—children charged with noncriminal misbehavior—in secure detention or correctional facilities intended for juvenile delinquents (7).

The combined effect of the introduction of due process protections into juvenile delinquency proceedings, due process restrictions on the transfer of serious offenders to adult courts, and the effective removal of status offenders from the court's delinquency jurisdiction, together with an apparent increase in the incidence of serious juvenile crime, have left the juvenile court with a clientele that is more violent, more disturbed, and less amenable to superficial therapeutic interventions than that envisioned by Jane Addams and her fellow child-savers. In the words of one juvenile court prosecutor,

> [The juvenile court is]a very depressing, horrible place. It's completely not in the real world . . . .How does this court think it's going to rehabilitate a fifteen-year-old who's lived in an entirely different society . . . .The Family

Court was made for the little newsboy who broke somebody's window with a stone. That's when the laws were made. Not for the fifteen-year-old who's into drugs and killing (8).

PRACTICE IN THE JUVENILE COURT

Mental health professionals are called upon by the juvenile court to perform evaluations, to make treatment and program recommendations, and to provide consultation and expert testimony (9). It is important that the clinician who chooses to work in the juvenile court be familiar with its procedures and specialized terminology.

A juvenile delinquency case normally begins with an arrest, referred to as an "apprehension." The juvenile is either released to the custody of his or her parent or held in a "detention center," the equivalent of an adult jail for pretrial detainees. If the child is to be detained, he or she is provided a "detention hearing" before a judge. The standard for detention is customarily whether detention is necessary for the protection of the community or is otherwise in the child's best interests. "Preventive detention," the practice of incarcerating juveniles prior to trial in order to prevent them from committing further delinquent acts during the pretrial period, was upheld as constitutional by the United States Supreme Court in a 1984 decision, *Schall v. Martin,* on the ground that "juveniles, unlike adults, are always in some form of custody" (10).

Whether or not a juvenile has been taken into custody, the child and his or her parents will normally be summoned to an intake interview with a court probation officer. At that stage, a decision is made whether to proceed "nonjudicially" by diverting the child to a community resource for services or to advance the case to the next stage of the process. This normally requires that the youngster "admit" (confess) to the charges and agree to participate in the treatment or program recommended by the probation officer.

In some jurisdictions the child is brought before a judge, either before, after, or instead of the intake meeting with the probation officer, in order to "admit" (plead guilty) or "deny" (plead not guilty) the allegations contained in a "petition" (indictment or complaint) alleging that the child has committed specified acts that if committed by an adult would constitute a crime. The court official—probation officer or prosecutor (in some jurisdictions euphemistically referred to by some title such as "court advocate")—who signs the petition, or the state, is called the "petitioner," and the child the "respondent." At that hearing, analogous to an adult arraignment, the judge informs the juvenile and his or her parents of their rights, including the right to counsel. If the family cannot afford to hire an attorney, the court appoints a public defender or private attorney paid by the court to represent the child.

If the juvenile is an older, repeat offender and is charged with a serious criminal offense, the probation officer or prosecutor may seek to have the case "waived" (transferred) to an adult criminal court on the ground that the respondent is "not amenable to treatment" as a juvenile. A hearing is then held by the court to determine whether the types of "dispositions" (sentences) available in the juvenile court are likely to be of benefit to the juvenile and sufficient for the protection of the community.

The juvenile delinquency proceeding itself is in two stages. First, there is an "adjudicatory hearing" (trial). If the child is found guilty, there is said to have been a "finding" or "adjudication" (conviction). Second, if there has been an adjudication, the case proceeds to the "dispositional" (sentencing) phase. Prior to disposition, a probation officer will conduct a predisposition investigation and prepare a dispositional recommendation. At the disposition hearing the judge will consider the recommendations of the probation officer, the child's attorney, and any other relevant information and impose a "disposition" (sentence), which may be supervised or unsupervised probation, including probationary conditions such as a curfew, school attendance, counseling, or psychotherapy; community service; or a residential program in a private residential school or treatment center or in a state "training school" (the equivalent of an adult correctional institution).

THE MENTAL HEALTH PROFESSIONAL IN THE JUVENILE COURT

The rehabilitative ideal continues to inspire the rhetoric and guide the practice in the juvenile court. Individualized justice and nonpunitive, treatment-oriented dispositions intended to help juvenile offenders and, in so doing, to protect society are the articulated goals, if not the reality, of the juvenile court. Forensic child clinicians are regularly called upon by the court to perform mental health evaluations and family assessments, to recommend and refer juveniles to treatment, to consult with court staff and the child's advocate, and to provide expert testimony.

Unlike the adult criminal justice system, where mental health professionals most frequently are called upon to offer expert opinions on issues of competency, insanity, and diminished capacity, in the juvenile justice system the principal mental health issue is "amenability to treatment." At both preadjudicatory and postadjudicatory stages of a juvenile delinquency proceeding, the need for treatment, the appropriate type of treatment, and the likelihood of benefit from treatment are central concerns.

At intake the probation officer must decide whether to handle ("adjust") the case "nonjudicially" by releasing the juvenile or diverting him or her to a community agency or to file a petition and seek an adjudication of delinquency and court-imposed disposition. At this stage "disposition bargaining," analogous to adult plea bargaining, is common. The juvenile's advocate, or the juvenile may attempt to avoid the risk of incarceration or other restrictive disposition by admitting to some or all of the facts in exchange for some less intrusive form of community-based treatment.

If the probation officer is persuaded that the juvenile is amenable to treatment by a community agency, and the juvenile admits some or all of the facts alleged as the basis for the arrest and agrees to accept the referral to the community agency and to cooperate in the proposed treatment, the juvenile will not be required to stand trial before a juvenile court judge and face the possibility of an adjudication and court-imposed disposition.

At the intake stage both the probation officer and the juvenile's advocate may seek an expert clinical opinion regarding the respondent's amenability to treatment as an alternative to incarceration or other court-imposed disposition.

The next point in the process at which amenability to treatment may be evaluated is the so-called "waiver hearing" at which a judge decides whether to transfer a juvenile to the adult court for criminal prosecution. Often, a juvenile considered for transfer will be an older, repeat offender, charged with a serious crime. The mental health professional asked to evaluate such a youngster's amenability to treatment will need to consider the youth's prior experience with juvenile court dispositions, whether there are appropriate dispositional alternatives available to the juvenile court that have not been tried, and the relative superiority of dispositional alternatives available in the criminal justice system to address the juvenile's problems.

If the juvenile is not diverted or transferred from the juvenile court and he or she is adjudicated a juvenile delinquent, the mental health professional may be called upon at the dispositional stage to assess the youngster's amenability to treatment by performing a mental health evaluation and recommending a particular type of therapeutic or rehabilitative disposition.

The most common disposition is probation, involving periodic meetings with a juvenile court probation officer, and special conditions of probation, which may include psychotherapy. If the juvenile is determined not to be amenable to treatment in the community; he or she may be incarcerated in a training school or "placed" in a residential treatment program. The court is frequently guided by the recommendations of mental health professionals in deciding which of these dispositions to impose.

Assessment of the need for and amenability to treatment and recommendation of appropriate dispositions is the principal function of the mental health professional in the juvenile court. This function can be carried out in different roles. The forensic child clinician may serve as an adjunct to the court, providing consultation (or testimony) for the judge, probation staff or prosecutor. The clinician may also assist the defense. In either role, the clinician may be able to provide expert assistance in diagnosing mental health problems and their relationship to the particular behavior at issue, in supporting or rebutting claims that individual juveniles are or are not amenable to treatment, in recommending treatment or other rehabilitative programs, and in evaluating previous efforts to treat or rehabilitate an individual juvenile.

EVALUATION AND TREATMENT IN THE JUVENILE JUSTICE SYSTEM

The term *treatment* is used broadly in the juvenile justice system. A child or adolescent may be considered to be in need of or amenable to treatment not only because of a psychiatric condition but also, and more often, because of behavioral problems that may not be treatable by psychotherapy alone, or at all. Consequently, "a thorough assessment of a juvenile's amenability to treatment should usually include an evaluation not only of personality functioning, but also of cognitive, educational, vocational, and social needs in the context of the various systems (e.g., family, school, neighborhood) of which he or she is a part" (11).

It is important for the clinician to appreciate that the juvenile court's rhetorical commitment to individualized treatment and the rehabilitative ideal tends to mask a law enforcement function. As a practical matter, the juvenile court is concerned with community protection, notwithstanding its child-saving rhetoric. Judges, probation officers, and prosecutors want to know not only whether a child or adolescent suffers from a mental health problem for which he or she should receive treatment but whether that problem is the cause of the misconduct and whether the proposed treatment is likely to prevent the juvenile from recidivating. Therefore, mental health professionals must take care that they are not co-opted into a system that may misuse their expertise and induce them to exceed the bounds of their professional competence.

It is often not possible for the clinician to establish a clear connection between a juvenile's mental or emotional problems and the specific offense charged, or to predict the efficacy of a treatment plan in preventing recidivism. Indeed, research on the effectiveness of "correctional treatment" shows that most interventions appear to have little positive effect on recidivism and many appear to exacerbate the problem (12). Nevertheless, the clinician should offer the court his or her expert opinion and clinical judgment about the child's treatment needs and leave it to the court to determine whether the recommendations, if followed, will strike the proper legal balance between promoting the best interests of the child and protecting the community from the child.

References

1. J. Addams, et al., eds., *The Child, the Clinic and the Court* (New York: New Republic, Inc. 1925). Two excellent histories of the American juvenile court movement are E. Ryerson, *The Best Laid Plans: America's Juvenile Court Experiment* (New York: Hill & Wang, 1978); and A. Platt, *The Child Savers: The Invention of Delinquency* (Chicago: University of Chicago Press, 1969). In addition to its delinquency jurisdiction, the juvenile court also has jurisdiction over proceedings against parents alleged to have neglected or abused their children. Consideration of the court's neglect and abuse jurisdiction is beyond the scope of this chapter. See generally, *Institute of Judicial Administration and American Bar Association Juvenile Justice Standards Project: Standards Relating to Abuse and Neglect* (Cambridge, Massachusetts: Ballinger, 1981); Goldstein, Freud & Solnit, *Before the Best Interests of the Child* (New York: Free Press, 1979).

2. Cook County [Illinois] Charity Service Report 253 (1920), cited in Twentieth Century Fund Task Force on Sentencing Policy Toward Young Offenders, Confronting Youth Crime 55 (1978).

3. D. Hamparian, ed., *Youth in Adult Courts: Between Two Worlds* (Columbus, Ohio Academy for Contemporary Problems, 1982), 97–100, 143.

4. See, e.g., President's Commission on Law Enforcement and Administration of Justice, Task Force Report: *Juvenile Delinquency and Youth Crime* (1967); F. Allen, *The Borderland of Criminal Justice* (Chicago: University of Chicago Press, 1964); J. Polier, *A View from the Bench*

(1964); P. Murphy, *Our Kindly Parent—The State: The Juvenile Justice System and How It Works* (New York: Viking Press, 1974); *Institute of Judicial Administration & American Bar Association, Juvenile Justice Standards Project: Standards Relating to Juvenile Delinquency and Sanctions, Dispositions, and Noncriminal Misbehavior* (Cambridge, Massachusetts: Ballinger, 1981). See also, Juvenile Justice and Delinquency Prevention Act of 1974, as amended, 42 US Code § 5601 et seq., at § 5601 (a)(2): "The Congress hereby finds that...understaffed, over-crowded juvenile courts, probation services, and correctional facilities and inadequately trained staff in such courts, services and facilities are not able to provide individualized justice or effective help."
5. 383 US 541, 554–555, 562 (1966).

6. 387 US 1 (1967).
7. 42 US Code § 5633 (12) (1977).
8. P. Prescott, *The Child Savers: Juvenile Justice Observed* (New York: Alfred A. Knopf 1981), p. 168.
9. For a detailed description of juvenile court practice, and of the mental health professional's role in the court, see G. Melton, et al., *Psychological Evaluations for the Courts: A Handbook for Mental Health Professionals and Lawyers* (New York: Guilford Press, 1987, chapter 11, "Juvenile Delinquency"). See also, E. Futterman, et al., The Psychiatrist and the Juvenile Justice System, Report of the American Psychiatric Association Task Force on Juvenile Justice Issues, (revised version, 10/88).
10. *Schall v. Martin,* 467 U.S. 253, 265 (1984).
11. G. Melton, et al., op. cit. supra, at 300. See also

Juvenile Justice and Delinquency Prevention Act of 1974, as amended, 42 US Code § 5601 et seq., at § 5603(15): The term "treatment" includes but is not limited to medical, educational, special education social, psychological and vocational services, corrective and preventive guidance and training, and other rehabilitative services designed to protect the public, including services designed to benefit addicts and other users by eliminating their dependence on alcohol or other addictive or nonaddictive drugs or by controlling their dependence and susceptibility to addiction or use.
12. J.T. Whitehead & S.P. Lab, "A Meta-Analysis of Juvenile Correctional Treatment," *Journal of Research in Crime and Delinquency,* v. 26, n. 3, pp. 276–295 (1989).

115 MALPRACTICE

Barry Nurcombe, M.D., F.R.A.C.P.

THE CURRENT SITUATION

All physicians feel the burden of malpractice insurance; many will be sued at some time in their careers. Child psychiatrists are not sued as often as physicians who rely heavily on technology; however, their involvement in the hospitalization and medication of severely disturbed patients makes it likely that the profession will be a target for litigation.

Since 1980, the overall size of malpractice awards has risen by 12.7% per year, nearly double that of the yearly increase in the cost of living, and more than double the average yearly rise in medical costs. This startling increase in malpractice awards is the result of vigorous and ingenious legal advocacy (Rosenberg, 1988). Medical malpractice claims produce higher awards than the usual civil liability suit but they are more difficult to win. Currently, the national average for recovery in medical malpractice suits is 46%, compared to 57% in civil liability actions. The average monetary award in psychiatric malpractice suits is $340,000, compared to about $1,100,000 in all medical malpractice.

Traditionally, emotional injury was not compensable, largely because authorities feared opening a floodgate of dubious, unassessable suits. However, the courts have begun to regard emotional injury more favorably, particularly if the defendant's breach was wanton, outrageous, or extreme. Moreover, the proposed limitation of monetary awards for "pain and suffering" has been struck down in several states as unconstitutional; and awards have been made in some jurisdictions for "hedonic damages" (i.e., for post-traumatic impairment in the capacity to enjoy life.)

The potentially lucrative nature of malpractice litigation crowds the field and makes it intensely competitive. Able lawyers keep current with the medical literature, brandish *DSM-IV* in the courtroom, and grill clinicians on the meaning of such terms as "reliability" and "validity." The clinician would be wise to understand the basis of malpractice law and to take steps to limit liability. On the other hand, despite the increasing regulation and legal scrutiny of medicine, it is imperative that the profession avoid defensive psychiatry with its interminable tests, therapeutic homeopathy, and unnecessarily prolonged hospitalization: paradoxically, excessive caution can also put the clinician at risk of an action for negligence (Simon, 1987).

THE ELEMENTS OF MALPRACTICE LAW

The term "malpractice" refers to an *act or omission* by a professional in the course of his or her *professional duty*, which *causes or aggravates* an injury to a patient or client, and which is *the consequence of a failure to exercise a reasonable degree of prudence, diligence, knowledge, or skill.* In other words, to be held liable for malpractice, one must do something one shouldn't do, or fail to do something one should, and the act or omission must represent a level of care which is demonstrably less prudent, less diligent, less informed, or less skillful than would be provided by the average practitioner of the same training, in the same circumstances. Furthermore, the substandard act or omission must cause the patient a demonstrable injury which is of a compensable nature.

In order to substantiate malpractice, the plaintiff must establish the following four points, by a preponderance of the evidence:

1. A relationship existed between the clinician and the patient such that the clinician owed *a duty of reasonable care* to the patient.
2. When judged by the standard of the average, prudent practitioner, the clinician *breached the duty of care.*
3. The patient sustained *compensable injury or harm.*
4. The said injury or harm was a *direct result* of the clinician's failure to exercise a reasonable standard of care; or, in other words, the clinician's dereliction was the *proximate cause* of the patient's injury.

Duty of Care

THE CONTRACTUAL RELATIONSHIP

The clinician owes a duty of reasonable care toward a patient when there is a professional relationship between them. This relationship is formed when a clinician explicitly or implicitly agrees to provide care to a patient. The clinician thus enters a contract which binds him to provide a reasonable level of care in return for a valuable consideration (the fee). Note that, unless the clinician has unwisely promised a cure, he is not bound to provide more than a reasonable level of care.

The doctor-patient relationship cannot be imposed upon a competent patient; nor can a doctor be forced to care for a patient. The most controversial situations arise when it is argued that a relationship has been implied by the physician's actions or words. For example, the discussion of a patient's condition by telephone prior to transfer to a different hospital has been held to imply a contractual relationship (*O'Neill v. Montefiore Hospital*, 1960). Payment is not necessary; gratuitous services attract a duty. The clinician should be careful about giving casual advice at cocktail parties and the like, lest it be construed that a contractual relationship has been formed.

On the other hand, a physician cannot be forced to treat patients who are unable to pay for services, or to use a treatment he or she is not competent to implement. The physician also has a legal (if not an ethical) right to refuse to give aid in an emergency. Good Samaritan laws have been enacted to protect from liability those physicians who do render emergency aid, unless they have been grossly negligent (e.g., abandoning a live patient who is still hemorrhaging).

After the termination of the contract, the physician owes no further obligation to the patient other than that of confidentiality. Physicians who terminate contracts unilaterally and without reasonable cause are at risk of actions for *abandonment*. The physician must give the patient due notice of termination and ensure that necessary arrangements are made for alternative care. If the patient resists termination, failure to refer to another physician may be construed as negligence.

Clinicians may examine people on behalf of a third party, such as a government agency, to whom they owe a contractual duty. However, if the examination causes the examinee harm, for example by failure to detect suicidality or the possibility of child abuse, the liability risk is ambiguous. Some courts have held that the clinician's duty is to the employer; others have held that, if the person being examined reasonably relied upon the examination for diagnosis, a duty might be owed. The physician is advised to inform the examinee that the examination is not therapeutic in purpose.

VICARIOUS LIABILITY

In accordance with the doctrine of *respondeat superior*, a physician is legally responsible for the negligent actions of employees or supervisees. Thus, a psychiatrist may be held liable for the actions of an intern, resident, or nurse on an inpatient service, or for the negligence or outrageous behavior of a nurse or assistant employed in his office.

THE FIDUCIARY RELATIONSHIP

The clinician's obligations toward his patient go beyond the duty to provide reasonable care. The relationship between psychiatrist and patient is analogous to that between guardian and ward. The patient has a right to expect the physician to show good faith, that is, to act in the patient's best interest. This, the physician's *fiduciary duty*, is especially onerous in psychiatry, because emotionally disturbed people share their most private experiences with their mental health clinicians, and are, thus, very vulnerable. Improper sexual contact, invasion of privacy, breach of confidentiality, outrageous manipulation of the patient's emotions, and the exploitation of patients for financial gain are all examples of *double agentry* and *breaches of fiduciary trust*. These *intentional torts* will be discussed later in this chapter.

CONFIDENTIALITY AND PRIVILEGE

By ethical code and law, the physician is precluded from divulging private matters revealed by the patient in the context of the doctor-patient relationship. *Privilege* is the patient's right to bar his physician from disclosing confidential matters in a court of law.

In most jurisdictions, testimonial privilege derives from statute. Physicians should consult their local statutes to understand the extent of this privilege and its exceptions. Confusion may occur when a clinician receives a *subpoena* to appear in court (with or without records). *A subpoena merely requires the clinician to appear in court. It does not compel him to testify about confidential matters unless the patient has specifically authorized him to do so, or has waived privilege, or unless the clinician is ordered to do so by the judge.* If the clinician is asked to disclose confidential matters in court, he should refrain from doing so and ask the judge for guidance.

Although the states vary somewhat in the *exceptions* allowed to the rule of privilege, the following are the most usual:

1. *Waiver of privilege.* The clinician should seek specific written authorization from the patient before disclosing confidential material in court or to other parties (such as other mental health agencies).

2. *The psychiatric evidence exclusion.* If a patient offers his or her mental health as evidence in litigation, he or she waives privilege concerning the specific issue in evidence. Similarly, if the patient pleads insanity as a criminal defense, the psychiatric examination conducted to evaluate that matter is not privileged (*Bremer v. State*, 1973).

3. *Evaluation for a reason other than psychiatric treatment.* For example, the psychiatric evaluation of a disputant in a child custody case is not privileged if the evaluation was conducted as part of the case. A similar exclusion applies to evaluations for the purpose of civil commitment.

4. *Duty to protect endangered third parties.* The *Tarasoff* exclusion applies when the community is endangered. It is discussed later in this chapter.

Standard of Care

In accordance with the contract inherent in the doctor-patient relationship, the physician is bound to provide a reasonable level of care. In other words, the physician contracts to provide reasonable, prudent, diligent, knowledgeable and skillful medical care. Unless the clinician has unwisely promised a cure, the contract does not call for exceptional care, only a level of expertise equivalent to that exercised under similar circumstances by the average practitioner in the same field of medicine. *The clinician is not liable for an error of judgment unless the error represented a substandard level of care.*

The considerable variation between clinicians in methods of treatment has made standards difficult to establish, particularly in regard to psychotherapy. On the other hand, the standard is tighter with regard to precautions against suicide or violence, or monitoring medication.

Breach of the Duty of Care

Malpractice suits are founded in the legal theories of intentional and negligent torts. An *intentional tort* involves deliberate intent on the part of the wrongdoer, or wrongful conduct that the wrongdoer ought to have known was unacceptable (in which case it is known as a *quasi-intentional tort*). Examples of intentional torts are assault, battery, false imprisonment, fraudulent commitment, defamation, invasion of privacy, sexual exploitation, and the intentional infliction of emotional distress. Expert testimony is not required to substantiate an intentional tort; and malpractice insurance may not cover it. A *negligent tort* involves an unintentional error which reflects a failure by the clinician to exercise a reasonable standard of medical care. Expert testimony is required for proof of negligence.

The standard of care is established by professional practice and traditionally required that the clinician be judged by the professional standard in that locality. However, the emergence of national standards has caused the courts to move in this direction, with allowance for the paucity of resources in some areas. The standard of care is also linked to the standard of professional practice at the time of the alleged breach of duty; clinicians are expected to stay abreast of developments. If a clinician practices medicine in a specialty area for which he is not trained, he is likely to be held to the standard applying to that speciality.

Harm, Injury, or Damage

Harm may be physical or psychological. As previously described, the courts have been reluctant to award damages for psychological injury, unless the wrongdoer's actions have been wanton or outrageous. Physical harm or damage resulting from negligence can vary: for example, side effects of medication (such as tardive dyskinesia), physical injury incurred when a patient is improperly restrained, or homicide or suicide occurring when a patient is negligently released from a hospital. All these situations will be discussed later in this chapter.

Proximate Cause

The plaintiff must substantiate that the defendant's wrongful act or omission directly caused or aggravated the patient's injury. In other words, it must be proven that, but for the wrongful conduct, the damage would not have occurred or would not have been aggravated, or that there was a direct, uninterrupted link or foreseeable chain of events between the wrongful conduct and the injury or its aggravation. The legal concept of "cause" is analogous to the psychiatric concept of "precipitation" or "aggravation."

If Dr. A misdiagnoses B's illness, B must prove that, if not misdiagnosed, he would have received treatment that would have alleviated his condition. If Dr. A is held negligent in prescribing treatment X rather than treatment Y, B must still prove that, more probably than not, treatment Y would have been successful.

Damages

If the defendant is found liable, the judge or jury may award damages. Damages are designed to be *compensatory*, that is, to recompense the victim for medical expenses, pain, suffering, loss of enjoyment of life, impairment of capacity, and future loss of earnings, and to restore the plaintiff to his original position, so far as money is able to do so. If the defendant's behavior has been egregiously outrageous, malicious or wanton, *punitive* damages may be imposed over and above compensatory damages. Psychiatric evidence may be required to inform the jury about the impact of an injury on the plaintiff's capacity to enjoy life. Injury to a parent or child may give rise to an action for loss of consortium, that is, the loss of the care, comfort, and society of a spouse, parent, or child.

CIRCUMSTANCES IN WHICH MALPRACTICE IS MOST LIKELY TO OCCUR

Child psychiatrists are most at risk of liability in particular circumstances. This section describes the most perilous situations and their attendant risks.

Hospitalization

During the past ten years, there has been an increase of psychiatric beds for children and adolescents, and more child psychiatrists have begun to work in inpatient settings. Hospitalization and medication, which are often combined, present a number of situations in which the clinician is at risk of liability.

ADMISSION

Negligent Failure to Admit

The physician may fail to admit a suicidal or violent patient who subsequently harms himself or others. Such an error might be actionable if the physician had failed to evaluate the patient adequately, for example, by assessing mental status or reviewing the patient's past history for dangerous behavior. The assessment of suicide or violence risk will be discussed later in this chapter.

Wrongful Commitment, False Imprisonment, and Fraud

A physician who causes a patient to be admitted to a psychiatric hospital without proper evaluation may be sued for *negligent diagnosis* or *false imprisonment*. A falsely imprisoned plaintiff may recover damages for *loss of dignity* and *emotional distress*. Ignorance of the Mental Health Act is no defense; failure to comply with statutory requirements could be actionable. For example, in *Johnson v. Greer* (1973), a patient recovered damages after being forcibly detained in hospital for several days beyond the 24 hours permitted on an Emergency Warrant. Malice, spite, ulterior motive, bad faith, or fraud during involuntary hospitalization could also result in damages for false imprisonment or *malicious prosecution*, as was the case in *Pendleton v. Burkhalter* (1968). Parents or guardians may admit unemancipated minors against their will, and health care providers should be able to rely on parental consent (*R.J.D.*

v. Vaughan Clinic, 1990). However, the psychiatric justification for admission should be carefully documented.

NEGLIGENT DIAGNOSIS

The failure to distinguish organic disease from psychiatric disorder, or to differentiate functional psychosis from other psychiatric disorder, or to discriminate between the major psychoses, could be actionable if it resulted from inadequate or inept diagnostic investigation and if it caused harm to the patient.

PATIENT MANAGEMENT

Failure to Protect or Control a Suicidal, Violent, or Sexually Aggressive Patient

Hospitals assume a duty of care toward patients with a potential for suicide or violence. The psychiatrist must carefully assess the potential for danger, and ensure that the hospital staff take adequate precautions to protect a suicidal or violent patient from doing harm to himself or others. Past medical records should be scrutinized, and referring agents and parents questioned, concerning suicide potential. In accordance with the imminence of the risk, housing in a secure unit, confinement to a room, close observation, a search of clothing and personal effects, and removal of all dangerous objects (e.g., belts, mirrors), may be required. If the patient is medicated, staff should check that medication is actually swallowed. It is essential that the degree and nature of risk be communicated to all staff who care for the patient. The importance of good medical recordkeeping cannot be overstressed. Timely, clear, legible, pertinent, thorough, dated, timed, and signed records are the key to communication and the best proof that hospital and staff have exercised reasonable care. In *Abille v. United States* (1980), after a psychiatrist transferred a patient from a suicidal status to a less dangerous status, the patient committed suicide. The finding of negligence against the defendant hinged upon the psychiatrist's failure to keep detailed records that explained his decision to transfer, even though it was conceded that, under the circumstances, the decision might have been a reasonable one.

What if the patient refuses to cooperate with the admitting psychiatrist who consequently does not elicit and diagnose imminent suicide risk? In *Skar v. City of Lincoln, Nebraska* (1979), a recalcitrant patient injured himself in a suicide attempt. The court found for the defendant, holding that the patient had a duty to cooperate with his physician as far as he was able. However, it is essential in such a case that the psychiatrist record the questions put to the patient and the patient's responses or failure to respond.

The prevalence of sexual abuse and its relationship to psychiatric disorder mean that many minors admitted to psychiatric hospitals are at risk of precocious sexual activity and unwanted pregnancy. Known perpetrators should be closely observed and housed in single rooms, if necessary. Actions may be brought against hospitals and physicians who fail to take reasonable precautions to protect other patients from sexual assault, sexual coercion, or illicit sexual activity. Similar strictures apply to a failure to take reasonable precautions to protect others from physically violent patients. However, the closeness of the observation possible decreases if the therapeutic environment is less restrictive, for example, in a residential treatment center.

Negligent Release or Discharge of a Suicidal or Violent Patient

A patient may harm himself or others while on pass in the grounds of the hospital, on leave with relatives or friends, after discharge, or after absconding from hospital. Was the tragedy foreseeable by a reasonably prudent psychiatrist? This is the question that the courts seek to answer. In doing so, they are aware that the safety of the public must be balanced against the need to rehabilitate patients, that reasonable, calculated risks must often be taken, and that bona fide errors of clinical judgment are unavoidable (*Higgins v. State*, 1965).

Increasing pressure by managed care organizations, Medicaid agencies, and insurers has raised the specter of premature discharge against medical advice forced by withdrawal of funding. The clinician should be aware that legal responsibility for any harm that consequently befalls the patient or community will be placed on his shoulders. Hospitals and private clinicians who collaborate with health maintenance organizations would be wise to draw the line. If premature discharge is forced against medical advice, the clinician should protest vigorously in the medical record and appeal by letter before allowing it. The risk may be so great that the hospital should bear the cost of continued hospitalization.

Failure to Protect Endangered Third Parties

If a patient absconds from hospital and there is reason to suspect that a third person or persons are placed in jeopardy thereby, it is the psychiatrist's duty to take whatever steps are required in order to protect the community. This duty, which emanates from the *Tarasoff* decision, will be discussed in more detail later.

Wrongful Injury, Assault and Battery

A patient injured by staff who use excessive force to subdue him or her may have a claim against the hospital for battery or wrongful injury. Wrongful injury may also be claimed when one patient is harmed by another whom the staff could not control; however, the plaintiff would have to establish that the hospital was derelict in its duty to control the violent patient.

Seclusion and restraint present serious liability risks. They may be legitimate management techniques when the risk of harm is imminent and there are no alternatives; but they should not be used in order to compensate for understaffing. Physical control should be time-limited, and the patient examined by a physician if the maximum permissible time (e.g., one hour) requires extension. Seclusion and restraint should never be ordered "p.r.n." Close quality assurance tracking is required in order to determine when the use of physical controls becomes excessive.

If the person causing the harm is a hospital employee, the hospital may be liable, particularly if it were known that the employee had a propensity for violence or sexual misbehavior (*Samuels v. Southern Baptist Hospital*, 1992). The hospital may also be liable for the misbehavior of physicians, agency nurses, or others who work in hospital but are not employed by it. State institutions may claim *sovereign immunity*, which precludes litigants from suing governmental institutions; however, most jurisdictions have greatly limited or abolished this doctrine.

IMPROPER TREATMENT

Treatment may be administered against the patient's will in an emergency, or if the patient has been adjudicated incompetent. In other circumstances, a mature minor and his or her legal guardian, or the legal guardian alone (in the case of immature minors), must give informed consent to treatment. This matter is discussed in more detail later in this chapter. Erroneous choice of treatment, the use of an unapproved treatment, and failure to monitor side effects are also discussed later in this chapter. The hospital will be liable for failure to provide adequate staffing, equipment, and support to manage the problems associated with the procedures it offers.

RECORDKEEPING

Improper Release of Information from Medical Records

The comments to be made in this section are relevant to both hospital and outpatient practice. Traditionally, privilege has applied to all private communications between patient and doctor, including the medical record. However, in recent times, the confidentiality of the medical

record has been "polluted," that is, invaded by a number of bodies. Third party insurers, for example, have access to patients' records in order to ensure that medical costs are legitimate. Nevertheless, the unauthorized disclosure of confidential information from a patient's record could be actionable on the ground of breach of confidentiality. Medical records should be kept in a locked place on the ward or in the medical records department, in order to bar access to unauthorized people. The patient or legal guardian must give written consent for the transfer of information to legitimate professionals or agencies (e.g., other involved clinicians, attorneys, hospitals, schools, social welfare departments, and insurance companies).

A subpoena merely compels the clinician to appear in court (with or without records); it does not compel him to disclose confidential information from the record unless the patient or guardian has previously given specific authorization or has waived privilege, or unless the judge orders the clinician to disclose the information. If a subpoena is served without the written consent of the patient or guardian, the clinician has three alternatives: to seek the patient's consent; to have a motion filed by an attorney to quash the subpoena; or to refuse to testify unless ordered by the judge to do so. If the clinician persists in refusing to testify despite the judge's instruction to do so, he or she may be held in contempt of court (*In re Lifschutz*, 1970).

Defamation

Defamation involves communication by one party about a second party to a third party which damages the reputation of the second party. Defamation is most likely to occur in child psychiatry when carelessly written medical records are released to third parties. For example, the patient may have been described in the record as a "psychopath" or "malingerer," labels which could be extremely damaging in the hands of employers or creditors. Clinicians who gossip about patients over coffee or in elevators put themselves at risk of liability on the grounds of defamation or breach of confidentiality.

Defenses against defamation include *substantial truth* and *conditional privilege*. For example, if Dr. A refers patient B to Dr. C, and C reports to A that B has antisocial personality disorder, A and C have a duty and interest to receive and report such matters. In other words, conditional privilege applies. No such privilege applies to those who have no such duty and interest. Testimony given in court or provided to the court in documents such as medical reports or medical records attract *absolute privilege* insofar as they refer to the broadly defined matter at issue.

Malice, if proven, destroys conditional privilege. Malice is substantiated by the author's evident self-interest, excessive distribution of the defamatory material, reckless disregard of the truth, or the vituperative style of any documents involved in the case.

Liability for Failure to Communicate Records

The courts have generally refused to find that patients have a property or constitutional right to their records. However, records may be made available on request for legitimate reasons such as litigation. Some states have enacted legislation to allow patients to have access to their mental health records. However, "personal notes" may be excised (e.g., confidential information, information potentially injurious to the recipient, and the therapist's speculations), thus limiting access to the official record only.

Medication

The points in the medication of a patient at which negligence is most likely to occur are as follows:

1. The diagnosis of the psychiatric disorder.
2. The adoption of an appropriate rationale for drug therapy.
3. The choice of a particular drug to treat the patient's psychiatric disorder.

4. Enquiry concerning a past history of excessive therapeutic response, severe side effects, or allergic reaction to the drug in question or to related drugs.
5. The search for coexistent medical conditions which would contraindicate the medication in question or indicate the need for caution in its use.
6. Obtaining informed consent.
7. The administration of an appropriate dose of the drug in question, by an approved route.
8. The prescription of drugs in combination, or the addition of a drug or drugs to an existing medication regime.
9. The choice of a drug not approved by the FDA, or the use of a drug in a way, or for a purpose, which deviates from that recommended in the package insert or *Physician's Desk Reference*.
10. Monitoring the therapeutic effect and side effects of the medication.
11. Ceasing the medication after a therapeutic effect has been achieved, or maintaining long-term medication at the lowest effective dosage.

DIAGNOSIS

The physician must distinguish organic disease from functional disorders, and, within the latter, differentiate the major psychoses from each other and from other Axis I and II conditions. The physician who admits patients to a psychiatric hospital must be alert for signs that could indicate a toxic condition. In *Hirschberg v. State* (1977), for example, a patient who had taken an overdose of salicylates died after having been hospitalized without adequate physical examination, special investigations, or proper precautions. The hospital was found liable.

The physician who fails to diagnose the patient accurately (for example by missing psychosis when it is present or by confusing bipolar disorder with schizophrenia) may found treatment on a false premise, and thus be open to a liability suit. However, there have been few actions on these grounds; lawyers are reluctant to pursue such cases in view of reputedly widely varying expert opinion concerning the most appropriate treatment for different psychiatric conditions. As child psychiatry becomes more empirically based, it is likely that such actions will increase in frequency.

DECISION TO MEDICATE

Failure to Medicate When It Is Appropriate to Do So

In *Osheroff v. Chestnut Lodge et al.* (1987), suit was brought against a private hospital for negligent failure to disclose all treatment alternatives. The plaintiff, who suffered from mixed affective and personality disorder, had been treated for several months with individual psychotherapy. After transfer to a different hospital, he responded to antidepressant medication within a few weeks. Several eminent psychiatrists testified for the plaintiff that antidepressant medication was the treatment of choice, and that the plaintiff had had insufficient opportunity to consider it as a treatment alternative. The suit was settled out of court in favor of the plaintiff. It is likely that this case, which became an ideological battlefield, foreshadows future actions of a similar nature.

Inappropriate Rationale for Treatment

Psychotropic drugs are sometimes prescribed in order to control inmates in correctional or mental retardation institutions. These situations warrant close scrutiny; the physician may have been induced to medicate the patient by the urgings of harassed staff, rather than the medical needs of the patient, a practice which has been specifically criticized in at least one class action suit (*Nelson v. Heyne*, 1972/1974) and one malpractice case (*Clites v. State of Iowa*, 1982).

The Choice of an Inappropriate or Unapproved Drug

This kind of error occurs when the physician orders a drug which is inadequate to treat the patient's disorder (e.g.,a benzodiazepam for major depressive disorder), or when the physician prescribes a drug for which there are less risky alternatives (e.g., a neuroleptic for anxiety disorder).

A different problem arises when the clinician prescribes a drug not approved by the FDA. Undoubtedly, the risk of malpractice is greater if approved guidelines have not been followed. The clinician should reserve unapproved drugs for cases in which conventional treatment has failed. In addition, he should document a risk-benefit analysis, seek expert consultation, and obtain specific informed consent before prescribing the unapproved drug.

Failure to Obtain a Medication History

The patient's past medication history should be ascertained by interview, by review of medical records, and by telephone contact, if required, with other clinicians. The physician may be held liable for excessive side effects, allergic reactions, idiosyncratic responses, or drug interactions, if these had been foreseeable.

Failure to Detect Contraindicative Conditions

The physician may fail to check for conditions or disorders that would render the patient vulnerable to severe side effects. For example, preexisting subthyroidism may be overlooked when lithium is prescribed. Each class of psychotropic drug requires a standard workup involving medical history, physical examination, review of past medical records, and special investigations. If a contraindicative condition is uncovered, but the medication is still considered advisable, a risk-benefit analysis should be documented, expert consultation obtained, and specific informed consent recorded. Hospitals should mandate as policy standard diagnostic workups for all psychotropic drugs.

Failure to Obtain Informed Consent

The doctrine of informed consent is founded on the constitutional right of the individual to control what is done to his or her own body (*Schloendorff v. Society of New York Hospital*, 1914). A patient cannot give informed consent unless he or she has (*a*) *sufficient information* upon which to base a decision; (*b*) *mental competency* to make a rational decision; and (*c*) freedom to exercise *voluntary choice*.

The physician must therefore disclose sufficient information to enable the patient to weigh all material pros and cons. How much is that? The earlier "professional" standard (*Natanson v. Kline*, 1960; *Aiken v. Clarey*, 1965) referred to *what a reasonable medical practitioner would disclose* under similar circumstances. Following two 1972 cases, *Canterbury v. Spence* and *Cobbs v. Grant*, some jurisdictions may have adopted the "patient" standard, that is, *as much information as a reasonable patient would require* to make a rational decision under similar circumstances. *Canterbury* and other cases indicate that the physician should discuss the following matters with the patient:

1. The nature of the condition that requires treatment.
2. The nature, purpose, and benefits of the proposed treatment, and the probability that it will succeed.
3. The risks and consequences of the proposed treatment.
4. Alternatives to the proposed treatment (including no treatment) and their attendant risks and consequences.
5. The prognosis with and without the proposed treatment.

The courts have held that *not all risks need be disclosed—only the material ones*. Unfortunately, there are no clear guidelines concerning what is "material" except to suggest that the more serious the risk, even if the likelihood be slight, the greater the probability that it should be discussed. A risk is material when a reasonable person would be likely to attach significance to the risk or cluster of risks. Risk is linked not only to the procedure but also to the physician and his competence to perform the procedure (e.g., if he is alcoholic or suffers from HIV infection). The plaintiff must prove that nondisclosure of material risk caused the injury of which he complains. Some courts require that the plaintiff prove that a reasonable person would have refused the procedure had the risks been disclosed.

Therapeutic privilege countervails the clinician's duty to disclose. The physician is obliged to protect a vulnerable patient from the emotional trauma that could be sustained if upsetting risks were prematurely revealed. However, therapeutic privilege should never be invoked merely because the clinician fears that, if apprised of the facts, the patient would reject a desirable treatment. If the clinician proposes to limit disclosure on the ground of therapeutic privilege, clear documentation and expert consultation is required concerning the patient's exceptional sensitivity.

Disclosure is not required for an emergency in which the harm from failure to treat is imminent and outweighs the potential danger of the treatment. However, if possible, a relative's consent should be obtained.

Patients beyond the age of majority are presumed competent to make decisions about their own treatment. Competence may also be extended to emancipated minors. When should an unemancipated minor be regarded as sufficiently mature to participate in health care decisions? A series of landmark decisions (e.g., *Planned Parenthood of Central Missouri v. Danforth*, 1976; *Bellotti v. Baird*, 1976) have extended to minors the right to make health decisions concerning abortion, and a number of states have enacted legislation with regard to mature minors and contraception, venereal disease, substance abuse, and emergency psychiatric care. The present situation is very confused (Wadlington, 1983), and the practitioner should ascertain the law on the matter in his or her own state. However, although it may not be legally required, the desirability of promoting a treatment alliance suggests that it is judicious to promote the understanding and cooperation of all minors mature enough to comprehend. For patients over 13 years of age, it would be prudent to obtain formal assent. Other than in emergencies, when minors are treated, parental consent is also required. However, according to Annas (1975), no court in recent years has found a physician liable for treating in good faith a consenting minor over 15 years of age in the absence of parental consent.

The third element of informed consent, *voluntariness*, is easily compromised. True voluntary consent requires that the patient be free of coercion. However, even a mature minor can be susceptible to threat, cajolement, bribery, or false inducement by parents, physicians, or hospital staff. The inmates of correctional institutions and psychiatric hospitals are particularly vulnerable to therapeutic coercion.

IMPLEMENTATION OF TREATMENT

Forcible Administration

The involuntary commitment of a patient to a psychiatric hospital does not permit involuntary medication except in narrowly defined circumstances. Forcible medication can place the practitioner at risk of an action for the intentional tort of battery. The legal doctrine most pertinent to this issue, *the right to refuse treatment*, has been most clearly articulated in two convoluted cases, *Rennie v. Klein* (1978/1979/1981/1982) and *Rogers v. Okin* (1979). In *Rennie*, a New Jersey case, it was determined that the mentally ill had a sufficient liberty interest to require due process before treatment was forcibly administered, but that due process was satisfied by an in-hospital review. In considering this case, the United States Supreme Court deferred to the professionalization standard articulated in *Youngberg v. Romeo* (1982), in effect declining to uphold a constitutional right to refuse treatment.

Rogers v. Okin (1979), a Massachusetts case, evolved into *Rogers v. Commissioner of Mental Health* (1983) and was reviewed by the United States Supreme Court as *Mills v. Rogers* (1982). The Massachusetts Supreme Court held that involuntarily committed patients should be presumed competent to refuse treatment except in emergencies. An "emergency" was defined as a situation fraught with the need to prevent violence, or associated with the likelihood that the patient's health would

significantly deteriorate without treatment. In non-emergency situations, forcible treatment might be administered only after a judicial hearing in which the court approved a "substituted judgment" treatment plan. "Substituted judgment" requires the court to determine what the patient would have decided if he or she were competent.

The failure of the Supreme Court to clarify this matter means that each state must make its own determination of the boundaries of the right to refuse treatment. The legal situation with regard to children is unclear. The right to refuse treatment apparently extends to the legal guardians of minors and to emancipated minors. What of the mature minor? Arguably, except in emergencies, the clinician should seek the consent of both mature minor and parent before starting treatment. If the mature minor refuses treatment, and the treatment is regarded vital, a judicial determination of competence should be requested.

Inappropriate Dosage or Route of Administration

The *Physician's Desk Reference* (*PDR*) includes the information found in all official drug package inserts, together with manufacturers' information concerning drug products which have no insert. In *Mulder v. Parke Davis & Co.* (1970), the court held that a departure from *PDR* guidelines represented a *prima facie* case of negligence unless the clinician could provide adequate reason for having done so. In order to protect themselves from liability claims, drug manufacturers publish information concerning all reported adverse reactions, however rare, and are conservative in the dosages they recommend. In some circumstances, it may be good clinical practice to regard the risk of particular adverse reactions as insignificant, or to exceed the recommended dosage. However, before doing so, it would be advisable for the clinician to document a risk-benefit analysis, seek a consultation, and locate references in the literature that would support the proposed medication regime.

An intravenous or intramuscular route of administration carries an increased risk of excessive or adverse response. This is particularly likely if the patient is predisposed to side effects as a result of hepatic, renal, cardiac, or brain dysfunction. The clinician should be cautious if such conditions are detected. Parenteral administration should generally be reserved for emergencies or long-term depot treatment.

Polypharmacy

Psychotropic cocktails increase the risk of adverse reactions. They are most likely to be prescribed when psychotic patients are slow to respond, or in general hospitals and residential centers that have inadequate structure or psychiatric nursing care. On the other hand, as Simon (1987) points out, drug combinations (e.g., of an antidepressant with a neuroleptic) are sometimes more efficacious than one drug alone. Nevertheless, the clinician should record a risk-benefit analysis before prescribing multiple psychotropics.

Failure to Monitor Treatment

The case of *Clites v. State of Iowa* (1982) illustrates negligent failure to monitor psychotropic medication, in addition to a number of other errors. The plaintiff, a mentally retarded patient, was admitted to a state residential facility at the age of 11 years. Between the ages of 17 and 22 years he was treated with various psychotropic drug combinations, until tardive dyskinesia was noticed. The appellate court held that the hospital had failed to document behavior sufficiently aggressive or self-abusive to warrant neuroleptic treatment; that the medication appeared to be designed primarily for the staff's convenience; that the practice of prescribing polypharmacy was substandard; that the treatment had not been monitored adequately by a physician; that "drug holidays" should have been employed; that the staff had been too slow in recognizing the patient's dyskinesia; and that informed consent had not been sought from the patient's parents. Damages of over $750,000 were affirmed.

Adequate monitoring of drug effects requires baseline and regular mental status examinations, physical examinations, vital signs, and laboratory testing, in accordance with pharmacology of the drug and its potential side effects. ''Drug holidays'' should be considered if long-term medication is required. Physicians run a serious risk if they write p.r.n. orders for potent drugs, ''phone in'' prescriptions without examining their patients, or provide multiple repeat refills.

Suicide

An action for wrongful death may be brought against the physician who prescribed a drug which was subsequently used to procure a suicide. The precautions which might prevent such a tragedy will be discussed later in this chapter. When the risk of suicide is significant, less lethal drugs should be prescribed, in small amounts. Blood levels should be regularly determined, in order to ensure that the patient is not hoarding the medication.

Psychotherapy

Psychiatrists are most at risk of liability when they terminate the treatment of patients without adequate safeguards, when they are unavailable and either no covering physician is provided or the covering physician has not been given sufficient information, or when adequate steps are not taken to protect endangered third parties. A therapist runs the risk of being held to have committed an intentional tort when he or she recklessly inflicts emotional distress upon, has improper sexual contact with, breaches the confidentiality of, or defames, a patient.

Unless the physician has behaved outrageously or recklessly, or unless the patient has committed suicide, it is difficult to prove harm as a result of negligent psychotherapy, for mental injury is hard to substantiate when the plaintiff was already emotionally disturbed before the alleged negligence. It can also be awkward to establish what is a reasonable standard of care, since there are so many schools of psychotherapy. Thus, most successful actions have alleged either negligence leading to suicide or outrageous conduct.

ABANDONMENT

The physician has the duty to provide continued care, as long as needed, until the doctor- patient relationship is terminated. This relationship may be severed by mutual consent or by the patient. However, unilateral termination of care by the clinician, if abrupt or premature, may put him at risk of breach of contract should harm (e.g., suicide) befall the patient. Failure to provide a telephone number for a disturbed patient to call, failure to provide adequate substitute care during absences, or failure to convey adequate precautionary information to a substitute physician may all be construed as abandonment if the patient is found to have suffered harm as a consequence. The absolute duty to provide continued care does not apply to a consultant who has been asked by a primary physician to render an opinion; that is, unless it has been agreed that the consultant will treat the patient.

When is the therapist warranted in unilaterally terminating the relationship? Lack of cooperation or threatening behavior may justify termination; failure to pay does not (Smith, 1986). If the clinician does decide to terminate the relationship, the following safeguards are required (Simon, 1987):

1. The reason for the termination should be discussed with the patient. The clinician should give at least one month's notice of termination in order to allow the patient to locate another therapist.
2. The patient should be provided with the names and telephone numbers of alternative therapists or agencies.
3. The clinician should mail to the patient a certified letter (return receipt requested) reflecting this discussion and containing the reasons for termination. The letter should also convey the names and telephone numbers of alternative clinicians or agencies.

These problems are most likely to occur in highly ambivalent adolescent patients with personality disorder whose suicide risk is aggravated by loss, separation, or rejection.

FAILURE TO PROTECT ENDANGERED THIRD PARTIES

This matter is discussed at this point, rather than under ''Hospitalization'' because it is with outpatients that the most problematic situations arise. The facts of the original case, *Tarasoff v. Regents of the University of California* (1974, 1976) illustrate the problems of deciding what to do when, during outpatient treatment, a patient threatens to harm a third person.

In the course of psychotherapy with a psychologist at a university health center, Prosenjit Poddar mentioned that he had fantasies of killing Tatiana Tarasoff, a young woman with whom he was infatuated. The therapist also learned from Poddar's roommate that Poddar had obtained a gun. After the patient unilaterally terminated treatment, the psychologist consulted a psychiatrist at the center who had previously evaluated Poddar. The clinicians decided to contact the campus police, informing them that Poddar met criteria for involuntary hospitalization on the ground of dangerousness. The campus police detained and questioned Poddar, but concluded that he was not dangerous and released him when he promised to stay away from Tatiana. Two months later Poddar stabbed Tatiana to death. Tatiana's parents brought suit against the University of California alleging that they were negligent in not hospitalizing Poddar, and in not safeguarding the public by warning the Tarasoff family.

The trial court dismissed the suit on the ground that there was no duty to warn. The case was appealed on two occasions, known as *Tarasoff I* (1974) and *Tarasoff II* (1976). In *Tarasoff I*, the California supreme court found that the defendants were not liable for failing to confine Poddar, but that a treating clinician bears *a duty to warn threatened persons of foreseeable danger arising from a patient's condition*. Damages were awarded to the Tarasoffs.

Concerned by the serious implications of this judgment for confidentiality, the American Psychiatric Association pressed the appellate court to reopen the case. In *Tarasoff II* the issue of failure to warn was debated. The court decided that there was a *duty to protect* rather than a duty to warn: if there is a serious danger of violence, the clinician must take reasonable care to protect the foreseeable victim. The court failed to define what constituted ''reasonable care,'' and how dangerous the patient must be before precautions should be taken.

Tarasoff spawned a number of progeny. In *McIntosh v. Milano* (1979), a New Jersey case, the Tarasoff standards were applied even though the patient had never actually been heard to utter threats against his victim. The psychiatrist was described as having a broadly based obligation to protect the welfare of the community. In *Lipari v. Sears, Roebuck & Co.* (1980), the Nebraska Court held that the duty to protect applies even when the potential victim is unknown or unidentifiable. It was not made clear how the duty to protect unknown third persons should be discharged, other than by detaining the patient or informing the police. In *Peck v. The Counseling Service of Addison County, Inc.* (1985) the Vermont court held that a community mental health clinic was liable for the destruction of a barn by a firesetting patient, thereby extending the *Tarasoff* doctrine to nonmedical therapists and to property damage as well as personal harm.

On the other hand, in *Thompson v. County of Alameda* (1980) and *Brady v. Hopper* (1983), the California and Colorado courts reaffirmed the *Tarasoff* holding that the duty to protect was precipitated only by *a specific threat to an identifiable third person*, a decision upheld subsequently in other states.

In *Bellah v. Greenson* (1978) and *Cole v. Taylor* (1981) the California and Iowa courts, respectively, held (*a*) that the *Tarasoff* duty to breach confidentiality and warn others did not apply when the patient threatened suicide; and (*b*) that a psychiatrist was not liable to pay damages to a patient who killed her husband, when the psychiatrist had allegedly failed to control her or to warn the victim. However, in a Pennsylvania case, *Hopewell v. Adebimpe* (1981), a psychiatrist who informed a third party considered to be endangered was found liable for breach of confidentiality. In those states which have a statute concerning privilege in the doctor-patient relationship, the requirement to maintain confidentiality may take precedence over the *Tarasoff* doctrine. The clinician should ascertain the situation in his or her own state.

In *Jablonski v. United States* (1983) and *Davis v. Lhim* (1983), the findings of negligence were based on such dubious evidence that it has been suggested that a doctrine of *strict liability* was applied (Smith, 1986; Simon, 1987). In other words, if a patient causes harm, his clinician must be culpable. Such broad interpretations of the *Tarasoff* doctrine appear to be founded on the myth that mental health clinicians are reliable predictors of violence, that they have the means of preventing violence in patients not under their direct control, and that "warnings" or other unspecified precautions (short of hospitalization) would protect the community. In fact, in *Lundgren v. Fultz* (1984) the Minnesota court regarded warnings as problematical, for they add to the stigma of mental illness while doing little to protect the community.

What, then, should a clinician do if a patient threatens violence? The following steps are recommended. First, undertake and document a violence risk-resource analysis. If the risk is serious, take precautions to protect endangered parties. Second, if the patient is already hospitalized voluntarily, consider whether civil commitment is required. Take precautions against elopement, consider limiting visitation and leave, and do not discharge the patient unless you are convinced that the risk of violence has diminished. Ask for a consultation if you are in doubt. Third, if a potentially violent hospitalized patient elopes or fails to return from leave, seek consultation from a colleague and from the hospital's attorney. If the risk of harm is significant, inform the local police and the police department of the area where the patient lives, by telephone and certified letter. If there are people (e.g., family, friends, or acquaintances) who could be in danger, warn them by telephone, through the police, and by certified letter. Fourth, if you warn a third party by telephone or letter, take care to divulge only as much as necessary to let them know they are at risk. For example:

> In the course of my professional duties, it has come to my attention that John Smith has feelings of anger towards you, and that he has made threats to harm you. On (date), John Smith eloped from this hospital and is at large in the community. I have informed the police at _____."

Fifth, if the patient is an outpatient, attempt to deal with the problem in therapy. Seek consultation from a colleague, and consult your attorney. If you regard the risk of violence as serious, consider hospitalizing the patient on a voluntary basis, or after emergency commitment. Consider whether close observation at home is preferable to hospitalization. Document the rationale for your final decision. Lastly, if the risk is serious but hospitalization not feasible, inform the police and the endangered third party by telephone and certified letter. Let the patient know that it is your professional and legal duty to do so. Try to enlist the patient's cooperation by allying yourself with his or her ego controls. For example, if possible, let the patient be present when you telephone the police and the third party, and allow him or her to read the contents of the letters sent to the endangered third party and the police.

In summary, the *Tarasoff* decision has created many problems for clinicians and the courts. The doctrine assumes that clinicians are reliable predictors of violence, that the threshold of risk that should precipitate reasonable precautions is clear, and that reasonable precautions are available and effective. The courts in different states have varied from requiring that a specific threat have been made against a foreseeable victim, to applying the doctrine when no specific threat had been made and the victim was unknown to the patient, to including property damage as well as personal injury, to holding that the doctrine of confidentiality takes precedence and eliminates *Tarasoff* obligations. Thus, contrary trends are operating in different jurisdictions, extending, limiting, or preempting the *Tarasoff* duty. Simon's (1987) recommendations can be summarized as follows:

1. In outpatient cases the courts have generally held that, unless there is a foreseeable victim, the clinician's control over the patient is insufficient to create a duty to protect. The danger of harm must be substantial (that is, involve bodily harm or death), and the evidence must be specific (that is, involve threats or acts of violence towards a third person) for the Tarasoff duty to apply.
2. In inpatient cases, if harm results following release or elopement, liability may be created by the duty to control, regardless of whether or not a victim was foreseeable. Continued dangerousness necessitates continued close observation.

If the situation is unclear in the home state, the clinician would be well advised to act as though the broadest interpretation of the doctrine applies. However, as Simon (1987) points out, one should not allow concern about *Tarasoff* liability to interfere with sound clinical practice. Instead, the clinician should make reasonable efforts to control potentially violent patients before resorting to warnings; and if warnings are required, they should be incorporated into treatment, whenever possible.

SEXUAL EXPLOITATION AND THE TORT OF OUTRAGE

Expert testimony is not required to substantiate the impropriety of sexually molesting a patient. As an intentional tort, *res ipsa loquitur* ("the thing speaks for itself"), and the burden of proof shifts to the defendant. In *Roy v. Hartogs* (1976), the court held that public policy protected patients from such malicious abuses of authority, power, and fiduciary trust. The perpetrator faces criminal sanctions for rape or aggravated assault, and civil actions for malpractice or battery (unconsented touching). He or she may not be insured against the costs of such an action. Liability for improper sexual relations may extend beyond the patient to others involved, such as spouses. Residual transference has persuaded courts that cessation of treatment does not open the door to a sexual relationship. Indeed, *negligent management of the transference* is often adopted as the theory behind the action for damages.

The tort of *outrage* refers to the intentional infliction of severe emotional distress upon a patient, as a result of reckless and intolerable behavior. For example, in *Abraham v. Zaslow* (1970), damages were awarded to a woman who had sustained bruising and renal failure following exposure to "rage-reduction therapy," an intrusive treatment involving several hours of physical restraint, poking, tickling, and verbal insult. Patients have a right to expect that clinicians will adhere to established methods of treatment. If exceptional methods are proposed, full informed consent is required, supportive consultation from a colleague would be advisable, and adequate reference to the scientific literature should be made.

Teaching, Research and Publication

The torts of *invasion of privacy*, *breach of confidentiality*, and *defamation* are the liability risks most commonly incurred by teachers, researchers and writers. The doctrine of informed consent is discussed earlier in this chapter.

These torts stem from the ethical, contractual and (in some jurisdictions) statutory obligation of the clinician not to disclose private information that should be kept within the doctor-patient relationship. In invasion of privacy, the plaintiff alleges that details from his or her private life have been publicized. This may occur, for example, if a clinician publishes an article in which the identity of the subject is insufficiently disguised. It has been held that a patient undergoing psychotherapy cannot give proper informed consent to the publication of a book concerning the treatment (*Jane Doe v. Joan Roe and Peter Poe*, 1977).

A patient has the right to bar nonessential onlookers when he or she is being examined or treated, or when his or her case is discussed. The teacher should seek informed consent before exposing patients to case conferences or discussing cases for teaching purposes. The use of videotapes for teaching necessitates written informed consent, the continuation of which should be requested on a yearly basis.

LIABILITY UNDER NEW COST-CONTAINMENT SYSTEMS

The current national preoccupation with cost containment by means of managed care and capitation puts the clinician at risk, particularly in the care of suicidal or dangerous patients. In *Wickline v. State of California* (1986), a Medi-Cal reviewer allowed only four extra days inpatient treatment, following an arterial graft, rather than the eight days requested by a vascular surgeon. The patient was duly discharged after four days, and complications cost her the leg. The patient sued the physician, the hospital, and the state of California. The court determined that the state, through Medi-Cal, owed the patient a duty of care in that it was bound by statute to evaluate the medical necessity of length of stay and level of care. However, in this case no breach of duty was found. The surgeon was found liable for having acceded without appeal to the Medi-Cal determination. On the other hand, in *Wilson v. Blue Cross of California* (1990), a suicidal patient was prematurely discharged from hospital, over his psychiatrist's protest. After the patient's death, an appeal court found the insurer liable in that the managed care firm contracted by the insurer to conduct utilization review had made a "medically insensitive" decision. However, in this case, the patient's insurance contract had contained no provision for managed care, and vexatious questions remain unanswered. Managed care reviewers often preface their denials of further hospitalization by saying that the physician or hospital is at liberty to continue to treat the patient gratuitously; and, in many cases, the patient should be kept safe pending appeal. Physicians who receive financial incentives for diverting patients from specialized care should reveal this to their patients. Any economic constraints that could modify a physician's medical judgment should be disclosed.

The failure to regulate managed care regulators is certain to generate future liability actions that will help to clarify some of the questions. However, managed care and capitation will continue. Physicians and hospitals should define their standards and not be pressed to sink below them.

THE ASSESSMENT OF VIOLENCE AND SUICIDE RISK

It is generally accepted that clinicians have little expertise in the long-term prediction of violence or suicide (Monahan, 1981). However, most of the research in this area comes from prison populations or from the long-term follow-up of involuntary psychiatric patients. There has been no research concerning the prediction of imminent risk, and such research will never be done. Faced with an uncontrollable, potentially self-destructive or assaultive patient in an emergency room, no clinician would be willing to assign the subject randomly to a no-treatment control group. Thus, although the accuracy of clinical predictions of imminent dangerousness is unknown, such predictions must and will be made. The following risk-resource analyses present a method of taking into account the factors which increase or mitigate risk.

Violence

A risk-resource analysis should be conducted whenever a patient presents a risk of violence. Such an assessment is most likely to be required in the following circumstances: when the risk of violence is raised during outpatient evaluation or treatment; when a potentially violent patient presents for admission to hospital; and when the leave or discharge from hospital of a potentially violent patient is being considered, or when such a patient elopes.

The factors to be considered can be grouped into the following areas: (*a*) demographic factors, (*b*) the violent threat, (*c*) past history, (*d*) psychological factors, (*e*) the social environment, and (*f*) the therapeutic alliance. Do not merely sum the positive and negative items; their weighting and combination will differ in different cases.

DEMOGRAPHIC FACTORS

Late adolescent, male, patients from *disadvantaged ethnic groups* which have a *cultural tradition of masculine defensiveness* are at greater risk of violence.

THE VIOLENT THREAT

Has the patient *directly expressed a violent threat* or threats toward another, by word or message? Does the potential victim have a *provocative relationship* with the patient which could provoke hostility? Does the patient have a *plan* for harming the victim, and does he have *access to lethal weapons*?

PAST HISTORY

Is there a *past history of violent threats or actions*? Does the patient have a *history of being victimized* in early life by child abuse? Has the patient a *history of serious head injury, epilepsy, or neurological impairment*? Does the patient have a *history of alcohol or drug abuse*?

PSYCHOLOGICAL FACTORS

Is the patient prone to cope with anxiety or hostility by *externalizing* or *projecting* it in the form of *impulsive, explosive actions, suspicious vigilance*, or frank *persecutory delusions*? Is there evidence for *command hallucinations* that instruct the patient to take violent action, or *that threaten violence* to the patient or his family? Are the patient's *inner controls* against violent actions subjectively or objectively reduced? Is there a *strong inner urge to be violent*? Is the patient's *intelligence below average*? Is there evidence of *impairment of the sensorium*? Is the patient subject to *alcohol or substance abuse*?

THE SOCIAL ENVIRONMENT

Are the patient's *family or caretakers able and willing to control* the patient? Is there evidence of family psychopathology in the form of *rejection, neglect, physical or sexual abuse*, or *family violence*? Is *parental mental or physical health* impaired?

THE THERAPEUTIC ALLIANCE

Has the patient *lost* or *terminated* a *therapeutic relationship*? Is he *competent* and *motivated* to enter into one?

RESOURCES

Factors which may protect against violence or enhance self-control are as follows: *Younger, female, caucasian, religious, middle class* patients are at less risk. If there has been a threat of violence, a *threat without plan or identified victim*, in a patient *without access to lethal means*, is of relatively lower concern, particularly if the patient has *obsessional traits, low subjective urge*, and *above average intelligence*. A *secure family* without major psychopathology or mental or physical ill health is protective, as is a *positive relationship with a therapist*, or the *motivation* and *competence* to enter into one.

A HYPOTHETICAL HIGH-RISK CASE

The patient is an intoxicated 17-year-old, male, Hispanic youth from an impoverished family living in an urban ghetto. He has been brought to the emergency room by police because he was acting belligerently in a local bar. During the interview, he threatens to kill his allegedly unfaithful fiancée and her lover by stabbing them to death. He has a history of several episodes of juvenile violence, and is known to be a user of alcohol and street drugs. He has access to knives and other weapons. At interview he is highly emotionally aroused, threatening, hostile, and suspicious. He says that he is directed by an inner voice to take vengeance for the insult to his honor. His family is chaotic and afraid of him. He has no therapist and, at the interview, no desire to seek help.

Suicide

A suicide risk-resource analysis is required when the clinician must decide whether the risk of suicide is *imminent* and *serious*. This decision is most often required in the following situations: when the possibility of suicide is raised in the course of ambulatory or inpatient treatment; when a new patient presents for voluntary or involuntary hospitalization; or when leave or the discharge of a potentially suicidal patient is being considered. In these circumstances, it is important for the clinician to record the pros and cons upon which the clinical decision is based.

The factors to be considered incorporate 25 items in six sections. These items cannot be equally weighted since their relative valence and combination will differ according to the particular circumstances and characteristics of each case. As with a violence risk resource analysis, do not merely sum the risks and resources. Consider their weight and combination in each case. The factors to be considered can be classified under six headings: (*a*) demographic factors, (*b*) the suicide attempt, (*c*) physical factors, (*d*) psychological factors, (*e*) the social environment, and (*f*) the therapeutic alliance.

DEMOGRAPHIC FACTORS

Older white males are at greater risk.

THE SUICIDE ATTEMPT

Pay close attention to the suicide attempt, if one has occurred. *Lethal means* involves hanging, gassing, jumping from a height, drowning, knife or gunshot wound, using a motor vehicle for suicidal purposes, self-poisoning, major overdose, or other concerted attempt at self- destruction. Remember that, to a child who is ignorant of pharmacology, 10 aspirins may represent a lethal dose.

Greater risk attaches to suicide attempts which were *planned* and *concealed*, although *impulsiveness* (e.g., drinking and driving wildly after an upset) can also be very dangerous.

The intent of the patient should be explored from suicide notes, prior conversations with family and friends, and the patient's recollection of the attempt. Did the patient truly *wish to die, sacrifice himself, expunge shame*, exit permanently from an *intolerable existence*, find peace, or *be reunited with a lost loved one*? Was the suicide attempt a response to *command hallucinations*? On the other hand, did the suicide attempt represent a communication of the *need for help* or a *desire to punish someone*? Is the patient *able to grasp the finality of death*? Does he or she fantasize that *resurrection* is possible?

PAST HISTORY

A history of a *previous attempt or attempts* adds to the risk of future suicide. The *means and intent of previous attempts* might also predict the seriousness of future attempts. Some patients have given up on the future as a result of *chronic illness or handicap*. *Alcohol and drug abuse* increase the risk potential of other factors since the intoxicated adolescent may take desperate risks or express suicidal impulses that would otherwise be controlled. Is the patient *intoxicated* at the time of the examination? Is he or she *likely to resort to drugs or alcohol* if you do not hospitalize them?

PSYCHOLOGICAL FACTORS

Does the mental status examination reveal or confirm the presence of *depressive affect, despair, hopelessness*, or the *vegetative signs* associated with *melancholia*? Is there evidence of *psychosis* with mental disorganization, abnormal perception, or delusional thinking? Can you detect evidence of *command hallucinations*, which instruct the patient to kill or injure himself or to take serious risks (e.g., to fly from the roof of a building)? Is there evidence of *mental confusion, obtundation*, or *delirium* suggestive of an organic confusion or acute psychotic condition? Does the patient's history indicate *poor internal controls* with impulsiveness or explosive behavior when under stress? Is the patient preoccupied with *suicidal ideation* or with the *desirability of death*?

THE SOCIAL ENVIRONMENT

The resources and deficiencies of the family or caretakers are very relevant to the determination of suicide risk. Are the family able to provide a *safe environment*? Are the parents able to cooperate with each other? Are they willing or competent to get rid of, or secure, all potentially lethal agents of suicide (e.g., prescription drugs, poisons, weapons)? Are they prepared or able to watch the patient closely, and be emotionally available to him in times of stress? On the other hand, is there evidence of *parental rejection, neglect, physical or sexual abuse, mental illness, severe personality disorder, substance abuse, or physical illness or handicap* of a severity that would render the caretakers unable to provide adequate security and emotional sustenance to an acutely disturbed child?

Has there been a recent *loss* or *the severance of an important relationship*, such as the death of a close relative or beloved family pet, loss of contact with a noncustodial parent, or the departure of a close older sibling or special friend? Such an event may represent the "last straw" to an isolated, troubled child. Pay special attention to *peer relations*. Particularly vulnerable is the isolated, alienated, persecuted, or rejected youngster, or the patient who has withdrawn from contact with peers. *Has a love relationship been threatened or severed*? Does the patient feel intolerably *guilty* or *ashamed* before his family or peers, as a result of some action or dereliction? *Shame toward the family* is a particularly powerful emotion in Asian patients.

Is there a *family history of suicide*? A positive family history may reflect a genetically transmitted psychiatric disorder which increases suicide risk, or a family tradition of committing or attempting suicide in stressful circumstances. Suicidal parents may unwittingly act as *suicide models*.

THE THERAPEUTIC ALLIANCE

It is crucial to determine whether the patient has, or has lost, an adequate *therapeutic relationship*. Is the patient capable of forming an alliance? Do you believe the patient, if he promises to cooperate? Has he been reliable in the past? Is he prepared to sign a "suicide contract"? Although such contracts have no legal status, they are a useful clinical index of the patient's cooperativeness.

RESOURCES

To some extent, the reverse of the risk factors can operate as mitigating factors. For example, a suicide attempt associated with the *desire to communicate a need for help* indicates that the patient is still potentially available to other people. A *competent family*, free of serious mental, physical, or personality disorder, is the most powerful protective factor. A *network of caring friends* who can be mobilized is also protective. The *capacity for internal control*, accentuated for example in obsessional patients, may impede direct suicidal action, and be activated if the patient has, or wants, a therapeutic relationship. Finally, an *existing adequate therapeutic alliance*, or the *competence or motivation to seek one*, are mitigating factors.

CIRCUMSTANCES OF EXTREME RISK

The following stereotype describes an extreme case. The patient is a 17-year-old caucasian male who was discovered making his second suicide attempt by hanging, while intoxicated, in a remote part of the woods near his home. His family is chaotic. The father is psychotic and alcoholic and the mother chronically physically ill. One sibling has died by suicide and one by accidental gunshot wound. The patient's suicide was planned, and he intended to do away with himself. He has no friends, is persecuted at school, and was recently greatly upset by the death of a beloved grandmother. Mental status examination reveals severe depression with agitation, despair, and vegetative signs. He is preoccupied with the idea of dying and joining his grandmother. At times, he hears the voice of his grandmother begging him to join her. He has had no recent mental health contact, and rejects the offer of therapy.

CIRCUMSTANCES OF LESS RISK

The patient is a 14-year-old girl who swallowed 10 aspirin tablets in the bathroom at home, following an argument with her mother about permission to go out with a boyfriend on a week night. She told her mother about the overdose an hour after it had occurred, and the mother brought her to the emergency room at once. The parents have been separated for three years, but both of them remain close to the patient, and neither suffers from serious mental, personality, or substance use disorder. The parents and child are in good physical health. The patient reveals no psychotic or melancholic symptoms. She says she did not really want to die, but that she was angry with her mother for not listening to her and for restricting her too much. She accepts the need for therapy, promises not to attempt suicide without calling you, and agrees to return for an outpatient appointment on the following day.

CONCLUSIONS

Clinical practice is fraught with error, and error can have serious consequences. Confronted by the catalogue of litigation in this chapter, even the insouciant might quail. However, defensive psychiatry is no answer, for over-timid treatment can also put the clinician at risk of negligent malpractice. What, then, is the best way to avoid litigation?

The best precaution is to practice careful medicine while fully apprising the patient and family of the diagnosis, the treatment plan, and the progress of therapy. Many malpractice suits arise from a neglect of this simple principle. Hospitals provide many opportunities for failed communication, particularly when the attending physician delegates to other members of the team the responsibility for keeping parents informed of their children's progress. A good therapeutic alliance is the key to good medicine and the avoidance of lawsuits. Used for this purpose, informed consent can be transformed from an empty legalism into the foundation of a true collaboration.

"If it wasn't written down, it didn't happen." The clinician should keep a good record of the rationale for treatment. Progress notes should be timely, regular, dated, and signed. Whenever a course of action is problematic, a risk-benefit analysis should be undertaken and documented, and a consultation obtained. If you disagree with the diagnosis, investigations, or treatment plan in the record, note that you disagree, and insert your amended diagnosis and plan. If you merely sign off on a trainee's notes, you could be concurring with erroneous observations, diagnosis, or treatment. One of the commonest errors is to raise a diagnostic question but not follow through by investigating it or, having ordered investigations, to lose sight of the results.

Note any discrepancies between the nurses', the therapist's, and the physician's progress notes. If there is such a discrepancy try to account for it. Do not allow a nursing progress note concerning suicide risk to go unremarked.

If you detect an error in your notes, do not erase it. Draw a line through the error, write "error," date and sign your correction in the margin. Do not criticize or argue with other professionals or agencies in your notes; and avoid gratuitous or extravagant commentary (e.g., "This child has had an appalling home life").

Before a particular treatment is commenced, be careful to check that the patient harbors no conditions and is taking no drugs that would contraindicate it, and enquire for previous allergic or idiosyncratic reactions to drugs. Avoid polypharmacy. Monitor the progress of medication regularly. In long-term medication, "drug holidays" should be considered. Follow recommended guidelines for dosage and administration, unless there are good reasons for departing from them. Avoid prescribing medication p.r.n., automatic refills, and be careful of telephone requests for repeat prescriptions. If the suicide risk is serious only small amounts of a potentially lethal drug should be prescribed. Hospitals should check that potentially suicidal patients are not cheating, concealing, and hoarding medication.

When a patient is admitted to hospital, the degree of risk of suicide or violence should be assessed, and each degree of risk should be linked to a set of nursing precautions which are automatically activated when the clinician indicates the degree of risk. Every attempt should be made to obtain past records and to scan them for risk factors.

If you are unavailable in case of emergency during treatment, the name of a fully informed substitute physician should be provided to the patient. Do not terminate treatment unilaterally without preparing the patient, giving adequate notice, and providing him or her with the names of other clinicians or agencies who could help.

In outpatient practice, the duty to protect is precipitated when the patient makes a specific threat to harm a specified victim. When possible, incorporate the protection in therapy. Psychotherapy, hospitalization and medication may be both more protective and more therapeutic than warning the foreseeable victim or alerting the police.

Do not record psychodynamic speculations in the clinical record; those unconscious incestuous strivings may come back to haunt you. You may consider keeping your psychotherapy *process notes* separate from the official record of therapy *progress notes*.

Be vigilant to avoid unauthorized disclosure of confidential information to external agencies, do not gossip about patients, and do not publish articles about patients without adequately disguising their identity. Obtain the parents' consent before releasing reports to external agencies. Blanket consent forms, obtained during the rush of admission, may not hold water, legally.

In conclusion, remember that the law has no wish to penalize physicians for honest errors. Its purpose is to protect patients from being harmed by reckless, careless, or incompetent clinical practice, and if they have been so harmed, to compensate them for injury. In most successful suits for negligent malpractice, the errors are glaring. Attention to the safeguards described in this chapter will protect clinicians from litigation, while allowing them to practice nondefensive psychiatry.

Selected Readings

This chapter has relied heavily on Smith's (1986) *Medical Malpractice: Psychiatric Care* which elaborates the legal principles of malpractice litigation, giving numerous case precedents, and on Simon's (1987) *Clinical Psychiatry & the Law*, which contains a detailed examination of malpractice liability from the clinician's viewpoint. Gutheil's (1980) article, "Paranoia and Progress Notes: A Guide to Forensically Informed Psychiatric Recordkeeping" is required reading for all psychiatric residents. Gutheil and Appelbaum's (1982) *Clinical Handbook of Psychiatry and the Law* contains an elegant analysis of the doctrine of informed consent within its chapter on malpractice.

References

Abille v. United States, 482 F Supp 703 (ND Cal 1980).

Abraham v. Zaslow, No 245862 (Santa Clara County Sup Ct October 26, 1970).

Aiken v. Clary, 396 SW 2d 668 (Mo 1965).

Annas GJ: *The Rights of Hospital Patients*. New York, Avon, 1975.

Bellah v. Greenson, 81 Cal App 3d 614, 146 Cal Rptr 535 (1978).

Bellotti v. Baird, 428 US 132 (1976).

Brady v. Hopper, 570 F Supp 1333 D Co (1983).

Bremer v. State, 18 Md App 291, 307 A 2d 503 (1973).

Canterbury v. Spence, 464 F 2d 772 (DC Cir 1973).

Clites v. State of Iowa, 322 NW 2d 917 (Iowa Ct App 1982), 247, 533 nn., 182, 187.

Cobbs v. Grant, 8 Cal 3d 229, 502 P 2d 1, 104 Cal Rptr 505 (1972).

Cole v. Taylor, 301 NW 2d 761 (Iowa 1981).

Davis v. Lhim, 124 Mich App 291, 335 NW 2d 481 (1983).

Gutheil, TG: Paranoia and progress notes: A guide to forensically informed psychiatric recordkeeping. *Hosp Community Psychiatry* 31:479–482, 1980.

Gutheil, TG, Appelbaum PS: *Clinical Handbook of Psychiatry and the Law*. New York, McGraw-Hill, 1982.

Higgins v. State, 24 AD 2d 147, 265 NYS 2d 254 (1965).

Hirschberg v. State, 91 Misc 2d 590, 398 NYS 2d 470 (1977).

Hopewell v. Adebimpe, 130 PHLJ 107 (Pa Ct Com Pl 1981).

Jablonski v. United States, 712 F 2d 391 (9th Cir 1983).

Jane Doe v. Joan Doe and Peter Poe, 400 NY Supp 2d 668 (1977).

Johnson v. Greer, 477 F 2d 101 (5th Cir 1973).

In re Lifschutz, 2 Cal 3d 415, 467 P 2d 557, 85 Cal Rptr 829 (1970).

Lipari v. Sears, Roebuck & Co., 497 F Supp 185 D Nev (1980).

Lundgren v. Fultz, 354 NW 2d 25 (Minn. 1984), 239, 531n 98.

McIntosh v. Milano, 168 NJ Super 466, 403 A 2d 500 (1979).

Mills v. Rogers, 457 US 291 (1982).

Monahan, J: *Predicting Violent Behavior: An Assessment of Clinical Techniques*. Beverly Hills, CA, Sage, 1981.

Mulder v. Parke Davis & Co., 288 Minn 332, 181 NW 2d 882 (1970).

Natanson v. Kline, 186 Kan 393, 350 P 2d 1093 (1960).

Nelson v. Heyne, 355 F Supp 451 (ND Ind, 1972), *affd*, 491 F 2d 352 (7th Cir), *cert denied*, 417 US 976 (1974).

O'Neill v. Montefiore Hospital, 11 AD 2d 132, 202 NYS 2d 436 (1960).

Osheroff v. Chestnut Lodge et al., Maryland Health Claims Arbitration #82-262 (1987).

Peck v. The Counseling Service of Addison County, Inc., Vt Sup Ct Docket 83-062 (June 14, 1985).

Pendleton v. Burkhalter, 432 SW 2d 724 (Tex Civ App 1968).

Planned Parenthood of Central Missouri v. Danforth, 428 US 52 (1976).

R.J.D. v. Vaughan Clinic, 572 So 2d 1225 (Ala 1990), 25, 536n 237.

Rennie v. Klein, 462 F Supp 1131 (DNJ 1978), *preliminary injunction denied*, 476 F Supp 1294 (DNJ 1979), *modified* 653 F 2d 836 (3d Cir 1981), *vacated*, 458 US 1119 (1982).

Rogers v. Okin, 478 F Supp 1342 (D Mass 1979), *affd in part, revd in part*, 634 F 2d 650 (1st Cir 1980), *vacated subnom*.

Rogers v. Commissioner of Mental Health, 458 N.E. 2d 308 (Mass. 1983), 33, 545 n. 92.

Rosenberg K: Workshop on the expert witness in psychic stress litigation. Presented at the annual conference of the American Association of Psychiatry and the Law, San Francisco, 1988.

Roy v. Hartogs, 81 Misc 2d 350, 366 NYS 2d 297 (1975). *affd*, 85 Misc 2d 891, 381 NYS 2d 587 (1976).

Samuels v. Southern Baptist Hospital, 594 So 2d 571 (La App 1992), 254, 536n 246.

Schloendorff v. New York Hospital, 211 NY 125, 105 NE 92 (1914).

Skar v. City of Lincoln, Nebraska, 599 F 2d 253 (8th Cir 1979).

Simon, RI: *Clinical Psychiatry & the Law*. Washington, DC, American Psychiatric Press, 1987.

Smith, JT: *Medical Malpractice: Psychiatric Care*. Colorado Springs, CO, Shepard's/McGraw-Hill, 1986.

Tarasoff v. Regents of the University of California, 529 P 2d 553, 118 Cal Rptr 129 (1974).

Tarasoff v. Regents of the University of California, 17 Cal 3d 425, 551 P 2d 334, 131 Cal Rptr 14 (1976).

Thompson v. County of Alameda, 27 Cal 3d 741, 614 P 2d 728, 167 Cal Rptr 70 (1980).

Wadlington WJ: Consent to medical care for minors: The legal framework. In: Melton GB, Koocher GP, Saks MJ (eds): *Children's Competence to Consent*. New York, Plenum Press, 1983.

Wickline v. State, 239 Cal Rptr 810 (Cal App 1986).

Wilson v. Blue Cross of California, 271 Cal Rptr 876 (Cal App 1990), 261, 538n 290.

Youngberg v. Romeo, 457 US 307 (1982).

116 LEGAL ISSUES IN PROFESSIONAL LIABILITY

Angela R. Holder, LL.M.

MALPRACTICE

Definition

Medical malpractice or negligence may be defined as failure to use due care in the diagnosis or treatment of a patient's illness or injury. All negligence actions—medical malpractice claims, malpractice claims against lawyers or engineers, automobile wreck claims, airplane crash claims—are varieties of tort law, which is defined as "a violation of duty imposed by general law or otherwise upon all persons occupying the relation to each other which is involved in a given transaction" (1). Negligence in particular is defined as "the omission to do something which a reasonable man, guided by those ordinary considerations which ordinarily regulate human affairs, would do, or the doing of something which a reasonable and prudent man would not do" (2). All negligence actions are predicated on the claim that the person who asserts that he or she was damaged was owed a duty by the other and that the duty was breached, causing harm. In a lawsuit involving a defendant in an automobile accident who is accused of having been driving while drunk, for example, the plaintiff will claim that the defendant had a duty to all other parties on the road to drive safely and that he or she breached it.

Standard of Care

In any type of professional negligence action, including those against physicians, lawyers, architects, engineers, and others, the concept of "the reasonable man" becomes the "duly careful member of the profession" (3). This means that the physician will behave as "the reasonably prudent physician or surgeon acting in the same or similar circumstances" (4).

The physician who holds himself or herself out to be a specialist would, of course, under this criterion, be measured against a standard of the reasonably careful specialist. This higher standard required of those who claim greater expertise than that demanded of physicians who claim more general skills seems quite fair. The definition of a "specialist," it should be noted, does not require board certification in a field. All that is demanded is that the physician *says* that he or she is a specialist.

The three elements of due care are skill, care, and knowledge. Knowledge is, basically, knowing what other physicians with the same training would know about the problem. If a patient comes to the physician with complaints of A, B, and C, does the physician order the tests that any careful physician would order for these symptoms? Skill is that element of care that, given the cognitive element of knowledge, results in correct resolution of the problem (e.g., the surgeon sutures the wound correctly). Skill usually involves the employment of proper technique and correct use of motor skills. Care means that once a physician knows what to do and has the skill to do it correctly, he or she is paying attention to what is happening and does not make the mistake of, for example, failing to notice that a scalpel is left in the patient's abdomen.

As long as a physician complies with these standards, he or she is not negligent as a matter of law, no matter how catastrophic the result of the treatment may be. No inference of negligence may ever be drawn from the fact that a patient did not improve or got worse (5). Moreover, in almost all malpractice cases, the plaintiff-patient must prove the defendant physician's negligence by presenting expert testimony from a physician who is knowledgeable in the field in question, including evidence of the applicable standard of care. The expert witness must also give his or her opinion that the evidence shows that the defendant departed from that standard (6).

The last element that must be proved in a malpractice claim is that the negligence is the proximate cause of harm to the patient. However careless a physician may be, if the patient does not suffer harm as a result, damages may not be awarded. In one famous case, for example, a child had an orthopaedic problem requiring a cast on one leg. The physician put the cast on the wrong leg, an example of fairly obvious negligence. However, since the child stayed in bed the entire time until the error was discovered, there was no evidence that his leg had gotten worse, and the court held that there was no proximate cause of damage (7). Within the setting of a hospital, one of the more obviously negligent and frequently lethal errors is to give one patient a blood transfusion intended for another patient. If, however, both are the same blood type, the recipient may suffer no harm at all and hence could not prove proximate cause in a malpractice action.

Malpractice in Child Psychiatry

Although the number of malpractice suits against psychiatrists is much lower than those filed against physicians in most other specialties, the issue of liability is a serious one.

The most frequent cause of malpractice suits against psychiatrists is drug reactions or side effects. In particular, patients who develop tardive dyskinesia (for obvious reasons) may be inclined to sue (8). The issue of liability in drug reaction cases tends to revolve around two questions: (*a*) Was the drug properly prescribed? (*b*) Was the patient (or the family, if the patient's condition was such that he or she could not give consent) warned about this possibility and given enough information to allow for a genuinely informed consent?

However carefully a drug may be administered, if it is an inappropriate one for relief of the patient's condition, liability is virtually automatic if the patient has a problem with side effects (9). Moreover, if giving an inappropriate drug that in itself does not hurt the patient delays recovery because the patient was deprived of a drug that would have made him or her well faster, there may also be liability (10).

The usual question raised by tardive dyskinesia claims is whether the patient's condition was sufficiently severe to justify prescription of the drug that caused it. Prescribing dangerous psychotropic drugs for mild complaints of depression or distress is likely to result in liability if the patient should develop permanent difficulties as a result (11).

If a patient's condition is such that drugs are necessary, the possibility of side effects should be explained. If the patient is too young or too impaired to understand the explanation, the family should be fully informed of the risks (12).

Another area in which prescription of drugs might cause legal problems for a child psychiatrist is the use of psychoactive medication in the treatment of the child with attention deficit hyperactivity disorder (ADHD). In viewing this condition as a legal, not medical, question, the first problem is that of making sure of the accuracy of the diagnosis. Even discounting those who think that treatment of this problem is "drugging children into submission," many other factors, such as hunger or poor teachers, may cause behavior problems at school for many children. Further, making a diagnosis of ADHD without adequate medical and psychiatric evaluation might result in failure to diagnose a serious, even life-threatening problem, such as a brain tumor. Thus, due skill, care, and knowledge are required in diagnosis as well as in treatment.

Particularly in prescription of Ritalin, due care mandates careful history taking (13). Since children with a history (or even a family history) of neurological problems may develop tics or other movement disorders from these drugs, failure to take an adequate history might well be the critical point of a malpractice claim if the child encounters difficulties.

An issue that presents itself in this circumstance but not in most other areas of use of medications is the child's or parent's right to refuse these drugs. In many instances, the child is a disturbance in the classroom and is referred to a psychiatrist by the school system and not because the parent perceives a need for treatment. Even if the parent accepts the diagnosis (and many do not), there may be many reasons why he or she does not wish the child to receive psychoactive medication. There could

be adherence to the Christian Science faith, concern about the side effects of these drugs, or just philosophical rejection of the idea of controlling children's behavior through medication. While private schools have much more control over admission and retention of students than do public schools, it is questionable that a private school could make medication for this purpose a condition of admission or of staying in the school, especially if a parent found a physician who would lend medically credible support to the refusal, and it is absolutely certain that no public school could do so (14). Since *Brown v. Board of Education* (15) outlawed segregation, courts have assumed that education is a fundamental right. A child may be expelled from public school only when the school is able to show that the protection of other children requires exclusion of the child (16). Moreover, the Education for All Handicapped Children Act (17) of 1975 and decisions interpreting it have made clear that a child with a handicap (retarded, hard of hearing, speech impaired, visually impaired, emotionally disturbed, orthopaedically impaired, or learning disabled) cannot be denied a public education suitable for his or her needs.

Evaluating a child who may need special education programs also raises legal issues. Placement in special education carries enormous significance for a child's future. Improper placement as the result of negligent diagnosis or evaluation can easily mean that once the error is discovered, the child is so far behind the regular classroom's work that he or she will never catch up (18). Further, special education placement may adversely affect a child's self-image. Numerous awards of very substantial damages have resulted from suits against physicians or psychologists who were negligent in evaluating children and did not notice before diagnosing the child as "retarded" that he or she was of normal intelligence but deaf or nearly blind (19). The standard of care applied to such an evaluation is the same degree of care expected in any diagnostic situation.

Another area in which numerous malpractice suits against psychiatrists have succeeded is liability claims based on the patient's violence directed toward himself or another person. In adult psychiatry, there is a clear legal duty to warn a person whom the psychiatrist believes to be at risk of harm from a patient (20). Generalized threats of violence normally do not impose such a duty (21), although credible threats, general or specific, may very well impose a duty to commit a violent person to a mental hospital (22). The problem, of course, is that of attempting to establish whether or not the patient actually intends harm to someone, but if the reasonable psychiatrist would have concluded that actual danger exists and the treating psychiatrist does nothing, the psychiatrist may be found liable in damages to the victim or the victim's survivors (23).

In dealing with children as patients, however, a parent's right to know is certainly less restricted than an adult patient's family's would be. If a child is threatening suicide or harm to himself or others, the parents have every right to know, since they can restrict the child's access to dangerous objects or keep him or her away from those persons who could be hurt. Any threat, even if the psychiatrist is not inclined to take it seriously, to hurt the parents should be reported to them (24).

CHILDREN AND ADOLESCENTS AND CONSENT TO TREATMENT

At common law, a minor child, which meant anyone under 21, not 18, was effectively a chattel of his or her father. A father had the right to sue a physician who treated a child without his permission, even if the treatment was appropriate and had a good result, because such intervention transgressed upon the father's right to control the child.

This is still the rule in a nonacute situation involving a young child. If for example, a 3-year-old is visiting his grandmother and she takes him to a plastic surgeon for repair of a birthmark his parents had decided to leave alone, the plastic surgeon would be at substantial risk if he operated without consent of the parents (25).

On the other hand, since at least the early 1950s, adolescents in our society have become increasingly independent, and courts have recognized and accepted this independence. It has been at least 40 years since a parent successfully sued a physician in this country for treating a minor 15 or over without parental consent (26). It should be remembered, however, that, except in emergency situations, a parent is not liable for the cost of medical care for a minor unless the parent consented to having that care provided (27).

Consent in Emergencies

In an emergency, a child of any age may be treated without parental consent if the parents cannot be located immediately (28). For this purpose, an ''emergency'' is any condition requiring prompt treatment, and not only a condition that may lead to the child's death or disability if untreated. For example, a small child who has an earache or a cut foot and is brought to an emergency room by a teenage baby sitter would constitute ''an emergency'' for this purpose.

Special Consent Statutes

Because physicians were concerned about treating adolescents without parental consent, beginning in the early 1950s state legislatures began enacting statutes permitting teenagers to consent to their own treatment for venereal disease (VD). It was perfectly evident to legislators as well as to physicians that, if parental consent to treatment were required, teenagers would simply not go for treatment, and the epidemic of VD in this population would get worse. All states have enacted VD treatment statutes (29); most, in fact, forbid the physician to tell the parent that the young person has been treated, and some specify that the parents may not be billed for the care (on the theory that, if the parent receives a bill, he or she will find out the purpose of the visits) (30). The next public health concern involving adolescents was drug and alcohol abuse. Most, if not all, states now have specific statutes covering consent to treatment for these problems. These disease-specific statutes do not have an age limit—a 9-year-old with a drinking problem is given the same right to confidential treatment as a 17-year-old with the same difficulty.

General Consent Statutes

Many states also enacted statutes that provide that a minor of a given age—usually 16, but some statutes provide for consent as early as 14—may consent to any and all medical treatment as if she or he were an adult. Some of these statutes specifically prohibit consent to abortion or organ donation without parental consent, but a physician in a state with such a statute may, in keeping with any limitations the statute imposes, treat a teenager without discussing the situation with parents (31).

Emancipation

For at least 200 years, courts in the Anglo-American system have recognized the concept of an ''emancipated minor.'' This means one who is living on his or her own (in the earlier days of the law, it was on *his* own), is self-supporting, and is not subject to parental control. The old concepts of emancipation included minors in the military (of which there were numerous when the age of majority was 21) (32) or married minors. The concept has evolved nowadays to include college students under 18, even when parents are completely responsible for paying the bills, or unmarried minor mothers (33), and in some states a pregnant minor is considered completely emancipated. A runaway is also considered an emancipated minor, no matter how young he or she may be.

The Mature Minor Rule

In addition to the exceptions to requirements of parental consent discussed above, courts in this country have bowed to modern reality,

and decisions all over the country apply what has come to be known as the ''mature minor rule'' (34). The legal principle now applied is that if a young person (of 14 or 15) understands the nature of a proposed treatment and its risks and can give the same degree of informed consent as an adult patient, and if the treatment does not involve very serious risks, the young person may give a valid consent. The age and maturity of the patient must be considered, but the nature of the illness and the risks of therapy are also relevant. A 14-year-old might be perfectly capable of consenting to treatment of a sprained ankle; no oncologist would consider treating the same patient for leukemia without his or her parents' knowledge.

In almost all cases, the issue of treatment without parental knowledge arises in the context of ambulatory care. Most hospitals refuse to admit minors for nonemergency treatment unless the parent, who almost always is the person with insurance (on which children are carried as dependents), signs financial responsibility and insurance forms.

Thus, as we can see, in terms of consent to general medical care, courts are granting much more autonomy to increasingly younger adolescents. Preadolescents, however, do not have a right to consent (35).

REFUSAL OF TREATMENT

If a minor has the right to consent to treatment, it is likely that he or she has the right to refuse treatment. It is therefore always a good idea, if dealing with an adolescent of 14 or over, to obtain the patient's consent, as well as that of his or her parents, to a procedure. In any purely elective situation (such as cosmetic surgery) where a parent wishes an adolescent to be treated but the patient refuses, a prudent physician would decline to treat the patient. In any situation where a minor can be treated at his or her own request and without knowledge of the parents, it is likely that the minor has the right to refuse, at least if the problem is not life threatening.

Since a younger child does not have the right to consent, he or she also does not have the right to refuse.

It is clear that a pregnant teenager has the right to refuse an abortion that her parents wish her to have (36). In situations such as requests for court orders for treatment of a minor over parental religious objection, judges usually consult adolescent patients about their views on the matter before treatment is ordered, particularly if the patient's lack of cooperation could affect the outcome of the intervention (37). These cases, however, usually do not involve life-threatening problems. Only one case can be located in which a court allowed an adolescent to refuse lifesaving treatment (38). A 16-year-old girl, who was the daughter of Jehovah's Witnesses, refused on religious grounds to have blood transfusions for leukemia. Her physicians and the hospital in which she was a patient asked the court for guidance on the legality of a minor's refusal of lifesaving treatment. The judge ruled, and his ruling was upheld on appeal, that once he had determined that her religious views were her own and that she was not being coerced by her parents, her knowledgeable refusal should be respected to the same extent that it would be if she were an adult. It is unlikely that any judge would give such credence to the views of a minor under 16; it is also not at all clear that courts in other states will follow the same reasoning and allow any minor to decide to die where successful treatment of the problem is available.

Freedom of Religion and Refusal of Treatment

A parent's failure to provide ''adequate'' medical care for a child is a criminal offense under all states' child neglect and abuse laws (39). Court intervention is an option in circumstances in which physicians and hospital administrators wish to invoke it. Until recently, court orders to treat were virtually automatic, and in almost all cases, that is still the case. Where, however, parental objection to treatment is based on a risk assessment of complex therapy or newly developed surgical intervention, courts appear to be willing to consider parental reservations. For example, if a court order for chemotherapy is sought by physicians and the parents' reason for refusing the treatment is that their child is, by all accounts, terminally ill and they wish to let her "die in peace," it is unlikely that a court would order administration of the drugs. When a treating physician asks for court-ordered treatment, orders are still virtually automatic, but increasingly, when requests are initiated by welfare agencies, police, or school personnel under circumstances in which the physician taking care of the child agrees with the parents' decision, parents do seem universally to prevail. For example, in the Babies Doe cases involving handicapped newborns, when the physicians agreed with the parents that surgery on the babies was undesirable and state or federal governmental entities tried to intervene to ask the courts to order treatment, in every instance the parents and treating physicians prevailed (40).

Although it is now clear that a competent adult has the right to refuse lifesaving treatment for himself or herself for religious or other reasons, in all states parents whose refusal to allow necessary treatment of their child is based on religious conviction are still found to be "neglectful" even though their right to religious freedom is protected by the First Amendment (41).

All courts have held that a Jehovah's Witness whose child's condition requires blood transfusions has no right to forbid them on the ground of religious conviction (42).

THE MINOR IN THE MENTAL HEALTH SYSTEM

The Minor in the Outpatient Psychiatric System

Since minor treatment statutes and the mature minor rule apply to all forms of care provided by physicians, one must assume, although there are no cases on the point, that the same legal rules apply to an adolescent who goes to see a psychiatrist as apply to a visit to a gynecologist. If the psychiatrist wishes to treat the teenager, it is difficult to see how a parent could object. Since private psychotherapy is, however, extremely expensive, the issue is most likely to be raised when the teenager goes to a mental health center or community counseling service. Where the community facility is one in which a qualified psychiatrist is on staff and other mental health professionals, such as psychologists, nurse clinicians, or psychiatric social workers, provide therapy as a team effort with physicians, there is little question that the minor has the right to seek treatment. There are, however, many so-called mental health facilities where no physicians are involved or available. In particular, many drug treatment centers provide therapists who are drug addicts themselves, and no medical backup is available. This may be a viable method of providing drug treatment or other specialized therapies, but it is not at all clear that the legal right of a minor to seek medical care necessarily applies to such facilities.

The intent of legislatures and courts who broadened the adolescent's right to seek medical care was to get young people to physicians, not to well-meaning but nonmedical counselors whose training may be questionable.

The issue of refusal of outpatient mental health treatment that the parent wishes the adolescent to have but the adolescent does not want is a legally fascinating one, but for very practical reasons not a real issue. If a parent takes a young person to a psychiatrist and the patient does not want to cooperate, all he or she has to do is refuse to talk to the psychiatrist. It is physically possible to hold someone down and administer medical care if one must do so; it is not possible to engage in psychotherapy with someone who refuses to talk.

COMMITMENT OF THE MINOR PATIENT

Adult mental patients have certain legal protections against unjustified or malicious commitments to mental hospitals that minors do not necessarily have. An adult may voluntarily go to a mental hospital and may also leave it if he or she wishes to, unless the hospital concludes that the patient is so ill that involuntary commitment is necessary. In

that case, the patient has a right to a judicial hearing. Commitment as an involuntary patient, if one is an adult, may only follow a judicial hearing at which one is, among other things, entitled to counsel. The standard of commitment of an adult is that he or she is dangerous to self or others or is gravely mentally disabled, meaning that the person is too mentally ill to provide himself or herself with the basic necessities of life (43).

Minors, however, fall into an entirely different category. Many states allow "voluntary" commitment of minors by their parents, which means that, although the young person cannot leave the hospital, he or she is considered a "voluntary" patient and has no right to a hearing at which a judge can rule on the merits of the commitment. If all families were healthy and happy, that might be a reasonable solution to the problem, but in any number of instances, minors have been "dumped" into mental hospitals by their parent, when the parent is probably the one who needed treatment (44).

Nowadays it seems that frightened parents, probably in good faith in most instances, are having teenagers in record numbers admitted to for-profit drug and alcohol hospitals and treatment centers in instances in which there may not be very clear indications that inpatient treatment is required and, if recent media reports are correct, where the quality of care and the training of therapists is open to very serious question (45). At least two states' courts have held that, since these facilities are not considered "mental hospitals," a minor admitted by parents has none of the due process rights or access to the legal system that would accrue to him or her if admitted to a psychiatric hospital (46).

Beginning in the 1960s, after a fair number of young people were literally committed to mental hospitals by parents who were upset with antiwar protests, long hair, and general hippiness, most states did enact statutes providing for judicial intervention in the commitment process when minors were patients. In other states, courts ruled that these minor patients had the right to some constitutional protections. In North Carolina, for example, it was held in a 1975 case that a 15-year-old boy who had been committed by his mother had a right to a hearing within 72 hours of admission, although the young person could still be signed in by a parent in an emergency (47). This decision was fairly typical of those in most other states' courts during this period.

Many of the states' new statutes provided that a child under 13 or 14 could be admitted by parents without judicial intervention. Most, however, specified that minors over that age might continue to be admitted by their parents, but once in the hospital, the patients had a right to prompt hearings with the assistance of counsel if they wished to object to their admissions. Many statutes also provided that teenagers could admit themselves to mental hospitals as voluntary patients. If they did so, however, they had the same right as adult patients to discharge themselves unless the hospitals were willing to ask courts for orders of involuntary commitment (48).

On June 20, 1979, however, the Supreme Court ruled (49) that if a state legislature did not choose to enact procedural rights for minor mental patients, minors' federal constitutional rights were not violated if their parents admitted them to a mental hospital over their objection.

Thus, the rights of children and adolescents committed to mental hospitals are, at this time, exclusively derived from state law, and no federal constitutional protections are given them.

THE CHILD PSYCHIATRIST IN COURT

A physician may appear in court as a witness for one party or the other, as a treating physician, or as an expert witness. A treating physician may be subpoenaed to testify about facts within his or her knowledge relevant to the case; however, expert opinion testimony may never be compelled from an unwilling witness (50). The expert, who may never have seen the patient but who has reviewed the medical records, usually testifies about his or her *opinion* of the situation—views on child placement, whether medical care met the requisite standard or was negligent, or the like.

In an increasing number of cases involving children, judges feel the need of objective expert medical advice and may use their discretion to appoint a physician to be an independent witness. The purpose of such an appointment may be to examine a party to the action or the children in a family, or, in most cases, it is to serve as a true advisor to the judge, providing assistance based on information already in evidence in the court and giving the judge professional analyses of that evidence. In any case in which a physician is a court-appointed witness asked to examine a party, his or her testimony about that examination is not covered by physician-patient privilege because he or she is not a "treating physician" for purposes of privilege statutes. His or her role as a court-appointed expert is to investigate, as "an arm of the court," those matters on which professional expertise is requested and not to represent the interests of any party (51). If one is the treating physician of either parent or child involved in a custody case, physician-patient privilege is considered much less important than are the best interests of the child, so the physician will usually be obliged to testify. However, disclosure of confidential psychiatric information without being ordered to do so by a court may subject the psychiatrist to a successful malpractice suit. No information should be disclosed, particularly to the adverse party or his or her attorney, without consent of the patient or the patient's parent who has asked the psychiatrist to treat the child. If testimony is needed, a judge can order it to be given, and until that time arrives, no information should be disclosed without the patient's consent (52).

Another sort of issue is presented in some cases involving subtle forms of child abuse. Children's protective agencies are not usually staffed by particularly well-educated workers, and even if they are, in all jurisdictions they are overworked and understaffed. Abuse that is primarily emotional in nature or, although physical, does not leave clear marks, fractures, or other undeniable signs on the child may, when reported, not impress the caseworker enough to result in any action. One sort of situation in which most child protective services workers are uncomfortable is in a case of Munchausen's by proxy, in which a parent is deliberately making a child ill in some way. (Actually, this is the wrong name for this situation. Munchausen's syndrome refers to a factitious illness; these children may be made critically ill.) Typically, the child with mysterious symptoms is admitted to the hospital, and it eventually becomes obvious to the caregivers that the child becomes worse when one or both parents are present and recovers when the parent or parents go away. Close observation short of witnessing the act may

convince everyone at the hospital that the parent is harming the child, but the child protective services worker says "prove it" and refuses to go forward with court proceedings in the absence of objective evidence. Obtaining such evidence may, in rare cases, demand a hidden video camera, taping the child's room and all activities therein.

While such taping raises clear-cut moral dilemmas about invasion of privacy, it is, when used as a last resort, legal. First, no such spying operation on a parent should be carried out within a hospital unless the suspected activity is or may be causing serious harm to the child. (If the child has been admitted to the hospital in the first place, however, the child is usually sufficiently ill that there is no question about the gravity of the situation.) Second, all other means of obtaining evidence should have been exhausted, and, third, the child protective services authorities should have been told of the suspicion and refused to act without the evidence provided by a tape. If all those factors are present, the important factor to remember is that the privacy rights involved are those of the patient (the child), not the patient's parent. Whatever privacy rights a young child may or may not have, they obviously are subservient to his or her rights to be protected from life-threatening or disabling abuse. From the constitutional perspective, the provisions of the Bill of Rights (such as protections from searches and seizures) apply only to state agencies and would not, therefore, be relevant to evidence gathered by a private hospital. Even where a public hospital is involved, however, a warrant to videotape would be granted on a showing of probable cause to believe that abuse is occurring within the hospital.

In many of these cases, before the evidence is gathered or, if gathered, before it is turned over to child protective services authorities, the pediatrician may ask a child psychiatrist to interview the parent. The issue then becomes whether the parent should be told the purpose of the interview. It would seem that in general the parent does have a right to know that the interview is not intended to be directly therapeutic for the child and therefore she or he should be told that the interview is to assist in establishing whether the parent is making the child ill.

Since state statutes on evidentiary matters and state constitutions' provisions on such issues as videotaping vary widely, under no circumstances should a physician or a hospital engage in this sort of evidence gathering without advice from the hospital's local attorney. If a child may die if unprotected, a judge will be available to help with these situations.

References

1. Coleman v. California Friends Church, 81 P 2d 469,470 Cal 1938.
2. Schneider v. Little Company, 151 NW 587, Mich 1915.
3. Pike v. Honsinger, 49 NE 760, NY 1898; Adkins v. Ropp, 14 NE 2d 727, Ind 1938.
4. Armstrong v. Svoboda, 49 Cal Rptr 701, Cal 1966; Betesh v. United States, 400 F Supp 238, DC DC 1974.
5. Teig v. St. John's Hospital, 387 P 2d 527, Wash 1963; Williams v. Chamberlain, 316 SW 2d 505, Mo 1958; Lane v. Calvert, 138 A 2d 902, MD 1958; Staloch v. Holm, 111 NW 264, Minn 1907.
6. Speer v. United States, 512 F Supp 679, DC Tex 1981; Rudy v. Meshorer, 706 P 2d 1234, Ariz 1985; Sharpe v. South Carolina Department of Mental Health, 354 SE 2d 778, SC 1987.
7. Reder v. Hanson, 338 F 2d 244, CCA 8, 1964.
8. E.g., Barclay v. Campbell, 704 SW 2d 8, Tex 1986; Clites v. State, 322 NW 2d 917, Iowa 1982.
9. Rotan v. Greenbaum, 273 F 2d 830, CA DC 1959; Naughton v. Bevilacqua, 458 F Supp 610, 458 F Supp 610, 605 F 2d 586, 1978.
10. E.g., Troppi v. Scarf 187 NW 2d 511, Mich 1971.
11. Clites v. State, 322 NW 2d 917, Iowa 1982.
12. Barclay v. Campbell, 704 SW 2d 8, Tex 1986.
13. E.g., Domina v. Pratt, 13 A 2d 198, Vt 1940.
14. Wells, William, W., Drug Control of School Children: The Child's Right to Choose, 46 *So Cal Law Rev* 585, 1973; Ireland, Roderick L., and Dimond, Paul R., Drugs and Hyperactivity: Process Is Due, 9 *Inequality in Education* 19, 1971.
15. Brown v. Board of Education, 347 US 483, 1954.
16. E.g., People v. Jackson, 319 NYS 2d 331, NY 1971.
17. PL 94-142, 20 USCA sections 1401–61.
18. E.g., Hobson v. Hanson, 408 F 2d 175, CA DC 1969; Larry P. v. Riles, 343 F Supp 1306, DC Cal 1972.
19. Hoffman v. Board of Education of the City of New York, 410 NYS 2d 99, NY 1978.
20. E.g., Tarasoff v. Board of Regents of the University of California, 118 Cal Rptr 129, Cal 1974; Peterson v. Washington, 671 P 2d 230, 1983.
21. Thompson v. County of Alameda, 614P 2d 728, Cal 1980; Brady v. Hopper, 751 F 2d 329, CCA 10 1984.
22. Currie v. United States, 644 F Supp 1074, DC NC 1986; Estate of Johnson by Johnson v. Village of Libertyville, 496 NE 2d 1219, Ill 1986.
23. Bradley Center v. Wessner, 287 SE 2d 716, Ga 1982.
24. Peck v. Counseling Service of Addison County, 499 A 2d 422, Vt 1985; Cairl v. State, 323 NW 2d 20, Minn 1982.
25. Bonnerv. Moran, 126 F 2d 121, CA DC 1941; Zaman v. Schultz, 19 Pa D & C 309, 1933.
26. E.g., Carter v. Cangello, 164 Cal Rptr 361, Cal 1980; Younts v. St. Francis Hospital and School of Nursing, 469 P 2d 330, Kans 1970; Lacey v. Laird, 139 NE 2d 25, Ohio 1956.
27. Accent Service Company v. Ebsen, 306 NW 2d 575, Neb 1981; Poudre Valley Hospital District v. Heckart, 491 P 2d 984, Colo 1971; Ison v. Florida Sanitarium and Benevolent Association, 302 So 2d 200, Fla 1974; Cidis v. White, 336 NYS 2d 362, NY 1972; Alamance County Hospital, Inc. v. Neighbors, 315 SE 2d 779, NC 1984; Altman v. Altman, 518 NYS 2d 763, NY 1987.
28. Luka v. Lowrie, 136 NW 1106, Mich 1912; Sullivan v. Montgomery, 279 NYS 575, NY 1935.
29. Holder, Angela R., Treating a Minor for Venereal Disease, 214 *JAMA* 1949, December 7, 1970.
30. E.g., *Connecticut General Statutes*, Title 19a, Section 216.
31. See, e.g. North Carolina General Statutes Section 90-21.1,47 *North Carolina Attorneys General Opinions* 83 (1977). For further reading on this topic, see Morrisey, J.M., Hofmann, A.D. and Thrope, J.C., *Consent and Confidentiality in the Health Care of Children and Adolescents: A Legal Guide*, New York, The Free Press, 1986; Holder, Angela Roddey, *Legal Issues in Pediatrics and Adolescent Medicine*, 2nd Edition, New

Haven, Yale University Press 1985, Chapter 5; Ewald, Linda Sorenson, Medical Decision-making for Children: An Analysis of Competing Interests, 25 *St Louis Law J* 689, 1982.

32. Yarborough v. Yarborough, 290 US 202, 1933; Swenson v. Swenson, 227 SW 2d 103, Mo 1950.

33. E.g., Bach v. Long Island Jewish Hospital, 267 NYS 2d 289, NY 1966.

34. Cardwell v. Bechtol, 724 SW 2d 739, Tenn 1987; Holder, Angela R., Informed Consent and the Adolescent Patient, *Malpractice Digest*, January 1980; Holder, Angela R., The Minor's Right to Consent to Medical Treatment, 41 *Conn Med* 579, 1977; Holder, Angela R., Minors' Rights to Consent to Medical Care, 257 *JAMA* 3400, 1987; Munson, Carol F., Toward A Standard of Informed Consent by the Adolescent in Medical Treatment Decisions, 8 *Dickenson Law Rev*, 431, 1981.

35. Plutshack v. The University of Minnesota Hospitals, 316 NW 2d 1, Minn 1982; Rothenberg, Karen H., Medical Decision-making for Children, in Childress, James F., King, Patricia A., Rothenberg, Karen Al. Wadlington, Walter J., and Gaare, Ruth D., Editors, *Biolaw: A Legal and Ethical Reporter on Medicine. Health Care and Bioengineering*, Frederick, Maryland, University Publications of America, 1986.

36. In re Smith, 295 A 2d 238, Md 1972; In re Mary P., 444 NYS 2d 545, NY 1981.

37. E.g., In re Seiferth, 127 NE 2d 820, NY 1955; In re Green, 292 A 2d 387, Pa 1972.

38. In the Interests of E.G., 161 Ill App 3d 765, 113 Ill Dec 477, 515 NE 2d 286, 1987.

39. Commonwealth v. Barnhart, 487A 2d 616, Pa 1985; In re Willman, 24 Ohio App 3d 191, 493

NE 2d 1380, 1986; In re Alyne E., 113 Misc 2d 387, 448 NYS 2d 984, 1982; In re Hamilton, 657 SW 2d 425, Tenn 1983.

40. E.g., In re Doe, Circuit Court for Monroe County, Indiana, order signed April 12, 1982. The court order is published at 47 *Connecticut Medicine* 409, July, 1983. The most famous of these cases was the Baby Jane Doe case, United States v. University Hospital at Stony Brook and the Parents of Baby Jane Doe, 575 F Supp 607, 729 F 2d 144, CCA 2, 1984.

41. E.g., In the Matter of the Appeal in Cochise County Juvenile Action, 650P 2d 459, Ariz 1982; In re D.L.E., 645P 2d 271, Colo 1982; In re Tolbert, 378 NE 2d 565, Ill 1978.

42. There are literally hundreds of cases involving court orders for blood transfusions of Jehovah's Witnesses children. This is clearly the most common form of parental objection to treatment. Some of the more recent cases are Muhlenberg Hospital v. Patterson, 320A 2d 518, NJ 1974 and those discussed in Holder, Angela R., Circumstances Warranting Court-Ordered Medical Treatment of Minors, 24 *POF* 2d 169.

43. O'Conner v. Donaldson, 422 US 563, 1975.

44. E.g., In re Sippy, 97A 2d 455, DC Mun Ct App 1953, In re 61., 104 Cal Rptr 585, Cal 1972; In re Anonymous, 248 NYS 2d 608, NY 1964. Koocher, Gerald P., Different Lenses: Psycho-Legal Perspectives on Children's Rights, 16 *Nova Law Rev* 711, 1992.

45. For example, there was a horrifying 20-minute segment about parental admission of teenagers to these facilities on the ABC television program "20/20" on August 21, 1986. See, e.g., Weithorn, Lois A., Mental Hospitalization of Trouble-

some Youth: An Analysis of Skyrocketing Admission Rates, 40 *Stan Law Rev* 773, 1988; Sperber, Marc N., Short-Sheeting the Psychiatric Bed: State-level Strategies to Curtail the Unnecessary Hospitalization of Adolescents in For-Profit Mental Health Facilities, 18 *AJLM* 251, 1992; Kinney, Eleanor D., Legal and Ethical Issues in Mental Health Care Delivery: Does Corporate Form Make a Difference, 28 *Houston Law Rev* 175, 1991; Smith, Steven R., Mental Health Malpractice in the 1990s, 28 *Houston Law Rev* 209, 1991. See also, Cowley, Geoffrey, Money Madness, *Newsweek*, November 4, 1991, pages 50–52; Darnton, Nina, Committed Youth, *Newsweek* July 31, 1989, pp 66–72.

46. Department of Health and Rehabilitative Services v. Straight, Inc., 497 So 2d 692, Fla App 1986. R.J.D. v. The Vaughn Clinic, 572 So 2d 1225, Ala 1990.

47. In re Long, 214 SE 2d 626, NC 1975.

48. E.g., Melville v. Sabbatino, 313A 2d 886, Conn 1973.

49. Parham v. J.R., 442 US 584, 1979. See also Tiano, Linda V., Parham v. J.R., "Voluntary" Commitment of Minors to Mental Institutions, 6 *Am J Law and Med* 125, 1980.

50. Kaufman v. Edelstein, 539 F 2d 811, CCA 2 1976; United States v. Allen, 494 F Supp 107, DC Wisc 1980; Buchanan v. American Motors Corporation, 697 F 2d 151, CCA 6 1983.

51. In re Blaine, 282 NYS 2d 359, NY 1967; Lincoln v. Lincoln, 247 NE 2d 659, NY 1969; Williams v. Congdon, 257 SE 2d 677, NC 1979; Bond v. Pecault, 561 F Supp 1037, DC Ill 1983.

52. Schaffer v. Schaffer, 215 NW 2d 134, SD 1974; Adams v. Perk, 403 A 2d 840, 415 A 2d 292, Md 1980.

117 TESTIFYING IN COURT

A/ A Psychiatrist's Viewpoint

Elissa P. Benedek, M.D.

The process of being an expert witness begins the moment one accepts a telephone call from an attorney or court and agrees to become involved in litigation, continues through report writing, and culminates in testifying in court.

The use and misuse of forensic reports and court testimony by mental health experts has been debated by professionals in the legal and mental health system (Bank and Poythress, 1982). Some experts argue that the psychiatrist has no place in the court room but should stay in the consulting room, the area of his or her expertise. Others argue that providing appropriate and meaningful input into the legal system is a legitimate and important role for the mental health professional and that to abrogate that role would be a dereliction of duty. I believe that providing mental health input and psychiatric testimony to bench and bar can be another form of clinical effectiveness. For example, in a child custody determination, a mental health professional can provide critical information that might prevent a young child from being raised by a physically, sexually, or emotionally abusive parent. Such information might not be known without a forensic evaluation and expert testimony.

INITIAL CONTACT

Initial contact with the court or private attorney generally begins with a letter or phone call. Here, the consultee asks the clinician if he

or she would be willing to review the materials and render an opinion. It is incumbent on the clinician to set forth the ground rules under which he or she will participate in such a consultation. Ground rules can include the following: First, the attorney must recognize from the beginning that the clinician will evaluate the materials in an objective manner. It is entirely possible that the opinion rendered by the clinician will not be favorable to the attorney's position. However, the clinician must make it clear from the onset that his or her objectivity and ethics will not be compromised. Second, the attorney must be willing to send all available documents to the clinician. Even the most competent attorney selecting materials from a file will be hard pressed to determine which materials are relevant and critical to the determination of clinical issues. In addition, there may be an unconscious temptation to select only those materials that will portray the attorney's client's position and to omit materials that would present additional important data but might not be favorable to the client's position. Third, in many situations it may be impossible to adequately assess, evaluate, and have personal contact with clients, but an attempt should be made to do so. For example, in a custody suit, attorneys often request clinicians to see only their client. They protest that the other parent is not available for evaluation or explain that their client will provide all needed data. The clinician must stand firm about the necessity of interviewing all relevant parties. If the clinician agrees to be an expert in a discrete area (e.g., effect of medication on depressed children), it may not be necessary to see the client. Fourth, if the questions by the attorney are outside the area of expertise of the clinician, it is incumbent upon the clinician not to be seduced by a request for expertise. It is enticing to be asked to be an expert, but no mental health clinician is authoritative on every aspect of the vast variety of knowledge currently encompassed by the field. If the area is outside one's expertise, one should decline the referral. Fifth, the clinician should reach agreement with the attorney about fees. Many clinicians are embarrassed to discuss payment in advance of an evaluation and testimony. Discussing payment does not mean that a report will be biased or prejudicial in favor of the attorney's client. It is one safeguard that the clinician will be paid for work. Attorneys are quite comfortable with discussions of retainers and like matters. Sixth, the clinician may offer to provide a "care package" to the attorney at this point. The care package might include relevant clinical articles that might serve to educate the attorney regarding focal issues of the case. For example, if the case dealt with the suicide of an adolescent, materials about prediction of suicide, high-risk groups, treatment of depressed patients, and developmental issues in adolescents might be useful. Providing educational materials to an attorney at the onset of the case saves valuable time as the case progresses and provides for some common language of discussion. Seventh and last, the clinician should discuss the pros and cons of a written report and come to a tentative agreement with referring counsel.

Other chapters in this book discuss the conduct of the clinical examination, which ultimately serves as the basis for expert testimony. The forensic clinical examination differs from the standard clinical examination in that questions that address the pertinent legal issues must be posed. Thus, the expert must know the legal standards embodied by statute or case law in his or her particular jurisdiction, relative to making a recommendation as to child custody, waiver, and termination of parental rights (Benedek and Benedek, 1980). The questions asked in the clinical examination are specifically designed to seek meaningful psychological insights that bear upon the pertinent legal issues. In addition to the standard diagnostic psychiatric examination, these issues must be explored during the interview.

PRELIMINARY REPORT OF FINDINGS

After the initial assessment has been completed, the clinician should contact the attorney and present an oral summary of pertinent findings. This summary must be presented in a logical, clear, and coherent fashion. The clinician should assume that the attorney has little knowledge of how a clinical examination is conducted. Therefore, he or she should present the findings that form the basis for an ultimate conclusion in regard to the legal issues. Both the law and medicine are replete with jargon, which may make it difficult to communicate. If standard psychiatric terms such as illusions, delusions, and mental state are used, they need to be clearly defined (Petrella and Poythress, 1983).

The attorney and clinician can discuss what further steps or tests need to be taken to complete the evaluation. At this point, additional parties may need to be seen, or other relevant documents, such as depositions, may now be available. The issue of a written report may be rediscussed. If the verbal report is unfavorable to the attorney's client, the attorney may not want a written report, and the consultation may terminate. Even if the verbal report is favorable, a written report may not be necessary. At the same time, a written report in a forensic evaluation may be critical; it may serve as the basis for mediation and obviate the need for a trial. Behavioral observations leading to the ultimate opinion of the professional as well as statements by the patient and his or her parents or significant others that support observations are important.

In the report, if at all possible, the mental health professional must also answer the ultimate legal question at issue. A mental status evaluation and diagnostic formulation, while interesting and necessary, are ordinarily insufficient. A well-written cogent report may eliminate the need for expert testimony in the courtroom. Opposing attorneys may stipulate to the contents of the report, and it may serve as a basis for negotiation or mediation. The clinician must bear in mind that a forensic report, once issued, may become public property and available not only to opposing attorneys but also opposing clients and their children.

In a recent custody case, an attorney mailed a copy of the expert's report to one of the families involved. The report by a thoroughly trained clinician, inexperienced in the forensic arena, noted that two children had latent homosexual tendencies. Imagine the trauma to the children when they opened the family's mail and read about their "tendencies."

Even more disconcerting, portions of the report may be picked up by the media and publicized in the local press or on television. Thus, psychospeculation and the clinician's fantasies do not belong in forensic reports. Attention to detail and accuracy of information are required. A poorly written report may become in the hands of a skillful lawyer an instrument used to discredit and embarrass the mental health professional who has written it (Melton et al., 1987).

It is difficult to develop a generic report formulation suitable for all child forensic evaluations. Melton and his colleagues identify certain items of information that they believe should be included in forensic reports (Melton et al., 1987, p. 351).

1. *Date and nature of clinical contents.* This section would list chronologically the examiner's contacts with the person and describe the nature of the contact, e.g., interview, psychological testing, family observation, etc.
2. *Data relied upon.* In this section, the clinician would identify sources of information other than the individual who was examined, e.g., third party interviewers, written material such as academic, medical, or employment records, etc.
3. *Circumstances of the referral.* Here the clinician would identify the referral source, legal issues addressed, and the circumstances leading to the clinical evaluation, e.g., a description of the ongoing litigation and custody, divorce, or criminal proceedings.
4. *Relevant personal background information.* Historical information about the client relevant to the clinical formulation would be stated here. This section might be extensive in some kinds of cases, e.g., a lengthy history of illness and treatment in a disability case, and extremely brief in others, e.g., an evaluation of competency to stand trial.
5. *Present clinical findings.* This section would summarize the clinician's own observations and test results. Observations about present mental functioning or, when appropriate, statements about diagnosis would be included here.
6. *Psycho-legal formulation.* In this section, the examiner would draw upon information reported in the previous sections and integrate the data using a logical or theoretical theme to indicate the possible relevance of clinical material to the legal issue being decided.

EXPERT TESTIMONY

Despite issuing a comprehensive, high-quality report, it is often necessary to testify. The clinician who devotes any time to child psychiatry will find that he or she is being asked to testify either as an expert or as a treating clinician. There are ethical and legal problems when the clinician is asked to testify as a treating physician. The problems involve role conflict, dual agency, and therapeutic alliance. Most experts suggest that the treating physician should therefore not also serve as an expert because of role conflict and a possible destruction of the therapeutic alliance.

The law does permit participation of two distinct kinds of witnesses, the ordinary witness or lay witness and the expert witness. In general, a lay witness can testify to facts—that which he or she has directly observed. The judge or jury hears the facts presented by this type of witness, assesses them, and determines their veracity by assessing the credibility of the witness and integrating the material presented into the total gestalt of the trial. Federal Rules of Evidence, particularly Article 7(2), have somewhat relaxed the role of the lay witness by allowing some expression of opinion or inference in describing what one has seen or heard, but opinion testimony of a lay witness must meet two requirements: (*a*) The opinion must be rationally based on the witness's own perception, that is, be firsthand knowledge, and (b) the opinion must be helpful either in understanding the witnesses' testimony or in determining a fact at issue (Benedek and Benedek, 1980).

Consideration pertaining to expert witness and expert opinion are, of course, entirely different. Two requirements must be present before one can be qualified as an expert witness (anyone can call himself or herself an expert, but the judge has to qualify a professional as an expert after a voir dire): (a) The subject matter of inference must be distinctly related to a professional beyond the ordinary knowledge of the average layman, and (b) the witness must be shown to be qualified in the profession. Testimony of the expert is governed by rules different from those that apply to the ordinary fact witness. Thus, the expert may present an opinion or conclusion to the court. Furthermore, he or she may utilize facts gathered by others in forming an opinion. For example, the expert may review school records, past medical records, past therapy records, speak with family members about the behavior of patient, speak with schoolteachers about a patient, and request that psychological testing be performed. Information gathered by others and communicated to the expert via medical records, interviews, psychological testing, and other laboratory testing may be used in formulating an opinion. After reviewing and analyzing the findings of others, the expert may be allowed to formulate an opinion using "hearsay" material.

If the clinician knows that testimony will be necessary, it is sensible to contact the attorney and attempt to arrange a mutually convenient time for testimony. The clinician must remember that he or she is now playing in someone else's ballpark, and although courts are reasonably flexible in terms of scheduling, there are many participants in every trial, and no one person's schedule is more important than another's. In addition, it is important to present evidence in a logical, sequential fashion, and although it may appear to the expert that calling him or her out of sequence may make no difference, it may indeed effect the outcome of the trial. It may be important for the judge or jurors to hear certain expert testimony at the end of the trial. It is, however, disconcerting to discover that one may be on call for testimony for 2 weeks to a month. Often no one can predict when testimony will be necessary. A subpoena may not be necessary if the attorneys can agree to negotiate the time of appearance of the expert. If the subpoena specifies an inconvenient or previously scheduled time, the attorneys or court may be quite flexible in changing date and/or time.

Once the clinician is apprised that testimony will be necessary in court, it is important once again to meet with the attorney. This formal meeting allows the clinician an opportunity once again to educate the attorney about the clinical issues in the case as the clinician sees them. Such a meeting is also valuable for planning a strategy and sequence of direct examination and for anticipating questions that may arise during cross-examination. In addition, the clinician has an opportunity to "psyche out" the attorney, and the attorney has an equal opportunity to evaluate the clinician. It is helpful to know and understand the players on a team before one starts the game.

In this pretrial conference, the attorney may have modified his or her theory of the case, or a new theory may present itself. The attorney should make clear to the clinician what the theory is and how the clinician's data fits into the theory, and the clinician in turn helps the attorney to understand possible weakness in the theory and the clinician's opinion. Together they explore the other side's case and possible weaknesses in that case. Often it is useful to develop a list of questions that will be asked on direct examination. It is not sensible or helpful to rehearse questions and answers. This leads to a stilted presentation at the time of trial, and judges and juries are quick to detect a mechanical presentation and to suspect coaching or dishonesty on the part of attorney and clinician. The credibility of the clinician may be impugned.

COURTROOM

If a clinician has never visited a courtroom before, it may be helpful to do so prior to testifying. A courtroom, like an operating room, can be a strange, bewildering, and forbidding place to the uninitiated. It may be helpful to ask a forensically sophisticated colleague if it would be possible to observe his or her testimony prior to an actual experience. It is sensible to ask that colleague to identify the various players in the courtroom—bailiff, court reporter, and other ancillary personnel—and to define their roles.

Dress and demeanor are important in testifying. We instruct clinicians to dress neatly and conservatively. Dress is a way of showing respect for oneself and for the legal process.

When one is called, the first step in the testimonial process is the voir dire (Cameron, 1979). Here, the attorney leads the witness through a standard series of questions designed to elicit for the judge and jury a history of the witness's education, training, professional experience, and particular expertise testifying in the instant case. If the clinician has prepared a curriculum vita and remembered to take it to court, it can be used by the attorney to qualify him or her. The curriculum vita will help the attorney to focus questions on significant aspects of education and training, as well as such special qualifications as forensic training, forensic expertise, publications, and memberships and offices in local and national organizations. Novices often express concern that they will be asked how often they have testified in court and then fail to qualify as experts because of their limited courtroom experience. This rarely happens to a physician or medical resident. Generally, attorneys are prepared to use a physician's background, training, and education as medical student and resident to qualify him or her as a special witness. Though a particular physician has never testified, he or she probably has seen many patients with problems similar to that of the instant patient. It is always wise to be supervised in one's first forensic evaluations and to ask the supervisor to be present as a second expert in the courtroom, to be used on an as-needed basis, and to provide needed moral support.

Following recital of credentials on direct questioning, the opposing attorney has an opportunity to voir dire further. The opposing attorney's emphasis will be on the weakest areas in the witnesses experience in training as such limited contact with a particular population (e.g., suicidal adolescence, use of a particular antidepressant, or inpatient experience). During one of the author's first voir dires, she was asked if she had ever lived in a ghetto in Detroit. The opposing attorney attempted to show that the author could not possibly understand the mental and emotional state of residents in a public housing area because she had never lived in public housing. Needless to say, the author was qualified as an expert. On other occasions, attorneys have attempted to disqualify the author as an expert by arguing that she either worked primarily with a population of mentally ill adults and thus was no longer knowledgeable about children, or worked with a population of mentally ill children and thus was no longer knowledgeable about adults. On one occasion, the author's 20-page curriculum vita was reviewed in detail. The opposing attorney noted that the author has four children and asked how she had time to have such an active professional life and care for her four children. Again, the author was qualified as an expert witness. The attorney attempts not only to discredit credentials but also to undermine credibility as a witness.

Voir dire testimony is not particularly difficult, traumatic, or challenging. There is an opportunity for the witness to assess and familiarize himself or herself with players in the courtroom scene. Often, the witness may get a feeling that the judge is "on her side" or may note the jury smiling or laughing as opposing counsel attempts to bully or intimidate. It is an opportunity to "speak up" and overcome natural initial nervousness and anxiety. I advise new experts to draw upon their experience in the doctor-patient relationship and to envision everyone in the courtroom as family members who are asking a psychiatrist to explain relevant diagnostic and treatment information to them. I encourage the novice expert to pay attention to this new, strange environment and begin coping with it during the voir dire.

DIRECT TESTIMONY

The next step following qualification is a direct examination of the witness. During this portion of the testimony, the witness will be asked first to identify the patient/defendant/plaintiff and to explain the facts and/or clinical examination on which his other opinion is based. It is helpful to bring relevant materials to the stand, including a DSM-IV and articles that may support one's position. Poythress (1980) suggests treating the body of testimony like an inverted pyramid, beginning with evaluation techniques and the data those techniques have produced, proceeding to inferences, and ending with the peak, the summary conclusions. It is important that the expert present all relevant data in an articulate, clear, logical, and coherent fashion. It is also important to speak in a forceful fashion and not be meek or hesitant in the presentation of an opinion (Bettinghaus, 1973). It is equally important that the expert avoid using jargon here. Terms such as affect, neologisms, loosening of associations, flight of ideas, and lability must be explained. In addition, any laboratory tests and their significance, such as the dexamethasone suppression test or a computer axial tomography scan, must be explained. The judge or jury have no natural understanding of the variety of psychological tests and what data might be elicited from each one of them, so terms such as Rorschach, TAT, WISC, and WRAT may simply be an alphabet soup to them.

An attorney may wish to use the clinician to establish the credibility of a client. Most courts today do not allow testimony in regard to client credibility. Courts assume that the average lay jury and judge can and should make their own determinations about credibility. Questions about credibility generally raise valid legal objections. As with all objections, the clinician should sit back, relax, and allow counsel to argue the merits of the objection and the court to rule upon it. Testimony is resumed when a judge rules upon the objection. The novice clinician finds it difficult to remember that the objection is not personal; it is not an objection to the clinician or his or her testimony. It is an objection based on legal precedents. If an objection is overruled, then testimony may proceed along prior lines. If an objection is sustained, the question should not be answered in open court. The witness should not attempt to interject the same data in another fashion. Judges are sensitive to expert witnesses who do not attend to objections and may chastise or censure them from the bench. Typical objections often center around possible hearsay evidence or admission or the lack of a proper foundation for data.

An attorney and clinician decide prior to the onset of the trial whether to bring out material that is inconsistent with the expert's ultimate conclusion during the direct examination, so as to diffuse a possible cross-examination. The ultimate decision in regard to strategy is, of course, counsel's. Despite the fact that the expert may feel that counsel's decisions will lead to disaster, the conduct of the case is ultimately the attorney's responsibility. While the expert may be correct in concluding that counsel has erred in a single particular decision, the expert should remember that his or her expertise is in clinical material, not the conduct of the trial, and that the attorney is dealing with a variety of considerations, many of which will be unfamiliar to the typical clinician. Second-guessing a counsel is poor clinical judgment.

CROSS-EXAMINATION

Following direct examination, cross-examination follows direct testimony. This stage of the trial is the most challenging for both the novice and the experienced forensic clinician. The attorney may question the witness's credentials on the basis of race, sex, age, training, theoretical orientation, experience, or any other number of criteria. The length and circumstances of the examination may be scrutinized, as well as the witnesses' biases or attitude toward the person examined. The source and amount of remuneration often becomes a focal point in the cross-examination. For example, the attorney may ask the clinician, "How much are you being paid for your opinion, Doctor?" The best way to diffuse that loaded question is to explain, "I'm being paid for my time, not for my opinion."

Another tactic on cross-examination is to ask the expert a series of questions that are clearly outside of his or her area of expertise. That

is, the child psychiatrist may be asked specific questions about research findings in biological psychiatry that deal with obscure points. The clinician need never be afraid to say, "I don't know," if in fact he or she does not know. Admitting fallibility only enhances credibility.

The attorney may attempt to box the clinician in by asking a series of questions and insisting that the clinician answer only with a yes or a no. The clinician can turn to the judge and say, "Your Honor, I believe that an answer of yes or no without an explanation would be misleading to the court." Judges generally do not like to be misled and may instruct the attorney to rephrase the question or allow the expert to answer in a more comprehensive fashion.

Many attorneys attempt to discredit an expert's opinion by asking if psychiatry is subjective or objective and if the clinician's opinion is objective or subjective. The attorney is attempting to impress upon the jury that a mental health clinician's formulations and opinions are simply subjective or "what the witness thinks," as opposed to having scientific legitimacy. The clinician should respond by repeating a brief statement of the scientific underpinning of his or her opinion and a modest statement about personal and professional integrity to the effect that because the clinician is a person with a particular personal set of values, he or she is careful in the collection and analysis of data to ascertain that his or her clinical formulations are consistent with known data or widely accepted theory.

It is also permissible for an attorney to pose a hypothetical question during cross-examination. The hypothetical question purports to summarize clinical data or factual data that is already in evidence. However, both the factual data and psychiatric clinical data contained in the hypothetical question often are different from those the expert has developed during a clinical examination and different from the facts as presented by the other attorney. It may be important to attempt first to point out how the hypothetical question differs from the case in point and then either to answer or not answer the hypothetical question. Pointing out first how it differs from the case in point allows opportunity for an objection. It is important to attempt to discriminate between the hypothetical case presented by the opposing attorney that presents his or her position in the best possible light and the real case as seen by the clinician.

One other specialized line of attack that mental health professionals find difficult to deal with concerns the learned treatise. In this form of cross-examination, the expert is first asked to authenticate a book or paper or DSM-IV as a recognized and standard authority on a subject. Then the contents of the book or paper or DSM-IV are read for the purpose of discrediting and contradicting the witness. There are a variety of techniques available for handling cross-examination on publications. These include denying the total authoritativeness of any publication, pointing out that a publication may be important but not authoritative about all issues, pointing out that a publication is outdated and no longer relevant if the rate of development of scientific literature has made a particular publication obsolete, or citing other publications that dispute a particular author's viewpoint. The learned treatise and an assault on it has been extensively discussed in the literature (Poythress, 1980). It is important for the witness to think clearly and carefully before answering any questions, particularly those posed during cross-examination. Stopping and thinking not only helps one to gain composure and think out answers in one's head, it decelerates the rate of cross-examination and allows a judge and jury to listen carefully to questions and answers.

During the cross-examination, the expert may feel harassed, badgered, angry, surprised, and confused. It is important to keep those affects and emotions private. The best appearance and demeanor is one of coolness under fire. The witness who remains calm when the attorney is clearly rattled is always in a good position. It is better to have an attorney called "badgering" than to be cited as an argumentative witness. As we've learned from many patients, many hostile remarks can be couched with a smile. Those techniques can be used to protect oneself during a cross-examination.

Most attorneys and mental health professionals agree that the expert should answer only the questions posed and that those questions should be developed ahead of time to focus on the important issues in the case. It is not the role of the expert to provide a minicourse in child psychiatry or to provide psychodynamic explanations in a case unless asked. Such display serves only to satisfy the narcissistic needs of the expert and at best confuses judges and juries; at worst, it makes the expert appear to be pompous and pedantic. It is important not to talk too much.

Legal procedure allows for redirect and recross. These procedures generally allow counselors to clarify material previously introduced. On redirect, the attorney who called the expert can allow the witness to expand on questions posed during cross-examination and to amplify. The opposing counsel is allowed the same opportunity in recross.

When testimony is completed, the witness may be excused by the judge. The witness must then decide if he or she wants to remain in the courtroom to listen to other expert testimony or to leave. Leaving makes one seem less involved, impartial, and less interested in the outcome of the case. Attorneys may request that the expert sit with them at the

counsel table and coach them while they question other witnesses. Although in some situations this may be acceptable, it is better to prepare the attorney for the cross-examination of other witnesses ahead of time, during pretrial conferences. Sitting at the table may make the expert witness appear biased.

If one contemplates testifying in court, the best preparation is to go to court with a skilled expert and to observe him or her during the testimonial process. Another useful additional training technique or practice is to participate in a mock trial at a training institution or law school. Often mock counsel, played by experienced forensic colleagues, are harder than real attorneys in real trials. Colleagues seem to take particular pleasure in embarrassing novices. If a novice can survive the challenge of a mock trial in a collegial atmosphere, a real court trial may seem tame in contrast. Videotapes of such mock trials are useful for ongoing critique and training. Participants are often surprised at their performances and learn a great deal from them.

References

Bank SC, Poythress NG: The elements of persuasion in expert testimony. *Psychiatry Law*, pp. 173–204, 1982.

Benedek RS, Benedek EP: The expert witness in child custody cases. In: Schetky DH, Benedek EP

(eds): *Child Psychiatry and the Law*. New York, Brunner/Mazel, 1980.

Bettinghaus E: *Persuasive Communication* (2nd ed). New York, Holt, Rinehart, & Winston, 1973.

Cameron R: The mental health expert: A guide to direct and cross-examination. *Criminal Justice J II*, pp. 299–311, 1979.

Melton G, Petrila J, Poythress NG, et al: Consul-

tation, report writing and expert testimony. In: *Psychological Evaluations for the Courts*. New York, Guilford Press, 1987, pp. 347–371.

Petrella R, Poythress N: The quality of forensic evaluations: An interdisciplinary study. *J Consult Psychol*, 1983.

Poythress N: Coping on the witness stand: Learned responses to "learning treatises." *Prof Psychol*, 1980.

B/ A Trial Lawyer's Perspective

David N. Rosen, LL.B.

What does it mean for a child psychiatrist to be an "expert witness?" On one hand, the phrase conjures images of a scientific demonstration by a chemist or fingerprint analyst. This conception is unlikely to seem appropriate because psychiatry does not lend itself to the seemingly unassailable conclusions of "hard" science. Alternatively, an invitation to testify may feel like being propositioned to be a hired gun and to do "junk science," appealing only to those who enjoy fighting or being on display. In fact, a child psychiatrist who testifies in court can be both effective and true to his or her understanding of the reality of the case. In order to do this, the prospective expert witness should think about the structure of a trial. Trials create a framework within which the expert's story will be told and evaluated, which creates a specific set of opportunities and hazards for an expert witness. This chapter discusses that framework and proposes that a child psychiatrist can be an effective witness by approaching testifying as an application or extension of his or her professional skills and activities. It is useful to consider separately direct examination and cross-examination, since these are very different activities and require the use of very different metaphors to understand and master. For direct examination, the first topic discussed in this chapter, a child psychiatrist must think about how to construct the most compelling story; while for cross-examination, he or she must cope with and learn to use the aggression inherent in the confrontation with the cross-examiner.

PART ONE: TELLING A STORY IN DIRECT EXAMINATION

A trial is not a direct reflection of reality. It is a reconstruction of reality. It might more accurately be called a *construction* of a reality of its own, since it has its own purpose and structure, created by the law. Even a straightforward-seeming criminal case does not address a question as simple as "Did A kill B?" The question is, rather, "Has the state proven beyond a reasonable doubt that A murdered B and, if so, was it murder in the first degree, or perhaps manslaughter?" Changing the question from "what happened?" to "what has been proven?" and introducing legal categories that may have little connection to how

anyone perceived events as they were occurring inevitably makes a trial different from, and more complex than, simply a search for truth. Additional complexity is added as the questions the trial seeks to address become forward looking, as in a custody case, where the issue is "where will it be in the child's best interest to live in the future?" In such a case there can be no pretense that the trial is simply finding a preexisting reality.

But in all cases the trial is a competition between versions or stories of what happened or will happen or should happen, a competition that is familiar to psychiatrists. Psychotherapy prominently includes formulating reconstructions of reality that "ring true" to a patient, or are useful to the patient. Inevitably such formulations are based on incomplete, perhaps fragmentary, evidence, but if they hang together and capture something important in the information the patient has been conveying, they can be persuasive and compelling. So it is in a trial, where the adversaries present competing stories, or versions, to the fact-finder, who must choose between them based on necessarily limited information.

As there may be formidable barriers to hearing a patient's story clearly and coherently, much about the structure of a trial makes it difficult to present a coherent narrative. One of the most striking features of most trials to any observer, and perhaps the most salient for a child psychiatrist contemplating testifying as an expert witness, is their fragmented, disjointed quality. Although trials make great subjects for stories and are often gripping drama, they are constantly subject to a variety of centrifugal forces that make them prone at any point to become incoherent. Since the expert's role in direct testimony is above all to counteract that incoherence and to provide order and a narrative thread to the case he or she is called to support, it is useful to identify the reasons trials are so much in need of the coherent unity effective expert testimony can provide.

Why are trials always in danger of becoming incoherent? First, because the adversary system entails by definition the clash of views. There are, at least, two sides to every story, and presentation of both sides almost invariably makes the narrative harder to follow. Moreover, in the adversary system, at every point confusion is likely to be in someone's interest. Ordinarily, when one side is presenting part of its case, it is in the other side's interest to disrupt the coherence of the presentation. As a result, one side is often doing what it can to interrupt the flow of the other side's presentation. And the rules of procedure offer many opportunities to do so, from objections to cross-examination to legal claims.

In addition to being under constant threat from the very nature of the adversary system, coherence of narrative is also jeopardized by features of the rules of procedure and evidence. For example, trials proceed by questions and answers, which tends to give testimony a staccato, as opposed to lyrical, quality. The lawyer and the witness are performing a duet, and if either gets out of step the narrative will quickly become choppy, entirely apart from interruptions by an adversary claiming that questions are improper or answers are nonresponsive or contain inadmissible material. Indeed, the basic rule that evidence must be presented through witnesses, each of whom is limited in the scope of his or her testimony, makes it harder to sustain a narrative thread. The story is told in pieces that come from different witnesses, and in real life the contributions of each witness cannot be entirely shaped by needs of dramatic effect. The areas about which any given witness may testify are not always adjacent to each other in the logical sequence in which one side's narrative unfolds. For example, in a trial for sexual abuse of a child, a teacher may be able to identify some relevant physical evidence such as the child's clothing, testify extensively about the child's behavior and condition at different times, and also testify about some contacts with the suspected abuser. The teacher's testimony about all these subjects will almost invariably be presented at once, rather than at different times according to the demands of dramatic narrative.

It is of course also the case that cross-examination of each witness follows the direct testimony of that witness, rather than, for example, beginning only after all witnesses have completed their direct testimony. Each witness, therefore, presents testimony that zigzags according to the competing dictates of the adversaries. Additionally, the scheduling difficulties and delay for which the legal system is justly notorious result in trials that are frequently interrupted, sometimes for long stretches, and in which witnesses cannot always testify in the sequence that would make for the most coherent narrative. Doctors in particular are often called "out of turn" to accommodate their schedules but, as a result, find themselves talking about evidence the court should logically have heard already but in fact has not. Finally, and most fundamentally, the story of a trial is told through witnesses, each of whom contributes only a part of the story. A case is built by weaving together the threads of the testimony of different witnesses or, to use another common metaphor, as a mosaic in which each exhibit and witness's testimony adds elements that together form a coherent pattern. In every case the task is to show that the elements form a coherent whole, and the danger is that they will be simply a jumble.

The trial lawyer's response to this problem is to develop and emphasize a theme for the case. It is a truism of trial advocacy that every successful case has a theme, a narrative structure on which the advocate tries to hang all the information the fact-finder receives. A theme provides clarity to a form of presentation that otherwise can easily dissolve into incoherence. A theme is the essence of one side's case boiled down to a clear, simple, attractive statement. In a murder case the prosecution's theme might be that the defendant was a violent, possessive husband who killed his wife in a jealous rage, while the defense's theme might be that a biased and sloppy police force fixated on the defendant and failed to perform the thorough investigation necessary to find the real killer—even more concisely: jealous rage versus rush to judgment. A theme is no less important in a civil case, such as a child custody dispute. One parent's theme might be "the child belongs with me because I was the one who raised her," while the other parent's theme may be, "the child belongs with the parent who is more stable and supportive now and promises to remain so in the future." While some might find this simplification frustratingly incomplete or even simple-minded, trial lawyers consider it distillation rather than distortion. The right theme captures the essence of one side's view of the truth, and it is often true that a case that cannot be summarized in a brief, clear, forceful way is not a very good case.

The child psychiatrist who is going to testify in court needs to understand how his or her testimony fits into the themes each side is presenting. If he or she is allied in some way with one side, as is common, he or she will want not only to understand but help shape the theme of that side's case. Like an actor in a play, a child psychiatrist witness must understand his or her role in the drama of the trial. Because, unlike an actor, the child psychiatrist's lines are limited not only by what is plausible but also but by what is actually true, the psychiatrist can help the lawyer and the patient/client by collaborating on identifying and formulating the essential theme of the entire presentation. In a child custody case, for example, the psychiatrist will ordinarily be giving an opinion about the ultimate issue in the case—what custody arrangement is in the best interest of the child. Before testifying, the psychiatrist should try to formulate the basis for her opinion as concisely as possible, ordinarily in a single, not overly complex sentence. Two examples were given above. Others might be "honoring the child's expressed desire to be with one parent is critical to giving the child a needed sense of autonomy" or "the child's most critical need is not to be separated from his or her half-sibling" or "that parent is dangerously unstable." These examples may or may not even count as good bases for a custody decision to some readers, but by virtue of being clear and simple themes, they will have force in a trial. Once having chosen a theme, a trial lawyer will throughout the trial look for opportunities to repeat it and point to evidence that supports it. In an important way, the trial will become about the theme, or competing themes, and the psychiatrist's role will be to testify about which theme is closer to the evidence and—what is more challenging—to critique one of the themes as, at least to some extent, shallow or irrelevant.

A child psychiatrist may protest that boiling the results of many hours of observation and years of training and experience into a phrase or a sentence trivializes any contribution he or she might make by substituting a slogan for an opinion. A trial lawyer would reply that simplicity is necessary because of the diffused and fractured nature of trials and also because the audience is either a lay jury or a judge who, whatever his or her experience with similar cases, is not a child psychiatrist. It is also common for experts to make a virtue of the necessity of simplicity in the courtroom. Boiling down opinions to their simplest and most direct expression can be a useful analytical as well as rhetorical device, and an expert who can summarize his or her most important point in a brief, direct sentence may find his or her ideas sharpened and improved as a result.

Having said this much about the virtues of simplicity and focus is not to say that there is no place for complexity. On the contrary. The issue is not whether complexity and nuance have a place in a trial and in the expert's testimony, but rather how to formulate and present complexity. Here the expert's model, like the trial lawyer's, should be the story. Fact-finders, like any audience, have tolerance, indeed an appetite, for complexity so long as it is presented within a narrative framework that holds it together.

The expert witness is privileged by the rules of evidence to tell a more complete and coherent story than other witnesses are allowed to tell. Experts can testify not only to their conclusions but, reasonably enough, to the basis for those conclusions. When explaining the basis for their conclusions, experts can, therefore, draw upon and restate other evidence. They therefore have a unique opportunity to draw the evidence together into a unified narrative. Moreover, in testifying about the basis for their conclusions, expert witnesses are not even limited to information that is admissible evidence. The rule is that they may rely on any information, even hearsay or other inadmissible evidence, so long as the expert affirms that the information is the type of material ordinarily relied on by experts in the field. Thus, the expert may testify about information he was given by a child's teacher even though the teacher does not himself come to court to verify the information. (It is, to be sure, important to take any reasonable steps to verify such information, particularly since it is a likely area for cross-examination.) The expert has an opportunity, then, to synthesize a lot of information and to communicate and discuss that information on the witness stand.

Robert Coles, a child psychiatrist, has written of "the call of stories." His view is that the clinician does well to eschew theoretical formulations of patients' psychodynamics, or at least keep them in their place, and focus primarily on the narratives, the stories, the patients will tell about themselves to those who want to listen. He argues, and demonstrates, that "a good deal of the time our patients' comments tell their own story, one that can be interpreted by us in ordinary language with no loss of psychological nuance and subtlety" (Coles, 1989, p. 27). This perspective is readily adaptable to trials and to expert testimony in particular. A child psychiatrist could present her conclusions by following a theoretical schema or reporting first test results, then the findings of a clinical examination, then conclusions, and so on. Ordinarily, however, a more compelling and persuasive method of presentation is to start wherever possible with a framework of the patient's story and to relate the details of findings and conclusions to the framework of a story that illustrates the expert's theme. Clinical observations and findings can be reported using this approach as illustrations of the themes of the story. Thus, the expert might begin testimony about her findings and conclusions as follows:

Q: Doctor, did you reach any conclusions concerning what custody arrangement would be in the best interests of the child?

A: Yes, I did.

Q: What conclusions did you reach?

A: My ultimate conclusion was that it would be in the best interest of the child for her mother to have custody of her.

Q: What is the basis for your conclusion?

A: [Introducing the theme] To put it as simply as possible, I found that this child's mother is the most important person in the world for her, and she needs to live with her mother to feel secure and protected.

Q: Can you explain what led you to this conclusion?

At this point the expert can try as best as he or she can to narrate the child's story and illustrate the theme in a nontechnical way. Rather than proceeding deductively by announcing the principle that the adult with whom the child has formed the closest bonds or who is appropriately designated the "psychological parent" should have custody, the story can properly revolve around the child's relationship with that adult. From the specifics of the child's life and relationship with that adult, the expert can then move convincingly to the observation that the child's experience of depending on and needing a sustained central relationship with the particular adult is just what the expert would expect. In fact, the expert can continue, everything we know about the way children develop is consistent with what this child's needs appeared to be from looking closely at her life story. This form of narration will ordinarily feel more "right" and persuasive to either a jury or a judge than one that begins with the generalizations of theory and then moves to apply theory to the particular case at hand.

As students of people and their life stories, psychiatrists are well trained to be expert witnesses. By focusing on the fundamental point they are going to make in their testimony, and how that point relates to the theme of the trial, and then allowing themselves to tell the story, with all its individual richness, that supports that theme, they can make a presentation on direct examination that feels right and consistent with their professional role and is at the same time highly effective in the courtroom.

PART TWO: THE USE AND MANAGEMENT OF AGGRESSION IN CROSS-EXAMINATION

What awaits a child psychiatrist who is to testify in court? The experience, particularly cross-examination, inevitably seems somewhat surreal: Anticipating a serious and consequential discussion about clinical issues, the psychiatrist instead may find himself or herself being hectored by an inquisitor who very evidently has no interest in either the truth or the best interests of the child whose welfare is ostensibly the purpose

of the proceeding. Equally disconcerting, the cross-examiner's questions may proceed from the assumption that the psychiatrist is dishonest or biased, leaving the psychiatrist feeling like a murder suspect protesting her innocence to a cynical police detective.

An important part of the difficulty many psychiatrists experience testifying in court is that they use the wrong model to understand it. A psychiatrist may imagine that testifying in court is more or less like giving an invited lecture. Using this model (or, laboring under this misapprehension), the psychiatrist will be likely to regard cross-examination as uninformed, distracting, and impertinent. Exchanges like the following will ensue:

Q: How much time did you spend reviewing the report of the family relations officer before you formed your opinion regarding custody?

A: I am afraid you didn't understand my earlier testimony. The report of the family relations officer has very little significance for me because I performed my own independent evaluation and spoke with all the people the family relations officer spoke to. In fact, I deliberately did not study that report because I did not want my own views to be biased by another professional's opinion.

Q: So the answer to my question is "none." Is that right?

A: You aren't taking into account the reason I didn't examine the report at that time.

Q: Is the answer to my question, "none?"

A: Yes.

Q: Thank you.

The witness would have done much better to respond as follows:

Q: How much time did you spend reviewing the report of the family relations officer before you formed your opinion regarding custody?

A: None; I read the report after I formed my opinion.

Or, simply,

A: None.

Somewhat similar results may occur when a psychiatrist-witness regards cross-examination as a debate or an argument; he or she will invite being viewed as biased, belligerent, or both and will have missed the opportunity to be an effective witness. For example:

Q: How much time did you spend reviewing the report of the family relations officer before you formed your opinion regarding custody?

A: None at all, which is probably fortunate, since when I ultimately did review it I found it very misleading.

Q: Was it misleading when it said the child has lived with her father for the past 6 months?

A: No, the part I was referring to is . . .

Q: [Interrupting] Please answer my question, Doctor. The answer to my question is, "No?"

A: Yes, but . . .

Q: Thank you. Now, was the report misleading when it said the child is doing well in school?

And so on. Again, the witness would have done better simply to answer the question and trust that subsequent redirect examination by the lawyer who originally had called her to testify would give her the opportunity to correct any misimpressions left by the cross-examination.

A more useful reference point is another form of dialogue with its own peculiar set of rules: the psychoanalytic session. Thinking about the similarities and differences between cross-examination of a witness and a psychoanalytic session is a helpful way to understand and therefore cope with the demands cross-examination places on a child psychiatrist testifying in court.

The lawyer's job, like the analyst's, is to lead a subject to the most difficult and painful topics and to peel away layers of rationalization or dissimulation to reveal a truth within. That is, not only are both psychoanalysis and cross-examination investigations, but they also both begin with the assumption that people's testimony should not be taken at face value, nor should their honesty be presumed. Thus, cross-examination has been described, in a phrase Freud might have used about psychoanalysis, as the greatest engine ever invented for the discovery of truth.

But while psychoanalysis depends upon the patient's free associating, saying whatever comes into his or her head without censoring any thoughts, in cross-examination the witness is entirely constrained and must answer precisely the question put by the cross-examiner. To a psychiatrist witness, used to a more discursive approach to the truth, this constraint can make cross-examination feel like the course in oral expression Holden Caulfield took in *The Catcher in the Rye* (1964), where each boy had to make a spontaneous speech in class:

> And if the boy digresses at all, you're supposed to yell 'Digression!' at him as fast as you can. It just about drove me crazy . . .. What I think is, you're supposed to leave somebody alone if he's at least being interesting and he's getting all excited about something.

That is not what cross-examiners think. What cross-examiners think is that their job is not so much to *discover* the truth as it is to *demonstrate* the truth, as they have been hired to see it, so that the judge or jury may discover it. Accordingly, the first rule of cross-examination is, never ask a question to which you do not know the answer. What this precept means in practice is that virtually all questions on cross-examination are closed-ended, and witnesses are very often merely foils whose role on cross-examination is simply to admit facts the examiner wants the judge or the jury to hear in the sequence the examiner has selected. For example, consider the following sequence:

Q: Doctor, how much time did you spend observing the mother and child interacting together?
A: One hour.
Q: And you have based your recommendation regarding custody primarily on your opinion about the relationship between the child and mother, isn't that right?
A: Yes.
Q: And that one hour was in your office, is that right?
A: Yes.
Q: And of course how people behave in your office when you are watching them may differ from how they behave at home when they are not being observed, isn't that right?
A: Yes.
Q: For example, the mother certainly may have been trying to impress you during that single one-hour session that you observed her with the child, isn't that right?
A: Yes.
Q: And that might affect her behavior, isn't that right?
A: I suppose so.
Q: So your only direct observation of the mother and child relating to each other was for a single hour, outside the home, under circumstances where the mother might be acting differently from the way she would before she came to your office and after she left it, isn't that right?
A: Yes.

And so on. Anticipating all of this, the psychiatrist may wish to respond by taking control of the conversation, for example as follows:

Q: How much time did you spend observing the child and her mother together?
A: I don't think that is what is important in making an evaluation concerning child custody in this case.

But she is not allowed to do so. If she does, the lawyer is entitled to say, "Please answer my question, Doctor," or even, "Are you willing to answer my question, Doctor?"

The psychiatrist cannot expose himself or herself to this line of questioning without damaging his or her credibility. The psychiatrist is not entitled to ignore the constraining rules of cross-examination and will score no points by attempting to do so. If the psychiatrist persists in trying to step outside the rules of cross-examination, she will be perceived, accurately, as breaking them.

Both court testimony and a psychoanalytic session are dialogues of a sort, but both are asymmetrical in important respects, in which the witness is analogous to the patient and the lawyer to the psychoanalyst. For example, they are asymmetrical with respect to disclosure. The central function of the witness or patient is to disclose information, freely and fully. On the other hand, the examiner and analyst need disclose nothing. In both settings this asymmetry can be frustrating; unlike an ordinary conversation, openness and candor in these settings cannot be expected to be reciprocated. So the witness, like patients, is vulnerable to feelings of powerlessness and loss of control.

These feelings may be intensified by the rule (or metarule) illustrated by the cross-examination excerpt above, but applicable to both settings, that the witness or patient cannot make the examiner or analyst step outside of his or her role. Thus, a patient who demands of an orthodox psychoanalyst, "What do *you* think" about this or that may get for a reply only "What do you think I think about it?" or silence. Likewise, a witness who demands of a cross-examiner, for example, "Don't you really think the child should stay with the parent who has been most involved with her up until now?" cannot expect to disarm the lawyer and get a straight, honest answer. Instead, the lawyer may reply: "Are you suggesting by that question, Doctor, that in your opinion the *character* of the parent is irrelevant to the best interest of the child?" The lawyer is *supposed* to respond only in whatever way he or she thinks is best calculated to advance a client's claim in the litigation, and this imperative will typically lead the lawyer to view a witness's appeal to step outside the game of the adversary system as simply another move in the game, calling for a countermove on the examiner's part.

These constraints on the witness suggest another, more fundamental asymmetry in cross-examination, which also has its counterpart in the psychoanalytic relationship. This is asymmetry with regard to aggression. Cross-examination is a weapon in the lawyer's arsenal within the adversary system. The lawyer uses it either to attack the witness or, perhaps, to turn the witness into a weapon directed at the adversary. But the witness is not supposed to be an adversary; the expert witness especially is supposed to be a representative in court of the commitment to truth. Thus, the cross-examiner properly regards the conversation, that is, the examination, as a form of warfare, but the witness cannot take this stance. The witness is required to treat the examination as a search for truth.

In this respect, the witness is analogous to the psychiatrist, not the patient, in the psychoanalytic relationship. While the lawyer is permitted to give more or less free rein to his or her aggression, the witness is required, no matter what accusations are leveled or what hostility expressed, not to retaliate in kind but to be the anchor of reason and to respond to hostility and aggression with understanding and without permitting himself or herself to be provoked to anger.

To understand why it is so important for the witness to preserve this asymmetry—not to respond in kind to the lawyer's aggression—consider that the expert witness, like the patient, is more knowledgeable about the subject matter of her testimony than the lawyer cross-examining her or the judge or jury evaluating her testimony. As the analyst, who has never met the patient's family and friends, evaluates the patient's narrative in part through careful attention to the patient's affect and with the aid of generous amounts of intuition rather than logical deduction or reference to externally acquired information, so the judge or jury evaluating the psychiatrist cannot be expected to learn as much as the psychiatrist knows about psychiatry. They do not perform a kind of peer review of the psychiatrist's testimony. Judges and particularly juries are lay people, not experts in any of the fields about which they may hear testimony. Indeed, people with special expertise in the area in which an expert will testify frequently are excluded as jurors, in order to prevent them from using their knowledge in a way that is not open to scrutiny and control by the court. Of course, one must ask on what basis, then, are judges and juries supposed to evaluate the conflicting testimony of experts?

The answer is that fact-finders in court, and particularly juries, evaluate an expert's conclusions based primarily upon their assessment of how the expert has handled the tension between the aggression of the cross-examiner and the witness's obligation to speak for scientific truth. That is, while judges or juries may well follow the substance of an expert's testimony carefully and attempt to evaluate it as a peer might, that is not the main thing they do, indeed not the main thing they are supposed to do. What courts and juries are designed to do is to evaluate the credibility of witnesses. And what this boils down to above all is evaluation of the witness's commitment to the value of truth when confronted with the aggression of the adversary system.

Coping with Aggression in Cross-examination

The way this process works in practice is that, to be persuasive, witnesses must accept and use the asymmetry of cross-examination. Like a psychiatrist with a belligerent patient (and in this way the psychiatrist witness is not switching roles but may call on familiar skills), the witness must be careful not to be provoked by the aggression of the cross-examiner. As the cross-examiner is aggressive, the witness succeeds by being gentle; the jury understands that, as aggression and an adversary stance are companions, so their opposites, gentleness and fidelity to truth, also go together. Thus, the cross-examiner marks it a success when he or she succeeds in getting under the skin of the witness, or in making the witness *blow up*. The successful witness, on the other hand, is one who *deflates* the cross-examiner.

Some examples of common lines of cross-examination show features of the adversary system in action and illustrate how the witness's use and management of the aggression inherent in the adversary system is the key to being an effective expert witness. Let us begin by imagining a case in which the psychiatrist who has treated a child for emotional problems arising from a physical injury is called to testify in a case seeking damages for the injury. Cross-examination begins as follows:

Q: You have seen the plaintiff as a patient for almost a year. Is that right?
A: Yes.
Q: In that time have you sent her family bills?
A: Yes.
Q: Have they paid the bills?
A: No.
Q: How do you expect to get paid?
A: They have agreed to pay me as they are able to do so.
Q: In fact, you expect to get paid out of the proceeds of this lawsuit don't you?
A: Well, yes.
Q: So you have a stake in the outcome of this lawsuit don't you?
A: I am being honest in my testimony.
Q: Isn't that for the jury to decide, Doctor?
A: Yes.
Q: My question was not: Are you being honest? It was: Don't you have a stake in the outcome of this lawsuit?
A: Well, not really.
Q: Don't you stand to get paid nearly $5000 if the plaintiffs win this lawsuit and little or nothing if they lose?
A: Yes.
Q: But $5000 is not a stake in this lawsuit, is that your testimony?

What is a witness to do about this sort of questioning? Clearly, the answer is not to say, for example, "Well, $5000 is not very much to me," or, "I wouldn't change my testimony for a million dollars." The

first is condescending, the second defensive. This is the sort of questioning against which the best inoculation is not the witness's protestations of innocence but rather her *demonstration* of lack of bias in her answers. The psychiatrist could answer as follows:

Q: How do you expect to get paid?
A: I suspect I will either get paid out of the proceeds of this lawsuit or not at all.

By anticipating the lawyer's point in her answer, the witness has taken much of the sting out of it. And when the lawyer asks the inevitable question, "So you have a stake in the outcome of this lawsuit, don't you," the better answer is simply, "To that extent I do, yes." By refusing to be put on the defensive—that is, refusing to resist a point that the examiner is going to make anyhow—the witness defuses the examiner's aggression. The point is *not* the witness's expectations regarding payment but whether the witness appears to be more concerned with accuracy than with preventing the examiner from scoring debating points.

Now consider an attack purportedly on the witness's expert knowledge, which again when looked at in action actually depends for its effectiveness not on the substance of the witness's answers but on how adversarial the witness is:

Q: Doctor, you diagnosed the patient as having posttraumatic stress disorder. What are the diagnostic criteria for posttraumatic stress disorder?
A: In my report I mention four basic diagnostic criteria.
Q: Can you name the criteria without looking at your report?
A: Well, (*a*) there must be a stressor, (*b*) the patient must reexperience the trauma, (*c*) there is a withdrawal from social engagement, and I am afraid that's all I can recall.
Q: You are not really an expert in the area of posttraumatic stress disorder, are you, Doctor?
A: Well, just because I don't remember all the criteria, that doesn't mean I'm not an expert. I have written in the area of schizophrenia and I couldn't recite all the diagnostic criteria for schizophrenia.
Q: But you have not written in the area of posttraumatic stress disorder, have you?
A: (Doesn't matter.)

The point about this line of questioning is that knowledge of the four diagnostic criteria may be elementary information or it may be arcane, but the jury does not know which it is, and even if they did know, they probably would not care. Their concern is with how the witness handles the questions, not with how high he or she scores on a pop quiz. The witness can defuse this line of questioning by refusing to take it as a challenge and at the same time staying within her role by not appearing to claim to judge the materiality of the question. For example,

Q: Can you name the four basic criteria without looking at your notes?
A: I don't think so.

By using a matter-of-fact, noncombative tone the witness has communicated all he or she needs to: This information is not something he or she needs to have memorized in order to feel capable of reaching whatever conclusions have been reached. Moreover, the witness is not acting like an adversary; implicitly, therefore, he or she is interested in the truth, not simply in winning. (If the psychiatrist can in fact name the criteria, the best answer is "Yes, I can." This answer is better than actually listing the criteria since it is not showing off and accordingly does not imply any agenda other than the accurate transmission of information.)

Likewise, to the inevitable question, "You are not really an expert in the area of posttraumatic stress disorder, are you?" a better answer is "Posttraumatic stress disorder is among the psychiatric disorders that I treat, but it is not an area of special expertise," or (if true), "No, I believe I am an expert in the area of posttraumatic stress disorder."

Special Problems of Child Psychiatrists

But all this is not to say that the testimony of a child psychiatrist must be or appear to be without feelings. On the contrary, to be persuasive a child psychiatrist must, like any expert, communicate commitment to the *field* and its values. In addition, as a child psychiatrist, the witness, unlike most expert witnesses, may properly, indeed must, communicate a form of partiality to the *welfare of the child* who is the subject of the court proceeding. But this is quite a different matter, indeed the reverse, of being adversarial or combative on one's own behalf or in order to score points. Consider the following exchange, from a child custody case before a judge without a jury:

Q: Doctor, if the mother is permitted to move far away with the child, it will be harder for the child to see her father, won't it?
A: Not if the father moves too.
Q: But don't you think if the mother wants to move away from the father now, she would just try to move again if he followed her?
A: Not necessarily.
Q: But you certainly aren't claiming that won't happen. Are you?
A: I don't think it's likely.
Q: But you really don't know one way or the other. Do you?
A: Of course not; no one can know for sure at this point.
Q: But if the court orders the mother not to move, then we would know for sure that the father will be nearby. Wouldn't we?

Here the psychiatrist, probably giving in to her frustration with the father, his lawyer, the legal system, or some combination of them, was unable in her answer to the first question to resist the impulse to be clever. Giving in to that impulse invariably gives the cross-examiner the opportunity to score points. If the witness had held her tongue, she would have had an opportunity to make her point not by being clever but simply by manifesting her commitment to the child's well-being:

Q: Doctor, if the mother is permitted to move far away with the child, it will be harder for the child to see her father, won't it?
A: It certainly may.
Q: There is no "may" about it, is there, Doctor?
A: Oh, I think it is far from certain that the mother's moving will necessarily have that effect. If the mother is permitted to move, she may feel more secure and be more open to the father's visitation; or, the father may even decide that being close to this child is so important that he will consider moving also.

The witness has in effect earned the right to give this answer by not jumping into combat with the examiner earlier. As a result, the effect of her testimony is fundamentally different from the effect of the first sequence.

Psychiatrists, particularly child psychiatrists, face a variety of other special problems as witnesses. The first of these is the plethora of experts who may be involved in a case. A child custody case may have testimony from psychiatrists retained by each of the parents, a court-appointed psychiatrist and/or one retained by counsel for the child, a court-employed family relations officer, and welfare department employees. To all these voices, frequently discordant, add those of counsel for the parents and the children, and the result can be that the competing opinions tend to cancel each other out, leaving the judge free to act on his or her impulses.

Moreover, confusion of roles is common in child custody cases (Goldstein et al., 1986). The child psychiatrist is ordinarily asked to testify concerning what custody arrangement is in the best interests of the child, the very same issue the judge will ultimately decide. (By contrast, an expert's testimony in a criminal case may establish that the bullet that struck the victim came from the defendant's gun, but that testimony is only one link in a chain needed to establish the defendant's guilt of a given crime.) As a result, it can be hard to distinguish the judge's role from the psychiatrist's. The psychiatrist may feel, and be treated by the parties, as if he or she is adjudicating competing claims. The psychiatrist may accordingly be subjected to criticism for not according one of the parties due process before deciding against that party, for example, by meeting with one side more than the other. The judge may also treat the child psychiatrist as the adjudicator and simply rubber-stamp his or her recommendation, particularly a psychiatrist retained by the court itself or by counsel for the child. More troubling from the point of view of the psychiatrist witness, the judge, like the parties, may evaluate the psychiatrist's work and testimony like a sort of court of appeals, asking not what is in the best interests of the child but whether the psychiatrist has been fair to all the parties. The psychiatrist, of course, is not trying to be fair to all the parties: At most, he or she is trying to determine what outcome will be in the best interests of the child. But because the psychiatrist is confused with a judge, he or she is liable to be criticized for not taking into account the interests of the disappointed parent.

Moreover, the judge, particularly in child custody cases, very frequently has had so much experience deciding such cases that he or she is convinced that the opinion of a child psychiatrist is superfluous. That is, the judge, not to mention the lawyers and other professionals, confuses his or her role with the psychiatrist's because, after all, in a way it is everyone's job to determine the best interests of the child. This confusion is exacerbated by the fact that many people, including many judges, do not believe child psychiatry has much special expertise to offer. Child psychiatrists thus encounter triple skepticism—as witnesses, as expert witnesses, and as specialists in a field that is viewed (as, say, surgery is not) with suspicion.

To be an effective witness under these circumstances, the child psychiatrist, even more than other expert witnesses, must not be inflamed by the aggression of cross-examination. The best defense of her expertise a child psychiatrist can offer as a witness is a demonstration of his or her therapeutic approach in the process of testifying. That is, the psychiatrist should let the court see how he or she operates as a therapist, not by practicing psychiatry in the courtroom but by showing a caring, gentle thoughtfulness rather than combativeness.

It is just this tone that makes for an effective witness: Any witness is more persuasive if he or she appears to treat the trial as a truth-seeking activity rather than as an arena. But for a psychiatrist a gentle, noncombative tone serves the additional function of illustrating the maturity and thoughtfulness that a court will recognize as characteristics of a good therapist. For example, consider the following exchange:

Q: Doctor, did you perform any formal psychological testing on your patient?
A: Certainly not. Psychological testing would have been a waste of time in this case.
Q: Isn't psychological testing recognized as an important diagnostic tool?
A: But I wasn't doing the kind of diagnosis that calls for psychological testing. I was investigating the question of custody, not doing a full-scale workup of a psychiatric patient.
Q: Wasn't this case just as important as a full-scale workup of a psychiatric patient?
A: As I just explained, it's not a question of importance, it's a question of whether psychological testing is going to be of any significant value in this context, and in my opinion it clearly isn't. What I did do was to talk at length with all the parties involved and observe the child interacting with each of her parents, and I think that was much more valuable than psychological testing could possibly be in this context.

Among the problems with this approach to testifying on cross-examination is that the witness does not sound like someone who is a gifted listener. A judge already somewhat skeptical of psychiatrists is unlikely to trust this witness. A better approach to the same line of questioning would be:

Q: Doctor, did you perform any formal psychological testing on your patient?

A: No, I didn't.

Q: Isn't psychological testing recognized as an important diagnostic tool?

A: Yes, it is.

Q: But you did not use that tool here, did you?

A: No, I didn't.

The witness is being used as a foil in this sequence, and instead of fighting that role, simply allows the lawyer to make points, patient or secure enough not to need to correct every misimpression right away. Such a witness will get an opportunity to say what he or she wants to say, either on direct examination or perhaps even, as in the following example, on cross-examination:

Q: So inasmuch as you did not do any psychological testing, you did not really do a thorough evaluation, did you?

A: No, I think my evaluation was thorough.

Q: But it would have been more thorough had you done psychological testing, wouldn't it?

A: No, the important issue that emerged in my evaluation was Mary's need to stay with her mother and her fears of losing the security her mother represents. And psychological testing would not really have added to my understanding of that issue.

Q: But it might have added to your understanding of other issues, isn't that right?

A: Yes, that is certainly true.

When and if the psychiatrist does get an opportunity like this one to say to the cross-examiner what he or she thinks is important about the case, the judge will be ready to listen, much readier than if the psychiatrist mistakenly believed that his or her job was to say what was necessary to say no matter what. (And if the psychiatrist does not get to say it on cross-examination, the other lawyers or even the judge will give him or her an opportunity when the cross-examination concludes.)

In short, the judge will be most likely to notice the psychiatrist's virtues as a therapist if some of them are shown as a witness. And, ultimately, the psychiatrist's professional skills—an ability to listen attentively and thoughtfully, to care about the well-being of patients, and to resist the urge to respond to aggression with aggression—will enable him or her to be a persuasive witness in court.

References

Coles R: *The Call of Stories*. Boston, Houghton Mifflin, 1989.

Goldstein J, Freud A, Solnit A, et al: *In the Best Interests of the Child*. New York, Free Press, 1986.

Salinger JD: *The Catcher in the Rye*. New York, Bantam, 1964.

118 THE ROLE OF THE CHILD EXPERT IN COURT-REQUESTED EVALUATIONS[a]

Barbara Nordhaus, M.S.W., L.C.S.W., and Albert J. Solnit, M.D.

In this chapter we explore the role of the child expert in court-contested child custody and placement conflicts. A child expert is a person who by training and experience has acquired and uses that body of knowledge referred to as clinical child development. There is no one discipline or profession that is the exclusive source of such knowledge and its applications; the professions of pediatrics, child psychiatry, child psychoanalysis, social work, and clinical child psychology all require a mastery of the theoretical and practice aspects of this body of knowledge as defined by state and national standards of academic and supervised training.

We assume that the knowledge used by child experts in the clinical evaluation, expert opinion and recommendations conveyed to the court about what will serve the child's best interests, is based on (*a*) the child's need for appropriate physical nurture and safety and (*b*) the child's need for a continuity of affectionate care by a limited number of adults who want to take care of the child on a permanent basis.

The child expert may be called upon to perform a clinical evaluation as part of a legal proceeding by agreement of the adult parties, by order of the court, or at the behest of one of the disputing parties. The legal conflict may stem from a custody or visitation dispute between divorcing parents or as part of a placement dispute between the child's parents and the state stemming from issues of neglect, abuse, or abandonment.

Divorce cases (issues of custody and visitation) are usually heard in family court, while placement cases are most often heard in juvenile court; guardianship and occasionally custody issues are determined in probate court. The most frequent request for clinical evaluations involves a legal decision about the child's custody and may include termination of parental rights. Although the principles of child development knowledge being applied are the same in evaluations regarding custody assignments and in state placement evaluations, the issues are considered separately in this chapter.

DIVORCE

After a rapid increase between 1960 and 1980, family disruption in our society is believed to have stabilized such that about half of couples married after 1970 will divorce at some point. Half of all children are likely to experience the divorce of their parents and go on to spend an average of 5 years in a single-parent household (Glick and Lin, 1986). Approximately 72% of divorced women and 80% of divorced men will remarry. The divorce rate for second marriages is greater than in first marriages. One of every 10 children will experience two or more divorces of the custodial parent before he or she becomes 16 (Furstenberg, 1988).

This year, and each year in the foreseeable future, more than one million American children are likely to be reared in families disrupted by separation and impending divorce (Maccoby and Mnookin, 1994). The authors note that no-fault divorce represents a judicial shift from the "tender years" doctrine, favoring mothers, to a "best interests of the child" standard. It also is associated with a preference for dispute resolution through mediation rather than litigation in the present divorce climate. The best interests standard not only places the child's needs at

---

[a] Editor's Note: Legal references in this chapter are listed numerically.

the center of custody decision-making, it also satisfies the requirements of our society for freedom from gender bias with respect to custody decisions. Programs to assist divorcing parents in dispute resolution typically offer parents information on the legal process for determining custody, visitation, and child support; the effects of divorce and separation on adults; and the effects of divorce and separation on children and how parents can help children cope with this difficult transition (Schepard, 1993).

Present knowledge about the impact of divorce on children suggests that it creates an immediate or short-term stressful challenge that may adversely effect the long-term development of the involved children. Wallerstein and Corbin (1991) note that "children of divorce are greatly overrepresented in outpatient psychiatric, family agency, and private practice populations relative to their presence within the general population" (p. 1108). Confirming this view, Maccoby commented on the Hetherington (1992) study stating, "A central finding is that the children in intact families were doing better at each assessment period than those living with divorced mothers who had either remained single or remarried. This finding is consistent with a considerable body of literature pointing to the disruptive effects of divorce (and/or the familial conditions that precede divorce) on children's functioning" (p. 231). There is no way to predict which children will be more vulnerable. Many clinicians believe that the single most corrosive element in the child's experience when parents divorce results from situations of unabated and intractable conflict. However, these inferences must remain tentative because there is no way at present of knowing whether it is the divorce or the influences of a child-disturbing marriage which are associated with these findings.

Nevertheless, many children and their reconfigured families will be able over time to achieve a progressive development and to restore an adequate sense of continuity and security. The parents' ability to resolve visitation and custody issues cooperatively either independently or with assistance (by family relations services of the court, mediation efforts, or voluntary mental health consultation) can be responsive to the child's needs for a sound unique relationship with each parent. Such effective collaboration after the divorce provides the conditions that enable parents de facto or de jure to create voluntary joint custody. The parents' ability, willingness, and motivation to cooperate enable the child to feel wanted and to trust and count on the parents to continue to provide nurture and guidance.

ROLE OF THE MENTAL HEALTH EXPERT

Most divorcing parents make their own custody arrangements. Statistical data on the percentage of divorces in which contested custody issues arise are estimated to be 5–8%. In their California study, Maccoby et al. (1994) found that only 1.5% of families actually relied upon the judge to decide the custody or visitation issue; another 2.2% went to trial but were able to settle during the trial. In the same study, 75% of families experienced negligible or mild conflict, while 25% experienced substantial or intense conflict.

When a mental health expert is consulted by divorcing parents on a voluntary basis, the usual rules of confidentiality apply. Some therapists make formal signed agreements with potentially litigious parents to emphasize the therapist's willingness to assist the parents to come to an agreement on a voluntary basis. Conversely, clinicians may not be willing to serve as experts in court if they already are committed to voluntary, confidential therapy. Usually a verbal understanding is sufficient. No agreement can completely shield the process from the possibility of a later subpoena by one of the parents. Most often in voluntary situations, the child is not seen; rather, the emphasis is on assisting the parents to maintain their relationship to their child in an affectionate and appropriately authoritative manner as the true experts on what the child needs.

When divorcing parents cannot agree about the custody and visitation arrangements for their child, the state temporarily becomes the parent in its parens patriae function. Once the parents cede their decision-making prerogative to the state and the court assumes the decision-making role, the atmosphere is likely to be charged with anger and conflict. In such instances the parents' disagreements are usually heightened, and there is a greater risk that psychological war will lead to emotional wounds, to feelings of betrayal and bitter rage that too often remain unhealed even after the judge has made a decision about custody and/or visitation. It is in connection with such cases that the child expert may be called upon to render an evaluation and recommendation that can be used in the court proceeding.

WHAT THE CLINICAL CHILD EXPERT SHOULD KEEP IN MIND ABOUT LEGAL CONSIDERATIONS

The child expert is frequently called upon in conflicted cases by one or both attorneys representing the parents. When the child has separate counsel, the child's lawyer may initiate or be involved in the designation of the child's clinical evaluation. Regardless of who hires the expert witness, the contribution of the child expert is as an advocate for the child's needs, i.e., for the "best interests of the child." The child expert translates this legal standard into clinical terms, meaning what is best or least harmful to the child, given her or his age, developmental level, special needs, and relationship with each parent. The child expert's recommendation to the court is based on a clinical evaluation of the child's development and attachments and on what can best facilitate the child's developmental progress.

From the legal side, the "best interests" standard is given lip service in most states, especially as the court's adversarial process forces into view the competing interests of the adults. In reality, concerns of fairness to adults and personal value biases of the individual judge or the society often prevail. In this sense all involved will verbalize their concern for the child's best interests but only a few will transcend their identification with the contending adults in a manner that makes the child's interests and needs paramount.

Lawyers and judges complain about the vagueness and indeterminacy of the "best interests" standard. While some experts advocate more rules and less discretion in custody decisions as a deterrent to litigation, the law as practiced requires a highly individualized determination of what is in the best interests of, or least detrimental to, each particular child (Mnookin, 1975).

Although the mental health practitioner is likely to be looked to by the court to assist in providing insight into the individual child's needs and the competing caretakers' capacities to meet the child's needs, increasingly the claims of these experts are being subject to question. Horner et al. (1991) believe " . . .by whatever processes of reasoning they use, clinicians predictably fail the most fundamental requirement of basic scientific inquiry, which is to achieve convincing demonstrations of interjudge reliabilities of perception and inference when the latter are applied to the same body of facts" (p. 170). We assume that experts disagree because their knowledge is not and cannot be precise. We respect the diversity of life styles and believe the community is best protected, not by experts, but by those who administer the rule of law, as imperfect as it is, to guide us in assuring parents and children of their constitutional rights.

DEVELOPMENTAL PRINCIPLES

Goldstein et al. (1973) have defined the central principle in custody and placement decisions, "the least detrimental available alternative," as " . . .that child placement and procedure for child placement which maximizes, in accord with the child's sense of time, the child's opportunity for being wanted and for maintaining a continuous, unconditional, and permanent basis . . .relationship with at least one adult who is or will become the child's psychological parent" (p. 99). The authors further explicate the child's sense of time as varying with the urgency of his or her instinctual and emotional needs: For example, separation from a central nurturing person is less tolerable to an infant or young child or a child with particular vulnerability or identified special need than to an older or sturdier child. The child needs to be wanted by at least one adult who offers safety, affection, and appropriate stimulation. The child's developmental needs are best met when there is opportunity to experience such an attachment to an adult in a continuing unconditional and permanent relationship. These principles offer the clinician a conceptual guide and frame of reference but are not meant to be formulaic.

The restoration of emotional security for that small number of children who are the subject of continued litigated custody disputes in postdivorce conflict often requires the difficult acknowledgment that, for the time being, the child's future is best safeguarded in the hands of one primary, custodial parent. The least detrimental alternative in extreme cases when parents are addicted to fighting and cannot tolerate the contact required by visitation is to support and protect the child's relationship with the custodial parent. Despite the flaws and imperfections in the relationship, the child can do reasonably well. Intervention by the court or other experts can risk undermining the custodial parent's security, sense of control, and effectiveness, often resulting in less cooperation between the parents (Nordhaus, 1991).

Noncustodial parents and those who consult with them would be well advised to emphasize how the noncustodial parent can persuade and make worthwhile voluntary agreements regarding visitation and other arrangements that will promote relatively conflict-free, sound relationships to both parents. For example, support by the noncustodial parent, not limited to money but including availability for child care, for doing errands, and for helping the custodial parent with various demands he or she confronts in maintaining the child's home can be very useful if presented as an attractive voluntary nonthreatening option.

CLINICAL EVALUATION

When the evaluation is for court purposes, what is the overall task of the child expert and how is the task accomplished? The clinical evaluation in custody or placement issues, while similar to the psychiatric evaluation, is different in its goals. The purpose of the psychiatric evaluation is to arrive at a psychodynamic formulation of the child's presenting problems, a diagnosis, and a treatment plan recommendation. Ordinarily it is conducted on a voluntary and confidential basis. In a custody evaluation the question is posed by the court. Usually a custody conflict requiring a court-ordered evaluation signifies that the parents are unable to cooperate voluntarily in planning for custody and visitation arrangements. The questions are: With whom should the child live? Which parent should have legal decision-making authority regarding education, medical decisions, religion, financial support, vacations, etc.? How can the opportunities for the child to maintain a useful and sound relationship with both parents be optimized?

Intractable postdivorce conflict usually has noxious and long-term negative impact on children (Emery, 1982). It is crucial that throughout the evaluation process the child expert support whatever capacity the parents have or can recover to resolve their own disputes, to diminish conflict, and to place themselves in the child's shoes in guiding themselves to be the best parents they can be for their child. Even experienced experts may find themselves unwittingly drawn into the family dispute because all adults, no matter how well trained, drift toward an identification with one of the conflicting adults. At times the evaluator may experience a resurgence of her or his own childhood family struggles, especially if divorce is a significant experience in his or her own past.

The first practical step is to clarify as much as possible the court's questions. In complex cases (particularly foster care placement cases), it is advisable to obtain a copy of the motion for evaluation. The evaluator can request that the court furnish the exact questions to be addressed in the evaluation. This phase of the process is significant, as it initiates the attempt at a dialogue between the professionals in two intersecting

fields. The law side usually values winning, establishing fault, being explicit, and meting out "justice"; mental health and developmental experts traditionally value helping and promoting understanding while tolerating ambiguity and ambivalence. During this phase it may be necessary for the clinician to explicate the nature and limits of his or her expertise to the court.

Some clinicians will agree to be retained by one side or the other in a case. There are several reasons to insist that the court order the evaluation. It enables the expert to state effectively that he or she serves as an expert on behalf of the child, striving to be neutral with respect to the adult because the child's interests are paramount. Court-ordered evaluations discourage multiple evaluations, which constitute an undesirable intrusion and burden for the child. When court-ordered, the report of the evaluation is sent to the court. Each court has its own policy with respect to making the report available to the lawyers in the case. Lawyers sometimes request that the consultant furnish them with the report even when this would be improper. When in doubt about any aspect of the legal proprieties, the court clerk is usually the appropriate person to consult.

Financial arrangements need to be attended to carefully. Many clinicians require a retainer fee before embarking on the evaluation, having learned that in adversarial settings the child expert's bill may be overlooked or deliberately left unpaid by disgruntled parents even when a court order obliges them to pay the costs. Whatever the fee arrangements, they should be clarified at the outset, including the charges for expenses entailed in reviewing case materials, preparing the report, and testifying in court.

Outside materials should not be utilized without signed permission of those involved or through approval by the court. In divorce cases, the child's pediatric and school records should be obtained, as they provide essential information including the child's educational, family, developmental, and health history. It is optimal if teachers or day care providers can write a paragraph about the child's school experience to supplement check list forms that are used by many experts. If the child is or has been in counselling or psychotherapy, a brief report with the informed consent of the parents should be requested to include the presenting complaint, diagnosis, and progress or termination summary. If such an intrusion into the confidentiality of an ongoing treatment would significantly disturb the treatment, the question should be raised as to whether the additional information is warranted considering the burden it would place on the child's or adult's treatment. All such reports should be in the form of written documents that can potentially be reviewed by anyone in the court proceeding. Verbal reports, i.e., hearsay, do not carry the same weight in court. Drug and alcohol treatment, psychiatric hospitalization, and criminal records concerning the adults are pertinent for review.

CLINICAL INTERVIEW

In preparing for the report and court testimony, the child expert evaluates the child's developmental and emotional level of functioning, describing what the child's needs are and whether there are special needs to be taken into account. The central issue is the child's relationship to the competing caregivers. As Anna Freud (1971) pointed out in her 1968 comment on the *Painter v. Bannister* case, "Clinical and analytic experience teaches us that children can fill many different roles in the emotional lives of their parents or of other adults. They may be no more for them than a piece of property which is valued egoistically as an extension of the adult's personality; when this happens they serve the adult's needs, while their own developmental needs remain unconsidered. In contrast to this, they may be loved unselfishly, as persons in their own right, with their own needs of paramount importance. Further, they may be no more than a pawn in a game, with no importance of their own, except that possession or dispossession of their persons signifies victory or defeat for the warring factions" (p. 251).

The task of staying focused on describing the child's needs in a custody case is difficult for all adults including the clinician. One significant source of difficulty is the adult's effort to identify with the child's sense of helplessness in the midst of unrelenting adult conflict. Because of the demanding nature of these cases, many clinicians pace themselves cautiously as to the number of custody evaluations they undertake. Specializing in such difficult work increases the risk that one's approach will become mechanical and superficial. Retaining a generalist's view lowers that risk, emphasizing that each case will be evaluated as unique.

In the consulting room with the family, it is useful and appropriate to review the purpose of the evaluation, its lack of confidentiality, the legal motives for the evaluation, and the requirement of submitting a written report to the court. Similarly, it is important to clarify that the report and testimony, where indicated, is designed to assist the judge since the judge, not the evaluator, has the authority and responsibility to make decisions.

The evaluator begins by meeting with the child's parents, usually individually. A sufficiently detailed history is taken to provide a general sense of the parent's own background, personality, and level of functioning. If severe character pathology or psychiatric illness that interferes with parenting is evident, a more systematic mental status examination and diagnosis may be desirable. This may indicate the need for further interviews and formal psychological testing. The parents are each asked to describe the child's developmental history, to explain how they get along with their child, and to discuss what the parent believes would be the best arrangement for the child. A discussion of the cause of the breakdown of the marriage and an idea of why the parents cannot cooperate with each other may provide further insight by which to gauge the intractibility of the conflict and to clarify what are realistic options for the child.

EVALUATING THE YOUNG CHILD

The child's age and developmental level influence the interviewing process. The appropriate method for assessment of children under 5 is through play and the administration of a developmental examination. A systematic developmental evaluation for younger children, such as the Yale Developmental Scales, provides an examination of five domains—gross motor, fine motor, speech and language, adaptive, and social functioning (see Chapter 38). Such an assessment affords a reliable method of determining the child's level of functioning as well as a way of screening for deviations and vulnerabilities. Constitutionally and environmentally generated difficulties can be identified in formulating a child's special needs.

From the history, the developmental examination, and the play situation with younger children, useful inferences can be made about the child's patterns of attachment, separation, mood regulation, and bodily functions. In this systematic way the clinical child expert prepares an inventory that becomes the basis for making recommendations to the court as well as for acknowledging the limits of what can be determined in such consultations. It is both tactful and useful in maintaining the primary focus on what is the least detrimental alternative for the child to avoid "scapegoating" the parent who the expert feels should not be the custodial parent.

The developmental and clinical (play) assessments are also used to explore how well each contending party meets the child's needs for feeling wanted; for providing continuity of affectionate care; for uplifting expectations; and for safety. Having at least one adult who meets these needs of the child is essential in supporting the child's capacities for self-regulation and in establishing development-promoting attachments. In turn, these capacities enhance the child's ability to be comforted and soothed, to engage in age-appropriate contacts with peers, and to feel comfortable in the care of substitute caregivers.

EVALUATING THE SCHOOL-AGE CHILD

Both the developmental and play assessment of a younger child usually occur in the presence of a parent, providing the opportunity to observe and differentiate the child's experience with each parent. The school-age and preadolescent child should be interviewed individually as well as together with each parent. Some evaluators find it useful to structure the interview with the parents to include a "task" the child and parent are asked to work on together. Leaving the interview unstructured can provide an opportunity to observe the child and parent in spontaneous interaction such as at play together, in conversation, in silence, and in conflict. In these observations, the quality of the child's relationship to the parent can be noted: Is he or she engaged, distant, apprehensive, responsive, avoidant, etc.?

The play interview is generally considered the most useful process in assessing a child of this age who has not yet developed the cognitive ability to rely on conceptual thinking and on language for full expression.

Discussion with the school-age child of the reasons for the evaluation, including the court's interest in the custody/visitation issue, can be informative and fruitful when comfortable and handled sensitively. The interview may include drawings, thematically developed play, and occasionally the opportunity to tactfully, often indirectly (e.g., "let's pretend"), evoke the child's opinions and desires with respect to the custody and visitation issues. Play and drawings are phenomena that may reflect a child's imagination, fantasies, conflicts, and life experiences, as well as developmental level and intelligence.

Direct questioning of the child about a preference in living arrangements is risky because it often increases the child's anxiety about loyalty conflicts. Asking the child to choose one parent over the other may increase the child's fear of losing the other parent, involving a painful confrontation with the child's strong wish to have the parents stay together—albeit more as mother and father than as husband and wife. When the child's preference can be determined, it is taken into account as an important but not decisive factor. The weight given to the school-age child's preference should be assessed individually in each case.

EVALUATING THE ADOLESCENT

Adolescents need not be seen routinely in custody assessments, as they are considered able to play an active and often decisive role in making their own choices. Occasionally in special circumstances where issues of physical safety, delinquent or behavioral problems, or a parent's mental illness are involved, an assessment may be required. Before the age of formal operational thought, which occurs around 11, children have limited ability to project the idea of themselves in the future and to sense how the past will influence the future. Beginning in early adolescence, cognitive and psychological development, including the push toward increased independence, enhance the adolescent's capacity to be more active in custody decisions. With support, the older child and adolescent can usually begin to assess his or her own needs and to form sound judgments based on actual life experiences about custody and visitation arrangements (Schowalter, 1979).

COURT REPORT

Once the clinical evaluation is completed, the report is prepared for the court. It reiterates the court's questions; cites all reviewed reports and documents; identifies all persons interviewed, specifying the dates and time spent in all interviews and reports; summarizes historical and clinical interview material; and concludes with a summary and recommendation. Court testimony is discussed in Chapter 117. In child custody and placement cases it is particularly important for the expert to review his or her testimony with the child's attorney when possible, to remain focused on the child's point of view, and not to go beyond professional expertise and knowledge. The Court's interpretation of a recent New Jersey statute, for example, requires the expert to testify to a prediction that a child's removal will cause irreparable harm. This poses a dilemma for the expert since no one can predict with accuracy the long-term future outcome of such a placement change or the development of future relationships (1). As child experts, it is essential and valid to use the capacity for short-term predictions to indicate what immediate psychological injuries can occur if the child's best interests are corroded by the passage of time. The child should not be exposed to the risk of avoidable injury in order to put fairness to the contending adults ahead of what would be least harmful to the child.

The nature of the child's relationship with each of the contending adults might enable the expert to document that one parent is more of a primary psychological parent than the other, despite socioeconomic consideration, or that each of the contending adults, for different reasons, is a primary psychological parent. In the latter instance if the parents cannot decide, preferring that a stranger, the judge, decide, the expert should indicate that each of the parents is a primary psychological parent, equally competent for different reasons. If the parents or contending adults cannot decide or agree, the court should use the principle of least detrimental alternative to meet the best interest standard of making a decision, not allowing the passage of time to be corrosive to the child while adults debate how to be fair to each other.

PLACEMENT EVALUATIONS

Unlike the desirability of private dispute resolution involved in divorce cases, foster care cases involving placement disputes are more regularly subject to court process and decision-making. The court regulates the functioning of the state child welfare bureaucracy by imposing time limitations on temporary custody arrangements, and through its termination of parental rights process, it legalizes permanent placements for children who cannot return to the care of their biological parents. The questions are: What is the best permanent placement for the child? Can the child ever be returned to the biological parents?

The child expert evaluating cases of abuse, neglect, or abandonment follows the previously discussed placement principles. The need for permanency and security is essential in these cases. While divorce conflict cases pose the difficulty of raw familial passions, the child welfare cases present a different challenge. Often the children to be evaluated have already suffered grave psychological damage as a result of chronic deprivation, multiple placements, and other conditions noxious to the developing child. It may be frustrating to the evaluator to recommend an outcome for the child that, while it may be the least detrimental, seems so far from ideal. An evaluator's inability to tolerate the available least detrimental alternative for the child can lead to harmful delays and postponements and recommendations for an unknown or unrealistic solution. Such delays and indecision can inflict further psychological damage on the child. The child's sense of time should be taken into account in not delaying, beyond the younger child's tolerance, the finding of at least one qualified adult who can provide the continuity of affectionate care as described above. It is important to observe the child's current realities and to make the best of what is available.

Evaluations involving allegations of sexual abuse, when there is a finding of physical damage, require the child to be assured of protection from further abuse (Solnit et al., 1992, p. 81). This means exclusion of the abuser, if that person can be identified, or a documented change in the child's circumstances that addresses the source and cause of the problem, as much as it can be determined. When there is no physical injury, the evaluator is unlikely to be able to know whether abuse occurred. Therefore, the mental health expert should not accept a request to determine whether sexual abuse has occurred, but should suggest the request be refocused to an assessment of the child's relationship to the caretakers for the purpose of determining placement, visitation, or custody issues.

CASE ILLUSTRATION: *Ireland v. Smith*

In this Michigan case a 15-year-old unmarried adolescent girl gave birth to a daughter who was raised in the mother's home with the mother as custodial parent assisted in child care by the maternal grandmother and the maternal aunt, while she completed her high school education. When the child was 1 year of age, the father, who had acknowledged paternity at birth, began to visit.

When the child was 3 years, 2 months of age, the mother filed a suit seeking the father's child support in preparation for her anticipated move to pursue a college education and to live independently with her daughter. The father then petitioned for custody of the child.

The judge found that the mother had established a custodial environment for the child, i.e., that the child looked to the mother for guidance, discipline, and the necessities of life. He found that the day-to-day care of the child was provided by the mother and that the child was acquainted with her father but in a way that was of necessity limited by the structure of the visiting relationship.

Comment

In this case the judge described himself as attempting to reach a decision that would represent "the child's best interest." He followed the state statute in examining the relative abilities of each parent to provide affection, guidance, and other material needs. He found the central issue to be maintaining continuity, but he construed continuity to mean of physical environment rather than of the child's primary tie to the mother. He wrote:

The mother's program would require that the child be in day care. The child was in a program at the University of Michigan which apparently was appropriate and resulted in the child having a meaningful experience. It would be the mother's intention to continue this on until such time as she either graduates, as previously stated, or her marital circumstances somehow change. For the purpose of deciding this case, the Court would have to assume that it is the mother's intention to maintain the child at the University of Michigan for some considerable number of years. This issue is pivotal.

The judge decided to intrude into and violate the integrity of this child's ongoing adequate family, concluding that the child's best interest was to be moved to the father because, during the day when the mother was in class, the paternal grandmother, a "blood relative," would be preferable to a day care program for the child. Thus, while espousing the central importance of the principle of continuity in the life of a young child who is developing well, he rendered a decision contrary to the principle. The judge did not make reference to any involvement by a child expert whose opinion might have assisted him to better accomplish his stated goal (2).

CASE ILLUSTRATION: *Prost v. Greene*

In the *Prost v. Greene* case, the parents separated after an 8½-year marriage, at first under the same roof and then 9 months later in separate domiciles when the mother received temporary physical custody with liberal visitation for the father. In a lengthy trial, each sought divorce, support, property, and custody of their sons 7 and 4 years of age. Despite the fact that the children were doing well in a custody arrangement that had been in place for over a year's time, the judge reversed the custody, awarding sole legal and physical custody to the father. In her opinion the judge wrote " . . .it is plain to the court (and should be to any other objective observer) that plaintiff (the mother) is simply more devoted to and absorbed by her work and her career than anything else in her life, including her health, her children and her family."

Comment

For the child expert, it is instructive to observe that the judge, finding the expert testimony of the child psychiatrist "unpersuasive," complained that the expert "seemed overly focused on the parents' emotional makeup and on the relationship/conflict between them, rather than on the best interest of the children as evidenced by their current psychological status and relationship to each parent." In the absence of convincing testimony explicating the developmental needs of each child and the nature of the children's relationship to each parent, the judge relied upon her own intuition, value judgments, and personal reactions to the parents' personalities.

Apparently the needs of Matthew, age 7, and Jeffrey, age 4, were not credibly articulated in the courtroom and therefore did not form the central consideration in the decision. Rather, the judge in this case wrote `` . . .children learn from the intensive presence, participation and involvement of a parent in their lives, from the frequent and sincere demonstrations of a parent's love and concern for them, from a parent's efforts to help them solve their problems, and from their observation that a parent enjoys being with them and, indeed, has fun with them. On all these fronts, the evidence is clear, defendant has it way over plaintiff.'' The judge's language demonstrated how in the powerful current of divorce conflict there is a tendency to be drawn into taking sides and to focus on the adults. The judge further overstepped the bounds of her role when she chided the parents, ``The parties should be ashamed of themselves, but it does not appear that they are.'' The judge's reproach of the parents prevented her from conveying the ``experience, wisdom, and compassion . . .to fashion an appropriate remedy'' (3).

CASE ILLUSTRATION: Baby Richard

In this case, Richard's parents began living together in the fall of 1989. Daniella, Richard's mother, became pregnant in June 1990, and Richard was born March 16, 1991. Otakar, Richard's father, lived with Daniella and provided for all of Daniella's expenses during her pregnancy until late January 1991, when he returned to his native Czechoslovakia to attend his gravely ill grandmother. Daniella was informed by a member of Otakar's family that he had reinvolved himself in a romantic relationship with a former girlfriend. Daniella felt so betrayed and distressed by this news that she fled the apartment she shared with Otakar, avoided contact with him, and then informed him that their baby had died. As a single mother, she executed a consent for adoption 4 days after Richard was born. Daniella refused to furnish Otakar's name to the adoptive parents or to their lawyer, although informing them that she knew his identity.

When Richard was 57 days of age, Otakar learned that Richard was alive and had been placed in adoption. He immediately began legal efforts to recover custody of his son. For the next 4 years, legal proceedings postponed the decision for Richard. First, the trial court ruled that Otakar did not show sufficient interest in

the child in his first 30 days of life, and therefore was found to be an ``unfit'' parent. As an ``unfit'' parent, Otakar's consent for adoption was not necessary. The appellate court then confirmed the trial court, citing a best interest standard that at age 2 years, 5 months Richard's adoptive parents were the only parents he had known. The judge wrote of Richard, ``He has not touched or seen Daniella since four days after his birth, and he has never spoken a word to her. Nor has he ever touched, seen, or communicated with Otakar. In fact, he is totally unaware of the existence of Daniella and Otakar.'' He further noted, ``Since Richard was a newborn, John and Jane Doe have done everything with Richard that is the essence of being parents, and Richard has done everything with them that is the essence of being a son.''

The Supreme Court of Illinois heard the appeal and reversed the decision of the trial and appeal courts, resulting in Richard's placement at 4 years of age with his biological parents, who were total strangers.

Comment

The psychologically distinctive role of the father begins early on with his anticipation of the child's birth. Through holding, feeding, protecting, and playfully interacting with the baby, he becomes a responsive and competent caretaker, central to the child. The father's presence is positively associated with the child's developmental progression (Pruett, 1987). Separation from such a parent to whom the child is emotionally tied can cause shattering loss, regression, and disruption to the child's sense of stability and security.

In the case of Richard, Otakar could not have been considered Richard's ``father'' in any but a biological sense. The legal system, by its delay of 4 years and by its awarding a child rather than other compensation to Otakar, failed to uphold its best interest standard. The court recognized that a grave injustice had been done to Otakar—first by Daniella, who concealed Richard's existence from Otakar; and then by the state, which concealed Otakar's identity and whereabouts from the adoptive parents and their lawyer; and then by the failure of the adoptive parents and the various legal representatives to make a decision based on the child's best interests. This case illustrates the way in which the child's best interest comes to be subordinate to the court's priority of fairness to an aggrieved adult (4).

The best guide for the child expert is: Put yourself in the place of the child.

References

Emery RE: Interparental conflict and the children of discord and divorce. *Psychol Bull* 92:310–330, 1982.

Freud A: *Problems of Psychoanalytic Training, Diagnosis, and the Technique of Therapy Writings* (Vol VII). New York, International University Press, 1971, p. 251.

Furstenberg FF: Child care after divorce and remarriage. In: Hetherington EM, Arasteh JD (eds): *Impact of Divorce, Single Parenting and Stepparenting on Children.* Hillsdale, NJ, Erlbaum, 1988, pp. 245–261.

Glick PC, Lin S: Recent changes in divorce and remarriage. *J Marriage Family* 737–747, 1986.

Goldstein J, Freud A, Solnit A: *Beyond the Best Interests of the Child.* London, Free Press, 1973, p. 99.

Horner T, Guyer M: Prediction, prevention, and clinical expertise in child custody cases in which allegations of child sexual abuse have been made. *Fam Law Q* XXV(2):170, 1991.

Maccoby E: Commentary. In: Hetherington EM, Clingempeel WG (eds): *Coping with Marital Transitions* (Vol 57, No. 2). Chicago, The University of Chicago Press, 1992, p. 231.

Maccoby E, Mnookin R (eds): *Dividing the Child.* Cambridge, MA, Harvard University Press, 1994.

Mnookin R: Child-custody adjudication: Judicial functions in the face of indeterminacy. In: *Children and the Law.* Durham, NC, Duke University School of Law, 1975, p. 227.

Nordhaus B: *Divorce—A Gordian Knot. The Psychoanalytic Study of the Child* (Vol. 46). New Haven, Yale University Press, 1991, pp. 381–391.

Pruett KD: *The Nurturing Father.* New York, Warner Books, 1987.

Schepard A: War and P.E.A.C.E.: A preliminary report and a model statute on an interdisciplinary educational program for divorcing and separating parents. *University of Michigan J Law Reform* 27(1):134, 1993.

Schowalter J: Views On The Role Of The Child's Preference In Custody Litigation. *Connecticut Bar J* 53:298, 1979.

Solnit AJ, Nordhaus B, Lord R: *When Home Is No Haven.* New Haven, CT, Yale University Press, 1992, p. 81.

Wallerstein JS, Corbin SB: The Child and the Vicissitudes of Divorce. In: Lewis M (ed): *Child and Adolescent Psychiatry: A Comprehensive Textbook.* Baltimore, Williams & Williams, 1991, p. 1108.

Legal References

1. 129 N.J. 1, Supreme Court 1992.
2. *Smith v. Smith*, Circuit Court, Macomb County, Michigan No. 93-385 D6, June 27, 1994.
3. *Prost v. Greene*, Superior Court District of Columbia Family Division, July 1994.
4. *Doe v. Kirchner* (Baby Richard Case) 254 Ill. App. 3d 405, 1994.

D/ Child and Adolescent Psychiatry and Public Health

119 EPIDEMIOLOGY

David R. Offord, M.D., and Jan E. Fleming, M.D.

Epidemiology is concerned with the study of both the distribution of a disease or physiological condition in human populations and the factors that influence that distribution (Lilienfeld, 1976). Kleinbaum et al. (1982) identify four aims of epidemiological research: (*a*) to *describe* the health status of populations by counting the number of occurrences of diseases in the population as a whole and in subgroups within it, and by monitoring trends over time; (*b*) to *explain* the etiology of diseases by discovering causal factors and understanding the mechanisms by which they operate; (*c*) to *predict* the number of disease occurrences in the population as a whole, and in high-risk groups; and (*d*) to *control* the distributions of diseases in the population by prevention of new occurrences, eradication of existing cases, prolongation of life with chronic disease, or otherwise improving the health status of afflicted persons.

Data from epidemiological studies have two uses, administrative (or services related) and scientific (Earls, 1989; Robins, 1978). Figure 119.1 illustrates these two uses. On the administrative side, the figure indicates where, in the development of a disease, the different intervention levels apply. Primary prevention comes into play before the initiation of the pathological processes when, without intervention, the onset of the disease is irreversible. Secondary prevention centers on altering the expression of disease after its onset. Tertiary prevention is concerned about minimizing the severity of disease and promoting recovery and remission. On the scientific side, the figure illustrates that epidemiology is concerned about factors associated with causes, initiation of the pathological processes and clinical detection, and those associated with resulting changes in health status.

Epidemiological studies are of two types, descriptive and experimental. Descriptive studies can answer a variety of questions depending on the sample and design used. For instance, large-scale cross-sectional community surveys of child and adolescent psychiatric disorders can provide data on the overall prevalence of disorder and on individual disorders. They can identify correlates of disorders in various domains, such as sociodemographic, familial, parental, and developmental, and discern associated features or consequences of disorders (e.g., impairments and utilization of services). Information from these studies can be helpful administratively by permitting the identification of geographic areas that are relatively underserved or overserved. The extent to which services are targeted accurately to those most in need can also be determined. Further, if population trends can be correctly predicted, it becomes feasible to plan future service needs in a more rational fashion.

Descriptive studies using a prospective design can address questions of outcome of disorders, identification of predictors or prognostic variables, and causal risk factors for disorders (e.g., Offord et al., 1992). Being able to distinguish between persistent and nonpersistent disorders allows the focusing of resources on the more chronic conditions. In addition, the identification of causal risk factors allows the formation of hypothesized causal chains for disorder. Table 119.1 presents an example of such a chain for antisocial behavior in childhood.

Various epidemiological research strategies have been proposed for demonstrating causation (Rutter, 1981b), and specific criteria have been published for evaluating the certainty with which a particular variable can be said to be etiologically linked to a disorder (Department of Clinical Epidemiology and Biostatistics, 1981a). The strongest design for evaluating causation (and the effectiveness of prevention and treatment programs) is a randomized controlled clinical trial where the assignment of subjects to the intervention and control groups is under the investigator's control and is carried out randomly (Department of Clinical Epidemiology and Biostatistics, 1981b). The rationale for a prevention or

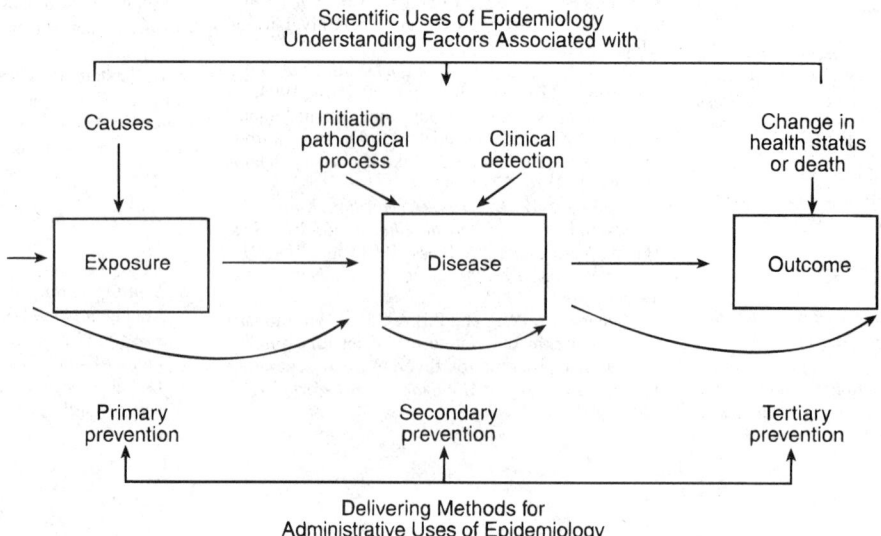

Figure 119.1. The uses of epidemiology.

Table 119.1. Hypothesized Causal Chain

(a) Learning disorders → (b) School failure → (c) Low self-esteem →
(d) Association with antisocial peer group → (e) Antisocial behavior

Adapted from Costello EJ, Burns BJ, Angold A, et al: How can epidemiology improve mental health services for children and adolescents? *J Am Acad Child Adol Psychiatry* 32:1106, 1993.

treatment program could be based on breaking a hypothesized casual chain at some point. In the example provided in Table 119.1, the prevention program for antisocial behavior could aim to break the causal chain at any of the points a through e. If an intervention program that reduced the incidence of school failure (point b) resulted in a reduction in the incidence of antisocial behavior, then this would provide strong evidence that school failure is a causal factor in the production of antisocial behavior. Such intervention studies have been termed experimental epidemiology (Robins, 1978) and are seen as the next phase of investigation in child psychiatric epidemiology (Earls, 1989).

The contents of this chapter have been selected so as not to duplicate information presented in other chapters. Thus, since the epidemiology of individual disorders is covered in the chapters focusing on these disorders, it is not reviewed in detail here. Rather, the chapter presents data on the epidemiology of one or more psychiatric disorders and uses data from individual disorders to illustrate findings in the field. It then identifies and discusses issues relevant to the epidemiology of virtually all the individual conditions. Data on four disorders—conduct disorder, hyperactivity, anxiety disorder, and affective disorder—are used to illustrate these topics. The chapter ends with a discussion of the implications of the findings in child psychiatric epidemiology for clinicians and policy makers and suggestions for future directions of the field.

ONE OR MORE PSYCHIATRIC DISORDERS

Prevalence

Prevalence rates of one or more psychiatric disorders in nonclinical samples of children and adolescents have been reviewed (Brandenburg et al., 1990; Costello, 1989). When DSM-III criteria (American Psychiatric Association, 1980) were employed, the prevalence rates in five community samples varied between 17.6% and 22% (Costello, 1989). The age ranges of the children and adolescents included in these studies also varied, with two studies including children as young as 4 years (Bird et al., 1989; Offord, Boyle, Szatmari, et al., 1987) and one including adolescents as old as 20 years (Velez et al., 1989). Another community study (Kashani et al., 1989) revealed rates of one or more disorders of between 31.4% and 41.4% for cohorts of boys and girls considered separately at ages 8, 12, and 17. Sources of the variability of the prevalence rates in these surveys include the characteristics of the target sample, the sampling method, number and types of disorders included, case definition, and assessment procedures. Case definition is particularly important; when it includes lax measures of severity or impairment, the prevalence rates can be high, (e.g., 26%) (Verhulst et al., 1985), and conversely, when the definition of disorder includes impaired functioning (Rutter and Graham, 1968) plus the need for treatment, the prevalence rate can drop dramatically, to as low as 5% (Vikan, 1985). The clinical consequences for children who meet diagnostic criteria for psychiatric disorder but who have minimal functional impairment is unknown (Weissman et al., 1990). Despite variations in the prevalence rates, it has been estimated that at the very least, 12% of children and adolescents have clinically important mental disorders, and at least half of them are deemed severely disordered or handicapped by their mental illness (Institute of Medicine, 1989).

Selected Correlates

INDIVIDUAL CHARACTERISTICS

Age and Sex

In community surveys, the prevalence of one or more disorders tends to be less in the younger (preadolescent) age group than in the older (adolescent) age group, and overall to be less common in boys than girls. In the Ontario Child Health Study (OCHS), a community prevalence survey of psychiatric disorders in children 4–16 years of age in the province, the prevalence of one or more disorders was significantly related to both age and sex (Offord, Boyle, Szatmari, et al., 1987). For children 4–11 years old, prevalence was higher among boys (19.5%) than girls (13.5%), while the reverse was true among children 12–16 years old (18.8% for boys versus 21.8% for girls). A recent report (Cohen et al., 1993) presents rates of individual disorders by sex for the age 10–20 range.

Racial and Ethnic Minorities

There is evidence from several community studies that the rate of emotional and behavioral problems varies by race or ethnic minority. For instance, a recent survey of high school students in New Mexico (924 Anglo and 1354 Mexican-American students) found that depressive symptoms were reported at a significantly higher rate in Mexican-Americans than Anglo students (Roberts and Chen, 1995). Further, in a total population survey of 10-year-old children in an inner London borough, children from West Indian immigrant families were compared with children from nonimmigrant families (Rutter et al., 1974). Teacher questionnaires were completed on all children, and interviews were conducted with a representative subsample. The methods and instruments used had been employed previously in the Isle of Wight study (Rutter, Tizard, and Whitemore, 1970). A major finding was that teachers reported, both on questionnaires and interviews, more behavioral problems in children from West Indian families. The higher rate did not apply to emotional or "internalizing" symptoms but did apply to antisocial symptoms of various kinds, and to both restlessness and poor concentration. Further, the behavioral differences between the two groups did not extend to parental reports but was restricted to teacher reports. An additional finding was that West Indian girls, compared to their nonimmigrant counterparts, showed a particularly marked increase in behavioral deviance based on teacher reports. For instance, on the teacher questionnaire, the percentage of West Indian Immigrant girls with "conduct" problems was 25.8; the corresponding percentage in nonimmigrant girls was 5.1. For boys, the percentages of conduct problems in West Indian and nonimmigrants were 40.1 and 14.1, respectively. A major factor involved in the etiology of the higher rate of behavioral problems in the school setting among children of West Indian families appeared to be the increased rate of educational retardation in this group (Yule et al., 1975). In addition, there was evidence that psychiatric disturbance in West Indian children was associated with many of the same variables, such as family disruption and dysfunction, that place children in nonimmigrant families at risk for psychiatric disorder.

Data from other studies in Great Britain make it clear that not all groups of nonwhite children have increased rates of mental disorders. For instance, children of Asian origin appear to have comparable rates or slightly reduced frequencies of psychiatric disorder compared to white children (Cochrane, 1979; Kallarackal and Herbert, 1976). Similarly, a recent study in the United States of 181 Chinese American children, ages 5–17, attending a Chinese school in New York City revealed that total problem, internalizing, and externalizing scores were significantly lower than Achenbach's American norms by age and sex (Chang et al., 1995). Within this population, recent immigrants did not have higher symptom scores. Among the individual scales, the Aggressive Behaviour scale scores were particularly depressed compared to American norms. The authors note that this may indicate that acting-out behavior is not tolerated by the Chinese families which emphasize self-control, respect, and obedience to authority. Major limitations of the work include the selection of only one school for inclusion in the study, and the low rate of response to the study (38%).

North American Indian children, compared to non-Indian children, have been reported to have higher rates of emotional and behavioral disturbance (Beiser, 1981; Beiser and Attneave, 1982; Green et al., 1981;

Yates, 1987). A recent study of Canadian Native children on two reserves in Southwestern Ontario indicates that adolescent girls are a particularly at-risk group with a prevalence rate of one or more disorders of 28.6% (Offord, Cadman, et al., 1990).

Three points should be noted about the finding of increased prevalence rates. First, the rates of emotional and behavioral problems in the Native children vary dramatically among tribes and among regions (Yates, 1987). Second, there is evidence that the rate of psychiatric disturbance among Indian children approximates that of majority culture children until about the age of 10, when it escalates disproportionately (Beiser and Attneave, 1982; Yates, 1987). This in turn may be related to the progressive increase in school difficulties of Indian children from the 3rd grade onward (Jensen et al., 1977; Saslow and Harrover, 1968; Yates, 1987). Lastly, in addition to their pattern of school difficulties, the circumstances of severe psychosocial disadvantage in which many of these children are raised also contribute to their increased rate of psychiatric disorder (Statistics Canada, 1984; US Department of Commerce, Census Bureau, 1973).

In the United States, work has been done on black-white differences in the rates of emotional and behavioral problems. For instance, there is evidence that blacks have higher rates than whites on self-report data of behavioral problems, especially for serious offenses involving violence against persons (Rutter and Giller, 1983). In addition, three studies have reported higher rates of depressive symptoms/syndromes in black as compared to white adolescents (Emslie et al., 1987; Garrison et al., 1985, 1989; Schoenbach et al., 1982), but no such differences exist in overall levels of anxiety or overanxious disorder (Bernstein et al., 1989; Costello et al., 1988; Velez et al., 1989).

Recently, Shaffer and colleagues (1994) examined adolescent suicide rates from 1986 to 1991 in the United States and drew from them three major conclusions: (*a*) the rate among females of all ethnic groups is stable and is much lower than the rate among males; (*b*) the rate among white male adolescents has stabilized in the past few years just below the peak rate in 1988; and (*c*) the rate in black and other minority males, previously both lower and more stable than that of white American males, has increased at a faster rate than the rate among whites. A number of hypotheses are offered for this increase in suicides among black adolescents including the possibility of ''imitation or identification'' with the predominant white culture as ''deculturation'' takes place in various parts of the United States.

In summary, the data show that the rates of child psychiatric disorder can vary by race and ethnic minority. The presence and pattern of variation is not constant across subgroups or across individual disorders. Difficulty performing satisfactorily in school and growing up in conditions of family adversity appear to be two major factors that place children in certain racial and ethnic groups at increased risk for emotional and behavioral problems (Offord, 1990).

Chronic Health Problems

A consistent finding in general population surveys of children is the increased rate of mental health and adjustment problems in children with chronic health problems, as compared to their healthy peers (Breslau, 1985; Pless, 1984; Satterwhite, 1978). Data from the OCHS show that the elevated rate of psychiatric disorder in children with chronic health problems applies to disorder in general and not a specific type of disorder (Cadman et al., 1987). Further, children with chronic medical conditions and associated disability—that is, limitations of usual childhood activities—were at a greater than three-fold risk for psychiatric disorders and at considerable risk for social adjustment problems (Cadman et al., 1987). Children with chronic medical conditions but no disability were at considerably less risk: About a two-fold increase in psychiatric disorders but little increased risk for social adjustment problems was observed. Knowledge about the causal mechanisms involved in producing the association between chronic health problems and psychiatric and social morbidity is incomplete. Possible etiological variables include low self-esteem, poor peer relationships, and poor school performance (Cadman et al., 1987).

This field of study has shown shifts at both the conceptual and research levels. For example, at the conceptual level, models aimed at understanding the impact of chronic disease have centered not only on children but also have included their families. In addition, they have begun to take into account the strengths of children and their families, in terms of coping and competence in dealing with chronic disease in the child (Eiser, 1990). This enlarged focus is justified by the uniform finding that most children with chronic medical illness are free of clinically important emotional and behavioral problems (Cadman et al., 1987; Perrin et al., 1987). Much research is now being carried out on single disease groups: for example, asthma (Perrin et al., 1989), cancer (Wasserman et al., 1987), and juvenile rheumatoid arthritis (Billings et al., 1987). There is no convincing evidence, however, that a certain type of disease is associated with a particular pattern of emotional and behavioral problems. However, there is universal agreement that diseases affecting cerebral functioning directly result in the highest prevalence rates of emotional and behavioral problems (Rutter, Tizard, and Whitmore, 1970) and within that group the highest susceptibility appears to be in cases of epilepsy (Hoare and Kerley, 1991).

Brain Disorder

Children with brain disorder are at increased risk for psychiatric disorder. In the Isle of Wight study, for example, the rate of psychiatric disorder was increased five times in youngsters with cerebral palsy, epilepsy, or some other disorder above the brainstem (Rutter, 1977). Further, different brain disorders resulted in different prevalence rates of psychiatric disorder (Rutter, Tizard, and Whitmore, 1970). For example, the rates of psychiatric disorder in children with uncomplicated epilepsy only, structural brain damage only, and both were 29%, 44%, and 58%, respectively. Several studies indicate that brain damage puts children at risk for psychiatric disorder in general rather than a specific type of disturbance (Brown et al., 1981; Rutter, 1977; 1981c). However, it should be noted that in the Isle of Wight study, hyperactivity was especially overrepresented in children with cerebral palsy and epilepsy (Rutter, Tizard, and Whitmore, 1970). In addition, there is preliminary evidence that unilateral damage to the dominant hemisphere (most often the left) results in more externalizing than internalizing symptoms, while damage to the other hemisphere results in the opposite pattern (Sollee and Kindlon, 1987).

The causal processes involved in producing increased rates of psychiatric disorder in brain-disordered children are not well understood. While there is some evidence that brain dysfunction may have a direct effect in producing psychiatric disorders (Breslau, 1990), the majority of the evidence indicates that the brain disorder is a vulnerability factor which operates through different mediating factors to produce the increased rates of psychiatric disorder. Potential mediating variables include psychosocial disadvantage (Brown et al., 1981; Shaffer et al., 1975); intellectual and cognitive disability, leading to poor school performance (Brown et al., 1981; Chadwick et al., 1981; Rutter, Tizard, and Whitemore, 1970; Shaffer et al., 1980); abnormal temperament (Offord and Waters, 1983; Ucko, 1965); and use of anticonvulsant drugs (Dodrill, 1975; Stores and Hart, 1976; Wolf and Forsythe, 1978). The relative strengths of the independent effects of these variables in accounting for the relationship between brain damage and psychiatric disorder is unknown, as is the presence of any significant interactions among them. An interesting prospective study found a relationship between certain soft neurological signs (those involving impairment in motor coordination) at age 7 and psychiatric disturbance at age 17, particularly affective and anxiety disorders in boys and anxiety disorders in girls (Shaffer et al., 1985). Again, the mechanisms underlying this association are unknown.

Temperament

It has become increasingly clear that individual children differ from one another in certain behavioral patterns such as activity level, behavioral inhibitions, and sociability (Rutter, 1987b). Not only can these behavioral patterns be measured with reasonable reliability, but they also predict emotional and behavioral disorders in both normal and high-risk samples. For instance, it has been shown that among community 2-year-olds, the temperamental characteristics of poor adaptability and high intensity of emotional expression more powerfully predicted behavior problems at age 3 than did indicators of interpersonal and material home environment (Earls and Jung, 1987). Similarly, it has been found that among a general population sample of children at age 7, those who were judged to be temperamentally difficult, compared to those with an easy temperament, had more psychiatric disorders at age 12 (Maziade et al., 1985). Further, a recent study used 164 children and their parents who participated as control subjects in the longitudinal Colorado Adoption Project to assess the longitudinal associations between temperament traits (emotionality-activity-sociability) assessed in infancy and early childhood, and specific behavioral syndromes in middle childhood (Rende, 1993). For boys, high emotionality in infancy and early childhood was associated with high scores on both the anxiety/depression and attention problem scales. For girls, both high emotionality and low sociability predicted high scores on the anxiety/depression scale. Finally, Hirshfield and colleagues (Hirshfield et al., 1992) examined children from the longitudinal study of Kagan and his group and found that children who were identified as behaviorally inhibited at 21 months of age and who remained inhibited at 4, $5\frac{1}{2}$ and $7\frac{1}{2}$ years had higher rates of anxiety disorders than children who were not consistently inhibited at those ages. It is evident from many studies that the cluster of behaviors that has been described as the ''difficult temperament'' has been shown to be positively associated with concurrent and future behavioral adjustment in children of varying ages, and social and ethnic groups (Prior, 1992). With respect to mechanisms, it is clear that children's temperamental characteristics affect the ways in which other people in and outside the family respond to them (Rutter, 1987b). In families with a mentally ill parent, for instance, children with a difficult temperament were more than twice as likely as children with an easy temperament to be the target of parental anger and criticism (Rutter and Quinton, 1984). Further, data indicate that the harmful effects of a difficult temperament on the adjustment of children are increased significantly if they live in dysfunctional families. Conversely, superior-functioning families reduce the risk associated with difficult temperament in terms, for instance, of a reduced rate of clinician-diagnosed psychiatric disorder (Maziade et al., 1985).

Many methodological issues remain to be sorted out in the study of temperament; four major ones are outlined below. First, there is a lack of agreement about the definition of temperament (Prior, 1992). For example, some investigators (e.g., Plomin, 1993; Plomin and Dunn, 1986) argue that the definition should be restricted to a limited number of constitutionally-determined, biologically-based characteristics with demonstrated heritability. However, others (e.g., Hinde in Goldsmith et al., 1989) argue that heritability should not form part of the definition of temperament. Second, instruments purporting to measure temperament must seek to operationalize the concept so it is separate from the measurement of psychopathology. Second, instruments measuring temperament must not only cover the negative aspects of the concept but also the positive ones as well. Third and last, the measurement of temperament cannot rely solely on parent reports. Parent-generated ratings of temperament appear to be less connected with the child's free play or peer-play behavior than they are to observed parent-child interactions (Dunn and Kendrick, 1980; Plomin, 1976; Plomin and Rowe, 1977). Comprehensive, critical reviews of the concept of temperament and its clinical applications are available (Garrison and Earls, 1987, Prior, 1992).

IQ, Learning Disorders, and Educational Retardation

Children who do poorly in school, whether because of low IQ or a specific learning disorder, are at increased risk for psychiatric disorders.

The increased risk applies to a wide range of conditions, including conduct disorder (Offord and Waters, 1983; Rutter, Tizard, and Whitemore, 1970), delinquency (West and Farrington, 1973), hyperactivity (Frick et al., 1991; Hinshaw, 1992; Hoy, et al., 1978; Minde et al.,1971), depressive symptoms in adolescents (Emslie et al., 1987; Fleming et al., 1989; Friedrich et al., 1988; Garrison et al., 1985; Hoberman et al., 1986; Reynolds and Coats, 1982; Teri, 1982), child reported anxiety disorders (Costello et al., 1988), over-anxious disorder but not separation anxiety disorder (Velez et al., 1989), and self-reported anxiety symptoms in 11-year-old girls (Williams et al., 1989). Poor school functioning, based on school reports of achievement test results and repeating a grade, was not associated with the presence of a depressive syndrome in preadolescents in the general population (Anderson et al., 1987; Costello et al., 1988; Kashani et al., 1983). On the other hand, 64% of students aged 6–15 attending a private school for learning-disabled children were found to have a depressive diagnosis (Weinberg et al., 1989); additionally, 36% of students aged 8–11 years with learning disabilities scored in the depressed range of a self-report depressive inventory (Wright-Strawderman and Watson, 1992). Finally, 10 out of 30 (33%) inpatient children aged 6–12 years with major depressive disorder had learning disabilities compared to the community base rate of 4.7% (Fristad et al., 1992). This finding is difficult to interpret due to the presence in over half of these children of comorbid diagnoses of conduct, oppositional defiant, and attention-deficit hyperactivity disorder.

The mechanisms by which poor school performance leads to increased rates of psychiatric disorder have been investigated most fully in the case of externalizing disorders, especially conduct disorder. There are four major hypotheses concerning the relationship between underachievement and externalizing behavior (Hinshaw, 1992): (a) externalizing behavior leads to underachievement; (b) underachievement leads to externalizing behavior; (c) each domain leads to the other; and (d) underlying variables (e.g., abnormal temperament [Offord and Waters, 1983; Rutter and Giller, 1983], cognitive deficits [Schonfeld et al., 1988]) are the actual cause in both domains. Not one of these four hypotheses can be discarded at this time, (Hinshaw, 1992) and additional research is needed to understand more thoroughly the causal processes involved in mediating the relationship between poor school performance and child psychiatric disorder.

PSYCHOSOCIAL FACTORS

Parental Psychopathology

Parental psychiatric disorder or deviance is associated with increased rates of emotional or behavioral problems in the offspring. This relationship can be investigated by collecting the initial sample at either the child or the parental level. For instance, there is evidence that children with various psychiatric disorders have parents with increased rates of psychiatric disability. Antisocial children or delinquents compared to their age-matched controls have parents with higher rates of severe psychiatric impairment, especially antisocial personality disorder and criminality (Farrington and West, 1981; Glueck and Glueck, 1950; Lewis and Balla, 1976; Offord, 1982). In addition, it has been reported that the parents of hyperactive children have increased rates of alcoholism, hysteria, antisocial personality, and hyperactivity (Gorenstein and Newman, 1980).

If the sample is drawn at the parental level, it is clear that parents with a variety of psychiatric disorders have offspring with increased rates of psychopathology (Rutter and Quinton, 1984). In a controlled family study, the frequency of psychiatric disorder in children of alcoholic parents was found to be higher than in children of nonalcoholic parents (Earls et al., 1988). The elevated rates of psychopathology applied to overall disorder and to behavioral disorders in particular, including conduct disorder, attention deficit disorder, and oppositional disorder. The rate of disorder in children of two alcoholic parents was higher than in those of one alcoholic parent. When children of antisocial parents (who usually also had alcoholism) were compared with children whose parents had alcoholism only, no significant differences in the rates of childhood disorder were found between the two groups.

Most studies of the offspring of depressed parents have been carried out in clinical samples of adults, and thus the results cannot be generalized to the community at large. Weissman and her colleagues (1987) found that the offspring, aged 6–23, of depressed parents had significantly higher rates of major depression, substance abuse, mean number of psychiatric diagnoses, psychiatric treatment, poor social functioning, and school problems, compared to the offspring of normal parents. Also, children of parents whose own depression had an early onset (before age 20) had the earliest mean age of onset of depression, suggesting the possibility that prepubertal-onset depression has the highest genetic loading (Weissman et al., 1988). Another study (Merikangas et al., 1988) found maternal alcoholism to be the strongest predictor of major depression in offspring. Also, parental concordance for diagnoses, especially for anxiety disorders, was found to increase significantly the risk of major depression in the children. Two other published studies were not restricted to clinical samples of depressed parents. One (Forehand and McCombs, 1988) recruited volunteers from the community, while the other (Beardslee et al., 1988) included families in a health maintenance organization (HMO). The first found that maternal depressive symptoms predicted self-reported adolescent depressive symptoms 1 year later, while the second study found that children of affectively disordered parents were at increased risk for depressive disorders.

Finally, there is evidence from clinic-based studies that parental psychiatric disorder, in particular affective and anxiety disorders, puts children at risk for developing anxiety disorders. The offspring of parents with panic disorder (PD) had more than a three-fold increased risk of separation anxiety disorder (SAD). Parents with PD and a major depression conferred a 10-fold increase in risk for their children. In these families over one-third of the offspring suffered from SAD (Leckman et al., 1985; Weissman et al., 1984). Finally, Turner and colleagues (1987) found that children of parents with agoraphobia or obsessive-compulsive disorder had significantly more child-reported DSM-III disorders, mostly anxiety disorders, than did children of normal parents. Children of parents with dysthymic disorder had fewer DSM-III disorders (all were anxiety disorders) than the children of anxious parents, but this difference was not statistically significant. In general, children of anxious parents were more impaired than children of depressed parents.

In summary, it is evident that parental mental disorder is associated with increased rates of child psychopathology in general. In addition, there is emerging evidence that specific parental psychiatric disorders are associated with increased rates of particular childhood disorders. For instance, parental alcoholism and antisocial behavior disorder are associated with increased rates of behavior disturbances in the offspring, parental depression with increased rates of depressive symptoms and disorder (especially in the adolescent age group), and parental anxiety disorders with increased rates of anxiety disorders, particularly SAD.

The mechanisms involved in the transmission of psychopathology from one generation to the next are not clear. Candidates include poor parenting practices resulting in harmful sequelae, such as poor supervision of the children and parental criticism and hostility; modeling by the child of deviant parental behavior; family dysfunction and marital discord; family disruption where the child is placed outside the home for a period of time; and genetic factors. The strength of the independent effects of these variables and their modes of interaction in producing childhood psychiatric disturbance in families with parental psychopathology are far from being completely understood (Offord and Waters, 1983; Rutter, 1989c; Rutter and Quinton, 1984).

Family Factors

Poor parenting, marital discord, and family dysfunction have all been associated with an increased rate of psychiatric disorder in children. For example, harsh and inconsistent parenting (Farrington and West, 1981), coercive interchanges between parent and child (Patterson, 1982), and marital discord (Earls and Jung, 1987; Emery and O'Leary, 1982; Rutter, 1981b) are all associated with antisocial behavior in children. The relationship between marital discord and behavior disorders is especially strong in boys. In the case of hyperactivity, family dysfunction has been found to be an independent predictor of disorder, but the relationship disappears when the co-occurrence of other disorders is taken into account (Szatmari et al., 1989). Depressive symptoms in adolescents have an increased prevalence in dysfunctional families (Friedrich et al., 1988; Garrison et al., 1985; Marton and Maharaj, 1992; Reynolds and Rob, 1988). Finally, child-identified but not parent-identified anxiety disorders have been reported to be significantly associated with family difficulties (Costello et al., 1988). The mediating processes involved in explaining the relationship between poor parenting, marital discord, and family dysfunction, on the one hand, and child psychiatric disorder, on the other, are probably similar to those hypothesized as accounting for the relationship between parental deviance and child psychiatric disorder (Offord and Waters, 1983; Rutter, 1989c; Rutter and Giller, 1983; Rutter and Quinton, 1984).

Finally, large family size (usually four or more children) has been associated with increased rates of conduct disorder and delinquency in boys (Farrington and West, 1981; Rutter, Tizard, and Whitemore, 1970) but not in girls (Jones et al., 1980). The results of the West and Farrington (1981) study of inner city boys indicate that large family size is related to antisocial behavior and delinquency, independent of sociodemographic and parental factors.

The causal processes underlying this association are not clear but indicate at least four possibilities. First, in a large family, maternal and parenting resources, especially among families already experiencing a good deal of family adversity, are stretched to the point that the parenting functions are seriously compromised. This hypothesis is supported by the finding that the relationship between large family size and delinquency is most marked in economically disadvantaged and disorganized families (Wadsworth, 1979; West and Farrington, 1973). A second possibility is that in large families there is a contagion effect where the presence of antisocial behavior in one child spreads to other members of the sibship (Robins et al., 1975). Third, it may be that there can be a potentiation of antisocial behavior among boys, especially in the absence of a female presence (Jones et al., 1980). It has been reported, for example, that the level of antisocial behavior among boys in a family was associated with the number of brothers in the family but not with the number of sisters (Jones et al., 1980). Indeed, when the number of brothers in the sibship was held constant, an increasing number of sisters was associated with a lower level of antisocial behavior among the brothers. The sisters appeared to suppress antisocial behavior among their brothers. A fourth possibility is that the relationship between large family size and antisocial behavior is accounted for by other, confounding variables, such as educational retardation and perhaps marital discord (Rutter and Giller, 1983). The evidence is firm that educational retardation is a risk factor for conduct disorder and delinquency and is associated with large family size. No information is available to allow a ranking in order of importance of these proposed mediating factors.

Social Class

The strength of the relationship between social class and child psychiatric disorder is dependent on both the measurement of social class and the measurement of psychiatric disorder. If occupational prestige (based on data obtained from the public on the social standing or prestige ranking of occupations [e.g., Siegel, 1971]) is used to operationalize social class, then there is a weak or nonexistent relationship between it and child psychiatric disorder. This finding holds for psychiatric disorder in general in preschool children (Earls, 1980; Richman et al., 1975) and school-age children (Achenbach and Edelbrock, 1981; Lapouse and Monk, 1964; Rutter, Tizard, and Whitemore, 1970) and for specific disorders such as hyperactivity (Boscoe and Robin, 1980), autism (Cox et al., 1975; Wing, 1980), and delinquency (Hindelang et al., 1981; Thornberry and Farnworth, 1982; Williams and Gold, 1972). In contrast, when social class is measured in terms of economic disadvantage, then there is a strong and consistent relationship between it and child psychiatric disorder (Anderson et al., 1989; Offord, 1990; Offord, Boyle, Jones, 1987; Offord, Boyle, et al., 1990; Raadal et al., 1994). For instance, in the OCHS, the rates of one or more psychiatric disorders in children, aged 4–16 whose parents were or were not on social assistance were 31.2% and 13.8%, respectively. Further, the relationship between economic disadvantage and child psychiatric disorder appears stronger in younger children than in adolescents (Lipman et al., 1994; Rutter, 1981a).

As far as the measurement of psychiatric disorder is concerned, the data indicate that the relationship between economic disadvantage and psychiatric disorder is stronger when disorders such as conduct disorder and hyperactivity are identified by teachers rather than by parents (Offord, Boyle, and Racine, 1989). The importance of informant or source in the identification of psychiatric disorders is addressed later in the chapter.

Finally, what are the mechanisms that put children living in economically disadvantaged families at increased risk for psychiatric disorder? Most of the evidence supports the contention that the relationship is mediated by parental and family characteristics, or attributes of the children associated with economic disadvantage, rather than economic disadvantage itself (Robins, 1979; Rutter and Giller, 1983). For example, economically disadvantaged families have higher rates of variables associated with child psychiatric disorder, such as low maternal education, marital discord, family dysfunction, and low intelligence in the children (Lipman et al., 1994; Robins, 1979; Rutter and Giller, 1983; West and Farrington, 1973).

Urban-Rural Residence

A number of studies have reported increased rates of child psychiatric disorder in urban as compared to rural settings (Lavik 1977; Offord, Boyle, and Szatmari, et al., 1987; Rutter, Cox, et al., 1975). These elevated rates are especially marked in preadolescents rather than adolescents (Rutter, Cox, et al., 1975) and apply particularly to chronic disorders of early onset (Rutter, 1981a), behavior disorders among boys (Lavik, 1977), and hyperactivity among boys and girls (Offord, Boyle, Szatmari, et al., 1987). Other conditions, including delinquency (Rutter and Giller, 1983), self-reports of antisocial behavior (Christie et al., 1965; Clark and Wenninger, 1962; Gold and Reimer, 1975), specific reading retardation and reading backwardness (Berger et al., 1975), and marijuana use (Boyle and Offord, 1986), have also been reported to be more common in children and adolescents in urban settings. However, it should be noted that not all types of psychiatric conditions in childhood or adolescence show increased rates in urban settings. For instance, the prevalence of parent-reported behavioral deviance in 6-year-olds in Denmark was not significantly different in an urban as compared to a rural setting (Kastrup, 1977). Similarly, in the OCHS, although elevated rates of marijuana use were associated with urban residence, (population >25,000) in 12- to 16-year-olds, other types of substance use in this adolescent population, such as occasional and regular use of tobacco, regular use of alcohol, and use of hard drugs, tended to be highest in small urban areas (population 3,000–25,000), and occasional use of alcohol and inhalants was highest in rural areas (population <3,000).

In a recent study of parent and teacher symptom reports from two epidemiological surveys of 2519 Connecticut children, certain rural-urban differences in childhood psychopathology were found (Zahner et al., 1993). Urban-rural variations reported by both parents and teachers included: among urban girls, higher rates of total disturbance and social withdrawal; among urban boys, trends indicating higher rates of emotional disturbance. In addition, the parent data indicated higher rates of all forms of behavioral disturbance for urban girls, and of schizoid anxiety for urban boys. Further, based on teacher reports, there was a trend

for higher rates of hyperactivity (inattention) among urban boys. The validity of the study results are weakened somewhat by the low response rate to the surveys. In the urban sample, the response rate for parental reports was 56%, and for teacher reports, 78% (of 56%). In the rural sample, the response rates were 71% and 78% (of 71%), respectively. There was no discussion of the possibility of selective loss biasing the findings, and perhaps not in the same ways, in the two samples.

Work has been done in understanding the mechanisms by which the urban environment is associated with increased rates of child psychiatric disorder. Mediating variables include parental and family variables, such as marital discord and parental deviance, disadvantaged social circumstances (e.g., large sibship size and overcrowding), and schools with undesirable characteristics such as high teacher turnover (Rutter, Yule, et al., 1975). In fact, in a comparison of the rates of child psychiatric disorder in the Isle of Wight (a predominantly rural setting) and an inner London borough (an inner city area), it was found that the two-fold increase in the prevalence of psychiatric disorder in the urban setting was accounted for entirely by the increased rates of psychosocial adversity and disadvantaged schools in the inner city area (Rutter and Quinton, 1977). Similarly, in the Connecticut study, when differences in culture, economy, and mobility were controlled, only two positive associations remained, both for girls: social withdrawal (reported by parents) and inattention (reported by teachers) (Zahner et al., 1993). Other characteristics of the urban environment, such as the physical design and layout of large housing complexes, which make it difficult to supervise children adequately, and the lack of social support for parents in this setting, may also contribute to the elevated rates of child psychiatric disturbance (Quinton, 1988).

Finally, the question of why parental and family pathology cluster in urban settings has not been completely answered. One possibility is that there is a migration into urban settings of disadvantaged families, and a migration out of the more advantaged families. This has clearly taken place in some urban areas in the United States (Wilson, 1987), but this selective migration did not account for the differences in the rates of psychiatric disorder in the Isle of Wight and in the inner London borough (Rutter, Cox, et al., 1975). Finally, it should be emphasized that the urban environment per se does not have to be invariably associated with increased rates of childhood psychopathology. It should be kept in mind that urban environments differ widely in the rates of maladjustment among their resident children.

PROTECTIVE FACTORS

Protective factors are defined as "those factors that modify, ameliorate or alter a person's response to some environmental hazard that predisposes to a maladaptive outcome" (Rutter, 1985). These factors are products of the interactions of the attributes of the child and the environment. They should not be seen primarily as existing in a cross-sectional snapshot, but they should be understood as processes having their effects perhaps in different ways at different points in the development of children and youth. Garmezy (1987) suggested that these variables can be classified into three broad categories: factors in the child, in the family, and in the wider community. Candidates for protective factors have been identified in each of these areas (Beardslee and Podorefsky, 1988; Fonagy et al., 1994; Offord, 1989, Rae-Grant, Thomas, et al., 1989; Rubenstein et al., 1989; Rutter, 1987a; Rutter and Giller, 1983). Female gender before adolescence, male gender after that, above-average IQ, easy temperament, and considerable self-understanding are examples of within-the-child factors. Family protective factors include a high degree of cohesiveness within the family and a good relationship with one parent. Examples of reported protective factors in the wider community are compensating good experiences outside the home, such as excellent schools and skill-development and recreational programs.

The important issues in this area are, first, the extent to which the concept of a protective factor is more than just the opposite of a risk factor and, second, the mediating mechanisms by which the protective factors have their effect. With respect to the first, Rutter (1987a) argues that it is helpful to conceptualize a protective factor as separate from the converse of a risk factor when the mechanism of action of the protective end of the variable is different from that of the risk end, or when the main effect is derived primarily from the positive end of the variable. For instance, with regard to the former, it has been reported that while shyness may protect against delinquency, an outgoing personality does not predispose toward delinquency (Farrington et al., 1988). With respect to the latter, in the study of institutionally-reared women, the presence of a supportive harmonious marital relationship had a marked protective effect on the quality of parenting, but a poor marital relationship was not as strongly related to poor parenting (Quinton et al., 1984). It could also be argued that these two criteria for the conceptualization of a protective factor can be subsumed under the concept of a single factor, with risk at one end and protective at the other, where the relationship with disorder can be linear or nonlinear. In the latter case, there could be evidence of a threshold effect where the strength of relationship between the factor and disorder changes abruptly at some point along the continuum of measurement of the variable. Finally, mediating mechanisms for protective factors include reducing the impact of risk factors on the individual, lessening a chain of negative events, and increasing the self-esteem and self-efficacy of the individual (Rutter, 1987a).

ISSUES

This portion of the chapter briefly discusses selected issues in child psychiatric epidemiology. Data on conduct disorder, hyperactivity, anxiety disorder, and affective disorder are used to illustrate the topics covered.

Measurement of Disorder

BOUNDARY BETWEEN NORMAL AND ABNORMAL

Many of the disorders in child psychiatry are based on data that appear to have strong dimensional characteristics; much conflict has arisen both inside and outside psychiatry about the meaningfulness of using a categorical systems to represent psychiatric disorder (Jensen et al; 1993; Meehl, 1992; Pichot, 1994). For instance, in the case of conduct disorder, most children have at least a few antisocial symptoms, and relatively few have a large number. When a count of symptoms from a larger pool is used to identify disorder, a central issue is where does one set the threshold that separates children into two categories, disordered (those above the threshold), and not disordered (those below the threshold). Changing the threshold slightly by requiring fewer or more symptoms can have a noticeable effect on prevalence of disorder when the variability among symptom counts is low (Robins, 1985). In this case, the symptom counts of many children are grouped closely around a threshold. Further, even small changes to defining the boundary between normal and abnormal can have a profound impact not only on prevalence but on patterns of comorbidity and associated features (Boyle et al., 1995).

Thresholds can be affected by altering the pool of symptoms used to measure a disorder, by changing the number or severity requirement of symptoms, or by modifying the needed criteria for associated impairments. For example, the decision in DSM-III-R (American Psychiatric Association, 1987) to require three symptoms for a diagnosis of conduct disorder versus the one symptom required in DSM-III (American Psychiatric Association, 1980) served to decrease the prevalence of conduct disorder (Robins, 1991). Conduct disorder also probably had a later onset and was more restricted to males. Two of the symptoms dropped in DSM-III-R, rule violation and academic underachievement, had typically been found to be the earliest symptoms of the disorder. Further, the dropped symptoms of previous use of alcohol and drugs, academic underachievement, early sexual experience, and rule violations were, along with running away, the symptoms in which the frequencies in girls came closest to the frequencies in boys (Robins, 1991).

Further, in the OCHS, altering the severity of symptoms required for the diagnosis of a major depressive syndrome resulted in a range of prevalence rates from 0.6% to 1.8% for preadolescents and adolescents, respectively, under conditions of high symptom severity, to rates of 17.5% and 43.9%, respectively, under conditions of low severity (Fleming et al., 1989). The requirement of additional impairment criteria lowered the prevalence rate of one or more DSM-III diagnoses among a sample of adolescents from 41.3% to 18.7% (Kashani et al., 1987). Similarly, in a large community sample of children and adolescents, the rate of one or more disorders dropped from 49.5% to 17.9% when impairment was considered (Bird et al., 1988).

A major lack in the area of thresholds for disorder is evidence that the thresholds that are set result in a meaningful division of children into disordered and nondisordered groups. It would be hoped, for instance, that children above the threshold, and thus disordered, would show independent evidence of impairment in their everyday functioning. Although it is accepted that the presence of impairment is an essential feature of psychiatric disorder (American Psychiatric Association, 1987), there is little systematic evidence to indicate that thresholds for individual disorders result in the identification of cases with clinically important impairments. In addition, the meaningfulness of a threshold would be supported if data on the relationship between symptom scores and associated features of disorder, such as correlates or need for treatment, show a discontinuity at the point of the threshold; that is, the relationships abruptly increase in strength when the threshold level is exceeded (Boyle, 1991). A major implication of the inability to provide firm data on which to justify thresholds for disorder is that the meaningfulness of disorders identified in community surveys is in question, especially as it relates to need for service.

BOUNDARY BETWEEN DISORDERS

Rates of co-occurrence of child psychiatric disorders, far in excess of chance, have been reported repeatedly in epidemiological studies of children in the general population (e.g., Anderson et al., 1987; Bird et al., 1993; Costello et al., 1988; Fergusson et al., 1993; Offord, Boyle, Szatmari, et al., 1987; Velez et al., 1989). In the OCHS, for instance, over two-thirds (68.2%) of the children aged 6–16 with a diagnosis of at least one of the four psychiatric disorders had one or more additional diagnoses (Offord, Boyle, and Fleming, 1989). Further, in the Puerto Rico study, of children aged 4–16 having one or more DSM-III diagnoses, 46.1% fell into two or more diagnostic categories (Bird et al., 1988). In the New Zealand study of a community sample of 11-year-olds, 55% of the cases identified occurred in combination with one or more other disorders (Anderson et al., 1987). Comorbidity is especially high between the externalizing disorders (conduct disorder and hyperactivity) (Szatmari et al., 1989; Taylor, 1989) and between the internalizing disorders (anxiety disorder and depressive disorder) (Kovacs et al., 1984; Strauss et al., 1988). However, there is a significant degree of comorbidity across these two major domains: for example, between conduct disorder and depressive conditions and between hyperactivity and depressive conditions (Fleming and Offord, 1990; Puig-Antich, 1982).

The high degree of overlap among some child psychiatric disorders is one of the factors that has brought into question the extent to which certain of these conditions are separate entities. Another factor contributing to this debate is the lack of consistent findings indicating that the various disorders have unique patterns of associated features. For example, in the New Zealand cohort, the cognitive and social correlates discriminated between externalizing and internalizing disorders but not between individual diagnostic categories (Anderson et al., 1989). Clearly, when the focus is on categories of disorder within the externalizing and internalizing domains, the evidence for discrete diagnostic entities with unique correlate patterns is not strong, especially if comparisons are made among diagnostic groups rather than between a diagnostic group and normal subjects (Werry et al., 1987). The high degree of comorbidity and the lack of distinctive features of many of the disorders, outside of the symptom patterns that define them, has led to a widespread recognition that the categories of disorder in existing schema are overrefined given existing levels of knowledge (Achenbach and Edelbrock, 1983; Boyle, 1980; Werry, 1985).

There are a variety of factors that can contribute to high rates of comorbidity (Achenbach, 1990/1991; Angold and Costello, 1993; Caron and Rutter, 1991). These include detection artefacts, (e.g., Berkson, 1946), problems of classification (e.g., the use of the same or similar symptoms to define different categories of disorder), and a situation where one disorder represents an early manifestation of another and both are found to co-exist in cross-sectional studies (Caron and Rutter, 1991; Rutter, 1989a). In any case, a major need in the field is for studies that will determine the extent to which diagnostic categories can be said to be separable because of distinctive patterns of etiology, prognosis, and response to treatment.

DISAGREEMENT AMONG INFORMANTS

A uniform finding in the literature is the low agreement among informants about children's behaviors. This finding holds for both self-administered problem checklists (Achenbach et al., 1987) and lay-administered structured interviews (Boyle et al., 1993b; Edelbrock et al., 1986). In the OCHS, for example, the two respondents, whether parent and teacher for children aged 4–11 years or parent and youth for those aged 12–16, identified the same children as having a particular disorder in a small minority of cases (Offord, Boyle, and Fleming, 1989). The highest percentage agreement (15.5%) was between parents and teachers on the diagnosis of hyperactivity in boys aged 4–11. In the cases of conduct disorder in girls age 4–11 and hyperactivity in girls age 12–16, no children were identified as having the disorder by the two respondents. These findings are consistent with a meta-analysis of child/adolescent behavioral and emotional problem ratings provided by different informants (Achenbach et al., 1987).

A corollary of the lack of agreement between informants is that case ascertainment depends heavily on who provides information for assessment. Prevalence rates of disorder and the patterns of associated features can vary depending on who identifies the child as having a disorder (Offord, Boyle, Racine, et al., 1989, 1995). For instance, in the OCHS, the prevalence of parent-identified conduct disorder among boys age 4–11 is 1.4%, while the prevalence of teacher-identified conduct disorder in the same children is 4.9% (Offord, Boyle, and Racine, 1989). Similarly, the prevalence of parent-identified emotional disorder in adolescent girls is 40%; the frequency of emotional disorder identified by the girls themselves is 9.8%. Further, not only do the prevalence rates differ depending on informant, but there is evidence that the associated features do as well. For example, in the OCHS, low family income (<$10,000) has a strong independent relationship with teacher-identified hyperactivity but not with parent-identified hyperactivity. Similarly, while parental arrest has a significant independent relationship with parent-identified conduct disorder, no such relationship exists for teacher-identified conduct disorder (Offord, Boyle, and Racine, 1989). In addition, several researchers have noted that the predictive value of assessment data used to classify disorder can vary by respondent (Boyle et al., 1993a; Loeber et al., 1991). The extent to which ratings provided by different informants classify children in a valid and useful way as judged by the usual criteria of etiology, prognosis, and response to treatment is unknown.

These findings taken as a whole suggest that the identification of childhood disorder is much influenced by the perception of informants and the contexts in which assessments are done. The factors that influence respondent judgments about emotional and behavioral problems of children are poorly understood. For instance, children tend to report more depressive and anxiety symptoms and disorders than their parents report about them (Angold et al., 1987; Edelbrock et al., 1986; Herjanic and Reich, 1982; Ivens and Rehm, 1988, Kashani et al., 1985; Reich et al., 1982; Silverman and Nelles, 1988; Weissman et al., 1987). To explain this, it has been hypothesized that parents are less aware of or less bothered by their children's internal feelings of discomfort than by their overt behaviors and are less likely to report them (e.g., Edelbrock et al., 1986; Kashani et al., 1985). On the other hand, as summarized by Richters and Pellegrini (1989), depressed mothers have been accused of overreporting depressive and other symptoms in children. But this assumption of misperception of their children has recently been challenged, and in fact, some evidence suggests that depressed mothers are more accurate than nondepressed mothers in assessing their children's emotional states (Conrad and Hammen, 1989; Richters and Pellegrini, 1989). Clearly, more work is needed on understanding factors that play a part in determining respondents' reporting of children's behaviors.

The dilemma of how to deal, in terms of classification, with the fact that different informants identify different children as disordered has not been solved. Strategies include (a) combining information, that is, giving value to any positive rating, regardless of informant; (b) giving priority to different informants about different kinds of behavior—for example, assigning priority to the child's report of internal mood and to the parent's report of behavior problems; (c) assigning a confidence rating to each behavior proportionate to the amount of agreement among observers; and (d) considering disorders as informant specific and making no attempt to combine reports from different informants to provide an overall classification (Institute of Medicine, 1989). It is not known which of these approaches is the most useful and valid, and clearly more research is needed on this important issue.

INSTRUMENTATION

There are two major types of instruments used to measure child psychiatric disorders in community surveys: structured interviews and problem checklists. The former offer many advantages, including the opportunity to clarify wording, to probe responses, to record observations, and to lead respondents through complex question sequences (Boyle, 1989). The main disadvantage of a structured interview is the requirement for personal data collection, which can result in considerable research costs and will add to respondent burden. Problem checklists, on the other hand, are much more efficient tools for data collection. They can be self-administered, the completion time can be relatively short, and there is the opportunity to use mail-backs or other less expensive forms of data retrieval.

Recent reviews of structured interview schedules (Edelbrock and Costello, 1988; Gutterman et al., 1987; Hodges, 1993) make it evident that while a good deal of information is available on reliability and on discrepancies between parent and child reports, data are lacking on the usefulness or validity of the resulting diagnostic categories. Further, with few exceptions (e.g., Sylvester et al., 1987), samples to evaluate these instruments have been drawn from children using psychiatric services; the instruments have not as yet been adequately evaluated in samples taken from the general population (Boyle, 1989). Recent reviews also exist of problem checklists (Barkley, 1988; Boyle, 1989). There is only one study in the literature that directly compares the classification of child psychiatric disorders by checklist data versus information obtained from structured interviews (Gould et al., 1993). There was no evidence of the superiority of either method in identifying valid diagnostic categories.

Two major issues in this area are the uncertainty about what to use as the "gold standard" in evaluating the validity of instruments and the problem of assessing psychopathology in the young child (under age 10). The most widely accepted standard for evaluating the validity of the diagnostic categories identified by these instruments is the clinician work-up. The content of the work-up can vary. It can consist, for example, of an unstructured interview, or a structured interview where the clinician has the opportunity to probe various responses to determine their clinical importance. In any case, a prerequisite for the acceptability of the clinical work-up as a standard is that it must have suitable levels of reliability.

The assessment of psychopathology in the child under age 10 is important because many child psychiatric disorders are first manifested during this period. It is of obvious importance to gain the child's view of his or her perceptions, emotional reactions, and feelings, which almost certainly cannot be accurately described by external observers such as parents, teachers, and researchers (Harter, 1982). Unfortunately, existing data indicate that the use of interview techniques among children under age 11 produces data that are highly unreliable (Achenbach et al., 1987; Edelbrock et al., 1985). Direct observation is one alternative, but data on the reliability and short-term stability of this technique are lacking, and there is generally poor agreement between direct observation of child behavior and parental report (Mash and Terdal, 1981).

There is, however, one instrument, the Dominic questionnaire which shows considerable promise as a standardized assessment instrument for children as young as 6 years of age (Valla et al., 1994). It is a structured pictorial instrument which takes 15–20 minutes to administer. Ninety-nine drawings represent situations corresponding to seven DSM-III-R-based diagnoses. The test has acceptable test-retest reliability and its validity, while not ideal, is encouraging.

Such advances in instrumentation are necessary to obtain reliable and useful subjective information directly from younger children. It should be kept in mind, however, that gains in the development and usefulness of instrumentation are dependent on increased understanding of the nature and classification of child psychiatric disorders.

Measurement of Other Variables

The preceding section of the chapter has focused on measurement concerns about disorder. It should be noted that the problems surrounding the measurement of disorder also apply to the measurement of other variables, such as correlates and associated features. Reliable and valid measures of correlates (e.g., family dysfunction) (Byles et al., 1988) are just as important as psychometrically sound measures of disorder if the aim is to describe accurately the strength of the relationship between disorder and correlates. Similarly, a major need in the field is to have reliable and valid measures of impairment conceptualized as a variable independent of disorder. Although there has been some progress in this area (e.g., John et al., 1987), unresolved issues remain. One is converting measures of impairment into meaningful dichotomies where children above the threshold have a degree of impairment that is clinically important. A second problem is that the measurement of impairment, like the evaluation of disorder, is highly situation specific (Boyle, 1980). Thus there is a high level of agreement, within informant or source, between measures of disorder and impairment, but a low level of agreement across informants. What is needed are reliable and useful measures of impairment that are independent of the usual informants, such as parents, teachers, or the child himself or herself.

Lack of Prospective Studies

Although there are now a number of large community studies of child psychiatric disorder (Brandenburg et al., 1990; Costello, 1989), most of them are cross-sectional. While such studies can make important contributions, there are many important questions that can only be answered adequately by prospective studies. Data on the incidence and duration of disorder can be addressed adequately only by longitudinal studies. In addition, although there is a considerable body of knowledge on the correlates of disorder, considerably less is known about risk factors (Offord, 1989). A risk factor must have a causal independent relationship with disorder. It therefore must precede the disorder itself. Data on the identification and strength of risk factors require prospective studies. Longitudinal studies can also provide information on prognostic factors, that is, variables that predict the outcome of disorders.

The modes of interaction among risk and protective factors need to be understood if valid causal chains for disorder are to be constructed. This task can only be accomplished successfully if the interactions

among these variables are understood over time as part of longitudinal studies (Rutter, 1988, 1989b). The New York State study, the New Zealand study, and the Oregon Adolescent Depression Project are all longitudinal projects and have begun to contribute much-needed information about risk factors, course, and persistence of symptoms and disorder (Chapel et al., 1982; Cohen and Brook, 1987; Cohen et al., 1989; Lewinsohn et al., 1993; McGee et al., 1984), but more work in this area is urgently needed.

IMPLICATIONS

Epidemiological data on psychiatric disorders of children and adolescents have implications for both clinicians and administrators or policy makers (Rae-Grant, Offord, et al., 1989). In the clinical area, the data illustrate the importance of eliciting information from multiple respondents when assessing and planning treatment for children with psychiatric disorder. Information from one informant only will almost always give an incomplete diagnostic picture. A second clinical implication arises from the finding of high rates of comorbidity of disorders in individual children. There is some evidence that when one disorder, for example, conduct disorder, co-occurs with another, for example, affective disorder, the successful treatment of the latter condition results in an improvement in the former (Puig-Antich, 1982). An adequate clinical work-up should include the determination of whether or not the criteria are met for a wide range of psychiatric disorders, not just those that appear to be most closely connected to the presenting symptoms.

A third implication of epidemiological data for clinicians centers on the importance of gathering information about a wide range of potential causal risk and protective factors. A treatment plan should be tied closely to these specific factors, bearing in mind that the evidence, limited as it is, suggests that increasing the strengths in the child may be as beneficial as decreasing the weaknesses or deficits. The aim is not necessarily to deal effectively with all weaknesses and strengths but to change the balance between the adverse effects of the weaknesses and the beneficial effects of the strengths (Offord and Waters, 1983; Rae-Grant, Thomas, et al., 1989).

The administrative implications of the epidemiological data are several. Although the clinical importance and the need for service of some of the disorders identified in community surveys are questionable, there is general agreement that at least 12% of children have clinically important psychiatric disorders (Institute of Medicine, 1989). Given this figure, it is unlikely that specialized mental health services will ever be able to deal adequately with children with psychiatric disorder. Family physicians, pediatricians, and school personnel will have to be important elements in the delivery of child mental health services (Offord, Boyle, Szatmari, et al., 1987). Second, the targeting of expensive specialized services becomes an issue of major concern (Ontario Ministry of Community and Social Services, 1988). The children (and their families) most in need of these services and most likely to benefit from them should be the priority group for receiving them. Finally, the enormity of the problem of child and adolescent psychiatric disorder makes it impossible to think that the burden of suffering from these conditions can ever be reduced significantly by seeing identified cases one at a time. A major need is for effective interventions of a primary prevention nature targeted at groups of children. Despite the extensive amount written about primary prevention, there is a paucity, but not an absence of proven effective programs (Offord, 1987).

FUTURE DIRECTIONS

Advances are being made along many fronts in child psychiatric epidemiology. Progress on the conceptualization, classification, and measurement of child psychiatric disorders and their associated features, including correlates, risk and protective factors, and impairments, will increase the value of epidemiological studies. On the other hand, the results of community epidemiological surveys will contribute to knowledge about these basic issues. Large-scale survey work in this field will continue to grow, and its contributions will be maximized if explicit scientific and policy objectives for each survey are spelled out in advance, and if a prospective dimension is built in from the beginning. Hopefully, the increased knowledge from this work will lead to rational, reasonably-priced intervention programs that will raise the life quality of groups of children and perhaps improve their life chances.

Acknowledgments. *The authors would like to thank Dr. Michael Boyle for his comments and suggestions on an earlier draft of the manuscript, and Ms. Cindy Edge for her exemplary work and good humor in typing various drafts of the chapter.*

References

Achenbach TM: ''Comorbidity'' in child and adolescent psychiatry: Categorical and quantitative perspectives. *J Child Adolesc Psychopharmacol* 1:271, 1990/1991.

Achenbach TM, Edelbrock CS: Behavioral problems and competencies by parents of normal and disturbed children aged four through sixteen. *Monogr Soc Res Child Dev* 46:1, 1981.

Achenbach TM, Edelbrock CS: Taxonomic issues in child psychopathology. In: Ollendick TN, Hersen M (eds): *Handbook of child psychopathology*. New York, Plenum, 1983, pp. 65–93.

Achenbach TM, Mcconaughy SH, Howell CT: Child/adolescent behavioral and emotional problems: Implications of cross-informant correlations for situational specificity. *Psychol Bull* 191:213, 1987.

American Psychiatric Association: *Diagnostic and Statistical Manual of Mental Disorders* (3rd ed). Washington, DC, American Psychiatric Association Press, 1980.

American Psychiatric Association: *Diagnostic and Statistical Manual of Mental Disorders* (3rd ed, rev). Washington, DC, American Psychiatric Association Press, 1987.

Anderson C, Williams S, McGee R, et al: DSM-III disorders in preadolescent children. *Arch Gen Psychiatry* 44:69, 1987.

Anderson J, Williams S, McGee R, et al: Cognitive and social correlates of DSM-III disorders in preadolescent children. *J Am Acad Child Adolesc Psychiatry* 28:842, 1989.

Angold A, Weissman MM, Karen J, et al: Parent and child reports of depressive symptoms in children at low and high risk of depression. *J Child Psychol Psychiatry* 28:901, 1987.

Angold A, Costello EJ: Depressive comorbidity in children and adolescents: Empirical, theoretical, and methodological issues. *Am J Psychiatry* 150: 1779,1993.

Barkley RA: Child behavior rating scales and checklists. In: Rutter M, Tuma AH, Lann IS (eds): *Assessment and diagnosis in child psychopathology*. New York, Guilford, 1988.

Beardslee WR, Keller MB, Lavori PW, et al: Psychiatric disorder in adolescent offspring of parents with affective disorder in a non-referred sample. *J Affective Disord* 15:313, 1988.

Beardslee WR, Podorefsky D: Resilient adolescents whose parents have serious affective and other psychiatric disorders: Importance of self-understanding and relationships. *Am J Psychiatry* 145:63, 1988.

Beiser M: Mental health of American Indian and Alaska Native children. *White Cloud J* 2:37, 1981.

Beiser M, Attneave CL: Mental disorder among Native American children: Rates and risk periods for entering treatment. *Am J Psychiatry* 139:193, 1982.

Berger M, Yule W, Rutter M: Attainment and adjustment in two geographical areas. II: The prevalence of specific reading retardation. *Br J Psychiatry* 126:510, 1975.

Berkson J: Limitations of the application of fourfold table analysis to hospital data. *Biometrics* 2: 47,1946.

Bernstein GA, Garfinkel BD, Hoberman NM: Self-reported anxiety in adolescents. *Am J Psychiatry* 146:384, 1989.

Billings AG, Moos RH, Miller JJ, et al. Psychosocial adaptation in juvenile rheumatic disease: a controlled evaluation. *Health Psychol* 6:343, 1987.

Bird HR, Canino G, Rubio-Stipec M, et al: Estimates of the prevalence of childhood maladjustment in a community survey in Puerto Rico. *Arch Gen Psychiatry* 45:1120, 1988.

Bird HR, Gould MS, Staghezza BM: Patterns of diagnostic comorbidity in a community sample of children aged 9 through 16 years. *J Am Acad Child Adolesc Psychiatry* 32:361, 1993.

Bird HR, Gould MS, Yager T, et al: Risk factors for maladjustment in Puerto Rican children. *J Am Acad Child Adolesc Psychiatry* 28:847, 1989.

Boscoe JJ, Robin SS: Hyperkinesis: Prevention and treatment. In: Whalen CK, Robin SS (eds): *Hyperactive children*. New York, Academic Press, 1980, pp. 173–187.

Boyle MH: *Evaluating scales to measure childhood psychiatric disorder: Findings on the Ontario Child Health Study.* Unpublished doctoral dissertation, University of Toronto, Toronto, Ontario, 1989.

Boyle MH: *Choosing instruments to assess emotional and behavioural disorders of childhood for use in primary prevention studies* (Report prepared for the Children's Services Branch, Community Services Division), Toronto, Ontario, Ministry of Community and Social Services, 1989.

Boyle MH: Children's mental health issues. In: Barnhorst D, Johnson L (eds): *Children, families and public policy in the 90's*. Toronto, Thompson Educational Publishing, 1991, pp. 92–116.

Boyle MH, Offord DR: Smoking, drinking, and use of illicit drugs among adolescents in Ontario: Prevalence, patterns of use and sociodemographic correlates. *Can Med Assoc J* 135:1113, 1986.

Boyle MH, Offord DR, Racine YA, et al: Predicting substance use in early adolescence based on parent and teacher assessments of childhood psychiatric disorders: Results from the Ontario Child Health Study follow-up. *J Child Psychol Psychiatry* 34:189, 1993a.

Boyle MH, Offord DR, Racine Y, et al: Evaluation of the Diagnostic Interview for Children and Adolescents for use in general population samples. *J Abnorm Child Psychol* 21:663, 1993b.

Boyle MH, Offord DR, Racine YA, et al: Identifying thresholds for psychiatric disorder: Issues and prospects. *J Am Acad Child Adolesc Psychiatry*, in press.

Brandenburg HA, Friedman RM, Silver SE: The epidemiology of childhood psychiatric disorders: Prevalence findings from recent studies. *J Am Acad Child Adolesc Psychiatry* 29:76, 1990.

Breslau N: Psychiatric disorder in children with disabilities. *J Am Acad Child Psychiatry* 24:87, 1985.

Breslau N: Does brain dysfunction increase children's vulnerability to environmental stress? *Arch Gen Psychiatry* 47:15, 1990.

Brown G, Chadwick O, Shaffer D, et al: A prospective study of children with head injuries. III: Psychiatric sequelae. *Psychol Med* 11:63, 1981.

Byles J, Byrne C, Boyle MS, et al: Ontario Child Health Study: Reliability and validity of the General Functioning Subscale of the McMaster Family Assessment Device. *Fam Process* 17:97, 1988.

Cadman D, Boyle M, Szatmari P, et al: Chronic illness, disability, and mental and social well-being: Findings of the Ontario Child Health Study. *Pediatrics* 79:805, 1987.

Caron C, Rutter M: Comorbidity in child psychopathology: Concepts, issues and research strategies. *J Child Psychol Psychiatry* 32:1063, 1991.

Chadwick O, Rutter M, Brown G, et al: A prospective study of children with head injuries. II: Cognitive sequelae. *Psychol Med* 11:49, 1981.

Chang L, Morrissey RF, Koplewicz HS: Prevalence of psychiatric symptoms and their relation to adjustment among Chinese-American youth. *J Am Acad Child Adolesc Psychiatry* 34:91, 1995.

Chapel JL, Robins AJ, McGee RO: A follow-up of inattentive and/or hyperactive children from birth to 7 years of age. *J Oper Psychiatry* 13:17, 1982.

Christie N, Adenaes J, Skirbekk S: A study of self-reported crime. *Scand Studies Criminal* 1:86, 1965.

Clark JP, Wenninger EP: Socioeconomic class and area as correlates of illegal behavior among juveniles. *Am Soc Rev* 27:826, 1962.

Cochrane R: Psychological and behavioral disturbance in West Indians, Indians and Pakistanis in Britain: A comparison of rates among children and adults. *Br J Psychiatry* 134:201, 1979.

Cohen P, Brook J: Family factors related to the persistence of psychopathology in childhood and adolescence. *Psychiatry* 50:332, 1987.

Cohen P, Velez CN, Brook J, et al: Mechanisms of the relation between perinatal problems, early childhood illness, and psychopathology in late childhood and adolescence. *Child Dev* 60:701, 1989.

Conrad M, Hammen C: Role of maternal depression in perceptions of child maladjustment. *J Consult Clin Psychol* 57:663, 1989.

Costello EJ: Developments in child psychiatric epidemiology. *J Am Acad Child Adolesc Psychiatry* 28:836, 1989.

Costello EJ, Costello AJ, Edelbrock C, et al: Psychiatric disorders in pediatric primary care. *Arch Gen Psychiatry* 45:1107, 1988.

Costello EJ, Burns BJ, Angold A, et al: How can epidemiology improve mental health services for children and adolescents? *J Am Acad Child Adol Psychiatry* 32:1106, 1993.

Cox A, Rutter M, Newman S, et al: A comparative study of infantile autism and specific developmental receptive language disorder. II: Parent characteristics. *Br J Psychiatry* 126:146, 1975.

Department of Clinical Epidemiology and Biostatistics, McMaster University Health Sciences Centre: Now to read clinical journals. IV: To determine etiology or causation. *Can Med Assoc J* 124: 985, 1981a.

Department of Clinical Epidemiology and Biostatistics, McMaster University Health Sciences Centre: How to read clinical journals. V: To distinguish useful from useless or even harmful therapy. *Can Med Assoc J* 124:1156, 1981b.

Dodrill CB: Diphenylhydantoin serum levels, toxicity and neuropsychological performance in patients with epilepsy. *Epilepsia* 16:593, 1975.

Dunn J, Kendrick C: Studying temperament and parent-child interaction: Comparison of interview and direct observation. *Dev Med Child Neurol* 22: 484, 1980.

Earls F: Prevalence of behavior problems in 3 year old children: A cross-national replication. *Arch Gen Psychiatry* 37:1153, 1980.

Earls F: Epidemiology and child psychiatry. *Am J Orthopsychiatry* 59: 279, 1989.

Earls F, Jung KG: Temperament and home environment characteristics as causal factors in the early development of childhood psychopathology. *J Am Acad Child Adolesc Psychiatry* 26:491, 1987.

Earls F, Reich W, Jung K, et al: Psychopathology in children of alcoholic and antisocial parents. *Alcohol Clin Exp Res* 12:481, 1988.

Edelbrock C, Costello AJ: A review of diagnostic interview schedules for children. In: Rutter M, Tuma AH, Lann IS (eds): *Assessment and diagnosis in child and adolescent psychopathology.* New York, Guilford, 1988, pp. 87–112.

Edelbrock C, Costello AJ, Dulcan MK, et al: Age differences in the reliability of the psychiatric interview of the child. *Child Dev* 56:265, 1985.

Edelbrock C, Costello AJ, Dulcan MK, et al: Parent-child agreement on child psychiatric symptoms assessed via structured interview. *J Child Psychol Psychiatry* 27:181, 1986.

Eiser C: Psychologic effects of chronic disease. *J Child Psychol Psychiatry* 31:85, 1990.

Emery RE, O'Leary KD: Children's perceptions of marital discord and behavioral problems of boys and girls. *J Abnorm Child Psychol* 10:11, 1982.

Emslie G, Rush AJ, Weinberg W, et al: Self-report of depressive symptoms in adolescents: Ethnic and sex differences. Paper presented at the annual meeting of the American Academy of Child and Adolescent Psychiatry, Washington, DC, 1987.

Farrington DP, Gallagher B, Morley L, et al: Are there successful men from criminologic backgrounds? *Psychiatry* 51:116, 1988.

Farrington DP, West DJ: The Cambridge study in delinquent development (United Kingdom). In: Mednick SA, Baert AE (eds): *Prospective longitudinal research: An empirical basis for the primary prevention of psychosocial disorders.* New York, Oxford University Press, 1981, pp. 137–145.

Fergusson DM, Horwood LJ, Lynskey MT: Prevalence and comorbidity of DSM-III-R diagnoses in a birth cohort of 15 year olds. *J Am Acad Child Adolesc Psychiatry* 32:1127, 1993.

Fleming JE, Offord DR: Epidemiology of childhood depressive disorders in the general population: A critical review. *J Am Acad Child Adolesc Psychiatry* 29:571, 1990.

Fleming JE, Offord DR, Boyle MH: Prevalence of childhood and adolescent depression in the community: Ontario Child Health Study. *Br J Psychiatry* 155:647, 1989.

Fonagy P, Steele M, Steele H, et al: The Emmanuel Miller Memorial Lecture 1992. The theory and practice of resilience. *J Child Psychol Psychiatry* 35:231, 1994.

Forehand R, McCombs A: Unravelling the antecedent-consequence conditions in maternal depression and adolescent functioning. *Behav Res Ther* 26:399, 1988.

Frick P, Kamphaus RW, Lahey RB, et al: Academic underachievement and the disruptive behavior disorders. *J Consult Clin Psychol* 59:289, 1991.

Friedrich WN, Reams R, Jacobs JH: Sex differences in depression in early adolescents. *Psychol Rep* 62:475, 1988.

Fristad MA, Topolosky S, Weller EB, et al: Depression and learning disabilities in children. *J Aff Dis* 26:53, 1992.

Garmezy N: Stress, competence and development: Continuities in the study of schizophrenic adults, children vulnerable to psychopathology, and the search for stress-resistant children. *Am J Orthopsychiatry* 57:159, 1987.

Garrison CZ, Schluchter MD, Schoenbach VJ, et al: Epidemiology of depressive symptoms in young adolescents. *J Am Acad Child Adolesc Psychiatry* 28: 343, 1989.

Garrison CZ, Schoenbach VJ, Kaplan BH: Depressive symptoms in early adolescence. In: Dean A (ed): *Depression in multidisciplinary perspective.* New York, Brunner-Mazel, 1985, pp. 60–82.

Garrison WT, Earls FJ: *Temperament and child psychopathology.* Beverly Hills, CA, Sage, 1987.

Glueck S, Glueck E: *Unravelling juvenile delinquency.* Cambridge, Harvard University Press, 1950.

Gold M, Reimer DJ: Changing patterns of delinquent behavior among Americans 13 through 16 years old: 1967–72. *Crime and Delinq Lit* 7:483, 1975.

Goldsmith HH, Buss AH, Plomin R, et al: Roundtable: What is temperament? Four approaches. *Child Dev* 58:505, 1987.

Gorenstein E, Newman J: Disinhibitory psychopathology: A new perspective and a model for research. *Psychol Rev* 87:301, 1980.

Gould MS, Bird H, Jaramillo BS: Correspondence between statistically derived behavior problem syndromes and child psychiatric diagnoses in a community sample. *J Abnorm Child Psychol* 21:287, 1993.

Green BE, Sack WH, Pambrun A: A review of child psychiatric epidemiology with special reference to American Indian and Alaskan Native children. *J White Cloud Indian Reservation Dev Centre* 2:22, 1981.

Gutterman EM, O'Brien JD, Young JG: Structured diagnostic interviews for children and adolescents: Current status and future directions. *J Am Acad Child Adolesc Psychiatry* 26:621, 1987.

Harter S: The Perceived Competence Scale for children. *Child Dev* 53:87, 1982.

Herjanic B, Reich W: Development of a structured psychiatric interview for children: Agreement between child and parent on individual symptoms. *J Abnorm Child Psychol* 10:307, 1982.

Hindelang MJ, Hirschi T, Weiss JG: *Measuring Delinquency.* Beverly Hills, CA, Sage, 1981.

Hinshaw SP: Externalizing behavior problems and academic underachievement in childhood and adolescence: Causal relationships and underlying mechanisms. *Psychol Bull* 111:127, 1992.

Hirshfield DR, Rosenbaum JF, Biederman J, et al: Stable behavioral inhibition and its association with anxiety disorder. *J Am Acad Child Adol Psychiatry* 31:103, 1992.

Hoare P, Kerley S: Psychosocial adjustment of children with chronic epilepsy and their families. *Dev Med Child Neurol* 33:201, 1991.

Hoberman HM, Garfinkel BD, Parsons JH. et al: Depression in a community sample of adolescents. Paper presented at the annual meeting of the American Academy of Child and Adolescent Psychiatry, Los Angeles, 1986.

Hodges, K: Structured interviews for assessing children. *J Child Psychol Psychiatry* 34:49,1993.

Hoy E, Weiss G. Minde K, et al: The hyperactive child at adolescence: Cognitive, emotional and social functioning. *J Abnorm Child Psychol* 6:311, 1978.

Institute of Medicine: *Research on children and adolescents with mental, behavioral and development disorders: Mobilizing a national initiative.* Washington, DC, National Academy Press, 1989.

Ivens C, Rehm LP: Assessment of childhood depression: Correspondence between reports by child, mother, and father. *J Am Acad Child Adolesc Psychiatry* 27:738, 1988.

Jensen GF, Strauss JH, Harris VH: Crime, delinquency and the American Indian. *Hum Organization* 36:252, 1977.

Jensen PS, Sulzberg AD, Richters, JE, et al: Scales, diagnoses, and child psychopathology: 1. CBCL and DISC relationships. *J Am Acad Child Adolesc Psychiatry* 32:397, 1993.

John K, Gammon GD, Prusoff BA, et al: Social Adjustment Inventory for Children and Adolescents (SAICA): Testing of a new semi-structured interview. *J Am Acad Child Adolesc Psychiatry* 26:898, 1987.

Jones MB, Offord DR, Abrams N: Brothers, sisters and antisocial behavior. *Br J Psychiatry* 136: 139, 1980.

Kallarackal AM, Herbert M: The happiness of Indian immigrant children. *New Soc* 35:422, 1976.

Kashani JH, Beck NC, Hoeper EW, et al: Psychiatric disorders in a community sample of adolescents. *Am J Psychiatry* 144:584, 1987.

Kashani JH, McGee RO, Clarkson SE, et al: Depression in a sample of 9-year-old children. *Arch Gen Psychiatry* 40:1217, 1983.

Kashani JH, Orvaschel H, Burk JP, et al: Informant variance: The issue of parent-child disagreement. *J Am Acad Child Psychiatry* 24:437, 1985.

Kashani JH, Orvaschel H, Rosenberg TK, et al: Psychopathology in a community sample of children and adolescents: A developmental perspective *J Am Acad Child Adolesc Psychiatry* 28:701, 1989.

Kastrup M: Urban-rural differences in 6 year olds. In: Graham PJ (ed): *Epidemiological approaches in child psychiatry.* London, Academic, 1977, pp. 181–194.

Kleinbaum DG, Kupper LL, Morgenstern H: *Epidemiologic research: Principles and quantitative methods.* Belmont, CA, Wadsworth, 1982.

Kovacs M, Feinberg TL, Crouse-Novak MA: Depressive disorders in childhood. I: A longitudinal prospective study of characteristics and recovery. *Arch Gen Psychiatry* 41:229, 1984.

Lapouse R, Monk MA: Behavior deviations in a representative sample of children: Variation by sex, race, social class, and family size. *Am J Orthopsychiatry* 34:436, 1964.

Lavik N: Urban-rural differences in rates of disorder. In: Graham PJ (ed): *Epidemiological approaches to child psychiatry.* London, Academic Press, 1977, pp. 223–251.

Leckman JF, Weissman MM, Merikangas KR, et al: Major depression and panic disorder. *Psychopharmacol Bull* 21:543, 1985.

Lewinsohn PM, Hops H, Roberts RE, et al: Adolescent psychopathology: 1. Prevalence and incidence of depression and other DSM-III-R disorders in high school students. *J Abnorm Psychol* 102:133, 1993.

Lewis DO, Balla DA: *Delinquency and psychopathology.* New York, Grune & Stratton, 1976.

Lilienfeld AM: *Foundations of epidemiology.* New York, Oxford University Press, 1976.

Lipman EL, Offord DR, Boyle MH: Relation between economic disadvantage and psychosocial morbidity in children. *Can Med Assoc J* 151:431, 1994.

Loeber R, Green SM, Lahey BB, et al: Differences and similarities between children, mothers, and teachers as informants on disruptive behavior disorders. *J Abnorm Child Psychol* 19:75, 1991.

Marton P, Maharaj S: Family factors in adolescent unipolar depression *Can J Psychiatry* 25:258, 1992.

Mash EJ, Terdal L (eds): *Behavioral assessment of childhood disorders.* New York, Guilford, 1981.

Maziade M, Caperaa P, Laplante B, et al: Value of difficult temperament among 7-year-olds in the general population for predicting psychiatric diagnosis at age 12. *Am J Psychiatry* 142:9443, 1985.

McGee R, Silva PA, Williams S: Perinatal, neurological, environmental and developmental characteristics of seven-year-old children with stable behavior problems. *J Child Psychol Psychiatry* 25:573, 1984.

Meehl, PE: Factors and taxa, traits and types, differences of degree and differences of kind. *J Personality* 60:117, 1992.

Merikangas KR, Prusoff BA, Weissman MM: Parental concordance for affective disorders: Psychopathology in offspring. *J Affective Disord* 15:279, 1988.

Minde K, Lewin D, Weiss G, et al: The hyperactive child in elementary school: A five-year controlled follow-up. *Except Child* 38:215, 1971.

Offord DR: Family backgrounds of male and female delinquents. In: Gunn J, Farrington DP (eds): *Delinquency and the criminal justice systems*. New York, John Wiley & Sons, 1982, pp. 121–151.

Offord DR: Prevention of behavioral and emotional disorders in children. *J Child Psychol Psychiatry* 28:9, 1987.

Offord DR: Conduct disorder: Risk factors and prevention. In: Shaffer D, Philips I, Enzer NB (eds): *Prevention of mental disorders, alcohol and other drug use in children and adolescents*. Rockville, MD, US Department of Health and Human Services, 1989, pp. 273–307.

Offord DR: Social factors in the aetiology of childhood disorders. In: Tonge B, Burrows G, Werry J (eds): *Handbook of studies on child psychiatry*. Amsterdam, The Netherlands, Elsevier, 1990, pp. 55–68.

Offord DR, Boyle MH, Fleming JE, et al: Ontario Child Health Study: Summary of selected results. *Can J Psychiatry* 34:483, 1989.

Offord DR, Boyle MH, Jones BA: Psychiatric disorder and poor school performance among welfare children in Ontario. *Can J Psychiatry* 32:518, 1987.

Offord DR, Boyle MH, Racine YA: Ontario Child Health Study: Correlates of disorder. *J Am Acad Child Adolesc Psychiatry* 28:856, 1989.

Offord DR, Boyle MH, Racine YA: *Ontario Child Health Study: Children at risk*. Toronto, Queen's Printer for Ontario, 1990.

Offord DR, Boyle MH, Racine YA: The epidemiology of antisocial behavior in childhood and adolescence: Findings from the Ontario Child Health Study. In: Pepler D, Rubin KH (eds): *The development and treatment of childhood aggression*. Hillsdale, NJ, Erlbaum, 1991, pp. 31–54.

Offord DR, Boyle MH, Racine YA, et al: Outcome, prognosis and risk in a longitudinal follow-up study. *J Am Acad Child Adol Psychiatry* 31:916, 1992.

Offord DR, Boyle MH, Racine YA, et al: Integrating assessment data from multiple informants. *J Am Acad Child Adolesc Psychiatry*, in press.

Offord DR, Boyle MH, Szatmari P, et al: Ontario Child Health Study. II: Six-month prevalence of disorder and rates of service utilization. *Arch Gen Psychiatry* 44:832, 1987.

Offord DR, Cadman D, Antone I, et al: *The First Nations Child Health Care Study: Final report*. Hamilton, Ontario, Centre for Studies of Children at Risk, 1990.

Offord DR, Waters BG: Socialization and its failure. In: Levine MD, Carey WB, Crocker AC, Gross RT (eds): *Developmental-behavioral pediatrics*. Philadelphia, Saunders, 1983, pp. 650–682.

Ontario Ministry of Community and Social Services: *Investing in Children* Toronto, Ontario, Ministry of Community and Social Services, 1988.

Patterson GR: *Coercive family process*. Eugene, Oregon, Castalia Publishing Company, 1982.

Perrin JM, MacLean WE, Perrin EC: Parental perceptions of health status and psychological adjustment of children with asthma. *Pediatrics* 83:26, 1989.

Perrin EC, Ramsey BK, Sandler HM: Competent kids: Children and adolescents with a chronic illness. *Child Care Health Dev* 13:13, 1987.

Pichot P: Nosological models in psychiatry. *Br J Psychiatry* 164:232, 1994.

Pless IB: Clinical assessment: Physical and psychological functioning. *Pediatr Clin North Am* 31:33, 1984.

Plomin R: Extraversion: Sociability and impulsivity. *J Pers Assess* 40:24, 1976.

Plomin R: Childhood temperament. *Ad Clin Child Psychol* 6:45, 1993.

Plomin R, Dunn J: *The study of temperament: Changes, continuities and challenges*. Hillsdale, NJ, Erlbaum, 1986.

Plomin R, Rowe DC: A twins study of temperament in young children. *J Child Psychol* 97:107, 1977.

Prior M: Childhood temperament. *J Child Psychol Psychiatry* 33:249, 1992.

Puig-Antich J: Major depression and conduct disorder in prepuberty. *J Am Acad Child Psychiatry* 21:118, 1982.

Quinton D: Urbanism and mental health. *J Child Psychol Psychiatry* 29:11, 1988.

Quinton D, Rutter M, Liddle C: Institutional rearing, parenting difficulties and marital support. *Psychol Med* 14:107, 1984.

Raadal M, Milgrom P, Cauce AM, et al: Behavior problems in 5- to 11-year-old children from low-income families. *J Am Acad Child Adolesc Psychiatry* 33:1017, 1994.

Rae-Grant N, Offord DR, Munroe-Blum H: Implications for clinical services, research and training. *Can J Psychiatry* 34:492, 1989.

Rae-Grant N, Thomas H, Offord DR, et al: Risk, protective factors and the prevalence of behavioral and emotional disorders in children and adolescents. *J Am Acad Child Adolesc Psychiatry* 28:262, 1989.

Reich W, Herjanic B, Weiner Z: Development of a structured psychiatric interview for children: Agreement on diagnosis comparing child and parent interviews. *J Abnorm Child Psychol* 10:325, 1982.

Rende RD: Longitudinal relations between temperament traits and behavioral syndromes in middle childhood. *J Am Acad Child Adolesc Psychiatry* 32:287, 1993.

Reynolds WM, Coats KI: *Depression in adolescents: Incidence, depth and correlates*. Paper presented at the 10th International Congress of the International Association of Child and Adolescent Psychiatry and Allied Professions, Dublin, Ireland, 1982.

Reynolds WM, Rob MI: The role of family difficulties in adolescent depression, drug-taking and other problem behaviors. *Med J Aust* 149:250, 1988.

Richman N, Stevenson JE, Graham PJ: Prevalence of behavior problems in 3-year-old children: An epidemiological study in a London borough. *J Child Psychol Psychiatry* 16:277, 1975.

Richters J, Pellegrini D: Depressed mothers' judgments about their children: An examination of the depression-distortion hypothesis. *Child Dev* 60:1068, 1989.

Roberts RE, Chen Y-W: Depressive symptoms and suicidal ideation among Mexican-Origin and Anglo adolescents *J Am Acad Child Adolesc Psychiatry* 34:81, 1995.

Robins LN: Psychiatric epidemiology. *Arch Gen Psychiatry* 35:697, 1978.

Robins LN: Longitudinal methods in the study of normal and pathological development. In: Kisker KP, Meyer JE, Muller C, et al. (eds): *Psychiatrie der Gugenwart. Band I: Grunlagen und Methoden der Psychiatrie*. Heidelberg, Springer-Verlag, 1979, pp. 627–685.

Robins LN: Reflections on testing the validity of psychiatric interviews. *Arch Gen Psychiatry* 42:918, 1985.

Robins LN: Conduct disorder. *J Child Psychol Psychiatry* 32:193, 1991.

Robins LN, West PA, Herjanic BL: Arrests and delinquency in two generations: A study of black urban families and their children. *J Child Psychol Psychiatry* 3:241, 1975.

Rubenstein JL, Heeren T, Housman D, et al: Suicidal behavior in "normal" adolescents: Risk and protective factors. *Am J Orthopsychiatry* 59:59, 1989.

Rutter M: Brain damage syndrome in childhood: Concepts and findings. *J Child Psychol Psychiatry* 18:1, 1977.

Rutter M: The city and the child. *Am J Orthopsychiatry* 51:610, 1981a.

Rutter M: Epidemiologic-longitudinal strategies and causal research in child psychiatry. *J Am Acad Child Psychiatry* 20:513, 1981b.

Rutter M: Psychological sequelae of brain damage in childhood. *Am J Psychiatry* 138:1533, 1981c.

Rutter M: Resilience in the face of adversity. *Br J Psychiatry* 147:596, 1985.

Rutter M: Psychosocial resilience and protective mechanisms. *Am J Orthopsychiatry* 57:316, 1987a.

Rutter M: Temperament, personality and personality disorder. *Br J Psychiatry* 150:443, 1987b.

Rutter M: Epidemiological approaches to developmental psychopathology. *Arch Gen Psychiatry* 45:486, 1988.

Rutter M: Isle of Wight revisited: Twenty-five years of child psychiatric epidemiology. *J Am Acad Child Adolesc Psychiatry* 28:633, 1989a.

Rutter M: Pathways from childhood to adult life. *J Child Psychol Psychiatry* 30:23, 1989b.

Rutter M: Psychiatric disorder in parents as a risk factor for children. In: Shaffer D, Philips I, Enzer NB (eds): *Prevention of mental disorders, alcohol and other drug use in children and adolescents*. Rockville, MD, US Department of Health and Human Services, 1989c, pp. 158–189.

Rutter M, Cox A, Tupling C, et al: Attainment and adjustment in two geographical areas. I: The prevalence of psychiatric disorder. *Br J Psychiatry* 126:493, 1975.

Rutter M, Giller H: *Juvenile delinquency: Trends and perspectives*. New York, Penguin Books, 1983.

Rutter M, Graham P: The reliability and validity of the psychiatric assessment of the child. *Br J Psychiatry* 114:563, 1968.

Rutter M, Graham P, Yule W: *A neuropsychiatric study in childhood*. Heinman, London, Clinics in Developmental Medicine 35/36, 1970.

Rutter M, Quinton D: Psychiatric disorder—ecological factors and concepts of causation. In: McGurk H (ed): *Ecological factors in human development*. Amsterdam, North-Holland, 1977, pp. 173–187.

Rutter M, Quinton D: Parental psychiatric disorder: Effects on children. *Psychol Med* 14:853, 1984.

Rutter M, Tizard I, Whitmore K: *Education, health and behaviour*. London, Longman, 1970.

Rutter M, Yule W, Berger M, et al: Children of West Indian immigrants. I: Rates of behavioral deviance and psychiatric disorder. *J Child Psychol Psychiatry* 15:241, 1974.

Rutter M, Yule B, Quinton D, et al: Attainment and adjustment in two geographical areas. 111: Some factors accounting for area differences. *Br J Psychiatry* 125:520, 1975.

Saslow HL, Harrover MJ: Research on psychosocial adjustment of Indian youth. *Am J Psychiatry* 125:224, 1968.

Satterwhite B: Impact of chronic illness on child and family: An overview based on five surveys. *Int J Rehabil Res* 1:7, 1978.

Schoenbach VJ, Kaplan BH, Grimson RC, et al: Use of a symptom scale to study the prevalence of a depressive syndrome in young adolescents. *Am J Epidemiol* 116:791, 1982.

Schonfeld IS, Shaffer D, O'Connor P, et al: Conduct disorder and cognitive functioning: Testing three causal hypotheses. *Child Dev* 59:993, 1988.

Shaffer D, Bijur P, Chadwick OF, et al: Head

injury and later reading disability. *J Am Acad Child Psychiatry* 19:592, 1980.

Shaffer D, Chadwick O, Rutter M: Psychiatric outcome of localized head injury in children. In: Porter R, Fitzsimons DW (eds): *Outcome of severe damage to the central nervous system* (Ciba Foundation no. 34). Amsterdam, Holland, Except Medica-North-Holland, 1975, pp. 191–214.

Shaffer D, Gould M, Hicks RC: Worsening suicide rate in black teenagers. *Am J Psychiatry* 151: 1810, 1994.

Shaffer D, Schonfeld IS, O'Connor PA, et al: Neurological soft signs: Their relationship to psychiatric disorder and intelligence in childhood and adolescence. *Arch Gen Psychiatry* 42:342, 1985.

Siegel PM: *Prestige in the American occupational structure.* Unpublished doctoral dissertation, Chicago, University of Chicago, 1971.

Silverman WK, Nelles WB: The Anxiety Disorders Interview Schedule for Children. *J Am Acad Child Adolesc Psychiatry* 27:772, 1988.

Sollee ND, Kindlon DJ: Lateralized brain injury and behavior problems in children. *J Abnorm Child Psychol* 15:479, 1987.

Statistics Canada: *Canada's native people 1981 census.* Ottawa, Canada, Minister of Supply and Services, 1984.

Stores G, Hart J: Reading skills of children with generalized and focal epilepsy attending ordinary schools. *Dev Med Child Neurol* 18:705, 1976.

Strauss CC, Last CG, Hersen M, et al: Association between anxiety and depression in children and adolescents with anxiety disorders. *J Abnorm Child Psychol* 16:57, 1988.

Sylvester LE, Hyde TS, Reichler RJ: The Diagnostic Interview for Children and Personality Interview for Children in studies of children at risk for anxiety disorders or depression. *J Am Acad Child Adolesc Psychiatry* 26:668, 1987.

Szatmari P, Boyle M, Offord DR: ADDH and conduct disorder: Degree of diagnostic overlap and differences among correlates. *J Am Acad Child Adolesc Psychiatry* 28:865, 1989.

Taylor E: On the epidemiology of hyperactivity. In: Sagvolden T Archer T (eds): *Attention deficit disorder and hyperkinetic syndrome.* Hillsdale, NJ, Erlbaum, 1989, pp. 31–52.

Teri L: The use of the Beck Depression Inventory with adolescents *J Abnorm Child Psychol* 10:277, 1982.

Thornberry TP, Farnworth M: Social correlates of criminal involvement: Further evidence on the relationship between social status and criminal behavior. *Am Soc Rev* 47:505, 1982.

Turner S, Beidel DC, Costello A: Psychopathology in the offspring of anxiety disorder patients. *J Consult Clin Psychol* 55:229, 1987.

Ucko LE: A comparative study of asphyxiated and non-asphyxiated boys from birth to 5 years. *Dev Med Child Neurol* 7:643, 1965.

US Department of Commerce, Census Bureau: *American Indians, Subject Report, 1970 Census of the Population: PC(2)-IF.* Washington, DC, US Department of Commerce, Census Bureau, 1973.

Valla JP, Bergeron L, Bérubé H, et al: A structured pictorial questionnaire to assess DSM-III-R-based diagnoses in children (6–11 years): Development, validity and reliability. *J Abnorm Child Psychol* 22:403, 1994.

Velez CN, Johnson J, Cohen P: A longitudinal analysis of selected risk factors for childhood psychopathology. *J Am Acad Child Adolesc Psychiatry* 28:861, 1989.

Verhulst FC, Berden GFG, Sanders-Woudstra JAR: Mental health in Dutch children. II: *Acta Psychiatr Scand* 72:1, 1985.

Vikan A: Psychiatric epidemiology in a sample of 1510 ten-year-old children, I: *J Child Psychol Psychiatry* 26:55, 1985.

Wadsworth M: Roots of delinquency. In: *Infancy, adolescence and crime.* Oxford, Martin Robertson, 1979.

Wasserman AL, Thompson EL, Wilimas JA: The psychological status of survivors of childhood/adolescent Hodgkin's disease. *Arch Dis Childhood* 141: 626, 1987.

Weinberg WA, McLean A, Snider RL: Depression, learning disability, and school behavior problems. *Psychol Rep* 64:275, 1989.

Weissman MM, Gammon D, John K, et al: Children of depressed parents: Increased psychopathology and early onset of major depression. *Arch Gen Psychiatry* 44:847, 1987.

Weissman MM, Merikangas KR, Gammon GD, et al: Depression and anxiety disorders in parents and children: Results from the Yale family study. *Arch Gen Psychiatry* 41:845, 1984.

Weissman MM, Warner V, Fendrich M: Applying impairment criteria to children's psychiatric diagnosis. *J Am Acad Child Adolesc Psychiatry* 29:789, 1990.

Weissman MM, Warner V, Wickramaratne P, et al: Early-onset major depression in parents and their children. *J Affect Dis* 15:269, 1988.

Werry JS: ICD-9 and DSM-III classification for clinicians. *J Child Psychol Psychiatry* 26:1, 1985.

Werry JS, Reeves JC, Elkind GS: Attention deficit, conduct, oppositional, and anxiety disorders in children. I: A review of research on differentiating characteristics. *J Am Acad Child Adolesc Psychiatry* 26:133, 1987.

West DJ, Farrington DP: *Who becomes delinquent?* London, Heinemann, 1973.

Williams JR, Gold M: From delinquent behavior to official delinquency. *Soc Prob* 20:209, 1972.

Williams S, McGee RO, Anderson J, et al: The structure and correlates of self-reported symptoms in 11-year-old children. *J Abnorm Child Psychol* 17: 55, 1989.

Wilson WJ: *The truly disadvantaged.* Chicago, University of Chicago Press, 1987.

Wing L: Childhood autism and social class: A question of selection? *Br J Psychiatry* 137:410, 1980.

Wolf SM, Forsythe A: Behavior disturbance, phenobarbital, and febrile seizures. *Pediatrics* 61: 728, 1978.

Wright-Strawderman C, Watson BL: The prevalence of depressive symptoms in children with learning disabilities. *J Learn Dis* 25:258, 1992.

Yates A: Current status and future directions of research on the American Indian child. *Am J Psychiatry* 144:1135, 1987.

Yule W, Berger M, Rutter M, Yule B: Children of West Indian Immigrants. II: Intellectual performance and reading attainment. *J Child Psychol Psychiatry* 16:1, 1975.

Zahner GEP, Jacobs JH, Freeman DH, et al: Rural-urban child psychopathology in a Northeastern U.S. State: 1986–1989. *J Am Acad Child Adolesc Psychiatry* 32:378, 1993.

120 EFFECTS OF HEALTH DELIVERY SYSTEMS ON CHILD AND ADOLESCENT MENTAL HEALTH CARE

Frank T. Rafferty, M.D.

The mental health of any given individual is a unique phenomenon. The therapist-patient dyad is the simplest of mental health delivery systems and has been the perennial favorite of child psychiatrists. A "system" is both a structural and functional concept that represents at least two or more components related in some measurable way. The parameters or variables that identify the components and specify the relationships between the components have to be named, described, explicated, and measured in a consensually valid manner before there is understanding of a specific system (Rafferty, 1978).

Much confusion is caused by the failure to understand and appreciate the hierarchical ordering and nesting of systems. The individual human being is the most frequent point of reference in ordinary discourse. The pronouns *I, she, he, him, her,* etc., unavoidably give a sense of unity and independence that is real and yet illusory. On the one hand, the individual is a clearly identifiable and measurable single unit, to be counted as a basic component of larger systems such as the family, group, clan, tribe, community, state, or nation. But on the other hand, the individual is already a most complicated array of organ systems (blood, cardiovascular, renal, central nervous, etc.). Within each organ system may nest other subordinate systems, which in turn are made up of thousands of cells, which in their turn are arrays of chemical systems, constructed and operated by genetic systems.

Fueling the operations of systems are the descriptive, explanatory, and analogous concepts of energy, money, and information. These are inventions of the human mind derived from the wonderful and poorly understood processes of cognition (Dewey and Bentley, 1949). Energy is a naturally occurring force, independent of the existence and experience of human beings. But everything we know about energy (uses, exchanges, transformations, measurements, etc.) is a product of human experience. The sciences devoted to understanding and using energy are chemistry, physics, and quantum mechanics. But for systems dedicated to achieving or improving the mental health of individuals or populations, the operant energy system is the individual workers or components of the system. Some of the disciplines working with this kind of energy are personnel management, human resources, and professional education.

A subtle but vital point is that the amount of energy in the world is limited, despite the fact that new energy is contributed from the sun each minute of the day. Furthermore, our limited knowledge of energy allows use of only a small part of what is available. And moreover, distribution of usable energy in a fair and just way is quite difficult. Distribution of energy requires the use of large amounts of energy. Frequently newspaper headlines scream about those who are starving while food is on the tarmac at a distant airport.

Each individual human being is the product of millions of years of evolution. The processes of evolution work through mechanisms that are biological, organismic solutions of environmental problems in processing, managing, and distributing energy. The most important, most uniquely evolved human traits are the capacities for cognition, language, social cooperation, and culture. Most people living daily lives within the constraints of time and space are only partially aware of and don't much care about how their species, their race, or their society achieved a particular position; they understandably attend to and focus on adaptation to the current stresses. Inevitably today's problems are part of yesterday's solutions. For example, a survey of today's mental health administrators and providers would surely elicit a "shortage of money" as their primary problem to solve. Yet money was invented by humans thousands of years ago, probably to solve problems of time and distance in the distribution of energy.

At the dawn of human culture, before the invention of a written language, humans had evolved simple mechanisms of human cooperation and communication. It is only speculation, but probably true, that sharing and trading of foodstuffs and assisting in providing shelter within family groups were among the earliest activities. Centuries later, perhaps after the invention of agriculture and stable domiciles, it must have become necessary and possible to trade these necessities of life over long distances. Sometime in the process, certain objects began to be used as symbols of the objects to be traded. Much later the ancient empires of China, Greece, and Rome had complicated domestic and long-distance systems of trading and well-developed practices of coinage and use of money (Encyclopedia Brittanica, 1972, "Money"). The cultural evolution of money and business continues actively to this day. Each new invention goes through decades, sometimes centuries, of trial and error to establish full economic, moral, and ethical acceptance (e.g., usury transformed into respectable interest). Today we struggle with credit cards, junk bonds, future contracts, and electronic markets.

After the invention of practical and scientific knowledge about energy and money, information is the third human cultural innovation that can be described as necessary for the function of any system. Formally discovered and mathematically described about 50 years ago with reference to radio wave conductance over bandwidth, information has come to dominate world culture. Like money and energy, information can be generated, transmitted, exchanged, transformed, stored, and used to shape the structural and functional properties of any system. The ubiquitous computer is an information machine. Although money would appear to be a totally human invention, information, like energy, occurs as a natural phenomenon but required human discovery, formulation, and measurement of its characteristics. The biological genetic code that determines the anatomical and physiological properties of living systems is a classic example of the role of information.

Although the computer and information theory are relatively new discoveries, information in the form of human knowledge has been a

crucial variable in the shaping of human experience, culture, and behavior. Knowledge is generated, exchanged, transmitted, and stored by virtue of the human mind. There has been lengthy debate about the nature of both knowledge and the human mind. The greatest scientific challenge of the future may be to understand the neurochemical and electrical functioning of the brain as it gives rise to complex thought and emotional processes. Psychiatric and mental health systems for caring for strangers and providing relief from pain and distress have developed with only limited information about the structure and function of the biological systems most involved. These caring disciplines have been shaped by the social contexts in which they function.

The history of medicine has emphasized that the first goal of the physician is to relieve the pain, suffering, and illness of the patient, and the second to seek to understand the scientific aspects of illness or disease. In many modern medical specialties, these goals can be dealt with in reverse order. Scientific understanding of the illness or disease can contribute to the relief of the pain and suffering. Psychiatric procedures and techniques have until recently been empirical mechanisms that have given promise of reducing the pain and suffering of patients and their families. The pharmacotherapies introduced in the late 1950s were initially empirical procedures that led to basic research techniques and theories that have now opened up new vistas in the management of mental illness. It is important in the examination of the mental health systems to be alert to the fundamental goal of the system.

THE CHILD GUIDANCE CLINIC

The American public, and frequently mental health professionals, tends to misunderstand and misuse the concept systems in the phrase *health care delivery systems*. The inferred meaning is that of an intentional, rationally planned, goal-directed, comprehensive organization that provides health care services to a defined population. There has never been such a system in the United States. Many people continue to wish for, to think about, and to lobby for some such organization.

Medical practice at the turn of the 20th century was not an inspiring sight. There were over 100,000 individually practicing physicians, dominated by 160, mostly proprietary, medical schools of uncertain quality. The profession was on the brink of the unity, cohesion, and public respect that would be achieved in the next 20 years. The American Medical Association (AMA) was just organizing as a national body. The move to state medical licensing boards has been a 20-year era of great divisiveness on issues of quality and sectarianism (Starr, 1982). In the midst of this creative foment came the first organizations dedicated to the care of disordered children. Terms such as *child psychiatry, mental health,* and *emotional disturbance* had yet to be invented.

The beginning came in the last decade of the 19th century, in a social movement of men and especially women concerned about the fate of children in the courts of the United States. Proposed legislation was introduced into the Illinois Assembly to create a special court to recognize the different needs of juveniles who were coming before the law. The original legislation (1895) contained provisions for diagnostic, probationary, and treatment services, including residential, but the legislation that was passed (1899) contained financial authorization for only the special juvenile court and judge (Lathrop, 1925). Note that the crucial determinism of money was present from the earliest beginning of child psychiatry.

Some 10 years later, financed by the personal fortune of Mrs. Elizabeth Dummer for the first 5 years, the clinical side of the original legislation came into existence as the Juvenile Psychopathic Institute (later to be the Institute for Juvenile Research). What were the energy and informational inputs to this new child care system? Perhaps four or five workers constituted the original staff, consisting of what would become the standard team of physician, psychologist, and social worker. The information resources were meager, consisting of the results of (*a*) the physical examination by the physician, organized around simple concepts of development and nutrition; (*b*) the newly formulated Binet intelligence test, administered by the psychologist; and (c) the detailed social and family history, taken by the social worker. Treatment consisted of coordinating the efforts of social agencies to restore each child to a normal, functioning relationship with the community.

This and similar organizations, known as child guidance clinics, survived and thrived through the 1950s. Private donations, philanthropic foundations, social service agencies, and eventually states and municipalities provided the money. Infusions of knowledge were received via the literatures of the three professional disciplines, and particularly from psychoanalysis, which eventually dominated the treatment techniques if not the theory of all three disciplines. Clinics with as many as 50–75 workers were located in the major metropolitan areas, and smaller clinics were spread throughout the states. Psychotherapy of child and mother became the preferred treatment technique. In 1946 the American Association of Psychiatric Clinics for Children established the standards for clinics and provided authorized training experiences for all disciplines. The training of the child psychiatrist became a dominant focus of clinic organization. The social workers outnumbered the psychiatrists or psychologists. However, all disciplines carefully deferred to the psychiatrist as director of the clinic.

UNIVERSITY CHILD PSYCHIATRY PROGRAMS

During the era of child guidance clinics, a great deal had been happening to the power and knowledge bases of medicine and psychiatry. Psychiatry had evolved in private and state-operated hospitals until World War II. Only psychiatry and the chronic infectious diseases of tuberculosis and leprosy had hospitals segregated from those of the other fields of medicine. The practice of medicine had become almost respectable, and medical education had moved to the university and had adopted an emphasis on the basic sciences. The reorganization of the AMA, the establishment of the Council on Medical Education, and publication of the Flexner Report of the Carnegie Foundation heralded a program of reform and consolidation of medical education. The Johns Hopkins University version of a research-oriented German university became the ideal, and medical education began to be more sharply differentiated from medical practice. The founding of medical specialty boards proceeded rapidly. The American Board of Psychiatry and Neurology was founded in 1938. Psychiatry was inexorably moving into mainstream medicine long before that target became a slogan. Could child psychiatry remain behind in this expansion of power and knowledge? Financial power was to come later.

By 1952 the American Academy of Child Psychiatry was founded as a medical organization to seek and, by 1960, to achieve specialty board recognition for child psychiatry. A few universities had had affiliations with famous child guidance clinics. In fact, a child guidance clinic had preceded the establishment of departments of psychiatry in some universities before World War II. But board recognition of child psychiatry and the university affiliation as a requirement for an accredited training program began a rapid movement of child psychiatry education to the universities, most often as divisions of the departments of psychiatry. The form of a predominantly outpatient clinic with a multidisciplinary treatment team was preserved. A few universities adopted the know-how of the social agency-operated residential treatment centers into the university hospital and thus began the (mostly under age 12) children's inpatient unit. This development of psychiatry and later of child psychiatry as medical specialties has had a profound effect on mental health delivery systems. Of prime importance is the sociopolitical reality that in the United States the social welfare system and the law enforcement/ corrections system went in a direction different from that of the medically oriented mental health systems. These later systems had and still have different sources of energy, money, and information. The problems of interagency conflict and different cultural worlds that are derived from these differences in social, political, scientific, and philosophical positions are as yet unresolved.

To a considerable degree, the financial support of the training and

research programs at the universities came from grants from the National Institute of Mental Health, although some states became interested in and generous about funding medical education. Despite the governmental capitalization of medical schools, hospitals, and medical research, the products from these activities moved rapidly into the private practice of medicine.

INSURANCE

The supply of money for medical services, education, and research has always been the first and most obvious limiting factor on the growth and the shape of health care delivery systems. For brief periods, as in the 1920s and 1960s, money flowed more freely, and shortages of trained personnel and information were the major constraints on the system. These personnel shortages seem to be more acceptable, generating complaints that are eased if not resolved by government targeting of more funds to the health and mental health professional disciplines. On the other hand a shortage of money is perceived to be due to the government's mean-spiritedness and unwillingness to nurture and succor its citizens.

Physicians' attitudes toward money have always been, and remain, profoundly problematic. The American physician has never been reluctant to accept a profit in the form of a fee. American medicine, with the possible exception of psychiatry, was a proprietary enterprise until the early years of this century (Starr, 1982). And now the income of the average physician is well within the upper 2% of incomes in the United States. But the American physician and, particularly, organized medicine has fought against any third-party effort to gain a position between the physician and the patient, especially any position that involved a profit for the third party.

Physicians disapproved of the friendly or fraternal societies that in the last decades of the 19th century introduced the concept of "sick benefits," in addition to the earlier concept of life insurance or "death benefits." At that time the major cost of being sick was the loss of wages rather than the cost of medical care. However, some of the fraternal societies, which were descendants of the old guilds and much stronger in Europe than in the United States, began to be direct providers of medical care, as well as of the funds to replace lost wages.

The sick benefits were perceived as preventive and were not necessarily medical services. Medicine had not yet achieved a monopoly, and there were competing nonmedical systems for the care of the sick. Contract physicians were paid a low fee and were looked down on by the rest of medicine, to the extent of being excluded from many local and state medical societies. Unions and large corporations also became direct providers of sick benefits. A measure of the extent of these services is the fact that the railroads in 1900 employed 20,000 surgeons as contract physicians (Starr, 1982).

Organized medicine disapproved of physicians' forming group practices despite the success of a number of such in the Midwest, which modeled themselves after the Mayo brothers and the Menningers. The new licensing laws and the reduction in numbers of medical schools from 360 proprietary schools to 70 more or less academically oriented schools in the early 1900s reduced the number of doctors available for low contract fees. This period of time, which came to a conclusion with the entry of the United States into World War I and the later prosperity of the 1920s, can be considered one of three major periods of heightened concern about the cost of medical care. The second period was during the depression of the 1930s, prior to World War II. The third period came in the early 1960s. A fourth period of even greater concern about health care costs began about 1980 and is at its peak as this is being written.

From the perspective of the present crisis, the most important question to ask history is: Why didn't the United States adopt national health insurance when all of the other major countries did between 1883 and 1910? Paul Starr (1982) provides an important, fascinating, complex, and lengthy analysis of the social, political, and economic phenomena of this period. Despite a great deal of interest, analysis, lobbying, and legislative effort, the American public rejected government-sponsored social insurance, including national health insurance. The opposition of organized medicine contributed to this rejection, but there were other forces that may have been crucial, including the absence of political unrest in the United States, as compared with Europe, and the widely dispersed, disparate, and decentralized state governments in this country, as opposed to the more authoritarian and centralized governments of Europe.

Child mental health services were barely bit players in this historical period. Children's problems were still the province of political and social concerns. Child labor, after a half century of agitation, was still a major problem in 1910 and after. The problems of orphans and other dependent and neglected children had occupied the attentions of volunteer social and church agencies for some time. It was feared that these problems were leading to delinquency in children, and it wasn't until the late 1960s that national legislation would attempt to separate, though not with complete success, the problems of dependency and delinquency. Mental illnesses in children and child psychiatry were yet to be described. Despite the occasional scattered case account of an interesting disordered child and the intense interest of psychoanalysis in the interior fantasy life of children, it was not until 1935 that Leo Kanner, M.D., introduced the first discussion of a clear-cut mental illness of children—early infantile autism—and identified the field of child psychiatry.

So during this first period of national concern about health care costs, when private health insurance, the quintessential American solution to health care costs, was invented, child psychiatry was still a peripheral concern, and it was not really a participant in setting health care economic policies during the next 50 years. The public's primary concern was about the cost of acute hospitalization, and the American public, speaking through business concerns, labor unions, politicians, and the AMA, again rejected national health insurance and opted for privately paid group health insurance. Later, the employer shared the expense with the worker, and still later, major tax incentives would be given both to employers who sponsored group health insurance and to the employees who were the beneficiaries. Neither had to pay taxes on these monies, and health care costs started on a long, wonderful, rising curve of expenditures, which for many years seemed to be a free ride in everybody's interest.

Organized medicine first opposed employer-sponsored group health insurance according to the principle of not allowing any third party between the doctor and the patient. Three general strategies developed for payment of health benefits:

1. Indemnity benefits, which reimburse the subscriber for medical expenses, though usually not the entire bill;
2. Service benefits, which guarantee payment for services directly to the physician or hospital, often covering the subscriber's bill in full;
3. Direct services, that is, the provision of health services to the subscriber by the organization receiving prepayment (Starr, 1982).

These three different strategies initiated different kinds of involvement for the intervention of third parties between the beneficiaries and the providers of health care.

Blue Cross usually dates its origin from late 1929 at Baylor University Hospital in Dallas, Texas. These plans evolved distinct from commercial indemnification insurance. They were locally organized and controlled, nonprofit, covered only hospital charges, provided free choice of physician and hospital, and required little start-up capital since the member hospitals guaranteed to provide the services regardless of the remuneration. The American Hospital Association played a major role in promoting community group health service plans to pay the costs of acute hospitalization. The AMA, throughout the mid-1930s, opposed the extension of payment to medical care. This established the split between payment for hospital care and payment for care by the physi-

cian, a topic to be revisited in the 1960s and the late 1980s. Simultaneously, the AMA was able to continue the essentially monopolistic control of the medical profession over the health care market and health institutions (Starr, 1982).

By 1940, commercial indemnification insurance carriers had about 3.7 million subscribers, whereas the 39 Blue Cross plans had 6 million total participants. More was to be heard from the direct service strategy later.

Despite the opposition of the AMA, the majority of doctors were able to support, and sought, political and legal protection for medical service plans that were under the control of the local medical societies. Thus, Blue Shield was born and by 1945 had 2 million subscribers, whereas its older Blue cousin had 19 million. So before World War II, health insurance was just emerging as a benefit of employment. In the late 1940s, unions sought and achieved protection for their right to collectively bargain over health benefits. By 1954 unions were negotiating the purchase of 25% of the health insurance in the United States (Starr, 1982). Such negotiations forced the naturally cautious and restricted coverage of insurance carriers to be extended. A landmark for psychiatric coverage was the American Auto Workers 1964 contract that extended coverage to 25 outpatient psychotherapy sessions.

In the early 1960s, child psychiatry began to ease into the world of insurance benefits through the poorly defined concept of "medical necessity." Early in the history of the insurance movement, when the approval and support of the medical profession were not assured, it was absolutely necessary to give control of the benefits to the physicians. Medical necessity was the felicitous phrase written into every insurance contract to say that the insurance carrier would pay for what the physician ordered. Similarly, the insurance carriers had found it politically unwise to question the quality of care provided by physicians. This resulted in a self-deceptive fiction that all physicians were equally well prepared and competent to perform any procedure included in the repertory of their specialty.

In any event, "medically necessary" became the route of entry for the newly confirmed medical specialty, child psychiatry. Also reasonably new in any numbers were psychiatric units in general hospitals. Throughout the next two decades, medical schools and university hospitals would train enough medical and surgical specialists that almost every community could have its own community hospital with a full array of specialists. Thus, the large university teaching hospitals produced their own competition. Child psychiatry began as a strictly outpatient endeavor, but gradually through the 1970s and 1980s learned the advantages of inpatient work, especially with adolescents.

With the financial support of insurance benefits and an untreated population, it did not take long for child psychiatry to become firmly established in the private sector. Psychologists and social workers also qualified for reimbursement from insurance contracts, as they became independent practitioners supported by antitrust legislation, as well as by laws that forbade restraint of trade. Competition in the private sector tended to weaken the traditional bonds between child psychiatrists and other members of the original child guidance team, and solo private practice became the preferred organizational style and delivery system for child psychiatry until the economic wars of the 1980s.

COMMUNITY MENTAL HEALTH

The election of John F. Kennedy in 1960 brought a new, liberal agenda into the eyes of the public. Health policy makers began criticizing the recent emphasis on hospitalization reflected in the Hill-Burton Act. The Kennedy Administration rediscovered the community and community participation. Waiting in the wings for some years had been a small group of psychiatrists who advocated "community psychiatry" to replace the old state hospital system. The Joint Commission on Mental Illness and Health (1955–1960) published a report calling for the federal government to fund clinical services in the same manner that it supported education and research (Joint Commission on Mental Illness and Health,

1961). In 1963 Congress approved legislation to fund the construction of community mental health centers, and 2 years later the funds for staffing grants were approved (Starr, 1982). Again, a new organization and a new system to deliver mental health services was initiated by a new source of money.

The new organizations were to be known as community mental health centers (CMHCs), and each one was to serve a catchment area of 250,000. Eventually about 750 centers were in operation. It seemed to many that there was an unacknowledged but obvious desire to reduce the influence of medicine in this new delivery system. Symbolically the ascendancy of the term *mental health* rather than the more medical *mental illness,* the use of *center* rather than *hospital,* and the emphasis on participation by the objects of the service tended to reduce the influence of scientific medicine. Indeed, this new, primarily ambulatory demonstration movement brought in new sources of money and energy but was woefully lacking in new information. The new organization was "meant to overcome the rigidities of the traditional social service agencies" (Starr, 1982, p. 366). It was left to the pioneers to find innovative new philosophies and practices. One of the most promising was Art Pearl's verbally transmitted aphorism that "in any helping organization, the one who gets the most help is the helper."

This philosophy led to widespread inclusion of community residents, patients, and expatients into the staffs of CMHCs. The Johnson administration had chosen the route of giving funds and control to local community agencies as a way of breaking through racial, class, and bureaucratic barriers. The War on Poverty had to be waged as if poverty were a disease. The pathology of poor people was the absence of money and the consequent inability to access the means of improving their own lot. The Peace Corps had pioneered methods to encourage the poor of foreign nations to be able to use instruction and seed money to overcome great obstacles. Most of the community programs of the War on Poverty tried to follow the example of the Peace Corps and to respect the dignity of poor people in the community and their ability to organize, learn, and work to solve their own problems. At times and in some places, the CMHCs looked like employment programs. A few traditional programs, such as the Philadelphia Child Guidance Clinic, made almost complete conversions. This clinic devoted much of its service effort to training local black residents to become family therapists. Needless to say, there was internal conflict with that portion of the program still dedicated to professional training and affiliated with the University of Pennsylvania. It took nearly 20 years to reintegrate the philosophical fragments.

Although some child psychiatrists, including the author, embraced community mental health (Rafferty, 1967, 1975), the profession as a whole was restrained in its enthusiasm. Child psychiatry had always been an outpatient specialty, and clinics that traveled into rural communities had been a feature of both the Institute for Juvenile Research and the University of Colorado since the late 1920s. As with family therapy, which also came into vogue at this time, many child psychiatrists thought that they already practiced community psychiatry. Some of the famous old child guidance clinics became incorporated into CMHCs. This was virtually the only way that a CMHC developed a strong child psychiatric component. Although child and adolescent mental health services were one of the five components (emergency, outpatient, inpatient, consultation, child) required for federal funding, these services were most often combined with consultation and seldom rose above that level unless some independent source of funds, such as from a preexisting child guidance clinic, was available.

The CMHC Act did encourage the development of consultative practices, especially in day care centers and schools (Rafferty and Mackie, 1967); so, although the CMHC did not appeal to the child psychiatrist with an exclusive commitment to long-term, dynamic psychotherapy, it did structure another clinical modality that could be used with many different clinical syndromes and in many situations where psychotherapy was not appropriate. Community psychiatry also had appeal for the child and adolescent psychiatrist who was concerned about mental health services for large populations and for those other than the middle and upper classes, who did not have broad insurance coverage.

For one brief shining moment in the history of CMHCs, Congress did establish Project F, a fund of a few million dollars for 50 states, dedicated to children. President Nixon promptly impounded the funds for a few years before he was forced by law to release the money. A number of small, innovative demonstration projects were developed, frequently involving early childhood education and treatment.

Many CMHCs developed affiliations with local or university community hospitals. Federal law permitted both facilities to access CMHC construction funds. Such units often provided a haven for psychiatrists fleeing the state hospital systems. These adult units were not of interest to the child or adolescent psychiatrist. Later, the development of adolescent units in private psychiatric hospitals and in general hospitals contributed to the growth of private sector child and adolescent psychiatric practice.

During the 1960s' rediscovery of community, there were comparable neighborhood programs for pediatrics and ambulatory family medicine. By 1966 there were eight neighborhood health centers under the sponsorship of the Office of Economic Opportunity and over 150 by 1971, counting those also started under Department of Health, Education, and Welfare (DHEW) planning grants. The objectives again emphasized indigenous competence and leadership. In the DHEW plans of the time, the neighborhood health center, rather than Medicaid, was to be the method of distribution of health care services to the poor (Starr, 1982).

The community mental health movement ran into the economic realities of most federal demonstration programs, which seldom secure state or local monies to follow the federal seed money. Some states did provide funds far in excess of the federal contribution, but they were subsequently confronted with the state budgetary realities that followed the OPEC oil crisis of the 1970s. It has always been difficult to identify within the large state mental health department budgets funds earmarked for child and adolescent services. Child psychiatrists have seldom been included within the power structure of these departments because units for children or adolescents were not part of the state hospital tradition. Even now, such units tend to be add-ons and grudgingly financed. Those few states that developed substantial regional and community child psychiatric programs experienced serious budgetary shortfalls through the 1970s and 1980s and were forced to curtail child and adolescent services.

MEDICARE AND MEDICAID

The liberal agenda of the Kennedy administration received a major impetus toward implementation and expansion by the succeeding president, Lyndon Baines Johnson. The interest in public discussion of national health care delivery systems was again aroused. Group health insurance had been a solution to the furor about health care costs in the 1930s. But the impoverishing expense of medical and hospital care was again newspaper headlines. The plight of the aged poor was particularly tragic. But there was also wide realization that although health insurance was wonderful, it did not provide access to health services for the poor and uninsured.

Even by 1958, still within the Eisenhower years, Medicare had become an overriding issue (Starr, 1982). A modest amendment to Social Security legislation had been introduced but had already drawn the wrath and well-financed political opposition of the AMA. It was not until 1964, amid the contagious excitement of the War on Poverty, that Medicare was again proposed to pay hospital costs for the aged. However, the excitement of the moment caught even the AMA, whose own survey showed that the people were solidly supportive of medical services for the poor. So in July 1965 President Johnson signed into law a three-part bill.

The three parts had different targets, different legislative histories, different constituencies, different sources of payment, and, not surprisingly, different fates 20 years later. Medicare Part A was a compulsory hospital insurance program for the aged under Social Security. Medicare Part B was a government-subsidized voluntary insurance to cover physicians' bills. Medicaid was a federal/state cost-sharing program that encouraged and assisted states to expand their programs of medical care for the poor, with special emphasis on pregnant women, dependent children, and the handicapped.

These pieces of legislation had tremendous impact on the development of the health care industry in the United States. They had little direct effect on the care of mentally ill children and adolescents. Psychiatry as a whole had only a small role in Medicare. Reimbursement for outpatient psychiatric services for the aged was severely limited for years to less than $500. Inpatient care was reimbursed in the same manner as for other illnesses. Medicaid had more promise, at least for the general health care of children and adolescents. But the promises went little fulfilled. There was tremendous variation in the way that different states bought into the Medicaid program. A few states, such as Pennsylvania and California, chose all of the options and set rates for diagnostic and treatment services comparable to customary doctors' fees. Some elected for a reasonable list of options but set fees in such a manner as to discourage the participation of physicians. Other states chose minimal options.

In those states where the volume of child and adolescent patients seen in solo office or clinic practice was significantly increased by the addition of poor people paid for by Medicaid, there was little effect on the shape or style of such practice. On the other hand, there was the introduction in a number of states of the 21-day period of hospitalization for children and adolescents. Until the introduction of Medicaid, the norm for inpatient care of children and adolescents had been set by the long-term tradition of the residential treatment centers. An occasional university hospital or children's hospital operated inpatient units for diagnosis only, but at that time, descriptive diagnoses for children and adolescents were not respected. For the occasional child psychiatrist who wanted to secure medical staff privileges in a general hospital, Medicaid provided a financial bonanza. The youngsters eligible for these units were the most severely damaged, with the least available family support, and they were usually unwelcome in school. It was amazing that some of these programs provided exemplary diagnostic and stabilization services. Thus, the brief length of stay (LOS) for children and adolescents is not an invention of the late 1980s. The term, borrowed from general medicine and surgery, *an acute hospital* stay was no more accurate then than now.

The state hospital systems were greatly helped by Medicare and especially by Medicaid. Up until then, the state hospital was rapidly filling up with the aged, who were not so much mentally ill as dependent and not well cared for anywhere, including the back wards of the hospitals. It quickly became possible to transfer these patients to nursing homes, thus accomplishing a significant part of the move to deinstitutionalization.

The importance of Medicare for the systems of delivering mental health to children and adolescents comes from an entirely different and indirect source. Until the advent of Medicare, the physician had been in total control of health care. Hospitals had become more necessary for the new, technically superior surgical procedures. Hospitals were the places where doctors worked. Legally, they were hotels or inns where physicians provided diagnostic and treatment services. It was frequently said that doctors had the ultimate legal responsibility and risk. Medicare changed much of that by significantly increasing the role of the hospital and simultaneously contributing to the development of a new health care industry in which there were many players. The profession of medicine was forced to share its status and power with many other players, including new, powerful hospital corporations, hospital administrators, and other professional disciplines.

Politically, the proponents of Medicare had to make some important accommodations and compromises. For physicians it was agreed to pay the usual, reasonable, and customary fees. For hospitals the legislation adopted the practice followed by Blue Cross of paying hospitals according to their costs and to pay depreciation on hospital assets on an accelerated basis (Starr, 1982). Medicare made an entirely new population of people eligible for reimbursed health care and provided a major infusion of capital into the system. Capital reimbursement and the erasing of the red ink of bad debt and uncompensated care enormously strengthened the financial position of hospitals, enabling them to qualify to accumulate and borrow capital on their own.

It was ironic that the liberal, quasi-welfare state agenda of the Kennedy and Johnson administrations was instrumental in privatizing the hospital industry and in establishing a competitive market for health care products. The private for-profit segment of the hospital industry was given great impetus by this explosion of financial resources and guaranteed profits. Nor would the effects of the monetarization of health care be limited to the for-profit hospital sector. Nonprofit hospitals quickly learned how to use surplus funds to expand their services, scope, and physical plants. The clinical laboratory industry, the pharmaceutical industry, the hospital supply industry, the manufacturers of hospital equipment and medical devices, the architects and hospital construction industry, and the labor unions all were able to join in on the establishment of a relatively free market in health care.

Members of the medical profession attributed their share in this good fortune to their personal skills, high-quality care, and their close relationships to their patients. Child and adolescent psychiatrists, as usual somewhat peripheral to the whole scene, were fundamentally preoccupied in the private and inward-looking intricacies of transferences and countertransferences, which could be managed only one at a time. The benefits of pharmacotherapies were not as apparent in child and adolescent patients. The presence of major affective disorders in adolescents was something yet to be appreciated.

So it was left to the for-profit hospital industry to recognize the unmet need of hospitalization for adolescents. Adolescence had, of course, been recognized as a stage of development by the ancient Greeks. But child guidance clinics and child psychiatry, though accepting adolescents as patients, had not deemed it necessary to differentiate them in their organizational names. It was those psychiatrists who had expanded from their training in adult psychiatry to an interest in the older adolescent and younger adult who demanded special recognition for the adolescent patient. The founding of the American Society for Adolescent Psychiatry (ASAP) in 1962 was a milestone in this process and preceded the growth of adolescent inpatient units. The primary focus of members of ASAP remained psychoanalysis and long-term psychotherapy. It was 25 years later that the American Academy of Child Psychiatry and the American Board of Psychiatry and Neurology saw fit to recognize adolescents in their official designations.

Eventually the adolescent inpatient unit would change the shape of the entire field from an almost exclusively outpatient specialty to one in which members increasingly recognized the professional, technical, and financial rewards of inpatient work. Few of those who made the shift appreciated the role of Medicare in their new opportunity. Nor did many understand the long, tortuous history of employer-sponsored group health insurance. Many child and adolescent psychiatrists trained after 1970 seemed to believe that reimbursement by insurance carriers was an inalienable right. These would be the ones who experienced the greatest shock and trauma when the cost of health care again became a topic of national debate.

DRG-HMO-IPO-RBRVS

The decade of the 1980s may well become known as the time when acronyms finally defeated doctors. It took only a few years of Medicare for health economists and federal budget watchers to know that serious trouble was inevitable. The American political system has never lent itself to systematic or comprehensive planning. Few industries in the United States participate in a true free market, certainly not the health care industry. But on the other hand, no industry in this country has ever been planned. So it should really be no surprise that planning of medical care and health care has never been successful despite the almost continuous existence of some planning group since the beginning of the 20th century. No major policy change in health care has ever been supported by the kind of informed, data-driven study that would permit accurate forecasting of the results. Every multimillion, or later multibillion, dollar change in the delivery systems has been an experiment, no matter how florid the rhetoric of planning.

The politics of Medicare and Medicaid had left control of medical and hospital services to the doctor and the hospital. These legislative actions have frequently been compared to giving doctors and hospitals blank, signed checks. Doctors, naturally, did not see anything wrong with a blank check. They believed they deserved and were entitled to such trust. Psychiatrists never fully appreciated this because they never were trusted with the blank check by either government or insurance carriers. By 1970 the health policy makers in the Nixon administration were desperately seeking a means of controlling health care costs, and by then they knew that this had to mean controlling the practice patterns of physicians and hospitals.

President Nixon delivered a special message in which he called for a new approach to "bring together a comprehensive range of medical services in a single organization so that a patient is assured of convenient access to all of them. And it [should provide] needed services for a fixed-contract fee which is paid in advance by all subscribers" (United States Congress, 1971). He called this organization a health maintenance organization (HMO) and identified the change in incentives for physician behavior. Physicians should be paid for reducing morbidity, for keeping people well, rather than for treating as many illnesses with as many different procedures as they could invent, in as many sick people as they could find. Health economists had discovered volume of care as a major villain (McKinlay, 1981).

The HMO was not new. The "friendly societies" that existed throughout Europe and to a lesser extent in the United States in the late 1800s and the large contract physician groups sponsored by industries such as the railroads and by such unions as the United Mine Workers at the turn of the century and into the early 1900s had been such organizations. A series of reports from 1927 to 1932 of the Committee on the Cost of Medical Care advocated prepayment and group practice (United States Congress, 1971). Most of the prototype organizations, including Kaiser Foundation Medical Care Program, had their origins in the years 1930–1940.

The crux of the HMO philosophy is to organize services in such a way that the participating physician is not rewarded for unnecessary referrals to specialists, unnecessary hospitalizations of patients, or unnecessary diagnostic tests or surgical procedures. The HMO is financed by capitation, that is, a prepaid, fixed fee per subscriber per year. The actual cost savings of an HMO are usually traced to the savings on the costs of hospitalization for the total population of subscribers.

Despite the enactment of encouraging legislation at both the state and local level in 1973–1974, the growth in HMOs was slow, but it was steady. The user of health care services is notoriously slow to change. The consumer is not knowledgeable enough about medical and health services to truly make an informed choice. Decisions seem to be made on the basis of familiarity and trust in the family physician (Mechanic, 1989). Since the prevailing fee-for-service system was left intact, there was no initial rush to the HMO. Legislation had established the criteria for a "federally certified HMO" and required all employers of a certain size to offer an HMO as an option to regular health insurance. Primarily the young, the unmarried, and those without an existing relationship with a physician elected the HMO option.

Despite the Kaiser-Permanente pattern of providing reasonable access to ambulatory psychiatric care, the federally certified HMO requirements did not include psychiatry. Clearly, HMO management was uncertain of its ability to control mental health services. Over the next 15 years, mental health services in HMOs would increase slightly. Primary care physicians had always treated a large proportion of patients with "nervous and mental disease." Even in fee-for-service practice, many primary care physicians preferred to hold on to the overall management of patients and to refer to social workers and psychologists for "the talking therapies." The development of mental health services in HMOs followed this pattern.

HMOs, from the beginning, developed in several different models. The Kaiser-Permanente closed staff version is the most successful in controlling costs. Kaiser-Permanente owns and operates its own hospitals. The medical staff belongs to a partnership group practice exclusively related to the HMO. Other closed staff models would utilize community hospitals, sometimes with a discounted contract and sometimes without. The medical staff could be on salary rather than being partners in a group practice.

There can be almost infinite variation, but preferred provider organizations (PPOs) and individual practice associations (IPAs) are common. The IPA represents an effort of the local medical societies to establish physician networks of their members in order to control the practices of a captive HMO. The PPO establishes a network of physicians and hospitals that have preferred provider status with the HMO. This model eventually represented about half of the HMOs. With a PPO, the subscriber would not have to change physicians if his or her personal physician was a member. Patients are seen in the doctor's office, thus avoiding the expense of building one or more physical plants. One of the biggest problems for an HMO is the start-up costs. The PPO arrangement minimizes these. In turn, the physician is not dependent on one organization and can run his or her office as usual and relate to a number of capitation arrangements. The office staff has the task of keeping track of which patient belongs to which PPO.

The key element of any HMO is the centralized and standardized control of the physician's pattern of practice. The closed staff model is the ideal but requires a total commitment on the part of the physician to the HMO and competes with the community of nonmember physicians. The PPO models sacrifice control and efficiency for the benefits of being better able to fit into the medical community. The individual physician might belong to several different PPOs, making it problematic for the PPO to have sufficient control. Control of the physician's pattern of practice became the key element in all efforts to control the rising costs of health care. "Managed care" became the generally accepted euphemism, and every later innovation or delivery system experiment was designed to adapt managed care for each corporation or insurance contract. Despite the dearth of psychiatry and child psychiatry in the HMOs and PPOs, these specialties after 1980 rapidly came under the purview of managed care.

Any economic system is, to a significant degree, a system for rewarding performance, to provide members of society with the incentives to behave in socially responsible ways. Performance, however, must be measured if it is to be rewarded (or in the case of socially undesirable behavior punished) and in many instances there are enormous difficulties in developing adequate operational measures of performance (Weisbrod, 1989).

Health economists have always understood that the control of costs depended on control of physicians' behavior. But there has never been any way to measure the productivity, efficiency, or efficacy of a physician. Each doctor is a rugged individualist, and organized medicine has fought for the principle that only other members of the profession could or should evaluate and control physicians. However, first health care and now mental health care have indisputably become of tremendous importance to the nation and too important to be left to the monopolistic control of physicians. The health care industry is a major contributor to the national GNP as well as a major expense to both government and corporate America.

The problem of measuring health care productivity, utilization, and quality had to be resolved. A breakthrough occurred when in 1980 two members of the Yale University School of Public Health developed computer software called the Grouper that could operate on national data provided by the Medicare Uniform Discharge data set on each hospitalized patient. The bare skeleton of diagnostic and demographic data, when aggregated into a database of over a million records, became a powerful tool to control the utilization of health care. The Grouper was able to formulate a list of Diagnostic Related Groups (DRGs) for medical and surgical procedures that permitted the establishment of a valid average length of stay for each category. Each DRG could be assigned an annually adjusted fixed fee.

Congress was fascinated with the concept and quickly installed in 1983 a prospective payment system (PPS) based on DRGs and providing for a fixed price to be paid for each of eventually 477 diagnostic groups. A complex mechanism to phase in regional and national prices was provided, along with accommodations in different kinds of hospitals: rural, urban, teaching, sole provider, etc. Medicare had learned from the HMOs that control of hospital costs was the way to save money, so the PPS applied only to hospitalized patients. Realistically, it was easier to control 11 million admissions to 7,000 hospitals for 477 DRGs than to monitor 350 million claims for 500,000 physicians for 7,000 different procedures (Roper, 1988).

The diagnostic and procedural categories for psychiatry, despite the progress made by the DSM-III, were too weak to support the operations of the Grouper, which utilized the International Classification of Diseases. For example, all child patients were aggregated in one general DRG. The American Psychiatric Association sponsored research on an even larger database and established that DRGs for psychiatry and child psychiatry explained less than 9% of the variance in length of hospital stay. With psychiatry representing only a small part of the Medicare market, Congress exempted both freestanding psychiatric hospitals and specialized psychiatric units in general hospitals.

From the perspective of Medicare, the PPS using DRGs was a great success. The hospital industry and the AMA did not strongly oppose DRGs. Some early windfall profits for hospitals and especially for teaching hospitals with special allowances for cost of residencies eased everybody into the system. For the first time the federal government had a handle on the distribution and financing of health care services. The data from hospitals began to reveal challenging variations in hospital costs, in utilization of specific procedures, in mortality data, and in professional profiles. Although still unable to directly control the pattern of medical practice, DRGs forced hospital administrations to manage their physicians as well as the mix of reimbursement sources, length of stay, and operating expenses. Annually the fate of hospitals rested on new regulations, the announcement of new DRG rates, and new market basket inflation-adjustment rates. According to a recent AMA survey, one of every eight physicians deliberately provided less care to Medicare patients. As a result of fee freezes and other controls on services, Medicare payment to physicians was from 10 to 20% below payment from other sources (*Health Week*, 1989). Rationing of health care services had become a reality.

The profit margin (surplus) for hospitals eroded drastically. With an oversupply of beds, many small rural hospitals closed, and mergers of two or more urban hospitals were common. The large hospital corporations reduced in size, sold off unprofitable facilities, and reorganized to reduce expenses, and some went out of business. Even the medical schools and university hospitals had to reorganize their budgets and the funding of their faculties. Indirectly the PPS gave every self-insured private corporation and every insurance carrier the incentive and the tools to control the cost of health care by managing the patterns of hospital and physician services. Managers concluded that many health care services were unnecessary, wasteful, of uncertain quality, and sometimes fraudulently provided. Gate keepers, managed care, outcome management, and physician networks selected by practice profiles became the rule for all of medicine.

By the end of the 1980s, the entire ambience of the practice of medicine had changed. Physicians were still nominally in control of their profession, but they had clearly lost control over the utilization of clinical services. Literally, for every patient, there was an applicable utilization review policy and some kind of review person on the telephone asking: "What?" "Why?" "How long?" and "How many?" Initially they asked questions. Then they began providing the answers.

But direct control of the physician's productivity and quality still temporarily eluded the regulators. There was no direct way of rewarding or punishing physicians for their productivity or lack of it. Since 1986 the Health Care Financing Agency (Medicare), the AMA, and most of the specialty societies had been cooperating with the Harvard School of Public Health to develop indices to relate the service procedures of one specialty to those of another. The indices, called Resource Based Relative Value Scales (RBRVS), were designed to reflect the actual resources of time, intensity, professional expenses, mental effort, knowledge base, and assumed risk consumed by the services. Full use of RBVRS will eventually facilitate measurement of a physician's productivity, the development of a national price scale, and the establishment of criteria for membership in provider networks or HMO staffs.

As the last decade of this century approached the midpoint, the ever-present and influential polls listed health care reform and control of crime as alternating number one and two topics of public concern, and political forces were again struggling to compile disparate ideas and philosophies into one complex piece of "reform" legislation.

CONCLUSIONS

In 1771 a Philadelphia Quaker physician, Thomas Bond, and his good friend Benjamin Franklin received a state charter to establish a place for the relief of the sick poor. This became the Pennsylvania Hospital and initiated the long march of medicine and hospitals through American history to the present (Rosenberg, 1987). Despite technological and organizational progress, the United States still has not found a way to care for the sick poor. The Constitution, the Bill of Rights, and the Declaration of Independence are the formal sources of documents of our political philosophy and system of governance. Just as these documents failed to address issues of race and gender, they also neglected the problems of the poor.

Under any system of government, the poor, by definition, do not have enough energy, money, or information. The poor do not have enough food, housing, fuel, transportation, education, legal services, or information. These services and products are as vital as health care. Nevertheless, health care has surfaced as the visible issue for political attention at this time, although one could suggest that control of much crime perhaps depends on control and amelioration of poverty.

The answers to race and gender are at least implied in the source documents. Not only are the poor not provided for, but acknowledgment of the poor is almost contravened by the basic assumption that individual responsibility and hard work properly exercised in a land of unfettered economic opportunity will provide for each citizen whatever is needed. There is no provision for failure, weakness, age, handicap, sheer misfortune, illness, or the side effect of technological innovations.

Presidents Roosevelt and Johnson led direct assaults against poverty in America with mixed results. Congress has passed incremental legislation such as the Social Security Act, Medicare, Medicaid, Aid for Dependent Children, etc. Legislation to address all citizens without a means test has historically been more acceptable than legislation that provides a transfer of wealth to a designated group or class. Many of the major efforts at social legislation have had serious unintended consequences on the national culture. Health care viewed as services or benefits to be universally provided would appear to be an area ripe for reform legislation. However, health care benefits provided to the complex varieties of uncovered poor presents serious problems in financing and transfer of wealth.

As to the potential of unintended consequences, there are two significant suspect areas. One is the area of expense to employers with the threat of loss of jobs, and the other is the health care industry itself. The health care industry in the United States comprises one-seventh of the nation's economy. A lot of people make their living from providing health care through the exercise of individual responsibility, hard work, and utilization of opportunity. They will not easily consent to a threat to their welfare.

Bumper sticker philosophy sums up the profound problem: "Where you stand on health care reform depends on whose ox is being gored."

References

Dewey J, Bentley A: *The Knowing and the Known*. Boston, Beacon, 1949.

Health Week, May 30, 1989.

Hospitals, August 20, 1988.

Joint Commission on Mental Illness and Health: *Action for Mental Health*. New York, Basic Books, 1961.

Kanner L: *Child Psychiatry*. Springfield, IL, Charles C Thomas, 1935.

Lathrop JC: *The Background of the Juvenile Court in Illinois: The Child, the Clinic and the Court*. New York, New Republic, 1925, pp. 290–295: cited in Bremmer RH: *Children and Youth in America*. Cambridge, Harvard University Press, 1971, pp. 504–506.

McKinlay JB (ed): *Health Maintenance Organizations*. Cambridge, MIT Press, 1981.

Mechanic D: Consumer choice among health insurance options. *Health Affairs*, Spring 1989, pp. 132–148.

Rafferty FT: Child psychiatry service for a total population. *J Am Acad Child Psychiatry* 6:295–308, 1967.

Rafferty FT: Community mental health centers and the criteria of quality and universality of services for children. *J Am Acad Child Psychiatry* 14:5–17, 1975.

Rafferty FT: A systems theory approach to understanding behavior. In: Balis GU (ed): *The Behavioral and Social Sciences and the Practice of Medicine*. Boston, Butterworth, 1978, pp. 327–336.

Rafferty FT, Mackie J: *The Diagnostic Check Point for Community Child Psychiatry* (Psychiatric Research Report 22). Washington, DC, American Psychiatric Association Press, 1967.

Roper WL: Perspectives on physician-payment reform. *N Engl J Med* 319:865–867, 1988.

Rosenberg CE: *The Care of Strangers: The Rise of America's Hospital System*. New York, Basic Books, 1987.

Starr P: *The Social Transformation of American Medicine*. New York, Basic Books, 1982, pp. 237–334, 366, 368, 371, 372, 375, 376, 487.

United States Congress: House Document no. 49. February 18, 1971.

Weisbrod BA: Rewarding performance that is hard to measure: The nonprofit sector. *Science* 244: 581, 1989.

121 NATIONAL POLICIES FOR CHILDREN, ADOLESCENTS, AND FAMILIES

Edward F. Zigler, Ph.D., and Matia Finn-Stevenson, Ph.D.

Researchers and clinicians in psychiatry, developmental psychology, and other disciplines related to mental health are becoming increasingly aware of the importance of policies to enhance family life, and of the need for legislative action to address the mental health problems of children and youth. The focus on legislative action on behalf of children is not new. As early as 1909, at the White House Conference on Children, policy recommendations for children's mental health care were made. At the numerous conferences, study panels, and commissions that have followed, children have been referred to as one of the most neglected groups in mental health, for whom appropriate policies and programs must be developed (e.g., Joint Commission on Mental Health of Children, 1969; President's Commission on Mental Health, 1978; Select Panel for the Promotion of Child Health, 1981). Although the concern for children is not new, it has taken on a different dimension in recent years, with mental health professionals demonstrating an avid interest in issues pertaining to social policy. Many of them are directing their work toward the understanding of how contemporary social problems contribute to mental dysfunction in children, not only reporting their research but also underscoring the policy implications inherent in their findings and suggesting a course of action.

The renewed interest in mental health policy issues is reflected in the contributions mental health professionals are making to the debate on health care reform. From the perspective of mental health, the proposed health care reform recommendations put forth by the White House hold much promise. If, on the basis of the recommendations, legislation is appropriately developed, it could lead to equating mental health with physical health and ensuring that children and adults have access to prevention and treatment options.

However, a careful scrutiny of developments thus far reveals potential problems. Solnit (1994) points out these concerns: (*a*) Mental health will not be on par with physical health until the turn of this century, and there will be copayment requirements that will discourage patients from seeking care. (*b*) In general, health care reform proposals focus on creating changes in health insurance with little or no concern for prevention practices that would promote the well-being of children and adults. This point is also made by Hamburg (1994) who notes that the underlying causes of mental health disorders, such as violence and poverty, are not addressed in the proposed health reforms. Failing to fully and appropriately address mental health needs will mean that children at risk for mental health disorders will not receive the preventive services they need and that many individuals with psychiatric disabilities will not have access to treatment.

In his analysis of the proposed health reform policies, Solnit (1994) not only points out potential problems, he also offers suggestions for change. He notes, for example, that one way to address the need for mental health services is to establish State Mental Health Authorities (SMHAs). The suggested SMHAs could be used to develop the various support systems, such as housing and social services, which are essential in the prevention of mental health disorders but which are now outside the scope of current discussions of health reform.

It is apparent, even in this brief review, that mental health can indeed become an integral and meaningful part of health reform in the United States, but this will only be achieved if mental health professionals become involved in the process, analyzing proposed plans and offering suggested changes. By participating in the development of policies in this way and by conducting studies relevant to social issues, mental health professionals not only can contribute to the accumulation of knowledge but also can act to improve the nation's capacity to address the needs of children and families.

In this chapter, we discuss the role of mental health professionals in the policy arena, as well as the possibilities and problems inherent in the utilization of mental health research in policy settings. Although a number of opportunities exist for mental health professionals to contribute to the development of policies for children and families, their effectiveness in this regard is dependent not only on their knowledge of scientific principles and findings from mental health research but also on their familiarity with the social policy process and their ability to work with policy makers.

THE FOCUS ON MENTAL HEALTH DISORDERS IN CHILDREN

The interest in social policy among mental health professionals was precipitated by a number of developments. One of these was the implementation during the 1960s and 1970s of federally sponsored social programs such as Project Head Start (Zigler and Berman, 1983; Zigler and Styfco, 1993; Zigler and Valentine, 1979). The proliferation of such programs, and the funds made available for them, enabled researchers and clinicians to apply their knowledge and training to such areas as program development and evaluation, which had not previously received their attention (Phillips, 1987; Salkind, 1983; Takanishi et al., 1983). Another development that fueled the interest in social policy was the recognition that children develop within the social context; they are influenced by various aspects of their immediate environment as well as by the more remote social institutions such as the school, the workplace, government, and the mass media, areas over which children and parents have little, if any, control (Bronfenbrenner, 1979). This realization gave impetus to a number of ecological studies and the compilation of information on children's behavior, achievement, and physical and mental health (Zill et al., 1983). On the basis of data generated by these efforts, it has become apparent that an ever-growing number of children and adolescents in the United States face serious problems that often result in mental dysfunction.

Scope of the Problem

This point is made in several documents, one of which is a report published by a committee of the Institute of Medicine (1989). The committee, convened at the request of the National Institute of Mental Health (NIMH), studied the mental health status of children and adolescents. It found that at least 12% of children under age 18 (7.5 million children) have a diagnosable mental illness and that many other children exhibit broader indicators of dysfunction, including substance abuse, teen pregnancy, and school drop-out, which the committee defines as consequences of or risk factors for developing mental disorders. Kazdin (1993), in a review of recent epidemiological studies, paints an even grimmer picture, noting that 17–22% of children under 18 suffer developmental, emotional, and behavioral problems, accounting for 11–14 million children.

These findings are not surprising. Similar findings are reported by the Children's Defense Fund in its analysis of children's mental health needs (Knitzer, 1982) and by the US House Select Committee on Children, Youth and Families (1987a), which held hearings on mental health issues. In both these analyses, it is noted that children experience mental disorders that vary widely in type and severity. The disorders encompass conditions ranging from serious depression or crippling states of anxiety to more moderate behavioral problems characterized by disruptive and antisocial acts. The consequences of such problems include suicide, serious harm to others, and the need to remove the children from their homes.

That so many children are affected by mental disorders suggests that the problem is of national concern. The costs involved in treating mental health disorders are difficult to estimate, in part because of comorbidity with other problems such as substance abuse, making it difficult to separate the costs of care associated with each disorder. Additionally, the information needed to calculate the personal, social, and other costs of childhood mental disorders has not been systematically collected (US House Select Committee on Children, Youth and Families, 1987a), thus rendering any current cost analysis preliminary at best. Even though they are as yet preliminary, the studies that are available suggest that the costs of childhood mental disorders are staggering. Rice et al. (1990) found that treatment services for mentally ill children aged 14 and under exceed $ 1.5 billion a year. Others suggest that the costs of mental illness in children are much higher since, besides treatment costs, there are indirect costs and costs for nonhealth services, which are borne by families, the schools, the juvenile justice system, and other social institutions (Office of Technology Assessment, 1986). Clearly, more definitive analyses are needed to establish the actual costs of childhood mental disorders, and such information is important if we are to have a context within which to make decisions about the care of mentally ill children and the allocation of funds to address their needs. But even in the absence of such data, it is evident that mental health disorders in children place a substantial burden on individuals, families, and society at large.

Contributing Factors

Perhaps even more significant than the findings on the prevalence and potential costs associated with childhood mental disorders are the findings on the factors that contribute to the development of such disorders. More research is needed to unravel the causes and determinants of childhood mental illness. However, much progress has been made in the past several decades, producing multiple lines of evidence which suggest that a variety of biological, psychological, social, and environmental factors are involved as causal agents, and that in some cases, an interaction between these factors exacerbates vulnerability to mental disorders. Of significance is the fact that in increasing numbers of children, social and environmental risk factors are implicated in the onset of mental dysfunction (Galston, 1993; Tuma, 1989). Included among these risk factors are prolonged separations between the parent and child (Tennant, 1988), physical or sexual abuse (Allen and Oliver, 1982; Kashani et al., 1987), poverty (Garmezy, 1985; Rutter, 1976), marital discord (Wallerstein, 1988), instability in the family environment (Rutter, 1987), and a variety of other stressors related to family life (American Psychiatric Association, 1987; Institute of Medicine, 1989; Tuma, 1989). Rutter (1980) points out that children who experience one of these risk factors may not be any more likely to suffer serious consequences than children with no risk factors. However, the more risks or stressors that are present in children's lives, the greater the probability of damaging outcomes.

It is also noted that some risk factors compound other problems, such as low birth weight and central nervous system difficulties, which, when they occur in isolation, may have no negative effects. Infant central nervous system difficulties, for example, may be overcome if the child is reared in a stable and supportive environment but are exacerbated if the child is raised in an unstable, poorly educated, low-income, or otherwise stressful family environment (Sameroff et al., 1987). Likewise, premature low birth weight babies, who are more vulnerable to environmental insufficiencies than are full-term babies, may experience developmental problems if they are reared by unresponsive adults but may suffer no negative consequences if they receive appropriate care.

Changes in Family Life

These findings raise concerns since many children today experience potentially damaging experiences that stem from difficult conditions in family life (Tuma, 1989). During the past 30 years, our society has undergone vast economic and social changes, which have transformed the structure of the family and the roles and responsibilities of men and women. These changes have made child rearing a more difficult task than it had been in the past and have created stressful conditions for children and adults.

Consider, for example, the increased fragmentation and isolation of the family. The growth in the number of single-parent families is particularly disturbing since it is often associated with multiple stressors for both parents and children. The presence of a female head of household, poverty, and the presence of young children are characteristic traits (although not ubiquitous ones) of single-parent families (US Bureau of the Census, 1988). Currently, one of every four children in the United States lives in a single-parent family, and among blacks the numbers are one of every two children (National Center for Children in Poverty, 1993). A related change in family life is the relative isolation and lack of social support that have occurred because of the increasing mobility of people in search of employment and other opportunities (S. McCullough, testimony presented to the US House Select Committee on Children, Youth and Families, 1987a: Packard, 1972). As a result, many families no longer live near or have access to the support and assistance of friends and relatives. Referred to by some as a decrease in "social capital" (Coleman, 1987), the lack of social support is notable, since having access to a support system often mediates the negative consequences of stress (Garmezy, 1985; Gore, 1980).

In addition to these changes in family life, an increasing number of families are experiencing serious economic problems; many of them are living in poverty. This is in part due to the growth in the number of single-parent households. Other contributing factors are cuts in public assistance and the decline in the real value of family income (Children's Defense Fund, 1993). In a report published by the Economic Policy Institute (1986) it is noted that between 1973 and 1984, weekly wages, adjusted for inflation, have declined by 14.5% and that hourly wages have declined by 10.1%. Reischauer (1987), in an analysis of the US job market, found that only one of three jobs pays enough to keep a family of four above the poverty line. With jobs paying so little, many women have had to join the labor force to supplement the family income. But even among dual-worker families, median family income, adjusted for inflation, has declined by 3.1% between 1973 and 1984 (Economic Policy Institute, 1986); had it not been for the additional money brought home by women, the drop in family income would have been even more severe: 9.5%.

The decline in real income and the increase in the number of families in poverty affect adults and children. However, for children the consequences are particularly serious in that a significant percentage of families in poverty are those with young children. According to the US Bureau of the Census (1988), the poverty rate of young families has almost doubled in the past 20 years. Currently, 32.6% of families where the primary breadwinner is 25 years of age or under are in poverty, and in families where the primary breadwinner is aged 30 or under, 21.6% are in poverty.

The ramifications of living in poverty are numerous and include assaults on children's physical and mental health. Margolis and Farran (1985) found that in many families, a drop in income leads to poor health care for the children. Klerman (1991) found that poor families have no access to health care and that other conditions associated with poverty, such as lack of money to spend on health-promoting activities, hunger, and lack of transportation and adequate housing further exacerbate the problem. As a result, poor children experience more health problems and have a higher mortality rate. In several other studies, it is indicated that there is a powerful albeit indirect link between poverty and mental health disorders, leading psychiatrists to the conclusion that poverty is one of the major risk factors in such disorders (Albee, 1986; Rutter, 1976). Although at one time mental dysfunction, low achievement, and other problems associated with poverty were discussed in terms of assumed negative traits of poor children, researchers now realize that the major sources of psychopathology associated with poverty stem from environmental stresses and feelings of powerlessness and frustration (Albee, 1986). It is further noted that, among poor families, there is a high incidence of poor prenatal care, low birth weight, and malnutrition (Brown et al., 1992), which are known to contribute to children's vulnerabilities to environmental stress (Institute of Medicine, 1989).

PREVENTING MENTAL HEALTH DISORDERS: POLICY DIRECTIONS

These stressful conditions are just a few examples of the changed circumstances under which many children live. Other potentially damaging conditions that result from marital discord, maternal employment, and the increasing reliance of families on child care are discussed later in the chapter. Although the majority of families are affected by these changes in family life, social policies in the United States have not kept pace with societal changes. Our society is, as a result, in a state of disequilibrium wherein social policies are not in synchrony with the realities of family life.

Contributions from Research

It is this disequilibrium that is creating difficulties for families. Not all mental health disorders in children stem from such difficulties. How-

ever, the stressful conditions under which many children live place a burden on children's ability to cope with the demands of school, the family, and relationships with peers. The problems that emanate from the changing conditions of family life touch on economic realities, traditions, and institutional structures, so solutions may be slow to evolve (Zeitlin, 1989). Nevertheless, mental health professionals can have a positive effect on family life: first, they can alert policy makers and the general public to how stress in families negatively affects the very core of society and, second, they can call for further studies of the conditions under which children now live and children's responses to these realities. This focus on research is important. It can deepen our understanding of how children are affected by different conditions and of why some children are able to cope with difficulties in their lives whereas other children succumb (Garmezy, 1985). The research can also enhance our understanding of the ways children cope with problems so that we can devise useful strategies for intervention and prevention. To illustrate how scientific research can be a constructive force in the policy process, we will discuss some of the studies related to major societal changes that have had a profound impact on family life.

MATERNAL EMPLOYMENT

One of the most critical and complex changes in our society has been the entry of a large number of women into the labor force. This phenomenon is especially apparent among women who have children. For women with school-age children, full-time employment has been relatively common for about two decades, with upwards of 70% of such mothers now working out of the home (Hoffman, 1989). Among women with infants and preschool children, more dramatic changes have taken place. In 1950 the percentage of women with children under age 6 who were working outside of the home was 11.9%; by 1987, it had grown to 56.8%. In 1987, less than 30% of women with infants 1 year old and under were working. A decade later it was found that 52% of these women are working (US Department of Labor, 1987, 1988), with many of them returning to work within a few weeks after the baby's birth.

The research on the effects of maternal employment on children has found that in and of itself maternal employment is not necessarily associated with either negative or positive effects (Greenberger, 1989; Hoffman, 1989). Rather, parental attitudes to the mother's employment are more significant in their effects on children than is employment itself (Hoffman, 1986, 1989). But researchers point out that although maternal employment appears to be benign in its effects on children, in many dual-worker families both the parents and the children experience an inordinate amount of stress. Although women have assumed new roles in the workplace, they have not abdicated their traditional responsibilities to family life and child rearing. This has resulted in role conflict and guilt among mothers in particular (Hoffman, 1989; Moen and Dempster, 1987), as well as changes in life-style and difficulties that permeate the whole family system. Studies have found that close to 40% of employed parents, both women and men, indicate that they experience severe conflict, guilt, and stress (Friedman, 1987). For children, this state of affairs means that not only do they have less time with their parents, but they are also affected by the fact that their parents are under stress from trying to do too much.

Not only families but also other institutions are affected by the increase in women's participation in the out-of-home labor force. Employers, concerned about worker productivity, are raising questions about women's juggling work and family responsibilities, and some of them are also beginning to realize that they may be losing valued female employees when child rearing conflicts with full-time work. There are also pressures on such institutions as the school, which have to implement changes in order to accommodate the needs of children not only during school hours but also before and after school (Zigler, 1987, 1989). Additionally, changes have occurred in some professions that were previously associated with flexible work schedules that enabled mothers to work and at the same time rear their children. Teachers, for example, are finding that they have to extend their workday and thus disrupt their own family life because many of their students' parents are working and unavailable for parent conferences and other school events during the day (Zeitlin, 1989).

Increased Demand for Child Care

Although numerous societal changes and problems are associated with women's participation in the labor force, none are as significant as the unprecedented demand for child care services.

Today, child care is one of the most widely recognized social problems. Virtually everyone, from working parents to chief executives of major corporations, is discussing the lack of good-quality, affordable child care services. Child care is the subject of debate at state and local level governments, where the need for child care services is noted. In a recent report on municipal problems in the United States, it was stated that the most important issue facing American cities is lack of child care. At the federal level, policy makers in both the US Senate and the House of Representatives are debating various policy approaches that may be implemented in an effort to address the problem (Zigler and Finn-Stevenson, 1989).

Two pieces of legislation have been enacted. One, the 1988 Family Support Act which, as part of an effort to reform welfare, includes child care assistance for women in school, training, or work. The other is the 1990 Child Care and Development Block Grant which, among other provisions, provides child care subsidies to low-income families. Although the provisions wherein these pieces of legislation may be considered a step in the right direction, there is just too little money involved (Children's Defense Fund, 1994a, 1994b). They may be considered, at best, only a partial solution to the problem.

This recent attention to the child care issue is not surprising, given the increase in the number of infants and children who need child care. However, it belies the fact that the child care problem is hardly new; it has been a major social problem for two decades. At the 1970 White House Conference on Children, the need for child care services was noted as the number one priority for the nation to address. However, two obstacles—ideological arguments against the use of child care as well as the lack of public awareness of the need for child care services—stood in the way of policy action on the issue (Nelson, 1982). As a result, the problem worsened, reaching crisis proportions before finally attracting national recognition.

Notwithstanding the attention that the issue now receives, child care continues to be regarded as an individual family problem to be addressed by parents. This is evident in that the majority of businesses do not make provisions to ease the stresses associated with balancing work and family life and that despite the enactment of the Family Support Act and the Child Care and Development Block Grant, we are still far short of having a comprehensive solution to the problem (Finn-Stevenson and Zigler, in press; Zigler and Lang, 1990).

There are numerous facets to the child care problem, one of these being the high cost of services. This is a major concern for parents, some of whom choose a child care facility solely on the basis of cost. This point is made by Hofferth and Wissoker (1992), who found that parents not only choose child care on the basis of cost, but also that they switch facilities if the price increases. Precise data on what families spend on child care are not available, but it is known that child care costs are anywhere between $ 1,500 and $ 10,000 a year, depending on the quality of care and the age of the children involved. It is estimated that full-time child care for preschoolers costs an average of $3000 a year, and that for infants the costs can exceed $9600 a year. With the cost of care being so prohibitive, it is not surprising that it is one of the major factors in choosing child care.

The high cost of care is significant for at least two reasons. First, child care costs are a major expenditure for families, and the amount of money families spend on child care is directly related to their income. Low-income families spend less on child care in absolute terms than do higher-income families, but the proportion of the family budget that is taken up by child care costs is greater among low-income families, who have to allocate as much as 25–30% of their earnings to child care (Friedman, 1987). Second, there is a relationship between the cost and quality of care, with good-quality care costing substantially more than poor quality, custodial care. This being the case, we may be witnessing the emergence of a two-tier system of child care in which the choices of care for low-income children are limited to low-cost and, potentially, low-quality care.

The fact that good-quality care is a privilege that only some children are enjoying is of concern because child care is an environment where children spend a large portion of every day. As such, it has significant effects on children's development and well-being. The long-term consequences of child care, especially for children who begin attending day care in infancy, are not yet known. In addition, the research on the topic is inconclusive, often yielding conflicting findings (Clarke-Stewart, 1989). However, there is consensus among researchers that children will be adversely affected by the child care experience unless they receive good-quality care (McCartney et al., 1982; National Center for Clinical Infant Programs, 1988).

In an attempt to define good-quality care, mental health professionals make a distinction between developmentally appropriate care that is responsive to the needs of children and care that is merely custodial in nature (Phillips, 1987). The determinants of good-quality care have been found to be an age-appropriate staff-child ratio, as well as the presence of providers who have knowledge of and training in child development (Roupp et al., 1979). Training in child development—rather than years of experience working with children—sets apart nurturing providers who respond to the varied and individual needs of young children from providers who are unable to provide children with appropriate experiences.

Having an appreciation for the importance of provider training, child development experts have taken steps to ensure that there are programs in place specifically designed to train child care providers. An example of one such national program is the Child Development Associate (CDA) National Credential Program, which was developed with initial funding from the US Office of Child Development (Ward, 1976). The CDA program provides competency-based training, assessment, and credentialing for child care workers. Although initially designed to meet the training needs of providers in child care centers for preschool children, it has expanded to include training for providers in infant day care centers and family day care homes.

In yet another effort, Provence (1982) has drawn upon research principles to provide guidelines for the operation of child care programs. Both this latter effort and the CDA program underscore two important points about the link between research and policy: (a) that research findings can be brought to bear on social problems and serve as the impetus for appropriate action (Zigler and Finn-Stevenson, 1987), and (b), that a thorough understanding of the problem—in this case, the factors that influence quality care—is essential if mental health researchers are to be able to make recommendations for appropriate action.

Research is also needed on the availability of care. There is little information on the number of child care facilities, level of quality, and staff qualifications. Additionally, although the information on the demand side—that is, who uses and needs child care—is better, that database also is inadequate; this results in some confusion and disagreement as to the issue of availability of care. Attempts to create a better national database on child care options and utilization have been made in recent years. In one such attempt, Kisker et al. (1991) found that although the supply of child care facilities for preschoolers has increased since 1977, there are still regions in the country where demand exceeds supply. Studies also suggest that the demand for child care is going to increase, given the growing presence of women in the labor force as well as other demographic factors and employment trends (Child Care Action Campaign, 1988). Additionally, it has been found that in two segments of child care, namely, child care for infants and toddlers (National Center for Clinical Infant Programs, 1988) and child care for school-age children, the demand far exceeds the supply (Seligson, 1989).

In terms of school-age children, it is noted that half the children who require child care services are school-age children between the ages of 5 and 12. An estimated 4–7 million of these children are left home alone before and after school and sometimes during school vacations as well (US House Select Committee on Children, Youth and Families, 1987b). As with other topics related to child care, research on the effects of being home alone is, as yet, in its infancy; very few studies examine the consequences on children of being left alone. On the basis of available studies, some researchers contend that there are no differences between children who are in self-care and children who are supervised when they are not in school (Rodman et al., 1985). However, there are many other researchers who are concerned that these children feel lonely and afraid and that they are at risk for injury (Garbarino, 1980; Long and Long, 1983). Additionally, in the most recent, wide-scale study on the topic, Richardson et al. (1989) found that among children and adolescents who are in self-care, there is greater prevalence of delinquency and drug and alcohol abuse than among children who are in programs before and after the school day.

Changes in the Workplace to Support Family Life

In addition to the possible harm to children, the lack of child care for school-age children is a source of concern and stress for parents. This has prompted discussions of the need to make changes in the workplace to create conditions that are supportive of family life. Several suggestions have been made, including corporate support of child care services. Although a few companies have developed on-site child care centers for their employees, and others partially offset the cost of child care for their employees or provide other supportive services, such as information and referral, the need for child care is too large for corporations to address alone. Corporate involvement can thus be conceived, at best, as only one part of a comprehensive solution to the child care problem.

However, there are other ways for corporations to support family life. For example, some corporations may be able to implement flexible schedules to allow employees time for child-rearing responsibilities (Bureau of National Affairs, 1986). Some corporations provide this option to their employees, but the majority do not (Friedman, 1987; Kamerman, 1983). In some businesses, flexible work schedules may prove to be counterproductive and therefore unworkable as a means to enhance family life. However, among some corporations, such changes can be effectively implemented if steps are taken to alert the corporate world to the need and importance of such changes in the workplace. It has been suggested that mental health researchers can help by engaging in relevant studies. Among the questions that need to be addressed, Stipek and McCroskey (1989) note that there is little research currently available on the different work schedules that support employees in their role as parents; the increased productivity, if any, associated with different work schedules; and other important questions, such as how do different work schedules for parents affect the frequency with which children are sent to school ill or are examined by a doctor? This latter research question is important in part because even in cases where parents have good child care arrangements, they need to be at home with their children when the children are ill. Parents' inability to take time off from work, however, has resulted not in any workplace policy changes but rather in the development of child care facilities that specialize in the care of sick children. This is disturbing, since children who are ill need to be with their parents. No studies are needed to establish this fact, but the American Academy of Pediatrics indicates that studies substantiate the fact that children's ability to overcome illness and benefit from medical treatment is directly related to their being with their parents during the illness. However, due to lack of advocacy on the issue, the policy response to the care of sick children has been child care for sick children rather than the institution of flexible work schedules for parents.

Related to flexible work schedules is the need for parental leave policies that would enable parents to spend time with their infants during the first several months after birth. The student in child psychiatry is well aware that the first few months of life represent a critical period for the development of attachment between parents and the infant and that within the context of a secure parent-infant relationship, the growing child thrives and is encouraged to become more autonomous (Ainsworth et al., 1978; Cicchetti et al., 1990). The first few months of life also represent a very stressful period of life that necessitates the adjustment of all family members to the newborn (Brazelton, 1985).

A Blue Ribbon Committee on Infant Care Leave studied the issue and found that an increasing number of women return to work very shortly after the birth of the baby. The committee recommended that in the interests of infant mental health as well as parents' well-being, one of the parents should be given the option of a paid leave of absence from work for the first 6 months after birth (Zigler and Frank, 1988). Although the importance of such leave is noted on the basis of medical and social science research (Hopper and Zigler, 1988), adequate parental leave is not available to most parents in the United States. Several states have enacted parental leave policies that offer, at best, six-months' unpaid leave over a two-year period for the birth of the baby or illness in the family (Finn-Stevenson and Trzcinski, 1991). In 1992, Congress passed family leave legislation which provides 12-weeks' leave for the birth of the baby or illness in the family. However, small businesses, which employ the majority of all workers, are exempt from the provisions of this act.

It is disheartening to note that the United States and South Africa are the only two industrialized nations that do not have a national parental leave policy. The business community is adamantly against any interference with their policies and has thus lobbied against any legislation that would mandate such a leave, which is why, in part, the family leave policy is so inadequate. However, the strong evidence from the research and the involvement of a number of psychiatrists, developmental psychologists, and pediatricians have together resulted in action on the issue at the state level (Finn-Stevenson and Trzcinski, 1991; Trzcinski and Finn-Stevenson, 1991; Zigler and Frank, 1988), causing employers to reflect seriously on the matter. As noted earlier, states have enacted a variety of leave policies; this action by the states served as a preface and perhaps the motivation behind the federal action on the issue (Finn-Stevenson and Trzcinski, 1991).

The above-stated policy changes are just a few examples of the many decisions that may be made to facilitate family life. Our discussion of such policy decisions is admittedly brief, but it illustrates the important role of scientific knowledge in identifying the needs of children and families and suggesting a course of action.

DIVORCE

Divorce is a fact of life for a significant number of families. The rate of divorce, particularly among families with children, rose dramatically between 1965 and 1979. Since 1979, the rate of divorce has declined and seems to have leveled off (Hernandez, 1988). Nevertheless, it is estimated that (a) about 50% of children born in the last decade will experience the divorce of their parents; (b) most of these children will experience the remarriage of one or both of their parents, and (c) after living for a period of time in a single-parent family, they will live in what has come to be known as a blended or reconstituted family (Hetherington et al., 1989).

In their investigations of children's responses to the divorce and remarriage of their parents, researchers found that for many children, divorce may have some benefits in that the children do not have to continue to experience unhealthy family relationships. Initially, however, most children experience changes in marital arrangements as stressful, and only some of them are able to cope with the changes and eventually adapt to their new family life (Hetherington et al., 1989). Many of the children suffer sustained developmental disruptions as a result of the changes in family life; some appear to adapt well in the early stages of family reorganization but show delayed negative effects (Wallerstein, 1988, 1991). Tschara et al. (1990), for example, found that children have difficulty adjusting to the divorce if they were older, had prior psychological problems, and had parents with more marital conflict. Hetherington et al. (1989) found that the long-term effects of divorce and remarriage appear to be related to a number of factors, including the child's developmental status, sex, and temperament; the quality of the home environment; and availability of support systems both to the parents and the child.

The number of stressors the child experiences is also a factor, since, as noted earlier, a single stress typically does not carry with it appreciable psychiatric risk, but multiple stressors increase the risk for mental dysfunction (Rutter, 1980). Particular concern is noted for children whose custodial parent experiences extreme economic difficulties for an extended period of time and/or whose noncustodial parent fails to pay for child support (Haskins et al., 1985). Children whose parents suffer emotional and psychological difficulties as a result of the divorce are also likely to experience multiple stressors. Researchers have found that when parents' distress is acute, the parents fail to attend to the needs of their children, they do not recognize the children's painful experience with the divorce, or they burden the children with their own adjustment difficulties (Kurdek and Blisk, 1983).

Also at substantial risk are children who are involved in prolonged custody fights. These children are the most vulnerable of children of divorce since custody battles can continue indefinitely. Judges attempt to make custody decisions on the basis of the best interests of the child. However, neither judges nor lawyers are prepared for the arduous task of determining the best interests of the child. Nor are they trained to interview the child, consider his or her needs and concerns, or weigh the urgency of the child's condition and circumstances (Wallerstein, 1986). Recognizing the child as the hidden client in divorce proceedings, Goldstein et al. (1973, 1979) have attempted to provide guidance to lawyers and judges by incorporating legal considerations within the framework of principles drawn from developmental psychology and psychiatry. They recommend that decisions regarding child custody be made quickly, that an effort be made to avoid prolonged proceedings, and that whatever decision is made have final effect that is not reversible. They further recommend that judges award full custody of the child to one "psychological parent." There is controversy surrounding this latter recommendation. Some psychiatrists emphasize the psychological value for some children of maintaining a close relationship with both parents, even those involved in a bitter dispute over custody issues (Guidibaldi et al., 1983). Although some of their recommendations are controversial, Goldstein et al. paved the way for other psychiatrists to think about the use of knowledge and theoretical principles in establishing criteria for practical decisions that involve children.

Mediating the Effects of Divorce

The need for mental health professionals to consider the policy implications of their work is underscored by Wallerstein (1986, 1988). Wallerstein further notes that although an increasing number of policy makers and legal professionals are seeking guidance from the mental health professions, the accumulation of psychological knowledge has not kept up with rapid changes that have occurred in family law. Hetherington and Camara (1984) make a similar point, indicating that the knowledge about the effects of divorce on children and postdivorce parent-child relationships is still fragmentary, with several important questions remaining to be addressed.

Although more research is needed, sufficient information currently exists for us to appreciate the widespread implications of the research and the opportunities that exist to mediate the consequences of divorce. In this regard, the knowledge of how divorce affects children and parents should be disseminated not only among mental health professionals but also among other professionals who work with children. Teachers, for

example, need to be alerted to these findings so they can be sensitive to any changes in children's behavior and offer them and their parents support and counsel about ways they can cope with the changes in their lives (Kurdek, 1981). Additionally, as noted earlier, the legal profession needs to be made aware of the research and its implications. Ideally, psychological support for parents and children should be made available immediately when the divorce proceedings begin. One important policy development has been the use of mediation services in divorce cases. These services are staffed by mental health professionals who have access to legal advice. Although initially begun as a way to curtail the high costs of divorce, families who have used mediation services note that one of the major benefits of the services is the availability of psychological support (Bahr, 1981).

The importance of psychological support for children of divorce should be made known to policy makers, who can make it a national priority to ensure that these children have access to support services. Several successful support programs for children of divorce have been developed in schools across the United States (Weiss, 1989). However, they are few in number and meet the needs of only a small percentage of the children who stand to benefit from such programs. Given the number of children who need such support, these programs should be made available in all schools, or at least in some schools in every community. The federal government can take a leadership role by making available funds that would finance the development of such programs.

OTHER EXAMPLES OF THE POSSIBILITIES INHERENT IN THE INTEGRATION OF RESEARCH AND POLICY

Development and Evaluation

The importance of support services is noted not only in reference to children and parents who experience divorce but also in reference to other individuals who encounter different types of stressful life events. Many families—for example, those who have premature or handicapped babies (Field et al., 1980; Goldberg and DiVitto, 1983) or who experience the illness or death of family members—have difficulty coping and are in need of some kind of support. Likewise, there are many people who need assistance with child rearing: many parents need help gaining the ability to simultaneously nurture and discipline children, or need assistance coping with transitional problems encountered during different stages of their children's development.

Support services are also needed to prevent chronic juvenile delinquency. Yoshikawa (1994) notes that there has been an increase in juvenile crime in the United States. There has been a 60.1% increase over a 10-year period in arrests of youths under age 18 for murder and manslaughter (Federal Bureau of Investigation, 1991). Juvenile crime is linked to the violence that has become part of the daily lives of families, especially those who are poor; it is experienced by increasingly younger children (Osofsky and Fenichel, 1994). Yoshikawa (1994) documents several factors that are predictive of chronic delinquency: low socioeconomic status, convicted parents, low intelligence, poor parental child rearing, troublesomeness, and conduct disorders. His review of the research further suggests that programs that combine early family support and education and which include, among several aspects, a parent-focused informational and emotional support component, represent a promising direction for the primary prevention of early-onset, chronic delinquency. Other studies (e.g., Zigler et al., 1992) suggest that early childhood intervention and support programs are linked to the prevention of juvenile delinquency.

FAMILY SUPPORT PROGRAMS

In response to the widespread need for such programs, a host of family support services has been developed and implemented in recent years. The programs range from informal, grass-roots, self-help services such as Parents Anonymous and Parents without Partners (Whittaker and Garbarino, 1983) to more formal types of services that include professional assistance. These programs have been referred to as a "new breed" of programs in that they are rooted in the premise that the most effective way to create and sustain benefits for children is to improve their families and communities. However, this premise is hardly new and can be traced to Project Head Start (Zigler and Freedman, 1987b). Project Head Start, along with other social programs, was initiated over two decades ago in an effort to enhance the lives of young children. It was, and continues to be, an innovative program that includes a cycle of experimentation and revision that helps ascertain which types of services are best suited for and have the most impact on children. As a result of this cycle of experimentation and revision, and of recent research interest in the ecological study of children, the conventional wisdom about how to address the needs of children has shifted from child-centered programs to programs that focus not only on the child but also on the family as a whole (Bronfenbrenner and Weiss, 1983; Zigler and Berman, 1983).

Although the development of family support programs is conceptually traced to previously developed social programs, they differ in a number of ways. Most important, many family support programs are nongovernmental initiatives. Rather, they began as grass-roots efforts, initiated and sustained by individuals in response to stressful situations in their lives, and in absence of any other form of social support. Although several states are beginning to initiate family support programs (Powell, 1991; Weiss, 1989), such programs are still characterized by the lack of government initiative. Another characteristic of family support programs is that although the programs are varied in the type of services rendered and the population served, they share a commitment to provide emotional, informational, and instrumental assistance to family members, thus enabling individuals to cope with whatever problems they may have (Zigler and Weiss, 1985).

Primary Prevention

In helping individuals in these ways, family support programs exemplify a primary prevention strategy that focuses on the prevention of mental health disorders (Caplan, 1974). As noted earlier in this chapter, there is a clear and consistent relation in research findings between adaptive difficulties and heightened levels of stress (Bloom, 1979; Cowen, 1980; Hamburg, 1982). Other studies have established that both personal and situational variables may mediate this reaction and enable individuals who are vulnerable to become better able to cope. One such variable is social support. Social support has been found to improve an individual's ability to withstand stress (Cassell, 1976), to mediate the consequences of life crises (Gore, 1980), and to enhance general adjustment and well-being. Social support systems, according to Caplan (1974), should not be conceived of as the propping up of someone who is in danger of falling. Rather, they refer to efforts to augment an individual's strengths in order to facilitate mastery of the environment. Caplan (1974) further points out that social support as a means of primary prevention in mental health should not be perceived as a one-time intervention but rather as an enduring pattern of continuous or intermittent ties that help maintain the psychological and physical integrity of the individual.

Families, like individuals, have a certain life course in which, at particular points, stresses and crises are a natural state of affairs. At those times, support programs can be invaluable in helping family members to utilize their strengths and rally to cope with the problem, thus warding off severe family dysfunction and mental health disorders (Riessman, 1986). Although family support programs have this primary prevention potential, the degree to which they are effective in preventing mental disorders is not yet known. This is due to the fact that the growth and proliferation of family support programs has not been matched by evaluations of their efficacy. The reason for this may be that the programs are grass-roots efforts that were not known to or recognized by many researchers in the field of mental health until recently (Weiss, 1984; Whittaker and Garbarino, 1983).

However, the lack of evaluation data is a characteristic not only of family support programs but of other types of primary prevention programs as well. Cowen (1986) notes that evaluation studies are needed to separate some of the good and effective prevention programs now being tried from others that are simply "maintained by inertia or falsely placed conviction." Addressing the problem caused by the lack of evaluation data, Zigler and Freedman (1987a) observe that although family support programs are proliferating, they are doing so without any clear indication as to the direction their course of growth should take. On a more practical level, Cowen (1986) notes that the future of prevention programs in general and family support programs in particular depends on evaluations of their effectiveness, since the funding and therefore the continued existence of many programs is often dependent on the answer to a single question: Are these programs beneficial and cost-effective?

The evaluation of family support programs, although important, is not a simple task. In many cases, the programs have no explicitly stated goals, thus rendering an evaluation difficult (Weiss and Jacobs, 1988). Additionally, many of these programs are in the formative stage, too early to evaulate results accurately (Campbell, 1987). These and other problems associated with the evaluation of programs are not insurmountable. Indeed, they are being addressed by many researchers in mental health, who are finding that by participating in program evaluation, they not only contribute to the development of more valid evaluation methodologies (Weiss and Jacobs, 1988), they are also contributing to a theoretical understanding of children's development, thereby opening up new vistas for research and practice (Travers and Light, 1982). For example, on the basis of a review of existing evaluations of family support programs, researchers have found that those that are successful in addressing the multiple needs of families have four common features: they are comprehensive; they are flexible; they are located in the community; and they are results oriented, their ultimate goal being to strengthen families (Carnegie Corporation of New York, 1994). These findings about family support services are useful, for they provide directions for implementation and the replication of the services on a wider scale.

Problems in the Use of Research in Policy

The contributions that mental health professionals can make and the benefits that they can realize are evident not only in the development and evaluation of family support programs but also in other types of programs (Price et al., 1988), including such programs as the Interpersonal Cognitive Problem Solving program developed by Shure and Spivak (1988), which is designed for schools. Numerous other school-based programs have been developed by psychiatrists such as James Comer in an effort to prevent affective disorders in children and ensure responsivity to children's mental health needs. Indeed, as a result of their involvement in program development and evaluation, mental health researchers have accumulated a vast amount of knowledge that "totally transforms the nation's capacity to improve outcomes for vulnerable children" (Schorr and Schorr, 1988). This knowledge, derived from over two decades of program development and evaluation, includes concrete evidence of the effectiveness of a number of programs that reduce the burdens of risk factors in childhood, thereby reducing the probability of later damage. For a review of effective programs see Schorr and Schorr (1988) and Price et al. (1988).

There is evidence that it is not necessary to change everything—the structure of opportunity, the neighborhood environment, and other aspects of the child's life—to make a crucial difference for children at risk. However, this knowledge is not being utilized to alter the life path of many of the children who are growing up under stressful conditions (D. Hamburg, testimony before the US House Select Committee on Children, Youth and Families, 1987a; Schorr and Schorr, 1988).

The failure to utilize knowledge from the research stems from several problems. One such problem is that the information on effective programs is generally not shared with the public or with policy makers (White, 1988). Thus these programs, many of them at the demonstration stage, fail to be replicated on a larger scale. Even in cases where programs' potential benefits are known, there is skepticism that such programs, once they are replicated, will continue to be effective. Although this is a valid concern, Schorr and Schorr (1988) note that successful programs can be built upon if we can attract and train enough skilled and committed personnel, if we devise a variety of replication strategies, and if we resist the lure of replication through dilution. In an effort to serve as many children as possible, programs are diluted, thus diminishing their quality and potential benefits. Zigler and Berman (1983) note that the inclusion of more children at the expense of program quality has occurred even in such well-known programs as Project Head Start. They suggest continued monitoring of programs as a means of ensuring their effectiveness.

This point needs to be conveyed to policy makers and others who are in charge of the allocation of funds for program development and replication. However, although an increasing number of mental health researchers are working in the policy arena, there is still a rather uneasy relationship between them and policy makers. Maccoby et al. (1983) note that policy makers often regard researchers as impractical. From their perspective, they may be skeptical of policy recommendations coming from researchers who do not seem to understand the complexities of achieving a consensus among rival constituencies. Researchers, on the other hand, seem to regard policy makers as disingenuous and too willing to compromise even when the research evidence does not justify such action. Meltsner (1986) also observes that part of the tension and mistrust between policy makers and mental health researchers emanates from the assumption that knowledge from research is value free whereas policies are made in a value-laden context. However, this characterization of research and policy is misleading. Often, scientific research takes on the values of the investigators, as is evident in the questions asked, methodologies employed, and the interpretation and presentation of the findings.

Problems such as these serve to impede the utilization of research in policy settings. The problems are further exacerbated by the fact that researchers are often perceived as unable to provide clear answers to policy questions, or, looked at from another perspective, that policy makers are unable to ask questions in a way that would lead to valid and reliable research (Maccoby et al., 1983). In part, this problem stems from the unrealistic expectations of policy makers and their inability to appreciate that single studies cannot, in and of themselves, provide definitive answers to questions. But researchers also contribute to the problem. Sheldon White (1988) notes that often researchers are unfamiliar with the policy process or are unable to ''read'' political issues. They hold to long, slow standards of proof and refutation that are, in the policy arena, ''obstructive and nihilistic.'' Thompson (1993) makes a similar point, noting that, often, policy issues do not lend themselves easily to research and that research findings are often limited in their applicability to policy because of sampling and measurement issues. Although it is imperative that researchers uphold their professional standards and credibility as scientists (Zigler and Finn-Stevenson, 1987), there are times when findings from the research, even if they are not entirely conclusive, can nonetheless provide a direction for policy. For example, the research on the effects of child care on children's development is as yet controversial, yielding conflicting findings that serve to confuse the public and policy makers (Clarke-Stewart, 1989). Although research on the topic continues, researchers were able to convene and come to a consensus that indicated that as long as young children are in a good-quality child care settings, they will not be adversely affected by their experiences in day care. This led to a policy recommendation for efforts to monitor the quality of care children receive and ensure that all children receive care that is conducive to optimal development (National Center for Clinical Infant Programs, 1988). It is apparent that there are circumstances, such as the increasing number of children in day care, when our awaiting definitive conclusions from the research is counterproductive, especially when action can be taken at the same time that research on a particular issue is continuing.

STRATEGIES FOR CHANGE

Understanding what impedes the use of research in policy is important if mental health researchers are to have an impact in the policy arena. Lindblom (1986) identified four general guidelines for researchers to follow in order to encourage the use of research in carving out policy directions: (a) that researchers be concerned in a nonpartisan way with the values and interests of society in general and children in particular, (b) that they take a practical approach and suggest policies that are feasible and have a chance of attracting widespread political and public support, (c) that they respond to the needs of policy makers and provide them with recommendations for action on the basis of research findings, and (d) that they become cognizant of and responsive to the policy process.

It is also suggested that researchers make serious attempts to disseminate the findings from the research, not only to policy makers but also to the general public. No society acts until it has a sense of the immediacy of the problem (Zigler and Finn, 1981). The Great Society programs of the 1960s illustrate this point. During that time, social issues were covered in major newspapers and were in the forefront of national attention. There were daily stories on welfare mothers, reports on poverty, and expositions on hunger in the United States. Hence there was sympathy for the poor and support for the War on Poverty (Zigler and Valentine, 1979).

Although for a time thereafter there was appreciably less interest in issues pertaining to children and families, there are indications that this is changing. First, developmental psychologists, psychiatrists, and other mental health professionals are becoming aware of the need for public education on the needs of children (McCall et al., 1984). And, in a departure from their past practices, many mental health professionals are no longer satisfied with simply sharing information with one another. Rather, they disseminate their knowledge not only by presenting their findings directly to policy makers but also by taking steps to ensure that the information is covered in the popular media. Indeed, the dissemination of research in the context of the popular media has come to be accepted as an important aspect of the training received by some professionals in the field of mental health (Stevenson and Siegel, 1984).

Many mental health professionals are also receiving training in the integration of child development research and social policy, learning not only about the policy process but also about some of the ways to merge their knowledge with that of policy makers in the formation of programs and policies for children. Over the past 10 years, for example, the Bush Centers in Child Development and Social Policy at Yale University, the University of North Carolina at Chapel Hill, the University of Michigan, and the University of California at Los Angeles have prepared doctoral students and postdoctoral fellows in a variety of disciplines related to mental health to apply their knowledge in the policy arena. The success of such efforts is evident in the numerous issues, such as child care, parental leave, and the need for family support services, that only a few years ago were not discussed but that now command national attention. The success of these efforts is further evident in the fact that an increasing number of policy makers are now acknowledging the importance of knowledge from the research in the formulation of policies and are actively seeking the collaboration of professionals in the field of mental health. If mental health professionals and policy makers continue to work together in this spirit of collaboration, we will be able to bring about much needed societal changes that will assist family life.

References

Ainsworth MDS, Blehar MC, Waters E, et al: *Patterns of attachment: A psychological study of the strange situation*. Hillsdale, NJ, Erlbaum, 1978.

Albee GW: Toward a just society: Lessons from observations on the primary prevention of psychopathology. *Am Psychol* 41:891–898, 1986.

Allen RE, Oliver JM: The effects of child maltreatment on language development. *Child Abuse Negl* 6:299–305, 1982.

American Psychiatric Association: *Diagnostic and Statistical Manual of Mental Disorders* (3rd ed, rev). Washington, DC, American Psychiatric Association Press, 1987.

Bahr SJ: Divorce mediation: An evaluation of an alternative divorce policy. *The Networker* 2:1, 1981. (Available from the Bush Center in Child Development and Social Policy, Yale University, New Haven, CT)

Bloom BL: Prevention of mental disorders: Recent advances in theory and practice. *Community Ment Health J* 15:179–191, 1979.

Brazelton TB: Issues for working parents. *Am J Orthopsychiatry* 56:14–25, 1985.

Bronfenbrenner U: *The ecology of human development*. Cambridge, MA, Harvard University Press, 1979.

Bronfenbrenner U, Weiss H: Beyond policies without people: An ecological perspective on child and family policy. In: Zigler E, Kagan SL, Klugman E (eds): *Children, families, and government: Perspectives on american policy*. Cambridge, MA, Harvard University Press, 1983.

Brown JL, Gershoff SN, Cook JT: The politics of hunger: When science and ideology clash. *Int J Health Sci* 22:44–60, 1992.

Bureau of National Affairs: *Special report. Work and family: A changing dynamic*. Rockville, MD, Bureau of National Affairs, 1986.

Campbell DT: An experimenting society in the interface between evaluation and service provider. In: Kagan S, Powell D, Weissbourd B, et al. (eds): *Family support programs: The state of the art*. New Haven, CT, Yale University Press. 1987.

Caplan G: *Support systems and community mental health*. New York, Behavioral Publications, 1974.

Carnegie Corporation of New York: Starting points: meeting the needs of our youngest children. Report of the Task Force on Meeting the Needs of Young Children. New York, Carnegie Corporation of New York, 1994.

Cassell J: The contributions of the social environment to host resistance. *Am J Epidemiol* 104:107–123, 1976.

Child Care Action Campaign: *Child care: the bottom line*. New York, Child Care Action Campaign, 1988.

Children's Defense Fund: State of America's Children. Washington, DC, Children's Defense Fund, 1993.

Children's Defense Fund: Protecting our children: State and federal policies for exempt child care settings. Washington, DC, Children's Defense Fund, 1994a.

Children's Defense Fund: Child care tradeoffs: States make painful choices. Washington, DC, Children's Defense Fund, 1994b.

Cicchetti D, Cummings M, Greenberg M, et al: An organizational perspective on attachment beyond infancy: Implications for theory, measurement, and research. In: Greenberg M, Cicchetti D, Cummings M (eds): *Attachment in the preschool years: Theory, research, and intervention*. Chicago, University of Chicago Press, 1990.

Clarke-Stewart KA: Infant day care: Maligned or malignant? *Am Psychol* 44:266–273, 1989.

Coleman JS: Families and schools. *Educ Researcher* 16:32, 1987.

Cowen EL: The wooing of primary prevention. *Am J Community Psychol* 5:258–284, 1980.

Cowen EL: Expanding horizons in prevention research. *Contemp Psychol* 31:260–261, 1986.

Economic Policy Institute: *Family income in America*. Washington, DC, Family Policy Institute, 1986.

Federal Bureau of Investigation: Uniform crime reports for the United States, 1990. Washington, DC, U.S. Government Printing Office, 1991.

Field TM, Goldberg S, Stern S, et al. (eds): *High-risk infants and children: Adult and peer interaction*. New York, Academic, 1980.

Finn-Stevenson M, Trzcinski E: Mandated leave: An analysis of federal and state legislation. *Am J Orthopsychiatry* 61:567–575, 1991.

Finn-Stevenson M, Zigler E: *Schools in the 21st century: Expanding the traditional mission of the press*. Denver, Westview Press, in press.

Friedman D: *Family supportive policies: The corporate decision making process*. New York, The Conference Board, 1987.

Galston W: Causes of declining well being among U.S. children. New York, Aspen Institute Quarterly, 1993.

Garbarino J: Latchkey children: Getting the short end of the stick? *Vital Issues* 30(3): 1–9, 1980.

Garmezy M: Stress resistant children: The search for protective factors. In: Stevenson JE (ed): *Recent research in developmental psychopathology*. Oxford, Pergamon, 1985, pp. 213–233.

Goldberg S, DiVitto BA: *Born too soon: Preterm birth and early development*. New York, Freeman, 1983.

Goldstein J, Freud A, Solnit A: *Beyond the best interests of the child*. New York, Free Press, 1973.

Goldstein J, Freud A, Solnit A: *Before the best interests of the child* (2nd ed). New York, Free Press, 1979.

Gore S: Stress-buffering functions of social supports: An appraisal and clarification of research models. In: Dohrenwend BS, Dohrenwend BP (eds): *Stressful life events: their nature and effects*. New York, Wiley, 1980.

Greenberger E: Bronfenbrenner et al revisited: Maternal employment and the perception of young children. Paper presented at the 97th annual convention of the American Psychological Association, New Orleans, August 11, 1989.

Guidibaldi J, Cleminshaw HK, Perry JD, et al: The effects of divorce on child development. *School Psychol Rev* 13:300–323, 1983.

Hamburg D: An outlook on stress research and health. In: Elliot G, Eisdorfer C (eds): *Stress and human health*. New York, Springer, 1982.

Hamburg D: *Contemporary intergroup violence*. New York, Carnegie Corporation of New York, 1994.

Haskins R, Schwartz JB, Akin JS, et al: How much support can absent fathers pay? *Policy Studies* 14:201, 1985.

Hernandez DJ: Demographic trends and the living arrangements of children. In: Hetherington EM, Arsteh ID (eds): *Impact of divorce, single-parenting, and stepparenting on children*. Hillsdale, NJ, Erlbaum, 1988.

Hetherington EM, Camara KA: Families in transition: The process of dissolution and reconstitution. In: Parke RD (ed): *Review of child development research. Vol 7: The family*. Chicago, University of Chicago Press, 1984.

Hetherington EM, Hagan MS, Anderson ER: Marital transition: A child's perspective. *Am Psychol* 44:303–312, 1989.

Hofferth SL, Wissoker DA: Price, quality, and income in child care choice. *J Hum Resources* 27:70–111, 1992.

Hoffman LW: Work, family and the child. In: Pallak MS, Perloff RO (eds): *Psychology and work: productivity, change and employment*. Washington, DC, American Psychological Association Press, 1986.

Hoffman LW: Effects of maternal employment in the two parent family. *Am Psychol* 44:283–292, 1989.

Hopper P, Zigler E: The medical and social science basis for a national infant care leave policy. *Am J Orthopsychiatry* 58:324–338, 1988.

Institute of Medicine: *Research on children and adolescents with mental, behavioral and developmental disorders*. Washington, DC, National Academy Press, 1989.

Joint Commission on Mental Health of Children: *Crisis in child mental health: challenge for the 1970's*. New York, Harper & Row, 1969.

Kamerman SB: Child care services: A national picture. *Monthly Labor Rev*, 448–464, 1983.

Kashani JH, Beck NC, Hoepper EW, et al: Psychiatric disorders in a community sample of adolescents. *Am J Psychiatry* 144:584–589, 1987.

Kazdin AE: Psychotherapy for children and adolescents: Current progress and future research directions. *Am Psychol* 48:644–657, 1993.

Kisker EE, Hofferth SL, Phillips DA, et al: *A profile of child care settings: early education and care in 1990*. Washington, DC, US Department of Education, 1991.

Klerman, L: *Alive and well? Health care for children in America*. New York, National Center for Children in Poverty, 1991.

Knitzer J: *Unclaimed children*. Washington, DC, Children's Defense Fund, 1982.

Kurdek LA: An integrative perspective on children's divorce adjustment. *Am Psychol* 36:856–866, 1981.

Kurdek LA, Blisk D: Dimensions and correlates of mothers' divorce experiences. *J Divorce* 6:1–24, 1983.

Lindblom CE: Who needs what social research for policy making? *Knowledge: Creation, Diffusion, Utilization* 7:345–366, 1986.

Long L, Long T: *The handbook for latchkey children and their parents*. New York, Arbor House, 1983.

Maccoby EE, Kahn Al, Everett BA: The role of psychology research in the formation of policies affecting children. *Am Psychol* 38:80–84, 1983.

Margolis L, Farran D: Consequences of unemployment. *The Networker* 4:1–3, 1985. (Available from the Bush Center in Child Development and Social Policy, Yale University, New Haven, CT)

McCall RB, Gregory TG, Murray JP: Community developmental research results to the general public through television. *Dev Psychol* 20:45–54, 1984.

McCartney K, Scarr S, Phillips D, et al: Environmental differences among day care centers and their effects on children's development. In: Zigler E, Gordon E (eds): *Day care: scientific and social policy issues*. Boston, Auburn House, 1982.

Meltsner AI: The seven deadly sins of policy analysis. *Knowledge: Creation, Diffusion, Utilization* 7:367–382, 1986.

Moen P, Dempster MC: Employed parents: Role strain, work time and preferences for working less. *J Marriage Fam* 49:579, 1987.

National Center for Children in Poverty: *Five million children: an update*. New York, National Center for Children in Poverty, 1993.

National Center for Clinical Infant Programs: *Who will mind the babies?* Washington, DC, National Center for Clinical Infant Programs, 1988.

Nelson JR Jr: The politics of federal day care regulation. In: Zigler E, Gordon E (eds): *Day care: scientific and social policy issues*. Boston, Auburn House, 1982.

Office of Technology Assessment: *Children's Mental Health: Problems and Services—A Background Paper* (publication no. OTA-BP-H33). Washington, DC, US Government Printing Office, 1986.

Osofsky J, Fenichel E (eds): Caring for infants and toddlers in violent environments: Hurt, healing and hope. Washington, DC, Zero to Three/National Center for Clinical Infant Programs, 1994.

Packard V: *A nation of strangers*. New York, Simon & Schuster, 1972.

Phillips D: *Quality child care: What does the research tell us?* Washington, DC, National Association for the Education of Young Children, 1987.

Powell DR: How schools support families. Critical policy tensions. *Elementary School Journal* 91: 307—319, 1991.

President's Commission on Mental Health: *Task panel reports submitted to the President's Commission on Mental Health* (Vols 1–4). Washington, DC, US Government Printing Office, 1978.

Price RH, Cowen EL, Lorion RP, et al (eds): *Fourteen ounces of prevention: A casebook for practitioners*. Washington, DC, American Psychological Association Press, 1988.

Provence S: Infant day care. The relationship between theory and practice. In: Zigler E, Gordon E (eds): *Day care: scientific and social policy issues*. Boston, Auburn House, 1982.

Reischauer R: *An analysis of the US job market*. Washington, DC, Congressional Budget Office, 1987.

Rice DP, Kelman S, Dunmeyer S: *The economic costs of alcohol and drug abuse and mental illness: 1985* (report to the Office of Financing and Coverage Policy, Alcohol, Drug Abuse and Mental Health Administration, US Department of Health and Human Services). San Francisco, Institutes for Health and Aging, University of California, 1990.

Richardson J, Dwyer K, McGuigan K, et al: Drug and alcohol use among eighth grade children who look after themselves after school. *Pediatrics* 84: 556–566, 1989.

Riessman F: Support groups as preventive intervention. In: Kessler M, Goldston SE (eds): *A decade of progress in primary prevention*. Hanover, NH, University Press of New England, 1986.

Rodman H, Pratt O, Nelson R: Child care arrangements and children's functioning: A comparison of self-care and adult care. *Dev Psychol* 21: 413–418, 1985.

Roupp R, Travers J, Glantz F, et al: *Children at the center: Final report of the National Day Care Study* (Vol 1). Cambridge, MA, Abt, 1979.

Rutter M: Institute of psychiatry department of child and adolescent psychiatry. *Psychol Med* 6: 505–516, 1976.

Rutter M: *Changing youth in a changing society*. Cambridge, MA, Harvard University Press, 1980.

Rutter M: Parental mental disorder as a psychiatric risk factor. In: Hales R, Frances A (eds): *American Psychiatric Association annual review* (Vol 6). Washington, DC, American Psychiatric Press, 1987, pp. 647–663.

Salkind NJ: The effectiveness of early intervention. In: Goets EM, Allen KE (eds): *Early childhood education: Special environmental, policy, and legal considerations*. Gaithersburg, MD, Aspen, 1983.

Sameroff AJ, Seifer R, Zax M, et al: Early indicators of developmental risk: The Rochester longitudinal study. *Schizophr Bull* 13:383–394, 1987.

Schorr LB, Schorr D: *Within our reach: Breaking the cycle of disadvantage*. New York, Doubleday, 1988.

Select Panel for the Promotion of Child Health: *Better health for our children: A national strategy*. Washington, DC, US Government Printing Office, 1981.

Seligson M: *School-age child care: Developmental and programmatic issues*. New Haven, CT, The Bush Center in Child Development and Social Policy, Yale University, 1989.

Shure M, Spivak G: Interpersonal cognitive problem solving. In: Price RH, Cowen EL, Lorion RP, et al. (eds): *Fourteen ounces of prevention: A casebook for practitioners*. Washington, DC, American Psychological Association Press, 1988.

Solnit AJ: Promise and risk in health care reform for the "public patient." *Yale Psychiatry*, p. 8, 1994.

Stevenson HW, Siegel AE (eds): *Child development research and social policy*. Chicago, University of Chicago Press, 1984.

Stipek D, McCroskey J: Investing in children: Government and workplace policies for parents. *Am Psychol* 44:416–432, 1989.

Takanishi R, DeLeon P, Pallack MS: Psychology and public policy affecting children, youth, and families. *Am Psychol* 38:67–69, 1983.

Tennant C: Parental loss in childhood. *Arch Gen Psychiatry* 45: 1045–1050, 1988.

Thompson R: Developmental research and legal policy: Toward a two-way street. In: Cicchetti D, Toth S (eds): *Child abuse, child development and social policy*. Norwood, NJ, Ablex, 1993.

Travers JR, Light RI: *Learning from experience: Evaluating early childhood demonstration programs*. Washington, DC, National Academy Press, 1982.

Trzcinski E, Finn-Stevenson M: A response to arguments against mandated parental leave: Findings from the Connecticut survey of parental leave policies. *J Marriage Fam* 53:445–460, 1991.

Tschara JM, Johnson JR, Kline M, et al: Conflict, loss, change and parent-child relationships: Predicting children's adjustment during divorce. *J Divorce* 13:1–22, 1990.

Tuma JM: Mental health services for children. *Am Psychol* 44:188–199, 1989.

US Bureau of the Census: *Money, income, and poverty status of families and persons in the United States* (Current Population Reports, p. 60). Washington, DC, US Bureau of the Census, 1988.

US Department of Labor: *Child care. A workforce issue*. Washington, DC, US Department of Labor, 1987.

US Department of Labor: Labor force participation among mothers with young children. In: *News*. Washington, DC, US Department of Labor, 88-431, 1988.

US House Select Committee on Children, Youth and Families: *Children's mental health: Promising responses to neglected problems: Hearing before the Select Committee on Children, Youth and Families*, 100th Congress, 1st session. Washington, DC, US Government Printing Office, 1987a.

US House Select Committee on Children, Youth and Families: *Hearings on Child Care* (report presented to the US House of Representatives). Washington, DC, US Government Printing Office, 1987b.

Wallerstein J: Child of divorce: An overview. *Behav Sci Law* 4:105–118, 1986.

Wallerstein JS: *Surviving the breakup*. New York, Basic Books, 1988.

Wallerstein JS: Tailoring the intervention to the child in the separating and divorced family. *Family-and-Conciliation-Courts-Rev* 29:448–459, 1991.

Ward EH: Credentialing for day care. *Voice for Children* 9:15, 1976.

Weiss HB: Introduction. In: Payne C (ed): *Programs to strengthen families: A resource guide*. Chicago, IL, Yale University and The Family Resource Coalition, 1984.

Weiss HB: *State leadership in family support programs*. Cambridge, MA, Harvard Family Research Project, Harvard University, 1989.

Weiss HB, Jacobs FH: *Evaluating family programs*. New York, Aldine De Gruyter, 1988.

White S: Review of *Within our reach. Young Children* September: 66–70, 1988.

Whittaker J, Garbarino J: *Social support networks: Informal helping in the human services*. New York, Aldine, 1983.

Yoshikawa H: Prevention as cumulative protection: Effects of early family support and education on chronic delinquency and its risks. *Psychol Bull* 115:28–54, 1994.

Zeitlin J: *Work and family responsibilities: Achieving a balance*. New York, Ford Foundation, 1989.

Zigler E: A solution to the nation's child care crisis: The school of the twenty-first century. In: Parents as Teachers' National Center (ed): *Investing in the beginning*. St. Louis, Parents as Teachers National Center, 1987.

Zigler E: The school of the 21st century. *Am J Orthopsychiatry* 36:31–32, 55–59, 1989.

Zigler E, Berman W: Discerning the future of early childhood intervention. *Am Psychol* 38: 894–906, 1983.

Zigler E, Finn M: From problem to solution: Changing public policy as it affects children and families. *Young Children* 36:31–32, 55–59, 1981.

Zigler E, Finn-Stevenson M: Applied developmental psychology. In: Lamb M, Bornstein M (eds): *Developmental psychology. An advanced textbook*. Hillsdale, NJ, Erlbaum, 1987.

Zigler E, Finn-Stevenson M: Child care in America: From problem to solution. *Educ Policy* 3: 313–329, 1989.

Zigler E, Frank M (eds): *The Parental leave crisis: Toward a national policy*. New Haven, CT Yale University Press, 1988.

Zigler E, Freedman J: Evaluating family support programs. In: Kagan S, Powell D, Weissbourd B, et al. (eds): *Family support programs: The state of the art*. New Haven, CT, Yale University Press, 1987a.

Zigler E, Freedman J: Head Start: A pioneer of family support. In: Kagan S, Powell D, Weissbourd B, et al (eds): *Family support programs: The state of the art*. New Haven, CT, Yale University Press, 1987b.

Zigler E, Lang M: *Child care choices: Balancing the needs of children, families, and society*. New York, Free Press, 1991.

Zigler E, Styfco S (eds): *Head Start and beyond: A national plan for extended childhood intervention*. New Haven, CT: Yale University Press, 1993.

Zigler E, Taussig C, Black K: Early childhood intervention: a promising preventative for juvenile delinquency. *Am Psychol* 47:997–1006, 1992.

Zigler E, Valentine J (eds): *Project Head Start: A legacy of the war on poverty*. New York, Free Press, 1979.

Zigler E, Weiss H: Family support systems: An ecological approach to child development. In: Rapoport N (ed): *Children, youth, and families: The action research relationship*. New York, Cambridge University Press, 1985.

Zill N, Sigal H, Brim OG Jr: Development of childhood social indicators. In: Zigler E, Kagan SL, Klugman E (eds): *Children, families, and government: Perspectives on American social policy*. New York, Cambridge University Press, 1983.

122 International Perspectives in Child Psychiatry

Felton Earls, M.D., and Leon Eisenberg, M.D.

Inexpensive and effective technologies now at hand are saving the lives of millions of the world's children each year (United Nations Children's Fund [UNICEF], 1993). Between 1975 and 1990, mortality under age 5 fell from 212 to 175 per 1000 live births in Sub-Saharan Africa, from 195 to 127 in India, from 85 to 43 in China, from 174 to 111 in the Middle Eastern Crescent and from 104 to 60 in Latin America and the Caribbean. Averages, however obscure substantial differences between and within countries. In 1960, one child in five died before reaching age 5 in both Indonesia and Ghana; by 1990, the rate had been cut in half in Indonesia (where Gross National Product per capita had undergone a 3.9% per annum growth) whereas it remained unchanged in Ghana where GNP per capita had shrunk by 0.3% per annum.

Indeed, the combination of family planning and low-cost health measures, such as vaccines for the common infectious diseases, the promotion of breast-feeding, growth monitoring, and oral rehydration therapy for diarrheal diseases of childhood, not only saves lives but also decreases morbidity. The extent to which these methods are made available for populations of children in developing countries is determined by political commitment, the economic priority given to the needs of children, and the emphasis given to primary care in national health planning. The full recognition of this new state of affairs in planning and providing for population health needs globally is captured by the term *health transition*, parallel to the expression *demographic transition*, which has been used to describe the economic, social, and cultural changes that accompanied the industrialization of Western societies. The advances made possible by these new technologies are of enormous potential benefit to children now, and to future generations of adults in the Third World.

Three conditions mark the context in which this potential societal benefit takes on significance for the mental health of children. First, the use of these technologies is dependent on the state of primary health care. In societies where primary care is underdeveloped, the existence of these measures provides a strong rationale to invigorate its growth and to expand the psychosocial skills of health workers (Chen, 1986). The inclusion of training modules in mental health is a prerequisite in this regard, since mental disorders form a substantial proportion of the complaints that bring adults and children to such facilities (Geil et al., 1981; Harding et al., 1980).

A second condition that necessitates the adoption of a mental health perspective is the ever greater importance placed on schooling. The social and academic demands in the school setting expose, and in some cases may create, behavioral and emotional problems in children. The percentage of children enrolled in school has increased from less than 30% in 1960 to more than 70% in 1990 in low-income countries (Carnegie Commission, 1992). Once again, however, variability is prominent. Of children enrolled in primary grades, only 45% reach grade four in the least developed of these countries whereas more than 80% do so in East Asia (UNICEF, 1993).

The third condition is a product of many other circumstances operating in countries undergoing rapid change. It stems from a growing desire on the part of parents for fewer children. As infant mortality rates decrease, parents no longer require high fertility to guarantee that some offspring will survive to lead productive lives and provide care for their parents in old age. However, more than the statistical reality of a falling infant death rate is needed to bring about a decrease in fertility rates.

Some measure of economic benefit must accompany improvements in the health status of children in order to accelerate the movement for fertility reduction (Nag et al., 1978). Whatever the precise circumstances for a given society, having smaller families permits parents to focus on the academic and social competence of their children to a greater extent than when the sibship is larger. This is evident today in the People's Republic of China (Lin and Eisenberg, 1985).

One final prefatory remark about long-term changes in mortality may be in order. Murray and Chen (1993) have identified an enigma: Mortality has continued to decline in the developing world over the past decade despite serious economic reversals in many countries. For example, mortality under age 5 declined substantially in Mali, Liberia, Senegal, Guatemala, Indonesia, and Kenya over the past decade and a half; yet, only Indonesia experienced a significant increase in GNP per capita over this time interval; the economies of Mali, Guatemala, Kenya and Senegal remained stagnant and that of Liberia grew substantially worse. Moreover, even in countries like Bangladesh where crises associated with famine and war led to an increase in under age 5 mortality over the short run, child mortality resumed the long-term declining secular trend line after the acute disruption was over. Although child mortality varies inversely with GNP when comparisons between nations are made (despite important exceptions), long-term trends remain surprisingly impervious to decade-long economic setbacks.

In trying to account for this discrepancy, Murray and Chen suggest that "health stocks" (by which they mean both physical and social assets) maintain the long-term momentum because of cumulative effects which override temporary reverses. The physical assets they tabulate as health stocks include the infrastructure of the health care system, schools, transportation, water supply, sanitation, and the like. The social assets are the greater human capabilities which have resulted from better education, improved health status, changed behavior, and new beliefs; these capabilities continue to have an impact on mortality. This concept argues that the policy of international aid agencies should be based on investing in social assets rather than targeting short-term goals. Murray and Chen (1993, p.152) suggest that "immunization campaigns may contribute less to the development of the health system than an equal investment in expanding access to maternal and child health services. Resources directed to primary schooling may contribute more to social assets than money spent on social marketing of a particular health message or product."

A recent report on *World Mental Health* (Desjarlais et al., 1995) has stressed that:

> World mental health is first and foremost a question of economic and political welfare. Although the links between social forces and ill health are complex and varied, mental health concerns almost always relate to more general concerns about the economic welfare of family and community, the environment in which a person lives, and the kinds of resources he or she can draw upon. Enduring political and economic structures contribute to the perpetuation of poverty, hunger and despair. Demographic and environmental pressures spark regional and intrastate conflicts, which lead to personal trauma, social demoralization and dislocation. The mental health problems associated with natural disasters, environmental scarcity, urbanization, and physical illness take a greater toll on poorer communities because of a lack of programs and services to lessen their impact . . ." (p. 15)

In this chapter, the current state and future needs of child and adolescent psychiatry will be appraised in global perspective. Children in developing countries not only constitute, by far, the majority of all children in the world (more than 80% at present) but also make up disproportionately high percentages of entire populations in many of these countries, compared to that of the technologically developed nations. The incongruity is that child psychiatry and specialized child mental health services are almost exclusively a product of the developed nations. Thus, a special sensitivity is needed to reach a common understanding on how best to build a relationship between Western child psychiatrists and those health workers in developing countries who will be central to meeting the mental health needs of children in the Third World.

It is well to start from a skeptical posture, that is, to doubt that notions about child mental health or the importance of psychiatric treatment hold much significance at all for children in the developing world. Our concerns may simply reflect the fact that child psychiatry, as it now exists, has its roots in the particular conditions under which Western societies have become industrialized over the past century. Mindless extrapolation of our own values to societies currently undergoing such changes smacks of cultural imperialism.

A quite different argument may also underpin a skeptical position. Here the concern is not so much the dangers of exporting health care practices from one society to another as the question of priorities. Why, it might be asked, should a country with limited resources and overwhelming physical health needs among its population devote any of those resources to child mental health care? The case for this argument is made more poignant when fiscal realities are considered. When a government is prepared to direct a greater share of its health budget for low-cost technologies to prevent death and preserve the health of children, additional monies for mental health services may simply be out of reach.

It is against the backdrop of these cultural and economic pressures that the mental health needs of children, as well as the justification for training child psychiatrists and other mental health professionals, must be assessed. These issues, covered in the remainder of this chapter, are organized around four topic headings: the current status of world child mental health; setting priorities; the role of the World Health Organization (WHO), the United Nations Children's Fund (UNICEF), and other international organizations in addressing child mental health needs; and future research directions.

CURRENT STATUS OF WORLD CHILD MENTAL HEALTH

The organization of child mental health services varies considerably by regions of the world, by individual societies, and within communities in a given society. The marked differences between the technologically developed and underdeveloped countries have already been mentioned. But among the developing countries, several currently have national plans in place to expand services. China introduced a system to train a sufficient number of child psychiatrists to serve as leaders to organize services in each of its provinces several years ago (Earls, 1987). Plans for India and Sri Lanka place emphasis on the training of primary health care workers in child mental health (Cox, 1989). The degree of organization within the countries of Latin America and the African continent vary considerably.

Variation among countries exists for developed and developing societies. Child mental health services operate on very limited manpower in all countries and are typically located in urban centers. Thus, the provision of services to rural populations is much less well developed than it is to city dwellers. Of equal concern is the way socioeconomic conditions (income, education) influence access to services. These problems are not unique to child psychiatry, but the sharp limits they place on resources and manpower may exert influences on who is seen, who is treated, and what kind of treatment is provided.

Over the past 25 years, investigations of the prevalence and distribution of child mental disorders in general population samples have been conducted in many parts of the world (Earls, 1985; Graham, 1980; Offord et al., 1987). The techniques used to define disorders have differed considerably. Yet despite variations in reported rates, there are some consistent patterns in the distribution of disorders.

Preadolescent boys are nearly always reported to have higher rates than girls. The types of disorders contributing to this sex difference are primarily confined to intellectual disorders (mental retardation, specific learning disabilities, and autism) and behavioral disorders (hyperactive and conduct). During adolescence, the gap in prevalence between boys and girls is closed by an increasing incidence of emotional (anxiety and depressive) disorders in girls. There has also been a consistent pattern by geographical area, with rates of ascertained disorders among city-dwelling children being higher than rates among children living in rural areas (Rutter et al., 1975).

Other indicators of the mental health of populations are found in mortality rates from suicide and homicide among adolescents. However, these data are likely to be too unreliable for international comparisons. Among the developed nations, there is evidence that the rate of suicide in adolescent males has tripled over the past 30 years (Eisenberg, 1980, Diekstra and Gulbinat, 1993). In the United States, the rate of suicide and homicide in young people varies by race, ethnicity, social status, and sex, limiting the usefulness of raw figures before disaggregation by group. For example, the suicide rate among Native American males under the age of 19 is estimated to be about 19 per 100,000, a rate more than 50% higher than that for white adolescent males (Earls et al., 1990). The homicide rate for black males in the United States (the peak age-specific mortality rate was 124 per 100,000 for 20–24-year-olds in 1980) is about seven times higher than for white males in the same age groups (Gulaid et al., 1988). Yet the rate of suicide among young Native American males and the homicide rate among black males show marked variation from one community to another. Thus, before generalizing from suicide and homicide rates even within race or ethnic groups in a single country, great caution is warranted. This leads to the conclusion that the level of aggregate national data provided by most countries is an inadequate basis for planning services at the local level. Put simply, there are no good indicators of the mental health of the population as a whole.

The results of local area studies have been more useful than aggregate data accumulated from total populations. Such studies have provided a varied picture of the burden of mental disorders in children and adolescents. Examples from studies done in different parts of the world serve to illustrate the point.

In a large sample of elementary school children in districts in and around Beijing, the prevalence of attention deficit disorder varied from 3% in urban areas to 7% in suburban and rural areas (Shen et al., 1985). This reversal of the typical urban/rural contrast was associated with the higher educational and occupational status of the parents in urban families. Despite this substantial effect of geographical area and parental education, the sex ratio and symptom pattern of the disorder was similar to that found in surveys in the United States and Western Europe.

Khartoum, Sudan, has been the setting for a study demonstrating the effects of urbanization and cultural change on the prevalence of psychiatric problems in cross-sectional samples of children between the ages of 3 and 15 over the 15-year period between 1965 and 1980 (Cederblad and Rahim, 1986; Rahim and Cederblad, 1984). The standard of living clearly improved over this interval, as did the physical health of the children; yet the prevalence of psychiatric problems increased. The proportion of children with severe disturbance increased from 8% to 13% in the total population, whereas the proportion of children rated as well adjusted decreased from 63% to 47%. The authors attributed their findings to modernization, during which new values and higher educational expectations of children led to the increase in the prevalence of psychiatric disorders.

Both the Beijing and the Khartoum studies underscore the importance of the interactions among geographical setting, culture change, parental education, and sex of the child in determining the observed prevalence of psychiatric disorders. If one extrapolates from these two carefully done local studies to other cities in the developing world, the expectation is that rates of psychiatric problems in children will continue to increase as these areas become more fully modernized.

Newcastle, England, the Hawaiian island of Kauai, and Dunedin, New Zealand, are local areas well known in child psychiatry because they have been the sites for birth cohort studies carried out over long intervals. The Newcastle study has shown that social deprivation experienced early in life is a contributing factor to the persistence of delinquency and criminal behavior well into the adult years (Kolvin et al., 1988). Much has been learned about the relative importance of biological (mainly perinatal) and social factors for the developmental paths followed by the 1200 children born on Kauai in 1958 and studied longitudinally over three decades by Werner and Smith (1977). Social factors appear to have been more powerful than perinatal factors during the early years of life in leading to behavioral problems. However, as the children grew into adolescence and began to have more complex problems, it became necessary to take into account not just the factors that were associated with difficulties but also the resiliency and relative immunity that many children showed in the face of misfortune (Werner and Smith, 1982). The Dunedin study provides one of the most closely followed birth cohort of any currently available and thus provides a detailed longitudinal picture of change and persistence in behavioral disorders from middle childhood to adolescence (Moffitt and Silva, 1988). An important contribution of this study is the demonstration that both preschool behavior and family characteristics present during this period reliably predict conduct disorder and persistent delinquency (White et al., 1991; Henry et al., 1993).

The investigation of youth suicide in different parts of the developing world offers another way of approaching the multifactorial contributions of gender, social setting, and cultural change to pathological behavior. Contrasts in the frequency of completed suicide between West Africa (Odejide et al., 1989), Algeria (Al-Issa, 1989), Sri Lanka (Ganesvaran et al., 1984), and Malaysia (Maniam, 1988) offer a complex picture in which social and cultural factors such as the status of women, caste membership, arranged marriages, and perceived educational failure may precipitate suicidal behavior.

High rates of suicide among youth are a matter of concern both in North and South. A longitudinal study of adolescents in the United States has demonstrated a relationship between suicidal ideation and prior depressive states (Garrison et al., 1991). Imitative suicides, that is, reports of one suicide that appear to motivate others, named the ''Werther Effect'' after the novel by Goethe, have led to concerns about sensational press coverage as a precipitating factor (Eisenberg, 1986; Gould and Shaffer, 1986; Phillips and Carstensen, 1986; Schmidtke and Hafner, 1988). Social researchers in Micronesia, Polynesia, and Melanesia have highlighted near epidemic levels of suicide in the region among youth, related to the dearth of economic opportunities and to important changes in social structure and family life (Rubinstein, 1992). Although suicide is recognized locally as a serious and mysterious problem, social analysis of suicidal behavior, in the Durkheim tradition, does not consider suicide a problem for medicine and the health system as distinct from the larger social context in which it occurs.

SETTING PRIORITIES

Based on current knowledge of child mental health, there are some general principles that should prove useful to governments and agencies interested in developing, or expanding, existing services.

First, a population-based approach to the development of services is required. Enough is known from existing studies to indicate which types of disorders are common and to estimate age and sex trends for those disorders.

Second, considerable caution should be exercised before transplanting diagnostic systems from one culture to another. This may be feasible in some cases; certainly, there is reason to hope that the system being devised for the 10th version of the ICD will prove acceptable to practitioners in most countries. Rather than relying solely on symptom clusters (the basis in most classification systems for the definition of disorders), it is important to go beyond the presence of symptoms to levels of impairment. School failure, inability to respond to customary disciplinary practices, lack of self-confidence, rejection by peers, and violent behavior are the types of dysfunctional patterns that can be expected to be associated with psychiatric disorder. True, it is possible to have such impairments without a disorder being present, but the diagnosis of a disorder does not make sense in the absence of impairment.

Third, prevention and early detection should be emphasized. Enough is known about the incidence of specific types of disorders to concentrate preventative efforts on the first 5 years of life for boys and on early adolescence for girls. It is unlikely that curative treatments, either psychological or pharmacological, will be discovered in the near future. Thus it is reasonable to focus on efforts to prevent problems such as hyperactivity, conduct disorder, mental retardation, depression, and anxiety disorders. For rare disorders, such as autism and Tourette's disorder, it is not feasible to justify, financially or scientifically, such an emphasis on prevention. In these cases child psychiatrists will have to continue to struggle with treatment approaches that appear efficacious. Beyond the concern with psychiatric disorders, promising interventions should be explored for such problems as substance abuse, early childbearing, sexually transmitted diseases, and intentional injuries due to suicidal and interpersonal violent behavior.

Finally, mental health services for children must become an integral component of primary care. Rather than having mental health distinguished from physical health in the organization of services, mental health should be viewed as an essential part of pediatrics. Particularly in developing countries where resources are limited, copying separately conceived and developed psychiatric services for children, based on Western models of child guidance centers, makes little sense. To create a secure base for child mental health services in primary care, pediatricians must be persuaded of their importance, however. The size of this task will vary with the level of training for pediatricians, local demand for health services, and available resources. Child psychiatrists must develop close working relationships with pediatricians to facilitate the integration of mental and physical health.

ROLE OF INTERNATIONAL ORGANIZATIONS IN CHILD MENTAL HEALTH

The Division of Mental Health of WHO in Geneva has been, and remains, the single most important agency in developing and coordinating multinational efforts in the field of mental health, including child mental health. The establishment of WHO itself in 1948 in the aftermath of World War II reflected a renewed commitment to human health the world over. The first director general of the organization was a psychiatrist, Dr. Brock Chisholm of Canada; the WHO charter defines health as ''a state of complete physical, mental and social well-being and not merely the absence of disease or infirmity'' and goes on to state that ''healthy development of the child is of basic importance; the ability to live harmoniously in a changing total environment is essential to such development.''

During the formative years of WHO, mental health had a relatively low priority; it was represented by an office, a bureaucratic entity less powerful than a division in the WHO organizational structure. One of the authors served as a member of a Scientific Group on Mental Health Research, which met in Geneva from April 6 to 10, 1964. The Scientific Group was chaired by Robert Felix, then director of the United States National Institute of Mental Health and included representatives from Africa, China, Latin America, the United States, the USSR, and Europe. Its formal report gave legitimacy to a mental health research agenda for WHO. After it was endorsed by the WHO Advisory Committee for Medical Research and formally approved by the WHO Executive Committee, mental health research under WHO auspices was set to go.

Appropriately, the first major effort of the new research program was in the field of nosology: the creation of successive international seminars, each on a major diagnostic grouping, to coordinate psychiatric diagnosis, classification, and statistics. The psychiatric disorders of childhood were reviewed at a meeting in Paris in 1967 (Rutter et al., 1969); the classification of mental retardation was the subject of a seminar in Washington in 1969 (Tarjan et al., 1972). Currently, in preparation for the 10th revision of the ICD (ICD-10), the American Psychiatric Association is cooperating with WHO in order to assure maximum compatibility between the DSM-IV and the ICD-10, while still allowing latitude for national variation. In preparation for ICD-10, the WHO Division of Mental Health mounted field trials in 40 countries (Sartorius et al., 1993).

The accomplishments in developing a common language and agreed-upon clinical criteria made possible a number of major multinational studies, summarized in a report by Norman Sartorius (1980), the director of the Division of Mental Health. A nine-nation study of schizophrenia (China, Colombia, Czechoslovakia, Denmark, India, Nigeria, the United Kingdom, the United States, and the USSR) demonstrated that similar schizophrenic syndromes exist in this diverse set of nations but that course and outcome differ significantly between countries, with more favorable outcomes observed in developing countries. Later, a cross-national study of the diagnostic criteria for depression and its course and outcome was inaugurated. A third major study in this series tabulated the frequency of mental disorders in primary health care in four developing countries (Colombia, India, the Sudan, and the Philippines). With stringent criteria for psychiatric morbidity, the overall frequency in some 1600 patients attending primary health facilities was about 14%; however, only a third of the psychiatric cases were detected by health workers using their customary assessment procedures (Harding et al., 1980).

In addition to its essential role in developing diagnostic criteria and classification systems to make international comparisons of the prevalence and treatment of psychiatric disorder possible, the Division of Mental Health has played a central role in assisting less-developed countries (LDCs) to establish central statistical systems, to analyze local variations in disease distribution, and to monitor changes in distribution over time within their own societies. This has included making on-site training opportunities available, both through training seminars in LDCs, by seconding central office staff to local governments for short periods of time, and providing fellowships for specialized study abroad for young professionals. When multinational research studies are undertaken, emphasis is given to the training of personnel in each collaborating center in order to develop an infrastructure able to continue to carry on local research after the initiating program has ended. In addition, WHO supplies travel funds for expert consultants requested at the local level, and it brings professionals from developed and less-developed countries together to develop consensus documents on mental health problems. An outstanding example of such publications is WHO technical report no. 613, entitled *Child Mental Health* and *Psychosocial Development*, prepared by a WHO expert committee in 1977.

In 1985 one of the authors served as a consultant to the WHO Division of Mental Health to prepare a draft paper on the prevention of mental, neurological, and psychosocial disorders (Eisenberg and Sartorius, 1988). That document was unanimously endorsed by the executive board of the World Health Assembly in January 1986 and then approved by the World Health Assembly without further revision in May 1986. It places major emphasis on primary prevention through improving provisions for maternal and child health, beginning with family planning and including prenatal and perinatal care, childhood immunizations, enriched day care, health education, and the teaching of parenting skills in public schools. It calls for the establishment in each nation of a coordinating group on mental health in order that health consequences be taken into account in planning for economic development, legislation, taxation, new housing, and the like. There is, of course, a very considerable gap between adopting a resolution that acknowledges the importance of prevention in principle and implementing national programs. None-

theless, the assembly resolution reflects international agreement on the proposition that preventing mental disorders merits higher priority on national agendas. The World Health Organization (1993) has issued four short documents on the prevention of mental, neurological, and psychosocial disorders, documents with separate fascicles intended for health professionals, mid-level health workers, and the general public.

UNICEF is the second major player in promoting international child health. Its major programmatic thrust is organized under the rubric of GOBI: growth monitoring, oral rehydration therapy (ORT), breast-feeding, and immunization. Systematic growth monitoring permits the detection of malnutrition in its early stages before irreversible changes have occurred and thus enables mothers and health workers to identify children at risk. ORT has been shown to be effective in markedly reducing the mortality that accompanies diarrhea in infants and young children in LDCs. Although ORT neither treats the underlying disease nor prevents its recurrence (inevitable as long as safe water is not available), it does contain morbidity and mortality. Breast-feeding not only ensures the transfer of maternal antibodies to the breast-fed infant but also reduces the likelihood of diarrhea from the contaminated water used in local preparation of infant formulas. The UNICEF immunization program has led to a remarkable increase in the uptake of vaccines by children in LDCs.

The significance of immunization in the prevention of brain damage in children is evident from an analysis based on the United States population. The administration of measles vaccine to the 3.5 million infants born in 1981 averted not only 3.3 million cases of measles and 360 deaths, but 1100 cases of measles encephalitis and 30 cases of subacute sclerosing panencephalitis. In the case of rubella vaccine, immunization avoided 1.5 million cases of rubella and 2000 cases of congenital rubella syndrome that would have resulted in 300 cases of mental retardation (Gruenberg et al., 1986). These figures, it should be noted, grossly *underestimate* the impact in LDCs where, for example, the mortality associated with measles in very young children may be as high as 10% because of comorbidity from malnutrition and parasitic diseases.

Tens of millions of children and adolescents are out of school before legal leaving age; they work, beg, or thieve on city streets in India, the Philippines, sub-Saharan Africa, and Latin America. While some are on the streets as a result of war, internal displacement or becoming refugees, most are on the streets because of rural migration to urban slums, inadequate housing and public services, family breakdown, and school failure. Some have given up on school, others have no school to go to and still others have been pushed out of school as "problems." The schools themselves are often grossly inadequate; increasingly, families see schooling as irrelevant because there are no jobs available at graduation; the regimentation and the bureaucratization in poorly run schools is the antithesis of the ways children live and learn in traditional communities. For families, the cost of keeping a child in school is no longer offset by higher wages after school completion.

Early indenture of children into wage earning roles is increasingly common in families that require additional income for their very survival. Children may be sold into virtual slavery in rug weaving factories where their small fingers and hands make it possible for them to do fine work. For 12–16 hours a day, 7 days a week, 52 weeks a year, "children as young as eight sit on rough planks knotting colored yarn around the stretched cords of the loom's warp, creating the carpets that India sells around the world" (Gargan, 1992). Estimates of the children's workforce in the Sewapuri area range from 300,000 to over a million.

According to a report by the International Labor Organization, India has 44 million child laborers nationwide. In most cities, the children who work in the carpet belt are purchased from their parents, or merely taken with promises of future payments. The vast majority come from the poorest parts of Bihar, the most impoverished state in India. "The going rate for an eight-year-old boy is 1,500 to 2,000 rupees ($50–66), a substantial sum for many families. Across India, in quarries, brass smelters, glass factories and match and explosive plants, children labor in dangerous, unhealthy and oppressive conditions, often against their will, sometimes with the consent of their parents. Child labor continues despite a 1976 law prohibiting all forms of bonded or slave labor and a 1986 act banning workers under the age of 14 from a broad range of industries.'' Yet children are forced into hazardous work places, sometimes with the connivance of the authorities, more often with their tacit acceptance. No one has ever gone to prison in India for using children as workers (Gargan, 1992). Those enslaved children who can escape to city streets; those who survive may be thrown on the streets when ill health, increasing size, ineptness at the job, or insubordination makes them undesirable.

Estimates of the number of youth who live on the streets in Brazil alone range up to 7 million! Many take to stealing and to exchanging sex for money. Most are initiated into sex by early adolescence; many have same sex as well as opposite sex partners. Few use condoms; most use drugs and alcohol; many contract STDs. They live in a world where sex meets multiple needs (survival, solidarity, pleasure, and dominance), where multiple partners predominate, and where dangerous sexual practices, such as anal intercourse and gang rape, are daily risks. Most of their sexual encounters are exploitative or coercive. They are at high risk for HIV infection in a sexual culture where male bisexuality is compatible with the designation of being macho (Raffaelli et al., 1993). Adding to the tenuousness of their lives is victimization by illegal police action. There have been many episodes in which off duty and out of uniform police, at the behest of, and in the pay of, local merchants, have summarily executed street youth in retribution for theft, alleged or real. An article published in the *Boston Globe* (1 February 1994) reported a statistic from Human Rights Watch/America, which claimed that 5,644 Brazilian children age 5–17 were murdered by death squads between 1988 and 1991.

Other nongovernmental international organizations play an important role. Professional organizations like the World Psychiatric Association and the International Association for Child Psychiatry and Allied Professions serve to promote collegial interchange between mental health workers in industrialized and developing countries. The World Federation for Mental Health mobilizes lay persons as well as professionals in the campaign against mental illness. In addition, alliances of former patients and the parents of patients, private foundations, and church groups play an important role in public education, lobbying for increased governmental expenditures for mental health, and the direct provision of funds to augment operating agency budgets.

FUTURE RESEARCH DIRECTIONS

Three strategies are recommended to encourage the continued development and refinement of child mental health services nationally and internationally. One, based on epidemiological concepts and methods that have proved useful in the past (Costello, 1989; Earls, 1979), involves studies to understand how changes in contemporary societies are reflected in the prevalence and incidence of child mental disorders. The second involves research that seeks to improve knowledge on the relationship of child-rearing methods to normal and deviant behavioral and emotional development. The third strategy involves research on the design and delivery of mental health services. Several examples will be given. In a final segment we attempt to animate these research issues with a travel experience that poignantly underscores what currently confronts the field in four markedly different nations: Sweden, South Africa, Brazil, and Mexico.

Incidence and Prevalence of Mental Disorders

The first question asks how the direction, pace, and types of changes under way in a given society relate to the incidence and prevalence of behavioral pathologies. If one divides societies into conventional strata based on levels of industrial or technological development, characteristics such as urbanization, compulsory schooling, and parental education may well be directly linked to the incidence of child mental disorder.

Societies undergoing rapid change in these characteristics would be expected to have higher incidence rates than those with a slower rate of change. Over fairly short intervals, they might attain the prevalence rates that exist in more highly developed societies. The rate of child mental disorder in the United States has been estimated to be in the range of 18–22% of the child population (Committee of the Institute of Medicine, 1989). This might be taken as an upper limit if the scale of technological development is, in fact, the critical factor it is thought to be in determining rates at the population level. Evidence for a lower limit is simply not available and perhaps less important since there is little reason to believe that it is less than 10%, based on recent surveys in rural parts of Norway (Vikan, 1985), Puerto Rico (Bird et al., 1988), and the Canadian province of Ontario (Offord et al., 1987). For example, Offord and his colleagues report a prevalence rate of 15% in rural Canadian children between the ages of 4 and 16, compared to a rate of 20% in urban children.

Assuming that the characteristics of city life, compulsory schooling, and social stratification are the factors that can double the rate of mental disorder in children, the key research issue is discovering how such risk conditions bring about increased rates of disorder. A number of possible mechanisms are suggested by past research: poor school environments, increased strain on marriages in urban environments, decreased social support, and increased opportunity to form bonds with deviant peers. Associated with these risk conditions may be new types of pathologies. Compulsory schooling inevitably leads to increasing saliency of learning disorders, a phenomenon recognized for several decades in the United States and recently gaining attention in China (Earls, 1987). Social stratification and urban environments are associated with conduct disorder, criminality, and violence. Ready availability of alcohol and drugs to youths makes abuse more likely. None of this is new, nor are causal roles implied by these associations. The research task is to unravel these associations within specific cultural contexts so that causal ordering can be established and rationally targeted preventive programs developed.

Technologically developed societies are also changing in their ethnic composition, due to migration within and between countries. For children a number of problems are associated with such social and cultural change. Their bicultural and bilingual status may produce problems related to identity and educational achievement (Diaz, 1983; Hakuta and Garcia, 1989). They may be victimized by prejudice, a condition that in itself can produce lowered self-esteem and underachievement. Even successful efforts at cultural assimilation on the part of children can produce friction with their parents. While remarkably successful children have emerged from disadvantaged immigrant groups and from families living in abject poverty, common experience also tells us that many children in these situations do poorly.

A second question is related to the first but is of particular import in developing societies. How is increasing survivorship, made possible by the growing success of WHO and UNICEF programs, translated into changes in the quality of life for children? Because of the enormous size of the populations undergoing such change, the problem is developing global dimensions. It affects countries where the mortality of children under 5 is falling, and highly developed societies as well.

Two issues need to be addressed. First, survivorship may be achieved at a cost to the health and vulnerability of children who would have succumbed had it not been for the intervention. The poor health associated with low birth weight, undernutrition, and unstimulating intellectual environments can result in poor school performance and reduced self-esteem, which in turn increase problem behaviors such as drug abuse and delinquency in adolescence. Mental disorders not previously recognized in developing societies (learning handicaps, mild mental retardation, and attentional problems) may well account for much of the difficulty experienced by these children. Thus epidemiological studies should be designed to detect the incidence of these disorders and to test their association with the various risk conditions.

The second issue associated with increasing survivorship stems from the limited economic resources of families. Low-cost health technologies that reduce the mortality rate of children under 5 are not correlated with improvements in the economic status of families in most developing countries. Parents necessarily experience economic stress when children survive in increasing numbers, but the resources required to raise healthy and successful children remain meager or even decline. How they cope with these trends and the extent to which they may make decisions to reduce fertility are largely unexplored. Cassidy (1987), in a provocative essay, distinguishes between "activist" and "adapter" orientations to intervention aimed at improving life in developing societies. The "activist" stance is predicated on the assumption that infant death is morally unjustifiable when methods exist to prevent it. Interventions organized from this perspective, it is argued, tend to be short-term and oriented toward individuals. The "adapter" perspective emphasizes the social and cultural evolution of communities and the continuity of groups over generations. Short-term efforts at increasing the survivorship of infants are of lesser import than enhancing the quality of life and the productivity of older members of the society.

An important contribution to this issue has been made by John C. Caldwell, an Australian demographer, who finds that infant mortality rates are more closely correlated with maternal education than with the more traditional measure of GNP (Caldwell, 1986). The implications of this finding are far-reaching; it suggests that the status of women in society, as reflected by their rate of literacy, is a more important predictor of the well-being of children than are economic indices such as the GNP. There are, however, several countries where fertility remains high despite increasing survivorship and rising rates of female literacy (Sindiga, 1985). Moreover, computed correlations between GNP per capita or maternal literacy rates and the indices of child survivorship should not be taken at face value. Unfortunately, the primary database for child mortality is of uncertain validity because of the limitations of the information systems in many LDCs. It is commonplace for international agencies, when data for a given nation are missing, to make estimates based on the experience of neighboring countries. Given the unreliability of the primary data, too close a reading of differences between correlation coefficients is not warranted. Nonetheless, it is a striking fact that oil-rich Arab countries, with high per capita incomes but low rates for maternal literacy, experience much worse child survivorship than countries such as Costa Rica and Sri Lanka and the state of Kerala in India, that have a much lower GNP per capita but higher levels of education for women.

More maternal education may translate into better child survival by the following paths (Hobcraft, 1993). Because women with more education marry later, have their first child later, and have fewer children, they are much less likely to die in childbirth. Therefore, they are less likely to leave their children orphaned; the magnitude of this effect in low-income countries where maternal mortality is high can reduce risk to less than one fifth (and potentially as low as one fiftieth) of the rate among uneducated mothers. Educated mothers are more likely to receive prenatal care, to have been given tetanus toxoid before delivery, and to have trained birth attendants at delivery. Thus, their perinatal morbidity and mortality is reduced. Their children are less likely to get diarrhea and more likely to be treated adequately for it if they do, because educated mothers are more responsive to modern hygienic practices. They have fewer stunted children. They are likely to marry more educated men, a further benefit to their children although the effect of paternal education is less than that of maternal education. These associations are remarkably robust in the data from the World Fertility Survey and the Demographic and Health Surveys. In some sub-Saharan African countries, correlations are weaker for reasons yet to be discovered.

Child Rearing and Developmental Studies

The disciplines of developmental psychology and anthropology are the principal basic social sciences of child mental health. Developmental psychology is concerned with patterns of normal and abnormal development and seeks to understand the mental, neural, and genetic bases of behavioral and emotional expression. Anthropology is chiefly concerned with the ways in which culture shapes human development in consonance with the customs and beliefs of a given society. Both perspectives are necessary to the understanding of the universal and the particular aspects of child rearing. Conceptual schemes are available to integrate these disciplines (Super and Harkness, 1986; Whiting, 1981), but more research is needed to inform mental health workers about how to distinguish growth-promoting from growth-damaging child-rearing practices. Rohner (1973) has proposed that child-rearing methods might be universally dimensionalized on an axis of parental acceptance and rejection, a reductionistic position that may appeal to those primarily interested in the development of psychopathology. However, field studies in which Western-trained scientists study parental behavior and children's development in non-Western societies are of dubious legitimacy.

Valuable leads arise from the current research literature. Sigman et al. (1988) recorded the verbal and social interactions between caretakers and infants in a Kenyan village and used the findings as predictors of subsequent cognitive development. It was not surprising to find that higher degrees of verbal and social stimulation were related to superior cognitive development. More interesting was the significant variability in levels of interaction between parents and infants in this small, culturally uniform, rural setting. It is apparent that caretaking practices valued in the West are present in a remote Kenyan village and operate in an expectable way. The study did not address the determinants of the extent to which parents in this setting emphasized high degrees of verbal and social stimulation as a cultural ideal.

Much effort has gone into development of standardized techniques to assess psychopathology in children. A number of structured interview methods are available to interview parents and children; checklists have been developed for parents and teachers. While the diagnostic categories yielded by these methods differ, they are useful in characterizing behavioral and emotional syndromes. The Child Behavior Checklist (CBCL) is one of the most carefully developed and widely used. Although developed and standardized on an American sample, it is now being used in many parts of the world. Weisz et al. (1987, 1989) compared Thai and American children on both the parent and teacher forms of the CBCL. The differences in parental reporting of child symptoms presumably reflect values and expectations that are specific to the two groups. Thai children are reported by their parents to have more overcontrolled behavior (shyness, anxiety, and depression) than children in the United States. Of equal interest is that Thai teachers reported more behavioral problems of all types than their counterparts in the United States. These studies represent a valuable beginning in efforts to learn how cultural differences in child rearing are translated into child psychopathology.

Mental Health Services Research

Quite different issues underlie the questions that must be addressed in mental health services research. They are so fundamental to the creation of any service that giving them priority on the research agenda may seem naive, yet there is surprisingly little information in the literature. They can be listed as follows:

1. What is the need for child mental health services in a given population?
2. How far does demand approximate the need?
3. How effective are services?
4. What resources should be allocated to them?

When resources are limited, as they are in all developing countries, a better way to put the last question is to ask, How might the available resources for mental health services best be distributed? This involves judgments about the settings in which mental health services will be placed, the relative importance to be given to primary versus hospital care, and the appropriate emphasis on prevention versus the provision of treatment (Eisenberg, 1992). Epidemiology is the linchpin for all of these goals (Costello et al., 1993).

Where the evidence to answer many of these questions is not available to administrators, emphasis must be given to the incorporation of ongoing research strategies into new and existing services so that data can be accumulated with time. That this is easier said than done will be readily endorsed by those who have been responsible for service delivery. Nevertheless, as the status of research and research training improves in our field, the capacity to address these simple questions will also be strengthened.

Three other issues should be placed on the agenda for mental health services research. First, there are special populations of children with unique mental health needs. Children who are victims of catastrophic events, torture, and other stressful and violent experiences often require treatment and less often rehabilitation. Data are only slowly emerging from current research, and it is still difficult to estimate their full public health dimensions of these problems (Earls et al., 1988; Terr, 1991; Jensen and Shaw, 1993). What we know gives reason for concern that large numbers of children will develop persisting symptoms of anxiety and depression in the aftermath of both natural and technological disasters.

Even more devastating is long-term exposure to warfare and racial oppression. Whole generations of children are at risk in countries such as Mozambique, Cambodia, and some parts of Eastern Europe (Cliff and Noormahomed, 1993; Zivcic, 1993). Substantial proportions of children in these areas are believed to have acquired behavioral and emotional impairment. Until now most societies seem to have assumed that children either are resilient in the face of adversity or are too naive to fully appreciate events that trouble adults. This view has little evidence to support it. Exposure to war is just one of the conditions that produce symptoms characteristic of posttraumatic stress disorder. The extent to which children develop the full clinical picture as described in adults is less important than judging how impaired are children experiencing even the partial syndrome. It may be the case that many children are able to do well even in circumstances that are devastating and inhumane. On the other hand, rates of disorder might be three and four times the expected rate and still involve less than half of all children.

The only way to address the needs of large numbers of children in such circumstances may be through the schools. Special schools or special services within existing schools may be necessary. Experience in training teachers to recognize the effects of torture in children and to provide interventions within the regular school environment is being gained in Mozambique, where pillaging of villages and murder and torture of adults and children have been widespread in recent years (N. Richman, N. Kanji, P. Zinkin, unpublished manuscript, 1988). The fact that the limited resources of schools in this very poor nation and the availability of child psychiatrists to train teachers have been directed to such children is a testament to the combined action of governmental support and international cooperation. The lesson is a valuable one for many other areas of the world.

A second target for research is the relationship between psychiatric disorder in parents and children. It is by now well established that some of most common psychiatric disorders cluster in families. Further, it is known that children of parents with depression and alcoholism have elevated rates of disorders themselves and are especially likely to have disorders that show similarity to those present in their parents (Beardslee et al., 1983). This opens important but neglected questions regarding the design and implementation of services for children. To what extent should child mental health services include systematic evaluation of parents' mental health? If an untreated disorder is discovered, should the program be prepared to treat or refer the parent for treatment? Many child services emphasize the central role played by parental psychopathology in the evaluation and treatment of children. Indeed, family therapy was created to address the mutual ways in which behavioral and emotional disturbances in parents and children have reciprocal influences. Yet from the service standpoint, little research has been done to document rates of diagnosable illness in parents and the impact of appropriate treatment of parents on alleviating distress in children.

The third issue concerns the costs and benefits of child mental health services. The research question is, Does the provision of mental health services to children improve their general health, enhance their school performance, and/or reduce family conflict? Answers to these questions would clearly be helpful in persuading skeptical planners and administrators of the utility of services for children. It is highly regrettable that such information is not already available. This implies that acquiring such data is difficult. For child mental health services to grow and prosper, particularly in societies with scarce resources for health care, it will be essential to be able to document their utility in actual practice.

Contemporary Contrasts in International Child Mental Health

In 1993, one of the authors visited large cities in four countries, Sweden, South Africa, Brazil, and Mexico, to gain fresh insights into children's mental health in markedly different social and political circumstances. In each country primary attention was directed towards urban children in disadvantaged contexts. The visits were facilitated by UNICEF's program on children in extremely difficult circumstances (Blanc, 1994). In the course of a few months the cities of Stockholm in Sweden, Johannesburg, Cape Town, Pietermaritzburg, and Durban in South Africa, Rio de Janeiro and Sao Paulo in Brazil, and Mexico City were toured. The framework for evaluating the status of children's mental health was organized around several issues, including efforts being made to locate and describe the needs of disadvantaged children, the role of governmental and nongovernmental agencies in providing services, and the availability of child mental health professionals to deliver the needed services.

Stockholm is a handsome metropolis of 700,000 persons. Over the course of the last half century, the social welfare system combined with other progressive policies has fostered a climate in which young children have prospered. It is difficult to imagine a large city where the quality of physical and social environment are more conducive to human growth. It represents an important point of reference in a journey to compare and contrast cities as habitats for children.

Stockholm's population represents something less than 10% of the country's eight million, yet nearly two thirds of the 300 child psychiatrists in the country are located there. As expected, the concentration of mental health services mirrors the abundance of child mental health professionals. With its well-organized mental health system, embracing schools, community clinics and hospitals, children with behavioral and emotional problems have access to appropriate services.

Despite these favorable conditions, delinquency and substance abuse among youth (particularly the use of tobacco, both in the form of cigarettes and snuff) represent serious problems in Stockholm. Though the prevalence and patterns of delinquency and juvenile crime appear to be similar to rates in other cities of Western Europe and North America, the overall severity of these problems may be less (Farrington and Wikstrom, 1994).

The challenge to this society rests in how well the existing high level of social welfare will be maintained as the population changes. Over the past decade the city has hosted significant numbers of immigrants from southern Europe and the Horn of Africa, many of whom plan to remain in Sweden. It is too soon to judge how well these immigrant families will be absorbed into Swedish urban society and how their children will fare socially and academically. There is some awareness of the risks that these children could learn to perceive themselves as depreciated by the larger society and indeed, this is accompanied by a pervasive sense of worry about the future.

South Africa is in the process of being transformed into a democratic society. Chief among the transformations already in progress is a dramatic migration of poor blacks from rural areas to the cities. It is difficult to estimate the present size of its three largest cities, Johannesburg, Durban, and Cape Town, because of the rapid growth of the townships that surround them. These cities are already experiencing increasing numbers of street children as a result of family dislocation and unemployment. When the effects of family stress are added to high levels of community violence and school non-attendance, the repercussions facing its new government's capacity to meet the needs of over 10 million children are foreboding.

A recent survey assessing the educational and social status of children produced a rather surprising result (Everatt and Sisulu, 1992). Only a small proportion of black children (about 6%) were thought to be seriously disconnected from their families and the larger society. Some four million (35–40%) however, were considered to be at risk of becoming disconnected or "marginalized." A focus of attention should be directed to stabilizing the lives of this group. But, to help accomplish this enormous task there are currently only about 12 child psychiatrists and a few hundred psychologists and social workers. These professionals are consumed with concerns about the consequences of children's exposure to violence. To adequately respond to the unmet mental health needs of this sort, this comparatively small cadre of child psychiatrists must reorganize services and develop new approaches to the training of health workers with competence in child mental health. Fortunately, these challenges are recognized and there were many examples witnessed during a three-week visit that reflected the initiatives that are being taken. It will be important to monitor the success of this effort over the next decade as the transition to a new society is completed.

The purpose of traveling to Brazil was to evaluate both governmental and nongovernmental responses to the welfare of the large number of youths who work and live on the streets. In reaction to rampant exploitation of street children and extreme episodes in which children were murdered, efforts to arouse many sectors of society and the children themselves was started in the mid-1980s. The movement was spurred by an opportunity to influence the drafting of a new constitution as the government made the transition from a military dictatorship to a democracy. The results for children are potentially far-reaching. An entire section of the constitution was formulated to provide a detailed description of the rights of children and the specific responsibilities that the government was charged with in taking steps to protect these rights. An important feature of this document is the way it transfers authority for developing programs and monitoring their implementation to local communities (Himes, 1992).

It is against the backdrop of such far-reaching constitutional reforms that one confronts the current status of children's welfare in Brazil's largest cities, Rio de Janeiro and Sao Paulo. Between them there are easily over 30 million people, 20% of the Brazilian population. In both cities there are programs and campaigns to protect these constitutional rights and promote the well being of children. For the most part, these efforts are supported by nongovernmental organizations. The reliance on such organizations is necessary since the government is repeatedly charged with corruption and the economy is experiencing a staggering degree of inflation. These organizations facilitate a "bottoms-up" approach in which community participation is fostered, as articulated in the constitution. In areas in which the local governments are engaged and cooperating with other organizations, the improvement in the status of children is obvious and gratifying.

Mexico City and Sao Paulo, two of the largest cities in the world, represent a striking contrast. Sao Paulo is jumbled in appearance and manifests much uninspired architecture, while the central districts of Mexico City reflect a level of grandeur in urban planning. At least as dramatic as the contrasts in urban environments is the social reality for children. The present Mexican government has made the improvement of child health a top priority and there is much evidence to underscore the seriousness of this commitment. Relatively few street children are encountered, many poor communities have been mobilized to solve local problems, and a nationwide census has been mounted to monitor the immunization records of children under age 5. Collectively, this "top-down" approach seems sufficiently well conceived to become an enduring policy to promote the health and welfare of children, although it is claimed that the centralized government does consult with local communities. Of significance is the virtual absence of nongovernmental organizations in this context.

The most important insights to be gained from this mission concerned the varying nature of societal response to children in difficult circumstances. Even in the contexts of South Africa, with its high level of violence and uncertainty about the future, and Brazil, with its unstable economy and uncontrolled urbanization, the numbers of children excluded from family and community life does not seem to be unmanageable. Indeed, the lesson to be learned in comparing Sao Paulo and Mexico City underscores just this fact. While a small proportion of children with serious social and behavioral problems in all of these societies need the help of child psychiatrists and other mental health professionals, the needs of a much larger group can be met through circumstances that generally increase the quality of life: adequate supports for families, communities that facilitate the growth of social bonds, and good schools.

Ideally, a combination of community mobilization and governmental financing is needed to design systems that function most efficiently for children. Stockholm comes close to this ideal, but they are not without the challenge of extending such benefits to new waves of immigrants. Perhaps the societal solutions being strived for in Brazilian and Mexican cities provide some glimpse of what life for children living in urban areas might be like in much of the world in the next century. Can Mexico City, with a population 25 times larger than Stockholm, aspire to be as wholesome an environment for the rearing of children? The problems of controlling the growth and scale of urban environments with human development, not just commerce, as the index of success is among the most challenging facing future societies throughout the world.

References

Al-Issa I: Psychiatry in Algeria. *Psychiatr Bull* 13:240–245, 1989.

Beardslee WR, Bemporad J, Keller MB, et al: Children of parents with affective disorder: A review. *Am J Psychiatry* 140:825–831, 1983.

Bird H, Canino G, Rubio-Stipec M, et al: Estimates of the prevalence of childhood maladjustment in a community survey in Puerto Rico: The use of combined measures. *Arch Gen Psychiatry* 45:1120–1126, 1988.

Blanc C: *Urban Children in Distress: Global Predicaments and Innovative Strategies.* Langhorne, PA, Gordon and Breach, 1994.

Caldwell JC: Routes to low mortality in poor countries. *Popul Dev Rev* 12:171–220, 1986.

Carnegie Commission: *Partnerships for Global Development: The clearing horizon.* New York, Carnegie Commission on Science, Technology and Government, 1992, p. 31.

Cassidy CM: World-view conflict and toddler malnutrition: Change agent dilemmas. In: Scheper-Hughes N (ed): *Child Survival.* Boston, D. Reidel, 1987, pp. 293–324.

Cederblad M, Rahim SA: Effects of rapid urbanization on child behavior and health in a part of Khartoum, Sudan. 1: Socio-economic changes 1965-1980. *Soc Sci Med* 22:713–721, 1986.

Chen LC: Primary health care in developing countries: Overcoming operational, technical, and social barriers. *Lancet* 2:1260–1265, 1986.

Cliff J, Noormahomed AR: The impact of war on children's health in Mozambique. *Soc Sci Med* 36:843–848, 1993.

Committee of the Institute of Medicine: *Research on Children and Adolescents with Mental, Behavioral, and Developmental Disorders: Mobilizing a National Initiative.* Washington, DC, National Academy Press, 1989.

Costello EJ: Developments in child psychiatric epidemiology. *J Am Acad Child Adolesc Psychiatry* 28:836–841, 1989.

Costello EJ, Burns BJ, Angold A, et al: How can epidemiology improve mental health services for adolescents? *J Am Acad Child Adolesc Psychiatry* 32:1106–1113, 1993.

Cox AD: Child and adolescent psychiatry. In: Holden N, Edwards G (eds): *Postgraduate Training in Psychiatry: Options for International Collaboration.* Geneva, World Health Organization, 1989.

Desjarlais R, Eisenberg L, Good B, et al: *World Mental Health: Problems and Priorities in Low- Income Countries.* New York, Oxford University Press, 1995.

Diaz RM: Thought and two languages: The impact of bilingualism on cognitive development. *Rev Res Educ* 10:23–54, 1983.

Diekstra RFW, Gulbinat W: The epidemiology of suicidal behavior: a review of three continents. *World Health Stat Q* 46:52–68, 1993.

Earls F: Epidemiology and child psychiatry: Historical and conceptual development. *Compr Psychiatry* 20:256–269, 1979.

Earls F: Epidemiology of psychiatric disorders in children and adolescents. In: Cavenar JO (ed): *Psychiatry* (Vol 3). Philadelphia, Lippincott, 1985, pp. 1–30.

Earls F: Child psychiatry in an international context: With remarks on the current status of child psychiatry in China. In: Super CM (ed): *The Role of Culture in Development Disorder*. New York, Academic, 1987, pp. 235–248.

Earls F, Escobar JI, Manson SM: Suicide in minority groups: Epidemiological and cultural perspectives. In: Blumenthal SJ, Kupfer DJ (eds): *Suicide Over the Life Cycle*. Washington, DC, American Psychiatric Press, 1990.

Earls F, Smith E, Reich W, et al: Investigating the psychopathological consequences of a disaster in children: A pilot study incorporating a structured diagnostic interview. *J Am Acad Child Adolesc Psychiatry* 27:90–95, 1988.

Eisenberg L: Adolescent suicide: On taking arms against a sea of troubles. *Pediatrics* 66:315–320, 1980.

Eisenberg L: Does bad news about suicide beget bad news? *N Engl J Med* 315:705–707, 1986.

Eisenberg L: Child mental health in the Americas: A public health approach. *Bull PAHO* 26(3): 230–241, 1992.

Eisenberg L, Sartorius N: Human ecology in the repertoire of health development. *World Health Forum* 9:564–568, 1988.

Everatt D, Sisulu E (eds.) *Black youth in crisis: Facing the future*. Braamfontein, South Africa, Raven Press, 1992.

Farrington DP, Wikstrom P-OH. Criminal careers in London and Stockholm: a cross-national comparative study: In: Weitekamp EGM, Kerner HJ (eds): *Cross-National Longitudinal Research on Human Development and Criminal Behavior*. Dordrecht, Netherlands, Kluwer, pp. 65–89, 1994.

Ganesvaran T, Subramaniam S, Mahadevan K: Suicide in a northern town of Sri Lanka. *Acta Psychiatr Scand* 69:420–425,1984.

Gargan, E. Bound to looms by poverty and fear, boys in India make a few men rich. *New York Times International*, July 9, 1992, A8.

Garrison CZ, Addy CL, Jackson KL, et al: A longitudinal study of suicidal ideation in young adolescents. *J Am Acad Child Adolesc Psychiatry* 30: 597–603, 1991.

Geil R, de Arango MV, Climent CE, et al: Childhood mental disorders in primary health care: Results of observations in four developing countries. *Pediatrics* 68:677–683, 1981.

Gould MS, Shaffer D: The impact of suicide in television movies: evidence of imitation. *N Engl J Med* 315:690–694, 1986.

Graham P: Epidemiological approaches to child mental health care in developing countries. In: Purcell EF (ed): *Psychopathology of Children and Youth: A Cross-Cultural Perspective*. New York, Josiah Macy, Jr., Foundation, 1980, pp. 28–45.

Gruenberg EM, Lewis C, Goldston SE (eds): *Vaccinating against Brain Syndromes: The Campaign Against Measles and Rubella*. New York, Oxford University Press, 1986.

Gulaid JA, Onwuachi-Saunders EC, Sacks JJ, et al: Differences in death rates due to injury among blacks and whites. *Morbid Mortal Weekly Rep* 37: 25–31, 1988.

Hakuta K, Garcia EE: Bilingualism and education. *Am Psychol* 44:374–379, 1989.

Harding TW, De Arango MV, Baltazar J, et al: Mental disorders in primary health care: A study of frequency and diagnosis in four developing countries. *Psychol Med* 10:231–241, 1980.

Henry B, Moffitt T, Robins L, et al: Early family predictors of child and adolescent antisocial behavior: Who are the mothers of delinquents? *Criminal Behavior and Mental Health* 3:97–118, 1993.

Himes JR: Implementing the United Nations Convention on the Rights of the Child: resource mobilization and the obligations of states parties. *Innocente Occasional Papers, Child Rights Series, No. 2*. Florence, Italy, UNICEF International Child Development Centre, 1992.

Hobcraft J: Women's education, child welfare and child survival: a review of the evidence. *Health Transition Review* 3:159–175, 1993.

Jensen PS, Shaw J: Children as victims of war: Current knowledge and future research needs. *J Am Acad Child Adolesc Psychiatry* 32:697–708, 1993.

Kolvin I, Miller FJW, Fleeting M, et al: Social and parenting factors affecting criminal-offence rates: Findings from the Newcastle Thousand Family Study (1947–1980). *Br J Psychiatry* 152:80–90, 1988.

Lin T-Y, Eisenberg L (eds): *Mental Health for One Billion People: A Chinese Perspective*. Vancouver, University of British Columbia Press, 1985.

Maniam T: Suicide and parasuicide in a hill resort in Malaysia. *Br J Psychiatry* 153:222–225, 1988.

Moffitt TE, Silva PA: Neuropsychological deficit and self-reported delinquency in an unselected birth cohort. *J Am Acad Child Adolesc Psychiatry* 27: 233–240, 1988.

Murray CJL, Chen, LC: In search of a contemporary theory for understanding mortality change. *Soc Sci Med* 36:143–155, 1993.

Nag M, White BNF, Peet RC: An anthropological approach to the study of the economic value of children in Java and Nepal. *Curr Anthropology* 19: 293–306, 1978.

Odejide AO, Oyewunmi LK, Ohaeri JU: Psychiatry in Africa: An overview. *Am J Psychiatry* 146: 708–716, 1989.

Offord DR, Boyle MN, Szatmari P: Ontario child health study: Six-month prevalence of disorder and rates of service utilization. *Arch Gen Psychiatry* 44: 832–836, 1987.

Phillips DP, Carstensen LL: Clustering of teenage suicides after television news stories about suicide. *N Engl J Med* 315:685–689, 1986.

Raffaelli M, Campos R, Merritt AP, et al.: Sexual practices and attitudes of street youth in Belo Horizonte, Brazil. *Soc Sci Med* 37:661–670, 1993.

Rahim SA, Cederblad M: Effects of rapid urbanization on child behavior in a part of Khartoum, Sudan. *J Child Psychol Psychiatry* 25:629–641, 1984.

Rohner RP: Parental acceptance-rejection and personality development: A universalist approach to behavioral science. In: Brislin N, Bochner I, Loner R (eds): *Cross-Cultural Perspectives on Learning*. New York, John Wiley & Sons, 1973.

Rubinstein DH: Suicide in Micronesia and Samoa: a critique of explanations. *Pacific Studies* 75: 51–75, 1992.

Rutter M, Cox A, Tepling C, et al: Attainment and adjustment in two geographical areas: The prevalence of psychiatric disorder. *Br J Psychiatry* 126: 493–509, 1975.

Rutter M, Lebovici S, Eisenberg L, et al: A triaxial classification of mental disorders in childhood. *J Child Psychol Psychiatry* 10:41–61, 1969.

Sartorius N: The research components of the WHO Mental Health Programme. *Psychol Med* 10: 175–185, 1980.

Sartorius N, Kelber CT, Cooper JE, et al: Progress toward achieving a common language in psychiatry. *Arch Gen Psychiatry* 50:115–124, 1993.

Schmidtke A, Hafner H: The Werther effect after television films: New evidence for an old hypothesis. *Psychol Med* 18:665–676, 1988.

Shen Y-C, Wang Y-F, Yang XL: An epidemiological investigation of minimal brain dysfunction in six elementary schools in Beijing. *J Child Psychol Psychiatry* 26:777–787, 1985.

Sigman M, Neumann C, Carter E, et al: Home interaction and the development of Embu toddlers in Kenya. *Child Dev* 59:1251–1261, 1988.

Sindiga I: The persistence of high fertility in Kenya. *Soc Sci Med* 20:71–84, 1985.

Super CM, Harkness S: The developmental niche: A conceptualization at the interface of child and culture. *Int J Behav Dev* 9:545–569, 1986.

Tarjan G, Tizard J, Rutter M, et al: Classification and mental retardation. *Am J Psychiatry* 128(suppl): 34–45, 1972.

Terr L: Childhood traumas. An outline and overview. *Am J Psychiatry* 148:10–20, 1991.

United Nations Children's Fund (UNICEF): *The State of the Worlds Children*. New York, Oxford University Press, 1993.

Vikan A: Psychiatric epidemiology in a sample of 1510 10-year-old children. I: Prevalence. *J Child Psychol Psychiatry* 26:85–109, 1985.

Weisz JR, Suwanlert S, Chaiyasit W, et al: Epidemiology of behavioral and emotional problems among Thai and American children: Parent reports for ages 6 to 11. *J Am Acad Child Adolesc Psychiatry* 26:890–897, 1987.

Weisz JR, Suwanlert S,Chaiyasit W, et al: Epidemiology of behavioral and emotional problems among Thai and American children: Teacher reports for ages 6–11. *J Child Psychol Psychiatry* 309: 471–484, 1989.

Werner EE, Smith RS: *Kauai's Children Come of Age*. Honolulu, University Press of Hawaii, 1977.

Werner EE, Smith RS: *Vulnerable But Invincible*. New York, McGraw-Hill, 1982.

White J, Moffitt T, Earls F, et al: How early can we tell? Predictors of conduct disorder and adolescent delinquency. *Criminology* 28:507–533m 1991.

Whiting JMW: Environmental constraints on infant care practices. In: Munroe RL, Whiting BB (eds): *Handbook of Cross-Cultural Human Development*. New York, Garland Press, 1981.

World Health Organization: *Guidelines for the Primary Prevention of Mental, Neurological and Psychosocial Disorders: 1 Principles; 2 Mental Retardation; 3 Epilepsy; 4 Suicide*. Geneva, WHO/MNH/MND 93.21-93.22-93.23-93.24, 1993.

Zivcic I: Emotional reactions of children to war stress in Croatia. *J Am Acad Child Adolesc Psychiatry* 32:709–713, 1993.

123 RECRUITMENT, TRAINING, AND CERTIFICATION IN CHILD AND ADOLESCENT PSYCHIATRY IN THE UNITED STATES

John E. Schowalter, M.D.

As we approach the 21st century, there are differing opinions about the number of recruits into child and adolescent psychiatry that is necessary to fulfill the research, educational, and service needs of the field and of society. While needs assessment studies routinely indicate that there should be four or more times the present number of practitioners and researchers, there is not evidence that society is willing to support many more than the current number of about 6000 subspecialists.

THE HISTORY OF TRAINING

Medicine began by being passed down as an apprentice-taught skill, not as a university-taught education. Even after the advent of schools of medicine, and up until this century, the science of medicine, learned at the university, was considered far less important than the art of medicine, learned from a more experienced colleague. It is because of this tradition that we still speak of residency training rather than residency education.

Child psychiatry in this country began during the first decade of the 20th century. The state of Illinois established in 1899 the Juvenile Court of Cook County, the first of its kind in the United States. As a means to study and treat delinquents, Dr. William Healy in 1909 formed a child guidance clinic, the Juvenile Psychopathic Institute in Chicago. This became the prototype for future clinics and employed a multidisciplinary staff that consisted of the so-called holy trinity: psychiatry, psychology, and social work. As child guidance clinics grew in numbers and in size during the second quarter of the century, it was increasingly necessary to train personnel for this new type of work. The clinics were typically headed by a psychiatrist, but the tasks accomplished by the staff of the three disciplines were often relatively interchangeable. It soon became clear that psychiatrists who worked with children must have training that was more extensive and specific than that obtained in their general psychiatry residency. Under the auspices of the Commonwealth Fund, a major conference was held in 1944 that provided an agreed-upon set of skill areas that should be mastered by psychiatrists who treat children and their families (Cohen, 1987). These skill areas included growth and development, psychodynamics, work with parents, administration, and community organization. The psychoanalytic viewpoint was by far the most prevalent nationally, but the emphasis of any particular clinic's training was unique to the beliefs of the director, the makeup of the staff, and the clinic's setting.

The year 1946 was a watershed one for child psychiatry training. World War II was over, psychiatry had proven itself as a useful medical specialty, and many psychiatrists returned to civilian life. There was a national thrust to do all that could be done to raise children to live in a better world tomorrow. The baby boom generation was born, and an optimistic American society wanted to be assured that this new postwar generation would grow up right. Included in the Mental Health Act of 1946 were monies for the training of child psychiatrists. Also in 1946, the child guidance clinics banded together in a confederation called the

American Association of Psychiatric Clinics for Children (AAPCC). The AAPCC set up a training committee. Clinics that wanted to offer approved training had to apply to the committee and be surveyed (Krug, 1969). This was a rigorous process, and only about one-half of the founding clinics were initially approved for training.

Scientific and training articles in the field of child psychiatry during this time tended to be published either in the *American Journal of Psychiatry*, the *American Journal of Orthopsychiatry*, *The Psychoanalytic Study of the Child*, or in pediatric journals. It became clear that child psychiatry needed its own forum, and in 1953 the American Academy of Child Psychiatry was established. This was a by-invitation-only organization for those who had made a "significant" contribution to the field. For the most part, membership in the Academy was synonymous with being a child psychiatry educator. One of the first tasks of the Academy, therefore, was to transfer training accreditation away from the clinic-based and multidisciplinary AAPCC and to an organization that was more medically oriented.

The American Board of Psychiatry and Neurology was established in 1934 and the American Board of Pediatrics in 1933. It was clear that recognition of child psychiatry as a medical subspecialty would better legitimize its status. Many of the early and influential Academy members were pediatricians originally, and there was vigorous debate whether child psychiatry would more appropriately be a subspecialty of pediatrics or of psychiatry. A mail poll was conducted of leading child psychiatrists, and the choice was made for psychiatry. However, the American Board of Pediatrics demanded, and received, the right in perpetuity to appoint a pediatrician member who would be part of the Committee on Certification in Child Psychiatry. With this stipulation, the American Board of Medical Specialties approved the petition, and the first subspecialty candidates in child psychiatry were examined in 1959.

Inextricably linked to subspecialty certification are standardized training criteria formulated through the Accreditation Council of Graduate Medical Education (ACGME). The ACGME Residency Review Committee (RRC) in Psychiatry oversees periodic surveys and decides whether or not to accredit and reaccredit each program for training (Schowalter, 1987). This approach was much more medically oriented than the AAPCC reviews. The ACGME demanded that child psychiatry training programs be linked to accredited general psychiatry residency programs and to medical centers approved by the Joint Commission on the Accreditation of Hospitals. These requirements forced the child guidance clinics interested in training to leave, at least somewhat, their community roots and to become more attached to medicine. It also stimulated the development of new child psychiatry training programs that were situated in medical centers rather than freestanding in the community. The relative equality between the "holy trinity" disciplines also shifted, since ACGME subspecialty training requirements with each new revision increasingly emphasized the necessity for child psychiatrists to receive the bulk of their training from child psychiatrists.

In 1969 the Academy opened its doors to all child psychiatrists who graduated from or who were in training in ACGME-approved programs. In this same year, the Society of Professors of Child Psychiatry was established. The membership of this organization was limited to chiefs of academic divisions of child psychiatry. Although not every division was accredited for training, the vast majority were, and the Society's relatively small membership made its meetings ideal forums for the discussion of training issues.

The American Association of Directors of Psychiatric Residency Training (AADPRT) and the Association for Academic Psychiatry are more recently formed organizations devoted to education and training. Although they began with an almost exclusive focus on general psychiatry, both organizations in the 1980s deliberately expanded their involvement with child psychiatry training and training directors.

PROGRAM ACCREDITATION

The ACGME consists of representatives from the American Medical Association, the American Board of Medical Specialties, the Association of American Medical Colleges, the American Hospital Association, and the Council of Medical Specialty Societies and is responsible for setting training requirements for all specialties and subspecialties approved by the American Board of Medical Specialties. There are two sets of requirements.

The General Requirements are generic and the same regardless of the specialty being reviewed. They are concerned less with the particular training area than with the overall support and surveillance provided by the medical center in which the training program is embedded. These issues include requirements for the selection of trainees and assurance that there are procedures for evaluation, evaluation feedback, grievance reporting, and due process. There must also be adequate compensation, an emphasis on education rather than on service, and acculturation help for those trainees who need it. Until the 1980s, the General Requirements were not stressed nearly as much as the Special Requirements. The ACGME site visitors, who usually survey a program every 3–5 years, have recently begun to very seriously query hospital officials about their involvement in and support of the individual program being reviewed. An individual program can be put on probation if the General Requirements are not fulfilled. More often, however, the threat of probation causes the medical center administration to become more forthcoming in its interest in and support of each of its training programs. It is the realization that many individual training programs falter because of supervisory and/or financial neglect by the central administration that caused the ACGME to place increasing emphasis on the General Requirements. Since hospitals and medical schools do not like to have their programs disaccredited, most program directors have found the General Requirements to be a useful lever whereby to obtain greater institutional support.

The Special Requirements are specific to a particular specialty or subspecialty. They are revised approximately every decade, although discrete changes may be made between revisions. The revisions of the Special Requirements and the evaluation of the ACGME surveys are the responsibility of the Residency Review Committee (RRC). There are RRCs for all accredited specialties, and the RRCs report to the ACGME. RRC members for psychiatry are nominated by three organizations: the American Medical Association (AMA), the American Board of Psychiatry and Neurology (ABPN), and the American Psychiatric Association (APA). There are now nine RRC members in general psychiatry and six members in child and adolescent psychiatry.

According to Residency Review Committee meeting minutes, the RRC for Psychiatry and Neurology was organized in Chicago in October, 1954. Members were chosen by the ABPN and by the AMA Council on Medical Education and Hospitals. At its October 1959 meeting, the RRC noted that the ABPN had developed a "sub-board in child psychia-

try," and the question arose whether to review child psychiatry training programs separately or at the same time as the survey of a general psychiatry residency. A decision was made in favor of the former. At the March 1960 meeting, the *Essentials for Child Psychiatry* was reviewed and subsequently approved. At the October 1960 meeting, a child psychiatrist, Dr. William Langford, was invited as a guest. He reviewed 17 programs and approved 11. Dr. Langford's recommendations needed an RRC vote to become official. This format of child psychiatry program review continued until in 1967 the Committee on Certification in Child Psychiatry of the ABPN petitioned for the position of a voting child psychiatrist member on the RRC. The RRC denied this petition at its April meeting, but for the October 1967 meeting listed the child psychiatrist as an "ex-officio member without vote," rather than "guest," as had been done before. This protocol continued unchallenged until the October 1978 meeting when the RRC expressed concern that child psychiatry program evaluation was in fact decided, if not voted, on by someone not part of the RRC. This seemed suspect functionally and legally, and the RRC requested that an official child psychiatry member be appointed by each of its two parent organizations. The ABPN approved, but the AMA Council on Medical Education refused. At the March 1979 meeting, the lone ex officio child psychiatrist reviewed 28 programs, while six general psychiatrist members reviewed 30 programs and six neurologist members reviewed only 15 programs. Since it was clear that more child psychiatry reviewers were needed, the RRC repeated even more strongly its request that two child psychiatrists be appointed as full Committee members. This second appeal was approved by both parent organizations, and at the March 1980 meeting two child psychiatrists attended as full Committee members. Two years later the RRC was restructured so that the neurology and psychiatry components met on separate occasions. It was also decided to include the American Psychiatric Association as a third parent organization for the RRC, and as part of its contribution the APA supported a third child psychiatrist member in 1983. Traditionally, the RRC Chair was from the ABPN and the Vice Chair was from the AMA Council on Medical Education. In 1985 the Committee appointed a child psychiatrist as Vice Chair, and this practice has been continued since. In 1989 it was decided to have each program's survey reviewed by two, rather than one, Committee member. This change required enlarging the RRC membership. In 1990 a fourth child psychiatrist was added, and in 1995 a fifth and sixth.

Although the initial draft of a Special Requirements revision for child and adolescent psychiatry is written by the RRC members, the draft is sent to the program directors of the approximately 115 accredited training sites and to the specialty's foremost national organizations for review. If major changes are made, the second draft is again sent for comment to program directors and to organizations. The revision process usually takes 2–3 years. The final approval of Special Requirements comes from the ACGME board. The most recent child and adolescent psychiatry Special Requirements revision went into effect in 1995. Although there are with each revision a greater number of requirements and a stricter enforcement of the requirements, the great majority of child and adolescent training directors have believed that the quality and quantity of requirements are fair and possible to do in the 2 years allotted (Schowalter, 1989). About a quarter of program directors surveyed in the late 1980s did believe that general psychiatry should be reduced to a single year of training, and approximately one-third believed that the child and adolescent psychiatry residency would have to be extended to 3 years before the end of the century.

Although there is a continuous debate as to whether or not child and adolescent psychiatry should, as did pediatrics from internal medicine, split from general psychiatry, the pressure for this is more through rhetoric than action. The majority of child and adolescent psychiatrists want the ability to also treat adults. And in practical terms, there are very few child and adolescent psychiatry training programs that have a faculty and financial base broad and deep enough to enable them to function as an autonomous department. One commonly raised proposal is to begin subspecialty training in the third postgraduate year and concentrate the next 3 years of residency on work with children and adolescents. This approach has found no support from either Directors of the ABPN or members of the general psychiatry RRC. These two bodies, crucial in the determination of any policy change, believe that less than 2 years of residency with adults is insufficient training to make one board-eligible in general psychiatry.

An innovative 5-year integrated training sequence in pediatrics, general psychiatry, and child and adolescent psychiatry, better known as the Triple Board, began as an experiment in 1985 and was approved nationwide as a combined residency in 1992 (Schowalter, 1993). This track is sponsored by the ABPN, the ABPN Committee on Certification in Child and Adolescent Psychiatry, and the American Board of Pediatrics. For trainees in approved programs, the sponsoring bodies waive the usual training periods required for eligibility for their certifying examinations.

INDIVIDUALS' CERTIFICATION

While it is the RRC's responsibility to accredit training programs, the ABPN certifies individuals as competent to practice as specialists. The ABPN determines the accuracy of the applicant's credentials in regard to schooling and residency. To be a candidate for certification in child and adolescent psychiatry, one must have completed at least 3 postgraduate years of ACGME-approved residency in general psychiatry and a 2-year approved residency in child and adolescent psychiatry. One must also have passed the written and oral ABPN examinations in general psychiatry. In 1987 the ABPN approved the expansion of the subspecialty of child psychiatry to child and adolescent psychiatry. This decision was based on the fact that the RRC Special Requirements for child psychiatry already mandated training with adolescents and that more than one-quarter of the content of the written and oral certifying examinations in child psychiatry were already devoted to the adolescent age range. An important impetus for the expansion was administrative. In the late 1980s, there was much interest in forming psychiatric subspecialties. This interest was based both on an expansion of the knowledge base in such areas as geriatric, forensic, and addiction psychiatry, and on a wish for subspecialty recognition for credentialing and differential remuneration. There was at this time also a move to form a separate subspecialty of adolescent psychiatry. By granting this age group to child psychiatry, where it was placed traditionally, the ABPN limited by one the number of subspecialties available for official recognition. Counterpressures to slow down the addition of psychiatric subspecialties picked up momentum in the early 1990s.

Another major decision in the late 1980s for the ABPN and the Committee on Certification in Child and Adolescent Psychiatry was to move toward time-limited certification. By this is meant that every 10 years the diplomate must meet a set of criteria in order to remain certified for the next decade. Not only must reassessment be meaningful, but it is also important to keep its cost and annoyance to a minimum. In November 1989, the ABPN decided to begin time-limited certification in both general psychiatry and in child and adolescent psychiatry beginning with examinations held after October 1, 1994. The first recertification examination will be held no later than January 1, 2000. The most likely recertification format will be cognitive and through modules. Modules will include general psychiatry, as well as modules in certain subspecialties. With this format, a child and adolescent psychiatrist would take a single recertification examination, but one that would include modules of both general and child and adolescent psychiatry.

Although there are increasing numbers of psychiatrists who take the certification examinations, both in general and in child and adolescent psychiatry, certification is technically voluntary. In point of fact, reimbursement and hospital credentialing are increasingly tied to specialty certification. Also, a number of state medical licensing boards have proposed legislation that ties medical relicensure with either the periodic passing of a state examination in general medicine or evidence within the time period of passage of a specialty board licensure or relicensure

examination. Therefore, although in psychiatry there will be a "grandfather" clause that will exclude the need for anyone certified prior to the onset of the time-limited certificate to be recertified, hospital credentials boards and state medical license boards may nonetheless require recertification as part of their requirements.

An ongoing challenge for all examining boards is how to provide a truly competence-based examination. It is relatively easy to obtain reliability in an examination, particularly a written one. To show validity (i.e., that the test performance is linked to actual clinical practice) is much more difficult. With any oral examination, the candidate always has the variability of hard or easy graders in the examiners he or she draws. To avoid these variables, the American Board of Internal Medicine dropped the oral examination in 1977, and the American Board of Pediatrics dropped it in 1989. The ABPN is the only board to still use live patients with an oral examination. In the child and adolescent psychiatry examination, there is an adolescent patient. With a patient interview, the candidate has the luck of the draw for both patient and examiner. While fairness and reliability are much surer for written examinations, especially with multiple choice questions, these questions cannot show a candidate's skill level in interacting with a patient. Actors who simulate patients, videotapes of patients, and written vignettes are all possible substitutes for live patients. Simulated patients come closest to the real thing and can provide a more standardized examination (Sanson-Fisher and Poole, 1980). They require, however, much time to train and are very expensive. Videotapes of patients are used by many boards, but some candidates seem unable to extract material well from a relatively lifeless tape. It is unfair to fail them at video-watching rather than clinical psychiatry. Written vignettes are usually brief and used more as a stimulus for discussion than as a substitute for a clinical interview. Written patient management problems help keep the focus of the examination on process rather than product (Langsley, 1986), but there is little evidence to prove that the ability to answer didactic questions about psychiatry is highly correlated to practicing well. In the future there will undoubtedly be an increased use of an examination format that uses personal computers, for example, with a CD-ROM format, especially for recertification. Other specialties have used office audits and even the videotaping of office examinations and procedures. These latter approaches are less applicable for psychiatry. A skill that is probably most difficult to assess is professional demeanor. To measure this is the main argument for the use of patients or patient simulators. Attitude does tend to be constant, although even here, a candidate's competence may vary enormously from interview to interview. It is known that attitudinal qualities are often judged by teachers and practitioners as equal to knowledge skills (Langsley and Yager, 1988). This is even true for much less patient-oriented specialties, such as radiology (Tarico et al., 1986).

It is clear that a continuum of evaluation is most accurate—a motion picture rather than a snapshot of a candidate's functioning. Program directors can be sources of information to the ABPN about a candidate's clinical and ethical behavior during residency, but the training director's understandable bias often renders such judgments unrealistically positive. There is pressure on the ABPN from the field to have residents take and pass the Part I written examination in the 3rd or 4th postgraduate year. This will probably not much affect child and adolescent psychiatry residencies, since many residents take this examination now during their subspecialty years. However, if a rule is made that residents cannot finish general psychiatry residency until they pass Part I, this could prove a complication for residents who were accepted for a child and adolescent psychiatry residency, failed Part I, and needed to take further general psychiatry training and a retest. These details have yet to be worked out.

Recertification provides an ideal opportunity to create a prospective, longitudinal research component to follow diplomates' careers and test results over time. Perhaps in this way it can be discovered how to better understand and test for competence as demonstrated in actual clinical performance. Although it is still not possible to prove a strong correlation between test scores and clinical performance, common sense suggests the likelihood of some correlation. Courts have accepted this common sense premise and have never overturned a specialty board's decision, except on procedural grounds.

RECRUITMENT

Child and adolescent psychiatry has a chronic recruitment problem. The Graduate Medical Education National Advisory Committee (GMENAC) Report of 1980 declared child psychiatry the least sufficiently staffed medical specialty and recommended that it triple its numbers from 3000 to 9000 in 10 years. The number was not even doubled in the time allotted. Surveys have shown a shortage of child and adolescent psychiatry trainees, faculty, and, especially, researchers (Beresin and Borus, 1989; Enzer, 1989; Institute of Medicine, 1989). In 1993 there were 807 positions offered at the 119 accredited residency programs in child and adolescent psychiatry (American Medical Association, 1993). Understandably, women and medical students interested in children are drawn to child and adolescent psychiatry, but less understandable is the frequent evidence that those not interested in research are attracted to the subspecialty (Haviland et al., 1988; Weissman and Bushook, 1987).

A national conference on recruitment for child and adolescent psychiatry was held in 1989. There was consensus that the greatest need was for more researchers and faculty. It was also acknowledged that improvement of the quantity and quality of residents was the best approach to enhance faculty recruitment. Deterrents to recruitment include a relatively long training period coupled with relatively low income. The latter is due to the high-ambulatory, low-procedure nature of work with patients whose families have not yet reached their earning capacity. In addition, researchers' training is extended, and their salaries tend to be lower than those of practitioners and clinically based faculty. The conference participants proposed a great number of suggestions, the foci of which extended from undergraduates and medical students to postfellowship researcher support (American Academy of Child and Adolescent Psychiatry, 1990). Personal contact is crucial for recruitment. This can be provided through the teaching of child development in college and medical schools, the organization of student child psychiatry clubs, and the provision of individual mentors for interested medical students and general psychiatry residents. Good communication must be established and maintained between child psychiatry and general psychiatry training directors. It is essential that child and adolescent psychiatry rotations be provided to general psychiatry residents before the time at which they must apply for subspecialty training. A greater emphasis on research should be added to the Special Requirements, and the RRC should be more vigorous and eliminate programs that cannot provide comprehensive training. More money is necessary from government, foundation, proprietary hospital, endowment, and other sources to better support child and adolescent researchers through their postresidency fellowships and early faculty years. Without more full-time researchers, there is little likelihood that investigative productivity can be substantially enhanced.

CONCLUSIONS

Child and adolescent psychiatry is the first subspecialty of psychiatry, and training has struggled with its level of interdependence with general psychiatry. This has been true for time allotment, faculty duties, standards, and recruitment. In a period when other psychiatric subspecialties are burgeoning, child and adolescent psychiatry's professional identity and goals must continue to be clarified and transmitted in a cogent manner. As research and clinical information accumulates, a decision will need to be made in regard to an expansion of training time, a rearrangement of general psychiatry and subspecialty time, a deletion of some present requirements, or a combination of these approaches. Such decisions can be made well only through a constant dialogue between the members of the American Academy of Child and Adolescent Psychiatry, the Society of Professors of Child and Adolescent Psychiatry, the Residency Review Committee, and the American Board of Psychiatry and Neurology. A permanent structure for this ongoing debate is necessary and should be developed.

Editor's Note: For discussion of antecedents of child and adolescent psychiatry found in historical accounts of the discovery of the child, see Chapter 127. For further discussion of the history of mental health delivery systems in the United States, see Chapter 120.

References

American Academy of Child and Adolescent Psychiatry: *Preparing for the Future: The 1989 Recruitment Conference on Child and Adolescent Psychiatry.* Washington, DC, American Academy of Child and Adolescent Psychiatry, 1990.

American Medical Association: *Graduate Medical Education Directory, 1993–1994.* Chicago, IL, American Medical Association, 1993.

Beresin EV, Borus JF: Child psychiatry fellowship training: A crisis in recruitment and manpower. *Am J Psychiatry* 146:759–763, 1989.

Cohen RL: The history of training in child and adolescent psychiatry. In: Cohen RL, Dulcan MK (eds): *Basic Handbook of Training in Child and Adolescent Psychiatry.* Springfield, IL, Charles C Thomas, 1987, pp. 10–23.

Enzer NB: Recent trends in the recruitment of child and adolescent psychiatrists: An overview of general and faculty needs. *Acad Psychiatry* 13: 176–188, 1989.

Graduate Medical Education National Advisory Committee: *Summary Report to the Secretary* (Vol. 1, publication on HRA 81-651). Washington, DC, US Department of Health and Human Services, 1980.

Haviland MG, Dial TH, Pincus HA: Characteristics of senior medical students planning to subspecialize in child psychiatry. *J Am Acad Child Adolesc Psychiatry* 27:404–407, 1988.

Institute of Medicine: *Research on Children and Adolescents with Mental, Behavioral, and Developmental Disorders: Mobilizing a National Initiative.* Washington, DC, National Academy of Sciences, 1989.

Krug O: Career training in child psychiatry and child psychiatry education in general psychiatry training. In: Adams P, Work H, Carmer J (eds): *Academic Child Psychiatry.* Gainesville, FL, Society of Professors of Child Psychiatry, 1969, pp. 59–80.

Langsley DG: Rating clinical skills of psychiatric residents. In: Lloyd JS, Langsley DG (eds): *How to Evaluate Residents.* Chicago, American Board of Medical Specialties, 1986, pp. 267–273.

Langsley DG, Yager J: The definition of a psychiatrist: Eight years later. *Am J Psychiatry* 45: 469–475, 1988.

Sanson-Fisher RW, Poole AD: Simulated patients and the assessment of medical students' interpersonal skills. *J Med Educ* 14:249–253, 1980.

Schowalter JE: Program accreditation. In: Cohen RL, Dulcan MK (eds): *Basic Handbook of Training in Child and Adolescent Psychiatry.* Springfield, IL, Charles C Thomas, 1987, pp. 391–401.

Schowalter JE: Child psychiatry program directors' ratings of residency experiences. *J Am Acad Child Adolesc Psychiatry* 28:124–129, 1989.

Schowalter JE: Tinker to Evers to Chance: Triple board update. *J Am Acad Child Adolesc Psychiatry* 32:243, 1993.

Tarico V, Smith WL, Altmaier E, et al: Critical incident interviewing in evaluation of resident performance. In: Lloyd JS, Langsley DG (eds): *How to Evaluate Residents.* Chicago, American Board of Medical Specialties, 1986, pp. 351–356.

Weissman SH, Bushook PG: Manpower and recruitment. In: Cohen RL, Dulcan MK (eds): *Basic Handbook of Training in Child and Adolescent Psychiatry.* Springfield, IL, Charles C Thomas, 1987, pp. 341–347.

124 THE DEVELOPING BRAIN AND MIND: ADVANCES IN RESEARCH TECHNIQUES

J. Gerald Young, M.D., James R. Brasic, M.D., M.P.H., Harry Ostrer, M.D.,
Diana Kaplan, Ph.D., Michael Will, M.D., E. Roy John, Ph.D., Leslie Prichep, Ph.D.,
and Monte Buchsbaum, M.D.

TECHNICAL ADVANCES ALTERING CLINICAL CARE IN CHILD AND ADOLESCENT PSYCHIATRY

The dizzying advances in genetics and the neurosciences leave clinicians and investigators puzzled. Which of the emerging technical methods are likely to enter into the mainstream of clinical practice? What should we know about these techniques? How do they alter clinical theory and practice? Predicting the future of clinically applicable technology is a humbling task. The most important clinical advances in the next decade might involve instrumental methods developed from physical or chemical principles that are remote from clinical application at the moment. However, technical methods emerging currently, but still developing and not yet widely available, can be considered.

Many categories of technical research methods could be described. Fortunately, there are more advances than can be reviewed, making us optimistic about future diagnostic and therapeutic progress. Rather than cataloging every new advance, examples of significant new techniques are reviewed in each section of this chapter.

BRAIN STRUCTURE: BRAIN IMAGING TECHNIQUES

Objectives of Neuroimaging

A wealth of brain imaging techniques are available whose validation through neuropathological, clinical, and alternative imaging methods has rapidly progressed. They are now applicable for clinical care or research and provide new explanations for behavioral abnormalities. Brain imaging techniques can be conceptually divided into those methods that demonstrate the brain structure or brain function, or both, as in Table 124.1. Neuroimaging methods are clinically utilized to search for demonstrable organic pathology that might contribute to the genesis of a disorder, i.e., a general medical condition that might be treatable. Neuroimaging cannot yet be routinely used clinically for the identification of abnormalities associated with a primary psychiatric disorder (e.g., depression) but increasing integration into the diagnostic process is anticipated in the near future.

X-ray Computed Tomography

Computerized axial tomography, or computed tomography (CT), became available in 1973 and was the first of the new brain imaging methods. Reconstruction imaging, central to the development of CT, is the foundation for many of the advances in brain imaging. The specific imaging technique determines the type of measurable parameter obtained for each unit of three-dimensional space (termed a ''voxel'') or two-dimensional space (a ''pixel''); in x-ray computed tomography it is multiple measurements of x-ray transmissions at different angles in a slice through the head. There is variable x-ray attenuation according to the properties of the tissue through which the x-rays pass. Computer methods are used to retrieve the resulting vast amounts of data; these data are the basis for reconstructing the image through additional computerized mathematical procedures.

A ring of beam generators and detectors images a single slice through the brain in the center of the ring. Sequential slices are obtained by advancing the patient through the gantry of the CT scanner after obtaining each slice. CT makes use of photomultiplier tubes as detectors, conferring much greater sensitivity than classical radiographic film. The detector converts the intensity of the x-ray beam into a proportional electrical impulse. By the time x-rays reach the detector, they are attenuated by a combination of scatter and absorption in tissue. When the x-ray beam passes through bone, there is high attenuation, and the bone appears white on the display; when it passes through air, there is minimal attenuation and the space is black in the image. Intermediate densities are represented as shades of gray.

The physical characteristics of the tissues, particularly their physical densities, are the primary influence on the degree of attenuation. Using multiple different angular projections, thousands of x-ray transmission measures are obtained. A computer digitizes the electrical impulses at the detector and generates a set of CT numbers associated with each voxel, with each number coding for the amount of attenuation associated with a given transmission. Such data sets are obtained for several cross-sectional planes (slices) and are then solved individually using one of several mathematical algorithms to produce a grey-scale image (Coffman, 1989), reflecting the different values of the measurable parameter. Color images can, alternatively, be generated to emphasize certain findings.

Rapid improvements in CT led to its wide dissemination and to its current place as the major brain imaging technique worldwide. It is well understood, relatively simple, and the cost is reasonable. It is useful for the detection of focal pathology (particularly calcific, hemorrhagic, and space-occupying lesions) where the x-ray density of the brain is changed, but it is relatively insensitive to gray/white matter boundaries. Its routine use in the evaluation of psychiatric patients is still controversial, as it appears not to meet the test of cost-benefit analysis. A contrast material can be injected intravenously to define vascular lesions and to identify abnormalities associated with blood-brain barrier disruption. Advantages and disadvantages of computed tomography are indicated in Table 124.2.

Major findings utilizing CT in psychiatric disorders have included ventricular enlargement and widened cortical sulci in schizophrenia, particularly associated with negative symptoms. However, these findings are nonspecific, because ventricular enlargement in patients with mood disorders with positive psychotic symptoms also has been described (Coffman, 1989).

The general pattern of CT findings in child and adolescent disorders has been a higher rate of abnormalities than comparison groups, but these are varying and nonspecific abnormalities that cannot yet be used diagnostically. Studies of autistic patients indicate subgroups with ventricular and/or subcortical abnormalities (Bauman and Kemper, 1985; Campbell et al., 1982; Caparulo et al., 1981). There may be abnormalities in a subgroup of patients with Tourette disorder (Caparulo et al., 1981), but no impairments were found in children with attention deficit hyperactivity disorder (Shaywitz et al., 1983). There is evidence for ventricular enlargement and reduced caudate volume in patients with childhood onset obsessive-compulsive disorder (Luxemberg et al., 1988).

CT is being replaced by magnetic resonance imaging (MRI) as a

Table 124.1. Brain Imaging Techniques

1. Structural techniques (to study brain structure and anatomy)
   a. Computed tomography (CT)
   b. Magnetic resonance imaging (MRI) (nuclear magnetic resonance, (NMR)
2. Functional/dynamic techniques (to study brain metabolism and regional variations in brain activity)
   a. Functional magnetic resonance imaging (fMRI)
   b. Quantitative electrophysiology (QEEG) (computerized mapping of the electrical activity of the brain)
   c. Single photon emission computerized tomography (SPECT)
   d. Positron emission tomography (PET)
   e. Magnetoencephalography (MEG)

Table 124.2. Computed Tomography

1. Advantages
   a. Most widely available imaging method
   b. Best understood imaging method
   c. Low to moderate cost
   d. Relative simplicity
   e. Brief scanning time
   f. Preferable for patients who might be adversely affected by the MRI magnetic field or instrument (e.g., pacemaker, aneurysm clip, claustrophobia, anxiety reactions)
   g. Can visualize materials with distinct x-ray attenuation properties (e.g., bony structures, fluid, gas) with excellent spatial resolution (<1 mm)
   h. Particularly useful for observing gross neuropathological conditions that affect tissue x-ray density
      Cortical atrophy
      Ventricular enlargement
      Calcified tissue
      Tumors
      Strokes
      Acute hemorrhage (less than 48–72 hours)
      Trauma, where tissue is grossly cut or removed
2. Disadvantages
   a. Uses ionizing radiation, although the dosage is low
   b. Limited to visualization of structures in transverse (axial) plane, so has limited capabilities for reconstructing three-dimensional anatomical images
   c. Poor contrast between gray matter and white matter; does not differentiate soft-tissue densities well, nor identify white matter lesions
   d. Soft-tissue imaging adjacent to bone is compromised by the beam-hardening artifact (especially in posterior fossa and cortex at highest levels above canthomeatal line)
   e. Utility apparently limited to the determination of focal pathology. It is less likely to be useful for the imaging of more subtle psychiatric brain abnormalities
   f. Possible idiosyncratic or chemotoxic allergic response to contrast material (intravenous iodine)
   g. More difficult to obtain normal controls, because of radiation exposure

high-resolution, anatomy-rich structural imaging technique that is coregistered to anchor functional imaging techniques in an anatomical template.

Magnetic Resonance Imaging

THEORETICAL AND TECHNICAL FOUNDATIONS OF MRI

MRI or nuclear magnetic resonance (NMR), as it was previously designated, is an imaging technique that utilizes manipulation and measurement of the electromagnetic properties of biologic tissues. Magnetic resonance relies upon the fact that certain species of atomic nuclei found in brain tissue behave as magnetic dipoles. These dipoles are randomly oriented at rest. By placing the head within a strong external homogeneous magnetic field, the dipoles align either with or against the field in one plane, producing a measurable, nonrandom, net magnetization (Fig. 124.1).

The magnetic field also induces each dipole to undergo a complex periodic movement (resonance), the frequency of which is specific for each nuclear species at a given field strength. A second, weaker gradient magnetic field is "pulsed" for a few milliseconds, creating a small but uniform gradation

of change across the main magnetic field and the associated frequencies. By applying a radio signal from a radio-frequency (RF) coil, tuned to the frequency of a particular species, a shift in the direction of the magnetic moment (resonance) is induced. Some lower energy nuclei absorb RF energy and align against the field (in phase). This phenomenon results in the emission of a radio-frequency signal that can be measured by the RF coil, which acts as a radio detector, or antenna. Upon turning off the RF pulse, nuclei at the higher energy level emit RF energy and return to the lower energy state, simultaneously aligning with the magnetic field (dephasing or decay of proton spins). A second RF pulse causes a progressive rephasing known as a spin-echo, and the RF coil detects this changing signal. The MR scanner generates spatial maps (images) of RF signals by applying magnetic field gradients during RF irradiation. Because of their abundance and high signal amplitude, hydrogen nuclei (protons) are the atomic species generally utilized for the creation of magnetic resonance images (Cox et al., 1994; Rauch and Renshaw, 1995).

The events involved in the measurement of nuclear magnetic resonance are complex, but certain properties related to the decay (or relaxation) of the resonant frequency signal are exploited to generate images based upon three different kinds of structurally relevant information, including two tissue relaxation times, T1 and T2 (Andreasen, 1989):

1. *Proton density weighted images:* images that display the quantity of hydrogen nuclei in a particular sample. The primary source of contrast in the MR image is the density of protons in the tissue, which are mostly in water. Pathological processes in the brain increase tissue free water content, enhancing signal intensity on these images.
2. *T1-weighted images:* images constructed from that aspect of resonance decay useful for displaying high contrast between white matter, gray matter, and CSF. T1 images are generally used to highlight normal cerebral anatomic relationships.
3. *T2-weighted images:* images constructed from that aspect of resonance decay useful for displaying pathologic structures. T2 images highlight regions of high free water content that are typical of many forms of cerebral pathology (e.g., demyelination, edema, infection, inflammation, or infarction).

The essential components of the MRI system include static and gradient magnets, a radio-frequency transmitter and receiver, a computer, and a display system. By varying the timing of the radio-frequency pulses used to stimulate nuclear magnetic resonance, the system operator can determine to what extent the resultant image will provide T1 information, T2 information, proton density information, or various weighted combinations of each. The most widely used scanning technique used today for routine clinical purposes is the "spin-echo" pulse sequence. Modifications of this basic pulse sequence can produce multislice images weighted to display almost any desired combination of T1, T2, or proton density weighting.

MR images have distinctly different appearances according to the pulse sequence employed, so it is necessary to have this information before an image can be interpreted (for example, see Figs. 124.2–124.7). While the manipulation of scanning sequences gives the flexibility to enhance different features of the image, it also makes the process more complex and requires that careful consideration be given to imaging objectives prior to the scan. The scanning procedure must be completed in a reasonable period of time for the patient, so selection of planes and pulse sequences requires a clinical decision at the outset (Andreasen, 1989). MRI parameters used to define pulse sequences are repetition time (TR) and echo time (TE).

Figure 124.1. **A,** How charged particles produce a magnetic field: the *Nuclear* in NMR. **B,** The effect of placing protons within an external magnetic field: the *Magnetic* in NMR. **C,** How an external field produces resonance (precession): the *Resonance* in NMR. **D,** The use of radio-frequency signals to shift the direction of the magnetic moment. (From Andreasen NC: Brain imaging: Applications in psychiatry. Washington, DC, American Psychiatric Press, 1989, pp. 70–72.)

A

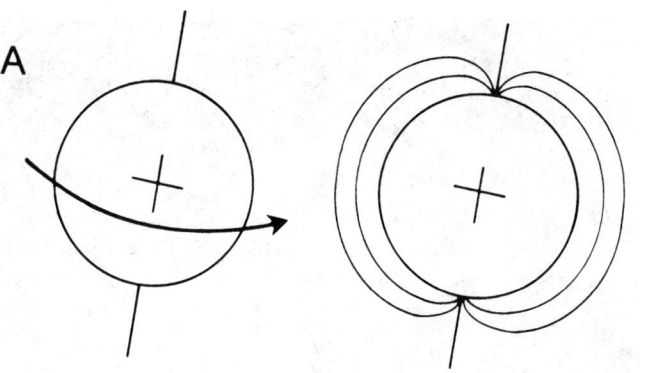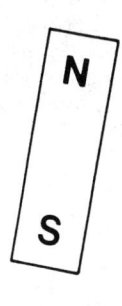

Spinning charged particles in the nuclei of atoms — induce a magentic moment — that acts like a tiny bar magnet.

B

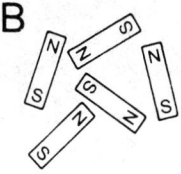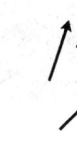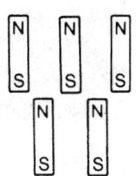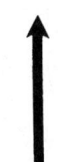

Without an external field the magnetic moments are random, — and therefore cancel one another and produce no net magnetization. — With an external magnetic field the protons are aligned and the magnetic moments concentrated, — producing a net positive magnetization.

WITHOUT AN EXTERNAL FIELD — WITH AN EXTERNAL FIELD

C

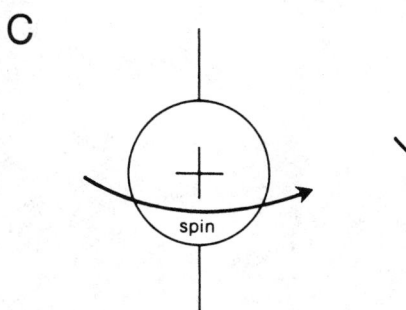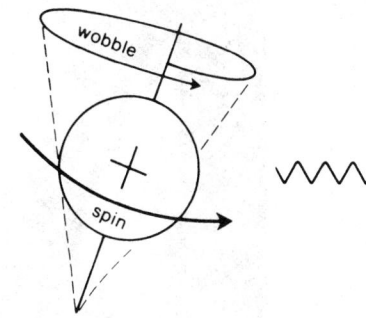

The spin is even. — The spin WOBBLES like a top, or precesses, with a resonant frequency specific to the nuclear species.

WITHOUT AN EXTERNAL FIELD — WITH AN EXTERNAL FIELD

D

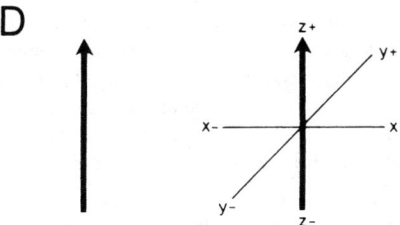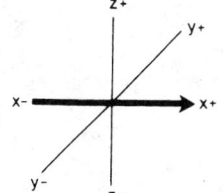

The net positive magnetic moment — is aligned in the Z axis (the direction of the external field). — But a radio frequency signal can be applied to give the protons extra energy, — which will tip them 90° into the X axis and change the direction of the net magnetic moment.

Figure 124.2. **A,** Inversion recovery image of a posterior fossa tumor. **B,** Spin-echo image of a posterior fossa tumor. (From Andreasen NC: Brain imaging: Applications in psychiatry. Washington, DC, American Psychiatric Press, 1989, p. 90.)

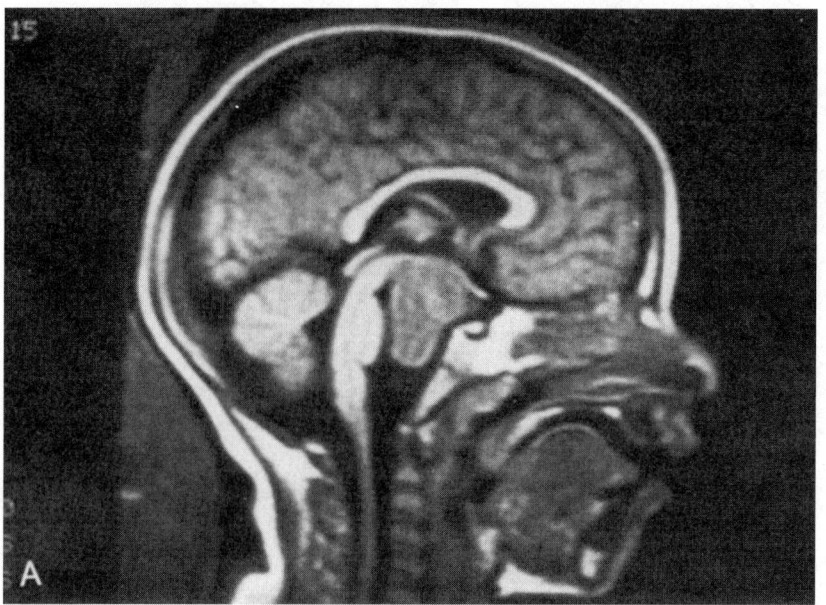

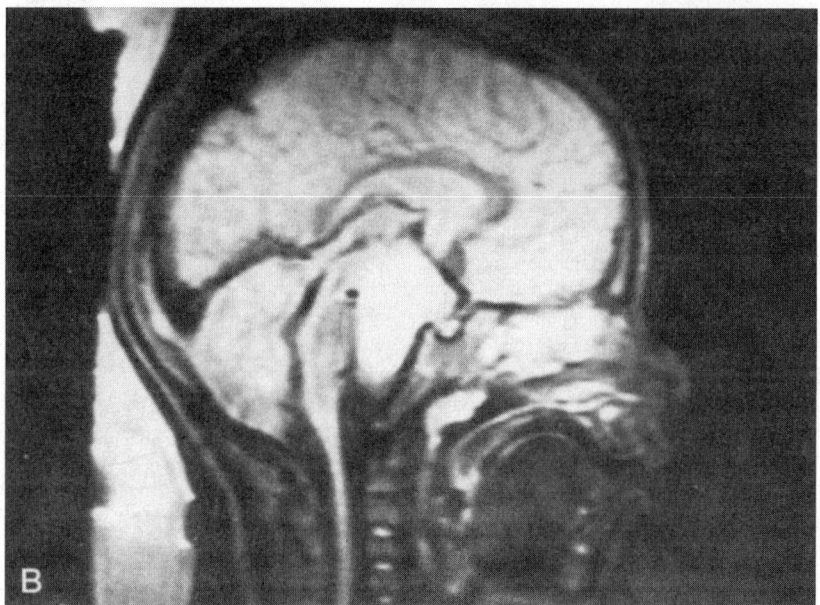

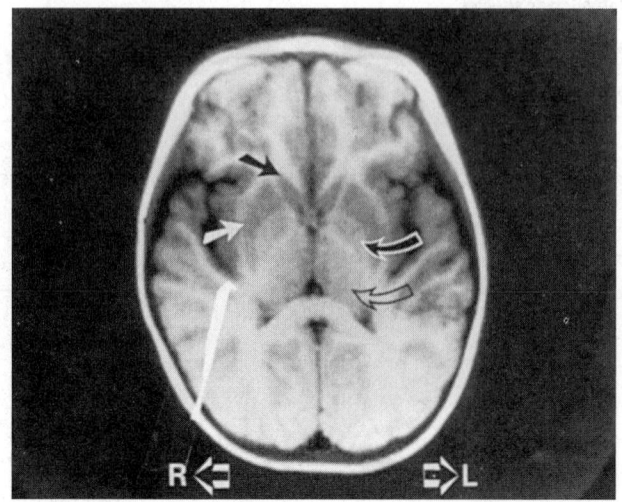

ADVANTAGES AND DISADVANTAGES OF MRI

MRI is generally viewed as a better imaging technique than CT (Table 124.3), due to the lack of ionizing radiation, capacity for imaging in several planes, improved tissue contrast with excellent differentiation of white matter and gray matter, heightened sensitivity for most pathological lesions, a capacity to image brain structures partly obscured by bone artifact interference in CT (e.g., the posterior fossa), and its ability to provide useful information concerning CSF and blood flow within normal and abnormal vascular structures. However, CT scans are several

Figure 124.3. Normal inversion recovery MRI. Note superb gray-white matter delineation. *Black arrow*, caudate. *White arrow*, putamen. *Black arrow with white border*, globus pallidus. *Black outlined arrow*, thalamus. (From Kuperman S, Gaffney GR, Hamdan-Allen, et al: Neuroimaging in child and adolescent psychiatry. *J Am Acad Child Adolesc Psychiatry* 29:161–162, 1990.)

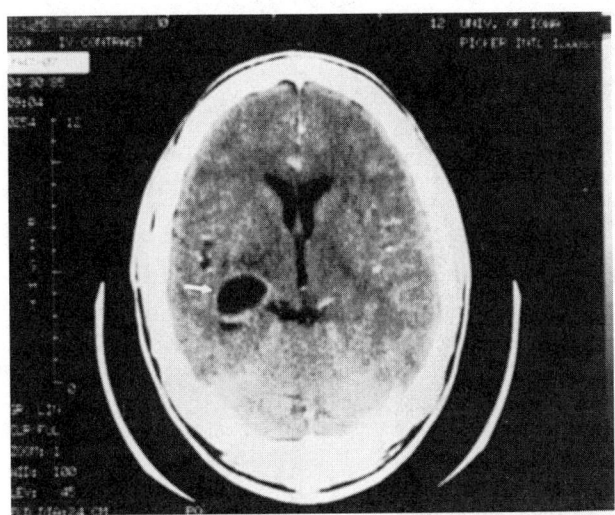

Figure 124.4. Axial CT scan with contrast of left basal ganglia glioma in a 19-year-old infantile-onset autistic patient. *White arrow,* basal ganglia glioma. (From Kupermen S, Gaffney GR, Hamdan-Allen G, et al: Neuroimaging in child and adolescent psychiatry. *J Am Acad Child Adolesc Psychiatry* 29:161–162, 1990.)

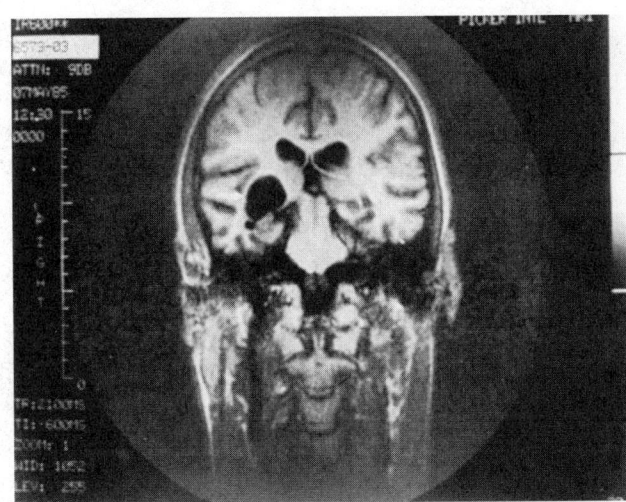

Figure 124.6. Same patient as in Figures 124.4 and 124.5, only coronal MRI. *White arrow,* basal ganglia glioma. (From Kuperman S, Gaffney GR, Hamdan-Allen G, et al: Neuroimaging in child and adolescent psychiatry. *J Am Acad Child Adolesc Psychiatry* 29:161–162, 1990.)

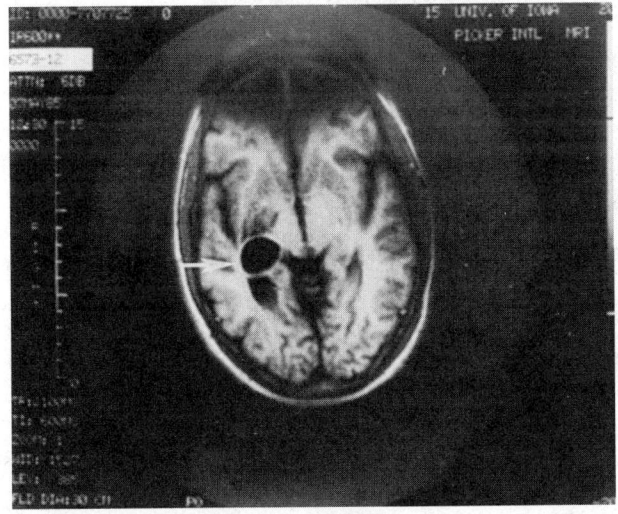

Figure 124.5. Axial scan MRI of same patient shown in Figure 124.4. Superior imaging of involved basal ganglia. *White arrow,* basal ganglia glioma. (From Kuperman S, Gaffney GR, Hamdan-Allen G, et al: Neuroimaging in child and adolescent psychiatry. *J Am Acad Child Adolesc Psychiatry* 29:161–162, 1990.)

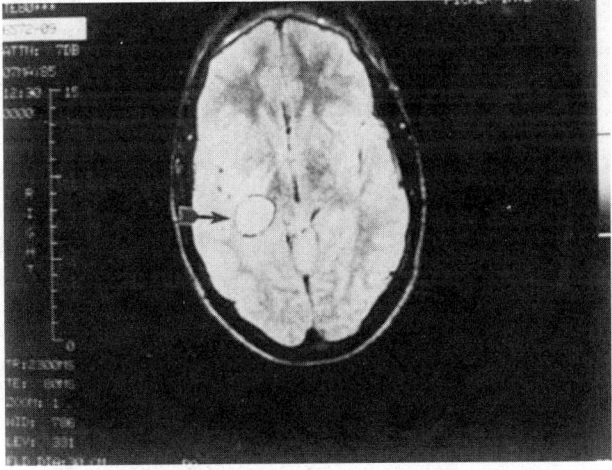

Figure 124.7. T2-weighted axial spin-echo MRI. *Black arrow,* basal ganglia glioma. Note how spin-echo MRI reveals that this lesion is not cystic. (From Kupermen S, Gaffney GR, Hamdan-Allen G, et al: Neuroimaging in child and adolescent psychiatry. *J Am Acad Child Adolesc Psychiatry* 29:161–162, 1990.)

hundred dollars cheaper and more widely available. The disadvantages associated with MRI usually are not significantly limiting in the clinical situation (Kuperman et al., 1990). However, the anxiety or claustrophobia spawned in some patients by the small, confined space within the instrument can be a problem. New instrument design and increasing familiarity with MRI by the public are helping to alleviate this problem.

The nuclei utilized for MRI must be abundant within the body and have a net charge that confers the necessary magnetic characteristics. Hydrogen fulfills these requirements and gives the best signal/noise ratio. However, other naturally occurring isotopes can be imaged, such as ^{23}Na, to generate scans that, while potentially providing useful diagnostic information, do so at the expense of image contrast and resolution. Contrast agents can increase the sensitivity and specificity of MRI for detecting and diagnosing some intracranial pathology. Paramagnetic isotopes (containing at least one unpaired electron, e.g., manganese), such as the intravenous con-

trast agent gadolinium diethylenetriaminepentaacetic acid (DTPA), alter the local magnetic environment and, therefore, tissue relaxation times. MR contrast agents rarely cause adverse reactions.

CLINICAL GOALS AND APPLICATIONS OF MRI

Two goals guide the development of MRI techniques for clinical brain research. The first is to develop and apply labeled compounds that monitor neurotransmission within specific neuronal tracts, but these substances are not yet available. The second goal is to enable magnetic resonance methods to achieve functional imaging, which has now been achieved.

Research on psychiatric disorders using MRI has produced increasingly reliable results. There are indications that there may be a reduction in the area of both the frontal lobes and general cerebral tissue in schizophrenic patients, as well as alterations in the corpus callosum that may imply impaired information transfer between the two lobes.

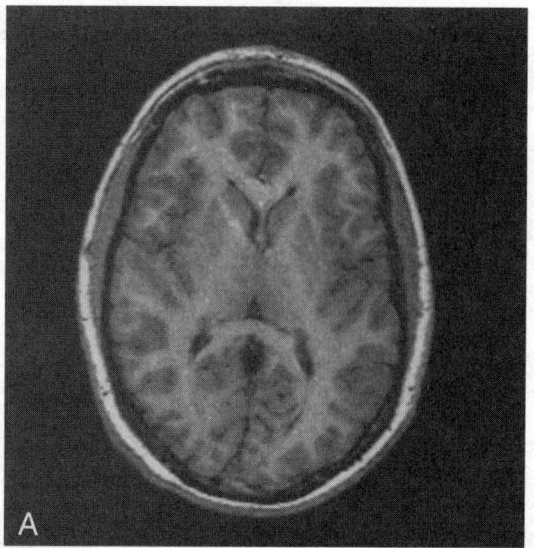

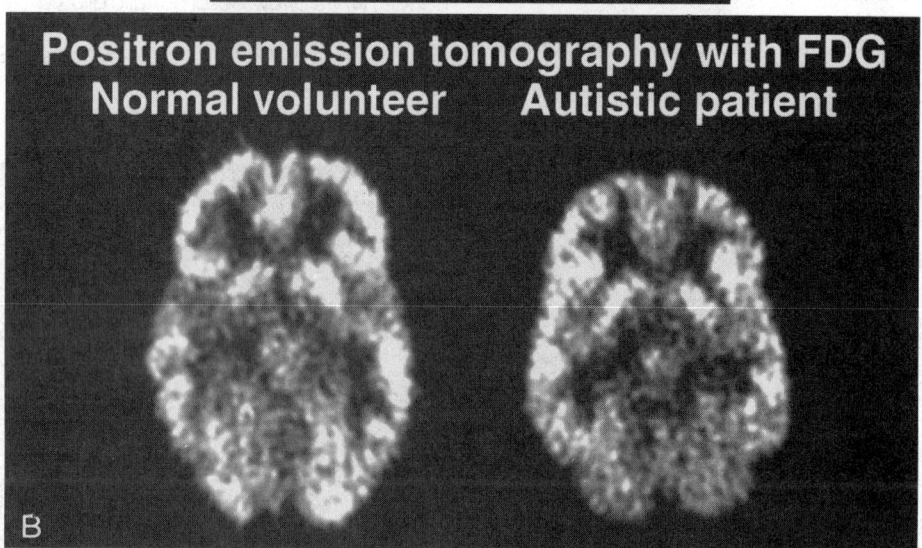

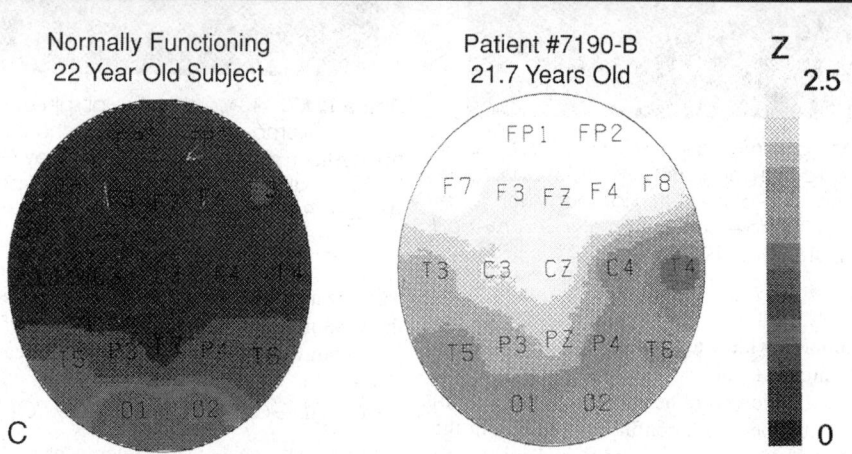

Figure 124.8.   Multimodal brain imaging in an adult with autistic disorder. **A,** *Axial MRI* of 21.7-year-old patient with autistic disorder. High-resolution MRI can be used to measure the volume of brain structures and assess regions hypothesized to be affected in autism. **B,** *Positron emission tomography scans* with ^{18}F-deoxyglucose (*FDG*) in normal volunteer and same adult patient with autism. Lower relative metabolic rate is seen in the medial frontal lobe and cingulate gyrus in the patient. This matches findings in Buchsbaum et al. (1992) and Siegel et al. (1992). **C,** *QEEG* topographic head maps (nose up) for Z absolute power in the theta frequency band (3.5–7.5 Hz),

for a normally functioning subject (*left map*) and same autistic Patient 7190-B (*right map*), both the same age. *Each map* represents the difference between the amount of absolute power in the theta band for the individual and that expected in the age-matched normal reference group, expressed in standard deviations of the normal distribution. Scale is in standard deviation steps corresponding to those shown on the *Z scale*, where ≥1.96 would be significant at the $P ≤ 0.05$ level. Few differences from expected normal values are seen in the normal subject, whereas significant deviations (especially in frontal polar and frontal regions) can be seen in the patient.

Table 124.3.   Magnetic Resonance Imaging

1. Advantages
   a. Does not use ionizing radiation
   b. Visualization of structures in a variety of planes (transverse, coronal, sagittal)
   c. Excellent tissue resolution, particularly differentiation of gray and white matter and soft-tissue contrast generally
   d. High sensitivity for detection of white matter lesions (e.g., multiple sclerosis plaques)
   e. Optimal for imaging pathological lesions
   f. Capable of imaging brain structures adjacent to bone (particularly important for posterior fossa structures)
   g. Injection of contrast material is not required, but can be utilized
   h. Flexible imaging measurement parameters
2. Disadvantages
   a. More expensive and less available than CT scans
   b. Limited by conditions adversely affected by the MRI magnetic field or instrument (e.g., pacemaker, aneurysm clip, claustrophobia, ferromagnetic foreign body)
   c. Possibility of toxicity if paramagnetic substances are injected as contrast materials
   d. Poor detection of acute hemorrhage, but good identification of subacute hemorrhage (>48–72 hours old)

Table 124.4.   Criteria for Identification of Receptors by Radioligand Binding Assays

1. Saturable, rapid, and reversible specific binding
2. Rank order of potency and stereospecificity of the ligands matches the rank order of potency and stereospecificity in pharmacological responses of the tissue
3. Linear increase in specific binding when tissue concentration is increased
4. Radioligand not degraded during the binding assay
5. Agreement of dissociation constants determined by independent methods

be examined by monitoring different proton-containing metabolic products. Several methods have been developed to determine the anatomical location of the source of the MR signal. Chemical compounds monitored in the brain include endogenous cerebral metabolites and psychoactive medications (Cox et al., 1994; Rauch and Renshaw, 1995).

These methods have been attempted with several compounds of interest to psychiatrists, using high field strength magnets. One example is the use of ^{31}P scanning to generate NMR spectra with peaks corresponding to metabolically interesting high-energy phosphate-containing compounds (such as phosphocreatine, ADP, ATP, and inorganic phosphate) or phospholipid metabolites. Relative quantification of these substances is important in experiments designed to monitor aspects of energy metabolism. Similarly, hydrogen (proton) MR spectra monitor signals from N-acetyl aspartate, a neuronal marker, or choline-containing compounds. Improved MRS methodology now makes it possible to study the weaker resonances of compounds such as glucose and glutamate. These methods permit measurement of rates of glucose transport across the blood-brain barrier, anaerobic glycolysis, and glutamate turnover to measure the tricarboxylic acid cycle rate (Shulman, 1994). Experiments can also be designed using exogenously administered compounds labeled with NMR excitable nuclei. For example, compounds labeled with ^{13}C or ^{19}F may be used as tracers for metabolic events. MRS techniques have been utilized in studies of several psychiatric disorders, suggesting differences in patient groups. More research is required in order to determine whether any of these new methods will attain a level of practical application in clinical psychiatry.

There are indications of posterior fossa (Gaffney et al., 1987a, 1987b, 1988) and subcortical abnormalities (Gaffney et al., 1989) in autism. One study of autistic patients suggested that the neocerebellar vermal lobules VI and VII were smaller in a group of 18 mostly high-functioning autistic patients of mixed ages than in normal control subjects. They judged this to be due to a developmental hypoplasia, rather than a degenerative process. The other anatomically and developmentally distinct vermal lobules were not reduced in size. They utilized a multisection spin-echo sequence in the axial and coronal planes and a multisection T1-weighted sequence in the sagittal plane (Courchesne et al., 1988). However, other MRI studies of autistic patients have not confirmed these results, suggesting that they might characterize a subgroup of autistic individuals (Gaffney and Tsai, 1987; Ritvo and Garber, 1988) or confounding factors (Piven et al., 1992). There are initial suggestions of similar findings in men with fragile X syndrome and autistic symptoms.

MRI studies of patients with Tourette syndrome (TS) demonstrate the potential utility of MRI. Spin-echo proton density-weighted images showed a reduction in the volume of the left lenticular nucleus and trends toward volume reduction in most TS basal ganglia structures (Peterson et al., 1993). Similar results have been reported in another MRI study, and a single photon emission computed tomography (SPECT) study showed a reduction in blood flow to the left lenticular nucleus.

Over the next decade, MRI studies of both normal and abnormal brain development will aid in our understanding of interacting molecular and cellular processes in brain development and related abnormalities in the developmental disorders (Barkovich and Wimberger, 1994).

MAGNETIC RESONANCE SPECTROSCOPY

Magnetic resonance spectroscopy (MRS) is a new technique finding initial applications in clinical research. MRS can provide a functional assessment of metabolic processes by yielding information on the relative abundance of various compounds containing NMR excitable nuclei within a preselected brain volume. The MR response of the nuclear spin system responds to both the physical microenvironment (as monitored in conventional MRI) and the chemical microenvironment. The latter is reflected in the property of chemical shift: The same nucleus is subjected to different local magnetic fields in different molecules because adjacent atoms in the same molecule provide different field-shielding. The offset from the expected resonance frequency is called the chemical shift, and this is the basis for assigning specific sites in different molecules.

MRS distinguishes protons or other nuclei in different molecules by exploiting these differences in chemical shift. Metabolic processes can

Quantitative Autoradiography

RECEPTOR BINDING MEASURES

Continuing study of receptors for neurotransmitters and neuromodulators is essential for the clinical understanding of brain function. Prior to the mid-1970s, the characteristics of receptor function were inferred from several indirect indices. Radioligand binding techniques now make it possible to assess specific features of receptor function directly. Radioligand binding studies allow identification of two critical indices for receptor function in cells, receptor affinity (the attraction existing between a neurotransmitter or hormone or other molecule and its specific receptor) and receptor number (the density of receptor sites on the surface membrane of the cell). Specific binding sites identified by radioligand binding studies are assumed to be identical with the actual receptor if certain criteria are satisfied (Table 124.4).

AUTORADIOGRAPHIC METHODS AND QUANTITATIVE TECHNIQUES

Autoradiographic methods permit the regional localization of specific receptor sites in the animal brain with great sensitivity. A radioactively tagged specific ligand is administered, and its binding at specific receptor sites in the animal brain is subsequently determined by exposure of radiation-sensitive film to the tissue. For in vitro quantitative autoradiography, tissue sections are incubated with the radiolabeled ligand, and unlabeled receptor-specific compounds can then be introduced in order to reliably identify the specific receptor distribution. In the in vivo procedure, radiolabeled ligand is administered to the animal before it is sacrificed. The brain is then sectioned and the slices are exposed to radiation-sensitive film.

These processes map the binding sites to neuronal systems, indicating the target systems for the ligand, which can be an endogenous substance (e.g., neurotransmitters or hormones) or a psychopharmacological agent. Autoradiography evolved from the development of biochemical methods for receptor binding and is now the principal method for receptor mapping in the brain. Used in tandem with histochemical techniques for defining the neuroanatomy of neurotransmitter-specific neuronal systems, it has moved neurobiology far ahead in the understanding of anatomical-functional correlates and has the potential to assist in improving the design of psychopharmacological agents. It provides a view of brain anatomy complementary to that of the classical delineation of gross neuroanatomical structures, cell groups, and fiber pathways delineated by tissue stains observable in the light microscope. Receptor mapping can achieve high sensitivity and excellent anatomical resolution. While it attains better resolution than dissection when film is used, true high resolution autoradiography is best achieved with emulsion or emulsion-coated cover slips. Film resolution is at the level of about 100 μm; emulsion reaches a resolution at the electron microscopy level. Immunohistochemical mapping of receptors has also been attempted, but it has been difficult to prepare antibodies to receptors. With the advent of increasing success in the purification of receptors, more success in antibody production to these receptors can be anticipated in the future (Holcomb et al., 1989; Kuhar and Goeders, 1987).

Earlier advances in receptor mapping were the development of quantitative methods for autoradiography and the application of receptor binding techniques to positron-emission tomography (PET) (discussed in a later section). Quantitative techniques for autoradiography utilize grain counting, densitometry, and photometry. However, these time-consuming, laborious techniques have been superseded by the use of computerized image analysis (Hibbard et al., 1987). The system instrumentation either analyzes optical densities in the image at lower magnification, or counts autoradiographic grains at higher magnification. Using a microcomputer and monitor, images are color coded to improve contrast, modify the image according to parameters utilized, compute average densities in a specific region, subtract one image from another, improve the precision of quantitative data, perform calculations, and store data. All of these activities can be performed much more rapidly than previously (Kuhar and Goeders, 1987).

Recent novel approaches include comparison of in vitro autoradiographic images with the results of fluorescence in situ hybridization. Complimentary RNA or DNA probes are labeled with a fluorescent marker and hybridized with receptor DNA or messenger RNA. This marker of receptor gene expression is compared with the distribution of ligand binding sites. Finally, confocal microscopy permits direct visualization of receptor binding and intracellular processes in living tissue.

BRAIN FUNCTION: BRAIN IMAGING TECHNIQUES

Functional Magnetic Resonance Imaging

The development of MRI as a functional brain imaging technique is at the forefront of clinical research efforts currently. Several *functional MRI (fMRI)* techniques are utilized.

One sector of techniques has been the development of *fast MRI*, in which images are obtained at subsecond resolution, permitting study of short-lived processes (e.g., functional activation of information processing) and less distortion by movement artifacts. A first type of fast MRI uses multiple RF excitations and is known as *fast spin-echo (FSE)* imaging; it functions in the "fast" range of seconds. A second type uses a single RF excitation and is known as *echo planar imaging (EPI)*; it functions in the "ultrafast" range of milliseconds. There is some compromise of spatial resolution in the fast MRI methods, because of a reduction in signal intensity (Rosen et al., 1994). FSE techniques employ a train of multiple spin-echoes, and imaging time is reduced. EPI appears

to have exceptional potential as a clinical fMRI technique. Requiring faster and stronger gradients, as well as faster data-sampling digitizers, technical development has only recently made it possible to apply EPI clinically. EPI involves the rapid acquisition of a train of gradient-recalled echoes. It is possible to obtain a series of images within seconds, so that blood flow patterns, contrast agents, and functional task activation can be monitored. Technical approaches to improving high-speed MRI and reducing scan times are under development, promising to improve temporal resolution. EPI is now capable of acquiring single-image planes in 50–100 msec.

Another sector of techniques employs *exogenous contrast agents*. For example, injection of a paramagnetic contrast agent (e.g., gadolinium DTPA) alters tissue magnetic susceptibility adjacent to the vessel and decreases the MR signal intensity. Functional activation, related to changing blood flow and blood volume (both closely coupled to local changes in neuronal activity), can be mapped by this method (Turner and Jezzard, 1994).

A final sector of techniques utilizes *no exogenous contrast agent*. Instead, noncontrast techniques use *endogenous high magnetic susceptibility contrast agents* to trace changes in cerebral activation as reflected in altered hemodynamic responses. *Deoxyhemoglobin* is the agent that has stimulated great excitement concerning this type of fMRI. An increase in brain blood flow without an accompanying increase in oxygen consumption leads to increased venous oxygen leaving the area of brain activation. (The brain utilizes anaerobic metabolism during spurts of neuronal activation.) When the oxygenation of hemoglobin is altered, its magnetic properties are affected, leading to increased contrast between brain and blood in the region activated: Function-related signals derived from these small magnetic fluctuations can be detected by MRI. T1-weighted pulse sequences monitor changes in blood flow. More often, T2-weighted pulse sequences monitor variations in the local concentration of paramagnetic deoxyhemoglobin, associated with changes in blood flow and blood volume.

This deoxyhemoglobin contrast fMRI technique has significant advantages. Functionally stimulated changes in the region are generated without the need for a radioactive or other exogenous agent. A major advantage is that both structural/anatomical and functional information is obtained. In addition, the spatial resolution is very good (1–2 mm), better than for PET. Finally, when combined with EPI, the oxygen signal accompanying blood flow changes can be measured in real time, suggesting the possibility of examining the timing of some brain functions (thousands of images can be obtained in less than 10 seconds). This type of fMRI was applied to the development of topographic maps in the human visual cortex as well as to studies of language organization in the brain (Raichle, 1994).

Quantitative Electrophysiology and Topographical Mapping

ELECTROPHYSIOLOGICAL METHODS

Recordings of the electrical activity of the brain have held great promise since first obtained in 1929, but technical limitations and the inability to determine the neural sources generating the electrical activity impeded progress. Marked improvement in technology, including better electroencephalography (EEG) amplifiers and remarkable progress in computer technology, has given new potential to electrophysiological methods, particularly their quantitative analysis. This is particularly evident in the increasing amount of clinical research utilizing computerized topographic mapping of brain electrical activity through EEG or modifications of EEG techniques such as evoked potential (EP) or event-related potential (ERP) recordings and multivariate analysis of quantitative descriptors extracted from EEG and ERP recordings. Nevertheless, the optimism engendered by these advances is tempered by the reservation that quantitative electrophysiology has only recently been demonstrated to have clinical advantages beyond the conventional EEG, sleep studies, telemetry, and evoked responses.

However, the emerging understanding of the relationship of the recording of surface electrical activity to the neural generators of this activity within the brain promises to bring new momentum to quantitative electrophysiology. It is increasingly evident that the EEG is the result of interactions of neural generator systems that can be described by equations. For example, two populations of pacemaker neurons have been suggested as candidates. One is a group of oscillator neurons in the thalamus that project to the cortex and are burst generating ("bursters"), escaping from hyperpolarization to fire. When hyperpolarized, the EEG is slowed. A second group consists of pyramidal cells deep in the cortex, which oscillate in the delta frequency band (McCormick, 1992; Steriade et al., 1990).

Quantitative electroencephalography (QEEG) utilizes techniques conventional for clinical EEGs, including standard electrode placement, and the waveforms generated by the electrical activity of the brain are amplified and recorded on magnetic tape or optical disk for off-line computer processing (including removal of artifacts: eye movements, eye blinks, muscle artifact, movement artifacts, and 60-Hz interference). Following analyses with the application of specific algorithms, an image (or "map") is formed by assigning different shades of gray or colors. These analyses include spectral analysis of conventional frequency bands (delta, theta, alpha, beta), through which brief periods of EEG data are transformed by algorithms to measure the average "power" in each band; this provides information concerning the relative local abundance of these frequency bands, which are the familiar constituents of classical electroencephalographic interpretation.

Similarly, quantitative electrophysiology can also include analysis of evoked potentials, the EEG response following presentations of visual, auditory, or somatosensory stimuli (QERP). Here, averaging of the brain wave response to multiple presentations of a stimulus enables the detection of an EEG change, contained within the background of brain electrical activity, that constitutes a specific response evoked by the stimulus. Such evoked potential studies provide information relevant to the temporal and topographic pattern of sensory information processing in the brain.

Therefore, QEEG utilizes a computerized EEG and evoked potential data acquisition and analysis system. Quantitative descriptors of resting EEG (QEEG) and event-related potentials (QERP) to visual and auditory stimuli are obtained from normal subjects and from various patient groups. In the typical clinical procedure, following placement of the scalp electrodes, 20 minutes of eyes closed, resting EEG data is obtained. Visual ERPs to 100 low contrast full field flashes, and auditory ERPs to 100 binaural randomized clicks delivered through loud speakers, are recorded. Visual editing is then used to select 1–2 minutes of artifact-free data for quantitative analysis. Quantitative features are extracted. In "neurometrics," one well-known QEEG method (John and Prichep, 1993), the data are transformed to assure gaussianity, and each feature compared with normative age-regression equations to obtain Z-scores. Z-scores indicate the probability that the patient's measured values are within the normal limits for a healthy individual his or her age.

Topographic mapping is accomplished through the addition of other specific methods to these conventional procedures. More scalp electrode sites are utilized, for example, 20 leads in one system and 32 in another. Statistical comparison of individual patient data to a normative group is often the final step, with statistical probabilities displayed in another color topographical map (Duffy, 1979; John et al., 1988).

ADVANTAGES AND DISADVANTAGES OF QUANTITATIVE ELECTROPHYSIOLOGY

Quantitative electrophysiology has several advantages as a clinical research technique when compared to PET and SPECT (Table 124.5). No radiation is used. The procedure is noninvasive, simple, and not uncomfortable for the patient, so evaluation sessions can be extended in length and repeated over time. While other images reflect brain activity averaged over 40 seconds to 30 minutes, QEEG and QERP sample activity every few milliseconds. This high temporal resolution makes it possible to identify specific phases of information processing. The cost of instrumentation, already much less than that for other imaging methods ($25,000–35,000), is steadily decreasing. In addition, QEEG requires no radioactive isotopes, eliminating an expensive recurring cost. The procedure itself requires little time with a cooperative patient, who sits in a chair in a dimly lit sound- and light-attenuated chamber.

Table 124.5. Quantitative Electrophysiology

1. Advantages
    a. Monitors changing patterns and regional variations in brain electrical activity
    b. No radiation exposure
    c. Noninvasive and requires minimal cooperation from patients, even those who are retarded and noncommunicative, and can be repeated many times
    d. Relatively easily administered, in a brief time period
    e. Relatively inexpensive
    f. Excellent time resolution (1 msec for EP, or 2 sec for spectral analysis), and well-adapted to repeated measures
    g. Easily quantifiable data
    h. Amenable to multivariate analysis
2. Disadvantages
    a. The data do not necessarily bear a specific relation to any brain structure, and knowledge about the neural generators and their interactions is only recently beginning to emerge.
    b. There are many possible artifacts that must be identified and edited.
    c. The effects of confounding variables, such as sex and handedness, are not yet known in detail.
    d. The use of computer programs for filtering and models carries assumptions and approximations that may be misleading.

QEEG procedures have demonstrated, using multiple independent populations and laboratories, that normally functioning individuals exhibit few values outside the normal range, and this is not affected by ethnic or cultural background. On the other hand, assessment of these features in large groups of patients with various neurological, cognitive, and psychiatric dysfunctions demonstrates the presence of a high proportion of abnormal values. These features are stable, being replicable within a test session and for intervals ranging from days to years (when there are no clinical changes). Significantly, the degree of QEEG abnormality increases with increasing levels of psychiatric/cognitive dysfunction.

However, there are also disadvantages. Various artifacts may contaminate QEEG results, particularly those due to eye movements, muscle activity, and 60-Hz interference, which require skillful editing to remove. This has led to extensive research attempting to define and filter these artifacts by using computer algorithms. Brain electrophysiological activity is quite sensitive to many medications that these patients have so often been taking; identification of medication effects is an ongoing challenge for all forms of functional brain imaging.

As the power of the computer is focused on these multiple problems, it is the source of both answers and further potential difficulties. All the programs used are the result of imperfect approximations whose strengths and weaknesses can then be exaggerated when the final data are produced. Another hazard is that both humans and computers involved in the data analysis may misconstrue significant data as artifact and thus edit out segments of raw EEG that contain potentially useful diagnostic information.

CLINICAL APPLICATIONS OF QEEG

Differential classification of some psychiatric disorders has been accomplished with considerable accuracy, providing independent criteria for diagnostic validity and treatment response research (John et al., 1988). The methodology has shown high discriminant accuracy in independent replications. The basis for comparison is a large database containing more than 12,000 evaluations of normal subjects and psychiatric and neurological patients. Multiple stepwise discriminant analysis has been used to construct classification functions. Discriminant functions have now been developed to evaluate the probability that an individual patient belongs to some particular DSM-III-R diagnostic group. For most major psychiatric disorders, these procedures achieve classification with good sensitivity and specificity (Prichep and John, 1992). Many categories of psychiatric patients are separated from normal subjects, as well as from each other. These disorders include major affective disorder, schizophrenia, dementia, obsessive-compulsive disorder, alcoholism, and learning disabilities. Unipolar and bipolar subtypes of depression can be differentiated. Cluster analysis has also been utilized to form subgroups of these diagnostic groups. QEEG methods are potentially important for the early diagnosis of disorders, identification of responders/nonresponders to treatments, and estimation of prognosis (John et al., 1994; Prichep and John, 1990; Prichep et al., 1993, 1995). Evidence has been presented indicating that members of different QEEG subtypes may display differential responses to treatment in attention deficit hyperactivity disorder (ADHD) (Prichep and Chabot, 1995), learning disability (Prichep and John, 1990), depression (Prichep et al., 1990), obsessive-compulsive disorder (Prichep et al., 1991, 1993), and schizophrenia (Czobor, 1991, 1993).

Within this context, there have been findings of interest in patients with several major psychiatric disorders. Using evoked potentials and information processing paradigms, investigators have developed generative models that may further define subsets of patients. Subgroups of children with developmental disorders, such as ADHD and Tourette disorder, have EEG abnormalities (Callaway et al., 1983; Satterfield et al., 1973; Waldo et al., 1978). Extensive comparative studies of attention deficit disorder (ADD), ADHD, SLD, and LD children (Ahn, 1980; Chabot, 1995; John, 1977, 1989; Kaye, 1981) have not only demonstrated a variety of QEEG abnormalities, but revealed characteristic and distinctive differences among these groups. Research on autistic patients has indicated a brainstem auditory evoked response abnormality, prolonged transmission time (Ornitz, 1985). More recent research has shown possible P300 abnormalities, differing in response to auditory and visual stimuli, that may reflect impaired orienting responses (Courchesne et al., 1985). New understanding of frontal lobe activation and asymmetries in children (Buchsbaum et al., 1992) hold promise for clinical application in the future. The results of quantitative evaluations of sensory evoked potentials and EEGs of over 1000 children have been accumulated by one investigative group (Chabot, 1995). The differences between normal and learning disabled groups in such studies might be the basis for practical subgrouping and examination of the clinical features of these subgroups in the future, as well as the specification of ability profiles for individual children (John et al., 1989).

Positron Emission Tomography

PET: BASIC PRINCIPLES AND TECHNIQUES

The development of PET brought within reach many of the goals long associated with brain research in psychiatry. On the other hand, formidable problems remain to be resolved before these objectives can be attained. This can be most easily appreciated when the complexity of PET techniques is recalled: PET techniques are derived from the application of concepts and methods from nuclear chemistry, physiology, biochemistry, metabolic modeling, digital image acquisition, and neuroscience. PET requires a cyclotron, a radiopharmaceutical laboratory, and an imaging unit.

PET is a functional imaging technique, such that the image can be obtained in relation to specific conditions, such as following the administration of a medication or in relation to simple or complex behaviors or emotional states. The image can be formed by monitoring any of several parameters in specific brain regions, such as metabolic activity, chemical composition, or receptors for specific neurotransmitters (e.g., dopamine or opiate binding sites blocked or unblocked by agonist or antagonist drugs).

PET utilizes a molecule labeled with a positron emitting element for whom the metabolic fate is known, including the physiological disposition of both the biologically active substance of interest and its metabolites. While ordinary chemical reactions involve changes in the outer electronic structure of atoms or molecules, nuclear reactions involve the conversion of one element to another. When a nuclear process results in a change in the number of protons in the nucleus, a new element of different atomic number is formed. Some nuclei are unstable; they decompose spontaneously and give off energy.

They have natural radioactivity. Radioisotopes are radioactive because they have unstable nuclei. The factor determining whether or not a radioisotope is stable is the ratio of protons to neutrons. Too many or too few neutrons can cause an unstable nucleus, which then loses energy by emitting radiation during the process of radioactive decay. A positron is an electron with a positive charge (an antimatter electron). Positron emission is never observed in natural radioactivity, but is a common mode of decay among radioactive isotopes produced in the laboratory (particularly with light isotopes, which have too few neutrons to be stable). The result of positron emission is the conversion of a proton in the nucleus to a neutron.

Bombarding particles used to induce nuclear reactions are of two types, neutrons and positive ions. A cyclotron accelerates charged particles, usually protons or deuterons, to high energies in a vacuum chamber. They are removed and caused to collide with a pure nonradioactive isotope. It is captured, raising the proton number so that the target is transmuted from one element to another. The cyclotron is used to produce short-lived radioisotopes for PET (^{15}O, ^{18}F, ^{11}C, ^{13}N). One of them is integrated into an appropriate molecule, which is injected intravenously. Sequential images are obtained immediately or a short time later. The detection of activity is based upon the use of unstable nuclides with an excess of protons in the nucleus; they undergo radioactive decay through positron emission, with a range of energies reaching a maximum characteristic of the radionuclide. A positron is a positively charged electron; the average positron energy is approximately one-third of the maximum. The positron may move several millimeters in the tissue, expending its energy until meeting an unbound (''free'') electron and causing mutual annihilation. Two 511-KeV gamma ray photons are emitted to obey the law of conservation of energy. They are emitted at 180° to one another and are the species detected in PET.

The PET scanner is a ring of radiation detectors that count the 511-KeV photons at a large number of angles surrounding the patient. PET detectors are crystals that give off light (scintillate) when energy is deposited in them through interactions between the molecules of the crystal lattice and the photons. Various generations of detectors have used sodium iodide, bismuth germinate, cesium fluoride, and barium fluoride crystals. The PET scanner detects the annihilation photons simultaneously emerging in opposite directions through the use of a coincidence circuit. Electronic coupling of the opposing detectors of the ring ''in coincidence'' enables detection of annihilation events along the line joining the detectors, and a large number of coincidence lines are accumulated to produce a PET scan. These data are then used to reconstruct a cross-sectional image of the distribution of the radiotracer in the patient, using a standard filtered back-projection algorithm. Modifications and refinements are utilized to correct for artifacts and various factors altering quantification (Buchsbaum, 1987; Holcomb et al., 1989).

PET MEASURES: REGIONAL METABOLIC ACTIVITY

The monitoring of regional metabolic activity is estimated indirectly by measurement of regional cerebral blood flow (rCBF) and is determined directly via measurement of regional cerebral glucose utilization (rCMRgl). The latter presumably gives an approximation of local neuronal synaptic activity, providing a view of regional function over the 30 minutes following administration of the tracer. Nerve terminals utilize glucose to generate the adenosine triphosphate (ATP) that maintains ionic gradients essential for neuronal signal function. It is this glucose utilization that is monitored in the radioactive deoxyglucose technique.

The method for in vivo measurement of energy metabolism in the brain that is most often used is the radioactive deoxyglucose technique (Sokoloff et al., 1977). This monitors local cerebral rates of glucose consumption. Measurement of a biochemical reaction involves the detection of the conversion of one molecule to another, usually through the determination of the rate of formation of product. Radiolabeling of a precursor molecule makes product measurement easier; it affects a relatively small number of molecules, not altering the kinetics of the overall reaction. Corrections are used to determine the rate of the reaction of the nonradioactive molecule. Careful biochemical techniques are required to assure that the species containing the radioactivity are well defined and limited to those accounted for in the calculations (Holcomb et al., 1989).

The analog of glucose, 2-deoxy-D-glucose (DG), is utilized as the labeled precursor for measuring local rates of glucose utilization, rather than glucose itself, because the label is known to be restricted to either of two species. They are unmetabolized deoxyglucose or the immediate metabolic product of the hexokinase catalyzed phosphorylation, deoxyglucose-6-phosphate (DG-6-P). This product accumulates and is trapped in brain tissue for a reasonable length of time, at least 45 minutes. On the other hand, if glucose is labeled, several metabolic products of glucose are produced, so that multiple products, depending on several reactions other than glucose metabolism, are produced and leave the tissue. A series of measures have been developed in the deoxyglucose technique to enable calculation of the amount of glucose phosphorylated during the same period, including the amount of labeled product formed (DG-6-P) and the integrated specific activity of the precursor, and various correction factors (Holcomb et al., 1989; Sokoloff et al., 1977).

In sum, the amount of DG-6-P retained in a cerebral region is a function of the rate of flux of glucose through the first step in glycolysis, the hexokinase-catalyzed phosphorylation of glucose. The rate through the overall metabolic pathway, at steady state, is the same as any step in the pathway, so this measure indicates the rate for the glycolytic pathway.

For human PET studies, the positron-emitting isotope used to label the DG is either ^{18}F or ^{11}C. The basic biochemical behavior of the molecule is not changed by the substitution of the very small fluorine atom for a hydrogen. The radiolabeled compound is administered intravenously; glucose and DG are competitive substrates for blood-brain transport. A single intravenous pulse of radiolabeled DG is followed by an interval of 30–45 minutes before measurement of the regional DG radioactivity level. This allows ample time for full conversion of free DG to DG-6-P or transport of DG back to the plasma. Thus, the detector measures the concentration of the product, DG-6-P, indicating the regional cerebral rates of glucose utilization (Buchsbaum, 1987; Holcomb et al., 1989).

Another technique for the measurement of brain energy metabolism is the steady state cerebral O_2-consumption method, providing blood flow, blood volume, and oxygen metabolism measurements. The nuclide ^{15}O is used to label circulating water as a tracer of cerebral perfusion. This method uses continuous administration of short half-life tracers to "freeze" the distribution of tracer in time. Inhalation of trace quantities of ^{15}O-labeled carbon dioxide ($C^{15}O_2$) is used for in vivo labeling of water in the pulmonary circulation in the continuous-inhalation CBF measurement technique. The rate of distribution of ^{15}O to cerebral tissue is dependent on CBF, and a series of measures and calculations enable measurement of oxygen metabolism. Other methods have also been devised (Holcomb et al., 1989). The images reflect neuronal activation, because blood flow is tightly coupled to neuronal activity. Because each scan requires only 1–2 minutes, scans can be obtained during a series of task activations.

PET MEASURES: RECEPTOR MAPPING

The application of PET that has caused the greatest excitement among psychiatric investigators is in vivo receptor mapping. The principles described for receptor binding methods and for quantitative autoradiography have been extended for use in PET. In this application, however, receptor mapping is accomplished in the living human brain. For example, substantial work has been undertaken toward dopamine receptor mapping by PET in several centers. An essential aspect of this work has been the development of more specific, higher-affinity ligands. Initial attempts to use ^{11}C-chlorpromazine as ligand for the dopamine receptors failed because of too high a level of nonspecific binding. A range of ligands has been investigated, and potent dopamine antagonists, such as spiperone and other butyrophenones and their derivatives (e.g., (^{11}C)-3-N-methylspiperone (NMSP), and ^{18}F-N-methylspiroperidol), or raclopride are examples of ligands investigated (Farde et al., 1985). Ligands for opiate, benzodiazepine, and other receptors have similarly been developed.

The development of optimal, specific ligands for receptor mapping continues to be a foremost goal. Specific criteria for these ligands have been devised, similar to those generally used in receptor binding studies (Table 124.4). Autoradiographic studies are the primary means for identifying the best ligands among those becoming available.

METHODOLOGICAL CHALLENGES FOR PET

Alongside the advances in PET methodology have been problems that continue to challenge investigators. Interpretation of the metabolic and functional images generated by PET is clouded by the poor delineation of anatomical landmarks of structures, particularly affecting reliability across patients. Stereotaxic methods have been applied as one solution to this problem; a face mask to stabilize the head and a standardized image reference system are used. Perhaps the most elegant and potentially useful solution to this problem is the use of computer algorithms for coregistering PET images with MRI or CT images from the same patient. Such techniques are now available and allow a precise unification of structural and functional data. The achievement of this goal will facilitate answers to such questions as what proportion of an observed reduction in glucose utilization is the result of tissue hypometabolism or tissue atrophy. Finally, time-consuming and expensive PET studies require a large staff and limit the number of patients in samples, so that small patient groups and the use of many intercorrelated measurements present significant statistical challenges. This problem is aggravated by the use of different methods and test conditions across PET centers, limiting comparability of data.

Test-retest designs have been increasingly used in order to control for the variance complicating group comparisons with small numbers of patients. Initial, control-condition scans are subtracted from a second scan including test conditions in which some type of activating stimulus is employed. The complex background patterns, partially specific to this individual, can be removed in this manner in order to specify the brain regions activated, and the amount of metabolic activity, associated with the given stimulus or task. This test-retest paradigm should also aid in developing an understanding of the interactional relationships between regions associated with stimuli and tasks. When elaborated into a series of related tasks, each dependent upon (and encompassing) the one before it, this has been described as the "hierarchical subtraction method" (Raichle, 1994).

PET STUDIES OF THE BRAIN PHYSIOLOGY ASSOCIATED WITH BEHAVIOR AND COGNITION

This type of study has produced interesting preliminary information concerning brain-behavior relations during specific tasks. Movements involve anatomically specific activation, such as the frontal eye fields for eye movements and the sensorimotor hand areas for finger movements; at the same time, the supplementary motor area and the cerebellum are activated for both eye and finger movements. The rate of visual stimulation has been shown to be associated with rCBF increase up to a maximum, followed by a decline with further increase in the stimulation rate. Another study demonstrated a specific regional activation within the somatosensory cortex by vibrotactile stimulation, differing in specific location according to whether it was applied to the lips, fingertips, or toes.

It has also been demonstrated that when the auditory cortex is activated by pure auditory tones, the specific site of activation in the auditory cortex is frequency-dependent: 4-kHz and 500-Hz tones activate slightly different areas. Another ^{18}F-deoxyglucose (FDG) project showed that verbal stimuli activated the thalamus bilaterally, but subjects who used visual imagery as a strategy to identify tone sequences activated the head of the left caudate. The verbal, unilateral presentation of a complicated story to normal subjects produced a strong contralateral increase in temporal lobe metabolic activity. Other task-specific studies have shown localizing results of similar interest. Regional specificity is evident when examined in the context of information processing sequences in behavior. Whereas passive sensory processing yields specific regional activation according to whether a visual or auditory mode was utilized, motor output programming (required for a motor response) and cognitive associations (involved in the extraction of meaning of a word) activate overlapping brain regions following either visual or auditory stimulation.

Considered at a more general cognitive level, strong correlations occur in the left para-Sylvian area between verbal IQ subtest scores and rCMRgl, as opposed to associations between performance IQ subtest scores and rCMRgl within the right posterior parietal area. A spatial task preferentially activates the right hemisphere homotopic region, whereas a verbal task activates Wernicke's region.

PET and other functional brain imaging techniques make profound contributions to our understanding of brain-behavior relationships, and findings alter the concepts and strategies initially used. When a hierarchical subtraction method was used in PET studies of lexical processing and verbal response selection, this strategy was anticipated to have the capacity to determine brain regions associated with increasingly complex verbal tasks presented to the subject: passive sensory processing, motor programming and articulatory output, and semantic analysis. While the brain regions participating in these tasks were identified, it was found that these brain regions dramatically changed as a result of practice. They demonstrated that two pathways were associated with this task, one for automatic processing and another for nonautomatic processing involving learning (Raichle, 1994). Such studies can be accomplished only with functional neuroimaging. They document the interactions of brain regions as the foundation of brain function and the essential differences between automatic processing and functions involving learning. Functional imaging will increasingly inform our understanding of brain regions participating in language (Frackowiak, 1994) and cognition (Sergent, 1994).

PET RESEARCH ON CLINICAL SYNDROMES

PET techniques have begun to elucidate the functional and biochemical neuroanatomy of clinical syndromes. In Parkinson's disease, regional cerebral oxygen utilization (rCMRoxy) and rCBF are elevated in the basal ganglia and reduced in the frontal cortex, both contralateral to the affected side of hemiparkinsonian patients. Other studies have indicated reduced CBF in the mesocortical areas contralateral to the affected side and increased rCMRgl in the lenticular and caudate nuclei.

While hypermetabolism has been demonstrated in subcortical and cortical areas during seizures, during interictal periods regions of hypometabolism are evident. The potential for clinical advantages from the application of PET is emphasized in results of research on Huntington's disease (HD). Several centers have suggested that patients at risk for HD show reduced caudate metabolic activity that precedes any CT signs (but not symptoms) of the illness.

The application of PET to psychiatric disorders has also produced illuminating data that generally corroborate other imaging data and clinical work indicating attentional and cognitive deficits. The CMRgl is reduced in the frontal lobes (generating a reduced anteroposterior gradient; Buchsbaum et al., 1982; Volkow et al., 1986b) and there are abnormal patterns following both sensory (Buchsbaum et al., 1983b) and cognitive challenges (Cohen et al., 1987) in schizophrenic patients. There is a reversal in the usual metabolic activity relations between cortical and subcortical regions (Gur et al., 1987; Volkow et al., 1986a). The effects of medications on regional metabolic activity in schizophrenic patients have begun to be elucidated; these include thiothixene (Volkow et al., 1986a) and other neuroleptics, amphetamine (Brodie et al., 1986), and cocaine. Research using D2 receptor ligands is still in a formative stage, with possibly conflicting results that need further clarification. Three biochemically distinct neuroleptics produced an 84–90% blockade of D2 receptors in the putamen, and D2 receptor occupancy was found to continue long after serum drug concentration had decreased significantly (Farde et al., 1988).

Basal ganglia CMRgl appears to be reduced in depressed patients (Baxter et al., 1985; Buchsbaum et al., 1986), while depression also is associated with high parietal CMRgl activity (Buchsbaum et al., 1985). PET rCMRgl changes during cycling in a bipolar patient have been recorded. There are interesting data showing higher metabolic activity in the right hemisphere in patients with anxiety and panic disorders; an inverted U-shaped relationship between anxiety level and frontal rCMRgl (increased metabolic activity with anxiety up to a peak, followed by a decrease in spite of higher anxiety) has been described by two centers.

PET studies of Tourette disorder suggest reduced rCMRgl in the frontal lobes, cingulate gyrus, and inferior corpus striatum, with an inverse correlation between the rates and vocal and motor tic severity (Chase et al., 1986; Singer et al, 1985). A more recent PET study of patients with Tourette syndrome using FDG suggested lower relative metabolic rates in inferior, limbic regions and higher relative metabolic rates in superior, sensorimotor cortices. The area that consistently distinguished these patients was the ventral striatum, and a reversal of its usual functional relationship with the sensorimotor cortices may characterize patients with Tourette syndrome (Stoetter et al., 1992). This may reflect a hypothesized dysregulation in circuits controlling voluntary motor function in Tourette syndrome (Shapiro et al., 1988).

Studies in patients with obsessive-compulsive disorder (OCD) exemplify the importance of the selection of varying PET techniques in relation to strategies for clarifying the pathophysiology of OCD. rCMRgl activities in the orbitofrontal cortex are consistently increased in these patients, with less consistent caudate and anterior cingulate abnormalities (Baxter et al., 1987, 1988; Nordahl et al., 1989). Such increased activities normalize in OCD patients who respond to drug treatment, both in adults (Baxter et al., 1992; Benkelfat et al., 1990) and in children (Swedo et al., 1992). In addition, this normalization also occurs in patients whose symptoms are reduced by behavior therapy (Baxter et al., 1992).

A more recent study used ^{15}O-CO_2 for repeated determinations of rCBF using PET during a resting state and a provoked state. During the provoked OCD symptomatic state, the rCBF increased (compared with that of the resting state) in the right caudate nucleus, left anterior cingulate cortex, and bilateral orbitofrontal cortex, as well as a trend in the left thalamus. OCD symptom scores were positively associated with activation of left anterior orbitofrontal cortex and negatively correlated with activation of right posterior orbitofrontal cortex, implying lateralized balancing and opposing modulation of OCD symptoms (Rauch et al., 1994). Interactions among brain regions have been further studied, and OCD patients differ from control subjects in their altered pattern of rCMRgl interdependencies, although this is not so after drug treatment. In fact, clinical responders can be predicted by individual differences in patterns of rCMRgl interactions. The involved regions are part of a hypothesized basal ganglia-limbic-thalamocortical functional circuit (Azari et al., 1993).

Research using PET in the study of autistic disorder shows that findings among patient groups may be more complex than anticipated and alter our understanding of an illness. As a developmental disorder with severe symptoms, autism stimulated anticipation that a discrete, definitive abnormality would be observed. Instead, the findings in a series of studies from several centers suggest a range of different abnormalities (see, e.g., Fig. 124.8). More variability and increases in CMRgl measures has been shown in autistic adults, but there were no absolute diffuse or local abnormalities (Herold et al., 1988; Rumsey et al., 1985). A PET study sought a metabolic abnormality in the cerebellum corresponding to the hypoplasia of the neocerebellar vermal lobules VI and VII identified by MRI. However, the mean cerebellar glucose metabolism of the adult autistic patients was not different than that of the control group (Heh et al., 1989).

Other PET studies also produced varied findings, typically abnormal metabolic activities in the basal ganglia and various cortical regions. More recent studies (Buchsbaum et al., 1992; Siegel et al., 1992) of high-functioning adults with a history of autistic disorder in childhood again found few differences between autistic and normal subjects. However, abnormal symmetry in the anterior rectal gyrus, low rCMRgl in the left posterior putamen, and high rCMRgl in the right posterior calcarine cortex and left inferior frontal cortex were observed. In addition, overall there were more brain regions in autistic subjects with rCMRgl more than 3 SD from the normal mean (outliers), similar to findings in an earlier study. Confounding variables might explain the cumulative results in all these studies, but another explanation has been suggested.

The data from PET research on autistic disorder may reflect the underlying etiological and neurophysiological heterogeneity of the disorder, overshadowing group comparisons. Abnormalities in brain func-

Table 124.6. Positron Emission Tomography

1. Advantages
   a. Capable of monitoring a broad range of biochemical processes
   b. Monitors brain metabolism and regional variations in brain activity
   c. Facilitates examination of brain neurotransmitter systems, particularly through receptor mapping
   d. Indicates sites of action of psychoactive drugs and can be used to monitor treatment
   e. Indicates brain activity during behavioral and cognitive functioning
   f. Good temporal resolution (less than 1 minute for ^{15}O, 30 minutes for FDG)
   g. Good spatial resolution of 2–5 mm
   h. Sensitive to cellular dysfunction without structural pathology, so may be useful for differential diagnosis and identification of patients at risk
2. Disadvantages
   a. Difficult to build, especially in urban areas
   b. High capital investment expense
   c. High recurring costs
   d. Limited clinical availability
   e. Radiation exposure (same or less than CT scan)

tion are evident, however, in the presence of more frequent outliers than expected, and in strong evidence for striatal and cortical abnormalities predicted by clinical symptoms (Siegel et al., 1992). A useful perspective is gained when we compare these varied abnormalities over multiple brain regions in adults with a *pervasive* developmental disorder with the finding of higher metabolic rates only in the medical temporal lobe in adults with dyslexia, a *specific* developmental disorder (Hagman et al., 1992).

PET: ADVANTAGES, DISADVANTAGES, AND GOALS

PET imaging provides some remarkable advantages (Table 124.6). The breadth of specific biochemical processes monitored is a particular strength: metabolism, enzymes, neurotransmitters, and receptors. It achieves good spatial resolution of 2–5 mm. The temporal resolution (less than a minute for a scan period is possible) is sufficient to encourage continuing attempts to utilize it for defining regional activation associated with sensory, association, motor, and more complex behavioral and cognitive processes. It is sensitive to pathological cellular dysfunction when structural abnormalities are not defined by other imaging techniques, and it provides accurate differentiating patterns when alternative diagnoses are being considered that other imaging techniques fail to distinguish. It appears that PET may be developed for future use in the evaluation and estimation of prognosis for patients at risk for certain illnesses, in improved classification and staging of disorders, and in the determination of treatment.

Regrettably, there are substantial disadvantages in the application of PET imaging. The initial costs of a PET facility are so prohibitive that there are only 100 in the United States. Each individual PET study is sufficiently expensive that the number of subjects and scans in a protocol is often less than optimal. Few medical centers in any region are likely to make the required capital investment in the cyclotron required for radionuclide production, and a unit staffed by chemists for the labeling of radiopharmaceuticals is also required. Finally, there is the diagnostic imaging unit itself. The large staff, supplies, additional equipment, and maintenance costs make the recurring annual costs great. However, there are great economies of scale and the incremental cost of the 200th scan at any center is comparable to MRI and quantitative SPECT. Advances in instrumentation and methods are now bringing PET spatial resolution to 2–4 mm and temporal resolution to under 1 minute. As investigators achieve new goals, new types of data are generated that become part of the information assembled into images. The demands for more sophisticated data reduction and analysis systems are unremitting. If this is not accomplished, the PET center will fail to utilize the data it has collected at great expense. Further development of data analysis systems continues to be a primary goal for PET investigators (Holcomb et al., 1989).

The sector of PET technology that possibly offers the most immediate

major research gains is the genesis of new ligands to be used as radiotracers. New opiate, serotonergic, cholinergic, dopaminergic, and adrenergic ligands may be successfully utilized in PET, as well as the imaging of presynaptic reuptake sites (Frost, 1992).

Single Photon Emission Computed Tomography

SPECT: BASIC PRINCIPLES AND METHODS

SPECT is the most rapidly developing technique for three-dimensional clinical imaging of brain function. SPECT (in addition to PET) is derived from the coupling of tomographic techniques for imaging brain structure with noninvasive methods for measuring brain blood flow. Brain blood flow was first determined by the use of the nitrous oxide technique (Kety and Schmidt, 1948), in which the difference between the arterial and venous outputs of an inert, freely diffusible substance was used to estimate the cellular uptake. Chemically inert radioisotopes were soon used, making possible regional detection, rather than whole brain measures. When Xe-133 became available, rCBF could be determined through the intact skull, and it became possible to switch from intraarterial injection to noninvasive techniques, either intravenous injection or inhalation (Devous et al., 1989).

Tomography is a process through which two-dimensional data can be used to reconstruct three-dimensional structures. When combined with the radiotracer measurement techniques of rCBF, it makes it possible to monitor physiologic events in the brain and use the data to project images of clinical utility. The initial techniques for tomographic imaging of rCBF with inert, diffusible elements (Kr-77 and Xe-133) evolved in the late 1970s. Problems were encountered, and they were superseded by radiotracers that are trapped in the brain. Their distribution remains stable over a sufficient period of time that they are considered statically distributed radiotracers. Radiotracers have now been extended from radioactive noble gases to labeled receptor agonists or antagonists.

While radiotracers employed in PET generate the simultaneous emission of two gamma rays in opposite directions, the radiotracers utilized in SPECT emit a single gamma ray. SPECT detectors are designed so as to detect gamma rays (photons) and to use these trajectories to determine their origins (Devous et al., 1989). In some cases radiotracer distribution is monitored simultaneously with its administration; an example is the determination of rCBF with Xe-133. However, a two-stage process is sometimes employed, in which there is a substantial time delay following the administration of the radiotracer and the imaging; here the example is labeled receptor ligands. For rCBF measures, the radiotracer is bound to a substance that enters the brain from arterial blood by crossing the blood-brain barrier according to the concentration gradient, theoretically with no other influences (such as active transport). High perfusion of a brain region would then be visible as an area with a high concentration of the radiotracer. The image is created by surrounding the head with detectors that record the gamma rays emitted by the radiotracer.

In order to localize the site emitting the gamma ray, a collimator is placed in front of the detectors. This is a lead screen thick enough to prevent gamma rays from reaching the detector. The long openings in the collimator allow only the aligned gamma rays to penetrate to the detector, in this way distinguishing those gamma rays on a line parallel with the collimator aperture. All gamma rays on lines enabling them to pass through any of the many holes in the collimator are detected simultaneously, generating a two-dimensional image. Gamma rays successfully traversing the collimator strike the detector, conventionally sodium iodide crystals, causing light to be emitted and detected by photomultiplier tubes. By utilizing detectors all around the brain, multiple two-dimensional projections are obtained, and computer algorithms produce a three-dimensional view of the radiotracer distribution. However, because of the difficulty achieving a display of a three-dimensional image, two-dimensional cross-sections are displayed instead.

SPECT instruments are of two types. Those that are for imaging static radiotracers utilize longer imaging times giving higher resolution (for example, 6–10 mm). Instruments using dynamic radiotracers that are redistributing are required to image quickly and repeatedly, reducing resolution (for example, to an optimum of 15 mm). Most instruments were capable of only static or dynamic imaging, although instruments now achieve both.

Once the image is generated, two methods of interpretation of the data are employed, each requiring attention to careful positioning of the patient and a technique for determining the relationship of the regions of the functional image to the anatomical structure of the brain. Quantitative methods have been developed, with either automatic or manual procedures, but all are imperfect. New methods are under development (Innis, 1992). This leaves a continuing role for visual interpretation of the images by expert clinicians. Surprisingly, visual inspection, if given the advantage of trained and experienced observers blind to the source of the image, can detect some image features (such as asymmetries) more accurately than quantitative techniques. Both methods are complicated by the question of the optimal state of the patients; at the present time, eyes and ears open in a situation of mild, stable background sensory stimulation appear to be superior to sensory deprivation, which seems to generate more variability that may reflect variable regional activation (Devous et al., 1989).

While the development of SPECT technology had lagged behind that of PET, which achieves superior spatial resolution, technical advances in recent years lifted SPECT into a more prominent position in functional neuroimaging:

1. Compounds used in SPECT imaging can be labeled with radiotracers that have longer half-lives, making their management prior to imaging easier (an on-site cyclotron is not required) and allowing monitoring of a neuropharmacologic probe over many hours. Improved radiopharmaceuticals are aiding enhanced spatial resolution. Two radiotracers for perfusion studies have been most commonly used. The first was an amphetamine labeled with iodine-123, I-123-*N*-isopropyl-iodoamphetamine (I-123 IMP). Its advantage is a higher energy level (providing improved spatial resolution) and a longer half-life (13 hours). The most commonly used radiotracer currently is technetium-99m hexamethylpropyleneamine oxime (Tc-99m HMPAO). It is stable and can be stored for months, preparation takes only a few minutes, it can be given in large doses that easily cross the blood-brain barrier, and imaging can begin as early as 15 minutes after injection. The pattern of the blood flow reflects the condition of the patient at the time of the injection earlier, which, for example, might have included a provocative cognitive test or medication (Reba, 1992; Schuckit, 1992; Van Heertum, 1992; Weinberger, 1992).

2. Single-detector technology currently is being displaced by multidetector instruments in which two or more detectors are used. This improves spatial resolution and reduces imaging time. These new systems are also more compact. Alternatively, new ring detector systems, though more expensive, permit even more rapid image acquisition and improved resolution (Van Heertum, 1992).

3. Reconstruction algorithms are continually improved.

4. SPECT receptor imaging is moving ahead rapidly, with improved ligands for a greater variety of receptors (Frost, 1992; Innis, 1992).

CLINICAL RESEARCH WITH SPECT

The bulk of SPECT research data is from Xe-133 rCBF imaging, because relatively little imaging research with other rCBF tracers or with labeled receptor agonists or antagonists was published until recently. The rCBF data for specific brain regions in normal subjects using alternative techniques are generally comparable. Flow in the right hemisphere is greater than in the left, except for the frontal and inferior temporal lobes, where flow is greater in the left hemisphere.

Sensory stimulation studies using PET or SPECT have provided fundamental validation of anatomical-functional correlations. Lesions of the visual system that fail to appear on x-ray CT scans are associated with metabolic abnormalities related to the clinical symptoms. Metabolic activation of the human visual cortex is systematically altered according to the region and size of retinal stimulation. Half of the input from each eye is distributed to each visual cortex. Stimulus complexity and stimulus rate each determine the amount of visual cortex glucose utilization or blood flow. Similar studies examining the metabolic topography of auditory stimulation of different types demonstrated a relation between the content of the stimulus and the regional pattern of glucose utilization.

When the stimulus is structured as a cognitive task, specific regional metabolic changes are observed. Many investigators have shown that speech in right-handed subjects is accompanied by increased rCBF in the left posterior inferior frontal area (Broca's area), while solving visual-spatial problems activates the posterior areas of the right hemisphere. Concentration, attention, and apprehension are associated with increased rCBF in the anterior frontal areas, especially on the left.

Analysis of the initial studies of patients with primary depression suggests that they have reduced global rCBF and focal reductions in the frontal and temporal lobes (Devous, 1992; George et al., 1993). Studies of schizophrenic patients utilizing several techniques for assessing rCBF are in general agreement that there is a reduction of frontal rCBF when compared to normal control subjects (Woods, 1992). There is some evidence that resting rCBF varies systematically: Higher flows are associated with positive symptoms (hallucinations, catatonic excitement, etc.), while lower flows occur in patients with negative symptoms (autism, inactivity, etc.). When performing a task related to frontal lobe function, the Wisconsin Card Sort Task (WCST), the frontal rCBF of schizophrenic patients increased less than that of normal control subjects (Weinberger et al., 1986). On the other hand, there are not rCBF differences between schizophrenic patients and normal control subjects when performing continuous performance tasks (CPT) requiring arousal, attention, vigilance, and mental effort, suggesting specificity for the changes in rCBF with the WCST. Drug effects do not appear to account for the frontal lobe metabolic abnormalities in schizophrenic patients, as they occur in unmedicated patients and may even improve toward normal with neuroleptic treatment.

SPECT studies of rCBF in schizophrenic patients confirm and extend some of the data derived from other methods of estimating rCBF. A bilateral reduction in frontal perfusion in schizophrenic patients appears to occur more commonly in the paranoid schizophrenic subgroup and to be more pronounced in the left frontal area (Devous et al., 1989). This is sometimes accompanied by temporal hypoperfusion. These results were analyzed in relation to their other data, which indicate that the frontal rCBF hypoperfusion in paranoid schizophrenic patients is accompanied by elevated hemispheric flow bilaterally, replicating the reduction in the anteroposterior rCBF gradient detected by other investigators and methods (Buchsbaum et al., 1984).

These regional metabolic abnormalities are related to altered performance on clinical neuropsychological testing: More global impairment on clinical testing and more errors on tests of frontal lobe function are associated with a decrease in left frontal rCBF. These findings are not affected by medication status. Overall, these results suggest that schizophrenic patients have generally increased metabolism and CBF, but frontal hypoperfusion that is more evident on the left side. The findings in the frontal areas are associated with cognitive functions traditionally associated with the frontal lobe.

Research with ADHD children suggests that they have reduced perfusion in the neostriatal and frontal areas and a relative increase in flow in the primary sensory region. This flow pattern was reversed by treatment with methylphenidate (Kuperman et al., 1990; Lou et al., 1989). A SPECT imaging study reported reduced HMPAO uptake in frontal cortical and basal ganglia regions in patients with Tourette syndrome, particularly in the left putamen and globus pallidus (Riddle et al., 1992). A subsequent MRI study of patients with Tourette syndrome by this group validated the SPECT results.

It is anticipated that activation studies, such as a challenge dose of a medication or a cognitive task, will be essential components of clinical SPECT research paradigms in the future.

ADVANTAGES AND DISADVANTAGES OF SPECT

At the present time it is possible to measure rCBF with SPECT and generate a set of three-dimensional measures for conversion to images. The spatial and temporal resolution of these studies is generally good (Table 124.7). The increasing use of labeled receptor ligands is a step that will lead to the realization of major diagnostic and treatment goals for the clinical neurosciences. Most importantly, SPECT instrumentation (typically the moderate resolution, rotating gamma cameras) is

Table 124.7. Single Photon Emission Computerized Tomography

1. Advantages
   a. Capable of monitoring a broad range of biochemical processes
   b. Monitors brain metabolism and regional variations in brain activity
   c. Instrumentation is widely available
   d. Relatively inexpensive in capital costs and recurring expenses
   e. Noninvasive, safe, and painless
   f. Radiation exposure similar to CT scan or PET
   g. Good temporal resolution
   h. Repeated measures within a short period possible
   i. Generates three-dimensional measures
   j. Facilitates examination of brain neurotransmitter systems, particularly through receptor mapping
   k. Indicates sites of action of psychoactive drugs and can be used to monitor treatment
   l. Indicates brain activity during behavioral and cognitive functioning
2. Disadvantages
   a. Limited spatial resolution (6–8 mm)
   b. Extracranial contamination from background radiation
   c. White matter lesions not easily detected
   d. Size of instrument and requirement for a dedicated scanner
   e. Cannot yet measure glucose metabolic rates
   f. Limited clinical experience
   g. Relative unavailability of radiotracers for other than perfusion studies currently

available in most nuclear medicine departments, and the quality of these instruments is improving (as more high resolution, dedicated SPECT instruments are available). Therefore, this is not an instance in which we are waiting for a projected period of technological breakthroughs or dropping instrument costs. The instrumentation and radiotracers required are available in standard nuclear medicine departments. For example, Tc-99m HMPAO and other radioisotopes require no cyclotron for production and are commercially available, as are SPECT instruments. In addition, a large staff is not required for operation, so reasonable operating costs can be anticipated and the imaging can be accomplished within a typical clinical setting. This suggests that substantial numbers of patients can be accommodated, giving much better potential for data analysis and interpretation than the small subject numbers typical for PET research (Devous et al., 1989).

The fundamental advantage of SPECT is that it provides functional brain imaging at a cost that can provide widespread clinical application in the near future. A major disadvantage of SPECT has been the problems in generating accurate *quantitative* information about the chemicophysiologic processes that it is currently being used to investigate. Data from SPECT scans are generally derived through visual inspection and subjective assessment. PET studies, however, result in images with local characteristics that can be directly converted into values representing, for instance, milliliters of blood flow/gram of brain tissue/minute or micromole of glucose consumed/100 grams of brain tissue/minute. PET is also able to provide detailed kinetic information about a variety of metabolic events. Techniques are currently being developed to improve SPECT's capacity to deliver quantitative data.

Comparison of the practical utility of SPECT with other imaging methods is instructive. Although controversial, most investigators remain unconvinced that PET will achieve broad use in the next decade. In contrast, SPECT instruments of reasonable sensitivity and resolution are now being commercially produced. These instruments are less expensive than those for CT, MRI, or PET. SPECT is already comparable or superior to PET for rCBF imaging.

The required instruments are available, and the development of radiotracers and acquisition of greater clinical experience with psychiatric disorders are the steps needed to realize the clinical potential of SPECT. This is in contrast to the remarkably high costs of PET scanning and its general unavailability. While PET, MRI, and CT instruments can cost $1–2 million, SPECT instruments, depending on quality, range from $200,000 to $700,000. The costs of SPECT radiotracers vary from inexpensive to moderate, so it can be expected that high quality SPECT images for a patient will soon have an expense equivalent to a CT

scan. Continuous advances in SPECT technology are improving spatial resolution to 6 mm and temporal resolution (imaging times for rCBF) to 2–3 minutes or less.

The neurotransmitter receptors accessible to SPECT imaging are now gaining breadth, with the extension of clinically available radiotracer ligands beyond the original research with muscarinic receptors to include dopaminergic, adrenergic, opiate, and other receptor agonists and antagonists. This gives SPECT extraordinary potential for unraveling questions concerning brain physiology and pathology. On the other hand, glucose metabolism cannot be measured by SPECT, because there is no radiotracer tied to regional glucose metabolism for SPECT at this time. The approximation to this through rCBF measurements (as an estimate of neuronal metabolism) reflects the very close relation between glucose metabolism and rCBF in most circumstances.

GOALS FOR SPECT RESEARCH

Further development of radiotracers for SPECT and the commercial production of labeled receptor ligands will play a central role in positioning SPECT as a major clinical brain imaging modality.

Occasional marked discrepancies between structural lesions and functional disturbances can be observed. Minimal structural alteration on a CT scan or MRI can be in contrast to a very substantial metabolic abnormality seen by SPECT. In some instances in which laboratory and imaging data fail to indicate the basis for marked symptomatology, a SPECT study may illuminate the diagnosis and lead to rational treatment planning. Just as PET holds promise for the identification of patients at risk for the development of pathology (as possibly may be true for Huntington's disease patients, as described above), SPECT may have a role in establishing risk and prognosis in neurological (such as stroke) and psychiatric disorders and determining treatment effects more accurately (Devous et al., 1989).

The experience gained through resting studies of normal subjects exposed to simple stimuli or asked to undertake simple to complex cognitive and motor tasks suggests that this alliance between information processing and topographical paradigms will have many advantages. In a similar way, activation with pharmacological probes will be very beneficial. This establishes the reserve and responsivity of specific neuronal systems and brain regions. It also indicates sites of action of drugs; this is essential to the development of targeted drugs specific to symptoms or disorders because it can facilitate the development of drugs tailored to receptors in a way that maximizes therapeutic effects and minimizes unwanted side effects.

Magnetoencephalography

MAGNETIC SOURCE IMAGING: PRINCIPLES AND METHODS

It has been known since the beginning of the 19th century that every confined electrical current is encircled by a magnetic field, oriented at right angles to the direction of the electrical current. It is possible to measure the small magnetic field produced by intraneuronal currents by magnetoencephalography (MEG). This predominately reflects currents in the proximal dendritic portions of cortical pyramidal cells. A sensory stimulus causes a volley of impulses to the cortex, simultaneously activating thousands of neurons and evoking a measurable and rapidly changing magnetic field over the head. In 1987 it was estimated that about 10,000 neurones must be simultaneously active in order to generate a magnetic field sufficient for measurement by instruments then available (Williamson and Kaufmann, 1987).

In spite of the fact that the extracranial magnetic fields reflecting brain magnetic activity are a billionfold weaker than the earth's background magnetic field, it is now possible to measure them noninvasively with a superconducting quantum interference device (SQUID). This specialized sensor utilizes detection coils sensitive to magnetic fields from proximate current sources in the head, while remaining much less sensitive to more distant sources, such as electrical equipment or elevators. These signals are then transformed into voltage. Liquid helium in a vacuum-insulated container (a "dewar") is used to maintain the SQUIDs and detection coils at a superconducting temperature (4.2°K). The SQUIDs are sensitive to either the full environmental magnetic field (a magnetometer) or to the gradient of the magnetic field (a gradiometer, which usually gives a better signal-to-noise ratio) (Hari and Lounasmaa, 1989; Reeve et al., 1989).

A major advantage of MEG is its capacity to localize signal sources more accurately than EEG. Although both methods generate information about neuronal currents, magnetic fields detected at the surface of the scalp are only minimally affected by brain, CSF, or scalp resistivity (unlike the EEG, which is affected by these different resistances). The spatial orientation of the neurons is a major influence on the localization of the signals from neuronal current dipoles. Those cells lying mostly on a radial axis drawn from the center of the head, generating radial current dipoles, tend to be those at the top of gyri; they dominate the EEG signal. Those cells positioned largely parallel to the scalp, producing tangential current dipoles, are those in the walls of sulci; they dominate the MEG (for complex reasons). Therefore, the EEG and MEG generate data concerning radial and tangential signal components that are complementary (Hari and Lounasmaa, 1989; Reeve et al., 1989; Reite et al., 1989).

Using a recording magnetometer at multiple points on the scalp, a contour map of the strengths of the magnetic fields is generated. Many technical problems must be considered in the interpretation of these data, however. In addition, so many recordings must be completed to map a magnetic field (each recording covering about 0.5 sq. in. of scalp) that several sessions of a few hours each may be required. Lying still for this long requires substantial cooperation. Other sources of magnetic fields are common in hospitals, so that a shielded room is necessary. An estimate of the cost of a shielded room and seven-channel magnetometer is close to $1 million. Finally, computer program models for localization of sources are used, and the validity and reliability of improved models are a continuing concern (Mondt, 1989; Reeve et al., 1989; Reite et al., 1989).

CLINICAL APPLICATIONS, ADVANTAGES, AND DISADVANTAGES OF MEG

Signal-noise differentiation is a problem in MEG, so the major work to date has examined phenomena involving clear signal activity, such as epileptic spikes and evoked potential signals averaged from hundreds or thousands of stimulus presentations. An example of the application of MEG in psychiatry is a study that examined MEG auditory evoked fields from the right and left hemispheres; they were recorded simultaneously with EEG recordings. A late auditory component (M100, corresponding to the EEG N100 signal) indicated a significantly different left hemisphere source orientation in six medicated paranoid schizophrenic patients when compared to six normal control subjects. This suggests abnormal function in the left hemisphere of these patients, or possibly abnormal structure (Reite et al., 1989).

The advantages of MEG (Table 124.8) are that it is capable of three-dimensional localization of the current sources following stimuli; the addition of the dimension of depth promises particularly illuminating findings from the clinical application of MEG. However, the MEG is not as sensitive to deep sources of activity as the EEG, because there is a rapid reduction in the magnetic field as the source moves closer to the center of the head. In contrast, the EEG gives some information about deep activity sources, including the brainstem. The spatial resolution of MEG can be as good as 1–2 mm for cortical sources, better than the EEG. The lack of homogeneity of the head causes distortions of electrical signals, interfering with source localization. However, magnetic fields are derived from currents in relatively homogeneous space that produce less distorted currents. A comparison of the different characteristics of EEG and MEG recordings is presented in Table 124.9 (Reite et al., 1989). Unlike CT, MRI, SPECT, and PET, MEG has the excellent time resolution characteristic of EEG: less than a millisecond, sufficient to monitor the spatiotemporal changes in neuronal signal processing of the brain. Clinical applications have included studies of attention, responses to speech sounds, and somatosensory research (Hari and Lounasmaa, 1989) and studies of cognitive processes using an information processing approach (Rogers, 1994). In the future, large multisensor arrays of more than 100 neuromagnetic sensors will significantly im-

Table 124.8. Magnetoencephalography

1. Advantages
   a. Capable of three-dimensional localization
   b. Excellent temporal resolution
   c. Very good spatial resolution
   d. Less interference with source localization by heterogeneity of tissue/structures in the head
   e. Relatively insensitive to muscle activity, so little muscle activity artifact
2. Disadvantages
   a. Less sensitive to deep sources of activity
   b. Limited signal/noise differentiation
   c. High capital investment for instrumentation and shielded room
   d. Necessitates several long recording sessions
   e. Not suitable for patients incapable of a high level of cooperation
   f. Further validation required for computer program models
   g. Available in very few centers

Table 124.9. Comparison of Several Characteristics of MEG and EEG Recordings

MEG	EEG
Reflects intracellular currents	Reflects extracellular volume currents
Maximally sensitive to tangential current sources	Maximally sensitive to radial current sources
Fields from deep-brain sources relatively unaffected by intervening tissue	Deep source activity smeared and/or altered by intervening tissue
True monopolar recording	Obligatorily referential recordings
No skin contact required	Skin contact required

From Reite M, Teale P, Goldstein L, et al: Late auditory magnetic sources may differ in the left hemisphere of schizophrenic patients. *Arch Gen Psychiatry* 46:565, 1989.

prove spatial resolution and temporal resolution in the production of three-dimensional images.

Multimodal Registration Techniques for Neuroimaging

Continuing research will pursue understanding of the relationships of brain structure and function, and alterations by pathology. However, some of the most important advances will occur in technical areas, such as the development of improved methods of coregistration of images from different modalities (e.g., PET and MRI). Data generated by differing modalities requires spatial alignment for proper interpretation of their meaning. The significance of these procedures is especially evident in our current need to superimpose functional images on the anatomical map of structural images, so that anatomical landmarks for the functional data are clear. Subsidiary problems evolve. What are the best methods for guiding registration to the elaborated database of a "brain atlas"? What standards can be agreed upon that will make it possible to examine an individual brain in reference to a "brain atlas? This question stimulates further work in morphometrics (the measurement of biological shape and shape change) and the varying procedures available for constructing a brain atlas (Bookstein, 1994; Ingvar et al., 1994; John et al., 1994).

BRAIN FUNCTION: NEUROCHEMICAL, PSYCHOPHARMACOLOGICAL, AND PSYCHOPHYSIOLOGICAL TECHNIQUES
Neurochemistry, Neuroendocrinology, and Neuropharmacology

Advances in neurochemistry, neuroendocrinology, psychopharmacology, and their clinical applications are reviewed elsewhere, but we briefly consider examples of directions such research is taking.

Clinical research is not focused so dominantly on classical adrenergic, dopaminergic, serotonergic, and cholinergic transmitters. A recent

Table 124.10. Autosomal Abnormalities Reported in the Pervasive Developmental Disorders

Aneuploidies
  Trisomy 6p partial
  Trisomy 8 mosaic
  Trisomy 21
  Trisomy 22
Structural abnormalities
  Deletions
    del(1)(p35), del(3), del(13), del(17)
  Duplications
    dup(3), dup(16)
  Fragile sites
    fra(2)(q13), fra(6)(q26), fra(16)(q23)
  Inversions
    inv(2)(p11q13), inv(3), inv(5)(p−q+)
    inv(9)(p11q12), inv(16)
  Translocations
    t(4p; + 9q−), t(7:20), t(22:13)
  Other structural abnormalities
    5p +, 9h+, Gp+

From Young JG, Brasic JR, Leven L: Genetic causes of autism and the pervasive developmental disorders. In: Deutsch S et al. (ed): *Application of Basic Neuroscience in Child Psychiatry.* New York, Plenum, 1990, p. 188.

Table 124.11. Sex Chromosomal Abnormalities Reported in the Pervasive Developmental Disorders

Aneuploidies
  XXX
  XXY
  XXYY
  XY mosaicism (long Y and short Y)
  XYY
Structural abnormalities
  Fragile sites
    fra(x)(p22)
    fra(x)(q27)
    fra(x)(q28)
  Other structural abnormalities
    long Y (Y = F)

From Young JG, Brasic JR, Leven L: Genetic causes of autism and the pervasive developmental disorders. In: Deutsch S et al. (ed): *Application of Basic Neuroscience to Child Psychiatry.* New York, Plenum Press, 1990, p. 188.

Table 124.12. Single-Gene Disorders Associated with the Autistic Syndrome

Autosomal-recessive disorders
  Disorders of purine metabolism
  Adenylosuccinate lyase deficiency
  Decreased adenosine deaminase activity
  Hyperuricosuria
  Increased phosphate 5-phosphoribosyl 1-pyrophosphate synthetase
  Histidinemia
  Neurolipidosis
  Phenylketonuria
  Oculocutaneous albinism
Autosomal-dominant disorders
  Neurofibromatosis
  Noonan syndrome
  Tuberous sclerosis

From Young JG, Brasic JR, Levin L: Genetic causes of autism and the pervasive developmental disorders. In: Deutsch S et al. (ed): *Application of Basic Neuroscience to Child Psychiatry.* New York, Plenum Press, 1990, p. 194.

example is evidence for altered concentrations of neuropeptide Y and peptide YY in anorexia and bulimia that appear to be associated with significant clinical symptoms in these illnesses (Kaye et al., 1990). More emphasis is given to clinical monitoring of the costorage and cotransmission of neurotransmitters and the function of receptors for multiple transmitters on a neuron. The possible contributions to pathophysiology of imbalances among these interacting systems is an important emerging clinical problem. Similarly, the effects of trophic factors on neuronal pathways is being examined, not only during development, but also in relation to neuronal sprouting and pathway formation in the adult nervous system adapting to the environment, particularly their role in the maintenance and regeneration of mature peripheral neurons. Mapping of these trophic factors in the brain is underway, and clarification of their potential roles in developmental disorders is a priority for investigators. The discovery of the large gene family of neurotrophins, related to nerve growth factor, exemplifies the richness of this research (Lindsay et al., 1994).

It is now possible to develop drugs to affect individual neuronal systems with increasing specificity, relatively uncomplicated by effects on other neuronal systems. For example, the relative serotoninergic and noradrenergic contributions to the pathogenesis of OCD have been clarified by a study of the clinical effects of the serotonin reuptake inhibitor fluvoxamine in contrast to the norepinephrine reuptake inhibitor desipramine. Fluvoxamine had a significantly greater effect reducing the severity of OCD symptoms than did desipramine, and 11 of 21 patients had a beneficial response to fluvoxamine, compared to 2 of 19 patients with a good response to desipramine. Fluvoxamine also led to improvement in ''secondary'' symptoms of depression, although the reduction in OCD symptoms was not associated with the baseline severity of depressive symptoms. These findings support the hypothesis that the anti-obsessive-compulsive efficacy of this class of drugs is related to the effects of the drug on acute serotonin reuptake. The design of this protocol exemplifies investigative approaches that are central to current clinical neurochemical and psychopharmacological research attempting to establish specificity of association among target neurotransmitter systems, drugs, and clinical disorders (Goodman et al., 1990). However, unraveling the basic neurochemical mechanisms of action that contribute to clinical effects continues to be a complex undertaking (Barr et al., 1994), in spite of extensive knowledge of the effects of a neurotransmitter (e.g., serotonin) on a target behavior (e.g., motor control) (Jacobs and Fornal, 1993). These systematic studies also more clearly identify nonresponders, stimulating investigators to apply clinical, genetic, and neurochemical knowledge to helping initial nonresponders achieve a better therapeutic

result (McDougle et al., 1994), for example, through addition of an agent affecting another receptor system (haloperidol and dopamine).

The influence of genetic research will be evident as families of proteins coded by genes with substantial segments of homologous DNA are identified. The response of these families of receptors and enzymes, many not previously understood to be related on a functional basis, will be clarified. For example, studies of genomic structure and sequence homologies are elucidating subfamilies of opioid-receptor genes that will have significant clinical implications (Uhl et al., 1994).

The cascade of molecular interactions responsible for membrane signal transduction are now well studied (Casey, 1995), and clinical application of this knowledge has begun. The similarity of transduction pathways in many types of cell receptor systems facilitates these efforts. One practical clinical outcome will be an enhanced capacity to manipulate receptor sensitivity when medications are administered, through receptor-receptor interactions and clarification of changes in receptor number or affinity. This, in turn, may be important in setting the balance between two types of related receptors, such as D1 and D2, and their contribution to symptom status and drug response. From the other direction, molecular biological research on receptors clarifies the existence of receptor subtypes previously not recognized. For example, such research points to the existence of at least five types of dopamine receptors (not two, as previously thought) in two families (Gingrich and Caron, 1993).

Applied Psychophysiology and Biofeedback

Psychophysiological measures of phenomena controlled by the autonomic nervous system provide indirect measures of brain function that have the advantage of being relatively simple techniques that utilize inexpensive and portable instrumentation. Their disadvantage is that they are nonspecifically associated with many phenomena, so that understanding of their meaning has been controversial. However, they continue to have significant potential for monitoring states of arousal and stress, as well as therapeutic utility for the patient through biofeedback procedures.

In recent years new technology, including the advent of microcomputers, has greatly enhanced the measurement of psychophysiological variables. ''Applied psychophysiology and biofeedback'' include a group of diagnostic and therapeutic procedures that utilize electronic instruments to measure, process, and ''feed back'' to a person information about his or her own physiological states. When used in research, the goals are to examine associations between diagnostic groups, symptoms, physiological states, or other clinical or neurobiological measures. Used therapeutically, the objectives are to help a person become aware of his or her normal or abnormal physiological processes, which are often involuntary, and when they are abnormal, to change them in a desired direction (Alson, 1987). A variety of biological processes, such as muscle tension, blood flow in the hands and feet, electrodermal activity, heart rate, blood volume pulse and pulse wave form, blood pressure, volume of air inspired, and brain electrical activity, can be monitored and amplified in the form of visual and auditory signals.

Muscle contraction is monitored through an electromyograph (EMG), which measures the electrical activity of the muscles. The EMG instrument utilizes surface sensors, which are placed above the muscle being measured, or needle electrodes, which penetrate the muscle and can measure single motor unit activity; the positioning of the sensors depends on the muscle being measured. EMG biofeedback allows a person to receive instant information about the state of his or her muscles. Its major application is in neuromuscular rehabilitation and anxiety reduction training, which has implications for psychological and physiological disorders.

The temperature instrument measures the peripheral temperature in the hands and feet and indirectly measures the degree of peripheral vasoconstriction, which is controlled by the sympathetic nervous system (SNS). As the blood vessels dilate, blood volume increases, and consequently the temperature in the hands or feet increases. Sensors are typically placed at points on the extremities, because the effects of vasoconstriction or vasodilation are more pronounced there. Vasoconstriction and vasodilation are associated with SNS activity, and when a person voluntarily produces an increase in temperature in the extremities, vascular relaxation and rebalancing often occur over the entire body. The major clinical applications are in treating circulatory disorders, such as Raynaud's disease and migraine headaches, as well as conditions in which sympathetic activation is implicated.

Galvanic skin response or skin conductance activity reflects an indirect measure of sweat gland activity and associated changes in the SNS. Increased sweat gland activity in response to SNS stimulation results in an increase in the level of conductance. Sympathetic activation and emotional arousal are related, although it is not yet possible to identify adequately the specific parameters of this relationship. The skin conductance response is, however, particularly sensitive to emotionally arousing stimuli and thus has applications to psychotherapy, as well as providing a general means of reducing sympathetic activation.

The pneumograph is a device that measures respiratory waves, as breath amplitude in the thoracic and abdominal regions, through sensors known as strain gauges. It also measures the number of breaths per minute. Both of these measures are used in biofeedback training. Major clinical applications are in a variety of respiratory disorders, for example, asthma or the hyperventilation syndrome.

Heart rate, blood volume pulse, and pulse wave form are measured by a plethysmograph. The sensor is placed on a finger and a small light beam is directed at the finger. The amount of light reflected is measured by a photocell also embedded in the sensor. The amount of light reflected is determined by the density of the blood, which gives an indirect measure of blood pulse. Heart rate is also measured on a beat-to-beat basis by a cardiotachometer. Feedback on the heart rate becomes particularly useful when working with arrhythmias. Blood volume is a measurement of the peak-to-peak amplitude of the pulse wave form. Blood volume and pulse are much more direct measures of the vascular system than peripheral temperature. Blood pressure is measured by a cuff that is automatically inflated through sensors in the cuff. It measures diastolic and systolic blood pressure once a minute.

In general, modern technology has expanded the possibilities for measuring multiple response systems with precision and expanding the modalities of the feedback stimulation. Current research monitors psychophysiologic indices in the context of more complex concepts of the regulatory control of these systems, elucidating causes for the apparent ''nonspecificity'' of many psychophysiological responses and the difficulties inherent in interpreting their meaning. There are many examples: Simple measures of the right-left forehead temperature asymmetry are related to an asymmetry in general sympathetic activity, to the asymmetry of frontal EEG activation, and to inhibited or uninhibited temperaments in preschool children (Kagan, 1994); a systematic series of studies has demonstrated the utility of cardiac vagal tone as an index of parasympathetic influences on emotion regulation, particularly restorative, self-regulatory processes (Porges et al., 1994); and drugs can be used to parse the varying exquisitely complex influences on basic psychophysiological parameters, such as heart rate, during fundamental psychological states (e.g., arousal or attention) (Middleton et al., 1994).

BRAIN DEVELOPMENT: MOLECULAR BIOLOGY AND BEHAVIORAL GENETICS

The search for genetic influences on disorders begins with a consideration of the type of genetic transmission being investigated: chromosomal abnormalities, single gene disorders, or polygenic/multifactorial disorders (multiple, small gene effects acting together with environmental factors). While most psychiatric disorders and normal behavioral characteristics are typically polygenic/multifactorial in origin (see discussion of behavioral genetics below), various disorders in the developmental period are caused by each of the three types of transmission. Therefore, a broad approach to clinical genetic research is essential to child and adolescent psychiatry; chromosomal and linkage studies are undertaken with the anticipation that not all disorders will be polygenic/multifactorial. For example, the causes of autistic disorder (Tables 124.10–124.12) include subgroups with chromosomal aberrations and single gene disorders (Young et al., 1990a).

Chromosomal Abnormalities

In spite of previous negative findings, occasional breakthroughs in the identification of chromosomal aberrations continue to illuminate the causes of developmental disorders in subgroups of children with these disorders. These advances tend to follow technical progress, such as novel culture techniques and high-resolution banding. Further improvements have come from the use of fluorescent-labeled molecular probes to identify chromosomal abnormalities. These techniques are known as *fluorescent in situ hybridization* (FISH), when probes for single regions of a chromosome are used, and as *chromosomal painting*, when probes corresponding to whole chromosomes are used (Sawyer et al., 1992). These techniques confer greater sensitivity. Deletions of chromosome 15 in the Prader-Willi and Angelman syndromes that cannot be seen by banding studies and light microscopy are readily detected by FISH. Low levels of chromosomal mosaicism can be detected by counting the chromosome painting signals in large numbers of interphase cells. These techniques also confer greater specificity. The origin of chromosomal fragments can now be readily identified by their annealing (reassociating) to specific DNA probes, even when their identities could not be readily established by the banding pattern (Rosenberg et al., 1992).

Single Gene Disorders and Linkage Analysis: The Clinical Applications of Gene Mapping

Single gene disorders are known to cause developmental disorders, and the search for single gene etiologies of common syndromes continues with the hope of improving diagnosis and enabling prevention. Phenylketonuria is a well-known example of a single gene disorder causing pervasive developmental disorders, some of whose symptoms are preventable if dietary treatment is initiated early. Clinical biochemical measures indicating abnormal enzyme or receptor function have been mainstays of such research, but linkage analysis and the candidate gene approach has moved to the forefront of investigations. It is largely applicable to single gene disorders.

Several fundamental principles of molecular biology are utilized in linkage analyses:

1. *Genes are distributed in a specific linear array on chromosomes.* The question arises how genetic differences between individuals might be demonstrated, short of determining the actual sequence of DNA bases in each chromosome of the individual. The arrangement of genes in a specific linear array on chromosomes has been described as resembling beads on a string. An exchange of genetic material between members of a chromosome pair, known as crossing over, occurs during meiosis. New combinations of linked genes occur following this crossover between loci, altering the linear sequence.

Following the rediscovery of Mendel's laws in the early part of this century, it was found that violations of mendelian patterns of inheritance occurred. Morgan completed experimental work that led him to attribute these unexpected differences to crossing over during meiosis (Vogel and Motulsky, 1986). Reasoning that genes were probably found on specific chromosomes, he investigated crossing-over events and demonstrated that genes are located in a linear order on the chromosomes; he accomplished the initial mapping of genes on chromosomes in *Drosophila* by measuring the frequency of crossovers. His principle was that more frequent crossover indicates a greater linear distance between the genes. It was a straightforward process to extend these techniques to other species, but application to human genetics was blocked by the inability to control matings, the unknown phase of the alleles (that is, whether the alleles in a doubly heterozygous parent are located in cis or in trans (MN on one chromosome and Mn on the other, or Mn and mN)), the presence of homozygous markers at certain locations, and small family size. Nevertheless, statistical techniques were eventually developed to give useful estimates of linkage from recombinant frequencies (Lathrop et al., 1985).

2. *Genes occur in alternative forms (alleles) at the same locus on homologous chromosomes.* This is the basis for both genetic variation and for genetic linkage analysis. A polymorphism is said to exist when two or more forms of a gene occur with appreciable frequency in a population. In practice, there is agreement about the meaning of "appreciable frequency": A polymorphism is arbitrarily defined to be present in a population when the most common allele at a locus accounts for fewer than 99% of the alleles (Thompson, 1986). Approximately 28% of human genes are polymorphic (as judged by analysis of the genes for soluble proteins), and more than 0.2% of the base pairs in DNA play a role in polymorphisms, so they are very common. Restriction enzyme analysis can be used to detect about 40% of these polymorphisms (approximately 1 of 1000 of the total base pairs in the human genome). Estimating the human genome to consist of 3 billion base pairs, it can be anticipated that several million polymorphisms can be identified as differences between individuals. It is important to recognize that most polymorphisms are benign and produce no phenotypic effects (White, 1984, 1985a, 1985b; White and Caskey, 1988; White and Lalouel, 1988).

3. *Base pairing within DNA determines the invariance of genetic transmission.* This is the foundation for molecular methods for linkage analysis. If two strands of the DNA double helix are separated, each strand is available to reanneal to one another: Single-stranded DNA lines up in close apposition to ("hybridizes" to) another single strand consisting of a complementary base sequence. Such hybridization takes place with the original complementary DNA strand and also occurs with any source of DNA or messenger RNA (mRNA) with a complementary base sequence. This is the basis for identifying complementary copies of a given DNA molecule.

When a strand of DNA is labeled, it is called a *gene probe*. Multiple copies of the labeled strand are then available for use to search for a complementary strand or strand fragment. This technique is used to demonstrate that genes identified by the probe are contained within DNA from another individual. However, in order to take advantage of this technical shortcut for finding genes, one of two pieces of information is needed to construct a gene probe. One method requires knowledge of a tissue in which the gene is expressed; mRNA extracted from that tissue can then be used as a template to construct a DNA probe that will be used to search for the gene in DNA obtained from the same or another individual. Another method for constructing a gene probe requires knowledge of the identity of the protein that the gene specifies; determination of its amino acid sequence is then used to predict the sequence in the mRNA and the gene.

4. *Determination of the tendency for two genetic traits (genes or polymorphisms) to remain together or recombine during meiosis is known as linkage analysis.* When the technique of linkage analysis is utilized, the clinical investigator seeks a trait that is genetically linked to polymorphic genetic markers. If they are located close enough together on the same chromosome, they will be exchanged together as a unit when the crossing over of genetic material occurs in meiosis. If the traits are separated by as little as 1 million base pairs, they will be linked 99% of the time and have a *recombinant fraction* of 1% (the percentage of individuals in which the two traits recombine and fail to be inherited together). When the recombinant fraction becomes 30% or greater, it cannot be distinguished from chance (50%). The acceptable recombinant fraction to determine the probability of linkage in most clinical genetic studies is not greater than 10% because of the possibility of chance association in the small subject samples typically used. A recombinant fraction of 10% corresponds to a distance of approximately 10 million base pairs (White, 1984, 1985a, 1985b; White and Caskey, 1988; White and Lalouel, 1988).

5. *Restriction enzymes strikingly increase the number of traits available for linkage analysis.* The ponderous methods of linking gene trait to gene trait previously used by clinical investigators were expanded initially by the use of restriction enzymes: enzymes from bacteria that cut DNA strands at specific "restriction sites" that range from four to eight bases in length. A restriction site polymorphism is simply a specific base sequence. Most are benign (e.g., point mutations affecting only a single base pair), but some restriction sites are pathogenic (e.g., causing splicing errors). Restriction enzymes can be used to examine about 40% of the base pairs in any gene because they are numerous and diverse. A polymorphism occurring within a gene might be detected by a restriction enzyme that would cut the DNA at a new locus (generating smaller DNA fragments identifiable on further analysis) or fail to cut DNA in the usual locus (leaving a longer DNA fragment). This is the basis for methods linking a gene of interest to one of the DNA polymorphisms that are common features of the human genome. The phenotype and specific *restriction fragment length polymorphisms* (RFLPs) travel together in a family pedigree if an appropriate RFLP is found and they are closely linked on the chromosome.

The method is powerful, but its clinical application is fraught with risk. Kidd (1987) delineated the requirements for successful linkage analysis research: standardized reliable diagnostic criteria; systematic symptom assessment methods; extended families with many affected individuals; polymorphic genetic loci densely distributed throughout the genome; and appropriate powerful statistical methods.

6. *Microsatellite DNA.* One of the problems of linkage analysis, that is, an absence of highly polymorphic markers dispersed at regular intervals throughout the genome, has been addressed by the identifica-

tion of microsatellite DNA sequences. These regions are comprised of short tandem repeats (STRs) of dinucleotide (CA), trinucleotide (CTG), or tetranucleotide (TGCA) sequences. The likelihood that the number of copies of these sequences at a given location will be different between an individual's two chromosomes is high. Whereas the microsatellite DNAs are dispersed throughout the genome, the regions that flank the microsatellites are unique. These unique regions are used as landmarks for recognizing a given microsatellite marker (Wilkie et al., 1992). Analysis of microsatellite markers lends itself well to automation. Robotic devices can label the microsatellites with fluorescent molecules. The sizes of the microsatellites can be analyzed with precision by automated DNA sequencers. In the past, linking a genetic trait to a specific DNA marker required months of work. Now this can be accomplished within a matter of weeks.

7. *Polymerase chain reaction.* A key step in improving the efficiency of genetic analysis has been the development of the polymerase chain reaction. This technique relies on using primers that are specific for a region of the genome to amplify short stretches of DNA. Two primers are used, priming the synthesis of opposite strands of the DNA molecule and 'pointing' toward each other. DNA is initiated from these primers in a series of rounds. In each round of DNA synthesis, the number of copies of the template DNA included between the primers is doubled. Following the first few rounds of synthesis, most of the amplified fragments are products of earlier DNA synthesis reactions rather than the sample DNA. These fragments have a single discrete size with common ends at the two primers, the size being determined by the distance between the two primers. Amplification of a single DNA molecule is possible, from such sources as a single sperm or hair follicle. Simultaneous PCR amplification may be applied to many regions of the genome or to two regions of different genes. The presence of a PCR product is diagnostic for a region between the two primers on at least one chromosome. Alteration in the size of the PCR product may indicate the presence of insertions or deletions.

PCR can be used in at least one of two ways for linkage analysis. First, the presence or absence of a polymorphic restriction site can be identified by whether the PCR product is digested with a restriction enzyme. Second, fluctuation in the number of short tandem repeats between the PCR primers can be detected as products whose lengths vary according to the number of repeats that are present (Gilliam, 1992; Hearne et al., 1992).

8. *Positional cloning and candidate genes.* After the gene for a trait has been mapped to a specific chromosomal location, it can be identified by using molecular techniques. One approach is known as *positional cloning* (Collins, 1990–1991; Parrish and Nelson, 1993). Fragments of DNA that span the region of interest are purified and studied for properties that are indicative of the presence of functional genes. These include: high concentration of CG dinucleotides (characteristic of the 5′ ends of genes), or presence of splice donor and splice acceptor sites, conservation in other species, or presence of complementary RNA molecules (all indicative of exons). Another method is known as the *candidate gene approach* (Gilliam, 1992; Parrish and Nelson, 1993). A gene becomes a candidate based on its mapping to the region of interest. The candidacy of the gene is proven by identifying mutations whose presence can be linked to the development of the phenotype.

Polygenic/Multifactorial Disorders and Behavioral Genetics

Behavioral genetics is challenged by several problems. First, behavior is the most complex set of phenotypes: It is the expression of the functional integration of all systems in the organism and varies dynamically in response to the environment. Advances in clinical operational definitions of specific behaviors and the use of reliable behavior rating instruments answer this problem to a significant degree, but gene-gene and gene-environment interactions entangle the best research efforts. Second, behavioral characteristics are not dichotomous but typically consist of features along a continuum. This complicates the designation of affected or nonaffected status and our understanding of gene expression and penetrance. Third, most behavioral traits are affected by multiple genes with small effects, rather than a single gene with an easily demonstrable effect. Fourth, there are strong nongenetic influences on behavior, reflecting both the anticipated gene-environment interaction and the special role of the nervous system in the coordination of adaptive responses to the environment (Plomin, 1990).

In order to unravel the roles of multiple genes and environment simultaneously affecting a set of behaviors, the techniques of quantitative genetics are employed. Classical mendelian laws are assumed to underlie the actions of each of these smaller gene effects. Quantitative genetics examines the total genetic determination of a behavior (heritability), whatever the genetic complexity, but does not attempt to determine the specific genes involved. Animal models of behavior have been utilized for the development of quantitative genetics. Studies of animals selected for breeding according to the presence of specific behaviors demonstrate that, whereas genetic influences on behavior are definite, heritability is less than 50%. In spite of a profound genetic contribution, most behavior has even greater nongenetic origins. In addition, it is clear that multiple genes influence behavior. Well-designed selection studies showing marked differences in a behavioral set after a few generations would demonstrate a ceiling on the specific behavioral change if only one or a few genes were involved. Continuing divergence of the specific behaviors of the two strains after many generations indicates the action of multiple genes. Animal research utilizing family studies, inbred strains, and the recombinant inbred strain method have generated similar results (Plomin et al., 1990).

Familial aggregation, twin, and adoption research designs have been used to examine the heritability of behavioral sets in humans. The results are similar. While the heritability of height, a complex physical trait, is about 90%, nongenetic influences are predominant for the determination of human behavior. Various studies indicate that the heritability of human behaviors is in the range of 5–50%, with substantial variation for any behavior set. This includes such behavioral characteristics as IQ and specific cognitive abilities (50%), personality (30%; for example, activity level, emotional reactivity, neuroticism, conscientiousness, agreeableness, openness, extroversion/introversion), and major psychopathological disorders (5–30%; for example, schizophrenia and mood disorders) (Bouchard, 1994; Plomin, 1990; Plomin et al., 1994).

If the heritability of behavior rests upon multiple genes, and nongenetic influences on behavior account for at least as much of the variance, then it appears that classical linkage studies will not be capable of identifying linkage. Neither the use of pedigrees of informative families nor the affected-sib-pair methods will be sufficient, because they are utilized to determine the chromosomal site of a single or few genes with powerful phenotypic effects whatever the environmental or genetic background. Failures to replicate apparent linkage marker findings for major psychiatric disorders suggest agreement with this point of view, and, again, investigators wonder if genetic heterogeneity is accountable and if families with the same spectrum illness might each have a distinct, specific causative familial gene. The expectation would be that the likelihood of a major gene effect in any of these families would be slim and that a significant principle of behavioral genetics will usually be active: "Although any one of many genes can disrupt behavioral development, the normal range of behavioral variation is orchestrated by a system of many genes, each with small effects" (Plomin, 1990).

In spite of these challenges to molecular biological methods for unraveling major problems in behavioral genetics, some methods are available using quantitative approaches. Studies of associations between multiple quantitative phenotypic traits and multiple genetic markers can be undertaken in larger samples and utilize the possible advantages of selecting candidate genes on the basis of their apparent neurobiological relevance (Plomin, 1990; Plomin et al., 1994). However, the advance that may aid in this research that is currently in the forefront of discussion and controversy is the mapping and sequencing of the human genome.

In this regard, significant discussion has been engendered by a recent study that demonstrated X-chromosomal linkage in some families with multiple homosexual members who had adopted a gay life style (Hamer et al., 1993).

The Human Genome Project

The Human Genome Project is now underway as a national effort of the United States, after several years of deliberation and preparation, under the guidance of the National Institutes of Health and the Department of Energy. It was the general consensus that in spite of controversy and the concern that other scientific projects would suffer because of the drain of large amounts of funds, there would be great advantages to having higher-resolution molecular genetic and physical maps of human DNA. They would be essential to locating human disease genes on the chromosomes and necessary for the next step of sequencing. Rather than rush to the effort at the outset of the project, however, it was judged more prudent to seek technological improvements that amplify the efficiency of gene mapping, sequencing, and data analysis activities. The first 5 years of this 15-year project were devoted to these technical goals. In addition, sequencing of model genomes (*Escherichia coli* and others) has been performed to facilitate similar work on the human genome. For example, informative advances nurtured by the use of model organisms may include the solution of technical problems impeding rapid sequencing, the delineation of genetic mechanisms controlling developmental processes, and the identification of sequence homologies both across and within species.

The first 7 years have led to the development of a human linkage map with a resolution of one cM (Anonymous, 1992, 1994). At the same time, fine-structure physical maps are being developed for each of the human chromosomes. All of these efforts will lead to cloning of various genes implicated in the cause of diseases, leading to new capacities to treat and prevent these afflictions (Cantor, 1990; Watson, 1990).

BRAIN DEVELOPMENT: DEVELOPMENTAL NEUROBIOLOGY

Developmental neuroscience has become the most rapidly expanding sector of the neurosciences, yet relatively little clinical application has emerged. Brief examples of imaginative, clinically informative research are discussed.

Genes controlling developmental sequence—the initiation or suppression of a genetically controlled path of development for a cell or tissue—are necessary because cells differentiate in spite of the fact that each contains the full genome. "Master control genes" that have the ability to induce a complete organ are now sought; they act as "developmental switches." Investigators identify them through their mutant phenotypes. The basic morphogenetic unit of embryonic insects is a segment, controlled by the expression of homeobox segment identity genes. Over the past years homeotic mutations have been the basis for identifying the master control genes that specify the body plan in the anteroposterior axis in *Drosophila* and the mouse. Homeotic transformations occur according to loss- or gain-of-function mutations in these genes. Manipulating these genes made it possible to generate mutants in which the body plan is altered so that body parts (e.g., middle legs) are located where other parts ought to be (e.g., antennae). More recently, ectopic eyes were induced in *Drosophila*, located on the wings, legs, and antennae. The appearance of the eyes was morphologically normal. Mammals and insects share the same master control gene for eye morphogenesis, and there is very substantial sequence conservation among *Drosophila*, mouse, and human genes. This suggests a much more universal control gene for eye morphogenesis than expected (Halder et al., 1995).

These discoveries are remarkable, but it is conceptually difficult to extend them to encompass the complexity of brain structures. How do we explain the leap from developmental regulatory genes to the developing brain, including cell migration, trophic factors, and competitive elimination of axons and neurons (see Chapters 1 and 2)? To what degree are these processes controlled by a genetic program? New research has begun to identify stages and structures of the process. The forebrain of mammals (thalamus, hypothalamus, basal ganglia, and cerebral cortex) has a complexity that matches the cognitive and other processes occurring there. Yet, investigators have determined a segmental structure in the forebrain, and more than 30 homeobox genes are among the many regulatory genes expressed according to regionally restricted patterns in the forebrain. Six forebrain segments, "prosomeres," have been proposed. The prosomeric model will be an important scaffold for determining the functions of the many novel developmental genes that are identified. These are basic first steps toward understanding the genetic control of the developing forebrain and its functions and the related developmental dysfunctions that we observe in the clinic (Puelles and Rubenstein, 1993; Rubenstein et al., 1994).

Just as it is necessary to dissect both the pattern of structural development of the forebrain and its multiple individual controlling factors, it is also essential that we parse the basic behaviors of the infant into replicable structures and seek individual regulatory influences. Social interactions are essential for humans, and mother-infant interactions have been the subject of intensive clinical attention. Yet, clinical emphasis on the significance of mother-infant attachment behaviors has been met with scepticism by some scientists who suspect more theory than fact. A series of animal studies over the past 20 years elucidated the regulators of infant physiology and behavior during attachment, putting attachment research on a firm biological base (Hofer, 1994). The behavioral and physiological responses of infant animals during separation and reunion were examined, and clear stages of protest and despair are present. The investigators demonstrated an array of regulators of biological and behavioral systems hidden within attachment behaviors observed between rats and their pups during the nursing period. The mother regulates specific behavioral and physiological response systems by having a specific mediator for each of these systems, including tactile stimuli, olfactory stimuli, gastric distention, gastric interoceptors, warmth, factors in milk, etc. When the infant is separated from its mother, all of these regulatory influences are lost, generating changes in each system released from its regulator. Following a long separation, the hypoactive rat pup, no longer hungry, alert, or interested in novelty, is characterized by a decrease in heart rate, body temperature, and growth and has increased oral activity and disrupted sleep. Now this familiar pattern is refocused by the recognition that it reflects release from multiple regulators that are available through the mother. This leads to a dysregulation of systems. Attachment is still proximity maintenance, but hidden within it are these regulators of infant behavior and biology. This mother-infant interaction, together with the emotions associated with regulation or dysregulation during attachment behaviors or separation, become the basic experiences that are the building blocks for mental representations (Hofer, 1994).

The comfort associated with mother-infant interactions now has a new meaning. It is no longer a vague term, but reflects the presence of necessary physiological regulators in the interaction. Comfort indicates the presence of affective attunement between mother and child. Clinical investigators have shown similar mechanisms to be involved as infants establish behavioral and physiological organization and develop emotion regulation within the context of mother-infant interactions. The roles of both infants and mothers necessary to achieve attunement and synchrony have been identified. The effects of the loss of the mother as a regulator—emotion dysregulation in the infant—have been documented (Field, 1994). Concurrent patterns of frontal EEG activation and asymmetries have been identified in the human infant during separation from the mother. Further studies of temperament, in particular the characteristic of a child being inhibited or uninhibited, have examined these features in relation to frontal EEG activation and asymmetries (Kagan, 1994). The pieces of the biological/psychological puzzle of the mother's influences on a child's emerging brain and behaviors are beginning to be put in place through laborious research by investigators using markedly different methods and strategies.

DEVELOPMENT AND DYSFUNCTION: THE PREVALENCE OF CHILD AND ADOLESCENT PSYCHIATRIC DISORDERS

Epidemiological Studies of Children and Adolescents

For epidemiological research, a subject in a population sample must be identified as affected or not affected by an illness. Difficulties assigning the presence or absence of psychiatric disorders in a subject were among the forces leading to improved clinical instruments for diagnosis, behavior ratings, and treatment response. As improved instruments were developed, the need for measures of characteristics, such as the consistency and stability of data, led to the application of increasingly refined procedures and methods, including the examination of nosology, criterion variance (leading to the use of specific diagnostic criteria and operational definitions), and information variance (spawning the use of structured interviews); the assessment of disagreement among informants (children, parents, teachers, and pediatricians); the determination of rates of comorbidity; and the study of various types of a best estimate diagnosis. Examples below indicate how a specific advance in epidemiology (the Epidemiological Catchment Area program) or statistics (the application of survival analysis techniques or logistic regression) is part of the current generative research developments of child and adolescent psychiatry (Brasic and Young, 1994).

Epidemiology, the study of the occurrence of disease in populations, is a powerful research tool to accurately estimate the number of affected children and adolescents (Gould et al., 1981) and the likely course of the illness (Costello et al., 1993; Dulcan, 1993; Offord, 1993; Robins, 1981). These results are crucial for mental health administrators planning services to meet the needs of the affected population and to determine the adequacy of current services (Costello et al., 1993; Zahner et al., 1992). For example, epidemiological approaches have been utilized to assess the extent of suicide and injury in adolescents to design prevention programs (Runyan and Gerken, 1989). Additionally, the Epidemiological Catchment Area program for children and adolescents was undertaken to obtain estimates of the numbers of individuals with psychiatric disorders in the general population since accurate data is not currently available.

A critical example of the purposes of epidemiological research is the determination of the cost-effectiveness of service programs for children and adolescents. Traditionally, epidemiological studies of children and adolescents provided a basis to request more services. The existence of many severely disturbed children in the community has been demonstrated through epidemiological studies, but the great cost of new drugs and other treatments may outweigh the benefits. For this reason epidemiological studies must be carried out to demonstrate the cost-effectiveness of innovative programs (Regier, 1993). Additionally once new programs are begun, evaluation research studies are required to substantiate the claims that innovative programs for the psychiatric care of children and adolescents are cost-effective.

Accurate epidemiological studies require reliable instruments to measure the existence and severity of psychiatric disorders in children and adolescents. The recent era of research in child and adolescent psychiatry has been characterized as a phase of method development (Young et al., 1987), resulting in the availability of rating scales and diagnostic interviews for children and adolescents. Key clinical techniques of child psychiatric epidemiology studies include accurate assessment of the child by both rating scales (Boyle et al., 1993b, 1993c; McConaughy et al., 1994; Shaffer et al., 1983) and diagnostic interviews (Boyle et al., 1993a; Shaffer et al., 1993; Young et al., 1987, 1990b).

Recognition of the need to know the prevalence and incidence of mental disorders in adults led to the National Institute of Mental Health (NIMH) Epidemiological Catchment Area (ECA) surveys, which resulted in several of the most important papers on the mental health of adults in this century. The NIMH Cooperative Agreement for Multi-Site Methodological Research for Multi-Site Epidemiological Surveys of Mental Disorders in Child and Adolescent Populations (MECA) (NIMH: RFA MH 8922) (Shaffer et al., 1993) study will utilize the best available rating scales and diagnostic interviews to determine the incidence and prevalence of psychiatric disorders in children and adolescents.

Although results of the MECA study have not been published, data concerning the prevalence of psychiatric disorders in children and adolescents from several epidemiological studies in several countries demonstrated that 5–18.7% of children and adolescents in the general population have psychiatric disorders (Kashani et al., 1987a; Weyerer et al., 1988). Rates are generally higher in adolescence than in childhood. Males have higher rates in childhood; females have higher rates in adolescence. Studies of adults found the highest prevalence of disorders to be in adolescence, with gradual declines in frequency of occurrence with increasing age (Kessler et al., 1994).

The ECA Program estimated the rates of mental disorders in adults in five regions of the United States (Eaton et al., 1984; Regier et al., 1984). Although children and adolescents were excluded from this study, information was obtained retrospectively from the adult subjects concerning the occurrence of symptoms earlier in life. The ECA results provide compelling evidence that children and adolescents experience considerable symptoms and signs of psychiatric disorders:

1. *Alcohol abuse or dependence.* The lifetime prevalence of alcohol abuse or dependence was 13.3% in the five sites of the ECA study. The ECA study indicates that the median age of onset of alcohol abuse or dependence is 21 years (Christie et al., 1988). The years of 15–19 are particularly important for the development of alcohol abuse and dependence (Burke et al., 1990).
2. *Antisocial personality disorder.* The ECA estimates that antisocial personality disorder (APD) occurred in 1.5% of the population of the United States and the 1-year estimate of the incidence of APD was 1.0%. APD is a chronic disorder with symptoms presenting before age 15 years, so this epidemiological study provides strong evidence that serious antisocial symptoms occur in a large group of children and adolescents in this country (Regier et al., 1993).
3. *Anxiety disorders.* A lifetime prevalence estimate of 14.6% for anxiety disorders occurred in the ECA study at the five sites. The median age at onset of anxiety disorders in the ECA study was 15 years (Christie et al., 1988).
4. *Drug abuse or dependence.* The estimate of lifetime prevalence of drug abuse or dependence in the five sites of the ECA was 5.9%. The ECA Program indicated that the median age of onset of drug abuse or dependence is 19 years of age (Christie et al., 1988); ages 15–19 years are important for the development of drug abuse or dependence (Burke et al., 1990).
5. *Phobias.* The median age of onset of agoraphobia, social phobia, and simple phobia is 13 years according to the ECA. The age range of 5–9 years is especially important for the development of these phobias (Burke et al., 1990).

Longitudinal Studies of Children and Adolescents

Prospective studies provide compelling evidence of the natural history of psychiatric disorders. Examples are the longitudinal studies of depression in children and adolescents (Geller, 1993). Separate longitudinal studies of depression in children and adolescents in different regions present evidence that individuals who experience depressive episodes in childhood and adolescence are likely to encounter later psychiatric and psychosocial impairments (Strober et al., 1993), including suicide attempts (Kovacs et al., 1993) and completed suicides (Rao et al., 1993).

New approaches to longitudinal studies are adapted to central problems for research on development and developmental psychopathology, such as the continuity of development, both adaptive and maladaptive. While strong stability has been demonstrated for behavioral characteristics beginning in middle childhood (e.g., for externalizing behaviors, such as aggression), in the preschool years this is true only when data are aggregated so that broad constructs can be used (e.g., ego control and ego resiliency). Similarly, using an organizational/adaptational perspective makes it possible to demonstrate continuity from infancy through childhood. This approach requires that significant issues be defined for each developmental period, so that the organization of the child's behavior in relation to each issue can be examined. Examples are quality of attachment in infancy or close friendships and effectiveness in the peer group in middle childhood. Preliminary research has successfully utilized this approach when following children from infancy to the preadolescent period. The identification of the continuity of such patterns of behavior across childhood is a novel goal for longitudinal studies and may generate new constructs for later epidemiological research (Urban et al., 1991).

An alternative approach is the examination of developmental sequences (developing in a domain of behavior, advancing to the next stage) in childhood in a more conventional sense, but allowing for the existence of more than one developmental pathway to a final behavioral set, such as disruptive behavior in children (Loeber et al., 1993).

Developments in Statistics Relevant to Child and Adolescent Psychiatry: Survival Analysis and Logistic Regression

Survival analysis examines the duration of time from the onset of a disorder to death. The life table techniques used by insurance companies to determine life insurance premiums is an example. Typically, a sample of a large cohort, say 100,000 persons, is followed from birth. The probability of dying at each age is calculated from this population, generating life tables. The Metropolitan Life Insurance Company has developed tables giving the likelihood of dying at different ages according to sex, ethnicity, and other demographic characteristics. These tables have long been the standard for comparison and analysis.

Although the life table traditionally considers death as the endpoint, other applications are relevant to mental disorders. For example, a cohort of persons hospitalized for a psychotic episode may be followed until the next hospitalization for a psychotic episode. Many mental disorders are episodic in nature, with long durations of normal functioning between breakdowns. Life table methodology is adapted to these conditions by considering the duration of the period of normal functioning until relapse as the "lifetime" studied in the life table analysis. Examples of this methodology in psychiatry include the time until recurrence in mood disorders in adults and the time until first depressive episode (Weissman et al., 1987) and first suicide attempt in children and adolescents (Kovacs et al., 1993). Additionally, the use of the life table and other techniques of survival analysis have been crucial for the ECA Program (Burke et al., 1990) and many other psychiatric epidemiological studies.

Epidemiological studies must contend with the possible presence of "red herrings," i.e., misleading influences that are irrelevant to the topic of study. Separation of the "noise" from the genuine effect may require extremely complex mathematical models that overwhelm the most sophisticated computers. Therefore, the technique of logistic regression

has been utilized with success to examine complicated relationships. The basic concept underlying logistic regression is simple. Special mathematical properties of the functions utilized in logistic regression permit the expression of complex mathematical ratios as sums that can be easily handled. Thus, complicated mathematical formulae that would challenge our best computers are transformed into equivalent simple mathematical expressions that can easily and quickly be solved. A textbook of logistic regression for self-study has recently been published to help make this subject accessible to psychiatrists and other clinicians with rudimentary statistical and epidemiological backgrounds (Kleinbaum, 1994).

Logistic regression is particularly useful for follow-up studies because one can readily compare rates of occurrence of disorders in the various groups. For example, suppose we want to compare the odds of suicide in groups of children who are depressed and not depressed. We perform an epidemiological study of a total population of children to determine those who are depressed and those who are not depressed. We let D equal the number of depressed children in the population and N equal the number of children in the population who are not depressed. We then determine the number of children in each group who commit suicide over a period of time. We define S_D to be the number of depressed children who commit suicide and S_N to be the number of nondepressed children who commit suicide.

An equation is generated that is a ratio of ratios, which may be difficult to compute, particularly if the individual terms of the fraction are themselves complex expressions. When logistic regression is utilized, this fraction can be expressed as a sum, resulting in a much easier mathematical representation. In practice, we may actually want to compare the odds ratio of suicide in depressed to nondepressed boys to the odds ratio of suicide in depressed to nondepressed girls, resulting in a ratio of ratios of ratios so the simplifications provided by this technique will reduce a formidable problem to an easy one. The logistic model is therefore well-suited to assess interactions and stratified analyses. It also readily analyzes the problem of one exposure variable and several extraneous variables (Kleinbaum et al., 1982). This technique has been applied in child and adolescent psychiatry to the assessment of lifetime report of major depression over time, demographic, psychosocial, family risk, and diagnostic variables.

ACCESS FOR CHILDREN AND ADOLESCENTS TO NEW RESEARCH TECHNIQUES

The simple existence of these new research methods by no means indicates that they will be applied soon on behalf of children, adolescents, or even adults with developmental disorders. Competition for resources is intense, and much of the capacity to utilize these advances will be determined by the concerted efforts of advocates for children working in clinical research policy and administration. Their success is essential to the realization of new strides forward in the prevention and treatment of childhood neuropsychiatric disorders and advances in the understanding of the developing brain and mind.

Acknowledgment. *This work was supported by the Medical Fellows Program of the New York State Office of Mental Retardation and Developmental Disabilities.*

References

Ahn H, Prichep LS, John ER, et al: Developmental equations reflect brain dysfunction. *Science* 210:1259–1262, 1980.

Alson PR: Definitions of biofeedback. In: Schwartz M (ed): *Biofeedback: A Practitioner's Guide.* New York, Guilford Press, 1987, pp. 33–38.

Andreasen NC: Nuclear magnetic resonance imaging. In: Andreasen NC (ed): *Brain Imaging: Applications in Psychiatry.* Washington, DC, American Psychiatric Press, 1989, pp. 67–121.

Anonymous: A comprehensive human linkage

map with centimorgan density. *Science* 265:2049–2054, 1994.

Anonymous: A comprehensive human linkage map with centimorgan density: NIH/CEPH Collaborative Mapping Group. *Science* 258:67–86, 1992.

Azari NP, Pietrini P, Horwitz B, et al: Individual differences in cerebral metabolic patterns during pharmacotherapy in obsessive-compulsive disorder: A multiple regression/discriminant analysis of positron emission tomographic data. *Biol Psychiatry* 34:798–809, 1993.

Barkovich AJ, Wimberger DM: Magnetic resonance of brain development. In: Kucharczyk J, Mose-

ley M, Barkovich AJ (eds): *Magnetic Resonance Neuroimaging.* Boca Raton, CRC Press, 1994.

Barr LC, Goodman WK, McDougle CJ, et al: Tryptophan depletion in patients with obsessive-compulsive disorder who respond to serotonin reuptake inhibitors. *Arch Gen Psychiatry* 51:309–317, 1994.

Bauman M, Kemper TL: Histoanatomic observations of the brain in early infantile autism. *Neurology* 35:866, 1985.

Baxter LR Jr, Phelps ME, Mazziotta JC, et al: Cerebral metabolic rates for glucose in mood disorders: Studies with positron emission tomography and fluorodeoxyglucose F-18. *Arch Gen Psychiatry* 42: 441–447, 1985.

Baxter LR, Phelps ME, Mazziotta JC, et al: Local cerebral glucose metabolic rates in obsessive-compulsive disorder: A comparison with rates in unipolar depression and in normal controls. *Arch Gen Psychiatry* 44:211–218, 1987.

Baxter LR Jr, Schwartz JM, Mazziotta JC, et al: Cerebral glucose metabolic rates in nondepressed patients with obsessive-compulsive disorder. *Am J Psychiatry* 145:1560–1563, 1988.

Baxter LR, Schwartz JM, Bergman KS, et al: Caudate glucose metabolic rate changes with both drug and behavior therapy for obsessive-compulsive disorder. *Arch Gen Psychiatry* 49:681–689, 1992.

Benkelfat C, Nordahl TE, Semple WE, et al: Local cerebral glucose metabolic rates in obsessive-compulsive disorder. *Arch Gen Psychiatry* 47: 840–848, 1990.

Bookstein FL: Landmarks, edges, morphometrics, and the brain atlas problem. In: Thatcher RW, Hallett M, Zeffiro T, et al (eds): *Functional Neuroimaging*. New York, Academic Press, 1994, pp. 107–119.

Bouchard TJ Jr: Genes, environment, and personality. *Science* 264:1700–1701, 1994.

Boyle MH, Offord DR, Racine Y, et al: Evaluation of the Diagnostic Interview for Children and Adolescents for use in general population samples. *J Abnorm Child Psychol* 21(6):663–681, 1993.

Brasic JR, Young JG: Research design, measures, and statistics. In: Robson KS (ed): *Manual of Clinical Child and Adolescent Psychiatry* (rev ed). Washington DC, American Psychiatric Press, 1994, pp. 435–463.

Brodie JD, Wolkin A, Angrist B, et al: Effects of amphetamine on local cerebral metabolism in normal and schizophrenic subjects as determined by positron emission tomography using (1-^{11}C)2-deoxy-D-glucose(^{11}C-2DG). *Nucl Med* 27:901, 1986.

Buchsbaum MS: Positron emission tomography in schizophrenia. In: Meltzer HY (ed): *Psychopharmacology: The Third Generation of Progress*. New York, Raven Press, 1987, pp. 783–792.

Buchsbaum MS, DeLisi L, Holcomb HH, et al: Cerebral glucography in schizophrenia. In: Greitz T, Ingvar DH, Widen L (eds): *The Metabolism of the Human Brain Studied with Positron Emission Tomography*. New York, Raven Press, 1985, pp. 471–484.

Buchsbaum MS, Ingvar DH, Kessler R, et al: Cerebral glucography with positron tomography: Use in normal subjects and in patients with schizophrenia. *Arch Gen Psychiatry* 39:251–259, 1982.

Buchsbaum MS, Mansour CS, Teng DG, et al: Adolescent developmental change in topography of EEG amplitude. *Schizophr Res* 7:101–107, 1992.

Buchsbaum MS, Siegel BV Jr, Wu JC, et al: Attention performance in autism and regional brain metabolic rate assessed by positron emission tomography. *J Autism Dev Disord* 22:115–125, 1992.

Buchsbaum MS, Wu J, DeLisi LE, et al: Frontal cortex and basal ganglia metabolic rates assessed by positron emission tomography with ^{18}F-2-deoxyglucose in affective illness. *J Affect Disord* 10:137–152, 1986.

Burke KC, Burke JC, Regier DA, et al: Age at onset of selected mental disorders in five community populations. *Arch Gen Psychiatry* 47:511–518, 1990.

Burns HD, Dannals RF, Langstrom B, et al: (3-N-[^{11}C] methyl)spiperone, a ligand binding to dopamine receptors: Radiochemical synthesis and biannual studies in mice. *J Nucl Med* 25:1222, 1984.

Callaway E, Halliday R, Naylor H: Hyperactive children's ERP's fail to support underarousal and maturational lag theories. *Arch Gen Psychiatry* 40: 1243, 1983.

Campbell M, Rosenbloom S, Perry R, et al: Computerized axial tomography in young autistic children. *Am J Psychiatry* 139:510, 1982.

Cantor CR: Orchestrating the Human Genome Project. *Science* 248:49, 1990.

Caparulo BK, Cohen DJ, Rothman SL, et al: Computed tomographic brain scanning in children with developmental neuropsychiatric disorders. *J Am Acad Child Adolesc Psychiatry* 20:338, 1981.

Casey PJ: Protein lipidation in cell signaling. *Science* 264:221–225, 1995.

Chabot RJ, Serfontein G: Quantitative EEG profiles of children with attention and learning problems. Submitted for publication, 1995.

Chase TN, Fedio P, Foster NL, et al: Wechsler Adult Intelligence Scale performance: Cortical localization by fluorodeoxyglucose F-18 positron emission tomography. *Arch Neurol* 41:1244, 1984.

Chase TN, Geofrey V, Gillespie M, et al: Structural and functional studies of Gilles de la Tourette syndrome. *Rev Neurol* 142:851, 1986.

Christie KA, Burke JD Jr, Regier DA, et al: Epidemiologic evidence for early onset of mental disorders and higher risk of drug abuse in young adults. *Am J Psychiatry* 145(8):971–975, 1988.

Coffman JA: Computer tomography. In: Andreasen NC (ed): *Brain Imaging: Applications in Psychiatry*. Washington, DC, American Psychiatric Press, 1989, pp. 1–65.

Cohen RM, Semple WE, Gross M, et al: Dysfunction in a prefrontal substrate of sustained attention in schizophrenia. *Life Sci* 40:2031–2039, 1987.

Collins FS: Identifying human disease genes by positional cloning. *Harvey Lect* 86:149–164, 1990–1991.

Costello EJ, Burns BJ, Angold A, et al: How can epidemiology improve mental health services for children and adolescents? *J Am Acad Child Adolesc Psychiatry* 32(6):1106–1113, 1993.

Courchesne E, Lincoln AJ, Kilman BA, et al: Event related brain potential correlates of the processing of novel visual and auditory information in autism. *J Autism Dev Disord* 15:55–76, 1985.

Cox IH, Roberts TPL, Moseley ME: Principles and techniques in neuroimaging. In: Kucharczyk J, Moseley M, Barkovich AJ (eds): *Magnetic Resonance Neuroimaging*. Boca Raton, CRC Press, 1994.

Czobor P, Volavka J: Pretreatment EEG predicts short-term response to haloperidol treatment. *Biol Psychiatry* 30:927–942, 1991.

Czobor P, Volavka J: Quantitative EEG electroencephalogram effect of risperidone in schizophrenic patients. *J Clin Psychopharmacol* 13:332–342, 1993.

Devous MD: Imaging brain function by single-photon emission computer tomography. In: Andreasen NC (ed): *Brain Imaging: Applications in Psychiatry*. Washington, DC, American Psychiatric Press, 1989, pp. 147–234.

Devous MD Sr: Comparison of SPECT applications in neurology and psychiatry. *J Clin Psychiatry* 53(11 suppl):13–19, 1992.

Eaton WW, Holzer CE III, Von Korff M, et al: The design of the Epidemiologic Catchment Area surveys: The control and measurement of error. *Arch Gen Psychiatry* 41:942–948, 1984.

Farde L, Ehrin E, Eriksson L, et al: Substituted benzamides as ligands for visualization of dopamine receptor binding in the human brain by positron emission tomography. *Proc Natl Acad Sci USA* 82:3863, 1985.

Farde L, Wiesel FA, Halldin C, et al: Central D2-dopamine receptor occupancy in schizophrenic patients treated with antipsychotic drugs. *Arch Gen Psychiatry* 45:71–76, 1988.

Field T: The effects of mother's physical and emotional unavailability on emotion regulation. *Monogr Soc Res Child Dev* 59(2–3)(Serial No. 240): 208–227, 1994.

Frackowiak RSJ: Functional mapping of verbal memory and language. *Trends Neurosci* 17(3): 109–115, 1994.

Frost JJ: Receptor imaging by positron emission tomography and single-photon emission computed tomography. *Invest Radiol* 27(suppl 2):S54–S58, 1992.

Gaffney GR, Tsai LY: Brief report: Magnetic resonance imaging of high level autism. *J Autism Dev Disord* 17(3):433, 1987.

Gaffney GR, Kuperman S, Tsai LY, et al: Midsagittal magnetic resonance imaging of autism. *Br J Psychiatry* 151:831, 1987a.

Gaffney GR, Kuperman K, Tsai LY, et al: Morphological evidence for brainstem involvement in infantile autism. *Biol Psychiatry* 24:578, 1988.

Gaffney GR, Kuperman S, Tsai LY, et al: Forebrain structure in infantile autism. *J Am Acad Child Adolesc Psychiatry* 28:534, 1989.

Gaffney GR, Tsai LY, Kuperman S, et al: Cerebellar structure in autism. *Am J Dis Child* 141:1330, 1987b.

Garber HJ, Weilburg JB, Boumanno FS, et al: Use of magnetic resonance imaging in psychiatry. *Am J Psychiatry* 145:164, 1988.

Geller B: Longitudinal studies of depressive disorders in children: Introduction. *J Am Acad Child Adolesc Psychiatry* 32(1):7, 1993.

George MS, Ketter TA, Post RM: SPECT and PET imaging in mood disorders. *J Clin Psychiatry* 54(11 suppl):6–13, 1993.

Gilliam TC: Mapping psychiatric disease genes: Impact of new molecular strategies. *J Psychiatr Res* 26:309–326, 1992.

Gingrich JA, Caron MG: Recent advances in the molecular biology of dopamine receptors. *Annu Rev Neurosci* 16:299–321, 1993.

Goodman WK, Price LH, Delgado PL, et al: Specificity of serotonin reuptake inhibitors in the treatment of obsessive-compulsive disorder: Comparison of fluvoxamine and desipramine. *Arch Gen Psychiatry* 47:577–585, 1990.

Gould MS, Wunsch-Hitzig R, Dohrenwend B: Estimating the prevalence of childhood psychopathology: A critical review. *J Am Acad Child Psychiatry* 20:462–476, 1981.

Hagman JO, Wood F, Buchsbaum MS, et al: Cerebral brain metabolism in adult dyslexic subjects assessed with positron emission tomography during performance of an auditory task. *Arch Neurol* 49: 734–739, 1992.

Harcherick DF, Cohen DJ, Ort S, et al: Computed tomographic brain scanning in four neuropsychiatric disorders of childhood. *Am J Psychiatry* 142:731, 1985.

Halder G, Callaerts P, Gehring WJ: Induction of ectopic eyes by targeted expression of the eyeless gene in drosophila. *Science* 267:1788–1792, 1995.

Hamer DH, Hu S, Magnuson VL, et al: A linkage between DNA markers on the X chromosome and male sexual orientation. *Science* 261:321–327, 1993.

Hari R, Loumasmaa OV: Recording and interpretation of cerebral magnetic fields. *Science* 244:432, 1989.

Hearne CM, Ghosh S, Todd JA: Microsatellites for linkage analysis of genetic traits. *Trends Genet* 8(8):288–294, 1992.

Heh WC, Smith R, Wu J, et al: Positron emission tomography of the cerebellum in autism. *Am J Psychiatry* 146:242–245, 1989.

Herold S, Frackowiak RSJ, LeCouteur A, et al: Cerebral blood flow and metabolism of oxygen and glucose in young autistic adults. *Psychol Med* 18: 823, 1988.

Hibbard LS, McGlone JS, Davis DW, et al: Three-dimensional representation and analysis of brain energy metabolism. *Science* 236:1641, 1987.

Hofer M: Hidden regulators in attachment, separation and loss. *Monogr Soc Res Child Dev* 59(2–3)(Serial No. 240):192–207, 1994.

Holcomb HH, Links J, Smith C, et al: Positron emission tomography: Measuring the metabolic and neurochemical characteristics of the living human nervous system. In: Andreasen NC (ed): *Brain Imaging: Applications in Psychiatry*. Washington, DC, American Psychiatric Press, 1989, pp. 235–370.

Ingvar M, Bohm C, Thurfjell L, et al: The role of a computerized, adjustable brain atlas for merging of data from examinations using PET, SPECT, MEG, CT, and MR images. In: Thatcher RW, Hallett M, Zeffiro T, et al (eds): *Functional Neuroimaging*. New York, Academic Press, 1994, pp. 209–215.

Innis RB: Neuroreceptor imaging with SPECT. *J Clin Psychiatry* 53(11 suppl):29–34, 1992.

Jacobs BL, Fornal CA: 5-HT and motor control: A hypothesis. *Trends Neurosci* 16(9):346–351, 1993.

John ER, Prichep LS: Principles of neurometric analysis of EEG and evoked potentials. In: Niedermeyer E, da Silva FL (eds): *Electroencephalography: Basic Principles, Clinical Applications and Related Fields*. Baltimore, Williams & Wilkins, 1993.

John ER, Chabot RJ, Prichep LS, et al: Real time intraoperative monitoring during neurosurgical and neuroradiological procedures. *J Clin Neurophysiology* 6:125–158, 1989.

John ER, Karmel BZ, Corning WC, et al: Neurometrics: Numerical taxonomy identifies different profiles of brain functions within groups of behaviorally similar people. *Science* 196:1383–1410, 1977.

John ER, Prichep LS, Ahn H, et al: *Neurometric Evaluation of Brain Function in Normal and Learning Disabled Children* (International Academy for Research in Learning Disabilities Monograph Series, no. 5). Ann Arbor, MI, The University of Michigan Press, 1989.

John ER, Prichep LS, Alper KR, et al: Quantitative electrophysiological characteristics and subtyping of schizophrenia. *Biol Psychiatry* 36:801–826, 1994.

John ER, Prichep LS, Fridman J, et al: Neurometrics: Computer-assisted differential diagnosis of brain dysfunctions. *Science* 239:162, 1988.

John ER, Zhang J-Z, Brodie JD, et al: Statistical probability mapping of brain function and structure. In: Thatcher RW, Hallett M, Zeffiro MH, et al (eds): *Functional Neuroimaging*. New York, Academic Press, 1994, pp. 137–143.

Kagan J: On the nature of emotion. *Monogr Soc Res Child Dev* 59(2–3)(Serial No. 240):7–24, 1994.

Kaye H, John ER, Ahn H, et al: Neurometric evaluation of learning disabled children. *Int J Neurosci* 13:15–25, 1881.

Kaye WH, Berretini W, Gwirtsman H, et al: Altered cerebrospinal neuropeptide Y and peptide YY immunoreactivity in anorexia and bulimia nervosa. *Arch Gen Psychiatry* 47:548–556, 1990.

Kalbfleisch JD, Prentice RL: *The Statistical Analysis of Failure Time Data*. New York, Wiley, 1980.

Kashani JH, Beck NC, Hoeper EW, et al: Psychiatric disorders in a community sample of adolescents. *Am J Psychiatry* 144(5):584–589, 1987.

Kessler RC, McGonagle KA, Zhao S, et al: Lifetime and 12-month prevalence of DSM-III-R psychiatric disorders in the United States: Results from the National Comorbidity Survey. *Arch Gen Psychiatry* 51:8–19, 1994.

Kleinbaum DG: *Logistic Regression: A Self-Learning Text*. New York, Springer-Verlag, 1994.

Kety SS, Schmidt CF: The nitrous oxide method for the quantitative determination of cerebral blood flow in man: Theory, procedure and normal values. *J Clin Invest* 27:476–483, 1948.

Kidd KK: Research design considerations for linkage studies of affective disorders using recombinant DNA markers. *J Psychiatry Res* 21:551–557, 1987.

Kleinbaum DG, Kupper LL, Morgenstern H: *Epidemiologic Research: Principles and Quantitative Methods*. Belmont, CA, Lifetime Learning Publications, Wadsworth, 1982.

Kovacs M, Goldston D, Gatsonis C: Suicidal behaviors and childhood-onset depressive disorders: A longitudinal investigation. *J Am Acad Child Adolesc Psychiatry* 32(1):8–20, 1993.

Kuhar MJ, Goeders NE: Receptor mapping in psychopharmacology. In: Meltzer HY (ed): *Psychopharmacology: The Third Generation of Progress*. New York, Raven Press, 1987, pp. 313–316.

Kuperman S, Gaffney GR, Hamdan-Allen G, et al: Neuroimaging in child and adolescent psychiatry. *J Am Acad Child Adolesc Psychiatry* 29(2):159–177, 1990.

Lathrop GM, Lalouel JM, Julier C, et al: Multilocus linkage analysis in humans: Detection of linkage and estimation of recombination. *Am J Hum Genet* 37:482–498, 1985.

Leckman JF: Genes and developmental neurobiology. In: Lewis M (ed): *Child and Adolescent Psychiatry: A Comprehensive Textbook*. Baltimore, Williams & Wilkins, 1991, pp. 3–11.

Lindsay RM, Wiegand SJ, Altar CJ, et al: Neurotrophic factors: From molecule to man. *Trends Neurosci* 17(5):182–189, 1994.

Loeber R, Wung P, Keenan K, et al: Developmental pathways in disruptive child behavior. *Dev Psychopathol* 5:103–133, 1993.

Lou HC, Henriksen L, Bruhn P, et al: Striatal dysfunction in attention deficit and hyperkinetic disorder. *Arch Neurol* 46:48–52, 1989.

Luxemberg JS, Swedo SE, Flament MF, et al: Neuroanatomical abnormalities in obsessive-compulsive disorder detected with quantitative x-ray computed tomography. *Am J Psychiatry* 145:1089, 1988.

McConaughy SH, Mattison RE, Peterson RL: Behavioral/emotional problems of children with serious emotional disturbances and learning disabilities. *School Psychol Rev* 23(1):81–98, 1994.

McCormick DA: Neurotransmitter actions in the thalamus and cerebral cortex and their role in neuromodulation of thalamocortical activity. *Prog Neurobiol* 39:337–388, 1992.

McDougle CJ, Goodman WK, Leckman JF, et al: Haloperidol addition in fluvoxamine-refractory obsessive-compulsive disorder. *Arch Gen Psychiatry* 51:302–308, 1994.

Middleton HC, Coull JT, Sahakian BJ, et al: Clonidine-induced changes in the spectral distribution of heart rate variability correlate with performance on a test of sustained attention. *J Psychopharmacology* 8(1):1–7, 1994.

Mondt JP: On the effects on source localisation of volume currents in neuroelectric and neuromagnetic signals. *Phys Med Biol* 34:1073, 1989.

Nordahl TE, Benkelfat C, Semple WE, et al: Cerebral glucose metabolic rates in obsessive compulsive disorder. *Neuropsychopharmacology* 2:23–28, 1989.

Offord DR: Discussion of "How can epidemiology improve mental health services for children and adolescents?" *J Am Acad Child Adolesc Psychiatry* 32(6):1116–1117, 1993.

Ornitz EM: Neurophysiology of infantile autism. *J Am Acad Child Psychiatry* 23:251, 1985.

Parrish JE, Nelson DL: Methods for finding genes: A major rate-limiting step in positional cloning. *Genet Anal Tech Appl* 10:29–41, 1993.

Peterson BS, Riddle MA, Cohen DJ, et al: Reduced basal ganglia volumes in Tourette's syndrome using 3-dimensional reconstruction techniques from magnetic resonance images. *Neurology* 43:941–949, 1993.

Piven J, Nehme E, Simon J, et al: Magnetic resonance imaging in autism: Measurement of the cerebellum, pons, and fourth ventricle. *Biol Psychiatry* 31:491–504, 1992.

Plomin R: The role of inheritance in behavior. *Science* 248:183, 1990.

Plomin R, DeFries JC, McClean GE: *Behavioral Genetics*. New York, Freeman, 1990.

Plomin R, Owen MJ, McGuffin P: The genetic basis of complex human behaviors. *Science* 264: 1733–1739, 1994.

Porges SE, Doussard-Roosevelt JA, Maiti AK: Vagal tone and the physiological regulation of emotion. *Monogr Soc Res Child Dev* 59(2–3) (Serial No. 240):167–186, 1994.

Prichep LS, Chabot RJ: QEEG subtyping of ADHD and treatment response. Submitted for publication, 1995.

Prichep LS, John ER: II. Neurometric studies of methylphenidate responders and non-responders. In: Pavlidis GTh (ed): *Perspectives on Dyslexia* (Vol 1). New York, Wiley, 1990, pp. 133–139.

Prichep LS, John ER: QEEG profiles of psychiatric disorders. *Brain Topogr* 4(4):249–257, 1992.

Prichep LS, John ER, Essig-Peppard T, et al: Neurometric subtyping of depressive disorders. In: Cazzullo CL, Invernizzi G, Sacchetti E, Vita A (eds): *Plasticity and Morphology of the Central Nervous System*. London, MTP Press, 1990.

Prichep LS, John ER, Reisberg B, et al: Quantitative EEG (QEEG) prediction of cognitive deterioration in normal subjectively impaired elderly: A longitudinal study. Submitted for publication, 1995.

Prichep LS, Mas F, John ER, et al: Neurometric subtyping of obsessive compulsive disorders. In: Stefanis CN, Rabavilas AD, Soldatos CR (eds): *Psychiatry: A World Perspective* (Vol I). Excerpta Medica. New York, Elsevier, 1991, pp. 557–562.

Prichep LS, Mas F, Hollander E, et al: Quantitative electroencephalographic (QEEG) subtyping of obsessive-compulsive disorder. *Psychiatry Res: Neuroimaging* 50(1):25–32, 1993.

Puelles L, Rubenstein JLR: Expression patterns of homeobox and other putative regulatory genes in the embryonic mouse forebrain suggest a neuromeric organization. *Trends Neurosci* 16(11):472–479, 1993.

Raichle ME: Images of the mind: Studies with modern imaging techniques. *Annu Rev Psychol* 45: 333–358, 1994.

Rakic P: Development of the primate cerebral cortex. In: Lewis M (ed): *Child and Adolescent Psychiatry: A Comprehensive Textbook*. Baltimore, Williams & Wilkins, 1991, pp. 11–28.

Rao U, Weissman MM, Martin JA, et al: Childhood depression and risk of suicide: A preliminary report of a longitudinal study. *J Am Acad Child Adolesc Psychiatry* 32(1):21–27, 1993.

Rauch SL, Renshaw PF: Clinical neuroimaging in psychiatry. *Harvard Rev Psychiatry* 2:297–312, 1995.

Rauch SL, Jenike MA, Alpert NM, et al: Regional cerebral blood flow measured during symptom provocation in obsessive-compulsive disorder using oxygen 15-labeled carbon dioxide and positron emission tomography. *Arch Gen Psychiatry* 51: 62–70, 1994.

Reba RC: PET and SPECT: Opportunities and challenges for psychiatry. *J Clin Psychiatry* 54(11 suppl):26–32, 1992.

Reeve A, Rose DF, Weinberger DR: Magnetoencephalography. *Arch Gen Psychiatry* 46:573, 1989.

Regier DA: The linkage of health care reform and

health services research (editorial). *Am J Psychiatry* 150(11):1613–1615, 1993.

Regier DA, Myers JK, Kramer M, et al: The NIMH Epidemiologic Catchment Area program: Historical context, major objectives, and study population characteristics. *Arch Gen Psychiatry* 41:934–941, 1984.

Regier DA, Narrow WE, Rae DS, et al: The de facto US Mental and Addictive Disorders Service System: Epidemiologic Catchment Area prospective 1-year prevalence rates of disorders and services. *Arch Gen Psychiatry* 50:85–94, 1993.

Reite M, Teale P, Goldstein L, et al: Late auditory magnetic sources may differ in the left hemisphere of schizophrenic patients. *Arch Gen Psychiatry* 46:565, 1989.

Riddle MA, Rasmusson AM, Woods SW, et al: SPECT imaging of cerebral blood flow in Tourette syndrome. *Adv Neurol* 58:207–211, 1992.

Ritvo ER, Garber HJ: Cerebellar hypoplasia and autism. *N Engl J Med* 319:1152, 1988.

Robins LN: Epidemiological approaches to natural history research: Antisocial disorders in children. *J Am Acad Child Psychiatry* 20:556–580, 1981.

Rogers RL: Magnetoencephalographic imaging of cognitive processes. In: Thatcher RW, Hallett M, Zeffiro T, et al (eds): *Functional Neuroimaging*. New York, Academic Press, 1994, pp. 289–297.

Rosen BR, Belliveau JW, Aronen HJ, et al: Functional neuroimaging. In: Kucharczyk, Mosely, Barkovich A (eds): *Magnetic Resonance Neuroimaging*. Boca Raton, CRC Press, 1994.

Rosenberg C, Blakemore KJ, Kearns WG, et al: Analysis of reciprocal translocations by chromosome painting: Applications and limitations of the technique. *Am J Hum Genet* 50:700–705, 1992.

Rubenstein JLR, Martinez S, Shimamura K, et al: The embryonic vertebrate forebrain: The prosomeric model. *Science* 266:578–580, 1994.

Rumsey JM, Duara R, Grady C, et al: Brain metabolism in autism: Resting cerebral glucose utilization rates as measured with positron emission tomography. *Arch Gen Psychiatry* 42:448–455, 1985.

Runyan CW, Gerken EA: Epidemiology and prevention of adolescent injury: A review and research agenda. *JAMA* 262(16):2273–2279, 1989.

Satterfield DH, Lisser LI, Saul RE, et al: EEG aspects of the diagnosis and treatment of minimal brain dysfunction. *Ann NY Acad Sci* 205:273, 1973.

Sawyer JR, Johnson MP, Miller OJ: Traditional and molecular cytogenetics. *J Reprod Med* 37:485–498, 1992.

Schuckit MA: An introduction and overview to clinical applications of neuroSPECT in psychiatry. *J Clin Psychiatry* 53(11 suppl):3–6, 1992.

Sergent J: Brain-imaging studies of cognitive functions. *Trends Neurosci* 17(6):221–226, 1994.

Shaffer D, Schwab-Stone M, Fisher P, et al: The Diagnostic Interview Schedule for Children—Revised version (DISC-R). I: Preparation, field testing, interrater reliability, and acceptability. *J Am Acad Child Adolesc Psychiatry* 32(3):643–650, 1993.

Shapiro AK, Shapiro ES, Young JG, et al: *Gilles de la Tourette Syndrome* (2nd ed). New York, Raven Press, 1988.

Shaffer D, Gould MS, Brasic JR, et al: A children's global assessment scale (CGAS). *Arch Gen Psychiatry* 40:1228–1231, 1983.

Shaywitz BA, Shaywitz SE, Byrne T, et al: Attention deficit disorder: Quantitative analysis of CT. *Neurology* 33:1500, 1983.

Shulman RG: Nuclear magnetic resonance imaging and spectroscopy of human brain function. *Proc Natl Acad Sci USA* 90:3127–3133, 1994.

Siegel BV Jr, Asarnow R, Tanguay P, et al: Regional cerebral glucose metabolism and attention in adults with a childhood history of autism. *J Neuropsychiatry Clin Neurosci* 4(4):406–414, 1992.

Singer HS, Wong DF, Tiemeyer M, et al: Pathophysiology of Tourette syndrome: A positron emission tomographic and postmortem analysis. *Ann Neurol* 18:416, 1985.

Sokoloff L, Reivich M, Kennedy C, et al: The (^{14}C) deoxyglucose method for the measurement of local cerebral glucose utilization: Theory, procedure, and normal values in the conscious and anesthetized albino rat. *J Neurochem* 28:897, 1977.

Steriade M, Gloor P, Llinas RR, et al: Report of the IFCN committee on basic mechanisms. *Electroencephalogr Clin Neurophysiol* 74:481–508, 1990.

Stoetter B, Braun AR, Randolph C, et al: Functional neuroanatomy of Tourette syndrome: Limbic-motor interactions studied with FDG PET. *Adv Neurol* 58:213–226, 1992.

Strober M, Lampert C, Schmidt S, et al: The course of major depressive disorder in adolescents. I: Recovery and risk of manic switching in a follow-up of psychotic and nonpsychotic subtypes. *J Am Acad Child Adolesc Psychiatry* 32(1):32–42, 1993.

Swedo SE, Pietrini P, Leonard HL, et al: Cerebral glucose metabolism in childhood-onset obsessive-compulsive disorder. *Arch Gen Psychiatry* 49:690–694, 1992.

Thompson JS, Thompson MW: *Genetics in Medicine* (4th ed). Philadelphia, Saunders, 1986.

Turner R, Jezzard P: Magnetic resonance studies of brain functional activation using echoplanar imaging. In: Thatcher RW, Hallet M, Zeffiro T, et al (eds): *Functional Neuroimaging: Technical Foundations*. San Diego, Academic Press, 1994, pp. 69–78, 1994

Uhl GR, Childers S, Pasternak G: An opiate-receptor gene family reunion. *Trends Neurosci* 17(3):89–93, 1994.

Urban J, Carlson E, Egeland B, et al: Patterns of individual adaptation across childhood. *Dev Psychopathol* 3:445–460, 1991.

Van Heertum RL: Brain SPECT imaging and psychiatry. *J Clin Psychiatry* 53(11 suppl):7–12, 1992.

Vogel F, Motulsky AG: *Human Genetics: Problems and Approaches* (2nd ed, rev) Berlin, Springer-Verlag, 1986.

Volkow ND, Brodie JD, Wolf AP, et al: Brain metabolism in patients with schizophrenia before and after acute neuroleptic administration. *J Neurol Neurosurg Psychiatry* 49:1199–1202, 1986a.

Volkow ND, Brodie JD, Wolf AP, et al: Brain organization in schizophrenia. *J Cereb Blood Flow Metab* 6:441–446, 1986b.

Waldo MC, Cohen DJ, Caparulo BS: EEG profiles of neuropsychiatrically disturbed children. *J Am Acad Child Psychiatry* 17:656–670, 1978.

Watson JD: The Human Genome Project: Past, present, and future. *Science* 248:44, 1990.

Weinberger DR: SPECT imaging in psychiatry: Introduction and overview. *J Clin Psychiatry* 54(11 suppl):3–5, 1993.

Weinberger DR, Berman KF, Zec RF: Physiologic dysfunction of dorsolateral prefrontal cortex in schizophrenia. I: Regional cerebral blood flow evidence. *Arch Gen Psychiatry* 43:114–125, 1986.

Weissman MM, Gammon GD, John K, et al: Children of depressed parents: Increased psychopathology and early onset of major depression. *Arch Gen Psychiatry* 44:847–853, 1987.

Weyerer S, Castell R, Biener A, et al: Prevalence and treatment of psychiatric disorders in 3 to 14 year-old children: Results of a representative field study in the small town rural region of Traunstein, Upper Bavaria. *Acta Psychiatr Scand* 77:290–296, 1988.

White RL: Human genetics. *Lancet* 2:1257–1262, 1984.

White RL: Diagnosis when the gene locus is unknown. *Hosp Pract* 20:103–112, 1985a.

White RL: DNA sequence polymorphisms revitalize linkage approaches in human genetics. *Trends Genet* 1:177–181, 1985b.

White R, Caskey DT: The human as experimental system in molecular genetics. *Science* 240:1483–1488, 1988.

White R, Lalouel J-M: Chromosome mapping with DNA markers. *Sci Am* 258:40–48, 1988.

Wilkie PJ, Ahmann PA, Hardacre J, et al: Application of microsatellite DNA polymorphisms to linkage mapping of Tourette syndrome gene(s). *Adv Neurol* 58:173–180, 1992.

Williamson S, Kaufman L: Analysis of neuromagnetic signals. In: Gevins AS, Remond A (eds): *Handbook of Electroencephalography and Clinical Neurophysiology*. New York, Elsevier, 1987, pp. 405–448.

Woods SW: Regional cerebral blood flow imaging with SPECT in psychiatric disease: Focus on schizophrenia, anxiety disorders, and substance abuse. *J Clin Psychiatry* 53(11 suppl):20–25, 1992.

Young JG, Brasic JR, Leven L: Genetic causes of autism and the pervasive developmental disorders. In: Deutsch SI, Weizman A, Weizman R (ed): *Application of Basic Neuroscience to Child Psychiatry*. New York, Plenum, 1990a, pp. 183–216.

Young JG, Leven L, Ludman W, et al: Interviewing children and adolescents. In: Garfinkel BD, Carlson GA, Weller EB (eds): *Psychiatric Disorders in Children and Adolescents*. Philadelphia, Saunders, pp. 443–468, 1990b.

Young JG, O'Brien JD, Gutterman EM, et al: Research on the clinical interview. *J Am Acad Child Adolesc Psychiatry* 26:613–620, 1987.

Zahner GEP, Pawelkiewicz W, DeFrancesco JJ, et al: Children's mental health service needs and utilization patterns in an urban community: An epidemiological assessment. *J Am Acad Child Adolesc Psychiatry* 31(5):951–960, 1992.

125 RESPECT FOR CHILDREN AS RESEARCH SUBJECTS

Robert J. Levine, M.D.

"So act as to treat humanity, whether in thine own person or in that of any other, in every case as an end withal, never as a means only." This formal statement of the ethical principle of respect for persons was provided by the German philosopher Immanuel Kant. Persons are to be regarded as ultimate values in and of themselves; they are not to be used merely as means to another's goals.

Those who conduct research involving human subjects first define their goals and then identify persons whom they use as means to accomplish these goals. This is not unethical. What is proscribed is the use of persons merely as means—"as means only." To avoid this, researchers are required both ethically and legally to secure through a process called informed consent the approval of persons to be used as research subjects. If this approval entails acceptance of the researcher's goals, then the subject is not used merely as a means. Rather, the subject freely chooses to embrace the goals as his or her own and thus remains an end.

This chapter is concerned with informed consent and other issues related to the principle of respect for persons (e.g., privacy and confidentiality) as they relate to the involvement as research subjects of adolescents and children of various ages.

ETHICAL PRINCIPLES

The basic ethical principles identified by the National Commission for the Protection of Human Subjects of Biomedical and Behavioral Research (1978) as those that should underlie the conduct of research involving human subjects are "respect for persons," "beneficence," and "justice." These principles were endorsed subsequently by the President's Commission for the Study of Ethical Problems in Medicine and Biomedical and Behavioral Research (President's Commission, 1983) as "basic values" for medical practice as well as for biomedical and behavioral research, calling them by somewhat different names, viz., "respect," "well-being," and "equity." According to these authoritative commissions, research involving human subjects should be conducted in accord with norms or rules designed to uphold and embody these basic principles or values. These rules are assembled in federal regulations for the "protection of human research subjects"; most relevant to the present concerns are those of the Department of Health and Human Services (Code of Federal Regulations, Title 45, Part 46; hereafter abbreviated as 45 CFR 46) and the Food and Drug Administration (Code of Federal Regulations, Title 21, Parts 50 and 56; hereafter abbreviated as 21 CFR 50 and 21 CFR 56).

In this chapter there are frequent references to federal regulations. This is not intended to suggest that all ethical considerations are reflected adequately in the law. Rather, the regulations in this field generally represent a broad social consensus about what ought and ought not to be done. Even for research not covered by the regulations, they have come to be regarded as establishing a community standard, departures from which require justification (Levine, 1986). The regulations include not only substantive rules that require specific actions regarding research subjects but also procedural rules. Of the latter, the most important is that plans to conduct research involving human subjects must be reviewed and approved by an institutional review board (IRB) (Levine, 1986).

According to the National Commission (1978), "Respect for persons incorporates at least two basic ethical convictions: First, that individuals should be treated as autonomous agents, and second, that persons with diminished autonomy and thus in need of protection are entitled to such protections."

An autonomous person is . . . an individual capable of deliberation about personal goals and of acting under the direction of such deliberation" (National Commission, 1978). To show respect for autonomous persons requires that we leave them alone, even to the point of allowing them to choose activities that might be harmful (e.g., hang gliding), unless they agree or consent that we may do otherwise. We are not to touch them or to encroach upon their private spaces unless such touching or encroachment is in accord with their wishes. Our actions should be designed to affirm their authority and enhance their capacity to be self-determining; we are not to obstruct their actions unless they are clearly detrimental to others. We show disrespect for autonomous persons when we either repudiate their considered judgments or deny them the freedom to act on those judgments in the absence of compelling reasons to do so.

Clearly, not every human being is capable of self-determination. The capacity for self-determination matures during a person's life; some lose this capacity partially or completely, owing to illness or mental disability or in situations that severely restrict liberty, such as prisons. Respect for the immature or the incapacitated may require one to offer protection to them as they mature or while they are incapacitated.

Because the central focus of this chapter is on respect for persons, it is necessary to emphasize that the other two principles are of equal importance in the sense that they have equal moral force. Research involving human subjects can be considered ethically justified if, and only if, it is adequately responsive to each of the three basic ethical principles (Levine, 1986). As we shall see, considerations of justice and beneficence place constraints on, for example, whom we can ask to serve as research subjects and how much risk we may ask them to accept in the interests of research.

INFORMED CONSENT

Principle I of the Nuremberg Code (1949) provides the definition of consent from which definitions supplied in all subsequent codes and regulations are derived:

The *voluntary* consent of the human subject is absolutely essential.

This means that the person involved should have *legal capacity* to give consent; should be so situated as to be able to exercise *free power of choice*, without the intervention of any element of force, fraud, deceit, duress, overreaching or other ulterior form of constraint or coercion; and should have sufficient *knowledge* and *comprehension* of the elements of the subject matter involved as to enable him to make an understanding and enlightened decision. (emphasis supplied)

Thus consent is recognized as valid if it has each of these four essential attributes: It must be competent (legally), voluntary, informed, and comprehending (or understanding).

It is through informed consent that the investigator and the subject enter into a relationship, defining mutual expectations and their limits. This relationship differs from ordinary commercial transactions in which each party is responsible for informing himself or herself of the terms and implications of any of their agreements. Professionals who intervene

Portions of this chapter are excerpted or adapted from Levine, RJ: *Ethics and Regulation of Clinical Research* (2nd ed). Baltimore: Urban & Schwarzenberg, 1986. Used with permission of the publisher.

in the lives of others are held to higher standards. They are obligated to inform the lay person of the consequences of their mutual agreements.

It is worth noticing that the Nuremberg Code defines and requires "voluntary consent." Since 1957 this term has been replaced by "informed consent," a term that reflects an idealized vision of the person as a rational, self-determining agent (Katz, 1984).

Federal regulations identify "elements" of information that must be transmitted during the negotiations for informed consent (45 CFR 46.116a); these are

1. A statement that the study involves research, an explanation of the purposes of the research and the expected duration of the subject's participation, a description of the procedures to be followed, and identification of any procedures which are experimental;
2. A description of any reasonably foreseeable risks or discomforts to the subject;
3. A description of any benefits to the subject or to others which may reasonably be expected from the research
4. A disclosure of appropriate alternative procedures or courses of treatment, if any, that might be advantageous to the subject;
5. A statement describing the extent, if any, to which confidentiality of records identifying the subject will be maintained;
6. For research involving more than minimal risk, an explanation as to whether any compensation and an explanation as to whether any medical treatments are available if injury occurs and, if so, what they may consist of or where further information may be obtained;
7. An explanation of whom to contact for answers to pertinent questions about the research and research subjects' rights, and whom to contact in the event of a research-related injury to the subject; and
8. A statement that participation is voluntary, refusal to participate will involve no penalty or loss of benefits to which the subject is otherwise entitled, and the subject may discontinue participation at any time without penalty or loss of benefits to which the subject is otherwise entitled.

In addition, according to the regulations, the following elements must be provided "when appropriate" (45 CFR 46.116b):

1. A statement that the particular treatment or procedure may involve risks to the subject (or to the embryo or fetus, if the subject is or may become pregnant) which are currently unforeseeable;
2. Anticipated circumstances under which the subject's participation may be terminated by the investigator without regard to the subject's consent;
3. Any additional costs to the subject that may result from participation in research;
4. The consequences of a subject's decision to withdraw from the research and procedures for orderly termination of participation by the subject;
5. A statement that significant new findings developed during the course of the research which may relate to the subject's willingness to continue participation will be provided to the subject; and
6. The approximate number of subjects involved in the study.

The regulations define only minimum standards for informed consent. In most cases it seems appropriate to supplement these basic requirements with additional elements of information (Levine, 1986). For example, prospective subjects should be told why they have been selected as invitees to participate in the research; ordinarily, this consists of a statement of the major inclusion and exclusion criteria for the protocol. In addition to the statement of "additional costs to the subject" required by the regulations, there should also be accurate statements of any cash payments or other economic advantages associated with participation in the research as a subject.

How does one determine whether any particular fact (e.g., any particular risk of injury) must be disclosed? The legal criterion for disclosure in the context of medical practice is "material risk"; that is, any fact that is material to the patient's decision must be disclosed (Holder, 1978; Levine, 1986). The determination of which risks are material in that they must be disclosed may be accomplished according to three different standards or tests (Curran, 1974; Levine, 1986). Until recently, the prevailing standard was that of the "reasonable physician"; the determination of whether any particular risk or other fact should be disclosed was made on the basis of whether it was customary to do so in the community of practicing physicians.

The standard that is applied most commonly is the "reasonable person" or "prudent patient" test. In the case of *Canterbury v. Spence* (1972), the court held that the disclosure required was determined by the "patient's right of self-decision," a right that can be

> effectively exercised only if the patient possesses enough information to enable an intelligent choice . . . A risk is thus material when a reasonable person, in what the physician knows or should know to be the patient's position, would be likely to attach significance to the risks or cluster of risks in deciding whether or not to forego the proposed therapy.

Some courts have adopted the rule that a risk is material if the particular patient making the choice or decision considers it material. Of the three standards, this rule, which some call the "idiosyncratic person" standard, is most responsive to the requirements of the ethical principle of respect for persons (Levine, 1986). It is, however, a highly impractical standard.

In the author's view, the minimum amount of information that should be imparted by the researcher to each and every prospective subject should be determined by the reasonable person standard. Then, in the course of the consent discussions, the researcher should attempt to learn from each prospective subject what more he or she would like to know.

Federal regulations permit "a consent procedure which does not include, or which alters, some or all of the elements of informed consent" or, in some cases, waiver of the entire requirement for informed consent, if "[a] The research involves no more than minimal risk to the subjects, [b] The waiver or alteration will not adversely affect the rights and welfare of the subjects, [c] The research could not practicably be carried out without the waiver or alteration, and [d] Whenever appropriate, the subjects will be provided with additional pertinent information after participation" (45 CFR 46.11 6d). Implicit in these conditions—particularly in the second condition—is a recognition of the standard of materiality. One may not withhold any material information without adversely affecting the rights of subjects. Waivers and alterations are commonly used in research involving medical records, "leftover" specimens of tissues and body fluids from which personal identifying information has been removed, survey research, and so on. It is more problematic when researchers propose to alter information for purposes of deceiving prospective research subjects (Levine, 1986).

The Department of Health and Human Services (DHHS) makes it clear that "Nothing in these regulations is intended to limit the authority of a physician to provide emergency medical care, to the extent the physician is permitted to do so under applicable federal, state, or local law" (45 CFR 46.116f). Implicit in this rule is a recognition of two exceptions to the legal requirement for informed consent: the emergency exception and therapeutic privilege.[a]

The Food and Drug Administration (FDA) permits waiver of the consent requirement only in "life-threatening situations" in which "informed consent cannot be obtained . . . because of an inability to communicate with, or obtain legally effective consent from, the subject" (21 CFR 50.23).[b]

---

[a] For an authoritative commentary on these two exceptions, the reader is referred to Appendix 1 of the President's Commission's report, Making Health Care Decisions, 1982, pp. 199–201. A more concise discussion may be found in Levine (1986, pp. 149–152).

[b] There are further conditions specified by FDA in its regulations; for further discussion see Levine (1986, pp. 150–152).

Consent Forms

Thus far we have been considering informed consent, a process designed to show respect for subjects, fostering their interests by empowering them to pursue and protect their own interests. The consent form, by contrast, is an instrument designed to protect the interests of researchers and their institutions by defending them against civil or criminal liability. I believe that one of the reasons there has been so little successful litigation against investigators, as compared with practicing physicians, is the very formal and thorough documentation of informed consent on consent forms. Consent forms may be detrimental to the subject's interests not only in adversary proceedings; signed consent forms in institutional records may lead to violations of privacy and confidentiality (Levine, 1986).

DHHS regulations require "A written consent document that embodies the elements of informed consent. . . . This form may be read to the subject or the subject's legally authorized representative, but, in any event, the investigator shall give either the subject or the representative adequate opportunity to read it before it is signed " (45 CFR 46.117).[c]

Although the primary purpose of the consent form is to protect the interests of researchers and their institutions, it is forbidden by federal regulations to "include any exculpatory language through which the subject or the representative is made to waive or appear to waive any of the subject's legal rights, or releases or appears to release the investigator, the sponsor, the institution or its agents from liability for negligence."[d]

DHHS requires that "[a] copy shall be given to the person signing the form" (45 CFR 46.117). The primary purpose of the form notwithstanding, it can and should be designed to be helpful to the subjects. Having a copy of the form will afford them an opportunity to continue to get more information as additional questions occur to them. It can also serve as a reminder of the plans they must follow in order to accomplish the purposes of research, of the symptoms they should watch for to protect their own safety, of the perils of omitting doses of drugs, and so on. It can serve as a guide to conversations they might choose to have with family, friends, personal doctors, and other trusted advisors about whether they should consent; in some cases such conversations should be recommended during the consent negotiations. In the use of these forms, however, the researcher should heed the words of the President's Commission (1982): "Ethically valid consent is a process of shared decision-making based upon mutual respect and participation, not a ritual to be equated with reciting the contents of a form that details the risks of particular treatments."

No consent form can be designed so as to anticipate all of any particular prospective subject's wishes to be informed. The consent form is most effective when it is viewed by the researcher as a guide to the negotiations with the prospective subject. The consent form should contain at least the minimum amount of information and advice that should be presented during the negotiations. If any substantive new understandings are developed in the process of negotiations that have any bearing on the prospective subject's willingness to participate, these should be added to the consent form signed by that individual.

DHHS regulations (45 CFR 46.117) permit waiver of the requirement for documentation of informed consent if either

1. . . . the only record linking the subject and the research would be the consent document and the principal risk would be potential harm resulting from a breach of confidentiality . . . or
2. . . . the research presents no more than minimal risk of harm to subjects and involves no procedures for which written consent is normally required outside of the research context.

In some cases in which the regulations permit waiver of the requirements for documentation, it may be advisable to provide subjects with information sheets. These documents provide a written account of all information that could serve subjects' interests in ways suggested earlier. They differ from consent forms primarily in that they are not signed by subjects and retained by researchers. Thus they afford limited protection to the researcher and the institution.

JUSTIFICATION OF RESEARCH INVOLVING CHILDREN

Children, as a class of persons, lack the legal capacity to consent. Moreover, many of them, particularly the younger ones, are not only incapable of sufficient comprehension to meet the Nuremberg Code's standard but are also not "so situated as to be able to exercise free power of choice." Since they cannot consent, it is necessary to rely on other devices to show respect for children. Two of these devices are permission and assent.

Permission of one or both parents or of the legal guardian is closely related to what was formerly called "proxy consent." With few exceptions, federal regulators regard permission as a necessary condition for authorizing the involvement of a child as a research subject; for children who cannot assent, it is usually a sufficient condition as well. The transactions involved in negotiating a valid permission are in all respects identical to those of informed consent.

Assent by the child should be as close an approximation of consent as the child's capabilities permit.

Before proceeding with our discussion of permission and assent, it is necessary to return to a consideration of the basic ethical principles.

Respect for persons requires that we treat individuals as autonomous agents only to the extent that they are autonomous. As noted earlier, "[p]ersons with diminished autonomy and thus in need of protection are entitled to such protections" (National Commission, 1978). In response to this ethical conviction, there is established in federal regulations a standard called "minimal risk," which "means that the probability and magnitude of harm or discomfort anticipated in the research are not greater in and of themselves than those ordinarily encountered in daily life or during the performance of routine physical or psychological examinations or tests" (45 CFR 46).[e] Minimal risk serves as a threshold standard in that plans to involve children in research that presents more than minimal risk require special justification and procedural protections.

But many therapeutic procedures present far more than minimal risk, and it is not customary to obstruct children's access to them by calling for special procedural protections. The regulations make it clear that the minimal risk standard is applicable only to procedures that do not "hold out the prospect of direct benefit for the individual subjects" (45 CFR 46.405). Therapeutic procedures, by contrast, are to be authorized and justified precisely as they are in the practice of medicine. That is to say, the risk of any procedure is justified in terms of the benefit expected for the individual child-subject who will bear that risk. Also, as in medical practice, the relationship of anticipated benefit to the risk presented by the procedure must be at least as advantageous to the subject as that presented by any available alternative, unless, of course, the subject (or his or her parents) has considered and refused to accept a superior alternative. These rules are responsive to the ethical principle of beneficence, which as articulated by the National Commission (1978) is expressed in the form of two general rules: "(1) Do no harm and (2) Maximize possible benefits and minimize possible harms."

Justice, as envisioned by the National Commission, requires a fair sharing of the burdens and benefits of society (Levine, 1986; National

---

[c] DHHS regulations also permit use of a "short form." Use of this form of documentation seems even more complicated and cumbersome than use of the standard consent form. Moreover, its use requires a witness to the consent discussion (Levine, 1986, pp. 134–135).

[d] Such language is also forbidden in the consent discussion (45 CFR 46.116).

[e] The term minimal risk presents many problems. As it is defined, it may be interpreted in several different ways. For a discussion of its deficiencies, see Levine (1986, p. 65) and Kopelman (1981, 1985). For an excellent discussion relating the concept of risk to the child's level of development, see Thompson (1990).

Commission, 1978). In the distribution of these burdens and benefits, special consideration is to be given to those who are vulnerable or disadvantaged. Because they lack the capacity to consent, children are considered vulnerable and are to be protected from exploitation. They are not to be involved in research that is irrelevant to the class of person of which they are representative. When appropriate, research should be done first on adults and then on older children before involving younger children and infants (Levine, 1986).

In summary, children and their parents are not completely free to do their own thing. There are constraints grounded in ethical considerations and enforced by regulations on whom researchers may invite to serve as subjects and how much risk they may be asked to assume for research purposes. With these constraints in mind, we now turn to further consideration of assent and permission.

Assent

Respect for children does not require that we leave them alone even to the point of allowing them to choose dangerous activities unless they agree that we may do otherwise. Young children have no such liberty rights. What they have instead is a right to custody (Freedman, 1975). We show respect for them by fostering their well-being, protecting them from harm, and guiding them to become "the right kind of people."

As we have already noticed, federal regulations reflect the obligation to protect children from harm and to secure their well-being. Let us now consider the obligation to guide their moral and social development—an obligation not recognized explicitly in the regulations.

In the 1970s there was a spirited debate over the legitimacy of using as research subjects persons who are incapable of consent ("unconsenting subjects"). Paul Ramsey (1976) argued that it is always morally wrong. Richard McCormick (1974), arguing the opposing viewpoint, pointed out that members of a moral community have certain obligations. One of these is to contribute to the general welfare when to do so requires little or no sacrifice. In the case of children, one may presume that they would consent if they could; he calls this a "correctly construed consent." In his view, when supplemented with parental permission, correctly construed consent authorized the use of children as subjects in research that fulfilled an important social need and involved "no discernible risk."

At this point, Terrence Ackerman (1979) entered the debate, arguing that we tend to fool ourselves with procedures designed to show respect for the child's very limited autonomy. He claims that the child tends to follow "the course of action that is recommended overtly or covertly by the adults who are responsible for the child's well-being." He further contends that, in general, this is as it ought to be. "Once we recognize our duty to guide the child and his inclination to be guided the task becomes that of guiding him in ways which will involve his well-being and contribute to his becoming the right kind of person."

Willard Gaylin (1982) tells the story of a man who acted in accord with Ackerman's position. After directing his 10-year-old son to cooperate with a venipuncture for research purposes, he explained that his direction arose from his perceived moral obligation to teach his child that there are certain things one does to serve the interests of others even if it does cause a bit of pain: "This is my child. I was less concerned with the research involved than with the kind of boy I was raising. I'll be damned if I was going to allow my child, because of some idiotic concept of children's rights, to assume that he was entitled to be a selfish, narcissistic little bastard."

Parenthetically, while it is appropriate to guide and persuade a 10-year-old boy to submit to a venipuncture for research purposes, it is not ethically defensible to command him to do so against his will; it is also contrary to the requirements of federal regulations. Guiding children to become the "right kind of persons" entails teaching them about and encouraging them to embrace the sense of obligation to the moral community discussed earlier. It further entails showing respect for their maturing capacities for self-determination; one hopes the child will learn

to choose to do unto others as the child would wish them to do unto her or him.

At what age does a child become capable of assent? Federal regulations specify no age, leaving it to the discretion of the IRB, taking into account not only the age but also the maturity and psychological state of the children involved.

As the assent regulation is written, it seems to reflect a presumption that the capability to assent is an all-or-none phenomenon; the child is either capable or incapable of assent. This presumption is incorrect (Weithorn, 1983a, 1983b) and, the author believes, unintended by the regulation writers. In the author's view the regulations are intended to be interpreted to permit a determination that prospective child-subjects may be capable of understanding some but not all of the elements of informed consent. Thus, for example, it may be appropriate to provide some children with "a description of any reasonably foreseeable risks or discomforts," without providing "an explanation as to whether any compensation [is] available if injury occurs."

It is possible to make some general comments on the capabilities to assent of children having normal cognitive development in various age groups. According to Lois Weithorn (1983a) who relates her empirical findings to Piaget's concepts of cognitive development,

> in general, developmental research suggests that most school-aged children are capable of meaningful assent for participation in most types of research studies. This means that the children probably are capable of comprehending the nature of the proposed procedures, the general purpose of the research, and of expressing a preference regarding participation. Research suggests that normal children ages 6 and older are quite capable of thoughtful and reasoned consideration of the types of information that investigators may provide.

Typically, at about age 11, children's cognitive development enters the "stage of formal operations," during which they become increasingly sophisticated in their capacities to reason about "possibility" and other abstract concepts. From ages 7 to 11, in the "stage of concrete operations," the child is more or less limited to thinking about matters that are not too far removed from concrete reality. Thus there are those who argue that the "age of assent" should be around 6 or 7, and others who say it should be around 11 or 12.[f]

Weithorn (1983a) continues:

> Early empirical findings also suggest that, although they may not be legally authorized to provide independent consent for treatment or research in most jurisdictions, normal adolescents age 14 and older may be as capable as adults of making competent decisions about such participation, according to the more stringent legal standards of competency.

The authority of mature and emancipated minors to consent will be discussed shortly. (See Chapter 116 for definitions of "mature minors" and "emancipated minors.")

Permission

Parental permission is envisioned by the National Commission as a reflection of the collective judgment of the family that an infant or child may participate in research (Levine, 1986; National Commission, 1977). In most cases the permission of one parent is sufficient; one may assume that he or she will represent the family's wishes satisfactorily.

When more than minimal risk is presented by a nontherapeutic procedure, the permission of both parents is required unless one is "deceased, unknown, incompetent, or not reasonably available, or when only one

---

[f] According to the National Commission (1977), a child with normal cognitive development becomes capable of meaningful assent at about the age of 7 years, although some may be younger and some older. DHHS did not accept this recommendation. Rather, at the time the proposed regulations were published, DHHS solicited public comment on which of three options it should adopt for nontherapeutic procedures: either age 7, age 12, or leaving the age to the discretion of the IRB. The final regulations reflect the third of these options.

person has legal responsibility for the care or custody of the child'' (45 CFR 46.408).

There are three additional criteria for justification of nontherapeutic procedures that present more than minimal risk (45 CFR 46.406): First, the degree of risk is limited to ''a minor increase over minimal risk.'' Second, the procedure or intervention must be ''likely to yield generalizable knowledge which is of vital importance for the understanding or amelioration of the subject's disorder or condition.''[g] Third, the procedure or intervention must present ''experiences to subjects that are reasonably commensurate with those inherent in their actual or expected medical, dental, psychological, social or educational situations.'' This means that the procedures must be ones that they or others with the specific disorder or condition under study will ordinarily experience by virtue of their having or being treated for that disorder or condition. Thus it might be appropriate to invite a child with leukemia who has had several bone marrow examinations to consider having another for research purposes.

The requirement of commensurability reflects the National Commission's judgment that children who have had a procedure performed upon them might be more capable than are those who are not so experienced of basing their assent on some familiarity with the procedure and its attendant discomforts; thus their decision to participate will be more knowledgeable.

Even though the parent gives permission, the child's refusal to assent to nontherapeutic interventions should be respected. Those who are incapable of assent may have some capacity to make their wishes known. The term *deliberate objection* is used to recognize that some children who are incapable of meaningful assent are able to communicate their disapproval or refusal of a proposed procedure. A 4-year-old may protest, ''No, I don't want to be stuck with a needle.'' However, an infant who might in certain circumstances cry or withdraw in response to almost any stimulus is not regarded as capable of deliberate objection. A child's deliberate objection usually should be regarded as a veto to his or her involvement in research (Levine, 1986; National Commission, 1977).

In the case of therapeutic interventions or procedures, the situation is much different. Federal regulations state simply, the assent of children is not a necessary condition (45 CFR 46.408). Parents have both the right and the responsibility to override the objection of school-age children to necessary therapy. With regard to teenagers, decisions regarding authorization of investigational therapies are about as complicated as they are in the practice of medicine. The law recognizes the authority of emancipated and some mature minors to consent to or refuse standard or accepted therapy; these rules are not recognized explicitly in federal regulations regarding investigational therapies.

In the practical world of decision making about who can authorize a therapeutic procedure, whether it be investigational or accepted, it rarely suffices to point to the law and thereby identify the person who has the legal right to make the decision. Many factors must be taken into account in reaching judgments about the capability of various persons to participate in and, in the event of irreconcilable disputes, to prevail in such choices. In general, these judgments become more complicated as the child gets older or as the stakes get higher (Gaylin, 1982; Thomasma and Mauer, 1982).

IRBs have the authority to waive the requirement for permission when ''it is not a reasonable requirement . . . provided an appropriate mechanism for protecting the children is substituted'' (45 CFR 46.408). The regulations suggest as an example of research in which a requirement for parental permission might not be reasonable is that on ''neglected or abused children.'' The National Commission (1977) specified several other examples:

Research designed to identify factors related to the incidence or treatment of certain conditions in adolescents for which, in certain jurisdictions, they may legally receive treatment without parental consent; research in which the subjects are ''mature minors'' and the procedures involved entail essentially no more than minimal risk that such individuals might reasonably assume on their own; research designed to meet the needs of children designated by their parents as ''in need of supervision,'' and research involving children whose parents are legally or functionally incompetent.

The National Commission (1977) further elaborates:

There is no single mechanism that can be substituted for parental permission in every instance. In some cases the consent of mature minors should be sufficient. In other cases court approval may be required. The mechanism involved will vary with the research and the age, status and condition of the prospective subject. . . .

Assent of . . . mature minors should be considered sufficient with respect to research about conditions for which they have the legal authority to consent on their own to treatment. An appropriate mechanism for protecting such subjects might be to require that a clinic nurse or physician, unrelated to the research, explain the nature and the purpose of the research . . . emphasizing that participation is unrelated to provision of care.

Another alternative might be to appoint a social worker, pediatric nurse, or physician to act as surrogate parent when the research is designed, for example, to study neglected or battered children. Such surrogate parents would be expected to participate not only in the process of soliciting the children's cooperation but also in the conduct of the research, in order to provide reassurance for the subject and to intervene or support their desires to withdraw if participation becomes too stressful.

In the 1990s there has been increasing interest in giving mature minors independent authority to authorize their own participation in certain types of research without requiring permission of their parents or guardians. To some extent this interest reflects a general trend in public policy toward facilitating inclusion as research subjects members of groups who were previously excluded (Levine, 1994). This interest also represents a pragmatic response to problems presented by the AIDS pandemic; specifically, many, and perhaps most, adolescents will not enroll as research subjects if this necessarily entails allowing their parents or guardians to learn or even suspect certain details of their sexual or drug taking experience (Rogers et al., 1994).

Most of the current federal regulations for the protection of human subjects reflect the attitude that prevailed in the 1960s and 1970s when they were written, that investigational drugs and participation in research were dangerous and that researchers were likely to exploit subjects. Since the mid-1980s, primarily as a consequence of the efforts of AIDS activists, this vision has been largely replaced by one that research participation and access to investigational drugs are both more beneficial than burdensome. As a result of this shift in perception, public policies that were designed to protect persons from harm and exploitation, particularly those persons who are considered vulnerable by reason of limitation in their capacity to give informed consent, are being reinterpreted or rewritten to assure the same classes of persons equitable access to the benefits of investigational drugs as well as to the benefits of participation in research (Levine, 1994).

At the time of this writing, federal policies have not been revised to permit involvement of mature minors as research subjects on their own authority except as discussed earlier in this chapter. However, it seems reasonable to predict that in the near future there could be such changes in the relevant policies or their interpretation. Examples of specific proposals have been published by Rogers et al. (1994) and Levine (1995).

Inclusion of children who are wards (e.g., of the state) in research in which more than minimal risk is presented by nontherapeutic interventions requires special procedural protections that are beyond the scope of this discussion (45 CFR 46.409; Levine, 1986). Many states and cities have regulations designed to protect the interests of foster children. Concern has been expressed recently that such regulations often create formidable bureaucratic barriers to involving such children in randomized clinical trials or to gaining them access to investigational drugs.

---

[g] What constitutes ''minor increase'' and ''vital importance'' is not defined in the regulations. Responsibility for deciding such matters in relation to particular research proposals is assigned to the IRB. If the IRB cannot decide or if it does decide that the degree of risk is more than a minor increase over minimal risk, it must refer the judgment to the Secretary of DHHS (Levine, 1986, pp. 247–250).

For two reasons this presents a special problem to children with AIDS: (*a*) a large percentage of such children are foster children, and (*b*) many apparently effective therapies for AIDS and its complications are investigational drugs (Secretary's Work Group on Pediatric HIV Infection and Disease, 1988).

DOCUMENTATION

The regulatory requirement for documentation of permission is exactly the same as it is for informed consent. In circumstances in which there is no requirement for permission because the minor is authorized to assent for himself or herself the same requirements for documentation obtain. Apart from this, when children are asked to sign forms, as they often and quite properly are, the principal purpose, in the author's view, is to enhance their sense of participation in the process.

PRIVACY AND CONFIDENTIALITY

Privacy is "the freedom of the individual to pick and choose for himself the time and circumstances under which, and most importantly, the extent to which, his attitudes, beliefs, behavior and opinions are to be shared with or withheld from others" (Kelman, 1977). Because this is the definition used in this chapter, some matters considered by the law to fall under the rubric of privacy are excluded (e.g., the right to abortion and contraception). In general, in clinical research, intrusions into individuals' privacy are permitted only with their informed consent. When an informed person allows a researcher into his or her private space, there is no invasion.

Confidentiality is a term that is all too often used interchangeably with *privacy*. *Confidentiality* refers to a mode of management of private information; if a subject shares private information with (confides in) a researcher, the researcher is expected to refrain from sharing this information with others without either the subject's authorization or some other justification.

The ethical grounding for the requirement to respect the privacy of persons may be found in the principle of respect for persons. The ethical justification for confidentiality, according to Sissela Bok (1982), is grounded in four premises, three of which support confidentiality in general; the fourth supports professional confidentiality in particular.

First and foremost, we must respect the individual's autonomy regarding personal information. To the extent they wish, and to the extent they are capable of doing so, they are entitled to have secrets. This facilitates their ability to live according to their own life plans.

Closely related is the second premise, which recognizes the legitimacy not only of having personal secrets but also of sharing them with whomever one chooses. This premise, which embodies an obligation to show respect for relationships among human beings and respect for intimacy, is exemplified by the marital privilege upheld in American law, according to which one spouse cannot be forced to testify against the other.

The third premise draws on the general requirement to keep promises. A pledge of confidentiality creates an obligation beyond the respect due to persons and existing relationships. Once we are bound by a promise, we may no longer be fully impartial in our dealings with the promisee.

These three premises, taken together, provides strong prima facie reasons to support confidentiality. That is to say, they are binding upon those who have accepted information in confidence unless there are sufficiently powerful reasons to do otherwise—as, for example, when maintaining confidentiality would cause serious harm to innocent third parties.

Bok's fourth premise adds strength to the pledge of silence given by professionals. The professional's duty to maintain confidentiality goes beyond ordinary loyalty "because of its utility to persons and to society. . . . Individuals benefit from such confidentiality because it allows them to seek help they might otherwise fear to ask for" from doctors or others who can provide it.

Investigators, of course, are not necessarily professionals to whom individuals turn for professional help. Thus only part of the fourth premise applies to investigators, that part which grounds the justification and requirement for confidentiality in its social utility. If researchers violated the confidence of their subjects, subjects would refuse to cooperate with them. This, in turn, would make it difficult, if not impossible, for researchers to contribute to the development of generalizable knowledge.

Over the millennia, the professions have viewed the obligation to maintain confidentiality as very important. The Hippocratic Oath requires "What I may see or hear in the course of the treatment or even outside the treatment in regard to the life of men, which on no account one must spread abroad, I will keep to myself holding such things shameful to be spoken about."

Thomas Percival's *Code of Medical Ethics* (1803), upon which was based the first code of ethics of the American Medical Association, incorporated the following exhortation: "Patients should be interrogated concerning their complaints in a tone of voice which cannot be overheard."

In all states, the law not only recognizes the obligation of physicians and many other professionals to maintain confidentiality, it requires it. In many states, there are statutes granting testimonial privilege to information secured by physicians from patients in the course of medical practice (Brennan, 1983). Testimonial privilege means that physicians cannot be compelled to disclose such information even under subpoena. Although the United States Supreme Court refused to extend the constitutional protections of privacy to physician-patient communications, the *Federal Rules of Evidence*, promulgated by the Judicial Conference, defer to state law on physician-patient privilege (Brennan, 1983).

Most state laws on physician-patient privilege contain various exceptions, including mandatory reporting of information regarding battered and abused children, various communicable diseases, gunshot wounds, and certain proceedings concerned with health issues, including workers' compensation and insurance claims (Brennan, 1983).

In 1974, in the case of *Tarasoff v. Board of Regents*, the supreme court of California ruled that a psychiatrist has a duty to protect the intended victim of a patient's threat of violence, if it is likely that such a threat would be carried out (Holder, 1985); this often but not always entails a duty to warn the intended victim. Subsequently, this duty has been recognized in many other states. The same principle is often invoked in debates over whether state laws should be changed to either permit or require doctors to warn lovers of persons infected with the HIV virus if they are unwilling to do so themselves (Gostin, 1989).

It must be recognized that the right to confidentiality or privilege belongs to the patient. The patient may authorize sharing of private information for whatever purposes he or she chooses. In civil or criminal litigation where the patient makes the information in his or her medical record material to the support of his or her position, as so often happens in child custody cases or in malpractice litigation, the court will usually require that the contents of the record be disclosed (Holder, 1985).

Confidentiality in Research

Most direct social injuries to research subjects result from breaches of confidentiality. An investigator may identify a subject as a drug or alcohol abuser, as a participant in various deviant sexual practices, as having any of a variety of diseases that may be deemed unacceptable by his or her family or social or political group, as having a higher or lower income than acquaintances might have predicted, as a felon, and so on. If such information becomes known to certain individuals, it might cost the subject his or her reputation, job, social standing, credit, or citizenship.

In recognition of these threats of social injury, federal regulations require the IRB to determine that "Where appropriate, there are adequate provisions to protect the privacy of subjects and to maintain the confidentiality of data" (45 CFR 46.111a).

How does one determine that provisions to maintain confidentiality are "adequate"? The first step is to become aware of the variety of factors that may pose threats to confidentiality in the research context. The second is to become aware of the various devices that are available to secure the confidentiality of research data.[h]

The National Commission (1978) offered some suggestions for safeguards of confidentiality: Depending upon the degree of sensitivity of the data, appropriate methods may include coding or removal of individual identifiers as soon as possible, limitation of access to data, or the use of locked file cabinets. Researchers occasionally collect data that, if disclosed, would put subjects in legal jeopardy. Because research records are subject to subpoena, the National Commission suggests that when the identity of subjects who have committed crimes is to be recorded, the study should be conducted under assurances of confidentiality that are available from DHHS as well as from the Department of Justice. For detailed information on these assurances of confidentiality, which provide immunity from subpoena, see Office for Protection from Research Risks (1993).

CONSENT

As mentioned earlier, informed consent regulations require "a statement describing the extent, if any, to which confidentiality of records identifying the subject will be maintained." Statements about confidentiality of research records should not promise more than the researchers can guarantee. For most studies in which the private information to be collected is not especially sensitive, it suffices to state that the researchers intend to maintain confidentiality, that they will take precautions against violations, and that all reports of the research will be in the form of aggregated data and devoid of identifiers. When dealing with more sensitive information, it may be useful to specify some of the precautions; for example, video tapes will be destroyed within 60 days or, if the subject so requests, earlier; data will be kept in locked files; individuals will be identified by a code and only a small number of researchers will have access to the key that links code numbers to identifiers.

Plans to incorporate data in the subjects' medical record should be made explicit. In general, when these data are relevant to patient management, they should be incorporated unless the subject objects. Incorporation of the results of nonvalidated diagnostic tests may lead to false diagnostic inferences, with adverse consequences to the patient's medical care or insurability. Most people do not understand the full implications of signing forms that release their medical records to insurance companies (Siegler, 1982).

It is essential to disclose all serious threats of confidentiality breaches that can be anticipated. One such disclosure was used in a study of devices designed to encourage young children who are thought to have been abused sexually to speak freely of their experiences. A portion of the permission form for the normal control subjects reads as follows (Levine, 1986).

> Because this study is not intended to be related to either diagnosis or therapy for you or your child, you are entitled to decide whether the information obtained during this study should be entered into the medical record. If, however, during your child's interview, his or her behavior raises a concern of sexual abuse, a clinical evaluation of your child will be performed. . . . If after that evaluation the suspicion of sexual abuse persists, the case will be reported as mandated by law.

FDA regulations require (21 CFR 50.25a) "a statement describing the extent, if any, to which confidentiality of records identifying the subject will be maintained and notes the possibility that the [FDA] may inspect the records."

As noted earlier, federal regulations permit waiver of the informed consent requirement under certain conditions. These conditions are usually but not invariably met in studies of medical records (given adequate safeguards of confidentiality) or of "leftover" specimens obtained at autopsy, surgery, or collection for diagnostic purposes of body fluids such as blood or urine. In general, use of tissues or fluids without consent is justified if two conditions are satisfied (Levine, 1986): (a) No more tissue or fluid is removed than the amount needed to accomplish the medically indicated purpose of removal, and (b) the specimens are obtained by the researcher under conditions of anonymity (that is, the diagnostic laboratory removes all personal identifiers before giving the specimens to the researcher).[i]

The practices just described are invasions of privacy. In such cases, patients are said to have a right of notice, that is, a right to be notified that such practices occur in the institution. These notices, which partially mitigate the invasion, are commonly printed in patient information brochures and on permission forms for surgery or autopsy. Although they are designed to afford patients opportunities to object, objections are rare. For examples of such notices, see Levine (1986, pp. 179–180).

In some cases, with suitable justification, even the right of notice may be waived. Examples of such activities include collections of cord blood from neonates under conditions of anonymity in a nationwide study to determine the prevalence of HIV antibodies (Levine, 1988); monitoring for compliance in some randomized clinical trials (Levine, 1986); and covert observation or recording of public behavior (Levine, 1986). Further discussion of these activities and their justification is beyond the scope of this chapter. It must be noted that covert observation is a mild form of deception. In some cases even stronger forms of deception may be justified (American Psychological Association, 1982; Levine, 1986).

Researchers commonly use medical or laboratory records to identify patients who might be suitable subjects for their studies. Having identified them, they then contact them by telephone or by mail with invitations to participate in research. Those who are contacted usually do not recall having read notices describing such activities in hospital brochures. Some will wonder why a stranger who knows his or her diagnosis is calling. Careful plans must be made to avoid offending patients in such activities (Levine, 1986).

CHILDREN AND PRIVACY

The concerns of young children about privacy are different from those of older children and adolescents (Thompson, 1990). Young children first develop territorial privacy ("This is my room") and possessional privacy ("This is my tricycle") and only later begin to develop informational privacy (concerns about others' knowledge of one's activities, associations, and interests). Thus young children may not know that what they say to others may be detrimental to the privacy interests of their families.

DHHS regulations are responsive to this concern. There are several classes of research that are generally considered so free of complicated ethical problems that they are exempted from coverage by the regulations (45 CFR 46. 101b). Two of these exemptions do not apply to research involving children: (a) research involving survey or interview procedures; (b) research involving observation of public behavior in which the researcher is a participant. These activities are not exempt in cases in which they "could reasonably place the subject at risk of criminal or civil liability or be damaging to the subject's financial standing or employability."

Researchers must often secure the approval of various custodians of children to involve them in research. Such custodians may be teachers, day care workers, camp counselors, and the like. At times it is important

---

[h] A full discussion of these threats and devices is beyond the scope of this chapter. A treatment of these topics adequate for the purposes of most clinical researchers is found in Levine (1986). Boruch and Cecil (1979) provide an excellent general overview directed primarily at social scientists, with particular concentration on the development of statistical methods for making the responses of any particular subject uninterpretable even if the research records are subpoenaed.

[i] In some cases it may be impossible to remove identifiers, as when the patient's physician is also the researcher. In such cases the requirement for consent may be waived if the research will not yield any information having diagnostic significance. For further discussion of this point, see Levine (1986, pp. 178–181).

to withhold or disguise some of the purposes of the research in order to protect the family's privacy or to avoid prejudicial treatment of children. For example, one would generally avoid telling teachers that the children are selected because they are offspring of parents with emotional disturbances.

As mentioned earlier, informed consent requires "an explanation of the purpose of research." Does this mean that parents must always receive a full disclosure of purposes? Suppose the purpose is—as it was in one study—to determine whether little boys with XYY chromosome patterns are more likely than those with XY patterns to develop violent behavior. Disclosure of such a purpose could become a self-fulfilling prophecy. For further discussion of withholding the purpose of research and its justification, see Levine (1986, p. 117).

As mentioned earlier, the requirement for parental permission may be waived in "research designed to identify factors related to the incidence or treatment of certain conditions in adolescents for which . . . they may legally receive treatment without parental consent." In general, the types of activities contemplated by this rule are treatment of sexually transmitted diseases, provision of contraceptive advice, and other matters that teenagers consider highly sensitive. We recognize the teenager's right to privacy, but how far should we go to protect it? Some of the factors that require consideration are illustrated in the following exchange.

Herceg-Baron (1981) published a case study in which she detailed some of the special problems involved in research in the field of family planning involving minors as subjects. Many adolescents wish to seek advice about such matters as contraception without the awareness of such others as their parents. She details her institution's policy for protecting the minors' confidentiality. For instance, with regard to follow-up, investigators are required to offer various options, for example, telephone calls during certain hours when the minor knows she will be at home alone; contacts through school personnel such as nurses, teachers, or counselors; contacts by mail containing no agency letterhead or other identifying information; or leaving messages with friends.

In commenting on this case study, Carol Levine (1981) raises several concerns. First, she suggests that many adolescents are ambivalent about clandestine sex and would, with some encouragement, welcome open discussion with their parents. The great concern with privacy seems to undermine the possibility for what could be valuable communication within the family. Levine is further concerned about the fact that the institution not only approves deception, it collaborates with the adolescent in deceiving her parents. This, she argues, sets a very poor example for the adolescent.

This brings us back to a point discussed earlier. Parents are not the only adults having responsibility for guiding the child to become the "right kind of person." Professionals must be aware of the fact that children see them as models of proper behavior. Consciously or otherwise, they provide examples that children will emulate. Accordingly, they should be especially careful not to suggest by example that promises (e.g., of confidentiality), truthfulness, and other ethical matters discussed in this chapter are to be taken lightly. In short, they should help children understand the importance of showing respect for persons.

References

Ackerman TF: Fooling ourselves with child autonomy and assent in nontherapeutic clinical research. *Clin Res* 27:345–348, 1979.

American Psychological Association: *Ethical Principles in the Conduct of Research with Human Participants*. Washington, DC, American Psychological Association, 1982.

Bok S: *Secrets: On the Ethics of Concealment and Revelation*. New York, Pantheon, 1982.

Boruch RF, Cecil JS: *Assuring the Confidentiality of Social Research Data*. Philadelphia, University of Pennsylvania Press, 1979.

Brennan TA: Research records. Litigation and confidentiality: The case of research on toxic substances. *IRB: Rev Hum Subjects Res* 5(5):6–9, 1983.

Curran WJ: Ethical issues in short term and long term psychiatric research. In: Ayd FJ (ed): *Medical, Moral, and Legal Issues in Mental Health Care*. Baltimore, Williams & Wilkins, 1974.

Canterbury v. Spence, 464 F 2d 72, CA DC 1972.

Freedman B: A moral theory of informed consent. *Hastings Center Rep* 5(4):32–39, 1975.

Gaylin W: Competence: No longer all or none. In: Gaylin W, Macklin R (eds): *Who Speaks for the Child?* New York, Plenum, 1982, pp. 27–54.

Gostin LD: Public health strategies for confronting AIDS: Legislative and regulatory policy in the United States, *JAMA* 261:1621–1630, 1989.

Herceg-Baron R: Parental consent and family planning research involving minors. *IRB: Rev Hum Subjects Res* 3(9):5–8, 1981.

Holder AR: *Medical Malpractice Law* (2nd ed). New York, Wiley, 1978.

Holder AR: *Legal Issues in Pediatrics and Adolescent Medicine* (2nd ed): New Haven, CT, Yale University Press, 1985.

Katz J: *The Silent World of Doctor and Patient*. New York, Free Press, 1984.

Kelman HC: Privacy and research with human beings. *J Soc Issues* 33:169–195, 1977.

Kopelman L: Estimating risk in human research. *Clin Res* 29:1–8, 1981.

Kopelman L: When is the risk minimal enough for children to be research subjects? In: Kopelman LM, Moskop JC (eds): *Children and Health Care: Moral and Social Issues*. Dordrecht, the Netherlands, Kluwer, 1989, pp. 89–99.

Levine C: Commentary: Teenagers, research and family involvement. *IRB: Rev Hum Subjects Res* 3(9):8, 1981.

Levine C: Has AIDS changed the ethics of human subjects research? *Law Med and Health Care* 16:167–173, 1988.

Levine RJ: *Ethics and Regulation of Clinical Research* (2nd ed). Baltimore, Urban & Schwarzenberg, 1986.

Levine RJ: The impact of HIV infection on society's perception of clinical trials. *Kennedy Inst Ethics J* 4:93–98, 1994.

Levine RJ: Adolescents as research subjects without permission of their parents or guardians: Ethical considerations. *J Adolesc Health* 17:287–297, 1995.

McCormick RA: Proxy consent in the experimentation situation. *Perspect Biol Med* 18:2–20, 1974.

National Commission for the Protection of Human Subjects of Biomedical and Behavioral Research. *Research Involving Children: Report and Recommendations* (DHEW publication no. [OS] 77-0004), Washington, DC, US Department of Health, Education, and Welfare, 1977.

National Commission for the Protection of Human Subjects of Biomedical and Behavioral Research. *Institutional Review Boards: Report and Recommendations* (DHEW publication no; [OS] 78-0010), Washington, DC, US Department of Health, Education, and Welfare, 1978.

Nuremberg Code (in) Trials of War Criminals before the Nuremberg Military Tribunals. Control Council Law no. 10 (Vol 2), Washington, DC, US Government Printing Office, 1949, pp. 181–182.

Office for Protection from Research Risks, National Institutes of Health: *Protecting Human Subjects: Institutional Review Board Guidebook*. U.S. Department of Health and Human Services, U.S.

Government Printing Office, Washington, DC, 1993, pages [3-31]–[3-33].

Percival T: *Medical Ethics*. London, Russell, 1803. Reprint edited by C.D. Leake, Baltimore, Williams & Wilkins, 1927.

President's Commission for the Study of Ethical Problems in Medicine and Biomedical and Behavioral Research. *Making Health Care Decisions: The Ethical and Legal Implications of Informed Consent in the Patient-Practitioner Relationship* (stock no. 040-000-00459-9). Washington, DC, US Government Printing Office, 1982.

President's Commission for the Study of Ethical Problems in Medicine and Biomedical and Behavioral Research. *Summing Up* (stock no. 040-000-00475-1). Washington, DC, US Government Printing Office, 1983.

Ramsey P: The enforcement of morals: Nontherapeutic research on children. *Hastings Center Rep* 6(4):21–30, 1976.

Rogers AS, D'Angelo L, and Futterman D for the Adolescent Scientific Committee of the Pediatric AIDS Clinical Trials Group: Guidelines for adolescent participation in research. *IRB: Rev Hum Subjects Res* 16(4):1–6, 1994.

Secretary's Work Group on Pediatric HIV Infection and Disease. *Final Report* (NIH Publication no. 89-3063). Washington, DC, Department of Health and Human Services, 1988.

Siegler M: Confidentiality in medicine—a decrepit concept. *N Engl J Med* 307:1518–1521, 1982.

Thomasma DC, Mauer AM: Ethical complications of clinical therapeutic research on children. *Soc Sci Med* 16:913–919, 1982.

Thompson RA: Behavioral research involving children: A developmental perspective on research risk. *IRB: Rev Hum Subjects Res*, 12(2):1–6, 1990.

Weithorn LA: Children's capacities to decide about participation in research. *IRB: Rev Hum Subjects Res* 5(5):1–5, 1983a.

Weithorn LA: Involving children in decisions involving their own welfare. In: Melton GB, Koocher GP, Saks MI (eds): *Children's Competence to Consent*. New York, Plenum, 1983b, pp. 235–260.

126 ETHICS IN THE PRACTICE OF CHILD AND ADOLESCENT PSYCHIATRY

Diane H. Schetky, M.D.

OVERVIEW

Ethical codes in medicine date back to the 5th century BC, yet they have received little attention in our medical literature until the last decade. Greater awareness and interest in ethics can be attributed to (*a*) heightened consumerism with increased emphasis on patient rights; (*b*) high technology medical developments that offer choices unheard of in the past and in turn introduce the need for health care rationing and decisions about prolonging life; and (*c*) changes in the delivery of health care that alter physician's autonomy, impose the role of gate keeper, and challenge our traditional ethical codes.

Ethical codes are not laws but standards of conduct expected from a professional. They exist to help professionals reconcile providing service while also earning a living from that service. In medicine, these codes define the norms, duties, and virtues expected in our professional work. As noted by Reiser et al. (1977), "Self-conscious reflection on standards of conduct is one of the defining characteristics of a profession." Ethical codes serve to protect the profession and benefit the patient and society as well. In maintaining the image and standard of conduct of the profession, they enable the patient to establish trust in the physician.

The Hippocratic Oath originated in the 5th century BC, but was not widely applied until the 10th century AD. It stressed the physician's power to heal and the need to divest this from killing. In doing so, as noted by Margaret Mead, the code clearly separated the physician from the sorcerer or shaman who had the power to both harm and cure. The Hippocratic Oath stressed the physician's obligation to the patient and the duty to keep confidences. It prohibited abortion, euthanasia, and sexual relationships with patients. Dyer (1988) notes that the Hippocratic tradition has come under scrutiny by critics who contend it is anachronistic. Critics argue that it does not deal with the technological advances in medicine nor with problems of cost containment. Many contend that it is too paternalistic and does not adequately address the rights of patients. Dyer (1988) recommends that we accept the oath "symbolically in terms of the intent and the concept of the profession it outlines."

Psychiatrists today follow the AMA's Principles of Medical Ethics with Annotations Especially Applicable to Psychiatry. These guidelines provide us with a way of thinking about ethical dilemmas, but do not necessarily solve them. Often competing ethical principles come in conflict, e.g., a woman's right to autonomy and to refuse a cesarean section versus her physician's concern for the welfare of her fetus. In order to understand these ethical guidelines, it is helpful to appreciate the ethical principles that underlie them. The four basic moral principles that guide use in medical research and health care are analyzed in great detail by Beauchamp and Childress (1989) and are briefly summarized here. *Autonomy* comes from the Greek words for self and rule and in medicine refers to the ability to make decisions for oneself without being controlled by others. Autonomy becomes the basis for informed consent and therapeutic privilege. *Nonmaleficence* is a concept derived from the Latin "primum non nocere," or first do no harm, and stems from the Hippocratic Oath, which states "I will use treatment to help the sick according to my ability and judgment, but I will never use it to injure or wrong them." The principle of *beneficence* refers to the obligation to help others further their legitimate interests and, more specifically, to promote the welfare of the patient. The principle of *justice* refers to offering fair treatment to all.

NATURE OF THE DOCTOR-PATIENT RELATIONSHIP

A fiduciary relationship is one in which one person receives the trust or confidence of another and is under a duty to act for the benefit of that person. Examples would include an attorney-client or broker-client relationship. Trust is the cornerstone of the fiduciary relationship that exists between physician and patient. The physician as fiduciary is expected to act for the benefit of the patient and not exploit that relationship for personal gain. Simon (1977) remainds us that the psychiatrist's main source of gratification should arise from the psychotherapeutic process and that his or her only material reward is payment for service.

Trust is essential to both evaluation and treatment. Without trust, patients would be loathe to divulge the intimate details about their lives that are often necessary to arrive at diagnoses and embark upon treatment. The fiduciary relationship is less clear cut in regard to children. Issues of trust and confidentiality are more complex in child and adolescent psychiatry because we must deal with parents as well as the child. Parents' rights to or need to know certain information about their child needs to be balanced with the child's interests. Further, the age and cognitive maturity of the child will have bearing on the child's ability to participate in decisions about treatment or medication, as well as disclosures to others.

Doctor-patient relationships are also defined by boundaries that keep us in our professional role and prevent us from exploiting patients. Boundaries provide a sense of security to both physician and patient. They help us maintain objectivity and allow us to focus on the patient's best interest. Boundaries discourage acting out by both patient and physician and foster respect for the patient's autonomy and dignity. The forces of both transference and countertransference threaten the therapist's neutrality and, if not recognized and resolved, may erode boundaries and undermine therapy. Straying from one's usual practices may be a warning sign of boundary violations. The psychiatrist who begins to see patients at unusual locales or times, who waives usual billing procedures, or finds himself or herself socializing with patients and their families may be on a slippery slope. He or she needs to reflect upon that behavior and consider the consequences, as seemingly benign boundary violations often lead to more serious ethical violations.

CONFIDENTIALITY

The terms *confidentiality* and *privilege* are often confused. Privilege, the narrower of the two terms, refers only to the disclosure of information obtained in treatment in judicial or quasi-judicial proceedings. Confidentiality, in contrast, refers to the disclosure of information learned in treatment to third parties. The physician's duty to maintain confidentiality is both a legal and an ethical one that derives from the right to privacy under common law and our ethical codes. Appelbaum and Gutheil (1991) note that the ethical foundations for confidentiality are 2-fold. First is the concern that without assurance of confidentiality patients would be reluctant to seek treatment. Second is the argument that, having implied that communications are confidential, mental health professionals must keep their implicit or explicit promise.

Privilege and confidentiality belong to the patient and may be waived by the patient only with certain exceptions. Generally, these include when the patient is in danger of harming himself or others, e.g., a sexually active HIV-positive male who refuses to take precautions or inform his sexual partners. Also, state laws mandate reporting a child abuse and may dictate reporting of other conditions as well, such as impaired physicians.

The psychiatrist may be faced with a moral dilemma when a subpoena demands patient records and their release is not in the best interest of that patient. The psychiatrist's conscience must guide him or her whether to defy the law or seek to quash the subpoena. For discussion of the legal ramifications of breach of confidentiality and consent issues see Chapter 115.

Consent

Minors, with some exceptions, are not competent to give consent to treatment, to medical research, or for release of medical information, but may be asked to give their assent in accord with their developmental age. Consent must be obtained from parents or guardians unless state law allows adolescents to consent to treatment or they are emancipated. For consent to be informed, parties must know the nature of the condition being treated, the risks and benefits of the proposed treatment, and what their choices are, and be free, i.e., without undue influence, to agree or disagree. It is advisable to get consent in writing for high risk treatments and release of records. If parents are separated or divorced, consent must be obtained from the custodial parent. If the child is in a shared custody arrangement, the psychiatrist should attempt to contact the other parent regarding treatment decisions, as joint decision-making on medical matters is usually part of shared custody arrangements.

The child psychiatrist, perhaps more so than the adult psychiatrist, faces many pressures to violate confidentiality owing to all the collateral contacts that arise during our work with children. These include parents, teachers, guidance counselors, other therapists involved with the family, day care providers, the child's physician, and sometimes personnel from protective services or other agencies. Even when there is consent for release of information, the psychiatrist must delicately balance how much; for instance, the school needs to know about a child's turbulent family life to help that child while respecting the family's wish for privacy. The child psychiatrist may need to decide when it is necessary to override a child's plea not to disclose certain information such as speaking to a teacher when parents have authorized such communication. The following case illustrates the many levels at which we must weigh decisions about confidentiality.

Sally Barnes, age 8, has been in treatment for an anxiety disorder that waxes and wanes. She lives with her recently widowed mother and younger sister. One day she is brought to her weekly appointment by her grandmother and tells her therapist, Dr. Coles, that her mother is home sick with the flu. Sally then reveals that her mother was drinking excessively the night before at a friend's house and drove Sally and her sister home while under the influence of alcohol. She heard her mother vomiting during the night, and in the morning her mother was so sick that she asked Sally to stay home to care for her little sister. Dr. Coles is faced with the issues of (a) using Sally's disclosures to confront Mrs. Barnes, (b) whether to share concerns with Sally's grandmother, (c) whether to contact Mrs. Barnes's therapist, and (d) whether to involve protective services. She chooses to say nothing to the grandmother as she does not have the mother's permission to speak with her. Sally is eager for her therapist to talk to her mother. Dr. Coles calls Mrs. Barnes who initially denies the allegations made by Sally, but then backs down and agrees to allow Dr. Coles to contact her therapist. Later, she admits that things are very out of control in her life, agrees to an inpatient admission, and approaches her mother to help care for the children. Dr. Coles does not feel the need to involve protective services at this juncture. The question of how much to tell the school and day care is discussed with Mrs. Barnes and left to her discretion. Sally might have

been afraid of Dr. Coles speaking to her mother about her drinking problem. In that case, she would have had to deal with Sally's fear around disclosing this secret and her rationale for overriding Sally's objections in taking the steps she did to ensure her welfare.

Limits of Confidentiality

Child psychiatrists need to define to both patient and parents the limits of confidentiality at the onset of evaluation and treatment. The extent to which communications from parent to therapist will be shared with the child should be discussed. If the psychiatrist needs to share the child's confidences with the parents, there are several options. The first would be to urge the child to do so or to meet jointly and discuss the issues. If this fails, the psychiatrist may then tell the child why he or she needs to share the information with the parents and what will be told.

In small, underserved communities the psychiatrist may, like it or not, have to medicate and sometimes treat more than one family member or friends of patients. This poses a challenge to the psychiatrist in terms of double bookkeeping, i.e., remembering what information was heard from whom and storing away what may have been heard but cannot be used because it was shared in confidence.

Double Agentry

Double agentry is a term that refers to serving two masters simultaneously. This is a potential problem that may arise from consultants when they are not clear about their roles. For instances, an adolescent may reveal to a consulting psychiatrist that he is dealing drugs in school. If the psychiatrist shares this with the school, the student is likely to be expelled. If she conceals this information, other students are at risk. The consultant needs to be clear that her duty is to the school, which hired her. Her dilemma could be minimized by informing the student at the onset of the evaluation as to the limits of confidentiality.

Double agentry may also arise when a therapist pursues the parents' agenda without regard to the child's best interests. For instance, Mr. and Mrs. Black seek help from Dr. White in regard to their 14-year-old son, Tom. They complain that he is defiant, questions his father, talks back, and refuses to attend services at their fundamentalist church. They hope Dr. White will render Tom more compliant and bring back their "good little boy." If Dr. White colludes with their agenda, he risks becoming their agent. Tom, on the other hand, doesn't see that he needs help other than using Dr. White's authority to get his parents off his back so he can gain more freedom. An overidentified therapist might be tempted to collude with Tom's agenda. Dr. White sympathizes with Tom's plight but sees his role as helping Tom separate and individuate from his family and develop responsible autonomy. Unless he spells out where he stands with the family, therapy is not likely to suceed.

Media

Child psychiatrists need to be on guard against violating confidences when giving press interviews. It is usually prudent to be circumspect and limit comments to what is already public knowledge and to comment on issues rather than specifics of a case. Parents may give consent for a therapist to talk with the media about their children in high profile custody and abuse cases. There is an unfortunate trend to try these cases in the media. Parents who are caught up in the heat of litigation are not always the best judges as to whether media attention will be harmful to their children.

The psychiatrist needs to guard against exploiting high profile cases for his or her own personal gain. Occasionally, psychiatrists may be tempted to go above the law and try to justify rash actions such as releasing confidential reports to the media as being in the child's best interests. Rarely can such actions be justified, and when closely examined they usually represent grandiosity, narcissism, and unchecked countertransference on the part of the psychiatrist.

Professional Presentations and Publications

Confidentiality must be preserved when we write about patients or present them or their artwork at conferences. One has the choice of sufficiently disguising material so as to preserve the patient's identity or seeking permission from the child and his parents to use the material. Therapists may be tempted to write books about their patients. It is difficult to reconcile this with keeping the patient's interests foremost, and such an agenda is likely to derail therapy. Literary exploitation of therapy in the mass media is unsettling to the public and does not promote trust in our profession. Even if this occurs with the patient's consent, questions may be raised about how informed the consent was, as in the case of author, Anne Sexton, whose psychiatrist released therapy tapes to her biographer following her death.

Dual Relationships

Dual relationships pose a challenge to maintaining confidentiality. Anyone practicing in close proximity to where they live or whose children attend the same school as their patients do is bound to encounter awkward situations. The child psychiatrist's children are unaware of who is or is not a patient of their parent. They may wish to invite patients to birthday parties, play at their homes, or share car pools. As the child psychiatrist's children grow older, attend larger schools, and engage in more extracurricular activities, it becomes increasingly difficult to screen patients for their potential ties to one's children. In small towns, one may end up evaluating or treating children of one's colleagues or one's children's teachers or future teachers. If there are no other resources, turning down requests for help in times of crises may be viewed as inhumane and does not help one's image. How well these dual relationships work often depends on the nature of the patient's disorder, the extent of family psychopathology, and the therapist's ability to maintain boundaries. Each new adult patient or parent of a child patient should be viewed as one less potential friend. The two-way give and take of friendships cannot exist in therapy, as the therapist may not use the relationship for his or her own personal needs. This should be explained to certain families at the onset of one's professional involvement with them.

The longer one is in practice, the more likely one is to run into patients all over town. The psychiatrist may need to patronize parents of patients, be they shop owners, pharmacists, plumbers, or restaurant owners. Adult patients and patients' parents may be appointed to boards one sits upon or join one's organizations. The child psychiatrist either learns to deal with these encounters or retreats to the high ground and becomes a recluse. There is much to be said for patients seeing their psychiatrists as a real person, whether at the dump on a Saturday morning or at the local high school basketball game. The trick is for the psychiatrist to become comfortable with his or her public persona, process these encounters, and maintain boundaries and confidentiality. In assessing how to address patients in public, one learns to take cues from patients. Children may be unabashed about seeing their therapist in the supermarket, whereas their parents may be less comfortable. Teenagers may shirk from public contact or surprise you by wanting to introduce their friends.

The Psychiatrist's Family

One learns to train family members not to ask "How do you know so and so?". Some psychiatrists develop nonverbal cues with spouses for handling awkward social situations. Should the psychiatrist's child learn the identity of a patient, he or she must appreciate that it is the patient's choice whether or not to disclose the psychiatrist-patient relationship. In some communities children may be quite comfortable telling a child that she is a patient of their parent. On the other hand, the author has had to curb her son's one-time enthusiasm for trying to refer classmates he thought were in need of help. Adult patients may deliberately attempt to become friends with their therapist's spouse, which becomes awkward if the professional relationship is not known to the

spouse. The therapist may have to intervene with the patient in such situations.

FORENSIC ISSUES

Forensic evaluations differ from regular diagnostic evaluations in that their intent is not therapeutic. Forensic evaluations are intended to help the court find the truth and address the legal question at hand. In order to do so, the forensic psychiatrist must strive for impartiality and avoid cases where prior ties, be they of a social or professional nature, might tinge objectivity or neutrality. Whenever possible, forensic examinations should be separated from treatment. Therapists inevitably become advocates for their patients and, in doing so, they may be less than objective. Another reason to avoid such a dual relationship is that confidentiality is compromised once the therapist has to testify in court. Attorneys may try to draw therapists into child custody battles. This complex issue is discussed extensively by Malmquist (1994).

The forensic psychiatrist needs to be clear with families from the start who has retained him and discuss the limits of confidentiality. It is not an unusual ploy for a parent to attempt to suppress an unfavorable report stating she went to the psychiatrist for therapy and that the therapist is therefore violating her confidences. When court appointed, the child psychiatrist may operate with quasi-judicial immunity, which protects the psychiatrist from liability (DePrato et al., 1993). Protection from liability is less certain in other situations.

The forensic psychiatrist should request payment up front in the form of a retainer. This assures payment and that one is being paid for one's time rather than for one's opinion. It is customary to charge more for forensic evaluations, as they require more expertise and can be very disruptive to one's practice. It is always unethical to accept a case on a contingency fee because this creates too much vested interest in the outcome of the case.

The child psychiatrist who practices forensic psychiatry needs to accept the limits of his or her experience, not inflate credentials, and avoid exceeding databases and making unsubstantiated statements. For further discussion of the pitfalls in these cases, see Schetky (1991) and Schetky and Benedek (1992).

DEALING WITH THIRD PARTY PAYERS

The down side of private practice is having to deal with third party payers and paper work. With the advent of managed care, voice mail, and the need for prior authorizations and written treatment plans, the task has become even more time consuming and distasteful. Ethical dilemmas arise when the patient's best interests and the psychiatrist's wish to get paid conflict with insurance companies' interest in minimizing cash outflow. This creates temptations on all sides to engage in unethical behaviors.

Insurance companies may deliberately lose or destroy claims, reject claims for spurious reasons, endlessly "research" disputed claims as a delaying tactic, or take deductibles out more than once a year. Noncustodial parents may pocket insurance payments. Patients or parents may request that diagnoses or codes be altered. This may be done because of concerns about confidentiality or so they can get better reimbursement.

The psychiatrist may be tempted to exaggerate the patient's condition in order to get needed services approved or higher reimbursement rates. There may be the temptation to alter dates of service, as when Medicaid will not pay for a parent visit on the same day the child is seen, regardless of how far they have traveled. A similar problem arises when only one psychiatric visit is allowed per day, even if the patient needs admission following an outpatient visit. Physicians may exaggerate duration of visits in order to compensate for low rates of reimbursement. Regardless of one's motives, these practices may be considered fraudulent and, as such, subject to criminal prosecution. The psychiatrist who engages in fraud may also be subject to ethical investigations and sanctions.

With the advent of health care rationing and a profit motive for managed care companies, serious concerns arise around who is responsible for the patient once a managed care company decides they will no longer pay for hospitalization or authorize further outpatient visits? Little regard is given to the impact on patients of forcing them to change therapists because their managed care company changes as a result of a job change or a takeover of a managed care organization. What are the ethics of managed care companies directing children of their subscribers to providers who lack adequate training in child therapy? Managed care further disrupts a practitioner's referral patterns if he or she is restricted to obtaining consults from a list of providers in a particular managed care company. Additional concerns arise over confidentiality as it becomes necessary to share more and more information about patients in order to justify ongoing treatment.

Managed care pressures physicians to become gatekeepers and consider not only the patient's needs but society's needs as well when it comes to allocation of health resources. Levinsky (1984) reminds us that this is an untenable position and that "physicians are required to do everything that they believe may benefit each patient without regard to costs or other societal considerations."

REPORTING ETHICAL VIOLATIONS

The AMA Principles of Medical Ethics, Section 2, states "A physician shall deal honestly with patients and colleagues and strive to expose those physicians deficient in character or competence, or who engage in fraud or deception." Reporting a colleague is a most unpleasant experience yet necessary to maintain the welfare of patients and the credibility of our profession. Ethical complaints may be filed with the district branch of the American Psychiatric Association (APA), with local medical societies, and/or with state licensing boards. Complaints are handled confidentially. Where appropriate, the psychiatrist should

urge patients to file a complaint. Following investigation, if an ethical violation is confirmed by the APA, there are four possible sanctions, ranging from admonishment or reprimand to suspension or expulsion from the APA. The defendant psychiatrist is entitled to appeal.

Reports of possible ethical violations may be based on our own observations, disclosures from patients, or extrinsic evidence. The psychiatrist may be reluctant to believe allegations by a patient, particularly if they involve sexual misconduct by a colleague known to the psychiatrist. The patient may feel protective of the abusing therapist or fearful of the investigation process and not wish to disclose. The treating psychiatrist may be reluctant to act contrary to his patient's wishes. Anonymous complaints by therapist or physician usually cannot be investigated. The APA Council on Ethical and Judicial Affairs (APA, 1991) believes that physicians must report sexual misconduct to the appropriate authorities. One should also be aware of state laws regarding the reporting of an impaired physician or one involved in abusive behavior.

Reports based on extrinsic evidence pertain to information a psychiatrist may have read in a newspaper or an event based on a legal fact, e.g., a psychiatrist adopts a patient. Filing a complaint allows the Ethics Committee to further look into the matter. Extrinsic evidence may also be used to bypass an ethics hearing if the facts speak for themselves.

SUMMARY

Child psychiatrists need to familiarize themselves with the ethical codes that govern their practices. They should not be pressured by patients or insurance companies, or influenced by their own needs, into acting in ways contrary to the patient's interests or our code of ethics. If in doubt as to whether a certain behavior is ethical, child psychiatrists may consult with the AACAP ethics committee or their APA district branch ethics committee.

References

American Academy of Child and Adolescent Psychiatry: *Annotations to AACAP Ethics Code with Special Reference to Evolving Health Care Delivery and Reimbursement Systems.* Washington, DC, American Academy of Child and Adolescent Psychiatry, 1995.

American Psychiatric Association: Reporting of unethical conduct. *Ethics Newslett.* VII(1), Washington, DC, American Psychiatric Association, 1991.

American Psychiatric Association: *The Principles of Medical Ethics.* Washington, DC, American Psychiatric Association, 1993.

Appelbaum P, Gutheil T: *Clinical Handbook of Psychiatry and the Law* (2nd ed). Baltimore, Williams & Wilkins, 1991.

Ayers W: Dilemmas and challenges: A clinician's perspective. Presidential address, American Academy of Child and Adolescent Psychiatry Oct 1993. *J Am Acad Child Adolesc Psychiatry* 33(2): 153–157, 1994.

Beauchamp T, Childress J: *Principles of Biomedical Ethics* (3rd ed). New York, Oxford Press, 1989.

DePrato D, Crane L, Zonana H: Immunity for psychiatrists: Protection from lawsuit. Presented at American Academy of Psychiatry and Law Annual Meeting, San Antonio, TX, October 1993.

Dyer AR: *Ethics and Psychiatry.* Washington, DC, American Psychiatric Press, 1988.

Jones WHS: *Hippocrates* (Vol I). Cambridge, Harvard University Press, 1923, p. 165.

Levinsky N: The doctor's master. N Engl J Med 311(24):1573–1575, 1984.

Malmquist C: Psychiatric confidentiality in child custody disputes. *J Am Acad Child Adolesc Psychiatry* 33(2):158–169, 1994.

Mead M: personal communication cited in Levine M: *Psychiatry and Ethics.* New York, George Brasilier, 1972, pp. 324–325.

Reiser S, Dyck A, Curran W: (eds): *Historical Perspectives and Contemporary Concerns.* Cambridge, MIT Press, 1977, p. 1.

Schetky DH: Ethical issues in forensic child psychiatry. *J Am Acad Child Adolesc Psychiatry* 31(3): 403–407, 1991.

Schetky DH, Benedek EP: *Clinical Handbook of Child Psychiatry and the Law* (2nd ed). Baltimore, Williams & Wilkins, 1992.

Simon R: *Clinical Psychiatry and the Law.* Washington, DC, APPI Press, 1987.

Simon R: *Clinical Psychiatry and the Law.* Washington, DC, APPI Press, 1987.

Appendix/Principles of Practice of Child Psychiatry

A child or adolescent and the family may expect the child psychiatrist to:

Have as primary concerns the welfare and the optimal development of the individual child or adolescent assessed in the context of the family, school, and community based upon scientific knowledge and collective and personal experience;

Foster the unique and nurturing relationship among the child or adolescent and the parents/caretakers, and the family;

Recognize the child's or adolescent's need for the support of adults;

Avoid all actions which may have a detrimental effect on the optimal development of the child;

Utilize his/her unique relationship with the child or adolescent and family to foster their well-being and optimal development;

Promote, by all appropriate means, the uniqueness of the individual;

Seek to develop with the child or adolescent as thorough an understanding as possible of the child psychiatrist's role, opinions, conclusions, and recommendations;

Protect specific confidences of the child or adolescent and the parents or guardians and others involved, unless this course would involve untenable risks or jeopardize care-taking responsibility;

Seek to develop with those involved in the care and/or treatment of the child or adolescent (parents or guardians, and where appropriate, the family, teacher and school, court or correctional agency, physician, and others) as thorough an understanding as possible of the child psychiatrist's role, opinions, conclusions, and recommendations;

Help the child or adolescent to recognize the influence of his/her own relationship to family members and the consequences of his/her decisions;

Help family members resolve differences in their views of professional judgments or recommendations;

Avoid acting solely as an agent of the parents, guardians, or agencies;

Maintain the integrity of professional judgments and behaviors independent of influence of the source of compensation.

Adapted from American Academy of Child Psychiatry Code of Ethics, May 16, 1982.

127 THE DISCOVERY OF THE CHILD: A HISTORICAL PERSPECTIVE ON CHILD AND ADOLESCENT PSYCHIATRY[a]

Dorothy M. Bernstein, M.D., M.A., M.S.

In the field of medicine, the specialty of child psychiatry is usually regarded as a 20th century innovation. Many psychiatrists place its beginning in the United States with William Healey's establishment of the Juvenile Psychopathic Institute at Chicago as a child guidance clinic serving the Juvenile Court of Cook County in 1909 (Schowalter, 1991). Others, such as Lawson Lowry in an address before the Centenary Meeting of the American Psychiatric Association in 1944, challenged that concept. In Lowry's opinion, child psychiatry lacked a sufficient scientific basis to be considered a medical subspecialty at that time (Lowry, 1944–1955).

It was not until the middle of the century that child psychiatry began to meet the requirements that George Tarjan later set forth as the necessary qualifications for professionalization of a medical specialty. In his Presidential Address in 1984 before the American Psychiatric Association, Tarjan proposed the idea that to gain recognition a medical specialty must have an adequate scientific foundation described with manifest conceptual clarity. Furthermore, such concepts should serve to form a framework that would fit in a medical curriculum. He added the imperative that the specialty should include a group of clinicians offering a unique set of knowledge and skills (Lewis, 1991).

Child psychiatry began to receive full recognition as a medical subspecialty when the mechanism was fully established by the American Board of Psychiatry and Neurology to examine its candidates for qualification in the field in 1957 (The History of the American Academy of Child Psychiatry, 1962). However, William Parry-Jones has pointed out that, unlike many other branches of medicine, advances in psychiatry have been slow and discontinuous (Parry-Jones, 1989). A historical examination of earlier issues and efforts might therefore clarify elements that contributed to this proposition as well as enhance our understanding of the origin of child psychiatry. Many of the preceding factors in the development of this field began to emerge in the 19th century. Among these factors were the changing views of child rearing and child development in the prevailing culture.

CHILDREN'S STATUS IN THE 18TH CENTURY

In earlier centuries, children were regarded as a homogeneous group subject to the rule and whim, and frequently abuse, of their parents. Adults were not interested in the developmental process of childhood, which was treated as a brief stage. In many cultures boys were attired in skirts until age 5, at which time parents dressed them in adultlike male clothing and gave them mature tasks to perform. Girls likewise were expected to perform adult domestic tasks.

Parents allotted little attention to child development, either normal or pathological. Often mothers were only peripherally involved in rearing their young children. In England, for example, in the mid- and late 18th century, middle class mothers invested little time and attention in their infants. Instead, to afford themselves social time, they yielded care and direction of their children to servants. Because of the formal structural relationship that existed between her and the servants, usually the mother asked only questions of formality and was not aware of the actual problems concerning the progress of her children. An authoritative nanny could be ruling the children by coercion and even abuse without the mother being aware.

Lower class English women had the opposite situation of almost no leisure time. Beset by many problems, these mothers tolerated child care as one among many burdens. They too were absent mothers. Economic necessity often forced them to delegate care of the children to older women in the family as the mothers left the household to assume a role in the small trade's and artisan's shops of their husbands.

In France as well as in England, it was considered bad taste for middle class women to nurse their own infants. Instead, women were expected to be available to engage in the many social activities during the day. It was a near universal custom for mothers in the city to send their infants to the country where professional wet nurses assumed their nurture. In the 1780s, more than 80% of the 21,000 babies born that year were so managed (Robertson, 1974). If a wet nurse found herself overstressed by numbers of charges with feeding or other problems, she was free to seek her own punitive means to handle the situation. Occupied by her other charges, often the wet nurse turned to other means, such as a goat's or cow's udder treated by boiling in lime water, for nourishment of her own offspring, thus removing her from that child's care.

Likewise in Italy, middle class women sent their infants away from the household to be managed by wet nurses. Mothers in Italy differed from mothers in France only in that they permitted their children to remain away for a far longer period of time. In Germany as well, middle and upper classes used wet nurses freely. It was rare to find a mother who nursed her own children (Baring-Gould, 1879). The German household differed from the English in that child care was delegated to servants in general and not to a single figure such as the nanny.

Among the affluent groups in the United States, development of young children was not under the direct purview of their mother. As cities began to grow on the eastern seaboard, farm girls from the villages and small towns went to the city seeking employment. Few positions were open to them other than that of domestics in the more flourishing

---

[a] Editor's Note: For history of health delivery systems, see Chapter 120. For history of training and certification, see Chapter 123.

households. There the more apt ones graduated from the position of scullery maid to upstairs nursemaid in charge of the children. As a group they represented the immaturity of youth in charge of the growth and development of the children.

Both in the United States and in England, the use of wet nurses was not as fashionable as it was on the continent. That did not mean that pregnancy and care of young children held a close and esteemed place in the lives of mothers. In England, childbirth was usually concealed. The event usually took place in a remote part of the household. The next morning the new member was introduced to the amazement of the other children of the household as if the infant arrived from nowhere. When bottles were developed by a midwife, Mme. Breton in Paris, they were quickly put to use. Manuals for mothers such as that written by a Mrs. Patten pointed out that nursing a child was not only painful but could lead to despair in middle age, might drive women to drink, and could even result in death. She advised mothers that it was much wiser and easier to train a child in good habits from the beginning by bottle-feeding (Robertson, 1974). The reality was that childbirth was a marked hazard because of the prevalence of postpartum sepsis, the etiology of which was unrecognized. Hence, pregnancy, childbirth, and its outcome were subject to superstition and speculative fears.

Another common practice that distanced mother from child, or nurse-maid from child, was that of swaddling. Everything about this procedure ensured minimal contact with the child. Bands of cloth were wound tightly around the child's body, confining its arms. It was difficult to hold a child bound like a mummy. In turn, the child so encased could not easily respond to the adult, if it were held. Thus, it was convenient, for instance, to hang the swaddled baby from a hook on a wall behind the stove for hours. Whenever the nurse decided the child needed changing, it was an uncomfortable process for the child and a difficult one for the nurse. This led to easy justification for infrequent handling and changing of the child. It was the general wisdom of the day that water, air, sunlight, and soap were harmful to the child. These superstitions were conveniently perpetuated by those nurses attuned to labor-saving practices. In England there arose a modified method of swaddling in which there were fastenings in the crotch, called culottes, making toilet training easier. This came to be known as the "English manner."

An autobiography of the period brings us a report: In England, where cold water was considered bracing, the usual morning routine was to bring the children from the nursery in the upstairs rooms down to the kitchen courtyard where a tub of water with a crust of ice awaited them, remove their thin cotton shirts, and plunge them into the ice water. Their protests and screams did not delay the process. After the immersion, they were dressed in light cotton clothing with no undershirt and served a stone cold breakfast. The father stood over them, and if they complained he did not hesitate to cut them with his whip (Smith, 1911).

In Italy it was reported that babies were wrapped so tightly in the process of swaddling that the pressure forced blood to their heads, causing their faces to turn purple. When more enlightened parents questioned the practice, the clergy opposed them. German babies were wrapped tighter and longer than others. The infant was pinioned and wrapped in yards of bandages that were unfolded once or at the most twice a day. The nursemaid rarely bathed the child. A later successor to the swaddling bands was a long bag lined with wadding in which the child was placed, confining its legs and body but not its arms. The nurse was told it was dangerous to pick up a child outside the bag since the child's bones were soft and unformed. Thus, the child lay isolated in the bag night and day for at least 6–8 weeks.

Changes began to take place when figures such as Rousseau and Pestalozzi, bearing the ideals of the Period of Enlightenment, began to speak out for a humane approach to the underprivileged of society (see Chapter 108). Jean Jacques Rousseau, the Swiss-French moralist, philosopher, and educator and one of the most eloquent and influential of the great rational thinkers of the 18th century, set forth principles in his two publications in 1762 including the young as the first stage of man. In the well-known first lines of his *Du Contrat Social* he states, "Man

is born free, and he is everywhere in chains." In *Emile*, he set forth the concept of the natural child possessed of self-direction and receptive to sensory training (Scheerenberger, 1983). He enunciated his beliefs in the following way:

> We are born capable of learning, but knowing nothing . . . since experiences are the raw material of thought, they should therefore, be presented to him [*Emile*] in a fitting order so that memory may at a future time present them in the same order to his understanding . . . between these sensations and the things which cause them (Rousseau, 1911).

Rousseau went on to state that the child needed to perceive directly heat, cold, hardness, softness, and heaviness or lightness of bodies by touching, looking, feeling, listening, and, above all, by comparing as he or she experienced these sensations. Rousseau cautioned parents not to check the child's movements when the child wished to explore. He was directing attention to his belief in the child's potential and its growth achieved by means of education.

A different goal for the child's education was held in colonial America, a view that was still adhered to at the end of the 18th century. For example, Hannah More (1820) set forth her belief that children were born bad, and before they could become acceptable adults it was necessary to break their will. She expressed her ideas thus:

> Is it not a fundamental error to consider children as innocent beings, whose little weaknesses may perhaps, want some correction, rather than as beings who bring into the world corrupt nature and evil dispositions which it should be the great end of education to rectify.

Nevertheless, Rousseau's work *Emile*, appearing when the principles of the Period of Enlightenment were becoming prevalent, had a great impact on education of the child. For the first time, children were being regarded as individuals with potential for growth and development. In that atmosphere, attention to the *tasks* of growth and development of childhood became possible.

19TH CENTURY ADVANCES

Nineteenth century educators such as Swiss-born Johann Pestalozzi contributed significantly to the change in how adults viewed childhood (see Chapter 108). Pestalozzi believed that there was order in the child's development, with an unfolding of potential according to definite stepwise laws (Scheerenberger, 1983). He thought this came about by repetitive exposure of the child to proper experiences. Development came from within the child and was not simply the product of inert exposure to external environmental influences. Teaching methods of engaging the child and encouraging expression of the child's basic possibilities as well as providing the proper schooling were now seen as necessary. Pestalozzi believed that the education of the individual child was not simply for vocational purposes but should serve a wide array of subjects basic to the child's development. He included topics such as geography, customs of the countries considered, nature study, math, drawing, reading, language usage, grammar, singing, and religion. The last was an essential element in the daily life of the populace at the time.

Pestalozzi in his writings made no gender distinction in setting forth his tenets for education of the young. This was an advanced idea, for this was a time when girls were not formally educated as boys were. Girls' instruction was from their mothers and focused on those areas preparing them for domestic and social pursuits. In middle class families boys received early education from their mothers at home and then proceeded to church schools or colleges, often at a young age. It was an accepted role for mothers to instill principles of virtue in their sons but they were not supposed to voice any political opinion.

According to Pestalozzi's plan, which encompassed education for both boys and girls, schools would be set in a family-like atmosphere. He believed that they should operate on the principle of mutual good will with cooperation between pupils and teacher. This was a distant cry from the educational regime of authority and strict discipline, enforced by punitive measures, that preceded Rousseau and Pestalozzi and which was the prevailing mode in colonial America.

The concepts of Rousseau and Pestalozzi began to exert considerable influence on childhood education early in the 19th century. Rousseau spoke out against the practices of wet nursing and swaddling. Mothers began to become more involved with their children and to attend to their children's early developmental stages more closely. This move was preceded by social and political events in Europe, such as the French Revolution and the Napoleonic Wars, which had served to reinforce domesticity. In England and the United States, the Industrial Revolution drew men into the work place, leaving their wives at home. A flood of religious and social sentiment was directed at women, reinforcing the concept that home life was their duty. Their role was postulated as creditable as men's but more sacred. Among the middle class there arose a new sense of commitment to the family with the creation of a new phase of development, namely, childhood. Children were no longer separated from their parents at birth, often not returning until adolescence. Mothers now began to note and encourage early signs of development in their young.

The novelist Elizabeth Cleghorn Gaskell is an example of a parent beginning to observe, participate in, and monitor the early development of her children (Robertson, 1974). She kept a journal recording the first years of her daughter, Marianne, born in September 1834. She noted such things as her first smile, the period when Marianne was suspicious of strangers, her beginning language, and her interaction with other children. However, Gaskell did not undertake a structured program of formalized teaching of the child. The parents did not plan to start lessons until Marianne reached age 4.

The parents were following the concepts of the early psychiatrists of the time, who held that until age 3 the child's brain was constantly on the verge of inflammation. Girls particularly were thought to be at greater risk of this deleterious effect than were boys, and this weakness might appear later in childhood as well. This belief hindered the future education of girls. The Victorian notion of ideal womanhood was that females were sensitive creatures and the keepers of virtue. Accompanying this concept was the idea that they were easily unbalanced physiologically and emotionally and this could occur with formal education.

Mothers following their children's development more closely began to turn to popular pamphlets for guidance. The early psychiatrists also began to make observations about child development and education and to include them in their writings. An example is Isaac Ray, the physician-superintendent at the Butler Hospital in Providence, Rhode Island. He was well-known for his significant contributions to forensic psychiatry as well as for numerous other additions to the fledgling field of psychiatry. In 1820 he produced a book directed to the instruction of youth. In the dedication he characterized his work as "a humble attempt to aid the cause of education, and aid the diffusion of useful knowledge" (Ray, 1829).

The form of the book was to present a dialogue between a fictitious early scientist, Dr. B., with a child, Emily, on the subject of the biologic or natural sciences. This was an area that increasingly captured the interest of adults of the time. In nine conversations with Emily, Dr. B. dealt in turn with the following subjects: (a) anatomy, both human and comparative; (b) digestion, or the passage of food through the alimentary canal; (c) chymification, or the digestion of food, with a comparison of that in humans to birds (he included the influence of the mind on digestion); (d) circulation of the blood, including influence of disease on the pulse; (e) respiration, including that of fish, reptiles, mollusks, and insects, as well as humans; (f) the nervous system, comparing the brain of humans to that of other animals, as well as touching on concepts of instinct and reason; (g) the senses, comparing their structure in humans to that in animals; (h) the muscles in all their actions, comparing those in humans to those in birds; and (I) sleep, commenting on the state of the brain during sleep, as well as dreaming and finally death.

In his introduction to the conversations between Emily and Dr. B. in this book, Dr. Ray was aware that it was not the custom to introduce children to the subjects he was presenting and that they might approach them with notions of "horrid ideas of dead bodies and mangled limbs." Thus, he sought to allay their anxieties by pointing out that Dr. B. would leave the explicit scenes of the anatomical dissecting room to the professional men and present the most interesting results of their researches without troubling Emily with the means and instruments of how they were obtained.

In another treatise, entitled *Mental Hygiene* published in 1863, Dr. Ray included children in his concepts about mental health. He is credited with being the first to use the term mental hygiene in print. He defined mental hygiene as "the art of preserving the mind against all the incidents and influences calculated to deteriorate its qualities, impair its energies or derange its movements" (Overholser, 1944). He saw the need for mental hygiene because of the diminished influence of the home as a source of education, a trend that was fast becoming evident at that time. Youths in great numbers were leaving the family farm in villages and towns to seek employment in the growing industrializing cities where they experienced a new freedom in life style.

Without parental guidance, Dr. Ray believed the young were susceptible to the strain and influences of the city and might evidence this in the deterioration of the health of their mind. He included children in his discourse. He believed that teachers had not sufficiently attended to the thin, weakly children in their classes. He thought there was a risk of overworking the mind of such children. On the other hand, firm and robust children of a sanguineous nature could meet the demands placed on their vital powers in more adequate fashion (Ray, 1863). Besides commenting on the mental health of children and its hazards, whether he was correct or not, Dr. Ray was elucidating a difference in temperament in children, a subject that was to be extensively studied in this century (see Chapter 13).

Other early psychiatrists of the 19th century such as Dr. Amariah Brigham, physician-superintendent of the State Lunatic Asylum at Utica, New York and editor of the *American Journal of Insanity*, the predecessor to the present-day *American Journal of Psychiatry*, began to make observations in his writings about education and its effect on the mental state of children. He published his book *Remarks on the Influence of Mental Cultivation and Mental Excitement Upon Health* as a guide to mental hygiene, stressing social influences (Brigham, 1845).

The object of Brigham's book was to awaken public attention to the importance of modifying the method of educating children. It was a popular attempt by one of the early psychiatrists to instruct the public in what he regarded as an erroneous view. The book was well received both in Britain and America. It first appeared in Edinburgh in 1836, in Glasgow in 1839, in America in 1845, and in London in 1865. One of the prevalent theories of mental illness at the time that Brigham fully embraced was that excess excitement and commotion of the brain could lead to mental derangement. For evidence Brigham pointed to the register of the Bicêtre, which showed that insanity was found chiefly among priests, painters, sculptors, poets, and musicians. There was no instance of the disease in naturalists, physicians, geometricians, and chemists. The latter group he thought exercised their minds only by calm inquiry (Hunter and Macalpine, 1963).

Brigham included children in his treatise, observing that children did not become insane often. However, if this did occur, he thought a prominent inciting cause was overly exercised mental excitement and injudicious development of the moral faculty. This was a time when many psychiatrists, following the tenets of phrenology, thought that the brain was made up of a number of mental faculties.

For children Brigham emphasized physical education and not overloading or overworking the brain. He specifically pointed to the city of Hartford where 1200 children between the ages of 4 and 16 attended religious school on the Sabbath both in the morning and afternoon. They went to church and school 6 hours on Sunday, and most of them attended school every other day of the week. He thought this confinement of the body and application of the mind was excessive and called for relief of their attending school on Sunday. Whether his theories proved correct in part or not, he was directing attention to the mental state of children and focusing on heretofore ignored problems in their developmental pattern.

Mental Disorders in Children and Juveniles

Early in the 19th century, parents overlooked or disregarded evidence of mental aberrations in their children. Mental disorders were regarded as instances of perverseness or wickedness on the part of the children and, consequently, they were severely chastised. If they were unable to function like other children, they were punished for idleness and, as described by a few perceptive early psychiatrists of the day, "grew up with many faults aggravated by severity" (Conolly, 1861). At age 14 or 15 if they remained difficult to manage, youths, including those of affluent families, were sent into the world with only minor protection and left to follow what was known as a "wayward course," committing mischievous acts and plaguing other families and neighborhoods. The parents in the poorer population, having fewer resources, would abandon their problem youths when hard pressed. The problem youths in turn became drifters and vagrants, often ending up in the jail of the town or village.

As the century progressed, humanitarian reforms were introduced for those considered to be on the periphery of society, e.g., adults who were beggars, paupers, or insane. Modes of thinking began to focus more closely on the individual person and his or her mind. The literature of the day espoused the idea that the mind was an attribute of value in every human being, and children came to be included in this viewpoint. John Conolly, the prominent English psychiatrist of the mid-19th century writing in the *American Journal of Insanity* in April 1862, noted that parents were slowly beginning to acknowledge this in their children.

Although they may have noted eccentricities or peculiarities in their children's early mental development, parents initially chose to ignore their presence. If by age 4 or 5 the symptoms persisted and increased, the parents developed sufficient anxiety to seek medical advice for their children. At first this centered around the most obviously mentally disabled children. As physicians and educators began to produce observable results with these children, parents noted the progress and began to seek medical advice about their other children with mental conditions that had bewildered them or that they had chosen to deny. Parents who were beginning to acknowledge and seek such aid were from the educated population.

By mid-19th century in England the literature of general psychiatry referred to psychiatric conditions in children regularly, although the number of cases presented was small. Writing in the *London Medical Times and Gazette* in 1862, Conolly described typical situations that the early English psychiatrists were likely to encounter. He pointed out that before that time medical practitioners rarely noted or mentioned instances of mental disturbance in young children. Both Dr. Pritchard's *Cyclopedia of Practical Medicine* and Dr. Copland's comprehensive essay on insanity in his *Dictionary* made little or no mention of insanity in children. By mid century, medical works began to refer to cases of insanity in children including suicide, although this occurred rarely. More frequently there were examples of mania in juveniles. Often psychiatrists associated these cases with hysteria. Statistical tables produced by early psychiatrists seldom included cases of juvenile insanity. Such data were compiled using the asylum population, and youths below the age of 15 usually were not admitted.

Conolly reflected the prevailing optimism among psychiatrists of the day about treatment and cure of patients with mental disorders, an optimism that predominated in the United States as well as England. His advice to parents was the following:

> If there have been convulsions in infancy, there are generally unmistakable appearances of an imbecility scarcely promising relief; but it is always to be remembered that the development of the brain may . . . be only retarded, so that, unless there is clear evidence of organic fault or change, hope of amendment should not be abandoned. No juvenile peculiarity, or waywardness or

violence, should induce despair. Both history and the experience . . . will furnish examples of very unmanageable boys becoming valuable and even distinguished men. (Conolly, 1861)

In addition to presentations in the literature about mental disorders in children and youth, a few individuals began to lecture on the subject. One notable example was Charles West, the founder and physician of the famous Hospital for Sick Children on Great Ormond Street in London. He included disorders of the mind in childhood in a series of lectures delivered in 1847 (West, 1854).

In the United States there were accounts of cases of mental disorders occurring in children and youth in the general psychiatric literature of the mid-19th century. These represented cases encountered by psychiatrists in the course of their practice and considered interesting and instructive enough to report at the annual meeting of the Association of Superintendents, the organization that was the predecessor to the present day American Psychiatric Association. Narrative presentations of such cases appeared intermittently in the *American Journal of Insanity*. There was no specific nomenclature for mental disorders of children. Treatment when available was described in terms of knowledge of the time as it applied to adults. Most cases were presented in a brief descriptive manner. A few were given with detailed observation and dynamics as understood at that time.

Statistics about the incidence of mental disorders in children and youth were not approached in an organized way and appeared only intermittently in the literature gathered from various sources. An example is the work of M. Brierre du Boismont, who in an 1860 publication turned to English, French, and American authors for information on the subject. He found that Aubanel and Thorpe had observed in the Bicêtre in 1839, 8 cases of mania in children and 1 of melancholia in the age group of 11–18 years. M. Boutteville found that 0.9% occurred in children from ages 5 to 9, 3.5% appeared from ages 11 to 18, and 20% from ages 15 to 19 years. He found that the maximum number of cases occurred not in childhood but between 30 and 34 years. He concluded that insanity in the young could not be ignored, as was the usual pattern.

The Mental Retardation Movement

There was one group of developmentally and emotionally disabled children and youth in the 19th century that psychiatrists and other allied groups, particularly educators, approached in a more systematic and remedial fashion than others. A movement began to center around the young with mental retardation. Interest in this group began in France and Switzerland in the first half of the century and spread to the rest of Europe and finally the United States. Interest grew because it involved a group of patients whose disabilities appeared early in childhood, were obvious to parents, and aroused the parents' anxiety, particularly that of parents who had become invested in following their children's development.

The mental retardation movement developed and was advanced in France early in the 19th century by two dedicated young men, Jean Itard and Edouard Seguin (see Chapters 45 and 108). Itard and Seguin persisted in their attempts to treat the young with mental retardation and other disabilities in spite of discouragement by their better known and well-respected mentors, Phillipe Pinel and Jean Etienne Esquirol. Pinel predicted that Itard's work with Victor, the feral child who was the object of Itard's major endeavors, would not succeed. Esquirol, although considered a friend of Seguin and supportive of Seguin's other works, was highly skeptical of the outcome of Sequin's efforts in this particular direction.

Both Itard and Seguin based their work on earlier efforts of Jacob Rodrigues Periere, a mid- and late 18th century educator with a background of studies in anatomy and physiology who had been actively interested in attempting to educate children who were congenitally deaf. Although Periere did not deal directly with children who were mentally retarded, his commitment to children with disabilities and the methods of his work were shaping factors for Itard's endeavors. In a 1904 monograph Barr pointed out that Itard's work would have been impossible without Periere's groundwork (Kanner, 1963).

Contributions of Itard

Jean Marc Gaspard Itard (1774–1838) was an assistant surgeon in a French military hospital who became so engrossed in his duties that he pursued the study of medicine upon discharge. After completing his studies, he joined the medical staff of the Institution for Deaf-mutes in Paris. There he directed his endeavors not only toward training the young children who were deaf, but he engaged in scientific study of the ear and organs of speech as well. In 1821 he published a treatise on diseases of the ear, which is regarded as a foundation of modern otology.

Soon after Itard began his duties at the Institution for Deaf-mutes, the Abbe Sicard Bonnaterre, Professor of Natural History at the Central School of the Department of Aveyron brought a young boy approximately 11 or 12 years of age to the institution for evaluation. The boy walked on all fours and took little notice of what was occurring around him. However, he bit and scratched anyone who came near him and interfered with his actions. He displayed no elements of language and instead uttered inarticulate sounds. He did so without any attempt to communicate with others around him. He was entirely unsocialized in his actions with no idea of appropriateness or modesty, relieving himself wherever he was. When offered food he refused all except chestnuts, acorns, and potatoes, which he preferred raw. He drank water while lying on his abdomen. He made no acknowledged response when spoken to. However, Itard noticed that he turned his head when anyone in the room exclaimed, "Oh!" After that Itard referred to him as Victor of Aveyron.

Scientists of the day became highly interested in Victor and classified him as *Juvenis averionensis*, a variety of the genus *Homo*. They spoke of him as a *Homo ferrus*, a wild child walking on all four limbs, mute and hirsute. There were different versions about his origin. P.J. Virey reported that he was found running naked in the woods of Cannes in the Department of Turn searching for food in the form of roots and acorns. A group of hunters caught him but he escaped. He was recaptured and taken to the Hospice St. Afrique. The naturalist Bonnaterre took charge of him and sought Itard's opinion about this youth.

After his assessment, Itard concluded the youth was mentally arrested because of social and educational neglect. He considered that this occurred following isolation and referred to Victor's state as one of mental atrophy resulting from disuse. Prominent scientists, physicians, educators, and philosophers were also interested in Victor's case and offered their opinion. Pinel examined him and concluded that Victor was irreversibly retarded and untreatable. However, Itard would not accept the finality of this prognosis.

Itard set forth five main goals he wished to attain in an attempt to transform Victor from a wild to a civilized state. The first of these was directed to Victor and his environment and relationships with those around him. The others were directed to Victor's personal development. Itard's objectives were:

1. To make social life Victor would encounter at the Institution initially as similar as possible to the wild life he had experienced;
2. To excite Victor's nervous sensibility with varied and energetic stimuli and supply his mind with the raw or basic impression of ideas;
3. To extend his range of ideas by creating new wants and expanding his relations with the world around him;
4. To lead Victor to the use of speech by initiating patterns that made it necessary for him to imitate;
5. To encourage Victor to respond with satisfaction to his growing physical wants and from this to lead him to a stage where he would apply his intelligence to the objects of instruction (Kanner, 1963).

Although his program for Victor was well-formulated, Itard felt that Victor was not responding as anticipated. After 5 years of laboring with the youth, Itard gave up his mission after Victor displayed an uncontrolled "wild storm of passion," which Itard attributed to puberty. After that, Victor lived with an elderly woman in custodial care until he died in 1828.

The French Academy of Science reviewed the case and was more laudatory about Itard's results. The members pointed out that Victor's progress should be compared only with himself and that he had advanced considerably from his basic starting point. He had learned to recognize objects, identify letters of the alphabet, comprehend the meaning of many words, apply names to objects and parts of objects, and make relatively fine sensory discriminations and he now preferred the social life of civilization to his former isolated existence in the wild. The members of the Academy commended Itard, stating that he had made a positive contribution to educational science (and, it could be added, to the developmental science of childhood, although this was not emphasized at the time). The Academy pointed out that Itard had made a series of fine judicious observations, used a combination of highly interactive processes, and furnished science with new data that would be extremely useful to all persons engaged in teaching the young. Itard had shown that even a child with severe mental deficits could be treated and improved by appropriate methods. In addition, he had engaged in an early form of psychotherapy with Victor.

The Work of Seguin

Another figure representing the French school who added to methods of investigation about children, their evaluation, learning possibilities, and the treatment of mental retardation in the early 19th century was Edouard Onesimus Seguin (1812–1880) (Kanner, 1964). Seguin had studied medicine and surgery under the tutelage of Itard, who encouraged him to focus on investigating and treating mental retardation. Seguin was aware of this strong influence but also acknowledged another, the principles of the Christian School, or Saint Simonism, which he embraced. The aim of this group was to apply the principles of the gospel for the most rapid evaluation of the poorest of the retarded populace by all means and institutions, particularly religious educational ones.

In 1837 at age 25, Seguin undertook the task of educating a boy with mental retardation who did not speak. Seguin worked with this child assiduously and consistently for 18 months, after which his pupil manifested an improvement in his cognitive state. He could speak, write, and count. In addition, he could remember the names of objects and could compare them. Before Seguin's attempt, Esquirol had discouraged him by declaring that "no means are known by which a larger amount of reason or intelligence can be bestowed upon the unhappy idiot, even for the briefest period." Nevertheless, Seguin, undaunted, proceeded with his efforts. Faced with evidence of Seguin's success, Esquirol in 1839 issued a statement giving credit to Seguin although Esquirol defended his earlier position by referring to the patient as an infant resembling an idiot.

Following his success with his first patient, Seguin began to treat other children with similar disabilities at the Hospice des Incurables and at the Bicêtre, one of the hospitals where Pinel had done his early work in "liberating" the mentally ill patients. (Pinel had liberated the mentally ill from being chained in the Bicêtre, which was a hospital for vagrants, thieves, various criminals, and the mentally ill. The last remained in the hospital but not whipped and chained.) By 1842 his reputation was growing and alienists, as psychiatrists were then called, came to Paris from near and far to view his work. At a session of the administrative council of hospitals in Paris in that year, a commission was appointed to report on the results of Seguin's work. Their conclusion was that he had contributed greatly toward the education of children with mental retardation, giving students of hygiene, medicine, and ethics a worthy example to follow.

In 1846, Seguin published his textbook, which is known as a classic discourse on the subject of mental retardation. In it he presented his method of combined physiological and moral instruction of this population group. Two years later when revolution erupted in France, he emigrated to the United States to begin a career there. He went successively from Cleveland, where he served as a general practitioner, to Portsmouth, Ohio, to Pennsylvania, where he was head of the Pennsylvania Training School for Idiots, and finally to New York. From his earliest days in the United States he played a major role as consultant to all interested in establishing new residential treatment facilities for mentally retarded children.

In 1873 he went to Europe as United States Commissioner on Education at the Vienna Universal Exposition and published a comprehensive report on his impressions of the contemporary ideas about child rearing, school education, and the care of handicapped children. In 1878 he was elected the first president of the Association of Medical Officers of American Institutions for Idiotic and Feeble Minded Persons, attesting to his prominence and recognition of his contributions in the field.

Spread of Treatment to the United States

Following its beginnings in Europe, interest in ameliorating the condition of people with mental retardation appeared in the United States in the mid-19th century. Previously, there was no public or private facility for the care of mentally retarded children on the North American continent. There was an early but limited attempt to offer them services in 1818 when the Asylum for the Deaf and Dumb was founded in Hartford, Connecticut. This was the first residential service intended for people with mental retardation (Scheerenberger, 1983). The asylum attempted to instruct children with mental retardation, achieving modest results. The physical condition of the children improved and a few who were unable to speak began to communicate in sign language. This program was the exception until the decade of the 1840s.

In July, 1848, Hervey Backus Wilbur (1820–1883) took the 7-year-old mentally retarded son of a distinguished lawyer into his home at Barre, Massachusetts for care and training. He followed this by accepting a group of similar children. In that same year Dr. Samuel Gridley Howe (1801–1876), the chairman of a committee appointed by the Massachusetts House of Representatives to inquire into the condition of the people with mental retardation in the commonwealth, submitted his report to that body. The committee's charge was to ascertain the number of people in the commonwealth who were mentally retarded and investigate whether there were any resources available to relieve their condition. The committee members visited 63 towns and personally examined the status of 574 persons. They concluded that this group had no resources and that they were "condemned to hopeless idiocy and left to their own brutishness" (Kanner, 1964).

Dr. Howe's report pointed out that the benefits that could be derived from establishing a school based on humane and scientific principles for these persons would be numerous. Not only would those who participated in the program benefit both mentally and physically but all others in the state and country would indirectly gain. Valuable information would be available to disseminate throughout the country demonstrating that no person with mental retardation need be confined or restrained by force. It would also become apparent that the children with mental retardation could be trained to be productive and orderly and would gain self-respect (self-esteem).

The report highly impressed the majority of the legislators. With only minimal dissent from their body, they allocated $2500 per annum for 3 years for teaching and training 10 children with mental retardation. On October 1, 1848, a wing opened at the Perkins Institution to serve as an experimental school. Toward the end of the 3-year period, the Joint Committee of Pyblic Charitable Institutions visited the facility and reported that the experiment was highly successful. The Committee suggested that the school be allocated a permanent status. The legislators heeded the recommendation and the school was established in South Boston in 1855 under the name of the Massachusetts School for Idiotic and Feeble-Minded Youth.

Dr. Howe involved himself extensively in the operation of the school and in the care of its pupils. He examined all candidates for admission and engaged all the officers. He had direct contact with all the pupils, making daily rounds and seeing each pupil. He prescribed their diets, established their daily regimen, formulated their rules and regulations, decided their discipline, and chose their exercises. In 1848 Seguin became the superintendent of the school. In 1887 the school was moved to Waltham, Massachusetts. Later it was renamed the Walter E. Fernald State School, in recognition of the long time services of its most distinguished superintendent.

Walter E. Fernald (1859–1924) obtained his medical degree from the Medical School of Maine. He was the first resident superintendent of the Massachusetts School for Idiotic and Feeble-Minded Youth and remained there, devoting his life to that and other facilities and educational programs for people with mental retardation. In his early years he expressed negative opinions about the attributes of, and possibilities of response to treatment for, that population. He characterized this group in the following way: "The brighter class of the feeble-minded with their weak will and deficient judgment are easily influenced for evil and are prone to become vagrants, drunkards and thieves" (Scheerenberger, 1983). Fernald was expressing an opinion commonly held by the general populace that people with mental retardation were responsible for crime. His remedy was to discipline the group in their early years and confine them to almshouses and hospitals and, if necessary, prisons when they reached adulthood. Fernald, however, grew in his understanding of the potentials of that group and just as assiduously spent the rest of his days in compensating for his early expressed critical views. In the end, his contributions and positive influence were great. As early as 1891, he was instrumental in the establishment of an outpatient psychiatric diagnostic clinic, one of the first such facilities in the United States. He sponsored a law permitting the parole of persons with mental retardation from state schools, a law recognizing delinquents who were mentally ill and making separate institutional provisions for them, a law requiring inquiry into the mental status of prisoners, and a law establishing psychiatric clinics for examining children who were mentally retarded in public schools (Lowry, 1944–1945).

Early Course of the Mental Retardation Movement

In his address at the Centenary Meeting of the American Psychiatric Association, Lawson Lowry designated the years from 1846 to 1909 as the period of time that mental retardation was the prominent area of focus in the origins of child psychiatry in the United States. Lowry based his date of 1846 on two events. That was the year that Seguin published his influential treatise on the education of children with mental retardation, and that was the time that the Massachusetts Legislature enacted their statute that established the Perkins Institute for the Blind, the first American experimental school for people with mental disabilities. This institution developed its services further when in 1850 it was incorporated as the Massachusetts School for Idiotic and Feeble-Minded Children.

The reason for the development of institutions in the various states in the 1840s was that they filled a void in an educational system that did not serve mentally retarded children. Hence, they were designated as schools. They were not established to contain these children away from the community but with the idea of returning them to their parental homes as quickly as they gained adequate skills. By the middle 1870s there were 7 states that recognized the need for such institutions, and physicians were placed in charge. Wylie (1930) reported that they cared for about 1300 persons, including adults that could not be discharged.

At the end of the 19th century a detrimental shift in attitude toward people with mental retardation took place. The Parisian school of psychiatry and neurology formulated a defect theory based on etiological factors and common inherited cerebral deficiency. The availability of the Binet Intelligence Test served to focus on the cognitive insufficiencies of people who were mentally retarded. This, along with the growing eugenics movement and misleading ideas of the potentials of this population, resulted in a trend toward institutionalization of persons who were mentally retarded, including those with only mild manifestations of the disorder. There followed a move toward sexual segregation and forced sterilization (Zigler and Hodapp, 1985). During this period, psychiatry paid little heed to this detrimental trend affecting mentally retarded persons, in part, because such persons were not viewed as proper candidates for the new discipline that had been discovered—psychoanalysis.

A number of decades in the 20th century passed before the current scientific understanding of and a more enlightened attitude toward the people with mental retardation began to prevail. Research in developmental psychology and later advances in child psychiatry in which a developmental point of view of children was formulated finally began to show that mentally retarded people mature along the same continuum as nonretarded individuals, albeit at a far slower rate. Mental retardation was then no longer considered as synonymous with psychopathology. This was ultimately affirmed in the *Diagnostic and Statistical Manual of Mental Disorders* (3rd ed) (DSM-III) in 1980. More recently, DSM-III-R (1987) and DSM-IV (1994) classified mental retardation as a developmental disorder. The current status of retarded persons was further advanced by the efforts of parents and other advocacy groups to ensure that retarded persons be permitted to live in the least restrictive environment and have access to educational services, which came to be mandated by federal law.

MAJOR TRENDS OF THE 20TH CENTURY

In the present century a number of other concepts and findings significant in the development of child psychiatry began to take place and accelerate its recognition as a medical subspecialty. In the early decades, noteworthy studies of juvenile delinquents began to appear where almost none were available before. These emerged between 1909 and 1919 when the neurologist William Healey began his work at the Juvenile Psychopathic Institute at Chicago, focusing on the problems of delinquent youths. Healey addressed the prevailing issue of the importance of organic versus environmental factors. Adherents on both sides of the nature versus nurture issue, as it came to be known, aired their views emphatically. Healy emphasized the latter.

When he began his work, Healy found that there were no comprehensive studies of the young population available. Physiological norms were not developed, standardized tests such as the Binet age level scale were not in use, and the importance of family relationships and attitudes was not yet affirmed. His book *The Individual Delinquent* when it appeared in 1915 was recognized as a monumental volume. His salient contribution to the developing concepts of child psychiatry lay in establishing the method of clinical case study of the young delinquent offender and developing a concept of the essentially dynamic character of the human personality. He encompassed all aspects of the child's state of health—physical, emotional, and intellectual.

In addition, Healy stimulated direct study by others so that by 1919 there was active commitment to the study of problems of delinquency. There was also interest in establishing norms for childhood as well as surveys of mental disorders. Furthermore, there was stress on the treatment of children's problems in a number of centers. Other active areas included the work of the National Committee for Mental Hygiene in defining a role in public education, the establishment of psychopathic hospitals and outpatient departments, and bringing child psychiatry into a relationship with problems and patterns of the social life of the community.

The quarter century of 1919–1944 began the era of child guidance with a rapid burgeoning of direct psychiatric work with children. Several distinct types of evolution appeared. The first was the development of state programs of child guidance clinics and the establishment of psychiatric units in the training schools for delinquents. New facilities of note were established, e.g., the Boston Psychopathic Hospital and the Phipps Psychiatric Clinic. Massachusetts founded clinics for children in connection with its state hospitals. These were later developed into mental hygiene clinics.

The second program of historical interest began with the opening of demonstration clinics operated by the National Committee of Mental Hygiene financed by the Commonwealth Fund. Growth of these clinics was rapid. The few clinics that were available to children in 1919 numbered 776 by 1939. The parent committee after changing its name to the Division on Community Clinics began making grants for specialized training in child psychiatry. These provided formal training to replace the system whereby professionals garnered experience on an individual basis wherever possible. During the period that child psychiatry was chiefly situated in the child guidance clinics, a trend away from institutional care for children was encouraged. Every effort was made to have children remain in their own homes or in foster homes with outpatient care if necessary. However, as the 1940s and 1950s approached, it became apparent that this too did not sufficiently meet the needs of children with major or acute emotional disorders. As a consequence, inpatient services in general hospitals began to proliferate, and hospital ward services for disturbed children appeared and developed. Special facilities such as the Children's Center associated with the Judge Baker Foundation in Boston and the Southard School of the Menninger Clinic at Topeka developed as well.

The rapid growth of all these centers made it clear that there had been a void in providing for the specialized psychiatric and emotional needs of children. Also it was apparent that there was a lack of clinical and academic training in facilities with adequate clinical standards and methods of delivering care to the young population with emotional problems. There followed a great expansion of child study institutes connected with universities. In addition, medical schools with departments of psychiatry added a division of child psychiatry. The first American textbook of child psychiatry was written by Leo Kanner in 1935. A basic curriculum of studies was developed. The divisions of child psychiatry began to offer specialized graduate training, and child psychiatry became a regular part of medical student education. Academia became defined as the place to develop future child psychiatrists as well as to ally the field to general medicine.

Introduction of Psychoanalysis

A major influence on the developing field of child psychiatry was the advent of psychoanalysis. In a 1907 paper presented before the New York Psychiatric Society, Dr. E. Stanley Abbott presented a number of case histories of paranoid patients in whom he believed their mental state was produced by purely mental causes, i.e., by conflicts and unhygienic ways of dealing with them (Hoch, 1907–1908). He stated his ideas were influenced by both Adolf Meyer and Sigmund Freud. Although Freud was well-known in Vienna, this is the first time his name was mentioned in the American literature. Interest in his work mounted after Stanley Hall and James Putnam invited Freud to lecture at Clarke University in Worchester, Massachusetts in 1909. This was followed by publication of Freud's account of the psychopathology and treatment of Little Hans, the 5-year-old phobic child, in the same year (Freud, 1955).

Freud's analysis of Little Hans was not an example of direct therapy in that the boy's father acted as an intermediary under the direction of Freud. Sandor Ferenczi in 1913 reported the first attempt at direct psychoanalysis of a child as a psychotherapeutic approach. Hug-Hellmuth, in Vienna in 1920, was the world's first child analyst to describe a technique of play in child analysis, especially in the preparatory phase, although she did not develop a concept of play in therapy. Melanie Klein, in Berlin, was the first to develop not only the extensive use of play with interpretation in child analysis, but also the concept of play in therapy. Melanie Klein used a wide range of small, single toys and wooden human figure representations. She read her first paper in Budapest in 1919, publishing it in the *International Zeitschrift fur Psychoanalyse* in 1920. Hug-Hellmuth's earliest account of all of the elements of child analysis were repeated by Anna Freud in 1927 (MacLean and Rappen, 1991). David Levy is credited with presenting the first report on play therapy at a scientific meeting in a paper he gave at the American Orthopsychiatric Association in 1925 (Harrison, 1980).

In England, Melanie Klein had a substantial number of followers and her theories about child psychoanalysis were influential (Bion et al., 1961; Grosskuth, 1986; Mora, 1980). Certain of her concepts differed from Freud's views. She was supported by Ernest Jones and had a considerable number of followers among members of the British Psychoanalytic Society. Later, dissension arose between the Kleinians and the Freudians close to Anna Freud, leading to "A" and "B" training programs in the British Psycho-Analytic Society in 1946.

Among Anna Freud's contributions to child psychiatry was her systematic and comprehensive account of the defenses used by the ego, presented in her classic monograph "The Ego and Mechanisms of Defense," first published in 1936 (Freud, 1946). In addition, she helped to clarify the importance of early developmental phases of childhood, a theme that Margaret Mahler used in developing her concept of separation-individuation in the child. Anna Freud also contributed to concepts of personality development as well as the role of bodily illness in childhood. Anna Freud founded the Hampstead Clinic and Child Training Center in London, where an index project was developed to categorize and classify many clinical syndromes. This provided material for diagnostic evaluation of children and assessment of their pathology and normality along developmental lines (Freud, 1965).

There followed many other British contributors to developmental theory now considered important in child psychiatry. Among these was Donald Winnicott, who introduced the concept of the transitional object in the early development of the child. Another was John Bowlby, known for his maternal deprivation studies and theories of attachment and loss.

Psychoanalysis, as a theory, a method of research, and a form of treatment hypothesized a number of psychodynamic "explanations" for numerous symptoms and behaviors, many of which were published in a new post-World War II annual series, the *Psychoanalytic Study of the Child*, which first appeared in 1945. The hypotheses were used at that time for the treatment of infants, children, and adolescents with such varied symptoms as failure to thrive, feeding and sleep difficulties, separation anxiety, bed-wetting, soiling, compulsions, conversion symptoms, depression, and even psychosis. Subsequently, newer hypotheses, especially biological and behavioral hypotheses based on findings derived from scientific research, gained prominence as a basis for a more effective clinical treatment of many of the above conditions.

The Pluralistic Approach

A pluralistic and multimodal approach to treatment, including cognitive, behavioral, psychodynamic, and psychopharmacologic methods gained widespread recognition and impetus in the 1960s and 1970s. This trend was accompanied by an acknowledgment that, until one comprehensive theory adequate to explain the full basis of child psychiatry arose, selection from or use of several systems or theories were necessary (Lewis and Vitulano, 1989).

The development of the *Journal of the American Academy of Child Psychiatry*, as it was first called, reflected this change. The first issue of this journal had appeared in 1962 under the editorship of Irene Josselyn and for several years published mostly papers derived from a psychodynamic perspective, which of course had been the dominant influence in the field at that time. Many papers on service delivery were published in the initial period of the Journal's life (American Academy of Child Psychiatry: A Plan for the Coming Decades, 1983, p. 22). Then, in the 1970s, multidisciplinary scientific research in child psychiatry began to soar, in part because of (a) more sophisticated research methodology and advanced statistical techniques; (b) the development of a standardized multiaxial classification system (DSM-III, which began in

1974); (c) discoveries in psychopharmacologic treatment; and (d) a change in the Journal, beginning in 1975. From the mid-1970s onward, the content of the *Journal of the American Academy of Child and Adolescent Psychiatry* (as it is now called) under the editorship of its third editor, Melvin Lewis, began to facilitate the multidisciplinary and multitheoretical research effort by publishing many more rigorously scientific research papers (Project Future, 1983).

At the same time, there were attempts to develop interactive models. One example is the goodness-of-fit pattern proposed by Alexander Thomas and Stella Chess in their study of temperament and development in children (Thomas and Chess, 1977). They considered that characteristic inborn behavior patterns were predisposing or contributory to the development of various conditions in the child. Genetic-familial factors and the demands of society figured as well. In the following year, Carey and McDevitt (1978) applied these concepts in considering attention deficit disorder.

Thomas and Chess, together with Herbert Birch, are known for their longitudinal study of temperament in children. They defined three common groups: the "easy child," found in 40% of children they studied; the "slow to warm up child," found in 20%; and the "difficult child," found in 10%. They examined each of these patterns in the context of the child's family and derived many different final expressions depending in part on "goodness-of-fit" (see Chapter 13).

Others followed with their version of a complex interactional model applied to such conditions as panic disorder, phobic disorder, pervasive developmental disorders, and obsessive-compulsive disorders. The components of the interaction model now include genetic, neuroanatomical, neurochemical, cognitive, developmental, psychodynamic, and socioenvironmental factors.

POSTSCRIPT

The antecedents of child psychiatry included social and cultural forces in the late 18th and 19th centuries that led to the recognition of children as individuals and then to the acknowledgment of emotional and behavioral problems in children. The mental retardation movement also began to be part of the early foundation of what would later be the field of child psychiatry. When psychoanalysis was discovered in the 20th century, it had a profound early influence for the first half of the century, but was overtaken by an enormous surge of advances in the neurosciences based on scientific research that took primacy and paved the way for the consolidation of child psychiatry as a specialty of medicine.

However, recently, other important economic, social, and political changes have arisen in the United States (and perhaps elsewhere) and have set the stage for a dramatic developmental shift in the way in which mental health care for children and their families might be delivered. Because of the prevailing sociopolitical climate in the United States, the driving force for health care delivery, including mental health care, now seems to be an ethos of cost avoidance by means of a corporate model of service delivery, which has now almost taken over in the country at large. While cost reduction (not improved health care) appears to be the primary goal for this mushrooming model of health care delivery, in many corporations the executive (nonmedical) group is highly paid (in the millions of dollars), and the corporation is extremely profit-oriented. This goal of cost reduction and corporate profits is achieved, in part, by strenuously driving down professional personnel and health care costs. The "consumer" is also usually faced with a restricted choice of specialist care and limited treatment.

In the case of children and their families who need mental health care, this restrictive corporate approach is having a particularly restrictive impact. Ironically, the impact occurs at a time when child psychiatry is exploring new frontiers based on advances in neuroscience.

References

American Academy of Child Psychiatry: *A Plan for the Coming Decades.* American Academy of Child Psychiatry, Washington, DC, 1983, p. 22.

Am J Insanity 54:309, 1901–1902.

Annual Meeting of the Association. *Am J Insanity* 15:122, 1858.

Baring-Gould S: *Germany: Present and Past* (Vol 2). London, CK Paul & Co, 1879, p. 274.

Bion WR, Rosenfeld H, Segal H, et al: Melanie Klein. *Int J Psychoanal* 42:4, 1961.

Brigham A: *Remarks on the Influence of Mental Cultivation and Mental Excitement upon Health.* Philadelphia, Lea & Blanchard, 1845, pp. 1–135.

Carey WB, McDevitt SC: Revision of the infant temperament questionnaire. *Pediatrics* 61:753, 1978.

Chipley WS: A warning to fathers, teachers and young men in relation to a fruitful cause of insanity and other serious disorders of youth. *Am J Insanity* 17:472–475, 1861.

Chipley WS: Feigned insanity. Motives. Special tests. *Am J Insanity* 22:5–13, 1865.

Conolly J: Juvenile insanity. *Am J Insanity* 18:395–403, 1861.

Freud A: *The Ego and the Mechanisms of Defense.* New York, International Universities Press, 1946.

Freud A: *Normality and Psychopathology.* New York, International Universities Press, 1965.

Freud S: Analysis of a phobia in a five-year old boy. In: Stachey J (ed): *The Standard Edition of the Complete Psychological Works of Sigmund Freud.* London, Hogarth Press, 1955, pp. 3–152.

Goldfarb W: Pervasive developmental disorders of childhood. In: Kaplan HI, Sadock BJ (eds): *Comprehensive Textbook of Psychiatry* (3rd ed). Baltimore, Williams & Wilkins, 1980, p. 2541.

Harrison SI: Individual psychotherapy. In: Kaplan HI, Sadock BJ (eds): *Comprehensive Textbook of Psychiatry* (3rd ed). Baltimore, Williams & Wilkins, 1980, pp. 2647–2667.

Hoch A: The psychogenetic factors in some paranoiac conditions with suggestion for prophylaxis and treatment. *Am J Insanity* 64:189, 1907–1908.

Hunter R, Macalpine I: Amariah Brigham (1798–1849). In: *Three Hundred Years of Psychiatry, 1535–1860.* London, Oxford University Press, 1963, pp. 821–823.

Kanner L: *A History of the Care and Study of the Mentally Retarded.* Springfield, IL, Charles C Thomas, 1964, pp. 9–44.

Lewis M, Vitulano L: A historical perspective on views of childhood psychopathology. In: Last CG, Hersen M (eds): *Handbook of Child Psychiatric Diagnosis.* New York, Wiley, 1989, pp. 3–11.

Lowry LG: Psychiatry for children. A brief history of developments. *Am J Psychiatry* 101:375–377, 1944–1945.

MacLean G, Rappen U: *Hermine Hug-Hellmuth.* New York, Routledge, 1991.

Mora G: Historical and theoretical trends in psychiatry. In: Kaplan HI, Sadock BJ (eds): *Comprehensive Textbook of Psychiatry* (3rd ed) Vol 1. Baltimore, Williams & Wilkins, 1980, pp. 86–87.

More H: Strictures on the modern system of female education. In: *Works* (Vol 6). New York, [sn] 1820, p. 36.

On the insanity of children. *Am J Insanity* 17:228–231, 1860.

Overholser W: The founding and founders of the Association. In: Hall JK (ed): *One Hundred Years of American Psychiatry.* New York, Columbia University Press, 1944, p. 69.

Parry-Jones WL: The history of child and adolescent psychiatry: Its present day relevance. *J Child Psychol Psychiatry* 30(1):3–11, 1989.

Ray I: *Conversations on the Animal Economy Designed for the Instruction of Youth and the Perusal of General Readers.* Portland, Shirley and Hyde, 1829, pp. 1–33.

Ray I: *Mental Hygiene.* Boston, Ticknor and Fields, 1863, p. 138.

Robertson P: Home as a nest: Middle class childhood in nineteenth century Europe. In: de Mause L (ed): *The History of Childhood.* New York, The Psychohistory Press, 1974, pp. 409–411, 413.

Rogeness GA, Javors MH, Tliszka SR: Neurochemistry and child and adolescent psychiatry. *J Am Acad Child Adolesc Psychiatry* 31:765–781, 1994.

Rousseau JJ: *Emile.* New York, EP Dutton, 1911, pp. 28, 32.

Scheerenberger RC: *A History of Mental Retardation.* Baltimore, Brookes, 1983, pp. 41–42, 48–49, 156–157.

Schowalter JE: Recruitment, training and certification in child and adolescent psychiatry in the United States. In: Lewis M (ed): *Child and Adolescent Psychiatry. A Comprehensive Textbook.* Baltimore, Williams & Wilkins, 1991, pp. 1197–1201.

Smith EG: *Memoirs of a Highland Lady: The Autobiography of Elizabeth Grant of Rothiemurchus, Afterwards Mrs. Smith of Baltiboys, 1797–1830.* Strachey L (ed), London, 1911.

Tarjan G: Foreword. In: Lewis M (ed): *Child and Adolescent Psychiatry. A Comprehensive Textbook.* Baltimore, Williams & Wilkins, 1991.

The History of the American Academy of Child Psychiatry. *J Am Acad Child Psychiatry* 1:196–202, 1962.

Thomas A, Chess S: *Temperament and Development.* New York, Brunner/Mazel, 1977.

van Praag H: *Psychotropic Drugs. A Guide for the Practitioner.* New York, Brunner/Mazel, 1978, p. 49.

West C: *Lectures on the Diseases of Infancy and Young Children.* London, Longman, 1854.

Wylie AR: Development of institutional care for the feebleminded. *Bull Mass Dept Ment Dis* 14:40–60, 1930.

Zeitlin H: *The Natural History of Psychiatric Disorder in Children.* Institute of Psychiatry Maudsley Monographs, No 29. New York, Oxford University Press, 1986, pp. 1–2.

Zigler E, Hodapp RM: In: Cavenar JO (ed): *Mental Retardation in Psychiatry* (Vol 2). Philadelphia, Lippincott, 1985.

INDEX

Page numbers in *italics* denote figures; those followed by "t" denote tables.

for hypersomnia, 719
violence and, 338
Amphotericin B, 985t
Amygdala
aggression and lesions in, 337
asymmetry in, 100
behavior and, 91
Amyl nitrate, 748
Amylophagia, 578
Amyotrophic lateral sclerosis, 7t, 647
Amytal interview, 698
Anafranil. *See* Clomipramine
Anal phase of development, 158–159, 229, 242
Analgesia
for burn injuries, 1017–1020, 1018t—1019t
for cancer pain, 960, 964
patient-controlled, 1019
for transplant patients, 977–978
Anatomically correct dolls, 1045
Anderson, J.R., 141–142, *142*
Anderson, Mike, 142–143, *143*
Androgens, 226–227, 272
aggressive and sexual behavior and, 335–336
prenatal, gender identity disorders and, 613–614
Anergia, 301
Angelman syndrome, 1, 7t, 992–993
Anhedonia, 301
Animal cruelty, 604
Animal phobias, 674
Animal studies
of aggressive behavior, 334–341
of classical and operant conditioning, 116–117
of preparedness theory, 296
of vicarious conditioning, 298
Anniversary reactions, 756
Anophthalmia, 25–26
Anorexia nervosa, 281, 586–592
age at onset of, 586, 587
amenorrhea in, 78, 588, 589
atypical forms of, 586
bupropion contraindicated in, 792
case illustration of, 592
clinical features of, 587–588
definition of, 78, 586
depression and, 581, 589
diagnostic criteria for, 586, 587t
differential diagnosis of, 590
directions for research in, 592
etiology and pathogenesis of, 588–590
biologic mechanisms and theories, 588–589
family and interpersonal dynamics, 589
genetic predisposition, 588–589
hypothalamic-pituitary-gonadal dysfunction, 78–79, 589
psychologic processes and theories, 589
historical descriptions of, 587
hospitalization for, 591
"infantile," 588
laboratory findings in, 590, 590t
medical complications of, 590
neurochemistry of, 589, 1225
outcome and follow-up data for, 591–592
premenarchial, 584, 586, 587
prevalence of, 587
psychologic testing in, 590
seasonal pattern of, 589
sex distribution of, 586, 587
subtypes of, 586
treatment of, 590–591
emergency management, 932
family therapy, 855
twin studies of, 588–589
Antabuse. *See* Disulfiram
Antibiotics, 985t
for meningitis, 369
Antibodies, 51–52
Anticipation, 204

Anticonvulsants, 640, 796–797
behavioral/emotional effects of, 638
benzodiazepines and, 640
dosage of, 769
effect on cognitive functioning, 637
half-lives of, 768t, 769
for Landau-Kleffner syndrome, 511
for mania, 654–655, 655t
methylphenidate and, 640
monitoring serum levels of, 640
pharmacokinetics of, 769
rate of metabolism of, 640
selection of, 640
Antidepressants, 662–663, 784–792
bupropion, 791–792
half-lives of, 768t
monoamine oxidase inhibitors, 663, 792
selective serotonin reuptake inhibitors, 663, 788–790
for symptoms of stimulant abstinence, 746
trazodone, 790–791
tricyclic, 662–663, 784–788
abrupt withdrawal of, 769, 785
for adolescents, 662–663
for attention deficit hyperactivity disorder, 33, 555
cardiotoxicity of, 555, 784–785
for child with cancer, 964
dosage of, 555, 769
ECG monitoring and, 659, 662, 678
half-lives of, 768t, 769
indications for, 784
metabolism in children, 555
monitoring blood levels of, 660, 776
pharmacokinetics of, 769
slow hydroxylators of, 769
for transplant recipients, 986t
treatment response to, 662, 662t
use in eating disorders, 591
use in epilepsy, 640
Antiepileptic drugs. *See* Anticonvulsants
Antigens, 51–52
Antipsychotics, 779–784
for attention deficit hyperactivity disorder, 556, 781
atypical, 782–784
clozapine, 782–784
risperidone, 784
for brain-injured child, 372
for burn patients, 1019
for child with mental retardation, 508, 779–780
discontinuation of, 776
dosage of, 769, 780t
extrapyramidal reactions to, 780t, 780–781
acute dystonic reaction, 780–781
akathisia, 781
neuroleptic malignant syndrome, 508, 781
parkinsonism, 781
rabbit syndrome, 781
tardive dyskinesia, 781
withdrawal dyskinesia, 776, 781
half-lives of, 768t
indications for, 779
pharmacokinetics of, 769
for schizophrenia, 633–634, 779
sedation induced by, 780t
side effects of, 627, 780t, 780–781
for Tourette's syndrome, 35, 556, 627
for transplant recipients, 986t
Antisocial behavior. *See also* Conduct disorder; Criminality
attention deficit hyperactivity disorder and, 544, 558–559
behavior therapy for, 573, 823
conduct disorder and, 566, 573
hypothesized causal chain for, 1167t
parental psychopathology and, 402–403, 1169

prevalence of, 1230
substance abuse and, 739
Anxiety
adjustment disorder with, 682, 728
bone marrow transplantation and, 983
in borderline disorders, 732–733
definition of, 674
development and, 674–675
hallucinations and, 449
management in transplant patients, 977–978
neurological soft signs and, 483
recurrent abdominal pain and, 1056
signs and symptoms of, 674t
stuttering and, 512
Anxiety disorders, 291–299, 674–683
assessment of, 676
associated with specific stressors, 682, 682t
attention deficit hyperactivity disorder and, 549
avoidant disorder, 682
classical conditioning and experimental neuroses, 118
communication disorders and, 510
comorbidity with other psychopathology, 674
conditioning and, 298–299, 676
current knowledge and research needs for, 683
with depressed mood, 660
diagnosis of, 674
differential diagnosis of, 676
directions for research on, 299
in DSM-IV and ICD-10, 428
ethological considerations in, 296
etiology and pathogenesis of, 675–676
biologic factors, 675
psychosocial factors, 676
family studies of, 291–295
bottom up studies, 292–295
genetic vs. environmental transmission, 295
top down studies, 291–292
generalized anxiety (overanxious) disorder, 678–680
genetic factors and, 675
historical classifications of, 675
panic disorder, 682–683
parental, 1170
phobias, 680–682
posttraumatic stress disorder, 682, 682t, 753–761
prevalence and epidemiology of, 291, 675, 1230
prognosis for, 674
psychoanalytic theories of, 299, 676
reactive attachment disorders, 498–501, 680
related to temperament and shyness, 296–298
in response to separation and deprivation, 386
among runaway youth, 1082
school phobia and, 1106
in school-age child, 277
separation anxiety disorder, 676–678
sex distribution of, 675
sexual abuse and, 1042, 1043
stressful life events and, 295–296
treatment of, 676
behavior therapy, 822
emergency management, 932
family therapy, 857
goals for, 676
medications, 793–796
Anxiolytics, 793–796
benzodiazepines, 793–795
buspirone, 795–796
for transplant recipients, 986t
Aphasia, 512–513. *See also* Language disorders
Appearance of child, 444
changes due to illness and medications, 977
sexual orientation and, 615
suggesting substance abuse, 749–750
Apperception, 181. *See also* Perception